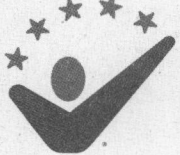

FIRST EDITION

HEALTHGRADES

★ GUIDE TO AMERICA'S ★
HOSPITALS AND DOCTORS

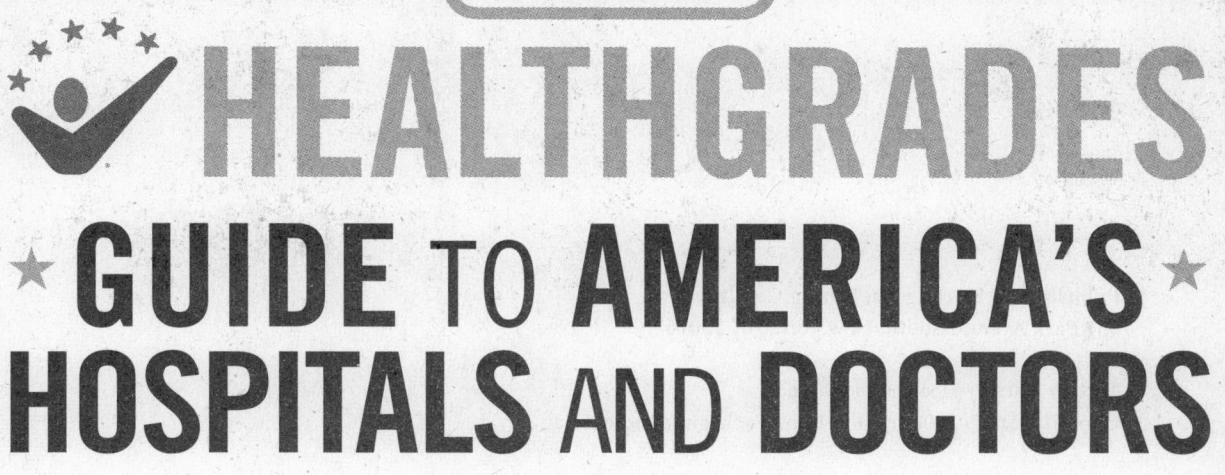

FIRST EDITION

HEALTHGRADES

★ GUIDE TO AMERICA'S ★ HOSPITALS AND DOCTORS

FROM HEALTHGRADES, THE LEADER IN HEALTHCARE RATINGS

WITH SAMANTHA L. COLLIER, MD, MBA, HEALTHGRADES' CHIEF MEDICAL OFFICER

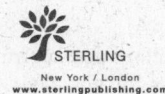

STERLING
New York / London
www.sterlingpublishing.com

Published by Sterling Publishing Co., Inc.
387 Park Avenue South, New York, NY 10016

Text © 2008 by HealthGrades, Inc.
Compilation © 2008 by D&J Book Packaging and Media

Distributed in Canada by Sterling Publishing
c/o Canadian Manda Group, 165 Dufferin Street,
Toronto, Ontario, Canada M6K 3H6

Distributed in the United Kingdom by GMC Distribution Services,
Castle Place, 166 High Street, Lewes, East Sussex, England BN7 1XU

Distributed in Australia by Capricorn Link (Australia) Pty. Ltd.
P.O. Box 704, Windsor, NSW 2756, Australia

Produced by D&J Book Packaging and Media

DESIGN BY: Laurie Dolphin and Allison Meierding
EDITOR: Jessica Dorfman Jones
COVER DESIGN BY: Laurie Dolphin and Allison Meierding

ISBN-13: 978-1-4351-0426-6
ISBN-10: 1-4351-0426-9

10 9 8 7 6 5 4 3 2 1

For information about custom editions, special sales, premium and corporate purchases, please
contact Sterling Special Sales Department at 800-805-5489 or specialsales@sterlingpub.com.

This book is dedicated to top performing hospitals and physicians nationwide, as well as those healthcare professionals and institutions that strive to improve the quality of medical care for the good of their patients.

CONTENTS

Foreword viii

Introduction xi

Chapter 1: How to Choose a Doctor 1

Chapter 2: How to Choose a Hospital 13

Chapter 3: Preparing for a Hospital Stay: What to Do, What to Expect 19

Chapter 4: Protecting Yourself and Your Loved Ones from Medical Errors ... 31

Chapter 5: Best Questions to Ask Before Common Procedures 39

Chapter 6: Hospital Ratings by Clinical Specialty 46

Chapter 7: Five Star Rated Hospitals 734

Chapter 8: Hospital Ratings by Procedure 826

Chapter 9: HealthGrades Top Doctors 1042

Appendix 1081

Index 1089

Acknowledgments 1118

About HealthGrades and About the Author 1119

The fifth leading cause of death in the United States is our healthcare system. Yes, there is a standing army, more than a million strong, of smart, dedicated, hard working doctors, nurses, and other providers, most of them armed to the teeth with the greatest medical technologies that money could buy. But still, hundreds of thousands of Americans die unnecessarily every year, not from accidents or disease, but from the often brutal side effects of entering a healthcare system that is not a system at all, but a public health disaster imploding in extremely slow motion. Healthcare in the United States may be the world's last best hope for finding and financing medical miracles and some of technology's greatest feats, but for the average patient seeking routine help, healthcare here is also a fragmented mess, designed by nobody, managed by nobody, and accountable, ultimately, to nobody.

The phenomenon of medical mistakes that contribute to healthcare being the fifth biggest killer in the United States is as old as the history of modern medicine itself. In 1910, what started out as an obscure academic study (the "Flexner Report") shocked the American public by describing the appalling conditions inside U.S. hospitals at the time. In the 1980s, another would-be obscure study ("Which Rate is Right?") made a stunning discovery: whether or not a patient has surgery for a wide variety of medical conditions has less to do with whether or not the patient actually needs the surgery and more to do with where the patient happens to live. In the 1990s, yet another would-be obscure study ("Crossing the Quality Chasm") found that more than 198,000 Americans die every year because of preventable medical errors

committed in hospitals. Sometimes, the treatment really is worse than the disease.

How did this happen? Why does the richest, most technically advanced medical infrastructure in the world produce such horrifying results? Books have been written trying to figure out why and proposing solutions for it, but at rock bottom, it comes down to this: the U.S. healthcare system is an economic, legal, and political free for all. We as a society cannot agree on the most basic ideas concerning how we want our healthcare system to work, and so our indecision has created an enormous vacuum. In this vacuum, there have been perennial power struggles—stretching back to the early 1900s—among hospitals, physicians, health insurers, drug companies, regulators, patient advocacy groups, and lawyers, lawyers, lawyers. And what is the end result? Medical care delivery in the United States is a miracle of disorganization held together through the sheer collective will of overworked professionals tasked with managing tens of millions of patients by memory, pen scrawls, sticky notes, and telephone calls. Indeed, it is overly generous to call this a system at all, when it more accurately resembles a chaos of small boats tossed about on a roiling sea of paper. The wonder of healthcare in the United States is not that so many patients fall through the cracks, fail to comply with medical orders, receive conflicting therapies, and so on. The greatest wonder, given the situation, is how *few* do.

Fragmentation, lack of integration, and absence of true accountability—these are what drive the enormous, inexplicable variations in the patterns of medical care Americans receive from their hospitals and doctors. Variations by region, type of physician, and especially the patient's financial and insurance status run wild across the entire spectrum of medical care: surgery vs. drugs for the same condition; hospital admission rates; hospital lengths of stay; traditional vs. leading-edge surgical technique; diagnostic imaging and lab testing frequency; specific drug selection; the list goes on, and on, and on. What drives it? The short answer is *money*. Variations in medical decision making, inefficiency in the system, and relying on insurers and other third parties to pay for most of our healthcare are all factors that have worked together to create the worst possible outcome: high rates of unnecessary and substandard medical care. More badly spent money flows through an already broken system when there is little or no patient information at the point of care or when the wrong drugs are prescribed. What patients really need, as anyone who has had to navigate healthcare in the United States can attest, takes a back seat to the system's bureaucracy.

I recently helped an obstetrician/gynecologist friend negotiate her employment contract with a new medical practice. Her contract included a modest base salary, but then dedicated five pages to describing in detail her opportunity to earn big monthly bonuses for what it called *production*. What exactly does production mean for today's OB/GYN in a busy private practice? It does *not* mean more and healthier babies and women, as you would imagine. Rather, it means more babies delivered via C-section, more hysterectomies, more procedures, more risky surgeries, and so on. In short, not only are we *not* paying our doctors (and our hospitals, and everybody else downstream in the system) to do the right things, we are paying them to do the most invasive, most expensive procedures. Small wonder our healthcare system is killing patients almost as

frequently as the diseases that drive them to that system for help.

The situation is not ideal for anyone, including most of the doctors and nurses trapped in a system they can't control. As a society, we believe in science; we believe in asking the hard questions of ourselves and each other; we believe in the power of information. As America's medical research establishment—a national treasure and the envy of the rest of the world—is built on a foundation of real science, so too should its practical application. Unfortunately, medical practice has evolved in a way that has isolated most of the system from the very scientific scrutiny that medicine supposedly represents. This isolation is finally coming to an end. In the 1990s and well into the 2000s, *managed care* was supposed to be the cure. Managed care was supposed to shed a white-hot light on all of these problems and use money—or the withholding of it—as the big stick needed to beat doctors and hospitals into line. For most of us, however, the managed care "cure" turned out to be worse than the disease, and in a few short years, Americans rejected most of its harsher forms and methods.

But two important things happened after managed care's false alarm to the healthcare system: we discovered the transformative power of money and the transformative power of information. In recent years, most health insurers have recognized that the best way to manage care is to allow patients to manage it themselves, by forcing them to shoulder more and more of the burden of paying for it. Motivated patients with suddenly high deductibles, ballooning co-payments, and slowly growing Health Savings Accounts would finally start to question decisions made by doctors and hospitals on their behalf. Is this procedure really necessary? Is there a cheaper drug? Do I really need the same test again that my other doctor already ordered?

The slow but steady economic revolution we are now experiencing in healthcare—with patients suddenly in charge of much of their own health spending—is coinciding perfectly with the information revolution we have been experiencing everywhere else. Ten and fifteen years ago, there was a wealth of data about which hospital would be the best place for a certain surgery and which hospital could end up costing you your life if you set foot in it. But that data was stashed away behind healthcare's wall of secrecy. Hospitals and doctors had a vested interest in keeping the information out of your hands. And so did health insurers, which for all their happy talk about promoting quality and caring about your health and well being, more often than not have always chosen hospitals and doctors for their networks based *not* on how well they take care of people, but on how low a price they would accept for that care. Your needs, the needs of the patient, have once again come last.

How far healthcare consumers have come in a few short years! You now have the Internet, and you now carry much of the economic burden for your own medical care. The combination of the two is turning healthcare upside down. This is why I am so pleased that HealthGrades is providing in this book a wealth of quality information about U.S. hospitals that, until recently, had been available only to insiders, the privileged few, the keepers of the dysfunctional healthcare system.

Because of books like this; because of Internet-era organizations like HealthGrades; and because of the difficult, diligent work that went into developing fair and useful quality information about the most important decisions you will ever make concerning your lives, healthcare in America will never be the same. And everyone can thank their lucky stars for that.

—J. D. Kleinke
Chairman and CEO
Omnimedix Institute
Portland, Oregon
August 1, 2007

WHY YOU SHOULD USE THIS BOOK

You are holding in your hands something that has never before been available in print: a guide, based on research and hard data, to choosing the best hospitals and doctors.

For too long, the best kept secret in healthcare has been that there are indisputable differences in quality between one doctor and another, and between one hospital and another. What's more, there are tangible differences in quality *within* a hospital, between one department and another. For instance, in your community, the best hospital in which to have your knee repaired may not be the best place in which to have bypass surgery.

This book is a result of HealthGrades' decade-long work to quantify those differences in quality, to turn vast amounts of data into star ratings that are easy to use for anyone facing or anticipating a medical condition. Through rigorous analysis of tens of millions of hospitalization records, HealthGrades has identified which hospitals outperform others and translated that into the star ratings you'll see in the chapters ahead. We've used those star ratings to identify top performing doctors as well.

That's a significant advance in comparison to what was possible a few short years ago. Think about it. The last time you chose a doctor, did you do it based on a word of mouth recommendation? If you had to go to the hospital for a procedure, did you go to that particular hospital simply because it was closest to your home?

Making your healthcare choices based only on reputation and geography is happening less and less these days as more information about the quality of specific healthcare providers is becoming public. The availability of this information has been driven by organizations like HealthGrades and the federal government.

You might ask why doing all this research and taking the extra steps to determine which doctor or hospital you should choose is so important. In recent years, study after study has shown that where you check in, and who provides your care, can seriously affect your recovery. In fact, it can truly be a life or death decision. So where should you go? Which doctor should you entrust with your health? And how can you maximize your chances for a successful outcome?

This book is designed to lead you through the process of choosing the people who are going to take care of you. Our goal is to arm you with the step-by-step guidance and hard data you need to get you and your loved ones the best care possible.

WHAT YOU'LL FIND IN THIS BOOK

The first section is a series of chapters written by Samantha Collier, MD, MBA, HealthGrades' chief medical officer. In these chapters, Dr. Collier demystifies and debunks commonly held beliefs about doctors, hospitals, and what you should expect if you're a patient. With a no-nonsense style, she explains everything you need to know to avoid feeling overwhelmed and victimized by the medical industry. She tells you how to accomplish such basic and vital tasks as finding the best doctor and hospital for your specific requirements, how to identify your own unique needs as a patient, and how to manage conversations and interactions within the healthcare community. Dr. Collier provides you with useful information such as specific questions to ask a doctor to determine if he or she is right for you, how to be an advocate for yourself or your loved ones, and what routine procedures to expect if you've been admitted to the hospital. In other words, Dr. Collier is your advocate as you learn how to become your own best healthcare advocate. These chapters help to take the usual fear and apprehension out of the healthcare process, and provide a look behind the curtain to give you the tools and confidence to demand the best care.

Following the chapters by Dr. Collier are HealthGrades' hospital ratings and top doctor lists, organized by state. These ratings are the essence of what HealthGrades has to offer and are the key to guiding you to the best healthcare you can find. These clearly defined, user friendly presentations of our ratings will show you which doctors and hospitals in each state have the best success rates in all of the most common areas of practice, and even a few uncommon ones too.

WHO IS HEALTHGRADES?

HealthGrades published the first hospital-quality ratings for consumers a decade ago. At the time, it was not widely known that doctor and hospital care varied dramatically from person to person and facility to facility. Additionally, most people didn't even know they had the ability to make choices regarding the hospitals they would attend. HealthGrades was invested in educating the public about its healthcare options so everyone would have a chance at receiving the best care possible. Extensive research was done into all aspects of physician and hospital care, from mortality and major complication rates to frequency of patient safety issues. The end result was a highly detailed body of information that made it clear which doctors and hospitals were making the grade and which were not.

Thanks to all that research, a few interesting facts came to light. Contrary to popular belief, it was clear that a doctor's or hospital's reputation could have very little to do with their overall performance. By using its fact-based research criteria such as actual patient outcomes, and ignoring word of mouth recommendations, HealthGrades found out that popular wisdom about doctors and hospitals actually held little water. For instance, they discovered that some highly reputable hospitals did not in fact have the superior patient outcomes you would suspect, while some smaller hospitals were performing at world-class levels in suburban or rural areas. HealthGrades learned that it would have to re-educate people about the basic ways in which they thought about their healthcare. Only then would they become better consumers.

Ten years ago, all of this peeling back of the healthcare veil was a revolutionary concept for the average person and more than a little bit scary for healthcare providers. Today, this groundbreaking idea of hard data based quality ratings for healthcare providers has been validated and accepted by peer-reviewed medical journals and is in widespread use by millions of consumers. In fact, it has become so accepted that the federal government, as well as various state governments, have followed HealthGrades' lead by rating hospitals in one way or another and providing statistics of their own.

In the ten years since its inception, HealthGrades has grown to be the leading healthcare ratings company in the nation, with more people, hospitals, companies, and health plans relying on HealthGrades' ratings than any other organization. Based in Golden, Colorado, HealthGrades employs statisticians, physicians, and data specialists of all stripes to gather and analyze data, largely from governmental sources.

As they have every year over the past decade, HealthGrades continues to push the limits on what consumers can expect from their healthcare by finding out which hospitals and doctors are excelling and which are not. HealthGrades analyzes tens of millions of hospitalization records, physician data, and more, from more than one hundred different sources. It's an enormous undertaking, and not only from a computing perspective. The hands-on human resources behind these ratings are striking, as each medical procedure is statistically analyzed in a variety of ways, relying on both statisticians and medical staff.

The result is the nation's most trusted healthcare rating system.

UNDERSTANDING OUR RATINGS

Throughout the book, you'll see simple star ratings for hospitals, like those used for hotels and restaurants.

All the star ratings in this book are based on *real patient outcomes*; we have analyzed the history of complication rates and death rates for patients at one hospital compared with another hospital over a period of three years. After compiling all of that information and determining the difference between the doctors and hospitals outcomes, we have identified the multiple levels of care and expertise available to healthcare consumers. We have grouped the doctors and hospitals according to their level of excellence and have assigned each one through five stars based on their performance.

A five star rating means the hospital performed among the best in the nation for a particular condition or procedure. A three star rating means the hospital performed as expected, or average. And a one star rating means the hospital performed worse than expected, or poorly, for a particular condition or procedure.

HealthGrades' star ratings reflect the complication rates and death rates for individual procedures and clinical specialty areas. So a five star rating for knee replacement means that complication rates for patients at that hospital are well below the national average for knee replacement. A one star rating would mean that the hospital's patients experienced more complications than other hospitals.

The difference between going to a five star hospital and a one star hospital can be striking. On average, death rates at one star hospitals are 64 percent higher than at five star hospitals for the procedures and treatments rated by HealthGrades. That is an enormous difference, underscoring the need for patients to do their homework before they check in.

If a hospital is not rated for a procedure or condition you are interested in researching, it is likely that the hospital either does not perform this procedure or did not have enough volume to be rated, which is a minimum of thirty cases over three years.

A NOTE ON COMPARING HOSPITALS FAIRLY

In order to make fair, apples-to-apples comparisons, HealthGrades uses a complex statistical formula called multivariate logistic regression to deal with the complex patients hospitals might receive. Some hospitals might get sicker patients than the hospital across town. For example, consider two sixty-five-year-old males admitted with pneumonia, but one has respiratory failure and one does not. Of the two men in this scenario, the man with respiratory failure will have the higher odds of dying in the hospital. Some hospitals may get more pneumonia patients who have respiratory failure, and some will get less. In order to be able to fairly compare the quality of each hospital's pneumonia care, it's imperative to level the playing field by adjusting for the different risks each patient has that would increase his or her chance of dying. HealthGrades has adjusted for these patient differences to fairly rate and compare hospitals for all the procedures and conditions listed in this book. The hospital ratings of five star, three star, and one star following this section are the end result of this adjustment.

WHERE SHOULD I START?

To find the best hospitals for you, first identify the state in which you need the doctor or hospital to be. Each state is represented by a chapter and each state chapter is divided into four sections:

- Hospital Ratings by Clinical Specialty
- Five Star Rated Hospitals
- HealthGrades Top Doctors
- Hospital Ratings by Procedure

Hospital Ratings by Clinical Specialty

To see an overview of hospitals, take a look at the Hospital Ratings by Clinical Specialty section. All of the hospitals listed are grouped by state for quick and easy reference. There, you'll find basic contact information for each hospital as well as overall ratings for clinical specialties, from gastrointestinal surgery to cardiac care. These star ratings are

summaries of the quality of care at each hospital for the individual procedures in that specialty area. For example, the cardiac clinical program rating is a summary of the hospital's star ratings across cardiac procedures and treatments, from bypass surgery to valve replacements.

Five Star Rated Hospitals

Within a state, you can quickly find which hospitals have HealthGrades' highest rating of five stars within a given procedure. For knee replacement surgery, maternity care, bypass surgery, and other specific procedures and treatments, five star rated hospitals are listed so that you can quickly have a baseline list of hospitals that have a track record of clinical excellence in that procedure.

HealthGrades Top Doctors

Consulting the Top Doctors section in this book will put you in the hands of physicians who perform procedures at highly rated hospitals.

The doctor lists in this book reflect the first time that highly performing physicians across the country have been identified based on objective data. You may be familiar with the "top doctors" editions of city news magazines. To put those together, magazines rely heavily on reputation—subjective surveys filled out by other doctors. HealthGrades' Top Doctors lists are very different from those that have come before them. By focusing on objective patient-outcome information, these doctors are, purely by the numbers, among the best in the nation.

Hospital Ratings by Procedure

Here you will find, in each state, all the Health-Grades star ratings for virtually every hospital in the country. There are two ways to view these pages: first, take a look at your local hospitals and track their star ratings across procedures and treatments. That will give you a good idea of each hospital's specific quality ratings across the board, from appendectomies to women's health. The second way to view these chapters is to look at the particular procedure or treatment in the top columns, and then follow that down the column and see the ratings for that particular procedure for each hospital in your state.

YOU'RE READY TO TAKE CONTROL OF YOUR WELL BEING

Using the tips learned in the chapters that follow, and the star ratings and Top Doctor lists that make up the bulk of this book, you will be equipped with a powerful set of information not available to individuals only a few years ago. But now, with HealthGrades as your guide, you can feel confident navigating the healthcare system and securing the highest quality care for yourself and your family.

CHAPTER 1

HOW TO CHOOSE A DOCTOR

The average American spends at least six hours a week shopping. Much of this time is spent researching the products and services we're interested in before we lay out our hard-earned money. We do this with everything from breakfast cereal to running shoes. Americans spend the most time researching automobiles because we want cars that will protect us, and maybe even save our lives should we ever be in an accident. Paradoxically, the one area in which we spend very little time and energy as consumers is when we decide which healthcare professionals to use. You might say, "Well, choosing a car is totally different from choosing a doctor." But consider the similarities. Each costs a lot of money, has to do a good job, and with both you are putting your life on the line.

The point is simply that we Americans should feel entitled to shift the way in which we view our healthcare—to view it the way any important purchase would be and to treat healthcare as our most important investment. Doctors aren't doing you a favor by performing their services, nor are they supposed to make you uncomfortable or frightened. You are paying them and, as a good consumer, you owe

> WE AMERICANS SHOULD FEEL entitled to shift the way in which we view our healthcare—to view it the way any important purchase would be and to treat healthcare as our most important investment.

it to yourself to learn how to get the best bang for your buck. It's the most important lesson you could ever learn. The mission of this book is to teach you how to be a savvy healthcare consumer; to optimize the healthcare that you and your loved ones receive.

This chapter is dedicated to teaching you the basic skills that go into effectively choosing a doctor. If you are going to put your life, or the life of a loved one, in the hands of a stranger, careful due diligence is paramount.

By following the simple and effective steps for finding a doctor outlined in this chapter, you will avoid situations that can lead to substandard care and you will maximize your chances of finding a healthy, comfortable, and long lasting relationship with a physician you and your family can trust.

STEP ONE: SPEAKING UP

The number one rule to remember as you embark on your search for the right doctor is to be proactive. Be sure to take charge and don't be afraid to speak up. Doctors and other medical professionals are busy people, but high quality clinicians will take the time to listen to their patients. An attentive physician will slow down to give you the answers you need to be a happy and satisfied patient because, ultimately, if you understand your own healthcare you have a better chance at contributing to maintaining your health. Any doctor who doesn't take the time to listen and respond is not providing top-notch care. And patients who don't ask questions risk finding themselves in an uncomfortable, if not dangerous, situation. It is your job to speak up.

If you're having a hard time picturing what is meant by being proactive versus being passive, imagine this scenario:

You are sitting in your physician's office after your annual exam, and a routine test has uncovered something unexpected: an unidentifiable spot on your lung that could be a tumor. The news stuns you and suddenly you feel helpless, afraid, and vulnerable. The white paper stretched tight along the exam table crinkles and sticks momentarily to your sweaty palms as you shift uncomfortably and ask in a barely audible voice, "A tumor?" Your mind is already forming what you can't yet voice, "Cancer? Lung cancer?"

You've never smoked cigarettes, but your husband is a pack-a-day smoker. In the back of your mind, you've seen this day coming for years. Your chest tightens.

"Well, we can't determine the exact nature of the abnormality at this point," the doctor says. "This type of imaging to find those spots just doesn't provide us with that level of detail. It may be nothing, but, I'll be honest with you, it may be an indication of something very serious. I'm recommending that you have a CT Scan as soon as possible. My office will call you to schedule the test."

Your head reeling, you barely hear the doctor ask if you have any more questions, as you struggle to your feet and walk numbly from the office to your car.

The next three weeks are agonizing. You check your voice mail messages every few hours. But there is no call from the doctor's office. You have already scoured the Internet, reading every symptom, prognosis, and death rate for lung cancer that you can find. You've prepared your family for the worst. You've even reviewed your will.

A few more days go by and you can't stand it anymore. You call the doctor's office. You get a nurse

DURING A RECENT ROUTINE EYE EXAM, the doctor mentioned a retinal abnormality. The patient was scared. "What does that mean?" he asked, while the doctor continued to examine his eye. "Do I have an emergency? Do I need to get this taken care of right now?"

It turned out that although the issue was minor and the patient—who also happened to be a doctor—didn't have to receive emergency care, he would have to see a specialist. Of course, the patient wanted to make sure he would be referred to the best specialist available. The eye doctor said, "There are a lot of good ones out there." But the other doctor pressed, "What do you mean by good?" He thought to himself, "Good golf handicap or good with my eyes?"

"Well, they all have a good reputation," he said.

The physician/patient was getting nowhere, so he finally asked, "Who would you go to?"

The eye doctor immediately responded, "Oh, I'd go to Dr. Milton."

who says he is busy, but assures you that someone will call you to schedule your CT Scan. You wait another two weeks. You make two more phone calls. Nothing.

Finally your daughter, exhausted by your emotional state and fed up with the lack of response from your doctor, convinces you to see a specialist recommended by a friend who is a physician.

"It's who she says she'd go to, mom," your daughter tells you.

The next Thursday, you see the doctor, who, during the visit, schedules a scan at the local hospital for Friday morning. Monday, at 4:30 p.m., you get the phone call.

"There is nothing to worry about," the doctor says. "It's just scar tissue from a past infection that resolved. Did you ever live in the southwest?" You quickly answer "yes" and he assures you that this type of scar tissue is common in people who lived in the southwest, as you once did, and there is nothing to worry about.

The preceding events happened to an older, female patient who endured weeks of emotional distress because of a preventable communication breakdown with her doctor. She could have avoided the confusion and miscommunication that lead to unnecessary pain and angst by being proactive and making as many calls as she needed to avoid waiting so long for results. As a passive patient, she assumed that her doctor was telling her everything she needed to know. She never thought of questioning her doctor, because to her, that would have been disrespectful. She was the type of patient who would have fared better in the care of an empowering and knowledgeable doctor, one who made a conscious effort to spend extra time listening to his or her patients and explaining diagnoses and treatments in layman's terms. She also may have been better matched with a physician in a smaller, less busy practice, who was diligent about following up on phone calls to patients.

Her physician, like many physicians working in overbooked, hectic practices, obviously failed to slow down long enough to realize that his strictly clinical explanation of her test results may not have addressed his patient's perfectly normal and human fears. He may have neglected to quickly schedule her CT Scan because he knew that the spots were probably nothing to worry about. Or, more likely, he simply forgot to follow up.

Either way, his brusque bedside manner didn't match up with his patient's need for a little extra time, thoughtful education, or communication.

Determining what kind of doctor-patient relationship you need is as simple as asking, "What kind of patient am I?" You must identify your personality and unique needs so you can communicate them to any potential doctor you may choose.

STEP TWO: DISCOVERING WHO YOU ARE AS A PATIENT

Choosing the right doctor is a lot like dating. The better you know yourself going into the process, the better your chances are for finding the perfect match. There are a lot of outstanding physicians out there who are capable of providing high quality

> DETERMINING WHAT KIND OF doctor-patient relationship you need is as simple as asking, "What kind of patient am I?" You must identify your personality and unique needs so you can communicate them to any potential doctor you may choose.

medical care, but if you are not comfortable enough to be open and honest with the one you choose, you could jeopardize your health. It is extremely important that you choose a doctor who puts you at ease and allows you to fully express yourself. It is essential that you feel comfortable being completely honest with your doctor, whether you are not taking your blood pressure medication, haven't given up your high fat diet, or have started smoking again.

It's completely normal to meet someone and think, "that person isn't for me." That applies to meeting a new doctor as well. The difference is that with doctors, unlike new acquaintances, you will be asked to share intimate details about your body, your health, and your habits. If your physician's social or cultural beliefs, age, gender, or bedside manner make you uncomfortable and you find you are less than forthright about your health habits, you could be preventing proper diagnosis and treatment by remaining silent in their presence. Don't worry about eliminating anyone from your list of potential doctors for any reason at all. Your comfort and health have to be your primary concern, not whether or not you're being "nice" or "fair" to a prospective doctor.

Figuring out what kind of patient you are is a task with which you're probably not very familiar. Here are a few questions that will help you better understand your patient profile so that you can choose the best doctor for you:

1. Do you feel more comfortable with a male or female physician? Some people are fine with either gender, while others are uncomfortable being examined or talking openly about their bodies with someone of the opposite—or the same—gender.

2. Do you value the wisdom and experience of an older doctor or the fresh, up-to-date perspective of a younger physician? If you lack respect for your doctor, you are less likely to take their advice, which can lead to poor health outcomes.

3. Is punctuality important to you? If so, you will easily grow frustrated and cranky with a doctor who routinely makes you wait half an hour in the waiting room and another twenty minutes in the exam room before each visit.

4. Are compassion and empathy important to you? If you're looking for a good listener, for example, research has shown you might be happier with a female doctor.

5. Do you value knowledge and intellectual prowess more than small talk and handholding? You may be more confident with a doctor who takes detailed notes and describes your diagnosis in clinical terms.

TOP FIVE TIPS FOR CHOOSING A DOCTOR

1. Do your research: check that the doctor is in good standing with state medical boards and see if they are board certified.

2. Ask to meet with and interview your doctor choices, free of charge. If they say "no," scratch them off your list of possibilities.

3. Imagine your ideal relationship with your future doctor. Write down these qualities in your ideal physician that bring out the best patient in you and use this as your checklist during your physician interviews.

4. Check out the doctor's office—is it organized or chaotic? Was the office staff attentive and courteous? Were you seen promptly? Were the reading materials up to date? If the answers are "yes," chances are your physician pays attention to details and will pay attention to you.

5. Find out how compulsive and thorough your doctor is by asking if they are ever afraid they might miss something. If they say "never," choose another doctor. If they say "sometimes," chances are, they will be thorough and compulsive with your care.

6. Do you expect your physician to always be available when you have an urgent or emergent medical need? If so, you may not be comfortable with a doctor who is part of a large group practice where the doctors share call.

Narrowing the Field

Now that you have a clearer idea of who you are and what you are looking for as a patient, you're ready to start searching for a compatible doctor. By now, you may even have a pretty good idea of the characteristics you're looking for.

If you have health insurance, the simplest place to start your search is by reviewing the list of doctors who are in your health plan's network. Most health plans offer quick access to physician directories on their Web sites. Or, you can request a paper version from your plan. If you do not have insurance, you can use a phone directory or a Web site that lists physicians by geographic area. You can quickly narrow your list by first looking for those doctors who practice within a few miles of your home or work. Remember, you want getting to the doctor to be

> BEFORE SEEKING TREATMENT FROM any doctor, check out his or her educational background and credentials; and use a credible source to do so.

convenient so you won't have excuses for missing appointments, or feel isolated from your doctor in an emergency.

Next, further hone your list by using what you learned about your personal preferences. For example, you might want to eliminate physicians of a certain gender or cross doctors off the list who are not in the age range that you prefer. It's interesting to note that healthcare providers' directories are starting to include detailed information about doctors, such as their age.

You should be able to identify a half dozen or so physicians who meet your initial criteria. For example: female pediatricians under age fifty who practice within ten miles of your child's daycare.

At this point, you may be tempted to call and schedule an appointment. But wait; with a little extra time and effort, you are going to make an informed and confident choice that will serve you well for years to come.

STEP THREE: THE BACKGROUND CHECK

The next step, the background check, is critical. Before seeking treatment from any doctor, check out his or her educational background and credentials; and use a credible source to do so. Most health plan directories provide only basic information, such as address, phone number, gender, and the name of the medical school from which the doctor graduated. You really can't tell much, if anything, about the quality of the doctor from this information. Unless you are an academic insider, you probably don't know, for example, which school houses the nation's best cardiology program or offers top-notch pediatrics training. Generally, doctors will tell you that the program he or she graduated from is the best. Don't believe them. Do your own research instead.

A more effective method of gauging the rigor of a physician's background is to use the physician pages in this book. If you search their name on the Web you can also find detailed reports on physicians' post-graduate training, such as residencies and fellowships, board certification, and other awards and professional honors. You can also find out if a doctor has had malpractice claims filed against him or her, or worse, been sanctioned by a state medical board.

What we're getting at here is that it is important to understand the meanings of the various academic achievements, training and credentials that your doctor may or may not have. Here are some critical questions for you to ask as you review the background of the doctors on your list:

1. Is the physician board certified? This can be more important in some specialty areas than others, but overall, being board certified means that the physician has taken and passed his or her medical specialty exam, which can be an indicator of doctor quality.

2. Has the physician ever paid out a large amount of money in a malpractice case? Unfortunately, these days even top-notch doctors can be the

TO BE OR NOT TO BE BOARD CERTIFIED

DOES BOARD CERTIFICATION REALLY MATTER? Yes and No.

Being board certified is a good indicator that a doctor has completed extensive training in their particular area of specialization, but it isn't a litmus test for quality in all cases. The significance of the certification really depends on the generation and on the doctor's area of specialty.

For example, many older doctors tend not to bother with getting board certified because the exam wasn't a prominent measure of quality when they began practicing. Plus, the two-day exam costs from $1,200 to $1,500 and many doctors just don't want to spend the time or money on something they aren't required to have.

Among younger physicians, board certification is a much clearer measure of quality, as the relevance of the designation has grown. Most accredited residency programs now require a passing score in order to successfully complete their program.

For specialties such as internal medicine, cardiology, pediatrics and gerontology, the exam is widely accepted as a necessary step to practicing medicine. However, in some specialties, like orthopedics and anesthesiology, board certification is not as common.

The bottom line is, ask any physician on your list who is not board certified why they are not. If they don't have a good answer or are evasive, it's probably best to move on.

DANGEROUS DOC OR FRIVOLOUS LAWSUIT?

MALPRACTICE LAWSUITS ARE A FACT OF life for physicians in today's litigation driven culture. So the presence of a malpractice claim or settlement on a doctor's record does not necessarily mean that physician is providing substandard care. As an informed patient, the easiest way for you to cut through the quagmire is to ask a physician about any high cost you found on his or her record. If the doctor gets defensive, refuses to answer your question, or says something that scares you, move on.

Sanctions are another matter altogether and should be treated like red flags. If you see a state sanction on a physician's record, you probably don't want this doctor to treat you.

Sanctions are disciplinary actions that come from a state board and they are serious. Sanctions don't get handed out because a few patients called the state medical board to complain. Events that lead to state sanctions are incredibly serious and have been investigated thoroughly. Not all investigations lead to official action, which means that if a doctor has been sanctioned, a board of doctors has reviewed the case and decided that serious errors were made.

MD vs. DO

DOCTORS OF MEDICINE (MDs) AND DOCTORS of Osteopathy (DOs) are both doctors, they just went to different types of medical schools. MDs graduate from allopathic medical schools, where each system of the body is studied separately. DOs graduate from osteopathic medical schools, where the body as a whole is emphasized.

There are far more MDs than DOs in the United States, but both MDs and DOs can become fully licensed physicians and surgeons. There are twenty-seven accredited osteopathic medical schools in the U.S. and 125 accredited U.S. allopathic (MD) medical schools.

Like an MD, an osteopath completes four years of medical school and can choose to practice in any specialty of medicine with further training, but most DOs choose to practice in the field of primary care.

Both curriculums are based in science. The treatment approach is a matter of your personal preference as a patient.

targets of frivolous malpractice lawsuits. The best indicator of whether or not a doctor has truly made a major mistake is a large payout ordered by the court.

3. Did the physician complete a residency in the area in which he or she is practicing? For example, if you plan to have cosmetic surgery, did the physician complete a residency training program in plastic surgery?

4. Is the physician an MD or a DO? An MD is a medical doctor, while a DO is a doctor of osteopathy. Each is equally well trained but has different philosophies for treating the human body. See "MD vs. DO" on this page for more details on MDs and DOs.

MEDICAL MYTHS: IT'S TIME TO DEBUNK THEM

Myth #1: Older is better

Don't count out the newbies. Recent medical school graduates have just experienced the intensity and rigors of training and may provide better care than you think. Conversely, the longer a doctor has been out of residency, the less familiar he or she is likely to be with the latest medical technology, cutting edge techniques, and treatment innovations.

Myth #2: The more tests the better

There's a fine line between the appropriate number of tests and too many. Just because your doctor orders more tests doesn't mean he or she is thorough. In fact, it may mean the doctor could be incompetent and doesn't know what's wrong with you, so he or she is trying to narrow it down by testing, testing, testing.

The majority of diagnoses usually are identified from your exam and medical history, not tests. Tests usually confirm or rule out a diagnosis. Basing a diagnosis solely on test results can be irresponsible because not only can a test yield false positives and cause undo anxiety, but they also can lead to more invasive testing and procedures for the patient.

Myth #3: Antibiotics kill just about everything

Don't mistake a prescription-happy doctor with a high quality one.

Just like lab tests, more prescriptions don't mean better care, especially when it comes to antibiotics. It can be hard to hear this when you've been sick as a dog for days, but antibiotics do not work on viral infections. No responsible physician will write a patient a prescription for antibiotics unless history, a physician exam, and sometimes tests prove the illness is caused by bacteria.

Many patients confuse viral illnesses with bacterial illnesses. For example, viruses cause the common cold and many upper respiratory ailments. Viruses do not respond to antibiotic medications. Bacteria do. Taking antibiotics when you do not need them can cause bacteria to mutate into drug-resistant monster strains that no drug can treat.

STEP FOUR: THE INTERVIEW

Now that you've determined what kind of patient you are, identified the traits you're looking for in a doctor, and screened out those doctors with troubling track records, you should have a handful of potentially high caliber candidates on your list. Now it's time to seal the deal. It is time to interview the doctors in person.

If you are tempted to skip this step, don't. You are going to entrust this total stranger with your health and well being. It is certainly worth sitting down face to face with him or her for twenty minutes, which is about all the time you'll need to make your decision.

Preparing for the Interview

Prepare for your interview visit just as you would if you were a manager at a big corporation scrutinizing a potential new hire. Get out a pen and paper or get on your computer and write down four or five key questions you want to ask the doctor. Remember to bring these with you to the interview! It's easy to get flustered in a new situation, and bringing that list of questions will ensure that you don't forget anything you want to ask. For some people, simply having a list makes them feel more authoritative, and therefore, more powerful. Let the list work for you.

The point of the prepared list of questions is to make sure you effectively communicate your expectations and needs and that your new doctor knows that he or she must live up to them. When you formulate your list, you should keep the attributes you identified in yourself as a patient in mind. Your patient profile will dictate your expectations and needs and will shape your questions. A few potential questions you might ask, regardless of your patient profile, are:

1. How far in advance do I need to call to make an appointment?
2. What if I have an urgent health need? Would you work me into your schedule the same day?

THE POINT OF THE prepared list of questions is to make sure you effectively communicate your expectations and needs and that your new doctor knows that he or she must live up to them.

3. If I have an emergency and go to the hospital, will you come to see me?
4. Can I bring my children to my appointments?
5. Will you respect and honor my dietary choices?
6. Will you work with me to create a health regimen that incorporates traditional as well as alternative therapies?
7. I have strong faith-based beliefs that could impact my care; are you willing to respect my wishes?

The Ultimate Question

And then there's the final, ultimate question; it's the tiebreaker. All top-notch doctors share one common characteristic. It may sound strange at first, but any doctor you ask, any good, honest doctor, will tell you it's true. The most diligent doctors share a near-compulsive attention to detail; constantly reviewing mental checklists, battling a nagging fear that something critical may have slipped by unnoticed in the chaos of the day. It's that nervous edge that keeps them sharp, alert, and focused. It is almost a constant fear of not getting it exactly right.

The way to discover if your doctor of choice is one of these doctors is to ask: "Do you ever worry?" If the answer is yes, chances are your doctor will tell you why and it will go something like this: "Yes, I worry sometimes that I may have missed some small detail, but that is why I may ask you a lot of questions that don't make sense to you right away. Medicine is an inexact science and so I'm always listening to my gut, listening to make sure I didn't miss something."

That sort of answer is honest and direct; a good bet for building a solid, trustworthy relationship that will last.

If the answer is a resounding no, then be wary. If the doctor isn't comfortable answering your questions now, he or she likely won't be a good fit for you in the future. There are plenty of doctors who will say yes.

Interview Time

It's best to call the doctor's office about two to three weeks before the date you'd like to schedule the interview. Physicians, especially good ones, can have schedules that are fully booked ahead for weeks or even months.

When you call the physician's office, tell the receptionist that you are a potential new patient and that you'd like to schedule a twenty-minute consultation to determine whether the doctor is right for you. Don't be shy. No truly attentive doctor wants to work with a patient who doesn't trust and respect him or her. If any doctor on your list refuses an introductory interview, scratch them off and move on.

Be aware that some physicians' practices may be closed to new patients, or closed to patients with certain types of insurance. If you do not have insurance, be sure to ask up front if the physician has a discount or charity care policy.

On the day of the interview, remember to bring a pen, paper, and the questions you've prepared in advance. The following are tips to help you get the most out of this all-important visit:

1. When you walk in the door, notice the environment of the physician's office. Is it clean? Is the staff friendly? Do the other patients look

MUST DO'S FOR YOUR FIRST VISIT WITH YOUR NEW DOCTOR

1. Have your medical records from your previous physician sent to your new physician one month before your scheduled visit. Ask and set the expectation that your new doctor will review these documents before your first visit.

2. Be prepared. Maximize your first visit by creating a list of no more than two to three symptomatic complaints and a document that includes your pertinent medical history, family history, last physical exam, significant lab tests, medical allergies, and medication list—with doses.

3. Discuss with your physician your hospital preference, who would make your medical decisions if you are incapacitated, and whether you would want to be resuscitated in the event you should stop breathing or your heart stops.

4. Bring a notebook so you can write down what the doctor says about any diagnoses and treatment plans. Make sure you completely understand the plan before your doctor leaves the room.

5. If you require any tests or specialist consultations, ask your doctor to call you for normal and abnormal results. Document these results in your notebook with the date and the reason for the test.

reasonably comfortable, or are they suffering in their seats because they've been waiting too long?

2. When you greet the doctor, is he or she attentive? Respectful?

3. As you conduct your interview, note the physician's communication style and body language. Is the doctor paying attention to you or is he or she simply reading the paperwork you just filled out or a medical chart?

4. When your twenty minutes is up, make sure to thank the doctor for his or her time and tell the doctor you will follow up later if you decide to schedule a medical exam.

STEP FIVE: REFERRALS— FINDING THAT EXTRA SPECIAL SPECIALIST

When your medical condition requires more advanced diagnosis or treatment than your primary care doctor can provide, you will need to see a specialist, such as a cardiologist, orthopedic surgeon, or gastroenterologist. While the steps already outlined in this chapter are designed not only to help you find the right primary care physician, but also guide you to quality specialty care, there are a few complicating factors to keep in mind when you need a referral.

Some types of health insurance plans allow patients to self-refer. If this is the case, or you plan to pay out of pocket for your care, you can follow the advice in this chapter to guide yourself to a specialist. However, if your insurance company requires what is

called a "referral" from your primary care physician, or if you'd simply like to get your family doctor's expert opinion, there are a few more issues to keep in mind.

Chances are that your primary care physician will recommend a few physicians for you to choose from. What you need to know is that while these may very well be top-notch physicians, they could also be golfing buddies or doctors who practice within the same medical office building who routinely refer each other business out of convenience and habit.

Or, your doctor may think he or she is doing you a favor by recommending a physician whose practice is located close to your home or work. Or he or she may choose to recommend only those doctors who are included in your health insurance plan's network, when, in fact, you want to know all the options available to you.

CHANCES ARE THAT YOUR primary care physician will recommend a few physicians for you to choose from. What you need to know is that while these very well may be top-notch physicians, they could also be golfing buddies or doctors who practice within the same medical office building who routinely refer each other business out of convenience and habit.

One of the best ways to guarantee that your doctor gives you the name of a truly top-notch specialist is to ask this one question: "Who would you go to?"

This almost always yields a decisive answer.

NOW WHAT?

Congratulations! Now that you've worked your way through the steps outlined in this chapter, you can be confident you've chosen a pretty great doctor. You're working with a physician who has a quality background and who listens to and respects you. Now it's up to you to keep your diligent, proactive approach during your first medical visit and all the visits that follow.

The most important thing to do once you start seeing your new doctor is to keep asking questions. If you have a health issue that is identified by your doctor, asking the following questions will help keep you on track as an empowered and informed patient:

1. What's my diagnosis?
2. What symptoms or health factors lead you to that diagnosis?
3. What is my treatment plan?
4. When will the results of my lab test be ready?
5. What happens after my test results come back?
6. Will you call me? When?
7. If I don't hear from you, is it okay for me to call your office?
8. With whom should I speak when I call for test results?

Make sure you understand each answer. Your physician should give you the information to feel empowered to take charge of your health.

Don't be passive. If you're not getting what you want, be clear about it.

Above all, you must trust your instincts about what's right for you. If you feel relaxed, empowered, and understood when you visit your doctor's office, you've chosen wisely and you'll most likely receive excellent healthcare. Remember that only you can know what's working for you and that a periodic assessment of the care you're getting will keep your doctor-patient relationship on track. To sum up the main lesson of this chapter: do your homework, trust your instincts, and then go with your gut.

WHEN TO BREAK UP WITH YOUR DOCTOR

THERE MAY BE A TIME WHEN it becomes clear that your doctor is not providing you with the best possible care. Leaving your doctor can be a difficult thing to do, especially if you have built a relationship with him or her over a long period of time. But for you own health and well being, the breakup is something you must do. Here are a few tips on how to recognize when it's time to move on:

1. Your physician does not return your calls in a timely manner, or isn't following up with you as discussed.

2. You feel like your physician doesn't care about you. A few signs may be: he or she isn't listening, isn't taking the time to answer your questions, allows frequent interruptions during your visit, or dismisses your complaints.

3. You feel like you can't trust or be honest with your physician.

4. You can't get an appointment when you need one.

5. Your physician received a disciplinary action/sanction from the state medical board.

Helpful Hint: *Before* "breaking up," make sure to get a complete copy of all of your outpatient medical records, including all physician notes, tests, X-rays, biopsies, and any other relevant medical information in your file. Also, out of courtesy, send a letter to your physician notifying them that you are changing physicians. You do not need to explain why. Follow the "Top Tips for Choosing a Doctor" in this section when selecting your new physician.

CHAPTER 2

HOW TO CHOOSE A HOSPITAL

Most people don't think about hospitals until they are faced with the prospect of having to check into one. Hospitals tend to make most people nervous at best, and panicky at worst. The result of this hospital-induced anxiety is that people don't spend any time thinking about the relative merits of the hospitals in their area and where they would go should they face an illness or emergency. If you fit this description, you risk winding up at a hospital wondering, "Is there a place out there that might be less (insert complaint here) than this one?" The answer is probably "yes." This chapter is dedicated to helping you choose the hospital that's right for you so that you can spend your time recovering, not worrying whether you are in the best place.

Most patients who have been admitted to a hospital have been directed there by the doctor who scheduled a procedure for them. People usually don't think twice about a referral to their doctor's hospital of choice and simply show up and check in. Although this is certainly one way to wind up at a good hospital, it's not necessarily the best.

Still, trusting your doctor's advice is a good place to start. But if you want to optimize the quality of medical care you receive, it's a good idea to learn how and why doctors send patients to certain hospitals, and how to identify which hospitals are likely to provide the best care in specific clinical areas. Then you can begin to think of the questions you should ask your doctor to ensure that you go to the hospital where you are most likely to get the highest possible quality of care. Contrary to most people's assumptions, very few hospitals are truly great at everything. Most specialize in one or two areas, such as treating heart attacks or repairing hips. It's vital to know whether or not that hospital is the best one for handling your specific procedure.

Choosing the right hospital is just as important as choosing the right doctor, since it can mean the difference between life and death. Consider these

> . . . IF YOU WANT to optimize the quality of medical care you receive, it's a good idea to learn how and why doctors send patients to certain hospitals, and how to identify which hospitals are likely to provide the best care in specific clinical areas.

startling statistics: HealthGrades' research has found that patients treated at top rated hospitals have nearly a one-third better chance of surviving, on average, than those admitted to all other hospitals. A patient who undergoes surgery at a high performing hospital also has an average of a five percent lower risk of complication during his or her stay.

If you want to ensure that you are getting the best possible care, it is imperative that you do your homework before being admitted to a hospital.

HOSPITAL 101

American hospitals come in all shapes and sizes, from small community hospitals which provide basic, emergency care, to urban medical centers specializing in a few clinical areas such as burn care or heart surgery. If you live in a large, urban area, you will have many options to choose from that are close to home. If you live in a more rural area, distance, travel conditions, and transportation options may play a large role in determining which hospital you choose.

Hospital policies and culture can also be influenced greatly by the hospital administration's choice of business model. For example, some hospitals are owned by large, for-profit, national corporations, while others are run by nonprofit groups such as local communities or faith-based organizations.

COMMON ASSUMPTIONS PATIENTS MAKE

1. **Nonprofit hospitals will take better care of me because it's their mission.** Not necessarily. While there are many high quality nonprofit hospitals nationwide, there are also many outstanding for-profit hospitals. Nonprofit hospitals have to watch their costs just as closely as for-profit hospitals; after all, they have a bottom line to protect as well.

2. **The longer my stay in the hospital, the better care I am getting.** In most cases, you will want to get out of the hospital as fast as you can. Hospital stays exceeding three or four days indicate serious illness or the occurrence of unexpected complications. Hospitals are full of germs and the longer you stay, the greater your chance of acquiring an infection or exposing yourself to a medication error or other risk.

There are academic medical centers that house teaching hospitals and there are small specialty hospitals owned and operated by physicians. All of these choices determine the amount of funding that the hospital has, the type of staff available, and the manner in which the hospital's patients are treated. Knowing your hospital's business model can provide a wealth of essential information and help steer you in the right direction in your quest for the optimal healthcare experience.

A hospital's reputation can frequently precede it, and the more recognizable the hospital's name, the more the average patient is likely to trust it. Frequently, a hospital's name or reputation is the only thing that will contribute to a patient's choice to entrust his or her care to that institution. It's very important to remember that, just like in other areas of life, reputation isn't everything. Just because you recognize a hospital's name, or your best friend's mother had a great experience getting her knee replaced at a particular hospital, doesn't necessarily mean the facility is a good one for you. Well known hospitals sometimes provide poor quality care and lesser known hospitals can provide excellent care. The resources in this book will help you take that all-important step toward identifying which hospitals excel in the treatment of your specific diagnosis or procedure, and will guide you in making the right decision for you and your loved ones.

HOW YOUR DOCTOR CAN HELP—OR HINDER— YOUR SEARCH FOR A TOP HOSPITAL

Many patients assume that their doctor will admit them to the best possible hospital for their needs. Don't make that mistake. You need to understand that you don't have to go to the first hospital, or to any hospital, your doctor recommends. In fact, going to the doctor-recommended hospital may not be in your best interest as a patient.

That said, your doctor may be a great resource in helping you identify a top quality institution. Knowing and asking the right questions will help you collaborate effectively with your doctor to find the right hospital for you.

There are two main assumptions that doctors make about their patients. The first is that patients want to go to the hospital that is located closest to home. That might be true for you, but remember: that hospital may not provide the best care for the treatment you need. Ask your physician for a list of the hospitals where he or she practices. Most physicians have what is called "admitting privileges" at multiple hospitals. You may find that you need to travel a bit farther for a place that best suits your needs.

The second assumption doctors frequently make is that patients want to be admitted to a hospital in their insurance plan network. While this is reasonable, because most health plans charge much more for care provided by out of network hospitals, it is still worth taking the extra time and effort to find the best hospital possible. Do your research and then determine your options: Don't reject anything out of hand, and don't fall into the trap of allowing your health insurance plan to tell you where to go—you may very well have choices. Besides, most major health insurance plans offer a network of hospitals from which to choose.

Finally don't forget to ask your doctor the all-important question: "If you had a choice of all the hospitals on this list, where would you go—and why?" This is one of the best ways to get a straight answer about what facility your doctor would choose if he or she wasn't imposing any assumptions about you and your needs on the situation.

HOSPITAL ASSESSMENT

Once you've gotten a short list of hospitals from your physician, your next step in identifying the best hospital for you is to check the quality rating of the hospitals on your list. Review the section of this book entitled Five Star Hospitals by Procedure

FROM DR. COLLIER'S FILES: REPUTATION WASN'T EVERYTHING

A PREVIOUSLY HEALTHY MAN NEEDED A total hip replacement. His primary care physician referred him to an orthopedic surgeon who recommended a very prestigious university hospital that had a well known international reputation for being a top institution. This man assumed that the excellent reputation of this hospital would guarantee a good outcome for what he considered a routine, elective surgery. He did not do any further research. He checked in for the surgery and wound up with a two-week ICU stay resulting from the development of a hospital-acquired pneumonia and a collapsed lung. After he recovered from these serious complications, he needed a re-operation to correct the new hip that was not working properly. Baffled that these things could happen at this well known university hospital, he politely asked to be discharged and decided he would seek another surgeon and hospital.

Lesson learned: had he checked out this hospital's HealthGrades ratings for total hip replacement, he would have found that this highly reputable university hospital was rated one star (complication rate worse than expected) for total hip replacement. Reputation does not guarantee quality. Do your homework!

and Diagnosis. You will find a chart that lists the top quality hospitals in your state, and in the specialty area for which you need care. For example, if you live in Tampa and need a hip replacement, you can search for hospitals in Florida that have been awarded five star ratings for hip replacement surgery. These hospitals may be different than those rated five stars for heart surgery or stroke care.

Five star hospitals are those that have demonstrated consistently lower complication and mortality rates than other hospitals year after year. Clearly, the more stars your hospital has been awarded in your specialty area, the better off you'll be!

Once you've narrowed your list to a few highly rated hospitals, it's time to pick up the phone. In Chapter 1 you learned to interview potential physicians. Now you will learn key questions you must ask hospital staff to find out if the hospital is consistently providing high quality medical care.

There is no need to be shy about calling and asking questions. Assertive, proactive patients are more likely to avoid poor quality care and potentially harmful situations. Top doctors and hospitals will always be forthright when it comes to talking to patients about their medical care.

Step One: Making the Call

Call the hospital's main number (listings are on pages 46–733), and tell the receptionist that you are a patient who may be admitted soon and tell him or her what procedure you will be having. Say you would like to learn more about the hospital before you check in. Ask to speak with someone in the quality department. If the person who answers the phone isn't sure where to transfer you, explain that you are shopping for the best hospital for your care

TEACHING HOSPITALS: KNOW BEFORE YOU GO

TEACHING HOSPITALS DEFINITELY HAVE THEIR PROS and cons. The benefit is you get access to cutting edge research, clinical trials, and studies you wouldn't get anywhere else. The downside can be that medical students will likely practice on you.

There is a big misconception about medical students training at teaching hospitals, however. Yes, students will be part of your care team, but they will not be the only ones involved. In some ways, academic teaching hospitals are among the best places to be because you will have access to a doctor in the hospital 24 hours a day. Medical students are supervised by residents who are supervised by a medical intern, all of whom report to the attending physician. In most cases, three physicians are scrutinizing the plan for the day. They are all watching you and there is always someone on call round the clock. In hospitals without teaching programs, there's often nobody around—especially at three in the morning.

That said, the teaching environment is not for everyone. If being treated by medical students would be stressful for you, don't go to a teaching hospital.

and that you have a few questions about clinical quality and safety you would like to have answered so that you can feel more comfortable during your stay.

Step Two: Asking the Right Questions

Once you get a knowledgeable person on the phone, here are some key questions to ask that will give you a good idea of whether or not the hospital is providing high quality care:

1. What are the complication and survival rates for the procedure or treatment you need? Are the rates better or worse than the national average?

2. What is the nurse to patient ratio for the department in which you will receive your care? The fewer number of patients to nurses the better.

3. What are the visiting hours? Will you be allowed to have a family member or friend with you (or at least in the waiting room) at all times to act as your advocate?

4. Has the hospital experienced any serious infectious outbreaks, such as sepsis, strep, or staph in the past six months? If so, what was done to remedy the situation, and what is the current risk of exposure?

If the hospital staff refuses to answer your questions, transfers you to someone else's voice mail, or sounds defensive, they might be covering up. Or worse, they don't know the answers because they aren't tracking these important quality measures. Top hospitals diligently track their rates and develop strategies to minimize the incidence of error at their facility. As a result, they are more than happy to discuss these efforts with potential patients. If a hospital won't share this information, it is likely that it's not of a sufficient caliber for your needs. Move on.

Step Three: The On Site Visit

Next, if your hospital stay is planned, and you know you might be there for several days, call ahead and schedule a time to tour the areas of the hospital where you will be treated and/or recovering.

Bear in mind that sometimes post-surgical floors or critical care units may be off limits to visitors because of concerns about patient privacy and care. As an alternative, you can always ask to visit an unoccupied room that will be most like the room where you will stay. Most hospitals will offer tours of labor and delivery departments to expectant parents, so this is a particularly easy request to make.

While touring the hospital, turn on your powers of observation: look, smell, listen. Here are a few things to tune in to:

1. Is the hospital cluttered and unclean, or is equipment tucked safely away with hallways free of carts and other unused items?

2. Does the hospital staff appear stressed out and overwhelmed, or are the nurses and doctors calm, collected, and cordial?

3. Do visiting family members look relatively calm, or is there a lot of noise and complaining?

4. Do you smell unpleasant odors such as urine, or is the air relatively fresh?

You may also want to ask about whether you will share your room with another patient, or if it will be private. Newer hospitals are converting to mostly private rooms, but older hospitals and some areas of newer hospitals still have double rooms. If you will be recovering from surgery, for example, and know you want to do so in a quiet area with lots of privacy, make sure you ask about the availability—and cost—of a private room. Many larger hospitals now offer private suites with sleeping areas for family members, and even gourmet menus and other amenities. This kind of service can improve the quality of your stay, but you will probably pay extra for the luxury.

Ultimately, there's no guarantee that your hospital stay will be problem-free, but by doing your homework and carefully choosing a hospital that consistently provides exceptional care to its patients, you will maximize your chances for a stay without complications. In the next chapter we'll review in detail what every patient needs to know—from admission through discharge—to help you avoid medical errors and poor quality care.

CHAPTER 3

PREPARING FOR A HOSPITAL STAY: WHAT TO DO, WHAT TO EXPECT

A hospital stay is generally due to unforeseen events, which is all the more reason to have a plan for yourself and your loved ones. Hospitals can be intimidating, especially if you don't know what to expect, what to ask, or how to make sure you are getting what you need. Compound this with the emotional and physical challenges of being a patient or the patient's loved one, and the situation can quickly become confusing and stressful. Being prepared and informed offers you an enormous advantage during this stressful time.

The most important thing you can train yourself to be, whether it's for yourself or a loved one, is a good patient advocate. A patient advocate is someone who can voice the patient's interests, issues, and concerns to hospital staff and make sure that all of the patient's needs are fulfilled. A good advocate also knows the patient's medical history and can communicate these facts effectively with the staff caring for the patient. The big question is, how do you become skilled in this particular way? How can you effectively advocate for yourself, a friend or a family member if you don't know the basics of what goes on in a hospital, not to mention your own medical history and those of your loved ones? Clearly, everything starts with being informed. You should not expect to get the best outcome unless you participate proactively, which is impossible to do if you don't have all the facts. As with all things in life, when you're in the hospital, knowledge is power.

Imagine the following scenario happening to you, and you will understand how being prepared can make all the difference.

It's 3:58 a.m. and your mother calls you on her way to the hospital. She's hysterical and sobbing something about your father passing out and not waking up. She says over and over that she doesn't know how she's going to live without him. You try to calm her down and get some information about your father's condition, but it's clear that she's too emotionally overwhelmed to tell you very much. You offer to come to the hospital as soon as possible.

You arrive at the hospital emergency room at 4:45 a.m., breathless and panicky, and are met by an uninterested desk clerk who asks if you are family. "Yes," you say, and are told to sit in the waiting room until further notice. You ask the clerk how your father is doing and you're told, "We are doing

> THE MOST IMPORTANT THING you can train yourself to be, whether it's for yourself or a loved one, is a good patient advocate. A patient advocate is someone who can voice the patient's interests, issues, and concerns to hospital staff and make sure that all of the patient's needs are fulfilled.

everything we can." This offers little comfort. You try to tell yourself that "everything will be all right" but deep down inside you know that this is serious. You feel helpless.

At 5:20 a.m., your father is still in the ER. Finally, a doctor comes out to the waiting area, and introduces himself as the cardiologist. Your heart sinks. He takes you to see your father while explaining that he has had a major heart attack and is unresponsive and your mother can't provide any meaningful information regarding your father's medical history or care directives. He's hopeful you can. He asks you basic questions about your father's health, told you about the results of his treadmill test. You start to think about your father dying and you begin to cry. The doctor tells you "We're doing everything we can," and walks away. You realize you are every bit as unprepared and overwhelmed as your mother.

The information that follows will help you avoid the helplessness and frustration of this situation.

THINKING THINGS THROUGH AHEAD of time will ensure that you will feel more in control of an otherwise seemingly uncontrollable experience. Preparation will give healthcare providers critical information that could make a big difference in your care and recovery rate.

This chapter is designed to empower you by providing crucial insight into the intimidating world of hospitals. You'll read about different circumstances under which you or your loved ones might enter a hospital and how to best handle the situation. It is information that will help you be the patient or advocate you need to be to get the best possible care.

medications, past hospitalizations, and allergies. You tell the doctor that you know he's taking a blue and a purple pill, but don't know why. You think he has some kind of indigestion problem and you know he had a treadmill test, but don't know when or the results of that test. While you are trying your hardest to remember all of this and trying to stay calm, the doctor is asking you if your father would want to be resuscitated in the event of a cardiopulmonary arrest. At the same time, your mother is hysterical, your father looks terrible, and all kinds of people are rushing in and out of the room doing tests and other unknown things, mumbling words and phrases that you don't understand and make you worry even more. You hear the doctor talk about intubations, mechanical ventilation, chest compressions, pressors, and cardioversion—more things you just don't understand. You are still trying to remember the names of those pills and whether or not your father

SCENARIO 1: THE SCHEDULED HOSPITAL STAY: WHEN YOU HAVE TIME TO PREPARE

If you know in advance that you will be admitted to the hospital—for a scheduled surgery, for example—you have time to get ready. There are several steps you need to take before your stay. Preparing in advance will also be invaluable should you or a family member ever experience a medical emergency. Thinking things through ahead of time will ensure that you will feel more in control of an otherwise seemingly uncontrollable experience. Preparation will give healthcare providers critical information that could make a big difference in your care and recovery rate.

Here are some essential steps you and your loved ones should take as you prepare for a hospital stay.

1. **Designate an advocate.** The advocate could be a primary family member, a more distant relative,

or even a close family friend. Choose someone who you know can stay cool and collected and can be trusted to carry out your wishes. Also designate a back-up advocate in the event the primary advocate is not available.

2. **Prepare documentation.** Document important medical information including past medical history, current medications, allergies, and any other pertinent history. Your physicians can help with this. Also, make a list of key contact information and include the location of important documents, both financial and legal.

3. **Create an Advance Directive (Living Will) and a Durable Power of Attorney (DPOA).** Asking the following questions of yourself or your loved ones may seem difficult, but it is much easier to think them through now than to make your family and friends guess at your wishes, or worse, fight over them, later.

Some questions to think about and discuss are:

1. In the event that you were unable to breathe on your own for a significant amount of time, would you want a machine to breathe for you? This is also known as being put on life support.

FROM DR. COLLIER'S FILES: HONORING THE PATIENT'S WISHES

MR. SMITH* IS A THIRTY-SIX-YEAR-OLD MAN who suffered a severe traumatic brain injury from a car accident. He has been in a vegetative coma ever since, requiring full life-support measures such as a breathing machine (ventilator) and feeding tubes. He now has a serious hospital-acquired bloodstream infection and ventilator-acquired pneumonia. He was most recently determined to be brain dead by a neurologist who performed an electroencephalography (EEG).

Mr. Smith was in excellent health prior to his accident. He has a wife, two young children, and his parents live in the same town. After learning of the EEG results, his wife wanted to take Mr. Smith off the breathing machine. She was sure that he would never want to live like this—just existing—and she was distraught over his continued suffering. Although Mr. Smith had no formal Advance Directive outlining his wishes for life sustaining measures, the state's law supported the next of kin to be his advocate and healthcare decision-maker, which would be his wife. Because Mr. Smith would surely die soon after being withdrawn from the ventilator, his wife brought their children to the hospital and asked her husband's parents to be at the bedside to say good-bye. When the parents learned of the decision to terminate life support,

they informed the doctor and nurses that they were against this decision and that their son would never want to give up, and so to honor him, they would "keep on fighting."

Shocked and overwhelmed, the patient's wife and parents began to argue over which decision was right and what Mr. Smith would want. Although he had the legal support of the next of kin, the physician did not want to withdraw care with this issue unresolved among the primary family members. So, the doctor kept on fighting the infections, renal failure, clogged feeding tubes, while the patient remained brain dead.

Three weeks later and still brain dead, Mr. Smith was now on dialysis three times a week for his renal failure, had a chest tube to drain infected fluid from his lung, and required IV medications to keep his blood pressure up. His case, considered futile by all the doctors and nurses, was taken to the hospital's ethics committee. It was decided that he was brain dead and all treatments were futile and that care should be withdrawn.

Mr. Smith's parents sued the hospital and refused to forgive his wife. This tragic situation could have been avoided had Mr. Smith had an Advance Directive.

*This patient's name has been changed.

If so, for how long? Is there a circumstance where you would want the breathing machine (life support) withdrawn?

2. Would you want a feeding tube placed in you if you couldn't swallow safely or were comatose? If so, for how long?

3. Are there situations in which you would not want a feeding tube?

4. Are there situations in which you would want the feeding tube withdrawn?

5. Would you want chest compressions if you went into cardiac arrest, but had a poor likelihood of meaningful recovery?

By discussing these things in advance, you may find out that your next of kin would not be able to honor your wishes. In that case, you need to find another advocate. If your healthcare advocate is going to be someone other than next of kin, you will need to get a legal document that formalizes this. This document is called a Durable Power of Attorney (DPOA). This will trump any existing state laws about the next of kin hierarchy regarding medical decision making. If you are married, don't assume your spouse would automatically be your DPOA. Once again, formalize your wishes with documentation.

Regardless of whom you choose to be your advocate, complete an Advance Directive form. This will serve as the legal document of your wishes about life support and artificial nutrition. Completing this form will let your loved ones know what you want and don't want, so they will be able to honor your wishes when you cannot honor them yourself. Taking this step can save your family unnecessary grief and turmoil.

4. **Review and Update.** Once you have compiled and formalized your choice of advocate, your medical history, your Advance Directive or Living Will, and list of key documents and contact numbers, the family should review this together with the advocate and then provide the advocate with a copy for your healthcare providers, should the need arise. These documents should be updated annually, or as needed.

SCENARIO 2: THE HOSPITAL'S REAL FRONT DOOR: THE EMERGENCY ROOM

The emergency room, commonly known as the ER, is often the first place, and sometimes the only place, patients go when they arrive at the hospital. The ER provides the initial treatment to patients with a broad spectrum of illnesses and injuries, some of which may be life threatening and require immediate attention. According to the American College of Emergency Physicians (ACEP) more than 100 million people go to the emergency room each year.

The good news is that most ERs are not as chaotic as depicted on NBC's famous show of the same name. Even so, before going to the ER, think about the urgency of your situation. More than half of all ER visits are unnecessary. Before calling an ambulance or getting in the car to drive there yourself, call your doctor, or have a loved one call to ask if he or she recommends that you go to the hospital.

If the answer is "no" and you go anyway, chances are you'll be put low down on the triage nurse's list of priorities and might spend several hours, if not the better part of your day or night waiting to be seen.

Getting Through the Inner Doors

Don't assume that the ER will be able to treat you right away. Many emergency rooms are experiencing overcrowding, as patients with non-emergent conditions use ERs for care. If you can, call ahead and check to see if the ER is on "divert." Divert means that they are sending ambulances to other hospitals because there are no available hospital beds, or more commonly, there are not enough nurses and therefore the hospital cannot accommodate any new patients. Federal law states that every hospital must allow walk-in patients into its ER—but if the hospital is diverting ambulance traffic, you may be in for a very, very long wait.

If you think you might need to be hospitalized after you are seen in the ER, it's a good idea to call ahead and check that the hospital has beds available. Otherwise, after the ER staff stabilizes you, you might be sent to another facility or worse, have to stay in the ER until a bed becomes available.

Once you arrive at the ER, you'll need to check in at the desk where someone will ask you for your name, address, billing, and insurance information, and collect any required co-payments. This person will also ask you about the illness or injury that prompted your ER visit and relay the information to a triage nurse whose responsibility it is to perform a cursory assessment of your symptoms and determine and prioritize the truly urgent and emergent cases from the non-urgent cases.

Once again, if you are going to the ER with a sore throat, you will be placed at the bottom of the patient list, following the people arriving with broken bones, chest pain, bleeding wounds and other, more severe medical issues.

Waiting, Waiting, and More Waiting

More than half of all ER visits are unnecessary. When people use the ER to seek treatment for non-emergency medical care, it ties up emergency rooms and personnel and delays the time it takes for you to be seen. That said, the total time you spend in the emergency room will depend on a lot of things. Medical emergencies are unpredictable. If you have to wait, you may be uncomfortable, but there is likely a good reason for the delay. Here are some other reasons you may have to wait:

MORE THAN HALF OF all ER visits are unnecessary. When people use the ER to seek treatment for non-emergency medical care, it ties up emergency rooms and personnel and delays the time it takes for you to be seen.

- Overcrowding due to epidemics, such as flu season, or serious accidents.
- Waiting for lab tests or X-rays to be completed.
- Waiting for a specialist consultation.
- If you need to be admitted to the hospital, sometimes there are no beds available.

How Long Is Too Long?

If you are one of the lucky ones in the ER to be determined not to have a serious or life threatening illness, reminding yourself of that while the time ticks away will help you stay calm. Although ER wait times can be notoriously long, most ERs have focused on improving their wait times and you should now expect an average ER wait time of forty-one minutes to see a doctor, according to the Centers for Disease Control. If your situation is found to be urgent or emergent, expect to be seen quickly and expect to get follow-up from an ER staff to let you know what's going on. If not, be assertive and ask what is causing the delay and when can you expect to see a doctor. If the cause of the delay or timeline is unacceptable to you, and you believe that waiting could have serious consequences, then let them know you are leaving to go to another emergency room. This usually gets their attention and you will most likely be seen within five minutes. Whatever you do, don't leave without getting medical attention, if at all possible. This could be extremely dangerous if the condition or injury that brought you to the hospital suddenly worsens after you leave. According to a study done by the U.S. General Accounting Office, as many as seven percent of emergency departments nationally have "leave without being seen" rates higher than five percent. In fact some emergency departments have reported rates as high as fifteen percent. Don't let you or your loved one be that statistic.

The ER Exam: What Happens Behind the Curtain?

Once you are finally escorted from the waiting room to an exam room, a nurse will come to your bedside to ask you about the illness or injury that prompted your ER visit. If you are fairly stable the nurse will likely check your vital signs—your breathing rate, temperature, and blood pressure.

If the ER is very busy, and your condition is not so serious that you need immediate medical intervention, expect to wait for a while before the doctor comes to examine you. Meanwhile, the nurse assigned to care for you will be there to help make

DOING YOUR HOMEWORK

DON'T ASSUME THAT ALL HOSPITALS ARE alike or that they are all equally good. Study after study has documented enormous quality and safety differences between hospitals. To maximize the likelihood of a safe hospitalization with a good outcome, you need to do your homework in advance to decide which hospital you or your loved ones will go to in the event of a planned or unplanned hospitalization. Chapter 2 discusses choosing the best hospital, but here is a summary of what you should research in advance of making your decision:

- Assessment of hospital quality and patient safety ratings. Visit www.healthgrades.com and check out chapter 2.

- Assessment of how good the hospital is in doing the right things at the right time for patients. Visit www.hospitalcompare.hhs.gov.

- Availability of Intensive Care Unit, ICU, and physicians who specialize in ICU medicine. Visit www.healthgrades.com or www.leapfroggroup.org, or contact the hospital medical staff office or quality management department.

- Number of patients for each nurse (including RNs). Contact the hospital's nursing administrator.

- Assessment of the strictness of medical staff rules as it relates to timeliness of physician evaluation. For example, how soon will you be seen by your doctor after you leave the ER? Contact the hospital medical staff department.

- Preference for teaching or non-teaching hospital. Contact the hospital's medical staff office to confirm teaching status.

- Distance from home.

- Does your physician have admitting privileges at your hospital of choice? Ask your physician.

you as comfortable as possible and answer any questions you might have.

Once the physician arrives, he or she will evaluate you to determine a diagnosis and whether or not your medical condition requires further medical attention. You may need to undergo diagnostic tests, such as X-rays or blood tests. Again, expect to wait a while before the doctor comes to tell you about the results. Based on his or her examination and any test results, the ER doctor will identify whether or not you need to be admitted to the hospital. If you are too sick or injured to go home, the doctor will also be working to determine what area of the hospital to admit you to, based on your specific medical needs. For example, if you are seriously ill you will likely go to the intensive care unit, and if you need surgery you will be admitted to the medical/surgical floor. If the doctor decides that your condition can be treated in the ER, you will be able to go directly home from the hospital.

and discussion with your admitting physician. An admitting physician is usually your regular physician, or in the event that he or she does not have admitting privileges at that particular hospital or they no longer take care of hospitalized patients, it may be a hospitalist. A hospitalist is a physician who specializes in hospital medicine and does not do outpatient work.

ALTHOUGH MOST ER PHYSICIANS are excellent diagnosticians, their preliminary diagnoses are just that, preliminary, and this could spell disaster if you are not reassessed quickly by a doctor more familiar with your medical history, especially if your condition is worsening.

SCENARIO 3: WHEN THE ER ISN'T ENOUGH: GETTING ADMITTED TO THE HOSPITAL

If the ER doctor determines that your medical condition requires further treatment, he or she will admit you to the hospital. In most cases this means you will be staying at least one night in the hospital. The ER doctor will ask you for the name of your regular physician, and he or she will call them, or whoever is on call for them, and tell them that you are being admitted to the hospital, share your diagnosis, and discuss initial treatments. The ER physician will then treat you based on that preliminary diagnosis

Behind the scenes, the ER staff is working hard to find you a bed. As discussed earlier, sometimes this wait can be very long. Make sure that appropriate treatments were initiated, and then try to relax. Once a bed has been found, you will be transported by wheel chair or stretcher to your hospital room. Then a nurse, who will be taking care of you for the remainder of her shift, will come do an intake of your medical history, allergies, religious beliefs, and any other information pertinent to your care. The nurse will also have your admitting physician paged to come admit you. This process requires that your admitting physician assess you, confirm or refute the ER doctor's diagnosis, and tailor the treatment plan accordingly.

There is an important difference in hospital admission policies that you need to be aware of. Some hospitals require the admitting physician to see you within four hours of admission, while others only require the admitting physician see you within twelve to twenty-four hours of admission. In this latter situation, it is typical for the ER doctor to make the diagnosis, write the "admit orders" and "tuck you in" for the night so that your admitting doctor can see you sometime the next day. Although most ER physicians are excellent diagnosticians, their preliminary diagnoses are just that, preliminary, and this could spell disaster if you are not reassessed quickly by a doctor more familiar with your medical history, especially if your condition is worsening.

The Hospital Stay

Being a patient is hard for most of us, and being sick in an unfamiliar place with a stranger seeing us in our most vulnerable state can be frightening. Chapter 4 will provide instructions on how to quell your fears and be more empowered. But to be fully informed, you first need to understand the day to day workings of inpatient care. The best place to start is by getting to know the people who will be caring for you and how they typically go about their jobs. If you know what to expect, you will feel more at ease, and be able to stay on top of whether or not your caregivers are doing everything they can to provide the best care possible.

Who's Who and What Do They Do?

PHYSICIANS

While you're in the hospital, your physician is required to see you every day. When this might happen is dependent upon your physician's own office or procedure schedule. However, it's pretty typical for physicians to see you early in the morning before they start seeing patients in their office. This usually means before 8 or 9 a.m. For cardiologists and other specialists, this could mean before 7 a.m. Although most of us do not like being awakened early in the morning from deep sleep to get poked and prodded and asked questions, you need to try to be awake when your doctor is there. This is likely the only time you are going to get any time with your physician and you should maximize the opportunity.

If not told, you should always ask for the day's goals and plans. Ask if he or she will be ordering any specialist consults or tests and if so, when and why. If you don't understand something your physician says, and he or she seems like they are in a hurry, ask the doctor to write it down so you can remember to ask your nurse to explain it to you.

FROM A PATIENT PERSPECTIVE, there are positive and negative aspects of teaching hospitals. Teaching hospitals usually are on the cutting edge of medicine, but are also obligated to train tomorrow's much needed physicians.

MEDICAL STUDENTS, RESIDENTS, AND FELLOWS

The most likely place you as a patient will encounter doctors in training is at an academic teaching hospital. This can be a university medical center, or a public hospital. From a patient perspective, there are positive and negative aspects of teaching hospitals. Teaching hospitals usually are on the cutting edge of medicine, but are also obligated to train tomorrow's much needed physicians. These physicians-in-training are usually available 24/7, whereas in non-teaching hospitals a physician may be sleeping at home when your condition changes. The medical students also provide a second opinion of sorts, not something you would routinely get at a non-teaching hospital.

Training requires practice and practice begins with the first procedure. Medical students, residents, and fellows are all in training. Medical students do not yet have their medical degree, but are in training for two years in hospitals as a requirement to graduate medical school. Residents have graduated medical school and have a medical degree, but aren't full fledged physicians in their specialty until they complete residency training, or post-graduate training. This can last three to five years depending on their specialty requirements, such as general surgery, internal medicine, or pediatrics. Fellows have finished their residency, but want to further specialize and require additional training, such as cardiology. They are usually supervised until they gain enough experience to supervise someone else. However, most residents and fellows have a mantra, "See one, do one, and teach one." They are under tremendous pressure to learn quickly without making mistakes. However, no physician is free from error.

If you do not want any medical students or "doctors in training," such as residents and fellows, evaluating you or managing your care, you should not go to a teaching hospital.

NURSES

Every shift, nurses are assigned six to ten patients. In states like California, there are state laws that mandate no more than six patients per nurse for patient safety reasons. Also, many nurses work twelve or more hours. You will want to check your state's laws regarding nurse to patient ratio. Be aware of "traveling nurses." These are nurses who are hired on a temporary basis and then move on. They are not employees of the hospital; rather, they are paid by a temp agency. While most traveling nurses are very good, some may not have incentive to perform at top level since they do not work directly for the hospital or live in its community.

In addition to the staff nurses, there is a charge nurse, or supervisor of the floor or medical unit you are in. He or she is responsible for managing all the nurses on that floor and may "float" and take care of you while your regular nurse is on a break or tied up with another patient.

> BE AWARE OF "TRAVELING nurses." These are nurses who are hired on a temporary basis and then move on. They are not employees of the hospital; rather, they are paid by a temp agency.

Nurses are made up of various qualifications from licensed practical nurses (LPN) to registered nurse (RN). The RN has more training, but may not have more experience. Experience and critical thinking are very important in patient care, and you want to make sure (as best you can) the charge nurse is very experienced.

Depending on the treatment plan ordered by your physician, nurses can be scheduled to come into your room usually every four to six hours to either check your vital signs (blood pressure, pulse, etc.) or give you any ordered medications. You will usually have at least two nurses a day—day shift and night shift. Make sure they are on the same page with each other about your condition and treatments.

REMEMBER TO COMMUNICATE WITH your loved ones, create documents so no one has to think on their feet in the middle of a crisis, and speak up once you're in the hospital.

They may have not seen or talked to your doctor that day. You need to ask. You can have your advocate speak with them, too.

OTHERS

Other hospital staff will come in and out of your room each day, too. These include lab personnel, radiology technicians, physical therapists, respiratory therapists, case managers, social workers, dieticians, housekeeping, and more. They each have an active role in your treatment plan. They usually knock, but you need to consider your room open access to anyone while you are there. If you want privacy, let the nurse know to shut the door and put a sign out to not be disturbed.

KNOWLEDGE IS POWER

Now that you know what you have to do to prepare for a hospital visit and are familiar with hospital procedures and who does what on staff, you are firmly on the road to being an empowered patient or patient advocate. Remember to communicate with your loved ones, create documents so no one has to think on their feet in the middle of a crisis, and speak up once you're in the hospital. As much as you would like to have others make decisions for you in times of crisis, being an active participant in your own care is the key to your good health and happiness.

CHAPTER 4

PROTECTING YOURSELF AND YOUR LOVED ONES FROM MEDICAL ERRORS

Despite the media's heightened focus on medical errors in recent years, hospitals are not getting any safer. Research shows that during the past three years, 247,662 patients died because of medical mistakes in hospitals; the equivalent of one jumbo jet crashing each week for a year. (HealthGrades 2007 Patient Safety Report). And, more than 7,000 of those deaths each year are related to medications. In other areas of our lives, it's possible to make a poor choice when purchasing goods and services, such as a new car or new refrigerator, and deal with the ramifications if and when they occur. When you're selecting your medical care, selecting poorly can have catastrophic, lifelong effects on you and your family members. Doing everything you can to avoid doctors and hospitals with a history of frequent medical errors is of unparalleled importance. It's time well spent on research that can save your life.

> When you're selecting your medical care, selecting poorly can have catastrophic, lifelong effects on you and your family members.

The reality is that in the frenzied environment of today's hospitals, mistakes are going to happen. We don't frequently hear about accidents and tragedies that nearly happened or were narrowly escaped, but they do happen as a regular part of life in many hospitals. Although it's impossible to avoid human error entirely as a patient, you can reduce your risk.

The first step you can take towards reducing your risk of medical error is not to assume all hospitals and healthcare providers are the same. In fact, you should assume that they are all potentially very different and it's your job to unearth the relative strengths and weaknesses of the hospitals and doctors you are considering consulting. This chapter outlines clear, proactive steps you can take to ensure you and your loved ones get the best possible quality of care. By taking these steps, you will be able to take comfort in knowing that you have done everything you can to prepare for the unexpected.

TALKING TO NURSES AND DOCTORS: YES, YOU DO HAVE A RIGHT TO ASK QUESTIONS

There's nothing more unsettling than not knowing what's going on when you are in the hospital, either as a patient or an advocate. This is particularly true when you are in a busy hospital. Medicine is a fast-paced business and doctors and nurses have a lot of patients to see and take care of, but you should expect undivided attention from your nurse and doctor each day. The number-one rule for avoiding being the victim of medical mistakes in this often chaotic environment is to keep asking questions so you or your advocate know what's going on during every step of your hospital stay.

Write It Down

The most common mistakes patients and advocates make is not being prepared with a list of organized questions and not being available when the doctor or nurse are making their rounds. The best way for you to prepare for the short time the caregiver is in the room is to sit down with the doctor and identify what you know and don't know. There are no dumb questions. If you don't know something, then you should ask. Develop a list of concise questions that you will ask the nurse or doctor when they come into the room. It's a good idea to find out each day when your doctor will be back again and advocates should plan to be there at the same time.

Strike the Right Tone

When talking with doctors and nurses it's a good idea to be assertive, but it is in your best interest not to be annoying! If you are overly critical, demanding, or hostile you will not get answers and you will have the unintended effect of interfering with the care you are getting. Being assertive means being organized, supportive, caring, and establishing appropriate expectations with healthcare providers.

Timing Is Everything

Another thing to keep in mind when interacting with doctors and nurses is to speak up and ask questions during the exam. Don't wait until the nurse or doctor is walking out of the room to let them know you have questions. By that point, he or she is already moving on to the next patient and you are likely to get only a short, cursory answer to what may be a very important question. Tell the nurse or doctor as soon as they walk in and greet you that you have a list of questions that you need answered. If they tell you that they don't have time to answer them now, get a confirmation of a time when they will review them with you and let them know you expect they will honor that commitment. Again, nurses and doctors are very busy and, while they care very much about providing the highest quality care to every patient, they are human too. They

MUST DO'S IF YOU NEED TO CHECK INTO THE HOSPITAL FOR AN ELECTIVE PROCEDURE

1. Do your research: make sure your doctor and hospital check out before checking in.

2. Ask your doctor what you can do before and after the procedure to improve your outcome and shorten your hospital stay.

3. Designate a healthcare advocate (usually a family member or close friend) who will be responsible for managing the information during your hospitalization. Make sure they know your wishes should you become incapacitated. Make this person the "go to" person for all healthcare providers and your family for information.

4. Make sure you or your healthcare advocate asks for the "plan for the day" when your doctor comes to see you each day.

5. Make sure you or your healthcare advocate follows up on the outstanding tests and specialist consultations.

can forget and overlook things. And they appreciate being reminded of the needs of their patient—you.

Now you are ready to start interacting with your care team. The following section outlines key questions every patient or family advocate should ask and will help you understand why these questions are so important. Depending on your particular medical condition, you may have other, more specific questions. It's a good idea to have your advocate take notes while the doctor or nurse is answering your questions so that you can review the information, which can be technical, later on. If you don't understand something they are saying, you should ask for clarification immediately. If you are afraid you will forget it, have the doctor or nurse write it down for you.

Key Questions

1. WHAT'S THE PLAN?

The first question you should ask every day is: "What is the goal for the day and the plan for the day?" If there is no goal or plan, then you need to question why you or your loved one is still in the hospital. It could be a sign that the doctors and nurses don't know what is going on.

2. WHAT'S THIS MEDICATION AND WHY DO I HAVE TO TAKE IT?

You should always know why you are taking a pill, why you are getting a test, and what the associated side effects or risks are. This is even more important when you are in the hospital, where the potential for a mix-up escalates.

Medication errors occur every day in hospitals. Fortunately, most do not cause any harm, but some result in disastrous outcomes. When the nurse brings you a little white cup with one or more medicines, you should ask her to identify each pill and why you are taking it. If something doesn't make sense to you or doesn't sound right, you should ask the nurse to double check that this is what the doctor ordered for you. If it still doesn't make sense, refuse to take the medication until you can speak to the doctor.

When you are told you will be getting a test or procedure, you need to check your daily goals and plan. Was it on the list? If not, ask who ordered it and why. If your doctor ordered it, but didn't tell you about it when you discussed your goals and plan for the day, refuse it until the doctor confirms directly with you the reason you need the test or procedure.

3. DID YOU WASH YOUR HANDS?

A recent studied identified that only 47% of physicians wash their hands before touching their patients. This means that as a patient you have slightly more than a 50% chance of acquiring the previous patients' germs. This can have serious consequences and even result in death.

With a surge in antibiotic resistant bacteria, hospitals are breeding grounds for just this kind of bacteria. It is therefore critical that all healthcare personnel wash their hands before touching you. Keeping your eye on them and requesting they wash their hands can save you from unnecessary severe infections and death. Don't know how to bring it up? Simply say, "Would you mind washing your hands? I have a policy that I need to see my caregivers wash their hands before treating me."

4. WHAT ARE ALL THESE TUBES?

Most hospitalized patients will have at least one tube or IV during their hospital stay. However, some patients can have five or more tubes and IVs at any given time. All of these go from the outside in—into veins, arteries, the bladder, the chest, the lungs, or the stomach. As such, they can be easy entry points for bacteria that can cause severe infections. Therefore, you should only have a tube or IV if you really need it.

Good nurses and doctors keep track of when the tubes and IVs were placed and know how long they have been in. However, this information may not always be documented in a central location for everyone to see. Consequently, many of your nurses and doctors many not know how long the tubes and IVs have been in place.

Additionally, nurses and physicians like tubes and IVs. It can make taking care of a patient easier, especially if a patient suddenly takes a turn for the worse, and no one wants to insert these tubes in an emergency situation. So, the tendency is to leave them in longer than they should.

Every day you need to ask why you still have the tube or IV and when it can be discontinued. Then you need to document that date and remind the healthcare team to remove the tube or IV when that day arrives.

5. WHO AM I?

Misidentifying patients occurs in hospitals every day. Most of the time, the mix-up will be caught and harm prevented, but if not caught, unnecessary surgeries, procedures, and medications could be given to you, resulting in great harm. Ask anyone who is putting something in your IV or your mouth or taking you for a test or procedure to state your name and the reason for the action in order to prevent a mishap.

MEDICAL ERRORS: HOW TO AVOID MISTAKES

1. Count the number of catheters. A catheter is a tube inserted into a body cavity to drain or inject fluids. It's important to keep track of these so they don't get overlooked. Open cavities in the body can invite infection.

2. Make sure everyone—nurses, doctors, even friends and family—washes their hands before they touch you.

3. Know your treatment plan for each day. For example, ask your nurse when you might be taken for tests and what those tests are meant to determine. Ask when the doctor will arrive to check on you. Be prepared for the doctor's visit as you would a professional meeting. Keep a note pad and write down questions and comments ahead of time. Doctors love that because it provides both you and your advocate with an efficient way to get your questions asked and answered. Write down what tests you've had each day and what the results were as you get them. Write down any procedures or test you are expecting the following day. Remind doctors of what they told you they would do.

4. If someone does something that is not in the plan, speak up and ask why.

5. Always ask the nurse or doctor to go over each pill or fluid and tell you what it is for.

6. Always ask nurses and doctors to address you by your name—nobody looks at the wristband—especially before they inject you or give you a pill.

7. Have a family member or friend with you as an advocate. This is no time to be shy; ask someone to be with you at all times. This person can help you direct your care and keep track of your treatment plan. This really keeps doctors on their toes. They've just been put on notice that you're watching every little thing that they do.

8. Ask for results of diagnostic tests. For example, ask if you can view your X-rays. If the doctor tells you that a test will be performed, make sure to ask, "Will you come back to talk to us about the results? Good. When?" You should get an answer within forty-eight hours; if you don't, ask why you haven't.

9. Be vocal. If you have strong negative feelings about the physician who is treating you, speak up and know that the doctor most likely won't take it personally if you ask for a new doctor. No physician wants to go through the headache and frustration of treating a patient who doesn't trust or respect his or her professional opinion.

10. If you don't like your doctor, just get a new one. Simply say, "I don't feel like you and I are a good fit. How can I get a new doctor?" or "I can't work with you. It's not personal."

6. TEST RESULTS, PLEASE?

Many medical mistakes are the result of inadequate or non-existent follow-up on consultations or test results. Without follow-up, accurate diagnoses and appropriate treatment plans may not be developed and could result in delayed recovery. You should keep track of all consultations and tests done and ask for follow-up, and keep track of the results and discuss the significance of the results with the doctor during your Q&A sessions. You also need to find out what test results are still pending at the time of your discharge from the hospital. Keep a list of these test results and at your post-hospital follow-up, ask your physician to review and interpret the results for you.

A WORD TO ADVOCATES: YOU DON'T HAVE TO FEEL HELPLESS

Sometimes, the way to avoid medical errors is to pay diligent attention to the patient on a regular basis. Doctors, nurses, and hospital staff are so harried they sometimes have a difficult time giving a patient's situation the scrutiny it deserves. As an advocate, you can achieve a lot by remaining vigilantly at the patient's side. The first goal you're accomplishing is making sure none of the patient's needs or changes in status go unnoticed. The second is that you can help to alleviate your own sense of helplessness, and sometimes, grief.

It's hard to have a loved one who is ill, but there are many things you can do to be an active participant in their care. Engaging in some of the simple tasks outlined below will keep you busy during what can be a very stressful time.

1. **Make the patient comfortable.** Ask the patient if they have everything they need to feel comfortable. Often, they will have left the house in a hurry and

> SOMETIMES, THE WAY TO avoid medical errors is to pay diligent attention to the patient on a regular basis. Doctors, nurses, and hospital staff are so harried they sometimes have a difficult time giving a patient's situation the scrutiny it deserves.

neglected to bring important items such as glasses, hearing aids, false teeth, or their favorite slippers. Find out what is missing and bring it to the hospital for them. Sometimes it helps to imagine what items would make you feel more at home, like a favorite photo or a soft sweater, and bring those too.

2. **Help keep boredom at bay.** Most hospitalized patients, if awake and alert, are bored and have little to do. It is very common that a patient's sleep/wake cycle gets reversed and they may sleep all day and be awake all night, requiring sleeping pills so they can get some rest. Sleeping pills in a hospitalized patient, especially an elderly and mildly confused patient, can spell disaster. You don't want them to take these unless all else has failed. You can help by visiting them during the day and coordinating a schedule of visits and activities to keep the patient occupied during the day and minimizing the need for potentially harmful sleeping pills at night.

3. **Keeping the status quo.** Sometimes basic activities of daily living get neglected. Nurses and doctors are occupied with taking care of many

critical patients at once. As such, they may not have the time for what may seem like very basic care, such as bathing, hair brushing, and assisting with feeding. These actions can be very comforting for the patient and are necessary elements to recovery. This is where you can step in and make a real difference.

PRIVACY LAWS: AVOIDING ROAD BLOCKS AND FRUSTRATION

One of the many ways that medical error can be avoided, if you're a patient advocate, is to have a full understanding of the patient's medical history. Having a grasp of the entire situation you're dealing with is the only way to achieve any kind of control over what can be a difficult situation to manage.

IF SOMEONE HAS DESIGNATED you as his or her advocate and you are not the legal guardian, it is imperative that you have what is called Durable Power of Attorney and that you or the patient has a legal document supporting that.

If you are acting as a patient advocate, you need to be aware that the patient's medical history and condition is legally protected information. Hospital and medical staff are strictly prohibited from discussing the specifics of the patient's medical condition to anyone except the legal guardian. If you are not the legal guardian, don't expect any details other than "he or she is in stable condition" or "he or she is doing okay today."

If someone has designated you as his or her advocate and you are not the legal guardian, it is imperative that you have what is called Durable Power of Attorney and that you or the patient has a legal document supporting that. This will allow you to gain access to any and all information about the patient, and allow you to make medical decisions in the event that the patient cannot.

If you are not a designated advocate, but would like to know about specific medical issues concerning your loved one, you should go directly to the patient or their advocate to get this information. If the patient is able, they can sign a release form to allow you to be privy to their confidential information.

Remember this simple rule: vigilance, a sense of entitlement, and using your voice to speak up if something doesn't look right are your best tools in avoiding medical error. If you don't get the response you want right off the bat, keep pushing. Everyone has a right to the best medical care available.

CHAPTER 5

BEST QUESTIONS TO ASK BEFORE COMMON PROCEDURES

There are tons of questions you should be asking when checking into a hospital. Earlier in this book, we discuss many of those general questions. In addition to those, in this chapter we provide useful procedure-specific questions you can ask (and answers to some questions you are too embarrassed to ask) for the three most common reasons for hospitalization: 1) giving birth, 2) getting a cardiac procedure, and 3) getting a knee or hip replaced.

GIVING BIRTH FOR THE FIRST TIME

Giving birth is a joyous occasion, but usually only after it's all over. Unlike many illnesses, giving birth is associated with a great deal of preparation. While most read up on the best crib and car seats to buy or the best schools, many do not prepare for all that's entailed in the actual delivery beyond Lamaze classes. Below are several questions you should be asking before having your baby.

1. I don't want an epidural, but what if I change my mind? Can I still get one at the last minute?
Maybe and maybe not. If you are past eight centimeters dilated, it may be too late because you'll likely deliver before the epidural effects kick in. Also, it can be more difficult to sit still for the epidural placement if you are writhing in labor pain. It's best to discuss this with your physician and ask him or her what your options are. You may want to sign your consent forms in advance of extreme pain, even if you don't plan to have one—just in case.

2. Do epidurals ever fail? If so, what else will be done to control my pain during labor?
Epidurals can sometimes not work. This can be due to incorrect placement, infusion, and other things. You should find out if the anesthesiologist (a doctor that specializes in pain control) has done many epidural placements during labor. You can probably find out by asking your obstetrician or midwife who they regularly use, and then calling the hospital to see how many he or she has done and how many didn't work.

3. What are typical scenarios for a Cesarean section after an attempt at normal vaginal delivery? What is the likelihood of that happening to me?
It is not atypical for a woman to need a Cesarean section after attempting vaginal delivery. While there are many reasons for requiring a Cesarean section after an attempt at vaginal delivery, some of the most common reasons for this are failure to progress—the cervix is just not dilating enough or timely enough—and fetal distress. Often it is difficult, if not impossible, to predict who will not progress or have fetal distress. The most important thing is to prepare yourself for the possibility of requiring a Cesarean section.

> I DON'T WANT AN epidural, but what if I change my mind? Can I still get one at the last minute?

4. How long would you make me labor after my water has broken before taking me for a Cesarean section? Will your partners follow the same plan?
Unfortunately, there is a lot of variation among physician thinking about how to best manage this

type of situation. The most important thing is that you discuss this with your physician in advance and make sure that his or her partners are on board with that plan because you do not want surprises in the delivery room.

While this event is one of the most exciting and celebrated times of your life, it can also be one of the most embarrassing. While you are not sick, you may still have concerns that cause you some anxiety, especially those that you think are too trivial or embarrassing to talk to your doctor about. We address those common concerns about giving birth below.

1. Is it a failure to need a Cesarean section after an attempt at vaginal delivery?

Absolutely not! The decision to have a Cesarean section after an attempt at vaginal delivery is a serious one and will be made based on clinical signs. These signs are not something you can change at will. If you have to go to Cesarean, focus on delivering a healthy baby quickly rather than not being able to deliver vaginally.

2. What will they really think about "down there?"

No one likes to get her Pap smear; now imagine that during a typical labor of fifteen hours there will be several people "down there." They will likely check on you hourly. This can mean fifteen or more examinations of your cervix and fetal position. Rest assured that this close up examination is a normal part of the doctor's job and the focus is exclusively on your health and the status of your baby.

3. I've read that squeezing my nipples can help labor progress by stimulating the contraction hormone, oxytocin. I'd like to do this, but am afraid that the medical staff might think I am weird. Am I?

While this act might be considered bizarre in every day public life, this is commonly witnessed in the labor rooms. Medical staffs have seen this practice before and do not find it odd or inappropriate at all. Squeeze away!

4. I've heard women who have had babies say that they pooped and/or peed during labor or pushing. Does this really happen?

Yes! Because of the location of the vaginal (birth) canal and the rectum, the pressure of the descending baby can cause a woman to have a bowel movement. The strain of the pelvic floor from carrying the baby for forty weeks along with pregnancy hormones can cause the pelvic floor to become weakened and urine can leak, especially during labor and delivery. This is very common and no nurse or physician thinks anything of it, except to sweep it away and make you comfortable.

5. If I get an epidural, when should I feel my legs?

It's a little different for everyone depending on how much of the anesthesia they received, but it typically takes a few hours after the epidural is discontinued before you start feeling like you can move your legs and stand. Ask to have someone with you during the time you are numb because you won't be able to get out of your bed.

6. Do I really want my partner "down there" during the delivery?

Maybe and maybe not. How comfortable are you with having someone see you in a very vulnerable position? Would you like that in your videotape? How much of it do you want them to see? Many partners like to be "down there" as the baby enters the world, and even want to cut the cord. However, many partners would rather not be "down there" when the physician/midwife is removing your placenta or stitching you up (if you have torn or had an episiotomy). Some partners may be turned off by this immediate post-delivery recovery. You should discuss this with your partner in advance and if you find out they are one of the turned-off variety, make sure to remind them to come stay with you at the head of the bed.

GETTING A CARDIAC PROCEDURE

Most cardiac procedures and surgeries start with understanding the anatomy and function of your coronaries (the arteries that supply blood to your heart that can get clogged and cause heart attacks) and heart muscle. This is usually done through a cardiac catheterization—a procedure that requires a skinny tube with a wire (catheter) to be inserted in the femoral artery in your groin. The cardiologist then threads this catheter up to your heart. Once there, they take pictures and then they are able to make a diagnosis and plan that is best for you. Sometimes this means getting a "stent," or device to open up your coronary artery. Some might need more invasive cardiac surgery to bypass the clogs in the coronary arteries, while others might be best left alone or with medications only.

1. My cardiologist/cardiac surgeon is the best in town. However, I heard on a recent news story that there can be big differences in survival among physicians. Is this true?
Yes! One of the most important things you can do to improve your survival is to check out your physician before checking in. Ask what the cardiologist or cardiac surgeon's volume, complications and survival rates are. Are you a typical patient, or a high risk patient? Is there anything you can do to

decrease your risk? Taking charge of who will perform procedures will empower you, make you feel good, and could save your life.

2. What if I get scared and don't understand the medical jargon my doctor is saying?
Don't be embarrassed to ask the doctor to explain or draw what they found and what the best treatment plan is. Keep asking until you can repeat it. Write it down so you can explain it later.

3. I am having angioplasty and a stent. I heard there are different kinds of stents. Does it matter which one I receive?
Yes. There are bare metal stents (BMS) and drug-eluting stents (DES). DES use is associated with less chance for clotting later on, but only in certain patients. In other patients, it may be associated with more. You should ask your cardiologist before your procedure if you would qualify. More importantly, you need to know which type you received for your future because the complications and management of these two types of stents are different.

TAKING CHARGE OF WHO will perform procedures will empower you, make you feel good, and could save your life.

4. Will I have to take medications after my angioplasty and stent or surgery?
If you do have coronary heart disease (clogged arteries), you will need to take prescriptions for the rest of your life, whether you have cardiac surgery or a stent. Some of these life saving medications can be very expensive and many patients cannot afford to

take them. More importantly, some of these costly drugs are absolutely critical to take every day, like a drug called Plavix (generic: clopidogrel), which is typically given to patients with heart attacks who are given a DES. Find out before you go for a cardiac catheterization if you can afford this drug, because you cannot have a drug-eluting stent in safely without daily Plavix.

5. If I can't afford Plavix, what can I do?

If you can't afford to buy Plavix for at least six to twelve months (and maybe life), it would be dangerous for you to receive a drug-eluting stent, so you need to tell your cardiologist before the catheterization. They may be able to put in a bare metal stent instead.

6. I've heard that there are bad side effects of the drugs used to treat heart disease. Is this true and what are those side effects?

Another class of drugs called beta blockers (metoprolol, atenolol, carvedilol) has been shown to improve survival in coronary artery disease; however, many people have side effects such as decreased sexual libido, fatigue, and depression. These side effects are quite common. They may, however, significantly distress patients, resulting in a self-discontinuation of this drug and the potential consequence of "rebound hypertension," which can cause a heart attack. If the side effects of beta blockers are unacceptable, you should discuss this with your doctor. Don't ever suddenly stop this drug without talking to your doctor first.

7. Are there any tricks on getting the cheapest price for my medications?

Prescription medications for the treatment of heart disease can be very expensive, especially if you have to pay for part or all of the cost. Always ask your doctor for the generic version and a ninety day supply, which usually is cheaper per month than just buying a one month supply with refills.

Also, shop around for the very best prices. Start on the Internet where there are sites that show you prices from various online stores. You can also use this information to call your local drugstores. Many drugstores run promotions to lure you into giving them your prescriptions. Ask if they will match competitor coupons and prices, then bargain with them. You can save a significant amount of money this way. See the example below of typical prescriptions for coronary heart disease and the variation in cost within one zip code in Denver, Colorado.

COMMONLY PRESCRIBED DRUGS FOR CORONARY HEART DISEASE	DRUG STORE IN THE ZIP CODE 80238 SEARCH AREA*				COST DIFFERENCE BETWEEN HIGHEST AND LOWEST
	Sam's Club	Walmart	Walgreens	Rite Aid	
Metoprolol 50 mg (#60)	$4.00	$4.00	$14.99	$18.99	$14.99
Simvistatin 80 mg (#30)	$52.54	$54.54	$64.99	$118.99	$66.45
Plavix 75 mg (#30)	$83.32	$138.84	$135.99	$151.99	$68.67
Total Cost of 1 Month Supply	$139.86	$197.38	$215.97	$289.97	$150.11

*Stores located nearest to 80238 (Denver, Colorado) were identified and contacted by phone. Prices were quoted 7/30/07.

These are life saving medications, but the reality is that you might not be able to afford the medications at Rite Aid® ; you may, however, be able to buy it at Sam's Club®. It literally pays to shop around.

GETTING YOUR KNEE OR HIP REPLACED

You've found out that your knee or hip needs to be replaced. You have friends that have gone through this—some claim it was easy while some claim they are suing. There is a lot of variation in how well a surgeon and hospital perform total knee and hip replacements. There may be a great hospital for treating a heart attack, but it may not be so good when it comes to replacing a knee or hip. While these two procedures require the skill of a good orthopedic surgeon, there are differences of which you need to be aware. Asking good questions is a way to find out and take charge.

1. My orthopedic surgeon is the best in town. However, I heard on a recent news story that there can be big differences in survival among physicians. Is this true?
Yes! One of the most important things you can do to improve your likelihood of an excellent outcome is to check out your physician before checking in. Ask what the orthopedic surgeon's volume, complications, and survival rates are. Are you a typical patient, or a high risk patient? Is there anything you can do to decrease your risk? Taking charge of who will perform procedures will empower you, make you feel good, and could save your life.

2. I have angina and I currently have diabetes. Am I a good candidate for surgery?
Possibly, so long as you are appropriately evaluated. You are a higher risk candidate than many, but you could reduce that risk with a thorough pre-operative evaluation and initiation of beta blockers (class of drug that slows the heart down and reduces blood pressure), which also decreases cardiac complications after joint replacement. Nothing can replace a thorough pre-operative risk assessment by a skilled internist or family practitioner. They may find things on the evaluation and assessment that warrant further investigation. Remember, your joint replacement is not an emergent or urgent surgery. If you have any risks (age, medical conditions, history of surgical complications in the past), it is prudent to do everything possible to reduce the risks before surgery to maximize the likelihood of a good outcome.

3. How should I prepare before my surgery to make sure I have the speediest recovery?
Most orthopedic surgeons have literature to give you that explains the surgery and answers many questions. You can also search the Internet for more information. Ask your surgeon if you can watch a video of what to expect before, during, and after the surgery and what milestones are typically

> MANY DRUGSTORES RUN PROMOTIONS to lure you into giving them your prescriptions. Ask if they will match competitor coupons and prices, then bargain with them.

achievable one, two, and three days after surgery. Knowing what to expect has been shown to accelerate your recovery.

4. I heard some of my friends received general anesthesia ("wake me up when it's all over") while others received an epidural or spinal block (awake during the procedure)? Is there a choice? Wouldn't everyone want to just wake up when it's all over?
This is an important discussion to have with your surgeon before scheduling surgery. General anesthesia, while associated with very low risk, has more risk than spinals or epidurals. General anesthesia acts on the brain and nervous system resulting in a very deep sleep, or unconsciousness. Because of this deep sleep and unconscious state, you cannot breathe on your own and need to have a breathing tube placed into your airway and have a breathing machine breathe for you during the surgery. Some patients with underlying chronic medical conditions should try to avoid general anesthesia if possible because they have a much higher risk of developing a major complication. Those who receive general anesthesia may experience more blood loss during surgery because of the effects of the anesthetic medication. You are also more likely to be groggy after the surgery, and some people may experience a longer recovery period.

Spinal and epidural blocks do not cause any change in your level of consciousness, so you are awake for the entire procedure (they don't make you watch unless you want to!). While there are still potential complications associated with spinal and epidural blocks compared to general anesthesia, studies have shown they are associated with less complications, like blood loss and clotting, but the pain control is still excellent.

5. I need both knees replaced. Can I get them done at the same time?
This is a possibility and many patients have had both knees done simultaneously, but not without significant risk. You must be in very good physical condition before the surgery because your recovery will be at least twice as difficult since you will not have a good leg to stand on! Surgeons understand that you might want to go through the surgical pain and recovery only once, but you need to understand that it can be twice the risk since your surgical and recovery time will be longer. Lastly, some surgeons will not perform two knee replacements at the same time.

HOSPITAL RATINGS BY CLINICAL SPECIALTY

HOSPITAL RATINGS BY CLINICAL SPECIALTY

HealthGrades' Hospital Ratings by Clinical Specialty provide you with in-depth profiles of hospital quality performance, based on HealthGrades' independent quality ratings. You'll find the hospitals listed by state and in alphabetical order. Each hospital's profile shows how that hospital performed in each of ten clinical specialties, such as gastrointestinal surgery or pulmonary care. Each one of those specialties is rated based on a summary of all the star ratings that particular hospital received in that general discipline. For example, a hospital's cardiac clinical program would be rated based on how many stars it received for its work in everything from bypass surgery to valve replacement.

In addition to the ten clinical specialties, we have included one extra category: patient safety. We have provided information on how each hospital rates for general patient safety, which is an essential part of any hospital stay. The rating takes into account avoiding incidents such as hospital-acquired infections, bed sores, and respiratory failure after surgery. Finally, we provide all the basic information for each hospital, including address and phone number.

Along with each hospital's star ratings, you will also find a list of HealthGrades awards. These are further indicators of top-quality clinical programs.

Note: Hospitals receive one, three, or five stars in each care category, indicating below-, at-, or above-average patient outcomes. Specialty Excellence Awards recipients are hospitals in the top 10 percent in the nation in terms of patient outcomes. Hospitals falling into that category can have ratings of either three or five stars.

Andalusia Regional Hospital

849 South Three Notch Street
Andalusia, AL 36420
(334) 222-8466

Overall patient safety: ★★★★★
Teaching: N

CLINICAL PROGRAM RATINGS:

CARDIAC	NR	ORTHOPEDICS	★★★
CRITICAL CARE	NR	PULMONARY	★★★
GASTROINTESTINAL	NR	STROKE	★★★
GENERAL SURGERY	NR	VASCULAR	NR
MATERNITY CARE	NR	WOMEN'S HEALTH	NR

HEALTHGRADES AWARDS

✓ DISTINGUISHED
HOSPITAL
• PATIENT SAFETY

Baptist Cherokee

400 Northwood Drive
Centre, AL 35960
(256) 927-5531

Overall patient safety: ★★★
Teaching: N

CLINICAL PROGRAM RATINGS:

CARDIAC	NR	ORTHOPEDICS	NR
CRITICAL CARE	NR	PULMONARY	★★★
GASTROINTESTINAL	NR	STROKE	NR
GENERAL SURGERY	NR	VASCULAR	NR
MATERNITY CARE	NR	WOMEN'S HEALTH	NR

HEALTHGRADES AWARDS

Athens-Limestone Hospital

700 West Market Street
Athens, AL 35611
(256) 233-9292

Overall patient safety: ★★★
Teaching: N

CLINICAL PROGRAM RATINGS:

CARDIAC	NR	ORTHOPEDICS	NR
CRITICAL CARE	NR	PULMONARY	★★★
GASTROINTESTINAL	★★★	STROKE	★★★
GENERAL SURGERY	NR	VASCULAR	NR
MATERNITY CARE	NR	WOMEN'S HEALTH	NR

HEALTHGRADES AWARDS

Baptist Citizens

604 Stone Avenue
Talladega, AL 35160
(256) 362-8111

Overall patient safety: ★★★
Teaching: N

CLINICAL PROGRAM RATINGS:

CARDIAC	NR	ORTHOPEDICS	NR
CRITICAL CARE	NR	PULMONARY	★★★
GASTROINTESTINAL	NR	STROKE	★★★
GENERAL SURGERY	NR	VASCULAR	NR
MATERNITY CARE	NR	WOMEN'S HEALTH	NR

HEALTHGRADES AWARDS

Atmore Community Hospital

401 Medical Parks Drive
Atmore, AL 36502
(251) 368-6362

Overall patient safety: ★★★
Teaching: N

CLINICAL PROGRAM RATINGS:

CARDIAC	NR	ORTHOPEDICS	NR
CRITICAL CARE	NR	PULMONARY	★★★
GASTROINTESTINAL	NR	STROKE	NR
GENERAL SURGERY	NR	VASCULAR	NR
MATERNITY CARE	NR	WOMEN'S HEALTH	NR

HEALTHGRADES AWARDS

Baptist Medical Center--Dekalb

200 Medical Center Drive
Fort Payne, AL 35968
(256) 845-3150

Overall patient safety: ★★★
Teaching: N

CLINICAL PROGRAM RATINGS:

CARDIAC	NR	ORTHOPEDICS	NR
CRITICAL CARE	NR	PULMONARY	★
GASTROINTESTINAL	NR	STROKE	★
GENERAL SURGERY	NR	VASCULAR	NR
MATERNITY CARE	NR	WOMEN'S HEALTH	NR

HEALTHGRADES AWARDS

KEY: ★★★★★ BEST   ★★★ AS EXPECTED   ★ POOR   NR NOT RATED BY HEALTHGRADES   For full definitions of ratings and awards, see Appendix.

Baptist Medical Center–East

400 Taylor Road
Montgomery, AL 36117
(334) 277-8330

Overall patient safety: ★★★
Teaching: N

CLINICAL PROGRAM RATINGS:

CARDIAC	NR	ORTHOPEDICS	NR
CRITICAL CARE	NR	PULMONARY	★★★
GASTROINTESTINAL	★★★	STROKE	★★★
GENERAL SURGERY	NR	VASCULAR	NR
MATERNITY CARE	NR	WOMEN'S HEALTH	NR

HEALTHGRADES AWARDS

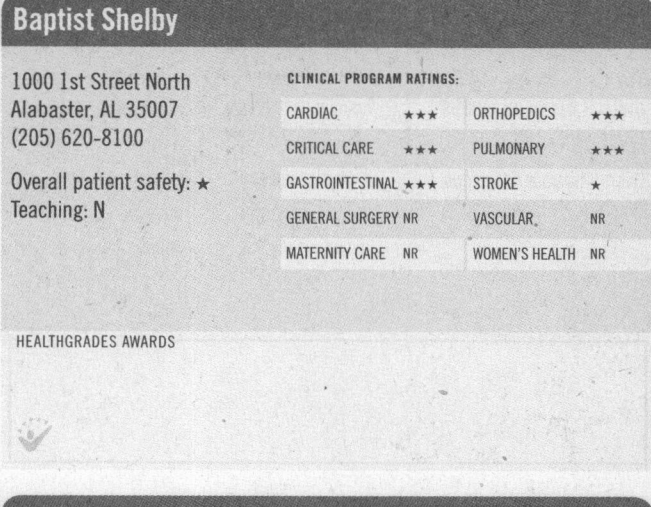

Baptist Shelby

1000 1st Street North
Alabaster, AL 35007
(205) 620-8100

Overall patient safety: ★
Teaching: N

CLINICAL PROGRAM RATINGS:

CARDIAC	★★★	ORTHOPEDICS	★★★
CRITICAL CARE	★★★	PULMONARY	★★★
GASTROINTESTINAL	★★★	STROKE	★
GENERAL SURGERY	NR	VASCULAR	NR
MATERNITY CARE	NR	WOMEN'S HEALTH	NR

HEALTHGRADES AWARDS

Baptist Medical Center–South

2105 East South Boulevard
Montgomery, AL 36116
(334) 288-2100

Overall patient safety: ★★★★★
Teaching: Y

CLINICAL PROGRAM RATINGS:

CARDIAC	★★★	ORTHOPEDICS	★
CRITICAL CARE	★	PULMONARY	★★★
GASTROINTESTINAL	★★★	STROKE	★
GENERAL SURGERY	NR	VASCULAR	★★★
MATERNITY CARE	NR	WOMEN'S HEALTH	NR

HEALTHGRADES AWARDS

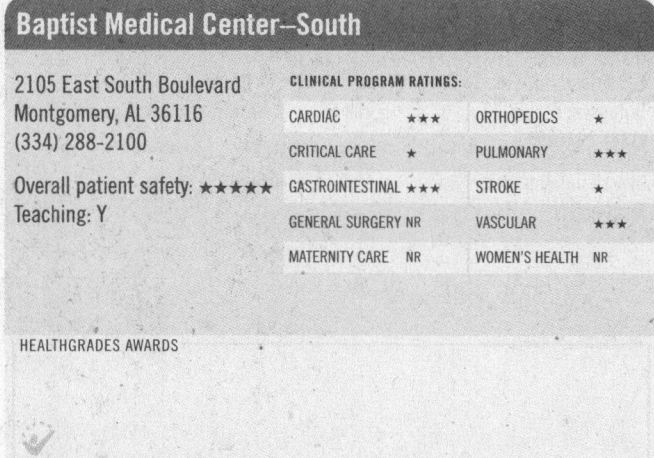

Brookwood Medical Center

2010 Brookwood Medical Center Drive
Birmingham, AL 35209
(205) 877-1000

Overall patient safety: ★
Teaching: N

CLINICAL PROGRAM RATINGS:

CARDIAC	★★★	ORTHOPEDICS	★★★
CRITICAL CARE	★★★	PULMONARY	★
GASTROINTESTINAL	★★★	STROKE	★★★
GENERAL SURGERY	NR	VASCULAR	NR
MATERNITY CARE	NR	WOMEN'S HEALTH	NR

HEALTHGRADES AWARDS

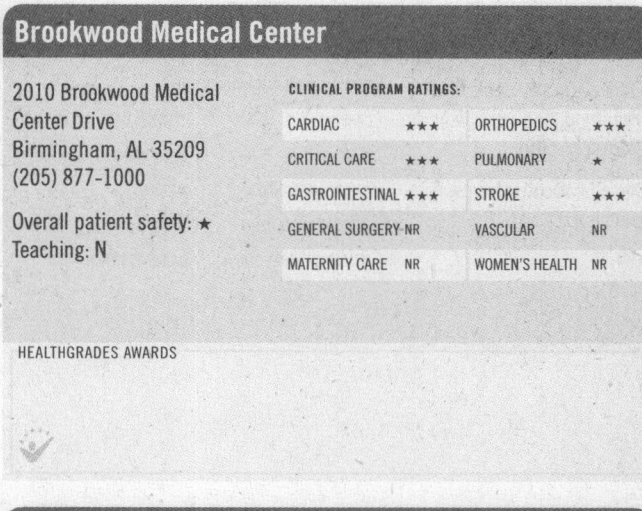

Baptist Princeton

701 Princeton Avenue Southwest
Birmingham, AL 35211
(205) 783-3000

Overall patient safety: ★
Teaching: Y

CLINICAL PROGRAM RATINGS:

CARDIAC	★	ORTHOPEDICS	★
CRITICAL CARE	★★★	PULMONARY	★★★★★
GASTROINTESTINAL	★★★	STROKE	★★★
GENERAL SURGERY	NR	VASCULAR	★★★
MATERNITY CARE	NR	WOMEN'S HEALTH	NR

HEALTHGRADES AWARDS

✓ SPECIALTY EXCELLENCE
• PULMONARY CARE

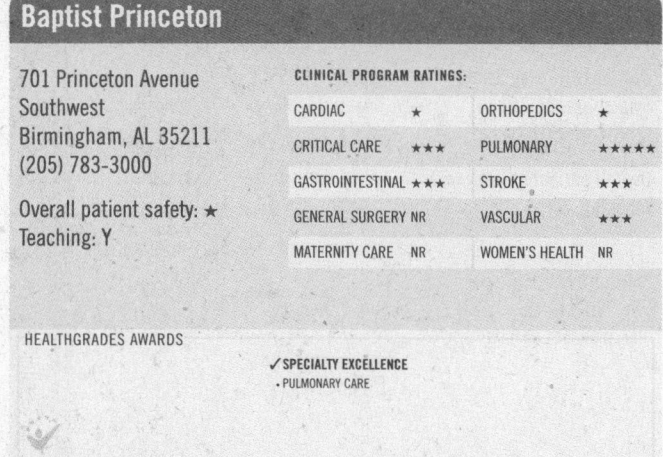

Bryan W. Whitfield Memorial Hospital

105 Highway 80 East
Demopolis, AL 36732
(334) 289-4000

Overall patient safety: ★★★
Teaching: N

CLINICAL PROGRAM RATINGS:

CARDIAC	NR	ORTHOPEDICS	NR
CRITICAL CARE	NR	PULMONARY	★
GASTROINTESTINAL	NR	STROKE	NR
GENERAL SURGERY	NR	VASCULAR	NR
MATERNITY CARE	NR	WOMEN'S HEALTH	NR

HEALTHGRADES AWARDS

ALABAMA HOSPITALS: RATINGS BY CLINICAL SPECIALTY

Bullock County Hospital

102 Conecuh Avenue West
Union Springs, AL 36089
(334) 738-2140

Overall patient safety: NR
Teaching: N

CLINICAL PROGRAM RATINGS:

CARDIAC	NR	ORTHOPEDICS	NR
CRITICAL CARE	NR	PULMONARY	★★★
GASTROINTESTINAL	NR	STROKE	NR
GENERAL SURGERY	NR	VASCULAR	NR
MATERNITY CARE	NR	WOMEN'S HEALTH	NR

HEALTHGRADES AWARDS

Clay County Hospital

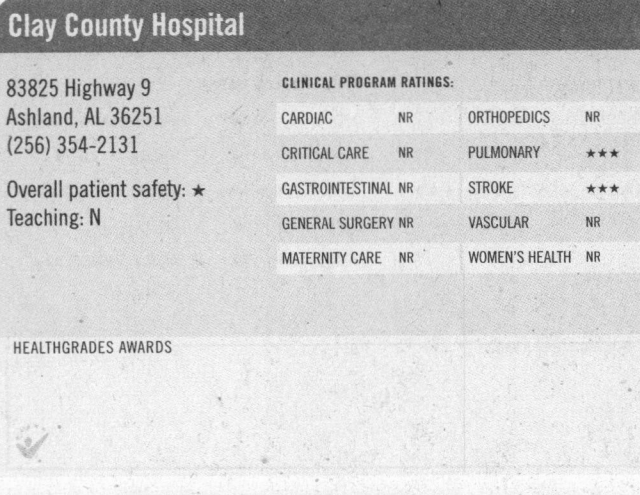

83825 Highway 9
Ashland, AL 36251
(256) 354-2131

Overall patient safety: ★
Teaching: N

CLINICAL PROGRAM RATINGS:

CARDIAC	NR	ORTHOPEDICS	NR
CRITICAL CARE	NR	PULMONARY	★★★
GASTROINTESTINAL	NR	STROKE	★★★
GENERAL SURGERY	NR	VASCULAR	NR
MATERNITY CARE	NR	WOMEN'S HEALTH	NR

HEALTHGRADES AWARDS

Carraway Methodist Medical Center

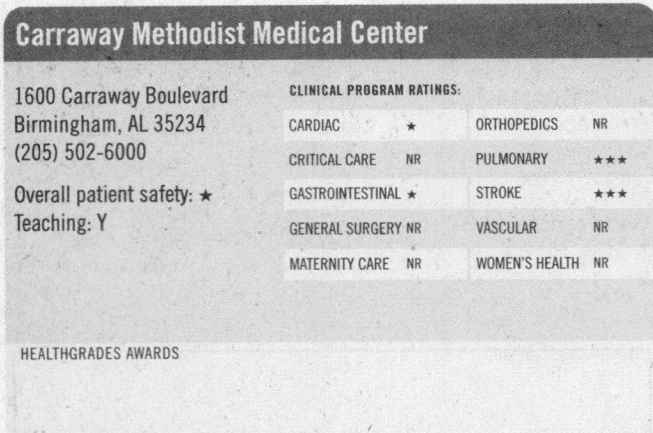

1600 Carraway Boulevard
Birmingham, AL 35234
(205) 502-6000

Overall patient safety: ★
Teaching: Y

CLINICAL PROGRAM RATINGS:

CARDIAC	★	ORTHOPEDICS	NR
CRITICAL CARE	NR	PULMONARY	★★★
GASTROINTESTINAL	★	STROKE	★★★
GENERAL SURGERY	NR	VASCULAR	NR
MATERNITY CARE	NR	WOMEN'S HEALTH	NR

HEALTHGRADES AWARDS

Community Hospital

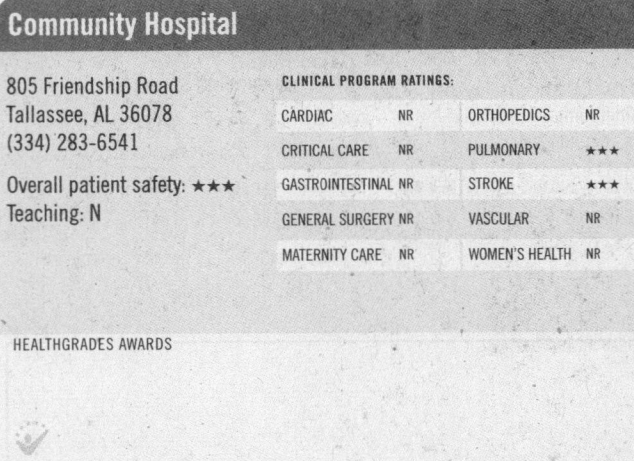

805 Friendship Road
Tallassee, AL 36078
(334) 283-6541

Overall patient safety: ★★★
Teaching: N

CLINICAL PROGRAM RATINGS:

CARDIAC	NR	ORTHOPEDICS	NR
CRITICAL CARE	NR	PULMONARY	★★★
GASTROINTESTINAL	NR	STROKE	★★★
GENERAL SURGERY	NR	VASCULAR	NR
MATERNITY CARE	NR	WOMEN'S HEALTH	NR

HEALTHGRADES AWARDS

Chilton Medical Center

1010 Lay Dam Road
Clanton, AL 35045
(205) 755-2500

Overall patient safety: ★★★
Teaching: N

CLINICAL PROGRAM RATINGS:

CARDIAC	NR	ORTHOPEDICS	NR
CRITICAL CARE	NR	PULMONARY	★★★
GASTROINTESTINAL	NR	STROKE	NR
GENERAL SURGERY	NR	VASCULAR	NR
MATERNITY CARE	NR	WOMEN'S HEALTH	NR

HEALTHGRADES AWARDS

Coosa Valley Medical Center

315 West Hickory Street
Sylacauga, AL 35150
(256) 249-5000

Overall patient safety: ★★★
Teaching: N

CLINICAL PROGRAM RATINGS:

CARDIAC	NR	ORTHOPEDICS	NR
CRITICAL CARE	NR	PULMONARY	★★★
GASTROINTESTINAL	NR	STROKE	★★★★★
GENERAL SURGERY	NR	VASCULAR	NR
MATERNITY CARE	NR	WOMEN'S HEALTH	NR

HEALTHGRADES AWARDS

✓ SPECIALTY EXCELLENCE
• STROKE CARE

KEY: ★★★★★ **BEST** ★★★ **AS EXPECTED** ★ **POOR** NR **NOT RATED BY HEALTHGRADES** For full definitions of ratings and awards, see Appendix.

Crenshaw Community Hospital

101 Hospital Circle
Luverne, AL 36049
(334) 335-1154

Overall patient safety: ★★★
Teaching: N

CLINICAL PROGRAM RATINGS:

CARDIAC	NR	ORTHOPEDICS	NR
CRITICAL CARE	NR	PULMONARY	★
GASTROINTESTINAL	NR	STROKE	★★★
GENERAL SURGERY	NR	VASCULAR	NR
MATERNITY CARE	NR	WOMEN'S HEALTH	NR

HEALTHGRADES AWARDS

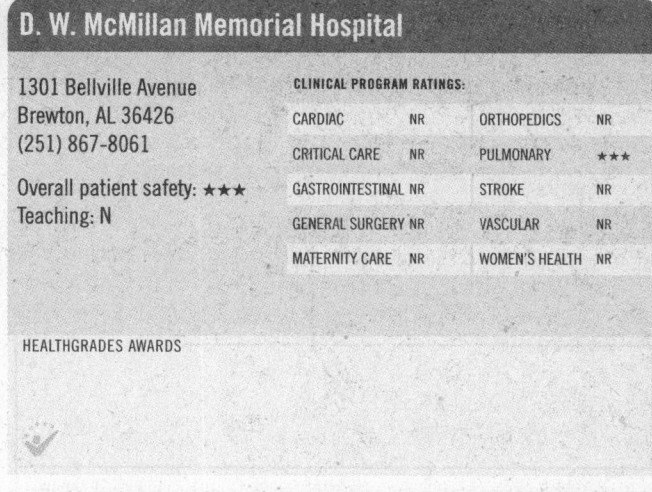

D. W. McMillan Memorial Hospital

1301 Bellville Avenue
Brewton, AL 36426
(251) 867-8061

Overall patient safety: ★★★
Teaching: N

CLINICAL PROGRAM RATINGS:

CARDIAC	NR	ORTHOPEDICS	NR
CRITICAL CARE	NR	PULMONARY	★★★
GASTROINTESTINAL	NR	STROKE	NR
GENERAL SURGERY	NR	VASCULAR	NR
MATERNITY CARE	NR	WOMEN'S HEALTH	NR

HEALTHGRADES AWARDS

Crestwood Medical Center

1 Hospital Drive
Huntsville, AL 35801
(256) 882-3100

Overall patient safety: ★★★
Teaching: N

CLINICAL PROGRAM RATINGS:

CARDIAC	NR	ORTHOPEDICS	★★★
CRITICAL CARE	NR	PULMONARY	★★★
GASTROINTESTINAL	★★★	STROKE	★★★
GENERAL SURGERY	NR	VASCULAR	NR
MATERNITY CARE	NR	WOMEN'S HEALTH	NR

HEALTHGRADES AWARDS

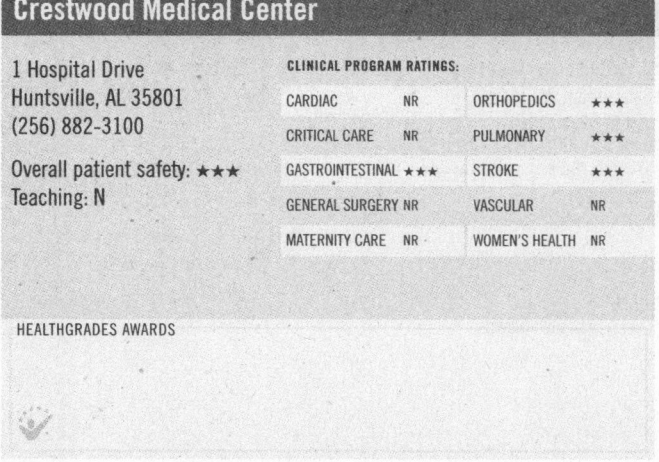

Dale Medical Center

126 Hospital Avenue
Ozark, AL 36360
(334) 774-2601

Overall patient safety: ★★★★★
Teaching: N

CLINICAL PROGRAM RATINGS:

CARDIAC	NR	ORTHOPEDICS	NR
CRITICAL CARE	NR	PULMONARY	★★★
GASTROINTESTINAL	NR	STROKE	★★★
GENERAL SURGERY	NR	VASCULAR	NR
MATERNITY CARE	NR	WOMEN'S HEALTH	NR

HEALTHGRADES AWARDS

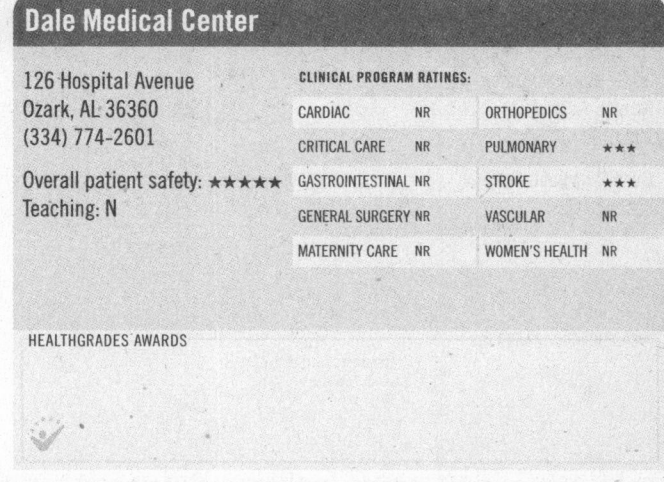

Cullman Regional Medical Center

1912 Alabama Highway 157
Cullman, AL 35058
(256) 737-2000

Overall patient safety: ★★★
Teaching: N

CLINICAL PROGRAM RATINGS:

CARDIAC	NR	ORTHOPEDICS	NR
CRITICAL CARE	★	PULMONARY	★★★
GASTROINTESTINAL	★★★	STROKE	★★★
GENERAL SURGERY	NR	VASCULAR	NR
MATERNITY CARE	NR	WOMEN'S HEALTH	NR

HEALTHGRADES AWARDS

DCH Regional Medical Center

809 University Boulevard East
Tuscaloosa, AL 35401
(205) 759-7111

Overall patient safety: ★★★
Teaching: Y

CLINICAL PROGRAM RATINGS:

CARDIAC	★★★	ORTHOPEDICS	★★★
CRITICAL CARE	★★★	PULMONARY	★★★★★
GASTROINTESTINAL	★★★	STROKE	★★★★★
GENERAL SURGERY	NR	VASCULAR	★★★
MATERNITY CARE	NR	WOMEN'S HEALTH	NR

HEALTHGRADES AWARDS

✓ DISTINGUISHED HOSPITAL • CLINICAL EXCELLENCE
✓ SPECIALTY EXCELLENCE • PULMONARY CARE • STROKE CARE

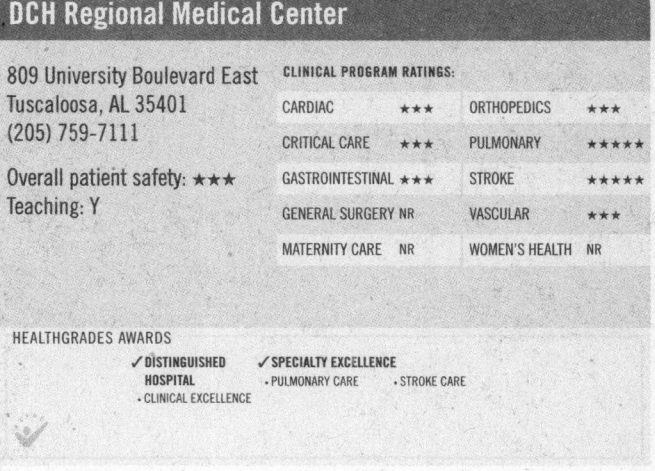

Decatur General Hospital

1201 7th Street Southeast
Decatur, AL 35601
(256) 341-2000

Overall patient safety: ★★★
Teaching: N

CLINICAL PROGRAM RATINGS:

CARDIAC	★★★	ORTHOPEDICS	NR
CRITICAL CARE	★	PULMONARY	★★★
GASTROINTESTINAL	★★★	STROKE	★★★
GENERAL SURGERY	NR	VASCULAR	★★★
MATERNITY CARE	NR	WOMEN'S HEALTH	NR

HEALTHGRADES AWARDS

Elmore Community Hospital

500 Hospital Drive
Wetumpka, AL 36092
(334) 567-4311

Overall patient safety: ★★★
Teaching: N

CLINICAL PROGRAM RATINGS:

CARDIAC	NR	ORTHOPEDICS	NR
CRITICAL CARE	NR	PULMONARY	★
GASTROINTESTINAL	NR	STROKE	★★★
GENERAL SURGERY	NR	VASCULAR	NR
MATERNITY CARE	NR	WOMEN'S HEALTH	NR

HEALTHGRADES AWARDS

East Alabama Medical Center and Skilled Nursing Facility

2000 Pepperell Parkway
Opelika, AL 36801
(334) 749-3411

Overall patient safety: ★
Teaching: N

CLINICAL PROGRAM RATINGS:

CARDIAC	★	ORTHOPEDICS	★★★★★
CRITICAL CARE	★★★	PULMONARY	★★★
GASTROINTESTINAL	★★★	STROKE	★★★
GENERAL SURGERY	NR	VASCULAR	NR
MATERNITY CARE	NR	WOMEN'S HEALTH	NR

HEALTHGRADES AWARDS

✓ SPECIALTY EXCELLENCE
· ORTHOPEDIC SURGERY

Evergreen Medical Center

101 Crestview Avenue
Evergreen, AL 36401
(251) 578-2480

Overall patient safety: ★★★
Teaching: N

CLINICAL PROGRAM RATINGS:

CARDIAC	NR	ORTHOPEDICS	NR
CRITICAL CARE	NR	PULMONARY	★★★
GASTROINTESTINAL	NR	STROKE	NR
GENERAL SURGERY	NR	VASCULAR	NR
MATERNITY CARE	NR	WOMEN'S HEALTH	NR

HEALTHGRADES AWARDS

Eliza Coffee Memorial Hospital

205 Marengo Street
Florence, AL 35630
(256) 768-9191

Overall patient safety: ★★★
Teaching: N

CLINICAL PROGRAM RATINGS:

CARDIAC	★★★	ORTHOPEDICS	★★★
CRITICAL CARE	★★★	PULMONARY	★★★★★
GASTROINTESTINAL	★★★	STROKE	★★★
GENERAL SURGERY	NR	VASCULAR	NR
MATERNITY CARE	NR	WOMEN'S HEALTH	NR

HEALTHGRADES AWARDS

✓ SPECIALTY EXCELLENCE
· PULMONARY CARE

Fayette Medical Center

1653 Temple Avenue North
Fayette, AL 35555
(205) 932-5966

Overall patient safety: ★★★
Teaching: N

CLINICAL PROGRAM RATINGS:

CARDIAC	NR	ORTHOPEDICS	NR
CRITICAL CARE	NR	PULMONARY	★★★
GASTROINTESTINAL	NR	STROKE	★★★
GENERAL SURGERY	NR	VASCULAR	NR
MATERNITY CARE	NR	WOMEN'S HEALTH	NR

HEALTHGRADES AWARDS

KEY: ★★★★★ BEST ★★★ AS EXPECTED ★ POOR NR NOT RATED BY HEALTHGRADES For full definitions of ratings and awards, see Appendix.

Flowers Hospital

4370 West Main Street
Dothan, AL 36305
(334) 793-5000

Overall patient safety: ★★★★★
Teaching: N

CLINICAL PROGRAM RATINGS:

CARDIAC	★★★	ORTHOPEDICS	★★★
CRITICAL CARE	★★★	PULMONARY	★★★★★
GASTROINTESTINAL	★★★	STROKE	★★★★★
GENERAL SURGERY	NR	VASCULAR	NR
MATERNITY CARE	NR	WOMEN'S HEALTH	NR

HEALTHGRADES AWARDS

✓ DISTINGUISHED HOSPITAL
• PATIENT SAFETY

✓ SPECIALTY EXCELLENCE
• PULMONARY CARE

Hale County Hospital

508 Green Street
Greensboro, AL 36744
(334) 624-3024

Overall patient safety: NR
Teaching: N

CLINICAL PROGRAM RATINGS:

CARDIAC	NR	ORTHOPEDICS	NR
CRITICAL CARE	NR	PULMONARY	★★★
GASTROINTESTINAL	NR	STROKE	NR
GENERAL SURGERY	NR	VASCULAR	NR
MATERNITY CARE	NR	WOMEN'S HEALTH	NR

HEALTHGRADES AWARDS

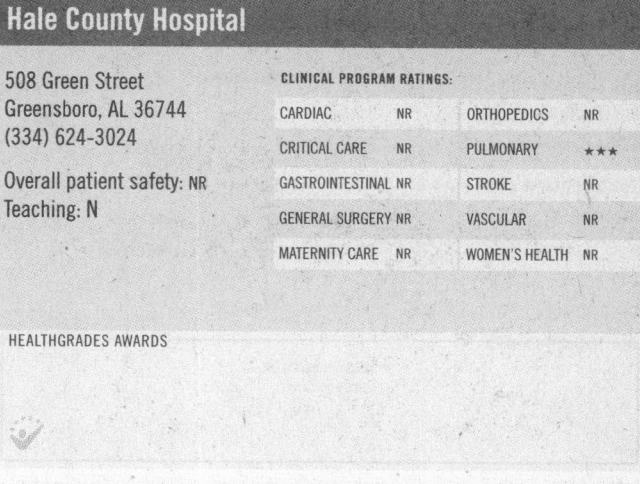

G. H. Lanier Memorial Hospital

4800 48th Street
Valley, AL 36854
(334) 756-9180

Overall patient safety: ★★★
Teaching: N

CLINICAL PROGRAM RATINGS:

CARDIAC	NR	ORTHOPEDICS	NR
CRITICAL CARE	NR	PULMONARY	★★★
GASTROINTESTINAL	NR	STROKE	★★★
GENERAL SURGERY	NR	VASCULAR	NR
MATERNITY CARE	NR	WOMEN'S HEALTH	NR

HEALTHGRADES AWARDS

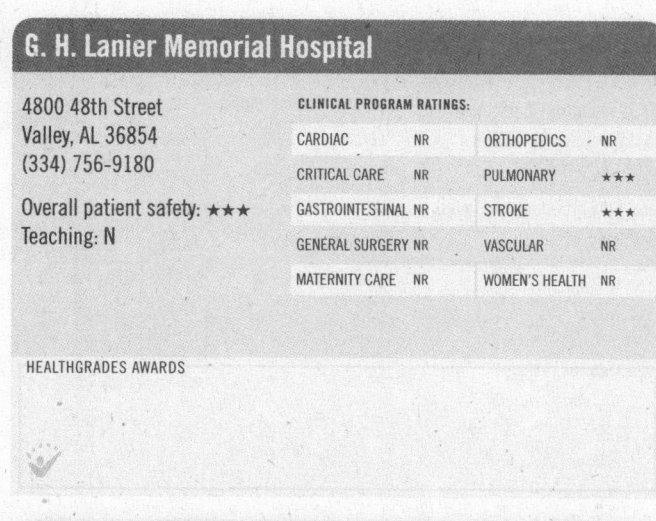

Hartselle Medical Center

201 Pine Street Northwest
Hartselle, AL 35640
(256) 751-3000

Overall patient safety: ★★★
Teaching: N

CLINICAL PROGRAM RATINGS:

CARDIAC	NR	ORTHOPEDICS	NR
CRITICAL CARE	NR	PULMONARY	★★★
GASTROINTESTINAL	NR	STROKE	★
GENERAL SURGERY	NR	VASCULAR	NR
MATERNITY CARE	NR	WOMEN'S HEALTH	NR

HEALTHGRADES AWARDS

Gadsden Regional Medical Center

1007 Goodyear Avenue
Gadsden, AL 35903
(256) 494-4000

Overall patient safety: ★★★
Teaching: N

CLINICAL PROGRAM RATINGS:

CARDIAC	★★★	ORTHOPEDICS	★★★
CRITICAL CARE	★★★	PULMONARY	★★★
GASTROINTESTINAL	★★★	STROKE	★★★
GENERAL SURGERY	NR	VASCULAR	NR
MATERNITY CARE	NR	WOMEN'S HEALTH	NR

HEALTHGRADES AWARDS

Helen Keller Hospital

1300 South Montgomery
Avenue
Sheffield, AL 35660
(256) 386-4196

Overall patient safety: ★★★
Teaching: N

CLINICAL PROGRAM RATINGS:

CARDIAC	NR	ORTHOPEDICS	★★★
CRITICAL CARE	NR	PULMONARY	★★★
GASTROINTESTINAL	★★★	STROKE	★★★
GENERAL SURGERY	NR	VASCULAR	NR
MATERNITY CARE	NR	WOMEN'S HEALTH	NR

HEALTHGRADES AWARDS

Huntsville Hospital

101 Sivley Road
Huntsville, AL 35801
(256) 265-1000

Overall patient safety: ★★★
Teaching: Y

CLINICAL PROGRAM RATINGS:

CARDIAC	★★★	ORTHOPEDICS	★★★
CRITICAL CARE	★	PULMONARY	★
GASTROINTESTINAL	★★★	STROKE	★
GENERAL SURGERY	NR	VASCULAR	★★★
MATERNITY CARE	NR	WOMEN'S HEALTH	NR

HEALTHGRADES AWARDS

✓ SPECIALTY EXCELLENCE
· CARDIAC SURGERY

Jackson Medical Center

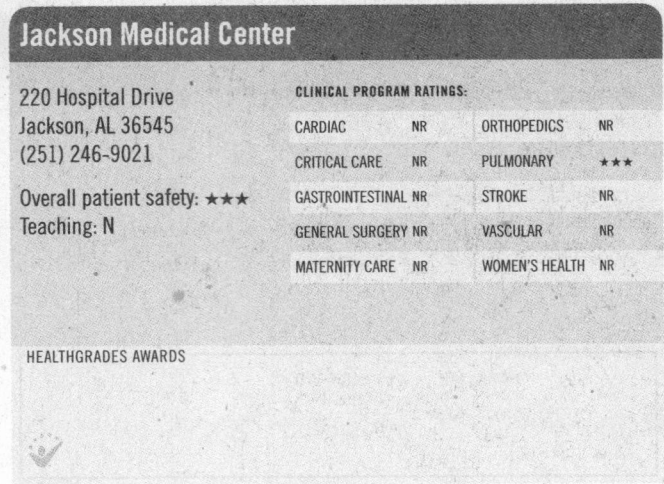

220 Hospital Drive
Jackson, AL 36545
(251) 246-9021

Overall patient safety: ★★★
Teaching: N

CLINICAL PROGRAM RATINGS:

CARDIAC	NR	ORTHOPEDICS	NR
CRITICAL CARE	NR	PULMONARY	★★★
GASTROINTESTINAL	NR	STROKE	NR
GENERAL SURGERY	NR	VASCULAR	NR
MATERNITY CARE	NR	WOMEN'S HEALTH	NR

HEALTHGRADES AWARDS

Jackson County Hospital

380 Woods Cove Road
Scottsboro, AL 35768
(256) 259-4444

Overall patient safety: ★★★
Teaching: N

CLINICAL PROGRAM RATINGS:

CARDIAC	NR	ORTHOPEDICS	NR
CRITICAL CARE	NR	PULMONARY	★★★
GASTROINTESTINAL	NR	STROKE	NR
GENERAL SURGERY	NR	VASCULAR	NR
MATERNITY CARE	NR	WOMEN'S HEALTH	NR

HEALTHGRADES AWARDS

Jacksonville Medical Center

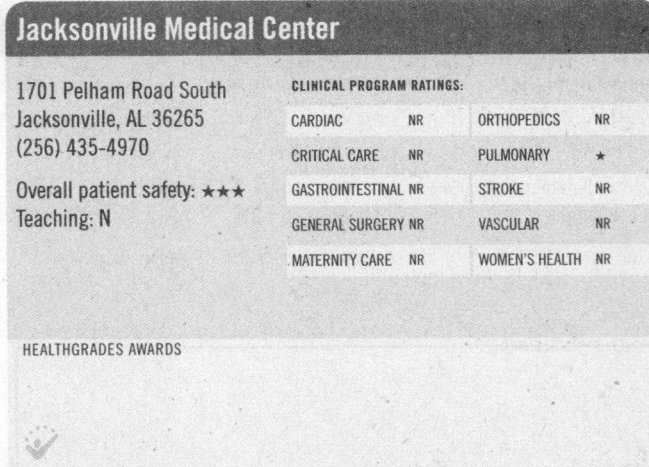

1701 Pelham Road South
Jacksonville, AL 36265
(256) 435-4970

Overall patient safety: ★★★
Teaching: N

CLINICAL PROGRAM RATINGS:

CARDIAC	NR	ORTHOPEDICS	NR
CRITICAL CARE	NR	PULMONARY	★
GASTROINTESTINAL	NR	STROKE	NR
GENERAL SURGERY	NR	VASCULAR	NR
MATERNITY CARE	NR	WOMEN'S HEALTH	NR

HEALTHGRADES AWARDS

Jackson Hospital and Clinic

1725 Pine Street
Montgomery, AL 36106
(334) 293-8000

Overall patient safety: ★
Teaching: N

CLINICAL PROGRAM RATINGS:

CARDIAC	★★★	ORTHOPEDICS	★★★★★
CRITICAL CARE	★	PULMONARY	★
GASTROINTESTINAL	★★★	STROKE	★
GENERAL SURGERY	NR	VASCULAR	NR
MATERNITY CARE	NR	WOMEN'S HEALTH	NR

HEALTHGRADES AWARDS

✓ SPECIALTY EXCELLENCE
· ORTHOPEDIC SURGERY

L. V. Stabler Memorial Hospital

29 L. V. Stabler Drive
Greenville, AL 36037
(334) 382-2671

Overall patient safety: ★★★
Teaching: N

CLINICAL PROGRAM RATINGS:

CARDIAC	NR	ORTHOPEDICS	NR
CRITICAL CARE	NR	PULMONARY	★★★
GASTROINTESTINAL	NR	STROKE	★★★
GENERAL SURGERY	NR	VASCULAR	NR
MATERNITY CARE	NR	WOMEN'S HEALTH	NR

HEALTHGRADES AWARDS

KEY: ★★★★★ BEST ★★★ AS EXPECTED ★ POOR NR NOT RATED BY HEALTHGRADES For full definitions of ratings and awards, see Appendix.

Lake Martin Community Hospital

201 Mariarden Road
Dadeville, AL 36853
(256) 825-7821

Overall patient safety: ★★★
Teaching: N

CLINICAL PROGRAM RATINGS:

CARDIAC	NR	ORTHOPEDICS	NR
CRITICAL CARE	NR	PULMONARY	★★★
GASTROINTESTINAL	NR	STROKE	NR
GENERAL SURGERY	NR	VASCULAR	NR
MATERNITY CARE	NR	WOMEN'S HEALTH	NR

HEALTHGRADES AWARDS

Lawrence Medical Center

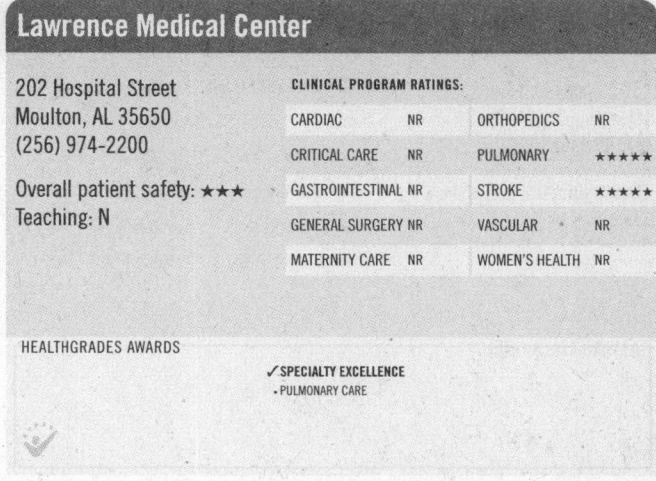

202 Hospital Street
Moulton, AL 35650
(256) 974-2200

Overall patient safety: ★★★
Teaching: N

CLINICAL PROGRAM RATINGS:

CARDIAC	NR	ORTHOPEDICS	NR
CRITICAL CARE	NR	PULMONARY	★★★★★
GASTROINTESTINAL	NR	STROKE	★★★★★
GENERAL SURGERY	NR	VASCULAR	NR
MATERNITY CARE	NR	WOMEN'S HEALTH	NR

HEALTHGRADES AWARDS

✓ **SPECIALTY EXCELLENCE**
• PULMONARY CARE

Lakeland Community Hospital

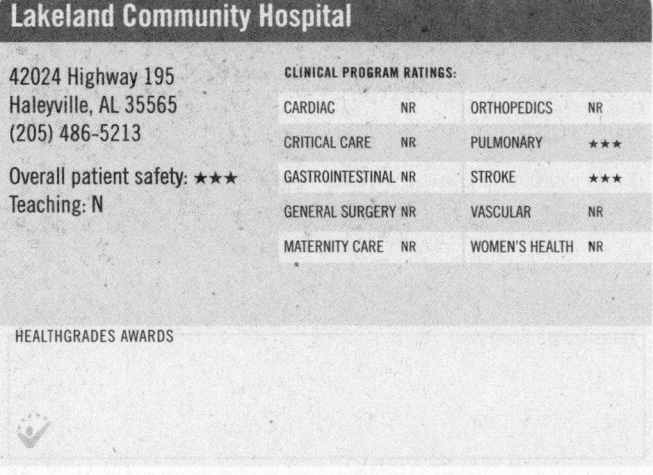

42024 Highway 195
Haleyville, AL 35565
(205) 486-5213

Overall patient safety: ★★★
Teaching: N

CLINICAL PROGRAM RATINGS:

CARDIAC	NR	ORTHOPEDICS	NR
CRITICAL CARE	NR	PULMONARY	★★★
GASTROINTESTINAL	NR	STROKE	★★★
GENERAL SURGERY	NR	VASCULAR	NR
MATERNITY CARE	NR	WOMEN'S HEALTH	NR

HEALTHGRADES AWARDS

LTC Hospital at Southeast Alabama Medical Center

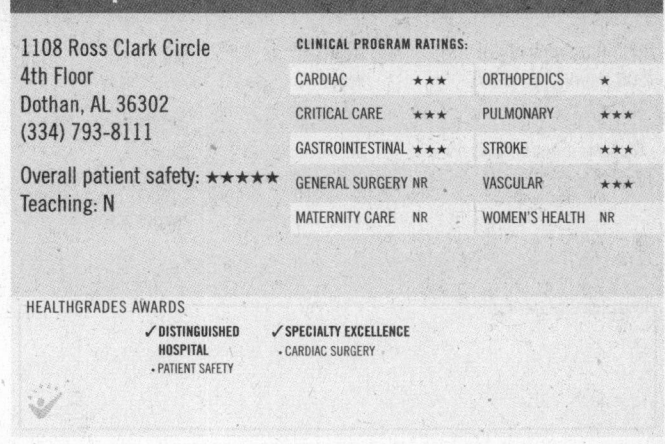

1108 Ross Clark Circle
4th Floor
Dothan, AL 36302
(334) 793-8111

Overall patient safety: ★★★★★
Teaching: N

CLINICAL PROGRAM RATINGS:

CARDIAC	★★★	ORTHOPEDICS	★
CRITICAL CARE	★★★	PULMONARY	★★★
GASTROINTESTINAL	★★★	STROKE	★★★
GENERAL SURGERY	NR	VASCULAR	★★★
MATERNITY CARE	NR	WOMEN'S HEALTH	NR

HEALTHGRADES AWARDS

✓ **DISTINGUISHED HOSPITAL**   ✓ **SPECIALTY EXCELLENCE**
• PATIENT SAFETY   • CARDIAC SURGERY

Lakeview Community Hospital

820 West Washington Street
Eufaula, AL 36027
(334) 688-7000

Overall patient safety: ★★★
Teaching: N

CLINICAL PROGRAM RATINGS:

CARDIAC	NR	ORTHOPEDICS	NR
CRITICAL CARE	NR	PULMONARY	★★★
GASTROINTESTINAL	NR	STROKE	★★★
GENERAL SURGERY	NR	VASCULAR	NR
MATERNITY CARE	NR	WOMEN'S HEALTH	NR

HEALTHGRADES AWARDS

LTC Hospital of Tuscaloosa

809 University Boulevard East
4th Floor
Tuscaloosa, AL 35401
(205) 759-7241

Overall patient safety: ★★★
Teaching: Y

CLINICAL PROGRAM RATINGS:

CARDIAC	★★★	ORTHOPEDICS	★★★
CRITICAL CARE	★★★	PULMONARY	★★★★★
GASTROINTESTINAL	★★★	STROKE	★★★★★
GENERAL SURGERY	NR	VASCULAR	★★★
MATERNITY CARE	NR	WOMEN'S HEALTH	NR

HEALTHGRADES AWARDS

✓ **SPECIALTY EXCELLENCE**
• PULMONARY CARE   • STROKE CARE

Marion Regional Medical Center

1256 Military Street South
Hamilton, AL 35570
(205) 921-6200

Overall patient safety: ★★★
Teaching: N

CLINICAL PROGRAM RATINGS:

CARDIAC	NR	ORTHOPEDICS	NR
CRITICAL CARE	NR	PULMONARY	★★★
GASTROINTESTINAL	NR	STROKE	★★★
GENERAL SURGERY	NR	VASCULAR	NR
MATERNITY CARE	NR	WOMEN'S HEALTH	NR

HEALTHGRADES AWARDS

Medical Center Enterprise

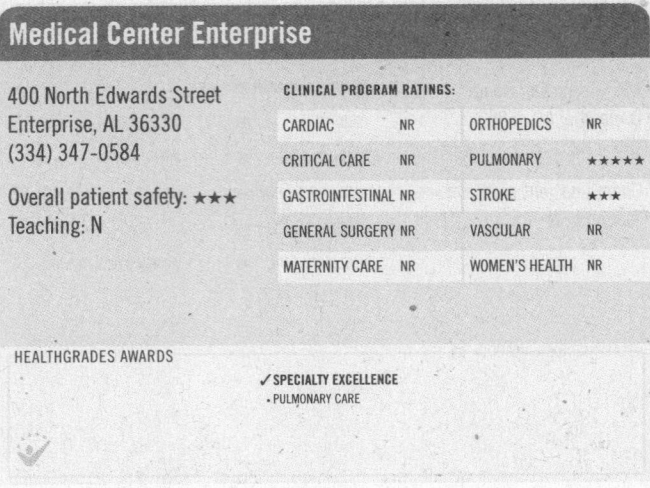

400 North Edwards Street
Enterprise, AL 36330
(334) 347-0584

Overall patient safety: ★★★
Teaching: N

CLINICAL PROGRAM RATINGS:

CARDIAC	NR	ORTHOPEDICS	NR
CRITICAL CARE	NR	PULMONARY	★★★★★
GASTROINTESTINAL	NR	STROKE	★★★
GENERAL SURGERY	NR	VASCULAR	NR
MATERNITY CARE	NR	WOMEN'S HEALTH	NR

HEALTHGRADES AWARDS

✓ SPECIALTY EXCELLENCE
· PULMONARY CARE

Marshall Medical Center—North

8000 Alabama Highway 69
Guntersville, AL 35976
(256) 753-8000

Overall patient safety: ★★★
Teaching: N

CLINICAL PROGRAM RATINGS:

CARDIAC	NR	ORTHOPEDICS	NR
CRITICAL CARE	NR	PULMONARY	★★★
GASTROINTESTINAL	★★★	STROKE	★★★
GENERAL SURGERY	NR	VASCULAR	NR
MATERNITY CARE	NR	WOMEN'S HEALTH	NR

HEALTHGRADES AWARDS

Mizell Memorial Hospital

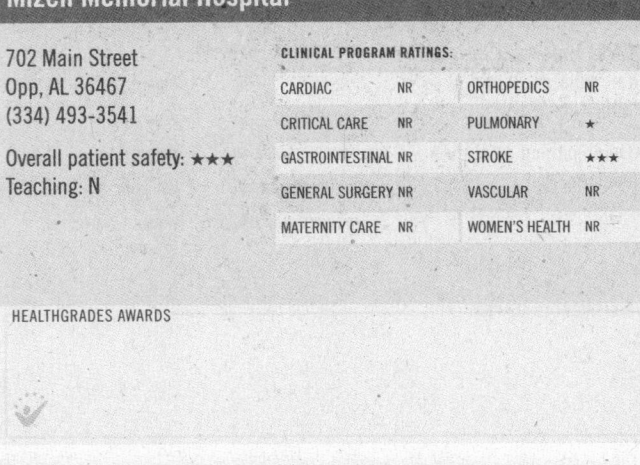

702 Main Street
Opp, AL 36467
(334) 493-3541

Overall patient safety: ★★★
Teaching: N

CLINICAL PROGRAM RATINGS:

CARDIAC	NR	ORTHOPEDICS	NR
CRITICAL CARE	NR	PULMONARY	★
GASTROINTESTINAL	NR	STROKE	★★★
GENERAL SURGERY	NR	VASCULAR	NR
MATERNITY CARE	NR	WOMEN'S HEALTH	NR

HEALTHGRADES AWARDS

Marshall Medical Center—South

2505 US Highway 431 North
Boaz, AL 35957
(256) 593-8310

Overall patient safety: ★
Teaching: N

CLINICAL PROGRAM RATINGS:

CARDIAC	NR	ORTHOPEDICS	NR
CRITICAL CARE	NR	PULMONARY	★★★
GASTROINTESTINAL	★★★	STROKE	★
GENERAL SURGERY	NR	VASCULAR	NR
MATERNITY CARE	NR	WOMEN'S HEALTH	NR

HEALTHGRADES AWARDS

Mobile Infirmary

5 Mobile Infirmary Circle
Mobile, AL 36607
(251) 435-2400

Overall patient safety: ★★★
Teaching: Y

CLINICAL PROGRAM RATINGS:

CARDIAC	★★★	ORTHOPEDICS	★★★
CRITICAL CARE	★★★	PULMONARY	★★★
GASTROINTESTINAL	★★★	STROKE	★
GENERAL SURGERY	NR	VASCULAR	★★★
MATERNITY CARE	NR	WOMEN'S HEALTH	NR

HEALTHGRADES AWARDS

✓ SPECIALTY EXCELLENCE
· VASCULAR SURGERY

KEY: ★★★★★ BEST ★★★ AS EXPECTED ★ POOR NR NOT RATED BY HEALTHGRADES For full definitions of ratings and awards, see Appendix.

Monroe County Hospital

2016 South Alabama Avenue
Monroeville, AL 36461
(251) 575-3111

Overall patient safety: ★★★
Teaching: N

CLINICAL PROGRAM RATINGS:

CARDIAC	NR	ORTHOPEDICS	NR
CRITICAL CARE	NR	PULMONARY	★
GASTROINTESTINAL	NR	STROKE	NR
GENERAL SURGERY	NR	VASCULAR	NR
MATERNITY CARE	NR	WOMEN'S HEALTH	NR

HEALTHGRADES AWARDS

Northport Medical Center

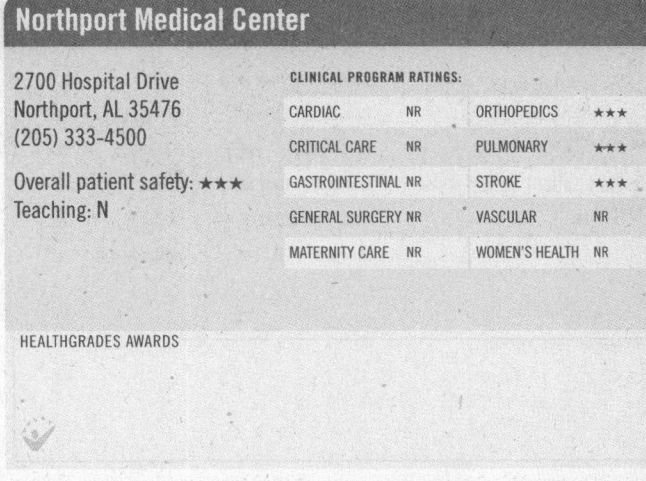

2700 Hospital Drive
Northport, AL 35476
(205) 333-4500

Overall patient safety: ★★★
Teaching: N

CLINICAL PROGRAM RATINGS:

CARDIAC	NR	ORTHOPEDICS	★★★
CRITICAL CARE	NR	PULMONARY	★★★
GASTROINTESTINAL	NR	STROKE	★★★
GENERAL SURGERY	NR	VASCULAR	NR
MATERNITY CARE	NR	WOMEN'S HEALTH	NR

HEALTHGRADES AWARDS

North Baldwin Infirmary

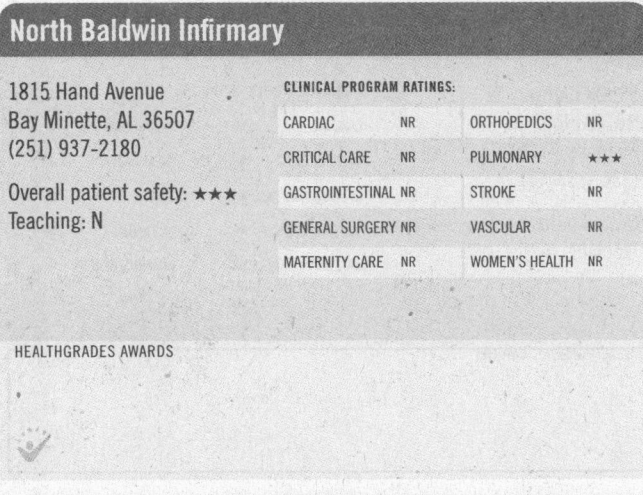

1815 Hand Avenue
Bay Minette, AL 36507
(251) 937-2180

Overall patient safety: ★★★
Teaching: N

CLINICAL PROGRAM RATINGS:

CARDIAC	NR	ORTHOPEDICS	NR
CRITICAL CARE	NR	PULMONARY	★★★
GASTROINTESTINAL	NR	STROKE	NR
GENERAL SURGERY	NR	VASCULAR	NR
MATERNITY CARE	NR	WOMEN'S HEALTH	NR

HEALTHGRADES AWARDS

Northwest Medical Center

1530 US Highway 43
Winfield, AL 35594
(205) 487-7000

Overall patient safety: ★★★★★
Teaching: N

CLINICAL PROGRAM RATINGS:

CARDIAC	NR	ORTHOPEDICS	NR
CRITICAL CARE	NR	PULMONARY	★★★
GASTROINTESTINAL	NR	STROKE	★★★
GENERAL SURGERY	NR	VASCULAR	NR
MATERNITY CARE	NR	WOMEN'S HEALTH	NR

HEALTHGRADES AWARDS

Northeast Alabama Regional Medical Center

400 East 10th Street
Anniston, AL 36207
(256) 235-5121

Overall patient safety: ★★★
Teaching: Y

CLINICAL PROGRAM RATINGS:

CARDIAC	★★★	ORTHOPEDICS	NR
CRITICAL CARE	★★★	PULMONARY	★★★★★
GASTROINTESTINAL	★★★	STROKE	★★★
GENERAL SURGERY	NR	VASCULAR	NR
MATERNITY CARE	NR	WOMEN'S HEALTH	NR

HEALTHGRADES AWARDS

✓ SPECIALTY EXCELLENCE
· PULMONARY CARE

Northwest Medical Center*

715 Highway 43 Northeast
Russellville, AL 35653
(205) 332-1611

Overall patient safety: ★★★
Teaching: N

CLINICAL PROGRAM RATINGS:

CARDIAC	NR	ORTHOPEDICS	NR
CRITICAL CARE	NR	PULMONARY	★
GASTROINTESTINAL	NR	STROKE	★★★
GENERAL SURGERY	NR	VASCULAR	NR
MATERNITY CARE	NR	WOMEN'S HEALTH	NR

HEALTHGRADES AWARDS

*This hospital reports its data to the federal government jointly with another hospital. Therefore the ratings and awards apply to multiple hospitals and this specific hospital may not provide all rated services.

ALABAMA HOSPITALS: RATINGS BY CLINICAL SPECIALTY

Parkway Medical Center Hospital

1874 Beltline Road Southwest
Decatur, AL 35601
(256) 350-2211

Overall patient safety: ★★★
Teaching: N

CLINICAL PROGRAM RATINGS:

CARDIAC	NR	ORTHOPEDICS	NR
CRITICAL CARE	NR	PULMONARY	★★★
GASTROINTESTINAL	NR	STROKE	★
GENERAL SURGERY	NR	VASCULAR	NR
MATERNITY CARE	NR	WOMEN'S HEALTH	NR

HEALTHGRADES AWARDS

Providence Hospital

6801 Airport Boulevard
Mobile, AL 36608
(251) 633-1000

Overall patient safety: ★★★
Teaching: N

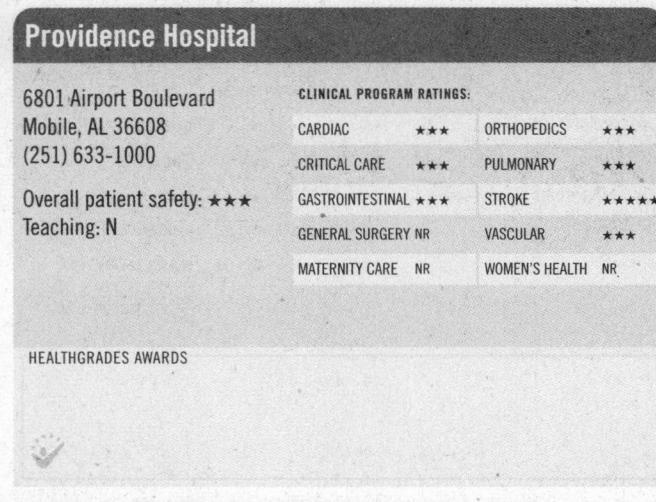

CLINICAL PROGRAM RATINGS:

CARDIAC	★★★	ORTHOPEDICS	★★★
CRITICAL CARE	★★★	PULMONARY	★★★
GASTROINTESTINAL	★★★	STROKE	★★★★★
GENERAL SURGERY	NR	VASCULAR	★★★
MATERNITY CARE	NR	WOMEN'S HEALTH	NR

HEALTHGRADES AWARDS

Pickens County Medical Center

241 Robert K. Wilson Drive
Carrollton, AL 35447
(205) 367-8111

Overall patient safety: ★★★
Teaching: N

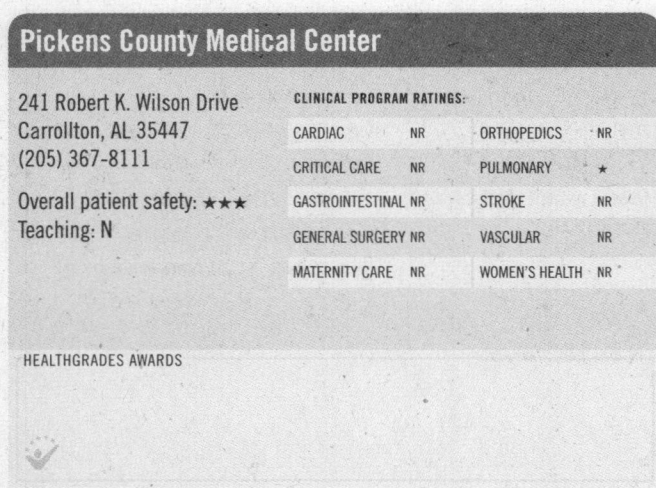

CLINICAL PROGRAM RATINGS:

CARDIAC	NR	ORTHOPEDICS	NR
CRITICAL CARE	NR	PULMONARY	★
GASTROINTESTINAL	NR	STROKE	NR
GENERAL SURGERY	NR	VASCULAR	NR
MATERNITY CARE	NR	WOMEN'S HEALTH	NR

HEALTHGRADES AWARDS

Randolph Medical Center

59928 Highway 22
P.O. Box 670
Roanoke, AL 36274
(334) 863-4111

Overall patient safety: ★★★
Teaching: N

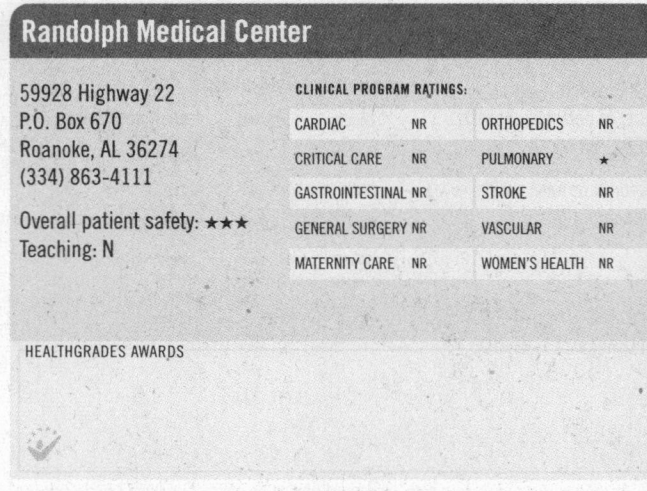

CLINICAL PROGRAM RATINGS:

CARDIAC	NR	ORTHOPEDICS	NR
CRITICAL CARE	NR	PULMONARY	★
GASTROINTESTINAL	NR	STROKE	NR
GENERAL SURGERY	NR	VASCULAR	NR
MATERNITY CARE	NR	WOMEN'S HEALTH	NR

HEALTHGRADES AWARDS

Prattville Baptist Hospital

124 South Memorial Drive
Prattville, AL 36067
(334) 365-0651

Overall patient safety: ★★★
Teaching: N

CLINICAL PROGRAM RATINGS:

CARDIAC	NR	ORTHOPEDICS	NR
CRITICAL CARE	NR	PULMONARY	★★★
GASTROINTESTINAL	NR	STROKE	★★★
GENERAL SURGERY	NR	VASCULAR	NR
MATERNITY CARE	NR	WOMEN'S HEALTH	NR

HEALTHGRADES AWARDS

Red Bay Hospital

211 Hospital Road
Red Bay, AL 35582
(256) 356-9532

Overall patient safety: NR
Teaching: N

CLINICAL PROGRAM RATINGS:

CARDIAC	NR	ORTHOPEDICS	NR
CRITICAL CARE	NR	PULMONARY	★
GASTROINTESTINAL	NR	STROKE	NR
GENERAL SURGERY	NR	VASCULAR	NR
MATERNITY CARE	NR	WOMEN'S HEALTH	NR

HEALTHGRADES AWARDS

KEY: ★★★★★ BEST ★★★ AS EXPECTED ★ POOR NR NOT RATED BY HEALTHGRADES For full definitions of ratings and awards, see Appendix.

Riverview Regional Medical Center

600 South 3rd Street
Gadsden, AL 35901
(256) 543-5200

Overall patient safety: ★★★
Teaching: N

CLINICAL PROGRAM RATINGS:

CARDIAC	★★★	ORTHOPEDICS	★★★
CRITICAL CARE	★★★	PULMONARY	★★★
GASTROINTESTINAL	★★★	STROKE	★★★★★
GENERAL SURGERY	NR	VASCULAR	NR
MATERNITY CARE	NR	WOMEN'S HEALTH	NR

HEALTHGRADES AWARDS

✓ SPECIALTY EXCELLENCE
• STROKE CARE

St. Vincent's—Birmingham

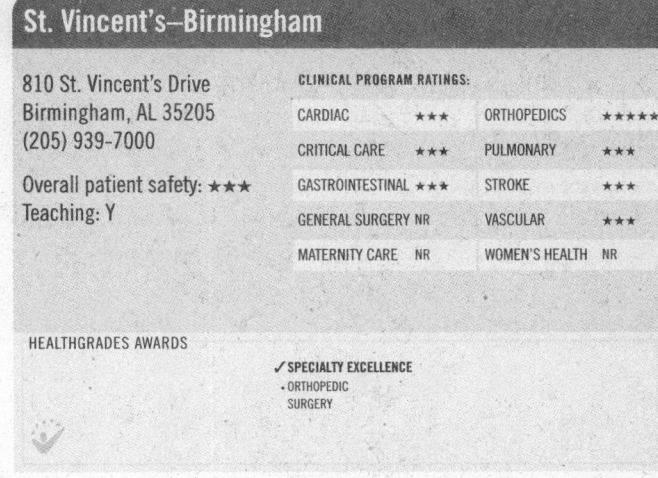

810 St. Vincent's Drive
Birmingham, AL 35205
(205) 939-7000

Overall patient safety: ★★★
Teaching: Y

CLINICAL PROGRAM RATINGS:

CARDIAC	★★★	ORTHOPEDICS	★★★★★
CRITICAL CARE	★★★	PULMONARY	★★★
GASTROINTESTINAL	★★★	STROKE	★★★
GENERAL SURGERY	NR	VASCULAR	★★★
MATERNITY CARE	NR	WOMEN'S HEALTH	NR

HEALTHGRADES AWARDS

✓ SPECIALTY EXCELLENCE
• ORTHOPEDIC SURGERY

Russell Medical Center

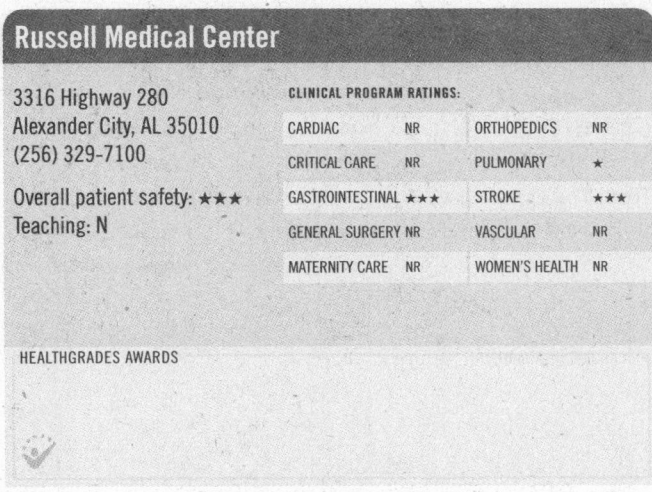

3316 Highway 280
Alexander City, AL 35010
(256) 329-7100

Overall patient safety: ★★★
Teaching: N

CLINICAL PROGRAM RATINGS:

CARDIAC	NR	ORTHOPEDICS	NR
CRITICAL CARE	NR	PULMONARY	★
GASTROINTESTINAL	★★★	STROKE	★★★
GENERAL SURGERY	NR	VASCULAR	NR
MATERNITY CARE	NR	WOMEN'S HEALTH	NR

HEALTHGRADES AWARDS

St. Vincent's—Blount

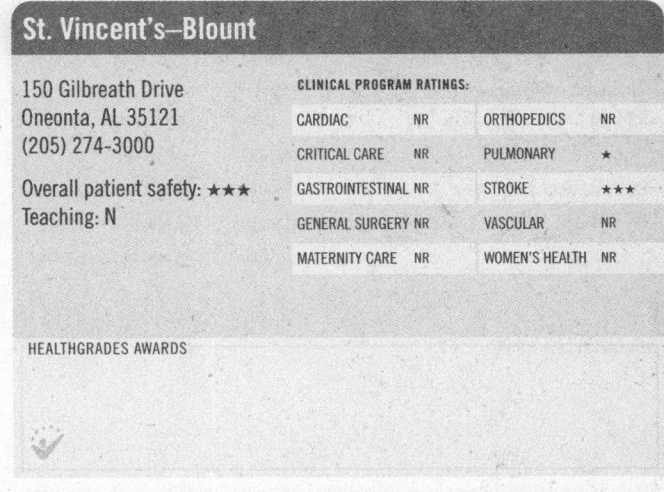

150 Gilbreath Drive
Oneonta, AL 35121
(205) 274-3000

Overall patient safety: ★★★
Teaching: N

CLINICAL PROGRAM RATINGS:

CARDIAC	NR	ORTHOPEDICS	NR
CRITICAL CARE	NR	PULMONARY	★
GASTROINTESTINAL	NR	STROKE	★★★
GENERAL SURGERY	NR	VASCULAR	NR
MATERNITY CARE	NR	WOMEN'S HEALTH	NR

HEALTHGRADES AWARDS

Russellville Hospital*

15155 Highway 43
Russellville, AL 35653
(256) 332-1611

Overall patient safety: ★★★
Teaching: N

CLINICAL PROGRAM RATINGS:

CARDIAC	NR	ORTHOPEDICS	NR
CRITICAL CARE	NR	PULMONARY	★
GASTROINTESTINAL	NR	STROKE	★★★
GENERAL SURGERY	NR	VASCULAR	NR
MATERNITY CARE	NR	WOMEN'S HEALTH	NR

HEALTHGRADES AWARDS

St. Vincent's—East

50 Medical Parks East Drive
Birmingham, AL 35235
(205) 838-3000

Overall patient safety: ★★★
Teaching: Y

CLINICAL PROGRAM RATINGS:

CARDIAC	★★★	ORTHOPEDICS	★★★
CRITICAL CARE	★	PULMONARY	★
GASTROINTESTINAL	★	STROKE	★
GENERAL SURGERY	NR	VASCULAR	★★★
MATERNITY CARE	NR	WOMEN'S HEALTH	NR

HEALTHGRADES AWARDS

ALABAMA HOSPITALS: RATINGS BY CLINICAL SPECIALTY

*This hospital reports its data to the federal government jointly with another hospital. Therefore the ratings and awards apply to multiple hospitals and this specific hospital may not provide all rated services.

St. Vincent's—St. Clair

2805 Dr. John Haynes Drive
Pell City, AL 35125
(205) 338-3301

Overall patient safety: ★
Teaching: N

CLINICAL PROGRAM RATINGS:

CARDIAC	NR	ORTHOPEDICS	NR
CRITICAL CARE	NR	PULMONARY	★★★
GASTROINTESTINAL	NR	STROKE	★
GENERAL SURGERY	NR	VASCULAR	NR
MATERNITY CARE	NR	WOMEN'S HEALTH	NR

HEALTHGRADES AWARDS

Southeast Alabama Medical Center

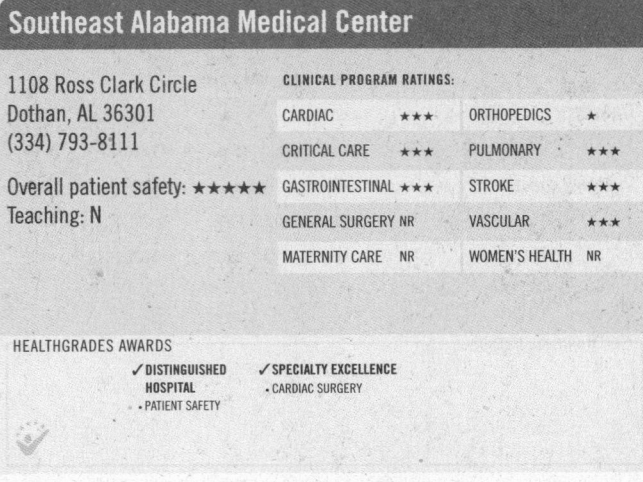

1108 Ross Clark Circle
Dothan, AL 36301
(334) 793-8111

Overall patient safety: ★★★★★
Teaching: N

CLINICAL PROGRAM RATINGS:

CARDIAC	★★★	ORTHOPEDICS	★
CRITICAL CARE	★★★	PULMONARY	★★★
GASTROINTESTINAL	★★★	STROKE	★★★
GENERAL SURGERY	NR	VASCULAR	★★★
MATERNITY CARE	NR	WOMEN'S HEALTH	NR

HEALTHGRADES AWARDS

✓ DISTINGUISHED HOSPITAL
• PATIENT SAFETY

✓ SPECIALTY EXCELLENCE
• CARDIAC SURGERY

Shoals Hospital

201 Avalon Avenue
Muscle Shoals, AL 35661
(256) 386-1600

Overall patient safety: ★
Teaching: N

CLINICAL PROGRAM RATINGS:

CARDIAC	NR	ORTHOPEDICS	NR
CRITICAL CARE	NR	PULMONARY	★★★
GASTROINTESTINAL	NR	STROKE	★★★
GENERAL SURGERY	NR	VASCULAR	NR
MATERNITY CARE	NR	WOMEN'S HEALTH	NR

HEALTHGRADES AWARDS

Southwest Alabama Medical Center

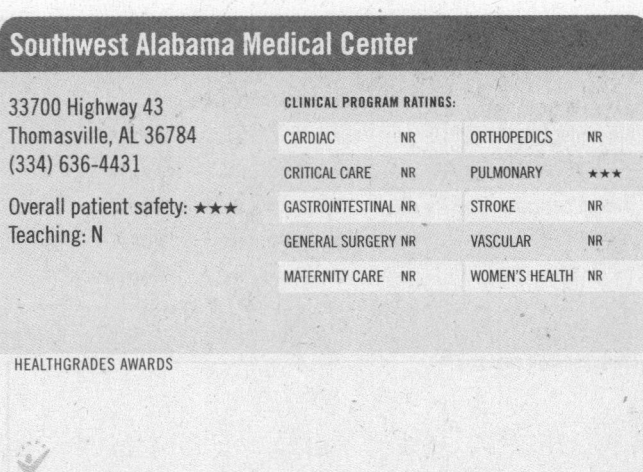

33700 Highway 43
Thomasville, AL 36784
(334) 636-4431

Overall patient safety: ★★★
Teaching: N

CLINICAL PROGRAM RATINGS:

CARDIAC	NR	ORTHOPEDICS	NR
CRITICAL CARE	NR	PULMONARY	★★★
GASTROINTESTINAL	NR	STROKE	NR
GENERAL SURGERY	NR	VASCULAR	NR
MATERNITY CARE	NR	WOMEN'S HEALTH	NR

HEALTHGRADES AWARDS

South Baldwin Regional Medical Center

1613 North McKenzie Street
Foley, AL 36535
(251) 952-3400

Overall patient safety: ★
Teaching: N

CLINICAL PROGRAM RATINGS:

CARDIAC	NR	ORTHOPEDICS	NR
CRITICAL CARE	NR	PULMONARY	★★★
GASTROINTESTINAL	★★★	STROKE	★★★
GENERAL SURGERY	NR	VASCULAR	NR
MATERNITY CARE	NR	WOMEN'S HEALTH	NR

HEALTHGRADES AWARDS

Springhill Medical Center

3719 Dauphin Street
Mobile, AL 36608
(251) 344-9630

Overall patient safety: ★★★
Teaching: Y

CLINICAL PROGRAM RATINGS:

CARDIAC	★★★	ORTHOPEDICS	★★★
CRITICAL CARE	★	PULMONARY	★★★
GASTROINTESTINAL	★★★	STROKE	★★★
GENERAL SURGERY	NR	VASCULAR	NR
MATERNITY CARE	NR	WOMEN'S HEALTH	NR

HEALTHGRADES AWARDS

KEY: ★★★★★ BEST   ★★★ AS EXPECTED   ★ POOR   NR NOT RATED BY HEALTHGRADES   For full definitions of ratings and awards, see Appendix.

Stringfellow Memorial Hospital

301 East 18th Street
Anniston, AL 36202
(256) 235-8900

Overall patient safety: ★★★
Teaching: N

CLINICAL PROGRAM RATINGS:

CARDIAC	NR	ORTHOPEDICS	NR
CRITICAL CARE	NR	PULMONARY	★★★
GASTROINTESTINAL	★★★	STROKE	★
GENERAL SURGERY	NR	VASCULAR	NR
MATERNITY CARE	NR	WOMEN'S HEALTH	NR

HEALTHGRADES AWARDS

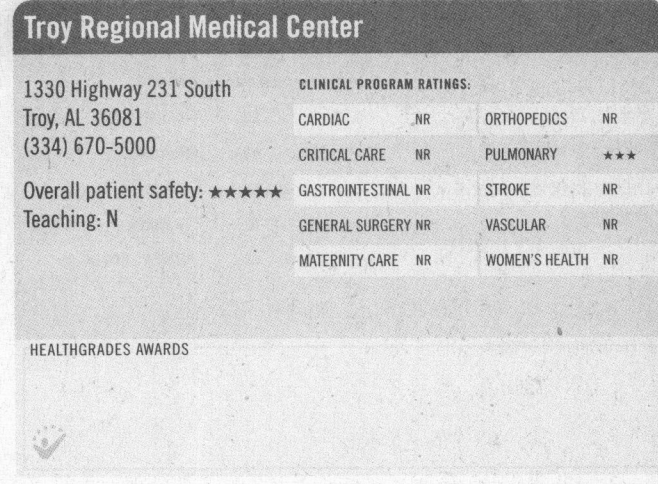

Troy Regional Medical Center

1330 Highway 231 South
Troy, AL 36081
(334) 670-5000

Overall patient safety: ★★★★★
Teaching: N

CLINICAL PROGRAM RATINGS:

CARDIAC	NR	ORTHOPEDICS	NR
CRITICAL CARE	NR	PULMONARY	★★★
GASTROINTESTINAL	NR	STROKE	NR
GENERAL SURGERY	NR	VASCULAR	NR
MATERNITY CARE	NR	WOMEN'S HEALTH	NR

HEALTHGRADES AWARDS

Thomas Hospital

750 Morphy Avenue
Fairhope, AL 36532
(251) 928-2375

Overall patient safety: ★★★
Teaching: N

CLINICAL PROGRAM RATINGS:

CARDIAC	★★★	ORTHOPEDICS	★★★
CRITICAL CARE	★★★	PULMONARY	★★★
GASTROINTESTINAL	★★★	STROKE	★★★
GENERAL SURGERY	NR	VASCULAR	NR
MATERNITY CARE	NR	WOMEN'S HEALTH	NR

HEALTHGRADES AWARDS

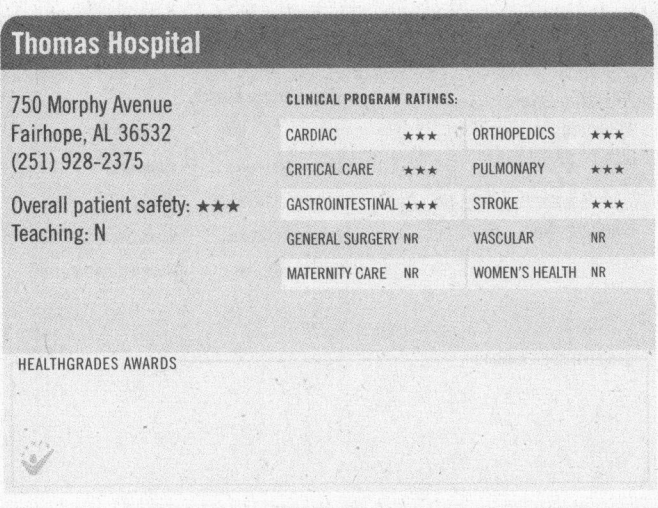

University of Alabama Hospital

619 South 19th Street
Birmingham, AL 35249
(205) 934-4011

Overall patient safety: ★
Teaching: Y

CLINICAL PROGRAM RATINGS:

CARDIAC	★★★	ORTHOPEDICS	★★★
CRITICAL CARE	★★★	PULMONARY	★
GASTROINTESTINAL	★★★	STROKE	★
GENERAL SURGERY	NR	VASCULAR	★★★
MATERNITY CARE	NR	WOMEN'S HEALTH	NR

HEALTHGRADES AWARDS

✓ SPECIALTY EXCELLENCE
· CARDIAC SURGERY

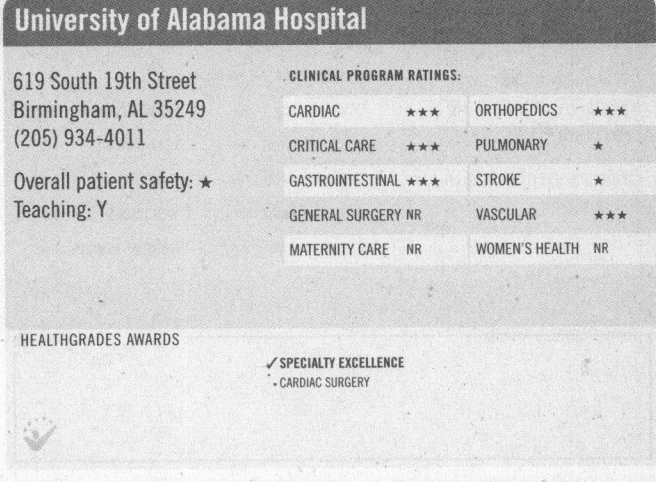

Trinity Medical Center

800 Montclair Road
Birmingham, AL 35213
(205) 592-1000

Overall patient safety: ★★★
Teaching: Y

CLINICAL PROGRAM RATINGS:

CARDIAC	★★★	ORTHOPEDICS	★★★
CRITICAL CARE	★★★	PULMONARY	★★★
GASTROINTESTINAL	★★★	STROKE	★★★
GENERAL SURGERY	NR	VASCULAR	★★★
MATERNITY CARE	NR	WOMEN'S HEALTH	NR

HEALTHGRADES AWARDS

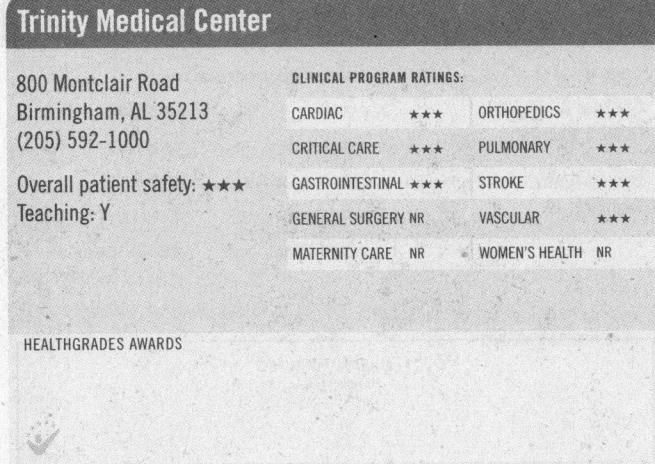

University of Alabama Medical West

US Highway 11 South
Bessemer, AL 35020
(205) 481-7000

Overall patient safety: ★★★
Teaching: N

CLINICAL PROGRAM RATINGS:

CARDIAC	NR	ORTHOPEDICS	NR
CRITICAL CARE	★★★	PULMONARY	★★★
GASTROINTESTINAL	★★★	STROKE	★★★
GENERAL SURGERY	NR	VASCULAR	NR
MATERNITY CARE	NR	WOMEN'S HEALTH	NR

HEALTHGRADES AWARDS

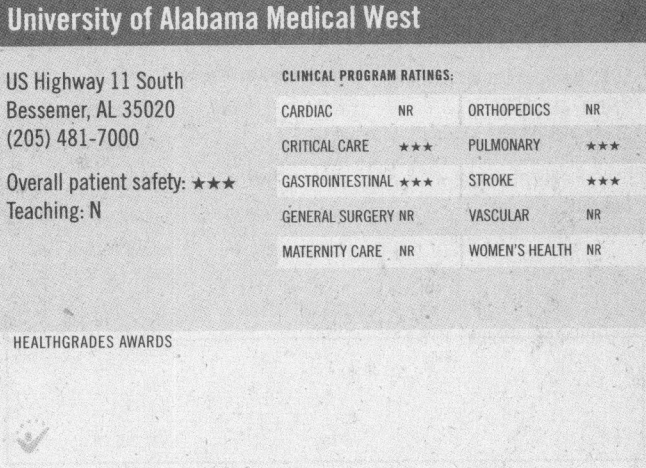

University of South Alabama Medical Center

2451 Fillingim Street
Mobile, AL 36617
(251) 471-7000

Overall patient safety: ★
Teaching: Y

CLINICAL PROGRAM RATINGS:

CARDIAC	NR	ORTHOPEDICS	NR
CRITICAL CARE	NR	PULMONARY	NR
GASTROINTESTINAL	NR	STROKE	★★★
GENERAL SURGERY	NR	VASCULAR	NR
MATERNITY CARE	NR	WOMEN'S HEALTH	NR

HEALTHGRADES AWARDS

Walker Baptist Medical Center

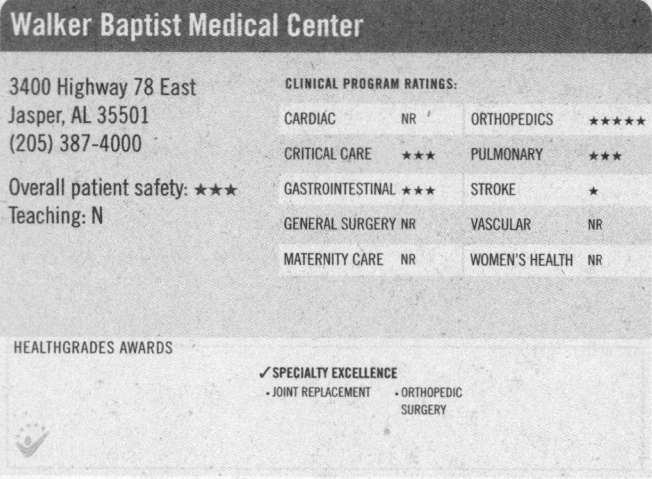

3400 Highway 78 East
Jasper, AL 35501
(205) 387-4000

Overall patient safety: ★★★
Teaching: N

CLINICAL PROGRAM RATINGS:

CARDIAC	NR	ORTHOPEDICS	★★★★★
CRITICAL CARE	★★★	PULMONARY	★★★
GASTROINTESTINAL	★★★	STROKE	★
GENERAL SURGERY	NR	VASCULAR	NR
MATERNITY CARE	NR	WOMEN'S HEALTH	NR

HEALTHGRADES AWARDS

✓ SPECIALTY EXCELLENCE
- JOINT REPLACEMENT
- ORTHOPEDIC SURGERY

University of South Alabama--Knollwood Hospital

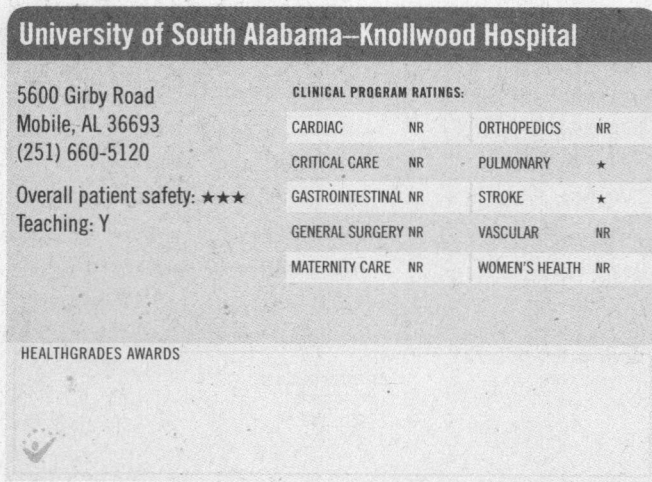

5600 Girby Road
Mobile, AL 36693
(251) 660-5120

Overall patient safety: ★★★
Teaching: Y

CLINICAL PROGRAM RATINGS:

CARDIAC	NR	ORTHOPEDICS	NR
CRITICAL CARE	NR	PULMONARY	★
GASTROINTESTINAL	NR	STROKE	★
GENERAL SURGERY	NR	VASCULAR	NR
MATERNITY CARE	NR	WOMEN'S HEALTH	NR

HEALTHGRADES AWARDS

Wedowee Hospital

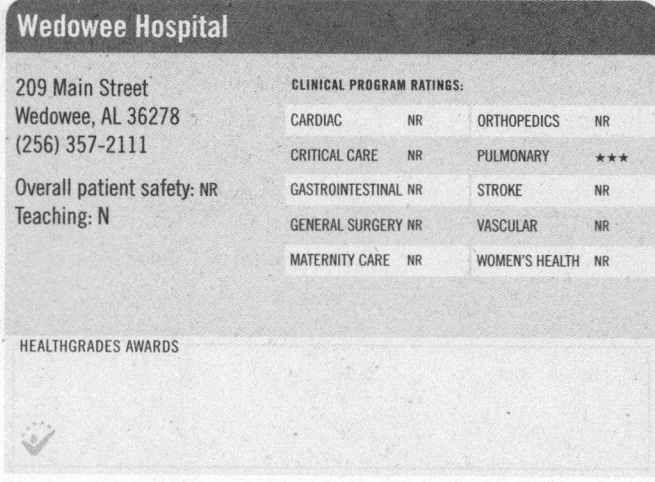

209 Main Street
Wedowee, AL 36278
(256) 357-2111

Overall patient safety: NR
Teaching: N

CLINICAL PROGRAM RATINGS:

CARDIAC	NR	ORTHOPEDICS	NR
CRITICAL CARE	NR	PULMONARY	★★★
GASTROINTESTINAL	NR	STROKE	NR
GENERAL SURGERY	NR	VASCULAR	NR
MATERNITY CARE	NR	WOMEN'S HEALTH	NR

HEALTHGRADES AWARDS

Vaughan Regional Medical Center--Parkway Campus

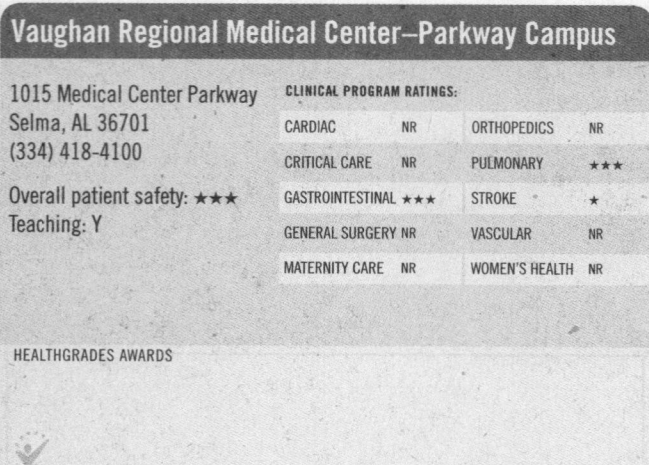

1015 Medical Center Parkway
Selma, AL 36701
(334) 418-4100

Overall patient safety: ★★★
Teaching: Y

CLINICAL PROGRAM RATINGS:

CARDIAC	NR	ORTHOPEDICS	NR
CRITICAL CARE	NR	PULMONARY	★★★
GASTROINTESTINAL	★★★	STROKE	★
GENERAL SURGERY	NR	VASCULAR	NR
MATERNITY CARE	NR	WOMEN'S HEALTH	NR

HEALTHGRADES AWARDS

Wiregrass Medical Center

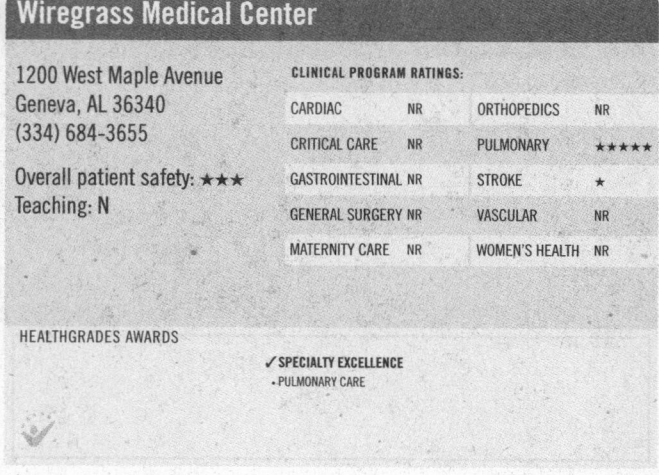

1200 West Maple Avenue
Geneva, AL 36340
(334) 684-3655

Overall patient safety: ★★★
Teaching: N

CLINICAL PROGRAM RATINGS:

CARDIAC	NR	ORTHOPEDICS	NR
CRITICAL CARE	NR	PULMONARY	★★★★★
GASTROINTESTINAL	NR	STROKE	★
GENERAL SURGERY	NR	VASCULAR	NR
MATERNITY CARE	NR	WOMEN'S HEALTH	NR

HEALTHGRADES AWARDS

✓ SPECIALTY EXCELLENCE
- PULMONARY CARE

KEY: ★★★★★ BEST ★★★ AS EXPECTED ★ POOR NR NOT RATED BY HEALTHGRADES For full definitions of ratings and awards, see Appendix.

Woodland Medical Center

1910 Cherokee Avenue
Southwest
Cullman, AL 35055
(256) 739-3500

Overall patient safety: ★★★
Teaching: N

CLINICAL PROGRAM RATINGS:

CARDIAC	NR	ORTHOPEDICS	NR
CRITICAL CARE	NR	PULMONARY	★
GASTROINTESTINAL	★★★	STROKE	★★★
GENERAL SURGERY	NR	VASCULAR	NR
MATERNITY CARE	NR	WOMEN'S HEALTH	NR

HEALTHGRADES AWARDS

ALASKA HOSPITALS: RATINGS BY CLINICAL SPECIALTY

Alaska Native Medical Center

4315 Tudor Centre Drive
Anchorage, AK 99508
(907) 563-2662

Overall patient safety: ★
Teaching: N

CLINICAL PROGRAM RATINGS:

CARDIAC	NR	ORTHOPEDICS	NR
CRITICAL CARE	NR	PULMONARY	★★★
GASTROINTESTINAL	NR	STROKE	★★★
GENERAL SURGERY	NR	VASCULAR	NR
MATERNITY CARE	NR	WOMEN'S HEALTH	NR

HEALTHGRADES AWARDS

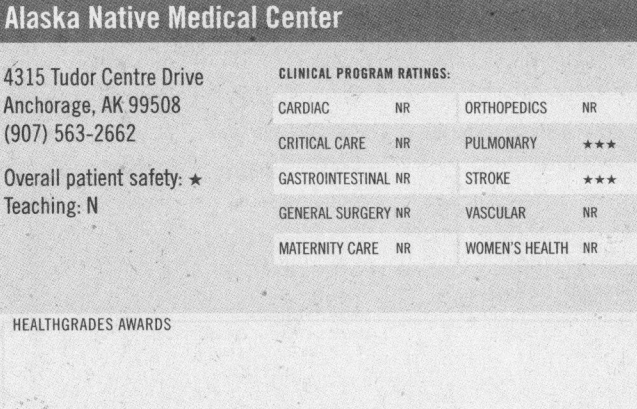

Bartlett Regional Hospital

3260 Hospital Drive
Juneau, AK 99801
(907) 796-8900

Overall patient safety: ★
Teaching: N

CLINICAL PROGRAM RATINGS:

CARDIAC	NR	ORTHOPEDICS	NR
CRITICAL CARE	NR	PULMONARY	★★★
GASTROINTESTINAL	NR	STROKE	★★★
GENERAL SURGERY	NR	VASCULAR	NR
MATERNITY CARE	NR	WOMEN'S HEALTH	NR

HEALTHGRADES AWARDS

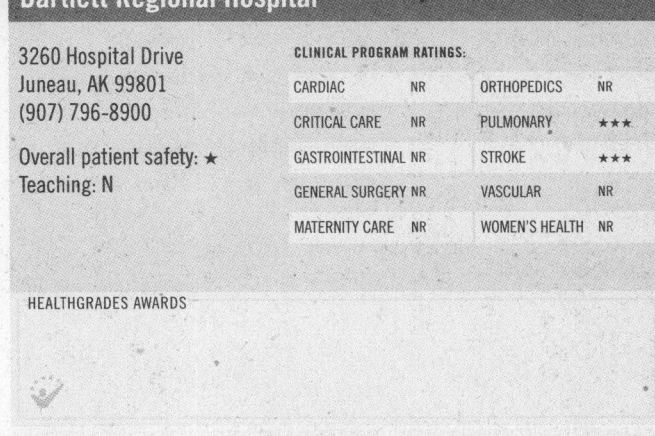

Alaska Regional Hospital

2801 Debarr Road
Anchorage, AK 99508
(907) 276-1131

Overall patient safety: ★★★
Teaching: N

CLINICAL PROGRAM RATINGS:

CARDIAC	★★★	ORTHOPEDICS	★★★
CRITICAL CARE	NR	PULMONARY	★★★
GASTROINTESTINAL	NR	STROKE	★★★
GENERAL SURGERY	NR	VASCULAR	NR
MATERNITY CARE	NR	WOMEN'S HEALTH	NR

HEALTHGRADES AWARDS

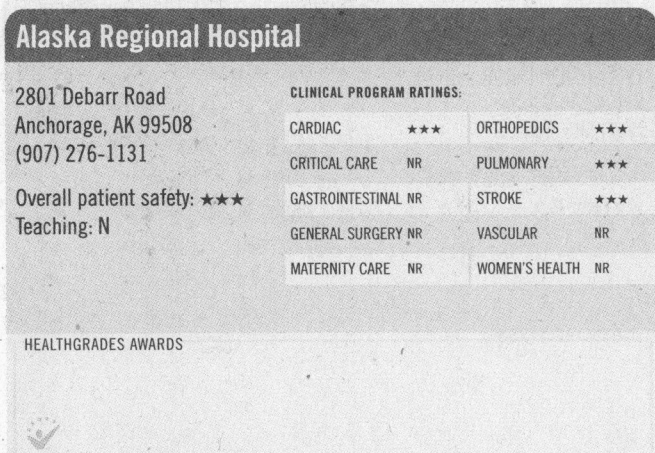

Central Peninsula General Hospital

250 Hospital Place
Soldotna, AK 99669
(907) 714-4721

Overall patient safety: ★★★
Teaching: N

CLINICAL PROGRAM RATINGS:

CARDIAC	NR	ORTHOPEDICS	NR
CRITICAL CARE	NR	PULMONARY	★★★
GASTROINTESTINAL	NR	STROKE	★★★
GENERAL SURGERY	NR	VASCULAR	NR
MATERNITY CARE	NR	WOMEN'S HEALTH	NR

HEALTHGRADES AWARDS

Fairbanks Memorial Hospital

1650 Cowles Street
Fairbanks, AK 99701
(907) 452-8181

Overall patient safety: ★
Teaching: N

CLINICAL PROGRAM RATINGS:

CARDIAC	NR	ORTHOPEDICS	NR
CRITICAL CARE	NR	PULMONARY	★★★
GASTROINTESTINAL	NR	STROKE	★★★
GENERAL SURGERY	NR	VASCULAR	NR
MATERNITY CARE	NR	WOMEN'S HEALTH	NR

HEALTHGRADES AWARDS

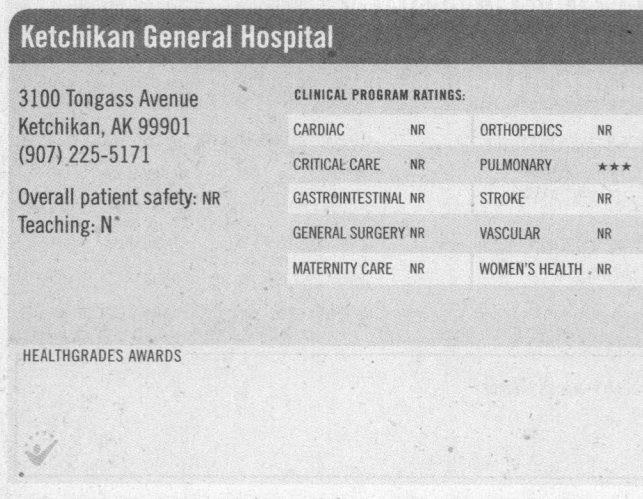

Mt. Edgecumbe Hospital

222 Tongass Drive
Sitka, AK 99835
(907) 966-2411

Overall patient safety: ★★★
Teaching: N

CLINICAL PROGRAM RATINGS:

CARDIAC	NR	ORTHOPEDICS	NR
CRITICAL CARE	NR	PULMONARY	★★★
GASTROINTESTINAL	NR	STROKE	NR
GENERAL SURGERY	NR	VASCULAR	NR
MATERNITY CARE	NR	WOMEN'S HEALTH	NR

HEALTHGRADES AWARDS

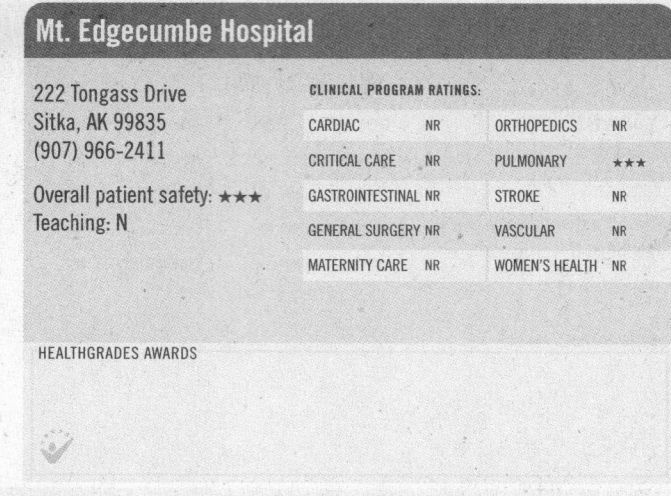

Ketchikan General Hospital

3100 Tongass Avenue
Ketchikan, AK 99901
(907) 225-5171

Overall patient safety: NR
Teaching: N

CLINICAL PROGRAM RATINGS:

CARDIAC	NR	ORTHOPEDICS	NR
CRITICAL CARE	NR	PULMONARY	★★★
GASTROINTESTINAL	NR	STROKE	NR
GENERAL SURGERY	NR	VASCULAR	NR
MATERNITY CARE	NR	WOMEN'S HEALTH	NR

HEALTHGRADES AWARDS

Providence Alaska Medical Center

3200 Providence Drive
Anchorage, AK 99508
(907) 562-2211

Overall patient safety: ★★★
Teaching: Y

CLINICAL PROGRAM RATINGS:

CARDIAC	★★★	ORTHOPEDICS	★★★
CRITICAL CARE	NR	PULMONARY	★★★★★
GASTROINTESTINAL	★★★	STROKE	★★★
GENERAL SURGERY	NR	VASCULAR	NR
MATERNITY CARE	NR	WOMEN'S HEALTH	NR

HEALTHGRADES AWARDS

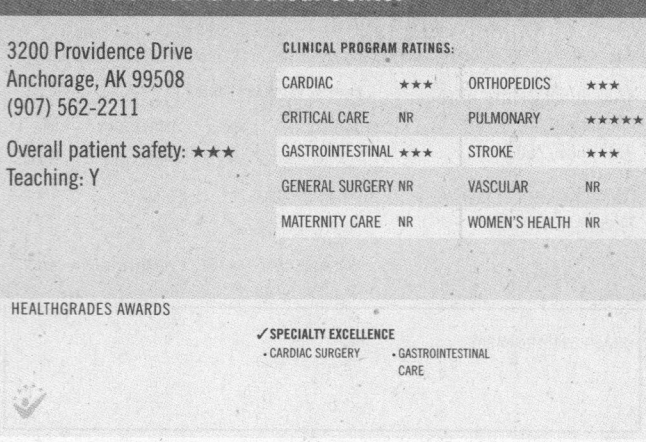

✓ SPECIALTY EXCELLENCE
- CARDIAC SURGERY
- GASTROINTESTINAL CARE

Mat-Su Regional Medical Center

515 East Dahlia
Palmer, AK 99645
(907) 746-8600

Overall patient safety: ★★★
Teaching: N

CLINICAL PROGRAM RATINGS:

CARDIAC	NR	ORTHOPEDICS	NR
CRITICAL CARE	NR	PULMONARY	★★★
GASTROINTESTINAL	NR	STROKE	★★★
GENERAL SURGERY	NR	VASCULAR	NR
MATERNITY CARE	NR	WOMEN'S HEALTH	NR

HEALTHGRADES AWARDS

Yukon Kuskokwim Delta Regional Hospital

700 Eddie Hoffman Highway
Bethel, AK 99559
(907) 543-6300

Overall patient safety: NR
Teaching: N

CLINICAL PROGRAM RATINGS:

CARDIAC	NR	ORTHOPEDICS	NR
CRITICAL CARE	NR	PULMONARY	★★★
GASTROINTESTINAL	NR	STROKE	NR
GENERAL SURGERY	NR	VASCULAR	NR
MATERNITY CARE	NR	WOMEN'S HEALTH	NR

HEALTHGRADES AWARDS

KEY: ★★★★★ BEST ★★★ AS EXPECTED ★ POOR NR NOT RATED BY HEALTHGRADES For full definitions of ratings and awards, see Appendix.

Arizona Heart Hospital

1930 East Thomas Road
Phoenix, AZ 85016
(602) 532-1000

Overall patient safety: ★★★★
Teaching: N

CLINICAL PROGRAM RATINGS:

CARDIAC	★★★	ORTHOPEDICS	NR
CRITICAL CARE	NR	PULMONARY	★★★
GASTROINTESTINAL	NR	STROKE	NR
GENERAL SURGERY	NR	VASCULAR	★★★
MATERNITY CARE	NR	WOMEN'S HEALTH	NR

HEALTHGRADES AWARDS

Banner Baywood Medical Center

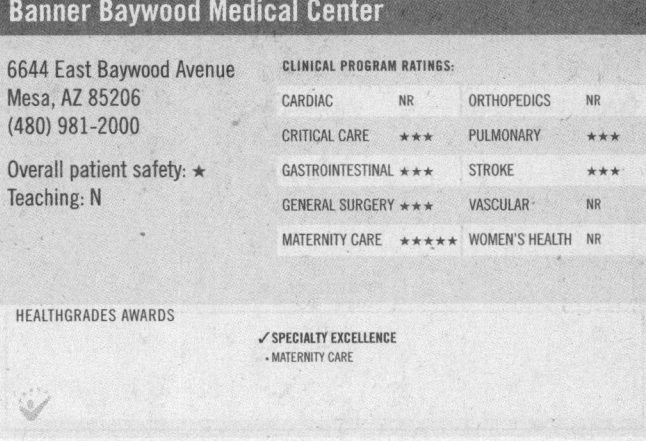

6644 East Baywood Avenue
Mesa, AZ 85206
(480) 981-2000

Overall patient safety: ★
Teaching: N

CLINICAL PROGRAM RATINGS:

CARDIAC	NR	ORTHOPEDICS	NR
CRITICAL CARE	★★★	PULMONARY	★★★
GASTROINTESTINAL	★★★	STROKE	★★★
GENERAL SURGERY	★★★	VASCULAR	NR
MATERNITY CARE	★★★★★	WOMEN'S HEALTH	NR

HEALTHGRADES AWARDS

✓ SPECIALTY EXCELLENCE
• MATERNITY CARE

Arrowhead Hospital

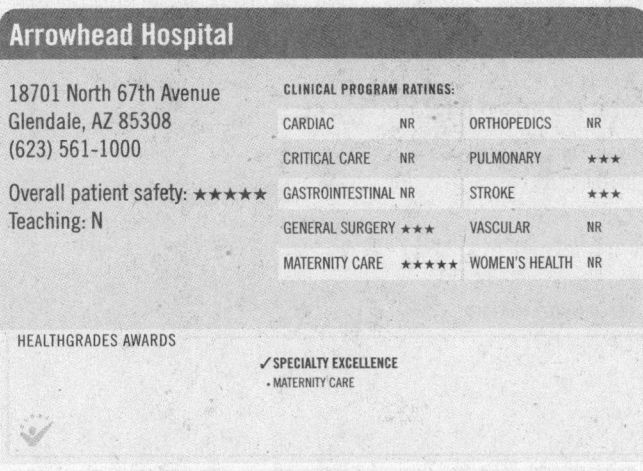

18701 North 67th Avenue
Glendale, AZ 85308
(623) 561-1000

Overall patient safety: ★★★★★
Teaching: N

CLINICAL PROGRAM RATINGS:

CARDIAC	NR	ORTHOPEDICS	NR
CRITICAL CARE	NR	PULMONARY	★★★
GASTROINTESTINAL	NR	STROKE	★★★
GENERAL SURGERY	★★★	VASCULAR	NR
MATERNITY CARE	★★★★★	WOMEN'S HEALTH	NR

HEALTHGRADES AWARDS

✓ SPECIALTY EXCELLENCE
• MATERNITY CARE

Banner Desert Medical Center

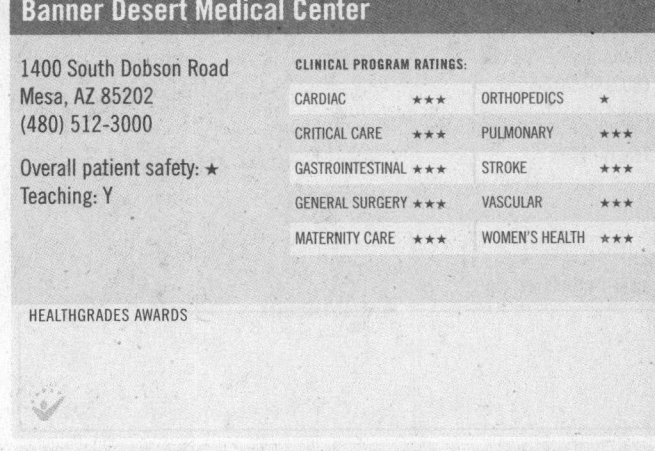

1400 South Dobson Road
Mesa, AZ 85202
(480) 512-3000

Overall patient safety: ★
Teaching: Y

CLINICAL PROGRAM RATINGS:

CARDIAC	★★★	ORTHOPEDICS	★
CRITICAL CARE	★★★	PULMONARY	★★★
GASTROINTESTINAL	★★★	STROKE	★★★
GENERAL SURGERY	★★★	VASCULAR	★★★
MATERNITY CARE	★★★	WOMEN'S HEALTH	★★★

HEALTHGRADES AWARDS

Banner Baywood Heart Hospital

6750 East Baywood Avenue
Mesa, AZ 85206
(480) 854-5050

Overall patient safety: ★★★★★
Teaching: N

CLINICAL PROGRAM RATINGS:

CARDIAC	★★★	ORTHOPEDICS	NR
CRITICAL CARE	NR	PULMONARY	★★★★★
GASTROINTESTINAL	NR	STROKE	★★★
GENERAL SURGERY	NR	VASCULAR	★★★
MATERNITY CARE	NR	WOMEN'S HEALTH	NR

HEALTHGRADES AWARDS

✓ SPECIALTY EXCELLENCE
• PULMONARY CARE

Banner Estrella Medical Center

9201 West Thomas Road
Phoenix, AZ 85037
(623) 327-5003

Overall patient safety: ★★★
Teaching: N

CLINICAL PROGRAM RATINGS:

CARDIAC	NR	ORTHOPEDICS	NR
CRITICAL CARE	NR	PULMONARY	★★★
GASTROINTESTINAL	NR	STROKE	NR
GENERAL SURGERY	NR	VASCULAR	NR
MATERNITY CARE	★★★	WOMEN'S HEALTH	NR

HEALTHGRADES AWARDS

Banner Good Samaritan Medical Center

1111 East McDowell Road
Phoenix, AZ 85006
(602) 239-2000

Overall patient safety: ★★★
Teaching: Y

CLINICAL PROGRAM RATINGS:

CARDIAC	★★★	ORTHOPEDICS	★
CRITICAL CARE	★★★	PULMONARY	★★★
GASTROINTESTINAL	★★★	STROKE	★★★★★
GENERAL SURGERY	★★★	VASCULAR	★★★
MATERNITY CARE	★★★	WOMEN'S HEALTH	★★★

HEALTHGRADES AWARDS

✓ SPECIALTY EXCELLENCE
· BARIATRIC SURGERY   · STROKE CARE

Carondelet St. Joseph's Hospital and Health Center

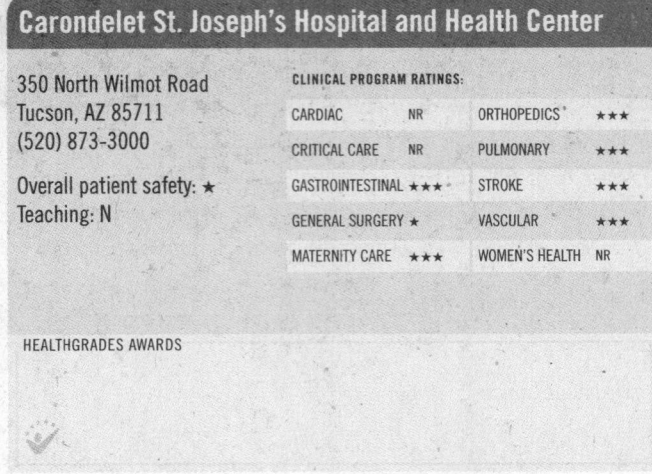

350 North Wilmot Road
Tucson, AZ 85711
(520) 873-3000

Overall patient safety: ★
Teaching: N

CLINICAL PROGRAM RATINGS:

CARDIAC	NR	ORTHOPEDICS	★★★
CRITICAL CARE	NR	PULMONARY	★★★
GASTROINTESTINAL	★★★	STROKE	★★★
GENERAL SURGERY	★	VASCULAR	★★★
MATERNITY CARE	★★★	WOMEN'S HEALTH	NR

HEALTHGRADES AWARDS

Banner Thunderbird Medical Center

5555 West Thunderbird Road
Glendale, AZ 85306
(602) 865-5555

Overall patient safety: ★★★
Teaching: Y

CLINICAL PROGRAM RATINGS:

CARDIAC	★★★	ORTHOPEDICS	★★★
CRITICAL CARE	★★★	PULMONARY	★★★
GASTROINTESTINAL	★★★	STROKE	★★★
GENERAL SURGERY	★★★	VASCULAR	★★★
MATERNITY CARE	★★★	WOMEN'S HEALTH	★★★

HEALTHGRADES AWARDS

✓ SPECIALTY EXCELLENCE
· CARDIAC CARE

Carondelet St. Mary's Hospital and Health Center

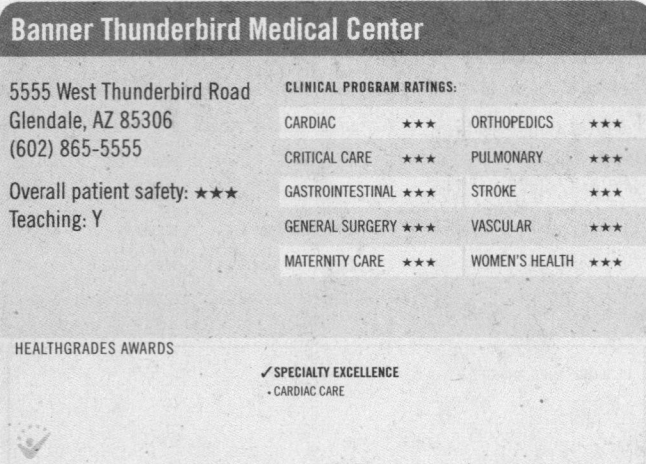

1601 West St. Mary's Road
Tucson, AZ 85745
(520) 872-3000

Overall patient safety: ★★★
Teaching: N

CLINICAL PROGRAM RATINGS:

CARDIAC	NR	ORTHOPEDICS	NR
CRITICAL CARE	NR	PULMONARY	★★★
GASTROINTESTINAL	★★★	STROKE	★★★★★
GENERAL SURGERY	★★★	VASCULAR	NR
MATERNITY CARE	NR	WOMEN'S HEALTH	NR

HEALTHGRADES AWARDS

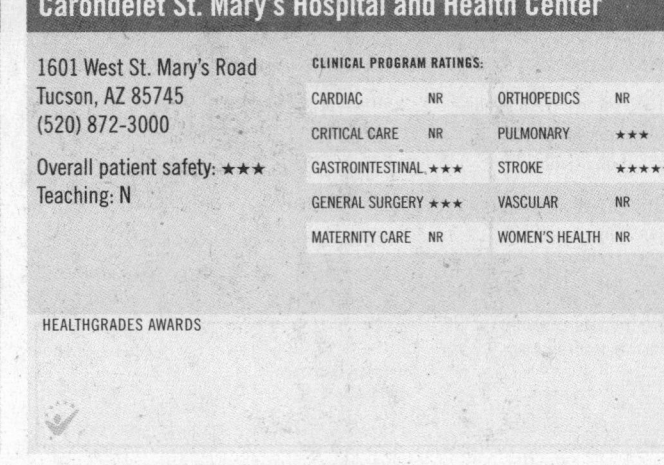

Carondelet Holy Cross Hospital

1171 West Target Range Road
Nogales, AZ 85621
(520) 285-3000

Overall patient safety: ★★★
Teaching: N

CLINICAL PROGRAM RATINGS:

CARDIAC	NR	ORTHOPEDICS	NR
CRITICAL CARE	NR	PULMONARY	★
GASTROINTESTINAL	NR	STROKE	NR
GENERAL SURGERY	NR	VASCULAR	NR
MATERNITY CARE	★★★★★	WOMEN'S HEALTH	NR

HEALTHGRADES AWARDS

✓ SPECIALTY EXCELLENCE
· MATERNITY CARE

Casa Grande Regional Medical Center

1800 East Florence Boulevard
Casa Grande, AZ 85222
(520) 381-6300

Overall patient safety: ★
Teaching: N

CLINICAL PROGRAM RATINGS:

CARDIAC	NR	ORTHOPEDICS	NR
CRITICAL CARE	NR	PULMONARY	★★★
GASTROINTESTINAL	★★★	STROKE	★★★
GENERAL SURGERY	★★★	VASCULAR	NR
MATERNITY CARE	★★★	WOMEN'S HEALTH	NR

HEALTHGRADES AWARDS

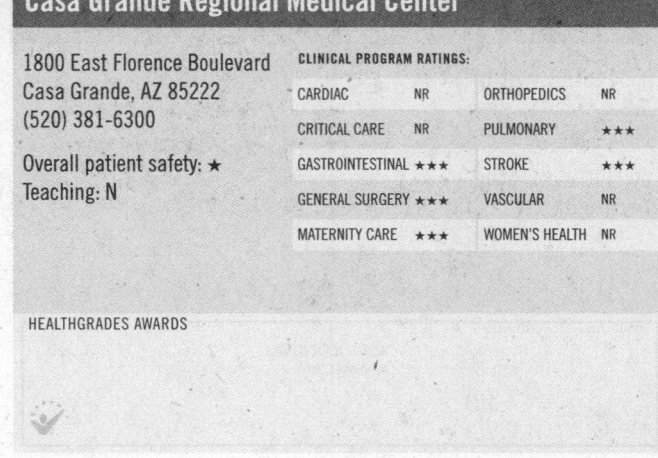

KEY: ★★★★★ BEST   ★★★ AS EXPECTED   ★ POOR   NR NOT RATED BY HEALTHGRADES   For full definitions of ratings and awards, see Appendix.

Chandler Regional Hospital

475 South Dobson Road
Chandler, AZ 85224
(480) 963-4561

Overall patient safety: ★★★
Teaching: N

CLINICAL PROGRAM RATINGS:

CARDIAC	★★★	ORTHOPEDICS	NR
CRITICAL CARE	★★★	PULMONARY	★★★
GASTROINTESTINAL	★★★	STROKE	★★★
GENERAL SURGERY	★	VASCULAR	NR
MATERNITY CARE	★★★	WOMEN'S HEALTH	★★★

HEALTHGRADES AWARDS

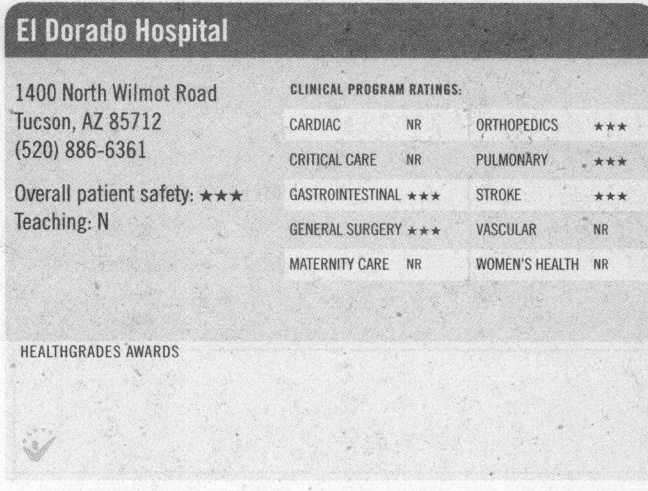

El Dorado Hospital

1400 North Wilmot Road
Tucson, AZ 85712
(520) 886-6361

Overall patient safety: ★★★
Teaching: N

CLINICAL PROGRAM RATINGS:

CARDIAC	NR	ORTHOPEDICS	★★★
CRITICAL CARE	NR	PULMONARY	★★★
GASTROINTESTINAL	★★★	STROKE	★★★
GENERAL SURGERY	★★★	VASCULAR	NR
MATERNITY CARE	NR	WOMEN'S HEALTH	NR

HEALTHGRADES AWARDS

Cobre Valley Community Hospital

5880 South Hospital Drive
Globe, AZ 85501
(928) 425-3261

Overall patient safety: ★
Teaching: N

CLINICAL PROGRAM RATINGS:

CARDIAC	NR	ORTHOPEDICS	NR
CRITICAL CARE	NR	PULMONARY	★
GASTROINTESTINAL	NR	STROKE	★
GENERAL SURGERY	NR	VASCULAR	NR
MATERNITY CARE	★★★	WOMEN'S HEALTH	NR

HEALTHGRADES AWARDS

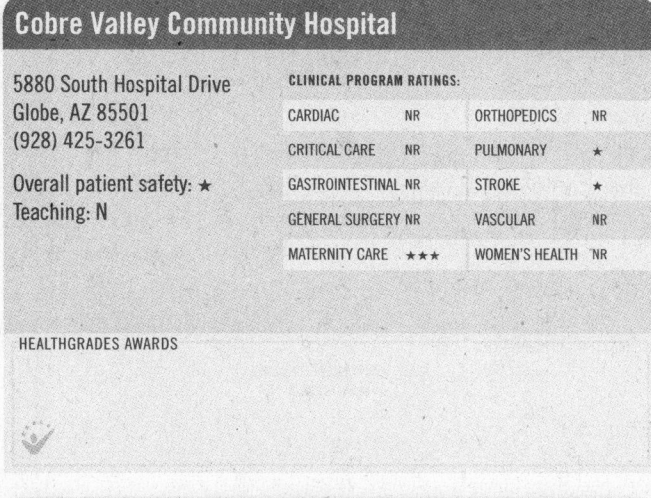

Flagstaff Medical Center

1200 North Beaver Street
Flagstaff, AZ 86001
(928) 779-3366

Overall patient safety: ★★★
Teaching: N

CLINICAL PROGRAM RATINGS:

CARDIAC	★★★	ORTHOPEDICS	★★★
CRITICAL CARE	NR	PULMONARY	★★★
GASTROINTESTINAL	★★★	STROKE	★★★★★
GENERAL SURGERY	★★★	VASCULAR	NR
MATERNITY CARE	★★★	WOMEN'S HEALTH	NR

HEALTHGRADES AWARDS

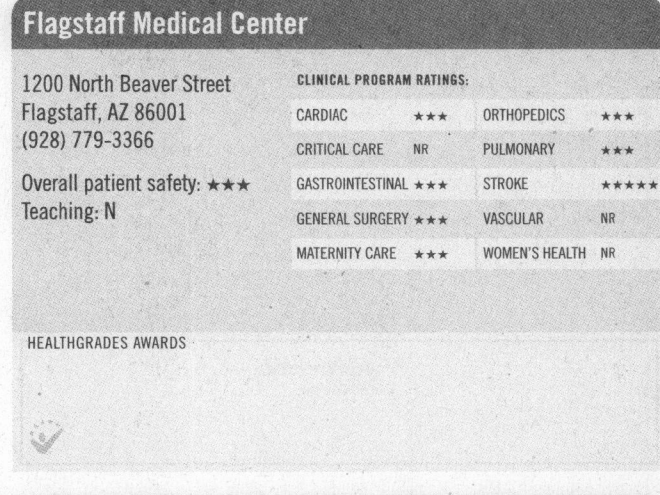

Del E. Webb Memorial Hospital

14502 West Meeker Boulevard
Sun City West, AZ 85375
(623) 214-4000

Overall patient safety: ★
Teaching: Y

CLINICAL PROGRAM RATINGS:

CARDIAC	NR	ORTHOPEDICS	NR
CRITICAL CARE	NR	PULMONARY	★★★★★
GASTROINTESTINAL	★★★	STROKE	★★★★★
GENERAL SURGERY	★★★	VASCULAR	NR
MATERNITY CARE	★★★	WOMEN'S HEALTH	NR

HEALTHGRADES AWARDS

✓DISTINGUISHED   ✓SPECIALTY EXCELLENCE
 HOSPITAL   · PULMONARY CARE   · STROKE CARE
· CLINICAL EXCELLENCE

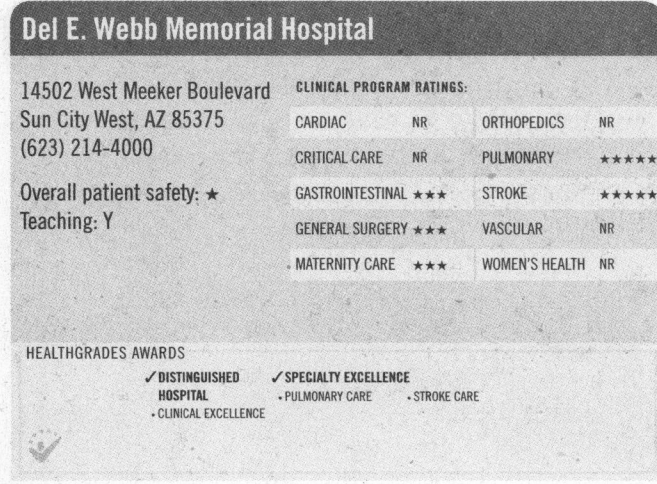

Fort Defiance Indian Hospital

Corner of Route 7 and Route 12
Fort Defiance, AZ 86504
(928) 729-5741

Overall patient safety: ★★★
Teaching: N

CLINICAL PROGRAM RATINGS:

CARDIAC	NR	ORTHOPEDICS	NR
CRITICAL CARE	NR	PULMONARY	NR
GASTROINTESTINAL	NR	STROKE	NR
GENERAL SURGERY	NR	VASCULAR	NR
MATERNITY CARE	NR	WOMEN'S HEALTH	NR

HEALTHGRADES AWARDS

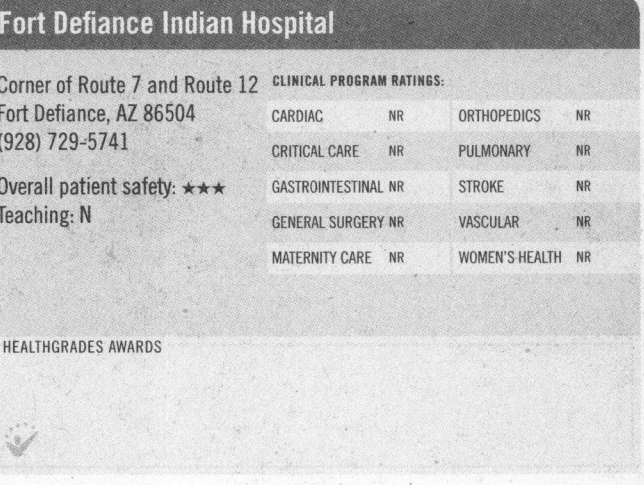

ARIZONA HOSPITALS: RATINGS BY CLINICAL SPECIALTY

Havasu Regional Medical Center

101 Civic Center Lane
Lake Havasu City, AZ 86403
(928) 855-8185

Overall patient safety: ★★★
Teaching: N

CLINICAL PROGRAM RATINGS:

CARDIAC	NR	ORTHOPEDICS	★★★
CRITICAL CARE	NR	PULMONARY	★
GASTROINTESTINAL	★★★	STROKE	★★★
GENERAL SURGERY	★★★	VASCULAR	NR
MATERNITY CARE	★★★	WOMEN'S HEALTH	NR

HEALTHGRADES AWARDS

Kingman Regional Medical Center

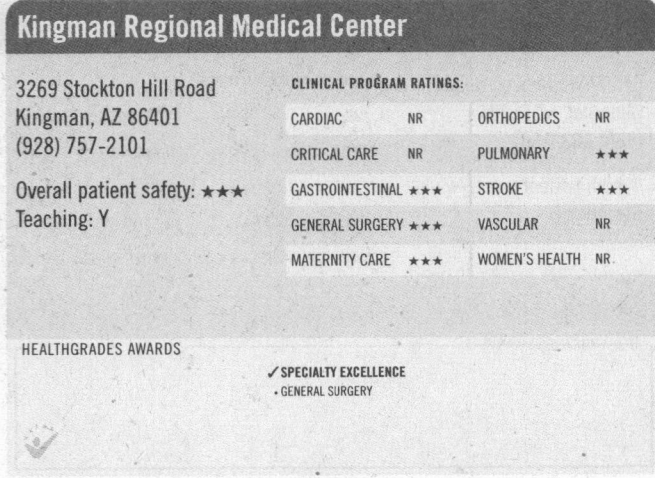

3269 Stockton Hill Road
Kingman, AZ 86401
(928) 757-2101

Overall patient safety: ★★★
Teaching: Y

CLINICAL PROGRAM RATINGS:

CARDIAC	NR	ORTHOPEDICS	NR
CRITICAL CARE	NR	PULMONARY	★★★
GASTROINTESTINAL	★★★	STROKE	★★★
GENERAL SURGERY	★★★	VASCULAR	NR
MATERNITY CARE	★★★	WOMEN'S HEALTH	NR

HEALTHGRADES AWARDS

✓ SPECIALTY EXCELLENCE
• GENERAL SURGERY

John C. Lincoln Deer Valley Hospital

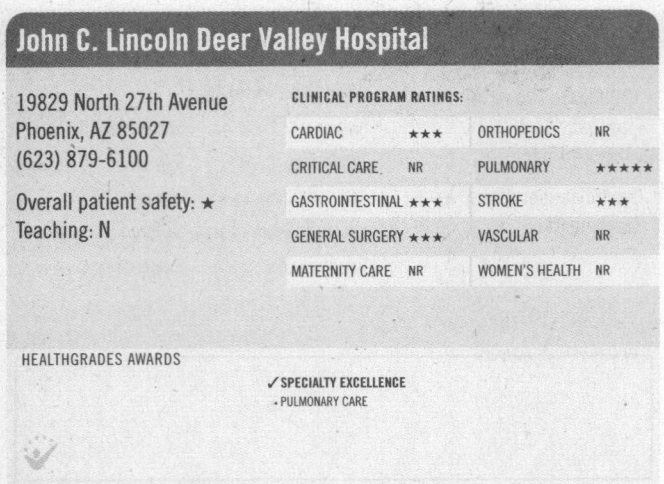

19829 North 27th Avenue
Phoenix, AZ 85027
(623) 879-6100

Overall patient safety: ★
Teaching: N

CLINICAL PROGRAM RATINGS:

CARDIAC	★★★	ORTHOPEDICS	NR
CRITICAL CARE	NR	PULMONARY	★★★★★
GASTROINTESTINAL	★★★	STROKE	★★★
GENERAL SURGERY	★★★	VASCULAR	NR
MATERNITY CARE	NR	WOMEN'S HEALTH	NR

HEALTHGRADES AWARDS

✓ SPECIALTY EXCELLENCE
• PULMONARY CARE

La Paz Regional Hospital

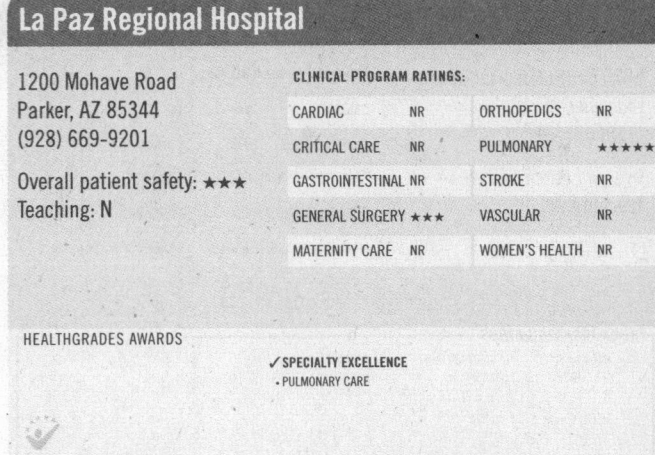

1200 Mohave Road
Parker, AZ 85344
(928) 669-9201

Overall patient safety: ★★★
Teaching: N

CLINICAL PROGRAM RATINGS:

CARDIAC	NR	ORTHOPEDICS	NR
CRITICAL CARE	NR	PULMONARY	★★★★★
GASTROINTESTINAL	NR	STROKE	NR
GENERAL SURGERY	★★★	VASCULAR	NR
MATERNITY CARE	NR	WOMEN'S HEALTH	NR

HEALTHGRADES AWARDS

✓ SPECIALTY EXCELLENCE
• PULMONARY CARE

John C. Lincoln North Mountain Hospital

250 East Dunlap Avenue
Phoenix, AZ 85020
(602) 943-2381

Overall patient safety: ★★★
Teaching: Y

CLINICAL PROGRAM RATINGS:

CARDIAC	★★★	ORTHOPEDICS	★★★
CRITICAL CARE	NR	PULMONARY	★★★
GASTROINTESTINAL	★★★	STROKE	★★★
GENERAL SURGERY	★★★	VASCULAR	NR
MATERNITY CARE	★★★★★	WOMEN'S HEALTH	★★★

HEALTHGRADES AWARDS

Maricopa Medical Center

2601 East Roosevelt Street
Phoenix, AZ 85008
(602) 344-5011

Overall patient safety: ★★★
Teaching: Y

CLINICAL PROGRAM RATINGS:

CARDIAC	NR	ORTHOPEDICS	NR
CRITICAL CARE	NR	PULMONARY	★★★
GASTROINTESTINAL	NR	STROKE	★★★
GENERAL SURGERY	NR	VASCULAR	NR
MATERNITY CARE	★	WOMEN'S HEALTH	NR

HEALTHGRADES AWARDS

KEY: ★★★★★ BEST ★★★ AS EXPECTED ★ POOR NR NOT RATED BY HEALTHGRADES For full definitions of ratings and awards, see Appendix.

Maryvale Hospital

5102 West Campbell Avenue
Phoenix, AZ 85031
(623) 848-5000

Overall patient safety: ★
Teaching: N

CLINICAL PROGRAM RATINGS:

CARDIAC	NR	ORTHOPEDICS	NR
CRITICAL CARE	NR	PULMONARY	★★★
GASTROINTESTINAL	NR	STROKE	★★★
GENERAL SURGERY	NR	VASCULAR	NR
MATERNITY CARE	★★★	WOMEN'S HEALTH	NR

HEALTHGRADES AWARDS

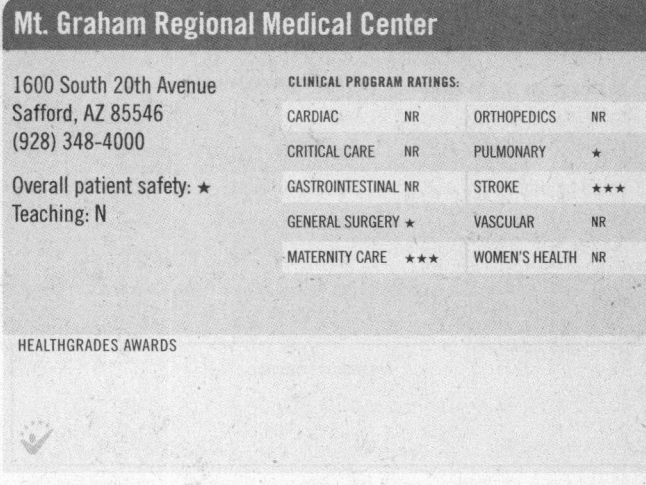

Mt. Graham Regional Medical Center

1600 South 20th Avenue
Safford, AZ 85546
(928) 348-4000

Overall patient safety: ★
Teaching: N

CLINICAL PROGRAM RATINGS:

CARDIAC	NR	ORTHOPEDICS	NR
CRITICAL CARE	NR	PULMONARY	★
GASTROINTESTINAL	NR	STROKE	★★★
GENERAL SURGERY	★	VASCULAR	NR
MATERNITY CARE	★★★	WOMEN'S HEALTH	NR

HEALTHGRADES AWARDS

Mayo Clinic Hospital

5777 East Mayo Boulevard
Phoenix, AZ 85054
(480) 515-6296

Overall patient safety: ★★★★★
Teaching: Y

CLINICAL PROGRAM RATINGS:

CARDIAC	★★★★★	ORTHOPEDICS	★★★
CRITICAL CARE	NR	PULMONARY	★★★★★
GASTROINTESTINAL	★★★	STROKE	★★★
GENERAL SURGERY	★★★	VASCULAR	★★★
MATERNITY CARE	NR	WOMEN'S HEALTH	NR

HEALTHGRADES AWARDS

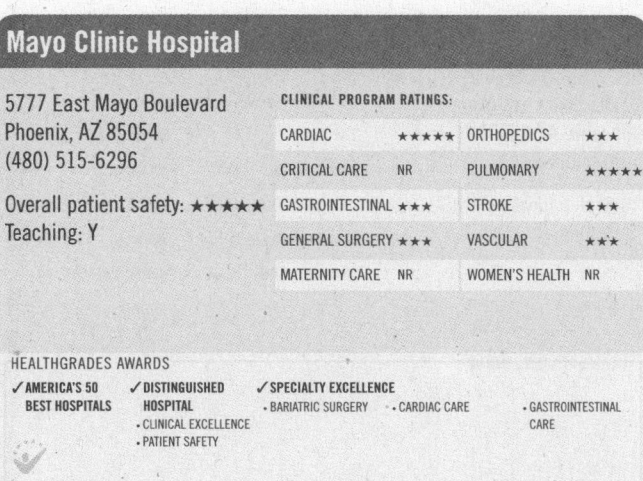

✓ AMERICA'S 50 BEST HOSPITALS
✓ DISTINGUISHED HOSPITAL
- CLINICAL EXCELLENCE
- PATIENT SAFETY
✓ SPECIALTY EXCELLENCE
- BARIATRIC SURGERY
- CARDIAC CARE
- GASTROINTESTINAL CARE

Navapache Regional Medical Center

2200 Show Low Lake Road
Show Low, AZ 85901
(928) 537-4375

Overall patient safety: ★★★
Teaching: N

CLINICAL PROGRAM RATINGS:

CARDIAC	NR	ORTHOPEDICS	NR
CRITICAL CARE	NR	PULMONARY	★★★
GASTROINTESTINAL	NR	STROKE	★★★
GENERAL SURGERY	★★★	VASCULAR	NR
MATERNITY CARE	★★★	WOMEN'S HEALTH	NR

HEALTHGRADES AWARDS

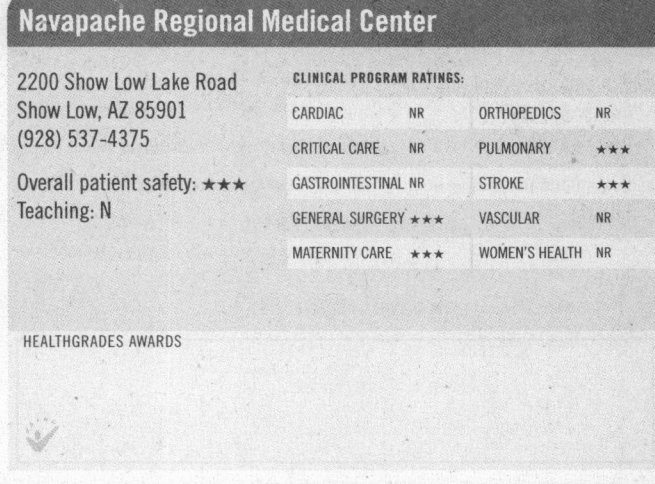

Mesa General Hospital

515 North Mesa Drive
Mesa, AZ 85201
(480) 969-9111

Overall patient safety: ★★★
Teaching: Y

CLINICAL PROGRAM RATINGS:

CARDIAC	★★★	ORTHOPEDICS	NR
CRITICAL CARE	NR	PULMONARY	★★★
GASTROINTESTINAL	NR	STROKE	★★★
GENERAL SURGERY	NR	VASCULAR	★★★
MATERNITY CARE	★★★	WOMEN'S HEALTH	★★★

HEALTHGRADES AWARDS

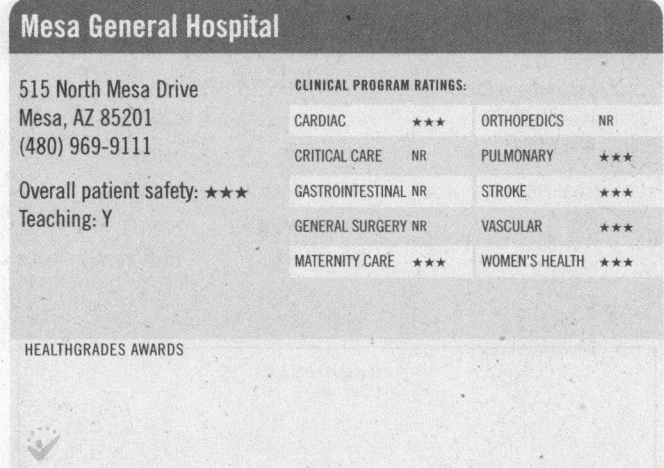

Northwest Medical Center

6200 North La Cholla
Boulevard
Tucson, AZ 85741
(520) 742-9000

Overall patient safety: ★★★
Teaching: N

CLINICAL PROGRAM RATINGS:

CARDIAC	★★★	ORTHOPEDICS	★★★
CRITICAL CARE	★★★	PULMONARY	★★★
GASTROINTESTINAL	★★★	STROKE	★★★
GENERAL SURGERY	★★★	VASCULAR	NR
MATERNITY CARE	★★★	WOMEN'S HEALTH	★★★★★

HEALTHGRADES AWARDS

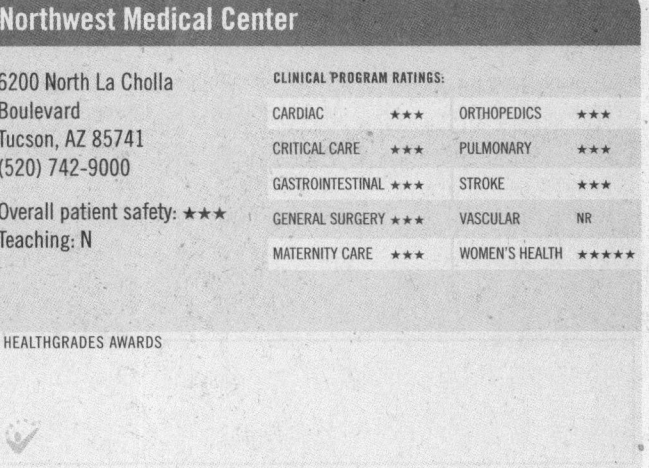

Northwest Medical Center—Oro Valley

1551 East Tangerine Road
Oro Valley, AZ 85755
5209013500

Overall patient safety: ★★★
Teaching: N

CLINICAL PROGRAM RATINGS:

CARDIAC	NR	ORTHOPEDICS	NR
CRITICAL CARE	NR	PULMONARY	★★★
GASTROINTESTINAL	NR	STROKE	★★★★★
GENERAL SURGERY	★★★	VASCULAR	NR
MATERNITY CARE	NR	WOMEN'S HEALTH	NR

HEALTHGRADES AWARDS

✓ SPECIALTY EXCELLENCE
· STROKE CARE

Phoenix Baptist Hospital

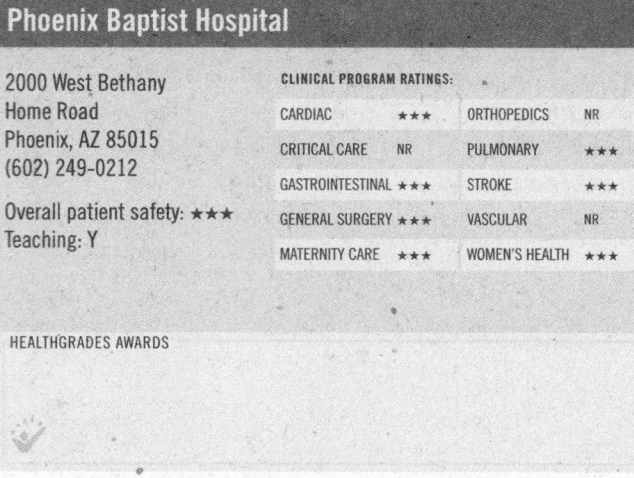

2000 West Bethany
Home Road
Phoenix, AZ 85015
(602) 249-0212

Overall patient safety: ★★★
Teaching: Y

CLINICAL PROGRAM RATINGS:

CARDIAC	★★★	ORTHOPEDICS	NR
CRITICAL CARE	NR	PULMONARY	★★★
GASTROINTESTINAL	★★★	STROKE	★★★
GENERAL SURGERY	★★★	VASCULAR	NR
MATERNITY CARE	★★★	WOMEN'S HEALTH	★★★

HEALTHGRADES AWARDS

Paradise Valley Hospital

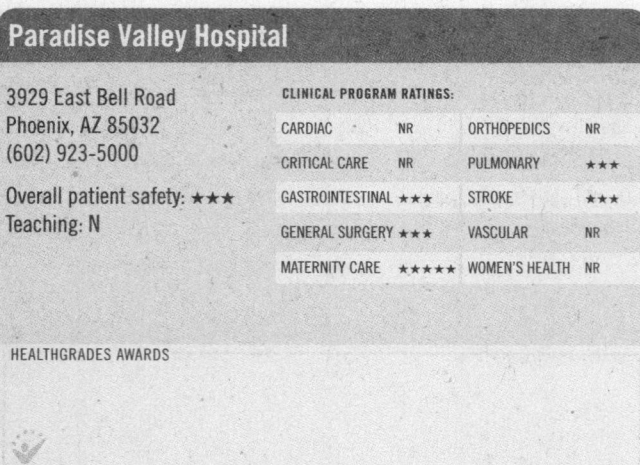

3929 East Bell Road
Phoenix, AZ 85032
(602) 923-5000

Overall patient safety: ★★★
Teaching: N

CLINICAL PROGRAM RATINGS:

CARDIAC	NR	ORTHOPEDICS	NR
CRITICAL CARE	NR	PULMONARY	★★★
GASTROINTESTINAL	★★★	STROKE	★★★
GENERAL SURGERY	★★★	VASCULAR	NR
MATERNITY CARE	★★★★★	WOMEN'S HEALTH	NR

HEALTHGRADES AWARDS

Phoenix Memorial Hospital

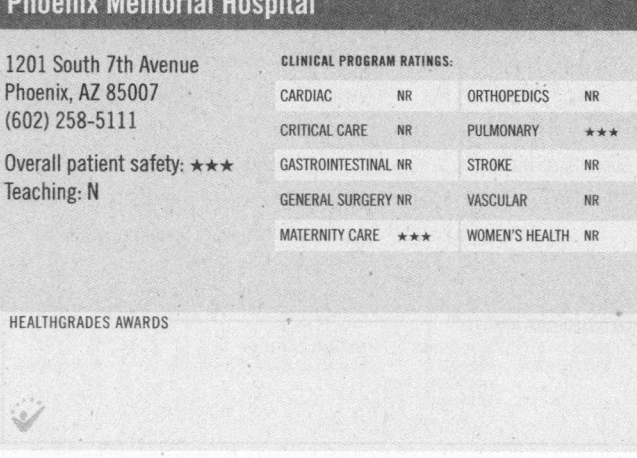

1201 South 7th Avenue
Phoenix, AZ 85007
(602) 258-5111

Overall patient safety: ★★★
Teaching: N

CLINICAL PROGRAM RATINGS:

CARDIAC	NR	ORTHOPEDICS	NR
CRITICAL CARE	NR	PULMONARY	★★★
GASTROINTESTINAL	NR	STROKE	NR
GENERAL SURGERY	NR	VASCULAR	NR
MATERNITY CARE	★★★	WOMEN'S HEALTH	NR

HEALTHGRADES AWARDS

Payson Regional Medical Center

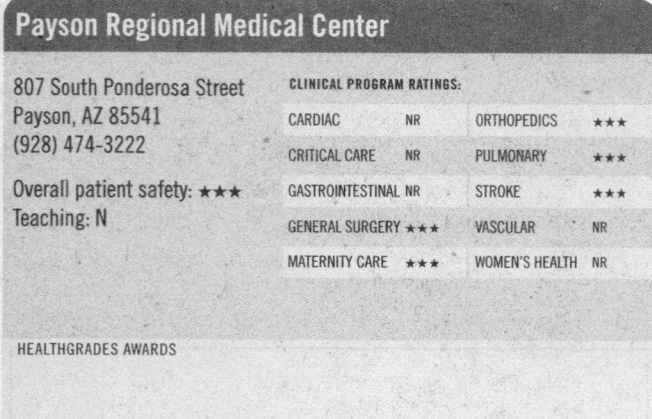

807 South Ponderosa Street
Payson, AZ 85541
(928) 474-3222

Overall patient safety: ★★★
Teaching: N

CLINICAL PROGRAM RATINGS:

CARDIAC	NR	ORTHOPEDICS	★★★
CRITICAL CARE	NR	PULMONARY	★★★
GASTROINTESTINAL	NR	STROKE	★★★
GENERAL SURGERY	★★★	VASCULAR	NR
MATERNITY CARE	★★★	WOMEN'S HEALTH	NR

HEALTHGRADES AWARDS

St. Joseph's Hospital and Medical Center

350 West Thomas Road
Phoenix, AZ 85013
(602) 406-3000

Overall patient safety: ★
Teaching: Y

CLINICAL PROGRAM RATINGS:

CARDIAC	★★★	ORTHOPEDICS	NR
CRITICAL CARE	NR	PULMONARY	★★★
GASTROINTESTINAL	NR	STROKE	★★★★★
GENERAL SURGERY	★	VASCULAR	NR
MATERNITY CARE	★	WOMEN'S HEALTH	★★★

HEALTHGRADES AWARDS

✓ SPECIALTY EXCELLENCE
· STROKE CARE

KEY: ★★★★★ BEST ★★★ AS EXPECTED ★ POOR NR NOT RATED BY HEALTHGRADES For full definitions of ratings and awards, see Appendix.

St. Luke's Behavioral Health Center*

P.O. Box 13609
Phoenix, AZ 85006
(602) 251-8484

Overall patient safety: NR
Teaching: N

CLINICAL PROGRAM RATINGS:

CARDIAC	★★★	ORTHOPEDICS	★★★
CRITICAL CARE	NR	PULMONARY	★★★
GASTROINTESTINAL	NR	STROKE	NR
GENERAL SURGERY	NR	VASCULAR	NR
MATERNITY CARE	NR	WOMEN'S HEALTH	NR

HEALTHGRADES AWARDS

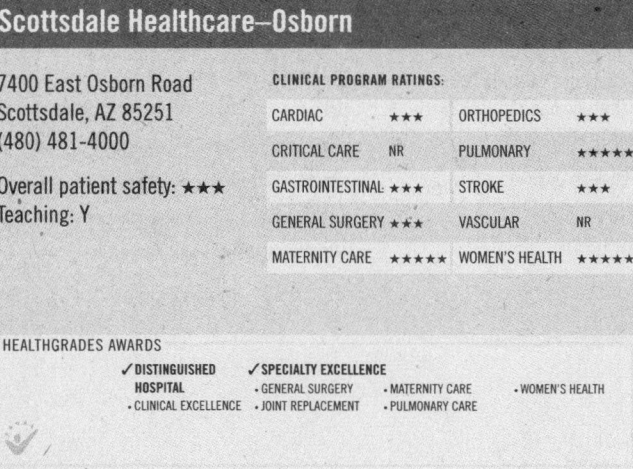

St. Luke's Medical Center*

1800 East Van Buren Street
Phoenix, AZ 85006
(602) 251-8100

Overall patient safety: ★
Teaching: N

CLINICAL PROGRAM RATINGS:

CARDIAC	★★★	ORTHOPEDICS	★★★
CRITICAL CARE	NR	PULMONARY	★★★
GASTROINTESTINAL	NR	STROKE	NR
GENERAL SURGERY	NR	VASCULAR	NR
MATERNITY CARE	NR	WOMEN'S HEALTH	NR

HEALTHGRADES AWARDS

Scottsdale Healthcare—Osborn

7400 East Osborn Road
Scottsdale, AZ 85251
(480) 481-4000

Overall patient safety: ★★★
Teaching: Y

CLINICAL PROGRAM RATINGS:

CARDIAC	★★★	ORTHOPEDICS	★★★
CRITICAL CARE	NR	PULMONARY	★★★★★
GASTROINTESTINAL	★★★	STROKE	★★★
GENERAL SURGERY	★★★	VASCULAR	NR
MATERNITY CARE	★★★★★	WOMEN'S HEALTH	★★★★★

HEALTHGRADES AWARDS

✓ **DISTINGUISHED HOSPITAL**
· CLINICAL EXCELLENCE

✓ **SPECIALTY EXCELLENCE**
· GENERAL SURGERY
· JOINT REPLACEMENT
· MATERNITY CARE
· PULMONARY CARE
· WOMEN'S HEALTH

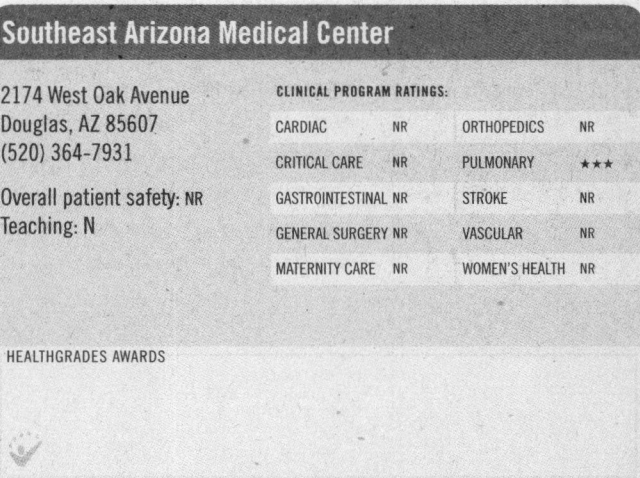

Scottsdale Healthcare–Shea

9003 East Shea Boulevard
Scottsdale, AZ 85260
(480) 323-3000

Overall patient safety: ★★★
Teaching: Y

CLINICAL PROGRAM RATINGS:

CARDIAC	★★★	ORTHOPEDICS	★★★
CRITICAL CARE	NR	PULMONARY	★★★
GASTROINTESTINAL	★★★	STROKE	★★★
GENERAL SURGERY	★★★	VASCULAR	NR
MATERNITY CARE	★★★	WOMEN'S HEALTH	★★★

HEALTHGRADES AWARDS

✓ **SPECIALTY EXCELLENCE**
· BARIATRIC SURGERY
· GENERAL SURGERY

Sierra Vista Regional Health Center

300 El Camino Real
Sierra Vista, AZ 85635
(520) 458-4641

Overall patient safety: ★★★
Teaching: N

CLINICAL PROGRAM RATINGS:

CARDIAC	NR	ORTHOPEDICS	NR
CRITICAL CARE	NR	PULMONARY	★★★
GASTROINTESTINAL	★★★	STROKE	★★★
GENERAL SURGERY	★★★	VASCULAR	NR
MATERNITY CARE	★★★	WOMEN'S HEALTH	NR

HEALTHGRADES AWARDS

Southeast Arizona Medical Center

2174 West Oak Avenue
Douglas, AZ 85607
(520) 364-7931

Overall patient safety: NR
Teaching: N

CLINICAL PROGRAM RATINGS:

CARDIAC	NR	ORTHOPEDICS	NR
CRITICAL CARE	NR	PULMONARY	★★★
GASTROINTESTINAL	NR	STROKE	NR
GENERAL SURGERY	NR	VASCULAR	NR
MATERNITY CARE	NR	WOMEN'S HEALTH	NR

HEALTHGRADES AWARDS

*This hospital reports its data to the federal government jointly with another hospital. Therefore the ratings and awards apply to multiple hospitals and this specific hospital may not provide all rated services.

ARIZONA HOSPITALS: RATINGS BY CLINICAL SPECIALTY

Tempe St. Luke's Hospital

1500 South Mill Avenue
Tempe, AZ 85281
(480) 784-5500

Overall patient safety: ★★★
Teaching: Y

CLINICAL PROGRAM RATINGS:

CARDIAC	NR	ORTHOPEDICS	NR
CRITICAL CARE	NR	PULMONARY	★★★
GASTROINTESTINAL	NR	STROKE	★★★
GENERAL SURGERY	NR	VASCULAR	NR
MATERNITY CARE	NR	WOMEN'S HEALTH	NR

HEALTHGRADES AWARDS

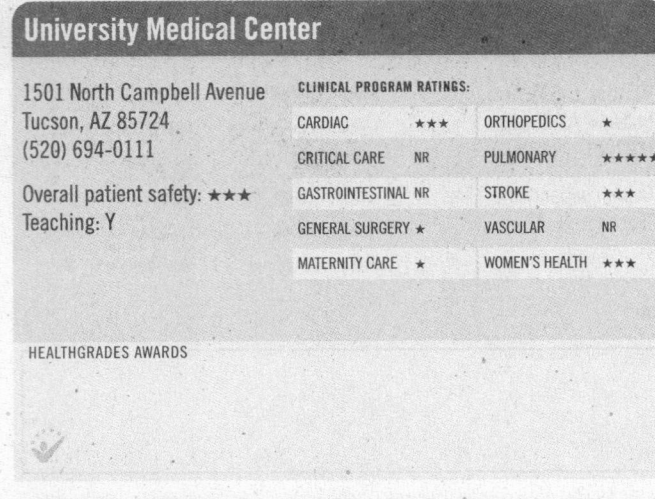

University Medical Center

1501 North Campbell Avenue
Tucson, AZ 85724
(520) 694-0111

Overall patient safety: ★★★
Teaching: Y

CLINICAL PROGRAM RATINGS:

CARDIAC	★★★	ORTHOPEDICS	★
CRITICAL CARE	NR	PULMONARY	★★★★★
GASTROINTESTINAL	NR	STROKE	★★★
GENERAL SURGERY	★	VASCULAR	NR
MATERNITY CARE	★	WOMEN'S HEALTH	★★★

HEALTHGRADES AWARDS

Tucson Heart Hospital

4888 North Stone Avenue
Tucson, AZ 85704
(520) 696-2328

Overall patient safety: ★★★★★
Teaching: N

CLINICAL PROGRAM RATINGS:

CARDIAC	★★★	ORTHOPEDICS	NR
CRITICAL CARE	NR	PULMONARY	★★★
GASTROINTESTINAL	NR	STROKE	★★★
GENERAL SURGERY	NR	VASCULAR	★★★
MATERNITY CARE	NR	WOMEN'S HEALTH	NR

HEALTHGRADES AWARDS

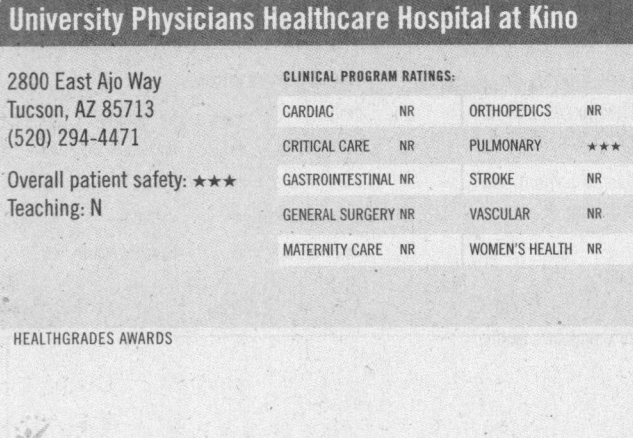

University Physicians Healthcare Hospital at Kino

2800 East Ajo Way
Tucson, AZ 85713
(520) 294-4471

Overall patient safety: ★★★
Teaching: N

CLINICAL PROGRAM RATINGS:

CARDIAC	NR	ORTHOPEDICS	NR
CRITICAL CARE	NR	PULMONARY	★★★
GASTROINTESTINAL	NR	STROKE	NR
GENERAL SURGERY	NR	VASCULAR	NR
MATERNITY CARE	NR	WOMEN'S HEALTH	NR

HEALTHGRADES AWARDS

Tucson Medical Center

5301 East Grant Road
Tucson, AZ 85712
(520) 327-5461

Overall patient safety: ★★★
Teaching: Y

CLINICAL PROGRAM RATINGS:

CARDIAC	★★★	ORTHOPEDICS	★★★
CRITICAL CARE	★★★	PULMONARY	★★★
GASTROINTESTINAL	★★★	STROKE	★★★★★
GENERAL SURGERY	★★★	VASCULAR	NR
MATERNITY CARE	★★★	WOMEN'S HEALTH	★★★

HEALTHGRADES AWARDS

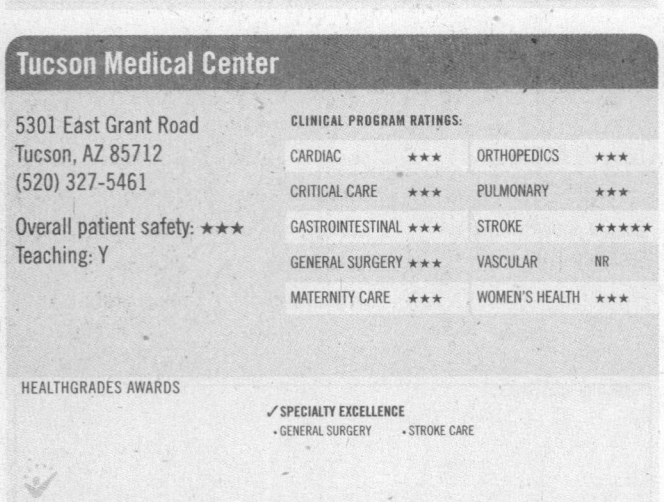

✓ SPECIALTY EXCELLENCE
· GENERAL SURGERY   · STROKE CARE

Verde Valley Medical Center

269 South Candy Lane
Cottonwood, AZ 86326
(928) 634-2251

Overall patient safety: ★★★
Teaching: N

CLINICAL PROGRAM RATINGS:

CARDIAC	NR	ORTHOPEDICS	NR
CRITICAL CARE	NR	PULMONARY	★
GASTROINTESTINAL	★★★	STROKE	★★★
GENERAL SURGERY	★★★	VASCULAR	NR
MATERNITY CARE	★★★★★	WOMEN'S HEALTH	NR

HEALTHGRADES AWARDS

KEY: ★★★★★ BEST   ★★★ AS EXPECTED   ★ POOR   NR NOT RATED BY HEALTHGRADES   For full definitions of ratings and awards, see Appendix.

Walter O. Boswell Memorial Hospital

10401 West Thunderbird
Boulevard
Sun City, AZ 85351
(623) 977-7211

Overall patient safety: ★★★
Teaching: Y

CLINICAL PROGRAM RATINGS:

CARDIAC	★★★	ORTHOPEDICS	★★★
CRITICAL CARE	NR	PULMONARY	★★★
GASTROINTESTINAL	★★★	STROKE	★★★
GENERAL SURGERY	★★★	VASCULAR	★★★
MATERNITY CARE	NR	WOMEN'S HEALTH	NR

HEALTHGRADES AWARDS

Winslow Memorial Hospital

1501 North Williamson Avenue
Winslow, AZ 86047
(928) 289-4691

Overall patient safety: ★★★
Teaching: N

CLINICAL PROGRAM RATINGS:

CARDIAC	NR	ORTHOPEDICS	NR
CRITICAL CARE	NR	PULMONARY	NR
GASTROINTESTINAL	NR	STROKE	NR
GENERAL SURGERY	NR	VASCULAR	NR
MATERNITY CARE	★★★	WOMEN'S HEALTH	NR

HEALTHGRADES AWARDS

West Valley Hospital

13677 West McDowell Road
Goodyear, AZ 85338
(623) 882-1500

Overall patient safety: ★★★
Teaching: N

CLINICAL PROGRAM RATINGS:

CARDIAC	★★★	ORTHOPEDICS	NR
CRITICAL CARE	NR	PULMONARY	★★★
GASTROINTESTINAL	NR	STROKE	★★★
GENERAL SURGERY	NR	VASCULAR	NR
MATERNITY CARE	★★★	WOMEN'S HEALTH	NR

HEALTHGRADES AWARDS

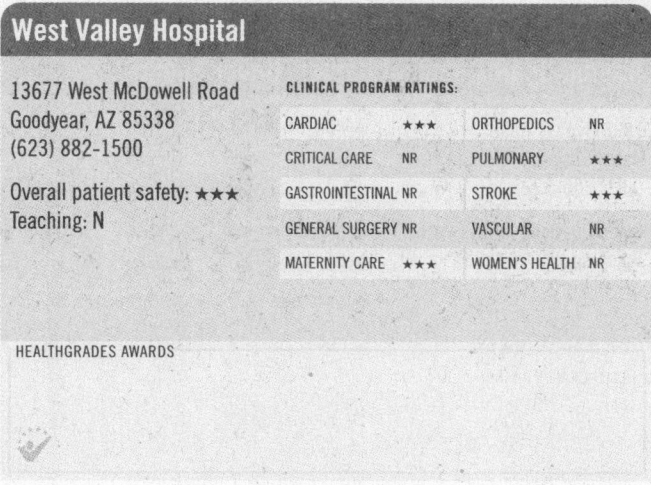

Yavapai Regional Medical Center

1003 Willow Creek Road
Prescott, AZ 86301
(928) 445-2700

Overall patient safety: ★★★★★
Teaching: N

CLINICAL PROGRAM RATINGS:

CARDIAC	NR	ORTHOPEDICS	NR
CRITICAL CARE	NR	PULMONARY	★★★
GASTROINTESTINAL	★★★	STROKE	★★★
GENERAL SURGERY	★★★★★	VASCULAR	NR
MATERNITY CARE	★★★	WOMEN'S HEALTH	NR

HEALTHGRADES AWARDS

✓ DISTINGUISHED HOSPITAL
- PATIENT SAFETY

✓ SPECIALTY EXCELLENCE
- GENERAL SURGERY   - JOINT REPLACEMENT

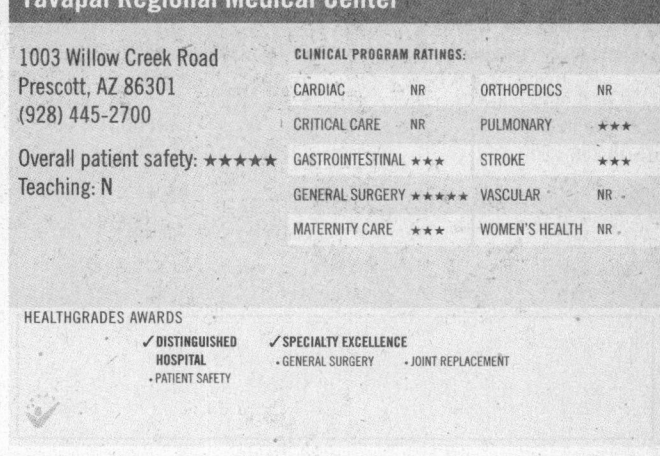

Western Arizona Regional Medical Center

2735 Silver Creek Road
Bullhead City, AZ 86442
(928) 763-2273

Overall patient safety: ★★★
Teaching: N

CLINICAL PROGRAM RATINGS:

CARDIAC	NR	ORTHOPEDICS	★★★
CRITICAL CARE	NR	PULMONARY	★★★
GASTROINTESTINAL	★★★	STROKE	★★★★★
GENERAL SURGERY	★	VASCULAR	★★★
MATERNITY CARE	★★★	WOMEN'S HEALTH	NR

HEALTHGRADES AWARDS

Yuma Regional Medical Center

2400 South Avenue A
Yuma, AZ 85364
(928) 344-2000

Overall patient safety: ★★★★★
Teaching: N

CLINICAL PROGRAM RATINGS:

CARDIAC	★★★	ORTHOPEDICS	★★★
CRITICAL CARE	NR	PULMONARY	★★★
GASTROINTESTINAL	★★★	STROKE	★★★
GENERAL SURGERY	★★★	VASCULAR	NR
MATERNITY CARE	★★★	WOMEN'S HEALTH	★★★★★

HEALTHGRADES AWARDS

✓ DISTINGUISHED HOSPITAL
- PATIENT SAFETY

Arkansas Heart Hospital

1701 South Shackleford Road
Little Rock, AR 72211
(501) 219-7000

Overall patient safety: ★★★
Teaching: N

CLINICAL PROGRAM RATINGS:

CARDIAC	★★★	ORTHOPEDICS	NR
CRITICAL CARE	NR	PULMONARY	★★★★★
GASTROINTESTINAL	NR	STROKE	★
GENERAL SURGERY	NR	VASCULAR	NR
MATERNITY CARE	NR	WOMEN'S HEALTH	NR

HEALTHGRADES AWARDS

✓ SPECIALTY EXCELLENCE
• CARDIAC CARE   • PULMONARY CARE

Baptist Health Medical Center—Arkadelphia

3050 Twin Rivers Drive
Arkadelphia, AR 71923
(870) 245-2622

Overall patient safety: ★★★
Teaching: N

CLINICAL PROGRAM RATINGS:

CARDIAC	NR	ORTHOPEDICS	NR
CRITICAL CARE	NR	PULMONARY	★
GASTROINTESTINAL	NR	STROKE	NR
GENERAL SURGERY	NR	VASCULAR	NR
MATERNITY CARE	NR	WOMEN'S HEALTH	NR

HEALTHGRADES AWARDS

Arkansas Methodist Medical Center

900 West Kingshighway
Paragould, AR 72450
(870) 239-7000

Overall patient safety: ★★★
Teaching: N

CLINICAL PROGRAM RATINGS:

CARDIAC	NR	ORTHOPEDICS	NR
CRITICAL CARE	NR	PULMONARY	★★★
GASTROINTESTINAL	★★★	STROKE	★★★
GENERAL SURGERY	NR	VASCULAR	NR
MATERNITY CARE	NR	WOMEN'S HEALTH	NR

HEALTHGRADES AWARDS

Baptist Health Medical Center—Heber Spings

1800 Bypass Road
Heber Springs, AR 72543
(501) 206-3221

Overall patient safety: ★★★
Teaching: N

CLINICAL PROGRAM RATINGS:

CARDIAC	NR	ORTHOPEDICS	NR
CRITICAL CARE	NR	PULMONARY	★★★
GASTROINTESTINAL	NR	STROKE	★★★
GENERAL SURGERY	NR	VASCULAR	NR
MATERNITY CARE	NR	WOMEN'S HEALTH	NR

HEALTHGRADES AWARDS

Ashley County Medical Center

1015 Unity Road
Crossett, AR 71635
(870) 364-4111

Overall patient safety: ★★★
Teaching: N

CLINICAL PROGRAM RATINGS:

CARDIAC	NR	ORTHOPEDICS	NR
CRITICAL CARE	NR	PULMONARY	★
GASTROINTESTINAL	NR	STROKE	★
GENERAL SURGERY	NR	VASCULAR	NR
MATERNITY CARE	NR	WOMEN'S HEALTH	NR

HEALTHGRADES AWARDS

Baptist Health Medical Center—Little Rock

9601 Interstate 630
Little Rock, AR 72205
(501) 202-2000

Overall patient safety: ★
Teaching: Y

CLINICAL PROGRAM RATINGS:

CARDIAC	★	ORTHOPEDICS	★★★
CRITICAL CARE	NR	PULMONARY	★★★
GASTROINTESTINAL	★★★	STROKE	★★★
GENERAL SURGERY	NR	VASCULAR	★★★
MATERNITY CARE	NR	WOMEN'S HEALTH	NR

HEALTHGRADES AWARDS

KEY: ★★★★★ BEST   ★★★ AS EXPECTED   ★ POOR   NR NOT RATED BY HEALTHGRADES   For full definitions of ratings and awards, see Appendix.

Baptist Health Medical Center–North Little Rock

3333 Springhill Drive
North Little Rock, AR 72117
(501) 202-3000

Overall patient safety: ★★★
Teaching: N

CLINICAL PROGRAM RATINGS:

CARDIAC	★★★	ORTHOPEDICS	★
CRITICAL CARE	NR	PULMONARY	★
GASTROINTESTINAL	★★★	STROKE	★★★
GENERAL SURGERY	NR	VASCULAR	NR
MATERNITY CARE	NR	WOMEN'S HEALTH	NR

HEALTHGRADES AWARDS

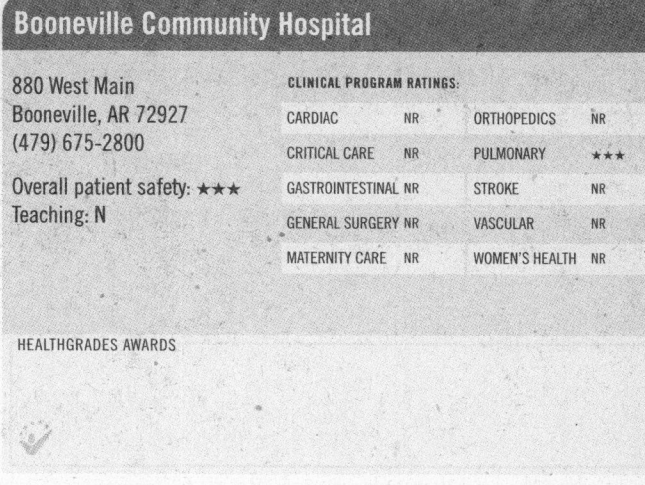

Booneville Community Hospital

880 West Main
Booneville, AR 72927
(479) 675-2800

Overall patient safety: ★★★
Teaching: N

CLINICAL PROGRAM RATINGS:

CARDIAC	NR	ORTHOPEDICS	NR
CRITICAL CARE	NR	PULMONARY	★★★
GASTROINTESTINAL	NR	STROKE	NR
GENERAL SURGERY	NR	VASCULAR	NR
MATERNITY CARE	NR	WOMEN'S HEALTH	NR

HEALTHGRADES AWARDS

Baptist Memorial Hospital–Forrest City

1601 New Castle Road
Forrest City, AR 72335
(870) 261-0000

Overall patient safety: ★
Teaching: N

CLINICAL PROGRAM RATINGS:

CARDIAC	NR	ORTHOPEDICS	NR
CRITICAL CARE	NR	PULMONARY	★★★
GASTROINTESTINAL	NR	STROKE	★★★
GENERAL SURGERY	NR	VASCULAR	NR
MATERNITY CARE	NR	WOMEN'S HEALTH	NR

HEALTHGRADES AWARDS

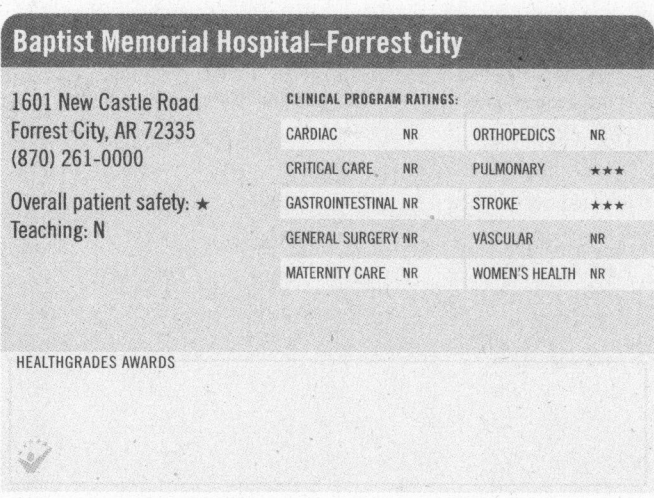

Bradley County Medical Center

404 South Bradley Street
Warren, AR 71671
(870) 226-3731

Overall patient safety: ★★★
Teaching: N

CLINICAL PROGRAM RATINGS:

CARDIAC	NR	ORTHOPEDICS	NR
CRITICAL CARE	NR	PULMONARY	★
GASTROINTESTINAL	NR	STROKE	NR
GENERAL SURGERY	NR	VASCULAR	NR
MATERNITY CARE	NR	WOMEN'S HEALTH	NR

HEALTHGRADES AWARDS

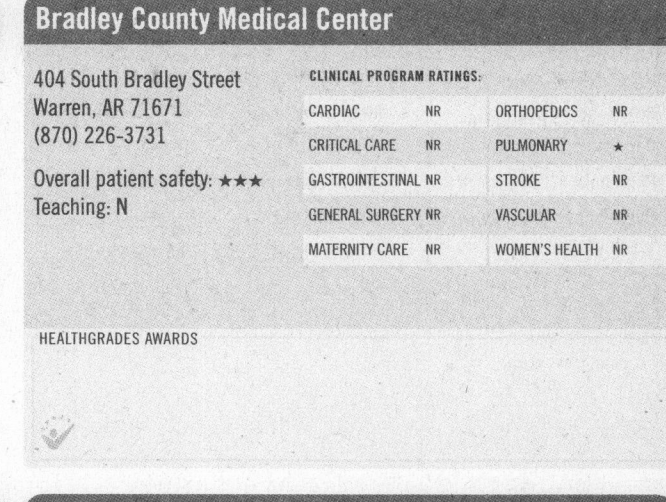

Baxter Regional Medical Center

624 Hospital Drive
Mountain Home, AR 72653
(870) 508-1000

Overall patient safety: ★★★★★
Teaching: N

CLINICAL PROGRAM RATINGS:

CARDIAC	★	ORTHOPEDICS	★
CRITICAL CARE	NR	PULMONARY	★
GASTROINTESTINAL	★★★	STROKE	★
GENERAL SURGERY	NR	VASCULAR	★★★
MATERNITY CARE	NR	WOMEN'S HEALTH	NR

HEALTHGRADES AWARDS

Chicot Memorial Hospital

2729 Highway 65 and
82 South
Lake Village, AR 71653
(870) 265-5351

Overall patient safety: ★★★
Teaching: N

CLINICAL PROGRAM RATINGS:

CARDIAC	NR	ORTHOPEDICS	NR
CRITICAL CARE	NR	PULMONARY	★
GASTROINTESTINAL	NR	STROKE	NR
GENERAL SURGERY	NR	VASCULAR	NR
MATERNITY CARE	NR	WOMEN'S HEALTH	NR

HEALTHGRADES AWARDS

Community Medical Center–Izard County

103 Grasse Street
Calico Rock, AR 72519
(870) 297-3726

Overall patient safety: ★★★
Teaching: N

CLINICAL PROGRAM RATINGS:

CARDIAC	NR	ORTHOPEDICS	NR
CRITICAL CARE	NR	PULMONARY	★
GASTROINTESTINAL	NR	STROKE	NR
GENERAL SURGERY	NR	VASCULAR	NR
MATERNITY CARE	NR	WOMEN'S HEALTH	NR

HEALTHGRADES AWARDS

De Queen Medical Center

1306 West Collin Raye Drive
De Queen, AR 71832
(870) 584-4111

Overall patient safety: ★★★
Teaching: N

CLINICAL PROGRAM RATINGS:

CARDIAC	NR	ORTHOPEDICS	NR
CRITICAL CARE	NR	PULMONARY	★
GASTROINTESTINAL	NR	STROKE	NR
GENERAL SURGERY	NR	VASCULAR	NR
MATERNITY CARE	NR	WOMEN'S HEALTH	NR

HEALTHGRADES AWARDS

Conway Regional Medical Center

2302 College Avenue
Conway, AR 72032
(501) 329-3831

Overall patient safety: ★★★
Teaching: N

CLINICAL PROGRAM RATINGS:

CARDIAC	★★★	ORTHOPEDICS	NR
CRITICAL CARE	NR	PULMONARY	★
GASTROINTESTINAL	★★★	STROKE	★
GENERAL SURGERY	NR	VASCULAR	NR
MATERNITY CARE	NR	WOMEN'S HEALTH	NR

HEALTHGRADES AWARDS

De Witt City Hospital

1641 Whitehead Drive
De Witt, AR 72042
(870) 946-3571

Overall patient safety: NR
Teaching: N

CLINICAL PROGRAM RATINGS:

CARDIAC	NR	ORTHOPEDICS	NR
CRITICAL CARE	NR	PULMONARY	★★★
GASTROINTESTINAL	NR	STROKE	★
GENERAL SURGERY	NR	VASCULAR	NR
MATERNITY CARE	NR	WOMEN'S HEALTH	NR

HEALTHGRADES AWARDS

Crittenden Regional Hospital

200 Tyler Avenue
West Memphis, AR 72301
(870) 735-1500

Overall patient safety: ★★★
Teaching: Y

CLINICAL PROGRAM RATINGS:

CARDIAC	NR	ORTHOPEDICS	NR
CRITICAL CARE	NR	PULMONARY	★★★
GASTROINTESTINAL	NR	STROKE	★
GENERAL SURGERY	NR	VASCULAR	NR
MATERNITY CARE	NR	WOMEN'S HEALTH	NR

HEALTHGRADES AWARDS

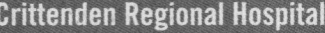

Delta Memorial Hospital Association

300 East Pickens
Dumas, AR 71639
(870) 382-4303

Overall patient safety: ★★★
Teaching: N

CLINICAL PROGRAM RATINGS:

CARDIAC	NR	ORTHOPEDICS	NR
CRITICAL CARE	NR	PULMONARY	NR
GASTROINTESTINAL	NR	STROKE	NR
GENERAL SURGERY	NR	VASCULAR	NR
MATERNITY CARE	NR	WOMEN'S HEALTH	NR

HEALTHGRADES AWARDS

KEY: ★★★★★ BEST   ★★★ AS EXPECTED   ★ POOR   NR NOT RATED BY HEALTHGRADES   For full definitions of ratings and awards, see Appendix.

Drew Memorial Hospital

778 Scogin Drive
Monticello, AR 71655
(870) 367-2411

Overall patient safety: ★
Teaching: N

CLINICAL PROGRAM RATINGS:

CARDIAC	NR	ORTHOPEDICS	NR
CRITICAL CARE	NR	PULMONARY	★★★
GASTROINTESTINAL	NR	STROKE	NR
GENERAL SURGERY	NR	VASCULAR	NR
MATERNITY CARE	NR	WOMEN'S HEALTH	NR

HEALTHGRADES AWARDS

Harris Hospital

1205 McLain Street
Newport, AR 72112
(870) 523-8911

Overall patient safety: ★★★
Teaching: N

CLINICAL PROGRAM RATINGS:

CARDIAC	NR	ORTHOPEDICS	NR
CRITICAL CARE	NR	PULMONARY	★★★★★
GASTROINTESTINAL	NR	STROKE	NR
GENERAL SURGERY	NR	VASCULAR	NR
MATERNITY CARE	NR	WOMEN'S HEALTH	NR

HEALTHGRADES AWARDS

Fulton County Hospital

679 North Main Street
Salem, AR 72576
(870) 895-2691

Overall patient safety: NR
Teaching: N

CLINICAL PROGRAM RATINGS:

CARDIAC	NR	ORTHOPEDICS	NR
CRITICAL CARE	NR	PULMONARY	★
GASTROINTESTINAL	NR	STROKE	NR
GENERAL SURGERY	NR	VASCULAR	NR
MATERNITY CARE	NR	WOMEN'S HEALTH	NR

HEALTHGRADES AWARDS

Helena Regional Medical Center

1801 Martin Luther
King Jr. Drive
Helena, AR 72342
(870) 338-5800

Overall patient safety: ★★★
Teaching: N

CLINICAL PROGRAM RATINGS:

CARDIAC	NR	ORTHOPEDICS	NR
CRITICAL CARE	NR	PULMONARY	★
GASTROINTESTINAL	NR	STROKE	★★★
GENERAL SURGERY	NR	VASCULAR	NR
MATERNITY CARE	NR	WOMEN'S HEALTH	NR

HEALTHGRADES AWARDS

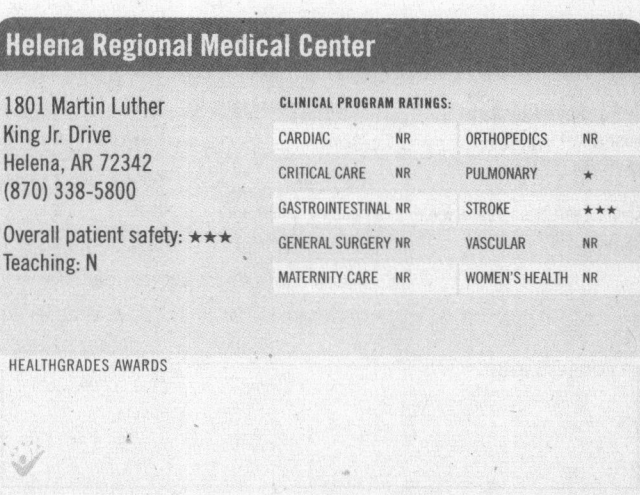

Great River Medical Center

1520 North Division Street
Blytheville, AR 72315
(870) 838-7300

Overall patient safety: ★
Teaching: N

CLINICAL PROGRAM RATINGS:

CARDIAC	NR	ORTHOPEDICS	NR
CRITICAL CARE	NR	PULMONARY	★
GASTROINTESTINAL	NR	STROKE	★
GENERAL SURGERY	NR	VASCULAR	NR
MATERNITY CARE	NR	WOMEN'S HEALTH	NR

HEALTHGRADES AWARDS

Hot Spring County Medical Center

1001 Schneider Drive
Malvern, AR 72104
(501) 332-1000

Overall patient safety: ★★★
Teaching: N

CLINICAL PROGRAM RATINGS:

CARDIAC	NR	ORTHOPEDICS	NR
CRITICAL CARE	NR	PULMONARY	★★★
GASTROINTESTINAL	NR	STROKE	★★★
GENERAL SURGERY	NR	VASCULAR	NR
MATERNITY CARE	NR	WOMEN'S HEALTH	NR

HEALTHGRADES AWARDS

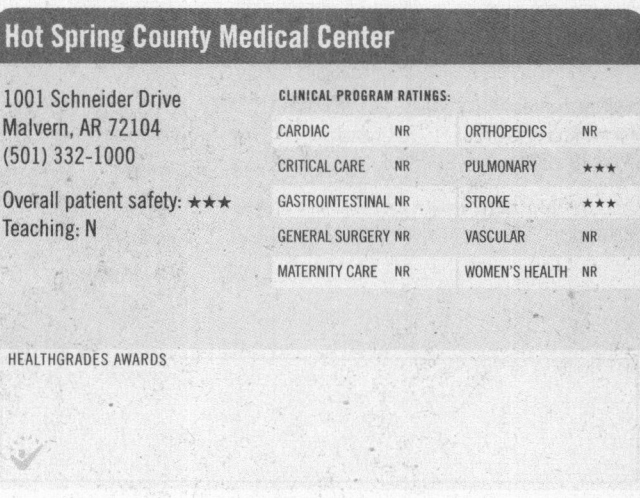

ARKANSAS HOSPITALS: RATINGS BY CLINICAL SPECIALTY

Howard Memorial Hospital

800 West Leslie Street
Nashville, AR 71852
(870) 845-4400

Overall patient safety: ★★★
Teaching: N

CLINICAL PROGRAM RATINGS:

CARDIAC	NR	ORTHOPEDICS	NR
CRITICAL CARE	NR	PULMONARY	★★★
GASTROINTESTINAL	NR	STROKE	NR
GENERAL SURGERY	NR	VASCULAR	NR
MATERNITY CARE	NR	WOMEN'S HEALTH	NR

HEALTHGRADES AWARDS

Johnson Regional Medical Center

1100 East Poplar Street
Clarksville, AR 72830
(479) 754-5454

Overall patient safety: ★★★
Teaching: Y

CLINICAL PROGRAM RATINGS:

CARDIAC	NR	ORTHOPEDICS	NR
CRITICAL CARE	NR	PULMONARY	★
GASTROINTESTINAL	NR	STROKE	★★★
GENERAL SURGERY	NR	VASCULAR	NR
MATERNITY CARE	NR	WOMEN'S HEALTH	NR

HEALTHGRADES AWARDS

Jefferson Regional Medical Center

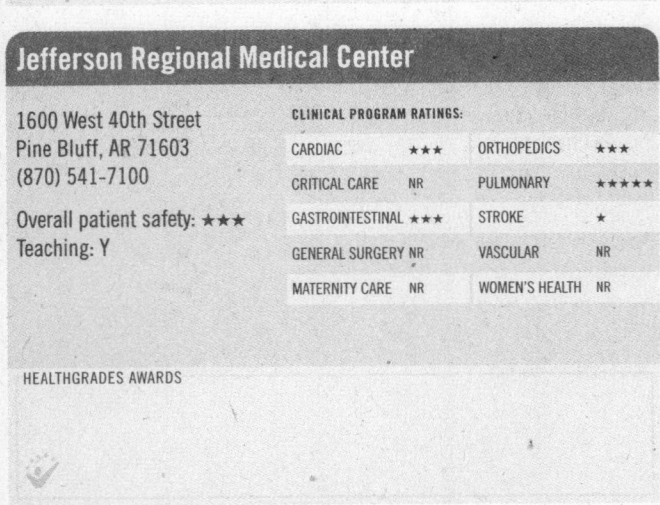

1600 West 40th Street
Pine Bluff, AR 71603
(870) 541-7100

Overall patient safety: ★★★
Teaching: Y

CLINICAL PROGRAM RATINGS:

CARDIAC	★★★	ORTHOPEDICS	★★★
CRITICAL CARE	NR	PULMONARY	★★★★★
GASTROINTESTINAL	★★★	STROKE	★
GENERAL SURGERY	NR	VASCULAR	NR
MATERNITY CARE	NR	WOMEN'S HEALTH	NR

HEALTHGRADES AWARDS

Little River Memorial Hospital

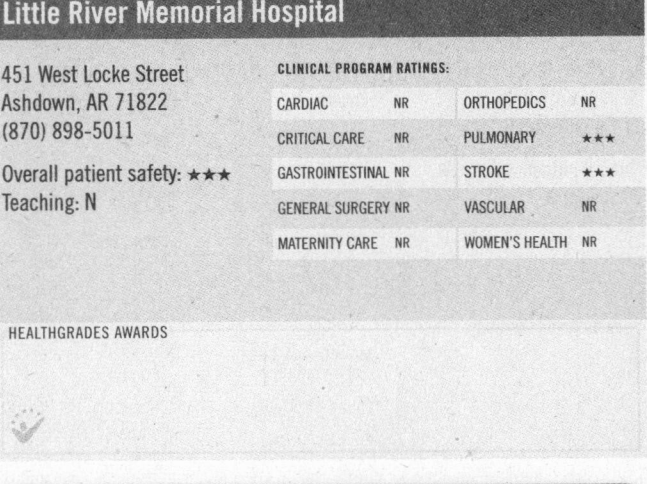

451 West Locke Street
Ashdown, AR 71822
(870) 898-5011

Overall patient safety: ★★★
Teaching: N

CLINICAL PROGRAM RATINGS:

CARDIAC	NR	ORTHOPEDICS	NR
CRITICAL CARE	NR	PULMONARY	★★★
GASTROINTESTINAL	NR	STROKE	★★★
GENERAL SURGERY	NR	VASCULAR	NR
MATERNITY CARE	NR	WOMEN'S HEALTH	NR

HEALTHGRADES AWARDS

John Ed Chambers Memorial Hospital

Highway 10 at Detroit Street
Danville, AR 72833
(479) 495-2241

Overall patient safety: ★★★★★
Teaching: N

CLINICAL PROGRAM RATINGS:

CARDIAC	NR	ORTHOPEDICS	NR
CRITICAL CARE	NR	PULMONARY	★★★
GASTROINTESTINAL	NR	STROKE	★
GENERAL SURGERY	NR	VASCULAR	NR
MATERNITY CARE	NR	WOMEN'S HEALTH	NR

HEALTHGRADES AWARDS

Magnolia Hospital

101 Hospital Drive
Magnolia, AR 71754
(870) 235-3000

Overall patient safety: ★★★
Teaching: N

CLINICAL PROGRAM RATINGS:

CARDIAC	NR	ORTHOPEDICS	NR
CRITICAL CARE	NR	PULMONARY	★★★
GASTROINTESTINAL	NR	STROKE	★★★
GENERAL SURGERY	NR	VASCULAR	NR
MATERNITY CARE	NR	WOMEN'S HEALTH	NR

HEALTHGRADES AWARDS

KEY: ★★★★★ BEST ★★★ AS EXPECTED ★ POOR NR NOT RATED BY HEALTHGRADES For full definitions of ratings and awards, see Appendix.

McGehee Desha County Hospital

900 South 3rd Street
McGehee, AR 71654
(870) 222-5600

Overall patient safety: NR
Teaching: N

CLINICAL PROGRAM RATINGS:

CARDIAC	NR	ORTHOPEDICS	NR
CRITICAL CARE	NR	PULMONARY	★
GASTROINTESTINAL	NR	STROKE	NR
GENERAL SURGERY	NR	VASCULAR	NR
MATERNITY CARE	NR	WOMEN'S HEALTH	NR

HEALTHGRADES AWARDS

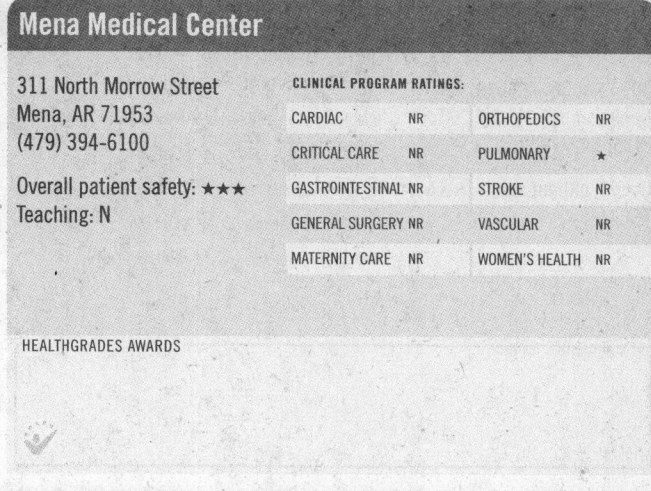

Mena Medical Center

311 North Morrow Street
Mena, AR 71953
(479) 394-6100

Overall patient safety: ★★★
Teaching: N

CLINICAL PROGRAM RATINGS:

CARDIAC	NR	ORTHOPEDICS	NR
CRITICAL CARE	NR	PULMONARY	★
GASTROINTESTINAL	NR	STROKE	NR
GENERAL SURGERY	NR	VASCULAR	NR
MATERNITY CARE	NR	WOMEN'S HEALTH	NR

HEALTHGRADES AWARDS

Medical Center—South Arkansas

700 West Grove
El Dorado, AR 71730
(870) 863-2000

Overall patient safety: ★
Teaching: Y

CLINICAL PROGRAM RATINGS:

CARDIAC	NR	ORTHOPEDICS	NR
CRITICAL CARE	NR	PULMONARY	★★★
GASTROINTESTINAL	★★★	STROKE	★
GENERAL SURGERY	NR	VASCULAR	NR
MATERNITY CARE	NR	WOMEN'S HEALTH	NR

HEALTHGRADES AWARDS

✓ SPECIALTY EXCELLENCE
· JOINT REPLACEMENT

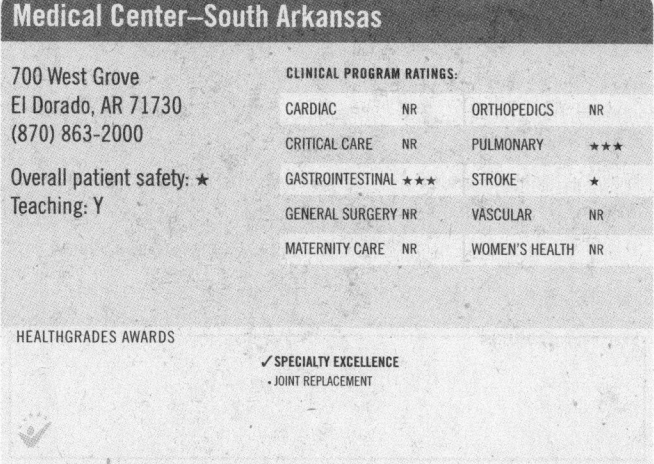

Mercy Hospital—Turner Memorial

801 West River Street
Ozark, AR 72949
(479) 314-6000

Overall patient safety: ★★★
Teaching: N

CLINICAL PROGRAM RATINGS:

CARDIAC	NR	ORTHOPEDICS	NR
CRITICAL CARE	NR	PULMONARY	★
GASTROINTESTINAL	NR	STROKE	NR
GENERAL SURGERY	NR	VASCULAR	NR
MATERNITY CARE	NR	WOMEN'S HEALTH	NR

HEALTHGRADES AWARDS

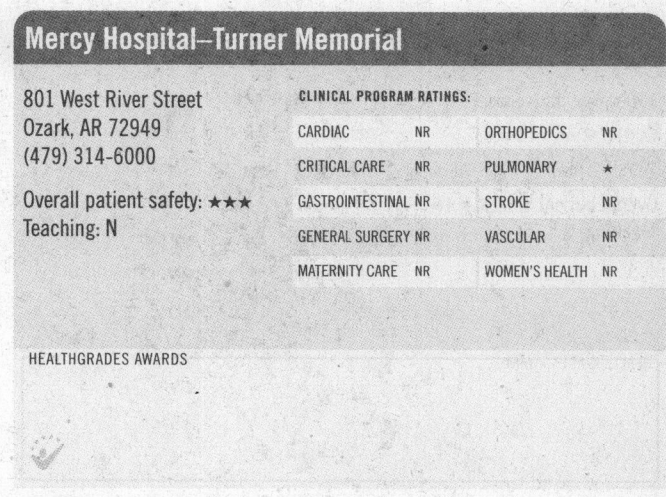

Medical Park Hospital

2001 South Main Street
Hope, AR 71801
(870) 777-2323

Overall patient safety: ★★★
Teaching: N

CLINICAL PROGRAM RATINGS:

CARDIAC	NR	ORTHOPEDICS	NR
CRITICAL CARE	NR	PULMONARY	★★★
GASTROINTESTINAL	NR	STROKE	★★★
GENERAL SURGERY	NR	VASCULAR	NR
MATERNITY CARE	NR	WOMEN'S HEALTH	NR

HEALTHGRADES AWARDS

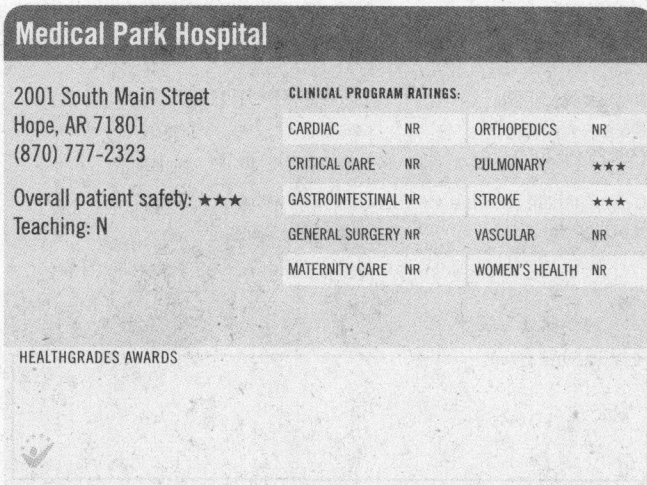

National Park Medical Center

1910 Malvern Avenue
Hot Springs, AR 71901
(501) 321-1000

Overall patient safety: ★
Teaching: N

CLINICAL PROGRAM RATINGS:

CARDIAC	★★★	ORTHOPEDICS	NR
CRITICAL CARE	NR	PULMONARY	★★★
GASTROINTESTINAL	NR	STROKE	★
GENERAL SURGERY	NR	VASCULAR	★
MATERNITY CARE	NR	WOMEN'S HEALTH	NR

HEALTHGRADES AWARDS

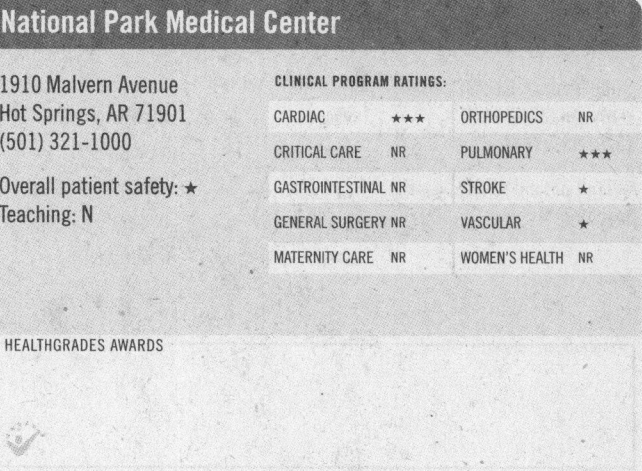

Nea Medical Center

3024 Stadium Boulevard
Jonesboro, AR 72401
(870) 972-7000

Overall patient safety: ★★★★★
Teaching: Y

CLINICAL PROGRAM RATINGS:

CARDIAC	★★★	ORTHOPEDICS	NR
CRITICAL CARE	NR	PULMONARY	★
GASTROINTESTINAL	NR	STROKE	★★★
GENERAL SURGERY	NR	VASCULAR	NR
MATERNITY CARE	NR	WOMEN'S HEALTH	NR

HEALTHGRADES AWARDS

Northwest Medical Center--Washington County*

609 West Maple Avenue
Springdale, AR 72764
(479) 751-5711

Overall patient safety: ★★★
Teaching: Y

CLINICAL PROGRAM RATINGS:

CARDIAC	★	ORTHOPEDICS	★★★
CRITICAL CARE	NR	PULMONARY	★★★
GASTROINTESTINAL	★★★	STROKE	★
GENERAL SURGERY	NR	VASCULAR	NR
MATERNITY CARE	NR	WOMEN'S HEALTH	NR

HEALTHGRADES AWARDS

North Arkansas Regional Medical Center

620 North Willow Street
Harrison, AR 72601
(870) 365-2000

Overall patient safety: ★★★
Teaching: N

CLINICAL PROGRAM RATINGS:

CARDIAC	NR	ORTHOPEDICS	NR
CRITICAL CARE	NR	PULMONARY	★★★
GASTROINTESTINAL	★★★	STROKE	★★★
GENERAL SURGERY	NR	VASCULAR	NR
MATERNITY CARE	NR	WOMEN'S HEALTH	NR

HEALTHGRADES AWARDS

Ouachita County Medical Center

638 California Avenue
Camden, AR 71701
(870) 836-1000

Overall patient safety: ★
Teaching: N

CLINICAL PROGRAM RATINGS:

CARDIAC	NR	ORTHOPEDICS	NR
CRITICAL CARE	NR	PULMONARY	★★★
GASTROINTESTINAL	NR	STROKE	★
GENERAL SURGERY	NR	VASCULAR	NR
MATERNITY CARE	NR	WOMEN'S HEALTH	NR

HEALTHGRADES AWARDS

Northwest Medical Center--Benton County

3000 Medical Center Parkway
Bentonville, AR 72712
(479) 553-1000

Overall patient safety: ★★★
Teaching: N

CLINICAL PROGRAM RATINGS:

CARDIAC	★★★	ORTHOPEDICS	★★★
CRITICAL CARE	NR	PULMONARY	★★★
GASTROINTESTINAL	★★★	STROKE	★
GENERAL SURGERY	NR	VASCULAR	NR
MATERNITY CARE	NR	WOMEN'S HEALTH	NR

HEALTHGRADES AWARDS

Ozark Health

Highway 65 South
Clinton, AR 72031
(501) 745-7000

Overall patient safety: ★★★
Teaching: N

CLINICAL PROGRAM RATINGS:

CARDIAC	NR	ORTHOPEDICS	NR
CRITICAL CARE	NR	PULMONARY	★★★
GASTROINTESTINAL	NR	STROKE	NR
GENERAL SURGERY	NR	VASCULAR	NR
MATERNITY CARE	NR	WOMEN'S HEALTH	NR

HEALTHGRADES AWARDS

KEY: ★★★★★ BEST ★★★ AS EXPECTED ★ POOR NR NOT RATED BY HEALTHGRADES For full definitions of ratings and awards, see Appendix.

Piggott Community Hospital

1206 Gordon Duckworth Drive
Piggott, AR 72454
(870) 598-3881

Overall patient safety: ★★★
Teaching: N

CLINICAL PROGRAM RATINGS:

CARDIAC	NR	ORTHOPEDICS	NR
CRITICAL CARE	NR	PULMONARY	★★★
GASTROINTESTINAL	NR	STROKE	★★★
GENERAL SURGERY	NR	VASCULAR	NR
MATERNITY CARE	NR	WOMEN'S HEALTH	NR

HEALTHGRADES AWARDS

Rebsamen Medical Center

1400 Braden Street
Jacksonville, AR 72076
(501) 985-7000

Overall patient safety: ★★★
Teaching: N

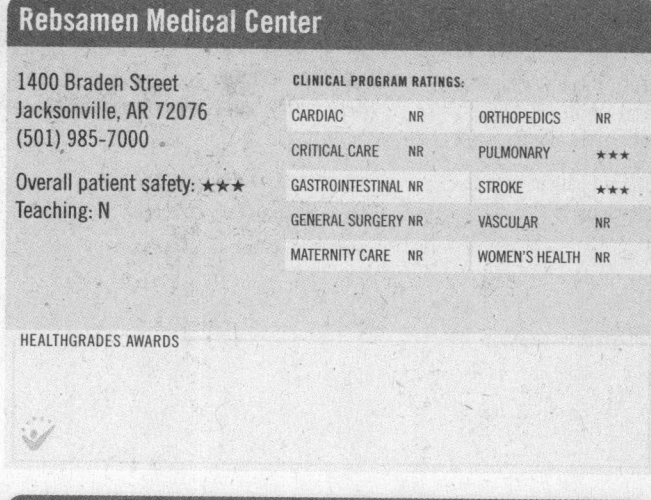

CLINICAL PROGRAM RATINGS:

CARDIAC	NR	ORTHOPEDICS	NR
CRITICAL CARE	NR	PULMONARY	★★★
GASTROINTESTINAL	NR	STROKE	★★★
GENERAL SURGERY	NR	VASCULAR	NR
MATERNITY CARE	NR	WOMEN'S HEALTH	NR

HEALTHGRADES AWARDS

Pike County Memorial Hospital

315 East 13th Street
Murfreesboro, AR 71958
(870) 285-3182

Overall patient safety: ★★★
Teaching: N

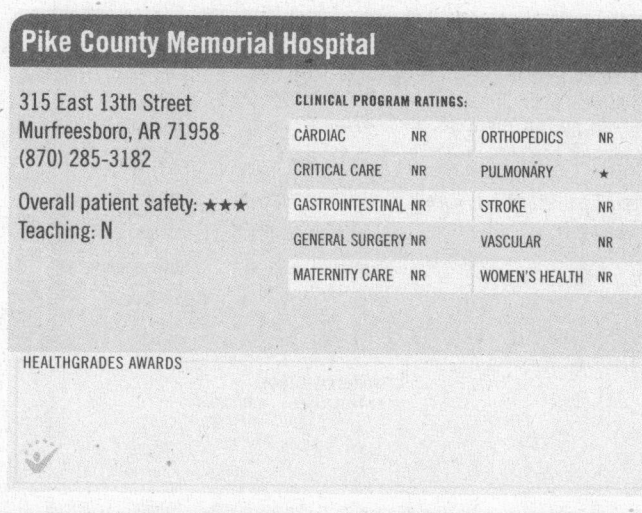

CLINICAL PROGRAM RATINGS:

CARDIAC	NR	ORTHOPEDICS	NR
CRITICAL CARE	NR	PULMONARY	★
GASTROINTESTINAL	NR	STROKE	NR
GENERAL SURGERY	NR	VASCULAR	NR
MATERNITY CARE	NR	WOMEN'S HEALTH	NR

HEALTHGRADES AWARDS

St. Anthony's Healthcare Center

4 Hospital Drive
Morrilton, AR 72110
(501) 977-2300

Overall patient safety: ★★★
Teaching: N

CLINICAL PROGRAM RATINGS:

CARDIAC	NR	ORTHOPEDICS	NR
CRITICAL CARE	NR	PULMONARY	★
GASTROINTESTINAL	NR	STROKE	NR
GENERAL SURGERY	NR	VASCULAR	NR
MATERNITY CARE	NR	WOMEN'S HEALTH	NR

HEALTHGRADES AWARDS

Randolph County Medical Center

2801 Medical Center Drive
Pocahontas, AR 72455
(870) 892-6000

Overall patient safety: ★★★
Teaching: N

CLINICAL PROGRAM RATINGS:

CARDIAC	NR	ORTHOPEDICS	NR
CRITICAL CARE	NR	PULMONARY	★★★
GASTROINTESTINAL	NR	STROKE	★★★
GENERAL SURGERY	NR	VASCULAR	NR
MATERNITY CARE	NR	WOMEN'S HEALTH	NR

HEALTHGRADES AWARDS

St. Bernards Medical Center

225 East Jackson
Jonesboro, AR 72401
(870) 972-4100

Overall patient safety: ★
Teaching: Y

CLINICAL PROGRAM RATINGS:

CARDIAC	★	ORTHOPEDICS	★★★
CRITICAL CARE	NR	PULMONARY	★
GASTROINTESTINAL	★	STROKE	★★★
GENERAL SURGERY	NR	VASCULAR	★★★
MATERNITY CARE	NR	WOMEN'S HEALTH	NR

HEALTHGRADES AWARDS

*This hospital reports its data to the federal government jointly with another hospital. Therefore the ratings and awards apply to multiple hospitals and this specific hospital may not provide all rated services.

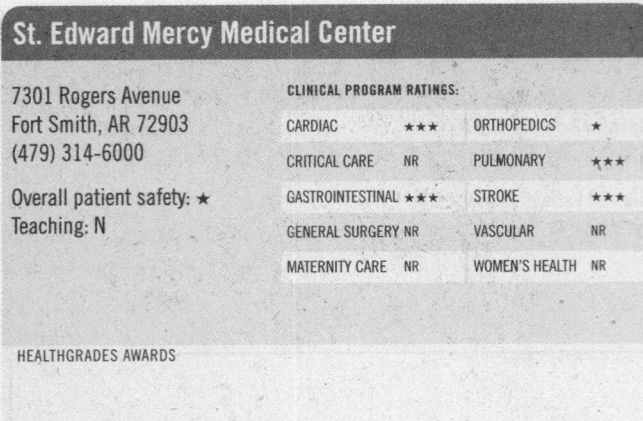

St. Edward Mercy Medical Center

7301 Rogers Avenue
Fort Smith, AR 72903
(479) 314-6000

Overall patient safety: ★
Teaching: N

CLINICAL PROGRAM RATINGS:

CARDIAC	★★★	ORTHOPEDICS	★
CRITICAL CARE	NR	PULMONARY	★★★
GASTROINTESTINAL	★★★	STROKE	★★★
GENERAL SURGERY	NR	VASCULAR	NR
MATERNITY CARE	NR	WOMEN'S HEALTH	NR

HEALTHGRADES AWARDS

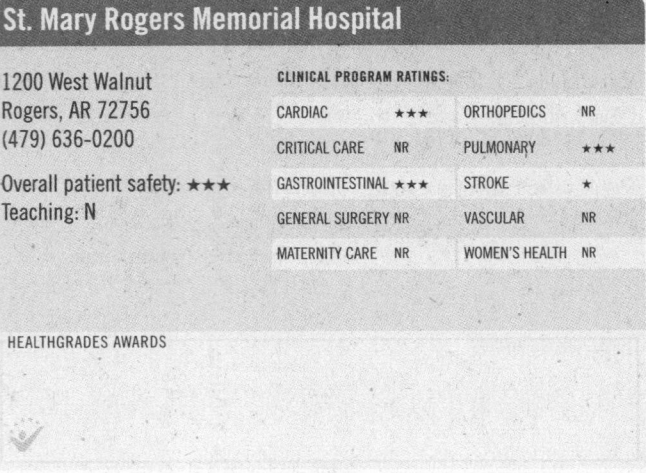

St. Mary Rogers Memorial Hospital

1200 West Walnut
Rogers, AR 72756
(479) 636-0200

Overall patient safety: ★★★
Teaching: N

CLINICAL PROGRAM RATINGS:

CARDIAC	★★★	ORTHOPEDICS	NR
CRITICAL CARE	NR	PULMONARY	★★★
GASTROINTESTINAL	★★★	STROKE	★
GENERAL SURGERY	NR	VASCULAR	NR
MATERNITY CARE	NR	WOMEN'S HEALTH	NR

HEALTHGRADES AWARDS

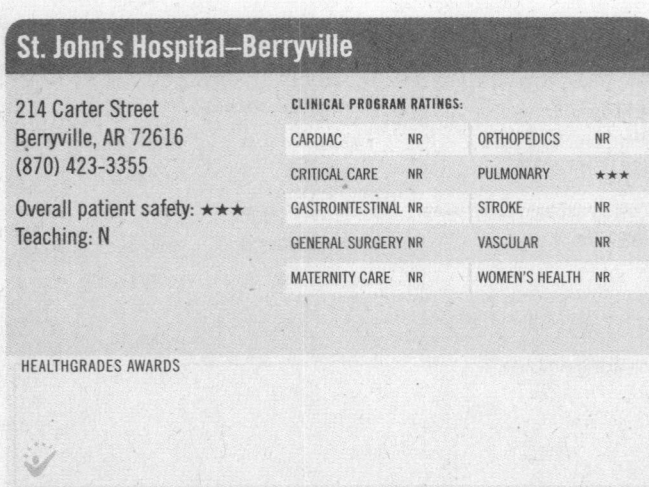

St. John's Hospital–Berryville

214 Carter Street
Berryville, AR 72616
(870) 423-3355

Overall patient safety: ★★★
Teaching: N

CLINICAL PROGRAM RATINGS:

CARDIAC	NR	ORTHOPEDICS	NR
CRITICAL CARE	NR	PULMONARY	★★★
GASTROINTESTINAL	NR	STROKE	NR
GENERAL SURGERY	NR	VASCULAR	NR
MATERNITY CARE	NR	WOMEN'S HEALTH	NR

HEALTHGRADES AWARDS

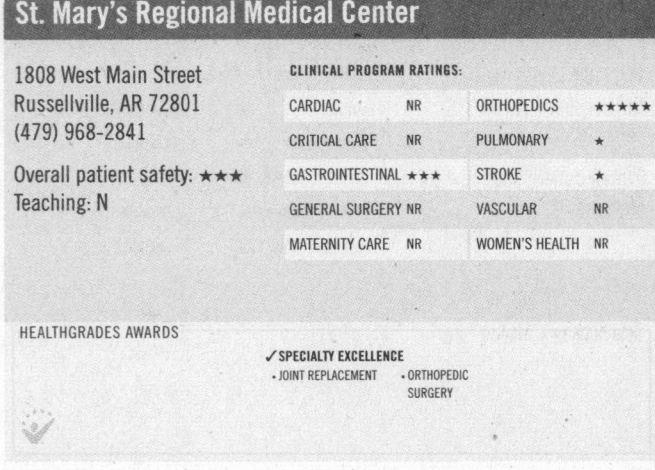

St. Mary's Regional Medical Center

1808 West Main Street
Russellville, AR 72801
(479) 968-2841

Overall patient safety: ★★★
Teaching: N

CLINICAL PROGRAM RATINGS:

CARDIAC	NR	ORTHOPEDICS	★★★★★
CRITICAL CARE	NR	PULMONARY	★
GASTROINTESTINAL	★★★	STROKE	★
GENERAL SURGERY	NR	VASCULAR	NR
MATERNITY CARE	NR	WOMEN'S HEALTH	NR

HEALTHGRADES AWARDS

✓ SPECIALTY EXCELLENCE
- JOINT REPLACEMENT
- ORTHOPEDIC SURGERY

St. Joseph's Mercy Health Center

300 Werner Street
Hot Springs, AR 71913
(501) 622-1000

Overall patient safety: ★★★
Teaching: N

CLINICAL PROGRAM RATINGS:

CARDIAC	★★★	ORTHOPEDICS	★★★★★
CRITICAL CARE	NR	PULMONARY	★★★★★
GASTROINTESTINAL	★★★	STROKE	★★★
GENERAL SURGERY	NR	VASCULAR	NR
MATERNITY CARE	NR	WOMEN'S HEALTH	NR

HEALTHGRADES AWARDS

✓ SPECIALTY EXCELLENCE
- ORTHOPEDIC SURGERY
- PULMONARY CARE

St. Vincent Doctors Hospital

6101 St. Vincent Circle
Little Rock, AR 72205
(501) 603-6000

Overall patient safety: ★★★★★
Teaching: Y

CLINICAL PROGRAM RATINGS:

CARDIAC	★★★	ORTHOPEDICS	★★★★★
CRITICAL CARE	NR	PULMONARY	★★★
GASTROINTESTINAL	★★★	STROKE	★★★
GENERAL SURGERY	NR	VASCULAR	★★★
MATERNITY CARE	NR	WOMEN'S HEALTH	NR

HEALTHGRADES AWARDS

✓ DISTINGUISHED HOSPITAL
- PATIENT SAFETY

✓ SPECIALTY EXCELLENCE
- JOINT REPLACEMENT
- ORTHOPEDIC SURGERY

KEY: ★★★★★ BEST   ★★★ AS EXPECTED   ★ POOR   NR NOT RATED BY HEALTHGRADES   For full definitions of ratings and awards, see Appendix.

St. Vincent Infirmary Medical Center

2 St. Vincent Circle
Little Rock, AR 72205
(501) 552-3000

Overall patient safety: ★★★★★
Teaching: Y

CLINICAL PROGRAM RATINGS:

CARDIAC	★★★	ORTHOPEDICS	★★★★★
CRITICAL CARE	NR	PULMONARY	★★★
GASTROINTESTINAL	★★★	STROKE	★★★
GENERAL SURGERY	NR	VASCULAR	★★★
MATERNITY CARE	NR	WOMEN'S HEALTH	NR

HEALTHGRADES AWARDS

✓ **DISTINGUISHED HOSPITAL**
• PATIENT SAFETY

✓ **SPECIALTY EXCELLENCE**
• JOINT REPLACEMENT
• ORTHOPEDIC SURGERY

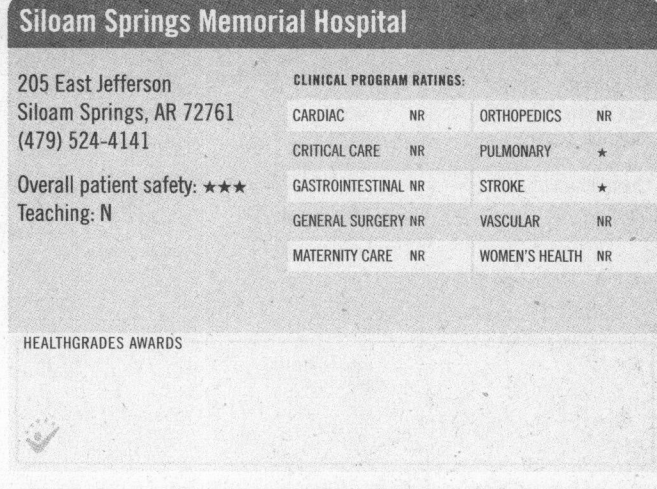

Siloam Springs Memorial Hospital

205 East Jefferson
Siloam Springs, AR 72761
(479) 524-4141

Overall patient safety: ★★★
Teaching: N

CLINICAL PROGRAM RATINGS:

CARDIAC	NR	ORTHOPEDICS	NR
CRITICAL CARE		PULMONARY	★
GASTROINTESTINAL	NR	STROKE	★
GENERAL SURGERY	NR	VASCULAR	NR
MATERNITY CARE	NR	WOMEN'S HEALTH	NR

HEALTHGRADES AWARDS

St. Vincent Medical Center–North

2215 Wildwood Avenue
Sherwood, AR 72120
(501) 552-7100

Overall patient safety: ★★★
Teaching: N

CLINICAL PROGRAM RATINGS:

CARDIAC	NR	ORTHOPEDICS	NR
CRITICAL CARE	NR	PULMONARY	★★★
GASTROINTESTINAL	NR	STROKE	★
GENERAL SURGERY	NR	VASCULAR	NR
MATERNITY CARE	NR	WOMEN'S HEALTH	NR

HEALTHGRADES AWARDS

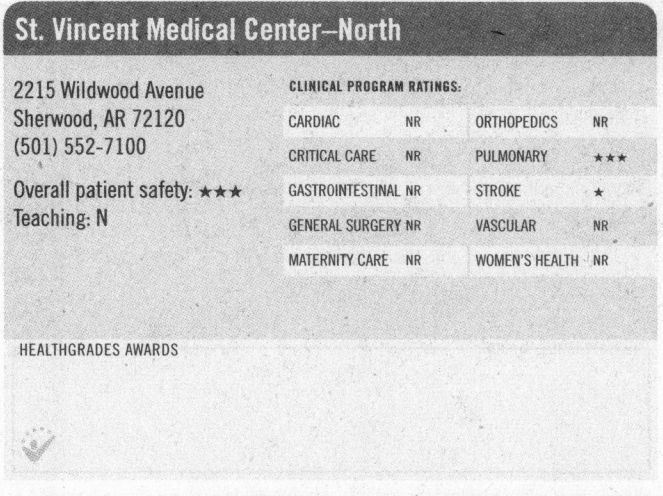

SMC Regional Medical Center

611 West Lee Avenue
Osceola, AR 72370
(870) 563-7000

Overall patient safety: ★★★
Teaching: N

CLINICAL PROGRAM RATINGS:

CARDIAC	NR	ORTHOPEDICS	NR
CRITICAL CARE	NR	PULMONARY	★
GASTROINTESTINAL	NR	STROKE	★★★
GENERAL SURGERY	NR	VASCULAR	NR
MATERNITY CARE	NR	WOMEN'S HEALTH	NR

HEALTHGRADES AWARDS

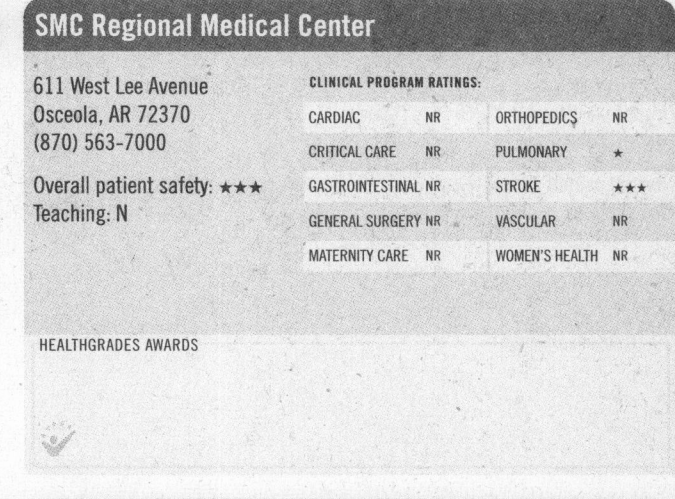

Saline Memorial Hospital

1 Medical Parks Drive
Benton, AR 72015
(501) 776-6000

Overall patient safety: ★★★
Teaching: N

CLINICAL PROGRAM RATINGS:

CARDIAC	NR	ORTHOPEDICS	NR
CRITICAL CARE	NR	PULMONARY	★
GASTROINTESTINAL	★★★	STROKE	★
GENERAL SURGERY	NR	VASCULAR	NR
MATERNITY CARE	NR	WOMEN'S HEALTH	NR

HEALTHGRADES AWARDS

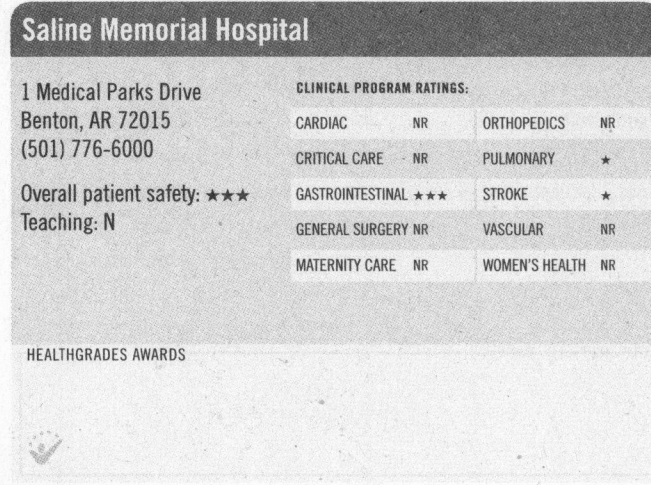

Southwest Regional Medical Center

11401 Interstate 30
Little Rock, AR 72209
(501) 455-7100

Overall patient safety: ★★★
Teaching: N

CLINICAL PROGRAM RATINGS:

CARDIAC	NR	ORTHOPEDICS	NR
CRITICAL CARE	NR	PULMONARY	★★★★★
GASTROINTESTINAL	NR	STROKE	NR
GENERAL SURGERY	NR	VASCULAR	NR
MATERNITY CARE	NR	WOMEN'S HEALTH	NR

HEALTHGRADES AWARDS

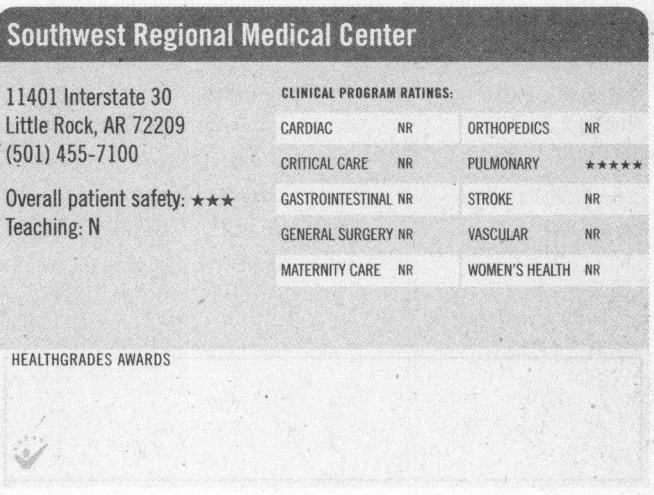

Sparks Regional Medical Center

1311 South I Street
Fort Smith, AR 72901
(479) 441-4000

Overall patient safety: ★★★
Teaching: Y

CLINICAL PROGRAM RATINGS:

CARDIAC	★	ORTHOPEDICS	★★★
CRITICAL CARE	NR	PULMONARY	★★★★★
GASTROINTESTINAL	★★★	STROKE	★★★
GENERAL SURGERY	NR	VASCULAR	★★★
MATERNITY CARE	NR	WOMEN'S HEALTH	NR

HEALTHGRADES AWARDS

✓ SPECIALTY EXCELLENCE
· PULMONARY CARE

Summit Medical Center

East Main and
South 20th Streets
Van Buren, AR 72956
(479) 474-3401

Overall patient safety: ★★★
Teaching: N

CLINICAL PROGRAM RATINGS:

CARDIAC	NR	ORTHOPEDICS	NR
CRITICAL CARE	NR	PULMONARY	★
GASTROINTESTINAL	NR	STROKE	NR
GENERAL SURGERY	NR	VASCULAR	NR
MATERNITY CARE	NR	WOMEN'S HEALTH	NR

HEALTHGRADES AWARDS

Stone County Medical Center

Highway 14 East
Mountain View, AR 72560
(870) 269-4361

Overall patient safety: ★★★
Teaching: N

CLINICAL PROGRAM RATINGS:

CARDIAC	NR	ORTHOPEDICS	NR
CRITICAL CARE	NR	PULMONARY	★★★
GASTROINTESTINAL	NR	STROKE	NR
GENERAL SURGERY	NR	VASCULAR	NR
MATERNITY CARE	NR	WOMEN'S HEALTH	NR

HEALTHGRADES AWARDS

UAMS Medical Center

4301 West Markham Street
Little Rock, AR 72205
(501) 686-7000

Overall patient safety: ★
Teaching: Y

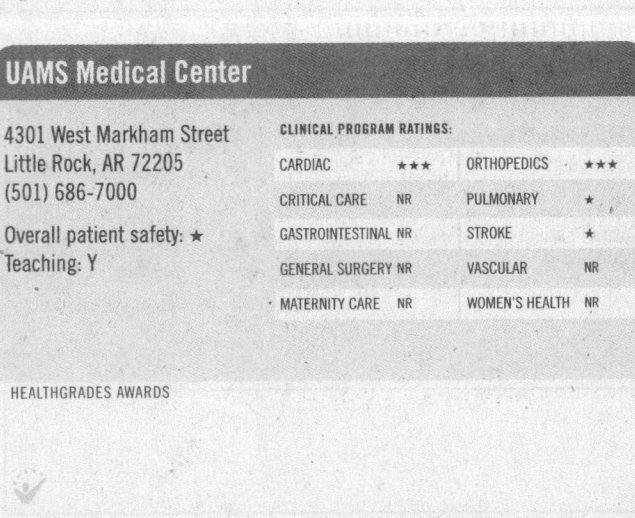

CLINICAL PROGRAM RATINGS:

CARDIAC	★★★	ORTHOPEDICS	★★★
CRITICAL CARE	NR	PULMONARY	★
GASTROINTESTINAL	NR	STROKE	★
GENERAL SURGERY	NR	VASCULAR	NR
MATERNITY CARE	NR	WOMEN'S HEALTH	NR

HEALTHGRADES AWARDS

Stuttgart Regional Medical Center

1703 North Buerkle Road
Stuttgart, AR 72160
(870) 673-3511

Overall patient safety: ★★★
Teaching: N

CLINICAL PROGRAM RATINGS:

CARDIAC	NR	ORTHOPEDICS	NR
CRITICAL CARE	NR	PULMONARY	★★★
GASTROINTESTINAL	NR	STROKE	★
GENERAL SURGERY	NR	VASCULAR	NR
MATERNITY CARE	NR	WOMEN'S HEALTH	NR

HEALTHGRADES AWARDS

Washington Regional Medical Center at North Hills

3215 North Hill Boulevard
Fayetteville, AR 72703
(479) 713-1000

Overall patient safety: ★★★
Teaching: Y

CLINICAL PROGRAM RATINGS:

CARDIAC	★★★	ORTHOPEDICS	★
CRITICAL CARE	NR	PULMONARY	★★★
GASTROINTESTINAL	★★★	STROKE	★★★
GENERAL SURGERY	NR	VASCULAR	★★★
MATERNITY CARE	NR	WOMEN'S HEALTH	NR

HEALTHGRADES AWARDS

KEY: ★★★★★ BEST   ★★★ AS EXPECTED   ★ POOR   NR NOT RATED BY HEALTHGRADES   For full definitions of ratings and awards, see Appendix.

White County Medical Center—North Campus

3214 East Race Street
Searcy, AR 72143
(501) 268-6121

Overall patient safety: ★★★
Teaching: N

CLINICAL PROGRAM RATINGS:

CARDIAC	★★★	ORTHOPEDICS	★★★
CRITICAL CARE	NR	PULMONARY	★★★
GASTROINTESTINAL	★★★	STROKE	★★★
GENERAL SURGERY	NR	VASCULAR	NR
MATERNITY CARE	NR	WOMEN'S HEALTH	NR

HEALTHGRADES AWARDS

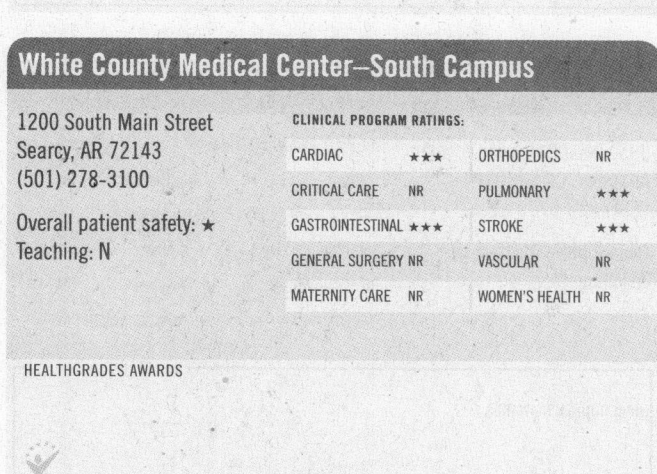

White River Medical Center

1710 Harrison Street
Batesville, AR 72501
(870) 793-1200

Overall patient safety: ★★★
Teaching: Y

CLINICAL PROGRAM RATINGS:

CARDIAC	NR	ORTHOPEDICS	NR
CRITICAL CARE	NR	PULMONARY	★★★
GASTROINTESTINAL	★★★	STROKE	★★★
GENERAL SURGERY	NR	VASCULAR	NR
MATERNITY CARE	NR	WOMEN'S HEALTH	NR

HEALTHGRADES AWARDS

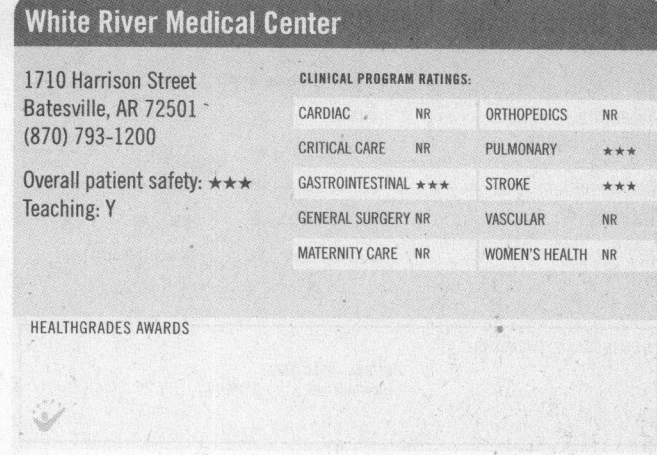

White County Medical Center—South Campus

1200 South Main Street
Searcy, AR 72143
(501) 278-3100

Overall patient safety: ★
Teaching: N

CLINICAL PROGRAM RATINGS:

CARDIAC	★★★	ORTHOPEDICS	NR
CRITICAL CARE	NR	PULMONARY	★★★
GASTROINTESTINAL	★★★	STROKE	★★★
GENERAL SURGERY	NR	VASCULAR	NR
MATERNITY CARE	NR	WOMEN'S HEALTH	NR

HEALTHGRADES AWARDS

CALIFORNIA HOSPITALS: RATINGS BY CLINICAL SPECIALTY

Alameda County Medical Center

15400 Foothill Boulevard
San Leandro, CA 94578
(510) 437-4800

Overall patient safety: ★
Teaching: Y

CLINICAL PROGRAM RATINGS:

CARDIAC	NR	ORTHOPEDICS	NR
CRITICAL CARE	NR	PULMONARY	★★★
GASTROINTESTINAL	NR	STROKE	★
GENERAL SURGERY	NR	VASCULAR	NR
MATERNITY CARE	★★★	WOMEN'S HEALTH	NR

HEALTHGRADES AWARDS

Alameda Hospital

2070 Clinton Avenue
Alameda, CA 94501
(510) 522-3700

Overall patient safety: ★
Teaching: N

CLINICAL PROGRAM RATINGS:

CARDIAC	NR	ORTHOPEDICS	NR
CRITICAL CARE	NR	PULMONARY	★★★
GASTROINTESTINAL	NR	STROKE	★★★
GENERAL SURGERY	NR	VASCULAR	NR
MATERNITY CARE	NR	WOMEN'S HEALTH	NR

HEALTHGRADES AWARDS

Alhambra Hospital and Medical Center

100 South Raymond Avenue
Alhambra, CA 91801
(626) 570-1606

Overall patient safety: ★★★★★
Teaching: N

CLINICAL PROGRAM RATINGS:

CARDIAC	NR	ORTHOPEDICS	NR
CRITICAL CARE	NR	PULMONARY	★★★★★
GASTROINTESTINAL	NR	STROKE	★★★★★
GENERAL SURGERY	NR	VASCULAR	NR
MATERNITY CARE	NR	WOMEN'S HEALTH	NR

HEALTHGRADES AWARDS

✓ SPECIALTY EXCELLENCE
· PULMONARY CARE   · STROKE CARE

Alvarado Hospital Medical Center

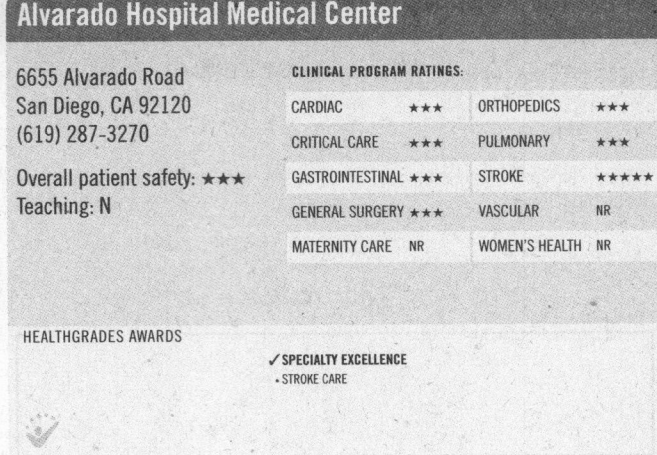

6655 Alvarado Road
San Diego, CA 92120
(619) 287-3270

Overall patient safety: ★★★
Teaching: N

CLINICAL PROGRAM RATINGS:

CARDIAC	★★★	ORTHOPEDICS	★★★
CRITICAL CARE	★★★	PULMONARY	★★★
GASTROINTESTINAL	★★★	STROKE	★★★★★
GENERAL SURGERY	★★★	VASCULAR	NR
MATERNITY CARE	NR	WOMEN'S HEALTH	NR

HEALTHGRADES AWARDS

✓ SPECIALTY EXCELLENCE
· STROKE CARE

Alta Bates Summit—Alta Bates Campus

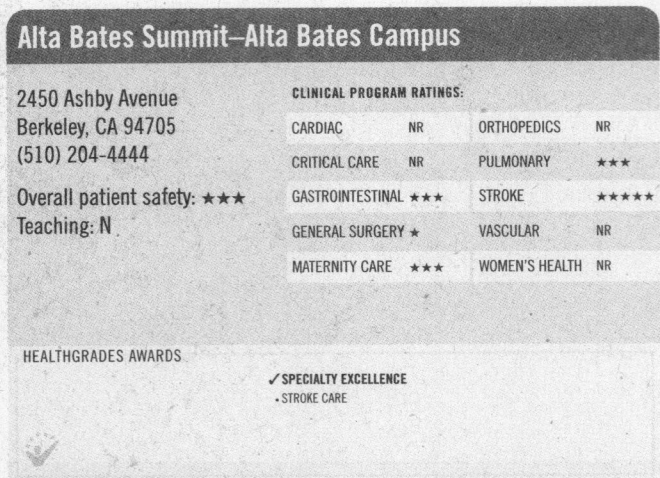

2450 Ashby Avenue
Berkeley, CA 94705
(510) 204-4444

Overall patient safety: ★★★
Teaching: N

CLINICAL PROGRAM RATINGS:

CARDIAC	NR	ORTHOPEDICS	NR
CRITICAL CARE	NR	PULMONARY	★★★
GASTROINTESTINAL	★★★	STROKE	★★★★★
GENERAL SURGERY	★	VASCULAR	NR
MATERNITY CARE	★★★	WOMEN'S HEALTH	NR

HEALTHGRADES AWARDS

✓ SPECIALTY EXCELLENCE
· STROKE CARE

Anaheim General Hospital

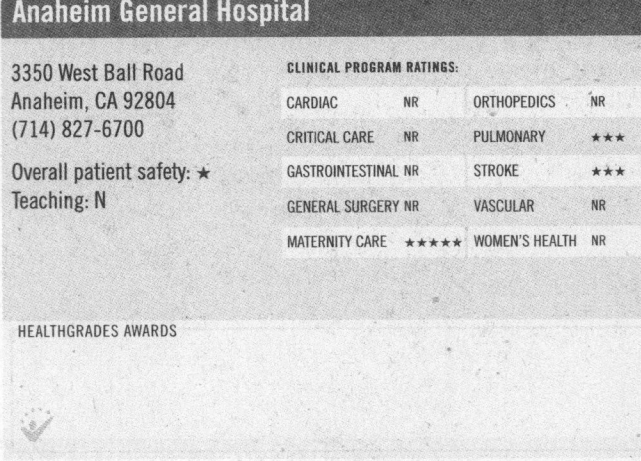

3350 West Ball Road
Anaheim, CA 92804
(714) 827-6700

Overall patient safety: ★
Teaching: N

CLINICAL PROGRAM RATINGS:

CARDIAC	NR	ORTHOPEDICS	NR
CRITICAL CARE	NR	PULMONARY	★★★
GASTROINTESTINAL	NR	STROKE	★★★
GENERAL SURGERY	NR	VASCULAR	NR
MATERNITY CARE	★★★★★	WOMEN'S HEALTH	NR

HEALTHGRADES AWARDS

Alta Bates Summit—Summit Campus

350 Hawthorne Avenue
Oakland, CA 94609
(510) 655-4000

Overall patient safety: ★★★
Teaching: Y

CLINICAL PROGRAM RATINGS:

CARDIAC	★★★	ORTHOPEDICS	NR
CRITICAL CARE	★★★★★	PULMONARY	★★★★★
GASTROINTESTINAL	★★★	STROKE	★★★★★
GENERAL SURGERY	★★★	VASCULAR	NR
MATERNITY CARE	NR	WOMEN'S HEALTH	NR

HEALTHGRADES AWARDS

✓ SPECIALTY EXCELLENCE
· CRITICAL CARE   · PULMONARY CARE   · STROKE CARE

Anaheim Memorial Hospital

1111 West La Palma Avenue
Anaheim, CA 92801
(714) 774-1450

Overall patient safety: ★★★
Teaching: N

CLINICAL PROGRAM RATINGS:

CARDIAC	★★★	ORTHOPEDICS	NR
CRITICAL CARE	NR	PULMONARY	★★★★★
GASTROINTESTINAL	★★★	STROKE	★★★
GENERAL SURGERY	★★★	VASCULAR	NR
MATERNITY CARE	★★★	WOMEN'S HEALTH	★★★

HEALTHGRADES AWARDS

✓ SPECIALTY EXCELLENCE
· CARDIAC SURGERY

KEY: ★★★★★ BEST   ★★★ AS EXPECTED   ★ POOR   NR NOT RATED BY HEALTHGRADES   For full definitions of ratings and awards, see Appendix.

Antelope Valley Hospital

1600 West Avenue J
Lancaster, CA 93534
(661) 949-5000

Overall patient safety: ★★★
Teaching: N

CLINICAL PROGRAM RATINGS:

CARDIAC	★★★	ORTHOPEDICS	NR
CRITICAL CARE	★★★	PULMONARY	★★★
GASTROINTESTINAL	★★★	STROKE	★★★★★
GENERAL SURGERY	★★★	VASCULAR	NR
MATERNITY CARE	★★★★★	WOMEN'S HEALTH	★★★

HEALTHGRADES AWARDS

✓ SPECIALTY EXCELLENCE
• MATERNITY CARE

Bakersfield Heart Hospital

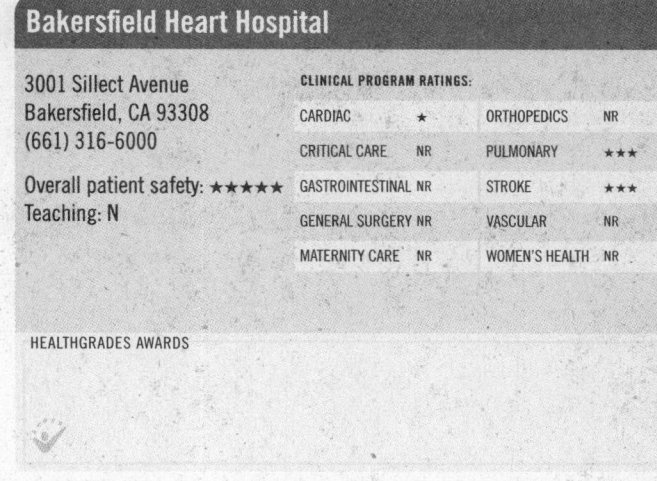

3001 Sillect Avenue
Bakersfield, CA 93308
(661) 316-6000

Overall patient safety: ★★★★★
Teaching: N

CLINICAL PROGRAM RATINGS:

CARDIAC	★	ORTHOPEDICS	NR
CRITICAL CARE	NR	PULMONARY	★★★
GASTROINTESTINAL	NR	STROKE	★★★
GENERAL SURGERY	NR	VASCULAR	NR
MATERNITY CARE	NR	WOMEN'S HEALTH	NR

HEALTHGRADES AWARDS

Arrowhead Regional Medical Center

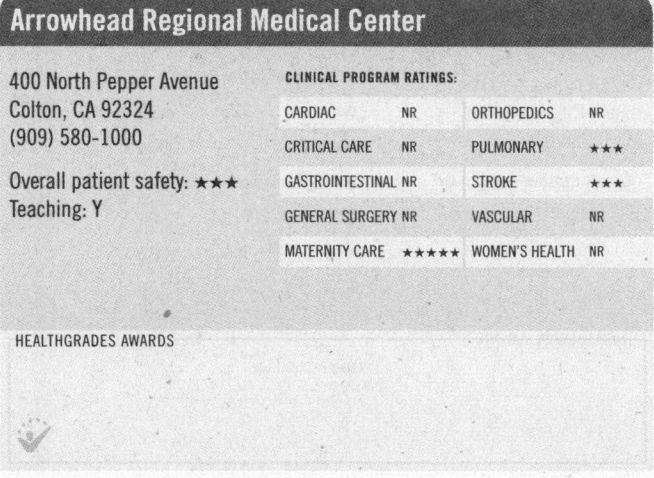

400 North Pepper Avenue
Colton, CA 92324
(909) 580-1000

Overall patient safety: ★★★
Teaching: Y

CLINICAL PROGRAM RATINGS:

CARDIAC	NR	ORTHOPEDICS	NR
CRITICAL CARE	NR	PULMONARY	★★★
GASTROINTESTINAL	NR	STROKE	★★★
GENERAL SURGERY	NR	VASCULAR	NR
MATERNITY CARE	★★★★★	WOMEN'S HEALTH	NR

HEALTHGRADES AWARDS

Bakersfield Memorial Hospital

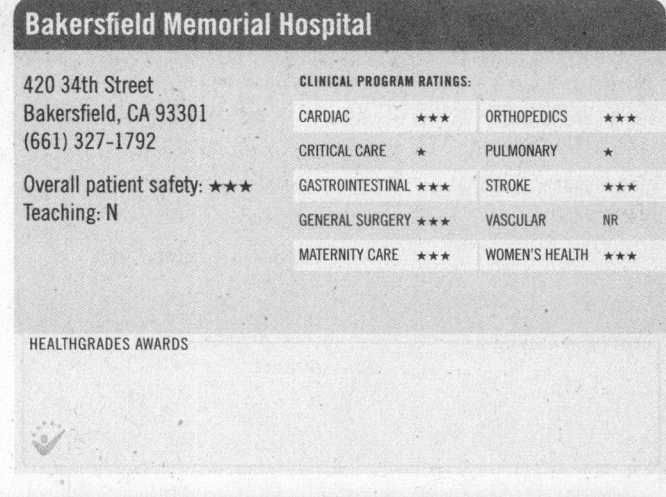

420 34th Street
Bakersfield, CA 93301
(661) 327-1792

Overall patient safety: ★★★
Teaching: N

CLINICAL PROGRAM RATINGS:

CARDIAC	★★★	ORTHOPEDICS	★★★
CRITICAL CARE	★	PULMONARY	★
GASTROINTESTINAL	★★★	STROKE	★★★
GENERAL SURGERY	★★★	VASCULAR	NR
MATERNITY CARE	★★★	WOMEN'S HEALTH	★★★

HEALTHGRADES AWARDS

Arroyo Grande Community Hospital

345 South Halcyon Road
Arroyo Grande, CA 93420
(805) 489-4261

Overall patient safety: ★★★
Teaching: N

CLINICAL PROGRAM RATINGS:

CARDIAC	NR	ORTHOPEDICS	NR
CRITICAL CARE	NR	PULMONARY	★
GASTROINTESTINAL	NR	STROKE	★★★
GENERAL SURGERY	★★★	VASCULAR	NR
MATERNITY CARE	NR	WOMEN'S HEALTH	NR

HEALTHGRADES AWARDS

Banner Lassen Medical Center

1800 Spring Ridge Drive
Susanville, CA 96130
(530) 252-2000

Overall patient safety: NR
Teaching: N

CLINICAL PROGRAM RATINGS:

CARDIAC	NR	ORTHOPEDICS	NR
CRITICAL CARE	NR	PULMONARY	★★★
GASTROINTESTINAL	NR	STROKE	★★★
GENERAL SURGERY	NR	VASCULAR	NR
MATERNITY CARE	NR	WOMEN'S HEALTH	NR

HEALTHGRADES AWARDS

Barstow Community Hospital

555 South 7th Avenue
Barstow, CA 92311
(760) 256-1761

Overall patient safety: ★★★
Teaching: N

CLINICAL PROGRAM RATINGS:

CARDIAC	NR	ORTHOPEDICS	NR
CRITICAL CARE	NR	PULMONARY	★★★
GASTROINTESTINAL	NR	STROKE	★★★
GENERAL SURGERY	★★★	VASCULAR	NR
MATERNITY CARE	★★★	WOMEN'S HEALTH	NR

HEALTHGRADES AWARDS

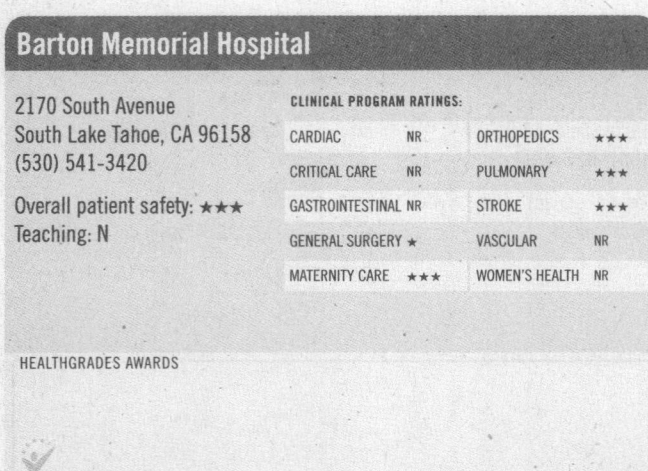

Beverly Hospital

309 West Beverly Boulevard
Montebello, CA 90640
(323) 726-1222

Overall patient safety: ★★★
Teaching: N

CLINICAL PROGRAM RATINGS:

CARDIAC	★★★	ORTHOPEDICS	NR
CRITICAL CARE	NR	PULMONARY	★★★★★
GASTROINTESTINAL	★★★	STROKE	★★★★★
GENERAL SURGERY	★★★	VASCULAR	NR
MATERNITY CARE	★★★	WOMEN'S HEALTH	NR

HEALTHGRADES AWARDS

✓ DISTINGUISHED HOSPITAL
· CLINICAL EXCELLENCE

✓ SPECIALTY EXCELLENCE
· PULMONARY CARE   · STROKE CARE

Barton Memorial Hospital

2170 South Avenue
South Lake Tahoe, CA 96158
(530) 541-3420

Overall patient safety: ★★★
Teaching: N

CLINICAL PROGRAM RATINGS:

CARDIAC	NR	ORTHOPEDICS	★★★
CRITICAL CARE	NR	PULMONARY	★★★
GASTROINTESTINAL	NR	STROKE	★★★
GENERAL SURGERY	★	VASCULAR	NR
MATERNITY CARE	★★★	WOMEN'S HEALTH	NR

HEALTHGRADES AWARDS

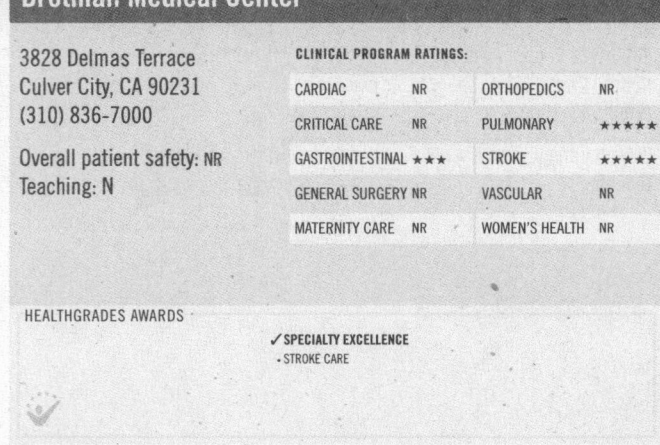

Brotman Medical Center

3828 Delmas Terrace
Culver City, CA 90231
(310) 836-7000

Overall patient safety: NR
Teaching: N

CLINICAL PROGRAM RATINGS:

CARDIAC	NR	ORTHOPEDICS	NR
CRITICAL CARE	NR	PULMONARY	★★★★★
GASTROINTESTINAL	★★★	STROKE	★★★★★
GENERAL SURGERY	NR	VASCULAR	NR
MATERNITY CARE	NR	WOMEN'S HEALTH	NR

HEALTHGRADES AWARDS

✓ SPECIALTY EXCELLENCE
· STROKE CARE

Bellflower Medical Center

9542 East Artesia Boulevard
Bellflower, CA 90706
(562) 925-8355

Overall patient safety: ★★★
Teaching: N

CLINICAL PROGRAM RATINGS:

CARDIAC	NR	ORTHOPEDICS	NR
CRITICAL CARE	NR	PULMONARY	★★★★★
GASTROINTESTINAL	NR	STROKE	NR
GENERAL SURGERY	NR	VASCULAR	NR
MATERNITY CARE	★★★	WOMEN'S HEALTH	NR

HEALTHGRADES AWARDS

✓ SPECIALTY EXCELLENCE
· PULMONARY CARE

California Hospital Medical Center--Los Angeles

1401 South Grand Avenue
Los Angeles, CA 90015
(213) 748-2411

Overall patient safety: ★
Teaching: Y

CLINICAL PROGRAM RATINGS:

CARDIAC	NR	ORTHOPEDICS	NR
CRITICAL CARE	NR	PULMONARY	★★★
GASTROINTESTINAL	NR	STROKE	★★★★★
GENERAL SURGERY	★★★	VASCULAR	NR
MATERNITY CARE	★★★	WOMEN'S HEALTH	NR

HEALTHGRADES AWARDS

✓ SPECIALTY EXCELLENCE
· STROKE CARE

KEY: ★★★★★ BEST   ★★★ AS EXPECTED   ★ POOR   NR NOT RATED BY HEALTHGRADES   For full definitions of ratings and awards, see Appendix.

California Pacific Medical Center*

3700 California Street
San Francisco, CA 94118
(415) 387-8700

Overall patient safety: ★★★
Teaching: Y

CLINICAL PROGRAM RATINGS:

CARDIAC	★★★	ORTHOPEDICS	★★★
CRITICAL CARE	★★★	PULMONARY	★★★★★
GASTROINTESTINAL	★★★	STROKE	★★★★★
GENERAL SURGERY	★★★	VASCULAR	★★★
MATERNITY CARE	★★★	WOMEN'S HEALTH	★★★

HEALTHGRADES AWARDS

✓ SPECIALTY EXCELLENCE
- JOINT REPLACEMENT   - PULMONARY CARE   - STROKE CARE

Cedars-Sinai Medical Center

8700 Beverly Boulevard
Los Angeles, CA 90048
(310) 423-3277

Overall patient safety: ★★★
Teaching: Y

CLINICAL PROGRAM RATINGS:

CARDIAC	★★★	ORTHOPEDICS	★★★
CRITICAL CARE	★★★★★	PULMONARY	★★★★★
GASTROINTESTINAL	★★★★★	STROKE	★★★★★
GENERAL SURGERY	★★★	VASCULAR	★★★
MATERNITY CARE	★★★	WOMEN'S HEALTH	★★★★★

HEALTHGRADES AWARDS

✓ AMERICA'S 50 BEST HOSPITALS   ✓ DISTINGUISHED HOSPITAL   ✓ SPECIALTY EXCELLENCE
- CLINICAL EXCELLENCE
- CARDIAC CARE   - GASTROINTESTINAL CARE   - PULMONARY CARE
- CARDIAC SURGERY   - GENERAL SURGERY   - STROKE CARE
- CRITICAL CARE

California Pacific Medical Center–Davies Campus

Castro at Duboce Streets
San Francisco, CA 94114
(415) 600-6000

Overall patient safety: ★★★
Teaching: N

CLINICAL PROGRAM RATINGS:

CARDIAC	NR	ORTHOPEDICS	NR
CRITICAL CARE	NR	PULMONARY	★★★
GASTROINTESTINAL	NR	STROKE	★★★
GENERAL SURGERY	NR	VASCULAR	NR
MATERNITY CARE	NR	WOMEN'S HEALTH	NR

HEALTHGRADES AWARDS

Centinela Freeman Regional Medical Center–Centinela

555 East Hardy Street
Inglewood, CA 90301
(310) 673-4660

Overall patient safety: ★
Teaching: Y

CLINICAL PROGRAM RATINGS:

CARDIAC	★★★	ORTHOPEDICS	★★★
CRITICAL CARE	★★★	PULMONARY	★★★
GASTROINTESTINAL	★★★	STROKE	★★★★★
GENERAL SURGERY	★★★	VASCULAR	NR
MATERNITY CARE	★★★	WOMEN'S HEALTH	★★★

HEALTHGRADES AWARDS

✓ SPECIALTY EXCELLENCE
- JOINT REPLACEMENT   - STROKE CARE

The Cancer Center at Riverside Community Hospital*

5900 Brockton Avenue
Riverside, CA 92506
(714) 788-3000

Overall patient safety: ★
Teaching: N

CLINICAL PROGRAM RATINGS:

CARDIAC	★★★	ORTHOPEDICS	★★★
CRITICAL CARE	NR	PULMONARY	★★★
GASTROINTESTINAL	★★★	STROKE	★★★
GENERAL SURGERY	★★★	VASCULAR	NR
MATERNITY CARE	★★★	WOMEN'S HEALTH	★★★

HEALTHGRADES AWARDS

Centinela Freeman Regional Medical Center–Marina

4650 Lincoln Boulevard
Marina Del Rey, CA 90291
(310) 823-8911

Overall patient safety: ★★★
Teaching: N

CLINICAL PROGRAM RATINGS:

CARDIAC	NR	ORTHOPEDICS	NR
CRITICAL CARE	NR	PULMONARY	★★★
GASTROINTESTINAL	NR	STROKE	★★★
GENERAL SURGERY	NR	VASCULAR	NR
MATERNITY CARE	NR	WOMEN'S HEALTH	NR

HEALTHGRADES AWARDS

---

*This hospital reports its data to the federal government jointly with another hospital. Therefore the ratings and awards apply to multiple hospitals and this specific hospital may not provide all rated services.

Centinela Freeman Regional Medical Center—Memorial

333 North Prairie Avenue
Inglewood, CA 90301
(310) 674-7050

Overall patient safety: ★
Teaching: N

CLINICAL PROGRAM RATINGS:

CARDIAC	NR	ORTHOPEDICS	NR
CRITICAL CARE	NR	PULMONARY	★★★★★
GASTROINTESTINAL	NR	STROKE	★★★★★
GENERAL SURGERY	NR	VASCULAR	NR
MATERNITY CARE	★★★	WOMEN'S HEALTH	NR

HEALTHGRADES AWARDS

✓ SPECIALTY EXCELLENCE
• PULMONARY CARE   • STROKE CARE

Chapman Medical Center

2601 East Chapman Avenue
Orange, CA 92869
(714) 633-0011

Overall patient safety: ★
Teaching: N

CLINICAL PROGRAM RATINGS:

CARDIAC	NR	ORTHOPEDICS	NR
CRITICAL CARE	NR	PULMONARY	★★★
GASTROINTESTINAL	NR	STROKE	NR
GENERAL SURGERY	NR	VASCULAR	NR
MATERNITY CARE	NR	WOMEN'S HEALTH	NR

HEALTHGRADES AWARDS

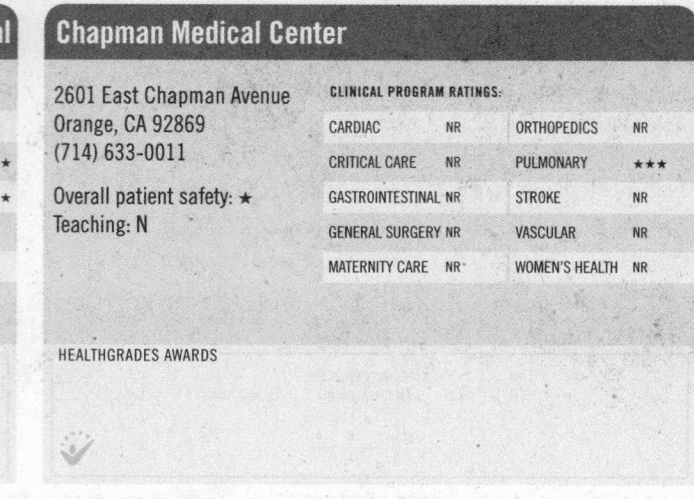

Central Valley General Hospital

1025 North Douty
Hanford, CA 93230
(559) 583-2100

Overall patient safety: ★★★
Teaching: N

CLINICAL PROGRAM RATINGS:

CARDIAC	NR	ORTHOPEDICS	NR
CRITICAL CARE	NR	PULMONARY	★
GASTROINTESTINAL	NR	STROKE	NR
GENERAL SURGERY	NR	VASCULAR	NR
MATERNITY CARE	★★★	WOMEN'S HEALTH	NR

HEALTHGRADES AWARDS

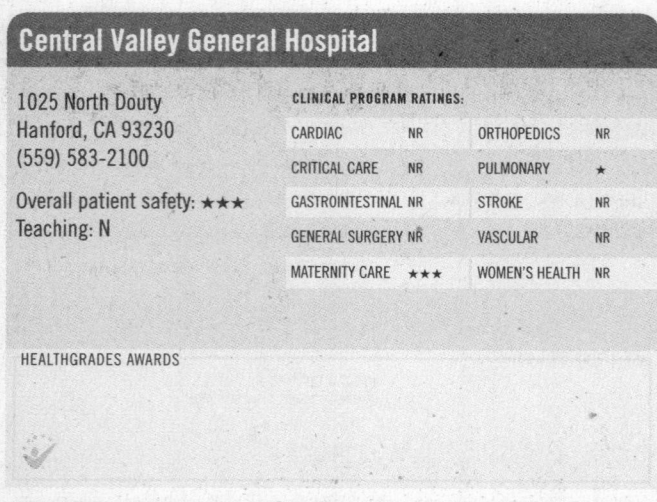

Chinese Hospital

845 Jackson Street
San Francisco, CA 94133
(415) 982-2400

Overall patient safety: ★★★
Teaching: N

CLINICAL PROGRAM RATINGS:

CARDIAC	NR	ORTHOPEDICS	NR
CRITICAL CARE	NR	PULMONARY	★★★
GASTROINTESTINAL	NR	STROKE	★★★
GENERAL SURGERY	★★★	VASCULAR	NR
MATERNITY CARE		WOMEN'S HEALTH	NR

HEALTHGRADES AWARDS

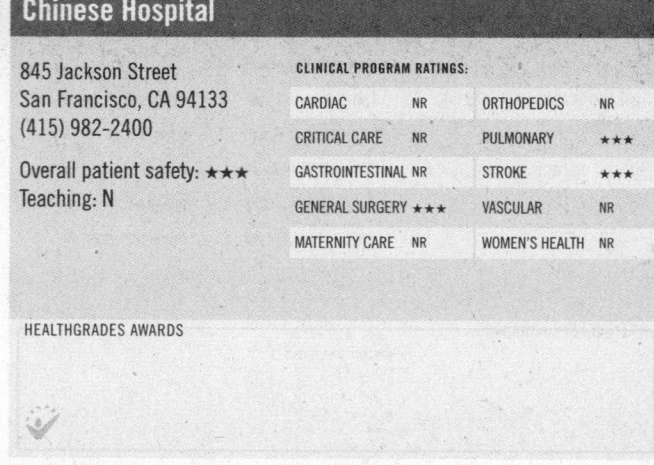

Century City Doctors Hospital

2070 Century Parks East
Los Angeles, CA 90067
(310) 772-4915

Overall patient safety: NR
Teaching: N

CLINICAL PROGRAM RATINGS:

CARDIAC	NR	ORTHOPEDICS	★
CRITICAL CARE	NR	PULMONARY	★★★
GASTROINTESTINAL	NR	STROKE	★★★★★
GENERAL SURGERY	NR	VASCULAR	NR
MATERNITY CARE	NR	WOMEN'S HEALTH	NR

HEALTHGRADES AWARDS

✓ SPECIALTY EXCELLENCE
• STROKE CARE

Chino Valley Medical Center

5451 Walnut Avenue
Chino, CA 91710
(909) 464-8600

Overall patient safety: ★★★★★
Teaching: Y

CLINICAL PROGRAM RATINGS:

CARDIAC	NR	ORTHOPEDICS	NR
CRITICAL CARE	NR	PULMONARY	★★★
GASTROINTESTINAL	NR	STROKE	★★★
GENERAL SURGERY	★★★	VASCULAR	NR
MATERNITY CARE	★★★★★	WOMEN'S HEALTH	NR

HEALTHGRADES AWARDS

✓ SPECIALTY EXCELLENCE
• MATERNITY CARE

KEY: ★★★★★ BEST   ★★★ AS EXPECTED   ★ POOR   NR NOT RATED BY HEALTHGRADES   For full definitions of ratings and awards, see Appendix.

Citrus Valley Medical Center–IC Campus

210 West San
Bernardino Road
Covina, CA 91723
(626) 331-7331

Overall patient safety: ★★★
Teaching: N

CLINICAL PROGRAM RATINGS:

CARDIAC	★★★	ORTHOPEDICS	NR
CRITICAL CARE	NR	PULMONARY	★★★
GASTROINTESTINAL	NR	STROKE	★★★★★
GENERAL SURGERY	★★★	VASCULAR	NR
MATERNITY CARE	NR	WOMEN'S HEALTH	NR

HEALTHGRADES AWARDS

✓ SPECIALTY EXCELLENCE
• STROKE CARE

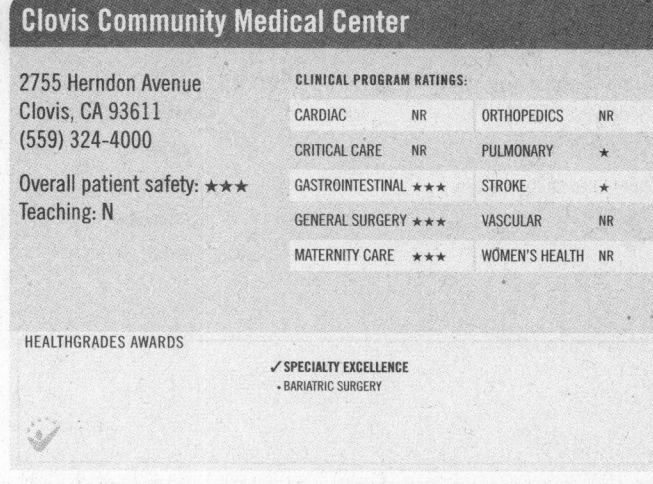

Clovis Community Medical Center

2755 Herndon Avenue
Clovis, CA 93611
(559) 324-4000

Overall patient safety: ★★★
Teaching: N

CLINICAL PROGRAM RATINGS:

CARDIAC	NR	ORTHOPEDICS	NR
CRITICAL CARE	NR	PULMONARY	★
GASTROINTESTINAL	★★★	STROKE	★
GENERAL SURGERY	★★★	VASCULAR	NR
MATERNITY CARE	★★★	WOMEN'S HEALTH	NR

HEALTHGRADES AWARDS

✓ SPECIALTY EXCELLENCE
• BARIATRIC SURGERY

Citrus Valley Medical Center–QV Campus

1115 Sunset Avenue
West Covina, CA 91790
(626) 962-4011

Overall patient safety: ★★★
Teaching: N

CLINICAL PROGRAM RATINGS:

CARDIAC	NR	ORTHOPEDICS	★★★
CRITICAL CARE	NR	PULMONARY	★★★★★
GASTROINTESTINAL	NR	STROKE	★★★★★
GENERAL SURGERY	★★★	VASCULAR	NR
MATERNITY CARE	★★★★★	WOMEN'S HEALTH	NR

HEALTHGRADES AWARDS

✓ SPECIALTY EXCELLENCE
• STROKE CARE

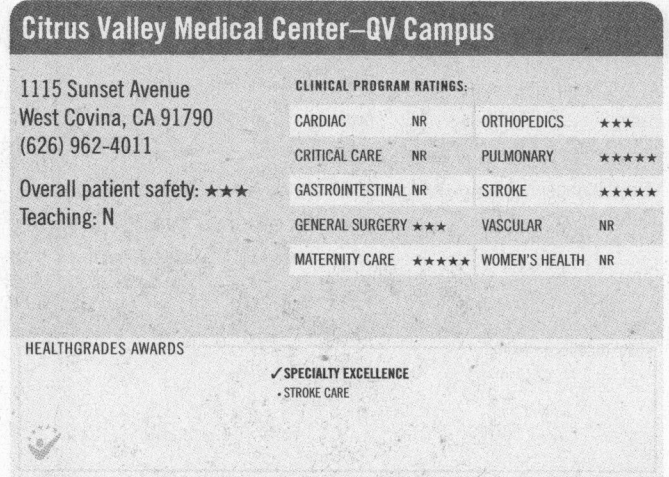

Coast Plaza Doctors Hospital

13100 Studebaker Road
Norwalk, CA 90650
(562) 868-3751

Overall patient safety: ★★★
Teaching: Y

CLINICAL PROGRAM RATINGS:

CARDIAC	NR	ORTHOPEDICS	NR
CRITICAL CARE	NR	PULMONARY	★★★
GASTROINTESTINAL	NR	STROKE	NR
GENERAL SURGERY	NR	VASCULAR	NR
MATERNITY CARE	NR	WOMEN'S HEALTH	NR

HEALTHGRADES AWARDS

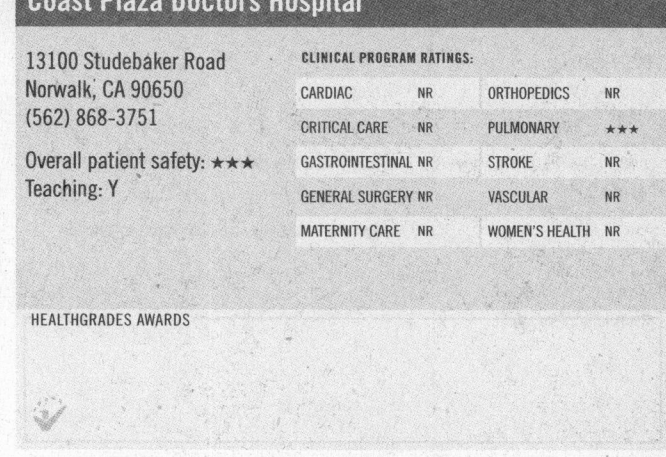

City of Angels Medical Center

1711 West Temple Street
Los Angeles, CA 90026
(213) 989-6100

Overall patient safety: ★★★
Teaching: Y

CLINICAL PROGRAM RATINGS:

CARDIAC	NR	ORTHOPEDICS	NR
CRITICAL CARE	NR	PULMONARY	★★★
GASTROINTESTINAL	NR	STROKE	★★★
GENERAL SURGERY	NR	VASCULAR	NR
MATERNITY CARE	NR	WOMEN'S HEALTH	NR

HEALTHGRADES AWARDS

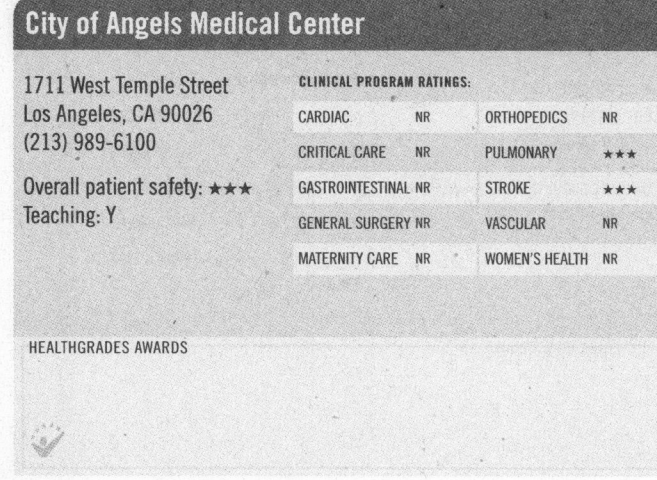

Coastal Communities Hospital

2701 South Bristol Street
Santa Ana, CA 92704
(714) 754-5454

Overall patient safety: ★
Teaching: N

CLINICAL PROGRAM RATINGS:

CARDIAC	NR	ORTHOPEDICS	NR
CRITICAL CARE	NR	PULMONARY	★★★
GASTROINTESTINAL	NR	STROKE	★★★
GENERAL SURGERY	NR	VASCULAR	NR
MATERNITY CARE	★★★	WOMEN'S HEALTH	NR

HEALTHGRADES AWARDS

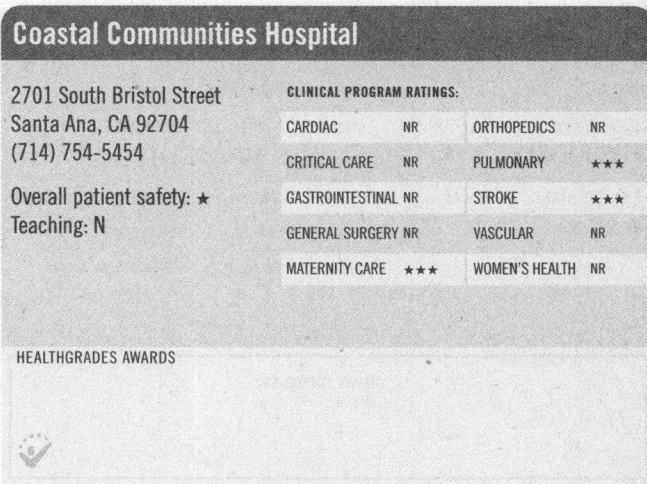

Colorado River Medical Center

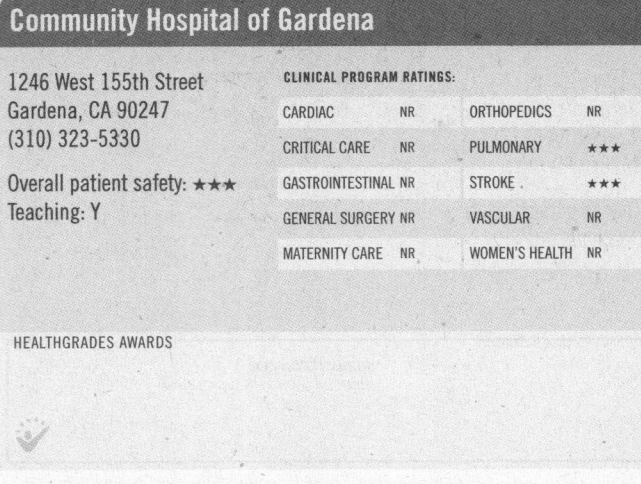

1401 Bailey Avenue
Needles, CA 92363
(619) 326-4531

Overall patient safety: ★★★
Teaching: N

CLINICAL PROGRAM RATINGS:

CARDIAC	NR	ORTHOPEDICS	NR
CRITICAL CARE	NR	PULMONARY	★★★
GASTROINTESTINAL	NR	STROKE	NR
GENERAL SURGERY	NR	VASCULAR	NR
MATERNITY CARE	★★★	WOMEN'S HEALTH	NR

HEALTHGRADES AWARDS

Community Hospital of Gardena

1246 West 155th Street
Gardena, CA 90247
(310) 323-5330

Overall patient safety: ★★★
Teaching: Y

CLINICAL PROGRAM RATINGS:

CARDIAC	NR	ORTHOPEDICS	NR
CRITICAL CARE	NR	PULMONARY	★★★
GASTROINTESTINAL	NR	STROKE	★★★
GENERAL SURGERY	NR	VASCULAR	NR
MATERNITY CARE	NR	WOMEN'S HEALTH	NR

HEALTHGRADES AWARDS

Colusa Regional Medical Center

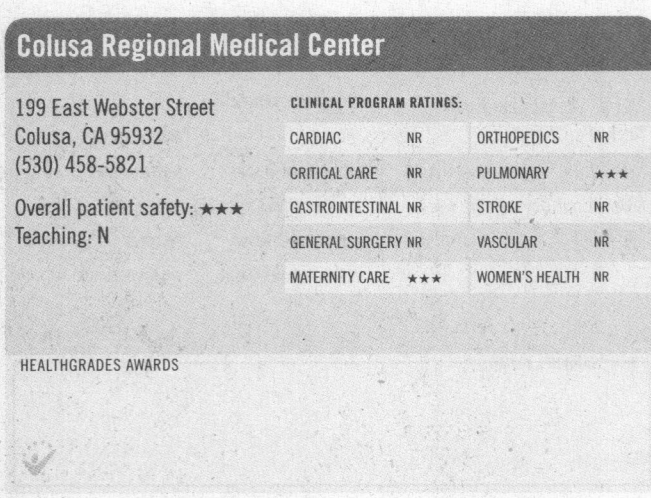

199 East Webster Street
Colusa, CA 95932
(530) 458-5821

Overall patient safety: ★★★
Teaching: N

CLINICAL PROGRAM RATINGS:

CARDIAC	NR	ORTHOPEDICS	NR
CRITICAL CARE	NR	PULMONARY	★★★
GASTROINTESTINAL	NR	STROKE	NR
GENERAL SURGERY	NR	VASCULAR	NR
MATERNITY CARE	★★★	WOMEN'S HEALTH	NR

HEALTHGRADES AWARDS

Community Hospital of Long Beach

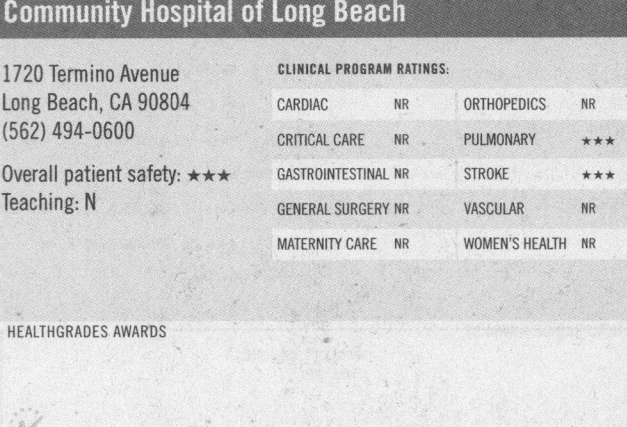

1720 Termino Avenue
Long Beach, CA 90804
(562) 494-0600

Overall patient safety: ★★★
Teaching: N

CLINICAL PROGRAM RATINGS:

CARDIAC	NR	ORTHOPEDICS	NR
CRITICAL CARE	NR	PULMONARY	★★★
GASTROINTESTINAL	NR	STROKE	★★★
GENERAL SURGERY	NR	VASCULAR	NR
MATERNITY CARE	NR	WOMEN'S HEALTH	NR

HEALTHGRADES AWARDS

Community and Mission Hospital of Huntington Park

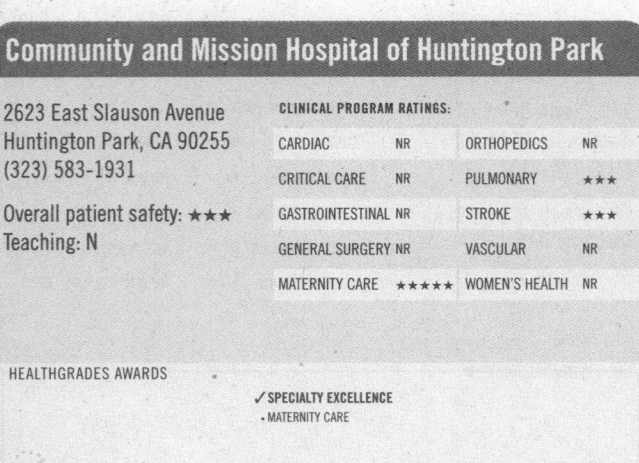

2623 East Slauson Avenue
Huntington Park, CA 90255
(323) 583-1931

Overall patient safety: ★★★
Teaching: N

CLINICAL PROGRAM RATINGS:

CARDIAC	NR	ORTHOPEDICS	NR
CRITICAL CARE	NR	PULMONARY	★★★
GASTROINTESTINAL	NR	STROKE	★★★
GENERAL SURGERY	NR	VASCULAR	NR
MATERNITY CARE	★★★★★	WOMEN'S HEALTH	NR

HEALTHGRADES AWARDS

✓ SPECIALTY EXCELLENCE
- MATERNITY CARE

Community Hospital of Los Gatos

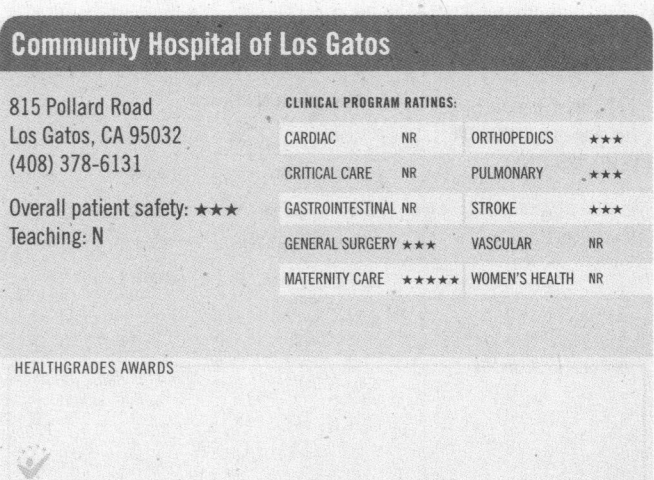

815 Pollard Road
Los Gatos, CA 95032
(408) 378-6131

Overall patient safety: ★★★
Teaching: N

CLINICAL PROGRAM RATINGS:

CARDIAC	NR	ORTHOPEDICS	★★★
CRITICAL CARE	NR	PULMONARY	★★★
GASTROINTESTINAL	NR	STROKE	★★★
GENERAL SURGERY	★★★	VASCULAR	NR
MATERNITY CARE	★★★★★	WOMEN'S HEALTH	NR

HEALTHGRADES AWARDS

KEY: ★★★★★ BEST   ★★★ AS EXPECTED   ★ POOR   NR NOT RATED BY HEALTHGRADES   For full definitions of ratings and awards, see Appendix.

Community Hospital of the Monterey Peninsula

23625 Holman Highway
Monterey, CA 93940
(831) 624-5311

Overall patient safety: ★★★★★
Teaching: N

CLINICAL PROGRAM RATINGS:

CARDIAC	NR	ORTHOPEDICS	★★★★★
CRITICAL CARE	★★★	PULMONARY	★★★
GASTROINTESTINAL	★★★	STROKE	★★★
GENERAL SURGERY	★★★	VASCULAR	NR
MATERNITY CARE	★★★	WOMEN'S HEALTH	NR

HEALTHGRADES AWARDS

✓ **DISTINGUISHED HOSPITAL**
- PATIENT SAFETY

✓ **SPECIALTY EXCELLENCE**
- GASTROINTESTINAL CARE
- GENERAL SURGERY
- JOINT REPLACEMENT
- ORTHOPEDIC SURGERY

Community Regional Medical Center*

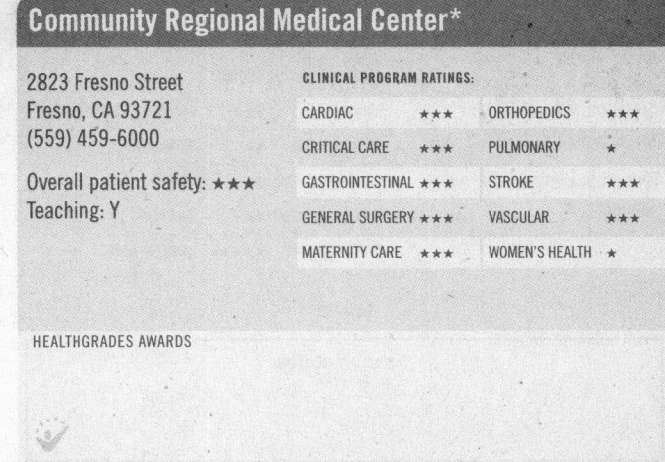

2823 Fresno Street
Fresno, CA 93721
(559) 459-6000

Overall patient safety: ★★★
Teaching: Y

CLINICAL PROGRAM RATINGS:

CARDIAC	★★★	ORTHOPEDICS	★★★
CRITICAL CARE	★★★	PULMONARY	★
GASTROINTESTINAL	★★★	STROKE	★★★
GENERAL SURGERY	★★★	VASCULAR	★★★
MATERNITY CARE	★★★	WOMEN'S HEALTH	★

HEALTHGRADES AWARDS

Community Hospital of San Bernardino

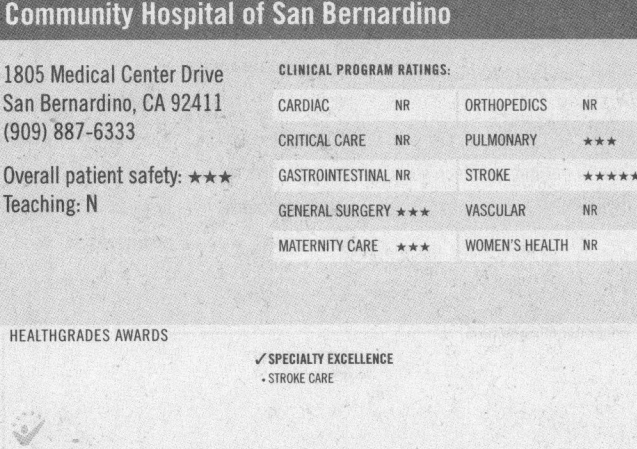

1805 Medical Center Drive
San Bernardino, CA 92411
(909) 887-6333

Overall patient safety: ★★★
Teaching: N

CLINICAL PROGRAM RATINGS:

CARDIAC	NR	ORTHOPEDICS	NR
CRITICAL CARE	NR	PULMONARY	★★★
GASTROINTESTINAL	NR	STROKE	★★★★★
GENERAL SURGERY	★★★	VASCULAR	NR
MATERNITY CARE	★★★	WOMEN'S HEALTH	NR

HEALTHGRADES AWARDS

✓ **SPECIALTY EXCELLENCE**
- STROKE CARE

Contra Costa Regional Medical Center

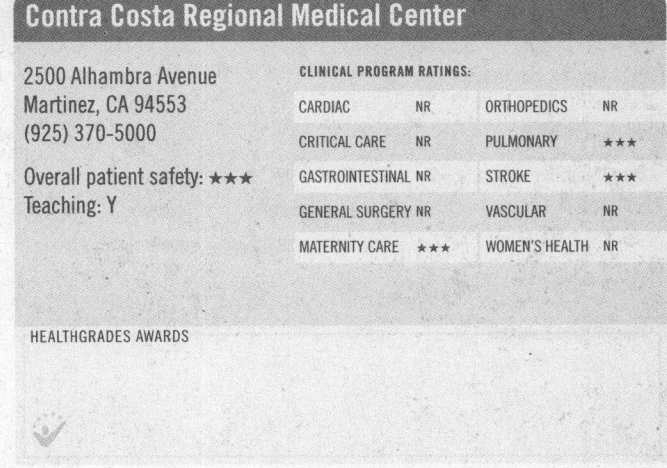

2500 Alhambra Avenue
Martinez, CA 94553
(925) 370-5000

Overall patient safety: ★★★
Teaching: Y

CLINICAL PROGRAM RATINGS:

CARDIAC	NR	ORTHOPEDICS	NR
CRITICAL CARE	NR	PULMONARY	★★★
GASTROINTESTINAL	NR	STROKE	★★★
GENERAL SURGERY	NR	VASCULAR	NR
MATERNITY CARE	★★★	WOMEN'S HEALTH	NR

HEALTHGRADES AWARDS

Community Memorial Hospital of San Buenaventura

147 North Brent
Ventura, CA 93003
(805) 652-5011

Overall patient safety: ★★★
Teaching: N

CLINICAL PROGRAM RATINGS:

CARDIAC	★★★	ORTHOPEDICS	★★★★★
CRITICAL CARE	★★★	PULMONARY	★★★
GASTROINTESTINAL	NR	STROKE	★★★
GENERAL SURGERY	★★★	VASCULAR	NR
MATERNITY CARE	★★★	WOMEN'S HEALTH	★★★★★

HEALTHGRADES AWARDS

✓ **SPECIALTY EXCELLENCE**
- ORTHOPEDIC SURGERY

Corona Regional Medical Center

800 South Main Street
Corona, CA 92882
(909) 737-4343

Overall patient safety: ★
Teaching: N

CLINICAL PROGRAM RATINGS:

CARDIAC	NR	ORTHOPEDICS	NR
CRITICAL CARE	NR	PULMONARY	★★★
GASTROINTESTINAL	★★★	STROKE	★★★
GENERAL SURGERY	★★★	VASCULAR	NR
MATERNITY CARE	★★★	WOMEN'S HEALTH	NR

HEALTHGRADES AWARDS

*This hospital reports its data to the federal government jointly with another hospital. Therefore the ratings and awards apply to multiple hospitals and this specific hospital may not provide all rated services.

Dameron Hospital Association

525 West Acacia Street
Stockton, CA 95203
(209) 944-5550

Overall patient safety: ★★★
Teaching: N

CLINICAL PROGRAM RATINGS:

CARDIAC	★★★	ORTHOPEDICS	★★★
CRITICAL CARE	NR	PULMONARY	★
GASTROINTESTINAL	NR	STROKE	★
GENERAL SURGERY	★★★	VASCULAR	NR
MATERNITY CARE	★★★★★	WOMEN'S HEALTH	★★★

HEALTHGRADES AWARDS

✓ SPECIALTY EXCELLENCE
• MATERNITY CARE

Desert Valley Hospital

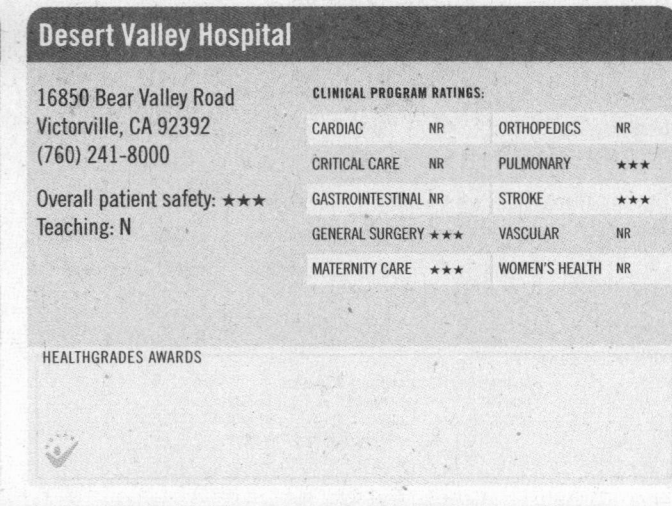

16850 Bear Valley Road
Victorville, CA 92392
(760) 241-8000

Overall patient safety: ★★★
Teaching: N

CLINICAL PROGRAM RATINGS:

CARDIAC	NR	ORTHOPEDICS	NR
CRITICAL CARE	NR	PULMONARY	★★★
GASTROINTESTINAL	NR	STROKE	★★★
GENERAL SURGERY	★★★	VASCULAR	NR
MATERNITY CARE	★★★	WOMEN'S HEALTH	NR

HEALTHGRADES AWARDS

Delano Regional Medical Center

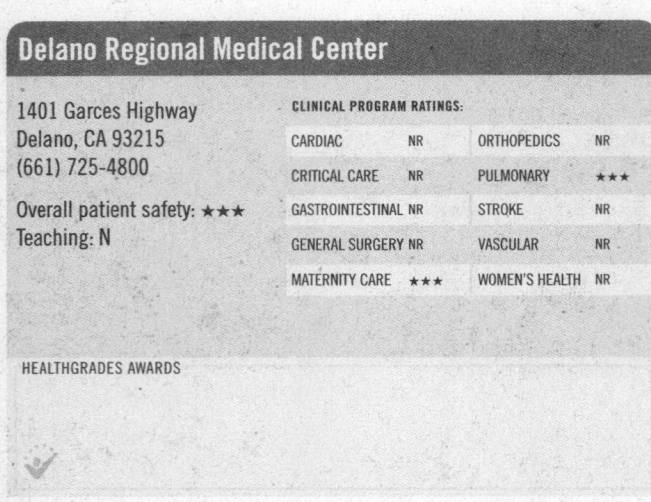

1401 Garces Highway
Delano, CA 93215
(661) 725-4800

Overall patient safety: ★★★
Teaching: N

CLINICAL PROGRAM RATINGS:

CARDIAC	NR	ORTHOPEDICS	NR
CRITICAL CARE	NR	PULMONARY	★★★
GASTROINTESTINAL	NR	STROKE	NR
GENERAL SURGERY	NR	VASCULAR	NR
MATERNITY CARE	★★★	WOMEN'S HEALTH	NR

HEALTHGRADES AWARDS

Doctor's Hospital Medical Center of Montclair

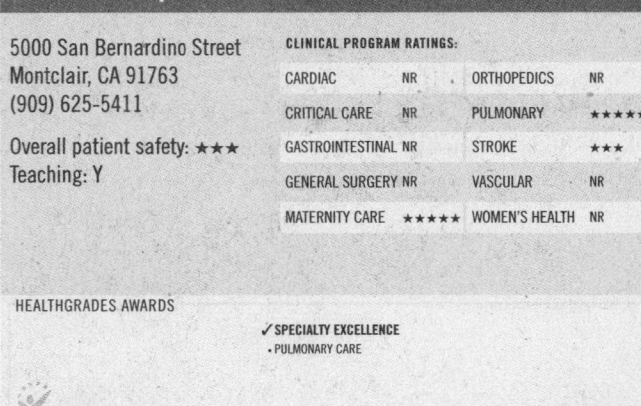

5000 San Bernardino Street
Montclair, CA 91763
(909) 625-5411

Overall patient safety: ★★★
Teaching: Y

CLINICAL PROGRAM RATINGS:

CARDIAC	NR	ORTHOPEDICS	NR
CRITICAL CARE	NR	PULMONARY	★★★★★
GASTROINTESTINAL	NR	STROKE	★★★
GENERAL SURGERY	NR	VASCULAR	NR
MATERNITY CARE	★★★★★	WOMEN'S HEALTH	NR

HEALTHGRADES AWARDS

✓ SPECIALTY EXCELLENCE
• PULMONARY CARE

Desert Regional Medical Center

1150 North Indian
Canyon Drive
Palm Springs, CA 92262
(760) 323-6511

Overall patient safety: ★★★
Teaching: N

CLINICAL PROGRAM RATINGS:

CARDIAC	★★★	ORTHOPEDICS	★★★★★
CRITICAL CARE	★★★	PULMONARY	★
GASTROINTESTINAL	★★★	STROKE	★
GENERAL SURGERY	★★★	VASCULAR	NR
MATERNITY CARE	★★★	WOMEN'S HEALTH	★★★

HEALTHGRADES AWARDS

✓ SPECIALTY EXCELLENCE
• ORTHOPEDIC SURGERY

Doctors Hospital of Manteca

1205 East North Street
Manteca, CA 95336
(209) 823-3111

Overall patient safety: ★★★
Teaching: N

CLINICAL PROGRAM RATINGS:

CARDIAC	NR	ORTHOPEDICS	NR
CRITICAL CARE	NR	PULMONARY	★★★
GASTROINTESTINAL	NR	STROKE	★★★
GENERAL SURGERY	★★★	VASCULAR	NR
MATERNITY CARE	★★★	WOMEN'S HEALTH	NR

HEALTHGRADES AWARDS

KEY: ★★★★★ BEST ★★★ AS EXPECTED ★ POOR NR NOT RATED BY HEALTHGRADES   For full definitions of ratings and awards, see Appendix.

Doctors Medical Center of Modesto

1441 Florida Avenue
Modesto, CA 95352
(209) 578-1211

Overall patient safety: ★★★
Teaching: Y

CLINICAL PROGRAM RATINGS:

CARDIAC	★★★	ORTHOPEDICS	★★★
CRITICAL CARE	★★★	PULMONARY	★
GASTROINTESTINAL	★★★	STROKE	★
GENERAL SURGERY	★★★	VASCULAR	★★★
MATERNITY CARE	★★★	WOMEN'S HEALTH	★★★

HEALTHGRADES AWARDS

Downey Regional Medical Center

11500 Brookshire Avenue
Downey, CA 90241
(562) 904-5000

Overall patient safety: ★★★
Teaching: Y

CLINICAL PROGRAM RATINGS:

CARDIAC	★★★	ORTHOPEDICS	NR
CRITICAL CARE	NR	PULMONARY	★★★
GASTROINTESTINAL	★★★	STROKE	★★★★★
GENERAL SURGERY	★★★	VASCULAR	NR
MATERNITY CARE	★★★★★	WOMEN'S HEALTH	★★★★★

HEALTHGRADES AWARDS

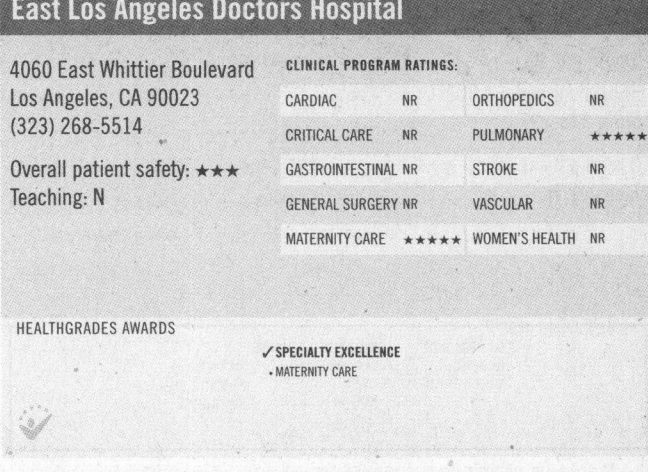

✓ SPECIALTY EXCELLENCE
• STROKE CARE   • WOMEN'S HEALTH

Doctors Medical Center—San Pablo/Pinole

2000 Vale Road
San Pablo, CA 94806
(510) 970-5000

Overall patient safety: ★★★
Teaching: N

CLINICAL PROGRAM RATINGS:

CARDIAC	★★★	ORTHOPEDICS	NR
CRITICAL CARE	★★★	PULMONARY	★★★
GASTROINTESTINAL	★★★	STROKE	★★★
GENERAL SURGERY	★★★	VASCULAR	NR
MATERNITY CARE	★★★	WOMEN'S HEALTH	★★★

HEALTHGRADES AWARDS

East Los Angeles Doctors Hospital

4060 East Whittier Boulevard
Los Angeles, CA 90023
(323) 268-5514

Overall patient safety: ★★★
Teaching: N

CLINICAL PROGRAM RATINGS:

CARDIAC	NR	ORTHOPEDICS	NR
CRITICAL CARE	NR	PULMONARY	★★★★★
GASTROINTESTINAL	NR	STROKE	NR
GENERAL SURGERY	NR	VASCULAR	NR
MATERNITY CARE	★★★★★	WOMEN'S HEALTH	NR

HEALTHGRADES AWARDS

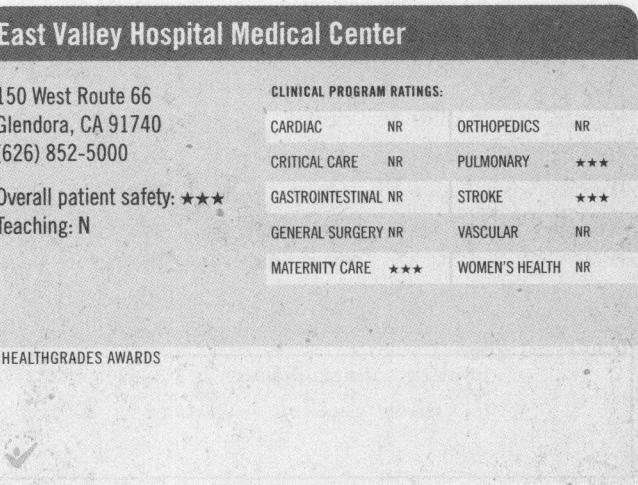

✓ SPECIALTY EXCELLENCE
• MATERNITY CARE

Dominican Hospital

1555 Soquel Drive
Santa Cruz, CA 95065
(831) 462-7700

Overall patient safety: ★★★
Teaching: N

CLINICAL PROGRAM RATINGS:

CARDIAC	★★★	ORTHOPEDICS	★★★
CRITICAL CARE	★★★	PULMONARY	★★★
GASTROINTESTINAL	★★★	STROKE	★★★
GENERAL SURGERY	★★★★★	VASCULAR	NR
MATERNITY CARE	★★★	WOMEN'S HEALTH	★★★

HEALTHGRADES AWARDS

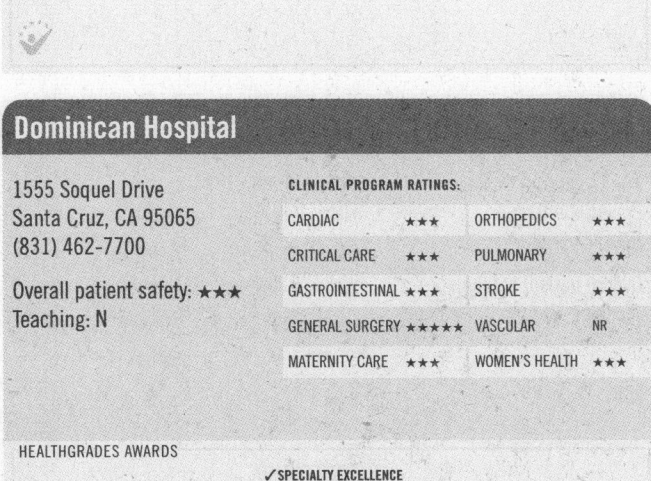

✓ SPECIALTY EXCELLENCE
• GENERAL SURGERY

East Valley Hospital Medical Center

150 West Route 66
Glendora, CA 91740
(626) 852-5000

Overall patient safety: ★★★
Teaching: N

CLINICAL PROGRAM RATINGS:

CARDIAC	NR	ORTHOPEDICS	NR
CRITICAL CARE	NR	PULMONARY	★★★
GASTROINTESTINAL	NR	STROKE	★★★
GENERAL SURGERY	NR	VASCULAR	NR
MATERNITY CARE	★★★	WOMEN'S HEALTH	NR

HEALTHGRADES AWARDS

CALIFORNIA HOSPITALS: RATINGS BY CLINICAL SPECIALTY

Eden Medical Center

20103 Lake Chabot Road
Castro Valley, CA 94546
(510) 537-1234

Overall patient safety: ★★★
Teaching: N

CLINICAL PROGRAM RATINGS:

CARDIAC	NR	ORTHOPEDICS	★★★
CRITICAL CARE	NR	PULMONARY	★★★
GASTROINTESTINAL	★★★	STROKE	★★★★★
GENERAL SURGERY	★★★	VASCULAR	NR
MATERNITY CARE	★★★	WOMEN'S HEALTH	NR

HEALTHGRADES AWARDS

✓ DISTINGUISHED HOSPITAL
- CLINICAL EXCELLENCE

✓ SPECIALTY EXCELLENCE
- STROKE CARE

El Centro Regional Medical Center

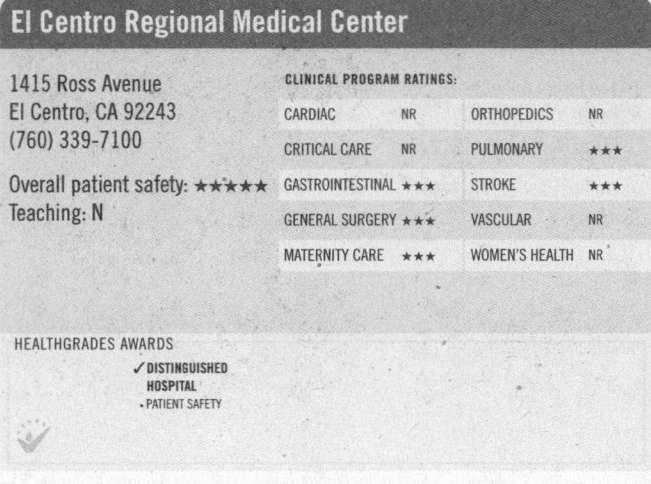

1415 Ross Avenue
El Centro, CA 92243
(760) 339-7100

Overall patient safety: ★★★★★
Teaching: N

CLINICAL PROGRAM RATINGS:

CARDIAC	NR	ORTHOPEDICS	NR
CRITICAL CARE	NR	PULMONARY	★★★
GASTROINTESTINAL	★★★	STROKE	★★★
GENERAL SURGERY	★★★	VASCULAR	NR
MATERNITY CARE	★★★	WOMEN'S HEALTH	NR

HEALTHGRADES AWARDS

✓ DISTINGUISHED HOSPITAL
- PATIENT SAFETY

Eisenhower Medical Center

39000 Bob Hope Drive
Rancho Mirage, CA 92270
(760) 340-3911

Overall patient safety: ★★★
Teaching: N

CLINICAL PROGRAM RATINGS:

CARDIAC	★★★	ORTHOPEDICS	★★★★★
CRITICAL CARE	★★★	PULMONARY	★★★
GASTROINTESTINAL	★★★	STROKE	★★★★★
GENERAL SURGERY	★★★	VASCULAR	★★★
MATERNITY CARE	NR	WOMEN'S HEALTH	NR

HEALTHGRADES AWARDS

✓ DISTINGUISHED HOSPITAL
- CLINICAL EXCELLENCE

✓ SPECIALTY EXCELLENCE
- GASTROINTESTINAL CARE
- JOINT REPLACEMENT
- ORTHOPEDIC SURGERY
- STROKE CARE

Emanuel Medical Center

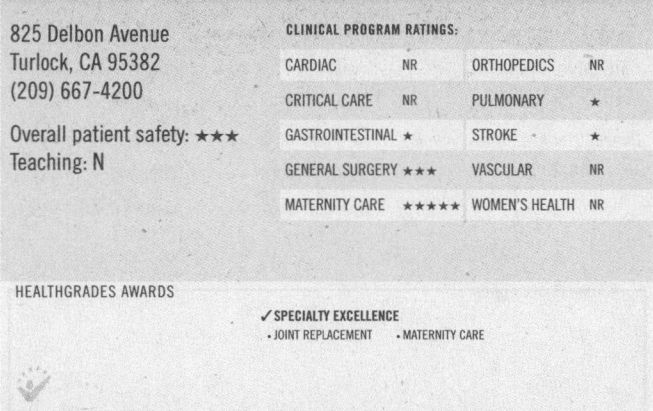

825 Delbon Avenue
Turlock, CA 95382
(209) 667-4200

Overall patient safety: ★★★
Teaching: N

CLINICAL PROGRAM RATINGS:

CARDIAC	NR	ORTHOPEDICS	NR
CRITICAL CARE	NR	PULMONARY	★
GASTROINTESTINAL	★	STROKE	★
GENERAL SURGERY	★★★	VASCULAR	NR
MATERNITY CARE	★★★★★	WOMEN'S HEALTH	NR

HEALTHGRADES AWARDS

✓ SPECIALTY EXCELLENCE
- JOINT REPLACEMENT
- MATERNITY CARE

El Camino Hospital

2500 Grant Road
Mountain View, CA 94040
(650) 940-7000

Overall patient safety: ★★★
Teaching: N

CLINICAL PROGRAM RATINGS:

CARDIAC	★★★★★	ORTHOPEDICS	★★★
CRITICAL CARE	★★★	PULMONARY	★★★★★
GASTROINTESTINAL	★★★	STROKE	★★★★★
GENERAL SURGERY	★★★	VASCULAR	NR
MATERNITY CARE	★★★	WOMEN'S HEALTH	★★★★★

HEALTHGRADES AWARDS

✓ DISTINGUISHED HOSPITAL
- CLINICAL EXCELLENCE

✓ SPECIALTY EXCELLENCE
- CARDIAC CARE
- PULMONARY CARE
- STROKE CARE
- WOMEN'S HEALTH

Encino-Tarzana Regional Medical Center

16237 Ventura Boulevard
Encino, CA 91436
(818) 881-0800

Overall patient safety: ★★★
Teaching: Y

CLINICAL PROGRAM RATINGS:

CARDIAC	NR	ORTHOPEDICS	NR
CRITICAL CARE	NR	PULMONARY	★★★
GASTROINTESTINAL	NR	STROKE	★★★
GENERAL SURGERY	NR	VASCULAR	NR
MATERNITY CARE	NR	WOMEN'S HEALTH	NR

HEALTHGRADES AWARDS

✓ SPECIALTY EXCELLENCE
- JOINT REPLACEMENT

KEY: ★★★★★ BEST   ★★★ AS EXPECTED   ★ POOR   NR NOT RATED BY HEALTHGRADES   For full definitions of ratings and awards, see Appendix.

96 CHAPTER 6: HOSPITAL RATINGS BY CLINICAL SPECIALTY

Encino-Tarzana Regional Medical Center–Tarzana Campus

18321 Clark Street
Tarzana, CA 91356
(818) 881-0800

Overall patient safety: ★★★
Teaching: Y

CLINICAL PROGRAM RATINGS:

CARDIAC	★★★	ORTHOPEDICS	NR
CRITICAL CARE	★★★	PULMONARY	★★★
GASTROINTESTINAL	★★★	STROKE	★★★★★
GENERAL SURGERY	★★★	VASCULAR	★★★
MATERNITY CARE	★★★★★	WOMEN'S HEALTH	★★★★★

HEALTHGRADES AWARDS

✓ SPECIALTY EXCELLENCE
- GASTROINTESTINAL CARE
- MATERNITY CARE
- STROKE CARE
- WOMEN'S HEALTH

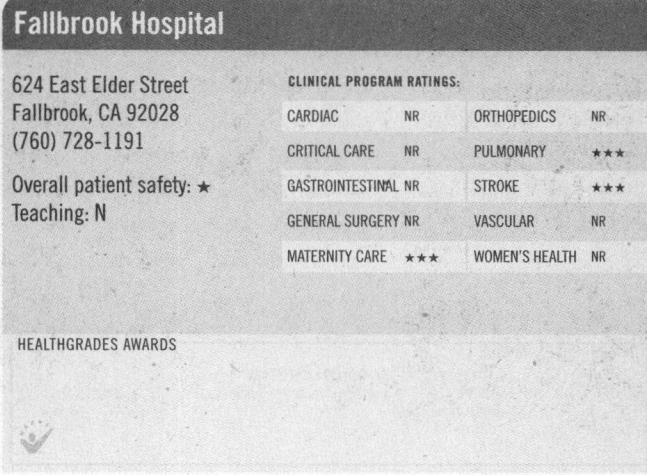

Fallbrook Hospital

624 East Elder Street
Fallbrook, CA 92028
(760) 728-1191

Overall patient safety: ★
Teaching: N

CLINICAL PROGRAM RATINGS:

CARDIAC	NR	ORTHOPEDICS	NR
CRITICAL CARE	NR	PULMONARY	★★★
GASTROINTESTINAL	NR	STROKE	★★★
GENERAL SURGERY	NR	VASCULAR	NR
MATERNITY CARE	★★★	WOMEN'S HEALTH	NR

HEALTHGRADES AWARDS

Enloe Medical Center*

1531 Esplanade
Chico, CA 95926
(530) 332-7300

Overall patient safety: ★★★
Teaching: N

CLINICAL PROGRAM RATINGS:

CARDIAC	★	ORTHOPEDICS	★★★
CRITICAL CARE	★★★	PULMONARY	★
GASTROINTESTINAL	★★★	STROKE	★★★
GENERAL SURGERY	★★★	VASCULAR	★★★
MATERNITY CARE	★★★	WOMEN'S HEALTH	★★★

HEALTHGRADES AWARDS

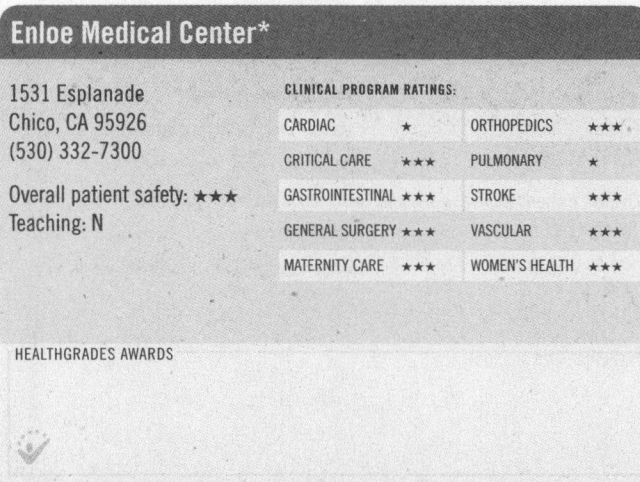

Feather River Hospital

5974 Pentz Road
Paradise, CA 95969
(530) 877-9361

Overall patient safety: ★★★
Teaching: N

CLINICAL PROGRAM RATINGS:

CARDIAC	NR	ORTHOPEDICS	NR
CRITICAL CARE	NR	PULMONARY	★★★
GASTROINTESTINAL	★★★	STROKE	★
GENERAL SURGERY	★★★	VASCULAR	NR
MATERNITY CARE	★★★	WOMEN'S HEALTH	NR

HEALTHGRADES AWARDS

✓ SPECIALTY EXCELLENCE
- JOINT REPLACEMENT

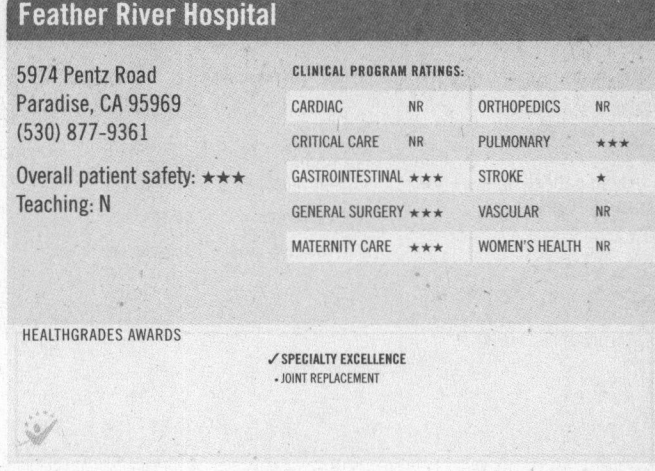

Fairchild Medical Center

444 Bruce Street
Yreka, CA 96097
(530) 842-4121

Overall patient safety: ★★★
Teaching: N

CLINICAL PROGRAM RATINGS:

CARDIAC	NR	ORTHOPEDICS	NR
CRITICAL CARE	NR	PULMONARY	★★★
GASTROINTESTINAL	NR	STROKE	★
GENERAL SURGERY	★★★	VASCULAR	NR
MATERNITY CARE	★★★	WOMEN'S HEALTH	NR

HEALTHGRADES AWARDS

Foothill Presbyterian Hospital

250 South Grand Avenue
Glendora, CA 91740
(626) 963-8411

Overall patient safety: ★★★
Teaching: N

CLINICAL PROGRAM RATINGS:

CARDIAC	NR	ORTHOPEDICS	NR
CRITICAL CARE	NR	PULMONARY	★★★
GASTROINTESTINAL	NR	STROKE	★★★
GENERAL SURGERY	NR	VASCULAR	NR
MATERNITY CARE	★★★	WOMEN'S HEALTH	NR

HEALTHGRADES AWARDS

*This hospital reports its data to the federal government jointly with another hospital. Therefore the ratings and awards apply to multiple hospitals and this specific hospital may not provide all rated services.

CALIFORNIA HOSPITALS: RATINGS BY CLINICAL SPECIALTY

Fountain Valley Regional Hospital and Medical Center

17100 Euclid Street
Fountain Valley, CA 92708
(714) 966-7200

Overall patient safety: ★★★
Teaching: Y

CLINICAL PROGRAM RATINGS:

CARDIAC	★★★	ORTHOPEDICS	★★★
CRITICAL CARE	NR	PULMONARY	★★★★★
GASTROINTESTINAL	★★★	STROKE	★★★★★
GENERAL SURGERY	★★★	VASCULAR	NR
MATERNITY CARE	★★★	WOMEN'S HEALTH	★★★★★

HEALTHGRADES AWARDS

✓ DISTINGUISHED HOSPITAL   ✓ SPECIALTY EXCELLENCE
· CLINICAL EXCELLENCE   · PULMONARY CARE   · STROKE CARE   · WOMEN'S HEALTH

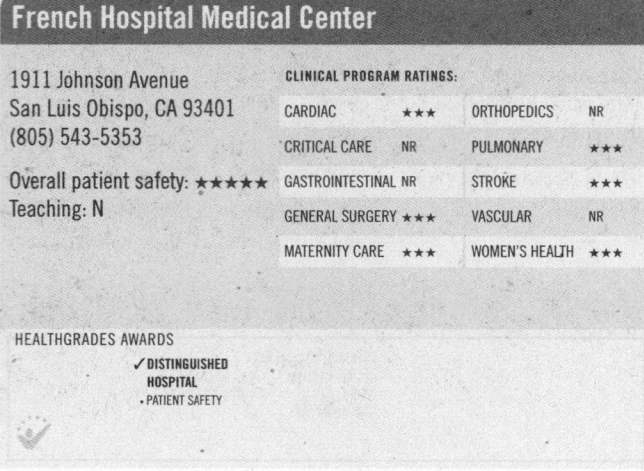

French Hospital Medical Center

1911 Johnson Avenue
San Luis Obispo, CA 93401
(805) 543-5353

Overall patient safety: ★★★★★
Teaching: N

CLINICAL PROGRAM RATINGS:

CARDIAC	★★★	ORTHOPEDICS	NR
CRITICAL CARE	NR	PULMONARY	★★★
GASTROINTESTINAL	NR	STROKE	★★★
GENERAL SURGERY	★★★	VASCULAR	NR
MATERNITY CARE	★★★	WOMEN'S HEALTH	★★★

HEALTHGRADES AWARDS

✓ DISTINGUISHED HOSPITAL
· PATIENT SAFETY

Frank R. Howard Memorial Hospital

1 Madrone Street
Willits, CA 95490
(707) 459-6801

Overall patient safety: ★★★
Teaching: N

CLINICAL PROGRAM RATINGS:

CARDIAC	NR	ORTHOPEDICS	NR
CRITICAL CARE	NR	PULMONARY	★★★
GASTROINTESTINAL	NR	STROKE	★
GENERAL SURGERY	NR	VASCULAR	NR
MATERNITY CARE	NR	WOMEN'S HEALTH	NR

HEALTHGRADES AWARDS

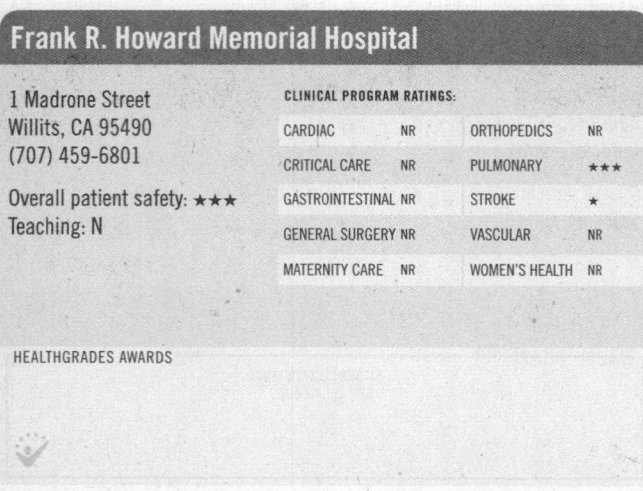

Fresno Heart and Surgical Hospital

15 East Audubon Drive
Fresno, CA 93720
(559) 433-8000

Overall patient safety: ★★★★★
Teaching: N

CLINICAL PROGRAM RATINGS:

CARDIAC	★★★	ORTHOPEDICS	NR
CRITICAL CARE	NR	PULMONARY	NR
GASTROINTESTINAL	NR	STROKE	NR
GENERAL SURGERY	NR	VASCULAR	NR
MATERNITY CARE	NR	WOMEN'S HEALTH	NR

HEALTHGRADES AWARDS

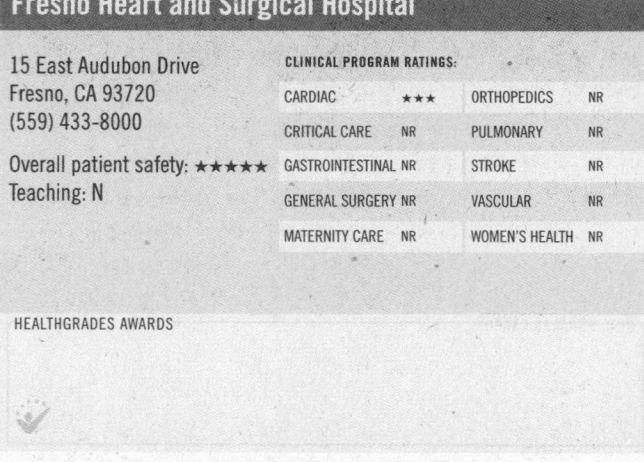

Fremont Medical Center*

970 Plumas Street
Yuba City, CA 95991
(530) 751-4000

Overall patient safety: ★★★
Teaching: Y

CLINICAL PROGRAM RATINGS:

CARDIAC	★★★	ORTHOPEDICS	★
CRITICAL CARE	★★★	PULMONARY	★★★
GASTROINTESTINAL	★★★	STROKE	★★★
GENERAL SURGERY	★★★	VASCULAR	NR
MATERNITY CARE	★★★	WOMEN'S HEALTH	★★★

HEALTHGRADES AWARDS

Garden Grove Hospital and Medical Center

12601 Garden Grove Boulevard
Garden Grove, CA 92843
(714) 537-5160

Overall patient safety: ★★★
Teaching: N

CLINICAL PROGRAM RATINGS:

CARDIAC	NR	ORTHOPEDICS	NR
CRITICAL CARE	NR	PULMONARY	★★★
GASTROINTESTINAL	NR	STROKE	★★★
GENERAL SURGERY	★★★	VASCULAR	NR
MATERNITY CARE	★★★★★	WOMEN'S HEALTH	NR

HEALTHGRADES AWARDS

✓ SPECIALTY EXCELLENCE
· MATERNITY CARE

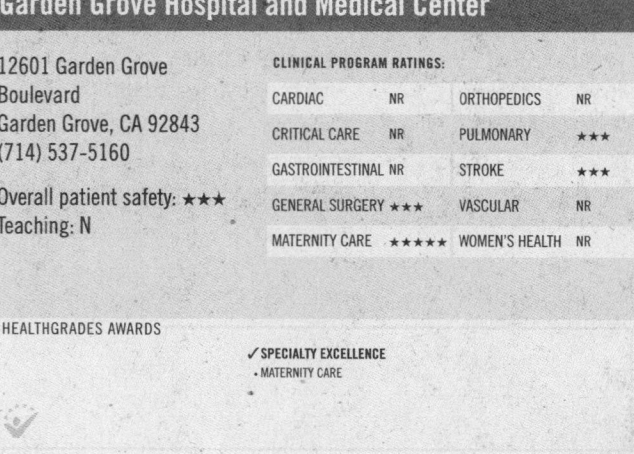

KEY: ★★★★★ BEST   ★★★ AS EXPECTED   ★ POOR   NR NOT RATED BY HEALTHGRADES   For full definitions of ratings and awards, see Appendix.

Garfield Medical Center

525 North Garfield Avenue
Monterey Park, CA 91754
(626) 573-2222

Overall patient safety: ★★★
Teaching: N

CLINICAL PROGRAM RATINGS:

CARDIAC	★★★★★	ORTHOPEDICS	NR
CRITICAL CARE	NR	PULMONARY	★★★★★
GASTROINTESTINAL	★★★	STROKE	★★★★★
GENERAL SURGERY	★★★★★	VASCULAR	NR
MATERNITY CARE	★★★	WOMEN'S HEALTH	★★★★★

HEALTHGRADES AWARDS

✓ DISTINGUISHED HOSPITAL
· CLINICAL EXCELLENCE

✓ SPECIALTY EXCELLENCE
· CARDIAC CARE
· GASTROINTESTINAL CARE
· GENERAL SURGERY
· PULMONARY CARE
· STROKE CARE
· WOMEN'S HEALTH

Glendale Memorial Hospital and Health Center

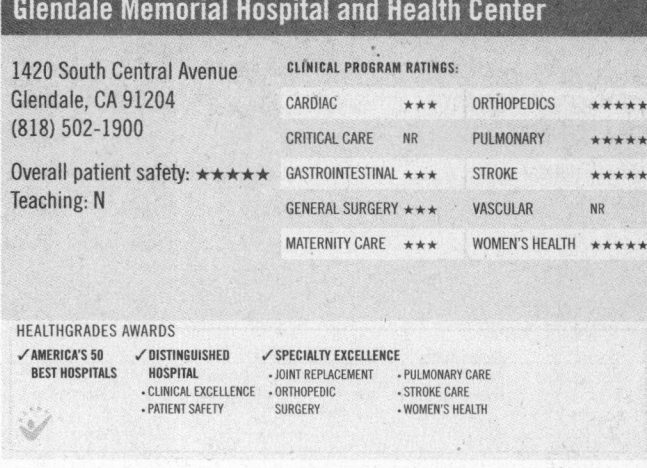

1420 South Central Avenue
Glendale, CA 91204
(818) 502-1900

Overall patient safety: ★★★★★
Teaching: N

CLINICAL PROGRAM RATINGS:

CARDIAC	★★★	ORTHOPEDICS	★★★★★
CRITICAL CARE	NR	PULMONARY	★★★★★
GASTROINTESTINAL	★★★	STROKE	★★★★★
GENERAL SURGERY	★★★	VASCULAR	NR
MATERNITY CARE	★★★	WOMEN'S HEALTH	★★★★★

HEALTHGRADES AWARDS

✓ AMERICA'S 50 BEST HOSPITALS

✓ DISTINGUISHED HOSPITAL
· CLINICAL EXCELLENCE
· PATIENT SAFETY

✓ SPECIALTY EXCELLENCE
· JOINT REPLACEMENT
· ORTHOPEDIC SURGERY
· PULMONARY CARE
· STROKE CARE
· WOMEN'S HEALTH

George L. Mee Memorial Hospital

300 Canal Street
King City, CA 93930
(831) 385-6000

Overall patient safety: ★★★
Teaching: N

CLINICAL PROGRAM RATINGS:

CARDIAC	NR	ORTHOPEDICS	NR
CRITICAL CARE	NR	PULMONARY	★★★
GASTROINTESTINAL	NR	STROKE	NR
GENERAL SURGERY	NR	VASCULAR	NR
MATERNITY CARE	★★★	WOMEN'S HEALTH	NR

HEALTHGRADES AWARDS

Goleta Valley Cottage Hospital

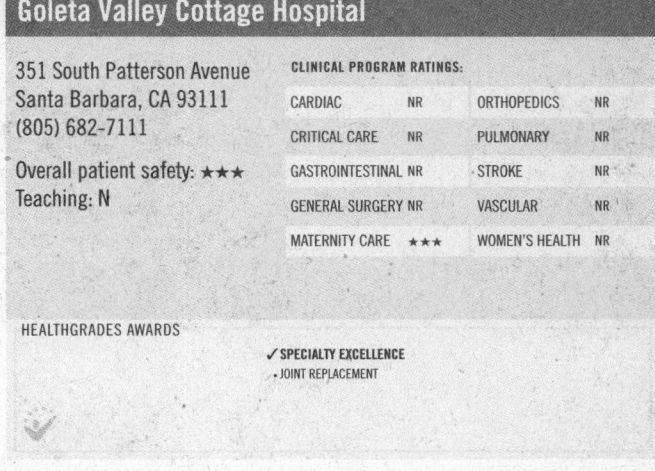

351 South Patterson Avenue
Santa Barbara, CA 93111
(805) 682-7111

Overall patient safety: ★★★
Teaching: N

CLINICAL PROGRAM RATINGS:

CARDIAC	NR	ORTHOPEDICS	NR
CRITICAL CARE	NR	PULMONARY	NR
GASTROINTESTINAL	NR	STROKE	NR
GENERAL SURGERY	NR	VASCULAR	NR
MATERNITY CARE	★★★	WOMEN'S HEALTH	NR

HEALTHGRADES AWARDS

✓ SPECIALTY EXCELLENCE
· JOINT REPLACEMENT

Glendale Adventist Medical Center

1509 Wilson Terrace
Glendale, CA 91206
(818) 409-8000

Overall patient safety: ★★★
Teaching: Y

CLINICAL PROGRAM RATINGS:

CARDIAC	★★★	ORTHOPEDICS	★★★
CRITICAL CARE	★★★★★	PULMONARY	★★★
GASTROINTESTINAL	★★★	STROKE	★★★★★
GENERAL SURGERY	★★★★★	VASCULAR	NR
MATERNITY CARE	★★★	WOMEN'S HEALTH	★★★★★

HEALTHGRADES AWARDS

✓ DISTINGUISHED HOSPITAL
· CLINICAL EXCELLENCE

✓ SPECIALTY EXCELLENCE
· CRITICAL CARE
· GASTROINTESTINAL CARE
· GENERAL SURGERY
· STROKE CARE

Good Samaritan Hospital

901 Olive Drive
Bakersfield, CA 93308
(661) 399-4461

Overall patient safety: ★★★
Teaching: N

CLINICAL PROGRAM RATINGS:

CARDIAC	NR	ORTHOPEDICS	NR
CRITICAL CARE	NR	PULMONARY	★★★
GASTROINTESTINAL	NR	STROKE	NR
GENERAL SURGERY	NR	VASCULAR	NR
MATERNITY CARE	NR	WOMEN'S HEALTH	NR

HEALTHGRADES AWARDS

*This hospital reports its data to the federal government jointly with another hospital. Therefore the ratings and awards apply to multiple hospitals and this specific hospital may not provide all rated services.

Good Samaritan Hospital

616 South Witmer
Los Angeles, CA 90017
(213) 977-2121

Overall patient safety: ★★★
Teaching: Y

CLINICAL PROGRAM RATINGS:

CARDIAC	★★★	ORTHOPEDICS	★★★
CRITICAL CARE	NR	PULMONARY	★★★★★
GASTROINTESTINAL	★★★	STROKE	★★★★★
GENERAL SURGERY	★★★	VASCULAR	NR
MATERNITY CARE	★★★★★	WOMEN'S HEALTH	★★★★★

HEALTHGRADES AWARDS

✓ AMERICA'S 50 BEST HOSPITALS
✓ DISTINGUISHED HOSPITAL
- CLINICAL EXCELLENCE
✓ SPECIALTY EXCELLENCE
- GASTROINTESTINAL CARE
- JOINT REPLACEMENT
- MATERNITY CARE
- PULMONARY CARE
- STROKE CARE
- WOMEN'S HEALTH

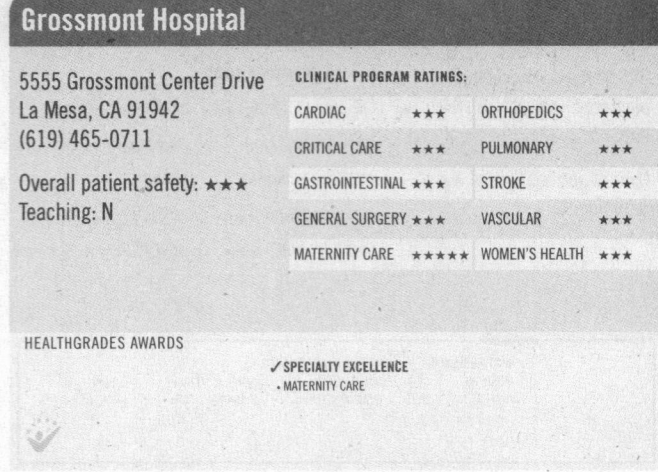

Grossmont Hospital

5555 Grossmont Center Drive
La Mesa, CA 91942
(619) 465-0711

Overall patient safety: ★★★
Teaching: N

CLINICAL PROGRAM RATINGS:

CARDIAC	★★★	ORTHOPEDICS	★★★
CRITICAL CARE	★★★	PULMONARY	★★★
GASTROINTESTINAL	★★★	STROKE	★★★
GENERAL SURGERY	★★★	VASCULAR	★★★
MATERNITY CARE	★★★★★	WOMEN'S HEALTH	★★★

HEALTHGRADES AWARDS

✓ SPECIALTY EXCELLENCE
- MATERNITY CARE

Good Samaritan Hospital

2425 Samaritan Drive
San Jose, CA 95124
(408) 559-2011

Overall patient safety: ★
Teaching: N

CLINICAL PROGRAM RATINGS:

CARDIAC	★★★	ORTHOPEDICS	★★★
CRITICAL CARE	★★★	PULMONARY	★★★
GASTROINTESTINAL	★★★	STROKE	★★★
GENERAL SURGERY	★★★★★	VASCULAR	NR
MATERNITY CARE	★★★	WOMEN'S HEALTH	★★★

HEALTHGRADES AWARDS

✓ SPECIALTY EXCELLENCE
- GENERAL SURGERY

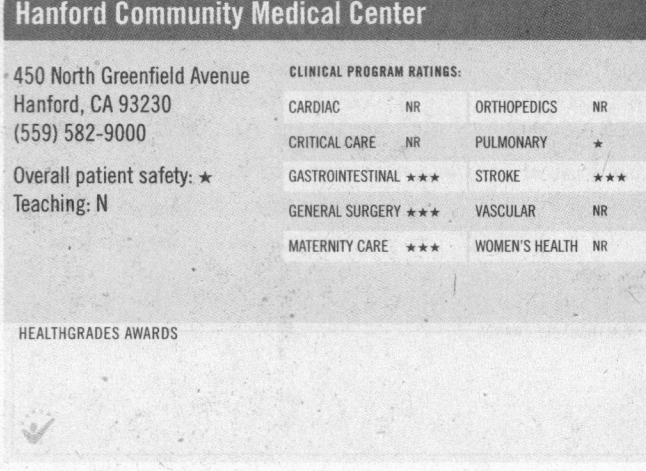

Hanford Community Medical Center

450 North Greenfield Avenue
Hanford, CA 93230
(559) 582-9000

Overall patient safety: ★
Teaching: N

CLINICAL PROGRAM RATINGS:

CARDIAC	NR	ORTHOPEDICS	NR
CRITICAL CARE	NR	PULMONARY	★
GASTROINTESTINAL	★★★	STROKE	★★★
GENERAL SURGERY	★★★	VASCULAR	NR
MATERNITY CARE	★★★	WOMEN'S HEALTH	NR

HEALTHGRADES AWARDS

Greater El Monte Community Hospital

1701 Santa Anita Avenue
South El Monte, CA 91733
(626) 350-7975

Overall patient safety: ★★★
Teaching: N

CLINICAL PROGRAM RATINGS:

CARDIAC	NR	ORTHOPEDICS	NR
CRITICAL CARE	NR	PULMONARY	★★★★★
GASTROINTESTINAL	NR	STROKE	NR
GENERAL SURGERY	NR	VASCULAR	NR
MATERNITY CARE	★★★★★	WOMEN'S HEALTH	NR

HEALTHGRADES AWARDS

✓ SPECIALTY EXCELLENCE
- MATERNITY CARE

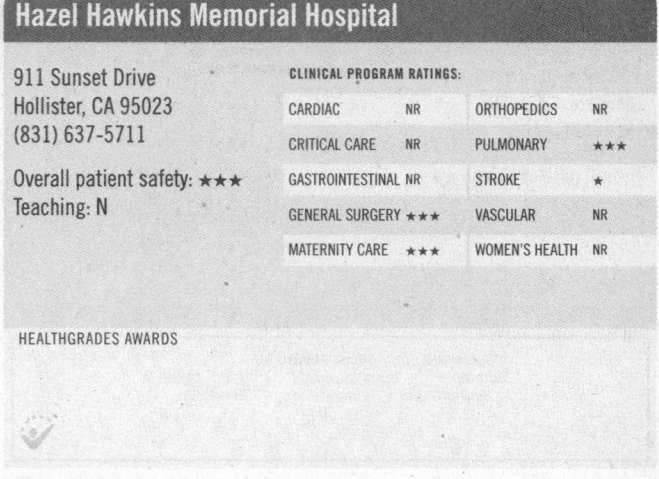

Hazel Hawkins Memorial Hospital

911 Sunset Drive
Hollister, CA 95023
(831) 637-5711

Overall patient safety: ★★★
Teaching: N

CLINICAL PROGRAM RATINGS:

CARDIAC	NR	ORTHOPEDICS	NR
CRITICAL CARE	NR	PULMONARY	★★★
GASTROINTESTINAL	NR	STROKE	★
GENERAL SURGERY	★★★	VASCULAR	NR
MATERNITY CARE	★★★	WOMEN'S HEALTH	NR

HEALTHGRADES AWARDS

KEY: ★★★★★ BEST ★★★ AS EXPECTED ★ POOR NR NOT RATED BY HEALTHGRADES For full definitions of ratings and awards, see Appendix.

Healdsburg District Hospital

1375 University Avenue
Healdsburg, CA 95448
(707) 431-6500

Overall patient safety: ★★★
Teaching: N

CLINICAL PROGRAM RATINGS:

CARDIAC	NR	ORTHOPEDICS	NR
CRITICAL CARE	NR	PULMONARY	NR
GASTROINTESTINAL	NR	STROKE	★★★
GENERAL SURGERY	NR	VASCULAR	NR
MATERNITY CARE	NR	WOMEN'S HEALTH	NR

HEALTHGRADES AWARDS

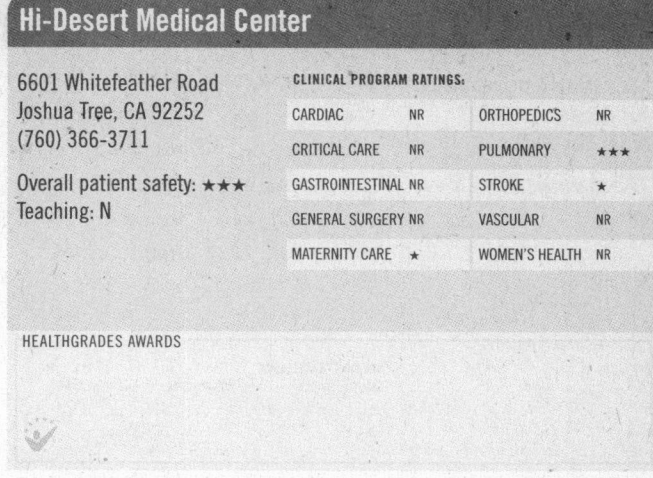

Hi-Desert Medical Center

6601 Whitefeather Road
Joshua Tree, CA 92252
(760) 366-3711

Overall patient safety: ★★★
Teaching: N

CLINICAL PROGRAM RATINGS:

CARDIAC	NR	ORTHOPEDICS	NR
CRITICAL CARE	NR	PULMONARY	★★★
GASTROINTESTINAL	NR	STROKE	★
GENERAL SURGERY	NR	VASCULAR	NR
MATERNITY CARE	★	WOMEN'S HEALTH	NR

HEALTHGRADES AWARDS

Hemet Valley Medical Center

1117 East Devonshire
Hemet, CA 92543
(909) 652-2811

Overall patient safety: ★
Teaching: N

CLINICAL PROGRAM RATINGS:

CARDIAC	NR	ORTHOPEDICS	NR
CRITICAL CARE	★	PULMONARY	★
GASTROINTESTINAL	★	STROKE	★★★
GENERAL SURGERY	★★★	VASCULAR	NR
MATERNITY CARE	★★★	WOMEN'S HEALTH	NR

HEALTHGRADES AWARDS

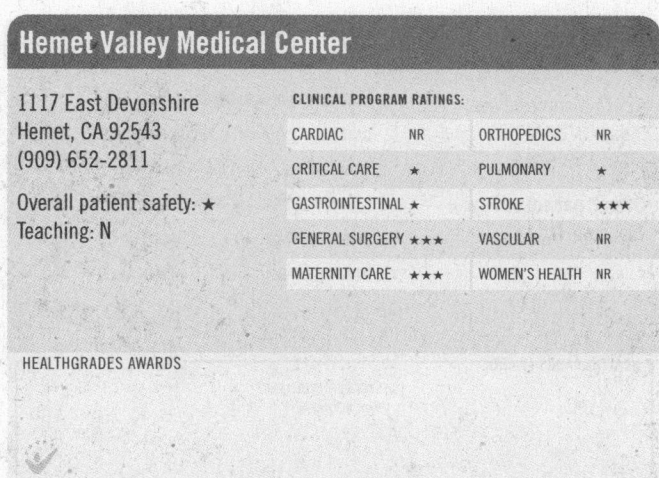

Hoag Memorial Hospital Presbyterian

One Hoag Drive
Newport Beach, CA 92663
(949) 764-4624

Overall patient safety: ★★★★★
Teaching: N

CLINICAL PROGRAM RATINGS:

CARDIAC	★★★	ORTHOPEDICS	★★★★★
CRITICAL CARE	★★★★★	PULMONARY	★★★
GASTROINTESTINAL	★★★	STROKE	★★★★★
GENERAL SURGERY	★★★	VASCULAR	NR
MATERNITY CARE	★★★	WOMEN'S HEALTH	★★★

HEALTHGRADES AWARDS

✓ **DISTINGUISHED HOSPITAL**
 · CLINICAL EXCELLENCE
 · PATIENT SAFETY

✓ **SPECIALTY EXCELLENCE**
 · CRITICAL CARE
 · GENERAL SURGERY
 · JOINT REPLACEMENT
 · ORTHOPEDIC SURGERY
 · STROKE CARE

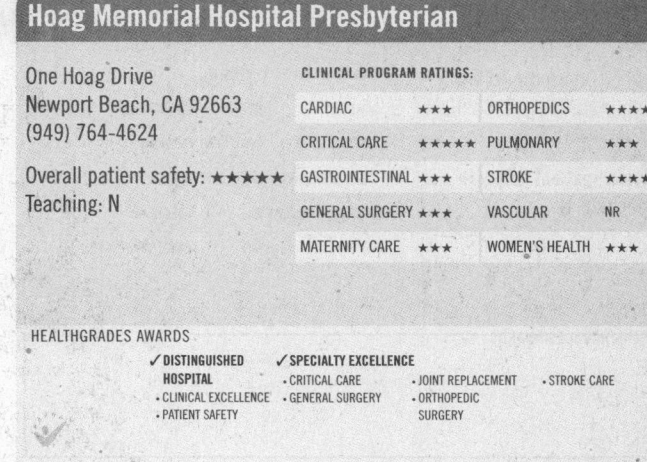

Henry Mayo Newhall Memorial Hospital

23845 McBean Parkway
Valencia, CA 91355
(661) 253-8000

Overall patient safety: ★
Teaching: N

CLINICAL PROGRAM RATINGS:

CARDIAC	NR	ORTHOPEDICS	NR
CRITICAL CARE	★★★	PULMONARY	★★★★★
GASTROINTESTINAL	NR	STROKE	★★★★★
GENERAL SURGERY	★★★	VASCULAR	NR
MATERNITY CARE	★★★	WOMEN'S HEALTH	NR

HEALTHGRADES AWARDS

✓ **SPECIALTY EXCELLENCE**
 · PULMONARY CARE
 · STROKE CARE

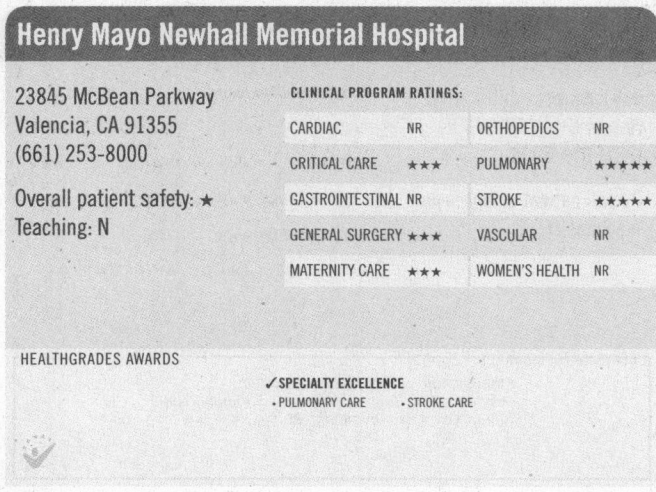

Hollywood Community Hospital

6245 De Longpre Avenue
Hollywood, CA 90028
(323) 462-2271

Overall patient safety: ★
Teaching: N

CLINICAL PROGRAM RATINGS:

CARDIAC	NR	ORTHOPEDICS	NR
CRITICAL CARE	NR	PULMONARY	★★★★★
GASTROINTESTINAL	NR	STROKE	★★★
GENERAL SURGERY	NR	VASCULAR	NR
MATERNITY CARE	NR	WOMEN'S HEALTH	NR

HEALTHGRADES AWARDS

✓ **SPECIALTY EXCELLENCE**
 · PULMONARY CARE

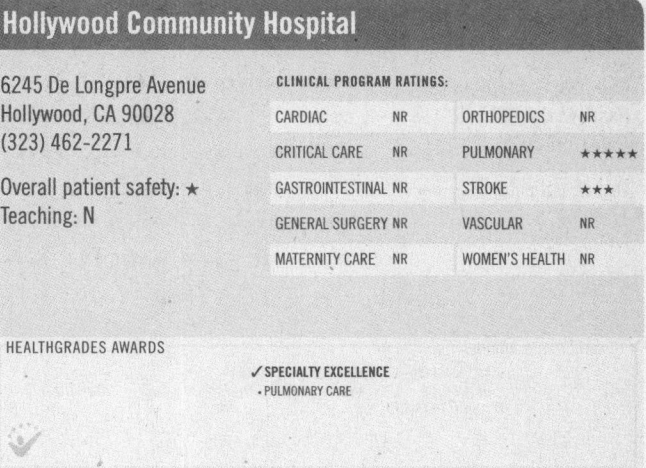

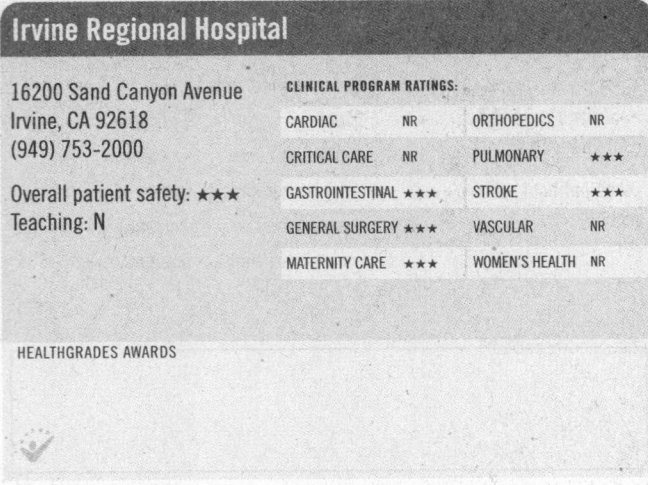

Hollywood Presbyterian Medical Center

1300 North Vermont Avenue
Los Angeles, CA 90027
(213) 413-3000

Overall patient safety: ★★★
Teaching: Y

CLINICAL PROGRAM RATINGS:

CARDIAC	NR	ORTHOPEDICS	★★★
CRITICAL CARE	NR	PULMONARY	★★★★★
GASTROINTESTINAL	NR	STROKE	★★★★★
GENERAL SURGERY	★★★	VASCULAR	NR
MATERNITY CARE	★★★	WOMEN'S HEALTH	NR

HEALTHGRADES AWARDS

✓ SPECIALTY EXCELLENCE
· GENERAL SURGERY   · PULMONARY CARE   · STROKE CARE

Irvine Regional Hospital

16200 Sand Canyon Avenue
Irvine, CA 92618
(949) 753-2000

Overall patient safety: ★★★
Teaching: N

CLINICAL PROGRAM RATINGS:

CARDIAC	NR	ORTHOPEDICS	NR
CRITICAL CARE	NR	PULMONARY	★★★
GASTROINTESTINAL	★★★	STROKE	★★★
GENERAL SURGERY	★★★	VASCULAR	NR
MATERNITY CARE	★★★	WOMEN'S HEALTH	NR

HEALTHGRADES AWARDS

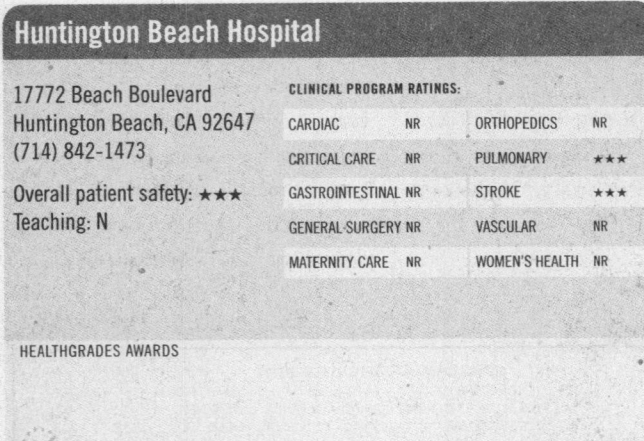

Huntington Beach Hospital

17772 Beach Boulevard
Huntington Beach, CA 92647
(714) 842-1473

Overall patient safety: ★★★
Teaching: N

CLINICAL PROGRAM RATINGS:

CARDIAC	NR	ORTHOPEDICS	NR
CRITICAL CARE	NR	PULMONARY	★★★
GASTROINTESTINAL	NR	STROKE	★★★
GENERAL SURGERY	NR	VASCULAR	NR
MATERNITY CARE	NR	WOMEN'S HEALTH	NR

HEALTHGRADES AWARDS

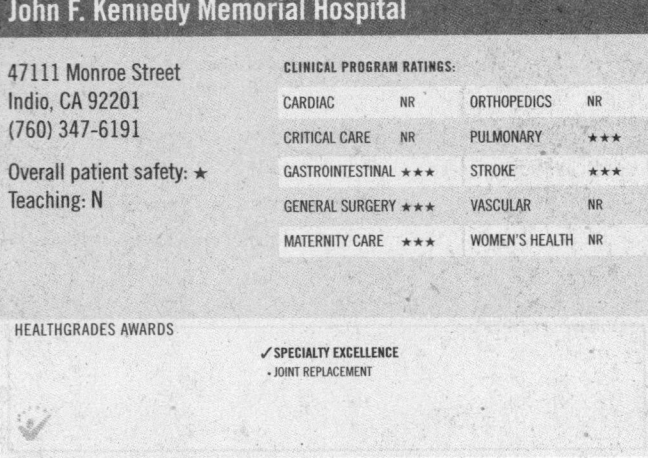

John F. Kennedy Memorial Hospital

47111 Monroe Street
Indio, CA 92201
(760) 347-6191

Overall patient safety: ★
Teaching: N

CLINICAL PROGRAM RATINGS:

CARDIAC	NR	ORTHOPEDICS	NR
CRITICAL CARE	NR	PULMONARY	★★★
GASTROINTESTINAL	★★★	STROKE	★★★
GENERAL SURGERY	★★★	VASCULAR	NR
MATERNITY CARE	★★★	WOMEN'S HEALTH	NR

HEALTHGRADES AWARDS

✓ SPECIALTY EXCELLENCE
· JOINT REPLACEMENT

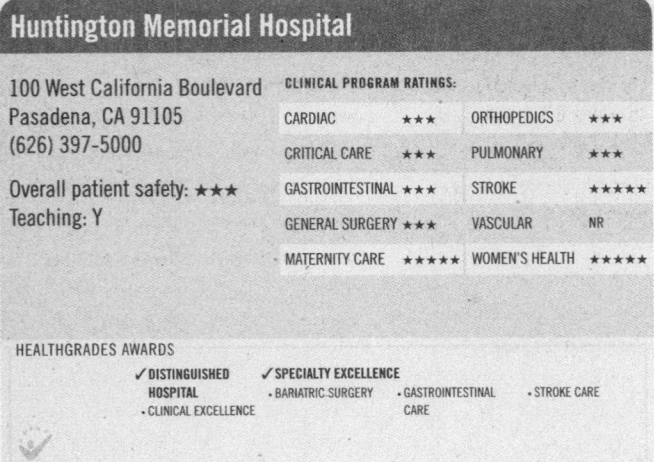

Huntington Memorial Hospital

100 West California Boulevard
Pasadena, CA 91105
(626) 397-5000

Overall patient safety: ★★★
Teaching: Y

CLINICAL PROGRAM RATINGS:

CARDIAC	★★★	ORTHOPEDICS	★★★
CRITICAL CARE	★★★	PULMONARY	★★★
GASTROINTESTINAL	★★★	STROKE	★★★★★
GENERAL SURGERY	★★★	VASCULAR	NR
MATERNITY CARE	★★★★★	WOMEN'S HEALTH	★★★★★

HEALTHGRADES AWARDS

✓ DISTINGUISHED HOSPITAL
· CLINICAL EXCELLENCE

✓ SPECIALTY EXCELLENCE
· BARIATRIC SURGERY   · GASTROINTESTINAL CARE   · STROKE CARE

John Muir Medical Center

1601 Ygnacio Valley Road
Walnut Creek, CA 94598
(925) 939-3000

Overall patient safety: ★★★
Teaching: N

CLINICAL PROGRAM RATINGS:

CARDIAC	NR	ORTHOPEDICS	★★★
CRITICAL CARE	★★★★★	PULMONARY	★★★★★
GASTROINTESTINAL	★★★★★	STROKE	★★★★★
GENERAL SURGERY	★★★	VASCULAR	NR
MATERNITY CARE	★★★	WOMEN'S HEALTH	NR

HEALTHGRADES AWARDS

✓ DISTINGUISHED HOSPITAL
· CLINICAL EXCELLENCE

✓ SPECIALTY EXCELLENCE
· CRITICAL CARE   · PULMONARY CARE
· GASTROINTESTINAL CARE   · STROKE CARE

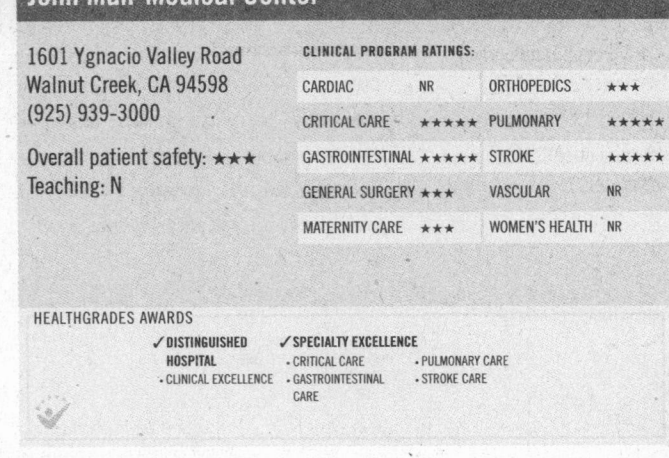

KEY: ★★★★★ BEST   ★★★ AS EXPECTED   ★ POOR   NR NOT RATED BY HEALTHGRADES   For full definitions of ratings and awards, see Appendix.

Kaiser Foundation Hospital

9400 East Rosecrans Avenue
Bellflower, CA 90706
(562) 461-3000

Overall patient safety: ★★★
Teaching: Y

CLINICAL PROGRAM RATINGS:

CARDIAC	NR	ORTHOPEDICS	NR
CRITICAL CARE	NR	PULMONARY	NR
GASTROINTESTINAL	NR	STROKE	NR
GENERAL SURGERY	NR	VASCULAR	NR
MATERNITY CARE	★★★	WOMEN'S HEALTH	NR

HEALTHGRADES AWARDS

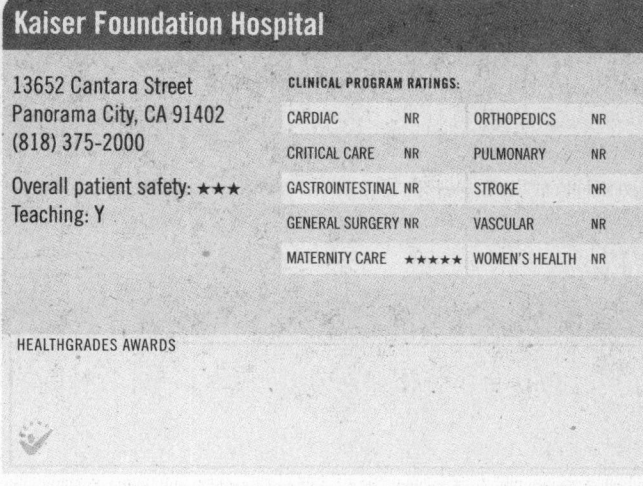

Kaiser Foundation Hospital

13652 Cantara Street
Panorama City, CA 91402
(818) 375-2000

Overall patient safety: ★★★
Teaching: Y

CLINICAL PROGRAM RATINGS:

CARDIAC	NR	ORTHOPEDICS	NR
CRITICAL CARE	NR	PULMONARY	NR
GASTROINTESTINAL	NR	STROKE	NR
GENERAL SURGERY	NR	VASCULAR	NR
MATERNITY CARE	★★★★★	WOMEN'S HEALTH	NR

HEALTHGRADES AWARDS

Kaiser Foundation Hospital

25825 South Vermont Avenue
Harbor City, CA 90710
(310) 325-5111

Overall patient safety: ★★★
Teaching: Y

CLINICAL PROGRAM RATINGS:

CARDIAC	NR	ORTHOPEDICS	NR
CRITICAL CARE	NR	PULMONARY	NR
GASTROINTESTINAL	NR	STROKE	NR
GENERAL SURGERY	NR	VASCULAR	NR
MATERNITY CARE	★★★	WOMEN'S HEALTH	NR

HEALTHGRADES AWARDS

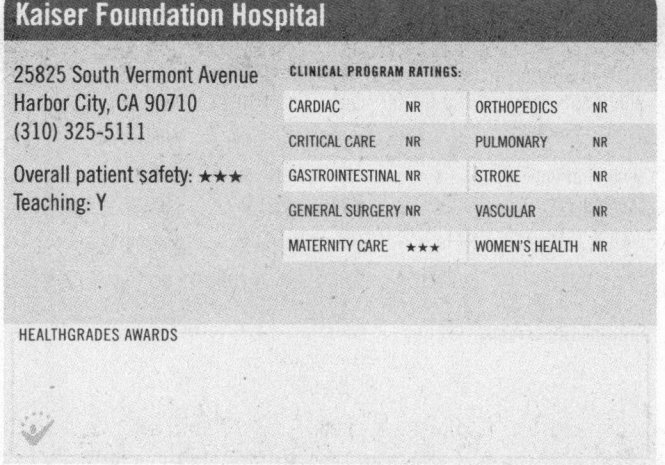

Kaiser Foundation Hospital

4647 Zion Avenue
San Diego, CA 92120
(619) 528-5000

Overall patient safety: ★★★
Teaching: Y

CLINICAL PROGRAM RATINGS:

CARDIAC	NR	ORTHOPEDICS	NR
CRITICAL CARE	NR	PULMONARY	★★★
GASTROINTESTINAL	NR	STROKE	★★★
GENERAL SURGERY	NR	VASCULAR	NR
MATERNITY CARE	★★★	WOMEN'S HEALTH	NR

HEALTHGRADES AWARDS

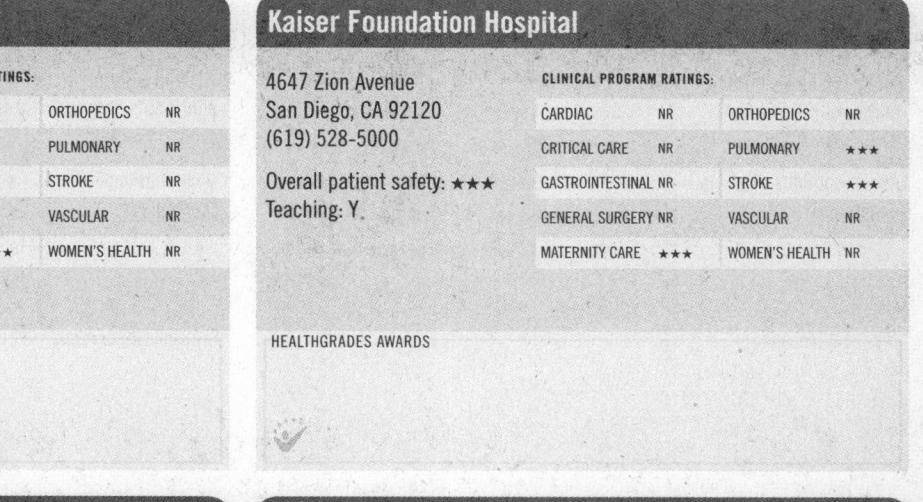

Kaiser Foundation Hospital

4867 Sunset Boulevard
Los Angeles, CA 90027
(323) 783-4011

Overall patient safety: ★★★
Teaching: Y

CLINICAL PROGRAM RATINGS:

CARDIAC	NR	ORTHOPEDICS	NR
CRITICAL CARE	NR	PULMONARY	NR
GASTROINTESTINAL	NR	STROKE	NR
GENERAL SURGERY	NR	VASCULAR	NR
MATERNITY CARE	★	WOMEN'S HEALTH	★★★

HEALTHGRADES AWARDS

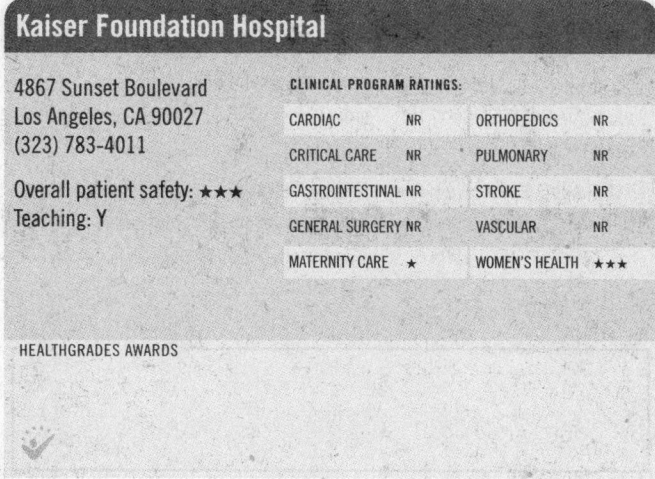

Kaiser Foundation Hospital--Anaheim

441 North Lakeview Avenue
Anaheim, CA 92807
(714) 279-4000

Overall patient safety: ★★★
Teaching: Y

CLINICAL PROGRAM RATINGS:

CARDIAC	NR	ORTHOPEDICS	NR
CRITICAL CARE	NR	PULMONARY	NR
GASTROINTESTINAL	NR	STROKE	NR
GENERAL SURGERY	NR	VASCULAR	NR
MATERNITY CARE	★★★	WOMEN'S HEALTH	NR

HEALTHGRADES AWARDS

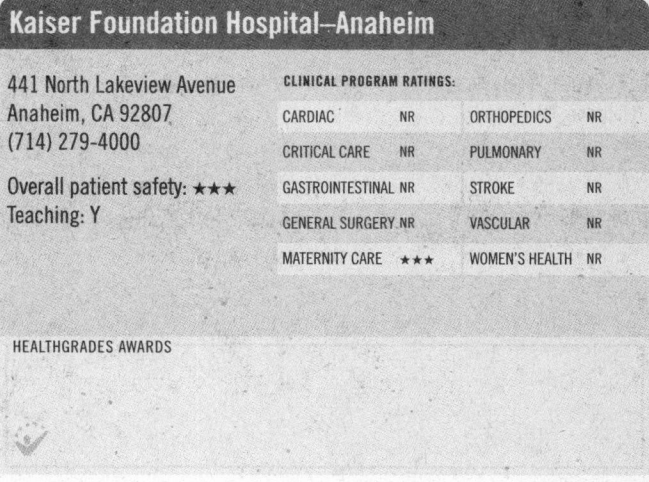

CALIFORNIA HOSPITALS: RATINGS BY CLINICAL SPECIALTY

Kaiser Foundation Hospital--Fontana

9961 Sierra Avenue
Fontana, CA 92335
(909) 427-5000

Overall patient safety: ★★★
Teaching: Y

CLINICAL PROGRAM RATINGS:

CARDIAC	NR	ORTHOPEDICS	NR
CRITICAL CARE	NR	PULMONARY	NR
GASTROINTESTINAL	NR	STROKE	NR
GENERAL SURGERY	NR	VASCULAR	NR
MATERNITY CARE	★★★	WOMEN'S HEALTH	NR

HEALTHGRADES AWARDS

Kaiser Foundation Hospital--Oakland/Richmond

280 West Macarthur Boulevard
Oakland, CA 94611
(510) 752-1000

Overall patient safety: ★★★
Teaching: Y

CLINICAL PROGRAM RATINGS:

CARDIAC	NR	ORTHOPEDICS	★★★
CRITICAL CARE	NR	PULMONARY	★★★
GASTROINTESTINAL	NR	STROKE	★★★
GENERAL SURGERY	NR	VASCULAR	NR
MATERNITY CARE	★	WOMEN'S HEALTH	NR

HEALTHGRADES AWARDS

Kaiser Foundation Hospital--Fremont/Hayward

27400 Hesperian Boulevard
Hayward, CA 94545
(510) 784-4000

Overall patient safety: ★★★
Teaching: Y

CLINICAL PROGRAM RATINGS:

CARDIAC	NR	ORTHOPEDICS	NR
CRITICAL CARE	NR	PULMONARY	★★★
GASTROINTESTINAL	NR	STROKE	★★★
GENERAL SURGERY	NR	VASCULAR	NR
MATERNITY CARE	★	WOMEN'S HEALTH	NR

HEALTHGRADES AWARDS

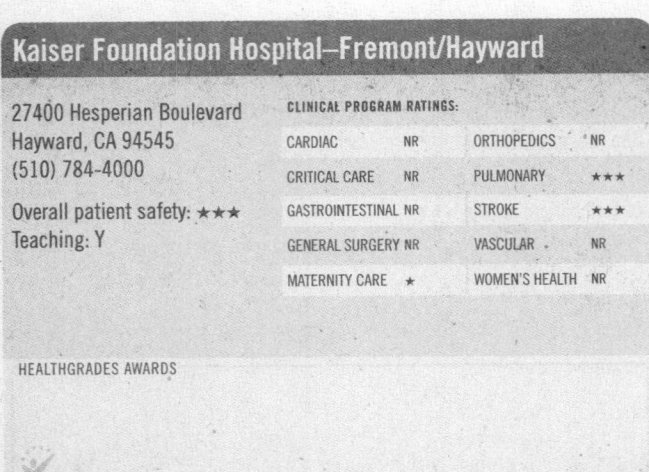

Kaiser Foundation Hospital--South San Francisco

1200 El Camino Real
South San Francisco, CA 94080
(650) 742-2000

Overall patient safety: ★★★
Teaching: N

CLINICAL PROGRAM RATINGS:

CARDIAC	NR	ORTHOPEDICS	NR
CRITICAL CARE	NR	PULMONARY	★★★
GASTROINTESTINAL	NR	STROKE	NR
GENERAL SURGERY	NR	VASCULAR	NR
MATERNITY CARE	NR	WOMEN'S HEALTH	NR

HEALTHGRADES AWARDS

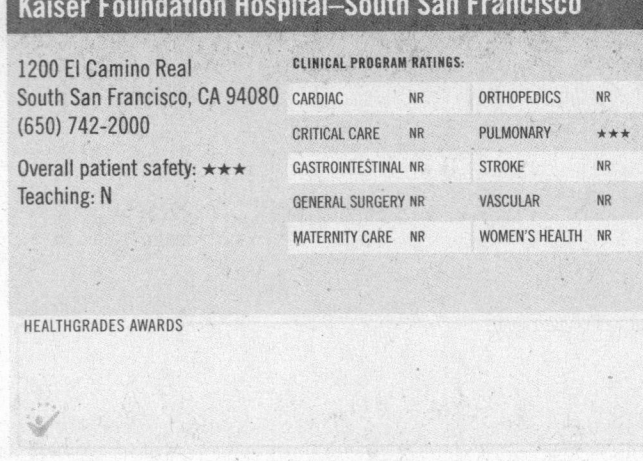

Kaiser Foundation Hospital--Manteca

1777 West Yosemite Avenue
Manteca, CA 95337
(209) 825-3700

Overall patient safety: NR
Teaching: N

CLINICAL PROGRAM RATINGS:

CARDIAC	NR	ORTHOPEDICS	NR
CRITICAL CARE	NR	PULMONARY	★★★
GASTROINTESTINAL	NR	STROKE	NR
GENERAL SURGERY	NR	VASCULAR	NR
MATERNITY CARE	NR	WOMEN'S HEALTH	NR

HEALTHGRADES AWARDS

Kaiser Foundation Hospital--Vallejo

975 Sereno Drive
Vallejo, CA 94590
(707) 651-1000

Overall patient safety: ★★★
Teaching: Y

CLINICAL PROGRAM RATINGS:

CARDIAC	NR	ORTHOPEDICS	NR
CRITICAL CARE	NR	PULMONARY	★★★
GASTROINTESTINAL	NR	STROKE	★★★
GENERAL SURGERY	NR	VASCULAR	NR
MATERNITY CARE	★★★	WOMEN'S HEALTH	NR

HEALTHGRADES AWARDS

KEY: ★★★★★ BEST ★★★ AS EXPECTED ★ POOR NR NOT RATED BY HEALTHGRADES   For full definitions of ratings and awards, see Appendix.

Kaiser Fresno Medical Center

7300 North Fresno Street
Fresno, CA 93720
(559) 448-4500

Overall patient safety: ★★★
Teaching: Y

CLINICAL PROGRAM RATINGS:

CARDIAC	NR	ORTHOPEDICS	NR
CRITICAL CARE	NR	PULMONARY	NR
GASTROINTESTINAL	NR	STROKE	NR
GENERAL SURGERY	NR	VASCULAR	NR
MATERNITY CARE	★★★	WOMEN'S HEALTH	NR

HEALTHGRADES AWARDS

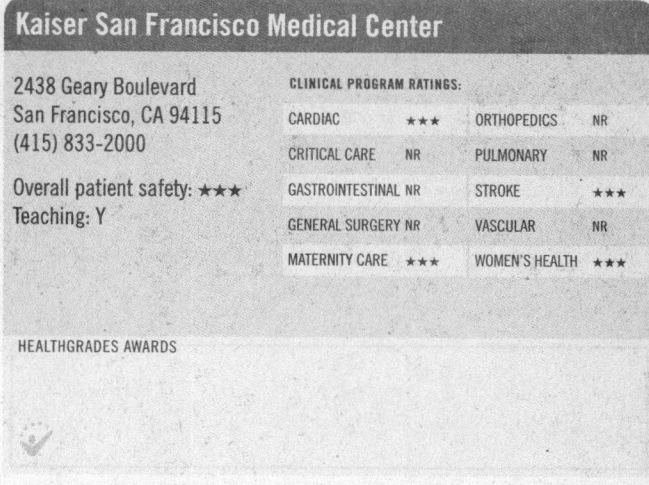

Kaiser San Francisco Medical Center

2438 Geary Boulevard
San Francisco, CA 94115
(415) 833-2000

Overall patient safety: ★★★
Teaching: Y

CLINICAL PROGRAM RATINGS:

CARDIAC	★★★	ORTHOPEDICS	NR
CRITICAL CARE	NR	PULMONARY	NR
GASTROINTESTINAL	NR	STROKE	★★★
GENERAL SURGERY	NR	VASCULAR	NR
MATERNITY CARE	★★★	WOMEN'S HEALTH	★★★

HEALTHGRADES AWARDS

Kaiser Redwood City Medical Center

1150 Veterans Boulevard
Redwood City, CA 94063
(650) 299-2000

Overall patient safety: ★★★
Teaching: N

CLINICAL PROGRAM RATINGS:

CARDIAC	NR	ORTHOPEDICS	NR
CRITICAL CARE	NR	PULMONARY	NR
GASTROINTESTINAL	NR	STROKE	NR
GENERAL SURGERY	NR	VASCULAR	NR
MATERNITY CARE	★★★	WOMEN'S HEALTH	NR

HEALTHGRADES AWARDS

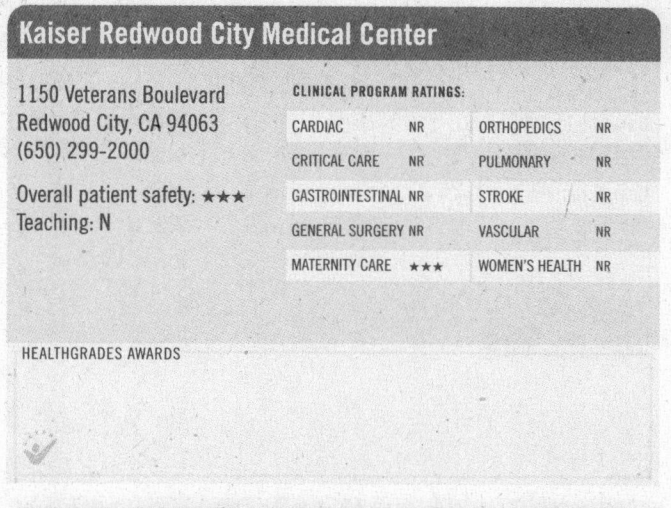

Kaiser San Rafael Medical Center

99 Montecillo Road
San Rafael, CA 94903
(415) 444-2000

Overall patient safety: ★★★
Teaching: N

CLINICAL PROGRAM RATINGS:

CARDIAC	NR	ORTHOPEDICS	NR
CRITICAL CARE	NR	PULMONARY	★★★
GASTROINTESTINAL	NR	STROKE	★★★
GENERAL SURGERY	NR	VASCULAR	NR
MATERNITY CARE	NR	WOMEN'S HEALTH	NR

HEALTHGRADES AWARDS

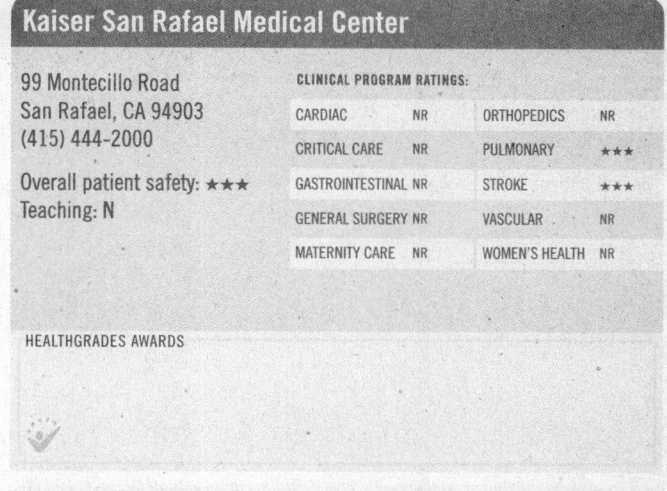

Kaiser Sacramento Medical Center

2025 Morse Avenue
Sacramento, CA 95825
(916) 973-5000

Overall patient safety: ★★★
Teaching: Y

CLINICAL PROGRAM RATINGS:

CARDIAC	NR	ORTHOPEDICS	★★★
CRITICAL CARE	NR	PULMONARY	★★★
GASTROINTESTINAL	NR	STROKE	★★★
GENERAL SURGERY	★★★	VASCULAR	NR
MATERNITY CARE	★	WOMEN'S HEALTH	NR

HEALTHGRADES AWARDS

Kaiser Santa Clara Medical Center

700 Lawrence Expy
Santa Clara, CA 95051
(408) 236-6400

Overall patient safety: ★★★
Teaching: Y

CLINICAL PROGRAM RATINGS:

CARDIAC	NR	ORTHOPEDICS	NR
CRITICAL CARE	NR	PULMONARY	★★★
GASTROINTESTINAL	NR	STROKE	★★★
GENERAL SURGERY	NR	VASCULAR	NR
MATERNITY CARE	★	WOMEN'S HEALTH	NR

HEALTHGRADES AWARDS

CALIFORNIA HOSPITALS: RATINGS BY CLINICAL SPECIALTY

Kaiser Santa Teresa Community Hospital

250 Hospital Parkway
San Jose, CA 95119
(408) 972-7000

Overall patient safety: ★★★
Teaching: N

CLINICAL PROGRAM RATINGS:

CARDIAC	NR	ORTHOPEDICS	NR
CRITICAL CARE	NR	PULMONARY	★★★
GASTROINTESTINAL	NR	STROKE	★★★
GENERAL SURGERY	NR	VASCULAR	NR
MATERNITY CARE	★★★	WOMEN'S HEALTH	NR

HEALTHGRADES AWARDS

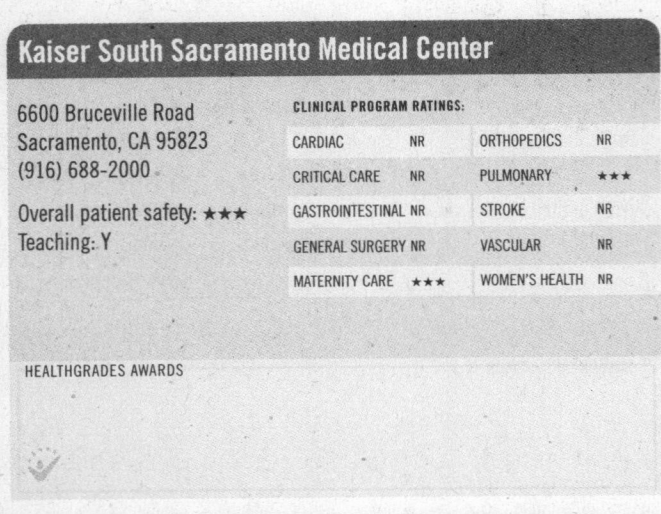

Kaweah Delta District Hospital

400 West Mineral King
Visalia, CA 93291
(559) 624-2000

Overall patient safety: ★
Teaching: N

CLINICAL PROGRAM RATINGS:

CARDIAC	★★★	ORTHOPEDICS	★★★★★
CRITICAL CARE	★	PULMONARY	★
GASTROINTESTINAL	★	STROKE	★
GENERAL SURGERY	★	VASCULAR	NR
MATERNITY CARE	★★★	WOMEN'S HEALTH	★★★

HEALTHGRADES AWARDS

✓ SPECIALTY EXCELLENCE
· ORTHOPEDIC
  SURGERY

Kaiser South Sacramento Medical Center

6600 Bruceville Road
Sacramento, CA 95823
(916) 688-2000

Overall patient safety: ★★★
Teaching: Y

CLINICAL PROGRAM RATINGS:

CARDIAC	NR	ORTHOPEDICS	NR
CRITICAL CARE	NR	PULMONARY	★★★
GASTROINTESTINAL	NR	STROKE	NR
GENERAL SURGERY	NR	VASCULAR	NR
MATERNITY CARE	★★★	WOMEN'S HEALTH	NR

HEALTHGRADES AWARDS

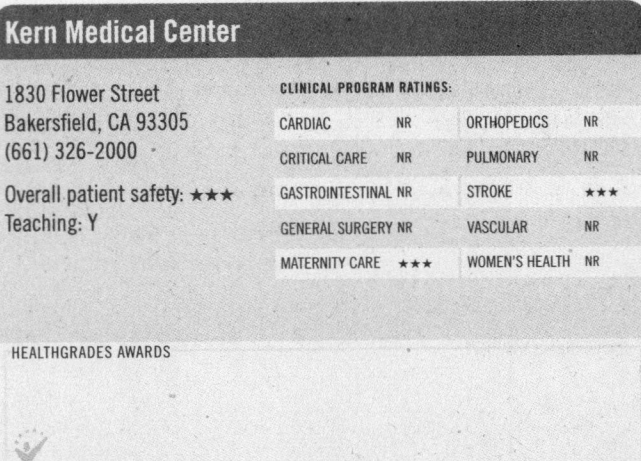

Kern Medical Center

1830 Flower Street
Bakersfield, CA 93305
(661) 326-2000

Overall patient safety: ★★★
Teaching: Y

CLINICAL PROGRAM RATINGS:

CARDIAC	NR	ORTHOPEDICS	NR
CRITICAL CARE	NR	PULMONARY	NR
GASTROINTESTINAL	NR	STROKE	★★★
GENERAL SURGERY	NR	VASCULAR	NR
MATERNITY CARE	★★★	WOMEN'S HEALTH	NR

HEALTHGRADES AWARDS

Kaiser Walnut Creek Medical Center

1425 South Main Street
Walnut Creek, CA 94596
(925) 295-4000

Overall patient safety: ★★★
Teaching: Y

CLINICAL PROGRAM RATINGS:

CARDIAC	NR	ORTHOPEDICS	NR
CRITICAL CARE	NR	PULMONARY	★★★
GASTROINTESTINAL	NR	STROKE	NR
GENERAL SURGERY	NR	VASCULAR	NR
MATERNITY CARE	★★★	WOMEN'S HEALTH	NR

HEALTHGRADES AWARDS

Kern Valley Healthcare District

6412 Laurel Avenue
Lake Isabella, CA 93240
(760) 379-2681

Overall patient safety: ★★★
Teaching: N

CLINICAL PROGRAM RATINGS:

CARDIAC	NR	ORTHOPEDICS	NR
CRITICAL CARE	NR	PULMONARY	★★★
GASTROINTESTINAL	NR	STROKE	NR
GENERAL SURGERY	NR	VASCULAR	NR
MATERNITY CARE	NR	WOMEN'S HEALTH	NR

HEALTHGRADES AWARDS

KEY: ★★★★★ BEST   ★★★ AS EXPECTED   ★ POOR   NR NOT RATED BY HEALTHGRADES   For full definitions of ratings and awards, see Appendix.

La Palma Intercommunity Hospital

7901 Walker Street
La Palma, CA 90623
(714) 670-7400

Overall patient safety: ★★★
Teaching: N

CLINICAL PROGRAM RATINGS:

CARDIAC	NR	ORTHOPEDICS	NR
CRITICAL CARE	NR	PULMONARY	★★★
GASTROINTESTINAL	NR	STROKE	★★★
GENERAL SURGERY	NR	VASCULAR	NR
MATERNITY CARE	★★★	WOMEN'S HEALTH	NR

HEALTHGRADES AWARDS

LAC Martin Luther King Jr. Multi Service Ambulatory Care Ctr.

12021 South Wilmington
Avenue
Los Angeles, CA 90059
(310) 668-4321

Overall patient safety: ★★★
Teaching: Y

CLINICAL PROGRAM RATINGS:

CARDIAC	NR	ORTHOPEDICS	NR
CRITICAL CARE	NR	PULMONARY	★★★
GASTROINTESTINAL	NR	STROKE	NR
GENERAL SURGERY	NR	VASCULAR	NR
MATERNITY CARE	★★★	WOMEN'S HEALTH	NR

HEALTHGRADES AWARDS

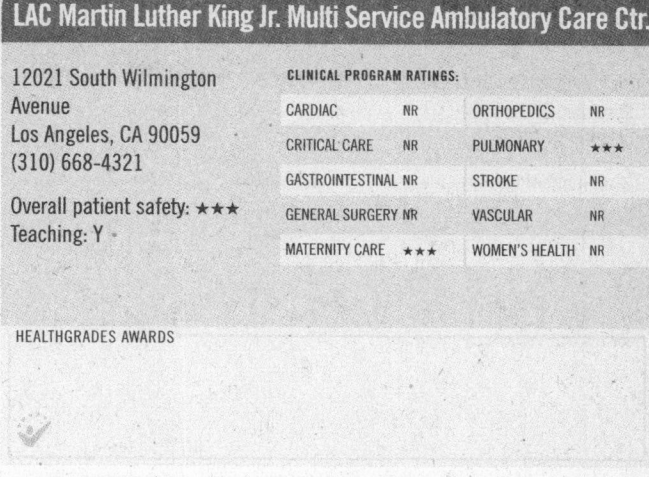

LAC+USC Medical Center

1200 North State Street
Los Angeles, CA 90033
(323) 226-2622

Overall patient safety: ★★★
Teaching: Y

CLINICAL PROGRAM RATINGS:

CARDIAC	NR	ORTHOPEDICS	NR
CRITICAL CARE	NR	PULMONARY	★★★
GASTROINTESTINAL	NR	STROKE	NR
GENERAL SURGERY	NR	VASCULAR	NR
MATERNITY CARE	★★★	WOMEN'S HEALTH	NR

HEALTHGRADES AWARDS

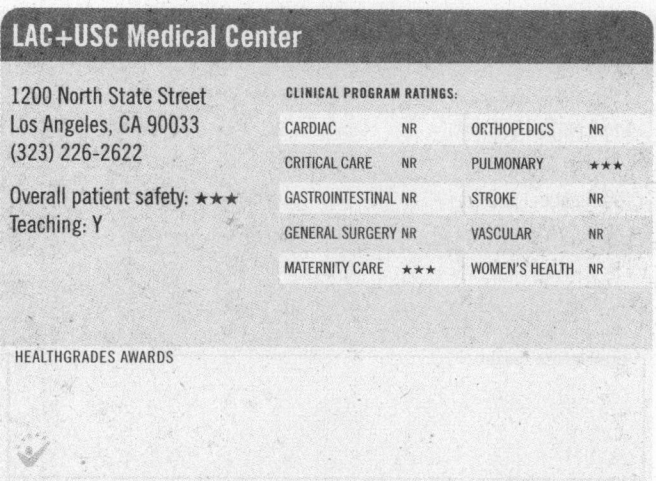

LAC Olive View-UCLA Medical Center

14445 Olive View Drive
Sylmar, CA 91342
(818) 364-1555

Overall patient safety: ★
Teaching: Y

CLINICAL PROGRAM RATINGS:

CARDIAC	NR	ORTHOPEDICS	NR
CRITICAL CARE	NR	PULMONARY	★★★
GASTROINTESTINAL	NR	STROKE	NR
GENERAL SURGERY	NR	VASCULAR	NR
MATERNITY CARE	★	WOMEN'S HEALTH	NR

HEALTHGRADES AWARDS

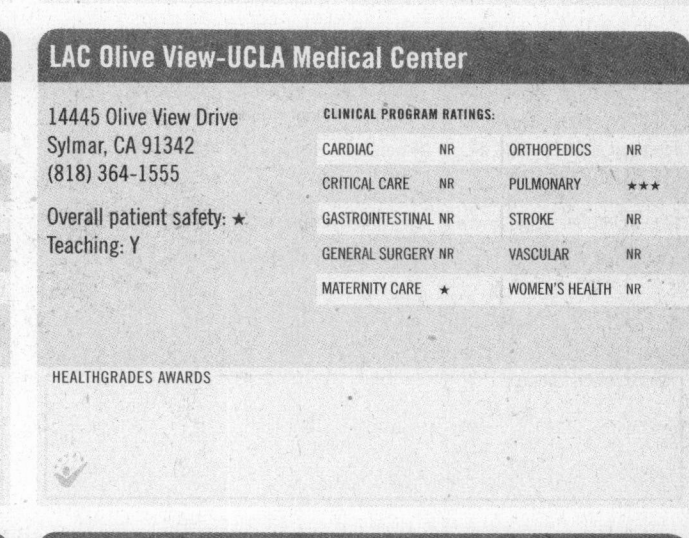

LAC Harbor-UCLA Medical Center

1000 West Carson Street
Torrance, CA 90509
(310) 222-2345

Overall patient safety: ★★★
Teaching: Y

CLINICAL PROGRAM RATINGS:

CARDIAC	NR	ORTHOPEDICS	NR
CRITICAL CARE	NR	PULMONARY	★★★
GASTROINTESTINAL	NR	STROKE	NR
GENERAL SURGERY	NR	VASCULAR	NR
MATERNITY CARE	★	WOMEN'S HEALTH	NR

HEALTHGRADES AWARDS

Lakewood Regional Medical Center

3700 East South Street
Lakewood, CA 90712
(562) 531-2550

Overall patient safety: ★★★
Teaching: Y

CLINICAL PROGRAM RATINGS:

CARDIAC	★★★	ORTHOPEDICS	NR
CRITICAL CARE	NR	PULMONARY	★★★
GASTROINTESTINAL	NR	STROKE	★★★
GENERAL SURGERY	★★★	VASCULAR	NR
MATERNITY CARE	NR	WOMEN'S HEALTH	NR

HEALTHGRADES AWARDS

Lancaster Community Hospital

43830 North 10th Street West
Lancaster, CA 93534
(661) 948-4781

Overall patient safety: ★★★
Teaching: N

CLINICAL PROGRAM RATINGS:

CARDIAC	NR	ORTHOPEDICS	NR
CRITICAL CARE	★★★	PULMONARY	★★★
GASTROINTESTINAL	NR	STROKE	★★★
GENERAL SURGERY	★★★	VASCULAR	NR
MATERNITY CARE	NR	WOMEN'S HEALTH	NR

HEALTHGRADES AWARDS

Lodi Memorial Hospital

975 South Fairmont Avenue
Lodi, CA 95240
(209) 334-3411

Overall patient safety: ★★★
Teaching: N

CLINICAL PROGRAM RATINGS:

CARDIAC	NR	ORTHOPEDICS	NR
CRITICAL CARE	★	PULMONARY	★
GASTROINTESTINAL	NR	STROKE	★
GENERAL SURGERY	★★★	VASCULAR	NR
MATERNITY CARE	★★★	WOMEN'S HEALTH	NR

HEALTHGRADES AWARDS

Little Company of Mary Hospital

4101 Torrance Boulevard
Torrance, CA 90503
(310) 540-7676

Overall patient safety: ★★★
Teaching: N

CLINICAL PROGRAM RATINGS:

CARDIAC	★	ORTHOPEDICS	★★★
CRITICAL CARE	★★★	PULMONARY	★★★
GASTROINTESTINAL	★★★	STROKE	★★★
GENERAL SURGERY	★★★	VASCULAR	NR
MATERNITY CARE	★★★	WOMEN'S HEALTH	★★★

HEALTHGRADES AWARDS

Loma Linda University Medical Center

11234 Anderson Street
Loma Linda, CA 92354
(909) 558-4000

Overall patient safety: ★
Teaching: Y

CLINICAL PROGRAM RATINGS:

CARDIAC	★★★	ORTHOPEDICS	★★★
CRITICAL CARE	★★★	PULMONARY	★
GASTROINTESTINAL	★★★	STROKE	★★★
GENERAL SURGERY	★★★	VASCULAR	NR
MATERNITY CARE	★	WOMEN'S HEALTH	★

HEALTHGRADES AWARDS

Little Company of Mary Hospital—San Pedro

1300 West 7th Street
San Pedro, CA 90732
(310) 832-3311

Overall patient safety: ★★★
Teaching: N

CLINICAL PROGRAM RATINGS:

CARDIAC	NR	ORTHOPEDICS	NR
CRITICAL CARE	NR	PULMONARY	★★★
GASTROINTESTINAL	NR	STROKE	★★★
GENERAL SURGERY	NR	VASCULAR	NR
MATERNITY CARE	★★★	WOMEN'S HEALTH	NR

HEALTHGRADES AWARDS

Lompoc Healthcare District

508 East Hickory
Lompoc, CA 93436
(805) 737-3300

Overall patient safety: ★★★
Teaching: N

CLINICAL PROGRAM RATINGS:

CARDIAC	NR	ORTHOPEDICS	NR
CRITICAL CARE	NR	PULMONARY	★
GASTROINTESTINAL	NR	STROKE	★
GENERAL SURGERY	NR	VASCULAR	NR
MATERNITY CARE	★★★	WOMEN'S HEALTH	NR

HEALTHGRADES AWARDS

KEY: ★★★★★ BEST   ★★★ AS EXPECTED   ★ POOR   NR NOT RATED BY HEALTHGRADES   For full definitions of ratings and awards, see Appendix.

Long Beach Memorial Medical Center

2801 Atlantic Avenue
Long Beach, CA 90801
(562) 933-2000

Overall patient safety: ★★★
Teaching: Y

CLINICAL PROGRAM RATINGS:

CARDIAC	★★★	ORTHOPEDICS	★★★
CRITICAL CARE	★★★	PULMONARY	★★★
GASTROINTESTINAL	★★★	STROKE	★★★★★
GENERAL SURGERY	★★★	VASCULAR	★★★
MATERNITY CARE	NR	WOMEN'S HEALTH	NR

HEALTHGRADES AWARDS

✓ SPECIALTY EXCELLENCE
· JOINT REPLACEMENT   · STROKE CARE

Los Angeles Metropolitan Medical Center

2231 South Western Avenue
Los Angeles, CA 90018
(323) 730-7300

Overall patient safety: ★
Teaching: N

CLINICAL PROGRAM RATINGS:

CARDIAC	NR	ORTHOPEDICS	NR
CRITICAL CARE	NR	PULMONARY	★★★★★
GASTROINTESTINAL	NR	STROKE	NR
GENERAL SURGERY	NR	VASCULAR	NR
MATERNITY CARE	★★★★★	WOMEN'S HEALTH	NR

HEALTHGRADES AWARDS

✓ SPECIALTY EXCELLENCE
· MATERNITY CARE   · PULMONARY CARE

Los Alamitos Medical Center

3751 Katella Avenue
Los Alamitos, CA 90720
(562) 598-1311

Overall patient safety: ★
Teaching: N

CLINICAL PROGRAM RATINGS:

CARDIAC	NR	ORTHOPEDICS	★★★
CRITICAL CARE	★★★	PULMONARY	★★★
GASTROINTESTINAL	NR	STROKE	★★★
GENERAL SURGERY	★★★	VASCULAR	NR
MATERNITY CARE	★★★	WOMEN'S HEALTH	NR

HEALTHGRADES AWARDS

Los Robles Regional Medical Center

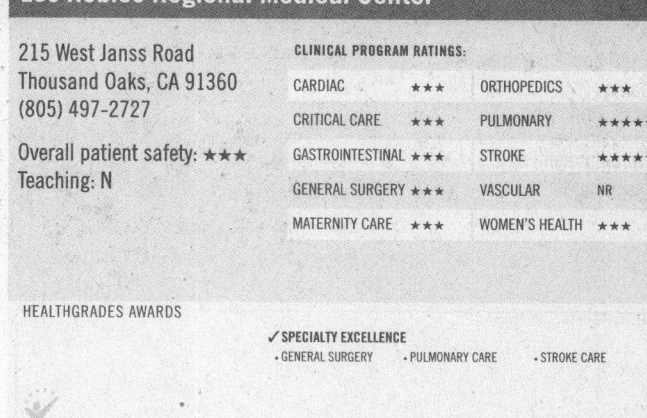

215 West Janss Road
Thousand Oaks, CA 91360
(805) 497-2727

Overall patient safety: ★★★
Teaching: N

CLINICAL PROGRAM RATINGS:

CARDIAC	★★★	ORTHOPEDICS	★★★
CRITICAL CARE	★★★	PULMONARY	★★★★★
GASTROINTESTINAL	★★★	STROKE	★★★★★
GENERAL SURGERY	★★★	VASCULAR	NR
MATERNITY CARE	★★★	WOMEN'S HEALTH	★★★

HEALTHGRADES AWARDS

✓ SPECIALTY EXCELLENCE
· GENERAL SURGERY   · PULMONARY CARE   · STROKE CARE

Los Angeles Community Hospital*

4081 East Olympic Boulevard
Los Angeles, CA 90023
(323) 267-0477

Overall patient safety: ★★★
Teaching: N

CLINICAL PROGRAM RATINGS:

CARDIAC	NR	ORTHOPEDICS	NR
CRITICAL CARE	NR	PULMONARY	★★★★★
GASTROINTESTINAL	NR	STROKE	★★★★★
GENERAL SURGERY	NR	VASCULAR	NR
MATERNITY CARE	★★★★★	WOMEN'S HEALTH	NR

HEALTHGRADES AWARDS

✓ SPECIALTY EXCELLENCE
· PULMONARY CARE   · STROKE CARE

Mad River Community Hospital

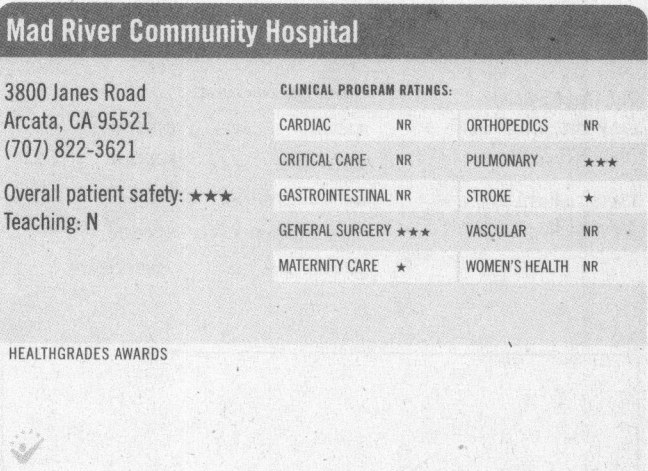

3800 Janes Road
Arcata, CA 95521
(707) 822-3621

Overall patient safety: ★★★
Teaching: N

CLINICAL PROGRAM RATINGS:

CARDIAC	NR	ORTHOPEDICS	NR
CRITICAL CARE	NR	PULMONARY	★★★
GASTROINTESTINAL	NR	STROKE	★
GENERAL SURGERY	★★★	VASCULAR	NR
MATERNITY CARE	★	WOMEN'S HEALTH	NR

HEALTHGRADES AWARDS

*This hospital reports its data to the federal government jointly with another hospital. Therefore the ratings and awards apply to multiple hospitals and this specific hospital may not provide all rated services.

Madera Community Hospital

1250 East Almond Avenue
Madera, CA 93637
(559) 675-5555

Overall patient safety: ★★★
Teaching: N

CLINICAL PROGRAM RATINGS:

CARDIAC	NR	ORTHOPEDICS	NR
CRITICAL CARE	NR	PULMONARY	★★★
GASTROINTESTINAL	★★★	STROKE	★
GENERAL SURGERY	★★★	VASCULAR	NR
MATERNITY CARE	★★★	WOMEN'S HEALTH	NR

HEALTHGRADES AWARDS

Mark Twain St. Joseph's Hospital

768 Mountain Ranch Road
San Andreas, CA 95249
(209) 754-3521

Overall patient safety: ★★★
Teaching: N

CLINICAL PROGRAM RATINGS:

CARDIAC	NR	ORTHOPEDICS	NR
CRITICAL CARE	NR	PULMONARY	★★★
GASTROINTESTINAL	NR	STROKE	★
GENERAL SURGERY	NR	VASCULAR	NR
MATERNITY CARE	★★★	WOMEN'S HEALTH	NR

HEALTHGRADES AWARDS

Marian Medical Center

1400 East Church Street
Santa Maria, CA 93454
(805) 739-3000

Overall patient safety: ★★★
Teaching: N

CLINICAL PROGRAM RATINGS:

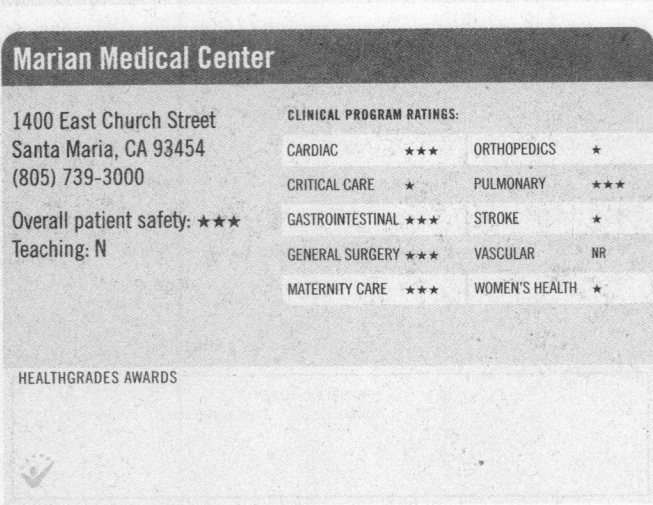

CARDIAC	★★★	ORTHOPEDICS	★
CRITICAL CARE	★	PULMONARY	★★★
GASTROINTESTINAL	★★★	STROKE	★
GENERAL SURGERY	★★★	VASCULAR	NR
MATERNITY CARE	★★★	WOMEN'S HEALTH	★

HEALTHGRADES AWARDS

Marshall Medical Center

1100 Marshall Way
Placerville, CA 95667
(530) 622-1441

Overall patient safety: ★★★
Teaching: N

CLINICAL PROGRAM RATINGS:

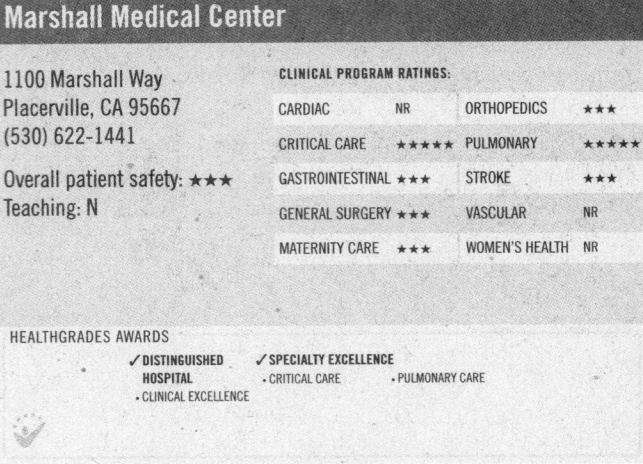

CARDIAC	NR	ORTHOPEDICS	★★★
CRITICAL CARE	★★★★★	PULMONARY	★★★★★
GASTROINTESTINAL	★★★	STROKE	★★★
GENERAL SURGERY	★★★	VASCULAR	NR
MATERNITY CARE	★★★	WOMEN'S HEALTH	NR

HEALTHGRADES AWARDS

✓ DISTINGUISHED HOSPITAL   ✓ SPECIALTY EXCELLENCE
• CLINICAL EXCELLENCE   • CRITICAL CARE   • PULMONARY CARE

Marin General Hospital

250 Bon Air Road
Greenbrae, CA 94904
(415) 925-7000

Overall patient safety: ★
Teaching: N

CLINICAL PROGRAM RATINGS:

CARDIAC	★★★	ORTHOPEDICS	★★★
CRITICAL CARE	★★★	PULMONARY	★★★
GASTROINTESTINAL	★★★	STROKE	★
GENERAL SURGERY	★★★	VASCULAR	NR
MATERNITY CARE	★★★	WOMEN'S HEALTH	NR

HEALTHGRADES AWARDS

Memorial Hospital of Gardena

1145 West Redondo
Beach Boulevard
Gardena, CA 90247
(310) 532-4200

Overall patient safety: ★★★
Teaching: N

CLINICAL PROGRAM RATINGS:

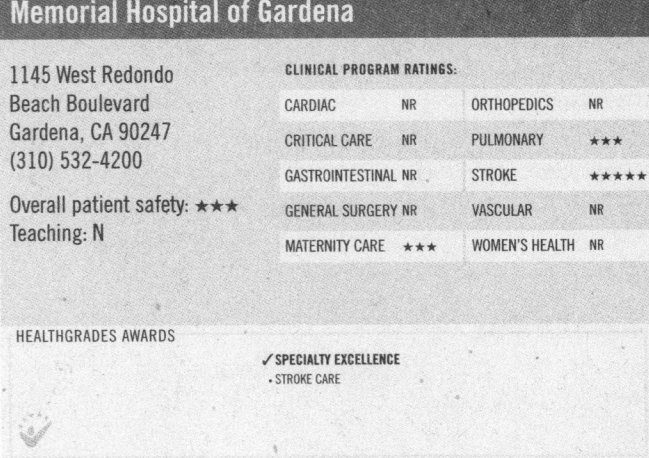

CARDIAC	NR	ORTHOPEDICS	NR
CRITICAL CARE	NR	PULMONARY	★★★
GASTROINTESTINAL	NR	STROKE	★★★★★
GENERAL SURGERY	NR	VASCULAR	NR
MATERNITY CARE	★★★	WOMEN'S HEALTH	NR

HEALTHGRADES AWARDS

✓ SPECIALTY EXCELLENCE
• STROKE CARE

KEY: ★★★★★ BEST   ★★★ AS EXPECTED   ★ POOR   NR NOT RATED BY HEALTHGRADES   For full definitions of ratings and awards, see Appendix.

Memorial Hospital–Los Banos

520 West I Street
Los Banos, CA 93635
(209) 826-0591

Overall patient safety: ★★★
Teaching: N

CLINICAL PROGRAM RATINGS:

CARDIAC	NR	ORTHOPEDICS	NR
CRITICAL CARE	NR	PULMONARY	★★★
GASTROINTESTINAL	NR	STROKE	★★★
GENERAL SURGERY	NR	VASCULAR	NR
MATERNITY CARE	★★★	WOMEN'S HEALTH	NR

HEALTHGRADES AWARDS

Menifee Valley Medical Center

28400 McCall Boulevard
Sun City, CA 92585
(909) 652-2811

Overall patient safety: ★
Teaching: N

CLINICAL PROGRAM RATINGS:

CARDIAC	NR	ORTHOPEDICS	NR
CRITICAL CARE	NR	PULMONARY	★
GASTROINTESTINAL	NR	STROKE	★★★
GENERAL SURGERY	NR	VASCULAR	NR
MATERNITY CARE	NR	WOMEN'S HEALTH	NR

HEALTHGRADES AWARDS

Memorial Medical Center

1700 Coffee Road
Modesto, CA 95355
(209) 526-4500

Overall patient safety: ★
Teaching: N

CLINICAL PROGRAM RATINGS:

CARDIAC	★★★	ORTHOPEDICS	★★★
CRITICAL CARE	NR	PULMONARY	★
GASTROINTESTINAL	★★★	STROKE	★
GENERAL SURGERY	★★★	VASCULAR	NR
MATERNITY CARE	★★★	WOMEN'S HEALTH	★★★

HEALTHGRADES AWARDS

Mercy General Hospital

4001 J Street
Sacramento, CA 95819
(916) 453-4545

Overall patient safety: ★★★★★
Teaching: Y

CLINICAL PROGRAM RATINGS:

CARDIAC	★★★	ORTHOPEDICS	★★★
CRITICAL CARE	★★★	PULMONARY	★★★
GASTROINTESTINAL	★★★	STROKE	★★★
GENERAL SURGERY	★★★	VASCULAR	★★★
MATERNITY CARE	★★★★★	WOMEN'S HEALTH	★★★

HEALTHGRADES AWARDS
✓ DISTINGUISHED
  HOSPITAL
  • PATIENT SAFETY

Mendocino Coast District Hospital

700 River Drive
Fort Bragg, CA 95437
(707) 961-1234

Overall patient safety: ★★★
Teaching: N

CLINICAL PROGRAM RATINGS:

CARDIAC	NR	ORTHOPEDICS	NR
CRITICAL CARE	NR	PULMONARY	★★★
GASTROINTESTINAL	NR	STROKE	★★★
GENERAL SURGERY	NR	VASCULAR	NR
MATERNITY CARE	★★★	WOMEN'S HEALTH	NR

HEALTHGRADES AWARDS

Mercy Hospital

2215 Truxtun Avenue
Bakersfield, CA 93301
(661) 632-5000

Overall patient safety: ★★★
Teaching: N

CLINICAL PROGRAM RATINGS:

CARDIAC	NR	ORTHOPEDICS	★★★
CRITICAL CARE	NR	PULMONARY	★
GASTROINTESTINAL	★★★	STROKE	★★★
GENERAL SURGERY	★	VASCULAR	NR
MATERNITY CARE	★★★	WOMEN'S HEALTH	NR

HEALTHGRADES AWARDS

Mercy Hospital of Folsom

1650 Creekside Drive
Folsom, CA 95630
(916) 983-7400

Overall patient safety: ★★★
Teaching: N

CLINICAL PROGRAM RATINGS:

CARDIAC	NR	ORTHOPEDICS	NR
CRITICAL-CARE	NR	PULMONARY	★
GASTROINTESTINAL	NR	STROKE	★★★
GENERAL SURGERY	★★★	VASCULAR	NR
MATERNITY CARE	★★★	WOMEN'S HEALTH	NR

HEALTHGRADES AWARDS

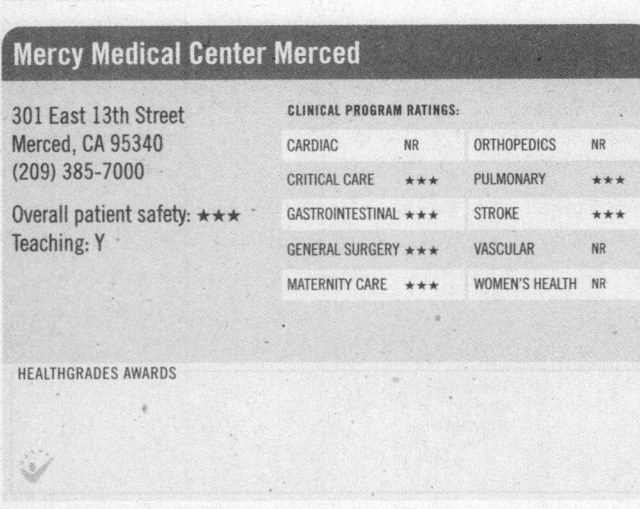

Mercy Medical Center Redding

2175 Rosaline Avenue,
Clairmont Heights
Redding, CA 96001
(530) 225-6000

Overall patient safety: ★★★
Teaching: Y

CLINICAL PROGRAM RATINGS:

CARDIAC	★★★	ORTHOPEDICS	★★★
CRITICAL CARE	★	PULMONARY	★
GASTROINTESTINAL	★	STROKE	★
GENERAL SURGERY	★★★	VASCULAR	★★★
MATERNITY CARE	★★★	WOMEN'S HEALTH	★

HEALTHGRADES AWARDS

✓ SPECIALTY EXCELLENCE
· JOINT REPLACEMENT

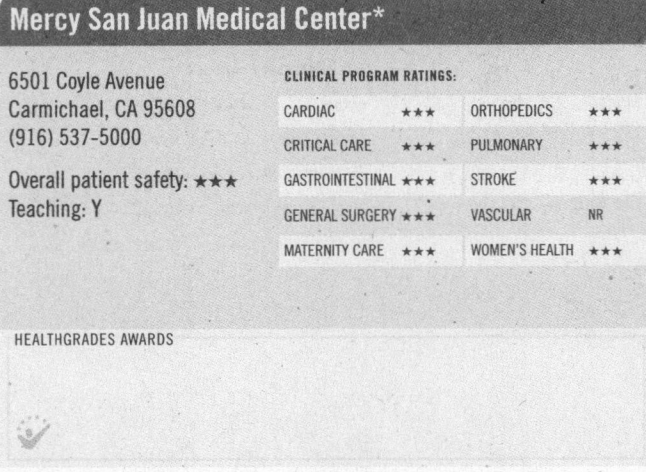

Mercy Medical Center Merced

301 East 13th Street
Merced, CA 95340
(209) 385-7000

Overall patient safety: ★★★
Teaching: Y

CLINICAL PROGRAM RATINGS:

CARDIAC	NR	ORTHOPEDICS	NR
CRITICAL CARE	★★★	PULMONARY	★★★
GASTROINTESTINAL	★★★	STROKE	★★★
GENERAL SURGERY	★★★	VASCULAR	NR
MATERNITY CARE	★★★	WOMEN'S HEALTH	NR

HEALTHGRADES AWARDS

Mercy San Juan Medical Center*

6501 Coyle Avenue
Carmichael, CA 95608
(916) 537-5000

Overall patient safety: ★★★
Teaching: Y

CLINICAL PROGRAM RATINGS:

CARDIAC	★★★	ORTHOPEDICS	★★★
CRITICAL CARE	★★★	PULMONARY	★★★
GASTROINTESTINAL	★★★	STROKE	★★★
GENERAL SURGERY	★★★	VASCULAR	NR
MATERNITY CARE	★★★	WOMEN'S HEALTH	★★★

HEALTHGRADES AWARDS

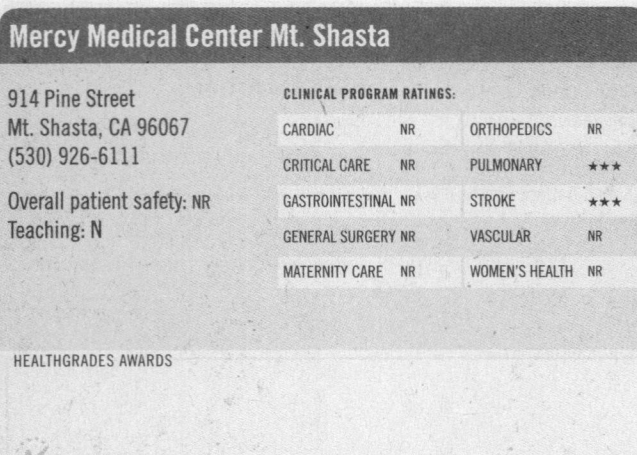

Mercy Medical Center Mt. Shasta

914 Pine Street
Mt. Shasta, CA 96067
(530) 926-6111

Overall patient safety: NR
Teaching: N

CLINICAL PROGRAM RATINGS:

CARDIAC	NR	ORTHOPEDICS	NR
CRITICAL CARE	NR	PULMONARY	★★★
GASTROINTESTINAL	NR	STROKE	★★★
GENERAL SURGERY	NR	VASCULAR	NR
MATERNITY CARE	NR	WOMEN'S HEALTH	NR

HEALTHGRADES AWARDS

Methodist Hospital

7500 Timberlake Way
Sacramento, CA 95823
(916) 423-3000

Overall patient safety: ★
Teaching: Y

CLINICAL PROGRAM RATINGS:

CARDIAC	NR	ORTHOPEDICS	NR
CRITICAL CARE	NR	PULMONARY	★★★
GASTROINTESTINAL	NR	STROKE	★★★
GENERAL SURGERY	★★★	VASCULAR	NR
MATERNITY CARE	★★★	WOMEN'S HEALTH	NR

HEALTHGRADES AWARDS

✓ SPECIALTY EXCELLENCE
· JOINT REPLACEMENT

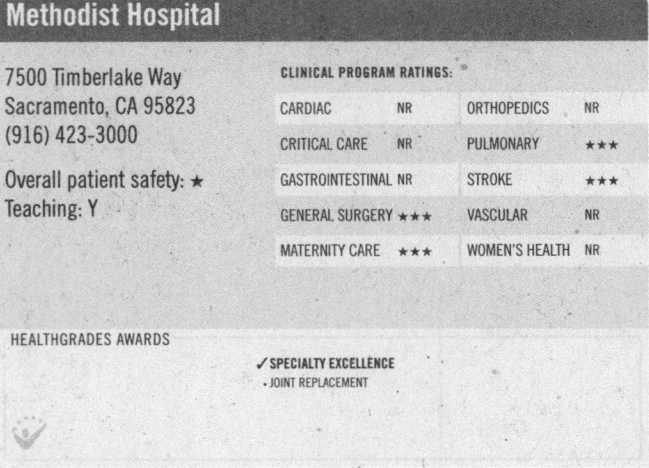

KEY: ★★★★★ BEST   ★★★ AS EXPECTED   ★ POOR   NR NOT RATED BY HEALTHGRADES   For full definitions of ratings and awards, see Appendix.

Methodist Hospital of Southern California

300 West Huntington Drive
Arcadia, CA 91007
(626) 898-8000

Overall patient safety: ★★★
Teaching: N

CLINICAL PROGRAM RATINGS:

CARDIAC	★★★	ORTHOPEDICS	★★★
CRITICAL CARE	★★★	PULMONARY	★★★
GASTROINTESTINAL	★★★	STROKE	★★★★★
GENERAL SURGERY	★★★	VASCULAR	NR
MATERNITY CARE	★★★	WOMEN'S HEALTH	★★★

HEALTHGRADES AWARDS

✓ SPECIALTY EXCELLENCE
· STROKE CARE

Mission Community Hospital–Panorama*

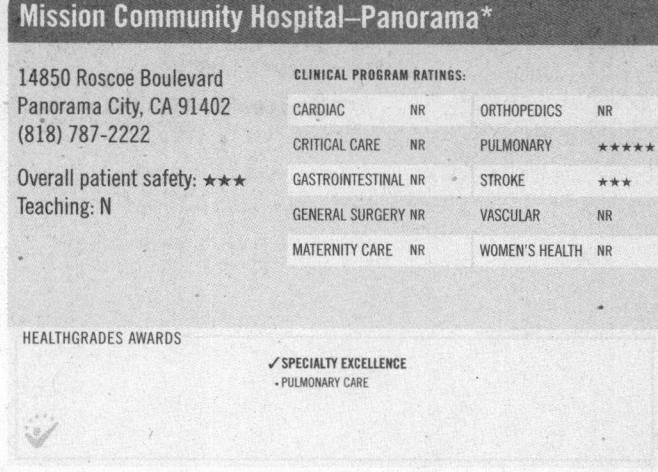

14850 Roscoe Boulevard
Panorama City, CA 91402
(818) 787-2222

Overall patient safety: ★★★
Teaching: N

CLINICAL PROGRAM RATINGS:

CARDIAC	NR	ORTHOPEDICS	NR
CRITICAL CARE	NR	PULMONARY	★★★★★
GASTROINTESTINAL	NR	STROKE	★★★
GENERAL SURGERY	NR	VASCULAR	NR
MATERNITY CARE	NR	WOMEN'S HEALTH	NR

HEALTHGRADES AWARDS

✓ SPECIALTY EXCELLENCE
· PULMONARY CARE

Mills Health Center*

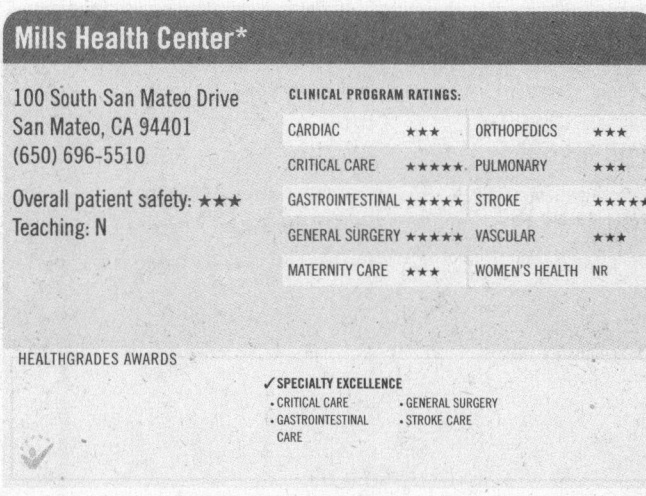

100 South San Mateo Drive
San Mateo, CA 94401
(650) 696-5510

Overall patient safety: ★★★
Teaching: N

CLINICAL PROGRAM RATINGS:

CARDIAC	★★★	ORTHOPEDICS	★★★
CRITICAL CARE	★★★★★	PULMONARY	★★★
GASTROINTESTINAL	★★★★★	STROKE	★★★★★
GENERAL SURGERY	★★★★★	VASCULAR	★★★
MATERNITY CARE	★★★	WOMEN'S HEALTH	NR

HEALTHGRADES AWARDS

✓ SPECIALTY EXCELLENCE
· CRITICAL CARE   · GENERAL SURGERY
· GASTROINTESTINAL   · STROKE CARE
  CARE

Mission Hospital Regional Medical Center

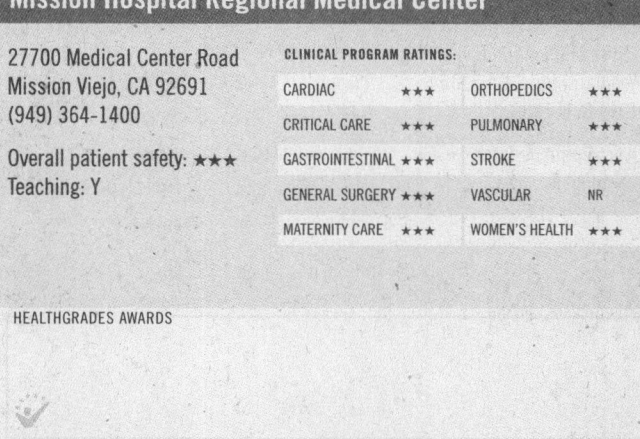

27700 Medical Center Road
Mission Viejo, CA 92691
(949) 364-1400

Overall patient safety: ★★★
Teaching: Y

CLINICAL PROGRAM RATINGS:

CARDIAC	★★★	ORTHOPEDICS	★★★
CRITICAL CARE	★★★	PULMONARY	★★★
GASTROINTESTINAL	★★★	STROKE	★★★
GENERAL SURGERY	★★★	VASCULAR	NR
MATERNITY CARE	★★★	WOMEN'S HEALTH	★★★

HEALTHGRADES AWARDS

Mills Peninsula Health Services*

1783 El Camino Real
Burlingame, CA 94010
(650) 696-4400

Overall patient safety: ★★★
Teaching: N

CLINICAL PROGRAM RATINGS:

CARDIAC	★★★	ORTHOPEDICS	★★★
CRITICAL CARE	★★★★★	PULMONARY	★★★
GASTROINTESTINAL	★★★★★	STROKE	★★★★★
GENERAL SURGERY	★★★★★	VASCULAR	★★★
MATERNITY CARE	★★★	WOMEN'S HEALTH	NR

HEALTHGRADES AWARDS

✓ DISTINGUISHED   ✓ SPECIALTY EXCELLENCE
  HOSPITAL   · CRITICAL CARE   · GENERAL SURGERY
· CLINICAL EXCELLENCE · GASTROINTESTINAL   · STROKE CARE
                         CARE

Monterey Park Hospital

900 South Atlantic Boulevard
Monterey Park, CA 91754
(626) 570-9000

Overall patient safety: ★★★
Teaching: Y

CLINICAL PROGRAM RATINGS:

CARDIAC	NR	ORTHOPEDICS	NR
CRITICAL CARE	NR	PULMONARY	★★★★★
GASTROINTESTINAL	NR	STROKE	★★★★★
GENERAL SURGERY	NR	VASCULAR	NR
MATERNITY CARE	★★★★★	WOMEN'S HEALTH	NR

HEALTHGRADES AWARDS

✓ SPECIALTY EXCELLENCE
· MATERNITY CARE   · PULMONARY CARE   · STROKE CARE

*This hospital reports its data to the federal government jointly with another hospital. Therefore the ratings and awards apply to multiple hospitals and this specific hospital may not provide all rated services.

Moreno Valley Medical Center

27300 Iris Avenue
Moreno Valley, CA 92555
(951) 243-0811

Overall patient safety: ★★★
Teaching: N

CLINICAL PROGRAM RATINGS:

CARDIAC	NR	ORTHOPEDICS	NR
CRITICAL CARE	NR	PULMONARY	★★★
GASTROINTESTINAL	NR	STROKE	NR
GENERAL SURGERY	★★★	VASCULAR	NR
MATERNITY CARE	★★★	WOMEN'S HEALTH	NR

HEALTHGRADES AWARDS

Natividad Medical Center

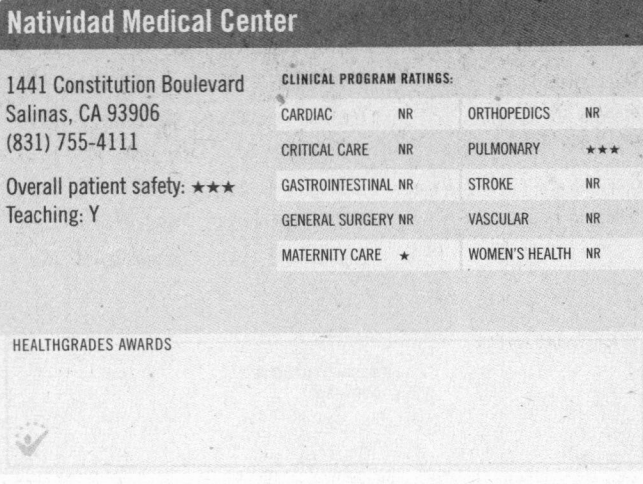

1441 Constitution Boulevard
Salinas, CA 93906
(831) 755-4111

Overall patient safety: ★★★
Teaching: Y

CLINICAL PROGRAM RATINGS:

CARDIAC	NR	ORTHOPEDICS	NR
CRITICAL CARE	NR	PULMONARY	★★★
GASTROINTESTINAL	NR	STROKE	NR
GENERAL SURGERY	NR	VASCULAR	NR
MATERNITY CARE	★	WOMEN'S HEALTH	NR

HEALTHGRADES AWARDS

Motion Picture and Television Hospital

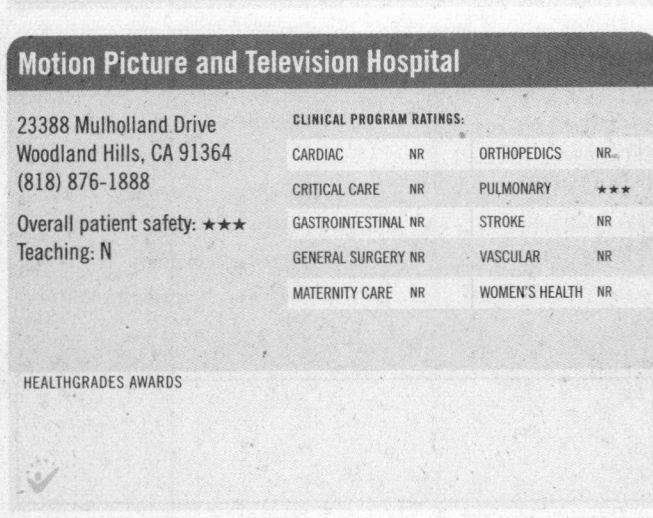

23388 Mulholland Drive
Woodland Hills, CA 91364
(818) 876-1888

Overall patient safety: ★★★
Teaching: N

CLINICAL PROGRAM RATINGS:

CARDIAC	NR	ORTHOPEDICS	NR
CRITICAL CARE	NR	PULMONARY	★★★
GASTROINTESTINAL	NR	STROKE	NR
GENERAL SURGERY	NR	VASCULAR	NR
MATERNITY CARE	NR	WOMEN'S HEALTH	NR

HEALTHGRADES AWARDS

NorthBay Medical Center

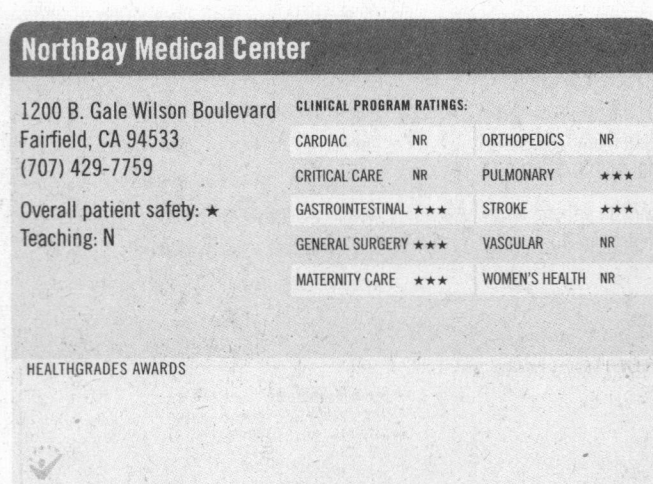

1200 B. Gale Wilson Boulevard
Fairfield, CA 94533
(707) 429-7759

Overall patient safety: ★
Teaching: N

CLINICAL PROGRAM RATINGS:

CARDIAC	NR	ORTHOPEDICS	NR
CRITICAL CARE	NR	PULMONARY	★★★
GASTROINTESTINAL	★★★	STROKE	★★★
GENERAL SURGERY	★★★	VASCULAR	NR
MATERNITY CARE	★★★	WOMEN'S HEALTH	NR

HEALTHGRADES AWARDS

Mt. Diablo Hospital Medical Center

2540 East Street
Concord, CA 94520
(925) 682-8200

Overall patient safety: ★★★
Teaching: N

CLINICAL PROGRAM RATINGS:

CARDIAC	★★★	ORTHOPEDICS	★★★
CRITICAL CARE	★★★	PULMONARY	★★★★★
GASTROINTESTINAL	★★★	STROKE	★★★★★
GENERAL SURGERY	★★★	VASCULAR	★★★
MATERNITY CARE	NR	WOMEN'S HEALTH	NR

HEALTHGRADES AWARDS

✓ DISTINGUISHED HOSPITAL
• CLINICAL EXCELLENCE

✓ SPECIALTY EXCELLENCE
• GASTROINTESTINAL CARE
• PULMONARY CARE
• STROKE CARE

NorthBay VacaValley Hospital

1000 Nut Tree Road
Vacaville, CA 95687
(707) 446-4000

Overall patient safety: ★
Teaching: N

CLINICAL PROGRAM RATINGS:

CARDIAC	NR	ORTHOPEDICS	NR
CRITICAL CARE	NR	PULMONARY	★★★
GASTROINTESTINAL	NR	STROKE	★★★
GENERAL SURGERY	NR	VASCULAR	NR
MATERNITY CARE	NR	WOMEN'S HEALTH	NR

HEALTHGRADES AWARDS

KEY: ★★★★★ BEST   ★★★ AS EXPECTED   ★ POOR   NR NOT RATED BY HEALTHGRADES   For full definitions of ratings and awards, see Appendix.

Northern Inyo Hospital

150 Pioneer Lane
Bishop, CA 93514
(760) 873-5811

Overall patient safety: ★★★
Teaching: N

CLINICAL PROGRAM RATINGS:

CARDIAC	NR	ORTHOPEDICS	NR
CRITICAL CARE	NR	PULMONARY	★★★
GASTROINTESTINAL	NR	STROKE	★★★
GENERAL SURGERY	NR	VASCULAR	NR
MATERNITY CARE	★	WOMEN'S HEALTH	NR

HEALTHGRADES AWARDS

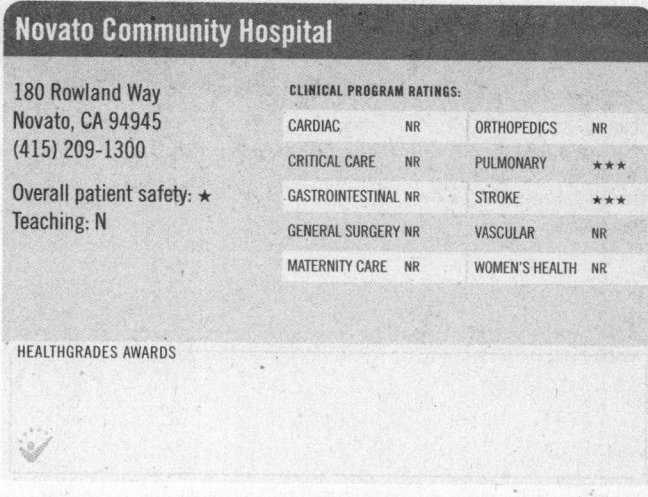

Novato Community Hospital

180 Rowland Way
Novato, CA 94945
(415) 209-1300

Overall patient safety: ★
Teaching: N

CLINICAL PROGRAM RATINGS:

CARDIAC	NR	ORTHOPEDICS	NR
CRITICAL CARE	NR	PULMONARY	★★★
GASTROINTESTINAL	NR	STROKE	★★★
GENERAL SURGERY	NR	VASCULAR	NR
MATERNITY CARE	NR	WOMEN'S HEALTH	NR

HEALTHGRADES AWARDS

Northridge Hospital Medical Center

18300 Roscoe Boulevard
Northridge, CA 91328
(818) 885-8500

Overall patient safety: ★
Teaching: Y

CLINICAL PROGRAM RATINGS:

CARDIAC	★★★	ORTHOPEDICS	★★★
CRITICAL CARE	★★★	PULMONARY	★★★★★
GASTROINTESTINAL	★★★	STROKE	★★★
GENERAL SURGERY	★★★	VASCULAR	NR
MATERNITY CARE	★★★★★	WOMEN'S HEALTH	★★★★★

HEALTHGRADES AWARDS

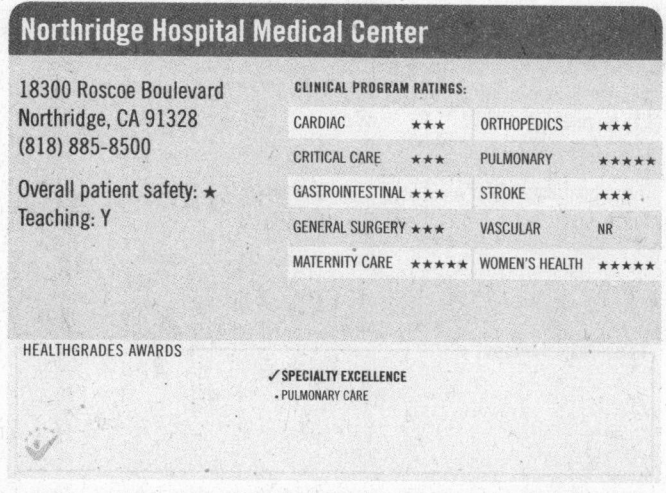

✓ SPECIALTY EXCELLENCE
· PULMONARY CARE

O'Connor Hospital

2105 Forest Avenue
San Jose, CA 95128
(408) 947-2500

Overall patient safety: ★★★★★
Teaching: N

CLINICAL PROGRAM RATINGS:

CARDIAC	★	ORTHOPEDICS	★★★
CRITICAL CARE	★★★	PULMONARY	★
GASTROINTESTINAL	★★★	STROKE	★★★★★
GENERAL SURGERY	★★★	VASCULAR	★★★
MATERNITY CARE	★★★★★	WOMEN'S HEALTH	★★★★★

HEALTHGRADES AWARDS

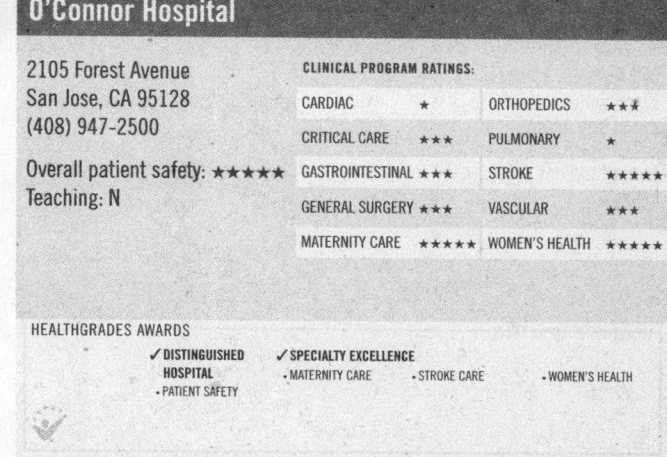

✓ DISTINGUISHED HOSPITAL
· PATIENT SAFETY

✓ SPECIALTY EXCELLENCE
· MATERNITY CARE · STROKE CARE · WOMEN'S HEALTH

Norwalk Community Hospital*

13222 Bloomfield Avenue
Norwalk, CA 90650
(562) 863-4763

Overall patient safety: ★★★
Teaching: N

CLINICAL PROGRAM RATINGS:

CARDIAC	NR	ORTHOPEDICS	NR
CRITICAL CARE	NR	PULMONARY	★★★★★
GASTROINTESTINAL	NR	STROKE	★★★★★
GENERAL SURGERY	NR	VASCULAR	NR
MATERNITY CARE	★★★★★	WOMEN'S HEALTH	NR

HEALTHGRADES AWARDS

✓ SPECIALTY EXCELLENCE
· PULMONARY CARE · STROKE CARE

Oak Valley District Hospital

350 South Oak Avenue
Oakdale, CA 95361
(209) 847-3011

Overall patient safety: ★★★
Teaching: N

CLINICAL PROGRAM RATINGS:

CARDIAC	NR	ORTHOPEDICS	NR
CRITICAL CARE	NR	PULMONARY	★★★
GASTROINTESTINAL	NR	STROKE	★
GENERAL SURGERY	NR	VASCULAR	NR
MATERNITY CARE	★★★	WOMEN'S HEALTH	NR

HEALTHGRADES AWARDS

*This hospital reports its data to the federal government jointly with another hospital. Therefore the ratings and awards apply to multiple hospitals and this specific hospital may not provide all rated services.

Ojai Valley Community Hospital

1306 Maricopa Highway
Ojai, CA 93023
(805) 646-1401

Overall patient safety: ★★★
Teaching: N

CLINICAL PROGRAM RATINGS:

CARDIAC	NR	ORTHOPEDICS	NR
CRITICAL CARE	NR	PULMONARY	★
GASTROINTESTINAL	NR	STROKE	★★★
GENERAL SURGERY	NR	VASCULAR	NR
MATERNITY CARE	NR	WOMEN'S HEALTH	NR

HEALTHGRADES AWARDS

Oroville Hospital

2767 Olive Highway
Oroville, CA 95966
(530) 533-8500

Overall patient safety: ★★★
Teaching: N

CLINICAL PROGRAM RATINGS:

CARDIAC	NR	ORTHOPEDICS	NR
CRITICAL CARE	★★★	PULMONARY	★★★★★
GASTROINTESTINAL	★★★	STROKE	★★★★★
GENERAL SURGERY	★	VASCULAR	NR
MATERNITY CARE	★★★	WOMEN'S HEALTH	NR

HEALTHGRADES AWARDS

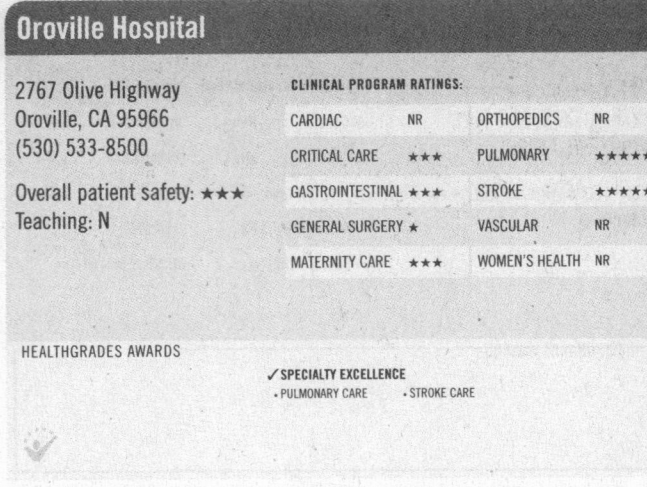

✓SPECIALTY EXCELLENCE
· PULMONARY CARE · STROKE CARE

Olympia Medical Center

5900 West Olympic Boulevard
Los Angeles, CA 90036
(310) 657-5900

Overall patient safety: ★★★
Teaching: Y

CLINICAL PROGRAM RATINGS:

CARDIAC	NR	ORTHOPEDICS	★★★
CRITICAL CARE	NR	PULMONARY	★★★★★
GASTROINTESTINAL	NR	STROKE	★★★
GENERAL SURGERY	NR	VASCULAR	NR
MATERNITY CARE	NR	WOMEN'S HEALTH	NR

HEALTHGRADES AWARDS

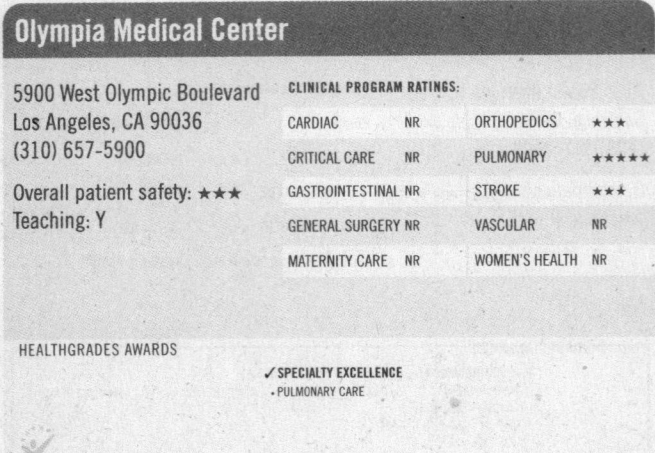

✓SPECIALTY EXCELLENCE
· PULMONARY CARE

Pacific Alliance Medical Center

531 West College Street
Los Angeles, CA 90012
(213) 624-8411

Overall patient safety: ★★★★★
Teaching: N

CLINICAL PROGRAM RATINGS:

CARDIAC	NR	ORTHOPEDICS	NR
CRITICAL CARE	NR	PULMONARY	★★★★★
GASTROINTESTINAL	NR	STROKE	★★★★★
GENERAL SURGERY	NR	VASCULAR	NR
MATERNITY CARE	★★★★★	WOMEN'S HEALTH	NR

HEALTHGRADES AWARDS

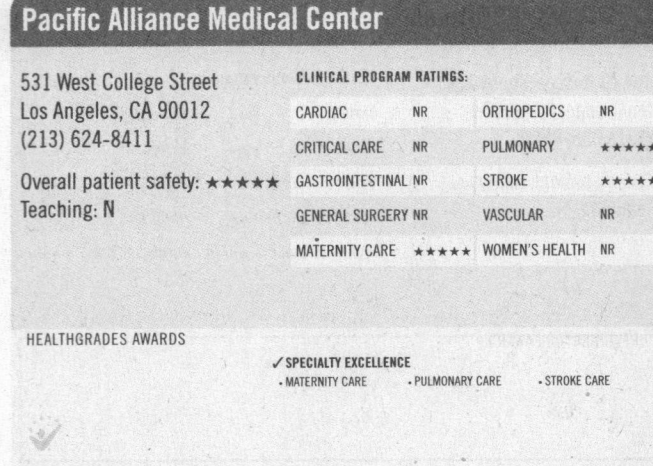

✓SPECIALTY EXCELLENCE
· MATERNITY CARE · PULMONARY CARE · STROKE CARE

Orange Coast Memorial Medical Center

9920 Talbert Avenue
Fountain Valley, CA 92708
(714) 378-7000

Overall patient safety: ★★★
Teaching: N

CLINICAL PROGRAM RATINGS:

CARDIAC	NR	ORTHOPEDICS	NR
CRITICAL CARE	NR	PULMONARY	★★★★★
GASTROINTESTINAL	NR	STROKE	★★★
GENERAL SURGERY	★★★	VASCULAR	NR
MATERNITY CARE	★★★	WOMEN'S HEALTH	NR

HEALTHGRADES AWARDS

Pacific Campus Hospital*

2333 Buchanan Street
San Francisco, CA 94115
(415) 600-6000

Overall patient safety: ★★★
Teaching: Y

CLINICAL PROGRAM RATINGS:

CARDIAC	★★★	ORTHOPEDICS	★★★
CRITICAL CARE	★★★	PULMONARY	★★★★★
GASTROINTESTINAL	★★★	STROKE	★★★★★
GENERAL SURGERY	★★★	VASCULAR	★★★
MATERNITY CARE	★★★	WOMEN'S HEALTH	★★★

HEALTHGRADES AWARDS

✓DISTINGUISHED
HOSPITAL
· CLINICAL EXCELLENCE

✓SPECIALTY EXCELLENCE
· JOINT REPLACEMENT · PULMONARY CARE · STROKE CARE

KEY: ★★★★★ BEST ★★★ AS EXPECTED ★ POOR NR NOT RATED BY HEALTHGRADES   For full definitions of ratings and awards, see Appendix.

Pacific Hospital of Long Beach

2776 Pacific Avenue
Long Beach, CA 90806
(562) 595-1911

Overall patient safety: ★★★
Teaching: Y

CLINICAL PROGRAM RATINGS:

CARDIAC	NR	ORTHOPEDICS	NR
CRITICAL CARE	NR	PULMONARY	★★★★★
GASTROINTESTINAL	NR	STROKE	NR
GENERAL SURGERY	NR	VASCULAR	NR
MATERNITY CARE	★★★	WOMEN'S HEALTH	NR

HEALTHGRADES AWARDS

Palo Verde Hospital

250 North 1st Street
Blythe, CA 92225
(760) 922-4115

Overall patient safety: ★★★
Teaching: N

CLINICAL PROGRAM RATINGS:

CARDIAC	NR	ORTHOPEDICS	NR
CRITICAL CARE	NR	PULMONARY	★
GASTROINTESTINAL	NR	STROKE	NR
GENERAL SURGERY	NR	VASCULAR	NR
MATERNITY CARE	★★★	WOMEN'S HEALTH	NR

HEALTHGRADES AWARDS

Pacifica Hospital of the Valley

9449 San Fernando Road
Sun Valley, CA 91352
(818) 767-3310

Overall patient safety: ★★★
Teaching: N

CLINICAL PROGRAM RATINGS:

CARDIAC	NR	ORTHOPEDICS	NR
CRITICAL CARE	NR	PULMONARY	★
GASTROINTESTINAL	NR	STROKE	★
GENERAL SURGERY	NR	VASCULAR	NR
MATERNITY CARE	★★★	WOMEN'S HEALTH	NR

HEALTHGRADES AWARDS

Palomar Medical Center

555 East Valley Parkway
Escondido, CA 92025
(760) 739-3000

Overall patient safety: ★
Teaching: Y

CLINICAL PROGRAM RATINGS:

CARDIAC	★★★	ORTHOPEDICS	★★★
CRITICAL CARE	★	PULMONARY	★
GASTROINTESTINAL	★★★	STROKE	★
GENERAL SURGERY	★★★	VASCULAR	NR
MATERNITY CARE	★★★	WOMEN'S HEALTH	★★★

HEALTHGRADES AWARDS

Palm Drive Hospital

501 Petaluma Avenue
Sebastopol, CA 95472
(707) 823-8511

Overall patient safety: ★★★
Teaching: N

CLINICAL PROGRAM RATINGS:

CARDIAC	NR	ORTHOPEDICS	NR
CRITICAL CARE	NR	PULMONARY	NR
GASTROINTESTINAL	NR	STROKE	★★★
GENERAL SURGERY	NR	VASCULAR	NR
MATERNITY CARE	NR	WOMEN'S HEALTH	NR

HEALTHGRADES AWARDS

Paradise Valley Hospital

2400 East 4th Street
National City, CA 91950
(619) 470-4321

Overall patient safety: ★
Teaching: N

CLINICAL PROGRAM RATINGS:

CARDIAC	NR	ORTHOPEDICS	NR
CRITICAL CARE	NR	PULMONARY	★★★★★
GASTROINTESTINAL	★★★	STROKE	★★★
GENERAL SURGERY	★★★	VASCULAR	NR
MATERNITY CARE	★★★★★	WOMEN'S HEALTH	NR

HEALTHGRADES AWARDS

✓ SPECIALTY EXCELLENCE
• PULMONARY CARE

*This hospital reports its data to the federal government jointly with another hospital. Therefore the ratings and awards apply to multiple hospitals and this specific hospital may not provide all rated services.

Parkview Community Hospital

3865 Jackson Street
Riverside, CA 92503
(909) 688-2211

Overall patient safety: ★★★
Teaching: N

CLINICAL PROGRAM RATINGS:

CARDIAC	NR	ORTHOPEDICS	NR
CRITICAL CARE	NR	PULMONARY	★★★
GASTROINTESTINAL	NR	STROKE	★★★
GENERAL SURGERY	NR	VASCULAR	NR
MATERNITY CARE	★★★★★	WOMEN'S HEALTH	NR

HEALTHGRADES AWARDS

✓ SPECIALTY EXCELLENCE
• MATERNITY CARE

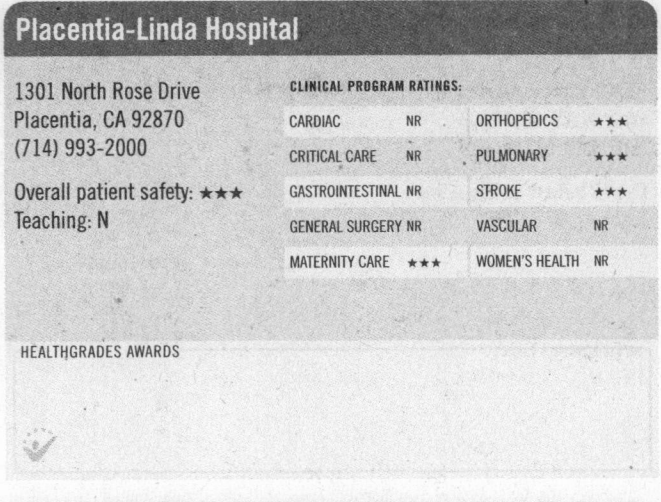

Placentia-Linda Hospital

1301 North Rose Drive
Placentia, CA 92870
(714) 993-2000

Overall patient safety: ★★★
Teaching: N

CLINICAL PROGRAM RATINGS:

CARDIAC	NR	ORTHOPEDICS	★★★
CRITICAL CARE	NR	PULMONARY	★★★
GASTROINTESTINAL	NR	STROKE	★★★
GENERAL SURGERY	NR	VASCULAR	NR
MATERNITY CARE	★★★	WOMEN'S HEALTH	NR

HEALTHGRADES AWARDS

Petaluma Valley Hospital

400 North McDowell Boulevard
Petaluma, CA 94954
(707) 778-1111

Overall patient safety: ★★★
Teaching: N

CLINICAL PROGRAM RATINGS:

CARDIAC	NR	ORTHOPEDICS	NR
CRITICAL CARE	NR	PULMONARY	★★★
GASTROINTESTINAL	NR	STROKE	★★★
GENERAL SURGERY	★★★	VASCULAR	NR
MATERNITY CARE	★★★	WOMEN'S HEALTH	NR

HEALTHGRADES AWARDS

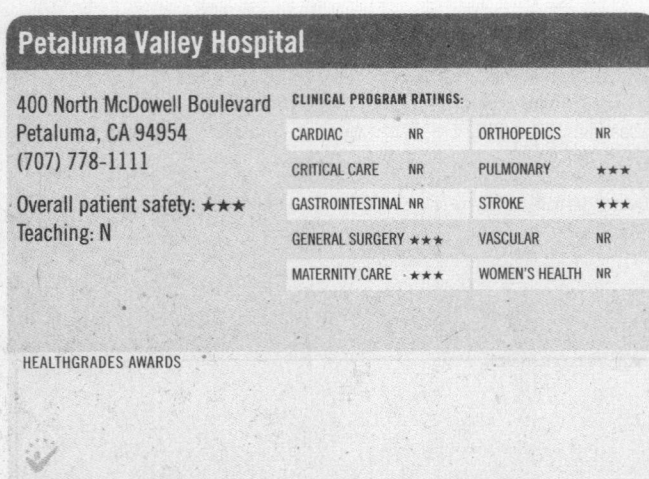

Pomerado Hospital

15615 Pomerado Road
Poway, CA 92064
(858) 613-4000

Overall patient safety: ★★★
Teaching: N

CLINICAL PROGRAM RATINGS:

CARDIAC	NR	ORTHOPEDICS	NR
CRITICAL CARE	★★★	PULMONARY	★★★
GASTROINTESTINAL	NR	STROKE	★★★
GENERAL SURGERY	★★★	VASCULAR	NR
MATERNITY CARE	★★★★★	WOMEN'S HEALTH	NR

HEALTHGRADES AWARDS

✓ SPECIALTY EXCELLENCE
• MATERNITY CARE

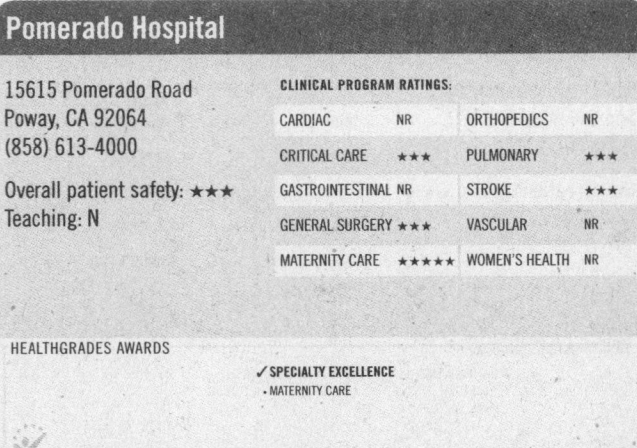

Pioneers Memorial Health Care District

207 West Legion Road
Brawley, CA 92227
(760) 351-3333

Overall patient safety: ★
Teaching: N

CLINICAL PROGRAM RATINGS:

CARDIAC	NR	ORTHOPEDICS	NR
CRITICAL CARE	NR	PULMONARY	★★★
GASTROINTESTINAL	NR	STROKE	★★★
GENERAL SURGERY	★★★	VASCULAR	NR
MATERNITY CARE	★★★★★	WOMEN'S HEALTH	NR

HEALTHGRADES AWARDS

✓ SPECIALTY EXCELLENCE
• MATERNITY CARE

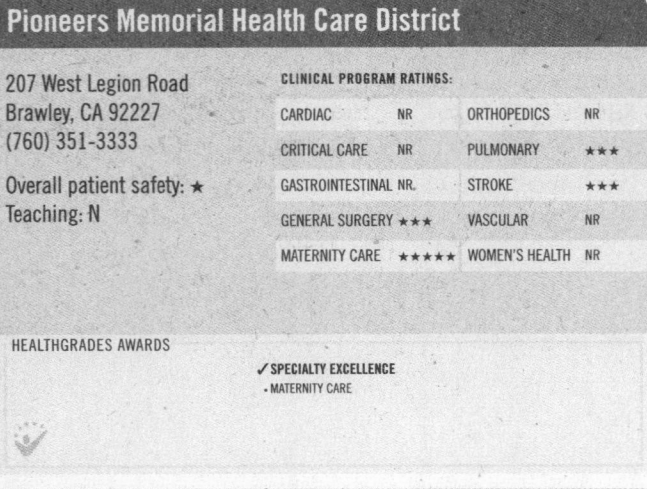

Pomona Valley Hospital Medical Center

1798 North Garey Avenue
Pomona, CA 91767
(909) 865-9500

Overall patient safety: ★★★
Teaching: Y

CLINICAL PROGRAM RATINGS:

CARDIAC	★★★	ORTHOPEDICS	★★★
CRITICAL CARE	NR	PULMONARY	★★★
GASTROINTESTINAL	★★★	STROKE	★★★★★
GENERAL SURGERY	★★★	VASCULAR	NR
MATERNITY CARE	★★★★★	WOMEN'S HEALTH	★★★

HEALTHGRADES AWARDS

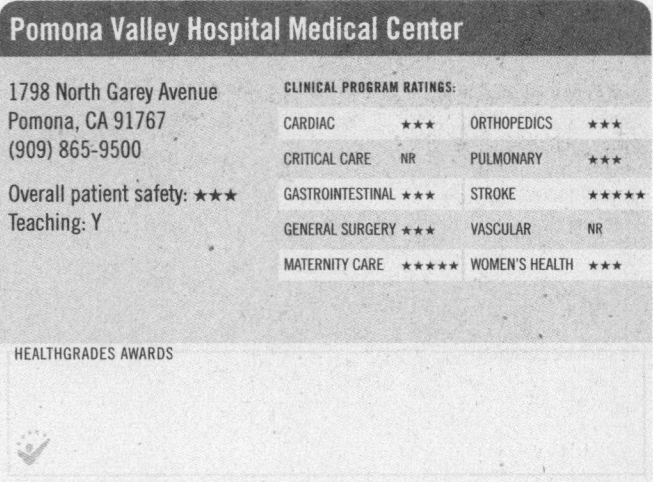

KEY: ★★★★★ BEST ★★★ AS EXPECTED ★ POOR NR NOT RATED BY HEALTHGRADES For full definitions of ratings and awards, see Appendix.

Presbyterian Intercommunity Hospital

12401 Washington Boulevard
Whittier, CA 90602
(562) 698-0811

Overall patient safety: ★★★
Teaching: Y

CLINICAL PROGRAM RATINGS:

CARDIAC	★★★	ORTHOPEDICS	★★★
CRITICAL CARE	NR	PULMONARY	★★★
GASTROINTESTINAL	★★★	STROKE	★★★★★
GENERAL SURGERY	★★★	VASCULAR	NR
MATERNITY CARE	★★★	WOMEN'S HEALTH	★★★

HEALTHGRADES AWARDS

✓ DISTINGUISHED HOSPITAL
• CLINICAL EXCELLENCE

✓ SPECIALTY EXCELLENCE
• CARDIAC SURGERY   • STROKE CARE

Queen of the Valley

1000 Trancas Street
Napa, CA 94558
(707) 252-4411

Overall patient safety: ★★★★★
Teaching: N

CLINICAL PROGRAM RATINGS:

CARDIAC	★★★	ORTHOPEDICS	★★★
CRITICAL CARE	NR	PULMONARY	★★★
GASTROINTESTINAL	★★★	STROKE	★★★
GENERAL SURGERY	★★★	VASCULAR	NR
MATERNITY CARE	★★★	WOMEN'S HEALTH	★★★

HEALTHGRADES AWARDS

✓ DISTINGUISHED HOSPITAL
• PATIENT SAFETY

Providence Holy Cross Medical Center

15031 Rinaldi Street
Mission Hills, CA 91346
(818) 365-8051

Overall patient safety: ★★★
Teaching: N

CLINICAL PROGRAM RATINGS:

CARDIAC	★★★	ORTHOPEDICS	NR
CRITICAL CARE	NR	PULMONARY	★★★★★
GASTROINTESTINAL	★★★	STROKE	★★★★★
GENERAL SURGERY	★★★	VASCULAR	NR
MATERNITY CARE	★★★	WOMEN'S HEALTH	★★★★★

HEALTHGRADES AWARDS

✓ DISTINGUISHED HOSPITAL
• CLINICAL EXCELLENCE

✓ SPECIALTY EXCELLENCE
• GASTROINTESTINAL CARE   • STROKE CARE
• PULMONARY CARE   • WOMEN'S HEALTH

Redbud Community Hospital

15630 18th Avenue
Clearlake, CA 95422
(707) 994-6486

Overall patient safety: ★★★
Teaching: N

CLINICAL PROGRAM RATINGS:

CARDIAC	NR	ORTHOPEDICS	NR
CRITICAL CARE	NR	PULMONARY	★★★
GASTROINTESTINAL	NR	STROKE	★
GENERAL SURGERY	NR	VASCULAR	NR
MATERNITY CARE	★★★	WOMEN'S HEALTH	NR

HEALTHGRADES AWARDS

Providence Saint Joseph Medical Center

501 South Buena Vista
Burbank, CA 91505
(818) 843-5111

Overall patient safety: ★
Teaching: N

CLINICAL PROGRAM RATINGS:

CARDIAC	★★★	ORTHOPEDICS	★★★
CRITICAL CARE	★★★	PULMONARY	★★★
GASTROINTESTINAL	★★★	STROKE	★★★★★
GENERAL SURGERY	★★★	VASCULAR	★★★
MATERNITY CARE	★★★★★	WOMEN'S HEALTH	★★★★★

HEALTHGRADES AWARDS

✓ SPECIALTY EXCELLENCE
• MATERNITY CARE   • STROKE CARE   • WOMEN'S HEALTH

Redlands Community Hospital

350 Terracina Boulevard
Redlands, CA 92373
(909) 335-5500

Overall patient safety: ★★★
Teaching: N

CLINICAL PROGRAM RATINGS:

CARDIAC	NR	ORTHOPEDICS	★★★
CRITICAL CARE	NR	PULMONARY	★
GASTROINTESTINAL	★★★	STROKE	★★★
GENERAL SURGERY	★★★	VASCULAR	NR
MATERNITY CARE	★★★	WOMEN'S HEALTH	NR

HEALTHGRADES AWARDS

Redwood Memorial Hospital

3300 Renner Drive
Fortuna, CA 95540
(707) 725-3361

Overall patient safety: NR
Teaching: N

CLINICAL PROGRAM RATINGS:

CARDIAC	NR	ORTHOPEDICS	NR
CRITICAL CARE	NR	PULMONARY	★★★
GASTROINTESTINAL	NR	STROKE	★
GENERAL SURGERY	NR	VASCULAR	NR
MATERNITY CARE	NR	WOMEN'S HEALTH	NR

HEALTHGRADES AWARDS

Ridgecrest Regional Hospital

1081 North China
Lake Boulevard
Ridgecrest, CA 93555
(760) 446-3551

Overall patient safety: ★★★
Teaching: N

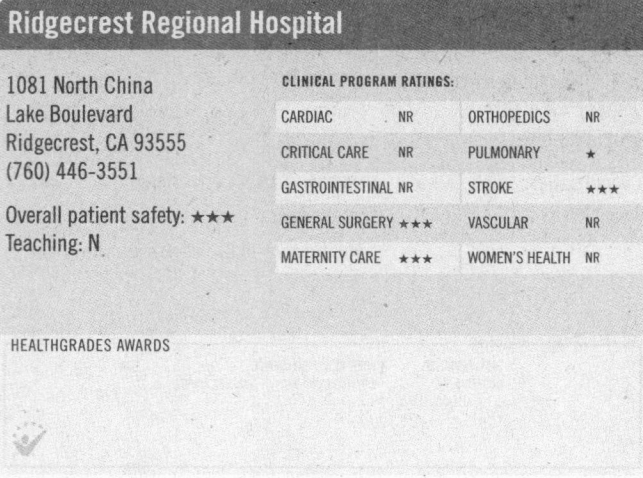

CLINICAL PROGRAM RATINGS:

CARDIAC	NR	ORTHOPEDICS	NR
CRITICAL CARE	NR	PULMONARY	★
GASTROINTESTINAL	NR	STROKE	★★★
GENERAL SURGERY	★★★	VASCULAR	NR
MATERNITY CARE	★★★	WOMEN'S HEALTH	NR

HEALTHGRADES AWARDS

Regional Medical Center of San Jose

225 North Jackson Avenue
San Jose, CA 95116
(408) 259-5000

Overall patient safety: ★★★
Teaching: Y

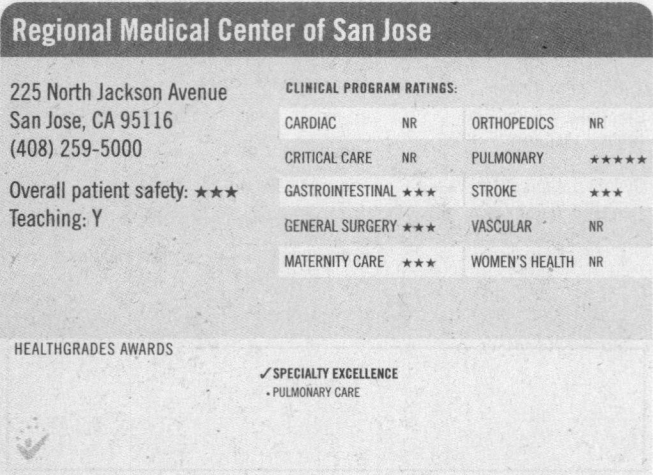

CLINICAL PROGRAM RATINGS:

CARDIAC	NR	ORTHOPEDICS	NR
CRITICAL CARE	NR	PULMONARY	★★★★★
GASTROINTESTINAL	★★★	STROKE	★★★
GENERAL SURGERY	★★★	VASCULAR	NR
MATERNITY CARE	★★★	WOMEN'S HEALTH	NR

HEALTHGRADES AWARDS

✓ SPECIALTY EXCELLENCE
• PULMONARY CARE

Riverside Community Hospital*

4445 Magnolia Avenue
Riverside, CA 92501
(951) 788-3000

Overall patient safety: ★
Teaching: N

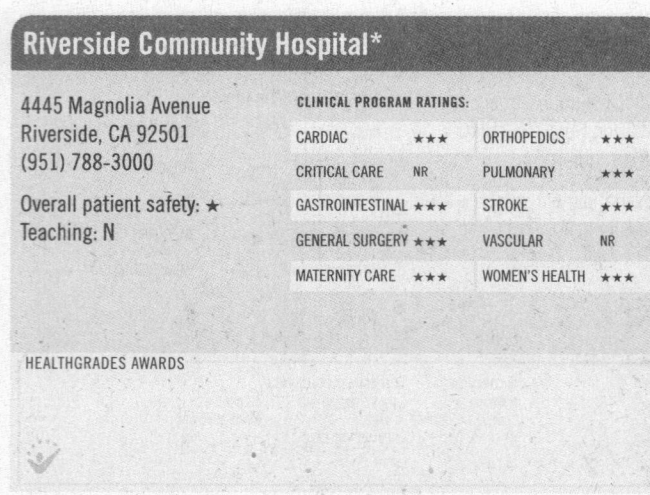

CLINICAL PROGRAM RATINGS:

CARDIAC	★★★	ORTHOPEDICS	★★★
CRITICAL CARE	NR	PULMONARY	★★★
GASTROINTESTINAL	★★★	STROKE	★★★
GENERAL SURGERY	★★★	VASCULAR	NR
MATERNITY CARE	★★★	WOMEN'S HEALTH	★★★

HEALTHGRADES AWARDS

Rideout Memorial Hospital*

726 4th Street
Marysville, CA 95901
(530) 749-4300

Overall patient safety: ★★★
Teaching: Y

CLINICAL PROGRAM RATINGS:

CARDIAC	★★★	ORTHOPEDICS	★
CRITICAL CARE	★★★	PULMONARY	★★★
GASTROINTESTINAL	★★★	STROKE	★★★
GENERAL SURGERY	★★★	VASCULAR	NR
MATERNITY CARE	★★★	WOMEN'S HEALTH	★★★

HEALTHGRADES AWARDS

Riverside County Regional Medical Center

26520 Cactus Avenue
Moreno Valley, CA 92555
(909) 486-4000

Overall patient safety: ★★★
Teaching: Y

CLINICAL PROGRAM RATINGS:

CARDIAC	NR	ORTHOPEDICS	NR
CRITICAL CARE	NR	PULMONARY	★★★
GASTROINTESTINAL	NR	STROKE	NR
GENERAL SURGERY	NR	VASCULAR	NR
MATERNITY CARE	★★★	WOMEN'S HEALTH	NR

HEALTHGRADES AWARDS

KEY: ★★★★★ BEST   ★★★ AS EXPECTED   ★ POOR   NR NOT RATED BY HEALTHGRADES   For full definitions of ratings and awards, see Appendix.

Saddleback Memorial Medical Center*

24451 Health Center Drive
Laguna Hills, CA 92653
(949) 837-4500

Overall patient safety: ★★★
Teaching: N

CLINICAL PROGRAM RATINGS:

CARDIAC	★★★	ORTHOPEDICS	★★★
CRITICAL CARE	★★★	PULMONARY	★★★
GASTROINTESTINAL	★★★	STROKE	★★★
GENERAL SURGERY	★★★	VASCULAR	NR
MATERNITY CARE	★★★	WOMEN'S HEALTH	★★★

HEALTHGRADES AWARDS

St. Bernardine Medical Center

2101 North Waterman Avenue
San Bernardino, CA 92404
(909) 883-8711

Overall patient safety: ★★★
Teaching: N

CLINICAL PROGRAM RATINGS:

CARDIAC	★	ORTHOPEDICS	★★★★★
CRITICAL CARE	NR	PULMONARY	★
GASTROINTESTINAL	★★★	STROKE	★★★
GENERAL SURGERY	★★★	VASCULAR	NR
MATERNITY CARE	★★★	WOMEN'S HEALTH	★★★

HEALTHGRADES AWARDS

✓ SPECIALTY EXCELLENCE
· JOINT REPLACEMENT   · ORTHOPEDIC
SURGERY

Saddleback Memorial Medical Center–San Clemente*

654 Camino De Los Mares
San Clemente, CA 92673
(949) 496-1122

Overall patient safety: ★★★
Teaching: N

CLINICAL PROGRAM RATINGS:

CARDIAC	★★★	ORTHOPEDICS	★★★
CRITICAL CARE	★★★	PULMONARY	★★★
GASTROINTESTINAL	★★★	STROKE	★★★
GENERAL SURGERY	★★★	VASCULAR	NR
MATERNITY CARE	★★★	WOMEN'S HEALTH	★★★

HEALTHGRADES AWARDS

St. Elizabeth Community Hospital

2550 Sister Mary
Columba Drive
Red Bluff, CA 96080
(530) 529-8000

Overall patient safety: ★★★★★
Teaching: N

CLINICAL PROGRAM RATINGS:

CARDIAC	NR	ORTHOPEDICS	NR
CRITICAL CARE	NR	PULMONARY	★
GASTROINTESTINAL	★★★	STROKE	★
GENERAL SURGERY	★★★	VASCULAR	NR
MATERNITY CARE	★★★	WOMEN'S HEALTH	NR

HEALTHGRADES AWARDS

✓ DISTINGUISHED   ✓ SPECIALTY EXCELLENCE
HOSPITAL   · JOINT REPLACEMENT
· PATIENT SAFETY

Saint Agnes Medical Center

1303 East Herndon Avenue
Fresno, CA 93720
(559) 450-3000

Overall patient safety: ★★★
Teaching: N

CLINICAL PROGRAM RATINGS:

CARDIAC	★★★	ORTHOPEDICS	★★★
CRITICAL CARE	★★★	PULMONARY	★★★
GASTROINTESTINAL	★★★	STROKE	★★★★★
GENERAL SURGERY	★★★	VASCULAR	NR
MATERNITY CARE	★★★★★	WOMEN'S HEALTH	★★★★★

HEALTHGRADES AWARDS

✓ SPECIALTY EXCELLENCE
· JOINT REPLACEMENT   · MATERNITY CARE

St. Francis Medical Center

3630 East Imperial Highway
Lynwood, CA 90262
(310) 900-8900

Overall patient safety: ★
Teaching: N

CLINICAL PROGRAM RATINGS:

CARDIAC	★★★	ORTHOPEDICS	NR
CRITICAL CARE	NR	PULMONARY	★★★
GASTROINTESTINAL	NR	STROKE	★★★★★
GENERAL SURGERY	★★★	VASCULAR	NR
MATERNITY CARE	★★★	WOMEN'S HEALTH	★★★

HEALTHGRADES AWARDS

✓ SPECIALTY EXCELLENCE
· STROKE CARE

*This hospital reports its data to the federal government jointly with another hospital. Therefore the ratings and awards apply to multiple hospitals and this specific hospital may not provide all rated services.

CALIFORNIA HOSPITALS: RATINGS BY CLINICAL SPECIALTY

Saint Francis Memorial Hospital

900 Hyde Street
San Francisco, CA 94109
(415) 353-6000

Overall patient safety: ★★★
Teaching: Y

CLINICAL PROGRAM RATINGS:

CARDIAC	NR	ORTHOPEDICS	★★★
CRITICAL CARE	NR	PULMONARY	★★★
GASTROINTESTINAL	NR	STROKE	★★★★★
GENERAL SURGERY	★★★	VASCULAR	NR
MATERNITY CARE	NR	WOMEN'S HEALTH	NR

HEALTHGRADES AWARDS

✓ SPECIALTY EXCELLENCE
· STROKE CARE

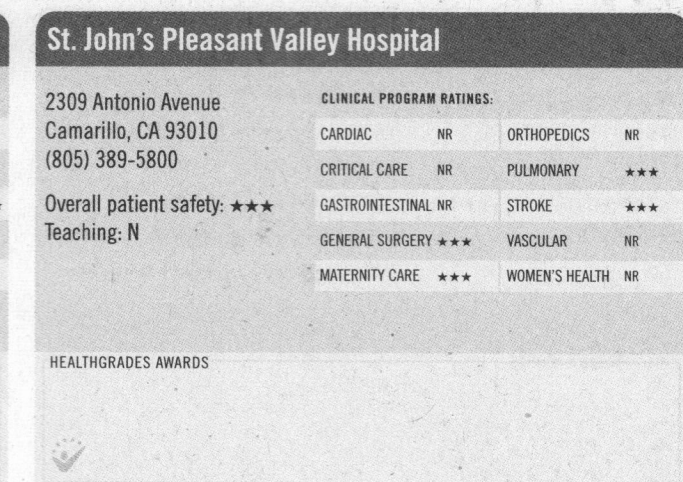

St. John's Pleasant Valley Hospital

2309 Antonio Avenue
Camarillo, CA 93010
(805) 389-5800

Overall patient safety: ★★★
Teaching: N

CLINICAL PROGRAM RATINGS:

CARDIAC	NR	ORTHOPEDICS	NR
CRITICAL CARE	NR	PULMONARY	★★★
GASTROINTESTINAL	NR	STROKE	★★★
GENERAL SURGERY	★★★	VASCULAR	NR
MATERNITY CARE	★★★	WOMEN'S HEALTH	NR

HEALTHGRADES AWARDS

St. Helena Hospital

10 Woodland Road
Deer Park, CA 94574
(707) 963-3611

Overall patient safety: ★★★
Teaching: N

CLINICAL PROGRAM RATINGS:

CARDIAC	★★★	ORTHOPEDICS	★★★
CRITICAL CARE	NR	PULMONARY	★★★
GASTROINTESTINAL	NR	STROKE	★★★
GENERAL SURGERY	NR	VASCULAR	NR
MATERNITY CARE	★★★	WOMEN'S HEALTH	★★★

HEALTHGRADES AWARDS

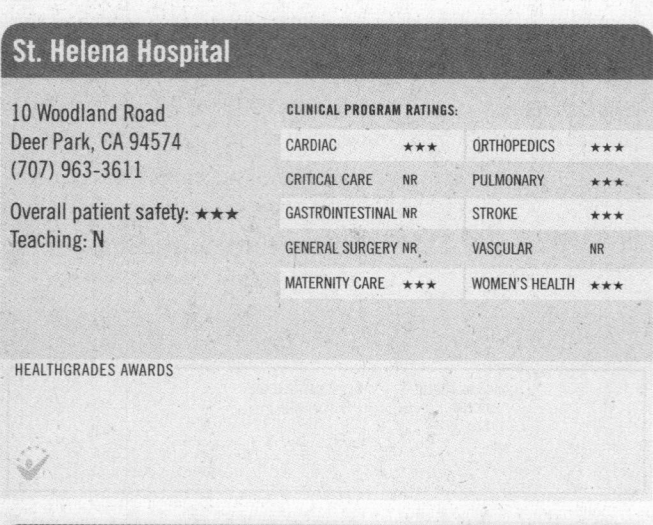

St. John's Regional Medical Center

1600 North Rose Avenue
Oxnard, CA 93030
(805) 988-2500

Overall patient safety: ★★★
Teaching: N

CLINICAL PROGRAM RATINGS:

CARDIAC	★★★	ORTHOPEDICS	★★★
CRITICAL CARE	★★★	PULMONARY	★★★
GASTROINTESTINAL	★★★	STROKE	★★★★★
GENERAL SURGERY	★★★	VASCULAR	NR
MATERNITY CARE	★★★	WOMEN'S HEALTH	★★★

HEALTHGRADES AWARDS

✓ DISTINGUISHED HOSPITAL ✓ SPECIALTY EXCELLENCE
· CLINICAL EXCELLENCE   · CARDIAC CARE   · CARDIAC SURGERY   · STROKE CARE

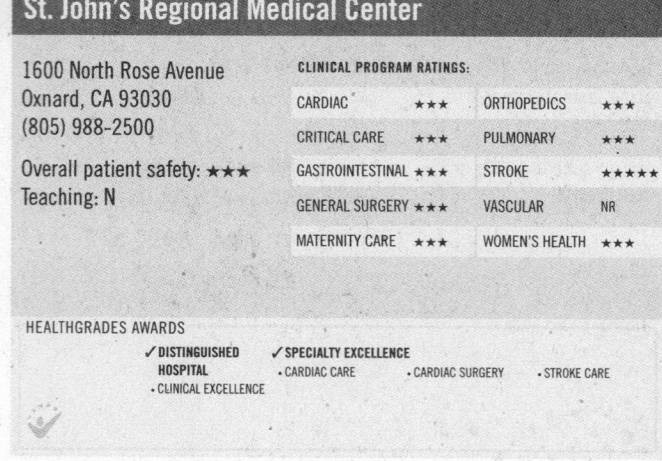

St. John's Health Center

1328 22nd Street
Santa Monica, CA 90404
(310) 829-5511

Overall patient safety: ★★★
Teaching: N

CLINICAL PROGRAM RATINGS:

CARDIAC	★★★	ORTHOPEDICS	★★★
CRITICAL CARE	★★★	PULMONARY	★★★★★
GASTROINTESTINAL	★★★	STROKE	★★★
GENERAL SURGERY	★★★	VASCULAR	NR
MATERNITY CARE	★★★	WOMEN'S HEALTH	★★★

HEALTHGRADES AWARDS

✓ AMERICA'S 50 BEST HOSPITALS ✓ DISTINGUISHED HOSPITAL ✓ SPECIALTY EXCELLENCE
· CLINICAL EXCELLENCE · GASTROINTESTINAL CARE · PULMONARY CARE

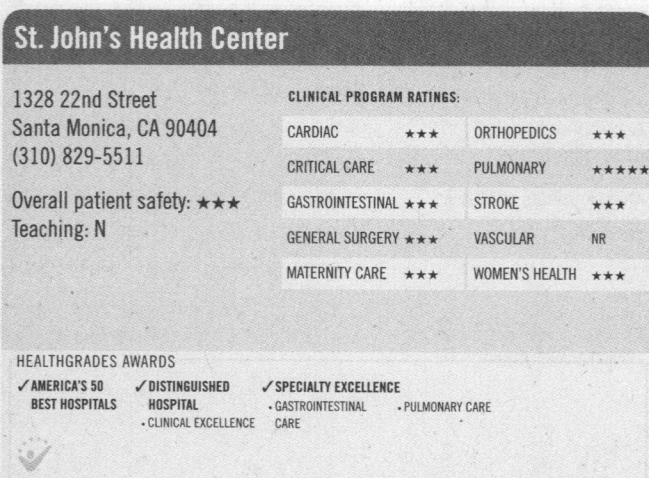

St. Joseph Hospital

2200 Harrison Avenue
Eureka, CA 95501
(707) 445-5111

Overall patient safety: ★
Teaching: N

CLINICAL PROGRAM RATINGS:

CARDIAC	★★★	ORTHOPEDICS	★★★
CRITICAL CARE	NR	PULMONARY	★
GASTROINTESTINAL	★★★	STROKE	★★★
GENERAL SURGERY	★★★	VASCULAR	NR
MATERNITY CARE	★★★	WOMEN'S HEALTH	★★★

HEALTHGRADES AWARDS

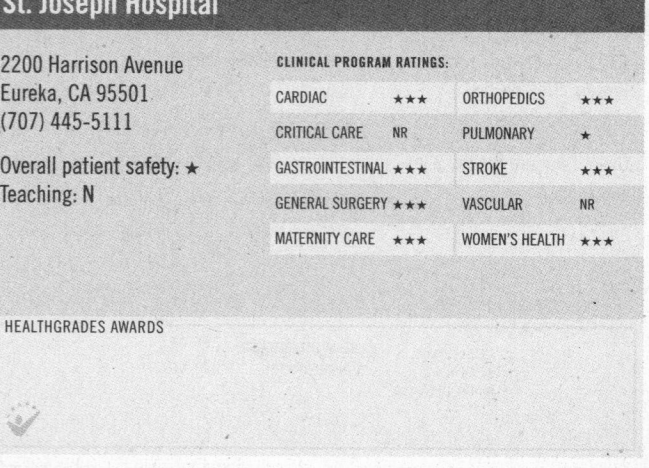

KEY: ★★★★★ BEST   ★★★ AS EXPECTED   ★ POOR   NR NOT RATED BY HEALTHGRADES   For full definitions of ratings and awards, see Appendix.

St. Joseph Hospital

1100 West Stewart Drive
Orange, CA 92868
(714) 633-9111

Overall patient safety: ★★★
Teaching: N

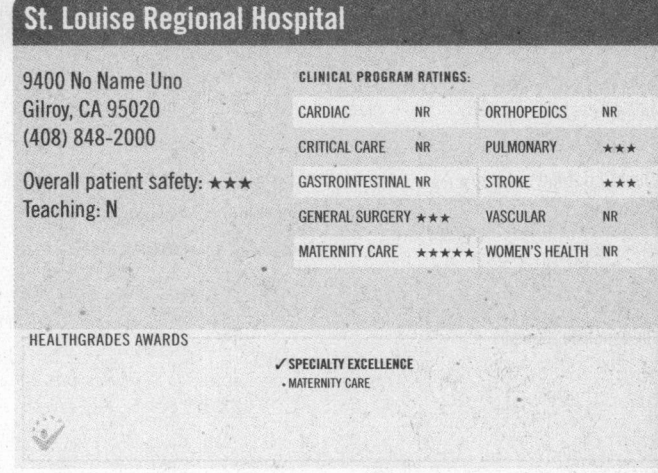

CLINICAL PROGRAM RATINGS:

CARDIAC	★★★	ORTHOPEDICS	★★★
CRITICAL CARE	★★★	PULMONARY	★
GASTROINTESTINAL	★★★	STROKE	★★★
GENERAL SURGERY	★★★★★	VASCULAR	★★★
MATERNITY CARE	★★★	WOMEN'S HEALTH	★★★

HEALTHGRADES AWARDS

✓ SPECIALTY EXCELLENCE
- GASTROINTESTINAL   - GENERAL SURGERY
  CARE

St. Louise Regional Hospital

9400 No Name Uno
Gilroy, CA 95020
(408) 848-2000

Overall patient safety: ★★★
Teaching: N

CLINICAL PROGRAM RATINGS:

CARDIAC	NR	ORTHOPEDICS	NR
CRITICAL CARE	NR	PULMONARY	★★★
GASTROINTESTINAL	NR	STROKE	★★★
GENERAL SURGERY	★★★	VASCULAR	NR
MATERNITY CARE	★★★★★	WOMEN'S HEALTH	NR

HEALTHGRADES AWARDS

✓ SPECIALTY EXCELLENCE
- MATERNITY CARE

St. Joseph's Medical Center of Stockton

1800 North California Street
Stockton, CA 95204
(209) 943-2000

Overall patient safety: ★★★
Teaching: N

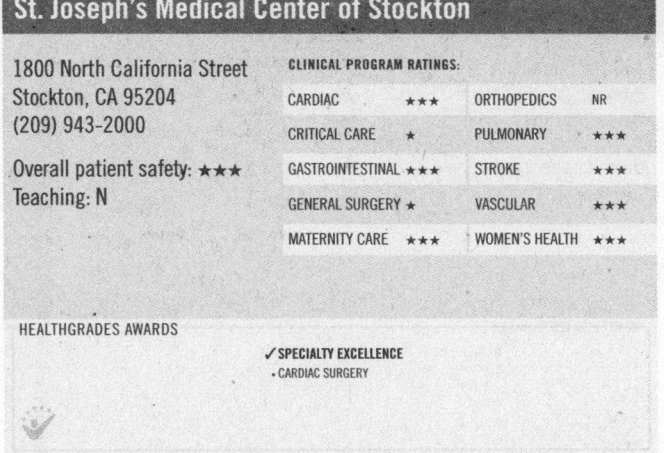

CLINICAL PROGRAM RATINGS:

CARDIAC	★★★	ORTHOPEDICS	NR
CRITICAL CARE	★	PULMONARY	★★★
GASTROINTESTINAL	★★★	STROKE	★★★
GENERAL SURGERY	★	VASCULAR	★★★
MATERNITY CARE	★★★	WOMEN'S HEALTH	★★★

HEALTHGRADES AWARDS

✓ SPECIALTY EXCELLENCE
- CARDIAC SURGERY

St. Luke's Hospital

3555 Cesar Chavez Street
San Francisco, CA 94110
(415) 641-6562

Overall patient safety: ★★★
Teaching: N

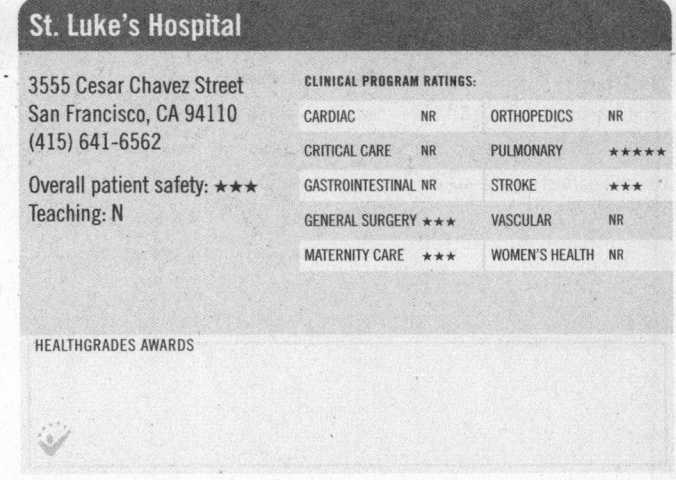

CLINICAL PROGRAM RATINGS:

CARDIAC	NR	ORTHOPEDICS	NR
CRITICAL CARE	NR	PULMONARY	★★★★★
GASTROINTESTINAL	NR	STROKE	★★★
GENERAL SURGERY	★★★	VASCULAR	NR
MATERNITY CARE	★★★	WOMEN'S HEALTH	NR

HEALTHGRADES AWARDS

St. Jude Medical Center

101 East Valencia Mesa Drive
Fullerton, CA 92835
(714) 992-3000

Overall patient safety: ★★★★★
Teaching: N

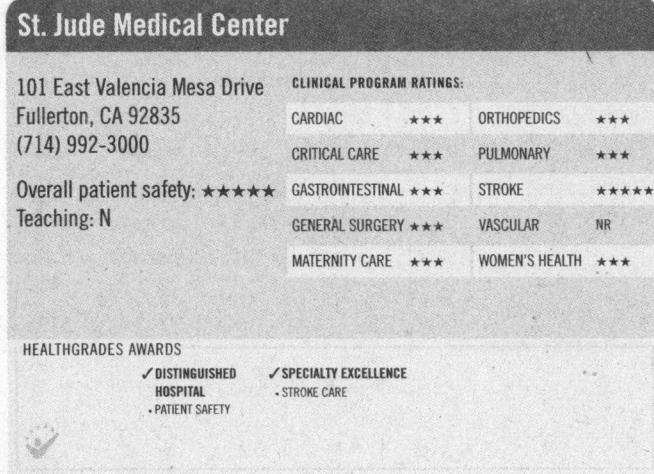

CLINICAL PROGRAM RATINGS:

CARDIAC	★★★	ORTHOPEDICS	★★★
CRITICAL CARE	★★★	PULMONARY	★★★
GASTROINTESTINAL	★★★	STROKE	★★★★★
GENERAL SURGERY	★★★	VASCULAR	NR
MATERNITY CARE	★★★	WOMEN'S HEALTH	★★★

HEALTHGRADES AWARDS

✓ DISTINGUISHED   ✓ SPECIALTY EXCELLENCE
  HOSPITAL   - STROKE CARE
- PATIENT SAFETY

St. Mary Medical Center

18300 Highway 18
Apple Valley, CA 92307
(760) 242-2311

Overall patient safety: ★
Teaching: N

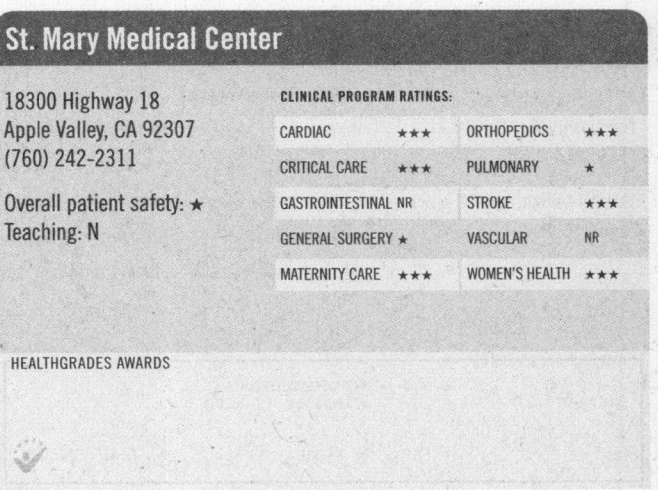

CLINICAL PROGRAM RATINGS:

CARDIAC	★★★	ORTHOPEDICS	★★★
CRITICAL CARE	★★★	PULMONARY	★
GASTROINTESTINAL	NR	STROKE	★★★
GENERAL SURGERY	★	VASCULAR	NR
MATERNITY CARE	★★★	WOMEN'S HEALTH	★★★

HEALTHGRADES AWARDS

St. Mary Medical Center

1050 Linden Avenue
Long Beach, CA 90813
(562) 491-9000

Overall patient safety: ★★★
Teaching: Y

CLINICAL PROGRAM RATINGS:

CARDIAC	★★★	ORTHOPEDICS	NR
CRITICAL CARE	NR	PULMONARY	★★★★★
GASTROINTESTINAL	NR	STROKE	★★★★★
GENERAL SURGERY	NR	VASCULAR	NR
MATERNITY CARE	★★★	WOMEN'S HEALTH	★★★★★

HEALTHGRADES AWARDS

✓ SPECIALTY EXCELLENCE
· PULMONARY CARE   · STROKE CARE   · WOMEN'S HEALTH

St. Vincent Medical Center

2131 West 3rd Street
Los Angeles, CA 90057
(213) 484-7111

Overall patient safety: ★★★
Teaching: Y

CLINICAL PROGRAM RATINGS:

CARDIAC	★★★	ORTHOPEDICS	NR
CRITICAL CARE	NR	PULMONARY	★★★★★
GASTROINTESTINAL	★★★	STROKE	★★★★★
GENERAL SURGERY	★★★	VASCULAR	NR
MATERNITY CARE	NR	WOMEN'S HEALTH	NR

HEALTHGRADES AWARDS

✓ DISTINGUISHED HOSPITAL   ✓ SPECIALTY EXCELLENCE
· CLINICAL EXCELLENCE   · PULMONARY CARE   · STROKE CARE

St. Mary's Medical Center

450 Stanyan Street
San Francisco, CA 94117
(415) 668-1000

Overall patient safety: ★★★
Teaching: Y

CLINICAL PROGRAM RATINGS:

CARDIAC	★★★	ORTHOPEDICS	★★★
CRITICAL CARE	NR	PULMONARY	★★★★★
GASTROINTESTINAL	★★★	STROKE	★★★
GENERAL SURGERY	★★★	VASCULAR	NR
MATERNITY CARE	NR	WOMEN'S HEALTH	NR

HEALTHGRADES AWARDS

Salinas Valley Memorial Health Care System

450 East Romie Lane
Salinas, CA 93901
(831) 757-4333

Overall patient safety: ★★★
Teaching: N

CLINICAL PROGRAM RATINGS:

CARDIAC	★★★	ORTHOPEDICS	★★★
CRITICAL CARE	★★★	PULMONARY	★
GASTROINTESTINAL	★★★	STROKE	★★★
GENERAL SURGERY	★★★	VASCULAR	★★★
MATERNITY CARE	★★★	WOMEN'S HEALTH	★★★

HEALTHGRADES AWARDS

St. Rose Hospital

27200 Calaroga Avenue
Hayward, CA 94545
(510) 264-4000

Overall patient safety: ★★★
Teaching: N

CLINICAL PROGRAM RATINGS:

CARDIAC	NR	ORTHOPEDICS	NR
CRITICAL CARE	NR	PULMONARY	★★★★★
GASTROINTESTINAL	★★★	STROKE	★★★
GENERAL SURGERY	★★★	VASCULAR	NR
MATERNITY CARE	★★★	WOMEN'S HEALTH	NR

HEALTHGRADES AWARDS

✓ SPECIALTY EXCELLENCE
· PULMONARY CARE

San Antonio Community Hospital

999 San Bernardino Road
Upland, CA 91786
(909) 985-2811

Overall patient safety: ★★★
Teaching: N

CLINICAL PROGRAM RATINGS:

CARDIAC	★★★	ORTHOPEDICS	★
CRITICAL CARE	★★★	PULMONARY	★★★
GASTROINTESTINAL	★★★	STROKE	★★★★★
GENERAL SURGERY	★★★	VASCULAR	NR
MATERNITY CARE	★★★★★	WOMEN'S HEALTH	★★★

HEALTHGRADES AWARDS

✓ SPECIALTY EXCELLENCE
· MATERNITY CARE   · STROKE CARE

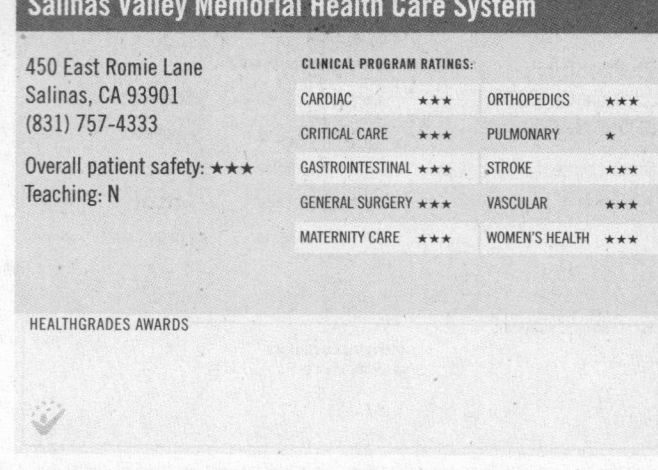

KEY: ★★★★★ BEST   ★★★ AS EXPECTED   ★ POOR   NR NOT RATED BY HEALTHGRADES   For full definitions of ratings and awards, see Appendix.

San Dimas Community Hospital

1350 West Covina Boulevard
San Dimas, CA 91773
(909) 599-6811

Overall patient safety: ★
Teaching: N

CLINICAL PROGRAM RATINGS:

CARDIAC	NR	ORTHOPEDICS	NR
CRITICAL CARE	NR	PULMONARY	★★★
GASTROINTESTINAL	NR	STROKE	★★★
GENERAL SURGERY	NR	VASCULAR	NR
MATERNITY CARE	★★★	WOMEN'S HEALTH	NR

HEALTHGRADES AWARDS

San Gabriel Valley Medical Center

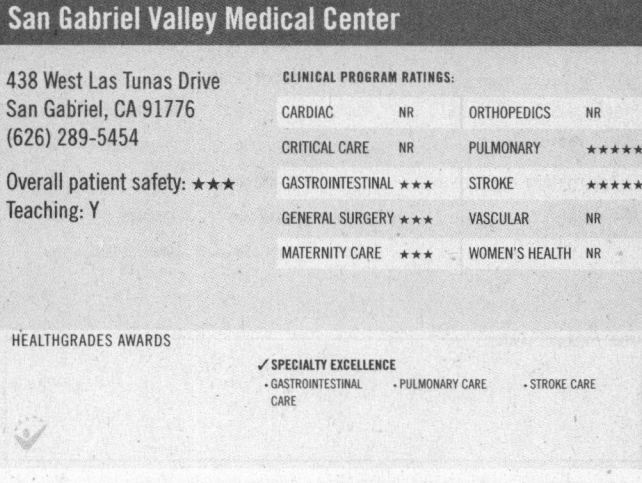

438 West Las Tunas Drive
San Gabriel, CA 91776
(626) 289-5454

Overall patient safety: ★★★
Teaching: Y

CLINICAL PROGRAM RATINGS:

CARDIAC	NR	ORTHOPEDICS	NR
CRITICAL CARE	NR	PULMONARY	★★★★★
GASTROINTESTINAL	★★★	STROKE	★★★★★
GENERAL SURGERY	★★★	VASCULAR	NR
MATERNITY CARE	★★★	WOMEN'S HEALTH	NR

HEALTHGRADES AWARDS

✓ SPECIALTY EXCELLENCE
• GASTROINTESTINAL CARE • PULMONARY CARE • STROKE CARE

San Fernando Community Hospital*

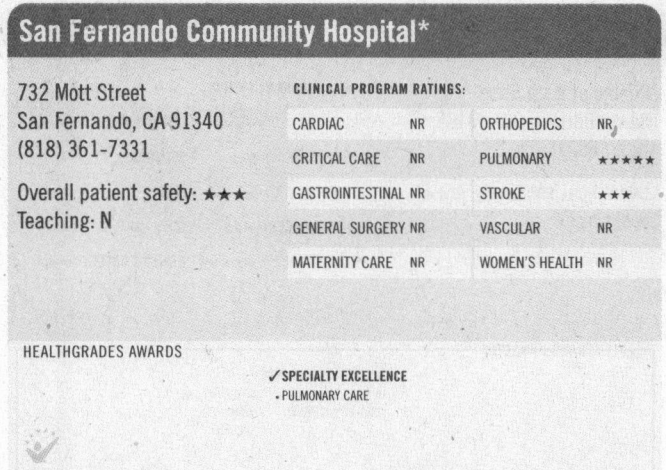

732 Mott Street
San Fernando, CA 91340
(818) 361-7331

Overall patient safety: ★★★
Teaching: N

CLINICAL PROGRAM RATINGS:

CARDIAC	NR	ORTHOPEDICS	NR
CRITICAL CARE	NR	PULMONARY	★★★★★
GASTROINTESTINAL	NR	STROKE	★★★
GENERAL SURGERY	NR	VASCULAR	NR
MATERNITY CARE	NR	WOMEN'S HEALTH	NR

HEALTHGRADES AWARDS

✓ SPECIALTY EXCELLENCE
• PULMONARY CARE

San Gorgonio Memorial Hospital

600 North Highland Springs Avenue
Banning, CA 92220
(951) 845-1121

Overall patient safety: ★★★
Teaching: N

CLINICAL PROGRAM RATINGS:

CARDIAC	NR	ORTHOPEDICS	NR
CRITICAL CARE	NR	PULMONARY	★
GASTROINTESTINAL	NR	STROKE	★★★
GENERAL SURGERY	NR	VASCULAR	NR
MATERNITY CARE	★	WOMEN'S HEALTH	NR

HEALTHGRADES AWARDS

San Francisco General Hospital

1001 Potrero Avenue
San Francisco, CA 94110
(415) 206-8000

Overall patient safety: ★
Teaching: Y

CLINICAL PROGRAM RATINGS:

CARDIAC	NR	ORTHOPEDICS	NR
CRITICAL CARE	NR	PULMONARY	★★★★★
GASTROINTESTINAL	NR	STROKE	★★★
GENERAL SURGERY	NR	VASCULAR	NR
MATERNITY CARE	★	WOMEN'S HEALTH	NR

HEALTHGRADES AWARDS

✓ SPECIALTY EXCELLENCE
• PULMONARY CARE

San Joaquin Community Hospital

2615 Eye Street
Bakersfield, CA 93301
(661) 395-3000

Overall patient safety: ★
Teaching: N

CLINICAL PROGRAM RATINGS:

CARDIAC	★★★	ORTHOPEDICS	NR
CRITICAL CARE	NR	PULMONARY	★★★
GASTROINTESTINAL	★★★	STROKE	★★★
GENERAL SURGERY	★★★	VASCULAR	NR
MATERNITY CARE	★★★★★	WOMEN'S HEALTH	★★★

HEALTHGRADES AWARDS

✓ SPECIALTY EXCELLENCE
• MATERNITY CARE

*This hospital reports its data to the federal government jointly with another hospital. Therefore the ratings and awards apply to multiple hospitals and this specific hospital may not provide all rated services.

San Joaquin General Hospital

500 West Hospital Road
French Camp, CA 95231
(209) 468-6000

Overall patient safety: ★
Teaching: Y

CLINICAL PROGRAM RATINGS:

CARDIAC	NR	ORTHOPEDICS	NR
CRITICAL CARE	NR	PULMONARY	★
GASTROINTESTINAL	NR	STROKE	★
GENERAL SURGERY	NR	VASCULAR	NR
MATERNITY CARE	★★★	WOMEN'S HEALTH	NR

HEALTHGRADES AWARDS

San Ramon Regional Medical Center

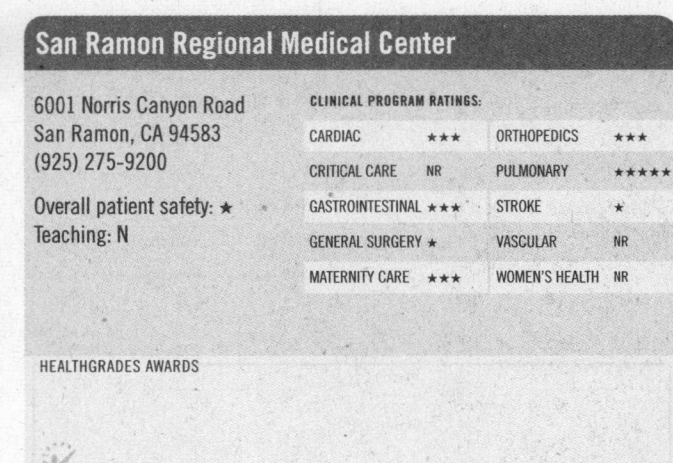

6001 Norris Canyon Road
San Ramon, CA 94583
(925) 275-9200

Overall patient safety: ★
Teaching: N

CLINICAL PROGRAM RATINGS:

CARDIAC	★★★	ORTHOPEDICS	★★★
CRITICAL CARE	NR	PULMONARY	★★★★★
GASTROINTESTINAL	★★★	STROKE	★
GENERAL SURGERY	★	VASCULAR	NR
MATERNITY CARE	★★★	WOMEN'S HEALTH	NR

HEALTHGRADES AWARDS

San Leandro Hospital

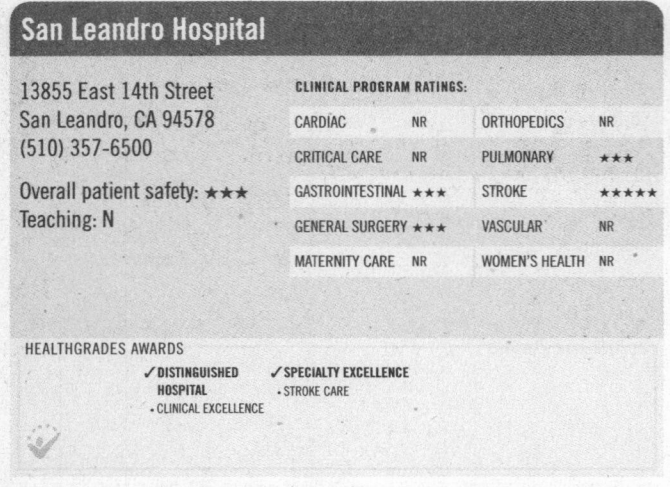

13855 East 14th Street
San Leandro, CA 94578
(510) 357-6500

Overall patient safety: ★★★
Teaching: N

CLINICAL PROGRAM RATINGS:

CARDIAC	NR	ORTHOPEDICS	NR
CRITICAL CARE	NR	PULMONARY	★★★
GASTROINTESTINAL	★★★	STROKE	★★★★★
GENERAL SURGERY	★★★	VASCULAR	NR
MATERNITY CARE	NR	WOMEN'S HEALTH	NR

HEALTHGRADES AWARDS

✓ DISTINGUISHED HOSPITAL
  - CLINICAL EXCELLENCE
✓ SPECIALTY EXCELLENCE
  - STROKE CARE

Santa Barbara Cottage Hospital

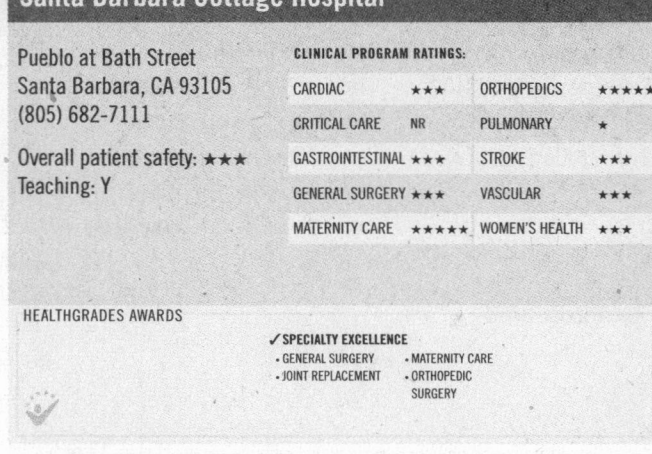

Pueblo at Bath Street
Santa Barbara, CA 93105
(805) 682-7111

Overall patient safety: ★★★
Teaching: Y

CLINICAL PROGRAM RATINGS:

CARDIAC	★★★	ORTHOPEDICS	★★★★★
CRITICAL CARE	NR	PULMONARY	★
GASTROINTESTINAL	★★★	STROKE	★★★
GENERAL SURGERY	★★★	VASCULAR	★★★
MATERNITY CARE	★★★★★	WOMEN'S HEALTH	★★★

HEALTHGRADES AWARDS

✓ SPECIALTY EXCELLENCE
  - GENERAL SURGERY
  - JOINT REPLACEMENT
  - MATERNITY CARE
  - ORTHOPEDIC SURGERY

San Mateo Medical Center

222 West 39th Avenue
San Mateo, CA 94403
(650) 573-2222

Overall patient safety: ★★★
Teaching: Y

CLINICAL PROGRAM RATINGS:

CARDIAC	NR	ORTHOPEDICS	NR
CRITICAL CARE	NR	PULMONARY	★★★
GASTROINTESTINAL	NR	STROKE	NR
GENERAL SURGERY	NR	VASCULAR	NR
MATERNITY CARE	NR	WOMEN'S HEALTH	NR

HEALTHGRADES AWARDS

Santa Clara Valley Medical Center

751 South Bascom Avenue
San Jose, CA 95128
(408) 885-5000

Overall patient safety: ★
Teaching: Y

CLINICAL PROGRAM RATINGS:

CARDIAC	NR	ORTHOPEDICS	NR
CRITICAL CARE	NR	PULMONARY	★★★
GASTROINTESTINAL	NR	STROKE	★★★
GENERAL SURGERY	★★★	VASCULAR	NR
MATERNITY CARE	★	WOMEN'S HEALTH	NR

HEALTHGRADES AWARDS

KEY: ★★★★★ BEST   ★★★ AS EXPECTED   ★ POOR   NR NOT RATED BY HEALTHGRADES   For full definitions of ratings and awards, see Appendix.

126   CHAPTER 6: HOSPITAL RATINGS BY CLINICAL SPECIALTY

Santa Monica–UCLA Medical Center

1250 16th Street
Santa Monica, CA 90404
(310) 319-4000

Overall patient safety: ★★★
Teaching: Y

CLINICAL PROGRAM RATINGS:

CARDIAC	NR	ORTHOPEDICS	★★★
CRITICAL CARE	★★★	PULMONARY	★★★
GASTROINTESTINAL	NR	STROKE	★★★
GENERAL SURGERY	NR	VASCULAR	NR
MATERNITY CARE	★★★	WOMEN'S HEALTH	NR

HEALTHGRADES AWARDS

Scripps Memorial Hospital–Encinitas

354 Santa Fe Drive
Encinitas, CA 92024
(760) 753-6501

Overall patient safety: ★★★
Teaching: N

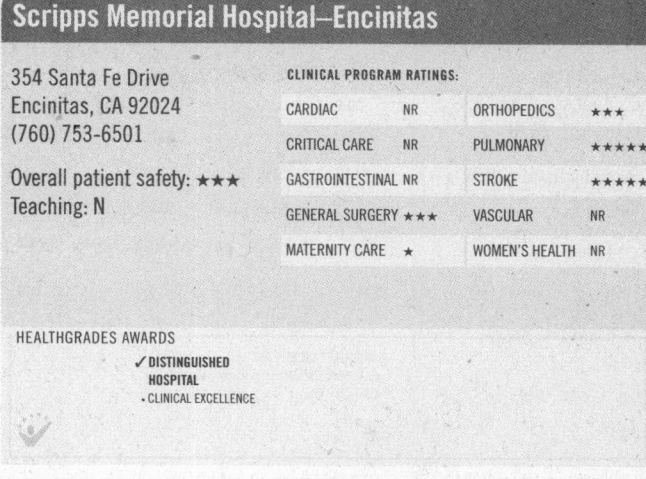

CLINICAL PROGRAM RATINGS:

CARDIAC	NR	ORTHOPEDICS	★★★
CRITICAL CARE	NR	PULMONARY	★★★★★
GASTROINTESTINAL	NR	STROKE	★★★★★
GENERAL SURGERY	★★★	VASCULAR	NR
MATERNITY CARE	★	WOMEN'S HEALTH	NR

HEALTHGRADES AWARDS

✓ DISTINGUISHED HOSPITAL
- CLINICAL EXCELLENCE

Santa Rosa Memorial Hospital

1165 Montgomery Drive
Santa Rosa, CA 95405
(707) 546-3210

Overall patient safety: ★★★
Teaching: N

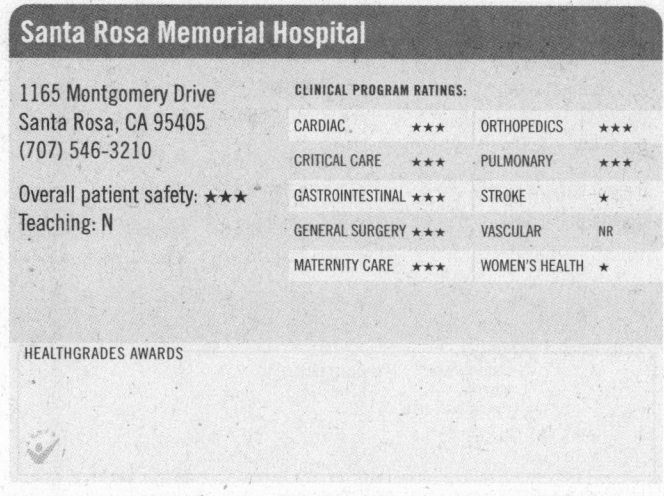

CLINICAL PROGRAM RATINGS:

CARDIAC	★★★	ORTHOPEDICS	★★★
CRITICAL CARE	★★★	PULMONARY	★★★
GASTROINTESTINAL	★★★	STROKE	★
GENERAL SURGERY	★★★	VASCULAR	NR
MATERNITY CARE	★★★	WOMEN'S HEALTH	★

HEALTHGRADES AWARDS

Scripps Memorial Hospital–La Jolla

9888 Genesee Avenue
La Jolla, CA 92037
(858) 457-4123

Overall patient safety: ★★★
Teaching: N

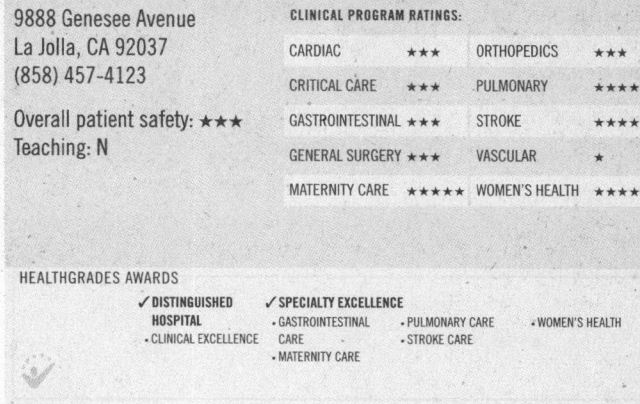

CLINICAL PROGRAM RATINGS:

CARDIAC	★★★	ORTHOPEDICS	★★★
CRITICAL CARE	★★★	PULMONARY	★★★★★
GASTROINTESTINAL	★★★	STROKE	★★★★★
GENERAL SURGERY	★★★	VASCULAR	★
MATERNITY CARE	★★★★★	WOMEN'S HEALTH	★★★★★

HEALTHGRADES AWARDS

✓ DISTINGUISHED HOSPITAL
- CLINICAL EXCELLENCE

✓ SPECIALTY EXCELLENCE
- GASTROINTESTINAL CARE
- MATERNITY CARE
- PULMONARY CARE
- STROKE CARE
- WOMEN'S HEALTH

Scripps Green Hospital

10666 North Torrey Pines Road
La Jolla, CA 92037
(858) 455-9100

Overall patient safety: ★★★
Teaching: Y

CLINICAL PROGRAM RATINGS:

CARDIAC	★★★	ORTHOPEDICS	★★★★★
CRITICAL CARE	NR	PULMONARY	★★★
GASTROINTESTINAL	NR	STROKE	★★★
GENERAL SURGERY	★★★	VASCULAR	★★★
MATERNITY CARE	NR	WOMEN'S HEALTH	NR

HEALTHGRADES AWARDS

✓ SPECIALTY EXCELLENCE
- JOINT REPLACEMENT
- ORTHOPEDIC SURGERY

Scripps Mercy Hospital*

4077 5th Avenue
San Diego, CA 92103
(619) 294-8111

Overall patient safety: ★★★
Teaching: Y

CLINICAL PROGRAM RATINGS:

CARDIAC	★★★	ORTHOPEDICS	★★★
CRITICAL CARE	★★★★★	PULMONARY	★★★★★
GASTROINTESTINAL	★★★	STROKE	★★★★★
GENERAL SURGERY	★★★	VASCULAR	NR
MATERNITY CARE	★★★★★	WOMEN'S HEALTH	★★★

HEALTHGRADES AWARDS

✓ DISTINGUISHED HOSPITAL
- CLINICAL EXCELLENCE

✓ SPECIALTY EXCELLENCE
- BARIATRIC SURGERY
- CRITICAL CARE
- PULMONARY CARE
- STROKE CARE

*This hospital reports its data to the federal government jointly with another hospital. Therefore the ratings and awards apply to multiple hospitals and this specific hospital may not provide all rated services.

Scripps Mercy Hospital–Chula Vista*

435 H Street
Chula Vista, CA 91910
(619) 691-7000

Overall patient safety: ★★★
Teaching: Y

CLINICAL PROGRAM RATINGS:

CARDIAC	★★★	ORTHOPEDICS	★★★
CRITICAL CARE	★★★★★	PULMONARY	★★★★★
GASTROINTESTINAL	★★★	STROKE	★★★★★
GENERAL SURGERY	★★★	VASCULAR	NR
MATERNITY CARE	★★★★★	WOMEN'S HEALTH	★★★

HEALTHGRADES AWARDS

✓ SPECIALTY EXCELLENCE
- BARIATRIC SURGERY   - PULMONARY CARE
- CRITICAL CARE   - STROKE CARE

Seton Medical Center*

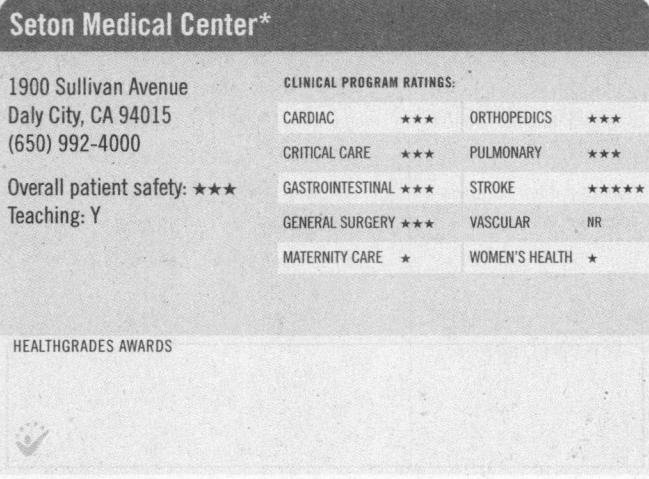

1900 Sullivan Avenue
Daly City, CA 94015
(650) 992-4000

Overall patient safety: ★★★
Teaching: Y

CLINICAL PROGRAM RATINGS:

CARDIAC	★★★	ORTHOPEDICS	★★★
CRITICAL CARE	★★★	PULMONARY	★★★
GASTROINTESTINAL	★★★	STROKE	★★★★★
GENERAL SURGERY	★★★	VASCULAR	NR
MATERNITY CARE	★	WOMEN'S HEALTH	★

HEALTHGRADES AWARDS

Selma Community Hospital

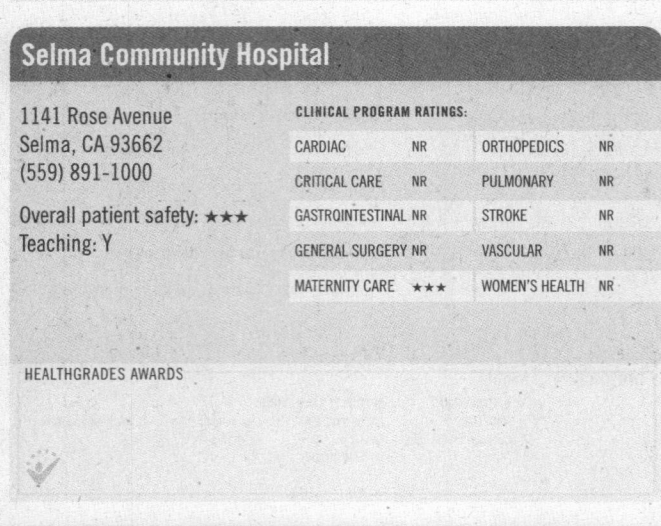

1141 Rose Avenue
Selma, CA 93662
(559) 891-1000

Overall patient safety: ★★★
Teaching: Y

CLINICAL PROGRAM RATINGS:

CARDIAC	NR	ORTHOPEDICS	NR
CRITICAL CARE	NR	PULMONARY	NR
GASTROINTESTINAL	NR	STROKE	NR
GENERAL SURGERY	NR	VASCULAR	NR
MATERNITY CARE	★★★	WOMEN'S HEALTH	NR

HEALTHGRADES AWARDS

Sharp Chula Vista Medical Center

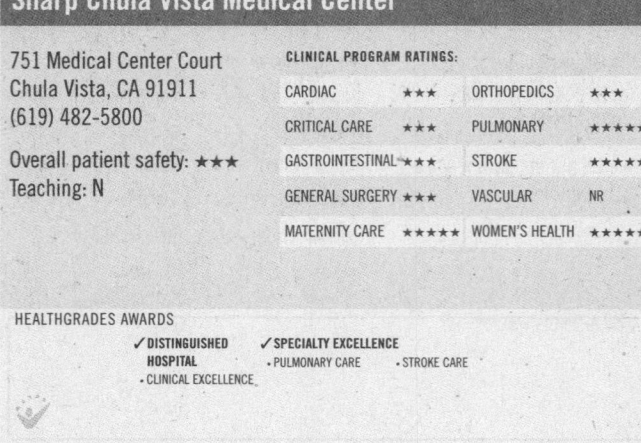

751 Medical Center Court
Chula Vista, CA 91911
(619) 482-5800

Overall patient safety: ★★★
Teaching: N

CLINICAL PROGRAM RATINGS:

CARDIAC	★★★	ORTHOPEDICS	★★★
CRITICAL CARE	★★★	PULMONARY	★★★★★
GASTROINTESTINAL	★★★	STROKE	★★★★★
GENERAL SURGERY	★★★	VASCULAR	NR
MATERNITY CARE	★★★★★	WOMEN'S HEALTH	★★★★★

HEALTHGRADES AWARDS

✓ DISTINGUISHED HOSPITAL   ✓ SPECIALTY EXCELLENCE
- CLINICAL EXCELLENCE   - PULMONARY CARE   - STROKE CARE

Sequoia Hospital

170 Alameda De Las Pulgas
Redwood City, CA 94062
(650) 369-5811

Overall patient safety: ★★★
Teaching: N

CLINICAL PROGRAM RATINGS:

CARDIAC	★★★★★	ORTHOPEDICS	★★★
CRITICAL CARE	★★★	PULMONARY	★★★
GASTROINTESTINAL	★★★	STROKE	★★★★★
GENERAL SURGERY	★★★	VASCULAR	★★★
MATERNITY CARE	★★★	WOMEN'S HEALTH	NR

HEALTHGRADES AWARDS

✓ DISTINGUISHED HOSPITAL   ✓ SPECIALTY EXCELLENCE
- CLINICAL EXCELLENCE   - CARDIAC CARE   - CARDIAC SURGERY   - STROKE CARE

Sharp Coronado Hospital and Healthcare Center

250 Prospect Place
Coronado, CA 92118
(619) 435-6251

Overall patient safety: ★★★
Teaching: N

CLINICAL PROGRAM RATINGS:

CARDIAC	NR	ORTHOPEDICS	NR
CRITICAL CARE	NR	PULMONARY	★★★
GASTROINTESTINAL	NR	STROKE	★★★
GENERAL SURGERY	NR	VASCULAR	NR
MATERNITY CARE	NR	WOMEN'S HEALTH	NR

HEALTHGRADES AWARDS

KEY: ★★★★★ BEST   ★★★ AS EXPECTED   ★ POOR   NR **NOT RATED BY HEALTHGRADES**   For full definitions of ratings and awards, see Appendix.

Sharp Memorial Hospital

7901 Frost Street
San Diego, CA 92123
(858) 541-3500

Overall patient safety: ★★★
Teaching: N

CLINICAL PROGRAM RATINGS:

CARDIAC	★★★	ORTHOPEDICS	★★★
CRITICAL CARE	★★★	PULMONARY	★★★
GASTROINTESTINAL	★★★	STROKE	★★★★★
GENERAL SURGERY	★★★	VASCULAR	NR
MATERNITY CARE	NR	WOMEN'S HEALTH	NR

HEALTHGRADES AWARDS

✓ SPECIALTY EXCELLENCE
• CARDIAC SURGERY   • STROKE CARE

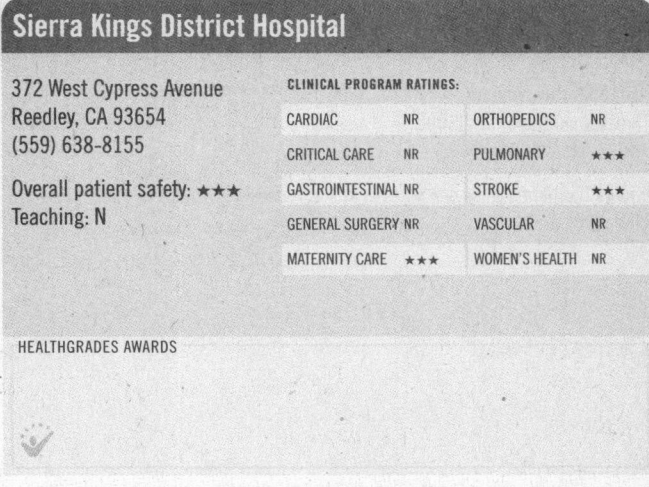

Sierra Kings District Hospital

372 West Cypress Avenue
Reedley, CA 93654
(559) 638-8155

Overall patient safety: ★★★
Teaching: N

CLINICAL PROGRAM RATINGS:

CARDIAC	NR	ORTHOPEDICS	NR
CRITICAL CARE	NR	PULMONARY	★★★
GASTROINTESTINAL	NR	STROKE	★★★
GENERAL SURGERY	NR	VASCULAR	NR
MATERNITY CARE	★★★	WOMEN'S HEALTH	NR

HEALTHGRADES AWARDS

Shasta Regional Medical Center

1100 Butte Street
Redding, CA 96001
(530) 244-5400

Overall patient safety: ★★★
Teaching: N

CLINICAL PROGRAM RATINGS:

CARDIAC	★★★	ORTHOPEDICS	★★★
CRITICAL CARE	★★★	PULMONARY	★
GASTROINTESTINAL	★★★	STROKE	★★★
GENERAL SURGERY	★★★	VASCULAR	NR
MATERNITY CARE	NR	WOMEN'S HEALTH	NR

HEALTHGRADES AWARDS

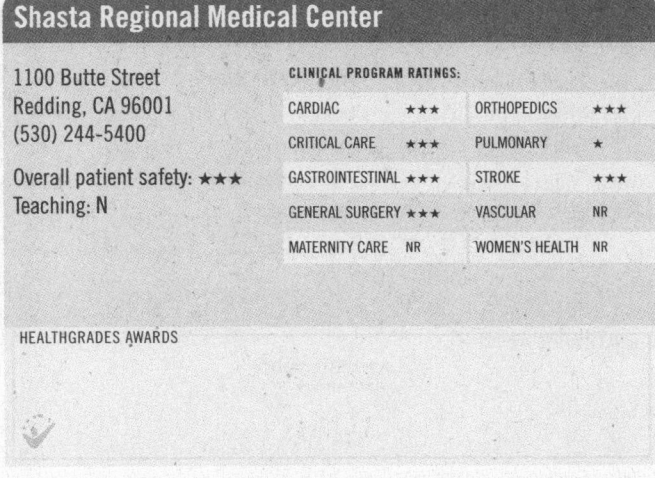

Sierra Nevada Memorial Hospital

155 Glasson Way
Grass Valley, CA 95945
(530) 274-6000

Overall patient safety: ★★★
Teaching: N

CLINICAL PROGRAM RATINGS:

CARDIAC	NR	ORTHOPEDICS	NR
CRITICAL CARE	NR	PULMONARY	★★★★★
GASTROINTESTINAL	★★★	STROKE	★★★★★
GENERAL SURGERY	★	VASCULAR	NR
MATERNITY CARE	★★★	WOMEN'S HEALTH	NR

HEALTHGRADES AWARDS

✓ SPECIALTY EXCELLENCE
• JOINT REPLACEMENT   • STROKE CARE

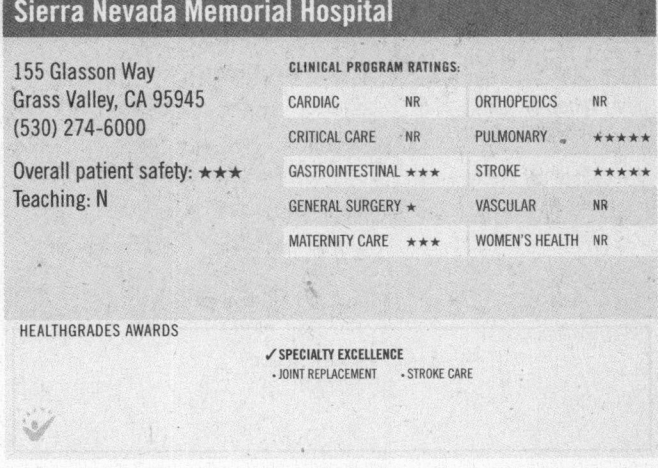

Sherman Oaks Hospital

4929 Van Nuys Boulevard
Sherman Oaks, CA 91403
(818) 981-7111

Overall patient safety: NR
Teaching: N

CLINICAL PROGRAM RATINGS:

CARDIAC	NR	ORTHOPEDICS	NR
CRITICAL CARE	NR	PULMONARY	★★★
GASTROINTESTINAL	NR	STROKE	★★★
GENERAL SURGERY	NR	VASCULAR	NR
MATERNITY CARE	NR	WOMEN'S HEALTH	NR

HEALTHGRADES AWARDS

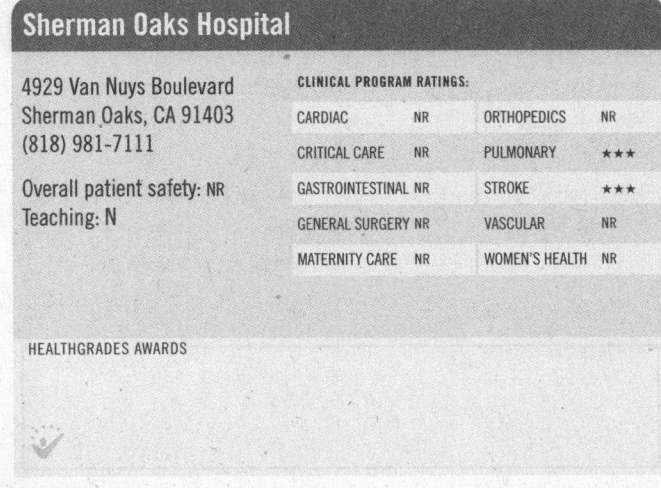

Sierra View District Hospital

465 West Putnam Avenue
Porterville, CA 93257
(559) 784-1110

Overall patient safety: ★★★
Teaching: N

CLINICAL PROGRAM RATINGS:

CARDIAC	NR	ORTHOPEDICS	NR
CRITICAL CARE	NR	PULMONARY	★★★
GASTROINTESTINAL	★★★	STROKE	★
GENERAL SURGERY	★★★	VASCULAR	NR
MATERNITY CARE	★★★	WOMEN'S HEALTH	NR

HEALTHGRADES AWARDS

*This hospital reports its data to the federal government jointly with another hospital. Therefore the ratings and awards apply to multiple hospitals and this specific hospital may not provide all rated services.

Sierra Vista Regional Medical Center

1010 Murray Avenue
San Luis Obispo, CA 93405
(805) 546-7600

Overall patient safety: ★★★
Teaching: N

CLINICAL PROGRAM RATINGS:

CARDIAC	★★★	ORTHOPEDICS	★★★★★
CRITICAL CARE	NR	PULMONARY	★★★
GASTROINTESTINAL	NR	STROKE	★
GENERAL SURGERY	★★★	VASCULAR	NR
MATERNITY CARE	★★★	WOMEN'S HEALTH	★

HEALTHGRADES AWARDS

Sonora Regional Medical Center

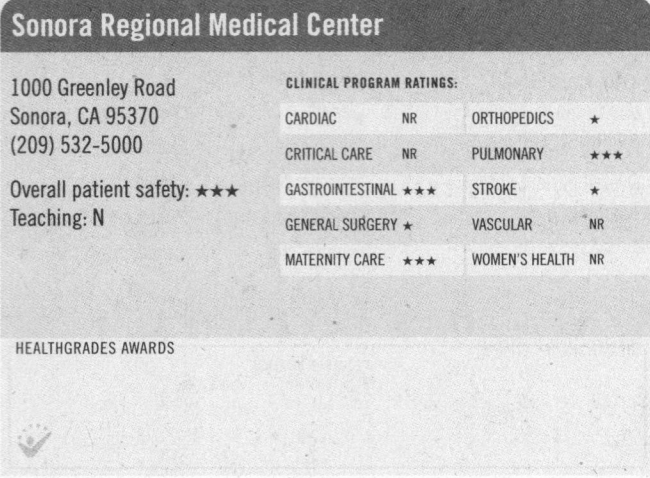

1000 Greenley Road
Sonora, CA 95370
(209) 532-5000

Overall patient safety: ★★★
Teaching: N

CLINICAL PROGRAM RATINGS:

CARDIAC	NR	ORTHOPEDICS	★
CRITICAL CARE	NR	PULMONARY	★★★
GASTROINTESTINAL	★★★	STROKE	★
GENERAL SURGERY	★	VASCULAR	NR
MATERNITY CARE	★★★	WOMEN'S HEALTH	NR

HEALTHGRADES AWARDS

Simi Valley Hospital and Health Care Service

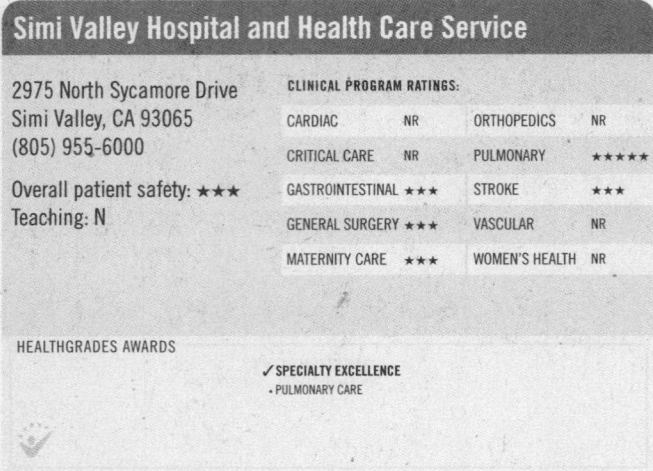

2975 North Sycamore Drive
Simi Valley, CA 93065
(805) 955-6000

Overall patient safety: ★★★
Teaching: N

CLINICAL PROGRAM RATINGS:

CARDIAC	NR	ORTHOPEDICS	NR
CRITICAL CARE	NR	PULMONARY	★★★★★
GASTROINTESTINAL	★★★	STROKE	★★★
GENERAL SURGERY	★★★	VASCULAR	NR
MATERNITY CARE	★★★	WOMEN'S HEALTH	NR

HEALTHGRADES AWARDS

✓ SPECIALTY EXCELLENCE
• PULMONARY CARE

South Coast Medical Center

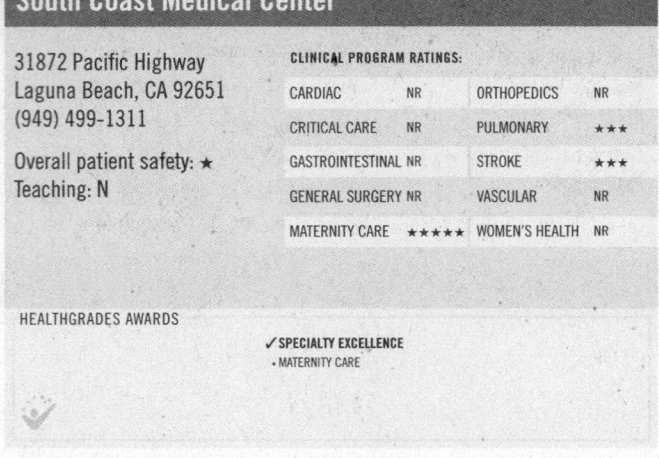

31872 Pacific Highway
Laguna Beach, CA 92651
(949) 499-1311

Overall patient safety: ★
Teaching: N

CLINICAL PROGRAM RATINGS:

CARDIAC	NR	ORTHOPEDICS	NR
CRITICAL CARE	NR	PULMONARY	★★★
GASTROINTESTINAL	NR	STROKE	★★★
GENERAL SURGERY	NR	VASCULAR	NR
MATERNITY CARE	★★★★★	WOMEN'S HEALTH	NR

HEALTHGRADES AWARDS

✓ SPECIALTY EXCELLENCE
• MATERNITY CARE

Sonoma Valley Hospital

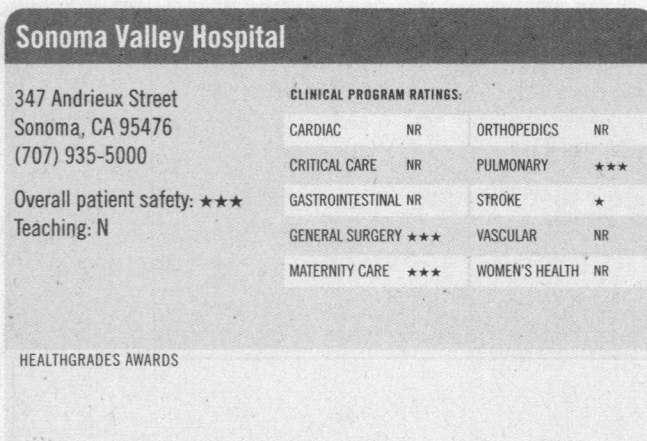

347 Andrieux Street
Sonoma, CA 95476
(707) 935-5000

Overall patient safety: ★★★
Teaching: N

CLINICAL PROGRAM RATINGS:

CARDIAC	NR	ORTHOPEDICS	NR
CRITICAL CARE	NR	PULMONARY	★★★
GASTROINTESTINAL	NR	STROKE	★
GENERAL SURGERY	★★★	VASCULAR	NR
MATERNITY CARE	★★★	WOMEN'S HEALTH	NR

HEALTHGRADES AWARDS

Southwest Healthcare System—Inland Valley Med. Ctr.*

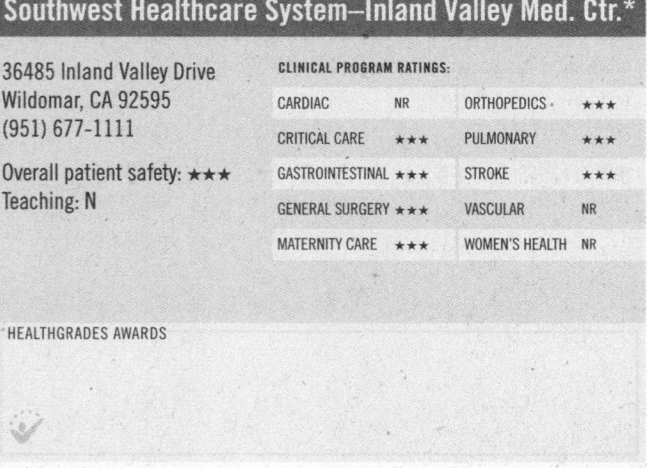

36485 Inland Valley Drive
Wildomar, CA 92595
(951) 677-1111

Overall patient safety: ★★★
Teaching: N

CLINICAL PROGRAM RATINGS:

CARDIAC	NR	ORTHOPEDICS	★★★
CRITICAL CARE	★★★	PULMONARY	★★★
GASTROINTESTINAL	★★★	STROKE	★★★
GENERAL SURGERY	★★★	VASCULAR	NR
MATERNITY CARE	★★★	WOMEN'S HEALTH	NR

HEALTHGRADES AWARDS

KEY: ★★★★★ BEST   ★★★ AS EXPECTED   ★ POOR   NR NOT RATED BY HEALTHGRADES   For full definitions of ratings and awards, see Appendix.

Southwest Healthcare System--Rancho Springs Med. Ctr.*

25500 Medical Center Drive
Murrieta, CA 92562
(909) 696-6000

Overall patient safety: ★★★
Teaching: N

CLINICAL PROGRAM RATINGS:

CARDIAC	NR	ORTHOPEDICS	★★★
CRITICAL CARE	★★★	PULMONARY	★★★
GASTROINTESTINAL	★★★	STROKE	★★★
GENERAL SURGERY	★★★	VASCULAR	NR
MATERNITY CARE	★★★	WOMEN'S HEALTH	NR

HEALTHGRADES AWARDS

Sutter Auburn Faith Hospital

11815 Education Street
Auburn, CA 95602
(530) 888-4500

Overall patient safety: ★★★
Teaching: N

CLINICAL PROGRAM RATINGS:

CARDIAC	NR	ORTHOPEDICS	NR
CRITICAL CARE	NR	PULMONARY	★★★
GASTROINTESTINAL	NR	STROKE	★★★
GENERAL SURGERY	★★★	VASCULAR	NR
MATERNITY CARE	★★★	WOMEN'S HEALTH	NR

HEALTHGRADES AWARDS

Stanford Hospital

300 Pasteur Drive
Stanford, CA 94305
(650) 723-4000

Overall patient safety: ★★★
Teaching: Y

CLINICAL PROGRAM RATINGS:

CARDIAC	★★★	ORTHOPEDICS	★★★
CRITICAL CARE	★★★	PULMONARY	★★★
GASTROINTESTINAL	★★★	STROKE	★★★
GENERAL SURGERY	★	VASCULAR	★★★
MATERNITY CARE	NR	WOMEN'S HEALTH	NR

HEALTHGRADES AWARDS

✓ SPECIALTY EXCELLENCE
· JOINT REPLACEMENT

Sutter Coast Hospital

800 East Washington
Boulevard
Crescent City, CA 95531
(707) 464-8511

Overall patient safety: ★★★
Teaching: N

CLINICAL PROGRAM RATINGS:

CARDIAC	NR	ORTHOPEDICS	NR
CRITICAL CARE	NR	PULMONARY	★★★
GASTROINTESTINAL	NR	STROKE	★★★
GENERAL SURGERY	★★★	VASCULAR	NR
MATERNITY CARE	★★★	WOMEN'S HEALTH	NR

HEALTHGRADES AWARDS

Sutter Amador Hospital

200 Mission Boulevard
Jackson, CA 95642
(209) 223-7500

Overall patient safety: ★★★
Teaching: N

CLINICAL PROGRAM RATINGS:

CARDIAC	NR	ORTHOPEDICS	NR
CRITICAL CARE	NR	PULMONARY	★★★
GASTROINTESTINAL	NR	STROKE	★
GENERAL SURGERY	★★★	VASCULAR	NR
MATERNITY CARE	★★★	WOMEN'S HEALTH	NR

HEALTHGRADES AWARDS

Sutter Davis Hospital

2000 Sutter Place
Davis, CA 95616
(530) 756-6440

Overall patient safety: ★★★
Teaching: Y

CLINICAL PROGRAM RATINGS:

CARDIAC	NR	ORTHOPEDICS	NR
CRITICAL CARE	NR	PULMONARY	★★★
GASTROINTESTINAL	NR	STROKE	★
GENERAL SURGERY	★★★	VASCULAR	NR
MATERNITY CARE	★★★	WOMEN'S HEALTH	NR

HEALTHGRADES AWARDS

*This hospital reports its data to the federal government jointly with another hospital. Therefore the ratings and awards apply to multiple hospitals and this specific hospital may not provide all rated services.

Sutter Delta Medical Center

3901 Lone Tree Way
Antioch, CA 94509
(925) 779-7200

Overall patient safety: ★★★
Teaching: N

CLINICAL PROGRAM RATINGS:

CARDIAC	NR	ORTHOPEDICS	NR
CRITICAL CARE	NR	PULMONARY	★★★
GASTROINTESTINAL	★★★	STROKE	★★★★★
GENERAL SURGERY	★★★	VASCULAR	NR
MATERNITY CARE	★★★	WOMEN'S HEALTH	NR

HEALTHGRADES AWARDS

✓ SPECIALTY EXCELLENCE
- STROKE CARE

Sutter Maternity and Surgery Center

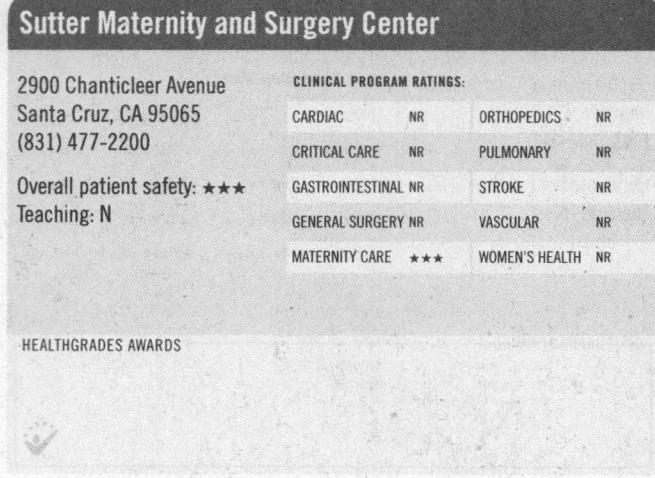

2900 Chanticleer Avenue
Santa Cruz, CA 95065
(831) 477-2200

Overall patient safety: ★★★
Teaching: N

CLINICAL PROGRAM RATINGS:

CARDIAC	NR	ORTHOPEDICS	NR
CRITICAL CARE	NR	PULMONARY	NR
GASTROINTESTINAL	NR	STROKE	NR
GENERAL SURGERY	NR	VASCULAR	NR
MATERNITY CARE	★★★	WOMEN'S HEALTH	NR

HEALTHGRADES AWARDS

Sutter General Hospital

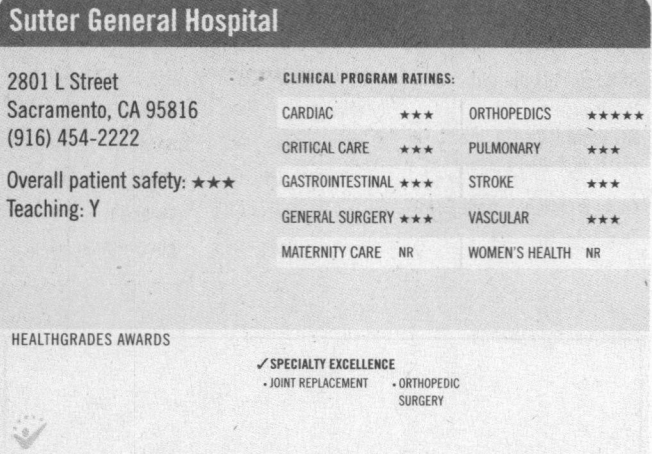

2801 L Street
Sacramento, CA 95816
(916) 454-2222

Overall patient safety: ★★★
Teaching: Y

CLINICAL PROGRAM RATINGS:

CARDIAC	★★★	ORTHOPEDICS	★★★★★
CRITICAL CARE	★★★	PULMONARY	★★★
GASTROINTESTINAL	★★★	STROKE	★★★
GENERAL SURGERY	★★★	VASCULAR	★★★
MATERNITY CARE	NR	WOMEN'S HEALTH	NR

HEALTHGRADES AWARDS

✓ SPECIALTY EXCELLENCE
- JOINT REPLACEMENT   - ORTHOPEDIC SURGERY

Sutter Medical Center of Santa Rosa—Chanate*

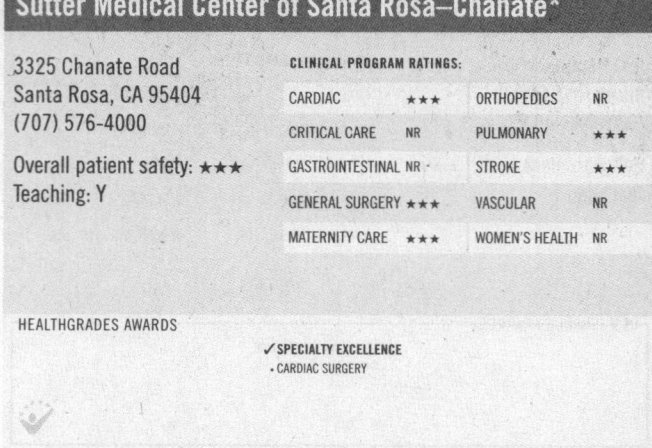

3325 Chanate Road
Santa Rosa, CA 95404
(707) 576-4000

Overall patient safety: ★★★
Teaching: Y

CLINICAL PROGRAM RATINGS:

CARDIAC	★★★	ORTHOPEDICS	NR
CRITICAL CARE	NR	PULMONARY	★★★
GASTROINTESTINAL	NR	STROKE	★★★
GENERAL SURGERY	★★★	VASCULAR	NR
MATERNITY CARE	★★★	WOMEN'S HEALTH	NR

HEALTHGRADES AWARDS

✓ SPECIALTY EXCELLENCE
- CARDIAC SURGERY

Sutter Lakeside Hospital

5176 Hill Road East
Lakeport, CA 95453
(707) 262-5000

Overall patient safety: ★
Teaching: N

CLINICAL PROGRAM RATINGS:

CARDIAC	NR	ORTHOPEDICS	NR
CRITICAL CARE	NR	PULMONARY	★★★
GASTROINTESTINAL	NR	STROKE	★★★
GENERAL SURGERY	★★★	VASCULAR	NR
MATERNITY CARE	★★★	WOMEN'S HEALTH	NR

HEALTHGRADES AWARDS

Sutter Memorial Hospital

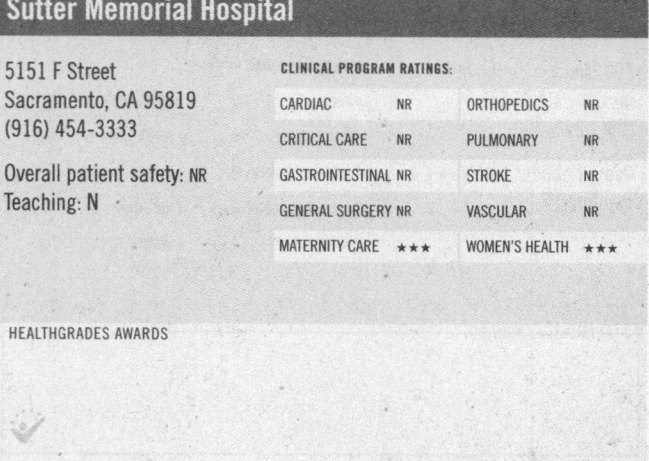

5151 F Street
Sacramento, CA 95819
(916) 454-3333

Overall patient safety: NR
Teaching: N

CLINICAL PROGRAM RATINGS:

CARDIAC	NR	ORTHOPEDICS	NR
CRITICAL CARE	NR	PULMONARY	NR
GASTROINTESTINAL	NR	STROKE	NR
GENERAL SURGERY	NR	VASCULAR	NR
MATERNITY CARE	★★★	WOMEN'S HEALTH	★★★

HEALTHGRADES AWARDS

KEY: ★★★★★ BEST ★★★ AS EXPECTED ★ POOR NR NOT RATED BY HEALTHGRADES For full definitions of ratings and awards, see Appendix.

Sutter Roseville Medical Center

1 Medical Plaza
Roseville, CA 95661
(916) 781-1000

Overall patient safety: ★★★
Teaching: N

CLINICAL PROGRAM RATINGS:

CARDIAC	NR	ORTHOPEDICS	★★★
CRITICAL CARE	★★★	PULMONARY	★★★
GASTROINTESTINAL	★★★	STROKE	★★★★★
GENERAL SURGERY	★★★	VASCULAR	NR
MATERNITY CARE	★★★	WOMEN'S HEALTH	NR

HEALTHGRADES AWARDS

✓ DISTINGUISHED HOSPITAL
- CLINICAL EXCELLENCE

✓ SPECIALTY EXCELLENCE
- STROKE CARE

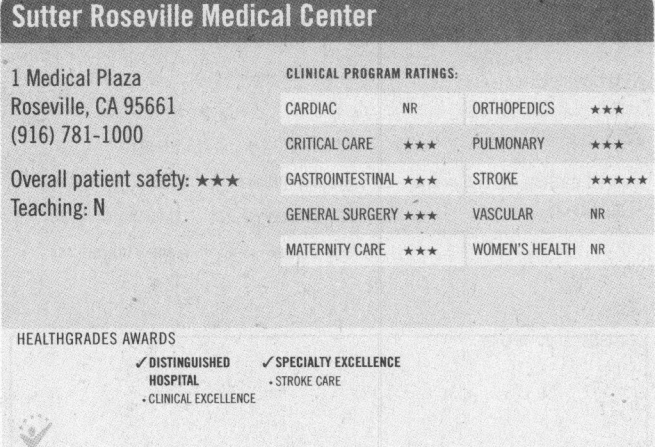

Sutter Warrack Hospital*

2449 Summerfield Road
Santa Rosa, CA 95405
(707) 542-9030

Overall patient safety: ★★★
Teaching: N

CLINICAL PROGRAM RATINGS:

CARDIAC	★★★	ORTHOPEDICS	NR
CRITICAL CARE	NR	PULMONARY	★★★
GASTROINTESTINAL	NR	STROKE	★★★
GENERAL SURGERY	★★★	VASCULAR	NR
MATERNITY CARE	NR	WOMEN'S HEALTH	NR

HEALTHGRADES AWARDS

✓ SPECIALTY EXCELLENCE
- CARDIAC SURGERY

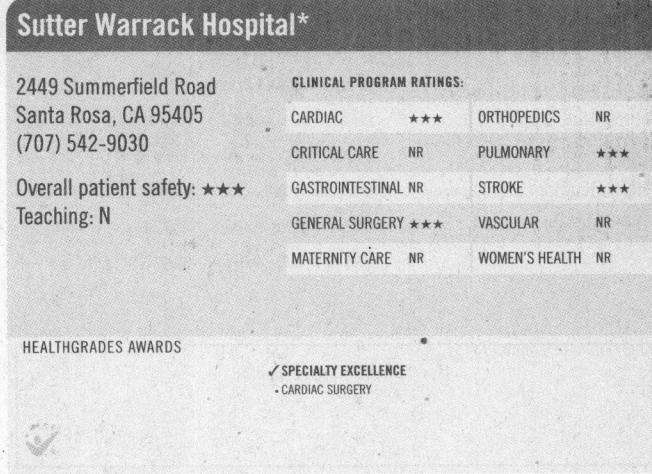

Sutter Solano Medical Center

300 Hospital Drive
Vallejo, CA 94589
(707) 554-4444

Overall patient safety: ★★★
Teaching: N

CLINICAL PROGRAM RATINGS:

CARDIAC	NR	ORTHOPEDICS	NR
CRITICAL CARE	NR	PULMONARY	★★★
GASTROINTESTINAL	NR	STROKE	★★★
GENERAL SURGERY	★★★	VASCULAR	NR
MATERNITY CARE	★★★	WOMEN'S HEALTH	NR

HEALTHGRADES AWARDS

Tahoe Forest Hospital District

10121 Pine Avenue
Truckee, CA 96161
(530) 587-6011

Overall patient safety: ★★★
Teaching: N

CLINICAL PROGRAM RATINGS:

CARDIAC	NR	ORTHOPEDICS	NR
CRITICAL CARE	NR	PULMONARY	NR
GASTROINTESTINAL	NR	STROKE	NR
GENERAL SURGERY	NR	VASCULAR	NR
MATERNITY CARE	★	WOMEN'S HEALTH	NR

HEALTHGRADES AWARDS

Sutter Tracy Community Hospital

1420 North Tracy Boulevard
Tracy, CA 95376
(209) 835-1500

Overall patient safety: ★
Teaching: N

CLINICAL PROGRAM RATINGS:

CARDIAC	NR	ORTHOPEDICS	NR
CRITICAL CARE	NR	PULMONARY	★★★
GASTROINTESTINAL	NR	STROKE	★★★
GENERAL SURGERY	★★★	VASCULAR	NR
MATERNITY CARE	★★★	WOMEN'S HEALTH	NR

HEALTHGRADES AWARDS

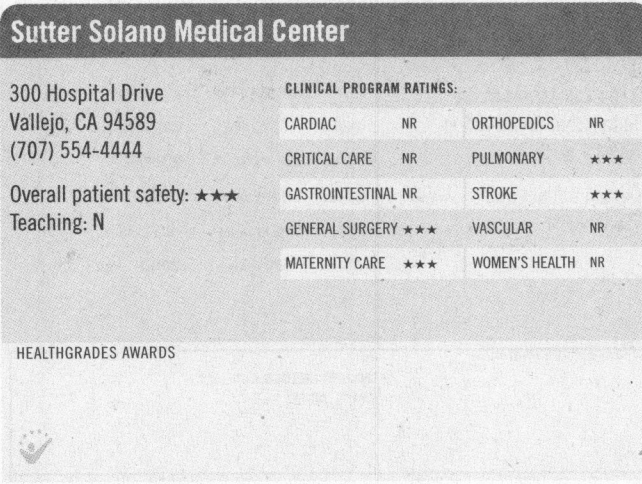

Temple Community Hospital

235 North Hoover Street
Los Angeles, CA 90004
(213) 382-7252

Overall patient safety: ★★★★★
Teaching: N

CLINICAL PROGRAM RATINGS:

CARDIAC	NR	ORTHOPEDICS	NR
CRITICAL CARE	NR	PULMONARY	★★★★★
GASTROINTESTINAL	NR	STROKE	★★★★★
GENERAL SURGERY	NR	VASCULAR	NR
MATERNITY CARE	NR	WOMEN'S HEALTH	NR

HEALTHGRADES AWARDS

✓ SPECIALTY EXCELLENCE
- PULMONARY CARE
- STROKE CARE

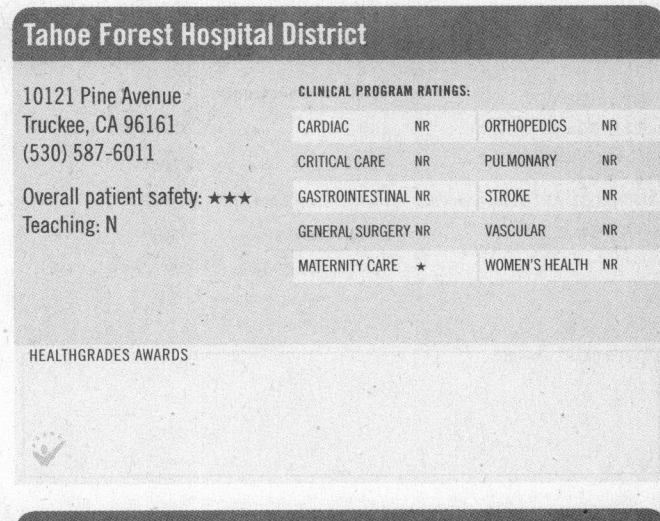

*This hospital reports its data to the federal government jointly with another hospital. Therefore the ratings and awards apply to multiple hospitals and this specific hospital may not provide all rated services.

Torrance Memorial Medical Center

.3330 West Lomita Boulevard
Torrance, CA 90505
(310) 325-9110

Overall patient safety: ★★★
Teaching: N

CLINICAL PROGRAM RATINGS:

CARDIAC	★★★	ORTHOPEDICS	★★★
CRITICAL CARE	★★★	PULMONARY	★★★
GASTROINTESTINAL	★★★	STROKE	★★★
GENERAL SURGERY	★★★	VASCULAR	NR
MATERNITY CARE	★★★	WOMEN'S HEALTH	★★★

HEALTHGRADES AWARDS

Tulare District Hospital

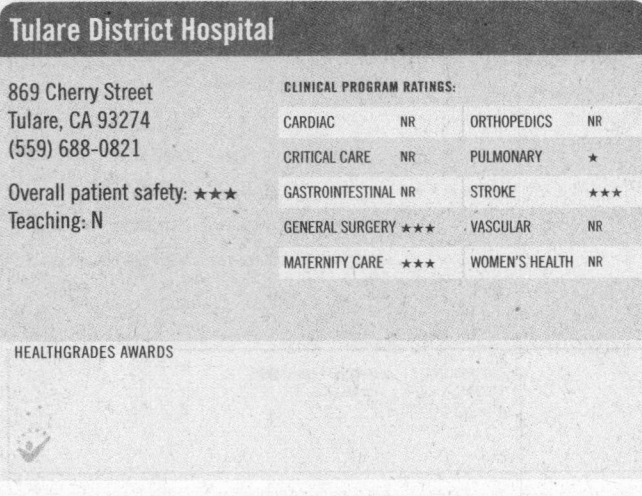

869 Cherry Street
Tulare, CA 93274
(559) 688-0821

Overall patient safety: ★★★
Teaching: N

CLINICAL PROGRAM RATINGS:

CARDIAC	NR	ORTHOPEDICS	NR
CRITICAL CARE	NR	PULMONARY	★
GASTROINTESTINAL	NR	STROKE	★★★
GENERAL SURGERY	★★★	VASCULAR	NR
MATERNITY CARE	★★★	WOMEN'S HEALTH	NR

HEALTHGRADES AWARDS

Tri-City Medical Center

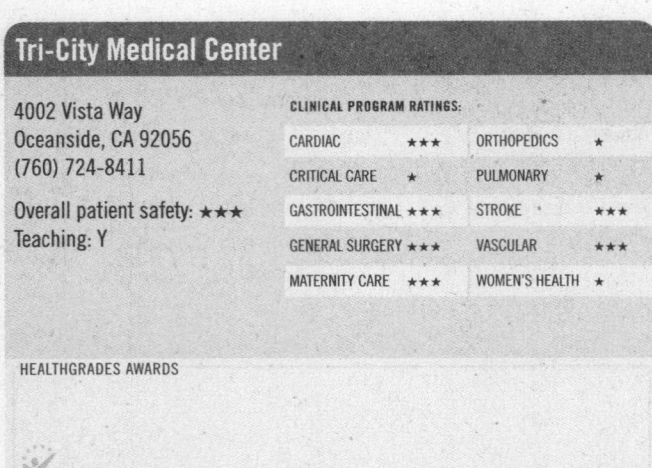

4002 Vista Way
Oceanside, CA 92056
(760) 724-8411

Overall patient safety: ★★★
Teaching: Y

CLINICAL PROGRAM RATINGS:

CARDIAC	★★★	ORTHOPEDICS	★
CRITICAL CARE	★	PULMONARY	★
GASTROINTESTINAL	★★★	STROKE	★★★
GENERAL SURGERY	★★★	VASCULAR	★★★
MATERNITY CARE	★★★	WOMEN'S HEALTH	★

HEALTHGRADES AWARDS

Twin Cities Community Hospital

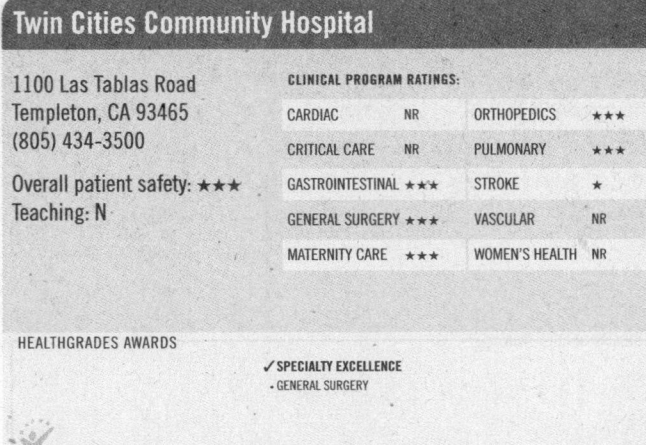

1100 Las Tablas Road
Templeton, CA 93465
(805) 434-3500

Overall patient safety: ★★★
Teaching: N

CLINICAL PROGRAM RATINGS:

CARDIAC	NR	ORTHOPEDICS	★★★
CRITICAL CARE	NR	PULMONARY	★★★
GASTROINTESTINAL	★★★	STROKE	★
GENERAL SURGERY	★★★	VASCULAR	NR
MATERNITY CARE	★★★	WOMEN'S HEALTH	NR

HEALTHGRADES AWARDS

✓ SPECIALTY EXCELLENCE
- GENERAL SURGERY

Tri-City Regional Medical Center

21530 South Pioneer Boulevard
Hawaiian Gardens, CA 90716
(562) 860-0401

Overall patient safety: ★
Teaching: N

CLINICAL PROGRAM RATINGS:

CARDIAC	NR	ORTHOPEDICS	NR
CRITICAL CARE	NR	PULMONARY	★★★★★
GASTROINTESTINAL	NR	STROKE	NR
GENERAL SURGERY	NR	VASCULAR	NR
MATERNITY CARE	NR	WOMEN'S HEALTH	NR

HEALTHGRADES AWARDS

✓ SPECIALTY EXCELLENCE
- PULMONARY CARE

UCLA Medical Center

10833 Le Conte Avenue
Los Angeles, CA 90095
(310) 825-9111

Overall patient safety: ★★★
Teaching: Y

CLINICAL PROGRAM RATINGS:

CARDIAC	★★★	ORTHOPEDICS	NR
CRITICAL CARE	★★★	PULMONARY	★★★★★
GASTROINTESTINAL	★★★	STROKE	★★★★★
GENERAL SURGERY	★★★	VASCULAR	★★★
MATERNITY CARE	★★★	WOMEN'S HEALTH	NR

HEALTHGRADES AWARDS

✓ DISTINGUISHED   ✓ SPECIALTY EXCELLENCE
   HOSPITAL   - CARDIAC CARE   - PULMONARY CARE
- CLINICAL EXCELLENCE   - CARDIAC SURGERY   - STROKE CARE

KEY: ★★★★★ BEST   ★★★ AS EXPECTED   ★ POOR   NR NOT RATED BY HEALTHGRADES   For full definitions of ratings and awards, see Appendix.

UCSF Medical Center

500 Parnassus Avenue
San Francisco, CA 94143
(415) 476-1000

Overall patient safety: ★★★
Teaching: Y

CLINICAL PROGRAM RATINGS:

CARDIAC	★★★	ORTHOPEDICS	★
CRITICAL CARE	★★★	PULMONARY	★★★★★
GASTROINTESTINAL	★★★	STROKE	★★★★★
GENERAL SURGERY	★★★	VASCULAR	★★★
MATERNITY CARE	★	WOMEN'S HEALTH	★★★

HEALTHGRADES AWARDS

✓ SPECIALTY EXCELLENCE
• PULMONARY CARE   • STROKE CARE

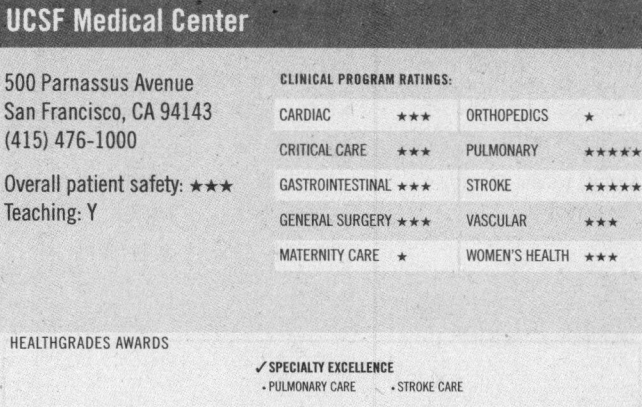

University of California—Davis Medical Center

2315 Stockton Boulevard
Sacramento, CA 95817
(916) 734-2011

Overall patient safety: ★
Teaching: Y

CLINICAL PROGRAM RATINGS:

CARDIAC	★★★	ORTHOPEDICS	★★★
CRITICAL CARE	★★★	PULMONARY	★★★
GASTROINTESTINAL	★★★	STROKE	★★★
GENERAL SURGERY	★★★	VASCULAR	NR
MATERNITY CARE	★	WOMEN'S HEALTH	★

HEALTHGRADES AWARDS

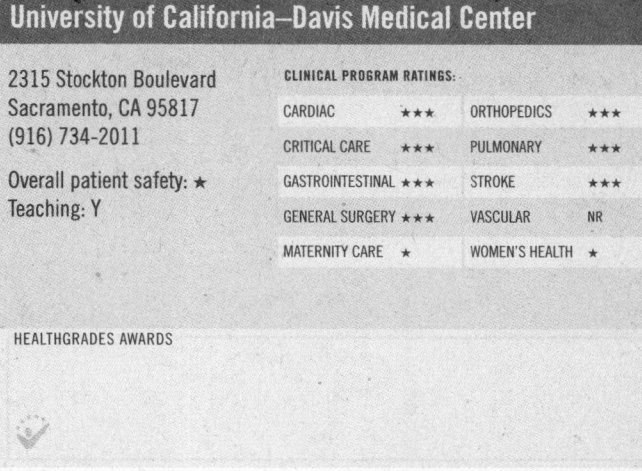

Ukiah Valley Medical Center

275 Hospital Drive
Ukiah, CA 95482
(707) 462-3111

Overall patient safety: ★
Teaching: N

CLINICAL PROGRAM RATINGS:

CARDIAC	NR	ORTHOPEDICS	NR
CRITICAL CARE	NR	PULMONARY	★★★
GASTROINTESTINAL	NR	STROKE	★
GENERAL SURGERY	★★★	VASCULAR	NR
MATERNITY CARE	★★★	WOMEN'S HEALTH	NR

HEALTHGRADES AWARDS

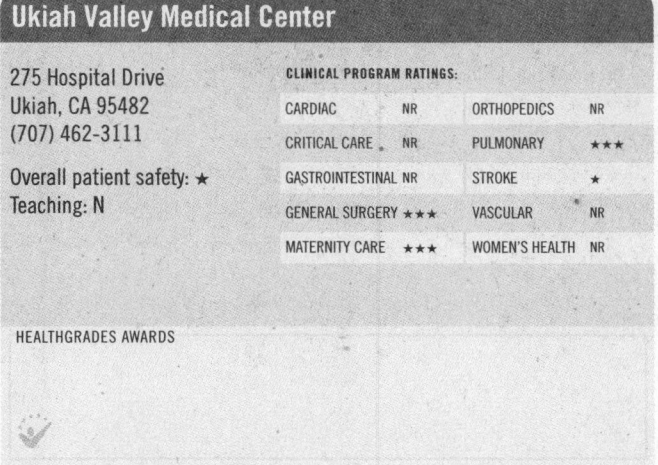

University of California—Irvine Medical Center

101 The City Drive
Orange, CA 92868
(714) 456-5678

Overall patient safety: ★★★
Teaching: Y

CLINICAL PROGRAM RATINGS:

CARDIAC	★★★	ORTHOPEDICS	★★★
CRITICAL CARE	NR	PULMONARY	★★★
GASTROINTESTINAL	★★★	STROKE	★★★
GENERAL SURGERY	★★★	VASCULAR	NR
MATERNITY CARE	★	WOMEN'S HEALTH	NR

HEALTHGRADES AWARDS

University Medical Center*

445 South Cedar Avenue
Fresno, CA 93702
(714) 670-7400

Overall patient safety: ★★★
Teaching: Y

CLINICAL PROGRAM RATINGS:

CARDIAC	★★★	ORTHOPEDICS	★★★
CRITICAL CARE	★★★	PULMONARY	★
GASTROINTESTINAL	★★★	STROKE	★★★
GENERAL SURGERY	★★★	VASCULAR	★★★
MATERNITY CARE	★★★	WOMEN'S HEALTH	★

HEALTHGRADES AWARDS

University of California—San Diego Medical Center

200 West Arbor Drive
San Diego, CA 92103
(619) 543-6222

Overall patient safety: ★
Teaching: Y

CLINICAL PROGRAM RATINGS:

CARDIAC	★★★	ORTHOPEDICS	★★★
CRITICAL CARE	NR	PULMONARY	★★★
GASTROINTESTINAL	NR	STROKE	★★★
GENERAL SURGERY	★★★	VASCULAR	NR
MATERNITY CARE	★	WOMEN'S HEALTH	★

HEALTHGRADES AWARDS

*This hospital reports its data to the federal government jointly with another hospital. Therefore the ratings and awards apply to multiple hospitals and this specific hospital may not provide all rated services.

USC University Hospital

1500 San Pablo
Los Angeles, CA 90033
(323) 442-8500

Overall patient safety: ★
Teaching: Y

CLINICAL PROGRAM RATINGS:

CARDIAC	★★★	ORTHOPEDICS	★
CRITICAL CARE	NR	PULMONARY	NR
GASTROINTESTINAL	NR	STROKE	★★★★★
GENERAL SURGERY	NR	VASCULAR	★★★
MATERNITY CARE	NR	WOMEN'S HEALTH	NR

HEALTHGRADES AWARDS

✓ SPECIALTY EXCELLENCE
· CARDIAC SURGERY   · STROKE CARE

Valley Presbyterian Hospital

15107 Vanowen St
Van Nuys, CA 91405
(818) 782-6600

Overall patient safety: ★★★
Teaching: N

CLINICAL PROGRAM RATINGS:

CARDIAC	NR	ORTHOPEDICS	★★★
CRITICAL CARE	NR	PULMONARY	★★★
GASTROINTESTINAL	NR	STROKE	★
GENERAL SURGERY	★★★	VASCULAR	NR
MATERNITY CARE	★★★★★	WOMEN'S HEALTH	NR

HEALTHGRADES AWARDS

Valley Care Medical Center*

5555 West Las
Positas Boulevard
Pleasanton, CA 94588
(925) 847-3000

Overall patient safety: ★
Teaching: N

CLINICAL PROGRAM RATINGS:

CARDIAC	NR	ORTHOPEDICS	★
CRITICAL CARE	NR	PULMONARY	★★★★★
GASTROINTESTINAL	★★★	STROKE	★★★
GENERAL SURGERY	★★★	VASCULAR	NR
MATERNITY CARE	★★★	WOMEN'S HEALTH	NR

HEALTHGRADES AWARDS

Ventura County Medical Center

3291 Loma Vista Road
Ventura, CA 93003
(805) 652-6000

Overall patient safety: ★★★
Teaching: Y

CLINICAL PROGRAM RATINGS:

CARDIAC	NR	ORTHOPEDICS	NR
CRITICAL CARE	NR	PULMONARY	★★★
GASTROINTESTINAL	NR	STROKE	★★★
GENERAL SURGERY	NR	VASCULAR	NR
MATERNITY CARE	★	WOMEN'S HEALTH	NR

HEALTHGRADES AWARDS

Valley Memorial Hospital*

1111 East Stanley Boulevard
Livermore, CA 94550
(925) 447-7000

Overall patient safety: ★
Teaching: N

CLINICAL PROGRAM RATINGS:

CARDIAC	NR	ORTHOPEDICS	★
CRITICAL CARE	NR	PULMONARY	★★★★★
GASTROINTESTINAL	★★★	STROKE	★★★
GENERAL SURGERY	★★★	VASCULAR	NR
MATERNITY CARE	★★★	WOMEN'S HEALTH	NR

HEALTHGRADES AWARDS

Verdugo Hills Hospital

1812 Verdugo Boulevard
Glendale, CA 91208
(818) 790-7100

Overall patient safety: ★★★
Teaching: N

CLINICAL PROGRAM RATINGS:

CARDIAC	NR	ORTHOPEDICS	NR
CRITICAL CARE	NR	PULMONARY	★★★
GASTROINTESTINAL	NR	STROKE	★★★
GENERAL SURGERY	NR	VASCULAR	NR
MATERNITY CARE	★★★★★	WOMEN'S HEALTH	NR

HEALTHGRADES AWARDS

KEY: ★★★★★ BEST   ★★★ AS EXPECTED   ★ POOR   NR NOT RATED BY HEALTHGRADES   For full definitions of ratings and awards, see Appendix.

Victor Valley Community Hospital

15248 11th Street
Victorville, CA 92395
(760) 245-8691

Overall patient safety: ★★★
Teaching: N

CLINICAL PROGRAM RATINGS:

CARDIAC	NR	ORTHOPEDICS	NR
CRITICAL CARE	NR	PULMONARY	★
GASTROINTESTINAL	NR	STROKE	★★★
GENERAL SURGERY	NR	VASCULAR	NR
MATERNITY CARE	★★★★★	WOMEN'S HEALTH	NR

HEALTHGRADES AWARDS

✓ SPECIALTY EXCELLENCE
• MATERNITY CARE

West Anaheim Medical Center

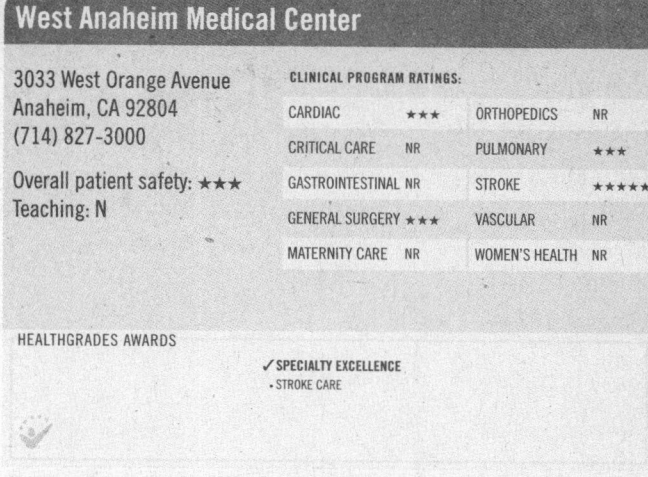

3033 West Orange Avenue
Anaheim, CA 92804
(714) 827-3000

Overall patient safety: ★★★
Teaching: N

CLINICAL PROGRAM RATINGS:

CARDIAC	★★★	ORTHOPEDICS	NR
CRITICAL CARE	NR	PULMONARY	★★★
GASTROINTESTINAL	NR	STROKE	★★★★★
GENERAL SURGERY	★★★	VASCULAR	NR
MATERNITY CARE	NR	WOMEN'S HEALTH	NR

HEALTHGRADES AWARDS

✓ SPECIALTY EXCELLENCE
• STROKE CARE

Washington Hospital Healthcare System

2000 Mowry Avenue
Fremont, CA 94538
(510) 797-1111

Overall patient safety: ★★★
Teaching: N

CLINICAL PROGRAM RATINGS:

CARDIAC	★★★	ORTHOPEDICS	★★★
CRITICAL CARE	★★★	PULMONARY	★★★
GASTROINTESTINAL	★★★	STROKE	★★★★★
GENERAL SURGERY	★★★	VASCULAR	NR
MATERNITY CARE	★★★	WOMEN'S HEALTH	★★★

HEALTHGRADES AWARDS

✓ SPECIALTY EXCELLENCE
• GENERAL SURGERY   • JOINT REPLACEMENT

West Hills Medical Center

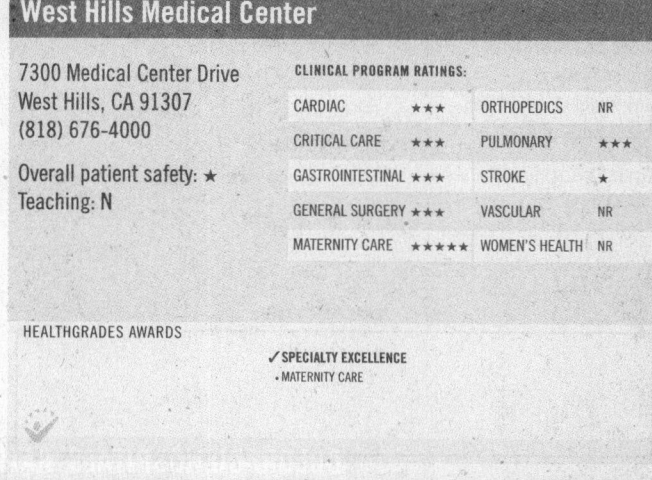

7300 Medical Center Drive
West Hills, CA 91307
(818) 676-4000

Overall patient safety: ★
Teaching: N

CLINICAL PROGRAM RATINGS:

CARDIAC	★★★	ORTHOPEDICS	NR
CRITICAL CARE	★★★	PULMONARY	★★★
GASTROINTESTINAL	★★★	STROKE	★
GENERAL SURGERY	★★★	VASCULAR	NR
MATERNITY CARE	★★★★★	WOMEN'S HEALTH	NR

HEALTHGRADES AWARDS

✓ SPECIALTY EXCELLENCE
• MATERNITY CARE

Watsonville Community Hospital

75 Nielson Street
Watsonville, CA 95076
(831) 724-4741

Overall patient safety: ★★★
Teaching: N

CLINICAL PROGRAM RATINGS:

CARDIAC	NR	ORTHOPEDICS	★★★
CRITICAL CARE	NR	PULMONARY	★★★
GASTROINTESTINAL	NR	STROKE	★★★
GENERAL SURGERY	★★★	VASCULAR	NR
MATERNITY CARE	★★★	WOMEN'S HEALTH	NR

HEALTHGRADES AWARDS

Western Medical Center Hospital Anaheim

1025 South Anaheim
Boulevard
Anaheim, CA 92805
(714) 533-6220

Overall patient safety: ★★★
Teaching: N

CLINICAL PROGRAM RATINGS:

CARDIAC	NR	ORTHOPEDICS	NR
CRITICAL CARE	NR	PULMONARY	★★★
GASTROINTESTINAL	NR	STROKE	★★★
GENERAL SURGERY	NR	VASCULAR	NR
MATERNITY CARE	★★★★★	WOMEN'S HEALTH	NR

HEALTHGRADES AWARDS

✓ SPECIALTY EXCELLENCE
• MATERNITY CARE

*This hospital reports its data to the federal government jointly with another hospital. Therefore the ratings and awards apply to multiple hospitals and this specific hospital may not provide all rated services.

Western Medical Center Santa Ana

1001 North Tustin Avenue
Santa Ana, CA 92705
(714) 953-3331

Overall patient safety: ★
Teaching: Y

CLINICAL PROGRAM RATINGS:

CARDIAC	★★★	ORTHOPEDICS	NR
CRITICAL CARE	NR	PULMONARY	★★★
GASTROINTESTINAL	NR	STROKE	★★★
GENERAL SURGERY	★★★	VASCULAR	NR
MATERNITY CARE	★★★	WOMEN'S HEALTH	★★★

HEALTHGRADES AWARDS

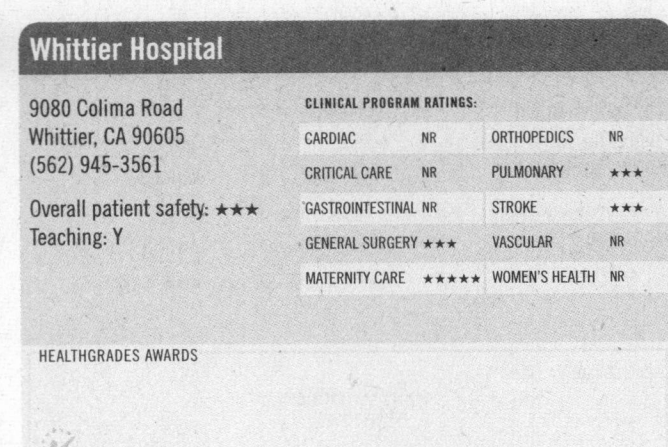

Whittier Hospital

9080 Colima Road
Whittier, CA 90605
(562) 945-3561

Overall patient safety: ★★★
Teaching: Y

CLINICAL PROGRAM RATINGS:

CARDIAC	NR	ORTHOPEDICS	NR
CRITICAL CARE	NR	PULMONARY	★★★
GASTROINTESTINAL	NR	STROKE	★★★
GENERAL SURGERY	★★★	VASCULAR	NR
MATERNITY CARE	★★★★★	WOMEN'S HEALTH	NR

HEALTHGRADES AWARDS

White Memorial Medical Center

1720 East Cesar
Chavez Avenue
Los Angeles, CA 90033
(323) 268-5000

Overall patient safety: ★★★
Teaching: Y

CLINICAL PROGRAM RATINGS:

CARDIAC	★★★	ORTHOPEDICS	NR
CRITICAL CARE	NR	PULMONARY	★★★★★
GASTROINTESTINAL	NR	STROKE	★★★★★
GENERAL SURGERY	★★★	VASCULAR	NR
MATERNITY CARE	★	WOMEN'S HEALTH	NR

HEALTHGRADES AWARDS

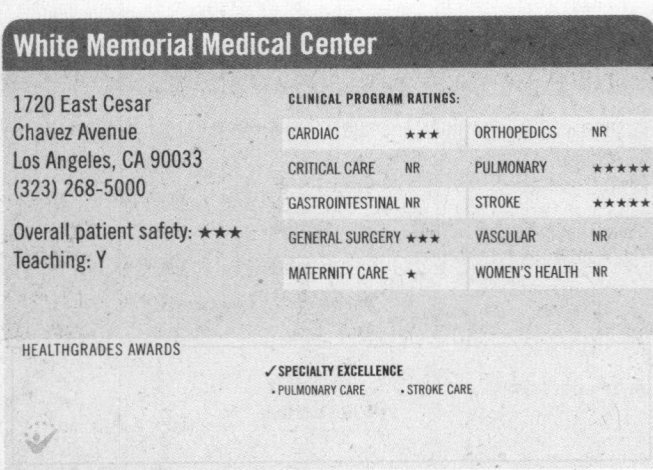

✓ SPECIALTY EXCELLENCE
· PULMONARY CARE · STROKE CARE

Woodland Memorial Hospital

1325 Cottonwood Street
Woodland, CA 95695
(530) 662-3961

Overall patient safety: ★★★
Teaching: N

CLINICAL PROGRAM RATINGS:

CARDIAC	NR	ORTHOPEDICS	NR
CRITICAL CARE	NR	PULMONARY	★
GASTROINTESTINAL	NR	STROKE	★★★
GENERAL SURGERY	★★★	VASCULAR	NR
MATERNITY CARE	★★★	WOMEN'S HEALTH	NR

HEALTHGRADES AWARDS

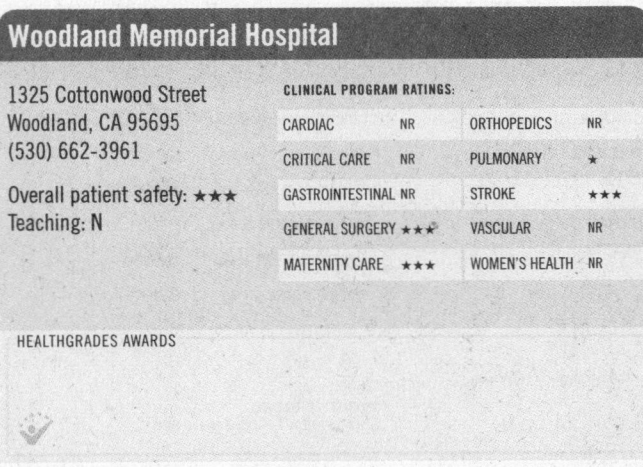

COLORADO HOSPITALS: RATINGS BY CLINICAL SPECIALTY

Arkansas Valley Regional Medical Center

1100 Carson Avenue
La Junta, CO 81050
(719) 383-6000

Overall patient safety: ★
Teaching: N

CLINICAL PROGRAM RATINGS:

CARDIAC	NR	ORTHOPEDICS	NR
CRITICAL CARE	NR	PULMONARY	★★★
GASTROINTESTINAL	NR	STROKE	★
GENERAL SURGERY	NR	VASCULAR	NR
MATERNITY CARE	NR	WOMEN'S HEALTH	NR

HEALTHGRADES AWARDS

Aspen Valley Hospital

0401 Castle Creek Road
Aspen, CO 81611
(970) 544-1261

Overall patient safety: ★★★
Teaching: N

CLINICAL PROGRAM RATINGS:

CARDIAC	NR	ORTHOPEDICS	NR
CRITICAL CARE	NR	PULMONARY	NR
GASTROINTESTINAL	NR	STROKE	NR
GENERAL SURGERY	NR	VASCULAR	NR
MATERNITY CARE	NR	WOMEN'S HEALTH	NR

HEALTHGRADES AWARDS

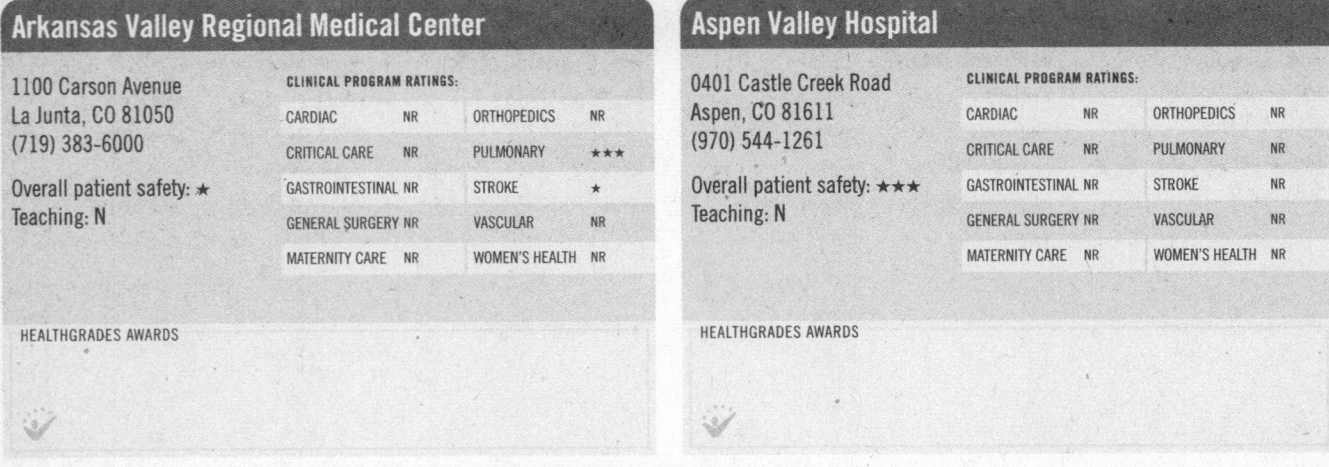

KEY: ★★★★★ BEST ★★★ AS EXPECTED ★ POOR NR NOT RATED BY HEALTHGRADES For full definitions of ratings and awards, see Appendix.

Boulder Community Hospital

311 Mapleton Avenue
Boulder, CO 80301
(303) 440-2273

Overall patient safety: ★★★
Teaching: N

CLINICAL PROGRAM RATINGS:

CARDIAC	★★★	ORTHOPEDICS	★★★
CRITICAL CARE	NR	PULMONARY	★★★
GASTROINTESTINAL	★★★	STROKE	★★★★★
GENERAL SURGERY	NR	VASCULAR	NR
MATERNITY CARE	NR	WOMEN'S HEALTH	NR

HEALTHGRADES AWARDS

✓ SPECIALTY EXCELLENCE
• STROKE CARE

Centura Health–Parker Adventist Hospital

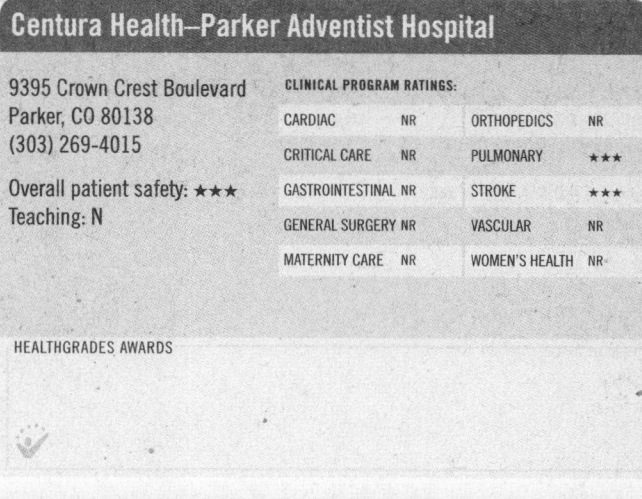

9395 Crown Crest Boulevard
Parker, CO 80138
(303) 269-4015

Overall patient safety: ★★★
Teaching: N

CLINICAL PROGRAM RATINGS:

CARDIAC	NR	ORTHOPEDICS	NR
CRITICAL CARE	NR	PULMONARY	★★★
GASTROINTESTINAL	NR	STROKE	★★★
GENERAL SURGERY	NR	VASCULAR	NR
MATERNITY CARE	NR	WOMEN'S HEALTH	NR

HEALTHGRADES AWARDS

Centura Health–Avista Adventist Hospital

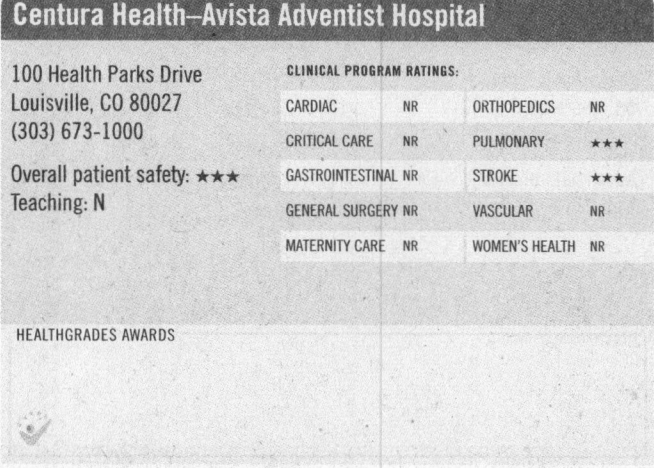

100 Health Parks Drive
Louisville, CO 80027
(303) 673-1000

Overall patient safety: ★★★
Teaching: N

CLINICAL PROGRAM RATINGS:

CARDIAC	NR	ORTHOPEDICS	NR
CRITICAL CARE	NR	PULMONARY	★★★
GASTROINTESTINAL	NR	STROKE	★★★
GENERAL SURGERY	NR	VASCULAR	NR
MATERNITY CARE	NR	WOMEN'S HEALTH	NR

HEALTHGRADES AWARDS

Centura Health–Penrose St. Francis Health Services

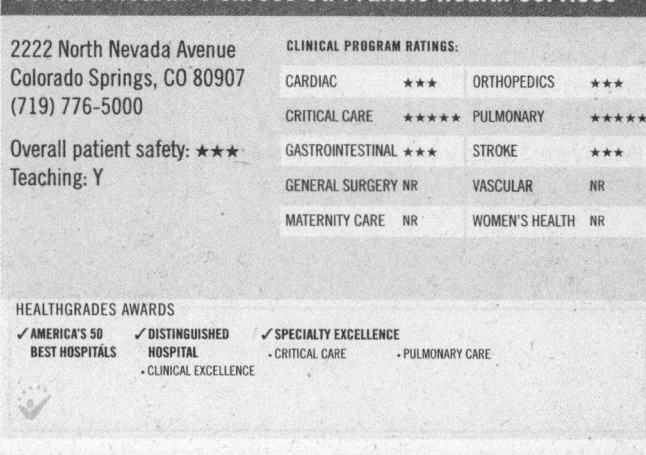

2222 North Nevada Avenue
Colorado Springs, CO 80907
(719) 776-5000

Overall patient safety: ★★★
Teaching: Y

CLINICAL PROGRAM RATINGS:

CARDIAC	★★★	ORTHOPEDICS	★★★
CRITICAL CARE	★★★★★	PULMONARY	★★★★★
GASTROINTESTINAL	★★★	STROKE	★★★
GENERAL SURGERY	NR	VASCULAR	NR
MATERNITY CARE	NR	WOMEN'S HEALTH	NR

HEALTHGRADES AWARDS

✓ AMERICA'S 50 BEST HOSPITALS
✓ DISTINGUISHED HOSPITAL
• CLINICAL EXCELLENCE
✓ SPECIALTY EXCELLENCE
• CRITICAL CARE
• PULMONARY CARE

Centura Health–Littleton Adventist Hospital

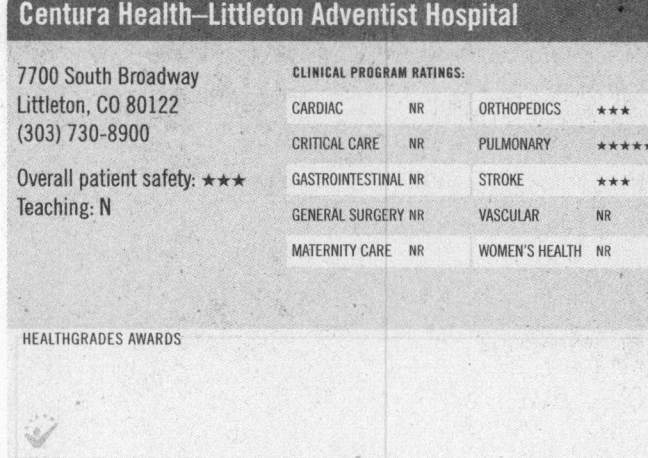

7700 South Broadway
Littleton, CO 80122
(303) 730-8900

Overall patient safety: ★★★
Teaching: N

CLINICAL PROGRAM RATINGS:

CARDIAC	NR	ORTHOPEDICS	★★★
CRITICAL CARE	NR	PULMONARY	★★★★★
GASTROINTESTINAL	NR	STROKE	★★★
GENERAL SURGERY	NR	VASCULAR	NR
MATERNITY CARE	NR	WOMEN'S HEALTH	NR

HEALTHGRADES AWARDS

Centura Health–Porter Adventist Hospital

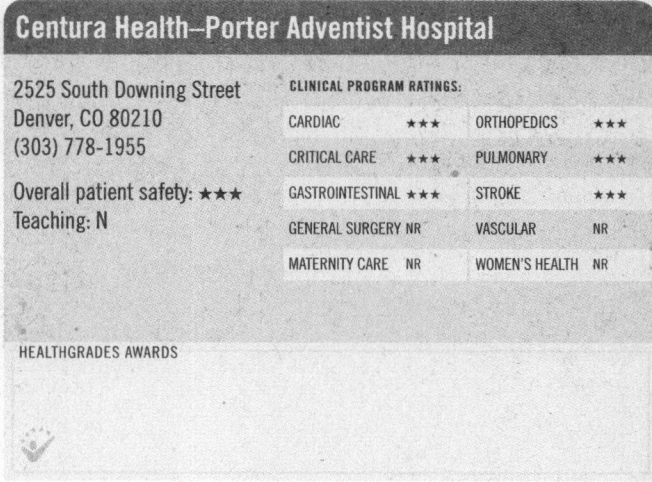

2525 South Downing Street
Denver, CO 80210
(303) 778-1955

Overall patient safety: ★★★
Teaching: N

CLINICAL PROGRAM RATINGS:

CARDIAC	★★★	ORTHOPEDICS	★★★
CRITICAL CARE	★★★	PULMONARY	★★★
GASTROINTESTINAL	★★★	STROKE	★★★
GENERAL SURGERY	NR	VASCULAR	NR
MATERNITY CARE	NR	WOMEN'S HEALTH	NR

HEALTHGRADES AWARDS

COLORADO HOSPITALS: RATINGS BY CLINICAL SPECIALTY

Centura Health—St. Anthony Central Hospital

4231 West 16th Avenue
Denver, CO 80204
(303) 629-3511

Overall patient safety: ★★★
Teaching: Y

CLINICAL PROGRAM RATINGS:

CARDIAC	★★★	ORTHOPEDICS	★★★
CRITICAL CARE	★★★	PULMONARY	★★★
GASTROINTESTINAL	★★★	STROKE	★★★
GENERAL SURGERY	NR	VASCULAR	NR
MATERNITY CARE	NR	WOMEN'S HEALTH	NR

HEALTHGRADES AWARDS

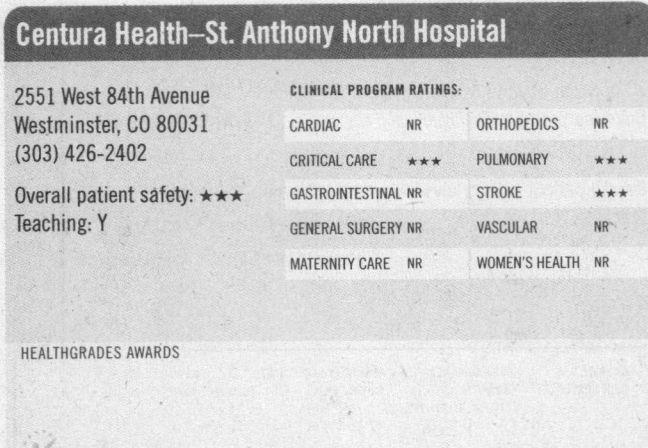

Centura Health—St. Thomas More Hospital*

1338 Phay Avenue
Canon City, CO 81212
(719) 285-2540

Overall patient safety: ★★★
Teaching: N

CLINICAL PROGRAM RATINGS:

CARDIAC	NR	ORTHOPEDICS	NR
CRITICAL CARE	NR	PULMONARY	★★★
GASTROINTESTINAL	NR	STROKE	★★★
GENERAL SURGERY	NR	VASCULAR	NR
MATERNITY CARE	NR	WOMEN'S HEALTH	NR

HEALTHGRADES AWARDS

Centura Health—St. Anthony North Hospital

2551 West 84th Avenue
Westminster, CO 80031
(303) 426-2402

Overall patient safety: ★★★
Teaching: Y

CLINICAL PROGRAM RATINGS:

CARDIAC	NR	ORTHOPEDICS	NR
CRITICAL CARE	★★★	PULMONARY	★★★
GASTROINTESTINAL	NR	STROKE	★★★
GENERAL SURGERY	NR	VASCULAR	NR
MATERNITY CARE	NR	WOMEN'S HEALTH	NR

HEALTHGRADES AWARDS

Colorado Plains Medical Center

1000 Lincoln Street
Fort Morgan, CO 80701
(970) 867-3391

Overall patient safety: ★★★
Teaching: N

CLINICAL PROGRAM RATINGS:

CARDIAC	NR	ORTHOPEDICS	NR
CRITICAL CARE	NR	PULMONARY	★★★
GASTROINTESTINAL	NR	STROKE	★★★
GENERAL SURGERY	NR	VASCULAR	NR
MATERNITY CARE	NR	WOMEN'S HEALTH	NR

HEALTHGRADES AWARDS

Centura Health—St. Mary Corwin Medical Center

1008 Minnequa Avenue
Pueblo, CO 81004
(719) 560-4000

Overall patient safety: ★★★
Teaching: Y

CLINICAL PROGRAM RATINGS:

CARDIAC	NR	ORTHOPEDICS	★★★
CRITICAL CARE	★★★	PULMONARY	★★★
GASTROINTESTINAL	★★★	STROKE	★★★
GENERAL SURGERY	NR	VASCULAR	NR
MATERNITY CARE	NR	WOMEN'S HEALTH	NR

HEALTHGRADES AWARDS

Community Hospital

2021 North 12th Street
Grand Junction, CO 81501
(970) 242-0920

Overall patient safety: ★★★
Teaching: N

CLINICAL PROGRAM RATINGS:

CARDIAC	NR	ORTHOPEDICS	★★★★★
CRITICAL CARE	NR	PULMONARY	★★★
GASTROINTESTINAL	NR	STROKE	★
GENERAL SURGERY	NR	VASCULAR	NR
MATERNITY CARE	NR	WOMEN'S HEALTH	NR

HEALTHGRADES AWARDS

KEY: ★★★★★ BEST   ★★★ AS EXPECTED   ★ POOR   NR NOT RATED BY HEALTHGRADES   For full definitions of ratings and awards, see Appendix.

Delta County Memorial Hospital

1501 East 3rd Street
Delta, CO 81416
(970) 874-7681

Overall patient safety: ★★★
Teaching: N

CLINICAL PROGRAM RATINGS:

CARDIAC	NR	ORTHOPEDICS	NR
CRITICAL CARE	NR	PULMONARY	★★★
GASTROINTESTINAL	NR	STROKE	★★★
GENERAL SURGERY	NR	VASCULAR	NR
MATERNITY CARE	NR	WOMEN'S HEALTH	NR

HEALTHGRADES AWARDS

Exempla Saint Joseph Hospital

1835 Franklin Street
Denver, CO 80218
(303) 837-7111

Overall patient safety: ★★★
Teaching: Y

CLINICAL PROGRAM RATINGS:

CARDIAC	★★★	ORTHOPEDICS	★★★
CRITICAL CARE	NR	PULMONARY	★★★
GASTROINTESTINAL	NR	STROKE	★★★
GENERAL SURGERY	NR	VASCULAR	NR
MATERNITY CARE	NR	WOMEN'S HEALTH	NR

HEALTHGRADES AWARDS

Denver Health Medical Center

777 Bannock Street
Denver, CO 80204
(303) 436-6000

Overall patient safety: ★★★
Teaching: Y

CLINICAL PROGRAM RATINGS:

CARDIAC	NR	ORTHOPEDICS	NR
CRITICAL CARE	NR	PULMONARY	★★★
GASTROINTESTINAL	NR	STROKE	★★★
GENERAL SURGERY	NR	VASCULAR	NR
MATERNITY CARE	NR	WOMEN'S HEALTH	NR

HEALTHGRADES AWARDS

Grand River Medical Center

501 Airport Road
Rifle, CO 81650
(970) 625-1510

Overall patient safety: ★★★
Teaching: N

CLINICAL PROGRAM RATINGS:

CARDIAC	NR	ORTHOPEDICS	NR
CRITICAL CARE	NR	PULMONARY	★★★
GASTROINTESTINAL	NR	STROKE	NR
GENERAL SURGERY	NR	VASCULAR	NR
MATERNITY CARE	NR	WOMEN'S HEALTH	NR

HEALTHGRADES AWARDS

Exempla Lutheran Medical Center

8300 West 38th Avenue
Wheat Ridge, CO 80033
(303) 425-4500

Overall patient safety: ★★★
Teaching: N

CLINICAL PROGRAM RATINGS:

CARDIAC	★★★	ORTHOPEDICS	★★★
CRITICAL CARE	★★★	PULMONARY	★★★★★
GASTROINTESTINAL	★★★	STROKE	★★★
GENERAL SURGERY	NR	VASCULAR	NR
MATERNITY CARE	NR	WOMEN'S HEALTH	NR

HEALTHGRADES AWARDS

✓ SPECIALTY EXCELLENCE
- PULMONARY CARE

Heart of the Rockies Regional Medical Center

448 East 1st Street
Salida, CO 81201
(719) 539-6661

Overall patient safety: ★★★
Teaching: N

CLINICAL PROGRAM RATINGS:

CARDIAC	NR	ORTHOPEDICS	NR
CRITICAL CARE	NR	PULMONARY	★★★
GASTROINTESTINAL	NR	STROKE	NR
GENERAL SURGERY	NR	VASCULAR	NR
MATERNITY CARE	NR	WOMEN'S HEALTH	NR

HEALTHGRADES AWARDS

*This hospital reports its data to the federal government jointly with another hospital. Therefore the ratings and awards apply to multiple hospitals and this specific hospital may not provide all rated services.

Longmont United Hospital

1950 Mountain View Avenue
Longmont, CO 80501
(303) 651-5111

Overall patient safety: ★★★
Teaching: N

CLINICAL PROGRAM RATINGS:

CARDIAC	★★★	ORTHOPEDICS	★★★
CRITICAL CARE	★★★	PULMONARY	★★★
GASTROINTESTINAL	★★★	STROKE	★★★
GENERAL SURGERY	NR	VASCULAR	NR
MATERNITY CARE	NR	WOMEN'S HEALTH	NR

HEALTHGRADES AWARDS

Memorial Hospital

1400 East Boulder Street
Colorado Springs, CO 80909
(719) 365-5000

Overall patient safety: ★★★
Teaching: N

CLINICAL PROGRAM RATINGS:

CARDIAC	★★★★★	ORTHOPEDICS	★★★
CRITICAL CARE	★★★	PULMONARY	★★★
GASTROINTESTINAL	★★★	STROKE	★★★
GENERAL SURGERY	NR	VASCULAR	★★★
MATERNITY CARE	NR	WOMEN'S HEALTH	NR

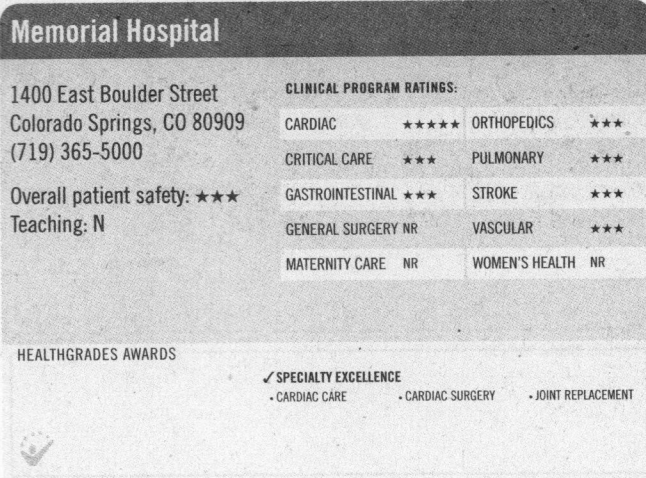

HEALTHGRADES AWARDS

✓ SPECIALTY EXCELLENCE
- CARDIAC CARE
- CARDIAC SURGERY
- JOINT REPLACEMENT

McKee Medical Center

2000 North Boise Avenue
Loveland, CO 80538
(970) 669-4640

Overall patient safety: ★★★
Teaching: N

CLINICAL PROGRAM RATINGS:

CARDIAC	NR	ORTHOPEDICS	★★★★★
CRITICAL CARE	NR	PULMONARY	★★★
GASTROINTESTINAL	★★★	STROKE	★★★
GENERAL SURGERY	NR	VASCULAR	NR
MATERNITY CARE	NR	WOMEN'S HEALTH	NR

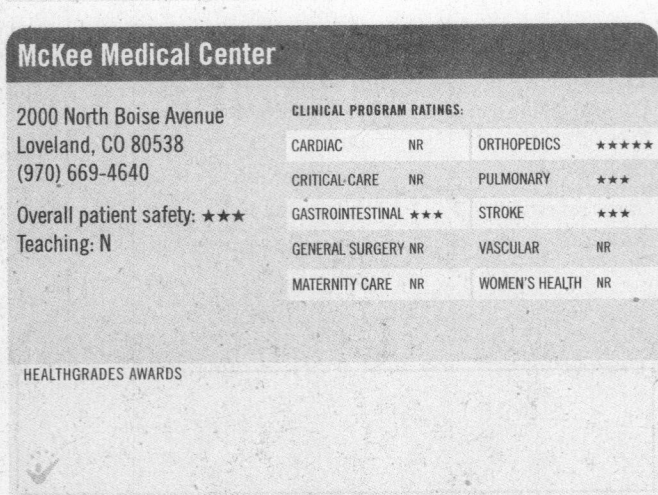

HEALTHGRADES AWARDS

Memorial Hospital

785 Russell Street
Craig, CO 81625
(970) 824-9411

Overall patient safety: ★★★
Teaching: N

CLINICAL PROGRAM RATINGS:

CARDIAC	NR	ORTHOPEDICS	NR
CRITICAL CARE	NR	PULMONARY	★★★
GASTROINTESTINAL	NR	STROKE	NR
GENERAL SURGERY	NR	VASCULAR	NR
MATERNITY CARE	NR	WOMEN'S HEALTH	NR

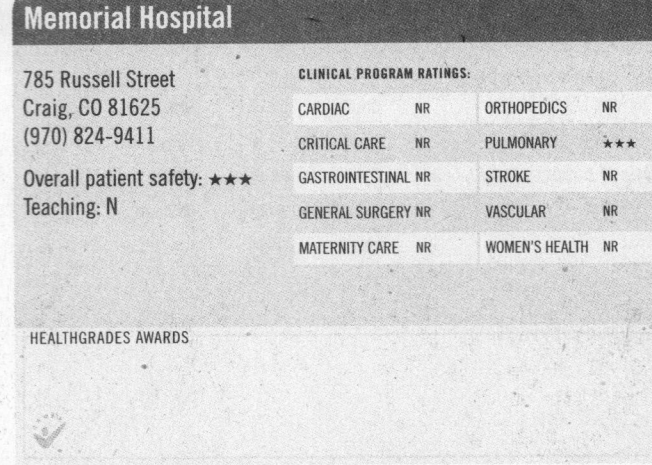

HEALTHGRADES AWARDS

Medical Center of Aurora

1501 South Potomac Street
Aurora, CO 80012
(303) 695-2600

Overall patient safety: ★★★
Teaching: Y

CLINICAL PROGRAM RATINGS:

CARDIAC	★★★	ORTHOPEDICS	★
CRITICAL CARE	★★★★★	PULMONARY	★★★★★
GASTROINTESTINAL	★★★	STROKE	★★★
GENERAL SURGERY	NR	VASCULAR	NR
MATERNITY CARE	NR	WOMEN'S HEALTH	NR

HEALTHGRADES AWARDS

✓ DISTINGUISHED HOSPITAL
- CLINICAL EXCELLENCE

✓ SPECIALTY EXCELLENCE
- CRITICAL CARE

Mercy Regional Medical Center

375 East Parks Avenue
Durango, CO 81301
(970) 247-4311

Overall patient safety: ★★★
Teaching: N

CLINICAL PROGRAM RATINGS:

CARDIAC	NR	ORTHOPEDICS	★★★
CRITICAL CARE	NR	PULMONARY	★★★
GASTROINTESTINAL	NR	STROKE	★★★
GENERAL SURGERY	NR	VASCULAR	NR
MATERNITY CARE	NR	WOMEN'S HEALTH	NR

HEALTHGRADES AWARDS

KEY: ★★★★★ BEST   ★★★ AS EXPECTED   ★ POOR   NR NOT RATED BY HEALTHGRADES   For full definitions of ratings and awards, see Appendix.

Montrose Memorial Hospital

800 South 3rd Street
Montrose, CO 81401
(970) 249-2211

Overall patient safety: ★★★
Teaching: N

CLINICAL PROGRAM RATINGS:

CARDIAC	NR	ORTHOPEDICS	NR
CRITICAL CARE	NR	PULMONARY	★★★
GASTROINTESTINAL	NR	STROKE	★★★
GENERAL SURGERY	NR	VASCULAR	NR
MATERNITY CARE	NR	WOMEN'S HEALTH	NR

HEALTHGRADES AWARDS

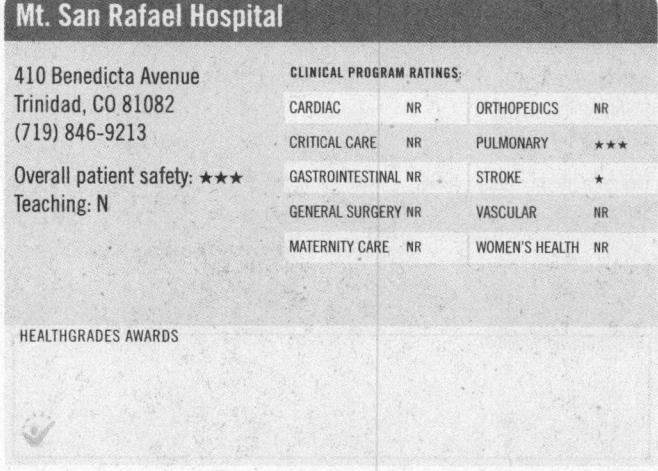

North Suburban Medical Center

9191 Grant Street
Thornton, CO 80229
(303) 451-7800

Overall patient safety: ★★★
Teaching: Y

CLINICAL PROGRAM RATINGS:

CARDIAC	NR	ORTHOPEDICS	★★★
CRITICAL CARE	NR	PULMONARY	★★★
GASTROINTESTINAL	NR	STROKE	★★★
GENERAL SURGERY	NR	VASCULAR	NR
MATERNITY CARE	NR	WOMEN'S HEALTH	NR

HEALTHGRADES AWARDS

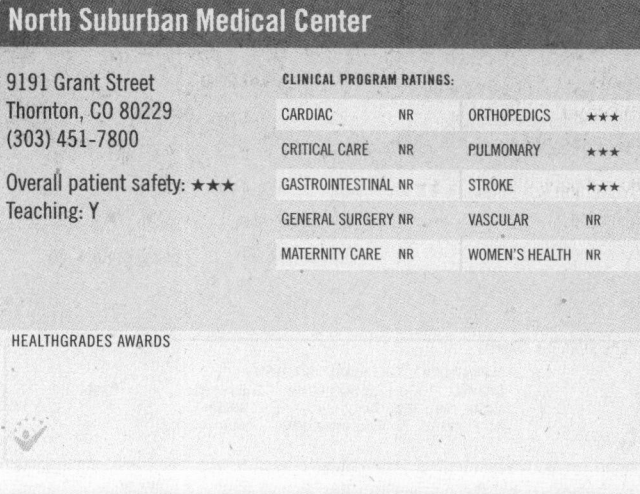

Mt. San Rafael Hospital

410 Benedicta Avenue
Trinidad, CO 81082
(719) 846-9213

Overall patient safety: ★★★
Teaching: N

CLINICAL PROGRAM RATINGS:

CARDIAC	NR	ORTHOPEDICS	NR
CRITICAL CARE	NR	PULMONARY	★★★
GASTROINTESTINAL	NR	STROKE	★
GENERAL SURGERY	NR	VASCULAR	NR
MATERNITY CARE	NR	WOMEN'S HEALTH	NR

HEALTHGRADES AWARDS

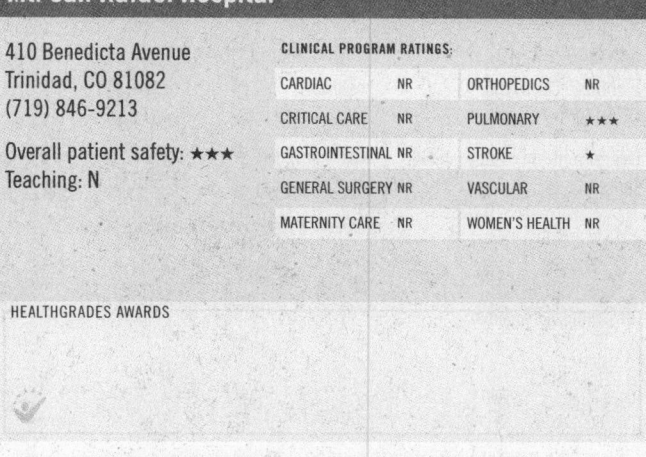

Parkview Medical Center

400 West 16th Street
Pueblo, CO 81003
(719) 584-4000

Overall patient safety: ★
Teaching: N

CLINICAL PROGRAM RATINGS:

CARDIAC	★★★	ORTHOPEDICS	★★★
CRITICAL CARE	★★★	PULMONARY	★★★
GASTROINTESTINAL	★★★	STROKE	★★★
GENERAL SURGERY	NR	VASCULAR	NR
MATERNITY CARE	NR	WOMEN'S HEALTH	NR

HEALTHGRADES AWARDS

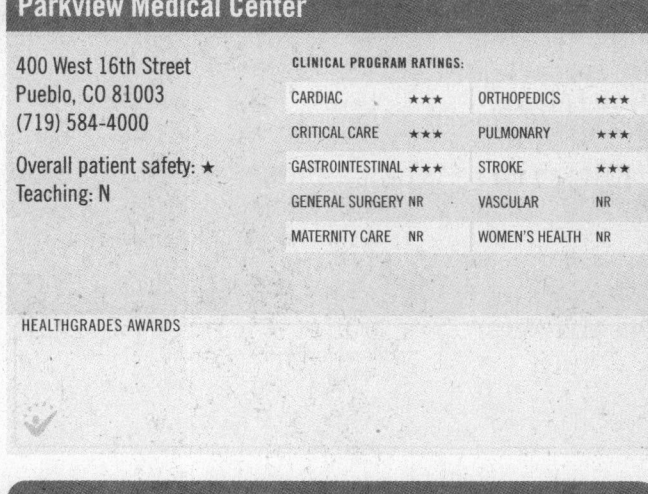

North Colorado Medical Center

1801 16th Street
Greeley, CO 80631
(970) 352-4121

Overall patient safety: ★★★
Teaching: Y

CLINICAL PROGRAM RATINGS:

CARDIAC	★★★	ORTHOPEDICS	★★★
CRITICAL CARE	★★★	PULMONARY	★★★
GASTROINTESTINAL	★★★	STROKE	★★★
GENERAL SURGERY	NR	VASCULAR	NR
MATERNITY CARE	NR	WOMEN'S HEALTH	NR

HEALTHGRADES AWARDS

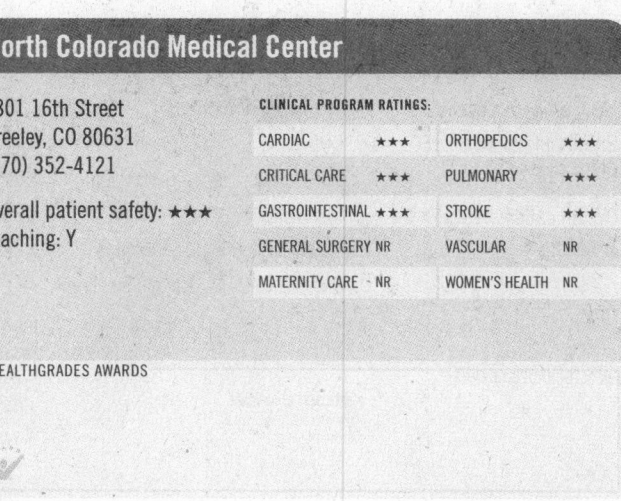

Platte Valley Medical Center

1600 Prairie Center Parkway
Brighton, CO 80601
(303) 498-1600

Overall patient safety: ★★★
Teaching: N

CLINICAL PROGRAM RATINGS:

CARDIAC	NR	ORTHOPEDICS	NR
CRITICAL CARE	NR	PULMONARY	★★★
GASTROINTESTINAL	NR	STROKE	NR
GENERAL SURGERY	NR	VASCULAR	NR
MATERNITY CARE	NR	WOMEN'S HEALTH	NR

HEALTHGRADES AWARDS

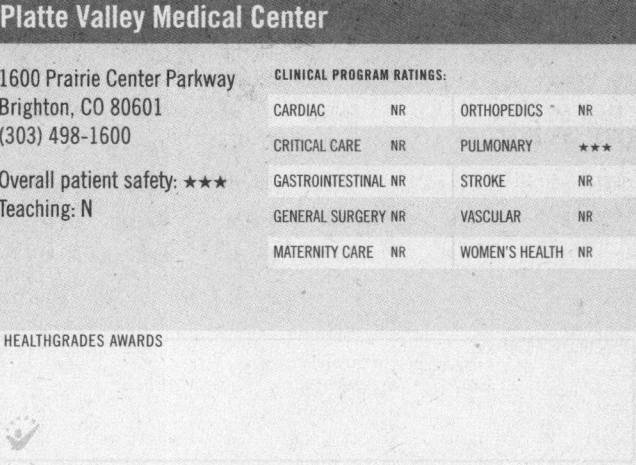

COLORADO HOSPITALS: RATINGS BY CLINICAL SPECIALTY

Poudre Valley Hospital

1024 South Lemay Avenue
Fort Collins, CO 80524
(970) 495-7000

Overall patient safety: ★★★★★
Teaching: Y

CLINICAL PROGRAM RATINGS:

CARDIAC	★★★	ORTHOPEDICS	★★★★★
CRITICAL CARE	★★★	PULMONARY	★★★★★
GASTROINTESTINAL	★★★	STROKE	★★★★★
GENERAL SURGERY	NR	VASCULAR	★★★
MATERNITY CARE	NR	WOMEN'S HEALTH	NR

HEALTHGRADES AWARDS

✓ DISTINGUISHED HOSPITAL
- CLINICAL EXCELLENCE
- PATIENT SAFETY

✓ SPECIALTY EXCELLENCE
- GASTROINTESTINAL CARE
- JOINT REPLACEMENT
- ORTHOPEDIC SURGERY
- PULMONARY CARE
- STROKE CARE

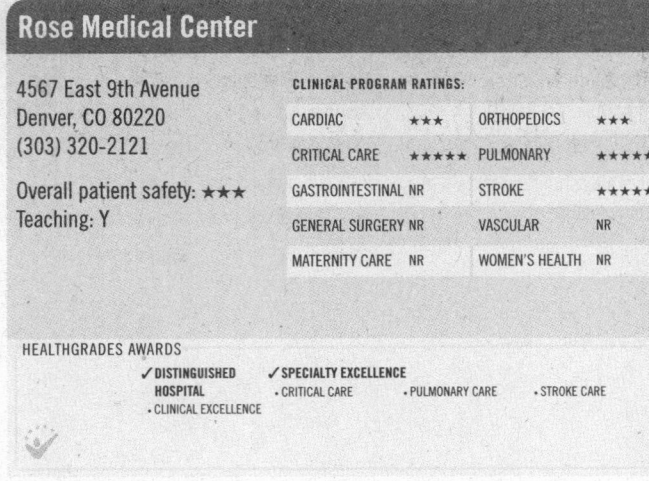

Rose Medical Center

4567 East 9th Avenue
Denver, CO 80220
(303) 320-2121

Overall patient safety: ★★★
Teaching: Y

CLINICAL PROGRAM RATINGS:

CARDIAC	★★★	ORTHOPEDICS	★★★
CRITICAL CARE	★★★★★	PULMONARY	★★★★★
GASTROINTESTINAL	NR	STROKE	★★★★★
GENERAL SURGERY	NR	VASCULAR	NR
MATERNITY CARE	NR	WOMEN'S HEALTH	NR

HEALTHGRADES AWARDS

✓ DISTINGUISHED HOSPITAL
- CLINICAL EXCELLENCE

✓ SPECIALTY EXCELLENCE
- CRITICAL CARE
- PULMONARY CARE
- STROKE CARE

Presbyterian/St. Luke's Medical Center

1719 East 19th Avenue
Denver, CO 80218
(303) 839-6100

Overall patient safety: ★★★
Teaching: Y

CLINICAL PROGRAM RATINGS:

CARDIAC	★★★	ORTHOPEDICS	★★★
CRITICAL CARE	★★★	PULMONARY	★★★
GASTROINTESTINAL	NR	STROKE	★★★★★
GENERAL SURGERY	NR	VASCULAR	★★★
MATERNITY CARE	NR	WOMEN'S HEALTH	NR

HEALTHGRADES AWARDS

✓ SPECIALTY EXCELLENCE
- STROKE CARE

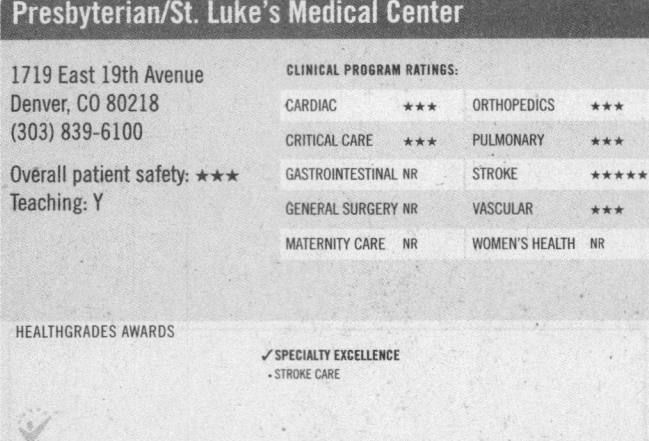

St. Joseph Hospital*

600 West 3rd Street
Florence, CO 81226
(719) 784-4891

Overall patient safety: ★★★
Teaching: N

CLINICAL PROGRAM RATINGS:

CARDIAC	NR	ORTHOPEDICS	NR
CRITICAL CARE	NR	PULMONARY	★★★
GASTROINTESTINAL	NR	STROKE	★★★
GENERAL SURGERY	NR	VASCULAR	NR
MATERNITY CARE	NR	WOMEN'S HEALTH	NR

HEALTHGRADES AWARDS

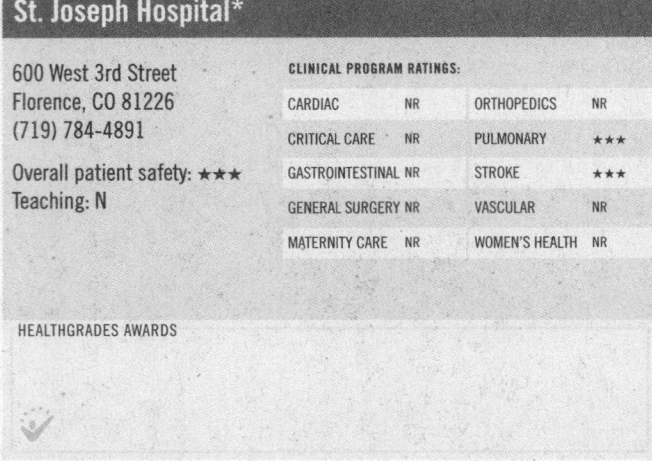

Prowers Medical Center

401 Kendall Drive
Lamar, CO 81052
(719) 336-4343

Overall patient safety: ★★★
Teaching: N

CLINICAL PROGRAM RATINGS:

CARDIAC	NR	ORTHOPEDICS	NR
CRITICAL CARE	NR	PULMONARY	★★★
GASTROINTESTINAL	NR	STROKE	★★★
GENERAL SURGERY	NR	VASCULAR	NR
MATERNITY CARE	NR	WOMEN'S HEALTH	NR

HEALTHGRADES AWARDS

St. Mary's Hospital and Medical Center

2635 North 7th Street
Grand Junction, CO 81501
(970) 244-2273

Overall patient safety: ★★★
Teaching: Y

CLINICAL PROGRAM RATINGS:

CARDIAC	★★★	ORTHOPEDICS	★★★★★
CRITICAL CARE	NR	PULMONARY	★★★
GASTROINTESTINAL	★★★	STROKE	★
GENERAL SURGERY	NR	VASCULAR	★★★
MATERNITY CARE	NR	WOMEN'S HEALTH	NR

HEALTHGRADES AWARDS

✓ SPECIALTY EXCELLENCE
- ORTHOPEDIC SURGERY

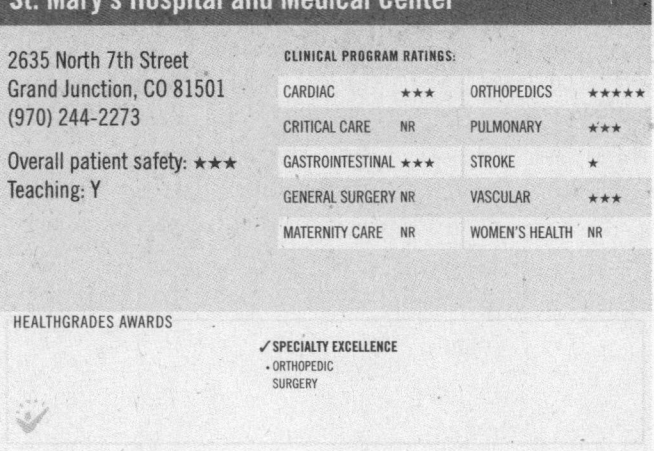

KEY: ★★★★★ BEST   ★★★ AS EXPECTED   ★ POOR   NR NOT RATED BY HEALTHGRADES   For full definitions of ratings and awards, see Appendix.

San Luis Valley Regional Medical Center

106 Blanca Avenue
Alamosa, CO 81101
(719) 589-2511

Overall patient safety: ★★★
Teaching: N

CLINICAL PROGRAM RATINGS:

CARDIAC	NR	ORTHOPEDICS	NR
CRITICAL CARE	NR	PULMONARY	★★★
GASTROINTESTINAL	NR	STROKE	★★★
GENERAL SURGERY	NR	VASCULAR	NR
MATERNITY CARE	NR	WOMEN'S HEALTH	NR

HEALTHGRADES AWARDS

Spanish Peaks Regional Health Center

23500 US Highway 160
Walsenburg, CO 81089
(719) 738-5000

Overall patient safety: ★★★
Teaching: N

CLINICAL PROGRAM RATINGS:

CARDIAC	NR	ORTHOPEDICS	NR
CRITICAL CARE	NR	PULMONARY	★★★
GASTROINTESTINAL	NR	STROKE	NR
GENERAL SURGERY	NR	VASCULAR	NR
MATERNITY CARE	NR	WOMEN'S HEALTH	NR

HEALTHGRADES AWARDS

Sky Ridge Medical Center

10101 Ridge Gate Parkway
Lone Tree, CO 80124
(720) 225-1000

Overall patient safety: ★★★
Teaching: N

CLINICAL PROGRAM RATINGS:

CARDIAC	NR	ORTHOPEDICS	★★★
CRITICAL CARE	NR	PULMONARY	★★★
GASTROINTESTINAL	★★★	STROKE	★★★
GENERAL SURGERY	NR	VASCULAR	NR
MATERNITY CARE	NR	WOMEN'S HEALTH	NR

HEALTHGRADES AWARDS

Sterling Regional Medical Center

615 Fairhurst Street
Sterling, CO 80751
(970) 521-3100

Overall patient safety: ★★★
Teaching: N

CLINICAL PROGRAM RATINGS:

CARDIAC	NR	ORTHOPEDICS	NR
CRITICAL CARE	NR	PULMONARY	★★★
GASTROINTESTINAL	NR	STROKE	★★★
GENERAL SURGERY	NR	VASCULAR	NR
MATERNITY CARE	NR	WOMEN'S HEALTH	NR

HEALTHGRADES AWARDS

Southwest Memorial Hospital

1311 North Mildred Road
Cortez, CO 81321
(970) 565-6666

Overall patient safety: ★★★
Teaching: Y

CLINICAL PROGRAM RATINGS:

CARDIAC	NR	ORTHOPEDICS	NR
CRITICAL CARE	NR	PULMONARY	★★★
GASTROINTESTINAL	NR	STROKE	★★★
GENERAL SURGERY	NR	VASCULAR	NR
MATERNITY CARE	NR	WOMEN'S HEALTH	NR

HEALTHGRADES AWARDS

Swedish Medical Center

501 East Hampden Avenue
Englewood, CO 80110
(303) 788-5000

Overall patient safety: ★★★
Teaching: Y

CLINICAL PROGRAM RATINGS:

CARDIAC	★★★	ORTHOPEDICS	★★★
CRITICAL CARE	★★★	PULMONARY	★★★
GASTROINTESTINAL	★★★	STROKE	★★★
GENERAL SURGERY	NR	VASCULAR	NR
MATERNITY CARE	NR	WOMEN'S HEALTH	NR

HEALTHGRADES AWARDS

*This hospital reports its data to the federal government jointly with another hospital. Therefore the ratings and awards apply to multiple hospitals and this specific hospital may not provide all rated services.

University of Colorado Hospital Authority

12605 East 16th Avenue
Aurora, CO 80045
(303) 372-0000

Overall patient safety: ★★★
Teaching: Y

CLINICAL PROGRAM RATINGS:

CARDIAC	★★★	ORTHOPEDICS	★★★
CRITICAL CARE	★★★	PULMONARY	★★★
GASTROINTESTINAL	NR	STROKE	★★★★★
GENERAL SURGERY	NR	VASCULAR	NR
MATERNITY CARE	NR	WOMEN'S HEALTH	NR

HEALTHGRADES AWARDS

✓ SPECIALTY EXCELLENCE
• STROKE CARE

Valley View Hospital Association

1906 Blake Avenue
Glenwood Springs, CO 81601
(970) 945-6535

Overall patient safety: ★★★
Teaching: N

CLINICAL PROGRAM RATINGS:

CARDIAC	NR	ORTHOPEDICS	NR
CRITICAL CARE	NR	PULMONARY	★★★
GASTROINTESTINAL	NR	STROKE	★★★
GENERAL SURGERY	NR	VASCULAR	NR
MATERNITY CARE	NR	WOMEN'S HEALTH	NR

HEALTHGRADES AWARDS

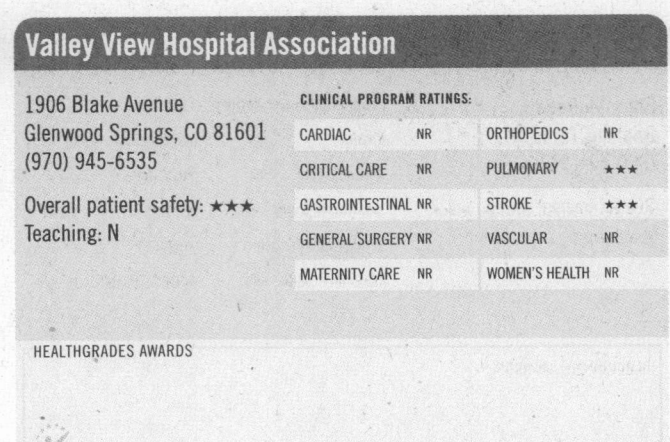

Vail Valley Medical Center

181 West Meadow Drive
Suite 100
Vail, CO 81657
(970) 476-2451

Overall patient safety: ★★★
Teaching: N

CLINICAL PROGRAM RATINGS:

CARDIAC	NR	ORTHOPEDICS	NR
CRITICAL CARE	NR	PULMONARY	NR
GASTROINTESTINAL	NR	STROKE	NR
GENERAL SURGERY	NR	VASCULAR	NR
MATERNITY CARE	NR	WOMEN'S HEALTH	NR

HEALTHGRADES AWARDS

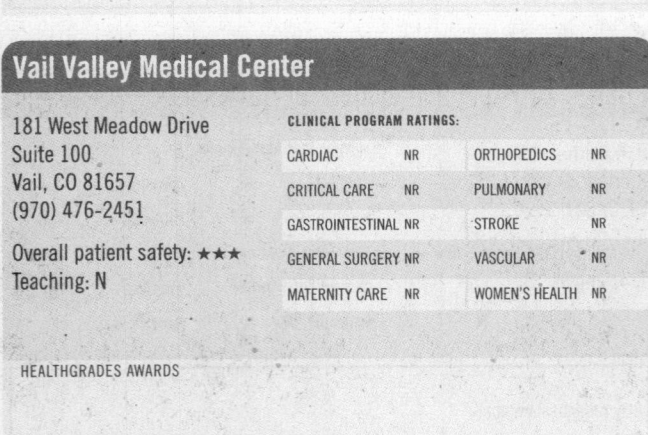

Yampa Valley Medical Center

1024 Central Parks Drive
Steamboat Springs, CO 80487
(970) 879-1322

Overall patient safety: ★★★
Teaching: N

CLINICAL PROGRAM RATINGS:

CARDIAC	NR	ORTHOPEDICS	NR
CRITICAL CARE	NR	PULMONARY	★★★
GASTROINTESTINAL	NR	STROKE	NR
GENERAL SURGERY	NR	VASCULAR	NR
MATERNITY CARE	NR	WOMEN'S HEALTH	NR

HEALTHGRADES AWARDS

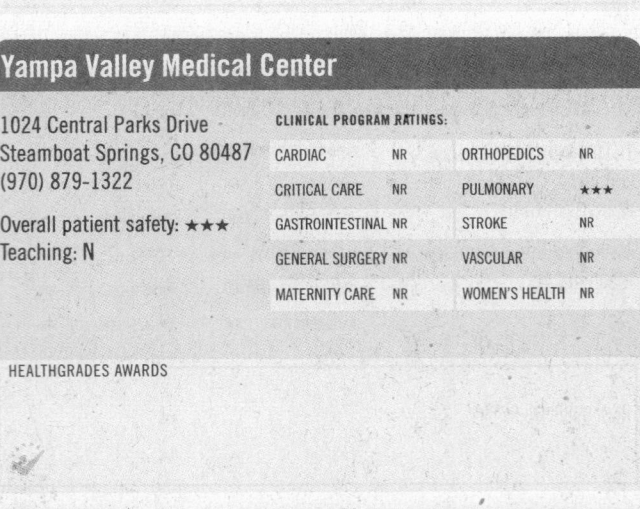

CONNECTICUT HOSPITALS: RATINGS BY CLINICAL SPECIALTY

Bradley Memorial Hospital and Health Center

81 Meriden Avenue
Southington, CT 06489
(860) 276-5000

Overall patient safety: ★★★
Teaching: N

CLINICAL PROGRAM RATINGS:

CARDIAC	NR	ORTHOPEDICS	NR
CRITICAL CARE	NR	PULMONARY	★
GASTROINTESTINAL	NR	STROKE	★★★
GENERAL SURGERY	NR	VASCULAR	NR
MATERNITY CARE	NR	WOMEN'S HEALTH	NR

HEALTHGRADES AWARDS

Bridgeport Hospital*

267 Grant Street
Bridgeport, CT 06610
(203) 384-3000

Overall patient safety: ★★★
Teaching: Y

CLINICAL PROGRAM RATINGS:

CARDIAC	★★★	ORTHOPEDICS	★★★
CRITICAL CARE	★★★	PULMONARY	★★★
GASTROINTESTINAL	★★★	STROKE	★★★
GENERAL SURGERY	NR	VASCULAR	NR
MATERNITY CARE	NR	WOMEN'S HEALTH	NR

HEALTHGRADES AWARDS

KEY: ★★★★★ BEST ★★★ AS EXPECTED ★ POOR NR NOT RATED BY HEALTHGRADES For full definitions of ratings and awards, see Appendix.

Bristol Hospital

Brewster Road
Bristol, CT 06010
(860) 585-3000

Overall patient safety: ★★★
Teaching: N

CLINICAL PROGRAM RATINGS:

CARDIAC	NR	ORTHOPEDICS	NR
CRITICAL CARE	NR	PULMONARY	★
GASTROINTESTINAL	★★★	STROKE	★★★
GENERAL SURGERY	NR	VASCULAR	NR
MATERNITY CARE	NR	WOMEN'S HEALTH	NR

HEALTHGRADES AWARDS

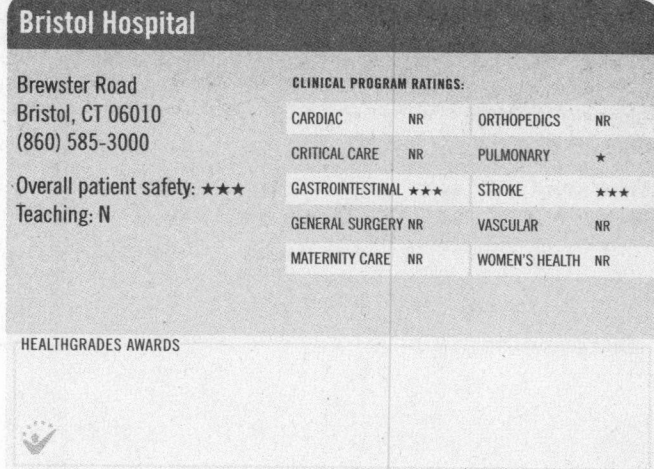

Day Kimball Hospital

320 Pomfret Street
Putnam, CT 06260
(860) 928-6541

Overall patient safety: ★★★
Teaching: N

CLINICAL PROGRAM RATINGS:

CARDIAC	NR	ORTHOPEDICS	NR
CRITICAL CARE	NR	PULMONARY	★
GASTROINTESTINAL	★★★	STROKE	★
GENERAL SURGERY	NR	VASCULAR	NR
MATERNITY CARE	NR	WOMEN'S HEALTH	NR

HEALTHGRADES AWARDS

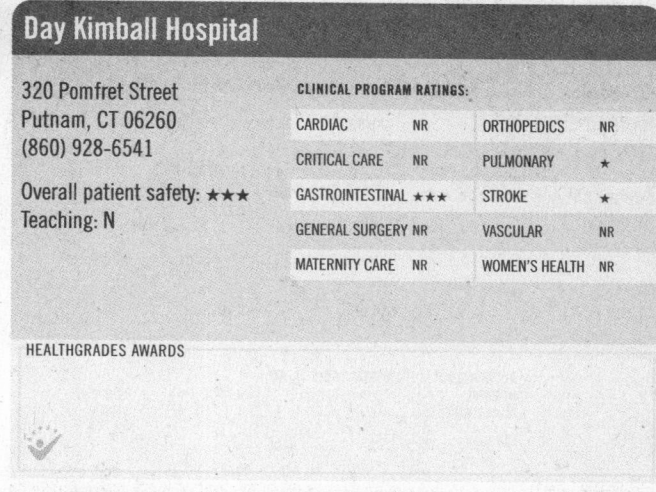

Charlotte Hungerford Hospital

540 Litchfield
Torrington, CT 06790
(860) 496-6666

Overall patient safety: ★★★
Teaching: N

CLINICAL PROGRAM RATINGS:

CARDIAC	NR	ORTHOPEDICS	★★★
CRITICAL CARE	★★★	PULMONARY	★★★
GASTROINTESTINAL	★★★	STROKE	★
GENERAL SURGERY	NR	VASCULAR	NR
MATERNITY CARE	NR	WOMEN'S HEALTH	NR

HEALTHGRADES AWARDS

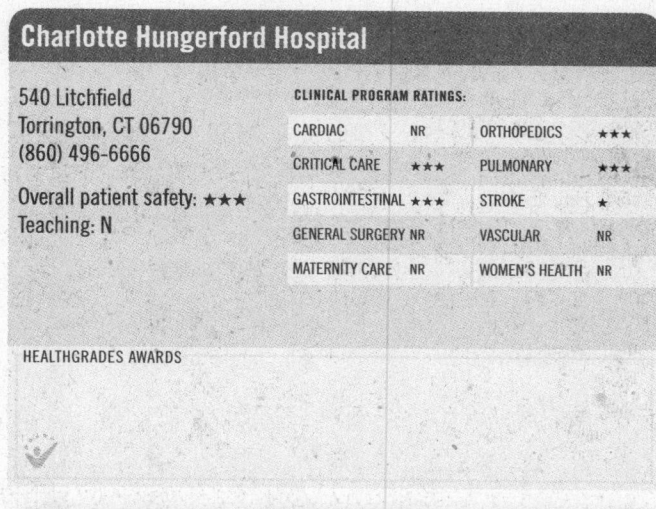

Greenwich Hospital Association

5 Perryridge Road
Greenwich, CT 06830
(203) 863-3000

Overall patient safety: ★★★
Teaching: Y

CLINICAL PROGRAM RATINGS:

CARDIAC	NR	ORTHOPEDICS	★★★
CRITICAL CARE	★★★	PULMONARY	★★★
GASTROINTESTINAL	★★★	STROKE	★★★
GENERAL SURGERY	NR	VASCULAR	NR
MATERNITY CARE	NR	WOMEN'S HEALTH	NR

HEALTHGRADES AWARDS

Danbury Hospital

24 Hospital Avenue
Danbury, CT 06810
(203) 797-7000

Overall patient safety: ★★★★★
Teaching: Y

CLINICAL PROGRAM RATINGS:

CARDIAC	★★★★★	ORTHOPEDICS	★★★
CRITICAL CARE	★★★	PULMONARY	★★★★★
GASTROINTESTINAL	★★★	STROKE	★★★★★
GENERAL SURGERY	NR	VASCULAR	★★★
MATERNITY CARE	NR	WOMEN'S HEALTH	NR

HEALTHGRADES AWARDS

✓ **DISTINGUISHED HOSPITAL**
- CLINICAL EXCELLENCE
- PATIENT SAFETY

✓ **SPECIALTY EXCELLENCE**
- CARDIAC CARE
- CARDIAC SURGERY
- GASTROINTESTINAL CARE
- PULMONARY CARE
- STROKE CARE

Griffin Hospital

130 Division Street
Derby, CT 06418
(203) 735-7421

Overall patient safety: ★★★
Teaching: Y

CLINICAL PROGRAM RATINGS:

CARDIAC	NR	ORTHOPEDICS	★★★
CRITICAL CARE	NR	PULMONARY	★★★★★
GASTROINTESTINAL	★★★	STROKE	★★★
GENERAL SURGERY	NR	VASCULAR	NR
MATERNITY CARE	NR	WOMEN'S HEALTH	NR

HEALTHGRADES AWARDS

✓ **SPECIALTY EXCELLENCE**
- PULMONARY CARE

*This hospital reports its data to the federal government jointly with another hospital. Therefore the ratings and awards apply to multiple hospitals and this specific hospital may not provide all rated services.

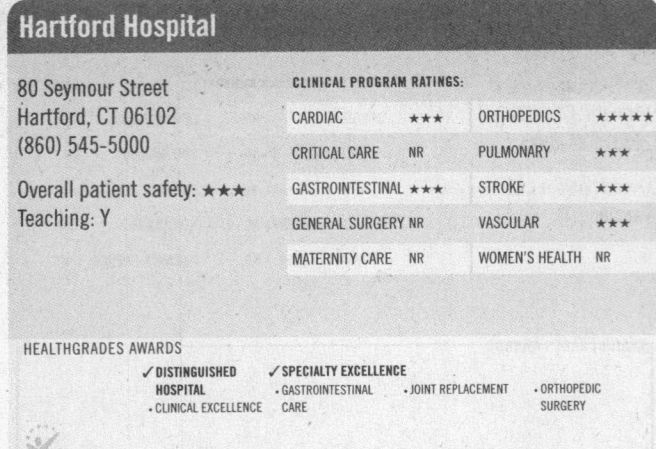

Hartford Hospital

80 Seymour Street
Hartford, CT 06102
(860) 545-5000

Overall patient safety: ★★★
Teaching: Y

CLINICAL PROGRAM RATINGS:

CARDIAC	★★★	ORTHOPEDICS	★★★★★
CRITICAL CARE	NR	PULMONARY	★★★
GASTROINTESTINAL	★★★	STROKE	★★★
GENERAL SURGERY	NR	VASCULAR	★★★
MATERNITY CARE	NR	WOMEN'S HEALTH	NR

HEALTHGRADES AWARDS

✓ DISTINGUISHED HOSPITAL
· CLINICAL EXCELLENCE

✓ SPECIALTY EXCELLENCE
· GASTROINTESTINAL CARE
· JOINT REPLACEMENT
· ORTHOPEDIC SURGERY

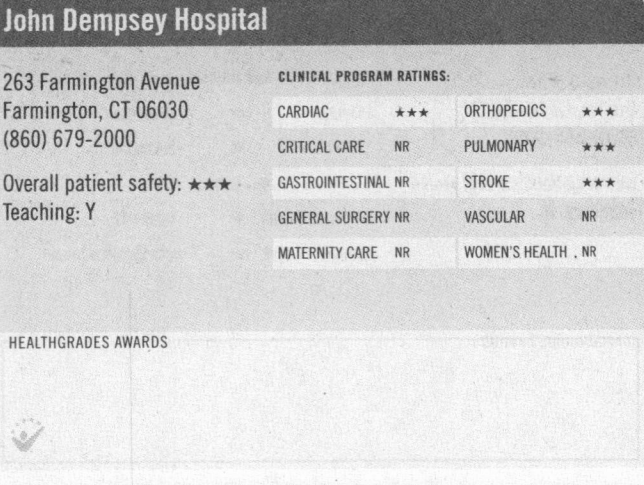

John Dempsey Hospital

263 Farmington Avenue
Farmington, CT 06030
(860) 679-2000

Overall patient safety: ★★★
Teaching: Y

CLINICAL PROGRAM RATINGS:

CARDIAC	★★★	ORTHOPEDICS	★★★
CRITICAL CARE	NR	PULMONARY	★★★
GASTROINTESTINAL	NR	STROKE	★★★
GENERAL SURGERY	NR	VASCULAR	NR
MATERNITY CARE	NR	WOMEN'S HEALTH	NR

HEALTHGRADES AWARDS

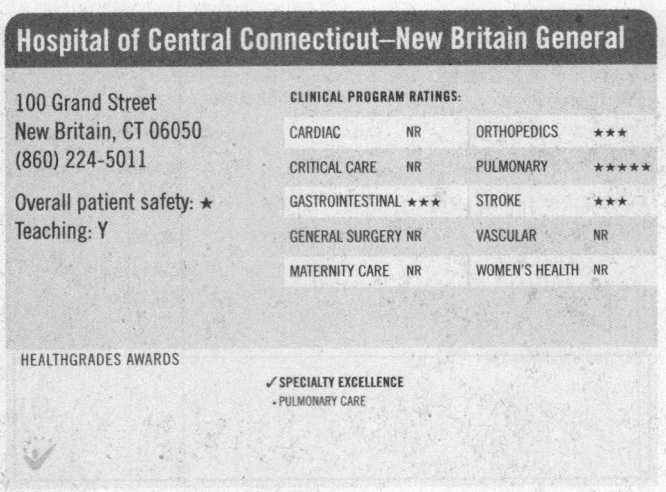

Hospital of Central Connecticut—New Britain General

100 Grand Street
New Britain, CT 06050
(860) 224-5011

Overall patient safety: ★
Teaching: Y

CLINICAL PROGRAM RATINGS:

CARDIAC	NR	ORTHOPEDICS	★★★
CRITICAL CARE	NR	PULMONARY	★★★★★
GASTROINTESTINAL	★★★	STROKE	★★★
GENERAL SURGERY	NR	VASCULAR	NR
MATERNITY CARE	NR	WOMEN'S HEALTH	NR

HEALTHGRADES AWARDS

✓ SPECIALTY EXCELLENCE
· PULMONARY CARE

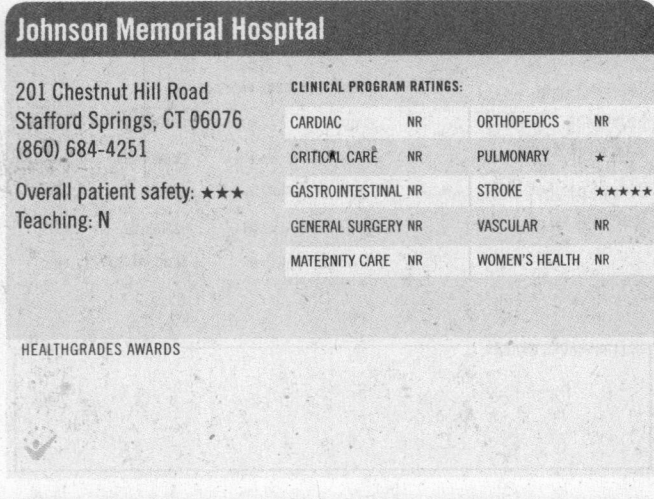

Johnson Memorial Hospital

201 Chestnut Hill Road
Stafford Springs, CT 06076
(860) 684-4251

Overall patient safety: ★★★
Teaching: N

CLINICAL PROGRAM RATINGS:

CARDIAC	NR	ORTHOPEDICS	NR
CRITICAL CARE	NR	PULMONARY	★
GASTROINTESTINAL	NR	STROKE	★★★★★
GENERAL SURGERY	NR	VASCULAR	NR
MATERNITY CARE	NR	WOMEN'S HEALTH	NR

HEALTHGRADES AWARDS

Hospital of St. Raphael

1450 Chapel Street
New Haven, CT 06511
(203) 789-3000

Overall patient safety: ★★★★★
Teaching: Y

CLINICAL PROGRAM RATINGS:

CARDIAC	★★★★★	ORTHOPEDICS	★★★
CRITICAL CARE	★★★	PULMONARY	★★★
GASTROINTESTINAL	★★★	STROKE	★★★
GENERAL SURGERY	NR	VASCULAR	★★★
MATERNITY CARE	NR	WOMEN'S HEALTH	NR

HEALTHGRADES AWARDS

✓ DISTINGUISHED HOSPITAL
· PATIENT SAFETY

✓ SPECIALTY EXCELLENCE
· CARDIAC CARE

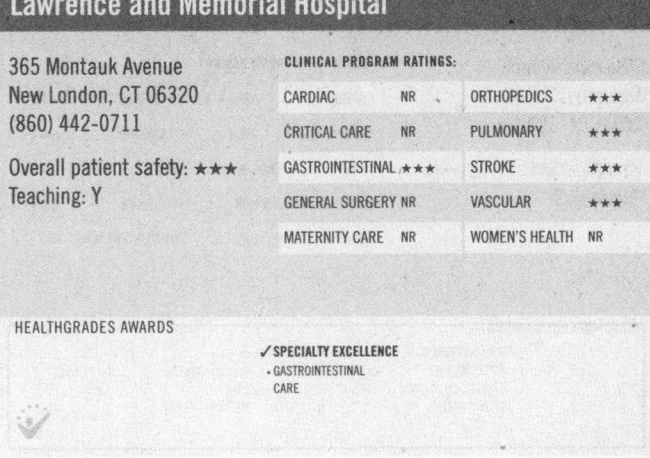

Lawrence and Memorial Hospital

365 Montauk Avenue
New London, CT 06320
(860) 442-0711

Overall patient safety: ★★★
Teaching: Y

CLINICAL PROGRAM RATINGS:

CARDIAC	NR	ORTHOPEDICS	★★★
CRITICAL CARE	NR	PULMONARY	★★★
GASTROINTESTINAL	★★★	STROKE	★★★
GENERAL SURGERY	NR	VASCULAR	★★★
MATERNITY CARE	NR	WOMEN'S HEALTH	NR

HEALTHGRADES AWARDS

✓ SPECIALTY EXCELLENCE
· GASTROINTESTINAL CARE

KEY: ★★★★★ BEST   ★★★ AS EXPECTED   ★ POOR   NR NOT RATED BY HEALTHGRADES   For full definitions of ratings and awards, see Appendix.

Manchester Memorial Hospital

71 Haynes Street
Manchester, CT 06040
(860) 646-1222

Overall patient safety: ★★★
Teaching: N

CLINICAL PROGRAM RATINGS:

CARDIAC	NR	ORTHOPEDICS	NR
CRITICAL CARE	NR	PULMONARY	★★★
GASTROINTESTINAL	★★★	STROKE	★★★
GENERAL SURGERY	NR	VASCULAR	NR
MATERNITY CARE	NR	WOMEN'S HEALTH	NR

HEALTHGRADES AWARDS

Milford Hospital

300 Seaside Avenue
Milford, CT 06460
(203) 876-4000

Overall patient safety: ★★★
Teaching: N

CLINICAL PROGRAM RATINGS:

CARDIAC	NR	ORTHOPEDICS	NR
CRITICAL CARE	★	PULMONARY	★★★
GASTROINTESTINAL	★★★	STROKE	★
GENERAL SURGERY	NR	VASCULAR	NR
MATERNITY CARE	NR	WOMEN'S HEALTH	NR

HEALTHGRADES AWARDS

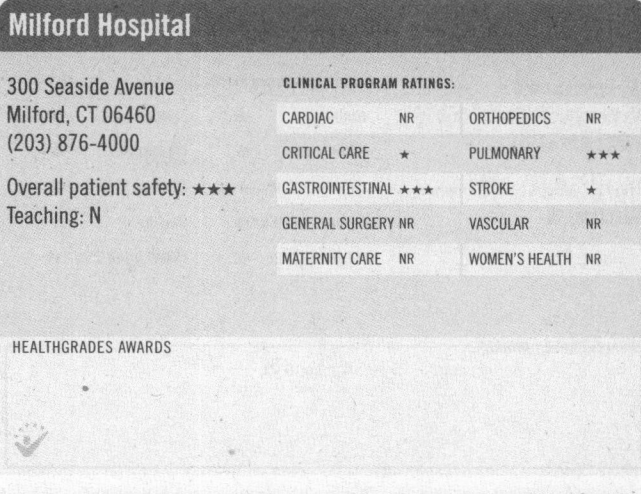

Middlesex Hospital

28 Crescent Street
Middletown, CT 06457
(860) 344-6000

Overall patient safety: ★★★
Teaching: Y

CLINICAL PROGRAM RATINGS:

CARDIAC	NR	ORTHOPEDICS	★★★
CRITICAL CARE	NR	PULMONARY	★★★★★
GASTROINTESTINAL	★★★	STROKE	★★★
GENERAL SURGERY	NR	VASCULAR	★★★
MATERNITY CARE	NR	WOMEN'S HEALTH	NR

HEALTHGRADES AWARDS

✓ DISTINGUISHED HOSPITAL
• CLINICAL EXCELLENCE

✓ SPECIALTY EXCELLENCE
• PULMONARY CARE

New Milford Hospital

21 Elm Street
New Milford, CT 06776
(860) 355-2611

Overall patient safety: ★★★
Teaching: N

CLINICAL PROGRAM RATINGS:

CARDIAC	NR	ORTHOPEDICS	★
CRITICAL CARE	NR	PULMONARY	★★★
GASTROINTESTINAL	NR	STROKE	★
GENERAL SURGERY	NR	VASCULAR	NR
MATERNITY CARE	NR	WOMEN'S HEALTH	NR

HEALTHGRADES AWARDS

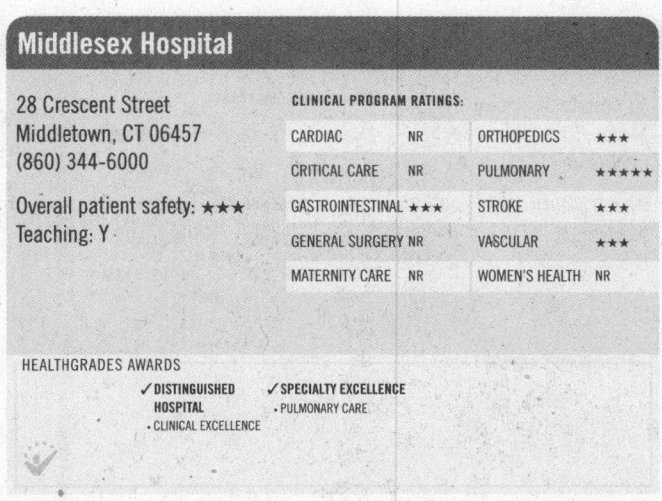

Midstate Medical Center*

435 Lewis Avenue
Meriden, CT 06451
(203) 694-8200

Overall patient safety: ★★★
Teaching: N

CLINICAL PROGRAM RATINGS:

CARDIAC	NR	ORTHOPEDICS	★★★
CRITICAL CARE	★	PULMONARY	★★★
GASTROINTESTINAL	★★★	STROKE	★★★
GENERAL SURGERY	NR	VASCULAR	NR
MATERNITY CARE	NR	WOMEN'S HEALTH	NR

HEALTHGRADES AWARDS

Norwalk Hospital Association

34 Maple Street
Norwalk, CT 06856
(203) 852-2000

Overall patient safety: ★★★
Teaching: Y

CLINICAL PROGRAM RATINGS:

CARDIAC	NR	ORTHOPEDICS	★★★★★
CRITICAL CARE	★	PULMONARY	★★★
GASTROINTESTINAL	★★★	STROKE	★★★★★
GENERAL SURGERY	NR	VASCULAR	NR
MATERNITY CARE	NR	WOMEN'S HEALTH	NR

HEALTHGRADES AWARDS

✓ SPECIALTY EXCELLENCE
• STROKE CARE

*This hospital reports its data to the federal government jointly with another hospital. Therefore the ratings and awards apply to multiple hospitals and this specific hospital may not provide all rated services.

Rockville General Hospital

31 Union Street
Vernon Rockville, CT 06066
(860) 872-0501

Overall patient safety: ★★★
Teaching: N

CLINICAL PROGRAM RATINGS:

CARDIAC	NR	ORTHOPEDICS	NR
CRITICAL CARE	NR	PULMONARY	★★★
GASTROINTESTINAL	★★★	STROKE	★★★
GENERAL SURGERY	NR	VASCULAR	NR
MATERNITY CARE	NR	WOMEN'S HEALTH	NR

HEALTHGRADES AWARDS

St. Vincent's Medical Center

2800 Main Street
Bridgeport, CT 06606
(203) 576-6000

Overall patient safety: ★★★
Teaching: Y

CLINICAL PROGRAM RATINGS:

CARDIAC	★★★	ORTHOPEDICS	★★★
CRITICAL CARE	★★★	PULMONARY	★★★
GASTROINTESTINAL	★★★	STROKE	★★★
GENERAL SURGERY	NR	VASCULAR	★★★
MATERNITY CARE	NR	WOMEN'S HEALTH	NR

HEALTHGRADES AWARDS

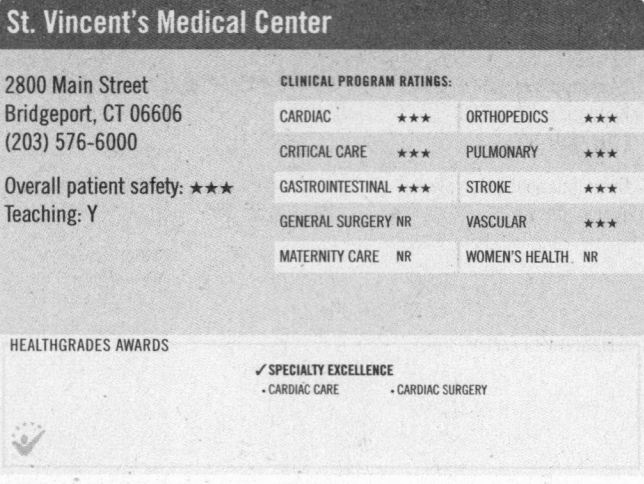

✓ SPECIALTY EXCELLENCE
- CARDIAC CARE   • CARDIAC SURGERY

St. Francis Hospital and Medical Center

114 Woodland Street
Hartford, CT 06105
(860) 714-4000

Overall patient safety: ★★★
Teaching: Y

CLINICAL PROGRAM RATINGS:

CARDIAC	★★★	ORTHOPEDICS	★★★★★
CRITICAL CARE	NR	PULMONARY	★★★
GASTROINTESTINAL	★★★	STROKE	★★★
GENERAL SURGERY	NR	VASCULAR	★★★
MATERNITY CARE	NR	WOMEN'S HEALTH	NR

HEALTHGRADES AWARDS

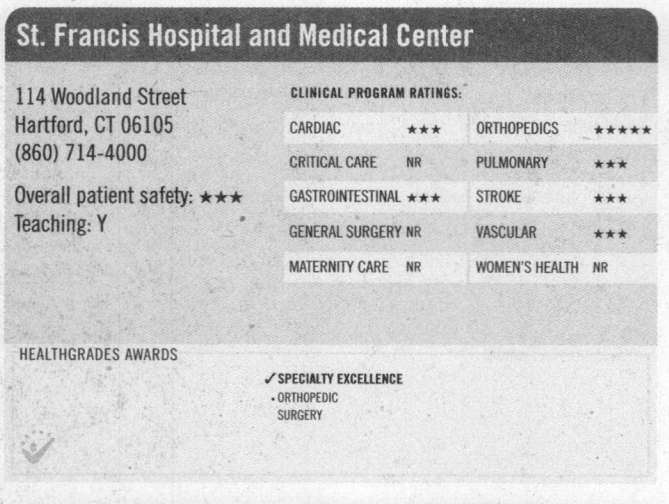

✓ SPECIALTY EXCELLENCE
- ORTHOPEDIC
  SURGERY

Sharon Hospital

50 Hospital Hill Road
Sharon, CT 06069
(860) 364-4141

Overall patient safety: ★★★
Teaching: N

CLINICAL PROGRAM RATINGS:

CARDIAC	NR	ORTHOPEDICS	NR
CRITICAL CARE	NR	PULMONARY	★★★
GASTROINTESTINAL	NR	STROKE	★★★
GENERAL SURGERY	NR	VASCULAR	NR
MATERNITY CARE	NR	WOMEN'S HEALTH	NR

HEALTHGRADES AWARDS

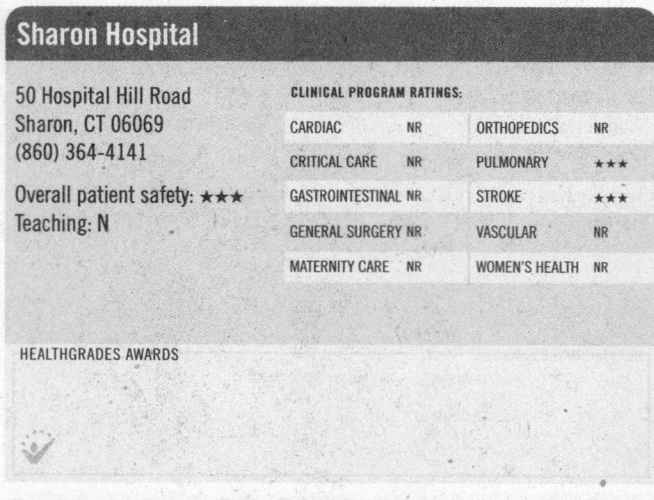

St. Mary's Hospital

56 Franklin Street
Waterbury, CT 06706
(203) 709-6000

Overall patient safety: ★★★
Teaching: Y

CLINICAL PROGRAM RATINGS:

CARDIAC	★★★	ORTHOPEDICS	★★★
CRITICAL CARE	★★★	PULMONARY	★★★
GASTROINTESTINAL	★★★	STROKE	★
GENERAL SURGERY	NR	VASCULAR	NR
MATERNITY CARE	NR	WOMEN'S HEALTH	NR

HEALTHGRADES AWARDS

Stamford Hospital

30 Shelburne Road
Stamford, CT 06902
(203) 276-1000

Overall patient safety: ★★★
Teaching: Y

CLINICAL PROGRAM RATINGS:

CARDIAC	NR	ORTHOPEDICS	★★★
CRITICAL CARE	★★★	PULMONARY	★★★
GASTROINTESTINAL	★★★	STROKE	★★★
GENERAL SURGERY	NR	VASCULAR	NR
MATERNITY CARE	NR	WOMEN'S HEALTH	NR

HEALTHGRADES AWARDS

KEY: ★★★★★ BEST   ★★★ AS EXPECTED   ★ POOR   NR NOT RATED BY HEALTHGRADES   For full definitions of ratings and awards, see Appendix.

Waterbury Hospital Health Center

64 Robbins Street
Waterbury, CT 06708
(203) 573-6000

Overall patient safety: ★★★
Teaching: Y

CLINICAL PROGRAM RATINGS:

CARDIAC	★★★	ORTHOPEDICS	★★★
CRITICAL CARE	★★★	PULMONARY	★★★
GASTROINTESTINAL	★★★	STROKE	★
GENERAL SURGERY	NR	VASCULAR	NR
MATERNITY CARE	NR	WOMEN'S HEALTH	NR

HEALTHGRADES AWARDS

✓ **SPECIALTY EXCELLENCE**
· JOINT REPLACEMENT

World War II Veterans Memorial Hospital*

883 Paddock Avenue
Meriden, CT 06450
(203) 630-5266

Overall patient safety: ★★★
Teaching: N

CLINICAL PROGRAM RATINGS:

CARDIAC	NR	ORTHOPEDICS	★★★
CRITICAL CARE	★	PULMONARY	★★★
GASTROINTESTINAL	★★★	STROKE	★★★
GENERAL SURGERY	NR	VASCULAR	NR
MATERNITY CARE	NR	WOMEN'S HEALTH	NR

HEALTHGRADES AWARDS

William W. Backus Hospital

326 Washington Street
Norwich, CT 06360
(860) 889-8331

Overall patient safety: ★★★
Teaching: N

CLINICAL PROGRAM RATINGS:

CARDIAC	NR	ORTHOPEDICS	★★★
CRITICAL CARE	NR	PULMONARY	★★★
GASTROINTESTINAL	★★★	STROKE	★★★
GENERAL SURGERY	NR	VASCULAR	NR
MATERNITY CARE	NR	WOMEN'S HEALTH	NR

HEALTHGRADES AWARDS

✓ **SPECIALTY EXCELLENCE**
· GASTROINTESTINAL CARE

Yale-New Haven Hospital

20 York Street
New Haven, CT 06510
(203) 688-4242

Overall patient safety: ★★★
Teaching: Y

CLINICAL PROGRAM RATINGS:

CARDIAC	★★★	ORTHOPEDICS	★★★
CRITICAL CARE	★★★	PULMONARY	★★★★★
GASTROINTESTINAL	★★★	STROKE	★★★
GENERAL SURGERY	NR	VASCULAR	★
MATERNITY CARE	NR	WOMEN'S HEALTH	NR

HEALTHGRADES AWARDS

✓ **DISTINGUISHED HOSPITAL**   ✓ **SPECIALTY EXCELLENCE**
· CLINICAL EXCELLENCE   · CARDIAC CARE   · PULMONARY CARE

Windham Community Memorial Hospital and Hatch Hospital

112 Mansfield Avenue
Willimantic, CT 06226
(860) 456-9116

Overall patient safety: ★★★
Teaching: N

CLINICAL PROGRAM RATINGS:

CARDIAC	NR	ORTHOPEDICS	NR
CRITICAL CARE	NR	PULMONARY	★★★
GASTROINTESTINAL	★★★	STROKE	★
GENERAL SURGERY	NR	VASCULAR	NR
MATERNITY CARE	NR	WOMEN'S HEALTH	NR

HEALTHGRADES AWARDS

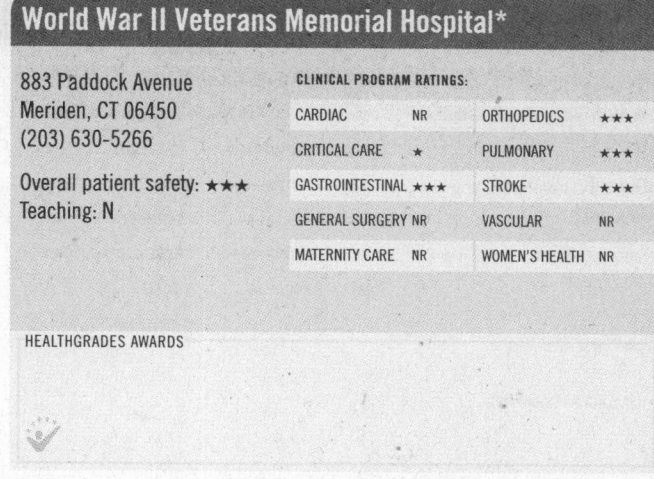

*This hospital reports its data to the federal government jointly with another hospital. Therefore the ratings and awards apply to multiple hospitals and this specific hospital may not provide all rated services.

Bayhealth Medical Center—Kent General Hospital*

640 South State Street
Dover, DE 19901
(302) 674-4700

Overall patient safety: ★★★
Teaching: N

CLINICAL PROGRAM RATINGS:

CARDIAC	★★★	ORTHOPEDICS	★
CRITICAL CARE	NR	PULMONARY	★★★
GASTROINTESTINAL	★★★	STROKE	★★★
GENERAL SURGERY	NR	VASCULAR	NR
MATERNITY CARE	NR	WOMEN'S HEALTH	NR

HEALTHGRADES AWARDS

Christiana Care Health System—Christiana Hospital

4755 Ogletown-Stanton Road
Newark, DE 19718
(302) 733-1000

Overall patient safety: ★★★
Teaching: Y

CLINICAL PROGRAM RATINGS:

CARDIAC	★★★	ORTHOPEDICS	★★★
CRITICAL CARE	NR	PULMONARY	★★★★★
GASTROINTESTINAL	★★★	STROKE	★★★
GENERAL SURGERY	NR	VASCULAR	★★★
MATERNITY CARE	NR	WOMEN'S HEALTH	NR

HEALTHGRADES AWARDS

✓ **DISTINGUISHED HOSPITAL**
- CLINICAL EXCELLENCE

✓ **SPECIALTY EXCELLENCE**
- GASTROINTESTINAL CARE
- PULMONARY CARE

Bayhealth Medical Center—Milford Memorial Campus*

21 West Clarke Avenue
Milford, DE 19963
(302) 422-3311

Overall patient safety: ★★★
Teaching: N

CLINICAL PROGRAM RATINGS:

CARDIAC	★★★	ORTHOPEDICS	★
CRITICAL CARE	NR	PULMONARY	★★★
GASTROINTESTINAL	★★★	STROKE	★★★
GENERAL SURGERY	NR	VASCULAR	NR
MATERNITY CARE	NR	WOMEN'S HEALTH	NR

HEALTHGRADES AWARDS

Nanticoke Memorial Hospital

801 Middleford Road
Seaford, DE 19973
(302) 629-6611

Overall patient safety: ★★★
Teaching: N

CLINICAL PROGRAM RATINGS:

CARDIAC	NR	ORTHOPEDICS	NR
CRITICAL CARE	NR	PULMONARY	★★★
GASTROINTESTINAL	★★★	STROKE	★
GENERAL SURGERY	NR	VASCULAR	NR
MATERNITY CARE	NR	WOMEN'S HEALTH	NR

HEALTHGRADES AWARDS

Beebe Medical Center

424 Savannah Road
Lewes, DE 19958
(302) 645-3100

Overall patient safety: ★★★
Teaching: N

CLINICAL PROGRAM RATINGS:

CARDIAC	NR	ORTHOPEDICS	★★★★★
CRITICAL CARE	NR	PULMONARY	★★★
GASTROINTESTINAL	★★★	STROKE	★★★
GENERAL SURGERY	NR	VASCULAR	★★★
MATERNITY CARE	NR	WOMEN'S HEALTH	NR

HEALTHGRADES AWARDS

✓ **SPECIALTY EXCELLENCE**
- ORTHOPEDIC SURGERY

St. Francis Hospital

7th and Clayton Streets
Wilmington, DE 19805
(302) 421-4100

Overall patient safety: ★★★
Teaching: Y

CLINICAL PROGRAM RATINGS:

CARDIAC	★★★	ORTHOPEDICS	NR
CRITICAL CARE	NR	PULMONARY	★★★
GASTROINTESTINAL	★★★	STROKE	★★★
GENERAL SURGERY	NR	VASCULAR	NR
MATERNITY CARE	NR	WOMEN'S HEALTH	NR

HEALTHGRADES AWARDS

✓ **SPECIALTY EXCELLENCE**
- JOINT REPLACEMENT

KEY: ★★★★★ BEST   ★★★ AS EXPECTED   ★ POOR   NR NOT RATED BY HEALTHGRADES   For full definitions of ratings and awards, see Appendix.

Wilmington Hospital

501 West 14th Street
Wilmington, DE 19801
(302) 733-1000

Overall patient safety: ★★★
Teaching: Y

CLINICAL PROGRAM RATINGS:

CARDIAC	★★★	ORTHOPEDICS	★★★
CRITICAL CARE	NR	PULMONARY	★★★★★
GASTROINTESTINAL	★★★	STROKE	★★★
GENERAL SURGERY	NR	VASCULAR	★★★
MATERNITY CARE	NR	WOMEN'S HEALTH	NR

HEALTHGRADES AWARDS

✓ **SPECIALTY EXCELLENCE**
· GASTROINTESTINAL   · PULMONARY CARE
  CARE

FLORIDA HOSPITALS: RATINGS BY CLINICAL SPECIALTY

Alachua General Hospital*

801 Southwest 2nd Avenue
Gainesville, FL 32601
(352) 372-4321

Overall patient safety: ★★★
Teaching: Y

CLINICAL PROGRAM RATINGS:

CARDIAC	★★★	ORTHOPEDICS	★★★
CRITICAL CARE	NR	PULMONARY	★★★
GASTROINTESTINAL	★★★	STROKE	★★★
GENERAL SURGERY	★★★	VASCULAR	★★★
MATERNITY CARE	★★★	WOMEN'S HEALTH	★★★

HEALTHGRADES AWARDS

Baptist Hospital of Miami

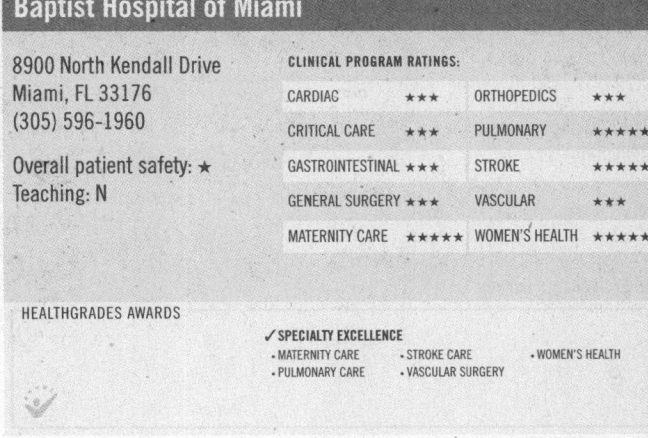

8900 North Kendall Drive
Miami, FL 33176
(305) 596-1960

Overall patient safety: ★
Teaching: N

CLINICAL PROGRAM RATINGS:

CARDIAC	★★★	ORTHOPEDICS	★★★
CRITICAL CARE	★★★	PULMONARY	★★★★★
GASTROINTESTINAL	★★★	STROKE	★★★★★
GENERAL SURGERY	★★★	VASCULAR	★★★
MATERNITY CARE	★★★★★	WOMEN'S HEALTH	★★★★★

HEALTHGRADES AWARDS

✓ **SPECIALTY EXCELLENCE**
· MATERNITY CARE   · STROKE CARE   · WOMEN'S HEALTH
· PULMONARY CARE   · VASCULAR SURGERY

Aventura Hospital and Medical Center

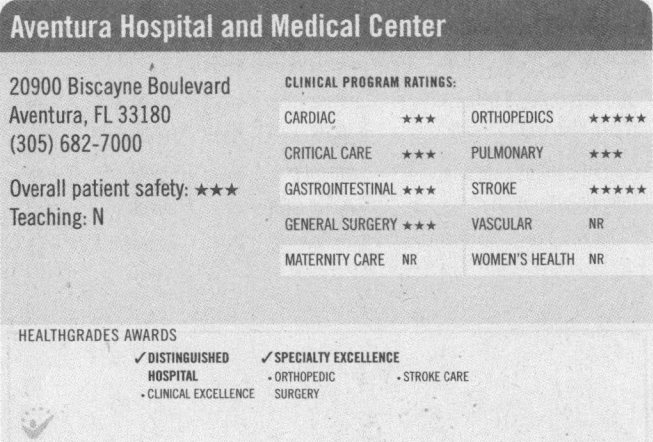

20900 Biscayne Boulevard
Aventura, FL 33180
(305) 682-7000

Overall patient safety: ★★★
Teaching: N

CLINICAL PROGRAM RATINGS:

CARDIAC	★★★	ORTHOPEDICS	★★★★★
CRITICAL CARE	★★★	PULMONARY	★★★
GASTROINTESTINAL	★★★	STROKE	★★★★★
GENERAL SURGERY	★★★	VASCULAR	NR
MATERNITY CARE	NR	WOMEN'S HEALTH	NR

HEALTHGRADES AWARDS

✓ **DISTINGUISHED**   ✓ **SPECIALTY EXCELLENCE**
   HOSPITAL   · ORTHOPEDIC   · STROKE CARE
· CLINICAL EXCELLENCE   SURGERY

Baptist Hospital Pensacola

1000 West Moreno Street
Pensacola, FL 32501
(850) 434-4011

Overall patient safety: ★★★
Teaching: N

CLINICAL PROGRAM RATINGS:

CARDIAC	★★★	ORTHOPEDICS	★★★
CRITICAL CARE	NR	PULMONARY	★★★
GASTROINTESTINAL	★★★	STROKE	★★★
GENERAL SURGERY	★★★	VASCULAR	★★★
MATERNITY CARE	★	WOMEN'S HEALTH	★★★

HEALTHGRADES AWARDS

---

*This hospital reports its data to the federal government jointly with another hospital. Therefore the ratings and awards apply to multiple hospitals and this specific hospital may not provide all rated services.

Baptist Medical Center

800 Prudential Drive
Jacksonville, FL 32207
(904) 202-2000

Overall patient safety: ★★★
Teaching: Y

CLINICAL PROGRAM RATINGS:

CARDIAC	★★★★★	ORTHOPEDICS	★
CRITICAL CARE	NR	PULMONARY	★★★★★
GASTROINTESTINAL	★★★	STROKE	★★★★★
GENERAL SURGERY	★★★	VASCULAR	★★★
MATERNITY CARE	★★★	WOMEN'S HEALTH	★★★

HEALTHGRADES AWARDS

✓ DISTINGUISHED HOSPITAL
• CLINICAL EXCELLENCE

✓ SPECIALTY EXCELLENCE
• CARDIAC CARE • PULMONARY CARE • STROKE CARE

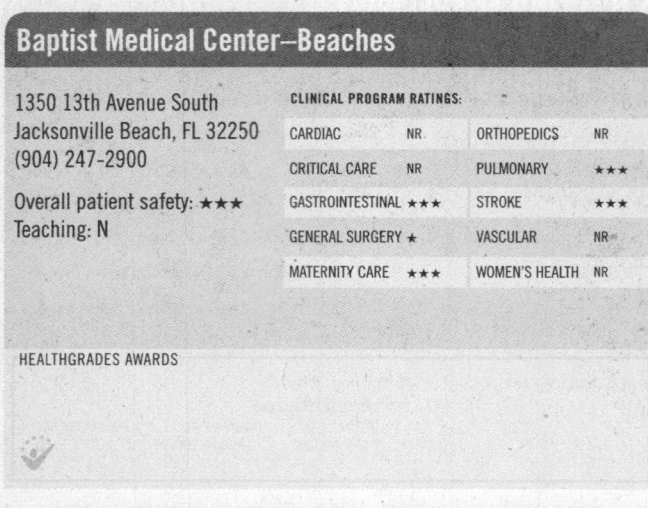

Bartow Regional Medical Center

2200 Osprey Boulevard
Bartow, FL 33830
(863) 519-1800

Overall patient safety: ★
Teaching: N

CLINICAL PROGRAM RATINGS:

CARDIAC	NR	ORTHOPEDICS	NR
CRITICAL CARE	NR	PULMONARY	★★★
GASTROINTESTINAL	NR	STROKE	★★★★★
GENERAL SURGERY	★★★	VASCULAR	NR
MATERNITY CARE	★★★★★	WOMEN'S HEALTH	NR

HEALTHGRADES AWARDS

Baptist Medical Center—Beaches

1350 13th Avenue South
Jacksonville Beach, FL 32250
(904) 247-2900

Overall patient safety: ★★★
Teaching: N

CLINICAL PROGRAM RATINGS:

CARDIAC	NR	ORTHOPEDICS	NR
CRITICAL CARE	NR	PULMONARY	★★★
GASTROINTESTINAL	★★★	STROKE	★★★
GENERAL SURGERY	★	VASCULAR	NR
MATERNITY CARE	★★★	WOMEN'S HEALTH	NR

HEALTHGRADES AWARDS

Bay Medical Center

615 North Bonita Avenue
Panama City, FL 32401
(850) 769-1511

Overall patient safety: ★★★★★
Teaching: N

CLINICAL PROGRAM RATINGS:

CARDIAC	★★★★★	ORTHOPEDICS	★★★
CRITICAL CARE	NR	PULMONARY	★★★★★
GASTROINTESTINAL	★★★	STROKE	★★★★★
GENERAL SURGERY	★★★	VASCULAR	NR
MATERNITY CARE	★★★	WOMEN'S HEALTH	★★★

HEALTHGRADES AWARDS

✓ AMERICA'S 50 BEST HOSPITALS

✓ DISTINGUISHED HOSPITAL
• CLINICAL EXCELLENCE • CARDIAC CARE
• PATIENT SAFETY

✓ SPECIALTY EXCELLENCE
• BARIATRIC SURGERY • GASTROINTESTINAL CARE • PULMONARY CARE
• GENERAL SURGERY • STROKE CARE

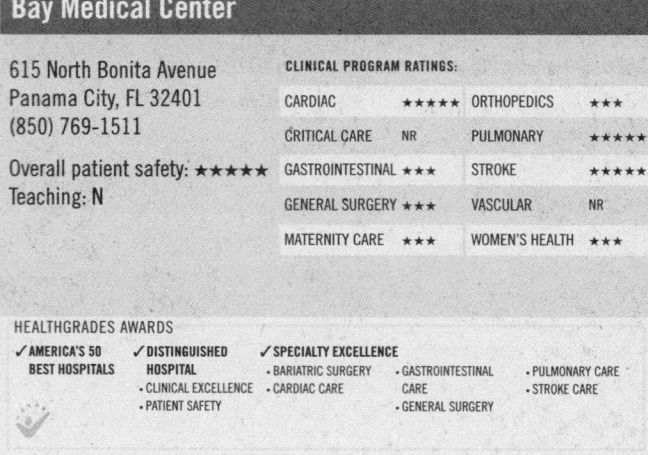

Baptist Medical Center—Nassau

1250 South 18th Street
Fernandina Beach, FL 32034
(904) 321-3500

Overall patient safety: ★★★
Teaching: N

CLINICAL PROGRAM RATINGS:

CARDIAC	NR	ORTHOPEDICS	NR
CRITICAL CARE	NR	PULMONARY	★
GASTROINTESTINAL	NR	STROKE	★★★
GENERAL SURGERY	NR	VASCULAR	NR
MATERNITY CARE	★★★	WOMEN'S HEALTH	NR

HEALTHGRADES AWARDS

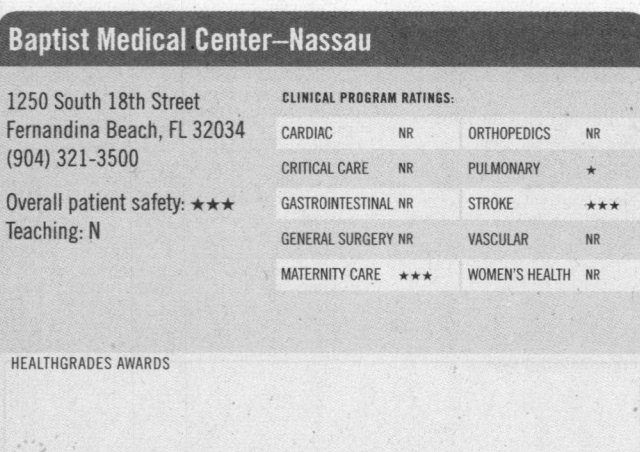

Bayfront Medical Center

701 6th Street South
St. Petersburg, FL 33701
(727) 893-6111

Overall patient safety: ★
Teaching: Y

CLINICAL PROGRAM RATINGS:

CARDIAC	★★★	ORTHOPEDICS	★★★
CRITICAL CARE	NR	PULMONARY	★★★
GASTROINTESTINAL	★★★	STROKE	★★★
GENERAL SURGERY	★★★	VASCULAR	NR
MATERNITY CARE	★★★	WOMEN'S HEALTH	★★★

HEALTHGRADES AWARDS

KEY: ★★★★★ **BEST** ★★★ **AS EXPECTED** ★ **POOR** NR **NOT RATED BY HEALTHGRADES** For full definitions of ratings and awards, see Appendix.

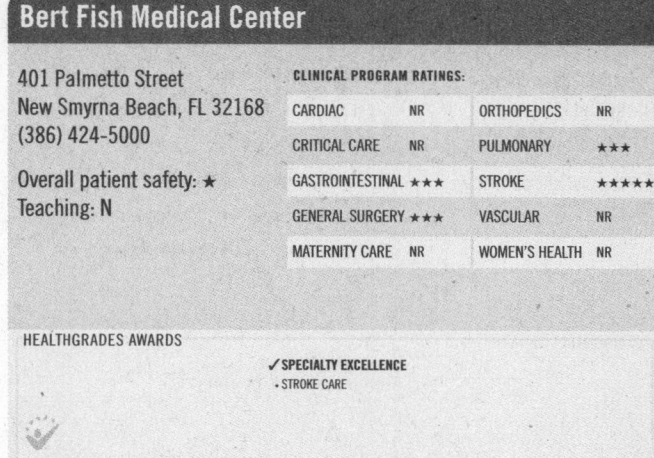

Bert Fish Medical Center

401 Palmetto Street
New Smyrna Beach, FL 32168
(386) 424-5000

Overall patient safety: ★
Teaching: N

CLINICAL PROGRAM RATINGS:

CARDIAC	NR	ORTHOPEDICS	NR
CRITICAL CARE	NR	PULMONARY	★★★
GASTROINTESTINAL	★★★	STROKE	★★★★★
GENERAL SURGERY	★★★	VASCULAR	NR
MATERNITY CARE	NR	WOMEN'S HEALTH	NR

HEALTHGRADES AWARDS

✓ SPECIALTY EXCELLENCE
- STROKE CARE

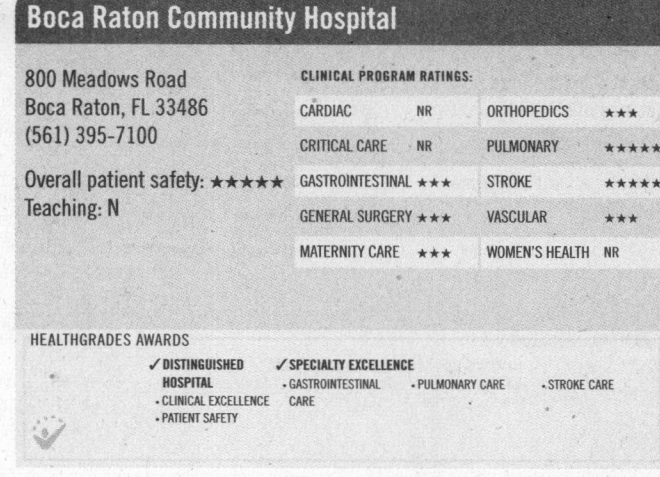

Boca Raton Community Hospital

800 Meadows Road
Boca Raton, FL 33486
(561) 395-7100

Overall patient safety: ★★★★★
Teaching: N

CLINICAL PROGRAM RATINGS:

CARDIAC	NR	ORTHOPEDICS	★★★
CRITICAL CARE	NR	PULMONARY	★★★★★
GASTROINTESTINAL	★★★	STROKE	★★★★★
GENERAL SURGERY	★★★	VASCULAR	★★★
MATERNITY CARE	★★★	WOMEN'S HEALTH	NR

HEALTHGRADES AWARDS

✓ DISTINGUISHED HOSPITAL
- CLINICAL EXCELLENCE
- PATIENT SAFETY

✓ SPECIALTY EXCELLENCE
- GASTROINTESTINAL CARE
- PULMONARY CARE
- STROKE CARE

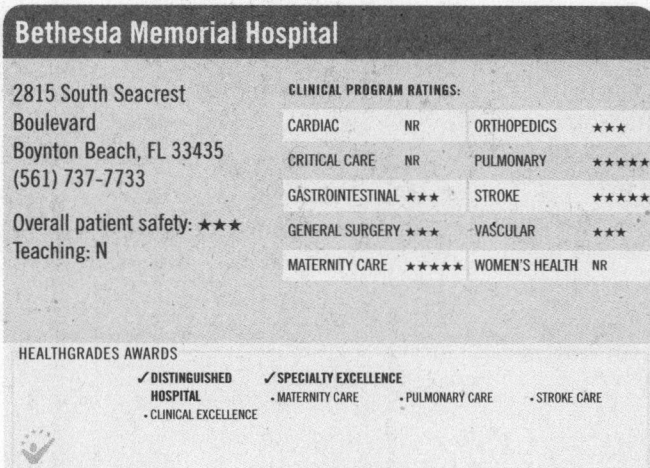

Bethesda Memorial Hospital

2815 South Seacrest Boulevard
Boynton Beach, FL 33435
(561) 737-7733

Overall patient safety: ★★★
Teaching: N

CLINICAL PROGRAM RATINGS:

CARDIAC	NR	ORTHOPEDICS	★★★
CRITICAL CARE	NR	PULMONARY	★★★★★
GASTROINTESTINAL	★★★	STROKE	★★★★★
GENERAL SURGERY	★★★	VASCULAR	★★★
MATERNITY CARE	★★★★★	WOMEN'S HEALTH	NR

HEALTHGRADES AWARDS

✓ DISTINGUISHED HOSPITAL
- CLINICAL EXCELLENCE

✓ SPECIALTY EXCELLENCE
- MATERNITY CARE
- PULMONARY CARE
- STROKE CARE

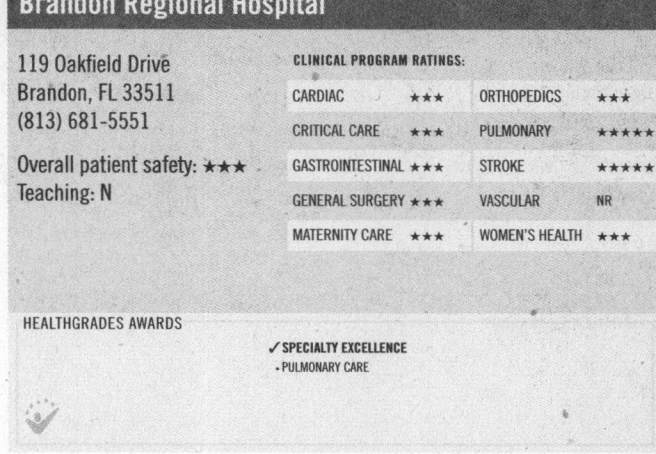

Brandon Regional Hospital

119 Oakfield Drive
Brandon, FL 33511
(813) 681-5551

Overall patient safety: ★★★
Teaching: N

CLINICAL PROGRAM RATINGS:

CARDIAC	★★★	ORTHOPEDICS	★★★
CRITICAL CARE	★★★	PULMONARY	★★★★★
GASTROINTESTINAL	★★★	STROKE	★★★★★
GENERAL SURGERY	★★★	VASCULAR	NR
MATERNITY CARE	★★★	WOMEN'S HEALTH	★★★

HEALTHGRADES AWARDS

✓ SPECIALTY EXCELLENCE
- PULMONARY CARE

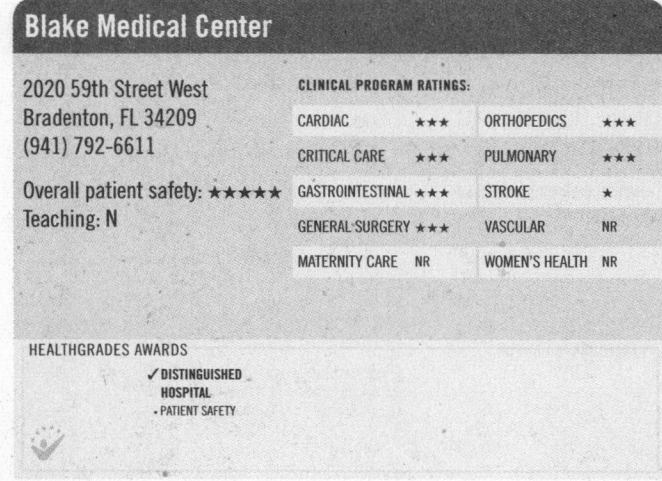

Blake Medical Center

2020 59th Street West
Bradenton, FL 34209
(941) 792-6611

Overall patient safety: ★★★★★
Teaching: N

CLINICAL PROGRAM RATINGS:

CARDIAC	★★★	ORTHOPEDICS	★★★
CRITICAL CARE	★★★	PULMONARY	★★★
GASTROINTESTINAL	★★★	STROKE	★
GENERAL SURGERY	★★★	VASCULAR	NR
MATERNITY CARE	NR	WOMEN'S HEALTH	NR

HEALTHGRADES AWARDS

✓ DISTINGUISHED HOSPITAL
- PATIENT SAFETY

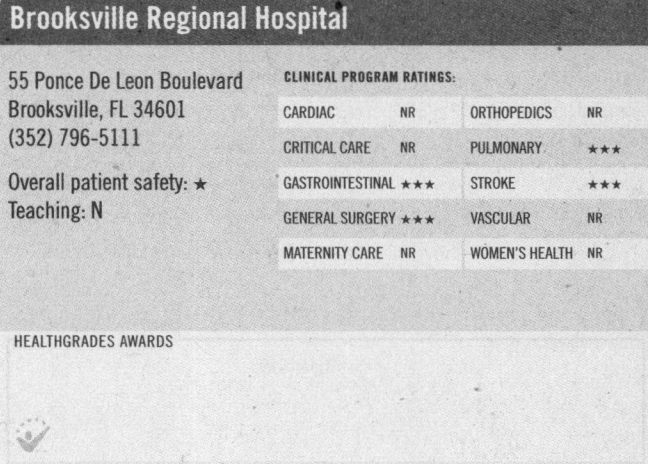

Brooksville Regional Hospital

55 Ponce De Leon Boulevard
Brooksville, FL 34601
(352) 796-5111

Overall patient safety: ★
Teaching: N

CLINICAL PROGRAM RATINGS:

CARDIAC	NR	ORTHOPEDICS	NR
CRITICAL CARE	NR	PULMONARY	★★★
GASTROINTESTINAL	★★★	STROKE	★★★
GENERAL SURGERY	★★★	VASCULAR	NR
MATERNITY CARE	NR	WOMEN'S HEALTH	NR

HEALTHGRADES AWARDS

Broward General Medical Center

1600 South Andrews Avenue
Fort Lauderdale, FL 33316
(954) 355-4400

Overall patient safety: ★★★
Teaching: Y

CLINICAL PROGRAM RATINGS:

CARDIAC	★★★	ORTHOPEDICS	★★★
CRITICAL CARE	NR	PULMONARY	★★★
GASTROINTESTINAL	★★★	STROKE	★★★
GENERAL SURGERY	★★★	VASCULAR	NR
MATERNITY CARE	★★★	WOMEN'S HEALTH	★★★★★

HEALTHGRADES AWARDS

✓ SPECIALTY EXCELLENCE
• WOMEN'S HEALTH

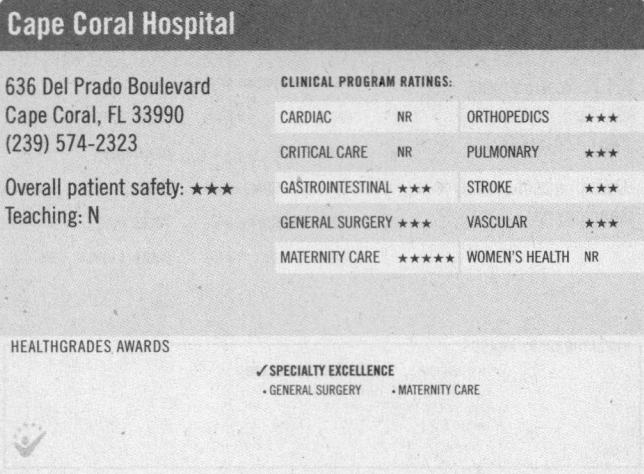

Cape Coral Hospital

636 Del Prado Boulevard
Cape Coral, FL 33990
(239) 574-2323

Overall patient safety: ★★★
Teaching: N

CLINICAL PROGRAM RATINGS:

CARDIAC	NR	ORTHOPEDICS	★★★
CRITICAL CARE	NR	PULMONARY	★★★
GASTROINTESTINAL	★★★	STROKE	★★★
GENERAL SURGERY	★★★	VASCULAR	★★★
MATERNITY CARE	★★★★★	WOMEN'S HEALTH	NR

HEALTHGRADES AWARDS

✓ SPECIALTY EXCELLENCE
• GENERAL SURGERY • MATERNITY CARE

Campbellton Graceville Hospital

5429 College Drive
Graceville, FL 32440
(850) 263-7201

Overall patient safety: NR
Teaching: N

CLINICAL PROGRAM RATINGS:

CARDIAC	NR	ORTHOPEDICS	NR
CRITICAL CARE	NR	PULMONARY	★★★
GASTROINTESTINAL	NR	STROKE	NR
GENERAL SURGERY	NR	VASCULAR	NR
MATERNITY CARE	NR	WOMEN'S HEALTH	NR

HEALTHGRADES AWARDS

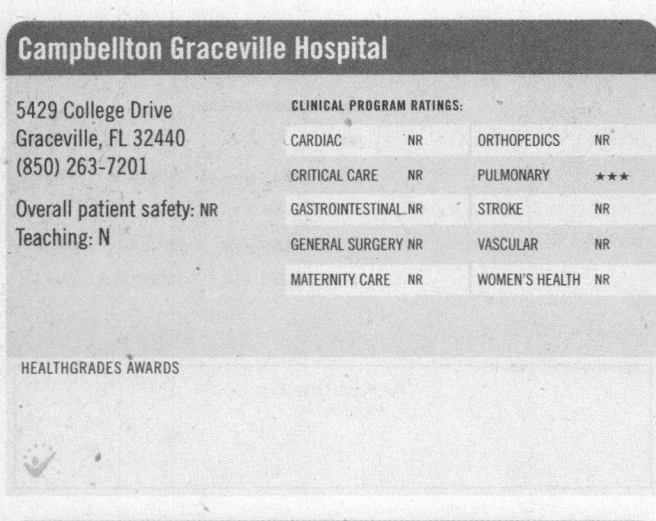

Capital Regional Medical Center

2626 Capital
Medical Boulevard
Tallahassee, FL 32308
(850) 656-5000

Overall patient safety: ★★★
Teaching: N

CLINICAL PROGRAM RATINGS:

CARDIAC	★★★	ORTHOPEDICS	★★★
CRITICAL CARE	★★★	PULMONARY	★★★
GASTROINTESTINAL	★★★	STROKE	★★★
GENERAL SURGERY	★★★	VASCULAR	NR
MATERNITY CARE	★★★	WOMEN'S HEALTH	★★★

HEALTHGRADES AWARDS

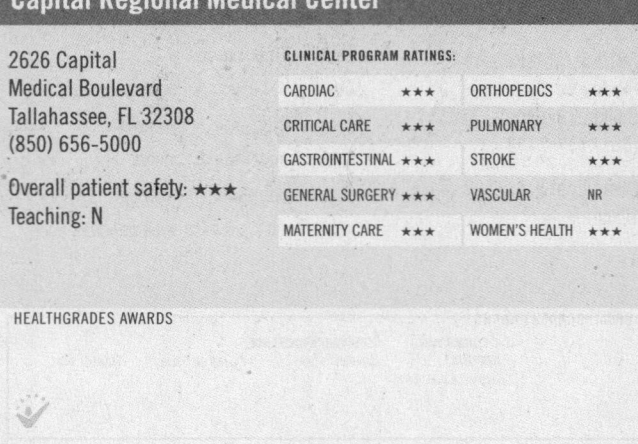

Cape Canaveral Hospital

701 West Cocoa
Beach Causeway
Cocoa Beach, FL 32931
(321) 799-7111

Overall patient safety: ★★★
Teaching: N

CLINICAL PROGRAM RATINGS:

CARDIAC	NR	ORTHOPEDICS	NR
CRITICAL CARE	★★★★★	PULMONARY	★★★
GASTROINTESTINAL	NR	STROKE	★★★★★
GENERAL SURGERY	★★★	VASCULAR	NR
MATERNITY CARE	★★★	WOMEN'S HEALTH	NR

HEALTHGRADES AWARDS

✓ SPECIALTY EXCELLENCE
• CRITICAL CARE • STROKE CARE

Cedars Medical Center

1400 Northwest 12th Avenue
Miami, FL 33136
(305) 325-5511

Overall patient safety: ★
Teaching: Y

CLINICAL PROGRAM RATINGS:

CARDIAC	★★★	ORTHOPEDICS	NR
CRITICAL CARE	★★★★★	PULMONARY	★★★★★
GASTROINTESTINAL	★★★	STROKE	★★★★★
GENERAL SURGERY	★★★	VASCULAR	NR
MATERNITY CARE	NR	WOMEN'S HEALTH	NR

HEALTHGRADES AWARDS

✓ SPECIALTY EXCELLENCE
• BARIATRIC SURGERY • PULMONARY CARE
• CRITICAL CARE • STROKE CARE

KEY: ★★★★★ BEST ★★★ AS EXPECTED ★ POOR NR NOT RATED BY HEALTHGRADES For full definitions of ratings and awards, see Appendix.

Central Florida Regional Hospital

1401 West Seminole Boulevard
Sanford, FL 32771
(407) 321-4500

Overall patient safety: ★★★★★
Teaching: N

CLINICAL PROGRAM RATINGS:

CARDIAC	★★★	ORTHOPEDICS	NR
CRITICAL CARE	★★★	PULMONARY	★★★
GASTROINTESTINAL	★★★	STROKE	★★★★★
GENERAL SURGERY	★★★	VASCULAR	NR
MATERNITY CARE	★★★	WOMEN'S HEALTH	★★★

HEALTHGRADES AWARDS

✓ DISTINGUISHED HOSPITAL
• CLINICAL EXCELLENCE
• PATIENT SAFETY

✓ SPECIALTY EXCELLENCE
• CARDIAC CARE

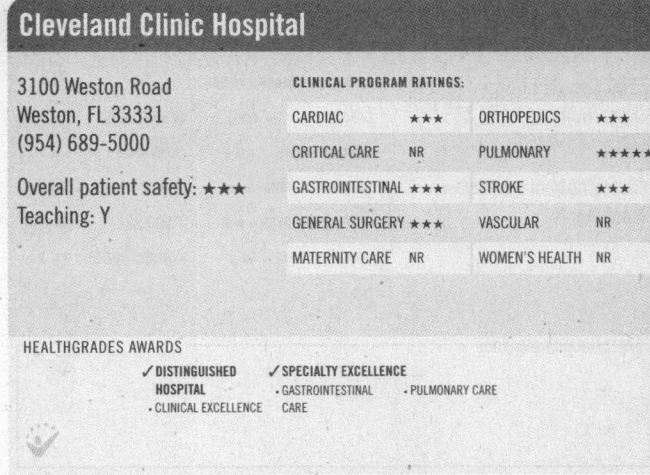

Cleveland Clinic Hospital

3100 Weston Road
Weston, FL 33331
(954) 689-5000

Overall patient safety: ★★★
Teaching: Y

CLINICAL PROGRAM RATINGS:

CARDIAC	★★★	ORTHOPEDICS	★★★
CRITICAL CARE	NR	PULMONARY	★★★★★
GASTROINTESTINAL	★★★	STROKE	★★★
GENERAL SURGERY	★★★	VASCULAR	NR
MATERNITY CARE	NR	WOMEN'S HEALTH	NR

HEALTHGRADES AWARDS

✓ DISTINGUISHED HOSPITAL
• CLINICAL EXCELLENCE

✓ SPECIALTY EXCELLENCE
• GASTROINTESTINAL CARE
• PULMONARY CARE

Charlotte Regional Medical Center

809 East Marion Avenue
Punta Gorda, FL 33950
(941) 639-3131

Overall patient safety: ★★★
Teaching: N

CLINICAL PROGRAM RATINGS:

CARDIAC	★★★★★	ORTHOPEDICS	★★★
CRITICAL CARE	NR	PULMONARY	★★★★★
GASTROINTESTINAL	★★★	STROKE	★★★
GENERAL SURGERY	★★★	VASCULAR	NR
MATERNITY CARE	NR	WOMEN'S HEALTH	NR

HEALTHGRADES AWARDS

✓ DISTINGUISHED HOSPITAL
• CLINICAL EXCELLENCE

✓ SPECIALTY EXCELLENCE
• CARDIAC CARE
• CARDIAC SURGERY

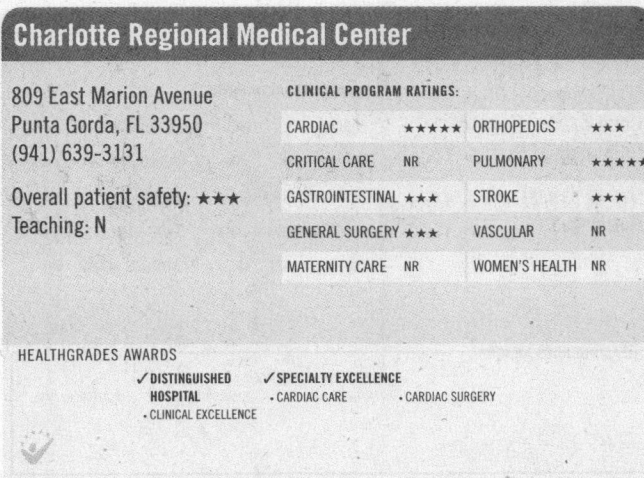
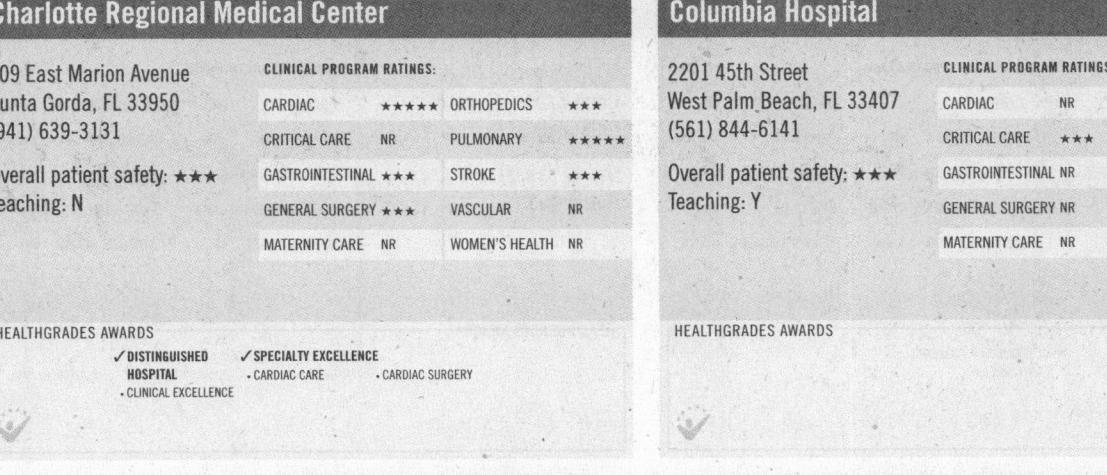

Columbia Hospital

2201 45th Street
West Palm Beach, FL 33407
(561) 844-6141

Overall patient safety: ★★★
Teaching: Y

CLINICAL PROGRAM RATINGS:

CARDIAC	NR	ORTHOPEDICS	NR
CRITICAL CARE	★★★	PULMONARY	★★★
GASTROINTESTINAL	NR	STROKE	★★★
GENERAL SURGERY	NR	VASCULAR	NR
MATERNITY CARE	NR	WOMEN'S HEALTH	NR

HEALTHGRADES AWARDS

Citrus Memorial Hospital

502 West Highland Boulevard
Inverness, FL 34452
(352) 726-1551

Overall patient safety: ★★★
Teaching: N

CLINICAL PROGRAM RATINGS:

CARDIAC	★★★	ORTHOPEDICS	★★★★★
CRITICAL CARE	NR	PULMONARY	★★★
GASTROINTESTINAL	★★★	STROKE	★★★
GENERAL SURGERY	★★★	VASCULAR	NR
MATERNITY CARE	★★★	WOMEN'S HEALTH	★★★

HEALTHGRADES AWARDS

✓ SPECIALTY EXCELLENCE
• JOINT REPLACEMENT
• ORTHOPEDIC SURGERY

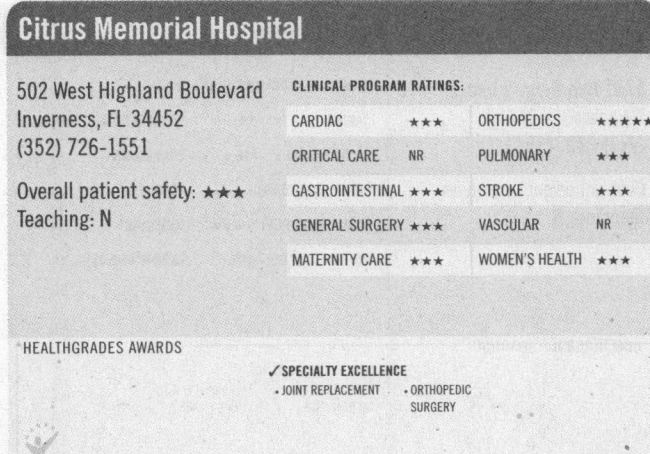

Community Hospital

5637 Marine Parkway
New Port Richey, FL 34652
(727) 848-1733

Overall patient safety: ★★★
Teaching: N

CLINICAL PROGRAM RATINGS:

CARDIAC	NR	ORTHOPEDICS	★
CRITICAL CARE	★★★	PULMONARY	★★★
GASTROINTESTINAL	★★★	STROKE	★★★
GENERAL SURGERY	★★★	VASCULAR	NR
MATERNITY CARE	★★★★★	WOMEN'S HEALTH	NR

HEALTHGRADES AWARDS

✓ SPECIALTY EXCELLENCE
• GASTROINTESTINAL CARE
• GENERAL SURGERY

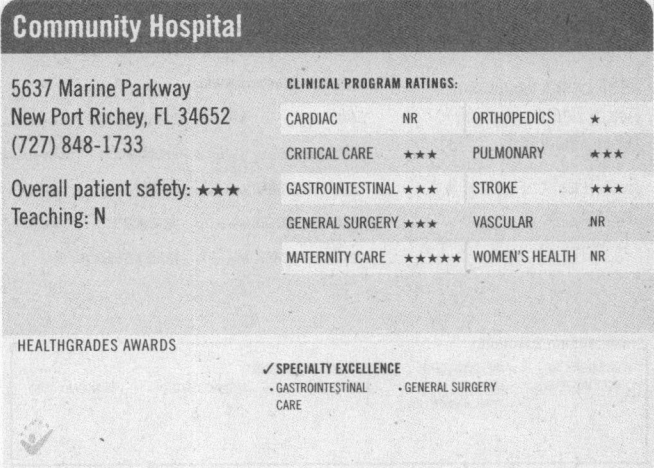

FLORIDA HOSPITALS: RATINGS BY CLINICAL SPECIALTY

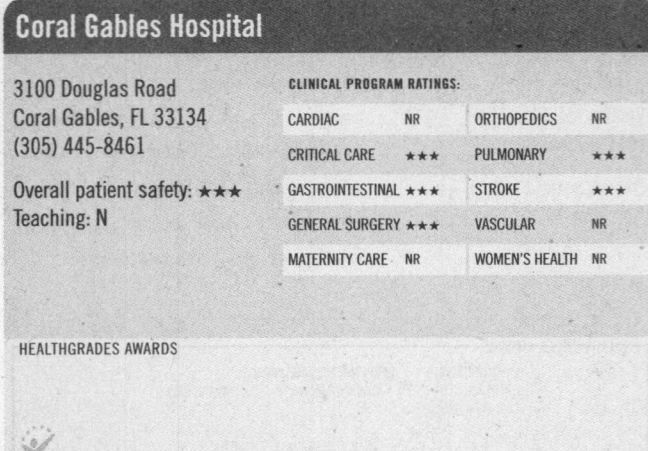

Coral Gables Hospital

3100 Douglas Road
Coral Gables, FL 33134
(305) 445-8461

Overall patient safety: ★★★
Teaching: N

CLINICAL PROGRAM RATINGS:

CARDIAC	NR	ORTHOPEDICS	NR
CRITICAL CARE	★★★	PULMONARY	★★★
GASTROINTESTINAL	★★★	STROKE	★★★
GENERAL SURGERY	★★★	VASCULAR	NR
MATERNITY CARE	NR	WOMEN'S HEALTH	NR

HEALTHGRADES AWARDS

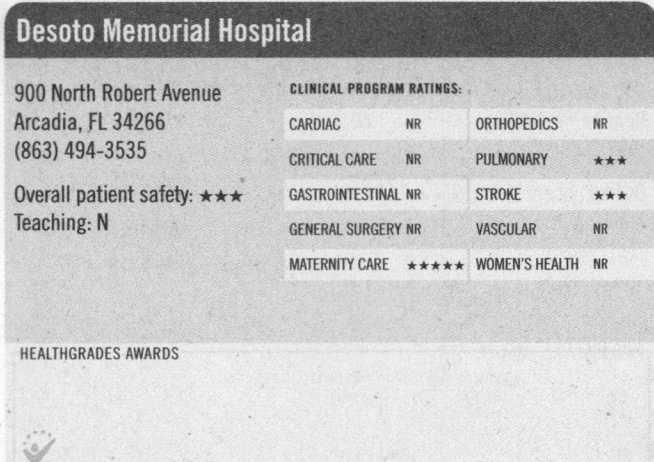

Desoto Memorial Hospital

900 North Robert Avenue
Arcadia, FL 34266
(863) 494-3535

Overall patient safety: ★★★
Teaching: N

CLINICAL PROGRAM RATINGS:

CARDIAC	NR	ORTHOPEDICS	NR
CRITICAL CARE	NR	PULMONARY	★★★
GASTROINTESTINAL	NR	STROKE	★★★
GENERAL SURGERY	NR	VASCULAR	NR
MATERNITY CARE	★★★★★	WOMEN'S HEALTH	NR

HEALTHGRADES AWARDS

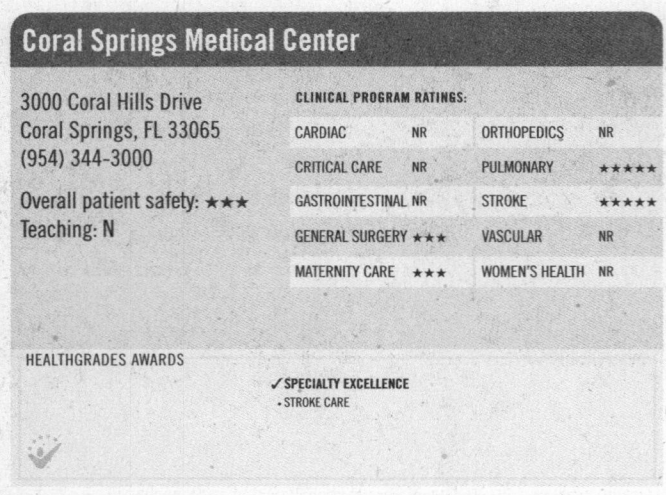

Coral Springs Medical Center

3000 Coral Hills Drive
Coral Springs, FL 33065
(954) 344-3000

Overall patient safety: ★★★
Teaching: N

CLINICAL PROGRAM RATINGS:

CARDIAC	NR	ORTHOPEDICS	NR
CRITICAL CARE	NR	PULMONARY	★★★★★
GASTROINTESTINAL	NR	STROKE	★★★★★
GENERAL SURGERY	★★★	VASCULAR	NR
MATERNITY CARE	★★★	WOMEN'S HEALTH	NR

HEALTHGRADES AWARDS

✓ SPECIALTY EXCELLENCE
• STROKE CARE

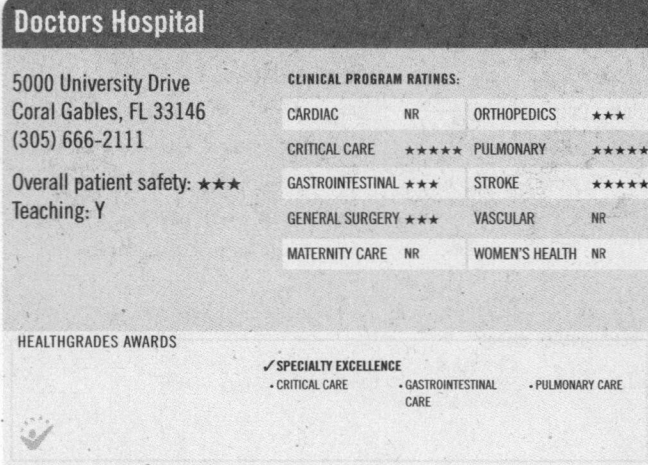

Doctors Hospital

5000 University Drive
Coral Gables, FL 33146
(305) 666-2111

Overall patient safety: ★★★
Teaching: Y

CLINICAL PROGRAM RATINGS:

CARDIAC	NR	ORTHOPEDICS	★★★
CRITICAL CARE	★★★★★	PULMONARY	★★★★★
GASTROINTESTINAL	★★★	STROKE	★★★★★
GENERAL SURGERY	★★★	VASCULAR	NR
MATERNITY CARE	NR	WOMEN'S HEALTH	NR

HEALTHGRADES AWARDS

✓ SPECIALTY EXCELLENCE
• CRITICAL CARE   • GASTROINTESTINAL CARE   • PULMONARY CARE

Delray Medical Center

5352 Linton Boulevard
Delray Beach, FL 33484
(561) 498-4440

Overall patient safety: ★★★
Teaching: N

CLINICAL PROGRAM RATINGS:

CARDIAC	★★★★★	ORTHOPEDICS	★★★
CRITICAL CARE	★★★	PULMONARY	★★★★★
GASTROINTESTINAL	★★★	STROKE	★★★
GENERAL SURGERY	★★★	VASCULAR	★★★
MATERNITY CARE	NR	WOMEN'S HEALTH	NR

HEALTHGRADES AWARDS

✓ AMERICA'S 50 BEST HOSPITALS   ✓ DISTINGUISHED HOSPITAL   ✓ SPECIALTY EXCELLENCE
• CLINICAL EXCELLENCE   • CARDIAC CARE   • CARDIAC SURGERY   • PULMONARY CARE

Doctors Hospital of Sarasota

5731 Bee Ridge Road
Sarasota, FL 34233
(941) 342-1100

Overall patient safety: ★★★
Teaching: N

CLINICAL PROGRAM RATINGS:

CARDIAC	NR	ORTHOPEDICS	★★★
CRITICAL CARE	NR	PULMONARY	★★★
GASTROINTESTINAL	★★★	STROKE	★★★
GENERAL SURGERY	★★★	VASCULAR	NR
MATERNITY CARE	NR	WOMEN'S HEALTH	NR

HEALTHGRADES AWARDS

KEY: ★★★★★ BEST   ★★★ AS EXPECTED   ★ POOR   NR NOT RATED BY HEALTHGRADES   For full definitions of ratings and awards, see Appendix.

FLORIDA HOSPITALS: RATINGS BY CLINICAL SPECIALTY

Doctors Memorial Hospital

401 East Byrd Avenue
Bonifay, FL 32425
(850) 547-1120

Overall patient safety: ★★★
Teaching: N

CLINICAL PROGRAM RATINGS:

CARDIAC	NR	ORTHOPEDICS	NR
CRITICAL CARE	NR	PULMONARY	★★★
GASTROINTESTINAL	NR	STROKE	NR
GENERAL SURGERY	NR	VASCULAR	NR
MATERNITY CARE	NR	WOMEN'S HEALTH	NR

HEALTHGRADES AWARDS

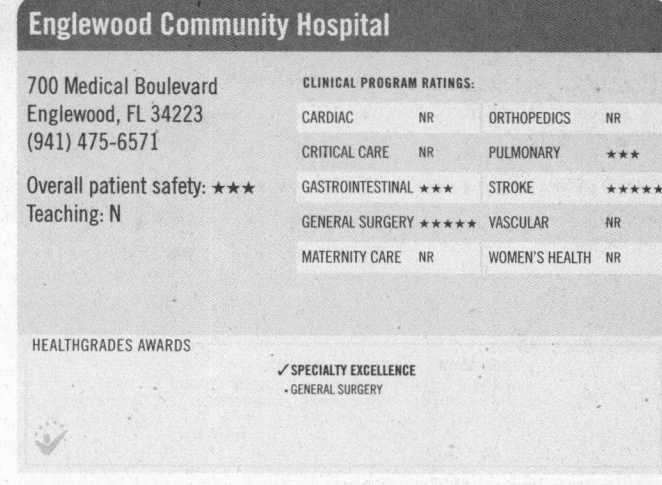

Englewood Community Hospital

700 Medical Boulevard
Englewood, FL 34223
(941) 475-6571

Overall patient safety: ★★★
Teaching: N

CLINICAL PROGRAM RATINGS:

CARDIAC	NR	ORTHOPEDICS	NR
CRITICAL CARE	NR	PULMONARY	★★★
GASTROINTESTINAL	★★★	STROKE	★★★★★
GENERAL SURGERY	★★★★★	VASCULAR	NR
MATERNITY CARE	NR	WOMEN'S HEALTH	NR

HEALTHGRADES AWARDS

✓ SPECIALTY EXCELLENCE
- GENERAL SURGERY

Doctors' Memorial Hospital

333 North Byron
Butler Parkway
Perry, FL 32347
(850) 584-0800

Overall patient safety: ★★★
Teaching: N

CLINICAL PROGRAM RATINGS:

CARDIAC	NR	ORTHOPEDICS	NR
CRITICAL CARE	NR	PULMONARY	★★★
GASTROINTESTINAL	NR	STROKE	NR
GENERAL SURGERY	★★★	VASCULAR	NR
MATERNITY CARE	★★★	WOMEN'S HEALTH	NR

HEALTHGRADES AWARDS

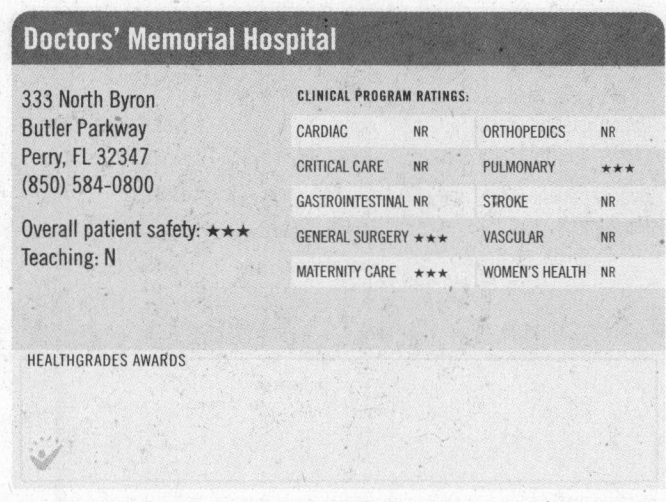

Fawcett Memorial Hospital

21298 Olean Boulevard
Port Charlotte, FL 33952
(941) 629-1181

Overall patient safety: ★★★
Teaching: N

CLINICAL PROGRAM RATINGS:

CARDIAC	NR	ORTHOPEDICS	★★★
CRITICAL CARE	★★★	PULMONARY	★★★★★
GASTROINTESTINAL	★★★	STROKE	★★★
GENERAL SURGERY	★★★	VASCULAR	★★★
MATERNITY CARE	NR	WOMEN'S HEALTH	NR

HEALTHGRADES AWARDS

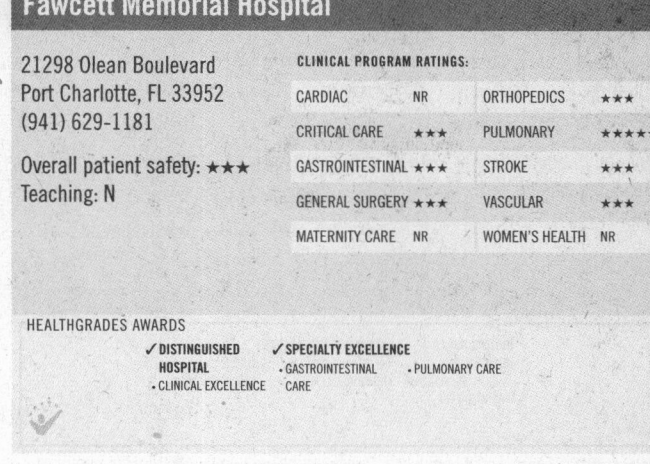

✓ DISTINGUISHED HOSPITAL
- CLINICAL EXCELLENCE

✓ SPECIALTY EXCELLENCE
- GASTROINTESTINAL CARE
- PULMONARY CARE

Edward White Hospital

2323 9th Avenue North
St. Petersburg, FL 33713
(727) 323-1111

Overall patient safety: ★★★
Teaching: N

CLINICAL PROGRAM RATINGS:

CARDIAC	NR	ORTHOPEDICS	NR
CRITICAL CARE	NR	PULMONARY	★★★
GASTROINTESTINAL	★★★	STROKE	★★★
GENERAL SURGERY	★★★	VASCULAR	NR
MATERNITY CARE	NR	WOMEN'S HEALTH	NR

HEALTHGRADES AWARDS

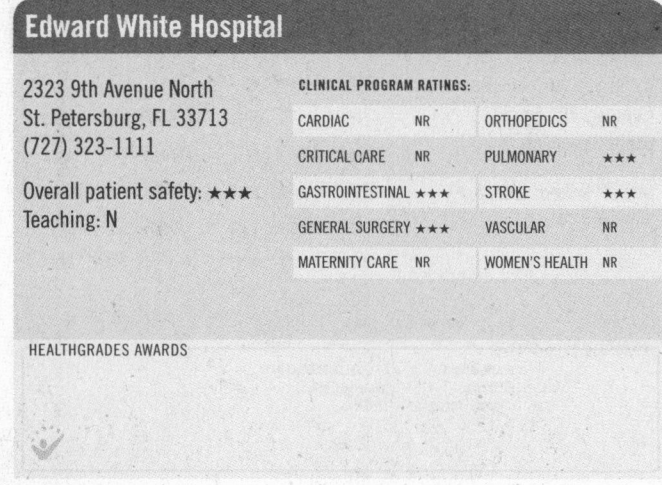

Fishermen's Hospital

3301 Overseas Highway
Marathon, FL 33050
(305) 743-5533

Overall patient safety: ★★★
Teaching: N

CLINICAL PROGRAM RATINGS:

CARDIAC	NR	ORTHOPEDICS	NR
CRITICAL CARE	NR	PULMONARY	★★★
GASTROINTESTINAL	NR	STROKE	NR
GENERAL SURGERY	NR	VASCULAR	NR
MATERNITY CARE	NR	WOMEN'S HEALTH	NR

HEALTHGRADES AWARDS

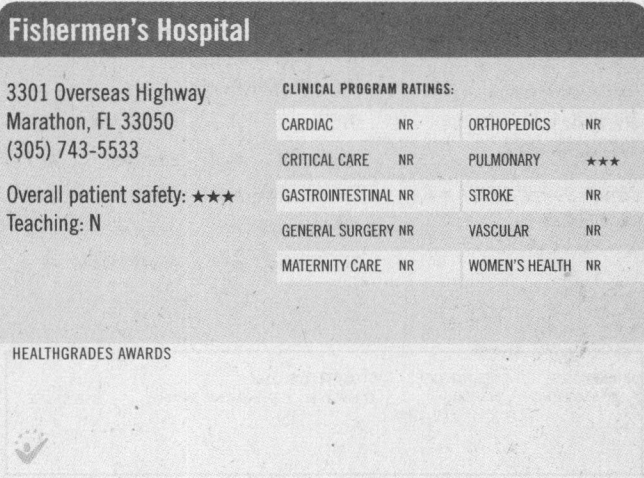

Flagler Hospital

400 Health Parks Boulevard
St. Augustine, FL 32086
(904) 829-5155

Overall patient safety: ★★★★★
Teaching: N

CLINICAL PROGRAM RATINGS:

CARDIAC	★★★★★	ORTHOPEDICS	★★★★★
CRITICAL CARE	NR	PULMONARY	★★★★★
GASTROINTESTINAL	★★★★★	STROKE	★★★★★
GENERAL SURGERY	★★★★★	VASCULAR	NR
MATERNITY CARE	★★★	WOMEN'S HEALTH	★★★★★

HEALTHGRADES AWARDS

✓ DISTINGUISHED HOSPITAL
- CLINICAL EXCELLENCE
- PATIENT SAFETY

✓ SPECIALTY EXCELLENCE
- CARDIAC CARE
- CARDIAC SURGERY
- GASTROINTESTINAL CARE
- GENERAL SURGERY
- ORTHOPEDIC SURGERY
- PULMONARY CARE
- STROKE CARE
- WOMEN'S HEALTH

Florida Hospital–Fish Memorial

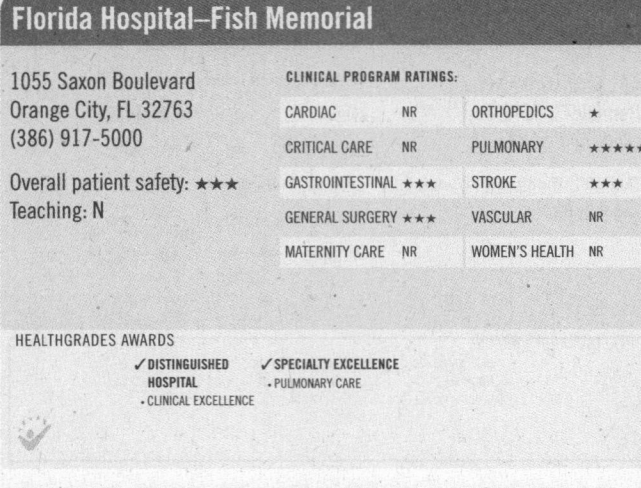

1055 Saxon Boulevard
Orange City, FL 32763
(386) 917-5000

Overall patient safety: ★★★
Teaching: N

CLINICAL PROGRAM RATINGS:

CARDIAC	NR	ORTHOPEDICS	★
CRITICAL CARE	NR	PULMONARY	★★★★★
GASTROINTESTINAL	★★★	STROKE	★★★
GENERAL SURGERY	★★★	VASCULAR	NR
MATERNITY CARE	NR	WOMEN'S HEALTH	NR

HEALTHGRADES AWARDS

✓ DISTINGUISHED HOSPITAL
- CLINICAL EXCELLENCE

✓ SPECIALTY EXCELLENCE
- PULMONARY CARE

Florida Hospital

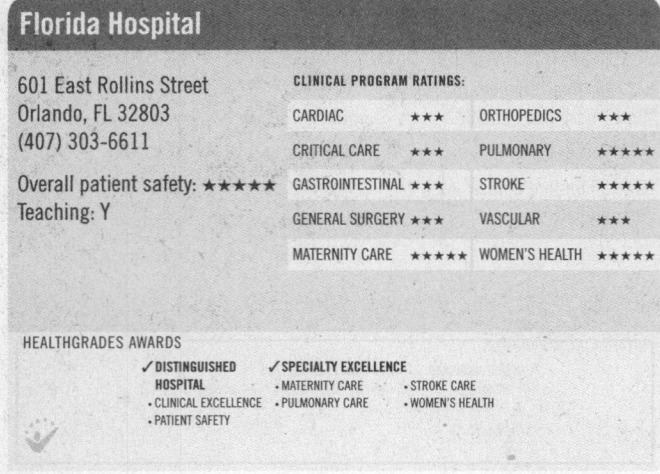

601 East Rollins Street
Orlando, FL 32803
(407) 303-6611

Overall patient safety: ★★★★★
Teaching: Y

CLINICAL PROGRAM RATINGS:

CARDIAC	★★★	ORTHOPEDICS	★★★
CRITICAL CARE	★★★	PULMONARY	★★★★★
GASTROINTESTINAL	★★★	STROKE	★★★★★
GENERAL SURGERY	★★★	VASCULAR	★★★
MATERNITY CARE	★★★★★	WOMEN'S HEALTH	★★★★★

HEALTHGRADES AWARDS

✓ DISTINGUISHED HOSPITAL
- CLINICAL EXCELLENCE
- PATIENT SAFETY

✓ SPECIALTY EXCELLENCE
- MATERNITY CARE
- PULMONARY CARE
- STROKE CARE
- WOMEN'S HEALTH

Florida Hospital–Flagler

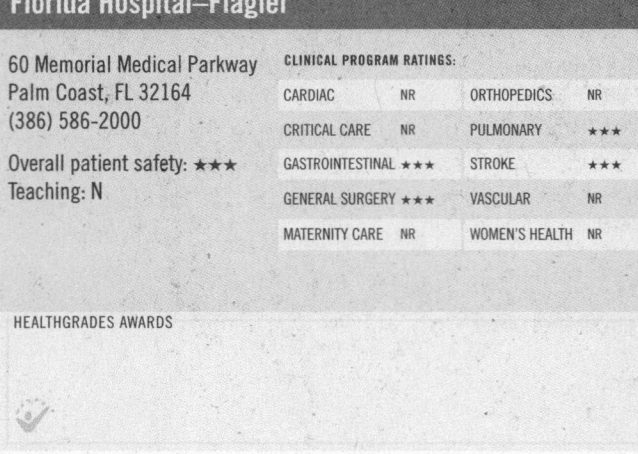

60 Memorial Medical Parkway
Palm Coast, FL 32164
(386) 586-2000

Overall patient safety: ★★★
Teaching: N

CLINICAL PROGRAM RATINGS:

CARDIAC	NR	ORTHOPEDICS	NR
CRITICAL CARE	NR	PULMONARY	★★★
GASTROINTESTINAL	★★★	STROKE	★★★
GENERAL SURGERY	★★★	VASCULAR	NR
MATERNITY CARE	NR	WOMEN'S HEALTH	NR

HEALTHGRADES AWARDS

Florida Hospital–Deland

701 West Plymouth Avenue
Deland, FL 32720
(386) 943-4522

Overall patient safety: ★★★
Teaching: N

CLINICAL PROGRAM RATINGS:

CARDIAC	NR	ORTHOPEDICS	NR
CRITICAL CARE	NR	PULMONARY	★★★
GASTROINTESTINAL	★★★	STROKE	★★★
GENERAL SURGERY	★★★	VASCULAR	NR
MATERNITY CARE	★★★	WOMEN'S HEALTH	NR

HEALTHGRADES AWARDS

Florida Hospital–Heartland Medical Center

4200 Sun 'n Lakes Boulevard
Sebring, FL 33871
(863) 314-4466

Overall patient safety: ★
Teaching: N

CLINICAL PROGRAM RATINGS:

CARDIAC	NR	ORTHOPEDICS	★★★
CRITICAL CARE	NR	PULMONARY	★★★★★
GASTROINTESTINAL	★★★	STROKE	★★★
GENERAL SURGERY	★★★	VASCULAR	NR
MATERNITY CARE	★★★	WOMEN'S HEALTH	NR

HEALTHGRADES AWARDS

✓ DISTINGUISHED HOSPITAL
- CLINICAL EXCELLENCE

✓ SPECIALTY EXCELLENCE
- GASTROINTESTINAL CARE

KEY: ★★★★★ BEST   ★★★ AS EXPECTED   ★ POOR   NR NOT RATED BY HEALTHGRADES   For full definitions of ratings and awards, see Appendix.

Florida Hospital—Oceanside*

875 Sterthaus Avenue
Ormond Beach, FL 32174
(386) 676-6000

Overall patient safety: ★★★
Teaching: N

CLINICAL PROGRAM RATINGS:

CARDIAC	★★★★★	ORTHOPEDICS	NR
CRITICAL CARE	NR	PULMONARY	★★★
GASTROINTESTINAL	★★★	STROKE	★★★
GENERAL SURGERY	★★★	VASCULAR	★★★
MATERNITY CARE	★★★	WOMEN'S HEALTH	★★★★★

HEALTHGRADES AWARDS

✓ DISTINGUISHED HOSPITAL
- CLINICAL EXCELLENCE

✓ SPECIALTY EXCELLENCE
- CARDIAC CARE
- GASTROINTESTINAL CARE
- GENERAL SURGERY
- WOMEN'S HEALTH

Florida Hospital—Zephyrhills

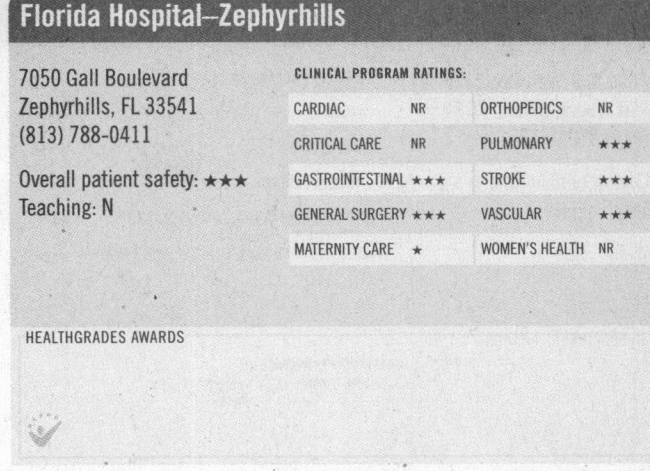

7050 Gall Boulevard
Zephyrhills, FL 33541
(813) 788-0411

Overall patient safety: ★★★
Teaching: N

CLINICAL PROGRAM RATINGS:

CARDIAC	NR	ORTHOPEDICS	NR
CRITICAL CARE	NR	PULMONARY	★★★
GASTROINTESTINAL	★★★	STROKE	★★★
GENERAL SURGERY	★★★	VASCULAR	★★★
MATERNITY CARE	★	WOMEN'S HEALTH	NR

HEALTHGRADES AWARDS

Florida Hospital—Ormond Beach*

264 South Atlantic Avenue
Ormond Beach, FL 32176
(386) 676-4200

Overall patient safety: ★★★
Teaching: N

CLINICAL PROGRAM RATINGS:

CARDIAC	★★★★★	ORTHOPEDICS	NR
CRITICAL CARE	NR	PULMONARY	★★★
GASTROINTESTINAL	★★★	STROKE	★★★
GENERAL SURGERY	★★★	VASCULAR	★★★
MATERNITY CARE	★★★	WOMEN'S HEALTH	★★★★★

HEALTHGRADES AWARDS

✓ SPECIALTY EXCELLENCE
- CARDIAC CARE
- GASTROINTESTINAL CARE
- GENERAL SURGERY
- WOMEN'S HEALTH

Florida Keys Memorial Hospital

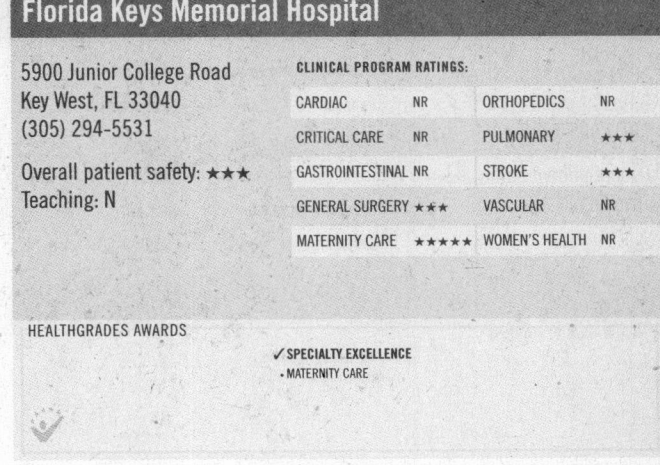

5900 Junior College Road
Key West, FL 33040
(305) 294-5531

Overall patient safety: ★★★
Teaching: N

CLINICAL PROGRAM RATINGS:

CARDIAC	NR	ORTHOPEDICS	NR
CRITICAL CARE	NR	PULMONARY	★★★
GASTROINTESTINAL	NR	STROKE	★★★
GENERAL SURGERY	★★★	VASCULAR	NR
MATERNITY CARE	★★★★★	WOMEN'S HEALTH	NR

HEALTHGRADES AWARDS

✓ SPECIALTY EXCELLENCE
- MATERNITY CARE

Florida Hospital—Waterman

1000 Waterman Way
Tavares, FL 32778
(352) 253-3333

Overall patient safety: ★★★
Teaching: N

CLINICAL PROGRAM RATINGS:

CARDIAC	NR	ORTHOPEDICS	★★★
CRITICAL CARE	★★★	PULMONARY	★★★★★
GASTROINTESTINAL	★★★	STROKE	★★★
GENERAL SURGERY	★★★	VASCULAR	NR
MATERNITY CARE	★★★	WOMEN'S HEALTH	NR

HEALTHGRADES AWARDS

✓ DISTINGUISHED HOSPITAL
- CLINICAL EXCELLENCE

✓ SPECIALTY EXCELLENCE
- PULMONARY CARE

Florida Medical Center

5000 West Oakland
Parks Boulevard
Fort Lauderdale, FL 33313
(954) 735-6000

Overall patient safety: ★★★
Teaching: N

CLINICAL PROGRAM RATINGS:

CARDIAC	★★★	ORTHOPEDICS	NR
CRITICAL CARE	★★★	PULMONARY	★★★★★
GASTROINTESTINAL	★★★	STROKE	★★★
GENERAL SURGERY	★★★	VASCULAR	NR
MATERNITY CARE	NR	WOMEN'S HEALTH	NR

HEALTHGRADES AWARDS

✓ SPECIALTY EXCELLENCE
- PULMONARY CARE

*This hospital reports its data to the federal government jointly with another hospital. Therefore the ratings and awards apply to multiple hospitals and this specific hospital may not provide all rated services.

FLORIDA HOSPITALS: RATINGS BY CLINICAL SPECIALTY

Fort Walton Beach Medical Center

1000 Mar-Walt Drive
Fort Walton Beach, FL 32547
(850) 862-1111

Overall patient safety: ★★★
Teaching: N

CLINICAL PROGRAM RATINGS:

CARDIAC	★★★	ORTHOPEDICS	★★★★★
CRITICAL CARE	★	PULMONARY	★★★
GASTROINTESTINAL	★★★	STROKE	★★★
GENERAL SURGERY	★★★★★	VASCULAR	★★★
MATERNITY CARE	★★★	WOMEN'S HEALTH	★★★

HEALTHGRADES AWARDS

✓ SPECIALTY EXCELLENCE
• GENERAL SURGERY • ORTHOPEDIC SURGERY

Gulf Breeze Hospital

1110 Gulf Breeze Parkway
Gulf Breeze, FL 32562
(850) 934-2000

Overall patient safety: ★★★
Teaching: N

CLINICAL PROGRAM RATINGS:

CARDIAC	NR	ORTHOPEDICS	NR
CRITICAL CARE	NR	PULMONARY	★★★
GASTROINTESTINAL	★★★	STROKE	★★★
GENERAL SURGERY	★★★	VASCULAR	NR
MATERNITY CARE	NR	WOMEN'S HEALTH	NR

HEALTHGRADES AWARDS

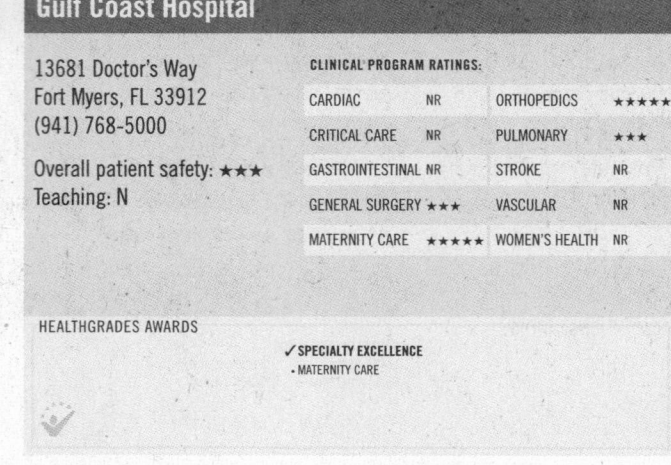

Glades General Hospital

1201 South Main Street
Belle Glade, FL 33430
(561) 996-6571

Overall patient safety: ★★★
Teaching: N

CLINICAL PROGRAM RATINGS:

CARDIAC	NR	ORTHOPEDICS	NR
CRITICAL CARE	NR	PULMONARY	★★★★★
GASTROINTESTINAL	NR	STROKE	NR
GENERAL SURGERY	NR	VASCULAR	NR
MATERNITY CARE	★★★	WOMEN'S HEALTH	NR

HEALTHGRADES AWARDS

✓ SPECIALTY EXCELLENCE
• PULMONARY CARE

Gulf Coast Hospital

13681 Doctor's Way
Fort Myers, FL 33912
(941) 768-5000

Overall patient safety: ★★★
Teaching: N

CLINICAL PROGRAM RATINGS:

CARDIAC	NR	ORTHOPEDICS	★★★★★
CRITICAL CARE	NR	PULMONARY	★★★
GASTROINTESTINAL	NR	STROKE	NR
GENERAL SURGERY	★★★	VASCULAR	NR
MATERNITY CARE	★★★★★	WOMEN'S HEALTH	NR

HEALTHGRADES AWARDS

✓ SPECIALTY EXCELLENCE
• MATERNITY CARE

Good Samaritan Medical Center

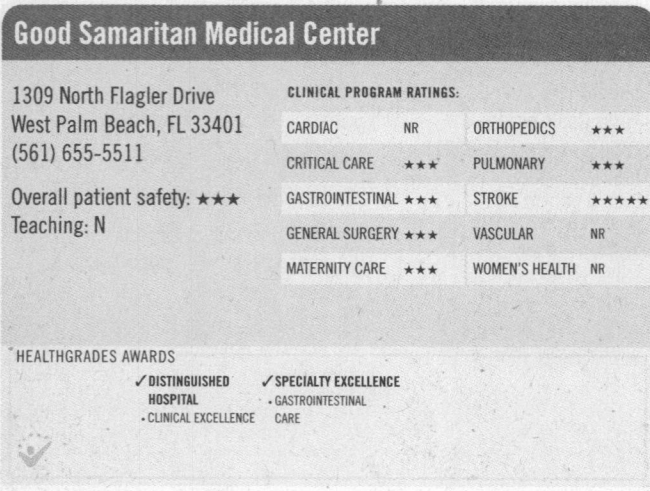

1309 North Flagler Drive
West Palm Beach, FL 33401
(561) 655-5511

Overall patient safety: ★★★
Teaching: N

CLINICAL PROGRAM RATINGS:

CARDIAC	NR	ORTHOPEDICS	★★★
CRITICAL CARE	★★★	PULMONARY	★★★
GASTROINTESTINAL	★★★	STROKE	★★★★★
GENERAL SURGERY	★★★	VASCULAR	NR
MATERNITY CARE	★★★	WOMEN'S HEALTH	NR

HEALTHGRADES AWARDS

✓ DISTINGUISHED HOSPITAL
• CLINICAL EXCELLENCE

✓ SPECIALTY EXCELLENCE
• GASTROINTESTINAL CARE

Gulf Coast Medical Center

449 West 23rd Street
Panama City, FL 32405
(850) 769-8341

Overall patient safety: ★★★★★
Teaching: N

CLINICAL PROGRAM RATINGS:

CARDIAC	NR	ORTHOPEDICS	★★★
CRITICAL CARE	★★★	PULMONARY	★★★★★
GASTROINTESTINAL	★★★	STROKE	★★★
GENERAL SURGERY	★★★	VASCULAR	NR
MATERNITY CARE	★★★	WOMEN'S HEALTH	NR

HEALTHGRADES AWARDS

✓ DISTINGUISHED HOSPITAL
• CLINICAL EXCELLENCE
• PATIENT SAFETY

✓ SPECIALTY EXCELLENCE
• BARIATRIC SURGERY   • GENERAL SURGERY
• GASTROINTESTINAL CARE   • PULMONARY CARE

KEY: ★★★★★ BEST   ★★★ AS EXPECTED   ★ POOR   NR NOT RATED BY HEALTHGRADES   For full definitions of ratings and awards, see Appendix.

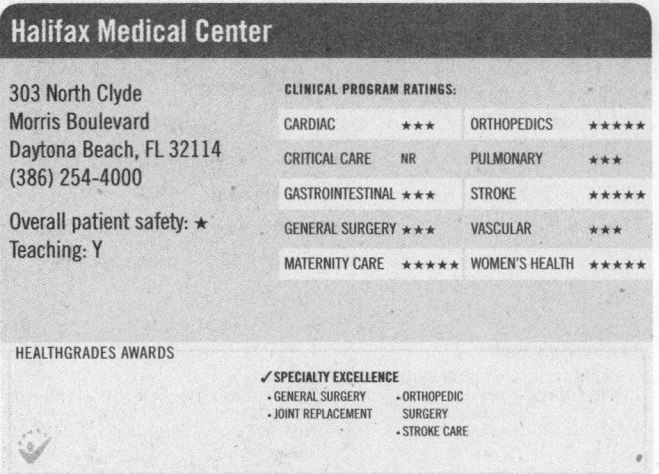

Halifax Medical Center

303 North Clyde
Morris Boulevard
Daytona Beach, FL 32114
(386) 254-4000

Overall patient safety: ★
Teaching: Y

CLINICAL PROGRAM RATINGS:

CARDIAC	★★★	ORTHOPEDICS	★★★★★
CRITICAL CARE	NR	PULMONARY	★★★
GASTROINTESTINAL	★★★	STROKE	★★★★★
GENERAL SURGERY	★★★	VASCULAR	★★★
MATERNITY CARE	★★★★★	WOMEN'S HEALTH	★★★★★

HEALTHGRADES AWARDS

✓ SPECIALTY EXCELLENCE
· GENERAL SURGERY   · ORTHOPEDIC
· JOINT REPLACEMENT   SURGERY
                     · STROKE CARE

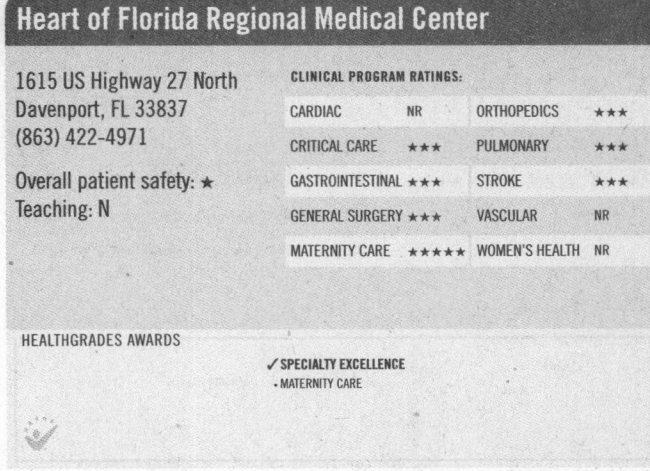

Heart of Florida Regional Medical Center

1615 US Highway 27 North
Davenport, FL 33837
(863) 422-4971

Overall patient safety: ★
Teaching: N

CLINICAL PROGRAM RATINGS:

CARDIAC	NR	ORTHOPEDICS	★★★
CRITICAL CARE	★★★	PULMONARY	★★★
GASTROINTESTINAL	★★★	STROKE	★★★
GENERAL SURGERY	★★★	VASCULAR	NR
MATERNITY CARE	★★★★★	WOMEN'S HEALTH	NR

HEALTHGRADES AWARDS

✓ SPECIALTY EXCELLENCE
· MATERNITY CARE

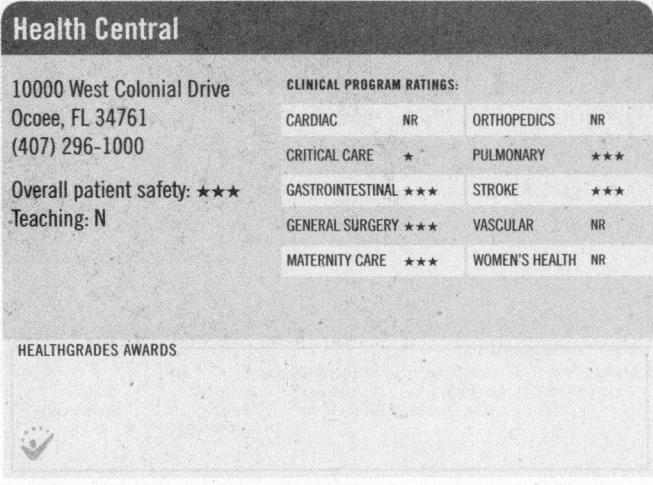

Health Central

10000 West Colonial Drive
Ocoee, FL 34761
(407) 296-1000

Overall patient safety: ★★★
Teaching: N

CLINICAL PROGRAM RATINGS:

CARDIAC	NR	ORTHOPEDICS	NR
CRITICAL CARE	★	PULMONARY	★★★
GASTROINTESTINAL	★★★	STROKE	★★★
GENERAL SURGERY	★★★	VASCULAR	NR
MATERNITY CARE	★★★	WOMEN'S HEALTH	NR

HEALTHGRADES AWARDS

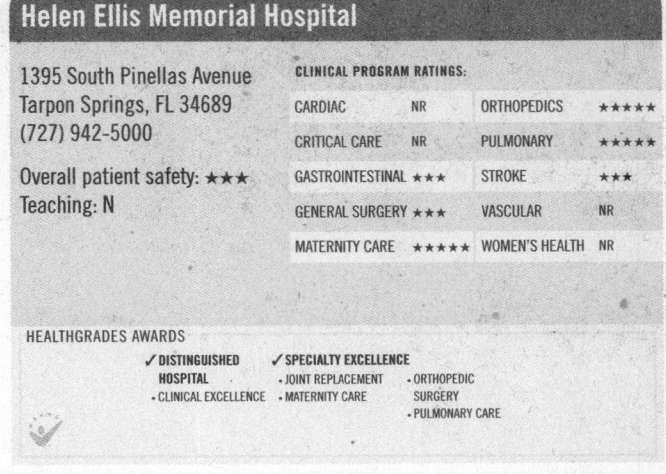

Helen Ellis Memorial Hospital

1395 South Pinellas Avenue
Tarpon Springs, FL 34689
(727) 942-5000

Overall patient safety: ★★★
Teaching: N

CLINICAL PROGRAM RATINGS:

CARDIAC	NR	ORTHOPEDICS	★★★★★
CRITICAL CARE	NR	PULMONARY	★★★★★
GASTROINTESTINAL	★★★	STROKE	★★★
GENERAL SURGERY	★★★	VASCULAR	NR
MATERNITY CARE	★★★★★	WOMEN'S HEALTH	NR

HEALTHGRADES AWARDS

✓ DISTINGUISHED   ✓ SPECIALTY EXCELLENCE
  HOSPITAL   · JOINT REPLACEMENT   · ORTHOPEDIC
· CLINICAL EXCELLENCE   · MATERNITY CARE   SURGERY
                                               · PULMONARY CARE

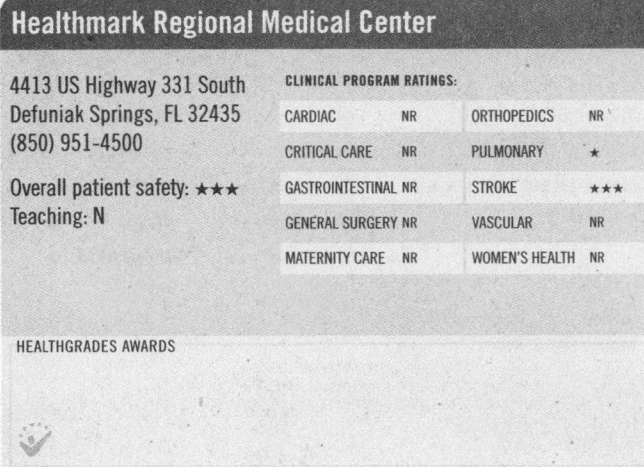

Healthmark Regional Medical Center

4413 US Highway 331 South
Defuniak Springs, FL 32435
(850) 951-4500

Overall patient safety: ★★★
Teaching: N

CLINICAL PROGRAM RATINGS:

CARDIAC	NR	ORTHOPEDICS	NR
CRITICAL CARE	NR	PULMONARY	★
GASTROINTESTINAL	NR	STROKE	★★★
GENERAL SURGERY	NR	VASCULAR	NR
MATERNITY CARE	NR	WOMEN'S HEALTH	NR

HEALTHGRADES AWARDS

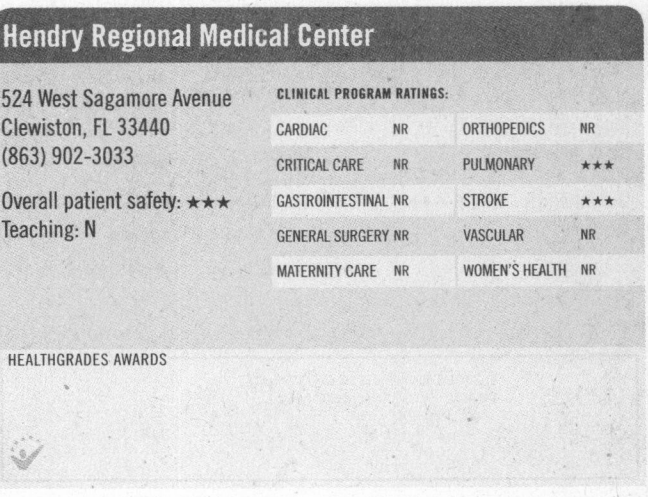

Hendry Regional Medical Center

524 West Sagamore Avenue
Clewiston, FL 33440
(863) 902-3033

Overall patient safety: ★★★
Teaching: N

CLINICAL PROGRAM RATINGS:

CARDIAC	NR	ORTHOPEDICS	NR
CRITICAL CARE	NR	PULMONARY	★★★
GASTROINTESTINAL	NR	STROKE	★★★
GENERAL SURGERY	NR	VASCULAR	NR
MATERNITY CARE	NR	WOMEN'S HEALTH	NR

HEALTHGRADES AWARDS

Hialeah Hospital

651 East 25th Street
Hialeah, FL 33013
(305) 693-6100

Overall patient safety: ★★★
Teaching: Y

CLINICAL PROGRAM RATINGS:

CARDIAC	NR	ORTHOPEDICS	NR
CRITICAL CARE	★★★	PULMONARY	★★★
GASTROINTESTINAL	NR	STROKE	★★★★★
GENERAL SURGERY	★★★	VASCULAR	NR
MATERNITY CARE	★★★★★	WOMEN'S HEALTH	NR

HEALTHGRADES AWARDS

✓ SPECIALTY EXCELLENCE
· BARIATRIC SURGERY · MATERNITY CARE · STROKE CARE

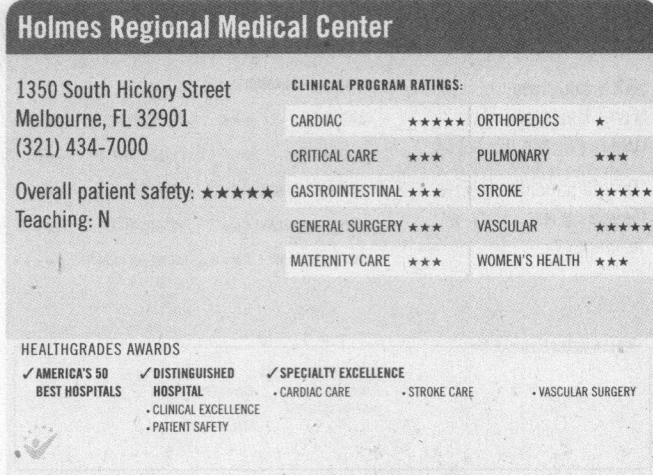

Holmes Regional Medical Center

1350 South Hickory Street
Melbourne, FL 32901
(321) 434-7000

Overall patient safety: ★★★★★
Teaching: N

CLINICAL PROGRAM RATINGS:

CARDIAC	★★★★★	ORTHOPEDICS	★
CRITICAL CARE	★★★	PULMONARY	★★★
GASTROINTESTINAL	★★★	STROKE	★★★★★
GENERAL SURGERY	★★★	VASCULAR	★★★★★
MATERNITY CARE	★★★	WOMEN'S HEALTH	★★★

HEALTHGRADES AWARDS

✓ AMERICA'S 50 BEST HOSPITALS ✓ DISTINGUISHED HOSPITAL · CLINICAL EXCELLENCE · PATIENT SAFETY ✓ SPECIALTY EXCELLENCE · CARDIAC CARE · STROKE CARE · VASCULAR SURGERY

Highlands Regional Medical Center

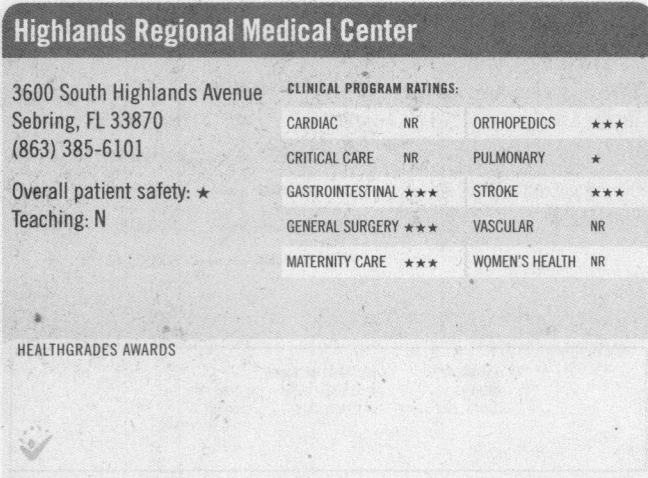

3600 South Highlands Avenue
Sebring, FL 33870
(863) 385-6101

Overall patient safety: ★
Teaching: N

CLINICAL PROGRAM RATINGS:

CARDIAC	NR	ORTHOPEDICS	★★★
CRITICAL CARE	NR	PULMONARY	★
GASTROINTESTINAL	★★★	STROKE	★★★
GENERAL SURGERY	★★★	VASCULAR	NR
MATERNITY CARE	★★★	WOMEN'S HEALTH	NR

HEALTHGRADES AWARDS

Holy Cross Hospital

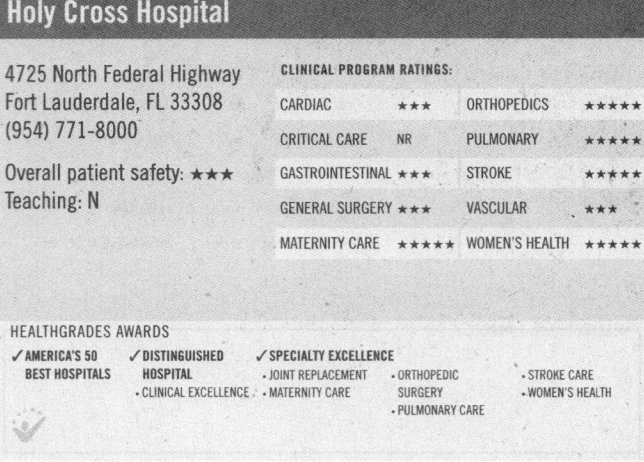

4725 North Federal Highway
Fort Lauderdale, FL 33308
(954) 771-8000

Overall patient safety: ★★★
Teaching: N

CLINICAL PROGRAM RATINGS:

CARDIAC	★★★	ORTHOPEDICS	★★★★★
CRITICAL CARE	NR	PULMONARY	★★★★★
GASTROINTESTINAL	★★★	STROKE	★★★★★
GENERAL SURGERY	★★★	VASCULAR	★★★
MATERNITY CARE	★★★★★	WOMEN'S HEALTH	★★★★★

HEALTHGRADES AWARDS

✓ AMERICA'S 50 BEST HOSPITALS ✓ DISTINGUISHED HOSPITAL · CLINICAL EXCELLENCE ✓ SPECIALTY EXCELLENCE · JOINT REPLACEMENT · MATERNITY CARE · ORTHOPEDIC SURGERY · PULMONARY CARE · STROKE CARE · WOMEN'S HEALTH

Hollywood Medical Center

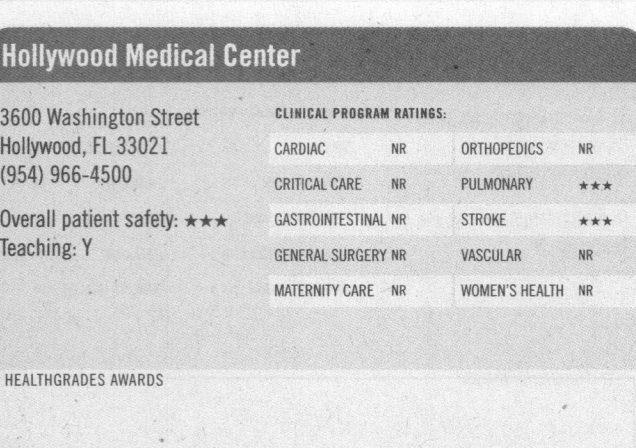

3600 Washington Street
Hollywood, FL 33021
(954) 966-4500

Overall patient safety: ★★★
Teaching: Y

CLINICAL PROGRAM RATINGS:

CARDIAC	NR	ORTHOPEDICS	NR
CRITICAL CARE	NR	PULMONARY	★★★
GASTROINTESTINAL	NR	STROKE	★★★
GENERAL SURGERY	NR	VASCULAR	NR
MATERNITY CARE	NR	WOMEN'S HEALTH	NR

HEALTHGRADES AWARDS

Homestead Hospital

975 Baptist Way
Homestead, FL 33030
(786) 243-8000

Overall patient safety: ★★★
Teaching: N

CLINICAL PROGRAM RATINGS:

CARDIAC	NR	ORTHOPEDICS	NR
CRITICAL CARE	NR	PULMONARY	★★★
GASTROINTESTINAL	NR	STROKE	★★★
GENERAL SURGERY	★★★	VASCULAR	NR
MATERNITY CARE	★★★	WOMEN'S HEALTH	NR

HEALTHGRADES AWARDS

KEY: ★★★★★ BEST ★★★ AS EXPECTED ★ POOR NR NOT RATED BY HEALTHGRADES For full definitions of ratings and awards, see Appendix.

Imperial Point Medical Center

6401 North Federal Highway
Fort Lauderdale, FL 33308
(954) 776-8500

Overall patient safety: ★
Teaching: N

CLINICAL PROGRAM RATINGS:

CARDIAC	NR	ORTHOPEDICS	NR
CRITICAL CARE	NR	PULMONARY	★★★
GASTROINTESTINAL	NR	STROKE	★★★
GENERAL SURGERY	★	VASCULAR	NR
MATERNITY CARE	NR	WOMEN'S HEALTH	NR

HEALTHGRADES AWARDS

Jackson Hospital

4250 Hospital Drive
Marianna, FL 32446
(850) 526-2200

Overall patient safety: ★★★
Teaching: N

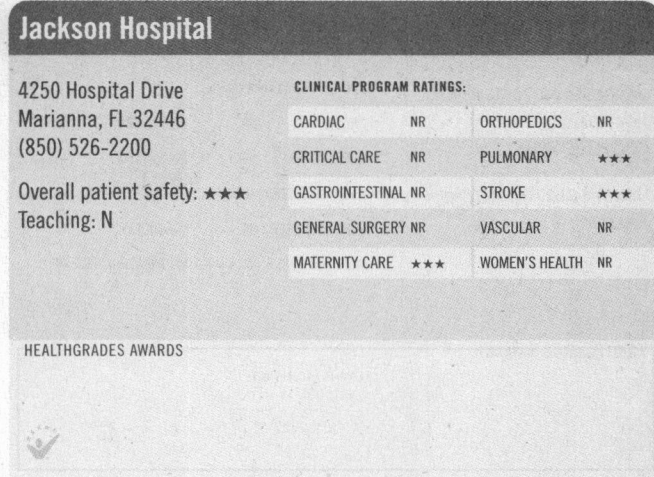

CLINICAL PROGRAM RATINGS:

CARDIAC	NR	ORTHOPEDICS	NR
CRITICAL CARE	NR	PULMONARY	★★★
GASTROINTESTINAL	NR	STROKE	★★★
GENERAL SURGERY	NR	VASCULAR	NR
MATERNITY CARE	★★★	WOMEN'S HEALTH	NR

HEALTHGRADES AWARDS

Indian River Medical Center

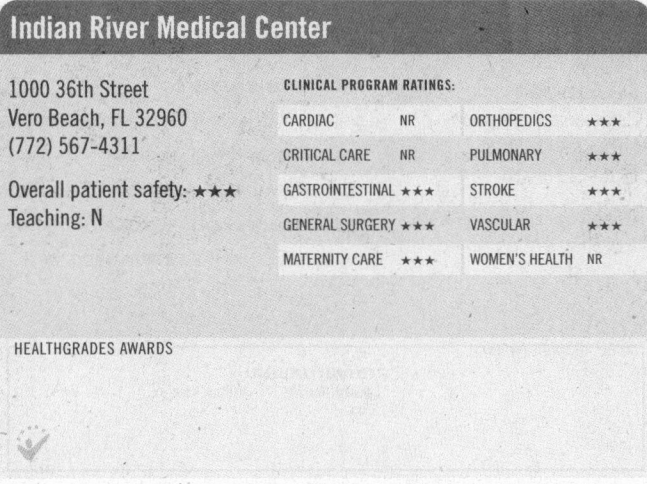

1000 36th Street
Vero Beach, FL 32960
(772) 567-4311

Overall patient safety: ★★★
Teaching: N

CLINICAL PROGRAM RATINGS:

CARDIAC	NR	ORTHOPEDICS	★★★
CRITICAL CARE	NR	PULMONARY	★★★
GASTROINTESTINAL	★★★	STROKE	★★★
GENERAL SURGERY	★★★	VASCULAR	★★★
MATERNITY CARE	★★★	WOMEN'S HEALTH	NR

HEALTHGRADES AWARDS

Jackson North Medical Center

160 Northwest 170th Street
North Miami Beach, FL 33169
(305) 651-1100

Overall patient safety: ★★★
Teaching: Y

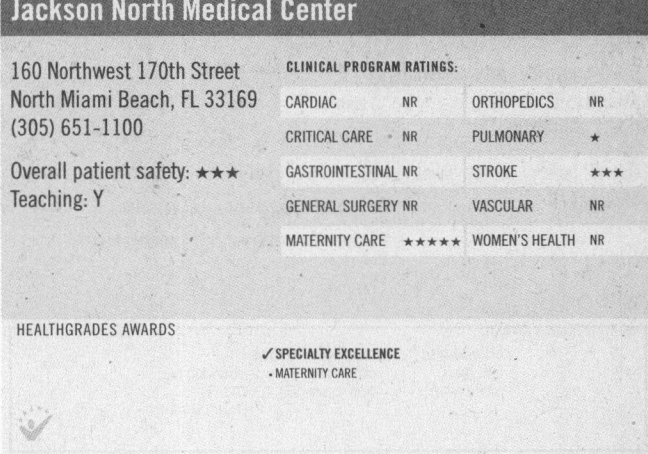

CLINICAL PROGRAM RATINGS:

CARDIAC	NR	ORTHOPEDICS	NR
CRITICAL CARE	NR	PULMONARY	★
GASTROINTESTINAL	NR	STROKE	★★★
GENERAL SURGERY	NR	VASCULAR	NR
MATERNITY CARE	★★★★★	WOMEN'S HEALTH	NR

HEALTHGRADES AWARDS

✓ SPECIALTY EXCELLENCE
· MATERNITY CARE

Jackson Health System*

1611 Northwest 12th Avenue
Miami, FL 33136
(305) 585-1111

Overall patient safety: ★
Teaching: Y

CLINICAL PROGRAM RATINGS:

CARDIAC	★★★	ORTHOPEDICS	NR
CRITICAL CARE	NR	PULMONARY	★★★
GASTROINTESTINAL	★★★	STROKE	★★★
GENERAL SURGERY	★★★	VASCULAR	NR
MATERNITY CARE	★★★	WOMEN'S HEALTH	★

HEALTHGRADES AWARDS

Jackson South Community Hospital*

9333 Southwest 152 Street
Miami, FL 33157
(305) 251-2500

Overall patient safety: ★
Teaching: Y

CLINICAL PROGRAM RATINGS:

CARDIAC	★★★	ORTHOPEDICS	NR
CRITICAL CARE	NR	PULMONARY	★★★
GASTROINTESTINAL	★★★	STROKE	★★★
GENERAL SURGERY	★★★	VASCULAR	NR
MATERNITY CARE	★★★	WOMEN'S HEALTH	★

HEALTHGRADES AWARDS

*This hospital reports its data to the federal government jointly with another hospital. Therefore the ratings and awards apply to multiple hospitals and this specific hospital may not provide all rated services.

FLORIDA HOSPITALS: RATINGS BY CLINICAL SPECIALTY

Jay Hospital

221 South Alabama Street
Jay, FL 32565
(850) 675-8000

Overall patient safety: ★★★
Teaching: N

CLINICAL PROGRAM RATINGS:

CARDIAC	NR	ORTHOPEDICS	NR
CRITICAL CARE	NR	PULMONARY	★★★
GASTROINTESTINAL	NR	STROKE	★★★
GENERAL SURGERY	NR	VASCULAR	NR
MATERNITY CARE	NR	WOMEN'S HEALTH	NR

HEALTHGRADES AWARDS

Kendall Regional Medical Center

11750 Bird Road
Miami, FL 33175
(305) 223-3000

Overall patient safety: ★★★
Teaching: Y

CLINICAL PROGRAM RATINGS:

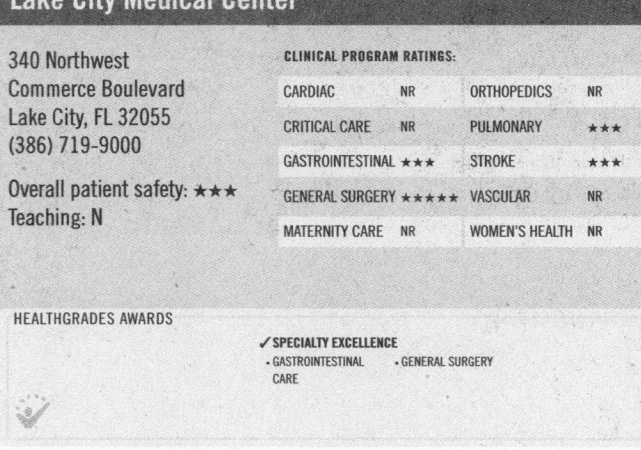

CARDIAC	★★★	ORTHOPEDICS	NR
CRITICAL CARE	★★★★★	PULMONARY	★★★★★
GASTROINTESTINAL	★★★	STROKE	★★★★★
GENERAL SURGERY	★★★	VASCULAR	NR
MATERNITY CARE	★★★★★	WOMEN'S HEALTH	★★★

HEALTHGRADES AWARDS

✓ DISTINGUISHED HOSPITAL
- CLINICAL EXCELLENCE

✓ SPECIALTY EXCELLENCE
- CRITICAL CARE
- MATERNITY CARE
- PULMONARY CARE
- STROKE CARE

JFK Medical Center

5301 South Congress Avenue
Atlantis, FL 33462
(561) 965-7300

Overall patient safety: ★★★★★
Teaching: Y

CLINICAL PROGRAM RATINGS:

CARDIAC	★★★	ORTHOPEDICS	★★★
CRITICAL CARE	★★★	PULMONARY	★★★
GASTROINTESTINAL	★★★	STROKE	★★★
GENERAL SURGERY	★★★★★	VASCULAR	★★★
MATERNITY CARE	NR	WOMEN'S HEALTH	NR

HEALTHGRADES AWARDS

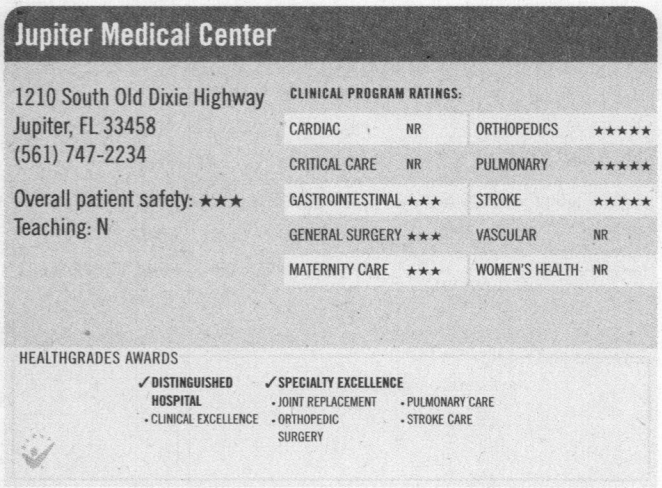

✓ DISTINGUISHED HOSPITAL
- PATIENT SAFETY

✓ SPECIALTY EXCELLENCE
- CARDIAC CARE
- CARDIAC SURGERY
- GASTROINTESTINAL CARE
- GENERAL SURGERY

Lake City Medical Center

340 Northwest
Commerce Boulevard
Lake City, FL 32055
(386) 719-9000

Overall patient safety: ★★★
Teaching: N

CLINICAL PROGRAM RATINGS:

CARDIAC	NR	ORTHOPEDICS	NR
CRITICAL CARE	NR	PULMONARY	★★★
GASTROINTESTINAL	★★★	STROKE	★★★
GENERAL SURGERY	★★★★★	VASCULAR	NR
MATERNITY CARE	NR	WOMEN'S HEALTH	NR

HEALTHGRADES AWARDS

✓ SPECIALTY EXCELLENCE
- GASTROINTESTINAL CARE
- GENERAL SURGERY

Jupiter Medical Center

1210 South Old Dixie Highway
Jupiter, FL 33458
(561) 747-2234

Overall patient safety: ★★★
Teaching: N

CLINICAL PROGRAM RATINGS:

CARDIAC	NR	ORTHOPEDICS	★★★★★
CRITICAL CARE	NR	PULMONARY	★★★★★
GASTROINTESTINAL	★★★	STROKE	★★★★★
GENERAL SURGERY	★★★	VASCULAR	NR
MATERNITY CARE	★★★	WOMEN'S HEALTH	NR

HEALTHGRADES AWARDS

✓ DISTINGUISHED HOSPITAL
- CLINICAL EXCELLENCE

✓ SPECIALTY EXCELLENCE
- JOINT REPLACEMENT
- ORTHOPEDIC SURGERY
- PULMONARY CARE
- STROKE CARE

Lake Wales Medical Center

410 South 11th Street
Lake Wales, FL 33853
(863) 676-1433

Overall patient safety: ★★★
Teaching: N

CLINICAL PROGRAM RATINGS:

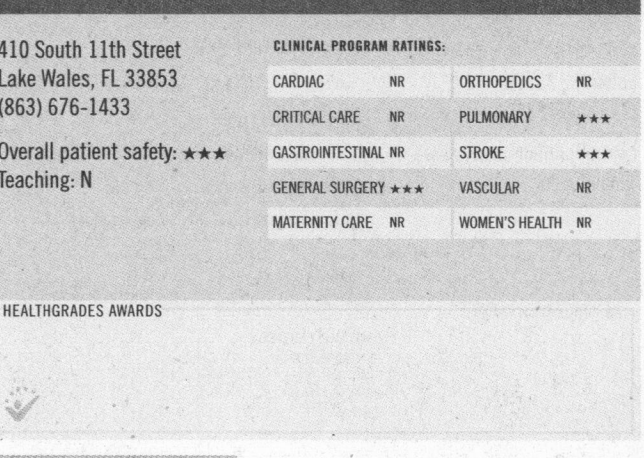

CARDIAC	NR	ORTHOPEDICS	NR
CRITICAL CARE	NR	PULMONARY	★★★
GASTROINTESTINAL	NR	STROKE	★★★
GENERAL SURGERY	★★★	VASCULAR	NR
MATERNITY CARE	NR	WOMEN'S HEALTH	NR

HEALTHGRADES AWARDS

KEY: ★★★★★ BEST   ★★★ AS EXPECTED   ★ POOR   NR NOT RATED BY HEALTHGRADES   For full definitions of ratings and awards, see Appendix.

Lakeland Regional Medical Center

1324 Lakeland Hill Boulevard
Lakeland, FL 33805
(863) 687-1100

Overall patient safety: ★
Teaching: N

CLINICAL PROGRAM RATINGS:

CARDIAC	★★★	ORTHOPEDICS	★★★
CRITICAL CARE	★★★	PULMONARY	★★★★★
GASTROINTESTINAL	★★★	STROKE	★
GENERAL SURGERY	★★★★★	VASCULAR	★★★
MATERNITY CARE	★★★	WOMEN'S HEALTH	★★★

HEALTHGRADES AWARDS

✓ SPECIALTY EXCELLENCE
- GENERAL SURGERY   - JOINT REPLACEMENT

Larkin Community Hospital

7031 Southwest 62nd Avenue
South Miami, FL 33143
(305) 284-7500

Overall patient safety: ★★★
Teaching: Y

CLINICAL PROGRAM RATINGS:

CARDIAC	NR	ORTHOPEDICS	NR
CRITICAL CARE	NR	PULMONARY	★★★
GASTROINTESTINAL	NR	STROKE	★★★
GENERAL SURGERY	NR	VASCULAR	NR
MATERNITY CARE	NR	WOMEN'S HEALTH	NR

HEALTHGRADES AWARDS

Lakewood Ranch Medical Center

8330 Lakewood
Ranch Boulevard
Bradenton, FL 34202
(941) 782-2100

Overall patient safety: ★★★
Teaching: N

CLINICAL PROGRAM RATINGS:

CARDIAC	NR	ORTHOPEDICS	NR
CRITICAL CARE	NR	PULMONARY	★★★
GASTROINTESTINAL	NR	STROKE	★★★
GENERAL SURGERY	NR	VASCULAR	NR
MATERNITY CARE	★★★	WOMEN'S HEALTH	NR

HEALTHGRADES AWARDS

Lawnwood Regional Medical Center and Heart Institute

1700 South 23rd Street
Fort Pierce, FL 34950
(772) 461-4000

Overall patient safety: ★★★★★
Teaching: N

CLINICAL PROGRAM RATINGS:

CARDIAC	★★★★★	ORTHOPEDICS	NR
CRITICAL CARE	★★★	PULMONARY	★★★
GASTROINTESTINAL	★★★	STROKE	★★★★★
GENERAL SURGERY	★★★	VASCULAR	NR
MATERNITY CARE	★★★	WOMEN'S HEALTH	★★★

HEALTHGRADES AWARDS

✓ AMERICA'S 50   ✓ DISTINGUISHED   ✓ SPECIALTY EXCELLENCE
BEST HOSPITALS   HOSPITAL   - CARDIAC CARE   - GENERAL SURGERY   - STROKE CARE
                   - CLINICAL EXCELLENCE
                   - PATIENT SAFETY

Largo Medical Center

201 14th Street Southwest
Largo, FL 33770
(727) 588-5200

Overall patient safety: ★★★
Teaching: N

CLINICAL PROGRAM RATINGS:

CARDIAC	★★★	ORTHOPEDICS	★★★★★
CRITICAL CARE	★★★	PULMONARY	★★★
GASTROINTESTINAL	★★★	STROKE	★★★
GENERAL SURGERY	★★★★★	VASCULAR	★★★★★
MATERNITY CARE	NR	WOMEN'S HEALTH	NR

HEALTHGRADES AWARDS

✓ SPECIALTY EXCELLENCE
- GASTROINTESTINAL   - JOINT REPLACEMENT   - VASCULAR SURGERY
  CARE   - ORTHOPEDIC
- GENERAL SURGERY   SURGERY

Lee Memorial Hospital

2776 Cleveland Avenue
Fort Myers, FL 33902
(239) 332-1111

Overall patient safety: ★★★★★
Teaching: N

CLINICAL PROGRAM RATINGS:

CARDIAC	★★★	ORTHOPEDICS	★★★
CRITICAL CARE	NR	PULMONARY	★★★★★
GASTROINTESTINAL	★★★	STROKE	★★★
GENERAL SURGERY	★★★	VASCULAR	★★★
MATERNITY CARE	★★★	WOMEN'S HEALTH	★★★★★

HEALTHGRADES AWARDS

✓ DISTINGUISHED   ✓ SPECIALTY EXCELLENCE
HOSPITAL   - PULMONARY CARE   - WOMEN'S HEALTH
- CLINICAL EXCELLENCE
- PATIENT SAFETY

Leesburg Regional Medical Center

600 East Dixie Avenue
Leesburg, FL 34748
(352) 323-5762

Overall patient safety: ★★★★★
Teaching: N

CLINICAL PROGRAM RATINGS:

CARDIAC	★★★	ORTHOPEDICS	★★★
CRITICAL CARE	★★★	PULMONARY	★★★
GASTROINTESTINAL	★★★	STROKE	★★★★★
GENERAL SURGERY	★★★	VASCULAR	★★★
MATERNITY CARE	★★★	WOMEN'S HEALTH	★★★

HEALTHGRADES AWARDS

✓ DISTINGUISHED HOSPITAL
• PATIENT SAFETY

✓ SPECIALTY EXCELLENCE
• STROKE CARE

Lucerne Medical Center*

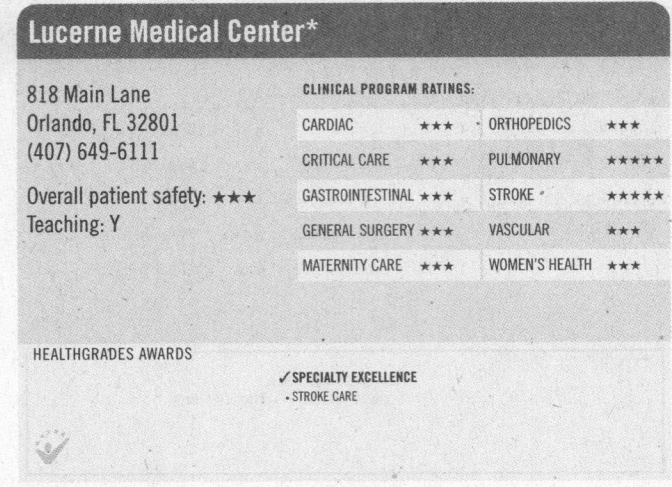

818 Main Lane
Orlando, FL 32801
(407) 649-6111

Overall patient safety: ★★★
Teaching: Y

CLINICAL PROGRAM RATINGS:

CARDIAC	★★★	ORTHOPEDICS	★★★
CRITICAL CARE	★★★	PULMONARY	★★★★★
GASTROINTESTINAL	★★★	STROKE	★★★★★
GENERAL SURGERY	★★★	VASCULAR	★★★
MATERNITY CARE	★★★	WOMEN'S HEALTH	★★★

HEALTHGRADES AWARDS

✓ SPECIALTY EXCELLENCE
• STROKE CARE

Lehigh Regional Medical Center

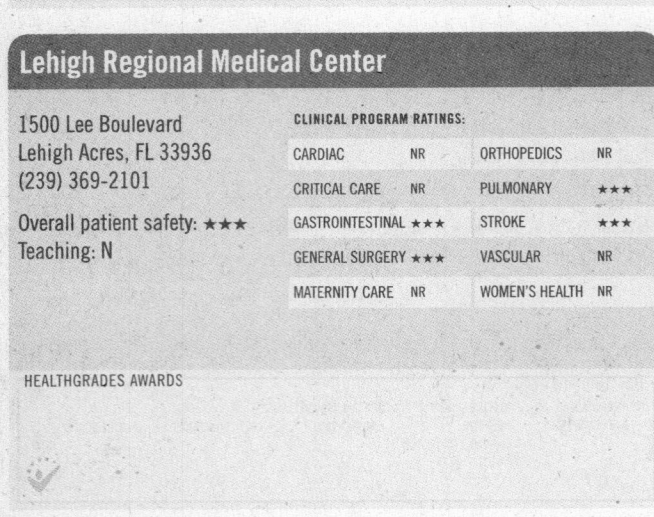

1500 Lee Boulevard
Lehigh Acres, FL 33936
(239) 369-2101

Overall patient safety: ★★★
Teaching: N

CLINICAL PROGRAM RATINGS:

CARDIAC	NR	ORTHOPEDICS	NR
CRITICAL CARE	NR	PULMONARY	★★★
GASTROINTESTINAL	★★★	STROKE	★★★
GENERAL SURGERY	★★★	VASCULAR	NR
MATERNITY CARE	NR	WOMEN'S HEALTH	NR

HEALTHGRADES AWARDS

Madison County Memorial Hospital

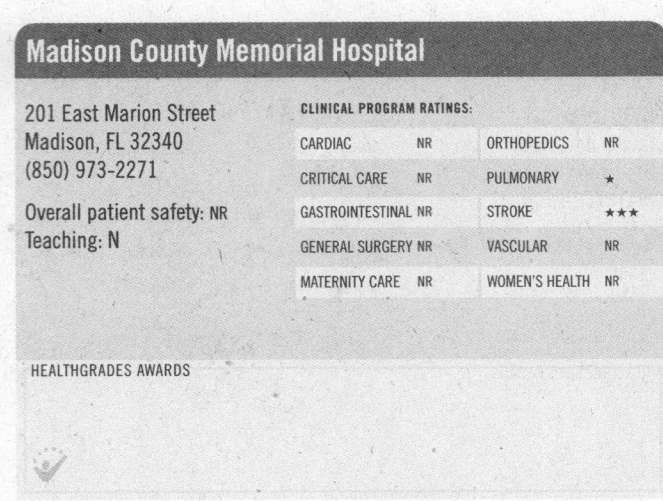

201 East Marion Street
Madison, FL 32340
(850) 973-2271

Overall patient safety: NR
Teaching: N

CLINICAL PROGRAM RATINGS:

CARDIAC	NR	ORTHOPEDICS	NR
CRITICAL CARE	NR	PULMONARY	★
GASTROINTESTINAL	NR	STROKE	★★★
GENERAL SURGERY	NR	VASCULAR	NR
MATERNITY CARE	NR	WOMEN'S HEALTH	NR

HEALTHGRADES AWARDS

Lower Keys Medical Center

5900 College Road
Key West, FL 33040
(305) 294-5531

Overall patient safety: ★★★
Teaching: N

CLINICAL PROGRAM RATINGS:

CARDIAC	NR	ORTHOPEDICS	NR
CRITICAL CARE	NR	PULMONARY	★★★
GASTROINTESTINAL	NR	STROKE	★★★
GENERAL SURGERY	★★★	VASCULAR	NR
MATERNITY CARE	★★★★★	WOMEN'S HEALTH	NR

HEALTHGRADES AWARDS

✓ SPECIALTY EXCELLENCE
• MATERNITY CARE

Manatee Memorial Hospital

206 2nd Street East
Bradenton, FL 34208
(941) 746-5111

Overall patient safety: ★★★★★
Teaching: N

CLINICAL PROGRAM RATINGS:

CARDIAC	★★★	ORTHOPEDICS	★★★
CRITICAL CARE	NR	PULMONARY	★★★
GASTROINTESTINAL	★★★	STROKE	★★★
GENERAL SURGERY	★★★	VASCULAR	★★★
MATERNITY CARE	★★★★★	WOMEN'S HEALTH	★★★

HEALTHGRADES AWARDS

✓ DISTINGUISHED HOSPITAL
• PATIENT SAFETY

✓ SPECIALTY EXCELLENCE
• MATERNITY CARE

KEY: ★★★★★ BEST   ★★★ AS EXPECTED   ★ POOR   NR NOT RATED BY HEALTHGRADES   For full definitions of ratings and awards, see Appendix.

Mariners Hospital

91500 Overseas Highway
Tavernier, FL 33070
(305) 434-3000

Overall patient safety: ★★★
Teaching: N

CLINICAL PROGRAM RATINGS:

CARDIAC	NR	ORTHOPEDICS	NR
CRITICAL CARE	NR	PULMONARY	★★★
GASTROINTESTINAL	NR	STROKE	★★★
GENERAL SURGERY	NR	VASCULAR	NR
MATERNITY CARE	NR	WOMEN'S HEALTH	NR

HEALTHGRADES AWARDS

Memorial Hospital—Jacksonville

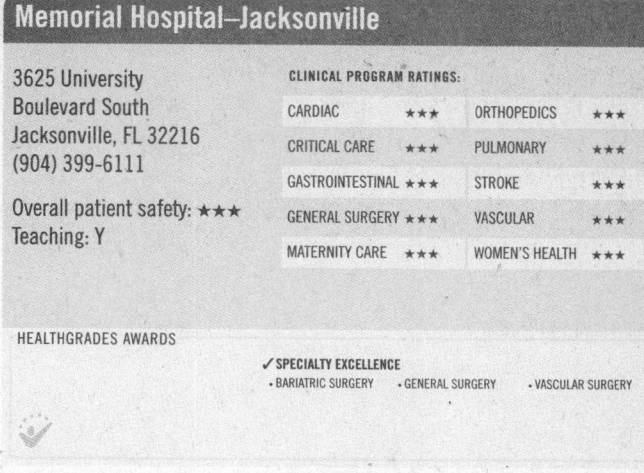

3625 University
Boulevard South
Jacksonville, FL 32216
(904) 399-6111

Overall patient safety: ★★★
Teaching: Y

CLINICAL PROGRAM RATINGS:

CARDIAC	★★★	ORTHOPEDICS	★★★
CRITICAL CARE	★★★	PULMONARY	★★★
GASTROINTESTINAL	★★★	STROKE	★★★
GENERAL SURGERY	★★★	VASCULAR	★★★
MATERNITY CARE	★★★	WOMEN'S HEALTH	★★★

HEALTHGRADES AWARDS

✓ **SPECIALTY EXCELLENCE**
· BARIATRIC SURGERY   · GENERAL SURGERY   · VASCULAR SURGERY

Martin Memorial Medical Center

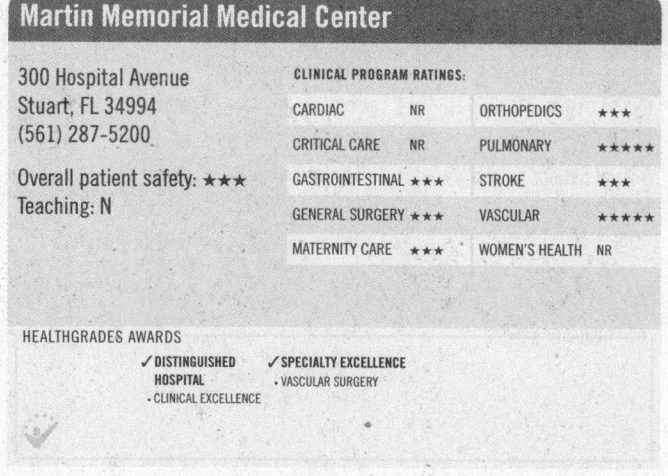

300 Hospital Avenue
Stuart, FL 34994
(561) 287-5200

Overall patient safety: ★★★
Teaching: N

CLINICAL PROGRAM RATINGS:

CARDIAC	NR	ORTHOPEDICS	★★★
CRITICAL CARE	NR	PULMONARY	★★★★★
GASTROINTESTINAL	★★★	STROKE	★★★
GENERAL SURGERY	★★★	VASCULAR	★★★★★
MATERNITY CARE	★★★	WOMEN'S HEALTH	NR

HEALTHGRADES AWARDS

✓ **DISTINGUISHED HOSPITAL**   ✓ **SPECIALTY EXCELLENCE**
· CLINICAL EXCELLENCE   · VASCULAR SURGERY

Memorial Hospital—Miramar

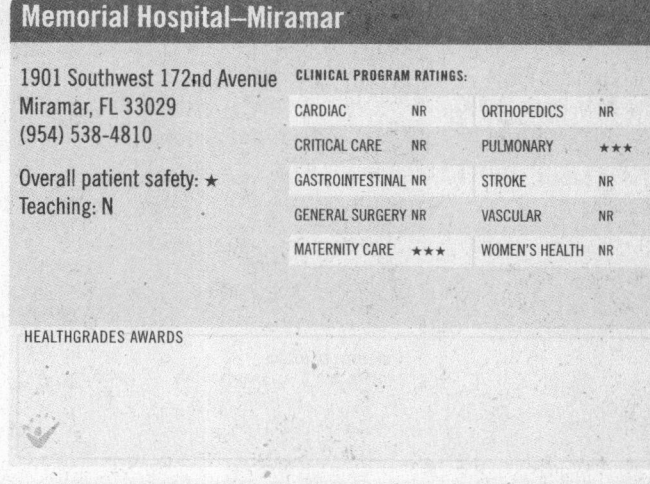

1901 Southwest 172nd Avenue
Miramar, FL 33029
(954) 538-4810

Overall patient safety: ★
Teaching: N

CLINICAL PROGRAM RATINGS:

CARDIAC	NR	ORTHOPEDICS	NR
CRITICAL CARE	NR	PULMONARY	★★★
GASTROINTESTINAL	NR	STROKE	NR
GENERAL SURGERY	NR	VASCULAR	NR
MATERNITY CARE	★★★	WOMEN'S HEALTH	NR

HEALTHGRADES AWARDS

Mease Healthcare Dunedin

601 Main Street
Dunedin, FL 34698
(727) 733-1111

Overall patient safety: ★★★
Teaching: N

CLINICAL PROGRAM RATINGS:

CARDIAC	NR	ORTHOPEDICS	★★★
CRITICAL CARE	NR	PULMONARY	★★★★★
GASTROINTESTINAL	★★★	STROKE	★★★
GENERAL SURGERY	★★★	VASCULAR	NR
MATERNITY CARE	★★★	WOMEN'S HEALTH	NR

HEALTHGRADES AWARDS

✓ **SPECIALTY EXCELLENCE**
· PULMONARY CARE

Memorial Hospital—Pembroke

7800 Sheridan Street
Pembroke Pines, FL 33024
(954) 962-9650

Overall patient safety: ★★★
Teaching: N

CLINICAL PROGRAM RATINGS:

CARDIAC	NR	ORTHOPEDICS	NR
CRITICAL CARE	NR	PULMONARY	★★★★★
GASTROINTESTINAL	NR	STROKE	★★★
GENERAL SURGERY	★★★	VASCULAR	NR
MATERNITY CARE	NR	WOMEN'S HEALTH	NR

HEALTHGRADES AWARDS

✓ **SPECIALTY EXCELLENCE**
· PULMONARY CARE

---

*This hospital reports its data to the federal government jointly with another hospital. Therefore the ratings and awards apply to multiple hospitals and this specific hospital may not provide all rated services.

FLORIDA HOSPITALS: RATINGS BY CLINICAL SPECIALTY

Memorial Hospital—Tampa

2901 Swann Avenue
Tampa, FL 33609
(813) 873-6400

Overall patient safety: ★★★
Teaching: N

CLINICAL PROGRAM RATINGS:

CARDIAC	NR	ORTHOPEDICS	NR
CRITICAL CARE	NR	PULMONARY	★★★★★
GASTROINTESTINAL	★★★	STROKE	★★★
GENERAL SURGERY	★★★	VASCULAR	NR
MATERNITY CARE	NR	WOMEN'S HEALTH	NR

HEALTHGRADES AWARDS

Mercy Hospital

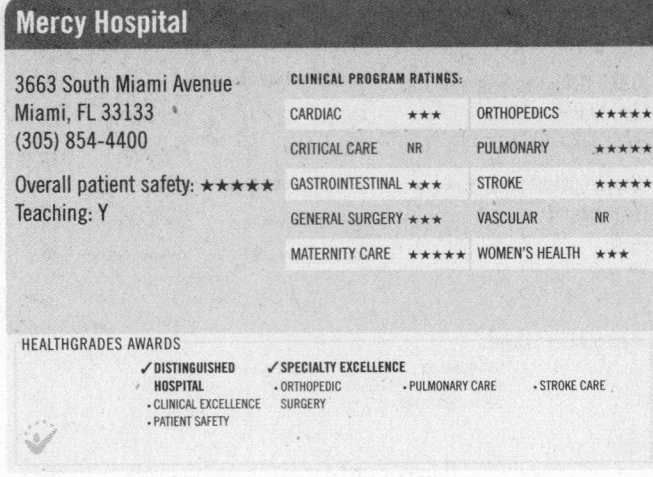

3663 South Miami Avenue
Miami, FL 33133
(305) 854-4400

Overall patient safety: ★★★★★
Teaching: Y

CLINICAL PROGRAM RATINGS:

CARDIAC	★★★	ORTHOPEDICS	★★★★★
CRITICAL CARE	NR	PULMONARY	★★★★★
GASTROINTESTINAL	★★★	STROKE	★★★★★
GENERAL SURGERY	★★★	VASCULAR	NR
MATERNITY CARE	★★★★★	WOMEN'S HEALTH	★★★

HEALTHGRADES AWARDS

✓ **DISTINGUISHED HOSPITAL**
· CLINICAL EXCELLENCE
· PATIENT SAFETY

✓ **SPECIALTY EXCELLENCE**
· ORTHOPEDIC SURGERY   · PULMONARY CARE   · STROKE CARE

Memorial Hospital—West

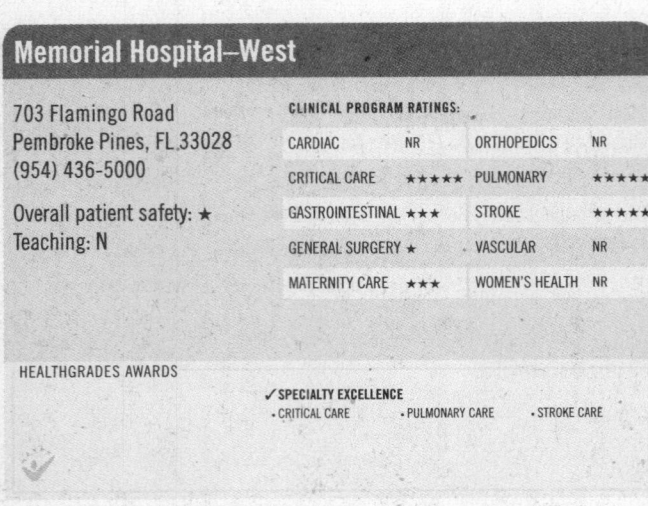

703 Flamingo Road
Pembroke Pines, FL 33028
(954) 436-5000

Overall patient safety: ★
Teaching: N

CLINICAL PROGRAM RATINGS:

CARDIAC	NR	ORTHOPEDICS	NR
CRITICAL CARE	★★★★★	PULMONARY	★★★★★
GASTROINTESTINAL	★★★	STROKE	★★★★★
GENERAL SURGERY	★	VASCULAR	NR
MATERNITY CARE	★★★	WOMEN'S HEALTH	NR

HEALTHGRADES AWARDS

✓ **SPECIALTY EXCELLENCE**
· CRITICAL CARE   · PULMONARY CARE   · STROKE CARE

Miami Beach Community Hospital*

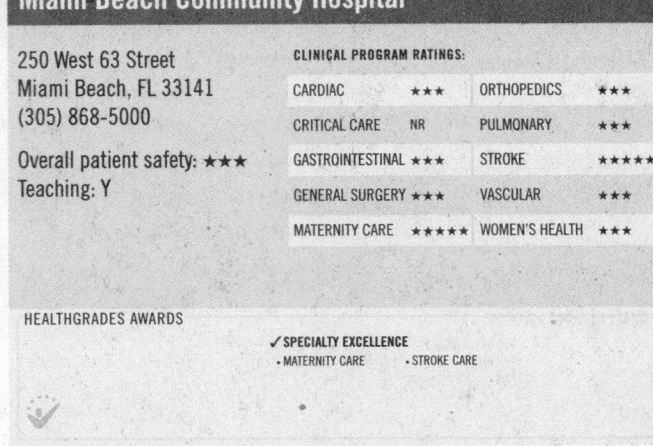

250 West 63 Street
Miami Beach, FL 33141
(305) 868-5000

Overall patient safety: ★★★
Teaching: Y

CLINICAL PROGRAM RATINGS:

CARDIAC	★★★	ORTHOPEDICS	★★★
CRITICAL CARE	NR	PULMONARY	★★★
GASTROINTESTINAL	★★★	STROKE	★★★★★
GENERAL SURGERY	★★★	VASCULAR	★★★
MATERNITY CARE	★★★★★	WOMEN'S HEALTH	★★★

HEALTHGRADES AWARDS

✓ **SPECIALTY EXCELLENCE**
· MATERNITY CARE   · STROKE CARE

Memorial Regional Hospital

3501 Johnson Street
Hollywood, FL 33021
(954) 987-2000

Overall patient safety: ★
Teaching: Y

CLINICAL PROGRAM RATINGS:

CARDIAC	★★★	ORTHOPEDICS	★★★
CRITICAL CARE	★★★★★	PULMONARY	★★★
GASTROINTESTINAL	★★★	STROKE	★★★
GENERAL SURGERY	★★★	VASCULAR	★★★
MATERNITY CARE	★★★★★	WOMEN'S HEALTH	★★★

HEALTHGRADES AWARDS

✓ **SPECIALTY EXCELLENCE**
· CRITICAL CARE   · MATERNITY CARE

Morton Plant Hospital

300 Pinellas Street
Clearwater, FL 33756
(727) 462-7000

Overall patient safety: ★★★★★
Teaching: Y

CLINICAL PROGRAM RATINGS:

CARDIAC	★★★	ORTHOPEDICS	★★★
CRITICAL CARE	NR	PULMONARY	★★★
GASTROINTESTINAL	★★★	STROKE	★★★
GENERAL SURGERY	★★★★★	VASCULAR	★★★
MATERNITY CARE	★★★	WOMEN'S HEALTH	★★★

HEALTHGRADES AWARDS

✓ **DISTINGUISHED HOSPITAL**
· PATIENT SAFETY

✓ **SPECIALTY EXCELLENCE**
· GASTROINTESTINAL CARE   · GENERAL SURGERY

KEY: ★★★★★ BEST   ★★★ AS EXPECTED   ★ POOR   NR NOT RATED BY HEALTHGRADES   For full definitions of ratings and awards, see Appendix.

Morton Plant Mease Healthcare Countryside

3231 McMullen Booth Road
Safety Harbor, FL 34695
(727) 725-6111

Overall patient safety: ★★★
Teaching: N

CLINICAL PROGRAM RATINGS:

CARDIAC	NR	ORTHOPEDICS	★★★★★
CRITICAL CARE	NR	PULMONARY	★★★★★
GASTROINTESTINAL	★★★	STROKE	★★★
GENERAL SURGERY	★★★	VASCULAR	★★★
MATERNITY CARE	★★★	WOMEN'S HEALTH	NR

HEALTHGRADES AWARDS

✓ **DISTINGUISHED HOSPITAL**
- CLINICAL EXCELLENCE

✓ **SPECIALTY EXCELLENCE**
- PULMONARY CARE

Mt. Sinai Medical Center and Miami Heart Institute*

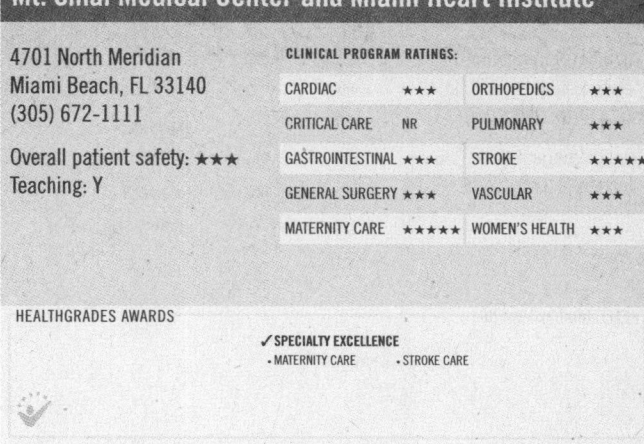

4701 North Meridian
Miami Beach, FL 33140
(305) 672-1111

Overall patient safety: ★★★
Teaching: Y

CLINICAL PROGRAM RATINGS:

CARDIAC	★★★	ORTHOPEDICS	★★★
CRITICAL CARE	NR	PULMONARY	★★★
GASTROINTESTINAL	★★★	STROKE	★★★★★
GENERAL SURGERY	★★★	VASCULAR	★★★
MATERNITY CARE	★★★★★	WOMEN'S HEALTH	★★★

HEALTHGRADES AWARDS

✓ **SPECIALTY EXCELLENCE**
- MATERNITY CARE
- STROKE CARE

Morton Plant North Bay Hospital

6600 Madison Street
New Port Richey, FL 34652
(727) 842-8468

Overall patient safety: ★
Teaching: N

CLINICAL PROGRAM RATINGS:

CARDIAC	NR	ORTHOPEDICS	NR
CRITICAL CARE	NR	PULMONARY	★★★
GASTROINTESTINAL	NR	STROKE	★★★
GENERAL SURGERY	★★★	VASCULAR	NR
MATERNITY CARE	NR	WOMEN'S HEALTH	NR

HEALTHGRADES AWARDS

Munroe Regional Medical Center

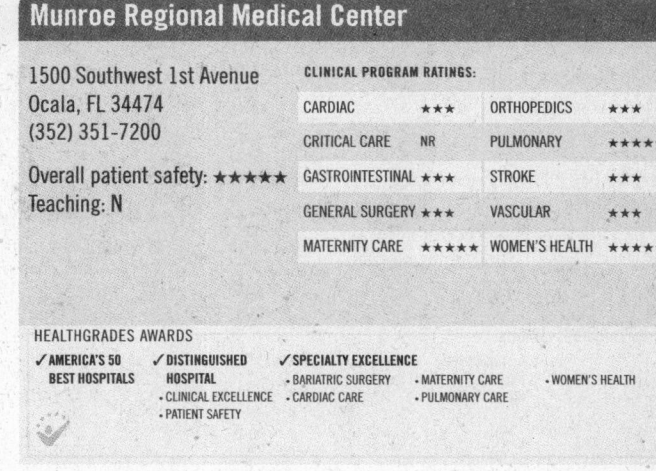

1500 Southwest 1st Avenue
Ocala, FL 34474
(352) 351-7200

Overall patient safety: ★★★★★
Teaching: N

CLINICAL PROGRAM RATINGS:

CARDIAC	★★★	ORTHOPEDICS	★★★
CRITICAL CARE	NR	PULMONARY	★★★★★
GASTROINTESTINAL	★★★	STROKE	★★★
GENERAL SURGERY	★★★	VASCULAR	★★★
MATERNITY CARE	★★★★★	WOMEN'S HEALTH	★★★★★

HEALTHGRADES AWARDS

✓ **AMERICA'S 50 BEST HOSPITALS**

✓ **DISTINGUISHED HOSPITAL**
- CLINICAL EXCELLENCE
- PATIENT SAFETY

✓ **SPECIALTY EXCELLENCE**
- BARIATRIC SURGERY
- CARDIAC CARE
- MATERNITY CARE
- PULMONARY CARE
- WOMEN'S HEALTH

Mt. Sinai Medical Center*

4300 Alton Road
Miami Beach, FL 33140
(305) 674-2121

Overall patient safety: ★★★
Teaching: Y

CLINICAL PROGRAM RATINGS:

CARDIAC	★★★	ORTHOPEDICS	★★★
CRITICAL CARE	NR	PULMONARY	★★★
GASTROINTESTINAL	★★★	STROKE	★★★★★
GENERAL SURGERY	★★★	VASCULAR	★★★
MATERNITY CARE	★★★★★	WOMEN'S HEALTH	★★★

HEALTHGRADES AWARDS

✓ **SPECIALTY EXCELLENCE**
- MATERNITY CARE
- STROKE CARE

NCH Healthcare System

350 7th Street North
Naples, FL 34102
(239) 436-5000

Overall patient safety: ★★★★★
Teaching: N

CLINICAL PROGRAM RATINGS:

CARDIAC	★★★★★	ORTHOPEDICS	★★★
CRITICAL CARE	NR	PULMONARY	★★★★★
GASTROINTESTINAL	★★★	STROKE	★★★
GENERAL SURGERY	★★★	VASCULAR	★★★
MATERNITY CARE	★★★★★	WOMEN'S HEALTH	★★★★★

HEALTHGRADES AWARDS

✓ **DISTINGUISHED HOSPITAL**
- CLINICAL EXCELLENCE
- PATIENT SAFETY

✓ **SPECIALTY EXCELLENCE**
- CARDIAC CARE
- CARDIAC SURGERY
- PULMONARY CARE
- WOMEN'S HEALTH

*This hospital reports its data to the federal government jointly with another hospital. Therefore the ratings and awards apply to multiple hospitals and this specific hospital may not provide all rated services.

FLORIDA HOSPITALS: RATINGS BY CLINICAL SPECIALTY

FLORIDA HOSPITALS: RATINGS BY CLINICAL SPECIALTY

North Broward Medical Center

201 East Sample Road
Deerfield Beach, FL 33064
(954) 941-8300

Overall patient safety: ★★★
Teaching: N

CLINICAL PROGRAM RATINGS:

CARDIAC	NR	ORTHOPEDICS	★★★
CRITICAL CARE	NR	PULMONARY	★★★
GASTROINTESTINAL	★★★	STROKE	★★★★★
GENERAL SURGERY	★★★	VASCULAR	NR
MATERNITY CARE	NR	WOMEN'S HEALTH	NR

HEALTHGRADES AWARDS

✓ SPECIALTY EXCELLENCE
• STROKE CARE

North Ridge Medical Center

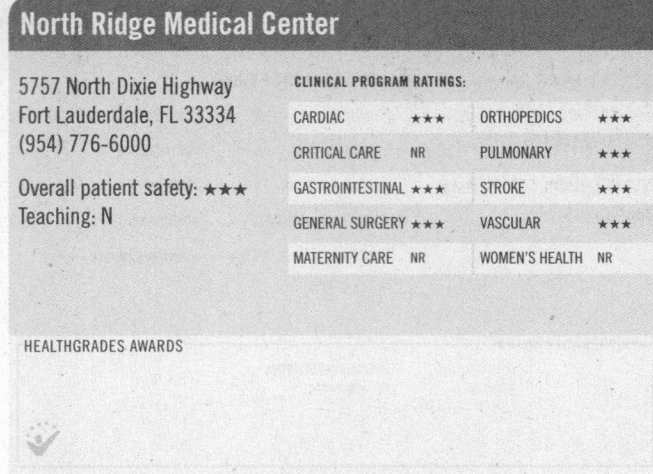

5757 North Dixie Highway
Fort Lauderdale, FL 33334
(954) 776-6000

Overall patient safety: ★★★
Teaching: N

CLINICAL PROGRAM RATINGS:

CARDIAC	★★★	ORTHOPEDICS	★★★
CRITICAL CARE	NR	PULMONARY	★★★
GASTROINTESTINAL	★★★	STROKE	★★★
GENERAL SURGERY	★★★	VASCULAR	★★★
MATERNITY CARE	NR	WOMEN'S HEALTH	NR

HEALTHGRADES AWARDS

North Florida Regional Medical Center

6500 Newberry Road
Gainesville, FL 32605
(352) 333-4000

Overall patient safety: ★★★★★
Teaching: N

CLINICAL PROGRAM RATINGS:

CARDIAC	★★★	ORTHOPEDICS	★★★
CRITICAL CARE	★★★	PULMONARY	★★★
GASTROINTESTINAL	★★★	STROKE	★★★
GENERAL SURGERY	★★★★★	VASCULAR	★★★
MATERNITY CARE	★★★	WOMEN'S HEALTH	★★★

HEALTHGRADES AWARDS

✓ DISTINGUISHED HOSPITAL
• PATIENT SAFETY

✓ SPECIALTY EXCELLENCE
• GENERAL SURGERY

North Shore Medical Center

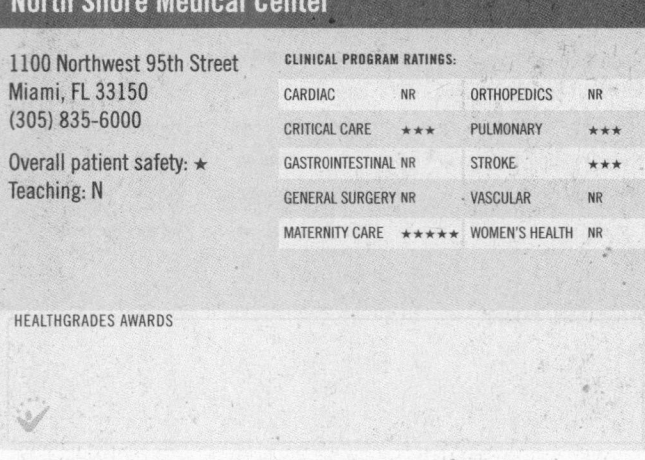

1100 Northwest 95th Street
Miami, FL 33150
(305) 835-6000

Overall patient safety: ★
Teaching: N

CLINICAL PROGRAM RATINGS:

CARDIAC	NR	ORTHOPEDICS	NR
CRITICAL CARE	★★★	PULMONARY	★★★
GASTROINTESTINAL	NR	STROKE	★★★
GENERAL SURGERY	NR	VASCULAR	NR
MATERNITY CARE	★★★★★	WOMEN'S HEALTH	NR

HEALTHGRADES AWARDS

North Okaloosa Medical Center

151 East Redstone Avenue
Crestview, FL 32539
(850) 689-8100

Overall patient safety: ★★★
Teaching: N

CLINICAL PROGRAM RATINGS:

CARDIAC	NR	ORTHOPEDICS	NR
CRITICAL CARE	NR	PULMONARY	★★★★★
GASTROINTESTINAL	NR	STROKE	★★★
GENERAL SURGERY	★★★	VASCULAR	NR
MATERNITY CARE	★	WOMEN'S HEALTH	NR

HEALTHGRADES AWARDS

✓ SPECIALTY EXCELLENCE
• PULMONARY CARE

Northside Hospital

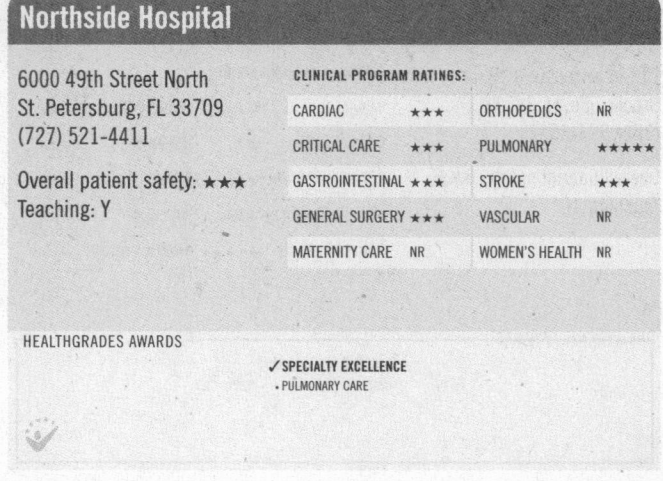

6000 49th Street North
St. Petersburg, FL 33709
(727) 521-4411

Overall patient safety: ★★★
Teaching: Y

CLINICAL PROGRAM RATINGS:

CARDIAC	★★★	ORTHOPEDICS	NR
CRITICAL CARE	★★★	PULMONARY	★★★★★
GASTROINTESTINAL	★★★	STROKE	★★★
GENERAL SURGERY	★★★	VASCULAR	NR
MATERNITY CARE	NR	WOMEN'S HEALTH	NR

HEALTHGRADES AWARDS

✓ SPECIALTY EXCELLENCE
• PULMONARY CARE

KEY: ★★★★★ BEST ★★★ AS EXPECTED ★ POOR NR NOT RATED BY HEALTHGRADES For full definitions of ratings and awards, see Appendix.

© Copyright 2008 HealthGrades, Inc. Use of this information is governed by the HealthGrades User Agreement, which can be viewed at www.healthgrades.com.

Northwest Florida Community Hospital

1360 Brickyard Road
Chipley, FL 32428
(850) 638-1610

Overall patient safety: ★★★
Teaching: N

CLINICAL PROGRAM RATINGS:

CARDIAC	NR	ORTHOPEDICS	NR
CRITICAL CARE	NR	PULMONARY	★
GASTROINTESTINAL	NR	STROKE	NR
GENERAL SURGERY	NR	VASCULAR	NR
MATERNITY CARE	NR	WOMEN'S HEALTH	NR

HEALTHGRADES AWARDS

Ocala Regional Medical Center

1431 Southwest 1st Avenue
Ocala, FL 34474
(352) 401-1000

Overall patient safety: ★★★
Teaching: N

CLINICAL PROGRAM RATINGS:

CARDIAC	★★★	ORTHOPEDICS	★★★
CRITICAL CARE	★★★	PULMONARY	★★★★★
GASTROINTESTINAL	★★★	STROKE	★★★
GENERAL SURGERY	★★★★★	VASCULAR	NR
MATERNITY CARE	★★★	WOMEN'S HEALTH	★★★

HEALTHGRADES AWARDS

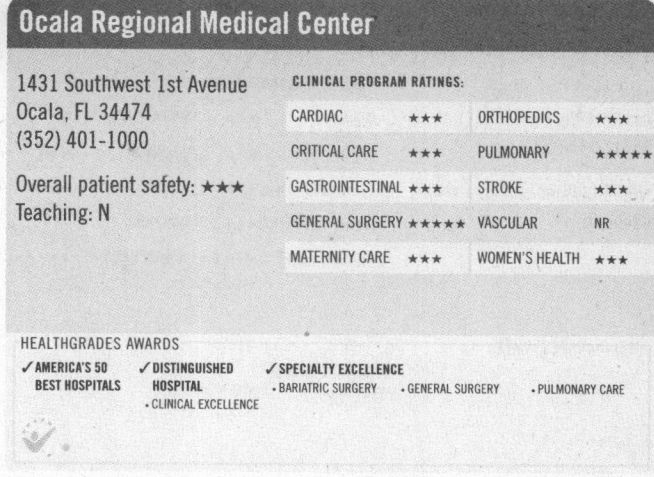

✓ AMERICA'S 50 BEST HOSPITALS   ✓ DISTINGUISHED HOSPITAL · CLINICAL EXCELLENCE   ✓ SPECIALTY EXCELLENCE · BARIATRIC SURGERY · GENERAL SURGERY · PULMONARY CARE

Northwest Medical Center

2801 North State Road 7
Margate, FL 33063
(954) 974-0400

Overall patient safety: ★★★
Teaching: Y

CLINICAL PROGRAM RATINGS:

CARDIAC	NR	ORTHOPEDICS	NR
CRITICAL CARE	★★★	PULMONARY	★★★
GASTROINTESTINAL	★★★	STROKE	★★★
GENERAL SURGERY	★★★	VASCULAR	NR
MATERNITY CARE	★★★★★	WOMEN'S HEALTH	NR

HEALTHGRADES AWARDS

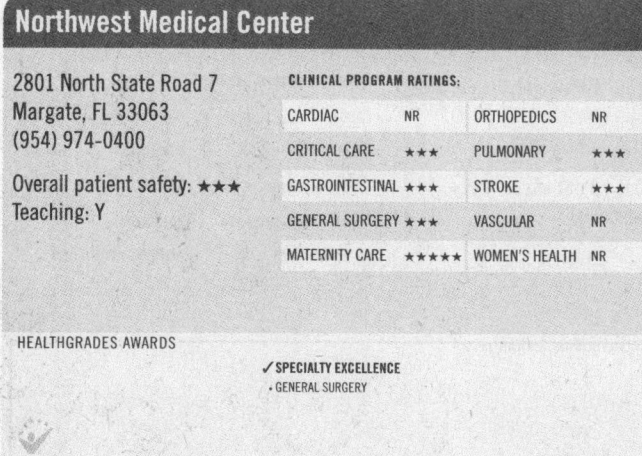

✓ SPECIALTY EXCELLENCE · GENERAL SURGERY

Orange Park Medical Center

2001 Kingsley Avenue
Orange Park, FL 32073
(904) 276-8500

Overall patient safety: ★★★
Teaching: N

CLINICAL PROGRAM RATINGS:

CARDIAC	NR	ORTHOPEDICS	★★★
CRITICAL CARE	★★★	PULMONARY	★★★★★
GASTROINTESTINAL	★★★	STROKE	★★★
GENERAL SURGERY	★★★	VASCULAR	NR
MATERNITY CARE	★★★★★	WOMEN'S HEALTH	NR

HEALTHGRADES AWARDS

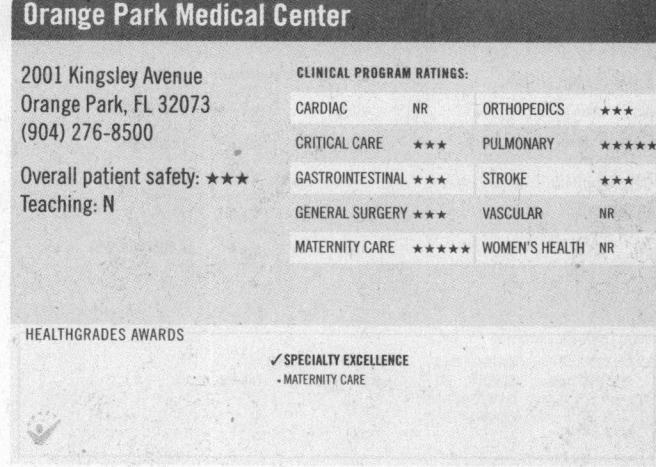

✓ SPECIALTY EXCELLENCE · MATERNITY CARE

Oak Hill Hospital

11375 Cortez Boulevard
Brooksville, FL 34613
(352) 596-6632

Overall patient safety: ★★★
Teaching: N

CLINICAL PROGRAM RATINGS:

CARDIAC	NR	ORTHOPEDICS	★★★
CRITICAL CARE	★★★	PULMONARY	★★★
GASTROINTESTINAL	★★★	STROKE	★★★★★
GENERAL SURGERY	★★★	VASCULAR	★★★
MATERNITY CARE	NR	WOMEN'S HEALTH	NR

HEALTHGRADES AWARDS

✓ SPECIALTY EXCELLENCE · STROKE CARE

Orlando Regional Healthcare*

1414 Kuhl Avenue
Orlando, FL 32806
(407) 841-5111

Overall patient safety: ★★★
Teaching: Y

CLINICAL PROGRAM RATINGS:

CARDIAC	★★★	ORTHOPEDICS	★★★
CRITICAL CARE	★★★	PULMONARY	★★★★★
GASTROINTESTINAL	★★★	STROKE	★★★★★
GENERAL SURGERY	★★★	VASCULAR	★★★
MATERNITY CARE	★★★	WOMEN'S HEALTH	★★★

HEALTHGRADES AWARDS

✓ SPECIALTY EXCELLENCE · STROKE CARE

*This hospital reports its data to the federal government jointly with another hospital. Therefore the ratings and awards apply to multiple hospitals and this specific hospital may not provide all rated services.

FLORIDA HOSPITALS: RATINGS BY CLINICAL SPECIALTY

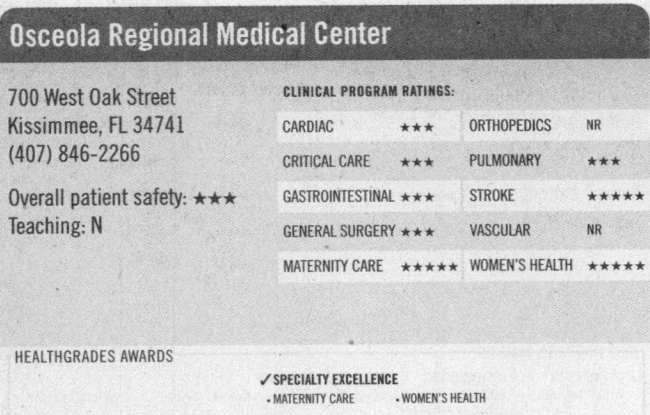

Osceola Regional Medical Center

700 West Oak Street
Kissimmee, FL 34741
(407) 846-2266

Overall patient safety: ★★★
Teaching: N

CLINICAL PROGRAM RATINGS:

CARDIAC	★★★	ORTHOPEDICS	NR
CRITICAL CARE	★★★	PULMONARY	★★★
GASTROINTESTINAL	★★★	STROKE	★★★★★
GENERAL SURGERY	★★★	VASCULAR	NR
MATERNITY CARE	★★★★★	WOMEN'S HEALTH	★★★★★

HEALTHGRADES AWARDS

✓ SPECIALTY EXCELLENCE
 · MATERNITY CARE   · WOMEN'S HEALTH

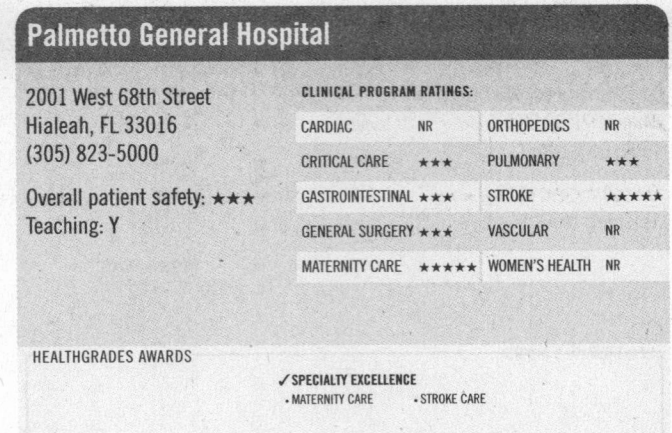

Palmetto General Hospital

2001 West 68th Street
Hialeah, FL 33016
(305) 823-5000

Overall patient safety: ★★★
Teaching: Y

CLINICAL PROGRAM RATINGS:

CARDIAC	NR	ORTHOPEDICS	NR
CRITICAL CARE	★★★	PULMONARY	★★★
GASTROINTESTINAL	★★★	STROKE	★★★★★
GENERAL SURGERY	★★★	VASCULAR	NR
MATERNITY CARE	★★★★★	WOMEN'S HEALTH	NR

HEALTHGRADES AWARDS

✓ SPECIALTY EXCELLENCE
 · MATERNITY CARE   · STROKE CARE

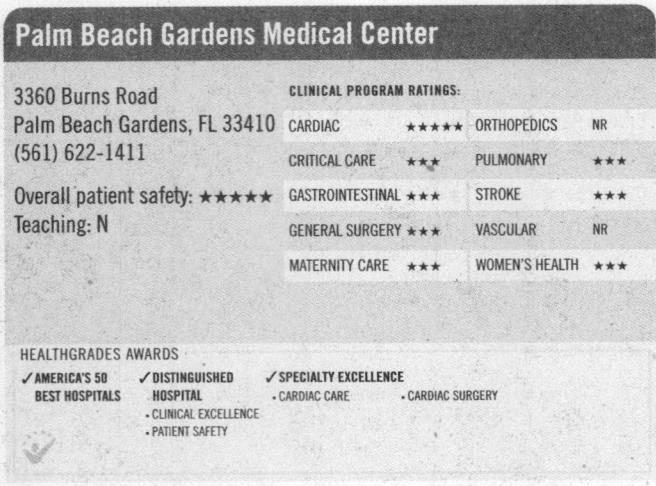

Palm Beach Gardens Medical Center

3360 Burns Road
Palm Beach Gardens, FL 33410
(561) 622-1411

Overall patient safety: ★★★★★
Teaching: N

CLINICAL PROGRAM RATINGS:

CARDIAC	★★★★★	ORTHOPEDICS	NR
CRITICAL CARE	★★★	PULMONARY	★★★
GASTROINTESTINAL	★★★	STROKE	★★★
GENERAL SURGERY	★★★	VASCULAR	NR
MATERNITY CARE	★★★	WOMEN'S HEALTH	★★★

HEALTHGRADES AWARDS

✓ AMERICA'S 50   ✓ DISTINGUISHED   ✓ SPECIALTY EXCELLENCE
  BEST HOSPITALS   HOSPITAL   · CARDIAC CARE   · CARDIAC SURGERY
                   · CLINICAL EXCELLENCE
                   · PATIENT SAFETY

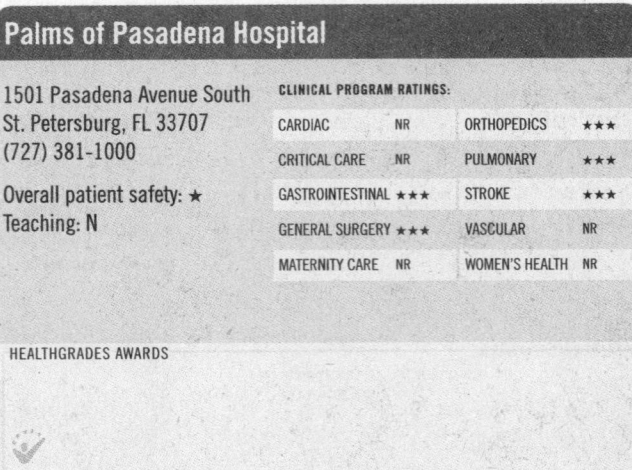

Palms of Pasadena Hospital

1501 Pasadena Avenue South
St. Petersburg, FL 33707
(727) 381-1000

Overall patient safety: ★
Teaching: N

CLINICAL PROGRAM RATINGS:

CARDIAC	NR	ORTHOPEDICS	★★★
CRITICAL CARE	NR	PULMONARY	★★★
GASTROINTESTINAL	★★★	STROKE	★★★
GENERAL SURGERY	★★★	VASCULAR	NR
MATERNITY CARE	NR	WOMEN'S HEALTH	NR

HEALTHGRADES AWARDS

Palm Springs General Hospital

1475 West 49th Street
Hialeah, FL 33012
(305) 558-2500

Overall patient safety: ★
Teaching: N

CLINICAL PROGRAM RATINGS:

CARDIAC	NR	ORTHOPEDICS	NR
CRITICAL CARE	NR	PULMONARY	★★★
GASTROINTESTINAL	★★★	STROKE	★★★★★
GENERAL SURGERY	★★★	VASCULAR	NR
MATERNITY CARE	NR	WOMEN'S HEALTH	NR

HEALTHGRADES AWARDS

✓ SPECIALTY EXCELLENCE
 · STROKE CARE

Palms West Hospital

13001 Southern Boulevard
Loxahatchee, FL 33470
(561) 798-3300

Overall patient safety: ★★★
Teaching: Y

CLINICAL PROGRAM RATINGS:

CARDIAC	NR	ORTHOPEDICS	NR
CRITICAL CARE	NR	PULMONARY	★★★
GASTROINTESTINAL	★★★	STROKE	★★★
GENERAL SURGERY	★★★	VASCULAR	NR
MATERNITY CARE	★★★★★	WOMEN'S HEALTH	NR

HEALTHGRADES AWARDS

✓ SPECIALTY EXCELLENCE
 · MATERNITY CARE

KEY: ★★★★★ BEST   ★★★ AS EXPECTED   ★ POOR   NR NOT RATED BY HEALTHGRADES   For full definitions of ratings and awards, see Appendix.

Pan American Hospital

5959 Northwest 7th Street
Miami, FL 33126
(305) 264-1000

Overall patient safety: ★★★
Teaching: N

CLINICAL PROGRAM RATINGS:

CARDIAC	NR	ORTHOPEDICS	NR
CRITICAL CARE	NR	PULMONARY	★★★★★
GASTROINTESTINAL	NR	STROKE	★★★
GENERAL SURGERY	★★★	VASCULAR	NR
MATERNITY CARE	NR	WOMEN'S HEALTH	NR

HEALTHGRADES AWARDS

✓ SPECIALTY EXCELLENCE
• PULMONARY CARE

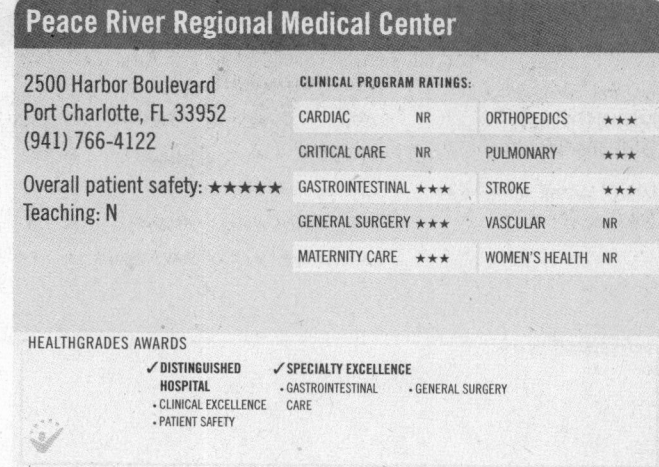

Peace River Regional Medical Center

2500 Harbor Boulevard
Port Charlotte, FL 33952
(941) 766-4122

Overall patient safety: ★★★★★
Teaching: N

CLINICAL PROGRAM RATINGS:

CARDIAC	NR	ORTHOPEDICS	★★★
CRITICAL CARE	NR	PULMONARY	★★★
GASTROINTESTINAL	★★★	STROKE	★★★
GENERAL SURGERY	★★★	VASCULAR	NR
MATERNITY CARE	★★★	WOMEN'S HEALTH	NR

HEALTHGRADES AWARDS

✓ DISTINGUISHED HOSPITAL
• CLINICAL EXCELLENCE
• PATIENT SAFETY

✓ SPECIALTY EXCELLENCE
• GASTROINTESTINAL CARE
• GENERAL SURGERY

Parrish Medical Center

951 North Washington Avenue
Titusville, FL 32796
(321) 268-6111

Overall patient safety: ★★★
Teaching: N

CLINICAL PROGRAM RATINGS:

CARDIAC	NR	ORTHOPEDICS	★★★
CRITICAL CARE	NR	PULMONARY	★★★
GASTROINTESTINAL	★★★	STROKE	★★★★★
GENERAL SURGERY	★★★	VASCULAR	NR
MATERNITY CARE	★★★	WOMEN'S HEALTH	NR

HEALTHGRADES AWARDS

✓ DISTINGUISHED HOSPITAL
• CLINICAL EXCELLENCE

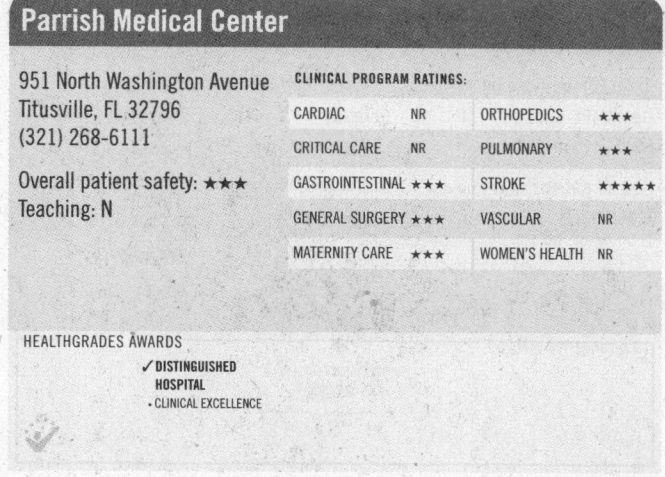

Physicians Regional Medical Center

6101 Pine Ridge Road
Naples, FL 34119
(239) 348-4000

Overall patient safety: ★★★★★
Teaching: N

CLINICAL PROGRAM RATINGS:

CARDIAC	NR	ORTHOPEDICS	★★★★★
CRITICAL CARE	NR	PULMONARY	★★★
GASTROINTESTINAL	★★★	STROKE	★★★
GENERAL SURGERY	★★★	VASCULAR	★★★
MATERNITY CARE	NR	WOMEN'S HEALTH	NR

HEALTHGRADES AWARDS

✓ DISTINGUISHED HOSPITAL
• CLINICAL EXCELLENCE
• PATIENT SAFETY

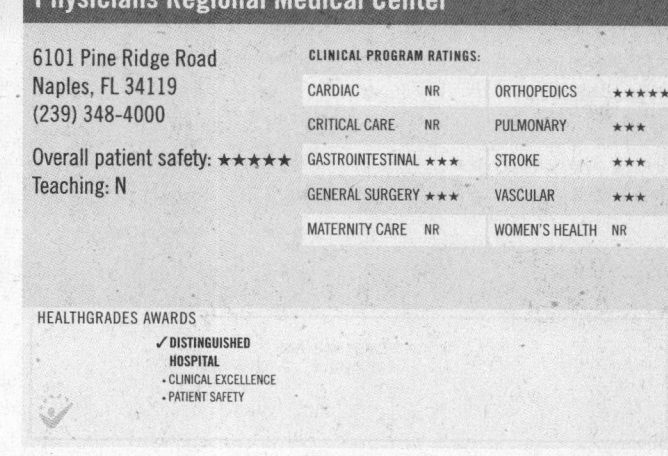

Pasco Regional Medical Center

13100 Fort King Road
Dade City, FL 33525
(352) 521-1100

Overall patient safety: ★★★
Teaching: N

CLINICAL PROGRAM RATINGS:

CARDIAC	NR	ORTHOPEDICS	NR
CRITICAL CARE	NR	PULMONARY	★★★
GASTROINTESTINAL	★★★	STROKE	★★★
GENERAL SURGERY	★★★★★	VASCULAR	NR
MATERNITY CARE	★★★	WOMEN'S HEALTH	NR

HEALTHGRADES AWARDS

✓ SPECIALTY EXCELLENCE
• GENERAL SURGERY

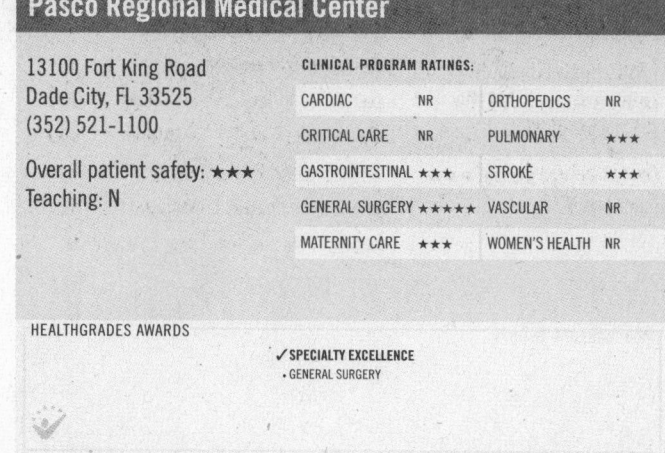

Plantation General Hospital

401 Northwest 42nd Avenue
Plantation, FL 33317
(954) 587-5010

Overall patient safety: ★★★
Teaching: Y

CLINICAL PROGRAM RATINGS:

CARDIAC	NR	ORTHOPEDICS	NR
CRITICAL CARE	NR	PULMONARY	★★★
GASTROINTESTINAL	NR	STROKE	★★★
GENERAL SURGERY	NR	VASCULAR	NR
MATERNITY CARE	★★★★★	WOMEN'S HEALTH	NR

HEALTHGRADES AWARDS

✓ SPECIALTY EXCELLENCE
• MATERNITY CARE

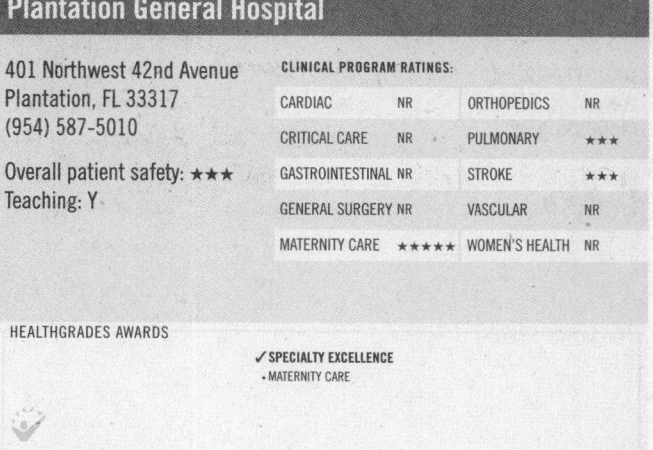

Putnam Community Medical Center

Highway 20 West
Palatka, FL 32177
(386) 328-5711

Overall patient safety: ★★★
Teaching: N

CLINICAL PROGRAM RATINGS:

CARDIAC	NR	ORTHOPEDICS	NR
CRITICAL CARE	NR	PULMONARY	★★★
GASTROINTESTINAL	★★★	STROKE	★★★
GENERAL SURGERY	★★★	VASCULAR	NR
MATERNITY CARE	★	WOMEN'S HEALTH	NR

HEALTHGRADES AWARDS

Sacred Heart Hospital

5150 North 9th Avenue
Pensacola, FL 32504
(850) 416-7000

Overall patient safety: ★★★
Teaching: Y

CLINICAL PROGRAM RATINGS:

CARDIAC	★★★	ORTHOPEDICS	★★★
CRITICAL CARE	NR	PULMONARY	★★★
GASTROINTESTINAL	★★★	STROKE	★★★
GENERAL SURGERY	★★★	VASCULAR	★★★
MATERNITY CARE	★★★	WOMEN'S HEALTH	★

HEALTHGRADES AWARDS

✓ SPECIALTY EXCELLENCE
- VASCULAR SURGERY

Raulerson Hospital

1796 Highway 441 North
Okeechobee, FL 34972
(863) 763-2151

Overall patient safety: ★★★
Teaching: N

CLINICAL PROGRAM RATINGS:

CARDIAC	NR	ORTHOPEDICS	NR
CRITICAL CARE	★★★	PULMONARY	★★★★★
GASTROINTESTINAL	★★★	STROKE	★★★
GENERAL SURGERY	★★★	VASCULAR	NR
MATERNITY CARE	NR	WOMEN'S HEALTH	NR

HEALTHGRADES AWARDS

✓ SPECIALTY EXCELLENCE
- GASTROINTESTINAL CARE
- PULMONARY CARE

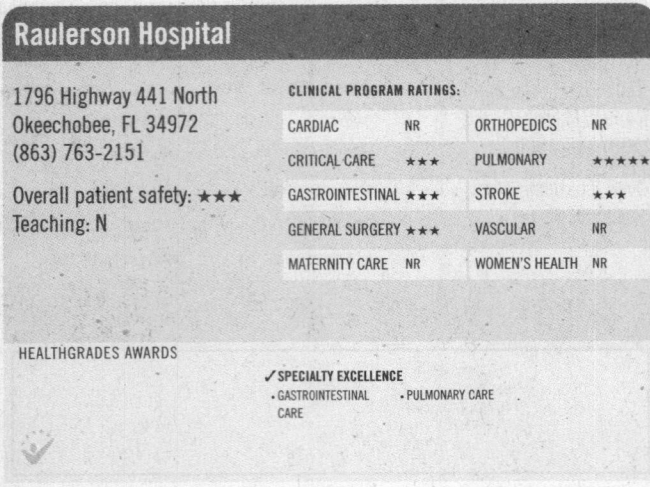

Sacred Heart Hospital at the Emerald Coast

7800 US Highway 90 West
Destin, FL 32550
(850) 278-3600

Overall patient safety: ★★★
Teaching: N

CLINICAL PROGRAM RATINGS:

CARDIAC	NR	ORTHOPEDICS	★★★
CRITICAL CARE	NR	PULMONARY	★★★
GASTROINTESTINAL	NR	STROKE	★★★
GENERAL SURGERY	★★★	VASCULAR	NR
MATERNITY CARE	NR	WOMEN'S HEALTH	NR

HEALTHGRADES AWARDS

✓ SPECIALTY EXCELLENCE
- GENERAL SURGERY

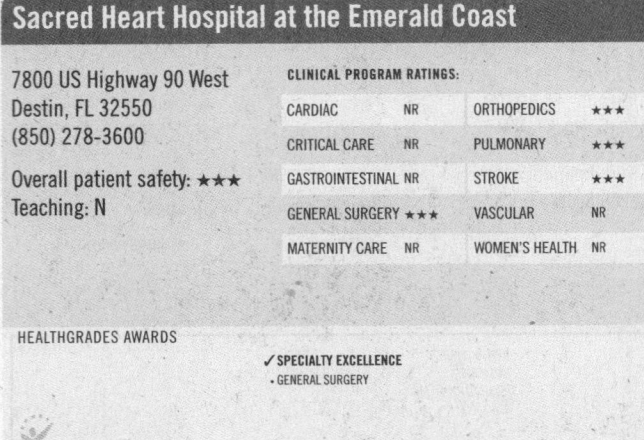

Regional Medical Center—Bayonet Point

14000 Fivay Road
Hudson, FL 34667
(727) 869-5400

Overall patient safety: ★★★
Teaching: N

CLINICAL PROGRAM RATINGS:

CARDIAC	★★★	ORTHOPEDICS	★★★
CRITICAL CARE	★★★	PULMONARY	★★★
GASTROINTESTINAL	★★★	STROKE	★★★
GENERAL SURGERY	★★★	VASCULAR	NR
MATERNITY CARE	NR	WOMEN'S HEALTH	NR

HEALTHGRADES AWARDS

St. Anthony's Hospital

1200 7th Avenue North
St. Petersburg, FL 33705
(727) 825-1100

Overall patient safety: ★★★
Teaching: N

CLINICAL PROGRAM RATINGS:

CARDIAC	NR	ORTHOPEDICS	★★★
CRITICAL CARE	NR	PULMONARY	★★★
GASTROINTESTINAL	★★★	STROKE	★★★★★
GENERAL SURGERY	★★★	VASCULAR	★★★
MATERNITY CARE	NR	WOMEN'S HEALTH	NR

HEALTHGRADES AWARDS

KEY: ★★★★★ BEST   ★★★ AS EXPECTED   ★ POOR   NR NOT RATED BY HEALTHGRADES   For full definitions of ratings and awards, see Appendix.

St. Cloud Regional Medical Center

2906 17th Street
St. Cloud, FL 34769
(407) 498-3432

Overall patient safety: NR
Teaching: N

CLINICAL PROGRAM RATINGS:

CARDIAC	NR	ORTHOPEDICS	NR
CRITICAL CARE	NR	PULMONARY	★★★
GASTROINTESTINAL	NR	STROKE	NR
GENERAL SURGERY	NR	VASCULAR	NR
MATERNITY CARE	NR	WOMEN'S HEALTH	NR

HEALTHGRADES AWARDS

St. Lucie Medical Center

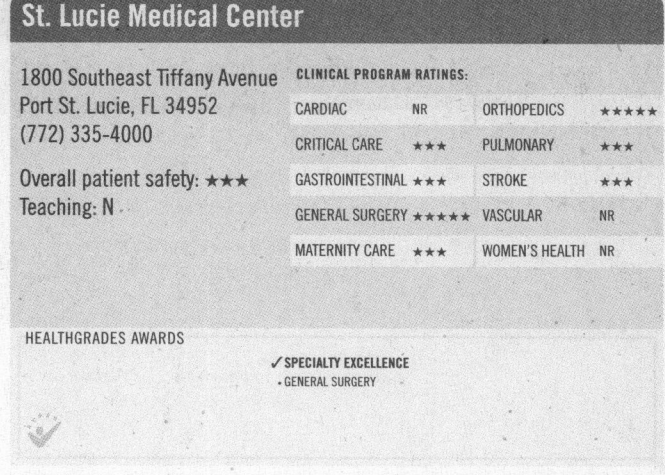

1800 Southeast Tiffany Avenue
Port St. Lucie, FL 34952
(772) 335-4000

Overall patient safety: ★★★
Teaching: N

CLINICAL PROGRAM RATINGS:

CARDIAC	NR	ORTHOPEDICS	★★★★★
CRITICAL CARE	★★★	PULMONARY	★★★
GASTROINTESTINAL	★★★	STROKE	★★★
GENERAL SURGERY	★★★★★	VASCULAR	NR
MATERNITY CARE	★★★	WOMEN'S HEALTH	NR

HEALTHGRADES AWARDS

✓ SPECIALTY EXCELLENCE
• GENERAL SURGERY

St. Joseph's Hospital*

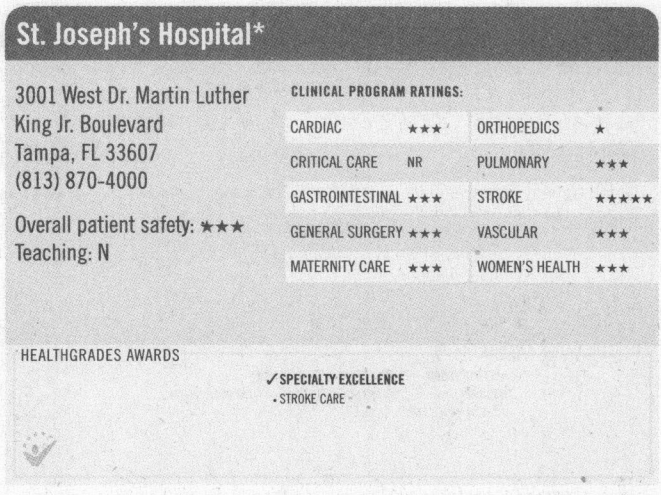

3001 West Dr. Martin Luther
King Jr. Boulevard
Tampa, FL 33607
(813) 870-4000

Overall patient safety: ★★★
Teaching: N

CLINICAL PROGRAM RATINGS:

CARDIAC	★★★	ORTHOPEDICS	★
CRITICAL CARE	NR	PULMONARY	★★★
GASTROINTESTINAL	★★★	STROKE	★★★★★
GENERAL SURGERY	★★★	VASCULAR	★★★
MATERNITY CARE	★★★	WOMEN'S HEALTH	★★★

HEALTHGRADES AWARDS

✓ SPECIALTY EXCELLENCE
• STROKE CARE

St. Luke's Hospital

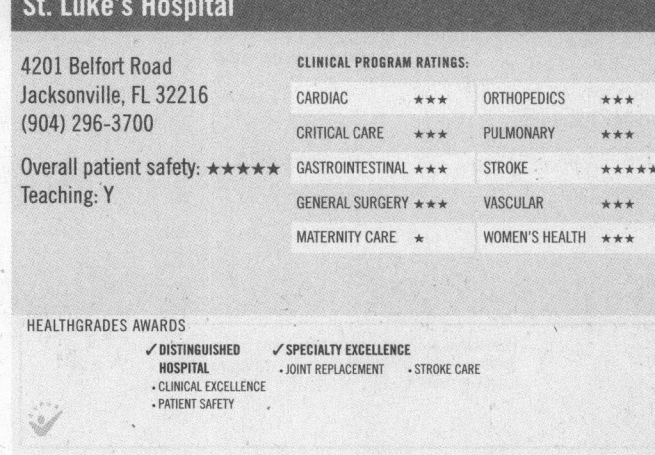

4201 Belfort Road
Jacksonville, FL 32216
(904) 296-3700

Overall patient safety: ★★★★★
Teaching: Y

CLINICAL PROGRAM RATINGS:

CARDIAC	★★★	ORTHOPEDICS	★★★
CRITICAL CARE	★★★	PULMONARY	★★★
GASTROINTESTINAL	★★★	STROKE	★★★★★
GENERAL SURGERY	★★★	VASCULAR	★★★
MATERNITY CARE	★	WOMEN'S HEALTH	★★★

HEALTHGRADES AWARDS

✓ DISTINGUISHED HOSPITAL
• CLINICAL EXCELLENCE
• PATIENT SAFETY

✓ SPECIALTY EXCELLENCE
• JOINT REPLACEMENT   • STROKE CARE

St. Joseph's Women's Hospital*

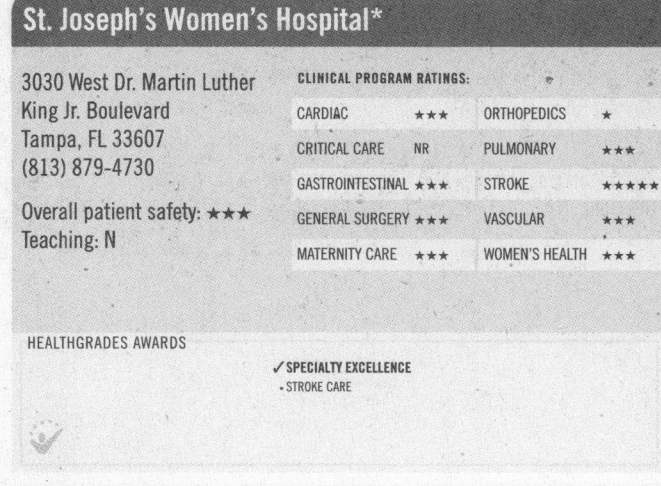

3030 West Dr. Martin Luther
King Jr. Boulevard
Tampa, FL 33607
(813) 879-4730

Overall patient safety: ★★★
Teaching: N

CLINICAL PROGRAM RATINGS:

CARDIAC	★★★	ORTHOPEDICS	★
CRITICAL CARE	NR	PULMONARY	★★★
GASTROINTESTINAL	★★★	STROKE	★★★★★
GENERAL SURGERY	★★★	VASCULAR	★★★
MATERNITY CARE	★★★	WOMEN'S HEALTH	★★★

HEALTHGRADES AWARDS

✓ SPECIALTY EXCELLENCE
• STROKE CARE

St. Mary's Medical Center

901 45th Street
West Palm Beach, FL 33407
(561) 844-6300

Overall patient safety: ★★★
Teaching: N

CLINICAL PROGRAM RATINGS:

CARDIAC	NR	ORTHOPEDICS	★★★
CRITICAL CARE	NR	PULMONARY	★★★
GASTROINTESTINAL	NR	STROKE	★★★
GENERAL SURGERY	NR	VASCULAR	NR
MATERNITY CARE	★★★	WOMEN'S HEALTH	NR

HEALTHGRADES AWARDS

*This hospital reports its data to the federal government jointly with another hospital. Therefore the ratings and awards apply to multiple hospitals and this specific hospital may not provide all rated services.

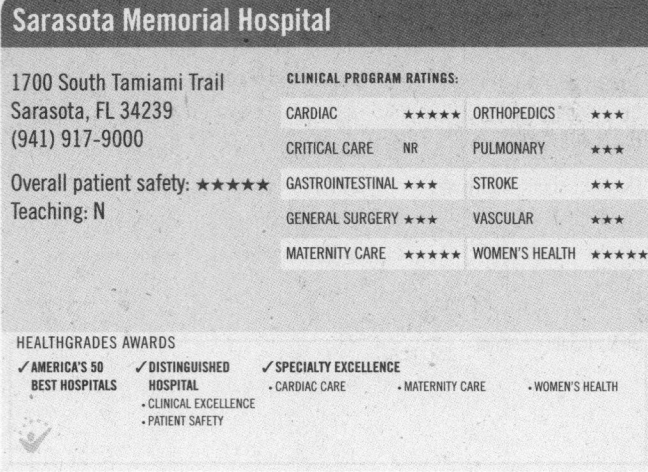

St. Petersburg General Hospital

6500 38th Avenue North
St. Petersburg, FL 33710
(727) 384-1414

Overall patient safety: ★★★
Teaching: N

CLINICAL PROGRAM RATINGS:

CARDIAC	NR	ORTHOPEDICS	NR
CRITICAL CARE	NR	PULMONARY	★★★★★
GASTROINTESTINAL	★★★	STROKE	★★★
GENERAL SURGERY	★★★	VASCULAR	NR
MATERNITY CARE	★★★★★	WOMEN'S HEALTH	NR

HEALTHGRADES AWARDS

✓ SPECIALTY EXCELLENCE
· GENERAL SURGERY   · MATERNITY CARE   · PULMONARY CARE

Sarasota Memorial Hospital

1700 South Tamiami Trail
Sarasota, FL 34239
(941) 917-9000

Overall patient safety: ★★★★★
Teaching: N

CLINICAL PROGRAM RATINGS:

CARDIAC	★★★★★	ORTHOPEDICS	★★★
CRITICAL CARE	NR	PULMONARY	★★★
GASTROINTESTINAL	★★★	STROKE	★★★
GENERAL SURGERY	★★★	VASCULAR	★★★
MATERNITY CARE	★★★★★	WOMEN'S HEALTH	★★★★★

HEALTHGRADES AWARDS

✓ AMERICA'S 50 BEST HOSPITALS   ✓ DISTINGUISHED HOSPITAL
· CLINICAL EXCELLENCE
· PATIENT SAFETY

✓ SPECIALTY EXCELLENCE
· CARDIAC CARE   · MATERNITY CARE   · WOMEN'S HEALTH

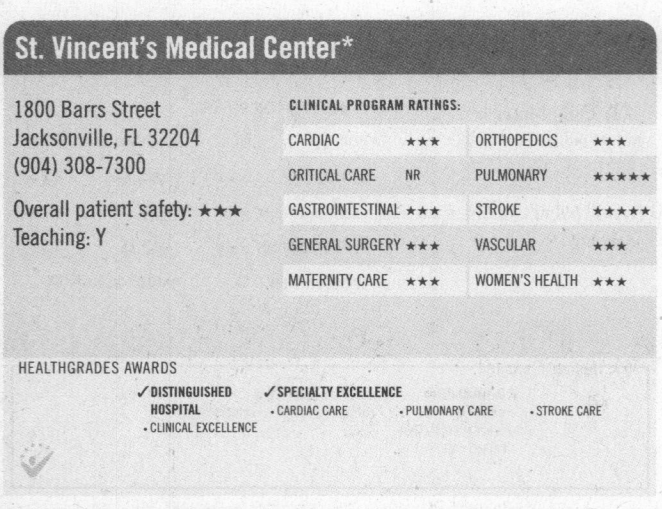

St. Vincent's Medical Center*

1800 Barrs Street
Jacksonville, FL 32204
(904) 308-7300

Overall patient safety: ★★★
Teaching: Y

CLINICAL PROGRAM RATINGS:

CARDIAC	★★★	ORTHOPEDICS	★★★
CRITICAL CARE	NR	PULMONARY	★★★★★
GASTROINTESTINAL	★★★	STROKE	★★★★★
GENERAL SURGERY	★★★	VASCULAR	★★★
MATERNITY CARE	★★★	WOMEN'S HEALTH	★★★

HEALTHGRADES AWARDS

✓ DISTINGUISHED HOSPITAL
· CLINICAL EXCELLENCE

✓ SPECIALTY EXCELLENCE
· CARDIAC CARE   · PULMONARY CARE   · STROKE CARE

Sebastian River Medical Center

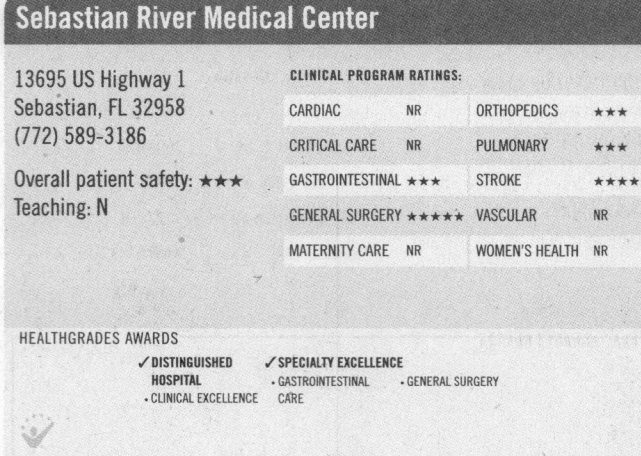

13695 US Highway 1
Sebastian, FL 32958
(772) 589-3186

Overall patient safety: ★★★
Teaching: N

CLINICAL PROGRAM RATINGS:

CARDIAC	NR	ORTHOPEDICS	★★★
CRITICAL CARE	NR	PULMONARY	★★★
GASTROINTESTINAL	★★★	STROKE	★★★★★
GENERAL SURGERY	★★★★★	VASCULAR	NR
MATERNITY CARE	NR	WOMEN'S HEALTH	NR

HEALTHGRADES AWARDS

✓ DISTINGUISHED HOSPITAL
· CLINICAL EXCELLENCE

✓ SPECIALTY EXCELLENCE
· GASTROINTESTINAL CARE   · GENERAL SURGERY

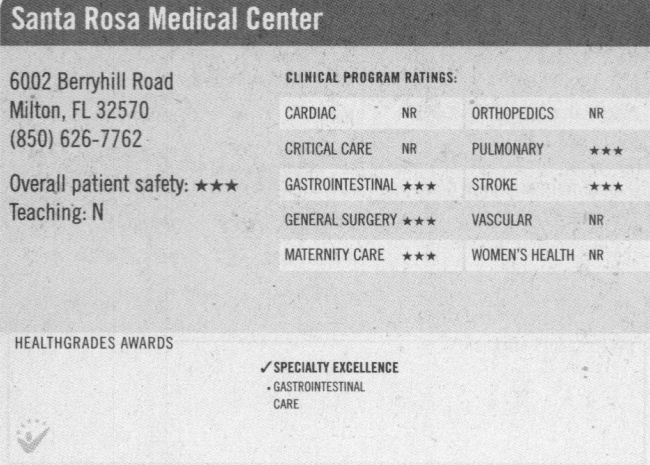

Santa Rosa Medical Center

6002 Berryhill Road
Milton, FL 32570
(850) 626-7762

Overall patient safety: ★★★
Teaching: N

CLINICAL PROGRAM RATINGS:

CARDIAC	NR	ORTHOPEDICS	NR
CRITICAL CARE	NR	PULMONARY	★★★
GASTROINTESTINAL	★★★	STROKE	★★★
GENERAL SURGERY	★★★	VASCULAR	NR
MATERNITY CARE	★★★	WOMEN'S HEALTH	NR

HEALTHGRADES AWARDS

✓ SPECIALTY EXCELLENCE
· GASTROINTESTINAL CARE

Seven Rivers Regional Medical Center

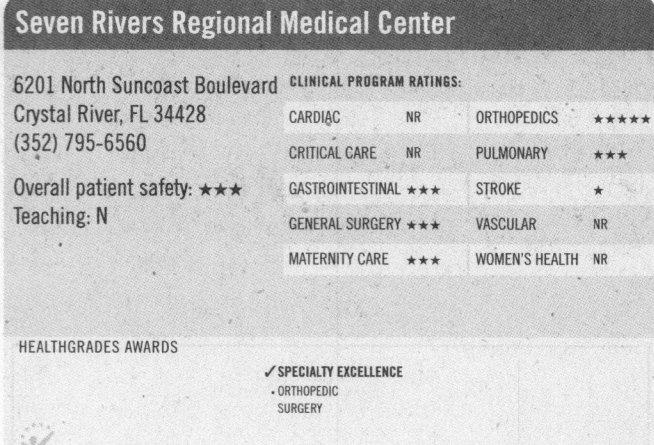

6201 North Suncoast Boulevard
Crystal River, FL 34428
(352) 795-6560

Overall patient safety: ★★★
Teaching: N

CLINICAL PROGRAM RATINGS:

CARDIAC	NR	ORTHOPEDICS	★★★★★
CRITICAL CARE	NR	PULMONARY	★★★
GASTROINTESTINAL	★★★	STROKE	★
GENERAL SURGERY	★★★	VASCULAR	NR
MATERNITY CARE	★★★	WOMEN'S HEALTH	NR

HEALTHGRADES AWARDS

✓ SPECIALTY EXCELLENCE
· ORTHOPEDIC SURGERY

KEY: ★★★★★ BEST   ★★★ AS EXPECTED   ★ POOR   NR NOT RATED BY HEALTHGRADES   For full definitions of ratings and awards, see Appendix.

Shands Hospital at the University of Florida*

1600 Southwest Archer Road
Gainesville, FL 32610
(352) 265-0111

Overall patient safety: ★★★
Teaching: Y

CLINICAL PROGRAM RATINGS:

CARDIAC	★★★	ORTHOPEDICS	★★★
CRITICAL CARE	NR	PULMONARY	★★★
GASTROINTESTINAL	★★★	STROKE	★★★
GENERAL SURGERY	★★★	VASCULAR	★★★
MATERNITY CARE	★★★	WOMEN'S HEALTH	★★★

HEALTHGRADES AWARDS

Shands Starke

922 East Call Street
Starke, FL 32091
(904) 368-2300

Overall patient safety: ★★★
Teaching: N

CLINICAL PROGRAM RATINGS:

CARDIAC	NR	ORTHOPEDICS	NR
CRITICAL CARE	NR	PULMONARY	★★★
GASTROINTESTINAL	NR	STROKE	NR
GENERAL SURGERY	NR	VASCULAR	NR
MATERNITY CARE	NR	WOMEN'S HEALTH	NR

HEALTHGRADES AWARDS

Shands Jacksonville*

655 West 8th Street
Jacksonville, FL 32209
(904) 244-0411

Overall patient safety: ★★★
Teaching: Y

CLINICAL PROGRAM RATINGS:

CARDIAC	★	ORTHOPEDICS	★★★
CRITICAL CARE	NR	PULMONARY	★★★
GASTROINTESTINAL	★★★	STROKE	★★★
GENERAL SURGERY	★★★	VASCULAR	NR
MATERNITY CARE	★	WOMEN'S HEALTH	★

HEALTHGRADES AWARDS

South Bay Hospital

4016 State Road 674
Sun City Center, FL 33573
(813) 634-3301

Overall patient safety: ★★★
Teaching: N

CLINICAL PROGRAM RATINGS:

CARDIAC	NR	ORTHOPEDICS	★★★
CRITICAL CARE	★★★	PULMONARY	★★★★★
GASTROINTESTINAL	★★★	STROKE	★★★
GENERAL SURGERY	★★★	VASCULAR	NR
MATERNITY CARE	NR	WOMEN'S HEALTH	NR

HEALTHGRADES AWARDS

✓ **DISTINGUISHED HOSPITAL**
• CLINICAL EXCELLENCE

✓ **SPECIALTY EXCELLENCE**
• GENERAL SURGERY   • PULMONARY CARE

Shands Lake Shore

560 East Franklin Street
Lake City, FL 32055
(386) 754-8000

Overall patient safety: ★★★
Teaching: N

CLINICAL PROGRAM RATINGS:

CARDIAC	NR	ORTHOPEDICS	NR
CRITICAL CARE	NR	PULMONARY	★★★★★
GASTROINTESTINAL	NR	STROKE	★★★★★
GENERAL SURGERY	★★★	VASCULAR	NR
MATERNITY CARE	★★★	WOMEN'S HEALTH	NR

HEALTHGRADES AWARDS

✓ **SPECIALTY EXCELLENCE**
• PULMONARY CARE   • STROKE CARE

South Beach Community Hospital

630 Alton Road
Miami Beach, FL 33139
(305) 672-2100

Overall patient safety: ★
Teaching: Y

CLINICAL PROGRAM RATINGS:

CARDIAC	NR	ORTHOPEDICS	NR
CRITICAL CARE	NR	PULMONARY	★★★
GASTROINTESTINAL	NR	STROKE	NR
GENERAL SURGERY	NR	VASCULAR	NR
MATERNITY CARE	NR	WOMEN'S HEALTH	NR

HEALTHGRADES AWARDS

*This hospital reports its data to the federal government jointly with another hospital. Therefore the ratings and awards apply to multiple hospitals and this specific hospital may not provide all rated services.

South Florida Baptist Hospital

301 North Alexander Street
Plant City, FL 33566
(813) 757-1200

Overall patient safety: ★
Teaching: N

CLINICAL PROGRAM RATINGS:

CARDIAC	NR	ORTHOPEDICS	NR
CRITICAL CARE	NR	PULMONARY	★★★
GASTROINTESTINAL	NR	STROKE	★★★
GENERAL SURGERY	★★★	VASCULAR	NR
MATERNITY CARE	★★★	WOMEN'S HEALTH	NR

HEALTHGRADES AWARDS

Southwest Florida Regional Medical Center

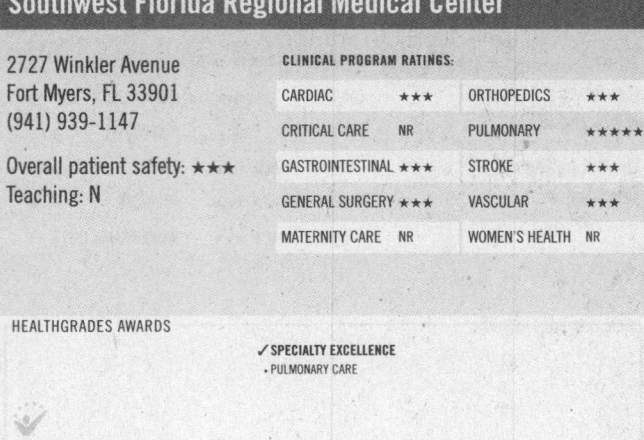

2727 Winkler Avenue
Fort Myers, FL 33901
(941) 939-1147

Overall patient safety: ★★★
Teaching: N

CLINICAL PROGRAM RATINGS:

CARDIAC	★★★	ORTHOPEDICS	★★★
CRITICAL CARE	NR	PULMONARY	★★★★★
GASTROINTESTINAL	★★★	STROKE	★★★
GENERAL SURGERY	★★★	VASCULAR	★★★
MATERNITY CARE	NR	WOMEN'S HEALTH	NR

HEALTHGRADES AWARDS

✓ SPECIALTY EXCELLENCE
- PULMONARY CARE

South Lake Hospital

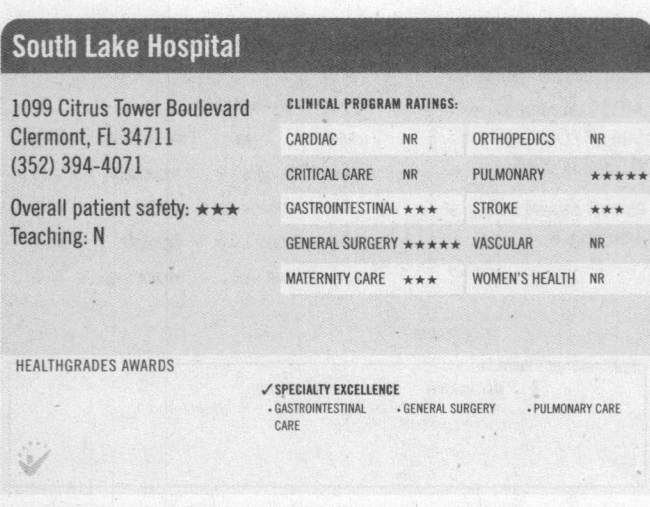

1099 Citrus Tower Boulevard
Clermont, FL 34711
(352) 394-4071

Overall patient safety: ★★★
Teaching: N

CLINICAL PROGRAM RATINGS:

CARDIAC	NR	ORTHOPEDICS	NR
CRITICAL CARE	NR	PULMONARY	★★★★★
GASTROINTESTINAL	★★★	STROKE	★★★
GENERAL SURGERY	★★★★★	VASCULAR	NR
MATERNITY CARE	★★★	WOMEN'S HEALTH	NR

HEALTHGRADES AWARDS

✓ SPECIALTY EXCELLENCE
- GASTROINTESTINAL CARE
- GENERAL SURGERY
- PULMONARY CARE

Sun Coast Hospital

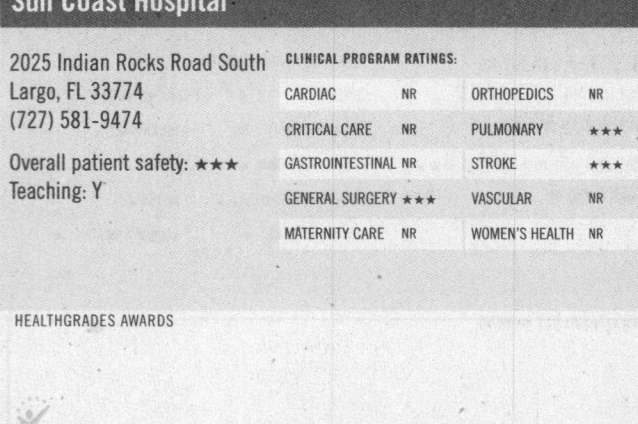

2025 Indian Rocks Road South
Largo, FL 33774
(727) 581-9474

Overall patient safety: ★★★
Teaching: Y

CLINICAL PROGRAM RATINGS:

CARDIAC	NR	ORTHOPEDICS	NR
CRITICAL CARE	NR	PULMONARY	★★★
GASTROINTESTINAL	NR	STROKE	★★★
GENERAL SURGERY	★★★	VASCULAR	NR
MATERNITY CARE	NR	WOMEN'S HEALTH	NR

HEALTHGRADES AWARDS

South Miami Hospital

6200 Southwest 73 Street
South Miami, FL 33143
(786) 662-4100

Overall patient safety: ★★★
Teaching: Y

CLINICAL PROGRAM RATINGS:

CARDIAC	★★★	ORTHOPEDICS	★★★
CRITICAL CARE	★★★	PULMONARY	★★★★★
GASTROINTESTINAL	★★★	STROKE	★★★★★
GENERAL SURGERY	★★★	VASCULAR	NR
MATERNITY CARE	★★★★★	WOMEN'S HEALTH	★★★★★

HEALTHGRADES AWARDS

✓ SPECIALTY EXCELLENCE
- MATERNITY CARE
- STROKE CARE
- WOMEN'S HEALTH

Tallahassee Memorial Healthcare

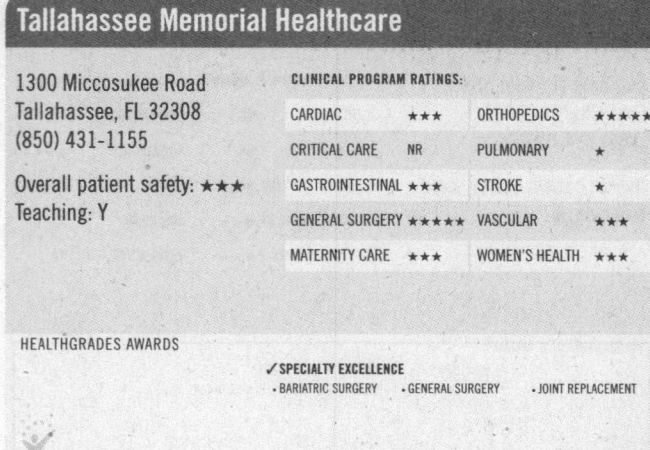

1300 Miccosukee Road
Tallahassee, FL 32308
(850) 431-1155

Overall patient safety: ★★★
Teaching: Y

CLINICAL PROGRAM RATINGS:

CARDIAC	★★★	ORTHOPEDICS	★★★★★
CRITICAL CARE	NR	PULMONARY	★
GASTROINTESTINAL	★★★	STROKE	★
GENERAL SURGERY	★★★★★	VASCULAR	★★★
MATERNITY CARE	★★★	WOMEN'S HEALTH	★★★

HEALTHGRADES AWARDS

✓ SPECIALTY EXCELLENCE
- BARIATRIC SURGERY
- GENERAL SURGERY
- JOINT REPLACEMENT

KEY: ★★★★★ BEST ★★★ AS EXPECTED ★ POOR NR NOT RATED BY HEALTHGRADES   For full definitions of ratings and awards, see Appendix.

Tampa General Hospital

2 Columbia Drive
Tampa, FL 33606
(813) 844-7000

Overall patient safety: ★
Teaching: Y

CLINICAL PROGRAM RATINGS:

CARDIAC	★★★	ORTHOPEDICS	★
CRITICAL CARE	★★★	PULMONARY	★★★
GASTROINTESTINAL	★★★	STROKE	★★★
GENERAL SURGERY	★★★	VASCULAR	★★★
MATERNITY CARE	★	WOMEN'S HEALTH	★

HEALTHGRADES AWARDS

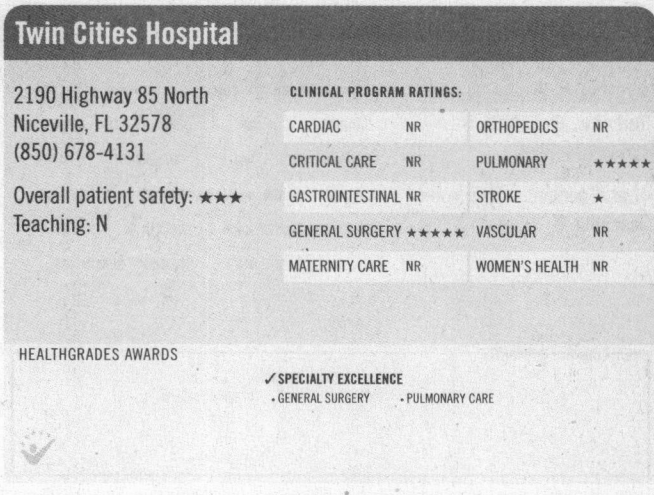

Twin Cities Hospital

2190 Highway 85 North
Niceville, FL 32578
(850) 678-4131

Overall patient safety: ★★★
Teaching: N

CLINICAL PROGRAM RATINGS:

CARDIAC	NR	ORTHOPEDICS	NR
CRITICAL CARE	NR	PULMONARY	★★★★★
GASTROINTESTINAL	NR	STROKE	★
GENERAL SURGERY	★★★★★	VASCULAR	NR
MATERNITY CARE	NR	WOMEN'S HEALTH	NR

HEALTHGRADES AWARDS

✓ **SPECIALTY EXCELLENCE**
• GENERAL SURGERY   • PULMONARY CARE

Town and Country Hospital

6001 Webb Road
Tampa, FL 33615
(813) 885-6666

Overall patient safety: ★★★
Teaching: N

CLINICAL PROGRAM RATINGS:

CARDIAC	NR	ORTHOPEDICS	NR
CRITICAL CARE	NR	PULMONARY	★★★
GASTROINTESTINAL	NR	STROKE	★★★
GENERAL SURGERY	★★★	VASCULAR	NR
MATERNITY CARE	NR	WOMEN'S HEALTH	NR

HEALTHGRADES AWARDS

✓ **SPECIALTY EXCELLENCE**
• BARIATRIC SURGERY

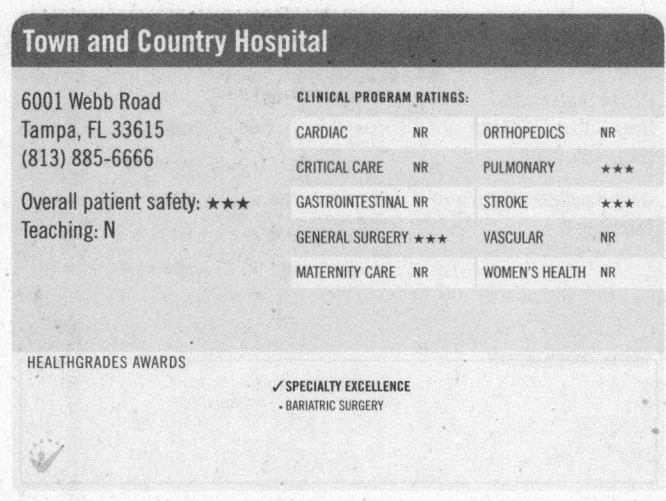

University Community Hospital

3100 East Fletcher Avenue
Tampa, FL 33613
(813) 971-6000

Overall patient safety: ★
Teaching: N

CLINICAL PROGRAM RATINGS:

CARDIAC	★★★	ORTHOPEDICS	★★★★★
CRITICAL CARE	NR	PULMONARY	★
GASTROINTESTINAL	★★★	STROKE	★★★
GENERAL SURGERY	★★★	VASCULAR	★★★
MATERNITY CARE	★★★	WOMEN'S HEALTH	★★★

HEALTHGRADES AWARDS

✓ **SPECIALTY EXCELLENCE**
• ORTHOPEDIC
SURGERY

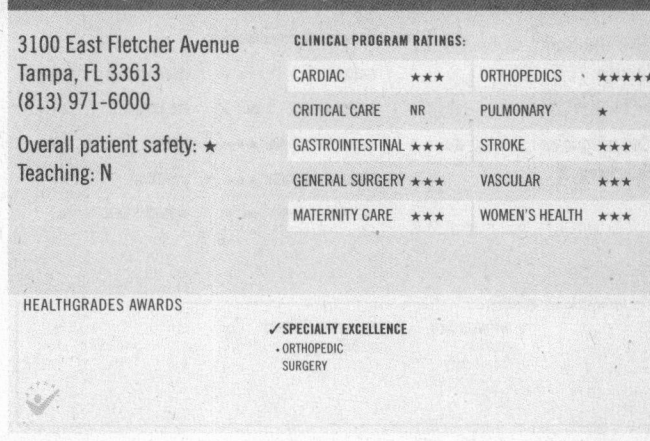

Trinity Community Hospital

506 Northwest 4th Street
Jasper, FL 32052
(386) 792-7200

Overall patient safety: ★★★
Teaching: N

CLINICAL PROGRAM RATINGS:

CARDIAC	NR	ORTHOPEDICS	NR
CRITICAL CARE	NR	PULMONARY	★★★
GASTROINTESTINAL	NR	STROKE	NR
GENERAL SURGERY	NR	VASCULAR	NR
MATERNITY CARE	NR	WOMEN'S HEALTH	NR

HEALTHGRADES AWARDS

University Community Hospital at Carrollwood

7171 North Dale Mabry
Tampa, FL 33614
(813) 932-2222

Overall patient safety: ★★★
Teaching: N

CLINICAL PROGRAM RATINGS:

CARDIAC	NR	ORTHOPEDICS	★★★
CRITICAL CARE	NR	PULMONARY	★★★★★
GASTROINTESTINAL	★★★	STROKE	★★★
GENERAL SURGERY	★★★	VASCULAR	NR
MATERNITY CARE	NR	WOMEN'S HEALTH	NR

HEALTHGRADES AWARDS

FLORIDA HOSPITALS: RATINGS BY CLINICAL SPECIALTY

University Hospital and Medical Center

7201 North University Drive
Tamarac, FL 33321
(954) 721-2200

Overall patient safety: ★★★
Teaching: N

CLINICAL PROGRAM RATINGS:

CARDIAC	NR	ORTHOPEDICS	NR
CRITICAL CARE	★★★	PULMONARY	★★★
GASTROINTESTINAL	★★★	STROKE	★★★
GENERAL SURGERY	★★★★★	VASCULAR	NR
MATERNITY CARE	NR	WOMEN'S HEALTH	NR

HEALTHGRADES AWARDS

✓ SPECIALTY EXCELLENCE
- BARIATRIC SURGERY   - GENERAL SURGERY

Wellington Regional Medical Center

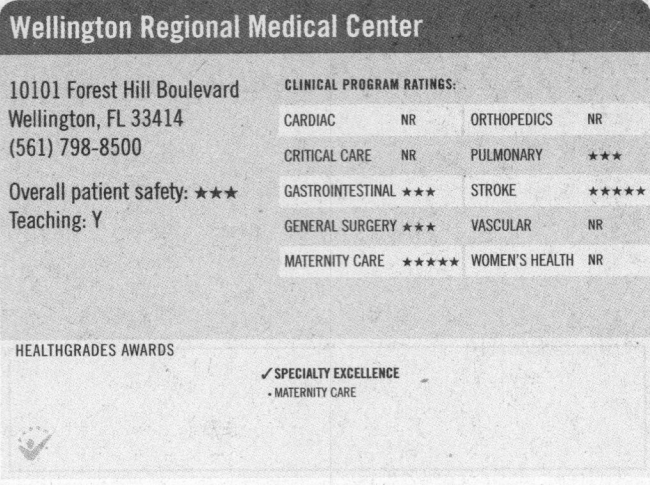

10101 Forest Hill Boulevard
Wellington, FL 33414
(561) 798-8500

Overall patient safety: ★★★
Teaching: Y

CLINICAL PROGRAM RATINGS:

CARDIAC	NR	ORTHOPEDICS	NR
CRITICAL CARE	NR	PULMONARY	★★★
GASTROINTESTINAL	★★★	STROKE	★★★★★
GENERAL SURGERY	★★★	VASCULAR	NR
MATERNITY CARE	★★★★★	WOMEN'S HEALTH	NR

HEALTHGRADES AWARDS

✓ SPECIALTY EXCELLENCE
- MATERNITY CARE

Venice Regional Medical Center

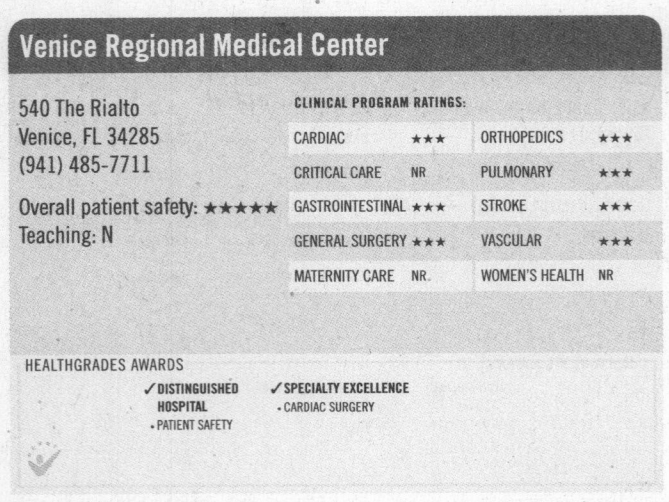

540 The Rialto
Venice, FL 34285
(941) 485-7711

Overall patient safety: ★★★★★
Teaching: N

CLINICAL PROGRAM RATINGS:

CARDIAC	★★★	ORTHOPEDICS	★★★
CRITICAL CARE	NR	PULMONARY	★★★
GASTROINTESTINAL	★★★	STROKE	★★★
GENERAL SURGERY	★★★	VASCULAR	★★★
MATERNITY CARE	NR.	WOMEN'S HEALTH	NR

HEALTHGRADES AWARDS

✓ DISTINGUISHED HOSPITAL
- PATIENT SAFETY

✓ SPECIALTY EXCELLENCE
- CARDIAC SURGERY

West Boca Medical Center

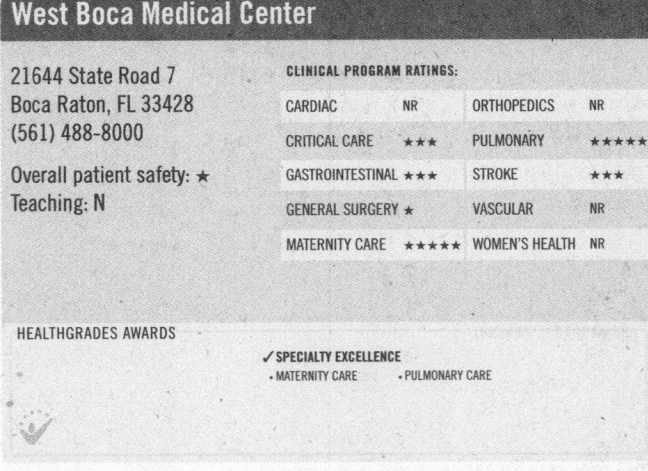

21644 State Road 7
Boca Raton, FL 33428
(561) 488-8000

Overall patient safety: ★
Teaching: N

CLINICAL PROGRAM RATINGS:

CARDIAC	NR	ORTHOPEDICS	NR
CRITICAL CARE	★★★	PULMONARY	★★★★★
GASTROINTESTINAL	★★★	STROKE	★★★
GENERAL SURGERY	★	VASCULAR	NR
MATERNITY CARE	★★★★★	WOMEN'S HEALTH	NR

HEALTHGRADES AWARDS

✓ SPECIALTY EXCELLENCE
- MATERNITY CARE   - PULMONARY CARE

Villages Regional Hospital

1451 El Camino Real
The Villages, FL 32159
(352) 751-8000

Overall patient safety: ★★★
Teaching: N

CLINICAL PROGRAM RATINGS:

CARDIAC	NR	ORTHOPEDICS	NR
CRITICAL CARE	NR	PULMONARY	★★★
GASTROINTESTINAL	★★★	STROKE	★★★
GENERAL SURGERY	★★★★★	VASCULAR	NR
MATERNITY CARE	NR	WOMEN'S HEALTH	NR

HEALTHGRADES AWARDS

✓ SPECIALTY EXCELLENCE
- GENERAL SURGERY

West Florida Hospital

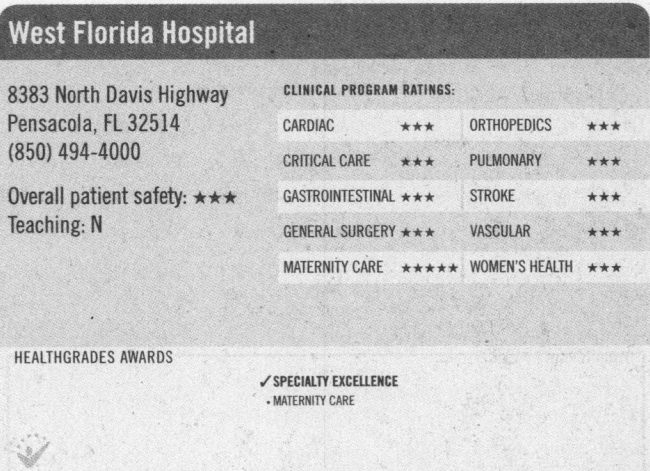

8383 North Davis Highway
Pensacola, FL 32514
(850) 494-4000

Overall patient safety: ★★★
Teaching: N

CLINICAL PROGRAM RATINGS:

CARDIAC	★★★	ORTHOPEDICS	★★★
CRITICAL CARE	★★★	PULMONARY	★★★
GASTROINTESTINAL	★★★	STROKE	★★★
GENERAL SURGERY	★★★	VASCULAR	★★★
MATERNITY CARE	★★★★★	WOMEN'S HEALTH	★★★

HEALTHGRADES AWARDS

✓ SPECIALTY EXCELLENCE
- MATERNITY CARE

KEY: ★★★★★ BEST   ★★★ AS EXPECTED   ★ POOR   NR NOT RATED BY HEALTHGRADES   For full definitions of ratings and awards, see Appendix.

Westchester General Hospital

2500 Southwest 75th Avenue
Miami, FL 33155
(305) 263-9270

Overall patient safety: ★★★
Teaching: Y

CLINICAL PROGRAM RATINGS:

CARDIAC	NR	ORTHOPEDICS	NR
CRITICAL CARE	NR	PULMONARY	★★★
GASTROINTESTINAL	NR	STROKE	★★★★★
GENERAL SURGERY	★★★	VASCULAR	NR
MATERNITY CARE	NR	WOMEN'S HEALTH	NR

HEALTHGRADES AWARDS

✓ SPECIALTY EXCELLENCE
· STROKE CARE

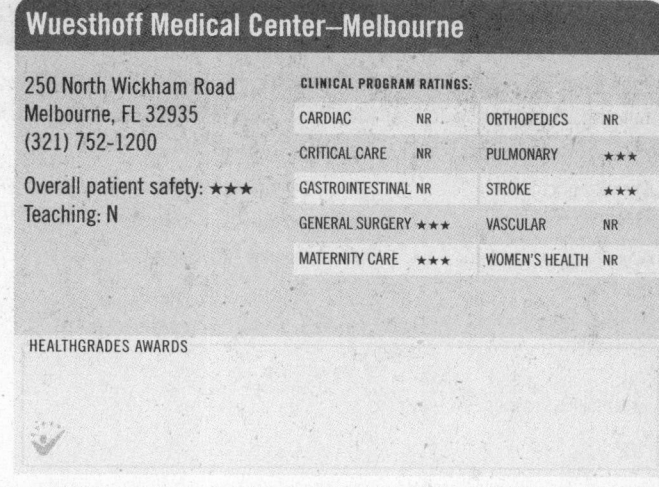

Wuesthoff Medical Center—Melbourne

250 North Wickham Road
Melbourne, FL 32935
(321) 752-1200

Overall patient safety: ★★★
Teaching: N

CLINICAL PROGRAM RATINGS:

CARDIAC	NR	ORTHOPEDICS	NR
CRITICAL CARE	NR	PULMONARY	★★★
GASTROINTESTINAL	NR	STROKE	★★★
GENERAL SURGERY	★★★	VASCULAR	NR
MATERNITY CARE	★★★	WOMEN'S HEALTH	NR

HEALTHGRADES AWARDS

Westside Regional Medical Center

8201 West Broward Boulevard
Plantation, FL 33324
(954) 473-6600

Overall patient safety: ★★★
Teaching: Y

CLINICAL PROGRAM RATINGS:

CARDIAC	★★★	ORTHOPEDICS	NR
CRITICAL CARE	★★★	PULMONARY	★★★
GASTROINTESTINAL	★★★	STROKE	★★★
GENERAL SURGERY	★★★	VASCULAR	NR
MATERNITY CARE	NR	WOMEN'S HEALTH	NR

HEALTHGRADES AWARDS

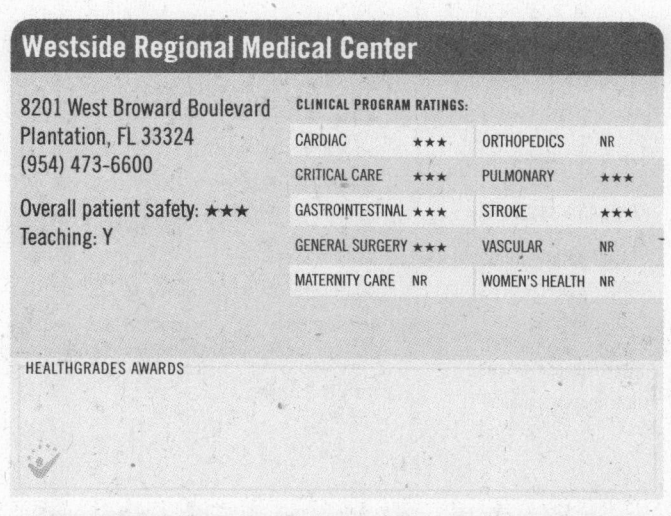

Wuesthoff Medical Center—Rockledge

110 Longwood Avenue
Rockledge, FL 32955
(321) 636-2211

Overall patient safety: ★★★★★
Teaching: N

CLINICAL PROGRAM RATINGS:

CARDIAC	★★★	ORTHOPEDICS	★★★
CRITICAL CARE	★★★	PULMONARY	★★★
GASTROINTESTINAL	★★★	STROKE	★★★
GENERAL SURGERY	★★★	VASCULAR	★★★
MATERNITY CARE	★★★	WOMEN'S HEALTH	★★★

HEALTHGRADES AWARDS

✓ DISTINGUISHED HOSPITAL
· PATIENT SAFETY

✓ SPECIALTY EXCELLENCE
· GASTROINTESTINAL CARE

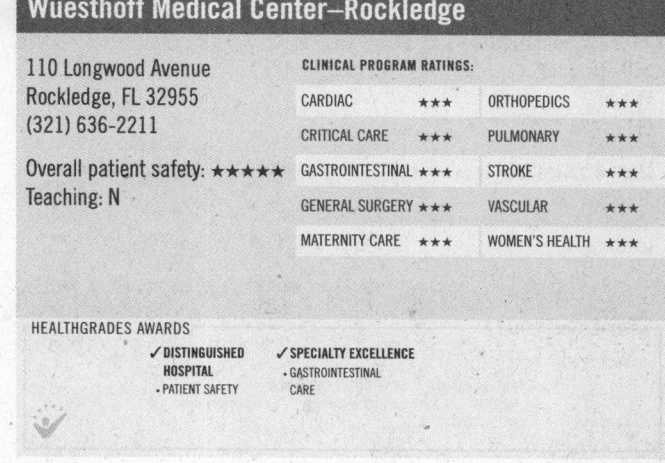

Winter Haven Hospital

200 Avenue F Northeast
Winter Haven, FL 33881
(863) 293-1121

Overall patient safety: ★
Teaching: N

CLINICAL PROGRAM RATINGS:

CARDIAC	★★★	ORTHOPEDICS	★★★
CRITICAL CARE	★	PULMONARY	★★★
GASTROINTESTINAL	★★★	STROKE	★★★
GENERAL SURGERY	★★★	VASCULAR	★★★
MATERNITY CARE	★★★	WOMEN'S HEALTH	NR

HEALTHGRADES AWARDS

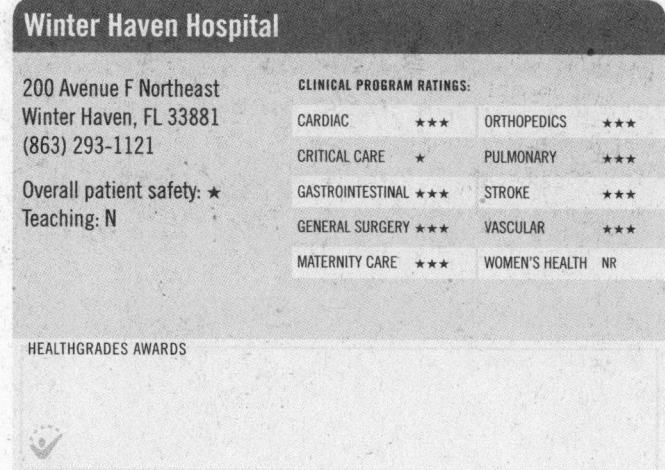

Appling Hospital

163 East Tollison Street
Baxley, GA 31513
(912) 367-9841

Overall patient safety: ★
Teaching: N

CLINICAL PROGRAM RATINGS:

CARDIAC	NR	ORTHOPEDICS	NR
CRITICAL CARE	NR	PULMONARY	★★★
GASTROINTESTINAL	NR	STROKE	★
GENERAL SURGERY	NR	VASCULAR	NR
MATERNITY CARE	NR	WOMEN'S HEALTH	NR

HEALTHGRADES AWARDS

Bacon County Hospital

302 South Wayne Street
Alma, GA 31510
(912) 632-8961

Overall patient safety: ★★★
Teaching: N

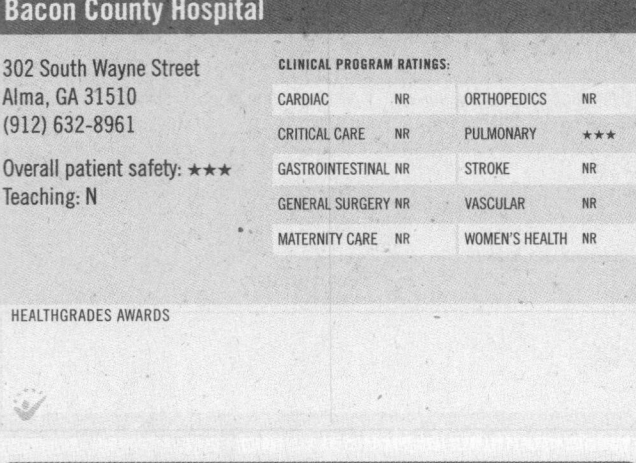

CLINICAL PROGRAM RATINGS:

CARDIAC	NR	ORTHOPEDICS	NR
CRITICAL CARE	NR	PULMONARY	★★★
GASTROINTESTINAL	NR	STROKE	NR
GENERAL SURGERY	NR	VASCULAR	NR
MATERNITY CARE	NR	WOMEN'S HEALTH	NR

HEALTHGRADES AWARDS

Athens Regional Medical Center

1199 Prince Avenue
Athens, GA 30606
(706) 475-7000

Overall patient safety: ★★★★★
Teaching: N

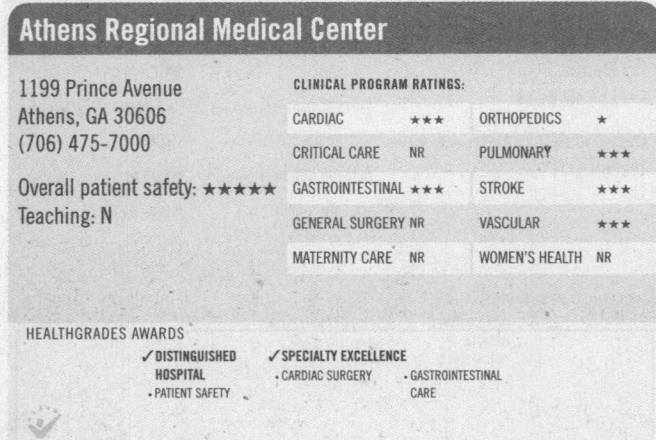

CLINICAL PROGRAM RATINGS:

CARDIAC	★★★	ORTHOPEDICS	★
CRITICAL CARE	NR	PULMONARY	★★★
GASTROINTESTINAL	★★★	STROKE	★★★
GENERAL SURGERY	NR	VASCULAR	★★★
MATERNITY CARE	NR	WOMEN'S HEALTH	NR

HEALTHGRADES AWARDS

✓ DISTINGUISHED HOSPITAL
· PATIENT SAFETY

✓ SPECIALTY EXCELLENCE
· CARDIAC SURGERY
· GASTROINTESTINAL CARE

Barrow Regional Medical Center

316 North Broad Street
Winder, GA 30680
(770) 867-3400

Overall patient safety: ★★★
Teaching: N

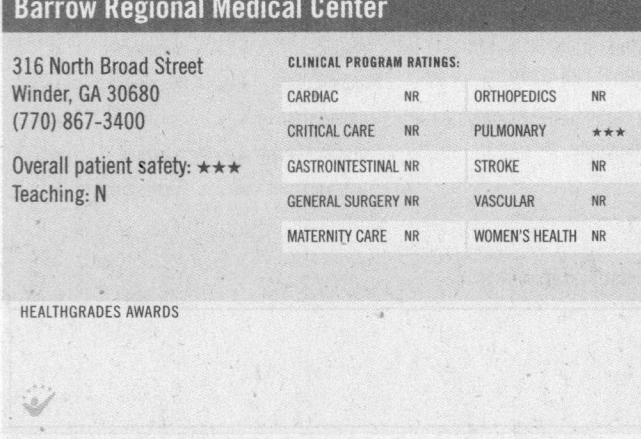

CLINICAL PROGRAM RATINGS:

CARDIAC	NR	ORTHOPEDICS	NR
CRITICAL CARE	NR	PULMONARY	★★★
GASTROINTESTINAL	NR	STROKE	NR
GENERAL SURGERY	NR	VASCULAR	NR
MATERNITY CARE	NR	WOMEN'S HEALTH	NR

HEALTHGRADES AWARDS

Atlanta Medical Center

303 Parkway Drive Northeast
Atlanta, GA 30312
(404) 265-4000

Overall patient safety: ★
Teaching: Y

CLINICAL PROGRAM RATINGS:

CARDIAC	★★★	ORTHOPEDICS	NR
CRITICAL CARE	NR	PULMONARY	★★★
GASTROINTESTINAL	NR	STROKE	★★★
GENERAL SURGERY	NR	VASCULAR	NR
MATERNITY CARE	NR	WOMEN'S HEALTH	NR

HEALTHGRADES AWARDS

Berrien County Hospital

1221 East McPherson Street
Nashville, GA 31639
(229) 543-7100

Overall patient safety: ★★★
Teaching: N

CLINICAL PROGRAM RATINGS:

CARDIAC	NR	ORTHOPEDICS	NR
CRITICAL CARE	NR	PULMONARY	★★★
GASTROINTESTINAL	NR	STROKE	★★★
GENERAL SURGERY	NR	VASCULAR	NR
MATERNITY CARE	NR	WOMEN'S HEALTH	NR

HEALTHGRADES AWARDS

KEY: ★★★★★ BEST   ★★★ AS EXPECTED   ★ POOR   NR NOT RATED BY HEALTHGRADES   For full definitions of ratings and awards, see Appendix.

BJC Medical Center

70 Medical Center Drive
Commerce, GA 30529
(706) 335-1000

Overall patient safety: ★★★
Teaching: N

CLINICAL PROGRAM RATINGS:

CARDIAC	NR	ORTHOPEDICS	NR
CRITICAL CARE	NR	PULMONARY	★★★
GASTROINTESTINAL	NR	STROKE	★★★
GENERAL SURGERY	NR	VASCULAR	NR
MATERNITY CARE	NR	WOMEN'S HEALTH	NR

HEALTHGRADES AWARDS

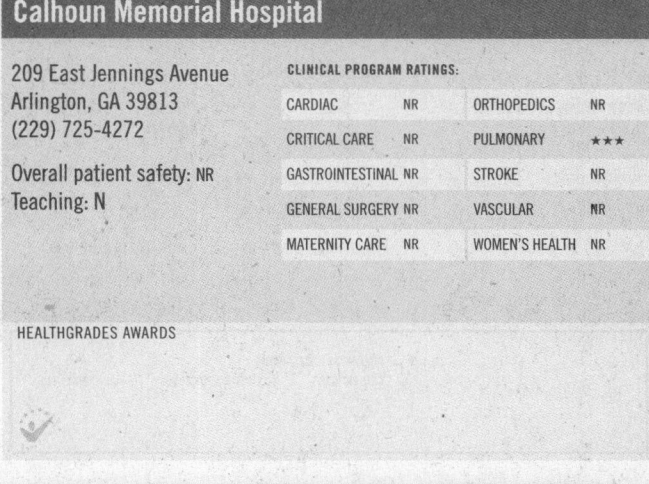

Calhoun Memorial Hospital

209 East Jennings Avenue
Arlington, GA 39813
(229) 725-4272

Overall patient safety: NR
Teaching: N

CLINICAL PROGRAM RATINGS:

CARDIAC	NR	ORTHOPEDICS	NR
CRITICAL CARE	NR	PULMONARY	★★★
GASTROINTESTINAL	NR	STROKE	NR
GENERAL SURGERY	NR	VASCULAR	NR
MATERNITY CARE	NR	WOMEN'S HEALTH	NR

HEALTHGRADES AWARDS

Brooks County Hospital

903 North Court Street
Quitman, GA 31643
(912) 263-4171

Overall patient safety: ★★★
Teaching: N

CLINICAL PROGRAM RATINGS:

CARDIAC	NR	ORTHOPEDICS	NR
CRITICAL CARE	NR	PULMONARY	★★★
GASTROINTESTINAL	NR	STROKE	NR
GENERAL SURGERY	NR	VASCULAR	NR
MATERNITY CARE	NR	WOMEN'S HEALTH	NR

HEALTHGRADES AWARDS

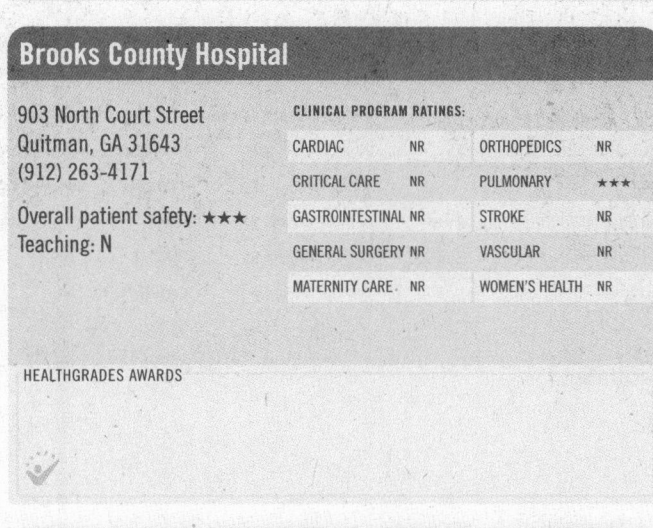

Camden Medical Center

2000 Dan Proctor Drive
St. Marys, GA 31558
(912) 576-6200

Overall patient safety: ★★★
Teaching: N

CLINICAL PROGRAM RATINGS:

CARDIAC	NR	ORTHOPEDICS	NR
CRITICAL CARE	NR	PULMONARY	★★★
GASTROINTESTINAL	NR	STROKE	NR
GENERAL SURGERY	NR	VASCULAR	NR
MATERNITY CARE	NR	WOMEN'S HEALTH	NR

HEALTHGRADES AWARDS

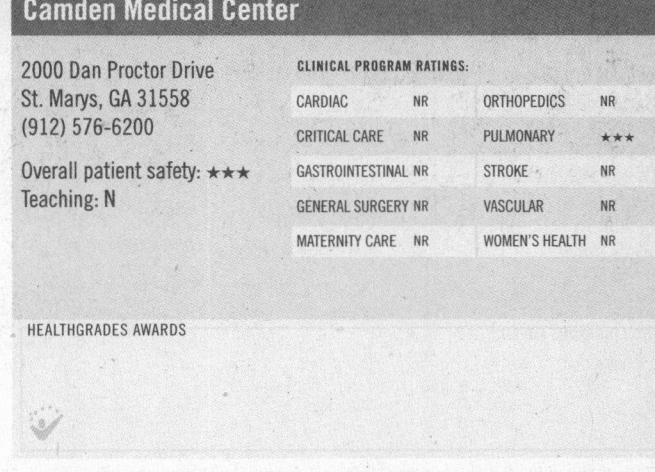

Burke Medical Center

351 Liberty Street
Waynesboro, GA 30830
(706) 554-4435

Overall patient safety: ★★★
Teaching: N

CLINICAL PROGRAM RATINGS:

CARDIAC	NR	ORTHOPEDICS	NR
CRITICAL CARE	NR	PULMONARY	★★★
GASTROINTESTINAL	NR	STROKE	★★★
GENERAL SURGERY	NR	VASCULAR	NR
MATERNITY CARE	NR	WOMEN'S HEALTH	NR

HEALTHGRADES AWARDS

Candler County Hospital

400 Cedar Street
Metter, GA 30439
(912) 685-5741

Overall patient safety: ★★★
Teaching: N

CLINICAL PROGRAM RATINGS:

CARDIAC	NR	ORTHOPEDICS	NR
CRITICAL CARE	NR	PULMONARY	★
GASTROINTESTINAL	NR	STROKE	NR
GENERAL SURGERY	NR	VASCULAR	NR
MATERNITY CARE	NR	WOMEN'S HEALTH	NR

HEALTHGRADES AWARDS

Candler Hospital

5353 Reynolds Street
Savannah, GA 31405
(912) 819-6000

Overall patient safety: ★★★
Teaching: N

CLINICAL PROGRAM RATINGS:

CARDIAC	NR	ORTHOPEDICS	NR
CRITICAL CARE	★★★★★	PULMONARY	★★★★★
GASTROINTESTINAL	★★★	STROKE	★★★
GENERAL SURGERY	NR	VASCULAR	NR
MATERNITY CARE	NR	WOMEN'S HEALTH	NR

HEALTHGRADES AWARDS

✓ SPECIALTY EXCELLENCE
· CRITICAL CARE
· GASTROINTESTINAL CARE
· PULMONARY CARE

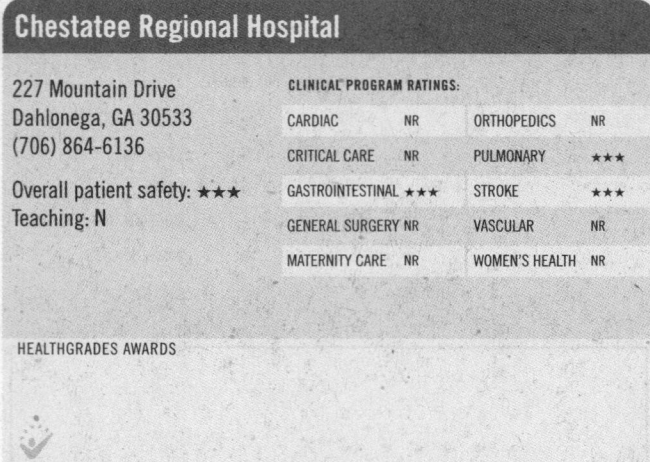

Chestatee Regional Hospital

227 Mountain Drive
Dahlonega, GA 30533
(706) 864-6136

Overall patient safety: ★★★
Teaching: N

CLINICAL PROGRAM RATINGS:

CARDIAC	NR	ORTHOPEDICS	NR
CRITICAL CARE	NR	PULMONARY	★★★
GASTROINTESTINAL	★★★	STROKE	★★★
GENERAL SURGERY	NR	VASCULAR	NR
MATERNITY CARE	NR	WOMEN'S HEALTH	NR

HEALTHGRADES AWARDS

Cartersville Medical Center

960 Joe Frank Harris Parkway
Cartersville, GA 30120
(770) 382-1530

Overall patient safety: ★★★
Teaching: N

CLINICAL PROGRAM RATINGS:

CARDIAC	NR	ORTHOPEDICS	★★★
CRITICAL CARE	★★★	PULMONARY	★★★
GASTROINTESTINAL	★★★	STROKE	★★★
GENERAL SURGERY	NR	VASCULAR	NR
MATERNITY CARE	NR	WOMEN'S HEALTH	NR

HEALTHGRADES AWARDS

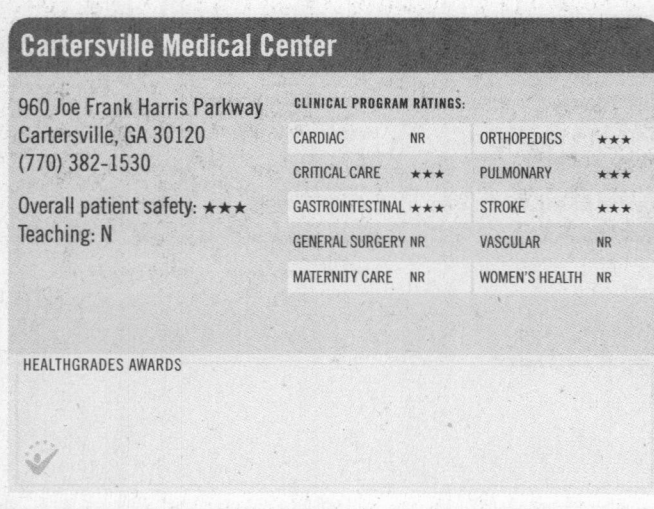

Cobb Memorial Hospital

577 Franklin Springs Street
Royston, GA 30662
(706) 245-5071

Overall patient safety: ★★★
Teaching: N

CLINICAL PROGRAM RATINGS:

CARDIAC	NR	ORTHOPEDICS	NR
CRITICAL CARE	NR	PULMONARY	★
GASTROINTESTINAL	NR	STROKE	NR
GENERAL SURGERY	NR	VASCULAR	NR
MATERNITY CARE	NR	WOMEN'S HEALTH	NR

HEALTHGRADES AWARDS

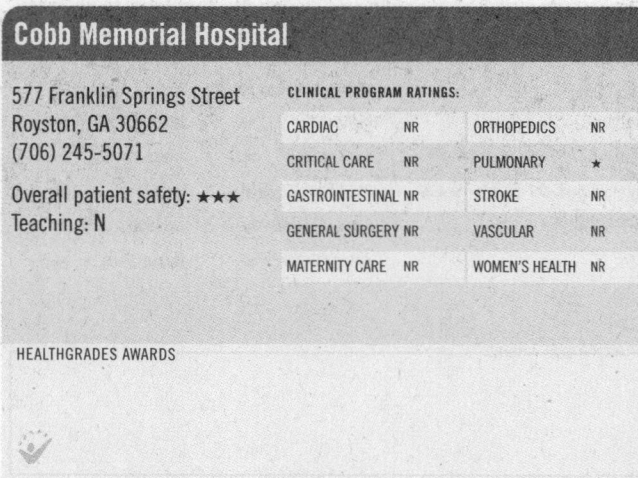

Chatuge Regional Hospital

110 East Main Street
Hiawassee, GA 30546
(706) 896-2222

Overall patient safety: NR
Teaching: N

CLINICAL PROGRAM RATINGS:

CARDIAC	NR	ORTHOPEDICS	NR
CRITICAL CARE	NR	PULMONARY	★★★
GASTROINTESTINAL	NR	STROKE	★
GENERAL SURGERY	NR	VASCULAR	NR
MATERNITY CARE	NR	WOMEN'S HEALTH	NR

HEALTHGRADES AWARDS

Coffee Regional Medical Center

1101 Ocilla Road
Douglas, GA 31533
(912) 384-1900

Overall patient safety: ★★★
Teaching: N

CLINICAL PROGRAM RATINGS:

CARDIAC	NR	ORTHOPEDICS	NR
CRITICAL CARE	NR	PULMONARY	★★★
GASTROINTESTINAL	NR	STROKE	★★★
GENERAL SURGERY	NR	VASCULAR	NR
MATERNITY CARE	NR	WOMEN'S HEALTH	NR

HEALTHGRADES AWARDS

KEY: ★★★★★ BEST   ★★★ AS EXPECTED   ★ POOR   NR NOT RATED BY HEALTHGRADES   For full definitions of ratings and awards, see Appendix.

Coliseum Medical Center

350 Hospital Drive
Macon, GA 31217
(478) 765-7000

Overall patient safety: ★
Teaching: N

CLINICAL PROGRAM RATINGS:

CARDIAC	★★★	ORTHOPEDICS	★★★
CRITICAL CARE	★★★	PULMONARY	★★★
GASTROINTESTINAL	★★★	STROKE	★★★
GENERAL SURGERY	NR	VASCULAR	NR
MATERNITY CARE	NR	WOMEN'S HEALTH	NR

HEALTHGRADES AWARDS

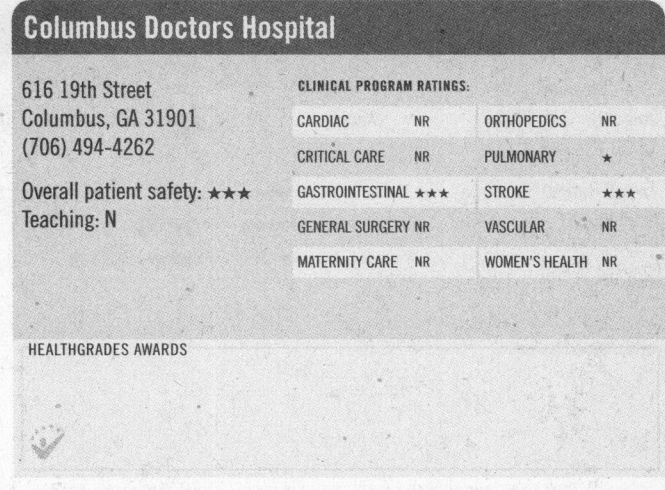

Columbus Doctors Hospital

616 19th Street
Columbus, GA 31901
(706) 494-4262

Overall patient safety: ★★★
Teaching: N

CLINICAL PROGRAM RATINGS:

CARDIAC	NR	ORTHOPEDICS	NR
CRITICAL CARE	NR	PULMONARY	★
GASTROINTESTINAL	★★★	STROKE	★★★
GENERAL SURGERY	NR	VASCULAR	NR
MATERNITY CARE	NR	WOMEN'S HEALTH	NR

HEALTHGRADES AWARDS

Coliseum Northside Hospital

400 Charter Boulevard
Macon, GA 31210
(478) 757-8200

Overall patient safety: ★★★
Teaching: N

CLINICAL PROGRAM RATINGS:

CARDIAC	NR	ORTHOPEDICS	NR
CRITICAL CARE	NR	PULMONARY	★★★
GASTROINTESTINAL	NR	STROKE	★★★
GENERAL SURGERY	NR	VASCULAR	NR
MATERNITY CARE	NR	WOMEN'S HEALTH	NR

HEALTHGRADES AWARDS

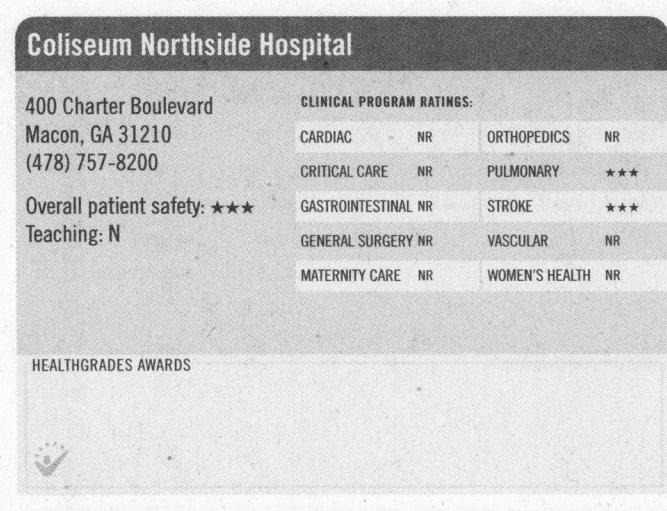

Crisp Regional Hospital

902 7th Street North
Cordele, GA 31015
(229) 276-3100

Overall patient safety: ★★★
Teaching: N

CLINICAL PROGRAM RATINGS:

CARDIAC	NR	ORTHOPEDICS	NR
CRITICAL CARE	NR	PULMONARY	★★★
GASTROINTESTINAL	NR	STROKE	★★★★★
GENERAL SURGERY	NR	VASCULAR	NR
MATERNITY CARE	NR	WOMEN'S HEALTH	NR

HEALTHGRADES AWARDS

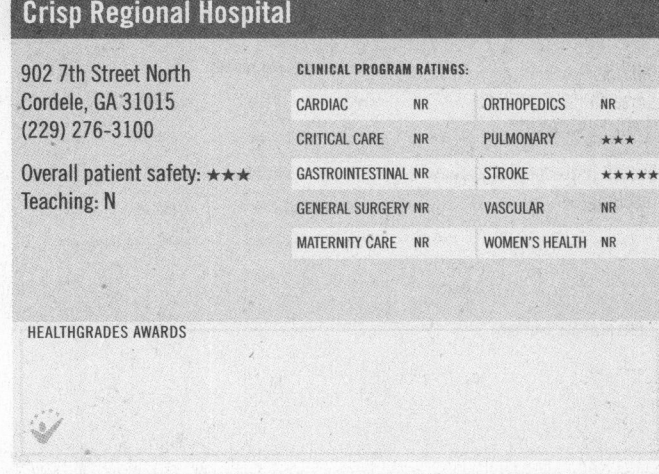

Colquitt Regional Medical Center

3131 South Main Street
Moultrie, GA 31768
(229) 985-3420

Overall patient safety: ★★★★★
Teaching: N

CLINICAL PROGRAM RATINGS:

CARDIAC	NR	ORTHOPEDICS	NR
CRITICAL CARE	NR	PULMONARY	★★★
GASTROINTESTINAL	★★★	STROKE	★★★
GENERAL SURGERY	NR	VASCULAR	NR
MATERNITY CARE	NR	WOMEN'S HEALTH	NR

HEALTHGRADES AWARDS

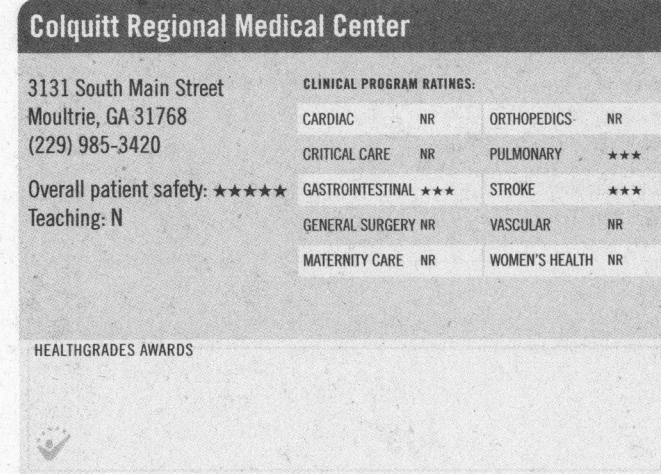

Dekalb Medical Center

2701 North Decatur Road
Decatur, GA 30033
(404) 501-1000

Overall patient safety: ★
Teaching: N

CLINICAL PROGRAM RATINGS:

CARDIAC	NR	ORTHOPEDICS	★★★
CRITICAL CARE	★★★	PULMONARY	★★★
GASTROINTESTINAL	★★★	STROKE	★★★
GENERAL SURGERY	NR	VASCULAR	NR
MATERNITY CARE	NR	WOMEN'S HEALTH	NR

HEALTHGRADES AWARDS

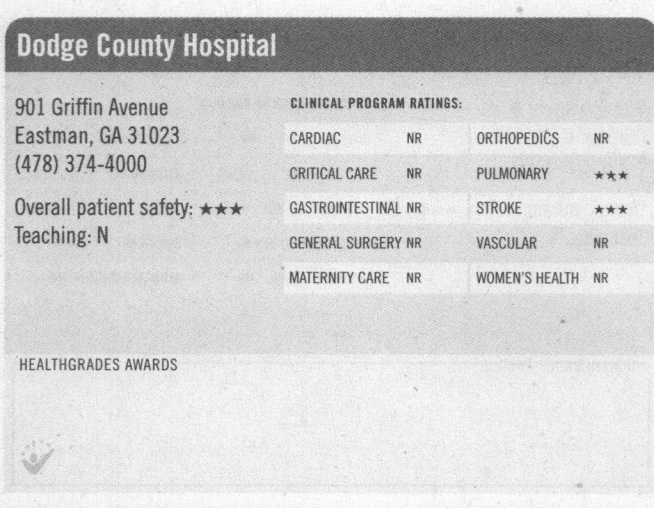

Doctors Hospital

3651 Wheeler Road
Augusta, GA 30909
(706) 651-3232

Overall patient safety: ★
Teaching: N

CLINICAL PROGRAM RATINGS:

CARDIAC	NR	ORTHOPEDICS	★★★
CRITICAL CARE	NR	PULMONARY	★★★
GASTROINTESTINAL	★★★	STROKE	★★★
GENERAL SURGERY	NR	VASCULAR	NR
MATERNITY CARE	NR	WOMEN'S HEALTH	NR

HEALTHGRADES AWARDS

Dorminy Medical Center

200 Perry House Road
Fitzgerald, GA 31750
(229) 424-7100

Overall patient safety: ★
Teaching: N

CLINICAL PROGRAM RATINGS:

CARDIAC	NR	ORTHOPEDICS	NR
CRITICAL CARE	NR	PULMONARY	★★★
GASTROINTESTINAL	NR	STROKE	NR
GENERAL SURGERY	NR	VASCULAR	NR
MATERNITY CARE	NR	WOMEN'S HEALTH	NR

HEALTHGRADES AWARDS

Dodge County Hospital

901 Griffin Avenue
Eastman, GA 31023
(478) 374-4000

Overall patient safety: ★★★
Teaching: N

CLINICAL PROGRAM RATINGS:

CARDIAC	NR	ORTHOPEDICS	NR
CRITICAL CARE	NR	PULMONARY	★★★
GASTROINTESTINAL	NR	STROKE	★★★
GENERAL SURGERY	NR	VASCULAR	NR
MATERNITY CARE	NR	WOMEN'S HEALTH	NR

HEALTHGRADES AWARDS

East Georgia Regional Medical Center

1499 Fair Road
Statesboro, GA 30458
(912) 486-1000

Overall patient safety: ★★★
Teaching: N

CLINICAL PROGRAM RATINGS:

CARDIAC	NR	ORTHOPEDICS	NR
CRITICAL CARE	NR	PULMONARY	★★★
GASTROINTESTINAL	NR	STROKE	★★★
GENERAL SURGERY	NR	VASCULAR	NR
MATERNITY CARE	NR	WOMEN'S HEALTH	NR

HEALTHGRADES AWARDS

Donalsonville Hospital

102 Hospital Circle
Donalsonville, GA 31745
(229) 524-5217

Overall patient safety: ★★★
Teaching: N

CLINICAL PROGRAM RATINGS:

CARDIAC	NR	ORTHOPEDICS	NR
CRITICAL CARE	NR	PULMONARY	★★★
GASTROINTESTINAL	NR	STROKE	NR
GENERAL SURGERY	NR	VASCULAR	NR
MATERNITY CARE	NR	WOMEN'S HEALTH	NR

HEALTHGRADES AWARDS

Elbert Memorial Hospital

4 Medical Drive
Elberton, GA 30635
(706) 283-3151

Overall patient safety: ★★★
Teaching: N

CLINICAL PROGRAM RATINGS:

CARDIAC	NR	ORTHOPEDICS	NR
CRITICAL CARE	NR	PULMONARY	★
GASTROINTESTINAL	NR	STROKE	★★★
GENERAL SURGERY	NR	VASCULAR	NR
MATERNITY CARE	NR	WOMEN'S HEALTH	NR

HEALTHGRADES AWARDS

GEORGIA HOSPITALS: RATINGS BY CLINICAL SPECIALTY

KEY: ★★★★★ BEST   ★★★ AS EXPECTED   ★ POOR   NR NOT RATED BY HEALTHGRADES   For full definitions of ratings and awards, see Appendix.

Emanuel County Hospital

117 Kite Road
Swainsboro, GA 30401
(478) 289-1100

Overall patient safety: ★★★
Teaching: N

CLINICAL PROGRAM RATINGS:

CARDIAC	NR	ORTHOPEDICS	NR
CRITICAL CARE	NR	PULMONARY	★★★
GASTROINTESTINAL	NR	STROKE	NR
GENERAL SURGERY	NR	VASCULAR	NR
MATERNITY CARE	NR	WOMEN'S HEALTH	NR

HEALTHGRADES AWARDS

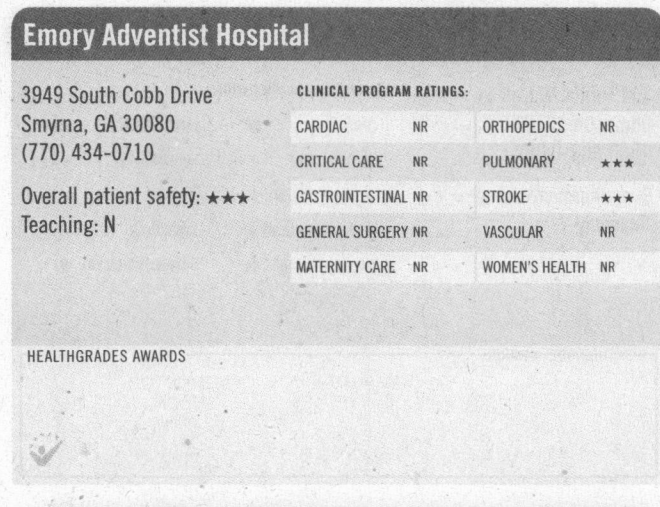

Emory Dunwoody Medical Center

4575 North Shallowford Road
Atlanta, GA 30338
(770) 454-2000

Overall patient safety: ★
Teaching: Y

CLINICAL PROGRAM RATINGS:

CARDIAC	NR	ORTHOPEDICS	NR
CRITICAL CARE	NR	PULMONARY	★★★
GASTROINTESTINAL	NR	STROKE	NR
GENERAL SURGERY	NR	VASCULAR	NR
MATERNITY CARE	NR	WOMEN'S HEALTH	NR

HEALTHGRADES AWARDS

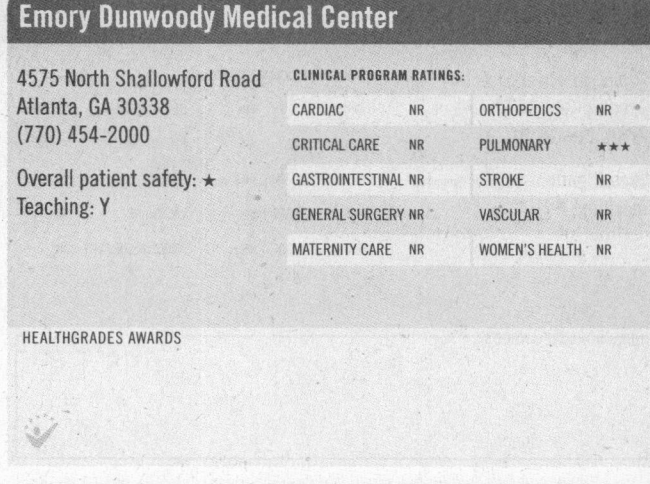

Emory Adventist Hospital

3949 South Cobb Drive
Smyrna, GA 30080
(770) 434-0710

Overall patient safety: ★★★
Teaching: N

CLINICAL PROGRAM RATINGS:

CARDIAC	NR	ORTHOPEDICS	NR
CRITICAL CARE	NR	PULMONARY	★★★
GASTROINTESTINAL	NR	STROKE	★★★
GENERAL SURGERY	NR	VASCULAR	NR
MATERNITY CARE	NR	WOMEN'S HEALTH	NR

HEALTHGRADES AWARDS

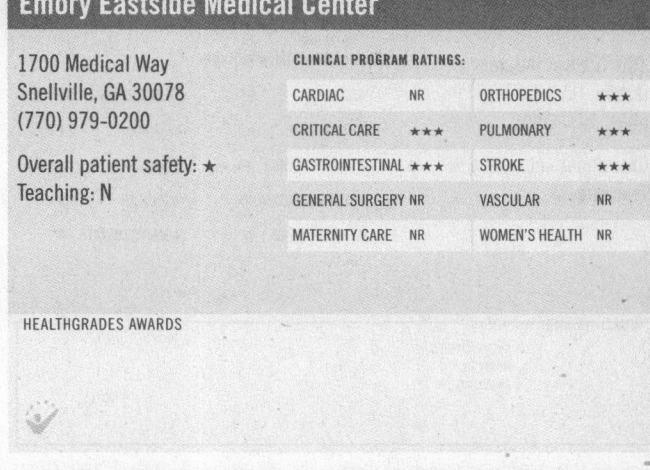

Emory Eastside Medical Center

1700 Medical Way
Snellville, GA 30078
(770) 979-0200

Overall patient safety: ★
Teaching: N

CLINICAL PROGRAM RATINGS:

CARDIAC	NR	ORTHOPEDICS	★★★
CRITICAL CARE	★★★	PULMONARY	★★★
GASTROINTESTINAL	★★★	STROKE	★★★
GENERAL SURGERY	NR	VASCULAR	NR
MATERNITY CARE	NR	WOMEN'S HEALTH	NR

HEALTHGRADES AWARDS

Emory Crawford Long Hospital

550 Peachtree Street Northeast
Atlanta, GA 30308
(404) 686-4411

Overall patient safety: ★★★
Teaching: Y

CLINICAL PROGRAM RATINGS:

CARDIAC	★★★	ORTHOPEDICS	★
CRITICAL CARE	★★★	PULMONARY	★★★
GASTROINTESTINAL	★★★	STROKE	★★★
GENERAL SURGERY	NR	VASCULAR	NR
MATERNITY CARE	NR	WOMEN'S HEALTH	NR

HEALTHGRADES AWARDS

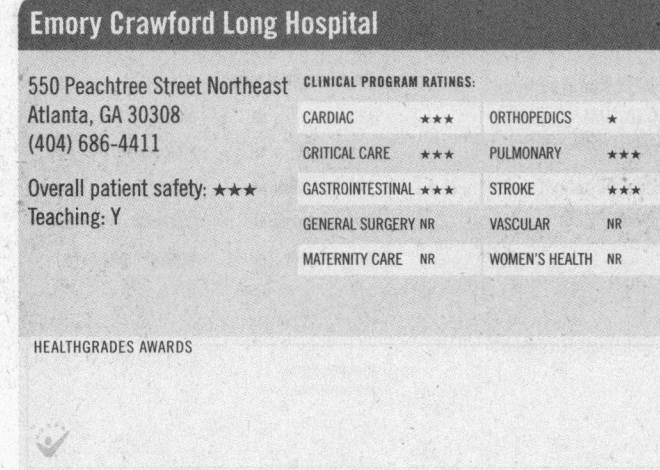

Emory University Hospital

1364 Clifton Road Northeast
Atlanta, GA 30322
(404) 712-7021

Overall patient safety: ★★★
Teaching: Y

CLINICAL PROGRAM RATINGS:

CARDIAC	★★★	ORTHOPEDICS	★
CRITICAL CARE	★	PULMONARY	★★★★★
GASTROINTESTINAL	★★★	STROKE	★★★
GENERAL SURGERY	NR	VASCULAR	★
MATERNITY CARE	NR	WOMEN'S HEALTH	NR

HEALTHGRADES AWARDS

Evans Memorial Hospital

200 North River Street
Claxton, GA 30417
(912) 739-2611

Overall patient safety: ★★★
Teaching: N

CLINICAL PROGRAM RATINGS:

CARDIAC	NR	ORTHOPEDICS	NR
CRITICAL CARE	NR	PULMONARY	★★★
GASTROINTESTINAL	NR	STROKE	NR
GENERAL SURGERY	NR	VASCULAR	NR
MATERNITY CARE	NR	WOMEN'S HEALTH	NR

HEALTHGRADES AWARDS

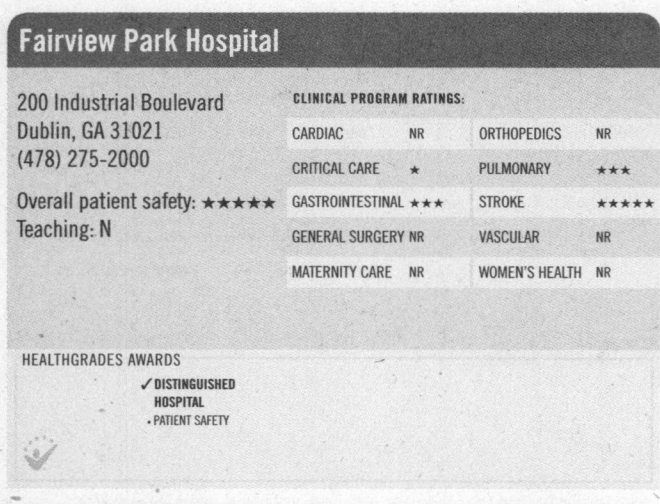

Flint River Hospital

509 Sumter Street
Montezuma, GA 31063
(478) 472-3100

Overall patient safety: ★★★
Teaching: N

CLINICAL PROGRAM RATINGS:

CARDIAC	NR	ORTHOPEDICS	NR
CRITICAL CARE	NR	PULMONARY	★★★
GASTROINTESTINAL	NR	STROKE	NR
GENERAL SURGERY	NR	VASCULAR	NR
MATERNITY CARE	NR	WOMEN'S HEALTH	NR

HEALTHGRADES AWARDS

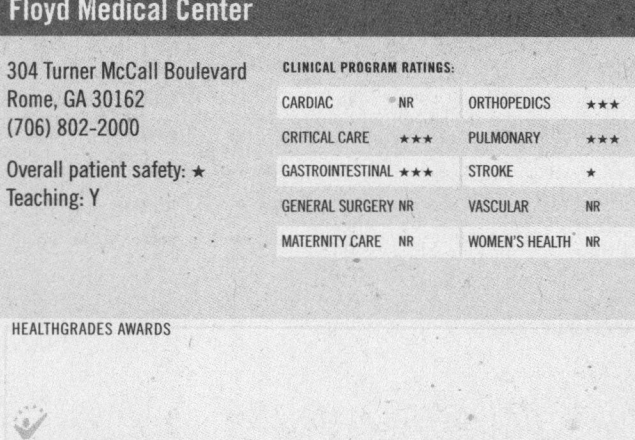

Fairview Park Hospital

200 Industrial Boulevard
Dublin, GA 31021
(478) 275-2000

Overall patient safety: ★★★★★
Teaching: N

CLINICAL PROGRAM RATINGS:

CARDIAC	NR	ORTHOPEDICS	NR
CRITICAL CARE	★	PULMONARY	★★★
GASTROINTESTINAL	★★★	STROKE	★★★★★
GENERAL SURGERY	NR	VASCULAR	NR
MATERNITY CARE	NR	WOMEN'S HEALTH	NR

HEALTHGRADES AWARDS

✓ DISTINGUISHED
HOSPITAL
• PATIENT SAFETY

Floyd Medical Center

304 Turner McCall Boulevard
Rome, GA 30162
(706) 802-2000

Overall patient safety: ★
Teaching: Y

CLINICAL PROGRAM RATINGS:

CARDIAC	NR	ORTHOPEDICS	★★★
CRITICAL CARE	★★★	PULMONARY	★★★
GASTROINTESTINAL	★★★	STROKE	★
GENERAL SURGERY	NR	VASCULAR	NR
MATERNITY CARE	NR	WOMEN'S HEALTH	NR

HEALTHGRADES AWARDS

Fannin Regional Hospital

2855 Old Highway 5
Blue Ridge, GA 30513
(706) 632-3711

Overall patient safety: ★★★★★
Teaching: N

CLINICAL PROGRAM RATINGS:

CARDIAC	NR	ORTHOPEDICS	NR
CRITICAL CARE	NR	PULMONARY	★
GASTROINTESTINAL	NR	STROKE	NR
GENERAL SURGERY	NR	VASCULAR	NR
MATERNITY CARE	NR	WOMEN'S HEALTH	NR

HEALTHGRADES AWARDS

Gordon Hospital

1035 Red Bud Road
Calhoun, GA 30701
(706) 629-2895

Overall patient safety: ★★★★★
Teaching: N

CLINICAL PROGRAM RATINGS:

CARDIAC	NR	ORTHOPEDICS	NR
CRITICAL CARE	NR	PULMONARY	★★★
GASTROINTESTINAL	NR	STROKE	★★★
GENERAL SURGERY	NR	VASCULAR	NR
MATERNITY CARE	NR	WOMEN'S HEALTH	NR

HEALTHGRADES AWARDS

KEY: ★★★★★ BEST   ★★★ AS EXPECTED   ★ POOR   NR NOT RATED BY HEALTHGRADES   For full definitions of ratings and awards, see Appendix.

Grady General Hospital

1155 5th Street Southeast
Cairo, GA 39828
(229) 377-1150

Overall patient safety: ★★★
Teaching: N

CLINICAL PROGRAM RATINGS:

CARDIAC	NR	ORTHOPEDICS	NR
CRITICAL CARE	NR	PULMONARY	★
GASTROINTESTINAL	NR	STROKE	★★★
GENERAL SURGERY	NR	VASCULAR	NR
MATERNITY CARE	NR	WOMEN'S HEALTH	NR

HEALTHGRADES AWARDS

Habersham County Medical Center

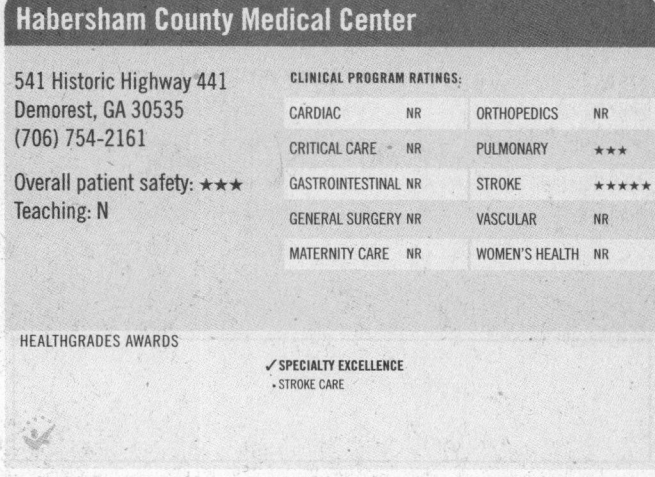

541 Historic Highway 441
Demorest, GA 30535
(706) 754-2161

Overall patient safety: ★★★
Teaching: N

CLINICAL PROGRAM RATINGS:

CARDIAC	NR	ORTHOPEDICS	NR
CRITICAL CARE	NR	PULMONARY	★★★
GASTROINTESTINAL	NR	STROKE	★★★★★
GENERAL SURGERY	NR	VASCULAR	NR
MATERNITY CARE	NR	WOMEN'S HEALTH	NR

HEALTHGRADES AWARDS

✓ SPECIALTY EXCELLENCE
• STROKE CARE

Grady Memorial Hospital

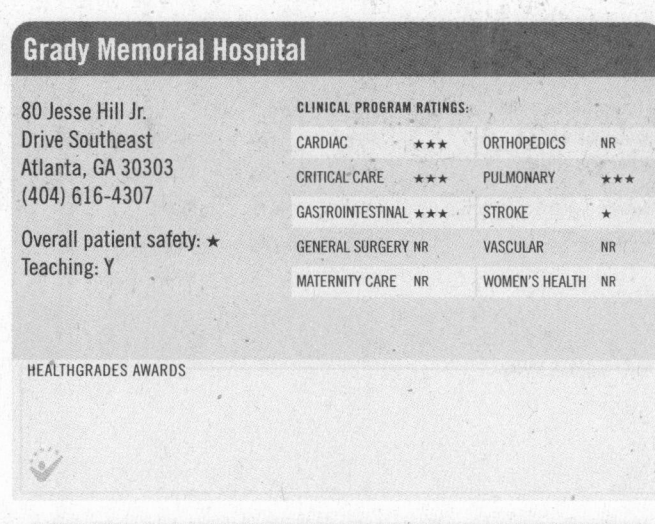

80 Jesse Hill Jr.
Drive Southeast
Atlanta, GA 30303
(404) 616-4307

Overall patient safety: ★
Teaching: Y

CLINICAL PROGRAM RATINGS:

CARDIAC	★★★	ORTHOPEDICS	NR
CRITICAL CARE	★★★	PULMONARY	★★★
GASTROINTESTINAL	★★★	STROKE	★
GENERAL SURGERY	NR	VASCULAR	NR
MATERNITY CARE	NR	WOMEN'S HEALTH	NR

HEALTHGRADES AWARDS

Hamilton Medical Center

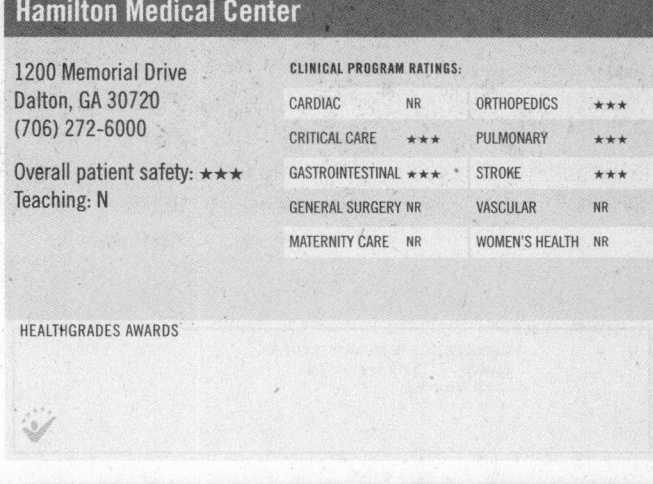

1200 Memorial Drive
Dalton, GA 30720
(706) 272-6000

Overall patient safety: ★★★
Teaching: N

CLINICAL PROGRAM RATINGS:

CARDIAC	NR	ORTHOPEDICS	★★★
CRITICAL CARE	★★★	PULMONARY	★★★
GASTROINTESTINAL	★★★	STROKE	★★★
GENERAL SURGERY	NR	VASCULAR	NR
MATERNITY CARE	NR	WOMEN'S HEALTH	NR

HEALTHGRADES AWARDS

Gwinnett Medical Center

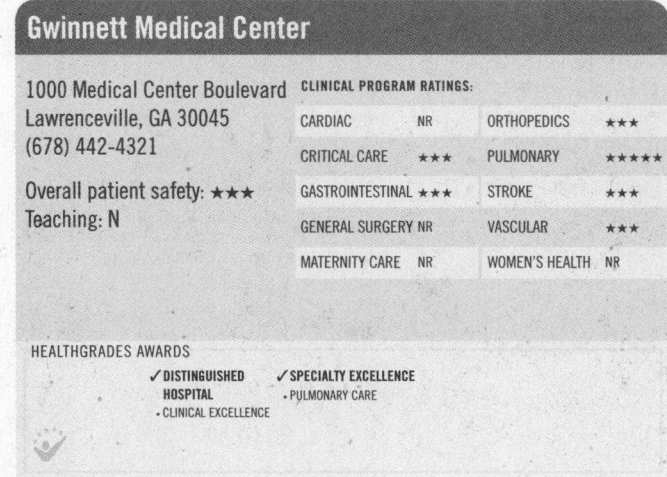

1000 Medical Center Boulevard
Lawrenceville, GA 30045
(678) 442-4321

Overall patient safety: ★★★
Teaching: N

CLINICAL PROGRAM RATINGS:

CARDIAC	NR	ORTHOPEDICS	★★★
CRITICAL CARE	★★★	PULMONARY	★★★★★
GASTROINTESTINAL	★★★	STROKE	★★★
GENERAL SURGERY	NR	VASCULAR	★★★
MATERNITY CARE	NR	WOMEN'S HEALTH	NR

HEALTHGRADES AWARDS

✓ DISTINGUISHED HOSPITAL
• CLINICAL EXCELLENCE

✓ SPECIALTY EXCELLENCE
• PULMONARY CARE

Hart County Hospital

138 West Gibson Street
Hartwell, GA 30643
(706) 856-6100

Overall patient safety: ★★★
Teaching: N

CLINICAL PROGRAM RATINGS:

CARDIAC	NR	ORTHOPEDICS	NR
CRITICAL CARE	NR	PULMONARY	★★★
GASTROINTESTINAL	NR	STROKE	★
GENERAL SURGERY	NR	VASCULAR	NR
MATERNITY CARE	NR	WOMEN'S HEALTH	NR

HEALTHGRADES AWARDS

Henry Medical Center

1133 Eagles Landing Parkway
Stockbridge, GA 30281
(770) 389-2200

Overall patient safety: ★★★
Teaching: N

CLINICAL PROGRAM RATINGS:

CARDIAC	NR	ORTHOPEDICS	★★★
CRITICAL CARE	NR	PULMONARY	★★★
GASTROINTESTINAL	★★★	STROKE	★★★
GENERAL SURGERY	NR	VASCULAR	NR
MATERNITY CARE	NR	WOMEN'S HEALTH	NR

HEALTHGRADES AWARDS

Hutcheson Medical Center

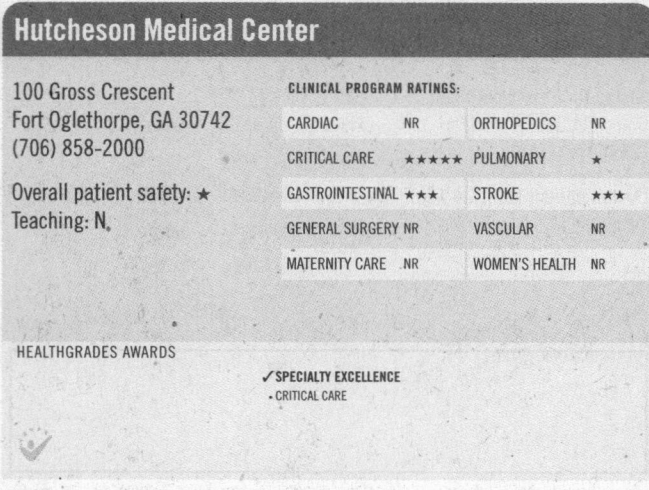

100 Gross Crescent
Fort Oglethorpe, GA 30742
(706) 858-2000

Overall patient safety: ★
Teaching: N

CLINICAL PROGRAM RATINGS:

CARDIAC	NR	ORTHOPEDICS	NR
CRITICAL CARE	★★★★★	PULMONARY	★
GASTROINTESTINAL	★★★	STROKE	★★★
GENERAL SURGERY	NR	VASCULAR	NR
MATERNITY CARE	NR	WOMEN'S HEALTH	NR

HEALTHGRADES AWARDS

✓ SPECIALTY EXCELLENCE
· CRITICAL CARE

Houston Medical Center

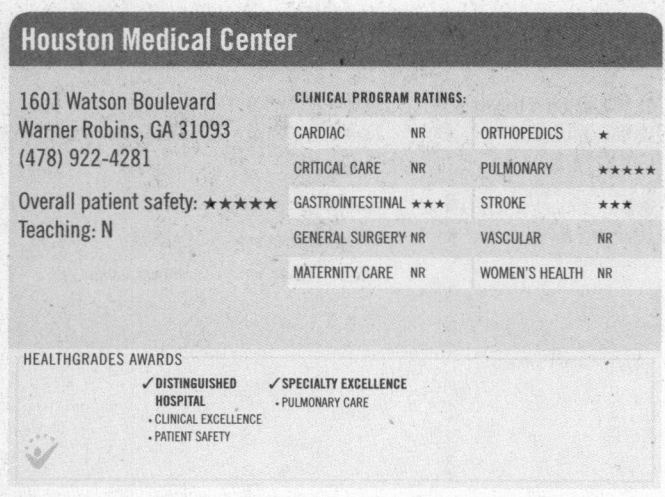

1601 Watson Boulevard
Warner Robins, GA 31093
(478) 922-4281

Overall patient safety: ★★★★★
Teaching: N

CLINICAL PROGRAM RATINGS:

CARDIAC	NR	ORTHOPEDICS	★
CRITICAL CARE	NR	PULMONARY	★★★★★
GASTROINTESTINAL	★★★	STROKE	★★★
GENERAL SURGERY	NR	VASCULAR	NR
MATERNITY CARE	NR	WOMEN'S HEALTH	NR

HEALTHGRADES AWARDS

✓ DISTINGUISHED HOSPITAL
· CLINICAL EXCELLENCE
· PATIENT SAFETY

✓ SPECIALTY EXCELLENCE
· PULMONARY CARE

Irwin County Hospital

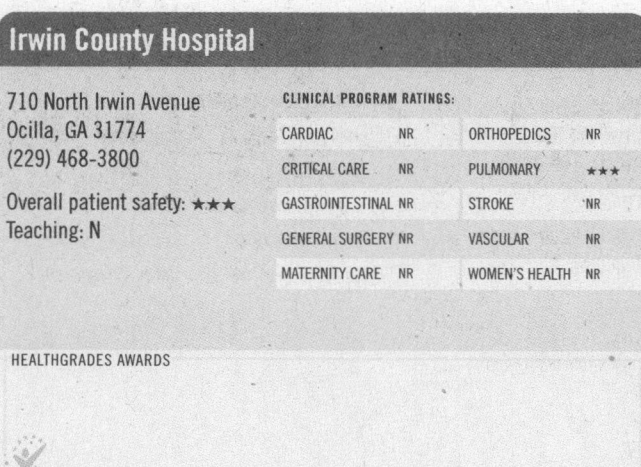

710 North Irwin Avenue
Ocilla, GA 31774
(229) 468-3800

Overall patient safety: ★★★
Teaching: N

CLINICAL PROGRAM RATINGS:

CARDIAC	NR	ORTHOPEDICS	NR
CRITICAL CARE	NR	PULMONARY	★★★
GASTROINTESTINAL	NR	STROKE	NR
GENERAL SURGERY	NR	VASCULAR	NR
MATERNITY CARE	NR	WOMEN'S HEALTH	NR

HEALTHGRADES AWARDS

Hughston Orthopedic Hospital

100 Frist Court
P.O. Box 7188
Columbus, GA 31908
(706) 494-2100

Overall patient safety: ★★★★
Teaching: N

CLINICAL PROGRAM RATINGS:

CARDIAC	NR	ORTHOPEDICS	★★★★★
CRITICAL CARE	NR	PULMONARY	NR
GASTROINTESTINAL	NR	STROKE	NR
GENERAL SURGERY	NR	VASCULAR	NR
MATERNITY CARE	NR	WOMEN'S HEALTH	NR

HEALTHGRADES AWARDS

✓ SPECIALTY EXCELLENCE
· JOINT REPLACEMENT

Jeff Davis Hospital

163 South Tallahassee Street
Hazlehurst, GA 31539
(912) 375-7781

Overall patient safety: ★
Teaching: N

CLINICAL PROGRAM RATINGS:

CARDIAC	NR	ORTHOPEDICS	NR
CRITICAL CARE	NR	PULMONARY	★
GASTROINTESTINAL	NR	STROKE	NR
GENERAL SURGERY	NR	VASCULAR	NR
MATERNITY CARE	NR	WOMEN'S HEALTH	NR

HEALTHGRADES AWARDS

KEY: ★★★★★ BEST   ★★★ AS EXPECTED   ★ POOR   NR NOT RATED BY HEALTHGRADES   For full definitions of ratings and awards, see Appendix.

Jefferson Hospital

1067 Peachtree Street
Louisville, GA 30434
(478) 625-7000

Overall patient safety: NR
Teaching: N

CLINICAL PROGRAM RATINGS:

CARDIAC	NR	ORTHOPEDICS	NR
CRITICAL CARE	NR	PULMONARY	★★★
GASTROINTESTINAL	NR	STROKE	NR
GENERAL SURGERY	NR	VASCULAR	NR
MATERNITY CARE	NR	WOMEN'S HEALTH	NR

HEALTHGRADES AWARDS

McDuffie Regional Medical Center

521 Hill Street Southwest
Thomson, GA 30824
(706) 595-1411

Overall patient safety: ★★★
Teaching: N

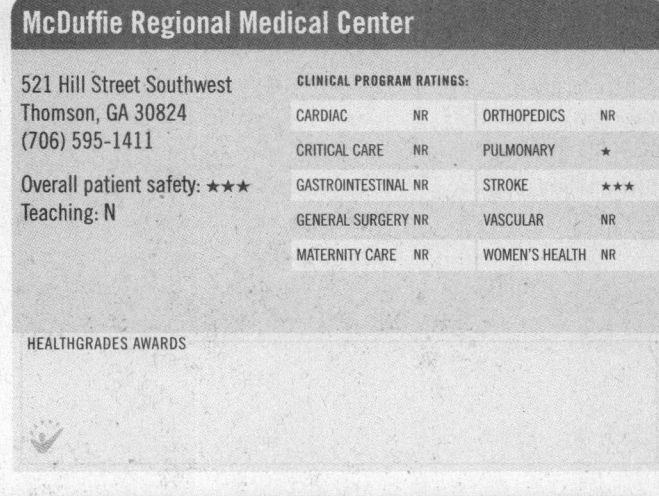

CLINICAL PROGRAM RATINGS:

CARDIAC	NR	ORTHOPEDICS	NR
CRITICAL CARE	NR	PULMONARY	★
GASTROINTESTINAL	NR	STROKE	★★★
GENERAL SURGERY	NR	VASCULAR	NR
MATERNITY CARE	NR	WOMEN'S HEALTH	NR

HEALTHGRADES AWARDS

John D. Archbold Memorial Hospital

Gordon Avenue at Mimosa Drive
Thomasville, GA 31792
(229) 228-2000

Overall patient safety: ★★★★★
Teaching: N

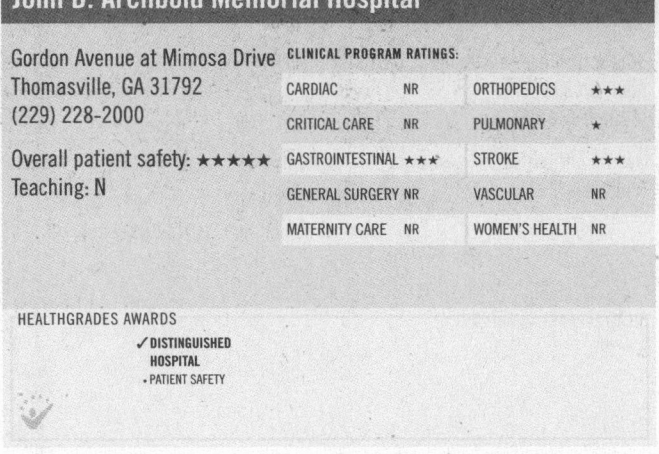

CLINICAL PROGRAM RATINGS:

CARDIAC	NR	ORTHOPEDICS	★★★
CRITICAL CARE	NR	PULMONARY	★
GASTROINTESTINAL	★★★	STROKE	★★★
GENERAL SURGERY	NR	VASCULAR	NR
MATERNITY CARE	NR	WOMEN'S HEALTH	NR

HEALTHGRADES AWARDS

✓ DISTINGUISHED HOSPITAL
• PATIENT SAFETY

Meadows Regional Medical Center

1703 Meadows Lane
P.O. Box 1048
Vidalia, GA 30474
(912) 537-8921

Overall patient safety: ★★★
Teaching: N

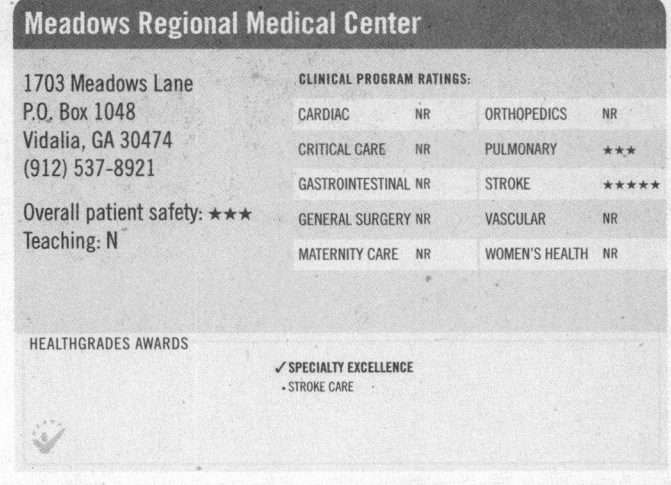

CLINICAL PROGRAM RATINGS:

CARDIAC	NR	ORTHOPEDICS	NR
CRITICAL CARE	NR	PULMONARY	★★★
GASTROINTESTINAL	NR	STROKE	★★★★★
GENERAL SURGERY	NR	VASCULAR	NR
MATERNITY CARE	NR	WOMEN'S HEALTH	NR

HEALTHGRADES AWARDS

✓ SPECIALTY EXCELLENCE
• STROKE CARE

Louis Smith Memorial Hospital

852 West Thigpen Avenue
Lakeland, GA 31635
(229) 482-2401

Overall patient safety: ★★★
Teaching: N

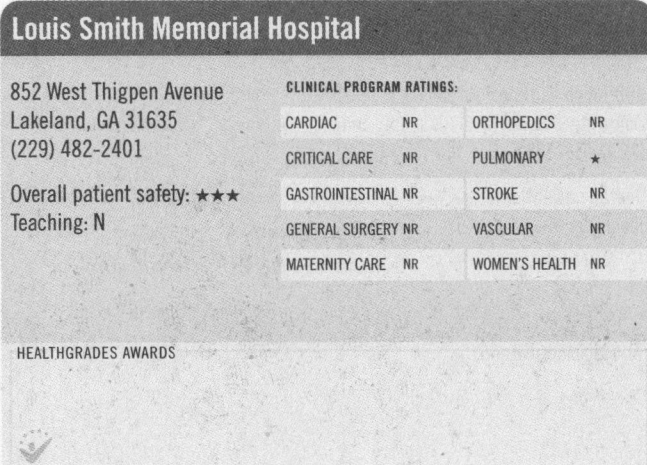

CLINICAL PROGRAM RATINGS:

CARDIAC	NR	ORTHOPEDICS	NR
CRITICAL CARE	NR	PULMONARY	★
GASTROINTESTINAL	NR	STROKE	NR
GENERAL SURGERY	NR	VASCULAR	NR
MATERNITY CARE	NR	WOMEN'S HEALTH	NR

HEALTHGRADES AWARDS

Medical College of Georgia Hospitals and Clinics

1120 15th Street
Augusta, GA 30912
(706) 721-0211

Overall patient safety: ★★★
Teaching: Y

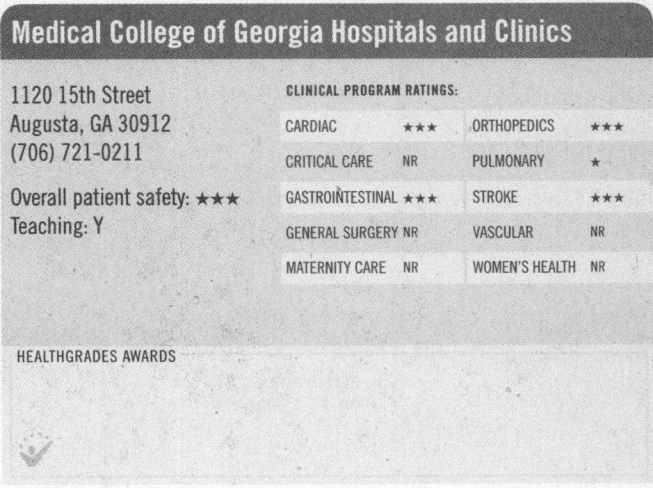

CLINICAL PROGRAM RATINGS:

CARDIAC	★★★	ORTHOPEDICS	★★★
CRITICAL CARE	NR	PULMONARY	★
GASTROINTESTINAL	★★★	STROKE	★★★
GENERAL SURGERY	NR	VASCULAR	NR
MATERNITY CARE	NR	WOMEN'S HEALTH	NR

HEALTHGRADES AWARDS

Medical Center

710 Center Street
Columbus, GA 31902
(706) 571-1000

Overall patient safety: ★
Teaching: Y

CLINICAL PROGRAM RATINGS:

CARDIAC	NR	ORTHOPEDICS	NR
CRITICAL CARE	NR	PULMONARY	★
GASTROINTESTINAL	★★★	STROKE	★★★
GENERAL SURGERY	NR	VASCULAR	NR
MATERNITY CARE	NR	WOMEN'S HEALTH	NR

HEALTHGRADES AWARDS

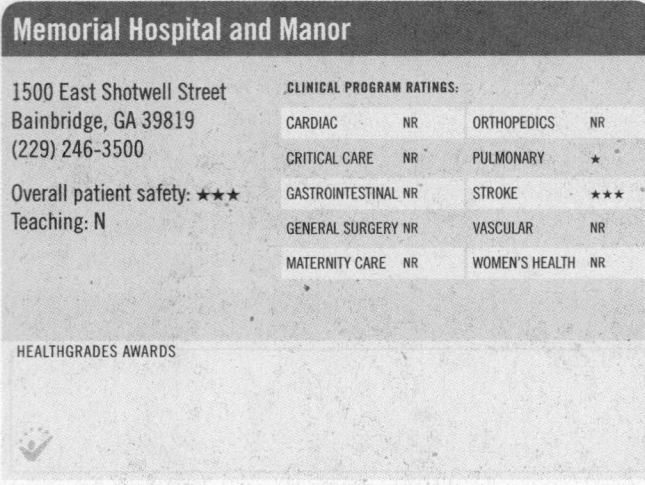

Memorial Hospital and Manor

1500 East Shotwell Street
Bainbridge, GA 39819
(229) 246-3500

Overall patient safety: ★★★
Teaching: N

CLINICAL PROGRAM RATINGS:

CARDIAC	NR	ORTHOPEDICS	NR
CRITICAL CARE	NR	PULMONARY	★
GASTROINTESTINAL	NR	STROKE	★★★
GENERAL SURGERY	NR	VASCULAR	NR
MATERNITY CARE	NR	WOMEN'S HEALTH	NR

HEALTHGRADES AWARDS

Medical Center of Central Georgia

777 Hemlock Street
Macon, GA 31201
(478) 633-1000

Overall patient safety: ★★★★★
Teaching: Y

CLINICAL PROGRAM RATINGS:

CARDIAC	★★★	ORTHOPEDICS	★★★
CRITICAL CARE	NR	PULMONARY	★
GASTROINTESTINAL	★	STROKE	★
GENERAL SURGERY	NR	VASCULAR	★★★
MATERNITY CARE	NR	WOMEN'S HEALTH	NR

HEALTHGRADES AWARDS

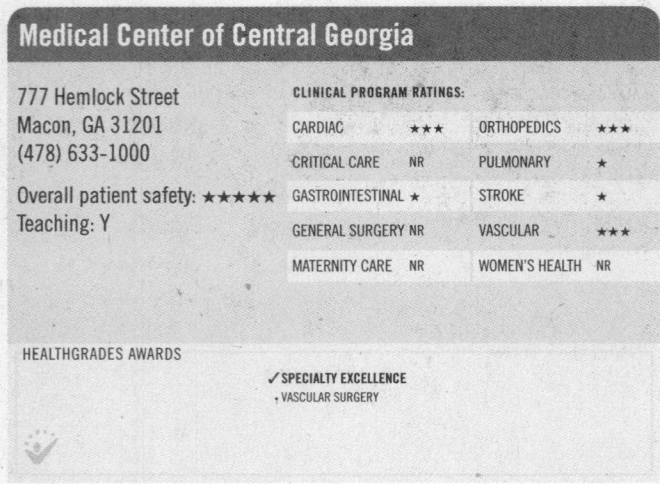

✓ SPECIALTY EXCELLENCE
 • VASCULAR SURGERY

Memorial Hospital of Adel

706 North Parrish Avenue
Adel, GA 31620
(229) 896-8000

Overall patient safety: ★★★
Teaching: N

CLINICAL PROGRAM RATINGS:

CARDIAC	NR	ORTHOPEDICS	NR
CRITICAL CARE	NR	PULMONARY	★★★
GASTROINTESTINAL	NR	STROKE	★★★
GENERAL SURGERY	NR	VASCULAR	NR
MATERNITY CARE	NR	WOMEN'S HEALTH	NR

HEALTHGRADES AWARDS

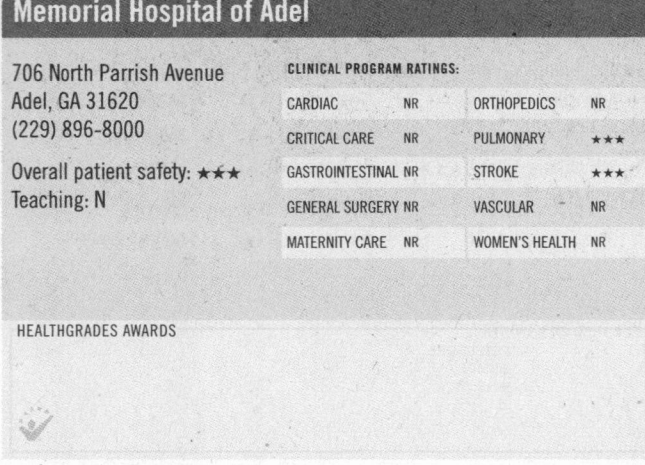

Memorial Health University Medical Center

4700 Waters Avenue
Savannah, GA 31404
(912) 350-8000

Overall patient safety: ★★★
Teaching: Y

CLINICAL PROGRAM RATINGS:

CARDIAC	★★★	ORTHOPEDICS	★★★
CRITICAL CARE	★★★★★	PULMONARY	★★★★★
GASTROINTESTINAL	★★★	STROKE	★★★
GENERAL SURGERY	NR	VASCULAR	★★★
MATERNITY CARE	NR	WOMEN'S HEALTH	NR

HEALTHGRADES AWARDS

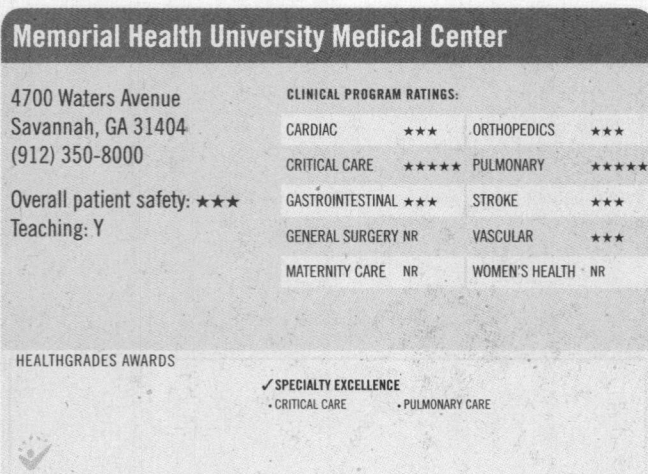

✓ SPECIALTY EXCELLENCE
 • CRITICAL CARE   • PULMONARY CARE

Miller County Hospital

209 North Cuthbert Street
Colquitt, GA 39837
(229) 758-3385

Overall patient safety: ★★★
Teaching: N

CLINICAL PROGRAM RATINGS:

CARDIAC	NR	ORTHOPEDICS	NR
CRITICAL CARE	NR	PULMONARY	NR
GASTROINTESTINAL	NR	STROKE	NR
GENERAL SURGERY	NR	VASCULAR	NR
MATERNITY CARE	NR	WOMEN'S HEALTH	NR

HEALTHGRADES AWARDS

KEY: ★★★★★ BEST   ★★★ AS EXPECTED   ★ POOR   NR NOT RATED BY HEALTHGRADES   For full definitions of ratings and awards, see Appendix.

Mitchell County Hospital

90 East Stephens
Camilla, GA 31730
(229) 336-5284

Overall patient safety: ★★★
Teaching: N

CLINICAL PROGRAM RATINGS:

CARDIAC	NR	ORTHOPEDICS	NR
CRITICAL CARE	NR	PULMONARY	NR
GASTROINTESTINAL	NR	STROKE	NR
GENERAL SURGERY	NR	VASCULAR	NR
MATERNITY CARE	NR	WOMEN'S HEALTH	NR

HEALTHGRADES AWARDS

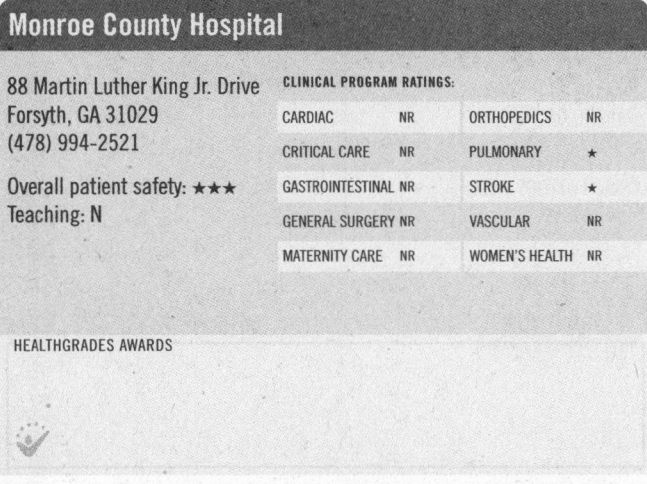

Murray Medical Center

707 Old Ellijay Road
Chatsworth, GA 30705
(706) 695-4564

Overall patient safety: ★★★
Teaching: N

CLINICAL PROGRAM RATINGS:

CARDIAC	NR	ORTHOPEDICS	NR
CRITICAL CARE	NR	PULMONARY	★★★
GASTROINTESTINAL	NR	STROKE	★★★
GENERAL SURGERY	NR	VASCULAR	NR
MATERNITY CARE	NR	WOMEN'S HEALTH	NR

HEALTHGRADES AWARDS

Monroe County Hospital

88 Martin Luther King Jr. Drive
Forsyth, GA 31029
(478) 994-2521

Overall patient safety: ★★★
Teaching: N

CLINICAL PROGRAM RATINGS:

CARDIAC	NR	ORTHOPEDICS	NR
CRITICAL CARE	NR	PULMONARY	★
GASTROINTESTINAL	NR	STROKE	★
GENERAL SURGERY	NR	VASCULAR	NR
MATERNITY CARE	NR	WOMEN'S HEALTH	NR

HEALTHGRADES AWARDS

Newton Medical Center

5126 Hospital Drive Northeast
Covington, GA 30014
(770) 786-7053

Overall patient safety: ★★★
Teaching: N

CLINICAL PROGRAM RATINGS:

CARDIAC	NR	ORTHOPEDICS	NR
CRITICAL CARE	★★★	PULMONARY	★
GASTROINTESTINAL	★★★	STROKE	★★★
GENERAL SURGERY	NR	VASCULAR	NR
MATERNITY CARE	NR	WOMEN'S HEALTH	NR

HEALTHGRADES AWARDS

Mountain Lakes Medical Center

196 Ridgecrest Circle
Clayton, GA 30525
(706) 782-4233

Overall patient safety: ★★★
Teaching: N

CLINICAL PROGRAM RATINGS:

CARDIAC	NR	ORTHOPEDICS	NR
CRITICAL CARE	NR	PULMONARY	★★★
GASTROINTESTINAL	NR	STROKE	NR
GENERAL SURGERY	NR	VASCULAR	NR
MATERNITY CARE	NR	WOMEN'S HEALTH	NR

HEALTHGRADES AWARDS

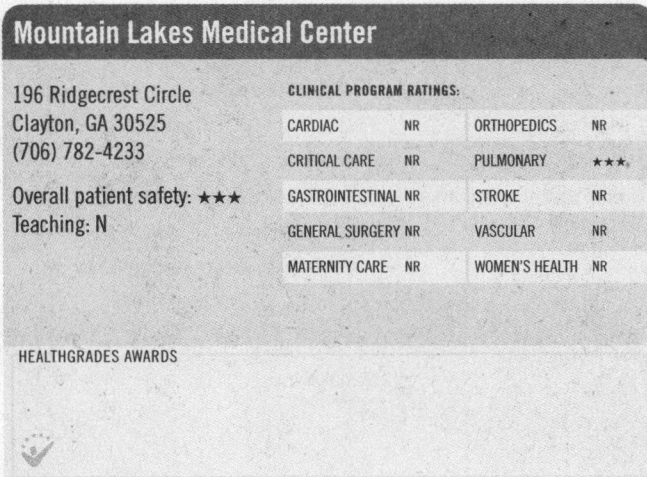

North Fulton Regional Hospital

3000 Hospital Boulevard
Roswell, GA 30076
(770) 751-2500

Overall patient safety: ★★★
Teaching: N

CLINICAL PROGRAM RATINGS:

CARDIAC	NR	ORTHOPEDICS	★★★
CRITICAL CARE	★★★★★	PULMONARY	★★★
GASTROINTESTINAL	★★★	STROKE	★★★
GENERAL SURGERY	NR	VASCULAR	NR
MATERNITY CARE	NR	WOMEN'S HEALTH	NR

HEALTHGRADES AWARDS

✓ SPECIALTY EXCELLENCE
· CRITICAL CARE

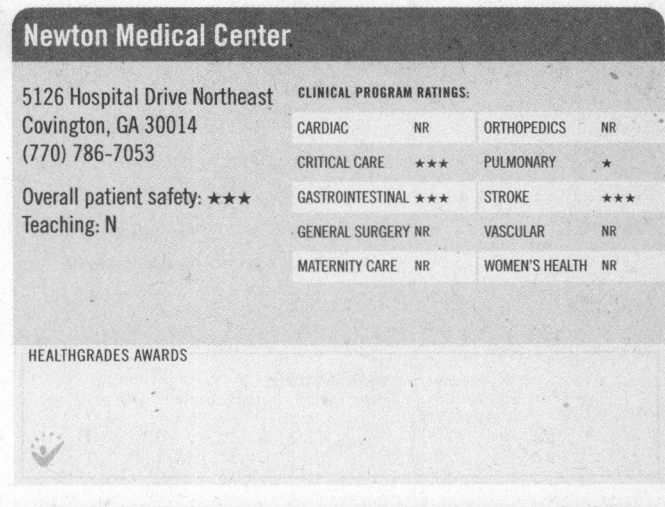

North Georgia Medical Center

1362 South Main Street
Ellijay, GA 30540
(706) 276-4741

Overall patient safety: ★★★
Teaching: N

CLINICAL PROGRAM RATINGS:

CARDIAC	NR	ORTHOPEDICS	NR
CRITICAL CARE	NR	PULMONARY	★★★
GASTROINTESTINAL	NR	STROKE	★★★
GENERAL SURGERY	NR	VASCULAR	NR
MATERNITY CARE	NR	WOMEN'S HEALTH	NR

HEALTHGRADES AWARDS

Northside Hospital

1000 Johnson Ferry
Road Northeast
Atlanta, GA 30342
(404) 851-8000

Overall patient safety: ★★★
Teaching: N

CLINICAL PROGRAM RATINGS:

CARDIAC	NR	ORTHOPEDICS	★★★
CRITICAL CARE	NR	PULMONARY	★★★
GASTROINTESTINAL	NR	STROKE	★★★
GENERAL SURGERY	NR	VASCULAR	NR
MATERNITY CARE	NR	WOMEN'S HEALTH	NR

HEALTHGRADES AWARDS

Northeast Georgia Medical Center*

743 Spring Street
Gainesville, GA 30501
(770) 535-3553

Overall patient safety: ★★★
Teaching: N

CLINICAL PROGRAM RATINGS:

CARDIAC	★★★★★	ORTHOPEDICS	★★★
CRITICAL CARE	★★★	PULMONARY	★★★
GASTROINTESTINAL	★★★	STROKE	★★★
GENERAL SURGERY	NR	VASCULAR	★★★
MATERNITY CARE	NR	WOMEN'S HEALTH	NR

HEALTHGRADES AWARDS

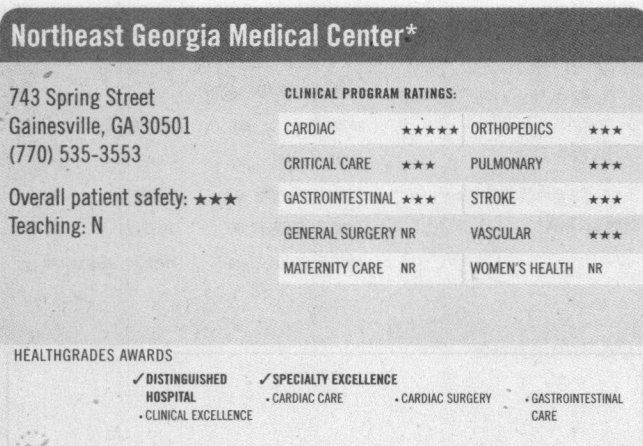

✓ DISTINGUISHED HOSPITAL
- CLINICAL EXCELLENCE

✓ SPECIALTY EXCELLENCE
- CARDIAC CARE
- CARDIAC SURGERY
- GASTROINTESTINAL CARE

Northside Hospital Cherokee

201 Hospital Road
Canton, GA 30114
(770) 720-5100

Overall patient safety: ★★★
Teaching: N

CLINICAL PROGRAM RATINGS:

CARDIAC	NR	ORTHOPEDICS	NR
CRITICAL CARE	NR	PULMONARY	★★★
GASTROINTESTINAL	NR	STROKE	★
GENERAL SURGERY	NR	VASCULAR	NR
MATERNITY CARE	NR	WOMEN'S HEALTH	NR

HEALTHGRADES AWARDS

Northeast Georgia Medical Center--Lanier Park Campus*

675 White Sulphur Road
Gainesville, GA 30501
(678) 343-4000

Overall patient safety: ★★★
Teaching: N

CLINICAL PROGRAM RATINGS:

CARDIAC	★★★★★	ORTHOPEDICS	★★★
CRITICAL CARE	★★★	PULMONARY	★★★
GASTROINTESTINAL	★★★	STROKE	★★★
GENERAL SURGERY	NR	VASCULAR	★★★
MATERNITY CARE	NR	WOMEN'S HEALTH	NR

HEALTHGRADES AWARDS

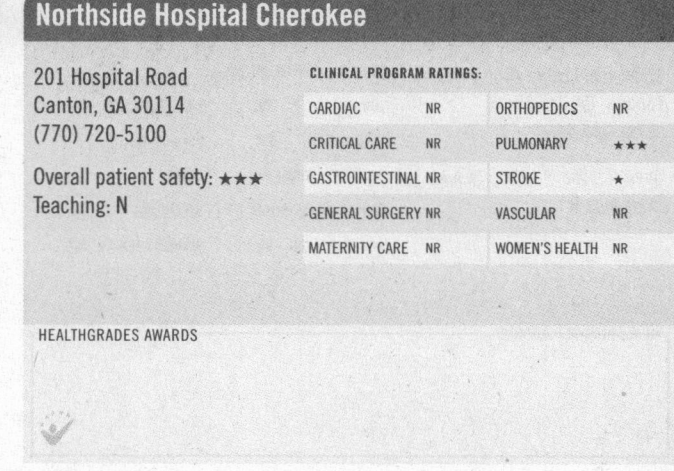

✓ SPECIALTY EXCELLENCE
- CARDIAC CARE
- CARDIAC SURGERY
- GASTROINTESTINAL CARE

Northside Hospital Forsyth

1200 Northside Forsyth Drive
Cumming, GA 30041
(770) 844-3200

Overall patient safety: ★★★
Teaching: N

CLINICAL PROGRAM RATINGS:

CARDIAC	NR	ORTHOPEDICS	★★★
CRITICAL CARE	★★★	PULMONARY	★★★★★
GASTROINTESTINAL	★★★	STROKE	★
GENERAL SURGERY	NR	VASCULAR	NR
MATERNITY CARE	NR	WOMEN'S HEALTH	NR

HEALTHGRADES AWARDS

✓ SPECIALTY EXCELLENCE
- PULMONARY CARE

KEY: ★★★★★ BEST   ★★★ AS EXPECTED   ★ POOR   NR NOT RATED BY HEALTHGRADES   For full definitions of ratings and awards, see Appendix.

Oconee Regional Medical Center

821 North Cobb Street
Milledgeville, GA 31061
(478) 454-3500

Overall patient safety: ★★★
Teaching: N

CLINICAL PROGRAM RATINGS:

CARDIAC	NR	ORTHOPEDICS	NR
CRITICAL CARE	NR	PULMONARY	★★★
GASTROINTESTINAL	★★★	STROKE	★★★
GENERAL SURGERY	NR	VASCULAR	NR
MATERNITY CARE	NR	WOMEN'S HEALTH	NR

HEALTHGRADES AWARDS

Perry General Hospital

1120 Morningside Drive
Perry, GA 31069
(478) 987-3600

Overall patient safety: ★★★
Teaching: N

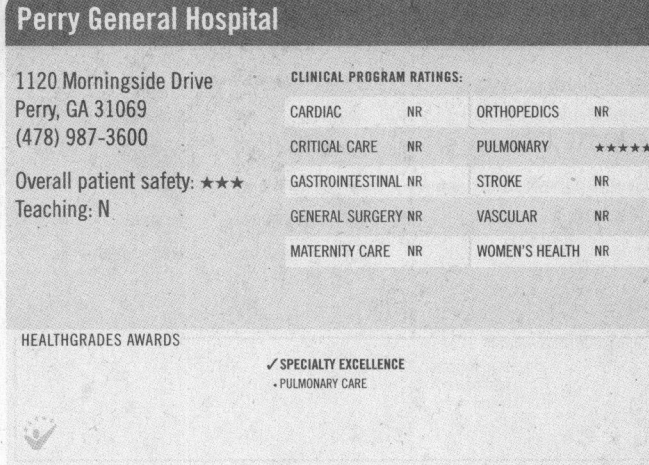

CLINICAL PROGRAM RATINGS:

CARDIAC	NR	ORTHOPEDICS	NR
CRITICAL CARE	NR	PULMONARY	★★★★★
GASTROINTESTINAL	NR	STROKE	NR
GENERAL SURGERY	NR	VASCULAR	NR
MATERNITY CARE	NR	WOMEN'S HEALTH	NR

HEALTHGRADES AWARDS

✓ SPECIALTY EXCELLENCE
• PULMONARY CARE

Palmyra Medical Center

2000 Palmyra Road
Albany, GA 31701
(229) 434-2000

Overall patient safety: ★★★
Teaching: N

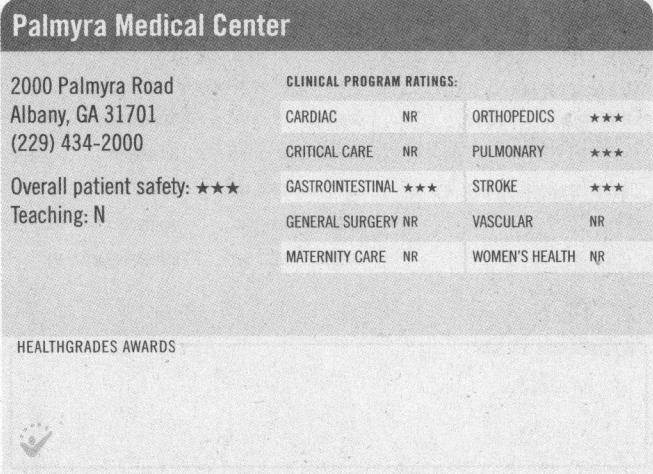

CLINICAL PROGRAM RATINGS:

CARDIAC	NR	ORTHOPEDICS	★★★
CRITICAL CARE	NR	PULMONARY	★★★
GASTROINTESTINAL	★★★	STROKE	★★★
GENERAL SURGERY	NR	VASCULAR	NR
MATERNITY CARE	NR	WOMEN'S HEALTH	NR

HEALTHGRADES AWARDS

Phoebe Putney Memorial Hospital

417 3rd Avenue
Albany, GA 31701
(229) 312-4100

Overall patient safety: ★★★
Teaching: Y

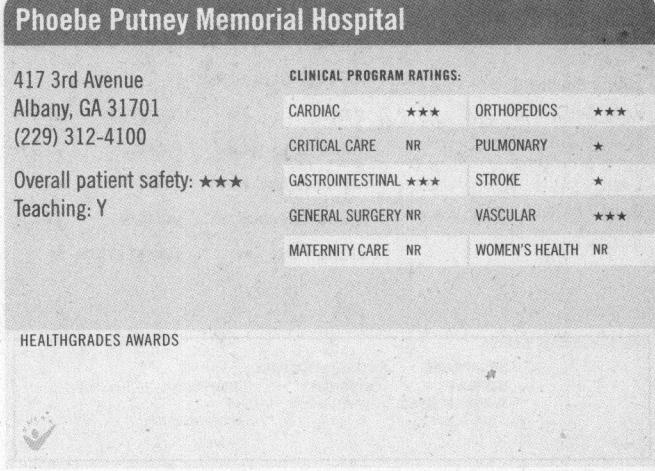

CLINICAL PROGRAM RATINGS:

CARDIAC	★★★	ORTHOPEDICS	★★★
CRITICAL CARE	NR	PULMONARY	★
GASTROINTESTINAL	★★★	STROKE	★
GENERAL SURGERY	NR	VASCULAR	★★★
MATERNITY CARE	NR	WOMEN'S HEALTH	NR

HEALTHGRADES AWARDS

Peach Regional Medical Center

601 Blue Bird Boulevard
Fort Valley, GA 31030
(478) 825-8691

Overall patient safety: ★★★
Teaching: N

CLINICAL PROGRAM RATINGS:

CARDIAC	NR	ORTHOPEDICS	NR
CRITICAL CARE	NR	PULMONARY	NR
GASTROINTESTINAL	NR	STROKE	NR
GENERAL SURGERY	NR	VASCULAR	NR
MATERNITY CARE	NR	WOMEN'S HEALTH	NR

HEALTHGRADES AWARDS

Phoebe Worth Medical Center

807 South Isabella Street
Sylvester, GA 31791
(229) 776-6961

Overall patient safety: ★★★
Teaching: N

CLINICAL PROGRAM RATINGS:

CARDIAC	NR	ORTHOPEDICS	NR
CRITICAL CARE	NR	PULMONARY	★★★
GASTROINTESTINAL	NR	STROKE	NR
GENERAL SURGERY	NR	VASCULAR	NR
MATERNITY CARE	NR	WOMEN'S HEALTH	NR

HEALTHGRADES AWARDS

*This hospital reports its data to the federal government jointly with another hospital. Therefore the ratings and awards apply to multiple hospitals and this specific hospital may not provide all rated services.

Piedmont Fayette Hospital

1255 Highway 54 West
Fayetteville, GA 30214
(770) 719-7070

Overall patient safety: ★★★★★
Teaching: N

CLINICAL PROGRAM RATINGS:

CARDIAC	NR	ORTHOPEDICS	NR
CRITICAL CARE	★★★	PULMONARY	★★★
GASTROINTESTINAL	★★★	STROKE	★★★
GENERAL SURGERY	NR	VASCULAR	NR
MATERNITY CARE	NR	WOMEN'S HEALTH	NR

HEALTHGRADES AWARDS

✓ DISTINGUISHED HOSPITAL
• PATIENT SAFETY

Piedmont Newnan Hospital

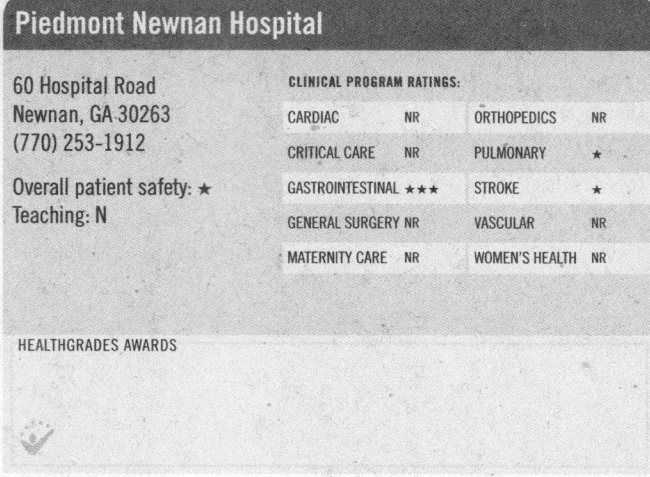

60 Hospital Road
Newnan, GA 30263
(770) 253-1912

Overall patient safety: ★
Teaching: N

CLINICAL PROGRAM RATINGS:

CARDIAC	NR	ORTHOPEDICS	NR
CRITICAL CARE	NR	PULMONARY	★
GASTROINTESTINAL	★★★	STROKE	★
GENERAL SURGERY	NR	VASCULAR	NR
MATERNITY CARE	NR	WOMEN'S HEALTH	NR

HEALTHGRADES AWARDS

Piedmont Hospital

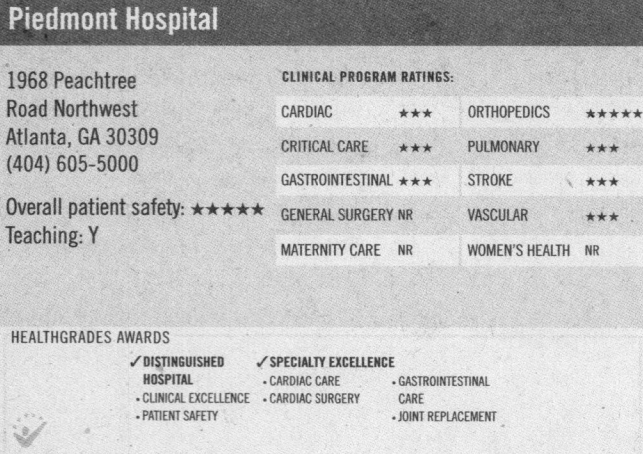

1968 Peachtree
Road Northwest
Atlanta, GA 30309
(404) 605-5000

Overall patient safety: ★★★★★
Teaching: Y

CLINICAL PROGRAM RATINGS:

CARDIAC	★★★	ORTHOPEDICS	★★★★★
CRITICAL CARE	★★★	PULMONARY	★★★
GASTROINTESTINAL	★★★	STROKE	★★★
GENERAL SURGERY	NR	VASCULAR	★★★
MATERNITY CARE	NR	WOMEN'S HEALTH	NR

HEALTHGRADES AWARDS

✓ DISTINGUISHED HOSPITAL
• CLINICAL EXCELLENCE
• PATIENT SAFETY

✓ SPECIALTY EXCELLENCE
• CARDIAC CARE
• CARDIAC SURGERY
• GASTROINTESTINAL CARE
• JOINT REPLACEMENT

Putnam General Hospital

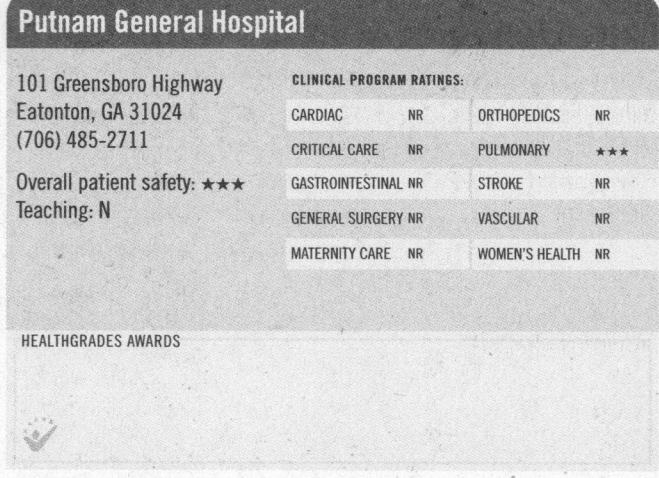

101 Greensboro Highway
Eatonton, GA 31024
(706) 485-2711

Overall patient safety: ★★★
Teaching: N

CLINICAL PROGRAM RATINGS:

CARDIAC	NR	ORTHOPEDICS	NR
CRITICAL CARE	NR	PULMONARY	★★★
GASTROINTESTINAL	NR	STROKE	NR
GENERAL SURGERY	NR	VASCULAR	NR
MATERNITY CARE	NR	WOMEN'S HEALTH	NR

HEALTHGRADES AWARDS

Piedmont Mountainside Hospital

1266 Highway 515 South
Jasper, GA 30143
(706) 301-5200

Overall patient safety: ★★★
Teaching: N

CLINICAL PROGRAM RATINGS:

CARDIAC	NR	ORTHOPEDICS	NR
CRITICAL CARE	NR	PULMONARY	★★★
GASTROINTESTINAL	NR	STROKE	★★★
GENERAL SURGERY	NR	VASCULAR	NR
MATERNITY CARE	NR	WOMEN'S HEALTH	NR

HEALTHGRADES AWARDS

Redmond Regional Medical Center

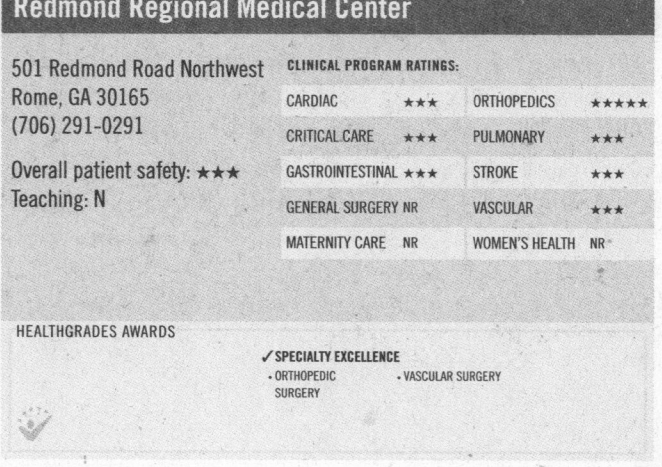

501 Redmond Road Northwest
Rome, GA 30165
(706) 291-0291

Overall patient safety: ★★★
Teaching: N

CLINICAL PROGRAM RATINGS:

CARDIAC	★★★	ORTHOPEDICS	★★★★★
CRITICAL CARE	★★★	PULMONARY	★★★
GASTROINTESTINAL	★★★	STROKE	★★★
GENERAL SURGERY	NR	VASCULAR	★★★
MATERNITY CARE	NR	WOMEN'S HEALTH	NR

HEALTHGRADES AWARDS

✓ SPECIALTY EXCELLENCE
• ORTHOPEDIC SURGERY
• VASCULAR SURGERY

KEY: ★★★★★ BEST   ★★★ AS EXPECTED   ★ POOR   NR NOT RATED BY HEALTHGRADES   For full definitions of ratings and awards, see Appendix.

Rockdale Medical Center

1412 Milstead Avenue
Northeast
Conyers, GA 30012
(770) 918-3000

Overall patient safety: ★★★
Teaching: N

CLINICAL PROGRAM RATINGS:

CARDIAC	NR	ORTHOPEDICS	★
CRITICAL CARE	★	PULMONARY	★★★
GASTROINTESTINAL	★★★	STROKE	★
GENERAL SURGERY	NR	VASCULAR	NR
MATERNITY CARE	NR	WOMEN'S HEALTH	NR

HEALTHGRADES AWARDS

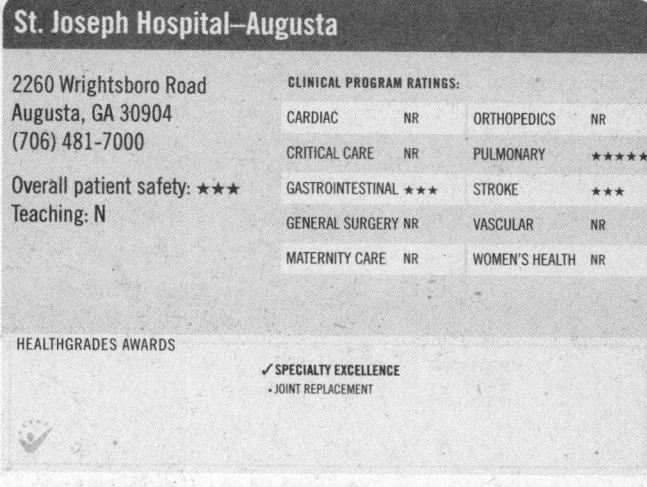

St. Joseph Hospital—Augusta

2260 Wrightsboro Road
Augusta, GA 30904
(706) 481-7000

Overall patient safety: ★★★
Teaching: N

CLINICAL PROGRAM RATINGS:

CARDIAC	NR	ORTHOPEDICS	NR
CRITICAL CARE	NR	PULMONARY	★★★★★
GASTROINTESTINAL	★★★	STROKE	★★★
GENERAL SURGERY	NR	VASCULAR	NR
MATERNITY CARE	NR	WOMEN'S HEALTH	NR

HEALTHGRADES AWARDS

✓ SPECIALTY EXCELLENCE
· JOINT REPLACEMENT

Roosevelt Warm Springs Rehabilitation Hospital*

6135 Roosevelt Highway
Warm Springs, GA 31830
(706) 655-5001

Overall patient safety: NR
Teaching: N

CLINICAL PROGRAM RATINGS:

CARDIAC	NR	ORTHOPEDICS	NR
CRITICAL CARE	NR	PULMONARY	★★★
GASTROINTESTINAL	NR	STROKE	NR
GENERAL SURGERY	NR	VASCULAR	NR
MATERNITY CARE	NR	WOMEN'S HEALTH	NR

HEALTHGRADES AWARDS

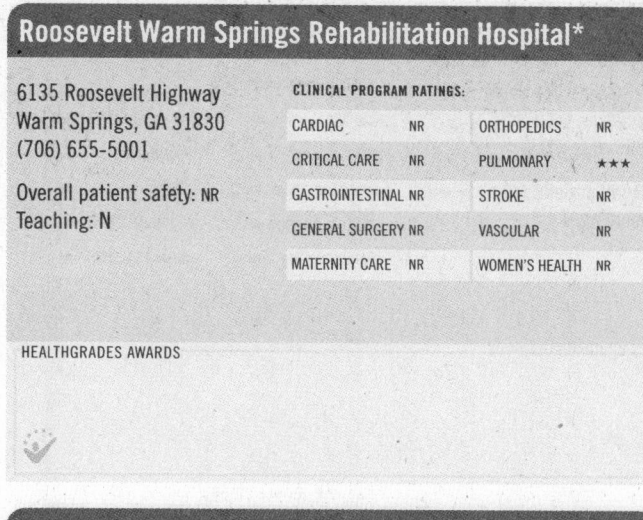

St. Joseph's Hospital

11705 Mercy Boulevard
Savannah, GA 31419
(912) 819-4100

Overall patient safety: ★★★
Teaching: N

CLINICAL PROGRAM RATINGS:

CARDIAC	★★★	ORTHOPEDICS	★★★
CRITICAL CARE	★★★★★	PULMONARY	★★★
GASTROINTESTINAL	★★★	STROKE	★
GENERAL SURGERY	NR	VASCULAR	★★★
MATERNITY CARE	NR	WOMEN'S HEALTH	NR

HEALTHGRADES AWARDS

✓ SPECIALTY EXCELLENCE
· CRITICAL CARE

St. Francis Hospital

2122 Manchester Expressway
Columbus, GA 31904
(706) 596-4000

Overall patient safety: ★★★
Teaching: N

CLINICAL PROGRAM RATINGS:

CARDIAC	★★★	ORTHOPEDICS	★★★
CRITICAL CARE	NR	PULMONARY	★★★
GASTROINTESTINAL	★★★	STROKE	★
GENERAL SURGERY	NR	VASCULAR	★★★
MATERNITY CARE	NR	WOMEN'S HEALTH	NR

HEALTHGRADES AWARDS

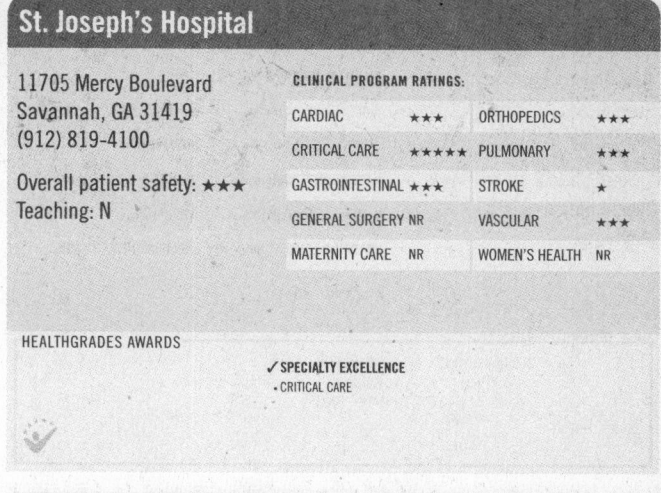

Saint Joseph's Hospital of Atlanta

5665 Peachtree Dunwoody
Road Northeast
Atlanta, GA 30342
(404) 851-7001

Overall patient safety: ★★★★★
Teaching: N

CLINICAL PROGRAM RATINGS:

CARDIAC	★★★	ORTHOPEDICS	★★★★★
CRITICAL CARE	★★★	PULMONARY	★★★
GASTROINTESTINAL	★★★★★	STROKE	★★★
GENERAL SURGERY	NR	VASCULAR	★★★★★
MATERNITY CARE	NR	WOMEN'S HEALTH	NR

HEALTHGRADES AWARDS

✓ AMERICA'S 50 BEST HOSPITALS

✓ DISTINGUISHED HOSPITAL
· CLINICAL EXCELLENCE
· PATIENT SAFETY

✓ SPECIALTY EXCELLENCE
· GASTROINTESTINAL CARE
· JOINT REPLACEMENT
· ORTHOPEDIC SURGERY
· VASCULAR SURGERY

---

*This hospital reports its data to the federal government jointly with another hospital. Therefore the ratings and awards apply to multiple hospitals and this specific hospital may not provide all rated services.

St. Mary's Hospital of Athens

1230 Baxter Street
Athens, GA 30606
(706) 548-7581

Overall patient safety: ★★★★★
Teaching: N

CLINICAL PROGRAM RATINGS:

CARDIAC	NR	ORTHOPEDICS	★★★
CRITICAL CARE	NR	PULMONARY	★★★
GASTROINTESTINAL	★★★	STROKE	★★★
GENERAL SURGERY	NR	VASCULAR	NR
MATERNITY CARE	NR	WOMEN'S HEALTH	NR

HEALTHGRADES AWARDS

✓ DISTINGUISHED
  HOSPITAL
- PATIENT SAFETY

Sempercare Hospital of Augusta

1350 Walton Way
7th Floor
Augusta, GA 30901
(706) 774-7101

Overall patient safety: ★★★
Teaching: N

CLINICAL PROGRAM RATINGS:

CARDIAC	★★★	ORTHOPEDICS	★★★
CRITICAL CARE	NR	PULMONARY	★
GASTROINTESTINAL	★★★	STROKE	★
GENERAL SURGERY	NR	VASCULAR	★★★
MATERNITY CARE	NR	WOMEN'S HEALTH	NR

HEALTHGRADES AWARDS

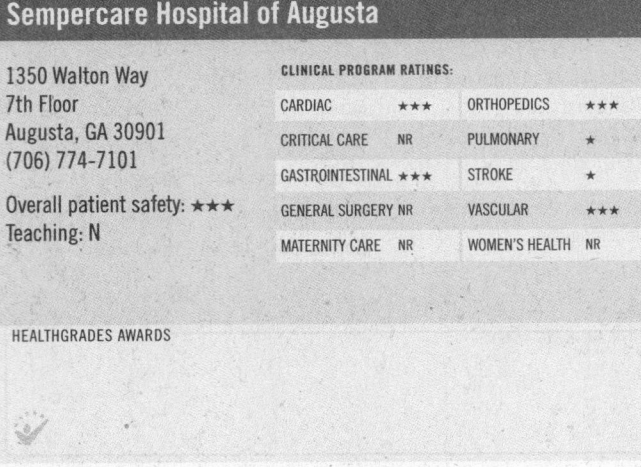

Satilla Regional Medical Center

410 Darling Avenue
Waycross, GA 31501
(912) 283-3030

Overall patient safety: ★★★
Teaching: Y

CLINICAL PROGRAM RATINGS:

CARDIAC	NR	ORTHOPEDICS	★★★
CRITICAL CARE	NR	PULMONARY	★★★
GASTROINTESTINAL	★★★	STROKE	★
GENERAL SURGERY	NR	VASCULAR	NR
MATERNITY CARE	NR	WOMEN'S HEALTH	NR

HEALTHGRADES AWARDS

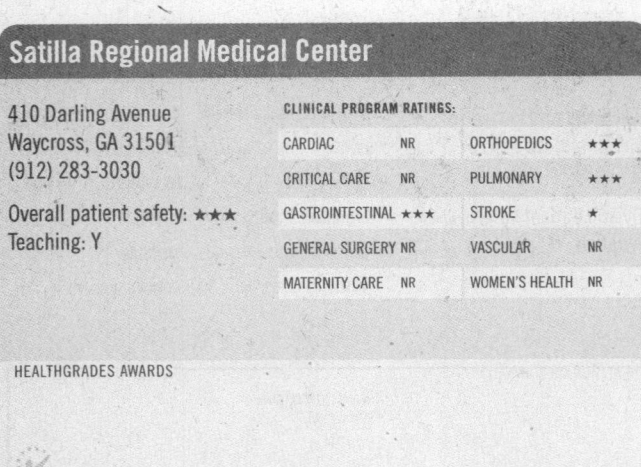

Smith Northview Hospital

4280 North Valdosta Road
Valdosta, GA 31602
(229) 671-2000

Overall patient safety: ★★★
Teaching: N

CLINICAL PROGRAM RATINGS:

CARDIAC	NR	ORTHOPEDICS	NR
CRITICAL CARE	NR	PULMONARY	★★★
GASTROINTESTINAL	NR	STROKE	NR
GENERAL SURGERY	NR	VASCULAR	NR
MATERNITY CARE	NR	WOMEN'S HEALTH	NR

HEALTHGRADES AWARDS

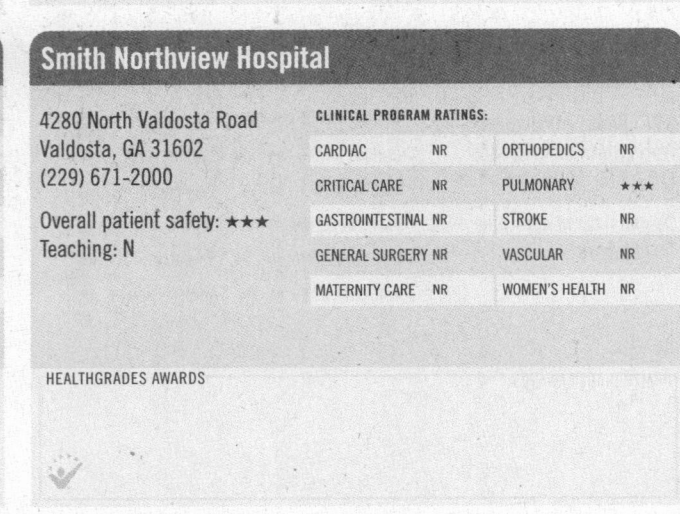

Screven County Hospital

215 Mims Road
Sylvania, GA 30467
(912) 564-7426

Overall patient safety: ★★★
Teaching: N

CLINICAL PROGRAM RATINGS:

CARDIAC	NR	ORTHOPEDICS	NR
CRITICAL CARE	NR	PULMONARY	★★★
GASTROINTESTINAL	NR	STROKE	NR
GENERAL SURGERY	NR	VASCULAR	NR
MATERNITY CARE	NR	WOMEN'S HEALTH	NR

HEALTHGRADES AWARDS

South Fulton Medical Center

1170 Cleveland Aveneue
East Point, GA 30344
(404) 466-1170

Overall patient safety: ★★★
Teaching: Y

CLINICAL PROGRAM RATINGS:

CARDIAC	NR	ORTHOPEDICS	NR
CRITICAL CARE	★★★	PULMONARY	★★★
GASTROINTESTINAL	★★★	STROKE	★★★★★
GENERAL SURGERY	NR	VASCULAR	NR
MATERNITY CARE	NR	WOMEN'S HEALTH	NR

HEALTHGRADES AWARDS

KEY: ★★★★★ **BEST**　★★★ **AS EXPECTED**　★ **POOR**　NR **NOT RATED BY HEALTHGRADES**　For full definitions of ratings and awards, see Appendix.

South Georgia Medical Center

2501 North Patterson Street
Valdosta, GA 31602
(229) 333-1000

Overall patient safety: ★★★
Teaching: N

CLINICAL PROGRAM RATINGS:

CARDIAC	★	ORTHOPEDICS	★★★
CRITICAL CARE	NR	PULMONARY	★★★
GASTROINTESTINAL	★★★	STROKE	★
GENERAL SURGERY	NR	VASCULAR	NR
MATERNITY CARE	NR	WOMEN'S HEALTH	NR

HEALTHGRADES AWARDS

Spalding Regional Medical Center

601 South 8th Street
Griffin, GA 30224
(770) 228-2721

Overall patient safety: ★★★
Teaching: N

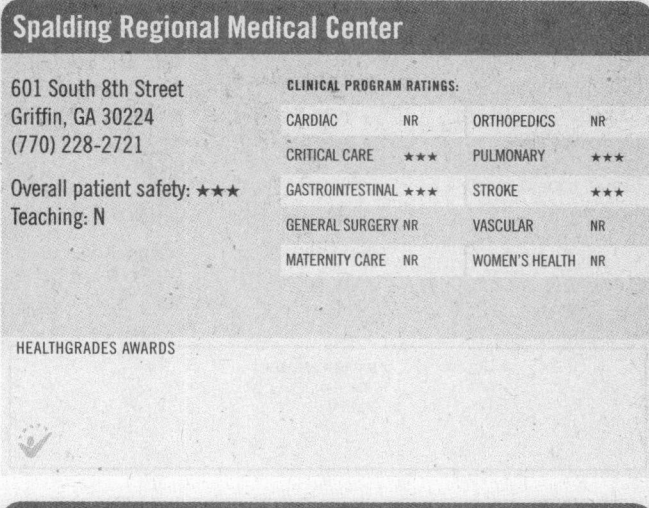

CLINICAL PROGRAM RATINGS:

CARDIAC	NR	ORTHOPEDICS	NR
CRITICAL CARE	★★★	PULMONARY	★★★
GASTROINTESTINAL	★★★	STROKE	★★★
GENERAL SURGERY	NR	VASCULAR	NR
MATERNITY CARE	NR	WOMEN'S HEALTH	NR

HEALTHGRADES AWARDS

Southeast Georgia Regional Medical Center

2415 Parkwood Drive
Brunswick, GA 31520
(912) 466-7000

Overall patient safety: ★★★
Teaching: N

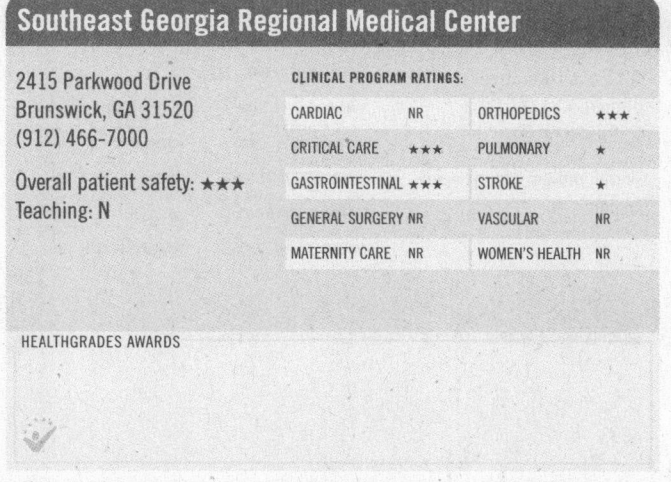

CLINICAL PROGRAM RATINGS:

CARDIAC	NR	ORTHOPEDICS	★★★
CRITICAL CARE	★★★	PULMONARY	★
GASTROINTESTINAL	★★★	STROKE	★
GENERAL SURGERY	NR	VASCULAR	NR
MATERNITY CARE	NR	WOMEN'S HEALTH	NR

HEALTHGRADES AWARDS

Stephens County Hospital

2003 Falls Road
Toccoa, GA 30577
(706) 282-4200

Overall patient safety: ★★★
Teaching: N

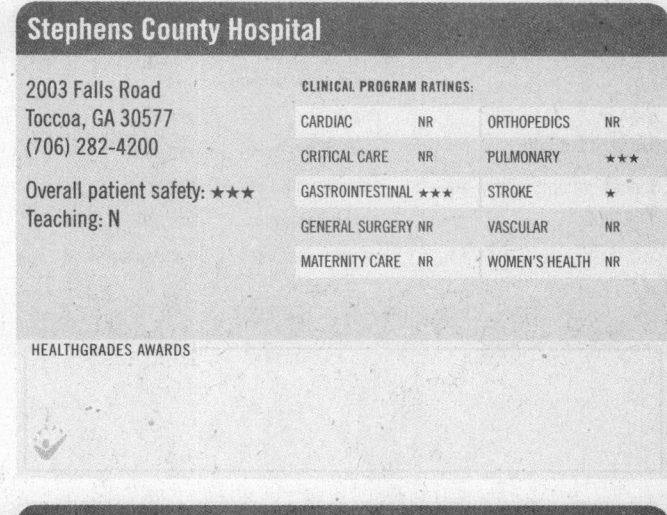

CLINICAL PROGRAM RATINGS:

CARDIAC	NR	ORTHOPEDICS	NR
CRITICAL CARE	NR	PULMONARY	★★★
GASTROINTESTINAL	★★★	STROKE	★
GENERAL SURGERY	NR	VASCULAR	NR
MATERNITY CARE	NR	WOMEN'S HEALTH	NR

HEALTHGRADES AWARDS

Southern Regional Medical Center

11 South West Upper
Riverdale Road
Riverdale, GA 30274
(770) 991-8000

Overall patient safety: ★★★
Teaching: N

CLINICAL PROGRAM RATINGS:

CARDIAC	NR	ORTHOPEDICS	NR
CRITICAL CARE	★★★	PULMONARY	★★★
GASTROINTESTINAL	★★★	STROKE	★★★
GENERAL SURGERY	NR	VASCULAR	NR
MATERNITY CARE	NR	WOMEN'S HEALTH	NR

HEALTHGRADES AWARDS

Stewart Webster Hospital

300 Alston Street
Richland, GA 31825
(229) 887-3366

Overall patient safety: ★★★
Teaching: N

CLINICAL PROGRAM RATINGS:

CARDIAC	NR	ORTHOPEDICS	NR
CRITICAL CARE	NR	PULMONARY	★
GASTROINTESTINAL	NR	STROKE	NR
GENERAL SURGERY	NR	VASCULAR	NR
MATERNITY CARE	NR	WOMEN'S HEALTH	NR

HEALTHGRADES AWARDS

Tanner Medical Center—Carrollton

705 Dixie Street
Carrollton, GA 30117
(770) 836-9666

Overall patient safety: ★★★
Teaching: N

CLINICAL PROGRAM RATINGS:

CARDIAC	NR	ORTHOPEDICS	★★★★★
CRITICAL CARE	★	PULMONARY	★★★
GASTROINTESTINAL	NR	STROKE	★★★
GENERAL SURGERY	NR	VASCULAR	NR
MATERNITY CARE	NR	WOMEN'S HEALTH	NR

HEALTHGRADES AWARDS

✓ SPECIALTY EXCELLENCE
  - ORTHOPEDIC SURGERY

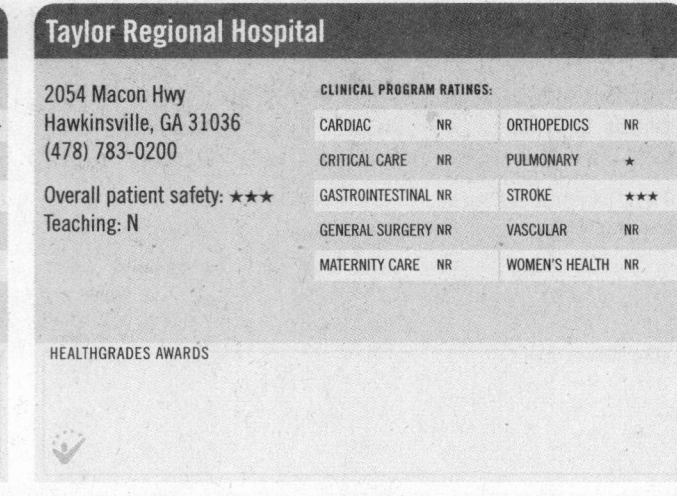

Taylor Regional Hospital

2054 Macon Hwy
Hawkinsville, GA 31036
(478) 783-0200

Overall patient safety: ★★★
Teaching: N

CLINICAL PROGRAM RATINGS:

CARDIAC	NR	ORTHOPEDICS	NR
CRITICAL CARE	NR	PULMONARY	★
GASTROINTESTINAL	NR	STROKE	★★★
GENERAL SURGERY	NR	VASCULAR	NR
MATERNITY CARE	NR	WOMEN'S HEALTH	NR

HEALTHGRADES AWARDS

Tanner Medical Center—Villa Rica

601 Dallas Highway
Villa Rica, GA 30180
(770) 456-3000

Overall patient safety: ★★★
Teaching: N

CLINICAL PROGRAM RATINGS:

CARDIAC	NR	ORTHOPEDICS	NR
CRITICAL CARE	NR	PULMONARY	★★★
GASTROINTESTINAL	NR	STROKE	★★★
GENERAL SURGERY	NR	VASCULAR	NR
MATERNITY CARE	NR	WOMEN'S HEALTH	NR

HEALTHGRADES AWARDS

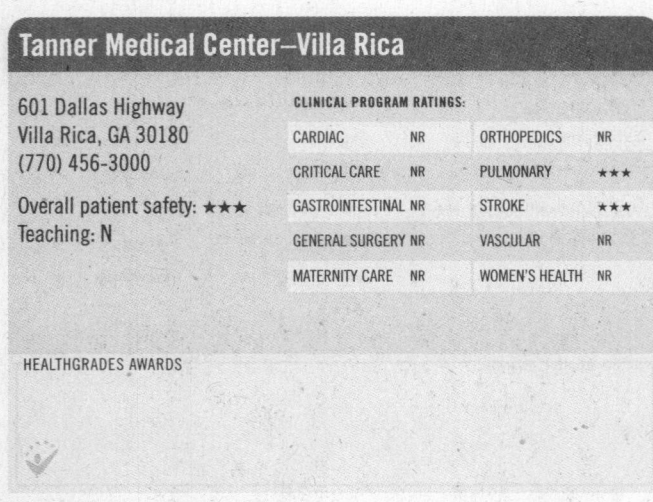

Tift Regional Medical Center

901 East 18th Street
Tifton, GA 31794
(229) 382-7120

Overall patient safety: ★★★
Teaching: N

CLINICAL PROGRAM RATINGS:

CARDIAC	NR	ORTHOPEDICS	★★★
CRITICAL CARE	NR	PULMONARY	★★★
GASTROINTESTINAL	★★★	STROKE	★
GENERAL SURGERY	NR	VASCULAR	NR
MATERNITY CARE	NR	WOMEN'S HEALTH	NR

HEALTHGRADES AWARDS

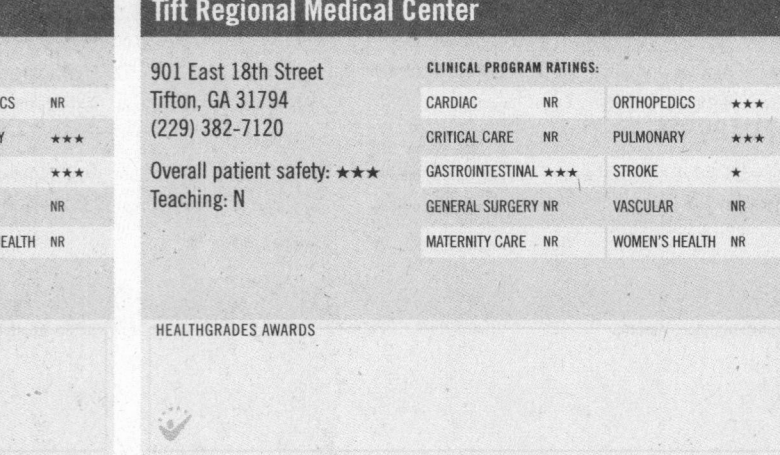

Tattnall Community Hospital

274 South Main Street
Reidsville, GA 30453
(912) 255-4731

Overall patient safety: ★★★
Teaching: N

CLINICAL PROGRAM RATINGS:

CARDIAC	NR	ORTHOPEDICS	NR
CRITICAL CARE	NR	PULMONARY	★
GASTROINTESTINAL	NR	STROKE	NR
GENERAL SURGERY	NR	VASCULAR	NR
MATERNITY CARE	NR	WOMEN'S HEALTH	NR

HEALTHGRADES AWARDS

Union General Hospital

214 Hospital Circle
Blairsville, GA 30512
(706) 745-2111

Overall patient safety: ★★★
Teaching: N

CLINICAL PROGRAM RATINGS:

CARDIAC	NR	ORTHOPEDICS	NR
CRITICAL CARE	NR	PULMONARY	★
GASTROINTESTINAL	NR	STROKE	★★★
GENERAL SURGERY	NR	VASCULAR	NR
MATERNITY CARE	NR	WOMEN'S HEALTH	NR

HEALTHGRADES AWARDS

KEY: ★★★★★ BEST ★★★ AS EXPECTED ★ POOR NR NOT RATED BY HEALTHGRADES For full definitions of ratings and awards, see Appendix.

University Hospital

1350 Walton Way
Augusta, GA 30901
(706) 722-9011

Overall patient safety: ★★★
Teaching: N

CLINICAL PROGRAM RATINGS:

CARDIAC	★★★	ORTHOPEDICS	★★★
CRITICAL CARE	NR	PULMONARY	★
GASTROINTESTINAL	★★★	STROKE	★
GENERAL SURGERY	NR	VASCULAR	★★★
MATERNITY CARE	NR	WOMEN'S HEALTH	NR

HEALTHGRADES AWARDS

Warm Springs Medical Center*

5995 Spring Street
Warm Springs, GA 31830
(706) 655-3331

Overall patient safety: ★★★
Teaching: N

CLINICAL PROGRAM RATINGS:

CARDIAC	NR	ORTHOPEDICS	NR
CRITICAL CARE	NR	PULMONARY	★★★
GASTROINTESTINAL	NR	STROKE	NR
GENERAL SURGERY	NR	VASCULAR	NR
MATERNITY CARE	NR	WOMEN'S HEALTH	NR

HEALTHGRADES AWARDS

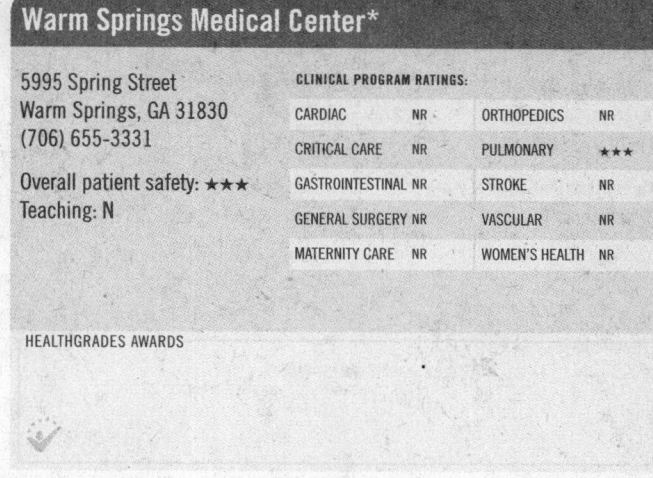

Upson Regional Medical Center

801 West Gordon Street
Thomaston, GA 30286
(706) 647-8111

Overall patient safety: ★★★
Teaching: N

CLINICAL PROGRAM RATINGS:

CARDIAC	NR	ORTHOPEDICS	NR
CRITICAL CARE	NR	PULMONARY	★★★
GASTROINTESTINAL	NR	STROKE	★
GENERAL SURGERY	NR	VASCULAR	NR
MATERNITY CARE	NR	WOMEN'S HEALTH	NR

HEALTHGRADES AWARDS

Washington County Regional Medical Center

610 Sparta Road
Sandersville, GA 31082
(478) 552-3901

Overall patient safety: ★★★
Teaching: N

CLINICAL PROGRAM RATINGS:

CARDIAC	NR	ORTHOPEDICS	NR
CRITICAL CARE	NR	PULMONARY	★
GASTROINTESTINAL	NR	STROKE	★★★
GENERAL SURGERY	NR	VASCULAR	NR
MATERNITY CARE	NR	WOMEN'S HEALTH	NR

HEALTHGRADES AWARDS

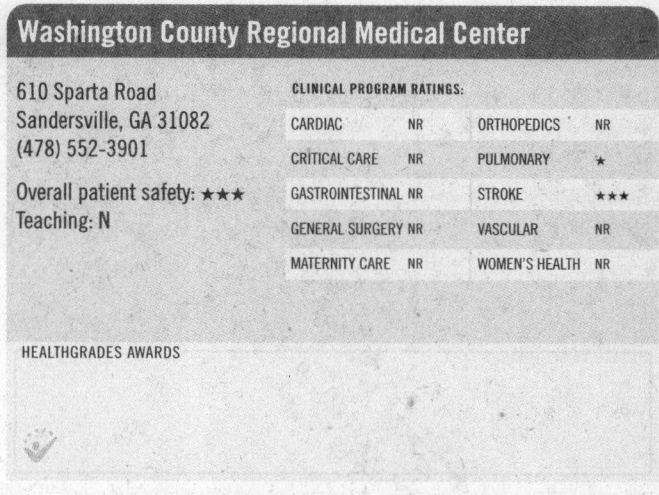

Walton Regional Medical Center

330 Alcovy Street
Monroe, GA 30655
(770) 267-8461

Overall patient safety: ★★★
Teaching: N

CLINICAL PROGRAM RATINGS:

CARDIAC	NR	ORTHOPEDICS	NR
CRITICAL CARE	NR	PULMONARY	★★★
GASTROINTESTINAL	★★★	STROKE	★★★
GENERAL SURGERY	NR	VASCULAR	NR
MATERNITY CARE	NR	WOMEN'S HEALTH	NR

HEALTHGRADES AWARDS

Wayne Memorial Hospital

865 South 1st Street
Jesup, GA 31545
(912) 427-6811

Overall patient safety: ★★★
Teaching: N

CLINICAL PROGRAM RATINGS:

CARDIAC	NR	ORTHOPEDICS	NR
CRITICAL CARE	NR	PULMONARY	★★★
GASTROINTESTINAL	NR	STROKE	NR
GENERAL SURGERY	NR	VASCULAR	NR
MATERNITY CARE	NR	WOMEN'S HEALTH	NR

HEALTHGRADES AWARDS

*This hospital reports its data to the federal government jointly with another hospital. Therefore the ratings and awards apply to multiple hospitals and this specific hospital may not provide all rated services.

GEORGIA HOSPITALS: RATINGS BY CLINICAL SPECIALTY

Wellstar Cobb Hospital

3950 Austell Road
Austell, GA 30106
(770) 732-4000

Overall patient safety: ★★★
Teaching: N

CLINICAL PROGRAM RATINGS:

CARDIAC	NR	ORTHOPEDICS	★★★
CRITICAL CARE	★	PULMONARY	★★★
GASTROINTESTINAL	★★★	STROKE	★★★★★
GENERAL SURGERY	NR	VASCULAR	★★★★★
MATERNITY CARE	NR	WOMEN'S HEALTH	NR

HEALTHGRADES AWARDS

✓ SPECIALTY EXCELLENCE
· STROKE CARE   · VASCULAR SURGERY

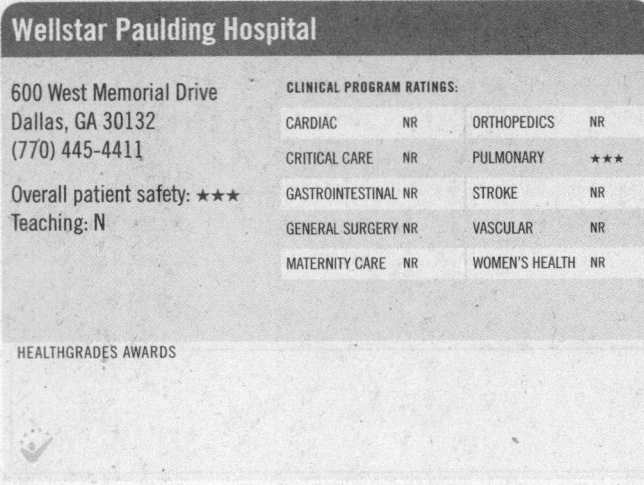

Wellstar Paulding Hospital

600 West Memorial Drive
Dallas, GA 30132
(770) 445-4411

Overall patient safety: ★★★
Teaching: N

CLINICAL PROGRAM RATINGS:

CARDIAC	NR	ORTHOPEDICS	NR
CRITICAL CARE	NR	PULMONARY	★★★
GASTROINTESTINAL	NR	STROKE	NR
GENERAL SURGERY	NR	VASCULAR	NR
MATERNITY CARE	NR	WOMEN'S HEALTH	NR

HEALTHGRADES AWARDS

Wellstar Douglas Hospital

8954 Hospital Drive
Douglasville, GA 30134
(770) 949-1500

Overall patient safety: ★★★
Teaching: N

CLINICAL PROGRAM RATINGS:

CARDIAC	NR	ORTHOPEDICS	NR
CRITICAL CARE	NR	PULMONARY	★★★
GASTROINTESTINAL	★★★	STROKE	★★★
GENERAL SURGERY	NR	VASCULAR	NR
MATERNITY CARE	NR	WOMEN'S HEALTH	NR

HEALTHGRADES AWARDS

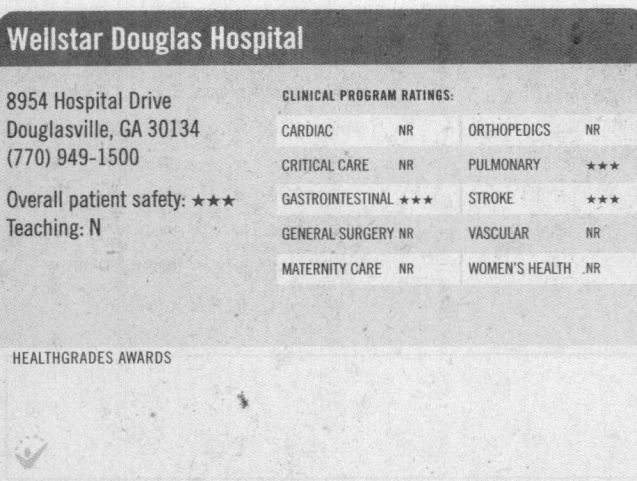

West Georgia Medical Center

1514 Vernon Road
Lagrange, GA 30240
(706) 882-1411

Overall patient safety: ★★★
Teaching: N

CLINICAL PROGRAM RATINGS:

CARDIAC	NR	ORTHOPEDICS	NR
CRITICAL CARE	★★★	PULMONARY	★★★
GASTROINTESTINAL	★★★	STROKE	★
GENERAL SURGERY	NR	VASCULAR	NR
MATERNITY CARE	NR	WOMEN'S HEALTH	NR

HEALTHGRADES AWARDS

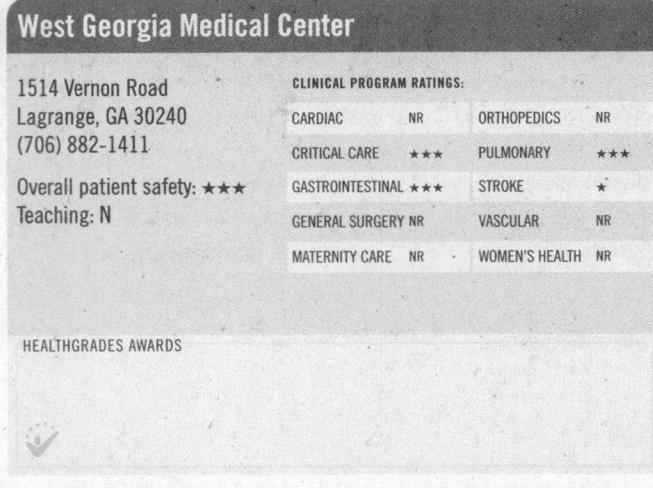

Wellstar Kennestone Hospital

677 Church Street
Marietta, GA 30060
(770) 793-5000

Overall patient safety: ★
Teaching: N

CLINICAL PROGRAM RATINGS:

CARDIAC	★★★	ORTHOPEDICS	★★★
CRITICAL CARE	★★★	PULMONARY	★★★
GASTROINTESTINAL	★★★	STROKE	★
GENERAL SURGERY	NR	VASCULAR	★★★
MATERNITY CARE	NR	WOMEN'S HEALTH	NR

HEALTHGRADES AWARDS

Wheeler County Hospital

Third Street
Glenwood, GA 30428
(912) 523-5113

Overall patient safety: ★★★
Teaching: N

CLINICAL PROGRAM RATINGS:

CARDIAC	NR	ORTHOPEDICS	NR
CRITICAL CARE	NR	PULMONARY	★★★★★
GASTROINTESTINAL	NR	STROKE	NR
GENERAL SURGERY	NR	VASCULAR	NR
MATERNITY CARE	NR	WOMEN'S HEALTH	NR

HEALTHGRADES AWARDS

KEY: ★★★★★ BEST   ★★★ AS EXPECTED   ★ POOR   NR NOT RATED BY HEALTHGRADES   For full definitions of ratings and awards, see Appendix.

Wills Memorial Hospital

120 Gordon Street
Washington, GA 30673
(706) 678-2151

Overall patient safety: ★★★
Teaching: N

CLINICAL PROGRAM RATINGS:

CARDIAC	NR	ORTHOPEDICS	NR
CRITICAL CARE	NR	PULMONARY	★★★
GASTROINTESTINAL	NR	STROKE	NR
GENERAL SURGERY	NR	VASCULAR	NR
MATERNITY CARE	NR	WOMEN'S HEALTH	NR

HEALTHGRADES AWARDS

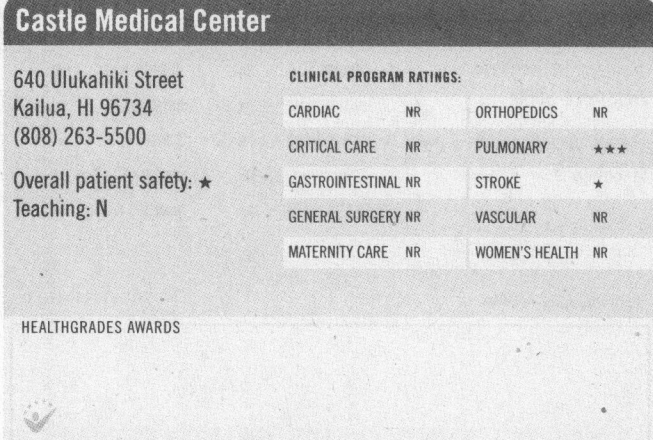

HAWAII HOSPITALS: RATINGS BY CLINICAL SPECIALTY

Castle Medical Center

640 Ulukahiki Street
Kailua, HI 96734
(808) 263-5500

Overall patient safety: ★
Teaching: N

CLINICAL PROGRAM RATINGS:

CARDIAC	NR	ORTHOPEDICS	NR
CRITICAL CARE	NR	PULMONARY	★★★
GASTROINTESTINAL	NR	STROKE	★
GENERAL SURGERY	NR	VASCULAR	NR
MATERNITY CARE	NR	WOMEN'S HEALTH	NR

HEALTHGRADES AWARDS

Hawaii Medical Center—West

912141 Fort Weaver Road
Ewa Beach, HI 96706
(808) 678-7000

Overall patient safety: ★
Teaching: N

CLINICAL PROGRAM RATINGS:

CARDIAC	NR	ORTHOPEDICS	NR
CRITICAL CARE	NR	PULMONARY	★
GASTROINTESTINAL	NR	STROKE	★★★★★
GENERAL SURGERY	NR	VASCULAR	NR
MATERNITY CARE	NR	WOMEN'S HEALTH	NR

HEALTHGRADES AWARDS

Hawaii Medical Center—East

2230 Liliha Street
Honolulu, HI 96817
(808) 547-6011

Overall patient safety: ★★★
Teaching: Y

CLINICAL PROGRAM RATINGS:

CARDIAC	★★★	ORTHOPEDICS	NR
CRITICAL CARE	NR	PULMONARY	★★★
GASTROINTESTINAL	NR	STROKE	★★★★★
GENERAL SURGERY	NR	VASCULAR	NR
MATERNITY CARE	NR	WOMEN'S HEALTH	NR

HEALTHGRADES AWARDS

✓ SPECIALTY EXCELLENCE
• STROKE CARE

Hilo Medical Center

1190 Waianuenue Avenue
Hilo, HI 96720
(808) 974-4700

Overall patient safety: ★★★
Teaching: N

CLINICAL PROGRAM RATINGS:

CARDIAC	NR	ORTHOPEDICS	NR
CRITICAL CARE	NR	PULMONARY	★★★
GASTROINTESTINAL	NR	STROKE	★★★
GENERAL SURGERY	NR	VASCULAR	NR
MATERNITY CARE	NR	WOMEN'S HEALTH	NR

HEALTHGRADES AWARDS

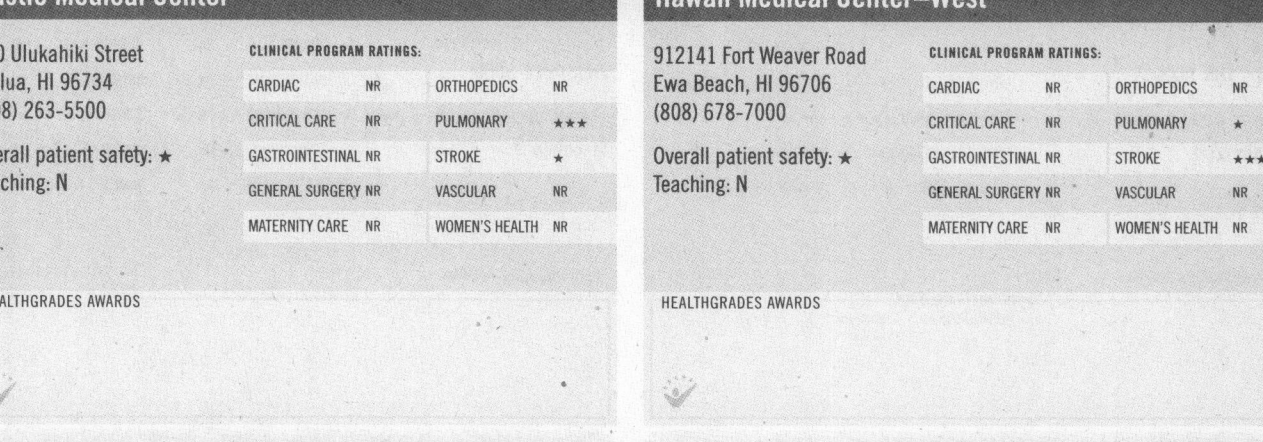

Kaiser Foundation Hospital

3288 Moanalua Road
Honolulu, HI 96819
(808) 432-0000

Overall patient safety: ★★★
Teaching: Y

CLINICAL PROGRAM RATINGS:

CARDIAC	★★★	ORTHOPEDICS	NR
CRITICAL CARE	NR	PULMONARY	★★★
GASTROINTESTINAL	NR	STROKE	★★★
GENERAL SURGERY	NR	VASCULAR	NR
MATERNITY CARE	NR	WOMEN'S HEALTH	NR

HEALTHGRADES AWARDS

Kuakini Medical Center

347 North Kuakini Street
Honolulu, HI 96817
(808) 536-2236

Overall patient safety: ★★★
Teaching: Y

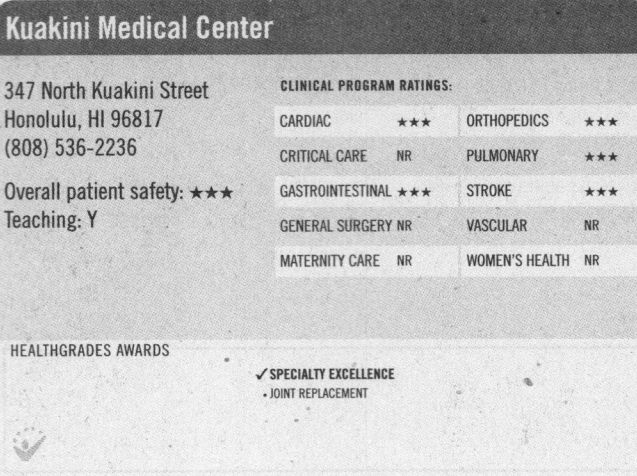

CLINICAL PROGRAM RATINGS:

CARDIAC	★★★	ORTHOPEDICS	★★★
CRITICAL CARE	NR	PULMONARY	★★★
GASTROINTESTINAL	★★★	STROKE	★★★
GENERAL SURGERY	NR	VASCULAR	NR
MATERNITY CARE	NR	WOMEN'S HEALTH	NR

HEALTHGRADES AWARDS

✓ SPECIALTY EXCELLENCE
• JOINT REPLACEMENT

Kapi'olani Medical Center at Pali Momi

98-1079 Moanalua Road
Aiea, HI 96701
(808) 486-6000

Overall patient safety: ★
Teaching: N

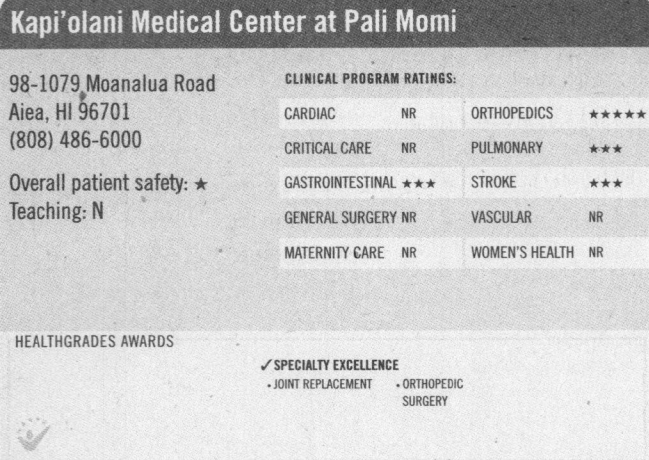

CLINICAL PROGRAM RATINGS:

CARDIAC	NR	ORTHOPEDICS	★★★★★
CRITICAL CARE	NR	PULMONARY	★★★
GASTROINTESTINAL	★★★	STROKE	★★★
GENERAL SURGERY	NR	VASCULAR	NR
MATERNITY CARE	NR	WOMEN'S HEALTH	NR

HEALTHGRADES AWARDS

✓ SPECIALTY EXCELLENCE
• JOINT REPLACEMENT   • ORTHOPEDIC SURGERY

Maui Memorial Medical Center

221 Mahalani Street
Wailuku, HI 96793
(808) 244-9056

Overall patient safety: ★★★
Teaching: N

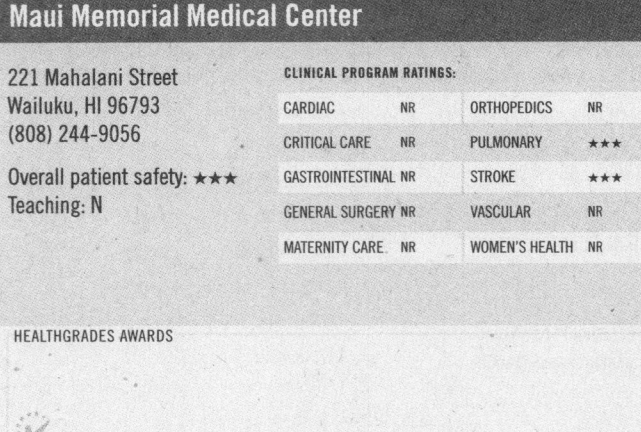

CLINICAL PROGRAM RATINGS:

CARDIAC	NR	ORTHOPEDICS	NR
CRITICAL CARE	NR	PULMONARY	★★★
GASTROINTESTINAL	NR	STROKE	★★★
GENERAL SURGERY	NR	VASCULAR	NR
MATERNITY CARE	NR	WOMEN'S HEALTH	NR

HEALTHGRADES AWARDS

Kona Community Hospital

79-1019 Haukapila Street
Kealakekua, HI 96750
(808) 322-9311

Overall patient safety: ★★★
Teaching: N

CLINICAL PROGRAM RATINGS:

CARDIAC	NR	ORTHOPEDICS	NR
CRITICAL CARE	NR	PULMONARY	★★★
GASTROINTESTINAL	NR	STROKE	★★★
GENERAL SURGERY	NR	VASCULAR	NR
MATERNITY CARE	NR	WOMEN'S HEALTH	NR

HEALTHGRADES AWARDS

North Hawaii Community Hospital

67-1125 Mamalahoa Highway
Kamuela, HI 96743
(808) 885-4444

Overall patient safety: ★★★
Teaching: N

CLINICAL PROGRAM RATINGS:

CARDIAC	NR	ORTHOPEDICS	NR
CRITICAL CARE	NR	PULMONARY	★★★
GASTROINTESTINAL	NR	STROKE	★★★
GENERAL SURGERY	NR	VASCULAR	NR
MATERNITY CARE	NR	WOMEN'S HEALTH	NR

HEALTHGRADES AWARDS

KEY: ★★★★★ BEST   ★★★ AS EXPECTED   ★ POOR   NR NOT RATED BY HEALTHGRADES   For full definitions of ratings and awards, see Appendix.

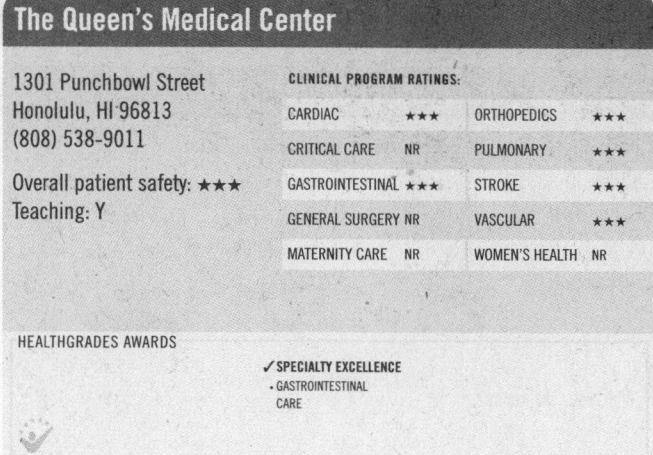

The Queen's Medical Center

1301 Punchbowl Street
Honolulu, HI 96813
(808) 538-9011

Overall patient safety: ★★★
Teaching: Y

CLINICAL PROGRAM RATINGS:

CARDIAC	★★★	ORTHOPEDICS	★★★
CRITICAL CARE	NR	PULMONARY	★★★
GASTROINTESTINAL	★★★	STROKE	★★★
GENERAL SURGERY	NR	VASCULAR	★★★
MATERNITY CARE	NR	WOMEN'S HEALTH	NR

HEALTHGRADES AWARDS

✓ **SPECIALTY EXCELLENCE**
• GASTROINTESTINAL
CARE

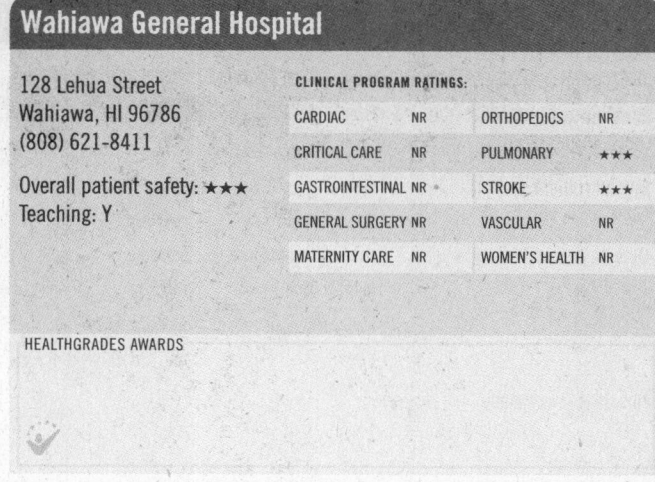

Wahiawa General Hospital

128 Lehua Street
Wahiawa, HI 96786
(808) 621-8411

Overall patient safety: ★★★
Teaching: Y

CLINICAL PROGRAM RATINGS:

CARDIAC	NR	ORTHOPEDICS	NR
CRITICAL CARE	NR	PULMONARY	★★★
GASTROINTESTINAL	NR	STROKE	★★★
GENERAL SURGERY	NR	VASCULAR	NR
MATERNITY CARE	NR	WOMEN'S HEALTH	NR

HEALTHGRADES AWARDS

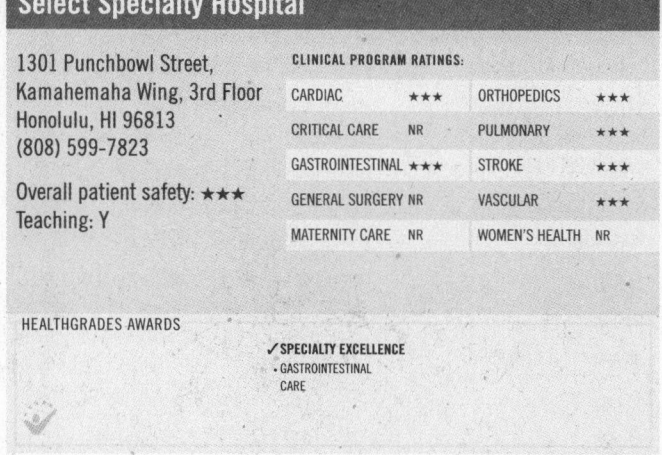

Select Specialty Hospital

1301 Punchbowl Street,
Kamahemaha Wing, 3rd Floor
Honolulu, HI 96813
(808) 599-7823

Overall patient safety: ★★★
Teaching: Y

CLINICAL PROGRAM RATINGS:

CARDIAC	★★★	ORTHOPEDICS	★★★
CRITICAL CARE	NR	PULMONARY	★★★
GASTROINTESTINAL	★★★	STROKE	★★★
GENERAL SURGERY	NR	VASCULAR	★★★
MATERNITY CARE	NR	WOMEN'S HEALTH	NR

HEALTHGRADES AWARDS

✓ **SPECIALTY EXCELLENCE**
• GASTROINTESTINAL
CARE

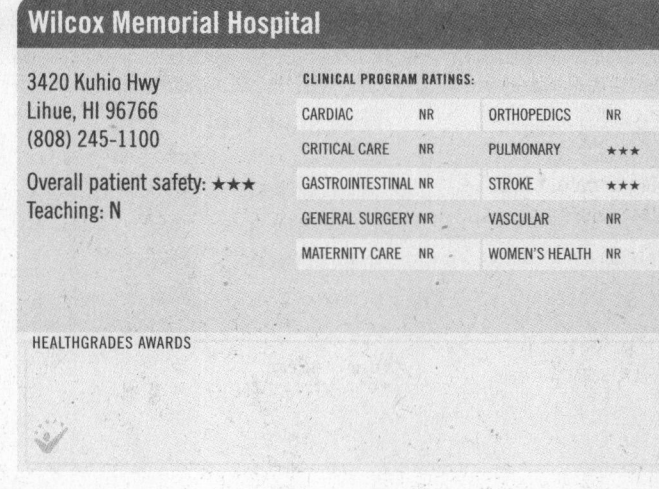

Wilcox Memorial Hospital

3420 Kuhio Hwy
Lihue, HI 96766
(808) 245-1100

Overall patient safety: ★★★
Teaching: N

CLINICAL PROGRAM RATINGS:

CARDIAC	NR	ORTHOPEDICS	NR
CRITICAL CARE	NR	PULMONARY	★★★
GASTROINTESTINAL	NR	STROKE	★★★
GENERAL SURGERY	NR	VASCULAR	NR
MATERNITY CARE	NR	WOMEN'S HEALTH	NR

HEALTHGRADES AWARDS

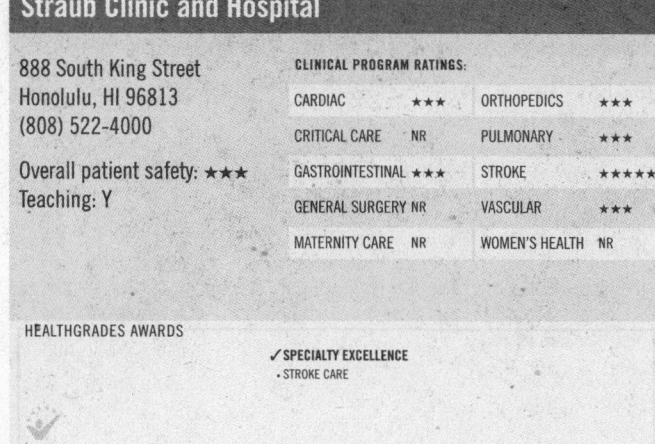

Straub Clinic and Hospital

888 South King Street
Honolulu, HI 96813
(808) 522-4000

Overall patient safety: ★★★
Teaching: Y

CLINICAL PROGRAM RATINGS:

CARDIAC	★★★	ORTHOPEDICS	★★★
CRITICAL CARE	NR	PULMONARY	★★★
GASTROINTESTINAL	★★★	STROKE	★★★★★
GENERAL SURGERY	NR	VASCULAR	★★★
MATERNITY CARE	NR	WOMEN'S HEALTH	NR

HEALTHGRADES AWARDS

✓ **SPECIALTY EXCELLENCE**
• STROKE CARE

HAWAII HOSPITALS: RATINGS BY CLINICAL SPECIALTY

Bear Lake Memorial Hospital

164 South 5th
Montpelier, ID 83254
(208) 847-1630

Overall patient safety: ★★★
Teaching: N

CLINICAL PROGRAM RATINGS:

CARDIAC	NR	ORTHOPEDICS	NR
CRITICAL CARE	NR	PULMONARY	★★★
GASTROINTESTINAL	NR	STROKE	NR
GENERAL SURGERY	NR	VASCULAR	NR
MATERNITY CARE	NR	WOMEN'S HEALTH	NR

HEALTHGRADES AWARDS

Cassia Regional Medical Center

1501 Hiland Avenue
Burley, ID 83318
(208) 678-4444

Overall patient safety: ★
Teaching: N

CLINICAL PROGRAM RATINGS:

CARDIAC	NR	ORTHOPEDICS	NR
CRITICAL CARE	NR	PULMONARY	★★★
GASTROINTESTINAL	NR	STROKE	★★★
GENERAL SURGERY	NR	VASCULAR	NR
MATERNITY CARE	NR	WOMEN'S HEALTH	NR

HEALTHGRADES AWARDS

Bingham Memorial Hospital

98 Poplar Street
P.O. Box 751
Blackfoot, ID 83221
(208) 785-4100

Overall patient safety: ★★★
Teaching: N

CLINICAL PROGRAM RATINGS:

CARDIAC	NR	ORTHOPEDICS	NR
CRITICAL CARE	NR	PULMONARY	★★★
GASTROINTESTINAL	NR	STROKE	NR
GENERAL SURGERY	NR	VASCULAR	NR
MATERNITY CARE	NR	WOMEN'S HEALTH	NR

HEALTHGRADES AWARDS

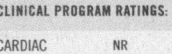

Eastern Idaho Regional Medical Center

3100 Channing Way
Idaho Falls, ID 83404
(208) 529-6111

Overall patient safety: ★
Teaching: N

CLINICAL PROGRAM RATINGS:

CARDIAC	★	ORTHOPEDICS	★
CRITICAL CARE	★★★	PULMONARY	★
GASTROINTESTINAL	★★★	STROKE	★
GENERAL SURGERY	NR	VASCULAR	NR
MATERNITY CARE	NR	WOMEN'S HEALTH	NR

HEALTHGRADES AWARDS

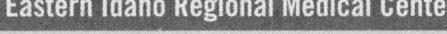

Bonner General Hospital

520 North 3rd Avenue
Sandpoint, ID 83864
(208) 263-1441

Overall patient safety: ★★★
Teaching: N

CLINICAL PROGRAM RATINGS:

CARDIAC	NR	ORTHOPEDICS	NR
CRITICAL CARE	NR	PULMONARY	★★★
GASTROINTESTINAL	NR	STROKE	★
GENERAL SURGERY	NR	VASCULAR	NR
MATERNITY CARE	NR	WOMEN'S HEALTH	NR

HEALTHGRADES AWARDS

Gritman Medical Center

700 South Main Street
Moscow, ID 83843
(208) 883-2220

Overall patient safety: ★★★
Teaching: N

CLINICAL PROGRAM RATINGS:

CARDIAC	NR	ORTHOPEDICS	NR
CRITICAL CARE	NR	PULMONARY	★★★
GASTROINTESTINAL	NR	STROKE	★
GENERAL SURGERY	NR	VASCULAR	NR
MATERNITY CARE	NR	WOMEN'S HEALTH	NR

HEALTHGRADES AWARDS

KEY: ★★★★★ BEST   ★★★ AS EXPECTED   ★ POOR   NR NOT RATED BY HEALTHGRADES   For full definitions of ratings and awards, see Appendix.

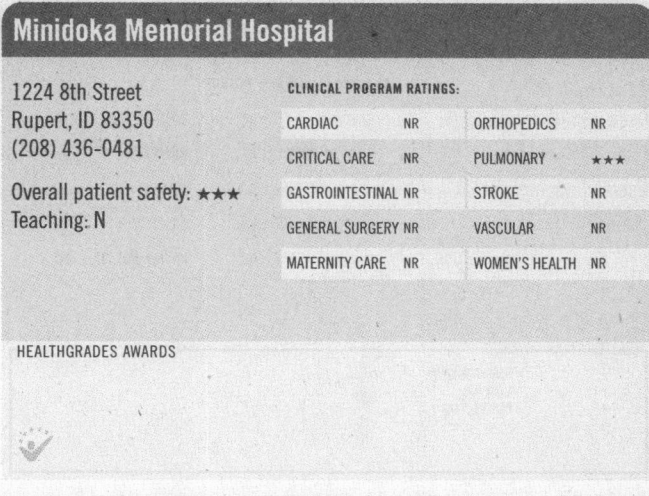

Kootenai Medical Center

2003 Lincoln Way
Coeur d'Alene, ID 83814
(208) 666-2000

Overall patient safety: ★★★
Teaching: N

CLINICAL PROGRAM RATINGS:

CARDIAC	★★★	ORTHOPEDICS	★★★
CRITICAL CARE	NR	PULMONARY	★
GASTROINTESTINAL	★★★	STROKE	★
GENERAL SURGERY	NR	VASCULAR	★★★
MATERNITY CARE	NR	WOMEN'S HEALTH	NR

HEALTHGRADES AWARDS

Minidoka Memorial Hospital

1224 8th Street
Rupert, ID 83350
(208) 436-0481

Overall patient safety: ★★★
Teaching: N

CLINICAL PROGRAM RATINGS:

CARDIAC	NR	ORTHOPEDICS	NR
CRITICAL CARE	NR	PULMONARY	★★★
GASTROINTESTINAL	NR	STROKE	NR
GENERAL SURGERY	NR	VASCULAR	NR
MATERNITY CARE	NR	WOMEN'S HEALTH	NR

HEALTHGRADES AWARDS

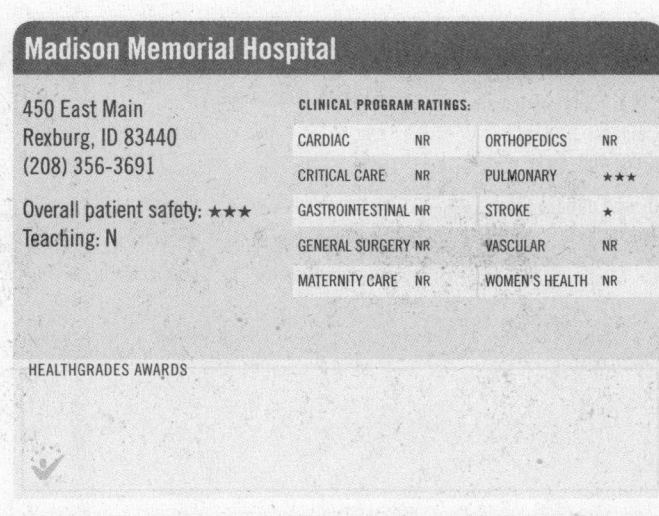

Madison Memorial Hospital

450 East Main
Rexburg, ID 83440
(208) 356-3691

Overall patient safety: ★★★
Teaching: N

CLINICAL PROGRAM RATINGS:

CARDIAC	NR	ORTHOPEDICS	NR
CRITICAL CARE	NR	PULMONARY	★★★
GASTROINTESTINAL	NR	STROKE	★
GENERAL SURGERY	NR	VASCULAR	NR
MATERNITY CARE	NR	WOMEN'S HEALTH	NR

HEALTHGRADES AWARDS

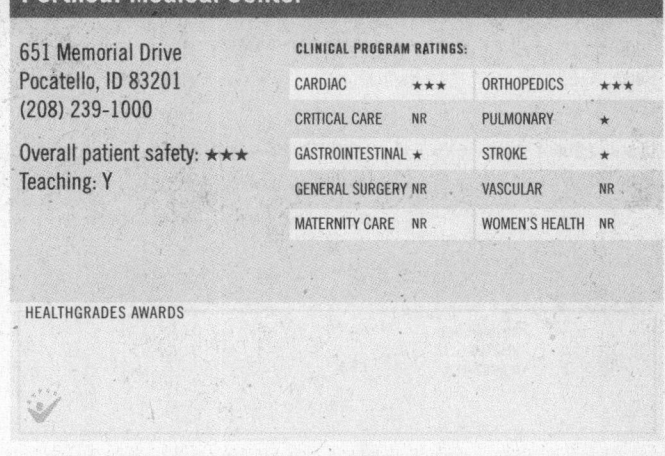

Portneuf Medical Center

651 Memorial Drive
Pocatello, ID 83201
(208) 239-1000

Overall patient safety: ★★★
Teaching: Y

CLINICAL PROGRAM RATINGS:

CARDIAC	★★★	ORTHOPEDICS	★★★
CRITICAL CARE	NR	PULMONARY	★
GASTROINTESTINAL	★	STROKE	★
GENERAL SURGERY	NR	VASCULAR	NR
MATERNITY CARE	NR	WOMEN'S HEALTH	NR

HEALTHGRADES AWARDS

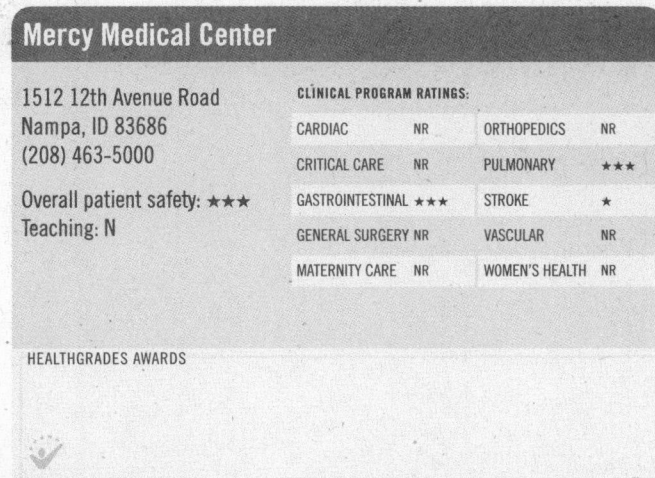

Mercy Medical Center

1512 12th Avenue Road
Nampa, ID 83686
(208) 463-5000

Overall patient safety: ★★★
Teaching: N

CLINICAL PROGRAM RATINGS:

CARDIAC	NR	ORTHOPEDICS	NR
CRITICAL CARE	NR	PULMONARY	★★★
GASTROINTESTINAL	★★★	STROKE	★
GENERAL SURGERY	NR	VASCULAR	NR
MATERNITY CARE	NR	WOMEN'S HEALTH	NR

HEALTHGRADES AWARDS

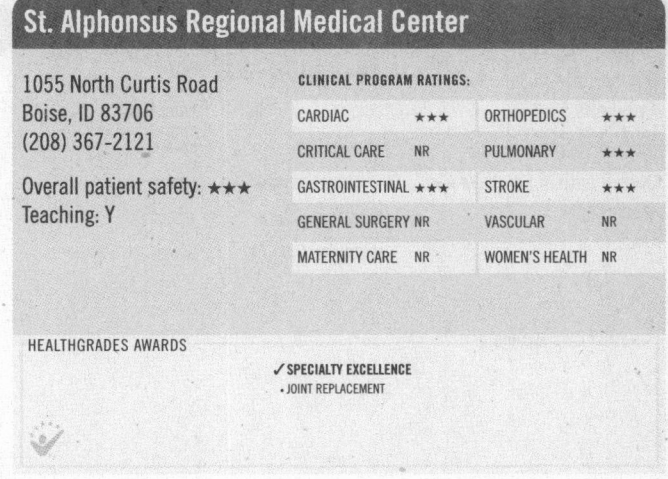

St. Alphonsus Regional Medical Center

1055 North Curtis Road
Boise, ID 83706
(208) 367-2121

Overall patient safety: ★★★
Teaching: Y

CLINICAL PROGRAM RATINGS:

CARDIAC	★★★	ORTHOPEDICS	★★★
CRITICAL CARE	NR	PULMONARY	★★★
GASTROINTESTINAL	★★★	STROKE	★★★
GENERAL SURGERY	NR	VASCULAR	NR
MATERNITY CARE	NR	WOMEN'S HEALTH	NR

HEALTHGRADES AWARDS

✓ SPECIALTY EXCELLENCE
• JOINT REPLACEMENT

St. Joseph Regional Medical Center

415 6th Street
Lewiston, ID 83501
(208) 743-2511

Overall patient safety: ★★★★★
Teaching: N

CLINICAL PROGRAM RATINGS:

CARDIAC	NR	ORTHOPEDICS	★★★
CRITICAL CARE	NR	PULMONARY	★★★
GASTROINTESTINAL	★★★	STROKE	★
GENERAL SURGERY	NR	VASCULAR	NR
MATERNITY CARE	NR	WOMEN'S HEALTH	NR

HEALTHGRADES AWARDS

✓ DISTINGUISHED HOSPITAL
• PATIENT SAFETY

St. Luke's Wood River Medical Center

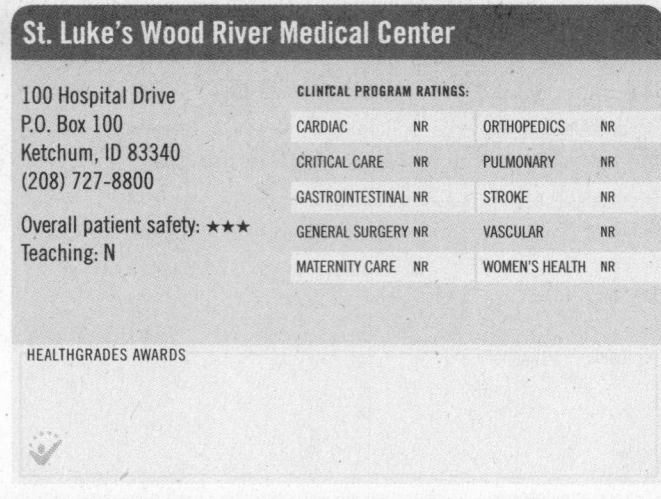

100 Hospital Drive
P.O. Box 100
Ketchum, ID 83340
(208) 727-8800

Overall patient safety: ★★★
Teaching: N

CLINICAL PROGRAM RATINGS:

CARDIAC	NR	ORTHOPEDICS	NR
CRITICAL CARE	NR	PULMONARY	NR
GASTROINTESTINAL	NR	STROKE	NR
GENERAL SURGERY	NR	VASCULAR	NR
MATERNITY CARE	NR	WOMEN'S HEALTH	NR

HEALTHGRADES AWARDS

St. Luke's Boise Medical Center

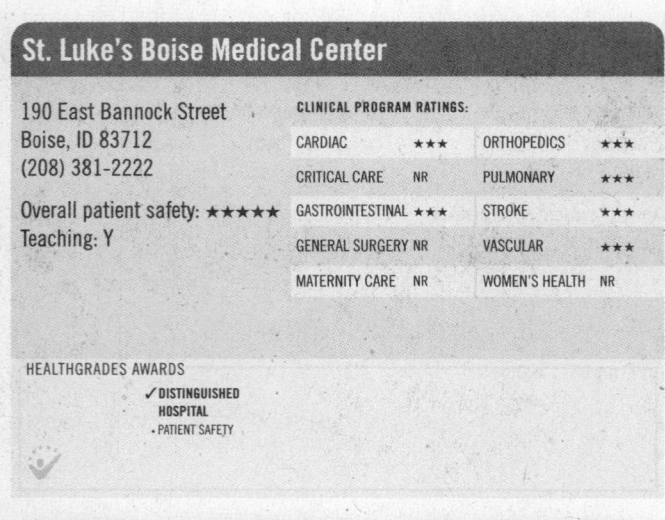

190 East Bannock Street
Boise, ID 83712
(208) 381-2222

Overall patient safety: ★★★★★
Teaching: Y

CLINICAL PROGRAM RATINGS:

CARDIAC	★★★	ORTHOPEDICS	★★★
CRITICAL CARE	NR	PULMONARY	★★★
GASTROINTESTINAL	★★★	STROKE	★★★
GENERAL SURGERY	NR	VASCULAR	★★★
MATERNITY CARE	NR	WOMEN'S HEALTH	NR

HEALTHGRADES AWARDS

✓ DISTINGUISHED HOSPITAL
• PATIENT SAFETY

West Valley Medical Center

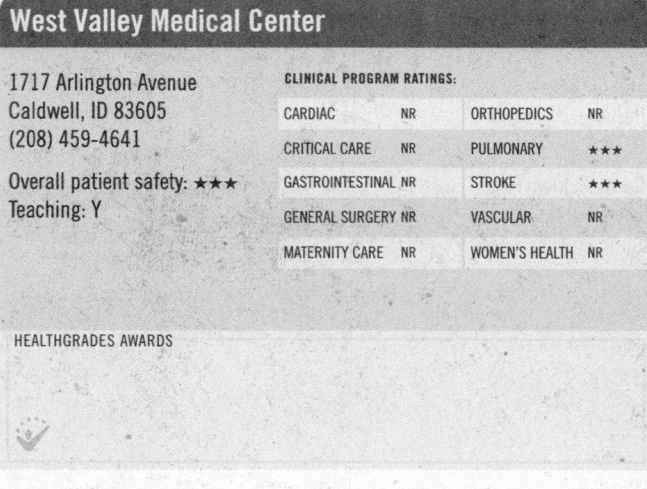

1717 Arlington Avenue
Caldwell, ID 83605
(208) 459-4641

Overall patient safety: ★★★
Teaching: Y

CLINICAL PROGRAM RATINGS:

CARDIAC	NR	ORTHOPEDICS	NR
CRITICAL CARE	NR	PULMONARY	★★★
GASTROINTESTINAL	NR	STROKE	★★★
GENERAL SURGERY	NR	VASCULAR	NR
MATERNITY CARE	NR	WOMEN'S HEALTH	NR

HEALTHGRADES AWARDS

St. Luke's Magic Valley Regional Medical Center

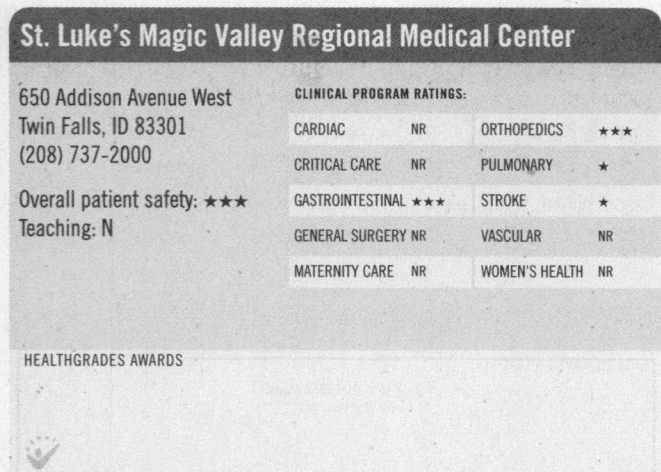

650 Addison Avenue West
Twin Falls, ID 83301
(208) 737-2000

Overall patient safety: ★★★
Teaching: N

CLINICAL PROGRAM RATINGS:

CARDIAC	NR	ORTHOPEDICS	★★★
CRITICAL CARE	NR	PULMONARY	★
GASTROINTESTINAL	★★★	STROKE	★
GENERAL SURGERY	NR	VASCULAR	NR
MATERNITY CARE	NR	WOMEN'S HEALTH	NR

HEALTHGRADES AWARDS

KEY: ★★★★★ BEST   ★★★ AS EXPECTED   ★ POOR   NR NOT RATED BY HEALTHGRADES   For full definitions of ratings and awards, see Appendix.

Abraham Lincoln Memorial Hospital

315 8th Street
Lincoln, IL 62656
(217) 732-2161

Overall patient safety: ★★★
Teaching: N

CLINICAL PROGRAM RATINGS:

CARDIAC	NR	ORTHOPEDICS	NR
CRITICAL CARE	NR	PULMONARY	★★★
GASTROINTESTINAL	NR	STROKE	★★★
GENERAL SURGERY	NR	VASCULAR	NR
MATERNITY CARE	NR	WOMEN'S HEALTH	NR

HEALTHGRADES AWARDS

Advocate Christ Hospital and Medical Center

4440 West 95th Street
Oak Lawn, IL 60453
(708) 425-8000

Overall patient safety: ★
Teaching: Y

CLINICAL PROGRAM RATINGS:

CARDIAC	★★★	ORTHOPEDICS	★★★
CRITICAL CARE	★★★	PULMONARY	★★★★★
GASTROINTESTINAL	★★★	STROKE	★★★★★
GENERAL SURGERY	NR	VASCULAR	★★★
MATERNITY CARE	NR	WOMEN'S HEALTH	NR

HEALTHGRADES AWARDS

✓ **SPECIALTY EXCELLENCE**
• PULMONARY CARE   • STROKE CARE

Adventist Glenoaks

701 Winthrop Avenue
Glendale Heights, IL 60139
(630) 545-8000

Overall patient safety: ★★★
Teaching: N

CLINICAL PROGRAM RATINGS:

CARDIAC	NR	ORTHOPEDICS	NR
CRITICAL CARE	NR	PULMONARY	★★★
GASTROINTESTINAL	NR	STROKE	★★★
GENERAL SURGERY	NR	VASCULAR	NR
MATERNITY CARE	NR	WOMEN'S HEALTH	NR

HEALTHGRADES AWARDS

Advocate Good Samaritan Hospital

3815 Highland Avenue
Downers Grove, IL 60515
(630) 275-5900

Overall patient safety: ★★★
Teaching: N

CLINICAL PROGRAM RATINGS:

CARDIAC	★★★	ORTHOPEDICS	★★★
CRITICAL CARE	★★★	PULMONARY	★★★★★
GASTROINTESTINAL	★★★	STROKE	★★★
GENERAL SURGERY	NR	VASCULAR	NR
MATERNITY CARE	NR	WOMEN'S HEALTH	NR

HEALTHGRADES AWARDS

✓ **DISTINGUISHED HOSPITAL**
• CLINICAL EXCELLENCE

✓ **SPECIALTY EXCELLENCE**
• GASTROINTESTINAL CARE   • PULMONARY CARE

Advocate Bethany Hospital

3435 West Van Buren Street
Chicago, IL 60624
(773) 265-7700

Overall patient safety: ★
Teaching: N

CLINICAL PROGRAM RATINGS:

CARDIAC	NR	ORTHOPEDICS	NR
CRITICAL CARE	NR-	PULMONARY	★★★
GASTROINTESTINAL	NR	STROKE	★★★
GENERAL SURGERY	NR	VASCULAR	NR
MATERNITY CARE	NR	WOMEN'S HEALTH	NR

HEALTHGRADES AWARDS

Advocate Good Shepherd Hospital

450 West Highway 22
Barrington, IL 60010
(847) 381-0123

Overall patient safety: ★★★
Teaching: N

CLINICAL PROGRAM RATINGS:

CARDIAC	★★★★★	ORTHOPEDICS	★
CRITICAL CARE	★★★	PULMONARY	★★★
GASTROINTESTINAL	★★★	STROKE	★★★
GENERAL SURGERY	NR	VASCULAR	NR
MATERNITY CARE	NR	WOMEN'S HEALTH	NR

HEALTHGRADES AWARDS

✓ **DISTINGUISHED HOSPITAL**
• CLINICAL EXCELLENCE

✓ **SPECIALTY EXCELLENCE**
• CARDIAC CARE   • GASTROINTESTINAL CARE

Advocate Illinois Masonic Medical Center

836 West Wellington Avenue
Chicago, IL 60657
(773) 975-1600

Overall patient safety: ★★★
Teaching: Y

CLINICAL PROGRAM RATINGS:

CARDIAC	★★★	ORTHOPEDICS	★★★
CRITICAL CARE	★★★	PULMONARY	★★★
GASTROINTESTINAL	NR	STROKE	★★★
GENERAL SURGERY	NR	VASCULAR	NR
MATERNITY CARE	NR	WOMEN'S HEALTH	NR

HEALTHGRADES AWARDS

Advocate Trinity Hospital

2320 East 93rd Street
Chicago, IL 60617
(773) 967-2000

Overall patient safety: ★★★
Teaching: Y

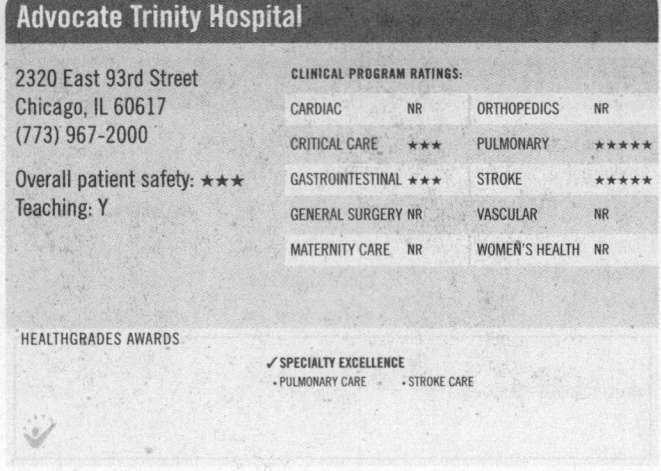

CLINICAL PROGRAM RATINGS:

CARDIAC	NR	ORTHOPEDICS	NR
CRITICAL CARE	★★★	PULMONARY	★★★★★
GASTROINTESTINAL	★★★	STROKE	★★★★★
GENERAL SURGERY	NR	VASCULAR	NR
MATERNITY CARE	NR	WOMEN'S HEALTH	NR

HEALTHGRADES AWARDS

✓ SPECIALTY EXCELLENCE
· PULMONARY CARE   · STROKE CARE

Advocate Lutheran General Hospital*

1775 West Dempster Street
Park Ridge, IL 60068
(847) 723-2210

Overall patient safety: ★★★
Teaching: Y

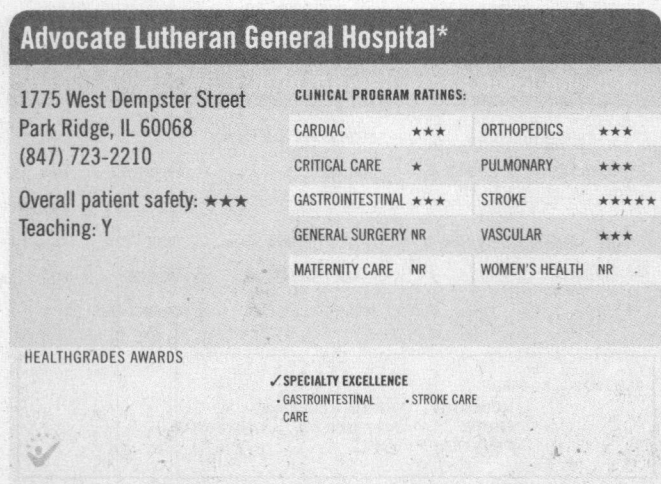

CLINICAL PROGRAM RATINGS:

CARDIAC	★★★	ORTHOPEDICS	★★★
CRITICAL CARE	★	PULMONARY	★★★
GASTROINTESTINAL	★★★	STROKE	★★★★★
GENERAL SURGERY	NR	VASCULAR	★★★
MATERNITY CARE	NR	WOMEN'S HEALTH	NR

HEALTHGRADES AWARDS

✓ SPECIALTY EXCELLENCE
· GASTROINTESTINAL   · STROKE CARE
CARE

Alexian Brothers Medical Center

800 Biesterfield Road
Elk Grove Village, IL 60007
(847) 437-5500

Overall patient safety: ★★★
Teaching: N

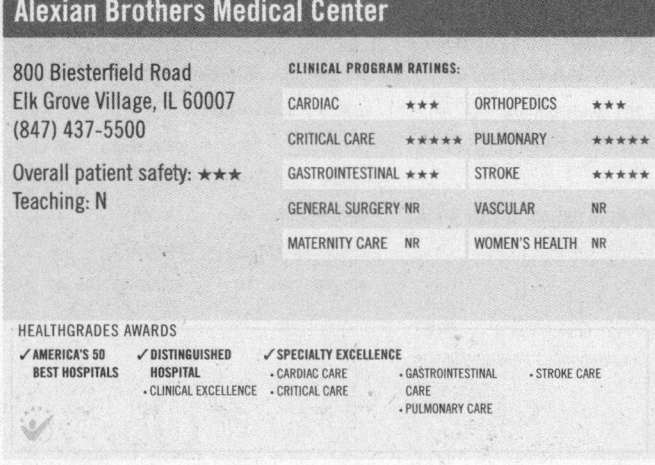

CLINICAL PROGRAM RATINGS:

CARDIAC	★★★	ORTHOPEDICS	★★★
CRITICAL CARE	★★★★★	PULMONARY	★★★★★
GASTROINTESTINAL	★★★	STROKE	★★★★★
GENERAL SURGERY	NR	VASCULAR	NR
MATERNITY CARE	NR	WOMEN'S HEALTH	NR

HEALTHGRADES AWARDS

✓ AMERICA'S 50   ✓ DISTINGUISHED   ✓ SPECIALTY EXCELLENCE
BEST HOSPITALS   HOSPITAL   · CARDIAC CARE   · GASTROINTESTINAL   · STROKE CARE
                     · CLINICAL EXCELLENCE · CRITICAL CARE   CARE
                                                              · PULMONARY CARE

Advocate South Suburban Hospital

17800 South Kedzie Avenue
Hazel Crest, IL 60429
(708) 799-8000

Overall patient safety: ★★★
Teaching: N

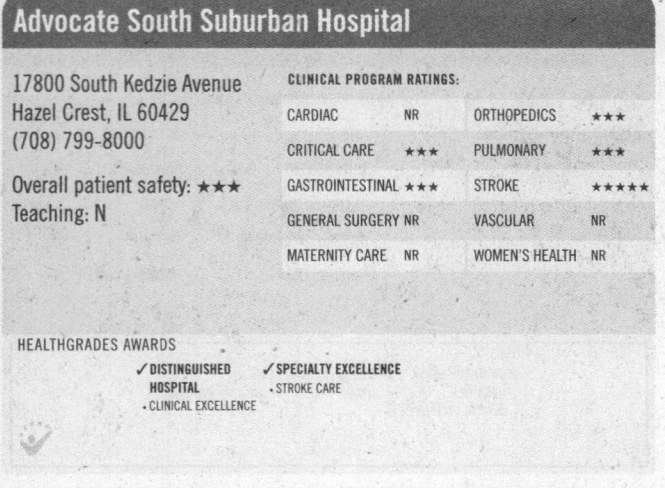

CLINICAL PROGRAM RATINGS:

CARDIAC	NR	ORTHOPEDICS	★★★
CRITICAL CARE	★★★	PULMONARY	★★★
GASTROINTESTINAL	★★★	STROKE	★★★★★
GENERAL SURGERY	NR	VASCULAR	NR
MATERNITY CARE	NR	WOMEN'S HEALTH	NR

HEALTHGRADES AWARDS

✓ DISTINGUISHED   ✓ SPECIALTY EXCELLENCE
HOSPITAL   · STROKE CARE
· CLINICAL EXCELLENCE

Alton Memorial Hospital

1 Memorial Drive
Alton, IL 62002
(618) 463-7311

Overall patient safety: ★★★
Teaching: N

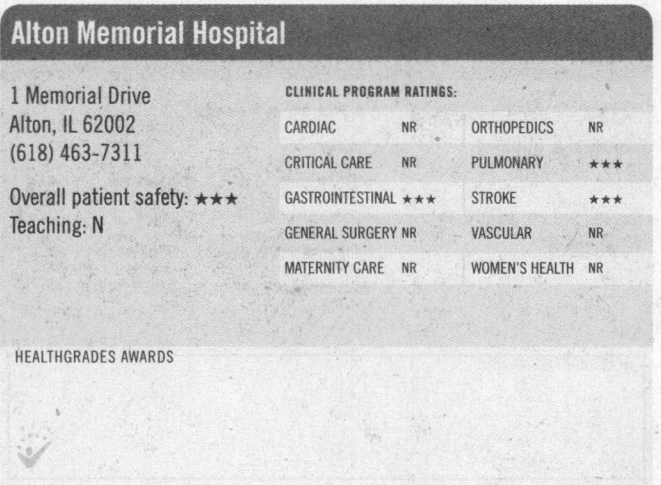

CLINICAL PROGRAM RATINGS:

CARDIAC	NR	ORTHOPEDICS	NR
CRITICAL CARE	NR	PULMONARY	★★★
GASTROINTESTINAL	★★★	STROKE	★★★
GENERAL SURGERY	NR	VASCULAR	NR
MATERNITY CARE	NR	WOMEN'S HEALTH	NR

HEALTHGRADES AWARDS

KEY: ★★★★★ BEST   ★★★ AS EXPECTED   ★ POOR   NR NOT RATED BY HEALTHGRADES   For full definitions of ratings and awards, see Appendix.

Anderson Hospital

6800 State Route 162
Maryville, IL 62062
(618) 288-5711

Overall patient safety: ★
Teaching: N

CLINICAL PROGRAM RATINGS:

CARDIAC	NR	ORTHOPEDICS	NR
CRITICAL CARE	★★★	PULMONARY	★★★
GASTROINTESTINAL	★	STROKE	★★★
GENERAL SURGERY	NR	VASCULAR	NR
MATERNITY CARE	NR	WOMEN'S HEALTH	NR

HEALTHGRADES AWARDS

Carle Foundation Hospital

611 West Parks Street
Urbana, IL 61801
(217) 383-3311

Overall patient safety: ★★★
Teaching: Y

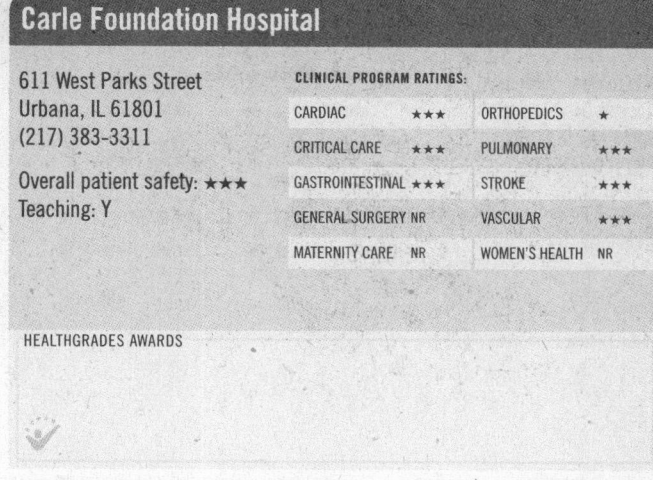

CLINICAL PROGRAM RATINGS:

CARDIAC	★★★	ORTHOPEDICS	★
CRITICAL CARE	★★★	PULMONARY	★★★
GASTROINTESTINAL	★★★	STROKE	★★★
GENERAL SURGERY	NR	VASCULAR	★★★
MATERNITY CARE	NR	WOMEN'S HEALTH	NR

HEALTHGRADES AWARDS

Blessing Hospital*

Broadway at 11th Street and
14th Street
Quincy, IL 62305
(217) 223-1200

Overall patient safety: ★★★★★
Teaching: Y

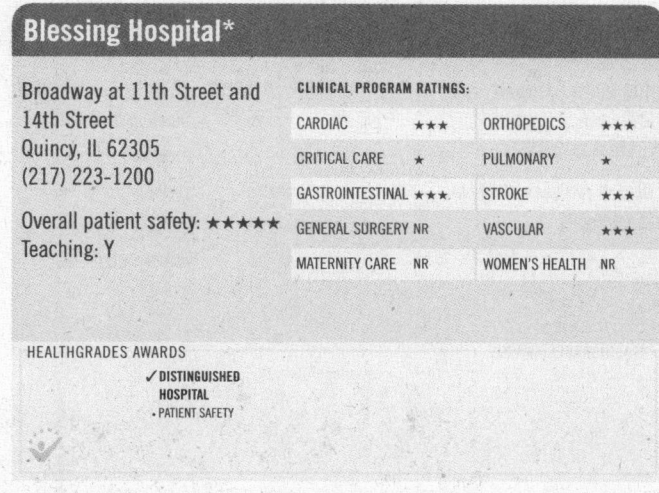

CLINICAL PROGRAM RATINGS:

CARDIAC	★★★	ORTHOPEDICS	★★★
CRITICAL CARE	★	PULMONARY	★
GASTROINTESTINAL	★★★	STROKE	★★★
GENERAL SURGERY	NR	VASCULAR	★★★
MATERNITY CARE	NR	WOMEN'S HEALTH	NR

HEALTHGRADES AWARDS

✓ DISTINGUISHED
HOSPITAL
• PATIENT SAFETY

Carlinville Area Hospital

1001 Morgan Street
Carlinville, IL 62626
(217) 854-3141

Overall patient safety: ★★★
Teaching: N

CLINICAL PROGRAM RATINGS:

CARDIAC	NR	ORTHOPEDICS	NR
CRITICAL CARE	NR	PULMONARY	★
GASTROINTESTINAL	NR	STROKE	★
GENERAL SURGERY	NR	VASCULAR	NR
MATERNITY CARE	NR	WOMEN'S HEALTH	NR

HEALTHGRADES AWARDS

Bromenn Healthcare

1304 Franklin Avenue
Normal, IL 61761
(309) 454-1400

Overall patient safety: ★★★
Teaching: Y

CLINICAL PROGRAM RATINGS:

CARDIAC	★★★	ORTHOPEDICS	★★★
CRITICAL CARE	NR	PULMONARY	★
GASTROINTESTINAL	★★★	STROKE	★★★
GENERAL SURGERY	NR	VASCULAR	NR
MATERNITY CARE	NR	WOMEN'S HEALTH	NR

HEALTHGRADES AWARDS

Centegra Memorial Medical Center

3701 Doty Road
Woodstock, IL 60098
(815) 338-2500

Overall patient safety: ★★★
Teaching: N

CLINICAL PROGRAM RATINGS:

CARDIAC	NR	ORTHOPEDICS	★★★
CRITICAL CARE	NR	PULMONARY	★★★★★
GASTROINTESTINAL	★★★	STROKE	★★★★★
GENERAL SURGERY	NR	VASCULAR	NR
MATERNITY CARE	NR	WOMEN'S HEALTH	NR

HEALTHGRADES AWARDS

✓ DISTINGUISHED   ✓ SPECIALTY EXCELLENCE
HOSPITAL   • PULMONARY CARE   • STROKE CARE
• CLINICAL EXCELLENCE

*This hospital reports its data to the federal government jointly with another hospital. Therefore the ratings and awards apply to multiple hospitals and this specific hospital may not provide all rated services.

Centegra Northern Illinois Medical Center

4201 West Medical
Center Drive
McHenry, IL 60050
(815) 344-5000

Overall patient safety: ★★★
Teaching: N

CLINICAL PROGRAM RATINGS:

CARDIAC	NR	ORTHOPEDICS	★★★
CRITICAL CARE	★★★	PULMONARY	★★★
GASTROINTESTINAL	★★★	STROKE	★
GENERAL SURGERY	NR	VASCULAR	NR
MATERNITY CARE	NR	WOMEN'S HEALTH	NR

HEALTHGRADES AWARDS

Community Hospital of Ottawa

1100 East Norris Drive
Ottawa, IL 61350
(815) 433-3100

Overall patient safety: ★★★
Teaching: N

CLINICAL PROGRAM RATINGS:

CARDIAC	NR	ORTHOPEDICS	NR
CRITICAL CARE	NR	PULMONARY	★
GASTROINTESTINAL	NR	STROKE	★★★
GENERAL SURGERY	NR	VASCULAR	NR
MATERNITY CARE	NR	WOMEN'S HEALTH	NR

HEALTHGRADES AWARDS

Central Dupage Hospital

25 North Winfield Road
Winfield, IL 60190
(630) 933-1600

Overall patient safety: ★★★★★
Teaching: N

CLINICAL PROGRAM RATINGS:

CARDIAC	★★★	ORTHOPEDICS	★★★
CRITICAL CARE	★★★★★	PULMONARY	★★★★★
GASTROINTESTINAL	★★★	STROKE	★★★★★
GENERAL SURGERY	NR	VASCULAR	NR
MATERNITY CARE	NR	WOMEN'S HEALTH	NR

HEALTHGRADES AWARDS

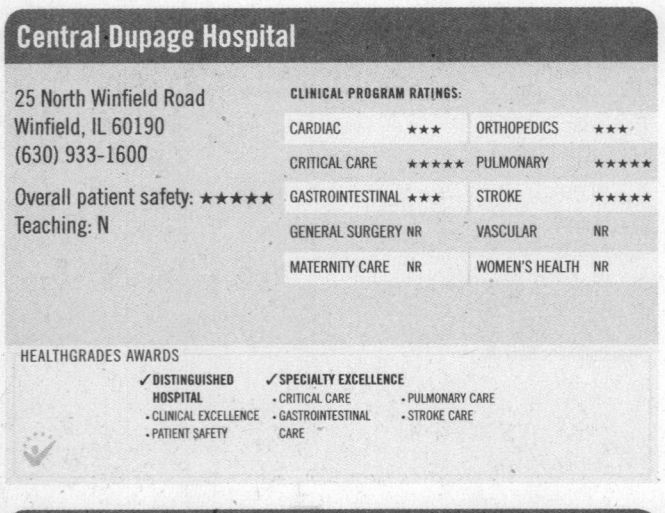

✓ DISTINGUISHED HOSPITAL
- CLINICAL EXCELLENCE
- PATIENT SAFETY

✓ SPECIALTY EXCELLENCE
- CRITICAL CARE
- GASTROINTESTINAL CARE
- PULMONARY CARE
- STROKE CARE

Community Memorial Hospital

400 North Caldwell Street
Staunton, IL 62088
(618) 635-2200

Overall patient safety: ★★★
Teaching: N

CLINICAL PROGRAM RATINGS:

CARDIAC	NR	ORTHOPEDICS	NR
CRITICAL CARE	NR	PULMONARY	★★★
GASTROINTESTINAL	NR	STROKE	NR
GENERAL SURGERY	NR	VASCULAR	NR
MATERNITY CARE	NR	WOMEN'S HEALTH	NR

HEALTHGRADES AWARDS

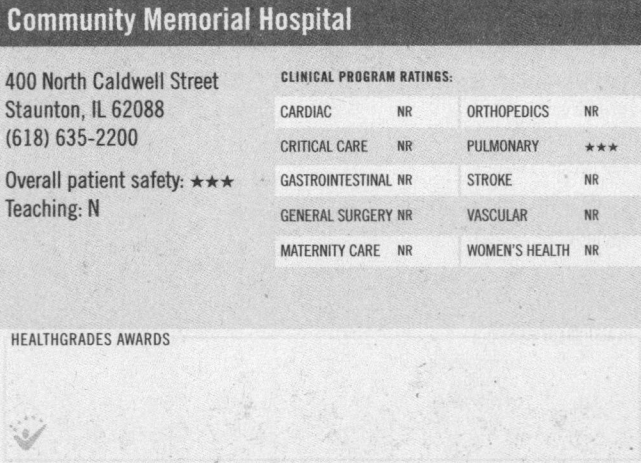

CGH Medical Center

100 East Lefevre Road
Sterling, IL 61081
(815) 625-0400

Overall patient safety: ★★★
Teaching: N

CLINICAL PROGRAM RATINGS:

CARDIAC	NR	ORTHOPEDICS	NR
CRITICAL CARE	★★★	PULMONARY	★★★
GASTROINTESTINAL	★★★	STROKE	★★★
GENERAL SURGERY	NR	VASCULAR	NR
MATERNITY CARE	NR	WOMEN'S HEALTH	NR

HEALTHGRADES AWARDS

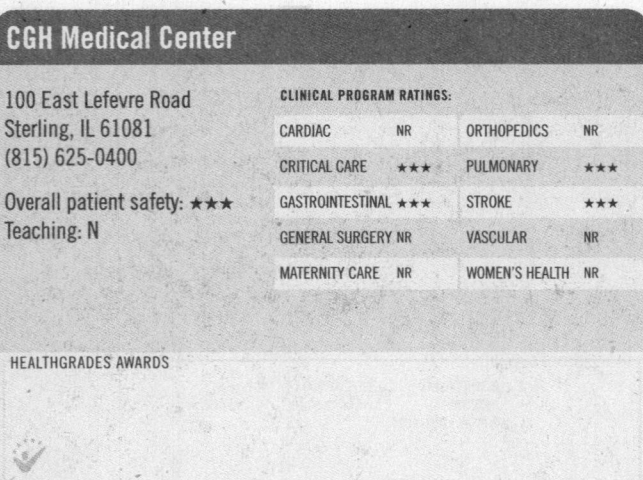

Condell Medical Center

801 South Milwaukee Avenue
Libertyville, IL 60048
(847) 362-2900

Overall patient safety: ★★★
Teaching: N

CLINICAL PROGRAM RATINGS:

CARDIAC	★★★	ORTHOPEDICS	★★★
CRITICAL CARE	★★★	PULMONARY	★★★
GASTROINTESTINAL	★★★	STROKE	★★★
GENERAL SURGERY	NR	VASCULAR	★★★
MATERNITY CARE	NR	WOMEN'S HEALTH	NR

HEALTHGRADES AWARDS

KEY: ★★★★★ BEST   ★★★ AS EXPECTED   ★ POOR   NR NOT RATED BY HEALTHGRADES   For full definitions of ratings and awards, see Appendix.

Crawford Memorial Hospital

1000 North Allen Street
Robinson, IL 62454
(618) 546-2514

Overall patient safety: ★★★
Teaching: N

CLINICAL PROGRAM RATINGS:

CARDIAC	NR	ORTHOPEDICS	NR
CRITICAL CARE	NR	PULMONARY	★
GASTROINTESTINAL	NR	STROKE	★
GENERAL SURGERY	NR	VASCULAR	NR
MATERNITY CARE	NR	WOMEN'S HEALTH	NR

HEALTHGRADES AWARDS

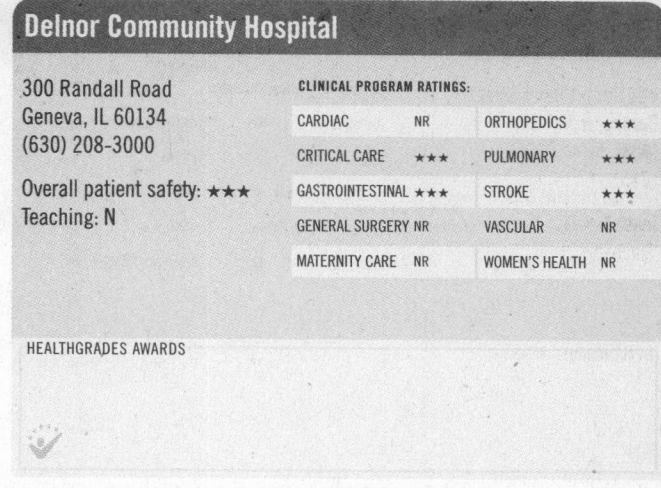

Delnor Community Hospital

300 Randall Road
Geneva, IL 60134
(630) 208-3000

Overall patient safety: ★★★
Teaching: N

CLINICAL PROGRAM RATINGS:

CARDIAC	NR	ORTHOPEDICS	★★★
CRITICAL CARE	★★★	PULMONARY	★★★
GASTROINTESTINAL	★★★	STROKE	★★★
GENERAL SURGERY	NR	VASCULAR	NR
MATERNITY CARE	NR	WOMEN'S HEALTH	NR

HEALTHGRADES AWARDS

Crossroads Community Hospital

8 Doctors Parks Road
Mount Vernon, IL 62864
(618) 244-5500

Overall patient safety: ★★★
Teaching: N

CLINICAL PROGRAM RATINGS:

CARDIAC	NR	ORTHOPEDICS	NR
CRITICAL CARE	NR	PULMONARY	★★★
GASTROINTESTINAL	NR	STROKE	★★★★★
GENERAL SURGERY	NR	VASCULAR	NR
MATERNITY CARE	NR	WOMEN'S HEALTH	NR

HEALTHGRADES AWARDS

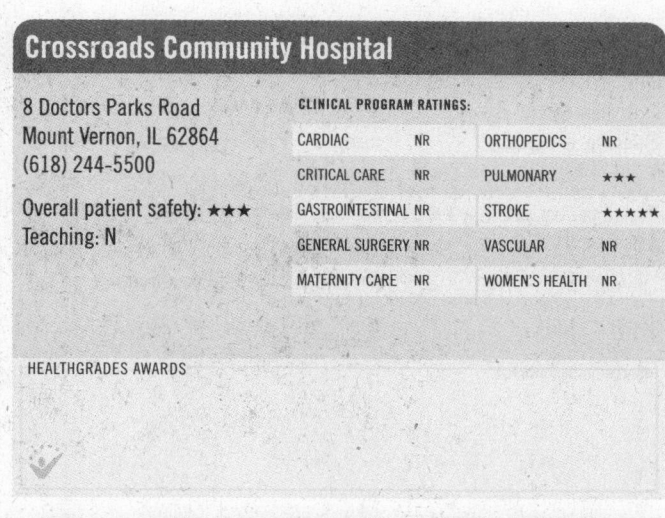

Edward Hospital

801 South Washington Street
Naperville, IL 60566
(630) 527-3000

Overall patient safety: ★★★
Teaching: N

CLINICAL PROGRAM RATINGS:

CARDIAC	★★★	ORTHOPEDICS	★★★
CRITICAL CARE	★★★	PULMONARY	★★★
GASTROINTESTINAL	★★★	STROKE	★★★★★
GENERAL SURGERY	NR	VASCULAR	NR
MATERNITY CARE	NR	WOMEN'S HEALTH	NR

HEALTHGRADES AWARDS

✓ SPECIALTY EXCELLENCE
• CARDIAC CARE   • STROKE CARE

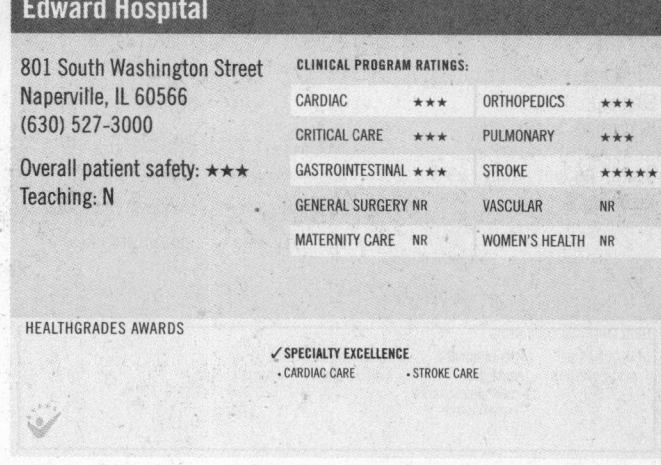

Decatur Memorial Hospital

2300 North Edward Street
Decatur, IL 62526
(217) 876-8121

Overall patient safety: ★★★★★
Teaching: Y

CLINICAL PROGRAM RATINGS:

CARDIAC	★★★	ORTHOPEDICS	★★★
CRITICAL CARE	★	PULMONARY	★
GASTROINTESTINAL	★★★	STROKE	★★★
GENERAL SURGERY	NR	VASCULAR	NR
MATERNITY CARE	NR	WOMEN'S HEALTH	NR

HEALTHGRADES AWARDS

✓ DISTINGUISHED HOSPITAL
• PATIENT SAFETY

✓ SPECIALTY EXCELLENCE
• CARDIAC SURGERY

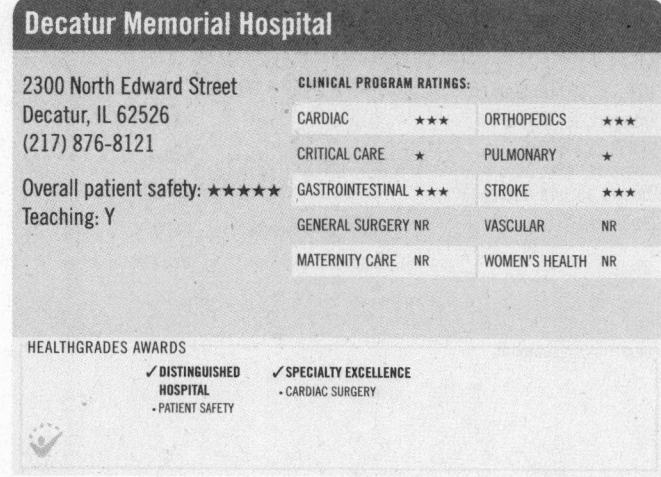

Elmhurst Memorial Hospital

200 Berteau Avenue
Elmhurst, IL 60126
(630) 833-1400

Overall patient safety: ★★★
Teaching: N

CLINICAL PROGRAM RATINGS:

CARDIAC	★★★	ORTHOPEDICS	★★★
CRITICAL CARE	★★★	PULMONARY	★★★
GASTROINTESTINAL	★★★	STROKE	★★★
GENERAL SURGERY	NR	VASCULAR	★★★
MATERNITY CARE	NR	WOMEN'S HEALTH	NR

HEALTHGRADES AWARDS

✓ DISTINGUISHED HOSPITAL
• CLINICAL EXCELLENCE

✓ SPECIALTY EXCELLENCE
• GASTROINTESTINAL CARE

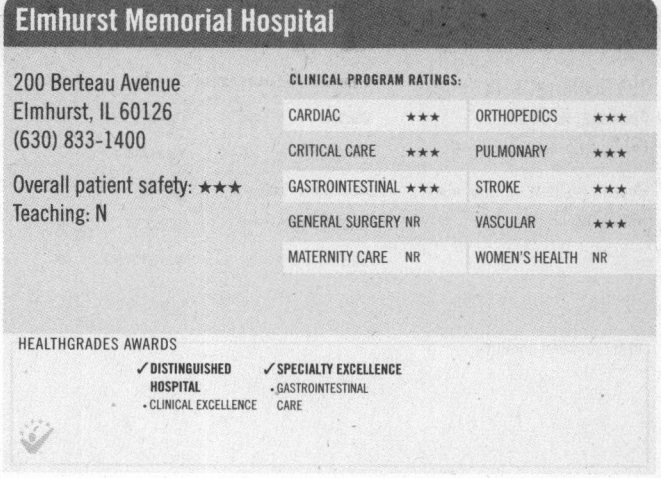

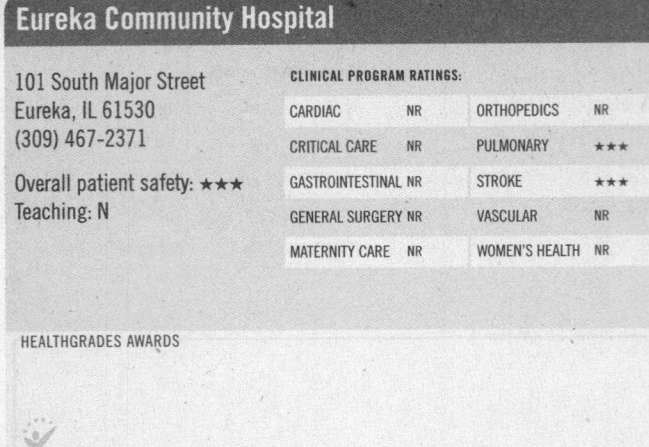

Eureka Community Hospital

101 South Major Street
Eureka, IL 61530
(309) 467-2371

Overall patient safety: ★★★
Teaching: N

CLINICAL PROGRAM RATINGS:

CARDIAC	NR	ORTHOPEDICS	NR
CRITICAL CARE	NR	PULMONARY	★★★
GASTROINTESTINAL	NR	STROKE	★★★
GENERAL SURGERY	NR	VASCULAR	NR
MATERNITY CARE	NR	WOMEN'S HEALTH	NR

HEALTHGRADES AWARDS

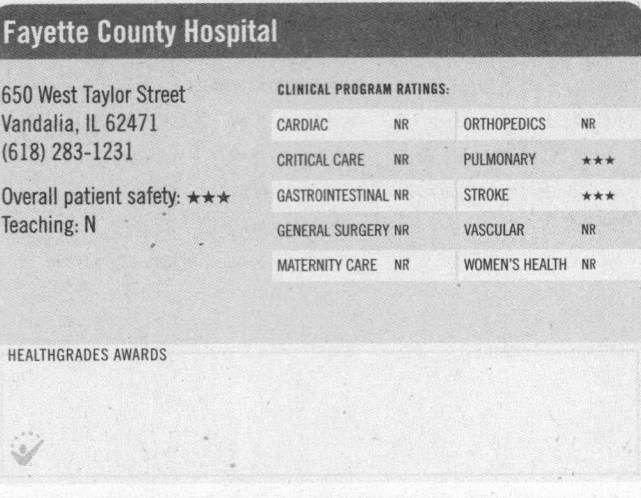

Fayette County Hospital

650 West Taylor Street
Vandalia, IL 62471
(618) 283-1231

Overall patient safety: ★★★
Teaching: N

CLINICAL PROGRAM RATINGS:

CARDIAC	NR	ORTHOPEDICS	NR
CRITICAL CARE	NR	PULMONARY	★★★
GASTROINTESTINAL	NR	STROKE	★★★
GENERAL SURGERY	NR	VASCULAR	NR
MATERNITY CARE	NR	WOMEN'S HEALTH	NR

HEALTHGRADES AWARDS

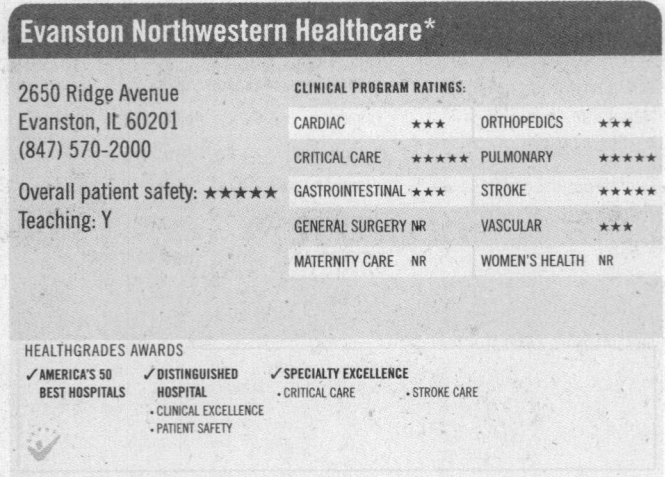

Evanston Northwestern Healthcare*

2650 Ridge Avenue
Evanston, IL 60201
(847) 570-2000

Overall patient safety: ★★★★★
Teaching: Y

CLINICAL PROGRAM RATINGS:

CARDIAC	★★★	ORTHOPEDICS	★★★
CRITICAL CARE	★★★★★	PULMONARY	★★★★★
GASTROINTESTINAL	★★★	STROKE	★★★★★
GENERAL SURGERY	NR	VASCULAR	★★★
MATERNITY CARE	NR	WOMEN'S HEALTH	NR

HEALTHGRADES AWARDS

✓ AMERICA'S 50 BEST HOSPITALS
✓ DISTINGUISHED HOSPITAL
· CLINICAL EXCELLENCE
· PATIENT SAFETY
✓ SPECIALTY EXCELLENCE
· CRITICAL CARE
· STROKE CARE

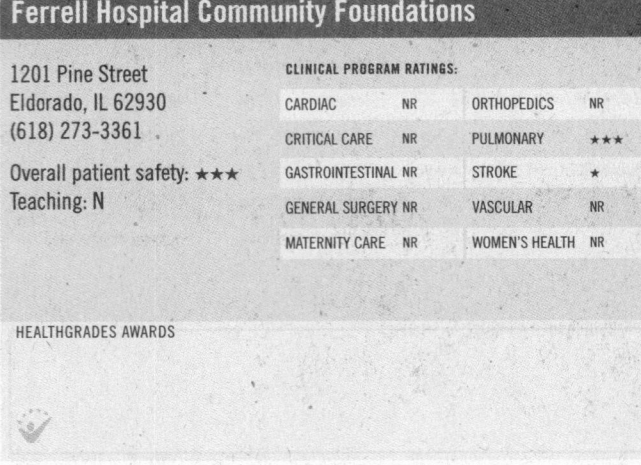

Ferrell Hospital Community Foundations

1201 Pine Street
Eldorado, IL 62930
(618) 273-3361

Overall patient safety: ★★★
Teaching: N

CLINICAL PROGRAM RATINGS:

CARDIAC	NR	ORTHOPEDICS	NR
CRITICAL CARE	NR	PULMONARY	★★★
GASTROINTESTINAL	NR	STROKE	★
GENERAL SURGERY	NR	VASCULAR	NR
MATERNITY CARE	NR	WOMEN'S HEALTH	NR

HEALTHGRADES AWARDS

Fairfield Memorial Hospital

303 Northwest 11th Street
Fairfield, IL 62837
(618) 842-2611

Overall patient safety: ★★★
Teaching: N

CLINICAL PROGRAM RATINGS:

CARDIAC	NR	ORTHOPEDICS	NR
CRITICAL CARE	NR	PULMONARY	★
GASTROINTESTINAL	NR	STROKE	NR
GENERAL SURGERY	NR	VASCULAR	NR
MATERNITY CARE	NR	WOMEN'S HEALTH	NR

HEALTHGRADES AWARDS

FHN Memorial Hospital

1045 West Stephenson
Freeport, IL 61032
(815) 599-6000

Overall patient safety: ★
Teaching: N

CLINICAL PROGRAM RATINGS:

CARDIAC	NR	ORTHOPEDICS	NR
CRITICAL CARE	★★★	PULMONARY	★★★★★
GASTROINTESTINAL	★★★	STROKE	★★★
GENERAL SURGERY	NR	VASCULAR	NR
MATERNITY CARE	NR	WOMEN'S HEALTH	NR

HEALTHGRADES AWARDS

✓ SPECIALTY EXCELLENCE
· PULMONARY CARE

KEY: ★★★★★ BEST ★★★ AS EXPECTED ★ POOR NR NOT RATED BY HEALTHGRADES · For full definitions of ratings and awards, see Appendix.

Franklin Hospital

201 Bailey Lane
Benton, IL 62812
(618) 439-3161

Overall patient safety: ★★★
Teaching: N

CLINICAL PROGRAM RATINGS:

CARDIAC	NR	ORTHOPEDICS	NR
CRITICAL CARE	NR	PULMONARY	★★★
GASTROINTESTINAL	NR	STROKE	★
GENERAL SURGERY	NR	VASCULAR	NR
MATERNITY CARE	NR	WOMEN'S HEALTH	NR

HEALTHGRADES AWARDS

Gibson Community Hospital

1120 North Melvin Street
Gibson City, IL 60936
(217) 784-4251

Overall patient safety: ★
Teaching: N

CLINICAL PROGRAM RATINGS:

CARDIAC	NR	ORTHOPEDICS	NR
CRITICAL CARE	NR	PULMONARY	★★★
GASTROINTESTINAL	NR	STROKE	NR
GENERAL SURGERY	NR	VASCULAR	NR
MATERNITY CARE	NR	WOMEN'S HEALTH	NR

HEALTHGRADES AWARDS

Galesburg Cottage Hospital

695 North Kellog Street
Galesburg, IL 61401
(309) 343-8131

Overall patient safety: ★★★
Teaching: N

CLINICAL PROGRAM RATINGS:

CARDIAC	NR	ORTHOPEDICS	NR
CRITICAL CARE	NR	PULMONARY	★★★
GASTROINTESTINAL	★★★	STROKE	★
GENERAL SURGERY	NR	VASCULAR	NR
MATERNITY CARE	NR	WOMEN'S HEALTH	NR

HEALTHGRADES AWARDS

Good Samaritan Regional Health Center

605 North 12th Street
Mount Vernon, IL 62864
(618) 242-4600

Overall patient safety: ★★★
Teaching: N

CLINICAL PROGRAM RATINGS:

CARDIAC	★★★	ORTHOPEDICS	NR
CRITICAL CARE	NR	PULMONARY	★★★
GASTROINTESTINAL	★★★	STROKE	★★★
GENERAL SURGERY	NR	VASCULAR	NR
MATERNITY CARE	NR	WOMEN'S HEALTH	NR

HEALTHGRADES AWARDS

Gateway Regional Medical Center

2100 Madison Avenue
Granite City, IL 62040
(618) 798-3000

Overall patient safety: ★★★
Teaching: N

CLINICAL PROGRAM RATINGS:

CARDIAC	NR	ORTHOPEDICS	NR
CRITICAL CARE	NR	PULMONARY	★
GASTROINTESTINAL	NR	STROKE	★★★
GENERAL SURGERY	NR	VASCULAR	NR
MATERNITY CARE	NR	WOMEN'S HEALTH	NR

HEALTHGRADES AWARDS

Gottlieb Memorial Hospital

701 West North Avenue
Melrose Park, IL 60160
(708) 681-3200

Overall patient safety: ★★★
Teaching: Y

CLINICAL PROGRAM RATINGS:

CARDIAC	★★★	ORTHOPEDICS	★★★
CRITICAL CARE	★★★	PULMONARY	★★★
GASTROINTESTINAL	★	STROKE	★★★
GENERAL SURGERY	NR	VASCULAR	NR
MATERNITY CARE	NR	WOMEN'S HEALTH	NR

HEALTHGRADES AWARDS

*This hospital reports its data to the federal government jointly with another hospital. Therefore the ratings and awards apply to multiple hospitals and this specific hospital may not provide all rated services.

Graham Hospital Association

210 West Walnut Street
Canton, IL 61520
(309) 647-5240

Overall patient safety: ★★★★★
Teaching: N

CLINICAL PROGRAM RATINGS:

CARDIAC	NR	ORTHOPEDICS	NR
CRITICAL CARE	NR	PULMONARY	★★★
GASTROINTESTINAL	NR	STROKE	★★★
GENERAL SURGERY	NR	VASCULAR	NR
MATERNITY CARE	NR	WOMEN'S HEALTH	NR

HEALTHGRADES AWARDS

Hammond Henry Hospital

600 North College Avenue
Geneseo, IL 61254
(309) 944-6431

Overall patient safety: ★★★
Teaching: N

CLINICAL PROGRAM RATINGS:

CARDIAC	NR	ORTHOPEDICS	NR
CRITICAL CARE	NR	PULMONARY	★★★
GASTROINTESTINAL	NR	STROKE	NR
GENERAL SURGERY	NR	VASCULAR	NR
MATERNITY CARE	NR	WOMEN'S HEALTH	NR

HEALTHGRADES AWARDS

Greenville Regional Hospital

200 Healthcare Drive
Greenville, IL 62246
(618) 664-1230

Overall patient safety: ★★★
Teaching: N

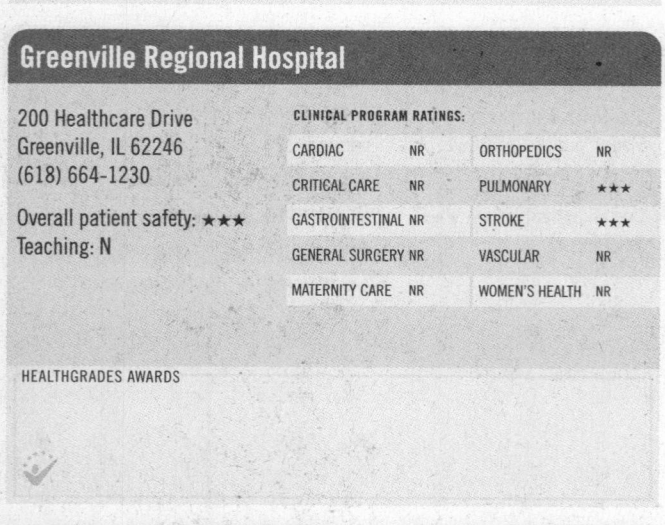

CLINICAL PROGRAM RATINGS:

CARDIAC	NR	ORTHOPEDICS	NR
CRITICAL CARE	NR	PULMONARY	★★★
GASTROINTESTINAL	NR	STROKE	★★★
GENERAL SURGERY	NR	VASCULAR	NR
MATERNITY CARE	NR	WOMEN'S HEALTH	NR

HEALTHGRADES AWARDS

Hardin County General Hospital

6 Ferrell Road
Rosiclare, IL 62982
(618) 285-6634

Overall patient safety: ★★★
Teaching: N

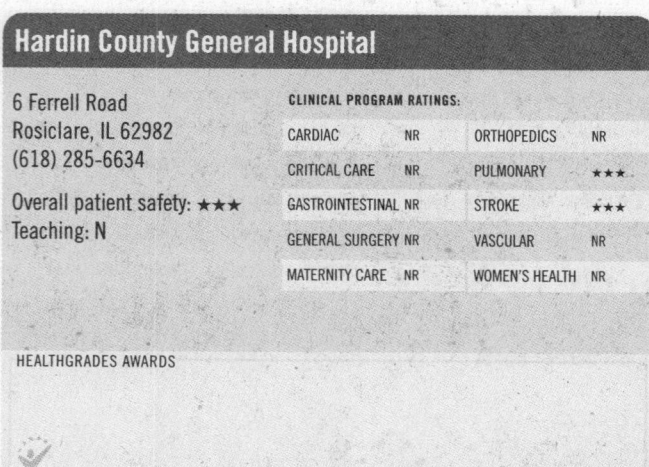

CLINICAL PROGRAM RATINGS:

CARDIAC	NR	ORTHOPEDICS	NR
CRITICAL CARE	NR	PULMONARY	★★★
GASTROINTESTINAL	NR	STROKE	★★★
GENERAL SURGERY	NR	VASCULAR	NR
MATERNITY CARE	NR	WOMEN'S HEALTH	NR

HEALTHGRADES AWARDS

Hamilton Memorial Hospital District

611 South Marshall Avenue
McLeansboro, IL 62859
(618) 643-2361

Overall patient safety: ★★★
Teaching: N

CLINICAL PROGRAM RATINGS:

CARDIAC	NR	ORTHOPEDICS	NR
CRITICAL CARE	NR	PULMONARY	★★★
GASTROINTESTINAL	NR	STROKE	NR
GENERAL SURGERY	NR	VASCULAR	NR
MATERNITY CARE	NR	WOMEN'S HEALTH	NR

HEALTHGRADES AWARDS

Harrisburg Medical Center

100 Hospital Drive
Harrisburg, IL 62946
(618) 253-7671

Overall patient safety: ★
Teaching: N

CLINICAL PROGRAM RATINGS:

CARDIAC	NR	ORTHOPEDICS	NR
CRITICAL CARE	NR	PULMONARY	★★★
GASTROINTESTINAL	NR	STROKE	★
GENERAL SURGERY	NR	VASCULAR	NR
MATERNITY CARE	NR	WOMEN'S HEALTH	NR

HEALTHGRADES AWARDS

KEY: ★★★★★ BEST   ★★★ AS EXPECTED   ★ POOR   NR NOT RATED BY HEALTHGRADES   For full definitions of ratings and awards, see Appendix.

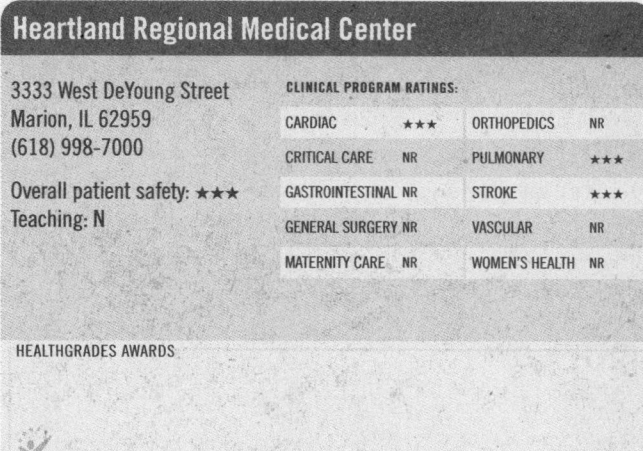

Heartland Regional Medical Center

3333 West DeYoung Street
Marion, IL 62959
(618) 998-7000

Overall patient safety: ★★★
Teaching: N

CLINICAL PROGRAM RATINGS:

CARDIAC	★★★	ORTHOPEDICS	NR
CRITICAL CARE	NR	PULMONARY	★★★
GASTROINTESTINAL	NR	STROKE	★★★
GENERAL SURGERY	NR	VASCULAR	NR
MATERNITY CARE	NR	WOMEN'S HEALTH	NR

HEALTHGRADES AWARDS

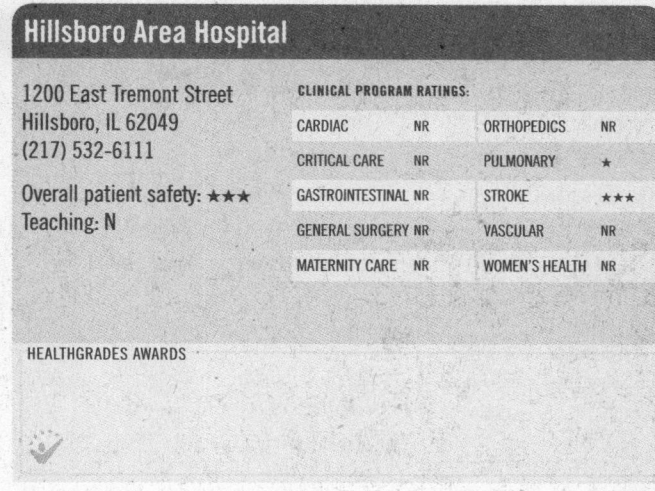

Hillsboro Area Hospital

1200 East Tremont Street
Hillsboro, IL 62049
(217) 532-6111

Overall patient safety: ★★★
Teaching: N

CLINICAL PROGRAM RATINGS:

CARDIAC	NR	ORTHOPEDICS	NR
CRITICAL CARE	NR	PULMONARY	★
GASTROINTESTINAL	NR	STROKE	★★★
GENERAL SURGERY	NR	VASCULAR	NR
MATERNITY CARE	NR	WOMEN'S HEALTH	NR

HEALTHGRADES AWARDS

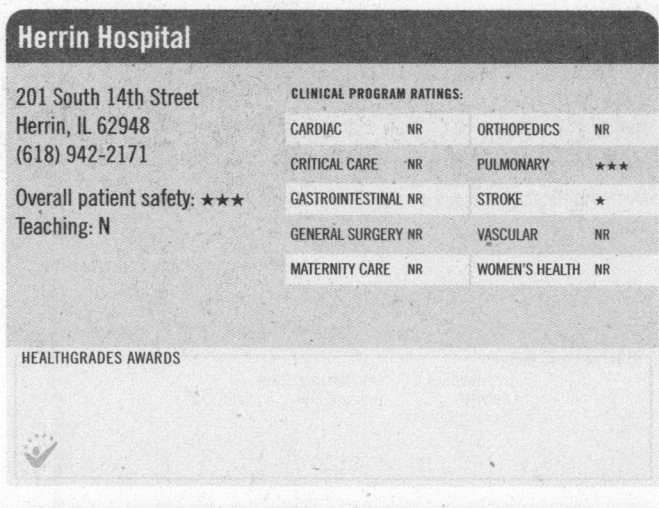

Herrin Hospital

201 South 14th Street
Herrin, IL 62948
(618) 942-2171

Overall patient safety: ★★★
Teaching: N

CLINICAL PROGRAM RATINGS:

CARDIAC	NR	ORTHOPEDICS	NR
CRITICAL CARE	NR	PULMONARY	★★★
GASTROINTESTINAL	NR	STROKE	★
GENERAL SURGERY	NR	VASCULAR	NR
MATERNITY CARE	NR	WOMEN'S HEALTH	NR

HEALTHGRADES AWARDS

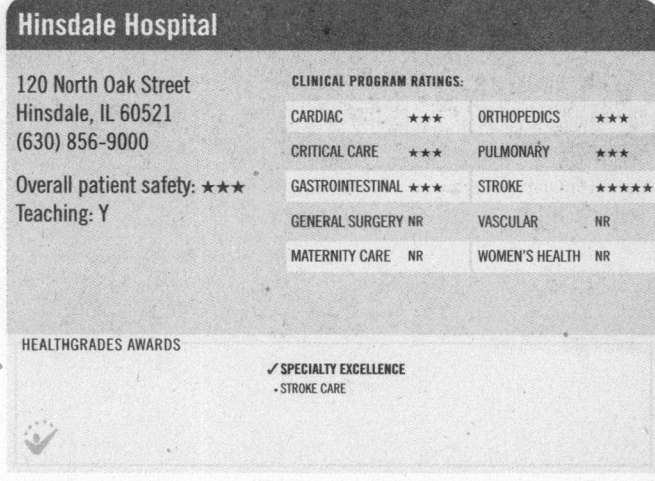

Hinsdale Hospital

120 North Oak Street
Hinsdale, IL 60521
(630) 856-9000

Overall patient safety: ★★★
Teaching: Y

CLINICAL PROGRAM RATINGS:

CARDIAC	★★★	ORTHOPEDICS	★★★
CRITICAL CARE	★★★	PULMONARY	★★★
GASTROINTESTINAL	★★★	STROKE	★★★★★
GENERAL SURGERY	NR	VASCULAR	NR
MATERNITY CARE	NR	WOMEN'S HEALTH	NR

HEALTHGRADES AWARDS

✓ SPECIALTY EXCELLENCE
• STROKE CARE

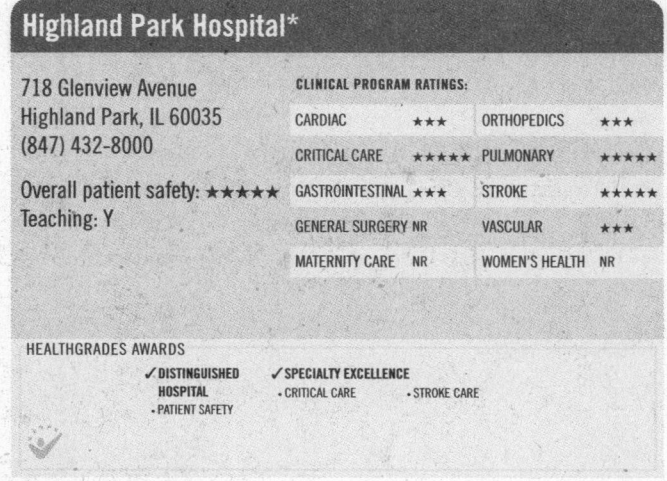

Highland Park Hospital*

718 Glenview Avenue
Highland Park, IL 60035
(847) 432-8000

Overall patient safety: ★★★★★
Teaching: Y

CLINICAL PROGRAM RATINGS:

CARDIAC	★★★	ORTHOPEDICS	★★★
CRITICAL CARE	★★★★★	PULMONARY	★★★★★
GASTROINTESTINAL	★★★	STROKE	★★★★★
GENERAL SURGERY	NR	VASCULAR	★★★
MATERNITY CARE	NR	WOMEN'S HEALTH	NR

HEALTHGRADES AWARDS

✓ DISTINGUISHED HOSPITAL
• PATIENT SAFETY

✓ SPECIALTY EXCELLENCE
• CRITICAL CARE   • STROKE CARE

Holy Cross Hospital

2701 West 68th Street
Chicago, IL 60629
(773) 884-9000

Overall patient safety: ★
Teaching: N

CLINICAL PROGRAM RATINGS:

CARDIAC	NR	ORTHOPEDICS	NR
CRITICAL CARE	★★★	PULMONARY	★★★
GASTROINTESTINAL	★★★	STROKE	★★★★★
GENERAL SURGERY	NR	VASCULAR	NR
MATERNITY CARE	NR	WOMEN'S HEALTH	NR

HEALTHGRADES AWARDS

*This hospital reports its data to the federal government jointly with another hospital. Therefore the ratings and awards apply to multiple hospitals and this specific hospital may not provide all rated services.

Hopedale Medical Complex

107 Tremont Street
Hopedale, IL 61747
(309) 449-3321

Overall patient safety: ★★★
Teaching: N

CLINICAL PROGRAM RATINGS:

CARDIAC	NR	ORTHOPEDICS	NR
CRITICAL CARE	NR	PULMONARY	★
GASTROINTESTINAL	NR	STROKE	NR
GENERAL SURGERY	NR	VASCULAR	NR
MATERNITY CARE	NR	WOMEN'S HEALTH	NR

HEALTHGRADES AWARDS

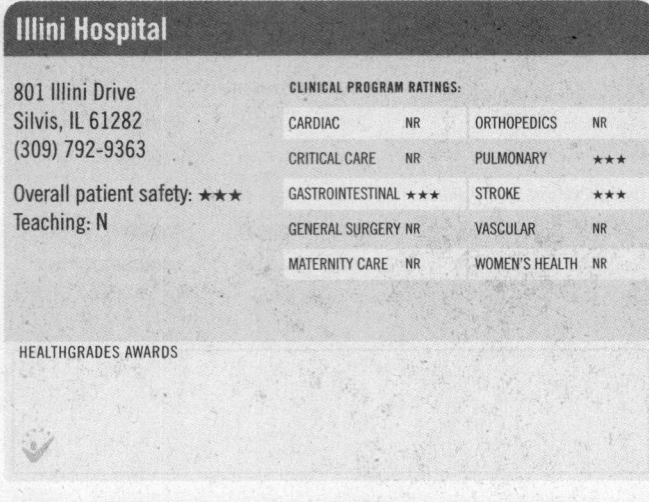

Illini Hospital

801 Illini Drive
Silvis, IL 61282
(309) 792-9363

Overall patient safety: ★★★
Teaching: N

CLINICAL PROGRAM RATINGS:

CARDIAC	NR	ORTHOPEDICS	NR
CRITICAL CARE	NR	PULMONARY	★★★
GASTROINTESTINAL	★★★	STROKE	★★★
GENERAL SURGERY	NR	VASCULAR	NR
MATERNITY CARE	NR	WOMEN'S HEALTH	NR

HEALTHGRADES AWARDS

Illinois Valley Community Hospital

925 West Street
Peru, IL 61354
(815) 223-3300

Overall patient safety: ★★★
Teaching: N

CLINICAL PROGRAM RATINGS:

CARDIAC	NR	ORTHOPEDICS	NR
CRITICAL CARE	NR	PULMONARY	★
GASTROINTESTINAL	NR	STROKE	★
GENERAL SURGERY	NR	VASCULAR	NR
MATERNITY CARE	NR	WOMEN'S HEALTH	NR

HEALTHGRADES AWARDS

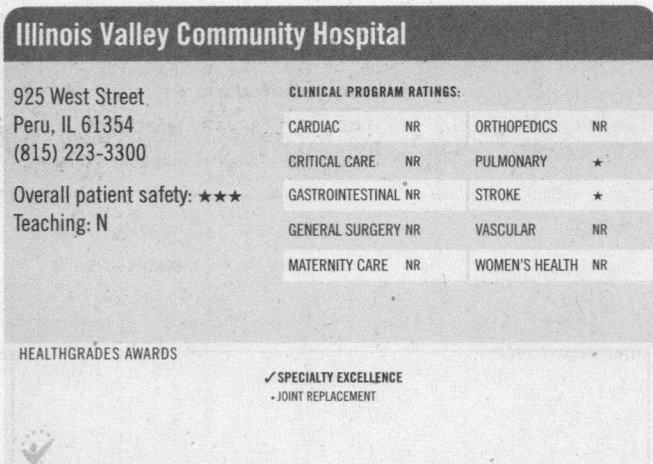

✓ SPECIALTY EXCELLENCE
• JOINT REPLACEMENT

Ingalls Memorial Hospital

1 Ingalls Drive
Harvey, IL 60426
(708) 333-2300

Overall patient safety: ★★★
Teaching: N

CLINICAL PROGRAM RATINGS:

CARDIAC	★★★	ORTHOPEDICS	★★★
CRITICAL CARE	★★★	PULMONARY	★★★★★
GASTROINTESTINAL	★★★	STROKE	★★★★★
GENERAL SURGERY	NR	VASCULAR	NR
MATERNITY CARE	NR	WOMEN'S HEALTH	NR

HEALTHGRADES AWARDS

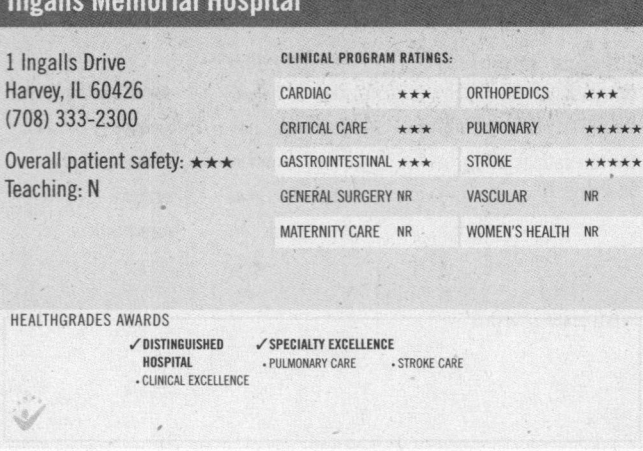

✓ DISTINGUISHED HOSPITAL   ✓ SPECIALTY EXCELLENCE
• CLINICAL EXCELLENCE   • PULMONARY CARE   • STROKE CARE

Illini Community Hospital

640 West Washington
Pittsfield, IL 62363
(217) 285-2113

Overall patient safety: ★★★
Teaching: N

CLINICAL PROGRAM RATINGS:

CARDIAC	NR	ORTHOPEDICS	NR
CRITICAL CARE	NR	PULMONARY	★★★
GASTROINTESTINAL	NR	STROKE	★
GENERAL SURGERY	NR	VASCULAR	NR
MATERNITY CARE	NR	WOMEN'S HEALTH	NR

HEALTHGRADES AWARDS

Iroquois Memorial Hospital

200 Fairman Avenue
Watseka, IL 60970
(815) 432-5841

Overall patient safety: ★★★
Teaching: N

CLINICAL PROGRAM RATINGS:

CARDIAC	NR	ORTHOPEDICS	NR
CRITICAL CARE	NR	PULMONARY	★★★
GASTROINTESTINAL	NR	STROKE	★★★★★
GENERAL SURGERY	NR	VASCULAR	NR
MATERNITY CARE	NR	WOMEN'S HEALTH	NR

HEALTHGRADES AWARDS

KEY: ★★★★★ BEST   ★★★ AS EXPECTED   ★ POOR   NR NOT RATED BY HEALTHGRADES   For full definitions of ratings and awards, see Appendix.

Jackson Park Hospital Foundation

7531 Stony Island Avenue
Chicago, IL 60649
(773) 947-7500

Overall patient safety: ★★★
Teaching: Y

CLINICAL PROGRAM RATINGS:

CARDIAC	NR	ORTHOPEDICS	NR
CRITICAL CARE	NR	PULMONARY	★★★
GASTROINTESTINAL	NR	STROKE	NR
GENERAL SURGERY	NR	VASCULAR	NR
MATERNITY CARE	NR	WOMEN'S HEALTH	NR

HEALTHGRADES AWARDS

Katherine Shaw Bethea Hospital

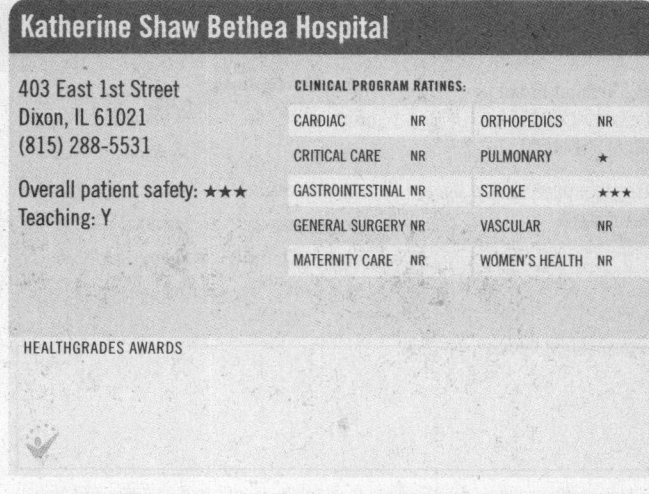

403 East 1st Street
Dixon, IL 61021
(815) 288-5531

Overall patient safety: ★★★
Teaching: Y

CLINICAL PROGRAM RATINGS:

CARDIAC	NR	ORTHOPEDICS	NR
CRITICAL CARE	NR	PULMONARY	★
GASTROINTESTINAL	NR	STROKE	★★★
GENERAL SURGERY	NR	VASCULAR	NR
MATERNITY CARE	NR	WOMEN'S HEALTH	NR

HEALTHGRADES AWARDS

Jersey Community Hospital

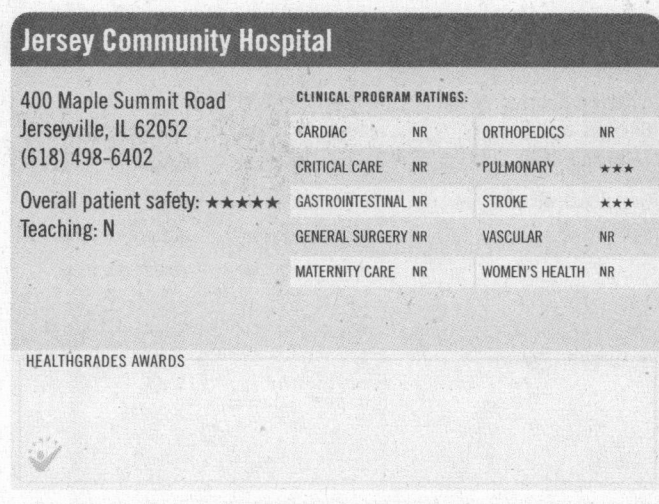

400 Maple Summit Road
Jerseyville, IL 62052
(618) 498-6402

Overall patient safety: ★★★★★
Teaching: N

CLINICAL PROGRAM RATINGS:

CARDIAC	NR	ORTHOPEDICS	NR
CRITICAL CARE	NR	PULMONARY	★★★
GASTROINTESTINAL	NR	STROKE	★★★
GENERAL SURGERY	NR	VASCULAR	NR
MATERNITY CARE	NR	WOMEN'S HEALTH	NR

HEALTHGRADES AWARDS

Kenneth Hall Regional Hospital

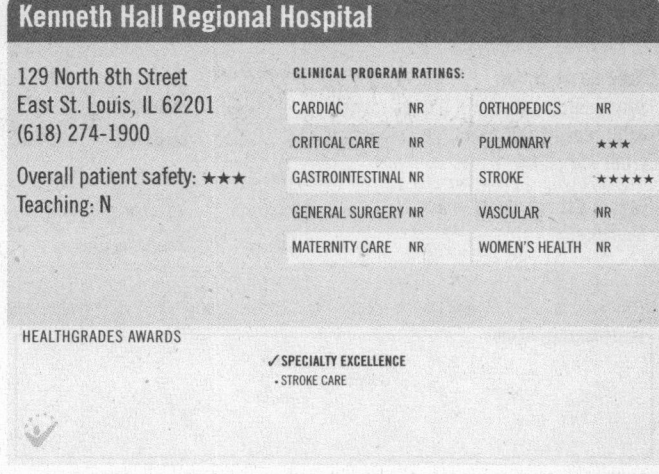

129 North 8th Street
East St. Louis, IL 62201
(618) 274-1900

Overall patient safety: ★★★
Teaching: N

CLINICAL PROGRAM RATINGS:

CARDIAC	NR	ORTHOPEDICS	NR
CRITICAL CARE	NR	PULMONARY	★★★
GASTROINTESTINAL	NR	STROKE	★★★★★
GENERAL SURGERY	NR	VASCULAR	NR
MATERNITY CARE	NR	WOMEN'S HEALTH	NR

HEALTHGRADES AWARDS

✓ SPECIALTY EXCELLENCE
· STROKE CARE

John H. Stroger Jr. Hospital

1901 West Harrison Street
Chicago, IL 60612
(312) 864-6000

Overall patient safety: ★★★
Teaching: Y

CLINICAL PROGRAM RATINGS:

CARDIAC	★★★	ORTHOPEDICS	NR
CRITICAL CARE	NR	PULMONARY	★★★
GASTROINTESTINAL	NR	STROKE	★★★
GENERAL SURGERY	NR	VASCULAR	NR
MATERNITY CARE	NR	WOMEN'S HEALTH	NR

HEALTHGRADES AWARDS

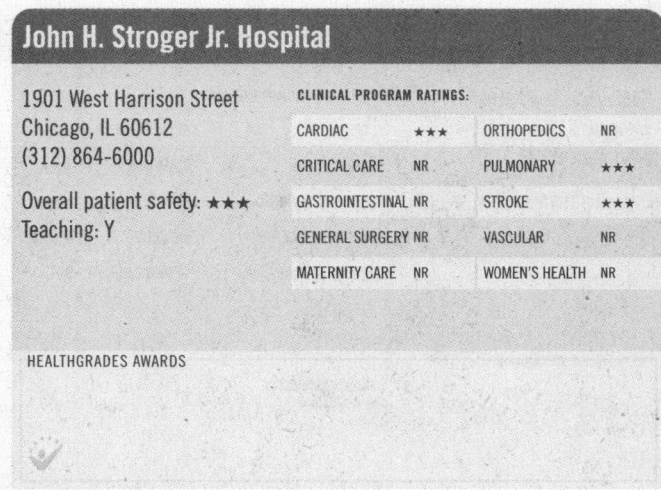

Kewanee Hospital

719 Elliott Street
Kewanee, IL 61443
(309) 853-3361

Overall patient safety: ★★★
Teaching: N

CLINICAL PROGRAM RATINGS:

CARDIAC	NR	ORTHOPEDICS	NR
CRITICAL CARE	NR	PULMONARY	★
GASTROINTESTINAL	NR	STROKE	NR
GENERAL SURGERY	NR	VASCULAR	NR
MATERNITY CARE	NR	WOMEN'S HEALTH	NR

HEALTHGRADES AWARDS

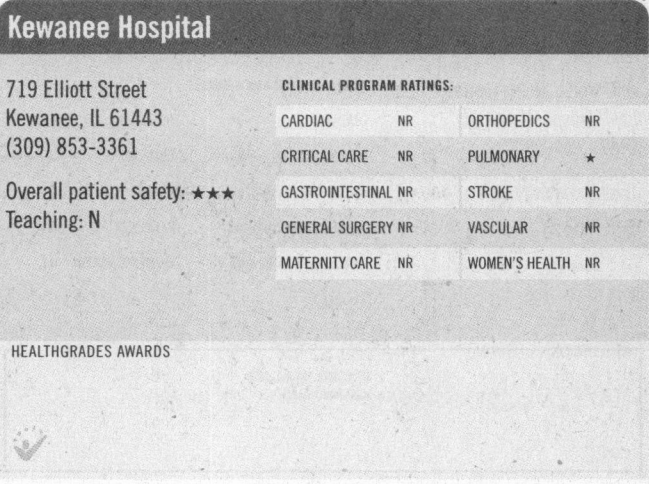

Kishwaukee Community Hospital

626 Bethany Road
DeKalb, IL 60115
(815) 756-1521

Overall patient safety: ★★★
Teaching: N

CLINICAL PROGRAM RATINGS:

CARDIAC	NR	ORTHOPEDICS	★★★
CRITICAL CARE	★★★	PULMONARY	★★★
GASTROINTESTINAL	NR	STROKE	★★★
GENERAL SURGERY	NR	VASCULAR	NR
MATERNITY CARE	NR	WOMEN'S HEALTH	NR

HEALTHGRADES AWARDS

Lawrence County Memorial Hospital

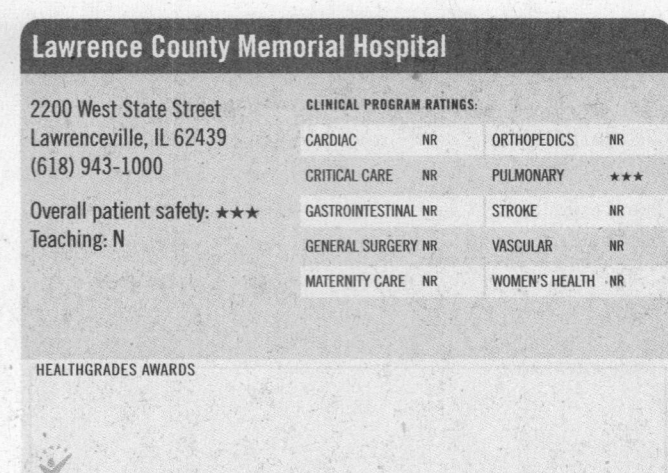

2200 West State Street
Lawrenceville, IL 62439
(618) 943-1000

Overall patient safety: ★★★
Teaching: N

CLINICAL PROGRAM RATINGS:

CARDIAC	NR	ORTHOPEDICS	NR
CRITICAL CARE	NR	PULMONARY	★★★
GASTROINTESTINAL	NR	STROKE	NR
GENERAL SURGERY	NR	VASCULAR	NR
MATERNITY CARE	NR	WOMEN'S HEALTH	NR

HEALTHGRADES AWARDS

La Grange Memorial Hospital

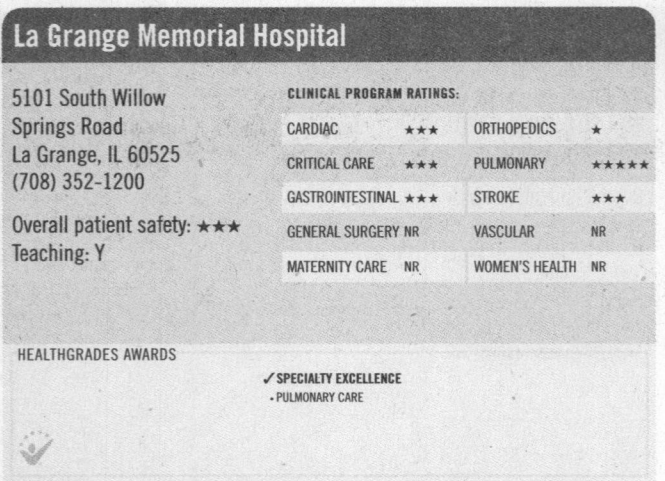

5101 South Willow
Springs Road
La Grange, IL 60525
(708) 352-1200

Overall patient safety: ★★★
Teaching: Y

CLINICAL PROGRAM RATINGS:

CARDIAC	★★★	ORTHOPEDICS	★
CRITICAL CARE	★★★	PULMONARY	★★★★★
GASTROINTESTINAL	★★★	STROKE	★★★
GENERAL SURGERY	NR	VASCULAR	NR
MATERNITY CARE	NR	WOMEN'S HEALTH	NR

HEALTHGRADES AWARDS

✓ SPECIALTY EXCELLENCE
• PULMONARY CARE

Lincoln Park Hospital

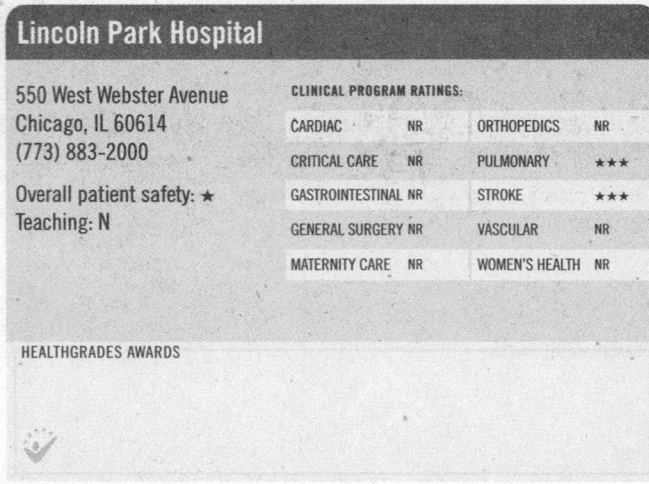

550 West Webster Avenue
Chicago, IL 60614
(773) 883-2000

Overall patient safety: ★
Teaching: N

CLINICAL PROGRAM RATINGS:

CARDIAC	NR	ORTHOPEDICS	NR
CRITICAL CARE	NR	PULMONARY	★★★
GASTROINTESTINAL	NR	STROKE	★★★
GENERAL SURGERY	NR	VASCULAR	NR
MATERNITY CARE	NR	WOMEN'S HEALTH	NR

HEALTHGRADES AWARDS

Lake Forest Hospital

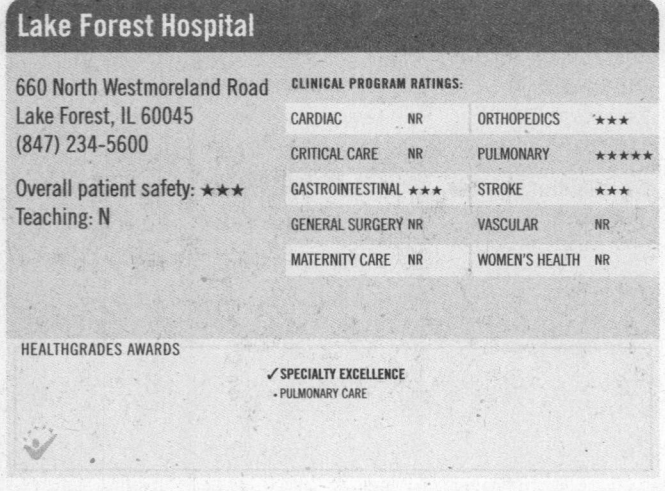

660 North Westmoreland Road
Lake Forest, IL 60045
(847) 234-5600

Overall patient safety: ★★★
Teaching: N

CLINICAL PROGRAM RATINGS:

CARDIAC	NR	ORTHOPEDICS	★★★
CRITICAL CARE	NR	PULMONARY	★★★★★
GASTROINTESTINAL	★★★	STROKE	★★★
GENERAL SURGERY	NR	VASCULAR	NR
MATERNITY CARE	NR	WOMEN'S HEALTH	NR

HEALTHGRADES AWARDS

✓ SPECIALTY EXCELLENCE
• PULMONARY CARE

Little Company of Mary Hospital

2800 West 95th Street
Evergreen Park, IL 60805
(708) 422-6200

Overall patient safety: ★★★
Teaching: Y

CLINICAL PROGRAM RATINGS:

CARDIAC	NR	ORTHOPEDICS	★★★
CRITICAL CARE	★★★	PULMONARY	★★★
GASTROINTESTINAL	★★★	STROKE	★★★
GENERAL SURGERY	NR	VASCULAR	NR
MATERNITY CARE	NR	WOMEN'S HEALTH	NR

HEALTHGRADES AWARDS

✓ SPECIALTY EXCELLENCE
• GASTROINTESTINAL
  CARE

KEY: ★★★★★ BEST   ★★★ AS EXPECTED   ★ POOR   NR NOT RATED BY HEALTHGRADES   For full definitions of ratings and awards, see Appendix.

Loretto Hospital

645 South Central Avenue
Chicago, IL 60644
(773) 626-4300

Overall patient safety: ★★★
Teaching: Y

CLINICAL PROGRAM RATINGS:

CARDIAC	NR	ORTHOPEDICS	NR
CRITICAL CARE	NR	PULMONARY	★★★
GASTROINTESTINAL	NR	STROKE	NR
GENERAL SURGERY	NR	VASCULAR	NR
MATERNITY CARE	NR	WOMEN'S HEALTH	NR

HEALTHGRADES AWARDS

MacNeal Hospital

3249 South Oak Parks
Avenue
Berwyn, IL 60402
(708) 783-9100

Overall patient safety: ★★★
Teaching: Y

CLINICAL PROGRAM RATINGS:

CARDIAC	★★★	ORTHOPEDICS	★★★
CRITICAL CARE	★★★	PULMONARY	★★★
GASTROINTESTINAL	★★★	STROKE	★★★★★
GENERAL SURGERY	NR	VASCULAR	NR
MATERNITY CARE	NR	WOMEN'S HEALTH	NR

HEALTHGRADES AWARDS

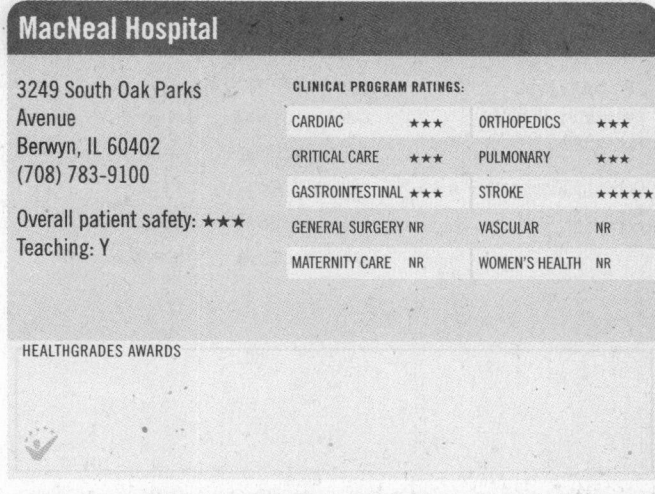

Louis A. Weiss Memorial Hospital

4646 North Marine Drive
Chicago, IL 60640
(773) 878-8700

Overall patient safety: ★
Teaching: Y

CLINICAL PROGRAM RATINGS:

CARDIAC	★★★	ORTHOPEDICS	NR
CRITICAL CARE	NR	PULMONARY	★★★
GASTROINTESTINAL	NR	STROKE	★★★
GENERAL SURGERY	NR	VASCULAR	NR
MATERNITY CARE	NR	WOMEN'S HEALTH	NR

HEALTHGRADES AWARDS

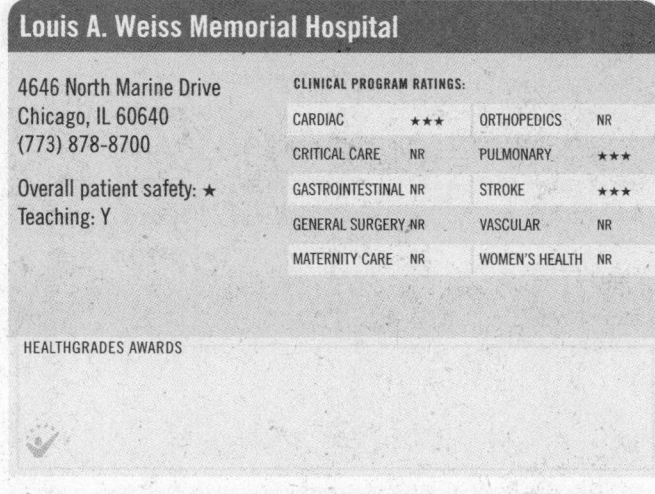

Marshall Browning Hospital

900 North Washington Street
DuQuoin, IL 62832
(618) 542-2146

Overall patient safety: ★★★
Teaching: N

CLINICAL PROGRAM RATINGS:

CARDIAC	NR	ORTHOPEDICS	NR
CRITICAL CARE	NR	PULMONARY	★★★
GASTROINTESTINAL	NR	STROKE	★★★
GENERAL SURGERY	NR	VASCULAR	NR
MATERNITY CARE	NR	WOMEN'S HEALTH	NR

HEALTHGRADES AWARDS

Loyola University Medical Center

2160 South 1st Avenue
Maywood, IL 60153
(708) 216-9000

Overall patient safety: ★★★
Teaching: Y

CLINICAL PROGRAM RATINGS:

CARDIAC	★★★	ORTHOPEDICS	★★★
CRITICAL CARE	★★★	PULMONARY	★★★
GASTROINTESTINAL	★★★	STROKE	★★★
GENERAL SURGERY	NR	VASCULAR	★★★
MATERNITY CARE	NR	WOMEN'S HEALTH	NR

HEALTHGRADES AWARDS

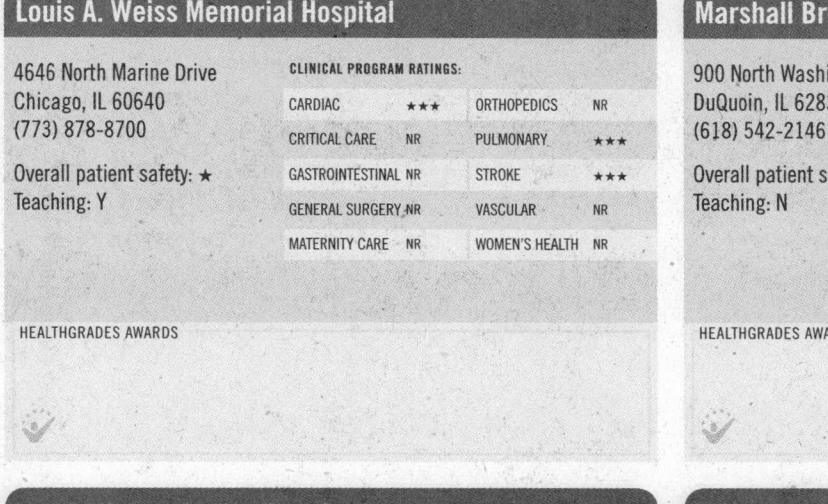

Mason District Hospital

615 North Promenade
Havana, IL 62644
(309) 543-4431

Overall patient safety: ★★★
Teaching: N

CLINICAL PROGRAM RATINGS:

CARDIAC	NR	ORTHOPEDICS	NR
CRITICAL CARE	NR	PULMONARY	★★★
GASTROINTESTINAL	NR	STROKE	NR
GENERAL SURGERY	NR	VASCULAR	NR
MATERNITY CARE	NR	WOMEN'S HEALTH	NR

HEALTHGRADES AWARDS

Massac Memorial Hospital

28 Chick Street
Metropolis, IL 62960
(618) 524-2176

Overall patient safety: ★★★
Teaching: N

CLINICAL PROGRAM RATINGS:

CARDIAC	NR	ORTHOPEDICS	NR
CRITICAL CARE	NR	PULMONARY	★★★
GASTROINTESTINAL	NR	STROKE	★★★
GENERAL SURGERY	NR	VASCULAR	NR
MATERNITY CARE	NR	WOMEN'S HEALTH	NR

HEALTHGRADES AWARDS

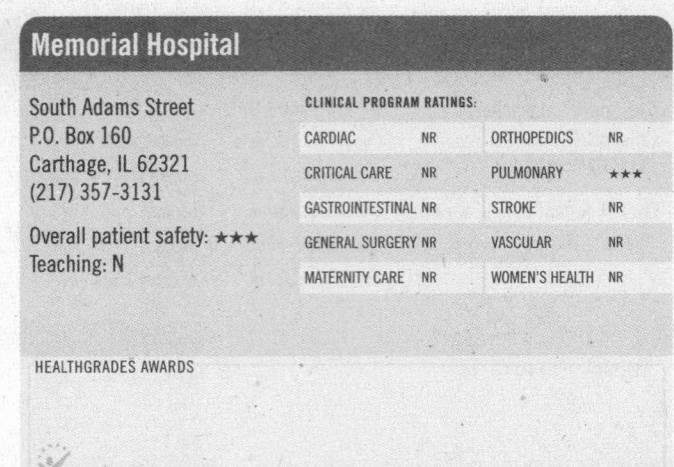

Memorial Hospital

South Adams Street
P.O. Box 160
Carthage, IL 62321
(217) 357-3131

Overall patient safety: ★★★
Teaching: N

CLINICAL PROGRAM RATINGS:

CARDIAC	NR	ORTHOPEDICS	NR
CRITICAL CARE	NR	PULMONARY	★★★
GASTROINTESTINAL	NR	STROKE	NR
GENERAL SURGERY	NR	VASCULAR	NR
MATERNITY CARE	NR	WOMEN'S HEALTH	NR

HEALTHGRADES AWARDS

McDonough District Hospital

525 East Grant Street
Macomb, IL 61455
(309) 833-4101

Overall patient safety: ★★★
Teaching: N

CLINICAL PROGRAM RATINGS:

CARDIAC	NR	ORTHOPEDICS	NR
CRITICAL CARE	NR	PULMONARY	★★★
GASTROINTESTINAL	★★★	STROKE	★★★
GENERAL SURGERY	NR	VASCULAR	NR
MATERNITY CARE	NR	WOMEN'S HEALTH	NR

HEALTHGRADES AWARDS

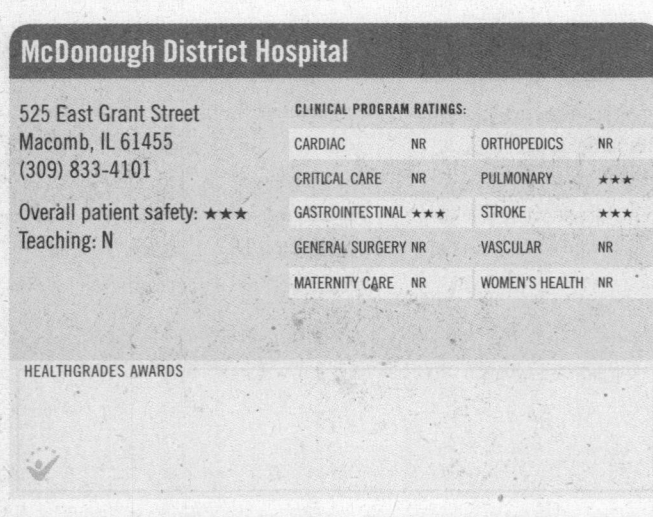

Memorial Hospital

1900 State Street
Chester, IL 62233
(618) 826-4581

Overall patient safety: ★★★
Teaching: N

CLINICAL PROGRAM RATINGS:

CARDIAC	NR	ORTHOPEDICS	NR
CRITICAL CARE	NR	PULMONARY	★★★
GASTROINTESTINAL	NR	STROKE	★★★
GENERAL SURGERY	NR	VASCULAR	NR
MATERNITY CARE	NR	WOMEN'S HEALTH	NR

HEALTHGRADES AWARDS

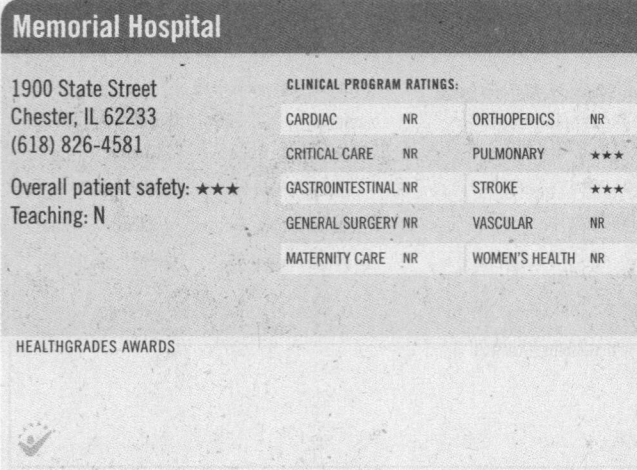

Memorial Hospital

4500 Memorial Drive
Belleville, IL 62226
(618) 233-7750

Overall patient safety: ★★★
Teaching: N

CLINICAL PROGRAM RATINGS:

CARDIAC	★★★	ORTHOPEDICS	★★★
CRITICAL CARE	★★★	PULMONARY	★★★
GASTROINTESTINAL	★★★	STROKE	★★★
GENERAL SURGERY	NR	VASCULAR	NR
MATERNITY CARE	NR	WOMEN'S HEALTH	NR

HEALTHGRADES AWARDS

✓ SPECIALTY EXCELLENCE
• JOINT REPLACEMENT

Memorial Hospital of Carbondale

405 West Jackson Street
Carbondale, IL 62901
(618) 549-0721

Overall patient safety: ★★★
Teaching: Y

CLINICAL PROGRAM RATINGS:

CARDIAC	★★★	ORTHOPEDICS	★★★
CRITICAL CARE	NR	PULMONARY	★
GASTROINTESTINAL	NR	STROKE	★★★
GENERAL SURGERY	NR	VASCULAR	NR
MATERNITY CARE	NR	WOMEN'S HEALTH	NR

HEALTHGRADES AWARDS

KEY: ★★★★★ BEST ★★★ AS EXPECTED ★ POOR NR NOT RATED BY HEALTHGRADES   For full definitions of ratings and awards, see Appendix.

Memorial Medical Center

701 North 1st Street
Springfield, IL 62781
(217) 788-3000

Overall patient safety: ★★★
Teaching: Y

CLINICAL PROGRAM RATINGS:

CARDIAC	★★★	ORTHOPEDICS	★★★★★
CRITICAL CARE	★	PULMONARY	★★★
GASTROINTESTINAL	★★★	STROKE	★★★
GENERAL SURGERY	NR	VASCULAR	★★★
MATERNITY CARE	NR	WOMEN'S HEALTH	NR

HEALTHGRADES AWARDS

✓ SPECIALTY EXCELLENCE
 · JOINT REPLACEMENT

Mercy Hospital and Medical Center

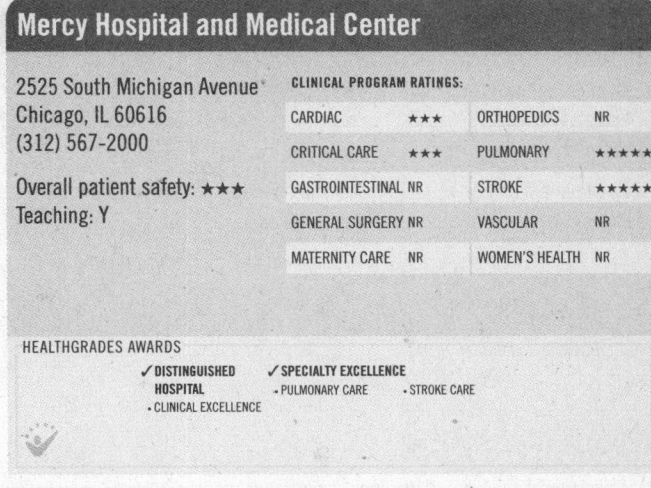

2525 South Michigan Avenue
Chicago, IL 60616
(312) 567-2000

Overall patient safety: ★★★
Teaching: Y

CLINICAL PROGRAM RATINGS:

CARDIAC	★★★	ORTHOPEDICS	NR
CRITICAL CARE	★★★	PULMONARY	★★★★★
GASTROINTESTINAL	NR	STROKE	★★★★★
GENERAL SURGERY	NR	VASCULAR	NR
MATERNITY CARE	NR	WOMEN'S HEALTH	NR

HEALTHGRADES AWARDS

✓ DISTINGUISHED   ✓ SPECIALTY EXCELLENCE
   HOSPITAL   · PULMONARY CARE   · STROKE CARE
 · CLINICAL EXCELLENCE

Mendota Community Hospital

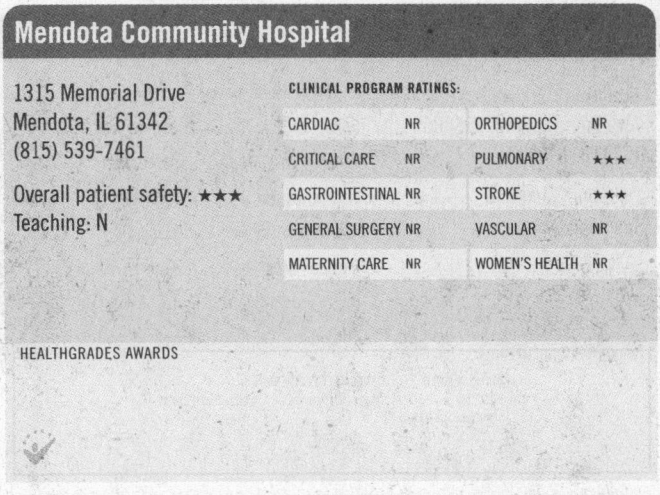

1315 Memorial Drive
Mendota, IL 61342
(815) 539-7461

Overall patient safety: ★★★
Teaching: N

CLINICAL PROGRAM RATINGS:

CARDIAC	NR	ORTHOPEDICS	NR
CRITICAL CARE	NR	PULMONARY	★★★
GASTROINTESTINAL	NR	STROKE	★★★
GENERAL SURGERY	NR	VASCULAR	NR
MATERNITY CARE	NR	WOMEN'S HEALTH	NR

HEALTHGRADES AWARDS

Methodist Hospital of Chicago

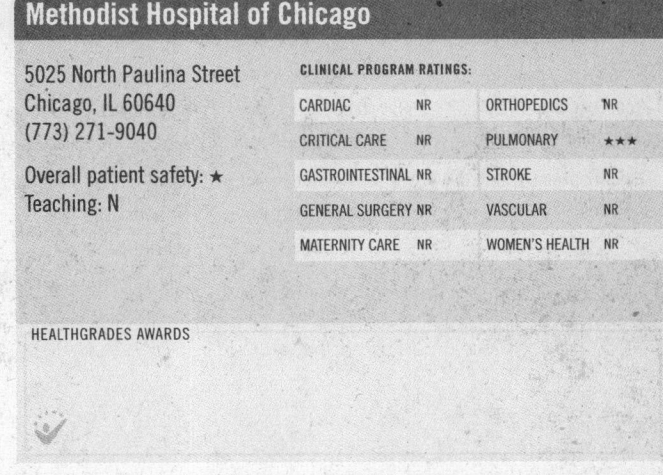

5025 North Paulina Street
Chicago, IL 60640
(773) 271-9040

Overall patient safety: ★
Teaching: N

CLINICAL PROGRAM RATINGS:

CARDIAC	NR	ORTHOPEDICS	NR
CRITICAL CARE	NR	PULMONARY	★★★
GASTROINTESTINAL	NR	STROKE	NR
GENERAL SURGERY	NR	VASCULAR	NR
MATERNITY CARE	NR	WOMEN'S HEALTH	NR

HEALTHGRADES AWARDS

Mercy Harvard Hospital

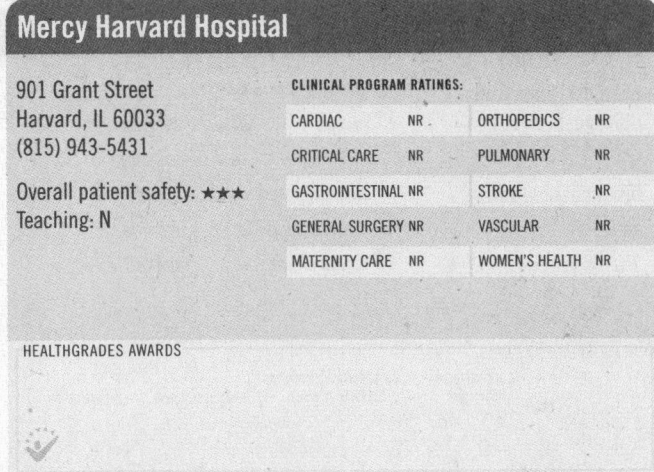

901 Grant Street
Harvard, IL 60033
(815) 943-5431

Overall patient safety: ★★★
Teaching: N

CLINICAL PROGRAM RATINGS:

CARDIAC	NR	ORTHOPEDICS	NR
CRITICAL CARE	NR	PULMONARY	NR
GASTROINTESTINAL	NR	STROKE	NR
GENERAL SURGERY	NR	VASCULAR	NR
MATERNITY CARE	NR	WOMEN'S HEALTH	NR

HEALTHGRADES AWARDS

Methodist Medical Center of Illinois

221 Northeast Glen
Oak Avenue
Peoria, IL 61636
(309) 672-5522

Overall patient safety: ★★★
Teaching: Y

CLINICAL PROGRAM RATINGS:

CARDIAC	★★★	ORTHOPEDICS	★★★
CRITICAL CARE	★★★	PULMONARY	★★★
GASTROINTESTINAL	★★★	STROKE	★★★
GENERAL SURGERY	NR	VASCULAR	NR
MATERNITY CARE	NR	WOMEN'S HEALTH	NR

HEALTHGRADES AWARDS

Michael Reese Hospital and Medical Center

2929 South Ellis Avenue
Chicago, IL 60616
(312) 791-2000

Overall patient safety: ★
Teaching: Y

CLINICAL PROGRAM RATINGS:

CARDIAC	NR	ORTHOPEDICS	NR
CRITICAL CARE	★★★	PULMONARY	★★★
GASTROINTESTINAL	NR	STROKE	★★★
GENERAL SURGERY	NR	VASCULAR	NR
MATERNITY CARE	NR	WOMEN'S HEALTH	NR

HEALTHGRADES AWARDS

Mt. Sinai Hospital Medical Center

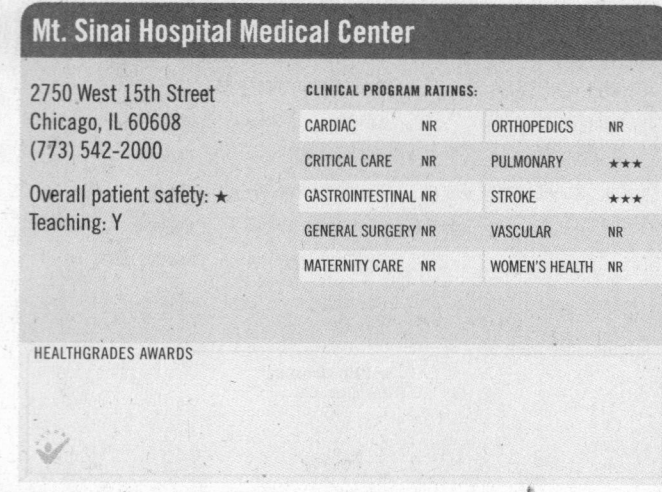

2750 West 15th Street
Chicago, IL 60608
(773) 542-2000

Overall patient safety: ★
Teaching: Y

CLINICAL PROGRAM RATINGS:

CARDIAC	NR	ORTHOPEDICS	NR
CRITICAL CARE	NR	PULMONARY	★★★
GASTROINTESTINAL	NR	STROKE	★★★
GENERAL SURGERY	NR	VASCULAR	NR
MATERNITY CARE	NR	WOMEN'S HEALTH	NR

HEALTHGRADES AWARDS

Midwestern Region Medical Center

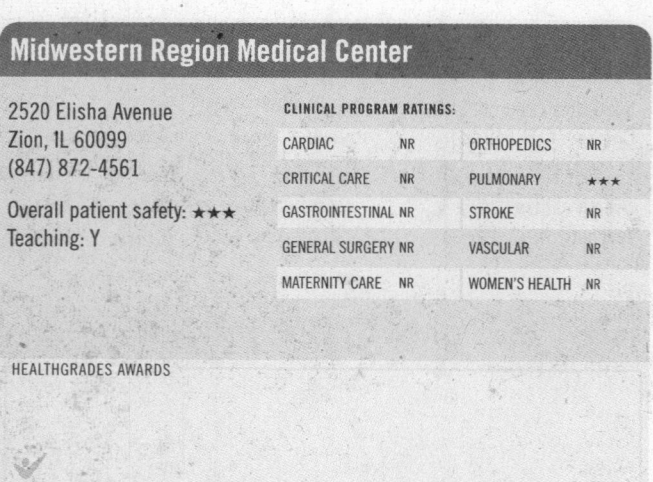

2520 Elisha Avenue
Zion, IL 60099
(847) 872-4561

Overall patient safety: ★★★
Teaching: Y

CLINICAL PROGRAM RATINGS:

CARDIAC	NR	ORTHOPEDICS	NR
CRITICAL CARE	NR	PULMONARY	★★★
GASTROINTESTINAL	NR	STROKE	NR
GENERAL SURGERY	NR	VASCULAR	NR
MATERNITY CARE	NR	WOMEN'S HEALTH	NR

HEALTHGRADES AWARDS

Northwest Community Hospital

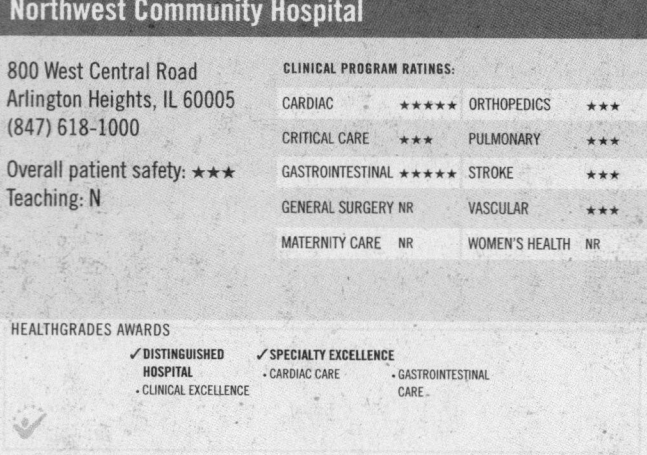

800 West Central Road
Arlington Heights, IL 60005
(847) 618-1000

Overall patient safety: ★★★
Teaching: N

CLINICAL PROGRAM RATINGS:

CARDIAC	★★★★★	ORTHOPEDICS	★★★
CRITICAL CARE	★★★	PULMONARY	★★★
GASTROINTESTINAL	★★★★★	STROKE	★★★
GENERAL SURGERY	NR	VASCULAR	★★★
MATERNITY CARE	NR	WOMEN'S HEALTH	NR

HEALTHGRADES AWARDS

✓ **DISTINGUISHED HOSPITAL**
• CLINICAL EXCELLENCE

✓ **SPECIALTY EXCELLENCE**
• CARDIAC CARE
• GASTROINTESTINAL CARE

Morris Hospital and Healthcare Center

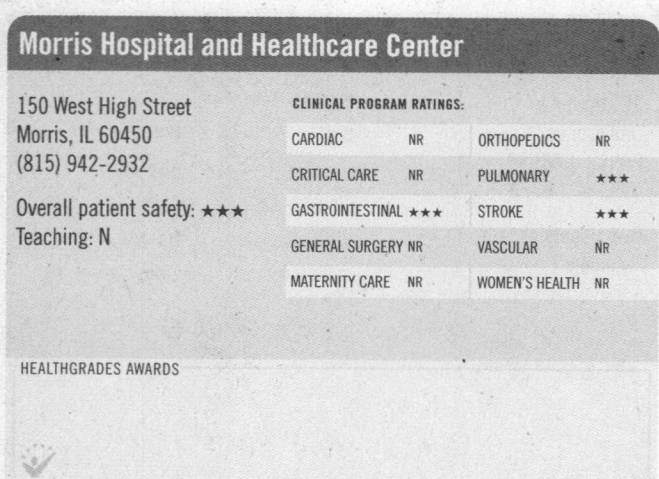

150 West High Street
Morris, IL 60450
(815) 942-2932

Overall patient safety: ★★★
Teaching: N

CLINICAL PROGRAM RATINGS:

CARDIAC	NR	ORTHOPEDICS	NR
CRITICAL CARE	NR	PULMONARY	★★★
GASTROINTESTINAL	★★★	STROKE	★★★
GENERAL SURGERY	NR	VASCULAR	NR
MATERNITY CARE	NR	WOMEN'S HEALTH	NR

HEALTHGRADES AWARDS

Northwestern Memorial Hospital

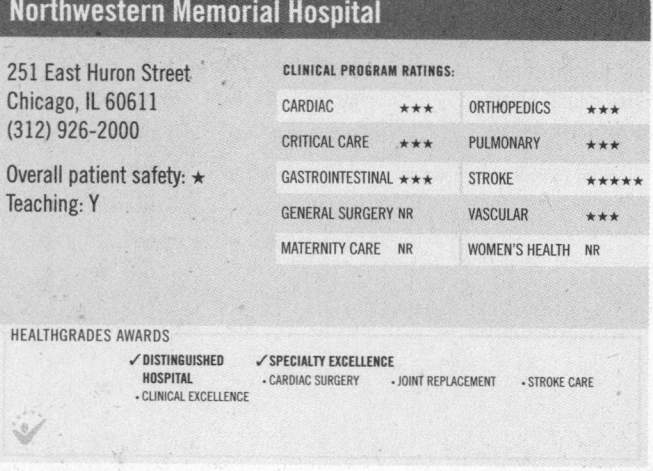

251 East Huron Street
Chicago, IL 60611
(312) 926-2000

Overall patient safety: ★
Teaching: Y

CLINICAL PROGRAM RATINGS:

CARDIAC	★★★	ORTHOPEDICS	★★★
CRITICAL CARE	★★★	PULMONARY	★★★
GASTROINTESTINAL	★★★	STROKE	★★★★★
GENERAL SURGERY	NR	VASCULAR	★★★
MATERNITY CARE	NR	WOMEN'S HEALTH	NR

HEALTHGRADES AWARDS

✓ **DISTINGUISHED HOSPITAL**
• CLINICAL EXCELLENCE

✓ **SPECIALTY EXCELLENCE**
• CARDIAC SURGERY
• JOINT REPLACEMENT
• STROKE CARE

KEY: ★★★★★ BEST ★★★ AS EXPECTED ★ POOR NR NOT RATED BY HEALTHGRADES For full definitions of ratings and awards, see Appendix.

Norwegian-American Hospital

1044 North Francisco Avenue
Chicago, IL 60622
(773) 292-8200

Overall patient safety: ★★★
Teaching: Y

CLINICAL PROGRAM RATINGS:

CARDIAC	NR	ORTHOPEDICS	NR
CRITICAL CARE	NR	PULMONARY	★★★
GASTROINTESTINAL	NR	STROKE	★★★
GENERAL SURGERY	NR	VASCULAR	NR
MATERNITY CARE	NR	WOMEN'S HEALTH	NR

HEALTHGRADES AWARDS

Our Lady of the Resurrection Medical Center

5645 West Addison Street
Chicago, IL 60634
(773) 282-7000

Overall patient safety: ★★★
Teaching: Y

CLINICAL PROGRAM RATINGS:

CARDIAC	NR	ORTHOPEDICS	NR
CRITICAL CARE	★★★★★	PULMONARY	★★★
GASTROINTESTINAL	★★★	STROKE	★★★★★
GENERAL SURGERY	NR	VASCULAR	NR
MATERNITY CARE	NR	WOMEN'S HEALTH	NR

HEALTHGRADES AWARDS

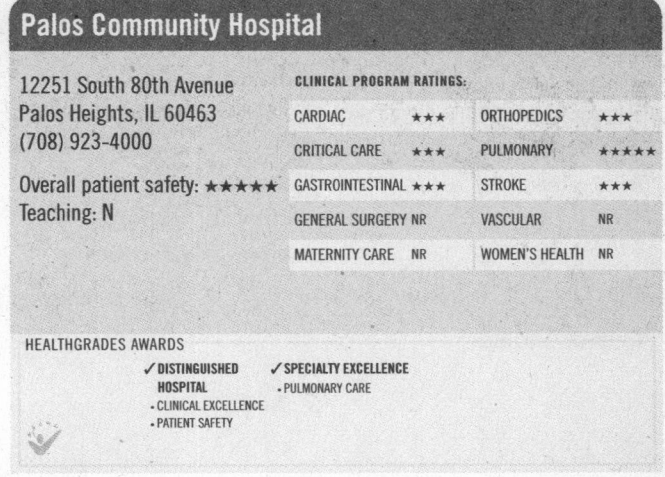

✓ DISTINGUISHED HOSPITAL
- CLINICAL EXCELLENCE

✓ SPECIALTY EXCELLENCE
- CRITICAL CARE
- STROKE CARE

Oak Forest Hospital

15900 Cicero Avenue
Oak Forest, IL 60452
(708) 687-7200

Overall patient safety: ★★★
Teaching: Y

CLINICAL PROGRAM RATINGS:

CARDIAC	NR	ORTHOPEDICS	NR
CRITICAL CARE	NR	PULMONARY	NR
GASTROINTESTINAL	NR	STROKE	NR
GENERAL SURGERY	NR	VASCULAR	NR
MATERNITY CARE	NR	WOMEN'S HEALTH	NR

HEALTHGRADES AWARDS

Palos Community Hospital

12251 South 80th Avenue
Palos Heights, IL 60463
(708) 923-4000

Overall patient safety: ★★★★★
Teaching: N

CLINICAL PROGRAM RATINGS:

CARDIAC	★★★	ORTHOPEDICS	★★★
CRITICAL CARE	★★★	PULMONARY	★★★★★
GASTROINTESTINAL	★★★	STROKE	★★★
GENERAL SURGERY	NR	VASCULAR	NR
MATERNITY CARE	NR	WOMEN'S HEALTH	NR

HEALTHGRADES AWARDS

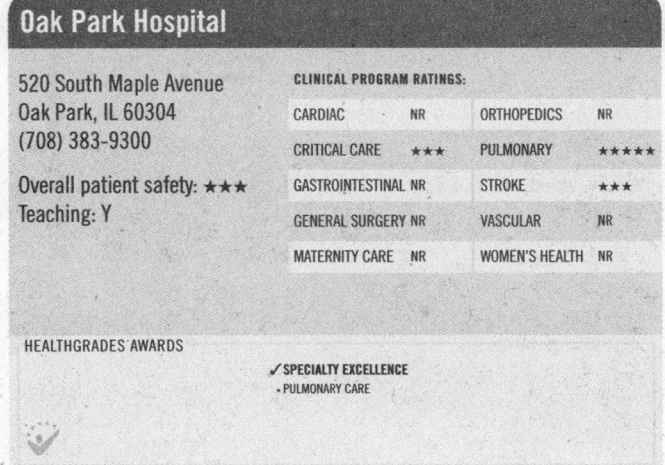

✓ DISTINGUISHED HOSPITAL
- CLINICAL EXCELLENCE
- PATIENT SAFETY

✓ SPECIALTY EXCELLENCE
- PULMONARY CARE

Oak Park Hospital

520 South Maple Avenue
Oak Park, IL 60304
(708) 383-9300

Overall patient safety: ★★★
Teaching: Y

CLINICAL PROGRAM RATINGS:

CARDIAC	NR	ORTHOPEDICS	NR
CRITICAL CARE	★★★	PULMONARY	★★★★★
GASTROINTESTINAL	NR	STROKE	★★★
GENERAL SURGERY	NR	VASCULAR	NR
MATERNITY CARE	NR	WOMEN'S HEALTH	NR

HEALTHGRADES AWARDS

✓ SPECIALTY EXCELLENCE
- PULMONARY CARE

Pana Community Hospital

101 East 9th Street
Pana, IL 62557
(217) 562-2131

Overall patient safety: ★★★
Teaching: N

CLINICAL PROGRAM RATINGS:

CARDIAC	NR	ORTHOPEDICS	NR
CRITICAL CARE	NR	PULMONARY	★
GASTROINTESTINAL	NR	STROKE	★★★
GENERAL SURGERY	NR	VASCULAR	NR
MATERNITY CARE	NR	WOMEN'S HEALTH	NR

HEALTHGRADES AWARDS

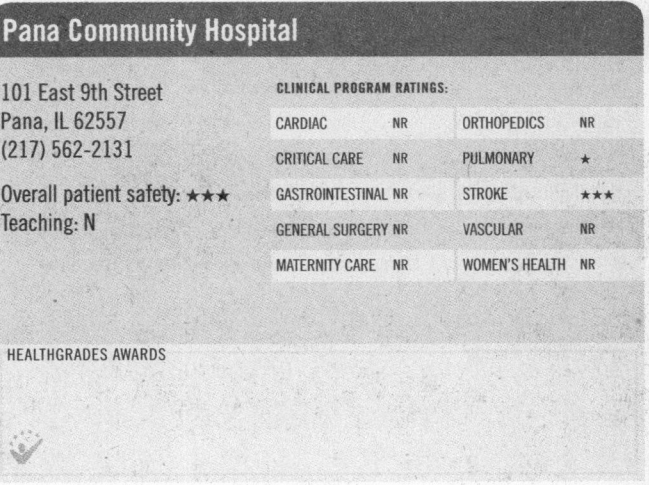

Paris Community Hospital

721 East Court Street
Paris, IL 61944
(217) 465-4141

Overall patient safety: ★★★
Teaching: N

CLINICAL PROGRAM RATINGS:

CARDIAC	NR	ORTHOPEDICS	NR
CRITICAL CARE	NR	PULMONARY	★
GASTROINTESTINAL	NR	STROKE	★
GENERAL SURGERY	NR	VASCULAR	NR
MATERNITY CARE	NR	WOMEN'S HEALTH	NR

HEALTHGRADES AWARDS

Perry Memorial Hospital

530 Parks Avenue East
Princeton, IL 61356
(815) 875-2811

Overall patient safety: ★★★★★
Teaching: N

CLINICAL PROGRAM RATINGS:

CARDIAC	NR	ORTHOPEDICS	NR
CRITICAL CARE	NR	PULMONARY	★
GASTROINTESTINAL	NR	STROKE	★
GENERAL SURGERY	NR	VASCULAR	NR
MATERNITY CARE	NR	WOMEN'S HEALTH	NR

HEALTHGRADES AWARDS

Passavant Area Hospital

1600 West Walnut Street
Jacksonville, IL 62650
(217) 245-9541

Overall patient safety: ★★★
Teaching: N

CLINICAL PROGRAM RATINGS:

CARDIAC	NR	ORTHOPEDICS	NR
CRITICAL CARE	NR	PULMONARY	★★★
GASTROINTESTINAL	★★★	STROKE	★★★
GENERAL SURGERY	NR	VASCULAR	NR
MATERNITY CARE	NR	WOMEN'S HEALTH	NR

HEALTHGRADES AWARDS

Pinckneyville Community Hospital

101 North Walnut
Pinckneyville, IL 62274
(618) 357-2187

Overall patient safety: ★★★
Teaching: N

CLINICAL PROGRAM RATINGS:

CARDIAC	NR	ORTHOPEDICS	NR
CRITICAL CARE	NR	PULMONARY	★★★
GASTROINTESTINAL	NR	STROKE	★
GENERAL SURGERY	NR	VASCULAR	NR
MATERNITY CARE	NR	WOMEN'S HEALTH	NR

HEALTHGRADES AWARDS

Pekin Memorial Hospital

600 South 13th Street
Pekin, IL 61554
(309) 347-1151

Overall patient safety: ★★★
Teaching: N

CLINICAL PROGRAM RATINGS:

CARDIAC	NR	ORTHOPEDICS	NR
CRITICAL CARE	NR	PULMONARY	★
GASTROINTESTINAL	★★★	STROKE	★
GENERAL SURGERY	NR	VASCULAR	NR
MATERNITY CARE	NR	WOMEN'S HEALTH	NR

HEALTHGRADES AWARDS

Proctor Hospital

5409 North Knoxville Avenue
Peoria, IL 61614
(309) 691-1000

Overall patient safety: ★★★
Teaching: N

CLINICAL PROGRAM RATINGS:

CARDIAC	★★★	ORTHOPEDICS	NR
CRITICAL CARE	★	PULMONARY	★
GASTROINTESTINAL	★★★	STROKE	★★★
GENERAL SURGERY	NR	VASCULAR	NR
MATERNITY CARE	NR	WOMEN'S HEALTH	NR

HEALTHGRADES AWARDS

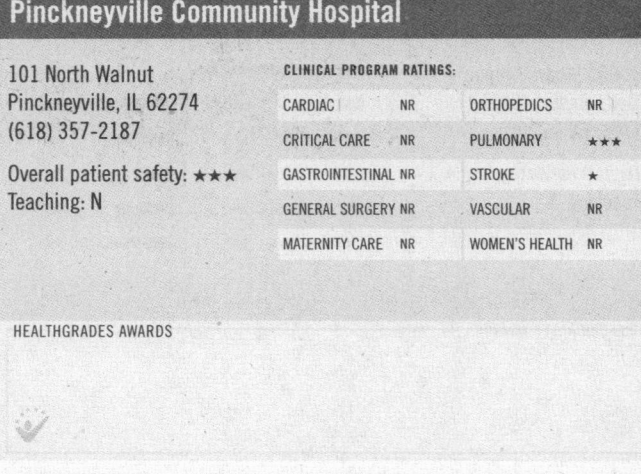
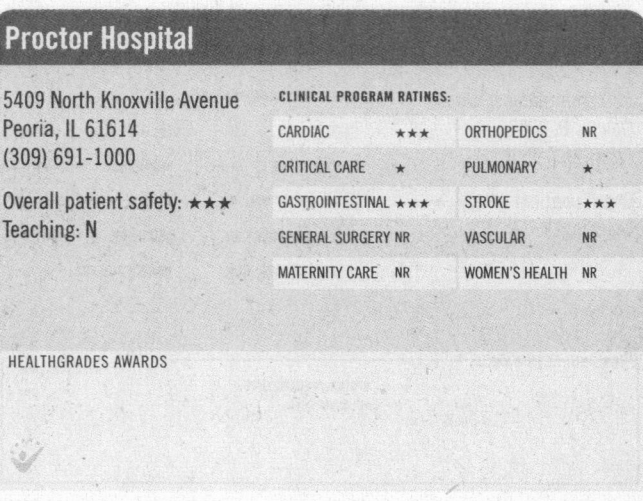

KEY: ★★★★★ BEST   ★★★ AS EXPECTED   ★ POOR   NR NOT RATED BY HEALTHGRADES   For full definitions of ratings and awards, see Appendix.

Provena Covenant Medical Center*

1400 West Parks Street
Urbana, IL 61801
(217) 337-2000

Overall patient safety: ★★★★★
Teaching: Y

CLINICAL PROGRAM RATINGS:

CARDIAC	★★★	ORTHOPEDICS	NR
CRITICAL CARE	★★★	PULMONARY	★★★
GASTROINTESTINAL	★★★	STROKE	★★★
GENERAL SURGERY	NR	VASCULAR	NR
MATERNITY CARE	NR	WOMEN'S HEALTH	NR

HEALTHGRADES AWARDS

✓ DISTINGUISHED
  HOSPITAL
  • PATIENT SAFETY

Provena St. Mary's Hospital

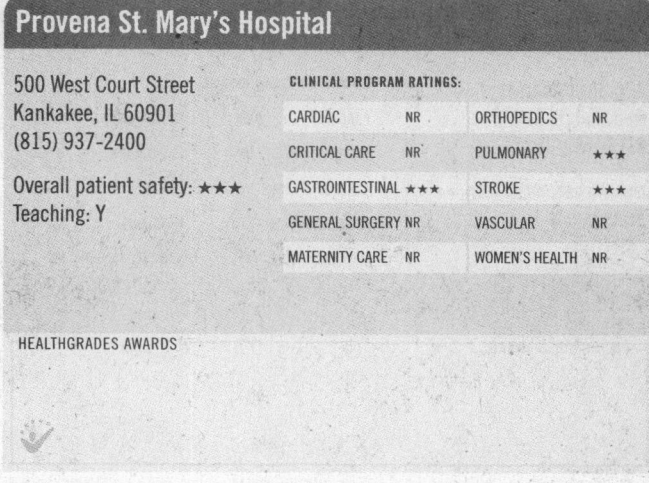

500 West Court Street
Kankakee, IL 60901
(815) 937-2400

Overall patient safety: ★★★
Teaching: Y

CLINICAL PROGRAM RATINGS:

CARDIAC	NR	ORTHOPEDICS	NR
CRITICAL CARE	NR	PULMONARY	★★★
GASTROINTESTINAL	★★★	STROKE	★★★
GENERAL SURGERY	NR	VASCULAR	NR
MATERNITY CARE	NR	WOMEN'S HEALTH	NR

HEALTHGRADES AWARDS

Provena Mercy Center

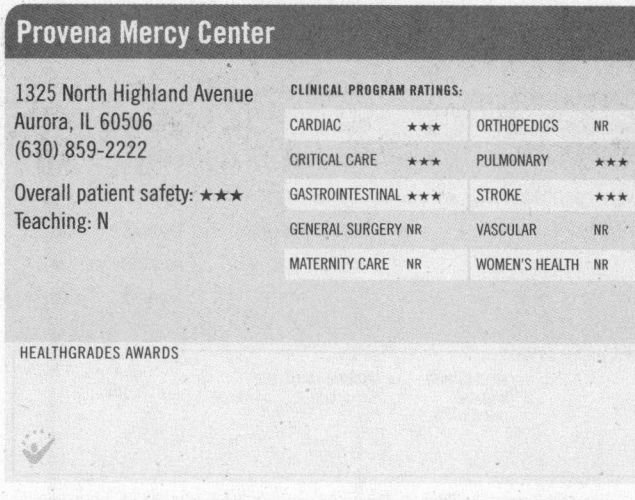

1325 North Highland Avenue
Aurora, IL 60506
(630) 859-2222

Overall patient safety: ★★★
Teaching: N

CLINICAL PROGRAM RATINGS:

CARDIAC	★★★	ORTHOPEDICS	NR
CRITICAL CARE	★★★	PULMONARY	★★★
GASTROINTESTINAL	★★★	STROKE	★★★
GENERAL SURGERY	NR	VASCULAR	NR
MATERNITY CARE	NR	WOMEN'S HEALTH	NR

HEALTHGRADES AWARDS

Provena United Samaritans Medical Center–Logan

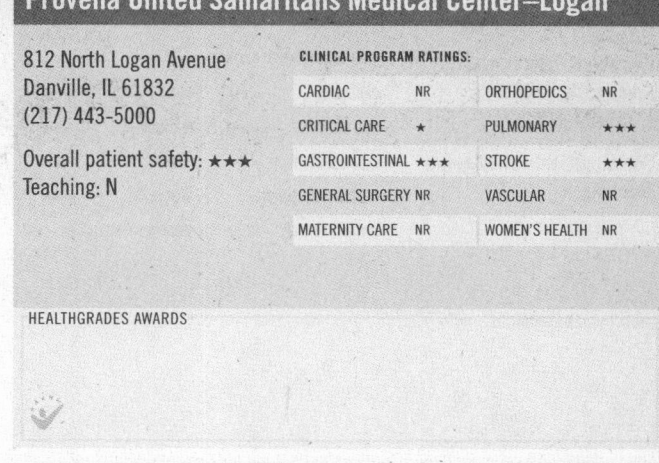

812 North Logan Avenue
Danville, IL 61832
(217) 443-5000

Overall patient safety: ★★★
Teaching: N

CLINICAL PROGRAM RATINGS:

CARDIAC	NR	ORTHOPEDICS	NR
CRITICAL CARE	★	PULMONARY	★★★
GASTROINTESTINAL	★★★	STROKE	★★★
GENERAL SURGERY	NR	VASCULAR	NR
MATERNITY CARE	NR	WOMEN'S HEALTH	NR

HEALTHGRADES AWARDS

Provena St. Joseph Medical Center

333 North Madison Street
Joliet, IL 60435
(815) 725-7133

Overall patient safety: ★★★
Teaching: N

CLINICAL PROGRAM RATINGS:

CARDIAC	★★★	ORTHOPEDICS	★★★
CRITICAL CARE	★★★	PULMONARY	★★★★★
GASTROINTESTINAL	★★★	STROKE	★★★
GENERAL SURGERY	NR	VASCULAR	★★★
MATERNITY CARE	NR	WOMEN'S HEALTH	NR

HEALTHGRADES AWARDS

✓ DISTINGUISHED   ✓ SPECIALTY EXCELLENCE
  HOSPITAL   • PULMONARY CARE
  • CLINICAL EXCELLENCE

Provident Hospital of Chicago

500 East 51st Street
Chicago, IL 60615
(312) 572-2000

Overall patient safety: ★★★
Teaching: Y

CLINICAL PROGRAM RATINGS:

CARDIAC	NR	ORTHOPEDICS	NR
CRITICAL CARE	NR	PULMONARY	★★★
GASTROINTESTINAL	NR	STROKE	NR
GENERAL SURGERY	NR	VASCULAR	NR
MATERNITY CARE	NR	WOMEN'S HEALTH	NR

HEALTHGRADES AWARDS

---

*This hospital reports its data to the federal government jointly with another hospital. Therefore the ratings and awards apply to multiple hospitals and this specific hospital may not provide all rated services.

Red Bud Regional Hospital

325 Spring Street
Red Bud, IL 62278
(618) 282-3831

Overall patient safety: ★★★
Teaching: N

CLINICAL PROGRAM RATINGS:

CARDIAC	NR	ORTHOPEDICS	NR
CRITICAL CARE	NR	PULMONARY	★★★
GASTROINTESTINAL	NR	STROKE	★★★
GENERAL SURGERY	NR	VASCULAR	NR
MATERNITY CARE	NR	WOMEN'S HEALTH	NR

HEALTHGRADES AWARDS

Richland Memorial Hospital

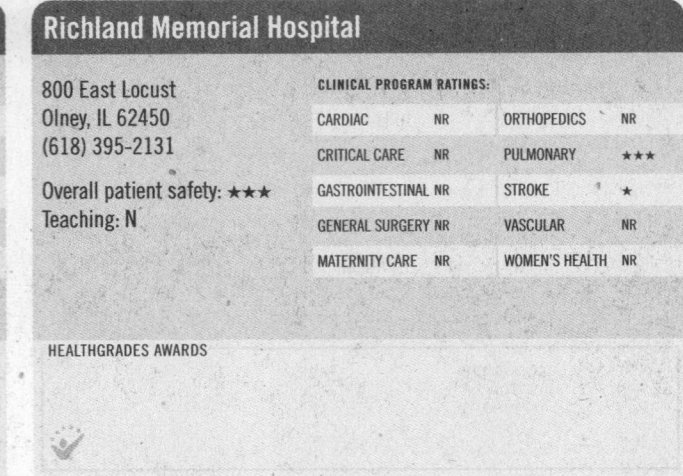

800 East Locust
Olney, IL 62450
(618) 395-2131

Overall patient safety: ★★★
Teaching: N

CLINICAL PROGRAM RATINGS:

CARDIAC	NR	ORTHOPEDICS	NR
CRITICAL CARE	NR	PULMONARY	★★★
GASTROINTESTINAL	NR	STROKE	★
GENERAL SURGERY	NR	VASCULAR	NR
MATERNITY CARE	NR	WOMEN'S HEALTH	NR

HEALTHGRADES AWARDS

Resurrection Medical Center

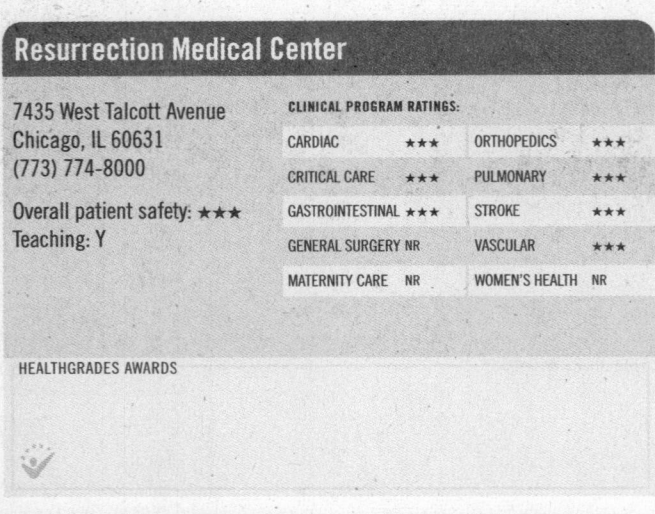

7435 West Talcott Avenue
Chicago, IL 60631
(773) 774-8000

Overall patient safety: ★★★
Teaching: Y

CLINICAL PROGRAM RATINGS:

CARDIAC	★★★	ORTHOPEDICS	★★★
CRITICAL CARE	★★★	PULMONARY	★★★
GASTROINTESTINAL	★★★	STROKE	★★★
GENERAL SURGERY	NR	VASCULAR	★★★
MATERNITY CARE	NR	WOMEN'S HEALTH	NR

HEALTHGRADES AWARDS

Riverside Medical Center

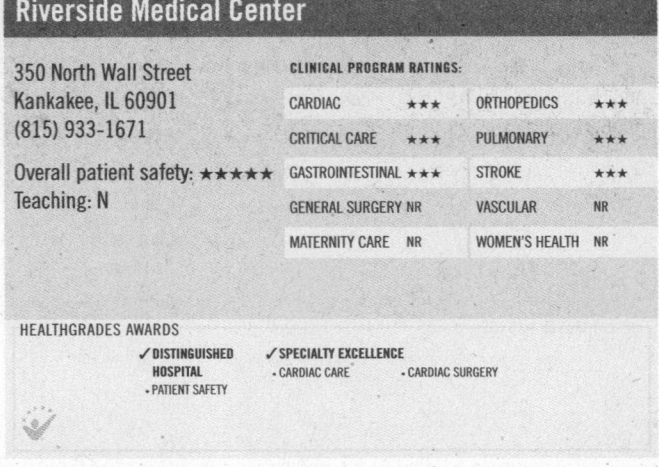

350 North Wall Street
Kankakee, IL 60901
(815) 933-1671

Overall patient safety: ★★★★★
Teaching: N

CLINICAL PROGRAM RATINGS:

CARDIAC	★★★	ORTHOPEDICS	★★★
CRITICAL CARE	★★★	PULMONARY	★★★
GASTROINTESTINAL	★★★	STROKE	★★★
GENERAL SURGERY	NR	VASCULAR	NR
MATERNITY CARE	NR	WOMEN'S HEALTH	NR

HEALTHGRADES AWARDS

✓ DISTINGUISHED HOSPITAL
- PATIENT SAFETY

✓ SPECIALTY EXCELLENCE
- CARDIAC CARE
- CARDIAC SURGERY

RHC St. Francis Hospital

355 Ridge Avenue
Evanston, IL 60202
(847) 316-4000

Overall patient safety: ★★★
Teaching: Y

CLINICAL PROGRAM RATINGS:

CARDIAC	★★★	ORTHOPEDICS	★★★
CRITICAL CARE	★★★	PULMONARY	★★★★★
GASTROINTESTINAL	★★★	STROKE	★★★
GENERAL SURGERY	NR	VASCULAR	NR
MATERNITY CARE	NR	WOMEN'S HEALTH	NR

HEALTHGRADES AWARDS

✓ SPECIALTY EXCELLENCE
- GASTROINTESTINAL CARE
- PULMONARY CARE

Rochelle Community Hospital

900 North 2nd Street
Rochelle, IL 61068
(815) 562-2181

Overall patient safety: ★★★
Teaching: N

CLINICAL PROGRAM RATINGS:

CARDIAC	NR	ORTHOPEDICS	NR
CRITICAL CARE	NR	PULMONARY	★★★
GASTROINTESTINAL	NR	STROKE	★★★
GENERAL SURGERY	NR	VASCULAR	NR
MATERNITY CARE	NR	WOMEN'S HEALTH	NR

HEALTHGRADES AWARDS

KEY: ★★★★★ BEST   ★★★ AS EXPECTED   ★ POOR   NR NOT RATED BY HEALTHGRADES   For full definitions of ratings and awards, see Appendix.

Rockford Memorial Hospital

2400 North Rockton Avenue
Rockford, IL 61103
(815) 971-5000

Overall patient safety: ★★★★★
Teaching: N

CLINICAL PROGRAM RATINGS:

CARDIAC	★★★	ORTHOPEDICS	★★★
CRITICAL CARE	★★★	PULMONARY	★★★
GASTROINTESTINAL	★★★	STROKE	★★★
GENERAL SURGERY	NR	VASCULAR	★★★
MATERNITY CARE	NR	WOMEN'S HEALTH	NR

HEALTHGRADES AWARDS

✓ DISTINGUISHED
   HOSPITAL
 • PATIENT SAFETY

Rush North Shore Medical Center

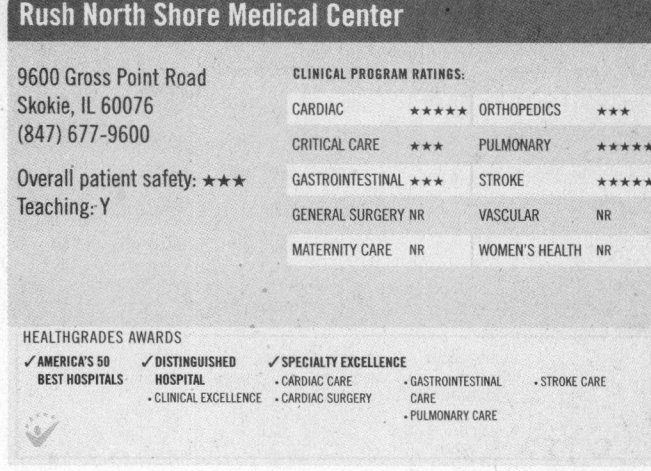

9600 Gross Point Road
Skokie, IL 60076
(847) 677-9600

Overall patient safety: ★★★
Teaching: Y

CLINICAL PROGRAM RATINGS:

CARDIAC	★★★★★	ORTHOPEDICS	★★★
CRITICAL CARE	★★★	PULMONARY	★★★★★
GASTROINTESTINAL	★★★	STROKE	★★★★★
GENERAL SURGERY	NR	VASCULAR	NR
MATERNITY CARE	NR	WOMEN'S HEALTH	NR

HEALTHGRADES AWARDS

✓ AMERICA'S 50   ✓ DISTINGUISHED   ✓ SPECIALTY EXCELLENCE
  BEST HOSPITALS   HOSPITAL   • CARDIAC CARE   • GASTROINTESTINAL   • STROKE CARE
                  • CLINICAL EXCELLENCE   • CARDIAC SURGERY   CARE
                                                        • PULMONARY CARE

Roseland Community Hospital

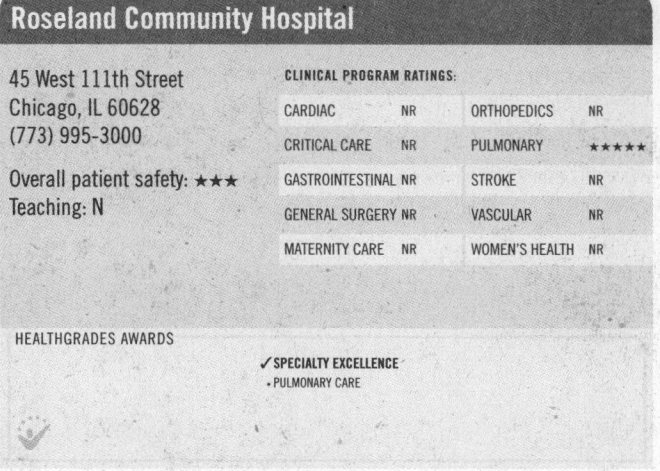

45 West 111th Street
Chicago, IL 60628
(773) 995-3000

Overall patient safety: ★★★
Teaching: N

CLINICAL PROGRAM RATINGS:

CARDIAC	NR	ORTHOPEDICS	NR
CRITICAL CARE	NR	PULMONARY	★★★★★
GASTROINTESTINAL	NR	STROKE	NR
GENERAL SURGERY	NR	VASCULAR	NR
MATERNITY CARE	NR	WOMEN'S HEALTH	NR

HEALTHGRADES AWARDS

✓ SPECIALTY EXCELLENCE
 • PULMONARY CARE

Rush University Medical Center

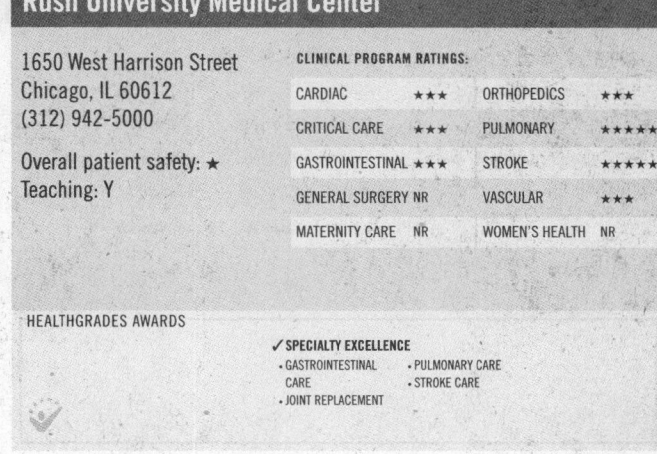

1650 West Harrison Street
Chicago, IL 60612
(312) 942-5000

Overall patient safety: ★
Teaching: Y

CLINICAL PROGRAM RATINGS:

CARDIAC	★★★	ORTHOPEDICS	★★★
CRITICAL CARE	★★★	PULMONARY	★★★★★
GASTROINTESTINAL	★★★	STROKE	★★★★★
GENERAL SURGERY	NR	VASCULAR	★★★
MATERNITY CARE	NR	WOMEN'S HEALTH	NR

HEALTHGRADES AWARDS

✓ SPECIALTY EXCELLENCE
 • GASTROINTESTINAL   • PULMONARY CARE
   CARE   • STROKE CARE
 • JOINT REPLACEMENT

Rush Copley Memorial Hospital

2000 Ogden Avenue
Aurora, IL 60504
(630) 978-6200

Overall patient safety: ★★★
Teaching: Y

CLINICAL PROGRAM RATINGS:

CARDIAC	★★★	ORTHOPEDICS	★★★
CRITICAL CARE	★★★	PULMONARY	★★★
GASTROINTESTINAL	★★★	STROKE	★★★
GENERAL SURGERY	NR	VASCULAR	NR
MATERNITY CARE	NR	WOMEN'S HEALTH	NR

HEALTHGRADES AWARDS

Sacred Heart Hospital

3240 West Franklin Boulevard
Chicago, IL 60624
(773) 722-3020

Overall patient safety: ★★★★★
Teaching: Y

CLINICAL PROGRAM RATINGS:

CARDIAC	NR	ORTHOPEDICS	NR
CRITICAL CARE	NR	PULMONARY	★★★
GASTROINTESTINAL	NR	STROKE	NR
GENERAL SURGERY	NR	VASCULAR	NR
MATERNITY CARE	NR	WOMEN'S HEALTH	NR

HEALTHGRADES AWARDS

ILLINOIS HOSPITALS: RATINGS BY CLINICAL SPECIALTY

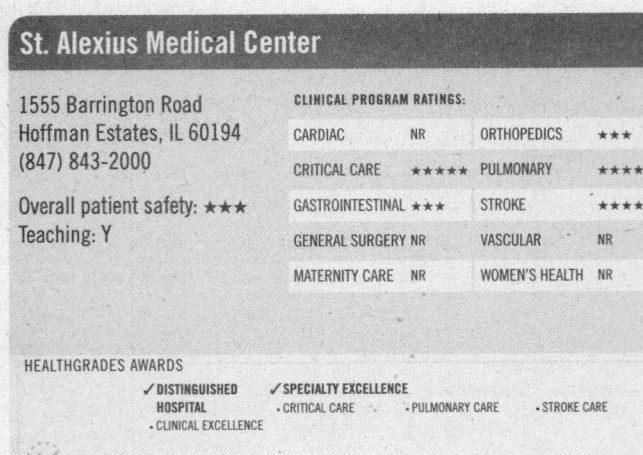

St. Alexius Medical Center

1555 Barrington Road
Hoffman Estates, IL 60194
(847) 843-2000

Overall patient safety: ★★★
Teaching: Y

CLINICAL PROGRAM RATINGS:

CARDIAC	NR	ORTHOPEDICS	★★★
CRITICAL CARE	★★★★★	PULMONARY	★★★★★
GASTROINTESTINAL	★★★	STROKE	★★★★★
GENERAL SURGERY	NR	VASCULAR	NR
MATERNITY CARE	NR	WOMEN'S HEALTH	NR

HEALTHGRADES AWARDS

✓ DISTINGUISHED HOSPITAL
- CLINICAL EXCELLENCE

✓ SPECIALTY EXCELLENCE
- CRITICAL CARE
- PULMONARY CARE
- STROKE CARE

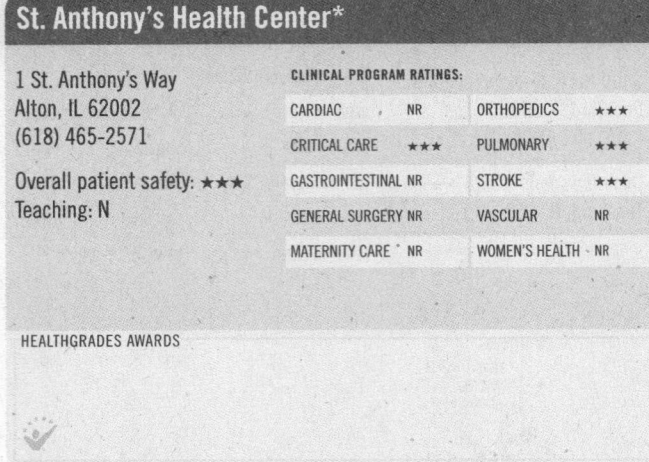

St. Anthony's Health Center*

1 St. Anthony's Way
Alton, IL 62002
(618) 465-2571

Overall patient safety: ★★★
Teaching: N

CLINICAL PROGRAM RATINGS:

CARDIAC	NR	ORTHOPEDICS	★★★
CRITICAL CARE	★★★	PULMONARY	★★★
GASTROINTESTINAL	NR	STROKE	★★★
GENERAL SURGERY	NR	VASCULAR	NR
MATERNITY CARE	NR	WOMEN'S HEALTH	NR

HEALTHGRADES AWARDS

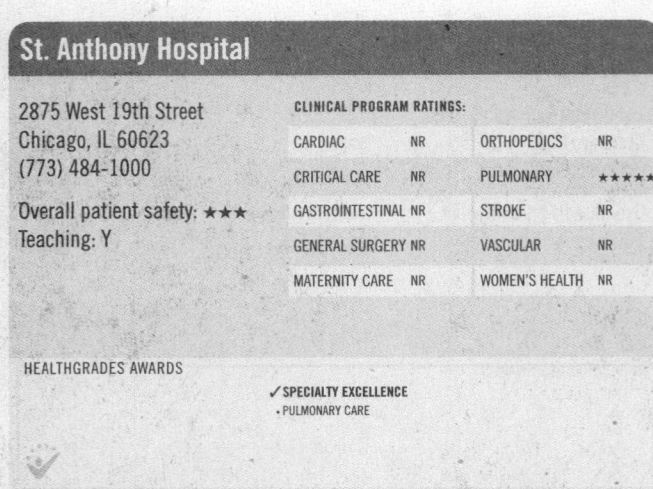

St. Anthony Hospital

2875 West 19th Street
Chicago, IL 60623
(773) 484-1000

Overall patient safety: ★★★
Teaching: Y

CLINICAL PROGRAM RATINGS:

CARDIAC	NR	ORTHOPEDICS	NR
CRITICAL CARE	NR	PULMONARY	★★★★★
GASTROINTESTINAL	NR	STROKE	NR
GENERAL SURGERY	NR	VASCULAR	NR
MATERNITY CARE	NR	WOMEN'S HEALTH	NR

HEALTHGRADES AWARDS

✓ SPECIALTY EXCELLENCE
- PULMONARY CARE

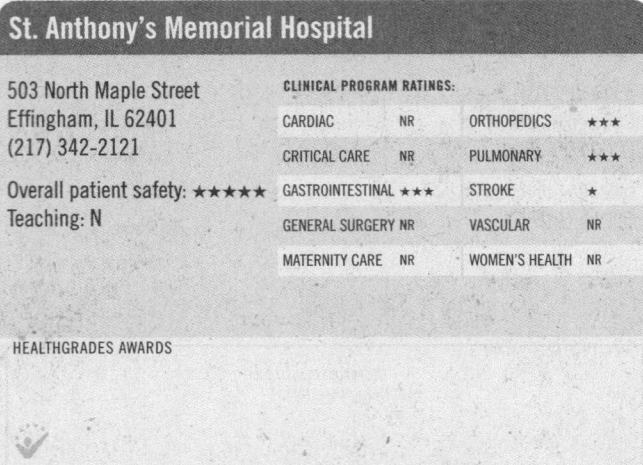

St. Anthony's Memorial Hospital

503 North Maple Street
Effingham, IL 62401
(217) 342-2121

Overall patient safety: ★★★★★
Teaching: N

CLINICAL PROGRAM RATINGS:

CARDIAC	NR	ORTHOPEDICS	★★★
CRITICAL CARE	NR	PULMONARY	★★★
GASTROINTESTINAL	★★★	STROKE	★
GENERAL SURGERY	NR	VASCULAR	NR
MATERNITY CARE	NR	WOMEN'S HEALTH	NR

HEALTHGRADES AWARDS

St. Anthony Medical Center

5666 East State Street
Rockford, IL 61108
(815) 226-2000

Overall patient safety: ★★★
Teaching: N

CLINICAL PROGRAM RATINGS:

CARDIAC	★★★	ORTHOPEDICS	★★★
CRITICAL CARE	★★★	PULMONARY	★★★★★
GASTROINTESTINAL	★★★	STROKE	★★★★★
GENERAL SURGERY	NR	VASCULAR	NR
MATERNITY CARE	NR	WOMEN'S HEALTH	NR

HEALTHGRADES AWARDS

✓ SPECIALTY EXCELLENCE
- STROKE CARE

St. Bernard Hospital

326 West 64th
Chicago, IL 60621
(773) 962-3900

Overall patient safety: ★
Teaching: Y

CLINICAL PROGRAM RATINGS:

CARDIAC	NR	ORTHOPEDICS	NR
CRITICAL CARE	NR	PULMONARY	★★★★★
GASTROINTESTINAL	NR	STROKE	NR
GENERAL SURGERY	NR	VASCULAR	NR
MATERNITY CARE	NR	WOMEN'S HEALTH	NR

HEALTHGRADES AWARDS

✓ SPECIALTY EXCELLENCE
- PULMONARY CARE

KEY: ★★★★★ BEST   ★★★ AS EXPECTED   ★ POOR   NR NOT RATED BY HEALTHGRADES   For full definitions of ratings and awards, see Appendix.

St. Elizabeth Hospital

211 South 3rd Street
Belleville, IL 62220
(618) 234-2120

Overall patient safety: ★★★
Teaching: Y

CLINICAL PROGRAM RATINGS:

CARDIAC	★★★	ORTHOPEDICS	NR
CRITICAL CARE	★★★	PULMONARY	★★★
GASTROINTESTINAL	★★★	STROKE	★★★
GENERAL SURGERY	NR	VASCULAR	NR
MATERNITY CARE	NR	WOMEN'S HEALTH	NR

HEALTHGRADES AWARDS

Saint Francis Medical Center

530 Northeast Glen
Oak Avenue
Peoria, IL 61637
(309) 655-2000

Overall patient safety: ★★★
Teaching: Y

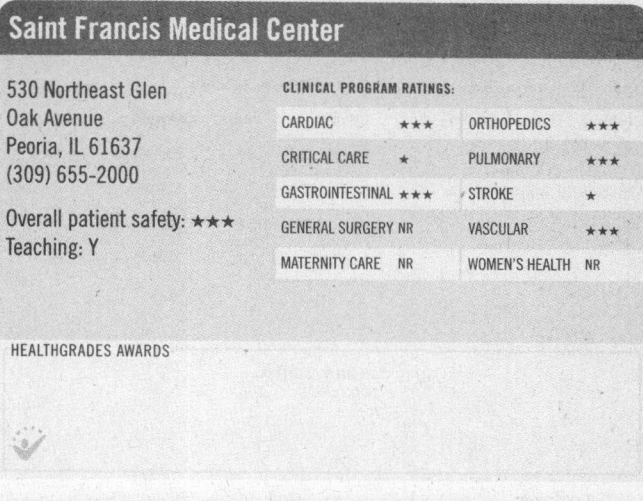

CLINICAL PROGRAM RATINGS:

CARDIAC	★★★	ORTHOPEDICS	★★★
CRITICAL CARE	★	PULMONARY	★★★
GASTROINTESTINAL	★★★	STROKE	★
GENERAL SURGERY	NR	VASCULAR	★★★
MATERNITY CARE	NR	WOMEN'S HEALTH	NR

HEALTHGRADES AWARDS

St. Francis Hospital

1215 Union Avenue
Litchfield, IL 62056
(217) 324-2191

Overall patient safety: ★★★
Teaching: N

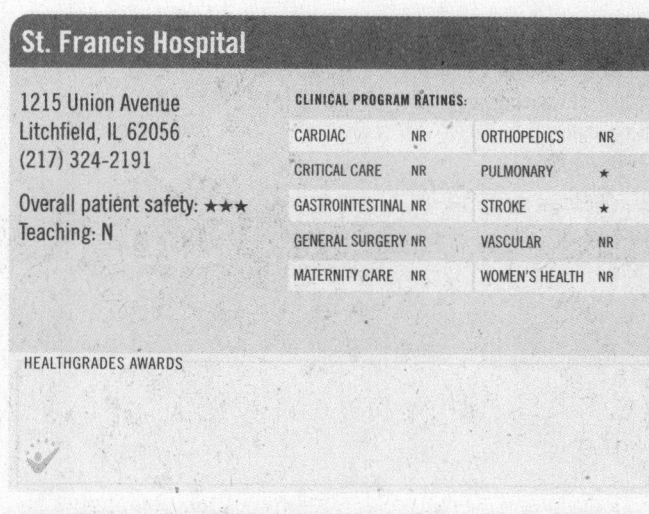

CLINICAL PROGRAM RATINGS:

CARDIAC	NR	ORTHOPEDICS	NR
CRITICAL CARE	NR	PULMONARY	★
GASTROINTESTINAL	NR	STROKE	★
GENERAL SURGERY	NR	VASCULAR	NR
MATERNITY CARE	NR	WOMEN'S HEALTH	NR

HEALTHGRADES AWARDS

Saint James Hospital

2500 West Reynolds Street
Pontiac, IL 61764
(815) 842-2828

Overall patient safety: ★★★
Teaching: N

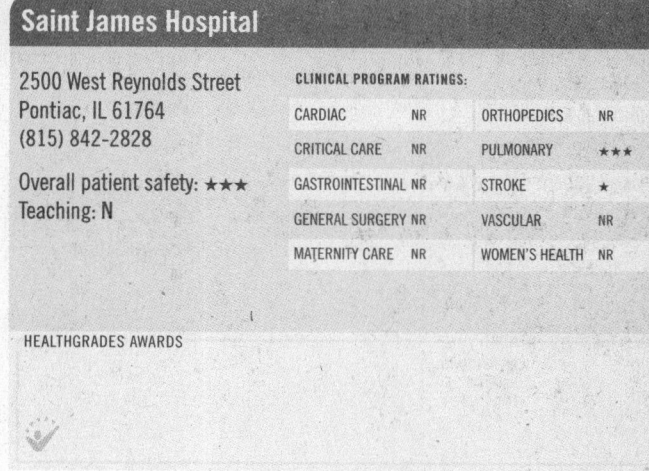

CLINICAL PROGRAM RATINGS:

CARDIAC	NR	ORTHOPEDICS	NR
CRITICAL CARE	NR	PULMONARY	★★★
GASTROINTESTINAL	NR	STROKE	★
GENERAL SURGERY	NR	VASCULAR	NR
MATERNITY CARE	NR	WOMEN'S HEALTH	NR

HEALTHGRADES AWARDS

St. Francis Hospital and Health Center

12935 South Gregory Street
Blue Island, IL 60406
(708) 597-2000

Overall patient safety: ★★★★★
Teaching: Y

CLINICAL PROGRAM RATINGS:

CARDIAC	★★★	ORTHOPEDICS	NR
CRITICAL CARE	★★★	PULMONARY	★★★★★
GASTROINTESTINAL	★★★	STROKE	★★★
GENERAL SURGERY	NR	VASCULAR	★★★
MATERNITY CARE	NR	WOMEN'S HEALTH	NR

HEALTHGRADES AWARDS

✓DISTINGUISHED HOSPITAL
· PATIENT SAFETY

✓SPECIALTY EXCELLENCE
· PULMONARY CARE

St. James Hospital and Health Center*

1423 Chicago Road
Chicago Heights, IL 60411
(708) 756-1000

Overall patient safety: ★
Teaching: Y

CLINICAL PROGRAM RATINGS:

CARDIAC	★★★	ORTHOPEDICS	★★★
CRITICAL CARE	★★★	PULMONARY	★★★
GASTROINTESTINAL	★★★	STROKE	★★★★★
GENERAL SURGERY	NR	VASCULAR	NR
MATERNITY CARE	NR	WOMEN'S HEALTH	NR

HEALTHGRADES AWARDS

✓SPECIALTY EXCELLENCE
· STROKE CARE

*This hospital reports its data to the federal government jointly with another hospital. Therefore the ratings and awards apply to multiple hospitals and this specific hospital may not provide all rated services.

St. James Hospital and Health Center—Olympia Fields*

20201 South Crawford Avenue
Olympia Fields, IL 60461
(708) 747-4000

Overall patient safety: ★
Teaching: Y

CLINICAL PROGRAM RATINGS:

CARDIAC	★★★	ORTHOPEDICS	★★★
CRITICAL CARE	★★★	PULMONARY	★★★
GASTROINTESTINAL	★★★	STROKE	★★★★★
GENERAL SURGERY	NR	VASCULAR	NR
MATERNITY CARE	NR	WOMEN'S HEALTH	NR

HEALTHGRADES AWARDS

✓ SPECIALTY EXCELLENCE
- STROKE CARE

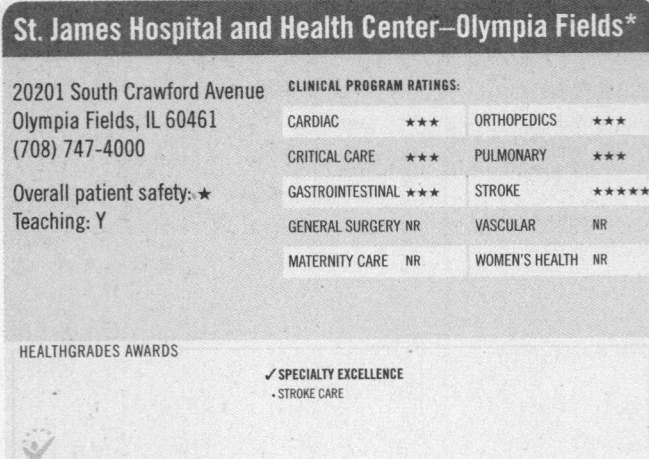

St. Joseph Hospital

77 North Airlite Street
Elgin, IL 60123
(847) 695-3200

Overall patient safety: ★★★
Teaching: N

CLINICAL PROGRAM RATINGS:

CARDIAC	★★★	ORTHOPEDICS	NR
CRITICAL CARE	NR	PULMONARY	★★★
GASTROINTESTINAL	NR	STROKE	★★★★★
GENERAL SURGERY	NR	VASCULAR	NR
MATERNITY CARE	NR	WOMEN'S HEALTH	NR

HEALTHGRADES AWARDS

✓ SPECIALTY EXCELLENCE
- CARDIAC SURGERY   - STROKE CARE

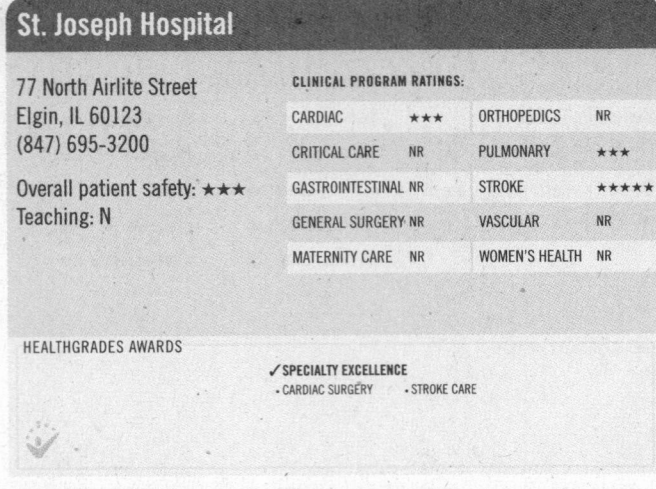

St. John's Hospital

800 East Carpenter
Springfield, IL 62769
(217) 544-6464

Overall patient safety: ★★★★★
Teaching: Y

CLINICAL PROGRAM RATINGS:

CARDIAC	★★★	ORTHOPEDICS	★★★
CRITICAL CARE	★★★	PULMONARY	★
GASTROINTESTINAL	★★★	STROKE	★★★
GENERAL SURGERY	NR	VASCULAR	★★★
MATERNITY CARE	NR	WOMEN'S HEALTH	NR

HEALTHGRADES AWARDS

✓ DISTINGUISHED
  HOSPITAL
- PATIENT SAFETY

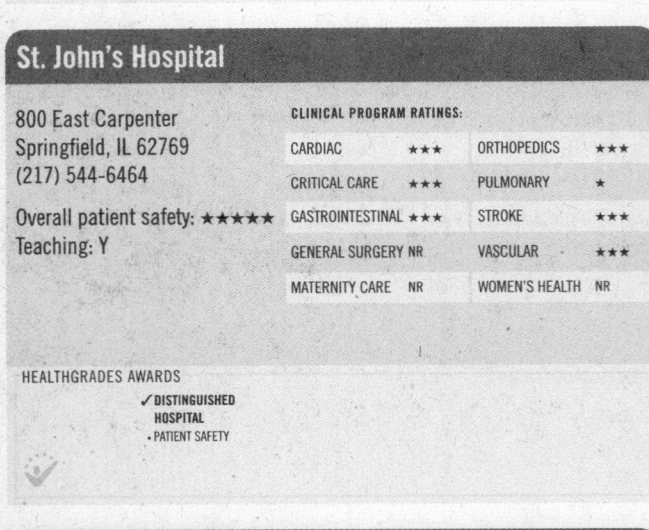

St. Joseph Medical Center

2200 East Washington Street
Bloomington, IL 61701
(309) 662-3311

Overall patient safety: ★★★
Teaching: N

CLINICAL PROGRAM RATINGS:

CARDIAC	★★★	ORTHOPEDICS	★★★
CRITICAL CARE	NR	PULMONARY	★★★
GASTROINTESTINAL	★★★	STROKE	★★★
GENERAL SURGERY	NR	VASCULAR	NR
MATERNITY CARE	NR	WOMEN'S HEALTH	NR

HEALTHGRADES AWARDS

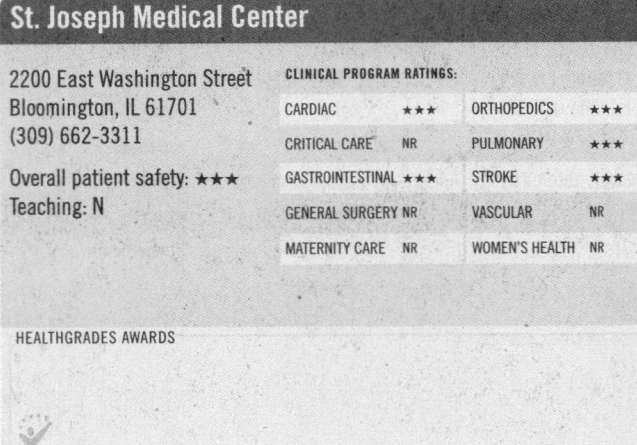

St. Joseph Hospital

2900 North Lake Shore Drive
Chicago, IL 60657
(773) 665-3000

Overall patient safety: ★★★★★
Teaching: Y

CLINICAL PROGRAM RATINGS:

CARDIAC	★★★★★	ORTHOPEDICS	★★★
CRITICAL CARE	★★★★★	PULMONARY	★★★★★
GASTROINTESTINAL	★★★	STROKE	★★★★★
GENERAL SURGERY	NR	VASCULAR	NR
MATERNITY CARE	NR	WOMEN'S HEALTH	NR

HEALTHGRADES AWARDS

✓ DISTINGUISHED   ✓ SPECIALTY EXCELLENCE
  HOSPITAL   - CARDIAC CARE   - PULMONARY CARE
- CLINICAL EXCELLENCE   - CRITICAL CARE   - STROKE CARE
- PATIENT SAFETY

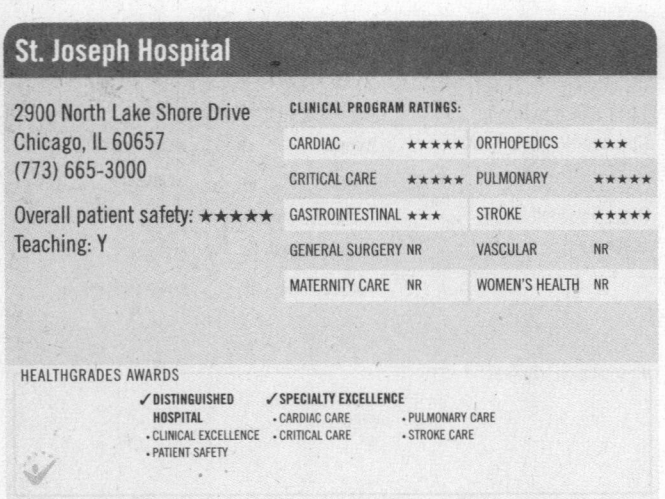

St. Joseph Memorial Hospital

2 South Hospital Drive
Murphysboro, IL 62966
(618) 684-3156

Overall patient safety: ★★★
Teaching: N

CLINICAL PROGRAM RATINGS:

CARDIAC	NR	ORTHOPEDICS	NR
CRITICAL CARE	NR	PULMONARY	★
GASTROINTESTINAL	NR	STROKE	★
GENERAL SURGERY	NR	VASCULAR	NR
MATERNITY CARE	NR	WOMEN'S HEALTH	NR

HEALTHGRADES AWARDS

KEY: ★★★★★ BEST   ★★★ AS EXPECTED   ★ POOR   NR NOT RATED BY HEALTHGRADES   For full definitions of ratings and awards, see Appendix.

St. Joseph's Hospital*

915 East 5th Street
Alton, IL 62002
(618) 463-5151

Overall patient safety: ★★★
Teaching: N

CLINICAL PROGRAM RATINGS:

CARDIAC	NR	ORTHOPEDICS	★★★
CRITICAL CARE	★★★	PULMONARY	★★★
GASTROINTESTINAL	NR	STROKE	★★★
GENERAL SURGERY	NR	VASCULAR	NR
MATERNITY CARE	NR	WOMEN'S HEALTH	NR

HEALTHGRADES AWARDS

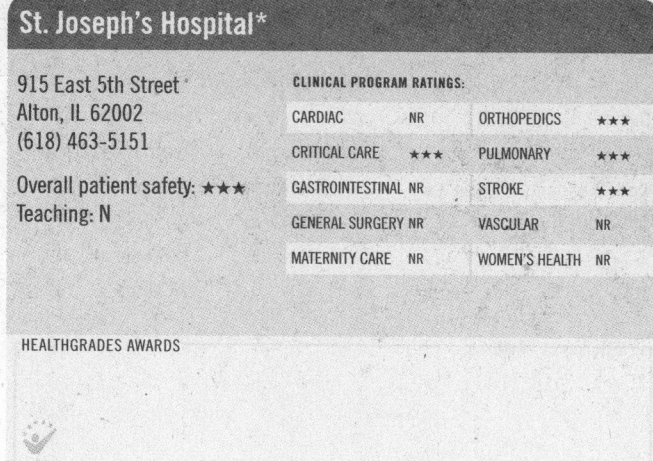

St. Margaret's Hospital

600 East 1st Street
Spring Valley, IL 61362
(815) 664-5311

Overall patient safety: ★★★
Teaching: N

CLINICAL PROGRAM RATINGS:

CARDIAC	NR	ORTHOPEDICS	NR
CRITICAL CARE	NR	PULMONARY	★★★
GASTROINTESTINAL	NR	STROKE	★★★★★
GENERAL SURGERY	NR	VASCULAR	NR
MATERNITY CARE	NR	WOMEN'S HEALTH	NR

HEALTHGRADES AWARDS

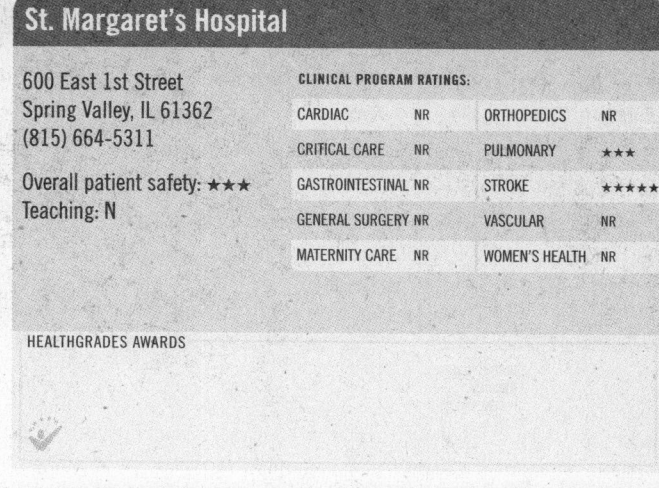

St. Joseph's Hospital

1915 Holy Cross Lane
Breese, IL 62230
(618) 526-4511

Overall patient safety: ★★★
Teaching: N

CLINICAL PROGRAM RATINGS:

CARDIAC	NR	ORTHOPEDICS	NR
CRITICAL CARE	NR	PULMONARY	★★★
GASTROINTESTINAL	NR	STROKE	★
GENERAL SURGERY	NR	VASCULAR	NR
MATERNITY CARE	NR	WOMEN'S HEALTH	NR

HEALTHGRADES AWARDS

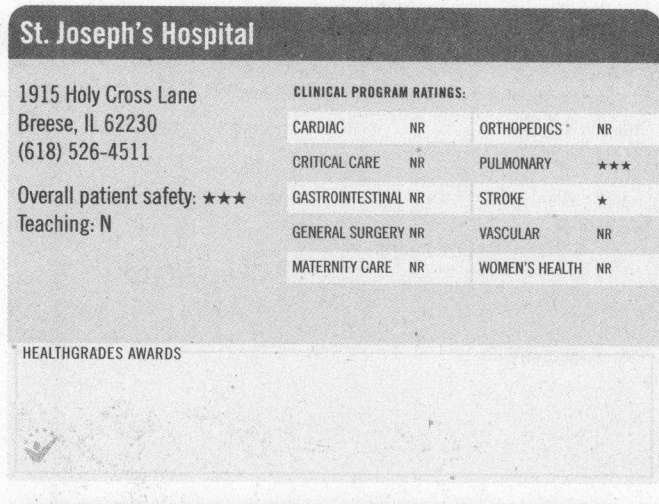

St. Mary and Elizabeth Medical Center—Claremont

1431 North Claremont Avenue
Chicago, IL 60622
(773) 278-2000

Overall patient safety: ★★★
Teaching: Y

CLINICAL PROGRAM RATINGS:

CARDIAC	NR	ORTHOPEDICS	NR
CRITICAL CARE	NR	PULMONARY	★★★
GASTROINTESTINAL	NR	STROKE	★★★★★
GENERAL SURGERY	NR	VASCULAR	NR
MATERNITY CARE	NR	WOMEN'S HEALTH	NR

HEALTHGRADES AWARDS

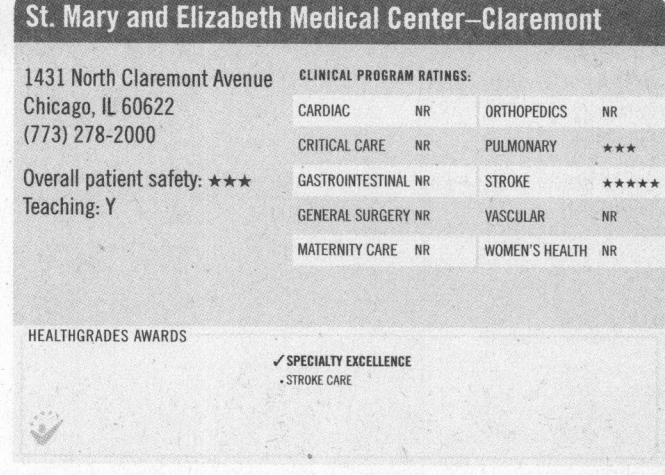

✓ **SPECIALTY EXCELLENCE**
• STROKE CARE

St. Joseph's Hospital

1515 Main Street
Highland, IL 62249
(618) 654-7421

Overall patient safety: ★★★
Teaching: N

CLINICAL PROGRAM RATINGS:

CARDIAC	NR	ORTHOPEDICS	NR
CRITICAL CARE	NR	PULMONARY	★
GASTROINTESTINAL	NR	STROKE	★
GENERAL SURGERY	NR	VASCULAR	NR
MATERNITY CARE	NR	WOMEN'S HEALTH	NR

HEALTHGRADES AWARDS

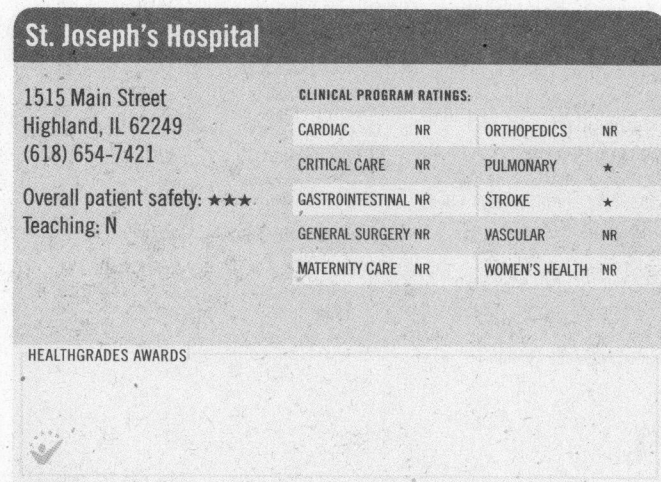

St. Mary and Elizabeth Medical Center—Division

2233 West Division Street
Chicago, IL 60622
(312) 770-2000

Overall patient safety: ★★★
Teaching: Y

CLINICAL PROGRAM RATINGS:

CARDIAC	★★★	ORTHOPEDICS	NR
CRITICAL CARE	NR	PULMONARY	★★★★★
GASTROINTESTINAL	★★★	STROKE	★★★
GENERAL SURGERY	NR	VASCULAR	NR
MATERNITY CARE	NR	WOMEN'S HEALTH	NR

HEALTHGRADES AWARDS

✓ **SPECIALTY EXCELLENCE**
• PULMONARY CARE

*This hospital reports its data to the federal government jointly with another hospital. Therefore the ratings and awards apply to multiple hospitals and this specific hospital may not provide all rated services.

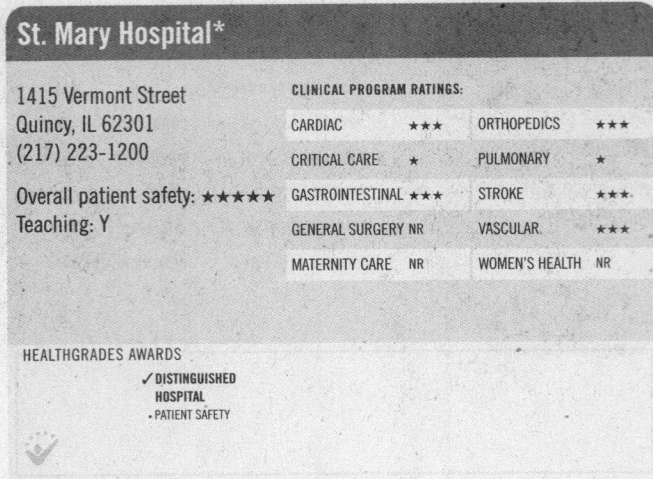

St. Mary Hospital*

1415 Vermont Street
Quincy, IL 62301
(217) 223-1200

Overall patient safety: ★★★★★
Teaching: Y

CLINICAL PROGRAM RATINGS:

CARDIAC	★★★	ORTHOPEDICS	★★★
CRITICAL CARE	★	PULMONARY	★
GASTROINTESTINAL	★★★	STROKE	★★★
GENERAL SURGERY	NR	VASCULAR	★★★
MATERNITY CARE	NR	WOMEN'S HEALTH	NR

HEALTHGRADES AWARDS

✓ DISTINGUISHED
HOSPITAL
- PATIENT SAFETY

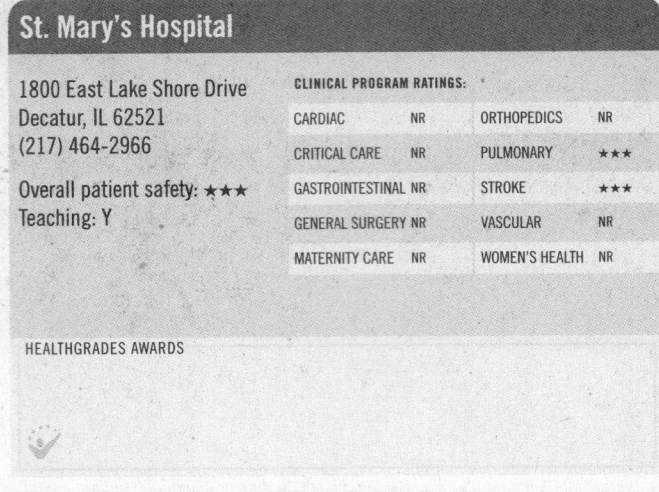

St. Mary's Hospital

1800 East Lake Shore Drive
Decatur, IL 62521
(217) 464-2966

Overall patient safety: ★★★
Teaching: Y

CLINICAL PROGRAM RATINGS:

CARDIAC	NR	ORTHOPEDICS	NR
CRITICAL CARE	NR	PULMONARY	★★★
GASTROINTESTINAL	NR	STROKE	★★★
GENERAL SURGERY	NR	VASCULAR	NR
MATERNITY CARE	NR	WOMEN'S HEALTH	NR

HEALTHGRADES AWARDS

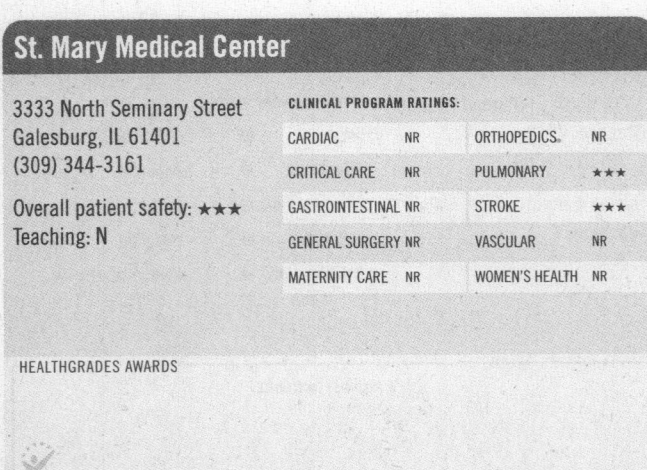

St. Mary Medical Center

3333 North Seminary Street
Galesburg, IL 61401
(309) 344-3161

Overall patient safety: ★★★
Teaching: N

CLINICAL PROGRAM RATINGS:

CARDIAC	NR	ORTHOPEDICS	NR
CRITICAL CARE	NR	PULMONARY	★★★
GASTROINTESTINAL	NR	STROKE	★★★
GENERAL SURGERY	NR	VASCULAR	NR
MATERNITY CARE	NR	WOMEN'S HEALTH	NR

HEALTHGRADES AWARDS

St. Mary's Hospital

111 Spring Street
Streator, IL 61364
(815) 673-2311

Overall patient safety: ★★★
Teaching: N

CLINICAL PROGRAM RATINGS:

CARDIAC	NR	ORTHOPEDICS	NR
CRITICAL CARE	NR	PULMONARY	★★★
GASTROINTESTINAL	NR	STROKE	★
GENERAL SURGERY	NR	VASCULAR	NR
MATERNITY CARE	NR	WOMEN'S HEALTH	NR

HEALTHGRADES AWARDS

St. Mary's Hospital

400 North Pleasant Avenue
Centralia, IL 62801
(618) 436-8000

Overall patient safety: ★★★
Teaching: N

CLINICAL PROGRAM RATINGS:

CARDIAC	NR	ORTHOPEDICS	NR
CRITICAL CARE	NR	PULMONARY	★★★
GASTROINTESTINAL	★★★	STROKE	★★★
GENERAL SURGERY	NR	VASCULAR	NR
MATERNITY CARE	NR	WOMEN'S HEALTH	NR

HEALTHGRADES AWARDS

Salem Township Hospital

1201 Ricker Drive
Salem, IL 62881
(618) 548-3194

Overall patient safety: ★★★
Teaching: N

CLINICAL PROGRAM RATINGS:

CARDIAC	NR	ORTHOPEDICS	NR
CRITICAL CARE	NR	PULMONARY	★★★
GASTROINTESTINAL	NR	STROKE	NR
GENERAL SURGERY	NR	VASCULAR	NR
MATERNITY CARE	NR	WOMEN'S HEALTH	NR

HEALTHGRADES AWARDS

ILLINOIS HOSPITALS: RATINGS BY CLINICAL SPECIALTY

Sarah Bush Lincoln Health Center

1000 Health Center Drive
Mattoon, IL 61938
(217) 258-2525

Overall patient safety: ★★★
Teaching: N

CLINICAL PROGRAM RATINGS:

CARDIAC	NR	ORTHOPEDICS	★★★
CRITICAL CARE	NR	PULMONARY	★★★
GASTROINTESTINAL	★★★	STROKE	★★★
GENERAL SURGERY	NR	VASCULAR	NR
MATERNITY CARE	NR	WOMEN'S HEALTH	NR

HEALTHGRADES AWARDS

✓ SPECIALTY EXCELLENCE
• JOINT REPLACEMENT

Sherman Hospital

934 Center Street
Elgin, IL 60120
(847) 742-9800

Overall patient safety: ★★★
Teaching: N

CLINICAL PROGRAM RATINGS:

CARDIAC	★★★	ORTHOPEDICS	NR
CRITICAL CARE	★★★	PULMONARY	★★★★★
GASTROINTESTINAL	★★★	STROKE	★★★
GENERAL SURGERY	NR	VASCULAR	NR
MATERNITY CARE	NR	WOMEN'S HEALTH	NR

HEALTHGRADES AWARDS

✓ SPECIALTY EXCELLENCE
• PULMONARY CARE

Sarah D. Culbertson Memorial Hospital

238 South Congress Street
Rushville, IL 62681
(217) 322-4321

Overall patient safety: ★★★
Teaching: N

CLINICAL PROGRAM RATINGS:

CARDIAC	NR	ORTHOPEDICS	NR
CRITICAL CARE	NR	PULMONARY	★★★
GASTROINTESTINAL	NR	STROKE	NR
GENERAL SURGERY	NR	VASCULAR	NR
MATERNITY CARE	NR	WOMEN'S HEALTH	NR

HEALTHGRADES AWARDS

Silver Cross Hospital

1200 Maple Road
Joliet, IL 60432
(815) 740-1100

Overall patient safety: ★★★
Teaching: N

CLINICAL PROGRAM RATINGS:

CARDIAC	NR	ORTHOPEDICS	NR
CRITICAL CARE	★★★	PULMONARY	★★★
GASTROINTESTINAL	★★★	STROKE	★★★
GENERAL SURGERY	NR	VASCULAR	NR
MATERNITY CARE	NR	WOMEN'S HEALTH	NR

HEALTHGRADES AWARDS

Shelby Memorial Hospital

200 South Cedar Street
Shelbyville, IL 62565
(217) 774-3961

Overall patient safety: ★★★
Teaching: N

CLINICAL PROGRAM RATINGS:

CARDIAC	NR	ORTHOPEDICS	NR
CRITICAL CARE	NR	PULMONARY	★★★★★
GASTROINTESTINAL	NR	STROKE	★
GENERAL SURGERY	NR	VASCULAR	NR
MATERNITY CARE	NR	WOMEN'S HEALTH	NR

HEALTHGRADES AWARDS

✓ SPECIALTY EXCELLENCE
• PULMONARY CARE

South Shore Hospital

8012 South Crandon Avenue
Chicago, IL 60617
(773) 768-0810

Overall patient safety: ★★★
Teaching: N

CLINICAL PROGRAM RATINGS:

CARDIAC	NR	ORTHOPEDICS	NR
CRITICAL CARE	NR	PULMONARY	★★★
GASTROINTESTINAL	NR	STROKE	NR
GENERAL SURGERY	NR	VASCULAR	NR
MATERNITY CARE	NR	WOMEN'S HEALTH	NR

HEALTHGRADES AWARDS

*This hospital reports its data to the federal government jointly with another hospital. Therefore the ratings and awards apply to multiple hospitals and this specific hospital may not provide all rated services.

Sparta Community Hospital

818 East Broadway
Sparta, IL 62286
(618) 443-2177

Overall patient safety: NR
Teaching: N

CLINICAL PROGRAM RATINGS:

CARDIAC	NR	ORTHOPEDICS	NR
CRITICAL CARE	NR	PULMONARY	★
GASTROINTESTINAL	NR	STROKE	★★★
GENERAL SURGERY	NR	VASCULAR	NR
MATERNITY CARE	NR	WOMEN'S HEALTH	NR

HEALTHGRADES AWARDS

Taylorville Memorial Hospital

201 East Pleasant Street
Taylorville, IL 62568
(217) 824-3331

Overall patient safety: ★★★
Teaching: N

CLINICAL PROGRAM RATINGS:

CARDIAC	NR	ORTHOPEDICS	NR
CRITICAL CARE	NR	PULMONARY	★
GASTROINTESTINAL	NR	STROKE	★★★
GENERAL SURGERY	NR	VASCULAR	NR
MATERNITY CARE	NR	WOMEN'S HEALTH	NR

HEALTHGRADES AWARDS

Swedish American Hospital

1401 East State Street
Rockford, IL 61104
(815) 968-4400

Overall patient safety: ★★★
Teaching: Y

CLINICAL PROGRAM RATINGS:

CARDIAC	★★★	ORTHOPEDICS	★★★
CRITICAL CARE	★★★	PULMONARY	★★★
GASTROINTESTINAL	★★★	STROKE	★★★
GENERAL SURGERY	NR	VASCULAR	NR
MATERNITY CARE	NR	WOMEN'S HEALTH	NR

HEALTHGRADES AWARDS

✓ SPECIALTY EXCELLENCE
- CARDIAC SURGERY

Thomas H. Boyd Memorial Hospital

800 School Street
Carrollton, IL 62016
(217) 942-6946

Overall patient safety: NR
Teaching: N

CLINICAL PROGRAM RATINGS:

CARDIAC	NR	ORTHOPEDICS	NR
CRITICAL CARE	NR	PULMONARY	★★★
GASTROINTESTINAL	NR	STROKE	NR
GENERAL SURGERY	NR	VASCULAR	NR
MATERNITY CARE	NR	WOMEN'S HEALTH	NR

HEALTHGRADES AWARDS

Swedish Covenant Hospital

5145 North California Avenue
Chicago, IL 60625
(773) 878-8200

Overall patient safety: ★★★
Teaching: Y

CLINICAL PROGRAM RATINGS:

CARDIAC	★★★	ORTHOPEDICS	NR
CRITICAL CARE	★★★	PULMONARY	★★★★★
GASTROINTESTINAL	★★★	STROKE	★★★★★
GENERAL SURGERY	NR	VASCULAR	NR
MATERNITY CARE	NR	WOMEN'S HEALTH	NR

HEALTHGRADES AWARDS

✓ DISTINGUISHED HOSPITAL
- CLINICAL EXCELLENCE

✓ SPECIALTY EXCELLENCE
- GASTROINTESTINAL CARE
- PULMONARY CARE
- STROKE CARE

Thorek Memorial Hospital

850 West Irving Park Road
Chicago, IL 60613
(773) 525-6780

Overall patient safety: ★★★
Teaching: Y

CLINICAL PROGRAM RATINGS:

CARDIAC	NR	ORTHOPEDICS	NR
CRITICAL CARE	NR	PULMONARY	★★★★★
GASTROINTESTINAL	NR	STROKE	★★★★★
GENERAL SURGERY	NR	VASCULAR	NR
MATERNITY CARE	NR	WOMEN'S HEALTH	NR

HEALTHGRADES AWARDS

KEY: ★★★★★ BEST   ★★★ AS EXPECTED   ★ POOR   NR NOT RATED BY HEALTHGRADES   For full definitions of ratings and awards, see Appendix.

Touchette Regional Hospital

5900 Bond Avenue
Centreville, IL 62207
(618) 332-3060

Overall patient safety: ★
Teaching: N

CLINICAL PROGRAM RATINGS:

CARDIAC	NR	ORTHOPEDICS	NR
CRITICAL CARE	NR	PULMONARY	★★★
GASTROINTESTINAL	NR	STROKE	NR
GENERAL SURGERY	NR	VASCULAR	NR
MATERNITY CARE	NR	WOMEN'S HEALTH	NR

HEALTHGRADES AWARDS

Union County Hospital District

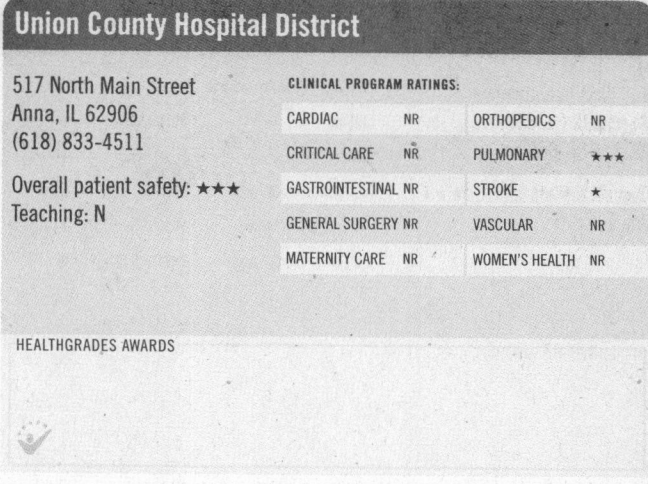

517 North Main Street
Anna, IL 62906
(618) 833-4511

Overall patient safety: ★★★
Teaching: N

CLINICAL PROGRAM RATINGS:

CARDIAC	NR	ORTHOPEDICS	NR
CRITICAL CARE	NR	PULMONARY	★★★
GASTROINTESTINAL	NR	STROKE	★
GENERAL SURGERY	NR	VASCULAR	NR
MATERNITY CARE	NR	WOMEN'S HEALTH	NR

HEALTHGRADES AWARDS

Trinity Medical Center—7th Street Campus*

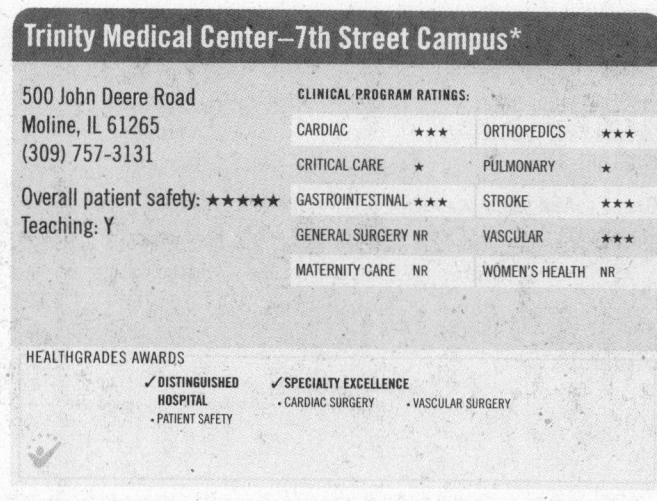

500 John Deere Road
Moline, IL 61265
(309) 757-3131

Overall patient safety: ★★★★★
Teaching: Y

CLINICAL PROGRAM RATINGS:

CARDIAC	★★★	ORTHOPEDICS	★★★
CRITICAL CARE	★	PULMONARY	★
GASTROINTESTINAL	★★★	STROKE	★★★
GENERAL SURGERY	NR	VASCULAR	★★★
MATERNITY CARE	NR	WOMEN'S HEALTH	NR

HEALTHGRADES AWARDS

✓ DISTINGUISHED HOSPITAL
- PATIENT SAFETY

✓ SPECIALTY EXCELLENCE
- CARDIAC SURGERY   - VASCULAR SURGERY

University of Chicago Medical Center

5841 South Maryland Avenue
Chicago, IL 60637
(773) 702-1000

Overall patient safety: ★
Teaching: Y

CLINICAL PROGRAM RATINGS:

CARDIAC	★★★	ORTHOPEDICS	★★★
CRITICAL CARE	★★★	PULMONARY	★★★
GASTROINTESTINAL	★★★	STROKE	★★★★★
GENERAL SURGERY	NR	VASCULAR	★★★
MATERNITY CARE	NR	WOMEN'S HEALTH	NR

HEALTHGRADES AWARDS

✓ SPECIALTY EXCELLENCE
- STROKE CARE

Trinity Medical Center—West Campus*

2701 17th Street
Rock Island, IL 61201
(309) 779-5000

Overall patient safety: ★★★★★
Teaching: Y

CLINICAL PROGRAM RATINGS:

CARDIAC	★★★	ORTHOPEDICS	★★★
CRITICAL CARE	★	PULMONARY	★
GASTROINTESTINAL	★★★	STROKE	★★★
GENERAL SURGERY	NR	VASCULAR	★★★
MATERNITY CARE	NR	WOMEN'S HEALTH	NR

HEALTHGRADES AWARDS

✓ DISTINGUISHED HOSPITAL
- PATIENT SAFETY

✓ SPECIALTY EXCELLENCE
- CARDIAC SURGERY   - VASCULAR SURGERY

University of Illinois Medical Center

1740 West Taylor Street
Chicago, IL 60612
(312) 996-7000

Overall patient safety: ★
Teaching: Y

CLINICAL PROGRAM RATINGS:

CARDIAC	★★★	ORTHOPEDICS	NR
CRITICAL CARE	★★★	PULMONARY	★★★
GASTROINTESTINAL	★★★	STROKE	★★★★★
GENERAL SURGERY	NR	VASCULAR	NR
MATERNITY CARE	NR	WOMEN'S HEALTH	NR

HEALTHGRADES AWARDS

*This hospital reports its data to the federal government jointly with another hospital. Therefore the ratings and awards apply to multiple hospitals and this specific hospital may not provide all rated services.

Valley West Community Hospital

11 East Pleasant Avenue
Sandwich, IL 60548
(815) 786-8484

Overall patient safety: ★★★
Teaching: N

CLINICAL PROGRAM RATINGS:

CARDIAC	NR	ORTHOPEDICS	NR
CRITICAL CARE	NR	PULMONARY	★★★
GASTROINTESTINAL	NR	STROKE	★★★
GENERAL SURGERY	NR	VASCULAR	NR
MATERNITY CARE	NR	WOMEN'S HEALTH	NR

HEALTHGRADES AWARDS

West Suburban Hospital Medical Center

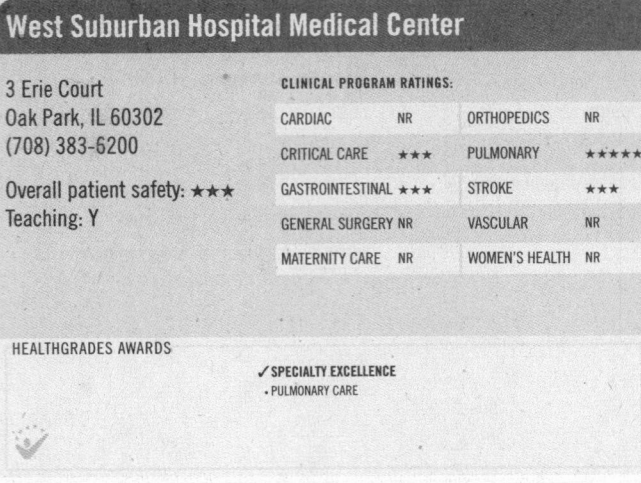

3 Erie Court
Oak Park, IL 60302
(708) 383-6200

Overall patient safety: ★★★
Teaching: Y

CLINICAL PROGRAM RATINGS:

CARDIAC	NR	ORTHOPEDICS	NR
CRITICAL CARE	★★★	PULMONARY	★★★★★
GASTROINTESTINAL	★★★	STROKE	★★★
GENERAL SURGERY	NR	VASCULAR	NR
MATERNITY CARE	NR	WOMEN'S HEALTH	NR

HEALTHGRADES AWARDS

✓ SPECIALTY EXCELLENCE
· PULMONARY CARE

Vista Medical Center—East

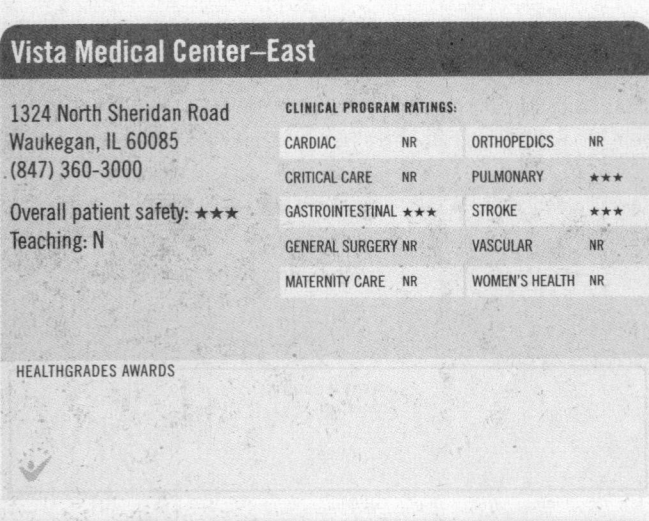

1324 North Sheridan Road
Waukegan, IL 60085
(847) 360-3000

Overall patient safety: ★★★
Teaching: N

CLINICAL PROGRAM RATINGS:

CARDIAC	NR	ORTHOPEDICS	NR
CRITICAL CARE	NR	PULMONARY	★★★
GASTROINTESTINAL	★★★	STROKE	★★★
GENERAL SURGERY	NR	VASCULAR	NR
MATERNITY CARE	NR	WOMEN'S HEALTH	NR

HEALTHGRADES AWARDS

Westlake Community Hospital

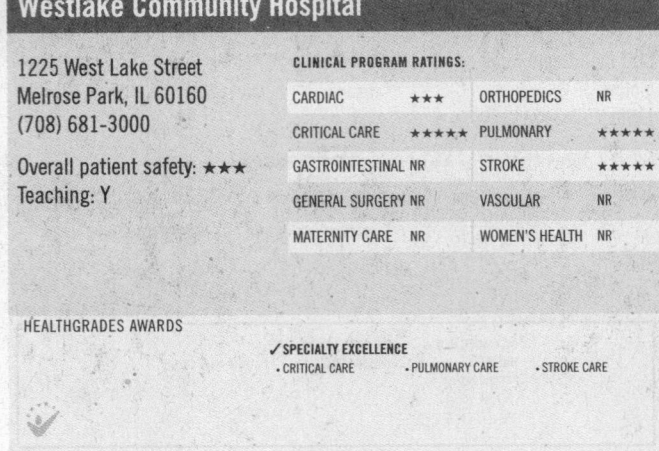

1225 West Lake Street
Melrose Park, IL 60160
(708) 681-3000

Overall patient safety: ★★★
Teaching: Y

CLINICAL PROGRAM RATINGS:

CARDIAC	★★★	ORTHOPEDICS	NR
CRITICAL CARE	★★★★★	PULMONARY	★★★★★
GASTROINTESTINAL	NR	STROKE	★★★★★
GENERAL SURGERY	NR	VASCULAR	NR
MATERNITY CARE	NR	WOMEN'S HEALTH	NR

HEALTHGRADES AWARDS

✓ SPECIALTY EXCELLENCE
· CRITICAL CARE   · PULMONARY CARE   · STROKE CARE

Wabash General Hospital

1418 College Drive
Mount Carmel, IL 62863
(618) 262-8621

Overall patient safety: ★★★
Teaching: N

CLINICAL PROGRAM RATINGS:

CARDIAC	NR	ORTHOPEDICS	NR
CRITICAL CARE	NR	PULMONARY	★★★
GASTROINTESTINAL	NR	STROKE	★★★
GENERAL SURGERY	NR	VASCULAR	NR
MATERNITY CARE	NR	WOMEN'S HEALTH	NR

HEALTHGRADES AWARDS

White County Medical Center

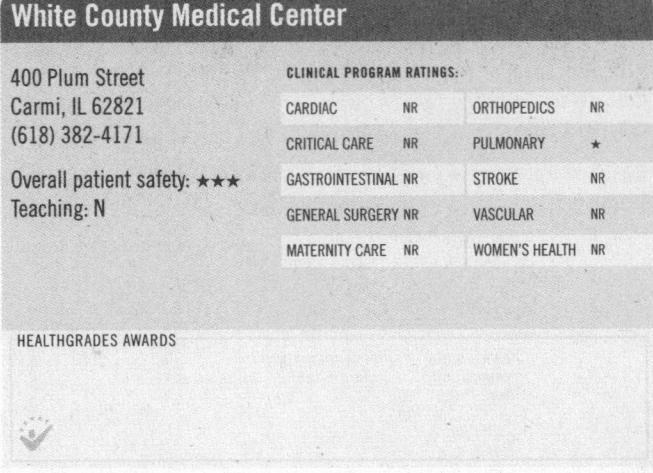

400 Plum Street
Carmi, IL 62821
(618) 382-4171

Overall patient safety: ★★★
Teaching: N

CLINICAL PROGRAM RATINGS:

CARDIAC	NR	ORTHOPEDICS	NR
CRITICAL CARE	NR	PULMONARY	★
GASTROINTESTINAL	NR	STROKE	NR
GENERAL SURGERY	NR	VASCULAR	NR
MATERNITY CARE	NR	WOMEN'S HEALTH	NR

HEALTHGRADES AWARDS

KEY: ★★★★★ BEST   ★★★ AS EXPECTED   ★ POOR   NR NOT RATED BY HEALTHGRADES   For full definitions of ratings and awards, see Appendix.

Adams County Memorial Hospital*

805 High Street
Decatur, IN 46733
(219) 724-2145

Overall patient safety: ★★★
Teaching: N

CLINICAL PROGRAM RATINGS:

CARDIAC	NR	ORTHOPEDICS	NR
CRITICAL CARE	NR	PULMONARY	★★★
GASTROINTESTINAL	NR	STROKE	★★★
GENERAL SURGERY	NR	VASCULAR	NR
MATERNITY CARE	NR	WOMEN'S HEALTH	NR

HEALTHGRADES AWARDS

Bedford Regional Medical Center

2900 West 16 Street
Bedford, IN 47421
(812) 275-1200

Overall patient safety: ★★★
Teaching: N

CLINICAL PROGRAM RATINGS:

CARDIAC	NR	ORTHOPEDICS	NR
CRITICAL CARE	NR	PULMONARY	★★★
GASTROINTESTINAL	NR	STROKE	★★★
GENERAL SURGERY	NR	VASCULAR	NR
MATERNITY CARE	NR	WOMEN'S HEALTH	NR

HEALTHGRADES AWARDS

Adams Memorial Hospital*

1100 Mercer Avenue
Decatur, IN 46733
(260) 724-2145

Overall patient safety: ★★★
Teaching: N

CLINICAL PROGRAM RATINGS:

CARDIAC	NR	ORTHOPEDICS	NR
CRITICAL CARE	NR	PULMONARY	★★★
GASTROINTESTINAL	NR	STROKE	★★★
GENERAL SURGERY	NR	VASCULAR	NR
MATERNITY CARE	NR	WOMEN'S HEALTH	NR

HEALTHGRADES AWARDS

Bloomington Hospital

601 West 2nd Street
Bloomington, IN 47403
(812) 336-6821

Overall patient safety: ★★★
Teaching: N

CLINICAL PROGRAM RATINGS:

CARDIAC	★★★	ORTHOPEDICS	★★★
CRITICAL CARE	★	PULMONARY	★★★
GASTROINTESTINAL	★★★	STROKE	★★★
GENERAL SURGERY	NR	VASCULAR	★★★
MATERNITY CARE	NR	WOMEN'S HEALTH	NR

HEALTHGRADES AWARDS

Ball Memorial Hospital

2401 West University Avenue
Muncie, IN 47303
(765) 747-3111

Overall patient safety: ★★★
Teaching: Y

CLINICAL PROGRAM RATINGS:

CARDIAC	★★★	ORTHOPEDICS	★★★
CRITICAL CARE	★★★	PULMONARY	★★★★★
GASTROINTESTINAL	★★★	STROKE	★★★
GENERAL SURGERY	NR	VASCULAR	★★★
MATERNITY CARE	NR	WOMEN'S HEALTH	NR

HEALTHGRADES AWARDS

✓ SPECIALTY EXCELLENCE
· CARDIAC SURGERY   · PULMONARY CARE

Bloomington Hospital of Orange County

642 West Hospital Road
Paoli, IN 47454
(812) 723-2811

Overall patient safety: ★★★
Teaching: N

CLINICAL PROGRAM RATINGS:

CARDIAC	NR	ORTHOPEDICS	NR
CRITICAL CARE	NR	PULMONARY	★
GASTROINTESTINAL	NR	STROKE	★★★
GENERAL SURGERY	NR	VASCULAR	NR
MATERNITY CARE	NR	WOMEN'S HEALTH	NR

HEALTHGRADES AWARDS

*This hospital reports its data to the federal government jointly with another hospital. Therefore the ratings and awards apply to multiple hospitals and this specific hospital may not provide all rated services.

Bluffton Regional Medical Center

303 South Main Street
Bluffton, IN 46714
(260) 824-3210

Overall patient safety: ★★★
Teaching: N

CLINICAL PROGRAM RATINGS:

CARDIAC	NR	ORTHOPEDICS	NR
CRITICAL CARE	NR	PULMONARY	★★★★★
GASTROINTESTINAL	★★★	STROKE	★★★
GENERAL SURGERY	NR	VASCULAR	NR
MATERNITY CARE	NR	WOMEN'S HEALTH	NR

HEALTHGRADES AWARDS

Clarian West Medical Center

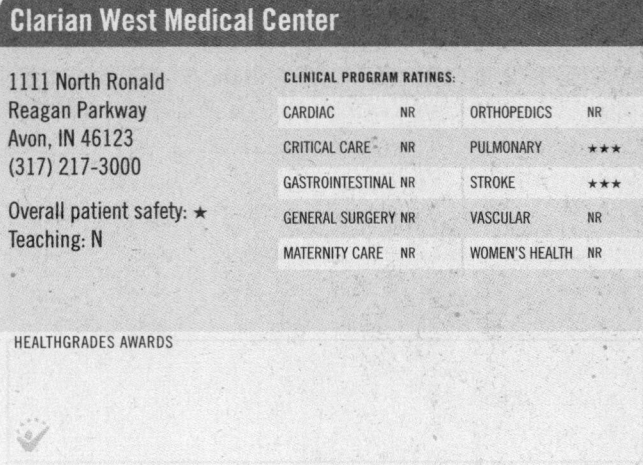

1111 North Ronald
Reagan Parkway
Avon, IN 46123
(317) 217-3000

Overall patient safety: ★
Teaching: N

CLINICAL PROGRAM RATINGS:

CARDIAC	NR	ORTHOPEDICS	NR
CRITICAL CARE	NR	PULMONARY	★★★
GASTROINTESTINAL	NR	STROKE	★★★
GENERAL SURGERY	NR	VASCULAR	NR
MATERNITY CARE	NR	WOMEN'S HEALTH	NR

HEALTHGRADES AWARDS

Cameron Memorial Community Hospital

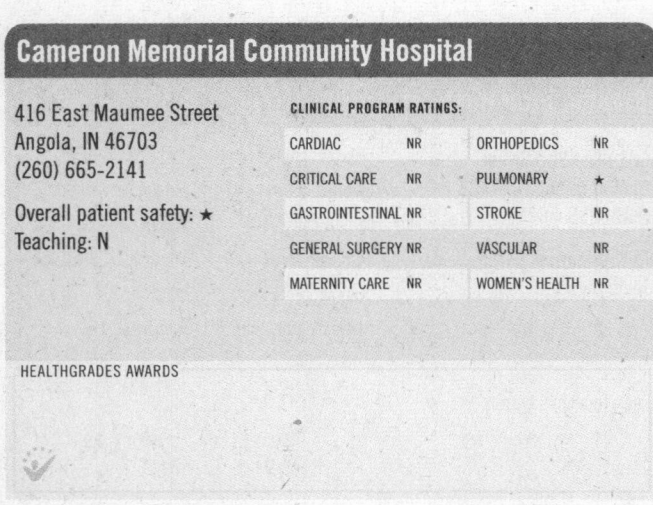

416 East Maumee Street
Angola, IN 46703
(260) 665-2141

Overall patient safety: ★
Teaching: N

CLINICAL PROGRAM RATINGS:

CARDIAC	NR	ORTHOPEDICS	NR
CRITICAL CARE	NR	PULMONARY	★
GASTROINTESTINAL	NR	STROKE	NR
GENERAL SURGERY	NR	VASCULAR	NR
MATERNITY CARE	NR	WOMEN'S HEALTH	NR

HEALTHGRADES AWARDS

Clark Memorial Hospital

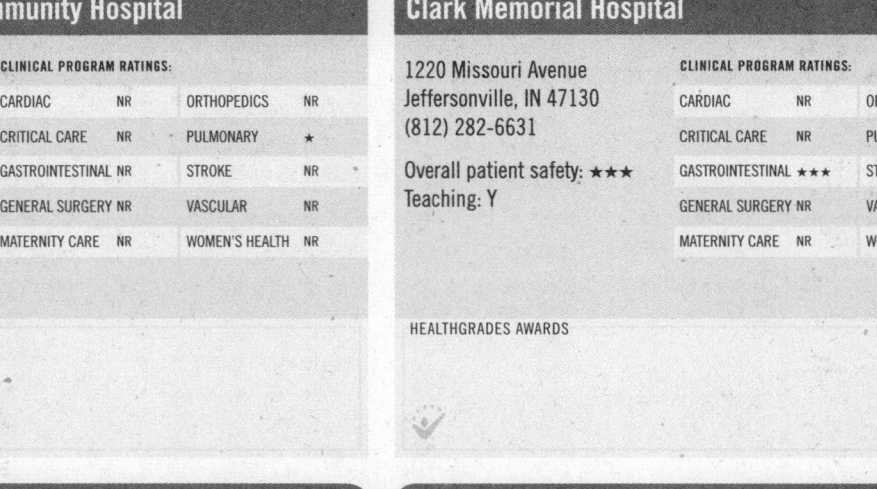

1220 Missouri Avenue
Jeffersonville, IN 47130
(812) 282-6631

Overall patient safety: ★★★
Teaching: Y

CLINICAL PROGRAM RATINGS:

CARDIAC	NR	ORTHOPEDICS	★
CRITICAL CARE	NR	PULMONARY	★★★
GASTROINTESTINAL	★★★	STROKE	★★★
GENERAL SURGERY	NR	VASCULAR	NR
MATERNITY CARE	NR	WOMEN'S HEALTH	NR

HEALTHGRADES AWARDS

Clarian Health Partners*

1701 North Senate Boulevard
Indianapolis, IN 46202
(317) 962-2000

Overall patient safety: ★
Teaching: Y

CLINICAL PROGRAM RATINGS:

CARDIAC	★★★	ORTHOPEDICS	★
CRITICAL CARE	★★★	PULMONARY	★★★★★
GASTROINTESTINAL	★★★	STROKE	★★★★★
GENERAL SURGERY	NR	VASCULAR	★★★
MATERNITY CARE	NR	WOMEN'S HEALTH	NR

HEALTHGRADES AWARDS

✓ SPECIALTY EXCELLENCE
• PULMONARY CARE   • STROKE CARE

Columbus Regional Hospital

2400 East 17th Street
Columbus, IN 47201
(812) 379-4441

Overall patient safety: ★★★
Teaching: N

CLINICAL PROGRAM RATINGS:

CARDIAC	★★★	ORTHOPEDICS	★★★
CRITICAL CARE	★★★	PULMONARY	★★★
GASTROINTESTINAL	★★★	STROKE	★★★
GENERAL SURGERY	NR	VASCULAR	NR
MATERNITY CARE	NR	WOMEN'S HEALTH	NR

HEALTHGRADES AWARDS

KEY: ★★★★★ BEST   ★★★ AS EXPECTED   ★ POOR   NR NOT RATED BY HEALTHGRADES   For full definitions of ratings and awards, see Appendix.

Community Hospital

901 MacArthur Boulevard
Munster, IN 46321
(219) 836-1600

Overall patient safety: ★★★★★
Teaching: N

CLINICAL PROGRAM RATINGS:

CARDIAC	★★★★★	ORTHOPEDICS	★★★★★
CRITICAL CARE	★★★	PULMONARY	★★★★★
GASTROINTESTINAL	★★★★★	STROKE	★★★
GENERAL SURGERY	NR	VASCULAR	★★★
MATERNITY CARE	NR	WOMEN'S HEALTH	NR

HEALTHGRADES AWARDS

✓AMERICA'S 50   ✓DISTINGUISHED   ✓SPECIALTY EXCELLENCE
  BEST HOSPITALS   HOSPITAL
- CLINICAL EXCELLENCE
- PATIENT SAFETY

- CARDIAC CARE
- CARDIAC SURGERY
- GASTROINTESTINAL CARE

- JOINT REPLACEMENT
- ORTHOPEDIC SURGERY

- PULMONARY CARE
- VASCULAR SURGERY

Community Hospital South

1402 East County Line Road
Indianapolis, IN 46227
(317) 887-7000

Overall patient safety: ★★★
Teaching: N

CLINICAL PROGRAM RATINGS:

CARDIAC	NR	ORTHOPEDICS	NR
CRITICAL CARE	NR	PULMONARY	★★★★★
GASTROINTESTINAL	★★★	STROKE	★★★
GENERAL SURGERY	NR	VASCULAR	NR
MATERNITY CARE	NR	WOMEN'S HEALTH	NR

HEALTHGRADES AWARDS

Community Hospital of Anderson and Madison County

1515 North Madison Avenue
Anderson, IN 46011
(765) 298-4242

Overall patient safety: ★★★
Teaching: N

CLINICAL PROGRAM RATINGS:

CARDIAC	NR	ORTHOPEDICS	NR
CRITICAL CARE	★	PULMONARY	★★★★★
GASTROINTESTINAL	★★★	STROKE	★★★
GENERAL SURGERY	NR	VASCULAR	NR
MATERNITY CARE	NR	WOMEN'S HEALTH	NR

HEALTHGRADES AWARDS

Community Hospitals Indianapolis

1500 North Ritter Avenue
Indianapolis, IN 46219
(317) 355-1411

Overall patient safety: ★★★
Teaching: Y

CLINICAL PROGRAM RATINGS:

CARDIAC	NR	ORTHOPEDICS	★★★
CRITICAL CARE	★★★	PULMONARY	★★★
GASTROINTESTINAL	★★★	STROKE	★★★
GENERAL SURGERY	NR	VASCULAR	NR
MATERNITY CARE	NR	WOMEN'S HEALTH	NR

HEALTHGRADES AWARDS

✓SPECIALTY EXCELLENCE
- GASTROINTESTINAL CARE

Community Hospital of Bremen

1020 High Road
Bremen, IN 46506
(574) 546-2211

Overall patient safety: ★★★
Teaching: N

CLINICAL PROGRAM RATINGS:

CARDIAC	NR	ORTHOPEDICS	NR
CRITICAL CARE	NR	PULMONARY	★★★
GASTROINTESTINAL	NR	STROKE	NR
GENERAL SURGERY	NR	VASCULAR	NR
MATERNITY CARE	NR	WOMEN'S HEALTH	NR

HEALTHGRADES AWARDS

Daviess Community Hospital

1314 Walnut Street
Washington, IN 47501
(812) 254-2760

Overall patient safety: ★★★
Teaching: N

CLINICAL PROGRAM RATINGS:

CARDIAC	NR	ORTHOPEDICS	NR
CRITICAL CARE	NR	PULMONARY	★★★
GASTROINTESTINAL	NR	STROKE	★★★★★
GENERAL SURGERY	NR	VASCULAR	NR
MATERNITY CARE	NR	WOMEN'S HEALTH	NR

HEALTHGRADES AWARDS

✓SPECIALTY EXCELLENCE
- STROKE CARE

*This hospital reports its data to the federal government jointly with another hospital. Therefore the ratings and awards apply to multiple hospitals and this specific hospital may not provide all rated services.

Deaconess Hospital

600 Mary Street
Evansville, IN 47747
(812) 450-5000

Overall patient safety: ★★★★★
Teaching: Y

CLINICAL PROGRAM RATINGS:

CARDIAC	★★★	ORTHOPEDICS	★
CRITICAL CARE	★★★	PULMONARY	★★★★★
GASTROINTESTINAL	★★★	STROKE	★★★
GENERAL SURGERY	NR	VASCULAR	★★★
MATERNITY CARE	NR	WOMEN'S HEALTH	NR

HEALTHGRADES AWARDS

✓ DISTINGUISHED HOSPITAL
  • PATIENT SAFETY

✓ SPECIALTY EXCELLENCE
  • PULMONARY CARE

DeKalb Memorial Hospital

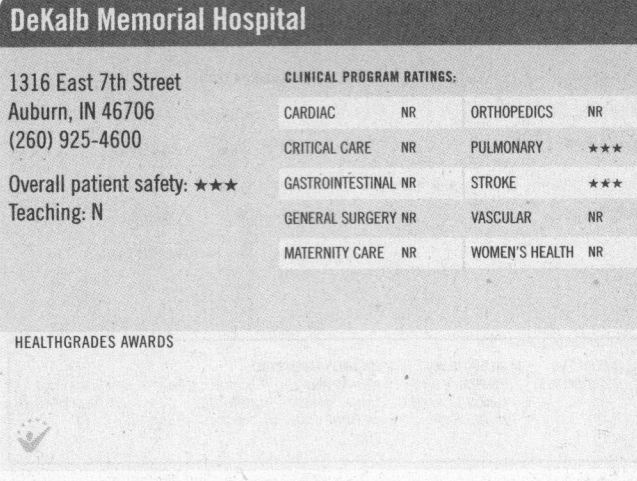

1316 East 7th Street
Auburn, IN 46706
(260) 925-4600

Overall patient safety: ★★★
Teaching: N

CLINICAL PROGRAM RATINGS:

CARDIAC	NR	ORTHOPEDICS	NR
CRITICAL CARE	NR	PULMONARY	★★★
GASTROINTESTINAL	NR	STROKE	★★★
GENERAL SURGERY	NR	VASCULAR	NR
MATERNITY CARE	NR	WOMEN'S HEALTH	NR

HEALTHGRADES AWARDS

Dearborn County Hospital

600 Wilson Creek Road
Lawrenceburg, IN 47025
(812) 537-1010

Overall patient safety: ★★★
Teaching: N

CLINICAL PROGRAM RATINGS:

CARDIAC	NR	ORTHOPEDICS	NR
CRITICAL CARE	NR	PULMONARY	★★★
GASTROINTESTINAL	★★★	STROKE	★★★
GENERAL SURGERY	NR	VASCULAR	NR
MATERNITY CARE	NR	WOMEN'S HEALTH	NR

HEALTHGRADES AWARDS

Dukes Memorial Hospital

275 West 12th Street
Peru, IN 46970
(765) 472-8000

Overall patient safety: ★★★
Teaching: N

CLINICAL PROGRAM RATINGS:

CARDIAC	NR	ORTHOPEDICS	NR
CRITICAL CARE	NR	PULMONARY	★★★
GASTROINTESTINAL	NR	STROKE	NR
GENERAL SURGERY	NR	VASCULAR	NR
MATERNITY CARE	NR	WOMEN'S HEALTH	NR

HEALTHGRADES AWARDS

Decatur County Memorial Hospital

720 North Lincoln Street
Greensburg, IN 47240
(812) 663-4331

Overall patient safety: ★★★
Teaching: N

CLINICAL PROGRAM RATINGS:

CARDIAC	NR	ORTHOPEDICS	NR
CRITICAL CARE	NR	PULMONARY	★★★
GASTROINTESTINAL	NR	STROKE	★★★
GENERAL SURGERY	NR	VASCULAR	NR
MATERNITY CARE	NR	WOMEN'S HEALTH	NR

HEALTHGRADES AWARDS

Dunn Memorial Hospital

1600 23rd Street
Bedford, IN 47421
(812) 275-3331

Overall patient safety: ★★★
Teaching: N

CLINICAL PROGRAM RATINGS:

CARDIAC	NR	ORTHOPEDICS	NR
CRITICAL CARE	NR	PULMONARY	★★★
GASTROINTESTINAL	NR	STROKE	★
GENERAL SURGERY	NR	VASCULAR	NR
MATERNITY CARE	NR	WOMEN'S HEALTH	NR

HEALTHGRADES AWARDS

KEY: ★★★★★ BEST   ★★★ AS EXPECTED   ★ POOR   NR NOT RATED BY HEALTHGRADES   For full definitions of ratings and awards, see Appendix.

Dupont Hospital

2520 East Dupont Road
Fort Wayne, IN 46825
(260) 416-3000

Overall patient safety: ★★★
Teaching: N

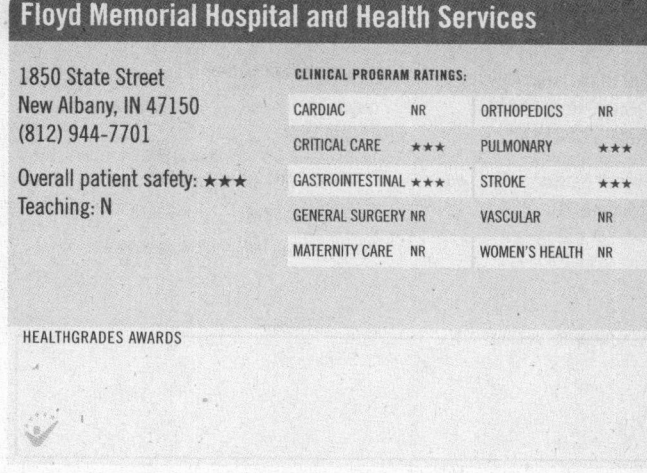

CLINICAL PROGRAM RATINGS:

CARDIAC	NR	ORTHOPEDICS	★★★
CRITICAL CARE	NR	PULMONARY	★★★★★
GASTROINTESTINAL	NR	STROKE	NR
GENERAL SURGERY	NR	VASCULAR	NR
MATERNITY CARE	NR	WOMEN'S HEALTH	NR

HEALTHGRADES AWARDS

✓ SPECIALTY EXCELLENCE
 • PULMONARY CARE

Floyd Memorial Hospital and Health Services

1850 State Street
New Albany, IN 47150
(812) 944-7701

Overall patient safety: ★★★
Teaching: N

CLINICAL PROGRAM RATINGS:

CARDIAC	NR	ORTHOPEDICS	NR
CRITICAL CARE	★★★	PULMONARY	★★★
GASTROINTESTINAL	★★★	STROKE	★★★
GENERAL SURGERY	NR	VASCULAR	NR
MATERNITY CARE	NR	WOMEN'S HEALTH	NR

HEALTHGRADES AWARDS

Elkhart General Hospital

600 East Boulevard
Elkhart, IN 46514
(574) 294-2621

Overall patient safety: ★★★★★
Teaching: N

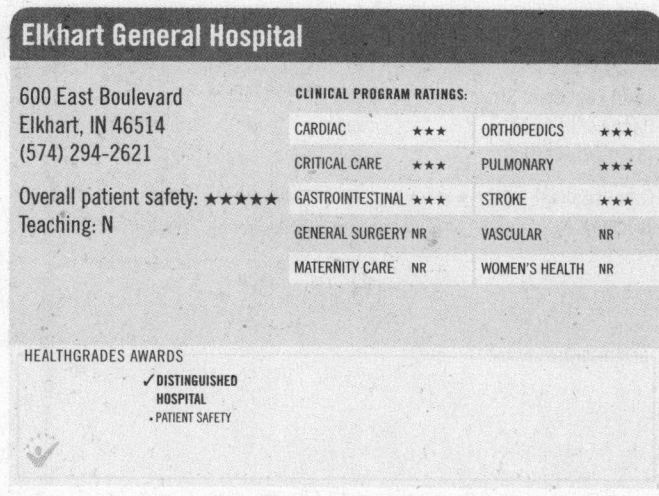

CLINICAL PROGRAM RATINGS:

CARDIAC	★★★	ORTHOPEDICS	★★★
CRITICAL CARE	★★★	PULMONARY	★★★
GASTROINTESTINAL	★★★	STROKE	★★★
GENERAL SURGERY	NR	VASCULAR	NR
MATERNITY CARE	NR	WOMEN'S HEALTH	NR

HEALTHGRADES AWARDS

✓ DISTINGUISHED HOSPITAL
 • PATIENT SAFETY

Gibson General Hospital

1808 Sherman Drive
Princeton, IN 47670
(812) 385-3401

Overall patient safety: ★★★
Teaching: N

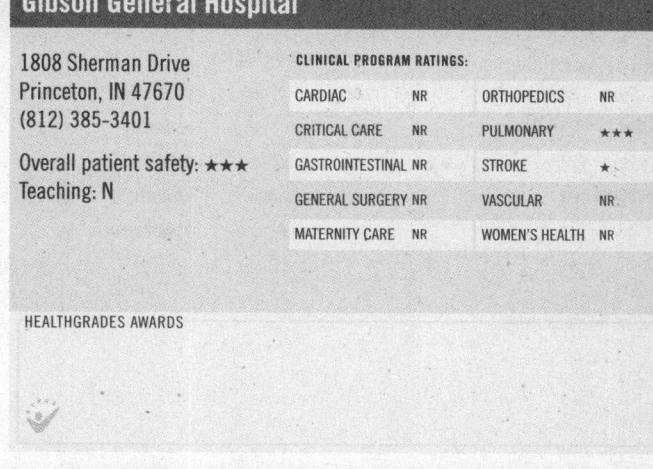

CLINICAL PROGRAM RATINGS:

CARDIAC	NR	ORTHOPEDICS	NR
CRITICAL CARE	NR	PULMONARY	★★★
GASTROINTESTINAL	NR	STROKE	★
GENERAL SURGERY	NR	VASCULAR	NR
MATERNITY CARE	NR	WOMEN'S HEALTH	NR

HEALTHGRADES AWARDS

Fayette Memorial Hospital

1941 Virginia Avenue
Connersville, IN 47331
(765) 825-5131

Overall patient safety: ★★★★★
Teaching: N

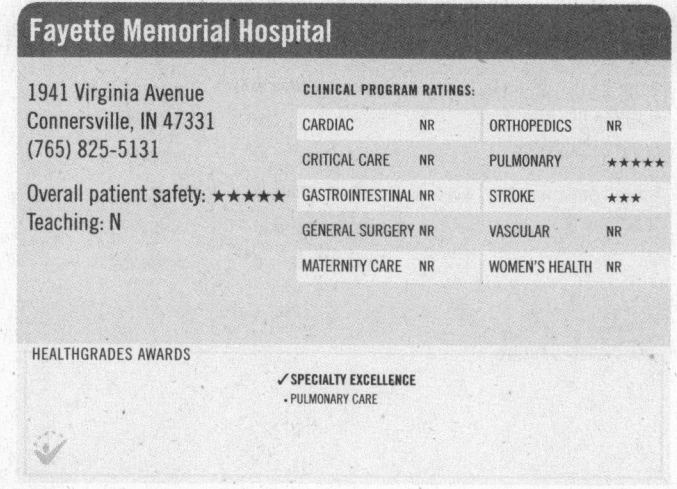

CLINICAL PROGRAM RATINGS:

CARDIAC	NR	ORTHOPEDICS	NR
CRITICAL CARE	NR	PULMONARY	★★★★★
GASTROINTESTINAL	NR	STROKE	★★★
GENERAL SURGERY	NR	VASCULAR	NR
MATERNITY CARE	NR	WOMEN'S HEALTH	NR

HEALTHGRADES AWARDS

✓ SPECIALTY EXCELLENCE
 • PULMONARY CARE

Good Samaritan Hospital

520 South 7th Street
Vincennes, IN 47591
(812) 882-5220

Overall patient safety: ★★★
Teaching: N

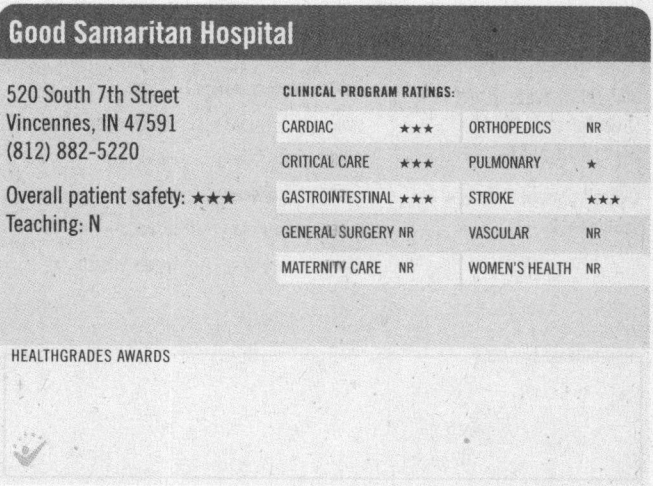

CLINICAL PROGRAM RATINGS:

CARDIAC	★★★	ORTHOPEDICS	NR
CRITICAL CARE	★★★	PULMONARY	★
GASTROINTESTINAL	★★★	STROKE	★★★
GENERAL SURGERY	NR	VASCULAR	NR
MATERNITY CARE	NR	WOMEN'S HEALTH	NR

HEALTHGRADES AWARDS

Goshen General Hospital

200 High Parks Avenue
Goshen, IN 46526
(574) 533-2141

Overall patient safety: ★★★
Teaching: N

CLINICAL PROGRAM RATINGS:

CARDIAC	NR	ORTHOPEDICS	NR
CRITICAL CARE	NR	PULMONARY	★
GASTROINTESTINAL	★★★	STROKE	★★★
GENERAL SURGERY	NR	VASCULAR	NR
MATERNITY CARE	NR	WOMEN'S HEALTH	NR

HEALTHGRADES AWARDS

Harrison County Hospital

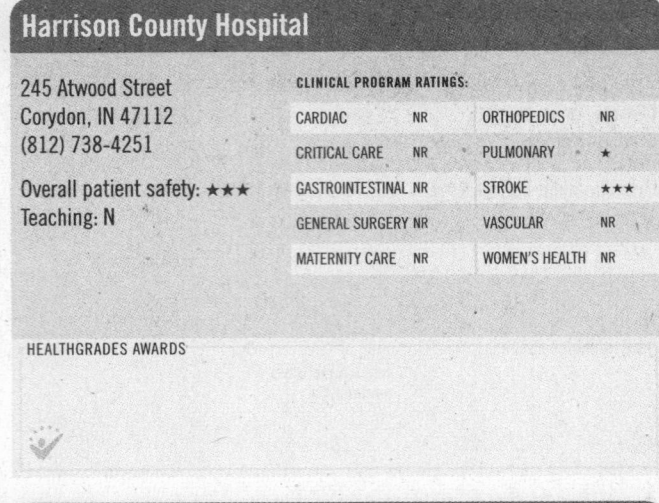

245 Atwood Street
Corydon, IN 47112
(812) 738-4251

Overall patient safety: ★★★
Teaching: N

CLINICAL PROGRAM RATINGS:

CARDIAC	NR	ORTHOPEDICS	NR
CRITICAL CARE	NR	PULMONARY	★
GASTROINTESTINAL	NR	STROKE	★★★
GENERAL SURGERY	NR	VASCULAR	NR
MATERNITY CARE	NR	WOMEN'S HEALTH	NR

HEALTHGRADES AWARDS

Greene County General Hospital

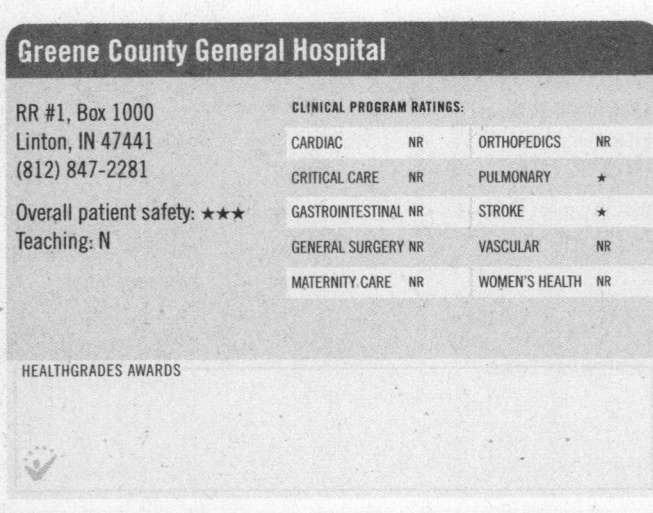

RR #1, Box 1000
Linton, IN 47441
(812) 847-2281

Overall patient safety: ★★★
Teaching: N

CLINICAL PROGRAM RATINGS:

CARDIAC	NR	ORTHOPEDICS	NR
CRITICAL CARE	NR	PULMONARY	★
GASTROINTESTINAL	NR	STROKE	★
GENERAL SURGERY	NR	VASCULAR	NR
MATERNITY CARE	NR	WOMEN'S HEALTH	NR

HEALTHGRADES AWARDS

Hendricks Regional Health

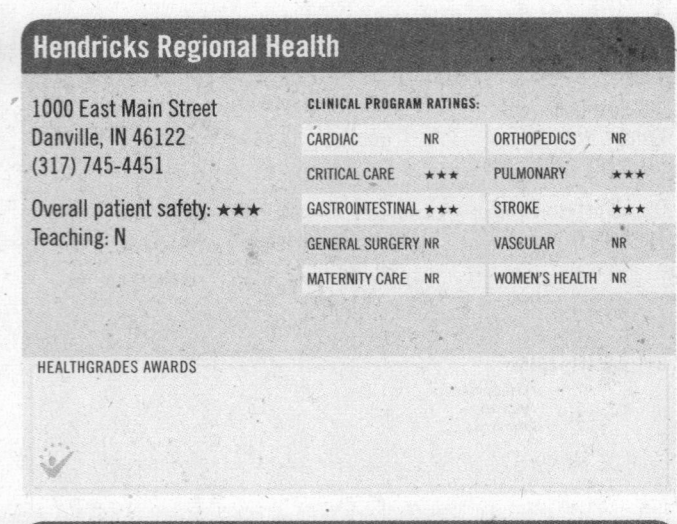

1000 East Main Street
Danville, IN 46122
(317) 745-4451

Overall patient safety: ★★★
Teaching: N

CLINICAL PROGRAM RATINGS:

CARDIAC	NR	ORTHOPEDICS	NR
CRITICAL CARE	★★★	PULMONARY	★★★
GASTROINTESTINAL	★★★	STROKE	★★★
GENERAL SURGERY	NR	VASCULAR	NR
MATERNITY CARE	NR	WOMEN'S HEALTH	NR

HEALTHGRADES AWARDS

Hancock Regional Hospital

801 North State Street
Greenfield, IN 46140
(317) 462-5544

Overall patient safety: ★★★
Teaching: N

CLINICAL PROGRAM RATINGS:

CARDIAC	NR	ORTHOPEDICS	NR
CRITICAL CARE	NR	PULMONARY	★★★
GASTROINTESTINAL	NR	STROKE	★★★
GENERAL SURGERY	NR	VASCULAR	NR
MATERNITY CARE	NR	WOMEN'S HEALTH	NR

HEALTHGRADES AWARDS

Henry County Memorial Hospital

1000 North 16th Street
New Castle, IN 47362
(765) 521-0890

Overall patient safety: ★★★
Teaching: N

CLINICAL PROGRAM RATINGS:

CARDIAC	NR	ORTHOPEDICS	NR
CRITICAL CARE	NR	PULMONARY	★
GASTROINTESTINAL	★★★	STROKE	★
GENERAL SURGERY	NR	VASCULAR	NR
MATERNITY CARE	NR	WOMEN'S HEALTH	NR

HEALTHGRADES AWARDS

KEY: ★★★★★ BEST ★★★ AS EXPECTED ★ POOR NR NOT RATED BY HEALTHGRADES   For full definitions of ratings and awards, see Appendix.

Howard Regional Health System

3500 South Lafountain Street
Kokomo, IN 46902
(765) 453-0702

Overall patient safety: ★★★
Teaching: N

CLINICAL PROGRAM RATINGS:

CARDIAC	NR	ORTHOPEDICS	NR
CRITICAL CARE	NR	PULMONARY	★★★
GASTROINTESTINAL	★★★	STROKE	★★★
GENERAL SURGERY	NR	VASCULAR	NR
MATERNITY CARE	NR	WOMEN'S HEALTH	NR

HEALTHGRADES AWARDS

Indiana University Medical Center*

550 University Boulevard
Indianapolis, IN 46202
(317) 274-4391

Overall patient safety: ★
Teaching: Y

CLINICAL PROGRAM RATINGS:

CARDIAC	★★★	ORTHOPEDICS	★
CRITICAL CARE	★★★	PULMONARY	★★★★★
GASTROINTESTINAL	★★★	STROKE	★★★★★
GENERAL SURGERY	NR	VASCULAR	★★★
MATERNITY CARE	NR	WOMEN'S HEALTH	NR

HEALTHGRADES AWARDS

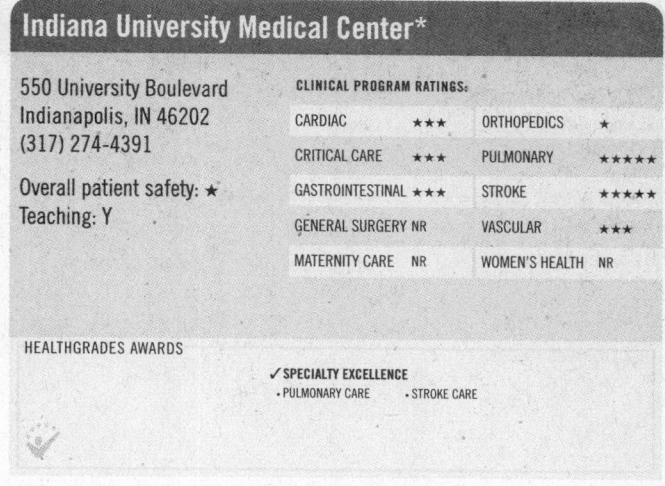

✓ SPECIALTY EXCELLENCE
• PULMONARY CARE   • STROKE CARE

Indiana Heart Hospital

8075 North Shadeland Avenue
Indianapolis, IN 46250
(317) 621-8061

Overall patient safety: ★★★
Teaching: N

CLINICAL PROGRAM RATINGS:

CARDIAC	★★★	ORTHOPEDICS	NR
CRITICAL CARE	NR	PULMONARY	NR
GASTROINTESTINAL	NR	STROKE	NR
GENERAL SURGERY	NR	VASCULAR	★★★
MATERNITY CARE	NR	WOMEN'S HEALTH	NR

HEALTHGRADES AWARDS

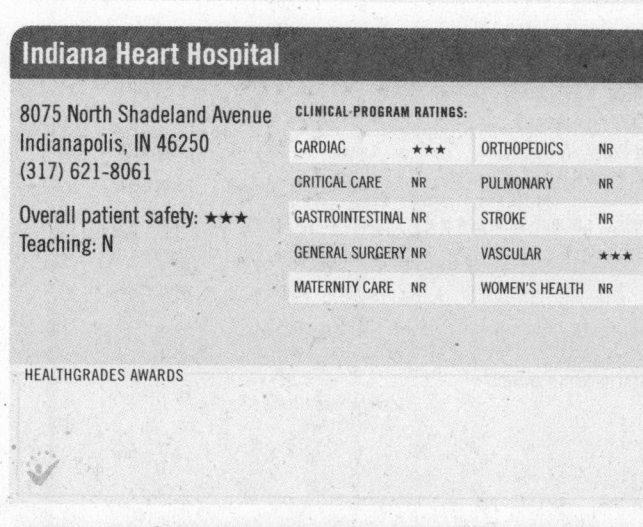

Jasper County Hospital

1104 East Grace Street
Rensselaer, IN 47978
(219) 866-5141

Overall patient safety: ★★★
Teaching: N

CLINICAL PROGRAM RATINGS:

CARDIAC	NR	ORTHOPEDICS	NR
CRITICAL CARE	NR	PULMONARY	★
GASTROINTESTINAL	NR	STROKE	★★★
GENERAL SURGERY	NR	VASCULAR	NR
MATERNITY CARE	NR	WOMEN'S HEALTH	NR

HEALTHGRADES AWARDS

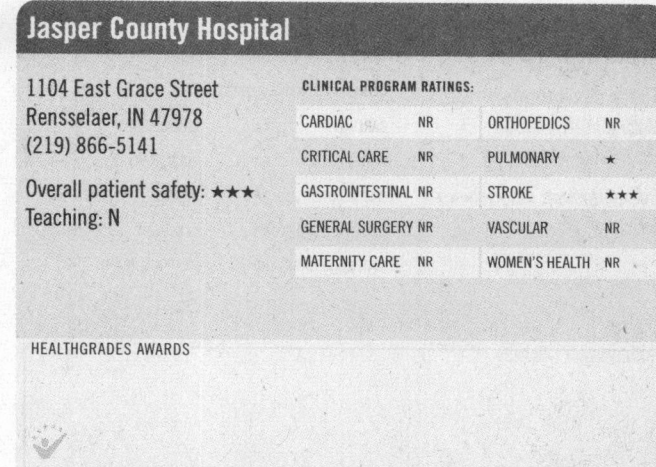

Indiana Orthopaedic Hospital

8400 Northwest Boulevard
Indianapolis, IN 46278
(317) 956-1000

Overall patient safety: ★★★
Teaching: N

CLINICAL PROGRAM RATINGS:

CARDIAC	NR	ORTHOPEDICS	NR
CRITICAL CARE	NR	PULMONARY	NR
GASTROINTESTINAL	NR	STROKE	NR
GENERAL SURGERY	NR	VASCULAR	NR
MATERNITY CARE	NR	WOMEN'S HEALTH	NR

HEALTHGRADES AWARDS

✓ SPECIALTY EXCELLENCE
• JOINT REPLACEMENT

Jay County Hospital

500 West Votaw Street
Portland, IN 47371
(260) 726-7131

Overall patient safety: ★★★
Teaching: N

CLINICAL PROGRAM RATINGS:

CARDIAC	NR	ORTHOPEDICS	NR
CRITICAL CARE	NR	PULMONARY	★★★
GASTROINTESTINAL	NR	STROKE	NR
GENERAL SURGERY	NR	VASCULAR	NR
MATERNITY CARE	NR	WOMEN'S HEALTH	NR

HEALTHGRADES AWARDS

*This hospital reports its data to the federal government jointly with another hospital. Therefore the ratings and awards apply to multiple hospitals and this specific hospital may not provide all rated services.

Johnson Memorial Hospital

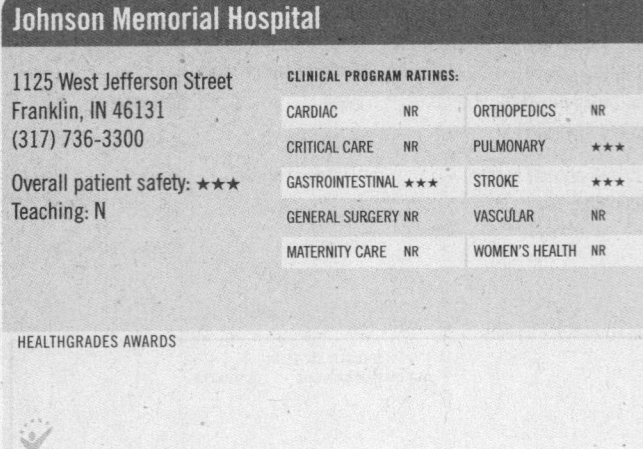

1125 West Jefferson Street
Franklin, IN 46131
(317) 736-3300

Overall patient safety: ★★★
Teaching: N

CLINICAL PROGRAM RATINGS:

CARDIAC	NR	ORTHOPEDICS	NR
CRITICAL CARE	NR	PULMONARY	★★★
GASTROINTESTINAL	★★★	STROKE	★★★
GENERAL SURGERY	NR	VASCULAR	NR
MATERNITY CARE	NR	WOMEN'S HEALTH	NR

HEALTHGRADES AWARDS

Lafayette Home Hospital

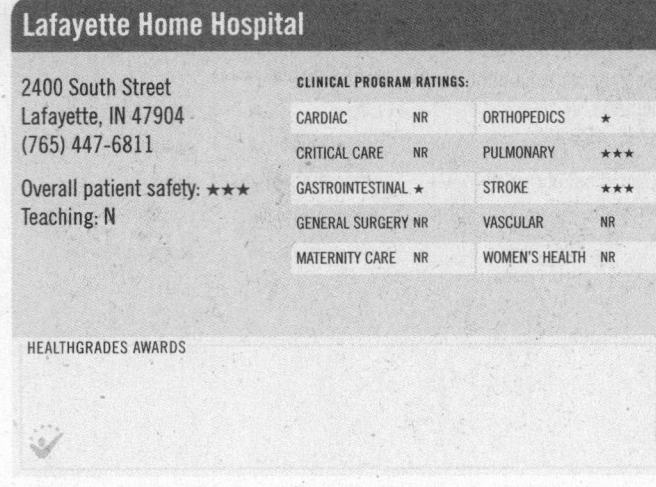

2400 South Street
Lafayette, IN 47904
(765) 447-6811

Overall patient safety: ★★★
Teaching: N

CLINICAL PROGRAM RATINGS:

CARDIAC	NR	ORTHOPEDICS	★
CRITICAL CARE	NR	PULMONARY	★★★
GASTROINTESTINAL	★	STROKE	★★★
GENERAL SURGERY	NR	VASCULAR	NR
MATERNITY CARE	NR	WOMEN'S HEALTH	NR

HEALTHGRADES AWARDS

The King's Daughters' Hospital and Health Services

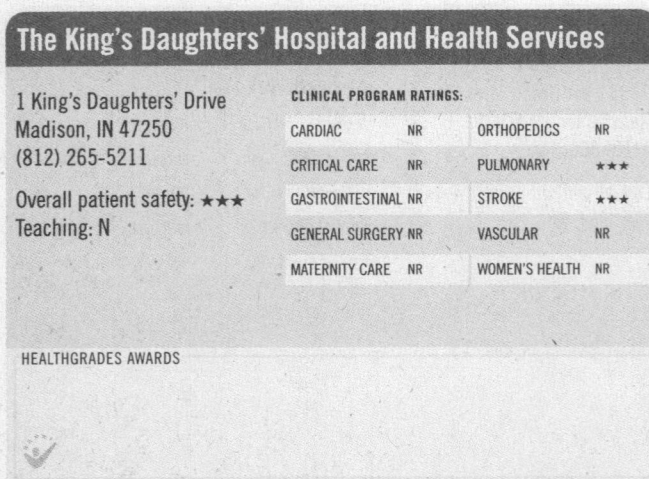

1 King's Daughters' Drive
Madison, IN 47250
(812) 265-5211

Overall patient safety: ★★★
Teaching: N

CLINICAL PROGRAM RATINGS:

CARDIAC	NR	ORTHOPEDICS	NR
CRITICAL CARE	NR	PULMONARY	★★★
GASTROINTESTINAL	NR	STROKE	★★★
GENERAL SURGERY	NR	VASCULAR	NR
MATERNITY CARE	NR	WOMEN'S HEALTH	NR

HEALTHGRADES AWARDS

Laporte Hospital and Health Services

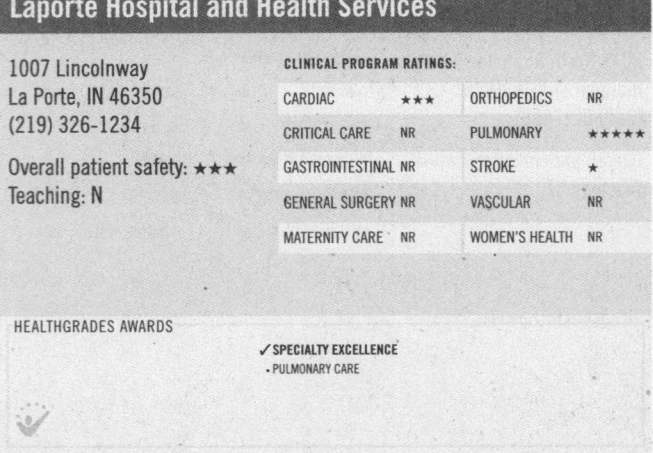

1007 Lincolnway
La Porte, IN 46350
(219) 326-1234

Overall patient safety: ★★★
Teaching: N

CLINICAL PROGRAM RATINGS:

CARDIAC	★★★	ORTHOPEDICS	NR
CRITICAL CARE	NR	PULMONARY	★★★★★
GASTROINTESTINAL	NR	STROKE	★
GENERAL SURGERY	NR	VASCULAR	NR
MATERNITY CARE	NR	WOMEN'S HEALTH	NR

HEALTHGRADES AWARDS

✓ SPECIALTY EXCELLENCE
- PULMONARY CARE

Kosciusko Community Hospital

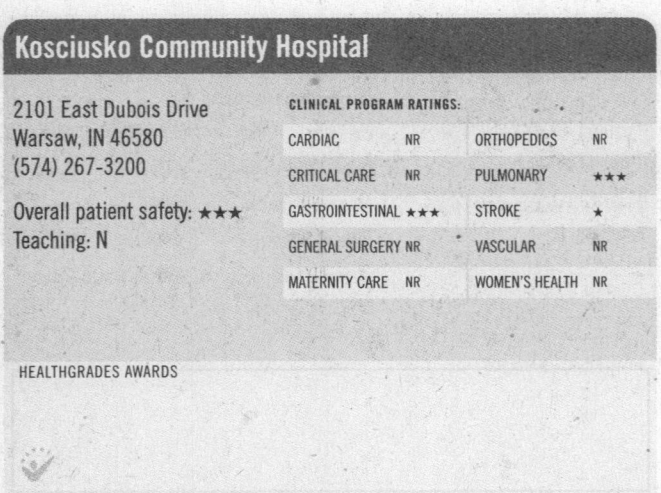

2101 East Dubois Drive
Warsaw, IN 46580
(574) 267-3200

Overall patient safety: ★★★
Teaching: N

CLINICAL PROGRAM RATINGS:

CARDIAC	NR	ORTHOPEDICS	NR
CRITICAL CARE	NR	PULMONARY	★★★
GASTROINTESTINAL	★★★	STROKE	★
GENERAL SURGERY	NR	VASCULAR	NR
MATERNITY CARE	NR	WOMEN'S HEALTH	NR

HEALTHGRADES AWARDS

Lutheran Hospital of Indiana

7950 West Jefferson Boulevard
Fort Wayne, IN 46804
(219) 435-7001

Overall patient safety: ★★★★★
Teaching: Y

CLINICAL PROGRAM RATINGS:

CARDIAC	★★★	ORTHOPEDICS	★★★
CRITICAL CARE	★★★	PULMONARY	★★★
GASTROINTESTINAL	★★★	STROKE	★★★
GENERAL SURGERY	NR	VASCULAR	★★★
MATERNITY CARE	NR	WOMEN'S HEALTH	NR

HEALTHGRADES AWARDS

✓ DISTINGUISHED
HOSPITAL
- PATIENT SAFETY

KEY: ★★★★★ BEST   ★★★ AS EXPECTED   ★ POOR   NR NOT RATED BY HEALTHGRADES   For full definitions of ratings and awards, see Appendix.

Major Hospital

150 West Washington Street
Shelbyville, IN 46176
(317) 392-3211

Overall patient safety: ★★★
Teaching: N

CLINICAL PROGRAM RATINGS:

CARDIAC	NR	ORTHOPEDICS	NR
CRITICAL CARE	NR	PULMONARY	★★★
GASTROINTESTINAL	NR	STROKE	★★★
GENERAL SURGERY	NR	VASCULAR	NR
MATERNITY CARE	NR	WOMEN'S HEALTH	NR

HEALTHGRADES AWARDS

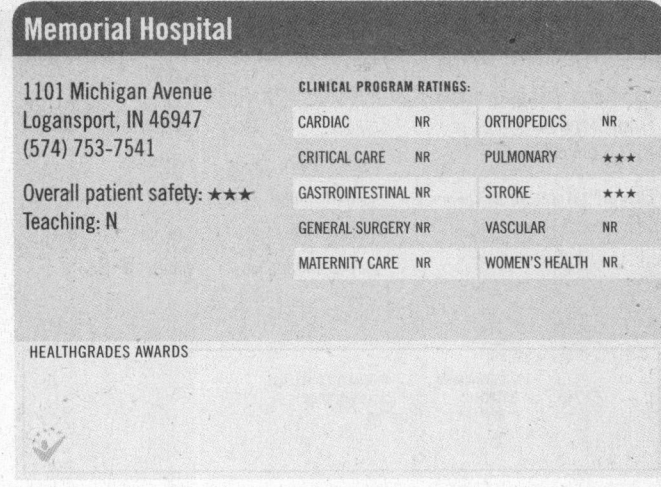

Memorial Hospital

1101 Michigan Avenue
Logansport, IN 46947
(574) 753-7541

Overall patient safety: ★★★
Teaching: N

CLINICAL PROGRAM RATINGS:

CARDIAC	NR	ORTHOPEDICS	NR
CRITICAL CARE	NR	PULMONARY	★★★
GASTROINTESTINAL	NR	STROKE	★★★
GENERAL SURGERY	NR	VASCULAR	NR
MATERNITY CARE	NR	WOMEN'S HEALTH	NR

HEALTHGRADES AWARDS

Margaret Mary Community Hospital

321 Mitchell Avenue
Batesville, IN 47006
(812) 934-6624

Overall patient safety: ★★★★★
Teaching: N

CLINICAL PROGRAM RATINGS:

CARDIAC	NR	ORTHOPEDICS	NR
CRITICAL CARE	NR	PULMONARY	★★★
GASTROINTESTINAL	NR	STROKE	★★★
GENERAL SURGERY	NR	VASCULAR	NR
MATERNITY CARE	NR	WOMEN'S HEALTH	NR

HEALTHGRADES AWARDS

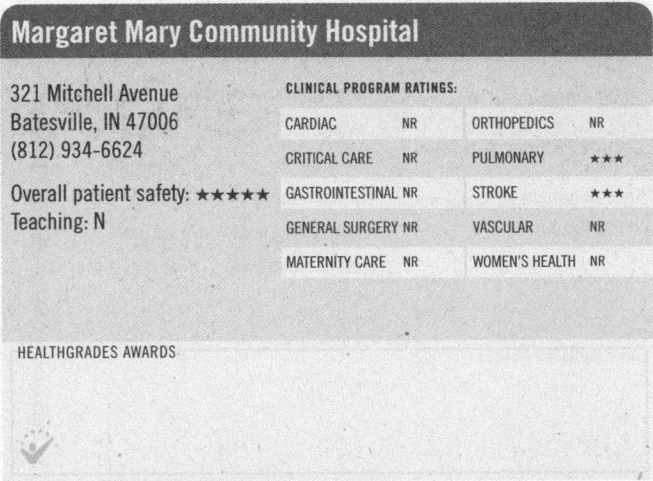

Memorial Hospital and Health Care Center

800 West 9th Street
Jasper, IN 47546
(812) 482-2345

Overall patient safety: ★★★
Teaching: N

CLINICAL PROGRAM RATINGS:

CARDIAC	NR	ORTHOPEDICS	NR
CRITICAL CARE	NR	PULMONARY	★★★
GASTROINTESTINAL	★★★	STROKE	★★★
GENERAL SURGERY	NR	VASCULAR	NR
MATERNITY CARE	NR	WOMEN'S HEALTH	NR

HEALTHGRADES AWARDS

Marion General Hospital

441 North Wabash Avenue
Marion, IN 46952
(765) 662-1441

Overall patient safety: ★★★
Teaching: N

CLINICAL PROGRAM RATINGS:

CARDIAC	NR	ORTHOPEDICS	★★★★★
CRITICAL CARE	NR	PULMONARY	★
GASTROINTESTINAL	★★★	STROKE	★
GENERAL SURGERY	NR	VASCULAR	NR
MATERNITY CARE	NR	WOMEN'S HEALTH	NR

HEALTHGRADES AWARDS

✓ **SPECIALTY EXCELLENCE**
• ORTHOPEDIC
  SURGERY

Memorial Hospital of Michigan City*

5th and Pine Streets
Michigan City, IN 46360
(219) 873-2491

Overall patient safety: ★★★
Teaching: N

CLINICAL PROGRAM RATINGS:

CARDIAC	NR	ORTHOPEDICS	★★★
CRITICAL CARE	NR	PULMONARY	★★★
GASTROINTESTINAL	NR	STROKE	★★★
GENERAL SURGERY	NR	VASCULAR	NR
MATERNITY CARE	NR	WOMEN'S HEALTH	NR

HEALTHGRADES AWARDS

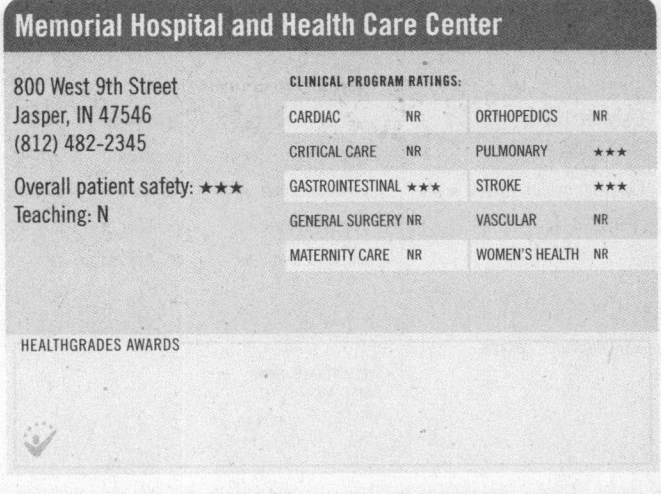

*This hospital reports its data to the federal government jointly with another hospital. Therefore the ratings and awards apply to multiple hospitals and this specific hospital may not provide all rated services.

INDIANA HOSPITALS: RATINGS BY CLINICAL SPECIALTY

Memorial Hospital of South Bend

615 North Michigan Street
South Bend, IN 46601
(574) 234-9041

Overall patient safety: ★★★★★
Teaching: Y

CLINICAL PROGRAM RATINGS:

CARDIAC	★★★	ORTHOPEDICS	★★★
CRITICAL CARE	★★★	PULMONARY	★★★
GASTROINTESTINAL	★★★	STROKE	★
GENERAL SURGERY	NR	VASCULAR	★★★
MATERNITY CARE	NR	WOMEN'S HEALTH	NR

HEALTHGRADES AWARDS

✓ DISTINGUISHED HOSPITAL
• PATIENT SAFETY

✓ SPECIALTY EXCELLENCE
• GASTROINTESTINAL CARE

Morgan Hospital and Medical Center

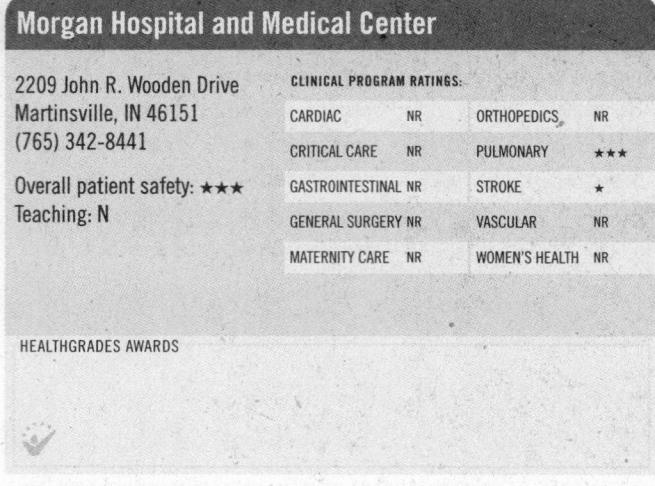

2209 John R. Wooden Drive
Martinsville, IN 46151
(765) 342-8441

Overall patient safety: ★★★
Teaching: N

CLINICAL PROGRAM RATINGS:

CARDIAC	NR	ORTHOPEDICS	NR
CRITICAL CARE	NR	PULMONARY	★★★
GASTROINTESTINAL	NR	STROKE	★
GENERAL SURGERY	NR	VASCULAR	NR
MATERNITY CARE	NR	WOMEN'S HEALTH	NR

HEALTHGRADES AWARDS

Methodist Hospital*

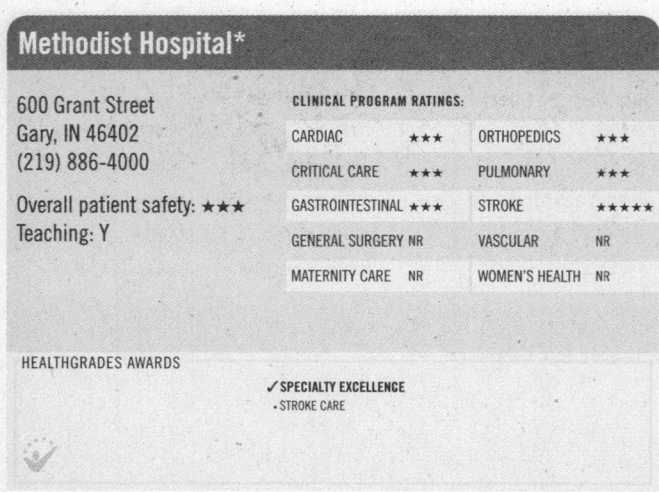

600 Grant Street
Gary, IN 46402
(219) 886-4000

Overall patient safety: ★★★
Teaching: Y

CLINICAL PROGRAM RATINGS:

CARDIAC	★★★	ORTHOPEDICS	★★★
CRITICAL CARE	★★★	PULMONARY	★★★
GASTROINTESTINAL	★★★	STROKE	★★★★★
GENERAL SURGERY	NR	VASCULAR	NR
MATERNITY CARE	NR	WOMEN'S HEALTH	NR

HEALTHGRADES AWARDS

✓ SPECIALTY EXCELLENCE
• STROKE CARE

Parkview Hospital

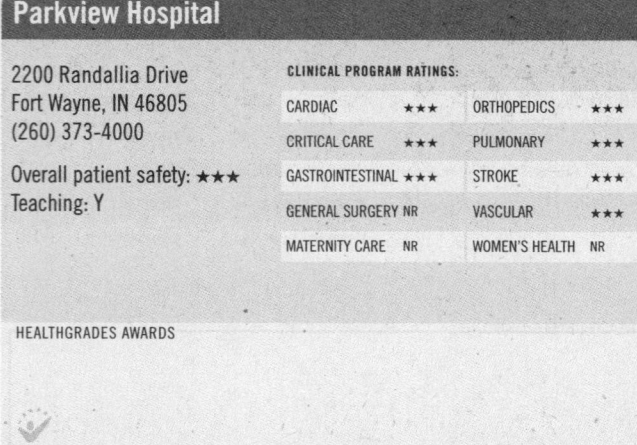

2200 Randallia Drive
Fort Wayne, IN 46805
(260) 373-4000

Overall patient safety: ★★★
Teaching: Y

CLINICAL PROGRAM RATINGS:

CARDIAC	★★★	ORTHOPEDICS	★★★
CRITICAL CARE	★★★	PULMONARY	★★★
GASTROINTESTINAL	★★★	STROKE	★★★
GENERAL SURGERY	NR	VASCULAR	★★★
MATERNITY CARE	NR	WOMEN'S HEALTH	NR

HEALTHGRADES AWARDS

Methodist Hospital Southlake*

8701 Broadway
Merrillville, IN 46410
(219) 738-5500

Overall patient safety: ★★★
Teaching: Y

CLINICAL PROGRAM RATINGS:

CARDIAC	★★★	ORTHOPEDICS	★★★
CRITICAL CARE	★★★	PULMONARY	★★★
GASTROINTESTINAL	★★★	STROKE	★★★★★
GENERAL SURGERY	NR	VASCULAR	NR
MATERNITY CARE	NR	WOMEN'S HEALTH	NR

HEALTHGRADES AWARDS

✓ SPECIALTY EXCELLENCE
• STROKE CARE

Parkview Huntington Hospital

2001 Stults Road
Huntington, IN 46750
(219) 355-3000

Overall patient safety: ★★★
Teaching: N

CLINICAL PROGRAM RATINGS:

CARDIAC	NR	ORTHOPEDICS	NR
CRITICAL CARE	NR	PULMONARY	★★★
GASTROINTESTINAL	NR	STROKE	★★★
GENERAL SURGERY	NR	VASCULAR	NR
MATERNITY CARE	NR	WOMEN'S HEALTH	NR

HEALTHGRADES AWARDS

KEY: ★★★★★ BEST   ★★★ AS EXPECTED   ★ POOR   NR NOT RATED BY HEALTHGRADES   For full definitions of ratings and awards, see Appendix.

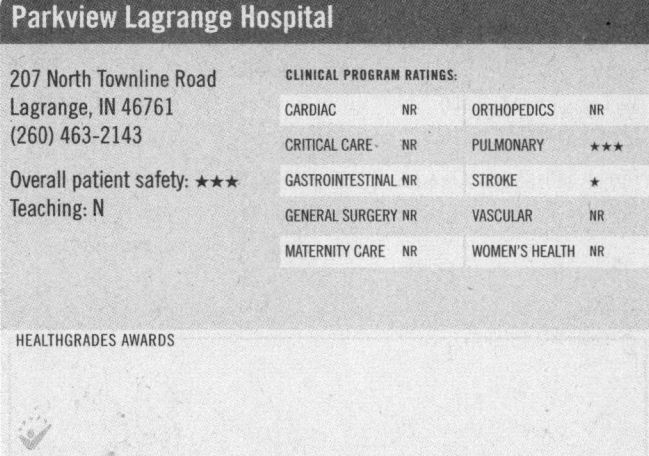

Parkview Lagrange Hospital

207 North Townline Road
Lagrange, IN 46761
(260) 463-2143

Overall patient safety: ★★★
Teaching: N

CLINICAL PROGRAM RATINGS:

CARDIAC	NR	ORTHOPEDICS	NR
CRITICAL CARE	NR	PULMONARY	★★★
GASTROINTESTINAL	NR	STROKE	★
GENERAL SURGERY	NR	VASCULAR	NR
MATERNITY CARE	NR	WOMEN'S HEALTH	NR

HEALTHGRADES AWARDS

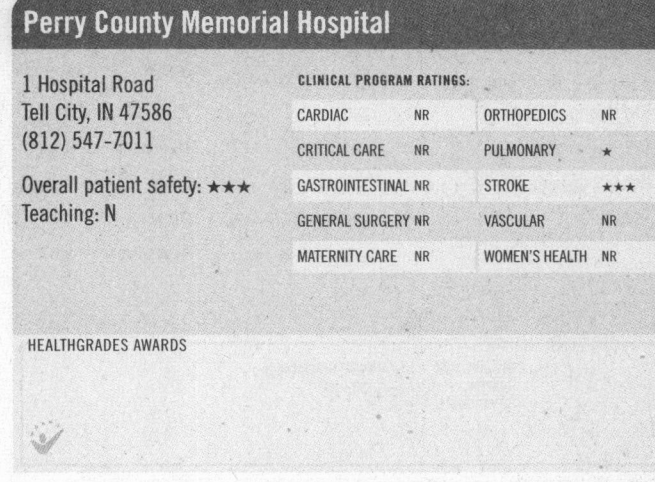

Perry County Memorial Hospital

1 Hospital Road
Tell City, IN 47586
(812) 547-7011

Overall patient safety: ★★★
Teaching: N

CLINICAL PROGRAM RATINGS:

CARDIAC	NR	ORTHOPEDICS	NR
CRITICAL CARE	NR	PULMONARY	★
GASTROINTESTINAL	NR	STROKE	★★★
GENERAL SURGERY	NR	VASCULAR	NR
MATERNITY CARE	NR	WOMEN'S HEALTH	NR

HEALTHGRADES AWARDS

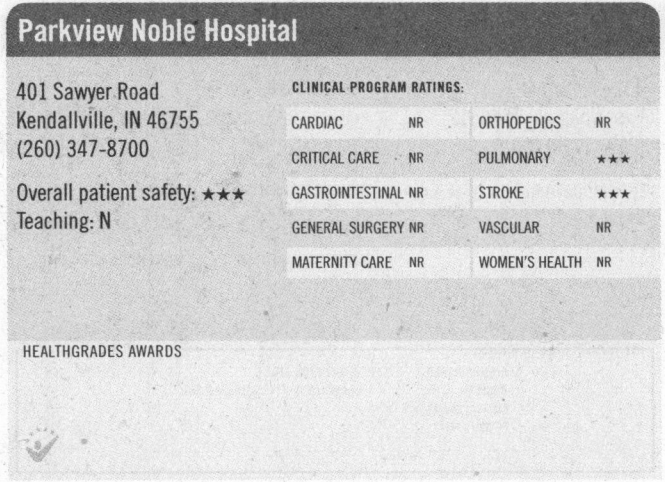

Parkview Noble Hospital

401 Sawyer Road
Kendallville, IN 46755
(260) 347-8700

Overall patient safety: ★★★
Teaching: N

CLINICAL PROGRAM RATINGS:

CARDIAC	NR	ORTHOPEDICS	NR
CRITICAL CARE	NR	PULMONARY	★★★
GASTROINTESTINAL	NR	STROKE	★★★
GENERAL SURGERY	NR	VASCULAR	NR
MATERNITY CARE	NR	WOMEN'S HEALTH	NR

HEALTHGRADES AWARDS

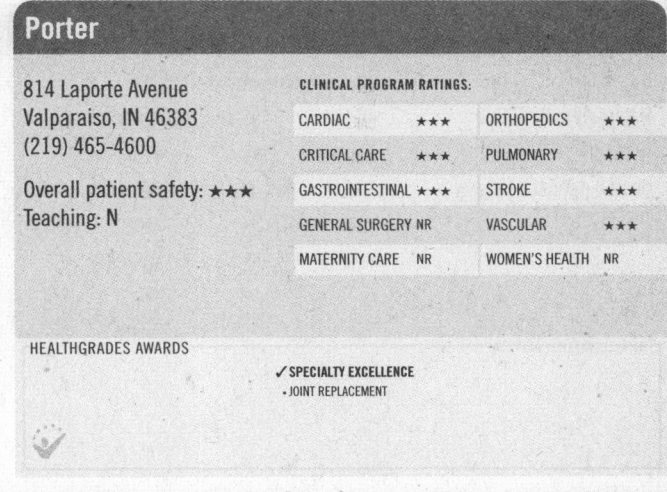

Porter

814 Laporte Avenue
Valparaiso, IN 46383
(219) 465-4600

Overall patient safety: ★★★
Teaching: N

CLINICAL PROGRAM RATINGS:

CARDIAC	★★★	ORTHOPEDICS	★★★
CRITICAL CARE	★★★	PULMONARY	★★★
GASTROINTESTINAL	★★★	STROKE	★★★
GENERAL SURGERY	NR	VASCULAR	★★★
MATERNITY CARE	NR	WOMEN'S HEALTH	NR

HEALTHGRADES AWARDS

✓ SPECIALTY EXCELLENCE
• JOINT REPLACEMENT

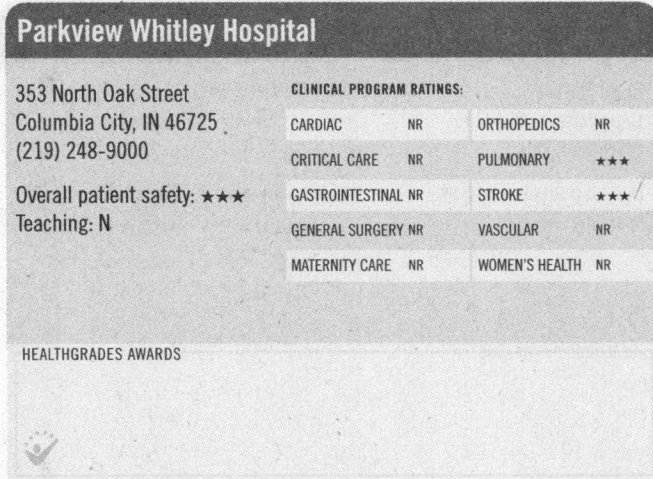

Parkview Whitley Hospital

353 North Oak Street
Columbia City, IN 46725
(219) 248-9000

Overall patient safety: ★★★
Teaching: N

CLINICAL PROGRAM RATINGS:

CARDIAC	NR	ORTHOPEDICS	NR
CRITICAL CARE	NR	PULMONARY	★★★
GASTROINTESTINAL	NR	STROKE	★★★
GENERAL SURGERY	NR	VASCULAR	NR
MATERNITY CARE	NR	WOMEN'S HEALTH	NR

HEALTHGRADES AWARDS

Putnam County Hospital

1542 South Blomington Street
Greencastle, IN 46135
(765) 655-2620

Overall patient safety: ★
Teaching: N

CLINICAL PROGRAM RATINGS:

CARDIAC	NR	ORTHOPEDICS	NR
CRITICAL CARE	NR	PULMONARY	★
GASTROINTESTINAL	NR	STROKE	NR
GENERAL SURGERY	NR	VASCULAR	NR
MATERNITY CARE	NR	WOMEN'S HEALTH	NR

HEALTHGRADES AWARDS

*This hospital reports its data to the federal government jointly with another hospital. Therefore the ratings and awards apply to multiple hospitals and this specific hospital may not provide all rated services.

INDIANA HOSPITALS: RATINGS BY CLINICAL SPECIALTY

Reid Hospital and Health Care Services

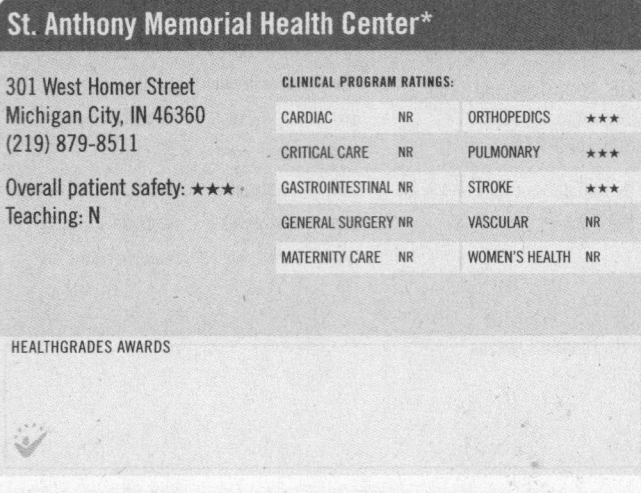

1401 Chester Boulevard
Richmond, IN 47374
(765) 983-3000

Overall patient safety: ★★★★★
Teaching: N

CLINICAL PROGRAM RATINGS:

CARDIAC	★★★	ORTHOPEDICS	★★★
CRITICAL CARE	NR	PULMONARY	★★★
GASTROINTESTINAL	★★★	STROKE	★★★★★
GENERAL SURGERY	NR	VASCULAR	★★★
MATERNITY CARE	NR	WOMEN'S HEALTH	NR

HEALTHGRADES AWARDS

✓ DISTINGUISHED HOSPITAL
 • PATIENT SAFETY

✓ SPECIALTY EXCELLENCE
 • STROKE CARE

St. Anthony Memorial Health Center*

301 West Homer Street
Michigan City, IN 46360
(219) 879-8511

Overall patient safety: ★★★
Teaching: N

CLINICAL PROGRAM RATINGS:

CARDIAC	NR	ORTHOPEDICS	★★★
CRITICAL CARE	NR	PULMONARY	★★★
GASTROINTESTINAL	NR	STROKE	★★★
GENERAL SURGERY	NR	VASCULAR	NR
MATERNITY CARE	NR	WOMEN'S HEALTH	NR

HEALTHGRADES AWARDS

Riverview Hospital

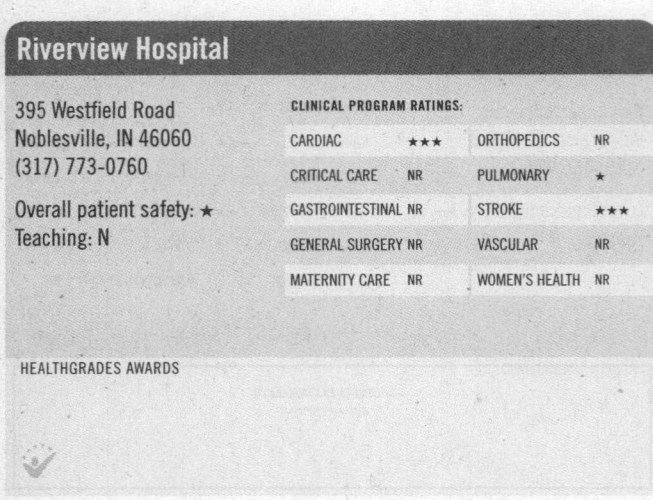

395 Westfield Road
Noblesville, IN 46060
(317) 773-0760

Overall patient safety: ★
Teaching: N

CLINICAL PROGRAM RATINGS:

CARDIAC	★★★	ORTHOPEDICS	NR
CRITICAL CARE	NR	PULMONARY	★
GASTROINTESTINAL	NR	STROKE	★★★
GENERAL SURGERY	NR	VASCULAR	NR
MATERNITY CARE	NR	WOMEN'S HEALTH	NR

HEALTHGRADES AWARDS

St. Catherine Hospital

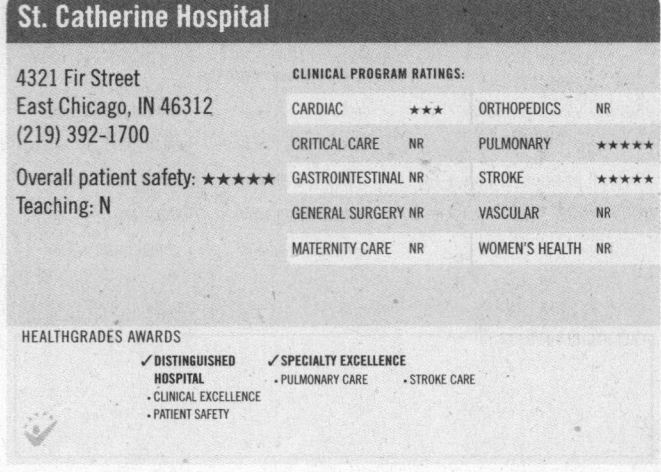

4321 Fir Street
East Chicago, IN 46312
(219) 392-1700

Overall patient safety: ★★★★★
Teaching: N

CLINICAL PROGRAM RATINGS:

CARDIAC	★★★	ORTHOPEDICS	NR
CRITICAL CARE	NR	PULMONARY	★★★★★
GASTROINTESTINAL	NR	STROKE	★★★★★
GENERAL SURGERY	NR	VASCULAR	NR
MATERNITY CARE	NR	WOMEN'S HEALTH	NR

HEALTHGRADES AWARDS

✓ DISTINGUISHED HOSPITAL
 • CLINICAL EXCELLENCE
 • PATIENT SAFETY

✓ SPECIALTY EXCELLENCE
 • PULMONARY CARE • STROKE CARE

St. Anthony Medical Center of Crown Point

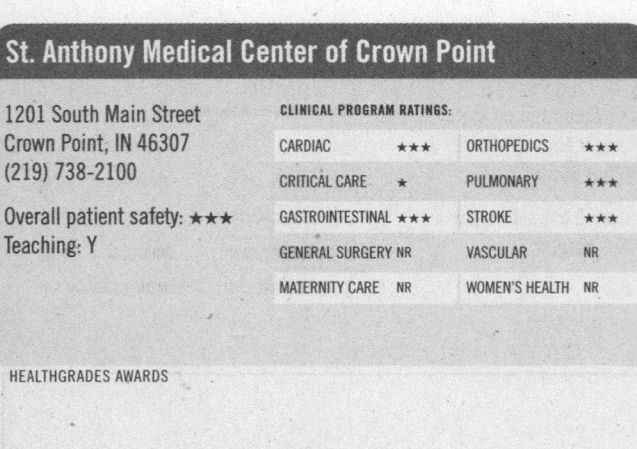

1201 South Main Street
Crown Point, IN 46307
(219) 738-2100

Overall patient safety: ★★★
Teaching: Y

CLINICAL PROGRAM RATINGS:

CARDIAC	★★★	ORTHOPEDICS	★★★
CRITICAL CARE	★	PULMONARY	★★★
GASTROINTESTINAL	★★★	STROKE	★★★
GENERAL SURGERY	NR	VASCULAR	NR
MATERNITY CARE	NR	WOMEN'S HEALTH	NR

HEALTHGRADES AWARDS

St. Catherine Regional Hospital

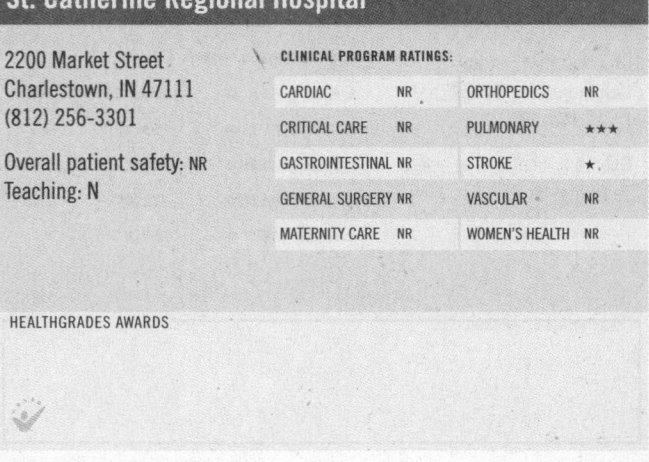

2200 Market Street
Charlestown, IN 47111
(812) 256-3301

Overall patient safety: NR
Teaching: N

CLINICAL PROGRAM RATINGS:

CARDIAC	NR	ORTHOPEDICS	NR
CRITICAL CARE	NR	PULMONARY	★★★
GASTROINTESTINAL	NR	STROKE	★
GENERAL SURGERY	NR	VASCULAR	NR
MATERNITY CARE	NR	WOMEN'S HEALTH	NR

HEALTHGRADES AWARDS

KEY: ★★★★★ BEST ★★★ AS EXPECTED ★ POOR NR NOT RATED BY HEALTHGRADES   For full definitions of ratings and awards, see Appendix.

St. Clare Medical Center

1710 Lafayette Road
Crawfordsville, IN 47933
(765) 362-2800

Overall patient safety: ★★★
Teaching: N

CLINICAL PROGRAM RATINGS:

CARDIAC	NR	ORTHOPEDICS	NR
CRITICAL CARE	NR	PULMONARY	★★★
GASTROINTESTINAL	NR	STROKE	★
GENERAL SURGERY	NR	VASCULAR	NR
MATERNITY CARE	NR	WOMEN'S HEALTH	NR

HEALTHGRADES AWARDS

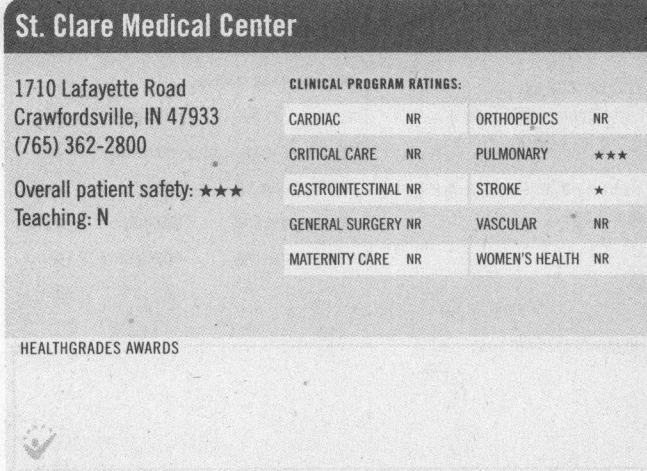

St. Elizabeth Medical Center

1501 Hartford Street
Lafayette, IN 47904
(765) 423-6011

Overall patient safety: ★★★
Teaching: N

CLINICAL PROGRAM RATINGS:

CARDIAC	★★★	ORTHOPEDICS	★★★
CRITICAL CARE	★★★	PULMONARY	★★★
GASTROINTESTINAL	★★★	STROKE	★
GENERAL SURGERY	NR	VASCULAR	NR
MATERNITY CARE	NR	WOMEN'S HEALTH	NR

HEALTHGRADES AWARDS

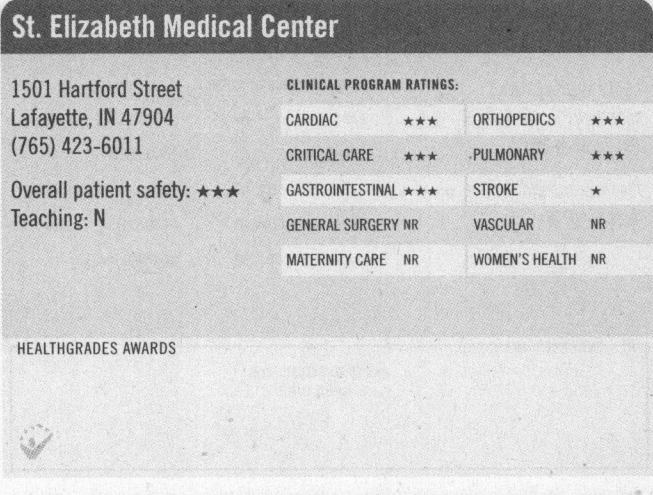

St. Elizabeth Ann Seton Hospital

1116 Millis Avenue
P.O. Box 290
Boonville, IN 47601
(812) 897-7400

Overall patient safety: ★★★
Teaching: N

CLINICAL PROGRAM RATINGS:

CARDIAC	NR	ORTHOPEDICS	NR
CRITICAL CARE	NR	PULMONARY	★★★
GASTROINTESTINAL	NR	STROKE	NR
GENERAL SURGERY	NR	VASCULAR	NR
MATERNITY CARE	NR	WOMEN'S HEALTH	NR

HEALTHGRADES AWARDS

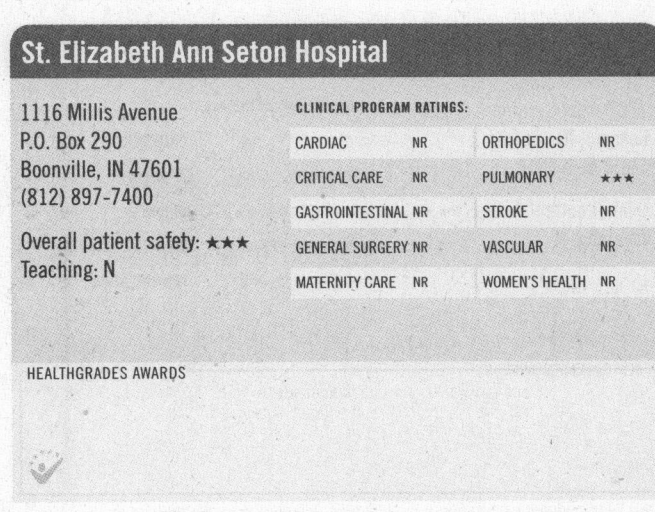

St. Francis Hospital and Health Center

1600 Albany Street
Beech Grove, IN 46107
(317) 787-3311

Overall patient safety: ★★★
Teaching: Y

CLINICAL PROGRAM RATINGS:

CARDIAC	★★★	ORTHOPEDICS	★★★★★
CRITICAL CARE	★★★	PULMONARY	★★★★★
GASTROINTESTINAL	★★★	STROKE	★★★★★
GENERAL SURGERY	NR	VASCULAR	★
MATERNITY CARE	NR	WOMEN'S HEALTH	NR

HEALTHGRADES AWARDS

✓ SPECIALTY EXCELLENCE
- JOINT REPLACEMENT   - ORTHOPEDIC SURGERY   - STROKE CARE

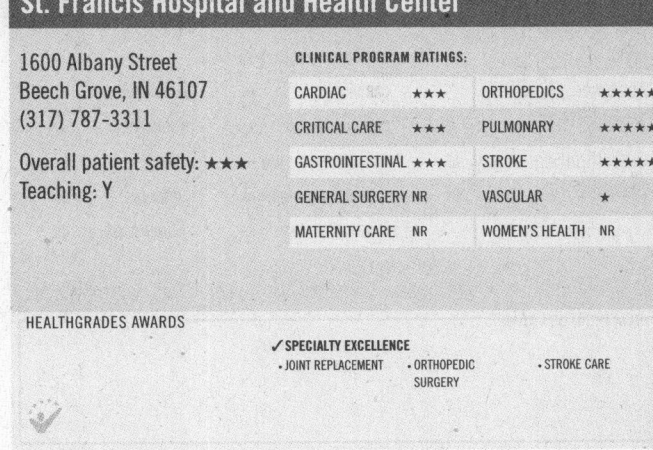

St. Elizabeth Ann Seton Speciality Care

13500 North Meridian
2nd Floor
Carmel, IN 46032
(317) 582-8500

Overall patient safety: ★★★
Teaching: N

CLINICAL PROGRAM RATINGS:

CARDIAC	NR	ORTHOPEDICS	★★★
CRITICAL CARE	NR	PULMONARY	★★★
GASTROINTESTINAL	NR	STROKE	★★★
GENERAL SURGERY	NR	VASCULAR	NR
MATERNITY CARE	NR	WOMEN'S HEALTH	NR

HEALTHGRADES AWARDS

✓ SPECIALTY EXCELLENCE
- JOINT REPLACEMENT

St. Francis Hospital and Health Center

8111 South Emerson Avenue
Indianapolis, IN 46237
(317) 865-5001

Overall patient safety: NR
Teaching: N

CLINICAL PROGRAM RATINGS:

CARDIAC	★★★	ORTHOPEDICS	NR
CRITICAL CARE	NR	PULMONARY	NR
GASTROINTESTINAL	NR	STROKE	NR
GENERAL SURGERY	NR	VASCULAR	NR
MATERNITY CARE	NR	WOMEN'S HEALTH	NR

HEALTHGRADES AWARDS

*This hospital reports its data to the federal government jointly with another hospital. Therefore the ratings and awards apply to multiple hospitals and this specific hospital may not provide all rated services.

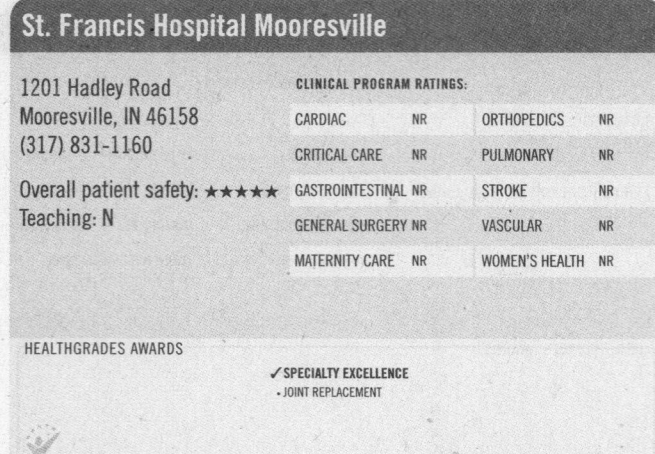

St. Francis Hospital Mooresville

1201 Hadley Road
Mooresville, IN 46158
(317) 831-1160

Overall patient safety: ★★★★★
Teaching: N

CLINICAL PROGRAM RATINGS:

CARDIAC	NR	ORTHOPEDICS	NR
CRITICAL CARE	NR	PULMONARY	NR
GASTROINTESTINAL	NR	STROKE	NR
GENERAL SURGERY	NR	VASCULAR	NR
MATERNITY CARE	NR	WOMEN'S HEALTH	NR

HEALTHGRADES AWARDS

✓ SPECIALTY EXCELLENCE
• JOINT REPLACEMENT

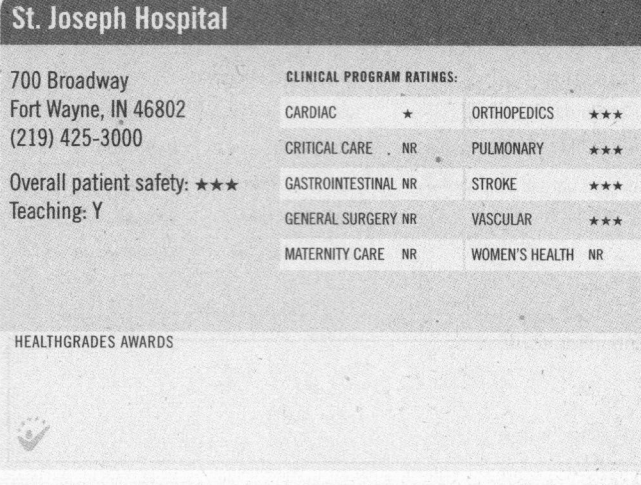

St. Joseph Hospital

700 Broadway
Fort Wayne, IN 46802
(219) 425-3000

Overall patient safety: ★★★
Teaching: Y

CLINICAL PROGRAM RATINGS:

CARDIAC	★	ORTHOPEDICS	★★★
CRITICAL CARE	NR	PULMONARY	★★★
GASTROINTESTINAL	NR	STROKE	★★★
GENERAL SURGERY	NR	VASCULAR	★★★
MATERNITY CARE	NR	WOMEN'S HEALTH	NR

HEALTHGRADES AWARDS

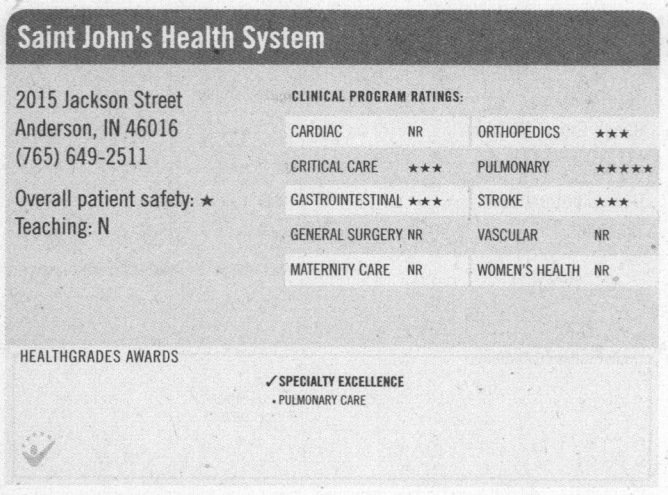

Saint John's Health System

2015 Jackson Street
Anderson, IN 46016
(765) 649-2511

Overall patient safety: ★
Teaching: N

CLINICAL PROGRAM RATINGS:

CARDIAC	NR	ORTHOPEDICS	★★★
CRITICAL CARE	★★★	PULMONARY	★★★★★
GASTROINTESTINAL	★★★	STROKE	★★★
GENERAL SURGERY	NR	VASCULAR	NR
MATERNITY CARE	NR	WOMEN'S HEALTH	NR

HEALTHGRADES AWARDS

✓ SPECIALTY EXCELLENCE
• PULMONARY CARE

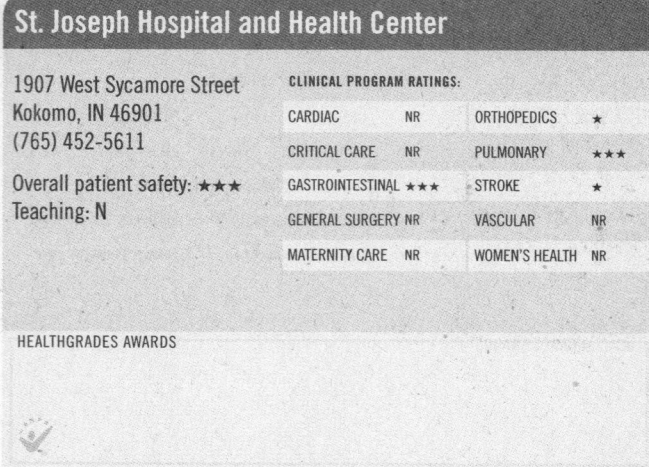

St. Joseph Hospital and Health Center

1907 West Sycamore Street
Kokomo, IN 46901
(765) 452-5611

Overall patient safety: ★★★
Teaching: N

CLINICAL PROGRAM RATINGS:

CARDIAC	NR	ORTHOPEDICS	★
CRITICAL CARE	NR	PULMONARY	★★★
GASTROINTESTINAL	★★★	STROKE	★
GENERAL SURGERY	NR	VASCULAR	NR
MATERNITY CARE	NR	WOMEN'S HEALTH	NR

HEALTHGRADES AWARDS

St. Joseph Community Hospital

215 West 4th Street
Mishawaka, IN 46544
(574) 259-2431

Overall patient safety: ★★★★★
Teaching: Y

CLINICAL PROGRAM RATINGS:

CARDIAC	NR	ORTHOPEDICS	NR
CRITICAL CARE	NR	PULMONARY	★
GASTROINTESTINAL	NR	STROKE	★★★
GENERAL SURGERY	NR	VASCULAR	NR
MATERNITY CARE	NR	WOMEN'S HEALTH	NR

HEALTHGRADES AWARDS

✓ DISTINGUISHED
HOSPITAL
• PATIENT SAFETY

St. Joseph Regional Medical Center

1915 Lake Avenue
Plymouth, IN 46563
(574) 936-3181

Overall patient safety: ★★★
Teaching: N

CLINICAL PROGRAM RATINGS:

CARDIAC	NR	ORTHOPEDICS	NR
CRITICAL CARE	NR	PULMONARY	★★★
GASTROINTESTINAL	NR	STROKE	★★★
GENERAL SURGERY	NR	VASCULAR	NR
MATERNITY CARE	NR	WOMEN'S HEALTH	NR

HEALTHGRADES AWARDS

KEY: ★★★★★ BEST   ★★★ AS EXPECTED   ★ POOR   NR NOT RATED BY HEALTHGRADES   For full definitions of ratings and awards, see Appendix.

St. Joseph Regional Medical Center–South Bend

801 East Lasalle Avenue
South Bend, IN 46617
(574) 237-7111

Overall patient safety: ★★★
Teaching: Y

CLINICAL PROGRAM RATINGS:

CARDIAC	★★★	ORTHOPEDICS	★★★★★
CRITICAL CARE	★★★	PULMONARY	★★★
GASTROINTESTINAL	★★★	STROKE	★★★
GENERAL SURGERY	NR	VASCULAR	NR
MATERNITY CARE	NR	WOMEN'S HEALTH	NR

HEALTHGRADES AWARDS

✓ SPECIALTY EXCELLENCE
- JOINT REPLACEMENT
- ORTHOPEDIC SURGERY

St. Mary's Medical Center–Evansville*

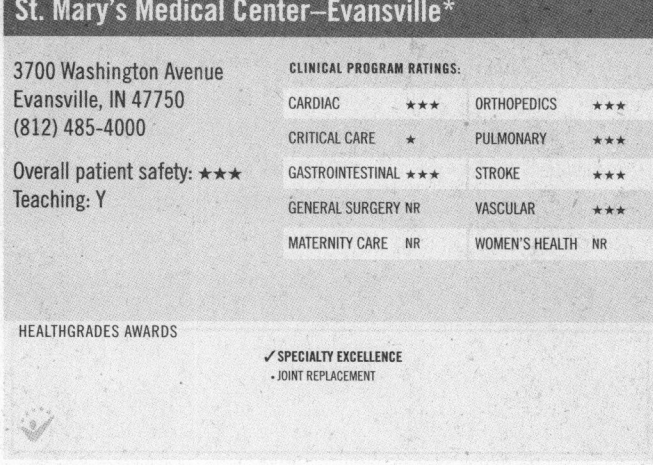

3700 Washington Avenue
Evansville, IN 47750
(812) 485-4000

Overall patient safety: ★★★
Teaching: Y

CLINICAL PROGRAM RATINGS:

CARDIAC	★★★	ORTHOPEDICS	★★★
CRITICAL CARE	★	PULMONARY	★★★
GASTROINTESTINAL	★★★	STROKE	★★★
GENERAL SURGERY	NR	VASCULAR	★★★
MATERNITY CARE	NR	WOMEN'S HEALTH	NR

HEALTHGRADES AWARDS

✓ SPECIALTY EXCELLENCE
- JOINT REPLACEMENT

St. Margaret Mercy Healthcare Center

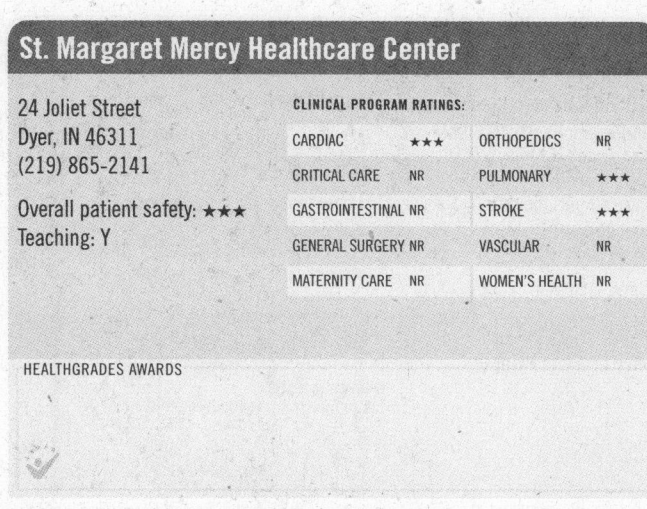

24 Joliet Street
Dyer, IN 46311
(219) 865-2141

Overall patient safety: ★★★
Teaching: Y

CLINICAL PROGRAM RATINGS:

CARDIAC	★★★	ORTHOPEDICS	NR
CRITICAL CARE	NR	PULMONARY	★★★
GASTROINTESTINAL	NR	STROKE	★★★
GENERAL SURGERY	NR	VASCULAR	NR
MATERNITY CARE	NR	WOMEN'S HEALTH	NR

HEALTHGRADES AWARDS

St. Mary's Medical Center–Hobart

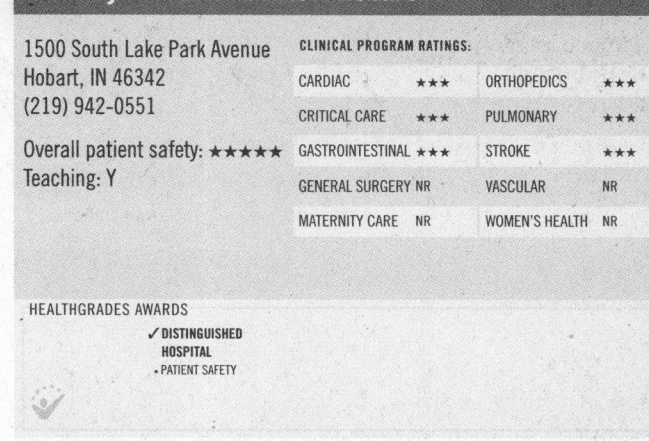

1500 South Lake Park Avenue
Hobart, IN 46342
(219) 942-0551

Overall patient safety: ★★★★★
Teaching: Y

CLINICAL PROGRAM RATINGS:

CARDIAC	★★★	ORTHOPEDICS	★★★
CRITICAL CARE	★★★	PULMONARY	★★★
GASTROINTESTINAL	★★★	STROKE	★★★
GENERAL SURGERY	NR	VASCULAR	NR
MATERNITY CARE	NR	WOMEN'S HEALTH	NR

HEALTHGRADES AWARDS

✓ DISTINGUISHED HOSPITAL
- PATIENT SAFETY

St. Margaret Mercy Healthcare Center

5454 Hohman Avenue
Hammond, IN 46320
(219) 932-2300

Overall patient safety: ★
Teaching: Y

CLINICAL PROGRAM RATINGS:

CARDIAC	★★★	ORTHOPEDICS	NR
CRITICAL CARE	★★★	PULMONARY	★★★
GASTROINTESTINAL	★★★	STROKE	★★★
GENERAL SURGERY	NR	VASCULAR	NR
MATERNITY CARE	NR	WOMEN'S HEALTH	NR

HEALTHGRADES AWARDS

St. Mary's Warrick

1116 Millis Avenue
Boonville, IN 47601
(812) 897-4800

Overall patient safety: ★★★
Teaching: N

CLINICAL PROGRAM RATINGS:

CARDIAC	NR	ORTHOPEDICS	NR
CRITICAL CARE	NR	PULMONARY	★★★
GASTROINTESTINAL	NR	STROKE	NR
GENERAL SURGERY	NR	VASCULAR	NR
MATERNITY CARE	NR	WOMEN'S HEALTH	NR

HEALTHGRADES AWARDS

*This hospital reports its data to the federal government jointly with another hospital. Therefore the ratings and awards apply to multiple hospitals and this specific hospital may not provide all rated services.

St. Vincent Carmel Hospital

13500 North Meridian Street
Carmel, IN 46032
(317) 582-7380

Overall patient safety: ★★★
Teaching: N

CLINICAL PROGRAM RATINGS:

CARDIAC	NR	ORTHOPEDICS	★★★
CRITICAL CARE	NR	PULMONARY	★★★
GASTROINTESTINAL	NR	STROKE	★★★
GENERAL SURGERY	NR	VASCULAR	NR
MATERNITY CARE	NR	WOMEN'S HEALTH	NR

HEALTHGRADES AWARDS

✓ SPECIALTY EXCELLENCE
· JOINT REPLACEMENT

St. Vincent Mercy Hospital

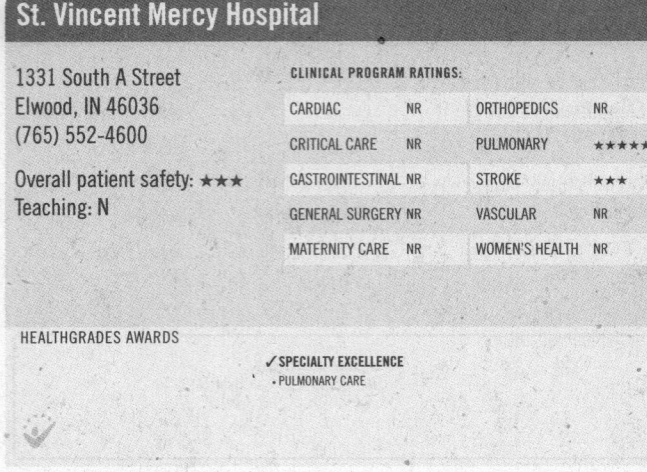

1331 South A Street
Elwood, IN 46036
(765) 552-4600

Overall patient safety: ★★★
Teaching: N

CLINICAL PROGRAM RATINGS:

CARDIAC	NR	ORTHOPEDICS	NR
CRITICAL CARE	NR	PULMONARY	★★★★★
GASTROINTESTINAL	NR	STROKE	★★★
GENERAL SURGERY	NR	VASCULAR	NR
MATERNITY CARE	NR	WOMEN'S HEALTH	NR

HEALTHGRADES AWARDS

✓ SPECIALTY EXCELLENCE
· PULMONARY CARE

St. Vincent Frankfort Hospital

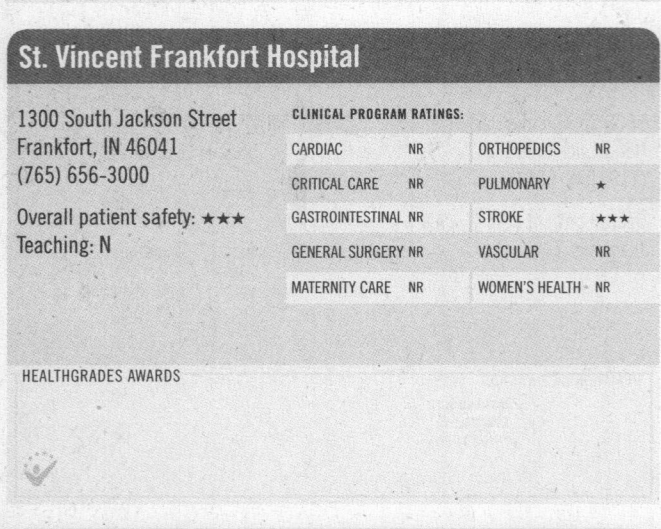

1300 South Jackson Street
Frankfort, IN 46041
(765) 656-3000

Overall patient safety: ★★★
Teaching: N

CLINICAL PROGRAM RATINGS:

CARDIAC	NR	ORTHOPEDICS	NR
CRITICAL CARE	NR	PULMONARY	★
GASTROINTESTINAL	NR	STROKE	★★★
GENERAL SURGERY	NR	VASCULAR	NR
MATERNITY CARE	NR	WOMEN'S HEALTH	NR

HEALTHGRADES AWARDS

St. Vincent Heart Center of Indiana

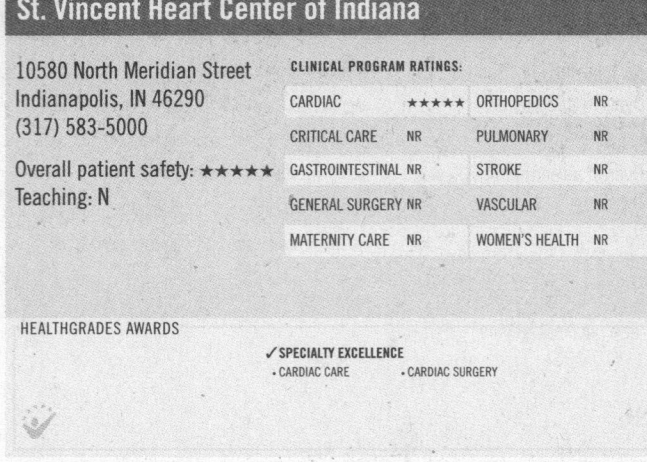

10580 North Meridian Street
Indianapolis, IN 46290
(317) 583-5000

Overall patient safety: ★★★★★
Teaching: N

CLINICAL PROGRAM RATINGS:

CARDIAC	★★★★★	ORTHOPEDICS	NR
CRITICAL CARE	NR	PULMONARY	NR
GASTROINTESTINAL	NR	STROKE	NR
GENERAL SURGERY	NR	VASCULAR	NR
MATERNITY CARE	NR	WOMEN'S HEALTH	NR

HEALTHGRADES AWARDS

✓ SPECIALTY EXCELLENCE
· CARDIAC CARE   · CARDIAC SURGERY

St. Vincent Hospital and Health Services

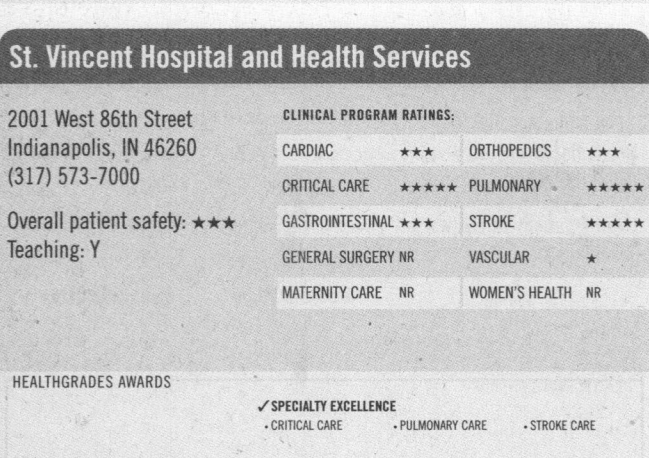

2001 West 86th Street
Indianapolis, IN 46260
(317) 573-7000

Overall patient safety: ★★★
Teaching: Y

CLINICAL PROGRAM RATINGS:

CARDIAC	★★★	ORTHOPEDICS	★★★
CRITICAL CARE	★★★★★	PULMONARY	★★★★★
GASTROINTESTINAL	★★★	STROKE	★★★★★
GENERAL SURGERY	NR	VASCULAR	★
MATERNITY CARE	NR	WOMEN'S HEALTH	NR

HEALTHGRADES AWARDS

✓ SPECIALTY EXCELLENCE
· CRITICAL CARE   · PULMONARY CARE   · STROKE CARE

Schneck Medical Center

411 West Tipton Street
Seymour, IN 47274
(812) 522-2349

Overall patient safety: ★★★
Teaching: N

CLINICAL PROGRAM RATINGS:

CARDIAC	NR	ORTHOPEDICS	NR
CRITICAL CARE	NR	PULMONARY	★★★
GASTROINTESTINAL	NR	STROKE	★
GENERAL SURGERY	NR	VASCULAR	NR
MATERNITY CARE	NR	WOMEN'S HEALTH	NR

HEALTHGRADES AWARDS

KEY: ★★★★★ BEST   ★★★ AS EXPECTED   ★ POOR   NR NOT RATED BY HEALTHGRADES   For full definitions of ratings and awards, see Appendix.

Scott Memorial Hospital

1451 North Gardner Street
Scottsburg, IN 47170
(812) 752-8500

Overall patient safety: NR
Teaching: N

CLINICAL PROGRAM RATINGS:

CARDIAC	NR	ORTHOPEDICS	NR
CRITICAL CARE	NR	PULMONARY	★★★
GASTROINTESTINAL	NR	STROKE	NR
GENERAL SURGERY	NR	VASCULAR	NR
MATERNITY CARE	NR	WOMEN'S HEALTH	NR

HEALTHGRADES AWARDS

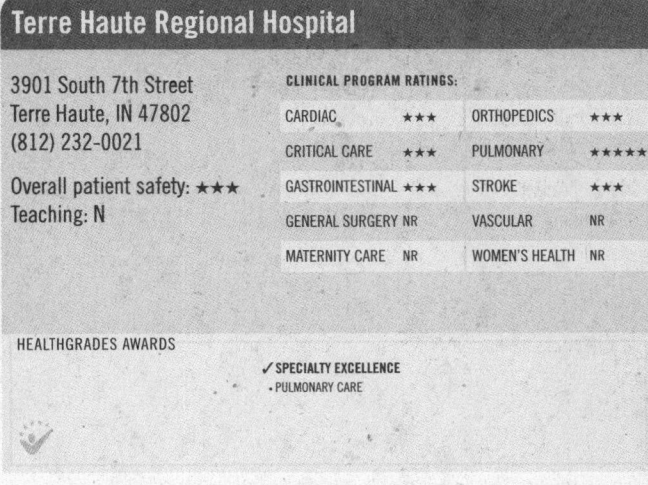

Terre Haute Regional Hospital

3901 South 7th Street
Terre Haute, IN 47802
(812) 232-0021

Overall patient safety: ★★★
Teaching: N

CLINICAL PROGRAM RATINGS:

CARDIAC	★★★	ORTHOPEDICS	★★★
CRITICAL CARE	★★★	PULMONARY	★★★★★
GASTROINTESTINAL	★★★	STROKE	★★★
GENERAL SURGERY	NR	VASCULAR	NR
MATERNITY CARE	NR	WOMEN'S HEALTH	NR

HEALTHGRADES AWARDS

✓ SPECIALTY EXCELLENCE
  • PULMONARY CARE

Starke Memorial Hospital

102 East Culver Road
Knox, IN 46534
(574) 772-6231

Overall patient safety: ★★★
Teaching: N

CLINICAL PROGRAM RATINGS:

CARDIAC	NR	ORTHOPEDICS	NR
CRITICAL CARE	NR	PULMONARY	★
GASTROINTESTINAL	NR	STROKE	★★★
GENERAL SURGERY	NR	VASCULAR	NR
MATERNITY CARE	NR	WOMEN'S HEALTH	NR

HEALTHGRADES AWARDS

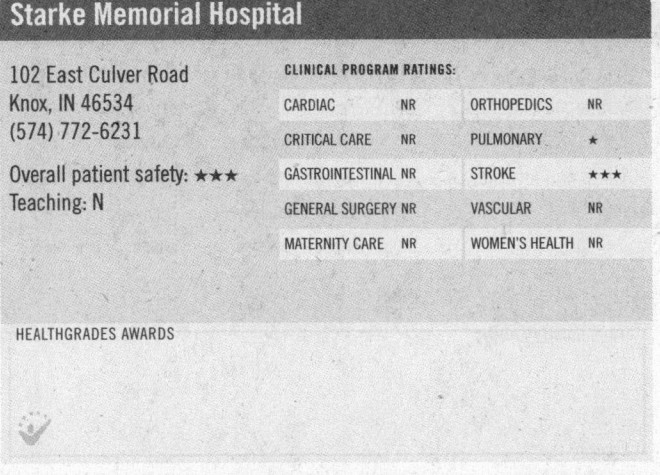

Tipton Hospital

1000 South Main Street
Tipton, IN 46072
(765) 675-8500

Overall patient safety: ★★★
Teaching: N

CLINICAL PROGRAM RATINGS:

CARDIAC	NR	ORTHOPEDICS	NR
CRITICAL CARE	NR	PULMONARY	★
GASTROINTESTINAL	NR	STROKE	★★★
GENERAL SURGERY	NR	VASCULAR	NR
MATERNITY CARE	NR	WOMEN'S HEALTH	NR

HEALTHGRADES AWARDS

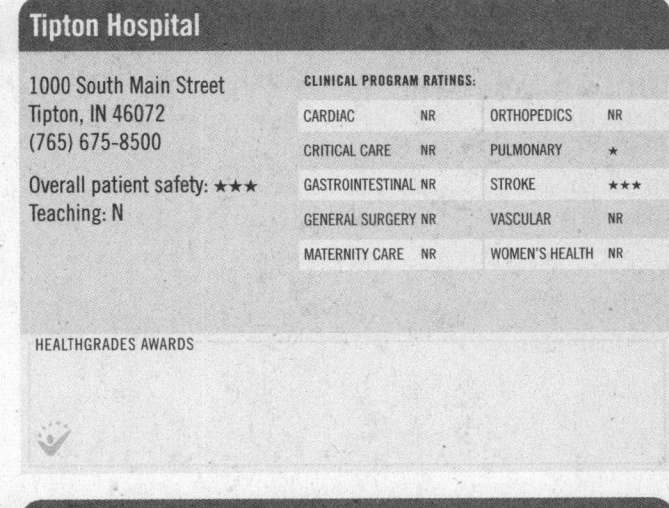

Sullivan County Community Hospital

2200 North Section Street
Sullivan, IN 47882
(812) 268-4311

Overall patient safety: ★★★
Teaching: N

CLINICAL PROGRAM RATINGS:

CARDIAC	NR	ORTHOPEDICS	NR
CRITICAL CARE	NR	PULMONARY	★★★
GASTROINTESTINAL	NR	STROKE	★★★
GENERAL SURGERY	NR	VASCULAR	NR
MATERNITY CARE	NR	WOMEN'S HEALTH	NR

HEALTHGRADES AWARDS

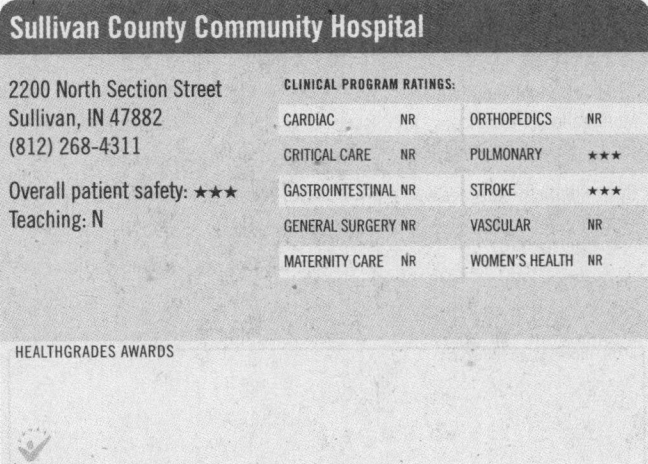

Union Hospital

1606 North 7th Street
Terre Haute, IN 47804
(812) 238-7000

Overall patient safety: ★★★
Teaching: Y

CLINICAL PROGRAM RATINGS:

CARDIAC	★★★	ORTHOPEDICS	★★★
CRITICAL CARE	★	PULMONARY	★
GASTROINTESTINAL	★	STROKE	★
GENERAL SURGERY	NR	VASCULAR	NR
MATERNITY CARE	NR	WOMEN'S HEALTH	NR

HEALTHGRADES AWARDS

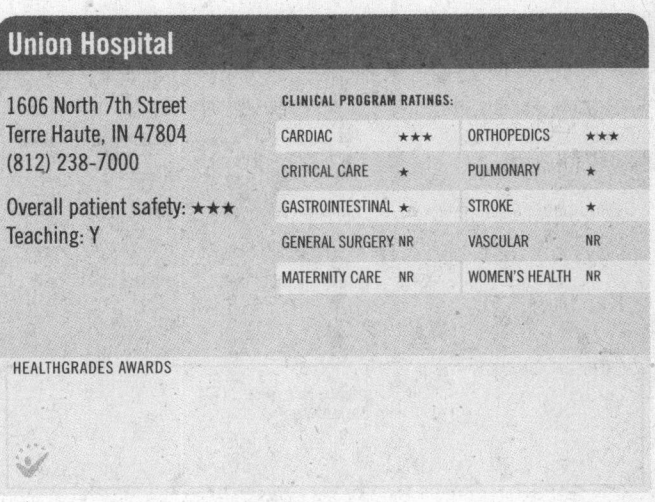

Wabash County Hospital

710 North East Street
Wabash, IN 46992
(260) 563-3131

Overall patient safety: ★★★
Teaching: N

CLINICAL PROGRAM RATINGS:

CARDIAC	NR	ORTHOPEDICS	NR
CRITICAL CARE	NR	PULMONARY	★★★
GASTROINTESTINAL	NR	STROKE	★★★
GENERAL SURGERY	NR	VASCULAR	NR
MATERNITY CARE	NR	WOMEN'S HEALTH	NR

HEALTHGRADES AWARDS

West Central Community Hospital

801 South Main Street
Clinton, IN 47842
(765) 832-1203

Overall patient safety: ★★★
Teaching: N

CLINICAL PROGRAM RATINGS:

CARDIAC	NR	ORTHOPEDICS	NR
CRITICAL CARE	NR	PULMONARY	★★★
GASTROINTESTINAL	NR	STROKE	★
GENERAL SURGERY	NR	VASCULAR	NR
MATERNITY CARE	NR	WOMEN'S HEALTH	NR

HEALTHGRADES AWARDS

Washington County Memorial Hospital

911 North Shelby Street
Salem, IN 47167
(812) 883-5881

Overall patient safety: ★
Teaching: N

CLINICAL PROGRAM RATINGS:

CARDIAC	NR	ORTHOPEDICS	NR
CRITICAL CARE	NR	PULMONARY	★
GASTROINTESTINAL	NR	STROKE	NR
GENERAL SURGERY	NR	VASCULAR	NR
MATERNITY CARE	NR	WOMEN'S HEALTH	NR

HEALTHGRADES AWARDS

Westview Hospital

3630 Guion Road
Indianapolis, IN 46222
(317) 924-6661

Overall patient safety: ★★★
Teaching: Y

CLINICAL PROGRAM RATINGS:

CARDIAC	NR	ORTHOPEDICS	NR
CRITICAL CARE	NR	PULMONARY	★★★
GASTROINTESTINAL	NR	STROKE	★★★
GENERAL SURGERY	NR	VASCULAR	NR
MATERNITY CARE	NR	WOMEN'S HEALTH	NR

HEALTHGRADES AWARDS

Welborn Baptist Hospital*

401 Southeast 6th Street
Evansville, IN 47713
(812) 426-8000

Overall patient safety: ★★★
Teaching: Y

CLINICAL PROGRAM RATINGS:

CARDIAC	★★★	ORTHOPEDICS	★★★
CRITICAL CARE	★	PULMONARY	★★★
GASTROINTESTINAL	★★★	STROKE	★★★
GENERAL SURGERY	NR	VASCULAR	★★★
MATERNITY CARE	NR	WOMEN'S HEALTH	NR

HEALTHGRADES AWARDS

✓ SPECIALTY EXCELLENCE
• JOINT REPLACEMENT

White County Memorial Hospital

1101 O'Connor Boulevard
Monticello, IN 47960
(574) 583-7111

Overall patient safety: ★★★
Teaching: N

CLINICAL PROGRAM RATINGS:

CARDIAC	NR	ORTHOPEDICS	NR
CRITICAL CARE	NR	PULMONARY	★
GASTROINTESTINAL	NR	STROKE	★
GENERAL SURGERY	NR	VASCULAR	NR
MATERNITY CARE	NR	WOMEN'S HEALTH	NR

HEALTHGRADES AWARDS

KEY: ★★★★★ BEST   ★★★ AS EXPECTED   ★ POOR   NR NOT RATED BY HEALTHGRADES   For full definitions of ratings and awards, see Appendix.

William N. Wishard Memorial Hospital

1001 West 10th Street
Indianapolis, IN 46202
(317) 639-6671

Overall patient safety: ★
Teaching: Y

CLINICAL PROGRAM RATINGS:

CARDIAC	NR	ORTHOPEDICS	NR
CRITICAL CARE	★★★	PULMONARY	★★★★★
GASTROINTESTINAL	NR	STROKE	★★★
GENERAL SURGERY	NR	VASCULAR	NR
MATERNITY CARE	NR	WOMEN'S HEALTH	NR

HEALTHGRADES AWARDS

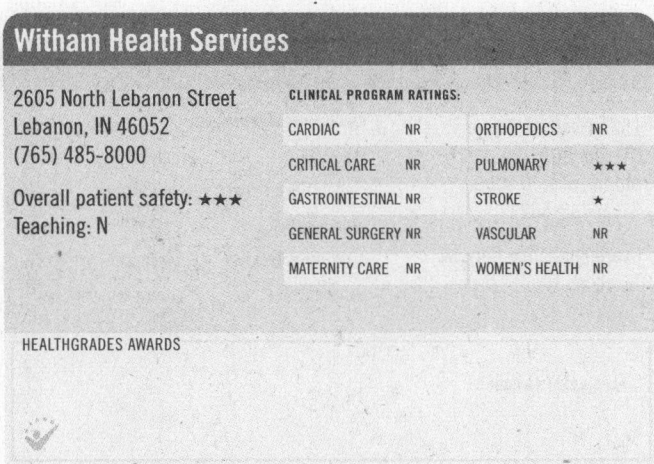

Woodlawn Hospital

1400 East 9th Street
Rochester, IN 46975
(574) 223-3141

Overall patient safety: ★★★
Teaching: N

CLINICAL PROGRAM RATINGS:

CARDIAC	NR	ORTHOPEDICS	NR
CRITICAL CARE	NR	PULMONARY	★
GASTROINTESTINAL	NR	STROKE	NR
GENERAL SURGERY	NR	VASCULAR	NR
MATERNITY CARE	NR	WOMEN'S HEALTH	NR

HEALTHGRADES AWARDS

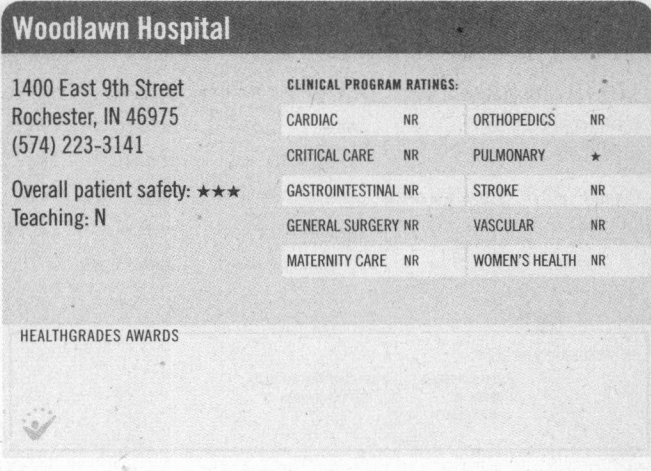

Witham Health Services

2605 North Lebanon Street
Lebanon, IN 46052
(765) 485-8000

Overall patient safety: ★★★
Teaching: N

CLINICAL PROGRAM RATINGS:

CARDIAC	NR	ORTHOPEDICS	NR
CRITICAL CARE	NR	PULMONARY	★★★
GASTROINTESTINAL	NR	STROKE	★
GENERAL SURGERY	NR	VASCULAR	NR
MATERNITY CARE	NR	WOMEN'S HEALTH	NR

HEALTHGRADES AWARDS

IOWA HOSPITALS: RATINGS BY CLINICAL SPECIALTY

Alegent Health Community Memorial Hospital

631 North 8th Street
Missouri Valley, IA 51555
(712) 642-2784

Overall patient safety: ★★★
Teaching: N

CLINICAL PROGRAM RATINGS:

CARDIAC	NR	ORTHOPEDICS	NR
CRITICAL CARE	NR	PULMONARY	★★★
GASTROINTESTINAL	NR	STROKE	★★★
GENERAL SURGERY	NR	VASCULAR	NR
MATERNITY CARE	NR	WOMEN'S HEALTH	NR

HEALTHGRADES AWARDS

Alegent Health Mercy Hospital

800 Mercy Drive
Council Bluffs, IA 51503
(712) 328-5000

Overall patient safety: ★★★
Teaching: N

CLINICAL PROGRAM RATINGS:

CARDIAC	NR	ORTHOPEDICS	★★★
CRITICAL CARE	NR	PULMONARY	★
GASTROINTESTINAL	★★★	STROKE	★
GENERAL SURGERY	★★★	VASCULAR	NR
MATERNITY CARE	★★★	WOMEN'S HEALTH	NR

HEALTHGRADES AWARDS

*This hospital reports its data to the federal government jointly with another hospital. Therefore the ratings and awards apply to multiple hospitals and this specific hospital may not provide all rated services.

Allen Memorial Hospital

1825 Logan Avenue
Waterloo, IA 50703
(319) 235-3941

Overall patient safety: ★★★★★
Teaching: Y

CLINICAL PROGRAM RATINGS:

CARDIAC	★★★	ORTHOPEDICS	★★★
CRITICAL CARE	NR	PULMONARY	★★★
GASTROINTESTINAL	★★★	STROKE	★★★
GENERAL SURGERY	★★★	VASCULAR	★★★★★
MATERNITY CARE	NR	WOMEN'S HEALTH	NR

HEALTHGRADES AWARDS

✓ DISTINGUISHED HOSPITAL
• PATIENT SAFETY

✓ SPECIALTY EXCELLENCE
• VASCULAR SURGERY

Buchanan County Health Center

1600 1st Street East
Independence, IA 50644
(319) 334-6071

Overall patient safety: ★★★
Teaching: N

CLINICAL PROGRAM RATINGS:

CARDIAC	NR	ORTHOPEDICS	NR
CRITICAL CARE	NR	PULMONARY	★★★
GASTROINTESTINAL	NR	STROKE	NR
GENERAL SURGERY	NR	VASCULAR	NR
MATERNITY CARE	★★★	WOMEN'S HEALTH	NR

HEALTHGRADES AWARDS

Boone County Hospital

1015 Union Street
Boone, IA 50036
(515) 432-3140

Overall patient safety: ★★★
Teaching: N

CLINICAL PROGRAM RATINGS:

CARDIAC	NR	ORTHOPEDICS	NR
CRITICAL CARE	NR	PULMONARY	★
GASTROINTESTINAL	NR	STROKE	★
GENERAL SURGERY	NR	VASCULAR	NR
MATERNITY CARE	★★★	WOMEN'S HEALTH	NR

HEALTHGRADES AWARDS

Buena Vista Regional Medical Center

1525 West 5th Street
P.O. Box 309
Storm Lake, IA 50588
(712) 732-5623

Overall patient safety: NR
Teaching: N

CLINICAL PROGRAM RATINGS:

CARDIAC	NR	ORTHOPEDICS	NR
CRITICAL CARE	NR	PULMONARY	★★★
GASTROINTESTINAL	NR	STROKE	★
GENERAL SURGERY	NR	VASCULAR	NR
MATERNITY CARE	NR	WOMEN'S HEALTH	NR

HEALTHGRADES AWARDS

Broadlawns Medical Center

1801 Hickman Road
Des Moines, IA 50314
(515) 282-2200

Overall patient safety: ★★★
Teaching: Y

CLINICAL PROGRAM RATINGS:

CARDIAC	NR	ORTHOPEDICS	NR
CRITICAL CARE	NR	PULMONARY	NR
GASTROINTESTINAL	NR	STROKE	NR
GENERAL SURGERY	NR	VASCULAR	NR
MATERNITY CARE	★★★	WOMEN'S HEALTH	NR

HEALTHGRADES AWARDS

Burgess Health Center

1600 Diamond Street
Onawa, IA 51040
(712) 423-2311

Overall patient safety: ★★★
Teaching: N

CLINICAL PROGRAM RATINGS:

CARDIAC	NR	ORTHOPEDICS	NR
CRITICAL CARE	NR	PULMONARY	★
GASTROINTESTINAL	NR	STROKE	NR
GENERAL SURGERY	NR	VASCULAR	NR
MATERNITY CARE	★	WOMEN'S HEALTH	NR

HEALTHGRADES AWARDS

KEY: ★★★★★ BEST ★★★ AS EXPECTED ★ POOR NR NOT RATED BY HEALTHGRADES For full definitions of ratings and awards, see Appendix.

Cass County Memorial Hospital

1501 East 10th Street
Atlantic, IA 50022
(712) 243-3250

Overall patient safety: NR
Teaching: N

CLINICAL PROGRAM RATINGS:

CARDIAC	NR	ORTHOPEDICS	NR
CRITICAL CARE	NR	PULMONARY	★
GASTROINTESTINAL	NR	STROKE	★★★
GENERAL SURGERY	NR	VASCULAR	NR
MATERNITY CARE	NR	WOMEN'S HEALTH	NR

HEALTHGRADES AWARDS

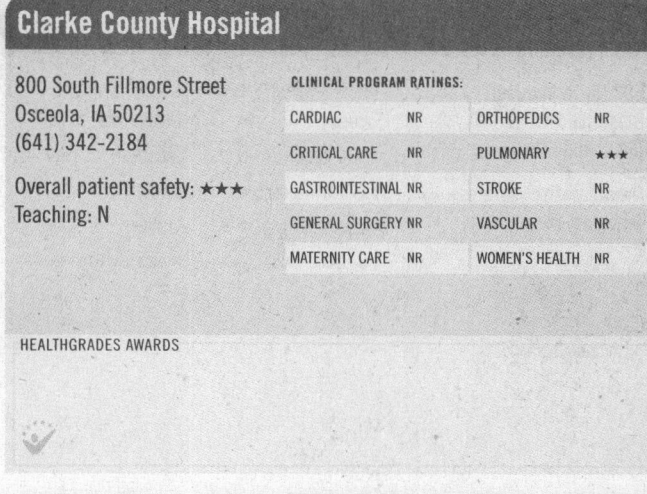

Clarke County Hospital

800 South Fillmore Street
Osceola, IA 50213
(641) 342-2184

Overall patient safety: ★★★
Teaching: N

CLINICAL PROGRAM RATINGS:

CARDIAC	NR	ORTHOPEDICS	NR
CRITICAL CARE	NR	PULMONARY	★★★
GASTROINTESTINAL	NR	STROKE	NR
GENERAL SURGERY	NR	VASCULAR	NR
MATERNITY CARE	NR	WOMEN'S HEALTH	NR

HEALTHGRADES AWARDS

Cherokee Regional Medical Center

300 Sioux Valley Drive
Cherokee, IA 51012
(712) 225-5101

Overall patient safety: ★★★
Teaching: N

CLINICAL PROGRAM RATINGS:

CARDIAC	NR	ORTHOPEDICS	NR
CRITICAL CARE	NR	PULMONARY	★★★
GASTROINTESTINAL	NR	STROKE	★★★
GENERAL SURGERY	NR	VASCULAR	NR
MATERNITY CARE	★★★	WOMEN'S HEALTH	NR

HEALTHGRADES AWARDS

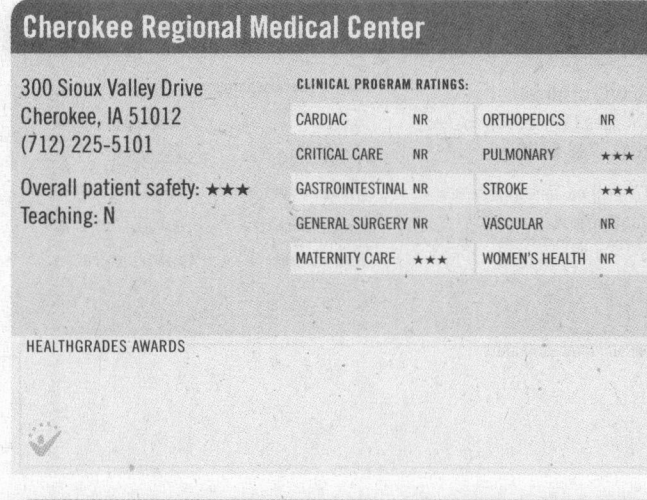

Covenant Medical Center

3421 West 9th Street
Waterloo, IA 50702
(319) 272-8000

Overall patient safety: ★★★
Teaching: Y

CLINICAL PROGRAM RATINGS:

CARDIAC	NR	ORTHOPEDICS	★★★
CRITICAL CARE	NR	PULMONARY	★★★
GASTROINTESTINAL	★★★	STROKE	★★★
GENERAL SURGERY	★★★	VASCULAR	NR
MATERNITY CARE	★★★	WOMEN'S HEALTH	NR

HEALTHGRADES AWARDS

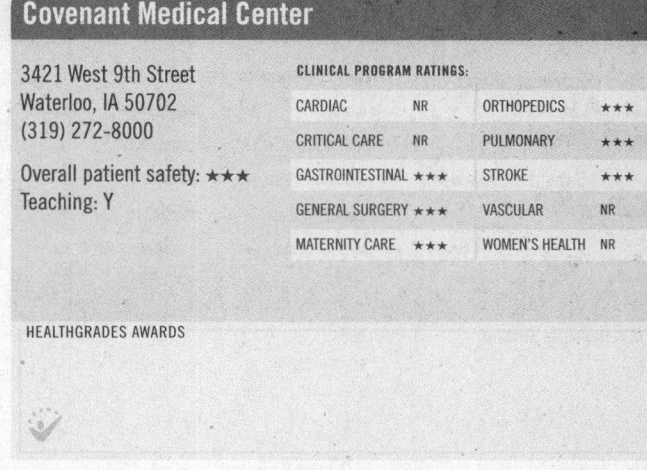

Clarinda Regional Health Center

823 South 17th
Clarinda, IA 51632
(712) 542-2176

Overall patient safety: ★★★
Teaching: N

CLINICAL PROGRAM RATINGS:

CARDIAC	NR	ORTHOPEDICS	NR
CRITICAL CARE	NR	PULMONARY	★
GASTROINTESTINAL	NR	STROKE	NR
GENERAL SURGERY	NR	VASCULAR	NR
MATERNITY CARE	NR	WOMEN'S HEALTH	NR

HEALTHGRADES AWARDS

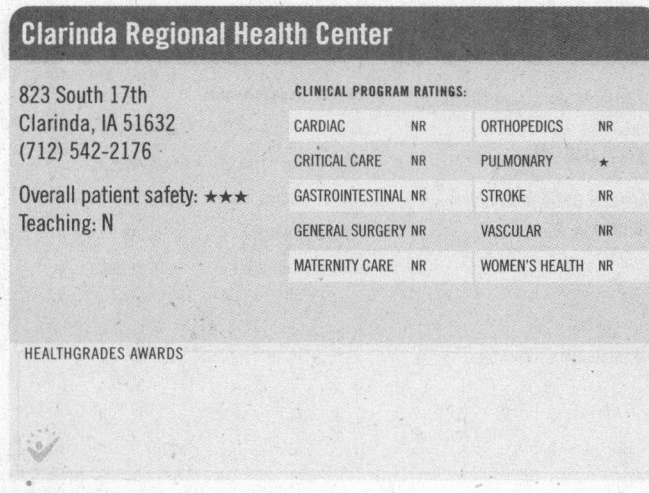

Crawford County Memorial Hospital

2020 1st Avenue South
Denison, IA 51442
(712) 263-5021

Overall patient safety: ★★★
Teaching: N

CLINICAL PROGRAM RATINGS:

CARDIAC	NR	ORTHOPEDICS	NR
CRITICAL CARE	NR	PULMONARY	★★★
GASTROINTESTINAL	NR	STROKE	★★★
GENERAL SURGERY	NR	VASCULAR	NR
MATERNITY CARE	★	WOMEN'S HEALTH	NR

HEALTHGRADES AWARDS

Davis County Hospital

507 North Madison
Bloomfield, IA 52537
(641) 664-2145

Overall patient safety: ★★★
Teaching: N

CLINICAL PROGRAM RATINGS:

CARDIAC	NR	ORTHOPEDICS	NR
CRITICAL CARE	NR	PULMONARY	★★★
GASTROINTESTINAL	NR	STROKE	★
GENERAL SURGERY	NR	VASCULAR	NR
MATERNITY CARE	★★★	WOMEN'S HEALTH	NR

HEALTHGRADES AWARDS

Finley Hospital

350 North Grandview Avenue
Dubuque, IA 52001
(563) 582-1881

Overall patient safety: ★★★
Teaching: N

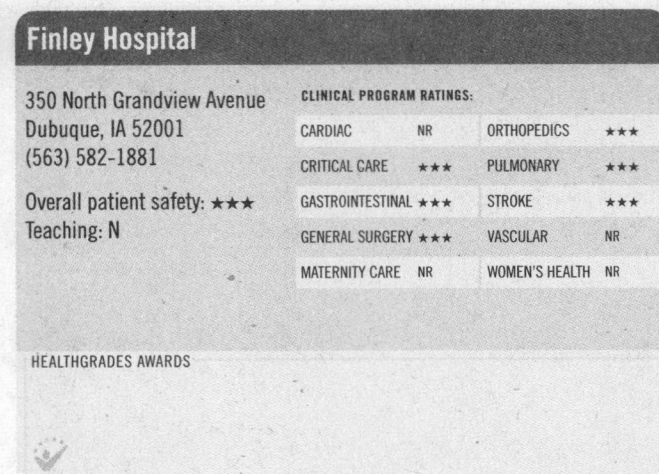

CLINICAL PROGRAM RATINGS:

CARDIAC	NR	ORTHOPEDICS	★★★
CRITICAL CARE	★★★	PULMONARY	★★★
GASTROINTESTINAL	★★★	STROKE	★★★
GENERAL SURGERY	★★★	VASCULAR	NR
MATERNITY CARE	NR	WOMEN'S HEALTH	NR

HEALTHGRADES AWARDS

Decatur County Hospital

1405 Northwest Church Street
Leon, IA 50144
(641) 446-4871

Overall patient safety: ★★★
Teaching: N

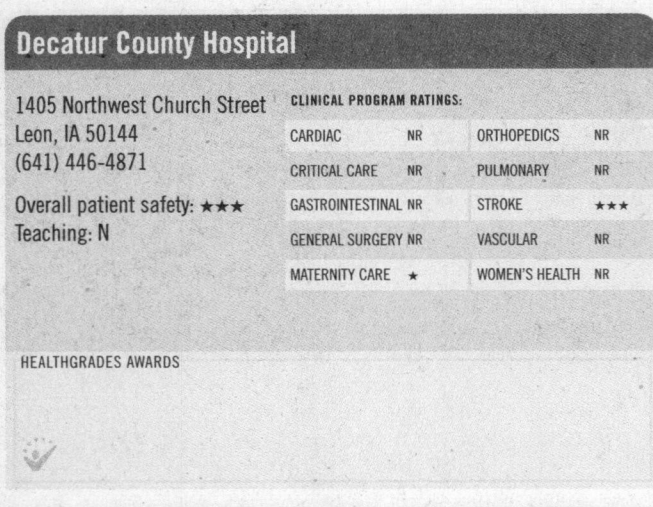

CLINICAL PROGRAM RATINGS:

CARDIAC	NR	ORTHOPEDICS	NR
CRITICAL CARE	NR	PULMONARY	NR
GASTROINTESTINAL	NR	STROKE	★★★
GENERAL SURGERY	NR	VASCULAR	NR
MATERNITY CARE	★	WOMEN'S HEALTH	NR

HEALTHGRADES AWARDS

Floyd County Memorial Hospital

800 11th Street
Charles City, IA 50616
(641) 228-6830

Overall patient safety: ★★★
Teaching: N

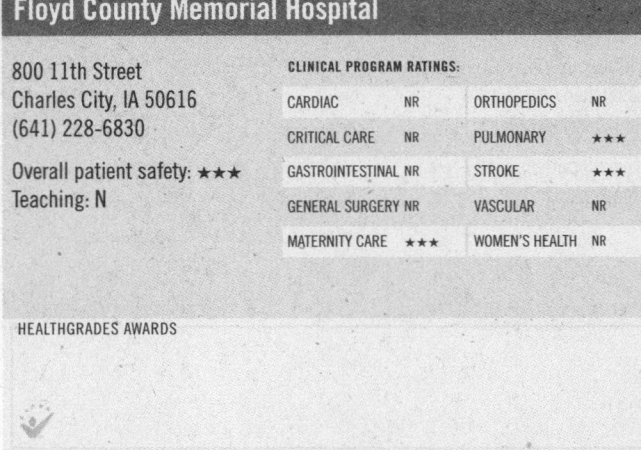

CLINICAL PROGRAM RATINGS:

CARDIAC	NR	ORTHOPEDICS	NR
CRITICAL CARE	NR	PULMONARY	★★★
GASTROINTESTINAL	NR	STROKE	★★★
GENERAL SURGERY	NR	VASCULAR	NR
MATERNITY CARE	★★★	WOMEN'S HEALTH	NR

HEALTHGRADES AWARDS

Ellsworth Municipal Hospital

110 Rocksylvania Avenue
Iowa Falls, IA 50126
(641) 648-4631

Overall patient safety: ★★★
Teaching: N

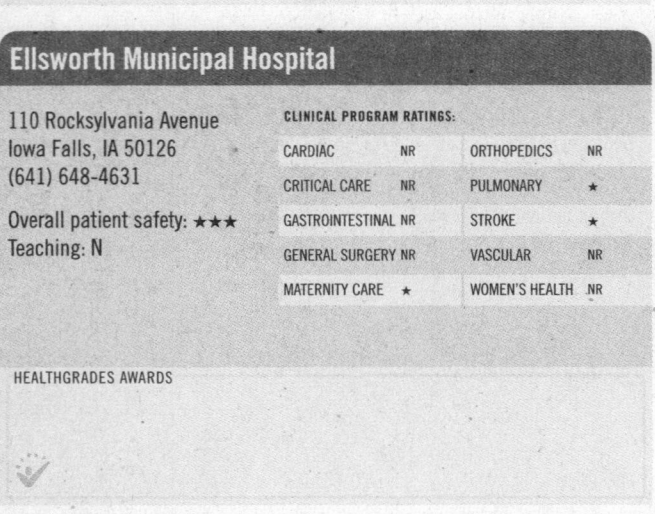

CLINICAL PROGRAM RATINGS:

CARDIAC	NR	ORTHOPEDICS	NR
CRITICAL CARE	NR	PULMONARY	★
GASTROINTESTINAL	NR	STROKE	★
GENERAL SURGERY	NR	VASCULAR	NR
MATERNITY CARE	★	WOMEN'S HEALTH	NR

HEALTHGRADES AWARDS

Floyd Valley Hospital

714 Lincoln Street Northeast
Le Mars, IA 51031
(712) 546-7871

Overall patient safety: ★★★
Teaching: N

CLINICAL PROGRAM RATINGS:

CARDIAC	NR	ORTHOPEDICS	NR
CRITICAL CARE	NR	PULMONARY	★★★
GASTROINTESTINAL	NR	STROKE	★★★
GENERAL SURGERY	★★★	VASCULAR	NR
MATERNITY CARE	★★★	WOMEN'S HEALTH	NR

HEALTHGRADES AWARDS

KEY: ★★★★★ BEST ★★★ AS EXPECTED ★ POOR NR NOT RATED BY HEALTHGRADES For full definitions of ratings and awards, see Appendix.

Fort Madison Community Hospital

5445 Avenue O
Fort Madison, IA 52627
(319) 372-6530

Overall patient safety: ★★★
Teaching: N

CLINICAL PROGRAM RATINGS:

CARDIAC	NR	ORTHOPEDICS	NR
CRITICAL CARE	NR	PULMONARY	★★★
GASTROINTESTINAL	NR	STROKE	★★★
GENERAL SURGERY	NR	VASCULAR	NR
MATERNITY CARE	★★★	WOMEN'S HEALTH	NR

HEALTHGRADES AWARDS

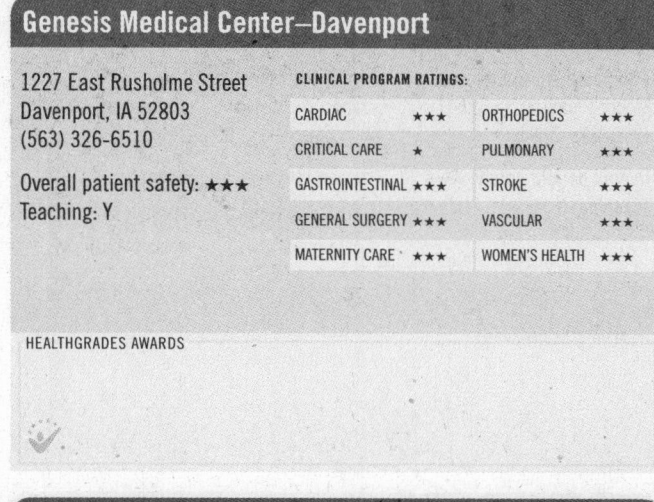

Great River Medical Center

1221 South Gear Avenue
West Burlington, IA 52655
(319) 768-1000

Overall patient safety: ★★★★★
Teaching: N

CLINICAL PROGRAM RATINGS:

CARDIAC	NR	ORTHOPEDICS	NR
CRITICAL CARE	NR	PULMONARY	★★★
GASTROINTESTINAL	NR	STROKE	★★★
GENERAL SURGERY	★★★	VASCULAR	NR
MATERNITY CARE	★	WOMEN'S HEALTH	NR

HEALTHGRADES AWARDS

✓ DISTINGUISHED
  HOSPITAL
· PATIENT SAFETY

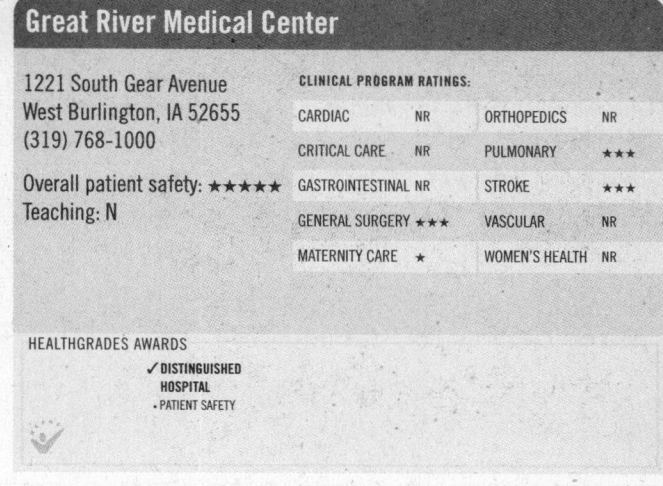

Genesis Medical Center–Davenport

1227 East Rusholme Street
Davenport, IA 52803
(563) 326-6510

Overall patient safety: ★★★
Teaching: Y

CLINICAL PROGRAM RATINGS:

CARDIAC	★★★	ORTHOPEDICS	★★★
CRITICAL CARE	★	PULMONARY	★★★
GASTROINTESTINAL	★★★	STROKE	★★★
GENERAL SURGERY	★★★	VASCULAR	★★★
MATERNITY CARE	★★★	WOMEN'S HEALTH	★★★

HEALTHGRADES AWARDS

Greater Community Hospital

1700 West Townline Road
Creston, IA 50801
(641) 782-3503

Overall patient safety: ★★★
Teaching: N

CLINICAL PROGRAM RATINGS:

CARDIAC	NR	ORTHOPEDICS	NR
CRITICAL CARE	NR	PULMONARY	★
GASTROINTESTINAL	NR	STROKE	★
GENERAL SURGERY	★★★	VASCULAR	NR
MATERNITY CARE	★★★	WOMEN'S HEALTH	NR

HEALTHGRADES AWARDS

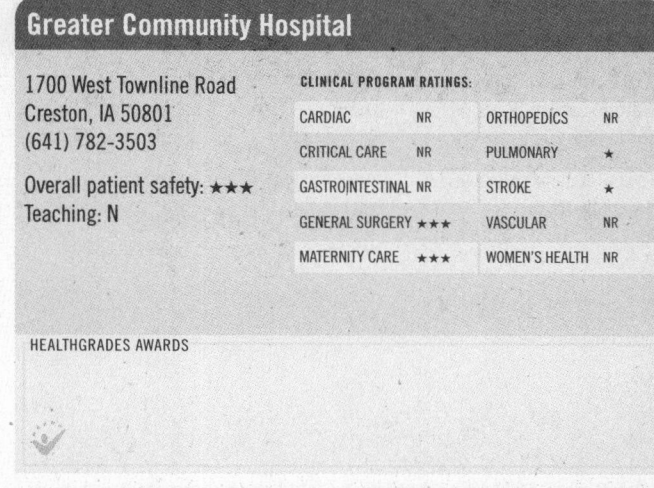

Grape Community Hospital

2959 US Highway 275
Hamburg, IA 51640
(712) 382-1515

Overall patient safety: ★★★
Teaching: N

CLINICAL PROGRAM RATINGS:

CARDIAC	NR	ORTHOPEDICS	NR
CRITICAL CARE	NR	PULMONARY	★★★
GASTROINTESTINAL	NR	STROKE	NR
GENERAL SURGERY	NR	VASCULAR	NR
MATERNITY CARE	NR	WOMEN'S HEALTH	NR

HEALTHGRADES AWARDS

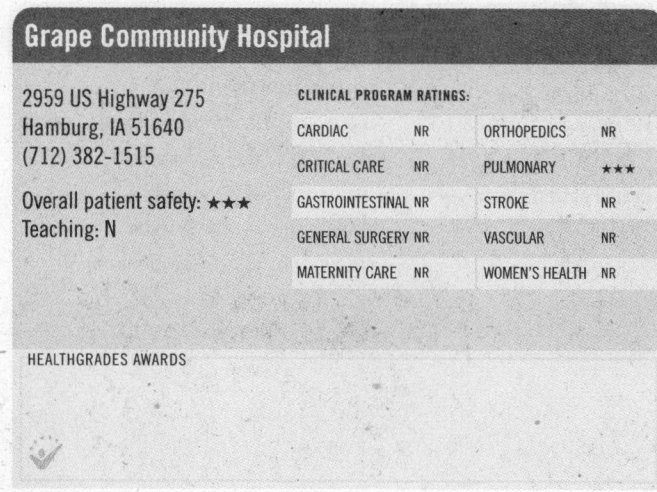

Greene County Medical Center

1000 West Lincolnway
Jefferson, IA 50129
(515) 386-2114

Overall patient safety: ★★★
Teaching: N

CLINICAL PROGRAM RATINGS:

CARDIAC	NR	ORTHOPEDICS	NR
CRITICAL CARE	NR	PULMONARY	★★★
GASTROINTESTINAL	NR	STROKE	★★★
GENERAL SURGERY	NR	VASCULAR	NR
MATERNITY CARE	★★★	WOMEN'S HEALTH	NR

HEALTHGRADES AWARDS

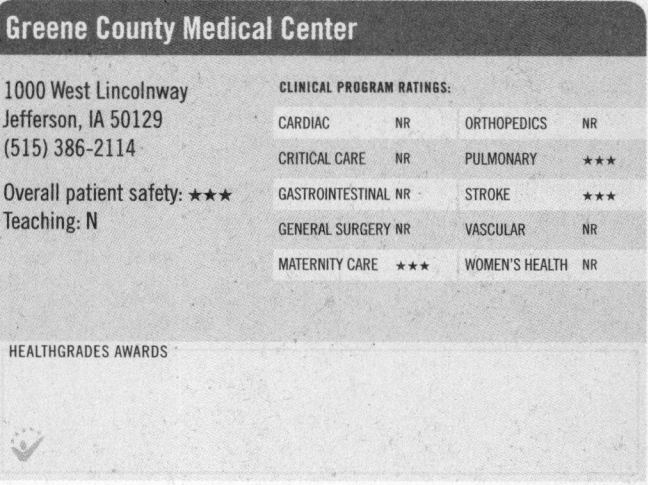

Grinnell Regional Medical Center

210 4th Avenue
Grinnell, IA 50112
(641) 236-7511

Overall patient safety: ★★★
Teaching: N

CLINICAL PROGRAM RATINGS:

CARDIAC	NR	ORTHOPEDICS	NR
CRITICAL CARE	NR	PULMONARY	★★★
GASTROINTESTINAL	NR	STROKE	★★★
GENERAL SURGERY	★	VASCULAR	NR
MATERNITY CARE	★	WOMEN'S HEALTH	NR

HEALTHGRADES AWARDS

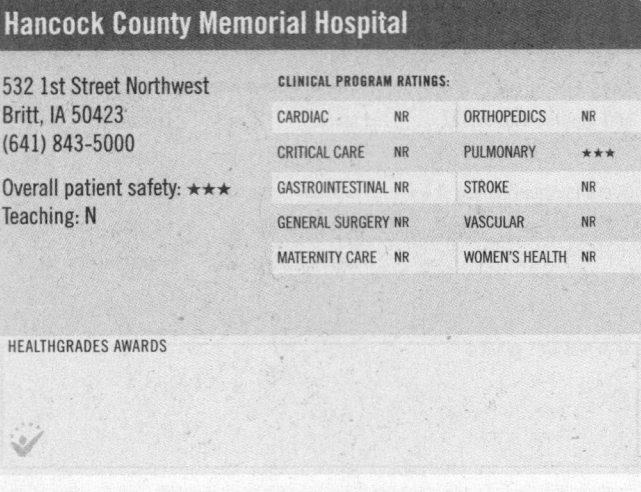

Hancock County Memorial Hospital

532 1st Street Northwest
Britt, IA 50423
(641) 843-5000

Overall patient safety: ★★★
Teaching: N

CLINICAL PROGRAM RATINGS:

CARDIAC	NR	ORTHOPEDICS	NR
CRITICAL CARE	NR	PULMONARY	★★★
GASTROINTESTINAL	NR	STROKE	NR
GENERAL SURGERY	NR	VASCULAR	NR
MATERNITY CARE	NR	WOMEN'S HEALTH	NR

HEALTHGRADES AWARDS

Guthrie County Hospital

710 North 12th Street
Guthrie Center, IA 50115
(641) 747-2001

Overall patient safety: ★★★
Teaching: N

CLINICAL PROGRAM RATINGS:

CARDIAC	NR	ORTHOPEDICS	NR
CRITICAL CARE	NR	PULMONARY	NR
GASTROINTESTINAL	NR	STROKE	★★★
GENERAL SURGERY	NR	VASCULAR	NR
MATERNITY CARE	NR	WOMEN'S HEALTH	NR

HEALTHGRADES AWARDS

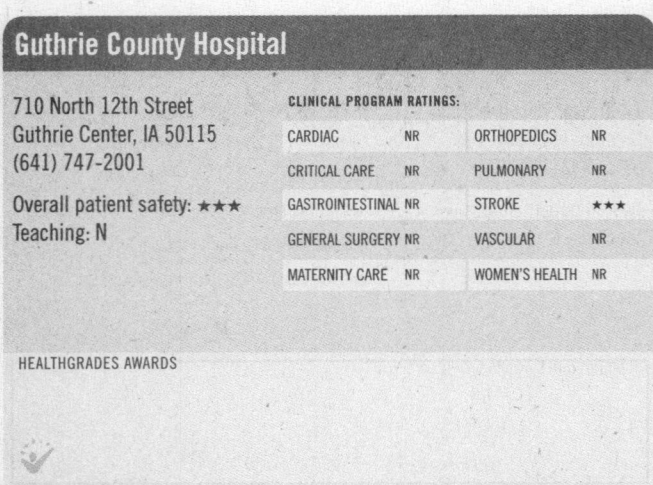

Henry County Health Center

407 South White Street
Mount Pleasant, IA 52641
(319) 385-3141

Overall patient safety: ★★★
Teaching: N

CLINICAL PROGRAM RATINGS:

CARDIAC	NR	ORTHOPEDICS	NR
CRITICAL CARE	NR	PULMONARY	★★★
GASTROINTESTINAL	NR	STROKE	★
GENERAL SURGERY	NR	VASCULAR	NR
MATERNITY CARE	★★★	WOMEN'S HEALTH	NR

HEALTHGRADES AWARDS

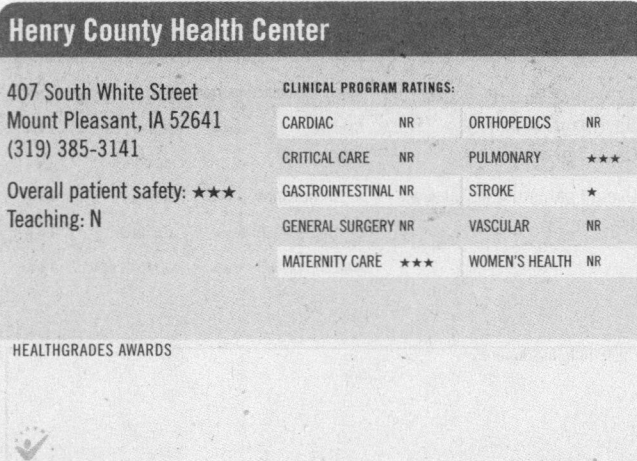

Hamilton County Public Hospital

800 Ohio Street
Webster City, IA 50595
(515) 832-9400

Overall patient safety: ★★★
Teaching: N

CLINICAL PROGRAM RATINGS:

CARDIAC	NR	ORTHOPEDICS	NR
CRITICAL CARE	NR	PULMONARY	★★★
GASTROINTESTINAL	NR	STROKE	NR
GENERAL SURGERY	NR	VASCULAR	NR
MATERNITY CARE	★★★	WOMEN'S HEALTH	NR

HEALTHGRADES AWARDS

Horn Memorial Hospital

701 East 2nd Street
Ida Grove, 1A 51445
(712) 364-3311

Overall patient safety: ★★★
Teaching: N

CLINICAL PROGRAM RATINGS:

CARDIAC	NR	ORTHOPEDICS	NR
CRITICAL CARE	NR	PULMONARY	★★★
GASTROINTESTINAL	NR	STROKE	NR
GENERAL SURGERY	NR	VASCULAR	NR
MATERNITY CARE	NR	WOMEN'S HEALTH	NR

HEALTHGRADES AWARDS

KEY: ★★★★★ BEST   ★★★ AS EXPECTED   ★ POOR   NR NOT RATED BY HEALTHGRADES   For full definitions of ratings and awards, see Appendix.

Iowa Lutheran Hospital

700 East University Avenue
Des Moines, IA 50316
(515) 263-5612

Overall patient safety: ★★★
Teaching: Y

CLINICAL PROGRAM RATINGS:

CARDIAC	★★★	ORTHOPEDICS	★★★
CRITICAL CARE	NR	PULMONARY	★★★
GASTROINTESTINAL	★★★	STROKE	★★★
GENERAL SURGERY	★★★	VASCULAR	NR
MATERNITY CARE	NR	WOMEN'S HEALTH	NR

HEALTHGRADES AWARDS

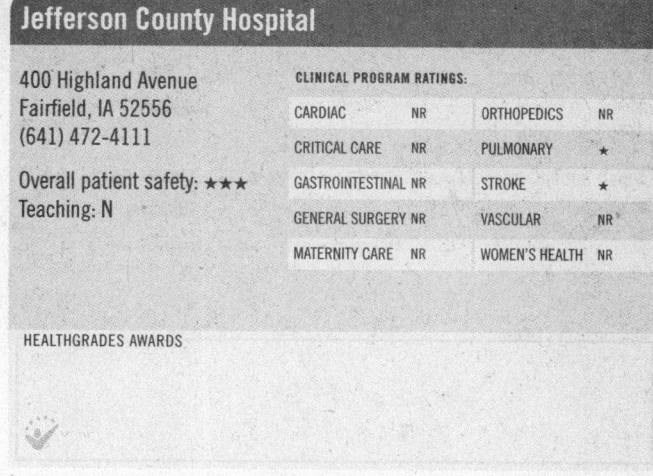

Jefferson County Hospital

400 Highland Avenue
Fairfield, IA 52556
(641) 472-4111

Overall patient safety: ★★★
Teaching: N

CLINICAL PROGRAM RATINGS:

CARDIAC	NR	ORTHOPEDICS	NR
CRITICAL CARE	NR	PULMONARY	★
GASTROINTESTINAL	NR	STROKE	★
GENERAL SURGERY	NR	VASCULAR	NR
MATERNITY CARE	NR	WOMEN'S HEALTH	NR

HEALTHGRADES AWARDS

Iowa Methodist Medical Center

1200 Pleasant Street
Des Moines, IA 50309
(515) 241-6212

Overall patient safety: ★★★★★
Teaching: Y

CLINICAL PROGRAM RATINGS:

CARDIAC	★★★	ORTHOPEDICS	★★★
CRITICAL CARE	NR	PULMONARY	★★★
GASTROINTESTINAL	★★★	STROKE	★★★
GENERAL SURGERY	★★★★★	VASCULAR	★★★
MATERNITY CARE	NR	WOMEN'S HEALTH	NR

HEALTHGRADES AWARDS

✓ DISTINGUISHED HOSPITAL
 • PATIENT SAFETY

✓ SPECIALTY EXCELLENCE
 • GENERAL SURGERY

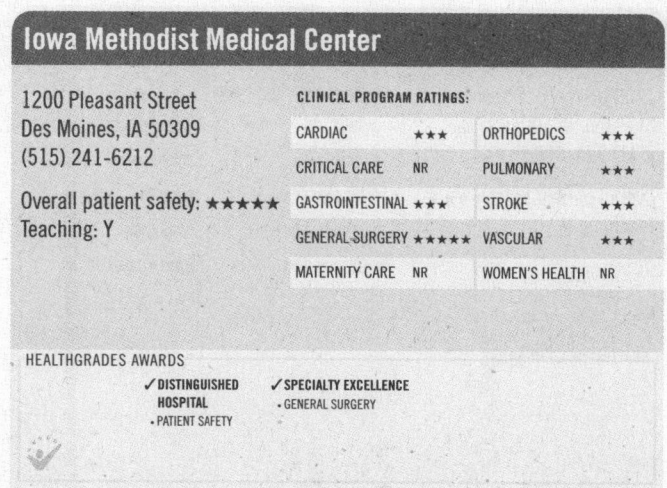

Jennie Edmundson Hospital

933 East Pierce Street
Council Bluffs, IA 51503
(712) 396-6000

Overall patient safety: ★★★
Teaching: Y

CLINICAL PROGRAM RATINGS:

CARDIAC	NR	ORTHOPEDICS	★★★
CRITICAL CARE	NR	PULMONARY	★
GASTROINTESTINAL	NR	STROKE	★
GENERAL SURGERY	★★★	VASCULAR	NR
MATERNITY CARE	★★★	WOMEN'S HEALTH	NR

HEALTHGRADES AWARDS

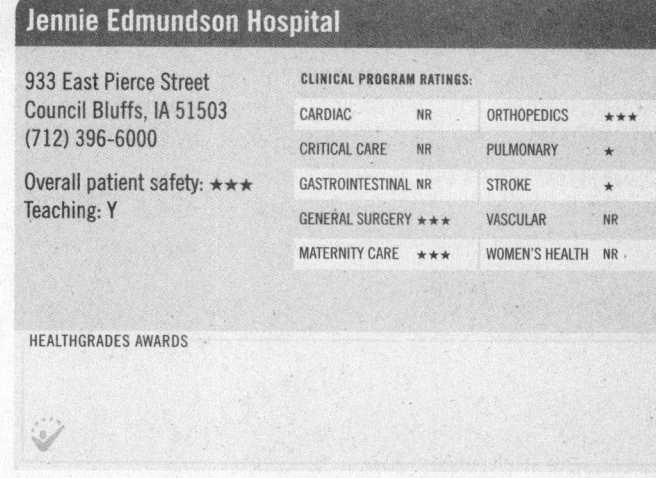

Jackson County Regional Health Center

700 West Grove Street
Maquoketa, IA 52060
(563) 652-2474

Overall patient safety: ★★★
Teaching: N

CLINICAL PROGRAM RATINGS:

CARDIAC	NR	ORTHOPEDICS	NR
CRITICAL CARE	NR	PULMONARY	★★★
GASTROINTESTINAL	NR	STROKE	NR
GENERAL SURGERY	NR	VASCULAR	NR
MATERNITY CARE	★★★	WOMEN'S HEALTH	NR

HEALTHGRADES AWARDS

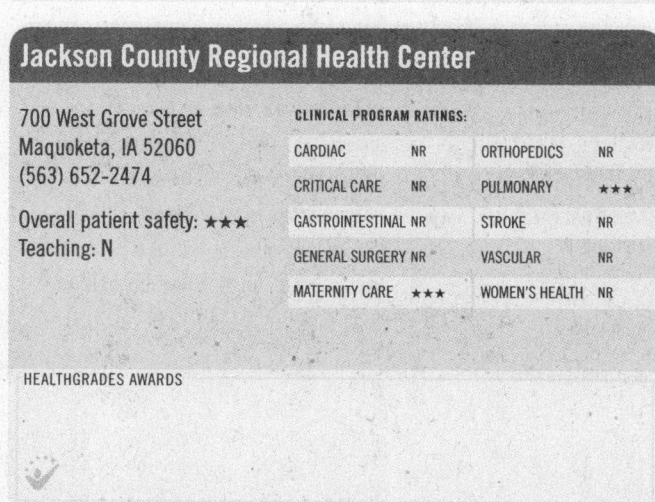

Jones Regional Medical Center

104 Broadway Place
Anamosa, IA 52205
(319) 462-6131

Overall patient safety: NR
Teaching: N

CLINICAL PROGRAM RATINGS:

CARDIAC	NR	ORTHOPEDICS	NR
CRITICAL CARE	NR	PULMONARY	★★★
GASTROINTESTINAL	NR	STROKE	NR
GENERAL SURGERY	NR	VASCULAR	NR
MATERNITY CARE	NR	WOMEN'S HEALTH	NR

HEALTHGRADES AWARDS

Keokuk Area Hospital

1600 Morgan Street
Keokuk, IA 52632
(319) 524-7150

Overall patient safety: ★★★
Teaching: N

CLINICAL PROGRAM RATINGS:

CARDIAC	NR	ORTHOPEDICS	NR
CRITICAL CARE	NR	PULMONARY	★★★
GASTROINTESTINAL	NR	STROKE	★★★
GENERAL SURGERY	NR	VASCULAR	NR
MATERNITY CARE	★★★	WOMEN'S HEALTH	NR

HEALTHGRADES AWARDS

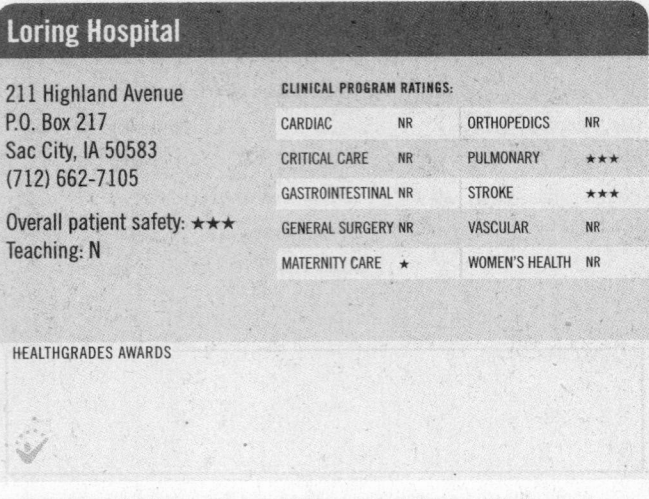

Loring Hospital

211 Highland Avenue
P.O. Box 217
Sac City, IA 50583
(712) 662-7105

Overall patient safety: ★★★
Teaching: N

CLINICAL PROGRAM RATINGS:

CARDIAC	NR	ORTHOPEDICS	NR
CRITICAL CARE	NR	PULMONARY	★★★
GASTROINTESTINAL	NR	STROKE	★★★
GENERAL SURGERY	NR	VASCULAR	NR
MATERNITY CARE	★	WOMEN'S HEALTH	NR

HEALTHGRADES AWARDS

Knoxville Hospital and Clinics

1002 South Lincoln
Knoxville, IA 50138
(641) 842-2151

Overall patient safety: ★★★
Teaching: N

CLINICAL PROGRAM RATINGS:

CARDIAC	NR	ORTHOPEDICS	NR
CRITICAL CARE	NR	PULMONARY	★★★
GASTROINTESTINAL	NR	STROKE	NR
GENERAL SURGERY	NR	VASCULAR	NR
MATERNITY CARE	★	WOMEN'S HEALTH	NR

HEALTHGRADES AWARDS

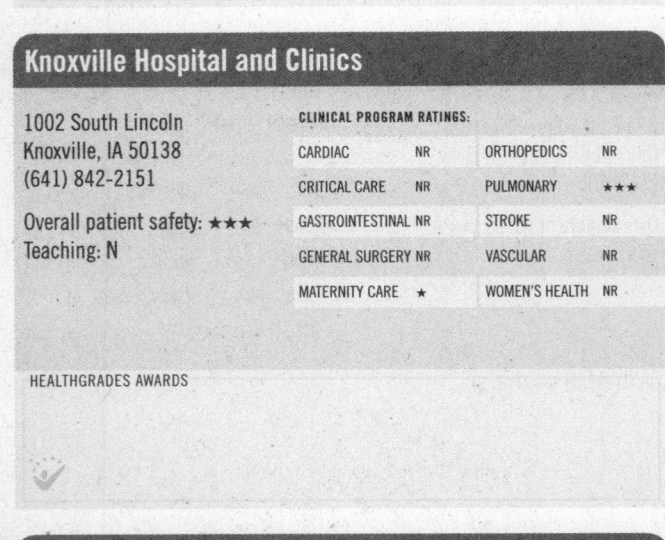

Lucas County Health Center

1200 North 7th Street
Chariton, IA 50049
(641) 774-3000

Overall patient safety: ★★★
Teaching: N

CLINICAL PROGRAM RATINGS:

CARDIAC	NR	ORTHOPEDICS	NR
CRITICAL CARE	NR	PULMONARY	★★★
GASTROINTESTINAL	NR	STROKE	NR
GENERAL SURGERY	NR	VASCULAR	NR
MATERNITY CARE	★★★	WOMEN'S HEALTH	NR

HEALTHGRADES AWARDS

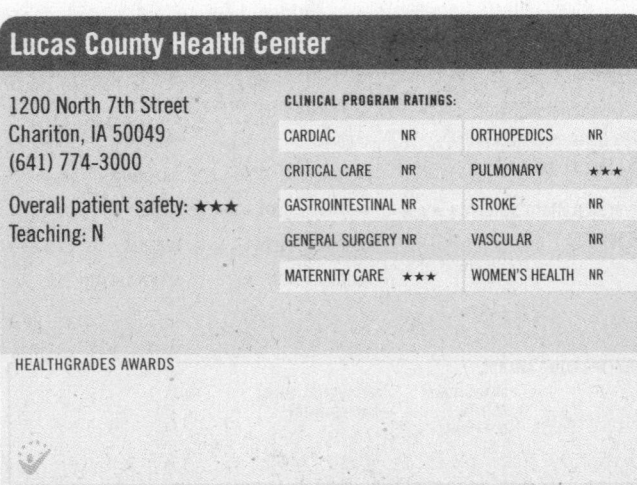

Lakes Regional Healthcare

Highway 71 South
Spirit Lake, IA 51360
(712) 336-1230

Overall patient safety: ★★★
Teaching: N

CLINICAL PROGRAM RATINGS:

CARDIAC	NR	ORTHOPEDICS	NR
CRITICAL CARE	NR	PULMONARY	★
GASTROINTESTINAL	NR	STROKE	★★★
GENERAL SURGERY	★★★	VASCULAR	NR
MATERNITY CARE	★★★	WOMEN'S HEALTH	NR

HEALTHGRADES AWARDS

Madison County Memorial Hospital

300 West Hutchings Street
Winterset, IA 50273
(515) 462-2373

Overall patient safety: ★★★
Teaching: N

CLINICAL PROGRAM RATINGS:

CARDIAC	NR	ORTHOPEDICS	NR
CRITICAL CARE	NR	PULMONARY	★
GASTROINTESTINAL	NR	STROKE	★★★
GENERAL SURGERY	NR	VASCULAR	NR
MATERNITY CARE	★	WOMEN'S HEALTH	NR

HEALTHGRADES AWARDS

KEY: ★★★★★ BEST   ★★★ AS EXPECTED   ★ POOR   NR NOT RATED BY HEALTHGRADES   For full definitions of ratings and awards, see Appendix.

Mahaska County Hospital

1229 C Avenue East
Oskaloosa, IA 52577
(641) 672-3100

Overall patient safety: ★★★
Teaching: N

CLINICAL PROGRAM RATINGS:

CARDIAC	NR	ORTHOPEDICS	NR
CRITICAL CARE	NR	PULMONARY	★
GASTROINTESTINAL	NR	STROKE	★
GENERAL SURGERY	NR	VASCULAR	NR
MATERNITY CARE	★★★	WOMEN'S HEALTH	NR

HEALTHGRADES AWARDS

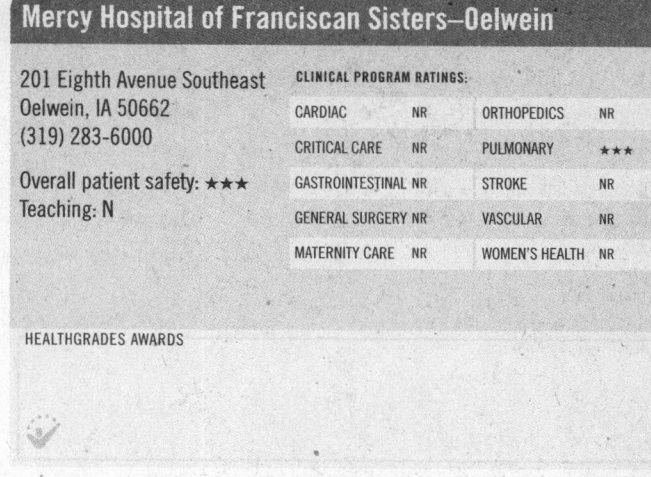

Mercy Hospital of Franciscan Sisters—Oelwein

201 Eighth Avenue Southeast
Oelwein, IA 50662
(319) 283-6000

Overall patient safety: ★★★
Teaching: N

CLINICAL PROGRAM RATINGS:

CARDIAC	NR	ORTHOPEDICS	NR
CRITICAL CARE	NR	PULMONARY	★★★
GASTROINTESTINAL	NR	STROKE	NR
GENERAL SURGERY	NR	VASCULAR	NR
MATERNITY CARE	NR	WOMEN'S HEALTH	NR

HEALTHGRADES AWARDS

Marshalltown Medical and Surgical Center

3 South 4th Avenue
Marshalltown, IA 50158
(641) 754-5151

Overall patient safety: ★★★
Teaching: N

CLINICAL PROGRAM RATINGS:

CARDIAC	NR	ORTHOPEDICS	NR
CRITICAL CARE	NR	PULMONARY	★★★
GASTROINTESTINAL	★★★	STROKE	★★★
GENERAL SURGERY	★	VASCULAR	NR
MATERNITY CARE	★	WOMEN'S HEALTH	NR

HEALTHGRADES AWARDS

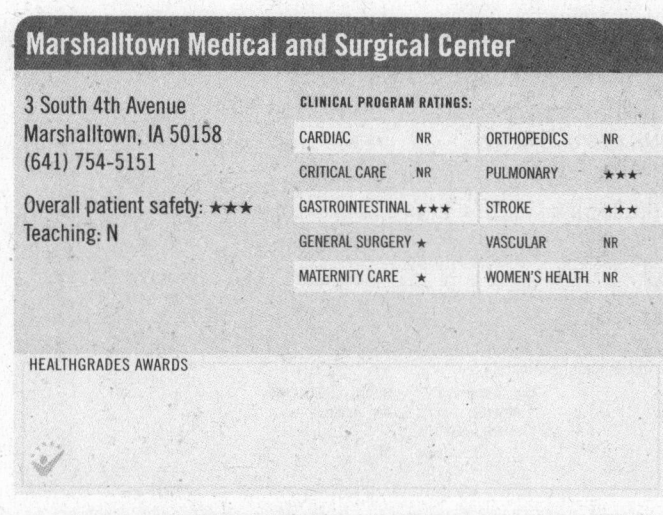

Mercy Hospital—Iowa City

500 East Market Street
Iowa City, IA 52245
(319) 339-0300

Overall patient safety: ★★★
Teaching: Y

CLINICAL PROGRAM RATINGS:

CARDIAC	★★★	ORTHOPEDICS	★★★
CRITICAL CARE	NR	PULMONARY	★★★
GASTROINTESTINAL	★★★	STROKE	★★★
GENERAL SURGERY	★★★	VASCULAR	NR
MATERNITY CARE	★★★	WOMEN'S HEALTH	★

HEALTHGRADES AWARDS

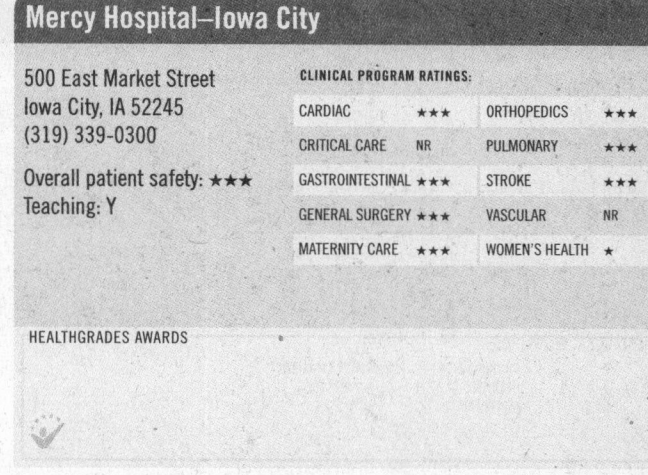

Mary Greeley Medical Center

1111 Duff Avenue
Ames, IA 50010
(515) 239-2011

Overall patient safety: ★★★★★
Teaching: N

CLINICAL PROGRAM RATINGS:

CARDIAC	NR	ORTHOPEDICS	★★★
CRITICAL CARE	NR	PULMONARY	★★★
GASTROINTESTINAL	★★★	STROKE	★★★
GENERAL SURGERY	★★★	VASCULAR	NR
MATERNITY CARE	★★★	WOMEN'S HEALTH	NR

HEALTHGRADES AWARDS

✓ DISTINGUISHED
HOSPITAL
• PATIENT SAFETY

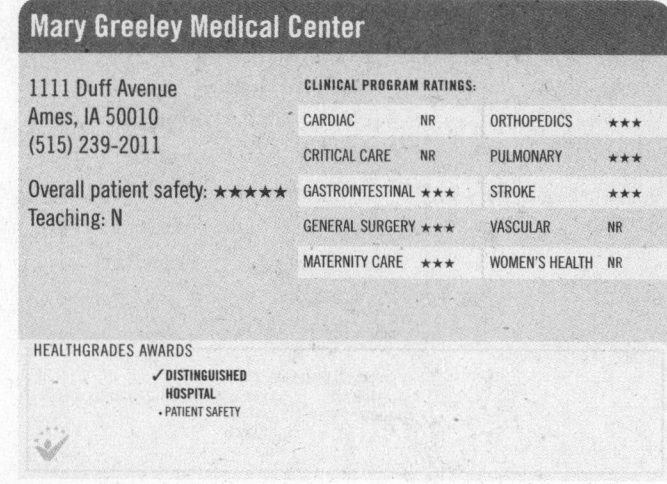

Mercy Medical Center—Cedar Rapids

701 10th Street Southeast
Cedar Rapids, IA 52403
(319) 398-6011

Overall patient safety: ★★★
Teaching: Y

CLINICAL PROGRAM RATINGS:

CARDIAC	NR	ORTHOPEDICS	★★★
CRITICAL CARE	NR	PULMONARY	★★★
GASTROINTESTINAL	★★★	STROKE	★★★
GENERAL SURGERY	★★★	VASCULAR	★★★
MATERNITY CARE	★★★	WOMEN'S HEALTH	NR

HEALTHGRADES AWARDS

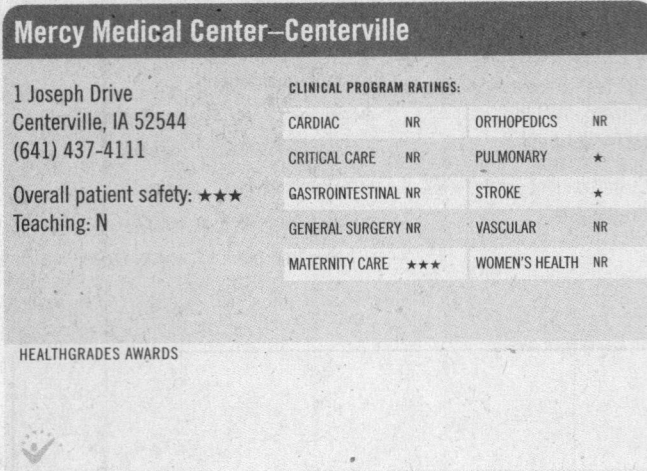

Mercy Medical Center—Centerville

1 Joseph Drive
Centerville, IA 52544
(641) 437-4111

Overall patient safety: ★★★
Teaching: N

CLINICAL PROGRAM RATINGS:

CARDIAC	NR	ORTHOPEDICS	NR
CRITICAL CARE	NR	PULMONARY	★
GASTROINTESTINAL	NR	STROKE	★
GENERAL SURGERY	NR	VASCULAR	NR
MATERNITY CARE	★★★	WOMEN'S HEALTH	NR

HEALTHGRADES AWARDS

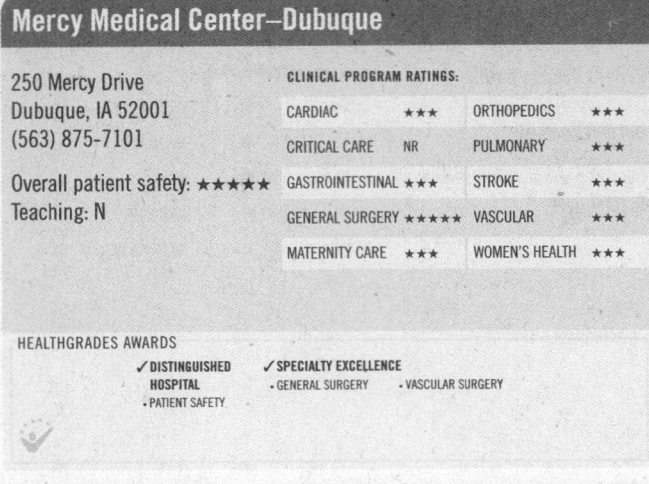

Mercy Medical Center—Dubuque

250 Mercy Drive
Dubuque, IA 52001
(563) 875-7101

Overall patient safety: ★★★★★
Teaching: N

CLINICAL PROGRAM RATINGS:

CARDIAC	★★★	ORTHOPEDICS	★★★
CRITICAL CARE	NR	PULMONARY	★★★
GASTROINTESTINAL	★★★	STROKE	★★★
GENERAL SURGERY	★★★★★	VASCULAR	★★★
MATERNITY CARE	★★★	WOMEN'S HEALTH	★★★

HEALTHGRADES AWARDS

✓ DISTINGUISHED HOSPITAL
· PATIENT SAFETY

✓ SPECIALTY EXCELLENCE
· GENERAL SURGERY   · VASCULAR SURGERY

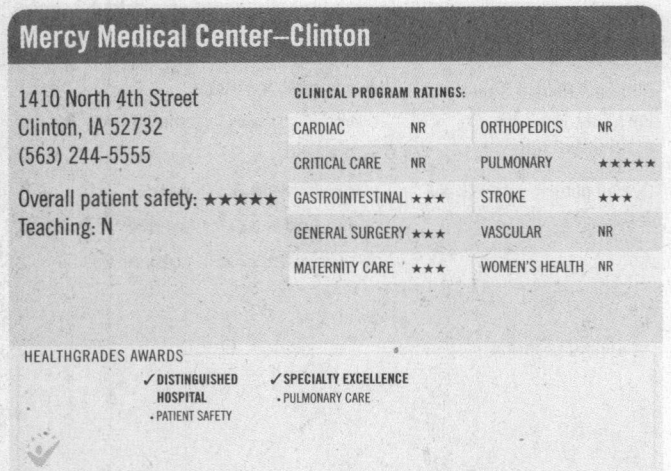

Mercy Medical Center—Clinton

1410 North 4th Street
Clinton, IA 52732
(563) 244-5555

Overall patient safety: ★★★★★
Teaching: N

CLINICAL PROGRAM RATINGS:

CARDIAC	NR	ORTHOPEDICS	NR
CRITICAL CARE	NR	PULMONARY	★★★★★
GASTROINTESTINAL	★★★	STROKE	★★★
GENERAL SURGERY	★★★	VASCULAR	NR
MATERNITY CARE	★★★	WOMEN'S HEALTH	NR

HEALTHGRADES AWARDS

✓ DISTINGUISHED HOSPITAL
· PATIENT SAFETY

✓ SPECIALTY EXCELLENCE
· PULMONARY CARE

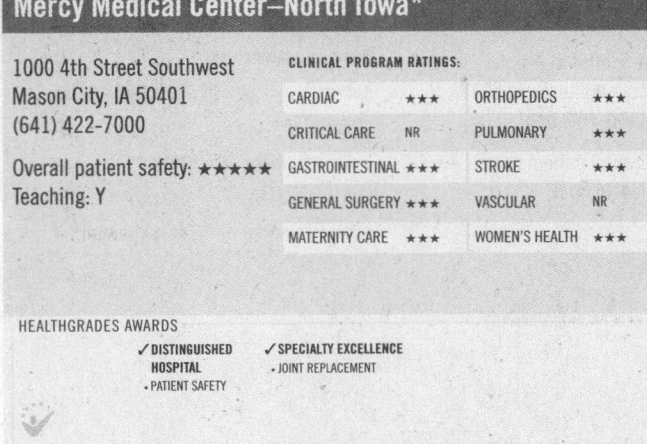

Mercy Medical Center—North Iowa*

1000 4th Street Southwest
Mason City, IA 50401
(641) 422-7000

Overall patient safety: ★★★★★
Teaching: Y

CLINICAL PROGRAM RATINGS:

CARDIAC	★★★	ORTHOPEDICS	★★★
CRITICAL CARE	NR	PULMONARY	★★★
GASTROINTESTINAL	★★★	STROKE	★★★
GENERAL SURGERY	★★★	VASCULAR	NR
MATERNITY CARE	★★★	WOMEN'S HEALTH	★★★

HEALTHGRADES AWARDS

✓ DISTINGUISHED HOSPITAL
· PATIENT SAFETY

✓ SPECIALTY EXCELLENCE
· JOINT REPLACEMENT

Mercy Medical Center—Des Moines*

1111 6th Avenue
Des Moines, IA 50314
(515) 247-3121

Overall patient safety: ★★★
Teaching: Y

CLINICAL PROGRAM RATINGS:

CARDIAC	★★★	ORTHOPEDICS	★★★
CRITICAL CARE	NR	PULMONARY	★★★★★
GASTROINTESTINAL	★★★	STROKE	★★★
GENERAL SURGERY	★★★	VASCULAR	★★★
MATERNITY CARE	★★★★★	WOMEN'S HEALTH	★★★★★

HEALTHGRADES AWARDS

✓ DISTINGUISHED HOSPITAL
· CLINICAL EXCELLENCE

✓ SPECIALTY EXCELLENCE
· PULMONARY CARE   · WOMEN'S HEALTH

Mercy Medical Center—Sioux City

801 5th Street
Sioux City, IA 51101
(712) 279-2010

Overall patient safety: ★★★
Teaching: Y

CLINICAL PROGRAM RATINGS:

CARDIAC	★★★	ORTHOPEDICS	★★★★★
CRITICAL CARE	NR	PULMONARY	★★★
GASTROINTESTINAL	★★★	STROKE	★★★
GENERAL SURGERY	★★★★★	VASCULAR	★★★
MATERNITY CARE	★★★	WOMEN'S HEALTH	★★★

HEALTHGRADES AWARDS

✓ SPECIALTY EXCELLENCE
· CARDIAC CARE   · JOINT REPLACEMENT   · VASCULAR SURGERY
· GENERAL SURGERY   · ORTHOPEDIC SURGERY

KEY: ★★★★★ BEST   ★★★ AS EXPECTED   ★ POOR   NR NOT RATED BY HEALTHGRADES   For full definitions of ratings and awards, see Appendix.

Metropolitan Medical Center*

603 East 12th Street
Des Moines, IA 50309
(515) 263-4200

Overall patient safety: ★★★
Teaching: Y

CLINICAL PROGRAM RATINGS:

CARDIAC	★★★	ORTHOPEDICS	★★★
CRITICAL CARE	NR	PULMONARY	★★★★★
GASTROINTESTINAL	★★★	STROKE	★★★
GENERAL SURGERY	★★★	VASCULAR	★★★
MATERNITY CARE	★★★★★	WOMEN'S HEALTH	★★★★★

HEALTHGRADES AWARDS

✓ SPECIALTY EXCELLENCE
- PULMONARY CARE   - WOMEN'S HEALTH

Northwest Iowa Health Center

118 North 7th Avenue
Sheldon, IA 51201
(712) 324-5041

Overall patient safety: NR
Teaching: N

CLINICAL PROGRAM RATINGS:

CARDIAC	NR	ORTHOPEDICS	NR
CRITICAL CARE	NR	PULMONARY	★★★
GASTROINTESTINAL	NR	STROKE	NR
GENERAL SURGERY	NR	VASCULAR	NR
MATERNITY CARE	NR	WOMEN'S HEALTH	NR

HEALTHGRADES AWARDS

Mitchell County Regional Health

616 North 8th Street
Osage, IA 50461
(641) 732-6000

Overall patient safety: ★★★
Teaching: N

CLINICAL PROGRAM RATINGS:

CARDIAC	NR	ORTHOPEDICS	NR
CRITICAL CARE	NR	PULMONARY	★★★
GASTROINTESTINAL	NR	STROKE	NR
GENERAL SURGERY	NR	VASCULAR	NR
MATERNITY CARE	★	WOMEN'S HEALTH	NR

HEALTHGRADES AWARDS

Orange City Area Health System

400 Central Avenue Northwest
Orange City, IA 51041
(712) 737-4984

Overall patient safety: ★★★
Teaching: N

CLINICAL PROGRAM RATINGS:

CARDIAC	NR	ORTHOPEDICS	NR
CRITICAL CARE	NR	PULMONARY	★★★
GASTROINTESTINAL	NR	STROKE	NR
GENERAL SURGERY	NR	VASCULAR	NR
MATERNITY CARE	★★★	WOMEN'S HEALTH	NR

HEALTHGRADES AWARDS

Montgomery County Memorial Hospital

2301 Eastern Avenue
Red Oak, IA 51566
(712) 623-7000

Overall patient safety: ★★★
Teaching: N

CLINICAL PROGRAM RATINGS:

CARDIAC	NR	ORTHOPEDICS	NR
CRITICAL CARE	NR	PULMONARY	★★★
GASTROINTESTINAL	NR	STROKE	★★★
GENERAL SURGERY	NR	VASCULAR	NR
MATERNITY CARE	★★★	WOMEN'S HEALTH	NR

HEALTHGRADES AWARDS

Osceola Community Hospital

600 9th Avenue North
Sibley, IA 51249
(712) 754-2574

Overall patient safety: ★★★
Teaching: N

CLINICAL PROGRAM RATINGS:

CARDIAC	NR	ORTHOPEDICS	NR
CRITICAL CARE	NR	PULMONARY	NR
GASTROINTESTINAL	NR	STROKE	NR
GENERAL SURGERY	NR	VASCULAR	NR
MATERNITY CARE	★★★	WOMEN'S HEALTH	NR

HEALTHGRADES AWARDS

*This hospital reports its data to the federal government jointly with another hospital. Therefore the ratings and awards apply to multiple hospitals and this specific hospital may not provide all rated services.

Ottumwa Regional Health Center

1001 Pennsylvania Avenue
Ottumwa, IA 52501
(641) 684-2300

Overall patient safety: ★★★
Teaching: N

CLINICAL PROGRAM RATINGS:

CARDIAC	NR	ORTHOPEDICS	NR
CRITICAL CARE	NR	PULMONARY	★★★★★
GASTROINTESTINAL	NR	STROKE	★★★
GENERAL SURGERY	★	VASCULAR	NR
MATERNITY CARE	NR	WOMEN'S HEALTH	NR

HEALTHGRADES AWARDS

✓ SPECIALTY EXCELLENCE
· PULMONARY CARE

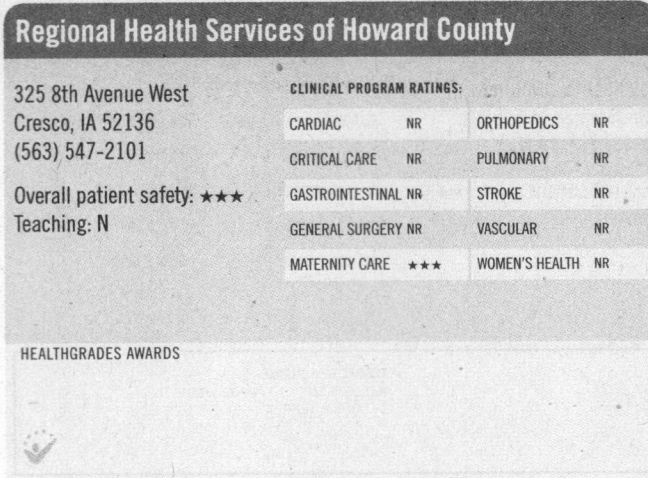

Regional Health Services of Howard County

325 8th Avenue West
Cresco, IA 52136
(563) 547-2101

Overall patient safety: ★★★
Teaching: N

CLINICAL PROGRAM RATINGS:

CARDIAC	NR	ORTHOPEDICS	NR
CRITICAL CARE	NR	PULMONARY	NR
GASTROINTESTINAL	NR	STROKE	NR
GENERAL SURGERY	NR	VASCULAR	NR
MATERNITY CARE	★★★	WOMEN'S HEALTH	NR

HEALTHGRADES AWARDS

Palmer Lutheran Health Center

112 Jefferson Street
West Union, IA 52175
(563) 422-3876

Overall patient safety: ★★★
Teaching: N

CLINICAL PROGRAM RATINGS:

CARDIAC	NR	ORTHOPEDICS	NR
CRITICAL CARE	NR	PULMONARY	★★★
GASTROINTESTINAL	NR	STROKE	NR
GENERAL SURGERY	NR	VASCULAR	NR
MATERNITY CARE	★★★	WOMEN'S HEALTH	NR

HEALTHGRADES AWARDS

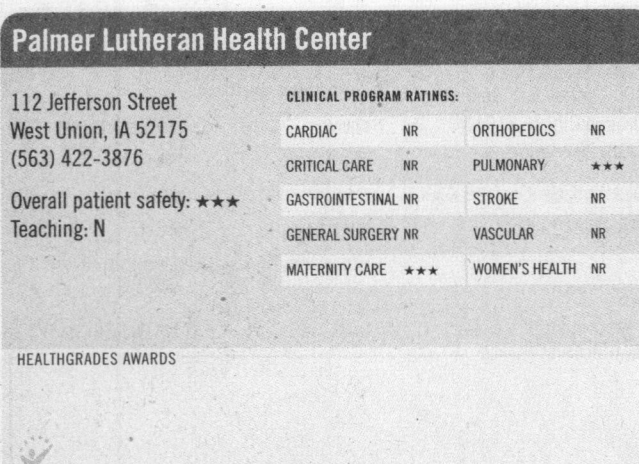

Regional Medical Center

709 West Main Street
Manchester, IA 52057
(563) 927-3232

Overall patient safety: ★★★
Teaching: N

CLINICAL PROGRAM RATINGS:

CARDIAC	NR	ORTHOPEDICS	NR
CRITICAL CARE	NR	PULMONARY	★★★
GASTROINTESTINAL	NR	STROKE	★★★
GENERAL SURGERY	NR	VASCULAR	NR
MATERNITY CARE	★	WOMEN'S HEALTH	NR

HEALTHGRADES AWARDS

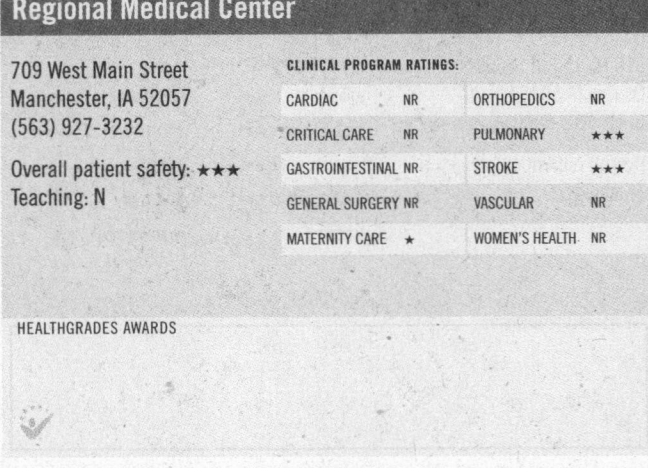

Pella Regional Health Center

404 Jefferson Street
Pella, IA 50219
(641) 628-3150

Overall patient safety: ★★★
Teaching: Y

CLINICAL PROGRAM RATINGS:

CARDIAC	NR	ORTHOPEDICS	NR
CRITICAL CARE	NR	PULMONARY	★★★
GASTROINTESTINAL	NR	STROKE	★★★
GENERAL SURGERY	NR	VASCULAR	NR
MATERNITY CARE	★	WOMEN'S HEALTH	NR

HEALTHGRADES AWARDS

Ringgold County Hospital

211 Shellway Drive
Mount Ayr, IA 50854
(641) 464-3226

Overall patient safety: ★★★
Teaching: N

CLINICAL PROGRAM RATINGS:

CARDIAC	NR	ORTHOPEDICS	NR
CRITICAL CARE	NR	PULMONARY	★★★
GASTROINTESTINAL	NR	STROKE	NR
GENERAL SURGERY	NR	VASCULAR	NR
MATERNITY CARE	NR	WOMEN'S HEALTH	NR

HEALTHGRADES AWARDS

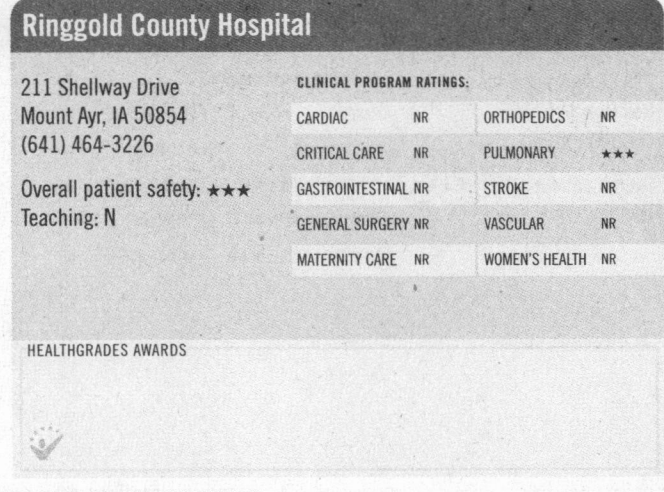

KEY: ★★★★★ BEST · ★★★ AS EXPECTED · ★ POOR NR NOT RATED BY HEALTHGRADES For full definitions of ratings and awards, see Appendix.

St. Anthony Regional Hospital

311 South Clark Street
Carroll, IA 51401
(712) 792-3581

Overall patient safety: ★★★
Teaching: N

CLINICAL PROGRAM RATINGS:

CARDIAC	NR	ORTHOPEDICS	NR
CRITICAL CARE	NR	PULMONARY	★
GASTROINTESTINAL	NR	STROKE	★★★
GENERAL SURGERY	NR	VASCULAR	NR
MATERNITY CARE	★★★	WOMEN'S HEALTH	NR

HEALTHGRADES AWARDS

Sartori Memorial Hospital

515 College Street
Cedar Falls, IA 50613
(319) 268-3000

Overall patient safety: ★★★
Teaching: N

CLINICAL PROGRAM RATINGS:

CARDIAC	NR	ORTHOPEDICS	NR
CRITICAL CARE	NR	PULMONARY	★★★
GASTROINTESTINAL	NR	STROKE	★★★
GENERAL SURGERY	★★★	VASCULAR	NR
MATERNITY CARE	NR	WOMEN'S HEALTH	NR

HEALTHGRADES AWARDS

St. Luke's Hospital

1026 A Avenue Northeast
Cedar Rapids, IA 52402
(319) 369-7211

Overall patient safety: ★★★
Teaching: Y

CLINICAL PROGRAM RATINGS:

CARDIAC	★★★	ORTHOPEDICS	★★★
CRITICAL CARE	NR	PULMONARY	★★★★★
GASTROINTESTINAL	★★★	STROKE	★★★
GENERAL SURGERY	★★★	VASCULAR	★★★
MATERNITY CARE	NR	WOMEN'S HEALTH	NR

HEALTHGRADES AWARDS

✓ DISTINGUISHED HOSPITAL
  • CLINICAL EXCELLENCE

✓ SPECIALTY EXCELLENCE
  • GASTROINTESTINAL CARE
  • GENERAL SURGERY
  • VASCULAR SURGERY

Shelby County Myrtue Memorial Hospital

1213 Garfield Avenue
Harlan, IA 51537
(712) 755-5161

Overall patient safety: ★★★
Teaching: N

CLINICAL PROGRAM RATINGS:

CARDIAC	NR	ORTHOPEDICS	NR
CRITICAL CARE	NR	PULMONARY	★★★
GASTROINTESTINAL	NR	STROKE	★★★
GENERAL SURGERY	NR	VASCULAR	NR
MATERNITY CARE	★	WOMEN'S HEALTH	NR

HEALTHGRADES AWARDS

St. Luke's Regional Medical Center

2720 Stone Park Boulevard
Sioux City, IA 51104
(712) 279-3500

Overall patient safety: ★★★
Teaching: Y

CLINICAL PROGRAM RATINGS:

CARDIAC	NR	ORTHOPEDICS	★
CRITICAL CARE	NR	PULMONARY	★★★
GASTROINTESTINAL	★★★	STROKE	★★★
GENERAL SURGERY	★★★	VASCULAR	NR
MATERNITY CARE	★★★	WOMEN'S HEALTH	NR

HEALTHGRADES AWARDS

Shenandoah Memorial Hospital

300 Pershing Avenue
Shenandoah, IA 51601
(712) 246-1230

Overall patient safety: ★★★
Teaching: N

CLINICAL PROGRAM RATINGS:

CARDIAC	NR	ORTHOPEDICS	NR
CRITICAL CARE	NR	PULMONARY	★★★
GASTROINTESTINAL	NR	STROKE	NR
GENERAL SURGERY	NR	VASCULAR	NR
MATERNITY CARE	★	WOMEN'S HEALTH	NR

HEALTHGRADES AWARDS

Skiff Medical Center

204 North 4th Avenue East
Newton, IA 50208
(641) 792-1273

Overall patient safety: ★★★
Teaching: N

CLINICAL PROGRAM RATINGS:

CARDIAC	NR	ORTHOPEDICS	NR
CRITICAL CARE	NR	PULMONARY	★★★
GASTROINTESTINAL	NR	STROKE	★★★
GENERAL SURGERY	NR	VASCULAR	NR
MATERNITY CARE	NR	WOMEN'S HEALTH	NR

HEALTHGRADES AWARDS

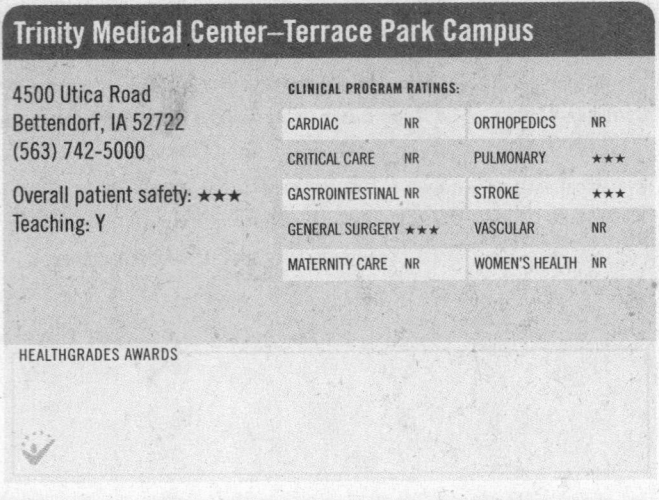

Trinity Medical Center—Terrace Park Campus

4500 Utica Road
Bettendorf, IA 52722
(563) 742-5000

Overall patient safety: ★★★
Teaching: Y

CLINICAL PROGRAM RATINGS:

CARDIAC	NR	ORTHOPEDICS	NR
CRITICAL CARE	NR	PULMONARY	★★★
GASTROINTESTINAL	NR	STROKE	★★★
GENERAL SURGERY	★★★	VASCULAR	NR
MATERNITY CARE	NR	WOMEN'S HEALTH	NR

HEALTHGRADES AWARDS

Spencer Municipal Hospital

1200 1st Avenue East
Spencer, IA 51301
(712) 264-6198

Overall patient safety: ★★★★★
Teaching: N

CLINICAL PROGRAM RATINGS:

CARDIAC	NR	ORTHOPEDICS	NR
CRITICAL CARE	NR	PULMONARY	★★★
GASTROINTESTINAL	NR	STROKE	★
GENERAL SURGERY	★★★	VASCULAR	NR
MATERNITY CARE	★	WOMEN'S HEALTH	NR

HEALTHGRADES AWARDS

✓ SPECIALTY EXCELLENCE
· JOINT REPLACEMENT

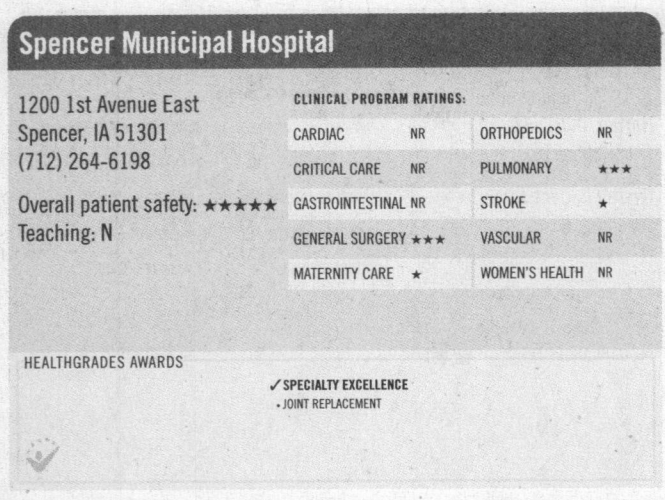

Trinity Regional Medical Center

802 Kenyon Road
Fort Dodge, IA 50501
(515) 573-3101

Overall patient safety: ★★★
Teaching: Y

CLINICAL PROGRAM RATINGS:

CARDIAC	★	ORTHOPEDICS	NR
CRITICAL CARE	NR	PULMONARY	★
GASTROINTESTINAL	★	STROKE	★
GENERAL SURGERY	★	VASCULAR	NR
MATERNITY CARE	NR	WOMEN'S HEALTH	NR

HEALTHGRADES AWARDS

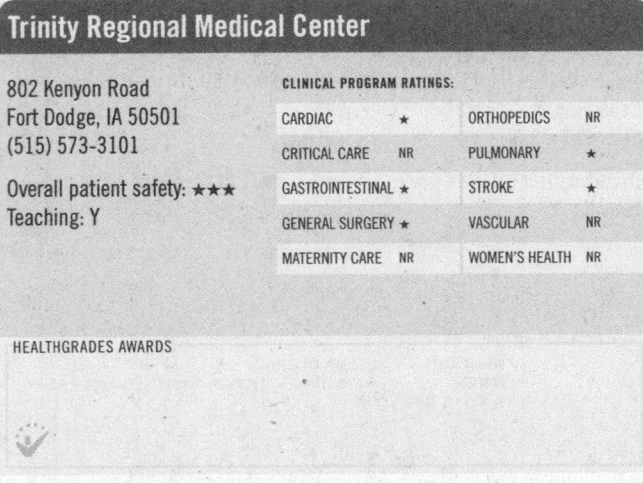

Stewart Memorial Community Hospital

1301 West Main Street
Lake City, IA 51449
(712) 464-3171

Overall patient safety: ★★★
Teaching: N

CLINICAL PROGRAM RATINGS:

CARDIAC	NR	ORTHOPEDICS	NR
CRITICAL CARE	NR	PULMONARY	★★★
GASTROINTESTINAL	NR	STROKE	NR
GENERAL SURGERY	NR	VASCULAR	NR
MATERNITY CARE	★★★	WOMEN'S HEALTH	NR

HEALTHGRADES AWARDS

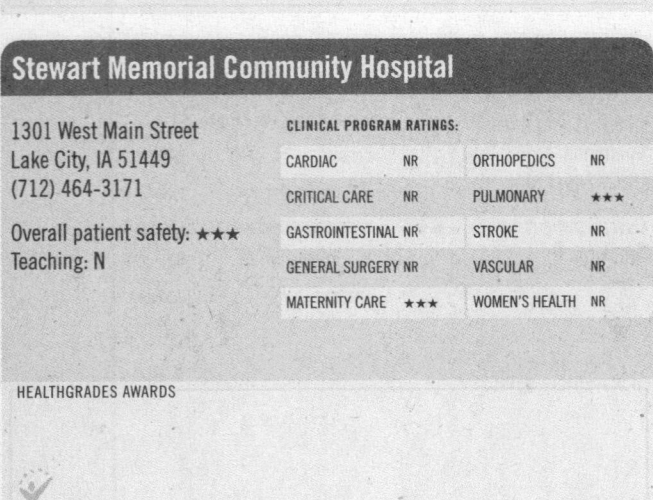

Unity Hospital

1518 Mulberry
Muscatine, IA 52761
(563) 264-9100

Overall patient safety: ★
Teaching: N

CLINICAL PROGRAM RATINGS:

CARDIAC	NR	ORTHOPEDICS	NR
CRITICAL CARE	NR	PULMONARY	★
GASTROINTESTINAL	NR	STROKE	★
GENERAL SURGERY	★★★	VASCULAR	NR
MATERNITY CARE	★	WOMEN'S HEALTH	NR

HEALTHGRADES AWARDS

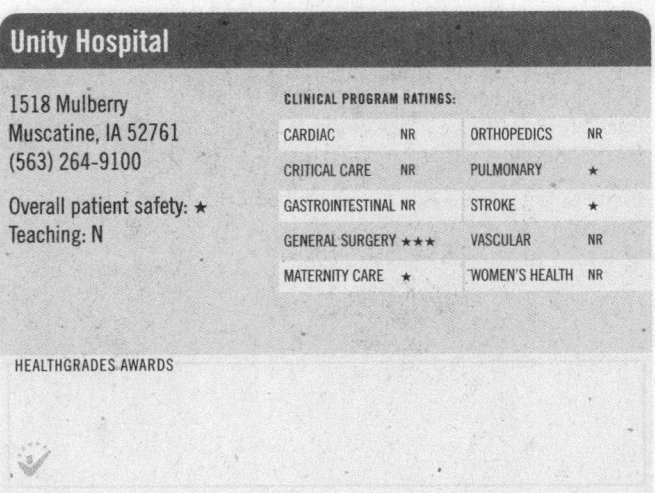

KEY: ★★★★★ BEST ★★★ AS EXPECTED ★ POOR NR NOT RATED BY HEALTHGRADES   For full definitions of ratings and awards, see Appendix.

University of Iowa Hospital and Clinics

200 Hawkins Drive
Iowa City, IA 52242
(319) 356-1616

Overall patient safety: ★
Teaching: Y

CLINICAL PROGRAM RATINGS:

CARDIAC	★★★	ORTHOPEDICS	★★★
CRITICAL CARE	NR	PULMONARY	★
GASTROINTESTINAL	★★★	STROKE	★★★
GENERAL SURGERY	★★★	VASCULAR	★★★
MATERNITY CARE	★	WOMEN'S HEALTH	★

HEALTHGRADES AWARDS

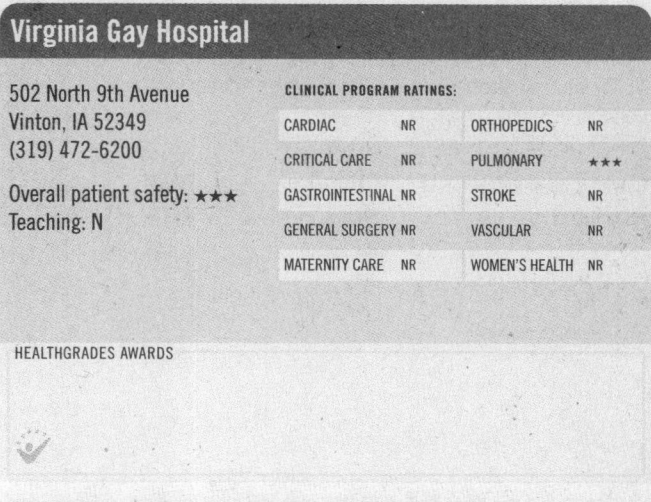

Virginia Gay Hospital

502 North 9th Avenue
Vinton, IA 52349
(319) 472-6200

Overall patient safety: ★★★
Teaching: N

CLINICAL PROGRAM RATINGS:

CARDIAC	NR	ORTHOPEDICS	NR
CRITICAL CARE	NR	PULMONARY	★★★
GASTROINTESTINAL	NR	STROKE	NR
GENERAL SURGERY	NR	VASCULAR	NR
MATERNITY CARE	NR	WOMEN'S HEALTH	NR

HEALTHGRADES AWARDS

Van Buren County Hospital

304 Franklin Street
Keosauqua, IA 52565
(319) 293-3171

Overall patient safety: ★★★
Teaching: N

CLINICAL PROGRAM RATINGS:

CARDIAC	NR	ORTHOPEDICS	NR
CRITICAL CARE	NR	PULMONARY	★★★
GASTROINTESTINAL	NR	STROKE	★★★
GENERAL SURGERY	NR	VASCULAR	NR
MATERNITY CARE	★	WOMEN'S HEALTH	NR

HEALTHGRADES AWARDS

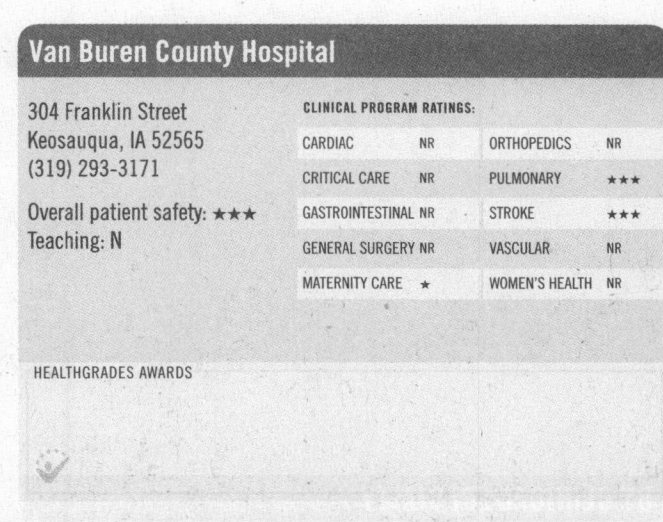

Washington County Hospital

400 East Polk Street
Washington, IA 52353
(319) 653-5481

Overall patient safety: ★★★
Teaching: N

CLINICAL PROGRAM RATINGS:

CARDIAC	NR	ORTHOPEDICS	NR
CRITICAL CARE	NR	PULMONARY	★★★
GASTROINTESTINAL	NR	STROKE	NR
GENERAL SURGERY	NR	VASCULAR	NR
MATERNITY CARE	★★★	WOMEN'S HEALTH	NR

HEALTHGRADES AWARDS

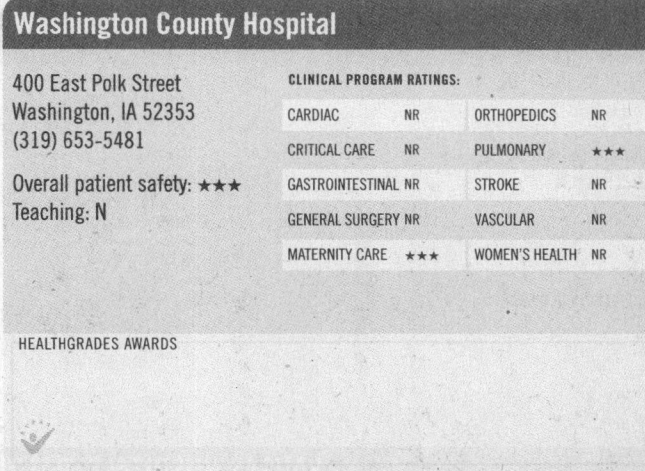

Veterans Memorial

40 1st Street Southeast
Waukon, IA 52172
(563) 568-3411

Overall patient safety: ★★★
Teaching: N

CLINICAL PROGRAM RATINGS:

CARDIAC	NR	ORTHOPEDICS	NR
CRITICAL CARE	NR	PULMONARY	★
GASTROINTESTINAL	NR	STROKE	★
GENERAL SURGERY	NR	VASCULAR	NR
MATERNITY CARE	★★★	WOMEN'S HEALTH	NR

HEALTHGRADES AWARDS

Waverly Health Center

3129th Street Southwest
Waverly, IA 50677
(319) 352-4120

Overall patient safety: ★★★
Teaching: N

CLINICAL PROGRAM RATINGS:

CARDIAC	NR	ORTHOPEDICS	NR
CRITICAL CARE	NR	PULMONARY	★★★
GASTROINTESTINAL	NR	STROKE	★
GENERAL SURGERY	NR	VASCULAR	NR
MATERNITY CARE	★★★	WOMEN'S HEALTH	NR

HEALTHGRADES AWARDS

Wayne County Hospital

417 South East Street
Corydon, IA 50060
(641) 872-2260

Overall patient safety: ★★★
Teaching: N

CLINICAL PROGRAM RATINGS:

CARDIAC	NR	ORTHOPEDICS	NR
CRITICAL CARE	NR	PULMONARY	★
GASTROINTESTINAL	NR	STROKE	★★★
GENERAL SURGERY	NR	VASCULAR	NR
MATERNITY CARE	★★★	WOMEN'S HEALTH	NR

HEALTHGRADES AWARDS

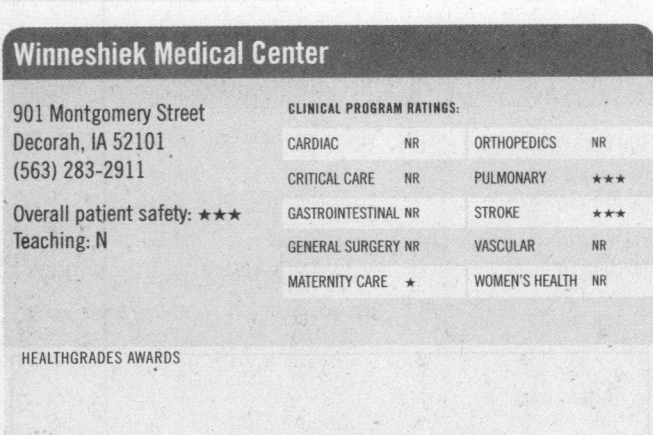

Wright Medical Center

1316 South Main Street
Clarion, IA 50525
(515) 532-2811

Overall patient safety: ★★★
Teaching: N

CLINICAL PROGRAM RATINGS:

CARDIAC	NR	ORTHOPEDICS	NR
CRITICAL CARE	NR	PULMONARY	★★★
GASTROINTESTINAL	NR	STROKE	NR
GENERAL SURGERY	NR	VASCULAR	NR
MATERNITY CARE	★★★	WOMEN'S HEALTH	NR

HEALTHGRADES AWARDS

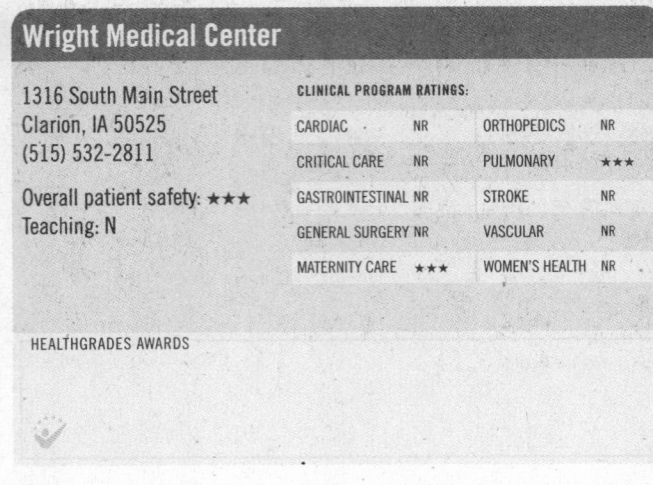

Winneshiek Medical Center

901 Montgomery Street
Decorah, IA 52101
(563) 283-2911

Overall patient safety: ★★★
Teaching: N

CLINICAL PROGRAM RATINGS:

CARDIAC	NR	ORTHOPEDICS	NR
CRITICAL CARE	NR	PULMONARY	★★★
GASTROINTESTINAL	NR	STROKE	★★★
GENERAL SURGERY	NR	VASCULAR	NR
MATERNITY CARE	★	WOMEN'S HEALTH	NR

HEALTHGRADES AWARDS

KANSAS HOSPITALS: RATINGS BY CLINICAL SPECIALTY

Allen County Hospital

101 South 1st Street
Iola, KS 66749
(620) 365-1020

Overall patient safety: ★★★
Teaching: N

CLINICAL PROGRAM RATINGS:

CARDIAC	NR	ORTHOPEDICS	NR
CRITICAL CARE	NR	PULMONARY	★
GASTROINTESTINAL	NR	STROKE	★★★
GENERAL SURGERY	NR	VASCULAR	NR
MATERNITY CARE	NR	WOMEN'S HEALTH	NR

HEALTHGRADES AWARDS

Atchison Hospital

1301 North 2nd Street
Atchison, KS 66002
(913) 367-6691

Overall patient safety: NR
Teaching: N

CLINICAL PROGRAM RATINGS:

CARDIAC	NR	ORTHOPEDICS	NR
CRITICAL CARE	NR	PULMONARY	★★★
GASTROINTESTINAL	NR	STROKE	NR
GENERAL SURGERY	NR	VASCULAR	NR
MATERNITY CARE	NR	WOMEN'S HEALTH	NR

HEALTHGRADES AWARDS

KEY: ★★★★★ BEST　★★★ AS EXPECTED　★ POOR　NR NOT RATED BY HEALTHGRADES　For full definitions of ratings and awards, see Appendix.

Bob Wilson Memorial Hospital

415 North Main Street
Ulysses, KS 67880
(620) 356-1266

Overall patient safety: ★★★
Teaching: N

CLINICAL PROGRAM RATINGS:

CARDIAC	NR	ORTHOPEDICS	NR
CRITICAL CARE	NR	PULMONARY	★★★
GASTROINTESTINAL	NR	STROKE	★★★
GENERAL SURGERY	NR	VASCULAR	NR
MATERNITY CARE	NR	WOMEN'S HEALTH	NR

HEALTHGRADES AWARDS

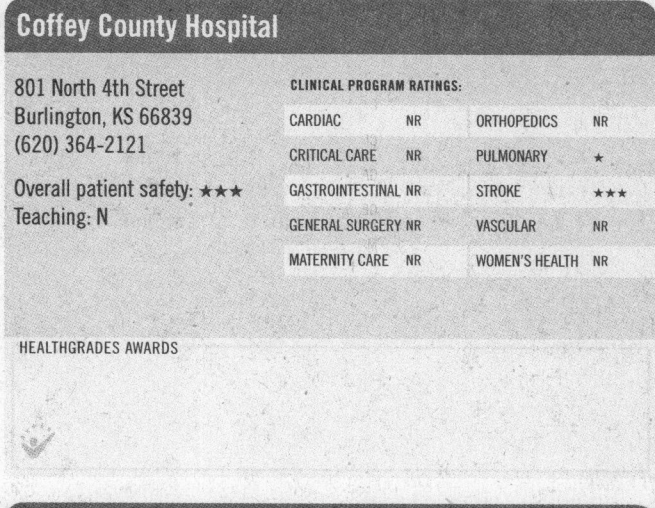

Coffey County Hospital

801 North 4th Street
Burlington, KS 66839
(620) 364-2121

Overall patient safety: ★★★
Teaching: N

CLINICAL PROGRAM RATINGS:

CARDIAC	NR	ORTHOPEDICS	NR
CRITICAL CARE	NR	PULMONARY	★
GASTROINTESTINAL	NR	STROKE	★★★
GENERAL SURGERY	NR	VASCULAR	NR
MATERNITY CARE	NR	WOMEN'S HEALTH	NR

HEALTHGRADES AWARDS

Central Kansas Medical Center

3515 Broadway
Great Bend, KS 67530
(620) 792-2511

Overall patient safety: ★★★
Teaching: N

CLINICAL PROGRAM RATINGS:

CARDIAC	NR	ORTHOPEDICS	NR
CRITICAL CARE	NR	PULMONARY	★
GASTROINTESTINAL	NR	STROKE	★★★
GENERAL SURGERY	NR	VASCULAR	NR
MATERNITY CARE	NR	WOMEN'S HEALTH	NR

HEALTHGRADES AWARDS

✓ SPECIALTY EXCELLENCE
• JOINT REPLACEMENT

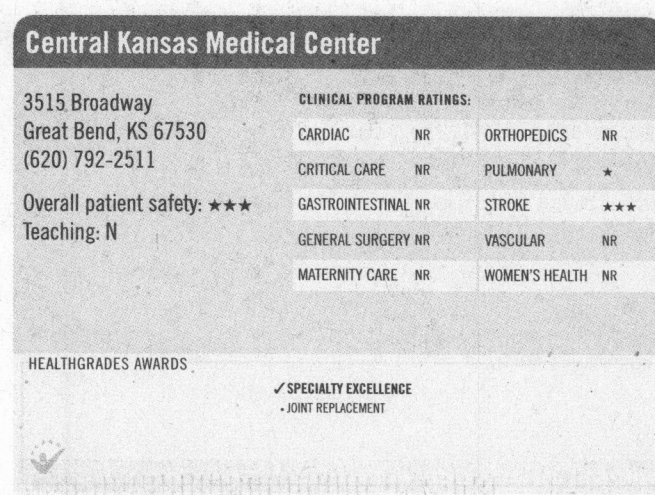

Coffeyville Regional Medical Center

1400 West 4th Street
Coffeyville, KS 67337
(620) 251-1200

Overall patient safety: ★★★
Teaching: N

CLINICAL PROGRAM RATINGS:

CARDIAC	NR	ORTHOPEDICS	NR
CRITICAL CARE	NR	PULMONARY	★★★★★
GASTROINTESTINAL	NR	STROKE	★★★
GENERAL SURGERY	NR	VASCULAR	NR
MATERNITY CARE	NR	WOMEN'S HEALTH	NR

HEALTHGRADES AWARDS

✓ SPECIALTY EXCELLENCE
• PULMONARY CARE

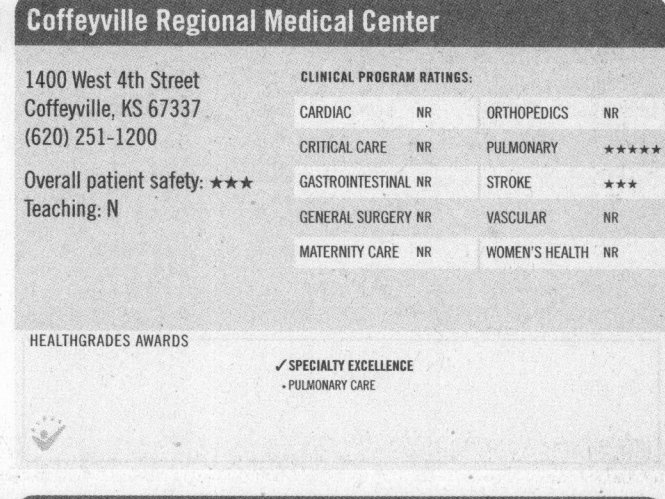

Clara Barton Hospital

250 West 9th Street
Hoisington, KS 67544
(620) 653-2114

Overall patient safety: ★★★
Teaching: N

CLINICAL PROGRAM RATINGS:

CARDIAC	NR	ORTHOPEDICS	NR
CRITICAL CARE	NR	PULMONARY	NR
GASTROINTESTINAL	NR	STROKE	NR
GENERAL SURGERY	NR	VASCULAR	NR
MATERNITY CARE	NR	WOMEN'S HEALTH	NR

HEALTHGRADES AWARDS

Community Hospital—Onaga

120 West 8th Street
Onaga, KS 66521
(785) 889-4272

Overall patient safety: ★★★
Teaching: N

CLINICAL PROGRAM RATINGS:

CARDIAC	NR	ORTHOPEDICS	NR
CRITICAL CARE	NR	PULMONARY	★★★
GASTROINTESTINAL	NR	STROKE	★★★
GENERAL SURGERY	NR	VASCULAR	NR
MATERNITY CARE	NR	WOMEN'S HEALTH	NR

HEALTHGRADES AWARDS

Community Memorial Healthcare

708 North 18th Street
Marysville, KS 66508
(785) 562-2311

Overall patient safety: ★★★
Teaching: N

CLINICAL PROGRAM RATINGS:

CARDIAC	NR	ORTHOPEDICS	NR
CRITICAL CARE	NR	PULMONARY	★
GASTROINTESTINAL	NR	STROKE	★★★
GENERAL SURGERY	NR	VASCULAR	NR
MATERNITY CARE	NR	WOMEN'S HEALTH	NR

HEALTHGRADES AWARDS

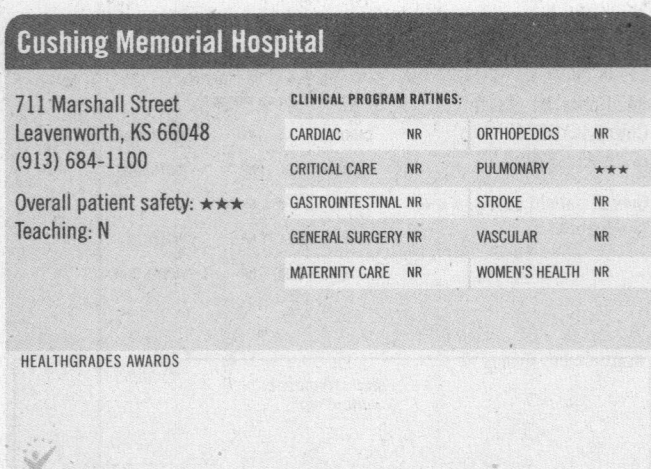

Galichia Heart Hospital

2610 North Woodlawn
Wichita, KS 67220
(316) 858-2608

Overall patient safety: ★★★★★
Teaching: N

CLINICAL PROGRAM RATINGS:

CARDIAC	★★★	ORTHOPEDICS	NR
CRITICAL CARE	NR	PULMONARY	★★★★★
GASTROINTESTINAL	NR	STROKE	★★★
GENERAL SURGERY	NR	VASCULAR	★★★
MATERNITY CARE	NR	WOMEN'S HEALTH	NR

HEALTHGRADES AWARDS

✓ SPECIALTY EXCELLENCE
• PULMONARY CARE

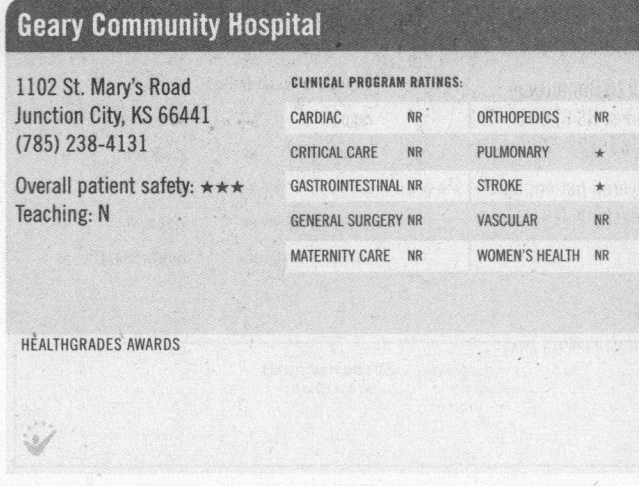

Cushing Memorial Hospital

711 Marshall Street
Leavenworth, KS 66048
(913) 684-1100

Overall patient safety: ★★★
Teaching: N

CLINICAL PROGRAM RATINGS:

CARDIAC	NR	ORTHOPEDICS	NR
CRITICAL CARE	NR	PULMONARY	★★★
GASTROINTESTINAL	NR	STROKE	NR
GENERAL SURGERY	NR	VASCULAR	NR
MATERNITY CARE	NR	WOMEN'S HEALTH	NR

HEALTHGRADES AWARDS

Geary Community Hospital

1102 St. Mary's Road
Junction City, KS 66441
(785) 238-4131

Overall patient safety: ★★★
Teaching: N

CLINICAL PROGRAM RATINGS:

CARDIAC	NR	ORTHOPEDICS	NR
CRITICAL CARE	NR	PULMONARY	★
GASTROINTESTINAL	NR	STROKE	★
GENERAL SURGERY	NR	VASCULAR	NR
MATERNITY CARE	NR	WOMEN'S HEALTH	NR

HEALTHGRADES AWARDS

Fredonia Regional Hospital

1527 Madison
P.O. Box 579
Fredonia, KS 66736
(620) 378-2121

Overall patient safety: ★★★
Teaching: N

CLINICAL PROGRAM RATINGS:

CARDIAC	NR	ORTHOPEDICS	NR
CRITICAL CARE	NR	PULMONARY	★★★
GASTROINTESTINAL	NR	STROKE	NR
GENERAL SURGERY	NR	VASCULAR	NR
MATERNITY CARE	NR	WOMEN'S HEALTH	NR

HEALTHGRADES AWARDS

Greenwood County Hospital

100 West 16th Street
Eureka, KS 67045
(620) 583-7451

Overall patient safety: NR
Teaching: N

CLINICAL PROGRAM RATINGS:

CARDIAC	NR	ORTHOPEDICS	NR
CRITICAL CARE	NR	PULMONARY	★★★
GASTROINTESTINAL	NR	STROKE	NR
GENERAL SURGERY	NR	VASCULAR	NR
MATERNITY CARE	NR	WOMEN'S HEALTH	NR

HEALTHGRADES AWARDS

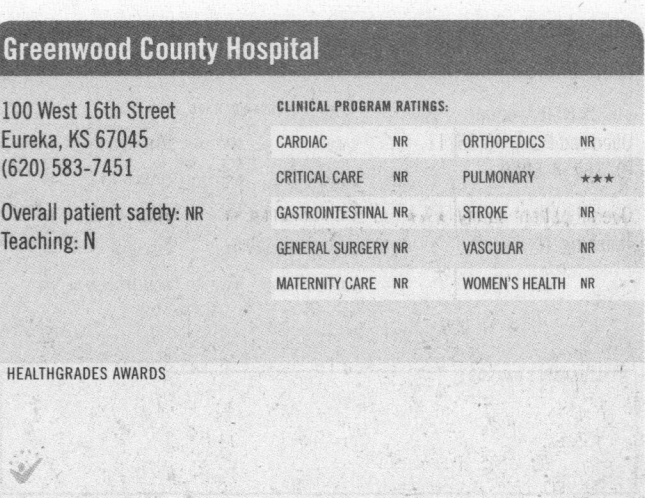

KEY: ★★★★★ BEST   ★★★ AS EXPECTED   ★ POOR   NR NOT RATED BY HEALTHGRADES   For full definitions of ratings and awards, see Appendix.

Harper Hospital District #5

1204 Maple Street
Harper, KS 67058
(620) 896-7324

Overall patient safety: ★★★
Teaching: N

CLINICAL PROGRAM RATINGS:

CARDIAC	NR	ORTHOPEDICS	NR
CRITICAL CARE	NR	PULMONARY	★★★
GASTROINTESTINAL	NR	STROKE	NR
GENERAL SURGERY	NR	VASCULAR	NR
MATERNITY CARE	NR	WOMEN'S HEALTH	NR

HEALTHGRADES AWARDS

Hiawatha Community Hospital

300 Utah Street
Hiawatha, KS 66434
(785) 742-2131

Overall patient safety: ★★★
Teaching: N

CLINICAL PROGRAM RATINGS:

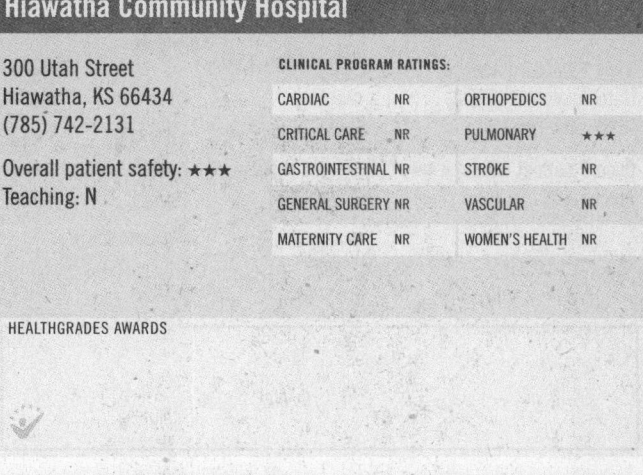

CARDIAC	NR	ORTHOPEDICS	NR
CRITICAL CARE	NR	PULMONARY	★★★
GASTROINTESTINAL	NR	STROKE	NR
GENERAL SURGERY	NR	VASCULAR	NR
MATERNITY CARE	NR	WOMEN'S HEALTH	NR

HEALTHGRADES AWARDS

Hays Medical Center

2220 Canterbury Road
Hays, KS 67601
(785) 623-5000

Overall patient safety: ★★★★★
Teaching: N

CLINICAL PROGRAM RATINGS:

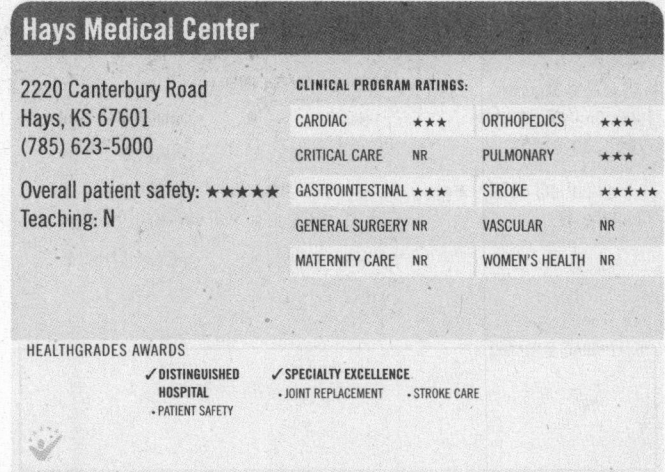

CARDIAC	★★★	ORTHOPEDICS	★★★
CRITICAL CARE	NR	PULMONARY	★★★
GASTROINTESTINAL	★★★	STROKE	★★★★★
GENERAL SURGERY	NR	VASCULAR	NR
MATERNITY CARE	NR	WOMEN'S HEALTH	NR

HEALTHGRADES AWARDS

✓ DISTINGUISHED HOSPITAL
· PATIENT SAFETY

✓ SPECIALTY EXCELLENCE
· JOINT REPLACEMENT   · STROKE CARE

Hospital District #1 of Crawford County

302 North Hospital Drive
Girard, KS 66743
(620) 724-8291

Overall patient safety: ★★★
Teaching: N

CLINICAL PROGRAM RATINGS:

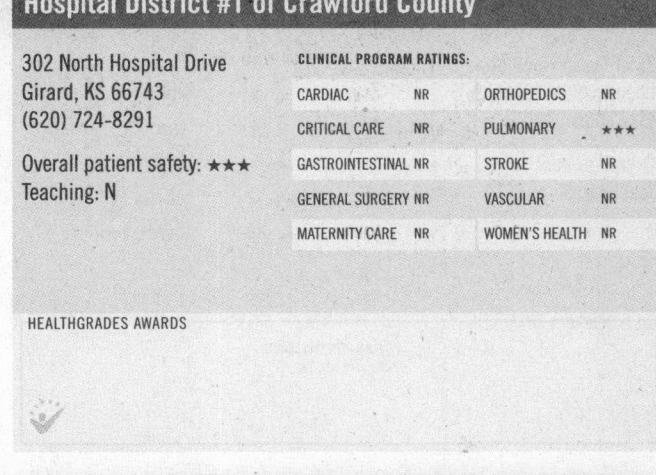

CARDIAC	NR	ORTHOPEDICS	NR
CRITICAL CARE	NR	PULMONARY	★★★
GASTROINTESTINAL	NR	STROKE	NR
GENERAL SURGERY	NR	VASCULAR	NR
MATERNITY CARE	NR	WOMEN'S HEALTH	NR

HEALTHGRADES AWARDS

Heartland Surgical Specialty Hospital

10720 Nall Avenue
Overland Park, KS 66211
(913) 754-5000

Overall patient safety: ★★★
Teaching: N

CLINICAL PROGRAM RATINGS:

CARDIAC	NR	ORTHOPEDICS	NR
CRITICAL CARE	NR	PULMONARY	NR
GASTROINTESTINAL	NR	STROKE	NR
GENERAL SURGERY	NR	VASCULAR	NR
MATERNITY CARE	NR	WOMEN'S HEALTH	NR

HEALTHGRADES AWARDS

Hospital District #1 of Rice County

619 South Clark Avenue
Lyons, KS 67554
(620) 257-5173

Overall patient safety: ★★★
Teaching: N

CLINICAL PROGRAM RATINGS:

CARDIAC	NR	ORTHOPEDICS	NR
CRITICAL CARE	NR	PULMONARY	★★★
GASTROINTESTINAL	NR	STROKE	NR
GENERAL SURGERY	NR	VASCULAR	NR
MATERNITY CARE	NR	WOMEN'S HEALTH	NR

HEALTHGRADES AWARDS

KANSAS HOSPITALS: RATINGS BY CLINICAL SPECIALTY

Hutchinson Hospital

1701 East 23rd Avenue
Hutchinson, KS 67502
(620) 665-2000

Overall patient safety: ★★★
Teaching: N

CLINICAL PROGRAM RATINGS:

CARDIAC	★★★	ORTHOPEDICS	★
CRITICAL CARE	NR	PULMONARY	★★★
GASTROINTESTINAL	★★★	STROKE	★★★
GENERAL SURGERY	NR	VASCULAR	NR
MATERNITY CARE	NR	WOMEN'S HEALTH	NR

HEALTHGRADES AWARDS

Labette Health

1902 South US Highway 59
Parsons, KS 67357
(316) 421-4880

Overall patient safety: ★★★
Teaching: N

CLINICAL PROGRAM RATINGS:

CARDIAC	NR	ORTHOPEDICS	★★★
CRITICAL CARE	NR	PULMONARY	★★★
GASTROINTESTINAL	NR	STROKE	★
GENERAL SURGERY	NR	VASCULAR	NR
MATERNITY CARE	NR	WOMEN'S HEALTH	NR

HEALTHGRADES AWARDS

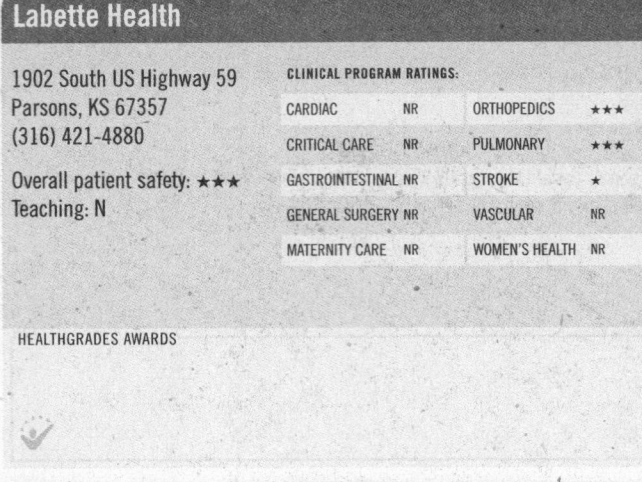

Kansas Heart Hospital

3601 North Webb Road
Wichita, KS 67226
(316) 630-5000

Overall patient safety: ★★★★★
Teaching: N

CLINICAL PROGRAM RATINGS:

CARDIAC	★★★	ORTHOPEDICS	NR
CRITICAL CARE	NR	PULMONARY	NR
GASTROINTESTINAL	NR	STROKE	NR
GENERAL SURGERY	NR	VASCULAR	★★★
MATERNITY CARE	NR	WOMEN'S HEALTH	NR

HEALTHGRADES AWARDS

✓ SPECIALTY EXCELLENCE
· VASCULAR SURGERY

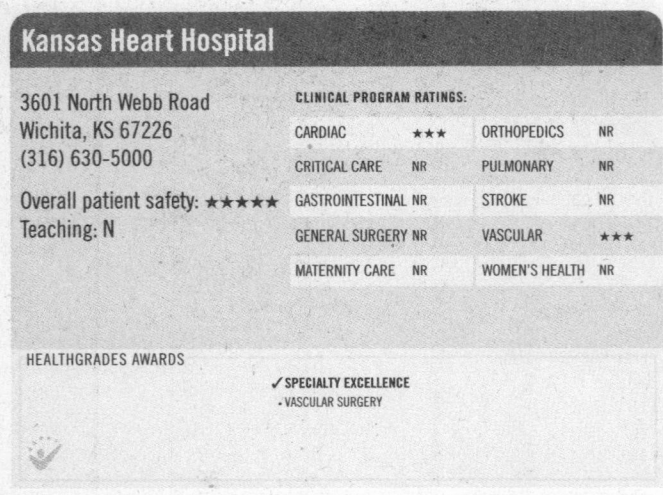

Lawrence Memorial Hospital

325 Maine Street
Lawrence, KS 66044
(785) 749-6100

Overall patient safety: ★★★
Teaching: N

CLINICAL PROGRAM RATINGS:

CARDIAC	NR	ORTHOPEDICS	NR
CRITICAL CARE	NR	PULMONARY	★
GASTROINTESTINAL	★★★	STROKE	★
GENERAL SURGERY	NR	VASCULAR	NR
MATERNITY CARE	NR	WOMEN'S HEALTH	NR

HEALTHGRADES AWARDS

Kingman Community Hospital

750 West Avenue D
Kingman, KS 67068
(620) 532-3147

Overall patient safety: ★
Teaching: N

CLINICAL PROGRAM RATINGS:

CARDIAC	NR	ORTHOPEDICS	NR
CRITICAL CARE	NR	PULMONARY	★★★
GASTROINTESTINAL	NR	STROKE	NR
GENERAL SURGERY	NR	VASCULAR	NR
MATERNITY CARE	NR	WOMEN'S HEALTH	NR

HEALTHGRADES AWARDS

Logan County Hospital

211 Cherry Avenue
Oakley, KS 67748
(785) 672-3211

Overall patient safety: ★★★
Teaching: N

CLINICAL PROGRAM RATINGS:

CARDIAC	NR	ORTHOPEDICS	NR
CRITICAL CARE	NR	PULMONARY	★★★
GASTROINTESTINAL	NR	STROKE	NR
GENERAL SURGERY	NR	VASCULAR	NR
MATERNITY CARE	NR	WOMEN'S HEALTH	NR

HEALTHGRADES AWARDS

KEY: ★★★★★ BEST   ★★★ AS EXPECTED   ★ POOR   NR NOT RATED BY HEALTHGRADES   For full definitions of ratings and awards, see Appendix.

Meade District Hospital

510 East Carthage
P.O. Box 680
Meade, KS 67864
(620) 873-2141

Overall patient safety: ★★★
Teaching: N

CLINICAL PROGRAM RATINGS:

CARDIAC	NR	ORTHOPEDICS	NR
CRITICAL CARE	NR	PULMONARY	★★★
GASTROINTESTINAL	NR	STROKE	NR
GENERAL SURGERY	NR	VASCULAR	NR
MATERNITY CARE	NR	WOMEN'S HEALTH	NR

HEALTHGRADES AWARDS

Memorial Hospital

1000 Hospital Drive
McPherson, KS 67460
(620) 241-2250

Overall patient safety: ★★★
Teaching: N

CLINICAL PROGRAM RATINGS:

CARDIAC	NR	ORTHOPEDICS	NR
CRITICAL CARE	NR	PULMONARY	★★★
GASTROINTESTINAL	NR	STROKE	★
GENERAL SURGERY	NR	VASCULAR	NR
MATERNITY CARE	NR	WOMEN'S HEALTH	NR

HEALTHGRADES AWARDS

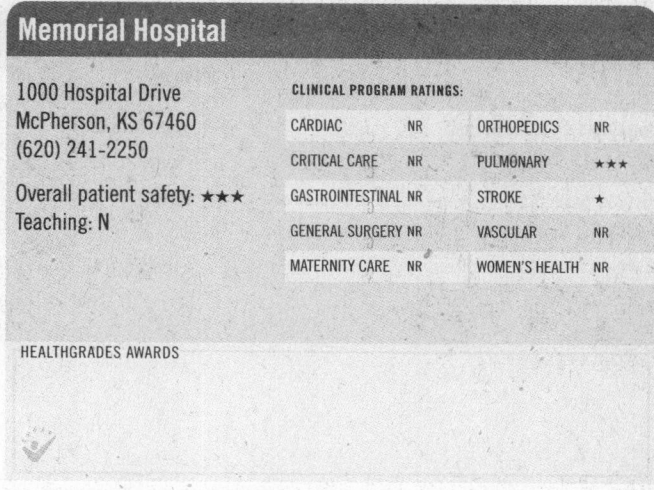

Medicine Lodge Memorial Hospital

710 North Walnut Street
Medicine Lodge, KS 67104
(620) 886-3771

Overall patient safety: ★★★
Teaching: N

CLINICAL PROGRAM RATINGS:

CARDIAC	NR	ORTHOPEDICS	NR
CRITICAL CARE	NR	PULMONARY	★★★
GASTROINTESTINAL	NR	STROKE	NR
GENERAL SURGERY	NR	VASCULAR	NR
MATERNITY CARE	NR	WOMEN'S HEALTH	NR

HEALTHGRADES AWARDS

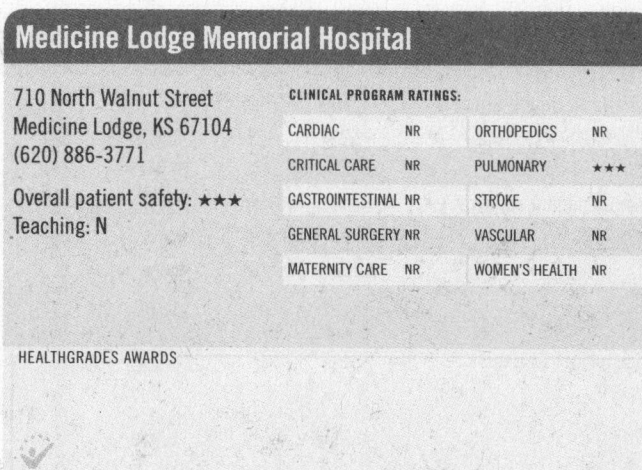

Menorah Medical Center*

5721 West 119th Street
Overland Park, KS 66209
(913) 498-6000

Overall patient safety: ★★★
Teaching: N

CLINICAL PROGRAM RATINGS:

CARDIAC	★★★	ORTHOPEDICS	★
CRITICAL CARE	NR	PULMONARY	★★★
GASTROINTESTINAL	★★★	STROKE	★★★
GENERAL SURGERY	NR	VASCULAR	NR
MATERNITY CARE	NR	WOMEN'S HEALTH	NR

HEALTHGRADES AWARDS

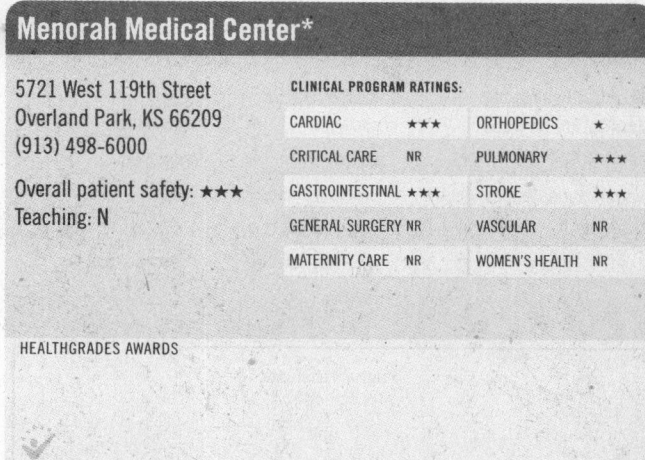

Memorial Hospital

511 North East 10th Street
Abilene, KS 67410
(620) 263-2100

Overall patient safety: NR
Teaching: N

CLINICAL PROGRAM RATINGS:

CARDIAC	NR	ORTHOPEDICS	NR
CRITICAL CARE	NR	PULMONARY	★★★
GASTROINTESTINAL	NR	STROKE	★★★
GENERAL SURGERY	NR	VASCULAR	NR
MATERNITY CARE	NR	WOMEN'S HEALTH	NR

HEALTHGRADES AWARDS

Mercy Health Center

401 Woodland Hills Boulevard
Fort Scott, KS 66701
(620) 223-2200

Overall patient safety: ★★★
Teaching: N

CLINICAL PROGRAM RATINGS:

CARDIAC	NR	ORTHOPEDICS	NR
CRITICAL CARE	NR	PULMONARY	★★★
GASTROINTESTINAL	NR	STROKE	★★★
GENERAL SURGERY	NR	VASCULAR	NR
MATERNITY CARE	NR	WOMEN'S HEALTH	NR

HEALTHGRADES AWARDS

*This hospital reports its data to the federal government jointly with another hospital. Therefore the ratings and awards apply to multiple hospitals and this specific hospital may not provide all rated services.

Mercy Hospital of Kansas Independence

800 West Myrtle Street
Independence, KS 67301
(620) 331-2200

Overall patient safety: ★★★
Teaching: N

CLINICAL PROGRAM RATINGS:

CARDIAC	NR	ORTHOPEDICS	NR
CRITICAL CARE	NR	PULMONARY	★★★
GASTROINTESTINAL	NR	STROKE	NR
GENERAL SURGERY	NR	VASCULAR	NR
MATERNITY CARE	NR	WOMEN'S HEALTH	NR

HEALTHGRADES AWARDS

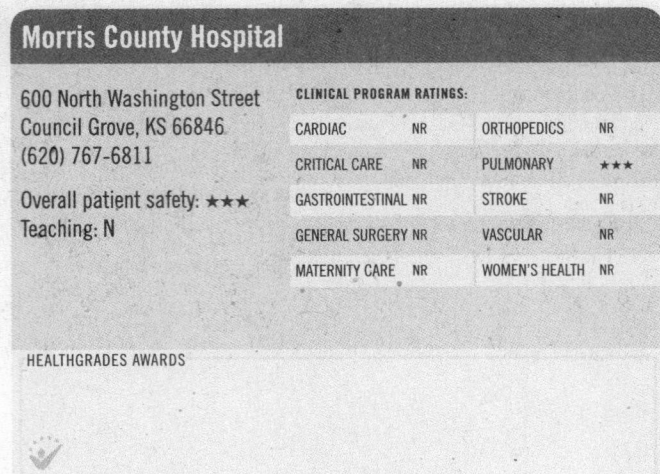

Morris County Hospital

600 North Washington Street
Council Grove, KS 66846
(620) 767-6811

Overall patient safety: ★★★
Teaching: N

CLINICAL PROGRAM RATINGS:

CARDIAC	NR	ORTHOPEDICS	NR
CRITICAL CARE	NR	PULMONARY	★★★
GASTROINTESTINAL	NR	STROKE	NR
GENERAL SURGERY	NR	VASCULAR	NR
MATERNITY CARE	NR	WOMEN'S HEALTH	NR

HEALTHGRADES AWARDS

Mercy Regional Health Center

1823 College Avenue
Manhattan, KS 66502
(785) 776-3322

Overall patient safety: ★★★
Teaching: N

CLINICAL PROGRAM RATINGS:

CARDIAC	NR	ORTHOPEDICS	★★★
CRITICAL CARE	NR	PULMONARY	★★★
GASTROINTESTINAL	NR	STROKE	★★★
GENERAL SURGERY	NR	VASCULAR	NR
MATERNITY CARE	NR	WOMEN'S HEALTH	NR

HEALTHGRADES AWARDS

✓ SPECIALTY EXCELLENCE
• JOINT REPLACEMENT

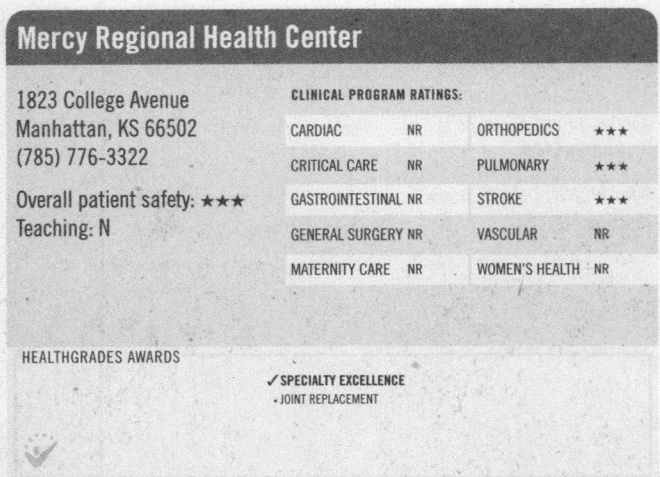

Morton County Hospital

445 North Hilltop Street
Elkhart, KS 67950
(620) 697-2141

Overall patient safety: ★★★
Teaching: N

CLINICAL PROGRAM RATINGS:

CARDIAC	NR	ORTHOPEDICS	NR
CRITICAL CARE	NR	PULMONARY	★★★
GASTROINTESTINAL	NR	STROKE	★★★
GENERAL SURGERY	NR	VASCULAR	NR
MATERNITY CARE	NR	WOMEN'S HEALTH	NR

HEALTHGRADES AWARDS

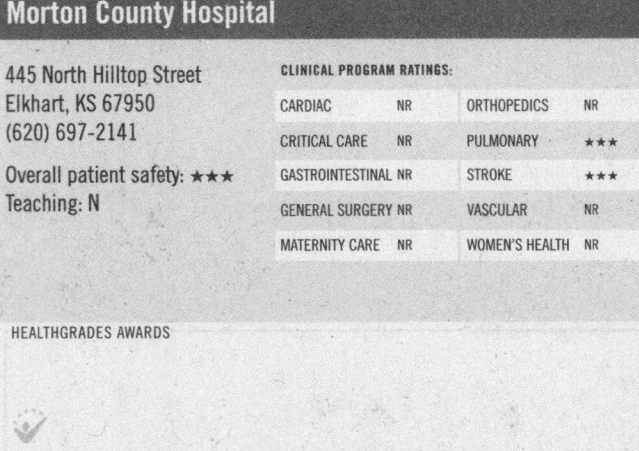

Mitchell County Hospital Health Systems

400 West 8th Street
Beloit, KS 67420
(785) 738-2266

Overall patient safety: ★★★
Teaching: Y

CLINICAL PROGRAM RATINGS:

CARDIAC	NR	ORTHOPEDICS	NR
CRITICAL CARE	NR	PULMONARY	★★★
GASTROINTESTINAL	NR	STROKE	★★★
GENERAL SURGERY	NR	VASCULAR	NR
MATERNITY CARE	NR	WOMEN'S HEALTH	NR

HEALTHGRADES AWARDS

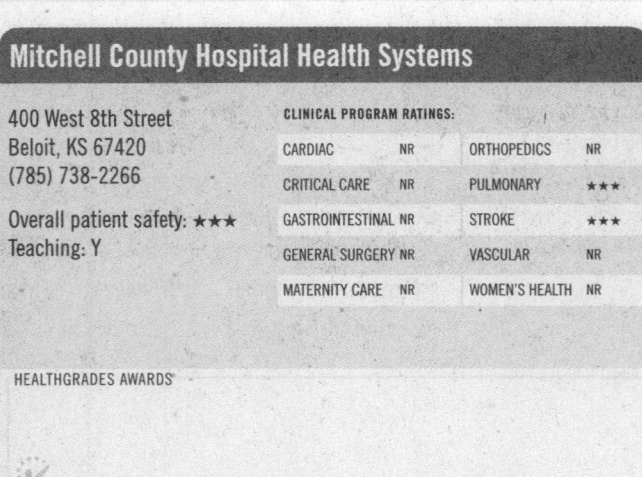

Mt. Carmel Regional Medical Center

1102 East Centennial Drive
Pittsburg, KS 66762
(620) 231-6100

Overall patient safety: ★★★
Teaching: N

CLINICAL PROGRAM RATINGS:

CARDIAC	NR	ORTHOPEDICS	NR
CRITICAL CARE	NR	PULMONARY	★★★
GASTROINTESTINAL	NR	STROKE	★★★
GENERAL SURGERY	NR	VASCULAR	NR
MATERNITY CARE	NR	WOMEN'S HEALTH	NR

HEALTHGRADES AWARDS

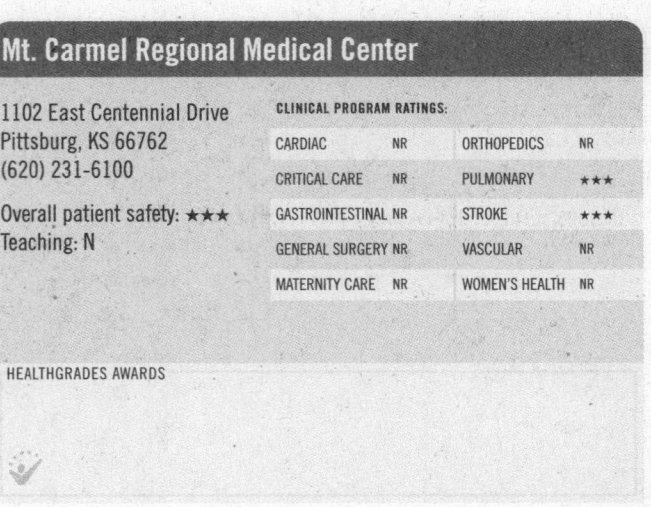

KEY: ★★★★★ BEST   ★★★ AS EXPECTED   ★ POOR   NR NOT RATED BY HEALTHGRADES   For full definitions of ratings and awards, see Appendix.

Neosho Memorial Regional Medical Center

629 South Plummer Avenue
Chanute, KS 66720
(620) 491-4000

Overall patient safety: ★★★
Teaching: N

CLINICAL PROGRAM RATINGS:

CARDIAC	NR	ORTHOPEDICS	NR
CRITICAL CARE	NR	PULMONARY	★★★
GASTROINTESTINAL	NR	STROKE	★★★
GENERAL SURGERY	NR	VASCULAR	NR
MATERNITY CARE	NR	WOMEN'S HEALTH	NR

HEALTHGRADES AWARDS

Norton County Hospital

102 East Holme Street
Norton, KS 67654
(785) 877-3351

Overall patient safety: ★★★
Teaching: N

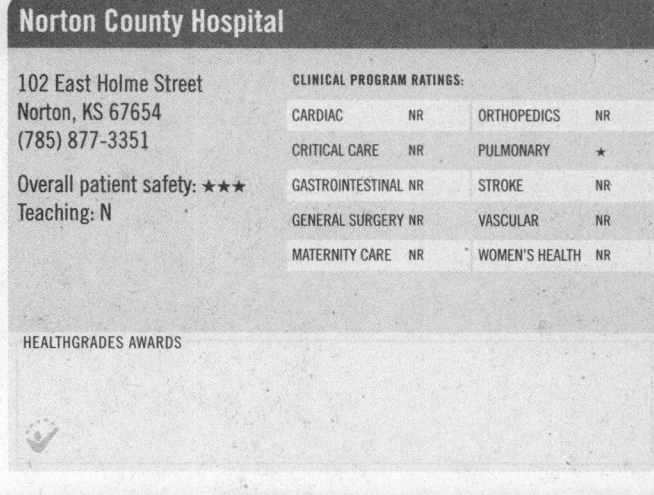

CLINICAL PROGRAM RATINGS:

CARDIAC	NR	ORTHOPEDICS	NR
CRITICAL CARE	NR	PULMONARY	★
GASTROINTESTINAL	NR	STROKE	NR
GENERAL SURGERY	NR	VASCULAR	NR
MATERNITY CARE	NR	WOMEN'S HEALTH	NR

HEALTHGRADES AWARDS

Newman Regional Health

1201 West 12th Avenue
Emporia, KS 66801
(620) 343-6800

Overall patient safety: ★★★
Teaching: N

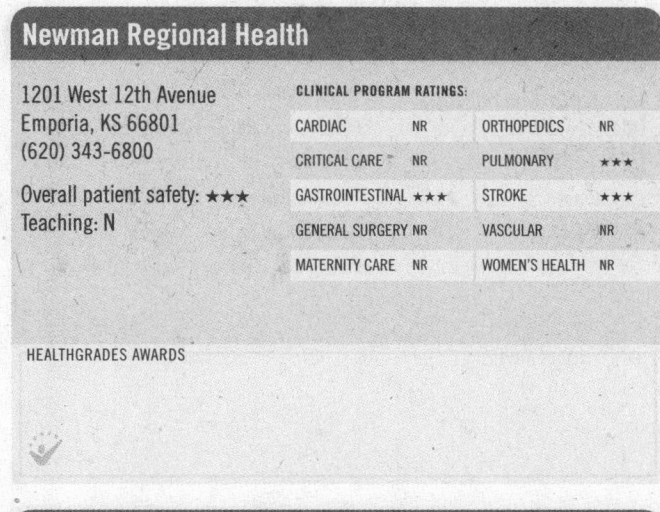

CLINICAL PROGRAM RATINGS:

CARDIAC	NR	ORTHOPEDICS	NR
CRITICAL CARE	NR	PULMONARY	★★★
GASTROINTESTINAL	★★★	STROKE	★★★
GENERAL SURGERY	NR	VASCULAR	NR
MATERNITY CARE	NR	WOMEN'S HEALTH	NR

HEALTHGRADES AWARDS

Olathe Medical Center

20333 West 151st Street
Olathe, KS 66061
(913) 791-4200

Overall patient safety: ★★★
Teaching: N

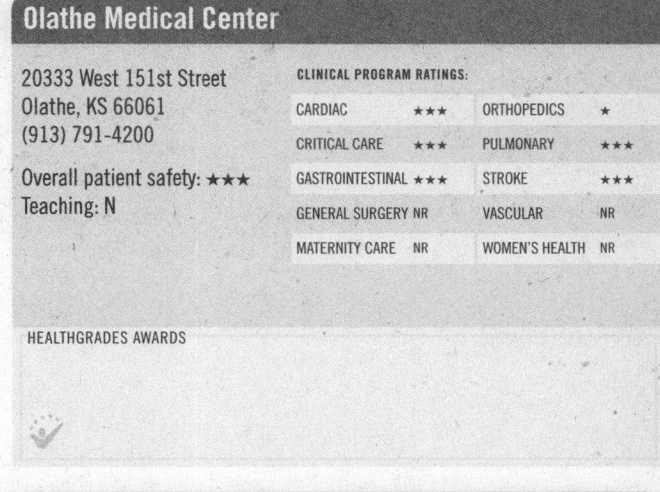

CLINICAL PROGRAM RATINGS:

CARDIAC	★★★	ORTHOPEDICS	★
CRITICAL CARE	★★★	PULMONARY	★★★
GASTROINTESTINAL	★★★	STROKE	★★★
GENERAL SURGERY	NR	VASCULAR	NR
MATERNITY CARE	NR	WOMEN'S HEALTH	NR

HEALTHGRADES AWARDS

Newton Medical Center

600 Medical Center Drive
Newton, KS 67114
(316) 283-2700

Overall patient safety: ★★★★★
Teaching: N

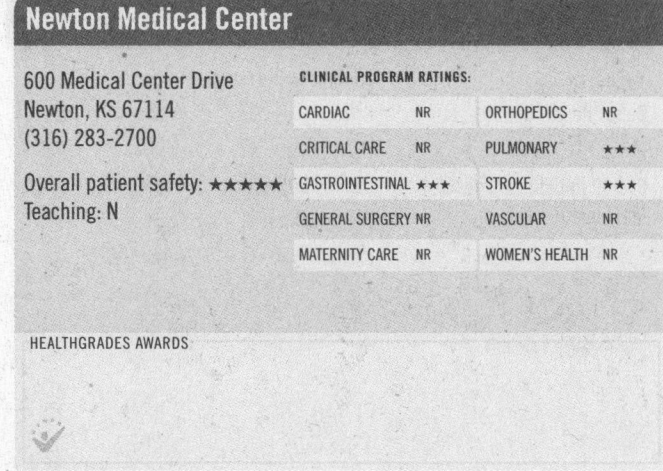

CLINICAL PROGRAM RATINGS:

CARDIAC	NR	ORTHOPEDICS	NR
CRITICAL CARE	NR	PULMONARY	★★★
GASTROINTESTINAL	★★★	STROKE	★★★
GENERAL SURGERY	NR	VASCULAR	NR
MATERNITY CARE	NR	WOMEN'S HEALTH	NR

HEALTHGRADES AWARDS

Ottawa County Health Center

215 East 8th Street
P.O. Box 290
Minneapolis, KS 67467
(785) 392-2122

Overall patient safety: NR
Teaching: N

CLINICAL PROGRAM RATINGS:

CARDIAC	NR	ORTHOPEDICS	NR
CRITICAL CARE	NR	PULMONARY	★
GASTROINTESTINAL	NR	STROKE	NR
GENERAL SURGERY	NR	VASCULAR	NR
MATERNITY CARE	NR	WOMEN'S HEALTH	NR

HEALTHGRADES AWARDS

Overland Park Regional Medical Center

10500 Quivira Road
Overland Park, KS 66215
(913) 541-5000

Overall patient safety: ★★★
Teaching: N

CLINICAL PROGRAM RATINGS:

CARDIAC	★★★	ORTHOPEDICS	★★★
CRITICAL CARE	NR	PULMONARY	★★★
GASTROINTESTINAL	NR	STROKE	★★★
GENERAL SURGERY	NR	VASCULAR	NR
MATERNITY CARE	NR	WOMEN'S HEALTH	NR

HEALTHGRADES AWARDS

Providence Medical Center

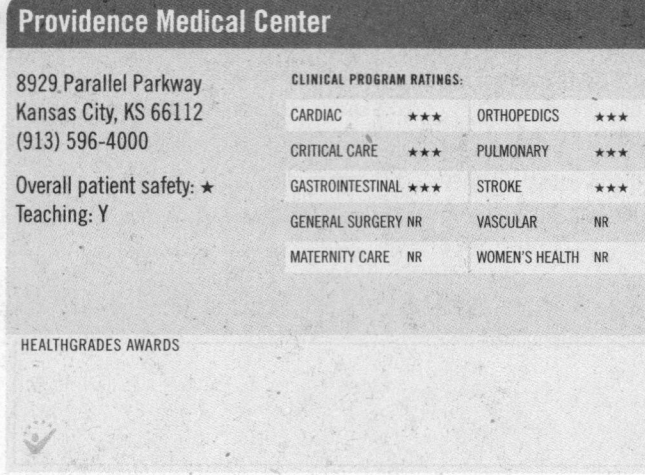

8929 Parallel Parkway
Kansas City, KS 66112
(913) 596-4000

Overall patient safety: ★
Teaching: Y

CLINICAL PROGRAM RATINGS:

CARDIAC	★★★	ORTHOPEDICS	★★★
CRITICAL CARE	★★★	PULMONARY	★★★
GASTROINTESTINAL	★★★	STROKE	★★★
GENERAL SURGERY	NR	VASCULAR	NR
MATERNITY CARE	NR	WOMEN'S HEALTH	NR

HEALTHGRADES AWARDS

Phillips County Hospital

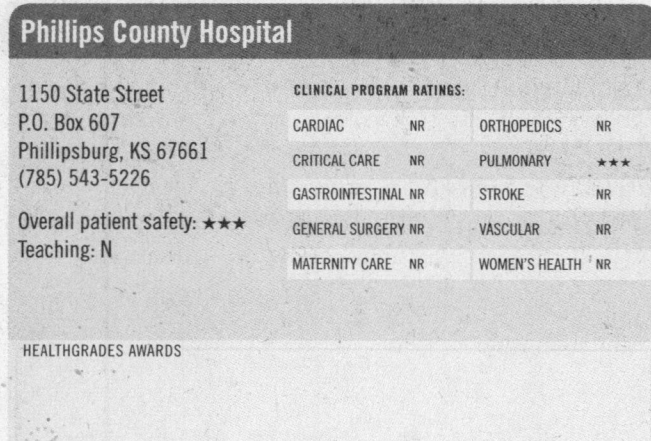

1150 State Street
P.O. Box 607
Phillipsburg, KS 67661
(785) 543-5226

Overall patient safety: ★★★
Teaching: N

CLINICAL PROGRAM RATINGS:

CARDIAC	NR	ORTHOPEDICS	NR
CRITICAL CARE	NR	PULMONARY	★★★
GASTROINTESTINAL	NR	STROKE	NR
GENERAL SURGERY	NR	VASCULAR	NR
MATERNITY CARE	NR	WOMEN'S HEALTH	NR

HEALTHGRADES AWARDS

Ransom Memorial Hospital

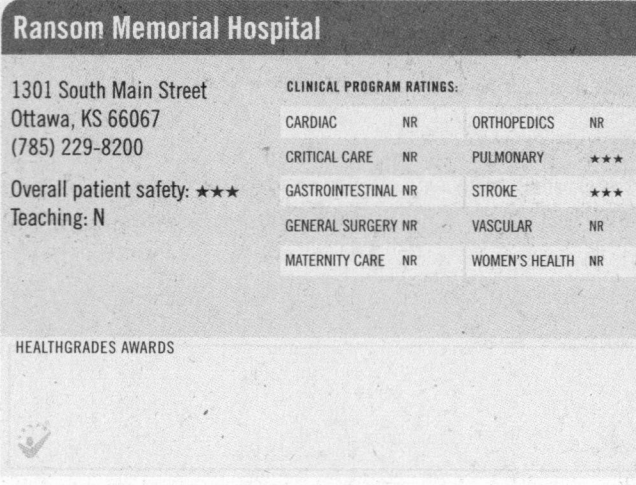

1301 South Main Street
Ottawa, KS 66067
(785) 229-8200

Overall patient safety: ★★★
Teaching: N

CLINICAL PROGRAM RATINGS:

CARDIAC	NR	ORTHOPEDICS	NR
CRITICAL CARE	NR	PULMONARY	★★★
GASTROINTESTINAL	NR	STROKE	★★★
GENERAL SURGERY	NR	VASCULAR	NR
MATERNITY CARE	NR	WOMEN'S HEALTH	NR

HEALTHGRADES AWARDS

Pratt Regional Medical Center

200 Commodore
Pratt, KS 67124
(620) 672-7451

Overall patient safety: ★★★
Teaching: N

CLINICAL PROGRAM RATINGS:

CARDIAC	NR	ORTHOPEDICS	NR
CRITICAL CARE	NR	PULMONARY	★★★
GASTROINTESTINAL	NR	STROKE	★★★
GENERAL SURGERY	NR	VASCULAR	NR
MATERNITY CARE	NR	WOMEN'S HEALTH	NR

HEALTHGRADES AWARDS

Republic County Hospital

2420 G Street
Belleville, KS 66935
(785) 527-2254

Overall patient safety: ★★★
Teaching: N

CLINICAL PROGRAM RATINGS:

CARDIAC	NR	ORTHOPEDICS	NR
CRITICAL CARE	NR	PULMONARY	★★★
GASTROINTESTINAL	NR	STROKE	★★★
GENERAL SURGERY	NR	VASCULAR	NR
MATERNITY CARE	NR	WOMEN'S HEALTH	NR

HEALTHGRADES AWARDS

KEY: ★★★★★ BEST   ★★★ AS EXPECTED   ★ POOR   NR NOT RATED BY HEALTHGRADES   For full definitions of ratings and awards, see Appendix.

St. Catherine Hospital

401 East Spruce Street
Garden City, KS 67846
(620) 272-2222

Overall patient safety: ★★★
Teaching: Y

CLINICAL PROGRAM RATINGS:

CARDIAC	NR	ORTHOPEDICS	NR
CRITICAL CARE	NR	PULMONARY	★
GASTROINTESTINAL	NR	STROKE	★★★
GENERAL SURGERY	NR	VASCULAR	NR
MATERNITY CARE	NR	WOMEN'S HEALTH	NR

HEALTHGRADES AWARDS

St. Johns Regional Health Center*

139 North Penn Street
Salina, KS 67401
(913) 827-5591

Overall patient safety: ★★★★★
Teaching: Y

CLINICAL PROGRAM RATINGS:

CARDIAC	★★★	ORTHOPEDICS	★
CRITICAL CARE	NR	PULMONARY	★
GASTROINTESTINAL	★★★	STROKE	★★★
GENERAL SURGERY	NR	VASCULAR	★★★
MATERNITY CARE	NR	WOMEN'S HEALTH	NR

HEALTHGRADES AWARDS

✓ DISTINGUISHED HOSPITAL
- PATIENT SAFETY

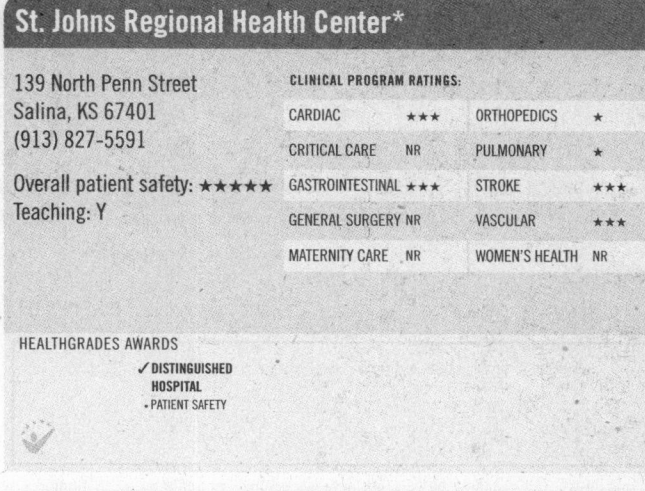

St. Francis Health Center

1700 Southwest 7th Street
Topeka, KS 66606
(785) 295-8000

Overall patient safety: ★★★
Teaching: Y

CLINICAL PROGRAM RATINGS:

CARDIAC	★★★	ORTHOPEDICS	★★★
CRITICAL CARE	NR	PULMONARY	★★★★★
GASTROINTESTINAL	★★★	STROKE	★★★
GENERAL SURGERY	NR	VASCULAR	★★★
MATERNITY CARE	NR	WOMEN'S HEALTH	NR

HEALTHGRADES AWARDS

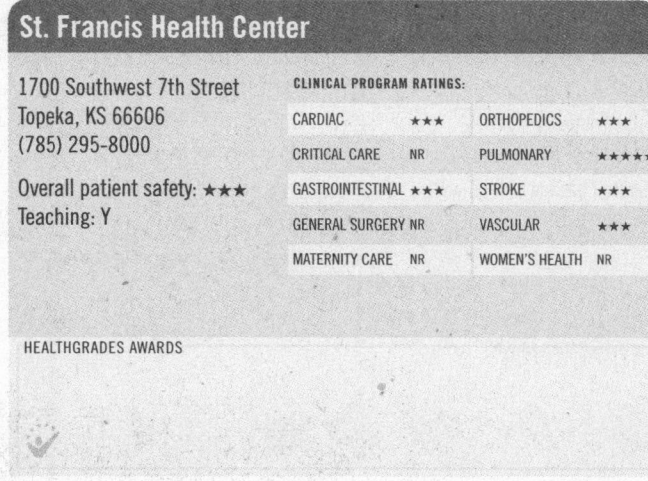

St. Joseph Medical Center*

3600 East Harry Street
Wichita, KS 67218
(316) 685-1111

Overall patient safety: ★★★
Teaching: Y

CLINICAL PROGRAM RATINGS:

CARDIAC	★★★	ORTHOPEDICS	★★★
CRITICAL CARE	★★★	PULMONARY	★★★★★
GASTROINTESTINAL	★★★	STROKE	★★★★★
GENERAL SURGERY	NR	VASCULAR	★★★
MATERNITY CARE	NR	WOMEN'S HEALTH	NR

HEALTHGRADES AWARDS

✓ SPECIALTY EXCELLENCE
- CARDIAC CARE   - PULMONARY CARE
- CARDIAC SURGERY   - STROKE CARE

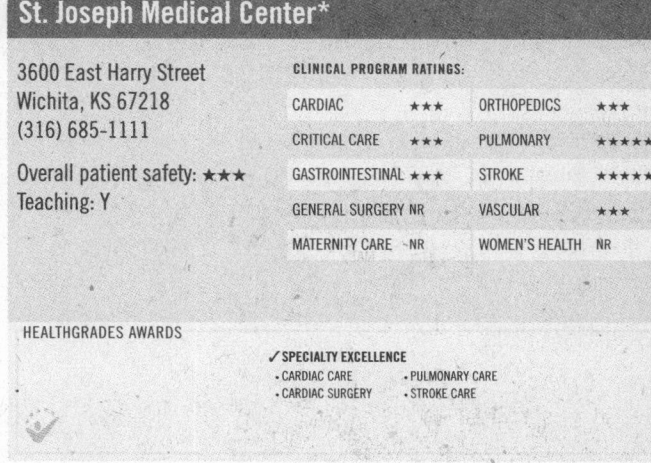

St. John Hospital

3500 South 4th Street
Leavenworth, KS 66048
(913) 680-6000

Overall patient safety: ★★★
Teaching: N

CLINICAL PROGRAM RATINGS:

CARDIAC	NR	ORTHOPEDICS	NR
CRITICAL CARE	NR	PULMONARY	★★★
GASTROINTESTINAL	NR	STROKE	★★★
GENERAL SURGERY	NR	VASCULAR	NR
MATERNITY CARE	NR	WOMEN'S HEALTH	NR

HEALTHGRADES AWARDS

St. Luke's South Hospital

12300 Metcalf Avenue
Overland Park, KS 66213
(913) 317-7000

Overall patient safety: ★★★
Teaching: N

CLINICAL PROGRAM RATINGS:

CARDIAC	NR	ORTHOPEDICS	NR
CRITICAL CARE	NR	PULMONARY	★★★
GASTROINTESTINAL	★★★	STROKE	★★★
GENERAL SURGERY	NR	VASCULAR	NR
MATERNITY CARE	NR	WOMEN'S HEALTH	NR

HEALTHGRADES AWARDS

*This hospital reports its data to the federal government jointly with another hospital. Therefore the ratings and awards apply to multiple hospitals and this specific hospital may not provide all rated services.

Salina Regional Health Center*

400 South Santa Fe Avenue
Salina, KS 67402
(785) 452-7000

Overall patient safety: ★★★★★
Teaching: Y

CLINICAL PROGRAM RATINGS:

CARDIAC	★★★	ORTHOPEDICS	★
CRITICAL CARE	NR	PULMONARY	★
GASTROINTESTINAL	★★★	STROKE	★★★
GENERAL SURGERY	NR	VASCULAR	★★★
MATERNITY CARE	NR	WOMEN'S HEALTH	NR

HEALTHGRADES AWARDS

✓ DISTINGUISHED
HOSPITAL
• PATIENT SAFETY

Shawnee Mission Medical Center

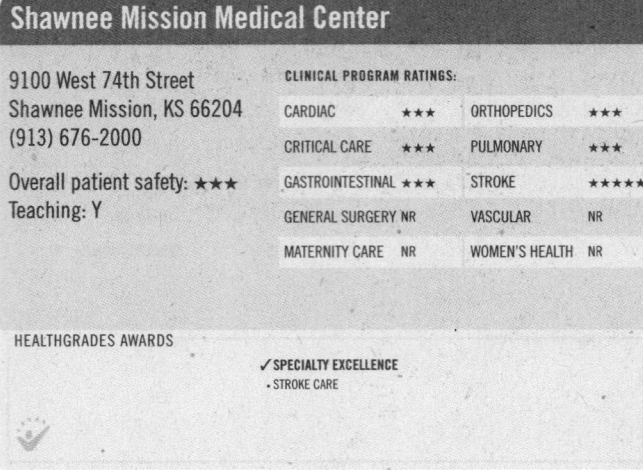

9100 West 74th Street
Shawnee Mission, KS 66204
(913) 676-2000

Overall patient safety: ★★★
Teaching: Y

CLINICAL PROGRAM RATINGS:

CARDIAC	★★★	ORTHOPEDICS	★★★
CRITICAL CARE	★★★	PULMONARY	★★★
GASTROINTESTINAL	★★★	STROKE	★★★★★
GENERAL SURGERY	NR	VASCULAR	NR
MATERNITY CARE	NR	WOMEN'S HEALTH	NR

HEALTHGRADES AWARDS

✓ SPECIALTY EXCELLENCE
• STROKE CARE

Scott County Hospital

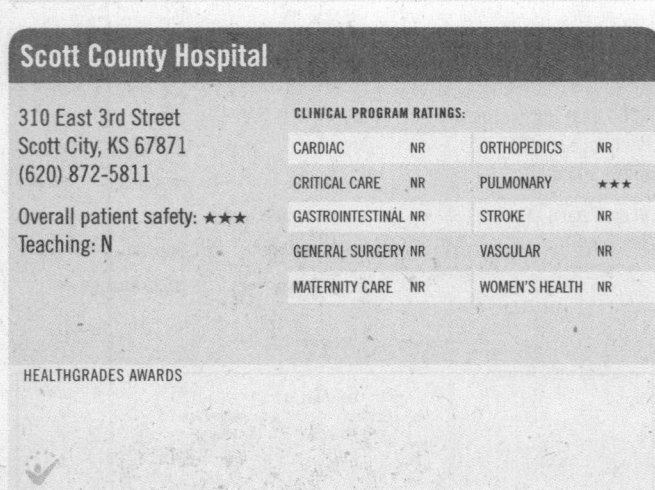

310 East 3rd Street
Scott City, KS 67871
(620) 872-5811

Overall patient safety: ★★★
Teaching: N

CLINICAL PROGRAM RATINGS:

CARDIAC	NR	ORTHOPEDICS	NR
CRITICAL CARE	NR	PULMONARY	★★★
GASTROINTESTINAL	NR	STROKE	NR
GENERAL SURGERY	NR	VASCULAR	NR
MATERNITY CARE	NR	WOMEN'S HEALTH	NR

HEALTHGRADES AWARDS

Smith County Memorial Hospital

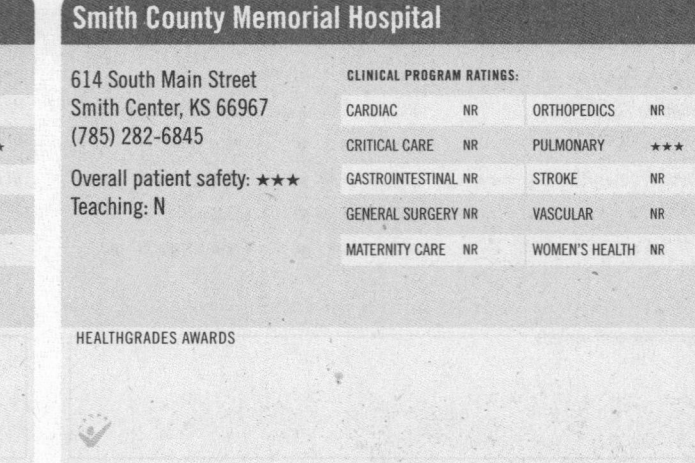

614 South Main Street
Smith Center, KS 66967
(785) 282-6845

Overall patient safety: ★★★
Teaching: N

CLINICAL PROGRAM RATINGS:

CARDIAC	NR	ORTHOPEDICS	NR
CRITICAL CARE	NR	PULMONARY	★★★
GASTROINTESTINAL	NR	STROKE	NR
GENERAL SURGERY	NR	VASCULAR	NR
MATERNITY CARE	NR	WOMEN'S HEALTH	NR

HEALTHGRADES AWARDS

Select Specialty Hospital Wichita

550 North Hillside Street
Wichita, KS 67214
(316) 688-3900

Overall patient safety: ★★★★★
Teaching: Y

CLINICAL PROGRAM RATINGS:

CARDIAC	★★★	ORTHOPEDICS	★★★
CRITICAL CARE	★	PULMONARY	★★★
GASTROINTESTINAL	★★★	STROKE	★★★
GENERAL SURGERY	NR	VASCULAR	★★★
MATERNITY CARE	NR	WOMEN'S HEALTH	NR

HEALTHGRADES AWARDS

✓ DISTINGUISHED
HOSPITAL
• PATIENT SAFETY

✓ SPECIALTY EXCELLENCE
• GASTROINTESTINAL
CARE

South Central Kansas Regional Medical Center

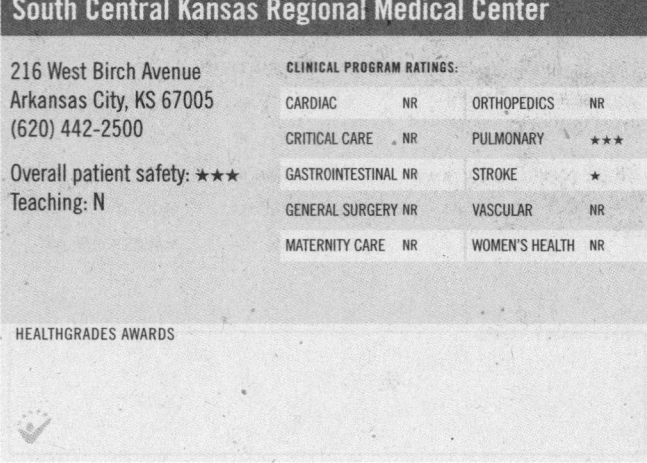

216 West Birch Avenue
Arkansas City, KS 67005
(620) 442-2500

Overall patient safety: ★★★
Teaching: N

CLINICAL PROGRAM RATINGS:

CARDIAC	NR	ORTHOPEDICS	NR
CRITICAL CARE	NR	PULMONARY	★★★
GASTROINTESTINAL	NR	STROKE	★
GENERAL SURGERY	NR	VASCULAR	NR
MATERNITY CARE	NR	WOMEN'S HEALTH	NR

HEALTHGRADES AWARDS

KEY: ★★★★★ BEST   ★★★ AS EXPECTED   ★ POOR   NR NOT RATED BY HEALTHGRADES   For full definitions of ratings and awards, see Appendix.

Southwest Medical Center

315 West 15th Street
Liberal, KS 67901
(620) 624-1651

Overall patient safety: ★★★
Teaching: N

CLINICAL PROGRAM RATINGS:

CARDIAC	NR	ORTHOPEDICS	NR
CRITICAL CARE	NR	PULMONARY	★★★
GASTROINTESTINAL	NR	STROKE	★
GENERAL SURGERY	NR	VASCULAR	NR
MATERNITY CARE	NR	WOMEN'S HEALTH	NR

HEALTHGRADES AWARDS

Susan B. Allen Memorial Hospital

720 West Central Avenue
El Dorado, KS 67042
(316) 321-3300

Overall patient safety: ★★★
Teaching: N

CLINICAL PROGRAM RATINGS:

CARDIAC	NR	ORTHOPEDICS	NR
CRITICAL CARE	NR	PULMONARY	★★★
GASTROINTESTINAL	NR	STROKE	★★★
GENERAL SURGERY	NR	VASCULAR	NR
MATERNITY CARE	NR	WOMEN'S HEALTH	NR

HEALTHGRADES AWARDS

Stormont-Vail Healthcare

1500 Southwest 10th Street
Topeka, KS 66604
(785) 354-6000

Overall patient safety: ★★★★★
Teaching: Y

CLINICAL PROGRAM RATINGS:

CARDIAC	★★★	ORTHOPEDICS	★★★
CRITICAL CARE	NR	PULMONARY	★★★
GASTROINTESTINAL	★★★	STROKE	★★★
GENERAL SURGERY	NR	VASCULAR	NR
MATERNITY CARE	NR	WOMEN'S HEALTH	NR

HEALTHGRADES AWARDS

✓ DISTINGUISHED
  HOSPITAL
• PATIENT SAFETY

Trego County Lemke Memorial Hospital

320 13th Street
WaKeeney, KS 67672
(785) 743-2182

Overall patient safety: ★★★
Teaching: N

CLINICAL PROGRAM RATINGS:

CARDIAC	NR	ORTHOPEDICS	NR
CRITICAL CARE	NR	PULMONARY	★★★
GASTROINTESTINAL	NR	STROKE	NR
GENERAL SURGERY	NR	VASCULAR	NR
MATERNITY CARE	NR	WOMEN'S HEALTH	NR

HEALTHGRADES AWARDS

Sumner Regional Medical Center

1323 North A Street
Wellington, KS 67152
(316) 326-7451

Overall patient safety: ★★★
Teaching: N

CLINICAL PROGRAM RATINGS:

CARDIAC	NR	ORTHOPEDICS	NR
CRITICAL CARE	NR	PULMONARY	★
GASTROINTESTINAL	NR	STROKE	★
GENERAL SURGERY	NR	VASCULAR	NR
MATERNITY CARE	NR	WOMEN'S HEALTH	NR

HEALTHGRADES AWARDS

University of Kansas Hospital

3901 Rainbow Boulevard
Kansas City, KS 66160
(913) 588-5000

Overall patient safety: ★★★
Teaching: Y

CLINICAL PROGRAM RATINGS:

CARDIAC	★★★	ORTHOPEDICS	★
CRITICAL CARE	★★★	PULMONARY	★★★
GASTROINTESTINAL	★★★	STROKE	★★★★★
GENERAL SURGERY	NR	VASCULAR	★★★
MATERNITY CARE	NR	WOMEN'S HEALTH	NR

HEALTHGRADES AWARDS

*This hospital reports its data to the federal government jointly with another hospital. Therefore the ratings and awards apply to multiple hospitals and this specific hospital may not provide all rated services.

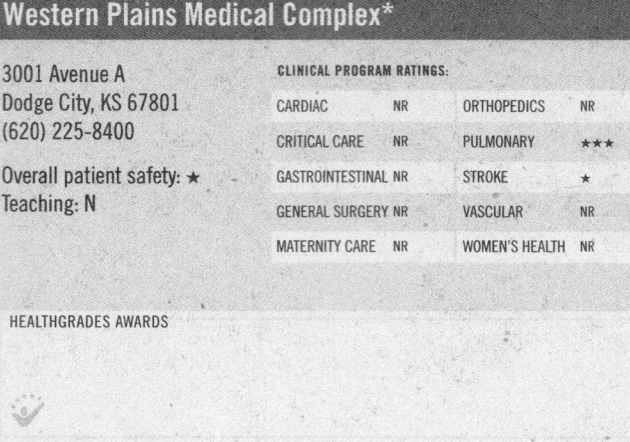

Via Christi Regional Medical Center*

929 North St. Francis Street
Wichita, KS 67214
(316) 268-5000

Overall patient safety: ★★★
Teaching: Y

CLINICAL PROGRAM RATINGS:

CARDIAC	★★★	ORTHOPEDICS	★★★
CRITICAL CARE	★★★	PULMONARY	★★★★★
GASTROINTESTINAL	★★★	STROKE	★★★★★
GENERAL SURGERY	NR	VASCULAR	★★★
MATERNITY CARE	NR	WOMEN'S HEALTH	NR

HEALTHGRADES AWARDS

✓ DISTINGUISHED HOSPITAL
- CLINICAL EXCELLENCE

✓ SPECIALTY EXCELLENCE
- CARDIAC CARE
- CARDIAC SURGERY
- PULMONARY CARE
- STROKE CARE

Western Plains Medical Complex*

3001 Avenue A
Dodge City, KS 67801
(620) 225-8400

Overall patient safety: ★
Teaching: N

CLINICAL PROGRAM RATINGS:

CARDIAC	NR	ORTHOPEDICS	NR
CRITICAL CARE	NR	PULMONARY	★★★
GASTROINTESTINAL	NR	STROKE	★
GENERAL SURGERY	NR	VASCULAR	NR
MATERNITY CARE	NR	WOMEN'S HEALTH	NR

HEALTHGRADES AWARDS

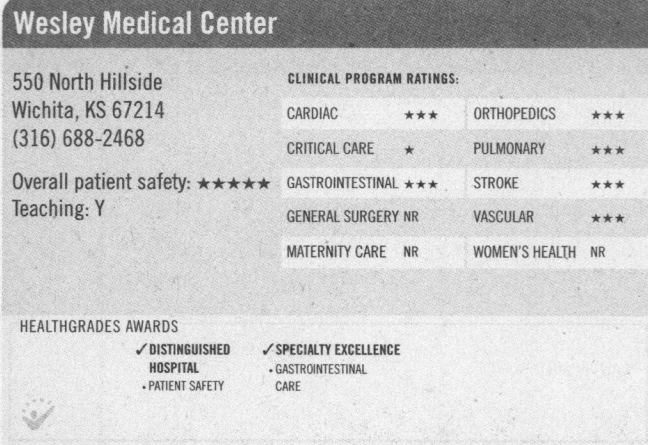

Wesley Medical Center

550 North Hillside
Wichita, KS 67214
(316) 688-2468

Overall patient safety: ★★★★★
Teaching: Y

CLINICAL PROGRAM RATINGS:

CARDIAC	★★★	ORTHOPEDICS	★★★
CRITICAL CARE	★	PULMONARY	★★★
GASTROINTESTINAL	★★★	STROKE	★★★
GENERAL SURGERY	NR	VASCULAR	★★★
MATERNITY CARE	NR	WOMEN'S HEALTH	NR

HEALTHGRADES AWARDS

✓ DISTINGUISHED HOSPITAL
- PATIENT SAFETY

✓ SPECIALTY EXCELLENCE
- GASTROINTESTINAL CARE

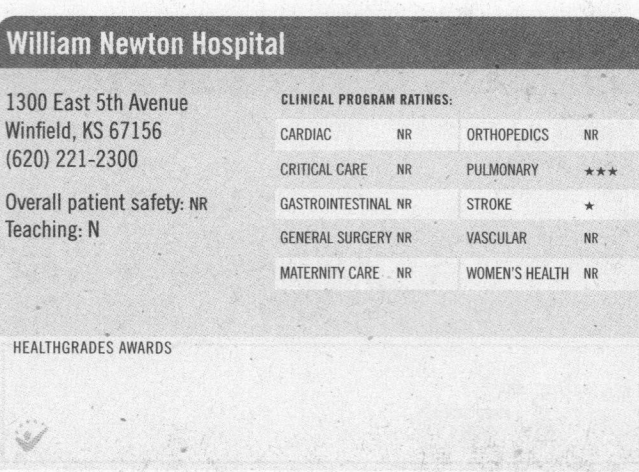

William Newton Hospital

1300 East 5th Avenue
Winfield, KS 67156
(620) 221-2300

Overall patient safety: NR
Teaching: N

CLINICAL PROGRAM RATINGS:

CARDIAC	NR	ORTHOPEDICS	NR
CRITICAL CARE	NR	PULMONARY	★★★
GASTROINTESTINAL	NR	STROKE	★
GENERAL SURGERY	NR	VASCULAR	NR
MATERNITY CARE	NR	WOMEN'S HEALTH	NR

HEALTHGRADES AWARDS

KENTUCKY HOSPITALS: RATINGS BY CLINICAL SPECIALTY

ARH Regional Medical Center—Hazard

100 Medical Center Drive
Hazard, KY 41701
(606) 439-6600

Overall patient safety: ★★★
Teaching: Y

CLINICAL PROGRAM RATINGS:

CARDIAC	NR	ORTHOPEDICS	NR
CRITICAL CARE	NR	PULMONARY	★★★★★
GASTROINTESTINAL	★★★	STROKE	★★★
GENERAL SURGERY	NR	VASCULAR	NR
MATERNITY CARE	NR	WOMEN'S HEALTH	NR

HEALTHGRADES AWARDS

✓ SPECIALTY EXCELLENCE
- PULMONARY CARE

Baptist Hospital East

4000 Kresge Way
Louisville, KY 40207
(502) 897-8100

Overall patient safety: ★★★★★
Teaching: N

CLINICAL PROGRAM RATINGS:

CARDIAC	★★★★★	ORTHOPEDICS	★★★★★
CRITICAL CARE	NR	PULMONARY	★★★★★
GASTROINTESTINAL	★★★	STROKE	★★★
GENERAL SURGERY	NR	VASCULAR	★★★
MATERNITY CARE	NR	WOMEN'S HEALTH	NR

HEALTHGRADES AWARDS

✓ AMERICA'S 50 BEST HOSPITALS

✓ DISTINGUISHED HOSPITAL
- CLINICAL EXCELLENCE
- PATIENT SAFETY

✓ SPECIALTY EXCELLENCE
- CARDIAC CARE
- CARDIAC SURGERY
- JOINT REPLACEMENT
- PULMONARY CARE

KEY: ★★★★★ BEST   ★★★ AS EXPECTED   ★ POOR   NR NOT RATED BY HEALTHGRADES   For full definitions of ratings and awards, see Appendix.

Baptist Hospital Northeast*

1025 New Moody Lane
La Grange, KY 40031
(502) 222-5388

Overall patient safety: ★★★
Teaching: N

CLINICAL PROGRAM RATINGS:

CARDIAC	NR	ORTHOPEDICS	NR
CRITICAL CARE	NR	PULMONARY	★★★
GASTROINTESTINAL	NR	STROKE	★★★★★
GENERAL SURGERY	NR	VASCULAR	NR
MATERNITY CARE	NR	WOMEN'S HEALTH	NR

HEALTHGRADES AWARDS

✓ SPECIALTY EXCELLENCE
• STROKE CARE

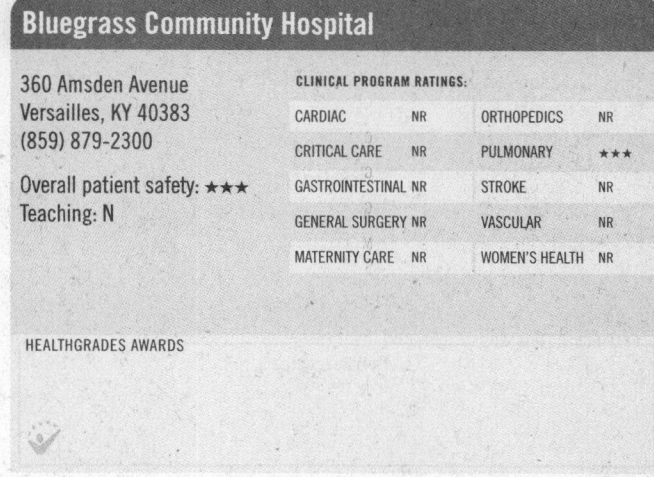

Bluegrass Community Hospital

360 Amsden Avenue
Versailles, KY 40383
(859) 879-2300

Overall patient safety: ★★★
Teaching: N

CLINICAL PROGRAM RATINGS:

CARDIAC	NR	ORTHOPEDICS	NR
CRITICAL CARE	NR	PULMONARY	★★★
GASTROINTESTINAL	NR	STROKE	NR
GENERAL SURGERY	NR	VASCULAR	NR
MATERNITY CARE	NR	WOMEN'S HEALTH	NR

HEALTHGRADES AWARDS

Baptist Regional Medical Center

1 Trillium Way
Corbin, KY 40701
(606) 528-1212

Overall patient safety: ★
Teaching: N

CLINICAL PROGRAM RATINGS:

CARDIAC	NR	ORTHOPEDICS	NR
CRITICAL CARE	NR	PULMONARY	★★★
GASTROINTESTINAL	★★★	STROKE	★★★
GENERAL SURGERY	NR	VASCULAR	NR
MATERNITY CARE	NR	WOMEN'S HEALTH	NR

HEALTHGRADES AWARDS

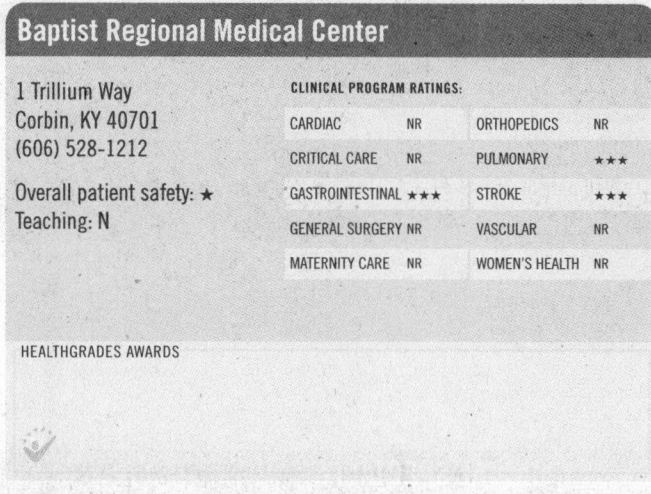

Bourbon Community Hospital

9 Linville Drive
Paris, KY 40361
(859) 987-3600

Overall patient safety: ★★★
Teaching: N

CLINICAL PROGRAM RATINGS:

CARDIAC	NR	ORTHOPEDICS	NR
CRITICAL CARE	NR	PULMONARY	★★★
GASTROINTESTINAL	NR	STROKE	NR
GENERAL SURGERY	NR	VASCULAR	NR
MATERNITY CARE	NR	WOMEN'S HEALTH	NR

HEALTHGRADES AWARDS

Berea Hospital

305 Estill Street
Berea, KY 40403
(859) 986-6500

Overall patient safety: ★★★
Teaching: N

CLINICAL PROGRAM RATINGS:

CARDIAC	NR	ORTHOPEDICS	NR
CRITICAL CARE	NR	PULMONARY	★★★
GASTROINTESTINAL	NR	STROKE	★★★
GENERAL SURGERY	NR	VASCULAR	NR
MATERNITY CARE	NR	WOMEN'S HEALTH	NR

HEALTHGRADES AWARDS

Caldwell County Hospital

101 Hospital Drive
Princeton, KY 42445
(270) 365-0300

Overall patient safety: ★★★
Teaching: N

CLINICAL PROGRAM RATINGS:

CARDIAC	NR	ORTHOPEDICS	NR
CRITICAL CARE	NR	PULMONARY	★
GASTROINTESTINAL	NR	STROKE	★
GENERAL SURGERY	NR	VASCULAR	NR
MATERNITY CARE	NR	WOMEN'S HEALTH	NR

HEALTHGRADES AWARDS

*This hospital reports its data to the federal government jointly with another hospital. Therefore the ratings and awards apply to multiple hospitals and this specific hospital may not provide all rated services.

Cardinal Hill Specialty Hospital

85 North Grand Avenue at
St. Luke Hospital East
Fort Thomas, KY 41075
(859) 572-3880

Overall patient safety: ★★★
Teaching: N

CLINICAL PROGRAM RATINGS:

CARDIAC	NR	ORTHOPEDICS	NR
CRITICAL CARE	NR	PULMONARY	★★★★★
GASTROINTESTINAL	★★★	STROKE	★★★
GENERAL SURGERY	NR	VASCULAR	NR
MATERNITY CARE	NR	WOMEN'S HEALTH	NR

HEALTHGRADES AWARDS

✓ **SPECIALTY EXCELLENCE**
· PULMONARY CARE

Central Baptist Hospital

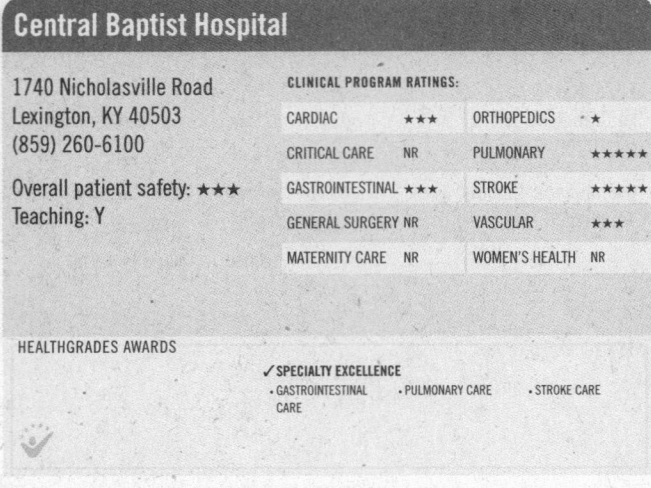

1740 Nicholasville Road
Lexington, KY 40503
(859) 260-6100

Overall patient safety: ★★★
Teaching: Y

CLINICAL PROGRAM RATINGS:

CARDIAC	★★★	ORTHOPEDICS	★
CRITICAL CARE	NR	PULMONARY	★★★★★
GASTROINTESTINAL	★★★	STROKE	★★★★★
GENERAL SURGERY	NR	VASCULAR	★★★
MATERNITY CARE	NR	WOMEN'S HEALTH	NR

HEALTHGRADES AWARDS

✓ **SPECIALTY EXCELLENCE**
· GASTROINTESTINAL   · PULMONARY CARE   · STROKE CARE
CARE

Carroll County Hospital

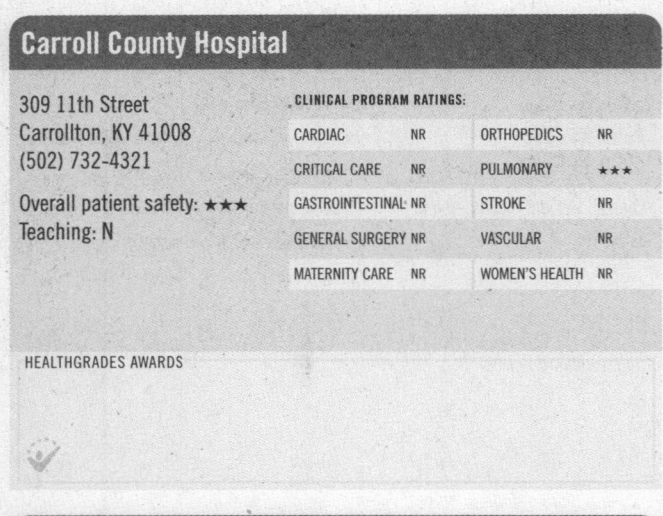

309 11th Street
Carrollton, KY 41008
(502) 732-4321

Overall patient safety: ★★★
Teaching: N

CLINICAL PROGRAM RATINGS:

CARDIAC	NR	ORTHOPEDICS	NR
CRITICAL CARE	NR	PULMONARY	★★★
GASTROINTESTINAL	NR	STROKE	NR
GENERAL SURGERY	NR	VASCULAR	NR
MATERNITY CARE	NR	WOMEN'S HEALTH	NR

HEALTHGRADES AWARDS

Clark Regional Medical Center

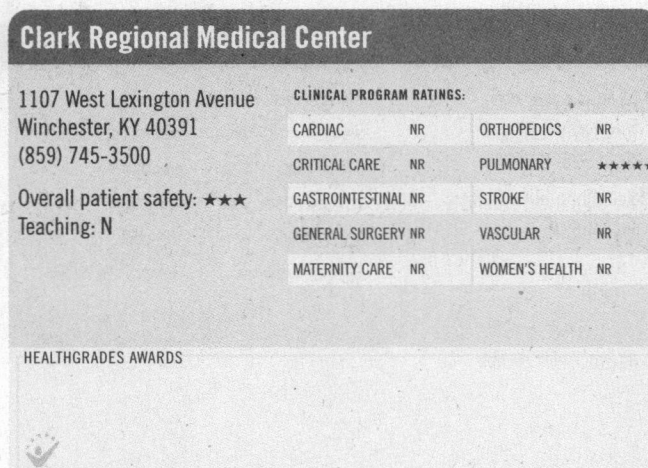

1107 West Lexington Avenue
Winchester, KY 40391
(859) 745-3500

Overall patient safety: ★★★
Teaching: N

CLINICAL PROGRAM RATINGS:

CARDIAC	NR	ORTHOPEDICS	NR
CRITICAL CARE	NR	PULMONARY	★★★★★
GASTROINTESTINAL	NR	STROKE	NR
GENERAL SURGERY	NR	VASCULAR	NR
MATERNITY CARE	NR	WOMEN'S HEALTH	NR

HEALTHGRADES AWARDS

Caverna Memorial Hospital

1501 South Dixie Street
Horse Cave, KY 42749
(270) 786-2191

Overall patient safety: ★★★
Teaching: N

CLINICAL PROGRAM RATINGS:

CARDIAC	NR	ORTHOPEDICS	NR
CRITICAL CARE	NR	PULMONARY	★
GASTROINTESTINAL	NR	STROKE	NR
GENERAL SURGERY	NR	VASCULAR	NR
MATERNITY CARE	NR	WOMEN'S HEALTH	NR

HEALTHGRADES AWARDS

Clinton County Hospital

723 Burkesville Road
Albany, KY 42602
(606) 387-6421

Overall patient safety: ★★★
Teaching: N

CLINICAL PROGRAM RATINGS:

CARDIAC	NR	ORTHOPEDICS	NR
CRITICAL CARE	NR	PULMONARY	★
GASTROINTESTINAL	NR	STROKE	★★★
GENERAL SURGERY	NR	VASCULAR	NR
MATERNITY CARE	NR	WOMEN'S HEALTH	NR

HEALTHGRADES AWARDS

KEY: ★★★★★ **BEST**   ★★★ **AS EXPECTED**   ★ **POOR**   NR **NOT RATED BY HEALTHGRADES**   For full definitions of ratings and awards, see Appendix.

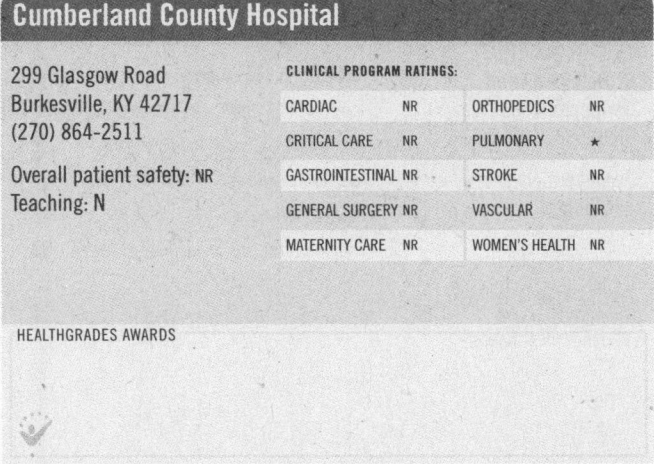

Crittenden Health Systems

520 West Gum Street
Marion, KY 42064
(270) 965-1018

Overall patient safety: ★★★
Teaching: N

CLINICAL PROGRAM RATINGS:

CARDIAC	NR	ORTHOPEDICS	NR
CRITICAL CARE	NR	PULMONARY	★★★
GASTROINTESTINAL	NR	STROKE	★★★
GENERAL SURGERY	NR	VASCULAR	NR
MATERNITY CARE	NR	WOMEN'S HEALTH	NR

HEALTHGRADES AWARDS

Flaget Memorial Hospital

4305 New Sheperd Villa Road
Bardstown, KY 40004
(502) 350-5000

Overall patient safety: ★★★
Teaching: N

CLINICAL PROGRAM RATINGS:

CARDIAC	NR	ORTHOPEDICS	NR
CRITICAL CARE	NR	PULMONARY	★★★
GASTROINTESTINAL	NR	STROKE	★
GENERAL SURGERY	NR	VASCULAR	NR
MATERNITY CARE	NR	WOMEN'S HEALTH	NR

HEALTHGRADES AWARDS

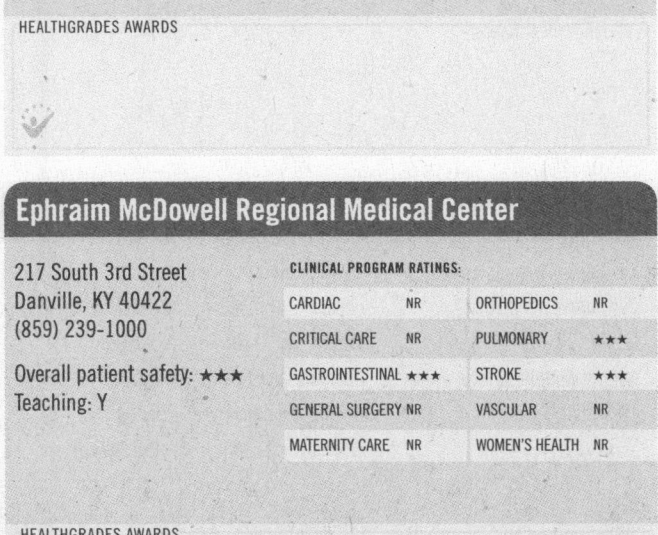

Cumberland County Hospital

299 Glasgow Road
Burkesville, KY 42717
(270) 864-2511

Overall patient safety: NR
Teaching: N

CLINICAL PROGRAM RATINGS:

CARDIAC	NR	ORTHOPEDICS	NR
CRITICAL CARE	NR	PULMONARY	★
GASTROINTESTINAL	NR	STROKE	NR
GENERAL SURGERY	NR	VASCULAR	NR
MATERNITY CARE	NR	WOMEN'S HEALTH	NR

HEALTHGRADES AWARDS

Fleming County Hospital

920 Elizaville Road
Flemingsburg, KY 41041
(606) 849-5000

Overall patient safety: ★★★
Teaching: N

CLINICAL PROGRAM RATINGS:

CARDIAC	NR	ORTHOPEDICS	NR
CRITICAL CARE	NR	PULMONARY	★★★
GASTROINTESTINAL	NR	STROKE	★★★
GENERAL SURGERY	NR	VASCULAR	NR
MATERNITY CARE	NR	WOMEN'S HEALTH	NR

HEALTHGRADES AWARDS

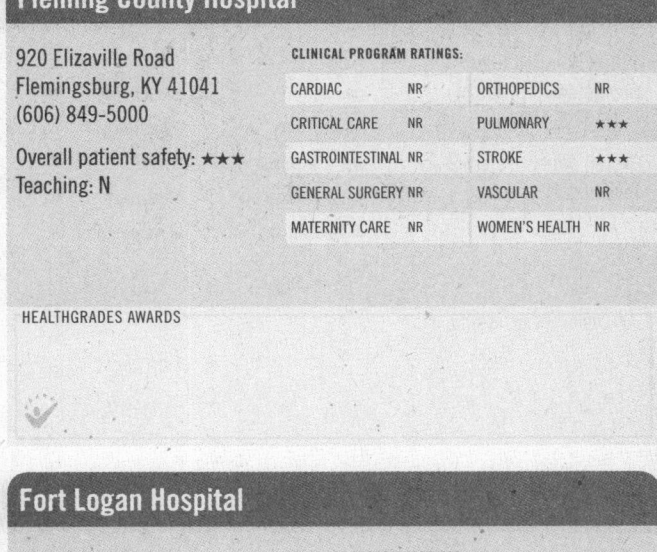

Ephraim McDowell Regional Medical Center

217 South 3rd Street
Danville, KY 40422
(859) 239-1000

Overall patient safety: ★★★
Teaching: Y

CLINICAL PROGRAM RATINGS:

CARDIAC	NR	ORTHOPEDICS	NR
CRITICAL CARE	NR	PULMONARY	★★★
GASTROINTESTINAL	★★★	STROKE	★★★
GENERAL SURGERY	NR	VASCULAR	NR
MATERNITY CARE	NR	WOMEN'S HEALTH	NR

HEALTHGRADES AWARDS

Fort Logan Hospital

124 Portman Avenue
Stanford, KY 40484
(606) 365-2187

Overall patient safety: ★★★
Teaching: N

CLINICAL PROGRAM RATINGS:

CARDIAC	NR	ORTHOPEDICS	NR
CRITICAL CARE	NR	PULMONARY	★★★
GASTROINTESTINAL	NR	STROKE	NR
GENERAL SURGERY	NR	VASCULAR	NR
MATERNITY CARE	NR	WOMEN'S HEALTH	NR

HEALTHGRADES AWARDS

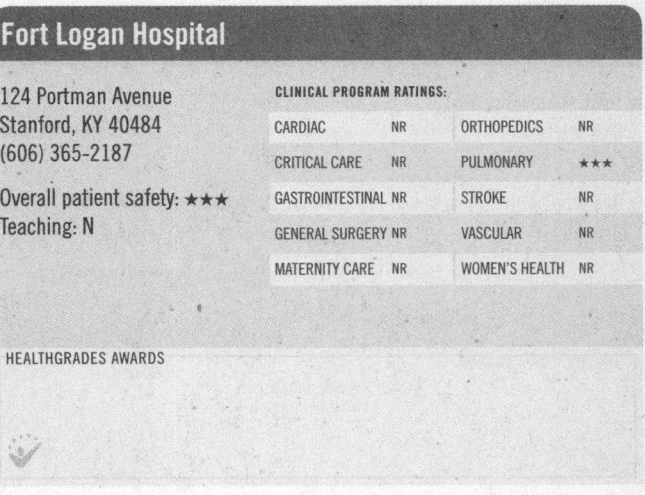

KENTUCKY HOSPITALS: RATINGS BY CLINICAL SPECIALTY

Frankfort Regional Medical Center

299 King's Daughters' Drive
Frankfort, KY 40601
(502) 875-5240

Overall patient safety: ★★★
Teaching: N

CLINICAL PROGRAM RATINGS:

CARDIAC	NR	ORTHOPEDICS	NR
CRITICAL CARE	NR	PULMONARY	★★★
GASTROINTESTINAL	★★★	STROKE	★★★
GENERAL SURGERY	NR	VASCULAR	NR
MATERNITY CARE	NR	WOMEN'S HEALTH	NR

HEALTHGRADES AWARDS

Hardin Memorial Hospital

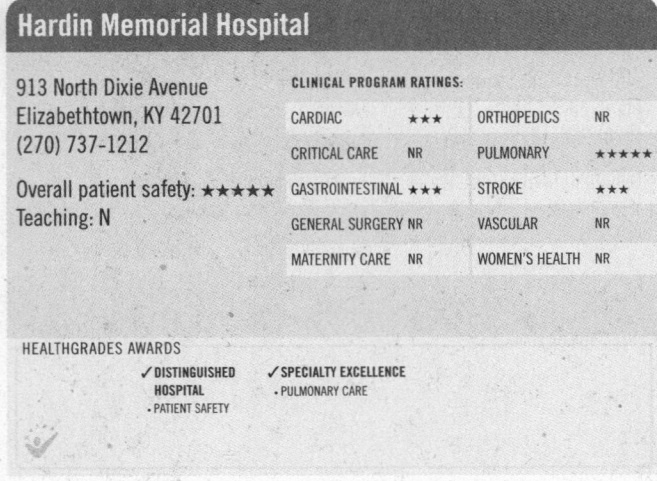

913 North Dixie Avenue
Elizabethtown, KY 42701
(270) 737-1212

Overall patient safety: ★★★★★
Teaching: N

CLINICAL PROGRAM RATINGS:

CARDIAC	★★★	ORTHOPEDICS	NR
CRITICAL CARE	NR	PULMONARY	★★★★★
GASTROINTESTINAL	★★★	STROKE	★★★
GENERAL SURGERY	NR	VASCULAR	NR
MATERNITY CARE	NR	WOMEN'S HEALTH	NR

HEALTHGRADES AWARDS

✓ **DISTINGUISHED HOSPITAL**
• PATIENT SAFETY

✓ **SPECIALTY EXCELLENCE**
• PULMONARY CARE

Georgetown Community Hospital

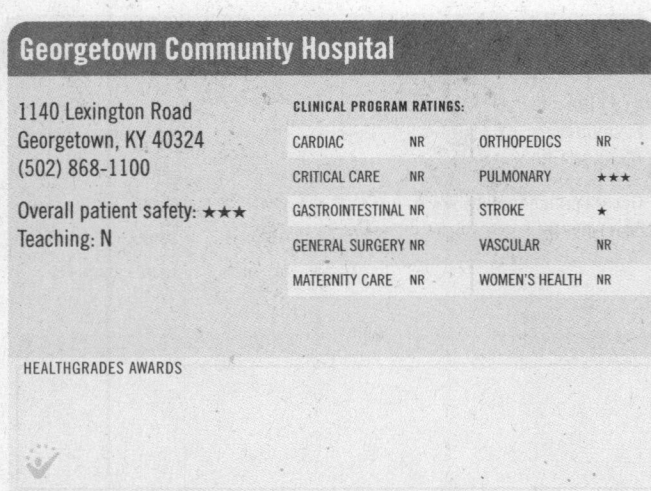

1140 Lexington Road
Georgetown, KY 40324
(502) 868-1100

Overall patient safety: ★★★
Teaching: N

CLINICAL PROGRAM RATINGS:

CARDIAC	NR	ORTHOPEDICS	NR
CRITICAL CARE	NR	PULMONARY	★★★
GASTROINTESTINAL	NR	STROKE	★
GENERAL SURGERY	NR	VASCULAR	NR
MATERNITY CARE	NR	WOMEN'S HEALTH	NR

HEALTHGRADES AWARDS

Harlan ARH Hospital

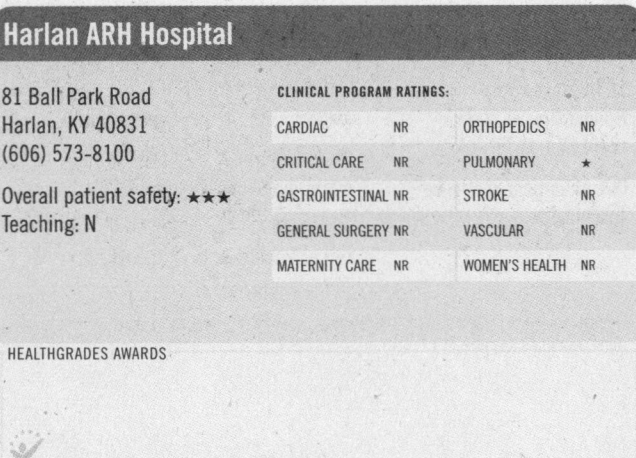

81 Ball Park Road
Harlan, KY 40831
(606) 573-8100

Overall patient safety: ★★★
Teaching: N

CLINICAL PROGRAM RATINGS:

CARDIAC	NR	ORTHOPEDICS	NR
CRITICAL CARE	NR	PULMONARY	★
GASTROINTESTINAL	NR	STROKE	NR
GENERAL SURGERY	NR	VASCULAR	NR
MATERNITY CARE	NR	WOMEN'S HEALTH	NR

HEALTHGRADES AWARDS

Greenview Regional Hospital

1801 Ashley Circle
Bowling Green, KY 42104
(270) 793-1000

Overall patient safety: ★★★
Teaching: N

CLINICAL PROGRAM RATINGS:

CARDIAC	NR	ORTHOPEDICS	★★★★★
CRITICAL CARE	NR	PULMONARY	★★★
GASTROINTESTINAL	★★★	STROKE	★★★
GENERAL SURGERY	NR	VASCULAR	NR
MATERNITY CARE	NR	WOMEN'S HEALTH	NR

HEALTHGRADES AWARDS

✓ **SPECIALTY EXCELLENCE**
• JOINT REPLACEMENT
• ORTHOPEDIC SURGERY

Harrison Memorial Hospital

1210 Key Highway 36 East
Cynthiana, KY 41031
(859) 234-2300

Overall patient safety: ★★★
Teaching: N

CLINICAL PROGRAM RATINGS:

CARDIAC	NR	ORTHOPEDICS	NR
CRITICAL CARE	NR	PULMONARY	★★★
GASTROINTESTINAL	NR	STROKE	★★★
GENERAL SURGERY	NR	VASCULAR	NR
MATERNITY CARE	NR	WOMEN'S HEALTH	NR

HEALTHGRADES AWARDS

KEY: ★★★★★ BEST   ★★★ AS EXPECTED   ★ POOR   NR NOT RATED BY HEALTHGRADES   For full definitions of ratings and awards, see Appendix.

Highlands Regional Medical Center

5000 Kentucky Route 321
Prestonsburg, KY 41653
(606) 886-8511

Overall patient safety: ★★★
Teaching: Y

CLINICAL PROGRAM RATINGS:

CARDIAC	NR	ORTHOPEDICS	NR
CRITICAL CARE	NR	PULMONARY	★★★
GASTROINTESTINAL	NR	STROKE	NR
GENERAL SURGERY	NR	VASCULAR	NR
MATERNITY CARE	NR	WOMEN'S HEALTH	NR

HEALTHGRADES AWARDS

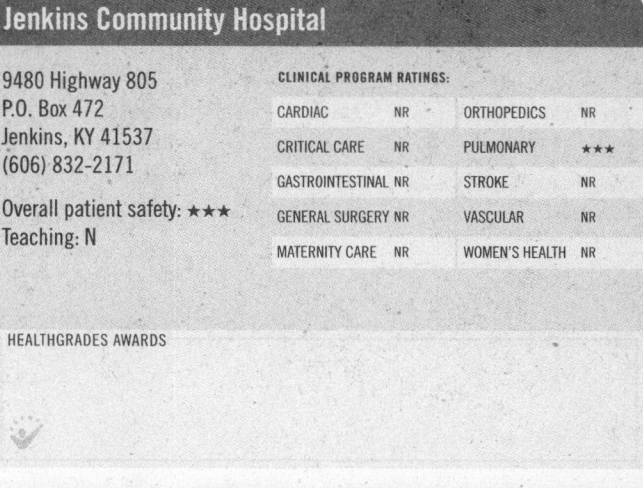

Jenkins Community Hospital

9480 Highway 805
P.O. Box 472
Jenkins, KY 41537
(606) 832-2171

Overall patient safety: ★★★
Teaching: N

CLINICAL PROGRAM RATINGS:

CARDIAC	NR	ORTHOPEDICS	NR
CRITICAL CARE	NR	PULMONARY	★★★
GASTROINTESTINAL	NR	STROKE	NR
GENERAL SURGERY	NR	VASCULAR	NR
MATERNITY CARE	NR	WOMEN'S HEALTH	NR

HEALTHGRADES AWARDS

Jackson Purchase Medical Center

1099 Medical Center Circle
Mayfield, KY 42066
(270) 251-4100

Overall patient safety: ★★★
Teaching: N

CLINICAL PROGRAM RATINGS:

CARDIAC	NR	ORTHOPEDICS	★★★
CRITICAL CARE	NR	PULMONARY	★★★
GASTROINTESTINAL	NR	STROKE	★★★
GENERAL SURGERY	NR	VASCULAR	NR
MATERNITY CARE	NR	WOMEN'S HEALTH	NR

HEALTHGRADES AWARDS

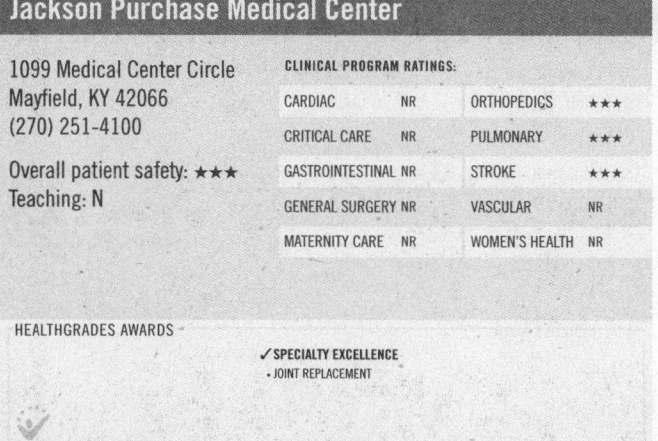

✓ SPECIALTY EXCELLENCE
• JOINT REPLACEMENT

Jennie Stuart Medical Center

320 West 18th Street
Hopkinsville, KY 42240
(270) 887-0100

Overall patient safety: ★★★
Teaching: N

CLINICAL PROGRAM RATINGS:

CARDIAC	NR	ORTHOPEDICS	NR
CRITICAL CARE	NR	PULMONARY	★★★
GASTROINTESTINAL	★★★	STROKE	★★★
GENERAL SURGERY	NR	VASCULAR	NR
MATERNITY CARE	NR	WOMEN'S HEALTH	NR

HEALTHGRADES AWARDS

James B. Haggin Memorial Hospital

464 Linden Avenue
Harrodsburg, KY 40330
(859) 734-5441

Overall patient safety: ★★★
Teaching: N

CLINICAL PROGRAM RATINGS:

CARDIAC	NR	ORTHOPEDICS	NR
CRITICAL CARE	NR	PULMONARY	★
GASTROINTESTINAL	NR	STROKE	NR
GENERAL SURGERY	NR	VASCULAR	NR
MATERNITY CARE	NR	WOMEN'S HEALTH	NR

HEALTHGRADES AWARDS

Jewish Hospital*

200 Abraham Flexner Way
Louisville, KY 40202
(502) 587-4011

Overall patient safety: ★★★
Teaching: Y

CLINICAL PROGRAM RATINGS:

CARDIAC	★★★	ORTHOPEDICS	★★★
CRITICAL CARE	NR	PULMONARY	★★★★★
GASTROINTESTINAL	★★★	STROKE	★★★★★
GENERAL SURGERY	NR	VASCULAR	★★★
MATERNITY CARE	NR	WOMEN'S HEALTH	NR

HEALTHGRADES AWARDS

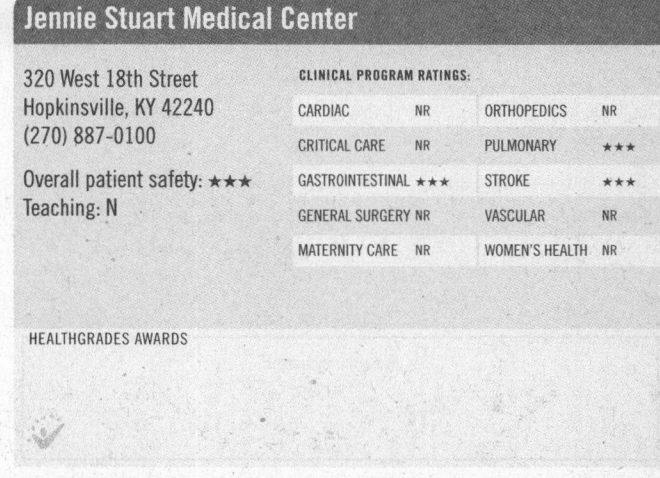

✓ AMERICA'S 50 BEST HOSPITALS
✓ DISTINGUISHED HOSPITAL
 • CLINICAL EXCELLENCE
✓ SPECIALTY EXCELLENCE
 • PULMONARY CARE • STROKE CARE

*This hospital reports its data to the federal government jointly with another hospital. Therefore the ratings and awards apply to multiple hospitals and this specific hospital may not provide all rated services.

Jewish Hospital--Shelbyville

727 Hospital Drive
Shelbyville, KY 40065
(502) 647-4000

Overall patient safety: ★★★
Teaching: N

CLINICAL PROGRAM RATINGS:

CARDIAC	NR	ORTHOPEDICS	NR
CRITICAL CARE	NR	PULMONARY	★★★
GASTROINTESTINAL	NR	STROKE	★
GENERAL SURGERY	NR	VASCULAR	NR
MATERNITY CARE	NR	WOMEN'S HEALTH	NR

HEALTHGRADES AWARDS

Knox County Hospital

80 Hospital Drive
Barbourville, KY 40906
(606) 546-4175

Overall patient safety: ★★★
Teaching: N

CLINICAL PROGRAM RATINGS:

CARDIAC	NR	ORTHOPEDICS	NR
CRITICAL CARE	NR	PULMONARY	★
GASTROINTESTINAL	NR	STROKE	NR
GENERAL SURGERY	NR	VASCULAR	NR
MATERNITY CARE	NR	WOMEN'S HEALTH	NR

HEALTHGRADES AWARDS

Kentucky River Medical Center

540 Jetts Drive
Jackson, KY 41339
(606) 666-6000

Overall patient safety: ★★★
Teaching: N

CLINICAL PROGRAM RATINGS:

CARDIAC	NR	ORTHOPEDICS	NR
CRITICAL CARE	NR	PULMONARY	★★★★★
GASTROINTESTINAL	NR	STROKE	NR
GENERAL SURGERY	NR	VASCULAR	NR
MATERNITY CARE	NR	WOMEN'S HEALTH	NR

HEALTHGRADES AWARDS

✓ SPECIALTY EXCELLENCE
· PULMONARY CARE

Lake Cumberland Regional Hospital

305 Langdon Street
Somerset, KY 42503
(606) 679-7441

Overall patient safety: ★★★
Teaching: N

CLINICAL PROGRAM RATINGS:

CARDIAC	★★★	ORTHOPEDICS	★★★★★
CRITICAL CARE	NR	PULMONARY	★
GASTROINTESTINAL	★★★	STROKE	★★★
GENERAL SURGERY	NR	VASCULAR	NR
MATERNITY CARE	NR	WOMEN'S HEALTH	NR

HEALTHGRADES AWARDS

✓ SPECIALTY EXCELLENCE
· ORTHOPEDIC
  SURGERY

King's Daughters Medical Center

2201 Lexington Avenue
Ashland, KY 41101
(606) 327-4000

Overall patient safety: ★★★
Teaching: N

CLINICAL PROGRAM RATINGS:

CARDIAC	★★★	ORTHOPEDICS	★★★
CRITICAL CARE	NR	PULMONARY	★★★
GASTROINTESTINAL	★★★	STROKE	★
GENERAL SURGERY	NR	VASCULAR	★★★
MATERNITY CARE	NR	WOMEN'S HEALTH	NR

HEALTHGRADES AWARDS

✓ SPECIALTY EXCELLENCE
· CARDIAC SURGERY

Livingston Hospital and Healthcare

131 Hospital Drive
Salem, KY 42078
(270) 988-2299

Overall patient safety: ★★★
Teaching: N

CLINICAL PROGRAM RATINGS:

CARDIAC	NR	ORTHOPEDICS	NR
CRITICAL CARE	NR	PULMONARY	★★★
GASTROINTESTINAL	NR	STROKE	NR
GENERAL SURGERY	NR	VASCULAR	NR
MATERNITY CARE	NR	WOMEN'S HEALTH	NR

HEALTHGRADES AWARDS

KEY: ★★★★★ BEST   ★★★ AS EXPECTED   ★ POOR   NR NOT RATED BY HEALTHGRADES   For full definitions of ratings and awards, see Appendix.

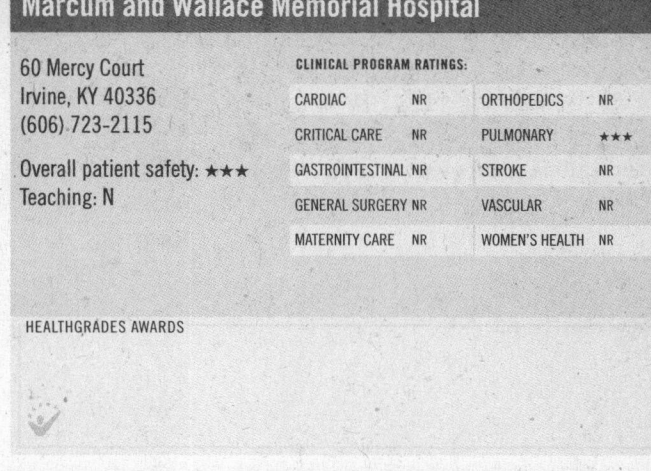

Logan Memorial Hospital

1625 South Nashville Road
Russellville, KY 42276
(270) 726-4011

Overall patient safety: ★★★
Teaching: N

CLINICAL PROGRAM RATINGS:

CARDIAC	NR	ORTHOPEDICS	NR
CRITICAL CARE	NR	PULMONARY	★★★
GASTROINTESTINAL	NR	STROKE	★★★
GENERAL SURGERY	NR	VASCULAR	NR
MATERNITY CARE	NR	WOMEN'S HEALTH	NR

HEALTHGRADES AWARDS

Marcum and Wallace Memorial Hospital

60 Mercy Court
Irvine, KY 40336
(606) 723-2115

Overall patient safety: ★★★
Teaching: N

CLINICAL PROGRAM RATINGS:

CARDIAC	NR	ORTHOPEDICS	NR
CRITICAL CARE	NR	PULMONARY	★★★
GASTROINTESTINAL	NR	STROKE	NR
GENERAL SURGERY	NR	VASCULAR	NR
MATERNITY CARE	NR	WOMEN'S HEALTH	NR

HEALTHGRADES AWARDS

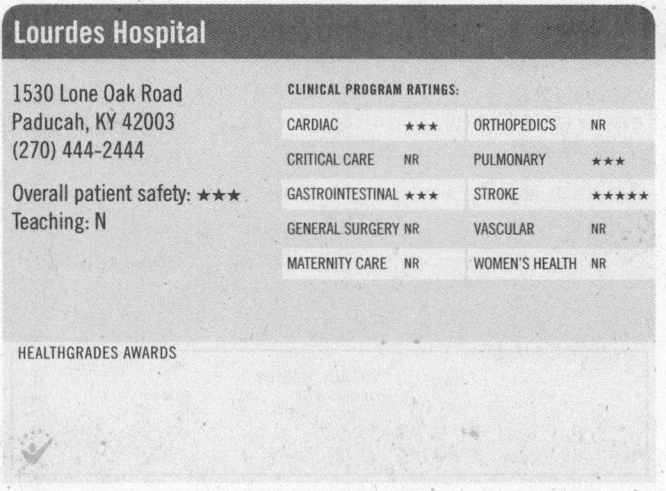

Lourdes Hospital

1530 Lone Oak Road
Paducah, KY 42003
(270) 444-2444

Overall patient safety: ★★★
Teaching: N

CLINICAL PROGRAM RATINGS:

CARDIAC	★★★	ORTHOPEDICS	NR
CRITICAL CARE	NR	PULMONARY	★★★
GASTROINTESTINAL	★★★	STROKE	★★★★★
GENERAL SURGERY	NR	VASCULAR	NR
MATERNITY CARE	NR	WOMEN'S HEALTH	NR

HEALTHGRADES AWARDS

Marshall County Hospital

503 George McClain Drive
Benton, KY 42025
(270) 527-4800

Overall patient safety: ★★★
Teaching: N

CLINICAL PROGRAM RATINGS:

CARDIAC	NR	ORTHOPEDICS	NR
CRITICAL CARE	NR	PULMONARY	★★★
GASTROINTESTINAL	NR	STROKE	★★★
GENERAL SURGERY	NR	VASCULAR	NR
MATERNITY CARE	NR	WOMEN'S HEALTH	NR

HEALTHGRADES AWARDS

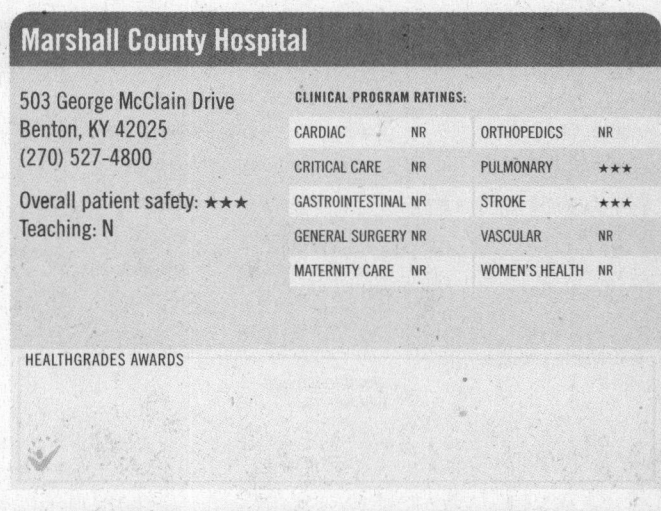

Manchester Memorial Hospital

401 Memorial Drive
Manchester, KY 40962
(606) 598-5104

Overall patient safety: ★★★
Teaching: N

CLINICAL PROGRAM RATINGS:

CARDIAC	NR	ORTHOPEDICS	NR
CRITICAL CARE	NR	PULMONARY	★★★★★
GASTROINTESTINAL	NR	STROKE	NR
GENERAL SURGERY	NR	VASCULAR	NR
MATERNITY CARE	NR	WOMEN'S HEALTH	NR

HEALTHGRADES AWARDS

✓ **SPECIALTY EXCELLENCE**
· PULMONARY CARE

Mary Breckinridge Hospital

130 Kate Ireland Drive
Hyden, KY 41749
(606) 672-2901

Overall patient safety: NR
Teaching: N

CLINICAL PROGRAM RATINGS:

CARDIAC	NR	ORTHOPEDICS	NR
CRITICAL CARE	NR	PULMONARY	★★★
GASTROINTESTINAL	NR	STROKE	NR
GENERAL SURGERY	NR	VASCULAR	NR
MATERNITY CARE	NR	WOMEN'S HEALTH	NR

HEALTHGRADES AWARDS

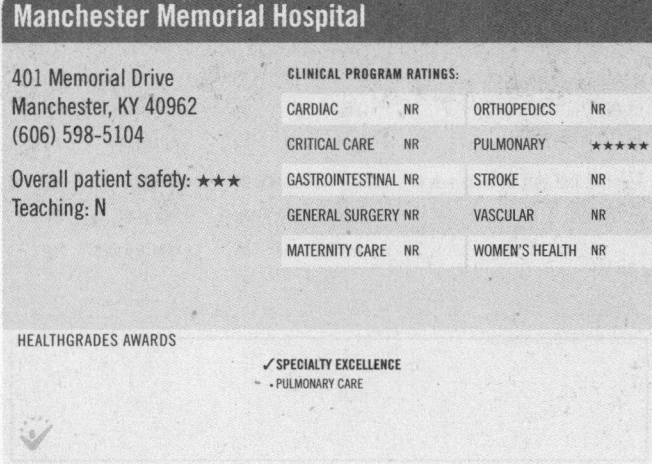

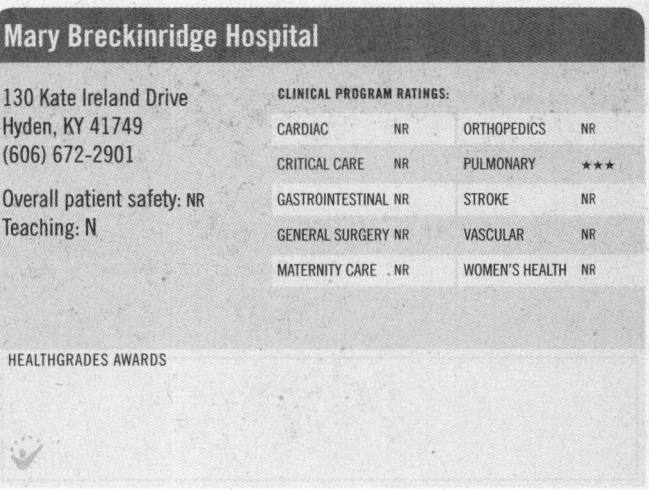

Mary Chiles Hospital

50 Sterling Avenue
Mount Sterling, KY 40353
(859) 498-1220

Overall patient safety: ★★★
Teaching: N

CLINICAL PROGRAM RATINGS:

CARDIAC	NR	ORTHOPEDICS	NR
CRITICAL CARE	NR	PULMONARY	★★★
GASTROINTESTINAL	NR	STROKE	★★★
GENERAL SURGERY	NR	VASCULAR	NR
MATERNITY CARE	NR	WOMEN'S HEALTH	NR

HEALTHGRADES AWARDS

Meadowview Regional Medical Center

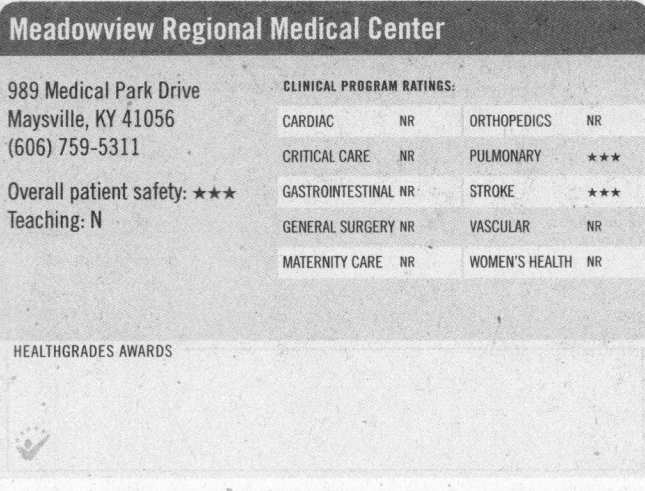

989 Medical Park Drive
Maysville, KY 41056
(606) 759-5311

Overall patient safety: ★★★
Teaching: N

CLINICAL PROGRAM RATINGS:

CARDIAC	NR	ORTHOPEDICS	NR
CRITICAL CARE	NR	PULMONARY	★★★
GASTROINTESTINAL	NR	STROKE	★★★
GENERAL SURGERY	NR	VASCULAR	NR
MATERNITY CARE	NR	WOMEN'S HEALTH	NR

HEALTHGRADES AWARDS

Marymount Medical Center

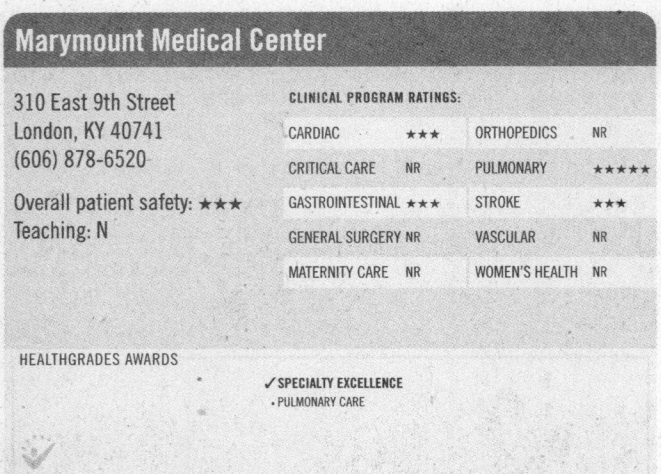

310 East 9th Street
London, KY 40741
(606) 878-6520

Overall patient safety: ★★★
Teaching: N

CLINICAL PROGRAM RATINGS:

CARDIAC	★★★	ORTHOPEDICS	NR
CRITICAL CARE	NR	PULMONARY	★★★★★
GASTROINTESTINAL	★★★	STROKE	★★★
GENERAL SURGERY	NR	VASCULAR	NR
MATERNITY CARE	NR	WOMEN'S HEALTH	NR

HEALTHGRADES AWARDS

✓ SPECIALTY EXCELLENCE
• PULMONARY CARE

Medical Center

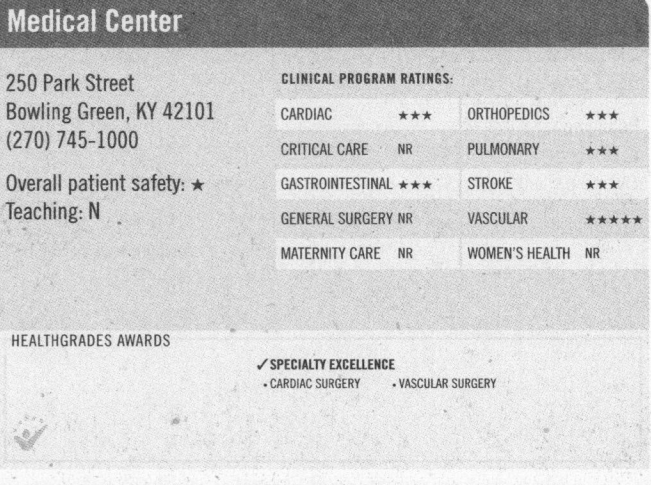

250 Park Street
Bowling Green, KY 42101
(270) 745-1000

Overall patient safety: ★
Teaching: N

CLINICAL PROGRAM RATINGS:

CARDIAC	★★★	ORTHOPEDICS	★★★
CRITICAL CARE	NR	PULMONARY	★★★
GASTROINTESTINAL	★★★	STROKE	★★★
GENERAL SURGERY	NR	VASCULAR	★★★★★
MATERNITY CARE	NR	WOMEN'S HEALTH	NR

HEALTHGRADES AWARDS

✓ SPECIALTY EXCELLENCE
• CARDIAC SURGERY   • VASCULAR SURGERY

McDowell ARH Hospital

9879 Kentucky Route 122
P.O. Box 247
McDowell, KY 41647
(606) 377-3400

Overall patient safety: ★★★
Teaching: N

CLINICAL PROGRAM RATINGS:

CARDIAC	NR	ORTHOPEDICS	NR
CRITICAL CARE	NR	PULMONARY	★★★
GASTROINTESTINAL	NR	STROKE	NR
GENERAL SURGERY	NR	VASCULAR	NR
MATERNITY CARE	NR	WOMEN'S HEALTH	NR

HEALTHGRADES AWARDS

Medical Center at Franklin

1100 Brookhaven Road
Franklin, KY 42135
(270) 598-4800

Overall patient safety: ★★★
Teaching: N

CLINICAL PROGRAM RATINGS:

CARDIAC	NR	ORTHOPEDICS	NR
CRITICAL CARE	NR	PULMONARY	★★★
GASTROINTESTINAL	NR	STROKE	NR
GENERAL SURGERY	NR	VASCULAR	NR
MATERNITY CARE	NR	WOMEN'S HEALTH	NR

HEALTHGRADES AWARDS

KEY: ★★★★★ **BEST**   ★★★ **AS EXPECTED**   ★ **POOR**   NR **NOT RATED BY HEALTHGRADES**   For full definitions of ratings and awards, see Appendix.

The Medical Center at Scottsville

456 Burnley Road
Scottsville, KY 42164
(270) 622-2800

Overall patient safety: NR
Teaching: N

CLINICAL PROGRAM RATINGS:

CARDIAC	NR	ORTHOPEDICS	NR
CRITICAL CARE	NR	PULMONARY	★
GASTROINTESTINAL	NR	STROKE	NR
GENERAL SURGERY	NR	VASCULAR	NR
MATERNITY CARE	NR	WOMEN'S HEALTH	NR

HEALTHGRADES AWARDS

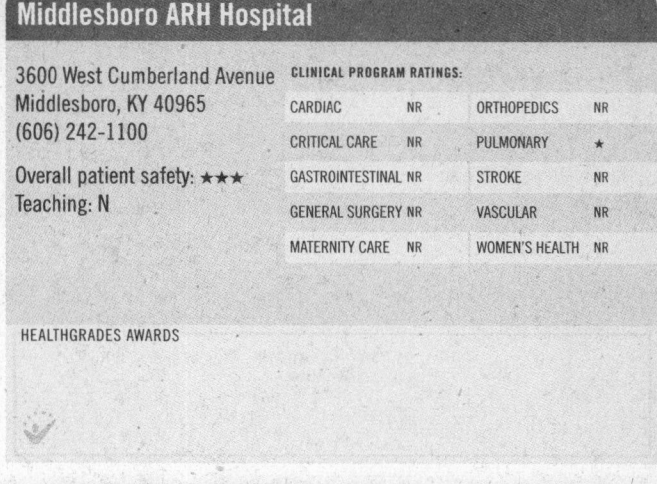

Middlesboro ARH Hospital

3600 West Cumberland Avenue
Middlesboro, KY 40965
(606) 242-1100

Overall patient safety: ★★★
Teaching: N

CLINICAL PROGRAM RATINGS:

CARDIAC	NR	ORTHOPEDICS	NR
CRITICAL CARE	NR	PULMONARY	★
GASTROINTESTINAL	NR	STROKE	NR
GENERAL SURGERY	NR	VASCULAR	NR
MATERNITY CARE	NR	WOMEN'S HEALTH	NR

HEALTHGRADES AWARDS

Methodist Hospital

1305 North Elm Street
Henderson, KY 42420
(270) 827-7700

Overall patient safety: ★★★
Teaching: Y

CLINICAL PROGRAM RATINGS:

CARDIAC	NR	ORTHOPEDICS	NR
CRITICAL CARE	NR	PULMONARY	★★★
GASTROINTESTINAL	NR	STROKE	★★★
GENERAL SURGERY	NR	VASCULAR	NR
MATERNITY CARE	NR	WOMEN'S HEALTH	NR

HEALTHGRADES AWARDS

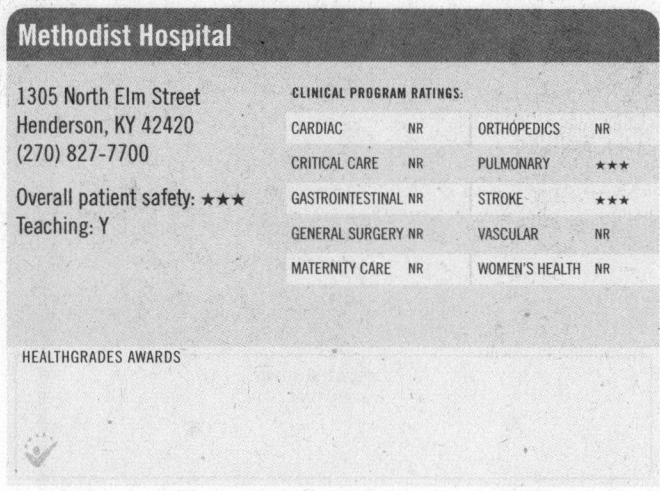

Monroe County Medical Center

529 Cap Harlan Road
Tompkinsville, KY 42167
(270) 487-9231

Overall patient safety: ★★★
Teaching: N

CLINICAL PROGRAM RATINGS:

CARDIAC	NR	ORTHOPEDICS	NR
CRITICAL CARE	NR	PULMONARY	★
GASTROINTESTINAL	NR	STROKE	NR
GENERAL SURGERY	NR	VASCULAR	NR
MATERNITY CARE	NR	WOMEN'S HEALTH	NR

HEALTHGRADES AWARDS

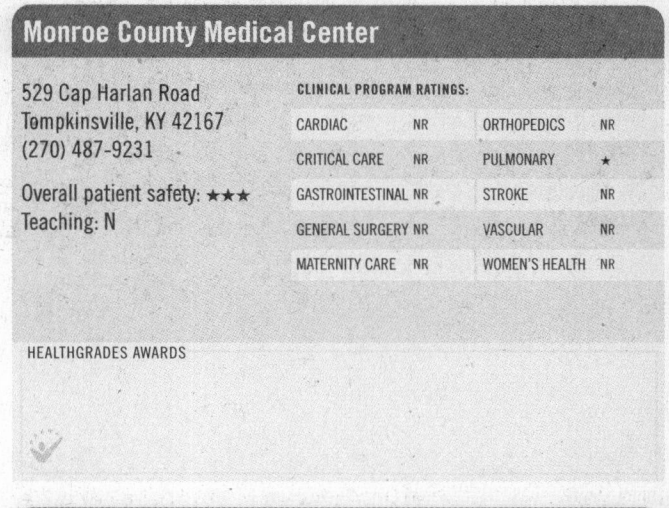

Methodist Hospital Union County

4604 US Highway 60 West
Morganfield, KY 42437
(270) 389-5000

Overall patient safety: ★★★
Teaching: N

CLINICAL PROGRAM RATINGS:

CARDIAC	NR	ORTHOPEDICS	NR
CRITICAL CARE	NR	PULMONARY	★★★
GASTROINTESTINAL	NR	STROKE	NR
GENERAL SURGERY	NR	VASCULAR	NR
MATERNITY CARE	NR	WOMEN'S HEALTH	NR

HEALTHGRADES AWARDS

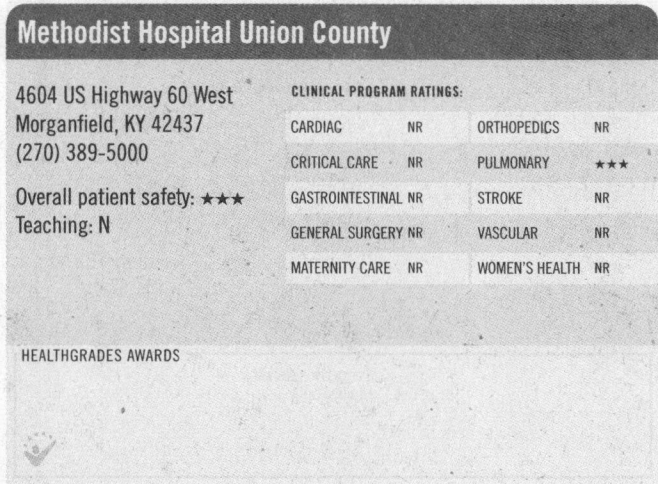

Muhlenberg Community Hospital

440 Hopkinsville Street
Greenville, KY 42345
(270) 338-8000

Overall patient safety: ★★★
Teaching: N

CLINICAL PROGRAM RATINGS:

CARDIAC	NR	ORTHOPEDICS	NR
CRITICAL CARE	NR	PULMONARY	★★★
GASTROINTESTINAL	★★★	STROKE	NR
GENERAL SURGERY	NR	VASCULAR	NR
MATERNITY CARE	NR	WOMEN'S HEALTH	NR

HEALTHGRADES AWARDS

Murray-Calloway County Hospital

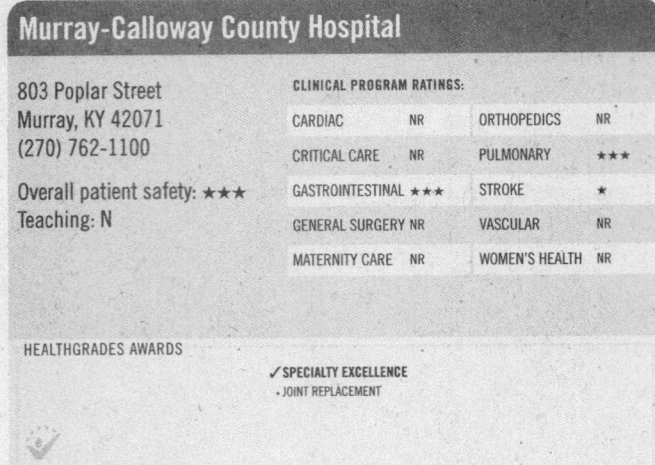

803 Poplar Street
Murray, KY 42071
(270) 762-1100

Overall patient safety: ★★★
Teaching: N

CLINICAL PROGRAM RATINGS:

CARDIAC	NR	ORTHOPEDICS	NR
CRITICAL CARE	NR	PULMONARY	★★★
GASTROINTESTINAL	★★★	STROKE	★
GENERAL SURGERY	NR	VASCULAR	NR
MATERNITY CARE	NR	WOMEN'S HEALTH	NR

HEALTHGRADES AWARDS

✓ SPECIALTY EXCELLENCE
• JOINT REPLACEMENT

Norton Hospital*

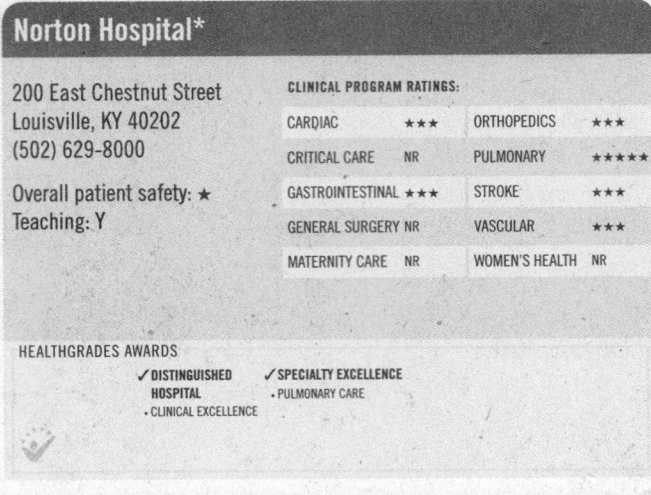

200 East Chestnut Street
Louisville, KY 40202
(502) 629-8000

Overall patient safety: ★
Teaching: Y

CLINICAL PROGRAM RATINGS:

CARDIAC	★★★	ORTHOPEDICS	★★★
CRITICAL CARE	NR	PULMONARY	★★★★★
GASTROINTESTINAL	★★★	STROKE	★★★
GENERAL SURGERY	NR	VASCULAR	★★★
MATERNITY CARE	NR	WOMEN'S HEALTH	NR

HEALTHGRADES AWARDS

✓ DISTINGUISHED HOSPITAL
• CLINICAL EXCELLENCE

✓ SPECIALTY EXCELLENCE
• PULMONARY CARE

New Horizons Health Systems

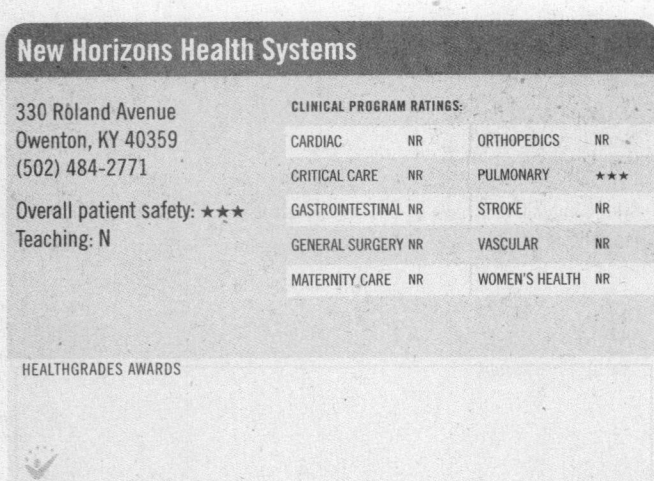

330 Roland Avenue
Owenton, KY 40359
(502) 484-2771

Overall patient safety: ★★★
Teaching: N

CLINICAL PROGRAM RATINGS:

CARDIAC	NR	ORTHOPEDICS	NR
CRITICAL CARE	NR	PULMONARY	★★★
GASTROINTESTINAL	NR	STROKE	NR
GENERAL SURGERY	NR	VASCULAR	NR
MATERNITY CARE	NR	WOMEN'S HEALTH	NR

HEALTHGRADES AWARDS

Norton Southwest Hospital*

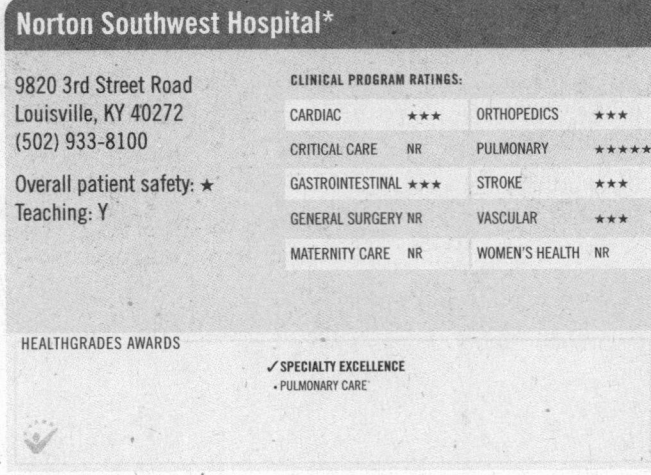

9820 3rd Street Road
Louisville, KY 40272
(502) 933-8100

Overall patient safety: ★
Teaching: Y

CLINICAL PROGRAM RATINGS:

CARDIAC	★★★	ORTHOPEDICS	★★★
CRITICAL CARE	NR	PULMONARY	★★★★★
GASTROINTESTINAL	★★★	STROKE	★★★
GENERAL SURGERY	NR	VASCULAR	★★★
MATERNITY CARE	NR	WOMEN'S HEALTH	NR

HEALTHGRADES AWARDS

✓ SPECIALTY EXCELLENCE
• PULMONARY CARE

Norton Audubon Hospital*

1 Audubon Plaza Drive
Louisville, KY 40217
(502) 636-7111

Overall patient safety: ★
Teaching: Y

CLINICAL PROGRAM RATINGS:

CARDIAC	★★★	ORTHOPEDICS	★★★
CRITICAL CARE	NR	PULMONARY	★★★★★
GASTROINTESTINAL	★★★	STROKE	★★★
GENERAL SURGERY	NR	VASCULAR	★★★
MATERNITY CARE	NR	WOMEN'S HEALTH	NR

HEALTHGRADES AWARDS

✓ SPECIALTY EXCELLENCE
• PULMONARY CARE

Norton Suburban Hospital*

4001 Dutchmans Lane
Louisville, KY 40207
(502) 893-1000

Overall patient safety: ★
Teaching: Y

CLINICAL PROGRAM RATINGS:

CARDIAC	★★★	ORTHOPEDICS	★★★
CRITICAL CARE	NR	PULMONARY	★★★★★
GASTROINTESTINAL	★★★	STROKE	★★★
GENERAL SURGERY	NR	VASCULAR	★★★
MATERNITY CARE	NR	WOMEN'S HEALTH	NR

HEALTHGRADES AWARDS

✓ SPECIALTY EXCELLENCE
• PULMONARY CARE

KEY: ★★★★★ BEST   ★★★ AS EXPECTED   ★ POOR   NR NOT RATED BY HEALTHGRADES   For full definitions of ratings and awards, see Appendix.

Oak Tree Hospital at Baptist Hospital Northeast*

1025 New Moody Lane
La Grange, KY 40031
(502) 222-8509

Overall patient safety: NR
Teaching: N

CLINICAL PROGRAM RATINGS:

CARDIAC	NR	ORTHOPEDICS	NR
CRITICAL CARE	NR	PULMONARY	★★★
GASTROINTESTINAL	NR	STROKE	★★★★★
GENERAL SURGERY	NR	VASCULAR	NR
MATERNITY CARE	NR	WOMEN'S HEALTH	NR

HEALTHGRADES AWARDS

✓ **SPECIALTY EXCELLENCE**
- STROKE CARE

Our Lady of Bellefonte Hospital

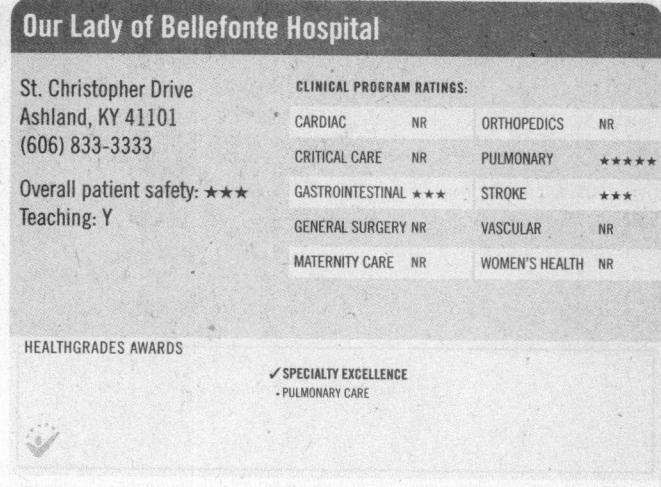

St. Christopher Drive
Ashland, KY 41101
(606) 833-3333

Overall patient safety: ★★★
Teaching: Y

CLINICAL PROGRAM RATINGS:

CARDIAC	NR	ORTHOPEDICS	NR
CRITICAL CARE	NR	PULMONARY	★★★★★
GASTROINTESTINAL	★★★	STROKE	★★★
GENERAL SURGERY	NR	VASCULAR	NR
MATERNITY CARE	NR	WOMEN'S HEALTH	NR

HEALTHGRADES AWARDS

✓ **SPECIALTY EXCELLENCE**
- PULMONARY CARE

Oak Tree Hospital at Baptist Regional Medical Center

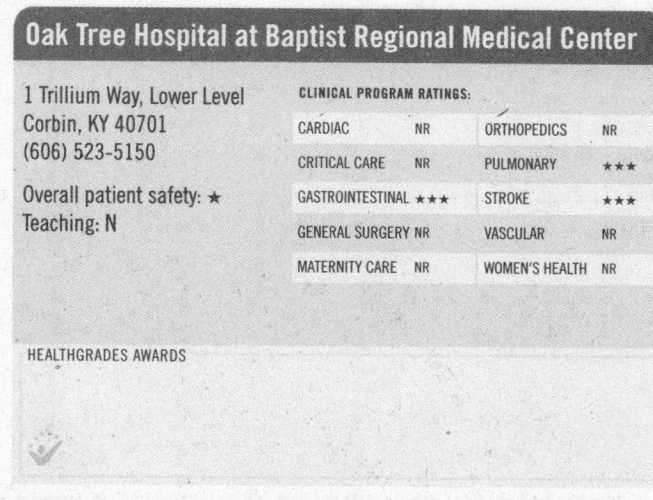

1 Trillium Way, Lower Level
Corbin, KY 40701
(606) 523-5150

Overall patient safety: ★
Teaching: N

CLINICAL PROGRAM RATINGS:

CARDIAC	NR	ORTHOPEDICS	NR
CRITICAL CARE	NR	PULMONARY	★★★
GASTROINTESTINAL	★★★	STROKE	★★★
GENERAL SURGERY	NR	VASCULAR	NR
MATERNITY CARE	NR	WOMEN'S HEALTH	NR

HEALTHGRADES AWARDS

Our Lady of the Way

11203 Main Street
Martin, KY 41649
(606) 285-5181

Overall patient safety: ★★★
Teaching: N

CLINICAL PROGRAM RATINGS:

CARDIAC	NR	ORTHOPEDICS	NR
CRITICAL CARE	NR	PULMONARY	★★★
GASTROINTESTINAL	NR	STROKE	NR
GENERAL SURGERY	NR	VASCULAR	NR
MATERNITY CARE	NR	WOMEN'S HEALTH	NR

HEALTHGRADES AWARDS

Ohio County Hospital

1211 Main Street
Hartford, KY 42347
(270) 298-7411

Overall patient safety: ★★★
Teaching: N

CLINICAL PROGRAM RATINGS:

CARDIAC	NR	ORTHOPEDICS	NR
CRITICAL CARE	NR	PULMONARY	★★★
GASTROINTESTINAL	NR	STROKE	NR
GENERAL SURGERY	NR	VASCULAR	NR
MATERNITY CARE	NR	WOMEN'S HEALTH	NR

HEALTHGRADES AWARDS

Owensboro Medical Health System*

811 East Parrish Avenue
Owensboro, KY 42303
(270) 688-2000

Overall patient safety: ★★★
Teaching: N

CLINICAL PROGRAM RATINGS:

CARDIAC	★★★	ORTHOPEDICS	★★★★★
CRITICAL CARE	★★★	PULMONARY	★★★
GASTROINTESTINAL	★★★	STROKE	★
GENERAL SURGERY	NR	VASCULAR	NR
MATERNITY CARE	NR	WOMEN'S HEALTH	NR

HEALTHGRADES AWARDS

✓ **SPECIALTY EXCELLENCE**
- GASTROINTESTINAL CARE
- JOINT REPLACEMENT
- ORTHOPEDIC SURGERY

*This hospital reports its data to the federal government jointly with another hospital. Therefore the ratings and awards apply to multiple hospitals and this specific hospital may not provide all rated services.

Owensboro Mercy Health System Ford*

1006 Ford Avenue
Owensboro, KY 42302
(502) 686-6100

Overall patient safety: ★★★
Teaching: N

CLINICAL PROGRAM RATINGS:

CARDIAC	★★★	ORTHOPEDICS	★★★★★
CRITICAL CARE	★★★	PULMONARY	★★★
GASTROINTESTINAL	★★★	STROKE	★
GENERAL SURGERY	NR	VASCULAR	NR
MATERNITY CARE	NR	WOMEN'S HEALTH	NR

HEALTHGRADES AWARDS

✓ SPECIALTY EXCELLENCE
- GASTROINTESTINAL CARE
- JOINT REPLACEMENT
- ORTHOPEDIC SURGERY

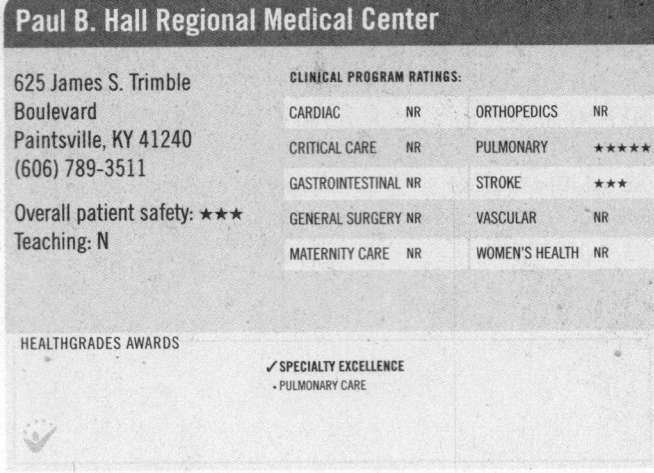

Paul B. Hall Regional Medical Center

625 James S. Trimble
Boulevard
Paintsville, KY 41240
(606) 789-3511

Overall patient safety: ★★★
Teaching: N

CLINICAL PROGRAM RATINGS:

CARDIAC	NR	ORTHOPEDICS	NR
CRITICAL CARE	NR	PULMONARY	★★★★★
GASTROINTESTINAL	NR	STROKE	★★★
GENERAL SURGERY	NR	VASCULAR	NR
MATERNITY CARE	NR	WOMEN'S HEALTH	NR

HEALTHGRADES AWARDS

✓ SPECIALTY EXCELLENCE
- PULMONARY CARE

Parkway Regional Hospital

2000 Holiday Lane
Fulton, KY 42041
(270) 472-2522

Overall patient safety: ★★★
Teaching: N

CLINICAL PROGRAM RATINGS:

CARDIAC	NR	ORTHOPEDICS	NR
CRITICAL CARE	NR	PULMONARY	★
GASTROINTESTINAL	NR	STROKE	★★★
GENERAL SURGERY	NR	VASCULAR	NR
MATERNITY CARE	NR	WOMEN'S HEALTH	NR

HEALTHGRADES AWARDS

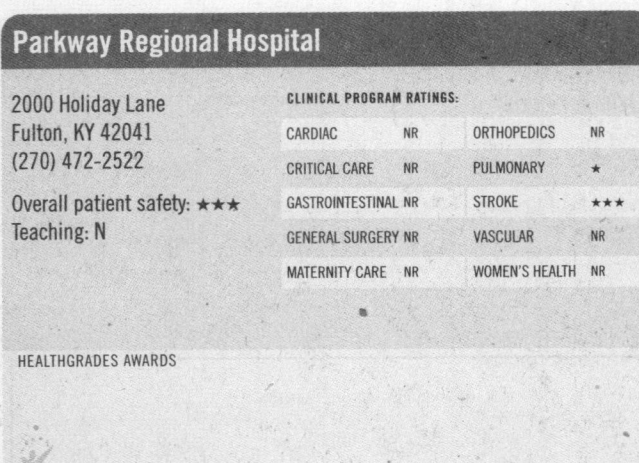

Pikeville Medical Center

911 South Bypass Road
Pikeville, KY 41501
(606) 218-3500

Overall patient safety: ★★★
Teaching: Y

CLINICAL PROGRAM RATINGS:

CARDIAC	★★★	ORTHOPEDICS	NR
CRITICAL CARE	NR	PULMONARY	★★★
GASTROINTESTINAL	★★★	STROKE	★★★
GENERAL SURGERY	NR	VASCULAR	NR
MATERNITY CARE	NR	WOMEN'S HEALTH	NR

HEALTHGRADES AWARDS

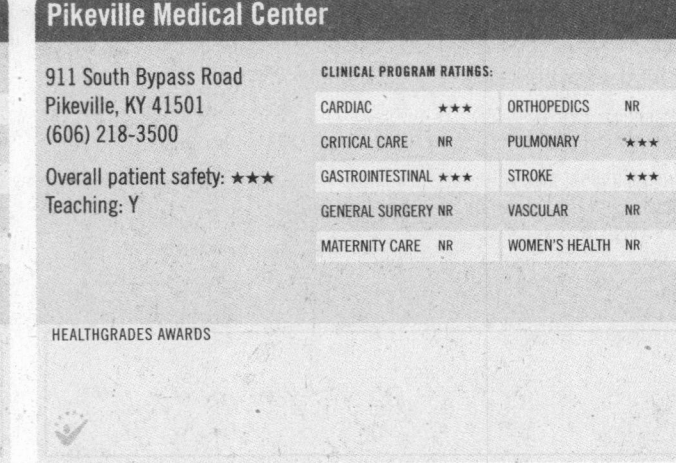

Pattie A. Clay Regional Medical Center

789 Eastern Bypass
Richmond, KY 40475
(859) 623-3131

Overall patient safety: ★★★
Teaching: N

CLINICAL PROGRAM RATINGS:

CARDIAC	NR	ORTHOPEDICS	NR
CRITICAL CARE	NR	PULMONARY	★★★★★
GASTROINTESTINAL	★★★	STROKE	NR
GENERAL SURGERY	NR	VASCULAR	NR
MATERNITY CARE	NR	WOMEN'S HEALTH	NR

HEALTHGRADES AWARDS

✓ SPECIALTY EXCELLENCE
- PULMONARY CARE

Pineville Community Hospital

850 Riverview Avenue
Pineville, KY 40977
(606) 337-3051

Overall patient safety: ★★★★★
Teaching: N

CLINICAL PROGRAM RATINGS:

CARDIAC	NR	ORTHOPEDICS	NR
CRITICAL CARE	NR	PULMONARY	★★★
GASTROINTESTINAL	NR	STROKE	★
GENERAL SURGERY	NR	VASCULAR	NR
MATERNITY CARE	NR	WOMEN'S HEALTH	NR

HEALTHGRADES AWARDS

KEY: ★★★★★ BEST   ★★★ AS EXPECTED   ★ POOR   NR NOT RATED BY HEALTHGRADES   For full definitions of ratings and awards, see Appendix.

Regional Medical Center

900 Hospital Drive
Madisonville, KY 42431
(270) 825-5100

Overall patient safety: ★★★
Teaching: Y

CLINICAL PROGRAM RATINGS:

CARDIAC	★★★	ORTHOPEDICS	★
CRITICAL CARE	NR	PULMONARY	★★★
GASTROINTESTINAL	★★★	STROKE	★★★
GENERAL SURGERY	NR	VASCULAR	NR
MATERNITY CARE	NR	WOMEN'S HEALTH	NR

HEALTHGRADES AWARDS

St. Claire Medical Center

222 Medical Circle
Morehead, KY 40351
(606) 783-6500

Overall patient safety: ★★★
Teaching: Y

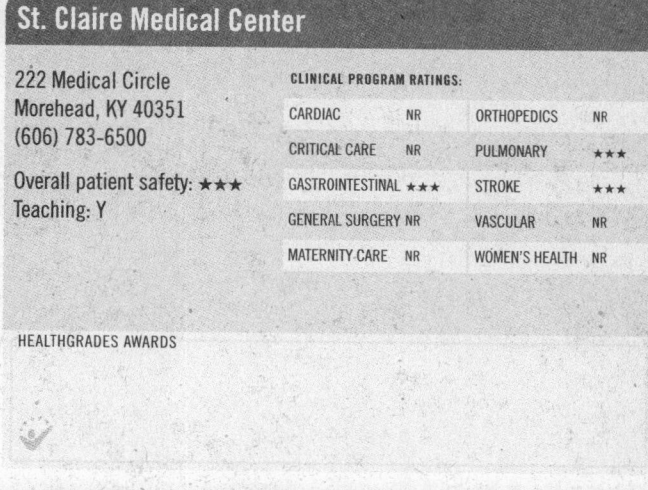

CLINICAL PROGRAM RATINGS:

CARDIAC	NR	ORTHOPEDICS	NR
CRITICAL CARE	NR	PULMONARY	★★★
GASTROINTESTINAL	★★★	STROKE	★★★
GENERAL SURGERY	NR	VASCULAR	NR
MATERNITY CARE	NR	WOMEN'S HEALTH	NR

HEALTHGRADES AWARDS

Rockcastle Hospital Respiratory Care Center

145 Newcomb Avenue
Mount Vernon, KY 40456
(606) 256-2195

Overall patient safety: ★
Teaching: N

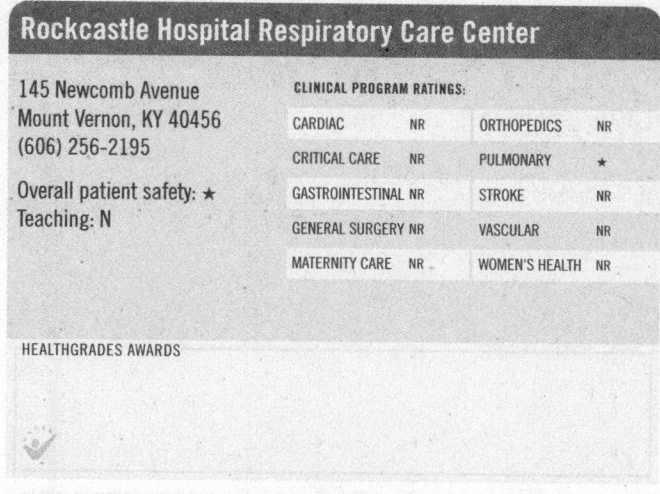

CLINICAL PROGRAM RATINGS:

CARDIAC	NR	ORTHOPEDICS	NR
CRITICAL CARE	NR	PULMONARY	★
GASTROINTESTINAL	NR	STROKE	NR
GENERAL SURGERY	NR	VASCULAR	NR
MATERNITY CARE	NR	WOMEN'S HEALTH	NR

HEALTHGRADES AWARDS

St. Elizabeth Medical Center—South

1 Medical Village Drive
Edgewood, KY 41017
(859) 344-2000

Overall patient safety: ★★★
Teaching: Y

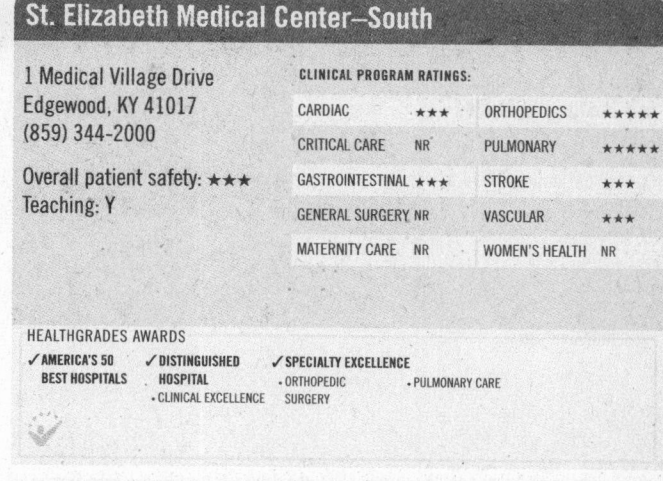

CLINICAL PROGRAM RATINGS:

CARDIAC	★★★	ORTHOPEDICS	★★★★★
CRITICAL CARE	NR	PULMONARY	★★★★★
GASTROINTESTINAL	★★★	STROKE	★★★
GENERAL SURGERY	NR	VASCULAR	★★★
MATERNITY CARE	NR	WOMEN'S HEALTH	NR

HEALTHGRADES AWARDS

✓ AMERICA'S 50 BEST HOSPITALS

✓ DISTINGUISHED HOSPITAL
· CLINICAL EXCELLENCE

✓ SPECIALTY EXCELLENCE
· ORTHOPEDIC SURGERY
· PULMONARY CARE

Russell County Hospital

153 Dowell Road
P.O. Box 1610
Russell Springs, KY 42642
(270) 866-4141

Overall patient safety: ★★★
Teaching: N

CLINICAL PROGRAM RATINGS:

CARDIAC	NR	ORTHOPEDICS	NR
CRITICAL CARE	NR	PULMONARY	★★★
GASTROINTESTINAL	NR	STROKE	★★★
GENERAL SURGERY	NR	VASCULAR	NR
MATERNITY CARE	NR	WOMEN'S HEALTH	NR

HEALTHGRADES AWARDS

St. Joseph East

150 North Eagle Creek Drive
Lexington, KY 40509
(859) 967-5000

Overall patient safety: ★★★
Teaching: N

CLINICAL PROGRAM RATINGS:

CARDIAC	NR	ORTHOPEDICS	★★★
CRITICAL CARE	NR	PULMONARY	★★★
GASTROINTESTINAL	★★★	STROKE	★★★
GENERAL SURGERY	NR	VASCULAR	NR
MATERNITY CARE	NR	WOMEN'S HEALTH	NR

HEALTHGRADES AWARDS

*This hospital reports its data to the federal government jointly with another hospital. Therefore the ratings and awards apply to multiple hospitals and this specific hospital may not provide all rated services.

St. Joseph Hospital

1 St. Joseph Drive
Lexington, KY 40504
(859) 313-1000

Overall patient safety: ★★★
Teaching: Y

CLINICAL PROGRAM RATINGS:

CARDIAC	★★★	ORTHOPEDICS	★★★
CRITICAL CARE	NR	PULMONARY	★★★
GASTROINTESTINAL	★★★	STROKE	★★★
GENERAL SURGERY	NR	VASCULAR	★★★
MATERNITY CARE	NR	WOMEN'S HEALTH	NR

HEALTHGRADES AWARDS

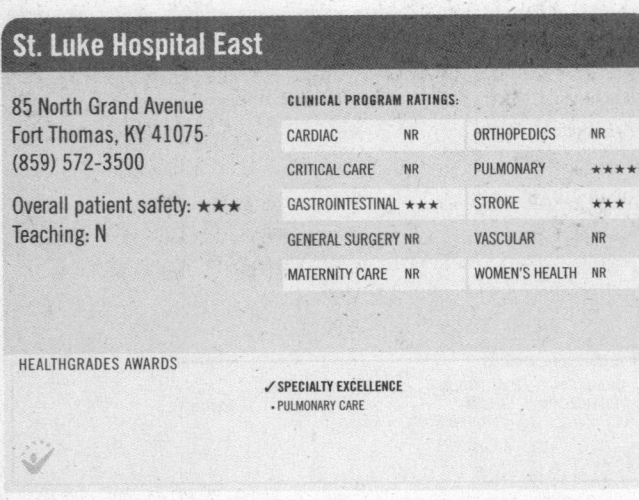

Sts. Mary and Elizabeth Hospital*

1850 Bluegrass Avenue
Louisville, KY 40215
(502) 361-6000

Overall patient safety: ★★★
Teaching: Y

CLINICAL PROGRAM RATINGS:

CARDIAC	★★★	ORTHOPEDICS	★★★
CRITICAL CARE	NR	PULMONARY	★★★★★
GASTROINTESTINAL	★★★	STROKE	★★★★★
GENERAL SURGERY	NR	VASCULAR	★★★
MATERNITY CARE	NR	WOMEN'S HEALTH	NR

HEALTHGRADES AWARDS

✓ SPECIALTY EXCELLENCE
• PULMONARY CARE   • STROKE CARE

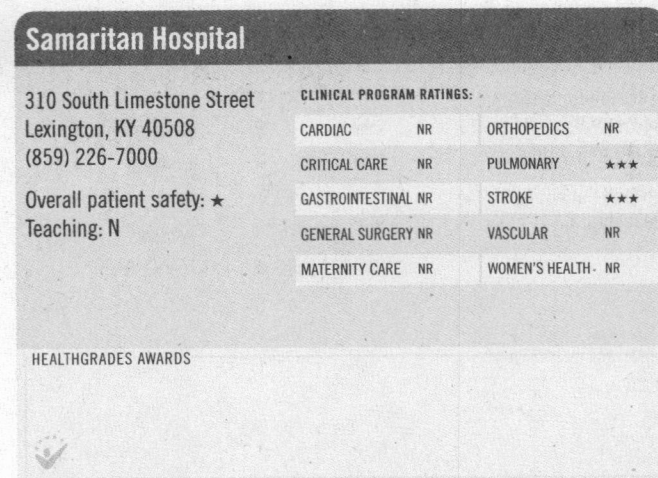

St. Luke Hospital East

85 North Grand Avenue
Fort Thomas, KY 41075
(859) 572-3500

Overall patient safety: ★★★
Teaching: N

CLINICAL PROGRAM RATINGS:

CARDIAC	NR	ORTHOPEDICS	NR
CRITICAL CARE	NR	PULMONARY	★★★★★
GASTROINTESTINAL	★★★	STROKE	★★★
GENERAL SURGERY	NR	VASCULAR	NR
MATERNITY CARE	NR	WOMEN'S HEALTH	NR

HEALTHGRADES AWARDS

✓ SPECIALTY EXCELLENCE
• PULMONARY CARE

Samaritan Hospital

310 South Limestone Street
Lexington, KY 40508
(859) 226-7000

Overall patient safety: ★
Teaching: N

CLINICAL PROGRAM RATINGS:

CARDIAC	NR	ORTHOPEDICS	NR
CRITICAL CARE	NR	PULMONARY	★★★
GASTROINTESTINAL	NR	STROKE	★★★
GENERAL SURGERY	NR	VASCULAR	NR
MATERNITY CARE	NR	WOMEN'S HEALTH	NR

HEALTHGRADES AWARDS

St. Luke Hospital West

7380 Turfway Road
Florence, KY 41042
(859) 962-5200

Overall patient safety: ★★★
Teaching: Y

CLINICAL PROGRAM RATINGS:

CARDIAC	NR	ORTHOPEDICS	NR
CRITICAL CARE	NR	PULMONARY	★★★
GASTROINTESTINAL	NR	STROKE	★★★
GENERAL SURGERY	NR	VASCULAR	NR
MATERNITY CARE	NR	WOMEN'S HEALTH	NR

HEALTHGRADES AWARDS

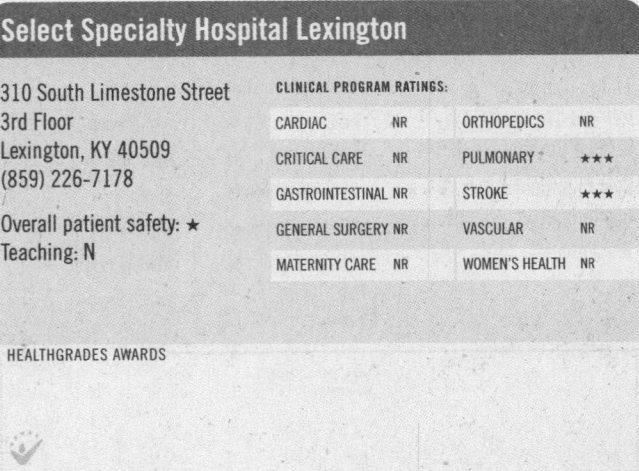

Select Specialty Hospital Lexington

310 South Limestone Street
3rd Floor
Lexington, KY 40509
(859) 226-7178

Overall patient safety: ★
Teaching: N

CLINICAL PROGRAM RATINGS:

CARDIAC	NR	ORTHOPEDICS	NR
CRITICAL CARE	NR	PULMONARY	★★★
GASTROINTESTINAL	NR	STROKE	★★★
GENERAL SURGERY	NR	VASCULAR	NR
MATERNITY CARE	NR	WOMEN'S HEALTH	NR

HEALTHGRADES AWARDS

KEY: ★★★★★ BEST   ★★★ AS EXPECTED   ★ POOR   NR NOT RATED BY HEALTHGRADES   For full definitions of ratings and awards, see Appendix.

Spring View Hospital

320 Loretto Road
Lebanon, KY 40033
(270) 692-3161

Overall patient safety: ★★★
Teaching: N

CLINICAL PROGRAM RATINGS:

CARDIAC	NR	ORTHOPEDICS	NR
CRITICAL CARE	NR	PULMONARY	★★★
GASTROINTESTINAL	NR	STROKE	NR
GENERAL SURGERY	NR	VASCULAR	NR
MATERNITY CARE	NR	WOMEN'S HEALTH	NR

HEALTHGRADES AWARDS

Three Rivers Medical Center

2483 Highway 644
Louisa, KY 41230
(606) 638-9451

Overall patient safety: ★★★
Teaching: N

CLINICAL PROGRAM RATINGS:

CARDIAC	NR	ORTHOPEDICS	NR
CRITICAL CARE	NR	PULMONARY	★★★
GASTROINTESTINAL	NR	STROKE	NR
GENERAL SURGERY	NR	VASCULAR	NR
MATERNITY CARE	NR	WOMEN'S HEALTH	NR

HEALTHGRADES AWARDS

T. J. Samson Community Hospital

1301 North Race Street
Glasgow, KY 42141
(270) 651-4444

Overall patient safety: ★★★★★
Teaching: Y

CLINICAL PROGRAM RATINGS:

CARDIAC	NR	ORTHOPEDICS	NR
CRITICAL CARE	NR	PULMONARY	★★★
GASTROINTESTINAL	★★★	STROKE	★★★
GENERAL SURGERY	NR	VASCULAR	NR
MATERNITY CARE	NR	WOMEN'S HEALTH	NR

HEALTHGRADES AWARDS

✓ DISTINGUISHED
　 HOSPITAL
・ PATIENT SAFETY

Trigg County Hospital

254 Main Street
Cadiz, KY 42211
(270) 522-3215

Overall patient safety: NR
Teaching: N

CLINICAL PROGRAM RATINGS:

CARDIAC	NR	ORTHOPEDICS	NR
CRITICAL CARE	NR	PULMONARY	★★★
GASTROINTESTINAL	NR	STROKE	NR
GENERAL SURGERY	NR	VASCULAR	NR
MATERNITY CARE	NR	WOMEN'S HEALTH	NR

HEALTHGRADES AWARDS

Taylor Regional Hospital

1700 Old Lebanon Road
Campbellsville, KY 42718
(270) 465-3561

Overall patient safety: ★★★
Teaching: N

CLINICAL PROGRAM RATINGS:

CARDIAC	NR	ORTHOPEDICS	NR
CRITICAL CARE	NR	PULMONARY	★★★★★
GASTROINTESTINAL	NR	STROKE	NR
GENERAL SURGERY	NR	VASCULAR	NR
MATERNITY CARE	NR	WOMEN'S HEALTH	NR

HEALTHGRADES AWARDS

✓ SPECIALTY EXCELLENCE
・ PULMONARY CARE

Twin Lakes Regional Medical Center

910 Wallace Avenue
Leitchfield, KY 42754
(270) 259-9400

Overall patient safety: ★★★
Teaching: N

CLINICAL PROGRAM RATINGS:

CARDIAC	NR	ORTHOPEDICS	NR
CRITICAL CARE	NR	PULMONARY	★★★
GASTROINTESTINAL	NR	STROKE	★★★
GENERAL SURGERY	NR	VASCULAR	NR
MATERNITY CARE	NR	WOMEN'S HEALTH	NR

HEALTHGRADES AWARDS

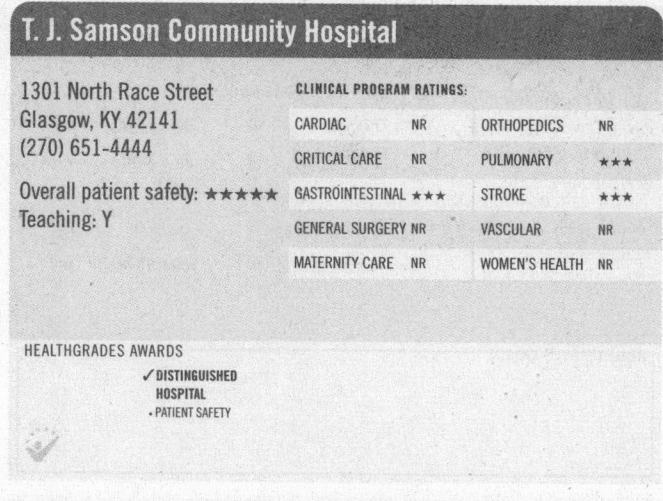

*This hospital reports its data to the federal government jointly with another hospital. Therefore the ratings and awards apply to multiple hospitals and this specific hospital may not provide all rated services.

University of Kentucky Hospital

800 Rose Street
Lexington, KY 40536
(859) 323-5000

Overall patient safety: ★
Teaching: Y

CLINICAL PROGRAM RATINGS:

CARDIAC	★	ORTHOPEDICS	★★★
CRITICAL CARE	NR	PULMONARY	★★★
GASTROINTESTINAL	★★★	STROKE	★
GENERAL SURGERY	NR	VASCULAR	★★★
MATERNITY CARE	NR	WOMEN'S HEALTH	NR

HEALTHGRADES AWARDS

Western Baptist Hospital

2501 Kentucky Avenue
Paducah, KY 42003
(270) 575-2100

Overall patient safety: ★★★
Teaching: N

CLINICAL PROGRAM RATINGS:

CARDIAC	★★★	ORTHOPEDICS	★
CRITICAL CARE	NR	PULMONARY	★★★
GASTROINTESTINAL	★★★	STROKE	★★★
GENERAL SURGERY	NR	VASCULAR	★★★
MATERNITY CARE	NR	WOMEN'S HEALTH	NR

HEALTHGRADES AWARDS

University of Louisville Hospital

530 South Jackson Street
Louisville, KY 40202
(502) 562-3000

Overall patient safety: ★
Teaching: Y

CLINICAL PROGRAM RATINGS:

CARDIAC	NR	ORTHOPEDICS	NR
CRITICAL CARE	NR	PULMONARY	★★★
GASTROINTESTINAL	NR	STROKE	★
GENERAL SURGERY	NR	VASCULAR	NR
MATERNITY CARE	NR	WOMEN'S HEALTH	NR

HEALTHGRADES AWARDS

Westlake Regional Hospital

901 Westlake Drive
P.O. Box 1269
Columbia, KY 42728
(270) 384-4753

Overall patient safety: ★★★
Teaching: N

CLINICAL PROGRAM RATINGS:

CARDIAC	NR	ORTHOPEDICS	NR
CRITICAL CARE	NR	PULMONARY	★★★
GASTROINTESTINAL	NR	STROKE	NR
GENERAL SURGERY	NR	VASCULAR	NR
MATERNITY CARE	NR	WOMEN'S HEALTH	NR

HEALTHGRADES AWARDS

Wayne County Hospital

166 Hospital Street
Monticello, KY 42633
(606) 348-9343

Overall patient safety: ★★★
Teaching: N

CLINICAL PROGRAM RATINGS:

CARDIAC	NR	ORTHOPEDICS	NR
CRITICAL CARE	NR	PULMONARY	★★★
GASTROINTESTINAL	NR	STROKE	NR
GENERAL SURGERY	NR	VASCULAR	NR
MATERNITY CARE	NR	WOMEN'S HEALTH	NR

HEALTHGRADES AWARDS

Whitesburg ARH Hospital

240 Hospital Road
Whitesburg, KY 41858
(606) 633-3500

Overall patient safety: ★★★
Teaching: N

CLINICAL PROGRAM RATINGS:

CARDIAC	NR	ORTHOPEDICS	NR
CRITICAL CARE	NR	PULMONARY	★★★
GASTROINTESTINAL	NR	STROKE	★★★
GENERAL SURGERY	NR	VASCULAR	NR
MATERNITY CARE	NR	WOMEN'S HEALTH	NR

HEALTHGRADES AWARDS

KEY: ★★★★★ BEST   ★★★ AS EXPECTED   ★ POOR   NR NOT RATED BY HEALTHGRADES   For full definitions of ratings and awards, see Appendix.

Williamson ARH Hospital

260 Hospital Drive
South Williamson, KY 41503
(606) 237-1700

Overall patient safety: ★★★
Teaching: N

CLINICAL PROGRAM RATINGS:

CARDIAC	NR	ORTHOPEDICS	NR
CRITICAL CARE	NR	PULMONARY	★★★
GASTROINTESTINAL	NR	STROKE	★★★
GENERAL SURGERY	NR	VASCULAR	NR
MATERNITY CARE	NR	WOMEN'S HEALTH	NR

HEALTHGRADES AWARDS

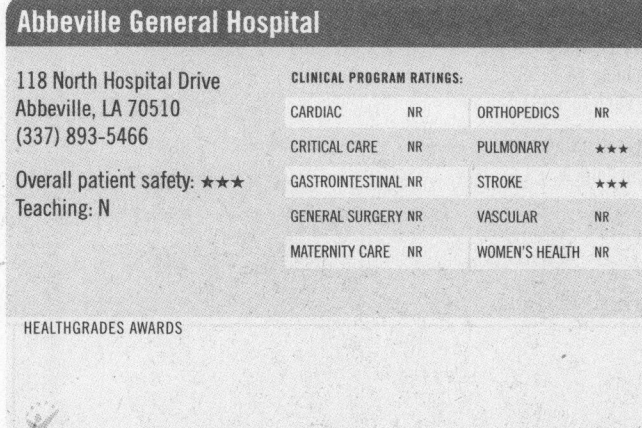

LOUISIANA HOSPITALS: RATINGS BY CLINICAL SPECIALTY

Abbeville General Hospital

118 North Hospital Drive
Abbeville, LA 70510
(337) 893-5466

Overall patient safety: ★★★
Teaching: N

CLINICAL PROGRAM RATINGS:

CARDIAC	NR	ORTHOPEDICS	NR
CRITICAL CARE	NR	PULMONARY	★★★
GASTROINTESTINAL	NR	STROKE	★★★
GENERAL SURGERY	NR	VASCULAR	NR
MATERNITY CARE	NR	WOMEN'S HEALTH	NR

HEALTHGRADES AWARDS

Acadian Medical Center

400 Moosa Boulevard
Eunice, LA 70535
(337) 457-5244

Overall patient safety: ★
Teaching: N

CLINICAL PROGRAM RATINGS:

CARDIAC	NR	ORTHOPEDICS	NR
CRITICAL CARE	NR	PULMONARY	★★★
GASTROINTESTINAL	NR	STROKE	NR
GENERAL SURGERY	NR	VASCULAR	NR
MATERNITY CARE	NR	WOMEN'S HEALTH	NR

HEALTHGRADES AWARDS

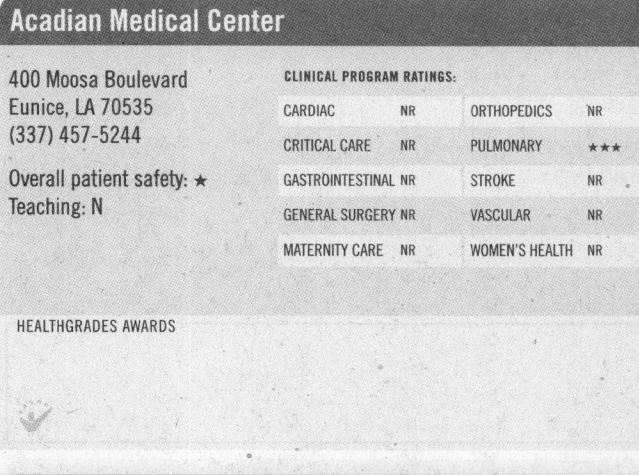

Abrom Kaplan Memorial Hospital

1310 West 7th Street
Kaplan, LA 70548
(337) 643-8300

Overall patient safety: ★★★
Teaching: N

CLINICAL PROGRAM RATINGS:

CARDIAC	NR	ORTHOPEDICS	NR
CRITICAL CARE	NR	PULMONARY	★★★
GASTROINTESTINAL	NR	STROKE	NR
GENERAL SURGERY	NR	VASCULAR	NR
MATERNITY CARE	NR	WOMEN'S HEALTH	NR

HEALTHGRADES AWARDS

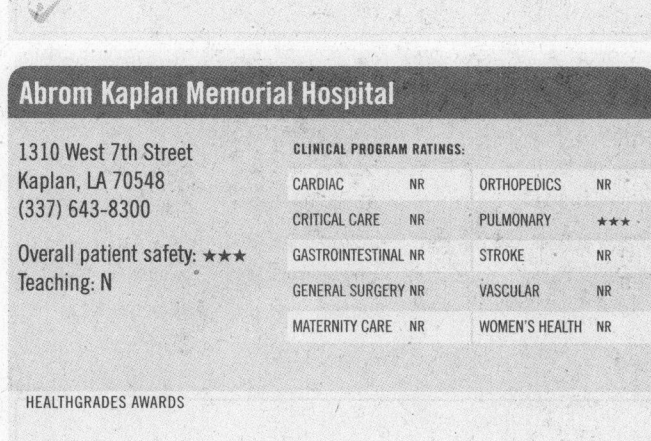

Allen Parish Hospital

108 6th Avenue
Kinder, LA 70648
(337) 738-2527

Overall patient safety: ★★★
Teaching: N

CLINICAL PROGRAM RATINGS:

CARDIAC	NR	ORTHOPEDICS	NR
CRITICAL CARE	NR	PULMONARY	★★★
GASTROINTESTINAL	NR	STROKE	NR
GENERAL SURGERY	NR	VASCULAR	NR
MATERNITY CARE	NR	WOMEN'S HEALTH	NR

HEALTHGRADES AWARDS

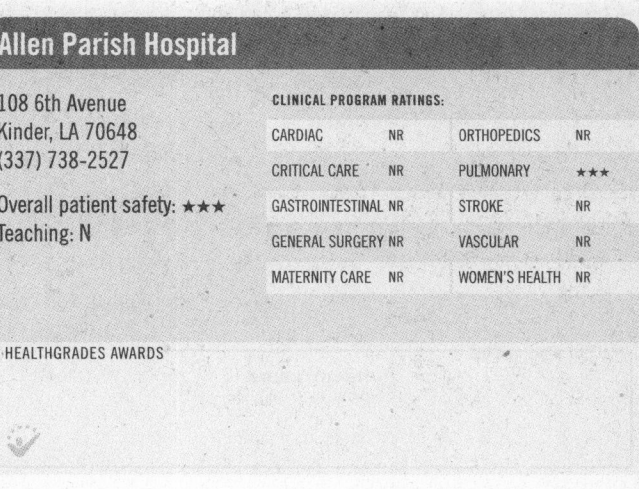

American Legion Hospital

1305 Crowley Rayne Highway
Crowley, LA 70526
(337) 783-3222

Overall patient safety: ★★★
Teaching: N

CLINICAL PROGRAM RATINGS:

CARDIAC	NR	ORTHOPEDICS	NR
CRITICAL CARE	NR	PULMONARY	★
GASTROINTESTINAL	NR	STROKE	★★★
GENERAL SURGERY	NR	VASCULAR	NR
MATERNITY CARE	NR	WOMEN'S HEALTH	NR

HEALTHGRADES AWARDS

Beauregard Memorial Hospital

600 South Pine
Deridder, LA 70634
(337) 462-7100

Overall patient safety: ★★★
Teaching: N

CLINICAL PROGRAM RATINGS:

CARDIAC	NR	ORTHOPEDICS	NR
CRITICAL CARE	NR	PULMONARY	★★★
GASTROINTESTINAL	NR	STROKE	★★★
GENERAL SURGERY	NR	VASCULAR	NR
MATERNITY CARE	NR	WOMEN'S HEALTH	NR

HEALTHGRADES AWARDS

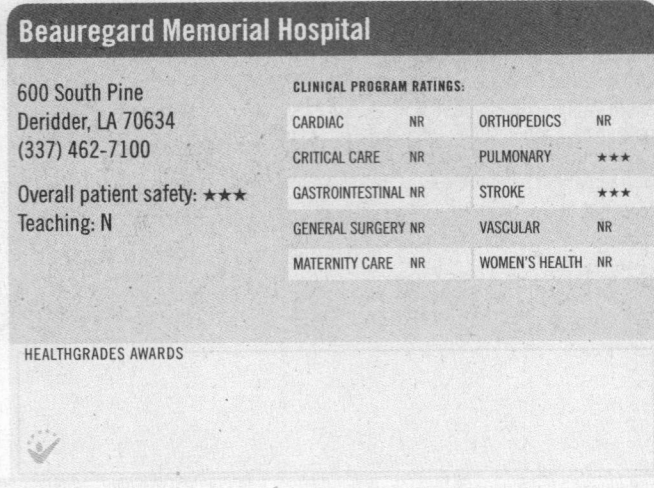

Avoyelles Hospital

4231 Highway 1192
Marksville, LA 71351
(318) 253-8611

Overall patient safety: ★★★
Teaching: N

CLINICAL PROGRAM RATINGS:

CARDIAC	NR	ORTHOPEDICS	NR
CRITICAL CARE	NR	PULMONARY	★★★
GASTROINTESTINAL	NR	STROKE	★★★
GENERAL SURGERY	NR	VASCULAR	NR
MATERNITY CARE	NR	WOMEN'S HEALTH	NR

HEALTHGRADES AWARDS

Bunkie General Hospital

427 Evergreen Street
Bunkie, LA 71322
(318) 346-6681

Overall patient safety: ★★★
Teaching: N

CLINICAL PROGRAM RATINGS:

CARDIAC	NR	ORTHOPEDICS	NR
CRITICAL CARE	NR	PULMONARY	★★★
GASTROINTESTINAL	NR	STROKE	NR
GENERAL SURGERY	NR	VASCULAR	NR
MATERNITY CARE	NR	WOMEN'S HEALTH	NR

HEALTHGRADES AWARDS

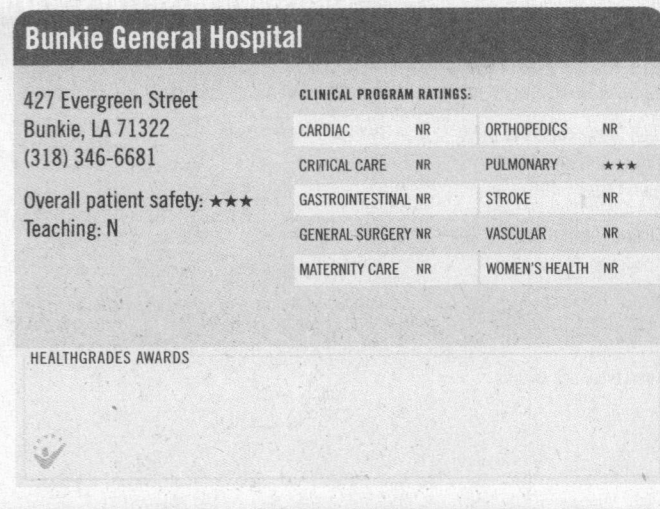

Baton Rouge General Medical Center

3600 Florida Boulevard
Baton Rouge, LA 70806
(225) 387-7000

Overall patient safety: ★★★
Teaching: Y

CLINICAL PROGRAM RATINGS:

CARDIAC	★★★	ORTHOPEDICS	NR
CRITICAL CARE	★★★★★	PULMONARY	★★★
GASTROINTESTINAL	★★★	STROKE	★★★
GENERAL SURGERY	NR	VASCULAR	NR
MATERNITY CARE	NR	WOMEN'S HEALTH	NR

HEALTHGRADES AWARDS

✓ SPECIALTY EXCELLENCE
· CRITICAL CARE

Byrd Regional Hospital

1020 Fertitta Boulevard
Leesville, LA 71446
(337) 239-5113

Overall patient safety: ★★★
Teaching: N

CLINICAL PROGRAM RATINGS:

CARDIAC	NR	ORTHOPEDICS	NR
CRITICAL CARE	NR	PULMONARY	★★★
GASTROINTESTINAL	NR	STROKE	★★★
GENERAL SURGERY	NR	VASCULAR	NR
MATERNITY CARE	NR	WOMEN'S HEALTH	NR

HEALTHGRADES AWARDS

KEY: ★★★★★ BEST   ★★★ AS EXPECTED   ★ POOR   NR NOT RATED BY HEALTHGRADES   For full definitions of ratings and awards, see Appendix.

Caldwell Memorial Hospital

411 Main Street
Columbia, LA 71418
(318) 649-6111

Overall patient safety: NR
Teaching: N

CLINICAL PROGRAM RATINGS:

CARDIAC	NR	ORTHOPEDICS	NR
CRITICAL CARE	NR	PULMONARY	★★★
GASTROINTESTINAL	NR	STROKE	NR
GENERAL SURGERY	NR	VASCULAR	NR
MATERNITY CARE	NR	WOMEN'S HEALTH	NR

HEALTHGRADES AWARDS

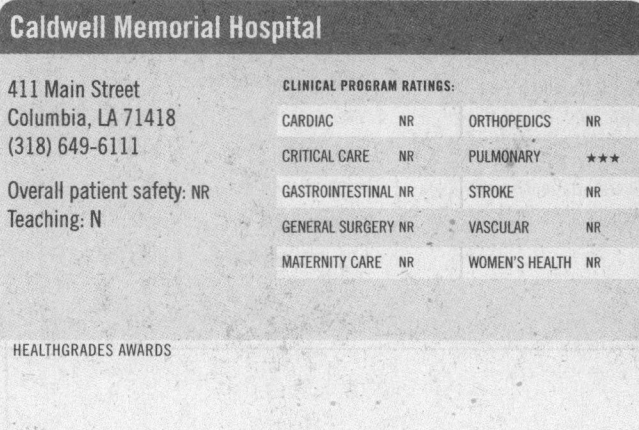

Christus Schumpert Health System

1 St. Mary Place
Shreveport, LA 71101
(318) 681-4500

Overall patient safety: ★★★
Teaching: Y

CLINICAL PROGRAM RATINGS:

CARDIAC	★★★	ORTHOPEDICS	★
CRITICAL CARE	NR	PULMONARY	★★★★★
GASTROINTESTINAL	★★★	STROKE	★★★
GENERAL SURGERY	NR	VASCULAR	★
MATERNITY CARE	NR	WOMEN'S HEALTH	NR

HEALTHGRADES AWARDS

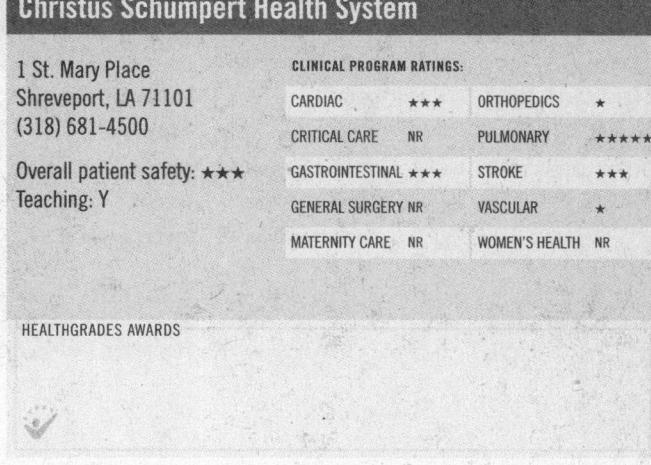

Christus Coushatta Health Care*

309 Marvelle Street
Coushatta, LA 71019
(318) 932-2000

Overall patient safety: NR
Teaching: N

CLINICAL PROGRAM RATINGS:

CARDIAC	NR	ORTHOPEDICS	NR
CRITICAL CARE	NR	PULMONARY	★★★
GASTROINTESTINAL	NR	STROKE	★★★
GENERAL SURGERY	NR	VASCULAR	NR
MATERNITY CARE	NR	WOMEN'S HEALTH	NR

HEALTHGRADES AWARDS

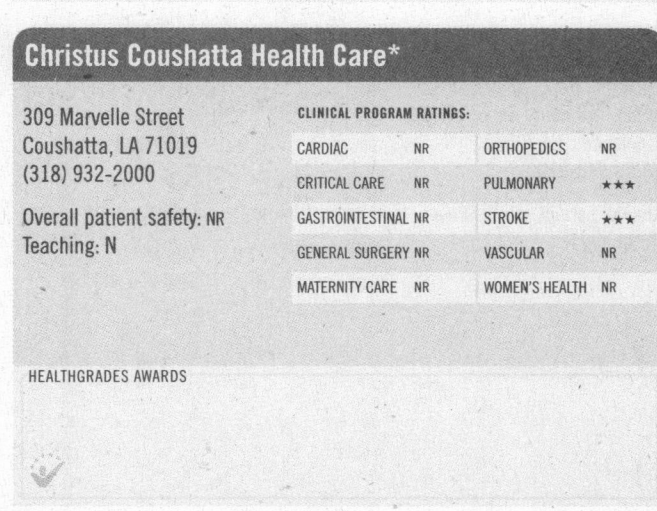

Christus St. Francis Cabrini Hospital

3330 Masonic Drive
Alexandria, LA 71301
(318) 487-1122

Overall patient safety: ★
Teaching: N

CLINICAL PROGRAM RATINGS:

CARDIAC	★★★	ORTHOPEDICS	★★★
CRITICAL CARE	NR	PULMONARY	★★★
GASTROINTESTINAL	★★★	STROKE	★★★
GENERAL SURGERY	NR	VASCULAR	NR
MATERNITY CARE	NR	WOMEN'S HEALTH	NR

HEALTHGRADES AWARDS

Christus Coushatta Health Care Center*

1635 Marvel Street
Coushatta, LA 71019
(318) 932-2199

Overall patient safety: ★★★
Teaching: N

CLINICAL PROGRAM RATINGS:

CARDIAC	NR	ORTHOPEDICS	NR
CRITICAL CARE	NR	PULMONARY	★★★
GASTROINTESTINAL	NR	STROKE	★★★
GENERAL SURGERY	NR	VASCULAR	NR
MATERNITY CARE	NR	WOMEN'S HEALTH	NR

HEALTHGRADES AWARDS

Christus St. Patrick Hospital

524 South Ryan Street
Lake Charles, LA 70601
(337) 436-2511

Overall patient safety: ★
Teaching: N

CLINICAL PROGRAM RATINGS:

CARDIAC	★★★	ORTHOPEDICS	★★★
CRITICAL CARE	NR	PULMONARY	★★★
GASTROINTESTINAL	★★★	STROKE	★★★
GENERAL SURGERY	NR	VASCULAR	NR
MATERNITY CARE	NR	WOMEN'S HEALTH	NR

HEALTHGRADES AWARDS

*This hospital reports its data to the federal government jointly with another hospital. Therefore the ratings and awards apply to multiple hospitals and this specific hospital may not provide all rated services.

LOUISIANA HOSPITALS: RATINGS BY CLINICAL SPECIALTY

Citizens Medical Center

7939 Highway 165 South
Columbia, LA 71418
(318) 649-6106

Overall patient safety: ★★★
Teaching: N

CLINICAL PROGRAM RATINGS:

CARDIAC	NR	ORTHOPEDICS	NR
CRITICAL CARE	NR	PULMONARY	★★★
GASTROINTESTINAL	NR	STROKE	NR
GENERAL SURGERY	NR	VASCULAR	NR
MATERNITY CARE	NR	WOMEN'S HEALTH	NR

HEALTHGRADES AWARDS

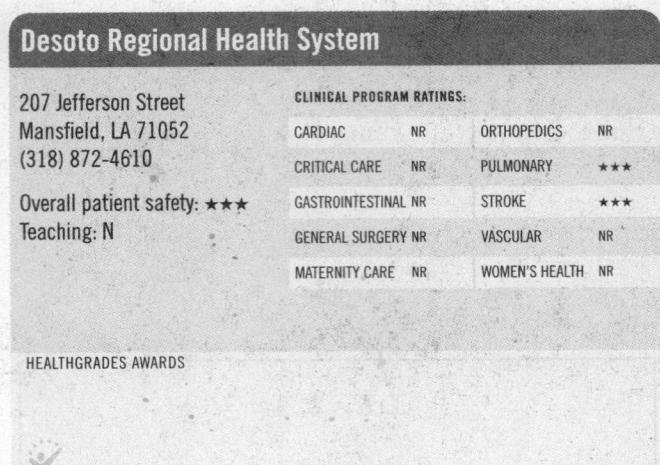

Desoto Regional Health System

207 Jefferson Street
Mansfield, LA 71052
(318) 872-4610

Overall patient safety: ★★★
Teaching: N

CLINICAL PROGRAM RATINGS:

CARDIAC	NR	ORTHOPEDICS	NR
CRITICAL CARE	NR	PULMONARY	★★★
GASTROINTESTINAL	NR	STROKE	★★★
GENERAL SURGERY	NR	VASCULAR	NR
MATERNITY CARE	NR	WOMEN'S HEALTH	NR

HEALTHGRADES AWARDS

Columbia Jefferson Medical Center*

1221 South Clearview Parkway
Jefferson, LA 70121
(504) 734-1900

Overall patient safety: ★
Teaching: Y

CLINICAL PROGRAM RATINGS:

CARDIAC	NR	ORTHOPEDICS	NR
CRITICAL CARE	NR	PULMONARY	★★★
GASTROINTESTINAL	NR	STROKE	★★★★★
GENERAL SURGERY	NR	VASCULAR	NR
MATERNITY CARE	NR	WOMEN'S HEALTH	NR

HEALTHGRADES AWARDS

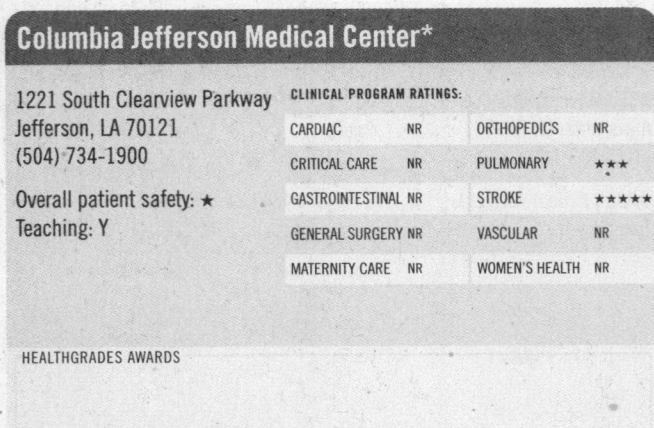

Doctors' Hospital of Opelousas

3983 I-49 South Service Road
Opelousas, LA 70570
(337) 948-2100

Overall patient safety: ★★★
Teaching: N

CLINICAL PROGRAM RATINGS:

CARDIAC	NR	ORTHOPEDICS	NR
CRITICAL CARE	NR	PULMONARY	★★★
GASTROINTESTINAL	NR	STROKE	★
GENERAL SURGERY	NR	VASCULAR	NR
MATERNITY CARE	NR	WOMEN'S HEALTH	NR

HEALTHGRADES AWARDS

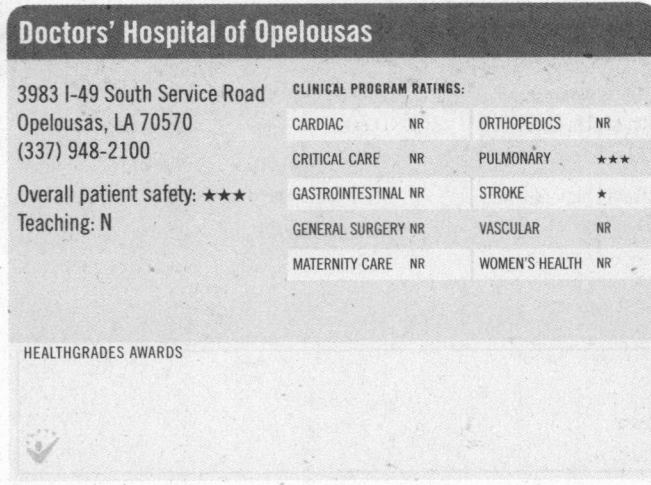

Dauterive Hospital

600 North Lewis Avenue
New Iberia, LA 70563
(337) 365-7311

Overall patient safety: ★★★
Teaching: N

CLINICAL PROGRAM RATINGS:

CARDIAC	NR	ORTHOPEDICS	NR
CRITICAL CARE	NR	PULMONARY	★★★
GASTROINTESTINAL	NR	STROKE	★
GENERAL SURGERY	NR	VASCULAR	NR
MATERNITY CARE	NR	WOMEN'S HEALTH	NR

HEALTHGRADES AWARDS

Doctors' Hospital of Shreveport

1130 Louisiana Avenue
Shreveport, LA 71101
(318) 227-1211

Overall patient safety: ★★★
Teaching: N

CLINICAL PROGRAM RATINGS:

CARDIAC	NR	ORTHOPEDICS	NR
CRITICAL CARE	NR	PULMONARY	★★★
GASTROINTESTINAL	NR	STROKE	★★★
GENERAL SURGERY	NR	VASCULAR	NR
MATERNITY CARE	NR	WOMEN'S HEALTH	NR

HEALTHGRADES AWARDS

KEY: ★★★★★ BEST   ★★★ AS EXPECTED   ★ POOR   NR NOT RATED BY HEALTHGRADES   For full definitions of ratings and awards, see Appendix.

Dubuis Hospital Continuing Care Shreveport

1 St. Mary Place
5th and 6th Floors
Shreveport, LA 71101
(318) 678-1000

Overall patient safety: ★★★
Teaching: Y

CLINICAL PROGRAM RATINGS:

CARDIAC	★★★	ORTHOPEDICS	★
CRITICAL CARE	NR	PULMONARY	★★★★★
GASTROINTESTINAL	★★★	STROKE	★★★
GENERAL SURGERY	NR	VASCULAR	★
MATERNITY CARE	NR	WOMEN'S HEALTH	NR

HEALTHGRADES AWARDS

Franklin Foundation Hospital

1501 Hospital Avenue
Franklin, LA 70538
(337) 828-0760

Overall patient safety: ★★★
Teaching: N

CLINICAL PROGRAM RATINGS:

CARDIAC	NR	ORTHOPEDICS	NR
CRITICAL CARE	NR	PULMONARY	★★★
GASTROINTESTINAL	NR	STROKE	NR
GENERAL SURGERY	NR	VASCULAR	NR
MATERNITY CARE	NR	WOMEN'S HEALTH	NR

HEALTHGRADES AWARDS

E. A. Conway Medical Center

4864 Jackson Street
Monroe, LA 71202
(318) 330-7000

Overall patient safety: ★★★
Teaching: Y

CLINICAL PROGRAM RATINGS:

CARDIAC	NR	ORTHOPEDICS	NR
CRITICAL CARE	NR	PULMONARY	★
GASTROINTESTINAL	NR	STROKE	★★★
GENERAL SURGERY	NR	VASCULAR	NR
MATERNITY CARE	NR	WOMEN'S HEALTH	NR

HEALTHGRADES AWARDS

Franklin Medical Center

2106 Loop Road
Winnsboro, LA 71295
(318) 435-9411

Overall patient safety: ★★★
Teaching: N

CLINICAL PROGRAM RATINGS:

CARDIAC	NR	ORTHOPEDICS	NR
CRITICAL CARE	NR	PULMONARY	★
GASTROINTESTINAL	NR	STROKE	NR
GENERAL SURGERY	NR	VASCULAR	NR
MATERNITY CARE	NR	WOMEN'S HEALTH	NR

HEALTHGRADES AWARDS

East Jefferson General Hospital

4200 Houma Boulevard
Metairie, LA 70006
(504) 454-4000

Overall patient safety: ★★★
Teaching: Y

CLINICAL PROGRAM RATINGS:

CARDIAC	★★★	ORTHOPEDICS	★★★
CRITICAL CARE	NR	PULMONARY	★★★★★
GASTROINTESTINAL	★★★	STROKE	★★★
GENERAL SURGERY	NR	VASCULAR	NR
MATERNITY CARE	NR	WOMEN'S HEALTH	NR

HEALTHGRADES AWARDS

✓ SPECIALTY EXCELLENCE
- CARDIAC SURGERY
- PULMONARY CARE

Glenwood Regional Medical Center

503 McMillan Road
West Monroe, LA 71291
(318) 329-4200

Overall patient safety: ★★★★★
Teaching: N

CLINICAL PROGRAM RATINGS:

CARDIAC	★★★	ORTHOPEDICS	★★★
CRITICAL CARE	NR	PULMONARY	★★★
GASTROINTESTINAL	★★★	STROKE	★★★
GENERAL SURGERY	NR	VASCULAR	NR
MATERNITY CARE	NR	WOMEN'S HEALTH	NR

HEALTHGRADES AWARDS

✓ DISTINGUISHED HOSPITAL
- CLINICAL EXCELLENCE
- PATIENT SAFETY

✓ SPECIALTY EXCELLENCE
- CARDIAC SURGERY
- JOINT REPLACEMENT

*This hospital reports its data to the federal government jointly with another hospital. Therefore the ratings and awards apply to multiple hospitals and this specific hospital may not provide all rated services.

Hardtner Medical Center

1102 North Pine Road
Olla, LA 71465
(318) 495-3131

Overall patient safety: ★★★
Teaching: N

CLINICAL PROGRAM RATINGS:

CARDIAC	NR	ORTHOPEDICS	NR
CRITICAL CARE	NR	PULMONARY	★★★
GASTROINTESTINAL	NR	STROKE	NR
GENERAL SURGERY	NR	VASCULAR	NR
MATERNITY CARE	NR	WOMEN'S HEALTH	NR

HEALTHGRADES AWARDS

Iberia Medical Center

2315 East Main Street
New Iberia, LA 70560
(337) 364-0441

Overall patient safety: ★★★
Teaching: N

CLINICAL PROGRAM RATINGS:

CARDIAC	NR	ORTHOPEDICS	NR
CRITICAL CARE	NR	PULMONARY	★★★
GASTROINTESTINAL	★★★	STROKE	★
GENERAL SURGERY	NR	VASCULAR	NR
MATERNITY CARE	NR	WOMEN'S HEALTH	NR

HEALTHGRADES AWARDS

Heart Hospital of Lafayette

1105 Kaliste Saloon Road
Lafayette, LA 70508
(337) 521-1000

Overall patient safety: ★★★
Teaching: N

CLINICAL PROGRAM RATINGS:

CARDIAC	★★★	ORTHOPEDICS	NR
CRITICAL CARE	NR	PULMONARY	NR
GASTROINTESTINAL	NR	STROKE	NR
GENERAL SURGERY	NR	VASCULAR	NR
MATERNITY CARE	NR	WOMEN'S HEALTH	NR

HEALTHGRADES AWARDS

Jackson Parish Hospital

165 Beech Springs Road
Jonesboro, LA 71251
(318) 259-4435

Overall patient safety: ★★★
Teaching: N

CLINICAL PROGRAM RATINGS:

CARDIAC	NR	ORTHOPEDICS	NR
CRITICAL CARE	NR	PULMONARY	★★★
GASTROINTESTINAL	NR	STROKE	★★★
GENERAL SURGERY	NR	VASCULAR	NR
MATERNITY CARE	NR	WOMEN'S HEALTH	NR

HEALTHGRADES AWARDS

Homer Memorial Hospital

620 East College
Homer, LA 71040
(318) 927-2024

Overall patient safety: ★★★
Teaching: N

CLINICAL PROGRAM RATINGS:

CARDIAC	NR	ORTHOPEDICS	NR
CRITICAL CARE	NR	PULMONARY	★★★
GASTROINTESTINAL	NR	STROKE	★★★
GENERAL SURGERY	NR	VASCULAR	NR
MATERNITY CARE	NR	WOMEN'S HEALTH	NR

HEALTHGRADES AWARDS

Jennings American Legion Hospital

1634 Elton Road
Jennings, LA 70546
(337) 616-7000

Overall patient safety: ★★★
Teaching: N

CLINICAL PROGRAM RATINGS:

CARDIAC	NR	ORTHOPEDICS	NR
CRITICAL CARE	NR	PULMONARY	★★★
GASTROINTESTINAL	NR	STROKE	★★★
GENERAL SURGERY	NR	VASCULAR	NR
MATERNITY CARE	NR	WOMEN'S HEALTH	NR

HEALTHGRADES AWARDS

KEY: ★★★★★ BEST   ★★★ AS EXPECTED   ★ POOR   NR NOT RATED BY HEALTHGRADES   For full definitions of ratings and awards, see Appendix.

LOUISIANA HOSPITALS: RATINGS BY CLINICAL SPECIALTY

Lady of the Sea General Hospital

200 West 134th Place
Cut Off, LA 70345
(985) 632-6401

Overall patient safety: NR
Teaching: N

CLINICAL PROGRAM RATINGS:

CARDIAC	NR	ORTHOPEDICS	NR
CRITICAL CARE	NR	PULMONARY	★★★
GASTROINTESTINAL	NR	STROKE	NR
GENERAL SURGERY	NR	VASCULAR	NR
MATERNITY CARE	NR	WOMEN'S HEALTH	NR

HEALTHGRADES AWARDS

Lakeview Regional Medical Center

95 East Fairway Center Drive
Covington, LA 70433
(985) 867-4444

Overall patient safety: ★★★
Teaching: N

CLINICAL PROGRAM RATINGS:

CARDIAC	★★★	ORTHOPEDICS	NR
CRITICAL CARE	NR	PULMONARY	★★★
GASTROINTESTINAL	★★★	STROKE	★★★
GENERAL SURGERY	NR	VASCULAR	NR
MATERNITY CARE	NR	WOMEN'S HEALTH	NR

HEALTHGRADES AWARDS

Lafayette General Medical Center

1214 Coolidge Boulevard
Lafayette, LA 70503
(337) 289-7991

Overall patient safety: ★★★
Teaching: N

CLINICAL PROGRAM RATINGS:

CARDIAC	★★★	ORTHOPEDICS	★★★
CRITICAL CARE	NR	PULMONARY	★★★
GASTROINTESTINAL	★★★	STROKE	★★★
GENERAL SURGERY	NR	VASCULAR	NR
MATERNITY CARE	NR	WOMEN'S HEALTH	NR

HEALTHGRADES AWARDS

Lallie Kemp Medical Center

52579 Highway 21 South
Independence, LA 70443
(985) 878-9421

Overall patient safety: ★★★
Teaching: N

CLINICAL PROGRAM RATINGS:

CARDIAC	NR	ORTHOPEDICS	NR
CRITICAL CARE	NR	PULMONARY	NR
GASTROINTESTINAL	NR	STROKE	NR
GENERAL SURGERY	NR	VASCULAR	NR
MATERNITY CARE	NR	WOMEN'S HEALTH	NR

HEALTHGRADES AWARDS

Lake Charles Memorial Hospital

1701 Oak Park Boulevard
Lake Charles, LA 70601
(337) 494-3000

Overall patient safety: ★★★
Teaching: Y

CLINICAL PROGRAM RATINGS:

CARDIAC	★	ORTHOPEDICS	★★★
CRITICAL CARE	NR	PULMONARY	★★★
GASTROINTESTINAL	★★★	STROKE	★★★
GENERAL SURGERY	NR	VASCULAR	NR
MATERNITY CARE	NR	WOMEN'S HEALTH	NR

HEALTHGRADES AWARDS

Lane Memorial Hospital

6300 Main Street
Zachary, LA 70791
(225) 658-4000

Overall patient safety: ★
Teaching: N

CLINICAL PROGRAM RATINGS:

CARDIAC	NR	ORTHOPEDICS	NR
CRITICAL CARE	NR	PULMONARY	★
GASTROINTESTINAL	NR	STROKE	★★★
GENERAL SURGERY	NR	VASCULAR	NR
MATERNITY CARE	NR	WOMEN'S HEALTH	NR

HEALTHGRADES AWARDS

Lasalle General Hospital

187 9th Street
Jena, LA 71342
(318) 992-9200

Overall patient safety: ★★★
Teaching: N

CLINICAL PROGRAM RATINGS:

CARDIAC	NR	ORTHOPEDICS	NR
CRITICAL CARE	NR	PULMONARY	★★★
GASTROINTESTINAL	NR	STROKE	★★★
GENERAL SURGERY	NR	VASCULAR	NR
MATERNITY CARE	NR	WOMEN'S HEALTH	NR

HEALTHGRADES AWARDS

Louisiana Heart Hospital

64030 Highway 434
Lacombe, LA 70445
(985) 690-7500

Overall patient safety: ★★★★★
Teaching: N

CLINICAL PROGRAM RATINGS:

CARDIAC	★★★	ORTHOPEDICS	NR
CRITICAL CARE	NR	PULMONARY	★★★
GASTROINTESTINAL	NR	STROKE	NR
GENERAL SURGERY	NR	VASCULAR	NR
MATERNITY CARE	NR	WOMEN'S HEALTH	NR

HEALTHGRADES AWARDS

Leonard J. Chabert Medical Center

1978 Industrial Boulevard
Houma, LA 70363
(985) 873-2200

Overall patient safety: ★★★
Teaching: Y

CLINICAL PROGRAM RATINGS:

CARDIAC	NR	ORTHOPEDICS	NR
CRITICAL CARE	NR	PULMONARY	★
GASTROINTESTINAL	NR	STROKE	NR
GENERAL SURGERY	NR	VASCULAR	NR
MATERNITY CARE	NR	WOMEN'S HEALTH	NR

HEALTHGRADES AWARDS

LSU Health Sciences Center--Shreveport

1501 Kings Highway
Shreveport, LA 71130
(318) 675-5000

Overall patient safety: ★★★
Teaching: Y

CLINICAL PROGRAM RATINGS:

CARDIAC	★★★	ORTHOPEDICS	NR
CRITICAL CARE	NR	PULMONARY	★★★
GASTROINTESTINAL	NR	STROKE	★
GENERAL SURGERY	NR	VASCULAR	NR
MATERNITY CARE	NR	WOMEN'S HEALTH	NR

HEALTHGRADES AWARDS

Lincoln General Hospital

401 East Vaughn Avenue
Ruston, LA 71270
(318) 254-2100

Overall patient safety: ★★★
Teaching: N

CLINICAL PROGRAM RATINGS:

CARDIAC	NR	ORTHOPEDICS	NR
CRITICAL CARE	NR	PULMONARY	★★★
GASTROINTESTINAL	★	STROKE	★★★
GENERAL SURGERY	NR	VASCULAR	NR
MATERNITY CARE	NR	WOMEN'S HEALTH	NR

HEALTHGRADES AWARDS

Madison Parish Hospital

900 Johnson Street
Tallulah, LA 71282
(318) 574-2374

Overall patient safety: NR
Teaching: N

CLINICAL PROGRAM RATINGS:

CARDIAC	NR	ORTHOPEDICS	NR
CRITICAL CARE	NR	PULMONARY	★
GASTROINTESTINAL	NR	STROKE	NR
GENERAL SURGERY	NR	VASCULAR	NR
MATERNITY CARE	NR	WOMEN'S HEALTH	NR

HEALTHGRADES AWARDS

KEY: ★★★★★ BEST   ★★★ AS EXPECTED   ★ POOR   NR NOT RATED BY HEALTHGRADES   For full definitions of ratings and awards, see Appendix.

Minden Medical Center

1 Medical Plaza
Minden, LA 71055
(318) 377-2321

Overall patient safety: ★★★
Teaching: N

CLINICAL PROGRAM RATINGS:

CARDIAC	NR	ORTHOPEDICS	NR
CRITICAL CARE	NR	PULMONARY	★★★
GASTROINTESTINAL	NR	STROKE	★
GENERAL SURGERY	NR	VASCULAR	NR
MATERNITY CARE	NR	WOMEN'S HEALTH	NR

HEALTHGRADES AWARDS

North Caddo Medical Center

1000 South Spruce Street
Vivian, LA 71082
(318) 375-3235

Overall patient safety: ★★★
Teaching: N

CLINICAL PROGRAM RATINGS:

CARDIAC	NR	ORTHOPEDICS	NR
CRITICAL CARE	NR	PULMONARY	★★★
GASTROINTESTINAL	NR	STROKE	NR
GENERAL SURGERY	NR	VASCULAR	NR
MATERNITY CARE	NR	WOMEN'S HEALTH	NR

HEALTHGRADES AWARDS

Morehouse General Hospital

323 West Walnut Avenue
Bastrop, LA 71220
(318) 283-3600

Overall patient safety: ★
Teaching: N

CLINICAL PROGRAM RATINGS:

CARDIAC	NR	ORTHOPEDICS	NR
CRITICAL CARE	NR	PULMONARY	★
GASTROINTESTINAL	NR	STROKE	★
GENERAL SURGERY	NR	VASCULAR	NR
MATERNITY CARE	NR	WOMEN'S HEALTH	NR

HEALTHGRADES AWARDS

North Oaks Medical Center North Campus*

1900 South Morrison Boulevard
Hammond, LA 70403
(504) 542-7777

Overall patient safety: ★★★
Teaching: N

CLINICAL PROGRAM RATINGS:

CARDIAC	★★★	ORTHOPEDICS	NR
CRITICAL CARE	NR	PULMONARY	★★★
GASTROINTESTINAL	★★★	STROKE	★★★
GENERAL SURGERY	NR	VASCULAR	★★★
MATERNITY CARE	NR	WOMEN'S HEALTH	NR

HEALTHGRADES AWARDS

Natchitoches Regional Medical Center

501 Keyser Avenue
Natchitoches, LA 71457
(318) 214-4200

Overall patient safety: ★★★
Teaching: N

CLINICAL PROGRAM RATINGS:

CARDIAC	NR	ORTHOPEDICS	NR
CRITICAL CARE	NR	PULMONARY	★★★
GASTROINTESTINAL	NR	STROKE	★★★
GENERAL SURGERY	NR	VASCULAR	NR
MATERNITY CARE	NR	WOMEN'S HEALTH	NR

HEALTHGRADES AWARDS

North Oaks Medical Center*

15790 Paul Vega, MD Drive
Hammond, LA 70403
(985) 345-2700

Overall patient safety: ★★★
Teaching: N

CLINICAL PROGRAM RATINGS:

CARDIAC	★★★	ORTHOPEDICS	NR
CRITICAL CARE	NR	PULMONARY	★★★
GASTROINTESTINAL	★★★	STROKE	★★★
GENERAL SURGERY	NR	VASCULAR	★★★
MATERNITY CARE	NR	WOMEN'S HEALTH	NR

HEALTHGRADES AWARDS

*This hospital reports its data to the federal government jointly with another hospital. Therefore the ratings and awards apply to multiple hospitals and this specific hospital may not provide all rated services.

Northshore Regional Medical Center

100 Medical Center Drive
Slidell, LA 70461
(985) 649-7070

Overall patient safety: ★★★
Teaching: N

CLINICAL PROGRAM RATINGS:

CARDIAC	★★★	ORTHOPEDICS	NR
CRITICAL CARE	NR	PULMONARY	★★★
GASTROINTESTINAL	NR	STROKE	★★★
GENERAL SURGERY	NR	VASCULAR	NR
MATERNITY CARE	NR	WOMEN'S HEALTH	NR

HEALTHGRADES AWARDS

Ochsner Medical Center--Baton Rouge

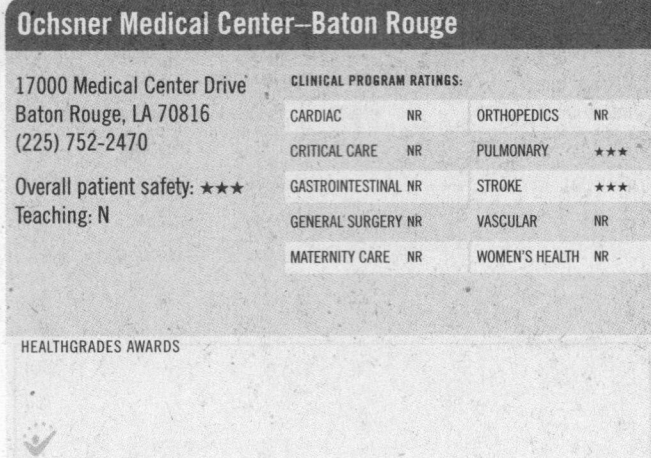

17000 Medical Center Drive
Baton Rouge, LA 70816
(225) 752-2470

Overall patient safety: ★★★
Teaching: N

CLINICAL PROGRAM RATINGS:

CARDIAC	NR	ORTHOPEDICS	NR
CRITICAL CARE	NR	PULMONARY	★★★
GASTROINTESTINAL	NR	STROKE	★★★
GENERAL SURGERY	NR	VASCULAR	NR
MATERNITY CARE	NR	WOMEN'S HEALTH	NR

HEALTHGRADES AWARDS

Oakdale Community Hospital

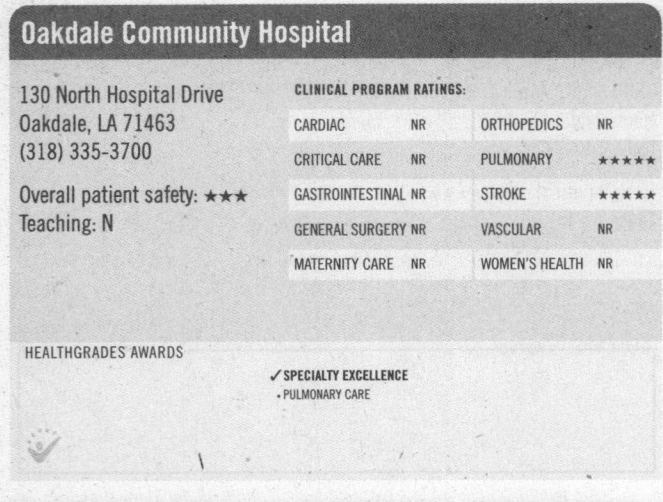

130 North Hospital Drive
Oakdale, LA 71463
(318) 335-3700

Overall patient safety: ★★★
Teaching: N

CLINICAL PROGRAM RATINGS:

CARDIAC	NR	ORTHOPEDICS	NR
CRITICAL CARE	NR	PULMONARY	★★★★★
GASTROINTESTINAL	NR	STROKE	★★★★★
GENERAL SURGERY	NR	VASCULAR	NR
MATERNITY CARE	NR	WOMEN'S HEALTH	NR

HEALTHGRADES AWARDS

✓ SPECIALTY EXCELLENCE
• PULMONARY CARE

Ochsner Medical Center--Kenner

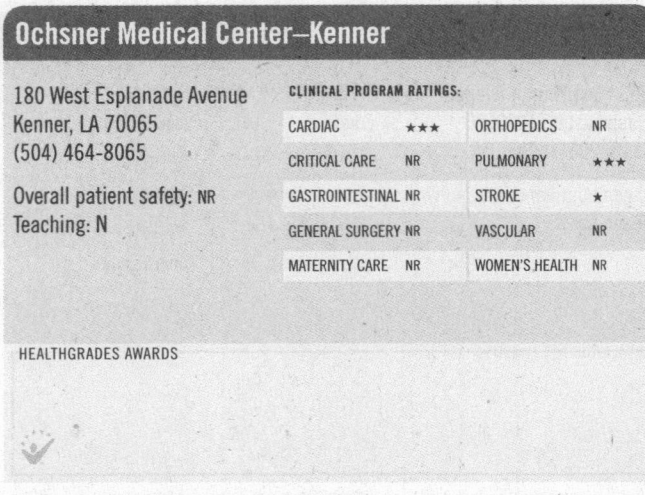

180 West Esplanade Avenue
Kenner, LA 70065
(504) 464-8065

Overall patient safety: NR
Teaching: N

CLINICAL PROGRAM RATINGS:

CARDIAC	★★★	ORTHOPEDICS	NR
CRITICAL CARE	NR	PULMONARY	★★★
GASTROINTESTINAL	NR	STROKE	★
GENERAL SURGERY	NR	VASCULAR	NR
MATERNITY CARE	NR	WOMEN'S HEALTH	NR

HEALTHGRADES AWARDS

Ochsner Clinic Foundation

1514 Jefferson Highway
New Orleans, LA 70121
(504) 842-3000

Overall patient safety: ★★★
Teaching: Y

CLINICAL PROGRAM RATINGS:

CARDIAC	★★★	ORTHOPEDICS	★
CRITICAL CARE	NR	PULMONARY	★★★
GASTROINTESTINAL	★★★	STROKE	★★★
GENERAL SURGERY	NR	VASCULAR	NR
MATERNITY CARE	NR	WOMEN'S HEALTH	NR

HEALTHGRADES AWARDS

Ochsner Medical Center--Westbank

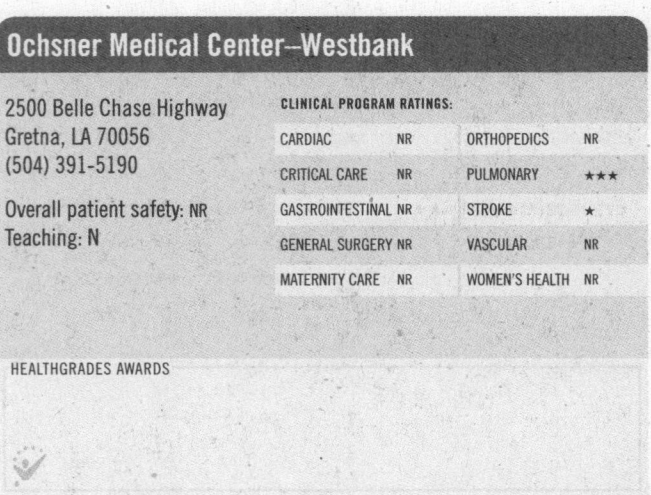

2500 Belle Chase Highway
Gretna, LA 70056
(504) 391-5190

Overall patient safety: NR
Teaching: N

CLINICAL PROGRAM RATINGS:

CARDIAC	NR	ORTHOPEDICS	NR
CRITICAL CARE	NR	PULMONARY	★★★
GASTROINTESTINAL	NR	STROKE	★
GENERAL SURGERY	NR	VASCULAR	NR
MATERNITY CARE	NR	WOMEN'S HEALTH	NR

HEALTHGRADES AWARDS

LOUISIANA HOSPITALS: RATINGS BY CLINICAL SPECIALTY

KEY: ★★★★★ **BEST**   ★★★ **AS EXPECTED**   ★ **POOR**   NR **NOT RATED BY HEALTHGRADES**   For full definitions of ratings and awards, see Appendix.

Ochsner St. Anne General Hospital

4608 Highway 1
Raceland, LA 70394
(985) 537-6841

Overall patient safety: NR
Teaching: N

CLINICAL PROGRAM RATINGS:

CARDIAC	NR	ORTHOPEDICS	NR
CRITICAL CARE	NR	PULMONARY	★★★
GASTROINTESTINAL	NR	STROKE	NR
GENERAL SURGERY	NR	VASCULAR	NR
MATERNITY CARE	NR	WOMEN'S HEALTH	NR

HEALTHGRADES AWARDS

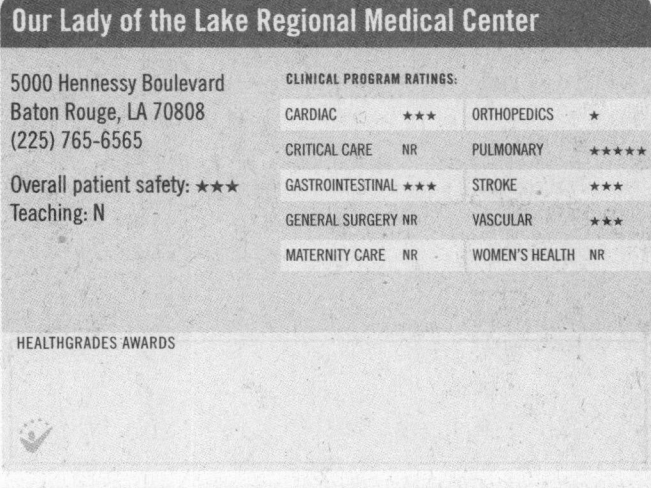

Our Lady of the Lake Regional Medical Center

5000 Hennessy Boulevard
Baton Rouge, LA 70808
(225) 765-6565

Overall patient safety: ★★★
Teaching: N

CLINICAL PROGRAM RATINGS:

CARDIAC	★★★	ORTHOPEDICS	★
CRITICAL CARE	NR	PULMONARY	★★★★★
GASTROINTESTINAL	★★★	STROKE	★★★
GENERAL SURGERY	NR	VASCULAR	★★★
MATERNITY CARE	NR	WOMEN'S HEALTH	NR

HEALTHGRADES AWARDS

Opelousas General Health System

539 East Prudhomme Lane
Opelousas, LA 70570
(337) 948-3011

Overall patient safety: ★★★
Teaching: N

CLINICAL PROGRAM RATINGS:

CARDIAC	NR	ORTHOPEDICS	★★★
CRITICAL CARE	NR	PULMONARY	★★★
GASTROINTESTINAL	★★★	STROKE	★★★
GENERAL SURGERY	NR	VASCULAR	NR
MATERNITY CARE	NR	WOMEN'S HEALTH	NR

HEALTHGRADES AWARDS

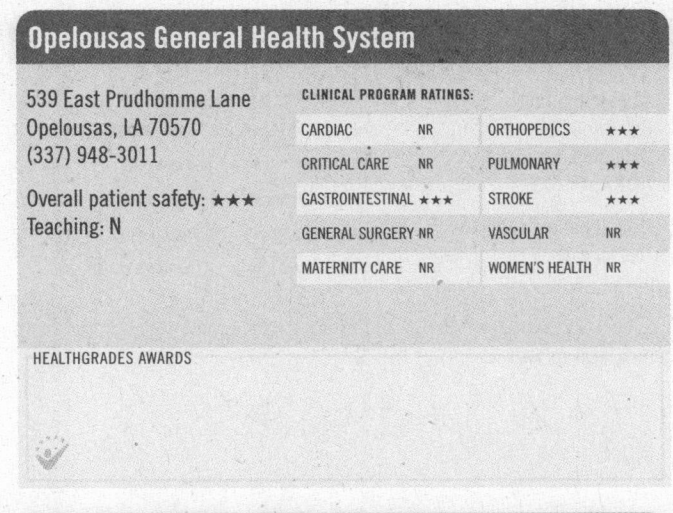

Pointe Coupee General Hospital

2202 False River Drive
New Roads, LA 70760
(225) 638-6331

Overall patient safety: NR
Teaching: N

CLINICAL PROGRAM RATINGS:

CARDIAC	NR	ORTHOPEDICS	NR
CRITICAL CARE	NR	PULMONARY	★★★
GASTROINTESTINAL	NR	STROKE	NR
GENERAL SURGERY	NR	VASCULAR	NR
MATERNITY CARE	NR	WOMEN'S HEALTH	NR

HEALTHGRADES AWARDS

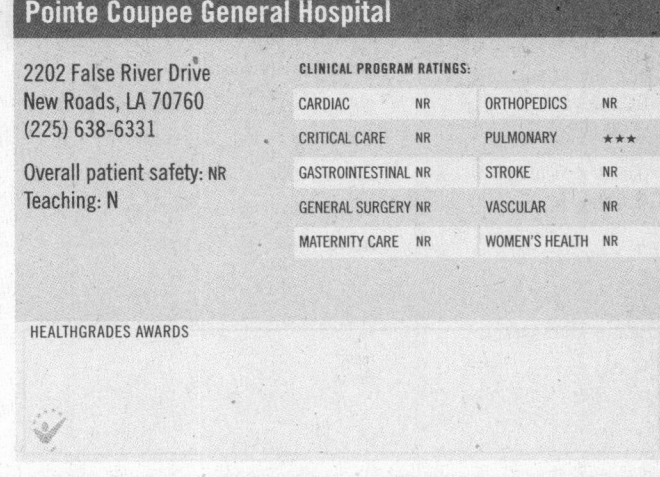

Our Lady of Lourdes Regional Medical Center

611 Street Landry Street
Lafayette, LA 70506
(337) 289-2000

Overall patient safety: ★★★
Teaching: N

CLINICAL PROGRAM RATINGS:

CARDIAC	★	ORTHOPEDICS	★★★
CRITICAL CARE	NR	PULMONARY	★★★
GASTROINTESTINAL	★★★	STROKE	★★★
GENERAL SURGERY	NR	VASCULAR	NR
MATERNITY CARE	NR	WOMEN'S HEALTH	NR

HEALTHGRADES AWARDS

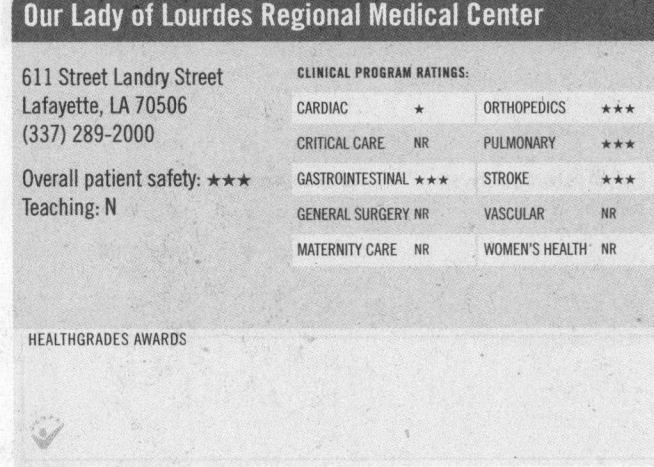

Rapides Regional Medical Center

211 4th Street
Alexandria, LA 71301
(318) 473-3000

Overall patient safety: ★★★★★
Teaching: N

CLINICAL PROGRAM RATINGS:

CARDIAC	★★★	ORTHOPEDICS	★★★
CRITICAL CARE	★★★	PULMONARY	★★★
GASTROINTESTINAL	★★★	STROKE	★★★
GENERAL SURGERY	NR	VASCULAR	★★★
MATERNITY CARE	NR	WOMEN'S HEALTH	NR

HEALTHGRADES AWARDS

✓ DISTINGUISHED
HOSPITAL
• PATIENT SAFETY

Richardson Medical Center

254 Highway 3048
Rayville, LA 71269
(318) 728-4181

Overall patient safety: ★★★
Teaching: N

CLINICAL PROGRAM RATINGS:

CARDIAC	NR	ORTHOPEDICS	NR
CRITICAL CARE	NR	PULMONARY	★
GASTROINTESTINAL	NR	STROKE	★★★
GENERAL SURGERY	NR	VASCULAR	NR
MATERNITY CARE	NR	WOMEN'S HEALTH	NR

HEALTHGRADES AWARDS

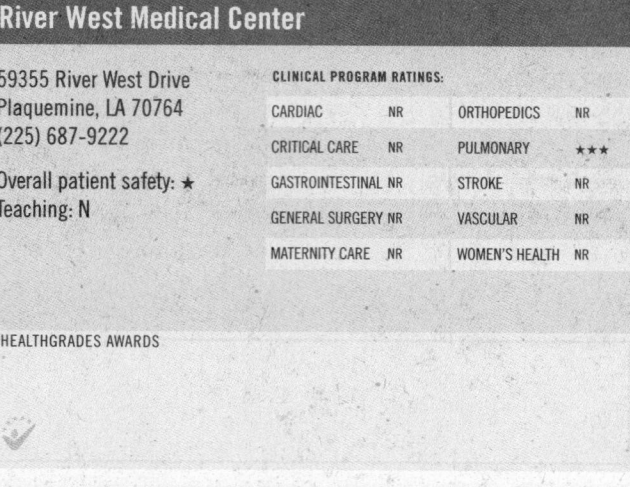

River West Medical Center

59355 River West Drive
Plaquemine, LA 70764
(225) 687-9222

Overall patient safety: ★
Teaching: N

CLINICAL PROGRAM RATINGS:

CARDIAC	NR	ORTHOPEDICS	NR
CRITICAL CARE	NR	PULMONARY	★★★
GASTROINTESTINAL	NR	STROKE	NR
GENERAL SURGERY	NR	VASCULAR	NR
MATERNITY CARE	NR	WOMEN'S HEALTH	NR

HEALTHGRADES AWARDS

Richland Parish Hospital Delhi

407 Cincinnati Street
Delhi, LA 71232
(318) 878-5171

Overall patient safety: ★★★
Teaching: N

CLINICAL PROGRAM RATINGS:

CARDIAC	NR	ORTHOPEDICS	NR
CRITICAL CARE	NR	PULMONARY	★★★
GASTROINTESTINAL	NR	STROKE	NR
GENERAL SURGERY	NR	VASCULAR	NR
MATERNITY CARE	NR	WOMEN'S HEALTH	NR

HEALTHGRADES AWARDS

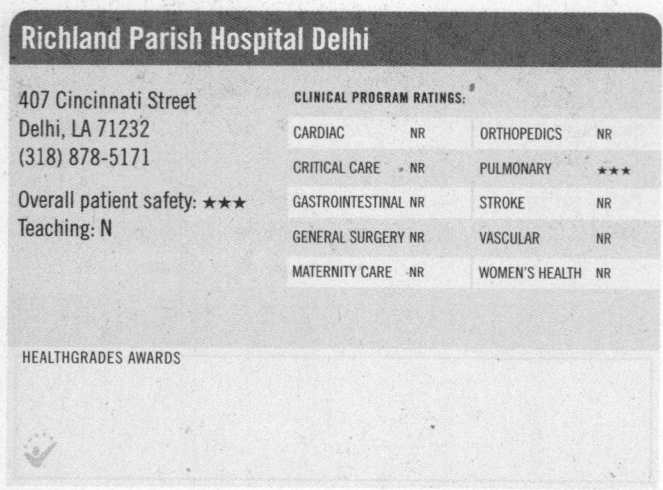

Riverbend Rehab Hospital

410 Main Street
P.O. Box 420
Columbia, LA 71418
(318) 649-6111

Overall patient safety: NR
Teaching: N

CLINICAL PROGRAM RATINGS:

CARDIAC	NR	ORTHOPEDICS	NR
CRITICAL CARE	NR	PULMONARY	★★★
GASTROINTESTINAL	NR	STROKE	NR
GENERAL SURGERY	NR	VASCULAR	NR
MATERNITY CARE	NR	WOMEN'S HEALTH	NR

HEALTHGRADES AWARDS

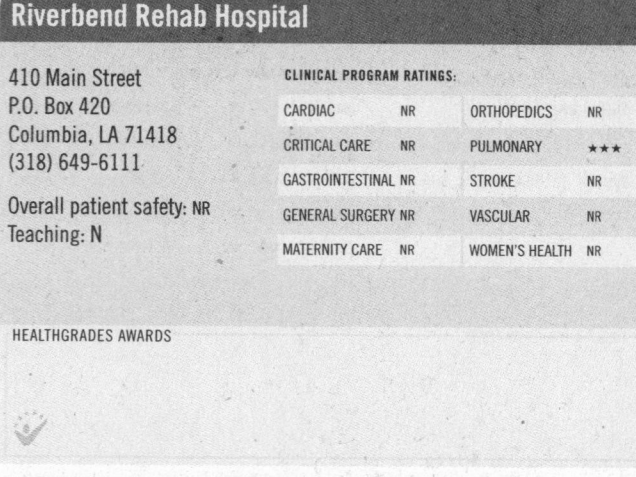

River Parishes Hospital

500 Rue De Sante
La Place, LA 70068
(985) 652-7000

Overall patient safety: ★★★
Teaching: N

CLINICAL PROGRAM RATINGS:

CARDIAC	NR	ORTHOPEDICS	NR
CRITICAL CARE	NR	PULMONARY	★★★
GASTROINTESTINAL	NR	STROKE	★★★
GENERAL SURGERY	NR	VASCULAR	NR
MATERNITY CARE	NR	WOMEN'S HEALTH	NR

HEALTHGRADES AWARDS

Riverland Medical Center

1700 Northeast Wallace Road
Ferriday, LA 71334
(318) 757-6551

Overall patient safety: ★★★
Teaching: N

CLINICAL PROGRAM RATINGS:

CARDIAC	NR	ORTHOPEDICS	NR
CRITICAL CARE	NR	PULMONARY	★★★
GASTROINTESTINAL	NR	STROKE	NR
GENERAL SURGERY	NR	VASCULAR	NR
MATERNITY CARE	NR	WOMEN'S HEALTH	NR

HEALTHGRADES AWARDS

KEY: ★★★★★ BEST   ★★★ AS EXPECTED   ★ POOR   NR NOT RATED BY HEALTHGRADES   For full definitions of ratings and awards, see Appendix.

Riverside Medical Center

1900 South Main Street
Franklinton, LA 70438
(985) 839-4431

Overall patient safety: ★★★
Teaching: N

CLINICAL PROGRAM RATINGS:

CARDIAC	NR	ORTHOPEDICS	NR
CRITICAL CARE	NR	PULMONARY	★★★
GASTROINTESTINAL	NR	STROKE	★★★
GENERAL SURGERY	NR	VASCULAR	NR
MATERNITY CARE	NR	WOMEN'S HEALTH	NR

HEALTHGRADES AWARDS

St. Charles Parish Hospital

1057 Paul Maillard Road
Luling, LA 70070
(985) 785-6242

Overall patient safety: ★★★
Teaching: N

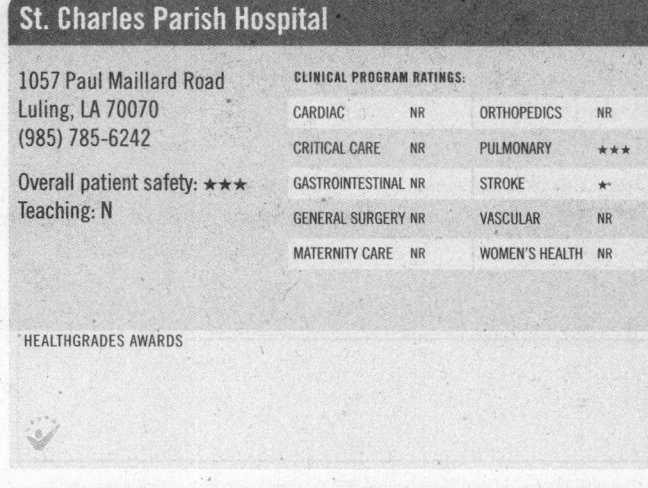

CLINICAL PROGRAM RATINGS:

CARDIAC	NR	ORTHOPEDICS	NR
CRITICAL CARE	NR	PULMONARY	★★★
GASTROINTESTINAL	NR	STROKE	★
GENERAL SURGERY	NR	VASCULAR	NR
MATERNITY CARE	NR	WOMEN'S HEALTH	NR

HEALTHGRADES AWARDS

Sabine Medical Center

240 Highland Drive
Many, LA 71449
(318) 256-5691

Overall patient safety: ★★★
Teaching: N

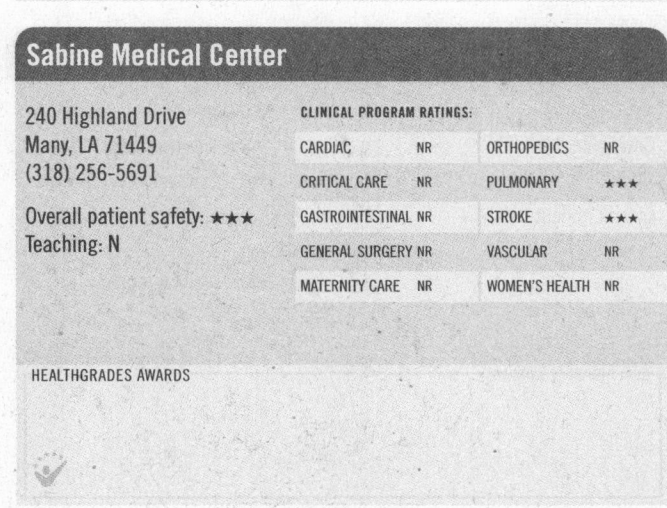

CLINICAL PROGRAM RATINGS:

CARDIAC	NR	ORTHOPEDICS	NR
CRITICAL CARE	NR	PULMONARY	★★★
GASTROINTESTINAL	NR	STROKE	★★★
GENERAL SURGERY	NR	VASCULAR	NR
MATERNITY CARE	NR	WOMEN'S HEALTH	NR

HEALTHGRADES AWARDS

St. Elizabeth Hospital

1125 West Highway 30
Gonzales, LA 70737
(225) 647-5000

Overall patient safety: ★★★
Teaching: N

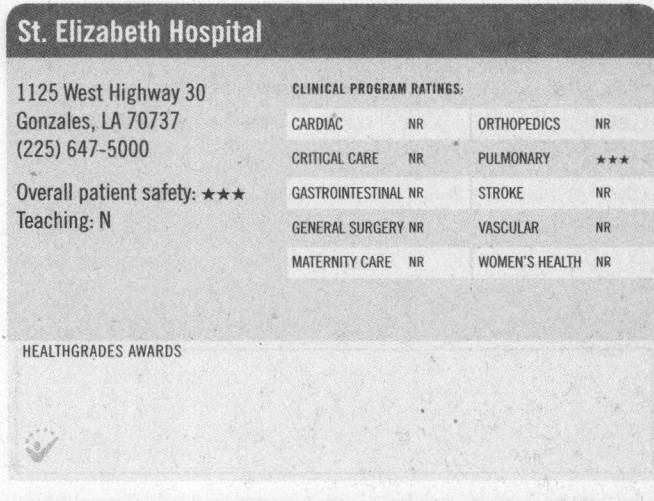

CLINICAL PROGRAM RATINGS:

CARDIAC	NR	ORTHOPEDICS	NR
CRITICAL CARE	NR	PULMONARY	★★★
GASTROINTESTINAL	NR	STROKE	NR
GENERAL SURGERY	NR	VASCULAR	NR
MATERNITY CARE	NR	WOMEN'S HEALTH	NR

HEALTHGRADES AWARDS

St. Brendan Rehab and Specialty Hospital

611 St. Landry Street
7th Floor
Lafayette, LA 70506
(318) 289-2240

Overall patient safety: ★★★
Teaching: N

CLINICAL PROGRAM RATINGS:

CARDIAC	★	ORTHOPEDICS	★★★
CRITICAL CARE	NR	PULMONARY	★★★
GASTROINTESTINAL	★★★	STROKE	★★★
GENERAL SURGERY	NR	VASCULAR	NR
MATERNITY CARE	NR	WOMEN'S HEALTH	NR

HEALTHGRADES AWARDS

St. Francis Medical Center

309 Jackson Street
Monroe, LA 71210
(318) 327-4000

Overall patient safety: ★★★★★
Teaching: N

CLINICAL PROGRAM RATINGS:

CARDIAC	★★★	ORTHOPEDICS	★★★
CRITICAL CARE	NR	PULMONARY	★★★
GASTROINTESTINAL	★★★	STROKE	★★★★★
GENERAL SURGERY	NR	VASCULAR	NR
MATERNITY CARE	NR	WOMEN'S HEALTH	NR

HEALTHGRADES AWARDS

✓ **DISTINGUISHED HOSPITAL**
· CLINICAL EXCELLENCE
· PATIENT SAFETY

✓ **SPECIALTY EXCELLENCE**
· CARDIAC SURGERY · STROKE CARE

St. Francis North Hospital

3421 Medical Parks Drive
Monroe, LA 71203
(318) 388-1946

Overall patient safety: ★★★
Teaching: N

CLINICAL PROGRAM RATINGS:

CARDIAC	★★★	ORTHOPEDICS	NR
CRITICAL CARE	NR	PULMONARY	★★★
GASTROINTESTINAL	★★★	STROKE	★★★
GENERAL SURGERY	NR	VASCULAR	NR
MATERNITY CARE	NR	WOMEN'S HEALTH	NR

HEALTHGRADES AWARDS

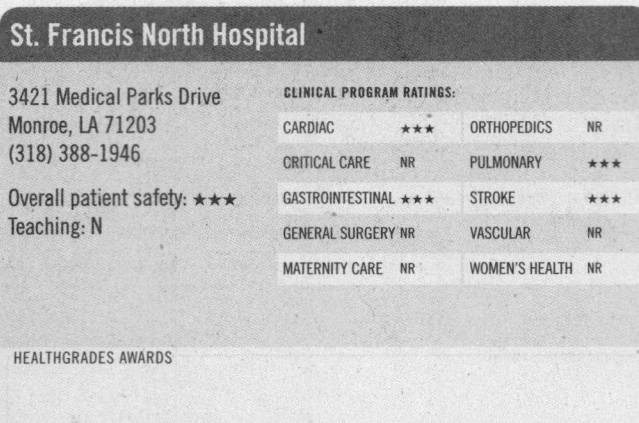

St. Martin Hospital

210 Champagne Boulevard
Breaux Bridge, LA 70517
(337) 332-2178

Overall patient safety: NR
Teaching: N

CLINICAL PROGRAM RATINGS:

CARDIAC	NR	ORTHOPEDICS	NR
CRITICAL CARE	NR	PULMONARY	★★★
GASTROINTESTINAL	NR	STROKE	NR
GENERAL SURGERY	NR	VASCULAR	NR
MATERNITY CARE	NR	WOMEN'S HEALTH	NR

HEALTHGRADES AWARDS

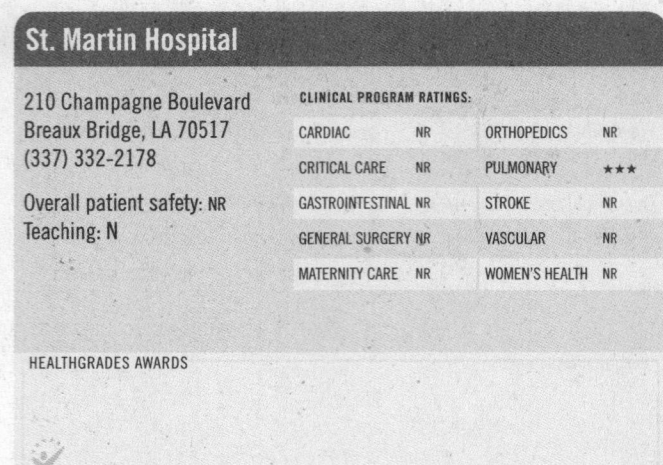

St. Helena Parish Hospital

Highway 43 North
Greensburg, LA 70441
(225) 222-6111

Overall patient safety: NR
Teaching: N

CLINICAL PROGRAM RATINGS:

CARDIAC	NR	ORTHOPEDICS	NR
CRITICAL CARE	NR	PULMONARY	★★★
GASTROINTESTINAL	NR	STROKE	NR
GENERAL SURGERY	NR	VASCULAR	NR
MATERNITY CARE	NR	WOMEN'S HEALTH	NR

HEALTHGRADES AWARDS

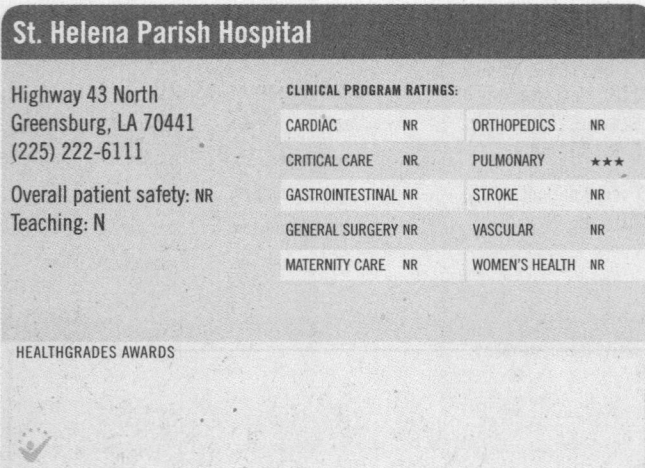

St. Tammany Parish Hospital

1202 South Tyler Street
Covington, LA 70433
(985) 898-4000

Overall patient safety: ★
Teaching: N

CLINICAL PROGRAM RATINGS:

CARDIAC	★★★	ORTHOPEDICS	★★★
CRITICAL CARE	NR	PULMONARY	★★★
GASTROINTESTINAL	★★★	STROKE	★
GENERAL SURGERY	NR	VASCULAR	NR
MATERNITY CARE	NR	WOMEN'S HEALTH	NR

HEALTHGRADES AWARDS

St. James Parish Hospital

2471 Louisiana Avenue
Lutcher, LA 70071
(225) 869-5512

Overall patient safety: ★★★
Teaching: N

CLINICAL PROGRAM RATINGS:

CARDIAC	NR	ORTHOPEDICS	NR
CRITICAL CARE	NR	PULMONARY	NR
GASTROINTESTINAL	NR	STROKE	NR
GENERAL SURGERY	NR	VASCULAR	NR
MATERNITY CARE	NR	WOMEN'S HEALTH	NR

HEALTHGRADES AWARDS

Savoy Medical Center

801 Poincianna Avenue
Mamou, LA 70554
(337) 468-5261

Overall patient safety: ★
Teaching: N

CLINICAL PROGRAM RATINGS:

CARDIAC	NR	ORTHOPEDICS	NR
CRITICAL CARE	NR	PULMONARY	★★★
GASTROINTESTINAL	NR	STROKE	★★★
GENERAL SURGERY	NR	VASCULAR	NR
MATERNITY CARE	NR	WOMEN'S HEALTH	NR

HEALTHGRADES AWARDS

KEY: ★★★★★ BEST   ★★★ AS EXPECTED   ★ POOR   NR NOT RATED BY HEALTHGRADES   For full definitions of ratings and awards, see Appendix.

Slidell Memorial Hospital

1001 Gause Boulevard
Slidell, LA 70458
(985) 643-2200

Overall patient safety: ★★★★★
Teaching: Y

CLINICAL PROGRAM RATINGS:

CARDIAC	★★★	ORTHOPEDICS	NR
CRITICAL CARE	NR	PULMONARY	★★★
GASTROINTESTINAL	★★★	STROKE	★★★
GENERAL SURGERY	NR	VASCULAR	NR
MATERNITY CARE	NR	WOMEN'S HEALTH	NR

HEALTHGRADES AWARDS

✓ DISTINGUISHED
HOSPITAL
• PATIENT SAFETY

Teche Regional Medical Center

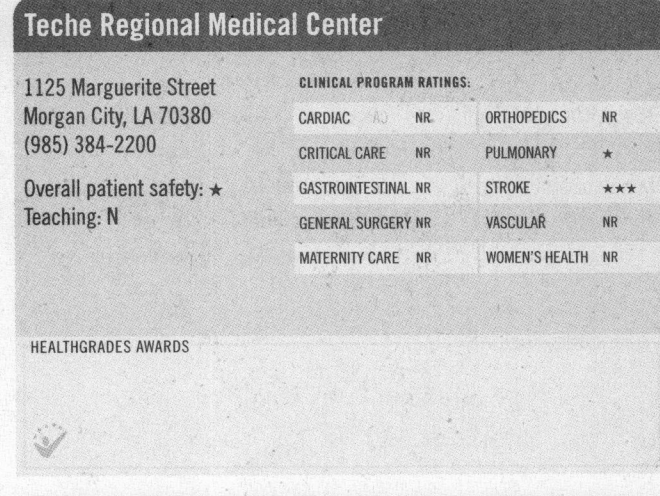

1125 Marguerite Street
Morgan City, LA 70380
(985) 384-2200

Overall patient safety: ★
Teaching: N

CLINICAL PROGRAM RATINGS:

CARDIAC	NR	ORTHOPEDICS	NR
CRITICAL CARE	NR	PULMONARY	★
GASTROINTESTINAL	NR	STROKE	★★★
GENERAL SURGERY	NR	VASCULAR	NR
MATERNITY CARE	NR	WOMEN'S HEALTH	NR

HEALTHGRADES AWARDS

Southwest Medical Center

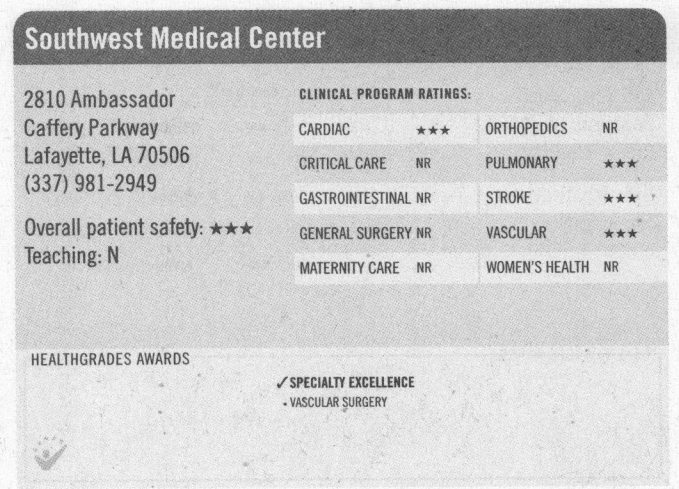

2810 Ambassador
Caffery Parkway
Lafayette, LA 70506
(337) 981-2949

Overall patient safety: ★★★
Teaching: N

CLINICAL PROGRAM RATINGS:

CARDIAC	★★★	ORTHOPEDICS	NR
CRITICAL CARE	NR	PULMONARY	★★★
GASTROINTESTINAL	NR	STROKE	★★★
GENERAL SURGERY	NR	VASCULAR	★★★
MATERNITY CARE	NR	WOMEN'S HEALTH	NR

HEALTHGRADES AWARDS

✓ SPECIALTY EXCELLENCE
• VASCULAR SURGERY

Terrebonne General Hospital

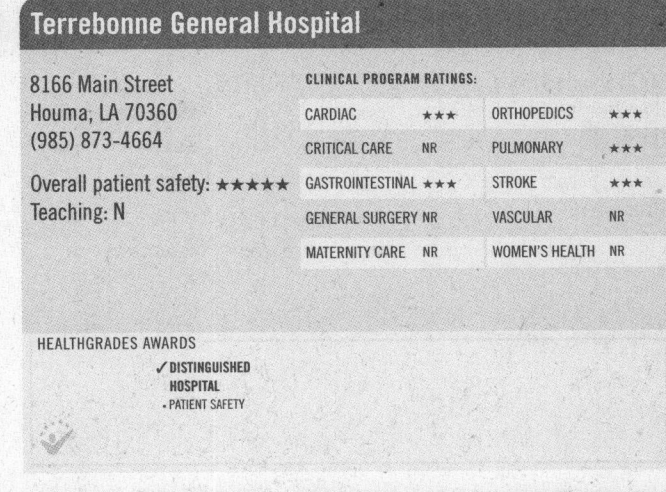

8166 Main Street
Houma, LA 70360
(985) 873-4664

Overall patient safety: ★★★★★
Teaching: N

CLINICAL PROGRAM RATINGS:

CARDIAC	★★★	ORTHOPEDICS	★★★
CRITICAL CARE	NR	PULMONARY	★★★
GASTROINTESTINAL	★★★	STROKE	★★★
GENERAL SURGERY	NR	VASCULAR	NR
MATERNITY CARE	NR	WOMEN'S HEALTH	NR

HEALTHGRADES AWARDS

✓ DISTINGUISHED
HOSPITAL
• PATIENT SAFETY

Springhill Medical Center

2001 Doctors Drive
Springhill, LA 71075
(318) 539-1000

Overall patient safety: ★★★
Teaching: N

CLINICAL PROGRAM RATINGS:

CARDIAC	NR	ORTHOPEDICS	NR
CRITICAL CARE	NR	PULMONARY	★★★
GASTROINTESTINAL	NR	STROKE	★★★
GENERAL SURGERY	NR	VASCULAR	NR
MATERNITY CARE	NR	WOMEN'S HEALTH	NR

HEALTHGRADES AWARDS

Thibodaux Regional Medical Center

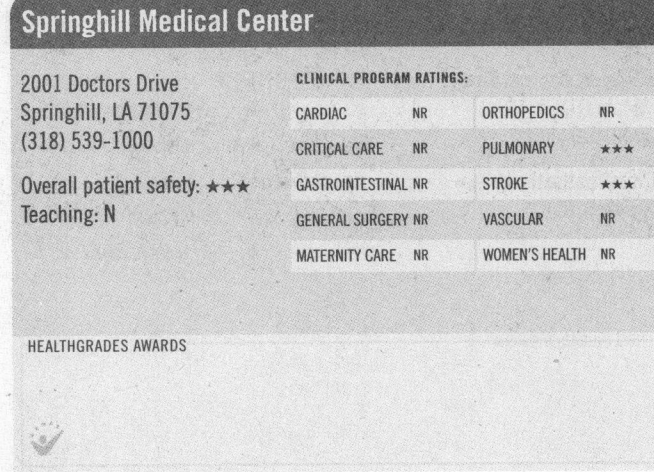

602 North Acadia Road
Thibodaux, LA 70301
(985) 447-5500

Overall patient safety: ★★★
Teaching: N

CLINICAL PROGRAM RATINGS:

CARDIAC	★★★	ORTHOPEDICS	NR
CRITICAL CARE	NR	PULMONARY	★★★
GASTROINTESTINAL	★★★	STROKE	★
GENERAL SURGERY	NR	VASCULAR	NR
MATERNITY CARE	NR	WOMEN'S HEALTH	NR

HEALTHGRADES AWARDS

✓ SPECIALTY EXCELLENCE
• GASTROINTESTINAL
CARE

Touro Infirmary

1401 Foucher Street
New Orleans, LA 70115
(504) 897-7011

Overall patient safety: ★
Teaching: Y

CLINICAL PROGRAM RATINGS:

CARDIAC	★★★	ORTHOPEDICS	★★★
CRITICAL CARE	NR	PULMONARY	★★★
GASTROINTESTINAL	NR	STROKE	★★★
GENERAL SURGERY	NR	VASCULAR	NR
MATERNITY CARE	NR	WOMEN'S HEALTH	NR

HEALTHGRADES AWARDS

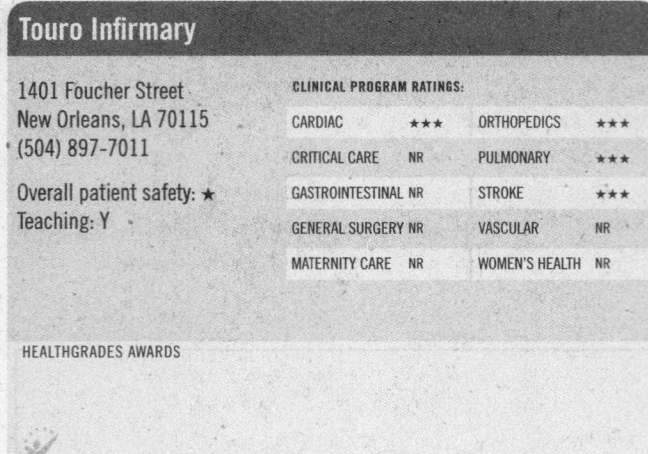

Ville Platte Medical Center

800 East Main Street
Ville Platte, LA 70586
(337) 363-5684

Overall patient safety: ★★★
Teaching: N

CLINICAL PROGRAM RATINGS:

CARDIAC	NR	ORTHOPEDICS	NR
CRITICAL CARE	NR	PULMONARY	★★★
GASTROINTESTINAL	NR	STROKE	★★★
GENERAL SURGERY	NR	VASCULAR	NR
MATERNITY CARE	NR	WOMEN'S HEALTH	NR

HEALTHGRADES AWARDS

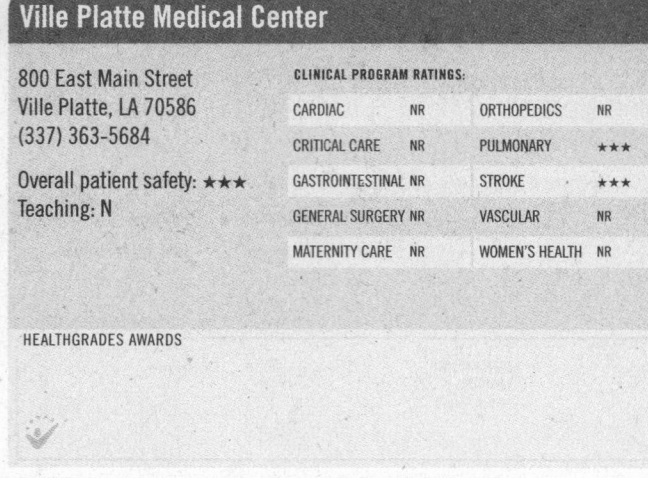

Tulane University Hospital*

1415 Tulane Avenue
New Orleans, LA 70112
(504) 588-5800

Overall patient safety: ★
Teaching: Y

CLINICAL PROGRAM RATINGS:

CARDIAC	NR	ORTHOPEDICS	NR
CRITICAL CARE	NR	PULMONARY	★★★
GASTROINTESTINAL	NR	STROKE	★★★★★
GENERAL SURGERY	NR	VASCULAR	NR
MATERNITY CARE	NR	WOMEN'S HEALTH	NR

HEALTHGRADES AWARDS

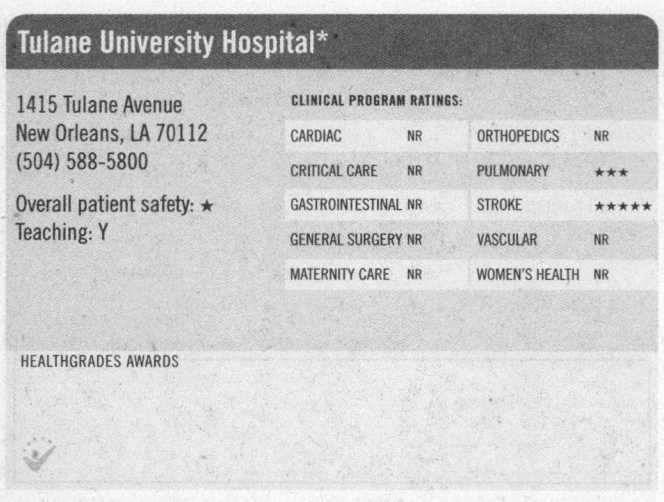

Washington St. Tammany Parish Medical Center

433 Plaza Street
Bogalusa, LA 70427
(985) 735-1322

Overall patient safety: ★★★
Teaching: N

CLINICAL PROGRAM RATINGS:

CARDIAC	NR	ORTHOPEDICS	NR
CRITICAL CARE	NR	PULMONARY	★★★
GASTROINTESTINAL	NR	STROKE	★★★
GENERAL SURGERY	NR	VASCULAR	NR
MATERNITY CARE	NR	WOMEN'S HEALTH	NR

HEALTHGRADES AWARDS

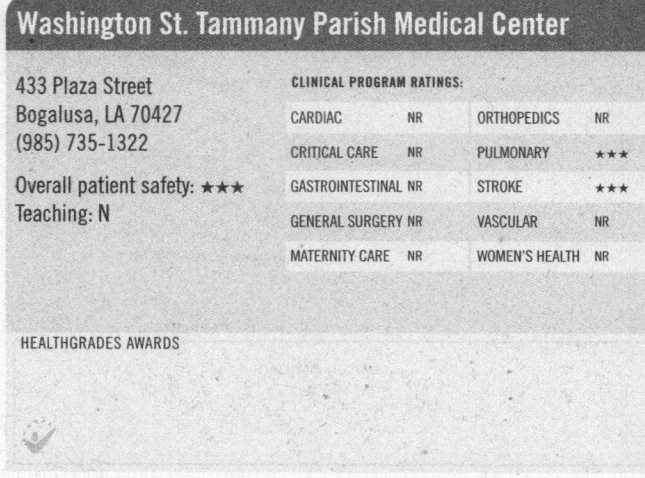

Union General Hospital

901 James Avenue
Farmerville, LA 71241
(318) 368-9751

Overall patient safety: NR
Teaching: N

CLINICAL PROGRAM RATINGS:

CARDIAC	NR	ORTHOPEDICS	NR
CRITICAL CARE	NR	PULMONARY	★
GASTROINTESTINAL	NR	STROKE	NR
GENERAL SURGERY	NR	VASCULAR	NR
MATERNITY CARE	NR	WOMEN'S HEALTH	NR

HEALTHGRADES AWARDS

West Calcasieu Cameron Hospital

701 East Cypress Street
Sulphur, LA 70663
(337) 527-7034

Overall patient safety: ★
Teaching: N

CLINICAL PROGRAM RATINGS:

CARDIAC	NR	ORTHOPEDICS	NR
CRITICAL CARE	NR	PULMONARY	★★★
GASTROINTESTINAL	NR	STROKE	★★★
GENERAL SURGERY	NR	VASCULAR	NR
MATERNITY CARE	NR	WOMEN'S HEALTH	NR

HEALTHGRADES AWARDS

KEY: ★★★★★ BEST   ★★★ AS EXPECTED   ★ POOR   NR NOT RATED BY HEALTHGRADES   For full definitions of ratings and awards, see Appendix.

West Carroll Memorial Hospital

522 Ross Street
Oak Grove, LA 71263
(318) 428-3237

Overall patient safety: NR
Teaching: N

CLINICAL PROGRAM RATINGS:

CARDIAC	NR	ORTHOPEDICS	NR
CRITICAL CARE	NR	PULMONARY	★★★
GASTROINTESTINAL	NR	STROKE	NR
GENERAL SURGERY	NR	VASCULAR	NR
MATERNITY CARE	NR	WOMEN'S HEALTH	NR

HEALTHGRADES AWARDS

Willis Knighton Medical Center

2600 Greenwood Road
Shreveport, LA 71103
(318) 212-4000

Overall patient safety: ★★★★★
Teaching: Y

CLINICAL PROGRAM RATINGS:

CARDIAC	★★★	ORTHOPEDICS	★★★
CRITICAL CARE	NR	PULMONARY	★★★★★
GASTROINTESTINAL	★★★	STROKE	★★★
GENERAL SURGERY	NR	VASCULAR	★★★
MATERNITY CARE	NR	WOMEN'S HEALTH	NR

HEALTHGRADES AWARDS

✓ **DISTINGUISHED HOSPITAL**
- CLINICAL EXCELLENCE
- PATIENT SAFETY

✓ **SPECIALTY EXCELLENCE**
- CARDIAC CARE
- GASTROINTESTINAL CARE
- PULMONARY CARE

West Jefferson Medical Center

1101 Medical Center Boulevard
Marrero, LA 70072
(504) 347-5511

Overall patient safety: ★
Teaching: N

CLINICAL PROGRAM RATINGS:

CARDIAC	★★★	ORTHOPEDICS	★★★
CRITICAL CARE	NR	PULMONARY	★★★
GASTROINTESTINAL	★★★	STROKE	★★★
GENERAL SURGERY	NR	VASCULAR	NR
MATERNITY CARE	NR	WOMEN'S HEALTH	NR

HEALTHGRADES AWARDS

Winn Parish Medical Center

301 West Boundary Street
Winnfield, LA 71483
(318) 628-2721

Overall patient safety: ★★★
Teaching: N

CLINICAL PROGRAM RATINGS:

CARDIAC	NR	ORTHOPEDICS	NR
CRITICAL CARE	NR	PULMONARY	★★★
GASTROINTESTINAL	NR	STROKE	NR
GENERAL SURGERY	NR	VASCULAR	NR
MATERNITY CARE	NR	WOMEN'S HEALTH	NR

HEALTHGRADES AWARDS

Willis Knighton Bossier Health Center

2400 Hospital Drive
Bossier City, LA 71111
(318) 212-7000

Overall patient safety: ★★★★★
Teaching: N

CLINICAL PROGRAM RATINGS:

CARDIAC	★★★	ORTHOPEDICS	★
CRITICAL CARE	NR	PULMONARY	★★★★★
GASTROINTESTINAL	★★★	STROKE	★★★
GENERAL SURGERY	NR	VASCULAR	NR
MATERNITY CARE	NR	WOMEN'S HEALTH	NR

HEALTHGRADES AWARDS

✓ **DISTINGUISHED HOSPITAL**
- CLINICAL EXCELLENCE
- PATIENT SAFETY

✓ **SPECIALTY EXCELLENCE**
- PULMONARY CARE

*This hospital reports its data to the federal government jointly with another hospital. Therefore the ratings and awards apply to multiple hospitals and this specific hospital may not provide all rated services.

Aroostook Medical Center

140 Academy Street
Presque Isle, ME 04769
(207) 768-4000

Overall patient safety: ★
Teaching: N

CLINICAL PROGRAM RATINGS:

CARDIAC	NR	ORTHOPEDICS	NR
CRITICAL CARE	NR	PULMONARY	★★★
GASTROINTESTINAL	NR	STROKE	★★★
GENERAL SURGERY	★★★	VASCULAR	NR
MATERNITY CARE	★	WOMEN'S HEALTH	NR

HEALTHGRADES AWARDS

Brighton Medical Center*

335 Brighton Avenue
Portland, ME 04101
(207) 879-8000

Overall patient safety: ★★★
Teaching: Y

CLINICAL PROGRAM RATINGS:

CARDIAC	★★★	ORTHOPEDICS	★★★
CRITICAL CARE	★★★	PULMONARY	★★★
GASTROINTESTINAL	★★★	STROKE	★★★
GENERAL SURGERY	★★★	VASCULAR	★★★
MATERNITY CARE	★	WOMEN'S HEALTH	★

HEALTHGRADES AWARDS

✓ SPECIALTY EXCELLENCE
- CARDIAC CARE   - JOINT REPLACEMENT

Blue Hill Memorial Hospital

57 Water Street
Blue Hill, ME 04614
(207) 374-2836

Overall patient safety: ★★★
Teaching: N

CLINICAL PROGRAM RATINGS:

CARDIAC	NR	ORTHOPEDICS	NR
CRITICAL CARE	NR	PULMONARY	★★★
GASTROINTESTINAL	NR	STROKE	★
GENERAL SURGERY	NR	VASCULAR	NR
MATERNITY CARE	★	WOMEN'S HEALTH	NR

HEALTHGRADES AWARDS

Calais Regional Hospital

22 Hospital Lane
Calais, ME 04619
(207) 454-7521

Overall patient safety: ★★★
Teaching: N

CLINICAL PROGRAM RATINGS:

CARDIAC	NR	ORTHOPEDICS	NR
CRITICAL CARE	NR	PULMONARY	★★★
GASTROINTESTINAL	NR	STROKE	★
GENERAL SURGERY	NR	VASCULAR	NR
MATERNITY CARE	★	WOMEN'S HEALTH	NR

HEALTHGRADES AWARDS

Bridgton Hospital

10 Hospital Drive
Bridgton, ME 04009
(207) 647-6000

Overall patient safety: ★★★
Teaching: N

CLINICAL PROGRAM RATINGS:

CARDIAC	NR	ORTHOPEDICS	NR
CRITICAL CARE	NR	PULMONARY	★★★
GASTROINTESTINAL	NR	STROKE	★★★
GENERAL SURGERY	NR	VASCULAR	NR
MATERNITY CARE	★★★	WOMEN'S HEALTH	NR

HEALTHGRADES AWARDS

Cary Medical Center

163 Van Buren Road
Suite 1
Caribou, ME 04736
(207) 498-3111

Overall patient safety: ★
Teaching: N

CLINICAL PROGRAM RATINGS:

CARDIAC	NR	ORTHOPEDICS	NR
CRITICAL CARE	NR	PULMONARY	★★★
GASTROINTESTINAL	NR	STROKE	★★★
GENERAL SURGERY	NR	VASCULAR	NR
MATERNITY CARE	★	WOMEN'S HEALTH	NR

HEALTHGRADES AWARDS

KEY: ★★★★★ BEST   ★★★ AS EXPECTED   ★ POOR   NR NOT RATED BY HEALTHGRADES   For full definitions of ratings and awards, see Appendix.

Central Maine Medical Center

300 Main Street
Lewiston, ME 04240
(207) 795-0111

Overall patient safety: ★★★
Teaching: Y

CLINICAL PROGRAM RATINGS:

CARDIAC	★★★	ORTHOPEDICS	★★★
CRITICAL CARE	★★★	PULMONARY	★★★
GASTROINTESTINAL	★★★	STROKE	★★★
GENERAL SURGERY	★★★	VASCULAR	NR
MATERNITY CARE	★★★	WOMEN'S HEALTH	★★★

HEALTHGRADES AWARDS

Franklin Memorial Hospital

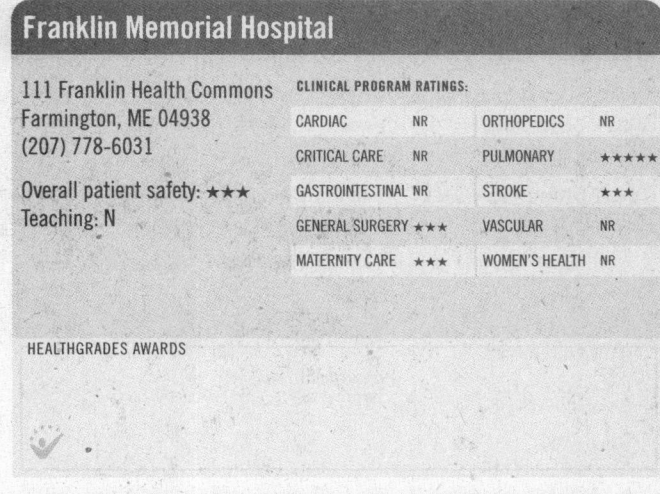

111 Franklin Health Commons
Farmington, ME 04938
(207) 778-6031

Overall patient safety: ★★★
Teaching: N

CLINICAL PROGRAM RATINGS:

CARDIAC	NR	ORTHOPEDICS	NR
CRITICAL CARE	NR	PULMONARY	★★★★★
GASTROINTESTINAL	NR	STROKE	★★★
GENERAL SURGERY	★★★	VASCULAR	NR
MATERNITY CARE	★★★	WOMEN'S HEALTH	NR

HEALTHGRADES AWARDS

Down East Community Hospital

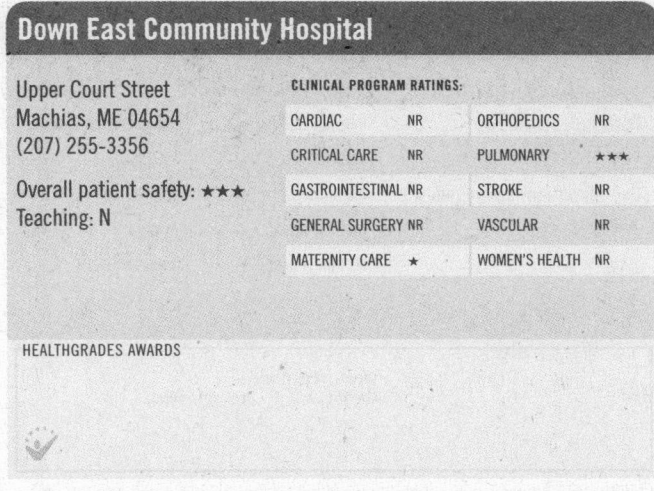

Upper Court Street
Machias, ME 04654
(207) 255-3356

Overall patient safety: ★★★
Teaching: N

CLINICAL PROGRAM RATINGS:

CARDIAC	NR	ORTHOPEDICS	NR
CRITICAL CARE	NR	PULMONARY	★★★
GASTROINTESTINAL	NR	STROKE	NR
GENERAL SURGERY	NR	VASCULAR	NR
MATERNITY CARE	★	WOMEN'S HEALTH	NR

HEALTHGRADES AWARDS

Henrietta D. Goodall Hospital

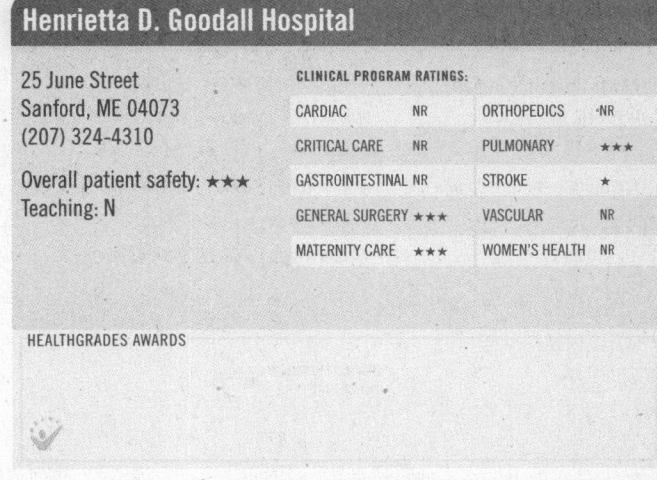

25 June Street
Sanford, ME 04073
(207) 324-4310

Overall patient safety: ★★★
Teaching: N

CLINICAL PROGRAM RATINGS:

CARDIAC	NR	ORTHOPEDICS	NR
CRITICAL CARE	NR	PULMONARY	★★★
GASTROINTESTINAL	NR	STROKE	★
GENERAL SURGERY	★★★	VASCULAR	NR
MATERNITY CARE	★★★	WOMEN'S HEALTH	NR

HEALTHGRADES AWARDS

Eastern Maine Medical Center

489 State Street
Bangor, ME 04402
(207) 973-7000

Overall patient safety: ★★★
Teaching: Y

CLINICAL PROGRAM RATINGS:

CARDIAC	★★★	ORTHOPEDICS	★★★
CRITICAL CARE	★★★	PULMONARY	★★★
GASTROINTESTINAL	★★★	STROKE	★★★★★
GENERAL SURGERY	★★★	VASCULAR	★★★
MATERNITY CARE	★★★	WOMEN'S HEALTH	★★★

HEALTHGRADES AWARDS

Houlton Regional Hospital

20 Hartford Street
Houlton, ME 04730
(207) 532-2900

Overall patient safety: ★★★
Teaching: N

CLINICAL PROGRAM RATINGS:

CARDIAC	NR	ORTHOPEDICS	NR
CRITICAL CARE	NR	PULMONARY	★★★
GASTROINTESTINAL	NR	STROKE	★
GENERAL SURGERY	NR	VASCULAR	NR
MATERNITY CARE	★★★	WOMEN'S HEALTH	NR

HEALTHGRADES AWARDS

*This hospital reports its data to the federal government jointly with another hospital. Therefore the ratings and awards apply to multiple hospitals and this specific hospital may not provide all rated services.

Inland Hospital

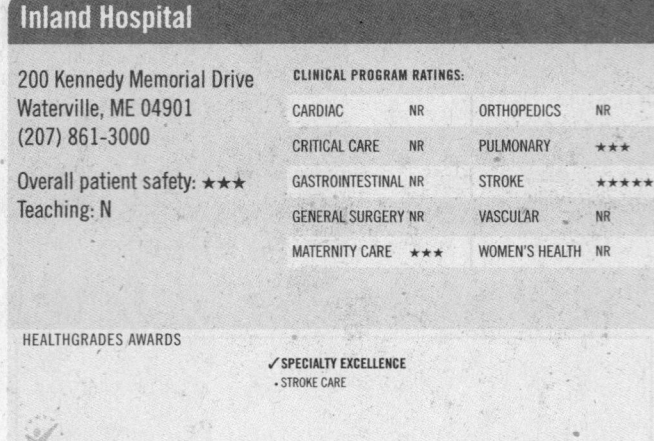

200 Kennedy Memorial Drive
Waterville, ME 04901
(207) 861-3000

Overall patient safety: ★★★
Teaching: N

CLINICAL PROGRAM RATINGS:

CARDIAC	NR	ORTHOPEDICS	NR
CRITICAL CARE	NR	PULMONARY	★★★
GASTROINTESTINAL	NR	STROKE	★★★★★
GENERAL SURGERY	NR	VASCULAR	NR
MATERNITY CARE	★★★	WOMEN'S HEALTH	NR

HEALTHGRADES AWARDS

✓ SPECIALTY EXCELLENCE
• STROKE CARE

Maine General Medical Center*

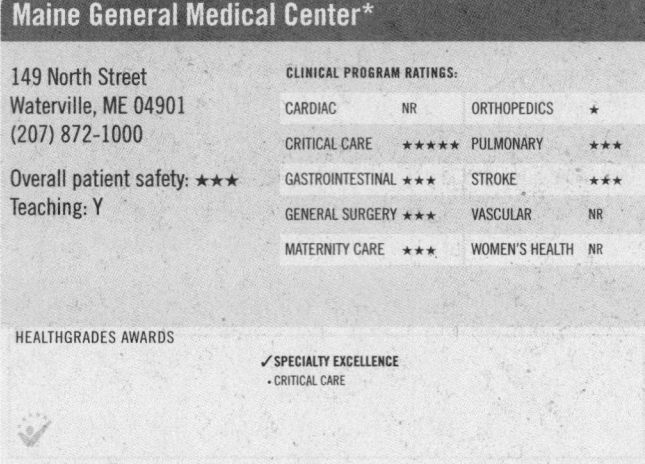

149 North Street
Waterville, ME 04901
(207) 872-1000

Overall patient safety: ★★★
Teaching: Y

CLINICAL PROGRAM RATINGS:

CARDIAC	NR	ORTHOPEDICS	★
CRITICAL CARE	★★★★★	PULMONARY	★★★
GASTROINTESTINAL	★★★	STROKE	★★★
GENERAL SURGERY	★★★	VASCULAR	NR
MATERNITY CARE	★★★	WOMEN'S HEALTH	NR

HEALTHGRADES AWARDS

✓ SPECIALTY EXCELLENCE
• CRITICAL CARE

Kennebec Valley Medical Center*

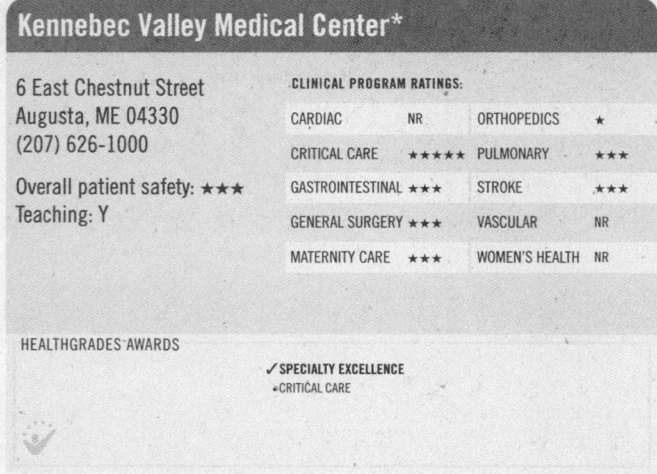

6 East Chestnut Street
Augusta, ME 04330
(207) 626-1000

Overall patient safety: ★★★
Teaching: Y

CLINICAL PROGRAM RATINGS:

CARDIAC	NR	ORTHOPEDICS	★
CRITICAL CARE	★★★★★	PULMONARY	★★★
GASTROINTESTINAL	★★★	STROKE	★★★
GENERAL SURGERY	★★★	VASCULAR	NR
MATERNITY CARE	★★★	WOMEN'S HEALTH	NR

HEALTHGRADES AWARDS

✓ SPECIALTY EXCELLENCE
• CRITICAL CARE

Maine Medical Center*

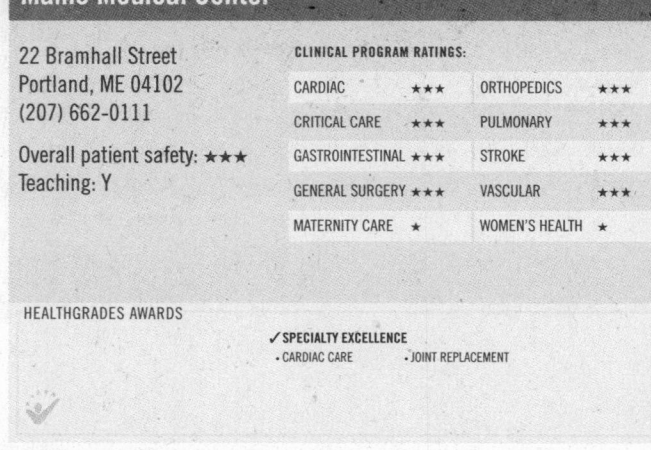

22 Bramhall Street
Portland, ME 04102
(207) 662-0111

Overall patient safety: ★★★
Teaching: Y

CLINICAL PROGRAM RATINGS:

CARDIAC	★★★	ORTHOPEDICS	★★★
CRITICAL CARE	★★★	PULMONARY	★★★
GASTROINTESTINAL	★★★	STROKE	★★★
GENERAL SURGERY	★★★	VASCULAR	★★★
MATERNITY CARE	★	WOMEN'S HEALTH	★

HEALTHGRADES AWARDS

✓ SPECIALTY EXCELLENCE
• CARDIAC CARE   • JOINT REPLACEMENT

Maine Coast Memorial Hospital

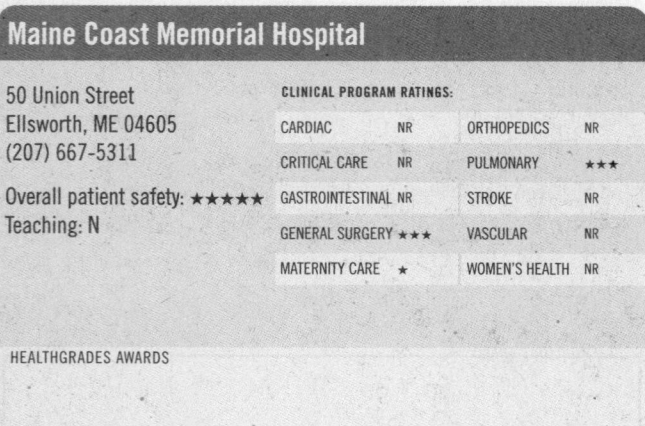

50 Union Street
Ellsworth, ME 04605
(207) 667-5311

Overall patient safety: ★★★★★
Teaching: N

CLINICAL PROGRAM RATINGS:

CARDIAC	NR	ORTHOPEDICS	NR
CRITICAL CARE	NR	PULMONARY	★★★
GASTROINTESTINAL	NR	STROKE	NR
GENERAL SURGERY	★★★	VASCULAR	NR
MATERNITY CARE	★	WOMEN'S HEALTH	NR

HEALTHGRADES AWARDS

Mayo Regional Hospital

75 West Main Street
Dover Foxcroft, ME 04426
(207) 564-4251

Overall patient safety: ★★★
Teaching: N

CLINICAL PROGRAM RATINGS:

CARDIAC	NR	ORTHOPEDICS	NR
CRITICAL CARE	NR	PULMONARY	★
GASTROINTESTINAL	NR	STROKE	NR
GENERAL SURGERY	NR	VASCULAR	NR
MATERNITY CARE	★★★	WOMEN'S HEALTH	NR

HEALTHGRADES AWARDS

KEY: ★★★★★ BEST   ★★★ AS EXPECTED   ★ POOR   NR NOT RATED BY HEALTHGRADES   For full definitions of ratings and awards, see Appendix.

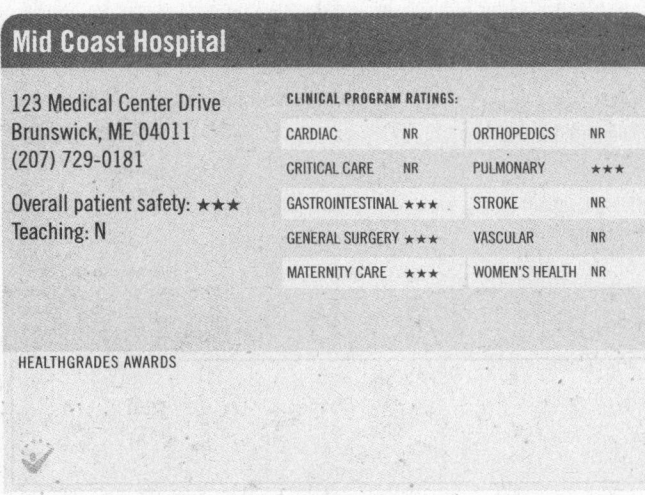

Mercy Hospital*

144 State Street
Portland, ME 04101
(207) 879-3000

Overall patient safety: ★★★
Teaching: Y

CLINICAL PROGRAM RATINGS:

CARDIAC	NR	ORTHOPEDICS	★★★
CRITICAL CARE	★★★	PULMONARY	★★★
GASTROINTESTINAL	★★★	STROKE	★
GENERAL SURGERY	★★★	VASCULAR	★★★
MATERNITY CARE	★★★	WOMEN'S HEALTH	NR

HEALTHGRADES AWARDS

Millinocket Regional Hospital

200 Somerset Street
Millinocket, ME 04462
(207) 723-5161

Overall patient safety: ★★★
Teaching: N

CLINICAL PROGRAM RATINGS:

CARDIAC	NR	ORTHOPEDICS	NR
CRITICAL CARE	NR	PULMONARY	★★★
GASTROINTESTINAL	NR	STROKE	NR
GENERAL SURGERY	NR	VASCULAR	NR
MATERNITY CARE	NR	WOMEN'S HEALTH	NR

HEALTHGRADES AWARDS

Mid Coast Hospital

123 Medical Center Drive
Brunswick, ME 04011
(207) 729-0181

Overall patient safety: ★★★
Teaching: N

CLINICAL PROGRAM RATINGS:

CARDIAC	NR	ORTHOPEDICS	NR
CRITICAL CARE	NR	PULMONARY	★★★
GASTROINTESTINAL	★★★	STROKE	NR
GENERAL SURGERY	★★★	VASCULAR	NR
MATERNITY CARE	★★★	WOMEN'S HEALTH	NR

HEALTHGRADES AWARDS

Mount Desert Island Hospital

10 Wayman Lane
P.O. Box 8
Bar Harbor, ME 04609
(207) 288-5081

Overall patient safety: ★★★
Teaching: N

CLINICAL PROGRAM RATINGS:

CARDIAC	NR	ORTHOPEDICS	NR
CRITICAL CARE	NR	PULMONARY	★★★
GASTROINTESTINAL	NR	STROKE	NR
GENERAL SURGERY	NR	VASCULAR	NR
MATERNITY CARE	★★★	WOMEN'S HEALTH	NR

HEALTHGRADES AWARDS

Miles Memorial Hospital

35 Miles Street
Damariscotta, ME 04543
(207) 563-1234

Overall patient safety: ★★★
Teaching: N

CLINICAL PROGRAM RATINGS:

CARDIAC	NR	ORTHOPEDICS	NR
CRITICAL CARE	NR	PULMONARY	★★★★★
GASTROINTESTINAL	NR	STROKE	NR
GENERAL SURGERY	NR	VASCULAR	NR
MATERNITY CARE	★	WOMEN'S HEALTH	NR

HEALTHGRADES AWARDS

✓ SPECIALTY EXCELLENCE
- PULMONARY CARE

Northern Maine Medical Center

194 East Main Street
Fort Kent, ME 04743
(207) 834-3155

Overall patient safety: ★★★
Teaching: N

CLINICAL PROGRAM RATINGS:

CARDIAC	NR	ORTHOPEDICS	NR
CRITICAL CARE	NR	PULMONARY	★★★
GASTROINTESTINAL	NR	STROKE	★★★
GENERAL SURGERY	NR	VASCULAR	NR
MATERNITY CARE	★★★	WOMEN'S HEALTH	NR

HEALTHGRADES AWARDS

*This hospital reports its data to the federal government jointly with another hospital. Therefore the ratings and awards apply to multiple hospitals and this specific hospital may not provide all rated services.

MAINE HOSPITALS: RATINGS BY CLINICAL SPECIALTY

Parkview Adventist Medical Center

329 Maine Street
Brunswick, ME 04011
(207) 373-2000

Overall patient safety: ★★★
Teaching: N

CLINICAL PROGRAM RATINGS:

CARDIAC	NR	ORTHOPEDICS	NR
CRITICAL CARE	NR	PULMONARY	★★★★★
GASTROINTESTINAL	NR	STROKE	★★★
GENERAL SURGERY	NR	VASCULAR	NR
MATERNITY CARE	★	WOMEN'S HEALTH	NR

HEALTHGRADES AWARDS

✓ SPECIALTY EXCELLENCE
• PULMONARY CARE

Redington Fairview General Hospital

Fairview Avenue
Skowhegan, ME 04976
(207) 474-5121

Overall patient safety: NR
Teaching: N

CLINICAL PROGRAM RATINGS:

CARDIAC	NR	ORTHOPEDICS	NR
CRITICAL CARE	NR	PULMONARY	★★★
GASTROINTESTINAL	NR	STROKE	★★★
GENERAL SURGERY	NR	VASCULAR	NR
MATERNITY CARE	NR	WOMEN'S HEALTH	NR

HEALTHGRADES AWARDS

Penobscot Bay Medical Center

6 Glen Cove Drive
Rockport, ME 04856
(207) 596-8000

Overall patient safety: ★★★
Teaching: N

CLINICAL PROGRAM RATINGS:

CARDIAC	NR	ORTHOPEDICS	NR
CRITICAL CARE	NR	PULMONARY	★★★
GASTROINTESTINAL	NR	STROKE	★★★
GENERAL SURGERY	★★★	VASCULAR	NR
MATERNITY CARE	★	WOMEN'S HEALTH	NR

HEALTHGRADES AWARDS

Rumford Hospital

420 Franklin Street
Rumford, ME 04276
(207) 369-1000

Overall patient safety: ★★★
Teaching: N

CLINICAL PROGRAM RATINGS:

CARDIAC	NR	ORTHOPEDICS	NR
CRITICAL CARE	NR	PULMONARY	★
GASTROINTESTINAL	NR	STROKE	★★★
GENERAL SURGERY	NR	VASCULAR	NR
MATERNITY CARE	★★★	WOMEN'S HEALTH	NR

HEALTHGRADES AWARDS

Penobscot Valley Hospital

7 Transalpine Road
Lincoln, ME 04457
(207) 794-3321

Overall patient safety: ★
Teaching: N

CLINICAL PROGRAM RATINGS:

CARDIAC	NR	ORTHOPEDICS	NR
CRITICAL CARE	NR	PULMONARY	★
GASTROINTESTINAL	NR	STROKE	★
GENERAL SURGERY	NR	VASCULAR	NR
MATERNITY CARE	★★★	WOMEN'S HEALTH	NR

HEALTHGRADES AWARDS

St. Andrews Hospital

6 St. Andrews Lane
Boothbay Harbor, ME 04538
(207) 633-2121

Overall patient safety: ★★★
Teaching: N

CLINICAL PROGRAM RATINGS:

CARDIAC	NR	ORTHOPEDICS	NR
CRITICAL CARE	NR	PULMONARY	★★★
GASTROINTESTINAL	NR	STROKE	NR
GENERAL SURGERY	NR	VASCULAR	NR
MATERNITY CARE	NR	WOMEN'S HEALTH	NR

HEALTHGRADES AWARDS

KEY: ★★★★★ BEST   ★★★ AS EXPECTED   ★ POOR   NR NOT RATED BY HEALTHGRADES   For full definitions of ratings and awards, see Appendix.

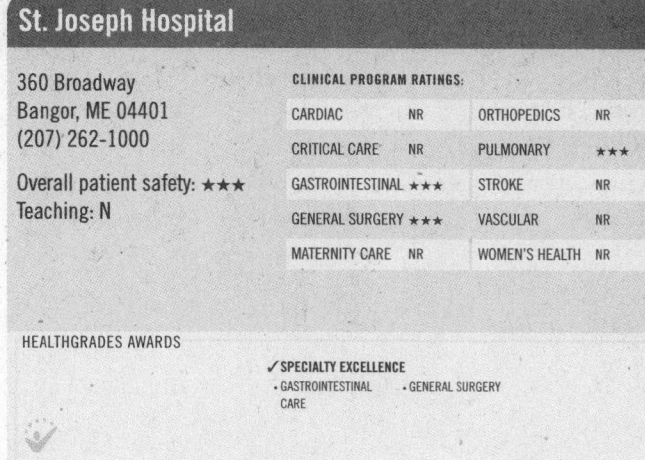

St. Joseph Hospital

360 Broadway
Bangor, ME 04401
(207) 262-1000

Overall patient safety: ★★★
Teaching: N

CLINICAL PROGRAM RATINGS:

CARDIAC	NR	ORTHOPEDICS	NR
CRITICAL CARE	NR	PULMONARY	★★★
GASTROINTESTINAL	★★★	STROKE	NR
GENERAL SURGERY	★★★	VASCULAR	NR
MATERNITY CARE	NR	WOMEN'S HEALTH	NR

HEALTHGRADES AWARDS

✓ SPECIALTY EXCELLENCE
• GASTROINTESTINAL   • GENERAL SURGERY
  CARE

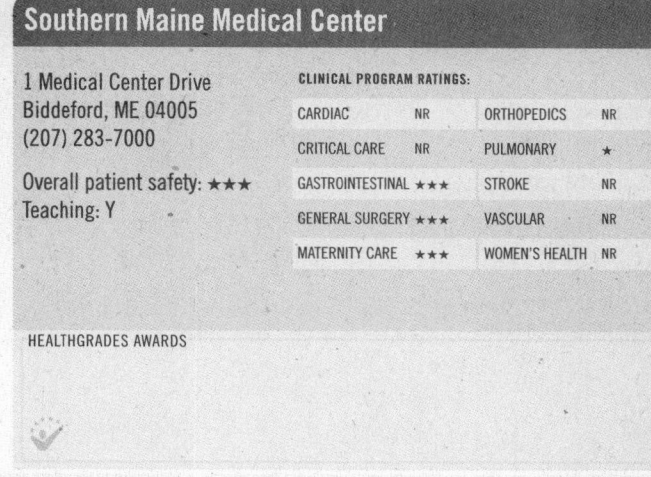

Southern Maine Medical Center

1 Medical Center Drive
Biddeford, ME 04005
(207) 283-7000

Overall patient safety: ★★★
Teaching: Y

CLINICAL PROGRAM RATINGS:

CARDIAC	NR	ORTHOPEDICS	NR
CRITICAL CARE	NR	PULMONARY	★
GASTROINTESTINAL	★★★	STROKE	NR
GENERAL SURGERY	★★★	VASCULAR	NR
MATERNITY CARE	★★★	WOMEN'S HEALTH	NR

HEALTHGRADES AWARDS

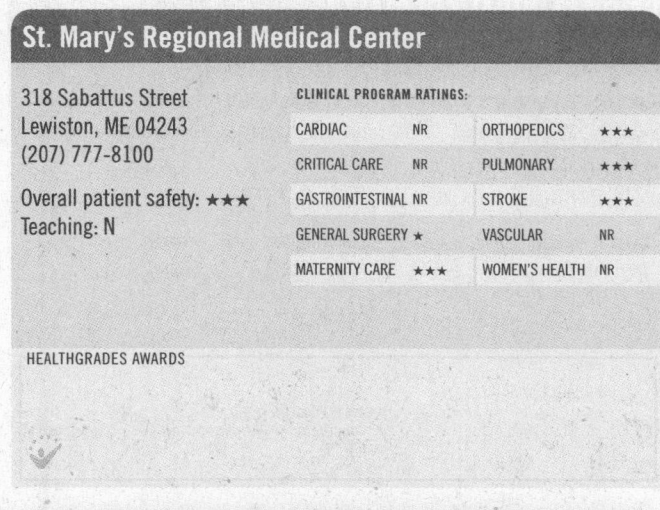

St. Mary's Regional Medical Center

318 Sabattus Street
Lewiston, ME 04243
(207) 777-8100

Overall patient safety: ★★★
Teaching: N

CLINICAL PROGRAM RATINGS:

CARDIAC	NR	ORTHOPEDICS	★★★
CRITICAL CARE	NR	PULMONARY	★★★
GASTROINTESTINAL	NR	STROKE	★★★
GENERAL SURGERY	★	VASCULAR	NR
MATERNITY CARE	★★★	WOMEN'S HEALTH	NR

HEALTHGRADES AWARDS

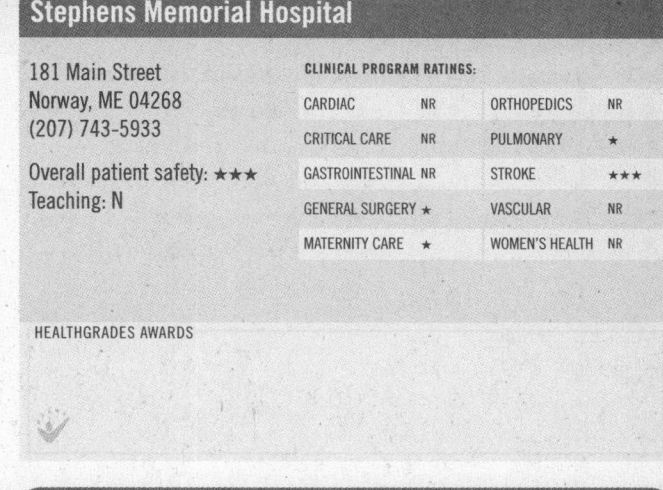

Stephens Memorial Hospital

181 Main Street
Norway, ME 04268
(207) 743-5933

Overall patient safety: ★★★
Teaching: N

CLINICAL PROGRAM RATINGS:

CARDIAC	NR	ORTHOPEDICS	NR
CRITICAL CARE	NR	PULMONARY	★
GASTROINTESTINAL	NR	STROKE	★★★
GENERAL SURGERY	★	VASCULAR	NR
MATERNITY CARE	★	WOMEN'S HEALTH	NR

HEALTHGRADES AWARDS

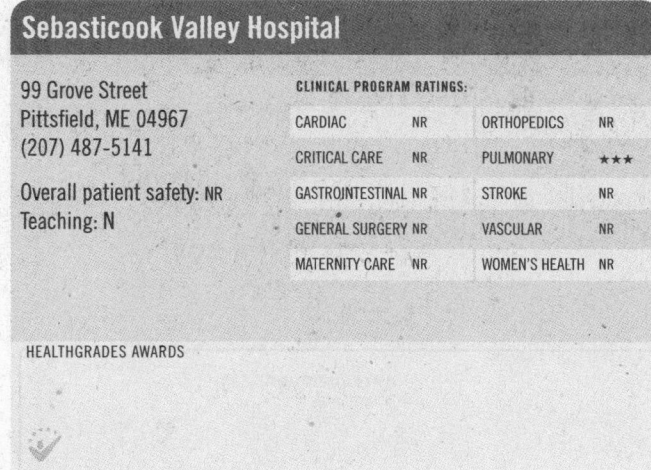

Sebasticook Valley Hospital

99 Grove Street
Pittsfield, ME 04967
(207) 487-5141

Overall patient safety: NR
Teaching: N

CLINICAL PROGRAM RATINGS:

CARDIAC	NR	ORTHOPEDICS	NR
CRITICAL CARE	NR	PULMONARY	★★★
GASTROINTESTINAL	NR	STROKE	NR
GENERAL SURGERY	NR	VASCULAR	NR
MATERNITY CARE	NR	WOMEN'S HEALTH	NR

HEALTHGRADES AWARDS

Waldo County General Hospital

118 Northport Avenue
Belfast, ME 04915
(207) 338-2500

Overall patient safety: ★
Teaching: N

CLINICAL PROGRAM RATINGS:

CARDIAC	NR	ORTHOPEDICS	NR
CRITICAL CARE	NR	PULMONARY	★
GASTROINTESTINAL	NR	STROKE	★
GENERAL SURGERY	NR	VASCULAR	NR
MATERNITY CARE	★★★	WOMEN'S HEALTH	NR

HEALTHGRADES AWARDS

Westbrook Community Hospital*

40 Park Road
Westbrook, ME 04092
(207) 857-8000

Overall patient safety: ★★★
Teaching: Y

CLINICAL PROGRAM RATINGS:

CARDIAC	NR	ORTHOPEDICS	★★★
CRITICAL CARE	★★★	PULMONARY	★★★
GASTROINTESTINAL	★★★	STROKE	★
GENERAL SURGERY	★★★	VASCULAR	★★★
MATERNITY CARE	★★★	WOMEN'S HEALTH	NR

HEALTHGRADES AWARDS

York Hospital

15 Hospital Drive
York, ME 03909
(207) 363-4321

Overall patient safety: ★★★
Teaching: N

CLINICAL PROGRAM RATINGS:

CARDIAC	NR	ORTHOPEDICS	NR
CRITICAL CARE	NR	PULMONARY	★★★
GASTROINTESTINAL	★★★	STROKE	★★★
GENERAL SURGERY	★★★	VASCULAR	NR
MATERNITY CARE	★★★	WOMEN'S HEALTH	NR

HEALTHGRADES AWARDS

MARYLAND HOSPITALS: RATINGS BY CLINICAL SPECIALTY

Anne Arundel Medical Center

2001 Medical Parkway
Annapolis, MD 21401
(443) 481-1000

Overall patient safety: ★★★
Teaching: N

CLINICAL PROGRAM RATINGS:

CARDIAC	NR	ORTHOPEDICS	★
CRITICAL CARE	★★★	PULMONARY	★★★
GASTROINTESTINAL	★★★	STROKE	★★★
GENERAL SURGERY	★	VASCULAR	★★★
MATERNITY CARE	★★★	WOMEN'S HEALTH	NR

HEALTHGRADES AWARDS

Baltimore Washington Medical Center

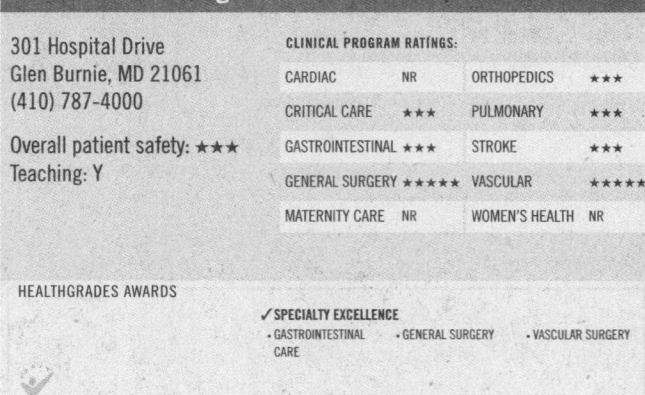

301 Hospital Drive
Glen Burnie, MD 21061
(410) 787-4000

Overall patient safety: ★★★
Teaching: Y

CLINICAL PROGRAM RATINGS:

CARDIAC	NR	ORTHOPEDICS	★★★
CRITICAL CARE	★★★	PULMONARY	★★★
GASTROINTESTINAL	★★★	STROKE	★★★
GENERAL SURGERY	★★★★★	VASCULAR	★★★★★
MATERNITY CARE	NR	WOMEN'S HEALTH	NR

HEALTHGRADES AWARDS

✓ SPECIALTY EXCELLENCE
· GASTROINTESTINAL · GENERAL SURGERY · VASCULAR SURGERY
  CARE

Atlantic General Hospital

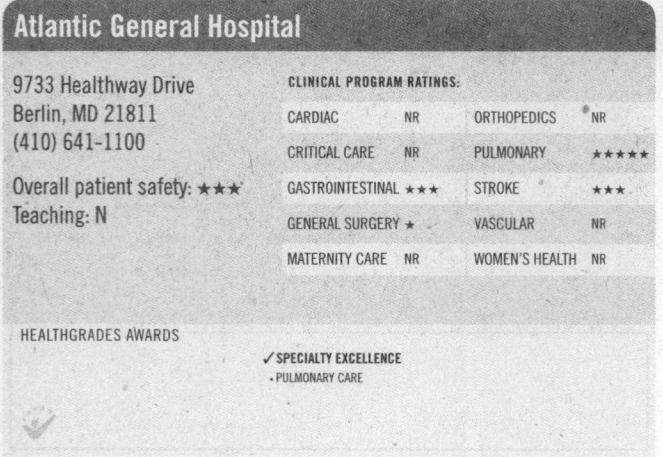

9733 Healthway Drive
Berlin, MD 21811
(410) 641-1100

Overall patient safety: ★★★
Teaching: N

CLINICAL PROGRAM RATINGS:

CARDIAC	NR	ORTHOPEDICS	NR
CRITICAL CARE	NR	PULMONARY	★★★★★
GASTROINTESTINAL	★★★	STROKE	★★★
GENERAL SURGERY	★	VASCULAR	NR
MATERNITY CARE	NR	WOMEN'S HEALTH	NR

HEALTHGRADES AWARDS

✓ SPECIALTY EXCELLENCE
· PULMONARY CARE

Bon Secours Hospital

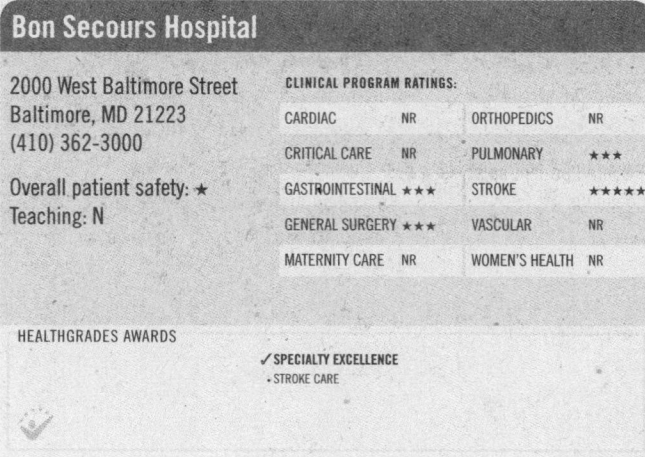

2000 West Baltimore Street
Baltimore, MD 21223
(410) 362-3000

Overall patient safety: ★
Teaching: N

CLINICAL PROGRAM RATINGS:

CARDIAC	NR	ORTHOPEDICS	NR
CRITICAL CARE	NR	PULMONARY	★★★
GASTROINTESTINAL	★★★	STROKE	★★★★★
GENERAL SURGERY	★★★	VASCULAR	NR
MATERNITY CARE	NR	WOMEN'S HEALTH	NR

HEALTHGRADES AWARDS

✓ SPECIALTY EXCELLENCE
· STROKE CARE

KEY: ★★★★★ BEST   ★★★ AS EXPECTED   ★ POOR   NR NOT RATED BY HEALTHGRADES   For full definitions of ratings and awards, see Appendix.

Calvert Memorial Hospital

100 Hospital Road
Prince Frederick, MD 20678
(410) 535-4000

Overall patient safety: ★
Teaching: N

CLINICAL PROGRAM RATINGS:

CARDIAC	NR	ORTHOPEDICS	★
CRITICAL CARE	★★★	PULMONARY	★★★★★
GASTROINTESTINAL	★★★	STROKE	★★★
GENERAL SURGERY	★★★	VASCULAR	NR
MATERNITY CARE	★★★	WOMEN'S HEALTH	NR

HEALTHGRADES AWARDS

✓ SPECIALTY EXCELLENCE
- GASTROINTESTINAL CARE
- PULMONARY CARE

Civista Medical Center

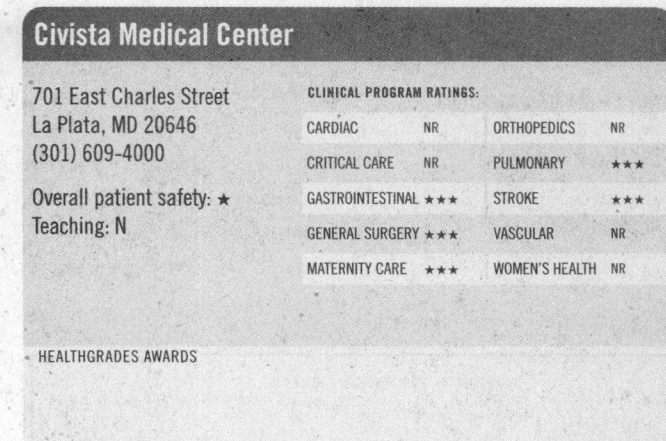

701 East Charles Street
La Plata, MD 20646
(301) 609-4000

Overall patient safety: ★
Teaching: N

CLINICAL PROGRAM RATINGS:

CARDIAC	NR	ORTHOPEDICS	NR
CRITICAL CARE	NR	PULMONARY	★★★
GASTROINTESTINAL	★★★	STROKE	★★★
GENERAL SURGERY	★★★	VASCULAR	NR
MATERNITY CARE	★★★	WOMEN'S HEALTH	NR

HEALTHGRADES AWARDS

Carroll Hospital Center

200 Memorial Avenue
Westminster, MD 21157
(410) 876-3000

Overall patient safety: ★★★
Teaching: N

CLINICAL PROGRAM RATINGS:

CARDIAC	NR	ORTHOPEDICS	★★★
CRITICAL CARE	★	PULMONARY	★★★
GASTROINTESTINAL	★★★	STROKE	★★★
GENERAL SURGERY	★★★	VASCULAR	★★★
MATERNITY CARE	★★★	WOMEN'S HEALTH	NR

HEALTHGRADES AWARDS

Doctors Community Hospital

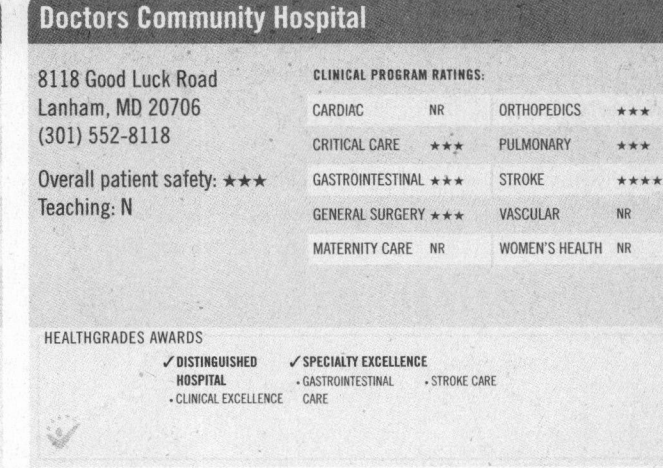

8118 Good Luck Road
Lanham, MD 20706
(301) 552-8118

Overall patient safety: ★★★
Teaching: N

CLINICAL PROGRAM RATINGS:

CARDIAC	NR	ORTHOPEDICS	★★★
CRITICAL CARE	★★★	PULMONARY	★★★
GASTROINTESTINAL	★★★	STROKE	★★★★★
GENERAL SURGERY	★★★	VASCULAR	NR
MATERNITY CARE	NR	WOMEN'S HEALTH	NR

HEALTHGRADES AWARDS

✓ DISTINGUISHED HOSPITAL
- CLINICAL EXCELLENCE

✓ SPECIALTY EXCELLENCE
- GASTROINTESTINAL CARE
- STROKE CARE

Chester River Hospital Center

100 Brown Street
Chestertown, MD 21620
(410) 778-3300

Overall patient safety: ★★★
Teaching: N

CLINICAL PROGRAM RATINGS:

CARDIAC	NR	ORTHOPEDICS	NR
CRITICAL CARE	NR	PULMONARY	★★★
GASTROINTESTINAL	★★★	STROKE	★★★
GENERAL SURGERY	★★★	VASCULAR	NR
MATERNITY CARE	★	WOMEN'S HEALTH	NR

HEALTHGRADES AWARDS

Fort Washington Hospital

11711 Livingston Road
Fort Washington, MD 20744
(301) 292-7000

Overall patient safety: ★★★
Teaching: N

CLINICAL PROGRAM RATINGS:

CARDIAC	NR	ORTHOPEDICS	NR
CRITICAL CARE	NR	PULMONARY	★★★
GASTROINTESTINAL	NR	STROKE	★★★
GENERAL SURGERY	★★★	VASCULAR	NR
MATERNITY CARE	NR	WOMEN'S HEALTH	NR

HEALTHGRADES AWARDS

*This hospital reports its data to the federal government jointly with another hospital. Therefore the ratings and awards apply to multiple hospitals and this specific hospital may not provide all rated services.

Franklin Square Hospital Center

9000 Franklin Square Drive
Baltimore, MD 21237
(443) 777-7000

Overall patient safety: ★★★
Teaching: Y

CLINICAL PROGRAM RATINGS:

CARDIAC	NR	ORTHOPEDICS	★★★
CRITICAL CARE	★★★	PULMONARY	★★★★★
GASTROINTESTINAL	★★★★★	STROKE	★★★
GENERAL SURGERY	★★★★★	VASCULAR	★★★
MATERNITY CARE	★	WOMEN'S HEALTH	NR

HEALTHGRADES AWARDS

✓ DISTINGUISHED HOSPITAL
- CLINICAL EXCELLENCE

✓ SPECIALTY EXCELLENCE
- GASTROINTESTINAL CARE
- GENERAL SURGERY
- PULMONARY CARE

Good Samaritan Hospital

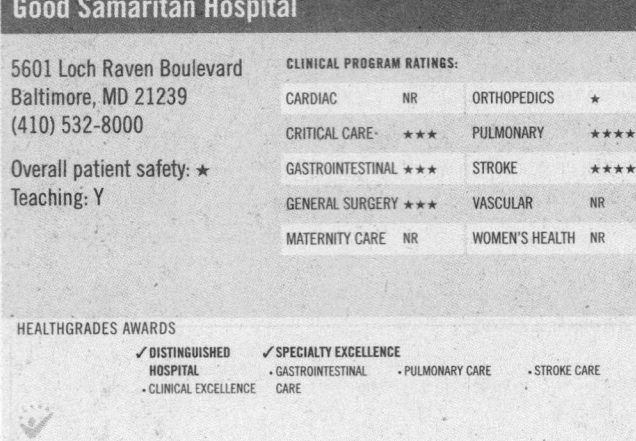

5601 Loch Raven Boulevard
Baltimore, MD 21239
(410) 532-8000

Overall patient safety: ★
Teaching: Y

CLINICAL PROGRAM RATINGS:

CARDIAC	NR	ORTHOPEDICS	★
CRITICAL CARE	★★★	PULMONARY	★★★★★
GASTROINTESTINAL	★★★	STROKE	★★★★★
GENERAL SURGERY	★★★	VASCULAR	NR
MATERNITY CARE	NR	WOMEN'S HEALTH	NR

HEALTHGRADES AWARDS

✓ DISTINGUISHED HOSPITAL
- CLINICAL EXCELLENCE

✓ SPECIALTY EXCELLENCE
- GASTROINTESTINAL CARE
- PULMONARY CARE
- STROKE CARE

Frederick Memorial Hospital

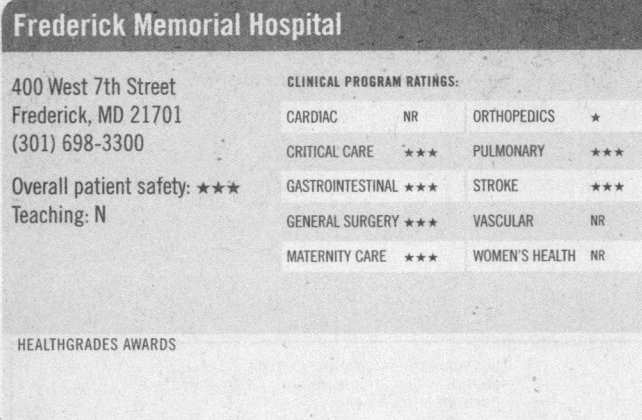

400 West 7th Street
Frederick, MD 21701
(301) 698-3300

Overall patient safety: ★★★
Teaching: N

CLINICAL PROGRAM RATINGS:

CARDIAC	NR	ORTHOPEDICS	★
CRITICAL CARE	★★★	PULMONARY	★★★
GASTROINTESTINAL	★★★	STROKE	★★★
GENERAL SURGERY	★★★	VASCULAR	NR
MATERNITY CARE	★★★	WOMEN'S HEALTH	NR

HEALTHGRADES AWARDS

Greater Baltimore Medical Center

6701 North Charles Street
Baltimore, MD 21204
(443) 849-2000

Overall patient safety: ★★★
Teaching: Y

CLINICAL PROGRAM RATINGS:

CARDIAC	NR	ORTHOPEDICS	★★★
CRITICAL CARE	★★★★★	PULMONARY	★★★★★
GASTROINTESTINAL	★★★★★	STROKE	★★★★★
GENERAL SURGERY	★★★	VASCULAR	★★★
MATERNITY CARE	★★★★★	WOMEN'S HEALTH	NR

HEALTHGRADES AWARDS

✓ DISTINGUISHED HOSPITAL
- CLINICAL EXCELLENCE

✓ SPECIALTY EXCELLENCE
- CRITICAL CARE
- GASTROINTESTINAL CARE
- MATERNITY CARE
- PULMONARY CARE
- STROKE CARE

Garrett County Memorial Hospital

251 North 4th Street
Oakland, MD 21550
(301) 533-4000

Overall patient safety: ★★★
Teaching: N

CLINICAL PROGRAM RATINGS:

CARDIAC	NR	ORTHOPEDICS	NR
CRITICAL CARE	NR	PULMONARY	★★★
GASTROINTESTINAL	NR	STROKE	★
GENERAL SURGERY	★★★	VASCULAR	NR
MATERNITY CARE	★★★	WOMEN'S HEALTH	NR

HEALTHGRADES AWARDS

Harbor Hospital

3001 South Hanover Street
Baltimore, MD 21225
(410) 350-3200

Overall patient safety: ★★★
Teaching: Y

CLINICAL PROGRAM RATINGS:

CARDIAC	NR	ORTHOPEDICS	★★★
CRITICAL CARE	★★★	PULMONARY	★★★★★
GASTROINTESTINAL	★★★	STROKE	★★★★★
GENERAL SURGERY	★★★	VASCULAR	NR
MATERNITY CARE	★★★	WOMEN'S HEALTH	NR

HEALTHGRADES AWARDS

✓ DISTINGUISHED HOSPITAL
- CLINICAL EXCELLENCE

✓ SPECIALTY EXCELLENCE
- STROKE CARE

KEY: ★★★★★ BEST   ★★★ AS EXPECTED   ★ POOR ◦ NR NOT RATED BY HEALTHGRADES   For full definitions of ratings and awards, see Appendix.

Harford Memorial Hospital

501 South Union Avenue
Havre De Grace, MD 21078
(443) 843-5000

Overall patient safety: ★★★
Teaching: N

CLINICAL PROGRAM RATINGS:

CARDIAC	NR	ORTHOPEDICS	NR
CRITICAL CARE	NR	PULMONARY	★★★
GASTROINTESTINAL	NR	STROKE	★★★
GENERAL SURGERY	★★★	VASCULAR	NR
MATERNITY CARE	NR	WOMEN'S HEALTH	NR

HEALTHGRADES AWARDS

Johns Hopkins Bayview Medical Center

4940 Eastern Avenue
Baltimore, MD 21224
(410) 550-0100

Overall patient safety: ★
Teaching: Y

CLINICAL PROGRAM RATINGS:

CARDIAC	NR	ORTHOPEDICS	★
CRITICAL CARE	★★★	PULMONARY	★★★★★
GASTROINTESTINAL	★★★	STROKE	★★★
GENERAL SURGERY	★	VASCULAR	NR
MATERNITY CARE	★★★	WOMEN'S HEALTH	NR

HEALTHGRADES AWARDS

✓ SPECIALTY EXCELLENCE
• BARIATRIC SURGERY • PULMONARY CARE

Holy Cross Hospital

1500 Forest Glen Road
Silver Spring, MD 20910
(301) 754-7000

Overall patient safety: ★★★
Teaching: Y

CLINICAL PROGRAM RATINGS:

CARDIAC	NR	ORTHOPEDICS	★
CRITICAL CARE	★★★	PULMONARY	★★★★★
GASTROINTESTINAL	★★★	STROKE	★★★★★
GENERAL SURGERY	★	VASCULAR	NR
MATERNITY CARE	★★★★★	WOMEN'S HEALTH	NR

HEALTHGRADES AWARDS

✓ SPECIALTY EXCELLENCE
• MATERNITY CARE • STROKE CARE

Johns Hopkins Hospital

600 North Wolfe Street
Baltimore, MD 21287
(410) 955-5000

Overall patient safety: ★
Teaching: Y

CLINICAL PROGRAM RATINGS:

CARDIAC	★★★	ORTHOPEDICS	NR
CRITICAL CARE	★★★	PULMONARY	★★★
GASTROINTESTINAL	★★★	STROKE	★★★
GENERAL SURGERY	★★★	VASCULAR	NR
MATERNITY CARE	★	WOMEN'S HEALTH	★★★

HEALTHGRADES AWARDS

Howard County General Hospital

5755 Cedar Lane
Columbia, MD 21044
(410) 740-7890

Overall patient safety: ★
Teaching: Y

CLINICAL PROGRAM RATINGS:

CARDIAC	NR	ORTHOPEDICS	★
CRITICAL CARE	★★★★★	PULMONARY	★★★★★
GASTROINTESTINAL	★★★	STROKE	★★★
GENERAL SURGERY	★	VASCULAR	NR
MATERNITY CARE	★★★	WOMEN'S HEALTH	NR

HEALTHGRADES AWARDS

✓ SPECIALTY EXCELLENCE
• CRITICAL CARE • PULMONARY CARE

Laurel Regional Hospital

7300 Van Dusen Road
Laurel, MD 20707
(301) 725-4300

Overall patient safety: ★★★
Teaching: N

CLINICAL PROGRAM RATINGS:

CARDIAC	NR	ORTHOPEDICS	NR
CRITICAL CARE	NR	PULMONARY	★★★
GASTROINTESTINAL	★★★	STROKE	★★★
GENERAL SURGERY	★★★	VASCULAR	NR
MATERNITY CARE	★★★	WOMEN'S HEALTH	NR

HEALTHGRADES AWARDS

MARYLAND HOSPITALS: RATINGS BY CLINICAL SPECIALTY

Maryland General Hospital

827 Linden Avenue
Baltimore, MD 21201
(410) 225-8000

Overall patient safety: ★★★
Teaching: Y

CLINICAL PROGRAM RATINGS:

CARDIAC	NR	ORTHOPEDICS	NR
CRITICAL CARE	NR	PULMONARY	★★★
GASTROINTESTINAL	NR	STROKE	★★★
GENERAL SURGERY	★★★	VASCULAR	NR
MATERNITY CARE	★	WOMEN'S HEALTH	NR

HEALTHGRADES AWARDS

Memorial Hospital at Easton

219 South Washington Street
Easton, MD 21601
(410) 822-1000

Overall patient safety: ★★★
Teaching: N

CLINICAL PROGRAM RATINGS:

CARDIAC	NR	ORTHOPEDICS	★
CRITICAL CARE	NR	PULMONARY	★★★
GASTROINTESTINAL	★★★	STROKE	★
GENERAL SURGERY	★★★	VASCULAR	NR
MATERNITY CARE	★★★	WOMEN'S HEALTH	NR

HEALTHGRADES AWARDS

McCready Memorial Hospital

201 Hall Highway
Crisfield, MD 21817
(410) 968-1200

Overall patient safety: ★★★
Teaching: N

CLINICAL PROGRAM RATINGS:

CARDIAC	NR	ORTHOPEDICS	NR
CRITICAL CARE	NR	PULMONARY	★★★
GASTROINTESTINAL	NR	STROKE	NR
GENERAL SURGERY	NR	VASCULAR	NR
MATERNITY CARE	NR	WOMEN'S HEALTH	NR

HEALTHGRADES AWARDS

Mercy Medical Center

301 St. Paul Place
Baltimore, MD 21202
(410) 332-9000

Overall patient safety: ★★★
Teaching: Y

CLINICAL PROGRAM RATINGS:

CARDIAC	NR	ORTHOPEDICS	★★★
CRITICAL CARE	★★★	PULMONARY	★★★★★
GASTROINTESTINAL	★★★	STROKE	★★★
GENERAL SURGERY	★★★	VASCULAR	★★★
MATERNITY CARE	★★★	WOMEN'S HEALTH	NR

HEALTHGRADES AWARDS

✓ SPECIALTY EXCELLENCE
• PULMONARY CARE

Memorial Hospital and Medical Center—Cumberland

600 Memorial Avenue
Cumberland, MD 21502
(301) 723-4000

Overall patient safety: ★
Teaching: N

CLINICAL PROGRAM RATINGS:

CARDIAC	NR	ORTHOPEDICS	★
CRITICAL CARE	NR	PULMONARY	★★★
GASTROINTESTINAL	★★★	STROKE	★★★
GENERAL SURGERY	★★★	VASCULAR	NR
MATERNITY CARE	★★★	WOMEN'S HEALTH	NR

HEALTHGRADES AWARDS

Montgomery General Hospital

18101 Prince Phillip Drive
Olney, MD 20832
(301) 774-8882

Overall patient safety: ★★★
Teaching: N

CLINICAL PROGRAM RATINGS:

CARDIAC	NR	ORTHOPEDICS	★★★
CRITICAL CARE	★★★	PULMONARY	★★★
GASTROINTESTINAL	★★★	STROKE	★
GENERAL SURGERY	★★★	VASCULAR	NR
MATERNITY CARE	★★★	WOMEN'S HEALTH	NR

HEALTHGRADES AWARDS

KEY: ★★★★★ BEST   ★★★ AS EXPECTED   ★ POOR   NR NOT RATED BY HEALTHGRADES   For full definitions of ratings and awards, see Appendix.

Northwest Hospital Center

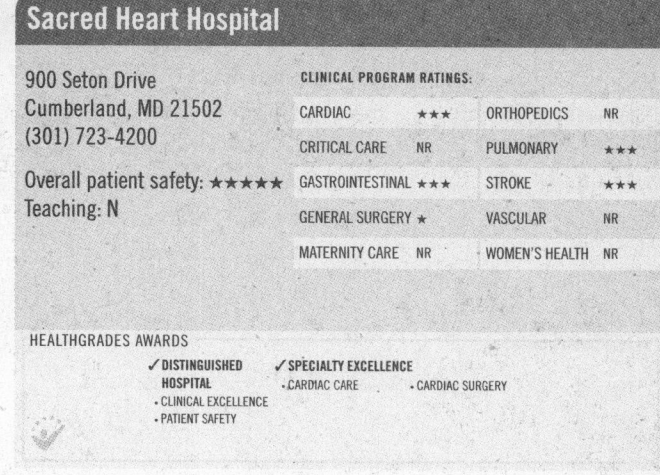

5401 Old Court Road
Randallstown, MD 21133
(410) 521-2200

Overall patient safety: ★★★
Teaching: N

CLINICAL PROGRAM RATINGS:

CARDIAC	NR	ORTHOPEDICS	★★★
CRITICAL CARE	★★★	PULMONARY	★★★★★
GASTROINTESTINAL	★★★	STROKE	★★★
GENERAL SURGERY	★★★	VASCULAR	NR
MATERNITY CARE	NR	WOMEN'S HEALTH	NR

HEALTHGRADES AWARDS

✓ SPECIALTY EXCELLENCE
· PULMONARY CARE

Sacred Heart Hospital

900 Seton Drive
Cumberland, MD 21502
(301) 723-4200

Overall patient safety: ★★★★★
Teaching: N

CLINICAL PROGRAM RATINGS:

CARDIAC	★★★	ORTHOPEDICS	NR
CRITICAL CARE	NR	PULMONARY	★★★
GASTROINTESTINAL	★★★	STROKE	★★★
GENERAL SURGERY	★	VASCULAR	NR
MATERNITY CARE	NR	WOMEN'S HEALTH	NR

HEALTHGRADES AWARDS

✓ DISTINGUISHED HOSPITAL
· CLINICAL EXCELLENCE
· PATIENT SAFETY

✓ SPECIALTY EXCELLENCE
· CARDIAC CARE   · CARDIAC SURGERY

Peninsula Regional Medical Center

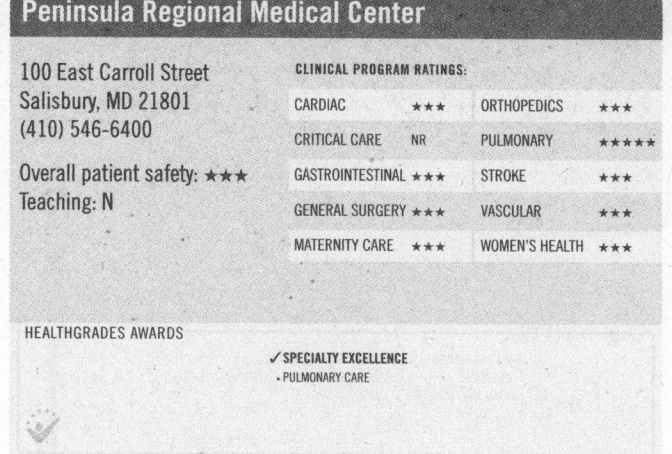

100 East Carroll Street
Salisbury, MD 21801
(410) 546-6400

Overall patient safety: ★★★
Teaching: N

CLINICAL PROGRAM RATINGS:

CARDIAC	★★★	ORTHOPEDICS	★★★
CRITICAL CARE	NR	PULMONARY	★★★★★
GASTROINTESTINAL	★★★	STROKE	★★★
GENERAL SURGERY	★★★	VASCULAR	★★★
MATERNITY CARE	★★★	WOMEN'S HEALTH	★★★

HEALTHGRADES AWARDS

✓ SPECIALTY EXCELLENCE
· PULMONARY CARE

St. Agnes Hospital

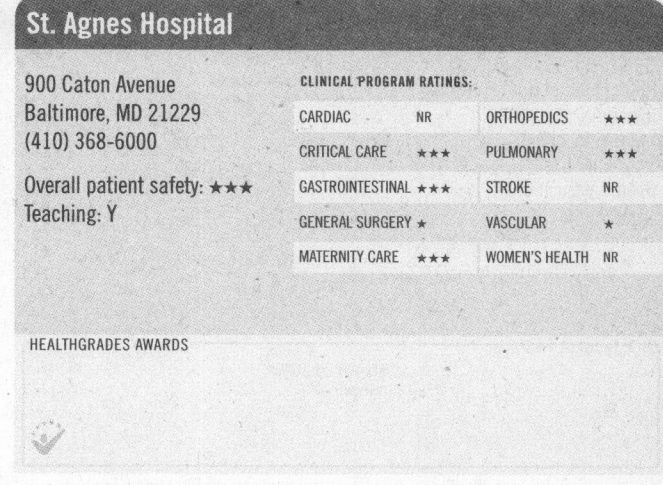

900 Caton Avenue
Baltimore, MD 21229
(410) 368-6000

Overall patient safety: ★★★
Teaching: Y

CLINICAL PROGRAM RATINGS:

CARDIAC	NR	ORTHOPEDICS	★★★
CRITICAL CARE	★★★	PULMONARY	★★★
GASTROINTESTINAL	★★★	STROKE	NR
GENERAL SURGERY	★	VASCULAR	★
MATERNITY CARE	★★★	WOMEN'S HEALTH	NR

HEALTHGRADES AWARDS

Prince George's Hospital Center

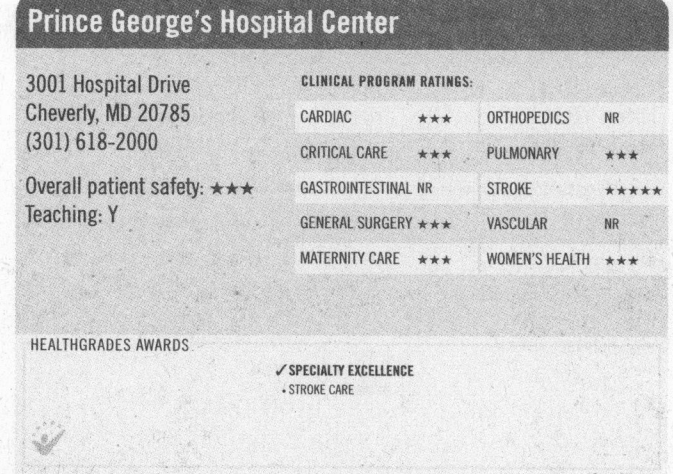

3001 Hospital Drive
Cheverly, MD 20785
(301) 618-2000

Overall patient safety: ★★★
Teaching: Y

CLINICAL PROGRAM RATINGS:

CARDIAC	★★★	ORTHOPEDICS	NR
CRITICAL CARE	★★★	PULMONARY	★★★
GASTROINTESTINAL	NR	STROKE	★★★★★
GENERAL SURGERY	★★★	VASCULAR	NR
MATERNITY CARE	★★★	WOMEN'S HEALTH	★★★

HEALTHGRADES AWARDS

✓ SPECIALTY EXCELLENCE
· STROKE CARE

St. Joseph Medical Center

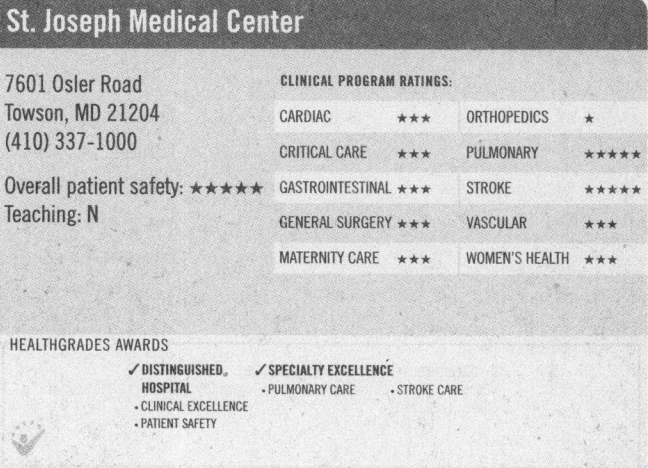

7601 Osler Road
Towson, MD 21204
(410) 337-1000

Overall patient safety: ★★★★★
Teaching: N

CLINICAL PROGRAM RATINGS:

CARDIAC	★★★	ORTHOPEDICS	★
CRITICAL CARE	★★★	PULMONARY	★★★★★
GASTROINTESTINAL	★★★	STROKE	★★★★★
GENERAL SURGERY	★★★	VASCULAR	★★★
MATERNITY CARE	★★★	WOMEN'S HEALTH	★★★

HEALTHGRADES AWARDS

✓ DISTINGUISHED HOSPITAL
· CLINICAL EXCELLENCE
· PATIENT SAFETY

✓ SPECIALTY EXCELLENCE
· PULMONARY CARE   · STROKE CARE

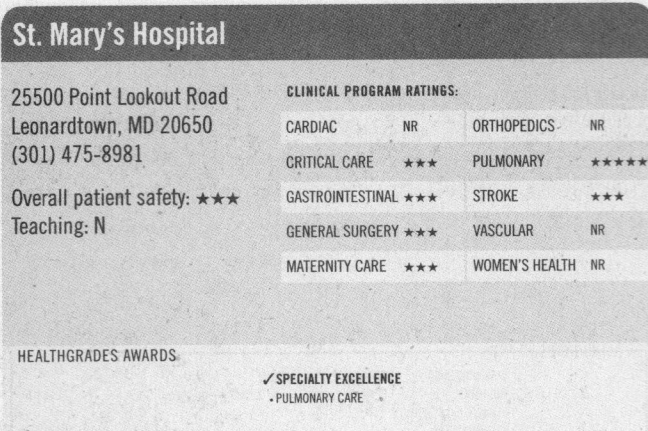

St. Mary's Hospital

25500 Point Lookout Road
Leonardtown, MD 20650
(301) 475-8981

Overall patient safety: ★★★
Teaching: N

CLINICAL PROGRAM RATINGS:

CARDIAC	NR	ORTHOPEDICS	NR
CRITICAL CARE	★★★	PULMONARY	★★★★★
GASTROINTESTINAL	★★★	STROKE	★★★
GENERAL SURGERY	★★★	VASCULAR	NR
MATERNITY CARE	★★★	WOMEN'S HEALTH	NR

HEALTHGRADES AWARDS

✓ SPECIALTY EXCELLENCE
· PULMONARY CARE

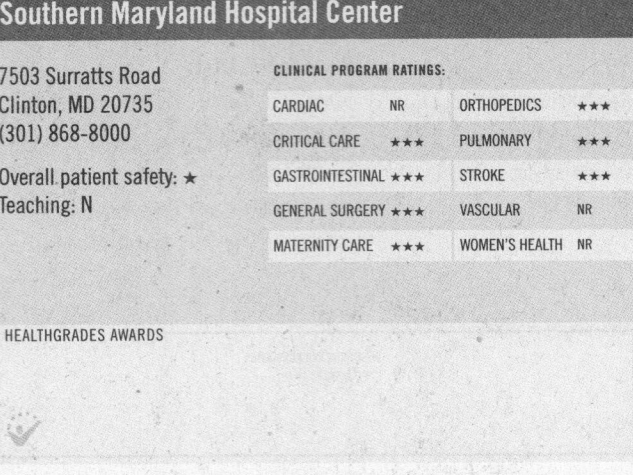

Southern Maryland Hospital Center

7503 Surratts Road
Clinton, MD 20735
(301) 868-8000

Overall patient safety: ★
Teaching: N

CLINICAL PROGRAM RATINGS:

CARDIAC	NR	ORTHOPEDICS	★★★
CRITICAL CARE	★★★	PULMONARY	★★★
GASTROINTESTINAL	★★★	STROKE	★★★
GENERAL SURGERY	★★★	VASCULAR	NR
MATERNITY CARE	★★★	WOMEN'S HEALTH	NR

HEALTHGRADES AWARDS

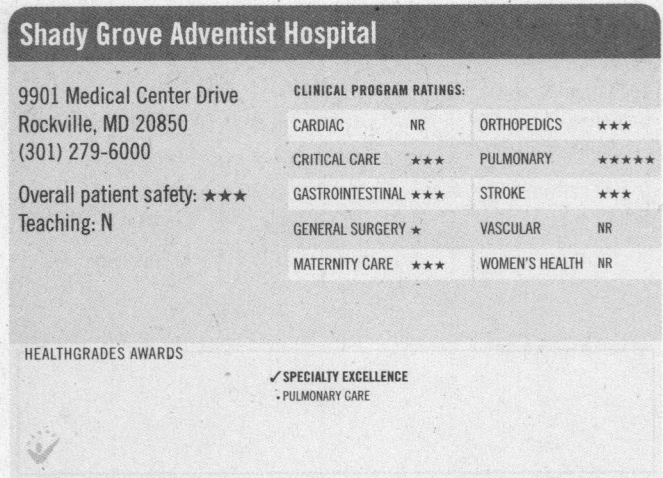

Shady Grove Adventist Hospital

9901 Medical Center Drive
Rockville, MD 20850
(301) 279-6000

Overall patient safety: ★★★
Teaching: N

CLINICAL PROGRAM RATINGS:

CARDIAC	NR	ORTHOPEDICS	★★★
CRITICAL CARE	★★★	PULMONARY	★★★★★
GASTROINTESTINAL	★★★	STROKE	★★★
GENERAL SURGERY	★	VASCULAR	NR
MATERNITY CARE	★★★	WOMEN'S HEALTH	NR

HEALTHGRADES AWARDS

✓ SPECIALTY EXCELLENCE
· PULMONARY CARE

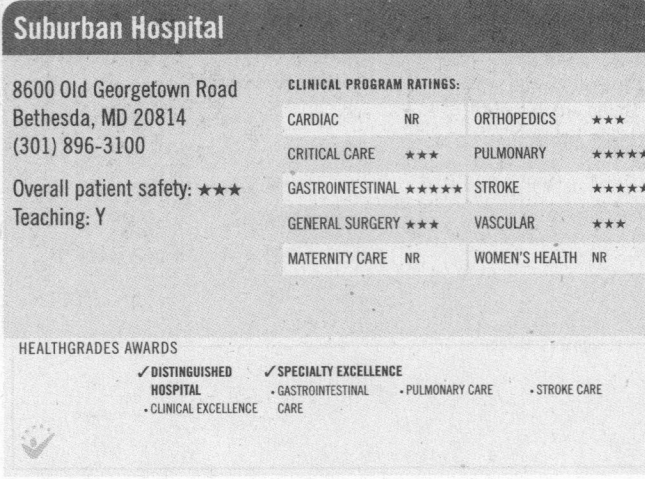

Suburban Hospital

8600 Old Georgetown Road
Bethesda, MD 20814
(301) 896-3100

Overall patient safety: ★★★
Teaching: Y

CLINICAL PROGRAM RATINGS:

CARDIAC	NR	ORTHOPEDICS	★★★
CRITICAL CARE	★★★	PULMONARY	★★★★★
GASTROINTESTINAL	★★★★★	STROKE	★★★★★
GENERAL SURGERY	★★★	VASCULAR	★★★
MATERNITY CARE	NR	WOMEN'S HEALTH	NR

HEALTHGRADES AWARDS

✓ DISTINGUISHED HOSPITAL
· CLINICAL EXCELLENCE

✓ SPECIALTY EXCELLENCE
· GASTROINTESTINAL CARE · PULMONARY CARE · STROKE CARE

Sinai Hospital of Baltimore

2401 West Belvedere Avenue
Baltimore, MD 21215
(410) 601-9000

Overall patient safety: ★
Teaching: Y

CLINICAL PROGRAM RATINGS:

CARDIAC	★★★	ORTHOPEDICS	★
CRITICAL CARE	★★★★★	PULMONARY	★★★
GASTROINTESTINAL	★★★	STROKE	★★★★★
GENERAL SURGERY	★★★	VASCULAR	NR
MATERNITY CARE	★★★	WOMEN'S HEALTH	★★★

HEALTHGRADES AWARDS

✓ DISTINGUISHED HOSPITAL
· CLINICAL EXCELLENCE

✓ SPECIALTY EXCELLENCE
· CRITICAL CARE · GASTROINTESTINAL CARE · STROKE CARE

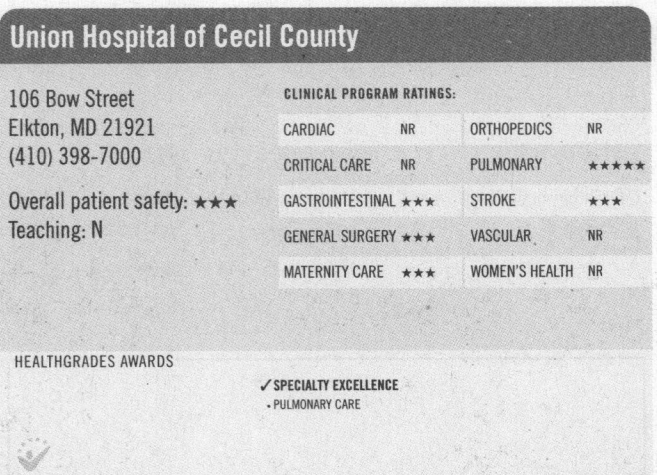

Union Hospital of Cecil County

106 Bow Street
Elkton, MD 21921
(410) 398-7000

Overall patient safety: ★★★
Teaching: N

CLINICAL PROGRAM RATINGS:

CARDIAC	NR	ORTHOPEDICS	NR
CRITICAL CARE	NR	PULMONARY	★★★★★
GASTROINTESTINAL	★★★	STROKE	★★★
GENERAL SURGERY	★★★	VASCULAR	NR
MATERNITY CARE	★★★	WOMEN'S HEALTH	NR

HEALTHGRADES AWARDS

✓ SPECIALTY EXCELLENCE
· PULMONARY CARE

KEY: ★★★★★ BEST ★★★ AS EXPECTED ★ POOR NR NOT RATED BY HEALTHGRADES For full definitions of ratings and awards, see Appendix.

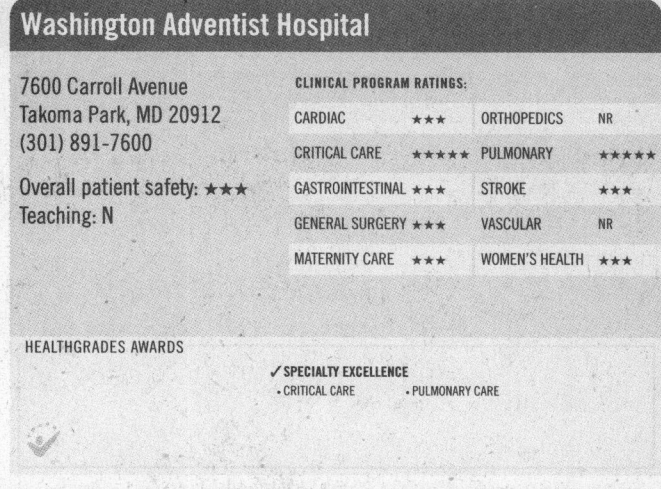

Union Memorial Hospital

201 East University Parkway
Baltimore, MD 21218
(410) 554-2000

Overall patient safety: ★★★
Teaching: Y

CLINICAL PROGRAM RATINGS:

CARDIAC	★★★	ORTHOPEDICS	★★★
CRITICAL CARE	★★★	PULMONARY	★★★
GASTROINTESTINAL	★★★	STROKE	★★★
GENERAL SURGERY	★★★	VASCULAR	★★★
MATERNITY CARE	NR	WOMEN'S HEALTH	NR

HEALTHGRADES AWARDS

Washington Adventist Hospital

7600 Carroll Avenue
Takoma Park, MD 20912
(301) 891-7600

Overall patient safety: ★★★
Teaching: N

CLINICAL PROGRAM RATINGS:

CARDIAC	★★★	ORTHOPEDICS	NR
CRITICAL CARE	★★★★★	PULMONARY	★★★★★
GASTROINTESTINAL	★★★	STROKE	★★★
GENERAL SURGERY	★★★	VASCULAR	NR
MATERNITY CARE	★★★	WOMEN'S HEALTH	★★★

HEALTHGRADES AWARDS

✓ SPECIALTY EXCELLENCE
- CRITICAL CARE   - PULMONARY CARE

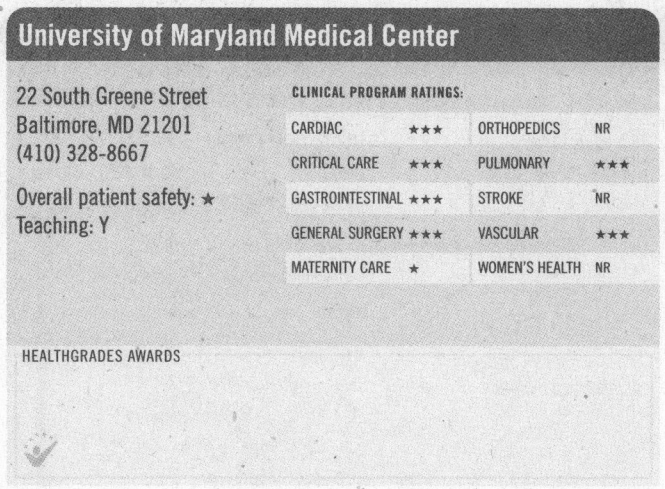

University of Maryland Medical Center

22 South Greene Street
Baltimore, MD 21201
(410) 328-8667

Overall patient safety: ★
Teaching: Y

CLINICAL PROGRAM RATINGS:

CARDIAC	★★★	ORTHOPEDICS	NR
CRITICAL CARE	★★★	PULMONARY	★★★
GASTROINTESTINAL	★★★	STROKE	NR
GENERAL SURGERY	★★★	VASCULAR	★★★
MATERNITY CARE	★	WOMEN'S HEALTH	NR

HEALTHGRADES AWARDS

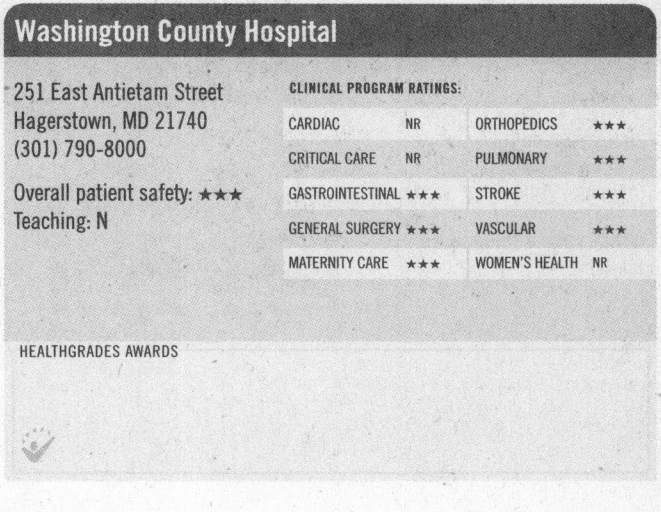

Washington County Hospital

251 East Antietam Street
Hagerstown, MD 21740
(301) 790-8000

Overall patient safety: ★★★
Teaching: N

CLINICAL PROGRAM RATINGS:

CARDIAC	NR	ORTHOPEDICS	★★★
CRITICAL CARE	NR	PULMONARY	★★★
GASTROINTESTINAL	★★★	STROKE	★★★
GENERAL SURGERY	★★★	VASCULAR	★★★
MATERNITY CARE	★★★	WOMEN'S HEALTH	NR

HEALTHGRADES AWARDS

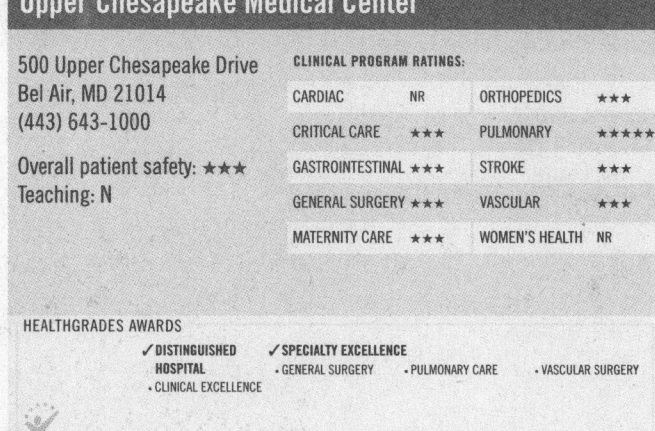

Upper Chesapeake Medical Center

500 Upper Chesapeake Drive
Bel Air, MD 21014
(443) 643-1000

Overall patient safety: ★★★
Teaching: N

CLINICAL PROGRAM RATINGS:

CARDIAC	NR	ORTHOPEDICS	★★★
CRITICAL CARE	★★★	PULMONARY	★★★★★
GASTROINTESTINAL	★★★	STROKE	★★★
GENERAL SURGERY	★★★	VASCULAR	★★★
MATERNITY CARE	★★★	WOMEN'S HEALTH	NR

HEALTHGRADES AWARDS

✓ DISTINGUISHED HOSPITAL
- CLINICAL EXCELLENCE

✓ SPECIALTY EXCELLENCE
- GENERAL SURGERY   - PULMONARY CARE   - VASCULAR SURGERY

Addison Gilbert Hospital*

298 Washington Street
Gloucester, MA 01930
(978) 283-4000

Overall patient safety: ★★★
Teaching: Y

CLINICAL PROGRAM RATINGS:

CARDIAC	NR	ORTHOPEDICS	NR
CRITICAL CARE	★★★	PULMONARY	★★★★★
GASTROINTESTINAL	★★★	STROKE	★★★
GENERAL SURGERY	★★★	VASCULAR	NR
MATERNITY CARE	★★★	WOMEN'S HEALTH	NR

HEALTHGRADES AWARDS

Atlanticare Medical Center—Union*

500 Lynnfield Street
Lynn, MA 01904
(781) 581-9200

Overall patient safety: ★★★★★
Teaching: Y

CLINICAL PROGRAM RATINGS:

CARDIAC	★★★	ORTHOPEDICS	★★★
CRITICAL CARE	★★★	PULMONARY	★★★★★
GASTROINTESTINAL	★★★	STROKE	★★★★★
GENERAL SURGERY	★★★	VASCULAR	★★★
MATERNITY CARE	★★★	WOMEN'S HEALTH	★★★

HEALTHGRADES AWARDS

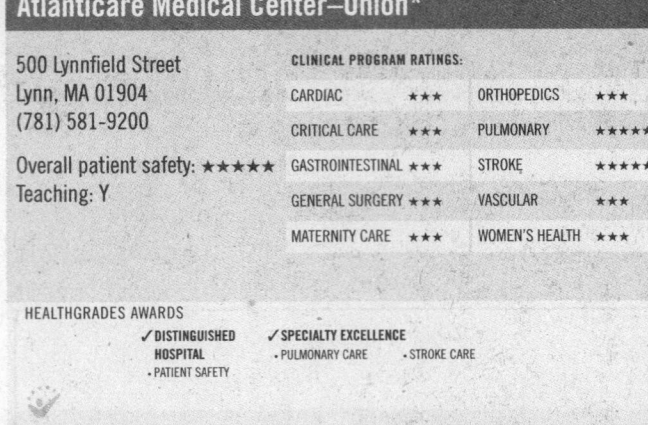

✓ DISTINGUISHED HOSPITAL · PATIENT SAFETY   ✓ SPECIALTY EXCELLENCE · PULMONARY CARE · STROKE CARE

Anna Jaques Hospital

25 Highland Avenue
Newburyport, MA 01950
(978) 463-1000

Overall patient safety: ★★★
Teaching: N

CLINICAL PROGRAM RATINGS:

CARDIAC	NR	ORTHOPEDICS	NR
CRITICAL CARE	NR	PULMONARY	★★★
GASTROINTESTINAL	NR	STROKE	★★★
GENERAL SURGERY	★★★	VASCULAR	NR
MATERNITY CARE	★★★	WOMEN'S HEALTH	NR

HEALTHGRADES AWARDS

Baystate Franklin Medical Center

164 High Street
Greenfield, MA 01301
(413) 773-0211

Overall patient safety: ★★★★★
Teaching: N

CLINICAL PROGRAM RATINGS:

CARDIAC	NR	ORTHOPEDICS	NR
CRITICAL CARE	NR	PULMONARY	★★★
GASTROINTESTINAL	NR	STROKE	★
GENERAL SURGERY	★★★	VASCULAR	NR
MATERNITY CARE	★★★	WOMEN'S HEALTH	NR

HEALTHGRADES AWARDS

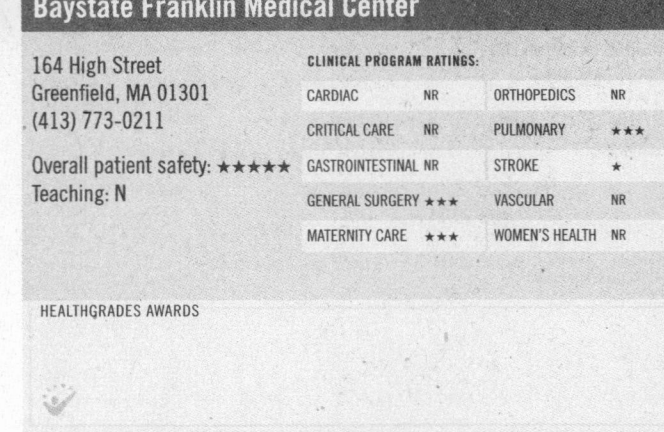

Athol Memorial Hospital

2033 Main Street
Athol, MA 01331
(978) 249-3511

Overall patient safety: ★★★
Teaching: N

CLINICAL PROGRAM RATINGS:

CARDIAC	NR	ORTHOPEDICS	NR
CRITICAL CARE	NR	PULMONARY	★★★
GASTROINTESTINAL	NR	STROKE	NR
GENERAL SURGERY	NR	VASCULAR	NR
MATERNITY CARE	NR	WOMEN'S HEALTH	NR

HEALTHGRADES AWARDS

Baystate Mary Lane Hospital

85 South Street
Ware, MA 01082
(413) 967-6211

Overall patient safety: ★★★
Teaching: N

CLINICAL PROGRAM RATINGS:

CARDIAC	NR	ORTHOPEDICS	NR
CRITICAL CARE	NR	PULMONARY	★★★
GASTROINTESTINAL	NR	STROKE	★★★
GENERAL SURGERY	NR	VASCULAR	NR
MATERNITY CARE	★	WOMEN'S HEALTH	NR

HEALTHGRADES AWARDS

KEY: ★★★★★ BEST   ★★★ AS EXPECTED   ★ POOR   NR NOT RATED BY HEALTHGRADES   For full definitions of ratings and awards, see Appendix.

Baystate Medical Center

759 Chestnut Street
Springfield, MA 01199
(413) 794-0000

Overall patient safety: ★★★
Teaching: Y

CLINICAL PROGRAM RATINGS:

CARDIAC	★★★★★	ORTHOPEDICS	★★★
CRITICAL CARE	★★★	PULMONARY	★★★
GASTROINTESTINAL	★★★	STROKE	★
GENERAL SURGERY	★★★	VASCULAR	★★★
MATERNITY CARE	★★★	WOMEN'S HEALTH	★★★

HEALTHGRADES AWARDS

✓ SPECIALTY EXCELLENCE
· CARDIAC CARE · CARDIAC SURGERY · VASCULAR SURGERY

Beth Israel Deaconess Medical Center

330 Brookline Avenue
Boston, MA 02215
(617) 667-7000

Overall patient safety: ★★★
Teaching: Y

CLINICAL PROGRAM RATINGS:

CARDIAC	★★★	ORTHOPEDICS	★
CRITICAL CARE	★★★	PULMONARY	★★★★★
GASTROINTESTINAL	★★★	STROKE	★★★
GENERAL SURGERY	★★★	VASCULAR	★★★
MATERNITY CARE	★★★	WOMEN'S HEALTH	★★★

HEALTHGRADES AWARDS

✓ SPECIALTY EXCELLENCE
· CARDIAC SURGERY

Berkshire Medical Center*

725 North Street
Pittsfield, MA 01201
(413) 447-2000

Overall patient safety: ★★★
Teaching: Y

CLINICAL PROGRAM RATINGS:

CARDIAC	NR	ORTHOPEDICS	★★★
CRITICAL CARE	★★★	PULMONARY	★★★
GASTROINTESTINAL	★★★	STROKE	★★★
GENERAL SURGERY	★★★	VASCULAR	NR
MATERNITY CARE	★★★	WOMEN'S HEALTH	NR

HEALTHGRADES AWARDS

Beverly Hospital*

85 Herrick Street
Beverly, MA 01915
(978) 922-3000

Overall patient safety: ★★★
Teaching: Y

CLINICAL PROGRAM RATINGS:

CARDIAC	NR	ORTHOPEDICS	NR
CRITICAL CARE	★★★	PULMONARY	★★★★★
GASTROINTESTINAL	★★★	STROKE	★★★
GENERAL SURGERY	★★★	VASCULAR	NR
MATERNITY CARE	★★★	WOMEN'S HEALTH	NR

HEALTHGRADES AWARDS

Beth Israel Deaconess Hospital—Needham

148 Chestnut Street
Needham, MA 02492
(781) 453-3000

Overall patient safety: ★★★
Teaching: Y

CLINICAL PROGRAM RATINGS:

CARDIAC	NR	ORTHOPEDICS	NR
CRITICAL CARE	NR	PULMONARY	★★★
GASTROINTESTINAL	NR	STROKE	NR
GENERAL SURGERY	NR	VASCULAR	NR
MATERNITY CARE	NR	WOMEN'S HEALTH	NR

HEALTHGRADES AWARDS

Boston Medical Center

1 Boston Medical Center Place
Boston, MA 02118
(617) 638-8000

Overall patient safety: ★★★
Teaching: Y

CLINICAL PROGRAM RATINGS:

CARDIAC	★★★	ORTHOPEDICS	★★★
CRITICAL CARE	★★★	PULMONARY	★★★★★
GASTROINTESTINAL	★★★	STROKE	★★★
GENERAL SURGERY	★★★	VASCULAR	★★★
MATERNITY CARE	★	WOMEN'S HEALTH	★

HEALTHGRADES AWARDS

*This hospital reports its data to the federal government jointly with another hospital. Therefore the ratings and awards apply to multiple hospitals and this specific hospital may not provide all rated services.

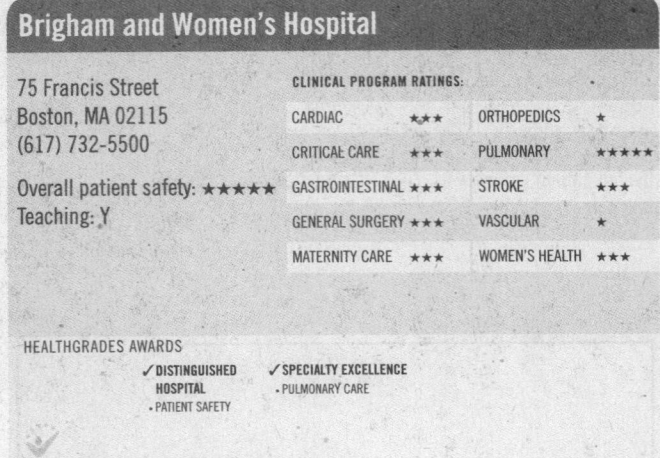

Brigham and Women's Hospital

75 Francis Street
Boston, MA 02115
(617) 732-5500

Overall patient safety: ★★★★★
Teaching: Y

CLINICAL PROGRAM RATINGS:

CARDIAC	★★★	ORTHOPEDICS	★
CRITICAL CARE	★★★	PULMONARY	★★★★★
GASTROINTESTINAL	★★★	STROKE	★★★
GENERAL SURGERY	★★★	VASCULAR	★
MATERNITY CARE	★★★	WOMEN'S HEALTH	★★★

HEALTHGRADES AWARDS

✓ DISTINGUISHED HOSPITAL
 • PATIENT SAFETY

✓ SPECIALTY EXCELLENCE
 • PULMONARY CARE

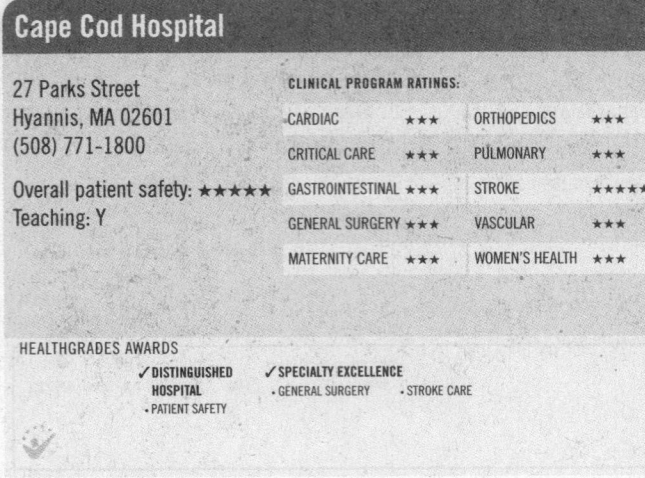

Cape Cod Hospital

27 Parks Street
Hyannis, MA 02601
(508) 771-1800

Overall patient safety: ★★★★★
Teaching: Y

CLINICAL PROGRAM RATINGS:

CARDIAC	★★★	ORTHOPEDICS	★★★
CRITICAL CARE	★★★	PULMONARY	★★★
GASTROINTESTINAL	★★★	STROKE	★★★★★
GENERAL SURGERY	★★★	VASCULAR	★★★
MATERNITY CARE	★★★	WOMEN'S HEALTH	★★★

HEALTHGRADES AWARDS

✓ DISTINGUISHED HOSPITAL
 • PATIENT SAFETY

✓ SPECIALTY EXCELLENCE
 • GENERAL SURGERY   • STROKE CARE

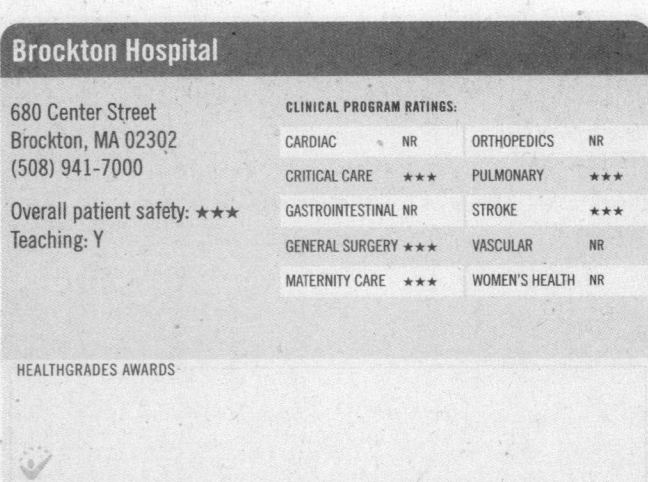

Brockton Hospital

680 Center Street
Brockton, MA 02302
(508) 941-7000

Overall patient safety: ★★★
Teaching: Y

CLINICAL PROGRAM RATINGS:

CARDIAC	NR	ORTHOPEDICS	NR
CRITICAL CARE	★★★	PULMONARY	★★★
GASTROINTESTINAL	NR	STROKE	★★★
GENERAL SURGERY	★★★	VASCULAR	NR
MATERNITY CARE	★★★	WOMEN'S HEALTH	NR

HEALTHGRADES AWARDS

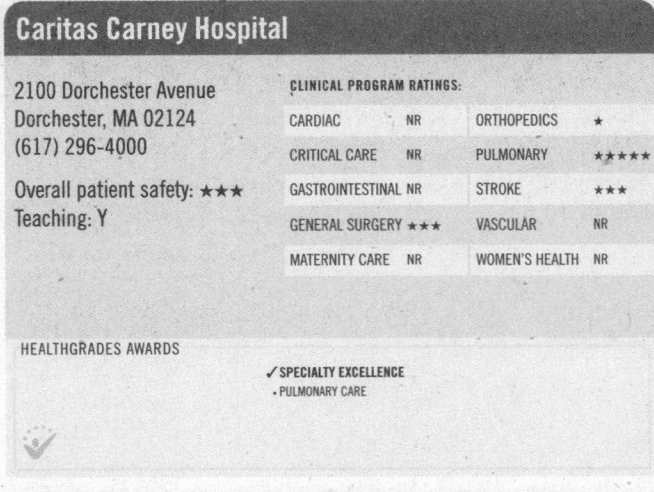

Caritas Carney Hospital

2100 Dorchester Avenue
Dorchester, MA 02124
(617) 296-4000

Overall patient safety: ★★★
Teaching: Y

CLINICAL PROGRAM RATINGS:

CARDIAC	NR	ORTHOPEDICS	★
CRITICAL CARE	NR	PULMONARY	★★★★★
GASTROINTESTINAL	NR	STROKE	★★★
GENERAL SURGERY	★★★	VASCULAR	NR
MATERNITY CARE	NR	WOMEN'S HEALTH	NR

HEALTHGRADES AWARDS

✓ SPECIALTY EXCELLENCE
 • PULMONARY CARE

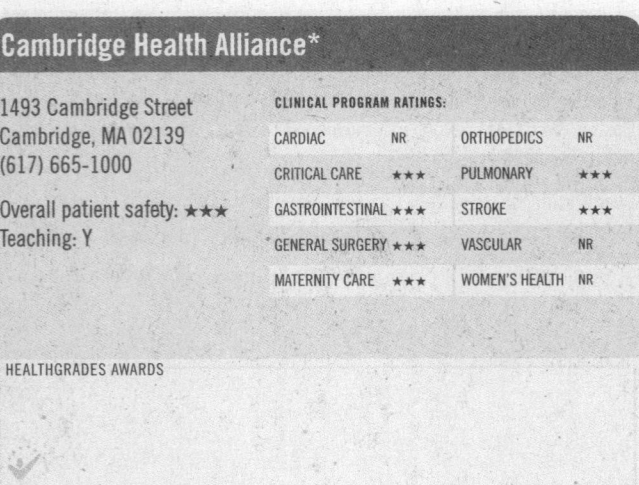

Cambridge Health Alliance*

1493 Cambridge Street
Cambridge, MA 02139
(617) 665-1000

Overall patient safety: ★★★
Teaching: Y

CLINICAL PROGRAM RATINGS:

CARDIAC	NR	ORTHOPEDICS	NR
CRITICAL CARE	★★★	PULMONARY	★★★
GASTROINTESTINAL	★★★	STROKE	★★★
GENERAL SURGERY	★★★	VASCULAR	NR
MATERNITY CARE	★★★	WOMEN'S HEALTH	NR

HEALTHGRADES AWARDS

Caritas Good Samaritan Medical Center

235 North Pearl Street
Brockton, MA 02301
(508) 427-3000

Overall patient safety: ★★★
Teaching: Y

CLINICAL PROGRAM RATINGS:

CARDIAC	NR	ORTHOPEDICS	NR
CRITICAL CARE	★★★	PULMONARY	★★★
GASTROINTESTINAL	★★★	STROKE	★★★
GENERAL SURGERY	★★★	VASCULAR	NR
MATERNITY CARE	★★★	WOMEN'S HEALTH	NR

HEALTHGRADES AWARDS

KEY: ★★★★★ BEST   ★★★ AS EXPECTED   ★ POOR   NR NOT RATED BY HEALTHGRADES   For full definitions of ratings and awards, see Appendix.

Caritas Holy Family Hospital and Medical Center

70 East Street
Methuen, MA 01844
(978) 687-0151

Overall patient safety: ★★★
Teaching: N

CLINICAL PROGRAM RATINGS:

CARDIAC	NR	ORTHOPEDICS	★★★
CRITICAL CARE	★	PULMONARY	★★★
GASTROINTESTINAL	★★★	STROKE	★
GENERAL SURGERY	★★★	VASCULAR	NR
MATERNITY CARE	★★★	WOMEN'S HEALTH	NR

HEALTHGRADES AWARDS

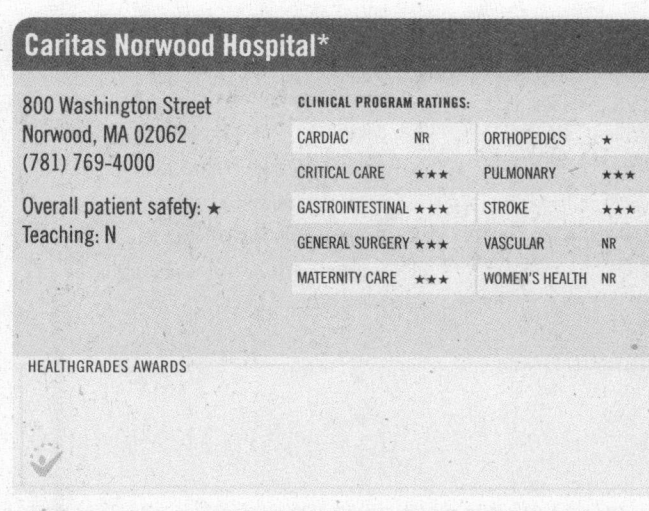

Caritas St. Elizabeth's Medical Center

736 Cambridge Street
Boston, MA 02135
(617) 789-3000

Overall patient safety: ★★★
Teaching: Y

CLINICAL PROGRAM RATINGS:

CARDIAC	★★★	ORTHOPEDICS	★★★
CRITICAL CARE	★★★	PULMONARY	★★★
GASTROINTESTINAL	★★★	STROKE	★★★
GENERAL SURGERY	★★★	VASCULAR	NR
MATERNITY CARE	★	WOMEN'S HEALTH	★

HEALTHGRADES AWARDS

Caritas Norwood Hospital*

800 Washington Street
Norwood, MA 02062
(781) 769-4000

Overall patient safety: ★
Teaching: N

CLINICAL PROGRAM RATINGS:

CARDIAC	NR	ORTHOPEDICS	★
CRITICAL CARE	★★★	PULMONARY	★★★
GASTROINTESTINAL	★★★	STROKE	★★★
GENERAL SURGERY	★★★	VASCULAR	NR
MATERNITY CARE	★★★	WOMEN'S HEALTH	NR

HEALTHGRADES AWARDS

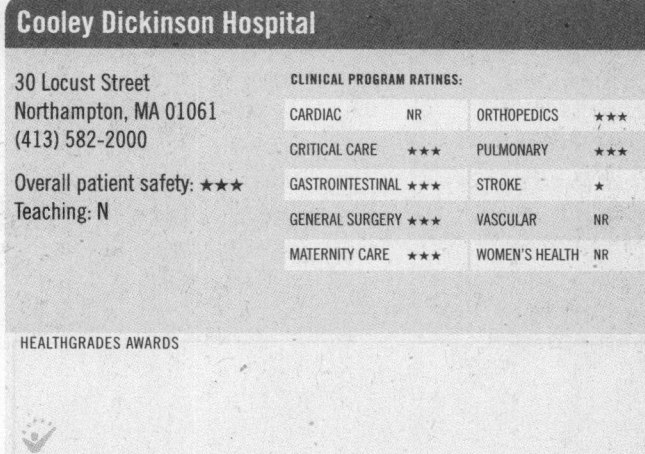

Cooley Dickinson Hospital

30 Locust Street
Northampton, MA 01061
(413) 582-2000

Overall patient safety: ★★★
Teaching: N

CLINICAL PROGRAM RATINGS:

CARDIAC	NR	ORTHOPEDICS	★★★
CRITICAL CARE	★★★	PULMONARY	★★★
GASTROINTESTINAL	★★★	STROKE	★
GENERAL SURGERY	★★★	VASCULAR	NR
MATERNITY CARE	★★★	WOMEN'S HEALTH	NR

HEALTHGRADES AWARDS

Caritas Southwood Hospital*

111 Dedham Street
Norfolk, MA 02056
(508) 668-0385

Overall patient safety: ★
Teaching: N

CLINICAL PROGRAM RATINGS:

CARDIAC	NR	ORTHOPEDICS	★
CRITICAL CARE	★★★	PULMONARY	★★★
GASTROINTESTINAL	★★★	STROKE	★★★
GENERAL SURGERY	★★★	VASCULAR	NR
MATERNITY CARE	★★★	WOMEN'S HEALTH	NR

HEALTHGRADES AWARDS

Emerson Hospital

133 Old Road to
Nine Acre Corner
Concord, MA 01742
(978) 369-1400

Overall patient safety: ★★★
Teaching: N

CLINICAL PROGRAM RATINGS:

CARDIAC	NR	ORTHOPEDICS	★★★
CRITICAL CARE	NR	PULMONARY	★★★
GASTROINTESTINAL	NR	STROKE	★★★★★
GENERAL SURGERY	★★★	VASCULAR	NR
MATERNITY CARE	★★★★★	WOMEN'S HEALTH	NR

HEALTHGRADES AWARDS

✓ SPECIALTY EXCELLENCE
• MATERNITY CARE • STROKE CARE

*This hospital reports its data to the federal government jointly with another hospital. Therefore the ratings and awards apply to multiple hospitals and this specific hospital may not provide all rated services.

Falmouth Hospital

100 Terrace Heun Drive
Falmouth, MA 02540
(508) 548-5300

Overall patient safety: ★★★
Teaching: N

CLINICAL PROGRAM RATINGS:

CARDIAC	NR	ORTHOPEDICS	NR
CRITICAL CARE	NR	PULMONARY	★★★
GASTROINTESTINAL	★★★	STROKE	★★★
GENERAL SURGERY	★★★	VASCULAR	NR
MATERNITY CARE	★★★	WOMEN'S HEALTH	NR

HEALTHGRADES AWARDS

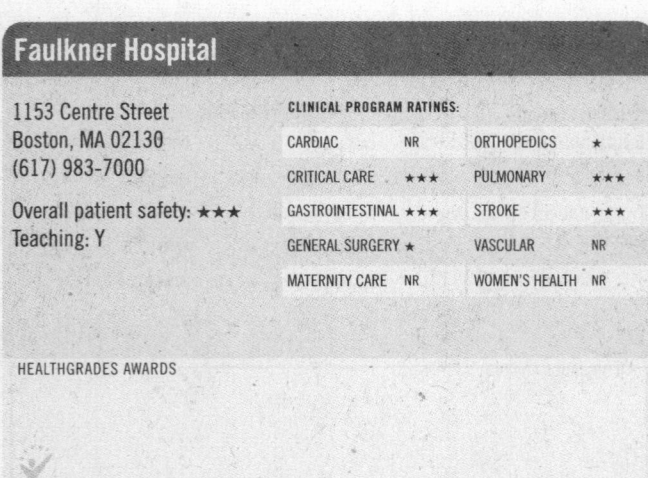

Harrington Memorial Hospital

100 South Street
Southbridge, MA 01550
(508) 765-9771

Overall patient safety: ★★★
Teaching: N

CLINICAL PROGRAM RATINGS:

CARDIAC	NR	ORTHOPEDICS	NR
CRITICAL CARE	NR	PULMONARY	★★★
GASTROINTESTINAL	NR	STROKE	★
GENERAL SURGERY	NR	VASCULAR	NR
MATERNITY CARE	★★★	WOMEN'S HEALTH	NR

HEALTHGRADES AWARDS

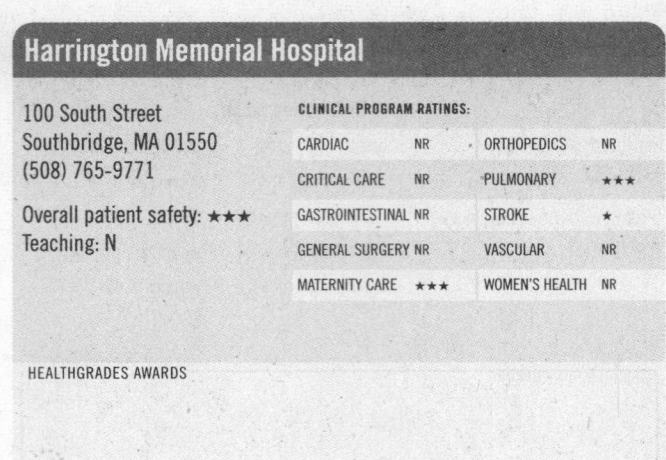

Faulkner Hospital

1153 Centre Street
Boston, MA 02130
(617) 983-7000

Overall patient safety: ★★★
Teaching: Y

CLINICAL PROGRAM RATINGS:

CARDIAC	NR	ORTHOPEDICS	★
CRITICAL CARE	★★★	PULMONARY	★★★
GASTROINTESTINAL	★★★	STROKE	★★★
GENERAL SURGERY	★	VASCULAR	NR
MATERNITY CARE	NR	WOMEN'S HEALTH	NR

HEALTHGRADES AWARDS

HealthAlliance Hospital Burbank Campus*

275 Nichols Road
Fitchburg, MA 01420
(978) 343-5000

Overall patient safety: ★★★
Teaching: Y

CLINICAL PROGRAM RATINGS:

CARDIAC	NR	ORTHOPEDICS	NR
CRITICAL CARE	NR	PULMONARY	★★★
GASTROINTESTINAL	NR	STROKE	★★★
GENERAL SURGERY	NR	VASCULAR	NR
MATERNITY CARE	★★★	WOMEN'S HEALTH	NR

HEALTHGRADES AWARDS

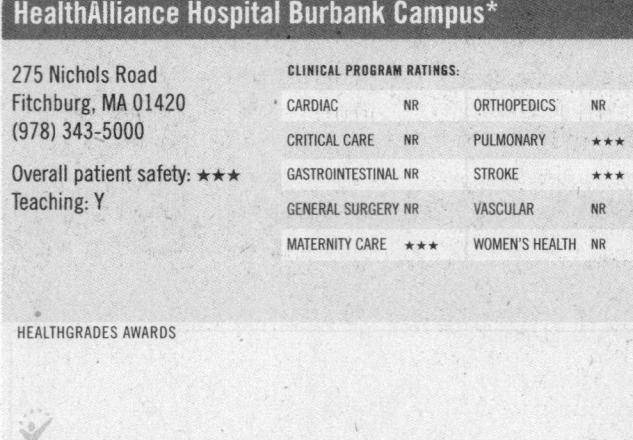

Hallmark Health*

170 Governors Avenue
Medford, MA 02155
(781) 306-6000

Overall patient safety: ★★★
Teaching: Y

CLINICAL PROGRAM RATINGS:

CARDIAC	NR	ORTHOPEDICS	★★★
CRITICAL CARE	★★★	PULMONARY	★★★
GASTROINTESTINAL	★★★	STROKE	★★★
GENERAL SURGERY	★★★	VASCULAR	NR
MATERNITY CARE	★★★★★	WOMEN'S HEALTH	NR

HEALTHGRADES AWARDS

✓ SPECIALTY EXCELLENCE
• MATERNITY CARE

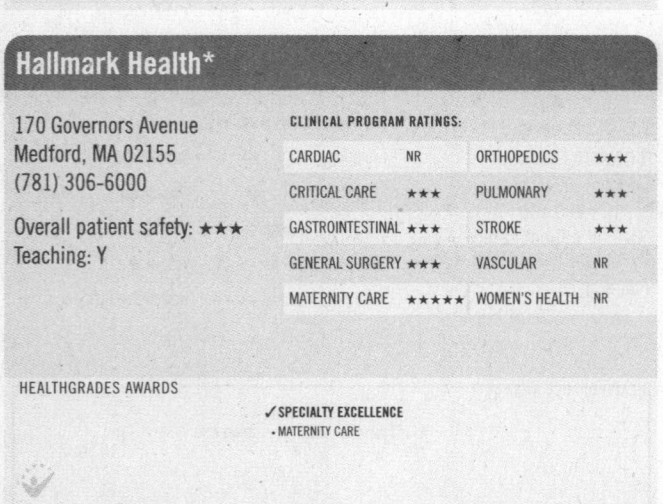

HealthAlliance Hospital Leominster Campus*

60 Hospital Road
Leominster, MA 01453
(978) 466-2000

Overall patient safety: ★★★
Teaching: Y

CLINICAL PROGRAM RATINGS:

CARDIAC	NR	ORTHOPEDICS	NR
CRITICAL CARE	NR	PULMONARY	★★★
GASTROINTESTINAL	NR	STROKE	★★★
GENERAL SURGERY	NR	VASCULAR	NR
MATERNITY CARE	★★★	WOMEN'S HEALTH	NR

HEALTHGRADES AWARDS

KEY: ★★★★★ BEST ★★★ AS EXPECTED ★ POOR NR NOT RATED BY HEALTHGRADES For full definitions of ratings and awards, see Appendix.

Heritage Hospital*

26 Central Street
Somerville, MA 02143
(617) 625-8900

Overall patient safety: ★★★
Teaching: Y

CLINICAL PROGRAM RATINGS:

CARDIAC	NR	ORTHOPEDICS	NR
CRITICAL CARE	★★★	PULMONARY	★★★
GASTROINTESTINAL	★★★	STROKE	★★★
GENERAL SURGERY	★★★	VASCULAR	NR
MATERNITY CARE	★★★	WOMEN'S HEALTH	NR

HEALTHGRADES AWARDS

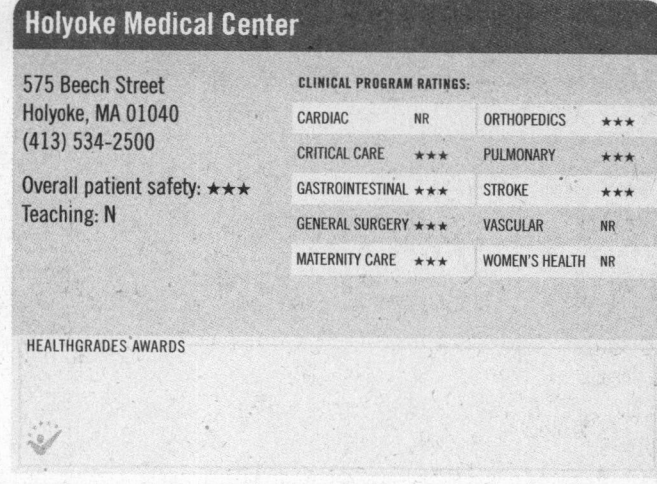

Holyoke Medical Center

575 Beech Street
Holyoke, MA 01040
(413) 534-2500

Overall patient safety: ★★★
Teaching: N

CLINICAL PROGRAM RATINGS:

CARDIAC	NR	ORTHOPEDICS	★★★
CRITICAL CARE	★★★	PULMONARY	★★★
GASTROINTESTINAL	★★★	STROKE	★★★
GENERAL SURGERY	★★★	VASCULAR	NR
MATERNITY CARE	★★★	WOMEN'S HEALTH	NR

HEALTHGRADES AWARDS

Heywood Hospital

242 Green Street
Gardner, MA 01440
(978) 632-3420

Overall patient safety: ★★★
Teaching: N

CLINICAL PROGRAM RATINGS:

CARDIAC	NR	ORTHOPEDICS	NR
CRITICAL CARE	NR	PULMONARY	★★★
GASTROINTESTINAL	NR	STROKE	★★★
GENERAL SURGERY	NR	VASCULAR	NR
MATERNITY CARE	★★★	WOMEN'S HEALTH	NR

HEALTHGRADES AWARDS

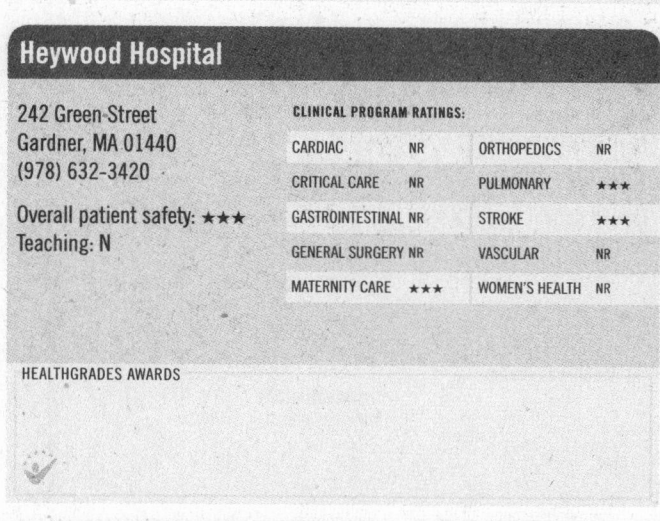

Jordan Hospital

275 Sandwich Street
Plymouth, MA 02360
(508) 746-2000

Overall patient safety: ★★★
Teaching: N

CLINICAL PROGRAM RATINGS:

CARDIAC	NR	ORTHOPEDICS	★★★
CRITICAL CARE	★	PULMONARY	★
GASTROINTESTINAL	★★★	STROKE	★★★
GENERAL SURGERY	★★★	VASCULAR	NR
MATERNITY CARE	★★★	WOMEN'S HEALTH	NR

HEALTHGRADES AWARDS

✓ SPECIALTY EXCELLENCE
· JOINT REPLACEMENT

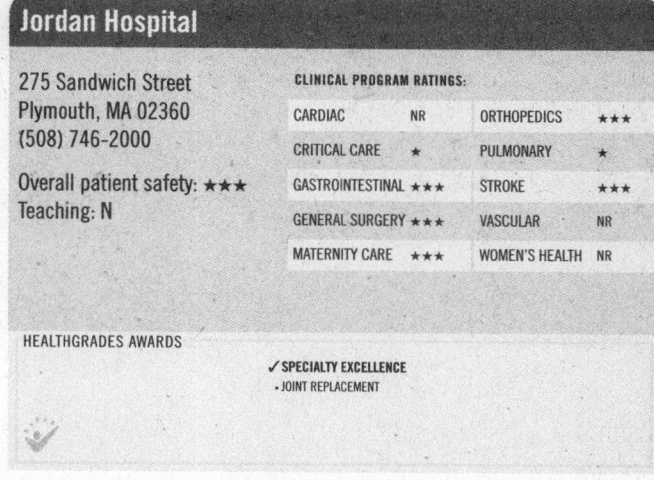

Hillcrest Hospital*

165 Tor Court
Pittsfield, MA 01201
(413) 443-4761

Overall patient safety: ★★★
Teaching: Y

CLINICAL PROGRAM RATINGS:

CARDIAC	NR	ORTHOPEDICS	★★★
CRITICAL CARE	★★★	PULMONARY	★★★
GASTROINTESTINAL	★★★	STROKE	★★★
GENERAL SURGERY	★★★	VASCULAR	NR
MATERNITY CARE	★★★	WOMEN'S HEALTH	NR

HEALTHGRADES AWARDS

Lawrence General Hospital

1 General Street
Lawrence, MA 01842
(978) 683-4000

Overall patient safety: ★★★
Teaching: Y

CLINICAL PROGRAM RATINGS:

CARDIAC	NR	ORTHOPEDICS	★★★
CRITICAL CARE	★★★	PULMONARY	★★★
GASTROINTESTINAL	★★★	STROKE	★★★
GENERAL SURGERY	★★★	VASCULAR	NR
MATERNITY CARE	★★★	WOMEN'S HEALTH	NR

HEALTHGRADES AWARDS

*This hospital reports its data to the federal government jointly with another hospital. Therefore the ratings and awards apply to multiple hospitals and this specific hospital may not provide all rated services.

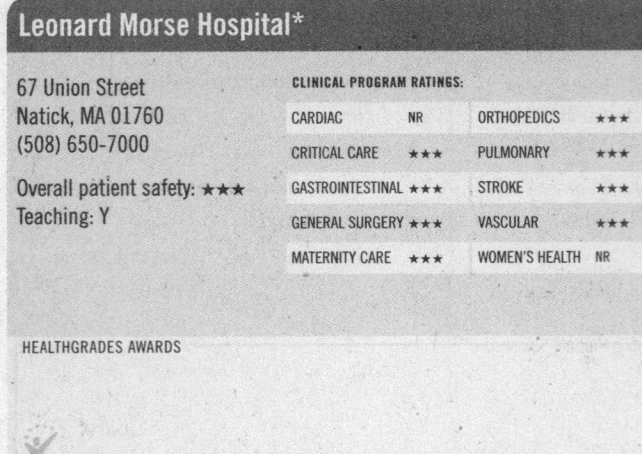

Leonard Morse Hospital*

67 Union Street
Natick, MA 01760
(508) 650-7000

Overall patient safety: ★★★
Teaching: Y

CLINICAL PROGRAM RATINGS:

CARDIAC	NR	ORTHOPEDICS	★★★
CRITICAL CARE	★★★	PULMONARY	★★★
GASTROINTESTINAL	★★★	STROKE	★★★
GENERAL SURGERY	★★★	VASCULAR	★★★
MATERNITY CARE	★★★	WOMEN'S HEALTH	NR

HEALTHGRADES AWARDS

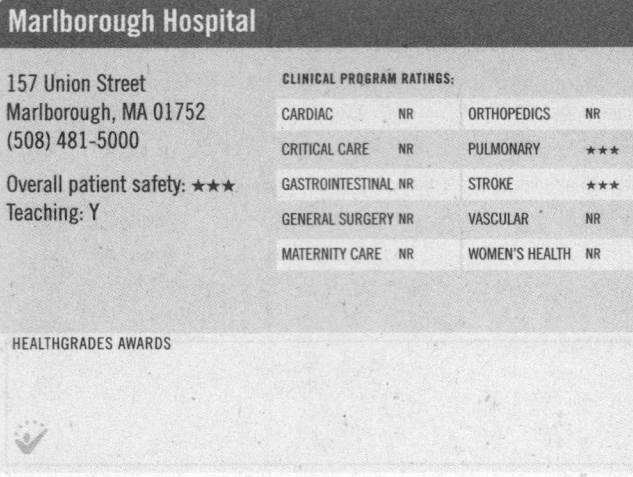

Marlborough Hospital

157 Union Street
Marlborough, MA 01752
(508) 481-5000

Overall patient safety: ★★★
Teaching: Y

CLINICAL PROGRAM RATINGS:

CARDIAC	NR	ORTHOPEDICS	NR
CRITICAL CARE	NR	PULMONARY	★★★
GASTROINTESTINAL	NR	STROKE	★★★
GENERAL SURGERY	NR	VASCULAR	NR
MATERNITY CARE	NR	WOMEN'S HEALTH	NR

HEALTHGRADES AWARDS

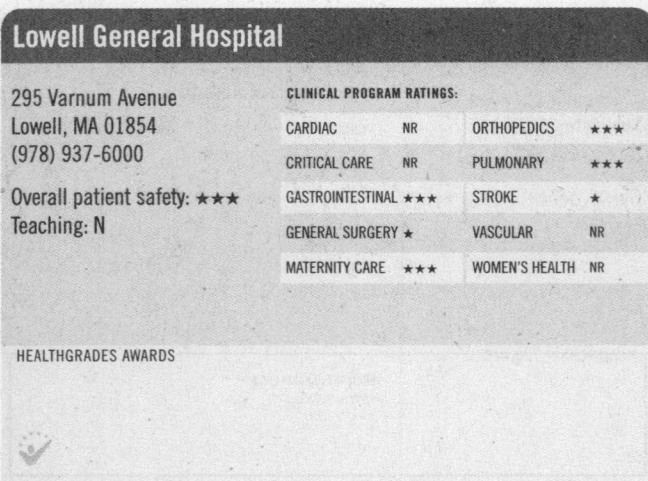

Lowell General Hospital

295 Varnum Avenue
Lowell, MA 01854
(978) 937-6000

Overall patient safety: ★★★
Teaching: N

CLINICAL PROGRAM RATINGS:

CARDIAC	NR	ORTHOPEDICS	★★★
CRITICAL CARE	NR	PULMONARY	★★★
GASTROINTESTINAL	★★★	STROKE	★
GENERAL SURGERY	★	VASCULAR	NR
MATERNITY CARE	★★★	WOMEN'S HEALTH	NR

HEALTHGRADES AWARDS

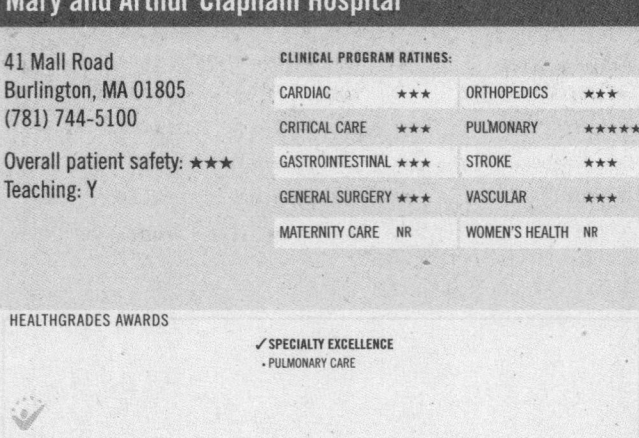

Mary and Arthur Clapham Hospital

41 Mall Road
Burlington, MA 01805
(781) 744-5100

Overall patient safety: ★★★
Teaching: Y

CLINICAL PROGRAM RATINGS:

CARDIAC	★★★	ORTHOPEDICS	★★★
CRITICAL CARE	★★★	PULMONARY	★★★★★
GASTROINTESTINAL	★★★	STROKE	★★★
GENERAL SURGERY	★★★	VASCULAR	★★★
MATERNITY CARE	NR	WOMEN'S HEALTH	NR

HEALTHGRADES AWARDS

✓ SPECIALTY EXCELLENCE
• PULMONARY CARE

Malden Hospital*

100 Hospital Road
Malden, MA 02148
(617) 322-7560

Overall patient safety: ★★★
Teaching: Y

CLINICAL PROGRAM RATINGS:

CARDIAC	NR	ORTHOPEDICS	★★★
CRITICAL CARE	★★★	PULMONARY	★★★
GASTROINTESTINAL	★★★	STROKE	★★★
GENERAL SURGERY	★★★	VASCULAR	NR
MATERNITY CARE	★★★★★	WOMEN'S HEALTH	NR

HEALTHGRADES AWARDS

✓ SPECIALTY EXCELLENCE
• MATERNITY CARE

Massachusetts General Hospital

55 Fruit Street
Boston, MA 02114
(617) 726-2000

Overall patient safety: ★★★
Teaching: Y

CLINICAL PROGRAM RATINGS:

CARDIAC	★★★★★	ORTHOPEDICS	★★★
CRITICAL CARE	★★★	PULMONARY	★★★★★
GASTROINTESTINAL	★★★	STROKE	★★★
GENERAL SURGERY	★★★	VASCULAR	★★★
MATERNITY CARE	★★★	WOMEN'S HEALTH	★★★

HEALTHGRADES AWARDS

✓ SPECIALTY EXCELLENCE
• CARDIAC CARE   • GASTROINTESTINAL
• CARDIAC SURGERY   CARE
                    • PULMONARY CARE

KEY: ★★★★★ BEST   ★★★ AS EXPECTED   ★ POOR   NR NOT RATED BY HEALTHGRADES   For full definitions of ratings and awards, see Appendix.

Melrose-Wakefield Hospital*

585 Lebanon Street
Melrose, MA 02176
(781) 979-3000

Overall patient safety: ★★★
Teaching: Y

CLINICAL PROGRAM RATINGS:

CARDIAC	NR	ORTHOPEDICS	★★★
CRITICAL CARE	★★★	PULMONARY	★★★
GASTROINTESTINAL	★★★	STROKE	★★★
GENERAL SURGERY	★★★	VASCULAR	NR
MATERNITY CARE	★★★★★	WOMEN'S HEALTH	NR

HEALTHGRADES AWARDS

✓ SPECIALTY EXCELLENCE
• MATERNITY CARE

MetroWest Medical Center*

115 Lincoln Street
Framingham, MA 01701
(508) 383-1000

Overall patient safety: ★★★
Teaching: Y

CLINICAL PROGRAM RATINGS:

CARDIAC	NR	ORTHOPEDICS	★★★
CRITICAL CARE	★★★	PULMONARY	★★★
GASTROINTESTINAL	★★★	STROKE	★★★
GENERAL SURGERY	★★★	VASCULAR	★★★
MATERNITY CARE	★★★	WOMEN'S HEALTH	NR

HEALTHGRADES AWARDS

Mercy Medical Center*

271 Carew Street
Springfield, MA 01104
(413) 748-9000

Overall patient safety: ★★★
Teaching: N

CLINICAL PROGRAM RATINGS:

CARDIAC	NR	ORTHOPEDICS	★
CRITICAL CARE	★	PULMONARY	★★★
GASTROINTESTINAL	★★★	STROKE	★★★
GENERAL SURGERY	★★★	VASCULAR	NR
MATERNITY CARE	★★★	WOMEN'S HEALTH	NR

HEALTHGRADES AWARDS

Milford Regional Medical Center

14 Prospect Street
Milford, MA 01757
(508) 473-1190

Overall patient safety: ★★★
Teaching: Y

CLINICAL PROGRAM RATINGS:

CARDIAC	NR	ORTHOPEDICS	★
CRITICAL CARE	★★★	PULMONARY	★★★★★
GASTROINTESTINAL	★★★	STROKE	★
GENERAL SURGERY	★	VASCULAR	NR
MATERNITY CARE	★★★	WOMEN'S HEALTH	NR

HEALTHGRADES AWARDS

✓ SPECIALTY EXCELLENCE
• PULMONARY CARE

Merrimack Valley Hospital

140 Lincoln Avenue
Haverhill, MA 01830
(978) 374-2000

Overall patient safety: ★★★
Teaching: N

CLINICAL PROGRAM RATINGS:

CARDIAC	NR	ORTHOPEDICS	NR
CRITICAL CARE	NR	PULMONARY	★★★
GASTROINTESTINAL	NR	STROKE	★★★
GENERAL SURGERY	★★★	VASCULAR	NR
MATERNITY CARE	NR	WOMEN'S HEALTH	NR

HEALTHGRADES AWARDS

Milton Hospital

92 Highland Street
Milton, MA 02186
(617) 696-4600

Overall patient safety: ★★★
Teaching: N

CLINICAL PROGRAM RATINGS:

CARDIAC	NR	ORTHOPEDICS	★★★
CRITICAL CARE	NR	PULMONARY	★★★
GASTROINTESTINAL	★★★	STROKE	★★★
GENERAL SURGERY	★★★	VASCULAR	NR
MATERNITY CARE	NR	WOMEN'S HEALTH	NR

HEALTHGRADES AWARDS

*This hospital reports its data to the federal government jointly with another hospital. Therefore the ratings and awards apply to multiple hospitals and this specific hospital may not provide all rated services.

MASSACHUSETTS HOSPITALS: RATINGS BY CLINICAL SPECIALTY

Morton Hospital and Medical Center

88 Washington Street
Taunton, MA 02780
(508) 828-7000

Overall patient safety: ★
Teaching: N

CLINICAL PROGRAM RATINGS:

CARDIAC	NR	ORTHOPEDICS	NR
CRITICAL CARE	★★★	PULMONARY	★★★
GASTROINTESTINAL	★★★	STROKE	★★★
GENERAL SURGERY	★★★	VASCULAR	NR
MATERNITY CARE	★	WOMEN'S HEALTH	NR

HEALTHGRADES AWARDS

New England Baptist Hospital

125 Parker Hill Avenue
Boston, MA 02120
(617) 754-5800

Overall patient safety: ★★★★★
Teaching: Y

CLINICAL PROGRAM RATINGS:

CARDIAC	NR	ORTHOPEDICS	★★★
CRITICAL CARE	NR	PULMONARY	★★★★★
GASTROINTESTINAL	NR	STROKE	NR
GENERAL SURGERY	★★★	VASCULAR	NR
MATERNITY CARE	NR	WOMEN'S HEALTH	NR

HEALTHGRADES AWARDS

✓ SPECIALTY EXCELLENCE
- JOINT REPLACEMENT   - PULMONARY CARE

Mount Auburn Hospital

330 Mount Auburn Street
Cambridge, MA 02138
(617) 492-3500

Overall patient safety: ★★★
Teaching: Y

CLINICAL PROGRAM RATINGS:

CARDIAC	★★★	ORTHOPEDICS	★★★
CRITICAL CARE	★★★	PULMONARY	★★★
GASTROINTESTINAL	★★★	STROKE	★
GENERAL SURGERY	★★★	VASCULAR	NR
MATERNITY CARE	★★★★★	WOMEN'S HEALTH	★★★

HEALTHGRADES AWARDS

✓ SPECIALTY EXCELLENCE
- CARDIAC SURGERY   - MATERNITY CARE

Newton-Wellesley Hospital

2014 Washington Street
Newton, MA 02462
(617) 243-5555

Overall patient safety: ★★★
Teaching: Y

CLINICAL PROGRAM RATINGS:

CARDIAC	NR	ORTHOPEDICS	★★★
CRITICAL CARE	★★★	PULMONARY	★★★
GASTROINTESTINAL	★★★★★	STROKE	★★★
GENERAL SURGERY	★★★★★	VASCULAR	NR
MATERNITY CARE	★★★★★	WOMEN'S HEALTH	NR

HEALTHGRADES AWARDS

✓ SPECIALTY EXCELLENCE
- BARIATRIC SURGERY   - GASTROINTESTINAL CARE   - GENERAL SURGERY

Nashoba Valley Medical Center

200 Groton Road
Ayer, MA 01432
(978) 784-9000

Overall patient safety: ★★★
Teaching: N

CLINICAL PROGRAM RATINGS:

CARDIAC	NR	ORTHOPEDICS	NR
CRITICAL CARE	NR	PULMONARY	★★★★★
GASTROINTESTINAL	NR	STROKE	NR
GENERAL SURGERY	NR	VASCULAR	NR
MATERNITY CARE	NR	WOMEN'S HEALTH	NR

HEALTHGRADES AWARDS

Noble Hospital

115 West Silver Street
Westfield, MA 01085
(413) 568-2811

Overall patient safety: ★
Teaching: N

CLINICAL PROGRAM RATINGS:

CARDIAC	NR	ORTHOPEDICS	NR
CRITICAL CARE	NR	PULMONARY	★★★
GASTROINTESTINAL	★★★	STROKE	★★★
GENERAL SURGERY	★★★	VASCULAR	NR
MATERNITY CARE	NR	WOMEN'S HEALTH	NR

HEALTHGRADES AWARDS

KEY: ★★★★★ BEST   ★★★ AS EXPECTED   ★ POOR   NR NOT RATED BY HEALTHGRADES   For full definitions of ratings and awards, see Appendix.

North Adams Regional Hospital

71 Hospital Avenue
North Adams, MA 01247
(413) 663-3701

Overall patient safety: ★★★
Teaching: N

CLINICAL PROGRAM RATINGS:

CARDIAC	NR	ORTHOPEDICS	NR
CRITICAL CARE	NR	PULMONARY	★
GASTROINTESTINAL	NR	STROKE	★★★
GENERAL SURGERY	★★★	VASCULAR	NR
MATERNITY CARE	★★★	WOMEN'S HEALTH	NR

HEALTHGRADES AWARDS

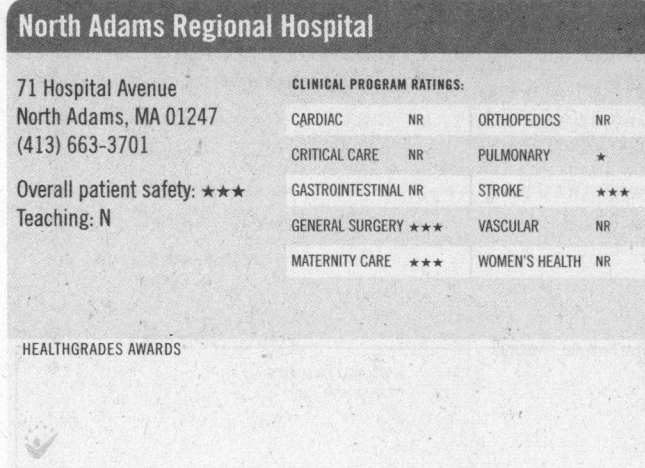

Quincy Medical Center

114 Whitwell Street
Quincy, MA 02169
(617) 773-6100

Overall patient safety: ★★★
Teaching: N

CLINICAL PROGRAM RATINGS:

CARDIAC	NR	ORTHOPEDICS	NR
CRITICAL CARE	NR	PULMONARY	★★★
GASTROINTESTINAL	NR	STROKE	★★★
GENERAL SURGERY	★★★	VASCULAR	NR
MATERNITY CARE	NR	WOMEN'S HEALTH	NR

HEALTHGRADES AWARDS

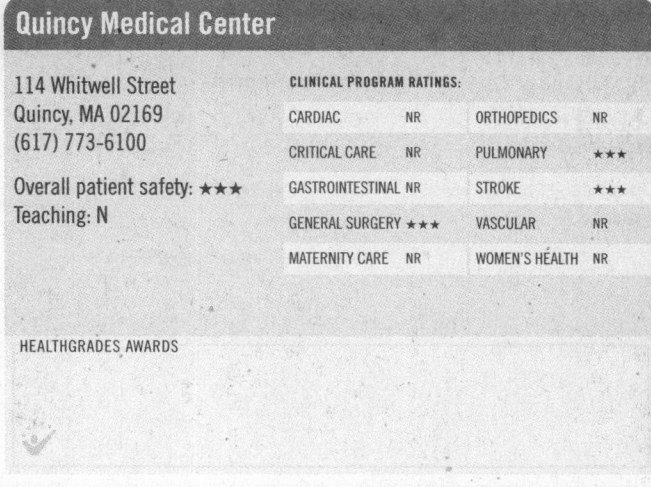

North Shore Medical Center*

81 Highland Avenue
Salem, MA 01970
(978) 741-1200

Overall patient safety: ★★★★★
Teaching: Y

CLINICAL PROGRAM RATINGS:

CARDIAC	★★★	ORTHOPEDICS	★★★
CRITICAL CARE	★★★	PULMONARY	★★★★★
GASTROINTESTINAL	★★★	STROKE	★★★★★
GENERAL SURGERY	★★★	VASCULAR	★★★
MATERNITY CARE	★★★	WOMEN'S HEALTH	★★★

HEALTHGRADES AWARDS

✓ DISTINGUISHED HOSPITAL
• CLINICAL EXCELLENCE
• PATIENT SAFETY

✓ SPECIALTY EXCELLENCE
• PULMONARY CARE   • STROKE CARE

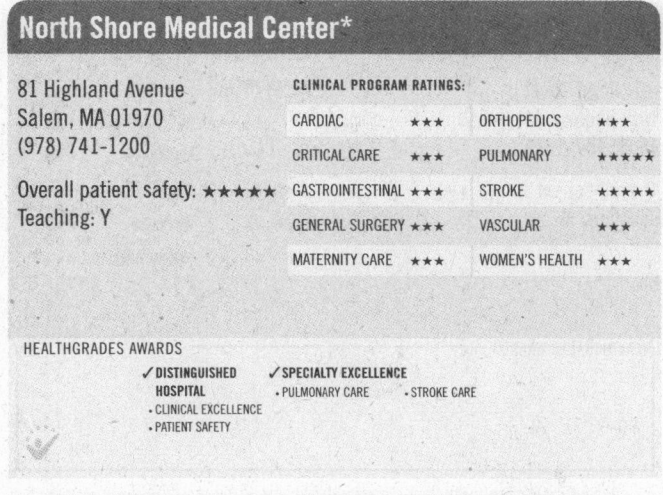

St. Anne's Hospital Corporation

795 Middle Street
Fall River, MA 02721
(508) 674-5741

Overall patient safety: ★★★
Teaching: Y

CLINICAL PROGRAM RATINGS:

CARDIAC	NR	ORTHOPEDICS	NR
CRITICAL CARE	★★★	PULMONARY	★★★★★
GASTROINTESTINAL	★★★	STROKE	★★★
GENERAL SURGERY	★	VASCULAR	NR
MATERNITY CARE	NR	WOMEN'S HEALTH	NR

HEALTHGRADES AWARDS

✓ SPECIALTY EXCELLENCE
• PULMONARY CARE

Providence Hospital*

1233 Main Street
Holyoke, MA 01040
(413) 536-5111

Overall patient safety: ★★★
Teaching: N

CLINICAL PROGRAM RATINGS:

CARDIAC	NR	ORTHOPEDICS	★
CRITICAL CARE	★	PULMONARY	★★★
GASTROINTESTINAL	★★★	STROKE	★★★
GENERAL SURGERY	★★★	VASCULAR	NR
MATERNITY CARE	★★★	WOMEN'S HEALTH	NR

HEALTHGRADES AWARDS

St. Vincent Hospital

20 Worcester Center Boulevard
Worcester, MA 01608
(508) 363-5000

Overall patient safety: ★★★
Teaching: Y

CLINICAL PROGRAM RATINGS:

CARDIAC	★★★	ORTHOPEDICS	★★★
CRITICAL CARE	★★★	PULMONARY	★
GASTROINTESTINAL	★★★	STROKE	★★★
GENERAL SURGERY	★★★	VASCULAR	NR
MATERNITY CARE	★★★	WOMEN'S HEALTH	★★★

HEALTHGRADES AWARDS

*This hospital reports its data to the federal government jointly with another hospital. Therefore the ratings and awards apply to multiple hospitals and this specific hospital may not provide all rated services.

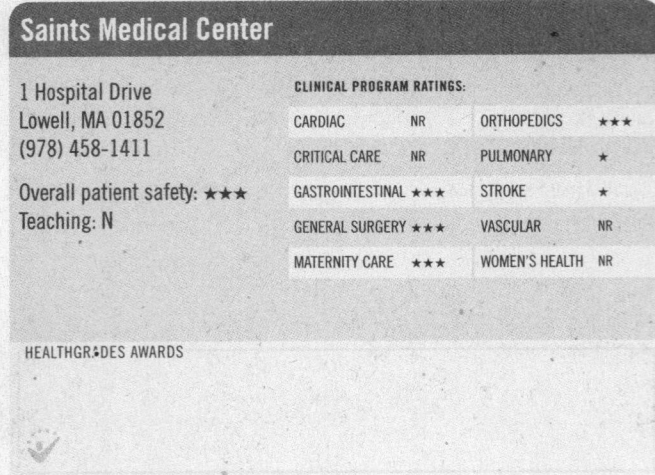

Saints Medical Center

1 Hospital Drive
Lowell, MA 01852
(978) 458-1411

Overall patient safety: ★★★
Teaching: N

CLINICAL PROGRAM RATINGS:

CARDIAC	NR	ORTHOPEDICS	★★★
CRITICAL CARE	NR	PULMONARY	★
GASTROINTESTINAL	★★★	STROKE	★
GENERAL SURGERY	★★★	VASCULAR	NR
MATERNITY CARE	★★★	WOMEN'S HEALTH	NR

HEALTHGRADES AWARDS

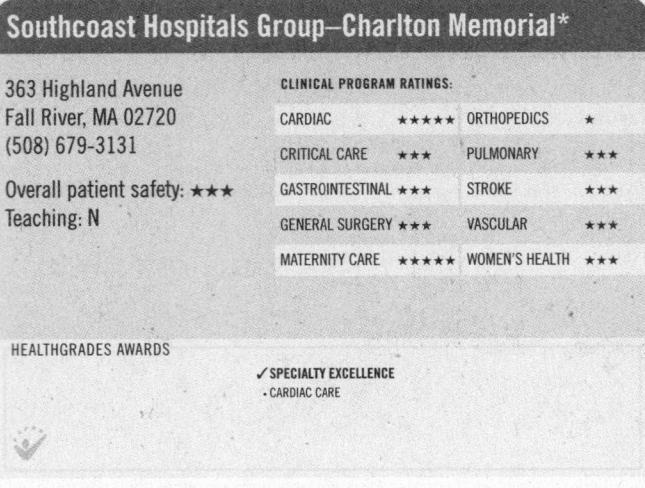

Southcoast Hospitals Group—Charlton Memorial*

363 Highland Avenue
Fall River, MA 02720
(508) 679-3131

Overall patient safety: ★★★
Teaching: N

CLINICAL PROGRAM RATINGS:

CARDIAC	★★★★★	ORTHOPEDICS	★
CRITICAL CARE	★★★	PULMONARY	★★★
GASTROINTESTINAL	★★★	STROKE	★★★
GENERAL SURGERY	★★★	VASCULAR	★★★
MATERNITY CARE	★★★★★	WOMEN'S HEALTH	★★★

HEALTHGRADES AWARDS

✓ SPECIALTY EXCELLENCE
• CARDIAC CARE

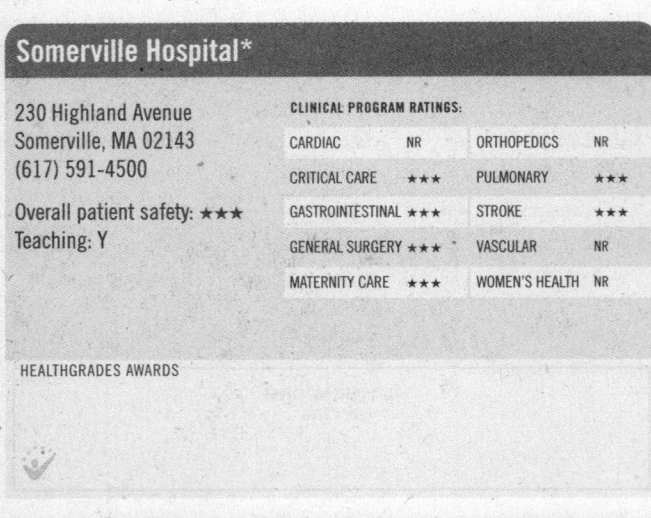

Somerville Hospital*

230 Highland Avenue
Somerville, MA 02143
(617) 591-4500

Overall patient safety: ★★★
Teaching: Y

CLINICAL PROGRAM RATINGS:

CARDIAC	NR	ORTHOPEDICS	NR
CRITICAL CARE	★★★	PULMONARY	★★★
GASTROINTESTINAL	★★★	STROKE	★★★
GENERAL SURGERY	★★★	VASCULAR	NR
MATERNITY CARE	★★★	WOMEN'S HEALTH	NR

HEALTHGRADES AWARDS

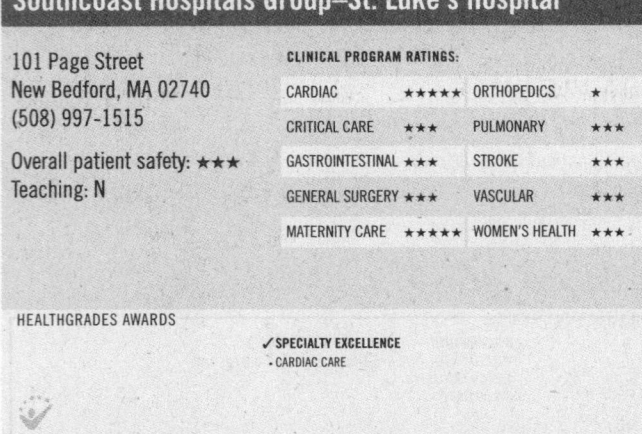

Southcoast Hospitals Group—St. Luke's Hospital*

101 Page Street
New Bedford, MA 02740
(508) 997-1515

Overall patient safety: ★★★
Teaching: N

CLINICAL PROGRAM RATINGS:

CARDIAC	★★★★★	ORTHOPEDICS	★
CRITICAL CARE	★★★	PULMONARY	★★★
GASTROINTESTINAL	★★★	STROKE	★★★
GENERAL SURGERY	★★★	VASCULAR	★★★
MATERNITY CARE	★★★★★	WOMEN'S HEALTH	★★★

HEALTHGRADES AWARDS

✓ SPECIALTY EXCELLENCE
• CARDIAC CARE

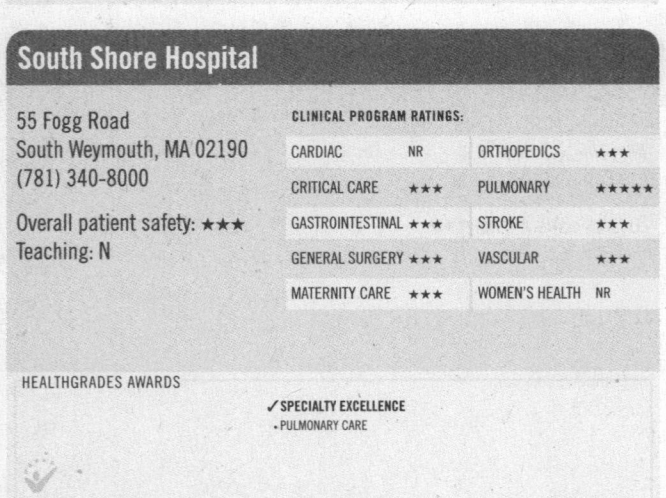

South Shore Hospital

55 Fogg Road
South Weymouth, MA 02190
(781) 340-8000

Overall patient safety: ★★★
Teaching: N

CLINICAL PROGRAM RATINGS:

CARDIAC	NR	ORTHOPEDICS	★★★
CRITICAL CARE	★★★	PULMONARY	★★★★★
GASTROINTESTINAL	★★★	STROKE	★★★
GENERAL SURGERY	★★★	VASCULAR	★★★
MATERNITY CARE	★★★	WOMEN'S HEALTH	NR

HEALTHGRADES AWARDS

✓ SPECIALTY EXCELLENCE
• PULMONARY CARE

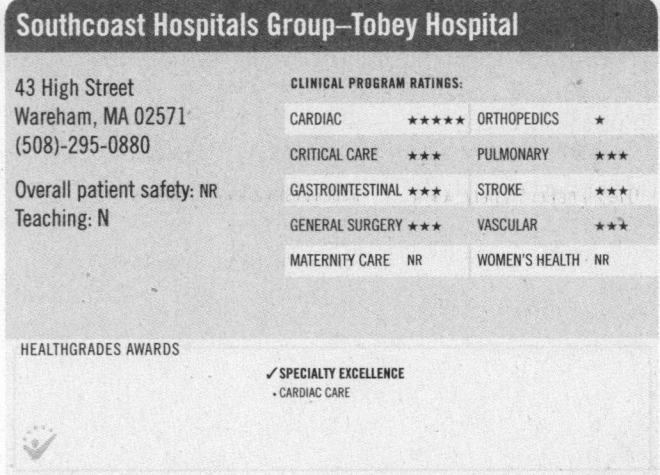

Southcoast Hospitals Group—Tobey Hospital

43 High Street
Wareham, MA 02571
(508)-295-0880

Overall patient safety: NR
Teaching: N

CLINICAL PROGRAM RATINGS:

CARDIAC	★★★★★	ORTHOPEDICS	★
CRITICAL CARE	★★★	PULMONARY	★★★
GASTROINTESTINAL	★★★	STROKE	★★★
GENERAL SURGERY	★★★	VASCULAR	★★★
MATERNITY CARE	NR	WOMEN'S HEALTH	NR

HEALTHGRADES AWARDS

✓ SPECIALTY EXCELLENCE
• CARDIAC CARE

KEY: ★★★★★ BEST   ★★★ AS EXPECTED   ★ POOR   NR NOT RATED BY HEALTHGRADES   For full definitions of ratings and awards, see Appendix.

Sturdy Memorial Hospital

211 Parks Street
Attleboro, MA 02703
(508) 222-5200

Overall patient safety: ★★★
Teaching: N

CLINICAL PROGRAM RATINGS:

CARDIAC	NR	ORTHOPEDICS	NR
CRITICAL CARE	NR	PULMONARY	★★★
GASTROINTESTINAL	★★★	STROKE	★★★
GENERAL SURGERY	★	VASCULAR	NR
MATERNITY CARE	★★★	WOMEN'S HEALTH	NR

HEALTHGRADES AWARDS

UMass Memorial Medical Center—Memorial Campus*

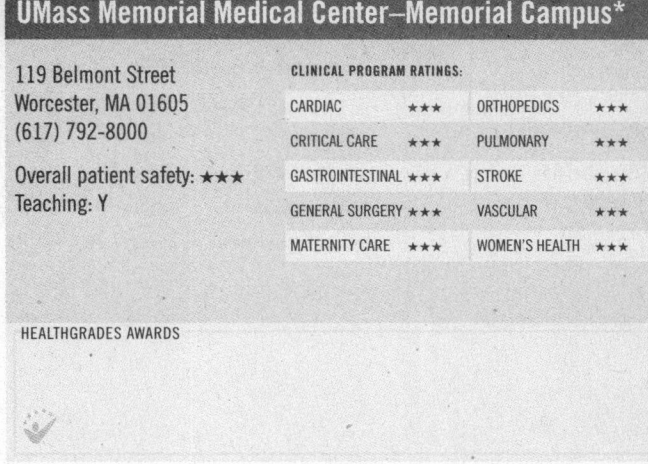

119 Belmont Street
Worcester, MA 01605
(617) 792-8000

Overall patient safety: ★★★
Teaching: Y

CLINICAL PROGRAM RATINGS:

CARDIAC	★★★	ORTHOPEDICS	★★★
CRITICAL CARE	★★★	PULMONARY	★★★
GASTROINTESTINAL	★★★	STROKE	★★★
GENERAL SURGERY	★★★	VASCULAR	★★★
MATERNITY CARE	★★★	WOMEN'S HEALTH	★★★

HEALTHGRADES AWARDS

Tufts-New England Medical Center

750 Washington Street
Boston, MA 02111
(617) 636-5000

Overall patient safety: ★
Teaching: Y

CLINICAL PROGRAM RATINGS:

CARDIAC	★★★	ORTHOPEDICS	★★★
CRITICAL CARE	★★★	PULMONARY	★★★
GASTROINTESTINAL	★★★	STROKE	★★★
GENERAL SURGERY	★★★	VASCULAR	★★★
MATERNITY CARE	★	WOMEN'S HEALTH	★★★

HEALTHGRADES AWARDS

Whidden Memorial Hospital*

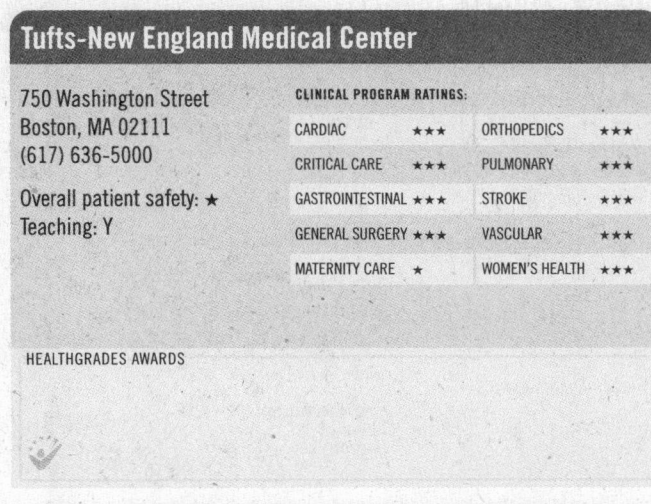

103 Garland Street
Everett, MA 02149
(617) 389-6270

Overall patient safety: ★★★
Teaching: Y

CLINICAL PROGRAM RATINGS:

CARDIAC	NR	ORTHOPEDICS	★★★
CRITICAL CARE	★★★	PULMONARY	★★★
GASTROINTESTINAL	★★★	STROKE	★★★
GENERAL SURGERY	★★★	VASCULAR	NR
MATERNITY CARE	★★★★★	WOMEN'S HEALTH	NR

HEALTHGRADES AWARDS

✓ SPECIALTY EXCELLENCE
• MATERNITY CARE

UMass Memorial Medical Center*

55 Lake Avenue North
Worcester, MA 01655
(508) 334-1000

Overall patient safety: ★★★
Teaching: Y

CLINICAL PROGRAM RATINGS:

CARDIAC	★★★	ORTHOPEDICS	★★★
CRITICAL CARE	★★★	PULMONARY	★★★
GASTROINTESTINAL	★★★	STROKE	★★★
GENERAL SURGERY	★★★	VASCULAR	★★★
MATERNITY CARE	★★★	WOMEN'S HEALTH	★★★

HEALTHGRADES AWARDS

Winchester Hospital

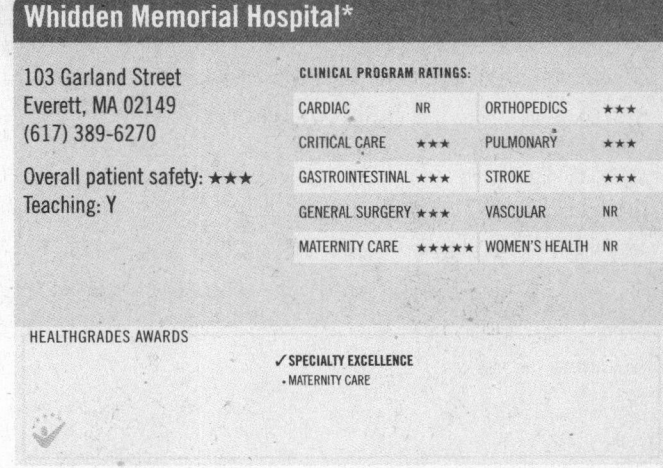

41 Highland Avenue
Winchester, MA 01890
(781) 729-9000

Overall patient safety: ★★★
Teaching: Y

CLINICAL PROGRAM RATINGS:

CARDIAC	NR	ORTHOPEDICS	NR
CRITICAL CARE	★★★	PULMONARY	★★★
GASTROINTESTINAL	★★★	STROKE	★★★
GENERAL SURGERY	★	VASCULAR	NR
MATERNITY CARE	★★★	WOMEN'S HEALTH	NR

HEALTHGRADES AWARDS

*This hospital reports its data to the federal government jointly with another hospital. Therefore the ratings and awards apply to multiple hospitals and this specific hospital may not provide all rated services.

MASSACHUSETTS HOSPITALS: RATINGS BY CLINICAL SPECIALTY

Wing Memorial Hospital and Medical Center

40 Wright Street
Palmer, MA 01069
(413) 283-7651

Overall patient safety: ★★★
Teaching: N

CLINICAL PROGRAM RATINGS:

CARDIAC	NR	ORTHOPEDICS	NR
CRITICAL CARE	NR	PULMONARY	★★★★★
GASTROINTESTINAL	NR	STROKE	★★★
GENERAL SURGERY	NR	VASCULAR	NR
MATERNITY CARE	NR	WOMEN'S HEALTH	NR

HEALTHGRADES AWARDS

MICHIGAN HOSPITALS: RATINGS BY CLINICAL SPECIALTY

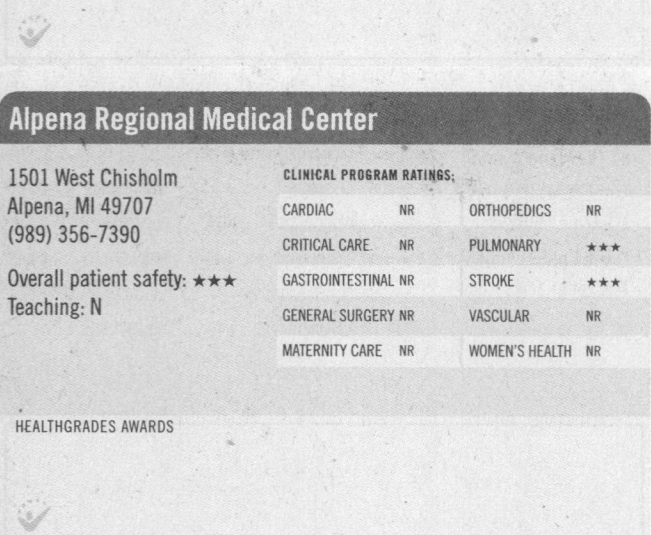

Allegan General Hospital

555 Linn Street
Allegan, MI 49010
(269) 686-4284

Overall patient safety: ★★★
Teaching: N

CLINICAL PROGRAM RATINGS:

CARDIAC	NR	ORTHOPEDICS	NR
CRITICAL CARE	NR	PULMONARY	★★★
GASTROINTESTINAL	NR	STROKE	★★★
GENERAL SURGERY	NR	VASCULAR	NR
MATERNITY CARE	NR	WOMEN'S HEALTH	NR

HEALTHGRADES AWARDS

Alpena Regional Medical Center

1501 West Chisholm
Alpena, MI 49707
(989) 356-7390

Overall patient safety: ★★★
Teaching: N

CLINICAL PROGRAM RATINGS:

CARDIAC	NR	ORTHOPEDICS	NR
CRITICAL CARE	NR	PULMONARY	★★★
GASTROINTESTINAL	NR	STROKE	★★★
GENERAL SURGERY	NR	VASCULAR	NR
MATERNITY CARE	NR	WOMEN'S HEALTH	NR

HEALTHGRADES AWARDS

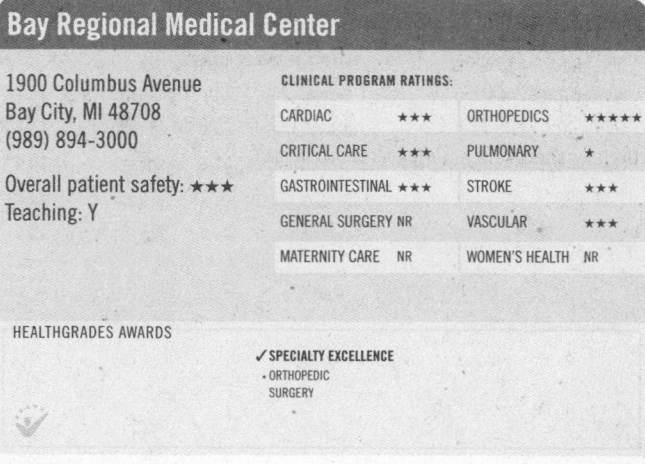

Battle Creek Health System

300 North Avenue
Battle Creek, MI 49016
(616) 966-8000

Overall patient safety: ★★★
Teaching: N

CLINICAL PROGRAM RATINGS:

CARDIAC	NR	ORTHOPEDICS	★★★★★
CRITICAL CARE	★★★	PULMONARY	★★★
GASTROINTESTINAL	★★★	STROKE	★
GENERAL SURGERY	NR	VASCULAR	★★★
MATERNITY CARE	NR	WOMEN'S HEALTH	NR

HEALTHGRADES AWARDS

✓ SPECIALTY EXCELLENCE
• ORTHOPEDIC
SURGERY

Bay Regional Medical Center

1900 Columbus Avenue
Bay City, MI 48708
(989) 894-3000

Overall patient safety: ★★★
Teaching: Y

CLINICAL PROGRAM RATINGS:

CARDIAC	★★★	ORTHOPEDICS	★★★★★
CRITICAL CARE	★★★	PULMONARY	★
GASTROINTESTINAL	★★★	STROKE	★★★
GENERAL SURGERY	NR	VASCULAR	★★★
MATERNITY CARE	NR	WOMEN'S HEALTH	NR

HEALTHGRADES AWARDS

✓ SPECIALTY EXCELLENCE
• ORTHOPEDIC
SURGERY

KEY: ★★★★★ BEST ★★★ AS EXPECTED ★ POOR NR NOT RATED BY HEALTHGRADES For full definitions of ratings and awards, see Appendix.

Beaumont Hospital—Grosse Pointe

468 Cadieux Road
Grosse Pointe, MI 48230
(313) 343-1000

Overall patient safety: ★★★
Teaching: Y

CLINICAL PROGRAM RATINGS:

CARDIAC	NR	ORTHOPEDICS	★★★★★
CRITICAL CARE	★★★	PULMONARY	★★★
GASTROINTESTINAL	★★★	STROKE	★★★★★
GENERAL SURGERY	NR	VASCULAR	★★★
MATERNITY CARE	NR	WOMEN'S HEALTH	NR

HEALTHGRADES AWARDS

✓ DISTINGUISHED HOSPITAL
- CLINICAL EXCELLENCE

✓ SPECIALTY EXCELLENCE
- ORTHOPEDIC SURGERY
- STROKE CARE

Bell Memorial Hospital

101 South 4th Street
Ishpeming, MI 49849
(906) 486-4431

Overall patient safety: ★★★
Teaching: N

CLINICAL PROGRAM RATINGS:

CARDIAC	NR	ORTHOPEDICS	NR
CRITICAL CARE	NR	PULMONARY	★★★
GASTROINTESTINAL	NR	STROKE	★★★
GENERAL SURGERY	NR	VASCULAR	NR
MATERNITY CARE	NR	WOMEN'S HEALTH	NR

HEALTHGRADES AWARDS

Beaumont Hospital—Royal Oak

3601 West Thirteen Mile Road
Royal Oak, MI 48073
(248) 551-5000

Overall patient safety: ★★★
Teaching: Y

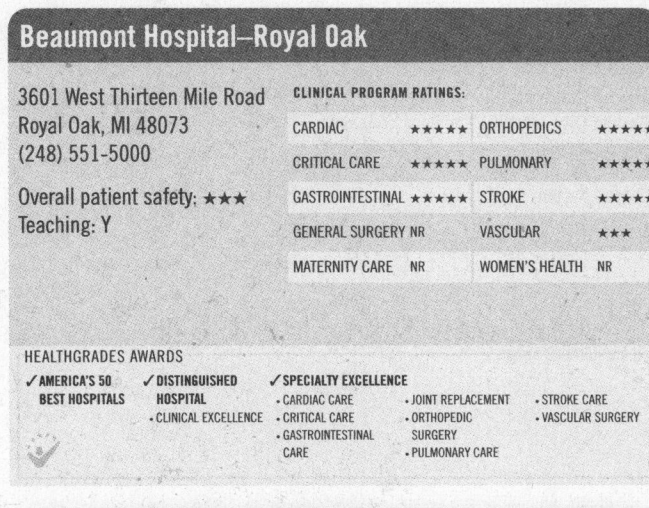

CLINICAL PROGRAM RATINGS:

CARDIAC	★★★★★	ORTHOPEDICS	★★★★★
CRITICAL CARE	★★★★★	PULMONARY	★★★★★
GASTROINTESTINAL	★★★★★	STROKE	★★★★★
GENERAL SURGERY	NR	VASCULAR	★★★
MATERNITY CARE	NR	WOMEN'S HEALTH	NR

HEALTHGRADES AWARDS

✓ AMERICA'S 50 BEST HOSPITALS

✓ DISTINGUISHED HOSPITAL
- CLINICAL EXCELLENCE

✓ SPECIALTY EXCELLENCE
- CARDIAC CARE
- CRITICAL CARE
- GASTROINTESTINAL CARE
- JOINT REPLACEMENT
- ORTHOPEDIC SURGERY
- PULMONARY CARE
- STROKE CARE
- VASCULAR SURGERY

Borgess Medical Center

1521 Gull Road
Kalamazoo, MI 49048
(269) 226-7000

Overall patient safety: ★★★
Teaching: Y

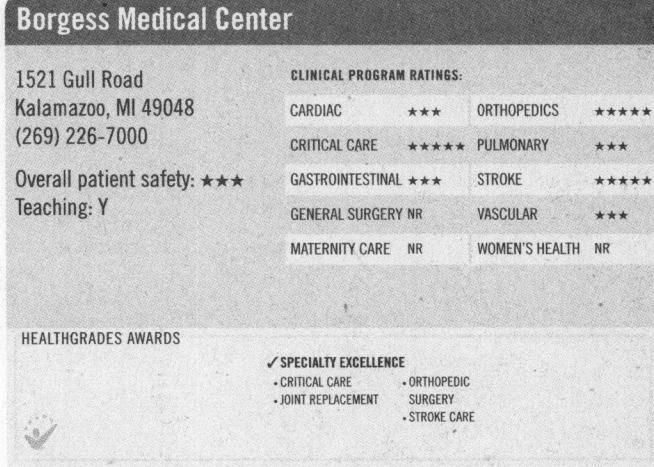

CLINICAL PROGRAM RATINGS:

CARDIAC	★★★	ORTHOPEDICS	★★★★★
CRITICAL CARE	★★★★★	PULMONARY	★★★
GASTROINTESTINAL	★★★	STROKE	★★★★★
GENERAL SURGERY	NR	VASCULAR	★★★
MATERNITY CARE	NR	WOMEN'S HEALTH	NR

HEALTHGRADES AWARDS

✓ SPECIALTY EXCELLENCE
- CRITICAL CARE
- JOINT REPLACEMENT
- ORTHOPEDIC SURGERY
- STROKE CARE

Beaumont Hospital—Troy

44201 Dequindre Road
Troy, MI 48085
(248) 964-5000

Overall patient safety: ★★★★★
Teaching: Y

CLINICAL PROGRAM RATINGS:

CARDIAC	★★★★★	ORTHOPEDICS	★★★★★
CRITICAL CARE	★★★	PULMONARY	★★★★★
GASTROINTESTINAL	★★★	STROKE	★★★★★
GENERAL SURGERY	NR	VASCULAR	★★★
MATERNITY CARE	NR	WOMEN'S HEALTH	NR

HEALTHGRADES AWARDS

✓ DISTINGUISHED HOSPITAL
- CLINICAL EXCELLENCE
- PATIENT SAFETY

✓ SPECIALTY EXCELLENCE
- CARDIAC CARE
- GASTROINTESTINAL CARE
- ORTHOPEDIC SURGERY
- PULMONARY CARE
- STROKE CARE
- VASCULAR SURGERY

Borgess Pipp Health Center

411 Naomi Street
Plainwell, MI 49080
(269) 685-0801

Overall patient safety: ★★★
Teaching: Y

CLINICAL PROGRAM RATINGS:

CARDIAC	★★★	ORTHOPEDICS	★★★★★
CRITICAL CARE	★★★★★	PULMONARY	★★★
GASTROINTESTINAL	★★★	STROKE	★★★★★
GENERAL SURGERY	NR	VASCULAR	★★★
MATERNITY CARE	NR	WOMEN'S HEALTH	NR

HEALTHGRADES AWARDS

✓ SPECIALTY EXCELLENCE
- CRITICAL CARE
- JOINT REPLACEMENT
- ORTHOPEDIC SURGERY
- STROKE CARE

Borgess-Lee Memorial Hospital

420 West High Street
Dowagiac, MI 49047
(269) 782-8681

Overall patient safety: ★★★
Teaching: N

CLINICAL PROGRAM RATINGS:

CARDIAC	NR	ORTHOPEDICS	NR
CRITICAL CARE	NR	PULMONARY	★★★
GASTROINTESTINAL	NR	STROKE	NR
GENERAL SURGERY	NR	VASCULAR	NR
MATERNITY CARE	NR	WOMEN'S HEALTH	NR

HEALTHGRADES AWARDS

Caro Community Hospital

401 North Hooper Street
Caro, MI 48723
(989) 673-3141

Overall patient safety: ★★★
Teaching: N

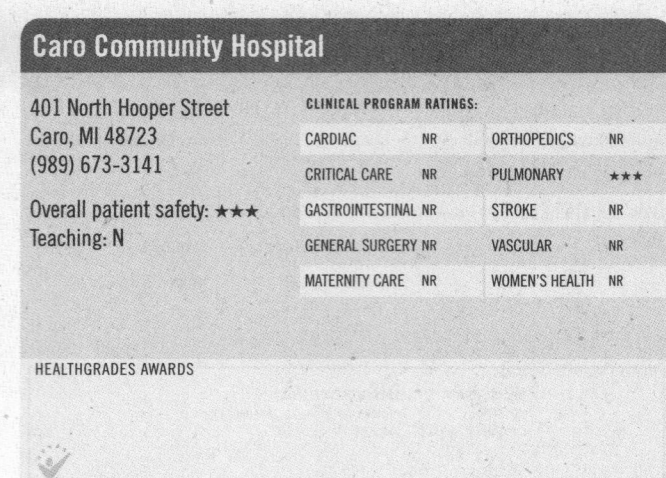

CLINICAL PROGRAM RATINGS:

CARDIAC	NR	ORTHOPEDICS	NR
CRITICAL CARE	NR	PULMONARY	★★★
GASTROINTESTINAL	NR	STROKE	NR
GENERAL SURGERY	NR	VASCULAR	NR
MATERNITY CARE	NR	WOMEN'S HEALTH	NR

HEALTHGRADES AWARDS

Botsford Hospital

28050 Grand Avenue
Farmington Hills, MI 48336
(248) 471-8000

Overall patient safety: ★★★★★
Teaching: Y

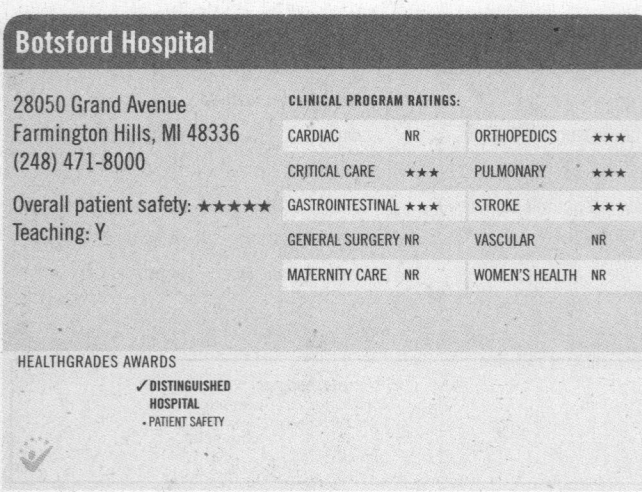

CLINICAL PROGRAM RATINGS:

CARDIAC	NR	ORTHOPEDICS	★★★
CRITICAL CARE	★★★	PULMONARY	★★★
GASTROINTESTINAL	★★★	STROKE	★★★
GENERAL SURGERY	NR	VASCULAR	NR
MATERNITY CARE	NR	WOMEN'S HEALTH	NR

HEALTHGRADES AWARDS

✓ DISTINGUISHED
  HOSPITAL
· PATIENT SAFETY

Carson City Hospital

406 East Elm Street
Carson City, MI 48811
(989) 584-3131

Overall patient safety: ★★★
Teaching: Y

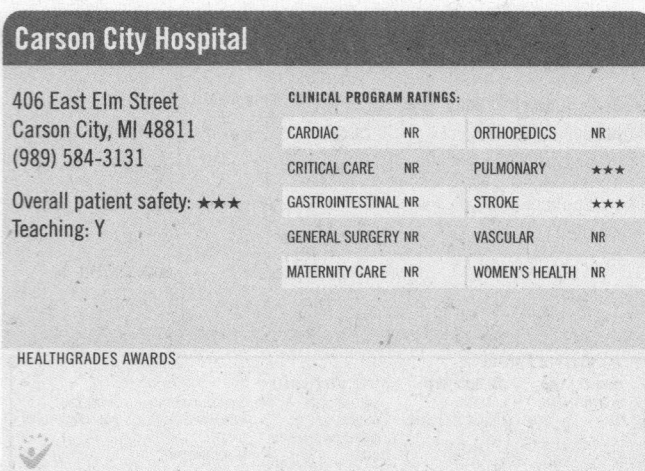

CLINICAL PROGRAM RATINGS:

CARDIAC	NR	ORTHOPEDICS	NR
CRITICAL CARE	NR	PULMONARY	★★★
GASTROINTESTINAL	NR	STROKE	★★★
GENERAL SURGERY	NR	VASCULAR	NR
MATERNITY CARE	NR	WOMEN'S HEALTH	NR

HEALTHGRADES AWARDS

Bronson Methodist Hospital

601 John Street
Kalamazoo, MI 49007
(269) 341-7654

Overall patient safety: ★★★
Teaching: Y

CLINICAL PROGRAM RATINGS:

CARDIAC	★★★	ORTHOPEDICS	★★★★★
CRITICAL CARE	★★★	PULMONARY	★★★
GASTROINTESTINAL	★★★	STROKE	★★★★★
GENERAL SURGERY	NR	VASCULAR	★★★
MATERNITY CARE	NR	WOMEN'S HEALTH	NR

HEALTHGRADES AWARDS

✓ SPECIALTY EXCELLENCE
· JOINT REPLACEMENT

Central Michigan Community Hospital

1221 South Drive
Mount Pleasant, MI 48858
(989) 772-6700

Overall patient safety: ★★★
Teaching: N

CLINICAL PROGRAM RATINGS:

CARDIAC	NR	ORTHOPEDICS	NR
CRITICAL CARE	NR	PULMONARY	★
GASTROINTESTINAL	★★★	STROKE	★★★
GENERAL SURGERY	NR	VASCULAR	NR
MATERNITY CARE	NR	WOMEN'S HEALTH	NR

HEALTHGRADES AWARDS

KEY: ★★★★★ BEST   ★★★ AS EXPECTED   ★ POOR   NR NOT RATED BY HEALTHGRADES   For full definitions of ratings and awards, see Appendix.

Charlevoix Area Hospital

14700 Lakeshore Drive
Charlevoix, MI 49720
(231) 547-4024

Overall patient safety: ★★★
Teaching: N

CLINICAL PROGRAM RATINGS:

CARDIAC	NR	ORTHOPEDICS	NR
CRITICAL CARE	NR	PULMONARY	★★★
GASTROINTESTINAL	NR	STROKE	★★★
GENERAL SURGERY	NR	VASCULAR	NR
MATERNITY CARE	NR	WOMEN'S HEALTH	NR

HEALTHGRADES AWARDS

Chippewa County War Memorial Hospital

500 Osborn Boulevard
Sault Ste. Marie, MI 49783
(906) 635-4460

Overall patient safety: ★★★
Teaching: N

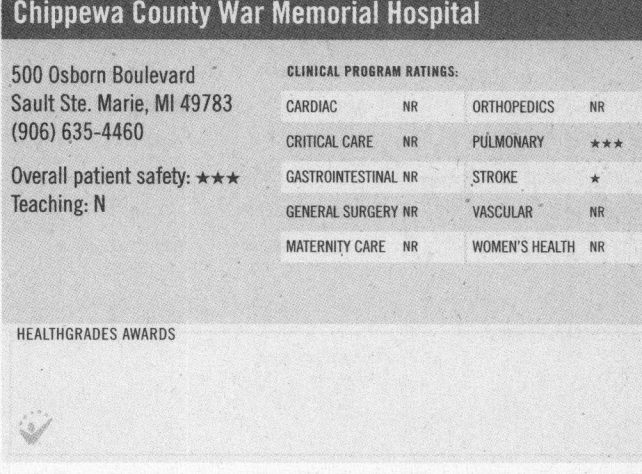

CLINICAL PROGRAM RATINGS:

CARDIAC	NR	ORTHOPEDICS	NR
CRITICAL CARE	NR	PULMONARY	★★★
GASTROINTESTINAL	NR	STROKE	★
GENERAL SURGERY	NR	VASCULAR	NR
MATERNITY CARE	NR	WOMEN'S HEALTH	NR

HEALTHGRADES AWARDS

Cheboygan Memorial Hospital

748 South Main Street
Cheboygan, MI 49721
(231) 627-5601

Overall patient safety: ★★★
Teaching: N

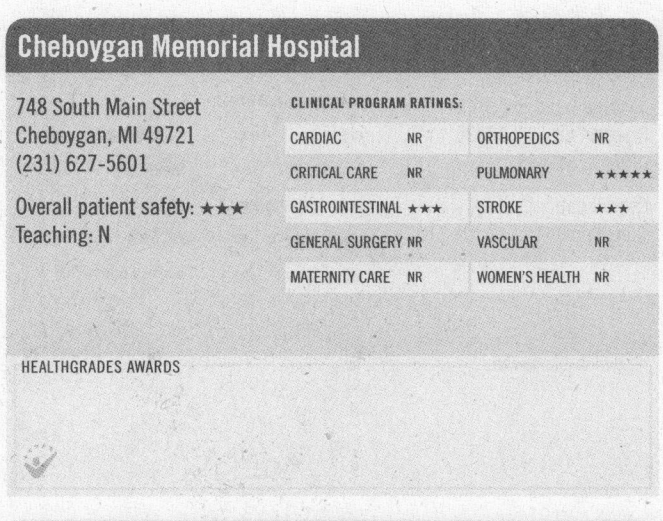

CLINICAL PROGRAM RATINGS:

CARDIAC	NR	ORTHOPEDICS	NR
CRITICAL CARE	NR	PULMONARY	★★★★★
GASTROINTESTINAL	★★★	STROKE	★★★
GENERAL SURGERY	NR	VASCULAR	NR
MATERNITY CARE	NR	WOMEN'S HEALTH	NR

HEALTHGRADES AWARDS

Clinton Memorial Hospital

805 South Oakland
St. Johns, MI 48879
(989) 224-6861

Overall patient safety: ★★★
Teaching: N

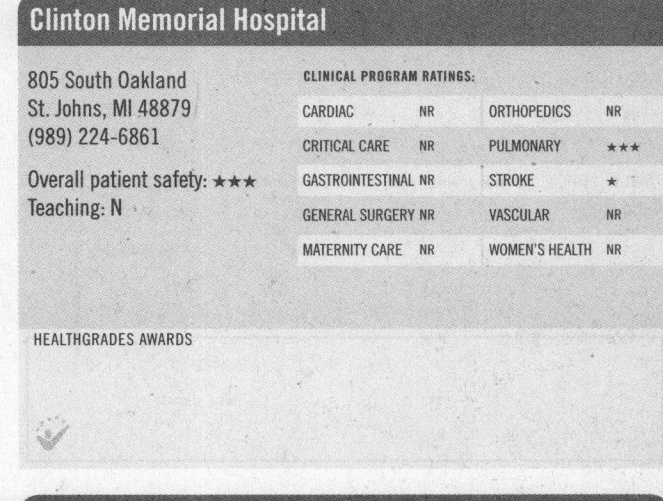

CLINICAL PROGRAM RATINGS:

CARDIAC	NR	ORTHOPEDICS	NR
CRITICAL CARE	NR	PULMONARY	★★★
GASTROINTESTINAL	NR	STROKE	★
GENERAL SURGERY	NR	VASCULAR	NR
MATERNITY CARE	NR	WOMEN'S HEALTH	NR

HEALTHGRADES AWARDS

Chelsea Community Hospital

775 South Main Street
Chelsea, MI 48118
(734) 475-1311

Overall patient safety: ★
Teaching: N

CLINICAL PROGRAM RATINGS:

CARDIAC	NR	ORTHOPEDICS	★★★
CRITICAL CARE	NR	PULMONARY	★★★
GASTROINTESTINAL	NR	STROKE	★★★★★
GENERAL SURGERY	NR	VASCULAR	NR
MATERNITY CARE	NR	WOMEN'S HEALTH	NR

HEALTHGRADES AWARDS

Community Health Center of Branch County

274 East Chicago Street
Coldwater, MI 49036
(517) 279-5489

Overall patient safety: ★★★
Teaching: Y

CLINICAL PROGRAM RATINGS:

CARDIAC	NR	ORTHOPEDICS	★★★
CRITICAL CARE	NR	PULMONARY	★★★
GASTROINTESTINAL	NR	STROKE	★★★
GENERAL SURGERY	NR	VASCULAR	NR
MATERNITY CARE	NR	WOMEN'S HEALTH	NR

HEALTHGRADES AWARDS

Community Hospital Foundation*

80650 North Van Dyke
Almont, MI 48003
(313) 798-8551

Overall patient safety: ★★★
Teaching: Y

CLINICAL PROGRAM RATINGS:

CARDIAC	★★★	ORTHOPEDICS	★★★
CRITICAL CARE	★★★★★	PULMONARY	★★★
GASTROINTESTINAL	★★★	STROKE	★★★★★
GENERAL SURGERY	NR	VASCULAR	NR
MATERNITY CARE	NR	WOMEN'S HEALTH	NR

HEALTHGRADES AWARDS

✓ SPECIALTY EXCELLENCE
- CRITICAL CARE   - STROKE CARE

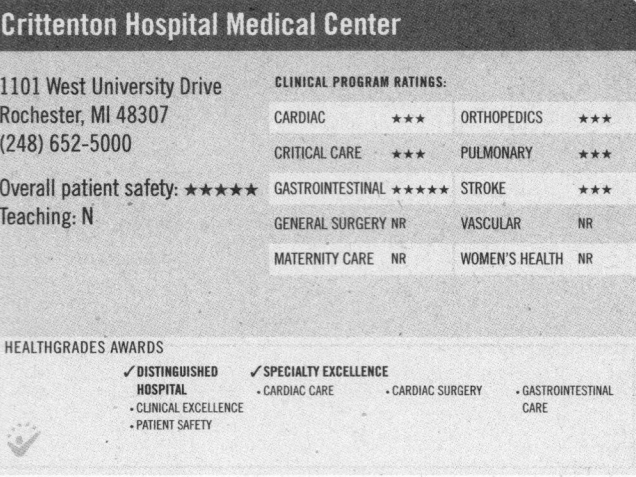

Crittenton Hospital Medical Center

1101 West University Drive
Rochester, MI 48307
(248) 652-5000

Overall patient safety: ★★★★★
Teaching: N

CLINICAL PROGRAM RATINGS:

CARDIAC	★★★	ORTHOPEDICS	★★★
CRITICAL CARE	★★★	PULMONARY	★★★
GASTROINTESTINAL	★★★★★	STROKE	★★★
GENERAL SURGERY	NR	VASCULAR	NR
MATERNITY CARE	NR	WOMEN'S HEALTH	NR

HEALTHGRADES AWARDS

✓ DISTINGUISHED   ✓ SPECIALTY EXCELLENCE
  HOSPITAL   - CARDIAC CARE   - CARDIAC SURGERY   - GASTROINTESTINAL
- CLINICAL EXCELLENCE   CARE
- PATIENT SAFETY

Community Hospital–Watervliet

400 Medical Parks Drive
Watervliet, MI 49098
(269) 463-3111

Overall patient safety: ★★★
Teaching: N

CLINICAL PROGRAM RATINGS:

CARDIAC	NR	ORTHOPEDICS	NR
CRITICAL CARE	NR	PULMONARY	★★★
GASTROINTESTINAL	NR	STROKE	NR
GENERAL SURGERY	NR	VASCULAR	NR
MATERNITY CARE	NR	WOMEN'S HEALTH	NR

HEALTHGRADES AWARDS

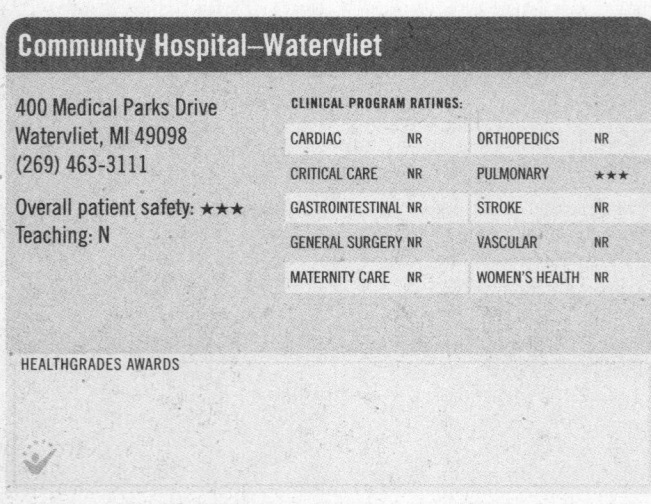

Crystal Falls Community Hospital*

Michigan and 3rd Street
Crystal Falls, MI 49920
(906) 875-6661

Overall patient safety: ★★★
Teaching: N

CLINICAL PROGRAM RATINGS:

CARDIAC	NR	ORTHOPEDICS	NR
CRITICAL CARE	NR	PULMONARY	★★★
GASTROINTESTINAL	NR	STROKE	★
GENERAL SURGERY	NR	VASCULAR	NR
MATERNITY CARE	NR	WOMEN'S HEALTH	NR

HEALTHGRADES AWARDS

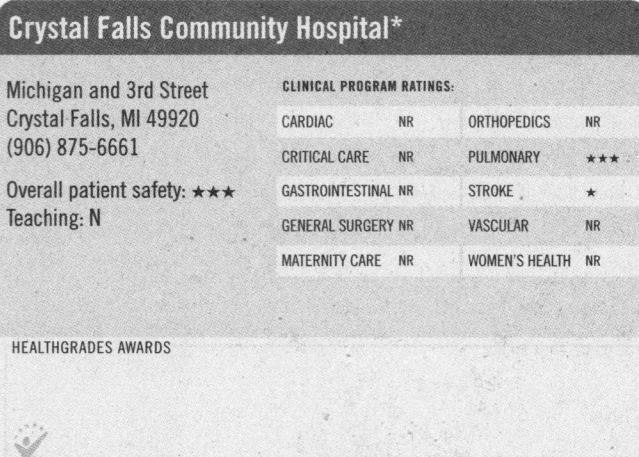

Covenant Medical Center

1447 North Harrison Street
Saginaw, MI 48602
(989) 583-4000

Overall patient safety: ★★★
Teaching: Y

CLINICAL PROGRAM RATINGS:

CARDIAC	★★★	ORTHOPEDICS	★★★★★
CRITICAL CARE	★★★	PULMONARY	★★★
GASTROINTESTINAL	★★★	STROKE	★★★
GENERAL SURGERY	NR	VASCULAR	★★★
MATERNITY CARE	NR	WOMEN'S HEALTH	NR

HEALTHGRADES AWARDS

✓ SPECIALTY EXCELLENCE
- JOINT REPLACEMENT   - ORTHOPEDIC
                         SURGERY

Detroit Receiving Hospital and University Health Center

4201 St. Antoine Boulevard
Detroit, MI 48201
(313) 745-3104

Overall patient safety: ★
Teaching: Y

CLINICAL PROGRAM RATINGS:

CARDIAC	NR	ORTHOPEDICS	NR
CRITICAL CARE	★★★	PULMONARY	★★★
GASTROINTESTINAL	★★★	STROKE	★★★★★
GENERAL SURGERY	NR	VASCULAR	NR
MATERNITY CARE	NR	WOMEN'S HEALTH	NR

HEALTHGRADES AWARDS

KEY: ★★★★★ BEST   ★★★ AS EXPECTED   ★ POOR   NR NOT RATED BY HEALTHGRADES   For full definitions of ratings and awards, see Appendix.

Dickinson County Healthcare System*

1721 South Stephenson
Iron Mountain, MI 49801
(906) 774-1313

Overall patient safety: ★★★
Teaching: N

CLINICAL PROGRAM RATINGS:

CARDIAC	NR	ORTHOPEDICS	NR
CRITICAL CARE	NR	PULMONARY	★★★
GASTROINTESTINAL	★★★	STROKE	★★★
GENERAL SURGERY	NR	VASCULAR	NR
MATERNITY CARE	NR	WOMEN'S HEALTH	NR

HEALTHGRADES AWARDS

Emma L. Bixby Medical Center*

818 Riverside Avenue
Adrian, MI 49221
(517) 265-0900

Overall patient safety: ★★★
Teaching: N

CLINICAL PROGRAM RATINGS:

CARDIAC	NR	ORTHOPEDICS	NR
CRITICAL CARE	NR	PULMONARY	★★★
GASTROINTESTINAL	NR	STROKE	★★★
GENERAL SURGERY	NR	VASCULAR	NR
MATERNITY CARE	NR	WOMEN'S HEALTH	NR

HEALTHGRADES AWARDS

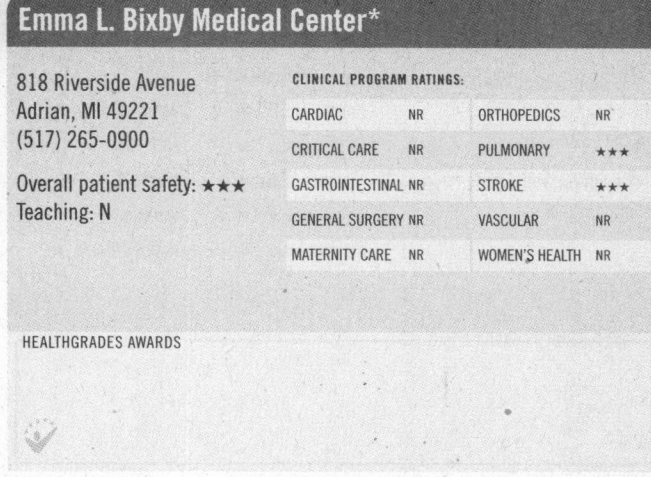

Eaton Rapids Medical Center

1500 South Main Street
Eaton Rapids, MI 48827
(517) 663-2671

Overall patient safety: ★★★
Teaching: N

CLINICAL PROGRAM RATINGS:

CARDIAC	NR	ORTHOPEDICS	NR
CRITICAL CARE	NR	PULMONARY	★★★
GASTROINTESTINAL	NR	STROKE	NR
GENERAL SURGERY	NR	VASCULAR	NR
MATERNITY CARE	NR	WOMEN'S HEALTH	NR

HEALTHGRADES AWARDS

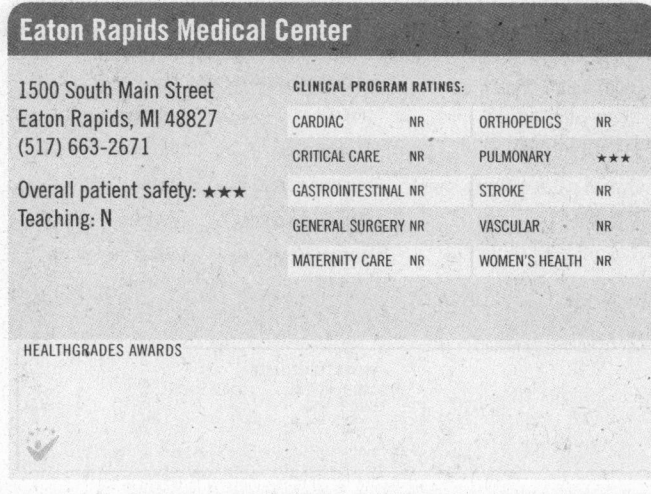

Garden City Osteopathic Hospital

6245 North Inkster Road
Garden City, MI 48135
(734) 421-3300

Overall patient safety: ★★★
Teaching: Y

CLINICAL PROGRAM RATINGS:

CARDIAC	NR	ORTHOPEDICS	★★★★★
CRITICAL CARE	★★★	PULMONARY	★★★
GASTROINTESTINAL	★★★	STROKE	★★★
GENERAL SURGERY	NR	VASCULAR	NR
MATERNITY CARE	NR	WOMEN'S HEALTH	NR

HEALTHGRADES AWARDS

✓ SPECIALTY EXCELLENCE
· JOINT REPLACEMENT   · ORTHOPEDIC SURGERY

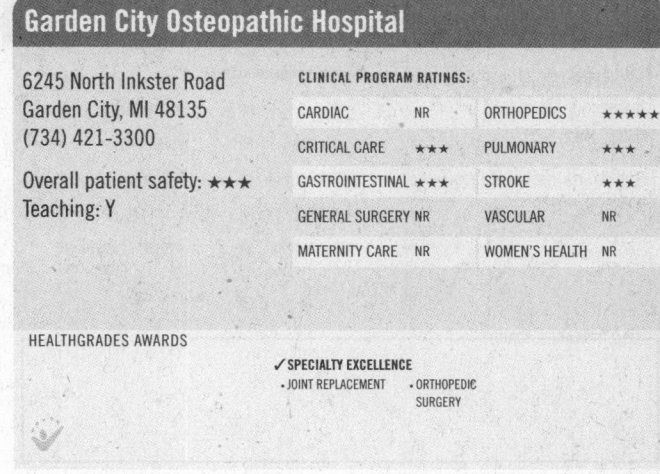

Edward W. Sparrow Hospital Association

1215 East Michigan Avenue
Lansing, MI 48909
(517) 364-1000

Overall patient safety: ★★★
Teaching: Y

CLINICAL PROGRAM RATINGS:

CARDIAC	★★★	ORTHOPEDICS	★★★
CRITICAL CARE	★	PULMONARY	★★★
GASTROINTESTINAL	★★★	STROKE	★★★
GENERAL SURGERY	NR	VASCULAR	NR
MATERNITY CARE	NR	WOMEN'S HEALTH	NR

HEALTHGRADES AWARDS

Genesys Regional Medical Center*

1 Genesys Parkway
Grand Blanc, MI 48439
(810) 606-5000

Overall patient safety: ★★★★★
Teaching: Y

CLINICAL PROGRAM RATINGS:

CARDIAC	★★★	ORTHOPEDICS	★★★
CRITICAL CARE	★★★★★	PULMONARY	★★★★★
GASTROINTESTINAL	★★★	STROKE	★★★★★
GENERAL SURGERY	NR	VASCULAR	★★★
MATERNITY CARE	NR	WOMEN'S HEALTH	NR

HEALTHGRADES AWARDS

✓ AMERICA'S 50 BEST HOSPITALS
· CLINICAL EXCELLENCE
· PATIENT SAFETY

✓ DISTINGUISHED HOSPITAL

✓ SPECIALTY EXCELLENCE
· CARDIAC CARE   · CRITICAL CARE   · PULMONARY CARE
· CARDIAC SURGERY   · GASTROINTESTINAL   · STROKE CARE
                      CARE

MICHIGAN HOSPITALS: RATINGS BY CLINICAL SPECIALTY

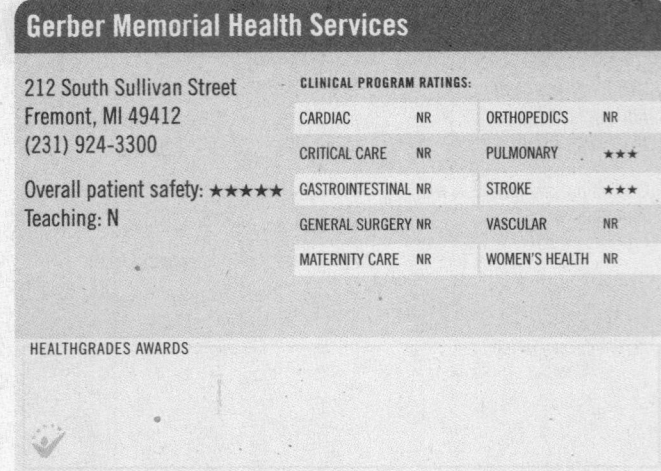

Gerber Memorial Health Services

212 South Sullivan Street
Fremont, MI 49412
(231) 924-3300

Overall patient safety: ★★★★★
Teaching: N

CLINICAL PROGRAM RATINGS:

CARDIAC	NR	ORTHOPEDICS	NR
CRITICAL CARE	NR	PULMONARY	★★★
GASTROINTESTINAL	NR	STROKE	★★★
GENERAL SURGERY	NR	VASCULAR	NR
MATERNITY CARE	NR	WOMEN'S HEALTH	NR

HEALTHGRADES AWARDS

Hackley Hospital

1700 Clinton Street
Muskegon, MI 49442
(231) 726-3511

Overall patient safety: ★★★★★
Teaching: N

CLINICAL PROGRAM RATINGS:

CARDIAC	NR	ORTHOPEDICS	★★★★★
CRITICAL CARE	NR	PULMONARY	★★★★★
GASTROINTESTINAL	★★★	STROKE	★★★
GENERAL SURGERY	NR	VASCULAR	NR
MATERNITY CARE	NR	WOMEN'S HEALTH	NR

HEALTHGRADES AWARDS

✓ DISTINGUISHED HOSPITAL
• CLINICAL EXCELLENCE
• PATIENT SAFETY

✓ SPECIALTY EXCELLENCE
• ORTHOPEDIC SURGERY
• PULMONARY CARE

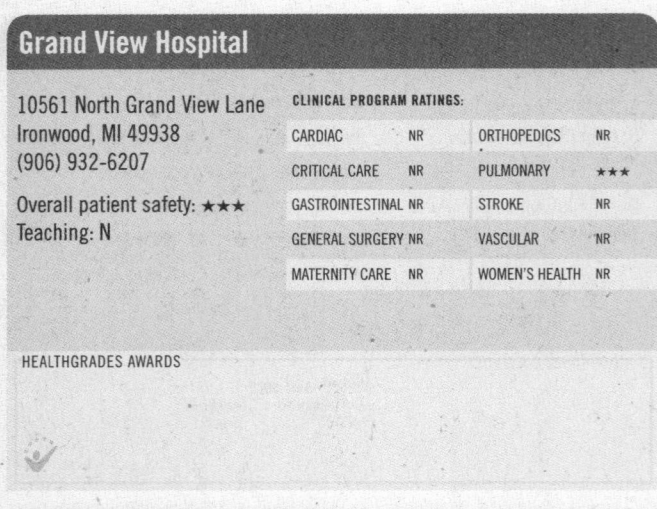

Grand View Hospital

10561 North Grand View Lane
Ironwood, MI 49938
(906) 932-6207

Overall patient safety: ★★★
Teaching: N

CLINICAL PROGRAM RATINGS:

CARDIAC	NR	ORTHOPEDICS	NR
CRITICAL CARE	NR	PULMONARY	★★★
GASTROINTESTINAL	NR	STROKE	NR
GENERAL SURGERY	NR	VASCULAR	NR
MATERNITY CARE	NR	WOMEN'S HEALTH	NR

HEALTHGRADES AWARDS

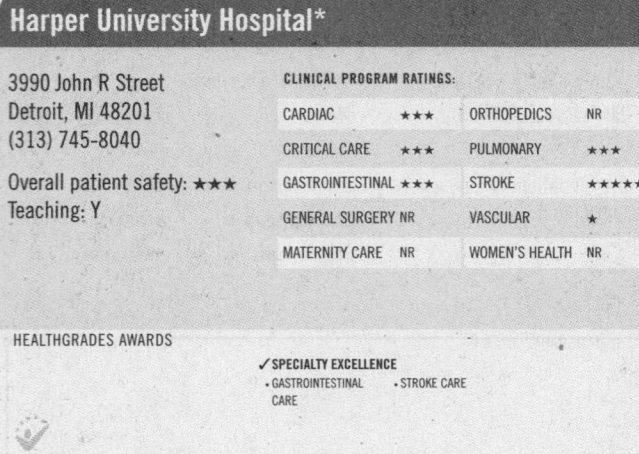

Harper University Hospital*

3990 John R Street
Detroit, MI 48201
(313) 745-8040

Overall patient safety: ★★★
Teaching: Y

CLINICAL PROGRAM RATINGS:

CARDIAC	★★★	ORTHOPEDICS	NR
CRITICAL CARE	★★★	PULMONARY	★★★
GASTROINTESTINAL	★★★	STROKE	★★★★★
GENERAL SURGERY	NR	VASCULAR	★
MATERNITY CARE	NR	WOMEN'S HEALTH	NR

HEALTHGRADES AWARDS

✓ SPECIALTY EXCELLENCE
• GASTROINTESTINAL CARE
• STROKE CARE

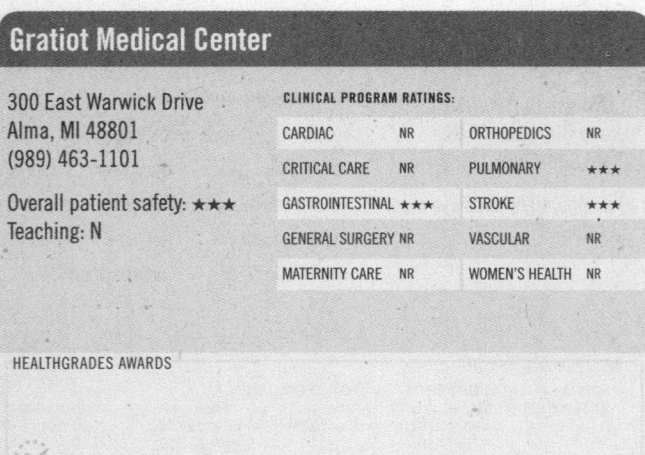

Gratiot Medical Center

300 East Warwick Drive
Alma, MI 48801
(989) 463-1101

Overall patient safety: ★★★
Teaching: N

CLINICAL PROGRAM RATINGS:

CARDIAC	NR	ORTHOPEDICS	NR
CRITICAL CARE	NR	PULMONARY	★★★
GASTROINTESTINAL	★★★	STROKE	★★★
GENERAL SURGERY	NR	VASCULAR	NR
MATERNITY CARE	NR	WOMEN'S HEALTH	NR

HEALTHGRADES AWARDS

Hayes Green Beach Memorial Hospital

321 East Harris Street
Charlotte, MI 48813
(517) 543-1050

Overall patient safety: ★★★
Teaching: N

CLINICAL PROGRAM RATINGS:

CARDIAC	NR	ORTHOPEDICS	NR
CRITICAL CARE	NR	PULMONARY	★★★
GASTROINTESTINAL	NR	STROKE	NR
GENERAL SURGERY	NR	VASCULAR	NR
MATERNITY CARE	NR	WOMEN'S HEALTH	NR

HEALTHGRADES AWARDS

KEY: ★★★★★ BEST   ★★★ AS EXPECTED   ★ POOR   NR NOT RATED BY HEALTHGRADES   For full definitions of ratings and awards, see Appendix.

Helen Newberry Joy Hospital

502 West Harrie Street
Newberry, MI 49868
(906) 293-9200

Overall patient safety: ★★★
Teaching: N

CLINICAL PROGRAM RATINGS:

CARDIAC	NR	ORTHOPEDICS	NR
CRITICAL CARE	NR	PULMONARY	★
GASTROINTESTINAL	NR	STROKE	NR
GENERAL SURGERY	NR	VASCULAR	NR
MATERNITY CARE	NR	WOMEN'S HEALTH	NR

HEALTHGRADES AWARDS

Henry Ford Macomb Hospital*

15815 Nineteen Mile Road
Clinton Township, MI 48038
(586) 263-2300

Overall patient safety: ★★★
Teaching: Y

CLINICAL PROGRAM RATINGS:

CARDIAC	★★★	ORTHOPEDICS	★★★
CRITICAL CARE	★★★★★	PULMONARY	★★★
GASTROINTESTINAL	★★★	STROKE	★★★★★
GENERAL SURGERY	NR	VASCULAR	NR
MATERNITY CARE	NR	WOMEN'S HEALTH	NR

HEALTHGRADES AWARDS

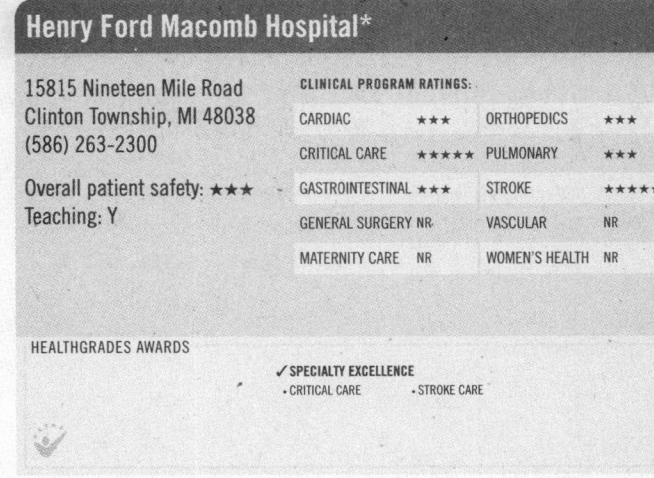

✓ SPECIALTY EXCELLENCE
• CRITICAL CARE   • STROKE CARE

Henry Ford Bi-County Hospital

13355 East Ten Mile Road
Warren, MI 48089
(586) 759-7500

Overall patient safety: ★★★
Teaching: Y

CLINICAL PROGRAM RATINGS:

CARDIAC	NR	ORTHOPEDICS	NR
CRITICAL CARE	NR	PULMONARY	★★★
GASTROINTESTINAL	★★★	STROKE	★★★
GENERAL SURGERY	NR	VASCULAR	NR
MATERNITY CARE	NR	WOMEN'S HEALTH	NR

HEALTHGRADES AWARDS

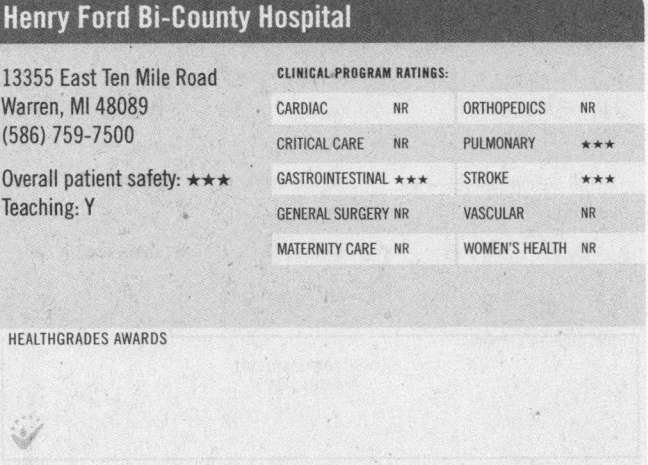

Henry Ford Wyandotte Hospital

2333 Biddle Avenue
Wyandotte, MI 48192
(734) 284-2400

Overall patient safety: ★★★
Teaching: Y

CLINICAL PROGRAM RATINGS:

CARDIAC	NR	ORTHOPEDICS	★★★★★
CRITICAL CARE	★★★	PULMONARY	★★★
GASTROINTESTINAL	★★★	STROKE	★★★★★
GENERAL SURGERY	NR	VASCULAR	NR
MATERNITY CARE	NR	WOMEN'S HEALTH	NR

HEALTHGRADES AWARDS

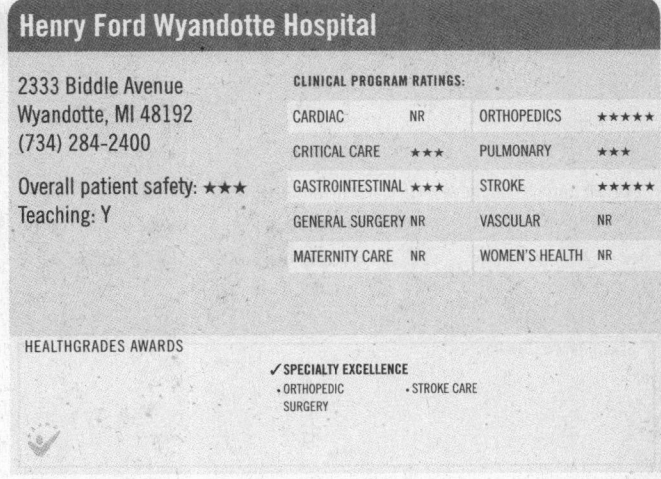

✓ SPECIALTY EXCELLENCE
• ORTHOPEDIC   • STROKE CARE
  SURGERY

Henry Ford Hospital

2799 West Grand Boulevard
Detroit, MI 48202
(313) 916-2600

Overall patient safety: ★
Teaching: Y

CLINICAL PROGRAM RATINGS:

CARDIAC	★★★	ORTHOPEDICS	★
CRITICAL CARE	★★★★★	PULMONARY	★★★★★
GASTROINTESTINAL	★★★	STROKE	★★★★★
GENERAL SURGERY	NR	VASCULAR	★★★
MATERNITY CARE	NR	WOMEN'S HEALTH	NR

HEALTHGRADES AWARDS

✓ SPECIALTY EXCELLENCE
• CRITICAL CARE   • PULMONARY CARE   • STROKE CARE

Herrick Memorial Hospital

500 East Pottawatamie Street
Tecumseh, MI 49286
(517) 265-0441

Overall patient safety: ★★★
Teaching: N

CLINICAL PROGRAM RATINGS:

CARDIAC	NR	ORTHOPEDICS	NR
CRITICAL CARE	NR	PULMONARY	★★★
GASTROINTESTINAL	NR	STROKE	★★★
GENERAL SURGERY	NR	VASCULAR	NR
MATERNITY CARE	NR	WOMEN'S HEALTH	NR

HEALTHGRADES AWARDS

---

*This hospital reports its data to the federal government jointly with another hospital. Therefore the ratings and awards apply to multiple hospitals and this specific hospital may not provide all rated services.

Hills and Dales General Hospital

4675 Hill Street
Cass City, MI 48726
(989) 872-2121

Overall patient safety: ★★★
Teaching: N

CLINICAL PROGRAM RATINGS:

CARDIAC	NR	ORTHOPEDICS	NR
CRITICAL CARE	NR	PULMONARY	★★★
GASTROINTESTINAL	NR	STROKE	NR
GENERAL SURGERY	NR	VASCULAR	NR
MATERNITY CARE	NR	WOMEN'S HEALTH	NR

HEALTHGRADES AWARDS

Hurley Medical Center

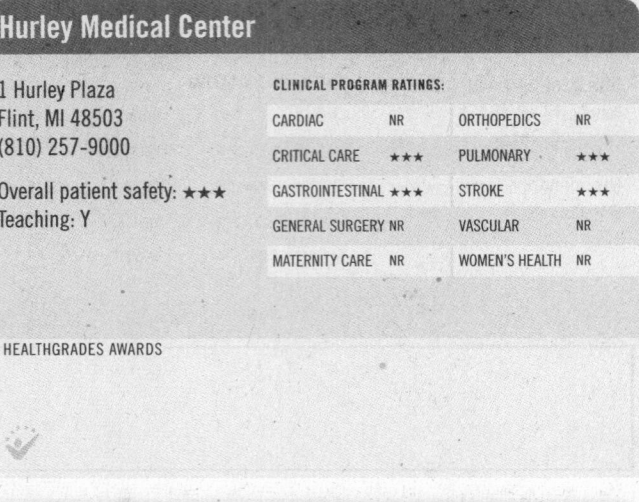

1 Hurley Plaza
Flint, MI 48503
(810) 257-9000

Overall patient safety: ★★★
Teaching: Y

CLINICAL PROGRAM RATINGS:

CARDIAC	NR	ORTHOPEDICS	NR
CRITICAL CARE	★★★	PULMONARY	★★★
GASTROINTESTINAL	★★★	STROKE	★★★
GENERAL SURGERY	NR	VASCULAR	NR
MATERNITY CARE	NR	WOMEN'S HEALTH	NR

HEALTHGRADES AWARDS

Hillsdale Community Health Center

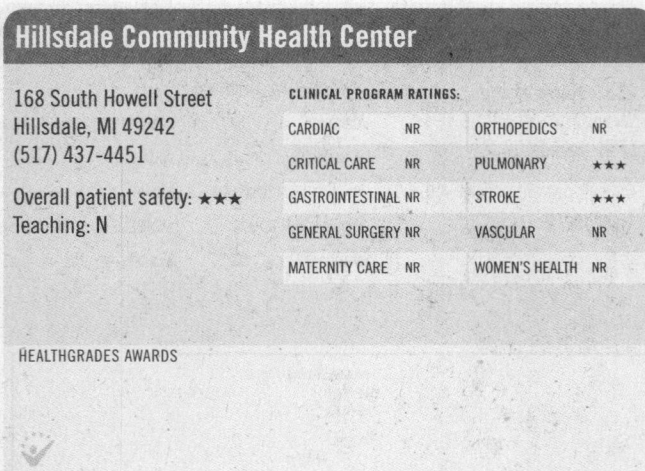

168 South Howell Street
Hillsdale, MI 49242
(517) 437-4451

Overall patient safety: ★★★
Teaching: N

CLINICAL PROGRAM RATINGS:

CARDIAC	NR	ORTHOPEDICS	NR
CRITICAL CARE	NR	PULMONARY	★★★
GASTROINTESTINAL	NR	STROKE	★★★
GENERAL SURGERY	NR	VASCULAR	NR
MATERNITY CARE	NR	WOMEN'S HEALTH	NR

HEALTHGRADES AWARDS

Huron Medical Center

1100 South Van Dyke
Bad Axe, MI 48413
(989) 269-9521

Overall patient safety: ★★★
Teaching: N

CLINICAL PROGRAM RATINGS:

CARDIAC	NR	ORTHOPEDICS	NR
CRITICAL CARE	NR	PULMONARY	★★★
GASTROINTESTINAL	NR	STROKE	★★★
GENERAL SURGERY	NR	VASCULAR	NR
MATERNITY CARE	NR	WOMEN'S HEALTH	NR

HEALTHGRADES AWARDS

✓ SPECIALTY EXCELLENCE
• JOINT REPLACEMENT

Holland Community Hospital

602 Michigan Avenue
Holland, MI 49423
(616) 392-5141

Overall patient safety: ★★★★★
Teaching: N

CLINICAL PROGRAM RATINGS:

CARDIAC	NR	ORTHOPEDICS	★★★
CRITICAL CARE	★★★	PULMONARY	★★★
GASTROINTESTINAL	★★★	STROKE	★★★
GENERAL SURGERY	NR	VASCULAR	NR
MATERNITY CARE	NR	WOMEN'S HEALTH	NR

HEALTHGRADES AWARDS

✓ DISTINGUISHED
  HOSPITAL
  • PATIENT SAFETY

Huron Valley Sinai Hospital

1 William Carls Drive
Commerce Township, MI 48382
(248) 937-3300

Overall patient safety: ★★★
Teaching: Y

CLINICAL PROGRAM RATINGS:

CARDIAC	NR	ORTHOPEDICS	★★★
CRITICAL CARE	★★★	PULMONARY	★★★
GASTROINTESTINAL	★★★	STROKE	★★★
GENERAL SURGERY	NR	VASCULAR	NR
MATERNITY CARE	NR	WOMEN'S HEALTH	NR

HEALTHGRADES AWARDS

✓ DISTINGUISHED
  HOSPITAL
  • CLINICAL EXCELLENCE

KEY: ★★★★★ BEST   ★★★ AS EXPECTED   ★ POOR   NR NOT RATED BY HEALTHGRADES   For full definitions of ratings and awards, see Appendix.

Hutzel Hospital*

3980 John R Street
Detroit, MI 48201
(313) 745-7552

Overall patient safety: ★★★
Teaching: Y

CLINICAL PROGRAM RATINGS:

CARDIAC	★★★	ORTHOPEDICS	NR
CRITICAL CARE	★★★	PULMONARY	★★★
GASTROINTESTINAL	★★★	STROKE	★★★★★
GENERAL SURGERY	NR	VASCULAR	★
MATERNITY CARE	NR	WOMEN'S HEALTH	NR

HEALTHGRADES AWARDS

✓ SPECIALTY EXCELLENCE
· GASTROINTESTINAL   · STROKE CARE
  CARE

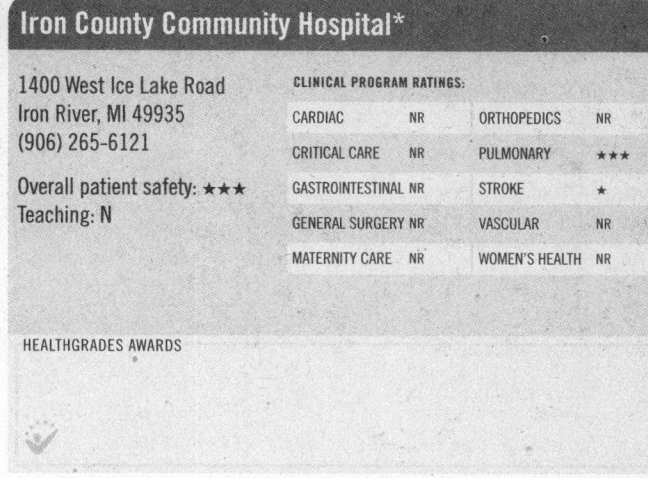

Iron County Community Hospital*

1400 West Ice Lake Road
Iron River, MI 49935
(906) 265-6121

Overall patient safety: ★★★
Teaching: N

CLINICAL PROGRAM RATINGS:

CARDIAC	NR	ORTHOPEDICS	NR
CRITICAL CARE	NR	PULMONARY	★★★
GASTROINTESTINAL	NR	STROKE	★
GENERAL SURGERY	NR	VASCULAR	NR
MATERNITY CARE	NR	WOMEN'S HEALTH	NR

HEALTHGRADES AWARDS

Ingham Regional Medical Center

401 West Greenlawn Avenue
Lansing, MI 48910
(517) 334-2967

Overall patient safety: ★★★
Teaching: Y

CLINICAL PROGRAM RATINGS:

CARDIAC	★★★	ORTHOPEDICS	★★★
CRITICAL CARE	★★★	PULMONARY	★★★
GASTROINTESTINAL	★★★	STROKE	★
GENERAL SURGERY	NR	VASCULAR	★★★★★
MATERNITY CARE	NR	WOMEN'S HEALTH	NR

HEALTHGRADES AWARDS

✓ SPECIALTY EXCELLENCE
· JOINT REPLACEMENT   · VASCULAR SURGERY

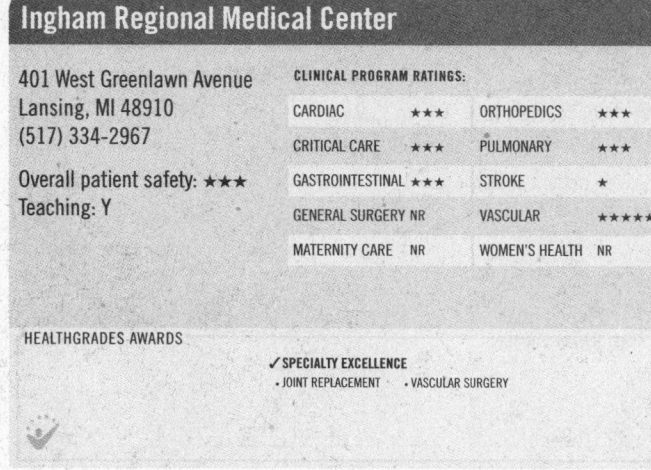

Keweenaw Memorial Medical Center

205 Osceola Street
Laurium, MI 49913
(906) 337-6543

Overall patient safety: ★★★
Teaching: N

CLINICAL PROGRAM RATINGS:

CARDIAC	NR	ORTHOPEDICS	NR
CRITICAL CARE	NR	PULMONARY	★★★
GASTROINTESTINAL	NR	STROKE	★★★
GENERAL SURGERY	NR	VASCULAR	NR
MATERNITY CARE	NR	WOMEN'S HEALTH	NR

HEALTHGRADES AWARDS

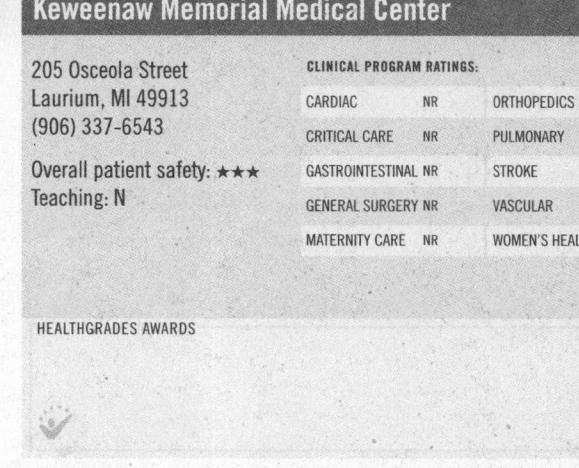

Ionia County Memorial Hospital

479 Lafayette Street
Ionia, MI 48846
(616) 527-4200

Overall patient safety: ★★★
Teaching: N

CLINICAL PROGRAM RATINGS:

CARDIAC	NR	ORTHOPEDICS	NR
CRITICAL CARE	NR	PULMONARY	★★★
GASTROINTESTINAL	NR	STROKE	★★★
GENERAL SURGERY	NR	VASCULAR	NR
MATERNITY CARE	NR	WOMEN'S HEALTH	NR

HEALTHGRADES AWARDS

Lakeland Hospital--St. Joseph*

1234 Napier Avenue
St. Joseph, MI 49085
(269) 983-8300

Overall patient safety: ★★★
Teaching: N

CLINICAL PROGRAM RATINGS:

CARDIAC	★★★	ORTHOPEDICS	★★★
CRITICAL CARE	★★★	PULMONARY	★★★
GASTROINTESTINAL	★★★	STROKE	★★★
GENERAL SURGERY	NR	VASCULAR	NR
MATERNITY CARE	NR	WOMEN'S HEALTH	NR

HEALTHGRADES AWARDS

*This hospital reports its data to the federal government jointly with another hospital. Therefore the ratings and awards apply to multiple hospitals and this specific hospital may not provide all rated services.

Lakeland Medical Center–Niles*

31 North St. Joseph Avenue
Niles, MI 49120
(269) 683-5510

Overall patient safety: ★★★
Teaching: N

CLINICAL PROGRAM RATINGS:

CARDIAC	★★★	ORTHOPEDICS	★★★
CRITICAL CARE	★★★	PULMONARY	★★★
GASTROINTESTINAL	★★★	STROKE	★★★
GENERAL SURGERY	NR	VASCULAR	NR
MATERNITY CARE	NR	WOMEN'S HEALTH	NR

HEALTHGRADES AWARDS

Madison Community Hospital*

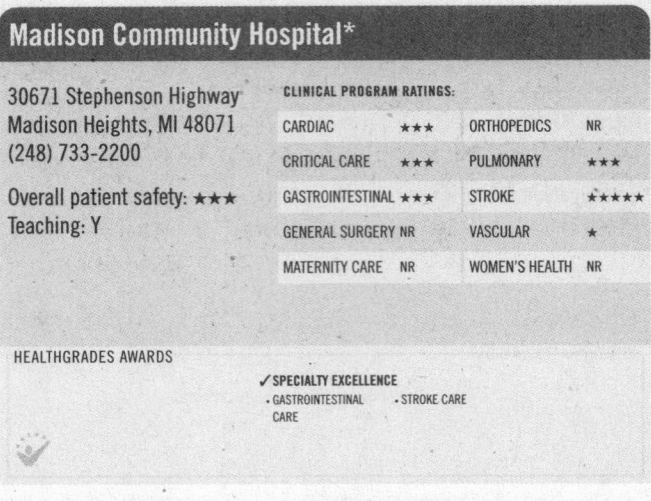

30671 Stephenson Highway
Madison Heights, MI 48071
(248) 733-2200

Overall patient safety: ★★★
Teaching: Y

CLINICAL PROGRAM RATINGS:

CARDIAC	★★★	ORTHOPEDICS	NR
CRITICAL CARE	★★★	PULMONARY	★★★
GASTROINTESTINAL	★★★	STROKE	★★★★★
GENERAL SURGERY	NR	VASCULAR	★
MATERNITY CARE	NR	WOMEN'S HEALTH	NR

HEALTHGRADES AWARDS

✓ **SPECIALTY EXCELLENCE**
• GASTROINTESTINAL   • STROKE CARE
  CARE

Lakeview Community Hospital

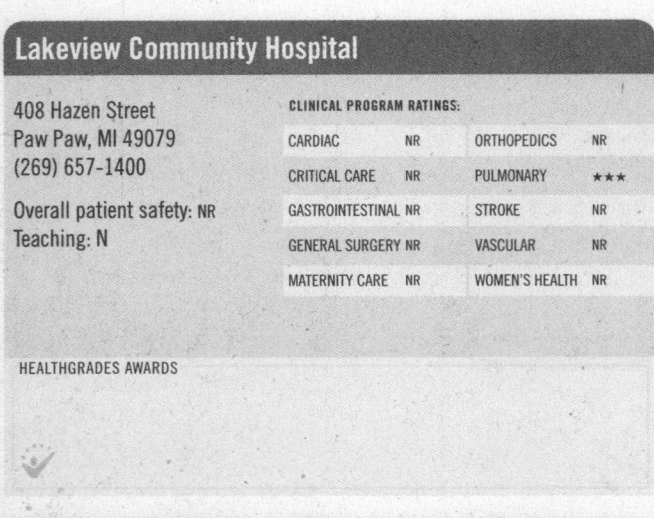

408 Hazen Street
Paw Paw, MI 49079
(269) 657-1400

Overall patient safety: NR
Teaching: N

CLINICAL PROGRAM RATINGS:

CARDIAC	NR	ORTHOPEDICS	NR
CRITICAL CARE	NR	PULMONARY	★★★
GASTROINTESTINAL	NR	STROKE	NR
GENERAL SURGERY	NR	VASCULAR	NR
MATERNITY CARE	NR	WOMEN'S HEALTH	NR

HEALTHGRADES AWARDS

Marlette Community Hospital

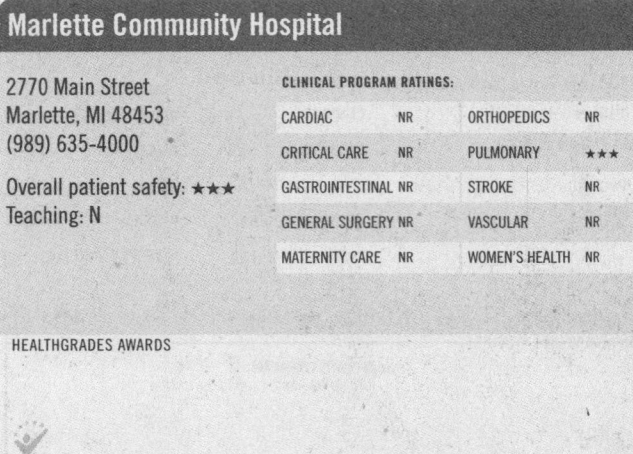

2770 Main Street
Marlette, MI 48453
(989) 635-4000

Overall patient safety: ★★★
Teaching: N

CLINICAL PROGRAM RATINGS:

CARDIAC	NR	ORTHOPEDICS	NR
CRITICAL CARE	NR	PULMONARY	★★★
GASTROINTESTINAL	NR	STROKE	NR
GENERAL SURGERY	NR	VASCULAR	NR
MATERNITY CARE	NR	WOMEN'S HEALTH	NR

HEALTHGRADES AWARDS

Lapeer Regional Medical Center

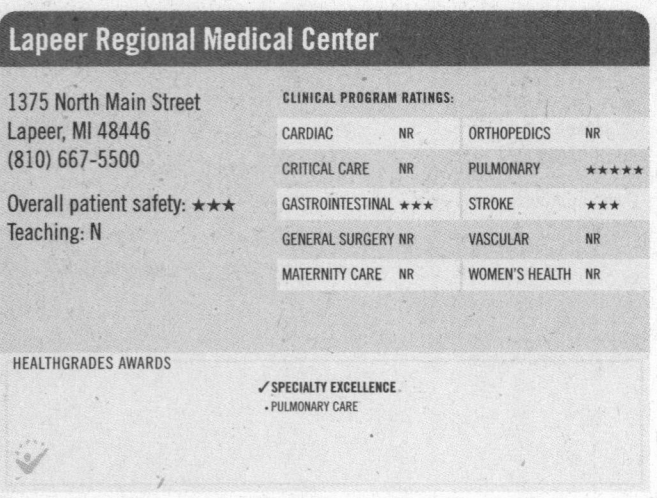

1375 North Main Street
Lapeer, MI 48446
(810) 667-5500

Overall patient safety: ★★★
Teaching: N

CLINICAL PROGRAM RATINGS:

CARDIAC	NR	ORTHOPEDICS	NR
CRITICAL CARE	NR	PULMONARY	★★★★★
GASTROINTESTINAL	★★★	STROKE	★★★
GENERAL SURGERY	NR	VASCULAR	NR
MATERNITY CARE	NR	WOMEN'S HEALTH	NR

HEALTHGRADES AWARDS

✓ **SPECIALTY EXCELLENCE**
• PULMONARY CARE

Marquette General Hospital

580 West College Avenue
Marquette, MI 49855
(906) 228-9440

Overall patient safety: ★★★★★
Teaching: Y

CLINICAL PROGRAM RATINGS:

CARDIAC	★★★	ORTHOPEDICS	★★★
CRITICAL CARE	NR	PULMONARY	★★★
GASTROINTESTINAL	★★★	STROKE	★★★
GENERAL SURGERY	NR	VASCULAR	★★★
MATERNITY CARE	NR	WOMEN'S HEALTH	NR

HEALTHGRADES AWARDS

✓ **DISTINGUISHED
  HOSPITAL**
• PATIENT SAFETY

KEY: ★★★★★ BEST   ★★★ AS EXPECTED   ★ POOR   NR NOT RATED BY HEALTHGRADES   For full definitions of ratings and awards, see Appendix.

McKenzie Memorial Hospital

120 Delaware Street
Sandusky, MI 48471
(810) 648-3770

Overall patient safety: ★★★
Teaching: N

CLINICAL PROGRAM RATINGS:

CARDIAC	NR	ORTHOPEDICS	NR
CRITICAL CARE	NR	PULMONARY	★★★
GASTROINTESTINAL	NR	STROKE	NR
GENERAL SURGERY	NR	VASCULAR	NR
MATERNITY CARE	NR	WOMEN'S HEALTH	NR

HEALTHGRADES AWARDS

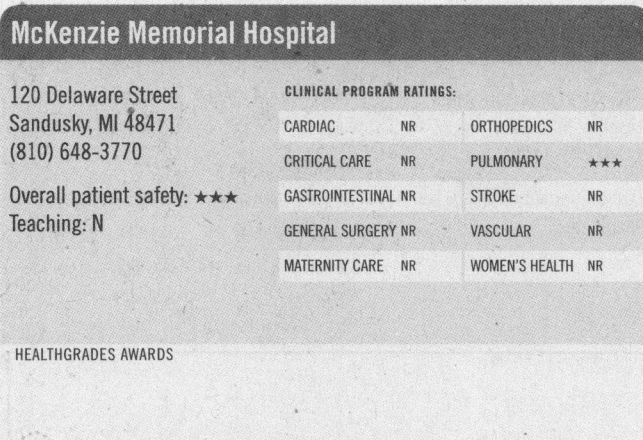

Memorial Healthcare Center

826 West King Street
Owosso, MI 48867
(989) 723-5211

Overall patient safety: ★★★
Teaching: N

CLINICAL PROGRAM RATINGS:

CARDIAC	NR	ORTHOPEDICS	NR
CRITICAL CARE	NR	PULMONARY	★★★
GASTROINTESTINAL	★★★	STROKE	★★★
GENERAL SURGERY	NR	VASCULAR	NR
MATERNITY CARE	NR	WOMEN'S HEALTH	NR

HEALTHGRADES AWARDS

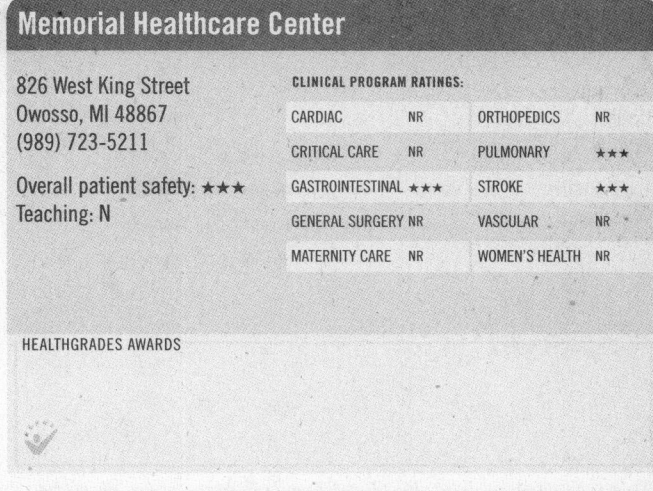

McLaren Regional Medical Center

401 South Ballenger Highway
Flint, MI 48532
(810) 342-2000

Overall patient safety: ★★★★★
Teaching: Y

CLINICAL PROGRAM RATINGS:

CARDIAC	★★★	ORTHOPEDICS	★★★
CRITICAL CARE	★★★	PULMONARY	★★★★★
GASTROINTESTINAL	★★★	STROKE	★★★
GENERAL SURGERY	NR	VASCULAR	★★★
MATERNITY CARE	NR	WOMEN'S HEALTH	NR

HEALTHGRADES AWARDS

✓ DISTINGUISHED HOSPITAL
- PATIENT SAFETY

✓ SPECIALTY EXCELLENCE
- PULMONARY CARE

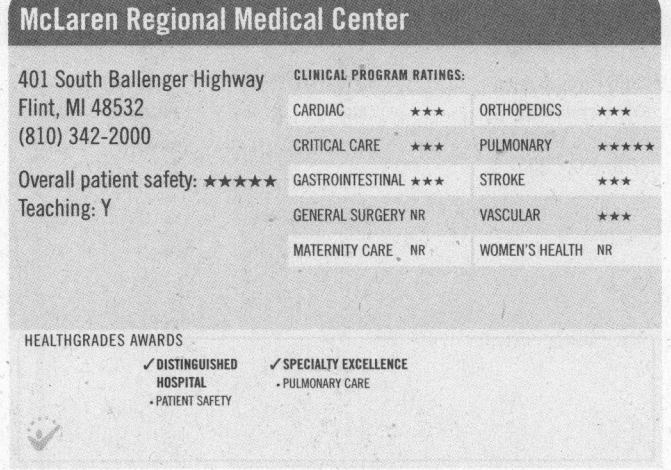

Memorial Medical Center of West Michigan

1 Atkinson Drive
Ludington, MI 49431
(231) 843-2591

Overall patient safety: ★★★★★
Teaching: N

CLINICAL PROGRAM RATINGS:

CARDIAC	NR	ORTHOPEDICS	NR
CRITICAL CARE	NR	PULMONARY	★★★
GASTROINTESTINAL	★★★	STROKE	★★★
GENERAL SURGERY	NR	VASCULAR	NR
MATERNITY CARE	NR	WOMEN'S HEALTH	NR

HEALTHGRADES AWARDS

Mecosta County Medical Center

605 Oak Street
Big Rapids, MI 49307
(231) 796-8691

Overall patient safety: ★★★★★
Teaching: N

CLINICAL PROGRAM RATINGS:

CARDIAC	NR	ORTHOPEDICS	NR
CRITICAL CARE	NR	PULMONARY	★★★
GASTROINTESTINAL	NR	STROKE	★★★
GENERAL SURGERY	NR	VASCULAR	NR
MATERNITY CARE	NR	WOMEN'S HEALTH	NR

HEALTHGRADES AWARDS

✓ SPECIALTY EXCELLENCE
- JOINT REPLACEMENT

Mercy General Health Partners

1500 Sherman Avenue
Muskegon, MI 49444
(231) 739-9341

Overall patient safety: ★★★★★
Teaching: Y

CLINICAL PROGRAM RATINGS:

CARDIAC	★★★	ORTHOPEDICS	★★★
CRITICAL CARE	★★★	PULMONARY	★★★
GASTROINTESTINAL	★★★	STROKE	★
GENERAL SURGERY	NR	VASCULAR	★★★★★
MATERNITY CARE	NR	WOMEN'S HEALTH	NR

HEALTHGRADES AWARDS

✓ DISTINGUISHED HOSPITAL
- PATIENT SAFETY

✓ SPECIALTY EXCELLENCE
- JOINT REPLACEMENT
- VASCULAR SURGERY

*This hospital reports its data to the federal government jointly with another hospital. Therefore the ratings and awards apply to multiple hospitals and this specific hospital may not provide all rated services.

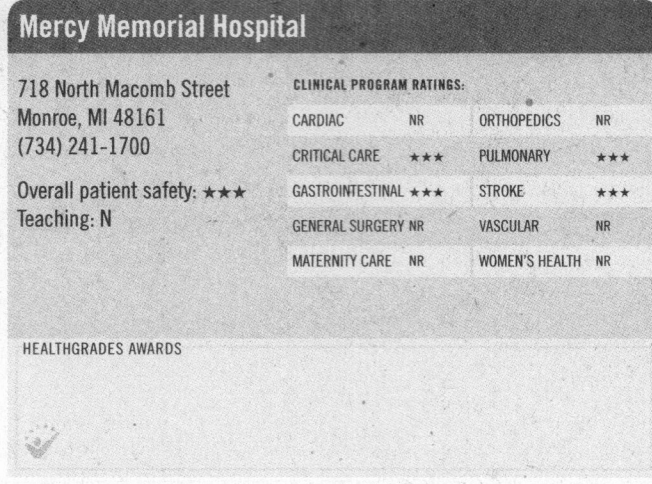

Mercy Hospital–Cadillac

400 Hobart Street
Cadillac, MI 49601
(231) 876-7200

Overall patient safety: ★★★
Teaching: N

CLINICAL PROGRAM RATINGS:

CARDIAC	NR	ORTHOPEDICS	NR
CRITICAL CARE	NR	PULMONARY	★★★
GASTROINTESTINAL	NR	STROKE	★★★
GENERAL SURGERY	NR	VASCULAR	NR
MATERNITY CARE	NR	WOMEN'S HEALTH	NR

HEALTHGRADES AWARDS

Mercy Memorial Hospital

718 North Macomb Street
Monroe, MI 48161
(734) 241-1700

Overall patient safety: ★★★
Teaching: N

CLINICAL PROGRAM RATINGS:

CARDIAC	NR	ORTHOPEDICS	NR
CRITICAL CARE	★★★	PULMONARY	★★★
GASTROINTESTINAL	★★★	STROKE	★★★
GENERAL SURGERY	NR	VASCULAR	NR
MATERNITY CARE	NR	WOMEN'S HEALTH	NR

HEALTHGRADES AWARDS

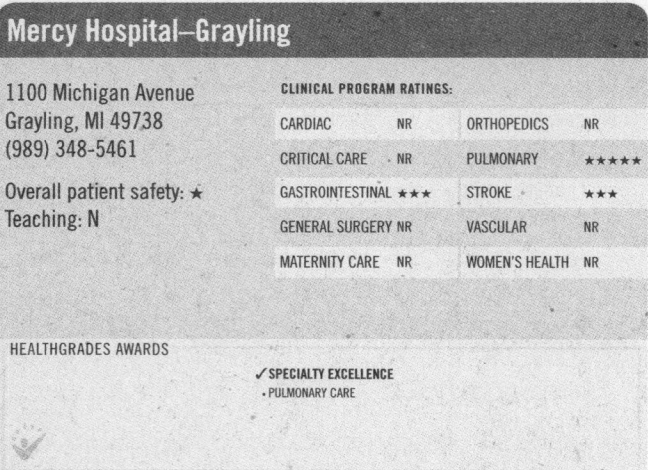

Mercy Hospital–Grayling

1100 Michigan Avenue
Grayling, MI 49738
(989) 348-5461

Overall patient safety: ★
Teaching: N

CLINICAL PROGRAM RATINGS:

CARDIAC	NR	ORTHOPEDICS	NR
CRITICAL CARE	NR	PULMONARY	★★★★★
GASTROINTESTINAL	★★★	STROKE	★★★
GENERAL SURGERY	NR	VASCULAR	NR
MATERNITY CARE	NR	WOMEN'S HEALTH	NR

HEALTHGRADES AWARDS

✓ SPECIALTY EXCELLENCE
· PULMONARY CARE

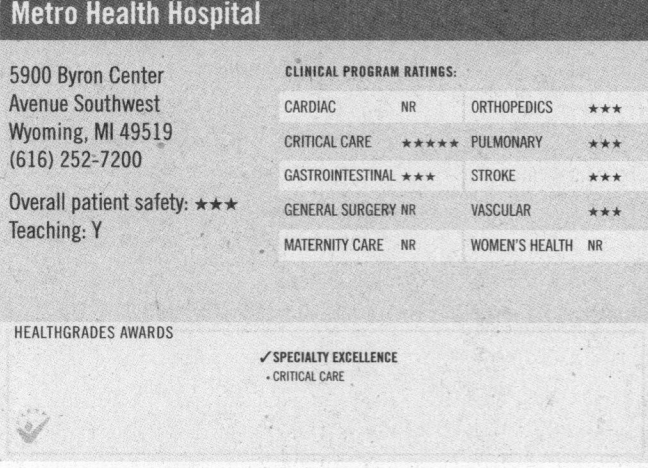

Metro Health Hospital

5900 Byron Center
Avenue Southwest
Wyoming, MI 49519
(616) 252-7200

Overall patient safety: ★★★
Teaching: Y

CLINICAL PROGRAM RATINGS:

CARDIAC	NR	ORTHOPEDICS	★★★
CRITICAL CARE	★★★★★	PULMONARY	★★★
GASTROINTESTINAL	★★★	STROKE	★★★
GENERAL SURGERY	NR	VASCULAR	★★★
MATERNITY CARE	NR	WOMEN'S HEALTH	NR

HEALTHGRADES AWARDS

✓ SPECIALTY EXCELLENCE
· CRITICAL CARE

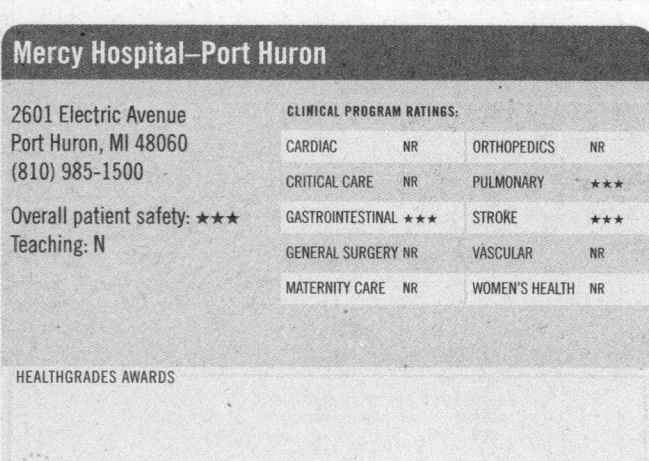

Mercy Hospital–Port Huron

2601 Electric Avenue
Port Huron, MI 48060
(810) 985-1500

Overall patient safety: ★★★
Teaching: N

CLINICAL PROGRAM RATINGS:

CARDIAC	NR	ORTHOPEDICS	NR
CRITICAL CARE	NR	PULMONARY	★★★
GASTROINTESTINAL	★★★	STROKE	★★★
GENERAL SURGERY	NR	VASCULAR	NR
MATERNITY CARE	NR	WOMEN'S HEALTH	NR

HEALTHGRADES AWARDS

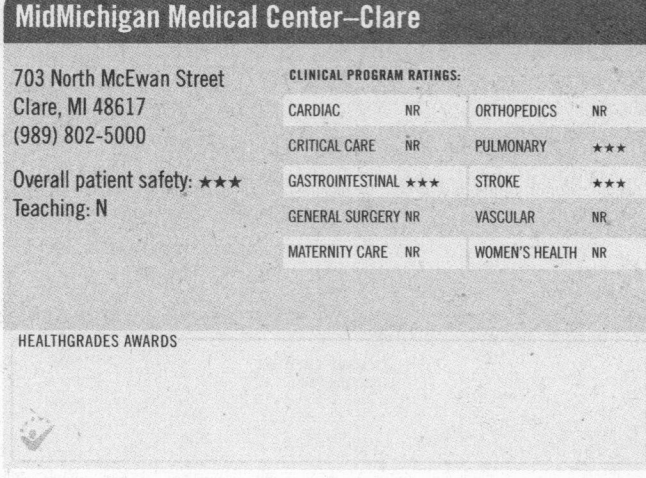

MidMichigan Medical Center–Clare

703 North McEwan Street
Clare, MI 48617
(989) 802-5000

Overall patient safety: ★★★
Teaching: N

CLINICAL PROGRAM RATINGS:

CARDIAC	NR	ORTHOPEDICS	NR
CRITICAL CARE	NR	PULMONARY	★★★
GASTROINTESTINAL	★★★	STROKE	★★★
GENERAL SURGERY	NR	VASCULAR	NR
MATERNITY CARE	NR	WOMEN'S HEALTH	NR

HEALTHGRADES AWARDS

KEY: ★★★★★ BEST   ★★★ AS EXPECTED   ★ POOR   NR NOT RATED BY HEALTHGRADES   For full definitions of ratings and awards, see Appendix.

MidMichigan Medical Center—Gladwin

515 Quarter Street
Gladwin, MI 48624
(989) 246-6200

Overall patient safety: ★★★
Teaching: N

CLINICAL PROGRAM RATINGS:

CARDIAC	NR	ORTHOPEDICS	NR
CRITICAL CARE	NR	PULMONARY	★★★★★
GASTROINTESTINAL	NR	STROKE	NR
GENERAL SURGERY	NR	VASCULAR	NR
MATERNITY CARE	NR	WOMEN'S HEALTH	NR

HEALTHGRADES AWARDS

✓ SPECIALTY EXCELLENCE
• PULMONARY CARE

Mount Clemens Regional Medical Center

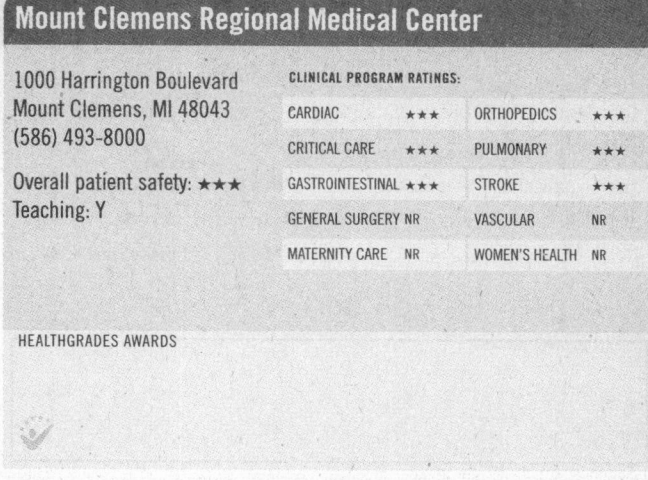

1000 Harrington Boulevard
Mount Clemens, MI 48043
(586) 493-8000

Overall patient safety: ★★★
Teaching: Y

CLINICAL PROGRAM RATINGS:

CARDIAC	★★★	ORTHOPEDICS	★★★
CRITICAL CARE	★★★	PULMONARY	★★★
GASTROINTESTINAL	★★★	STROKE	★★★
GENERAL SURGERY	NR	VASCULAR	NR
MATERNITY CARE	NR	WOMEN'S HEALTH	NR

HEALTHGRADES AWARDS

MidMichigan Medical Center—Midland

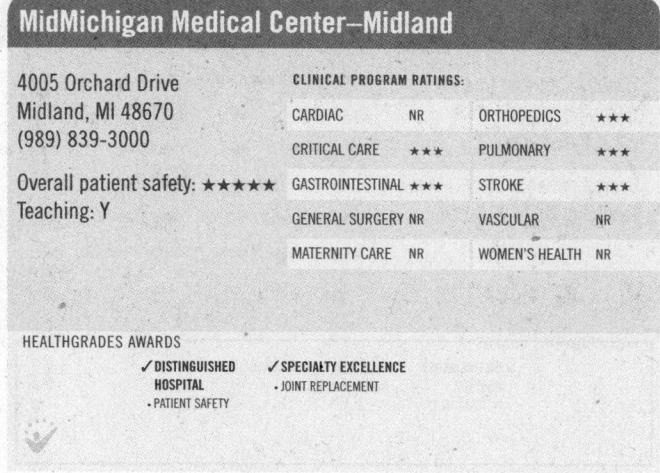

4005 Orchard Drive
Midland, MI 48670
(989) 839-3000

Overall patient safety: ★★★★★
Teaching: Y

CLINICAL PROGRAM RATINGS:

CARDIAC	NR	ORTHOPEDICS	★★★
CRITICAL CARE	★★★	PULMONARY	★★★
GASTROINTESTINAL	★★★	STROKE	★★★
GENERAL SURGERY	NR	VASCULAR	NR
MATERNITY CARE	NR	WOMEN'S HEALTH	NR

HEALTHGRADES AWARDS

✓ DISTINGUISHED HOSPITAL
• PATIENT SAFETY

✓ SPECIALTY EXCELLENCE
• JOINT REPLACEMENT

Munson Medical Center*

1105 6th Street
Traverse City, MI 49684
(231) 935-5000

Overall patient safety: ★★★★★
Teaching: Y

CLINICAL PROGRAM RATINGS:

CARDIAC	★★★	ORTHOPEDICS	★★★★★
CRITICAL CARE	NR	PULMONARY	★★★★★
GASTROINTESTINAL	★★★★★	STROKE	★★★
GENERAL SURGERY	NR	VASCULAR	★★★
MATERNITY CARE	NR	WOMEN'S HEALTH	NR

HEALTHGRADES AWARDS

✓ AMERICA'S 50 BEST HOSPITALS

✓ DISTINGUISHED HOSPITAL
• CLINICAL EXCELLENCE
• PATIENT SAFETY

✓ SPECIALTY EXCELLENCE
• GASTROINTESTINAL CARE
• JOINT REPLACEMENT
• ORTHOPEDIC SURGERY
• PULMONARY CARE

Morenci Area Hospital*

13101 Sims Highway
Morenci, MI 49256
(517) 458-2236

Overall patient safety: ★★★
Teaching: N

CLINICAL PROGRAM RATINGS:

CARDIAC	NR	ORTHOPEDICS	NR
CRITICAL CARE	NR	PULMONARY	★★★
GASTROINTESTINAL	NR	STROKE	★★★
GENERAL SURGERY	NR	VASCULAR	NR
MATERNITY CARE	NR	WOMEN'S HEALTH	NR

HEALTHGRADES AWARDS

North Oakland Medical Center

461 West Huron Street
Pontiac, MI 48341
(248) 857-7200

Overall patient safety: ★★★
Teaching: Y

CLINICAL PROGRAM RATINGS:

CARDIAC	NR	ORTHOPEDICS	NR
CRITICAL CARE	NR	PULMONARY	★★★
GASTROINTESTINAL	★★★	STROKE	★★★
GENERAL SURGERY	NR	VASCULAR	NR
MATERNITY CARE	NR	WOMEN'S HEALTH	NR

HEALTHGRADES AWARDS

*This hospital reports its data to the federal government jointly with another hospital. Therefore the ratings and awards apply to multiple hospitals and this specific hospital may not provide all rated services.

North Ottawa Community Hospital

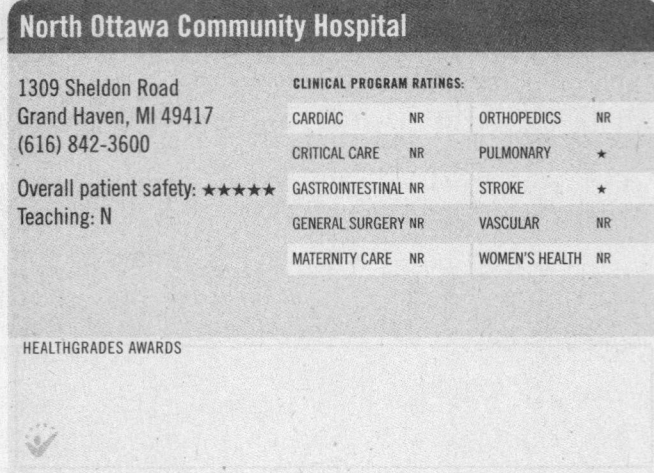

1309 Sheldon Road
Grand Haven, MI 49417
(616) 842-3600

Overall patient safety: ★★★★★
Teaching: N

CLINICAL PROGRAM RATINGS:

CARDIAC	NR	ORTHOPEDICS	NR
CRITICAL CARE	NR	PULMONARY	★
GASTROINTESTINAL	NR	STROKE	★
GENERAL SURGERY	NR	VASCULAR	NR
MATERNITY CARE	NR	WOMEN'S HEALTH	NR

HEALTHGRADES AWARDS

Oakwood Annapolis Hospital

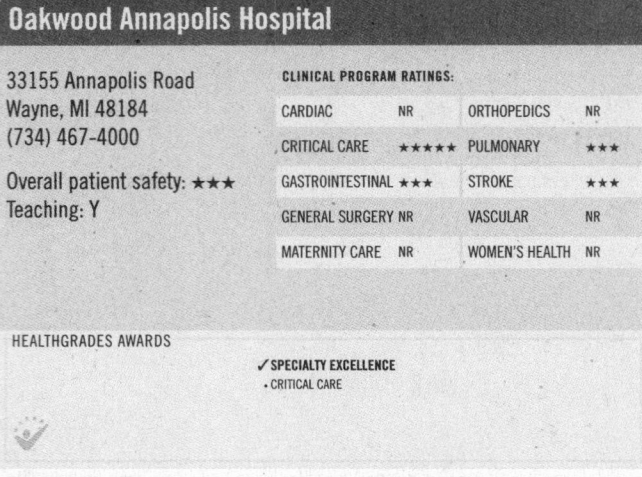

33155 Annapolis Road
Wayne, MI 48184
(734) 467-4000

Overall patient safety: ★★★
Teaching: Y

CLINICAL PROGRAM RATINGS:

CARDIAC	NR	ORTHOPEDICS	NR
CRITICAL CARE	★★★★★	PULMONARY	★★★
GASTROINTESTINAL	★★★	STROKE	★★★
GENERAL SURGERY	NR	VASCULAR	NR
MATERNITY CARE	NR	WOMEN'S HEALTH	NR

HEALTHGRADES AWARDS
✓ SPECIALTY EXCELLENCE
• CRITICAL CARE

Northern Michigan Hospital

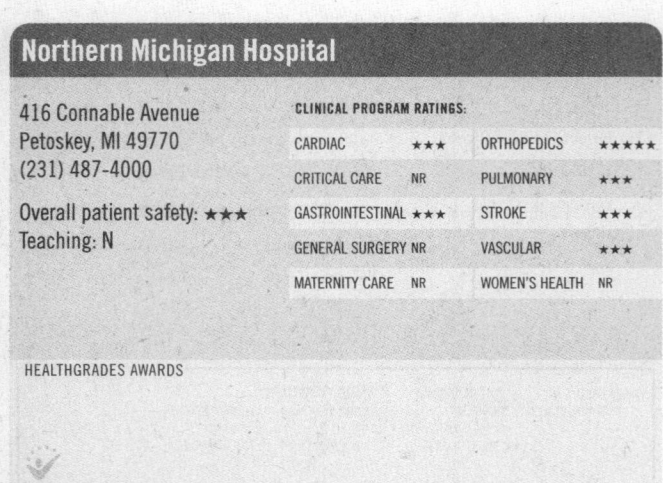

416 Connable Avenue
Petoskey, MI 49770
(231) 487-4000

Overall patient safety: ★★★
Teaching: N

CLINICAL PROGRAM RATINGS:

CARDIAC	★★★	ORTHOPEDICS	★★★★★
CRITICAL CARE	NR	PULMONARY	★★★
GASTROINTESTINAL	★★★	STROKE	★★★
GENERAL SURGERY	NR	VASCULAR	★★★
MATERNITY CARE	NR	WOMEN'S HEALTH	NR

HEALTHGRADES AWARDS

Oakwood Heritage Hospital

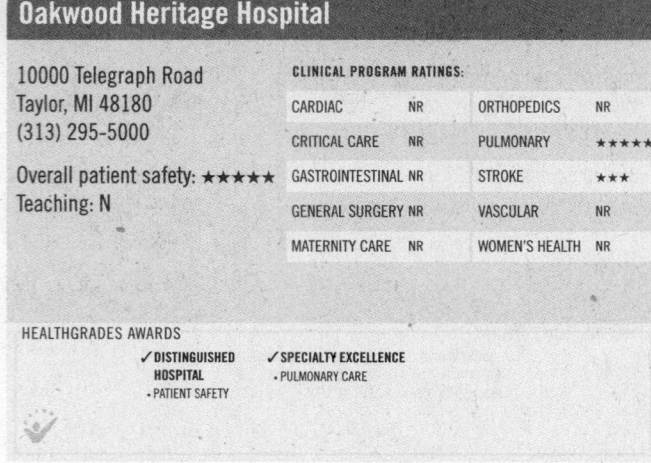

10000 Telegraph Road
Taylor, MI 48180
(313) 295-5000

Overall patient safety: ★★★★★
Teaching: N

CLINICAL PROGRAM RATINGS:

CARDIAC	NR	ORTHOPEDICS	NR
CRITICAL CARE	NR	PULMONARY	★★★★★
GASTROINTESTINAL	NR	STROKE	★★★
GENERAL SURGERY	NR	VASCULAR	NR
MATERNITY CARE	NR	WOMEN'S HEALTH	NR

HEALTHGRADES AWARDS
✓ DISTINGUISHED HOSPITAL
• PATIENT SAFETY
✓ SPECIALTY EXCELLENCE
• PULMONARY CARE

Oaklawn Hospital

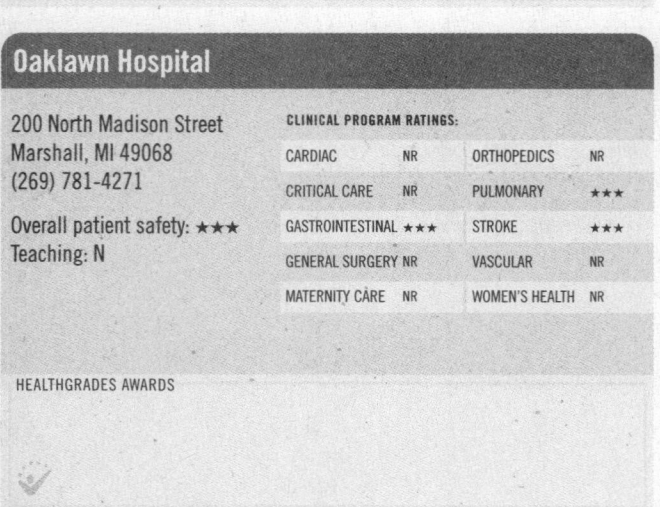

200 North Madison Street
Marshall, MI 49068
(269) 781-4271

Overall patient safety: ★★★
Teaching: N

CLINICAL PROGRAM RATINGS:

CARDIAC	NR	ORTHOPEDICS	NR
CRITICAL CARE	NR	PULMONARY	★★★
GASTROINTESTINAL	★★★	STROKE	★★★
GENERAL SURGERY	NR	VASCULAR	NR
MATERNITY CARE	NR	WOMEN'S HEALTH	NR

HEALTHGRADES AWARDS

Oakwood Hospital and Medical Center--Dearborn

18101 Oakwood Boulevard
Dearborn, MI 48124
(313) 593-7000

Overall patient safety: ★★★★★
Teaching: Y

CLINICAL PROGRAM RATINGS:

CARDIAC	★★★	ORTHOPEDICS	★★★★★
CRITICAL CARE	★★★	PULMONARY	★★★★★
GASTROINTESTINAL	★★★	STROKE	★★★★★
GENERAL SURGERY	NR	VASCULAR	★
MATERNITY CARE	NR	WOMEN'S HEALTH	NR

HEALTHGRADES AWARDS
✓ DISTINGUISHED HOSPITAL
• PATIENT SAFETY
✓ SPECIALTY EXCELLENCE
• JOINT REPLACEMENT • ORTHOPEDIC SURGERY • PULMONARY CARE

KEY: ★★★★★ BEST   ★★★ AS EXPECTED   ★ POOR   NR NOT RATED BY HEALTHGRADES   For full definitions of ratings and awards, see Appendix.

Oakwood Southshore Medical Center

5450 Fort Street
Trenton, MI 48183
(734) 671-3800

Overall patient safety: ★★★
Teaching: Y

CLINICAL PROGRAM RATINGS:

CARDIAC	NR	ORTHOPEDICS	NR
CRITICAL CARE	★★★	PULMONARY	★★★★★
GASTROINTESTINAL	★★★★★	STROKE	★★★
GENERAL SURGERY	NR	VASCULAR	NR
MATERNITY CARE	NR	WOMEN'S HEALTH	NR

HEALTHGRADES AWARDS

✓ **DISTINGUISHED HOSPITAL**
- CLINICAL EXCELLENCE

✓ **SPECIALTY EXCELLENCE**
- GASTROINTESTINAL CARE
- PULMONARY CARE

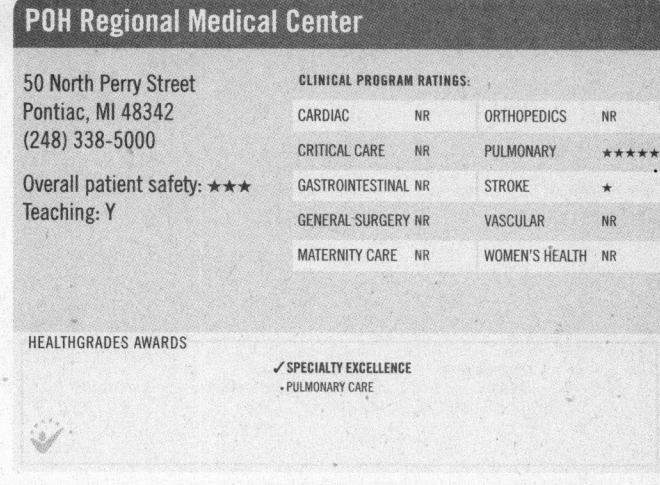

POH Regional Medical Center

50 North Perry Street
Pontiac, MI 48342
(248) 338-5000

Overall patient safety: ★★★
Teaching: Y

CLINICAL PROGRAM RATINGS:

CARDIAC	NR	ORTHOPEDICS	NR
CRITICAL CARE	NR	PULMONARY	★★★★★
GASTROINTESTINAL	NR	STROKE	★
GENERAL SURGERY	NR	VASCULAR	NR
MATERNITY CARE	NR	WOMEN'S HEALTH	NR

HEALTHGRADES AWARDS

✓ **SPECIALTY EXCELLENCE**
- PULMONARY CARE

Otsego Memorial Hospital

825 North Center Street
Gaylord, MI 49735
(989) 731-2100

Overall patient safety: ★★★
Teaching: N

CLINICAL PROGRAM RATINGS:

CARDIAC	NR	ORTHOPEDICS	NR
CRITICAL CARE	NR	PULMONARY	★★★
GASTROINTESTINAL	NR	STROKE	★★★
GENERAL SURGERY	NR	VASCULAR	NR
MATERNITY CARE	NR	WOMEN'S HEALTH	NR

HEALTHGRADES AWARDS

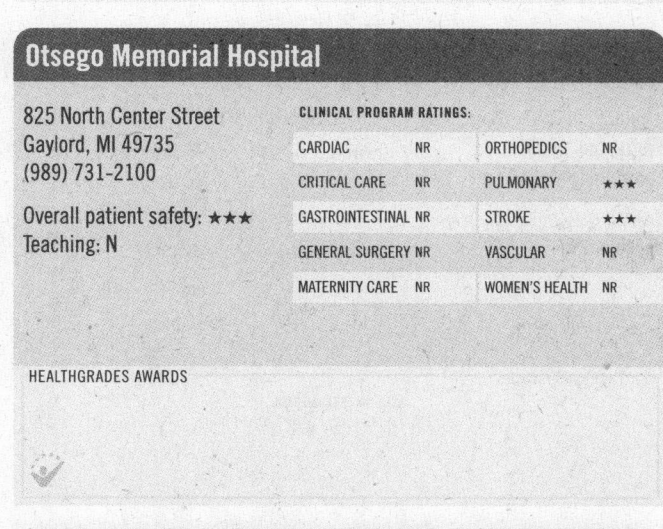

Port Huron Hospital

1221 Pine Grove Avenue
Port Huron, MI 48060
(810) 987-5000

Overall patient safety: ★★★
Teaching: N

CLINICAL PROGRAM RATINGS:

CARDIAC	★★★	ORTHOPEDICS	★★★
CRITICAL CARE	★★★	PULMONARY	★★★★★
GASTROINTESTINAL	★★★	STROKE	★★★
GENERAL SURGERY	NR	VASCULAR	NR
MATERNITY CARE	NR	WOMEN'S HEALTH	NR

HEALTHGRADES AWARDS

✓ **DISTINGUISHED HOSPITAL**
- CLINICAL EXCELLENCE

✓ **SPECIALTY EXCELLENCE**
- GASTROINTESTINAL CARE

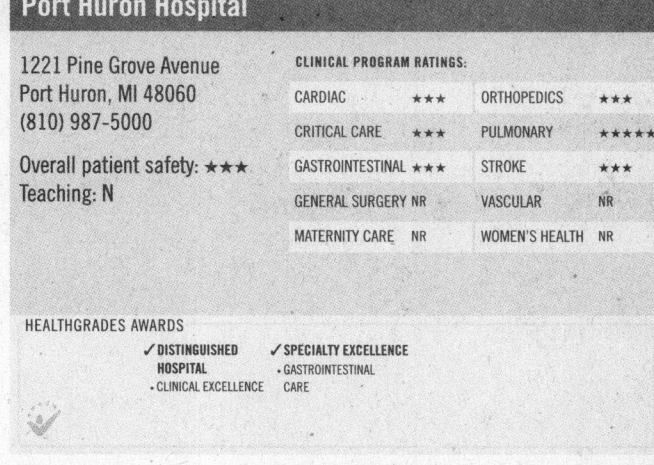

Pennock Hospital

1009 West Green Street
Hastings, MI 49058
(269) 945-3451

Overall patient safety: ★★★
Teaching: N

CLINICAL PROGRAM RATINGS:

CARDIAC	NR	ORTHOPEDICS	NR
CRITICAL CARE	NR	PULMONARY	★
GASTROINTESTINAL	★★★	STROKE	★
GENERAL SURGERY	NR	VASCULAR	NR
MATERNITY CARE	NR	WOMEN'S HEALTH	NR

HEALTHGRADES AWARDS

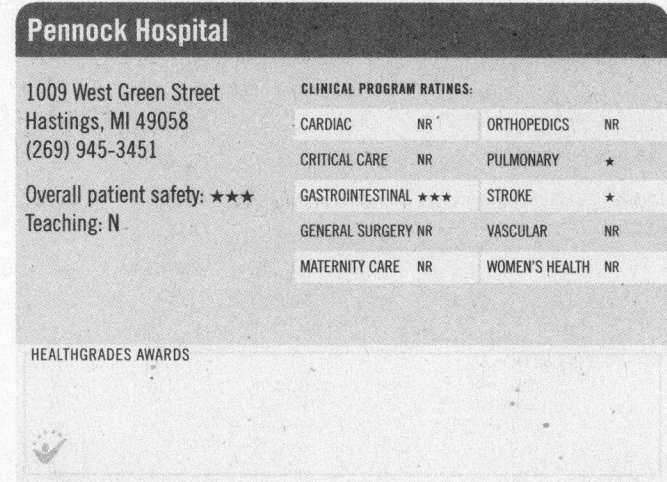

Portage Health System

500 Campus Drive
Hancock, MI 49930
(906) 483-1000

Overall patient safety: ★★★
Teaching: N

CLINICAL PROGRAM RATINGS:

CARDIAC	NR	ORTHOPEDICS	NR
CRITICAL CARE	NR	PULMONARY	★★★
GASTROINTESTINAL	NR	STROKE	★★★
GENERAL SURGERY	NR	VASCULAR	NR
MATERNITY CARE	NR	WOMEN'S HEALTH	NR

HEALTHGRADES AWARDS

Providence Hospital

16001 West Nine Mile Road
Southfield, MI 48075
(248) 424-3000

Overall patient safety: ★★★
Teaching: Y

CLINICAL PROGRAM RATINGS:

CARDIAC	★★★	ORTHOPEDICS	★★★
CRITICAL CARE	★★★★★	PULMONARY	★★★★★
GASTROINTESTINAL	★★★★★	STROKE	★★★★★
GENERAL SURGERY	NR	VASCULAR	★★★
MATERNITY CARE	NR	WOMEN'S HEALTH	NR

HEALTHGRADES AWARDS

✓ **DISTINGUISHED HOSPITAL**
- CLINICAL EXCELLENCE

✓ **SPECIALTY EXCELLENCE**
- CARDIAC SURGERY
- CRITICAL CARE
- GASTROINTESTINAL CARE
- PULMONARY CARE
- STROKE CARE

St. John Hospital and Medical Center

22101 Moross Road
Detroit, MI 48236
(313) 343-4000

Overall patient safety: ★★★
Teaching: Y

CLINICAL PROGRAM RATINGS:

CARDIAC	★★★	ORTHOPEDICS	★★★
CRITICAL CARE	★★★	PULMONARY	★★★★★
GASTROINTESTINAL	★★★	STROKE	★★★★★
GENERAL SURGERY	NR	VASCULAR	★★★
MATERNITY CARE	NR	WOMEN'S HEALTH	NR

HEALTHGRADES AWARDS

✓ **SPECIALTY EXCELLENCE**
- PULMONARY CARE
- STROKE CARE

St. Francis Hospital

3401 Ludington Street
Escanaba, MI 49829
(906) 786-3311

Overall patient safety: ★★★
Teaching: N

CLINICAL PROGRAM RATINGS:

CARDIAC	NR	ORTHOPEDICS	NR
CRITICAL CARE	NR	PULMONARY	★★★
GASTROINTESTINAL	★★★	STROKE	★★★
GENERAL SURGERY	NR	VASCULAR	NR
MATERNITY CARE	NR	WOMEN'S HEALTH	NR

HEALTHGRADES AWARDS

St. John Macomb Hospital

11800 East Twelve Mile Road
Warren, MI 48093
(586) 573-5000

Overall patient safety: ★★★
Teaching: Y

CLINICAL PROGRAM RATINGS:

CARDIAC	★★★	ORTHOPEDICS	★★★★★
CRITICAL CARE	★★★	PULMONARY	★★★
GASTROINTESTINAL	★★★	STROKE	★★★★★
GENERAL SURGERY	NR	VASCULAR	NR
MATERNITY CARE	NR	WOMEN'S HEALTH	NR

HEALTHGRADES AWARDS

✓ **SPECIALTY EXCELLENCE**
- ORTHOPEDIC SURGERY
- STROKE CARE

St. John Detroit Riverview Hospital

7733 East Jefferson Avenue
Detroit, MI 48214
(313) 499-4000

Overall patient safety: ★★★
Teaching: Y

CLINICAL PROGRAM RATINGS:

CARDIAC	NR	ORTHOPEDICS	NR
CRITICAL CARE	NR	PULMONARY	★★★★★
GASTROINTESTINAL	★★★	STROKE	★★★★★
GENERAL SURGERY	NR	VASCULAR	NR
MATERNITY CARE	NR	WOMEN'S HEALTH	NR

HEALTHGRADES AWARDS

✓ **SPECIALTY EXCELLENCE**
- PULMONARY CARE
- STROKE CARE

St. John Oakland Hospital

27351 Dequindre Road
Madison Heights, MI 48071
(248) 967-7000

Overall patient safety: ★★★
Teaching: Y

CLINICAL PROGRAM RATINGS:

CARDIAC	NR	ORTHOPEDICS	NR
CRITICAL CARE	NR	PULMONARY	★★★
GASTROINTESTINAL	★★★	STROKE	★★★
GENERAL SURGERY	NR	VASCULAR	NR
MATERNITY CARE	NR	WOMEN'S HEALTH	NR

HEALTHGRADES AWARDS

KEY: ★★★★★ BEST   ★★★ AS EXPECTED   ★ POOR   NR NOT RATED BY HEALTHGRADES   For full definitions of ratings and awards, see Appendix.

St. John River District Hospital

4100 South River Road
East China, MI 48054
(810) 329-7111

Overall patient safety: ★★★
Teaching: Y

CLINICAL PROGRAM RATINGS:

CARDIAC	NR	ORTHOPEDICS	NR
CRITICAL CARE	NR	PULMONARY	★★★
GASTROINTESTINAL	NR	STROKE	★★★
GENERAL SURGERY	NR	VASCULAR	NR
MATERNITY CARE	NR	WOMEN'S HEALTH	NR

HEALTHGRADES AWARDS

St. Joseph Mercy Livingston Hospital

620 Byron Road
Howell, MI 48843
(517) 545-6000

Overall patient safety: ★
Teaching: N

CLINICAL PROGRAM RATINGS:

CARDIAC	NR	ORTHOPEDICS	NR
CRITICAL CARE	NR	PULMONARY	★★★
GASTROINTESTINAL	★★★	STROKE	★
GENERAL SURGERY	NR	VASCULAR	NR
MATERNITY CARE	NR	WOMEN'S HEALTH	NR

HEALTHGRADES AWARDS

St. Joseph Health System—Tawas

200 Hemlock Street
Tawas City, MI 48764
(989) 362-3411

Overall patient safety: ★★★
Teaching: N

CLINICAL PROGRAM RATINGS:

CARDIAC	NR	ORTHOPEDICS	NR
CRITICAL CARE	NR	PULMONARY	★
GASTROINTESTINAL	NR	STROKE	★
GENERAL SURGERY	NR	VASCULAR	NR
MATERNITY CARE	NR	WOMEN'S HEALTH	NR

HEALTHGRADES AWARDS

St. Joseph Mercy Oakland

44405 Woodward Avenue
Pontiac, MI 48341
(248) 858-3000

Overall patient safety: ★★★
Teaching: Y

CLINICAL PROGRAM RATINGS:

CARDIAC	★★★	ORTHOPEDICS	★★★
CRITICAL CARE	★★★★★	PULMONARY	★★★★★
GASTROINTESTINAL	★★★	STROKE	★★★
GENERAL SURGERY	NR	VASCULAR	★★★
MATERNITY CARE	NR	WOMEN'S HEALTH	NR

HEALTHGRADES AWARDS

✓ DISTINGUISHED HOSPITAL
• CLINICAL EXCELLENCE

✓ SPECIALTY EXCELLENCE
• CARDIAC SURGERY • CRITICAL CARE • JOINT REPLACEMENT

St. Joseph Mercy Hospital

5301 East Huron River Drive
Ypsilanti, MI 48197
(734) 712-3456

Overall patient safety: ★★★★★
Teaching: Y

CLINICAL PROGRAM RATINGS:

CARDIAC	★★★	ORTHOPEDICS	★
CRITICAL CARE	★	PULMONARY	★★★
GASTROINTESTINAL	★★★	STROKE	★★★
GENERAL SURGERY	NR	VASCULAR	★★★
MATERNITY CARE	NR	WOMEN'S HEALTH	NR

HEALTHGRADES AWARDS

✓ DISTINGUISHED HOSPITAL
• PATIENT SAFETY

St. Joseph Mercy Saline Hospital

400 Russell Street
Saline, MI 48176
(734) 429-1500

Overall patient safety: ★★★
Teaching: N

CLINICAL PROGRAM RATINGS:

CARDIAC	NR	ORTHOPEDICS	NR
CRITICAL CARE	NR	PULMONARY	★★★
GASTROINTESTINAL	NR	STROKE	★★★
GENERAL SURGERY	NR	VASCULAR	NR
MATERNITY CARE	NR	WOMEN'S HEALTH	NR

HEALTHGRADES AWARDS

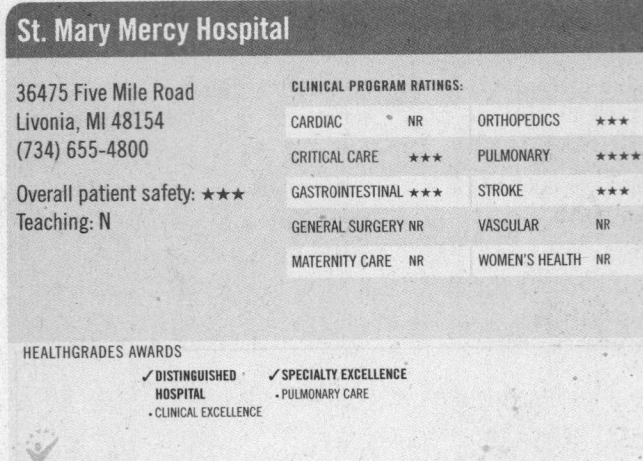

St. Mary Mercy Hospital

36475 Five Mile Road
Livonia, MI 48154
(734) 655-4800

Overall patient safety: ★★★
Teaching: N

CLINICAL PROGRAM RATINGS:

CARDIAC	NR	ORTHOPEDICS	★★★
CRITICAL CARE	★★★	PULMONARY	★★★★★
GASTROINTESTINAL	★★★	STROKE	★★★
GENERAL SURGERY	NR	VASCULAR	NR
MATERNITY CARE	NR	WOMEN'S HEALTH	NR

HEALTHGRADES AWARDS

✓ DISTINGUISHED HOSPITAL
- CLINICAL EXCELLENCE

✓ SPECIALTY EXCELLENCE
- PULMONARY CARE

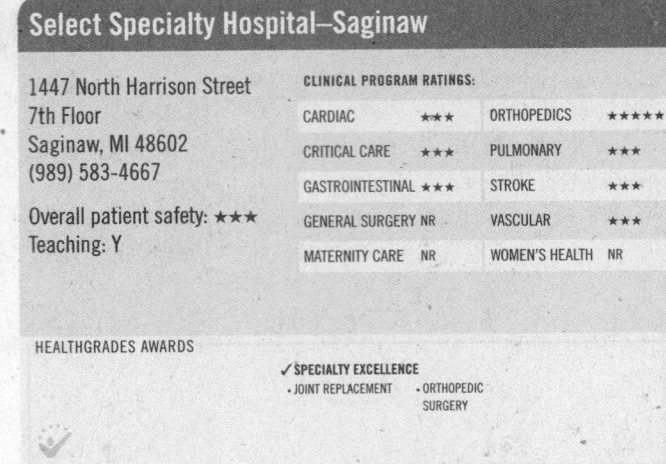

Select Specialty Hospital—Saginaw

1447 North Harrison Street
7th Floor
Saginaw, MI 48602
(989) 583-4667

Overall patient safety: ★★★
Teaching: Y

CLINICAL PROGRAM RATINGS:

CARDIAC	★★★	ORTHOPEDICS	★★★★★
CRITICAL CARE	★★★	PULMONARY	★★★
GASTROINTESTINAL	★★★	STROKE	★★★
GENERAL SURGERY	NR	VASCULAR	★★★
MATERNITY CARE	NR	WOMEN'S HEALTH	NR

HEALTHGRADES AWARDS

✓ SPECIALTY EXCELLENCE
- JOINT REPLACEMENT
- ORTHOPEDIC SURGERY

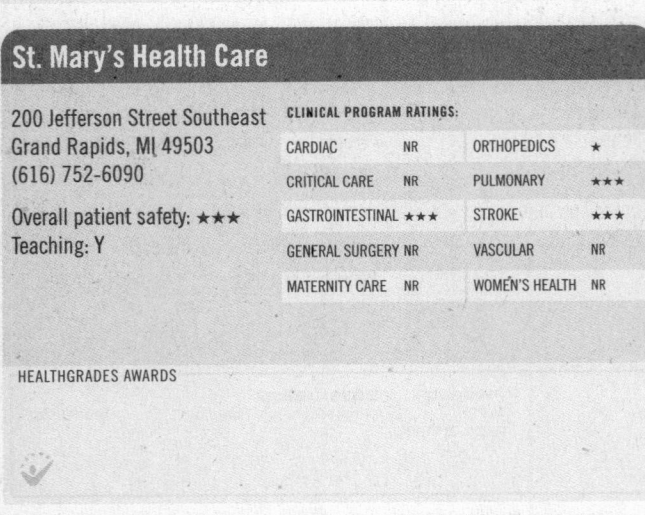

St. Mary's Health Care

200 Jefferson Street Southeast
Grand Rapids, MI 49503
(616) 752-6090

Overall patient safety: ★★★
Teaching: Y

CLINICAL PROGRAM RATINGS:

CARDIAC	NR	ORTHOPEDICS	★
CRITICAL CARE	NR	PULMONARY	★★★
GASTROINTESTINAL	★★★	STROKE	★★★
GENERAL SURGERY	NR	VASCULAR	NR
MATERNITY CARE	NR	WOMEN'S HEALTH	NR

HEALTHGRADES AWARDS

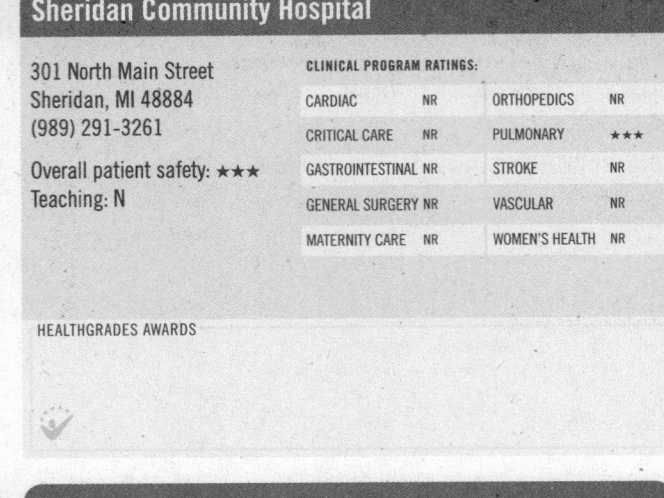

Sheridan Community Hospital

301 North Main Street
Sheridan, MI 48884
(989) 291-3261

Overall patient safety: ★★★
Teaching: N

CLINICAL PROGRAM RATINGS:

CARDIAC	NR	ORTHOPEDICS	NR
CRITICAL CARE	NR	PULMONARY	★★★
GASTROINTESTINAL	NR	STROKE	NR
GENERAL SURGERY	NR	VASCULAR	NR
MATERNITY CARE	NR	WOMEN'S HEALTH	NR

HEALTHGRADES AWARDS

St. Mary's of Michigan Medical Center

800 South Washington Avenue
Saginaw, MI 48601
(989) 776-8000

Overall patient safety: ★★★
Teaching: Y

CLINICAL PROGRAM RATINGS:

CARDIAC	★★★	ORTHOPEDICS	★★★★★
CRITICAL CARE	★★★	PULMONARY	★★★
GASTROINTESTINAL	★★★	STROKE	★★★
GENERAL SURGERY	NR	VASCULAR	★★★
MATERNITY CARE	NR	WOMEN'S HEALTH	NR

HEALTHGRADES AWARDS

✓ SPECIALTY EXCELLENCE
- ORTHOPEDIC SURGERY

Sinai-Grace Hospital

6071 West Outer Drive
Detroit, MI 48235
(313) 966-3300

Overall patient safety: ★
Teaching: Y

CLINICAL PROGRAM RATINGS:

CARDIAC	★★★	ORTHOPEDICS	NR
CRITICAL CARE	★★★★★	PULMONARY	★★★
GASTROINTESTINAL	★★★	STROKE	★★★★★
GENERAL SURGERY	NR	VASCULAR	NR
MATERNITY CARE	NR	WOMEN'S HEALTH	NR

HEALTHGRADES AWARDS

✓ SPECIALTY EXCELLENCE
- CRITICAL CARE
- STROKE CARE

KEY: ★★★★★ BEST   ★★★ AS EXPECTED   ★ POOR   NR NOT RATED BY HEALTHGRADES   For full definitions of ratings and awards, see Appendix.

MICHIGAN HOSPITALS: RATINGS BY CLINICAL SPECIALTY

South Haven Community Hospital

955 South Bailey Avenue
South Haven, MI 49090
(269) 637-5271

Overall patient safety: ★
Teaching: N

CLINICAL PROGRAM RATINGS:

CARDIAC	NR	ORTHOPEDICS	NR
CRITICAL CARE	NR	PULMONARY	★★★
GASTROINTESTINAL	NR	STROKE	NR
GENERAL SURGERY	NR	VASCULAR	NR
MATERNITY CARE	NR	WOMEN'S HEALTH	NR

HEALTHGRADES AWARDS

Standish Community Hospital

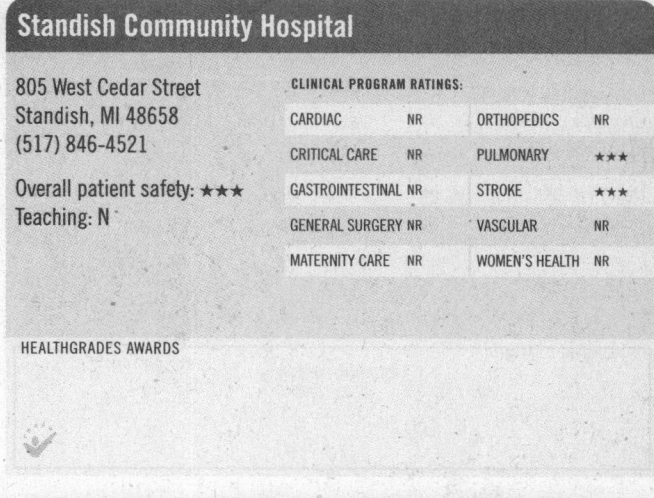

805 West Cedar Street
Standish, MI 48658
(517) 846-4521

Overall patient safety: ★★★
Teaching: N

CLINICAL PROGRAM RATINGS:

CARDIAC	NR	ORTHOPEDICS	NR
CRITICAL CARE	NR	PULMONARY	★★★
GASTROINTESTINAL	NR	STROKE	★★★
GENERAL SURGERY	NR	VASCULAR	NR
MATERNITY CARE	NR	WOMEN'S HEALTH	NR

HEALTHGRADES AWARDS

Spectrum Health Hospitals

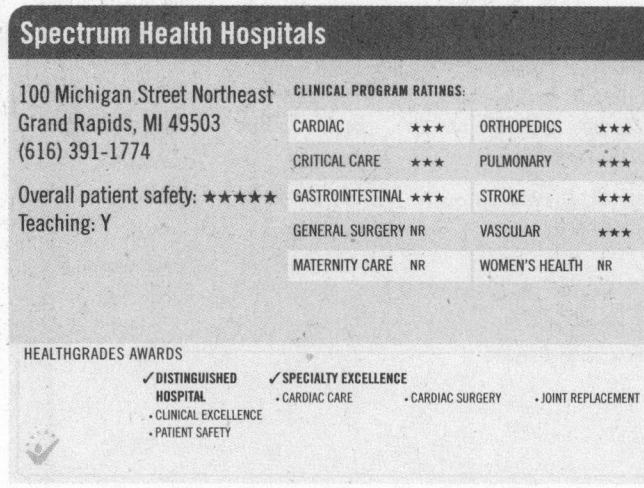

100 Michigan Street Northeast
Grand Rapids, MI 49503
(616) 391-1774

Overall patient safety: ★★★★★
Teaching: Y

CLINICAL PROGRAM RATINGS:

CARDIAC	★★★	ORTHOPEDICS	★★★
CRITICAL CARE	★★★	PULMONARY	★★★
GASTROINTESTINAL	★★★	STROKE	★★★
GENERAL SURGERY	NR	VASCULAR	★★★
MATERNITY CARE	NR	WOMEN'S HEALTH	NR

HEALTHGRADES AWARDS

✓ DISTINGUISHED HOSPITAL
- CLINICAL EXCELLENCE
- PATIENT SAFETY

✓ SPECIALTY EXCELLENCE
- CARDIAC CARE
- CARDIAC SURGERY
- JOINT REPLACEMENT

Sturgis Hospital

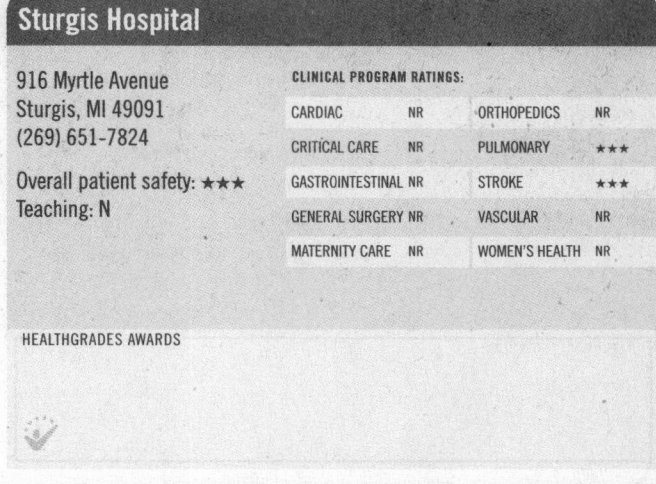

916 Myrtle Avenue
Sturgis, MI 49091
(269) 651-7824

Overall patient safety: ★★★
Teaching: N

CLINICAL PROGRAM RATINGS:

CARDIAC	NR	ORTHOPEDICS	NR
CRITICAL CARE	NR	PULMONARY	★★★
GASTROINTESTINAL	NR	STROKE	★★★
GENERAL SURGERY	NR	VASCULAR	NR
MATERNITY CARE	NR	WOMEN'S HEALTH	NR

HEALTHGRADES AWARDS

Spectrum Health—Reed City Campus

300 North Patterson Road
Reed City, MI 49677
(231) 832-7159

Overall patient safety: ★★★
Teaching: N

CLINICAL PROGRAM RATINGS:

CARDIAC	NR	ORTHOPEDICS	NR
CRITICAL CARE	NR	PULMONARY	★★★
GASTROINTESTINAL	NR	STROKE	NR
GENERAL SURGERY	NR	VASCULAR	NR
MATERNITY CARE	NR	WOMEN'S HEALTH	NR

HEALTHGRADES AWARDS

Three Rivers Health

701 South Health Parkway
Three Rivers, MI 49093
(269) 278-1145

Overall patient safety: ★★★
Teaching: N

CLINICAL PROGRAM RATINGS:

CARDIAC	NR	ORTHOPEDICS	NR
CRITICAL CARE	NR	PULMONARY	★★★
GASTROINTESTINAL	NR	STROKE	NR
GENERAL SURGERY	NR	VASCULAR	NR
MATERNITY CARE	NR	WOMEN'S HEALTH	NR

HEALTHGRADES AWARDS

United Memorial Health Center

615 South Bower Street
Greenville, MI 48838
(616) 754-4691

Overall patient safety: ★★★
Teaching: N

CLINICAL PROGRAM RATINGS:

CARDIAC	NR	ORTHOPEDICS	NR
CRITICAL CARE	NR	PULMONARY	★★★
GASTROINTESTINAL	NR	STROKE	★★★
GENERAL SURGERY	NR	VASCULAR	NR
MATERNITY CARE	NR	WOMEN'S HEALTH	NR

HEALTHGRADES AWARDS

West Branch Regional Medical Center

2463 South M-30
West Branch, MI 48661
(989) 345-3660

Overall patient safety: ★
Teaching: N

CLINICAL PROGRAM RATINGS:

CARDIAC	NR	ORTHOPEDICS	NR
CRITICAL CARE	NR	PULMONARY	★
GASTROINTESTINAL	NR	STROKE	★★★
GENERAL SURGERY	NR	VASCULAR	NR
MATERNITY CARE	NR	WOMEN'S HEALTH	NR

HEALTHGRADES AWARDS

University of Michigan Hospital

1500 East Medical
Center Drive
Ann Arbor, MI 48109
(734) 936-4000

Overall patient safety: ★★★
Teaching: Y

CLINICAL PROGRAM RATINGS:

CARDIAC	★★★	ORTHOPEDICS	★
CRITICAL CARE	★★★	PULMONARY	★★★
GASTROINTESTINAL	★★★	STROKE	★★★
GENERAL SURGERY	NR	VASCULAR	★★★
MATERNITY CARE	NR	WOMEN'S HEALTH	NR

HEALTHGRADES AWARDS

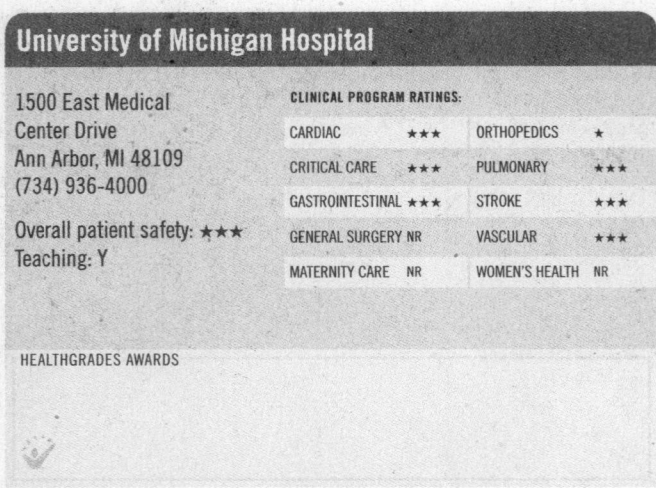

West Shore Hospital

1465 East Parkdale Avenue
Manistee, MI 49660
(231) 398-1000

Overall patient safety: ★★★
Teaching: N

CLINICAL PROGRAM RATINGS:

CARDIAC	NR	ORTHOPEDICS	NR
CRITICAL CARE	NR	PULMONARY	★★★
GASTROINTESTINAL	NR	STROKE	★
GENERAL SURGERY	NR	VASCULAR	NR
MATERNITY CARE	NR	WOMEN'S HEALTH	NR

HEALTHGRADES AWARDS

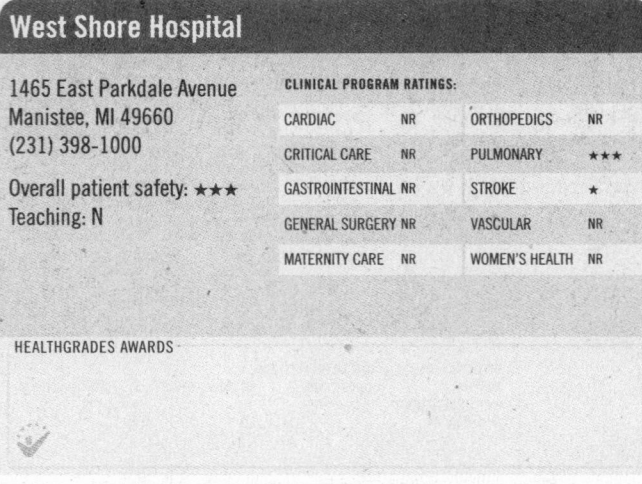

Wa Foote Hospital

205 North East Avenue
Jackson, MI 49201
(517) 788-4800

Overall patient safety: ★★★
Teaching: N

CLINICAL PROGRAM RATINGS:

CARDIAC	NR	ORTHOPEDICS	★★★
CRITICAL CARE	★★★	PULMONARY	★★★
GASTROINTESTINAL	★★★	STROKE	★★★
GENERAL SURGERY	NR	VASCULAR	NR
MATERNITY CARE	NR	WOMEN'S HEALTH	NR

HEALTHGRADES AWARDS

Zeeland Community Hospital

8333 Felch Street
Zeeland, MI 49464
(616) 772-4644

Overall patient safety: ★★★
Teaching: N

CLINICAL PROGRAM RATINGS:

CARDIAC	NR	ORTHOPEDICS	NR
CRITICAL CARE	NR	PULMONARY	★★★
GASTROINTESTINAL	NR	STROKE	★★★
GENERAL SURGERY	NR	VASCULAR	NR
MATERNITY CARE	NR	WOMEN'S HEALTH	NR

HEALTHGRADES AWARDS

KEY: ★★★★★ BEST ★★★ AS EXPECTED ★ POOR NR NOT RATED BY HEALTHGRADES   For full definitions of ratings and awards, see Appendix.

Abbott-Northwestern Hospital

800 East 28th Street
Minneapolis, MN 55407
(612) 863-4000

Overall patient safety: ★★★★★
Teaching: Y

CLINICAL PROGRAM RATINGS:

CARDIAC	★★★	ORTHOPEDICS	★
CRITICAL CARE	★★★	PULMONARY	★★★
GASTROINTESTINAL	★★★	STROKE	★★★★★
GENERAL SURGERY	NR	VASCULAR	★★★
MATERNITY CARE	NR	WOMEN'S HEALTH	NR

HEALTHGRADES AWARDS

✓ DISTINGUISHED HOSPITAL
• PATIENT SAFETY

✓ SPECIALTY EXCELLENCE
• GASTROINTESTINAL CARE
• STROKE CARE

Avera Marshall Regional Medical Center

300 South Bruce Street
Marshall, MN 56258
(507) 532-9661

Overall patient safety: ★★★
Teaching: N

CLINICAL PROGRAM RATINGS:

CARDIAC	NR	ORTHOPEDICS	NR
CRITICAL CARE	NR	PULMONARY	★★★
GASTROINTESTINAL	NR	STROKE	★★★
GENERAL SURGERY	NR	VASCULAR	NR
MATERNITY CARE	NR	WOMEN'S HEALTH	NR

HEALTHGRADES AWARDS

Albert Lea Medical Center--Mayo Health System

404 West Fountain Street
Albert Lea, MN 56007
(507) 373-2384

Overall patient safety: ★★★
Teaching: N

CLINICAL PROGRAM RATINGS:

CARDIAC	NR	ORTHOPEDICS	NR
CRITICAL CARE	NR	PULMONARY	★★★
GASTROINTESTINAL	NR	STROKE	★
GENERAL SURGERY	NR	VASCULAR	NR
MATERNITY CARE	NR	WOMEN'S HEALTH	NR

HEALTHGRADES AWARDS

Buffalo Hospital

303 Catlin Street
Buffalo, MN 55313
(763) 682-1212

Overall patient safety: ★★★
Teaching: N

CLINICAL PROGRAM RATINGS:

CARDIAC	NR	ORTHOPEDICS	NR
CRITICAL CARE	NR	PULMONARY	★★★
GASTROINTESTINAL	NR	STROKE	★★★
GENERAL SURGERY	NR	VASCULAR	NR
MATERNITY CARE	NR	WOMEN'S HEALTH	NR

HEALTHGRADES AWARDS

Austin Medical Center

1000 1st Drive Northwest
Austin, MN 55912
(507) 433-7351

Overall patient safety: ★★★
Teaching: N

CLINICAL PROGRAM RATINGS:

CARDIAC	NR	ORTHOPEDICS	NR
CRITICAL CARE	NR	PULMONARY	★★★★★
GASTROINTESTINAL	NR	STROKE	★★★
GENERAL SURGERY	NR	VASCULAR	NR
MATERNITY CARE	NR	WOMEN'S HEALTH	NR

HEALTHGRADES AWARDS

✓ SPECIALTY EXCELLENCE
• PULMONARY CARE

Cambridge Medical Center

701 South Dellwood Street
Cambridge, MN 55008
(763) 689-7700

Overall patient safety: ★★★★★
Teaching: N

CLINICAL PROGRAM RATINGS:

CARDIAC	NR	ORTHOPEDICS	NR
CRITICAL CARE	NR	PULMONARY	★★★★★
GASTROINTESTINAL	NR	STROKE	★★★
GENERAL SURGERY	NR	VASCULAR	NR
MATERNITY CARE	NR	WOMEN'S HEALTH	NR

HEALTHGRADES AWARDS

✓ SPECIALTY EXCELLENCE
• PULMONARY CARE

Chippewa County Hospital

824 North 11th Street
Montevideo, MN 56265
(320) 269-8878

Overall patient safety: ★★★
Teaching: N

CLINICAL PROGRAM RATINGS:

CARDIAC	NR	ORTHOPEDICS	NR
CRITICAL CARE	NR	PULMONARY	★
GASTROINTESTINAL	NR	STROKE	★
GENERAL SURGERY	NR	VASCULAR	NR
MATERNITY CARE	NR	WOMEN'S HEALTH	NR

HEALTHGRADES AWARDS

Cuyuna Regional Medical Center

320 East Main Street
Crosby, MN 56441
(218) 546-7000

Overall patient safety: ★★★
Teaching: N

CLINICAL PROGRAM RATINGS:

CARDIAC	NR	ORTHOPEDICS	NR
CRITICAL CARE	NR	PULMONARY	★★★
GASTROINTESTINAL	NR	STROKE	★★★
GENERAL SURGERY	NR	VASCULAR	NR
MATERNITY CARE	NR	WOMEN'S HEALTH	NR

HEALTHGRADES AWARDS

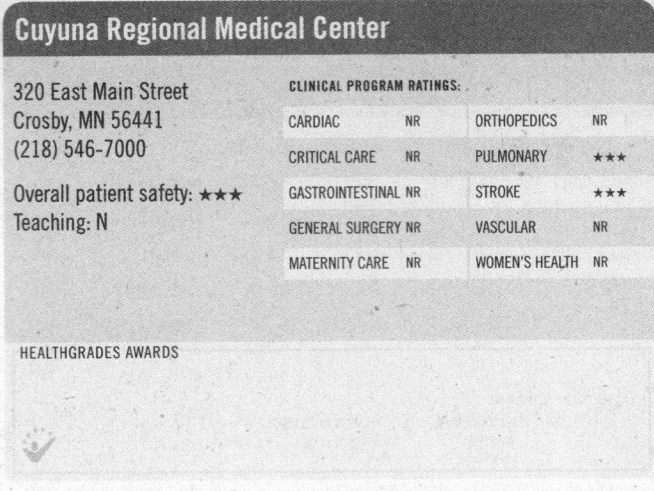

Clearwater Health Services

203 4th Street Northwest
Bagley, MN 56621
(218) 694-6501

Overall patient safety: ★★★
Teaching: N

CLINICAL PROGRAM RATINGS:

CARDIAC	NR	ORTHOPEDICS	NR
CRITICAL CARE	NR	PULMONARY	★★★
GASTROINTESTINAL	NR	STROKE	NR
GENERAL SURGERY	NR	VASCULAR	NR
MATERNITY CARE	NR	WOMEN'S HEALTH	NR

HEALTHGRADES AWARDS

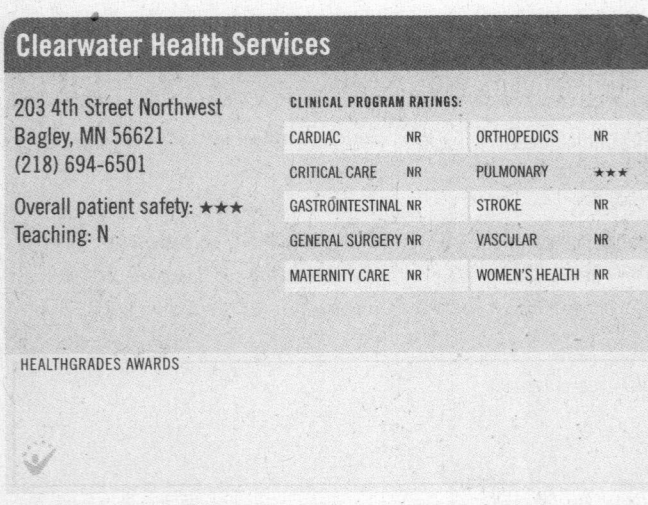

Douglas County Hospital

111 17th Avenue East
Alexandria, MN 56308
(320) 762-1511

Overall patient safety: ★★★
Teaching: N

CLINICAL PROGRAM RATINGS:

CARDIAC	NR	ORTHOPEDICS	★★★
CRITICAL CARE	NR	PULMONARY	★★★
GASTROINTESTINAL	★★★	STROKE	★
GENERAL SURGERY	NR	VASCULAR	NR
MATERNITY CARE	NR	WOMEN'S HEALTH	NR

HEALTHGRADES AWARDS

✓ SPECIALTY EXCELLENCE
· GASTROINTESTINAL
CARE

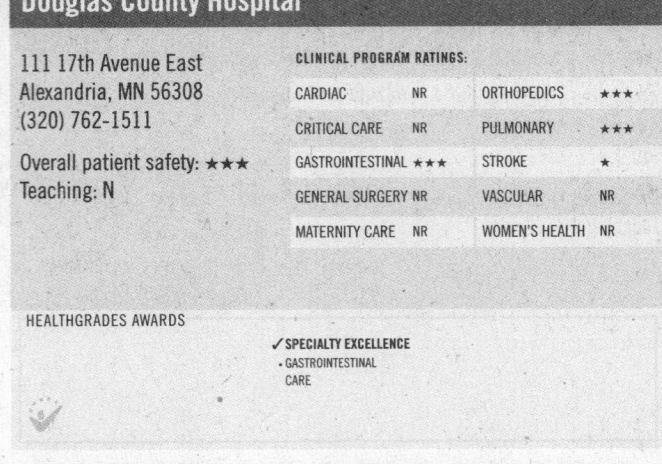

Community Memorial Hospital

512 Skyline Boulevard
Cloquet, MN 55720
(218) 879-4641

Overall patient safety: ★★★
Teaching: N

CLINICAL PROGRAM RATINGS:

CARDIAC	NR	ORTHOPEDICS	NR
CRITICAL CARE	NR	PULMONARY	★
GASTROINTESTINAL	NR	STROKE	★★★
GENERAL SURGERY	NR	VASCULAR	NR
MATERNITY CARE	NR	WOMEN'S HEALTH	NR

HEALTHGRADES AWARDS

Ely Bloomenson Community Hospital

328 West Conan Street
Ely, MN 55731
(218) 365-3271

Overall patient safety: NR
Teaching: N

CLINICAL PROGRAM RATINGS:

CARDIAC	NR	ORTHOPEDICS	NR
CRITICAL CARE	NR	PULMONARY	★★★
GASTROINTESTINAL	NR	STROKE	NR
GENERAL SURGERY	NR	VASCULAR	NR
MATERNITY CARE	NR	WOMEN'S HEALTH	NR

HEALTHGRADES AWARDS

KEY: ★★★★★ BEST   ★★★ AS EXPECTED   ★ POOR   NR NOT RATED BY HEALTHGRADES   For full definitions of ratings and awards, see Appendix.

Fairmont Medical Center

800 Medical Center Drive
Fairmont, MN 56031
(507) 238-8101

Overall patient safety: ★★★
Teaching: N

CLINICAL PROGRAM RATINGS:

CARDIAC	NR	ORTHOPÉDICS	★
CRITICAL CARE	NR	PULMONARY	★★★
GASTROINTESTINAL	NR	STROKE	★★★
GENERAL SURGERY	NR	VASCULAR	NR
MATERNITY CARE	NR	WOMEN'S HEALTH	NR

HEALTHGRADES AWARDS

Fairview Northland Regional Hospital

911 Northland Drive
Princeton, MN 55371
(763) 389-1313

Overall patient safety: ★★★
Teaching: N

CLINICAL PROGRAM RATINGS:

CARDIAC	NR	ORTHOPEDICS	NR
CRITICAL CARE	NR	PULMONARY	★★★
GASTROINTESTINAL	NR	STROKE	★★★
GENERAL SURGERY	NR	VASCULAR	NR
MATERNITY CARE	NR	WOMEN'S HEALTH	NR

HEALTHGRADES AWARDS

Fairview Hospital Chisago Lakes*

11685 Lake Boulevard North
Chisago City, MN 55013
(612) 257-8400

Overall patient safety: ★★★
Teaching: N

CLINICAL PROGRAM RATINGS:

CARDIAC	NR	ORTHOPEDICS	NR
CRITICAL CARE	NR	PULMONARY	★★★
GASTROINTESTINAL	NR	STROKE	★★★
GENERAL SURGERY	NR	VASCULAR	NR
MATERNITY CARE	NR	WOMEN'S HEALTH	NR

HEALTHGRADES AWARDS

Fairview Red Wing Hospital

1407 West 4th Street
Red Wing, MN 55066
(651) 267-5000

Overall patient safety: ★★★★★
Teaching: N

CLINICAL PROGRAM RATINGS:

CARDIAC	NR	ORTHOPEDICS	★
CRITICAL CARE	NR	PULMONARY	★★★
GASTROINTESTINAL	NR	STROKE	★★★
GENERAL SURGERY	NR	VASCULAR	NR
MATERNITY CARE	NR	WOMEN'S HEALTH	NR

HEALTHGRADES AWARDS

Fairview Lakes Health Services*

5200 Fairview Boulevard
Wyoming, MN 55092
(651) 982-7000

Overall patient safety: ★★★
Teaching: N

CLINICAL PROGRAM RATINGS:

CARDIAC	NR	ORTHOPEDICS	NR
CRITICAL CARE	NR	PULMONARY	★★★
GASTROINTESTINAL	NR	STROKE	★★★
GENERAL SURGERY	NR	VASCULAR	NR
MATERNITY CARE	NR	WOMEN'S HEALTH	NR

HEALTHGRADES AWARDS

Fairview Ridges Hospital

201 East Nicollet Boulevard
Burnsville, MN 55337
(952) 892-2000

Overall patient safety: ★
Teaching: N

CLINICAL PROGRAM RATINGS:

CARDIAC	NR	ORTHOPEDICS	NR
CRITICAL CARE	★★★	PULMONARY	★★★★★
GASTROINTESTINAL	★★★	STROKE	★★★
GENERAL SURGERY	NR	VASCULAR	NR
MATERNITY CARE	NR	WOMEN'S HEALTH	NR

HEALTHGRADES AWARDS

*This hospital reports its data to the federal government jointly with another hospital. Therefore the ratings and awards apply to multiple hospitals and this specific hospital may not provide all rated services.

Fairview Southdale Hospital

6401 France Avenue South
Edina, MN 55435
(952) 924-5000

Overall patient safety: ★★★★★
Teaching: N

CLINICAL PROGRAM RATINGS:

CARDIAC	★★★★★	ORTHOPEDICS	★★★
CRITICAL CARE	★★★★★	PULMONARY	★★★★★
GASTROINTESTINAL	★★★	STROKE	★★★★★
GENERAL SURGERY	NR	VASCULAR	★★★
MATERNITY CARE	NR	WOMEN'S HEALTH	NR

HEALTHGRADES AWARDS

✓ **DISTINGUISHED HOSPITAL**
· CLINICAL EXCELLENCE
· PATIENT SAFETY

✓ **SPECIALTY EXCELLENCE**
· CARDIAC CARE
· CRITICAL CARE
· PULMONARY CARE
· STROKE CARE

Glacial Ridge Hospital

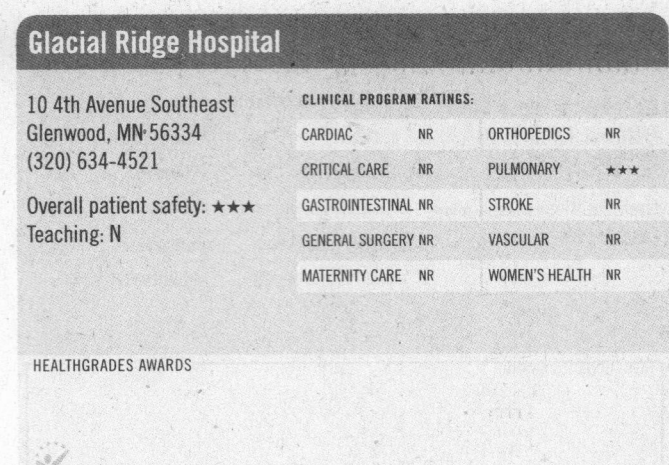

10 4th Avenue Southeast
Glenwood, MN 56334
(320) 634-4521

Overall patient safety: ★★★
Teaching: N

CLINICAL PROGRAM RATINGS:

CARDIAC	NR	ORTHOPEDICS	NR
CRITICAL CARE	NR	PULMONARY	★★★
GASTROINTESTINAL	NR	STROKE	NR
GENERAL SURGERY	NR	VASCULAR	NR
MATERNITY CARE	NR	WOMEN'S HEALTH	NR

HEALTHGRADES AWARDS

Falls Memorial Hospital

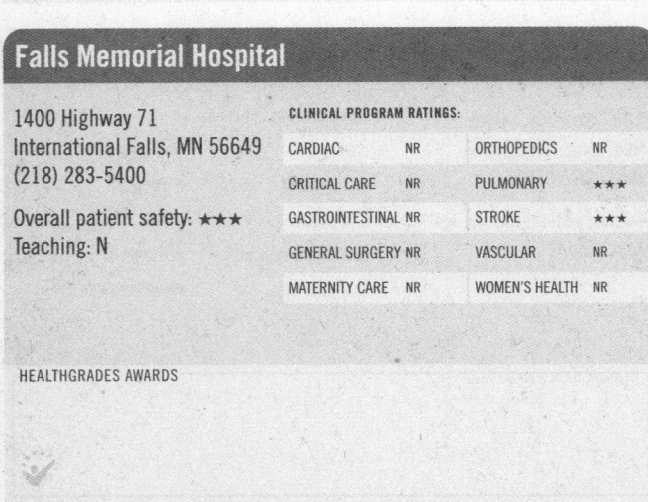

1400 Highway 71
International Falls, MN 56649
(218) 283-5400

Overall patient safety: ★★★
Teaching: N

CLINICAL PROGRAM RATINGS:

CARDIAC	NR	ORTHOPEDICS	NR
CRITICAL CARE	NR	PULMONARY	★★★
GASTROINTESTINAL	NR	STROKE	★★★
GENERAL SURGERY	NR	VASCULAR	NR
MATERNITY CARE	NR	WOMEN'S HEALTH	NR

HEALTHGRADES AWARDS

Glencoe Regional Health Services

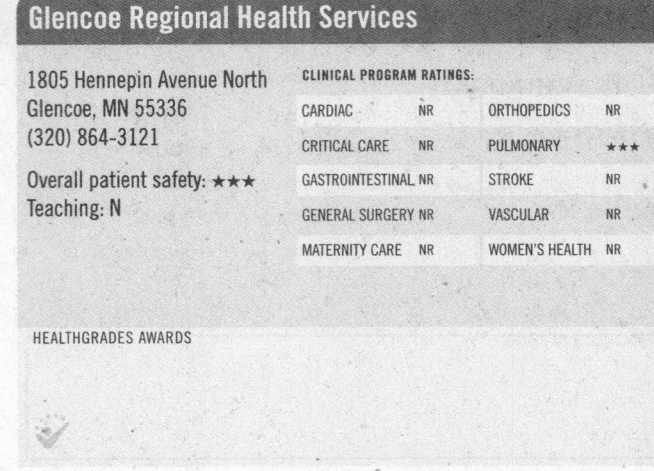

1805 Hennepin Avenue North
Glencoe, MN 55336
(320) 864-3121

Overall patient safety: ★★★
Teaching: N

CLINICAL PROGRAM RATINGS:

CARDIAC	NR	ORTHOPEDICS	NR
CRITICAL CARE	NR	PULMONARY	★★★
GASTROINTESTINAL	NR	STROKE	NR
GENERAL SURGERY	NR	VASCULAR	NR
MATERNITY CARE	NR	WOMEN'S HEALTH	NR

HEALTHGRADES AWARDS

First Care Medical Services

900 Hilligoss Boulevard
Southeast
Fosston, MN 56542
(218) 435-1133

Overall patient safety: ★
Teaching: N

CLINICAL PROGRAM RATINGS:

CARDIAC	NR	ORTHOPEDICS	NR
CRITICAL CARE	NR	PULMONARY	★★★
GASTROINTESTINAL	NR	STROKE	★★★
GENERAL SURGERY	NR	VASCULAR	NR
MATERNITY CARE	NR	WOMEN'S HEALTH	NR

HEALTHGRADES AWARDS

Grand Itasca Clinic and Hospital

1601 Golf Course Road
Grand Rapids, MN 55744
(218) 326-3401

Overall patient safety: ★★★
Teaching: N

CLINICAL PROGRAM RATINGS:

CARDIAC	NR	ORTHOPEDICS	NR
CRITICAL CARE	NR	PULMONARY	★★★
GASTROINTESTINAL	NR	STROKE	★★★
GENERAL SURGERY	NR	VASCULAR	NR
MATERNITY CARE	NR	WOMEN'S HEALTH	NR

HEALTHGRADES AWARDS

KEY: ★★★★★ BEST ★★★ AS EXPECTED ★ POOR NR NOT RATED BY HEALTHGRADES For full definitions of ratings and awards, see Appendix.

Healtheast St. John's Hospital

1575 Beam Avenue
Maplewood, MN 55109
(651) 232-7000

Overall patient safety: ★★★★★
Teaching: Y

CLINICAL PROGRAM RATINGS:

CARDIAC	NR	ORTHOPEDICS	★★★★★
CRITICAL CARE	★★★	PULMONARY	★★★
GASTROINTESTINAL	★★★	STROKE	★★★
GENERAL SURGERY	NR	VASCULAR	NR
MATERNITY CARE	NR	WOMEN'S HEALTH	NR

HEALTHGRADES AWARDS

✓ DISTINGUISHED HOSPITAL
- CLINICAL EXCELLENCE
- PATIENT SAFETY

✓ SPECIALTY EXCELLENCE
- ORTHOPEDIC SURGERY

Hutchinson Area Health Care

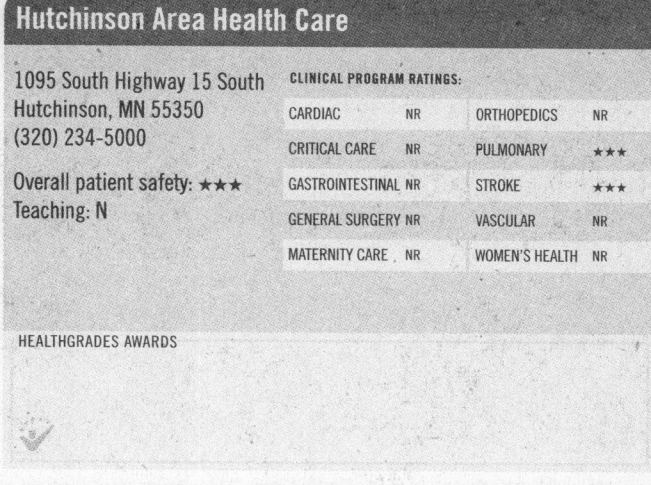

1095 South Highway 15 South
Hutchinson, MN 55350
(320) 234-5000

Overall patient safety: ★★★
Teaching: N

CLINICAL PROGRAM RATINGS:

CARDIAC	NR	ORTHOPEDICS	NR
CRITICAL CARE	NR	PULMONARY	★★★
GASTROINTESTINAL	NR	STROKE	★★★
GENERAL SURGERY	NR	VASCULAR	NR
MATERNITY CARE	NR	WOMEN'S HEALTH	NR

HEALTHGRADES AWARDS

Healtheast Woodwinds Hospital

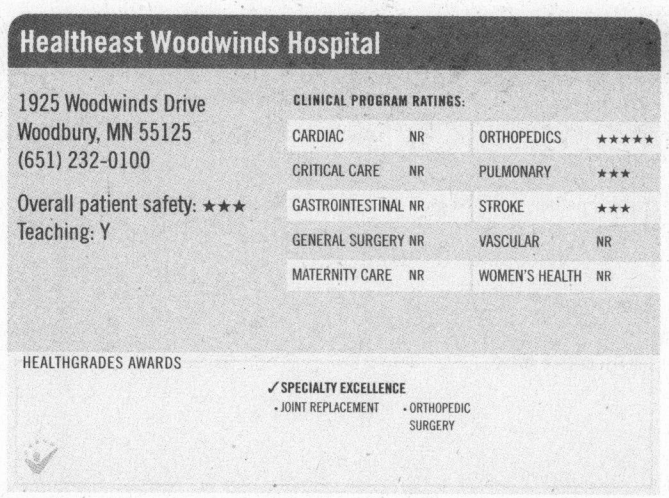

1925 Woodwinds Drive
Woodbury, MN 55125
(651) 232-0100

Overall patient safety: ★★★
Teaching: Y

CLINICAL PROGRAM RATINGS:

CARDIAC	NR	ORTHOPEDICS	★★★★★
CRITICAL CARE	NR	PULMONARY	★★★
GASTROINTESTINAL	NR	STROKE	★★★
GENERAL SURGERY	NR	VASCULAR	NR
MATERNITY CARE	NR	WOMEN'S HEALTH	NR

HEALTHGRADES AWARDS

✓ SPECIALTY EXCELLENCE
- JOINT REPLACEMENT
- ORTHOPEDIC SURGERY

Immanuel St. Joseph's—Mayo Health System

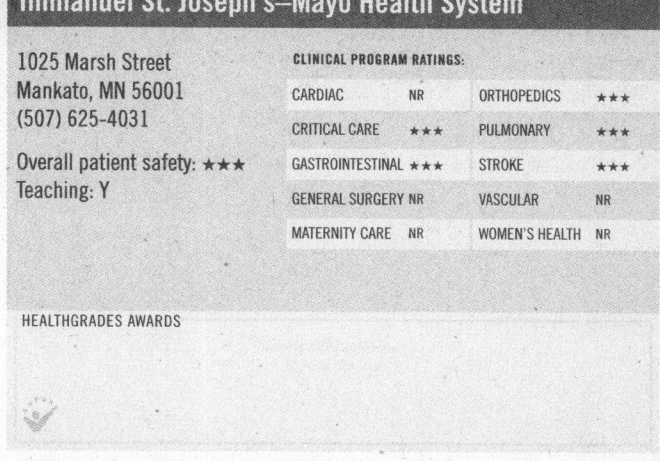

1025 Marsh Street
Mankato, MN 56001
(507) 625-4031

Overall patient safety: ★★★
Teaching: Y

CLINICAL PROGRAM RATINGS:

CARDIAC	NR	ORTHOPEDICS	★★★
CRITICAL CARE	★★★	PULMONARY	★★★
GASTROINTESTINAL	★★★	STROKE	★★★
GENERAL SURGERY	NR	VASCULAR	NR
MATERNITY CARE	NR	WOMEN'S HEALTH	NR

HEALTHGRADES AWARDS

Hennepin County Medical Center

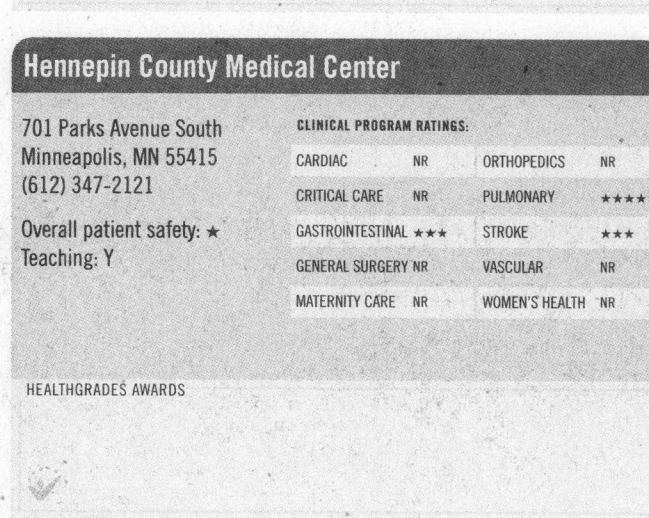

701 Parks Avenue South
Minneapolis, MN 55415
(612) 347-2121

Overall patient safety: ★
Teaching: Y

CLINICAL PROGRAM RATINGS:

CARDIAC	NR	ORTHOPEDICS	NR
CRITICAL CARE	NR	PULMONARY	★★★★★
GASTROINTESTINAL	★★★	STROKE	★★★
GENERAL SURGERY	NR	VASCULAR	NR
MATERNITY CARE	NR	WOMEN'S HEALTH	NR

HEALTHGRADES AWARDS

Kanabec Hospital

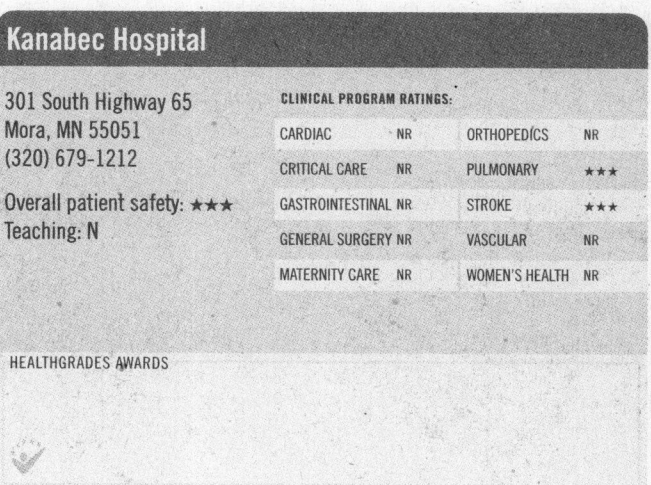

301 South Highway 65
Mora, MN 55051
(320) 679-1212

Overall patient safety: ★★★
Teaching: N

CLINICAL PROGRAM RATINGS:

CARDIAC	NR	ORTHOPEDICS	NR
CRITICAL CARE	NR	PULMONARY	★★★
GASTROINTESTINAL	NR	STROKE	★★★
GENERAL SURGERY	NR	VASCULAR	NR
MATERNITY CARE	NR	WOMEN'S HEALTH	NR

HEALTHGRADES AWARDS

Lake Region Healthcare Corporation

712 Cascade Street South
Fergus Falls, MN 56537
(218) 736-8000

Overall patient safety: ★
Teaching: N

CLINICAL PROGRAM RATINGS:

CARDIAC	NR	ORTHOPEDICS	NR
CRITICAL CARE	NR	PULMONARY	★★★
GASTROINTESTINAL	★★★	STROKE	★★★
GENERAL SURGERY	NR	VASCULAR	NR
MATERNITY CARE	NR	WOMEN'S HEALTH	NR

HEALTHGRADES AWARDS

Luverne Community Hospital

305 East Luverne Street
P.O. Box 1019
Luverne, MN 56156
(507) 283-2321

Overall patient safety: ★
Teaching: N

CLINICAL PROGRAM RATINGS:

CARDIAC	NR	ORTHOPEDICS	NR
CRITICAL CARE	NR	PULMONARY	★★★
GASTROINTESTINAL	NR	STROKE	★★★
GENERAL SURGERY	NR	VASCULAR	NR
MATERNITY CARE	NR	WOMEN'S HEALTH	NR

HEALTHGRADES AWARDS

Lakeview Hospital

927 West Churchill Street
Stillwater, MN 55082
(651) 439-5330

Overall patient safety: ★★★
Teaching: N

CLINICAL PROGRAM RATINGS:

CARDIAC	NR	ORTHOPEDICS	★★★★★
CRITICAL CARE	NR	PULMONARY	★★★
GASTROINTESTINAL	NR	STROKE	★★★
GENERAL SURGERY	NR	VASCULAR	NR
MATERNITY CARE	NR	WOMEN'S HEALTH	NR

HEALTHGRADES AWARDS

✓ SPECIALTY EXCELLENCE
• JOINT REPLACEMENT • ORTHOPEDIC SURGERY

Madison Hospital

820 3rd Avenue
Madison, MN 56256
(320) 598-7556

Overall patient safety: ★★★
Teaching: N

CLINICAL PROGRAM RATINGS:

CARDIAC	NR	ORTHOPEDICS	NR
CRITICAL CARE	NR	PULMONARY	NR
GASTROINTESTINAL	NR	STROKE	NR
GENERAL SURGERY	NR	VASCULAR	NR
MATERNITY CARE	NR	WOMEN'S HEALTH	NR

HEALTHGRADES AWARDS

Lakewood Health System

401 Prairie Avenue Northeast
Staples, MN 56479
(218) 894-1515

Overall patient safety: ★★★
Teaching: N

CLINICAL PROGRAM RATINGS:

CARDIAC	NR	ORTHOPEDICS	NR
CRITICAL CARE	NR	PULMONARY	★★★
GASTROINTESTINAL	NR	STROKE	NR
GENERAL SURGERY	NR	VASCULAR	NR
MATERNITY CARE	NR	WOMEN'S HEALTH	NR

HEALTHGRADES AWARDS

Meeker County Memorial Hospital

612 South Sibley Avenue
Litchfield, MN 55355
(320) 693-3242

Overall patient safety: ★★★
Teaching: N

CLINICAL PROGRAM RATINGS:

CARDIAC	NR	ORTHOPEDICS	NR
CRITICAL CARE	NR	PULMONARY	★★★
GASTROINTESTINAL	NR	STROKE	★
GENERAL SURGERY	NR	VASCULAR	NR
MATERNITY CARE	NR	WOMEN'S HEALTH	NR

HEALTHGRADES AWARDS

KEY: ★★★★★ BEST ★★★ AS EXPECTED ★ POOR NR NOT RATED BY HEALTHGRADES For full definitions of ratings and awards, see Appendix.

Melrose Area Hospital Centracare

11 North 5th Avenue West
Melrose, MN 56352
(320) 256-4231

Overall patient safety: ★★★
Teaching: N

CLINICAL PROGRAM RATINGS:

CARDIAC	NR	ORTHOPEDICS	NR
CRITICAL CARE	NR	PULMONARY	★★★
GASTROINTESTINAL	NR	STROKE	NR
GENERAL SURGERY	NR	VASCULAR	NR
MATERNITY CARE	NR	WOMEN'S HEALTH	NR

HEALTHGRADES AWARDS

Methodist Hospital

6500 Excelsior Boulevard
Minneapolis, MN 55426
(952) 993-5000

Overall patient safety: ★★★★★
Teaching: Y

CLINICAL PROGRAM RATINGS:

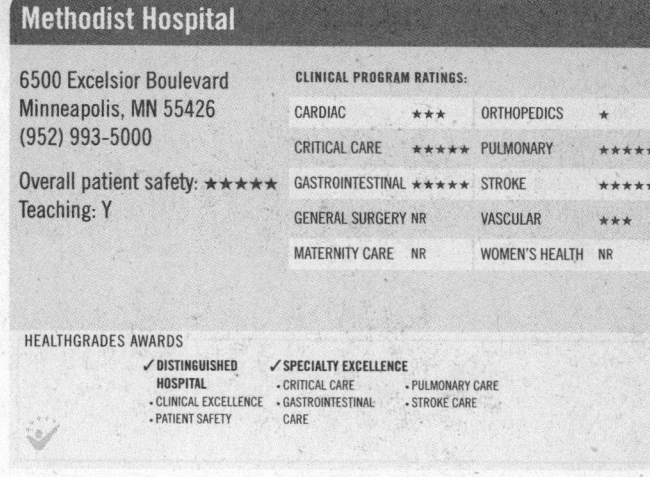

CARDIAC	★★★	ORTHOPEDICS	★
CRITICAL CARE	★★★★★	PULMONARY	★★★★★
GASTROINTESTINAL	★★★★★	STROKE	★★★★★
GENERAL SURGERY	NR	VASCULAR	★★★
MATERNITY CARE	NR	WOMEN'S HEALTH	NR

HEALTHGRADES AWARDS

✓ **DISTINGUISHED HOSPITAL**
- CLINICAL EXCELLENCE
- PATIENT SAFETY

✓ **SPECIALTY EXCELLENCE**
- CRITICAL CARE
- GASTROINTESTINAL CARE
- PULMONARY CARE
- STROKE CARE

Mercy Hospital

4050 Coon Rapids Boulevard
Coon Rapids, MN 55433
(763) 236-6000

Overall patient safety: ★★★★★
Teaching: Y

CLINICAL PROGRAM RATINGS:

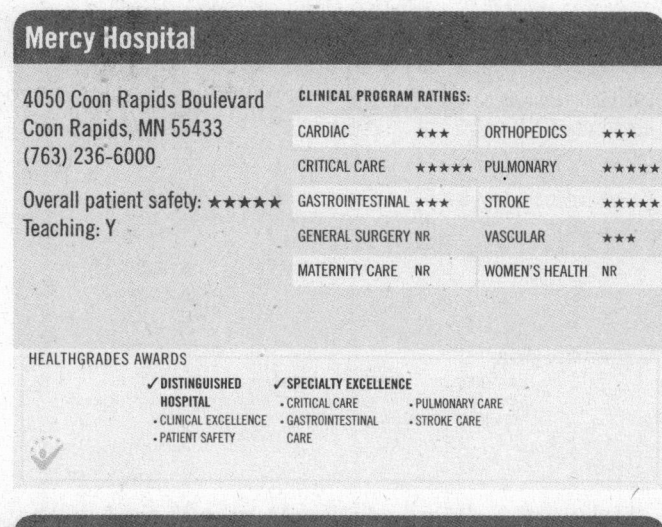

CARDIAC	★★★	ORTHOPEDICS	★★★
CRITICAL CARE	★★★★★	PULMONARY	★★★★★
GASTROINTESTINAL	★★★	STROKE	★★★★★
GENERAL SURGERY	NR	VASCULAR	★★★
MATERNITY CARE	NR	WOMEN'S HEALTH	NR

HEALTHGRADES AWARDS

✓ **DISTINGUISHED HOSPITAL**
- CLINICAL EXCELLENCE
- PATIENT SAFETY

✓ **SPECIALTY EXCELLENCE**
- CRITICAL CARE
- GASTROINTESTINAL CARE
- PULMONARY CARE
- STROKE CARE

Mille Lacs Health System

200 North Elm Street
Onamia, MN 56359
(320) 532-8020

Overall patient safety: ★★★
Teaching: N

CLINICAL PROGRAM RATINGS:

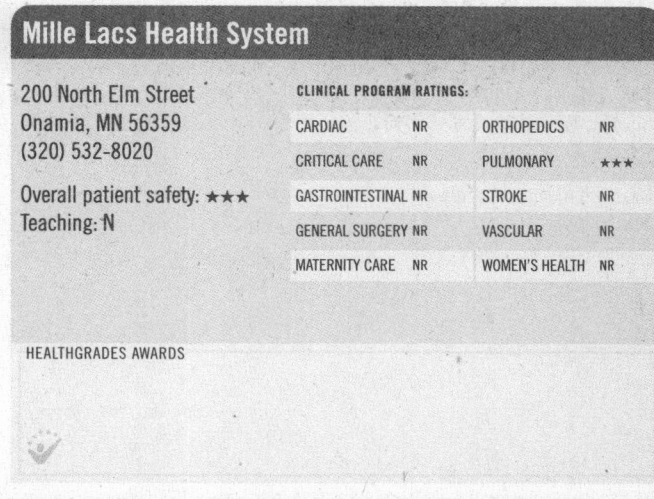

CARDIAC	NR	ORTHOPEDICS	NR
CRITICAL CARE	NR	PULMONARY	★★★
GASTROINTESTINAL	NR	STROKE	NR
GENERAL SURGERY	NR	VASCULAR	NR
MATERNITY CARE	NR	WOMEN'S HEALTH	NR

HEALTHGRADES AWARDS

Mercy Hospital and Health Care Center

710 Kenwood Avenue
Moose Lake, MN 55767
(218) 485-4481

Overall patient safety: ★★★
Teaching: N

CLINICAL PROGRAM RATINGS:

CARDIAC	NR	ORTHOPEDICS	NR
CRITICAL CARE	NR	PULMONARY	★★★
GASTROINTESTINAL	NR	STROKE	★★★
GENERAL SURGERY	NR	VASCULAR	NR
MATERNITY CARE	NR	WOMEN'S HEALTH	NR

HEALTHGRADES AWARDS

Monticello-Big Lake Community Hospital

1013 Hart Boulevard
Monticello, MN 55362
(763) 295-2945

Overall patient safety: ★★★
Teaching: N

CLINICAL PROGRAM RATINGS:

CARDIAC	NR	ORTHOPEDICS	NR
CRITICAL CARE	NR	PULMONARY	★★★
GASTROINTESTINAL	NR	STROKE	NR
GENERAL SURGERY	NR	VASCULAR	NR
MATERNITY CARE	NR	WOMEN'S HEALTH	NR

HEALTHGRADES AWARDS

Municipal Hospital and Granite Manor

345 10th Avenue
Granite Falls, MN 56241
(320) 564-3111

Overall patient safety: ★★★
Teaching: N

CLINICAL PROGRAM RATINGS:

CARDIAC	NR	ORTHOPEDICS	NR
CRITICAL CARE	NR	PULMONARY	★★★
GASTROINTESTINAL	NR	STROKE	★★★
GENERAL SURGERY	NR	VASCULAR	NR
MATERNITY CARE	NR	WOMEN'S HEALTH	NR

HEALTHGRADES AWARDS

North Country Regional Hospital

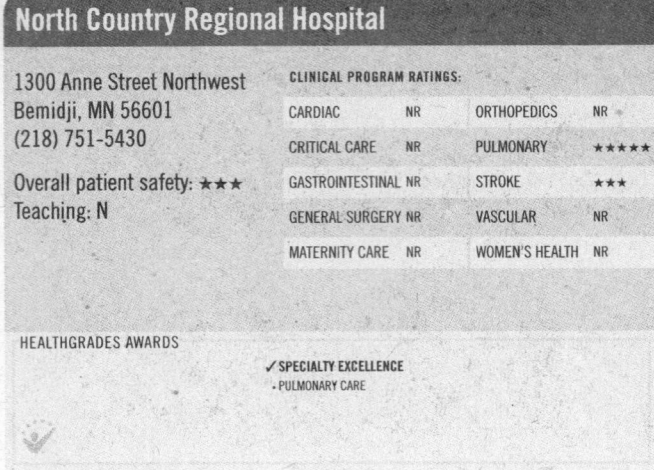

1300 Anne Street Northwest
Bemidji, MN 56601
(218) 751-5430

Overall patient safety: ★★★
Teaching: N

CLINICAL PROGRAM RATINGS:

CARDIAC	NR	ORTHOPEDICS	NR
CRITICAL CARE	NR	PULMONARY	★★★★★
GASTROINTESTINAL	NR	STROKE	★★★
GENERAL SURGERY	NR	VASCULAR	NR
MATERNITY CARE	NR	WOMEN'S HEALTH	NR

HEALTHGRADES AWARDS

✓ SPECIALTY EXCELLENCE
· PULMONARY CARE

Murray County Memorial Hospital

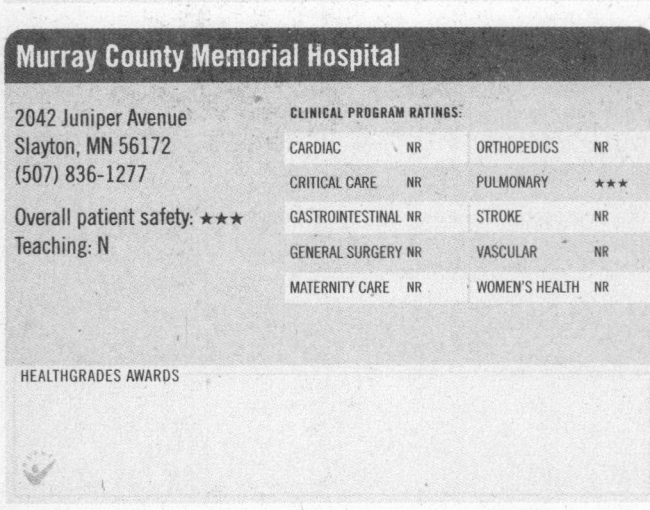

2042 Juniper Avenue
Slayton, MN 56172
(507) 836-1277

Overall patient safety: ★★★
Teaching: N

CLINICAL PROGRAM RATINGS:

CARDIAC	NR	ORTHOPEDICS	NR
CRITICAL CARE	NR	PULMONARY	★★★
GASTROINTESTINAL	NR	STROKE	NR
GENERAL SURGERY	NR	VASCULAR	NR
MATERNITY CARE	NR	WOMEN'S HEALTH	NR

HEALTHGRADES AWARDS

North Memorial Health Care

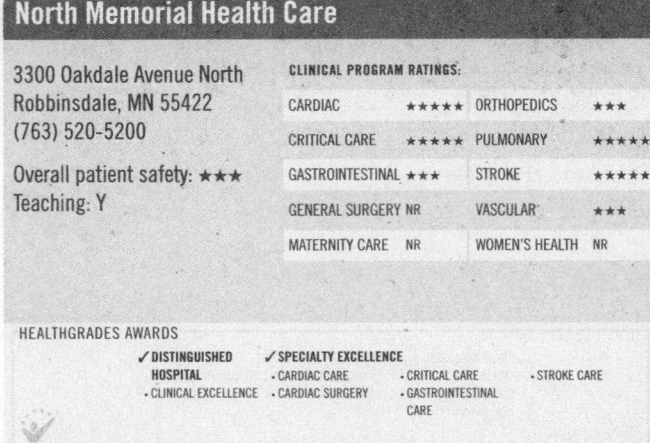

3300 Oakdale Avenue North
Robbinsdale, MN 55422
(763) 520-5200

Overall patient safety: ★★★
Teaching: Y

CLINICAL PROGRAM RATINGS:

CARDIAC	★★★★★	ORTHOPEDICS	★★★
CRITICAL CARE	★★★★★	PULMONARY	★★★★★
GASTROINTESTINAL	★★★	STROKE	★★★★★
GENERAL SURGERY	NR	VASCULAR	★★★
MATERNITY CARE	NR	WOMEN'S HEALTH	NR

HEALTHGRADES AWARDS

✓ DISTINGUISHED HOSPITAL	✓ SPECIALTY EXCELLENCE		
· CLINICAL EXCELLENCE	· CARDIAC CARE	· CRITICAL CARE	· STROKE CARE
	· CARDIAC SURGERY	· GASTROINTESTINAL CARE	

New Ulm Medical Center

1324 5th North Street
New Ulm, MN 56073
(507) 233-1281

Overall patient safety: ★★★
Teaching: N

CLINICAL PROGRAM RATINGS:

CARDIAC	NR	ORTHOPEDICS	NR
CRITICAL CARE	NR	PULMONARY	★★★
GASTROINTESTINAL	NR	STROKE	★★★
GENERAL SURGERY	NR	VASCULAR	NR
MATERNITY CARE	NR	WOMEN'S HEALTH	NR

HEALTHGRADES AWARDS

Northfield Hospital

2000 North Avenue
Northfield, MN 55057
(507) 646-1000

Overall patient safety: ★★★
Teaching: N

CLINICAL PROGRAM RATINGS:

CARDIAC	NR	ORTHOPEDICS	NR
CRITICAL CARE	NR	PULMONARY	★★★
GASTROINTESTINAL	NR	STROKE	NR
GENERAL SURGERY	NR	VASCULAR	NR
MATERNITY CARE	NR	WOMEN'S HEALTH	NR

HEALTHGRADES AWARDS

KEY: ★★★★★ BEST   ★★★ AS EXPECTED   ★ POOR   NR NOT RATED BY HEALTHGRADES   For full definitions of ratings and awards, see Appendix.

Northwest Medical Center

120 Labree Avenue South
Thief River Falls, MN 56701
(218) 681-4240

Overall patient safety: ★★★
Teaching: N

CLINICAL PROGRAM RATINGS:

CARDIAC	NR	ORTHOPEDICS	NR
CRITICAL CARE	NR	PULMONARY	★★★
GASTROINTESTINAL	NR	STROKE	★
GENERAL SURGERY	NR	VASCULAR	NR
MATERNITY CARE	NR	WOMEN'S HEALTH	NR

HEALTHGRADES AWARDS

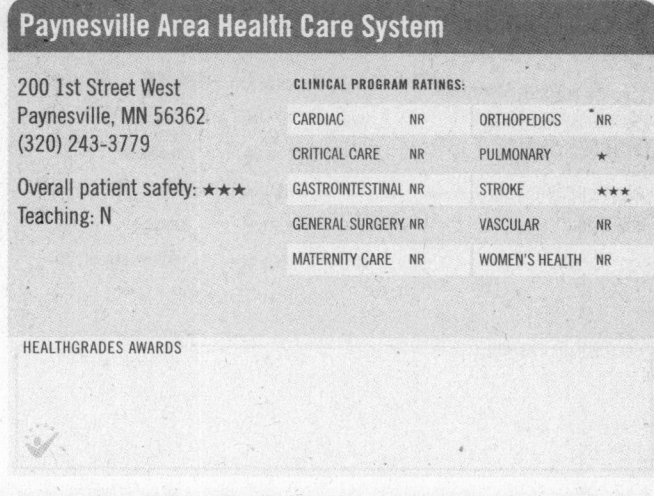

Paynesville Area Health Care System

200 1st Street West
Paynesville, MN 56362
(320) 243-3779

Overall patient safety: ★★★
Teaching: N

CLINICAL PROGRAM RATINGS:

CARDIAC	NR	ORTHOPEDICS	NR
CRITICAL CARE	NR	PULMONARY	★
GASTROINTESTINAL	NR	STROKE	★★★
GENERAL SURGERY	NR	VASCULAR	NR
MATERNITY CARE	NR	WOMEN'S HEALTH	NR

HEALTHGRADES AWARDS

Olmsted Medical Center

1650 4th Street Southeast
Rochester, MN 55904
(507) 288-3443

Overall patient safety: ★★★
Teaching: N

CLINICAL PROGRAM RATINGS:

CARDIAC	NR	ORTHOPEDICS	NR
CRITICAL CARE	NR	PULMONARY	★★★
GASTROINTESTINAL	NR	STROKE	NR
GENERAL SURGERY	NR	VASCULAR	NR
MATERNITY CARE	NR	WOMEN'S HEALTH	NR

HEALTHGRADES AWARDS

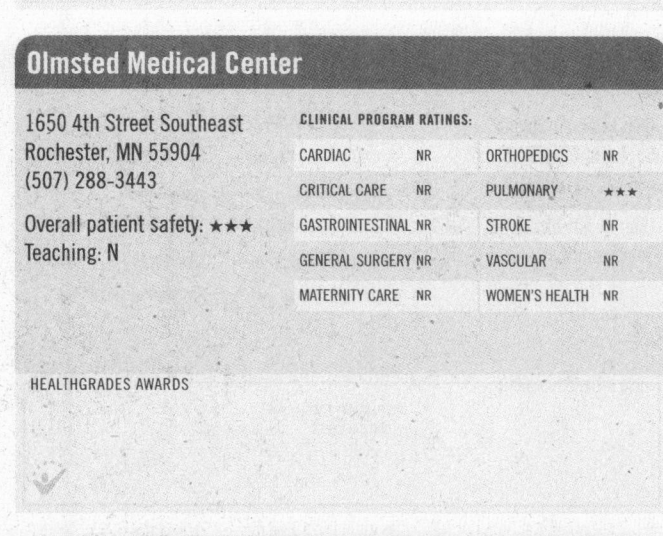

Perham Memorial Hospital and Home

665 3rd Street Southwest
Perham, MN 56573
(218) 346-4500

Overall patient safety: NR
Teaching: N

CLINICAL PROGRAM RATINGS:

CARDIAC	NR	ORTHOPEDICS	NR
CRITICAL CARE	NR	PULMONARY	★★★
GASTROINTESTINAL	NR	STROKE	NR
GENERAL SURGERY	NR	VASCULAR	NR
MATERNITY CARE	NR	WOMEN'S HEALTH	NR

HEALTHGRADES AWARDS

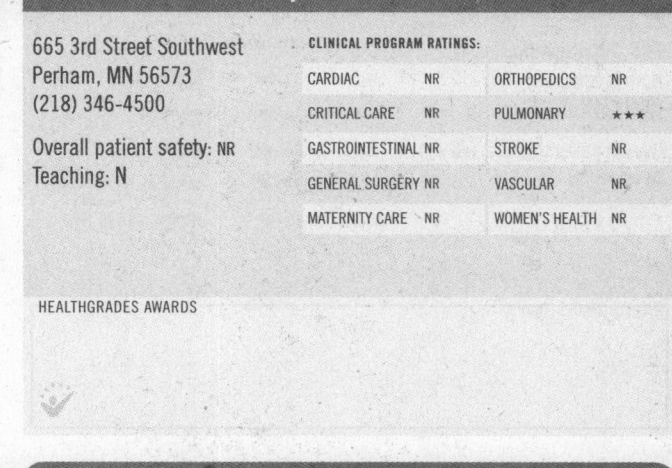

Owatonna Hospital

903 South Oak Avenue
Owatonna, MN 55060
(507) 451-3850

Overall patient safety: ★★★
Teaching: N

CLINICAL PROGRAM RATINGS:

CARDIAC	NR	ORTHOPEDICS	NR
CRITICAL CARE	NR	PULMONARY	★★★
GASTROINTESTINAL	NR	STROKE	★★★
GENERAL SURGERY	NR	VASCULAR	NR
MATERNITY CARE	NR	WOMEN'S HEALTH	NR

HEALTHGRADES AWARDS

Pine Medical Center

109 Court Avenue South
Sandstone, MN 55072
(320) 245-2212

Overall patient safety: NR
Teaching: N

CLINICAL PROGRAM RATINGS:

CARDIAC	NR	ORTHOPEDICS	NR
CRITICAL CARE	NR	PULMONARY	★★★
GASTROINTESTINAL	NR	STROKE	NR
GENERAL SURGERY	NR	VASCULAR	NR
MATERNITY CARE	NR	WOMEN'S HEALTH	NR

HEALTHGRADES AWARDS

Pipestone County Medical Center Ashton Care Center

916 4th Avenue Southwest
Pipestone, MN 56164
(507) 825-5811

Overall patient safety: ★★★
Teaching: N

CLINICAL PROGRAM RATINGS:

CARDIAC	NR	ORTHOPEDICS	NR
CRITICAL CARE	NR	PULMONARY	NR
GASTROINTESTINAL	NR	STROKE	★★★
GENERAL SURGERY	NR	VASCULAR	NR
MATERNITY CARE	NR	WOMEN'S HEALTH	NR

HEALTHGRADES AWARDS

Regina Medical Center

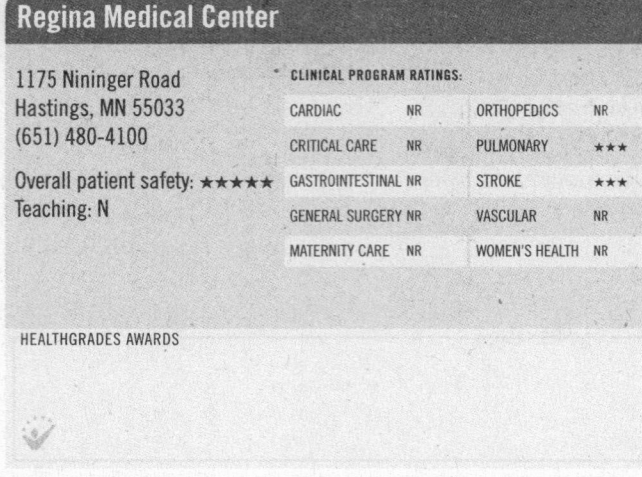

1175 Nininger Road
Hastings, MN 55033
(651) 480-4100

Overall patient safety: ★★★★★
Teaching: N

CLINICAL PROGRAM RATINGS:

CARDIAC	NR	ORTHOPEDICS	NR
CRITICAL CARE	NR	PULMONARY	★★★
GASTROINTESTINAL	NR	STROKE	★★★
GENERAL SURGERY	NR	VASCULAR	NR
MATERNITY CARE	NR	WOMEN'S HEALTH	NR

HEALTHGRADES AWARDS

Queen of Peace Hospital

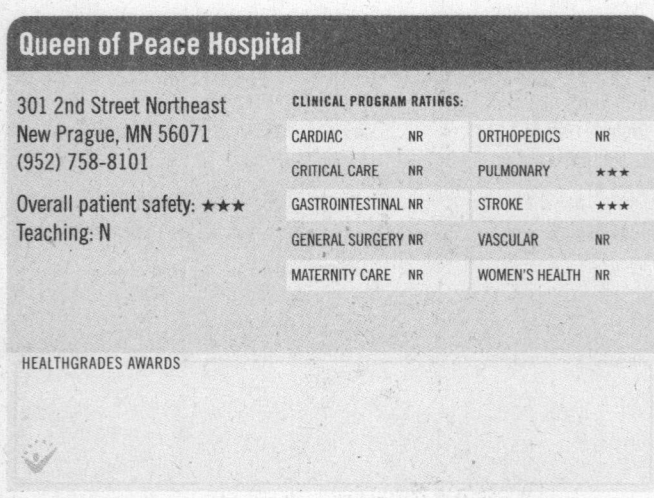

301 2nd Street Northeast
New Prague, MN 56071
(952) 758-8101

Overall patient safety: ★★★
Teaching: N

CLINICAL PROGRAM RATINGS:

CARDIAC	NR	ORTHOPEDICS	NR
CRITICAL CARE	NR	PULMONARY	★★★
GASTROINTESTINAL	NR	STROKE	★★★
GENERAL SURGERY	NR	VASCULAR	NR
MATERNITY CARE	NR	WOMEN'S HEALTH	NR

HEALTHGRADES AWARDS

Regions Hospital

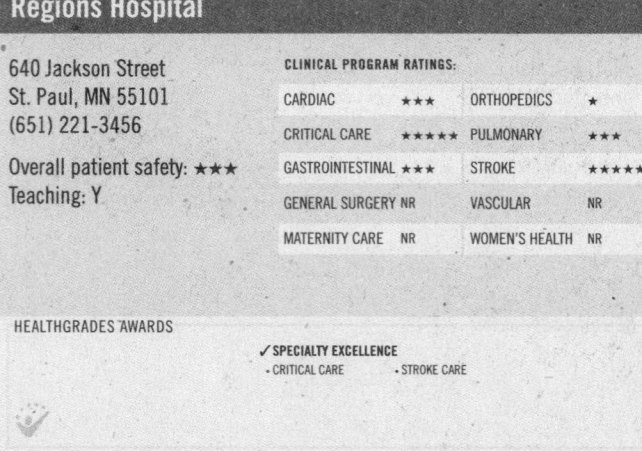

640 Jackson Street
St. Paul, MN 55101
(651) 221-3456

Overall patient safety: ★★★
Teaching: Y

CLINICAL PROGRAM RATINGS:

CARDIAC	★★★	ORTHOPEDICS	★
CRITICAL CARE	★★★★★	PULMONARY	★★★
GASTROINTESTINAL	★★★	STROKE	★★★★★
GENERAL SURGERY	NR	VASCULAR	NR
MATERNITY CARE	NR	WOMEN'S HEALTH	NR

HEALTHGRADES AWARDS

✓ SPECIALTY EXCELLENCE
· CRITICAL CARE · STROKE CARE

Redwood Area Hospital

100 Fallwood Road
Redwood Falls, MN 56283
(507) 637-4500

Overall patient safety: ★★★
Teaching: N

CLINICAL PROGRAM RATINGS:

CARDIAC	NR	ORTHOPEDICS	NR
CRITICAL CARE	NR	PULMONARY	★★★
GASTROINTESTINAL	NR	STROKE	★
GENERAL SURGERY	NR	VASCULAR	NR
MATERNITY CARE	NR	WOMEN'S HEALTH	NR

HEALTHGRADES AWARDS

Rice County District One Hospital

200 State Avenue
Faribault, MN 55021
(507) 334-6451

Overall patient safety: ★★★
Teaching: N

CLINICAL PROGRAM RATINGS:

CARDIAC	NR	ORTHOPEDICS	NR
CRITICAL CARE	NR	PULMONARY	★★★
GASTROINTESTINAL	NR	STROKE	★★★
GENERAL SURGERY	NR	VASCULAR	NR
MATERNITY CARE	NR	WOMEN'S HEALTH	NR

HEALTHGRADES AWARDS

KEY: ★★★★★ BEST   ★★★ AS EXPECTED   ★ POOR   NR NOT RATED BY HEALTHGRADES   For full definitions of ratings and awards, see Appendix.

Rice Memorial Hospital

301 Becker Avenue
Willmar, MN 56201
(320) 235-4543

Overall patient safety: ★★★
Teaching: N

CLINICAL PROGRAM RATINGS:

CARDIAC	NR	ORTHOPEDICS	NR
CRITICAL CARE	NR	PULMONARY	★★★
GASTROINTESTINAL	NR	STROKE	★★★
GENERAL SURGERY	NR	VASCULAR	NR
MATERNITY CARE	NR	WOMEN'S HEALTH	NR

HEALTHGRADES AWARDS

✓ SPECIALTY EXCELLENCE
• JOINT REPLACEMENT

Rochester Methodist Hospital

201 West Center Street
Rochester, MN 55902
(507) 284-2511

Overall patient safety: ★★★
Teaching: Y

CLINICAL PROGRAM RATINGS:

CARDIAC	NR	ORTHOPEDICS	NR
CRITICAL CARE	NR	PULMONARY	★★★
GASTROINTESTINAL	NR	STROKE	NR
GENERAL SURGERY	NR	VASCULAR	NR
MATERNITY CARE	NR	WOMEN'S HEALTH	NR

HEALTHGRADES AWARDS

Ridgeview Medical Center

500 South Maple Street
Waconia, MN 55387
(952) 442-2191

Overall patient safety: ★★★
Teaching: N

CLINICAL PROGRAM RATINGS:

CARDIAC	NR	ORTHOPEDICS	★★★
CRITICAL CARE	NR	PULMONARY	★
GASTROINTESTINAL	★★★	STROKE	★★★
GENERAL SURGERY	NR	VASCULAR	NR
MATERNITY CARE	NR	WOMEN'S HEALTH	NR

HEALTHGRADES AWARDS

Roseau Area Hospital and Homes

715 Delmore Drive
Roseau, MN 56751
(218) 463-2500

Overall patient safety: ★★★
Teaching: N

CLINICAL PROGRAM RATINGS:

CARDIAC	NR	ORTHOPEDICS	NR
CRITICAL CARE	NR	PULMONARY	★★★
GASTROINTESTINAL	NR	STROKE	NR
GENERAL SURGERY	NR	VASCULAR	NR
MATERNITY CARE	NR	WOMEN'S HEALTH	NR

HEALTHGRADES AWARDS

Riverview Hospital

323 South Minnesota
Crookston, MN 56716
(218) 281-9200

Overall patient safety: ★★★
Teaching: N

CLINICAL PROGRAM RATINGS:

CARDIAC	NR	ORTHOPEDICS	NR
CRITICAL CARE	NR	PULMONARY	★★★
GASTROINTESTINAL	NR	STROKE	★
GENERAL SURGERY	NR	VASCULAR	NR
MATERNITY CARE	NR	WOMEN'S HEALTH	NR

HEALTHGRADES AWARDS

Rush City Hospital*

760 West 4th Street
Rush City, MN 55069
(612) 358-4708

Overall patient safety: ★★★
Teaching: N

CLINICAL PROGRAM RATINGS:

CARDIAC	NR	ORTHOPEDICS	NR
CRITICAL CARE	NR	PULMONARY	★★★
GASTROINTESTINAL	NR	STROKE	★★★
GENERAL SURGERY	NR	VASCULAR	NR
MATERNITY CARE	NR	WOMEN'S HEALTH	NR

HEALTHGRADES AWARDS

*This hospital reports its data to the federal government jointly with another hospital. Therefore the ratings and awards apply to multiple hospitals and this specific hospital may not provide all rated services.

St. Cloud Hospital

1406 6th Avenue North
St. Cloud, MN 56303
(320) 251-2700

Overall patient safety: ★★★★★
Teaching: Y

CLINICAL PROGRAM RATINGS:

CARDIAC	★★★	ORTHOPEDICS	★★★
CRITICAL CARE	★★★	PULMONARY	★★★
GASTROINTESTINAL	★★★	STROKE	★★★
GENERAL SURGERY	NR	VASCULAR	★★★
MATERNITY CARE	NR	WOMEN'S HEALTH	NR

HEALTHGRADES AWARDS

✓ DISTINGUISHED HOSPITAL
- CLINICAL EXCELLENCE
- PATIENT SAFETY

✓ SPECIALTY EXCELLENCE
- CARDIAC CARE - CARDIAC SURGERY - JOINT REPLACEMENT

St. Francis Regional Medical Center

1455 Street Francis Avenue
Shakopee, MN 55379
(952) 403-3000

Overall patient safety: ★★★
Teaching: N

CLINICAL PROGRAM RATINGS:

CARDIAC	NR	ORTHOPEDICS	NR
CRITICAL CARE	NR	PULMONARY	★★★
GASTROINTESTINAL	NR	STROKE	★★★
GENERAL SURGERY	NR	VASCULAR	NR
MATERNITY CARE	NR	WOMEN'S HEALTH	NR

HEALTHGRADES AWARDS

St. Elizabeth Medical Center

1200 Grant Boulevard West
Wabasha, MN 55981
(651) 565-4531

Overall patient safety: ★★★
Teaching: N

CLINICAL PROGRAM RATINGS:

CARDIAC	NR	ORTHOPEDICS	NR
CRITICAL CARE	NR	PULMONARY	NR
GASTROINTESTINAL	NR	STROKE	NR
GENERAL SURGERY	NR	VASCULAR	NR
MATERNITY CARE	NR	WOMEN'S HEALTH	NR

HEALTHGRADES AWARDS

St. Gabriel's Hospital

815 Southeast 2nd Street
Little Falls, MN 56345
(320) 632-5441

Overall patient safety: ★
Teaching: N

CLINICAL PROGRAM RATINGS:

CARDIAC	NR	ORTHOPEDICS	NR
CRITICAL CARE	NR	PULMONARY	★★★
GASTROINTESTINAL	NR	STROKE	★★★
GENERAL SURGERY	NR	VASCULAR	NR
MATERNITY CARE	NR	WOMEN'S HEALTH	NR

HEALTHGRADES AWARDS

St. Francis Medical Center

2400 St. Francis Drive
Breckenridge, MN 56520
(218) 643-3000

Overall patient safety: ★★★
Teaching: N

CLINICAL PROGRAM RATINGS:

CARDIAC	NR	ORTHOPEDICS	NR
CRITICAL CARE	NR	PULMONARY	★★★
GASTROINTESTINAL	NR	STROKE	★★★
GENERAL SURGERY	NR	VASCULAR	NR
MATERNITY CARE	NR	WOMEN'S HEALTH	NR

HEALTHGRADES AWARDS

St. James Health Services

1207 6th Avenue South
St. James, MN 56081
(507) 375-3261

Overall patient safety: ★★★
Teaching: N

CLINICAL PROGRAM RATINGS:

CARDIAC	NR	ORTHOPEDICS	NR
CRITICAL CARE	NR	PULMONARY	★★★
GASTROINTESTINAL	NR	STROKE	NR
GENERAL SURGERY	NR	VASCULAR	NR
MATERNITY CARE	NR	WOMEN'S HEALTH	NR

HEALTHGRADES AWARDS

KEY: ★★★★★ BEST ★★★ AS EXPECTED ★ POOR NR NOT RATED BY HEALTHGRADES For full definitions of ratings and awards, see Appendix.

St. Joseph's Hospital

69 West Exchange Street
St. Paul, MN 55102
(651) 232-3000

Overall patient safety: ★★★★★
Teaching: Y

CLINICAL PROGRAM RATINGS:

CARDIAC	★★★	ORTHOPEDICS	★★★★★
CRITICAL CARE	★★★	PULMONARY	★★★
GASTROINTESTINAL	★★★	STROKE	★★★
GENERAL SURGERY	NR	VASCULAR	NR
MATERNITY CARE	NR	WOMEN'S HEALTH	NR

HEALTHGRADES AWARDS

✓ DISTINGUISHED HOSPITAL
· CLINICAL EXCELLENCE
· PATIENT SAFETY

St. Luke's Hospital

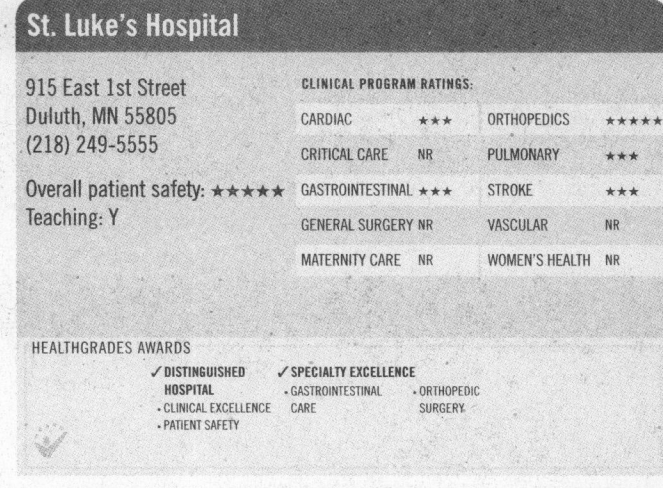

915 East 1st Street
Duluth, MN 55805
(218) 249-5555

Overall patient safety: ★★★★★
Teaching: Y

CLINICAL PROGRAM RATINGS:

CARDIAC	★★★	ORTHOPEDICS	★★★★★
CRITICAL CARE	NR	PULMONARY	★★★
GASTROINTESTINAL	★★★	STROKE	★★★
GENERAL SURGERY	NR	VASCULAR	NR
MATERNITY CARE	NR	WOMEN'S HEALTH	NR

HEALTHGRADES AWARDS

✓ DISTINGUISHED HOSPITAL
· CLINICAL EXCELLENCE
· PATIENT SAFETY

✓ SPECIALTY EXCELLENCE
· GASTROINTESTINAL CARE
· ORTHOPEDIC SURGERY

St. Joseph's Area Health Services

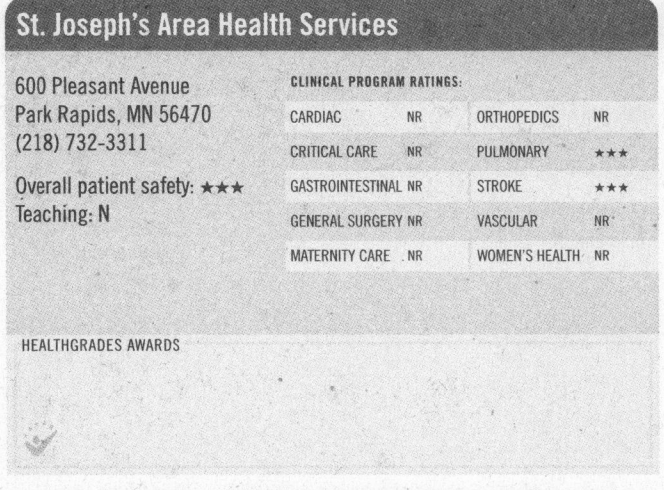

600 Pleasant Avenue
Park Rapids, MN 56470
(218) 732-3311

Overall patient safety: ★★★
Teaching: N

CLINICAL PROGRAM RATINGS:

CARDIAC	NR	ORTHOPEDICS	NR
CRITICAL CARE	NR	PULMONARY	★★★
GASTROINTESTINAL	NR	STROKE	★★★
GENERAL SURGERY	NR	VASCULAR	NR
MATERNITY CARE	NR	WOMEN'S HEALTH	NR

HEALTHGRADES AWARDS

St. Mary's Duluth Clinic

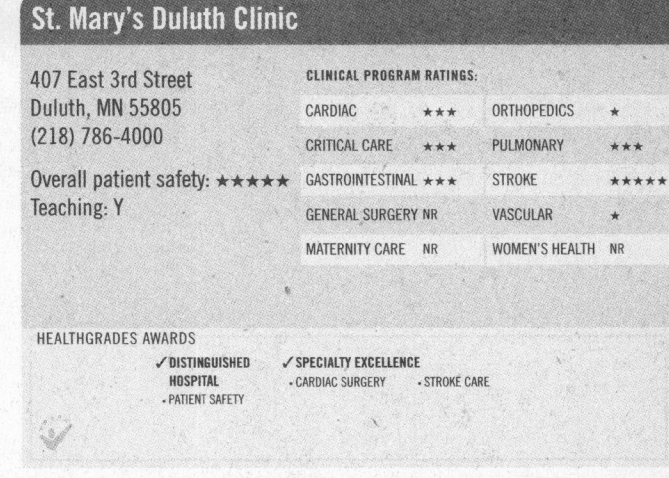

407 East 3rd Street
Duluth, MN 55805
(218) 786-4000

Overall patient safety: ★★★★★
Teaching: Y

CLINICAL PROGRAM RATINGS:

CARDIAC	★★★	ORTHOPEDICS	★
CRITICAL CARE	★★★	PULMONARY	★★★
GASTROINTESTINAL	★★★	STROKE	★★★★★
GENERAL SURGERY	NR	VASCULAR	★
MATERNITY CARE	NR	WOMEN'S HEALTH	NR

HEALTHGRADES AWARDS

✓ DISTINGUISHED HOSPITAL
· PATIENT SAFETY

✓ SPECIALTY EXCELLENCE
· CARDIAC SURGERY
· STROKE CARE

St. Joseph's Medical Center

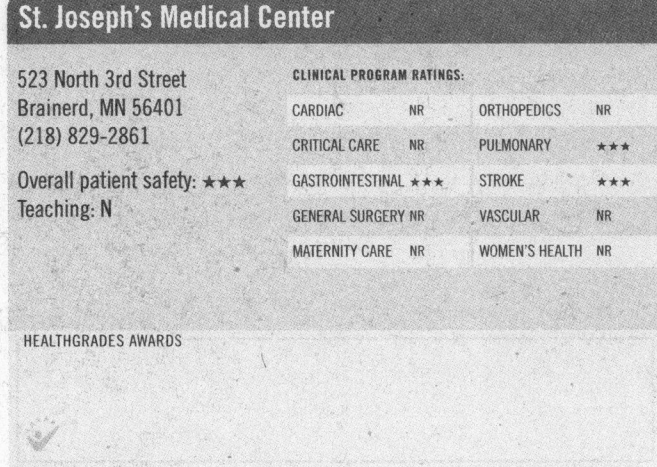

523 North 3rd Street
Brainerd, MN 56401
(218) 829-2861

Overall patient safety: ★★★
Teaching: N

CLINICAL PROGRAM RATINGS:

CARDIAC	NR	ORTHOPEDICS	NR
CRITICAL CARE	NR	PULMONARY	★★★
GASTROINTESTINAL	★★★	STROKE	★★★
GENERAL SURGERY	NR	VASCULAR	NR
MATERNITY CARE	NR	WOMEN'S HEALTH	NR

HEALTHGRADES AWARDS

St. Marys Hospital

1216 2nd Street Southwest
Rochester, MN 55902
(507) 285-5123

Overall patient safety: ★★★
Teaching: Y

CLINICAL PROGRAM RATINGS:

CARDIAC	★★★★★	ORTHOPEDICS	★
CRITICAL CARE	★★★★★	PULMONARY	★★★★★
GASTROINTESTINAL	★★★	STROKE	★★★★★
GENERAL SURGERY	NR	VASCULAR	★
MATERNITY CARE	NR	WOMEN'S HEALTH	NR

HEALTHGRADES AWARDS

✓ AMERICA'S 50 BEST HOSPITALS

✓ DISTINGUISHED HOSPITAL
· CLINICAL EXCELLENCE

✓ SPECIALTY EXCELLENCE
· CARDIAC CARE
· CARDIAC SURGERY
· CRITICAL CARE
· GASTROINTESTINAL CARE
· PULMONARY CARE
· STROKE CARE

St. Mary's Regional Health Center

1027 Washington Avenue
Detroit Lakes, MN 56501
(218) 847-5611

Overall patient safety: ★★★
Teaching: N

CLINICAL PROGRAM RATINGS:

CARDIAC	NR	ORTHOPEDICS	NR
CRITICAL CARE	NR	PULMONARY	★
GASTROINTESTINAL	NR	STROKE	★
GENERAL SURGERY	NR	VASCULAR	NR
MATERNITY CARE	NR	WOMEN'S HEALTH	NR

HEALTHGRADES AWARDS

Sioux Valley Canby Campus

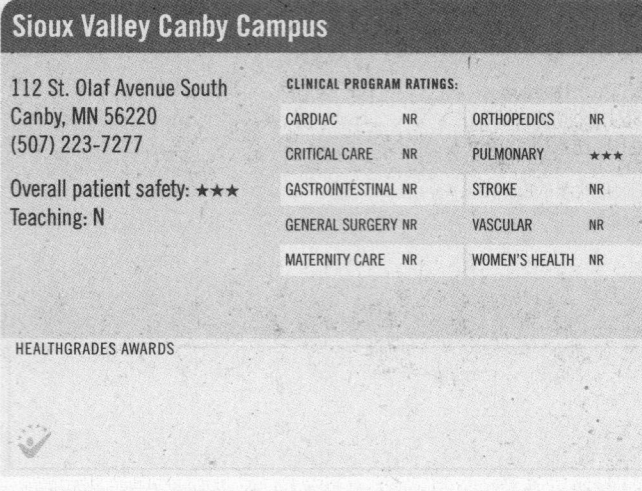

112 St. Olaf Avenue South
Canby, MN 56220
(507) 223-7277

Overall patient safety: ★★★
Teaching: N

CLINICAL PROGRAM RATINGS:

CARDIAC	NR	ORTHOPEDICS	NR
CRITICAL CARE	NR	PULMONARY	★★★
GASTROINTESTINAL	NR	STROKE	NR
GENERAL SURGERY	NR	VASCULAR	NR
MATERNITY CARE	NR	WOMEN'S HEALTH	NR

HEALTHGRADES AWARDS

St. Michael's Hospital and Nursing Home

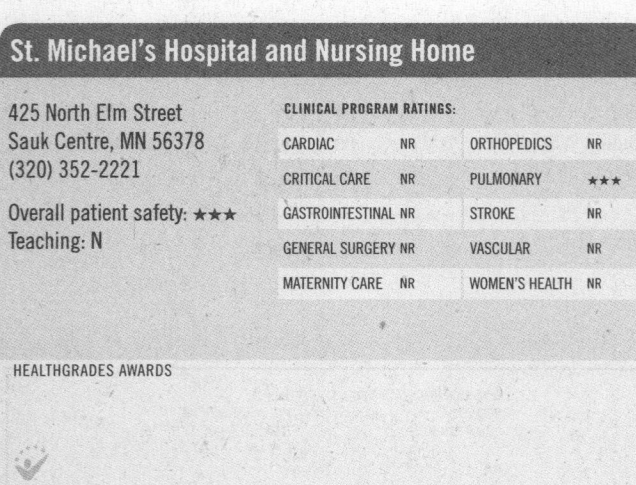

425 North Elm Street
Sauk Centre, MN 56378
(320) 352-2221

Overall patient safety: ★★★
Teaching: N

CLINICAL PROGRAM RATINGS:

CARDIAC	NR	ORTHOPEDICS	NR
CRITICAL CARE	NR	PULMONARY	★★★
GASTROINTESTINAL	NR	STROKE	NR
GENERAL SURGERY	NR	VASCULAR	NR
MATERNITY CARE	NR	WOMEN'S HEALTH	NR

HEALTHGRADES AWARDS

Stevens Community Medical Center

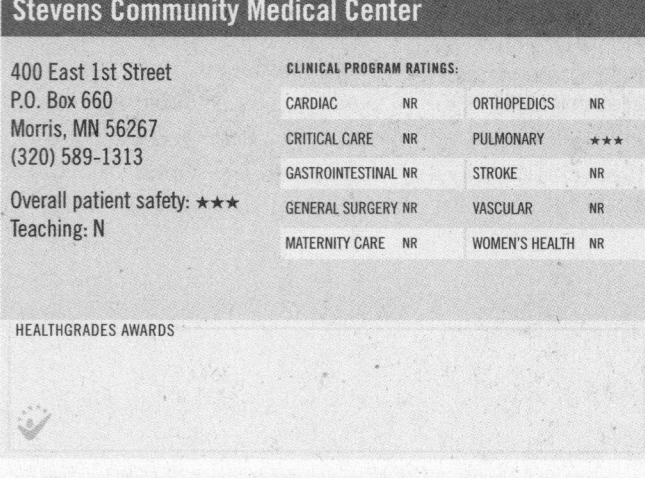

400 East 1st Street
P.O. Box 660
Morris, MN 56267
(320) 589-1313

Overall patient safety: ★★★
Teaching: N

CLINICAL PROGRAM RATINGS:

CARDIAC	NR	ORTHOPEDICS	NR
CRITICAL CARE	NR	PULMONARY	★★★
GASTROINTESTINAL	NR	STROKE	NR
GENERAL SURGERY	NR	VASCULAR	NR
MATERNITY CARE	NR	WOMEN'S HEALTH	NR

HEALTHGRADES AWARDS

St. Peter Community Hospital

1900 North Sunrise Drive
St. Peter, MN 56082
(507) 931-2200

Overall patient safety: ★★★
Teaching: N

CLINICAL PROGRAM RATINGS:

CARDIAC	NR	ORTHOPEDICS	NR
CRITICAL CARE	NR	PULMONARY	★★★
GASTROINTESTINAL	NR	STROKE	NR
GENERAL SURGERY	NR	VASCULAR	NR
MATERNITY CARE	NR	WOMEN'S HEALTH	NR

HEALTHGRADES AWARDS

Swift County Benson Hospital

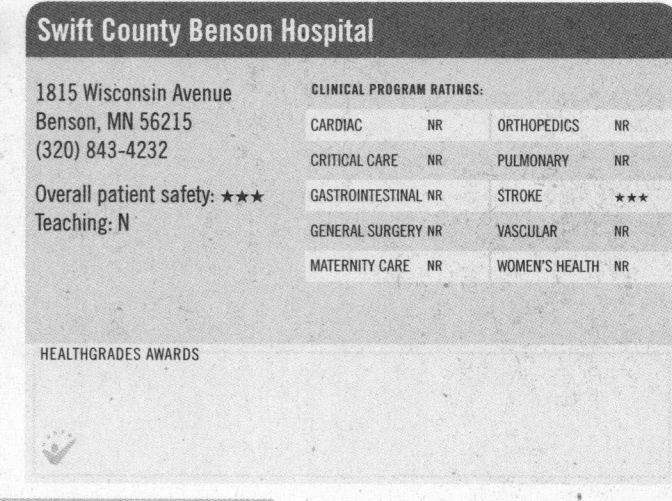

1815 Wisconsin Avenue
Benson, MN 56215
(320) 843-4232

Overall patient safety: ★★★
Teaching: N

CLINICAL PROGRAM RATINGS:

CARDIAC	NR	ORTHOPEDICS	NR
CRITICAL CARE	NR	PULMONARY	NR
GASTROINTESTINAL	NR	STROKE	★★★
GENERAL SURGERY	NR	VASCULAR	NR
MATERNITY CARE	NR	WOMEN'S HEALTH	NR

HEALTHGRADES AWARDS

KEY: ★★★★★ BEST   ★★★ AS EXPECTED   ★ POOR   NR NOT RATED BY HEALTHGRADES   For full definitions of ratings and awards, see Appendix.

Tracy Area Medical Services

251 5th Street East
Tracy, MN 56175
(507) 629-3200

Overall patient safety: ★★★
Teaching: N

CLINICAL PROGRAM RATINGS:

CARDIAC	NR	ORTHOPEDICS	NR
CRITICAL CARE	NR	PULMONARY	★★★
GASTROINTESTINAL	NR	STROKE	NR
GENERAL SURGERY	NR	VASCULAR	NR
MATERNITY CARE	NR	WOMEN'S HEALTH	NR

HEALTHGRADES AWARDS

United Hospitals

333 North Smith Avenue
St. Paul, MN 55102
(651) 220-8000

Overall patient safety: ★★★★★
Teaching: Y

CLINICAL PROGRAM RATINGS:

CARDIAC	★★★★★	ORTHOPEDICS	★
CRITICAL CARE	★★★★★	PULMONARY	★★★★★
GASTROINTESTINAL	★★★	STROKE	★★★
GENERAL SURGERY	NR	VASCULAR	★★★
MATERNITY CARE	NR	WOMEN'S HEALTH	NR

HEALTHGRADES AWARDS

✓ DISTINGUISHED HOSPITAL
 • CLINICAL EXCELLENCE
 • PATIENT SAFETY

✓ SPECIALTY EXCELLENCE
 • CARDIAC CARE   • CRITICAL CARE   • PULMONARY CARE

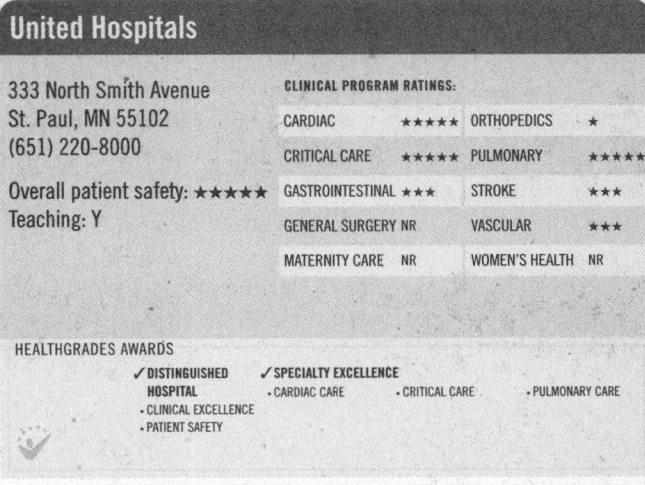

Tri-County Hospital

415 North Jefferson Street
Wadena, MN 56482
(218) 631-3510

Overall patient safety: ★★★
Teaching: N

CLINICAL PROGRAM RATINGS:

CARDIAC	NR	ORTHOPEDICS	NR
CRITICAL CARE	NR	PULMONARY	★★★
GASTROINTESTINAL	NR	STROKE	★★★
GENERAL SURGERY	NR	VASCULAR	NR
MATERNITY CARE	NR	WOMEN'S HEALTH	NR

HEALTHGRADES AWARDS

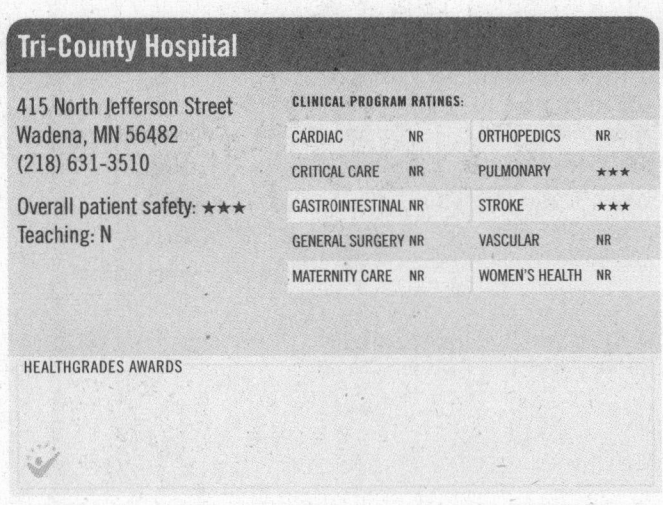

Unity Hospital

550 Osborne Road
Fridley, MN 55432
(763) 236-5000

Overall patient safety: ★★★
Teaching: Y

CLINICAL PROGRAM RATINGS:

CARDIAC	NR	ORTHOPEDICS	★
CRITICAL CARE	★★★★★	PULMONARY	★★★
GASTROINTESTINAL	★★★	STROKE	★★★
GENERAL SURGERY	NR	VASCULAR	NR
MATERNITY CARE	NR	WOMEN'S HEALTH	NR

HEALTHGRADES AWARDS

✓ DISTINGUISHED HOSPITAL
 • CLINICAL EXCELLENCE

✓ SPECIALTY EXCELLENCE
 • CRITICAL CARE

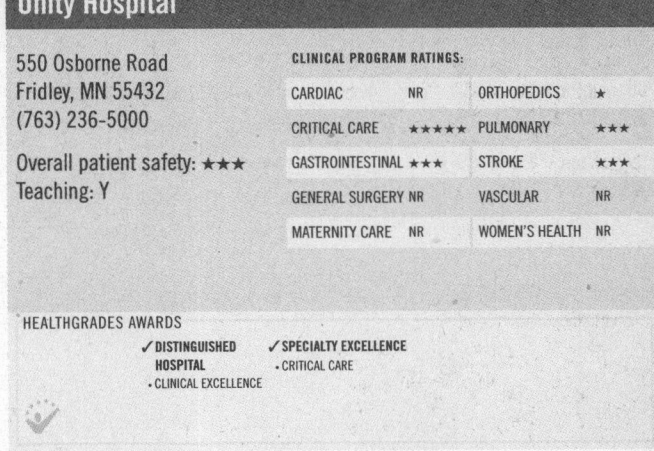

United Hospital District

515 South Moore Street
P.O. Box 160
Blue Earth, MN 56013
(507) 526-3273

Overall patient safety: ★★★
Teaching: N

CLINICAL PROGRAM RATINGS:

CARDIAC	NR	ORTHOPEDICS	NR
CRITICAL CARE	NR	PULMONARY	★★★
GASTROINTESTINAL	NR	STROKE	NR
GENERAL SURGERY	NR	VASCULAR	NR
MATERNITY CARE	NR	WOMEN'S HEALTH	NR

HEALTHGRADES AWARDS

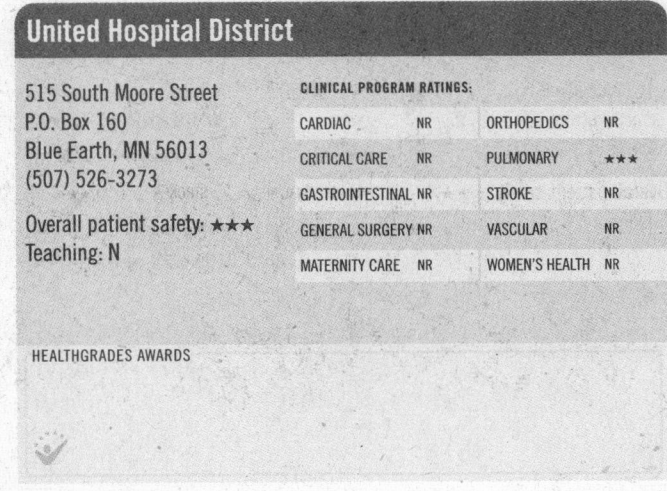

University Medical Center—Mesabi

750 East 34th Street
Hibbing, MN 55746
(218) 262-4881

Overall patient safety: ★★★
Teaching: N

CLINICAL PROGRAM RATINGS:

CARDIAC	NR	ORTHOPEDICS	NR
CRITICAL CARE	NR	PULMONARY	★★★
GASTROINTESTINAL	★★★	STROKE	★★★★★
GENERAL SURGERY	NR	VASCULAR	NR
MATERNITY CARE	NR	WOMEN'S HEALTH	NR

HEALTHGRADES AWARDS

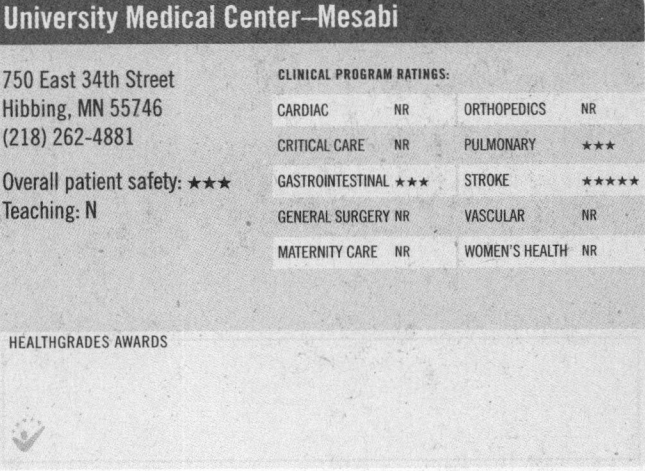

University of Minnesota Hospital and Clinic*

420 Delaware Street Southeast
Minneapolis, MN 55455
(612) 273-3000

Overall patient safety: ★★★
Teaching: Y

CLINICAL PROGRAM RATINGS:

CARDIAC	★★★	ORTHOPEDICS	★
CRITICAL CARE	NR	PULMONARY	★★★
GASTROINTESTINAL	★★★	STROKE	★★★
GENERAL SURGERY	NR	VASCULAR	NR
MATERNITY CARE	NR	WOMEN'S HEALTH	NR

HEALTHGRADES AWARDS

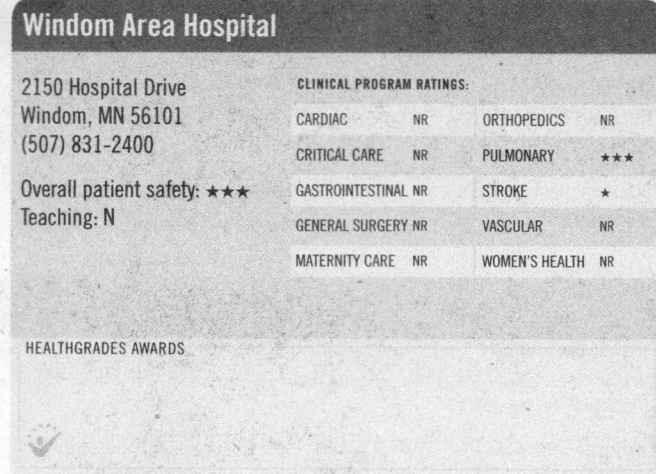

Windom Area Hospital

2150 Hospital Drive
Windom, MN 56101
(507) 831-2400

Overall patient safety: ★★★
Teaching: N

CLINICAL PROGRAM RATINGS:

CARDIAC	NR	ORTHOPEDICS	NR
CRITICAL CARE	NR	PULMONARY	★★★
GASTROINTESTINAL	NR	STROKE	★
GENERAL SURGERY	NR	VASCULAR	NR
MATERNITY CARE	NR	WOMEN'S HEALTH	NR

HEALTHGRADES AWARDS

University of Minnesota Medical Center–Fairview*

2450 Riverside Avenue
Minneapolis, MN 55454
(612) 672-6000

Overall patient safety: ★★★
Teaching: Y

CLINICAL PROGRAM RATINGS:

CARDIAC	★★★	ORTHOPEDICS	★
CRITICAL CARE	NR	PULMONARY	★★★
GASTROINTESTINAL	★★★	STROKE	★★★
GENERAL SURGERY	NR	VASCULAR	NR
MATERNITY CARE	NR	WOMEN'S HEALTH	NR

HEALTHGRADES AWARDS

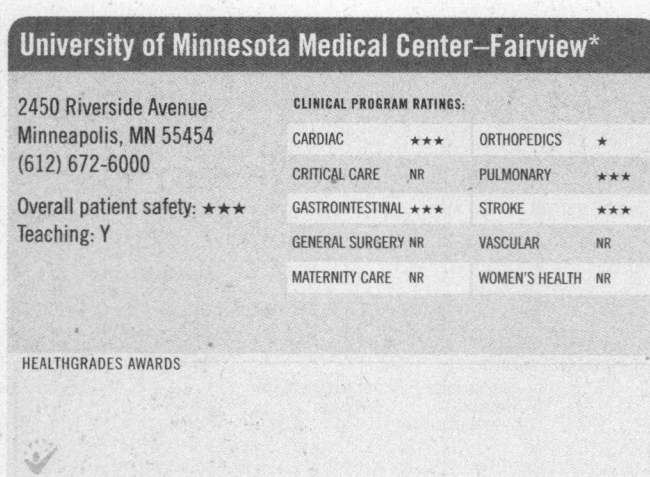

Winona Community Memorial Hospital

855 Mankato Avenue
Winona, MN 55987
(507) 454-3650

Overall patient safety: ★★★
Teaching: N

CLINICAL PROGRAM RATINGS:

CARDIAC	NR	ORTHOPEDICS	NR
CRITICAL CARE	NR	PULMONARY	★★★
GASTROINTESTINAL	NR	STROKE	★★★
GENERAL SURGERY	NR	VASCULAR	NR
MATERNITY CARE	NR	WOMEN'S HEALTH	NR

HEALTHGRADES AWARDS

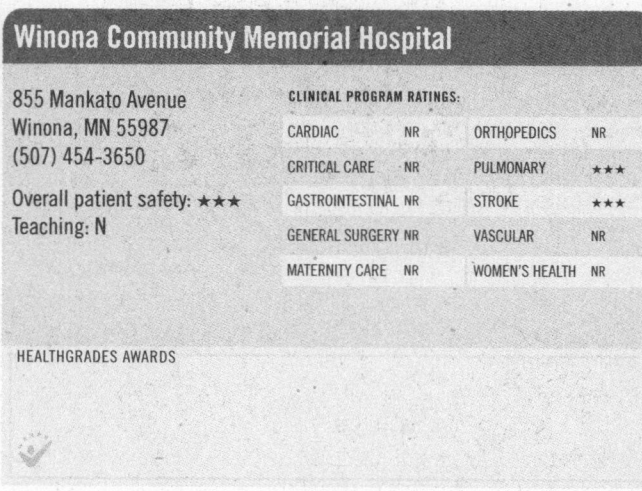

Virginia Regional Medical Center

901 9th Street North
Virginia, MN 55792
(218) 741-3340

Overall patient safety: ★★★
Teaching: N

CLINICAL PROGRAM RATINGS:

CARDIAC	NR	ORTHOPEDICS	NR
CRITICAL CARE	NR	PULMONARY	★★★
GASTROINTESTINAL	NR	STROKE	★★★
GENERAL SURGERY	NR	VASCULAR	NR
MATERNITY CARE	NR	WOMEN'S HEALTH	NR

HEALTHGRADES AWARDS

Worthington Regional Hospital

1018 6th Avenue
Worthington, MN 56187
(507) 372-2941

Overall patient safety: ★★★
Teaching: N

CLINICAL PROGRAM RATINGS:

CARDIAC	NR	ORTHOPEDICS	NR
CRITICAL CARE	NR	PULMONARY	★★★
GASTROINTESTINAL	NR	STROKE	NR
GENERAL SURGERY	NR	VASCULAR	NR
MATERNITY CARE	NR	WOMEN'S HEALTH	NR

HEALTHGRADES AWARDS

KEY: ★★★★★ BEST   ★★★ AS EXPECTED   ★ POOR   NR NOT RATED BY HEALTHGRADES   For full definitions of ratings and awards, see Appendix.

Baptist Memorial Hospital—Booneville

100 Hospital Street
Booneville, MS 38829
(662) 720-5000

Overall patient safety: ★★★
Teaching: N

CLINICAL PROGRAM RATINGS:

CARDIAC	NR	ORTHOPEDICS	NR
CRITICAL CARE	NR	PULMONARY	★★★
GASTROINTESTINAL	NR	STROKE	★
GENERAL SURGERY	NR	VASCULAR	NR
MATERNITY CARE	NR	WOMEN'S HEALTH	NR

HEALTHGRADES AWARDS

Baptist Memorial Hospital—North Mississippi

2301 South Lamar Boulevard
Oxford, MS 38655
(662) 232-8100

Overall patient safety: ★
Teaching: N

CLINICAL PROGRAM RATINGS:

CARDIAC	★★★	ORTHOPEDICS	★★★
CRITICAL CARE	NR	PULMONARY	★
GASTROINTESTINAL	★★★	STROKE	★
GENERAL SURGERY	NR	VASCULAR	NR
MATERNITY CARE	NR	WOMEN'S HEALTH	NR

HEALTHGRADES AWARDS

Baptist Memorial Hospital—De Soto

7601 Southcrest Parkway
Southaven, MS 38671
(662) 349-4000

Overall patient safety: ★★★
Teaching: Y

CLINICAL PROGRAM RATINGS:

CARDIAC	★★★	ORTHOPEDICS	★★★
CRITICAL CARE	★★★	PULMONARY	★★★
GASTROINTESTINAL	★★★	STROKE	★★★
GENERAL SURGERY	NR	VASCULAR	NR
MATERNITY CARE	NR	WOMEN'S HEALTH	NR

HEALTHGRADES AWARDS

Baptist Memorial Hospital—Union County

200 Highway 30 West
New Albany, MS 38652
(662) 538-7631

Overall patient safety: ★★★
Teaching: N

CLINICAL PROGRAM RATINGS:

CARDIAC	NR	ORTHOPEDICS	NR
CRITICAL CARE	NR	PULMONARY	★
GASTROINTESTINAL	NR	STROKE	★★★
GENERAL SURGERY	NR	VASCULAR	NR
MATERNITY CARE	NR	WOMEN'S HEALTH	NR

HEALTHGRADES AWARDS

Baptist Memorial Hospital—Golden Triangle

2520 5th Street North
Columbus, MS 39703
(662) 244-1000

Overall patient safety: ★★★
Teaching: N

CLINICAL PROGRAM RATINGS:

CARDIAC	★★★	ORTHOPEDICS	★★★
CRITICAL CARE	NR	PULMONARY	★
GASTROINTESTINAL	★★★	STROKE	★★★
GENERAL SURGERY	NR	VASCULAR	NR
MATERNITY CARE	NR	WOMEN'S HEALTH	NR

HEALTHGRADES AWARDS

Batesville Specialty Hospital*

303 Medical Center Drive
Batesville, MS 38606
(662) 712-2367

Overall patient safety: NR
Teaching: N

CLINICAL PROGRAM RATINGS:

CARDIAC	NR	ORTHOPEDICS	NR
CRITICAL CARE	NR	PULMONARY	★★★
GASTROINTESTINAL	NR	STROKE	NR
GENERAL SURGERY	NR	VASCULAR	NR
MATERNITY CARE	NR	WOMEN'S HEALTH	NR

HEALTHGRADES AWARDS

*This hospital reports its data to the federal government jointly with another hospital. Therefore the ratings and awards apply to multiple hospitals and this specific hospital may not provide all rated services.

Beacham Memorial

203 North Cherry Street
Magnolia, MS 39652
(601) 783-2351

Overall patient safety: NR
Teaching: N

CLINICAL PROGRAM RATINGS:

CARDIAC	NR	ORTHOPEDICS	NR
CRITICAL CARE	NR	PULMONARY	★★★
GASTROINTESTINAL	NR	STROKE	★★★
GENERAL SURGERY	NR	VASCULAR	NR
MATERNITY CARE	NR	WOMEN'S HEALTH	NR

HEALTHGRADES AWARDS

Central Mississippi Medical Center

1850 Chadwick Drive
Jackson, MS 39204
(601) 376-1000

Overall patient safety: ★★★
Teaching: N

CLINICAL PROGRAM RATINGS:

CARDIAC	★★★	ORTHOPEDICS	NR
CRITICAL CARE	NR	PULMONARY	★
GASTROINTESTINAL	★★★	STROKE	★★★
GENERAL SURGERY	NR	VASCULAR	NR
MATERNITY CARE	NR	WOMEN'S HEALTH	NR

HEALTHGRADES AWARDS

Biloxi Regional Medical Center

150 Reynoir Street
Biloxi, MS 39530
(228) 432-1571

Overall patient safety: ★
Teaching: N

CLINICAL PROGRAM RATINGS:

CARDIAC	NR	ORTHOPEDICS	NR
CRITICAL CARE	NR	PULMONARY	★★★
GASTROINTESTINAL	NR	STROKE	★★★
GENERAL SURGERY	NR	VASCULAR	NR
MATERNITY CARE	NR	WOMEN'S HEALTH	NR

HEALTHGRADES AWARDS

Clay County Medical Center

835 Medical Center Drive
West Point, MS 39773
(662) 495-2300

Overall patient safety: ★★★
Teaching: N

CLINICAL PROGRAM RATINGS:

CARDIAC	NR	ORTHOPEDICS	NR
CRITICAL CARE	NR	PULMONARY	★★★
GASTROINTESTINAL	NR	STROKE	★★★
GENERAL SURGERY	NR	VASCULAR	NR
MATERNITY CARE	NR	WOMEN'S HEALTH	NR

HEALTHGRADES AWARDS

Bolivar Medical Center

901 Highway 8 East
Cleveland, MS 38732
(662) 846-0061

Overall patient safety: ★★★
Teaching: N

CLINICAL PROGRAM RATINGS:

CARDIAC	NR	ORTHOPEDICS	NR
CRITICAL CARE	NR	PULMONARY	★★★
GASTROINTESTINAL	NR	STROKE	★★★
GENERAL SURGERY	NR	VASCULAR	NR
MATERNITY CARE	NR	WOMEN'S HEALTH	NR

HEALTHGRADES AWARDS

Covington County Hospital

701 South Holly Avenue
Collins, MS 39428
(601) 765-6711

Overall patient safety: ★★★
Teaching: N

CLINICAL PROGRAM RATINGS:

CARDIAC	NR	ORTHOPEDICS	NR
CRITICAL CARE	NR	PULMONARY	★
GASTROINTESTINAL	NR	STROKE	NR
GENERAL SURGERY	NR	VASCULAR	NR
MATERNITY CARE	NR	WOMEN'S HEALTH	NR

HEALTHGRADES AWARDS

KEY: ★★★★★ BEST   ★★★ AS EXPECTED   ★ POOR   NR NOT RATED BY HEALTHGRADES   For full definitions of ratings and awards, see Appendix.

Delta Regional Medical Center*

1400 East Union Street
Greenville, MS 38703
(662) 378-3873

Overall patient safety: ★★★
Teaching: N

CLINICAL PROGRAM RATINGS:

CARDIAC	★★★	ORTHOPEDICS	NR
CRITICAL CARE	NR	PULMONARY	★
GASTROINTESTINAL	★★★	STROKE	★★★
GENERAL SURGERY	NR	VASCULAR	NR
MATERNITY CARE	NR	WOMEN'S HEALTH	NR

HEALTHGRADES AWARDS

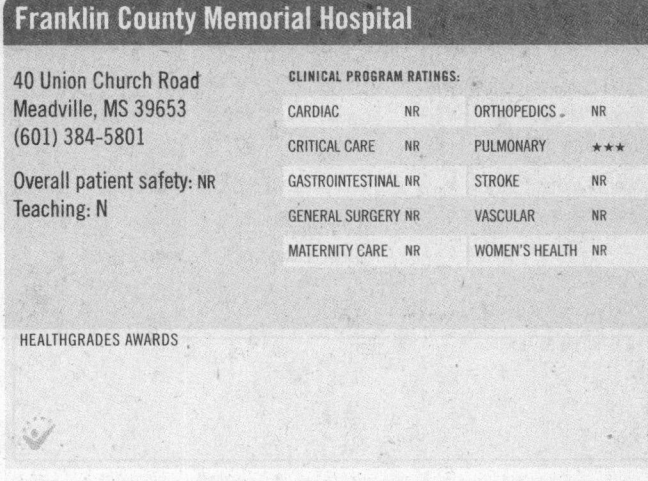

Franklin County Memorial Hospital

40 Union Church Road
Meadville, MS 39653
(601) 384-5801

Overall patient safety: NR
Teaching: N

CLINICAL PROGRAM RATINGS:

CARDIAC	NR	ORTHOPEDICS	NR
CRITICAL CARE	NR	PULMONARY	★★★
GASTROINTESTINAL	NR	STROKE	NR
GENERAL SURGERY	NR	VASCULAR	NR
MATERNITY CARE	NR	WOMEN'S HEALTH	NR

HEALTHGRADES AWARDS

Field Memorial Community Hospital

270 West Main Street
P.O. Box 639
Centreville, MS 39631
(601) 645-5221

Overall patient safety: ★★★
Teaching: N

CLINICAL PROGRAM RATINGS:

CARDIAC	NR	ORTHOPEDICS	NR
CRITICAL CARE	NR	PULMONARY	★
GASTROINTESTINAL	NR	STROKE	★
GENERAL SURGERY	NR	VASCULAR	NR
MATERNITY CARE	NR	WOMEN'S HEALTH	NR

HEALTHGRADES AWARDS

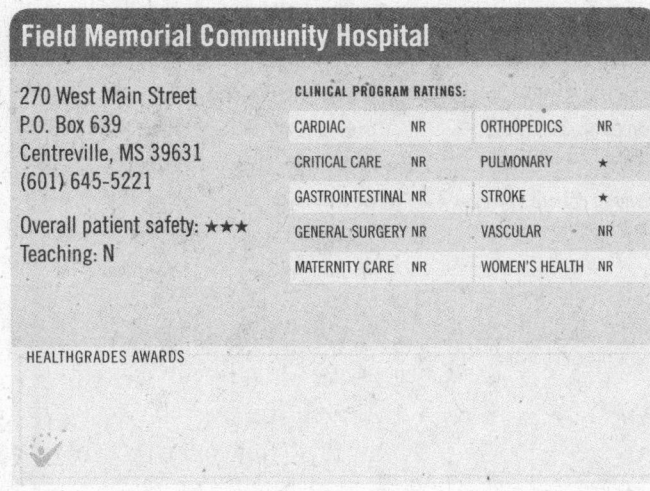

Garden Park Medical Center

15200 Community Road
Gulfport, MS 39503
(228) 575-7000

Overall patient safety: ★
Teaching: N

CLINICAL PROGRAM RATINGS:

CARDIAC	NR	ORTHOPEDICS	★★★
CRITICAL CARE	NR	PULMONARY	★★★
GASTROINTESTINAL	NR	STROKE	★★★
GENERAL SURGERY	NR	VASCULAR	NR
MATERNITY CARE	NR	WOMEN'S HEALTH	NR

HEALTHGRADES AWARDS

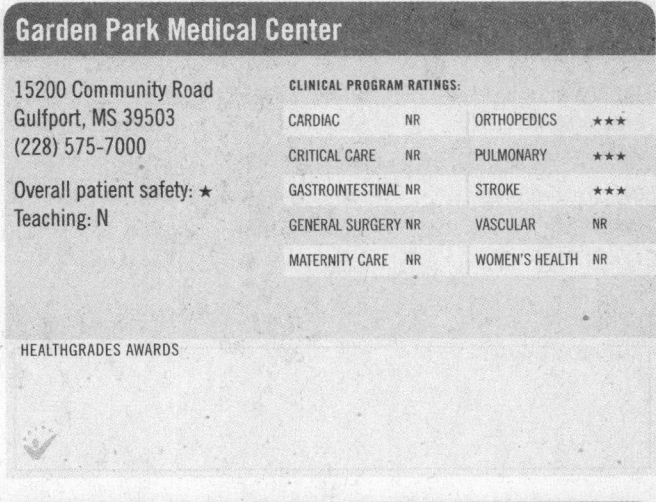

Forrest General Hospital

6051 US Highway 49 South
Hattiesburg, MS 39401
(601) 288-7000

Overall patient safety: ★
Teaching: N

CLINICAL PROGRAM RATINGS:

CARDIAC	★★★	ORTHOPEDICS	★★★★★
CRITICAL CARE	NR	PULMONARY	★★★
GASTROINTESTINAL	★★★	STROKE	★★★
GENERAL SURGERY	NR	VASCULAR	★★★★★
MATERNITY CARE	NR	WOMEN'S HEALTH	NR

HEALTHGRADES AWARDS

✓ SPECIALTY EXCELLENCE
· Vascular Surgery

George Regional Health System

859 Winter Street
Lucedale, MS 39452
(601) 947-3161

Overall patient safety: ★★★
Teaching: N

CLINICAL PROGRAM RATINGS:

CARDIAC	NR	ORTHOPEDICS	NR
CRITICAL CARE	NR	PULMONARY	★
GASTROINTESTINAL	NR	STROKE	★
GENERAL SURGERY	NR	VASCULAR	NR
MATERNITY CARE	NR	WOMEN'S HEALTH	NR

HEALTHGRADES AWARDS

*This hospital reports its data to the federal government jointly with another hospital. Therefore the ratings and awards apply to multiple hospitals and this specific hospital may not provide all rated services.

Gilmore Memorial Hospital

1105 Earl Frye Boulevard
Amory, MS 38821
(662) 256-7111

Overall patient safety: ★★★
Teaching: N

CLINICAL PROGRAM RATINGS:

CARDIAC	NR	ORTHOPEDICS	NR
CRITICAL CARE	NR	PULMONARY	★
GASTROINTESTINAL	NR	STROKE	★★★
GENERAL SURGERY	NR	VASCULAR	NR
MATERNITY CARE	NR	WOMEN'S HEALTH	NR

HEALTHGRADES AWARDS

Gulf Coast Medical Center

180 DeBuys Road
Biloxi, MS 39531
(228) 388-6711

Overall patient safety: ★★★
Teaching: N

CLINICAL PROGRAM RATINGS:

CARDIAC	NR	ORTHOPEDICS	★★★★★
CRITICAL CARE	NR	PULMONARY	★★★
GASTROINTESTINAL	NR	STROKE	★★★
GENERAL SURGERY	NR	VASCULAR	NR
MATERNITY CARE	NR	WOMEN'S HEALTH	NR

HEALTHGRADES AWARDS

✓ **SPECIALTY EXCELLENCE**
· JOINT REPLACEMENT   · ORTHOPEDIC SURGERY

Greenwood Leflore Hospital

1401 River Road
Greenwood, MS 38930
(662) 459-7000

Overall patient safety: ★
Teaching: N

CLINICAL PROGRAM RATINGS:

CARDIAC	NR	ORTHOPEDICS	NR
CRITICAL CARE	NR	PULMONARY	★★★
GASTROINTESTINAL	★★★	STROKE	★★★
GENERAL SURGERY	NR	VASCULAR	NR
MATERNITY CARE	NR	WOMEN'S HEALTH	NR

HEALTHGRADES AWARDS

H. C. Watkins Memorial Hospital

605 South Archusa Avenue
Quitman, MS 39355
(601) 776-6925

Overall patient safety: ★★★
Teaching: N

CLINICAL PROGRAM RATINGS:

CARDIAC	NR	ORTHOPEDICS	NR
CRITICAL CARE	NR	PULMONARY	★★★
GASTROINTESTINAL	NR	STROKE	NR
GENERAL SURGERY	NR	VASCULAR	NR
MATERNITY CARE	NR	WOMEN'S HEALTH	NR

HEALTHGRADES AWARDS

Grenada Lake Medical Center

960 Avent Drive
Grenada, MS 38901
(662) 227-7000

Overall patient safety: ★
Teaching: N

CLINICAL PROGRAM RATINGS:

CARDIAC	NR	ORTHOPEDICS	NR
CRITICAL CARE	NR	PULMONARY	★
GASTROINTESTINAL	NR	STROKE	★
GENERAL SURGERY	NR	VASCULAR	NR
MATERNITY CARE	NR	WOMEN'S HEALTH	NR

HEALTHGRADES AWARDS

Hancock Medical Center

149 Drinkwater Boulevard
Bay St. Louis, MS 39521
(228) 467-8600

Overall patient safety: NR
Teaching: N

CLINICAL PROGRAM RATINGS:

CARDIAC	NR	ORTHOPEDICS	NR
CRITICAL CARE	NR	PULMONARY	★★★
GASTROINTESTINAL	NR	STROKE	★★★
GENERAL SURGERY	NR	VASCULAR	NR
MATERNITY CARE	NR	WOMEN'S HEALTH	NR

HEALTHGRADES AWARDS

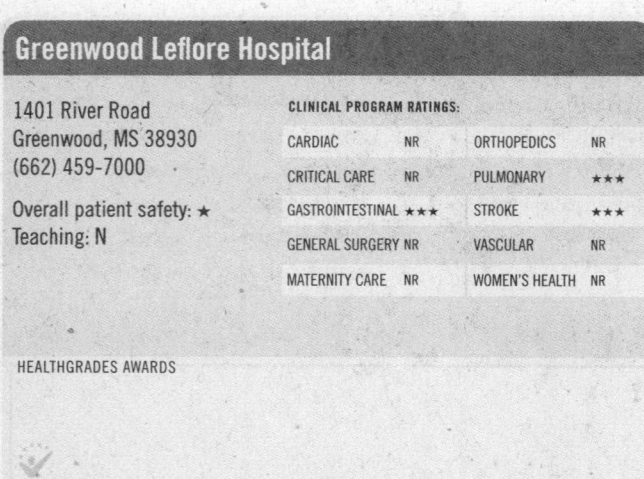
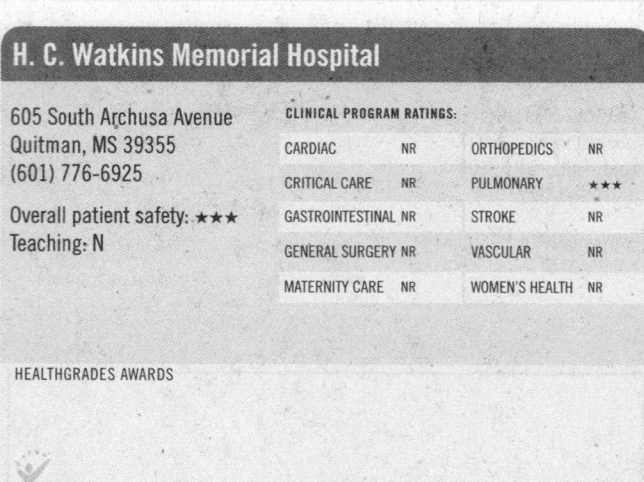

KEY: ★★★★★ BEST   ★★★ AS EXPECTED   ★ POOR   NR **NOT RATED BY HEALTHGRADES**   For full definitions of ratings and awards, see Appendix.

Hardy Wilson Memorial Hospital

233 Magnolia Street
Hazlehurst, MS 39083
(601) 894-4541

Overall patient safety: NR
Teaching: N

CLINICAL PROGRAM RATINGS:

CARDIAC	NR	ORTHOPEDICS	NR
CRITICAL CARE	NR	PULMONARY	★
GASTROINTESTINAL	NR	STROKE	NR
GENERAL SURGERY	NR	VASCULAR	NR
MATERNITY CARE	NR	WOMEN'S HEALTH	NR

HEALTHGRADES AWARDS

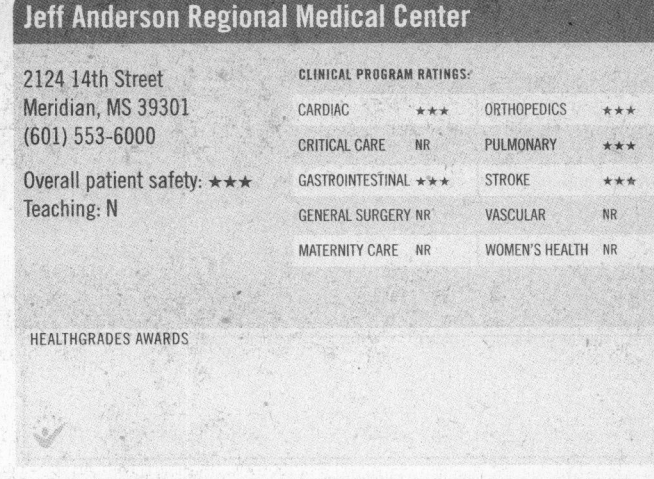

Jeff Anderson Regional Medical Center

2124 14th Street
Meridian, MS 39301
(601) 553-6000

Overall patient safety: ★★★
Teaching: N

CLINICAL PROGRAM RATINGS:

CARDIAC	★★★	ORTHOPEDICS	★★★
CRITICAL CARE	NR	PULMONARY	★★★
GASTROINTESTINAL	★★★	STROKE	★★★
GENERAL SURGERY	NR	VASCULAR	NR
MATERNITY CARE	NR	WOMEN'S HEALTH	NR

HEALTHGRADES AWARDS

Highland Community Hospital

801 Goodyear Boulevard
Picayune, MS 39466
(601) 798-4711

Overall patient safety: ★★★
Teaching: N

CLINICAL PROGRAM RATINGS:

CARDIAC	NR	ORTHOPEDICS	NR
CRITICAL CARE	NR	PULMONARY	★★★
GASTROINTESTINAL	NR	STROKE	★
GENERAL SURGERY	NR	VASCULAR	NR
MATERNITY CARE	NR	WOMEN'S HEALTH	NR

HEALTHGRADES AWARDS

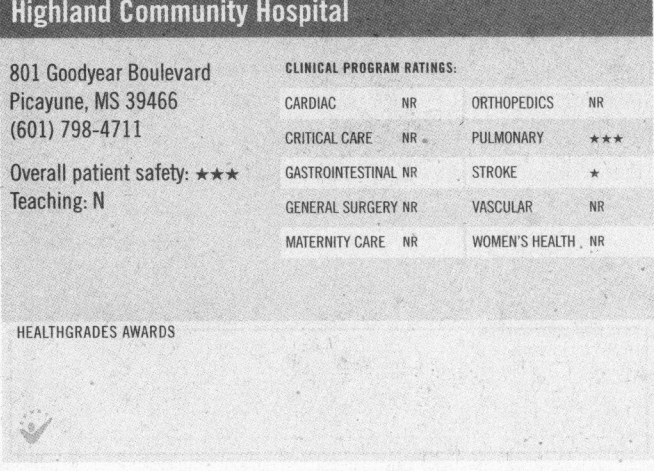

Jefferson Davis Community Hospital

1102 Rose Street
Prentiss, MS 39474
(601) 792-4276

Overall patient safety: NR
Teaching: N

CLINICAL PROGRAM RATINGS:

CARDIAC	NR	ORTHOPEDICS	NR
CRITICAL CARE	NR	PULMONARY	★★★
GASTROINTESTINAL	NR	STROKE	NR
GENERAL SURGERY	NR	VASCULAR	NR
MATERNITY CARE	NR	WOMEN'S HEALTH	NR

HEALTHGRADES AWARDS

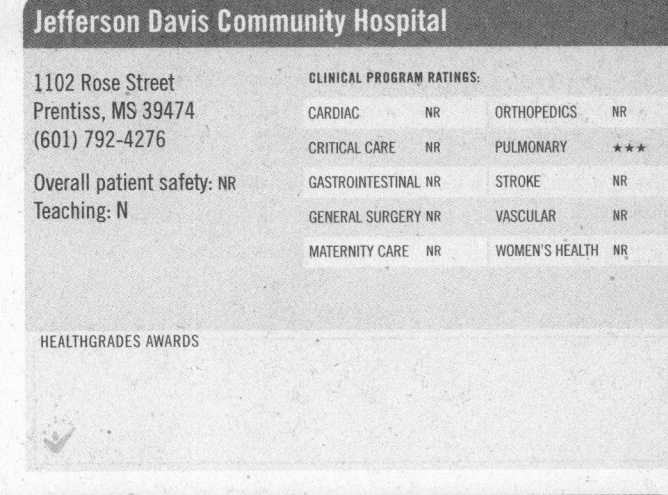

Humphreys County Memorial Hospital

500 Centre Road
Belzoni, MS 39038
(662) 247-3831

Overall patient safety: NR
Teaching: N

CLINICAL PROGRAM RATINGS:

CARDIAC	NR	ORTHOPEDICS	NR
CRITICAL CARE	NR	PULMONARY	★
GASTROINTESTINAL	NR	STROKE	NR
GENERAL SURGERY	NR	VASCULAR	NR
MATERNITY CARE	NR	WOMEN'S HEALTH	NR

HEALTHGRADES AWARDS

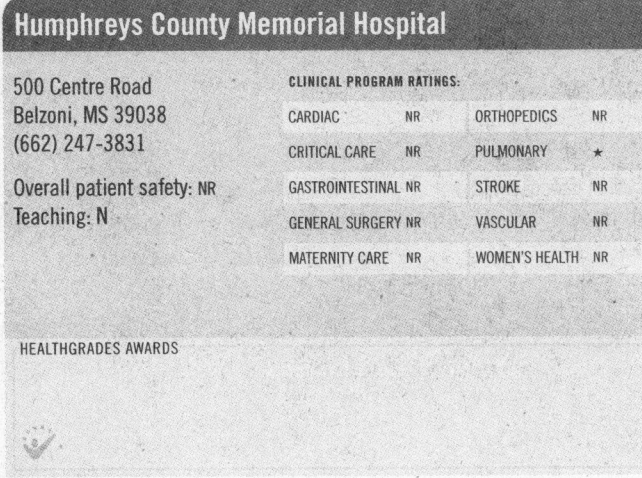

King's Daughters Medical Center–Brookhaven

427 Highway 51 North
Brookhaven, MS 39601
(601) 833-6011

Overall patient safety: ★★★
Teaching: N

CLINICAL PROGRAM RATINGS:

CARDIAC	NR	ORTHOPEDICS	NR
CRITICAL CARE	NR	PULMONARY	★★★
GASTROINTESTINAL	NR	STROKE	★
GENERAL SURGERY	NR	VASCULAR	NR
MATERNITY CARE	NR	WOMEN'S HEALTH	NR

HEALTHGRADES AWARDS

King's Daughters Hospital

823 Grand Avenue
Yazoo City, MS 39194
(662) 746-2261

Overall patient safety: ★★★
Teaching: N

CLINICAL PROGRAM RATINGS:

CARDIAC	NR	ORTHOPEDICS	NR
CRITICAL CARE	NR	PULMONARY	★★★
GASTROINTESTINAL	NR	STROKE	★★★
GENERAL SURGERY	NR	VASCULAR	NR
MATERNITY CARE	NR	WOMEN'S HEALTH	NR

HEALTHGRADES AWARDS

Laird Hospital

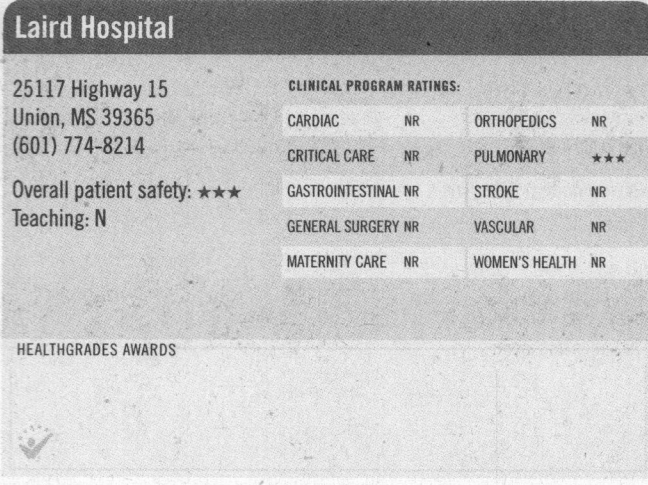

25117 Highway 15
Union, MS 39365
(601) 774-8214

Overall patient safety: ★★★
Teaching: N

CLINICAL PROGRAM RATINGS:

CARDIAC	NR	ORTHOPEDICS	NR
CRITICAL CARE	NR	PULMONARY	★★★
GASTROINTESTINAL	NR	STROKE	NR
GENERAL SURGERY	NR	VASCULAR	NR
MATERNITY CARE	NR	WOMEN'S HEALTH	NR

HEALTHGRADES AWARDS

King's Daughters Hospital—Greenville*

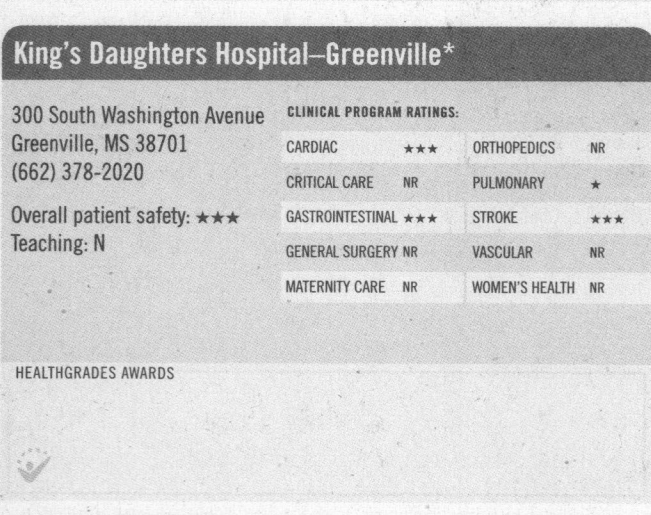

300 South Washington Avenue
Greenville, MS 38701
(662) 378-2020

Overall patient safety: ★★★
Teaching: N

CLINICAL PROGRAM RATINGS:

CARDIAC	★★★	ORTHOPEDICS	NR
CRITICAL CARE	NR	PULMONARY	★
GASTROINTESTINAL	★★★	STROKE	★★★
GENERAL SURGERY	NR	VASCULAR	NR
MATERNITY CARE	NR	WOMEN'S HEALTH	NR

HEALTHGRADES AWARDS

Lawrence County Hospital

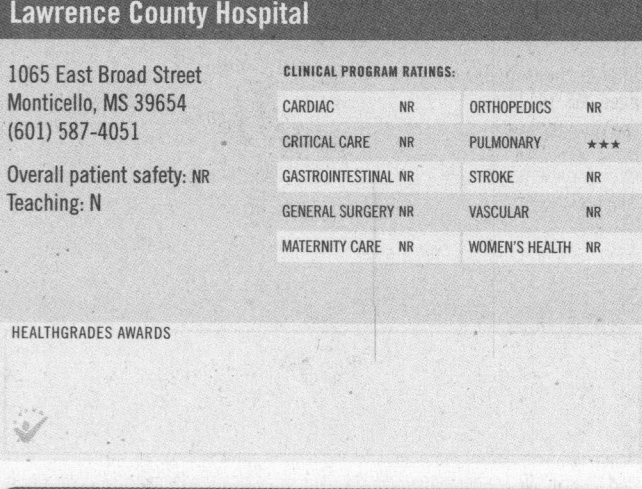

1065 East Broad Street
Monticello, MS 39654
(601) 587-4051

Overall patient safety: NR
Teaching: N

CLINICAL PROGRAM RATINGS:

CARDIAC	NR	ORTHOPEDICS	NR
CRITICAL CARE	NR	PULMONARY	★★★
GASTROINTESTINAL	NR	STROKE	NR
GENERAL SURGERY	NR	VASCULAR	NR
MATERNITY CARE	NR	WOMEN'S HEALTH	NR

HEALTHGRADES AWARDS

Lackey Memorial Hospital

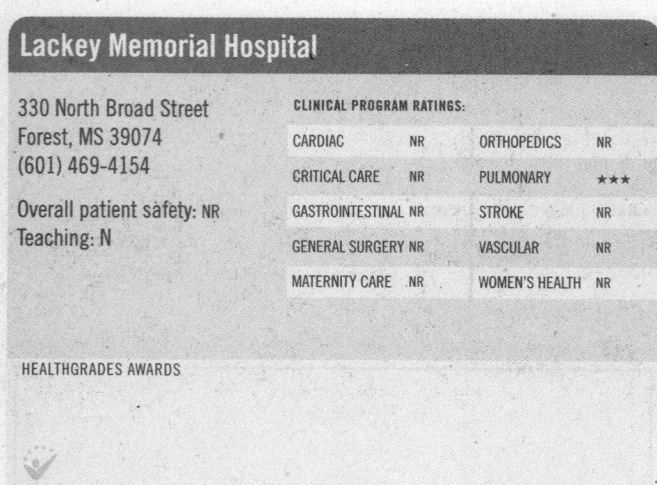

330 North Broad Street
Forest, MS 39074
(601) 469-4154

Overall patient safety: NR
Teaching: N

CLINICAL PROGRAM RATINGS:

CARDIAC	NR	ORTHOPEDICS	NR
CRITICAL CARE	NR	PULMONARY	★★★
GASTROINTESTINAL	NR	STROKE	NR
GENERAL SURGERY	NR	VASCULAR	NR
MATERNITY CARE	NR	WOMEN'S HEALTH	NR

HEALTHGRADES AWARDS

Leake County Memorial Hospital

310 Ellis Street
Carthage, MS 39051
(601) 267-1100

Overall patient safety: NR
Teaching: N

CLINICAL PROGRAM RATINGS:

CARDIAC	NR	ORTHOPEDICS	NR
CRITICAL CARE	NR	PULMONARY	★
GASTROINTESTINAL	NR	STROKE	★★★
GENERAL SURGERY	NR	VASCULAR	NR
MATERNITY CARE	NR	WOMEN'S HEALTH	NR

HEALTHGRADES AWARDS

KEY: ★★★★★ BEST ★★★ AS EXPECTED ★ POOR NR NOT RATED BY HEALTHGRADES For full definitions of ratings and awards, see Appendix.

Madison Regional Medical Center

1421 East Peace Street
Canton, MS 39046
(601) 859-1331

Overall patient safety: ★★★
Teaching: N

CLINICAL PROGRAM RATINGS:

CARDIAC	NR	ORTHOPEDICS	NR
CRITICAL CARE	NR	PULMONARY	★★★
GASTROINTESTINAL	NR	STROKE	NR
GENERAL SURGERY	NR	VASCULAR	NR
MATERNITY CARE	NR	WOMEN'S HEALTH	NR

HEALTHGRADES AWARDS

Marion General Hospital

1560 Sumrall Road
Columbia, MS 39429
(601) 736-6303

Overall patient safety: ★★★
Teaching: N

CLINICAL PROGRAM RATINGS:

CARDIAC	NR	ORTHOPEDICS	NR
CRITICAL CARE	NR	PULMONARY	★
GASTROINTESTINAL	NR	STROKE	NR
GENERAL SURGERY	NR	VASCULAR	NR
MATERNITY CARE	NR	WOMEN'S HEALTH	NR

HEALTHGRADES AWARDS

Magee General Hospital

300 3rd Avenue Southeast
Magee, MS 39111
(601) 849-5070

Overall patient safety: ★★★
Teaching: N

CLINICAL PROGRAM RATINGS:

CARDIAC	NR	ORTHOPEDICS	NR
CRITICAL CARE	NR	PULMONARY	★
GASTROINTESTINAL	NR	STROKE	NR
GENERAL SURGERY	NR	VASCULAR	NR
MATERNITY CARE	NR	WOMEN'S HEALTH	NR

HEALTHGRADES AWARDS

Memorial Hospital at Gulfport

4500 13th Street
Gulfport, MS 39501
(228) 867-4000

Overall patient safety: ★★★
Teaching: N

CLINICAL PROGRAM RATINGS:

CARDIAC	★	ORTHOPEDICS	★★★
CRITICAL CARE	NR	PULMONARY	★★★
GASTROINTESTINAL	★★★	STROKE	★★★
GENERAL SURGERY	NR	VASCULAR	★★★
MATERNITY CARE	NR	WOMEN'S HEALTH	NR

HEALTHGRADES AWARDS

Magnolia Regional Health Center

611 Alcorn Drive
Corinth, MS 38834
(662) 293-7660

Overall patient safety: ★★★
Teaching: N

CLINICAL PROGRAM RATINGS:

CARDIAC	NR	ORTHOPEDICS	NR
CRITICAL CARE	NR	PULMONARY	★
GASTROINTESTINAL	★★★	STROKE	★★★
GENERAL SURGERY	NR	VASCULAR	NR
MATERNITY CARE	NR	WOMEN'S HEALTH	NR

HEALTHGRADES AWARDS

Mississippi Baptist Medical Center

1225 North State Street
Jackson, MS 39202
(601) 968-1000

Overall patient safety: ★★★★★
Teaching: Y

CLINICAL PROGRAM RATINGS:

CARDIAC	★★★	ORTHOPEDICS	★★★
CRITICAL CARE	NR	PULMONARY	★★★
GASTROINTESTINAL	★★★	STROKE	★★★
GENERAL SURGERY	NR	VASCULAR	★★★★★
MATERNITY CARE	NR	WOMEN'S HEALTH	NR

HEALTHGRADES AWARDS

✓ DISTINGUISHED HOSPITAL
- PATIENT SAFETY

✓ SPECIALTY EXCELLENCE
- GASTROINTESTINAL CARE
- VASCULAR SURGERY

*This hospital reports its data to the federal government jointly with another hospital. Therefore the ratings and awards apply to multiple hospitals and this specific hospital may not provide all rated services.

Montfort Jones Memorial Hospital

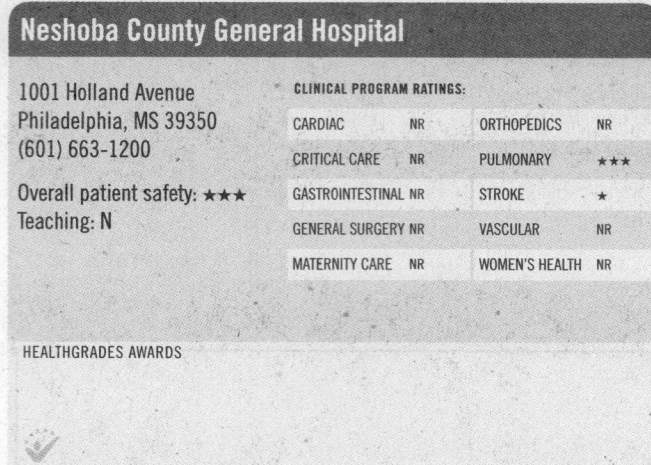

220 Highway 12 West
Kosciusko, MS 39090
(662) 289-4311

Overall patient safety: ★★★
Teaching: N

CLINICAL PROGRAM RATINGS:

CARDIAC	NR	ORTHOPEDICS	NR
CRITICAL CARE	NR	PULMONARY	★
GASTROINTESTINAL	NR	STROKE	★
GENERAL SURGERY	NR	VASCULAR	NR
MATERNITY CARE	NR	WOMEN'S HEALTH	NR

HEALTHGRADES AWARDS

Neshoba County General Hospital

1001 Holland Avenue
Philadelphia, MS 39350
(601) 663-1200

Overall patient safety: ★★★
Teaching: N

CLINICAL PROGRAM RATINGS:

CARDIAC	NR	ORTHOPEDICS	NR
CRITICAL CARE	NR	PULMONARY	★★★
GASTROINTESTINAL	NR	STROKE	★
GENERAL SURGERY	NR	VASCULAR	NR
MATERNITY CARE	NR	WOMEN'S HEALTH	NR

HEALTHGRADES AWARDS

Natchez Community Hospital

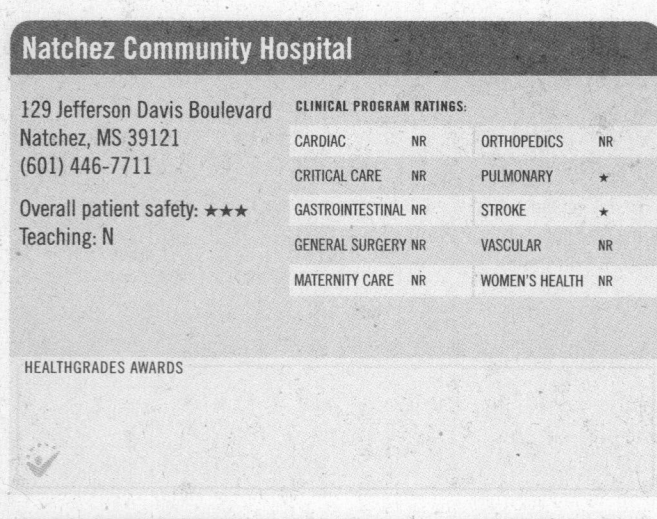

129 Jefferson Davis Boulevard
Natchez, MS 39121
(601) 446-7711

Overall patient safety: ★★★
Teaching: N

CLINICAL PROGRAM RATINGS:

CARDIAC	NR	ORTHOPEDICS	NR
CRITICAL CARE	NR	PULMONARY	★
GASTROINTESTINAL	NR	STROKE	★
GENERAL SURGERY	NR	VASCULAR	NR
MATERNITY CARE	NR	WOMEN'S HEALTH	NR

HEALTHGRADES AWARDS

Newton Regional Hospital

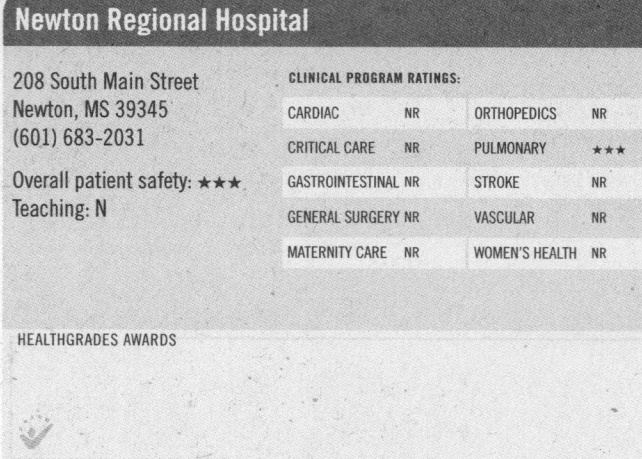

208 South Main Street
Newton, MS 39345
(601) 683-2031

Overall patient safety: ★★★
Teaching: N

CLINICAL PROGRAM RATINGS:

CARDIAC	NR	ORTHOPEDICS	NR
CRITICAL CARE	NR	PULMONARY	★★★
GASTROINTESTINAL	NR	STROKE	NR
GENERAL SURGERY	NR	VASCULAR	NR
MATERNITY CARE	NR	WOMEN'S HEALTH	NR

HEALTHGRADES AWARDS

Natchez Regional Medical Center

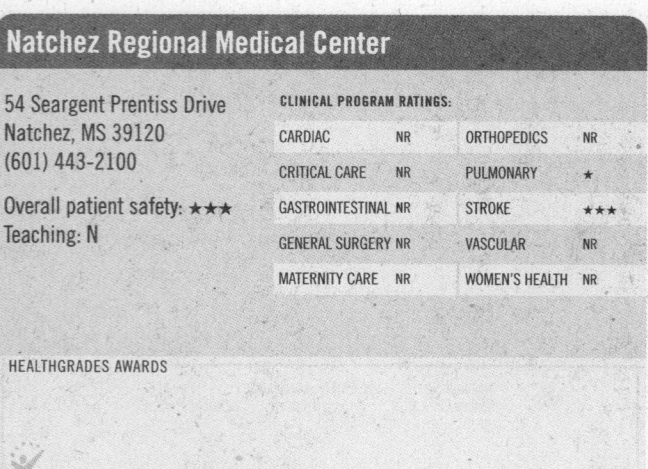

54 Seargent Prentiss Drive
Natchez, MS 39120
(601) 443-2100

Overall patient safety: ★★★
Teaching: N

CLINICAL PROGRAM RATINGS:

CARDIAC	NR	ORTHOPEDICS	NR
CRITICAL CARE	NR	PULMONARY	★
GASTROINTESTINAL	NR	STROKE	★★★
GENERAL SURGERY	NR	VASCULAR	NR
MATERNITY CARE	NR	WOMEN'S HEALTH	NR

HEALTHGRADES AWARDS

North Mississippi Medical Center

830 South Gloster Street
Tupelo, MS 38801
(662) 377-3000

Overall patient safety: ★★★★★
Teaching: Y

CLINICAL PROGRAM RATINGS:

CARDIAC	★★★	ORTHOPEDICS	★★★
CRITICAL CARE	NR	PULMONARY	★★★
GASTROINTESTINAL	★★★	STROKE	★★★
GENERAL SURGERY	NR	VASCULAR	★★★
MATERNITY CARE	NR	WOMEN'S HEALTH	NR

HEALTHGRADES AWARDS

KEY: ★★★★★ BEST   ★★★ AS EXPECTED   ★ POOR   NR NOT RATED BY HEALTHGRADES   For full definitions of ratings and awards, see Appendix.

North Oak Regional Medical Center

401 Getwell Drive
Senatobia, MS 38668
(662) 562-3100

Overall patient safety: ★★★
Teaching: N

CLINICAL PROGRAM RATINGS:

CARDIAC	NR	ORTHOPEDICS	NR
CRITICAL CARE	NR	PULMONARY	★★★
GASTROINTESTINAL	NR	STROKE	NR
GENERAL SURGERY	NR	VASCULAR	NR
MATERNITY CARE	NR	WOMEN'S HEALTH	NR

HEALTHGRADES AWARDS

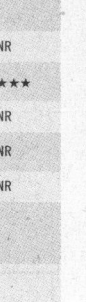

Northwest Mississippi Regional Medical Center

1970 Hospital Drive
Clarksdale, MS 38614
(662) 627-3211

Overall patient safety: ★★★
Teaching: N

CLINICAL PROGRAM RATINGS:

CARDIAC	NR	ORTHOPEDICS	NR
CRITICAL CARE	NR	PULMONARY	★★★
GASTROINTESTINAL	NR	STROKE	★★★
GENERAL SURGERY	NR	VASCULAR	NR
MATERNITY CARE	NR	WOMEN'S HEALTH	NR

HEALTHGRADES AWARDS

North Sunflower Medical Center

840 North Oak Avenue
P.O. Box 369
Ruleville, MS 38771
(662) 756-2711

Overall patient safety: NR
Teaching: N

CLINICAL PROGRAM RATINGS:

CARDIAC	NR	ORTHOPEDICS	NR
CRITICAL CARE	NR	PULMONARY	★★★
GASTROINTESTINAL	NR	STROKE	★
GENERAL SURGERY	NR	VASCULAR	NR
MATERNITY CARE	NR	WOMEN'S HEALTH	NR

HEALTHGRADES AWARDS

Oktibbeha County Hospital

400 Hospital Road
Starkville, MS 39759
(662) 323-4320

Overall patient safety: ★★★
Teaching: N

CLINICAL PROGRAM RATINGS:

CARDIAC	NR	ORTHOPEDICS	NR
CRITICAL CARE	NR	PULMONARY	★★★
GASTROINTESTINAL	NR	STROKE	★★★
GENERAL SURGERY	NR	VASCULAR	NR
MATERNITY CARE	NR	WOMEN'S HEALTH	NR

HEALTHGRADES AWARDS

Noxubee General Critical Access Hospital

606 North Jefferson Street
Macon, MS 39341
(662) 726-4231

Overall patient safety: NR
Teaching: N

CLINICAL PROGRAM RATINGS:

CARDIAC	NR	ORTHOPEDICS	NR
CRITICAL CARE	NR	PULMONARY	★★★
GASTROINTESTINAL	NR	STROKE	NR
GENERAL SURGERY	NR	VASCULAR	NR
MATERNITY CARE	NR	WOMEN'S HEALTH	NR

HEALTHGRADES AWARDS

Parkview Regional Medical Center*

100 McAuley Drive
Vicksburg, MS 39180
(601) 231-2131

Overall patient safety: ★
Teaching: N

CLINICAL PROGRAM RATINGS:

CARDIAC	★★★	ORTHOPEDICS	NR
CRITICAL CARE	NR	PULMONARY	★
GASTROINTESTINAL	★★★	STROKE	★★★
GENERAL SURGERY	NR	VASCULAR	NR
MATERNITY CARE	NR	WOMEN'S HEALTH	NR

HEALTHGRADES AWARDS

*This hospital reports its data to the federal government jointly with another hospital. Therefore the ratings and awards apply to multiple hospitals and this specific hospital may not provide all rated services.

Rankin Medical Center

350 Crossgates Boulevard
Brandon, MS 39042
(601) 825-2811

Overall patient safety: ★
Teaching: N

CLINICAL PROGRAM RATINGS:

CARDIAC	NR	ORTHOPEDICS	NR
CRITICAL CARE	NR	PULMONARY	★★★
GASTROINTESTINAL	NR	STROKE	★
GENERAL SURGERY	NR	VASCULAR	NR
MATERNITY CARE	NR	WOMEN'S HEALTH	NR

HEALTHGRADES AWARDS

River Region Health System*

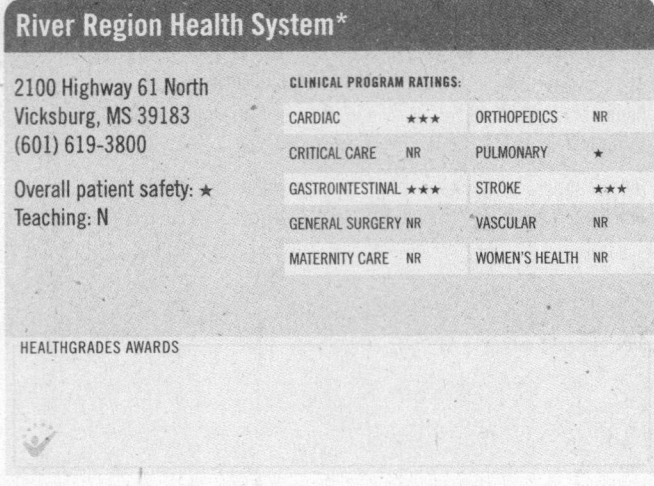

2100 Highway 61 North
Vicksburg, MS 39183
(601) 619-3800

Overall patient safety: ★
Teaching: N

CLINICAL PROGRAM RATINGS:

CARDIAC	★★★	ORTHOPEDICS	NR
CRITICAL CARE	NR	PULMONARY	★
GASTROINTESTINAL	★★★	STROKE	★★★
GENERAL SURGERY	NR	VASCULAR	NR
MATERNITY CARE	NR	WOMEN'S HEALTH	NR

HEALTHGRADES AWARDS

Riley Hospital

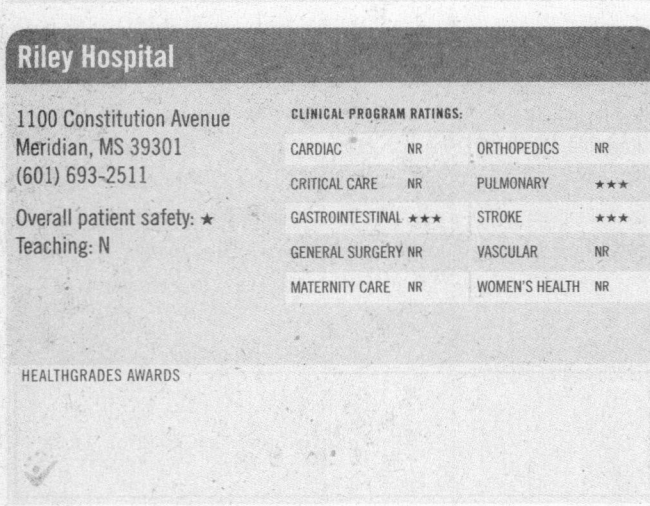

1100 Constitution Avenue
Meridian, MS 39301
(601) 693-2511

Overall patient safety: ★
Teaching: N

CLINICAL PROGRAM RATINGS:

CARDIAC	NR	ORTHOPEDICS	NR
CRITICAL CARE	NR	PULMONARY	★★★
GASTROINTESTINAL	★★★	STROKE	★★★
GENERAL SURGERY	NR	VASCULAR	NR
MATERNITY CARE	NR	WOMEN'S HEALTH	NR

HEALTHGRADES AWARDS

Rush Foundation Hospital

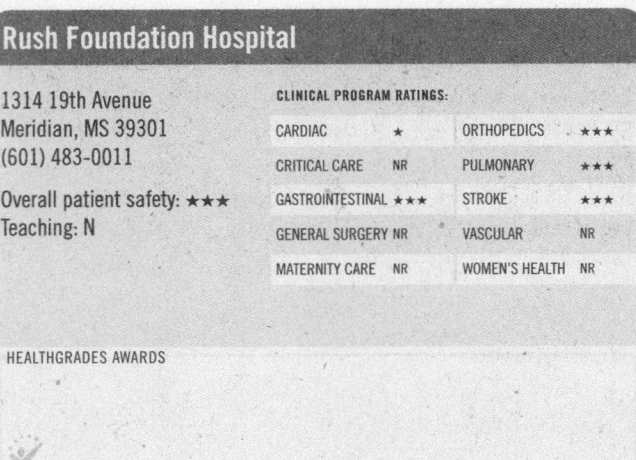

1314 19th Avenue
Meridian, MS 39301
(601) 483-0011

Overall patient safety: ★★★
Teaching: N

CLINICAL PROGRAM RATINGS:

CARDIAC	★	ORTHOPEDICS	★★★
CRITICAL CARE	NR	PULMONARY	★★★
GASTROINTESTINAL	★★★	STROKE	★★★
GENERAL SURGERY	NR	VASCULAR	NR
MATERNITY CARE	NR	WOMEN'S HEALTH	NR

HEALTHGRADES AWARDS

River Oaks Hospital

1030 River Oaks Drive
Jackson, MS 39232
(601) 932-1030

Overall patient safety: ★★★
Teaching: N

CLINICAL PROGRAM RATINGS:

CARDIAC	NR	ORTHOPEDICS	★★★
CRITICAL CARE	NR	PULMONARY	★★★
GASTROINTESTINAL	★★★	STROKE	★★★
GENERAL SURGERY	NR	VASCULAR	NR
MATERNITY CARE	NR	WOMEN'S HEALTH	NR

HEALTHGRADES AWARDS

St. Dominic-Jackson Memorial Hospital

969 Lakeland Drive
Jackson, MS 39216
(601) 200-2000

Overall patient safety: ★★★
Teaching: N

CLINICAL PROGRAM RATINGS:

CARDIAC	★★★	ORTHOPEDICS	★
CRITICAL CARE	NR	PULMONARY	★★★
GASTROINTESTINAL	★★★	STROKE	★★★★★
GENERAL SURGERY	NR	VASCULAR	★★★
MATERNITY CARE	NR	WOMEN'S HEALTH	NR

HEALTHGRADES AWARDS

✓ SPECIALTY EXCELLENCE
• STROKE CARE

KEY: ★★★★★ BEST   ★★★ AS EXPECTED   ★ POOR   NR NOT RATED BY HEALTHGRADES   For full definitions of ratings and awards, see Appendix.

Simpson General Hospital

1842 Simpson Highway 149
Mendenhall, MS 39114
(601) 847-2221

Overall patient safety: ★
Teaching: N

CLINICAL PROGRAM RATINGS:

CARDIAC	NR	ORTHOPEDICS	NR
CRITICAL CARE	NR	PULMONARY	★
GASTROINTESTINAL	NR	STROKE	NR
GENERAL SURGERY	NR	VASCULAR	NR
MATERNITY CARE	NR	WOMEN'S HEALTH	NR

HEALTHGRADES AWARDS

South Sunflower County Hospital

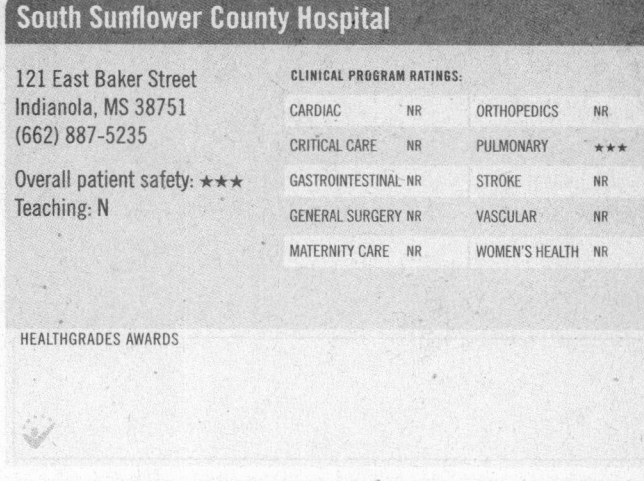

121 East Baker Street
Indianola, MS 38751
(662) 887-5235

Overall patient safety: ★★★
Teaching: N

CLINICAL PROGRAM RATINGS:

CARDIAC	NR	ORTHOPEDICS	NR
CRITICAL CARE	NR	PULMONARY	★★★
GASTROINTESTINAL	NR	STROKE	NR
GENERAL SURGERY	NR	VASCULAR	NR
MATERNITY CARE	NR	WOMEN'S HEALTH	NR

HEALTHGRADES AWARDS

Singing River Hospital System

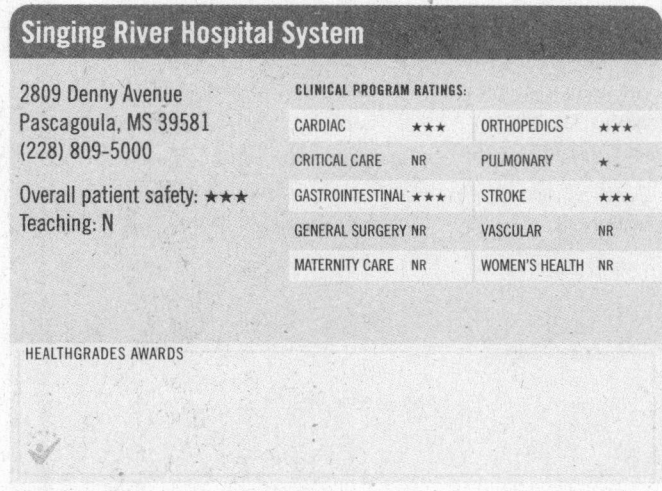

2809 Denny Avenue
Pascagoula, MS 39581
(228) 809-5000

Overall patient safety: ★★★
Teaching: N

CLINICAL PROGRAM RATINGS:

CARDIAC	★★★	ORTHOPEDICS	★★★
CRITICAL CARE	NR	PULMONARY	★
GASTROINTESTINAL	★★★	STROKE	★★★
GENERAL SURGERY	NR	VASCULAR	NR
MATERNITY CARE	NR	WOMEN'S HEALTH	NR

HEALTHGRADES AWARDS

Southwest Mississippi Regional Medical Center

215 Marion Avenue
McComb, MS 39648
(601) 249-5500

Overall patient safety: ★★★
Teaching: N

CLINICAL PROGRAM RATINGS:

CARDIAC	★	ORTHOPEDICS	NR
CRITICAL CARE	NR	PULMONARY	★★★
GASTROINTESTINAL	★	STROKE	★★★
GENERAL SURGERY	NR	VASCULAR	NR
MATERNITY CARE	NR	WOMEN'S HEALTH	NR

HEALTHGRADES AWARDS

South Central Regional Medical Center

1220 Jefferson Street
Laurel, MS 39440
(601) 426-4000

Overall patient safety: ★★★
Teaching: N

CLINICAL PROGRAM RATINGS:

CARDIAC	NR	ORTHOPEDICS	NR
CRITICAL CARE	NR	PULMONARY	★
GASTROINTESTINAL	★★★	STROKE	★★★★★
GENERAL SURGERY	NR	VASCULAR	NR
MATERNITY CARE	NR	WOMEN'S HEALTH	NR

HEALTHGRADES AWARDS

Stone County Hospital

1434 East Central Avenue
Wiggins, MS 39577
(601) 928-6600

Overall patient safety: NR
Teaching: N

CLINICAL PROGRAM RATINGS:

CARDIAC	NR	ORTHOPEDICS	NR
CRITICAL CARE	NR	PULMONARY	★
GASTROINTESTINAL	NR	STROKE	NR
GENERAL SURGERY	NR	VASCULAR	NR
MATERNITY CARE	NR	WOMEN'S HEALTH	NR

HEALTHGRADES AWARDS

*This hospital reports its data to the federal government jointly with another hospital. Therefore the ratings and awards apply to multiple hospitals and this specific hospital may not provide all rated services.

Tippah County Hospital

1005 City Avenue North
Ripley, MS 38663
(662) 837-9221

Overall patient safety: ★★★
Teaching: N

CLINICAL PROGRAM RATINGS:

CARDIAC	NR	ORTHOPEDICS	NR
CRITICAL CARE	NR	PULMONARY	★★★
GASTROINTESTINAL	NR	STROKE	★
GENERAL SURGERY	NR	VASCULAR	NR
MATERNITY CARE	NR	WOMEN'S HEALTH	NR

HEALTHGRADES AWARDS

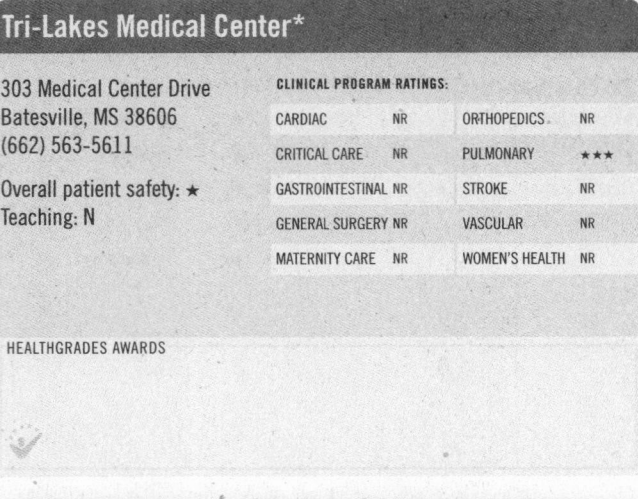

Tri-Lakes Medical Center*

303 Medical Center Drive
Batesville, MS 38606
(662) 563-5611

Overall patient safety: ★
Teaching: N

CLINICAL PROGRAM RATINGS:

CARDIAC	NR	ORTHOPEDICS	NR
CRITICAL CARE	NR	PULMONARY	★★★
GASTROINTESTINAL	NR	STROKE	NR
GENERAL SURGERY	NR	VASCULAR	NR
MATERNITY CARE	NR	WOMEN'S HEALTH	NR

HEALTHGRADES AWARDS

Tishomingo Health Services

1777 Curtis Drive
Iuka, MS 38852
(662) 423-6051

Overall patient safety: ★★★
Teaching: N

CLINICAL PROGRAM RATINGS:

CARDIAC	NR	ORTHOPEDICS	NR
CRITICAL CARE	NR	PULMONARY	★★★
GASTROINTESTINAL	NR	STROKE	★★★
GENERAL SURGERY	NR	VASCULAR	NR
MATERNITY CARE	NR	WOMEN'S HEALTH	NR

HEALTHGRADES AWARDS

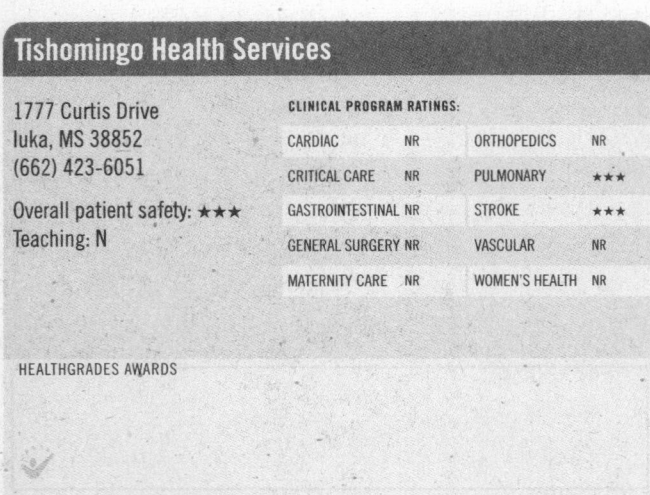

Tyler Holmes Memorial Hospital

409 Tyler Holmes Drive
Winona, MS 38967
(662) 283-4114

Overall patient safety: NR
Teaching: N

CLINICAL PROGRAM RATINGS:

CARDIAC	NR	ORTHOPEDICS	NR
CRITICAL CARE	NR	PULMONARY	★
GASTROINTESTINAL	NR	STROKE	★★★
GENERAL SURGERY	NR	VASCULAR	NR
MATERNITY CARE	NR	WOMEN'S HEALTH	NR

HEALTHGRADES AWARDS

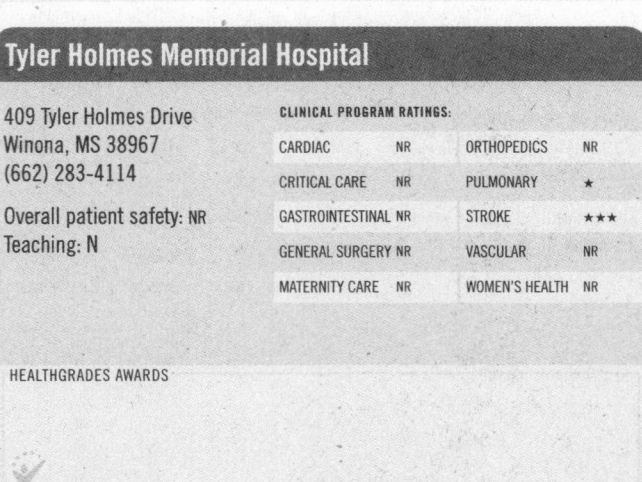

Trace Regional Hospital and Swing Bed

Highway 8 East
Houston, MS 38851
(662) 456-3700

Overall patient safety: ★★★
Teaching: N

CLINICAL PROGRAM RATINGS:

CARDIAC	NR	ORTHOPEDICS	NR
CRITICAL CARE	NR	PULMONARY	★★★★★
GASTROINTESTINAL	NR	STROKE	NR
GENERAL SURGERY	NR	VASCULAR	NR
MATERNITY CARE	NR	WOMEN'S HEALTH	NR

HEALTHGRADES AWARDS

✓ SPECIALTY EXCELLENCE
• PULMONARY CARE

University Hospital and Clinics–Holmes County

239 Bowling Green Road
Lexington, MS 39095
(662) 834-1321

Overall patient safety: ★★★
Teaching: N

CLINICAL PROGRAM RATINGS:

CARDIAC	NR	ORTHOPEDICS	NR
CRITICAL CARE	NR	PULMONARY	★★★
GASTROINTESTINAL	NR	STROKE	★
GENERAL SURGERY	NR	VASCULAR	NR
MATERNITY CARE	NR	WOMEN'S HEALTH	NR

HEALTHGRADES AWARDS

KEY: ★★★★★ BEST   ★★★ AS EXPECTED   ★ POOR   NR NOT RATED BY HEALTHGRADES   For full definitions of ratings and awards, see Appendix.

University of Mississippi Medical Center

2500 North State Street
Jackson, MS 39216
(601) 984-1000

Overall patient safety: ★★★
Teaching: Y

CLINICAL PROGRAM RATINGS:

CARDIAC	★★★	ORTHOPEDICS	★★★
CRITICAL CARE	NR	PULMONARY	★★★
GASTROINTESTINAL	NR	STROKE	★★★
GENERAL SURGERY	NR	VASCULAR	NR
MATERNITY CARE	NR	WOMEN'S HEALTH	NR

HEALTHGRADES AWARDS

Webster General Hospital

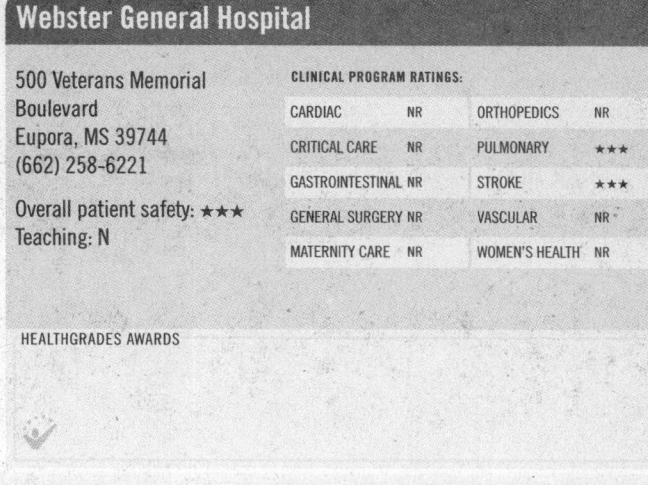

500 Veterans Memorial
Boulevard
Eupora, MS 39744
(662) 258-6221

Overall patient safety: ★★★
Teaching: N

CLINICAL PROGRAM RATINGS:

CARDIAC	NR	ORTHOPEDICS	NR
CRITICAL CARE	NR	PULMONARY	★★★
GASTROINTESTINAL	NR	STROKE	★★★
GENERAL SURGERY	NR	VASCULAR	NR
MATERNITY CARE	NR	WOMEN'S HEALTH	NR

HEALTHGRADES AWARDS

Walthall County General Hospital

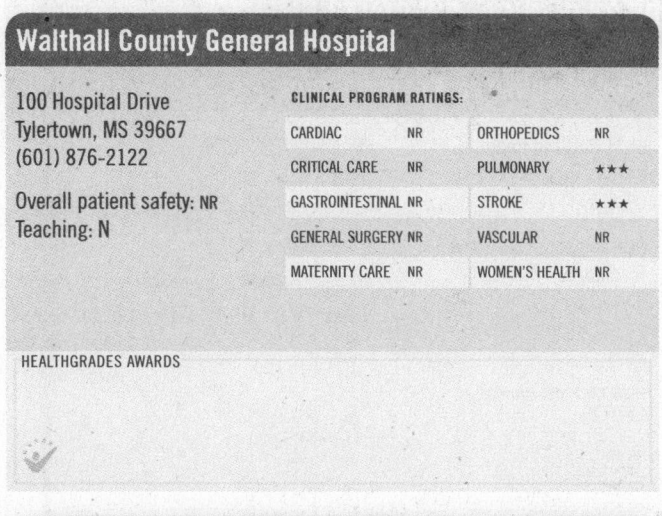

100 Hospital Drive
Tylertown, MS 39667
(601) 876-2122

Overall patient safety: NR
Teaching: N

CLINICAL PROGRAM RATINGS:

CARDIAC	NR	ORTHOPEDICS	NR
CRITICAL CARE	NR	PULMONARY	★★★
GASTROINTESTINAL	NR	STROKE	★★★
GENERAL SURGERY	NR	VASCULAR	NR
MATERNITY CARE	NR	WOMEN'S HEALTH	NR

HEALTHGRADES AWARDS

Wesley Medical Center

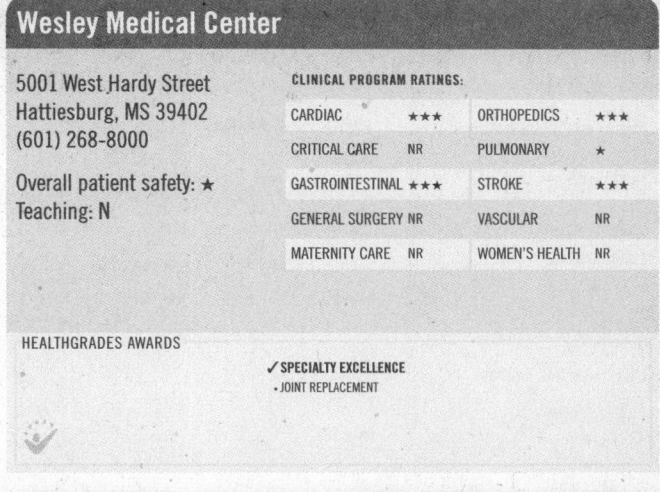

5001 West Hardy Street
Hattiesburg, MS 39402
(601) 268-8000

Overall patient safety: ★
Teaching: N

CLINICAL PROGRAM RATINGS:

CARDIAC	★★★	ORTHOPEDICS	★★★
CRITICAL CARE	NR	PULMONARY	★
GASTROINTESTINAL	★★★	STROKE	★★★
GENERAL SURGERY	NR	VASCULAR	NR
MATERNITY CARE	NR	WOMEN'S HEALTH	NR

HEALTHGRADES AWARDS

✓ SPECIALTY EXCELLENCE
· JOINT REPLACEMENT

Wayne General Hospital

950 Matthew Drive
Waynesboro, MS 39367
(601) 735-5151

Overall patient safety: ★★★
Teaching: N

CLINICAL PROGRAM RATINGS:

CARDIAC	NR	ORTHOPEDICS	NR
CRITICAL CARE	NR	PULMONARY	★
GASTROINTESTINAL	NR	STROKE	★
GENERAL SURGERY	NR	VASCULAR	NR
MATERNITY CARE	NR	WOMEN'S HEALTH	NR

HEALTHGRADES AWARDS

Winston Medical Center

562 East Main Street
Louisville, MS 39339
(662) 773-6211

Overall patient safety: ★★★
Teaching: N

CLINICAL PROGRAM RATINGS:

CARDIAC	NR	ORTHOPEDICS	NR
CRITICAL CARE	NR	PULMONARY	★
GASTROINTESTINAL	NR	STROKE	★★★
GENERAL SURGERY	NR	VASCULAR	NR
MATERNITY CARE	NR	WOMEN'S HEALTH	NR

HEALTHGRADES AWARDS

*This hospital reports its data to the federal government jointly with another hospital. Therefore the ratings and awards apply to multiple hospitals and this specific hospital may not provide all rated services.

Yalobusha General Hospital

Highway 7 South
Water Valley, MS 38965
(601) 473-1411

Overall patient safety: NR
Teaching: N

CLINICAL PROGRAM RATINGS:

CARDIAC	NR	ORTHOPEDICS	NR
CRITICAL CARE	NR	PULMONARY	★
GASTROINTESTINAL	NR	STROKE	NR
GENERAL SURGERY	NR	VASCULAR	NR
MATERNITY CARE	NR	WOMEN'S HEALTH	NR

HEALTHGRADES AWARDS

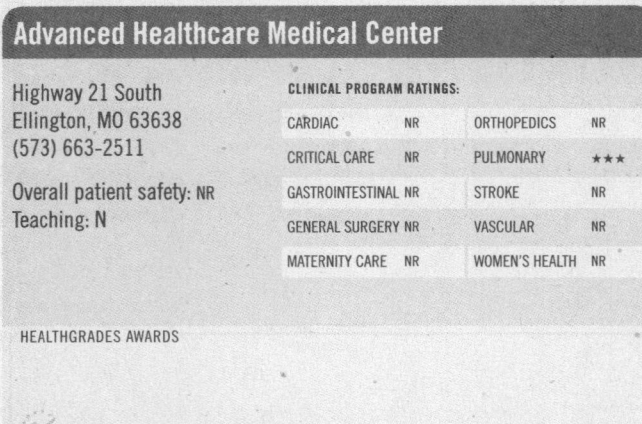

Advanced Healthcare Medical Center

Highway 21 South
Ellington, MO 63638
(573) 663-2511

Overall patient safety: NR
Teaching: N

CLINICAL PROGRAM RATINGS:

CARDIAC	NR	ORTHOPEDICS	NR
CRITICAL CARE	NR	PULMONARY	★★★
GASTROINTESTINAL	NR	STROKE	NR
GENERAL SURGERY	NR	VASCULAR	NR
MATERNITY CARE	NR	WOMEN'S HEALTH	NR

HEALTHGRADES AWARDS

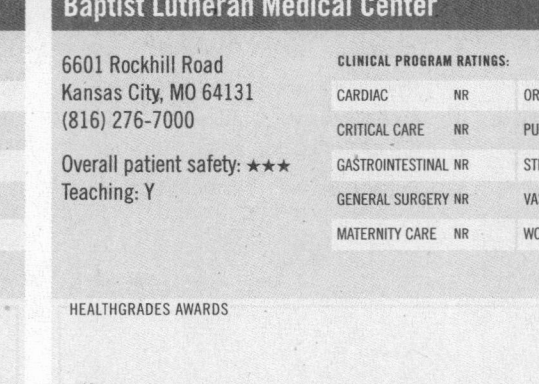

Baptist Lutheran Medical Center

6601 Rockhill Road
Kansas City, MO 64131
(816) 276-7000

Overall patient safety: ★★★
Teaching: Y

CLINICAL PROGRAM RATINGS:

CARDIAC	NR	ORTHOPEDICS	NR
CRITICAL CARE	NR	PULMONARY	★★★
GASTROINTESTINAL	NR	STROKE	★★★
GENERAL SURGERY	NR	VASCULAR	NR
MATERNITY CARE	NR	WOMEN'S HEALTH	NR

HEALTHGRADES AWARDS

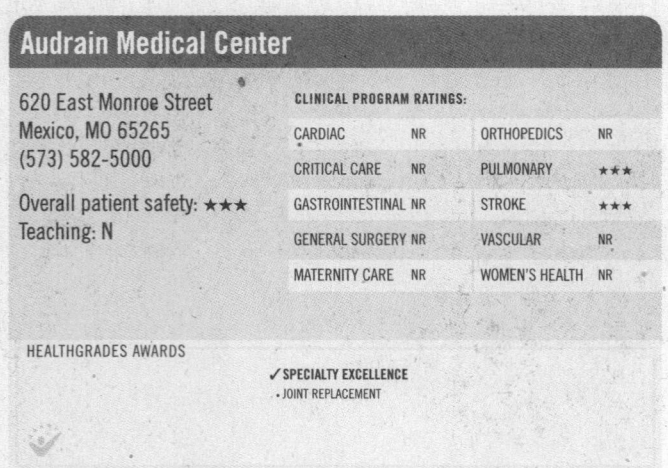

Audrain Medical Center

620 East Monroe Street
Mexico, MO 65265
(573) 582-5000

Overall patient safety: ★★★
Teaching: N

CLINICAL PROGRAM RATINGS:

CARDIAC	NR	ORTHOPEDICS	NR
CRITICAL CARE	NR	PULMONARY	★★★
GASTROINTESTINAL	NR	STROKE	★★★
GENERAL SURGERY	NR	VASCULAR	NR
MATERNITY CARE	NR	WOMEN'S HEALTH	NR

HEALTHGRADES AWARDS

✓ SPECIALTY EXCELLENCE
· JOINT REPLACEMENT

Barnes Hospital*

216 South Kingshighway
Boulevard
St. Louis, MO 63110
(314) 747-3000

Overall patient safety: ★
Teaching: Y

CLINICAL PROGRAM RATINGS:

CARDIAC	★★★	ORTHOPEDICS	★★★
CRITICAL CARE	★★★	PULMONARY	★★★
GASTROINTESTINAL	★★★	STROKE	★★★
GENERAL SURGERY	NR	VASCULAR	★★★
MATERNITY CARE	NR	WOMEN'S HEALTH	NR

HEALTHGRADES AWARDS

✓ SPECIALTY EXCELLENCE
· CARDIAC CARE · GASTROINTESTINAL CARE

KEY: ★★★★★ BEST   ★★★ AS EXPECTED   ★ POOR   NR NOT RATED BY HEALTHGRADES   For full definitions of ratings and awards, see Appendix.

Barnes-Jewish Hospital*

1 Barnes-Jewish
Hospital Plaza
St. Louis, MO 63110
(314) 747-3000

Overall patient safety: ★
Teaching: Y

CLINICAL PROGRAM RATINGS:

CARDIAC	★★★	ORTHOPEDICS	★★★
CRITICAL CARE	★★★	PULMONARY	★★★
GASTROINTESTINAL	★★★	STROKE	★★★
GENERAL SURGERY	NR	VASCULAR	★★★
MATERNITY CARE	NR	WOMEN'S HEALTH	NR

HEALTHGRADES AWARDS

✓ SPECIALTY EXCELLENCE
• CARDIAC CARE
• GASTROINTESTINAL CARE

Barton County Memorial Hospital

2nd and Gulf Streets
Lamar, MO 64759
(417) 682-6081

Overall patient safety: ★★★
Teaching: N

CLINICAL PROGRAM RATINGS:

CARDIAC	NR	ORTHOPEDICS	NR
CRITICAL CARE	NR	PULMONARY	★★★
GASTROINTESTINAL	NR	STROKE	★★★
GENERAL SURGERY	NR	VASCULAR	NR
MATERNITY CARE	NR	WOMEN'S HEALTH	NR

HEALTHGRADES AWARDS

Barnes-Jewish St. Peters Hospital

10 Hospital Drive
St. Peters, MO 63376
(636) 916-9000

Overall patient safety: ★★★
Teaching: Y

CLINICAL PROGRAM RATINGS:

CARDIAC	NR	ORTHOPEDICS	★★★
CRITICAL CARE	NR	PULMONARY	★★★
GASTROINTESTINAL	★★★	STROKE	★★★
GENERAL SURGERY	NR	VASCULAR	NR
MATERNITY CARE	NR	WOMEN'S HEALTH	NR

HEALTHGRADES AWARDS

Bates County Memorial Hospital

615 West Nursery Street
Butler, MO 64730
(660) 679-4135

Overall patient safety: ★★★
Teaching: N

CLINICAL PROGRAM RATINGS:

CARDIAC	NR	ORTHOPEDICS	NR
CRITICAL CARE	NR	PULMONARY	★★★
GASTROINTESTINAL	NR	STROKE	★★★
GENERAL SURGERY	NR	VASCULAR	NR
MATERNITY CARE	NR	WOMEN'S HEALTH	NR

HEALTHGRADES AWARDS

Barnes-Jewish West County Hospital

12634 Olive Boulevard
St. Louis, MO 63141
(314) 996-8000

Overall patient safety: ★★★
Teaching: Y

CLINICAL PROGRAM RATINGS:

CARDIAC	NR	ORTHOPEDICS	★★★
CRITICAL CARE	NR	PULMONARY	★★★
GASTROINTESTINAL	NR	STROKE	NR
GENERAL SURGERY	NR	VASCULAR	NR
MATERNITY CARE	NR	WOMEN'S HEALTH	NR

HEALTHGRADES AWARDS

Bonne Terre Hospital*

10 Lake Drive
Bonne Terre, MO 63628
(314) 358-2211

Overall patient safety: ★★★
Teaching: N

CLINICAL PROGRAM RATINGS:

CARDIAC	NR	ORTHOPEDICS	NR
CRITICAL CARE	NR	PULMONARY	★★★
GASTROINTESTINAL	NR	STROKE	★★★
GENERAL SURGERY	NR	VASCULAR	NR
MATERNITY CARE	NR	WOMEN'S HEALTH	NR

HEALTHGRADES AWARDS

*This hospital reports its data to the federal government jointly with another hospital. Therefore the ratings and awards apply to multiple hospitals and this specific hospital may not provide all rated services.

Boone Hospital Center

1600 East Broadway
Columbia, MO 65201
(573) 815-8000

Overall patient safety: ★★★★★
Teaching: N

CLINICAL PROGRAM RATINGS:

CARDIAC	★★★	ORTHOPEDICS	★★★★★
CRITICAL CARE	NR	PULMONARY	★★★
GASTROINTESTINAL	★★★	STROKE	★★★
GENERAL SURGERY	NR	VASCULAR	★★★★★
MATERNITY CARE	NR	WOMEN'S HEALTH	NR

HEALTHGRADES AWARDS

✓ DISTINGUISHED HOSPITAL
· PATIENT SAFETY

✓ SPECIALTY EXCELLENCE
· JOINT REPLACEMENT
· ORTHOPEDIC SURGERY
· VASCULAR SURGERY

Cameron Regional Medical Center

1600 East Evergreen Street
Cameron, MO 64429
(816) 632-2101

Overall patient safety: ★★★
Teaching: N

CLINICAL PROGRAM RATINGS:

CARDIAC	NR	ORTHOPEDICS	NR
CRITICAL CARE	NR	PULMONARY	★
GASTROINTESTINAL	NR	STROKE	★★★
GENERAL SURGERY	NR	VASCULAR	NR
MATERNITY CARE	NR	WOMEN'S HEALTH	NR

HEALTHGRADES AWARDS

Bothwell Regional Health Center

601 East 14th Street
Sedalia, MO 65301
(660) 826-8833

Overall patient safety: ★★★
Teaching: N

CLINICAL PROGRAM RATINGS:

CARDIAC	NR	ORTHOPEDICS	NR
CRITICAL CARE	NR	PULMONARY	★★★
GASTROINTESTINAL	★★★	STROKE	★★★★★
GENERAL SURGERY	NR	VASCULAR	NR
MATERNITY CARE	NR	WOMEN'S HEALTH	NR

HEALTHGRADES AWARDS

Capital Region Medical Center

1125 Madison Street
Jefferson City, MO 65102
(573) 632-5000

Overall patient safety: ★★★
Teaching: Y

CLINICAL PROGRAM RATINGS:

CARDIAC	★★★	ORTHOPEDICS	★★★
CRITICAL CARE	NR	PULMONARY	★★★
GASTROINTESTINAL	★★★	STROKE	★★★
GENERAL SURGERY	NR	VASCULAR	NR
MATERNITY CARE	NR	WOMEN'S HEALTH	NR

HEALTHGRADES AWARDS

Callaway Community Hospital

10 South Hospital Drive
Fulton, MO 65251
(573) 642-3376

Overall patient safety: ★★★
Teaching: Y

CLINICAL PROGRAM RATINGS:

CARDIAC	NR	ORTHOPEDICS	NR
CRITICAL CARE	NR	PULMONARY	★★★
GASTROINTESTINAL	NR	STROKE	NR
GENERAL SURGERY	NR	VASCULAR	NR
MATERNITY CARE	NR	WOMEN'S HEALTH	NR

HEALTHGRADES AWARDS

Carroll County Memorial Hospital

1502 North Jefferson Street
Carrollton, MO 64633
(660) 542-1695

Overall patient safety: NR
Teaching: N

CLINICAL PROGRAM RATINGS:

CARDIAC	NR	ORTHOPEDICS	NR
CRITICAL CARE	NR	PULMONARY	★★★
GASTROINTESTINAL	NR	STROKE	★★★
GENERAL SURGERY	NR	VASCULAR	NR
MATERNITY CARE	NR	WOMEN'S HEALTH	NR

HEALTHGRADES AWARDS

KEY: ★★★★★ BEST   ★★★ AS EXPECTED   ★ POOR   NR NOT RATED BY HEALTHGRADES   For full definitions of ratings and awards, see Appendix.

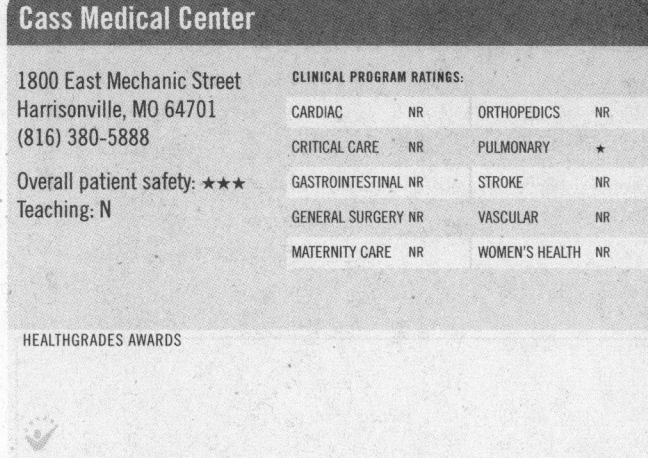

Cass Medical Center

1800 East Mechanic Street
Harrisonville, MO 64701
(816) 380-5888

Overall patient safety: ★★★
Teaching: N

CLINICAL PROGRAM RATINGS:

CARDIAC	NR	ORTHOPEDICS	NR
CRITICAL CARE	NR	PULMONARY	★
GASTROINTESTINAL	NR	STROKE	NR
GENERAL SURGERY	NR	VASCULAR	NR
MATERNITY CARE	NR	WOMEN'S HEALTH	NR

HEALTHGRADES AWARDS

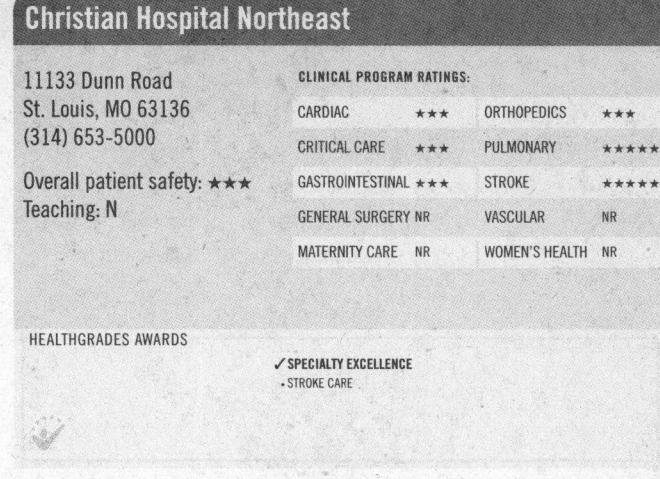

Christian Hospital Northeast

11133 Dunn Road
St. Louis, MO 63136
(314) 653-5000

Overall patient safety: ★★★
Teaching: N

CLINICAL PROGRAM RATINGS:

CARDIAC	★★★	ORTHOPEDICS	★★★
CRITICAL CARE	★★★	PULMONARY	★★★★★
GASTROINTESTINAL	★★★	STROKE	★★★★★
GENERAL SURGERY	NR	VASCULAR	NR
MATERNITY CARE	NR	WOMEN'S HEALTH	NR

HEALTHGRADES AWARDS

✓ SPECIALTY EXCELLENCE
• STROKE CARE

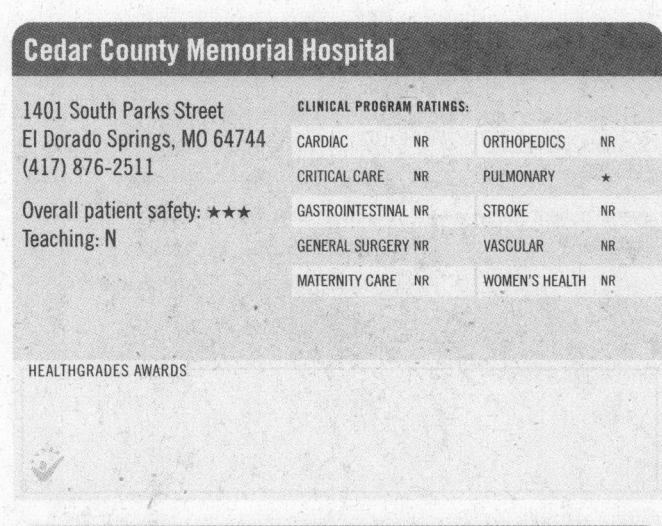

Cedar County Memorial Hospital

1401 South Parks Street
El Dorado Springs, MO 64744
(417) 876-2511

Overall patient safety: ★★★
Teaching: N

CLINICAL PROGRAM RATINGS:

CARDIAC	NR	ORTHOPEDICS	NR
CRITICAL CARE	NR	PULMONARY	★
GASTROINTESTINAL	NR	STROKE	NR
GENERAL SURGERY	NR	VASCULAR	NR
MATERNITY CARE	NR	WOMEN'S HEALTH	NR

HEALTHGRADES AWARDS

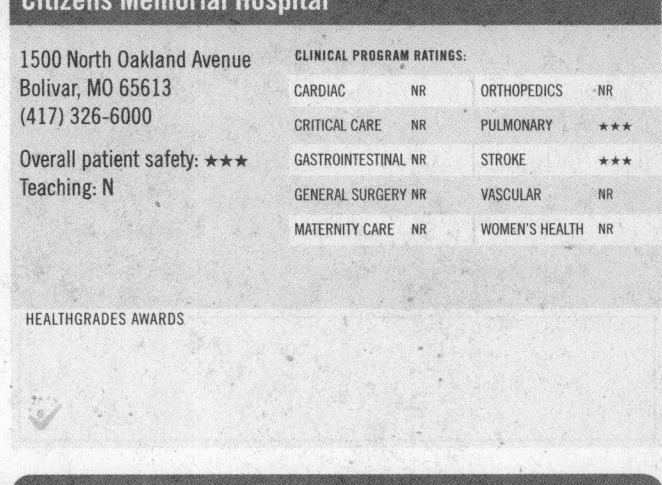

Citizens Memorial Hospital

1500 North Oakland Avenue
Bolivar, MO 65613
(417) 326-6000

Overall patient safety: ★★★
Teaching: N

CLINICAL PROGRAM RATINGS:

CARDIAC	NR	ORTHOPEDICS	NR
CRITICAL CARE	NR	PULMONARY	★★★
GASTROINTESTINAL	NR	STROKE	★★★
GENERAL SURGERY	NR	VASCULAR	NR
MATERNITY CARE	NR	WOMEN'S HEALTH	NR

HEALTHGRADES AWARDS

Centerpoint Medical Center

19600 East 39th Street
Independence, MO 64057
(816) 698-7000

Overall patient safety: ★★★
Teaching: Y

CLINICAL PROGRAM RATINGS:

CARDIAC	★★★	ORTHOPEDICS	★★★
CRITICAL CARE	NR	PULMONARY	★★★
GASTROINTESTINAL	★	STROKE	★
GENERAL SURGERY	NR	VASCULAR	NR
MATERNITY CARE	NR	WOMEN'S HEALTH	NR

HEALTHGRADES AWARDS

Columbia Regional Hospital

404 Keene Street
Columbia, MO 65201
(573) 875-9200

Overall patient safety: ★★★★★
Teaching: N

CLINICAL PROGRAM RATINGS:

CARDIAC	NR	ORTHOPEDICS	★★★
CRITICAL CARE	NR	PULMONARY	★★★
GASTROINTESTINAL	NR	STROKE	★★★
GENERAL SURGERY	NR	VASCULAR	NR
MATERNITY CARE	NR	WOMEN'S HEALTH	NR

HEALTHGRADES AWARDS

✓ DISTINGUISHED HOSPITAL
• PATIENT SAFETY

✓ SPECIALTY EXCELLENCE
• JOINT REPLACEMENT

Community Hospital Association

405 East Main
Fairfax, MO 64446
(660) 686-2211

Overall patient safety: ★★★
Teaching: N

CLINICAL PROGRAM RATINGS:

CARDIAC	NR	ORTHOPEDICS	NR
CRITICAL CARE	NR	PULMONARY	★
GASTROINTESTINAL	NR	STROKE	★★★
GENERAL SURGERY	NR	VASCULAR	NR
MATERNITY CARE	NR	WOMEN'S HEALTH	NR

HEALTHGRADES AWARDS

Cox Monett Hospital

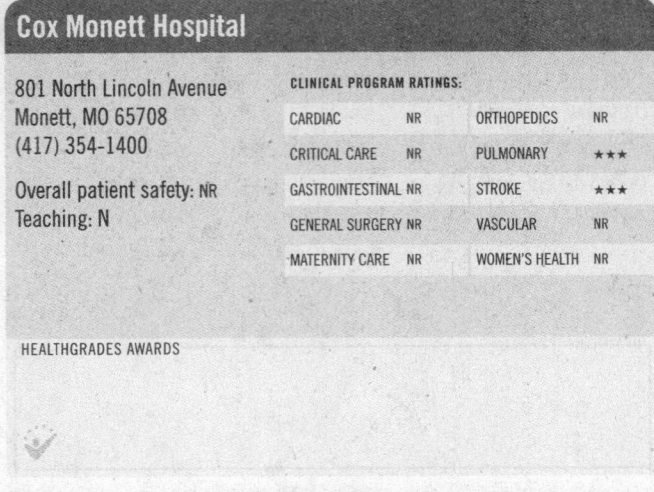

801 North Lincoln Avenue
Monett, MO 65708
(417) 354-1400

Overall patient safety: NR
Teaching: N

CLINICAL PROGRAM RATINGS:

CARDIAC	NR	ORTHOPEDICS	NR
CRITICAL CARE	NR	PULMONARY	★★★
GASTROINTESTINAL	NR	STROKE	★★★
GENERAL SURGERY	NR	VASCULAR	NR
MATERNITY CARE	NR	WOMEN'S HEALTH	NR

HEALTHGRADES AWARDS

Cooper County Memorial Hospital

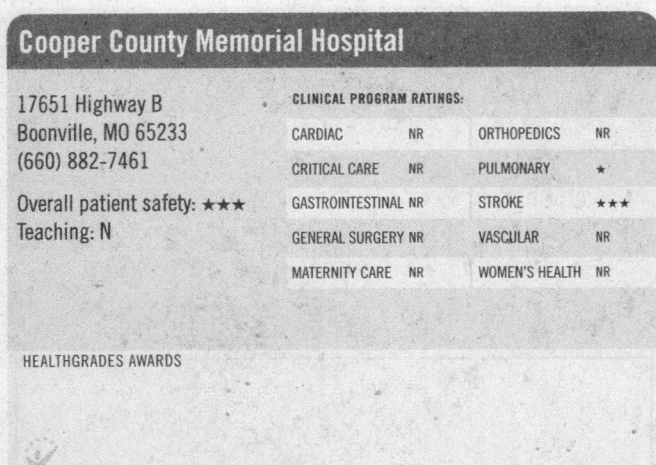

17651 Highway B
Boonville, MO 65233
(660) 882-7461

Overall patient safety: ★★★
Teaching: N

CLINICAL PROGRAM RATINGS:

CARDIAC	NR	ORTHOPEDICS	NR
CRITICAL CARE	NR	PULMONARY	★
GASTROINTESTINAL	NR	STROKE	★★★
GENERAL SURGERY	NR	VASCULAR	NR
MATERNITY CARE	NR	WOMEN'S HEALTH	NR

HEALTHGRADES AWARDS

Des Peres Hospital

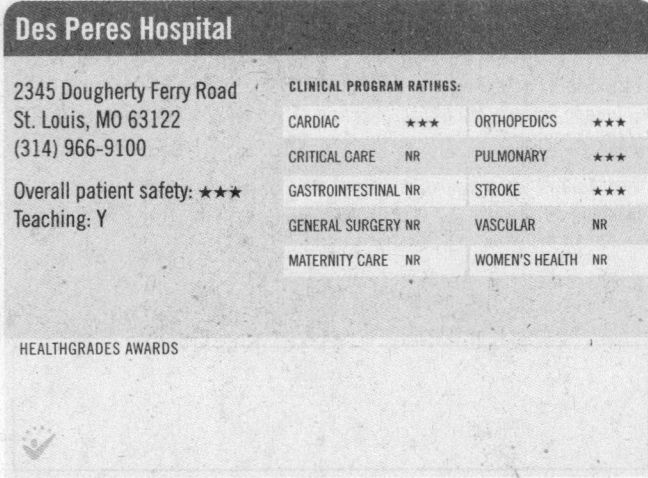

2345 Dougherty Ferry Road
St. Louis, MO 63122
(314) 966-9100

Overall patient safety: ★★★
Teaching: Y

CLINICAL PROGRAM RATINGS:

CARDIAC	★★★	ORTHOPEDICS	★★★
CRITICAL CARE	NR	PULMONARY	★★★
GASTROINTESTINAL	NR	STROKE	★★★
GENERAL SURGERY	NR	VASCULAR	NR
MATERNITY CARE	NR	WOMEN'S HEALTH	NR

HEALTHGRADES AWARDS

Cox Medical Center

1423 North Jefferson Avenue
Springfield, MO 65802
(417) 269-3000

Overall patient safety: ★★★
Teaching: Y

CLINICAL PROGRAM RATINGS:

CARDIAC	★★★	ORTHOPEDICS	★
CRITICAL CARE	NR	PULMONARY	★★★
GASTROINTESTINAL	★★★	STROKE	★★★
GENERAL SURGERY	NR	VASCULAR	★
MATERNITY CARE	NR	WOMEN'S HEALTH	NR

HEALTHGRADES AWARDS

Ellett Memorial Hospital

610 North Ohio Avenue
Appleton City, MO 64724
(660) 476-2111

Overall patient safety: NR
Teaching: N

CLINICAL PROGRAM RATINGS:

CARDIAC	NR	ORTHOPEDICS	NR
CRITICAL CARE	NR	PULMONARY	★★★
GASTROINTESTINAL	NR	STROKE	NR
GENERAL SURGERY	NR	VASCULAR	NR
MATERNITY CARE	NR	WOMEN'S HEALTH	NR

HEALTHGRADES AWARDS

KEY: ★★★★★ BEST   ★★★ AS EXPECTED   ★ POOR   NR NOT RATED BY HEALTHGRADES   For full definitions of ratings and awards, see Appendix.

Excelsior Springs Medical Center

1700 Rainbow Boulevard
Excelsior Springs, MO 64024
(816) 630-6081

Overall patient safety: ★★★
Teaching: N

CLINICAL PROGRAM RATINGS:

CARDIAC	NR	ORTHOPEDICS	NR
CRITICAL CARE	NR	PULMONARY	★★★
GASTROINTESTINAL	NR	STROKE	NR
GENERAL SURGERY	NR	VASCULAR	NR
MATERNITY CARE	NR	WOMEN'S HEALTH	NR

HEALTHGRADES AWARDS

Freeman Health System

1102 West 32nd Street
Joplin, MO 64804
(417) 347-1111

Overall patient safety: ★★★
Teaching: Y

CLINICAL PROGRAM RATINGS:

CARDIAC	★★★	ORTHOPEDICS	★★★
CRITICAL CARE	NR	PULMONARY	★★★
GASTROINTESTINAL	★★★	STROKE	★★★
GENERAL SURGERY	NR	VASCULAR	★★★
MATERNITY CARE	NR	WOMEN'S HEALTH	NR

HEALTHGRADES AWARDS

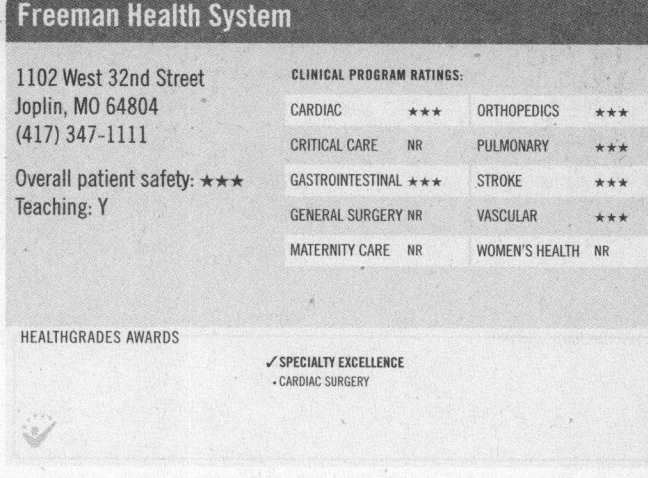

✓ SPECIALTY EXCELLENCE
• CARDIAC SURGERY

Fitzgibbon Memorial Hospital

2305 South 65 Highway
Marshall, MO 65340
(660) 886-7431

Overall patient safety: ★★★★★
Teaching: N

CLINICAL PROGRAM RATINGS:

CARDIAC	NR	ORTHOPEDICS	NR
CRITICAL CARE	NR	PULMONARY	★★★
GASTROINTESTINAL	NR	STROKE	★★★
GENERAL SURGERY	NR	VASCULAR	NR
MATERNITY CARE	NR	WOMEN'S HEALTH	NR

HEALTHGRADES AWARDS

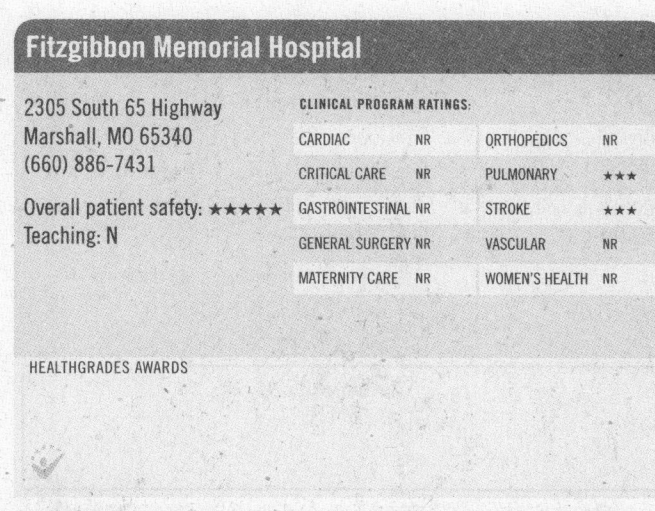

Freeman Neosho Hospital

113 West Hickory Street
Neosho, MO 64850
(417) 451-1234

Overall patient safety: NR
Teaching: N

CLINICAL PROGRAM RATINGS:

CARDIAC	NR	ORTHOPEDICS	NR
CRITICAL CARE	NR	PULMONARY	★★★
GASTROINTESTINAL	NR	STROKE	★★★
GENERAL SURGERY	NR	VASCULAR	NR
MATERNITY CARE	NR	WOMEN'S HEALTH	NR

HEALTHGRADES AWARDS

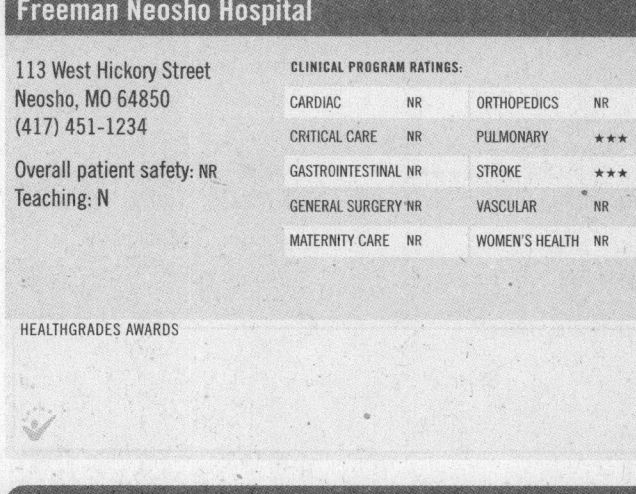

Forest Park Community Hospital

6150 Oakland Avenue
St. Louis, MO 63139
(314) 768-3000

Overall patient safety: ★
Teaching: Y

CLINICAL PROGRAM RATINGS:

CARDIAC	★	ORTHOPEDICS	NR
CRITICAL CARE	NR	PULMONARY	★★★
GASTROINTESTINAL	★★★	STROKE	★★★
GENERAL SURGERY	NR	VASCULAR	NR
MATERNITY CARE	NR	WOMEN'S HEALTH	NR

HEALTHGRADES AWARDS

Golden Valley Memorial Hospital

1600 North 2nd Street
Clinton, MO 64735
(660) 885-5511

Overall patient safety: ★★★
Teaching: N

CLINICAL PROGRAM RATINGS:

CARDIAC	NR	ORTHOPEDICS	NR
CRITICAL CARE	NR	PULMONARY	★★★
GASTROINTESTINAL	★★★	STROKE	★★★
GENERAL SURGERY	NR	VASCULAR	NR
MATERNITY CARE	NR	WOMEN'S HEALTH	NR

HEALTHGRADES AWARDS

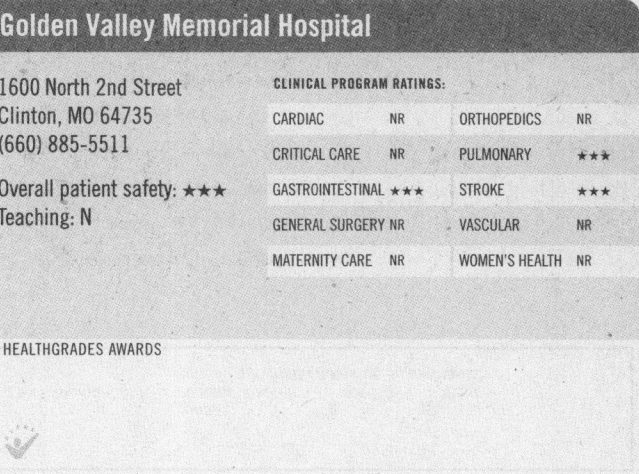

Grim-Smith Hospital and Clinic*

112 East Patterson Avenue
Kirksville, MO 63501
(816) 665-7241

Overall patient safety: ★★★★★
Teaching: Y

CLINICAL PROGRAM RATINGS:

CARDIAC	NR	ORTHOPEDICS	NR
CRITICAL CARE	NR	PULMONARY	★★★
GASTROINTESTINAL	★★★	STROKE	★★★
GENERAL SURGERY	NR	VASCULAR	NR
MATERNITY CARE	NR	WOMEN'S HEALTH	NR

HEALTHGRADES AWARDS

Hermann Area District Hospital

509 West 18th Street
Hermann, MO 65041
(573) 486-2191

Overall patient safety: ★★★
Teaching: N

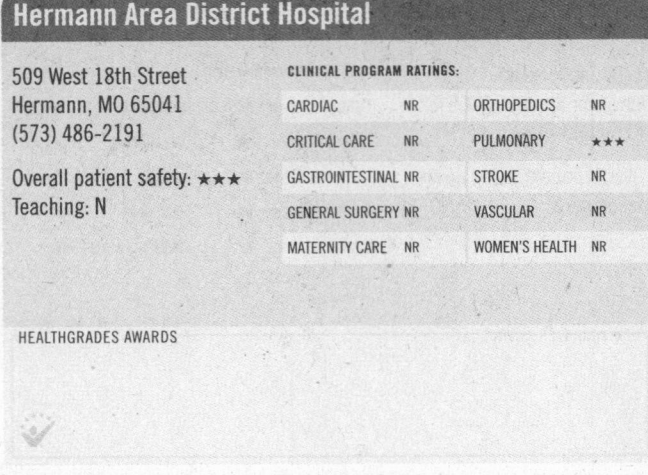

CLINICAL PROGRAM RATINGS:

CARDIAC	NR	ORTHOPEDICS	NR
CRITICAL CARE	NR	PULMONARY	★★★
GASTROINTESTINAL	NR	STROKE	NR
GENERAL SURGERY	NR	VASCULAR	NR
MATERNITY CARE	NR	WOMEN'S HEALTH	NR

HEALTHGRADES AWARDS

Hannibal Regional Hospital

Highway 36 West
Hannibal, MO 63401
(573) 248-1300

Overall patient safety: ★★★
Teaching: N

CLINICAL PROGRAM RATINGS:

CARDIAC	NR	ORTHOPEDICS	★★★
CRITICAL CARE	NR	PULMONARY	★★★
GASTROINTESTINAL	NR	STROKE	★★★
GENERAL SURGERY	NR	VASCULAR	NR
MATERNITY CARE	NR	WOMEN'S HEALTH	NR

HEALTHGRADES AWARDS

Jefferson Memorial Hospital

1400 US Highway 61 South
Crystal City, MO 63019
(636) 933-1000

Overall patient safety: ★
Teaching: N

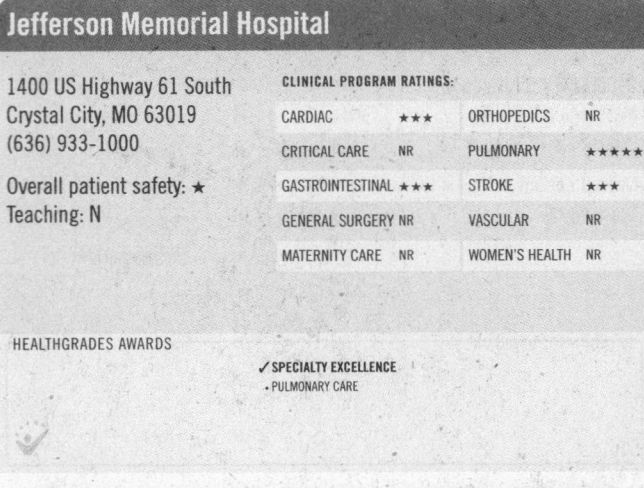

CLINICAL PROGRAM RATINGS:

CARDIAC	★★★	ORTHOPEDICS	NR
CRITICAL CARE	NR	PULMONARY	★★★★★
GASTROINTESTINAL	★★★	STROKE	★★★
GENERAL SURGERY	NR	VASCULAR	NR
MATERNITY CARE	NR	WOMEN'S HEALTH	NR

HEALTHGRADES AWARDS

✓ SPECIALTY EXCELLENCE
• PULMONARY CARE

Heartland Regional Medical Center

5325 Faraon Street
St. Joseph, MO 64506
(816) 271-6000

Overall patient safety: ★★★★★
Teaching: N

CLINICAL PROGRAM RATINGS:

CARDIAC	★★★	ORTHOPEDICS	★★★★★
CRITICAL CARE	★★★	PULMONARY	★★★★★
GASTROINTESTINAL	★★★	STROKE	★★★
GENERAL SURGERY	NR	VASCULAR	★★★
MATERNITY CARE	NR	WOMEN'S HEALTH	NR

HEALTHGRADES AWARDS

✓ DISTINGUISHED HOSPITAL
• PATIENT SAFETY

✓ SPECIALTY EXCELLENCE
• JOINT REPLACEMENT   • ORTHOPEDIC SURGERY   • PULMONARY CARE

Lafayette Regional Health Center

1500 State Street
Lexington, MO 64067
(660) 259-2203

Overall patient safety: ★★★
Teaching: N

CLINICAL PROGRAM RATINGS:

CARDIAC	NR	ORTHOPEDICS	NR
CRITICAL CARE	NR	PULMONARY	★
GASTROINTESTINAL	NR	STROKE	★
GENERAL SURGERY	NR	VASCULAR	NR
MATERNITY CARE	NR	WOMEN'S HEALTH	NR

HEALTHGRADES AWARDS

KEY: ★★★★★ BEST   ★★★ AS EXPECTED   ★ POOR   NR NOT RATED BY HEALTHGRADES   For full definitions of ratings and awards, see Appendix.

Lake Regional Health System

54 Hospital Drive
Osage Beach, MO 65065
(573) 348-8000

Overall patient safety: ★★★
Teaching: N

CLINICAL PROGRAM RATINGS:

CARDIAC	★★★	ORTHOPEDICS	NR
CRITICAL CARE	NR	PULMONARY	★★★
GASTROINTESTINAL	★★★	STROKE	★★★
GENERAL SURGERY	NR	VASCULAR	NR
MATERNITY CARE	NR	WOMEN'S HEALTH	NR

HEALTHGRADES AWARDS

Lincoln County Medical Center

1000 East Cherry Street
Troy, MO 63379
(636) 528-8551

Overall patient safety: ★★★
Teaching: N

CLINICAL PROGRAM RATINGS:

CARDIAC	NR	ORTHOPEDICS	NR
CRITICAL CARE	NR	PULMONARY	★★★
GASTROINTESTINAL	NR	STROKE	★
GENERAL SURGERY	NR	VASCULAR	NR
MATERNITY CARE	NR	WOMEN'S HEALTH	NR

HEALTHGRADES AWARDS

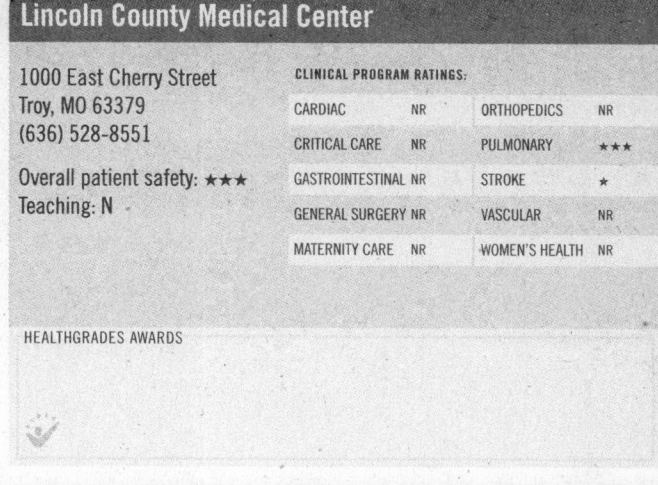

Lee's Summit Medical Center

2100 Southeast Blue Parkway
Lee's Summit, MO 64081
(816) 969-6000

Overall patient safety: ★
Teaching: N

CLINICAL PROGRAM RATINGS:

CARDIAC	NR	ORTHOPEDICS	NR
CRITICAL CARE	NR	PULMONARY	★
GASTROINTESTINAL	★★★	STROKE	★★★
GENERAL SURGERY	NR	VASCULAR	NR
MATERNITY CARE	NR	WOMEN'S HEALTH	NR

HEALTHGRADES AWARDS

Macon County Samaritan Memorial Hospital

1205 North Missouri Street
Macon, MO 63552
(660) 385-8700

Overall patient safety: ★★★
Teaching: N

CLINICAL PROGRAM RATINGS:

CARDIAC	NR	ORTHOPEDICS	NR
CRITICAL CARE	NR	PULMONARY	★★★
GASTROINTESTINAL	NR	STROKE	NR
GENERAL SURGERY	NR	VASCULAR	NR
MATERNITY CARE	NR	WOMEN'S HEALTH	NR

HEALTHGRADES AWARDS

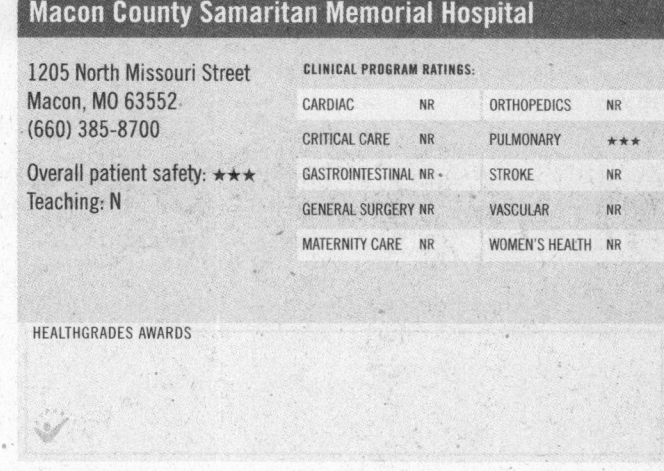

Liberty Hospital

2525 Glenn Hendren Drive
Liberty, MO 64068
(816) 781-7200

Overall patient safety: ★
Teaching: N

CLINICAL PROGRAM RATINGS:

CARDIAC	NR	ORTHOPEDICS	★
CRITICAL CARE	★★★	PULMONARY	★★★★★
GASTROINTESTINAL	★★★	STROKE	★★★
GENERAL SURGERY	NR	VASCULAR	NR
MATERNITY CARE	NR	WOMEN'S HEALTH	NR

HEALTHGRADES AWARDS

Madison Medical Center

611 West Main Street
Fredericktown, MO 63645
(573) 781-3341

Overall patient safety: ★★★
Teaching: N

CLINICAL PROGRAM RATINGS:

CARDIAC	NR	ORTHOPEDICS	NR
CRITICAL CARE	NR	PULMONARY	★★★
GASTROINTESTINAL	NR	STROKE	NR
GENERAL SURGERY	NR	VASCULAR	NR
MATERNITY CARE	NR	WOMEN'S HEALTH	NR

HEALTHGRADES AWARDS

*This hospital reports its data to the federal government jointly with another hospital. Therefore the ratings and awards apply to multiple hospitals and this specific hospital may not provide all rated services.

McCune-Brooks Hospital

627 West Centennial Street
Carthage, MO 64836
(417) 358-8121

Overall patient safety: ★★★
Teaching: N

CLINICAL PROGRAM RATINGS:

CARDIAC	NR	ORTHOPEDICS	NR
CRITICAL CARE	NR	PULMONARY	★★★
GASTROINTESTINAL	NR	STROKE	★★★
GENERAL SURGERY	NR	VASCULAR	NR
MATERNITY CARE	NR	WOMEN'S HEALTH	NR

HEALTHGRADES AWARDS

Missouri Baptist Hospital Sullivan

751 Sappington Bridge Road
Sullivan, MO 63080
(573) 468-4186

Overall patient safety: ★★★
Teaching: N

CLINICAL PROGRAM RATINGS:

CARDIAC	NR	ORTHOPEDICS	NR
CRITICAL CARE	NR	PULMONARY	★★★
GASTROINTESTINAL	NR	STROKE	★
GENERAL SURGERY	NR	VASCULAR	NR
MATERNITY CARE	NR	WOMEN'S HEALTH	NR

HEALTHGRADES AWARDS

Menorah Medical Center*

4949 Rockhill Road
Kansas City, MO 64110
(816) 276-8000

Overall patient safety: ★★★
Teaching: N

CLINICAL PROGRAM RATINGS:

CARDIAC	★★★	ORTHOPEDICS	★
CRITICAL CARE	NR	PULMONARY	★★★
GASTROINTESTINAL	★★★	STROKE	★★★
GENERAL SURGERY	NR	VASCULAR	NR
MATERNITY CARE	NR	WOMEN'S HEALTH	NR

HEALTHGRADES AWARDS

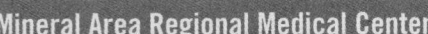

Missouri Baptist Medical Center

3015 North Ballas Road
St. Louis, MO 63131
(314) 996-5000

Overall patient safety: ★★★
Teaching: Y

CLINICAL PROGRAM RATINGS:

CARDIAC	★★★	ORTHOPEDICS	★
CRITICAL CARE	★★★	PULMONARY	★★★★★
GASTROINTESTINAL	★★★	STROKE	★★★★★
GENERAL SURGERY	NR	VASCULAR	★★★
MATERNITY CARE	NR	WOMEN'S HEALTH	NR

HEALTHGRADES AWARDS

✓ SPECIALTY EXCELLENCE
- PULMONARY CARE   - STROKE CARE

Mineral Area Regional Medical Center

1212 Weber Road
Farmington, MO 63640
(573) 756-4581

Overall patient safety: ★★★
Teaching: Y

CLINICAL PROGRAM RATINGS:

CARDIAC	NR	ORTHOPEDICS	NR
CRITICAL CARE	NR	PULMONARY	★
GASTROINTESTINAL	NR	STROKE	★★★
GENERAL SURGERY	NR	VASCULAR	NR
MATERNITY CARE	NR	WOMEN'S HEALTH	NR

HEALTHGRADES AWARDS

Missouri Delta Medical Center

1008 North Main Street
Sikeston, MO 63801
(573) 471-1600

Overall patient safety: ★★★
Teaching: N

CLINICAL PROGRAM RATINGS:

CARDIAC	NR	ORTHOPEDICS	NR
CRITICAL CARE	NR	PULMONARY	★
GASTROINTESTINAL	★★★	STROKE	★★★
GENERAL SURGERY	NR	VASCULAR	NR
MATERNITY CARE	NR	WOMEN'S HEALTH	NR

HEALTHGRADES AWARDS

KEY: ★★★★★ BEST   ★★★ AS EXPECTED   ★ POOR   NR NOT RATED BY HEALTHGRADES   For full definitions of ratings and awards, see Appendix.

Missouri Southern Healthcare

1200 North One Mile Road
Dexter, MO 63841
(573) 624-5566

Overall patient safety: ★★★
Teaching: N

CLINICAL PROGRAM RATINGS:

CARDIAC	NR	ORTHOPEDICS	NR
CRITICAL CARE	NR	PULMONARY*	★★★
GASTROINTESTINAL	NR	STROKE	★★★
GENERAL SURGERY	NR	VASCULAR	NR
MATERNITY CARE	NR	WOMEN'S HEALTH	NR

HEALTHGRADES AWARDS

North Kansas City Hospital

2800 Clay Edwards Drive
North Kansas City, MO 64116
(816) 691-2000

Overall patient safety: ★★★
Teaching: N

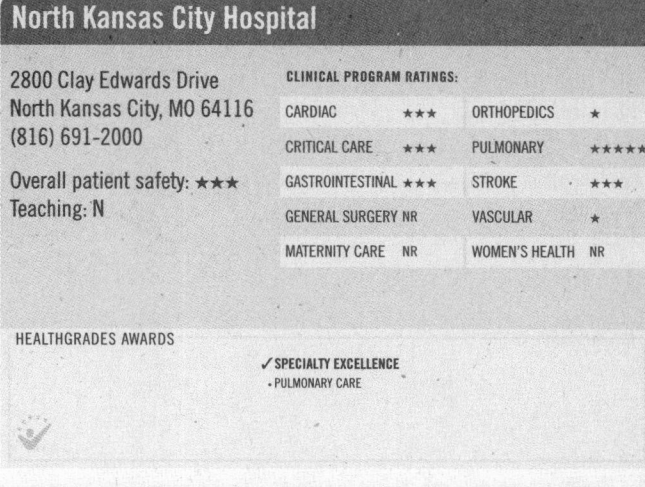

CLINICAL PROGRAM RATINGS:

CARDIAC	★★★	ORTHOPEDICS	★
CRITICAL CARE	★★★	PULMONARY	★★★★★
GASTROINTESTINAL	★★★	STROKE	★★★
GENERAL SURGERY	NR	VASCULAR	★
MATERNITY CARE	NR	WOMEN'S HEALTH	NR

HEALTHGRADES AWARDS

✓ SPECIALTY EXCELLENCE
- PULMONARY CARE

Moberly Regional Medical Center

1515 Union Avenue
Moberly, MO 65270
(660) 263-8400

Overall patient safety: ★★★
Teaching: Y

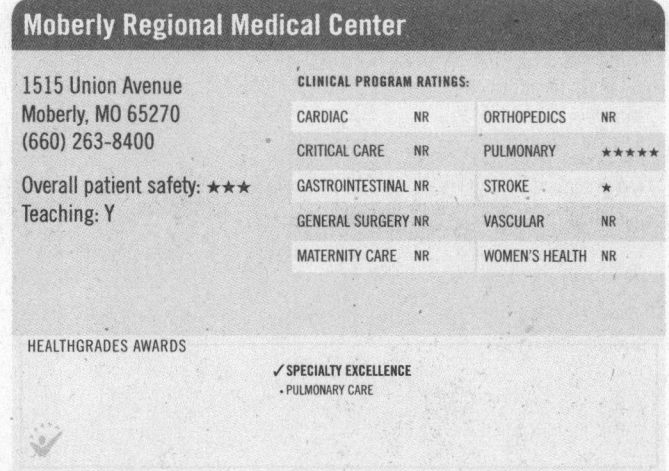

CLINICAL PROGRAM RATINGS:

CARDIAC	NR	ORTHOPEDICS	NR
CRITICAL CARE	NR	PULMONARY	★★★★★
GASTROINTESTINAL	NR	STROKE	★
GENERAL SURGERY	NR	VASCULAR	NR
MATERNITY CARE	NR	WOMEN'S HEALTH	NR

HEALTHGRADES AWARDS

✓ SPECIALTY EXCELLENCE
- PULMONARY CARE

Northeast Regional Medical Center*

315 South Osteopathy Street
Kirksville, MO 63501
(660) 785-1000

Overall patient safety: ★★★★★
Teaching: Y

CLINICAL PROGRAM RATINGS:

CARDIAC	NR	ORTHOPEDICS	NR
CRITICAL CARE	NR	PULMONARY	★★★
GASTROINTESTINAL	★★★	STROKE	★★★
GENERAL SURGERY	NR	VASCULAR	NR
MATERNITY CARE	NR	WOMEN'S HEALTH	NR

HEALTHGRADES AWARDS

Nevada Regional Medical Center

800 South Ash Street
Nevada, MO 64772
(417) 667-3355

Overall patient safety: ★★★
Teaching: N

CLINICAL PROGRAM RATINGS:

CARDIAC	NR	ORTHOPEDICS	NR
CRITICAL CARE	NR	PULMONARY	★★★
GASTROINTESTINAL	NR	STROKE	★
GENERAL SURGERY	NR	VASCULAR	NR
MATERNITY CARE	NR	WOMEN'S HEALTH	NR

HEALTHGRADES AWARDS

Northwest Medical Center

705 North College Street
Albany, MO 64402
(660) 726-3941

Overall patient safety: NR
Teaching: N

CLINICAL PROGRAM RATINGS:

CARDIAC	NR	ORTHOPEDICS	NR
CRITICAL CARE	NR	PULMONARY	★★★
GASTROINTESTINAL	NR	STROKE	NR
GENERAL SURGERY	NR	VASCULAR	NR
MATERNITY CARE	NR	WOMEN'S HEALTH	NR

HEALTHGRADES AWARDS

*This hospital reports its data to the federal government jointly with another hospital. Therefore the ratings and awards apply to multiple hospitals and this specific hospital may not provide all rated services.

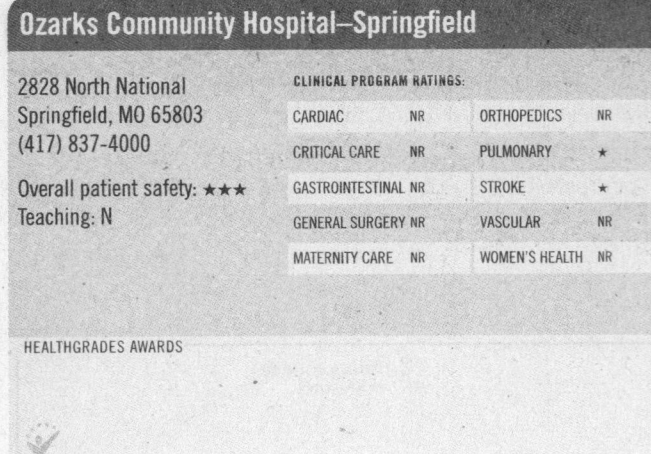

Ozarks Community Hospital—Springfield

2828 North National
Springfield, MO 65803
(417) 837-4000

Overall patient safety: ★★★
Teaching: N

CLINICAL PROGRAM RATINGS:

CARDIAC	NR	ORTHOPEDICS	NR
CRITICAL CARE	NR	PULMONARY	★
GASTROINTESTINAL	NR	STROKE	★
GENERAL SURGERY	NR	VASCULAR	NR
MATERNITY CARE	NR	WOMEN'S HEALTH	NR

HEALTHGRADES AWARDS

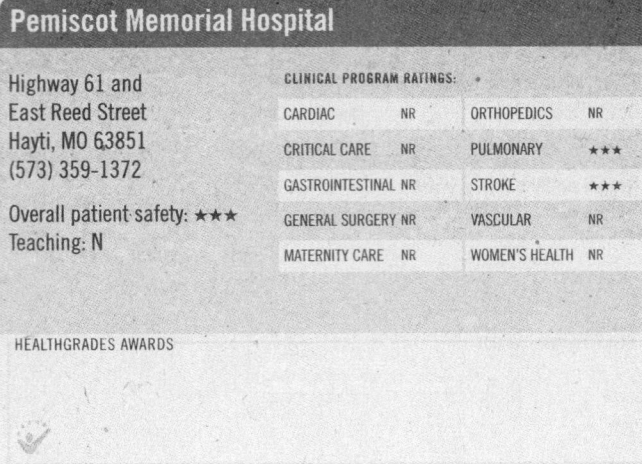

Pemiscot Memorial Hospital

Highway 61 and
East Reed Street
Hayti, MO 63851
(573) 359-1372

Overall patient safety: ★★★
Teaching: N

CLINICAL PROGRAM RATINGS:

CARDIAC	NR	ORTHOPEDICS	NR
CRITICAL CARE	NR	PULMONARY	★★★
GASTROINTESTINAL	NR	STROKE	★★★
GENERAL SURGERY	NR	VASCULAR	NR
MATERNITY CARE	NR	WOMEN'S HEALTH	NR

HEALTHGRADES AWARDS

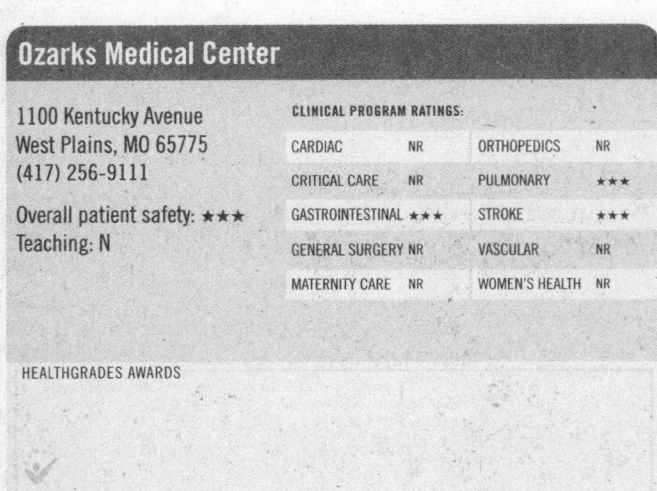

Ozarks Medical Center

1100 Kentucky Avenue
West Plains, MO 65775
(417) 256-9111

Overall patient safety: ★★★
Teaching: N

CLINICAL PROGRAM RATINGS:

CARDIAC	NR	ORTHOPEDICS	NR
CRITICAL CARE	NR	PULMONARY	★★★
GASTROINTESTINAL	★★★	STROKE	★★★
GENERAL SURGERY	NR	VASCULAR	NR
MATERNITY CARE	NR	WOMEN'S HEALTH	NR

HEALTHGRADES AWARDS

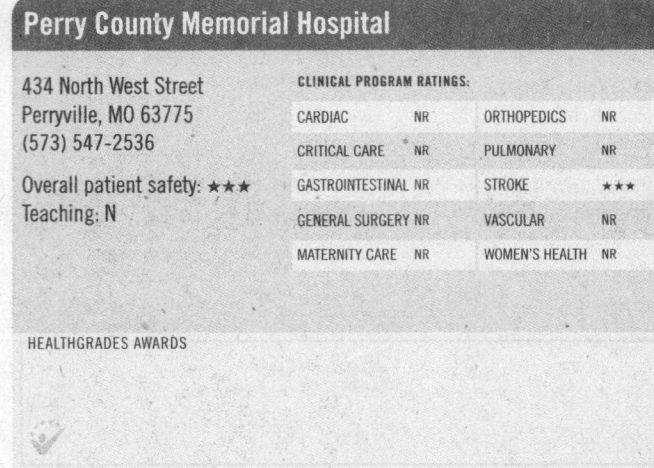

Perry County Memorial Hospital

434 North West Street
Perryville, MO 63775
(573) 547-2536

Overall patient safety: ★★★
Teaching: N

CLINICAL PROGRAM RATINGS:

CARDIAC	NR	ORTHOPEDICS	NR
CRITICAL CARE	NR	PULMONARY	NR
GASTROINTESTINAL	NR	STROKE	★★★
GENERAL SURGERY	NR	VASCULAR	NR
MATERNITY CARE	NR	WOMEN'S HEALTH	NR

HEALTHGRADES AWARDS

Parkland Health Center*

1101 West Liberty Street
Farmington, MO 63640
(573) 756-6451

Overall patient safety: ★★★
Teaching: N

CLINICAL PROGRAM RATINGS:

CARDIAC	NR	ORTHOPEDICS	NR
CRITICAL CARE	NR	PULMONARY	★★★
GASTROINTESTINAL	NR	STROKE	★★★
GENERAL SURGERY	NR	VASCULAR	NR
MATERNITY CARE	NR	WOMEN'S HEALTH	NR

HEALTHGRADES AWARDS

Pershing Memorial Hospital

130 East Lockling Avenue
Brookfield, MO 64628
(660) 258-2222

Overall patient safety: ★★★
Teaching: N

CLINICAL PROGRAM RATINGS:

CARDIAC	NR	ORTHOPEDICS	NR
CRITICAL CARE	NR	PULMONARY	★★★
GASTROINTESTINAL	NR	STROKE	NR
GENERAL SURGERY	NR	VASCULAR	NR
MATERNITY CARE	NR	WOMEN'S HEALTH	NR

HEALTHGRADES AWARDS

KEY: ★★★★★ BEST   ★★★ AS EXPECTED   ★ POOR   NR NOT RATED BY HEALTHGRADES   For full definitions of ratings and awards, see Appendix.

Phelps County Regional Medical Center

1000 West 10th Street
Rolla, MO 65401
(573) 364-8899

Overall patient safety: ★★★
Teaching: N

CLINICAL PROGRAM RATINGS:

CARDIAC	NR	ORTHOPEDICS	NR
CRITICAL CARE	NR	PULMONARY	★★★
GASTROINTESTINAL	★★★	STROKE	★★★
GENERAL SURGERY	NR	VASCULAR	NR
MATERNITY CARE	NR	WOMEN'S HEALTH	NR

HEALTHGRADES AWARDS

Ray County Memorial Hospital

904 Wollard Boulevard
Richmond, MO 64085
(816) 470-5432

Overall patient safety: ★★★
Teaching: N

CLINICAL PROGRAM RATINGS:

CARDIAC	NR	ORTHOPEDICS	NR
CRITICAL CARE	NR	PULMONARY	★★★
GASTROINTESTINAL	NR	STROKE	NR
GENERAL SURGERY	NR	VASCULAR	NR
MATERNITY CARE	NR	WOMEN'S HEALTH	NR

HEALTHGRADES AWARDS

Pike County Memorial Hospital

2305 West Georgia Street
Louisiana, MO 63353
(573) 754-5531

Overall patient safety: NR
Teaching: N

CLINICAL PROGRAM RATINGS:

CARDIAC	NR	ORTHOPEDICS	NR
CRITICAL CARE	NR	PULMONARY	★★★
GASTROINTESTINAL	NR	STROKE	NR
GENERAL SURGERY	NR	VASCULAR	NR
MATERNITY CARE	NR	WOMEN'S HEALTH	NR

HEALTHGRADES AWARDS

Research Belton Hospital

17065 South 71 Highway
Belton, MO 64012
(816) 348-1236

Overall patient safety: ★★★
Teaching: N

CLINICAL PROGRAM RATINGS:

CARDIAC	NR	ORTHOPEDICS	NR
CRITICAL CARE	NR	PULMONARY	★★★
GASTROINTESTINAL	NR	STROKE	NR
GENERAL SURGERY	NR	VASCULAR	NR
MATERNITY CARE	NR	WOMEN'S HEALTH	NR

HEALTHGRADES AWARDS

Poplar Bluff Regional Medical Center

2620 North Westwood
Boulevard
Poplar Bluff, MO 63901
(573) 785-7721

Overall patient safety: ★★★
Teaching: N

CLINICAL PROGRAM RATINGS:

CARDIAC	★★★	ORTHOPEDICS	NR
CRITICAL CARE	NR	PULMONARY	★
GASTROINTESTINAL	★	STROKE	★
GENERAL SURGERY	NR	VASCULAR	NR
MATERNITY CARE	NR	WOMEN'S HEALTH	NR

HEALTHGRADES AWARDS

Research Medical Center

2316 East Meyer Boulevard
Kansas City, MO 64132
(816) 276-4000

Overall patient safety: ★
Teaching: Y

CLINICAL PROGRAM RATINGS:

CARDIAC	★★★	ORTHOPEDICS	★★★
CRITICAL CARE	★★★	PULMONARY	★★★
GASTROINTESTINAL	★★★	STROKE	★★★
GENERAL SURGERY	NR	VASCULAR	★★★
MATERNITY CARE	NR	WOMEN'S HEALTH	NR

HEALTHGRADES AWARDS

*This hospital reports its data to the federal government jointly with another hospital. Therefore the ratings and awards apply to multiple hospitals and this specific hospital may not provide all rated services.

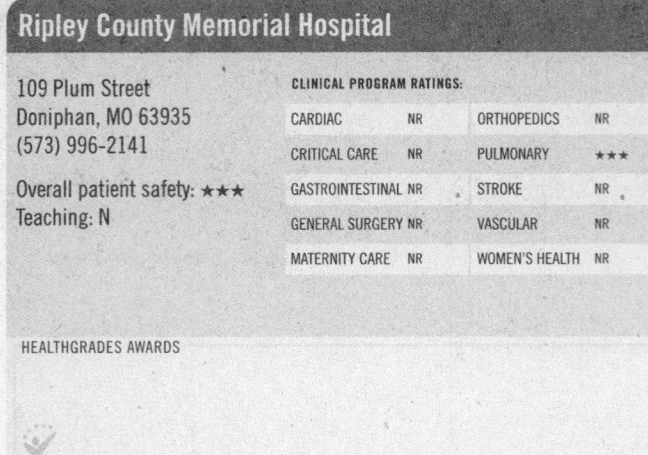

Ripley County Memorial Hospital

109 Plum Street
Doniphan, MO 63935
(573) 996-2141

Overall patient safety: ★★★
Teaching: N

CLINICAL PROGRAM RATINGS:

CARDIAC	NR	ORTHOPEDICS	NR
CRITICAL CARE	NR	PULMONARY	★★★
GASTROINTESTINAL	NR	STROKE	NR
GENERAL SURGERY	NR	VASCULAR	NR
MATERNITY CARE	NR	WOMEN'S HEALTH	NR

HEALTHGRADES AWARDS

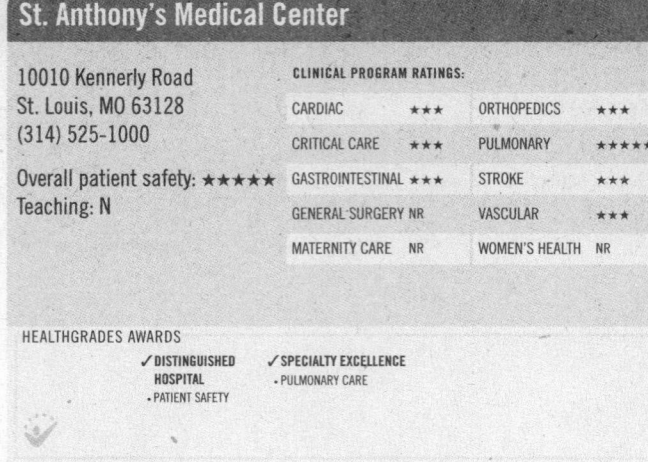

St. Anthony's Medical Center

10010 Kennerly Road
St. Louis, MO 63128
(314) 525-1000

Overall patient safety: ★★★★★
Teaching: N

CLINICAL PROGRAM RATINGS:

CARDIAC	★★★	ORTHOPEDICS	★★★
CRITICAL CARE	★★★	PULMONARY	★★★★★
GASTROINTESTINAL	★★★	STROKE	★★★
GENERAL SURGERY	NR	VASCULAR	★★★
MATERNITY CARE	NR	WOMEN'S HEALTH	NR

HEALTHGRADES AWARDS

✓ DISTINGUISHED HOSPITAL
- PATIENT SAFETY

✓ SPECIALTY EXCELLENCE
- PULMONARY CARE

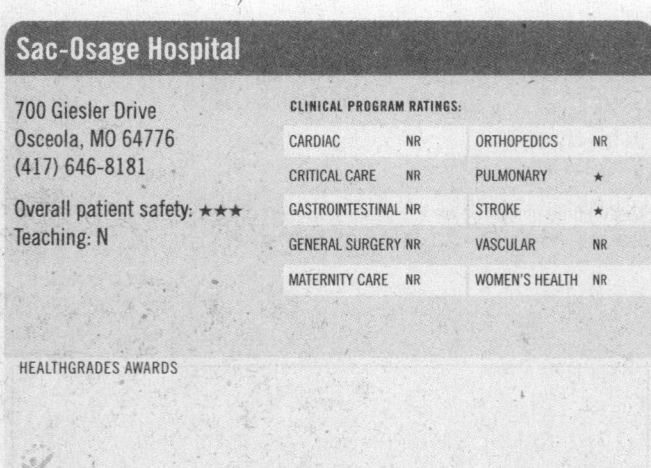

Sac-Osage Hospital

700 Giesler Drive
Osceola, MO 64776
(417) 646-8181

Overall patient safety: ★★★
Teaching: N

CLINICAL PROGRAM RATINGS:

CARDIAC	NR	ORTHOPEDICS	NR
CRITICAL CARE	NR	PULMONARY	★
GASTROINTESTINAL	NR	STROKE	★
GENERAL SURGERY	NR	VASCULAR	NR
MATERNITY CARE	NR	WOMEN'S HEALTH	NR

HEALTHGRADES AWARDS

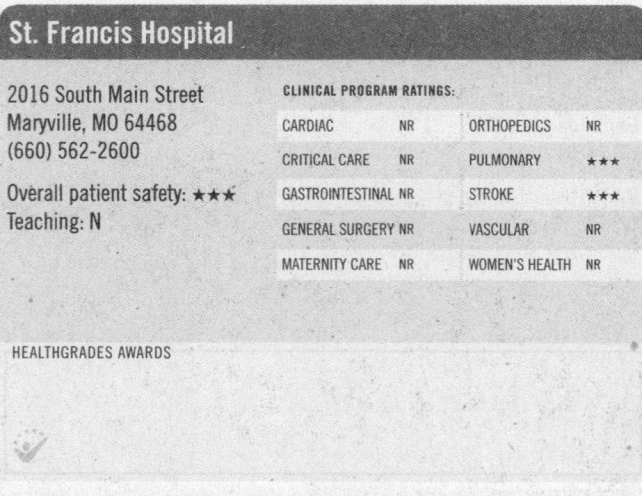

St. Francis Hospital

2016 South Main Street
Maryville, MO 64468
(660) 562-2600

Overall patient safety: ★★★
Teaching: N

CLINICAL PROGRAM RATINGS:

CARDIAC	NR	ORTHOPEDICS	NR
CRITICAL CARE	NR	PULMONARY	★★★
GASTROINTESTINAL	NR	STROKE	★★★
GENERAL SURGERY	NR	VASCULAR	NR
MATERNITY CARE	NR	WOMEN'S HEALTH	NR

HEALTHGRADES AWARDS

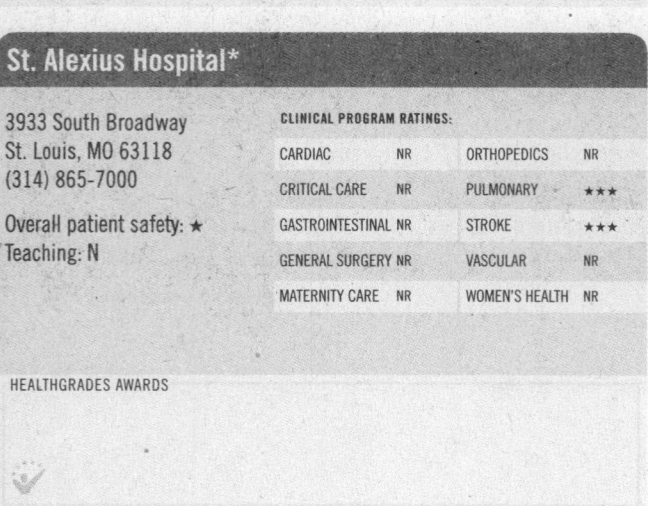

St. Alexius Hospital*

3933 South Broadway
St. Louis, MO 63118
(314) 865-7000

Overall patient safety: ★
Teaching: N

CLINICAL PROGRAM RATINGS:

CARDIAC	NR	ORTHOPEDICS	NR
CRITICAL CARE	NR	PULMONARY	★★★
GASTROINTESTINAL	NR	STROKE	★★★
GENERAL SURGERY	NR	VASCULAR	NR
MATERNITY CARE	NR	WOMEN'S HEALTH	NR

HEALTHGRADES AWARDS

St. Francis Medical Center

211 St. Francis Drive
Cape Girardeau, MO 63703
(573) 331-3000

Overall patient safety: ★
Teaching: N

CLINICAL PROGRAM RATINGS:

CARDIAC	★★★	ORTHOPEDICS	★★★
CRITICAL CARE	NR	PULMONARY	★★★
GASTROINTESTINAL	★★★	STROKE	★★★
GENERAL SURGERY	NR	VASCULAR	★★★
MATERNITY CARE	NR	WOMEN'S HEALTH	NR

HEALTHGRADES AWARDS

✓ SPECIALTY EXCELLENCE
- VASCULAR SURGERY

KEY: ★★★★★ BEST   ★★★ AS EXPECTED   ★ POOR   NR NOT RATED BY HEALTHGRADES   For full definitions of ratings and awards, see Appendix.

St. John's Hospital—Aurora

500 Porter Avenue
Aurora, MO 65605
(417) 678-2122

Overall patient safety: ★★★
Teaching: N

CLINICAL PROGRAM RATINGS:

CARDIAC	NR	ORTHOPEDICS	NR
CRITICAL CARE	NR	PULMONARY	★★★
GASTROINTESTINAL	NR	STROKE	NR
GENERAL SURGERY	NR	VASCULAR	NR
MATERNITY CARE	NR	WOMEN'S HEALTH	NR

HEALTHGRADES AWARDS

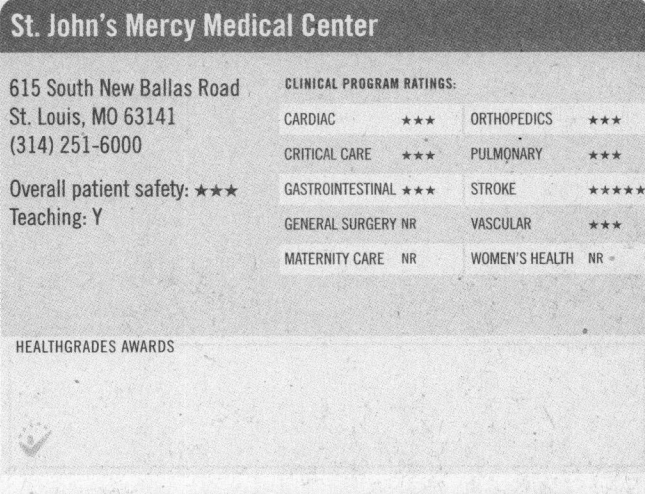

St. John's Mercy Medical Center

615 South New Ballas Road
St. Louis, MO 63141
(314) 251-6000

Overall patient safety: ★★★
Teaching: Y

CLINICAL PROGRAM RATINGS:

CARDIAC	★★★	ORTHOPEDICS	★★★
CRITICAL CARE	★★★	PULMONARY	★★★
GASTROINTESTINAL	★★★	STROKE	★★★★★
GENERAL SURGERY	NR	VASCULAR	★★★
MATERNITY CARE	NR	WOMEN'S HEALTH	NR *

HEALTHGRADES AWARDS

St. John's Hospital—Lebanon

100 Hospital Drive
Lebanon, MO 65536
(417) 533-6100

Overall patient safety: ★★★
Teaching: N

CLINICAL PROGRAM RATINGS:

CARDIAC	NR	ORTHOPEDICS	NR
CRITICAL CARE	NR	PULMONARY	★
GASTROINTESTINAL	NR	STROKE	★
GENERAL SURGERY	NR	VASCULAR	NR
MATERNITY CARE	NR	WOMEN'S HEALTH	NR

HEALTHGRADES AWARDS

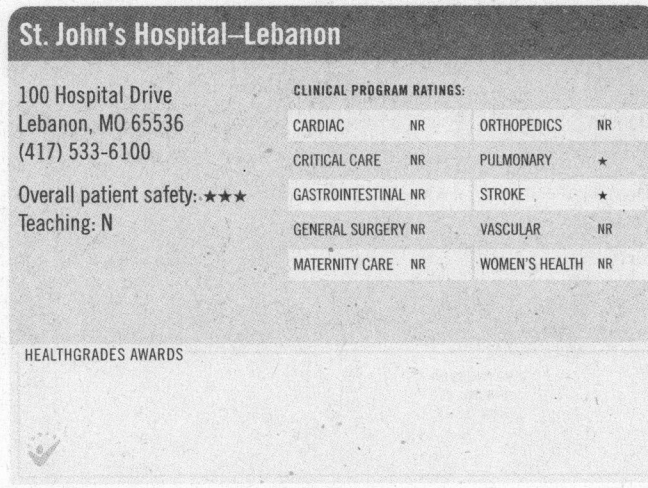

St. John's Regional Health Center

1235 East Cherokee Street
Springfield, MO 65804
(417) 885-2000

Overall patient safety: ★★★
Teaching: N

CLINICAL PROGRAM RATINGS:

CARDIAC	★	ORTHOPEDICS	★★★
CRITICAL CARE	NR	PULMONARY	★★★
GASTROINTESTINAL	★★★	STROKE	★
GENERAL SURGERY	NR	VASCULAR	★★★
MATERNITY CARE	NR	WOMEN'S HEALTH	NR

HEALTHGRADES AWARDS

✓ **SPECIALTY EXCELLENCE**
- JOINT REPLACEMENT

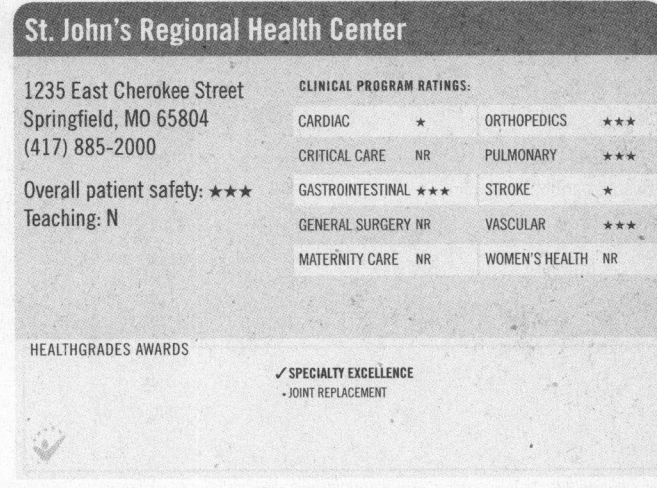

St. John's Mercy Hospital

901 East 5th Street
Washington, MO 63090
(636) 239-8000

Overall patient safety: ★★★★★
Teaching: N

CLINICAL PROGRAM RATINGS:

CARDIAC	NR	ORTHOPEDICS	NR
CRITICAL CARE	NR	PULMONARY	★★★
GASTROINTESTINAL	NR	STROKE	★★★
GENERAL SURGERY	NR	VASCULAR	NR
MATERNITY CARE	NR	WOMEN'S HEALTH	NR

HEALTHGRADES AWARDS

✓ **DISTINGUISHED HOSPITAL**
- PATIENT SAFETY

St. John's Regional Medical Center

2727 McClelland Boulevard
Joplin, MO 64804
(417) 781-2727

Overall patient safety: ★★★
Teaching: N

CLINICAL PROGRAM RATINGS:

CARDIAC	★★★	ORTHOPEDICS	★★★
CRITICAL CARE	NR	PULMONARY	★★★
GASTROINTESTINAL	★★★	STROKE	★
GENERAL SURGERY	NR	VASCULAR	★★★
MATERNITY CARE	NR	WOMEN'S HEALTH	NR

HEALTHGRADES AWARDS

✓ **SPECIALTY EXCELLENCE**
- JOINT REPLACEMENT

*This hospital reports its data to the federal government jointly with another hospital. Therefore the ratings and awards apply to multiple hospitals and this specific hospital may not provide all rated services.

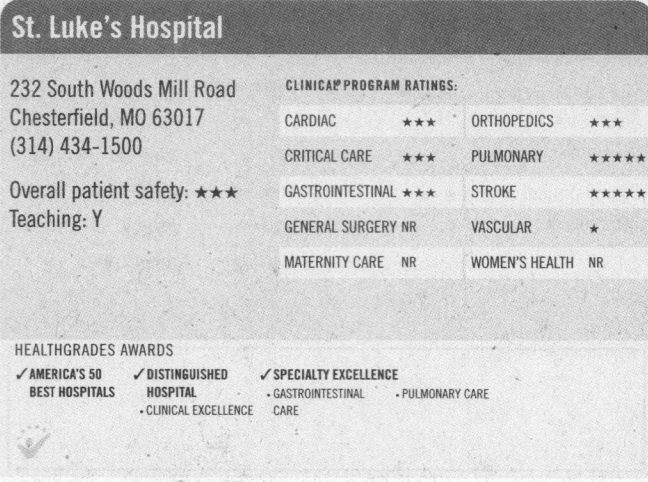

St. Joseph Medical Center

1000 Carondelet Drive
Kansas City, MO 64114
(816) 942-4400

Overall patient safety: ★★★
Teaching: Y

CLINICAL PROGRAM RATINGS:

CARDIAC	★★★	ORTHOPEDICS	★★★
CRITICAL CARE	★★★	PULMONARY	★★★
GASTROINTESTINAL	★★★	STROKE	★★★
GENERAL SURGERY	NR	VASCULAR	★★★
MATERNITY CARE	NR	WOMEN'S HEALTH	NR

HEALTHGRADES AWARDS

St. Luke's Hospital

232 South Woods Mill Road
Chesterfield, MO 63017
(314) 434-1500

Overall patient safety: ★★★
Teaching: Y

CLINICAL PROGRAM RATINGS:

CARDIAC	★★★	ORTHOPEDICS	★★★
CRITICAL CARE	★★★	PULMONARY	★★★★★
GASTROINTESTINAL	★★★	STROKE	★★★★★
GENERAL SURGERY	NR	VASCULAR	★
MATERNITY CARE	NR	WOMEN'S HEALTH	NR

HEALTHGRADES AWARDS

✓ AMERICA'S 50 BEST HOSPITALS ✓ DISTINGUISHED HOSPITAL · CLINICAL EXCELLENCE ✓ SPECIALTY EXCELLENCE · GASTROINTESTINAL CARE · PULMONARY CARE

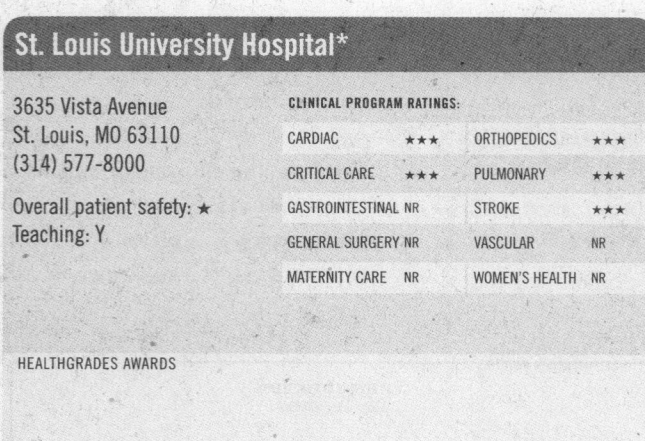

St. Louis University Hospital*

3635 Vista Avenue
St. Louis, MO 63110
(314) 577-8000

Overall patient safety: ★
Teaching: Y

CLINICAL PROGRAM RATINGS:

CARDIAC	★★★	ORTHOPEDICS	★★★
CRITICAL CARE	★★★	PULMONARY	★★★
GASTROINTESTINAL	NR	STROKE	★★★
GENERAL SURGERY	NR	VASCULAR	NR
MATERNITY CARE	NR	WOMEN'S HEALTH	NR

HEALTHGRADES AWARDS

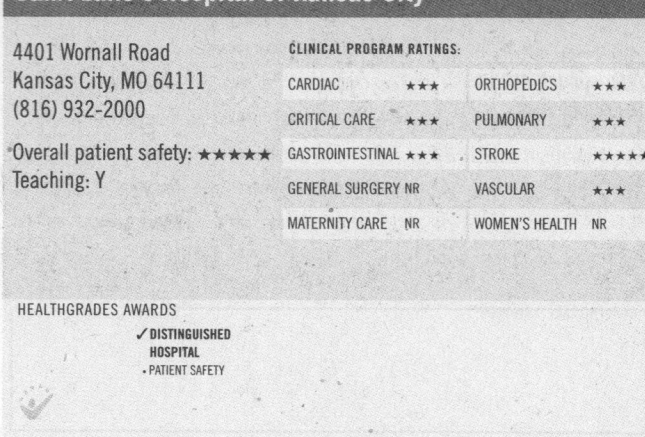

Saint Luke's Hospital of Kansas City

4401 Wornall Road
Kansas City, MO 64111
(816) 932-2000

Overall patient safety: ★★★★★
Teaching: Y

CLINICAL PROGRAM RATINGS:

CARDIAC	★★★	ORTHOPEDICS	★★★
CRITICAL CARE	★★★	PULMONARY	★★★
GASTROINTESTINAL	★★★	STROKE	★★★★★
GENERAL SURGERY	NR	VASCULAR	★★★
MATERNITY CARE	NR	WOMEN'S HEALTH	NR

HEALTHGRADES AWARDS

✓ DISTINGUISHED HOSPITAL · PATIENT SAFETY

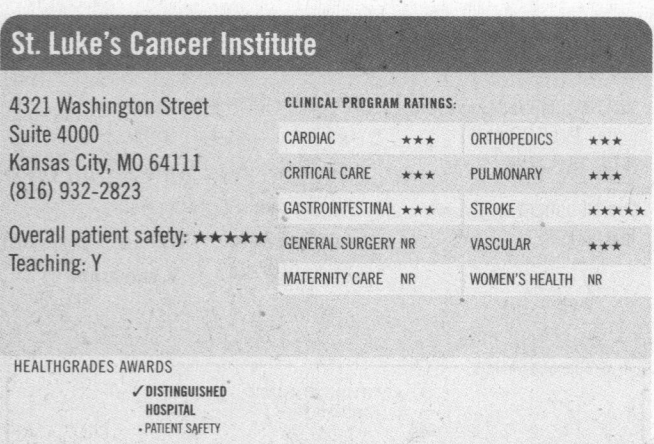

St. Luke's Cancer Institute

4321 Washington Street
Suite 4000
Kansas City, MO 64111
(816) 932-2823

Overall patient safety: ★★★★★
Teaching: Y

CLINICAL PROGRAM RATINGS:

CARDIAC	★★★	ORTHOPEDICS	★★★
CRITICAL CARE	★★★	PULMONARY	★★★
GASTROINTESTINAL	★★★	STROKE	★★★★★
GENERAL SURGERY	NR	VASCULAR	★★★
MATERNITY CARE	NR	WOMEN'S HEALTH	NR

HEALTHGRADES AWARDS

✓ DISTINGUISHED HOSPITAL · PATIENT SAFETY

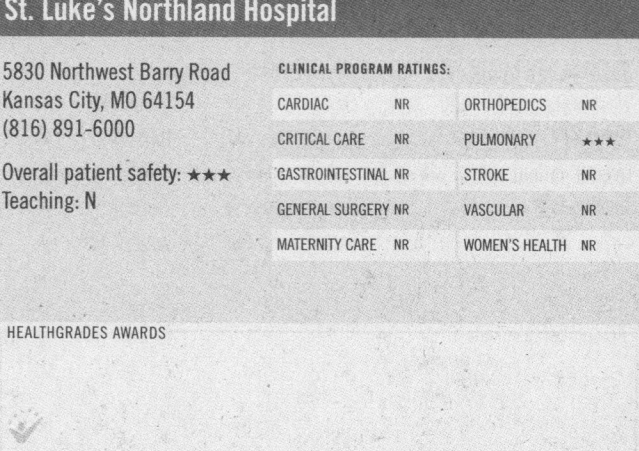

St. Luke's Northland Hospital

5830 Northwest Barry Road
Kansas City, MO 64154
(816) 891-6000

Overall patient safety: ★★★
Teaching: N

CLINICAL PROGRAM RATINGS:

CARDIAC	NR	ORTHOPEDICS	NR
CRITICAL CARE	NR	PULMONARY	★★★
GASTROINTESTINAL	NR	STROKE	NR
GENERAL SURGERY	NR	VASCULAR	NR
MATERNITY CARE	NR	WOMEN'S HEALTH	NR

HEALTHGRADES AWARDS

KEY: ★★★★★ BEST ★★★ AS EXPECTED ★ POOR NR NOT RATED BY HEALTHGRADES For full definitions of ratings and awards, see Appendix.

MISSOURI HOSPITALS: RATINGS BY CLINICAL SPECIALTY

St. Mary's Health Center

100 St. Mary's Medical Plaza
Jefferson City, MO 65101
(573) 761-7000

Overall patient safety: ★★★
Teaching: N

CLINICAL PROGRAM RATINGS:

CARDIAC	★★★	ORTHOPEDICS	★★★
CRITICAL CARE	NR	PULMONARY	★★★
GASTROINTESTINAL	★★★	STROKE	★★★
GENERAL SURGERY	NR	VASCULAR	NR
MATERNITY CARE	NR	WOMEN'S HEALTH	NR

HEALTHGRADES AWARDS

Scotland County Memorial Hospital

Route 1 Box 53
Memphis, MO 63555
(660) 465-8511

Overall patient safety: ★★★
Teaching: N

CLINICAL PROGRAM RATINGS:

CARDIAC	NR	ORTHOPEDICS	NR
CRITICAL CARE	NR	PULMONARY	★★★
GASTROINTESTINAL	NR	STROKE	NR
GENERAL SURGERY	NR	VASCULAR	NR
MATERNITY CARE	NR	WOMEN'S HEALTH	NR

HEALTHGRADES AWARDS

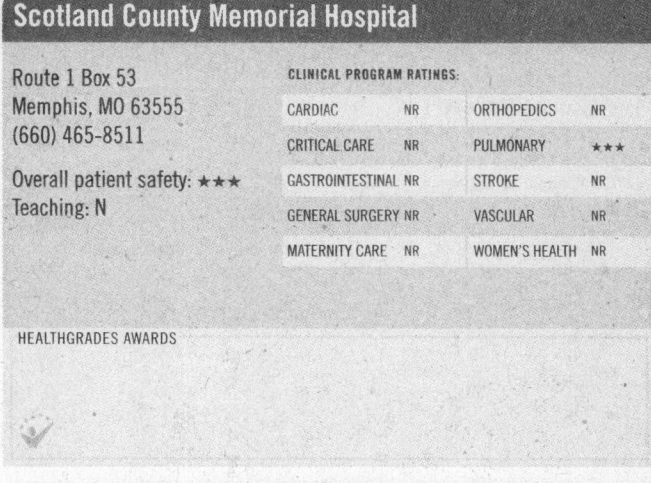

St. Mary's Medical Center

201 West R D Mize Road
Blue Springs, MO 64014
(816) 228-5900

Overall patient safety: ★
Teaching: Y

CLINICAL PROGRAM RATINGS:

CARDIAC	NR	ORTHOPEDICS	NR
CRITICAL CARE	★	PULMONARY	★★★
GASTROINTESTINAL	★★★	STROKE	★★★
GENERAL SURGERY	NR	VASCULAR	NR
MATERNITY CARE	NR	WOMEN'S HEALTH	NR

HEALTHGRADES AWARDS

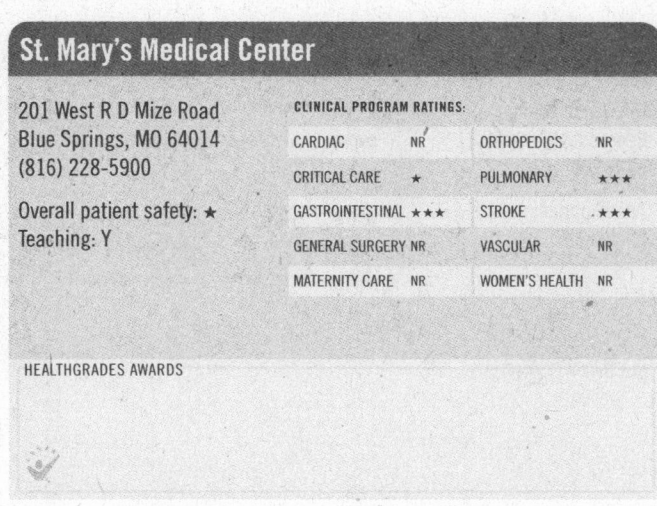

Skaggs Community Health Center

North Business 65 and
Skaggs Road
Branson, MO 65615
(417) 335-7000

Overall patient safety: ★★★
Teaching: N

CLINICAL PROGRAM RATINGS:

CARDIAC	★★★	ORTHOPEDICS	NR
CRITICAL CARE	NR	PULMONARY	★★★
GASTROINTESTINAL	★★★	STROKE	★★★★★
GENERAL SURGERY	NR	VASCULAR	NR
MATERNITY CARE	NR	WOMEN'S HEALTH	NR

HEALTHGRADES AWARDS

✓ DISTINGUISHED HOSPITAL   ✓ SPECIALTY EXCELLENCE
· CLINICAL EXCELLENCE   · STROKE CARE

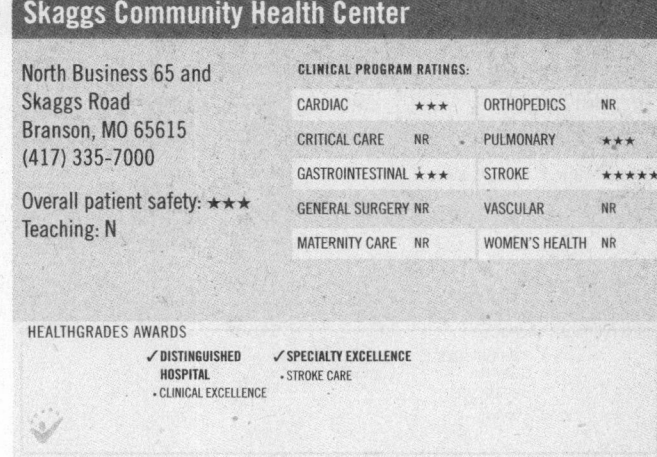

Ste. Genevieve County Memorial Hospital

800 Ste. Genevieve Drive
Ste. Genevieve, MO 63670
(573) 883-2751

Overall patient safety: ★★★
Teaching: N

CLINICAL PROGRAM RATINGS:

CARDIAC	NR	ORTHOPEDICS	NR
CRITICAL CARE	NR	PULMONARY	★★★
GASTROINTESTINAL	NR	STROKE	NR
GENERAL SURGERY	NR	VASCULAR	NR
MATERNITY CARE	NR	WOMEN'S HEALTH	NR

HEALTHGRADES AWARDS

South Point Hospital*

2639 Miami Street
St. Louis, MO 63118
(314) 772-1456

Overall patient safety: ★
Teaching: N

CLINICAL PROGRAM RATINGS:

CARDIAC	NR	ORTHOPEDICS	NR
CRITICAL CARE	NR	PULMONARY	★★★
GASTROINTESTINAL	NR	STROKE	★★★
GENERAL SURGERY	NR	VASCULAR	NR
MATERNITY CARE	NR	WOMEN'S HEALTH	NR

HEALTHGRADES AWARDS

*This hospital reports its data to the federal government jointly with another hospital. Therefore the ratings and awards apply to multiple hospitals and this specific hospital may not provide all rated services.

Southeast Missouri Hospital

1701 Lacey Street
Cape Girardeau, MO 63701
(573) 334-4822

Overall patient safety: ★★★
Teaching: N

CLINICAL PROGRAM RATINGS:

CARDIAC	★★★	ORTHOPEDICS	★★★
CRITICAL CARE	NR	PULMONARY	★★★
GASTROINTESTINAL	★★★	STROKE	★★★
GENERAL SURGERY	NR	VASCULAR	★★★
MATERNITY CARE	NR	WOMEN'S HEALTH	NR

HEALTHGRADES AWARDS

✓ SPECIALTY EXCELLENCE
· CARDIAC SURGERY

SSM St. Joseph Health Center—Wentzville*

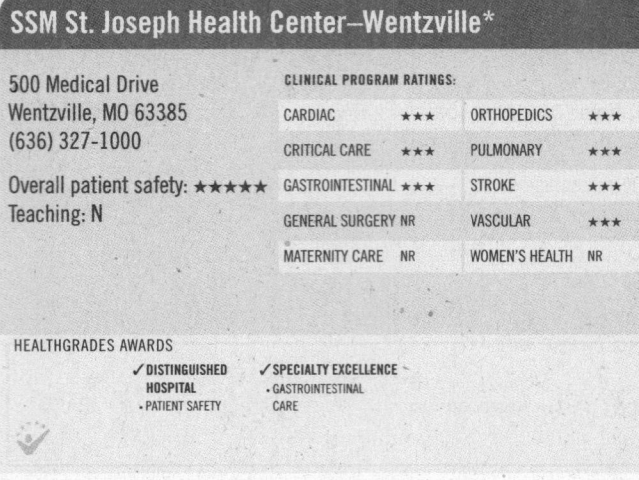

500 Medical Drive
Wentzville, MO 63385
(636) 327-1000

Overall patient safety: ★★★★★
Teaching: N

CLINICAL PROGRAM RATINGS:

CARDIAC	★★★	ORTHOPEDICS	★★★
CRITICAL CARE	★★★	PULMONARY	★★★
GASTROINTESTINAL	★★★	STROKE	★★★
GENERAL SURGERY	NR	VASCULAR	★★★
MATERNITY CARE	NR	WOMEN'S HEALTH	NR

HEALTHGRADES AWARDS

✓ DISTINGUISHED HOSPITAL
· PATIENT SAFETY

✓ SPECIALTY EXCELLENCE
· GASTROINTESTINAL CARE

SSM DePaul Health Center

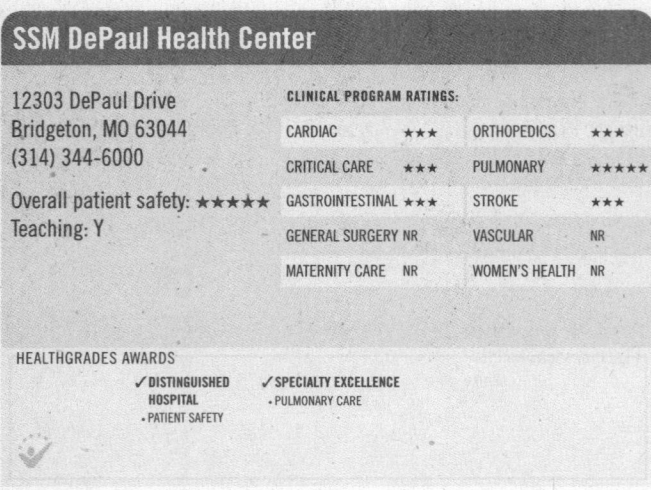

12303 DePaul Drive
Bridgeton, MO 63044
(314) 344-6000

Overall patient safety: ★★★★★
Teaching: Y

CLINICAL PROGRAM RATINGS:

CARDIAC	★★★	ORTHOPEDICS	★★★
CRITICAL CARE	★★★	PULMONARY	★★★★★
GASTROINTESTINAL	★★★	STROKE	★★★
GENERAL SURGERY	NR	VASCULAR	NR
MATERNITY CARE	NR	WOMEN'S HEALTH	NR

HEALTHGRADES AWARDS

✓ DISTINGUISHED HOSPITAL
· PATIENT SAFETY

✓ SPECIALTY EXCELLENCE
· PULMONARY CARE

SSM St. Joseph Hospital of Kirkwood

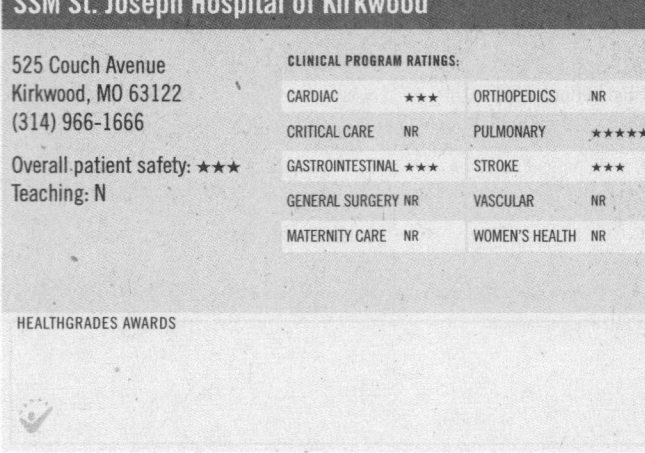

525 Couch Avenue
Kirkwood, MO 63122
(314) 966-1666

Overall patient safety: ★★★
Teaching: N

CLINICAL PROGRAM RATINGS:

CARDIAC	★★★	ORTHOPEDICS	NR
CRITICAL CARE	NR	PULMONARY	★★★★★
GASTROINTESTINAL	★★★	STROKE	★★★
GENERAL SURGERY	NR	VASCULAR	NR
MATERNITY CARE	NR	WOMEN'S HEALTH	NR

HEALTHGRADES AWARDS

SSM St. Joseph Health Center*

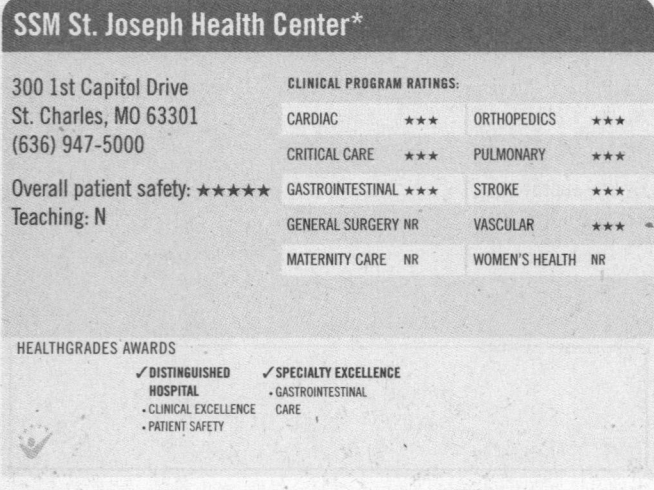

300 1st Capitol Drive
St. Charles, MO 63301
(636) 947-5000

Overall patient safety: ★★★★★
Teaching: N

CLINICAL PROGRAM RATINGS:

CARDIAC	★★★	ORTHOPEDICS	★★★
CRITICAL CARE	★★★	PULMONARY	★★★
GASTROINTESTINAL	★★★	STROKE	★★★
GENERAL SURGERY	NR	VASCULAR	★★★
MATERNITY CARE	NR	WOMEN'S HEALTH	NR

HEALTHGRADES AWARDS

✓ DISTINGUISHED HOSPITAL
· CLINICAL EXCELLENCE
· PATIENT SAFETY

✓ SPECIALTY EXCELLENCE
· GASTROINTESTINAL CARE

SSM St. Joseph Hospital West

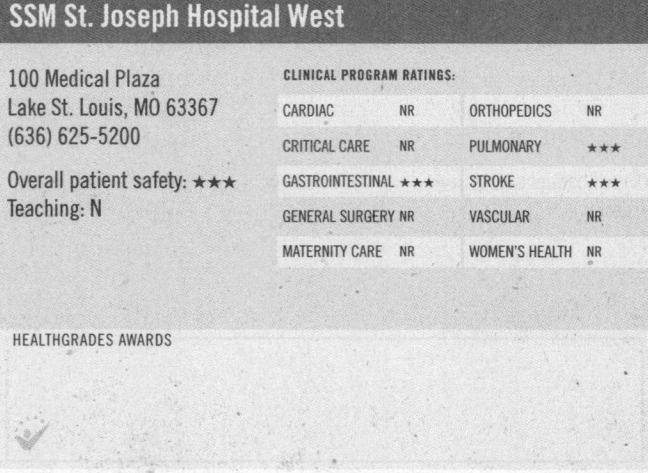

100 Medical Plaza
Lake St. Louis, MO 63367
(636) 625-5200

Overall patient safety: ★★★
Teaching: N

CLINICAL PROGRAM RATINGS:

CARDIAC	NR	ORTHOPEDICS	NR
CRITICAL CARE	NR	PULMONARY	★★★
GASTROINTESTINAL	★★★	STROKE	★★★
GENERAL SURGERY	NR	VASCULAR	NR
MATERNITY CARE	NR	WOMEN'S HEALTH	NR

HEALTHGRADES AWARDS

KEY: ★★★★★ BEST   ★★★ AS EXPECTED   ★ POOR   NR NOT RATED BY HEALTHGRADES   For full definitions of ratings and awards, see Appendix.

SSM St. Mary's Health Center

6420 Clayton Road
St. Louis, MO 63117
(314) 768-8000

Overall patient safety: ★★★
Teaching: Y

CLINICAL PROGRAM RATINGS:

CARDIAC	★★★	ORTHOPEDICS	★★★
CRITICAL CARE	★★★	PULMONARY	★★★
GASTROINTESTINAL	★★★	STROKE	★★★★★
GENERAL SURGERY	NR	VASCULAR	★★★
MATERNITY CARE	NR	WOMEN'S HEALTH	NR

HEALTHGRADES AWARDS

✓ DISTINGUISHED HOSPITAL
· CLINICAL EXCELLENCE

✓ SPECIALTY EXCELLENCE
· STROKE CARE

Truman Medical Center—Lakewood

7900 Lee's Summit Road
Kansas City, MO 64139
(816) 404-7000

Overall patient safety: ★★★
Teaching: Y

CLINICAL PROGRAM RATINGS:

CARDIAC	NR	ORTHOPEDICS	NR
CRITICAL CARE	NR	PULMONARY	★★★
GASTROINTESTINAL	NR	STROKE	NR
GENERAL SURGERY	NR	VASCULAR	NR
MATERNITY CARE	NR	WOMEN'S HEALTH	NR

HEALTHGRADES AWARDS

Texas County Memorial Hospital

1333 South Sam
Houston Boulevard
Houston, MO 65483
(417) 967-3311

Overall patient safety: ★★★
Teaching: N

CLINICAL PROGRAM RATINGS:

CARDIAC	NR	ORTHOPEDICS	NR
CRITICAL CARE	NR	PULMONARY	★★★
GASTROINTESTINAL	NR	STROKE	★★★
GENERAL SURGERY	NR	VASCULAR	NR
MATERNITY CARE	NR	WOMEN'S HEALTH	NR

HEALTHGRADES AWARDS

Twin Rivers Regional Medical Center

1301 1st Street
Kennett, MO 63857
(573) 888-4522

Overall patient safety: ★★★
Teaching: N

CLINICAL PROGRAM RATINGS:

CARDIAC	NR	ORTHOPEDICS	NR
CRITICAL CARE	NR	PULMONARY	★★★
GASTROINTESTINAL	NR	STROKE	★
GENERAL SURGERY	NR	VASCULAR	NR
MATERNITY CARE	NR	WOMEN'S HEALTH	NR

HEALTHGRADES AWARDS

Truman Medical Center—Hospital Hill

2301 Holmes Street
Kansas City, MO 64108
(816) 404-1000

Overall patient safety: ★★★
Teaching: Y

CLINICAL PROGRAM RATINGS:

CARDIAC	NR	ORTHOPEDICS	NR
CRITICAL CARE	NR	PULMONARY	★★★★★
GASTROINTESTINAL	NR	STROKE	★★★
GENERAL SURGERY	NR	VASCULAR	NR
MATERNITY CARE	NR	WOMEN'S HEALTH	NR

HEALTHGRADES AWARDS

✓ SPECIALTY EXCELLENCE
· PULMONARY CARE

University of Missouri Hospital and Clinics

1 Hospital Drive
Columbia, MO 65212
(573) 882-4141

Overall patient safety: ★
Teaching: Y

CLINICAL PROGRAM RATINGS:

CARDIAC	★★★	ORTHOPEDICS	NR
CRITICAL CARE	NR	PULMONARY	★
GASTROINTESTINAL	★★★	STROKE	★★★
GENERAL SURGERY	NR	VASCULAR	NR
MATERNITY CARE	NR	WOMEN'S HEALTH	NR

HEALTHGRADES AWARDS

*This hospital reports its data to the federal government jointly with another hospital. Therefore the ratings and awards apply to multiple hospitals and this specific hospital may not provide all rated services.

Washington County Memorial Hospital

300 Health Way
Potosi, MO 63664
(573) 438-5451

Overall patient safety: ★★★
Teaching: N

CLINICAL PROGRAM RATINGS:

CARDIAC	NR	ORTHOPEDICS	NR
CRITICAL CARE	NR	PULMONARY	★★★
GASTROINTESTINAL	NR	STROKE	NR
GENERAL SURGERY	NR	VASCULAR	NR
MATERNITY CARE	NR	WOMEN'S HEALTH	NR

HEALTHGRADES AWARDS

Whispering Oaks Hospital

1314 West Edgewood Drive
Jefferson City, MO 65101
(314) 634-5000

Overall patient safety: ★★★
Teaching: N

CLINICAL PROGRAM RATINGS:

CARDIAC	★★★	ORTHOPEDICS	★★★
CRITICAL CARE	NR	PULMONARY	★★★
GASTROINTESTINAL	★★★	STROKE	★★★
GENERAL SURGERY	NR	VASCULAR	NR
MATERNITY CARE	NR	WOMEN'S HEALTH	NR

HEALTHGRADES AWARDS

Western Missouri Medical Center

403 Burkarth Road
Warrensburg, MO 64093
(660) 747-2500

Overall patient safety: ★★★
Teaching: N

CLINICAL PROGRAM RATINGS:

CARDIAC	NR	ORTHOPEDICS	NR
CRITICAL CARE	NR	PULMONARY	★★★
GASTROINTESTINAL	NR	STROKE	★★★
GENERAL SURGERY	NR	VASCULAR	NR
MATERNITY CARE	NR	WOMEN'S HEALTH	NR

HEALTHGRADES AWARDS

MONTANA HOSPITALS: RATINGS BY CLINICAL SPECIALTY

Benefis Healthcare

1101 26th Street South
Great Falls, MT 59405
(406) 455-5000

Overall patient safety: ★★★★★
Teaching: N

CLINICAL PROGRAM RATINGS:

CARDIAC	★★★	ORTHOPEDICS	★★★
CRITICAL CARE	NR	PULMONARY	★★★
GASTROINTESTINAL	★★★	STROKE	★★★★★
GENERAL SURGERY	NR	VASCULAR	NR
MATERNITY CARE	NR	WOMEN'S HEALTH	NR

HEALTHGRADES AWARDS

✓ DISTINGUISHED HOSPITAL
- CLINICAL EXCELLENCE
- PATIENT SAFETY

✓ SPECIALTY EXCELLENCE
- STROKE CARE

Billings Clinic

2800 10th Avenue North
Billings, MT 59101
(406) 657-4000

Overall patient safety: ★★★★★
Teaching: Y

CLINICAL PROGRAM RATINGS:

CARDIAC	★★★	ORTHOPEDICS	★★★★★
CRITICAL CARE	NR	PULMONARY	★★★
GASTROINTESTINAL	★★★	STROKE	★★★
GENERAL SURGERY	NR	VASCULAR	★★★★★
MATERNITY CARE	NR	WOMEN'S HEALTH	NR

HEALTHGRADES AWARDS

✓ DISTINGUISHED HOSPITAL
- PATIENT SAFETY

✓ SPECIALTY EXCELLENCE
- JOINT REPLACEMENT
- ORTHOPEDIC SURGERY
- VASCULAR SURGERY

KEY: ★★★★★ BEST   ★★★ AS EXPECTED   ★ POOR   NR NOT RATED BY HEALTHGRADES   For full definitions of ratings and awards, see Appendix.

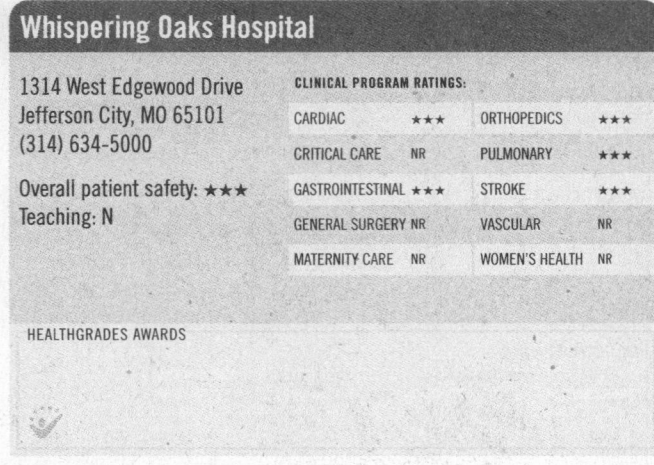
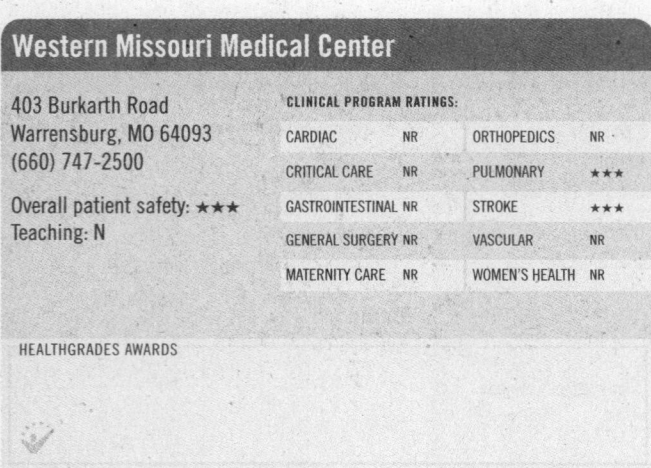

Bozeman Deaconess Hospital

915 Highland Boulevard
Bozeman, MT 59715
(406) 585-5000

Overall patient safety: ★★★
Teaching: N

CLINICAL PROGRAM RATINGS:

CARDIAC	NR	ORTHOPEDICS	★★★
CRITICAL CARE	NR	PULMONARY	★★★
GASTROINTESTINAL	★★★	STROKE	★★★
GENERAL SURGERY	NR	VASCULAR	NR
MATERNITY CARE	NR	WOMEN'S HEALTH	NR

HEALTHGRADES AWARDS

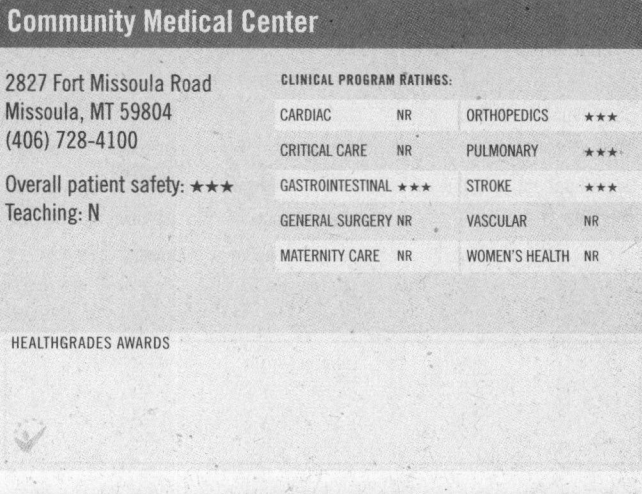

Community Medical Center

2827 Fort Missoula Road
Missoula, MT 59804
(406) 728-4100

Overall patient safety: ★★★
Teaching: N

CLINICAL PROGRAM RATINGS:

CARDIAC	NR	ORTHOPEDICS	★★★
CRITICAL CARE	NR	PULMONARY	★★★
GASTROINTESTINAL	★★★	STROKE	★★★
GENERAL SURGERY	NR	VASCULAR	NR
MATERNITY CARE	NR	WOMEN'S HEALTH	NR

HEALTHGRADES AWARDS

Central Montana Medical Center

408 Wendell Avenue
Lewistown, MT 59457
(406) 538-7711

Overall patient safety: ★★★★★
Teaching: N

CLINICAL PROGRAM RATINGS:

CARDIAC	NR	ORTHOPEDICS	NR
CRITICAL CARE	NR	PULMONARY	★★★
GASTROINTESTINAL	NR	STROKE	★★★
GENERAL SURGERY	NR	VASCULAR	NR
MATERNITY CARE	NR	WOMEN'S HEALTH	NR

HEALTHGRADES AWARDS

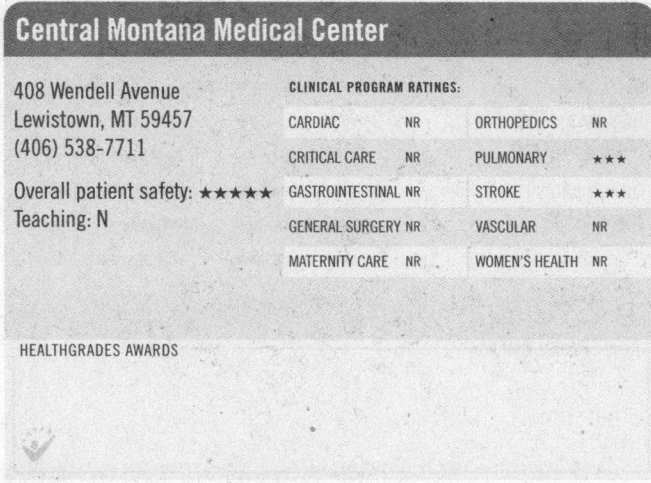

Holy Rosary Healthcare

2600 Wilson Avenue
Miles City, MT 59301
(406) 233-2600

Overall patient safety: ★★★
Teaching: N

CLINICAL PROGRAM RATINGS:

CARDIAC	NR	ORTHOPEDICS	NR
CRITICAL CARE	NR	PULMONARY	★★★
GASTROINTESTINAL	NR	STROKE	NR
GENERAL SURGERY	NR	VASCULAR	NR
MATERNITY CARE	NR	WOMEN'S HEALTH	NR

HEALTHGRADES AWARDS

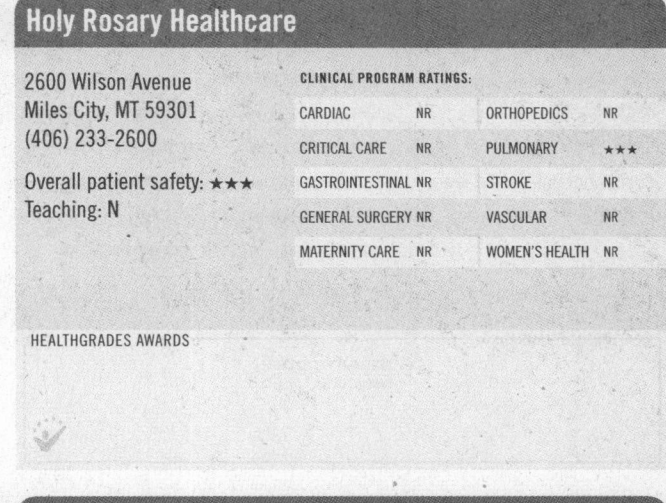

Community Hospital of Anaconda

401 West Pennsylvania Street
Anaconda, MT 59711
(406) 563-8500

Overall patient safety: ★★★
Teaching: N

CLINICAL PROGRAM RATINGS:

CARDIAC	NR	ORTHOPEDICS	NR
CRITICAL CARE	NR	PULMONARY	★
GASTROINTESTINAL	NR	STROKE	NR
GENERAL SURGERY	NR	VASCULAR	NR
MATERNITY CARE	NR	WOMEN'S HEALTH	NR

HEALTHGRADES AWARDS

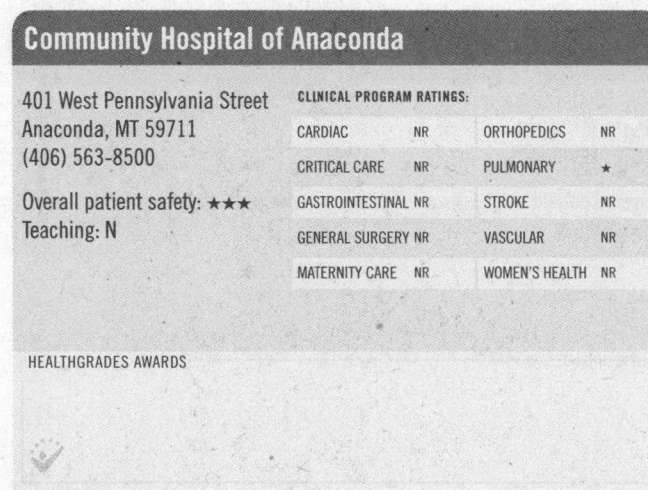

Kalispell Regional Hospital

310 Sunnyview Lane
Kalispell, MT 59901
(406) 752-5111

Overall patient safety: ★★★
Teaching: N

CLINICAL PROGRAM RATINGS:

CARDIAC	★★★	ORTHOPEDICS	★★★
CRITICAL CARE	NR	PULMONARY	★★★
GASTROINTESTINAL	★★★	STROKE	★★★
GENERAL SURGERY	NR	VASCULAR	NR
MATERNITY CARE	NR	WOMEN'S HEALTH	NR

HEALTHGRADES AWARDS

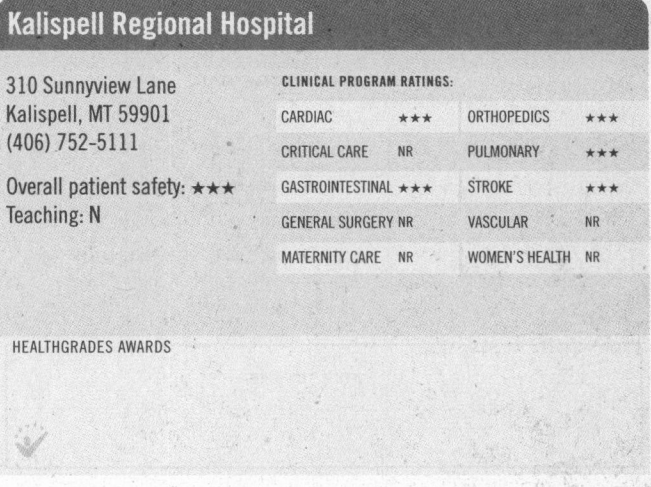

Marcus Daly Memorial Hospital

1200 Westwood Drive
Hamilton, MT 59840
(406) 363-2211

Overall patient safety: ★★★
Teaching: N

CLINICAL PROGRAM RATINGS:

CARDIAC	NR	ORTHOPEDICS	NR
CRITICAL CARE	NR	PULMONARY	★★★
GASTROINTESTINAL	NR	STROKE	★★★
GENERAL SURGERY	NR	VASCULAR	NR
MATERNITY CARE	NR	WOMEN'S HEALTH	NR

HEALTHGRADES AWARDS

Northern Montana Hospital

30 13th Street
Havre, MT 59501
(406) 265-2211

Overall patient safety: ★★★
Teaching: N

CLINICAL PROGRAM RATINGS:

CARDIAC	NR	ORTHOPEDICS	NR
CRITICAL CARE	NR	PULMONARY	★★★
GASTROINTESTINAL	NR	STROKE	★
GENERAL SURGERY	NR	VASCULAR	NR
MATERNITY CARE	NR	WOMEN'S HEALTH	NR

HEALTHGRADES AWARDS

Missoula General Hospital*

900 North Orange Street
Missoula, MT 59802
(406) 542-2191

Overall patient safety: ★★★
Teaching: N

CLINICAL PROGRAM RATINGS:

CARDIAC	★★★	ORTHOPEDICS	★★★
CRITICAL CARE	NR	PULMONARY	★
GASTROINTESTINAL	★★★	STROKE	★
GENERAL SURGERY	NR	VASCULAR	★★★
MATERNITY CARE	NR	WOMEN'S HEALTH	NR

HEALTHGRADES AWARDS

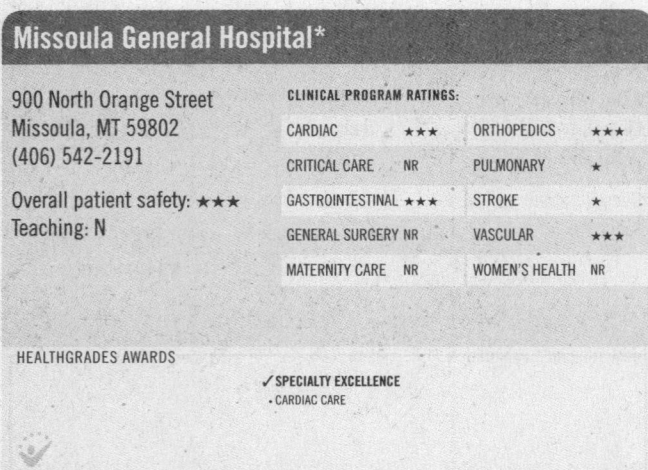

✓ SPECIALTY EXCELLENCE
• CARDIAC CARE

PHS Indian Hospital—Browning

North Piegan Street
Browning, MT 59417
(406) 338-6100

Overall patient safety: NR
Teaching: N

CLINICAL PROGRAM RATINGS:

CARDIAC	NR	ORTHOPEDICS	NR
CRITICAL CARE	NR	PULMONARY	★★★
GASTROINTESTINAL	NR	STROKE	NR
GENERAL SURGERY	NR	VASCULAR	NR
MATERNITY CARE	NR	WOMEN'S HEALTH	NR

HEALTHGRADES AWARDS

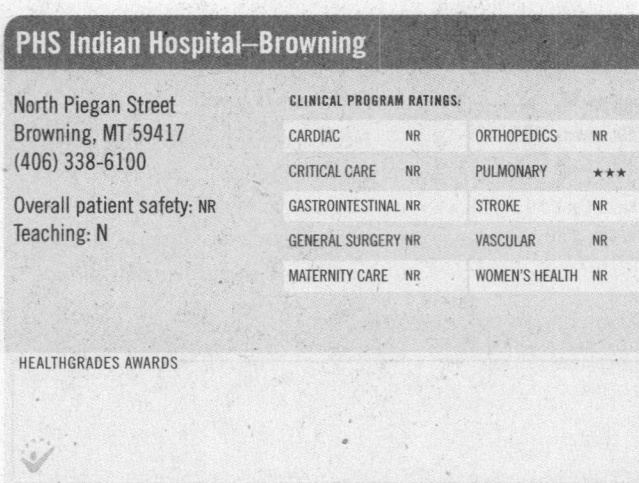

North Valley Hospital

1600 Hospital Way
Whitefish, MT 59937
(406) 863-3500

Overall patient safety: ★★★
Teaching: N

CLINICAL PROGRAM RATINGS:

CARDIAC	NR	ORTHOPEDICS	NR
CRITICAL CARE	NR	PULMONARY	★★★
GASTROINTESTINAL	NR	STROKE	★★★
GENERAL SURGERY	NR	VASCULAR	NR
MATERNITY CARE	NR	WOMEN'S HEALTH	NR

HEALTHGRADES AWARDS

St. James Healthcare

400 South Clark Street
Butte, MT 59701
(406) 723-2500

Overall patient safety: ★★★
Teaching: N

CLINICAL PROGRAM RATINGS:

CARDIAC	NR	ORTHOPEDICS	★
CRITICAL CARE	NR	PULMONARY	★
GASTROINTESTINAL	NR	STROKE	★
GENERAL SURGERY	NR	VASCULAR	NR
MATERNITY CARE	NR	WOMEN'S HEALTH	NR

HEALTHGRADES AWARDS

KEY: ★★★★★ BEST ★★★ AS EXPECTED ★ POOR NR NOT RATED BY HEALTHGRADES   For full definitions of ratings and awards, see Appendix.

St. Patrick Hospital and Health Sciences Center*

500 West Broadway
Missoula, MT 59802
(406) 543-7271

Overall patient safety: ★★★
Teaching: N

CLINICAL PROGRAM RATINGS:

CARDIAC	★★★	ORTHOPEDICS	★★★
CRITICAL CARE	NR	PULMONARY	★
GASTROINTESTINAL	★★★	STROKE	★
GENERAL SURGERY	NR	VASCULAR	★★★
MATERNITY CARE	NR	WOMEN'S HEALTH	NR

HEALTHGRADES AWARDS

✓ SPECIALTY EXCELLENCE
- CARDIAC CARE

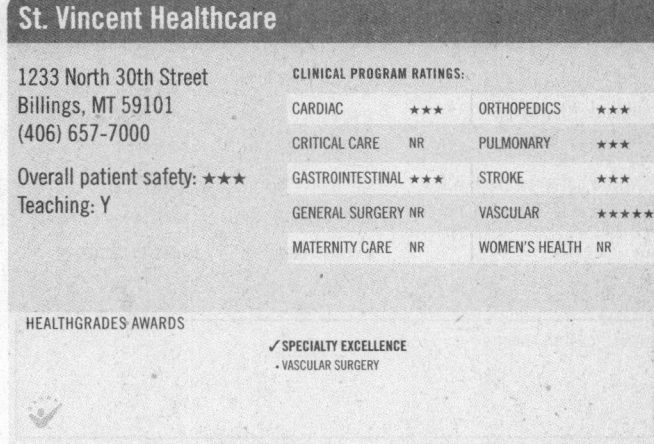

St. Vincent Healthcare

1233 North 30th Street
Billings, MT 59101
(406) 657-7000

Overall patient safety: ★★★
Teaching: Y

CLINICAL PROGRAM RATINGS:

CARDIAC	★★★	ORTHOPEDICS	★★★
CRITICAL CARE	NR	PULMONARY	★★★
GASTROINTESTINAL	★★★	STROKE	★★★
GENERAL SURGERY	NR	VASCULAR	★★★★★
MATERNITY CARE	NR	WOMEN'S HEALTH	NR

HEALTHGRADES AWARDS

✓ SPECIALTY EXCELLENCE
- VASCULAR SURGERY

St. Peter's Hospital

2475 Broadway Street
Helena, MT 59601
(406) 442-2480

Overall patient safety: ★★★
Teaching: N

CLINICAL PROGRAM RATINGS:

CARDIAC	NR	ORTHOPEDICS	★★★
CRITICAL CARE	NR	PULMONARY	★
GASTROINTESTINAL	★★★	STROKE	★
GENERAL SURGERY	NR	VASCULAR	NR
MATERNITY CARE	NR	WOMEN'S HEALTH	NR

HEALTHGRADES AWARDS

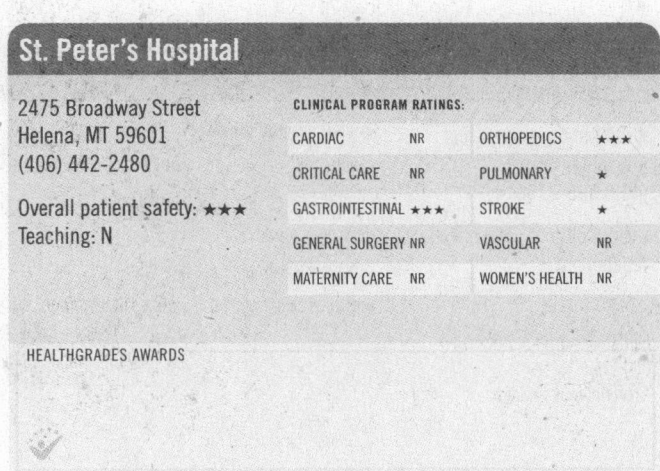

Sidney Health Center

216 14th Avenue Southwest
Sidney, MT 59270
(406) 488-2100

Overall patient safety: ★★★
Teaching: N

CLINICAL PROGRAM RATINGS:

CARDIAC	NR	ORTHOPEDICS	NR
CRITICAL CARE	NR	PULMONARY	★★★
GASTROINTESTINAL	NR	STROKE	★★★
GENERAL SURGERY	NR	VASCULAR	NR
MATERNITY CARE	NR	WOMEN'S HEALTH	NR

HEALTHGRADES AWARDS

NEBRASKA HOSPITALS: RATINGS BY CLINICAL SPECIALTY

Alegent Health—Bergan Mercy Medical Center

7500 Mercy Road
Omaha, NE 68124
(402) 398-6060

Overall patient safety: ★★★
Teaching: Y

CLINICAL PROGRAM RATINGS:

CARDIAC	★★★	ORTHOPEDICS	★★★
CRITICAL CARE	NR	PULMONARY	★★★★★
GASTROINTESTINAL	★★★	STROKE	★★★
GENERAL SURGERY	NR	VASCULAR	★★★
MATERNITY CARE	NR	WOMEN'S HEALTH	NR

HEALTHGRADES AWARDS

✓ SPECIALTY EXCELLENCE
- PULMONARY CARE

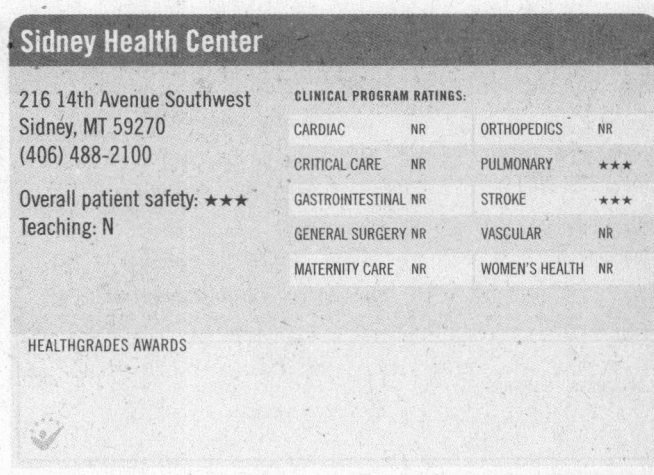

Alegent Health—Immanuel Medical Center

6901 North 72nd Street
Omaha, NE 68122
(402) 572-2121

Overall patient safety: ★★★
Teaching: Y

CLINICAL PROGRAM RATINGS:

CARDIAC	★★★	ORTHOPEDICS	★★★★★
CRITICAL CARE	NR	PULMONARY	★★★
GASTROINTESTINAL	★★★	STROKE	★★★
GENERAL SURGERY	NR	VASCULAR	NR
MATERNITY CARE	NR	WOMEN'S HEALTH	NR

HEALTHGRADES AWARDS

✓ SPECIALTY EXCELLENCE
- ORTHOPEDIC SURGERY

*This hospital reports its data to the federal government jointly with another hospital. Therefore the ratings and awards apply to multiple hospitals and this specific hospital may not provide all rated services.

Alegent Health–Lakeside Hospital

16901 Lakeside Hills Court
Omaha, NE 68130
(402) 717-8000

Overall patient safety: ★★★
Teaching: N

CLINICAL PROGRAM RATINGS:

CARDIAC	NR	ORTHOPEDICS	NR
CRITICAL CARE	NR	PULMONARY	★★★
GASTROINTESTINAL	NR	STROKE	★★★
GENERAL SURGERY	NR	VASCULAR	NR
MATERNITY CARE	NR	WOMEN'S HEALTH	NR

HEALTHGRADES AWARDS

Beatrice Community Hospital and Health Center

1110 North 10th Street
P.O. Box 278
Beatrice, NE 68310
(402) 228-3344

Overall patient safety: ★★★
Teaching: N

CLINICAL PROGRAM RATINGS:

CARDIAC	NR	ORTHOPEDICS	NR
CRITICAL CARE	NR	PULMONARY	★★★
GASTROINTESTINAL	NR	STROKE	★
GENERAL SURGERY	NR	VASCULAR	NR
MATERNITY CARE	NR	WOMEN'S HEALTH	NR

HEALTHGRADES AWARDS

Alegent Health–Midlands Community Hospital

11111 South 84th Street
Papillion, NE 68046
(402) 593-3000

Overall patient safety: ★
Teaching: N

CLINICAL PROGRAM RATINGS:

CARDIAC	NR	ORTHOPEDICS	NR
CRITICAL CARE	NR	PULMONARY	★★★
GASTROINTESTINAL	★★★	STROKE	★
GENERAL SURGERY	NR	VASCULAR	NR
MATERNITY CARE	NR	WOMEN'S HEALTH	NR

HEALTHGRADES AWARDS

Boone County Health Center

723 West Fairview Street
Albion, NE 68620
(402) 395-2191

Overall patient safety: ★★★
Teaching: N

CLINICAL PROGRAM RATINGS:

CARDIAC	NR	ORTHOPEDICS	NR
CRITICAL CARE	NR	PULMONARY	★★★
GASTROINTESTINAL	NR	STROKE	★
GENERAL SURGERY	NR	VASCULAR	NR
MATERNITY CARE	NR	WOMEN'S HEALTH	NR

HEALTHGRADES AWARDS

Avera St. Anthony's Hospital

300 North 2nd Street
Oneill, NE 68763
(402) 336-2611

Overall patient safety: ★★★
Teaching: N

CLINICAL PROGRAM RATINGS:

CARDIAC	NR	ORTHOPEDICS	NR
CRITICAL CARE	NR	PULMONARY	★
GASTROINTESTINAL	NR	STROKE	★
GENERAL SURGERY	NR	VASCULAR	NR
MATERNITY CARE	NR	WOMEN'S HEALTH	NR

HEALTHGRADES AWARDS

Box Butte General Hospital

2101 Box Butte Avenue
Alliance, NE 69301
(308) 762-6660

Overall patient safety: ★★★
Teaching: N

CLINICAL PROGRAM RATINGS:

CARDIAC	NR	ORTHOPEDICS	NR
CRITICAL CARE	NR	PULMONARY	★★★
GASTROINTESTINAL	NR	STROKE	NR
GENERAL SURGERY	NR	VASCULAR	NR
MATERNITY CARE	NR	WOMEN'S HEALTH	NR

HEALTHGRADES AWARDS

KEY: ★★★★★ BEST   ★★★ AS EXPECTED   ★ POOR   NR NOT RATED BY HEALTHGRADES   For full definitions of ratings and awards, see Appendix.

Brodstone Memorial Nuckolls County Hospital

520 East 10th Street
Superior, NE 68978
(402) 879-3281

Overall patient safety: ★★★
Teaching: N

CLINICAL PROGRAM RATINGS:

CARDIAC	NR	ORTHOPEDICS	NR
CRITICAL CARE	NR	PULMONARY	★★★
GASTROINTESTINAL	NR	STROKE	★★★
GENERAL SURGERY	NR	VASCULAR	NR
MATERNITY CARE	NR	WOMEN'S HEALTH	NR

HEALTHGRADES AWARDS

Butler County Health Care Center

372 South 9th Street
David City, NE 68632
(402) 367-1200

Overall patient safety: ★★★
Teaching: N

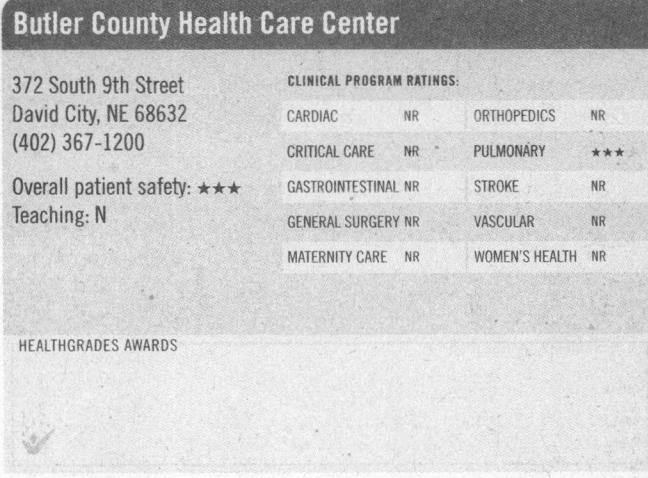

CLINICAL PROGRAM RATINGS:

CARDIAC	NR	ORTHOPEDICS	NR
CRITICAL CARE	NR	PULMONARY	★★★
GASTROINTESTINAL	NR	STROKE	NR
GENERAL SURGERY	NR	VASCULAR	NR
MATERNITY CARE	NR	WOMEN'S HEALTH	NR

HEALTHGRADES AWARDS

Bryanlgh Medical Center*

1600 South 48th Street
Lincoln, NE 68506
(402) 489-0200

Overall patient safety: ★★★
Teaching: Y

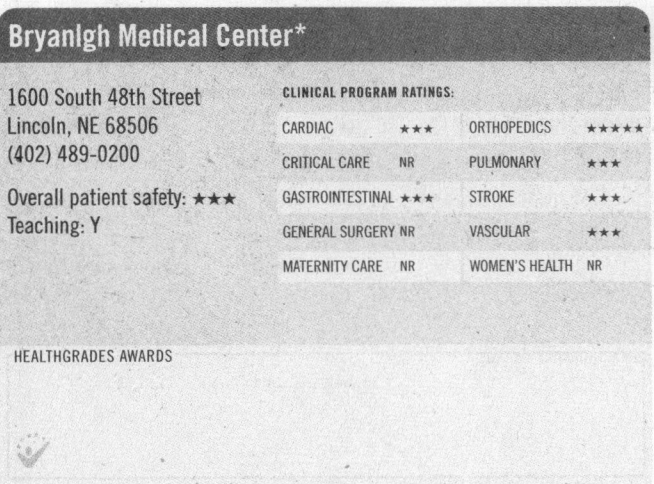

CLINICAL PROGRAM RATINGS:

CARDIAC	★★★	ORTHOPEDICS	★★★★★
CRITICAL CARE	NR	PULMONARY	★★★
GASTROINTESTINAL	★★★	STROKE	★★★
GENERAL SURGERY	NR	VASCULAR	★★★
MATERNITY CARE	NR	WOMEN'S HEALTH	NR

HEALTHGRADES AWARDS

Chase County Community Hospital

600 West 12th Street
Imperial, NE 69033
(308) 882-7111

Overall patient safety: ★★★
Teaching: N

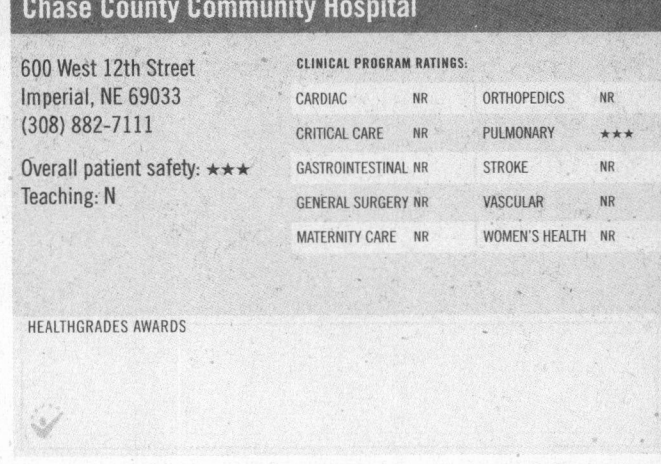

CLINICAL PROGRAM RATINGS:

CARDIAC	NR	ORTHOPEDICS	NR
CRITICAL CARE	NR	PULMONARY	★★★
GASTROINTESTINAL	NR	STROKE	NR
GENERAL SURGERY	NR	VASCULAR	NR
MATERNITY CARE	NR	WOMEN'S HEALTH	NR

HEALTHGRADES AWARDS

Bryanlgh Medical Center—West*

2300 South 16th Street
Lincoln, NE 68502
(402) 475-1011

Overall patient safety: ★★★
Teaching: Y

CLINICAL PROGRAM RATINGS:

CARDIAC	★★★	ORTHOPEDICS	★★★★★
CRITICAL CARE	NR	PULMONARY	★★★
GASTROINTESTINAL	★★★	STROKE	★★★
GENERAL SURGERY	NR	VASCULAR	★★★
MATERNITY CARE	NR	WOMEN'S HEALTH	NR

HEALTHGRADES AWARDS

Clarkson Bishop Memorial Hospital*

Dewey Avenue at 44th Street
Omaha, NE 68105
(402) 559-3203

Overall patient safety: ★★★
Teaching: Y

CLINICAL PROGRAM RATINGS:

CARDIAC	★★★	ORTHOPEDICS	★★★
CRITICAL CARE	NR	PULMONARY	★
GASTROINTESTINAL	★★★	STROKE	★★★
GENERAL SURGERY	NR	VASCULAR	★★★
MATERNITY CARE	NR	WOMEN'S HEALTH	NR

HEALTHGRADES AWARDS

*This hospital reports its data to the federal government jointly with another hospital. Therefore the ratings and awards apply to multiple hospitals and this specific hospital may not provide all rated services.

Columbus Community Hospital

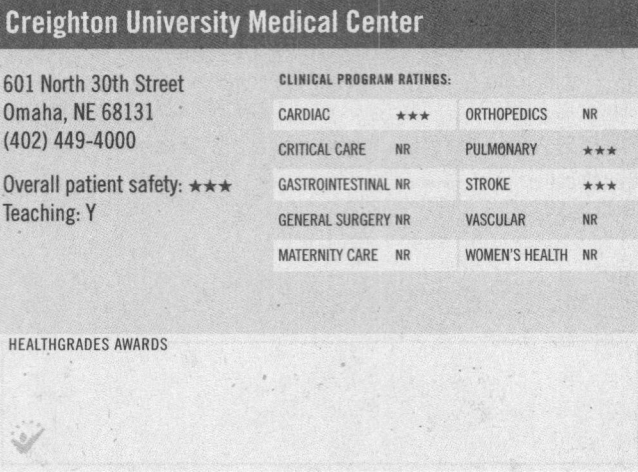

3020 38th Street
Columbus, NE 68601
(402) 564-7118

Overall patient safety: ★★★
Teaching: N

CLINICAL PROGRAM RATINGS:

CARDIAC	NR	ORTHOPEDICS	NR
CRITICAL CARE	NR	PULMONARY	★
GASTROINTESTINAL	NR	STROKE	★★★
GENERAL SURGERY	NR	VASCULAR	NR
MATERNITY CARE	NR	WOMEN'S HEALTH	NR

HEALTHGRADES AWARDS

Creighton University Medical Center

601 North 30th Street
Omaha, NE 68131
(402) 449-4000

Overall patient safety: ★★★
Teaching: Y

CLINICAL PROGRAM RATINGS:

CARDIAC	★★★	ORTHOPEDICS	NR
CRITICAL CARE	NR	PULMONARY	★★★
GASTROINTESTINAL	NR	STROKE	★★★
GENERAL SURGERY	NR	VASCULAR	NR
MATERNITY CARE	NR	WOMEN'S HEALTH	NR

HEALTHGRADES AWARDS

Community Hospital

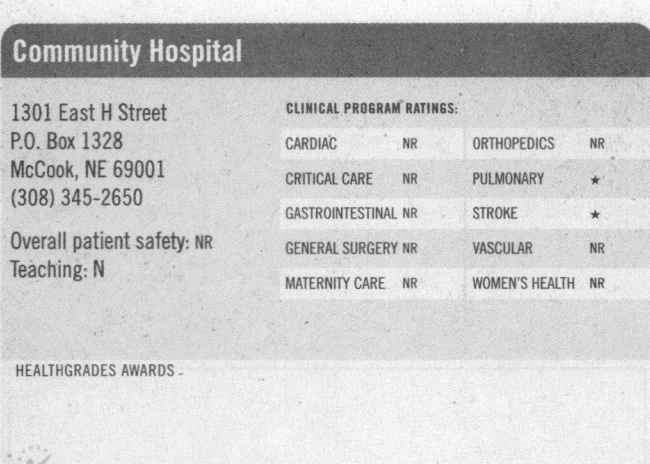

1301 East H Street
P.O. Box 1328
McCook, NE 69001
(308) 345-2650

Overall patient safety: NR
Teaching: N

CLINICAL PROGRAM RATINGS:

CARDIAC	NR	ORTHOPEDICS	NR
CRITICAL CARE	NR	PULMONARY	★
GASTROINTESTINAL	NR	STROKE	★
GENERAL SURGERY	NR	VASCULAR	NR
MATERNITY CARE	NR	WOMEN'S HEALTH	NR

HEALTHGRADES AWARDS

Faith Regional Health Services*

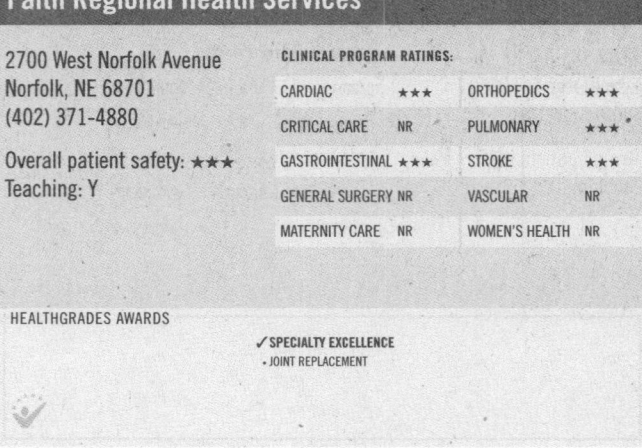

2700 West Norfolk Avenue
Norfolk, NE 68701
(402) 371-4880

Overall patient safety: ★★★
Teaching: Y

CLINICAL PROGRAM RATINGS:

CARDIAC	★★★	ORTHOPEDICS	★★★
CRITICAL CARE	NR	PULMONARY	★★★
GASTROINTESTINAL	★★★	STROKE	★★★
GENERAL SURGERY	NR	VASCULAR	NR
MATERNITY CARE	NR	WOMEN'S HEALTH	NR

HEALTHGRADES AWARDS

✓ SPECIALTY EXCELLENCE
• JOINT REPLACEMENT

Community Medical Center

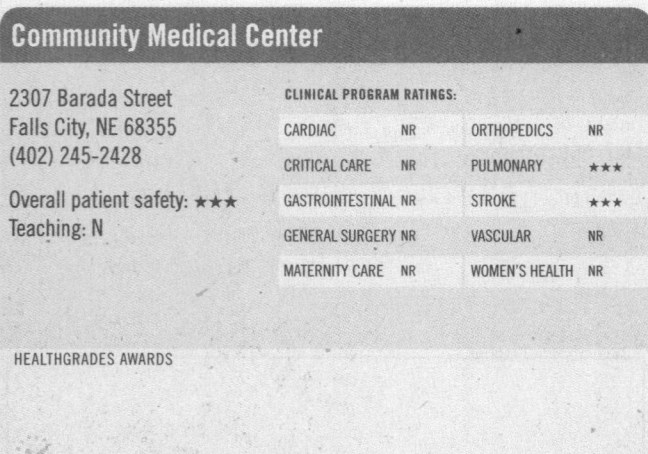

2307 Barada Street
Falls City, NE 68355
(402) 245-2428

Overall patient safety: ★★★
Teaching: N

CLINICAL PROGRAM RATINGS:

CARDIAC	NR	ORTHOPEDICS	NR
CRITICAL CARE	NR	PULMONARY	★★★
GASTROINTESTINAL	NR	STROKE	★★★
GENERAL SURGERY	NR	VASCULAR	NR
MATERNITY CARE	NR	WOMEN'S HEALTH	NR

HEALTHGRADES AWARDS

Fremont Area Medical Center

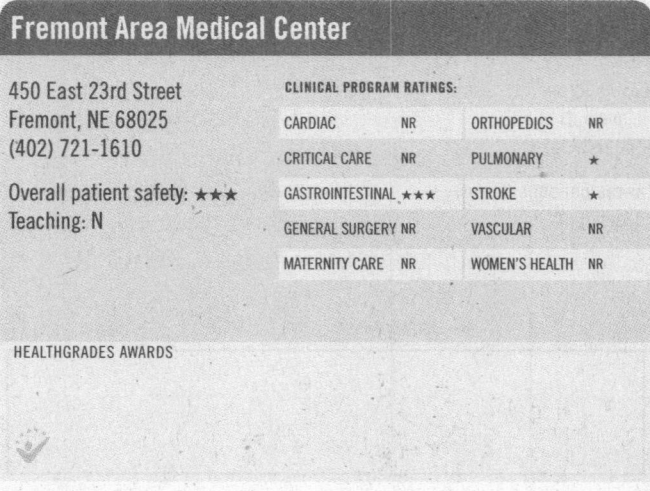

450 East 23rd Street
Fremont, NE 68025
(402) 721-1610

Overall patient safety: ★★★
Teaching: N

CLINICAL PROGRAM RATINGS:

CARDIAC	NR	ORTHOPEDICS	NR
CRITICAL CARE	NR	PULMONARY	★
GASTROINTESTINAL	★★★	STROKE	★
GENERAL SURGERY	NR	VASCULAR	NR
MATERNITY CARE	NR	WOMEN'S HEALTH	NR

HEALTHGRADES AWARDS

KEY: ★★★★★ BEST   ★★★ AS EXPECTED   ★ POOR   NR NOT RATED BY HEALTHGRADES   For full definitions of ratings and awards, see Appendix.

Good Samaritan Hospital

10 East 31st Street
Kearney, NE 68847
(308) 865-7100

Overall patient safety: ★★★
Teaching: Y

CLINICAL PROGRAM RATINGS:

CARDIAC	★★★	ORTHOPEDICS	★★★
CRITICAL CARE	NR	PULMONARY	★
GASTROINTESTINAL	★★★	STROKE	★★★
GENERAL SURGERY	NR	VASCULAR	NR
MATERNITY CARE	NR	WOMEN'S HEALTH	NR

HEALTHGRADES AWARDS

Jefferson Community Health Center

2200 North H Street
Fairbury, NE 68352
(402) 729-3351

Overall patient safety: ★★★
Teaching: N

CLINICAL PROGRAM RATINGS:

CARDIAC	NR	ORTHOPEDICS	NR
CRITICAL CARE	NR	PULMONARY	★★★
GASTROINTESTINAL	NR	STROKE	NR
GENERAL SURGERY	NR	VASCULAR	NR
MATERNITY CARE	NR	WOMEN'S HEALTH	NR

HEALTHGRADES AWARDS

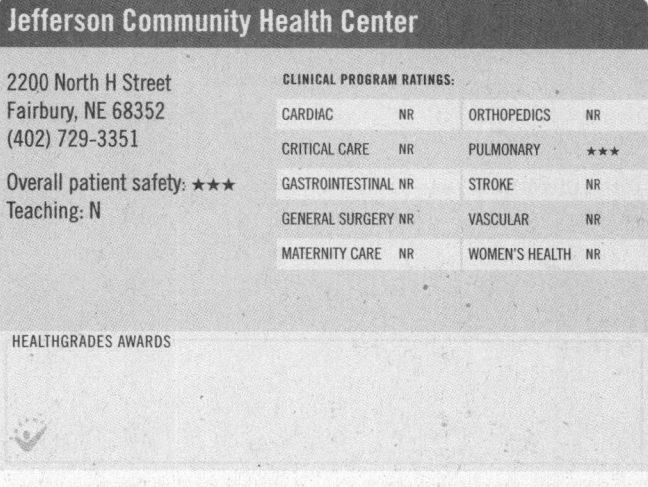

Great Plains Regional Medical Center

601 West Leota Street
North Platte, NE 69101
(308) 534-9310

Overall patient safety: ★★★
Teaching: Y

CLINICAL PROGRAM RATINGS:

CARDIAC	NR	ORTHOPEDICS	NR
CRITICAL CARE	NR	PULMONARY	★★★
GASTROINTESTINAL	NR	STROKE	★
GENERAL SURGERY	NR	VASCULAR	NR
MATERNITY CARE	NR	WOMEN'S HEALTH	NR

HEALTHGRADES AWARDS

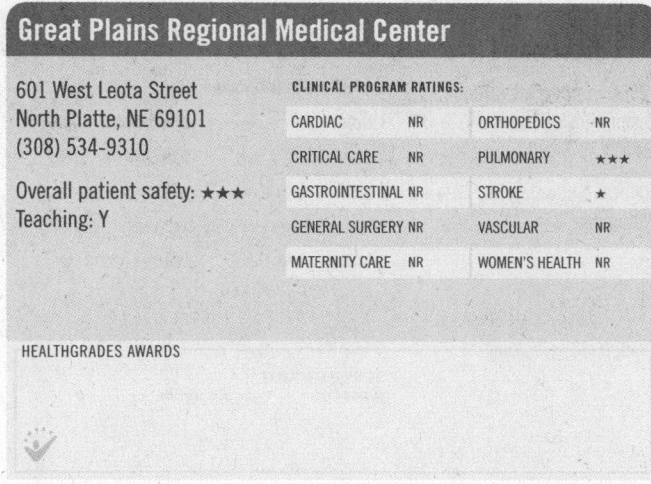

Jennie M. Melham Memorial Medical Center

145 Memorial Drive
Broken Bow, NE 68822
(308) 872-6891

Overall patient safety: ★★★
Teaching: N

CLINICAL PROGRAM RATINGS:

CARDIAC	NR	ORTHOPEDICS	NR
CRITICAL CARE	NR	PULMONARY	★★★
GASTROINTESTINAL	NR	STROKE	NR
GENERAL SURGERY	NR	VASCULAR	NR
MATERNITY CARE	NR	WOMEN'S HEALTH	NR

HEALTHGRADES AWARDS

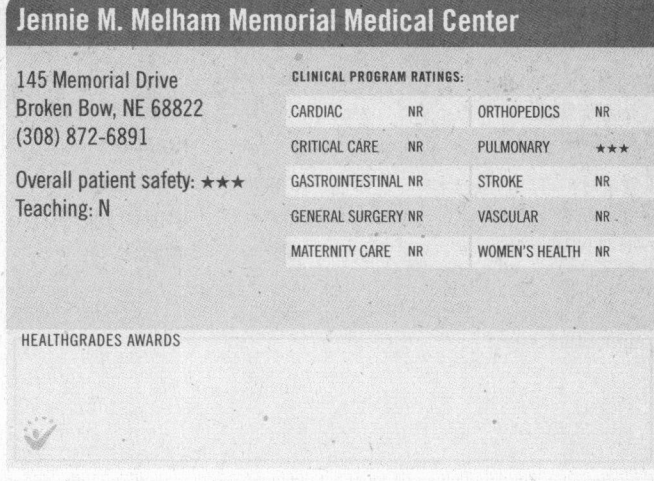

Howard County Community Hospital

1113 Sherman Street
St. Paul, NE 68873
(308) 754-4421

Overall patient safety: ★★★
Teaching: N

CLINICAL PROGRAM RATINGS:

CARDIAC	NR	ORTHOPEDICS	NR
CRITICAL CARE	NR	PULMONARY	★★★
GASTROINTESTINAL	NR	STROKE	NR
GENERAL SURGERY	NR	VASCULAR	NR
MATERNITY CARE	NR	WOMEN'S HEALTH	NR

HEALTHGRADES AWARDS

Lutheran Community Hospital*

2700 Norfolk Avenue
Norfolk, NE 68701
(402) 644-7528

Overall patient safety: ★★★
Teaching: Y

CLINICAL PROGRAM RATINGS:

CARDIAC	★★★	ORTHOPEDICS	★★★
CRITICAL CARE	NR	PULMONARY	★★★
GASTROINTESTINAL	★★★	STROKE	★★★
GENERAL SURGERY	NR	VASCULAR	NR
MATERNITY CARE	NR	WOMEN'S HEALTH	NR

HEALTHGRADES AWARDS

✓ SPECIALTY EXCELLENCE
· JOINT REPLACEMENT

*This hospital reports its data to the federal government jointly with another hospital. Therefore the ratings and awards apply to multiple hospitals and this specific hospital may not provide all rated services.

Mary Lanning Memorial Hospital

715 North St. Joseph Avenue
Hastings, NE 68901
(402) 463-4521

Overall patient safety: ★★★
Teaching: N

CLINICAL PROGRAM RATINGS:

CARDIAC	NR	ORTHOPEDICS	★
CRITICAL CARE	NR	PULMONARY	★★★
GASTROINTESTINAL	★★★	STROKE	★★★
GENERAL SURGERY	NR	VASCULAR	NR
MATERNITY CARE	NR	WOMEN'S HEALTH	NR

HEALTHGRADES AWARDS

Memorial Hospital

1423 7th Street
Aurora, NE 68818
(402) 694-3171

Overall patient safety: ★★★
Teaching: N

CLINICAL PROGRAM RATINGS:

CARDIAC	NR	ORTHOPEDICS	NR
CRITICAL CARE	NR	PULMONARY	★
GASTROINTESTINAL	NR	STROKE	NR
GENERAL SURGERY	NR	VASCULAR	NR
MATERNITY CARE	NR	WOMEN'S HEALTH	NR

HEALTHGRADES AWARDS

Memorial Community Hospital

810 North 22nd Street
Blair, NE 68008
(402) 426-1199

Overall patient safety: ★★★
Teaching: N

CLINICAL PROGRAM RATINGS:

CARDIAC	NR	ORTHOPEDICS	NR
CRITICAL CARE	NR	PULMONARY	★
GASTROINTESTINAL	NR	STROKE	★★★
GENERAL SURGERY	NR	VASCULAR	NR
MATERNITY CARE	NR	WOMEN'S HEALTH	NR

HEALTHGRADES AWARDS

Nebraska Heart Hospital

7500 South 91st Street
Lincoln, NE 68526
(402) 327-2700

Overall patient safety: ★★★★★
Teaching: N

CLINICAL PROGRAM RATINGS:

CARDIAC	★★★	ORTHOPEDICS	NR
CRITICAL CARE	NR	PULMONARY	NR
GASTROINTESTINAL	NR	STROKE	NR
GENERAL SURGERY	NR	VASCULAR	★★★
MATERNITY CARE	NR	WOMEN'S HEALTH	NR

HEALTHGRADES AWARDS

✓ SPECIALTY EXCELLENCE
- CARDIAC CARE   - VASCULAR SURGERY

Memorial Health Care Systems

300 North Columbia Avenue
Seward, NE 68434
(402) 643-2971

Overall patient safety: ★★★
Teaching: N

CLINICAL PROGRAM RATINGS:

CARDIAC	NR	ORTHOPEDICS	NR
CRITICAL CARE	NR	PULMONARY	NR
GASTROINTESTINAL	NR	STROKE	★
GENERAL SURGERY	NR	VASCULAR	NR
MATERNITY CARE	NR	WOMEN'S HEALTH	NR

HEALTHGRADES AWARDS

Nebraska Medical Center*

4350 Dewey Avenue
Omaha, NE 68198
(402) 559-2000

Overall patient safety: ★★★
Teaching: Y

CLINICAL PROGRAM RATINGS:

CARDIAC	★★★	ORTHOPEDICS	★★★
CRITICAL CARE	NR	PULMONARY	★
GASTROINTESTINAL	★★★	STROKE	★★★
GENERAL SURGERY	NR	VASCULAR	★★★
MATERNITY CARE	NR	WOMEN'S HEALTH	NR

HEALTHGRADES AWARDS

KEY: ★★★★★ BEST   ★★★ AS EXPECTED   ★ POOR   NR NOT RATED BY HEALTHGRADES   For full definitions of ratings and awards, see Appendix.

Nebraska Methodist Hospital

8303 Dodge Street
Omaha, NE 68114
(402) 354-4000

Overall patient safety: ★★★
Teaching: Y

CLINICAL PROGRAM RATINGS:

CARDIAC	★★★	ORTHOPEDICS	★
CRITICAL CARE	NR	PULMONARY	★★★
GASTROINTESTINAL	★★★	STROKE	★★★
GENERAL SURGERY	NR	VASCULAR	★★★
MATERNITY CARE	NR	WOMEN'S HEALTH	NR

HEALTHGRADES AWARDS

Pender Community Hospital

603 Earl Street
Pender, NE 68047
(402) 385-3083

Overall patient safety: ★
Teaching: N

CLINICAL PROGRAM RATINGS:

CARDIAC	NR	ORTHOPEDICS	NR
CRITICAL CARE	NR	PULMONARY	NR
GASTROINTESTINAL	NR	STROKE	★★★
GENERAL SURGERY	NR	VASCULAR	NR
MATERNITY CARE	NR	WOMEN'S HEALTH	NR

HEALTHGRADES AWARDS

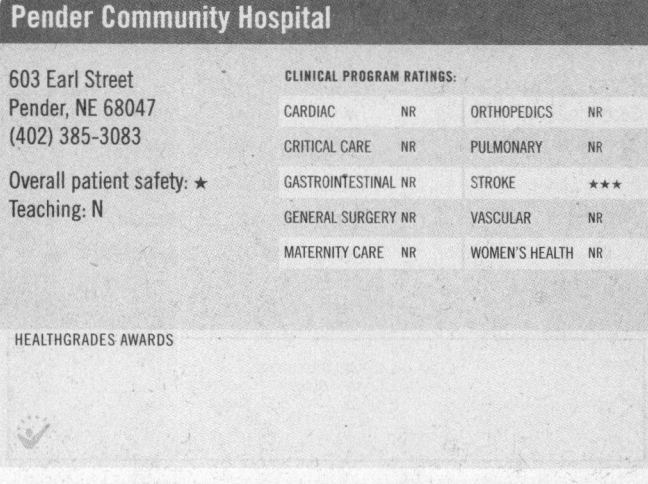

Osmond General Hospital

5th and Maple Streets
Osmond, NE 68765
(402) 748-3393

Overall patient safety: ★★★
Teaching: N

CLINICAL PROGRAM RATINGS:

CARDIAC	NR	ORTHOPEDICS	NR
CRITICAL CARE	NR	PULMONARY	NR
GASTROINTESTINAL	NR	STROKE	★★★
GENERAL SURGERY	NR	VASCULAR	NR
MATERNITY CARE	NR	WOMEN'S HEALTH	NR

HEALTHGRADES AWARDS

Phelps Memorial Health Center

1215 Tibbals Street
Holdrege, NE 68949
(308) 995-2211

Overall patient safety: NR
Teaching: N

CLINICAL PROGRAM RATINGS:

CARDIAC	NR	ORTHOPEDICS	NR
CRITICAL CARE	NR	PULMONARY	★
GASTROINTESTINAL	NR	STROKE	NR
GENERAL SURGERY	NR	VASCULAR	NR
MATERNITY CARE	NR	WOMEN'S HEALTH	NR

HEALTHGRADES AWARDS

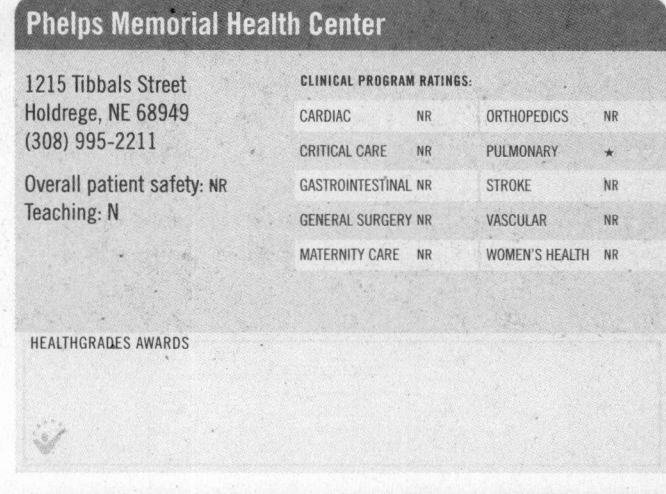

Our Lady of Lourdes Hospital*

1500 Koenigstein Avenue
Norfolk, NE 68701
(402) 371-4880

Overall patient safety: ★★★
Teaching: Y

CLINICAL PROGRAM RATINGS:

CARDIAC	★★★	ORTHOPEDICS	★★★
CRITICAL CARE	NR	PULMONARY	★★★
GASTROINTESTINAL	★★★	STROKE	★★★
GENERAL SURGERY	NR	VASCULAR	NR
MATERNITY CARE	NR	WOMEN'S HEALTH	NR

HEALTHGRADES AWARDS

✓ SPECIALTY EXCELLENCE
· JOINT REPLACEMENT

Providence Medical Center

1200 Providence Road
Wayne, NE 68787
(402) 375-3800

Overall patient safety: ★★★
Teaching: N

CLINICAL PROGRAM RATINGS:

CARDIAC	NR	ORTHOPEDICS	NR
CRITICAL CARE	NR	PULMONARY	★★★
GASTROINTESTINAL	NR	STROKE	NR
GENERAL SURGERY	NR	VASCULAR	NR
MATERNITY CARE	NR	WOMEN'S HEALTH	NR

HEALTHGRADES AWARDS

*This hospital reports its data to the federal government jointly with another hospital. Therefore the ratings and awards apply to multiple hospitals and this specific hospital may not provide all rated services.

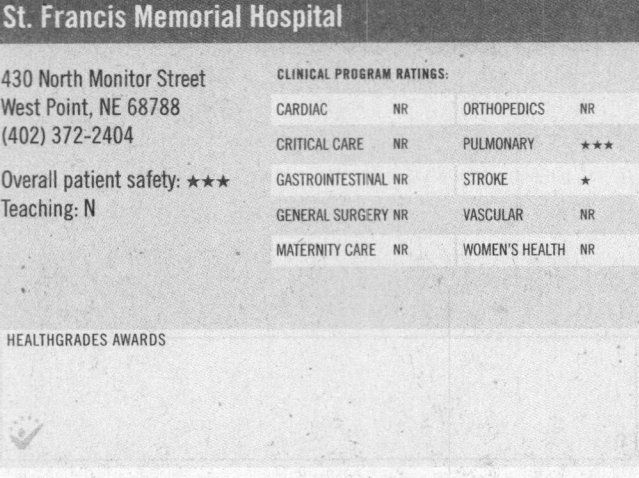

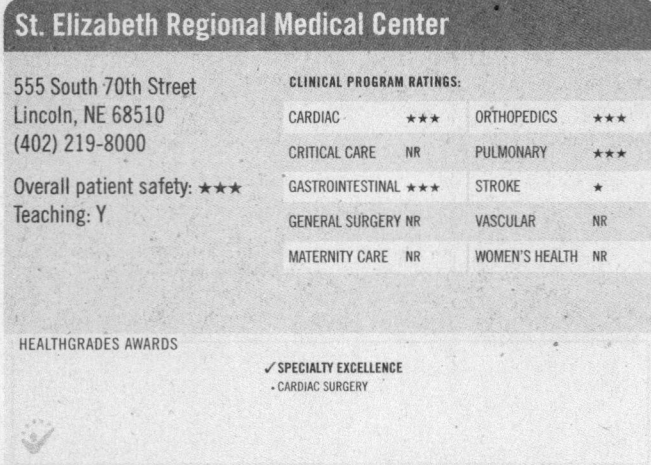

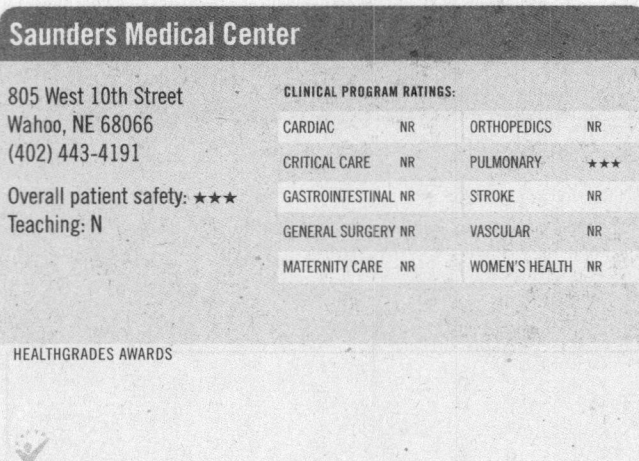

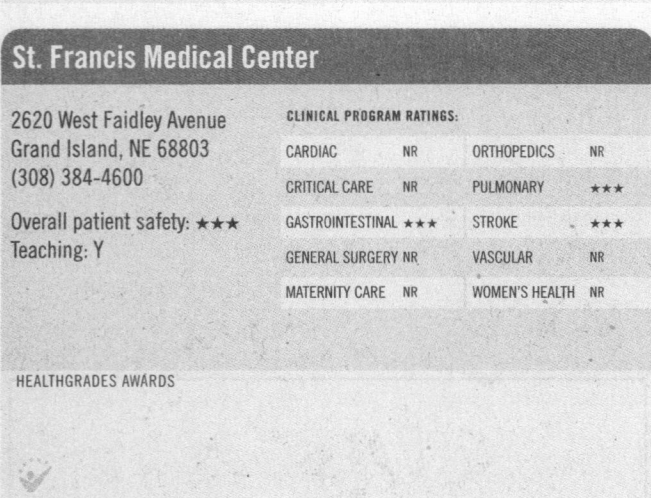

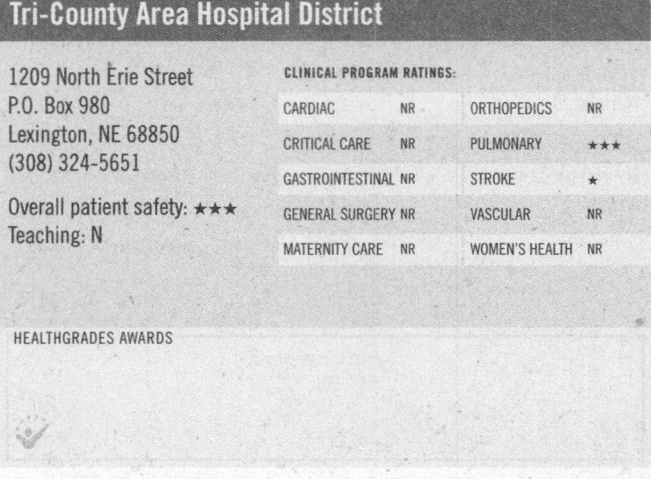

Regional West Medical Center

4021 Avenue B
Scottsbluff, NE 69361
(308) 635-3711

Overall patient safety: ★★★
Teaching: Y

CLINICAL PROGRAM RATINGS:

CARDIAC	NR	ORTHOPEDICS	★★★★★
CRITICAL CARE	NR	PULMONARY	★
GASTROINTESTINAL	★★★	STROKE	★★★
GENERAL SURGERY	NR	VASCULAR	NR
MATERNITY CARE	NR	WOMEN'S HEALTH	NR

HEALTHGRADES AWARDS

✓ SPECIALTY EXCELLENCE
· JOINT REPLACEMENT · ORTHOPEDIC SURGERY

St. Francis Memorial Hospital

430 North Monitor Street
West Point, NE 68788
(402) 372-2404

Overall patient safety: ★★★
Teaching: N

CLINICAL PROGRAM RATINGS:

CARDIAC	NR	ORTHOPEDICS	NR
CRITICAL CARE	NR	PULMONARY	★★★
GASTROINTESTINAL	NR	STROKE	★
GENERAL SURGERY	NR	VASCULAR	NR
MATERNITY CARE	NR	WOMEN'S HEALTH	NR

HEALTHGRADES AWARDS

St. Elizabeth Regional Medical Center

555 South 70th Street
Lincoln, NE 68510
(402) 219-8000

Overall patient safety: ★★★
Teaching: Y

CLINICAL PROGRAM RATINGS:

CARDIAC	★★★	ORTHOPEDICS	★★★
CRITICAL CARE	NR	PULMONARY	★★★
GASTROINTESTINAL	★★★	STROKE	★
GENERAL SURGERY	NR	VASCULAR	NR
MATERNITY CARE	NR	WOMEN'S HEALTH	NR

HEALTHGRADES AWARDS

✓ SPECIALTY EXCELLENCE
· CARDIAC SURGERY

Saunders Medical Center

805 West 10th Street
Wahoo, NE 68066
(402) 443-4191

Overall patient safety: ★★★
Teaching: N

CLINICAL PROGRAM RATINGS:

CARDIAC	NR	ORTHOPEDICS	NR
CRITICAL CARE	NR	PULMONARY	★★★
GASTROINTESTINAL	NR	STROKE	NR
GENERAL SURGERY	NR	VASCULAR	NR
MATERNITY CARE	NR	WOMEN'S HEALTH	NR

HEALTHGRADES AWARDS

St. Francis Medical Center

2620 West Faidley Avenue
Grand Island, NE 68803
(308) 384-4600

Overall patient safety: ★★★
Teaching: Y

CLINICAL PROGRAM RATINGS:

CARDIAC	NR	ORTHOPEDICS	NR
CRITICAL CARE	NR	PULMONARY	★★★
GASTROINTESTINAL	★★★	STROKE	★★★
GENERAL SURGERY	NR	VASCULAR	NR
MATERNITY CARE	NR	WOMEN'S HEALTH	NR

HEALTHGRADES AWARDS

Tri-County Area Hospital District

1209 North Erie Street
P.O. Box 980
Lexington, NE 68850
(308) 324-5651

Overall patient safety: ★★★
Teaching: N

CLINICAL PROGRAM RATINGS:

CARDIAC	NR	ORTHOPEDICS	NR
CRITICAL CARE	NR	PULMONARY	★★★
GASTROINTESTINAL	NR	STROKE	★
GENERAL SURGERY	NR	VASCULAR	NR
MATERNITY CARE	NR	WOMEN'S HEALTH	NR

HEALTHGRADES AWARDS

NEBRASKA HOSPITALS: RATINGS BY CLINICAL SPECIALTY

KEY: ★★★★★ BEST   ★★★ AS EXPECTED   ★ POOR   NR NOT RATED BY HEALTHGRADES   For full definitions of ratings and awards, see Appendix.

York General Hospital

2222 Lincoln Avenue
York, NE 68467
(402) 362-6671

Overall patient safety: ★★★
Teaching: N

CLINICAL PROGRAM RATINGS:

CARDIAC	NR	ORTHOPEDICS	NR
CRITICAL CARE	NR	PULMONARY	★
GASTROINTESTINAL	NR	STROKE	NR
GENERAL SURGERY	NR	VASCULAR	NR
MATERNITY CARE	NR	WOMEN'S HEALTH	NR

HEALTHGRADES AWARDS

NEVADA HOSPITALS: RATINGS BY CLINICAL SPECIALTY

Carson Tahoe Regional Medical Center

775 Fleischmann Way
Carson City, NV 89703
(775) 882-1361

Overall patient safety: ★★★
Teaching: N

CLINICAL PROGRAM RATINGS:

CARDIAC	NR	ORTHOPEDICS	★
CRITICAL CARE	★★★	PULMONARY	★★★
GASTROINTESTINAL	★★★	STROKE	★
GENERAL SURGERY	★★★	VASCULAR	NR
MATERNITY CARE	★★★	WOMEN'S HEALTH	NR

HEALTHGRADES AWARDS

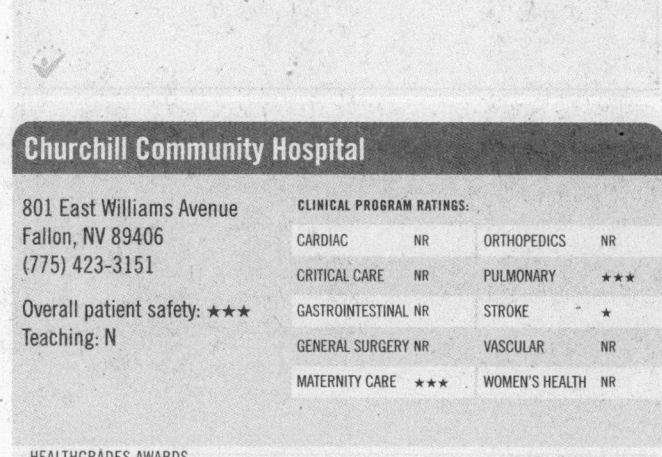

Desert Springs Hospital

2075 East Flamingo Road
Las Vegas, NV 89119
(702) 369-7610

Overall patient safety: ★
Teaching: N

CLINICAL PROGRAM RATINGS:

CARDIAC	★★★	ORTHOPEDICS	NR
CRITICAL CARE	★★★	PULMONARY	★★★
GASTROINTESTINAL	★★★	STROKE	★★★
GENERAL SURGERY	★★★	VASCULAR	NR
MATERNITY CARE	NR	WOMEN'S HEALTH	NR

HEALTHGRADES AWARDS

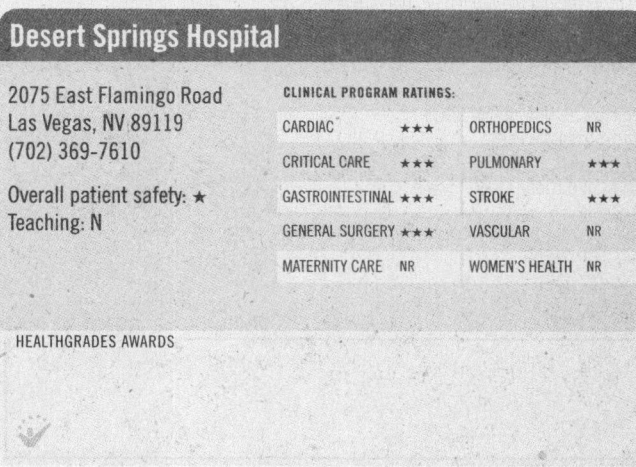

Churchill Community Hospital

801 East Williams Avenue
Fallon, NV 89406
(775) 423-3151

Overall patient safety: ★★★
Teaching: N

CLINICAL PROGRAM RATINGS:

CARDIAC	NR	ORTHOPEDICS	NR
CRITICAL CARE	NR	PULMONARY	★★★
GASTROINTESTINAL	NR	STROKE	★
GENERAL SURGERY	NR	VASCULAR	NR
MATERNITY CARE	★★★	WOMEN'S HEALTH	NR

HEALTHGRADES AWARDS

Mesa View Regional Hospital

1299 Bertha Howe Avenue
Mesquite, NV 89027
(702) 346-8040

Overall patient safety: ★★★
Teaching: N

CLINICAL PROGRAM RATINGS:

CARDIAC	NR	ORTHOPEDICS	NR
CRITICAL CARE	NR	PULMONARY	★★★
GASTROINTESTINAL	NR	STROKE	NR
GENERAL SURGERY	NR	VASCULAR	NR
MATERNITY CARE	★★★	WOMEN'S HEALTH	NR

HEALTHGRADES AWARDS

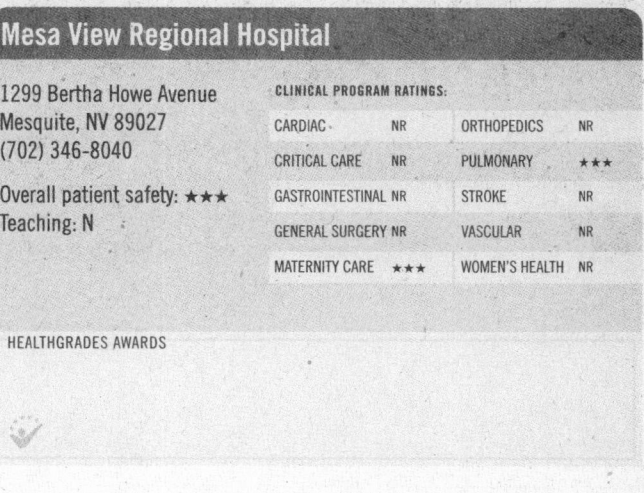

Mountainview Hospital

3100 North Tenaya Way
Las Vegas, NV 89128
(702) 255-5000

Overall patient safety: ★
Teaching: N

CLINICAL PROGRAM RATINGS:

CARDIAC	★	ORTHOPEDICS	★★★
CRITICAL CARE	★	PULMONARY	★★★
GASTROINTESTINAL	★★★	STROKE	★★★
GENERAL SURGERY	★★★	VASCULAR	NR
MATERNITY CARE	★★★★★	WOMEN'S HEALTH	★★★

HEALTHGRADES AWARDS

Northern Nevada Medical Center

2375 East Prater Way
Sparks, NV 89434
(775) 331-7000

Overall patient safety: ★
Teaching: N

CLINICAL PROGRAM RATINGS:

CARDIAC	NR	ORTHOPEDICS	★★★
CRITICAL CARE	NR	PULMONARY	★★★
GASTROINTESTINAL	NR	STROKE	★★★
GENERAL SURGERY	★	VASCULAR	NR
MATERNITY CARE	NR	WOMEN'S HEALTH	NR

HEALTHGRADES AWARDS

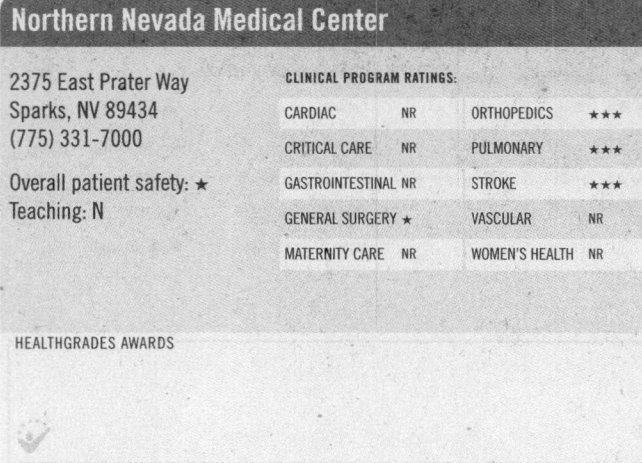

North Vista Hospital

1409 East Lake
Mead Boulevard
North Las Vegas, NV 89030
(702) 649-7711

Overall patient safety: ★★★
Teaching: Y

CLINICAL PROGRAM RATINGS:

CARDIAC	NR	ORTHOPEDICS	NR
CRITICAL CARE	NR	PULMONARY	★★★
GASTROINTESTINAL	NR	STROKE	★★★
GENERAL SURGERY	NR	VASCULAR	NR
MATERNITY CARE	★★★★★	WOMEN'S HEALTH	NR

HEALTHGRADES AWARDS

✓ SPECIALTY EXCELLENCE
· BARIATRIC SURGERY   · MATERNITY CARE

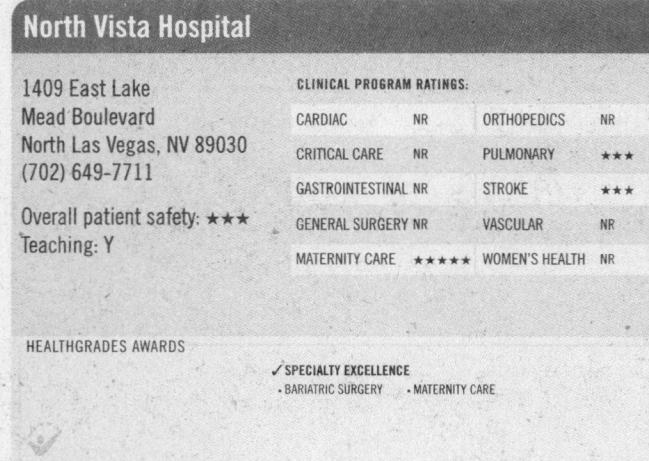

Renown Regional Medical Center

77 Pringle Way
Reno, NV 89502
(775) 982-4100

Overall patient safety: ★
Teaching: Y

CLINICAL PROGRAM RATINGS:

CARDIAC	★★★	ORTHOPEDICS	★
CRITICAL CARE	★★★	PULMONARY	★★★
GASTROINTESTINAL	★★★	STROKE	★★★
GENERAL SURGERY	★★★	VASCULAR	★★★
MATERNITY CARE	★★★	WOMEN'S HEALTH	★★★

HEALTHGRADES AWARDS

✓ SPECIALTY EXCELLENCE
· BARIATRIC SURGERY

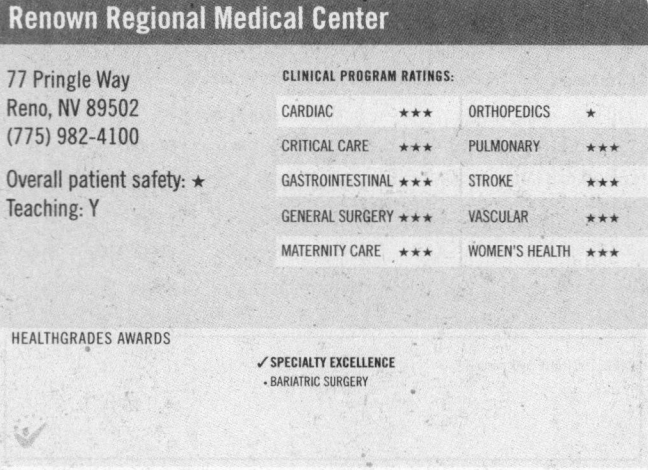

Northeastern Nevada Regional Hospital

2001 Errecart Boulevard
Elko, NV 89801
(775) 738-5151

Overall patient safety: ★★★
Teaching: N

CLINICAL PROGRAM RATINGS:

CARDIAC	NR	ORTHOPEDICS	NR
CRITICAL CARE	NR	PULMONARY	★★★
GASTROINTESTINAL	NR	STROKE	★
GENERAL SURGERY	★★★	VASCULAR	NR
MATERNITY CARE	★★★	WOMEN'S HEALTH	NR

HEALTHGRADES AWARDS

Renown South Meadows Medical Center

10101 Double R Boulevard
Reno, NV 89502
(772) 985-7000

Overall patient safety: ★★★
Teaching: N

CLINICAL PROGRAM RATINGS:

CARDIAC	NR	ORTHOPEDICS	NR
CRITICAL CARE	NR	PULMONARY	★★★
GASTROINTESTINAL	NR	STROKE	NR
GENERAL SURGERY	NR	VASCULAR	NR
MATERNITY CARE	NR	WOMEN'S HEALTH	NR

HEALTHGRADES AWARDS

KEY: ★★★★★ BEST   ★★★ AS EXPECTED   ★ POOR   NR NOT RATED BY HEALTHGRADES   For full definitions of ratings and awards, see Appendix.

St. Mary's Regional Medical Center

235 West 6th Street
Reno, NV 89503
(775) 770-3000

Overall patient safety: ★★★
Teaching: N

CLINICAL PROGRAM RATINGS:

CARDIAC	★★★	ORTHOPEDICS	★★★
CRITICAL CARE	NR	PULMONARY	★★★
GASTROINTESTINAL	★★★	STROKE	★
GENERAL SURGERY	★	VASCULAR	NR
MATERNITY CARE	★★★★★	WOMEN'S HEALTH	★★★

HEALTHGRADES AWARDS

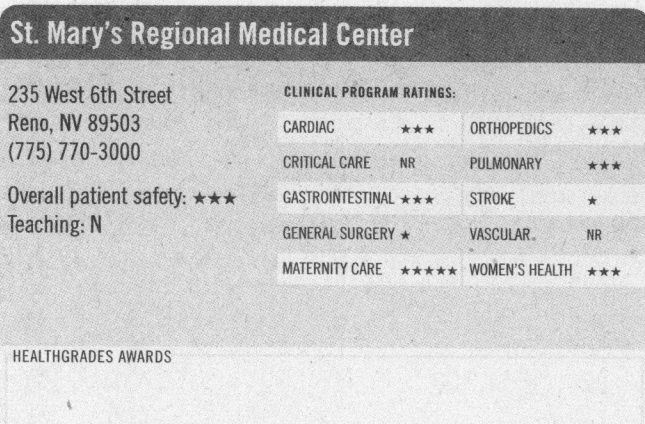

Southern Hills Hospital and Medical Center

9300 West Sunset
Las Vegas, NV 89148
(702) 880-2100

Overall patient safety: ★
Teaching: N

CLINICAL PROGRAM RATINGS:

CARDIAC	NR	ORTHOPEDICS	NR
CRITICAL CARE	NR	PULMONARY	★★★
GASTROINTESTINAL	NR	STROKE	★★★
GENERAL SURGERY	NR	VASCULAR	NR
MATERNITY CARE	★	WOMEN'S HEALTH	NR

HEALTHGRADES AWARDS

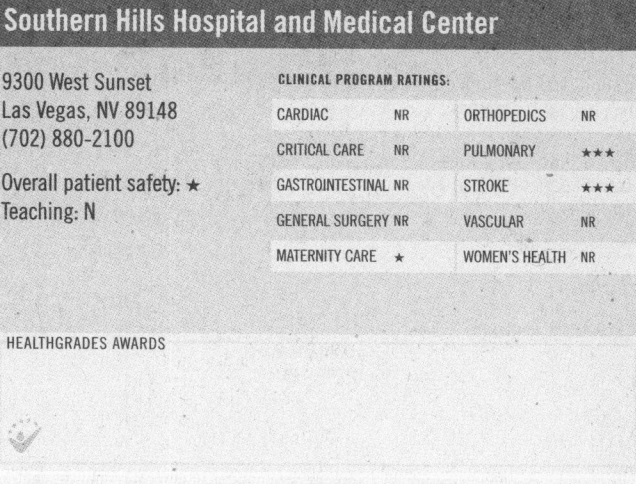

St. Rose Dominican Hospital

102 East Lake Mead Parkway
Henderson, NV 89015
(702) 616-5000

Overall patient safety: ★★★
Teaching: N

CLINICAL PROGRAM RATINGS:

CARDIAC	NR	ORTHOPEDICS	NR
CRITICAL CARE	NR	PULMONARY	★★★
GASTROINTESTINAL	★★★	STROKE	★★★
GENERAL SURGERY	★★★	VASCULAR	NR
MATERNITY CARE	★	WOMEN'S HEALTH	NR

HEALTHGRADES AWARDS

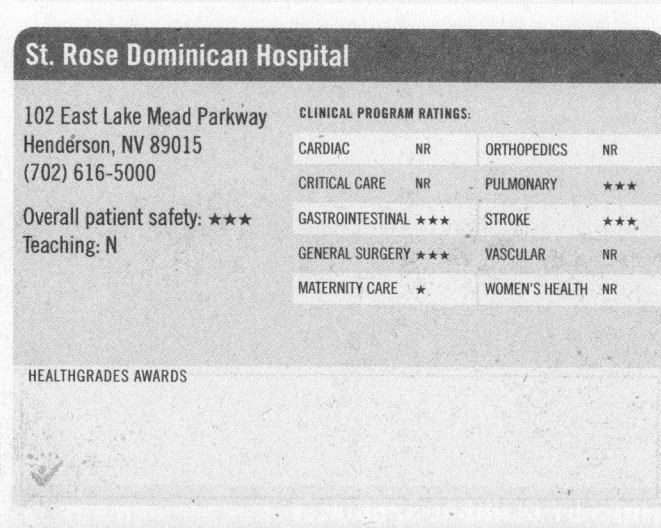

Spring Valley Hospital

5400 South Rainbow Boulevard
Las Vegas, NV 89118
(702) 853-3000

Overall patient safety: ★★★
Teaching: N

CLINICAL PROGRAM RATINGS:

CARDIAC	NR	ORTHOPEDICS	NR
CRITICAL CARE	NR	PULMONARY	★★★
GASTROINTESTINAL	NR	STROKE	★★★
GENERAL SURGERY	★★★	VASCULAR	NR
MATERNITY CARE	★★★	WOMEN'S HEALTH	NR

HEALTHGRADES AWARDS

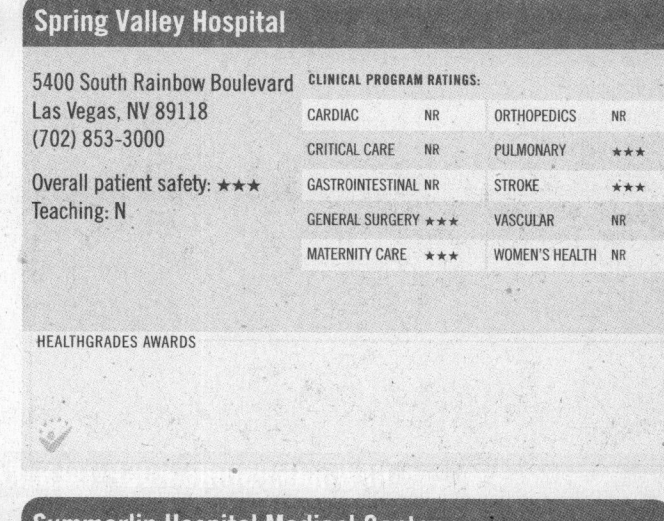

St. Rose Dominican Hospital—Siena Campus

3001 St. Rose Parkway
Henderson, NV 89015
(702) 616-5000

Overall patient safety: ★
Teaching: N

CLINICAL PROGRAM RATINGS:

CARDIAC	★★★	ORTHOPEDICS	★★★
CRITICAL CARE	★★★	PULMONARY	★★★
GASTROINTESTINAL	★★★	STROKE	★★★
GENERAL SURGERY	★	VASCULAR	NR
MATERNITY CARE	★★★	WOMEN'S HEALTH	★★★

HEALTHGRADES AWARDS

Summerlin Hospital Medical Center

657 Town Center Drive
Las Vegas, NV 89144
(702) 233-7000

Overall patient safety: ★
Teaching: N

CLINICAL PROGRAM RATINGS:

CARDIAC	NR	ORTHOPEDICS	NR
CRITICAL CARE	★★★	PULMONARY	★★★
GASTROINTESTINAL	★★★	STROKE	★
GENERAL SURGERY	★★★	VASCULAR	NR
MATERNITY CARE	★★★	WOMEN'S HEALTH	NR

HEALTHGRADES AWARDS

Sunrise Hospital and Medical Center

3186 South Maryland Parkway
Las Vegas, NV 89109
(702) 731-8000

Overall patient safety: ★★★
Teaching: Y

CLINICAL PROGRAM RATINGS:

CARDIAC	★★★	ORTHOPEDICS	★★★
CRITICAL CARE	★★★	PULMONARY	★★★★★
GASTROINTESTINAL	★★★	STROKE	★★★
GENERAL SURGERY	★	VASCULAR	★★★
MATERNITY CARE	★★★	WOMEN'S HEALTH	★★★

HEALTHGRADES AWARDS

✓ SPECIALTY EXCELLENCE
  • PULMONARY CARE

Valley Hospital Medical Center

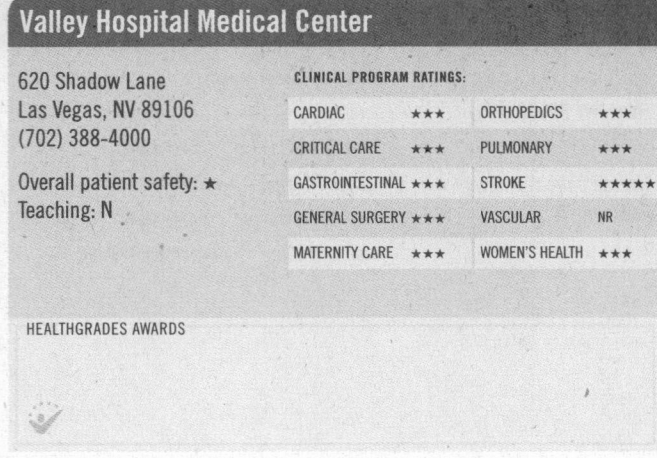

620 Shadow Lane
Las Vegas, NV 89106
(702) 388-4000

Overall patient safety: ★
Teaching: N

CLINICAL PROGRAM RATINGS:

CARDIAC	★★★	ORTHOPEDICS	★★★
CRITICAL CARE	★★★	PULMONARY	★★★
GASTROINTESTINAL	★★★	STROKE	★★★★★
GENERAL SURGERY	★★★	VASCULAR	NR
MATERNITY CARE	★★★	WOMEN'S HEALTH	★★★

HEALTHGRADES AWARDS

UMC of Southern Nevada

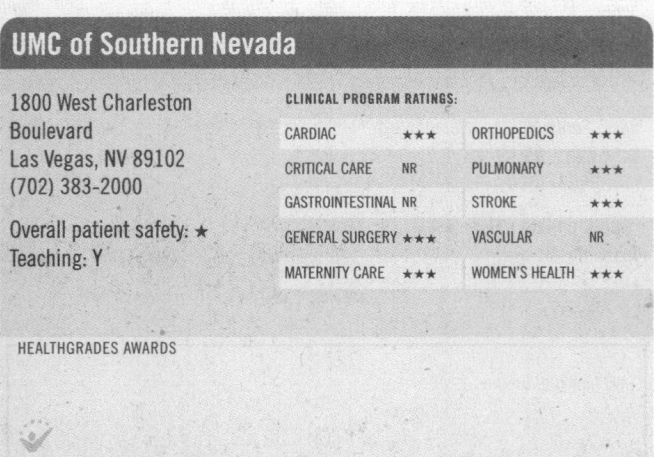

1800 West Charleston
Boulevard
Las Vegas, NV 89102
(702) 383-2000

Overall patient safety: ★
Teaching: Y

CLINICAL PROGRAM RATINGS:

CARDIAC	★★★	ORTHOPEDICS	★★★
CRITICAL CARE	NR	PULMONARY	★★★
GASTROINTESTINAL	NR	STROKE	★★★
GENERAL SURGERY	★★★	VASCULAR	NR
MATERNITY CARE	★★★	WOMEN'S HEALTH	★★★

HEALTHGRADES AWARDS

NEW HAMPSHIRE HOSPITALS: RATINGS BY CLINICAL SPECIALTY

Alice Peck Day Memorial Hospital

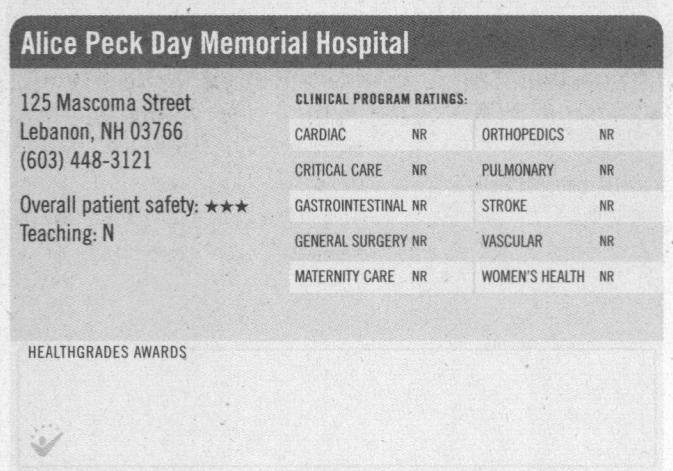

125 Mascoma Street
Lebanon, NH 03766
(603) 448-3121

Overall patient safety: ★★★
Teaching: N

CLINICAL PROGRAM RATINGS:

CARDIAC	NR	ORTHOPEDICS	NR
CRITICAL CARE	NR	PULMONARY	NR
GASTROINTESTINAL	NR	STROKE	NR
GENERAL SURGERY	NR	VASCULAR	NR
MATERNITY CARE	NR	WOMEN'S HEALTH	NR

HEALTHGRADES AWARDS

Androscoggin Valley Hospital

59 Page Hill Road
Berlin, NH 03570
(603) 752-2200

Overall patient safety: ★★★
Teaching: N

CLINICAL PROGRAM RATINGS:

CARDIAC	NR	ORTHOPEDICS	NR
CRITICAL CARE	NR	PULMONARY	★★★
GASTROINTESTINAL	NR	STROKE	★★★
GENERAL SURGERY	NR	VASCULAR	NR
MATERNITY CARE	NR	WOMEN'S HEALTH	NR

HEALTHGRADES AWARDS

KEY: ★★★★★ BEST ★★★ AS EXPECTED ★ POOR NR NOT RATED BY HEALTHGRADES For full definitions of ratings and awards, see Appendix.

Catholic Medical Center

100 McGregor Street
Manchester, NH 03102
(603) 668-3545

Overall patient safety: ★★★
Teaching: N

CLINICAL PROGRAM RATINGS:

CARDIAC	★★★	ORTHOPEDICS	★★★
CRITICAL CARE	NR	PULMONARY	★★★
GASTROINTESTINAL	★★★	STROKE	★★★
GENERAL SURGERY	NR	VASCULAR	★★★
MATERNITY CARE	NR	WOMEN'S HEALTH	NR

HEALTHGRADES AWARDS

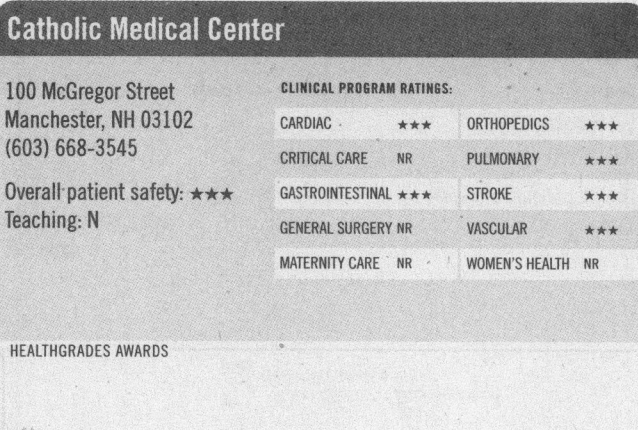

Cottage Hospital

90 Swiftwater Road
Woodsville, NH 03785
(603) 747-9000

Overall patient safety: ★★★
Teaching: N

CLINICAL PROGRAM RATINGS:

CARDIAC	NR	ORTHOPEDICS	NR
CRITICAL CARE	NR	PULMONARY	★
GASTROINTESTINAL	NR	STROKE	★
GENERAL SURGERY	NR	VASCULAR	NR
MATERNITY CARE	NR	WOMEN'S HEALTH	NR

HEALTHGRADES AWARDS

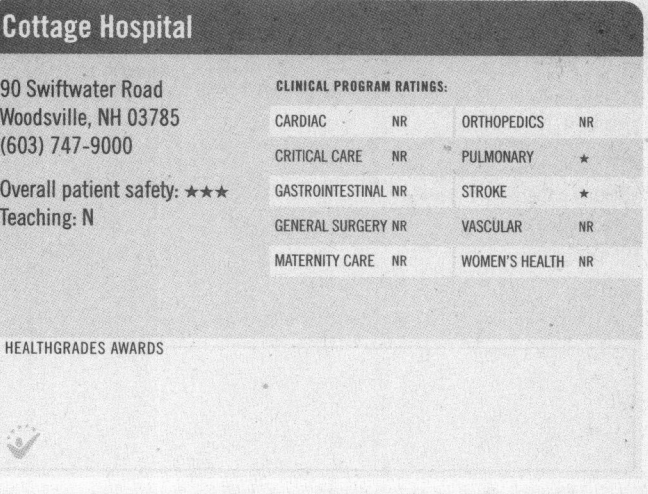

Cheshire Medical Center

580 Court Street
Keene, NH 03431
(603) 354-5400

Overall patient safety: ★★★
Teaching: N

CLINICAL PROGRAM RATINGS:

CARDIAC	NR	ORTHOPEDICS	NR
CRITICAL CARE	NR	PULMONARY	★★★
GASTROINTESTINAL	★★★	STROKE	★★★
GENERAL SURGERY	NR	VASCULAR	NR
MATERNITY CARE	NR	WOMEN'S HEALTH	NR

HEALTHGRADES AWARDS

✓ SPECIALTY EXCELLENCE
· JOINT REPLACEMENT

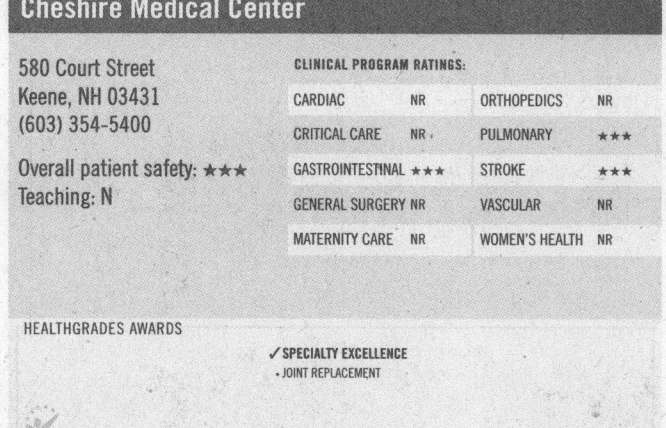

Elliot Hospital

1 Elliot Way
Manchester, NH 03103
(603) 669-5300

Overall patient safety: ★★★
Teaching: N

CLINICAL PROGRAM RATINGS:

CARDIAC	NR	ORTHOPEDICS	★
CRITICAL CARE	NR	PULMONARY	★
GASTROINTESTINAL	★★★	STROKE	★★★
GENERAL SURGERY	NR	VASCULAR	NR
MATERNITY CARE	NR	WOMEN'S HEALTH	NR

HEALTHGRADES AWARDS

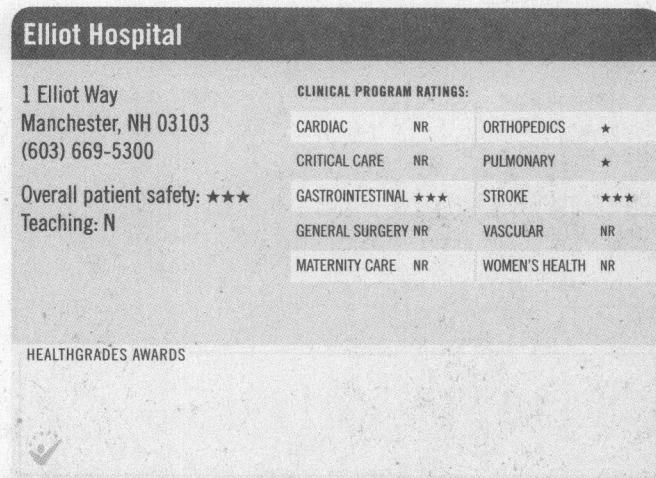

Concord Hospital

250 Pleasant Street
Concord, NH 03301
(603) 225-2711

Overall patient safety: ★★★
Teaching: Y

CLINICAL PROGRAM RATINGS:

CARDIAC	★★★	ORTHOPEDICS	★★★★★
CRITICAL CARE	★	PULMONARY	★
GASTROINTESTINAL	★★★	STROKE	★★★
GENERAL SURGERY	NR	VASCULAR	NR
MATERNITY CARE	NR	WOMEN'S HEALTH	NR

HEALTHGRADES AWARDS

✓ SPECIALTY EXCELLENCE
· JOINT REPLACEMENT

Exeter Hospital

5 Alumni Drive
Exeter, NH 03833
(603) 778-7311

Overall patient safety: ★★★
Teaching: N

CLINICAL PROGRAM RATINGS:

CARDIAC	NR	ORTHOPEDICS	NR
CRITICAL CARE	NR	PULMONARY	★★★
GASTROINTESTINAL	★★★	STROKE	★★★
GENERAL SURGERY	NR	VASCULAR	NR
MATERNITY CARE	NR	WOMEN'S HEALTH	NR

HEALTHGRADES AWARDS

Franklin Regional Hospital

15 Aiken Avenue
Franklin, NH 03235
(603) 934-2060

Overall patient safety: ★★★
Teaching: N

CLINICAL PROGRAM RATINGS:

CARDIAC	NR	ORTHOPEDICS	NR
CRITICAL CARE	NR	PULMONARY	★★★
GASTROINTESTINAL	NR	STROKE	★
GENERAL SURGERY	NR	VASCULAR	NR
MATERNITY CARE	NR	WOMEN'S HEALTH	NR

HEALTHGRADES AWARDS

Lakes Region General Hospital

80 Highland Street
Laconia, NH 03246
(603) 524-3211

Overall patient safety: ★★★
Teaching: N

CLINICAL PROGRAM RATINGS:

CARDIAC	NR	ORTHOPEDICS	★★★
CRITICAL CARE	NR	PULMONARY	★
GASTROINTESTINAL	★★★	STROKE	★★★
GENERAL SURGERY	NR	VASCULAR	NR
MATERNITY CARE	NR	WOMEN'S HEALTH	NR

HEALTHGRADES AWARDS

Frisbie Memorial Hospital

11 Whitehall Road
Rochester, NH 03867
(603) 332-5211

Overall patient safety: ★
Teaching: N

CLINICAL PROGRAM RATINGS:

CARDIAC	NR	ORTHOPEDICS	NR
CRITICAL CARE	NR	PULMONARY	★
GASTROINTESTINAL	NR	STROKE	★
GENERAL SURGERY	NR	VASCULAR	NR
MATERNITY CARE	NR	WOMEN'S HEALTH	NR

HEALTHGRADES AWARDS

Littleton Regional Hospital

600 St. Johnsbury Road
Littleton, NH 03561
(603) 444-9000

Overall patient safety: ★★★
Teaching: N

CLINICAL PROGRAM RATINGS:

CARDIAC	NR	ORTHOPEDICS	NR
CRITICAL CARE	NR	PULMONARY	★★★
GASTROINTESTINAL	NR	STROKE	★★★
GENERAL SURGERY	NR	VASCULAR	NR
MATERNITY CARE	NR	WOMEN'S HEALTH	NR

HEALTHGRADES AWARDS

Huggins Hospital

240 South Main Street
Wolfeboro, NH 03894
(603) 569-7500

Overall patient safety: ★★★
Teaching: N

CLINICAL PROGRAM RATINGS:

CARDIAC	NR	ORTHOPEDICS	NR
CRITICAL CARE	NR	PULMONARY	★★★
GASTROINTESTINAL	NR	STROKE	★★★
GENERAL SURGERY	NR	VASCULAR	NR
MATERNITY CARE	NR	WOMEN'S HEALTH	NR

HEALTHGRADES AWARDS

Mary Hitchcock Memorial Hospital

1 Medical Center Drive
Lebanon, NH 03756
(603) 650-5000

Overall patient safety: ★★★
Teaching: Y

CLINICAL PROGRAM RATINGS:

CARDIAC	★★★	ORTHOPEDICS	★★★
CRITICAL CARE	NR	PULMONARY	★★★★★
GASTROINTESTINAL	★★★	STROKE	★★★★★
GENERAL SURGERY	NR	VASCULAR	★★★
MATERNITY CARE	NR	WOMEN'S HEALTH	NR

HEALTHGRADES AWARDS

✓ DISTINGUISHED HOSPITAL
· CLINICAL EXCELLENCE

✓ SPECIALTY EXCELLENCE
· GASTROINTESTINAL CARE
· STROKE CARE

KEY: ★★★★★ BEST ★★★ AS EXPECTED ★ POOR NR NOT RATED BY HEALTHGRADES   For full definitions of ratings and awards, see Appendix.

Memorial Hospital

3073 White Mountain Highway
North Conway, NH 03860
(603) 356-5461

Overall patient safety: ★★★
Teaching: N

CLINICAL PROGRAM RATINGS:

CARDIAC	NR	ORTHOPEDICS	NR
CRITICAL CARE	NR	PULMONARY	★★★
GASTROINTESTINAL	NR	STROKE	★★★
GENERAL SURGERY	NR	VASCULAR	NR
MATERNITY CARE	NR	WOMEN'S HEALTH	NR

HEALTHGRADES AWARDS

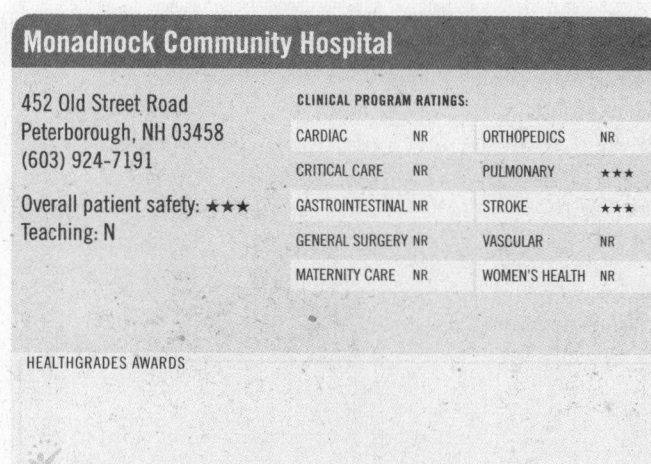

Portsmouth Regional Hospital

333 Borthwick Avenue
Suite 100
Portsmouth, NH 03801
(603) 436-5110

Overall patient safety: ★★★
Teaching: N

CLINICAL PROGRAM RATINGS:

CARDIAC	★★★	ORTHOPEDICS	★
CRITICAL CARE	NR	PULMONARY	★★★
GASTROINTESTINAL	★★★	STROKE	★★★
GENERAL SURGERY	NR	VASCULAR	NR
MATERNITY CARE	NR	WOMEN'S HEALTH	NR

HEALTHGRADES AWARDS

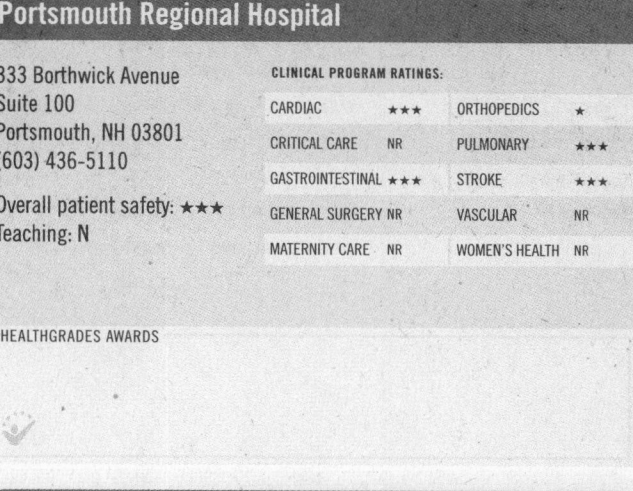

Monadnock Community Hospital

452 Old Street Road
Peterborough, NH 03458
(603) 924-7191

Overall patient safety: ★★★
Teaching: N

CLINICAL PROGRAM RATINGS:

CARDIAC	NR	ORTHOPEDICS	NR
CRITICAL CARE	NR	PULMONARY	★★★
GASTROINTESTINAL	NR	STROKE	★★★
GENERAL SURGERY	NR	VASCULAR	NR
MATERNITY CARE	NR	WOMEN'S HEALTH	NR

HEALTHGRADES AWARDS

St. Joseph Hospital

172 Kinsley Street
Nashua, NH 03060
(603) 882-3000

Overall patient safety: ★
Teaching: N

CLINICAL PROGRAM RATINGS:

CARDIAC	NR	ORTHOPEDICS	NR
CRITICAL CARE	NR	PULMONARY	★
GASTROINTESTINAL	NR	STROKE	★
GENERAL SURGERY	NR	VASCULAR	NR
MATERNITY CARE	NR	WOMEN'S HEALTH	NR

HEALTHGRADES AWARDS

Parkland Medical Center

1 Parkland Drive
Derry, NH 03038
(603) 432-1500

Overall patient safety: ★★★
Teaching: N

CLINICAL PROGRAM RATINGS:

CARDIAC	NR	ORTHOPEDICS	NR
CRITICAL CARE	NR	PULMONARY	★★★
GASTROINTESTINAL	NR	STROKE	★★★
GENERAL SURGERY	NR	VASCULAR	NR
MATERNITY CARE	NR	WOMEN'S HEALTH	NR

HEALTHGRADES AWARDS

Southern New Hampshire Medical Center

8 Prospect Street
Nashua, NH 03060
(603) 577-2000

Overall patient safety: ★★★
Teaching: Y

CLINICAL PROGRAM RATINGS:

CARDIAC	NR	ORTHOPEDICS	NR
CRITICAL CARE	NR	PULMONARY	★★★
GASTROINTESTINAL	★★★	STROKE	★★★
GENERAL SURGERY	NR	VASCULAR	NR
MATERNITY CARE	NR	WOMEN'S HEALTH	NR

HEALTHGRADES AWARDS

Speare Memorial Hospital

16 Hospital Road
Plymouth, NH 03264
(603) 536-1120

Overall patient safety: ★★★
Teaching: N

CLINICAL PROGRAM RATINGS:

CARDIAC	NR	ORTHOPEDICS	NR
CRITICAL CARE	NR	PULMONARY	★
GASTROINTESTINAL	NR	STROKE	★★★
GENERAL SURGERY	NR	VASCULAR	NR
MATERNITY CARE	NR	WOMEN'S HEALTH	NR

HEALTHGRADES AWARDS

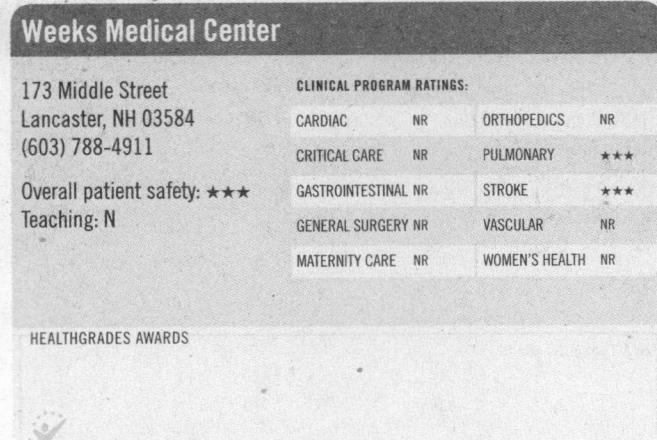

Weeks Medical Center

173 Middle Street
Lancaster, NH 03584
(603) 788-4911

Overall patient safety: ★★★
Teaching: N

CLINICAL PROGRAM RATINGS:

CARDIAC	NR	ORTHOPEDICS	NR
CRITICAL CARE	NR	PULMONARY	★★★
GASTROINTESTINAL	NR	STROKE	★★★
GENERAL SURGERY	NR	VASCULAR	NR
MATERNITY CARE	NR	WOMEN'S HEALTH	NR

HEALTHGRADES AWARDS

Valley Regional Hospital

243 Elm Street
Claremont, NH 03743
(603) 542-7771

Overall patient safety: ★★★
Teaching: N

CLINICAL PROGRAM RATINGS:

CARDIAC	NR	ORTHOPEDICS	NR
CRITICAL CARE	NR	PULMONARY	★★★
GASTROINTESTINAL	NR	STROKE	★★★
GENERAL SURGERY	NR	VASCULAR	NR
MATERNITY CARE	NR	WOMEN'S HEALTH	NR

HEALTHGRADES AWARDS

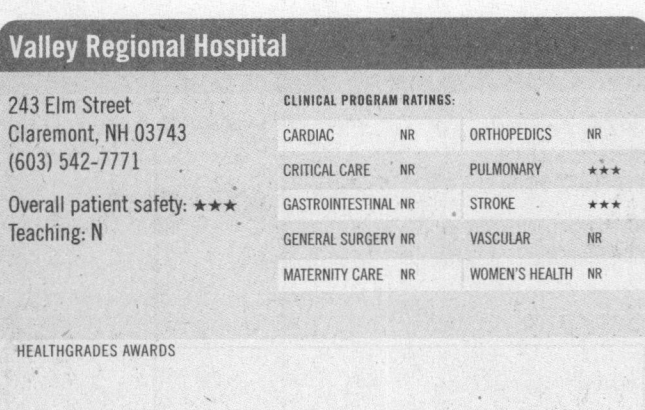

Wentworth-Douglass Hospital

789 Central Avenue
Dover, NH 03820
(603) 742-5252

Overall patient safety: ★★★
Teaching: N

CLINICAL PROGRAM RATINGS:

CARDIAC	NR	ORTHOPEDICS	★
CRITICAL CARE	★★★	PULMONARY	★★★
GASTROINTESTINAL	NR	STROKE	★★★
GENERAL SURGERY	NR	VASCULAR	★★★
MATERNITY CARE	NR	WOMEN'S HEALTH	NR

HEALTHGRADES AWARDS

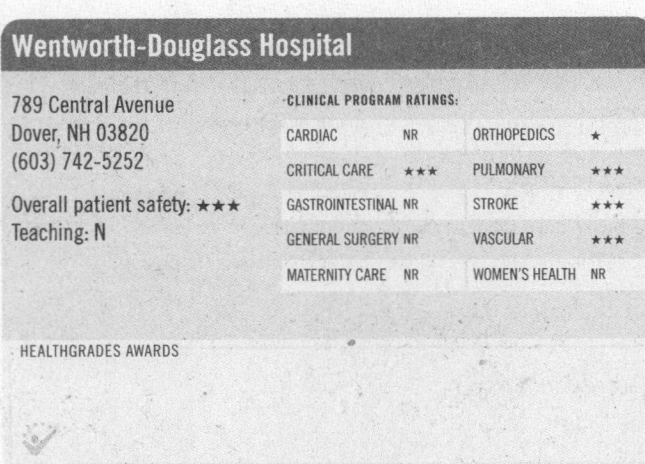

NEW JERSEY HOSPITALS: RATINGS BY CLINICAL SPECIALTY

Atlanticare Regional Medical Center

1925 Pacific Avenue
Atlantic City, NJ 08401
(609) 345-4000

Overall patient safety: ★★★
Teaching: Y

CLINICAL PROGRAM RATINGS:

CARDIAC	★★★	ORTHOPEDICS	★★★
CRITICAL CARE	★★★	PULMONARY	★★★
GASTROINTESTINAL	★★★	STROKE	★★★★★
GENERAL SURGERY	★★★	VASCULAR	NR
MATERNITY CARE	★★★	WOMEN'S HEALTH	★★★

HEALTHGRADES AWARDS
✓ DISTINGUISHED
HOSPITAL
· CLINICAL EXCELLENCE ·

Barnert Hospital

680 Broadway
Paterson, NJ 07514
(973) 977-6600

Overall patient safety: ★★★
Teaching: Y

CLINICAL PROGRAM RATINGS:

CARDIAC	NR	ORTHOPEDICS	NR
CRITICAL CARE	NR	PULMONARY	★★★
GASTROINTESTINAL	NR	STROKE	★★★
GENERAL SURGERY	NR	VASCULAR	NR
MATERNITY CARE	★★★	WOMEN'S HEALTH	NR

HEALTHGRADES AWARDS

KEY: ★★★★★ BEST   ★★★ AS EXPECTED   ★ POOR   NR NOT RATED BY HEALTHGRADES   For full definitions of ratings and awards, see Appendix.

Bayonne Hospital

29 East 29th Street
Bayonne, NJ 07002
(201) 858-5000

Overall patient safety: ★
Teaching: N

CLINICAL PROGRAM RATINGS:

CARDIAC	NR	ORTHOPEDICS	NR
CRITICAL CARE	★★★	PULMONARY	★★★
GASTROINTESTINAL	★★★	STROKE	★★★★★
GENERAL SURGERY	★★★	VASCULAR	NR
MATERNITY CARE	★★★	WOMEN'S HEALTH	NR

HEALTHGRADES AWARDS

✓ SPECIALTY EXCELLENCE
· STROKE CARE

Cape Regional Medical Center

2 Stone Harbour Boulevard
Cape May Court House, NJ
08210
(609) 463-2000

Overall patient safety: ★★★
Teaching: N

CLINICAL PROGRAM RATINGS:

CARDIAC	NR	ORTHOPEDICS	NR
CRITICAL CARE	NR	PULMONARY	★★★
GASTROINTESTINAL	★	STROKE	★★★
GENERAL SURGERY	★	VASCULAR	NR
MATERNITY CARE	★★★	WOMEN'S HEALTH	NR

HEALTHGRADES AWARDS

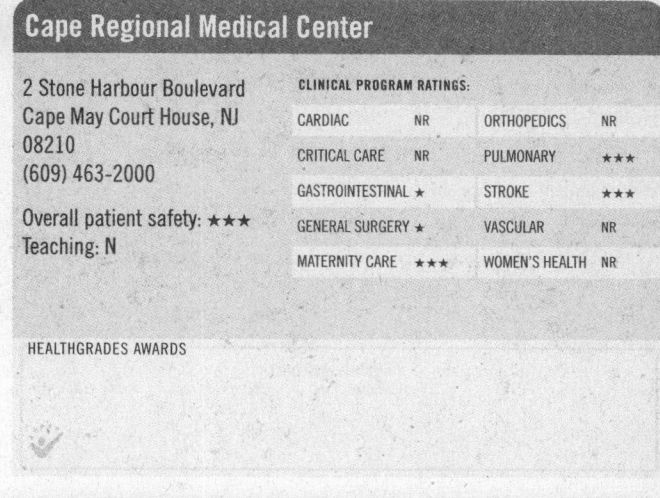

Bayshore Community Hospital

727 North Beers Street
Holmdel, NJ 07733
(732) 739-5900

Overall patient safety: ★★★
Teaching: N

CLINICAL PROGRAM RATINGS:

CARDIAC	NR	ORTHOPEDICS	NR
CRITICAL CARE	★★★	PULMONARY	★★★
GASTROINTESTINAL	★★★	STROKE	★★★
GENERAL SURGERY	★★★	VASCULAR	NR
MATERNITY CARE	NR	WOMEN'S HEALTH	NR

HEALTHGRADES AWARDS

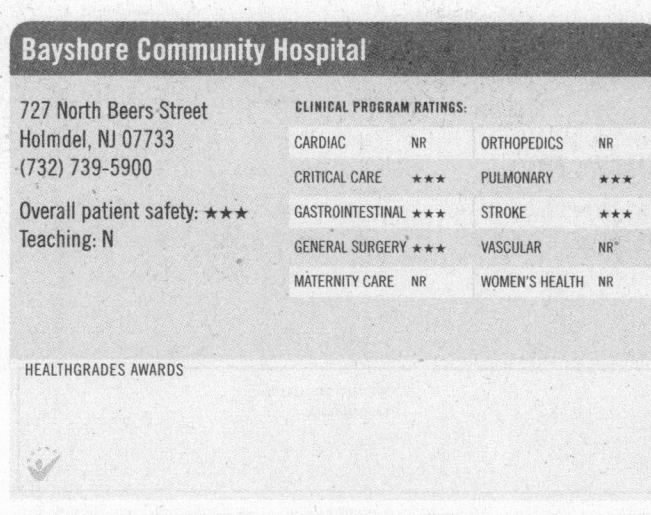

Capital Health System—Fuld Campus

750 Brunswick Avenue
Trenton, NJ 08638
(609) 394-6000

Overall patient safety: ★★★
Teaching: Y

CLINICAL PROGRAM RATINGS:

CARDIAC	NR	ORTHOPEDICS	NR
CRITICAL CARE	★★★	PULMONARY	★★★★★
GASTROINTESTINAL	NR	STROKE	★★★★★
GENERAL SURGERY	★★★	VASCULAR	NR
MATERNITY CARE	NR	WOMEN'S HEALTH	NR

HEALTHGRADES AWARDS

✓ SPECIALTY EXCELLENCE
· PULMONARY CARE   · STROKE CARE

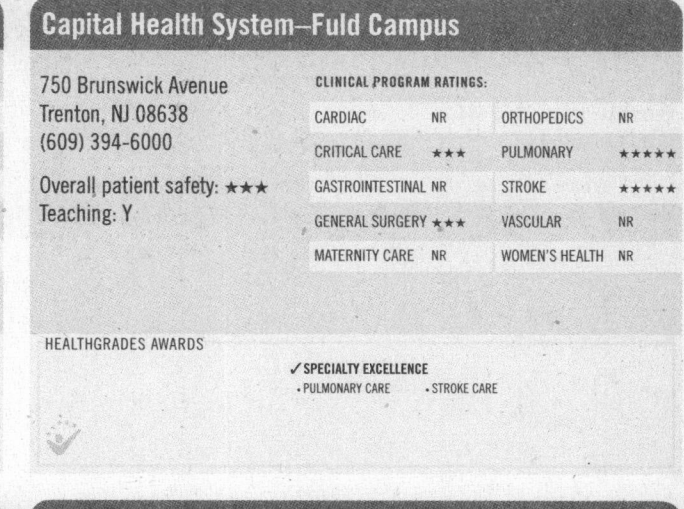

Bergen Regional Medical Center

230 East Ridgewood Avenue
Paramus, NJ 07652
(201) 967-4000

Overall patient safety: ★★★
Teaching: Y

CLINICAL PROGRAM RATINGS:

CARDIAC	NR	ORTHOPEDICS	NR
CRITICAL CARE	NR	PULMONARY	★
GASTROINTESTINAL	NR	STROKE	NR
GENERAL SURGERY	NR	VASCULAR	NR
MATERNITY CARE	NR	WOMEN'S HEALTH	NR

HEALTHGRADES AWARDS

Capital Health System—Mercer Campus

446 Bellevue Avenue
Trenton, NJ 08618
(609) 394-4000

Overall patient safety: ★★★
Teaching: N

CLINICAL PROGRAM RATINGS:

CARDIAC	NR	ORTHOPEDICS	★
CRITICAL CARE	★★★	PULMONARY	★★★
GASTROINTESTINAL	NR	STROKE	★★★
GENERAL SURGERY	★★★	VASCULAR	NR
MATERNITY CARE	★★★	WOMEN'S HEALTH	NR

HEALTHGRADES AWARDS

Centrastate Medical Center

901 West Main Street
Freehold, NJ 07728
(732) 431-2000

Overall patient safety: ★★★
Teaching: N

CLINICAL PROGRAM RATINGS:

CARDIAC	NR	ORTHOPEDICS	NR
CRITICAL CARE	★★★	PULMONARY	★★★★★
GASTROINTESTINAL	★★★	STROKE	★★★★★
GENERAL SURGERY	★★★	VASCULAR	NR
MATERNITY CARE	★★★★★	WOMEN'S HEALTH	NR

HEALTHGRADES AWARDS

✓ SPECIALTY EXCELLENCE
• MATERNITY CARE   • PULMONARY CARE   • STROKE CARE

Clara Maass Medical Center

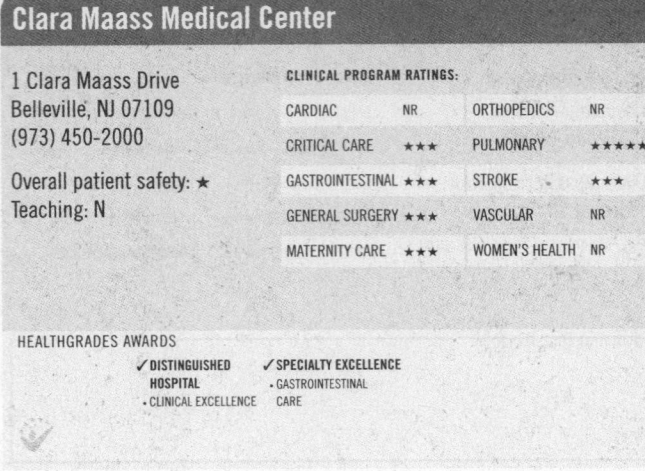

1 Clara Maass Drive
Belleville, NJ 07109
(973) 450-2000

Overall patient safety: ★
Teaching: N

CLINICAL PROGRAM RATINGS:

CARDIAC	NR	ORTHOPEDICS	NR
CRITICAL CARE	★★★	PULMONARY	★★★★★
GASTROINTESTINAL	★★★	STROKE	★★★
GENERAL SURGERY	★★★	VASCULAR	NR
MATERNITY CARE	★★★	WOMEN'S HEALTH	NR

HEALTHGRADES AWARDS

✓ DISTINGUISHED HOSPITAL
• CLINICAL EXCELLENCE

✓ SPECIALTY EXCELLENCE
• GASTROINTESTINAL CARE

Chilton Memorial Hospital

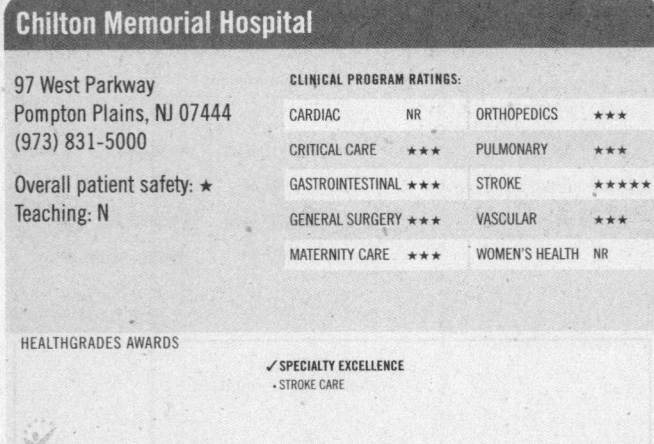

97 West Parkway
Pompton Plains, NJ 07444
(973) 831-5000

Overall patient safety: ★
Teaching: N

CLINICAL PROGRAM RATINGS:

CARDIAC	NR	ORTHOPEDICS	★★★
CRITICAL CARE	★★★	PULMONARY	★★★
GASTROINTESTINAL	★★★	STROKE	★★★★★
GENERAL SURGERY	★★★	VASCULAR	★★★
MATERNITY CARE	★★★	WOMEN'S HEALTH	NR

HEALTHGRADES AWARDS

✓ SPECIALTY EXCELLENCE
• STROKE CARE

Columbus Hospital

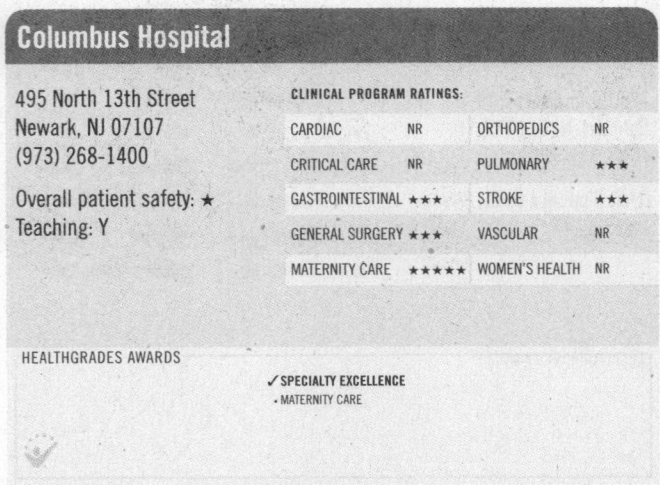

495 North 13th Street
Newark, NJ 07107
(973) 268-1400

Overall patient safety: ★
Teaching: Y

CLINICAL PROGRAM RATINGS:

CARDIAC	NR	ORTHOPEDICS	NR
CRITICAL CARE	NR	PULMONARY	★★★
GASTROINTESTINAL	★★★	STROKE	★★★
GENERAL SURGERY	★★★	VASCULAR	NR
MATERNITY CARE	★★★★★	WOMEN'S HEALTH	NR

HEALTHGRADES AWARDS

✓ SPECIALTY EXCELLENCE
• MATERNITY CARE

Christ Hospital

176 Palisade Avenue
Jersey City, NJ 07306
(201) 795-8200

Overall patient safety: ★
Teaching: Y

CLINICAL PROGRAM RATINGS:

CARDIAC	NR	ORTHOPEDICS	NR
CRITICAL CARE	NR	PULMONARY	★★★
GASTROINTESTINAL	★★★	STROKE	★★★
GENERAL SURGERY	★★★	VASCULAR	NR
MATERNITY CARE	★★★★★	WOMEN'S HEALTH	NR

HEALTHGRADES AWARDS

✓ SPECIALTY EXCELLENCE
• MATERNITY CARE

Community Medical Center

99 Highway 37 West
Toms River, NJ 08755
(732) 557-8000

Overall patient safety: ★★★★★
Teaching: N

CLINICAL PROGRAM RATINGS:

CARDIAC	NR	ORTHOPEDICS	★★★★★
CRITICAL CARE	★★★	PULMONARY	★★★★★
GASTROINTESTINAL	★★★	STROKE	★★★
GENERAL SURGERY	★★★	VASCULAR	★★★
MATERNITY CARE	★★★★★	WOMEN'S HEALTH	NR

HEALTHGRADES AWARDS

✓ DISTINGUISHED HOSPITAL
• CLINICAL EXCELLENCE
• PATIENT SAFETY

✓ SPECIALTY EXCELLENCE
• ORTHOPEDIC SURGERY   • PULMONARY CARE

KEY: ★★★★★ BEST   ★★★ AS EXPECTED   ★ POOR   NR NOT RATED BY HEALTHGRADES   For full definitions of ratings and awards, see Appendix.

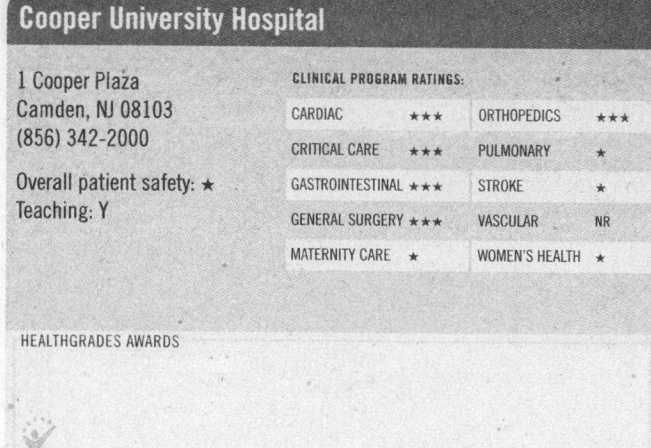

Cooper University Hospital

1 Cooper Plaza
Camden, NJ 08103
(856) 342-2000

Overall patient safety: ★
Teaching: Y

CLINICAL PROGRAM RATINGS:

CARDIAC	★★★	ORTHOPEDICS	★★★
CRITICAL CARE	★★★	PULMONARY	★
GASTROINTESTINAL	★★★	STROKE	★
GENERAL SURGERY	★★★	VASCULAR	NR
MATERNITY CARE	★	WOMEN'S HEALTH	★

HEALTHGRADES AWARDS

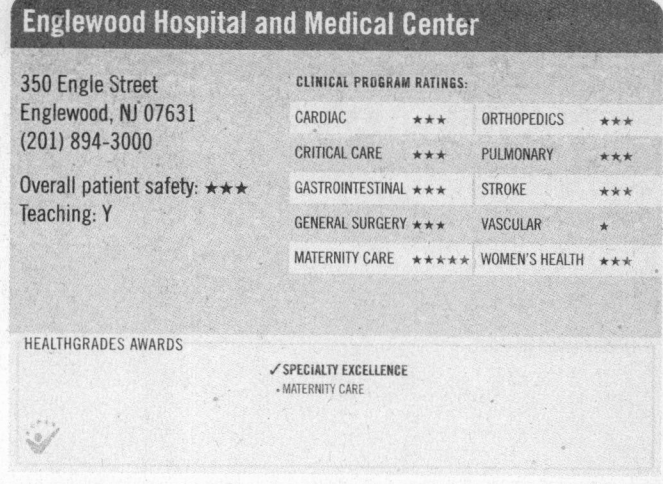

Englewood Hospital and Medical Center

350 Engle Street
Englewood, NJ 07631
(201) 894-3000

Overall patient safety: ★★★
Teaching: Y

CLINICAL PROGRAM RATINGS:

CARDIAC	★★★	ORTHOPEDICS	★★★
CRITICAL CARE	★★★	PULMONARY	★★★
GASTROINTESTINAL	★★★	STROKE	★★★
GENERAL SURGERY	★★★	VASCULAR	★
MATERNITY CARE	★★★★★	WOMEN'S HEALTH	★★★

HEALTHGRADES AWARDS

✓ SPECIALTY EXCELLENCE
- MATERNITY CARE

Deborah Heart and Lung Center

200 Trenton Road
Browns Mills, NJ 08015
(609) 893-6611

Overall patient safety: ★★★
Teaching: Y

CLINICAL PROGRAM RATINGS:

CARDIAC	★★★	ORTHOPEDICS	NR
CRITICAL CARE	NR	PULMONARY	NR
GASTROINTESTINAL	NR	STROKE	NR
GENERAL SURGERY	NR	VASCULAR	NR
MATERNITY CARE	NR	WOMEN'S HEALTH	NR

HEALTHGRADES AWARDS

✓ SPECIALTY EXCELLENCE
- CARDIAC SURGERY

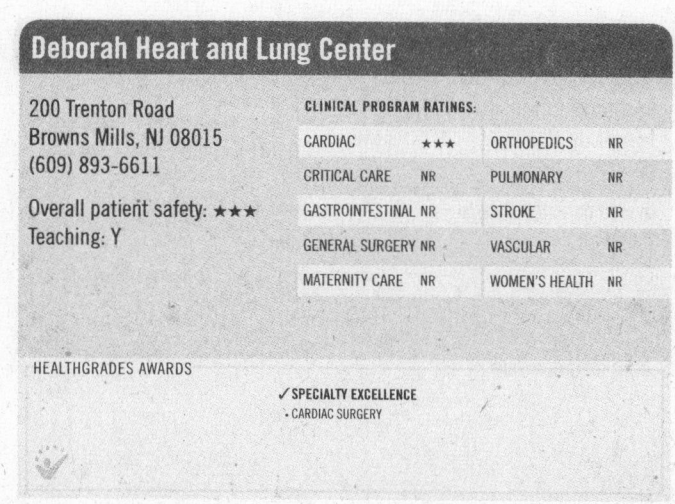

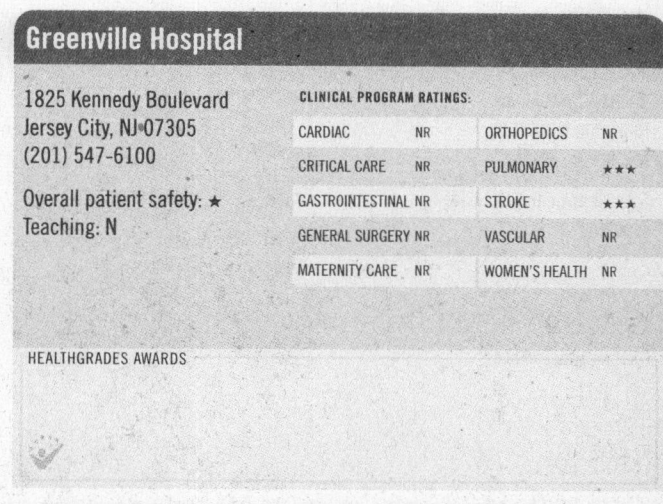

Greenville Hospital

1825 Kennedy Boulevard
Jersey City, NJ 07305
(201) 547-6100

Overall patient safety: ★
Teaching: N

CLINICAL PROGRAM RATINGS:

CARDIAC	NR	ORTHOPEDICS	NR
CRITICAL CARE	NR	PULMONARY	★★★
GASTROINTESTINAL	NR	STROKE	★★★
GENERAL SURGERY	NR	VASCULAR	NR
MATERNITY CARE	NR	WOMEN'S HEALTH	NR

HEALTHGRADES AWARDS

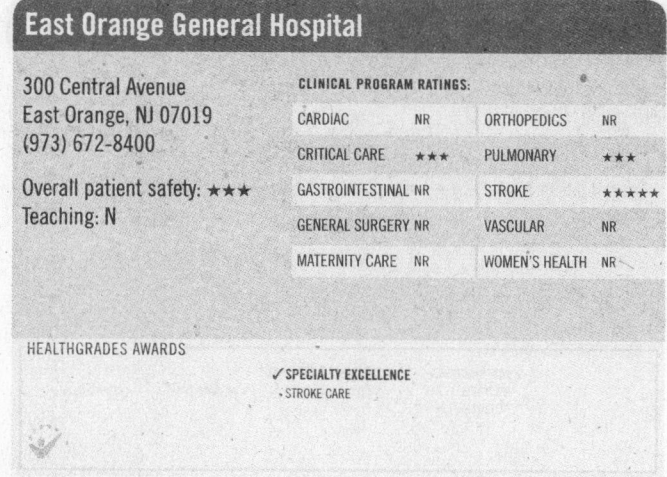

East Orange General Hospital

300 Central Avenue
East Orange, NJ 07019
(973) 672-8400

Overall patient safety: ★★★
Teaching: N

CLINICAL PROGRAM RATINGS:

CARDIAC	NR	ORTHOPEDICS	NR
CRITICAL CARE	★★★	PULMONARY	★★★
GASTROINTESTINAL	NR	STROKE	★★★★★
GENERAL SURGERY	NR	VASCULAR	NR
MATERNITY CARE	NR	WOMEN'S HEALTH	NR

HEALTHGRADES AWARDS

✓ SPECIALTY EXCELLENCE
- STROKE CARE

Hackensack University Medical Center

30 Prospect Avenue
Hackensack, NJ 07601
(201) 996-2000

Overall patient safety: ★
Teaching: Y

CLINICAL PROGRAM RATINGS:

CARDIAC	★★★★★	ORTHOPEDICS	★★★★★
CRITICAL CARE	★★★	PULMONARY	★★★★★
GASTROINTESTINAL	★★★	STROKE	★★★★★
GENERAL SURGERY	★★★★★	VASCULAR	★★★
MATERNITY CARE	★★★	WOMEN'S HEALTH	★★★★★

HEALTHGRADES AWARDS

✓ AMERICA'S 50 BEST HOSPITALS

✓ DISTINGUISHED HOSPITAL
- CLINICAL EXCELLENCE

✓ SPECIALTY EXCELLENCE
- BARIATRIC SURGERY
- CARDIAC CARE
- CARDIAC SURGERY
- GASTROINTESTINAL CARE
- GENERAL SURGERY
- ORTHOPEDIC SURGERY
- PULMONARY CARE
- STROKE CARE
- WOMEN'S HEALTH

Hackettstown Community Hospital

651 Willow Grove Street
Hackettstown, NJ 07840
(908) 852-5100

Overall patient safety: ★★★
Teaching: N

CLINICAL PROGRAM RATINGS:

CARDIAC	NR	ORTHOPEDICS	NR
CRITICAL CARE	NR	PULMONARY	★★★
GASTROINTESTINAL	★★★	STROKE	★★★
GENERAL SURGERY	★★★	VASCULAR	NR
MATERNITY CARE	★★★★★	WOMEN'S HEALTH	NR

HEALTHGRADES AWARDS

Hunterdon Medical Center

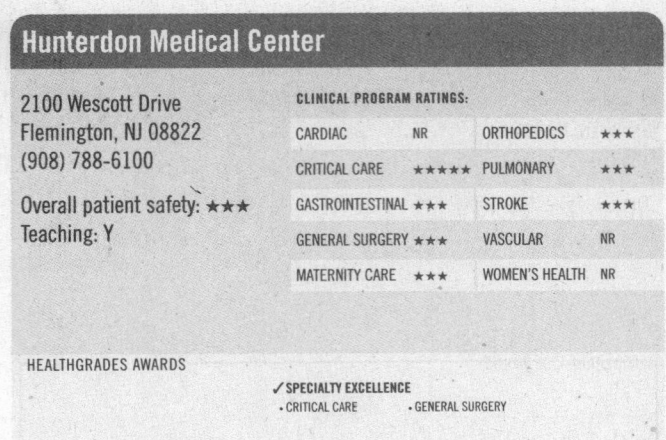

2100 Wescott Drive
Flemington, NJ 08822
(908) 788-6100

Overall patient safety: ★★★
Teaching: Y

CLINICAL PROGRAM RATINGS:

CARDIAC	NR	ORTHOPEDICS	★★★
CRITICAL CARE	★★★★★	PULMONARY	★★★
GASTROINTESTINAL	★★★	STROKE	★★★
GENERAL SURGERY	★★★	VASCULAR	NR
MATERNITY CARE	★★★	WOMEN'S HEALTH	NR

HEALTHGRADES AWARDS

✓ SPECIALTY EXCELLENCE
• CRITICAL CARE • GENERAL SURGERY

Hoboken University Medical Center

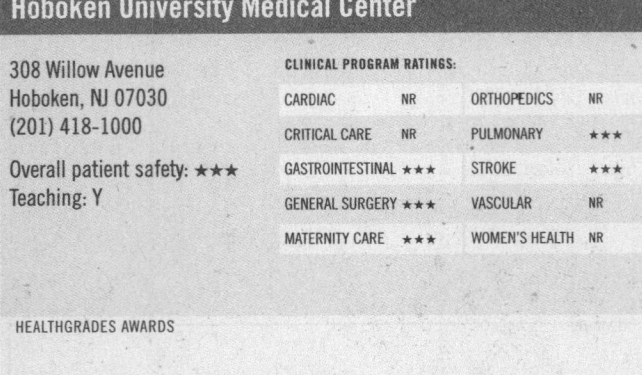

308 Willow Avenue
Hoboken, NJ 07030
(201) 418-1000

Overall patient safety: ★★★
Teaching: Y

CLINICAL PROGRAM RATINGS:

CARDIAC	NR	ORTHOPEDICS	NR
CRITICAL CARE	NR	PULMONARY	★★★
GASTROINTESTINAL	★★★	STROKE	★★★
GENERAL SURGERY	★★★	VASCULAR	NR
MATERNITY CARE	★★★	WOMEN'S HEALTH	NR

HEALTHGRADES AWARDS

Jersey City Medical Center

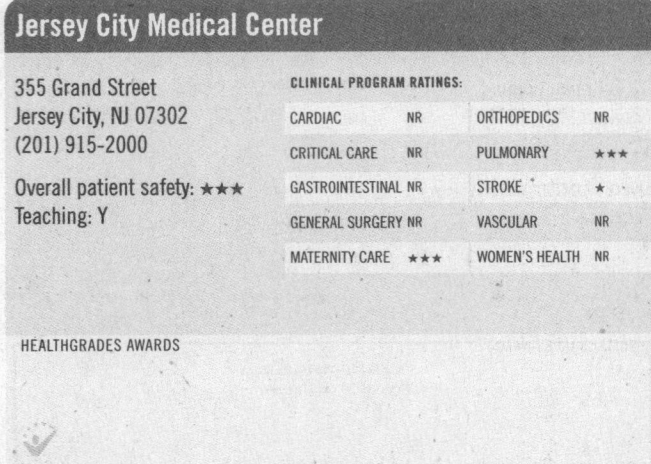

355 Grand Street
Jersey City, NJ 07302
(201) 915-2000

Overall patient safety: ★★★
Teaching: Y

CLINICAL PROGRAM RATINGS:

CARDIAC	NR	ORTHOPEDICS	NR
CRITICAL CARE	NR	PULMONARY	★★★
GASTROINTESTINAL	NR	STROKE	★
GENERAL SURGERY	NR	VASCULAR	NR
MATERNITY CARE	★★★	WOMEN'S HEALTH	NR

HEALTHGRADES AWARDS

Holy Name Hospital

718 Teaneck Road
Teaneck, NJ 07666
(201) 833-3000

Overall patient safety: ★
Teaching: N

CLINICAL PROGRAM RATINGS:

CARDIAC	NR	ORTHOPEDICS	★★★
CRITICAL CARE	★★★	PULMONARY	★★★★★
GASTROINTESTINAL	★★★	STROKE	★★★★★
GENERAL SURGERY	★★★	VASCULAR	NR
MATERNITY CARE	★★★★★	WOMEN'S HEALTH	NR

HEALTHGRADES AWARDS

✓ DISTINGUISHED HOSPITAL
• CLINICAL EXCELLENCE

✓ SPECIALTY EXCELLENCE
• GASTROINTESTINAL CARE • PULMONARY CARE • STROKE CARE

Jersey Shore University Medical Center

1945 State Route 33
Neptune, NJ 07753
(732) 775-5500

Overall patient safety: ★★★★★
Teaching: Y

CLINICAL PROGRAM RATINGS:

CARDIAC	★★★	ORTHOPEDICS	★★★
CRITICAL CARE	★★★	PULMONARY	★★★★★
GASTROINTESTINAL	★★★	STROKE	★★★★★
GENERAL SURGERY	★★★	VASCULAR	★★★
MATERNITY CARE	★★★	WOMEN'S HEALTH	★★★

HEALTHGRADES AWARDS

✓ DISTINGUISHED HOSPITAL
• PATIENT SAFETY

✓ SPECIALTY EXCELLENCE
• CARDIAC SURGERY • PULMONARY CARE • STROKE CARE

KEY: ★★★★★ BEST ★★★ AS EXPECTED ★ POOR NR NOT RATED BY HEALTHGRADES   For full definitions of ratings and awards, see Appendix.

JFK Medical Center

65 James Street
Edison, NJ 08818
(732) 321-7000

Overall patient safety: ★
Teaching: Y

CLINICAL PROGRAM RATINGS:

CARDIAC	NR	ORTHOPEDICS	★
CRITICAL CARE	★★★	PULMONARY	★★★
GASTROINTESTINAL	★★★	STROKE	★★★★★
GENERAL SURGERY	★★★	VASCULAR	★
MATERNITY CARE	★★★	WOMEN'S HEALTH	NR

HEALTHGRADES AWARDS

✓ SPECIALTY EXCELLENCE
• STROKE CARE

Kimball Medical Center

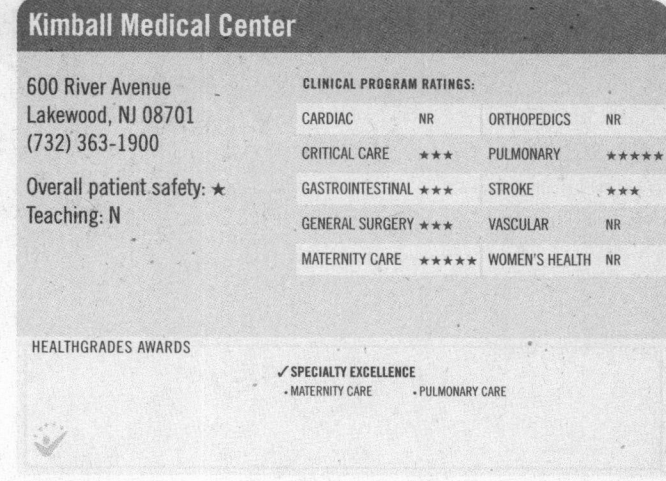

600 River Avenue
Lakewood, NJ 08701
(732) 363-1900

Overall patient safety: ★
Teaching: N

CLINICAL PROGRAM RATINGS:

CARDIAC	NR	ORTHOPEDICS	NR
CRITICAL CARE	★★★	PULMONARY	★★★★★
GASTROINTESTINAL	★★★	STROKE	★★★
GENERAL SURGERY	★★★	VASCULAR	NR
MATERNITY CARE	★★★★★	WOMEN'S HEALTH	NR

HEALTHGRADES AWARDS

✓ SPECIALTY EXCELLENCE
• MATERNITY CARE   • PULMONARY CARE

Kennedy Memorial Hospitals—Stratford

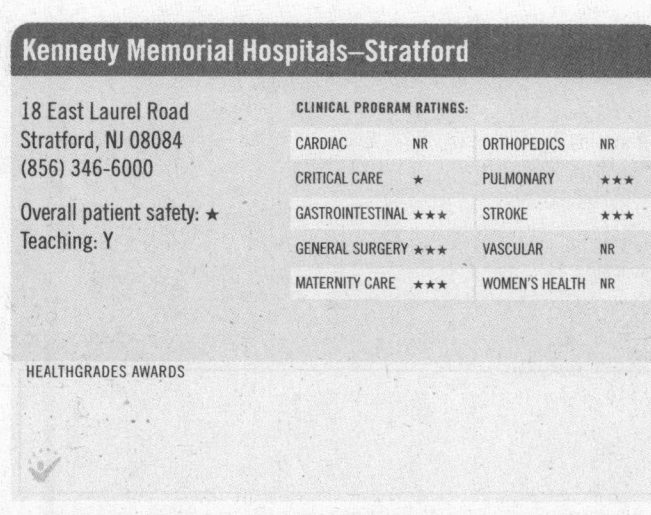

18 East Laurel Road
Stratford, NJ 08084
(856) 346-6000

Overall patient safety: ★
Teaching: Y

CLINICAL PROGRAM RATINGS:

CARDIAC	NR	ORTHOPEDICS	NR
CRITICAL CARE	★	PULMONARY	★★★
GASTROINTESTINAL	★★★	STROKE	★★★
GENERAL SURGERY	★★★	VASCULAR	NR
MATERNITY CARE	★★★	WOMEN'S HEALTH	NR

HEALTHGRADES AWARDS

Lourdes Medical Center of Burlington County

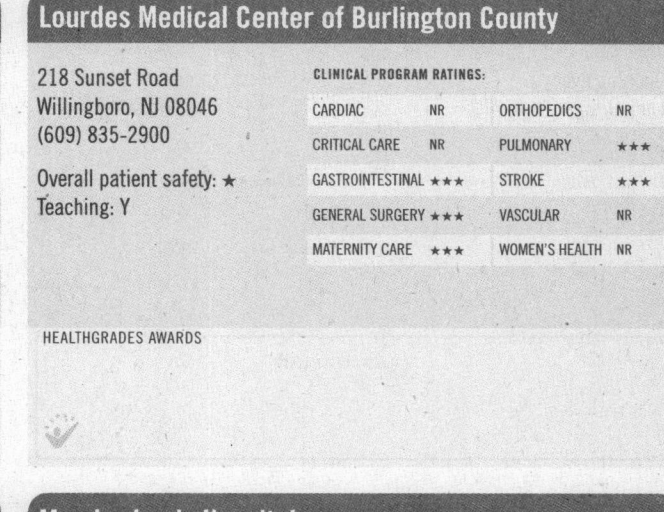

218 Sunset Road
Willingboro, NJ 08046
(609) 835-2900

Overall patient safety: ★
Teaching: Y

CLINICAL PROGRAM RATINGS:

CARDIAC	NR	ORTHOPEDICS	NR
CRITICAL CARE	NR	PULMONARY	★★★
GASTROINTESTINAL	★★★	STROKE	★★★
GENERAL SURGERY	★★★	VASCULAR	NR
MATERNITY CARE	★★★	WOMEN'S HEALTH	NR

HEALTHGRADES AWARDS

Kessler Memorial Hospital

600 South White Horse Pike
Hammonton, NJ 08037
(609) 561-6700

Overall patient safety: ★★★
Teaching: Y

CLINICAL PROGRAM RATINGS:

CARDIAC	NR	ORTHOPEDICS	NR
CRITICAL CARE	NR	PULMONARY	★★★
GASTROINTESTINAL	NR	STROKE	★★★
GENERAL SURGERY	★★★	VASCULAR	NR
MATERNITY CARE	NR	WOMEN'S HEALTH	NR

HEALTHGRADES AWARDS

Meadowlands Hospital

55 Meadowlands Parkway
Secaucus, NJ 07096
(201) 392-3100

Overall patient safety: ★
Teaching: N

CLINICAL PROGRAM RATINGS:

CARDIAC	NR	ORTHOPEDICS	NR
CRITICAL CARE	NR	PULMONARY	★★★
GASTROINTESTINAL	NR	STROKE	★★★
GENERAL SURGERY	★★★	VASCULAR	NR
MATERNITY CARE	★★★★★	WOMEN'S HEALTH	NR

HEALTHGRADES AWARDS

✓ SPECIALTY EXCELLENCE
• MATERNITY CARE

Memorial Hospital of Salem County

310 Woodstown Road
Salem, NJ 08079
(856) 935-1000

Overall patient safety: ★
Teaching: N

CLINICAL PROGRAM RATINGS:

CARDIAC	NR	ORTHOPEDICS	NR
CRITICAL CARE	★★★	PULMONARY	★★★★★
GASTROINTESTINAL	★★★	STROKE	★★★
GENERAL SURGERY	★★★	VASCULAR	NR
MATERNITY CARE	★★★	WOMEN'S HEALTH	NR

HEALTHGRADES AWARDS

✓ SPECIALTY EXCELLENCE
- GENERAL SURGERY

Mountainside Hospital

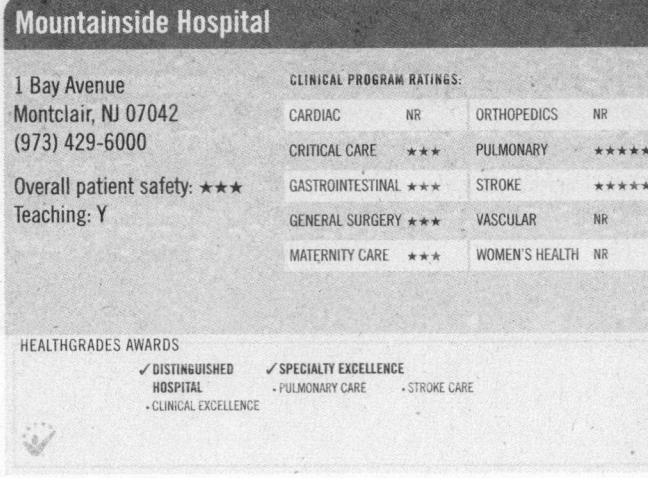

1 Bay Avenue
Montclair, NJ 07042
(973) 429-6000

Overall patient safety: ★★★
Teaching: Y

CLINICAL PROGRAM RATINGS:

CARDIAC	NR	ORTHOPEDICS	NR
CRITICAL CARE	★★★	PULMONARY	★★★★★
GASTROINTESTINAL	★★★	STROKE	★★★★★
GENERAL SURGERY	★★★	VASCULAR	NR
MATERNITY CARE	★★★	WOMEN'S HEALTH	NR

HEALTHGRADES AWARDS

✓ DISTINGUISHED HOSPITAL
- CLINICAL EXCELLENCE

✓ SPECIALTY EXCELLENCE
- PULMONARY CARE   - STROKE CARE

Monmouth Medical Center

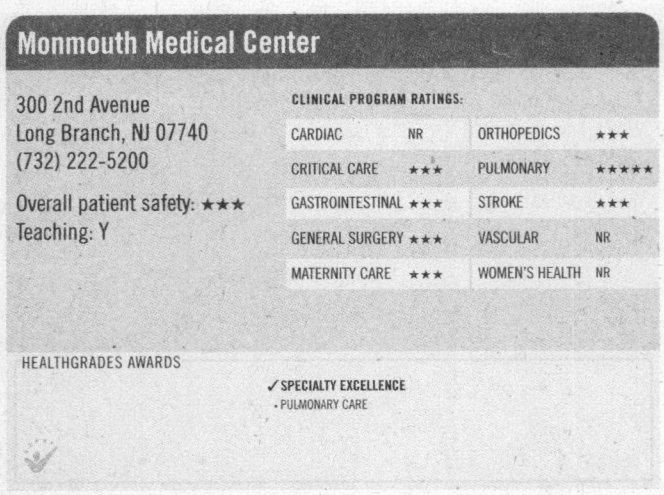

300 2nd Avenue
Long Branch, NJ 07740
(732) 222-5200

Overall patient safety: ★★★
Teaching: Y

CLINICAL PROGRAM RATINGS:

CARDIAC	NR	ORTHOPEDICS	★★★
CRITICAL CARE	★★★	PULMONARY	★★★★★
GASTROINTESTINAL	★★★	STROKE	★★★
GENERAL SURGERY	★★★	VASCULAR	NR
MATERNITY CARE	★★★	WOMEN'S HEALTH	NR

HEALTHGRADES AWARDS

✓ SPECIALTY EXCELLENCE
- PULMONARY CARE

Muhlenberg Regional Medical Center

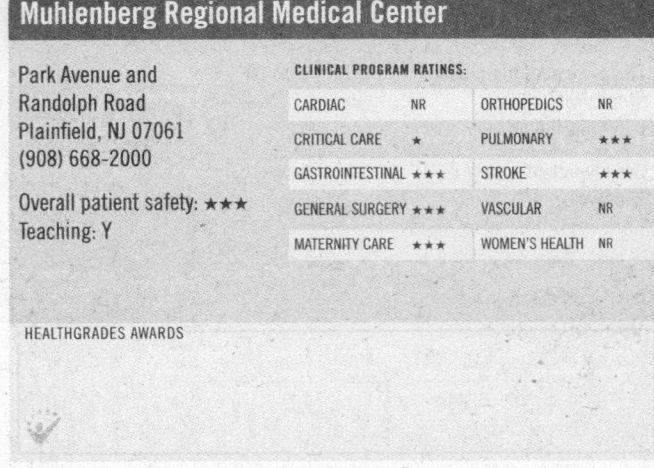

Park Avenue and
Randolph Road
Plainfield, NJ 07061
(908) 668-2000

Overall patient safety: ★★★
Teaching: Y

CLINICAL PROGRAM RATINGS:

CARDIAC	NR	ORTHOPEDICS	NR
CRITICAL CARE	★	PULMONARY	★★★
GASTROINTESTINAL	★★★	STROKE	★★★
GENERAL SURGERY	★★★	VASCULAR	NR
MATERNITY CARE	★★★	WOMEN'S HEALTH	NR

HEALTHGRADES AWARDS

Morristown Memorial Hospital

100 Madison Avenue
Morristown, NJ 07960
(973) 971-5000

Overall patient safety: ★★★
Teaching: Y

CLINICAL PROGRAM RATINGS:

CARDIAC	★★★	ORTHOPEDICS	★★★
CRITICAL CARE	★★★	PULMONARY	★★★
GASTROINTESTINAL	★★★	STROKE	★★★
GENERAL SURGERY	★★★	VASCULAR	★★★
MATERNITY CARE	★★★★★	WOMEN'S HEALTH	★★★

HEALTHGRADES AWARDS

✓ SPECIALTY EXCELLENCE
- BARIATRIC SURGERY

Newark Beth Israel Medical Center

201 Lyons Avenue
Newark, NJ 07112
(973) 926-7000

Overall patient safety: ★★★
Teaching: Y

CLINICAL PROGRAM RATINGS:

CARDIAC	★★★	ORTHOPEDICS	NR
CRITICAL CARE	★★★	PULMONARY	★★★
GASTROINTESTINAL	★★★	STROKE	★★★
GENERAL SURGERY	★★★	VASCULAR	★★★
MATERNITY CARE	★★★★★	WOMEN'S HEALTH	★★★★★

HEALTHGRADES AWARDS

✓ SPECIALTY EXCELLENCE
- MATERNITY CARE

KEY: ★★★★★ BEST   ★★★ AS EXPECTED   ★ POOR   NR NOT RATED BY HEALTHGRADES   For full definitions of ratings and awards, see Appendix.

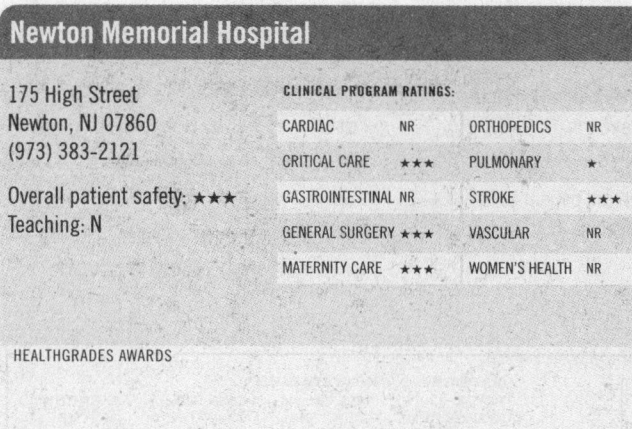

Newton Memorial Hospital

175 High Street
Newton, NJ 07860
(973) 383-2121

Overall patient safety: ★★★
Teaching: N

CLINICAL PROGRAM RATINGS:

CARDIAC	NR	ORTHOPEDICS	NR
CRITICAL CARE	★★★	PULMONARY	★
GASTROINTESTINAL	NR	STROKE	★★★
GENERAL SURGERY	★★★	VASCULAR	NR
MATERNITY CARE	★★★	WOMEN'S HEALTH	NR

HEALTHGRADES AWARDS

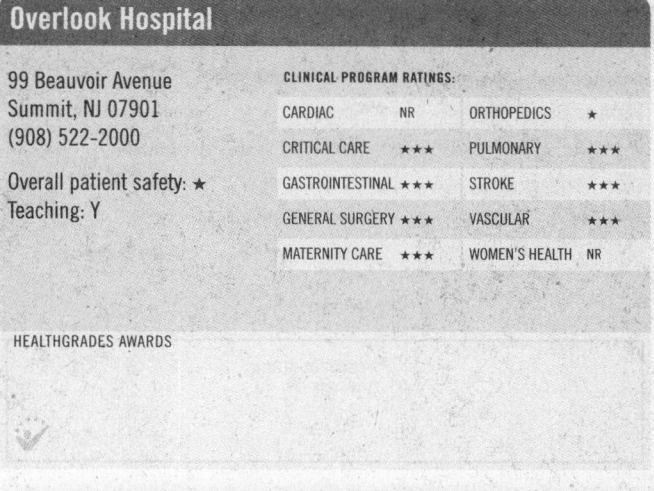

Overlook Hospital

99 Beauvoir Avenue
Summit, NJ 07901
(908) 522-2000

Overall patient safety: ★
Teaching: Y

CLINICAL PROGRAM RATINGS:

CARDIAC	NR	ORTHOPEDICS	★
CRITICAL CARE	★★★	PULMONARY	★★★
GASTROINTESTINAL	★★★	STROKE	★★★
GENERAL SURGERY	★★★	VASCULAR	★★★
MATERNITY CARE	★★★	WOMEN'S HEALTH	NR

HEALTHGRADES AWARDS

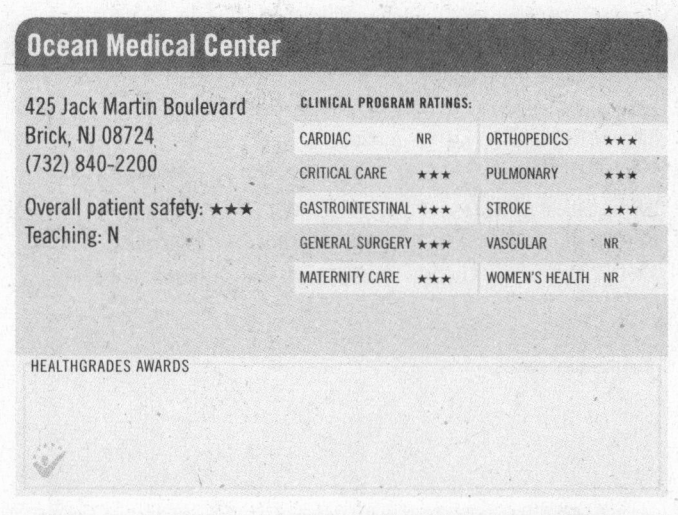

Ocean Medical Center

425 Jack Martin Boulevard
Brick, NJ 08724
(732) 840-2200

Overall patient safety: ★★★
Teaching: N

CLINICAL PROGRAM RATINGS:

CARDIAC	NR	ORTHOPEDICS	★★★
CRITICAL CARE	★★★	PULMONARY	★★★
GASTROINTESTINAL	★★★	STROKE	★★★
GENERAL SURGERY	★★★	VASCULAR	NR
MATERNITY CARE	★★★	WOMEN'S HEALTH	NR

HEALTHGRADES AWARDS

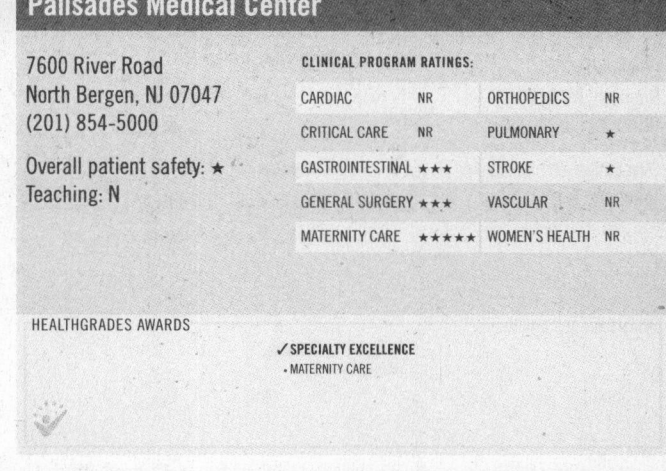

Palisades Medical Center

7600 River Road
North Bergen, NJ 07047
(201) 854-5000

Overall patient safety: ★
Teaching: N

CLINICAL PROGRAM RATINGS:

CARDIAC	NR	ORTHOPEDICS	NR
CRITICAL CARE	NR	PULMONARY	★
GASTROINTESTINAL	★★★	STROKE	★
GENERAL SURGERY	★★★	VASCULAR	NR
MATERNITY CARE	★★★★★	WOMEN'S HEALTH	NR

HEALTHGRADES AWARDS

✓ SPECIALTY EXCELLENCE
• MATERNITY CARE

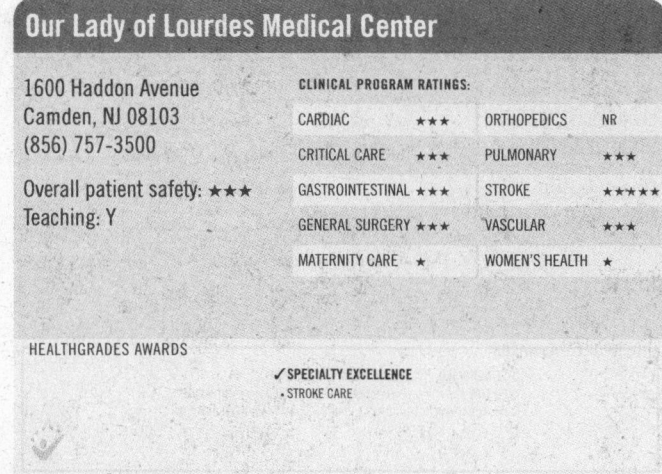

Our Lady of Lourdes Medical Center

1600 Haddon Avenue
Camden, NJ 08103
(856) 757-3500

Overall patient safety: ★★★
Teaching: Y

CLINICAL PROGRAM RATINGS:

CARDIAC	★★★	ORTHOPEDICS	NR
CRITICAL CARE	★★★	PULMONARY	★★★
GASTROINTESTINAL	★★★	STROKE	★★★★★
GENERAL SURGERY	★★★	VASCULAR	★★★
MATERNITY CARE	★	WOMEN'S HEALTH	★

HEALTHGRADES AWARDS

✓ SPECIALTY EXCELLENCE
• STROKE CARE

Pascack Valley Hospital

250 Old Hook Road
Westwood, NJ 07675
(201) 358-3000

Overall patient safety: ★★★
Teaching: Y

CLINICAL PROGRAM RATINGS:

CARDIAC	NR	ORTHOPEDICS	★★★
CRITICAL CARE	★★★	PULMONARY	★★★
GASTROINTESTINAL	★★★	STROKE	★★★
GENERAL SURGERY	★★★	VASCULAR	NR
MATERNITY CARE	★★★	WOMEN'S HEALTH	NR

HEALTHGRADES AWARDS

Raritan Bay Medical Center

530 New Brunswick Avenue
Perth Amboy, NJ 08861
(732) 442-3700

Overall patient safety: ★★★
Teaching: Y

CLINICAL PROGRAM RATINGS:

CARDIAC	NR	ORTHOPEDICS	NR
CRITICAL CARE	★★★	PULMONARY	★★★
GASTROINTESTINAL	★★★	STROKE	★★★★★
GENERAL SURGERY	★★★	VASCULAR	NR
MATERNITY CARE	★★★	WOMEN'S HEALTH	NR

HEALTHGRADES AWARDS

✓ SPECIALTY EXCELLENCE
· STROKE CARE

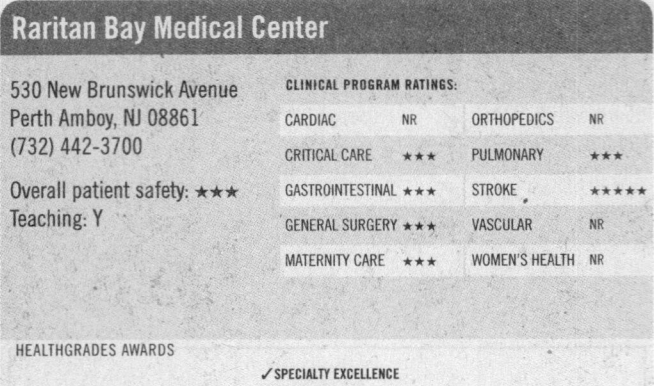

Robert Wood Johnson University Hospital at Hamilton

1 Hamilton Health Place
Hamilton, NJ 08690
(609) 586-7900

Overall patient safety: ★★★
Teaching: N

CLINICAL PROGRAM RATINGS:

CARDIAC	NR	ORTHOPEDICS	★★★
CRITICAL CARE	★★★★★	PULMONARY	★★★★★
GASTROINTESTINAL	★★★	STROKE	★★★★★
GENERAL SURGERY	★★★★★	VASCULAR	NR
MATERNITY CARE	★★★★★	WOMEN'S HEALTH	NR

HEALTHGRADES AWARDS

✓ DISTINGUISHED HOSPITAL
· CLINICAL EXCELLENCE

✓ SPECIALTY EXCELLENCE
· CRITICAL CARE
· GASTROINTESTINAL CARE
· GENERAL SURGERY
· MATERNITY CARE
· PULMONARY CARE
· STROKE CARE

Riverside Hospital*

Powerville Road Box 59
Boonton, NJ 07005
(201) 334-5000

Overall patient safety: ★
Teaching: N

CLINICAL PROGRAM RATINGS:

CARDIAC	NR	ORTHOPEDICS	★★★
CRITICAL CARE	★	PULMONARY	★
GASTROINTESTINAL	★★★	STROKE	★★★
GENERAL SURGERY	★★★	VASCULAR	NR
MATERNITY CARE	★★★★★	WOMEN'S HEALTH	NR

HEALTHGRADES AWARDS

✓ SPECIALTY EXCELLENCE
· MATERNITY CARE

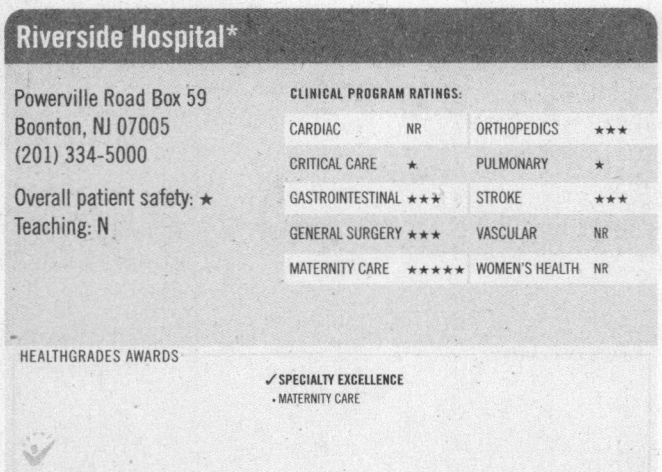

Robert Wood Johnson University Hospital—Rahway

865 Stone Street
Rahway, NJ 07065
(732) 381-4200

Overall patient safety: ★
Teaching: N

CLINICAL PROGRAM RATINGS:

CARDIAC	NR	ORTHOPEDICS	NR
CRITICAL CARE	NR	PULMONARY	★★★
GASTROINTESTINAL	★★★	STROKE	★★★★★
GENERAL SURGERY	★★★	VASCULAR	NR
MATERNITY CARE	NR	WOMEN'S HEALTH	NR

HEALTHGRADES AWARDS

Riverview Medical Center

1 Riverview Plaza
Red Bank, NJ 07701
(732) 741-2700

Overall patient safety: ★★★
Teaching: N

CLINICAL PROGRAM RATINGS:

CARDIAC	NR	ORTHOPEDICS	★
CRITICAL CARE	★★★	PULMONARY	★★★★★
GASTROINTESTINAL	★★★	STROKE	★★★
GENERAL SURGERY	★	VASCULAR	NR
MATERNITY CARE	★★★★★	WOMEN'S HEALTH	NR

HEALTHGRADES AWARDS

✓ SPECIALTY EXCELLENCE
· MATERNITY CARE   · PULMONARY CARE

St. Barnabas Medical Center

94 Old Short Hills Road
Livingston, NJ 07039
(973) 322-5000

Overall patient safety: ★★★
Teaching: Y

CLINICAL PROGRAM RATINGS:

CARDIAC	★★★★★	ORTHOPEDICS	★★★
CRITICAL CARE	★★★	PULMONARY	★★★
GASTROINTESTINAL	★★★	STROKE	★★★
GENERAL SURGERY	★★★	VASCULAR	★★★
MATERNITY CARE	★★★★★	WOMEN'S HEALTH	★★★★★

HEALTHGRADES AWARDS

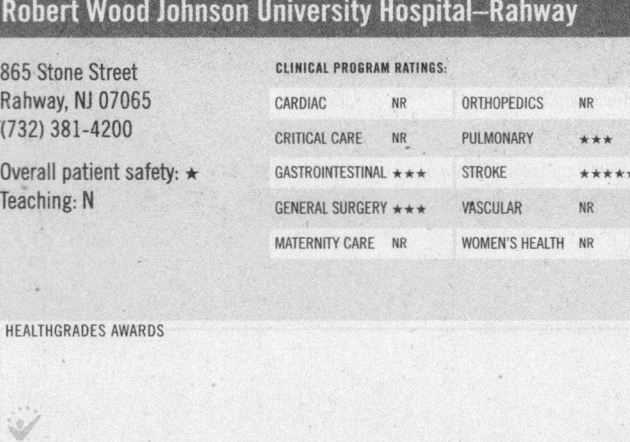

✓ DISTINGUISHED HOSPITAL
· CLINICAL EXCELLENCE

✓ SPECIALTY EXCELLENCE
· BARIATRIC SURGERY
· CARDIAC CARE
· MATERNITY CARE
· WOMEN'S HEALTH

KEY: ★★★★★ **BEST** ★★★ **AS EXPECTED** ★ **POOR** NR **NOT RATED BY HEALTHGRADES** For full definitions of ratings and awards, see Appendix.

440 CHAPTER 6: HOSPITAL RATINGS BY CLINICAL SPECIALTY

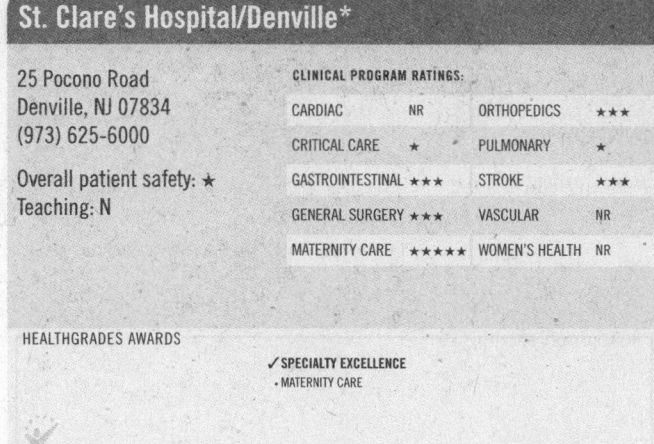

St. Clare's Hospital/Denville*

25 Pocono Road
Denville, NJ 07834
(973) 625-6000

Overall patient safety: ★
Teaching: N

CLINICAL PROGRAM RATINGS:

CARDIAC	NR	ORTHOPEDICS	★★★
CRITICAL CARE	★	PULMONARY	★
GASTROINTESTINAL	★★★	STROKE	★★★
GENERAL SURGERY	★★★	VASCULAR	NR
MATERNITY CARE	★★★★★	WOMEN'S HEALTH	NR

HEALTHGRADES AWARDS

✓ SPECIALTY EXCELLENCE
- MATERNITY CARE

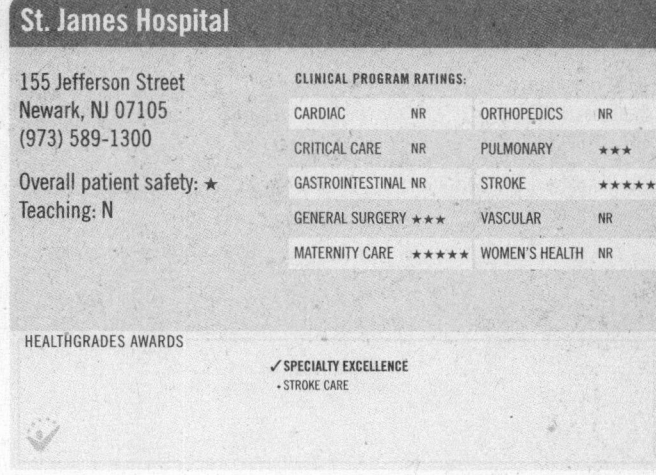

St. James Hospital

155 Jefferson Street
Newark, NJ 07105
(973) 589-1300

Overall patient safety: ★
Teaching: N

CLINICAL PROGRAM RATINGS:

CARDIAC	NR	ORTHOPEDICS	NR
CRITICAL CARE	NR	PULMONARY	★★★
GASTROINTESTINAL	NR	STROKE	★★★★★
GENERAL SURGERY	★★★	VASCULAR	NR
MATERNITY CARE	★★★★★	WOMEN'S HEALTH	NR

HEALTHGRADES AWARDS

✓ SPECIALTY EXCELLENCE
- STROKE CARE

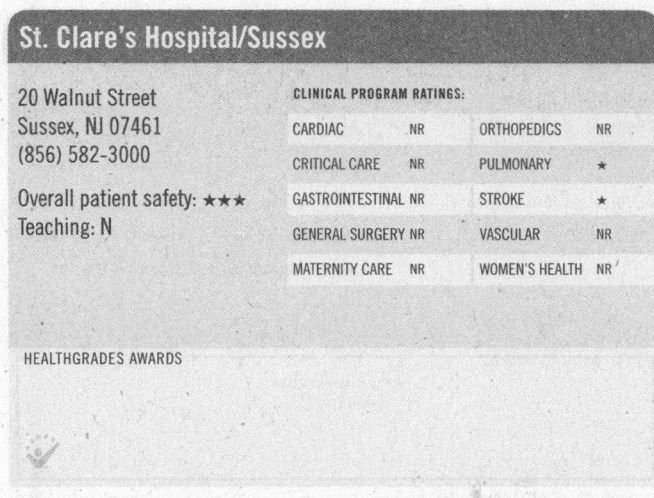

St. Clare's Hospital/Sussex

20 Walnut Street
Sussex, NJ 07461
(856) 582-3000

Overall patient safety: ★★★
Teaching: N

CLINICAL PROGRAM RATINGS:

CARDIAC	NR	ORTHOPEDICS	NR
CRITICAL CARE	NR	PULMONARY	★
GASTROINTESTINAL	NR	STROKE	★
GENERAL SURGERY	NR	VASCULAR	NR
MATERNITY CARE	NR	WOMEN'S HEALTH	NR

HEALTHGRADES AWARDS

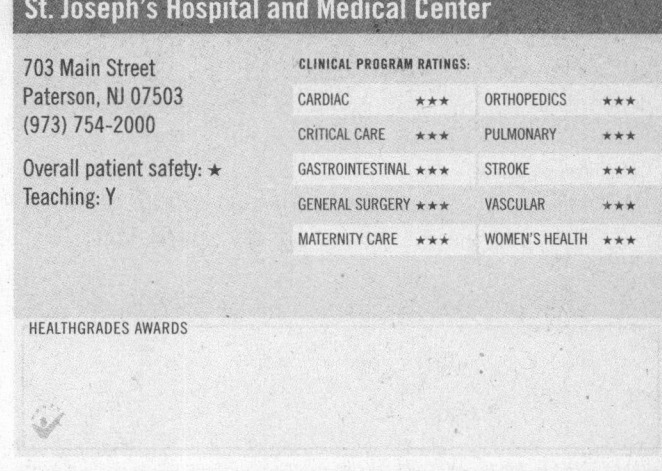

St. Joseph's Hospital and Medical Center

703 Main Street
Paterson, NJ 07503
(973) 754-2000

Overall patient safety: ★
Teaching: Y

CLINICAL PROGRAM RATINGS:

CARDIAC	★★★	ORTHOPEDICS	★★★
CRITICAL CARE	★★★	PULMONARY	★★★
GASTROINTESTINAL	★★★	STROKE	★★★
GENERAL SURGERY	★★★	VASCULAR	★★★
MATERNITY CARE	★★★	WOMEN'S HEALTH	★★★

HEALTHGRADES AWARDS

St. Francis Medical Center

601 Hamilton Avenue
Trenton, NJ 08629
(609) 599-5000

Overall patient safety: ★
Teaching: Y

CLINICAL PROGRAM RATINGS:

CARDIAC	★★★	ORTHOPEDICS	NR
CRITICAL CARE	NR	PULMONARY	★★★
GASTROINTESTINAL	NR	STROKE	★★★
GENERAL SURGERY	★★★	VASCULAR	NR
MATERNITY CARE	NR	WOMEN'S HEALTH	NR

HEALTHGRADES AWARDS

St. Joseph's Wayne Hospital

224 Hamburg Turnpike
Wayne, NJ 07470
(973) 942-6900

Overall patient safety: ★
Teaching: N

CLINICAL PROGRAM RATINGS:

CARDIAC	NR	ORTHOPEDICS	NR
CRITICAL CARE	★★★	PULMONARY	★★★
GASTROINTESTINAL	★★★	STROKE	★★★
GENERAL SURGERY	★★★	VASCULAR	NR
MATERNITY CARE	NR	WOMEN'S HEALTH	NR

HEALTHGRADES AWARDS

*This hospital reports its data to the federal government jointly with another hospital. Therefore the ratings and awards apply to multiple hospitals and this specific hospital may not provide all rated services.

St. Mary's Hospital*

350 Boulevard
Passaic, NJ 07055
(973) 470-3000

Overall patient safety: ★★★
Teaching: N

CLINICAL PROGRAM RATINGS:

CARDIAC	★★★	ORTHOPEDICS	NR
CRITICAL CARE	★	PULMONARY	★
GASTROINTESTINAL	★★★	STROKE	★★★★★
GENERAL SURGERY	★★★	VASCULAR	NR
MATERNITY CARE	★★★★★	WOMEN'S HEALTH	NR

HEALTHGRADES AWARDS

✓ SPECIALTY EXCELLENCE
• MATERNITY CARE   • STROKE CARE

Shore Memorial Hospital

1 East New York Avenue
Somers Point, NJ 08244
(609) 653-3500

Overall patient safety: ★★★
Teaching: N

CLINICAL PROGRAM RATINGS:

CARDIAC	NR	ORTHOPEDICS	★★★
CRITICAL CARE	★★★	PULMONARY	★★★
GASTROINTESTINAL	★★★	STROKE	★★★
GENERAL SURGERY	★	VASCULAR	NR
MATERNITY CARE	★★★	WOMEN'S HEALTH	NR

HEALTHGRADES AWARDS

St. Michael's Medical Center

111 Central Avenue
Newark, NJ 07102
(973) 877-5000

Overall patient safety: ★★★
Teaching: Y

CLINICAL PROGRAM RATINGS:

CARDIAC	★★★	ORTHOPEDICS	NR
CRITICAL CARE	NR	PULMONARY	★★★
GASTROINTESTINAL	NR	STROKE	★
GENERAL SURGERY	★★★	VASCULAR	NR
MATERNITY CARE	NR	WOMEN'S HEALTH	NR

HEALTHGRADES AWARDS

Somerset Medical Center

110 Rehill Avenue
Somerville, NJ 08876
(908) 685-2200

Overall patient safety: ★
Teaching: Y

CLINICAL PROGRAM RATINGS:

CARDIAC	NR	ORTHOPEDICS	★★★★★
CRITICAL CARE	★★★	PULMONARY	★★★
GASTROINTESTINAL	★★★	STROKE	★★★★★
GENERAL SURGERY	★★★	VASCULAR	NR
MATERNITY CARE	★★★	WOMEN'S HEALTH	NR

HEALTHGRADES AWARDS

✓ SPECIALTY EXCELLENCE
• STROKE CARE

St. Peter's University Hospital

254 Easton Avenue
New Brunswick, NJ 08901
(732) 745-8600

Overall patient safety: ★
Teaching: Y

CLINICAL PROGRAM RATINGS:

CARDIAC	NR	ORTHOPEDICS	★★★
CRITICAL CARE	★★★	PULMONARY	★★★
GASTROINTESTINAL	★★★	STROKE	★★★★★
GENERAL SURGERY	★★★	VASCULAR	★★★
MATERNITY CARE	★★★	WOMEN'S HEALTH	NR

HEALTHGRADES AWARDS

South Jersey Healthcare Regional Medical Center

1505 West Sherman Avenue
Vineland, NJ 08360
(856) 641-8000

Overall patient safety: ★
Teaching: N

CLINICAL PROGRAM RATINGS:

CARDIAC	NR	ORTHOPEDICS	★★★
CRITICAL CARE	★	PULMONARY	★
GASTROINTESTINAL	★★★	STROKE	★★★
GENERAL SURGERY	★★★	VASCULAR	NR
MATERNITY CARE	★★★	WOMEN'S HEALTH	NR

HEALTHGRADES AWARDS

KEY: ★★★★★ BEST   ★★★ AS EXPECTED   ★ POOR   NR NOT RATED BY HEALTHGRADES   For full definitions of ratings and awards, see Appendix.

South Jersey Hospital–Elmer Division

1090 West Front Street
Elmer, NJ 08318
(856) 363-1000

Overall patient safety: ★
Teaching: N

CLINICAL PROGRAM RATINGS:

CARDIAC	NR	ORTHOPEDICS	★★★
CRITICAL CARE	NR	PULMONARY	★★★
GASTROINTESTINAL	NR	STROKE	★
GENERAL SURGERY	★★★	VASCULAR	NR
MATERNITY CARE	★★★	WOMEN'S HEALTH	NR

HEALTHGRADES AWARDS

UMDNJ-University Hospital

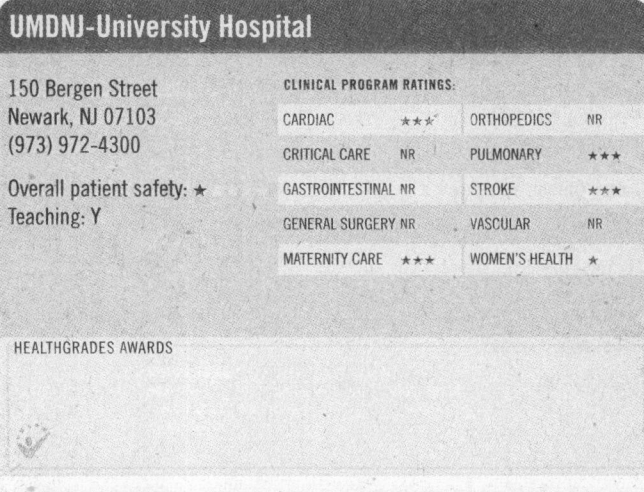

150 Bergen Street
Newark, NJ 07103
(973) 972-4300

Overall patient safety: ★
Teaching: Y

CLINICAL PROGRAM RATINGS:

CARDIAC	★★★	ORTHOPEDICS	NR
CRITICAL CARE	NR	PULMONARY	★★★
GASTROINTESTINAL	NR	STROKE	★★★
GENERAL SURGERY	NR	VASCULAR	NR
MATERNITY CARE	★★★	WOMEN'S HEALTH	★

HEALTHGRADES AWARDS

Southern Ocean County Hospital

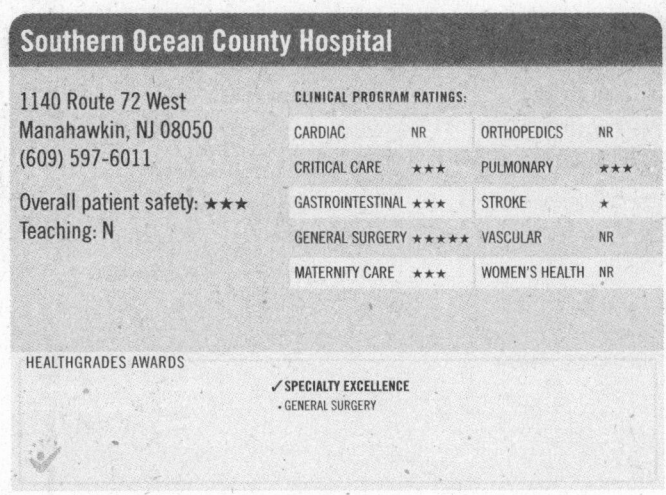

1140 Route 72 West
Manahawkin, NJ 08050
(609) 597-6011

Overall patient safety: ★★★
Teaching: N

CLINICAL PROGRAM RATINGS:

CARDIAC	NR	ORTHOPEDICS	NR
CRITICAL CARE	★★★	PULMONARY	★★★
GASTROINTESTINAL	★★★	STROKE	★
GENERAL SURGERY	★★★★★	VASCULAR	NR
MATERNITY CARE	★★★	WOMEN'S HEALTH	NR

HEALTHGRADES AWARDS

✓ SPECIALTY EXCELLENCE
• GENERAL SURGERY

Underwood Memorial Hospital

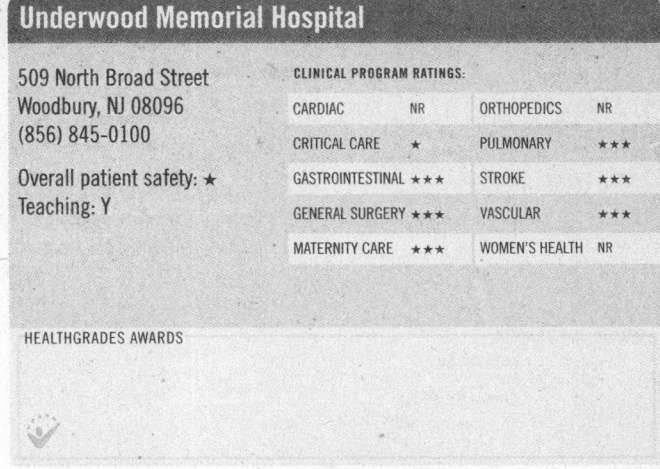

509 North Broad Street
Woodbury, NJ 08096
(856) 845-0100

Overall patient safety: ★
Teaching: Y

CLINICAL PROGRAM RATINGS:

CARDIAC	NR	ORTHOPEDICS	NR
CRITICAL CARE	★	PULMONARY	★★★
GASTROINTESTINAL	★★★	STROKE	★★★
GENERAL SURGERY	★★★	VASCULAR	★★★
MATERNITY CARE	★★★	WOMEN'S HEALTH	NR

HEALTHGRADES AWARDS

Trinitas Hospital–Williamson*

225 Williamson Street
Elizabeth, NJ 07207
(908) 994-5000

Overall patient safety: ★★★
Teaching: Y

CLINICAL PROGRAM RATINGS:

CARDIAC	NR	ORTHOPEDICS	NR
CRITICAL CARE	NR	PULMONARY	★
GASTROINTESTINAL	★★★	STROKE	★
GENERAL SURGERY	★★★	VASCULAR	NR
MATERNITY CARE	★★★	WOMEN'S HEALTH	NR

HEALTHGRADES AWARDS

Union Hospital

1000 Galloping Hill Road
Union, NJ 07083
(908) 687-1900

Overall patient safety: ★★★
Teaching: Y

CLINICAL PROGRAM RATINGS:

CARDIAC	NR	ORTHOPEDICS	★★★
CRITICAL CARE	NR	PULMONARY	★
GASTROINTESTINAL	★★★	STROKE	★★★
GENERAL SURGERY	★★★	VASCULAR	NR
MATERNITY CARE	NR	WOMEN'S HEALTH	NR

HEALTHGRADES AWARDS

*This hospital reports its data to the federal government jointly with another hospital. Therefore the ratings and awards apply to multiple hospitals and this specific hospital may not provide all rated services.

University Medical Center at Princeton

253 Witherspoon Street
Princeton, NJ 08540
(609) 497-4000

Overall patient safety: ★★★
Teaching: Y

CLINICAL PROGRAM RATINGS:

CARDIAC	NR	ORTHOPEDICS	★★★
CRITICAL CARE	★★★	PULMONARY	★★★
GASTROINTESTINAL	★★★	STROKE	★
GENERAL SURGERY	★★★	VASCULAR	★★★
MATERNITY CARE	★★★★★	WOMEN'S HEALTH	NR

HEALTHGRADES AWARDS

✓ SPECIALTY EXCELLENCE
· MATERNITY CARE

Virtua West Jersey Hospital—Berlin*

Whitehorse Pike and
Townsend Avenue
Berlin, NJ 08009
(856) 322-3000

Overall patient safety: ★
Teaching: Y

CLINICAL PROGRAM RATINGS:

CARDIAC	NR	ORTHOPEDICS	★★★
CRITICAL CARE	★	PULMONARY	★★★
GASTROINTESTINAL	★★★	STROKE	★★★
GENERAL SURGERY	★★★	VASCULAR	★★★
MATERNITY CARE	★★★	WOMEN'S HEALTH	NR

HEALTHGRADES AWARDS

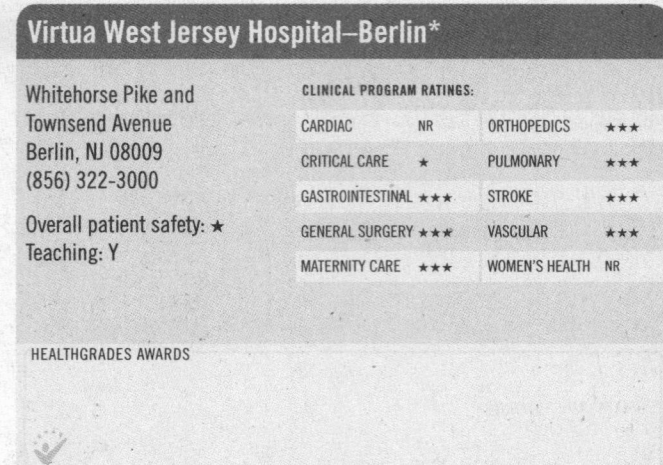

Valley Hospital

223 North Van Dien Avenue
Ridgewood, NJ 07450
(201) 447-8000

Overall patient safety: ★
Teaching: N

CLINICAL PROGRAM RATINGS:

CARDIAC	★★★	ORTHOPEDICS	★★★
CRITICAL CARE	★★★	PULMONARY	★★★
GASTROINTESTINAL	★★★	STROKE	★★★★★
GENERAL SURGERY	★★★	VASCULAR	★
MATERNITY CARE	★★★★★	WOMEN'S HEALTH	★★★★★

HEALTHGRADES AWARDS

✓ DISTINGUISHED   ✓ SPECIALTY EXCELLENCE
   HOSPITAL   · MATERNITY CARE
· CLINICAL EXCELLENCE

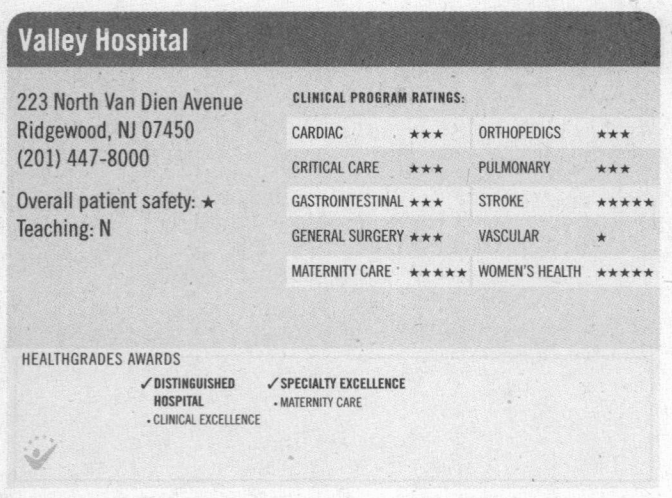

Virtua West Jersey Hospital—Marlton*

90 Brick Road
Marlton, NJ 08053
(856) 355-6000

Overall patient safety: ★
Teaching: Y

CLINICAL PROGRAM RATINGS:

CARDIAC	NR	ORTHOPEDICS	★★★
CRITICAL CARE	★	PULMONARY	★★★
GASTROINTESTINAL	★★★	STROKE	★★★
GENERAL SURGERY	★★★	VASCULAR	★★★
MATERNITY CARE	★★★	WOMEN'S HEALTH	NR

HEALTHGRADES AWARDS

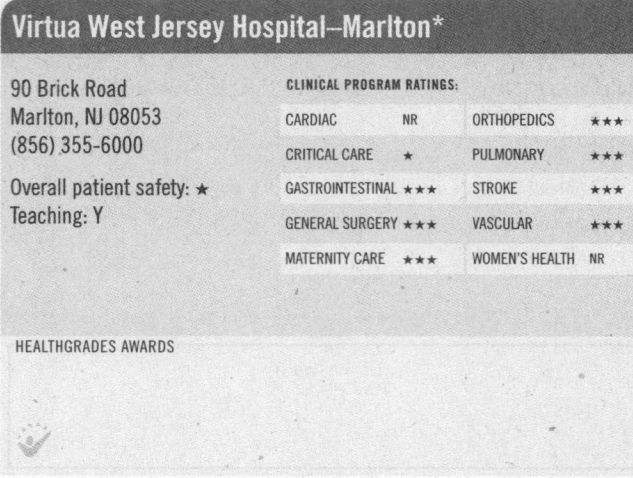

Virtua Memorial Hospital—Burlington County

175 Madison Avenue
Mount Holly, NJ 08060
(609) 267-0700

Overall patient safety: ★★★
Teaching: Y

CLINICAL PROGRAM RATINGS:

CARDIAC	NR	ORTHOPEDICS	★
CRITICAL CARE	★	PULMONARY	★★★
GASTROINTESTINAL	★★★	STROKE	★★★
GENERAL SURGERY	★★★	VASCULAR	NR
MATERNITY CARE	★★★	WOMEN'S HEALTH	NR

HEALTHGRADES AWARDS

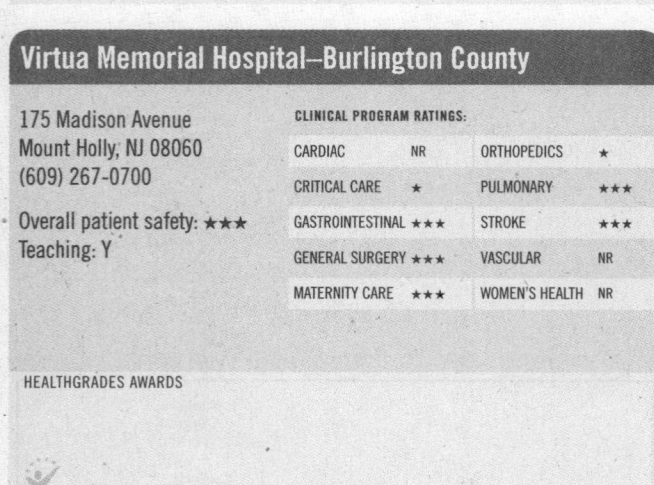

Warren Hospital

185 Roseberry Street
Phillipsburg, NJ 08865
(908) 859-6700

Overall patient safety: ★★★
Teaching: Y

CLINICAL PROGRAM RATINGS:

CARDIAC	NR	ORTHOPEDICS	★★★
CRITICAL CARE	★★★	PULMONARY	★
GASTROINTESTINAL	★★★	STROKE	★★★
GENERAL SURGERY	★★★	VASCULAR	NR
MATERNITY CARE	★★★	WOMEN'S HEALTH	NR

HEALTHGRADES AWARDS

✓ SPECIALTY EXCELLENCE
· GASTROINTESTINAL
  CARE

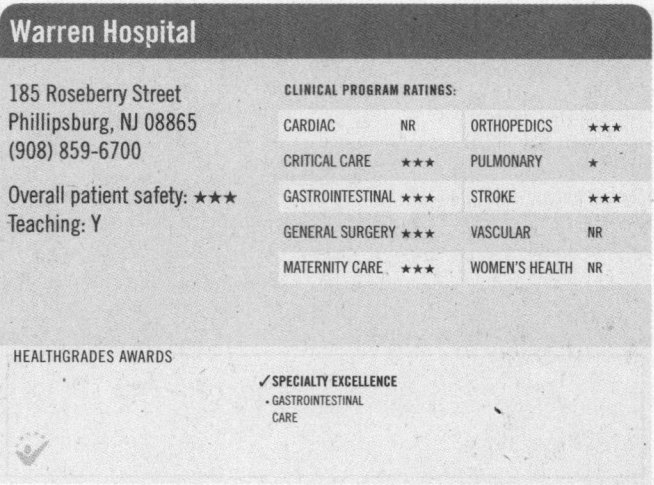

KEY: ★★★★★ BEST   ★★★ AS EXPECTED   ★ POOR   NR NOT RATED BY HEALTHGRADES   For full definitions of ratings and awards, see Appendix.

Alta Vista Regional Hospital

104 Legion Drive
Las Vegas, NM 87701
(505) 426-3500

Overall patient safety: ★★★
Teaching: N

CLINICAL PROGRAM RATINGS:

CARDIAC	NR	ORTHOPEDICS	NR
CRITICAL CARE	NR	PULMONARY	★★★
GASTROINTESTINAL	NR	STROKE	★★★
GENERAL SURGERY	NR	VASCULAR	NR
MATERNITY CARE	NR	WOMEN'S HEALTH	NR

HEALTHGRADES AWARDS

Cibola General Hospital

1016 Roosevelt Avenue
Grants, NM 87020
(505) 287-4446

Overall patient safety: ★★★
Teaching: N

CLINICAL PROGRAM RATINGS:

CARDIAC	NR	ORTHOPEDICS	NR
CRITICAL CARE	NR	PULMONARY	★★★
GASTROINTESTINAL	NR	STROKE	NR
GENERAL SURGERY	NR	VASCULAR	NR
MATERNITY CARE	NR	WOMEN'S HEALTH	NR

HEALTHGRADES AWARDS

Artesia General Hospital

702 North 13th Street
Artesia, NM 88210
(505) 748-3333

Overall patient safety: ★★★
Teaching: N

CLINICAL PROGRAM RATINGS:

CARDIAC	NR	ORTHOPEDICS	NR
CRITICAL CARE	NR	PULMONARY	★★★
GASTROINTESTINAL	NR	STROKE	★★★
GENERAL SURGERY	NR	VASCULAR	NR
MATERNITY CARE	NR	WOMEN'S HEALTH	NR

HEALTHGRADES AWARDS

Dr. Dan C. Trigg Memorial Hospital

301 East Miel De Luna
P.O. Box 608
Tucumcari, NM 88401
(505) 461-0141

Overall patient safety: ★★★
Teaching: N

CLINICAL PROGRAM RATINGS:

CARDIAC	NR	ORTHOPEDICS	NR
CRITICAL CARE	NR	PULMONARY	★★★
GASTROINTESTINAL	NR	STROKE	NR
GENERAL SURGERY	NR	VASCULAR	NR
MATERNITY CARE	NR	WOMEN'S HEALTH	NR

HEALTHGRADES AWARDS

Carlsbad Medical Center

2430 West Pierce Street
Carlsbad, NM 88220
(505) 887-4100

Overall patient safety: ★★★
Teaching: N

CLINICAL PROGRAM RATINGS:

CARDIAC	NR	ORTHOPEDICS	NR
CRITICAL CARE	NR	PULMONARY	★★★
GASTROINTESTINAL	★★★	STROKE	★★★
GENERAL SURGERY	NR	VASCULAR	NR
MATERNITY CARE	NR	WOMEN'S HEALTH	NR

HEALTHGRADES AWARDS

Eastern New Mexico Medical Center

405 West Country Club Road
Roswell, NM 88201
(505) 622-8170

Overall patient safety: ★★★
Teaching: Y

CLINICAL PROGRAM RATINGS:

CARDIAC	NR	ORTHOPEDICS	★★★
CRITICAL CARE	NR	PULMONARY	★★★
GASTROINTESTINAL	★★★	STROKE	★★★
GENERAL SURGERY	NR	VASCULAR	NR
MATERNITY CARE	NR	WOMEN'S HEALTH	NR

HEALTHGRADES AWARDS

*This hospital reports its data to the federal government jointly with another hospital. Therefore the ratings and awards apply to multiple hospitals and this specific hospital may not provide all rated services.

Española Hospital

1010 Spruce Street
Española, NM 87532
(505) 753-7111

Overall patient safety: ★
Teaching: N

CLINICAL PROGRAM RATINGS:

CARDIAC	NR	ORTHOPEDICS	NR
CRITICAL CARE	NR	PULMONARY	★★★
GASTROINTESTINAL	NR	STROKE	NR
GENERAL SURGERY	NR	VASCULAR	NR
MATERNITY CARE	NR	WOMEN'S HEALTH	NR

HEALTHGRADES AWARDS

Gila Regional Medical Center

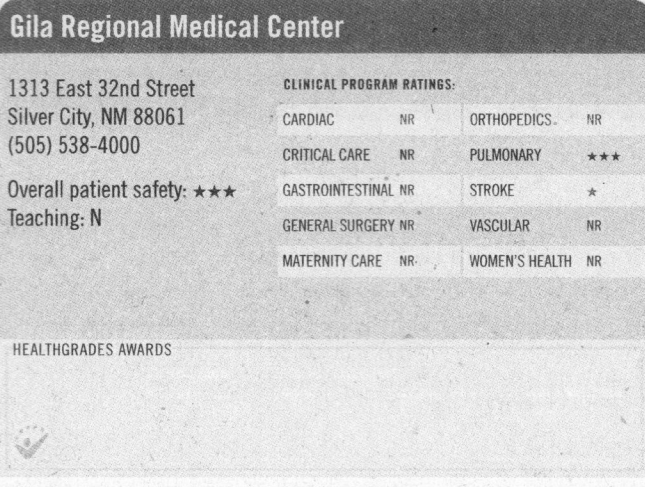

1313 East 32nd Street
Silver City, NM 88061
(505) 538-4000

Overall patient safety: ★★★
Teaching: N

CLINICAL PROGRAM RATINGS:

CARDIAC	NR	ORTHOPEDICS	NR
CRITICAL CARE	NR	PULMONARY	★★★
GASTROINTESTINAL	NR	STROKE	★
GENERAL SURGERY	NR	VASCULAR	NR
MATERNITY CARE	NR	WOMEN'S HEALTH	NR

HEALTHGRADES AWARDS

Gallup Indian Medical Center

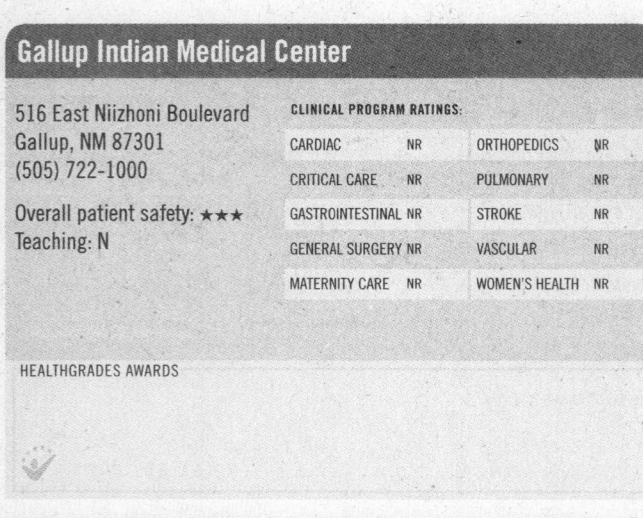

516 East Niizhoni Boulevard
Gallup, NM 87301
(505) 722-1000

Overall patient safety: ★★★
Teaching: N

CLINICAL PROGRAM RATINGS:

CARDIAC	NR	ORTHOPEDICS	NR
CRITICAL CARE	NR	PULMONARY	NR
GASTROINTESTINAL	NR	STROKE	NR
GENERAL SURGERY	NR	VASCULAR	NR
MATERNITY CARE	NR	WOMEN'S HEALTH	NR

HEALTHGRADES AWARDS

Heart Hospital of New Mexico

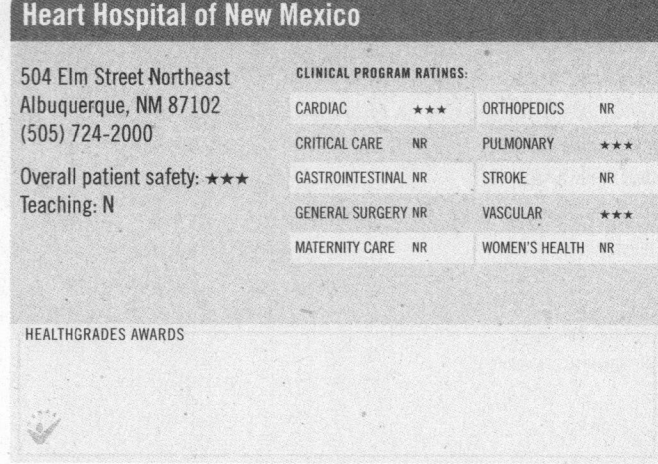

504 Elm Street Northeast
Albuquerque, NM 87102
(505) 724-2000

Overall patient safety: ★★★
Teaching: N

CLINICAL PROGRAM RATINGS:

CARDIAC	★★★	ORTHOPEDICS	NR
CRITICAL CARE	NR	PULMONARY	★★★
GASTROINTESTINAL	NR	STROKE	NR
GENERAL SURGERY	NR	VASCULAR	★★★
MATERNITY CARE	NR	WOMEN'S HEALTH	NR

HEALTHGRADES AWARDS

Gerald Champion Regional Medical Center

2669 North Scenic Drive
Alamogordo, NM 88310
(505) 439-6100

Overall patient safety: ★★★
Teaching: N

CLINICAL PROGRAM RATINGS:

CARDIAC	NR	ORTHOPEDICS	★★★
CRITICAL CARE	NR	PULMONARY	★★★
GASTROINTESTINAL	★★★	STROKE	★
GENERAL SURGERY	NR	VASCULAR	NR
MATERNITY CARE	NR	WOMEN'S HEALTH	NR

HEALTHGRADES AWARDS

Holy Cross Hospital

1397 Weimer Road
Taos, NM 87571
(505) 758-8883

Overall patient safety: ★★★
Teaching: N

CLINICAL PROGRAM RATINGS:

CARDIAC	NR	ORTHOPEDICS	NR
CRITICAL CARE	NR	PULMONARY	★★★
GASTROINTESTINAL	NR	STROKE	NR
GENERAL SURGERY	NR	VASCULAR	NR
MATERNITY CARE	NR	WOMEN'S HEALTH	NR

HEALTHGRADES AWARDS

KEY: ★★★★★ BEST   ★★★ AS EXPECTED   ★ POOR   NR NOT RATED BY HEALTHGRADES   For full definitions of ratings and awards, see Appendix.

Lea Regional Hospital

5419 North Lovington Highway
Hobbs, NM 88240
(505) 492-5000

Overall patient safety: ★
Teaching: N

CLINICAL PROGRAM RATINGS:

CARDIAC	NR	ORTHOPEDICS	NR
CRITICAL CARE	NR	PULMONARY	★★★★★
GASTROINTESTINAL	NR	STROKE	NR
GENERAL SURGERY	NR	VASCULAR	NR
MATERNITY CARE	NR	WOMEN'S HEALTH	NR

HEALTHGRADES AWARDS

✓ SPECIALTY EXCELLENCE
• PULMONARY CARE

Lovelace Medical Center—Gibson

5400 Gibson Boulevard
Southeast
Albuquerque, NM 87108
(505) 262-7000

Overall patient safety: ★
Teaching: Y

CLINICAL PROGRAM RATINGS:

CARDIAC	NR	ORTHOPEDICS	★★★
CRITICAL CARE	NR	PULMONARY	★
GASTROINTESTINAL	NR	STROKE	★
GENERAL SURGERY	NR	VASCULAR	NR
MATERNITY CARE	NR	WOMEN'S HEALTH	NR

HEALTHGRADES AWARDS

Los Alamos Medical Center

3917 West Road
Los Alamos, NM 87544
(505) 662-4201

Overall patient safety: ★★★
Teaching: N

CLINICAL PROGRAM RATINGS:

CARDIAC	NR	ORTHOPEDICS	NR
CRITICAL CARE	NR	PULMONARY	NR
GASTROINTESTINAL	NR	STROKE	NR
GENERAL SURGERY	NR	VASCULAR	NR
MATERNITY CARE	NR	WOMEN'S HEALTH	NR

HEALTHGRADES AWARDS

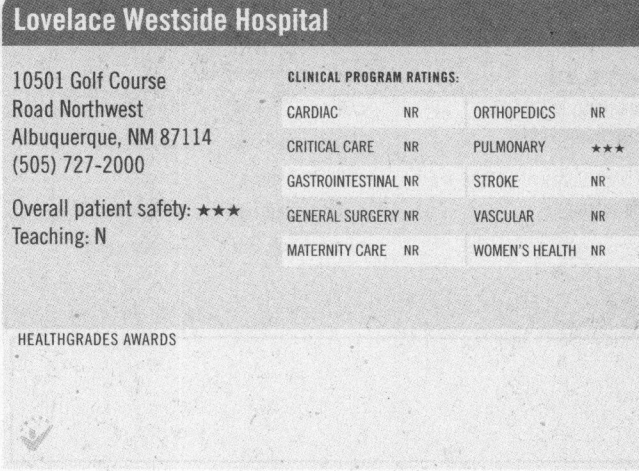

Lovelace Westside Hospital

10501 Golf Course
Road Northwest
Albuquerque, NM 87114
(505) 727-2000

Overall patient safety: ★★★
Teaching: N

CLINICAL PROGRAM RATINGS:

CARDIAC	NR	ORTHOPEDICS	NR
CRITICAL CARE	NR	PULMONARY	★★★
GASTROINTESTINAL	NR	STROKE	NR
GENERAL SURGERY	NR	VASCULAR	NR
MATERNITY CARE	NR	WOMEN'S HEALTH	NR

HEALTHGRADES AWARDS

Lovelace Medical Center—Downtown

601 Martin Luther
King Drive Northeast
Albuquerque, NM 87102
(505) 727-8000

Overall patient safety: ★
Teaching: N

CLINICAL PROGRAM RATINGS:

CARDIAC	NR	ORTHOPEDICS	★★★
CRITICAL CARE	NR	PULMONARY	★★★
GASTROINTESTINAL	★★★	STROKE	★
GENERAL SURGERY	NR	VASCULAR	NR
MATERNITY CARE	NR	WOMEN'S HEALTH	NR

HEALTHGRADES AWARDS

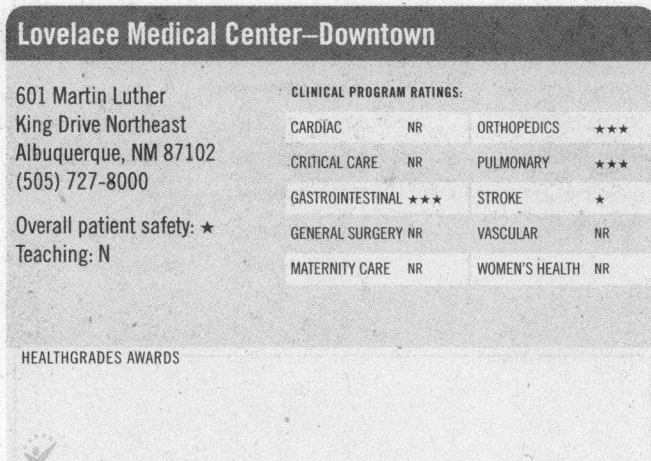

Lovelace Women's Hospital

4701 Montgomery Northeast
Albuquerque, NM 87109
(505) 727-7800

Overall patient safety: ★★★
Teaching: Y

CLINICAL PROGRAM RATINGS:

CARDIAC	NR	ORTHOPEDICS	NR
CRITICAL CARE	NR	PULMONARY	★★★
GASTROINTESTINAL	NR	STROKE	NR
GENERAL SURGERY	NR	VASCULAR	NR
MATERNITY CARE	NR	WOMEN'S HEALTH	NR

HEALTHGRADES AWARDS

Memorial Medical Center

2450 South Telshor Boulevard
Las Cruces, NM 88011
(505) 522-8641

Overall patient safety: ★★★
Teaching: Y

CLINICAL PROGRAM RATINGS:

CARDIAC	★★★	ORTHOPEDICS	NR
CRITICAL CARE	NR	PULMONARY	★
GASTROINTESTINAL	★★★	STROKE	★★★
GENERAL SURGERY	NR	VASCULAR	NR
MATERNITY CARE	NR	WOMEN'S HEALTH	NR

HEALTHGRADES AWARDS

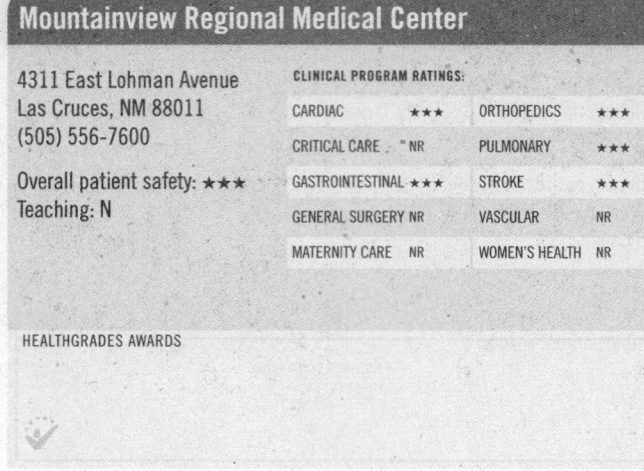

Mountainview Regional Medical Center

4311 East Lohman Avenue
Las Cruces, NM 88011
(505) 556-7600

Overall patient safety: ★★★
Teaching: N

CLINICAL PROGRAM RATINGS:

CARDIAC	★★★	ORTHOPEDICS	★★★
CRITICAL CARE	NR	PULMONARY	★★★
GASTROINTESTINAL	★★★	STROKE	★★★
GENERAL SURGERY	NR	VASCULAR	NR
MATERNITY CARE	NR	WOMEN'S HEALTH	NR

HEALTHGRADES AWARDS

Mimbres Memorial Hospital

900 West Ash Street
Deming, NM 88030
(505) 546-5800

Overall patient safety: ★★★
Teaching: N

CLINICAL PROGRAM RATINGS:

CARDIAC	NR	ORTHOPEDICS	NR
CRITICAL CARE	NR	PULMONARY	★★★
GASTROINTESTINAL	NR	STROKE	★★★
GENERAL SURGERY	NR	VASCULAR	NR
MATERNITY CARE	NR	WOMEN'S HEALTH	NR

HEALTHGRADES AWARDS

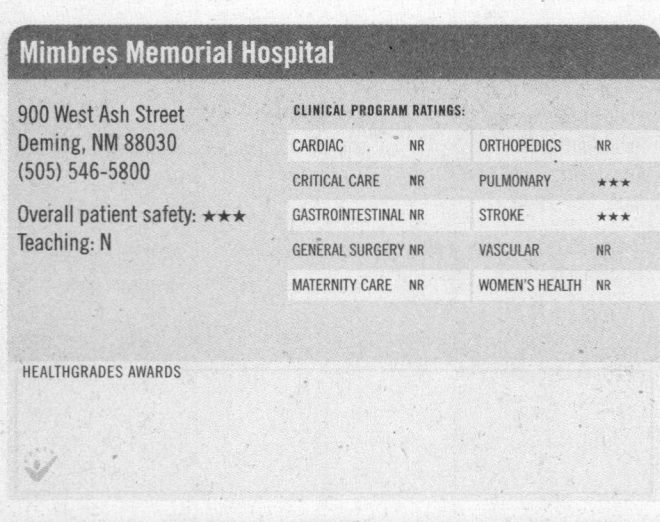

Nor Lea General Hospital

1600 North Main
Lovington, NM 88260
(505) 396-6611

Overall patient safety: ★★★
Teaching: N

CLINICAL PROGRAM RATINGS:

CARDIAC	NR	ORTHOPEDICS	NR
CRITICAL CARE	NR	PULMONARY	★★★
GASTROINTESTINAL	NR	STROKE	NR
GENERAL SURGERY	NR	VASCULAR	NR
MATERNITY CARE	NR	WOMEN'S HEALTH	NR

HEALTHGRADES AWARDS

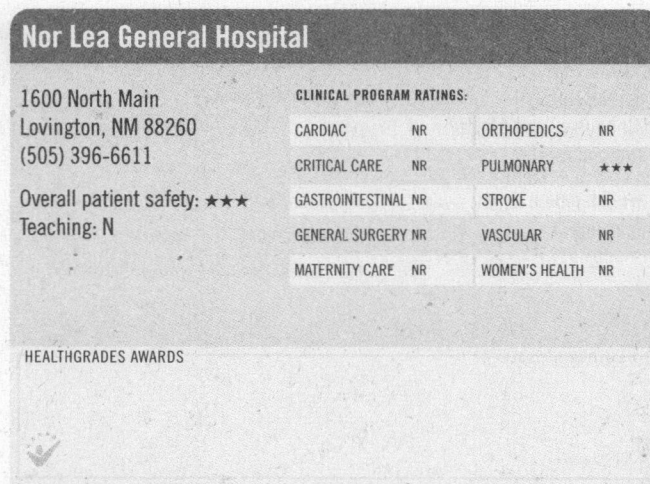

Miners' Colfax Medical Center

200 Hospital Drive
Raton, NM 87740
(505) 445-3661

Overall patient safety: ★★★
Teaching: N

CLINICAL PROGRAM RATINGS:

CARDIAC	NR	ORTHOPEDICS	NR
CRITICAL CARE	NR	PULMONARY	★★★
GASTROINTESTINAL	NR	STROKE	★★★
GENERAL SURGERY	NR	VASCULAR	NR
MATERNITY CARE	NR	WOMEN'S HEALTH	NR

HEALTHGRADES AWARDS

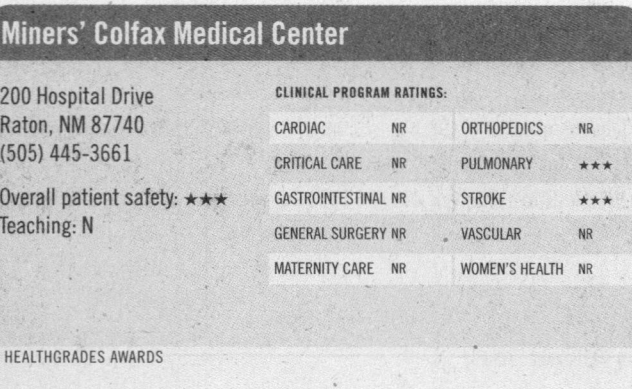

Northern Navajo Physicians Indian Hospital

P.O. Box 160
Shiprock, NM 87420
(505) 368-6001

Overall patient safety: ★★★
Teaching: N

CLINICAL PROGRAM RATINGS:

CARDIAC	NR	ORTHOPEDICS	NR
CRITICAL CARE	NR	PULMONARY	NR
GASTROINTESTINAL	NR	STROKE	NR
GENERAL SURGERY	NR	VASCULAR	NR
MATERNITY CARE	NR	WOMEN'S HEALTH	NR

HEALTHGRADES AWARDS

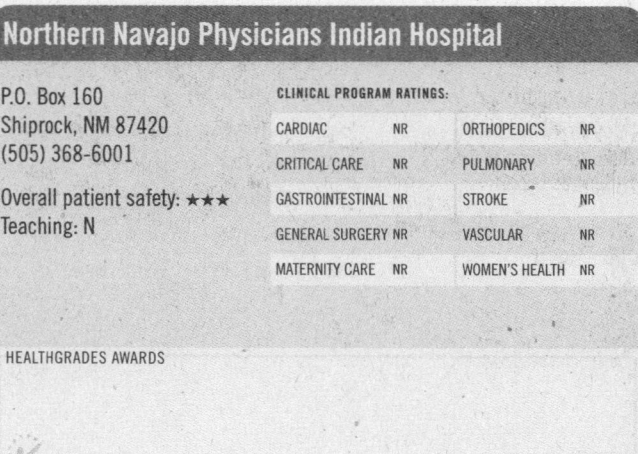

KEY: ★★★★★ BEST   ★★★ AS EXPECTED   ★ POOR   NR NOT RATED BY HEALTHGRADES   For full definitions of ratings and awards, see Appendix.

Plains Regional Medical Center–Clovis

2100 North Dr. Martin Luther
King Jr. Boulevard
Clovis, NM 88101
(505) 769-2141

Overall patient safety: ★
Teaching: N

CLINICAL PROGRAM RATINGS:

CARDIAC	NR	ORTHOPEDICS	NR
CRITICAL CARE	NR	PULMONARY	★
GASTROINTESTINAL	NR	STROKE	★★★
GENERAL SURGERY	NR	VASCULAR	NR
MATERNITY CARE	NR	WOMEN'S HEALTH	NR

HEALTHGRADES AWARDS

Rehoboth McKinley Christian Health Services

1901 Red Rock Drive
Gallup, NM 87301
(505) 863-7000

Overall patient safety: ★★★
Teaching: N

CLINICAL PROGRAM RATINGS:

CARDIAC	NR	ORTHOPEDICS	NR
CRITICAL CARE	NR	PULMONARY	★★★
GASTROINTESTINAL	NR	STROKE	★★★
GENERAL SURGERY	NR	VASCULAR	NR
MATERNITY CARE	NR	WOMEN'S HEALTH	NR

HEALTHGRADES AWARDS

Presbyterian Hospital

1100 Central Avenue Southeast
Albuquerque, NM 87106
(505) 841-1234

Overall patient safety: ★
Teaching: Y

CLINICAL PROGRAM RATINGS:

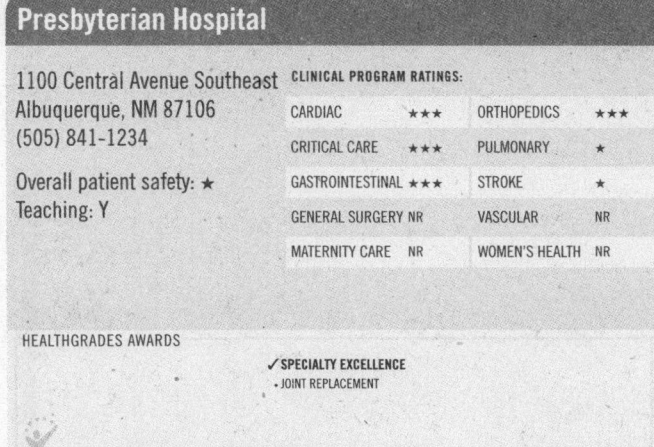

CARDIAC	★★★	ORTHOPEDICS	★★★
CRITICAL CARE	★★★	PULMONARY	★
GASTROINTESTINAL	★★★	STROKE	★
GENERAL SURGERY	NR	VASCULAR	NR
MATERNITY CARE	NR	WOMEN'S HEALTH	NR

HEALTHGRADES AWARDS

✓ SPECIALTY EXCELLENCE
• JOINT REPLACEMENT

St. Vincent Hospital

455 St. Michael's Drive
Santa Fe, NM 87505
(505) 983-3361

Overall patient safety: ★★★
Teaching: Y

CLINICAL PROGRAM RATINGS:

CARDIAC	NR	ORTHOPEDICS	★★★
CRITICAL CARE	NR	PULMONARY	★★★
GASTROINTESTINAL	★★★	STROKE	★★★
GENERAL SURGERY	NR	VASCULAR	NR
MATERNITY CARE	NR	WOMEN'S HEALTH	NR

HEALTHGRADES AWARDS

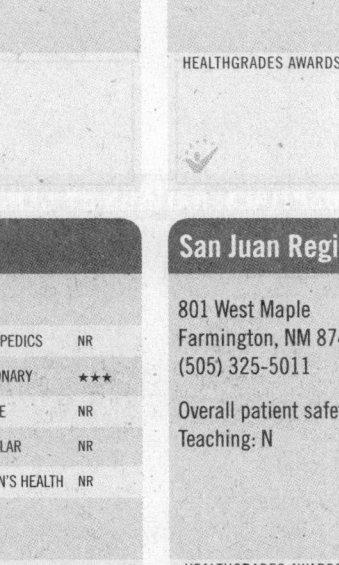

Presbyterian Kaseman Hospital

8300 Constitution Avenue
Northeast
Albuquerque, NM 87110
(505) 291-2000

Overall patient safety: ★★★
Teaching: N

CLINICAL PROGRAM RATINGS:

CARDIAC	NR	ORTHOPEDICS	NR
CRITICAL CARE	NR	PULMONARY	★★★
GASTROINTESTINAL	NR	STROKE	NR
GENERAL SURGERY	NR	VASCULAR	NR
MATERNITY CARE	NR	WOMEN'S HEALTH	NR

HEALTHGRADES AWARDS

San Juan Regional Medical Center

801 West Maple
Farmington, NM 87401
(505) 325-5011

Overall patient safety: ★★★
Teaching: N

CLINICAL PROGRAM RATINGS:

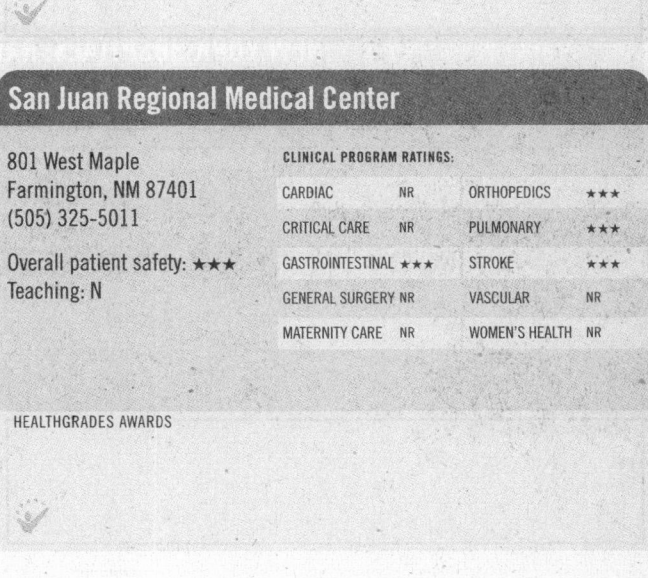

CARDIAC	NR	ORTHOPEDICS	★★★
CRITICAL CARE	NR	PULMONARY	★★★
GASTROINTESTINAL	★★★	STROKE	★★★
GENERAL SURGERY	NR	VASCULAR	NR
MATERNITY CARE	NR	WOMEN'S HEALTH	NR

HEALTHGRADES AWARDS

Sierra Vista Hospital

800 East 9th Avenue
Truth Or Consequences, NM
87901
(505) 894-2111

Overall patient safety: ★★★
Teaching: N

CLINICAL PROGRAM RATINGS:

CARDIAC	NR	ORTHOPEDICS	NR
CRITICAL CARE	NR	PULMONARY	★★★
GASTROINTESTINAL	NR	STROKE	NR
GENERAL SURGERY	NR	VASCULAR	NR
MATERNITY CARE	NR	WOMEN'S HEALTH	NR

HEALTHGRADES AWARDS

University of New Mexico Hospital

2211 Lomas Boulevard
Northeast
Albuquerque, NM 87106
(505) 272-2121

Overall patient safety: ★★★
Teaching: Y

CLINICAL PROGRAM RATINGS:

CARDIAC	★★★	ORTHOPEDICS	★★★
CRITICAL CARE	NR	PULMONARY	★
GASTROINTESTINAL	★★★	STROKE	★★★
GENERAL SURGERY	NR	VASCULAR	NR
MATERNITY CARE	NR	WOMEN'S HEALTH	NR

HEALTHGRADES AWARDS

Union County General Hospital

301 Harding Street
Clayton, NM 88415
(505) 374-2585

Overall patient safety: ★★★
Teaching: N

CLINICAL PROGRAM RATINGS:

CARDIAC	NR	ORTHOPEDICS	NR
CRITICAL CARE	NR	PULMONARY	★★★
GASTROINTESTINAL	NR	STROKE	NR
GENERAL SURGERY	NR	VASCULAR	NR
MATERNITY CARE	NR	WOMEN'S HEALTH	NR

HEALTHGRADES AWARDS

NEW YORK HOSPITALS: RATINGS BY CLINICAL SPECIALTY

Adirondack Medical Center

2233 State Route 86
Saranac Lake, NY 12983
(518) 891-4141

Overall patient safety: ★★★
Teaching: N

CLINICAL PROGRAM RATINGS:

CARDIAC	NR	ORTHOPEDICS	NR
CRITICAL CARE	NR	PULMONARY	★★★
GASTROINTESTINAL	NR	STROKE	★
GENERAL SURGERY	★★★	VASCULAR	NR
MATERNITY CARE	★★★	WOMEN'S HEALTH	NR

HEALTHGRADES AWARDS

Albany Medical Center Hospital

43 New Scotland Avenue
Albany, NY 12209
(518) 262-3125

Overall patient safety: ★
Teaching: Y

CLINICAL PROGRAM RATINGS:

CARDIAC	★★★	ORTHOPEDICS	★★★
CRITICAL CARE	★	PULMONARY	★★★
GASTROINTESTINAL	★★★	STROKE	★★★
GENERAL SURGERY	★★★	VASCULAR	★★★
MATERNITY CARE	★★★	WOMEN'S HEALTH	★★★

HEALTHGRADES AWARDS

✓ SPECIALTY EXCELLENCE
· CARDIAC SURGERY   · JOINT REPLACEMENT

KEY: ★★★★★ BEST   ★★★ AS EXPECTED   ★ POOR   NR NOT RATED BY HEALTHGRADES   For full definitions of ratings and awards, see Appendix.

Albany Memorial Hospital

600 Northern Boulevard
Albany, NY 12204
(518) 471-3221

Overall patient safety: ★★★
Teaching: N

CLINICAL PROGRAM RATINGS:

CARDIAC	NR	ORTHOPEDICS	★
CRITICAL CARE	NR	PULMONARY	★★★
GASTROINTESTINAL	★★★	STROKE	★★★
GENERAL SURGERY	★★★	VASCULAR	NR
MATERNITY CARE	NR	WOMEN'S HEALTH	NR

HEALTHGRADES AWARDS

Arnot Ogden Medical Center

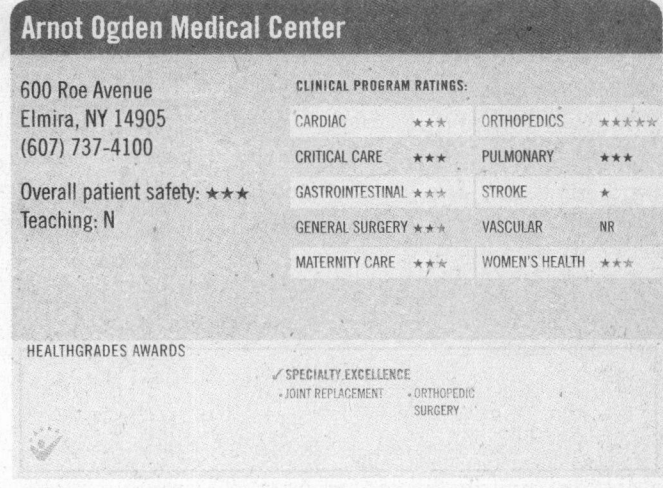

600 Roe Avenue
Elmira, NY 14905
(607) 737-4100

Overall patient safety: ★★★
Teaching: N

CLINICAL PROGRAM RATINGS:

CARDIAC	★★★	ORTHOPEDICS	★★★★★
CRITICAL CARE	★★★	PULMONARY	★★★
GASTROINTESTINAL	★★★	STROKE	★
GENERAL SURGERY	★★★	VASCULAR	NR
MATERNITY CARE	★★★	WOMEN'S HEALTH	★★★

HEALTHGRADES AWARDS

✓ SPECIALTY EXCELLENCE
• JOINT REPLACEMENT • ORTHOPEDIC SURGERY

Albert Lindley Lee Memorial Hospital

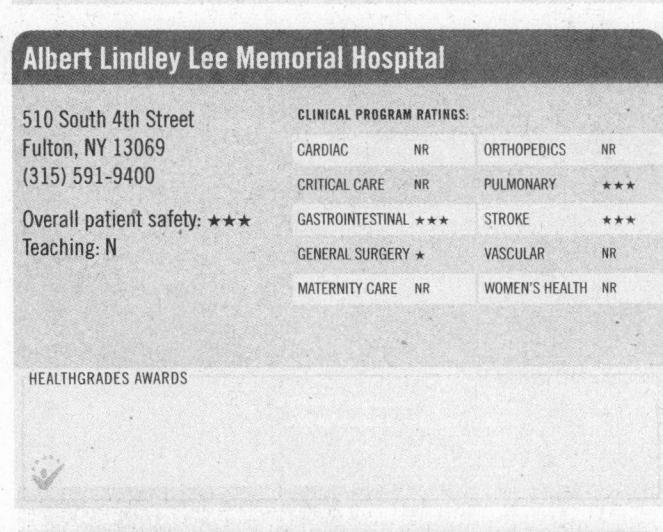

510 South 4th Street
Fulton, NY 13069
(315) 591-9400

Overall patient safety: ★★★
Teaching: N

CLINICAL PROGRAM RATINGS:

CARDIAC	NR	ORTHOPEDICS	NR
CRITICAL CARE	NR	PULMONARY	★★★
GASTROINTESTINAL	★★★	STROKE	★★★
GENERAL SURGERY	★	VASCULAR	NR
MATERNITY CARE	NR	WOMEN'S HEALTH	NR

HEALTHGRADES AWARDS

Auburn Memorial Hospital

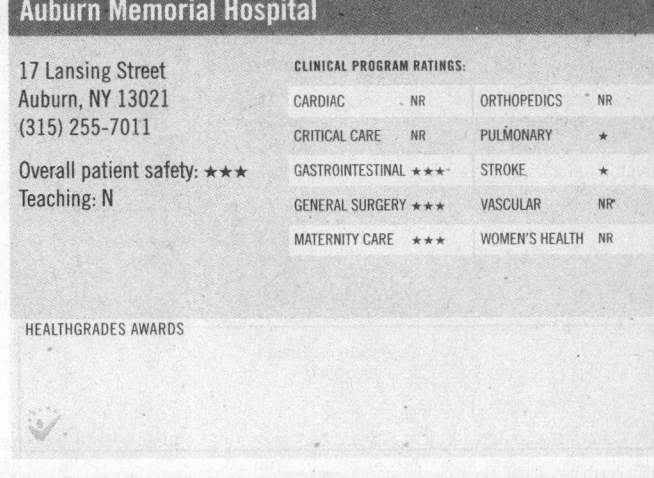

17 Lansing Street
Auburn, NY 13021
(315) 255-7011

Overall patient safety: ★★★
Teaching: N

CLINICAL PROGRAM RATINGS:

CARDIAC	NR	ORTHOPEDICS	NR
CRITICAL CARE	NR	PULMONARY	★
GASTROINTESTINAL	★★★	STROKE	★
GENERAL SURGERY	★★★	VASCULAR	NR
MATERNITY CARE	★★★	WOMEN'S HEALTH	NR

HEALTHGRADES AWARDS

Alice Hyde Medical Center

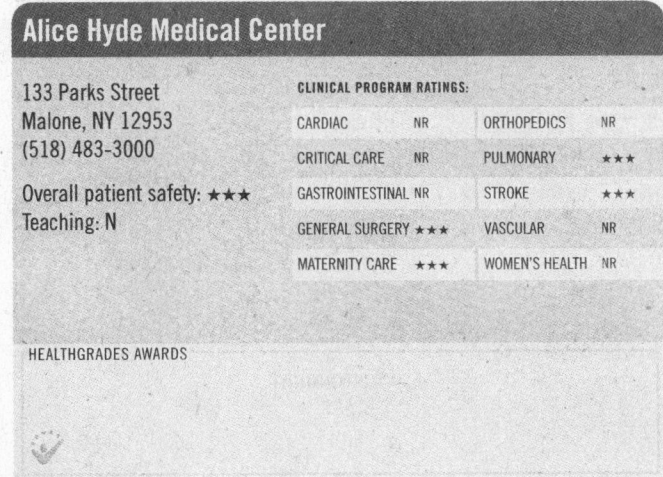

133 Parks Street
Malone, NY 12953
(518) 483-3000

Overall patient safety: ★★★
Teaching: N

CLINICAL PROGRAM RATINGS:

CARDIAC	NR	ORTHOPEDICS	NR
CRITICAL CARE	NR	PULMONARY	★★★
GASTROINTESTINAL	NR	STROKE	★★★
GENERAL SURGERY	★★★	VASCULAR	NR
MATERNITY CARE	★★★	WOMEN'S HEALTH	NR

HEALTHGRADES AWARDS

Aurelia Osborn Fox Memorial Hospital

1 Norton Avenue
Oneonta, NY 13820
(607) 432-2000

Overall patient safety: ★★★
Teaching: N

CLINICAL PROGRAM RATINGS:

CARDIAC	NR	ORTHOPEDICS	NR
CRITICAL CARE	NR	PULMONARY	★★★
GASTROINTESTINAL	NR	STROKE	★★★
GENERAL SURGERY	★★★	VASCULAR	NR
MATERNITY CARE	NR	WOMEN'S HEALTH	NR

HEALTHGRADES AWARDS

Bassett Hospital of Schoharie County

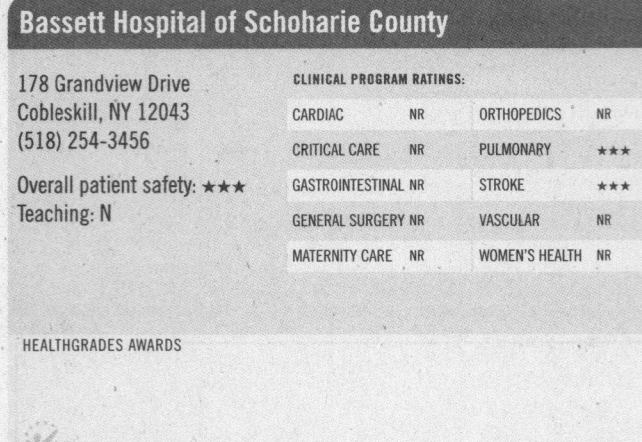

178 Grandview Drive
Cobleskill, NY 12043
(518) 254-3456

Overall patient safety: ★★★
Teaching: N

CLINICAL PROGRAM RATINGS:

CARDIAC	NR	ORTHOPEDICS	NR
CRITICAL CARE	NR	PULMONARY	★★★
GASTROINTESTINAL	NR	STROKE	★★★
GENERAL SURGERY	NR	VASCULAR	NR
MATERNITY CARE	NR	WOMEN'S HEALTH	NR

HEALTHGRADES AWARDS

Benedictine Hospital

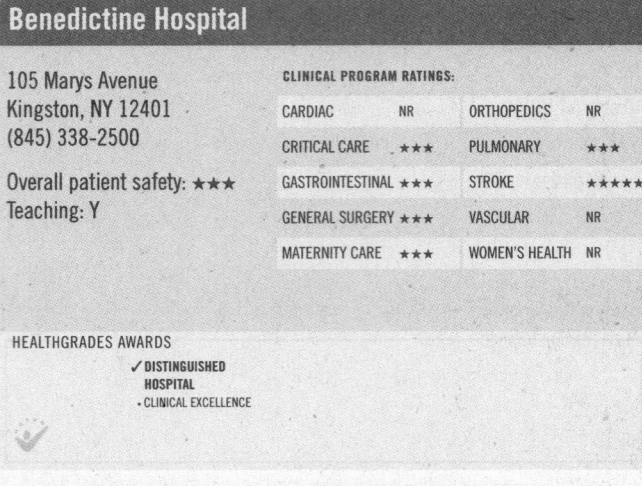

105 Marys Avenue
Kingston, NY 12401
(845) 338-2500

Overall patient safety: ★★★
Teaching: Y

CLINICAL PROGRAM RATINGS:

CARDIAC	NR	ORTHOPEDICS	NR
CRITICAL CARE	★★★	PULMONARY	★★★
GASTROINTESTINAL	★★★	STROKE	★★★★★
GENERAL SURGERY	★★★	VASCULAR	NR
MATERNITY CARE	★★★	WOMEN'S HEALTH	NR

HEALTHGRADES AWARDS

✓ DISTINGUISHED
 HOSPITAL
• CLINICAL EXCELLENCE

Bayley Seton Hospital*

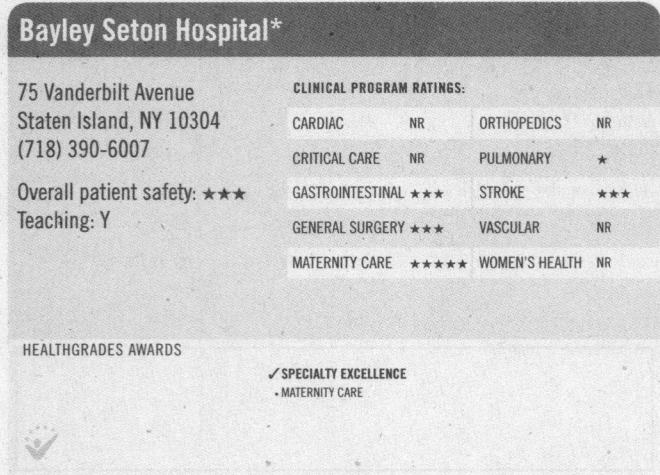

75 Vanderbilt Avenue
Staten Island, NY 10304
(718) 390-6007

Overall patient safety: ★★★
Teaching: Y

CLINICAL PROGRAM RATINGS:

CARDIAC	NR	ORTHOPEDICS	NR
CRITICAL CARE	NR	PULMONARY	★
GASTROINTESTINAL	★★★	STROKE	★★★
GENERAL SURGERY	★★★	VASCULAR	NR
MATERNITY CARE	★★★★★	WOMEN'S HEALTH	NR

HEALTHGRADES AWARDS

✓ SPECIALTY EXCELLENCE
• MATERNITY CARE

Bertrand Chaffee Hospital

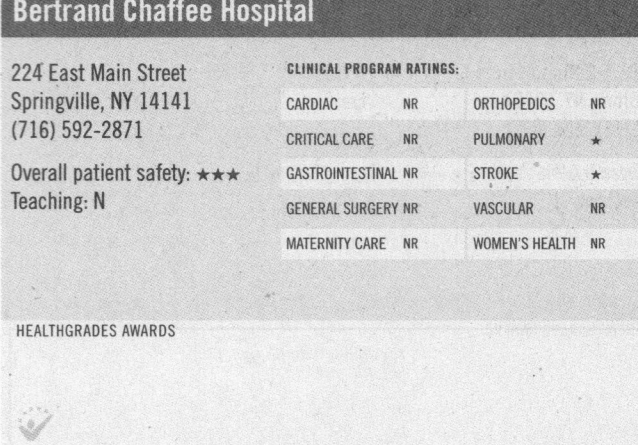

224 East Main Street
Springville, NY 14141
(716) 592-2871

Overall patient safety: ★★★
Teaching: N

CLINICAL PROGRAM RATINGS:

CARDIAC	NR	ORTHOPEDICS	NR
CRITICAL CARE	NR	PULMONARY	★
GASTROINTESTINAL	NR	STROKE	★
GENERAL SURGERY	NR	VASCULAR	NR
MATERNITY CARE	NR	WOMEN'S HEALTH	NR

HEALTHGRADES AWARDS

Bellevue Hospital Center

462 1st Avenue
New York, NY 10016
(212) 562-4516

Overall patient safety: ★
Teaching: Y

CLINICAL PROGRAM RATINGS:

CARDIAC	★★★	ORTHOPEDICS	NR
CRITICAL CARE	NR	PULMONARY	★★★
GASTROINTESTINAL	NR	STROKE	★★★★★
GENERAL SURGERY	★★★	VASCULAR	NR
MATERNITY CARE	★	WOMEN'S HEALTH	★

HEALTHGRADES AWARDS

Beth Israel Medical Center*

1st Avenue at East 16th Street
New York, NY 10003
(212) 420-2000

Overall patient safety: ★★★
Teaching: Y

CLINICAL PROGRAM RATINGS:

CARDIAC	★★★	ORTHOPEDICS	★★★★★
CRITICAL CARE	★★★	PULMONARY	★★★
GASTROINTESTINAL	★★★	STROKE	★★★
GENERAL SURGERY	★★★	VASCULAR	NR
MATERNITY CARE	★★★★★	WOMEN'S HEALTH	★★★

HEALTHGRADES AWARDS

✓ SPECIALTY EXCELLENCE
• ORTHOPEDIC
 SURGERY

KEY: ★★★★★ BEST ★★★ AS EXPECTED ★ POOR NR NOT RATED BY HEALTHGRADES For full definitions of ratings and awards, see Appendix.

Bon Secours Community Hospital

160 East Main Street
Port Jervis, NY 12771
(845) 858-7000

Overall patient safety: ★★★
Teaching: N

CLINICAL PROGRAM RATINGS:

CARDIAC	NR	ORTHOPEDICS	NR
CRITICAL CARE	NR	PULMONARY	★★★
GASTROINTESTINAL	NR	STROKE	★★★
GENERAL SURGERY	★★★	VASCULAR	NR
MATERNITY CARE	★★★	WOMEN'S HEALTH	NR

HEALTHGRADES AWARDS

Brookhaven Memorial Hospital Medical Center

101 Hospital Road
Patchogue, NY 11772
(631) 654-7100

Overall patient safety: ★★★
Teaching: N

CLINICAL PROGRAM RATINGS:

CARDIAC	NR	ORTHOPEDICS	★★★
CRITICAL CARE	★★★	PULMONARY	★★★
GASTROINTESTINAL	★★★	STROKE	★★★
GENERAL SURGERY	★	VASCULAR	NR
MATERNITY CARE	★★★	WOMEN'S HEALTH	NR

HEALTHGRADES AWARDS

Bronx-Lebanon Hospital Center

1276 Fulton Avenue
Bronx, NY 10457
(718) 590-1800

Overall patient safety: ★★★
Teaching: Y

CLINICAL PROGRAM RATINGS:

CARDIAC	NR	ORTHOPEDICS	NR
CRITICAL CARE	NR	PULMONARY	★★★
GASTROINTESTINAL	NR	STROKE	★★★
GENERAL SURGERY	★★★	VASCULAR	NR
MATERNITY CARE	★★★★★	WOMEN'S HEALTH	NR

HEALTHGRADES AWARDS

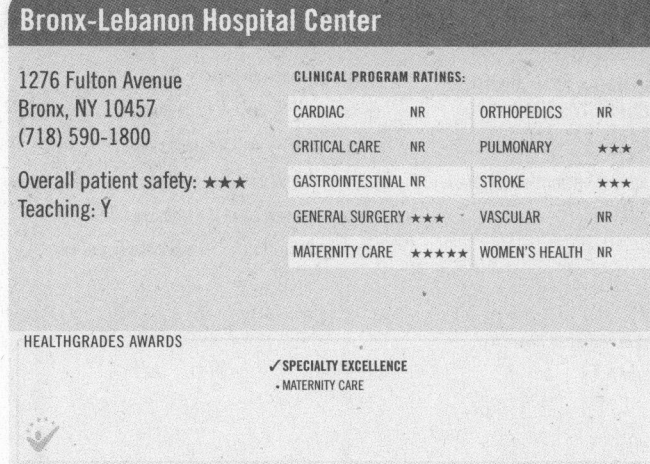

✓ SPECIALTY EXCELLENCE
- MATERNITY CARE

Brooklyn Hospital Center at Downtown Campus

121 Dekalb Avenue
Brooklyn, NY 11201
(718) 250-8000

Overall patient safety: ★
Teaching: Y

CLINICAL PROGRAM RATINGS:

CARDIAC	NR	ORTHOPEDICS	NR
CRITICAL CARE	★★★	PULMONARY	★★★★★
GASTROINTESTINAL	NR	STROKE	★★★★★
GENERAL SURGERY	★★★	VASCULAR	NR
MATERNITY CARE	★★★	WOMEN'S HEALTH	NR

HEALTHGRADES AWARDS

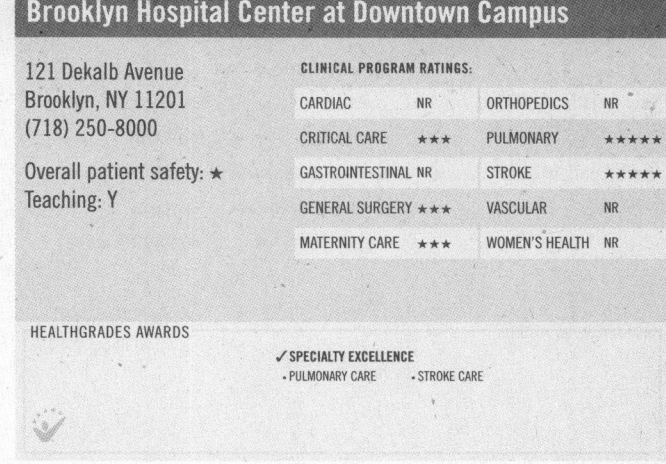

✓ SPECIALTY EXCELLENCE
- PULMONARY CARE   - STROKE CARE

Brookdale Hospital Medical Center

1 Brookdale Plaza
Brooklyn, NY 11212
(718) 240-5000

Overall patient safety: ★★★
Teaching: Y

CLINICAL PROGRAM RATINGS:

CARDIAC	NR	ORTHOPEDICS	NR
CRITICAL CARE	★★★	PULMONARY	★★★
GASTROINTESTINAL	★★★	STROKE	★★★
GENERAL SURGERY	★★★	VASCULAR	NR
MATERNITY CARE	★★★	WOMEN'S HEALTH	NR

HEALTHGRADES AWARDS

Brooks Memorial Hospital

529 Central Avenue
Dunkirk, NY 14048
(716) 366-1111

Overall patient safety: ★
Teaching: N

CLINICAL PROGRAM RATINGS:

CARDIAC	NR	ORTHOPEDICS	NR
CRITICAL CARE	NR	PULMONARY	★★★
GASTROINTESTINAL	NR	STROKE	★★★
GENERAL SURGERY	NR	VASCULAR	NR
MATERNITY CARE	★★★	WOMEN'S HEALTH	NR

HEALTHGRADES AWARDS

*This hospital reports its data to the federal government jointly with another hospital. Therefore the ratings and awards apply to multiple hospitals and this specific hospital may not provide all rated services.

Buffalo General Hospital—Kaleida Health*

100 High Street
Buffalo, NY 14203
(716) 859-5600

Overall patient safety: ★
Teaching: Y

CLINICAL PROGRAM RATINGS:

CARDIAC	★★★	ORTHOPEDICS	★★★
CRITICAL CARE	★	PULMONARY	★
GASTROINTESTINAL	★★★	STROKE	★★★
GENERAL SURGERY	★★★	VASCULAR	★★★
MATERNITY CARE	★★★	WOMEN'S HEALTH	★★★

HEALTHGRADES AWARDS

✓ SPECIALTY EXCELLENCE
• CARDIAC SURGERY

Carthage Area Hospital

1001 West Street Road
Carthage, NY 13619
(315) 493-1000

Overall patient safety: ★★★
Teaching: N

CLINICAL PROGRAM RATINGS:

CARDIAC	NR	ORTHOPEDICS	NR
CRITICAL CARE	NR	PULMONARY	★★★
GASTROINTESTINAL	NR	STROKE	★★★
GENERAL SURGERY	NR	VASCULAR	NR
MATERNITY CARE	★★★	WOMEN'S HEALTH	NR

HEALTHGRADES AWARDS

Cabrini Medical Center

227 East 19th Street
New York, NY 10003
(212) 995-6000

Overall patient safety: ★★★
Teaching: Y

CLINICAL PROGRAM RATINGS:

CARDIAC	NR	ORTHOPEDICS	NR
CRITICAL CARE	NR	PULMONARY	★★★
GASTROINTESTINAL	★★★	STROKE	★★★
GENERAL SURGERY	★★★	VASCULAR	NR
MATERNITY CARE	NR	WOMEN'S HEALTH	NR

HEALTHGRADES AWARDS

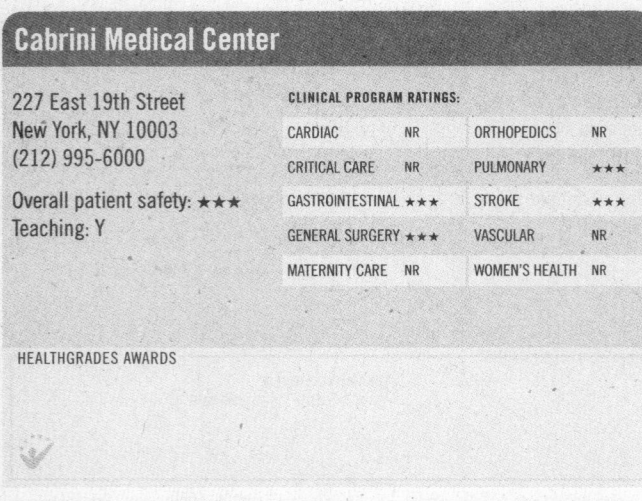

Catskill Regional Medical Center

68 Harris Bushville Road
Harris, NY 12742
(845) 794-3300

Overall patient safety: ★★★
Teaching: N

CLINICAL PROGRAM RATINGS:

CARDIAC	NR	ORTHOPEDICS	NR
CRITICAL CARE	NR	PULMONARY	★★★
GASTROINTESTINAL	NR	STROKE	★★★
GENERAL SURGERY	★★★	VASCULAR	NR
MATERNITY CARE	★★★	WOMEN'S HEALTH	NR

HEALTHGRADES AWARDS

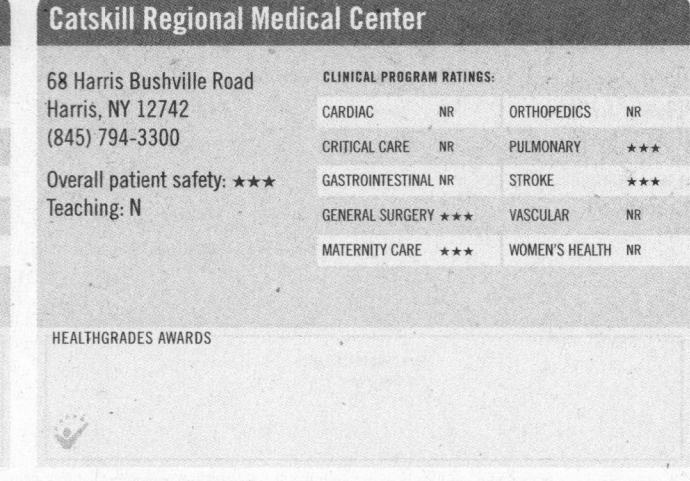

Canton-Potsdam Hospital

50 Leroy Street
Potsdam, NY 13676
(315) 265-3300

Overall patient safety: ★★★
Teaching: N

CLINICAL PROGRAM RATINGS:

CARDIAC	NR	ORTHOPEDICS	NR
CRITICAL CARE	NR	PULMONARY	★★★
GASTROINTESTINAL	NR	STROKE	★★★
GENERAL SURGERY	NR	VASCULAR	NR
MATERNITY CARE	★★★	WOMEN'S HEALTH	NR

HEALTHGRADES AWARDS

Cayuga Medical Center at Ithaca

101 Dates Drive
Ithaca, NY 14850
(607) 274-4011

Overall patient safety: ★★★
Teaching: N

CLINICAL PROGRAM RATINGS:

CARDIAC	NR	ORTHOPEDICS	★★★
CRITICAL CARE	NR	PULMONARY	★★★
GASTROINTESTINAL	★★★	STROKE	★
GENERAL SURGERY	★★★	VASCULAR	NR
MATERNITY CARE	★★★★★	WOMEN'S HEALTH	NR

HEALTHGRADES AWARDS

✓ SPECIALTY EXCELLENCE
• JOINT REPLACEMENT   • MATERNITY CARE

KEY: ★★★★★ BEST   ★★★ AS EXPECTED   ★ POOR   NR NOT RATED BY HEALTHGRADES   For full definitions of ratings and awards, see Appendix.

Champlain Valley Physicians Hospital Medical Center

75 Beekman Street
Plattsburgh, NY 12901
(518) 561-2000

Overall patient safety: ★★★
Teaching: N

CLINICAL PROGRAM RATINGS:

CARDIAC	★★★	ORTHOPEDICS	NR
CRITICAL CARE	NR	PULMONARY	★
GASTROINTESTINAL	★★★	STROKE	★★★
GENERAL SURGERY	★★★★★	VASCULAR	NR
MATERNITY CARE	★★★	WOMEN'S HEALTH	NR

HEALTHGRADES AWARDS

✓ SPECIALTY EXCELLENCE
- GENERAL SURGERY

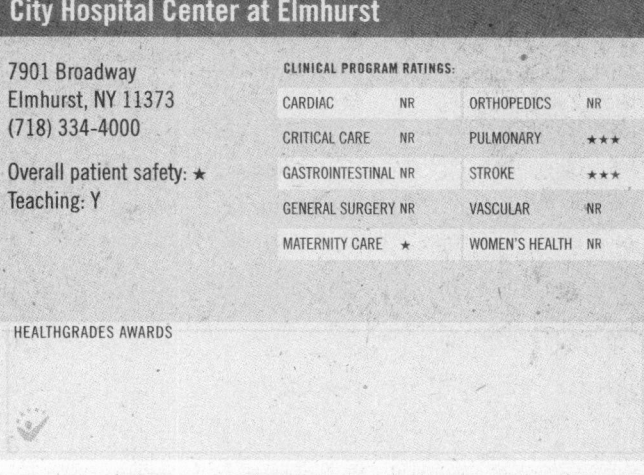

City Hospital Center at Elmhurst

7901 Broadway
Elmhurst, NY 11373
(718) 334-4000

Overall patient safety: ★
Teaching: Y

CLINICAL PROGRAM RATINGS:

CARDIAC	NR	ORTHOPEDICS	NR
CRITICAL CARE	NR	PULMONARY	★★★
GASTROINTESTINAL	NR	STROKE	★★★
GENERAL SURGERY	NR	VASCULAR	NR
MATERNITY CARE	★	WOMEN'S HEALTH	NR

HEALTHGRADES AWARDS

Chenango Memorial Hospital

179 North Broad Street
Norwich, NY 13815
(607) 337-4111

Overall patient safety: ★
Teaching: N

CLINICAL PROGRAM RATINGS:

CARDIAC	NR	ORTHOPEDICS	NR
CRITICAL CARE	NR	PULMONARY	★★★
GASTROINTESTINAL	NR	STROKE	★★★
GENERAL SURGERY	NR	VASCULAR	NR
MATERNITY CARE	★★★	WOMEN'S HEALTH	NR

HEALTHGRADES AWARDS

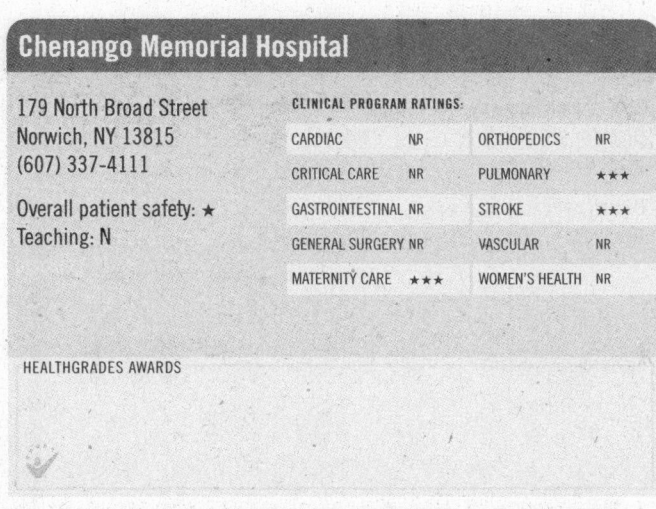

Claxton-Hepburn Medical Center

214 King Street
Ogdensburg, NY 13669
(315) 393-3600

Overall patient safety: ★★★
Teaching: N

CLINICAL PROGRAM RATINGS:

CARDIAC	NR	ORTHOPEDICS	NR
CRITICAL CARE	NR	PULMONARY	★
GASTROINTESTINAL	NR	STROKE	★★★
GENERAL SURGERY	★★★	VASCULAR	NR
MATERNITY CARE	★★★	WOMEN'S HEALTH	NR

HEALTHGRADES AWARDS

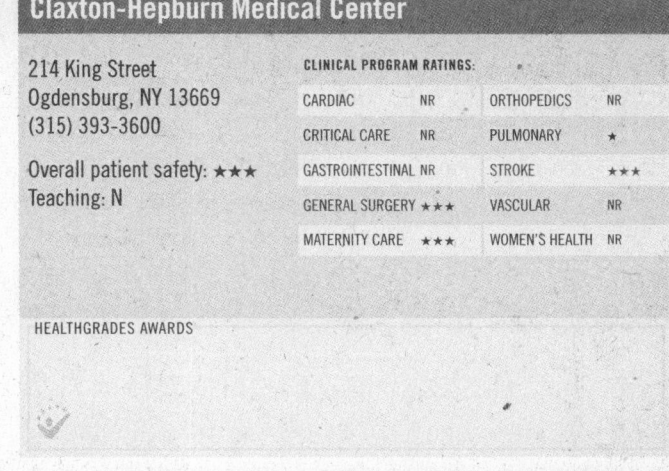

Children's Hospital Rehab Center*

1675 Bennett Street
Utica, NY 13502
(315) 724-5101

Overall patient safety: ★★★
Teaching: Y

CLINICAL PROGRAM RATINGS:

CARDIAC	NR	ORTHOPEDICS	★★★
CRITICAL CARE	★	PULMONARY	★
GASTROINTESTINAL	★★★	STROKE	★★★
GENERAL SURGERY	★★★	VASCULAR	NR
MATERNITY CARE	★★★★★	WOMEN'S HEALTH	NR

HEALTHGRADES AWARDS

✓ SPECIALTY EXCELLENCE
- MATERNITY CARE

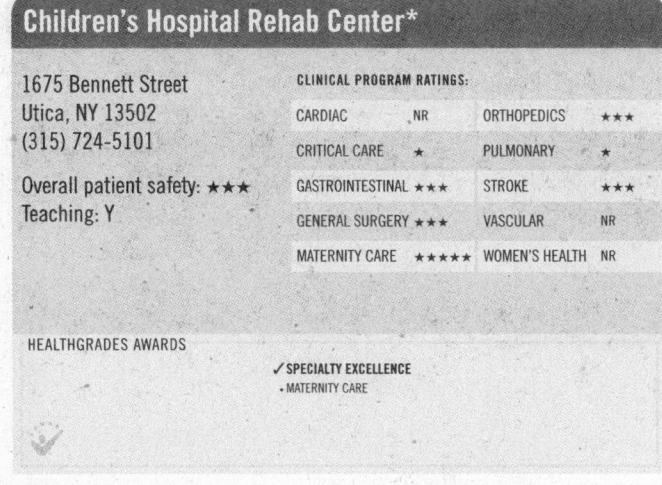

Clifton Springs Hospital and Clinic

2 Coulter Road
Clifton Springs, NY 14432
(315) 462-9561

Overall patient safety: ★★★
Teaching: N

CLINICAL PROGRAM RATINGS:

CARDIAC	NR	ORTHOPEDICS	NR
CRITICAL CARE	NR	PULMONARY	★★★
GASTROINTESTINAL	NR	STROKE	★★★
GENERAL SURGERY	NR	VASCULAR	NR
MATERNITY CARE	NR	WOMEN'S HEALTH	NR

HEALTHGRADES AWARDS

*This hospital reports its data to the federal government jointly with another hospital. Therefore the ratings and awards apply to multiple hospitals and this specific hospital may not provide all rated services.

Columbia Memorial Hospital

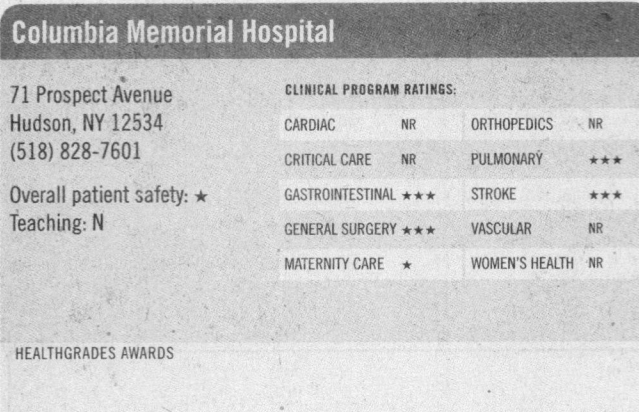

71 Prospect Avenue
Hudson, NY 12534
(518) 828-7601

Overall patient safety: ★
Teaching: N

CLINICAL PROGRAM RATINGS:

CARDIAC	NR	ORTHOPEDICS	NR
CRITICAL CARE	NR	PULMONARY	★★★
GASTROINTESTINAL	★★★	STROKE	★★★
GENERAL SURGERY	★★★	VASCULAR	NR
MATERNITY CARE	★	WOMEN'S HEALTH	NR

HEALTHGRADES AWARDS

Community-General Hospital of Greater Syracuse

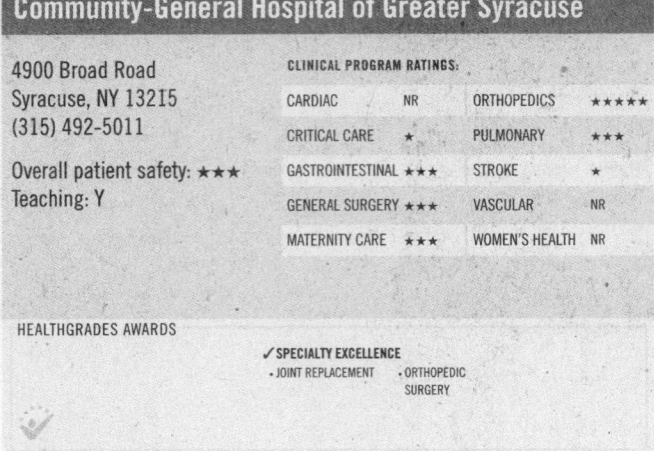

4900 Broad Road
Syracuse, NY 13215
(315) 492-5011

Overall patient safety: ★★★
Teaching: Y

CLINICAL PROGRAM RATINGS:

CARDIAC	NR	ORTHOPEDICS	★★★★★
CRITICAL CARE	★	PULMONARY	★★★
GASTROINTESTINAL	★★★	STROKE	★
GENERAL SURGERY	★★★	VASCULAR	NR
MATERNITY CARE	★★★	WOMEN'S HEALTH	NR

HEALTHGRADES AWARDS

✓ SPECIALTY EXCELLENCE
· JOINT REPLACEMENT · ORTHOPEDIC SURGERY

Community Hospital at Dobbs Ferry

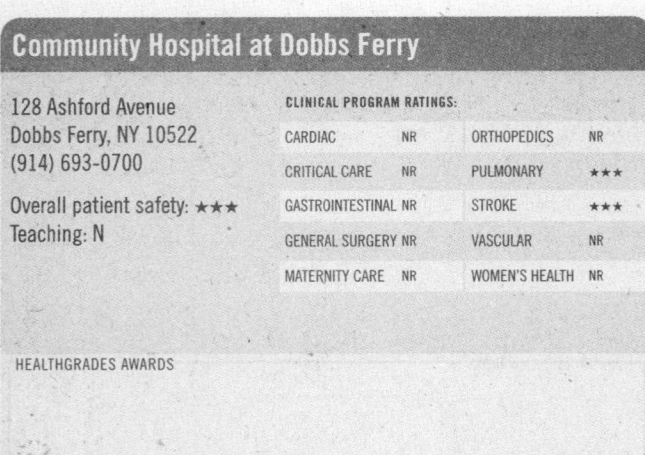

128 Ashford Avenue
Dobbs Ferry, NY 10522
(914) 693-0700

Overall patient safety: ★★★
Teaching: N

CLINICAL PROGRAM RATINGS:

CARDIAC	NR	ORTHOPEDICS	NR
CRITICAL CARE	NR	PULMONARY	★★★
GASTROINTESTINAL	NR	STROKE	★★★
GENERAL SURGERY	NR	VASCULAR	NR
MATERNITY CARE	NR	WOMEN'S HEALTH	NR

HEALTHGRADES AWARDS

Coney Island Hospital

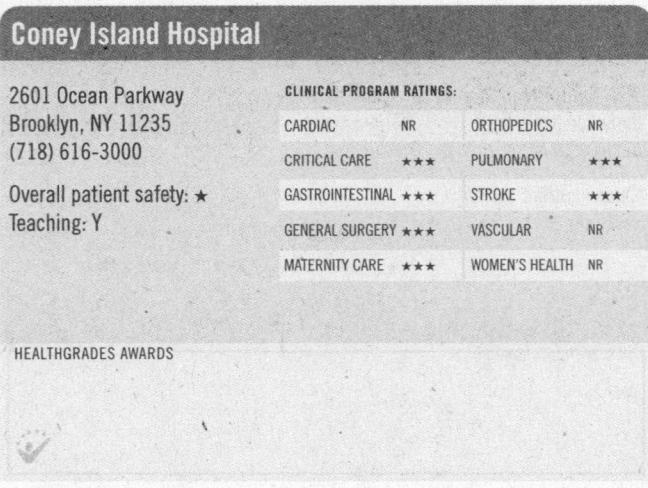

2601 Ocean Parkway
Brooklyn, NY 11235
(718) 616-3000

Overall patient safety: ★
Teaching: Y

CLINICAL PROGRAM RATINGS:

CARDIAC	NR	ORTHOPEDICS	NR
CRITICAL CARE	★★★	PULMONARY	★★★
GASTROINTESTINAL	★★★	STROKE	★★★
GENERAL SURGERY	★★★	VASCULAR	NR
MATERNITY CARE	★★★	WOMEN'S HEALTH	NR

HEALTHGRADES AWARDS

Community Memorial Hospital

150 Broad Street
Hamilton, NY 13346
(315) 824-1100

Overall patient safety: ★★★
Teaching: N

CLINICAL PROGRAM RATINGS:

CARDIAC	NR	ORTHOPEDICS	★★★
CRITICAL CARE	NR	PULMONARY	★★★
GASTROINTESTINAL	NR	STROKE	★★★
GENERAL SURGERY	NR	VASCULAR	NR
MATERNITY CARE	★★★	WOMEN'S HEALTH	NR

HEALTHGRADES AWARDS

✓ SPECIALTY EXCELLENCE
· JOINT REPLACEMENT

Corning Hospital

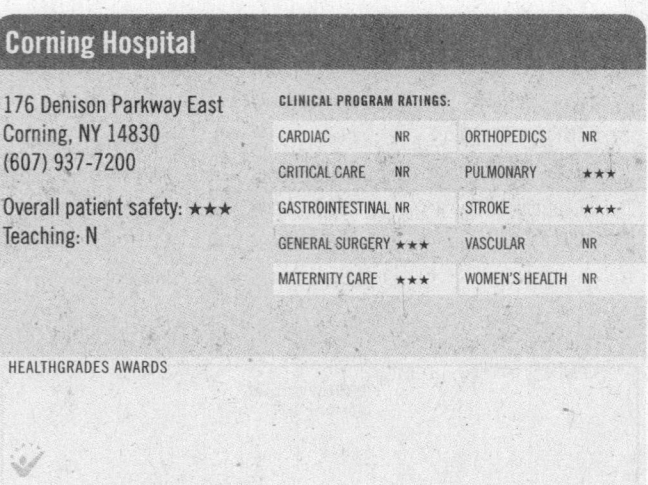

176 Denison Parkway East
Corning, NY 14830
(607) 937-7200

Overall patient safety: ★★★
Teaching: N

CLINICAL PROGRAM RATINGS:

CARDIAC	NR	ORTHOPEDICS	NR
CRITICAL CARE	NR	PULMONARY	★★★
GASTROINTESTINAL	NR	STROKE	★★★
GENERAL SURGERY	★★★	VASCULAR	NR
MATERNITY CARE	★★★	WOMEN'S HEALTH	NR

HEALTHGRADES AWARDS

KEY: ★★★★★ BEST   ★★★ AS EXPECTED   ★ POOR   NR NOT RATED BY HEALTHGRADES   For full definitions of ratings and awards, see Appendix.

Cortland Regional Medical Center

134 Homer Avenue
Cortland, NY 13045
(607) 756-3500

Overall patient safety: ★★★
Teaching: N

CLINICAL PROGRAM RATINGS:

CARDIAC	NR	ORTHOPEDICS	NR
CRITICAL CARE	NR	PULMONARY	★
GASTROINTESTINAL	NR	STROKE	★
GENERAL SURGERY	★★★	VASCULAR	NR
MATERNITY CARE	★★★	WOMEN'S HEALTH	NR

HEALTHGRADES AWARDS

Delaware Valley Hospital

1 Titus Place
Walton, NY 13856
(607) 865-2100

Overall patient safety: ★★★
Teaching: N

CLINICAL PROGRAM RATINGS:

CARDIAC	NR	ORTHOPEDICS	NR
CRITICAL CARE	NR	PULMONARY	★★★★★
GASTROINTESTINAL	NR	STROKE	NR
GENERAL SURGERY	NR	VASCULAR	NR
MATERNITY CARE	NR	WOMEN'S HEALTH	NR

HEALTHGRADES AWARDS

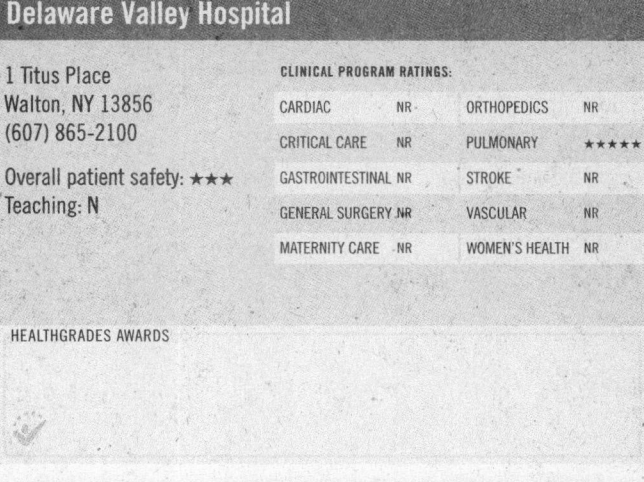

Crouse Hospital

736 Irving Avenue
Syracuse, NY 13210
(315) 470-7111

Overall patient safety: ★
Teaching: Y

CLINICAL PROGRAM RATINGS:

CARDIAC	NR	ORTHOPEDICS	★★★
CRITICAL CARE	★★★	PULMONARY	★★★
GASTROINTESTINAL	★★★	STROKE	★★★
GENERAL SURGERY	★★★	VASCULAR	★★★
MATERNITY CARE	★★★	WOMEN'S HEALTH	NR

HEALTHGRADES AWARDS

Eastern Long Island Hospital

201 Manor Place
Greenport, NY 11944
(631) 477-1000

Overall patient safety: ★
Teaching: N

CLINICAL PROGRAM RATINGS:

CARDIAC	NR	ORTHOPEDICS	NR
CRITICAL CARE	NR	PULMONARY	★★★
GASTROINTESTINAL	NR	STROKE	★★★
GENERAL SURGERY	★★★	VASCULAR	NR
MATERNITY CARE	NR	WOMEN'S HEALTH	NR

HEALTHGRADES AWARDS

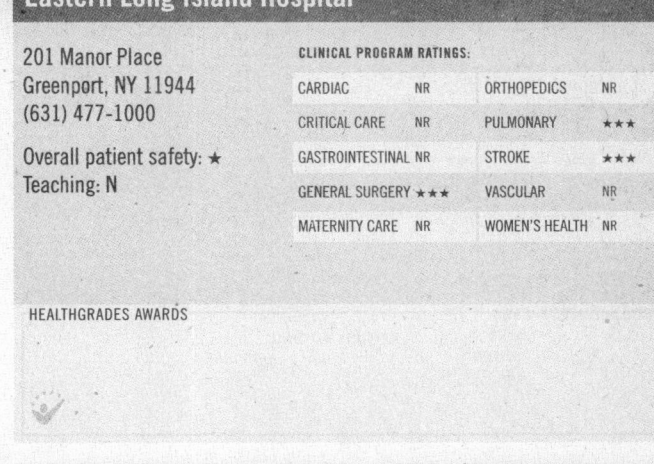

Degraff Memorial Hospital*

445 Tremont Street
North Tonawanda, NY 14120
(716) 694-4500

Overall patient safety: ★
Teaching: Y

CLINICAL PROGRAM RATINGS:

CARDIAC	★★★	ORTHOPEDICS	★★★
CRITICAL CARE	★	PULMONARY	★
GASTROINTESTINAL	★★★	STROKE	★★★
GENERAL SURGERY	★★★	VASCULAR	★★★
MATERNITY CARE	★★★	WOMEN'S HEALTH	★★★

HEALTHGRADES AWARDS

✓ SPECIALTY EXCELLENCE
• CARDIAC SURGERY

Edward John Noble Hospital of Gouverneur

77 West Barney Street
Gouverneur, NY 13642
(315) 287-1000

Overall patient safety: ★★★
Teaching: N

CLINICAL PROGRAM RATINGS:

CARDIAC	NR	ORTHOPEDICS	NR
CRITICAL CARE	NR	PULMONARY	★★★
GASTROINTESTINAL	NR	STROKE	★★★
GENERAL SURGERY	NR	VASCULAR	NR
MATERNITY CARE	★	WOMEN'S HEALTH	NR

HEALTHGRADES AWARDS

*This hospital reports its data to the federal government jointly with another hospital. Therefore the ratings and awards apply to multiple hospitals and this specific hospital may not provide all rated services.

Elizabethtown Community Hospital

75 Parks Street
Elizabethtown, NY 12932
(518) 873-6377

Overall patient safety: NR
Teaching: N

CLINICAL PROGRAM RATINGS:

CARDIAC	NR	ORTHOPEDICS	NR
CRITICAL CARE	NR	PULMONARY	★★★
GASTROINTESTINAL	NR	STROKE	NR
GENERAL SURGERY	NR	VASCULAR	NR
MATERNITY CARE	NR	WOMEN'S HEALTH	NR

HEALTHGRADES AWARDS

F. F. Thompson Hospital

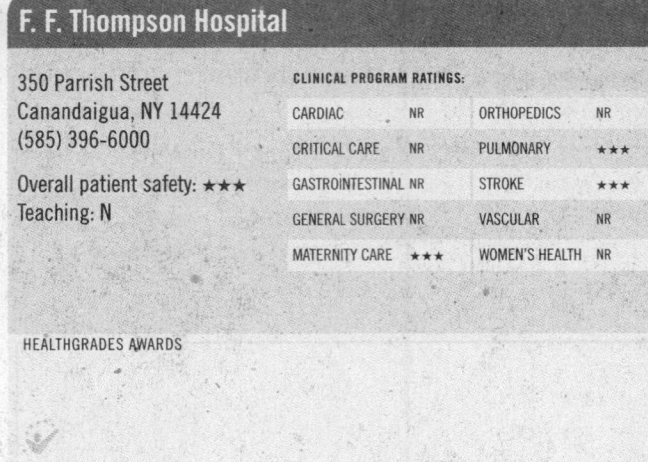

350 Parrish Street
Canandaigua, NY 14424
(585) 396-6000

Overall patient safety: ★★★
Teaching: N

CLINICAL PROGRAM RATINGS:

CARDIAC	NR	ORTHOPEDICS	NR
CRITICAL CARE	NR	PULMONARY	★★★
GASTROINTESTINAL	NR	STROKE	★★★
GENERAL SURGERY	NR	VASCULAR	NR
MATERNITY CARE	★★★	WOMEN'S HEALTH	NR

HEALTHGRADES AWARDS

Ellis Hospital

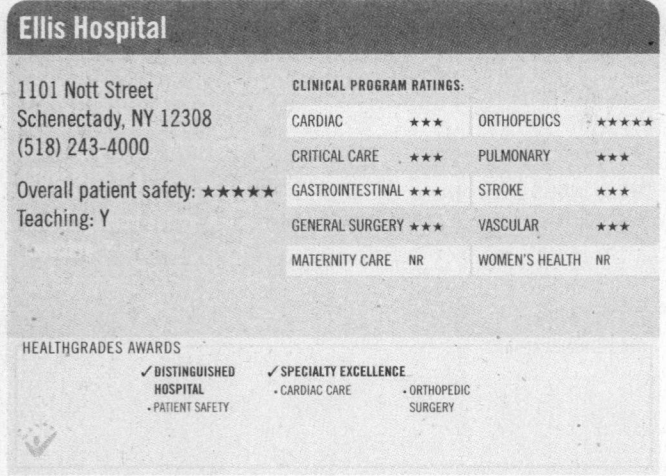

1101 Nott Street
Schenectady, NY 12308
(518) 243-4000

Overall patient safety: ★★★★★
Teaching: Y

CLINICAL PROGRAM RATINGS:

CARDIAC	★★★	ORTHOPEDICS	★★★★★
CRITICAL CARE	★★★	PULMONARY	★★★
GASTROINTESTINAL	★★★	STROKE	★★★
GENERAL SURGERY	★★★	VASCULAR	★★★
MATERNITY CARE	NR	WOMEN'S HEALTH	NR

HEALTHGRADES AWARDS

✓ DISTINGUISHED HOSPITAL
  • PATIENT SAFETY

✓ SPECIALTY EXCELLENCE
  • CARDIAC CARE
  • ORTHOPEDIC SURGERY

Faxton-Childrens Hospital*

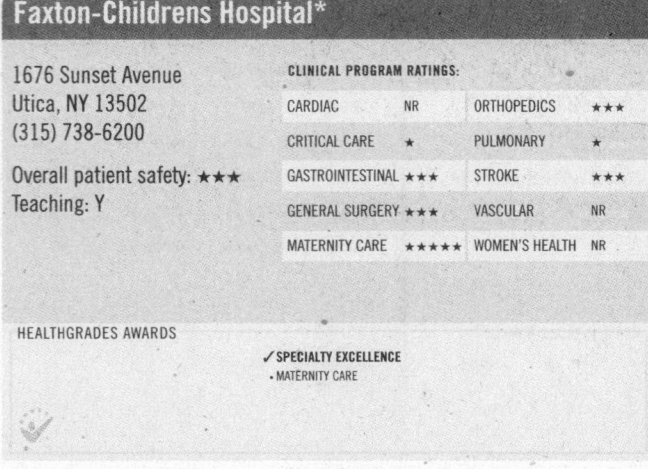

1676 Sunset Avenue
Utica, NY 13502
(315) 738-6200

Overall patient safety: ★★★
Teaching: Y

CLINICAL PROGRAM RATINGS:

CARDIAC	NR	ORTHOPEDICS	★★★
CRITICAL CARE	★	PULMONARY	★
GASTROINTESTINAL	★★★	STROKE	★★★
GENERAL SURGERY	★★★	VASCULAR	NR
MATERNITY CARE	★★★★★	WOMEN'S HEALTH	NR

HEALTHGRADES AWARDS

✓ SPECIALTY EXCELLENCE
  • MATERNITY CARE

Erie County Medical Center

462 Grider Street
Buffalo, NY 14215
(716) 898-3000

Overall patient safety: ★
Teaching: Y

CLINICAL PROGRAM RATINGS:

CARDIAC	★★★	ORTHOPEDICS	★★★
CRITICAL CARE	★	PULMONARY	★
GASTROINTESTINAL	NR	STROKE	★
GENERAL SURGERY	NR	VASCULAR	NR
MATERNITY CARE	NR	WOMEN'S HEALTH	NR

HEALTHGRADES AWARDS

Faxton-St. Luke's Healthcare*

1656 Champlin Avenue
Utica, NY 13502
(315) 624-5200

Overall patient safety: ★★★
Teaching: Y

CLINICAL PROGRAM RATINGS:

CARDIAC	NR	ORTHOPEDICS	★★★
CRITICAL CARE	★	PULMONARY	★
GASTROINTESTINAL	★★★	STROKE	★★★
GENERAL SURGERY	★★★	VASCULAR	NR
MATERNITY CARE	★★★★★	WOMEN'S HEALTH	NR

HEALTHGRADES AWARDS

✓ SPECIALTY EXCELLENCE
  • MATERNITY CARE

KEY: ★★★★★ BEST ★★★ AS EXPECTED ★ POOR NR NOT RATED BY HEALTHGRADES For full definitions of ratings and awards, see Appendix.

Flushing Hospital Medical Center

4500 Parsons Boulevard
Flushing, NY 11355
(718) 670-5000

Overall patient safety: ★
Teaching: Y

CLINICAL PROGRAM RATINGS:

CARDIAC	NR	ORTHOPEDICS	NR
CRITICAL CARE	NR	PULMONARY	★
GASTROINTESTINAL	NR	STROKE	★
GENERAL SURGERY	★★★	VASCULAR	NR
MATERNITY CARE	★★★★★	WOMEN'S HEALTH	NR

HEALTHGRADES AWARDS

✓ SPECIALTY EXCELLENCE
• MATERNITY CARE

Geneva General Hospital*

196 North Street
Geneva, NY 14456
(315) 787-4000

Overall patient safety: ★★★★★
Teaching: N

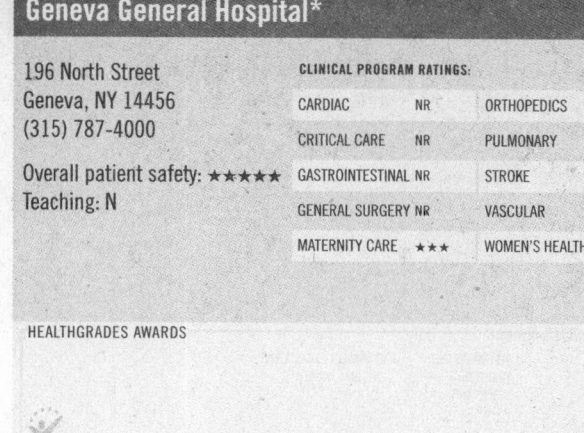

CLINICAL PROGRAM RATINGS:

CARDIAC	NR	ORTHOPEDICS	★★★
CRITICAL CARE	NR	PULMONARY	★★★
GASTROINTESTINAL	NR	STROKE	★★★
GENERAL SURGERY	NR	VASCULAR	NR
MATERNITY CARE	★★★	WOMEN'S HEALTH	NR

HEALTHGRADES AWARDS

Forest Hills Hospital

10201 66th Road
Forest Hills, NY 11375
(718) 830-4000

Overall patient safety: ★★★
Teaching: Y

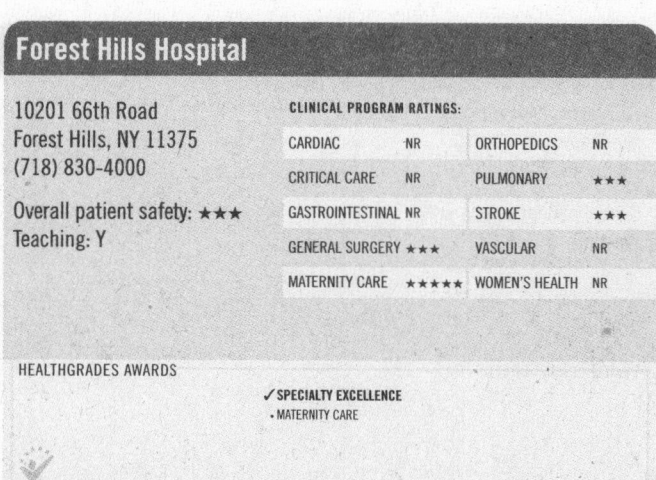

CLINICAL PROGRAM RATINGS:

CARDIAC	NR	ORTHOPEDICS	NR
CRITICAL CARE	NR	PULMONARY	★★★
GASTROINTESTINAL	NR	STROKE	★★★
GENERAL SURGERY	★★★	VASCULAR	NR
MATERNITY CARE	★★★★★	WOMEN'S HEALTH	NR

HEALTHGRADES AWARDS

✓ SPECIALTY EXCELLENCE
• MATERNITY CARE

Glen Cove Hospital

101 St. Andrews Lane
Glen Cove, NY 11542
(516) 674-7300

Overall patient safety: ★★★
Teaching: Y

CLINICAL PROGRAM RATINGS:

CARDIAC	NR	ORTHOPEDICS	★★★
CRITICAL CARE	★	PULMONARY	★★★
GASTROINTESTINAL	★★★	STROKE	★★★
GENERAL SURGERY	★★★	VASCULAR	NR
MATERNITY CARE	NR	WOMEN'S HEALTH	NR

HEALTHGRADES AWARDS

Franklin Hospital

900 Franklin Avenue
Valley Stream, NY 11580
(516) 256-6000

Overall patient safety: ★
Teaching: Y

CLINICAL PROGRAM RATINGS:

CARDIAC	NR	ORTHOPEDICS	NR
CRITICAL CARE	★★★	PULMONARY	★★★
GASTROINTESTINAL	★★★	STROKE	★★★
GENERAL SURGERY	★★★	VASCULAR	NR
MATERNITY CARE	★★★	WOMEN'S HEALTH	NR

HEALTHGRADES AWARDS

Glens Falls Hospital

100 Parks Street
Glens Falls, NY 12801
(518) 926-1000

Overall patient safety: ★★★
Teaching: N

CLINICAL PROGRAM RATINGS:

CARDIAC	NR	ORTHOPEDICS	★
CRITICAL CARE	★★★	PULMONARY	★★★
GASTROINTESTINAL	★★★	STROKE	★★★
GENERAL SURGERY	★★★	VASCULAR	NR
MATERNITY CARE	★★★★★	WOMEN'S HEALTH	NR

HEALTHGRADES AWARDS

✓ SPECIALTY EXCELLENCE
• GENERAL SURGERY   • MATERNITY CARE

*This hospital reports its data to the federal government jointly with another hospital. Therefore the ratings and awards apply to multiple hospitals and this specific hospital may not provide all rated services.

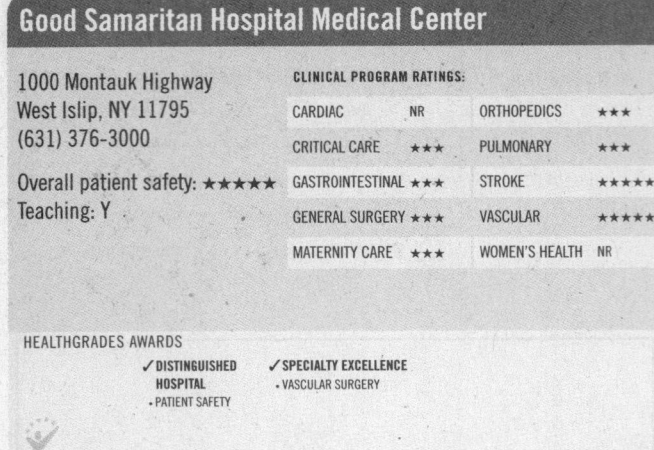

Good Samaritan Hospital Medical Center

1000 Montauk Highway
West Islip, NY 11795
(631) 376-3000

Overall patient safety: ★★★★★
Teaching: Y

CLINICAL PROGRAM RATINGS:

CARDIAC	NR	ORTHOPEDICS	★★★
CRITICAL CARE	★★★	PULMONARY	★★★
GASTROINTESTINAL	★★★	STROKE	★★★★★
GENERAL SURGERY	★★★	VASCULAR	★★★★★
MATERNITY CARE	★★★	WOMEN'S HEALTH	NR

HEALTHGRADES AWARDS

✓ DISTINGUISHED HOSPITAL
· PATIENT SAFETY

✓ SPECIALTY EXCELLENCE
· VASCULAR SURGERY

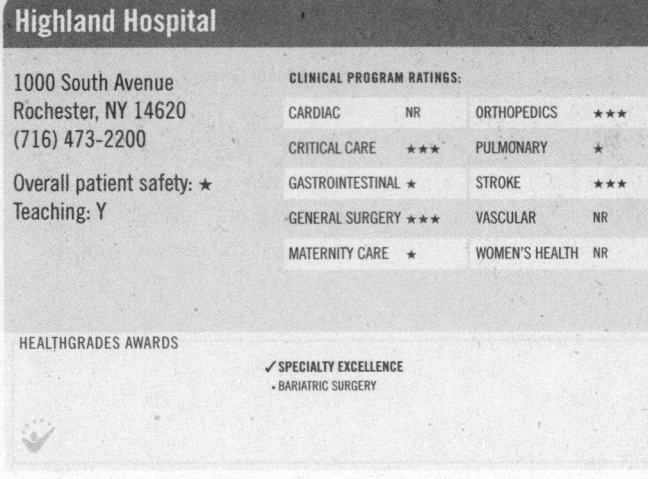

Highland Hospital

1000 South Avenue
Rochester, NY 14620
(716) 473-2200

Overall patient safety: ★
Teaching: Y

CLINICAL PROGRAM RATINGS:

CARDIAC	NR	ORTHOPEDICS	★★★
CRITICAL CARE	★★★	PULMONARY	★
GASTROINTESTINAL	★	STROKE	★★★
GENERAL SURGERY	★★★	VASCULAR	NR
MATERNITY CARE	★	WOMEN'S HEALTH	NR

HEALTHGRADES AWARDS

✓ SPECIALTY EXCELLENCE
· BARIATRIC SURGERY

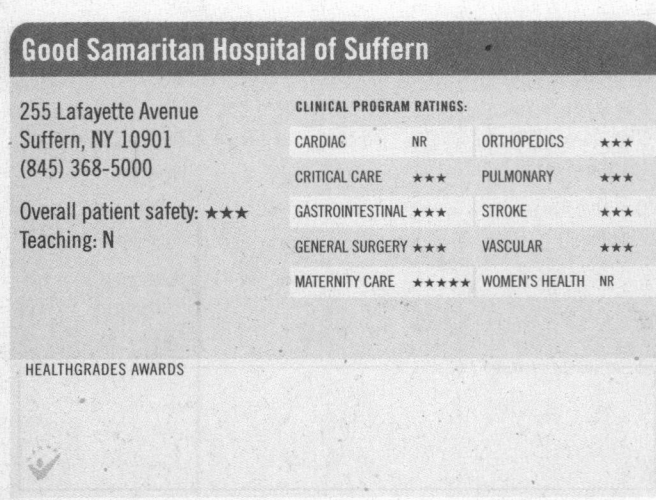

Good Samaritan Hospital of Suffern

255 Lafayette Avenue
Suffern, NY 10901
(845) 368-5000

Overall patient safety: ★★★
Teaching: N

CLINICAL PROGRAM RATINGS:

CARDIAC	NR	ORTHOPEDICS	★★★
CRITICAL CARE	★★★	PULMONARY	★★★
GASTROINTESTINAL	★★★	STROKE	★★★
GENERAL SURGERY	★★★	VASCULAR	★★★
MATERNITY CARE	★★★★★	WOMEN'S HEALTH	NR

HEALTHGRADES AWARDS

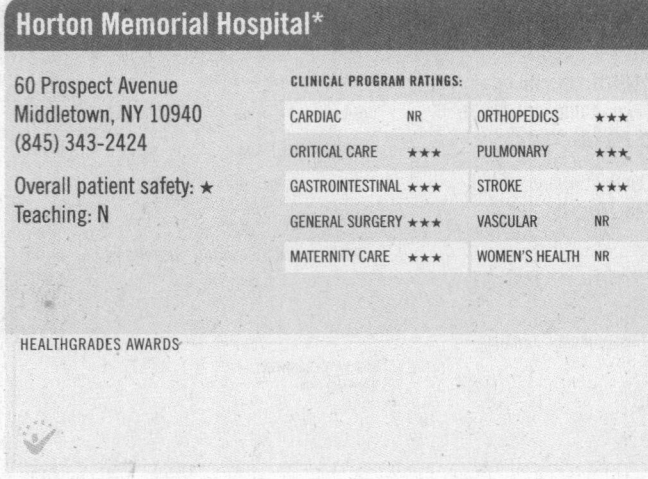

Horton Memorial Hospital*

60 Prospect Avenue
Middletown, NY 10940
(845) 343-2424

Overall patient safety: ★
Teaching: N

CLINICAL PROGRAM RATINGS:

CARDIAC	NR	ORTHOPEDICS	★★★
CRITICAL CARE	★★★	PULMONARY	★★★
GASTROINTESTINAL	★★★	STROKE	★★★
GENERAL SURGERY	★★★	VASCULAR	NR
MATERNITY CARE	★★★	WOMEN'S HEALTH	NR

HEALTHGRADES AWARDS

Harlem Hospital Center

506 Lenox Avenue
New York, NY 10037
(212) 939-1000

Overall patient safety: ★★★
Teaching: Y

CLINICAL PROGRAM RATINGS:

CARDIAC	NR	ORTHOPEDICS	NR
CRITICAL CARE	NR	PULMONARY	★★★
GASTROINTESTINAL	NR	STROKE	★★★
GENERAL SURGERY	NR	VASCULAR	NR
MATERNITY CARE	★	WOMEN'S HEALTH	NR

HEALTHGRADES AWARDS

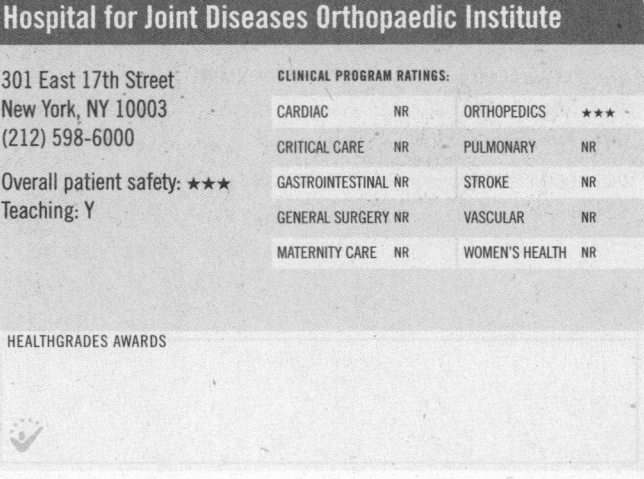

Hospital for Joint Diseases Orthopaedic Institute

301 East 17th Street
New York, NY 10003
(212) 598-6000

Overall patient safety: ★★★
Teaching: Y

CLINICAL PROGRAM RATINGS:

CARDIAC	NR	ORTHOPEDICS	★★★
CRITICAL CARE	NR	PULMONARY	NR
GASTROINTESTINAL	NR	STROKE	NR
GENERAL SURGERY	NR	VASCULAR	NR
MATERNITY CARE	NR	WOMEN'S HEALTH	NR

HEALTHGRADES AWARDS

KEY: ★★★★★ BEST   ★★★ AS EXPECTED   ★ POOR   NR NOT RATED BY HEALTHGRADES   For full definitions of ratings and awards, see Appendix.

Hospital for Special Surgery

535 East 70th Street
New York, NY 10021
(800) 676-0084

Overall patient safety: ★★★
Teaching: Y

CLINICAL PROGRAM RATINGS:

CARDIAC	NR	ORTHOPEDICS	★★★
CRITICAL CARE	NR	PULMONARY	NR
GASTROINTESTINAL	NR	STROKE	NR
GENERAL SURGERY	NR	VASCULAR	NR
MATERNITY CARE	NR	WOMEN'S HEALTH	NR

HEALTHGRADES AWARDS

✓ SPECIALTY EXCELLENCE
- JOINT REPLACEMENT

Inter-Community Memorial Hospital at Newfane

2600 William Street
Newfane, NY 14108
(716) 778-5111

Overall patient safety: ★★★
Teaching: N

CLINICAL PROGRAM RATINGS:

CARDIAC	NR	ORTHOPEDICS	NR
CRITICAL CARE	NR	PULMONARY	★
GASTROINTESTINAL	NR	STROKE	★★★
GENERAL SURGERY	NR	VASCULAR	NR
MATERNITY CARE	★★★	WOMEN'S HEALTH	NR

HEALTHGRADES AWARDS

Hudson Valley Hospital Center

1980 Crompond Road
Cortlandt Manor, NY 10567
(914) 737-9000

Overall patient safety: ★★★
Teaching: N

CLINICAL PROGRAM RATINGS:

CARDIAC	NR	ORTHOPEDICS	NR
CRITICAL CARE	★★★	PULMONARY	★★★★★
GASTROINTESTINAL	★★★	STROKE	★★★★★
GENERAL SURGERY	★	VASCULAR	NR
MATERNITY CARE	★★★	WOMEN'S HEALTH	NR

HEALTHGRADES AWARDS

✓ SPECIALTY EXCELLENCE
- PULMONARY CARE

Interfaith Medical Center

1545 Atlantic Avenue
Brooklyn, NY 11213
(718) 613-4000

Overall patient safety: ★
Teaching: Y

CLINICAL PROGRAM RATINGS:

CARDIAC	NR	ORTHOPEDICS	NR
CRITICAL CARE	NR	PULMONARY	★★★
GASTROINTESTINAL	NR	STROKE	★★★
GENERAL SURGERY	NR	VASCULAR	NR
MATERNITY CARE	★★★	WOMEN'S HEALTH	NR

HEALTHGRADES AWARDS

Huntington Hospital

270 Parks Avenue
Huntington, NY 11743
(631) 351-2000

Overall patient safety: ★★★
Teaching: Y

CLINICAL PROGRAM RATINGS:

CARDIAC	NR	ORTHOPEDICS	★★★
CRITICAL CARE	★★★	PULMONARY	★★★
GASTROINTESTINAL	★★★	STROKE	★★★★★
GENERAL SURGERY	★★★	VASCULAR	NR
MATERNITY CARE	★★★	WOMEN'S HEALTH	NR

HEALTHGRADES AWARDS

✓ SPECIALTY EXCELLENCE
- STROKE CARE

Ira Davenport Memorial Hospital

7571 State Route 54
Bath, NY 14810
(607) 776-8500

Overall patient safety: ★★★
Teaching: N

CLINICAL PROGRAM RATINGS:

CARDIAC	NR	ORTHOPEDICS	NR
CRITICAL CARE	NR	PULMONARY	★★★
GASTROINTESTINAL	NR	STROKE	★★★
GENERAL SURGERY	NR	VASCULAR	NR
MATERNITY CARE	★	WOMEN'S HEALTH	NR

HEALTHGRADES AWARDS

*This hospital reports its data to the federal government jointly with another hospital. Therefore the ratings and awards apply to multiple hospitals and this specific hospital may not provide all rated services.

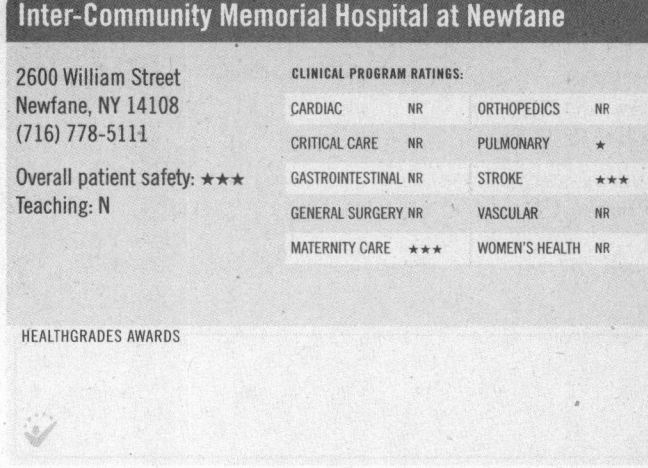

NEW YORK HOSPITALS: RATINGS BY CLINICAL SPECIALTY

Jacobi Medical Center

1400 Pelham Parkway South
Bronx, NY 10461
(718) 918-5000

Overall patient safety: ★★★
Teaching: Y

CLINICAL PROGRAM RATINGS:

CARDIAC	NR	ORTHOPEDICS	NR
CRITICAL CARE	NR	PULMONARY	★★★
GASTROINTESTINAL	NR	STROKE	★★★
GENERAL SURGERY	★★★	VASCULAR	NR
MATERNITY CARE	★	WOMEN'S HEALTH	NR

HEALTHGRADES AWARDS

Jones Memorial Hospital

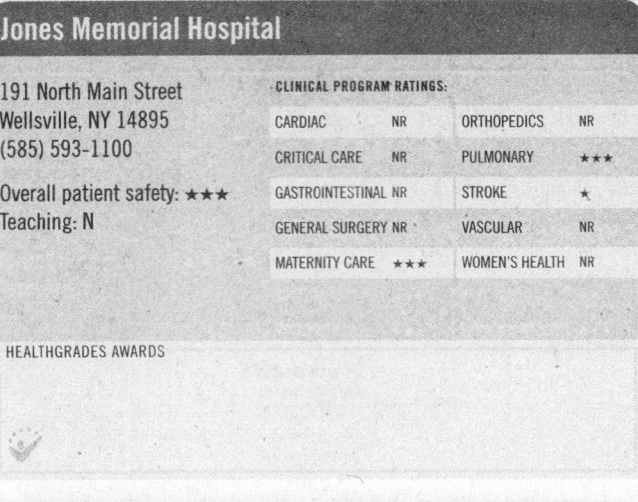

191 North Main Street
Wellsville, NY 14895
(585) 593-1100

Overall patient safety: ★★★
Teaching: N

CLINICAL PROGRAM RATINGS:

CARDIAC	NR	ORTHOPEDICS	NR
CRITICAL CARE	NR	PULMONARY	★★★
GASTROINTESTINAL	NR	STROKE	★
GENERAL SURGERY	NR	VASCULAR	NR
MATERNITY CARE	★★★	WOMEN'S HEALTH	NR

HEALTHGRADES AWARDS

Jamaica Hospital Medical Center

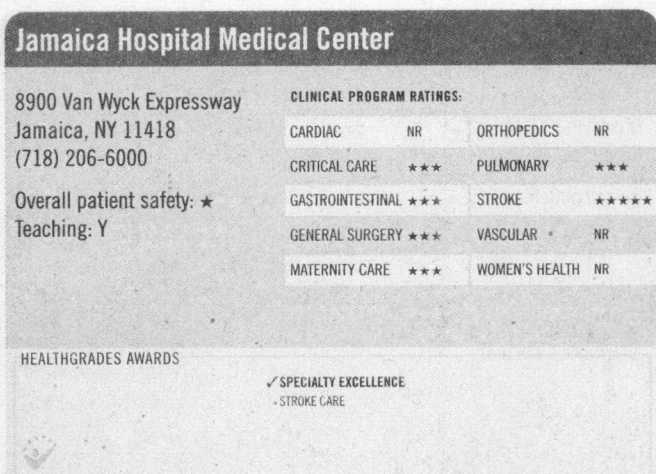

8900 Van Wyck Expressway
Jamaica, NY 11418
(718) 206-6000

Overall patient safety: ★
Teaching: Y

CLINICAL PROGRAM RATINGS:

CARDIAC	NR	ORTHOPEDICS	NR
CRITICAL CARE	★★★	PULMONARY	★★★
GASTROINTESTINAL	★★★	STROKE	★★★★★
GENERAL SURGERY	★★★	VASCULAR	NR
MATERNITY CARE	★★★	WOMEN'S HEALTH	NR

HEALTHGRADES AWARDS

✓ SPECIALTY EXCELLENCE
• STROKE CARE

Kenmore Mercy Hospital

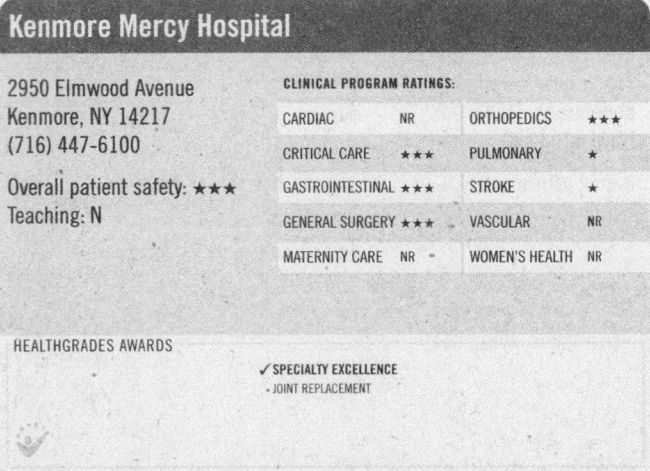

2950 Elmwood Avenue
Kenmore, NY 14217
(716) 447-6100

Overall patient safety: ★★★
Teaching: N

CLINICAL PROGRAM RATINGS:

CARDIAC	NR	ORTHOPEDICS	★★★
CRITICAL CARE	★★★	PULMONARY	★
GASTROINTESTINAL	★★★	STROKE	★
GENERAL SURGERY	★★★	VASCULAR	NR
MATERNITY CARE	NR	WOMEN'S HEALTH	NR

HEALTHGRADES AWARDS

✓ SPECIALTY EXCELLENCE
• JOINT REPLACEMENT

John T. Mather Memorial Hospital of Port Jefferson

75 North Country Road
Port Jefferson, NY 11777
(631) 473-1320

Overall patient safety: ★
Teaching: N

CLINICAL PROGRAM RATINGS:

CARDIAC	NR	ORTHOPEDICS	NR
CRITICAL CARE	★★★	PULMONARY	★★★★★
GASTROINTESTINAL	★★★	STROKE	★★★
GENERAL SURGERY	★★★★★	VASCULAR	★★★
MATERNITY CARE	NR	WOMEN'S HEALTH	NR

HEALTHGRADES AWARDS

✓ SPECIALTY EXCELLENCE
• GENERAL SURGERY   • PULMONARY CARE

Kings County Hospital Center

451 Clarkson Avenue
Brooklyn, NY 11203
(718) 245-3900

Overall patient safety: ★★★
Teaching: Y

CLINICAL PROGRAM RATINGS:

CARDIAC	NR	ORTHOPEDICS	NR
CRITICAL CARE	NR	PULMONARY	★★★
GASTROINTESTINAL	NR	STROKE	★★★
GENERAL SURGERY	NR	VASCULAR	NR
MATERNITY CARE	★★★	WOMEN'S HEALTH	NR

HEALTHGRADES AWARDS

KEY: ★★★★★ BEST   ★★★ AS EXPECTED   ★ POOR   NR NOT RATED BY HEALTHGRADES   For full definitions of ratings and awards, see Appendix.

Kings Highway Hospital*

3201 Kings Highway
Brooklyn, NY 11234
(718) 252-3000

Overall patient safety: ★★★
Teaching: Y

CLINICAL PROGRAM RATINGS:

CARDIAC	★★★	ORTHOPEDICS	★★★★★
CRITICAL CARE	★★★	PULMONARY	★★★
GASTROINTESTINAL	★★★	STROKE	★★★
GENERAL SURGERY	★★★	VASCULAR	NR
MATERNITY CARE	★★★★★	WOMEN'S HEALTH	★★★

HEALTHGRADES AWARDS

✓ SPECIALTY EXCELLENCE
• ORTHOPEDIC SURGERY

Lake Shore Hospital*

845 Routes 5 and 20
Irving, NY 14081
(716) 951-7000

Overall patient safety: ★★★
Teaching: N

CLINICAL PROGRAM RATINGS:

CARDIAC	NR	ORTHOPEDICS	NR
CRITICAL CARE	NR	PULMONARY	★
GASTROINTESTINAL	NR	STROKE	★★★
GENERAL SURGERY	NR	VASCULAR	NR
MATERNITY CARE	NR	WOMEN'S HEALTH	NR

HEALTHGRADES AWARDS

Kingsbrook Jewish Medical Center

585 Schenectady Avenue
Brooklyn, NY 11203
(718) 604-5000

Overall patient safety: ★
Teaching: Y

CLINICAL PROGRAM RATINGS:

CARDIAC	NR	ORTHOPEDICS	NR
CRITICAL CARE	NR	PULMONARY	★★★
GASTROINTESTINAL	NR	STROKE	★★★
GENERAL SURGERY	★★★	VASCULAR	NR
MATERNITY CARE	NR	WOMEN'S HEALTH	NR

HEALTHGRADES AWARDS

Lakeside Memorial Hospital

156 West Avenue
Brockport, NY 14420
(716) 395-6095

Overall patient safety: ★
Teaching: N

CLINICAL PROGRAM RATINGS:

CARDIAC	NR	ORTHOPEDICS	NR
CRITICAL CARE	NR	PULMONARY	★★★
GASTROINTESTINAL	NR	STROKE	★★★
GENERAL SURGERY	NR	VASCULAR	NR
MATERNITY CARE	★★★	WOMEN'S HEALTH	NR

HEALTHGRADES AWARDS

Kingston Hospital

396 Broadway
Kingston, NY 12401
(845) 331-3131

Overall patient safety: ★★★
Teaching: Y

CLINICAL PROGRAM RATINGS:

CARDIAC	NR	ORTHOPEDICS	NR
CRITICAL CARE	NR	PULMONARY	★★★
GASTROINTESTINAL	★★★	STROKE	★★★
GENERAL SURGERY	★★★	VASCULAR	NR
MATERNITY CARE	★★★	WOMEN'S HEALTH	NR

HEALTHGRADES AWARDS

Lawrence Hospital Center

55 Palmer Avenue
Bronxville, NY 10708
(914) 787-1000

Overall patient safety: ★★★
Teaching: N

CLINICAL PROGRAM RATINGS:

CARDIAC	NR	ORTHOPEDICS	NR
CRITICAL CARE	NR	PULMONARY	★★★
GASTROINTESTINAL	NR	STROKE	★★★★★
GENERAL SURGERY	★★★	VASCULAR	NR
MATERNITY CARE	★★★	WOMEN'S HEALTH	NR

HEALTHGRADES AWARDS

*This hospital reports its data to the federal government jointly with another hospital. Therefore the ratings and awards apply to multiple hospitals and this specific hospital may not provide all rated services.

Lenox Hill Hospital

100 East 77th Street
New York, NY 10021
(212) 434-2000

Overall patient safety: ★★★
Teaching: Y

CLINICAL PROGRAM RATINGS:

CARDIAC	★★★	ORTHOPEDICS	★★★
CRITICAL CARE	★★★	PULMONARY	★★★
GASTROINTESTINAL	★★★	STROKE	★★★
GENERAL SURGERY	★★★	VASCULAR	★★★
MATERNITY CARE	★★★★★	WOMEN'S HEALTH	★★★

HEALTHGRADES AWARDS

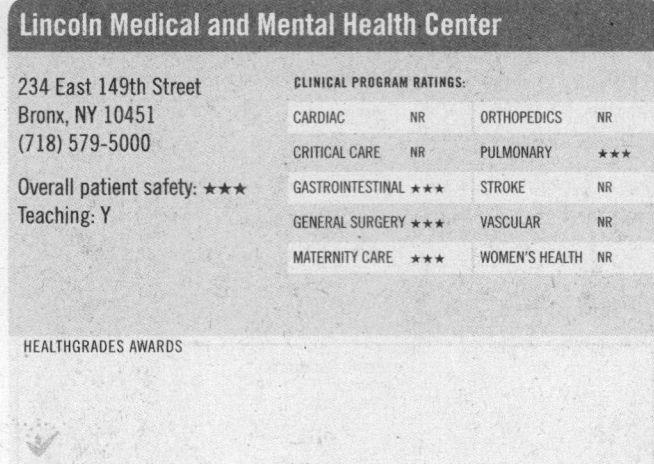

✓ SPECIALTY EXCELLENCE
• CARDIAC CARE   • MATERNITY CARE

Lincoln Medical and Mental Health Center

234 East 149th Street
Bronx, NY 10451
(718) 579-5000

Overall patient safety: ★★★
Teaching: Y

CLINICAL PROGRAM RATINGS:

CARDIAC	NR	ORTHOPEDICS	NR
CRITICAL CARE	NR	PULMONARY	★★★
GASTROINTESTINAL	★★★	STROKE	NR
GENERAL SURGERY	★★★	VASCULAR	NR
MATERNITY CARE	★★★	WOMEN'S HEALTH	NR

HEALTHGRADES AWARDS

Leonard Hospital*

74 New Turnpike Road
Troy, NY 12182
(518) 235-0310

Overall patient safety: ★★★
Teaching: N

CLINICAL PROGRAM RATINGS:

CARDIAC	NR	ORTHOPEDICS	★★★
CRITICAL CARE	NR	PULMONARY	★★★
GASTROINTESTINAL	★★★	STROKE	★★★
GENERAL SURGERY	★★★	VASCULAR	NR
MATERNITY CARE	★★★	WOMEN'S HEALTH	NR

HEALTHGRADES AWARDS

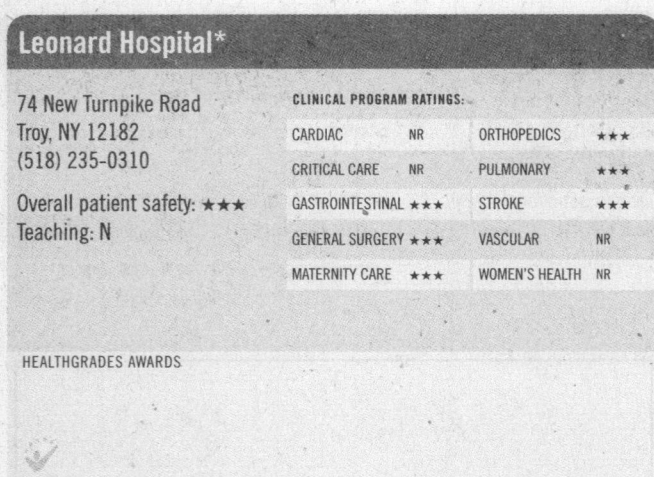

Little Falls Hospital

140 Burwell Street
Little Falls, NY 13365
(315) 823-5261

Overall patient safety: ★★★
Teaching: N

CLINICAL PROGRAM RATINGS:

CARDIAC	NR	ORTHOPEDICS	NR
CRITICAL CARE	NR	PULMONARY	★
GASTROINTESTINAL	NR	STROKE	NR
GENERAL SURGERY	NR	VASCULAR	NR
MATERNITY CARE	NR	WOMEN'S HEALTH	NR

HEALTHGRADES AWARDS

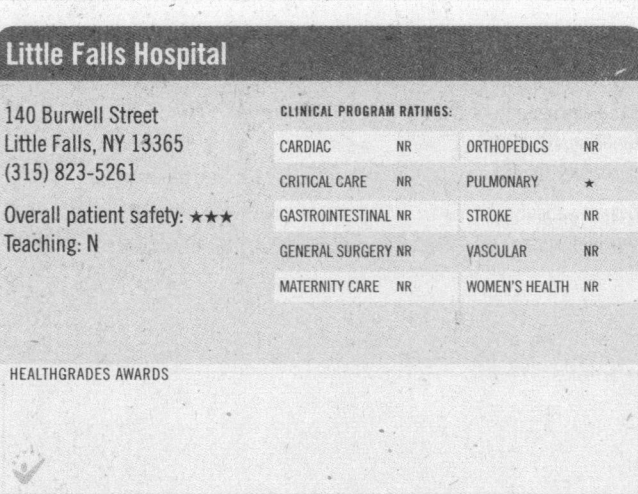

Lewis County General Hospital

7785 North State Street
Lowville, NY 13367
(315) 376-5200

Overall patient safety: ★★★
Teaching: N

CLINICAL PROGRAM RATINGS:

CARDIAC	NR	ORTHOPEDICS	NR
CRITICAL CARE	NR	PULMONARY	★★★
GASTROINTESTINAL	NR	STROKE	★★★
GENERAL SURGERY	★★★	VASCULAR	NR
MATERNITY CARE	★	WOMEN'S HEALTH	NR

HEALTHGRADES AWARDS

Lockport Memorial Hospital

521 East Avenue
Lockport, NY 14094
(716) 514-5700

Overall patient safety: ★★★
Teaching: N

CLINICAL PROGRAM RATINGS:

CARDIAC	NR	ORTHOPEDICS	NR
CRITICAL CARE	NR	PULMONARY	★
GASTROINTESTINAL	NR	STROKE	★★★
GENERAL SURGERY	★★★	VASCULAR	NR
MATERNITY CARE	★★★	WOMEN'S HEALTH	NR

HEALTHGRADES AWARDS

KEY: ★★★★★ **BEST**   ★★★ **AS EXPECTED**   ★ **POOR**   NR **NOT RATED BY HEALTHGRADES**   For full definitions of ratings and awards, see Appendix.

Long Beach Medical Center

455 East Bay Drive
Long Beach, NY 11561
(516) 897-1000

Overall patient safety: ★
Teaching: Y

CLINICAL PROGRAM RATINGS:

CARDIAC	NR	ORTHOPEDICS	NR
CRITICAL CARE	NR	PULMONARY	★★★
GASTROINTESTINAL	NR	STROKE	★★★
GENERAL SURGERY	★★★	VASCULAR	NR
MATERNITY CARE	NR	WOMEN'S HEALTH	NR

HEALTHGRADES AWARDS

Lutheran Medical Center

150 55th Street
Brooklyn, NY 11220
(718) 630-7000

Overall patient safety: ★★★
Teaching: Y

CLINICAL PROGRAM RATINGS:

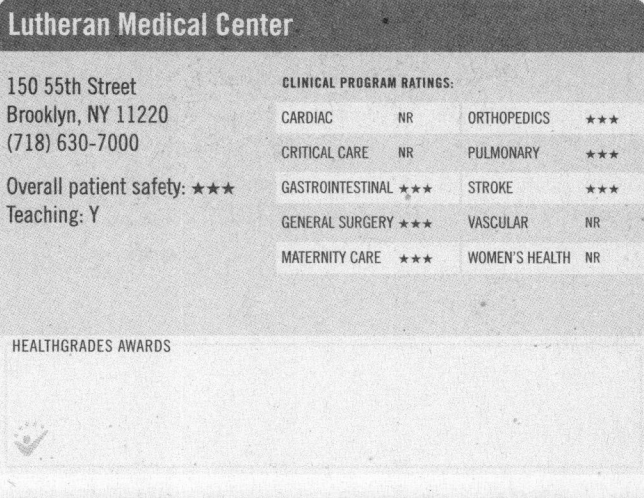

CARDIAC	NR	ORTHOPEDICS	★★★
CRITICAL CARE	NR	PULMONARY	★★★
GASTROINTESTINAL	★★★	STROKE	★★★
GENERAL SURGERY	★★★	VASCULAR	NR
MATERNITY CARE	★★★	WOMEN'S HEALTH	NR

HEALTHGRADES AWARDS

Long Island College Hospital

339 Hicks Street
Brooklyn, NY 11201
(718) 780-1000

Overall patient safety: ★★★
Teaching: Y

CLINICAL PROGRAM RATINGS:

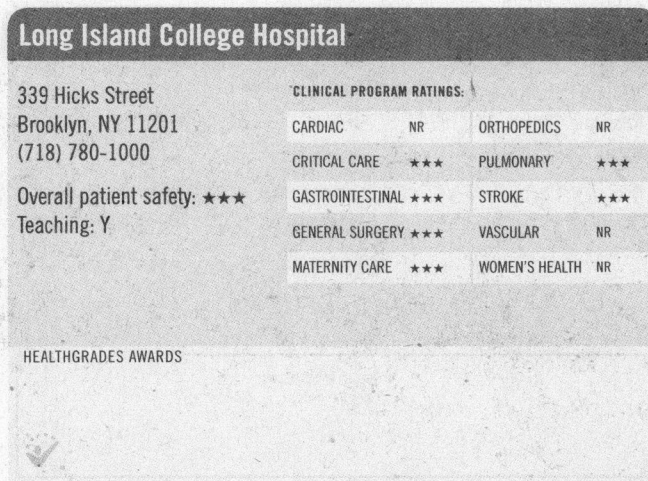

CARDIAC	NR	ORTHOPEDICS	NR
CRITICAL CARE	★★★	PULMONARY	★★★
GASTROINTESTINAL	★★★	STROKE	★★★
GENERAL SURGERY	★★★	VASCULAR	NR
MATERNITY CARE	★★★	WOMEN'S HEALTH	NR

HEALTHGRADES AWARDS

Maimonides Medical Center

4802 10th Avenue
Brooklyn, NY 11219
(718) 283-6000

Overall patient safety: ★
Teaching: Y

CLINICAL PROGRAM RATINGS:

CARDIAC	★★★	ORTHOPEDICS	★★★
CRITICAL CARE	★★★★★	PULMONARY	★★★
GASTROINTESTINAL	★★★	STROKE	★★★★★
GENERAL SURGERY	★★★	VASCULAR	★
MATERNITY CARE	★★★★★	WOMEN'S HEALTH	★★★★★

HEALTHGRADES AWARDS

✓ SPECIALTY EXCELLENCE
• CRITICAL CARE   • STROKE CARE   • WOMEN'S HEALTH

Long Island Jewish Medical Center

27005 76th Avenue
New Hyde Park, NY 11040
(718) 470-7000

Overall patient safety: ★
Teaching: Y

CLINICAL PROGRAM RATINGS:

CARDIAC	★★★	ORTHOPEDICS	★
CRITICAL CARE	★	PULMONARY	★
GASTROINTESTINAL	★★★	STROKE	★★★
GENERAL SURGERY	★★★	VASCULAR	★
MATERNITY CARE	★★★	WOMEN'S HEALTH	★★★

HEALTHGRADES AWARDS

Mary Immaculate Hospital*

15211 89th Avenue
Jamaica, NY 11432
(718) 558-2000

Overall patient safety: ★
Teaching: Y

CLINICAL PROGRAM RATINGS:

CARDIAC	NR	ORTHOPEDICS	NR
CRITICAL CARE	★	PULMONARY	★
GASTROINTESTINAL	★★★	STROKE	★★★
GENERAL SURGERY	★★★★★	VASCULAR	NR
MATERNITY CARE	★★★★★	WOMEN'S HEALTH	NR

HEALTHGRADES AWARDS

✓ SPECIALTY EXCELLENCE
• GENERAL SURGERY

*This hospital reports its data to the federal government jointly with another hospital. Therefore the ratings and awards apply to multiple hospitals and this specific hospital may not provide all rated services.

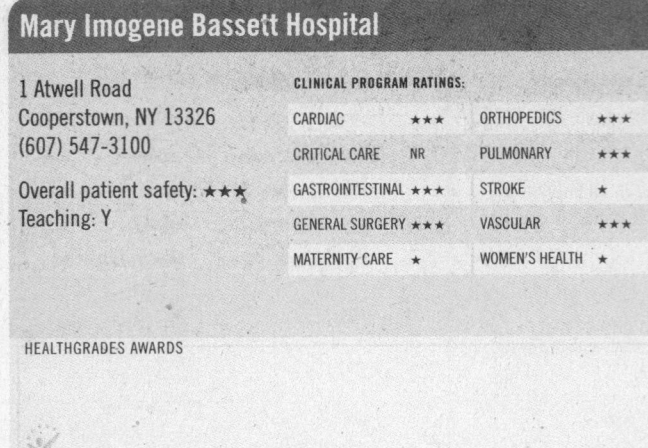

Mary Imogene Bassett Hospital

1 Atwell Road
Cooperstown, NY 13326
(607) 547-3100

Overall patient safety: ★★★
Teaching: Y

CLINICAL PROGRAM RATINGS:

CARDIAC	★★★	ORTHOPEDICS	★★★
CRITICAL CARE	NR	PULMONARY	★★★
GASTROINTESTINAL	★★★	STROKE	★
GENERAL SURGERY	★★★	VASCULAR	★★★
MATERNITY CARE	★	WOMEN'S HEALTH	★

HEALTHGRADES AWARDS

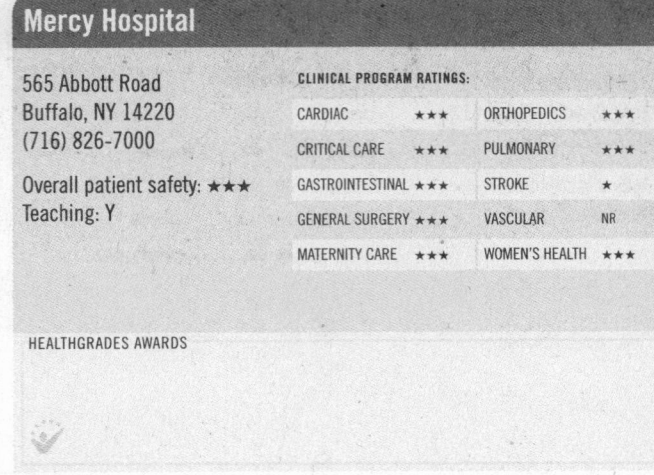

Mercy Hospital

565 Abbott Road
Buffalo, NY 14220
(716) 826-7000

Overall patient safety: ★★★
Teaching: Y

CLINICAL PROGRAM RATINGS:

CARDIAC	★★★	ORTHOPEDICS	★★★
CRITICAL CARE	★★★	PULMONARY	★★★
GASTROINTESTINAL	★★★	STROKE	★
GENERAL SURGERY	★★★	VASCULAR	NR
MATERNITY CARE	★★★	WOMEN'S HEALTH	★★★

HEALTHGRADES AWARDS

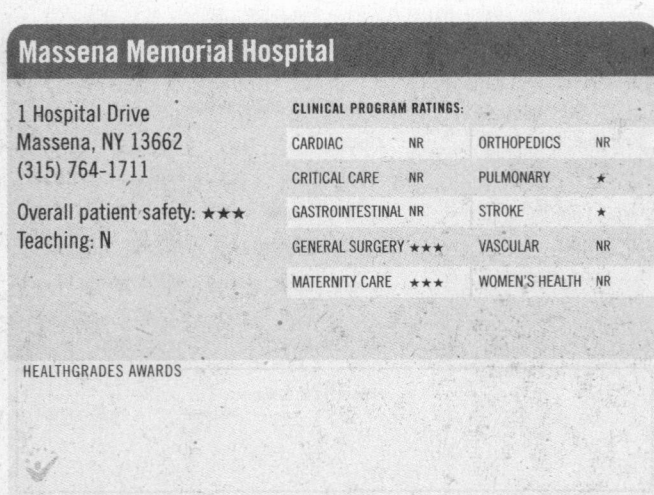

Massena Memorial Hospital

1 Hospital Drive
Massena, NY 13662
(315) 764-1711

Overall patient safety: ★★★
Teaching: N

CLINICAL PROGRAM RATINGS:

CARDIAC	NR	ORTHOPEDICS	NR
CRITICAL CARE	NR	PULMONARY	★
GASTROINTESTINAL	NR	STROKE	★
GENERAL SURGERY	★★★	VASCULAR	NR
MATERNITY CARE	★★★	WOMEN'S HEALTH	NR

HEALTHGRADES AWARDS

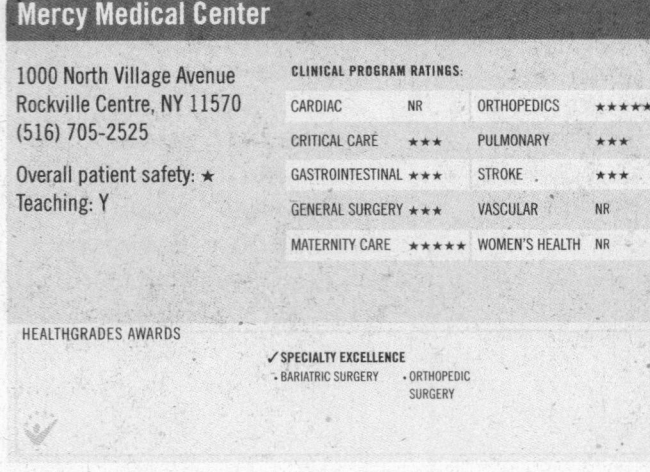

Mercy Medical Center

1000 North Village Avenue
Rockville Centre, NY 11570
(516) 705-2525

Overall patient safety: ★
Teaching: Y

CLINICAL PROGRAM RATINGS:

CARDIAC	NR	ORTHOPEDICS	★★★★★
CRITICAL CARE	★★★	PULMONARY	★★★
GASTROINTESTINAL	★★★	STROKE	★★★
GENERAL SURGERY	★★★	VASCULAR	NR
MATERNITY CARE	★★★★★	WOMEN'S HEALTH	NR

HEALTHGRADES AWARDS

✓ SPECIALTY EXCELLENCE
• BARIATRIC SURGERY • ORTHOPEDIC SURGERY

Medina Memorial Hospital

200 Ohio Street
Medina, NY 14103
(585) 798-2000

Overall patient safety: ★★★
Teaching: N

CLINICAL PROGRAM RATINGS:

CARDIAC	NR	ORTHOPEDICS	NR
CRITICAL CARE	NR	PULMONARY	★
GASTROINTESTINAL	NR	STROKE	★
GENERAL SURGERY	NR	VASCULAR	NR
MATERNITY CARE	★★★	WOMEN'S HEALTH	NR

HEALTHGRADES AWARDS

Metropolitan Hospital Center

1901 1st Avenue
New York, NY 10029
(212) 423-6262

Overall patient safety: ★★★
Teaching: Y

CLINICAL PROGRAM RATINGS:

CARDIAC	NR	ORTHOPEDICS	NR
CRITICAL CARE	NR	PULMONARY	★★★
GASTROINTESTINAL	NR	STROKE	★★★
GENERAL SURGERY	NR	VASCULAR	NR
MATERNITY CARE	★★★	WOMEN'S HEALTH	NR

HEALTHGRADES AWARDS

KEY: ★★★★★ BEST   ★★★ AS EXPECTED   ★ POOR   NR NOT RATED BY HEALTHGRADES   For full definitions of ratings and awards, see Appendix.

Millard Fillmore Hospital*

3 Gates Circle
Buffalo, NY 14209
(716) 887-4600

Overall patient safety: ★
Teaching: Y

CLINICAL PROGRAM RATINGS:

CARDIAC	★★★	ORTHOPEDICS	★★★
CRITICAL CARE	★	PULMONARY	★
GASTROINTESTINAL	★★★	STROKE	★★★
GENERAL SURGERY	★★★	VASCULAR	★★★
MATERNITY CARE	★★★	WOMEN'S HEALTH	★★★

HEALTHGRADES AWARDS

✓ SPECIALTY EXCELLENCE
- CARDIAC SURGERY

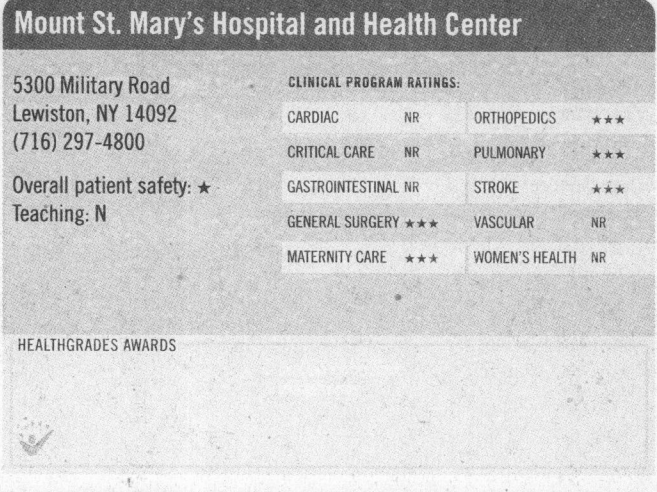

Mount St. Mary's Hospital and Health Center

5300 Military Road
Lewiston, NY 14092
(716) 297-4800

Overall patient safety: ★
Teaching: N

CLINICAL PROGRAM RATINGS:

CARDIAC	NR	ORTHOPEDICS	★★★
CRITICAL CARE	NR	PULMONARY	★★★
GASTROINTESTINAL	NR	STROKE	★★★
GENERAL SURGERY	★★★	VASCULAR	NR
MATERNITY CARE	★★★	WOMEN'S HEALTH	NR

HEALTHGRADES AWARDS

Mohawk Valley General Hospital*

295 West Main Street
Ilion, NY 13357
(315) 895-7474

Overall patient safety: ★★★
Teaching: Y

CLINICAL PROGRAM RATINGS:

CARDIAC	NR	ORTHOPEDICS	★★★
CRITICAL CARE	★	PULMONARY	★
GASTROINTESTINAL	★★★	STROKE	★★★
GENERAL SURGERY	★★★	VASCULAR	NR
MATERNITY CARE	★★★★★	WOMEN'S HEALTH	NR

HEALTHGRADES AWARDS

✓ SPECIALTY EXCELLENCE
- MATERNITY CARE

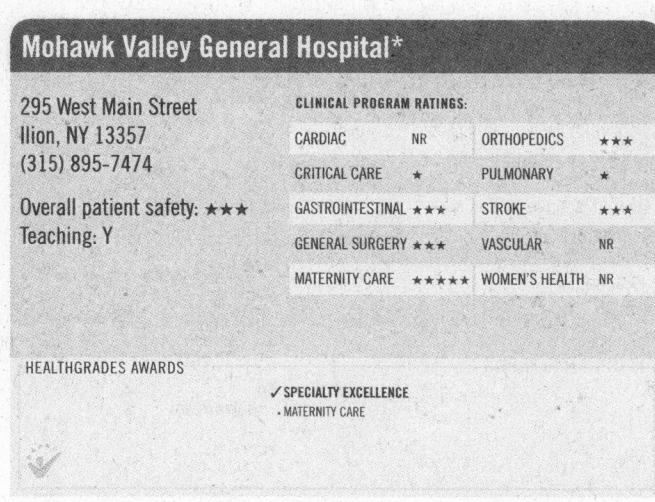

Mount Sinai Hospital

1 Gustave L. Levy Place
New York, NY 10029
(212) 241-6500

Overall patient safety: ★
Teaching: Y

CLINICAL PROGRAM RATINGS:

CARDIAC	★★★	ORTHOPEDICS	★★★
CRITICAL CARE	★★★	PULMONARY	★★★
GASTROINTESTINAL	★★★	STROKE	★★★★★
GENERAL SURGERY	★★★	VASCULAR	★
MATERNITY CARE	★	WOMEN'S HEALTH	★★★

HEALTHGRADES AWARDS

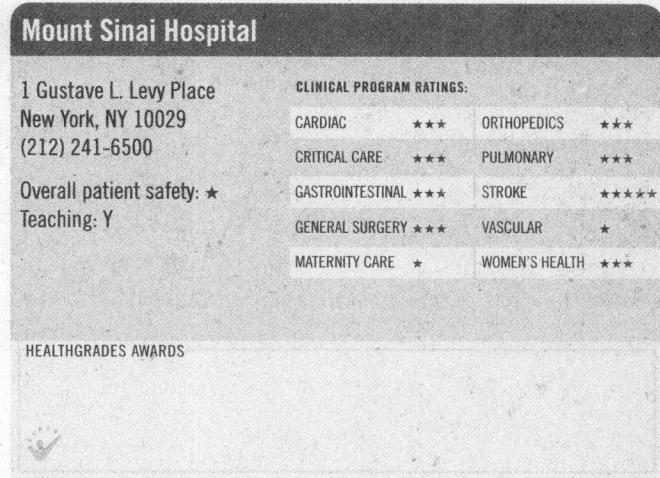

Montefiore Medical Center

111 East 210th Street
Bronx, NY 10467
(718) 920-4321

Overall patient safety: ★★★
Teaching: Y

CLINICAL PROGRAM RATINGS:

CARDIAC	★★★	ORTHOPEDICS	★
CRITICAL CARE	★★★	PULMONARY	★
GASTROINTESTINAL	★★★	STROKE	★★★
GENERAL SURGERY	★	VASCULAR	★
MATERNITY CARE	★★★	WOMEN'S HEALTH	★

HEALTHGRADES AWARDS

Mount Vernon Hospital

12 North 7th Avenue
Mount Vernon, NY 10550
(914) 664-8000

Overall patient safety: ★★★
Teaching: Y

CLINICAL PROGRAM RATINGS:

CARDIAC	NR	ORTHOPEDICS	NR
CRITICAL CARE	NR	PULMONARY	★★★
GASTROINTESTINAL	NR	STROKE	★★★
GENERAL SURGERY	NR	VASCULAR	NR
MATERNITY CARE	NR	WOMEN'S HEALTH	NR

HEALTHGRADES AWARDS

NEW YORK HOSPITALS: RATINGS BY CLINICAL SPECIALTY

Nassau University Medical Center

2201 Hempstead Turnpike
East Meadow, NY 11554
(516) 572-0123

Overall patient safety: ★
Teaching: Y

CLINICAL PROGRAM RATINGS:

CARDIAC	NR	ORTHOPEDICS	NR
CRITICAL CARE	★	PULMONARY	★★★
GASTROINTESTINAL	NR	STROKE	★
GENERAL SURGERY	NR	VASCULAR	NR
MATERNITY CARE	★★★	WOMEN'S HEALTH	NR

HEALTHGRADES AWARDS

New York Community Hospital of Brooklyn

2525 Kings Highway
Brooklyn, NY 11229
(718) 692-5300

Overall patient safety: ★★★
Teaching: N

CLINICAL PROGRAM RATINGS:

CARDIAC	NR	ORTHOPEDICS	NR
CRITICAL CARE	NR	PULMONARY	★★★
GASTROINTESTINAL	★★★	STROKE	★★★
GENERAL SURGERY	★★★	VASCULAR	NR
MATERNITY CARE	NR	WOMEN'S HEALTH	NR

HEALTHGRADES AWARDS

Nathan Littauer Hospital

99 East State Street
Gloversville, NY 12078
(518) 725-8621

Overall patient safety: ★
Teaching: N

CLINICAL PROGRAM RATINGS:

CARDIAC	NR	ORTHOPEDICS	NR
CRITICAL CARE	NR	PULMONARY	★★★
GASTROINTESTINAL	NR	STROKE	★★★
GENERAL SURGERY	★★★	VASCULAR	NR
MATERNITY CARE	★★★	WOMEN'S HEALTH	NR

HEALTHGRADES AWARDS

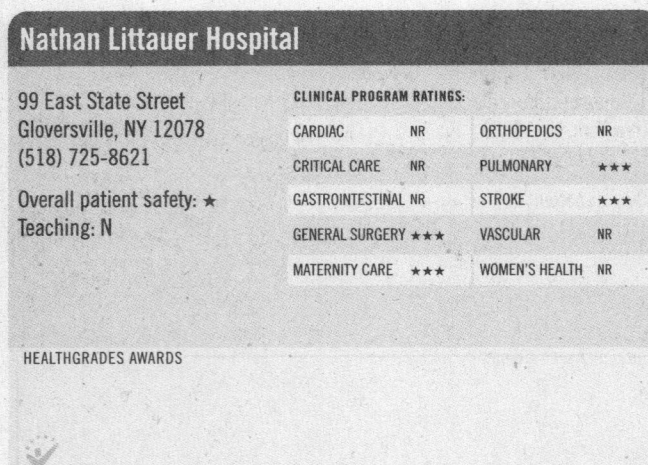

New York Downtown Hospital

170 William Street
New York, NY 10038
(212) 312-5000

Overall patient safety: ★★★
Teaching: Y

CLINICAL PROGRAM RATINGS:

CARDIAC	NR	ORTHOPEDICS	NR
CRITICAL CARE	NR	PULMONARY	★★★
GASTROINTESTINAL	NR	STROKE	★★★
GENERAL SURGERY	★★★★★	VASCULAR	NR
MATERNITY CARE	★★★★★	WOMEN'S HEALTH	NR

HEALTHGRADES AWARDS

✓ SPECIALTY EXCELLENCE
• GENERAL SURGERY   • MATERNITY CARE

New Island Hospital

4295 Hempstead Turnpike
Bethpage, NY 11714
(516) 579-6000

Overall patient safety: ★★★
Teaching: Y

CLINICAL PROGRAM RATINGS:

CARDIAC	NR	ORTHOPEDICS	NR
CRITICAL CARE	NR	PULMONARY	★★★
GASTROINTESTINAL	★★★	STROKE	★★★
GENERAL SURGERY	★★★	VASCULAR	NR
MATERNITY CARE	NR	WOMEN'S HEALTH	NR

HEALTHGRADES AWARDS

New York Hospital Medical Center of Queens

5645 Main Street
Flushing, NY 11355
(718) 670-1231

Overall patient safety: ★★★
Teaching: Y

CLINICAL PROGRAM RATINGS:

CARDIAC	★★★	ORTHOPEDICS	NR
CRITICAL CARE	★★★	PULMONARY	★
GASTROINTESTINAL	★★★	STROKE	★★★
GENERAL SURGERY	★★★	VASCULAR	NR
MATERNITY CARE	★★★★★	WOMEN'S HEALTH	★★★

HEALTHGRADES AWARDS

✓ SPECIALTY EXCELLENCE
• MATERNITY CARE

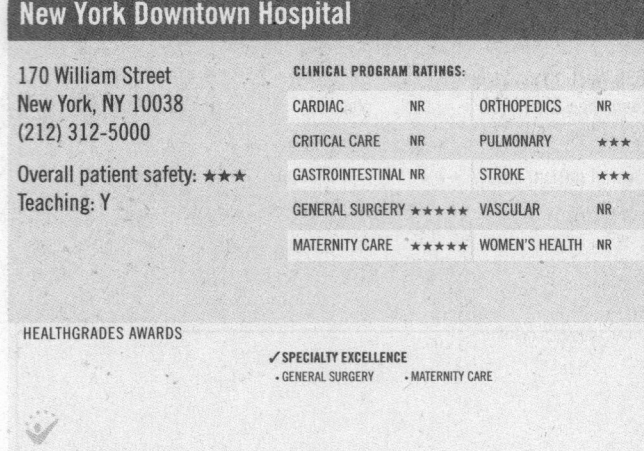

KEY: ★★★★★ BEST   ★★★ AS EXPECTED   ★ POOR   NR NOT RATED BY HEALTHGRADES   For full definitions of ratings and awards, see Appendix.

New York Methodist Hospital

506 6th Street
Brooklyn, NY 11215
(718) 780-3000

Overall patient safety: ★
Teaching: Y

CLINICAL PROGRAM RATINGS:

CARDIAC	★★★	ORTHOPEDICS	★★★
CRITICAL CARE	★	PULMONARY	★★★
GASTROINTESTINAL	★★★	STROKE	★★★★★
GENERAL SURGERY	★★★	VASCULAR	NR
MATERNITY CARE	★★★	WOMEN'S HEALTH	★★★

HEALTHGRADES AWARDS

✓ **SPECIALTY EXCELLENCE**
· STROKE CARE

New York Westchester Square Medical Center

2475 St. Raymond Avenue
Bronx, NY 10461
(718) 430-7300

Overall patient safety: ★
Teaching: N

CLINICAL PROGRAM RATINGS:

CARDIAC	NR	ORTHOPEDICS	NR
CRITICAL CARE	NR	PULMONARY	★★★
GASTROINTESTINAL	★★★	STROKE	★★★
GENERAL SURGERY	★★★	VASCULAR	NR
MATERNITY CARE	NR	WOMEN'S HEALTH	NR

HEALTHGRADES AWARDS

New York Presbyterian—Columbia*

630 West 168th Street
New York, NY 10032
(212) 305-2500

Overall patient safety: ★★★
Teaching: Y

CLINICAL PROGRAM RATINGS:

CARDIAC	★★★	ORTHOPEDICS	★★★
CRITICAL CARE	★★★	PULMONARY	★★★★★
GASTROINTESTINAL	★★★	STROKE	★★★★★
GENERAL SURGERY	★★★	VASCULAR	★★★
MATERNITY CARE	★★★	WOMEN'S HEALTH	★★★

HEALTHGRADES AWARDS

✓ **SPECIALTY EXCELLENCE**
· CARDIAC CARE   · PULMONARY CARE   · STROKE CARE

New York-Presbyterian/Weill Cornell*

525 East 68th Street
New York, NY 10021
(212) 746-5454

Overall patient safety: ★★★
Teaching: Y

CLINICAL PROGRAM RATINGS:

CARDIAC	★★★	ORTHOPEDICS	★★★
CRITICAL CARE	★★★	PULMONARY	★★★★★
GASTROINTESTINAL	★★★	STROKE	★★★★★
GENERAL SURGERY	★★★	VASCULAR	★★★
MATERNITY CARE	★★★	WOMEN'S HEALTH	★★★

HEALTHGRADES AWARDS

✓ **DISTINGUISHED HOSPITAL**   ✓ **SPECIALTY EXCELLENCE**
· CLINICAL EXCELLENCE   · CARDIAC CARE   · PULMONARY CARE   · STROKE CARE

New York University Medical Center—Tisch Hospital

560 1st Avenue
New York, NY 10016
(212) 263-7300

Overall patient safety: ★
Teaching: Y

CLINICAL PROGRAM RATINGS:

CARDIAC	★★★	ORTHOPEDICS	★
CRITICAL CARE	★★★	PULMONARY	★★★
GASTROINTESTINAL	★★★	STROKE	★★★★★
GENERAL SURGERY	★★★	VASCULAR	★
MATERNITY CARE	★★★	WOMEN'S HEALTH	★★★

HEALTHGRADES AWARDS

✓ **SPECIALTY EXCELLENCE**
· BARIATRIC SURGERY   · STROKE CARE

Newark-Wayne Community Hospital*

1200 Driving Park Avenue
Newark, NY 14513
(315) 332-2022

Overall patient safety: ★
Teaching: N

CLINICAL PROGRAM RATINGS:

CARDIAC	NR	ORTHOPEDICS	NR
CRITICAL CARE	NR	PULMONARY	★
GASTROINTESTINAL	NR	STROKE	★★★
GENERAL SURGERY	NR	VASCULAR	NR
MATERNITY CARE	★★★	WOMEN'S HEALTH	NR

HEALTHGRADES AWARDS

*This hospital reports its data to the federal government jointly with another hospital. Therefore the ratings and awards apply to multiple hospitals and this specific hospital may not provide all rated services.

Niagara Falls Memorial Medical Center

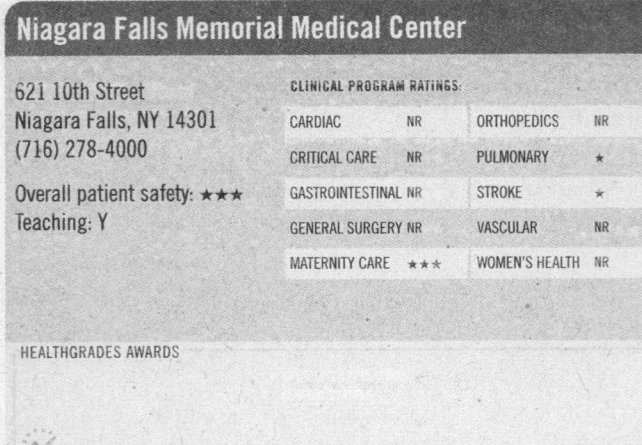

621 10th Street
Niagara Falls, NY 14301
(716) 278-4000

Overall patient safety: ★★★
Teaching: Y

CLINICAL PROGRAM RATINGS:

CARDIAC	NR	ORTHOPEDICS	NR
CRITICAL CARE	NR	PULMONARY	★
GASTROINTESTINAL	NR	STROKE	★
GENERAL SURGERY	NR	VASCULAR	NR
MATERNITY CARE	★★★	WOMEN'S HEALTH	NR

HEALTHGRADES AWARDS

North General Hospital

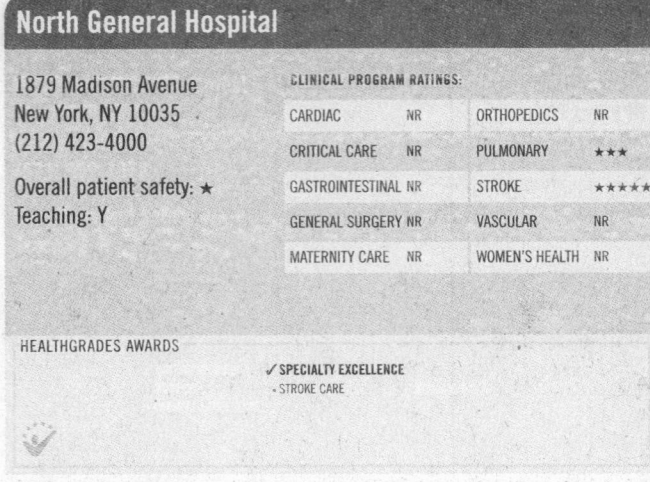

1879 Madison Avenue
New York, NY 10035
(212) 423-4000

Overall patient safety: ★
Teaching: Y

CLINICAL PROGRAM RATINGS:

CARDIAC	NR	ORTHOPEDICS	NR
CRITICAL CARE	NR	PULMONARY	★★★
GASTROINTESTINAL	NR	STROKE	★★★★★
GENERAL SURGERY	NR	VASCULAR	NR
MATERNITY CARE	NR	WOMEN'S HEALTH	NR

HEALTHGRADES AWARDS

✓ SPECIALTY EXCELLENCE
- STROKE CARE

Nicholas H. Noyes Memorial Hospital

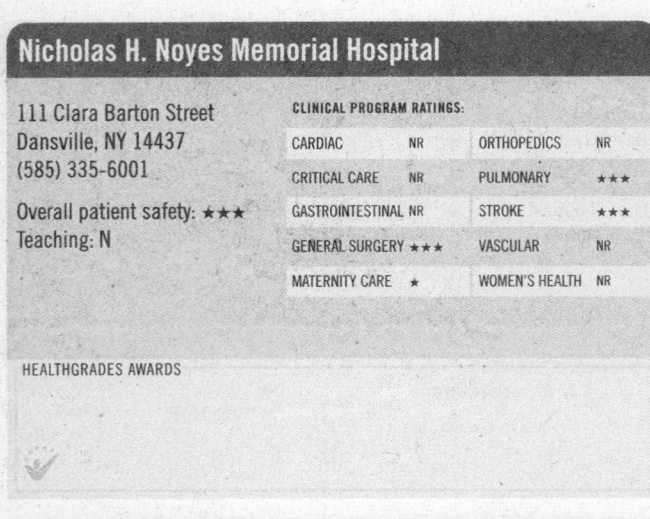

111 Clara Barton Street
Dansville, NY 14437
(585) 335-6001

Overall patient safety: ★★★
Teaching: N

CLINICAL PROGRAM RATINGS:

CARDIAC	NR	ORTHOPEDICS	NR
CRITICAL CARE	NR	PULMONARY	★★★
GASTROINTESTINAL	NR	STROKE	★★★
GENERAL SURGERY	★★★	VASCULAR	NR
MATERNITY CARE	★	WOMEN'S HEALTH	NR

HEALTHGRADES AWARDS

North Shore University Hospital*

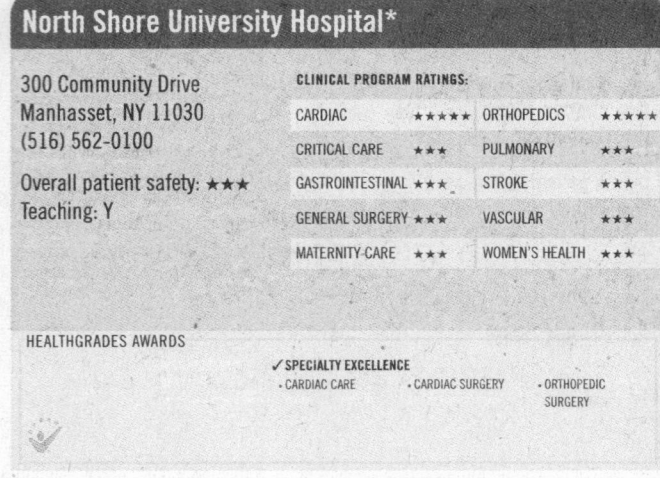

300 Community Drive
Manhasset, NY 11030
(516) 562-0100

Overall patient safety: ★★★
Teaching: Y

CLINICAL PROGRAM RATINGS:

CARDIAC	★★★★★	ORTHOPEDICS	★★★★★
CRITICAL CARE	★★★	PULMONARY	★★★
GASTROINTESTINAL	★★★	STROKE	★★★
GENERAL SURGERY	★★★	VASCULAR	★★★
MATERNITY CARE	★★★	WOMEN'S HEALTH	★★★

HEALTHGRADES AWARDS

✓ SPECIALTY EXCELLENCE
- CARDIAC CARE · CARDIAC SURGERY · ORTHOPEDIC SURGERY

North Central Bronx Hospital

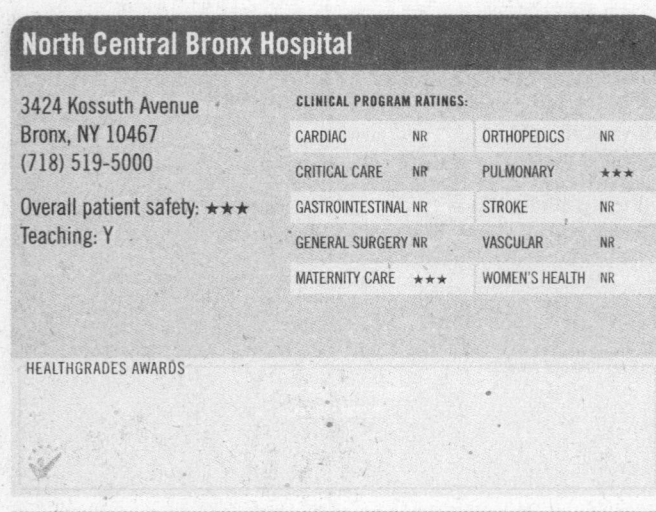

3424 Kossuth Avenue
Bronx, NY 10467
(718) 519-5000

Overall patient safety: ★★★
Teaching: Y

CLINICAL PROGRAM RATINGS:

CARDIAC	NR	ORTHOPEDICS	NR
CRITICAL CARE	NR	PULMONARY	★★★
GASTROINTESTINAL	NR	STROKE	NR
GENERAL SURGERY	NR	VASCULAR	NR
MATERNITY CARE	★★★	WOMEN'S HEALTH	NR

HEALTHGRADES AWARDS

North Shore University Hospital Syosset*

221 Jericho Turnpike
Syosset, NY 11791
(516) 496-6400

Overall patient safety: ★★★
Teaching: Y

CLINICAL PROGRAM RATINGS:

CARDIAC	★★★★★	ORTHOPEDICS	★★★★★
CRITICAL CARE	★★★	PULMONARY	★★★
GASTROINTESTINAL	★★★	STROKE	★★★
GENERAL SURGERY	★★★	VASCULAR	★★★
MATERNITY CARE	★★★	WOMEN'S HEALTH	★★★

HEALTHGRADES AWARDS

✓ SPECIALTY EXCELLENCE
- CARDIAC CARE · CARDIAC SURGERY · ORTHOPEDIC SURGERY

KEY: ★★★★★ BEST   ★★★ AS EXPECTED   ★ POOR   NR NOT RATED BY HEALTHGRADES   For full definitions of ratings and awards, see Appendix.

Northern Dutchess Hospital

6511 Springbrook Avenue
Rhinebeck, NY 12572
(845) 876-3001

Overall patient safety: ★★★
Teaching: N

CLINICAL PROGRAM RATINGS:

CARDIAC	NR	ORTHOPEDICS	NR
CRITICAL CARE	NR	PULMONARY	★
GASTROINTESTINAL	NR	STROKE	★★★
GENERAL SURGERY	★★★	VASCULAR	NR
MATERNITY CARE	★★★★★	WOMEN'S HEALTH	NR

HEALTHGRADES AWARDS

✓ SPECIALTY EXCELLENCE
• MATERNITY CARE

Olean General Hospital

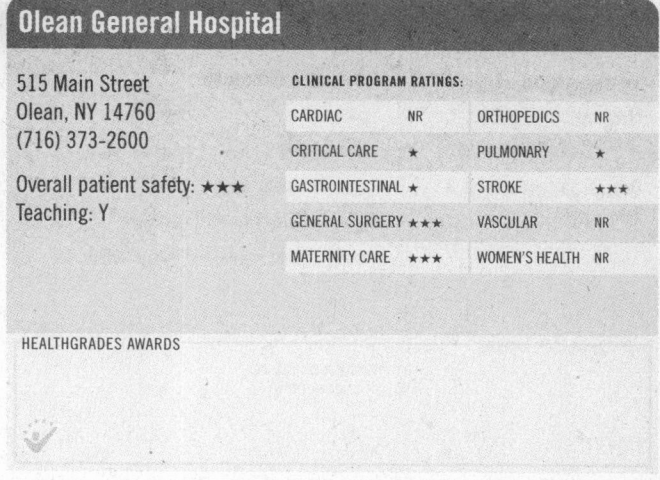

515 Main Street
Olean, NY 14760
(716) 373-2600

Overall patient safety: ★★★
Teaching: Y

CLINICAL PROGRAM RATINGS:

CARDIAC	NR	ORTHOPEDICS	NR
CRITICAL CARE	★	PULMONARY	★
GASTROINTESTINAL	★	STROKE	★★★
GENERAL SURGERY	★★★	VASCULAR	NR
MATERNITY CARE	★★★	WOMEN'S HEALTH	NR

HEALTHGRADES AWARDS

Northern Westchester Hospital

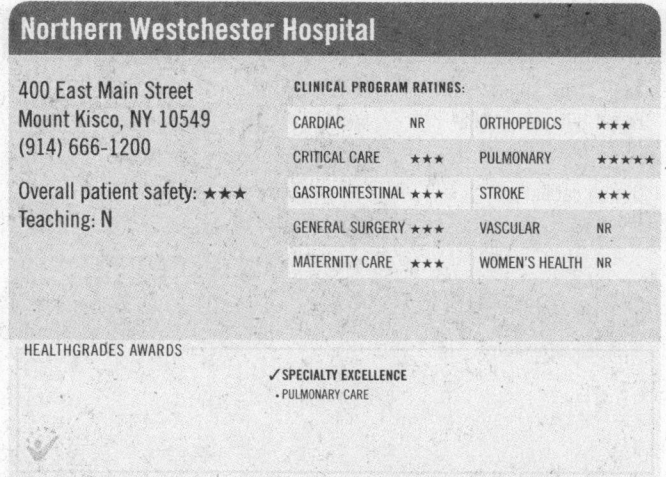

400 East Main Street
Mount Kisco, NY 10549
(914) 666-1200

Overall patient safety: ★★★
Teaching: N

CLINICAL PROGRAM RATINGS:

CARDIAC	NR	ORTHOPEDICS	★★★
CRITICAL CARE	★★★	PULMONARY	★★★★★
GASTROINTESTINAL	★★★	STROKE	★★★
GENERAL SURGERY	★★★	VASCULAR	NR
MATERNITY CARE	★★★	WOMEN'S HEALTH	NR

HEALTHGRADES AWARDS

✓ SPECIALTY EXCELLENCE
• PULMONARY CARE

Oneida Healthcare Center

321 Genesee Street
Oneida, NY 13421
(315) 363-6000

Overall patient safety: ★★★
Teaching: N

CLINICAL PROGRAM RATINGS:

CARDIAC	NR	ORTHOPEDICS	NR
CRITICAL CARE	NR	PULMONARY	★
GASTROINTESTINAL	NR	STROKE	★
GENERAL SURGERY	★★★	VASCULAR	NR
MATERNITY CARE	★★★	WOMEN'S HEALTH	NR

HEALTHGRADES AWARDS

Nyack Hospital

160 North Midland Avenue
Nyack, NY 10960
(845) 348-2000

Overall patient safety: ★★★
Teaching: Y

CLINICAL PROGRAM RATINGS:

CARDIAC	NR	ORTHOPEDICS	NR
CRITICAL CARE	★★★	PULMONARY	★★★
GASTROINTESTINAL	★★★	STROKE	★★★
GENERAL SURGERY	★★★	VASCULAR	★★★
MATERNITY CARE	★★★★★	WOMEN'S HEALTH	NR

HEALTHGRADES AWARDS

✓ SPECIALTY EXCELLENCE
• MATERNITY CARE

Orange Regional Medical Center*

4 Harriman Drive
Goshen, NY 10924
(845) 294-5441

Overall patient safety: ★
Teaching: N

CLINICAL PROGRAM RATINGS:

CARDIAC	NR	ORTHOPEDICS	★★★
CRITICAL CARE	★★★	PULMONARY	★★★
GASTROINTESTINAL	★★★	STROKE	★★★
GENERAL SURGERY	★★★	VASCULAR	NR
MATERNITY CARE	★★★	WOMEN'S HEALTH	NR

HEALTHGRADES AWARDS

---

*This hospital reports its data to the federal government jointly with another hospital. Therefore the ratings and awards apply to multiple hospitals and this specific hospital may not provide all rated services.

Osteopathic Hospital Clinic of New York*

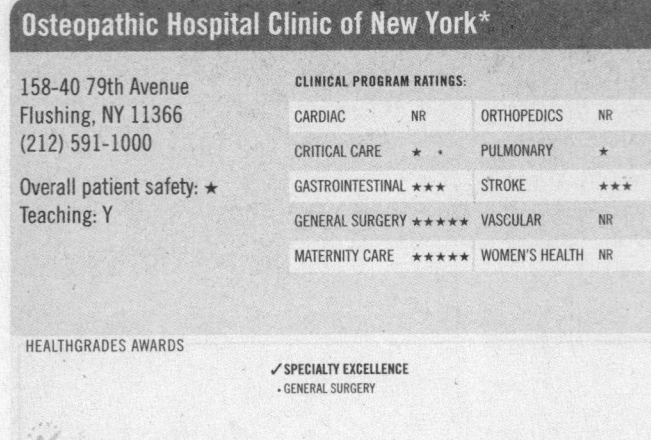

158-40 79th Avenue
Flushing, NY 11366
(212) 591-1000

Overall patient safety: ★
Teaching: Y

CLINICAL PROGRAM RATINGS:

CARDIAC	NR	ORTHOPEDICS	NR
CRITICAL CARE	★ ·	PULMONARY	★
GASTROINTESTINAL	★★★	STROKE	★★★
GENERAL SURGERY	★★★★★	VASCULAR	NR
MATERNITY CARE	★★★★★	WOMEN'S HEALTH	NR

HEALTHGRADES AWARDS

✓ SPECIALTY EXCELLENCE
· GENERAL SURGERY

Our Lady of Mercy Medical Center

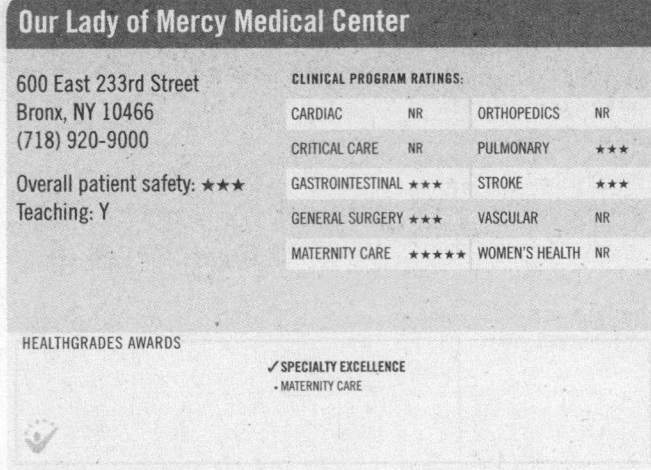

600 East 233rd Street
Bronx, NY 10466
(718) 920-9000

Overall patient safety: ★★★
Teaching: Y

CLINICAL PROGRAM RATINGS:

CARDIAC	NR	ORTHOPEDICS	NR
CRITICAL CARE	NR	PULMONARY	★★★
GASTROINTESTINAL	★★★	STROKE	★★★
GENERAL SURGERY	★★★	VASCULAR	NR
MATERNITY CARE	★★★★★	WOMEN'S HEALTH	NR

HEALTHGRADES AWARDS

✓ SPECIALTY EXCELLENCE
· MATERNITY CARE

Oswego Hospital

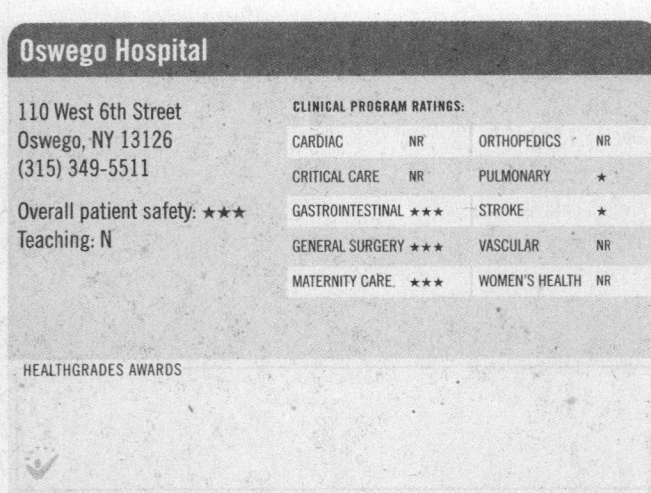

110 West 6th Street
Oswego, NY 13126
(315) 349-5511

Overall patient safety: ★★★
Teaching: N

CLINICAL PROGRAM RATINGS:

CARDIAC	NR	ORTHOPEDICS	NR
CRITICAL CARE	NR	PULMONARY	★
GASTROINTESTINAL	★★★	STROKE	★
GENERAL SURGERY	★★★	VASCULAR	NR
MATERNITY CARE	★★★	WOMEN'S HEALTH	NR

HEALTHGRADES AWARDS

Parkway Hospital

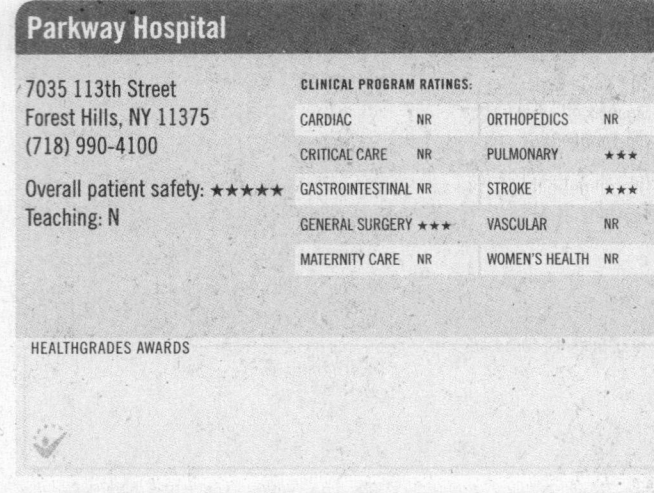

7035 113th Street
Forest Hills, NY 11375
(718) 990-4100

Overall patient safety: ★★★★★
Teaching: N

CLINICAL PROGRAM RATINGS:

CARDIAC	NR	ORTHOPEDICS	NR
CRITICAL CARE	NR	PULMONARY	★★★
GASTROINTESTINAL	NR	STROKE	★★★
GENERAL SURGERY	★★★	VASCULAR	NR
MATERNITY CARE	NR	WOMEN'S HEALTH	NR

HEALTHGRADES AWARDS

Our Lady of Lourdes Memorial Hospital

169 Riverside Drive
Binghamton, NY 13905
(607) 798-5111

Overall patient safety: ★★★
Teaching: Y

CLINICAL PROGRAM RATINGS:

CARDIAC	NR	ORTHOPEDICS	★★★
CRITICAL CARE	★★★	PULMONARY	★★★
GASTROINTESTINAL	★★★	STROKE	★★★
GENERAL SURGERY	★★★	VASCULAR	★★★
MATERNITY CARE	★★★	WOMEN'S HEALTH	NR

HEALTHGRADES AWARDS

Peconic Bay Medical Center

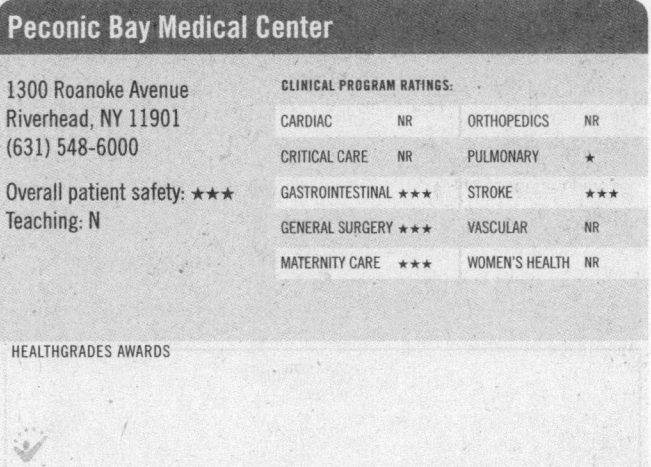

1300 Roanoke Avenue
Riverhead, NY 11901
(631) 548-6000

Overall patient safety: ★★★
Teaching: N

CLINICAL PROGRAM RATINGS:

CARDIAC	NR	ORTHOPEDICS	NR
CRITICAL CARE	NR	PULMONARY	★
GASTROINTESTINAL	★★★	STROKE	★★★
GENERAL SURGERY	★★★	VASCULAR	NR
MATERNITY CARE	★★★	WOMEN'S HEALTH	NR

HEALTHGRADES AWARDS

KEY: ★★★★★ **BEST** ★★★ **AS EXPECTED** ★ **POOR** NR **NOT RATED BY HEALTHGRADES** For full definitions of ratings and awards, see Appendix.

Peninsula Hospital Center

5115 Beach Channel Drive
Far Rockaway, NY 11691
(718) 734-2000

Overall patient safety: ★
Teaching: Y

CLINICAL PROGRAM RATINGS:

CARDIAC	NR	ORTHOPEDICS	NR
CRITICAL CARE	NR	PULMONARY	★★★
GASTROINTESTINAL	★★★	STROKE	★★★
GENERAL SURGERY	★★★	VASCULAR	NR
MATERNITY CARE	NR	WOMEN'S HEALTH	NR

HEALTHGRADES AWARDS

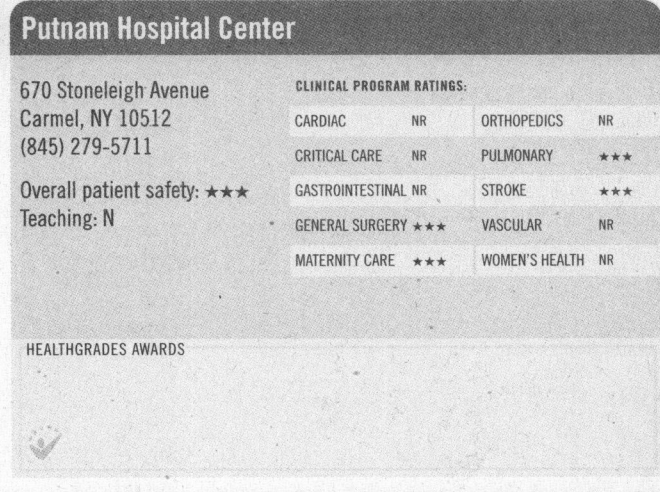

Putnam Hospital Center

670 Stoneleigh Avenue
Carmel, NY 10512
(845) 279-5711

Overall patient safety: ★★★
Teaching: N

CLINICAL PROGRAM RATINGS:

CARDIAC	NR	ORTHOPEDICS	NR
CRITICAL CARE	NR	PULMONARY	★★★
GASTROINTESTINAL	NR	STROKE	★★★
GENERAL SURGERY	★★★	VASCULAR	NR
MATERNITY CARE	★★★	WOMEN'S HEALTH	NR

HEALTHGRADES AWARDS

Phelps Memorial Hospital Association

701 North Broadway
Sleepy Hollow, NY 10591
(914) 366-3000

Overall patient safety: ★★★
Teaching: N

CLINICAL PROGRAM RATINGS:

CARDIAC	NR	ORTHOPEDICS	★★★
CRITICAL CARE	NR	PULMONARY	★
GASTROINTESTINAL	★★★	STROKE	★★★
GENERAL SURGERY	★★★	VASCULAR	NR
MATERNITY CARE	★★★	WOMEN'S HEALTH	NR

HEALTHGRADES AWARDS

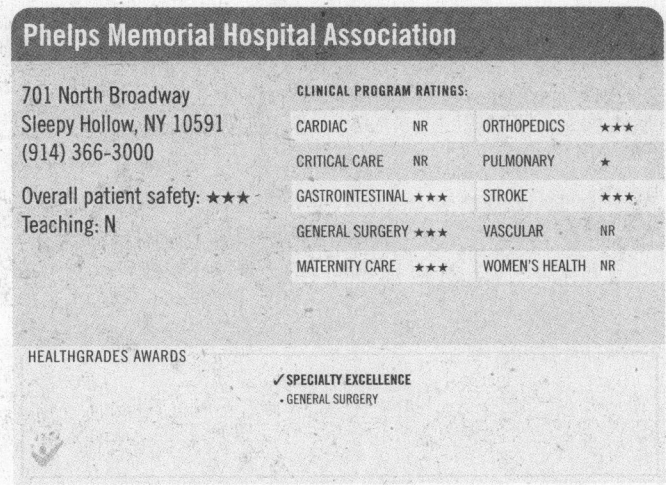

✓ SPECIALTY EXCELLENCE
• GENERAL SURGERY

Queens Hospital Center

8268 164th Street
Jamaica, NY 11432
(718) 883-3000

Overall patient safety: ★★★
Teaching: Y

CLINICAL PROGRAM RATINGS:

CARDIAC	NR	ORTHOPEDICS	NR
CRITICAL CARE	NR	PULMONARY	★★★
GASTROINTESTINAL	NR	STROKE	★★★
GENERAL SURGERY	NR	VASCULAR	NR
MATERNITY CARE	★★★	WOMEN'S HEALTH	NR

HEALTHGRADES AWARDS

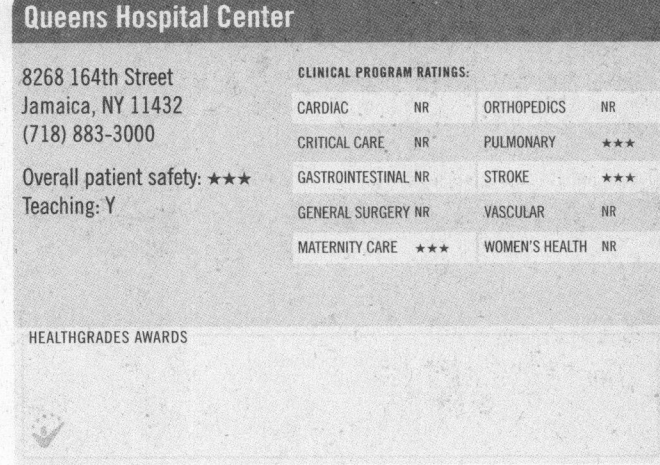

Plainview Hospital

888 Old Country Road
Plainview, NY 11803
(516) 719-3000

Overall patient safety: ★
Teaching: Y

CLINICAL PROGRAM RATINGS:

CARDIAC	NR	ORTHOPEDICS	NR
CRITICAL CARE	★	PULMONARY	★
GASTROINTESTINAL	★★★	STROKE	★★★
GENERAL SURGERY	★★★	VASCULAR	NR
MATERNITY CARE	★★★★★	WOMEN'S HEALTH	NR

HEALTHGRADES AWARDS

✓ SPECIALTY EXCELLENCE
• MATERNITY CARE

Rochester General Hospital

1425 Portland Avenue
Rochester, NY 14621
(585) 922-4000

Overall patient safety: ★★★
Teaching: Y

CLINICAL PROGRAM RATINGS:

CARDIAC	★★★	ORTHOPEDICS	★★★
CRITICAL CARE	★★★	PULMONARY	★★★
GASTROINTESTINAL	★★★	STROKE	★★★
GENERAL SURGERY	★★★	VASCULAR	★★★
MATERNITY CARE	★★★	WOMEN'S HEALTH	★★★

HEALTHGRADES AWARDS

*This hospital reports its data to the federal government jointly with another hospital. Therefore the ratings and awards apply to multiple hospitals and this specific hospital may not provide all rated services.

NEW YORK HOSPITALS: RATINGS BY CLINICAL SPECIALTY

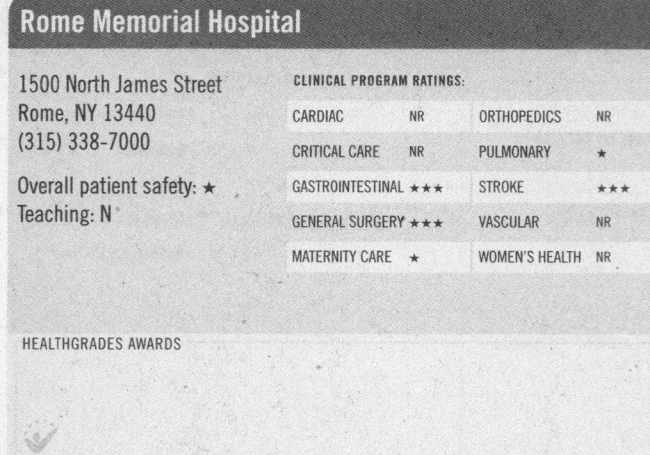

Rome Memorial Hospital

1500 North James Street
Rome, NY 13440
(315) 338-7000

Overall patient safety: ★
Teaching: N

CLINICAL PROGRAM RATINGS:

CARDIAC	NR	ORTHOPEDICS	NR
CRITICAL CARE	NR	PULMONARY	★
GASTROINTESTINAL	★★★	STROKE	★★★
GENERAL SURGERY	★★★	VASCULAR	NR
MATERNITY CARE	★	WOMEN'S HEALTH	NR

HEALTHGRADES AWARDS

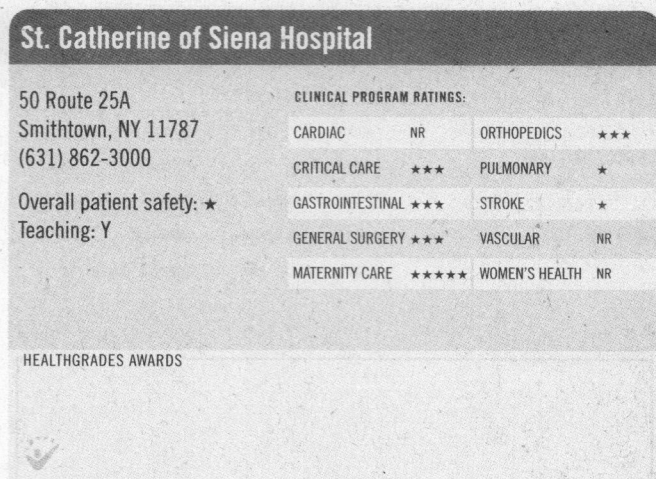

St. Catherine of Siena Hospital

50 Route 25A
Smithtown, NY 11787
(631) 862-3000

Overall patient safety: ★
Teaching: Y

CLINICAL PROGRAM RATINGS:

CARDIAC	NR	ORTHOPEDICS	★★★
CRITICAL CARE	★★★	PULMONARY	★
GASTROINTESTINAL	★★★	STROKE	★
GENERAL SURGERY	★★★	VASCULAR	NR
MATERNITY CARE	★★★★★	WOMEN'S HEALTH	NR

HEALTHGRADES AWARDS

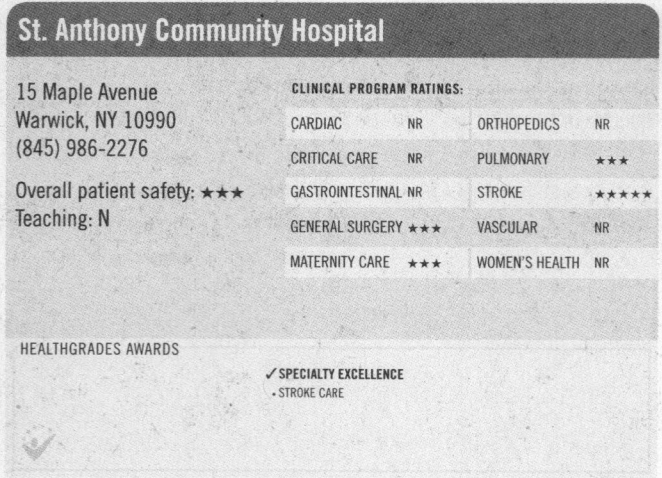

St. Anthony Community Hospital

15 Maple Avenue
Warwick, NY 10990
(845) 986-2276

Overall patient safety: ★★★
Teaching: N

CLINICAL PROGRAM RATINGS:

CARDIAC	NR	ORTHOPEDICS	NR
CRITICAL CARE	NR	PULMONARY	★★★
GASTROINTESTINAL	NR	STROKE	★★★★★
GENERAL SURGERY	★★★	VASCULAR	NR
MATERNITY CARE	★★★	WOMEN'S HEALTH	NR

HEALTHGRADES AWARDS

✓ SPECIALTY EXCELLENCE
· STROKE CARE

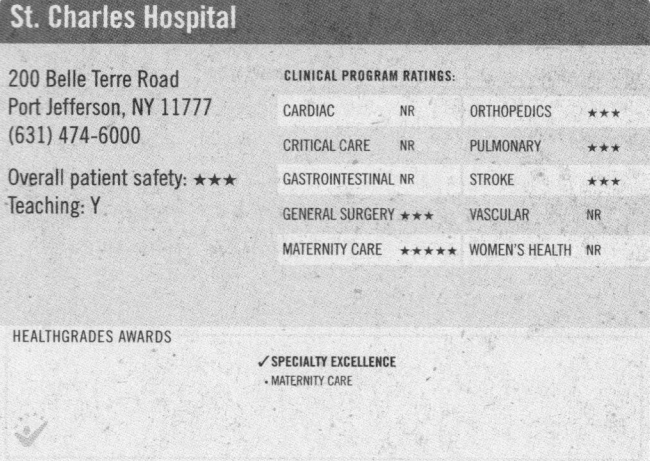

St. Charles Hospital

200 Belle Terre Road
Port Jefferson, NY 11777
(631) 474-6000

Overall patient safety: ★★★
Teaching: Y

CLINICAL PROGRAM RATINGS:

CARDIAC	NR	ORTHOPEDICS	★★★
CRITICAL CARE	NR	PULMONARY	★★★
GASTROINTESTINAL	NR	STROKE	★★★
GENERAL SURGERY	★★★	VASCULAR	NR
MATERNITY CARE	★★★★★	WOMEN'S HEALTH	NR

HEALTHGRADES AWARDS

✓ SPECIALTY EXCELLENCE
· MATERNITY CARE

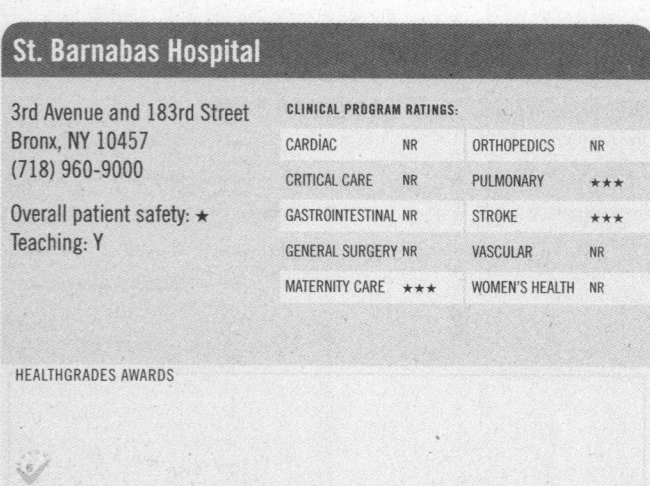

St. Barnabas Hospital

3rd Avenue and 183rd Street
Bronx, NY 10457
(718) 960-9000

Overall patient safety: ★
Teaching: Y

CLINICAL PROGRAM RATINGS:

CARDIAC	NR	ORTHOPEDICS	NR
CRITICAL CARE	NR	PULMONARY	★★★
GASTROINTESTINAL	NR	STROKE	★★★
GENERAL SURGERY	NR	VASCULAR	NR
MATERNITY CARE	★★★	WOMEN'S HEALTH	NR

HEALTHGRADES AWARDS

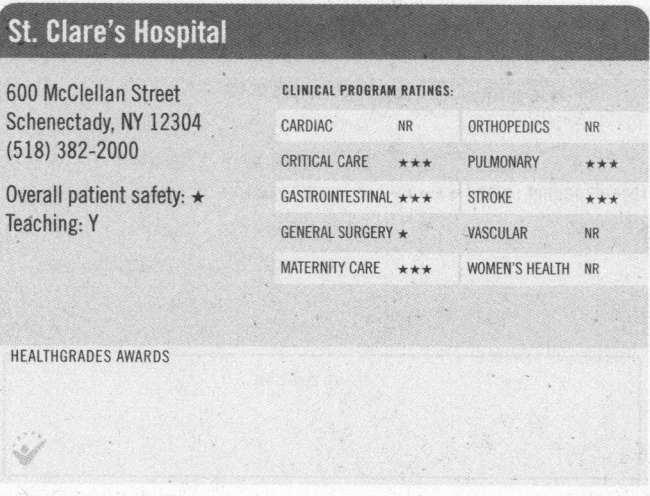

St. Clare's Hospital

600 McClellan Street
Schenectady, NY 12304
(518) 382-2000

Overall patient safety: ★
Teaching: Y

CLINICAL PROGRAM RATINGS:

CARDIAC	NR	ORTHOPEDICS	NR
CRITICAL CARE	★★★	PULMONARY	★★★
GASTROINTESTINAL	★★★	STROKE	★★★
GENERAL SURGERY	★	VASCULAR	NR
MATERNITY CARE	★★★	WOMEN'S HEALTH	NR

HEALTHGRADES AWARDS

KEY: ★★★★★ **BEST** ★★★ **AS EXPECTED** ★ **POOR** NR **NOT RATED BY HEALTHGRADES** For full definitions of ratings and awards, see Appendix.

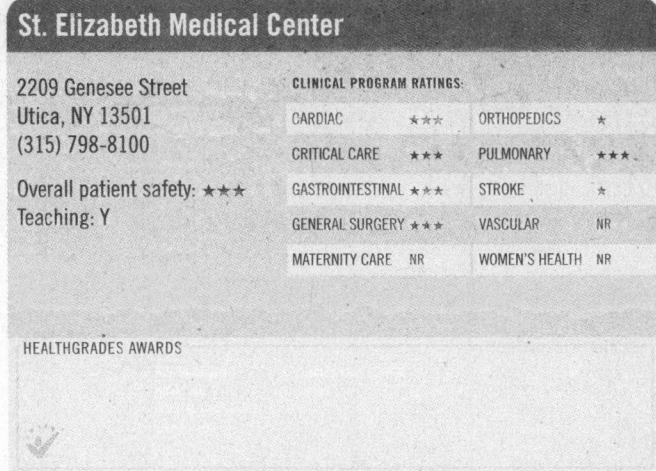

St. Elizabeth Medical Center

2209 Genesee Street
Utica, NY 13501
(315) 798-8100

Overall patient safety: ★★★
Teaching: Y

CLINICAL PROGRAM RATINGS:

CARDIAC	★★★	ORTHOPEDICS	★
CRITICAL CARE	★★★	PULMONARY	★★★
GASTROINTESTINAL	★★★	STROKE	★
GENERAL SURGERY	★★★	VASCULAR	NR
MATERNITY CARE	NR	WOMEN'S HEALTH	NR

HEALTHGRADES AWARDS

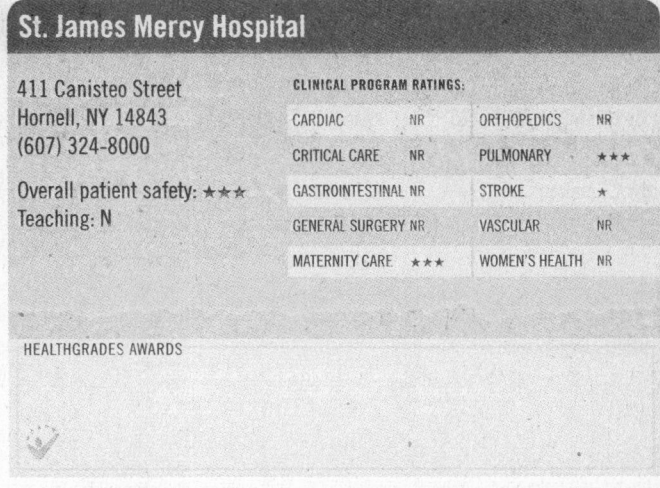

St. James Mercy Hospital

411 Canisteo Street
Hornell, NY 14843
(607) 324-8000

Overall patient safety: ★★★
Teaching: N

CLINICAL PROGRAM RATINGS:

CARDIAC	NR	ORTHOPEDICS	NR
CRITICAL CARE	NR	PULMONARY	★★★
GASTROINTESTINAL	NR	STROKE	★
GENERAL SURGERY	NR	VASCULAR	NR
MATERNITY CARE	★★★	WOMEN'S HEALTH	NR

HEALTHGRADES AWARDS

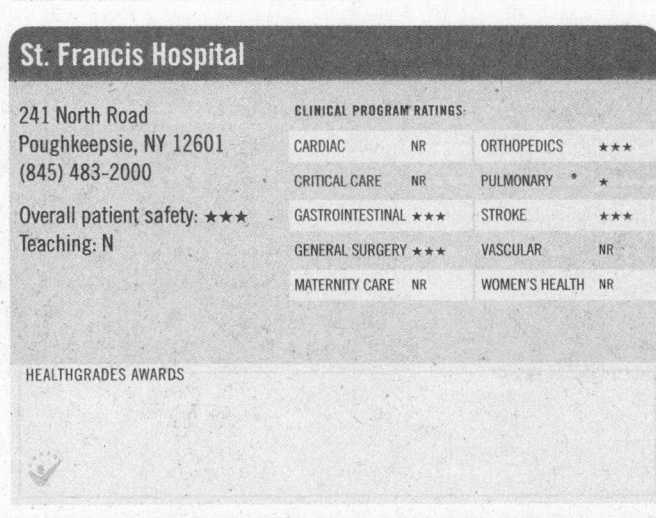

St. Francis Hospital

241 North Road
Poughkeepsie, NY 12601
(845) 483-2000

Overall patient safety: ★★★
Teaching: N

CLINICAL PROGRAM RATINGS:

CARDIAC	NR	ORTHOPEDICS	★★★
CRITICAL CARE	NR	PULMONARY	★
GASTROINTESTINAL	★★★	STROKE	★★★
GENERAL SURGERY	★★★	VASCULAR	NR
MATERNITY CARE	NR	WOMEN'S HEALTH	NR

HEALTHGRADES AWARDS

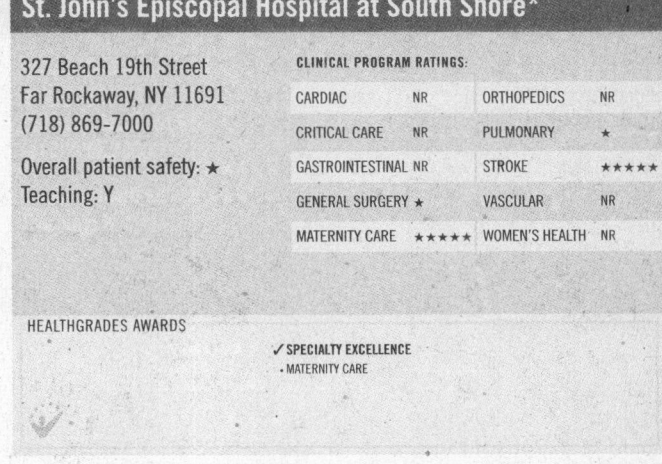

St. John's Episcopal Hospital at South Shore*

327 Beach 19th Street
Far Rockaway, NY 11691
(718) 869-7000

Overall patient safety: ★
Teaching: Y

CLINICAL PROGRAM RATINGS:

CARDIAC	NR	ORTHOPEDICS	NR
CRITICAL CARE	NR	PULMONARY	★
GASTROINTESTINAL	NR	STROKE	★★★★★
GENERAL SURGERY	★	VASCULAR	NR
MATERNITY CARE	★★★★★	WOMEN'S HEALTH	NR

HEALTHGRADES AWARDS

✓ SPECIALTY EXCELLENCE
· MATERNITY CARE

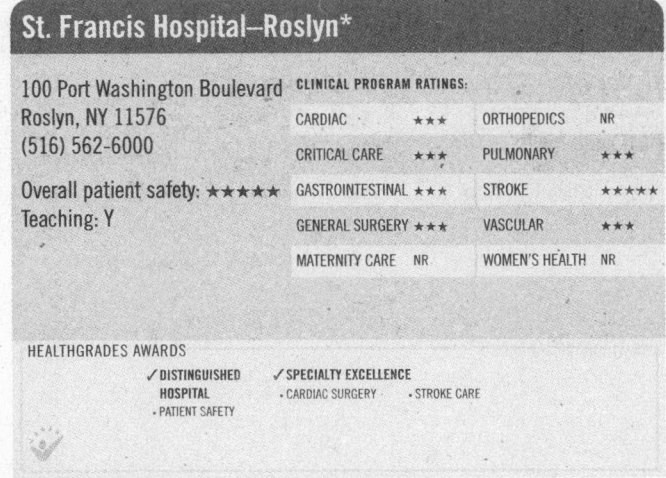

St. Francis Hospital–Roslyn*

100 Port Washington Boulevard
Roslyn, NY 11576
(516) 562-6000

Overall patient safety: ★★★★★
Teaching: Y

CLINICAL PROGRAM RATINGS:

CARDIAC	★★★	ORTHOPEDICS	NR
CRITICAL CARE	★★★	PULMONARY	★★★
GASTROINTESTINAL	★★★	STROKE	★★★★★
GENERAL SURGERY	★★★	VASCULAR	★★★
MATERNITY CARE	NR	WOMEN'S HEALTH	NR

HEALTHGRADES AWARDS

✓ DISTINGUISHED
  HOSPITAL
· PATIENT SAFETY

✓ SPECIALTY EXCELLENCE
· CARDIAC SURGERY   · STROKE CARE

St. John's Riverside Hospital*

967 North Broadway
Yonkers, NY 10701
(914) 964-4444

Overall patient safety: ★
Teaching: N

CLINICAL PROGRAM RATINGS:

CARDIAC	NR	ORTHOPEDICS	NR
CRITICAL CARE	NR	PULMONARY	★★★
GASTROINTESTINAL	★★★	STROKE	★★★★★
GENERAL SURGERY	★★★	VASCULAR	NR
MATERNITY CARE	★★★★★	WOMEN'S HEALTH	NR

HEALTHGRADES AWARDS

✓ SPECIALTY EXCELLENCE
· MATERNITY CARE

*This hospital reports its data to the federal government jointly with another hospital. Therefore the ratings and awards apply to multiple hospitals and this specific hospital may not provide all rated services.

St. Joseph Hospital of Cheektowaga New York

2605 Harlem Road
Cheektowaga, NY 14225
(716) 891-2400

Overall patient safety: ★★★
Teaching: N

CLINICAL PROGRAM RATINGS:

CARDIAC	NR	ORTHOPEDICS	★★★
CRITICAL CARE	★★★	PULMONARY	★★★
GASTROINTESTINAL	NR	STROKE	★★★
GENERAL SURGERY	★★★	VASCULAR	NR
MATERNITY CARE	NR	WOMEN'S HEALTH	NR

HEALTHGRADES AWARDS

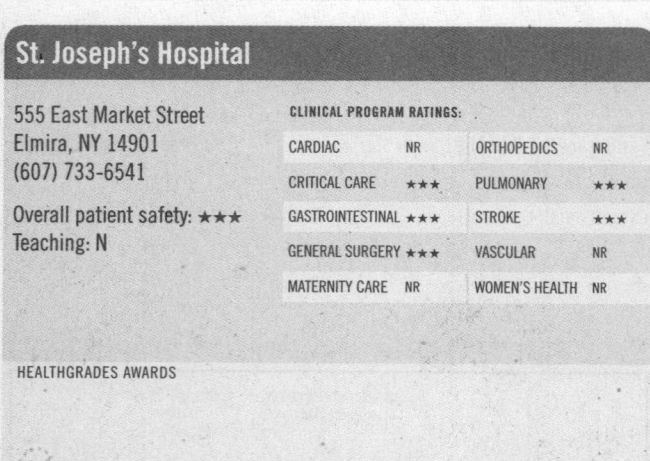

St. Joseph's Hospital Yonkers

127 South Broadway
Yonkers, NY 10701
(914) 378-7000

Overall patient safety: ★★★
Teaching: Y

CLINICAL PROGRAM RATINGS:

CARDIAC	NR	ORTHOPEDICS	NR
CRITICAL CARE	NR	PULMONARY	★
GASTROINTESTINAL	NR	STROKE	★★★
GENERAL SURGERY	★	VASCULAR	NR
MATERNITY CARE	NR	WOMEN'S HEALTH	NR

HEALTHGRADES AWARDS

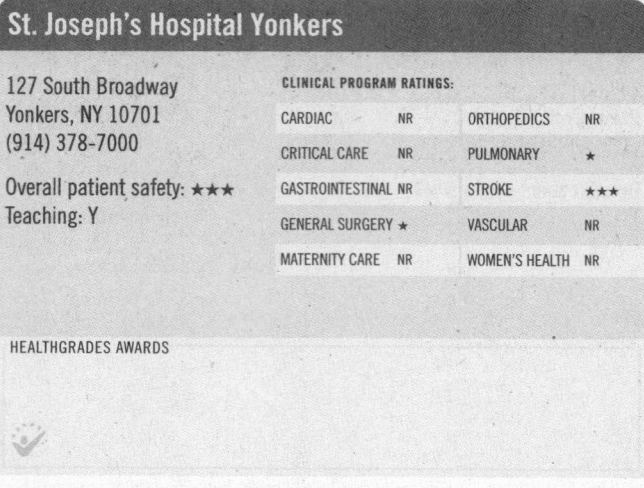

St. Joseph's Hospital

555 East Market Street
Elmira, NY 14901
(607) 733-6541

Overall patient safety: ★★★
Teaching: N

CLINICAL PROGRAM RATINGS:

CARDIAC	NR	ORTHOPEDICS	NR
CRITICAL CARE	★★★	PULMONARY	★★★
GASTROINTESTINAL	★★★	STROKE	★★★
GENERAL SURGERY	★★★	VASCULAR	NR
MATERNITY CARE	NR	WOMEN'S HEALTH	NR

HEALTHGRADES AWARDS

St. Luke's Cornwall Hospital

19 Laurel Avenue
Cornwall, NY 12518
(845) 534-7711

Overall patient safety: ★★★★★
Teaching: N

CLINICAL PROGRAM RATINGS:

CARDIAC	NR	ORTHOPEDICS	★★★★★
CRITICAL CARE	★★★★★	PULMONARY	★★★★★
GASTROINTESTINAL	★★★	STROKE	★★★
GENERAL SURGERY	★★★	VASCULAR	NR
MATERNITY CARE	★★★★★	WOMEN'S HEALTH	NR

HEALTHGRADES AWARDS

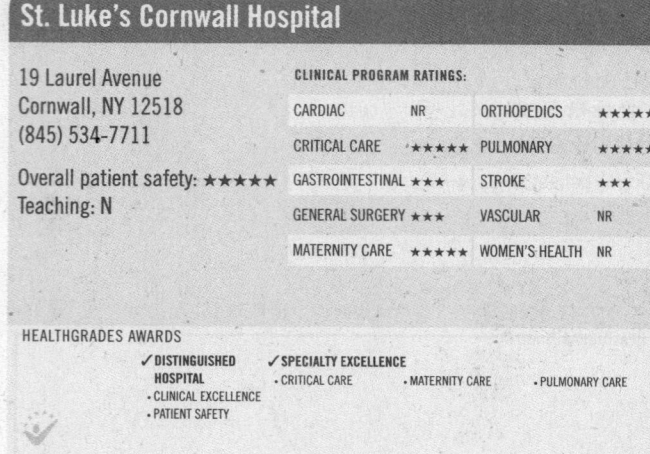

✓ DISTINGUISHED HOSPITAL
• CLINICAL EXCELLENCE
• PATIENT SAFETY

✓ SPECIALTY EXCELLENCE
• CRITICAL CARE   • MATERNITY CARE   • PULMONARY CARE

St. Joseph's Hospital Health Center

301 Prospect Avenue
Syracuse, NY 13203
(315) 448-5111

Overall patient safety: ★★★
Teaching: Y

CLINICAL PROGRAM RATINGS:

CARDIAC	★★★★★	ORTHOPEDICS	★★★
CRITICAL CARE	★★★	PULMONARY	★
GASTROINTESTINAL	★★★	STROKE	★
GENERAL SURGERY	★★★	VASCULAR	★★★
MATERNITY CARE	★★★	WOMEN'S HEALTH	★★★

HEALTHGRADES AWARDS

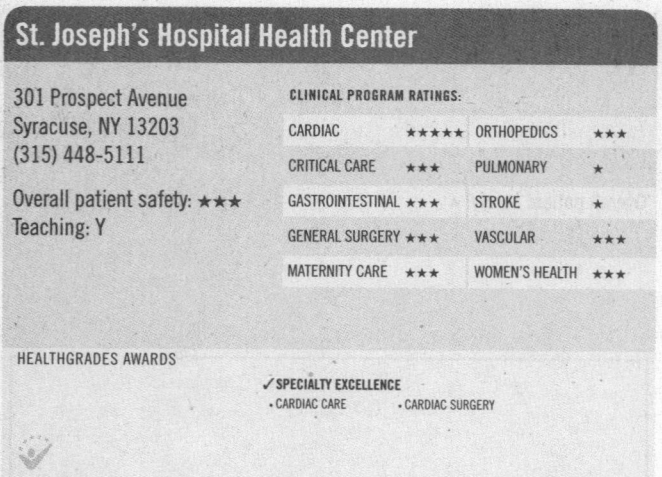

✓ SPECIALTY EXCELLENCE
• CARDIAC CARE   • CARDIAC SURGERY

St. Luke's Roosevelt Hospital

1111 Amsterdam Avenue
New York, NY 10025
(212) 523-4000

Overall patient safety: ★
Teaching: Y

CLINICAL PROGRAM RATINGS:

CARDIAC	★★★	ORTHOPEDICS	★★★
CRITICAL CARE	★	PULMONARY	★★★
GASTROINTESTINAL	★★★	STROKE	★★★
GENERAL SURGERY	★	VASCULAR	★★★
MATERNITY CARE	★★★	WOMEN'S HEALTH	★

HEALTHGRADES AWARDS

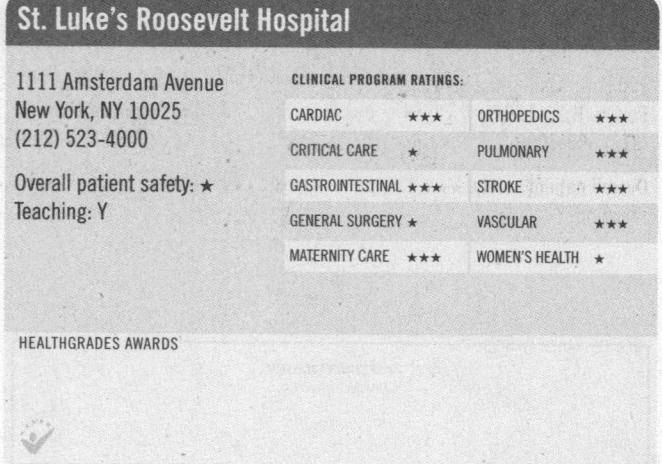

KEY: ★★★★★ BEST   ★★★ AS EXPECTED   ★ POOR   NR NOT RATED BY HEALTHGRADES   For full definitions of ratings and awards, see Appendix.

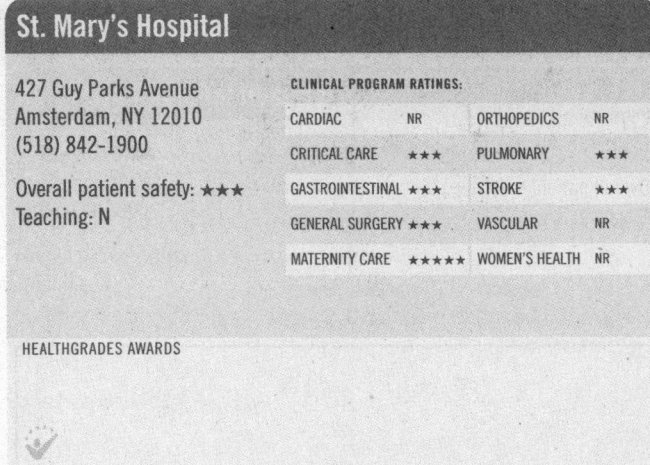

St. Mary's Hospital

427 Guy Parks Avenue
Amsterdam, NY 12010
(518) 842-1900

Overall patient safety: ★★★
Teaching: N

CLINICAL PROGRAM RATINGS:

CARDIAC	NR	ORTHOPEDICS	NR
CRITICAL CARE	★★★	PULMONARY	★★★
GASTROINTESTINAL	★★★	STROKE	★★★
GENERAL SURGERY	★★★	VASCULAR	NR
MATERNITY CARE	★★★★★	WOMEN'S HEALTH	NR

HEALTHGRADES AWARDS

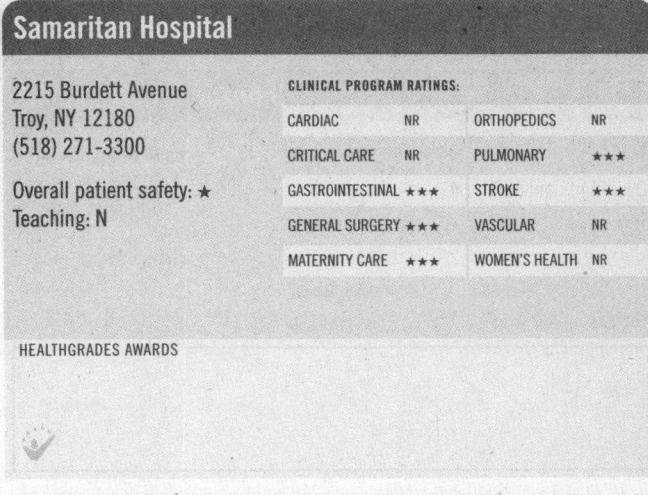

Samaritan Hospital

2215 Burdett Avenue
Troy, NY 12180
(518) 271-3300

Overall patient safety: ★
Teaching: N

CLINICAL PROGRAM RATINGS:

CARDIAC	NR	ORTHOPEDICS	NR
CRITICAL CARE	NR	PULMONARY	★★★
GASTROINTESTINAL	★★★	STROKE	★★★
GENERAL SURGERY	★★★	VASCULAR	NR
MATERNITY CARE	★★★	WOMEN'S HEALTH	NR

HEALTHGRADES AWARDS

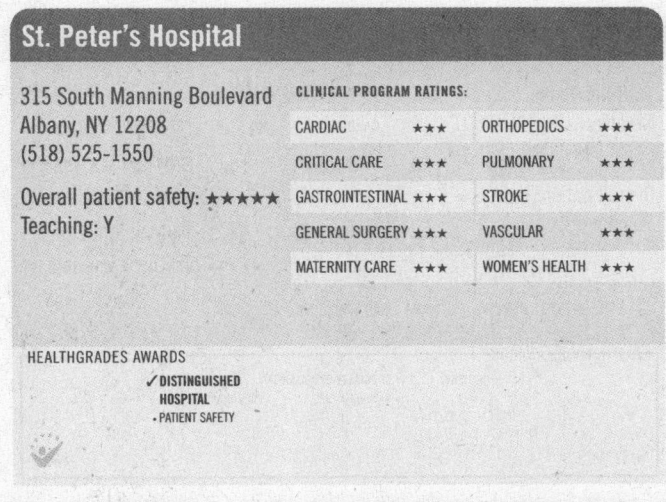

St. Peter's Hospital

315 South Manning Boulevard
Albany, NY 12208
(518) 525-1550

Overall patient safety: ★★★★★
Teaching: Y

CLINICAL PROGRAM RATINGS:

CARDIAC	★★★	ORTHOPEDICS	★★★
CRITICAL CARE	★★★	PULMONARY	★★★
GASTROINTESTINAL	★★★	STROKE	★★★
GENERAL SURGERY	★★★	VASCULAR	★★★
MATERNITY CARE	★★★	WOMEN'S HEALTH	★★★

HEALTHGRADES AWARDS

✓ DISTINGUISHED
HOSPITAL
• PATIENT SAFETY

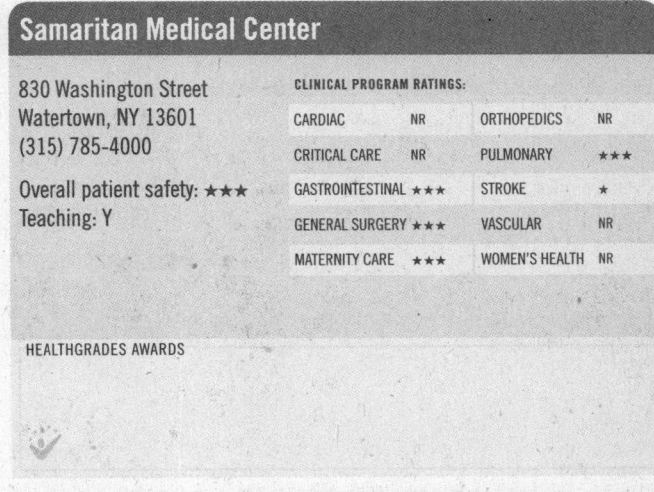

Samaritan Medical Center

830 Washington Street
Watertown, NY 13601
(315) 785-4000

Overall patient safety: ★★★
Teaching: Y

CLINICAL PROGRAM RATINGS:

CARDIAC	NR	ORTHOPEDICS	NR
CRITICAL CARE	NR	PULMONARY	★★★
GASTROINTESTINAL	★★★	STROKE	★
GENERAL SURGERY	★★★	VASCULAR	NR
MATERNITY CARE	★★★	WOMEN'S HEALTH	NR

HEALTHGRADES AWARDS

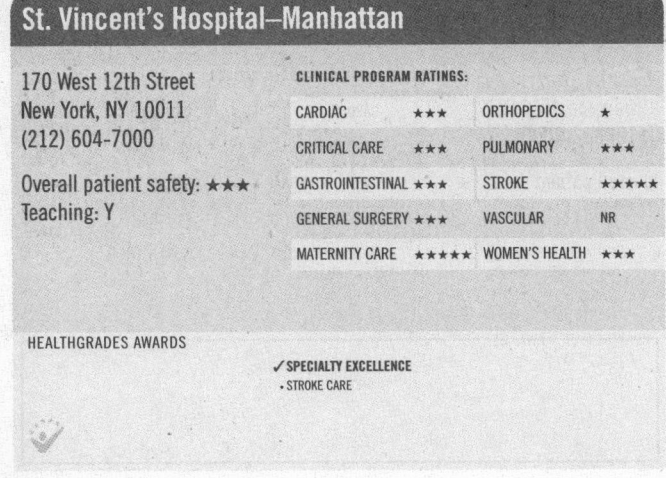

St. Vincent's Hospital–Manhattan

170 West 12th Street
New York, NY 10011
(212) 604-7000

Overall patient safety: ★★★
Teaching: Y

CLINICAL PROGRAM RATINGS:

CARDIAC	★★★	ORTHOPEDICS	★
CRITICAL CARE	★★★	PULMONARY	★★★
GASTROINTESTINAL	★★★	STROKE	★★★★★
GENERAL SURGERY	★★★	VASCULAR	NR
MATERNITY CARE	★★★★★	WOMEN'S HEALTH	★★★

HEALTHGRADES AWARDS

✓ SPECIALTY EXCELLENCE
• STROKE CARE

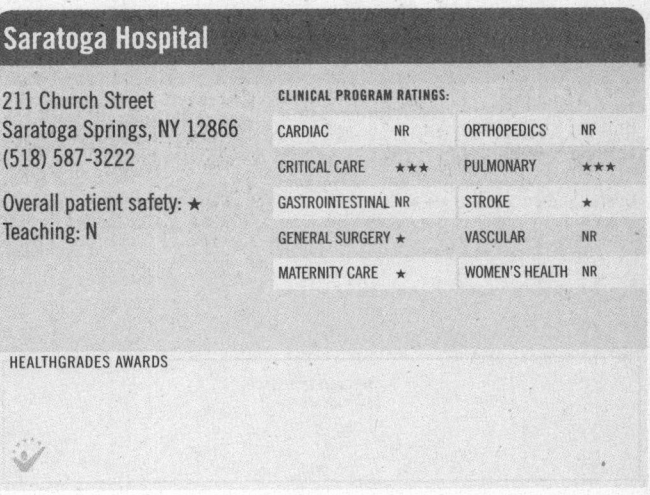

Saratoga Hospital

211 Church Street
Saratoga Springs, NY 12866
(518) 587-3222

Overall patient safety: ★
Teaching: N

CLINICAL PROGRAM RATINGS:

CARDIAC	NR	ORTHOPEDICS	NR
CRITICAL CARE	★★★	PULMONARY	★★★
GASTROINTESTINAL	NR	STROKE	★
GENERAL SURGERY	★	VASCULAR	NR
MATERNITY CARE	★	WOMEN'S HEALTH	NR

HEALTHGRADES AWARDS

Schuyler Hospital

220 Steuben Street
Montour Falls, NY 14865
(607) 530-7121

Overall patient safety: NR
Teaching: N

CLINICAL PROGRAM RATINGS:

CARDIAC	NR	ORTHOPEDICS	NR
CRITICAL CARE	NR	PULMONARY	★★★
GASTROINTESTINAL	NR	STROKE	NR
GENERAL SURGERY	NR	VASCULAR	NR
MATERNITY CARE	NR	WOMEN'S HEALTH	NR

HEALTHGRADES AWARDS

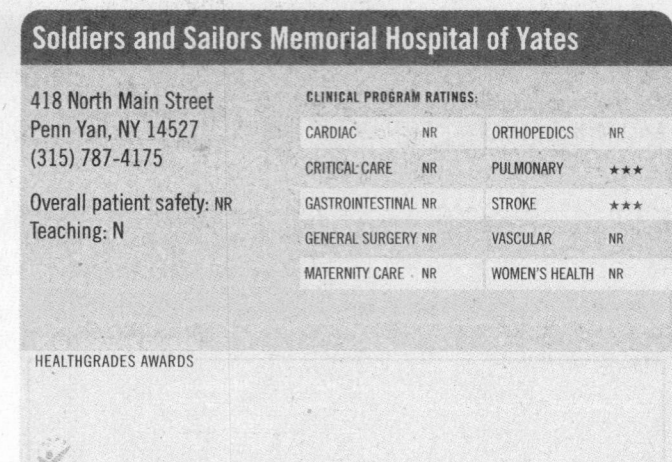

Soldiers and Sailors Memorial Hospital of Yates

418 North Main Street
Penn Yan, NY 14527
(315) 787-4175

Overall patient safety: NR
Teaching: N

CLINICAL PROGRAM RATINGS:

CARDIAC	NR	ORTHOPEDICS	NR
CRITICAL CARE	NR	PULMONARY	★★★
GASTROINTESTINAL	NR	STROKE	★★★
GENERAL SURGERY	NR	VASCULAR	NR
MATERNITY CARE	NR	WOMEN'S HEALTH	NR

HEALTHGRADES AWARDS

Seton Health System—St. Mary's Campus*

1300 Massachusetts Avenue
Troy, NY 12180
(518) 268-5000

Overall patient safety: ★★★
Teaching: N

CLINICAL PROGRAM RATINGS:

CARDIAC	NR	ORTHOPEDICS	★★★
CRITICAL CARE	NR	PULMONARY	★★★
GASTROINTESTINAL	★★★	STROKE	★★★
GENERAL SURGERY	★★★	VASCULAR	NR
MATERNITY CARE	★★★	WOMEN'S HEALTH	NR

HEALTHGRADES AWARDS

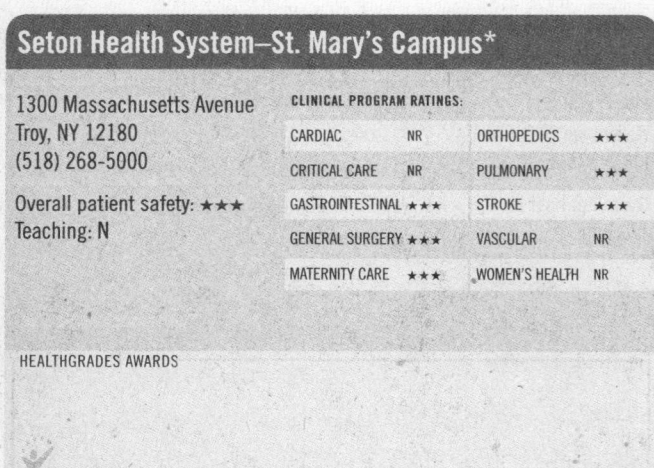

Sound Shore Medical Center of Westchester

16 Guion Place
New Rochelle, NY 10801
(914) 632-5000

Overall patient safety: ★
Teaching: Y

CLINICAL PROGRAM RATINGS:

CARDIAC	NR	ORTHOPEDICS	★★★
CRITICAL CARE	★★★	PULMONARY	★★★★★
GASTROINTESTINAL	NR	STROKE	★★★
GENERAL SURGERY	★★★	VASCULAR	NR
MATERNITY CARE	★★★★★	WOMEN'S HEALTH	NR

HEALTHGRADES AWARDS

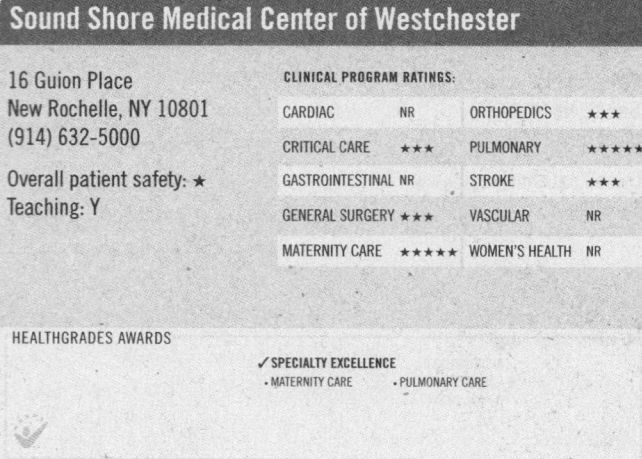

✓ SPECIALTY EXCELLENCE
- MATERNITY CARE   - PULMONARY CARE

Sisters of Charity Hospital

2157 Main Street
Buffalo, NY 14214
(716) 862-1000

Overall patient safety: ★★★
Teaching: Y

CLINICAL PROGRAM RATINGS:

CARDIAC	NR	ORTHOPEDICS	★★★
CRITICAL CARE	★★★	PULMONARY	★★★
GASTROINTESTINAL	★★★	STROKE	★★★
GENERAL SURGERY	★★★	VASCULAR	★★★
MATERNITY CARE	★★★	WOMEN'S HEALTH	NR

HEALTHGRADES AWARDS

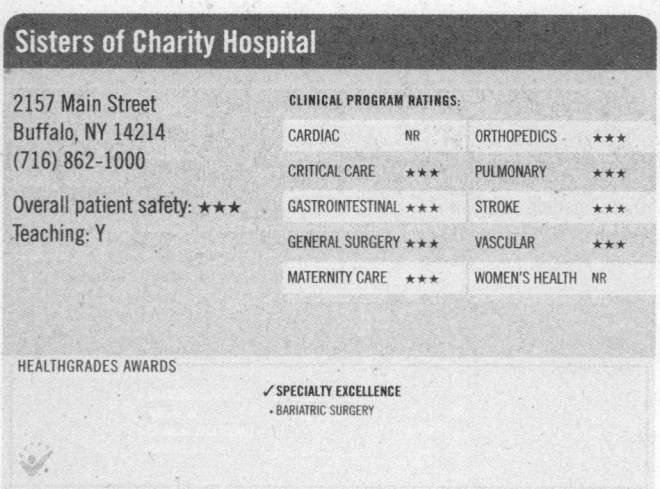

✓ SPECIALTY EXCELLENCE
- BARIATRIC SURGERY

South Nassau Communities Hospital

1 Healthy Way
Oceanside, NY 11572
(516) 632-3000

Overall patient safety: ★
Teaching: Y

CLINICAL PROGRAM RATINGS:

CARDIAC	NR	ORTHOPEDICS	★
CRITICAL CARE	★★★	PULMONARY	★★★
GASTROINTESTINAL	★★★	STROKE	★★★★★
GENERAL SURGERY	★	VASCULAR	NR
MATERNITY CARE	★★★★★	WOMEN'S HEALTH	NR

HEALTHGRADES AWARDS

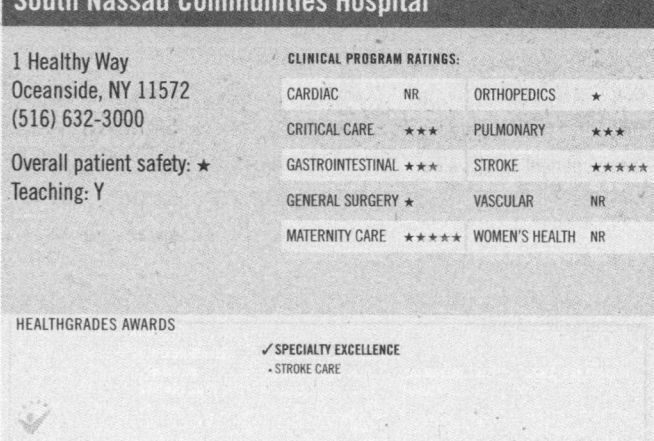

✓ SPECIALTY EXCELLENCE
- STROKE CARE

KEY: ★★★★★ BEST   ★★★ AS EXPECTED   ★ POOR   NR NOT RATED BY HEALTHGRADES   For full definitions of ratings and awards, see Appendix.

478   CHAPTER 6: HOSPITAL RATINGS BY CLINICAL SPECIALTY

Southampton Hospital

240 Meeting House Lane
Southampton, NY 11968
(631) 726-8200

Overall patient safety: ★★★
Teaching: N

CLINICAL PROGRAM RATINGS:

CARDIAC	NR	ORTHOPEDICS	NR
CRITICAL CARE	NR	PULMONARY	★★★
GASTROINTESTINAL	NR	STROKE	★★★
GENERAL SURGERY	★★★	VASCULAR	NR
MATERNITY CARE	★★★★★	WOMEN'S HEALTH	NR

HEALTHGRADES AWARDS

✓ SPECIALTY EXCELLENCE
• MATERNITY CARE

Stony Brook University Medical Center

Nicolls Road and Health
Sciences Drive
Stony Brook, NY 11794
(631) 444-4000

Overall patient safety: ★
Teaching: Y

CLINICAL PROGRAM RATINGS:

CARDIAC	★★★	ORTHOPEDICS	★
CRITICAL CARE	★★★	PULMONARY	★★★
GASTROINTESTINAL	★★★	STROKE	★★★
GENERAL SURGERY	★★★	VASCULAR	★★★
MATERNITY CARE	★★★	WOMEN'S HEALTH	★★★

HEALTHGRADES AWARDS

Southside Hospital

301 East Main Street
Bay Shore, NY 11706
(631) 968-3000

Overall patient safety: ★
Teaching: Y

CLINICAL PROGRAM RATINGS:

CARDIAC	NR	ORTHOPEDICS	NR
CRITICAL CARE	★	PULMONARY	★★★
GASTROINTESTINAL	★★★	STROKE	★★★
GENERAL SURGERY	★★★	VASCULAR	NR
MATERNITY CARE	★★★★★	WOMEN'S HEALTH	NR

HEALTHGRADES AWARDS

✓ SPECIALTY EXCELLENCE
• BARIATRIC SURGERY   • MATERNITY CARE

Strong Memorial Hospital

601 Elmwood Avenue
Rochester, NY 14642
(585) 275-2100

Overall patient safety: ★★★
Teaching: Y

CLINICAL PROGRAM RATINGS:

CARDIAC	★★★	ORTHOPEDICS	NR
CRITICAL CARE	★★★	PULMONARY	★★★
GASTROINTESTINAL	★★★	STROKE	★
GENERAL SURGERY	★★★	VASCULAR	★
MATERNITY CARE	★	WOMEN'S HEALTH	★

HEALTHGRADES AWARDS

Staten Island University Hospital*

475 Seaview Avenue
Staten Island, NY 10305
(718) 226-2000

Overall patient safety: ★★★
Teaching: Y

CLINICAL PROGRAM RATINGS:

CARDIAC	★★★	ORTHOPEDICS	NR
CRITICAL CARE	★	PULMONARY	★
GASTROINTESTINAL	★★★	STROKE	★★★
GENERAL SURGERY	★★★	VASCULAR	★★★
MATERNITY CARE	★★★	WOMEN'S HEALTH	★★★

HEALTHGRADES AWARDS

✓ SPECIALTY EXCELLENCE
• GENERAL SURGERY

SVCMC—St. Vincent's Hospital Staten Island*

355 Bard Avenue
Staten Island, NY 10310
(718) 818-1234

Overall patient safety: ★★★
Teaching: Y

CLINICAL PROGRAM RATINGS:

CARDIAC	NR	ORTHOPEDICS	NR
CRITICAL CARE	NR	PULMONARY	★
GASTROINTESTINAL	★★★	STROKE	★★★
GENERAL SURGERY	★★★	VASCULAR	NR
MATERNITY CARE	★★★★★	WOMEN'S HEALTH	NR

HEALTHGRADES AWARDS

✓ SPECIALTY EXCELLENCE
• MATERNITY CARE

*This hospital reports its data to the federal government jointly with another hospital. Therefore the ratings and awards apply to multiple hospitals and this specific hospital may not provide all rated services.

Taylor Brown Memorial Hospital* (Closed)

East Main Street
Waterloo, NY 13165
(315) 539-9204

Overall patient safety: ★★★★★
Teaching: N

CLINICAL PROGRAM RATINGS:

CARDIAC	NR	ORTHOPEDICS	★★★
CRITICAL CARE	NR	PULMONARY	★★★
GASTROINTESTINAL	NR	STROKE	★★★
GENERAL SURGERY	NR	VASCULAR	NR
MATERNITY CARE	★★★	WOMEN'S HEALTH	NR

HEALTHGRADES AWARDS

United Memorial Medical Center*

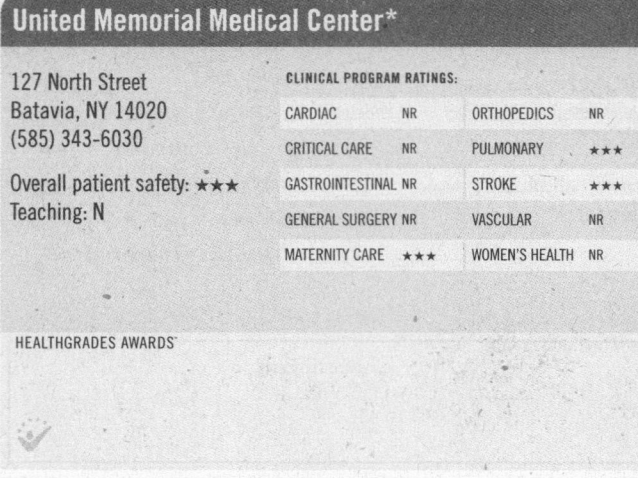

127 North Street
Batavia, NY 14020
(585) 343-6030

Overall patient safety: ★★★
Teaching: N

CLINICAL PROGRAM RATINGS:

CARDIAC	NR	ORTHOPEDICS	NR
CRITICAL CARE	NR	PULMONARY	★★★
GASTROINTESTINAL	NR	STROKE	★★★
GENERAL SURGERY	NR	VASCULAR	NR
MATERNITY CARE	★★★	WOMEN'S HEALTH	NR

HEALTHGRADES AWARDS

TLC Health Network*

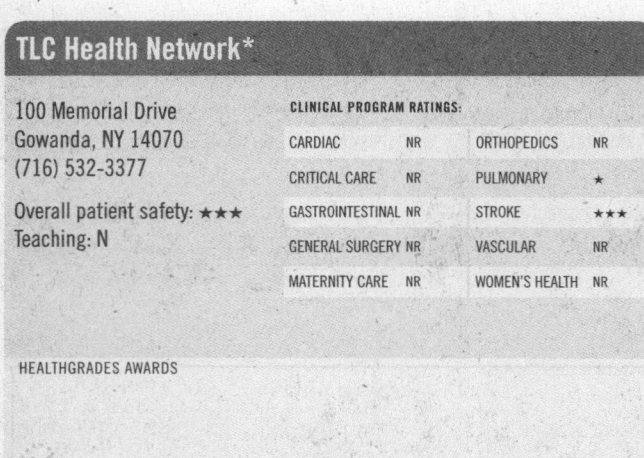

100 Memorial Drive
Gowanda, NY 14070
(716) 532-3377

Overall patient safety: ★★★
Teaching: N

CLINICAL PROGRAM RATINGS:

CARDIAC	NR	ORTHOPEDICS	NR
CRITICAL CARE	NR	PULMONARY	★
GASTROINTESTINAL	NR	STROKE	★★★
GENERAL SURGERY	NR	VASCULAR	NR
MATERNITY CARE	NR	WOMEN'S HEALTH	NR

HEALTHGRADES AWARDS

Unity Hospital*

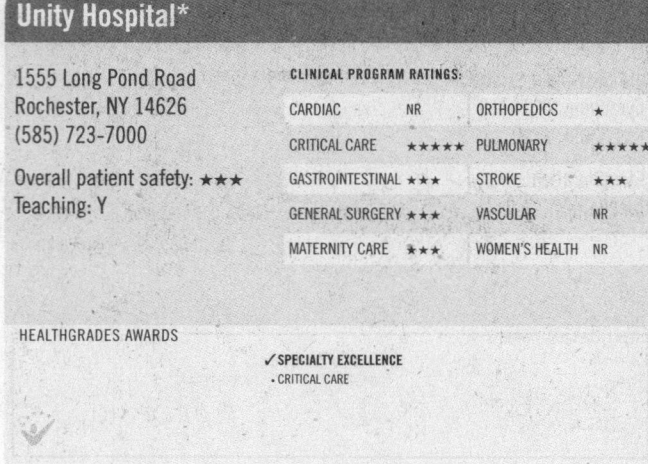

1555 Long Pond Road
Rochester, NY 14626
(585) 723-7000

Overall patient safety: ★★★
Teaching: Y

CLINICAL PROGRAM RATINGS:

CARDIAC	NR	ORTHOPEDICS	★
CRITICAL CARE	★★★★★	PULMONARY	★★★★★
GASTROINTESTINAL	★★★	STROKE	★★★
GENERAL SURGERY	★★★	VASCULAR	NR
MATERNITY CARE	★★★	WOMEN'S HEALTH	NR

HEALTHGRADES AWARDS

✓ SPECIALTY EXCELLENCE
- CRITICAL CARE

United Health Services Hospitals

10-42 Mitchell Avenue
Binghamton, NY 13903
(607) 762-2200

Overall patient safety: ★★★
Teaching: Y

CLINICAL PROGRAM RATINGS:

CARDIAC	★★★	ORTHOPEDICS	★★★
CRITICAL CARE	★	PULMONARY	★★★
GASTROINTESTINAL	★★★	STROKE	★★★
GENERAL SURGERY	★★★	VASCULAR	★★★
MATERNITY CARE	★★★	WOMEN'S HEALTH	★★★

HEALTHGRADES AWARDS

Unity St. Mary's Campus*

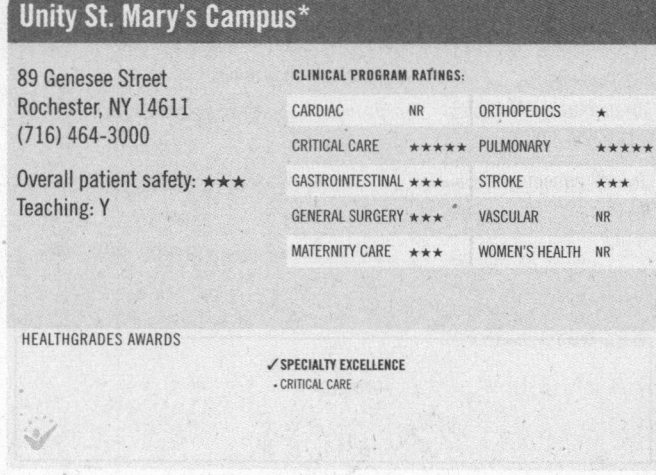

89 Genesee Street
Rochester, NY 14611
(716) 464-3000

Overall patient safety: ★★★
Teaching: Y

CLINICAL PROGRAM RATINGS:

CARDIAC	NR	ORTHOPEDICS	★
CRITICAL CARE	★★★★★	PULMONARY	★★★★★
GASTROINTESTINAL	★★★	STROKE	★★★
GENERAL SURGERY	★★★	VASCULAR	NR
MATERNITY CARE	★★★	WOMEN'S HEALTH	NR

HEALTHGRADES AWARDS

✓ SPECIALTY EXCELLENCE
- CRITICAL CARE

KEY: ★★★★★ BEST   ★★★ AS EXPECTED   ★ POOR   NR NOT RATED BY HEALTHGRADES   For full definitions of ratings and awards, see Appendix.

University Hospital of Brooklyn—Downstate

445 Lenox Road
Brooklyn, NY 11203
(718) 270-1000

Overall patient safety: ★★★
Teaching: Y

CLINICAL PROGRAM RATINGS:

CARDIAC	★★★	ORTHOPEDICS	NR
CRITICAL CARE	NR	PULMONARY	★★★
GASTROINTESTINAL	NR	STROKE	★★★
GENERAL SURGERY	NR	VASCULAR	NR
MATERNITY CARE	★★★	WOMEN'S HEALTH	★★★

HEALTHGRADES AWARDS

Victory Memorial Hospital

699 92nd Street
Brooklyn, NY 11228
(718) 567-1234

Overall patient safety: ★★★
Teaching: N

CLINICAL PROGRAM RATINGS:

CARDIAC	NR	ORTHOPEDICS	NR
CRITICAL CARE	NR	PULMONARY	★
GASTROINTESTINAL	★★★	STROKE	★★★
GENERAL SURGERY	★★★	VASCULAR	NR
MATERNITY CARE	★★★	WOMEN'S HEALTH	NR

HEALTHGRADES AWARDS

University Hospital SUNY Upstate Medical University

750 East Adams Street
Syracuse, NY 13210
(315) 464-5540

Overall patient safety: ★
Teaching: Y

CLINICAL PROGRAM RATINGS:

CARDIAC	★★★	ORTHOPEDICS	★★★
CRITICAL CARE	★★★	PULMONARY	★★★
GASTROINTESTINAL	★★★	STROKE	★★★
GENERAL SURGERY	★	VASCULAR	NR
MATERNITY CARE	NR	WOMEN'S HEALTH	NR

HEALTHGRADES AWARDS

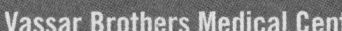

Westchester Medical Center

Valhalla Campus
Valhalla, NY 10595
(914) 493-7000

Overall patient safety: ★★★
Teaching: Y

CLINICAL PROGRAM RATINGS:

CARDIAC	★★★	ORTHOPEDICS	★★★
CRITICAL CARE	NR	PULMONARY	★★★
GASTROINTESTINAL	★★★	STROKE	★★★
GENERAL SURGERY	★	VASCULAR	★★★
MATERNITY CARE	★	WOMEN'S HEALTH	★★★

HEALTHGRADES AWARDS

✓ SPECIALTY EXCELLENCE
· BARIATRIC SURGERY   · CARDIAC CARE

Vassar Brothers Medical Center

45 Reade Place
Poughkeepsie, NY 12601
(845) 454-8500

Overall patient safety: ★★★
Teaching: N

CLINICAL PROGRAM RATINGS:

CARDIAC	★★★	ORTHOPEDICS	NR
CRITICAL CARE	★★★	PULMONARY	★
GASTROINTESTINAL	★★★	STROKE	★★★
GENERAL SURGERY	★★★	VASCULAR	★★★
MATERNITY CARE	★★★	WOMEN'S HEALTH	★★★

HEALTHGRADES AWARDS

✓ SPECIALTY EXCELLENCE
· CARDIAC CARE   · CARDIAC SURGERY

Westfield Memorial Hospital

189 East Main Street
Westfield, NY 14787
(718) 584-9000

Overall patient safety: ★★★
Teaching: N

CLINICAL PROGRAM RATINGS:

CARDIAC	NR	ORTHOPEDICS	NR
CRITICAL CARE	NR	PULMONARY	★
GASTROINTESTINAL	NR	STROKE	NR
GENERAL SURGERY	NR	VASCULAR	NR
MATERNITY CARE	★★★	WOMEN'S HEALTH	NR

HEALTHGRADES AWARDS

*This hospital reports its data to the federal government jointly with another hospital. Therefore the ratings and awards apply to multiple hospitals and this specific hospital may not provide all rated services.

White Plains Hospital Center

Davis Avenue at East Post Road
White Plains, NY 10601
(914) 681-0600

Overall patient safety: ★
Teaching: N

CLINICAL PROGRAM RATINGS:

CARDIAC	NR	ORTHOPEDICS	★
CRITICAL CARE	★★★	PULMONARY	★★★★★
GASTROINTESTINAL	★★★	STROKE	★★★★★
GENERAL SURGERY	★★★	VASCULAR	NR
MATERNITY CARE	★★★★★	WOMEN'S HEALTH	NR

HEALTHGRADES AWARDS

✓ SPECIALTY EXCELLENCE
- MATERNITY CARE - PULMONARY CARE

Woodhull Medical and Mental Health Center

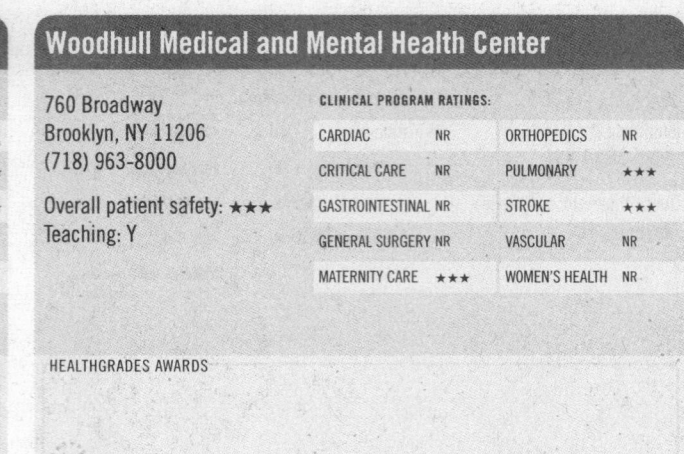

760 Broadway
Brooklyn, NY 11206
(718) 963-8000

Overall patient safety: ★★★
Teaching: Y

CLINICAL PROGRAM RATINGS:

CARDIAC	NR	ORTHOPEDICS	NR
CRITICAL CARE	NR	PULMONARY	★★★
GASTROINTESTINAL	NR	STROKE	★★★
GENERAL SURGERY	NR	VASCULAR	NR
MATERNITY CARE	★★★	WOMEN'S HEALTH	NR

HEALTHGRADES AWARDS

Winthrop-University Hospital

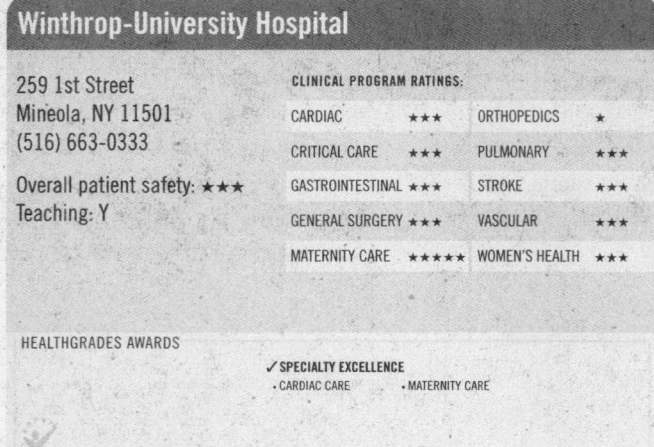

259 1st Street
Mineola, NY 11501
(516) 663-0333

Overall patient safety: ★★★
Teaching: Y

CLINICAL PROGRAM RATINGS:

CARDIAC	★★★	ORTHOPEDICS	★
CRITICAL CARE	★★★	PULMONARY	★★★
GASTROINTESTINAL	★★★	STROKE	★★★
GENERAL SURGERY	★★★	VASCULAR	★★★
MATERNITY CARE	★★★★★	WOMEN'S HEALTH	★★★

HEALTHGRADES AWARDS

✓ SPECIALTY EXCELLENCE
- CARDIAC CARE - MATERNITY CARE

Wyckoff Heights Medical Center

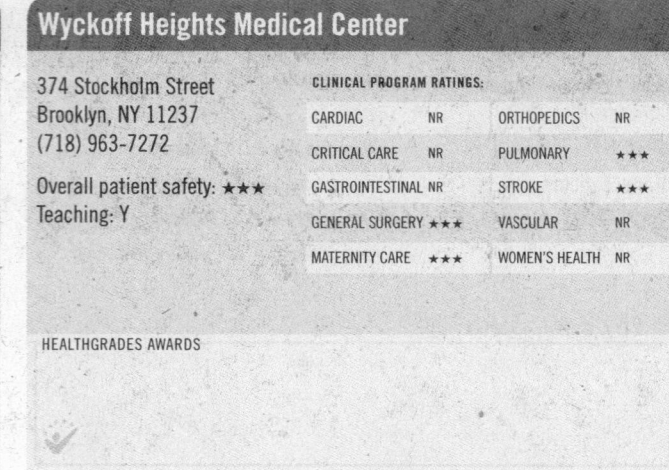

374 Stockholm Street
Brooklyn, NY 11237
(718) 963-7272

Overall patient safety: ★★★
Teaching: Y

CLINICAL PROGRAM RATINGS:

CARDIAC	NR	ORTHOPEDICS	NR
CRITICAL CARE	NR	PULMONARY	★★★
GASTROINTESTINAL	NR	STROKE	★★★
GENERAL SURGERY	★★★	VASCULAR	NR
MATERNITY CARE	★★★	WOMEN'S HEALTH	NR

HEALTHGRADES AWARDS

Woman's Christian Association

207 Foote Avenue
Jamestown, NY 14701
(716) 487-0141

Overall patient safety: ★★★
Teaching: N

CLINICAL PROGRAM RATINGS:

CARDIAC	NR	ORTHOPEDICS	★★★
CRITICAL CARE	NR	PULMONARY	★★★
GASTROINTESTINAL	★★★	STROKE	★★★
GENERAL SURGERY	★★★	VASCULAR	NR
MATERNITY CARE	★★★	WOMEN'S HEALTH	NR

HEALTHGRADES AWARDS

Wyoming County Community Hospital

400 North Main Street
Warsaw, NY 14569
(585) 786-2233

Overall patient safety: ★★★
Teaching: N

CLINICAL PROGRAM RATINGS:

CARDIAC	NR	ORTHOPEDICS	NR
CRITICAL CARE	NR	PULMONARY	★★★
GASTROINTESTINAL	NR	STROKE	★★★
GENERAL SURGERY	NR	VASCULAR	NR
MATERNITY CARE	★★★	WOMEN'S HEALTH	NR

HEALTHGRADES AWARDS

KEY: ★★★★★ BEST   ★★★ AS EXPECTED   ★ POOR   NR NOT RATED BY HEALTHGRADES   For full definitions of ratings and awards, see Appendix.

Yonkers General Hospital*

Two Parks Avenue
Yonkers, NY 10703
(914) 964-7300

Overall patient safety: ★
Teaching: N

CLINICAL PROGRAM RATINGS:

CARDIAC	NR	ORTHOPEDICS	NR
CRITICAL CARE	NR	PULMONARY	★★★
GASTROINTESTINAL	★★★	STROKE	★★★★★
GENERAL SURGERY	★★★	VASCULAR	NR
MATERNITY CARE	★★★★★	WOMEN'S HEALTH	NR

HEALTHGRADES AWARDS

✓ SPECIALTY EXCELLENCE
• MATERNITY CARE

NORTH CAROLINA HOSPITALS: RATINGS BY CLINICAL SPECIALTY

Alamance Regional Medical Center

1240 Huffman Mill Road
Burlington, NC 27216
(336) 538-7000

Overall patient safety: ★★★
Teaching: N

CLINICAL PROGRAM RATINGS:

CARDIAC	NR	ORTHOPEDICS	★★★★★
CRITICAL CARE	NR	PULMONARY	★★★
GASTROINTESTINAL	★★★	STROKE	★
GENERAL SURGERY	★★★	VASCULAR	NR
MATERNITY CARE	★★★	WOMEN'S HEALTH	NR

HEALTHGRADES AWARDS

✓ SPECIALTY EXCELLENCE
• ORTHOPEDIC SURGERY

Angel Medical Center

120 Riverview Street
Franklin, NC 28734
(828) 369-4211

Overall patient safety: ★★★
Teaching: N

CLINICAL PROGRAM RATINGS:

CARDIAC	NR	ORTHOPEDICS	NR
CRITICAL CARE	NR	PULMONARY	★
GASTROINTESTINAL	NR	STROKE	★★★
GENERAL SURGERY	NR	VASCULAR	NR
MATERNITY CARE	★★★	WOMEN'S HEALTH	NR

HEALTHGRADES AWARDS

Albemarle Hospital Authority

1144 North Road Street
Elizabeth City, NC 27909
(252) 335-0531

Overall patient safety: ★★★
Teaching: N

CLINICAL PROGRAM RATINGS:

CARDIAC	NR	ORTHOPEDICS	★★★
CRITICAL CARE	NR	PULMONARY	★
GASTROINTESTINAL	★★★	STROKE	★★★
GENERAL SURGERY	★★★	VASCULAR	NR
MATERNITY CARE	★	WOMEN'S HEALTH	NR

HEALTHGRADES AWARDS

Annie Penn Memorial Hospital*

618 South Main Street
Reidsville, NC 27320
(336) 951-4000

Overall patient safety: ★★★
Teaching: Y

CLINICAL PROGRAM RATINGS:

CARDIAC	★★★	ORTHOPEDICS	★★★
CRITICAL CARE	NR	PULMONARY	★★★
GASTROINTESTINAL	★★★	STROKE	★★★
GENERAL SURGERY	★★★★★	VASCULAR	★★★
MATERNITY CARE	★★★	WOMEN'S HEALTH	★★★

HEALTHGRADES AWARDS

✓ SPECIALTY EXCELLENCE
• GENERAL SURGERY

---

*This hospital reports its data to the federal government jointly with another hospital. Therefore the ratings and awards apply to multiple hospitals and this specific hospital may not provide all rated services.

Anson Community Hospital

500 Morven Road
Wadesboro, NC 28170
(704) 694-5131

Overall patient safety: ★★★
Teaching: N

CLINICAL PROGRAM RATINGS:

CARDIAC	NR	ORTHOPEDICS	NR
CRITICAL CARE	NR	PULMONARY	★★★★★
GASTROINTESTINAL	NR	STROKE	★★★
GENERAL SURGERY	NR	VASCULAR	NR
MATERNITY CARE	NR	WOMEN'S HEALTH	NR

HEALTHGRADES AWARDS

Betsy Johnson Memorial Hospital

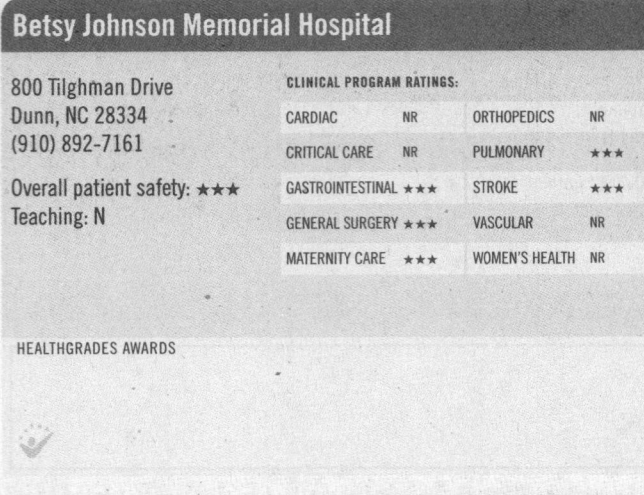

800 Tilghman Drive
Dunn, NC 28334
(910) 892-7161

Overall patient safety: ★★★
Teaching: N

CLINICAL PROGRAM RATINGS:

CARDIAC	NR	ORTHOPEDICS	NR
CRITICAL CARE	NR	PULMONARY	★★★
GASTROINTESTINAL	★★★	STROKE	★★★
GENERAL SURGERY	★★★	VASCULAR	NR
MATERNITY CARE	★★★	WOMEN'S HEALTH	NR

HEALTHGRADES AWARDS

Ashe Memorial Hospital

200 Hospital Avenue
Jefferson, NC 28640
(336) 246-7101

Overall patient safety: ★★★
Teaching: N

CLINICAL PROGRAM RATINGS:

CARDIAC	NR	ORTHOPEDICS	NR
CRITICAL CARE	NR	PULMONARY	★★★
GASTROINTESTINAL	NR	STROKE	★
GENERAL SURGERY	★★★	VASCULAR	NR
MATERNITY CARE	★	WOMEN'S HEALTH	NR

HEALTHGRADES AWARDS

Bladen County Hospital

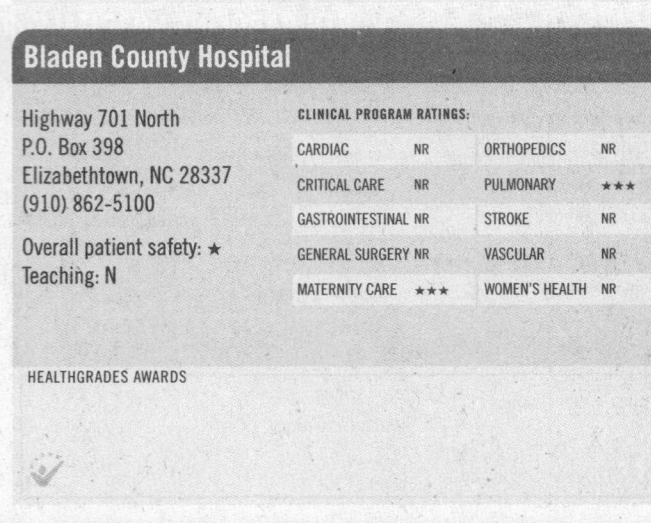

Highway 701 North
P.O. Box 398
Elizabethtown, NC 28337
(910) 862-5100

Overall patient safety: ★
Teaching: N

CLINICAL PROGRAM RATINGS:

CARDIAC	NR	ORTHOPEDICS	NR
CRITICAL CARE	NR	PULMONARY	★★★
GASTROINTESTINAL	NR	STROKE	NR
GENERAL SURGERY	NR	VASCULAR	NR
MATERNITY CARE	★★★	WOMEN'S HEALTH	NR

HEALTHGRADES AWARDS

Beaufort County Hospital

628 East 12th Street
Washington, NC 27889
(252) 975-4100

Overall patient safety: ★★★
Teaching: N

CLINICAL PROGRAM RATINGS:

CARDIAC	NR	ORTHOPEDICS	NR
CRITICAL CARE	NR	PULMONARY	★★★
GASTROINTESTINAL	NR	STROKE	NR
GENERAL SURGERY	★★★	VASCULAR	NR
MATERNITY CARE	★★★	WOMEN'S HEALTH	NR

HEALTHGRADES AWARDS

Brunswick Community Hospital

1 Medical Center Drive
Supply, NC 28462
(910) 755-8121

Overall patient safety: ★★★
Teaching: N

CLINICAL PROGRAM RATINGS:

CARDIAC	NR	ORTHOPEDICS	NR
CRITICAL CARE	NR	PULMONARY	★★★
GASTROINTESTINAL	★★★	STROKE	★★★
GENERAL SURGERY	★★★	VASCULAR	NR
MATERNITY CARE	★★★	WOMEN'S HEALTH	NR

HEALTHGRADES AWARDS

KEY: ★★★★★ BEST   ★★★ AS EXPECTED   ★ POOR   NR NOT RATED BY HEALTHGRADES   For full definitions of ratings and awards, see Appendix.

Caldwell Memorial Hospital

321 Mulberry Street Southwest
Lenoir, NC 28645
(828) 757-5100

Overall patient safety: ★★★
Teaching: N

CLINICAL PROGRAM RATINGS:

CARDIAC	NR	ORTHOPEDICS	NR
CRITICAL CARE	NR	PULMONARY	★★★
GASTROINTESTINAL	★★★	STROKE	★★★
GENERAL SURGERY	★★★	VASCULAR	NR
MATERNITY CARE	★★★	WOMEN'S HEALTH	NR

HEALTHGRADES AWARDS

Carolinas Medical Center

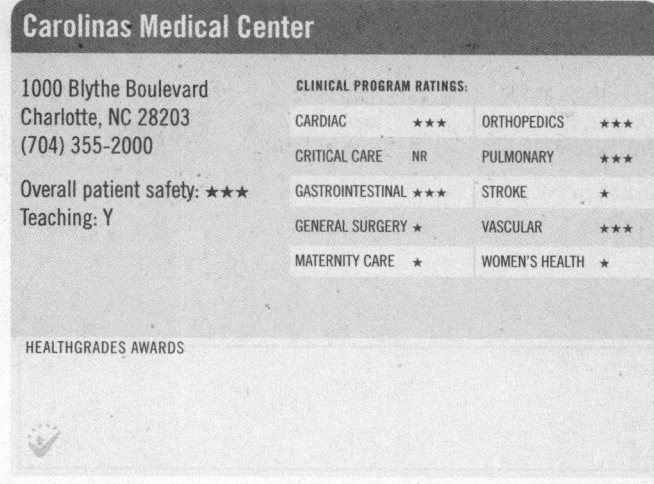

1000 Blythe Boulevard
Charlotte, NC 28203
(704) 355-2000

Overall patient safety: ★★★
Teaching: Y

CLINICAL PROGRAM RATINGS:

CARDIAC	★★★	ORTHOPEDICS	★★★
CRITICAL CARE	NR	PULMONARY	★★★
GASTROINTESTINAL	★★★	STROKE	★
GENERAL SURGERY	★	VASCULAR	★★★
MATERNITY CARE	★	WOMEN'S HEALTH	★

HEALTHGRADES AWARDS

Cape Fear Hospital*

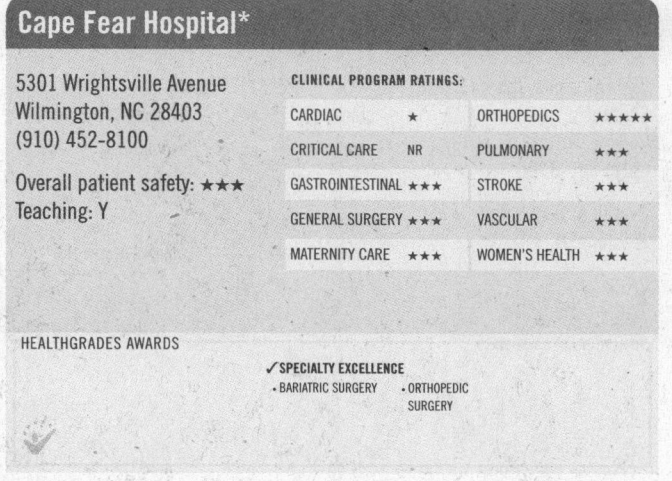

5301 Wrightsville Avenue
Wilmington, NC 28403
(910) 452-8100

Overall patient safety: ★★★
Teaching: Y

CLINICAL PROGRAM RATINGS:

CARDIAC	★	ORTHOPEDICS	★★★★★
CRITICAL CARE	NR	PULMONARY	★★★
GASTROINTESTINAL	★★★	STROKE	★★★
GENERAL SURGERY	★★★	VASCULAR	★★★
MATERNITY CARE	★★★	WOMEN'S HEALTH	★★★

HEALTHGRADES AWARDS

✓ SPECIALTY EXCELLENCE
- BARIATRIC SURGERY
- ORTHOPEDIC SURGERY

Carolinas Medical Center--Lincoln

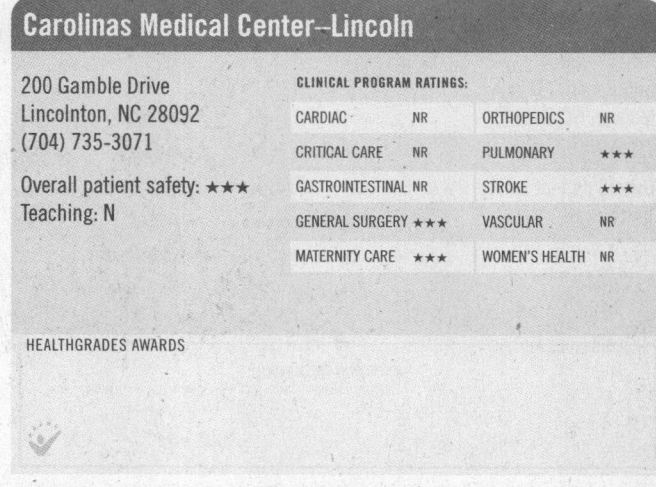

200 Gamble Drive
Lincolnton, NC 28092
(704) 735-3071

Overall patient safety: ★★★
Teaching: N

CLINICAL PROGRAM RATINGS:

CARDIAC	NR	ORTHOPEDICS	NR
CRITICAL CARE	NR	PULMONARY	★★★
GASTROINTESTINAL	NR	STROKE	★★★
GENERAL SURGERY	★★★	VASCULAR	NR
MATERNITY CARE	★★★	WOMEN'S HEALTH	NR

HEALTHGRADES AWARDS

Cape Fear Valley Medical Center

1638 Owen Drive
Fayetteville, NC 28304
(910) 609-4000

Overall patient safety: ★★★★★
Teaching: Y

CLINICAL PROGRAM RATINGS:

CARDIAC	★★★	ORTHOPEDICS	★★★
CRITICAL CARE	NR	PULMONARY	★★★★★
GASTROINTESTINAL	★★★	STROKE	★★★★★
GENERAL SURGERY	★★★	VASCULAR	★★★
MATERNITY CARE	★★★	WOMEN'S HEALTH	★★★

HEALTHGRADES AWARDS

✓ DISTINGUISHED HOSPITAL
- PATIENT SAFETY

✓ SPECIALTY EXCELLENCE
- PULMONARY CARE

Carolinas Medical Center--Mercy

2001 Vail Avenue
Charlotte, NC 28207
(704) 379-5000

Overall patient safety: ★
Teaching: N

CLINICAL PROGRAM RATINGS:

CARDIAC	★★★	ORTHOPEDICS	★★★
CRITICAL CARE	NR	PULMONARY	★★★
GASTROINTESTINAL	★★★	STROKE	★★★
GENERAL SURGERY	★★★	VASCULAR	NR
MATERNITY CARE	★★★	WOMEN'S HEALTH	★★★

HEALTHGRADES AWARDS

---

*This hospital reports its data to the federal government jointly with another hospital. Therefore the ratings and awards apply to multiple hospitals and this specific hospital may not provide all rated services.

Carolinas Medical Center—NorthEast

920 Church Street North
Concord, NC 28025
(704) 783-3000

Overall patient safety: ★★★
Teaching: Y

CLINICAL PROGRAM RATINGS:

CARDIAC	★★★	ORTHOPEDICS	★
CRITICAL CARE	NR	PULMONARY	★★★
GASTROINTESTINAL	★★★	STROKE	★★★
GENERAL SURGERY	★★★	VASCULAR	★★★
MATERNITY CARE	★★★	WOMEN'S HEALTH	★★★

HEALTHGRADES AWARDS

Carteret General Hospital

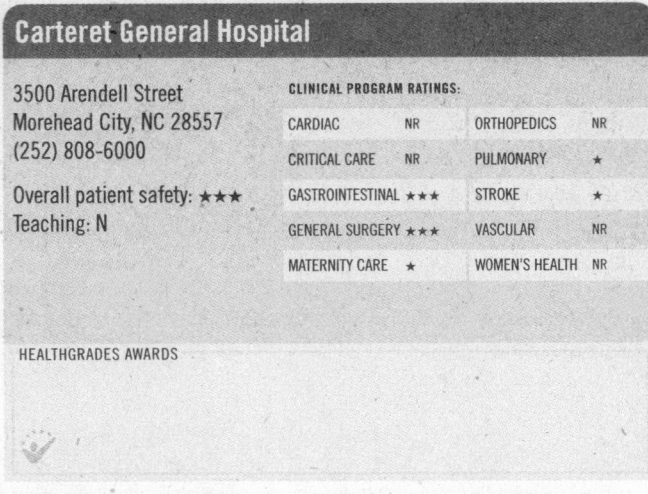

3500 Arendell Street
Morehead City, NC 28557
(252) 808-6000

Overall patient safety: ★★★
Teaching: N

CLINICAL PROGRAM RATINGS:

CARDIAC	NR	ORTHOPEDICS	NR
CRITICAL CARE	NR	PULMONARY	★
GASTROINTESTINAL	★★★	STROKE	★
GENERAL SURGERY	★★★	VASCULAR	NR
MATERNITY CARE	★	WOMEN'S HEALTH	NR

HEALTHGRADES AWARDS

Carolinas Medical Center—Union

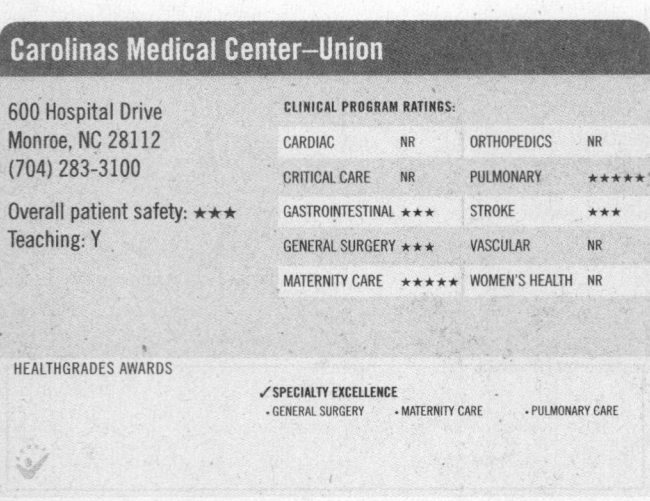

600 Hospital Drive
Monroe, NC 28112
(704) 283-3100

Overall patient safety: ★★★
Teaching: Y

CLINICAL PROGRAM RATINGS:

CARDIAC	NR	ORTHOPEDICS	NR
CRITICAL CARE	NR	PULMONARY	★★★★★
GASTROINTESTINAL	★★★	STROKE	★★★
GENERAL SURGERY	★★★	VASCULAR	NR
MATERNITY CARE	★★★★★	WOMEN'S HEALTH	NR

HEALTHGRADES AWARDS

✓ SPECIALTY EXCELLENCE
· GENERAL SURGERY   · MATERNITY CARE   · PULMONARY CARE

Catawba Valley Medical Center

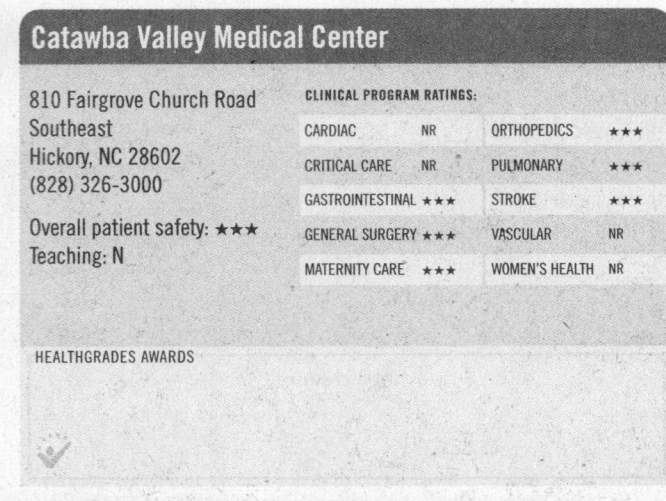

810 Fairgrove Church Road
Southeast
Hickory, NC 28602
(828) 326-3000

Overall patient safety: ★★★
Teaching: N

CLINICAL PROGRAM RATINGS:

CARDIAC	NR	ORTHOPEDICS	★★★
CRITICAL CARE	NR	PULMONARY	★★★
GASTROINTESTINAL	★★★	STROKE	★★★
GENERAL SURGERY	★★★	VASCULAR	NR
MATERNITY CARE	★★★	WOMEN'S HEALTH	NR

HEALTHGRADES AWARDS

Carolinas Medical Center—University

8800 North Tryon Street
Charlotte, NC 28262
(704) 548-6000

Overall patient safety: ★★★
Teaching: N

CLINICAL PROGRAM RATINGS:

CARDIAC	NR	ORTHOPEDICS	NR
CRITICAL CARE	NR	PULMONARY	★★★
GASTROINTESTINAL	NR	STROKE	★★★
GENERAL SURGERY	★★★	VASCULAR	NR
MATERNITY CARE	★★★	WOMEN'S HEALTH	NR

HEALTHGRADES AWARDS

Central Carolina Hospital

1135 Carthage Street
Sanford, NC 27330
(919) 774-2100

Overall patient safety: ★
Teaching: N

CLINICAL PROGRAM RATINGS:

CARDIAC	NR	ORTHOPEDICS	NR
CRITICAL CARE	★★★	PULMONARY	★
GASTROINTESTINAL	★	STROKE	★★★
GENERAL SURGERY	★★★	VASCULAR	NR
MATERNITY CARE	★	WOMEN'S HEALTH	NR

HEALTHGRADES AWARDS

KEY: ★★★★★ BEST   ★★★ AS EXPECTED   ★ POOR   NR NOT RATED BY HEALTHGRADES   For full definitions of ratings and awards, see Appendix.

Charles A. Cannon Jr. Memorial Hospital

P.O. Box 767
Linville, NC 28646
(828) 737-7000

Overall patient safety: ★★★★★
Teaching: N

CLINICAL PROGRAM RATINGS:

CARDIAC	NR	ORTHOPEDICS	NR
CRITICAL CARE	NR	PULMONARY	★
GASTROINTESTINAL	NR	STROKE	★
GENERAL SURGERY	★★★	VASCULAR	NR
MATERNITY CARE	★	WOMEN'S HEALTH	NR

HEALTHGRADES AWARDS

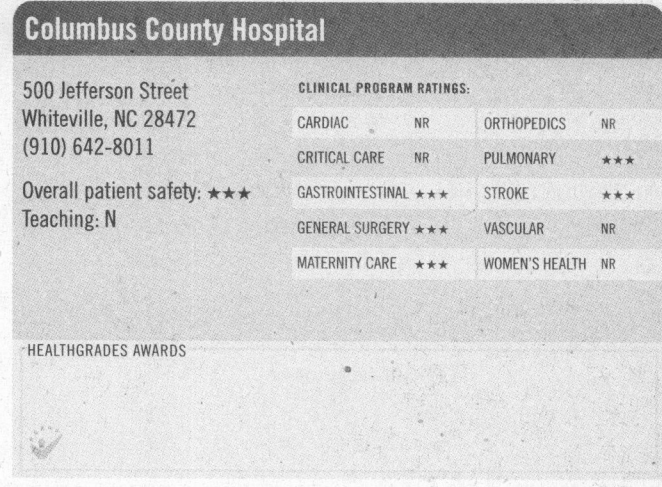

Columbus County Hospital

500 Jefferson Street
Whiteville, NC 28472
(910) 642-8011

Overall patient safety: ★★★
Teaching: N

CLINICAL PROGRAM RATINGS:

CARDIAC	NR	ORTHOPEDICS	NR
CRITICAL CARE	NR	PULMONARY	★★★
GASTROINTESTINAL	★★★	STROKE	★★★
GENERAL SURGERY	★★★	VASCULAR	NR
MATERNITY CARE	★★★	WOMEN'S HEALTH	NR

HEALTHGRADES AWARDS

Chowan Hospital

211 Virginia Road
Edenton, NC 27932
(252) 482-8451

Overall patient safety: ★★★
Teaching: N

CLINICAL PROGRAM RATINGS:

CARDIAC	NR	ORTHOPEDICS	NR
CRITICAL CARE	NR	PULMONARY	★
GASTROINTESTINAL	NR	STROKE	★★★
GENERAL SURGERY	★★★	VASCULAR	NR
MATERNITY CARE	★★★	WOMEN'S HEALTH	NR

HEALTHGRADES AWARDS

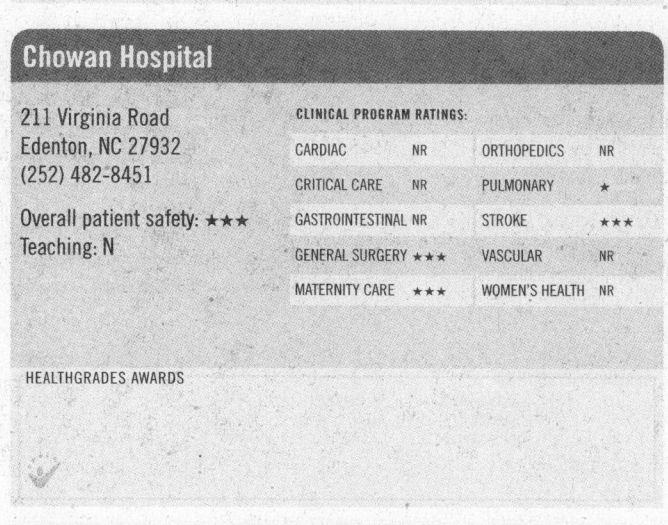

Craven Regional Medical Center

2000 Neuse Boulevard
New Bern, NC 28560
(252) 633-8111

Overall patient safety: ★★★
Teaching: N

CLINICAL PROGRAM RATINGS:

CARDIAC	★★★	ORTHOPEDICS	★★★
CRITICAL CARE	NR	PULMONARY	★★★
GASTROINTESTINAL	★★★	STROKE	★★★
GENERAL SURGERY	★★★	VASCULAR	★★★
MATERNITY CARE	★★★	WOMEN'S HEALTH	★★★

HEALTHGRADES AWARDS

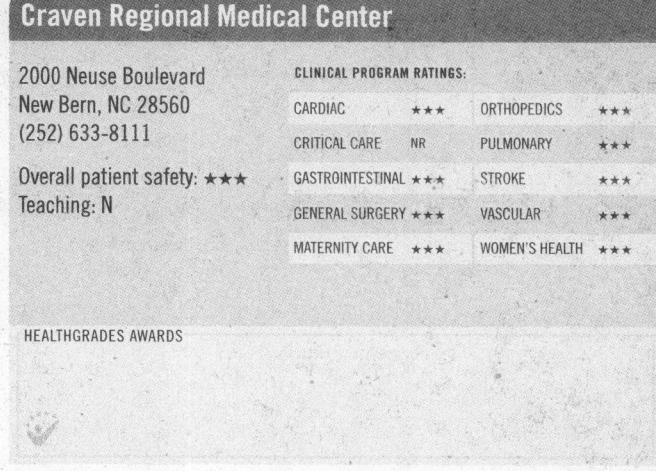

Cleveland Regional Medical Center

201 East Grover Street
Shelby, NC 28150
(704) 487-3000

Overall patient safety: ★★★
Teaching: N

CLINICAL PROGRAM RATINGS:

CARDIAC	NR	ORTHOPEDICS	NR
CRITICAL CARE	NR	PULMONARY	★★★
GASTROINTESTINAL	★★★	STROKE	★★★
GENERAL SURGERY	★★★	VASCULAR	NR
MATERNITY CARE	★★★★★	WOMEN'S HEALTH	NR

HEALTHGRADES AWARDS

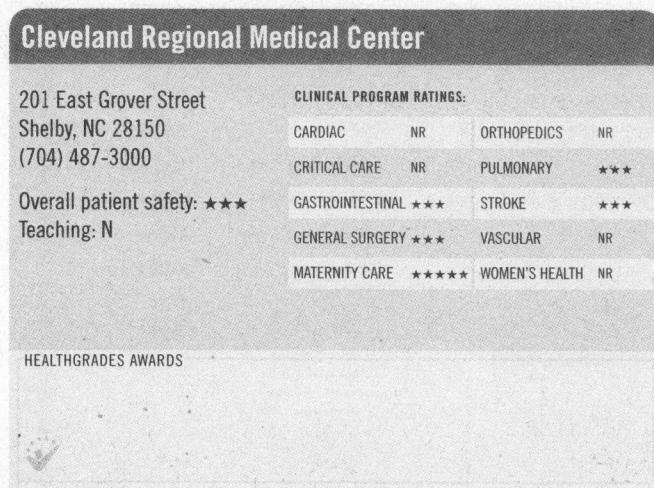

Davis Regional Medical Center

218 Old Mocksville Road
Statesville, NC 28625
(704) 873-0281

Overall patient safety: ★★★
Teaching: N

CLINICAL PROGRAM RATINGS:

CARDIAC	NR	ORTHOPEDICS	★★★
CRITICAL CARE	NR	PULMONARY	★★★★★
GASTROINTESTINAL	NR	STROKE	★★★
GENERAL SURGERY	★★★	VASCULAR	NR
MATERNITY CARE	★★★	WOMEN'S HEALTH	NR

HEALTHGRADES AWARDS

✓ SPECIALTY EXCELLENCE
• PULMONARY CARE

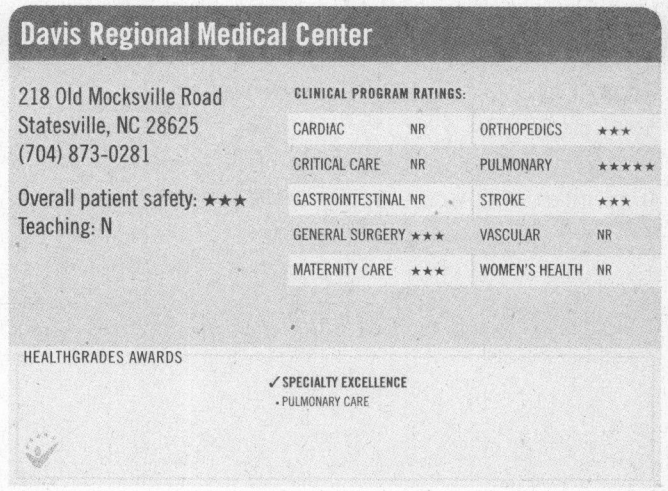

Duke Health Raleigh Hospital

3400 Wake Forest Road
Raleigh, NC 27609
(919) 954-3000

Overall patient safety: ★★★
Teaching: N

CLINICAL PROGRAM RATINGS:

CARDIAC	NR	ORTHOPEDICS	★★★
CRITICAL CARE	NR	PULMONARY	★★★
GASTROINTESTINAL	NR	STROKE	★★★
GENERAL SURGERY	★★★★★	VASCULAR	NR
MATERNITY CARE	★★★	WOMEN'S HEALTH	NR

HEALTHGRADES AWARDS

✓ SPECIALTY EXCELLENCE
- GENERAL SURGERY

Durham Regional Hospital

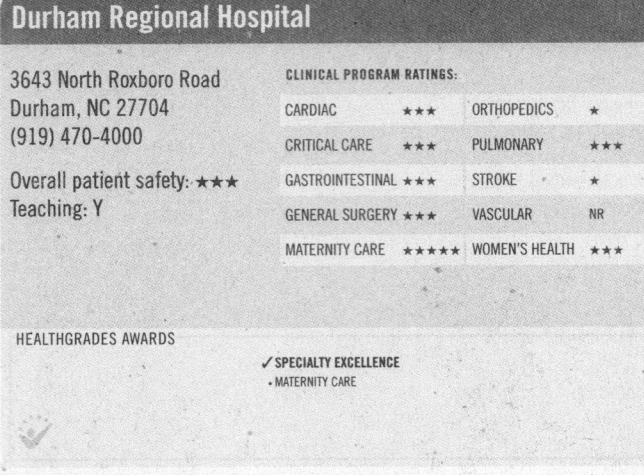

3643 North Roxboro Road
Durham, NC 27704
(919) 470-4000

Overall patient safety: ★★★
Teaching: Y

CLINICAL PROGRAM RATINGS:

CARDIAC	★★★	ORTHOPEDICS	★
CRITICAL CARE	★★★	PULMONARY	★★★
GASTROINTESTINAL	★★★	STROKE	★
GENERAL SURGERY	★★★	VASCULAR	NR
MATERNITY CARE	★★★★★	WOMEN'S HEALTH	★★★

HEALTHGRADES AWARDS

✓ SPECIALTY EXCELLENCE
- MATERNITY CARE

Duke University Hospital

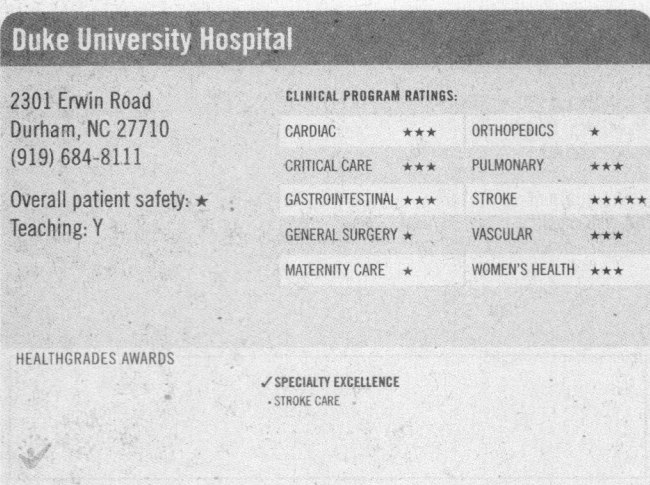

2301 Erwin Road
Durham, NC 27710
(919) 684-8111

Overall patient safety: ★
Teaching: Y

CLINICAL PROGRAM RATINGS:

CARDIAC	★★★	ORTHOPEDICS	★
CRITICAL CARE	★★★	PULMONARY	★★★
GASTROINTESTINAL	★★★	STROKE	★★★★★
GENERAL SURGERY	★	VASCULAR	★★★
MATERNITY CARE	★	WOMEN'S HEALTH	★★★

HEALTHGRADES AWARDS

✓ SPECIALTY EXCELLENCE
- STROKE CARE

FirstHealth Moore Regional Hospital

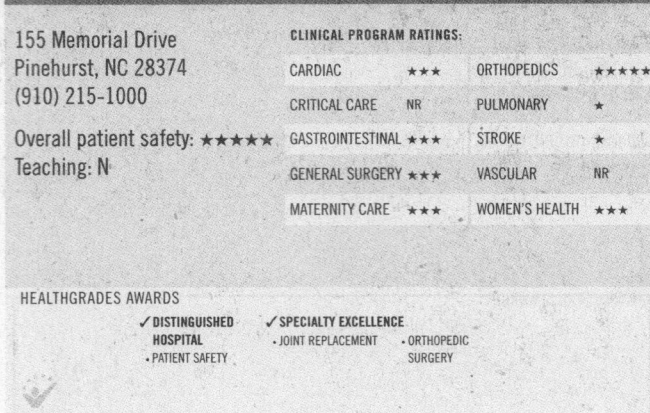

155 Memorial Drive
Pinehurst, NC 28374
(910) 215-1000

Overall patient safety: ★★★★★
Teaching: N

CLINICAL PROGRAM RATINGS:

CARDIAC	★★★	ORTHOPEDICS	★★★★★
CRITICAL CARE	NR	PULMONARY	★
GASTROINTESTINAL	★★★	STROKE	★
GENERAL SURGERY	★★★	VASCULAR	NR
MATERNITY CARE	★★★	WOMEN'S HEALTH	★★★

HEALTHGRADES AWARDS

✓ DISTINGUISHED HOSPITAL
- PATIENT SAFETY

✓ SPECIALTY EXCELLENCE
- JOINT REPLACEMENT
- ORTHOPEDIC SURGERY

Duplin General Hospital

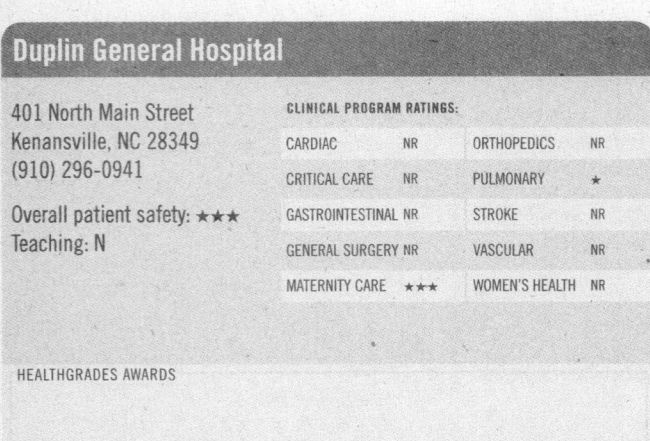

401 North Main Street
Kenansville, NC 28349
(910) 296-0941

Overall patient safety: ★★★
Teaching: N

CLINICAL PROGRAM RATINGS:

CARDIAC	NR	ORTHOPEDICS	NR
CRITICAL CARE	NR	PULMONARY	★
GASTROINTESTINAL	NR	STROKE	NR
GENERAL SURGERY	NR	VASCULAR	NR
MATERNITY CARE	★★★	WOMEN'S HEALTH	NR

HEALTHGRADES AWARDS

FirstHealth Richmond Memorial Hospital

925 Long Drive
Rockingham, NC 28379
(910) 417-3000

Overall patient safety: ★★★
Teaching: N

CLINICAL PROGRAM RATINGS:

CARDIAC	NR	ORTHOPEDICS	NR
CRITICAL CARE	NR	PULMONARY	★★★
GASTROINTESTINAL	NR	STROKE	NR
GENERAL SURGERY	★★★	VASCULAR	NR
MATERNITY CARE	★	WOMEN'S HEALTH	NR

HEALTHGRADES AWARDS

KEY: ★★★★★ BEST ★★★ AS EXPECTED ★ POOR NR NOT RATED BY HEALTHGRADES For full definitions of ratings and awards, see Appendix.

Forsyth Memorial Hospital

3333 Silas Creek Parkway
Winston-Salem, NC 27103
(336) 718-5000

Overall patient safety: ★
Teaching: Y

CLINICAL PROGRAM RATINGS:

CARDIAC	★★★	ORTHOPEDICS	★★★★★
CRITICAL CARE	NR	PULMONARY	★
GASTROINTESTINAL	★★★	STROKE	★★★
GENERAL SURGERY	★★★	VASCULAR	★★★
MATERNITY CARE	★★★	WOMEN'S HEALTH	★

HEALTHGRADES AWARDS

✓ SPECIALTY EXCELLENCE
- JOINT REPLACEMENT   - ORTHOPEDIC SURGERY

Gaston Memorial Hospital

2525 Court Drive
Gastonia, NC 28054
(704) 834-2000

Overall patient safety: ★★★
Teaching: N

CLINICAL PROGRAM RATINGS:

CARDIAC	★★★	ORTHOPEDICS	★★★
CRITICAL CARE	NR	PULMONARY	★★★
GASTROINTESTINAL	★★★	STROKE	★★★
GENERAL SURGERY	★★★	VASCULAR	★★★
MATERNITY CARE	★★★	WOMEN'S HEALTH	★★★

HEALTHGRADES AWARDS

Franklin Regional Medical Center

100 Hospital Drive
Louisburg, NC 27549
(919) 496-5131

Overall patient safety: ★★★
Teaching: N

CLINICAL PROGRAM RATINGS:

CARDIAC	NR	ORTHOPEDICS	NR
CRITICAL CARE	NR	PULMONARY	★★★
GASTROINTESTINAL	NR	STROKE	★
GENERAL SURGERY	★★★	VASCULAR	NR
MATERNITY CARE	NR	WOMEN'S HEALTH	NR

HEALTHGRADES AWARDS

Good Hope Hospital

410 Denim Drive
Erwin, NC 28339
(910) 897-6151

Overall patient safety: ★★★
Teaching: N

CLINICAL PROGRAM RATINGS:

CARDIAC	NR	ORTHOPEDICS	NR
CRITICAL CARE	NR	PULMONARY	★★★
GASTROINTESTINAL	NR	STROKE	NR
GENERAL SURGERY	NR	VASCULAR	NR
MATERNITY CARE	NR	WOMEN'S HEALTH	NR

HEALTHGRADES AWARDS

Frye Regional Medical Center

420 North Center Street
Hickory, NC 28601
(828) 315-5000

Overall patient safety: ★
Teaching: N

CLINICAL PROGRAM RATINGS:

CARDIAC	★★★	ORTHOPEDICS	★★★
CRITICAL CARE	★★★	PULMONARY	★
GASTROINTESTINAL	★★★	STROKE	★
GENERAL SURGERY	★★★	VASCULAR	★★★
MATERNITY CARE	★★★	WOMEN'S HEALTH	★★★

HEALTHGRADES AWARDS

Grace Hospital

2201 South Sterling Street
Morganton, NC 28655
(828) 580-5000

Overall patient safety: ★★★
Teaching: N

CLINICAL PROGRAM RATINGS:

CARDIAC	NR	ORTHOPEDICS	NR
CRITICAL CARE	NR	PULMONARY	★★★
GASTROINTESTINAL	★★★	STROKE	★★★
GENERAL SURGERY	★★★	VASCULAR	NR
MATERNITY CARE	★★★★★	WOMEN'S HEALTH	NR

HEALTHGRADES AWARDS

✓ SPECIALTY EXCELLENCE
- MATERNITY CARE

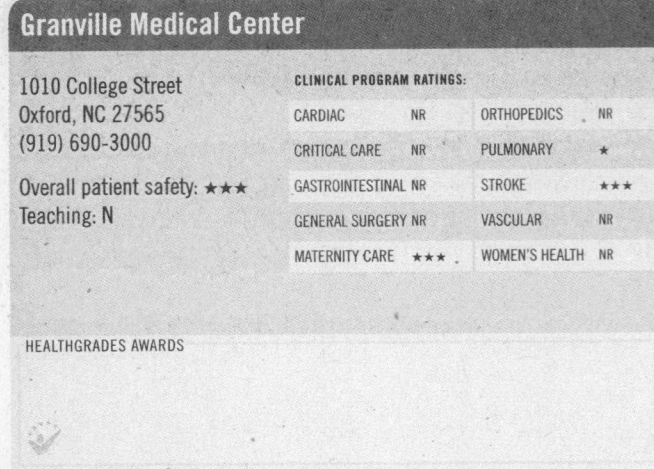

Granville Medical Center

1010 College Street
Oxford, NC 27565
(919) 690-3000

Overall patient safety: ★★★
Teaching: N

CLINICAL PROGRAM RATINGS:

CARDIAC	NR	ORTHOPEDICS	NR
CRITICAL CARE	NR	PULMONARY	★
GASTROINTESTINAL	NR	STROKE	★★★
GENERAL SURGERY	NR	VASCULAR	NR
MATERNITY CARE	★★★	WOMEN'S HEALTH	NR

HEALTHGRADES AWARDS

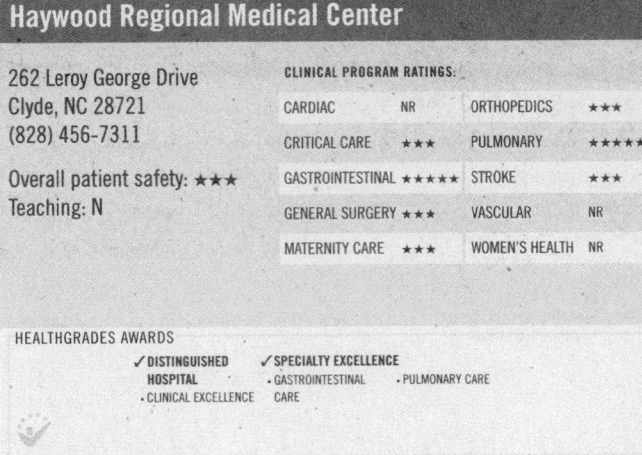

Haywood Regional Medical Center

262 Leroy George Drive
Clyde, NC 28721
(828) 456-7311

Overall patient safety: ★★★
Teaching: N

CLINICAL PROGRAM RATINGS:

CARDIAC	NR	ORTHOPEDICS	★★★
CRITICAL CARE	★★★	PULMONARY	★★★★★
GASTROINTESTINAL	★★★★★	STROKE	★★★
GENERAL SURGERY	★★★	VASCULAR	NR
MATERNITY CARE	★★★	WOMEN'S HEALTH	NR

HEALTHGRADES AWARDS

✓ DISTINGUISHED HOSPITAL
- CLINICAL EXCELLENCE

✓ SPECIALTY EXCELLENCE
- GASTROINTESTINAL CARE
- PULMONARY CARE

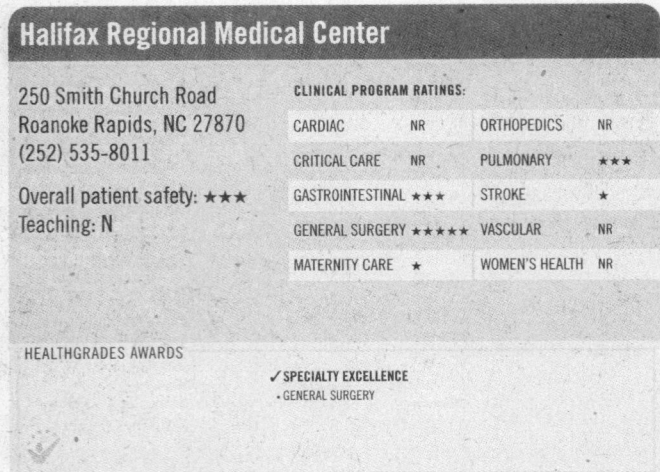

Halifax Regional Medical Center

250 Smith Church Road
Roanoke Rapids, NC 27870
(252) 535-8011

Overall patient safety: ★★★
Teaching: N

CLINICAL PROGRAM RATINGS:

CARDIAC	NR	ORTHOPEDICS	NR
CRITICAL CARE	NR	PULMONARY	★★★
GASTROINTESTINAL	★★★	STROKE	★
GENERAL SURGERY	★★★★★	VASCULAR	NR
MATERNITY CARE	★	WOMEN'S HEALTH	NR

HEALTHGRADES AWARDS

✓ SPECIALTY EXCELLENCE
- GENERAL SURGERY

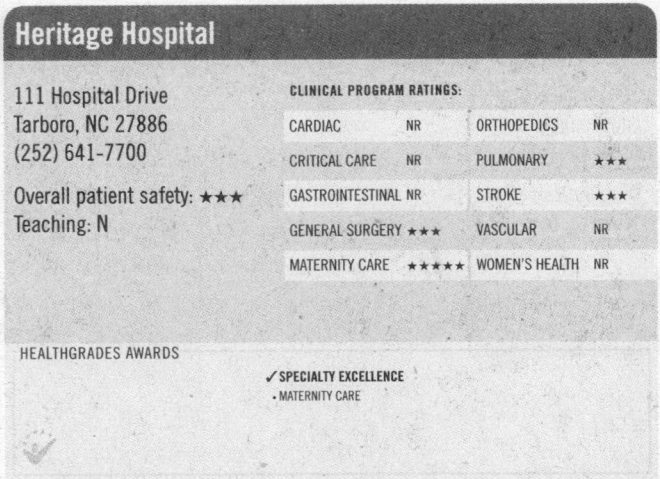

Heritage Hospital

111 Hospital Drive
Tarboro, NC 27886
(252) 641-7700

Overall patient safety: ★★★
Teaching: N

CLINICAL PROGRAM RATINGS:

CARDIAC	NR	ORTHOPEDICS	NR
CRITICAL CARE	NR	PULMONARY	★★★
GASTROINTESTINAL	NR	STROKE	★★★
GENERAL SURGERY	★★★	VASCULAR	NR
MATERNITY CARE	★★★★★	WOMEN'S HEALTH	NR

HEALTHGRADES AWARDS

✓ SPECIALTY EXCELLENCE
- MATERNITY CARE

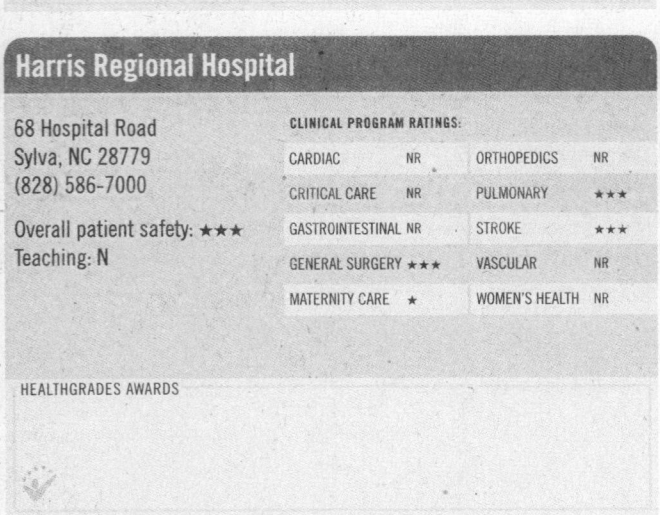

Harris Regional Hospital

68 Hospital Road
Sylva, NC 28779
(828) 586-7000

Overall patient safety: ★★★
Teaching: N

CLINICAL PROGRAM RATINGS:

CARDIAC	NR	ORTHOPEDICS	NR
CRITICAL CARE	NR	PULMONARY	★★★
GASTROINTESTINAL	NR	STROKE	★★★
GENERAL SURGERY	★★★	VASCULAR	NR
MATERNITY CARE	★	WOMEN'S HEALTH	NR

HEALTHGRADES AWARDS

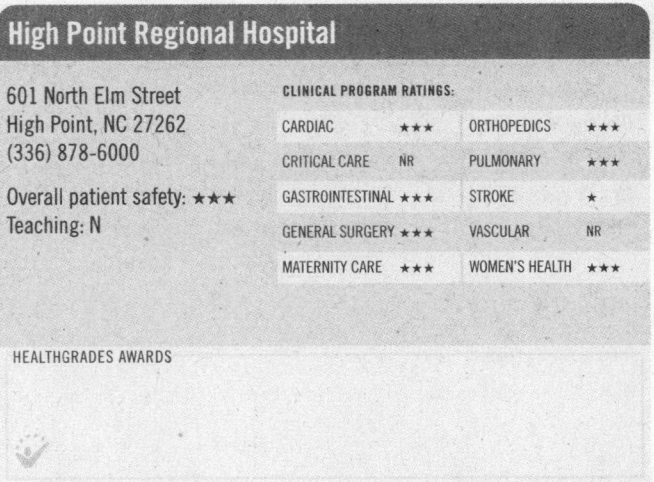

High Point Regional Hospital

601 North Elm Street
High Point, NC 27262
(336) 878-6000

Overall patient safety: ★★★
Teaching: N

CLINICAL PROGRAM RATINGS:

CARDIAC	★★★	ORTHOPEDICS	★★★
CRITICAL CARE	NR	PULMONARY	★★★
GASTROINTESTINAL	★★★	STROKE	★
GENERAL SURGERY	★★★	VASCULAR	NR
MATERNITY CARE	★★★	WOMEN'S HEALTH	★★★

HEALTHGRADES AWARDS

KEY: ★★★★★ BEST   ★★★ AS EXPECTED   ★ POOR   NR NOT RATED BY HEALTHGRADES   For full definitions of ratings and awards, see Appendix.

Hugh Chatham Memorial Hospital

180 Parkwood Drive
Elkin, NC 28621
(336) 527-7000

Overall patient safety: ★★★
Teaching: N

CLINICAL PROGRAM RATINGS:

CARDIAC	NR	ORTHOPEDICS	NR
CRITICAL CARE	NR	PULMONARY	★★★
GASTROINTESTINAL	NR	STROKE	★★★
GENERAL SURGERY	★★★	VASCULAR	NR
MATERNITY CARE	★★★	WOMEN'S HEALTH	NR

HEALTHGRADES AWARDS

Johnston Memorial Hospital

509 North Bright
Leaf Boulevard
Smithfield, NC 27577
(919) 934-8171

Overall patient safety: ★
Teaching: N

CLINICAL PROGRAM RATINGS:

CARDIAC	NR	ORTHOPEDICS	NR
CRITICAL CARE	NR	PULMONARY	★★★
GASTROINTESTINAL	★★★	STROKE	★★★
GENERAL SURGERY	★★★	VASCULAR	NR
MATERNITY CARE	★★★	WOMEN'S HEALTH	NR

HEALTHGRADES AWARDS

Iredell Memorial Hospital

557 Brookdale Drive
Statesville, NC 28677
(704) 873-5661

Overall patient safety: ★★★
Teaching: N

CLINICAL PROGRAM RATINGS:

CARDIAC	NR	ORTHOPEDICS	★★★
CRITICAL CARE	NR	PULMONARY	★★★
GASTROINTESTINAL	★★★	STROKE	★★★
GENERAL SURGERY	★★★	VASCULAR	NR
MATERNITY CARE	★★★	WOMEN'S HEALTH	NR

HEALTHGRADES AWARDS

Kings Mountain Hospital

706 West King Street
Kings Mountain, NC 28086
(704) 739-3601

Overall patient safety: ★★★
Teaching: N

CLINICAL PROGRAM RATINGS:

CARDIAC	NR	ORTHOPEDICS	NR
CRITICAL CARE	NR	PULMONARY	★★★
GASTROINTESTINAL	NR	STROKE	★★★
GENERAL SURGERY	★★★	VASCULAR	NR
MATERNITY CARE	NR	WOMEN'S HEALTH	NR

HEALTHGRADES AWARDS

J. Arthur Dosher Memorial Hospital

924 North Howe Street
Southport, NC 28461
(910) 457-3800

Overall patient safety: ★★★
Teaching: N

CLINICAL PROGRAM RATINGS:

CARDIAC	NR	ORTHOPEDICS	NR
CRITICAL CARE	NR	PULMONARY	★
GASTROINTESTINAL	NR	STROKE	★
GENERAL SURGERY	★★★	VASCULAR	NR
MATERNITY CARE	NR	WOMEN'S HEALTH	NR

HEALTHGRADES AWARDS

Lake Norman Regional Medical Center

171 Fairview Road
Mooresville, NC 28117
(704) 660-4000

Overall patient safety: ★★★
Teaching: N

CLINICAL PROGRAM RATINGS:

CARDIAC	NR	ORTHOPEDICS	NR
CRITICAL CARE	NR	PULMONARY	★★★
GASTROINTESTINAL	★★★	STROKE	★★★
GENERAL SURGERY	★★★	VASCULAR	NR
MATERNITY CARE	★★★	WOMEN'S HEALTH	NR

HEALTHGRADES AWARDS

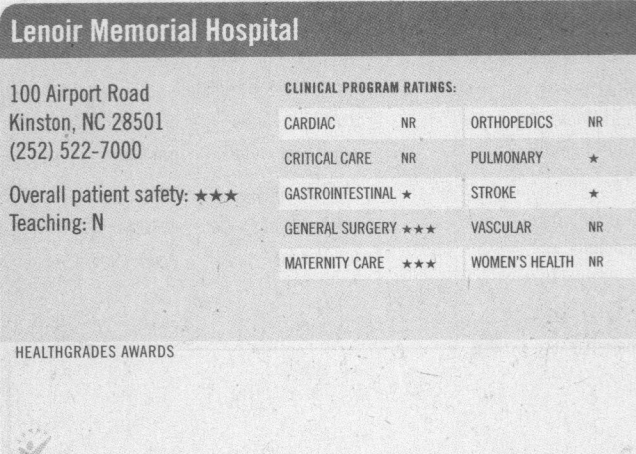

Lenoir Memorial Hospital

100 Airport Road
Kinston, NC 28501
(252) 522-7000

Overall patient safety: ★★★
Teaching: N

CLINICAL PROGRAM RATINGS:

CARDIAC	NR	ORTHOPEDICS	NR
CRITICAL CARE	NR	PULMONARY	★
GASTROINTESTINAL	★	STROKE	★
GENERAL SURGERY	★★★	VASCULAR	NR
MATERNITY CARE	★★★	WOMEN'S HEALTH	NR

HEALTHGRADES AWARDS

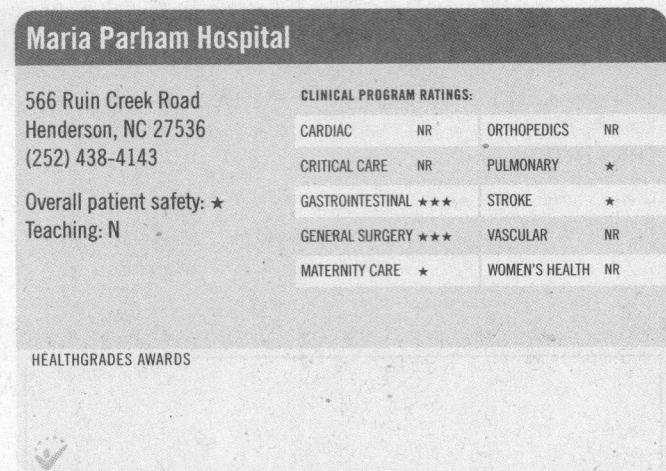

Maria Parham Hospital

566 Ruin Creek Road
Henderson, NC 27536
(252) 438-4143

Overall patient safety: ★
Teaching: N

CLINICAL PROGRAM RATINGS:

CARDIAC	NR	ORTHOPEDICS	NR
CRITICAL CARE	NR	PULMONARY	★
GASTROINTESTINAL	★★★	STROKE	★
GENERAL SURGERY	★★★	VASCULAR	NR
MATERNITY CARE	★	WOMEN'S HEALTH	NR

HEALTHGRADES AWARDS

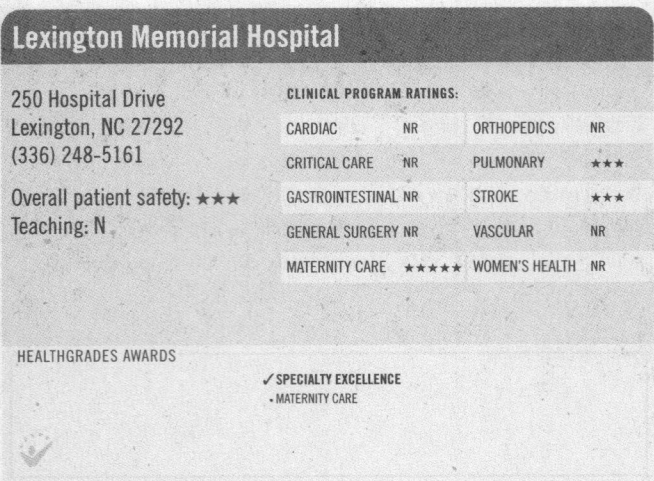

Lexington Memorial Hospital

250 Hospital Drive
Lexington, NC 27292
(336) 248-5161

Overall patient safety: ★★★
Teaching: N

CLINICAL PROGRAM RATINGS:

CARDIAC	NR	ORTHOPEDICS	NR
CRITICAL CARE	NR	PULMONARY	★★★
GASTROINTESTINAL	NR	STROKE	★★★
GENERAL SURGERY	NR	VASCULAR	NR
MATERNITY CARE	★★★★★	WOMEN'S HEALTH	NR

HEALTHGRADES AWARDS

✓ SPECIALTY EXCELLENCE
- MATERNITY CARE

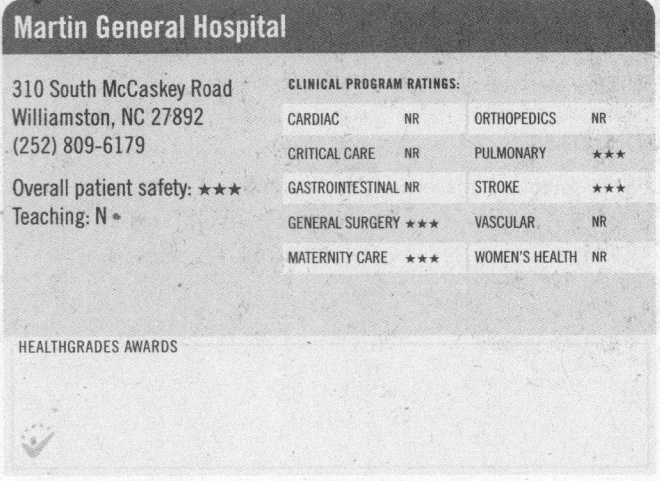

Martin General Hospital

310 South McCaskey Road
Williamston, NC 27892
(252) 809-6179

Overall patient safety: ★★★
Teaching: N

CLINICAL PROGRAM RATINGS:

CARDIAC	NR	ORTHOPEDICS	NR
CRITICAL CARE	NR	PULMONARY	★★★
GASTROINTESTINAL	NR	STROKE	★★★
GENERAL SURGERY	★★★	VASCULAR	NR
MATERNITY CARE	★★★	WOMEN'S HEALTH	NR

HEALTHGRADES AWARDS

Margaret R. Pardee Memorial Hospital

800 North Justice Street
Hendersonville, NC 28791
(828) 696-1000

Overall patient safety: ★★★
Teaching: Y

CLINICAL PROGRAM RATINGS:

CARDIAC	NR	ORTHOPEDICS	NR
CRITICAL CARE	★★★	PULMONARY	★★★
GASTROINTESTINAL	★★★	STROKE	★★★
GENERAL SURGERY	★★★	VASCULAR	NR
MATERNITY CARE	★★★	WOMEN'S HEALTH	NR

HEALTHGRADES AWARDS

✓ SPECIALTY EXCELLENCE
- JOINT REPLACEMENT

McDowell Hospital

430 Rankin Drive
Marion, NC 28752
(828) 659-5000

Overall patient safety: ★★★
Teaching: N

CLINICAL PROGRAM RATINGS:

CARDIAC	NR	ORTHOPEDICS	NR
CRITICAL CARE	NR	PULMONARY	★★★
GASTROINTESTINAL	NR	STROKE	★★★
GENERAL SURGERY	★★★	VASCULAR	NR
MATERNITY CARE	★	WOMEN'S HEALTH	NR

HEALTHGRADES AWARDS

KEY: ★★★★★ BEST ★★★ AS EXPECTED ★ POOR NR NOT RATED BY HEALTHGRADES For full definitions of ratings and awards, see Appendix.

Medical Park Hospital

1950 South Hawthorne Road
Winston-Salem, NC 27103
(336) 718-0600

Overall patient safety: ★★★★★
Teaching: N

CLINICAL PROGRAM RATINGS:

CARDIAC	NR	ORTHOPEDICS	NR
CRITICAL CARE	NR	PULMONARY	NR
GASTROINTESTINAL	NR	STROKE	NR
GENERAL SURGERY	NR	VASCULAR	NR
MATERNITY CARE	NR	WOMEN'S HEALTH	NR

HEALTHGRADES AWARDS

Moses H. Cone Memorial Hospital*

1200 North Elm Street
Greensboro, NC 27401
(336) 832-7000

Overall patient safety: ★★★
Teaching: Y

CLINICAL PROGRAM RATINGS:

CARDIAC	★★★	ORTHOPEDICS	★★★
CRITICAL CARE	NR	PULMONARY	★★★
GASTROINTESTINAL	★★★	STROKE	★★★
GENERAL SURGERY	★★★★★	VASCULAR	★★★
MATERNITY CARE	★★★	WOMEN'S HEALTH	★★★

HEALTHGRADES AWARDS

✓ SPECIALTY EXCELLENCE
- GENERAL SURGERY

Mission Hospitals—Memorial Campus*

509 Biltmore Avenue
Asheville, NC 28801
(828) 213-1111

Overall patient safety: ★★★★★
Teaching: Y

CLINICAL PROGRAM RATINGS:

CARDIAC	★★★	ORTHOPEDICS	★★★
CRITICAL CARE	★★★	PULMONARY	★★★★★
GASTROINTESTINAL	★★★★★	STROKE	★★★
GENERAL SURGERY	★★★	VASCULAR	★★★
MATERNITY CARE	★	WOMEN'S HEALTH	★★★

HEALTHGRADES AWARDS

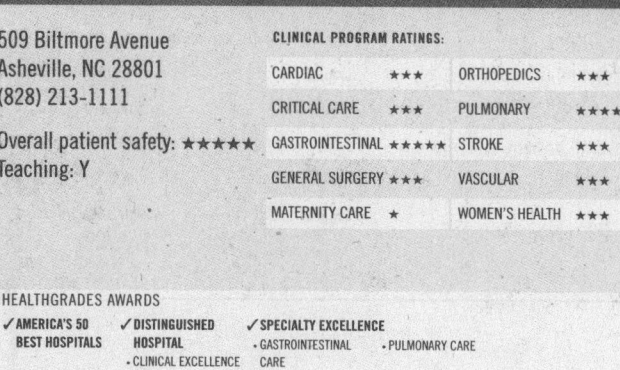

✓ AMERICA'S 50 BEST HOSPITALS

✓ DISTINGUISHED HOSPITAL
- CLINICAL EXCELLENCE
- PATIENT SAFETY

✓ SPECIALTY EXCELLENCE
- GASTROINTESTINAL CARE
- PULMONARY CARE

Murphy Medical Center

4130 US Highway 64 East
Murphy, NC 28906
(828) 837-8161

Overall patient safety: ★★★
Teaching: N

CLINICAL PROGRAM RATINGS:

CARDIAC	NR	ORTHOPEDICS	NR
CRITICAL CARE	NR	PULMONARY	★★★
GASTROINTESTINAL	NR	STROKE	★★★
GENERAL SURGERY	★	VASCULAR	NR
MATERNITY CARE	★	WOMEN'S HEALTH	NR

HEALTHGRADES AWARDS

Morehead Memorial Hospital

117 East Kings Highway
Eden, NC 27288
(336) 623-9711

Overall patient safety: ★★★
Teaching: N

CLINICAL PROGRAM RATINGS:

CARDIAC	NR	ORTHOPEDICS	NR
CRITICAL CARE	NR	PULMONARY	★★★
GASTROINTESTINAL	NR	STROKE	★
GENERAL SURGERY	★★★	VASCULAR	NR
MATERNITY CARE	★★★	WOMEN'S HEALTH	NR

HEALTHGRADES AWARDS

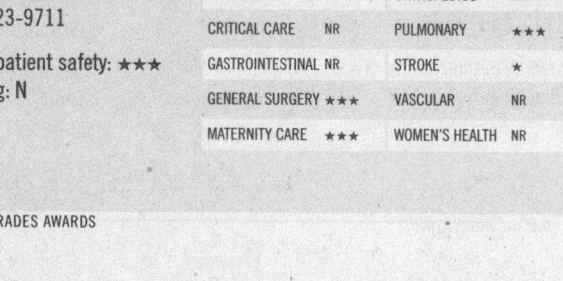

Nash General Hospital

2460 Curtis Ellis Drive
Rocky Mount, NC 27804
(252) 443-8000

Overall patient safety: ★★★
Teaching: N

CLINICAL PROGRAM RATINGS:

CARDIAC	NR	ORTHOPEDICS	★★★
CRITICAL CARE	NR	PULMONARY	★★★
GASTROINTESTINAL	★★★	STROKE	★★★
GENERAL SURGERY	★★★	VASCULAR	NR
MATERNITY CARE	★★★	WOMEN'S HEALTH	NR

HEALTHGRADES AWARDS

✓ DISTINGUISHED HOSPITAL
- CLINICAL EXCELLENCE

*This hospital reports its data to the federal government jointly with another hospital. Therefore the ratings and awards apply to multiple hospitals and this specific hospital may not provide all rated services.

New Hanover Regional Medical Center*

2131 South 17th Street
Wilmington, NC 28401
(910) 343-7000

Overall patient safety: ★★★
Teaching: Y

CLINICAL PROGRAM RATINGS:

CARDIAC	★	ORTHOPEDICS	★★★★★
CRITICAL CARE	NR	PULMONARY	★★★
GASTROINTESTINAL	★★★	STROKE	★★★
GENERAL SURGERY	★★★	VASCULAR	★★★
MATERNITY CARE	★★★	WOMEN'S HEALTH	★★★

HEALTHGRADES AWARDS

✓ SPECIALTY EXCELLENCE
- BARIATRIC SURGERY
- ORTHOPEDIC SURGERY

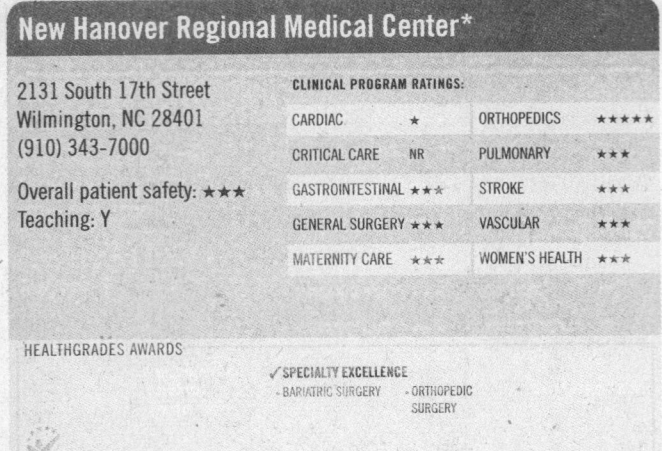

Onslow Memorial Hospital

317 Western Boulevard
Jacksonville, NC 28541
(910) 577-2345

Overall patient safety: ★
Teaching: N

CLINICAL PROGRAM RATINGS:

CARDIAC	NR	ORTHOPEDICS	NR
CRITICAL CARE	NR	PULMONARY	★
GASTROINTESTINAL	★★★	STROKE	★
GENERAL SURGERY	★★★	VASCULAR	NR
MATERNITY CARE	★★★★★	WOMEN'S HEALTH	NR

HEALTHGRADES AWARDS

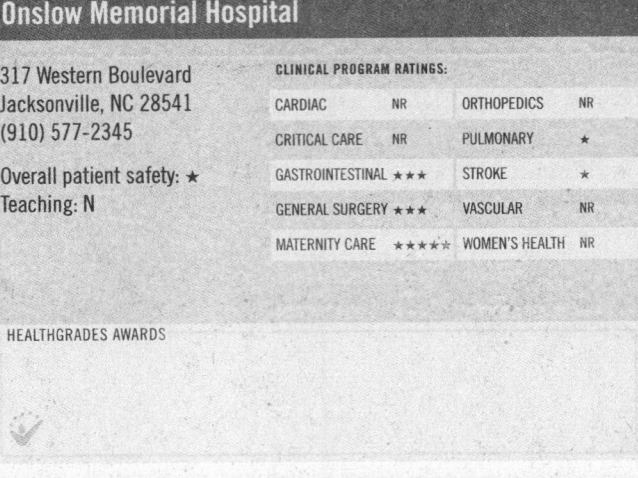

North Carolina Baptist Hospital

Medical Center Boulevard
Winston-Salem, NC 27157
(336) 716-2011

Overall patient safety: ★
Teaching: Y

CLINICAL PROGRAM RATINGS:

CARDIAC	★★★	ORTHOPEDICS	★★★
CRITICAL CARE	NR	PULMONARY	★★★★★
GASTROINTESTINAL	★★★	STROKE	★★★★★
GENERAL SURGERY	★★★	VASCULAR	★★★
MATERNITY CARE	NR	WOMEN'S HEALTH	NR

HEALTHGRADES AWARDS

✓ SPECIALTY EXCELLENCE
- PULMONARY CARE

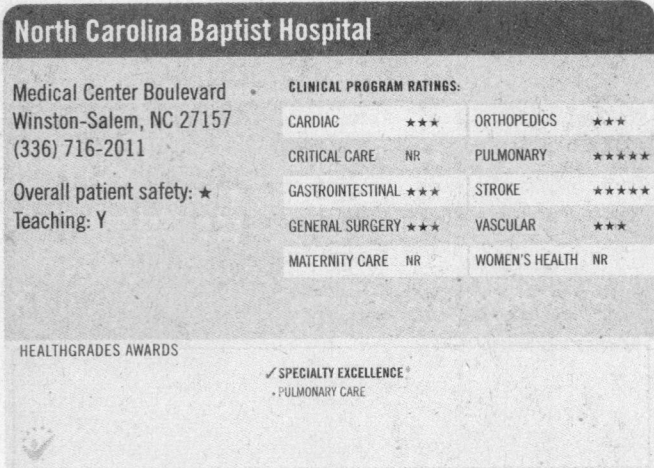

Park Ridge Hospital

Naples Road
Fletcher, NC 28732
(828) 684-8501

Overall patient safety: ★★★
Teaching: N

CLINICAL PROGRAM RATINGS:

CARDIAC	NR	ORTHOPEDICS	★★★
CRITICAL CARE	NR	PULMONARY	★★★
GASTROINTESTINAL	NR	STROKE	★★★
GENERAL SURGERY	★★★	VASCULAR	NR
MATERNITY CARE	★★★	WOMEN'S HEALTH	NR

HEALTHGRADES AWARDS

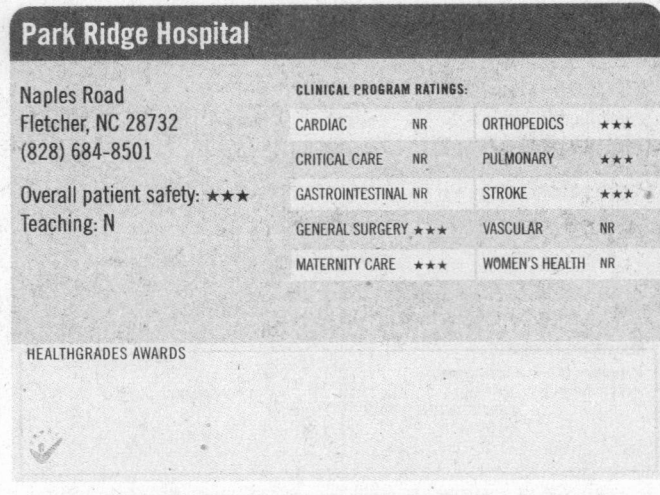

Northern Hospital of Surry County

830 Rockford Street
Mount Airy, NC 27030
(336) 719-7000

Overall patient safety: ★★★
Teaching: N

CLINICAL PROGRAM RATINGS:

CARDIAC	NR	ORTHOPEDICS	NR
CRITICAL CARE	NR	PULMONARY	★★★★★
GASTROINTESTINAL	NR	STROKE	★★★
GENERAL SURGERY	★★★	VASCULAR	NR
MATERNITY CARE	★★★	WOMEN'S HEALTH	NR

HEALTHGRADES AWARDS

✓ SPECIALTY EXCELLENCE
- PULMONARY CARE

Pender Memorial Hospital

507 East Fremont Street
Burgaw, NC 28425
(910) 259-5451

Overall patient safety: ★★★
Teaching: N

CLINICAL PROGRAM RATINGS:

CARDIAC	NR	ORTHOPEDICS	NR
CRITICAL CARE	NR	PULMONARY	★★★
GASTROINTESTINAL	NR	STROKE	NR
GENERAL SURGERY	NR	VASCULAR	NR
MATERNITY CARE	NR	WOMEN'S HEALTH	NR

HEALTHGRADES AWARDS

KEY: ★★★★★ BEST   ★★★ AS EXPECTED   ★ POOR   NR NOT RATED BY HEALTHGRADES   For full definitions of ratings and awards, see Appendix.

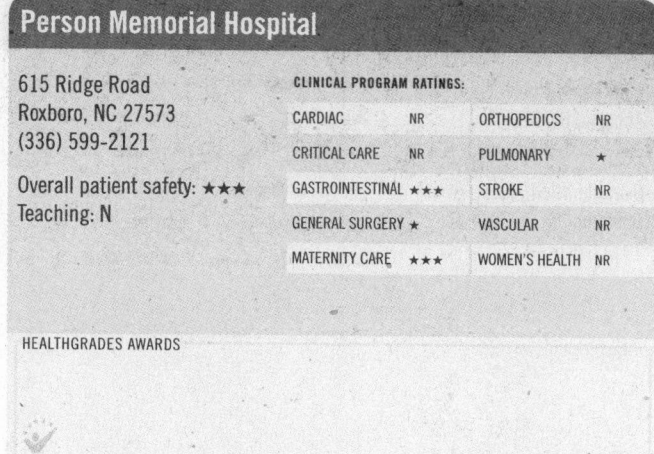

Person Memorial Hospital

615 Ridge Road
Roxboro, NC 27573
(336) 599-2121

Overall patient safety: ★★★
Teaching: N

CLINICAL PROGRAM RATINGS:

CARDIAC	NR	ORTHOPEDICS	NR
CRITICAL CARE	NR	PULMONARY	★
GASTROINTESTINAL	★★★	STROKE	NR
GENERAL SURGERY	★	VASCULAR	NR
MATERNITY CARE	★★★	WOMEN'S HEALTH	NR

HEALTHGRADES AWARDS

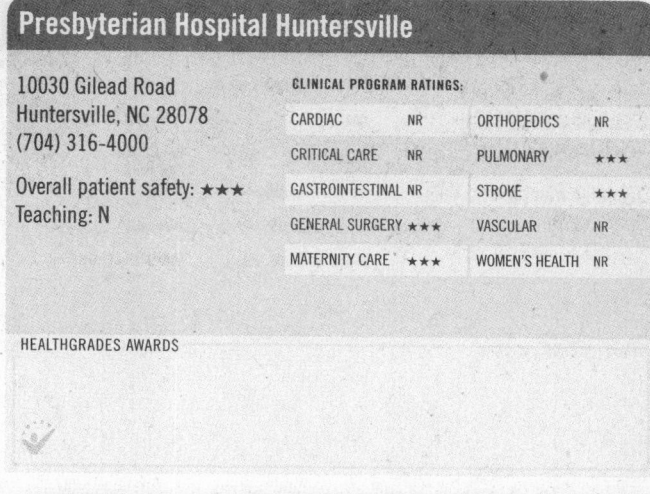

Presbyterian Hospital Huntersville

10030 Gilead Road
Huntersville, NC 28078
(704) 316-4000

Overall patient safety: ★★★
Teaching: N

CLINICAL PROGRAM RATINGS:

CARDIAC	NR	ORTHOPEDICS	NR
CRITICAL CARE	NR	PULMONARY	★★★
GASTROINTESTINAL	NR	STROKE	★★★
GENERAL SURGERY	★★★	VASCULAR	NR
MATERNITY CARE	★★★	WOMEN'S HEALTH	NR

HEALTHGRADES AWARDS

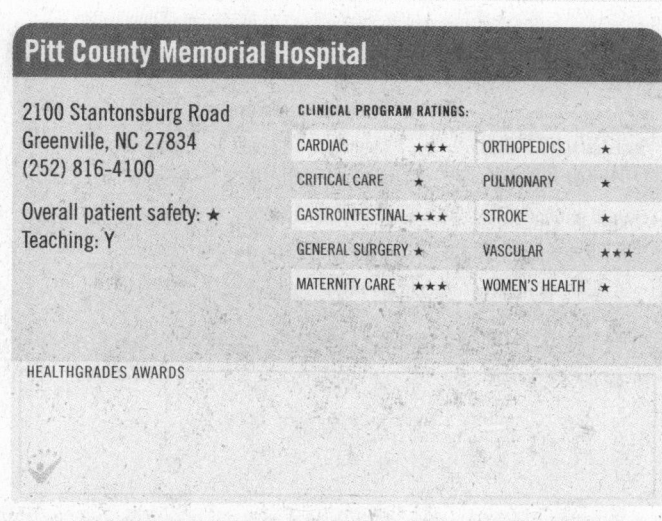

Pitt County Memorial Hospital

2100 Stantonsburg Road
Greenville, NC 27834
(252) 816-4100

Overall patient safety: ★
Teaching: Y

CLINICAL PROGRAM RATINGS:

CARDIAC	★★★	ORTHOPEDICS	★
CRITICAL CARE	★	PULMONARY	★
GASTROINTESTINAL	★★★	STROKE	★
GENERAL SURGERY	★	VASCULAR	★★★
MATERNITY CARE	★★★	WOMEN'S HEALTH	★

HEALTHGRADES AWARDS

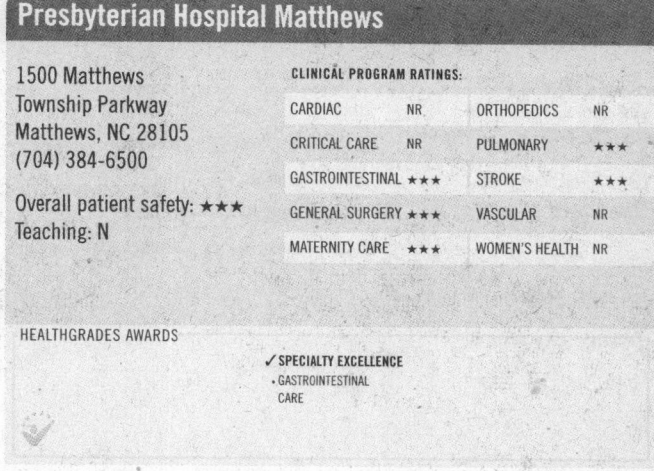

Presbyterian Hospital Matthews

1500 Matthews
Township Parkway
Matthews, NC 28105
(704) 384-6500

Overall patient safety: ★★★
Teaching: N

CLINICAL PROGRAM RATINGS:

CARDIAC	NR	ORTHOPEDICS	NR
CRITICAL CARE	NR	PULMONARY	★★★
GASTROINTESTINAL	★★★	STROKE	★★★
GENERAL SURGERY	★★★	VASCULAR	NR
MATERNITY CARE	★★★	WOMEN'S HEALTH	NR

HEALTHGRADES AWARDS

✓ SPECIALTY EXCELLENCE
• GASTROINTESTINAL
  CARE

Presbyterian Hospital

200 Hawthorne Lane
Charlotte, NC 28204
(704) 384-4000

Overall patient safety: ★★★
Teaching: N

CLINICAL PROGRAM RATINGS:

CARDIAC	★★★	ORTHOPEDICS	NR
CRITICAL CARE	NR	PULMONARY	★★★
GASTROINTESTINAL	★★★	STROKE	★★★
GENERAL SURGERY	★★★	VASCULAR	★★★
MATERNITY CARE	★	WOMEN'S HEALTH	★

HEALTHGRADES AWARDS

Presbyterian Orthopaedic Hospital

1901 Randolph Road
Charlotte, NC 28207
(704) 375-6792

Overall patient safety: ★★★★★
Teaching: N

CLINICAL PROGRAM RATINGS:

CARDIAC	NR	ORTHOPEDICS	★★★★★
CRITICAL CARE	NR	PULMONARY	NR
GASTROINTESTINAL	NR	STROKE	NR
GENERAL SURGERY	NR	VASCULAR	NR
MATERNITY CARE	NR	WOMEN'S HEALTH	NR

HEALTHGRADES AWARDS

✓ SPECIALTY EXCELLENCE
• JOINT REPLACEMENT

*This hospital reports its data to the federal government jointly with another hospital. Therefore the ratings and awards apply to multiple hospitals and this specific hospital may not provide all rated services.

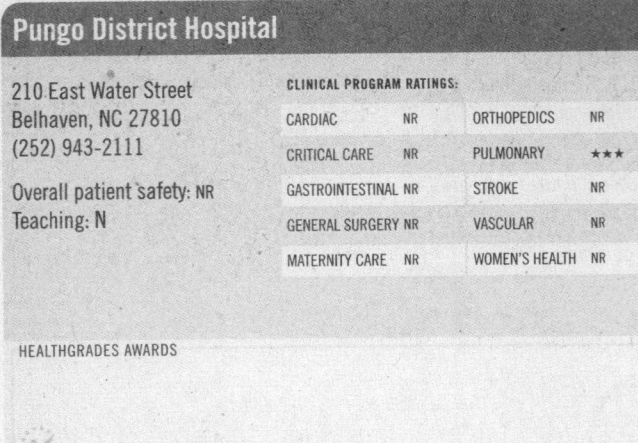

Pungo District Hospital

210 East Water Street
Belhaven, NC 27810
(252) 943-2111

Overall patient safety: NR
Teaching: N

CLINICAL PROGRAM RATINGS:

CARDIAC	NR	ORTHOPEDICS	NR
CRITICAL CARE	NR	PULMONARY	★★★
GASTROINTESTINAL	NR	STROKE	NR
GENERAL SURGERY	NR	VASCULAR	NR
MATERNITY CARE	NR	WOMEN'S HEALTH	NR

HEALTHGRADES AWARDS

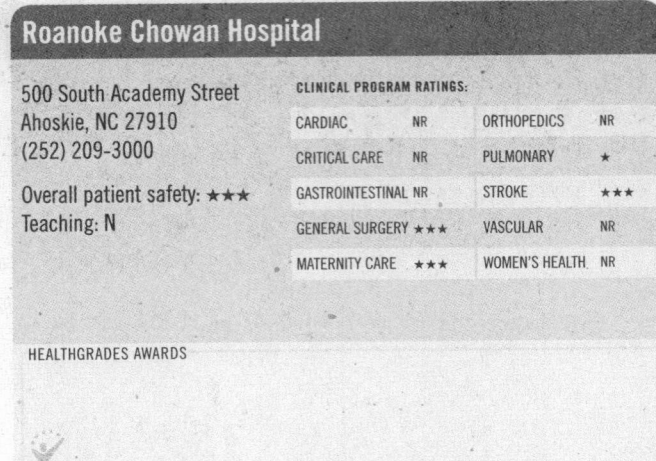

Roanoke Chowan Hospital

500 South Academy Street
Ahoskie, NC 27910
(252) 209-3000

Overall patient safety: ★★★
Teaching: N

CLINICAL PROGRAM RATINGS:

CARDIAC	NR	ORTHOPEDICS	NR
CRITICAL CARE	NR	PULMONARY	★
GASTROINTESTINAL	NR	STROKE	★★★
GENERAL SURGERY	★★★	VASCULAR	NR
MATERNITY CARE	★★★	WOMEN'S HEALTH	NR

HEALTHGRADES AWARDS

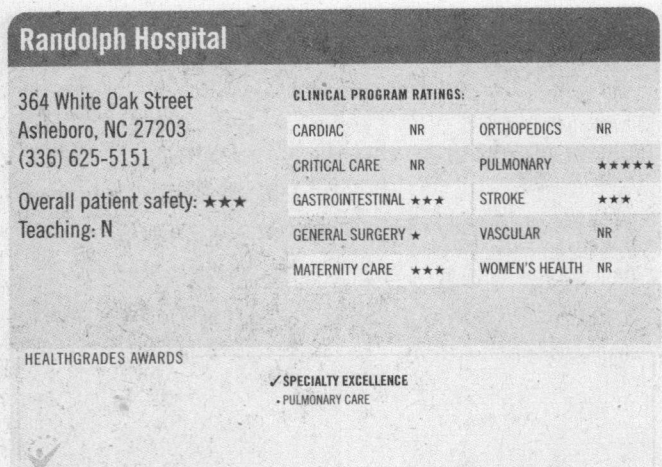

Randolph Hospital

364 White Oak Street
Asheboro, NC 27203
(336) 625-5151

Overall patient safety: ★★★
Teaching: N

CLINICAL PROGRAM RATINGS:

CARDIAC	NR	ORTHOPEDICS	NR
CRITICAL CARE	NR	PULMONARY	★★★★★
GASTROINTESTINAL	★★★	STROKE	★★★
GENERAL SURGERY	★	VASCULAR	NR
MATERNITY CARE	★★★	WOMEN'S HEALTH	NR

HEALTHGRADES AWARDS

✓ SPECIALTY EXCELLENCE
- PULMONARY CARE

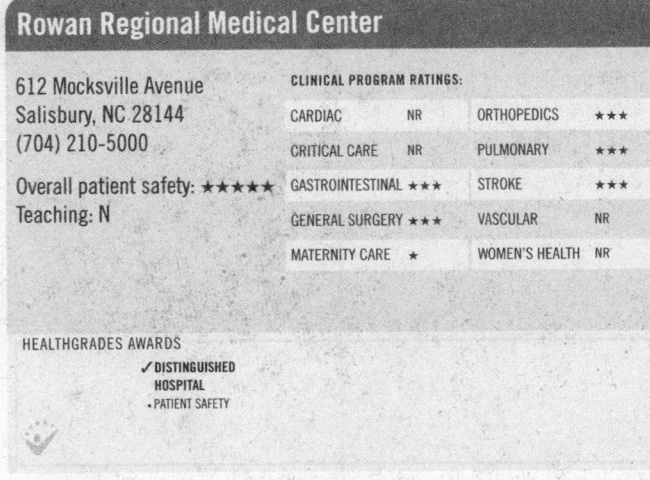

Rowan Regional Medical Center

612 Mocksville Avenue
Salisbury, NC 28144
(704) 210-5000

Overall patient safety: ★★★★★
Teaching: N

CLINICAL PROGRAM RATINGS:

CARDIAC	NR	ORTHOPEDICS	★★★
CRITICAL CARE	NR	PULMONARY	★★★
GASTROINTESTINAL	★★★	STROKE	★★★
GENERAL SURGERY	★★★	VASCULAR	NR
MATERNITY CARE	★	WOMEN'S HEALTH	NR

HEALTHGRADES AWARDS

✓ DISTINGUISHED
  HOSPITAL
- PATIENT SAFETY

Rex Hospital

4420 Lake Boone Trail
Raleigh, NC 27607
(919) 784-3100

Overall patient safety: ★★★★★
Teaching: N

CLINICAL PROGRAM RATINGS:

CARDIAC	★★★	ORTHOPEDICS	★
CRITICAL CARE	★★★	PULMONARY	★★★★★
GASTROINTESTINAL	★★★	STROKE	★★★★★
GENERAL SURGERY	★★★	VASCULAR	★★★
MATERNITY CARE	★★★	WOMEN'S HEALTH	NR

HEALTHGRADES AWARDS

✓ DISTINGUISHED   ✓ SPECIALTY EXCELLENCE
  HOSPITAL   - GASTROINTESTINAL   - PULMONARY CARE   - STROKE CARE
- CLINICAL EXCELLENCE   CARE
- PATIENT SAFETY

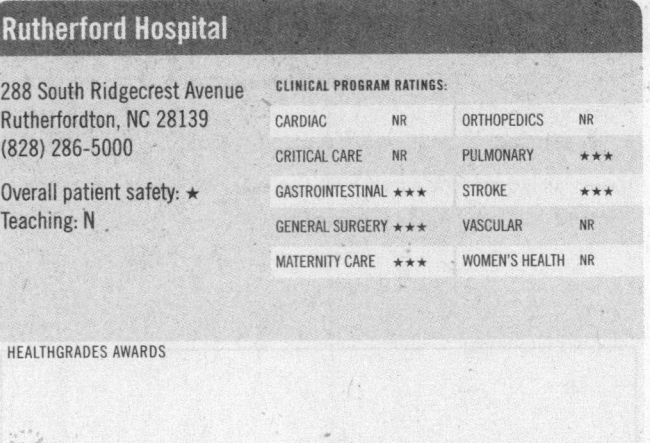

Rutherford Hospital

288 South Ridgecrest Avenue
Rutherfordton, NC 28139
(828) 286-5000

Overall patient safety: ★
Teaching: N

CLINICAL PROGRAM RATINGS:

CARDIAC	NR	ORTHOPEDICS	NR
CRITICAL CARE	NR	PULMONARY	★★★
GASTROINTESTINAL	★★★	STROKE	★★★
GENERAL SURGERY	★★★	VASCULAR	NR
MATERNITY CARE	★★★	WOMEN'S HEALTH	NR

HEALTHGRADES AWARDS

KEY: ★★★★★ BEST   ★★★ AS EXPECTED   ★ POOR   NR NOT RATED BY HEALTHGRADES   For full definitions of ratings and awards, see Appendix.

St. Joseph's Hospital*

428 Biltmore Avenue
Asheville, NC 28801
(828) 213-1111

Overall patient safety: ★★★
Teaching: N

CLINICAL PROGRAM RATINGS:

CARDIAC	★★★	ORTHOPEDICS	★★★
CRITICAL CARE	★★★	PULMONARY	★★★★★
GASTROINTESTINAL	★★★★★	STROKE	★★★
GENERAL SURGERY	★★★	VASCULAR	★★★
MATERNITY CARE	NR	WOMEN'S HEALTH	NR

HEALTHGRADES AWARDS

✓ SPECIALTY EXCELLENCE
• GASTROINTESTINAL   • PULMONARY CARE
CARE

St. Luke's Hospital

101 Hospital Drive
Columbus, NC 28722
(828) 894-3311

Overall patient safety: ★★★
Teaching: N

CLINICAL PROGRAM RATINGS:

CARDIAC	NR	ORTHOPEDICS	NR
CRITICAL CARE	NR	PULMONARY	★★★
GASTROINTESTINAL	NR	STROKE	★★★
GENERAL SURGERY	★★★	VASCULAR	NR
MATERNITY CARE	NR	WOMEN'S HEALTH	NR

HEALTHGRADES AWARDS

Sampson Regional Medical Center

607 Beaman Street
Clinton, NC 28328
(910) 592-8511

Overall patient safety: ★★★
Teaching: N

CLINICAL PROGRAM RATINGS:

CARDIAC	NR	ORTHOPEDICS	NR
CRITICAL CARE	NR	PULMONARY	★
GASTROINTESTINAL	★★★	STROKE	★★★
GENERAL SURGERY	★★★	VASCULAR	NR
MATERNITY CARE	★★★	WOMEN'S HEALTH	NR

HEALTHGRADES AWARDS

Sandhills Regional Medical Center

1000 West Hamlet Avenue
Hamlet, NC 28345
(910) 205-8000

Overall patient safety: ★★★
Teaching: N

CLINICAL PROGRAM RATINGS:

CARDIAC	NR	ORTHOPEDICS	NR
CRITICAL CARE	NR	PULMONARY	★
GASTROINTESTINAL	NR	STROKE	★
GENERAL SURGERY	★★★	VASCULAR	NR
MATERNITY CARE	NR	WOMEN'S HEALTH	NR

HEALTHGRADES AWARDS

Scotland Memorial Hospital

500 Lauchwood Drive
Laurinburg, NC 28352
(910) 291-7000

Overall patient safety: ★★★
Teaching: N

CLINICAL PROGRAM RATINGS:

CARDIAC	NR	ORTHOPEDICS	NR
CRITICAL CARE	NR	PULMONARY	★★★
GASTROINTESTINAL	NR	STROKE	★
GENERAL SURGERY	NR	VASCULAR	NR
MATERNITY CARE	★★★	WOMEN'S HEALTH	NR

HEALTHGRADES AWARDS

Southeastern Regional Medical Center

300 West 27th Street
Lumberton, NC 28358
(910) 671-5000

Overall patient safety: ★★★
Teaching: N

CLINICAL PROGRAM RATINGS:

CARDIAC	NR	ORTHOPEDICS	★★★
CRITICAL CARE	NR	PULMONARY	★★★
GASTROINTESTINAL	★★★	STROKE	★★★
GENERAL SURGERY	★	VASCULAR	NR
MATERNITY CARE	★★★	WOMEN'S HEALTH	NR

HEALTHGRADES AWARDS

*This hospital reports its data to the federal government jointly with another hospital. Therefore the ratings and awards apply to multiple hospitals and this specific hospital may not provide all rated services.

Spruce Pine Community Hospital

125 Hospital Drive
Spruce Pine, NC 28777
(828) 765-4201

Overall patient safety: ★★★
Teaching: N

CLINICAL PROGRAM RATINGS:

CARDIAC	NR	ORTHOPEDICS	NR
CRITICAL CARE	NR	PULMONARY	★★★
GASTROINTESTINAL	NR	STROKE	★
GENERAL SURGERY	NR	VASCULAR	NR
MATERNITY CARE	★	WOMEN'S HEALTH	NR

HEALTHGRADES AWARDS

Swain County Hospital

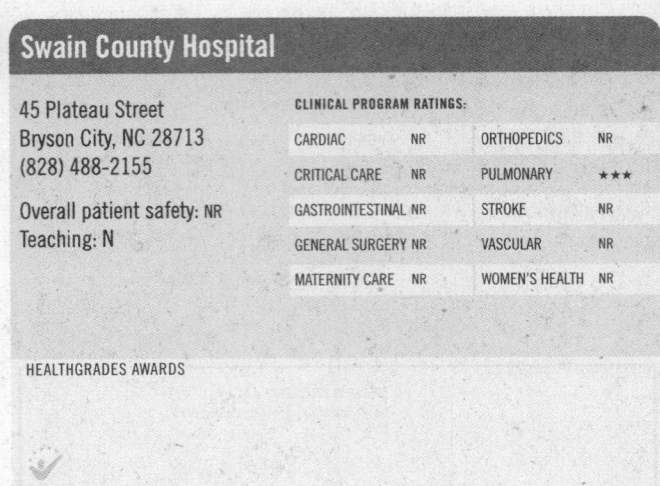

45 Plateau Street
Bryson City, NC 28713
(828) 488-2155

Overall patient safety: NR
Teaching: N

CLINICAL PROGRAM RATINGS:

CARDIAC	NR	ORTHOPEDICS	NR
CRITICAL CARE	NR	PULMONARY	★★★
GASTROINTESTINAL	NR	STROKE	NR
GENERAL SURGERY	NR	VASCULAR	NR
MATERNITY CARE	NR	WOMEN'S HEALTH	NR

HEALTHGRADES AWARDS

Stanly Memorial Hospital

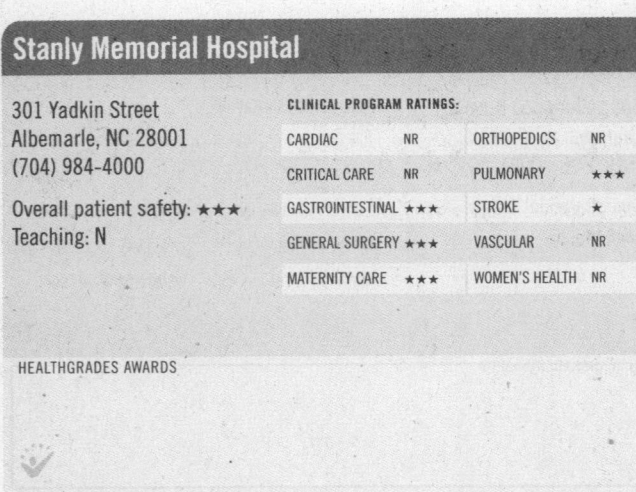

301 Yadkin Street
Albemarle, NC 28001
(704) 984-4000

Overall patient safety: ★★★
Teaching: N

CLINICAL PROGRAM RATINGS:

CARDIAC	NR	ORTHOPEDICS	NR
CRITICAL CARE	NR	PULMONARY	★★★
GASTROINTESTINAL	★★★	STROKE	★
GENERAL SURGERY	★★★	VASCULAR	NR
MATERNITY CARE	★★★	WOMEN'S HEALTH	NR

HEALTHGRADES AWARDS

Thomasville Medical Center

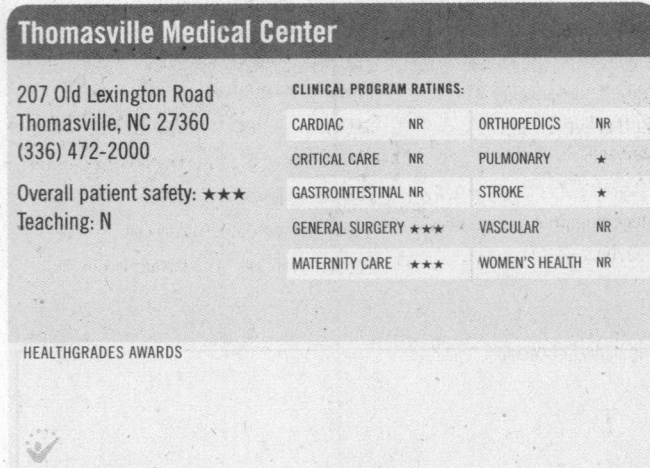

207 Old Lexington Road
Thomasville, NC 27360
(336) 472-2000

Overall patient safety: ★★★
Teaching: N

CLINICAL PROGRAM RATINGS:

CARDIAC	NR	ORTHOPEDICS	NR
CRITICAL CARE	NR	PULMONARY	★
GASTROINTESTINAL	NR	STROKE	★
GENERAL SURGERY	★★★	VASCULAR	NR
MATERNITY CARE	★★★	WOMEN'S HEALTH	NR

HEALTHGRADES AWARDS

Stokes-Reynolds Memorial Hospital

1570 NC 8 and Highway 89
North
Danbury, NC 27016
(336) 593-2831

Overall patient safety: ★★★
Teaching: N

CLINICAL PROGRAM RATINGS:

CARDIAC	NR	ORTHOPEDICS	NR
CRITICAL CARE	NR	PULMONARY	★★★
GASTROINTESTINAL	NR	STROKE	NR
GENERAL SURGERY	NR	VASCULAR	NR
MATERNITY CARE	NR	WOMEN'S HEALTH	NR

HEALTHGRADES AWARDS

Transylvania Community Hospital

90 Hospital Drive
Brevard, NC 28712
(828) 884-9111

Overall patient safety: ★★★
Teaching: N

CLINICAL PROGRAM RATINGS:

CARDIAC	NR	ORTHOPEDICS	NR
CRITICAL CARE	NR	PULMONARY	★★★
GASTROINTESTINAL	NR	STROKE	★
GENERAL SURGERY	★★★	VASCULAR	NR
MATERNITY CARE	★★★	WOMEN'S HEALTH	NR

HEALTHGRADES AWARDS

KEY: ★★★★★ BEST   ★★★ AS EXPECTED   ★ POOR   NR NOT RATED BY HEALTHGRADES   For full definitions of ratings and awards, see Appendix.

University of North Carolina Hospital

101 Manning Drive
Chapel Hill, NC 27514
(919) 966-4131

Overall patient safety: ★
Teaching: Y

CLINICAL PROGRAM RATINGS:

CARDIAC	★★★	ORTHOPEDICS	★★★
CRITICAL CARE	★★★	PULMONARY	★★★
GASTROINTESTINAL	★★★	STROKE	★★★
GENERAL SURGERY	★	VASCULAR	★★★
MATERNITY CARE	★	WOMEN'S HEALTH	★

HEALTHGRADES AWARDS

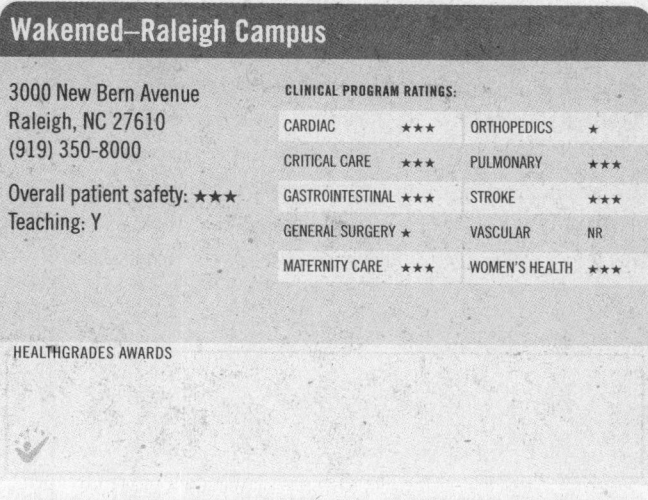

Wakemed—Raleigh Campus

3000 New Bern Avenue
Raleigh, NC 27610
(919) 350-8000

Overall patient safety: ★★★
Teaching: Y

CLINICAL PROGRAM RATINGS:

CARDIAC	★★★	ORTHOPEDICS	★
CRITICAL CARE	★★★	PULMONARY	★★★
GASTROINTESTINAL	★★★	STROKE	★★★
GENERAL SURGERY	★	VASCULAR	NR
MATERNITY CARE	★★★	WOMEN'S HEALTH	★★★

HEALTHGRADES AWARDS

Valdese General Hospital

720 Malcolm Boulevard
Rutherford College
Valdese, NC 28690
(828) 874-2251

Overall patient safety: ★★★
Teaching: N

CLINICAL PROGRAM RATINGS:

CARDIAC	NR	ORTHOPEDICS	NR
CRITICAL CARE	NR	PULMONARY	★★★
GASTROINTESTINAL	★★★	STROKE	★★★
GENERAL SURGERY	★★★	VASCULAR	NR
MATERNITY CARE	NR	WOMEN'S HEALTH	NR

HEALTHGRADES AWARDS

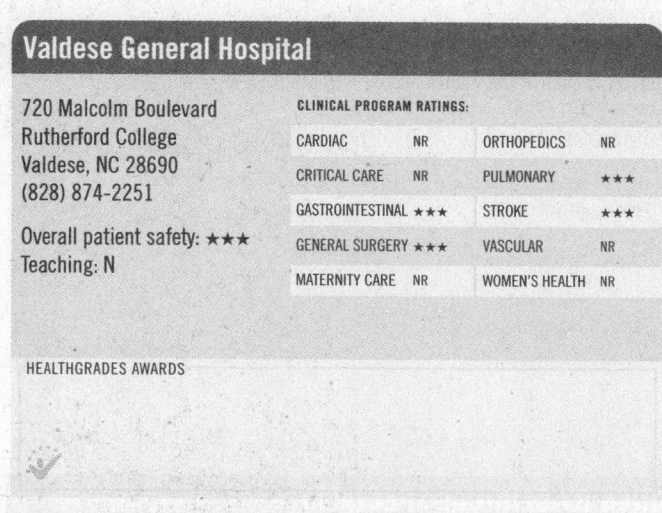

Washington County Hospital

958 US Highway 64 East
Plymouth, NC 27962
(252) 793-4135

Overall patient safety: ★★★
Teaching: N

CLINICAL PROGRAM RATINGS:

CARDIAC	NR	ORTHOPEDICS	NR
CRITICAL CARE	NR	PULMONARY	★★★
GASTROINTESTINAL	NR	STROKE	NR
GENERAL SURGERY	NR	VASCULAR	NR
MATERNITY CARE	NR	WOMEN'S HEALTH	NR

HEALTHGRADES AWARDS

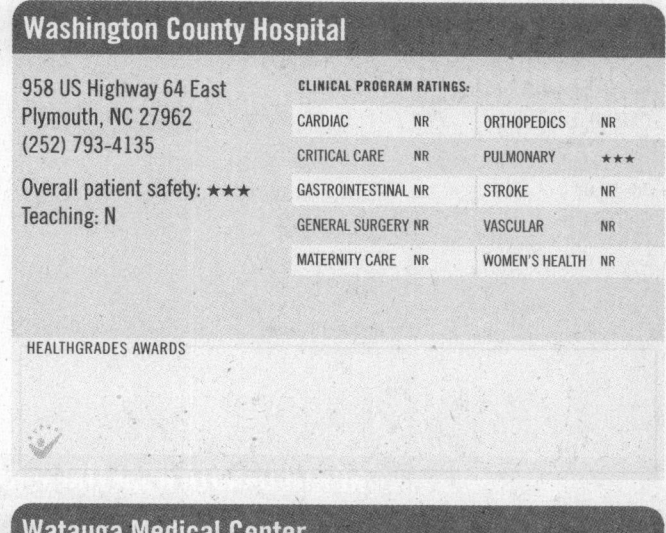

Wakemed Cary Hospital

1900 Kildare Farm Road
Cary, NC 27511
(919) 350-2300

Overall patient safety: ★★★
Teaching: N

CLINICAL PROGRAM RATINGS:

CARDIAC	NR	ORTHOPEDICS	NR
CRITICAL CARE	★★★	PULMONARY	★★★
GASTROINTESTINAL	★★★	STROKE	★★★
GENERAL SURGERY	★★★	VASCULAR	NR
MATERNITY CARE	★★★★★	WOMEN'S HEALTH	NR

HEALTHGRADES AWARDS

Watauga Medical Center

336 Deerfield Road
Boone, NC 28607
(828) 262-4100

Overall patient safety: ★★★★★
Teaching: N

CLINICAL PROGRAM RATINGS:

CARDIAC	NR	ORTHOPEDICS	NR
CRITICAL CARE	NR	PULMONARY	★★★
GASTROINTESTINAL	★★★	STROKE	★★★
GENERAL SURGERY	★★★	VASCULAR	NR
MATERNITY CARE	★★★	WOMEN'S HEALTH	NR

HEALTHGRADES AWARDS

✓ DISTINGUISHED
HOSPITAL
• PATIENT SAFETY

Wayne Memorial Hospital

2700 Wayne Memorial Drive
Goldsboro, NC 27534
(919) 736-1110

Overall patient safety: ★
Teaching: N

CLINICAL PROGRAM RATINGS:

CARDIAC	NR	ORTHOPEDICS	★★★
CRITICAL CARE	NR	PULMONARY	★
GASTROINTESTINAL	★★★	STROKE	★
GENERAL SURGERY	★★★	VASCULAR	NR
MATERNITY CARE	★★★	WOMEN'S HEALTH	NR

HEALTHGRADES AWARDS

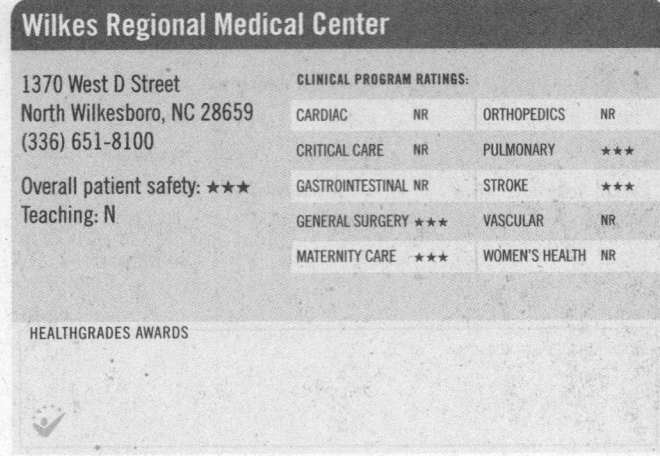

Wilkes Regional Medical Center

1370 West D Street
North Wilkesboro, NC 28659
(336) 651-8100

Overall patient safety: ★★★
Teaching: N

CLINICAL PROGRAM RATINGS:

CARDIAC	NR	ORTHOPEDICS	NR
CRITICAL CARE	NR	PULMONARY	★★★
GASTROINTESTINAL	NR	STROKE	★★★
GENERAL SURGERY	★★★	VASCULAR	NR
MATERNITY CARE	★★★	WOMEN'S HEALTH	NR

HEALTHGRADES AWARDS

Wesley Long Community Hospital*

501 North Elam Avenue
Greensboro, NC 27403
(336) 832-1000

Overall patient safety: ★★★
Teaching: Y

CLINICAL PROGRAM RATINGS:

CARDIAC	★★★	ORTHOPEDICS	★★★
CRITICAL CARE	NR	PULMONARY	★★★
GASTROINTESTINAL	★★★	STROKE	★★★
GENERAL SURGERY	★★★★★	VASCULAR	★★★
MATERNITY CARE	★★★	WOMEN'S HEALTH	★★★

HEALTHGRADES AWARDS

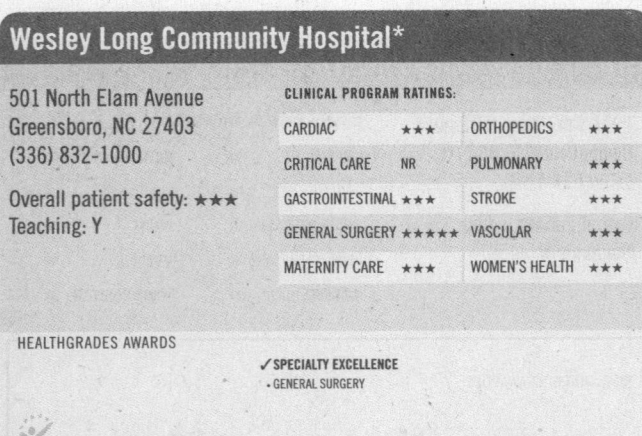

✓ SPECIALTY EXCELLENCE
- GENERAL SURGERY

Wilson Medical Center

1705 Tarboro Street Southwest
Wilson, NC 27893
(252) 399-8040

Overall patient safety: ★
Teaching: N

CLINICAL PROGRAM RATINGS:

CARDIAC	NR	ORTHOPEDICS	NR
CRITICAL CARE	NR	PULMONARY	★★★
GASTROINTESTINAL	★★★	STROKE	★★★
GENERAL SURGERY	★★★	VASCULAR	NR
MATERNITY CARE	★★★	WOMEN'S HEALTH	NR

HEALTHGRADES AWARDS

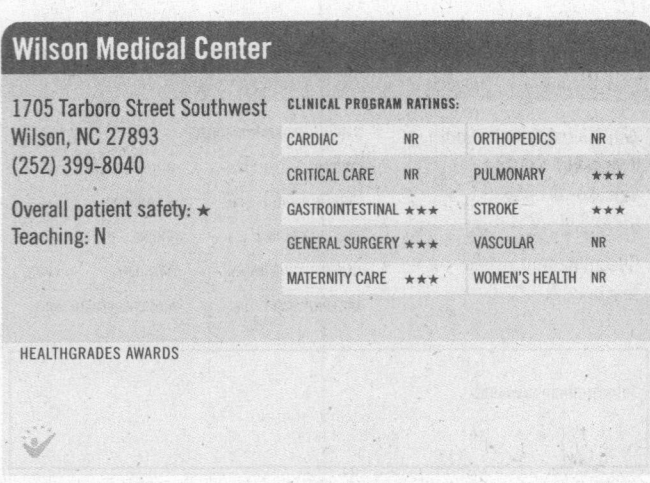

NORTH DAKOTA HOSPITALS: RATINGS BY CLINICAL SPECIALTY

Altru Hospital

1200 South Columbia Road
Grand Forks, ND 58201
(701) 780-5000

Overall patient safety: ★★★
Teaching: Y

CLINICAL PROGRAM RATINGS:

CARDIAC	★★★	ORTHOPEDICS	★★★★★
CRITICAL CARE	NR	PULMONARY	★★★★★
GASTROINTESTINAL	★★★	STROKE	★★★
GENERAL SURGERY	NR	VASCULAR	NR
MATERNITY CARE	NR	WOMEN'S HEALTH	NR

HEALTHGRADES AWARDS

✓ SPECIALTY EXCELLENCE
- PULMONARY CARE

Carrington Health Center

P.O. Box 461
Carrington, ND 58421
(701) 652-3141

Overall patient safety: ★★★
Teaching: N

CLINICAL PROGRAM RATINGS:

CARDIAC	NR	ORTHOPEDICS	NR
CRITICAL CARE	NR	PULMONARY	★★★
GASTROINTESTINAL	NR	STROKE	NR
GENERAL SURGERY	NR	VASCULAR	NR
MATERNITY CARE	NR	WOMEN'S HEALTH	NR

HEALTHGRADES AWARDS

KEY: ★★★★★ BEST　★★★ AS EXPECTED　★ POOR　NR NOT RATED BY HEALTHGRADES　For full definitions of ratings and awards, see Appendix.

Heart of America Medical Center

800 South Main Avenue
Rugby, ND 58368
(701) 776-5261

Overall patient safety: ★★★
Teaching: N

CLINICAL PROGRAM RATINGS:

CARDIAC	NR	ORTHOPEDICS	NR
CRITICAL CARE	NR	PULMONARY	★★★
GASTROINTESTINAL	NR	STROKE	★★★
GENERAL SURGERY	NR	VASCULAR	NR
MATERNITY CARE	NR	WOMEN'S HEALTH	NR

HEALTHGRADES AWARDS

Medcenter One

300 North 7th Street
Bismarck, ND 58501
(701) 323-6000

Overall patient safety: ★★★
Teaching: Y

CLINICAL PROGRAM RATINGS:

CARDIAC	★★★	ORTHOPEDICS	★★★
CRITICAL CARE	NR	PULMONARY	★★★
GASTROINTESTINAL	★★★	STROKE	★★★
GENERAL SURGERY	NR	VASCULAR	★★★
MATERNITY CARE	NR	WOMEN'S HEALTH	NR

HEALTHGRADES AWARDS

Innovis Health

3000 32nd Avenue South
Fargo, ND 58103
(701) 364-8050

Overall patient safety: ★★★
Teaching: N

CLINICAL PROGRAM RATINGS:

CARDIAC	★★★	ORTHOPEDICS	★★★
CRITICAL CARE	NR	PULMONARY	★★★★★
GASTROINTESTINAL	★★★	STROKE	★★★
GENERAL SURGERY	NR	VASCULAR	★★★
MATERNITY CARE	NR	WOMEN'S HEALTH	NR

HEALTHGRADES AWARDS

✓ SPECIALTY EXCELLENCE
 • PULMONARY CARE

Mercy Hospital

1031 7th Street Northeast
Devils Lake, ND 58301
(701) 662-2131

Overall patient safety: ★★★
Teaching: N

CLINICAL PROGRAM RATINGS:

CARDIAC	NR	ORTHOPEDICS	NR
CRITICAL CARE	NR	PULMONARY	★★★
GASTROINTESTINAL	NR	STROKE	★★★
GENERAL SURGERY	NR	VASCULAR	NR
MATERNITY CARE	NR	WOMEN'S HEALTH	NR

HEALTHGRADES AWARDS

Jamestown Hospital

419 5th Street Northeast
Jamestown, ND 58401
(701) 252-1050

Overall patient safety: ★★★★★
Teaching: N

CLINICAL PROGRAM RATINGS:

CARDIAC	NR	ORTHOPEDICS	NR
CRITICAL CARE	NR	PULMONARY	★★★
GASTROINTESTINAL	NR	STROKE	NR
GENERAL SURGERY	NR	VASCULAR	NR
MATERNITY CARE	NR	WOMEN'S HEALTH	NR

HEALTHGRADES AWARDS

Mercy Hospital of Valley City

570 Chautauqua Boulevard
Valley City, ND 58072
(701) 845-6400

Overall patient safety: ★★★
Teaching: N

CLINICAL PROGRAM RATINGS:

CARDIAC	NR	ORTHOPEDICS	NR
CRITICAL CARE	NR	PULMONARY	★★★★★
GASTROINTESTINAL	NR	STROKE	★
GENERAL SURGERY	NR	VASCULAR	NR
MATERNITY CARE	NR	WOMEN'S HEALTH	NR

HEALTHGRADES AWARDS

*This hospital reports its data to the federal government jointly with another hospital. Therefore the ratings and awards apply to multiple hospitals and this specific hospital may not provide all rated services.

Mercy Medical Center

1301 15th Avenue West
Williston, ND 58801
(701) 774-7400

Overall patient safety: ★★★
Teaching: N

CLINICAL PROGRAM RATINGS:

CARDIAC	NR	ORTHOPEDICS	NR
CRITICAL CARE	NR	PULMONARY	★★★
GASTROINTESTINAL	NR	STROKE	★★★
GENERAL SURGERY	NR	VASCULAR	NR
MATERNITY CARE	NR	WOMEN'S HEALTH	NR

HEALTHGRADES AWARDS

Pembina County Memorial Hospital

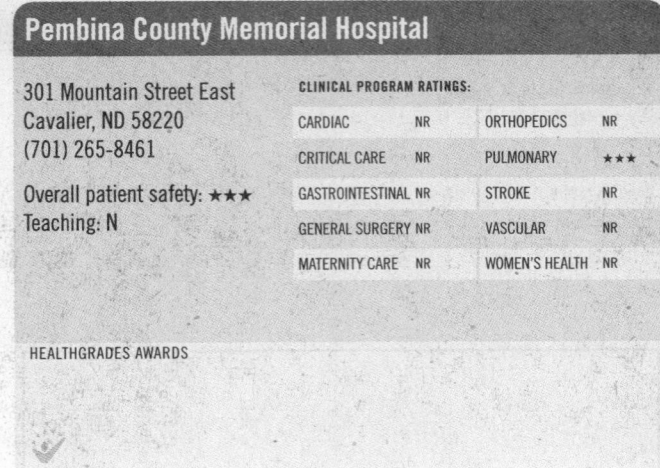

301 Mountain Street East
Cavalier, ND 58220
(701) 265-8461

Overall patient safety: ★★★
Teaching: N

CLINICAL PROGRAM RATINGS:

CARDIAC	NR	ORTHOPEDICS	NR
CRITICAL CARE	NR	PULMONARY	★★★
GASTROINTESTINAL	NR	STROKE	NR
GENERAL SURGERY	NR	VASCULAR	NR
MATERNITY CARE	NR	WOMEN'S HEALTH	NR

HEALTHGRADES AWARDS

Meritcare Health System

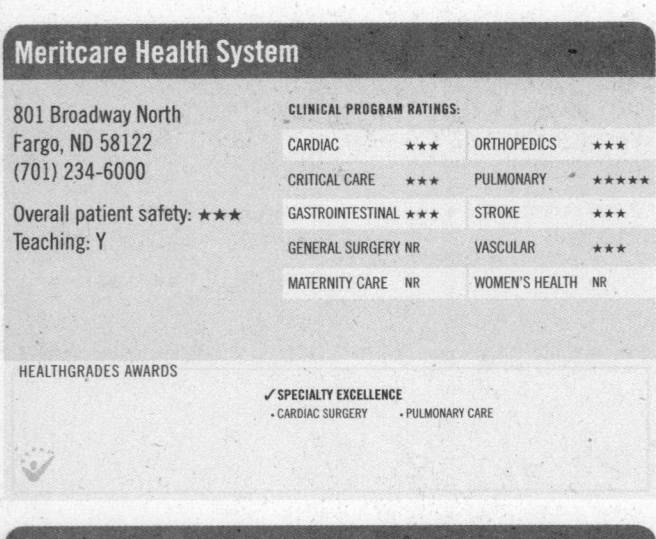

801 Broadway North
Fargo, ND 58122
(701) 234-6000

Overall patient safety: ★★★
Teaching: Y

CLINICAL PROGRAM RATINGS:

CARDIAC	★★★	ORTHOPEDICS	★★★
CRITICAL CARE	★★★	PULMONARY	★★★★★
GASTROINTESTINAL	★★★	STROKE	★★★
GENERAL SURGERY	NR	VASCULAR	★★★
MATERNITY CARE	NR	WOMEN'S HEALTH	NR

HEALTHGRADES AWARDS

✓ SPECIALTY EXCELLENCE
- CARDIAC SURGERY - PULMONARY CARE

PHS Indian Hospital at Belcourt-Quentin N. Burdick Memorial

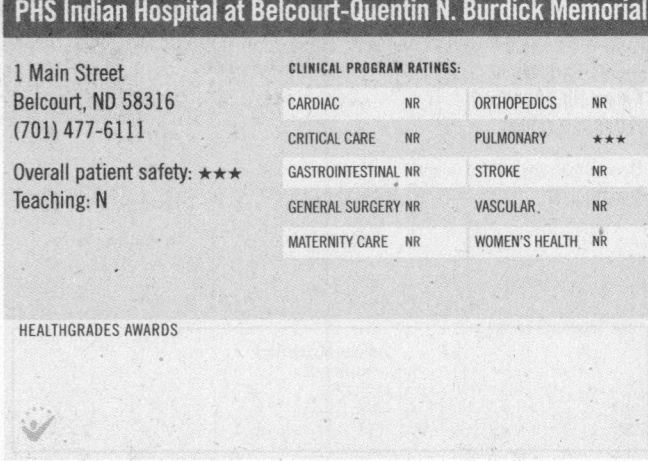

1 Main Street
Belcourt, ND 58316
(701) 477-6111

Overall patient safety: ★★★
Teaching: N

CLINICAL PROGRAM RATINGS:

CARDIAC	NR	ORTHOPEDICS	NR
CRITICAL CARE	NR	PULMONARY	★★★
GASTROINTESTINAL	NR	STROKE	NR
GENERAL SURGERY	NR	VASCULAR	NR
MATERNITY CARE	NR	WOMEN'S HEALTH	NR

HEALTHGRADES AWARDS

Oakes Community Hospital

314 South 8th Street
Oakes, ND 58474
(701) 742-3291

Overall patient safety: ★★★
Teaching: N

CLINICAL PROGRAM RATINGS:

CARDIAC	NR	ORTHOPEDICS	NR
CRITICAL CARE	NR	PULMONARY	★★★
GASTROINTESTINAL	NR	STROKE	NR
GENERAL SURGERY	NR	VASCULAR	NR
MATERNITY CARE	NR	WOMEN'S HEALTH	NR

HEALTHGRADES AWARDS

St. Alexius Medical Center

900 East Broadway
Bismarck, ND 58501
(701) 530-7000

Overall patient safety: ★★★
Teaching: Y

CLINICAL PROGRAM RATINGS:

CARDIAC	★★★★★	ORTHOPEDICS	★★★★★
CRITICAL CARE	NR	PULMONARY	★★★
GASTROINTESTINAL	★★★	STROKE	★★★
GENERAL SURGERY	NR	VASCULAR	NR
MATERNITY CARE	NR	WOMEN'S HEALTH	NR

HEALTHGRADES AWARDS

✓ DISTINGUISHED HOSPITAL
- CLINICAL EXCELLENCE

✓ SPECIALTY EXCELLENCE
- CARDIAC CARE
- CARDIAC SURGERY
- GASTROINTESTINAL CARE
- JOINT REPLACEMENT

KEY: ★★★★★ BEST ★★★ AS EXPECTED ★ POOR NR NOT RATED BY HEALTHGRADES   For full definitions of ratings and awards, see Appendix.

St. Aloisius Medical Center

325 East Brewster Street
Harvey, ND 58341
(701) 324-4651

Overall patient safety: ★★★
Teaching: N

CLINICAL PROGRAM RATINGS:

CARDIAC	NR	ORTHOPEDICS	NR
CRITICAL CARE	NR	PULMONARY	★★★
GASTROINTESTINAL	NR	STROKE	NR
GENERAL SURGERY	NR	VASCULAR	NR
MATERNITY CARE	NR	WOMEN'S HEALTH	NR

HEALTHGRADES AWARDS

Tioga Medical Center

810 North Welo Street
Tioga, ND 58852
(701) 664-3305

Overall patient safety: NR
Teaching: N

CLINICAL PROGRAM RATINGS:

CARDIAC	NR	ORTHOPEDICS	NR
CRITICAL CARE	NR	PULMONARY	★★★
GASTROINTESTINAL	NR	STROKE	NR
GENERAL SURGERY	NR	VASCULAR	NR
MATERNITY CARE	NR	WOMEN'S HEALTH	NR

HEALTHGRADES AWARDS

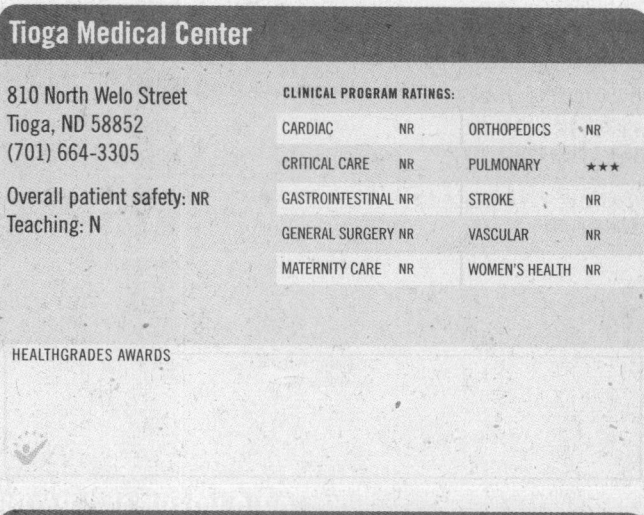

St. Joseph's Hospital and Health Center

30 West 7th Street
Dickinson, ND 58601
(701) 456-4000

Overall patient safety: ★★★
Teaching: N

CLINICAL PROGRAM RATINGS:

CARDIAC	NR	ORTHOPEDICS	NR
CRITICAL CARE	NR	PULMONARY	★★★
GASTROINTESTINAL	NR	STROKE	★★★
GENERAL SURGERY	NR	VASCULAR	NR
MATERNITY CARE	NR	WOMEN'S HEALTH	NR

HEALTHGRADES AWARDS

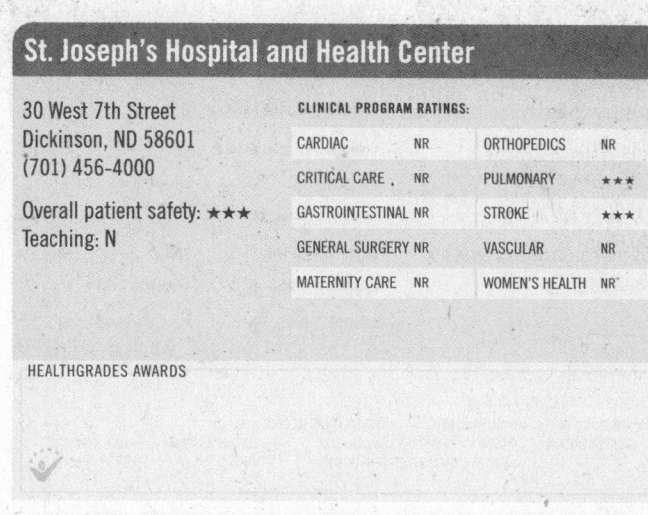

Trinity Hospitals*

407 3rd Street Southeast
Minot, ND 58701
(701) 857-2000

Overall patient safety: ★★★★★
Teaching: Y

CLINICAL PROGRAM RATINGS:

CARDIAC	★★★	ORTHOPEDICS	NR
CRITICAL CARE	NR	PULMONARY	★★★
GASTROINTESTINAL	★★★	STROKE	★★★
GENERAL SURGERY	NR	VASCULAR	NR
MATERNITY CARE	NR	WOMEN'S HEALTH	NR

HEALTHGRADES AWARDS

✓ DISTINGUISHED HOSPITAL
• PATIENT SAFETY

✓ SPECIALTY EXCELLENCE
• JOINT REPLACEMENT

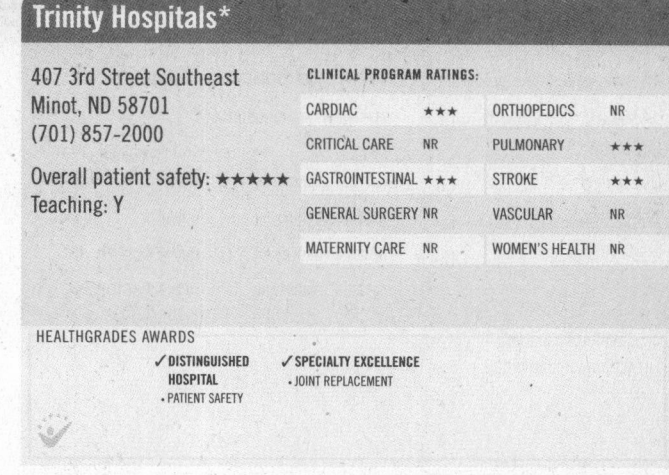

St. Luke's Hospital

702 1st Street Southwest
Crosby, ND 58730
(701) 965-6384

Overall patient safety: NR
Teaching: N

CLINICAL PROGRAM RATINGS:

CARDIAC	NR	ORTHOPEDICS	NR
CRITICAL CARE	NR	PULMONARY	★★★
GASTROINTESTINAL	NR	STROKE	NR
GENERAL SURGERY	NR	VASCULAR	NR
MATERNITY CARE	NR	WOMEN'S HEALTH	NR

HEALTHGRADES AWARDS

Trinity Medical Center*

1 Burdick Expressway West
Minot, ND 58702
(701) 857-5000

Overall patient safety: ★★★★★
Teaching: Y

CLINICAL PROGRAM RATINGS:

CARDIAC	★★★	ORTHOPEDICS	NR
CRITICAL CARE	NR	PULMONARY	★★★
GASTROINTESTINAL	★★★	STROKE	★★★
GENERAL SURGERY	NR	VASCULAR	NR
MATERNITY CARE	NR	WOMEN'S HEALTH	NR

HEALTHGRADES AWARDS

✓ DISTINGUISHED HOSPITAL
• PATIENT SAFETY

✓ SPECIALTY EXCELLENCE
• JOINT REPLACEMENT

*This hospital reports its data to the federal government jointly with another hospital. Therefore the ratings and awards apply to multiple hospitals and this specific hospital may not provide all rated services.

West River Regional Medical Center

1000 Highway 12
Hettinger, ND 58639
(701) 567-4561

Overall patient safety: ★★★
Teaching: N

CLINICAL PROGRAM RATINGS:

CARDIAC	NR	ORTHOPEDICS	NR
CRITICAL CARE	NR	PULMONARY	★★★★★
GASTROINTESTINAL	NR	STROKE	NR
GENERAL SURGERY	NR	VASCULAR	NR
MATERNITY CARE	NR	WOMEN'S HEALTH	NR

HEALTHGRADES AWARDS

✓ SPECIALTY EXCELLENCE
  - PULMONARY CARE

OHIO HOSPITALS: RATINGS BY CLINICAL SPECIALTY

Adams County Regional Medical Center

230 Medical Center Drive
Seaman, OH 45679
(937) 544-5571

Overall patient safety: ★★★
Teaching: N

CLINICAL PROGRAM RATINGS:

CARDIAC	NR	ORTHOPEDICS	NR
CRITICAL CARE	NR	PULMONARY	★
GASTROINTESTINAL	NR	STROKE	★★★
GENERAL SURGERY	NR	VASCULAR	NR
MATERNITY CARE	NR	WOMEN'S HEALTH	NR

HEALTHGRADES AWARDS

Akron General Medical Center

400 Wabash Avenue
Akron, OH 44307
(330) 344-6000

Overall patient safety: ★★★
Teaching: Y

CLINICAL PROGRAM RATINGS:

CARDIAC	★★★★★	ORTHOPEDICS	★
CRITICAL CARE	★★★★★	PULMONARY	★★★★★
GASTROINTESTINAL	★★★	STROKE	★★★★★
GENERAL SURGERY	NR	VASCULAR	★★★
MATERNITY CARE	NR	WOMEN'S HEALTH	NR

HEALTHGRADES AWARDS

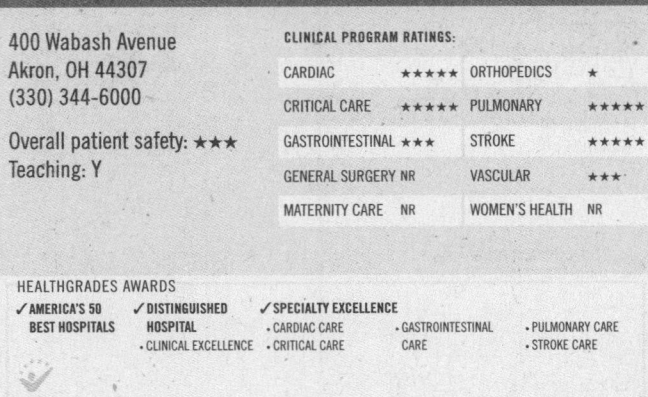

✓ AMERICA'S 50 BEST HOSPITALS
✓ DISTINGUISHED HOSPITAL
  - CLINICAL EXCELLENCE
✓ SPECIALTY EXCELLENCE
  - CARDIAC CARE
  - CRITICAL CARE
  - GASTROINTESTINAL CARE
  - PULMONARY CARE
  - STROKE CARE

Adena Regional Medical Center

272 Hospital Road
Chillicothe, OH 45601
(740) 779-7500

Overall patient safety: ★★★★★
Teaching: N

CLINICAL PROGRAM RATINGS:

CARDIAC	NR	ORTHOPEDICS	NR
CRITICAL CARE	★★★	PULMONARY	★★★★★
GASTROINTESTINAL	★★★	STROKE	★
GENERAL SURGERY	NR	VASCULAR	NR
MATERNITY CARE	NR	WOMEN'S HEALTH	NR

HEALTHGRADES AWARDS

✓ DISTINGUISHED HOSPITAL
  - PATIENT SAFETY

Allen Medical Center

200 West Lorain Street
Oberlin, OH 44074
(440) 776-7047

Overall patient safety: ★★★
Teaching: N

CLINICAL PROGRAM RATINGS:

CARDIAC	NR	ORTHOPEDICS	NR
CRITICAL CARE	NR	PULMONARY	★★★
GASTROINTESTINAL	NR	STROKE	★★★
GENERAL SURGERY	NR	VASCULAR	NR
MATERNITY CARE	NR	WOMEN'S HEALTH	NR

HEALTHGRADES AWARDS

KEY: ★★★★★ BEST   ★★★ AS EXPECTED   ★ POOR   NR NOT RATED BY HEALTHGRADES   For full definitions of ratings and awards, see Appendix.

Alliance Community Hospital

264 East Rice Street
Alliance, OH 44601
(330) 829-4000

Overall patient safety: ★
Teaching: Y

CLINICAL PROGRAM RATINGS:

CARDIAC	NR	ORTHOPEDICS	NR
CRITICAL CARE	NR	PULMONARY	★★★
GASTROINTESTINAL	★★★	STROKE	★★★
GENERAL SURGERY	NR	VASCULAR	NR
MATERNITY CARE	NR	WOMEN'S HEALTH	NR

HEALTHGRADES AWARDS

Barberton Citizens Hospital

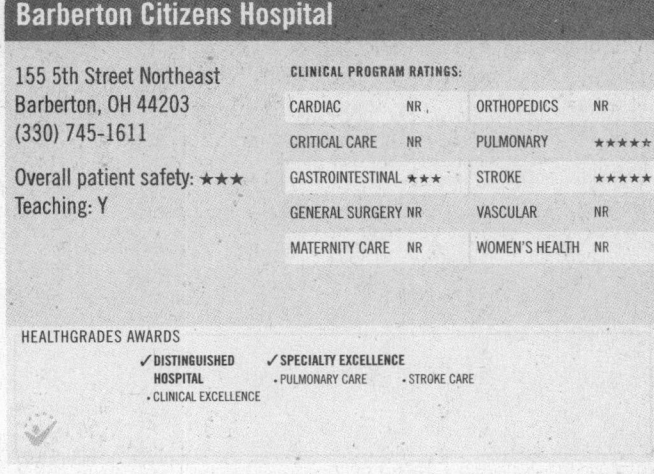

155 5th Street Northeast
Barberton, OH 44203
(330) 745-1611

Overall patient safety: ★★★
Teaching: Y

CLINICAL PROGRAM RATINGS:

CARDIAC	NR	ORTHOPEDICS	NR
CRITICAL CARE	NR	PULMONARY	★★★★★
GASTROINTESTINAL	★★★	STROKE	★★★★★
GENERAL SURGERY	NR	VASCULAR	NR
MATERNITY CARE	NR	WOMEN'S HEALTH	NR

HEALTHGRADES AWARDS

✓ DISTINGUISHED HOSPITAL
  • CLINICAL EXCELLENCE

✓ SPECIALTY EXCELLENCE
  • PULMONARY CARE   • STROKE CARE

Ashtabula County Medical Center

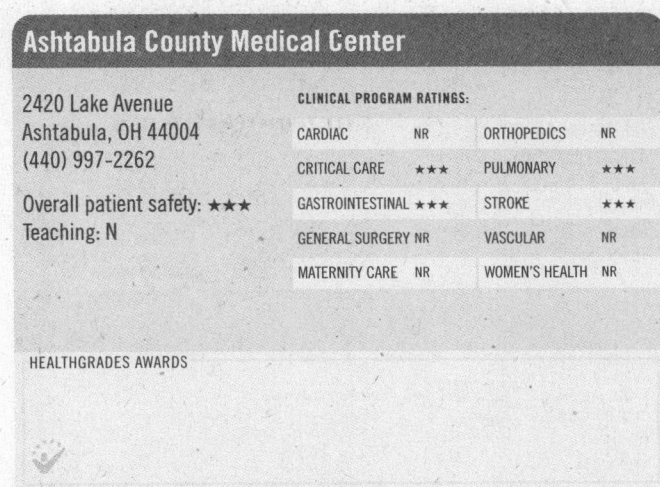

2420 Lake Avenue
Ashtabula, OH 44004
(440) 997-2262

Overall patient safety: ★★★
Teaching: N

CLINICAL PROGRAM RATINGS:

CARDIAC	NR	ORTHOPEDICS	NR
CRITICAL CARE	★★★	PULMONARY	★★★
GASTROINTESTINAL	★★★	STROKE	★★★
GENERAL SURGERY	NR	VASCULAR	NR
MATERNITY CARE	NR	WOMEN'S HEALTH	NR

HEALTHGRADES AWARDS

Barnesville Hospital Association

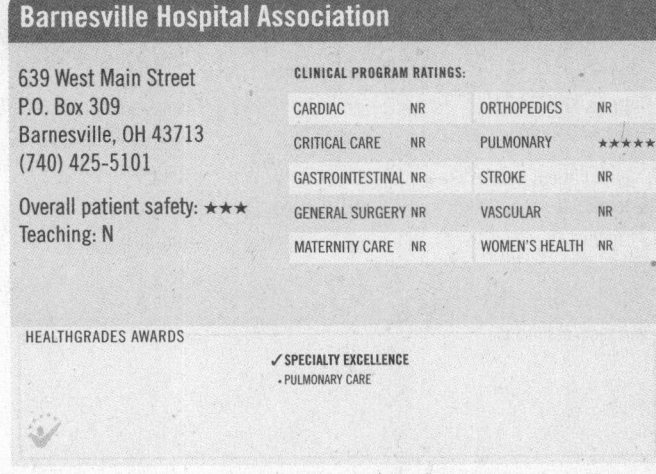

639 West Main Street
P.O. Box 309
Barnesville, OH 43713
(740) 425-5101

Overall patient safety: ★★★
Teaching: N

CLINICAL PROGRAM RATINGS:

CARDIAC	NR	ORTHOPEDICS	NR
CRITICAL CARE	NR	PULMONARY	★★★★★
GASTROINTESTINAL	NR	STROKE	NR
GENERAL SURGERY	NR	VASCULAR	NR
MATERNITY CARE	NR	WOMEN'S HEALTH	NR

HEALTHGRADES AWARDS

✓ SPECIALTY EXCELLENCE
  • PULMONARY CARE

Aultman Hospital

2600 6th Street Southwest
Canton, OH 44710
(330) 452-9911

Overall patient safety: ★★★
Teaching: Y

CLINICAL PROGRAM RATINGS:

CARDIAC	★★★	ORTHOPEDICS	★★★
CRITICAL CARE	NR	PULMONARY	★★★
GASTROINTESTINAL	★★★	STROKE	★★★
GENERAL SURGERY	NR	VASCULAR	★★★★★
MATERNITY CARE	NR	WOMEN'S HEALTH	NR

HEALTHGRADES AWARDS

✓ DISTINGUISHED HOSPITAL
  • CLINICAL EXCELLENCE

✓ SPECIALTY EXCELLENCE
  • CARDIAC SURGERY   • GASTROINTESTINAL CARE   • VASCULAR SURGERY

Bay Park Community Hospital

2801 Bay Parks Drive
Oregon, OH 43616
(419) 690-7900

Overall patient safety: ★★★
Teaching: N

CLINICAL PROGRAM RATINGS:

CARDIAC	NR	ORTHOPEDICS	NR
CRITICAL CARE	NR	PULMONARY	★★★
GASTROINTESTINAL	NR	STROKE	★★★
GENERAL SURGERY	NR	VASCULAR	NR
MATERNITY CARE	NR	WOMEN'S HEALTH	NR

HEALTHGRADES AWARDS

Bellevue Hospital

1400 West Main Street
Bellevue, OH 44811
(419) 483-4040

Overall patient safety: ★★★
Teaching: N

CLINICAL PROGRAM RATINGS:

CARDIAC	NR	ORTHOPEDICS	NR
CRITICAL CARE	NR	PULMONARY	★★★
GASTROINTESTINAL	NR	STROKE	★★★
GENERAL SURGERY	NR	VASCULAR	NR
MATERNITY CARE	NR	WOMEN'S HEALTH	NR

HEALTHGRADES AWARDS

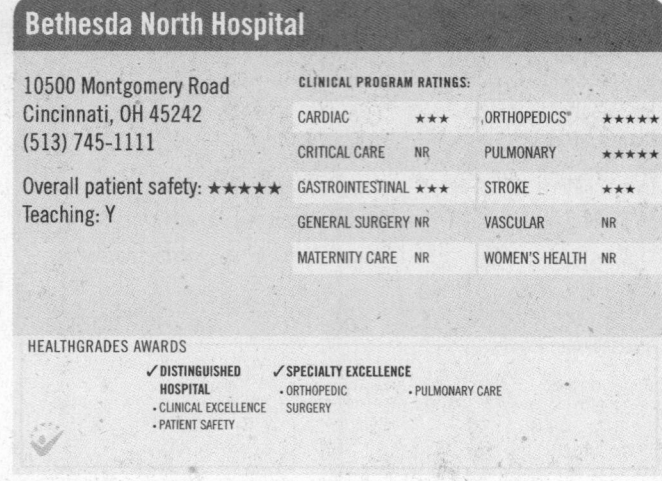

Bethesda North Hospital

10500 Montgomery Road
Cincinnati, OH 45242
(513) 745-1111

Overall patient safety: ★★★★★
Teaching: Y

CLINICAL PROGRAM RATINGS:

CARDIAC	★★★	ORTHOPEDICS	★★★★★
CRITICAL CARE	NR	PULMONARY	★★★★★
GASTROINTESTINAL	★★★	STROKE	★★★
GENERAL SURGERY	NR	VASCULAR	NR
MATERNITY CARE	NR	WOMEN'S HEALTH	NR

HEALTHGRADES AWARDS

✓ **DISTINGUISHED HOSPITAL**
- CLINICAL EXCELLENCE
- PATIENT SAFETY

✓ **SPECIALTY EXCELLENCE**
- ORTHOPEDIC SURGERY
- PULMONARY CARE

Belmont Community Hospital

4697 Harrison Street
Bellaire, OH 43906
(740) 671-1200

Overall patient safety: ★★★
Teaching: N

CLINICAL PROGRAM RATINGS:

CARDIAC	NR	ORTHOPEDICS	NR
CRITICAL CARE	NR	PULMONARY	★★★
GASTROINTESTINAL	NR	STROKE	NR
GENERAL SURGERY	NR	VASCULAR	NR
MATERNITY CARE	NR	WOMEN'S HEALTH	NR

HEALTHGRADES AWARDS

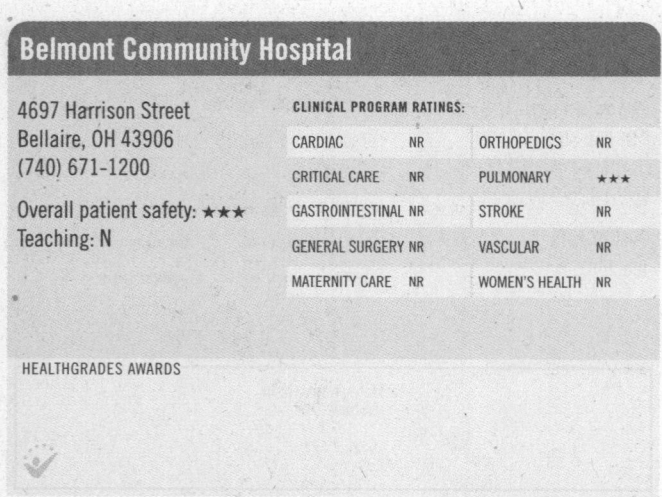

Blanchard Valley Regional Health Center

145 West Wallace Street
Findlay, OH 45840
(419) 423-4500

Overall patient safety: ★★★★★
Teaching: N

CLINICAL PROGRAM RATINGS:

CARDIAC	★★★	ORTHOPEDICS	★★★
CRITICAL CARE	NR	PULMONARY	★★★
GASTROINTESTINAL	★★★	STROKE	★★★
GENERAL SURGERY	NR	VASCULAR	NR
MATERNITY CARE	NR	WOMEN'S HEALTH	NR

HEALTHGRADES AWARDS

✓ **DISTINGUISHED HOSPITAL**
- PATIENT SAFETY

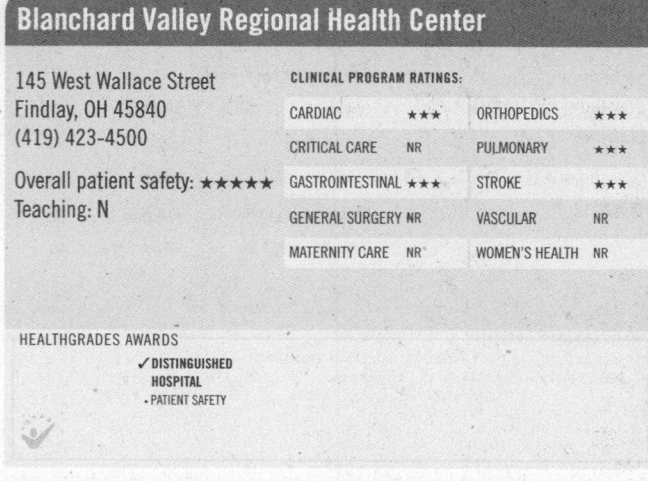

Berger Hospital

600 North Pickaway Street
Circleville, OH 43113
(740) 474-2126

Overall patient safety: ★★★
Teaching: N

CLINICAL PROGRAM RATINGS:

CARDIAC	NR	ORTHOPEDICS	NR
CRITICAL CARE	NR	PULMONARY	★★★
GASTROINTESTINAL	NR	STROKE	★★★
GENERAL SURGERY	NR	VASCULAR	NR
MATERNITY CARE	NR	WOMEN'S HEALTH	NR

HEALTHGRADES AWARDS

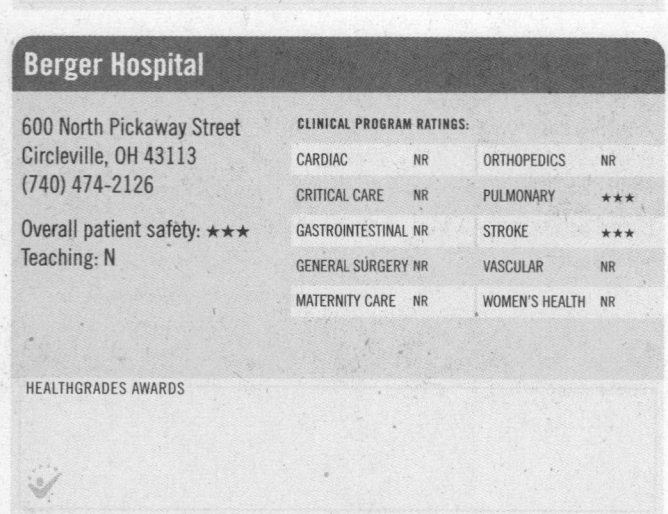

Brown County Hospital

425 Home Street
Georgetown, OH 45121
(937) 378-7500

Overall patient safety: ★★★
Teaching: N

CLINICAL PROGRAM RATINGS:

CARDIAC	NR	ORTHOPEDICS	NR
CRITICAL CARE	NR	PULMONARY	★★★
GASTROINTESTINAL	NR	STROKE	★★★
GENERAL SURGERY	NR	VASCULAR	NR
MATERNITY CARE	NR	WOMEN'S HEALTH	NR

HEALTHGRADES AWARDS

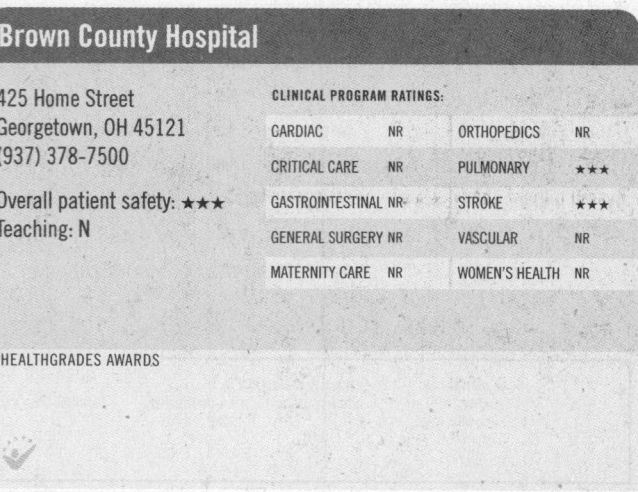

KEY: ★★★★★ BEST   ★★★ AS EXPECTED   ★ POOR   NR NOT RATED BY HEALTHGRADES   For full definitions of ratings and awards, see Appendix.

Christ Hospital

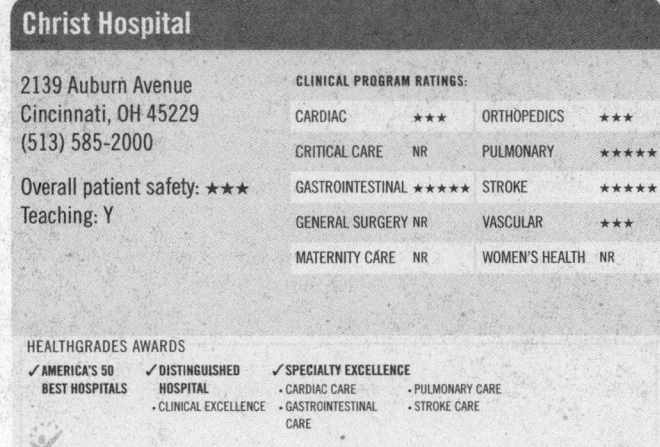

2139 Auburn Avenue
Cincinnati, OH 45229
(513) 585-2000

Overall patient safety: ★★★
Teaching: Y

CLINICAL PROGRAM RATINGS:

CARDIAC	★★★	ORTHOPEDICS	★★★
CRITICAL CARE	NR	PULMONARY	★★★★★
GASTROINTESTINAL	★★★★★	STROKE	★★★★★
GENERAL SURGERY	NR	VASCULAR	★★★
MATERNITY CARE	NR	WOMEN'S HEALTH	NR

HEALTHGRADES AWARDS

✓ AMERICA'S 50 BEST HOSPITALS
✓ DISTINGUISHED HOSPITAL
· CLINICAL EXCELLENCE
✓ SPECIALTY EXCELLENCE
· CARDIAC CARE
· GASTROINTESTINAL CARE
· PULMONARY CARE
· STROKE CARE

Community Health Partners of Ohio—West

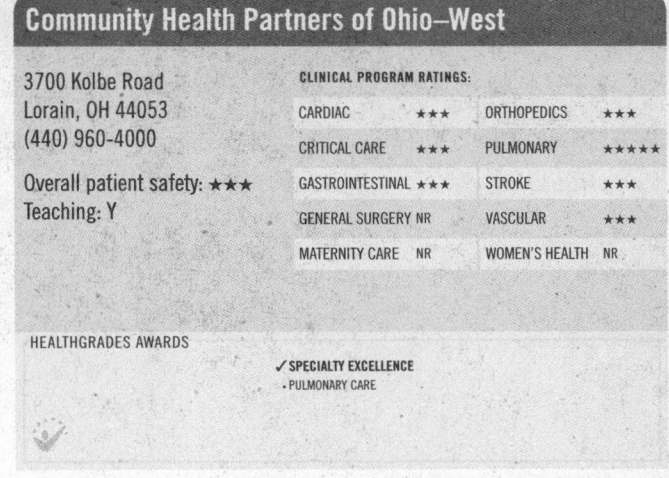

3700 Kolbe Road
Lorain, OH 44053
(440) 960-4000

Overall patient safety: ★★★
Teaching: Y

CLINICAL PROGRAM RATINGS:

CARDIAC	★★★	ORTHOPEDICS	★★★
CRITICAL CARE	★★★	PULMONARY	★★★★★
GASTROINTESTINAL	★★★	STROKE	★★★
GENERAL SURGERY	NR	VASCULAR	★★★
MATERNITY CARE	NR	WOMEN'S HEALTH	NR

HEALTHGRADES AWARDS

✓ SPECIALTY EXCELLENCE
· PULMONARY CARE

Cleveland Clinic

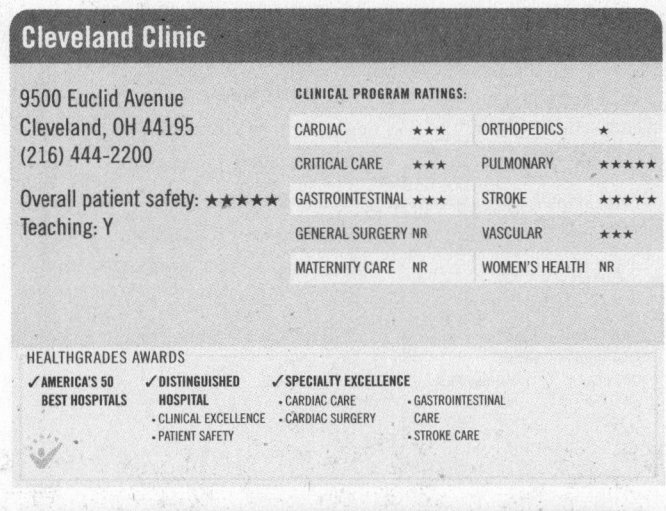

9500 Euclid Avenue
Cleveland, OH 44195
(216) 444-2200

Overall patient safety: ★★★★★
Teaching: Y

CLINICAL PROGRAM RATINGS:

CARDIAC	★★★	ORTHOPEDICS	★
CRITICAL CARE	★★★	PULMONARY	★★★★★
GASTROINTESTINAL	★★★	STROKE	★★★★★
GENERAL SURGERY	NR	VASCULAR	★★★
MATERNITY CARE	NR	WOMEN'S HEALTH	NR

HEALTHGRADES AWARDS

✓ AMERICA'S 50 BEST HOSPITALS
✓ DISTINGUISHED HOSPITAL
· CLINICAL EXCELLENCE
· PATIENT SAFETY
✓ SPECIALTY EXCELLENCE
· CARDIAC CARE
· CARDIAC SURGERY
· GASTROINTESTINAL CARE
· STROKE CARE

Community Hospital of Springfield and Clark County

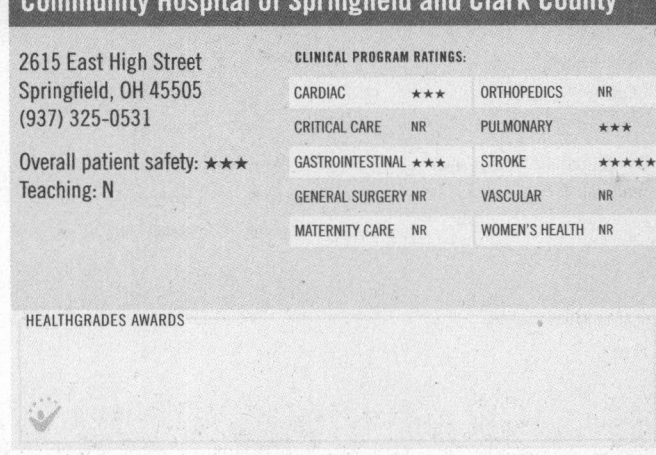

2615 East High Street
Springfield, OH 45505
(937) 325-0531

Overall patient safety: ★★★
Teaching: N

CLINICAL PROGRAM RATINGS:

CARDIAC	★★★	ORTHOPEDICS	NR
CRITICAL CARE	NR	PULMONARY	★★★
GASTROINTESTINAL	★★★	STROKE	★★★★★
GENERAL SURGERY	NR	VASCULAR	NR
MATERNITY CARE	NR	WOMEN'S HEALTH	NR

HEALTHGRADES AWARDS

Clinton Memorial Hospital

610 West Main Street
Wilmington, OH 45177
(937) 382-6611

Overall patient safety: ★★★
Teaching: Y

CLINICAL PROGRAM RATINGS:

CARDIAC	NR	ORTHOPEDICS	NR
CRITICAL CARE	NR	PULMONARY	★★★
GASTROINTESTINAL	★★★	STROKE	★★★★★
GENERAL SURGERY	NR	VASCULAR	NR
MATERNITY CARE	NR	WOMEN'S HEALTH	NR

HEALTHGRADES AWARDS

Community Hospital

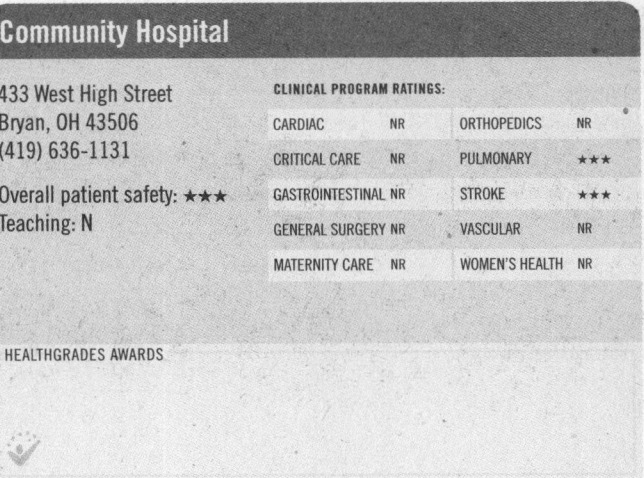

433 West High Street
Bryan, OH 43506
(419) 636-1131

Overall patient safety: ★★★
Teaching: N

CLINICAL PROGRAM RATINGS:

CARDIAC	NR	ORTHOPEDICS	NR
CRITICAL CARE	NR	PULMONARY	★★★
GASTROINTESTINAL	NR	STROKE	★★★
GENERAL SURGERY	NR	VASCULAR	NR
MATERNITY CARE	NR	WOMEN'S HEALTH	NR

HEALTHGRADES AWARDS

Community Memorial Hospital

208 North Columbus Street
Hicksville, OH 43526
(419) 542-6692

Overall patient safety: NR
Teaching: N

CLINICAL PROGRAM RATINGS:

CARDIAC	NR	ORTHOPEDICS	NR
CRITICAL CARE	NR	PULMONARY	★★★
GASTROINTESTINAL	NR	STROKE	NR
GENERAL SURGERY	NR	VASCULAR	NR
MATERNITY CARE	NR	WOMEN'S HEALTH	NR

HEALTHGRADES AWARDS

Dayton Heart Hospital

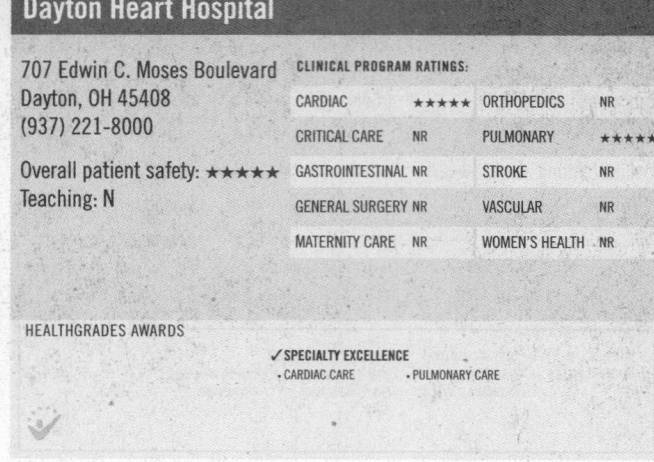

707 Edwin C. Moses Boulevard
Dayton, OH 45408
(937) 221-8000

Overall patient safety: ★★★★
Teaching: N

CLINICAL PROGRAM RATINGS:

CARDIAC	★★★★★	ORTHOPEDICS	NR
CRITICAL CARE	NR	PULMONARY	★★★★★
GASTROINTESTINAL	NR	STROKE	NR
GENERAL SURGERY	NR	VASCULAR	NR
MATERNITY CARE	NR	WOMEN'S HEALTH	NR

HEALTHGRADES AWARDS

✓ SPECIALTY EXCELLENCE
- CARDIAC CARE - PULMONARY CARE

Coshocton County Memorial Hospital

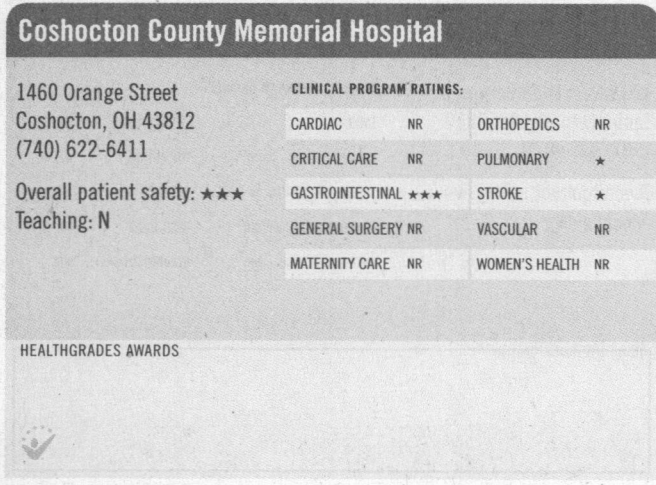

1460 Orange Street
Coshocton, OH 43812
(740) 622-6411

Overall patient safety: ★★★
Teaching: N

CLINICAL PROGRAM RATINGS:

CARDIAC	NR	ORTHOPEDICS	NR
CRITICAL CARE	NR	PULMONARY	★
GASTROINTESTINAL	★★★	STROKE	★
GENERAL SURGERY	NR	VASCULAR	NR
MATERNITY CARE	NR	WOMEN'S HEALTH	NR

HEALTHGRADES AWARDS

Deaconess Hospital

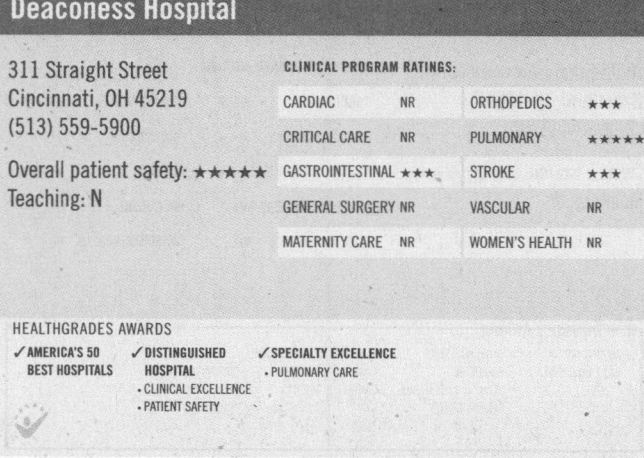

311 Straight Street
Cincinnati, OH 45219
(513) 559-5900

Overall patient safety: ★★★★★
Teaching: N

CLINICAL PROGRAM RATINGS:

CARDIAC	NR	ORTHOPEDICS	★★★
CRITICAL CARE	NR	PULMONARY	★★★★★
GASTROINTESTINAL	★★★	STROKE	★★★
GENERAL SURGERY	NR	VASCULAR	NR
MATERNITY CARE	NR	WOMEN'S HEALTH	NR

HEALTHGRADES AWARDS

✓ AMERICA'S 50 BEST HOSPITALS ✓ DISTINGUISHED HOSPITAL - CLINICAL EXCELLENCE - PATIENT SAFETY ✓ SPECIALTY EXCELLENCE - PULMONARY CARE

Cuyahoga Falls General Hospital

1900 23rd Street
Cuyahoga Falls, OH 44223
(330) 971-7000

Overall patient safety: ★★★
Teaching: Y

CLINICAL PROGRAM RATINGS:

CARDIAC	NR	ORTHOPEDICS	NR
CRITICAL CARE	NR	PULMONARY	★★★
GASTROINTESTINAL	★★★	STROKE	★★★
GENERAL SURGERY	NR	VASCULAR	NR
MATERNITY CARE	NR	WOMEN'S HEALTH	NR

HEALTHGRADES AWARDS

Defiance Regional Medical Center

1200 Ralston Avenue
Defiance, OH 43512
(419) 783-6955

Overall patient safety: ★★★
Teaching: N

CLINICAL PROGRAM RATINGS:

CARDIAC	NR	ORTHOPEDICS	NR
CRITICAL CARE	NR	PULMONARY	★
GASTROINTESTINAL	★★★	STROKE	★
GENERAL SURGERY	NR	VASCULAR	NR
MATERNITY CARE	NR	WOMEN'S HEALTH	NR

HEALTHGRADES AWARDS

KEY: ★★★★★ BEST ★★★ AS EXPECTED ★ POOR NR NOT RATED BY HEALTHGRADES For full definitions of ratings and awards, see Appendix.

Doctors Hospital of Nelsonville

1950 Mount St. Marys Drive
Nelsonville, OH 45764
(740) 753-1931

Overall patient safety: ★★★
Teaching: N

CLINICAL PROGRAM RATINGS:

CARDIAC	NR	ORTHOPEDICS	NR
CRITICAL CARE	NR	PULMONARY	★★★
GASTROINTESTINAL	NR	STROKE	NR
GENERAL SURGERY	NR	VASCULAR	NR
MATERNITY CARE	NR	WOMEN'S HEALTH	NR

HEALTHGRADES AWARDS

Dunlap Memorial Hospital

832 South Main Street
Orrville, OH 44667
(330) 682-3010

Overall patient safety: ★★★
Teaching: N

CLINICAL PROGRAM RATINGS:

CARDIAC	NR	ORTHOPEDICS	NR
CRITICAL CARE	NR	PULMONARY	★★★
GASTROINTESTINAL	NR	STROKE	★★★
GENERAL SURGERY	NR	VASCULAR	NR
MATERNITY CARE	NR	WOMEN'S HEALTH	NR

HEALTHGRADES AWARDS

Doctors Hospital of Stark County

400 Austin Avenue Northwest
Massillon, OH 44646
(330) 837-7200

Overall patient safety: ★★★
Teaching: Y

CLINICAL PROGRAM RATINGS:

CARDIAC	★★★	ORTHOPEDICS	★★★
CRITICAL CARE	NR	PULMONARY	★★★
GASTROINTESTINAL	NR	STROKE	★★★
GENERAL SURGERY	NR	VASCULAR	NR
MATERNITY CARE	NR	WOMEN'S HEALTH	NR

HEALTHGRADES AWARDS

East Liverpool City Hospital

425 West 5th Street
East Liverpool, OH 43920
(330) 385-7200

Overall patient safety: ★★★★★
Teaching: N

CLINICAL PROGRAM RATINGS:

CARDIAC	NR	ORTHOPEDICS	NR
CRITICAL CARE	NR	PULMONARY	★★★
GASTROINTESTINAL	NR	STROKE	★★★
GENERAL SURGERY	NR	VASCULAR	NR
MATERNITY CARE	NR	WOMEN'S HEALTH	NR

HEALTHGRADES AWARDS

Doctors Hospital Ohio Health

5100 West Broad Street
Columbus, OH 43228
(614) 544-1000

Overall patient safety: ★★★
Teaching: Y

CLINICAL PROGRAM RATINGS:

CARDIAC	★★★	ORTHOPEDICS	NR
CRITICAL CARE	NR	PULMONARY	★★★
GASTROINTESTINAL	NR	STROKE	★★★
GENERAL SURGERY	NR	VASCULAR	NR
MATERNITY CARE	NR	WOMEN'S HEALTH	NR

HEALTHGRADES AWARDS

East Ohio Regional Hospital

90 North 4th Street
Martins Ferry, OH 43935
(740) 633-1100

Overall patient safety: ★★★
Teaching: N

CLINICAL PROGRAM RATINGS:

CARDIAC	NR	ORTHOPEDICS	NR
CRITICAL CARE	NR	PULMONARY	★
GASTROINTESTINAL	NR	STROKE	★★★
GENERAL SURGERY	NR	VASCULAR	NR
MATERNITY CARE	NR	WOMEN'S HEALTH	NR

HEALTHGRADES AWARDS

Emh Regional Medical Center

630 East River Street
Elyria, OH 44035
(440) 329-7500

Overall patient safety: ★★★★★
Teaching: N

CLINICAL PROGRAM RATINGS:

CARDIAC	★★★	ORTHOPEDICS	★★★
CRITICAL CARE	★★★	PULMONARY	★★★★★
GASTROINTESTINAL	★★★	STROKE	★★★
GENERAL SURGERY	NR	VASCULAR	★★★
MATERNITY CARE	NR	WOMEN'S HEALTH	NR

HEALTHGRADES AWARDS

✓ DISTINGUISHED HOSPITAL
- CLINICAL EXCELLENCE
- PATIENT SAFETY

✓ SPECIALTY EXCELLENCE
- CARDIAC CARE
- PULMONARY CARE

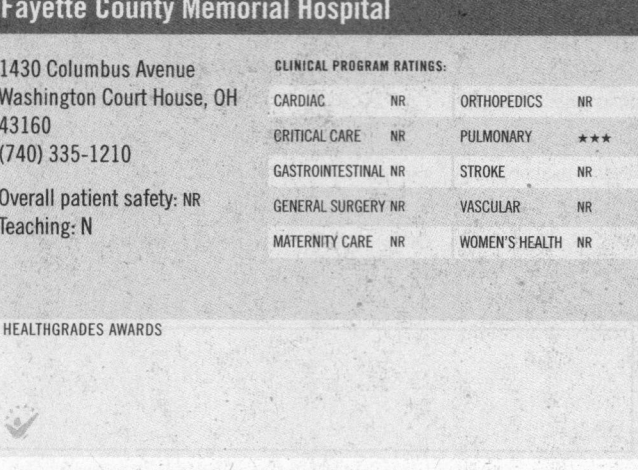

Fayette County Memorial Hospital

1430 Columbus Avenue
Washington Court House, OH 43160
(740) 335-1210

Overall patient safety: NR
Teaching: N

CLINICAL PROGRAM RATINGS:

CARDIAC	NR	ORTHOPEDICS	NR
CRITICAL CARE	NR	PULMONARY	★★★
GASTROINTESTINAL	NR	STROKE	NR
GENERAL SURGERY	NR	VASCULAR	NR
MATERNITY CARE	NR	WOMEN'S HEALTH	NR

HEALTHGRADES AWARDS

Fairfield Medical Center

401 North Ewing Street
Lancaster, OH 43130
(740) 687-8000

Overall patient safety: ★★★
Teaching: N

CLINICAL PROGRAM RATINGS:

CARDIAC	★★★	ORTHOPEDICS	★★★
CRITICAL CARE	★★★	PULMONARY	★★★
GASTROINTESTINAL	★★★	STROKE	★
GENERAL SURGERY	NR	VASCULAR	NR
MATERNITY CARE	NR	WOMEN'S HEALTH	NR

HEALTHGRADES AWARDS

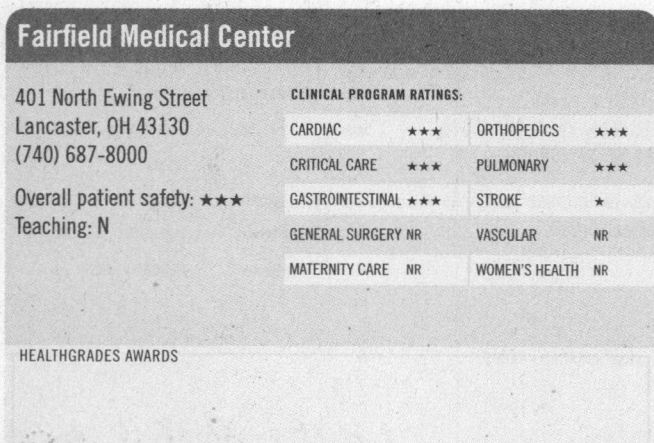

Firelands Regional Medical Center--Main Campus

1101 Decatur Street
Sandusky, OH 44870
(419) 626-7400

Overall patient safety: ★★★
Teaching: Y

CLINICAL PROGRAM RATINGS:

CARDIAC	★★★	ORTHOPEDICS	★★★
CRITICAL CARE	NR	PULMONARY	★
GASTROINTESTINAL	★★★	STROKE	★★★
GENERAL SURGERY	NR	VASCULAR	★★★
MATERNITY CARE	NR	WOMEN'S HEALTH	NR

HEALTHGRADES AWARDS

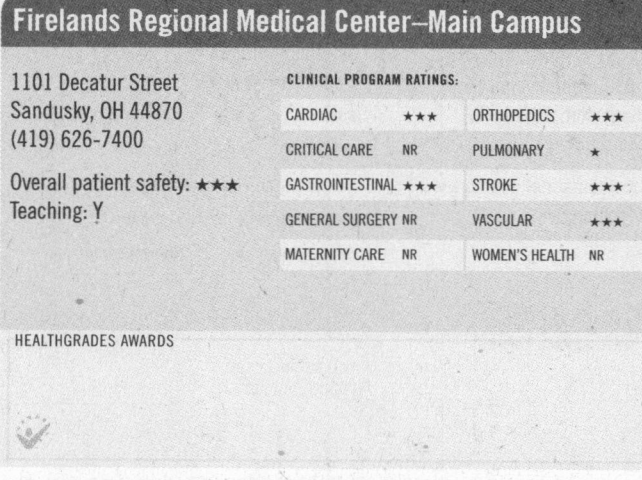

Fairview Hospital

18101 Lorain Avenue
Cleveland, OH 44111
(216) 476-7000

Overall patient safety: ★★★
Teaching: Y

CLINICAL PROGRAM RATINGS:

CARDIAC	★★★★★	ORTHOPEDICS	★★★
CRITICAL CARE	★★★	PULMONARY	★★★★★
GASTROINTESTINAL	★★★	STROKE	★★★★★
GENERAL SURGERY	NR	VASCULAR	NR
MATERNITY CARE	NR	WOMEN'S HEALTH	NR

HEALTHGRADES AWARDS

✓ AMERICA'S 50 BEST HOSPITALS

✓ DISTINGUISHED HOSPITAL
- CLINICAL EXCELLENCE

✓ SPECIALTY EXCELLENCE
- CARDIAC CARE
- CARDIAC SURGERY
- PULMONARY CARE
- STROKE CARE

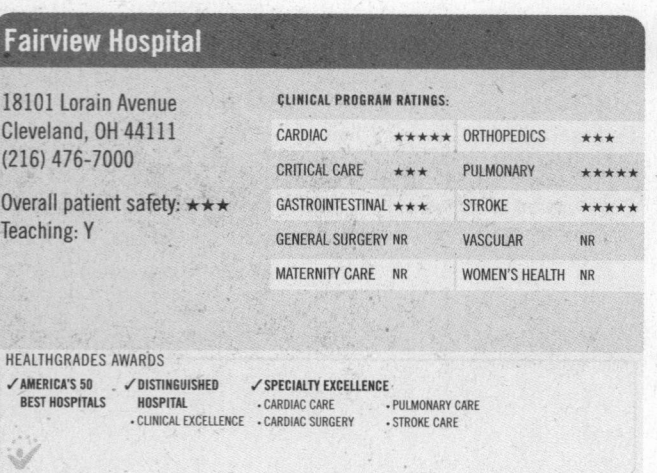

Fisher Titus Memorial Hospital

272 Benedict Avenue
Norwalk, OH 44857
(419) 668-8101

Overall patient safety: ★★★
Teaching: N

CLINICAL PROGRAM RATINGS:

CARDIAC	NR	ORTHOPEDICS	NR
CRITICAL CARE	NR	PULMONARY	★★★
GASTROINTESTINAL	NR	STROKE	★★★
GENERAL SURGERY	NR	VASCULAR	NR
MATERNITY CARE	NR	WOMEN'S HEALTH	NR

HEALTHGRADES AWARDS

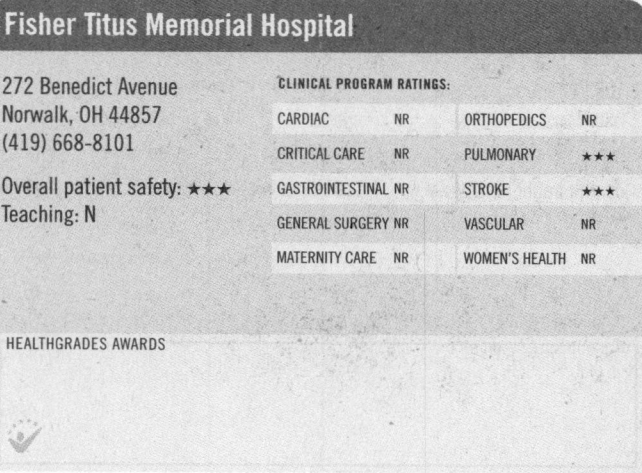

KEY: ★★★★★ BEST ★★★ AS EXPECTED ★ POOR NR NOT RATED BY HEALTHGRADES For full definitions of ratings and awards, see Appendix.

Flower Hospital

5200 Harroun Road
Sylvania, OH 43560
(419) 824-1444

Overall patient safety: ★★★
Teaching: Y

CLINICAL PROGRAM RATINGS:

CARDIAC	NR	ORTHOPEDICS	NR
CRITICAL CARE	NR	PULMONARY	★★★
GASTROINTESTINAL	★★★	STROKE	★★★
GENERAL SURGERY	NR	VASCULAR	NR
MATERNITY CARE	NR	WOMEN'S HEALTH	NR

HEALTHGRADES AWARDS

Fulton County Health Center

725 South Shoop Avenue
Wauseon, OH 43567
(419) 335-2015

Overall patient safety: ★★★
Teaching: N

CLINICAL PROGRAM RATINGS:

CARDIAC	NR	ORTHOPEDICS	NR
CRITICAL CARE	NR	PULMONARY	★
GASTROINTESTINAL	NR	STROKE	★★★
GENERAL SURGERY	NR	VASCULAR	NR
MATERNITY CARE	NR	WOMEN'S HEALTH	NR

HEALTHGRADES AWARDS

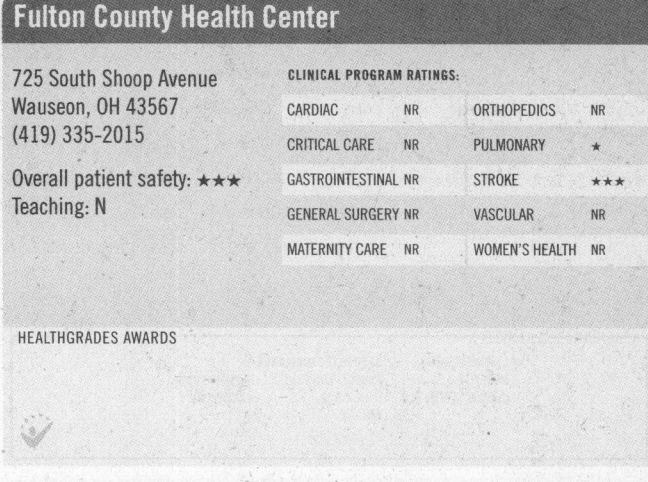

Fort Hamilton Hughes Memorial Hospital

630 Eaton Avenue
Hamilton, OH 45013
(513) 867-2000

Overall patient safety: ★
Teaching: N

CLINICAL PROGRAM RATINGS:

CARDIAC	NR	ORTHOPEDICS	NR
CRITICAL CARE	NR	PULMONARY	★★★★★
GASTROINTESTINAL	★★★	STROKE	★★★
GENERAL SURGERY	NR	VASCULAR	NR
MATERNITY CARE	NR	WOMEN'S HEALTH	NR

HEALTHGRADES AWARDS

✓ DISTINGUISHED HOSPITAL   ✓ SPECIALTY EXCELLENCE
· CLINICAL EXCELLENCE   · PULMONARY CARE

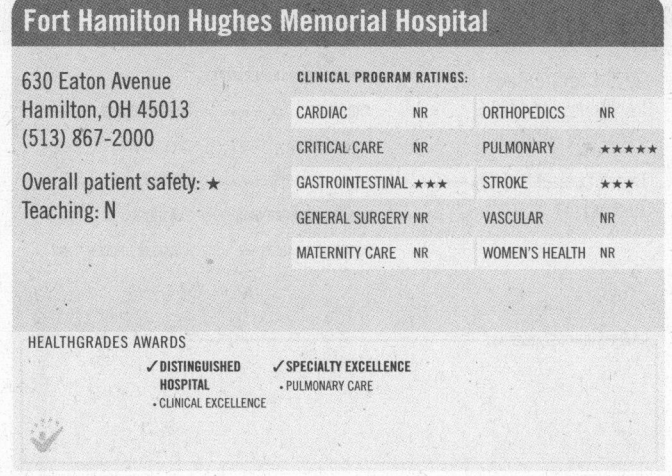

Galion Community Hospital

269 Portland Way South
Galion, OH 44833
(419) 468-4841

Overall patient safety: ★★★
Teaching: N

CLINICAL PROGRAM RATINGS:

CARDIAC	NR	ORTHOPEDICS	NR
CRITICAL CARE	NR	PULMONARY	★★★
GASTROINTESTINAL	NR	STROKE	★
GENERAL SURGERY	NR	VASCULAR	NR
MATERNITY CARE	NR	WOMEN'S HEALTH	NR

HEALTHGRADES AWARDS

Fostoria Community Hospital

501 Van Buren Street
Fostoria, OH 44830
(419) 435-7734

Overall patient safety: ★
Teaching: N

CLINICAL PROGRAM RATINGS:

CARDIAC	NR	ORTHOPEDICS	NR
CRITICAL CARE	NR	PULMONARY	★★★
GASTROINTESTINAL	NR	STROKE	★★★
GENERAL SURGERY	NR	VASCULAR	NR
MATERNITY CARE	NR	WOMEN'S HEALTH	NR

HEALTHGRADES AWARDS

Genesis Healthcare System

800 Forest Avenue
Zanesville, OH 43701
(740) 454-5000

Overall patient safety: ★★★
Teaching: N

CLINICAL PROGRAM RATINGS:

CARDIAC	★★★	ORTHOPEDICS	★★★
CRITICAL CARE	NR	PULMONARY	★★★★★
GASTROINTESTINAL	★★★	STROKE	★★★
GENERAL SURGERY	NR	VASCULAR	★★★
MATERNITY CARE	NR	WOMEN'S HEALTH	NR

HEALTHGRADES AWARDS

✓ SPECIALTY EXCELLENCE
· PULMONARY CARE

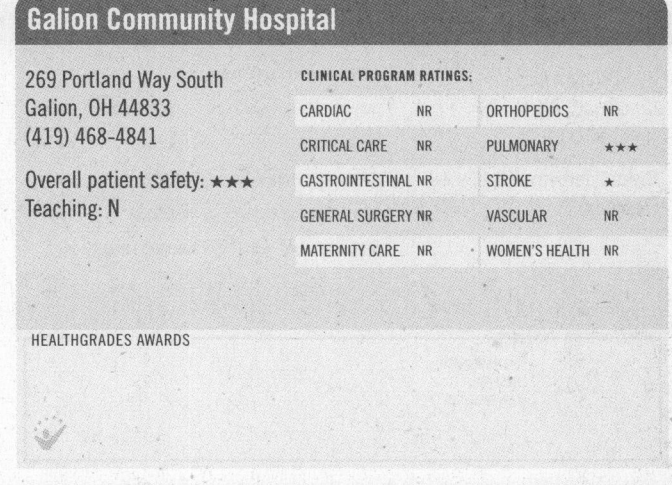

Good Samaritan Hospital

2222 Philadelphia Drive
Dayton, OH 45406
(937) 278-2612

Overall patient safety: ★★★
Teaching: Y

CLINICAL PROGRAM RATINGS:

CARDIAC	★★★	ORTHOPEDICS	★★★★★
CRITICAL CARE	NR	PULMONARY	★★★★★
GASTROINTESTINAL	★★★	STROKE	★★★★★
GENERAL SURGERY	NR	VASCULAR	★★★
MATERNITY CARE	NR	WOMEN'S HEALTH	NR

HEALTHGRADES AWARDS

✓ DISTINGUISHED HOSPITAL
 · CLINICAL EXCELLENCE

✓ SPECIALTY EXCELLENCE
 · JOINT REPLACEMENT
 · ORTHOPEDIC SURGERY
 · PULMONARY CARE
 · STROKE CARE

Grandview Medical Center

405 West Grand Avenue
Dayton, OH 45405
(937) 226-3200

Overall patient safety: ★★★
Teaching: Y

CLINICAL PROGRAM RATINGS:

CARDIAC	★★★	ORTHOPEDICS	★★★
CRITICAL CARE	NR	PULMONARY	★★★★★
GASTROINTESTINAL	★★★	STROKE	★★★
GENERAL SURGERY	NR	VASCULAR	NR
MATERNITY CARE	NR	WOMEN'S HEALTH	NR

HEALTHGRADES AWARDS

✓ DISTINGUISHED HOSPITAL
 · CLINICAL EXCELLENCE

✓ SPECIALTY EXCELLENCE
 · PULMONARY CARE

Good Samaritan Hospital

375 Dixmyth Avenue
Cincinnati, OH 45220
(513) 872-1400

Overall patient safety: ★★★
Teaching: Y

CLINICAL PROGRAM RATINGS:

CARDIAC	★★★	ORTHOPEDICS	★★★
CRITICAL CARE	NR	PULMONARY	★★★
GASTROINTESTINAL	★★★	STROKE	★★★
GENERAL SURGERY	NR	VASCULAR	★★★
MATERNITY CARE	NR	WOMEN'S HEALTH	NR

HEALTHGRADES AWARDS

✓ DISTINGUISHED HOSPITAL
 · CLINICAL EXCELLENCE

Grant Medical Center

111 South Grant Avenue
Columbus, OH 43215
(614) 566-9000

Overall patient safety: ★★★
Teaching: Y

CLINICAL PROGRAM RATINGS:

CARDIAC	★★★	ORTHOPEDICS	★
CRITICAL CARE	★★★	PULMONARY	★★★
GASTROINTESTINAL	★★★	STROKE	★★★
GENERAL SURGERY	NR	VASCULAR	NR
MATERNITY CARE	NR	WOMEN'S HEALTH	NR

HEALTHGRADES AWARDS

Grady Memorial Hospital

561 West Central Avenue
Delaware, OH 43015
(740) 369-8711

Overall patient safety: ★★★
Teaching: N

CLINICAL PROGRAM RATINGS:

CARDIAC	NR	ORTHOPEDICS	NR
CRITICAL CARE	NR	PULMONARY	★★★
GASTROINTESTINAL	NR	STROKE	★★★
GENERAL SURGERY	NR	VASCULAR	NR
MATERNITY CARE	NR	WOMEN'S HEALTH	NR

HEALTHGRADES AWARDS

Greene Memorial Hospital

1141 North Monroe Drive
Xenia, OH 45385
(937) 372-8011

Overall patient safety: ★★★
Teaching: Y

CLINICAL PROGRAM RATINGS:

CARDIAC	NR	ORTHOPEDICS	NR
CRITICAL CARE	NR	PULMONARY	★★★
GASTROINTESTINAL	★★★	STROKE	★★★
GENERAL SURGERY	NR	VASCULAR	NR
MATERNITY CARE	NR	WOMEN'S HEALTH	NR

HEALTHGRADES AWARDS

KEY: ★★★★★ **BEST**   ★★★ **AS EXPECTED**   ★ **POOR**   NR **NOT RATED BY HEALTHGRADES**   For full definitions of ratings and awards, see Appendix.

Greenfield Area Medical Center

550 Mirabeau Street
Greenfield, OH 45123
(937) 981-9400

Overall patient safety: NR
Teaching: N

CLINICAL PROGRAM RATINGS:

CARDIAC	NR	ORTHOPEDICS	NR
CRITICAL CARE	NR	PULMONARY	★★★
GASTROINTESTINAL	NR	STROKE	NR
GENERAL SURGERY	NR	VASCULAR	NR
MATERNITY CARE	NR	WOMEN'S HEALTH	NR

HEALTHGRADES AWARDS

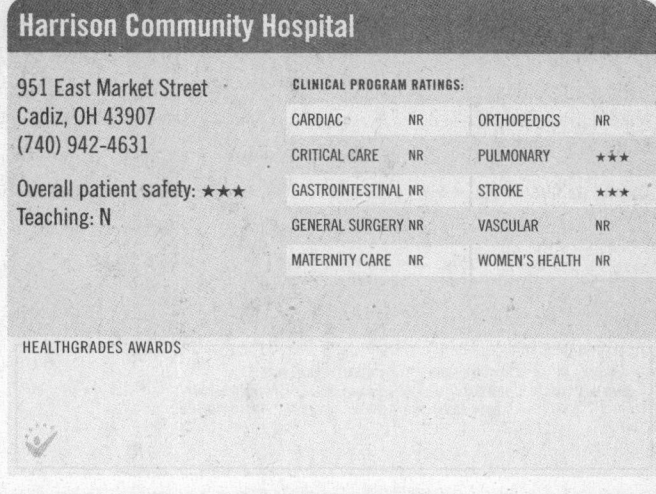

Harrison Community Hospital

951 East Market Street
Cadiz, OH 43907
(740) 942-4631

Overall patient safety: ★★★
Teaching: N

CLINICAL PROGRAM RATINGS:

CARDIAC	NR	ORTHOPEDICS	NR
CRITICAL CARE	NR	PULMONARY	★★★
GASTROINTESTINAL	NR	STROKE	★★★
GENERAL SURGERY	NR	VASCULAR	NR
MATERNITY CARE	NR	WOMEN'S HEALTH	NR

HEALTHGRADES AWARDS

H. B. Magruder Memorial Hospital

615 Fulton Street
Port Clinton, OH 43452
(419) 734-3131

Overall patient safety: ★
Teaching: N

CLINICAL PROGRAM RATINGS:

CARDIAC	NR	ORTHOPEDICS	NR
CRITICAL CARE	NR	PULMONARY	★★★
GASTROINTESTINAL	NR	STROKE	★★★
GENERAL SURGERY	NR	VASCULAR	NR
MATERNITY CARE	NR	WOMEN'S HEALTH	NR

HEALTHGRADES AWARDS

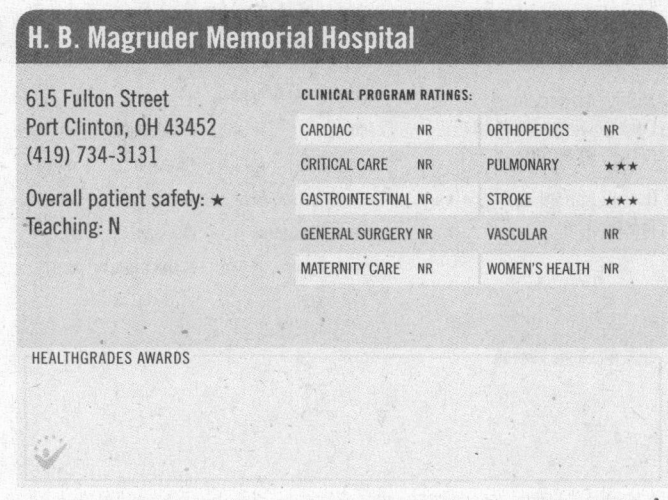

Henry County Hospital

11600 State Route 424
Napoleon, OH 43545
(419) 591-3844

Overall patient safety: ★★★
Teaching: N

CLINICAL PROGRAM RATINGS:

CARDIAC	NR	ORTHOPEDICS	NR
CRITICAL CARE	NR	PULMONARY	★
GASTROINTESTINAL	NR	STROKE	NR
GENERAL SURGERY	NR	VASCULAR	NR
MATERNITY CARE	NR	WOMEN'S HEALTH	NR

HEALTHGRADES AWARDS

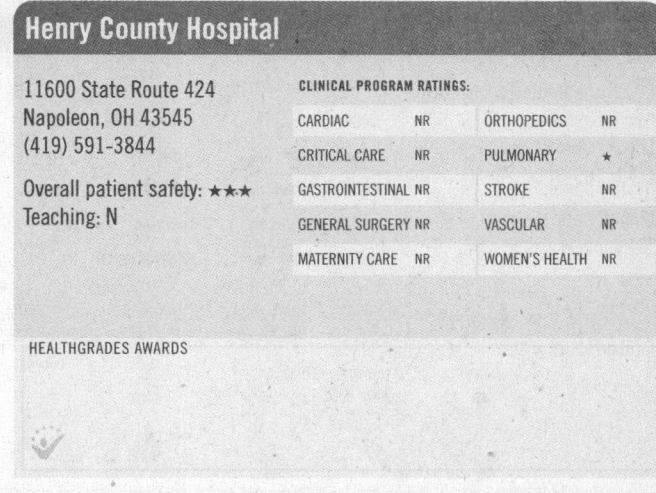

Hardin Memorial Hospital

921 East Franklin Street
Kenton, OH 43326
(419) 673-0761

Overall patient safety: ★★★
Teaching: N

CLINICAL PROGRAM RATINGS:

CARDIAC	NR	ORTHOPEDICS	NR
CRITICAL CARE	NR	PULMONARY	★
GASTROINTESTINAL	NR	STROKE	★
GENERAL SURGERY	NR	VASCULAR	NR
MATERNITY CARE	NR	WOMEN'S HEALTH	NR

HEALTHGRADES AWARDS

Highland District Hospital

1275 North High Street
Hillsboro, OH 45133
(937) 393-6100

Overall patient safety: NR
Teaching: N

CLINICAL PROGRAM RATINGS:

CARDIAC	NR	ORTHOPEDICS	NR
CRITICAL CARE	NR	PULMONARY	★
GASTROINTESTINAL	NR	STROKE	★★★
GENERAL SURGERY	NR	VASCULAR	NR
MATERNITY CARE	NR	WOMEN'S HEALTH	NR

HEALTHGRADES AWARDS

Hillcrest Hospital

6780 Mayfield Road
Mayfield Heights, OH 44124
(440) 449-4500

Overall patient safety: ★★★
Teaching: Y

CLINICAL PROGRAM RATINGS:

CARDIAC	★★★★★	ORTHOPEDICS	★★★
CRITICAL CARE	★★★★★	PULMONARY	★★★★★
GASTROINTESTINAL	★★★	STROKE	★★★★★
GENERAL SURGERY	NR	VASCULAR	★★★
MATERNITY CARE	NR	WOMEN'S HEALTH	NR

HEALTHGRADES AWARDS

✓ AMERICA'S 50   ✓ DISTINGUISHED   ✓ SPECIALTY EXCELLENCE
   BEST HOSPITALS   HOSPITAL   · CARDIAC CARE   · CRITICAL CARE   · STROKE CARE
              · CLINICAL EXCELLENCE   · CARDIAC SURGERY   · PULMONARY CARE

Hospital for Orthopaedic and Specialty Service

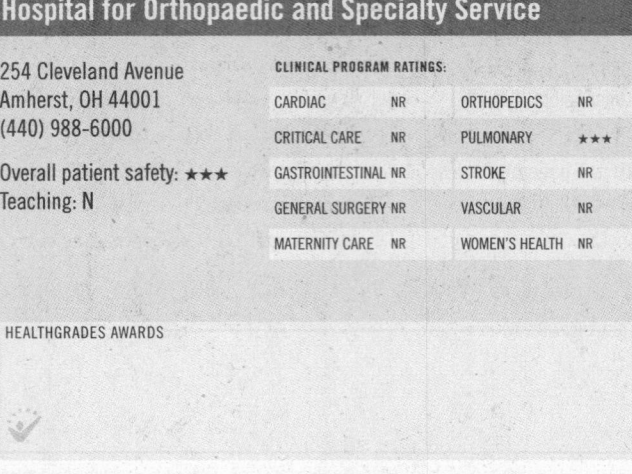

254 Cleveland Avenue
Amherst, OH 44001
(440) 988-6000

Overall patient safety: ★★★
Teaching: N

CLINICAL PROGRAM RATINGS:

CARDIAC	NR	ORTHOPEDICS	NR
CRITICAL CARE	NR	PULMONARY	★★★
GASTROINTESTINAL	NR	STROKE	NR
GENERAL SURGERY	NR	VASCULAR	NR
MATERNITY CARE	NR	WOMEN'S HEALTH	NR

HEALTHGRADES AWARDS

Hocking Valley Community Hospital

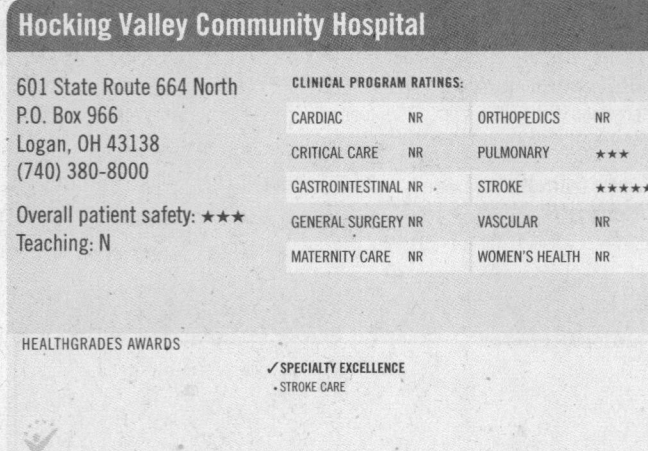

601 State Route 664 North
P.O. Box 966
Logan, OH 43138
(740) 380-8000

Overall patient safety: ★★★
Teaching: N

CLINICAL PROGRAM RATINGS:

CARDIAC	NR	ORTHOPEDICS	NR
CRITICAL CARE	NR	PULMONARY	★★★
GASTROINTESTINAL	NR	STROKE	★★★★★
GENERAL SURGERY	NR	VASCULAR	NR
MATERNITY CARE	NR	WOMEN'S HEALTH	NR

HEALTHGRADES AWARDS

✓ SPECIALTY EXCELLENCE
· STROKE CARE

Huron Hospital

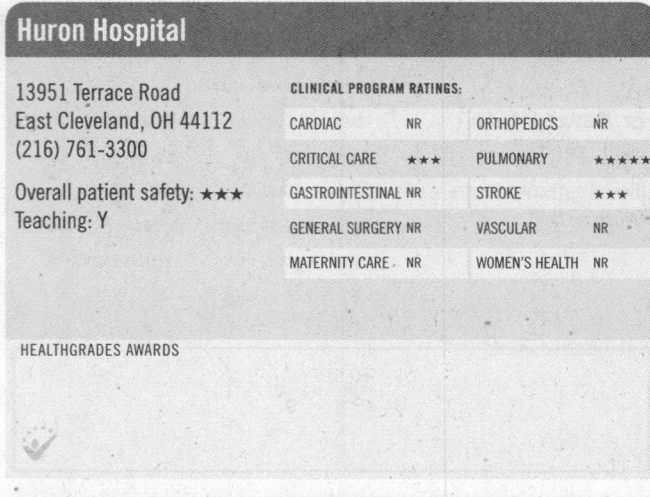

13951 Terrace Road
East Cleveland, OH 44112
(216) 761-3300

Overall patient safety: ★★★
Teaching: Y

CLINICAL PROGRAM RATINGS:

CARDIAC	NR	ORTHOPEDICS	NR
CRITICAL CARE	★★★	PULMONARY	★★★★★
GASTROINTESTINAL	NR	STROKE	★★★
GENERAL SURGERY	NR	VASCULAR	NR
MATERNITY CARE	NR	WOMEN'S HEALTH	NR

HEALTHGRADES AWARDS

Holzer Medical Center

100 Jackson Pike
Gallipolis, OH 45631
(740) 446-5000

Overall patient safety: ★★★
Teaching: N

CLINICAL PROGRAM RATINGS:

CARDIAC	★★★	ORTHOPEDICS	NR
CRITICAL CARE	NR	PULMONARY	★★★★★
GASTROINTESTINAL	★★★	STROKE	NR
GENERAL SURGERY	NR	VASCULAR	NR
MATERNITY CARE	NR	WOMEN'S HEALTH	NR

HEALTHGRADES AWARDS

Jewish Hospital

4777 East Galbraith Road
Cincinnati, OH 45236
(513) 686-3000

Overall patient safety: ★★★
Teaching: Y

CLINICAL PROGRAM RATINGS:

CARDIAC	★★★	ORTHOPEDICS	★★★
CRITICAL CARE	NR	PULMONARY	★★★
GASTROINTESTINAL	★★★	STROKE	★★★
GENERAL SURGERY	NR	VASCULAR	★★★
MATERNITY CARE	NR	WOMEN'S HEALTH	NR

HEALTHGRADES AWARDS

✓ DISTINGUISHED
   HOSPITAL
· CLINICAL EXCELLENCE

KEY: ★★★★★ BEST   ★★★ AS EXPECTED   ★ POOR   NR NOT RATED BY HEALTHGRADES   For full definitions of ratings and awards, see Appendix.

Joel Pomerene Memorial Hospital

981 Wooster Road
Millersburg, OH 44654
(330) 674-1015

Overall patient safety: ★★★
Teaching: N

CLINICAL PROGRAM RATINGS:

CARDIAC	NR	ORTHOPEDICS	NR
CRITICAL CARE	NR	PULMONARY	★
GASTROINTESTINAL	NR	STROKE	★★★
GENERAL SURGERY	NR	VASCULAR	NR
MATERNITY CARE	NR	WOMEN'S HEALTH	NR

HEALTHGRADES AWARDS

Joint Township District Memorial Hospital

200 St. Clair Street
St. Marys, OH 45885
(419) 394-3335

Overall patient safety: ★★★
Teaching: Y

CLINICAL PROGRAM RATINGS:

CARDIAC	NR	ORTHOPEDICS	NR
CRITICAL CARE	NR	PULMONARY	★★★★★
GASTROINTESTINAL	NR	STROKE	★★★
GENERAL SURGERY	NR	VASCULAR	NR
MATERNITY CARE	NR	WOMEN'S HEALTH	NR

HEALTHGRADES AWARDS

✓ SPECIALTY EXCELLENCE
· PULMONARY CARE

Kettering Medical Center

3535 Southern Boulevard
Kettering, OH 45429
(937) 298-4331

Overall patient safety: ★★★
Teaching: Y

CLINICAL PROGRAM RATINGS:

CARDIAC	★★★	ORTHOPEDICS	★★★
CRITICAL CARE	NR	PULMONARY	★★★★★
GASTROINTESTINAL	★★★	STROKE	★★★
GENERAL SURGERY	NR	VASCULAR	★★★
MATERNITY CARE	NR	WOMEN'S HEALTH	NR

HEALTHGRADES AWARDS

✓ DISTINGUISHED   ✓ SPECIALTY EXCELLENCE
   HOSPITAL   · GASTROINTESTINAL   · PULMONARY CARE
· CLINICAL EXCELLENCE   CARE

Kettering Medical Center--Sycamore

2150 Leiter Road
Miamisburg, OH 45342
(937) 384-8760

Overall patient safety: ★★★
Teaching: Y

CLINICAL PROGRAM RATINGS:

CARDIAC	NR	ORTHOPEDICS	NR
CRITICAL CARE	NR	PULMONARY	★★★
GASTROINTESTINAL	★★★	STROKE	★★★
GENERAL SURGERY	NR	VASCULAR	NR
MATERNITY CARE	NR	WOMEN'S HEALTH	NR

HEALTHGRADES AWARDS

Kettering-Mohican Area Medical Center*

546 North Union Street
Loudonville, OH 44842
(419) 358-9010

Overall patient safety: ★★★
Teaching: N

CLINICAL PROGRAM RATINGS:

CARDIAC	NR	ORTHOPEDICS	NR
CRITICAL CARE	NR	PULMONARY	★★★
GASTROINTESTINAL	★★★	STROKE	★★★
GENERAL SURGERY	NR	VASCULAR	NR
MATERNITY CARE	NR	WOMEN'S HEALTH	NR

HEALTHGRADES AWARDS

Knox Community Hospital

1330 Coshocton Road
Mount Vernon, OH 43050
(740) 393-9000

Overall patient safety: ★★★
Teaching: N

CLINICAL PROGRAM RATINGS:

CARDIAC	NR	ORTHOPEDICS	NR
CRITICAL CARE	NR	PULMONARY	★★★
GASTROINTESTINAL	★★★	STROKE	★★★
GENERAL SURGERY	NR	VASCULAR	NR
MATERNITY CARE	NR	WOMEN'S HEALTH	NR

HEALTHGRADES AWARDS

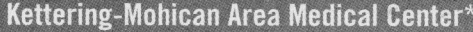

*This hospital reports its data to the federal government jointly with another hospital. Therefore the ratings and awards apply to multiple hospitals and this specific hospital may not provide all rated services.

Lake Hospital System

10 East Washington Street
Painesville, OH 44077
(440) 354-2400

Overall patient safety: ★★★
Teaching: N

CLINICAL PROGRAM RATINGS:

CARDIAC	★★★★★	ORTHOPEDICS	★★★
CRITICAL CARE	★★★	PULMONARY	★★★
GASTROINTESTINAL	★★★	STROKE	★★★
GENERAL SURGERY	NR	VASCULAR	★★★
MATERNITY CARE	NR	WOMEN'S HEALTH	NR

HEALTHGRADES AWARDS

✓ SPECIALTY EXCELLENCE
· CARDIAC CARE   · CARDIAC SURGERY

Lima Memorial Health System

1001 Bellefontaine Avenue
Lima, OH 45804
(419) 228-3335

Overall patient safety: ★★★
Teaching: N

CLINICAL PROGRAM RATINGS:

CARDIAC	★★★	ORTHOPEDICS	★★★
CRITICAL CARE	NR	PULMONARY	★★★
GASTROINTESTINAL	★★★	STROKE	★★★
GENERAL SURGERY	NR	VASCULAR	★★★
MATERNITY CARE	NR	WOMEN'S HEALTH	NR

HEALTHGRADES AWARDS

Lakewood Hospital

14519 Detroit Avenue
Lakewood, OH 44107
(216) 521-4200

Overall patient safety: ★★★
Teaching: N

CLINICAL PROGRAM RATINGS:

CARDIAC	★★★	ORTHOPEDICS	★★★
CRITICAL CARE	★★★	PULMONARY	★★★★★
GASTROINTESTINAL	★★★	STROKE	★★★★★
GENERAL SURGERY	NR	VASCULAR	NR
MATERNITY CARE	NR	WOMEN'S HEALTH	NR

HEALTHGRADES AWARDS

✓ DISTINGUISHED   ✓ SPECIALTY EXCELLENCE
  HOSPITAL   · GASTROINTESTINAL   · PULMONARY CARE   · STROKE CARE
· CLINICAL EXCELLENCE   CARE

Lutheran Hospital

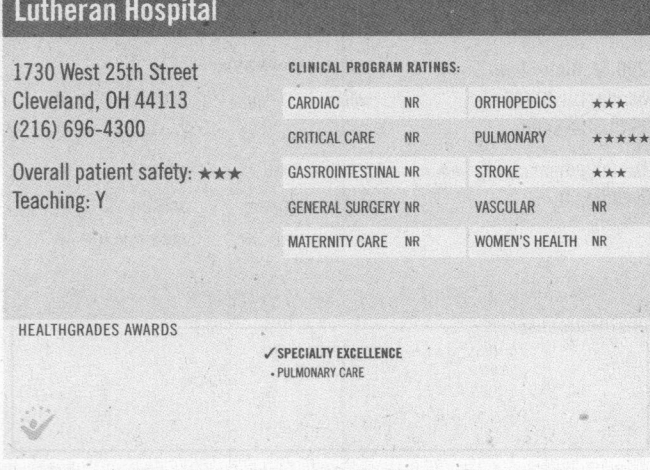

1730 West 25th Street
Cleveland, OH 44113
(216) 696-4300

Overall patient safety: ★★★
Teaching: Y

CLINICAL PROGRAM RATINGS:

CARDIAC	NR	ORTHOPEDICS	★★★
CRITICAL CARE	NR	PULMONARY	★★★★★
GASTROINTESTINAL	NR	STROKE	★★★
GENERAL SURGERY	NR	VASCULAR	NR
MATERNITY CARE	NR	WOMEN'S HEALTH	NR

HEALTHGRADES AWARDS

✓ SPECIALTY EXCELLENCE
· PULMONARY CARE

Licking Memorial Hospital

1320 West Main Street
Newark, OH 43055
(740) 348-4000

Overall patient safety: ★★★
Teaching: N

CLINICAL PROGRAM RATINGS:

CARDIAC	NR	ORTHOPEDICS	NR
CRITICAL CARE	★★★	PULMONARY	★★★
GASTROINTESTINAL	★★★	STROKE	★★★
GENERAL SURGERY	NR	VASCULAR	NR
MATERNITY CARE	NR	WOMEN'S HEALTH	NR

HEALTHGRADES AWARDS

Madison County Hospital

210 North Main Street
London, OH 43140
(740) 845-7000

Overall patient safety: ★★★
Teaching: N

CLINICAL PROGRAM RATINGS:

CARDIAC	NR	ORTHOPEDICS	NR
CRITICAL CARE	NR	PULMONARY	★★★
GASTROINTESTINAL	NR	STROKE	NR
GENERAL SURGERY	NR	VASCULAR	NR
MATERNITY CARE	NR	WOMEN'S HEALTH	NR

HEALTHGRADES AWARDS

KEY: ★★★★★ BEST   ★★★ AS EXPECTED   ★ POOR   NR NOT RATED BY HEALTHGRADES   For full definitions of ratings and awards, see Appendix.

Marietta Memorial Hospital

401 Matthew Street
Marietta, OH 45750
(740) 374-1400

Overall patient safety: ★★★
Teaching: N

CLINICAL PROGRAM RATINGS:

CARDIAC	NR	ORTHOPEDICS	★★★
CRITICAL CARE	NR	PULMONARY	★★★
GASTROINTESTINAL	★★★	STROKE	★★★
GENERAL SURGERY	NR	VASCULAR	NR
MATERNITY CARE	NR	WOMEN'S HEALTH	NR

HEALTHGRADES AWARDS

✓ SPECIALTY EXCELLENCE
- GASTROINTESTINAL CARE

Marymount Hospital

12300 MacCracken Road
Garfield Heights, OH 44125
(216) 581-0500

Overall patient safety: ★★★
Teaching: N

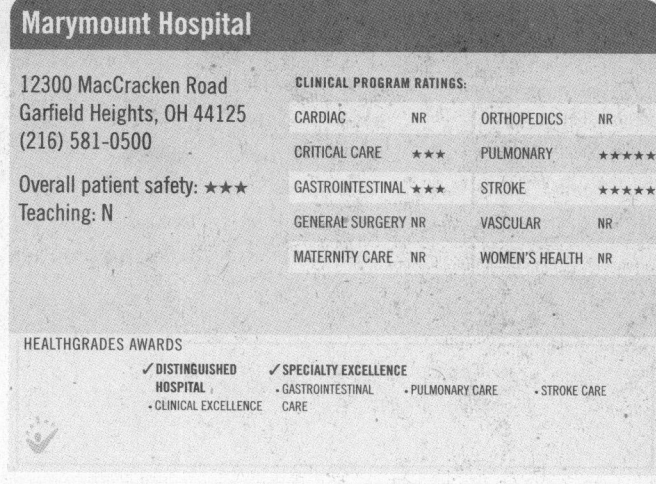

CLINICAL PROGRAM RATINGS:

CARDIAC	NR	ORTHOPEDICS	NR
CRITICAL CARE	★★★	PULMONARY	★★★★★
GASTROINTESTINAL	★★★	STROKE	★★★★★
GENERAL SURGERY	NR	VASCULAR	NR
MATERNITY CARE	NR	WOMEN'S HEALTH	NR

HEALTHGRADES AWARDS

✓ DISTINGUISHED HOSPITAL
- CLINICAL EXCELLENCE

✓ SPECIALTY EXCELLENCE
- GASTROINTESTINAL CARE · PULMONARY CARE · STROKE CARE

Marion General Hospital*

1000 McKinley Park Drive
Marion, OH 43302
(740) 383-8400

Overall patient safety: ★★★★★
Teaching: N

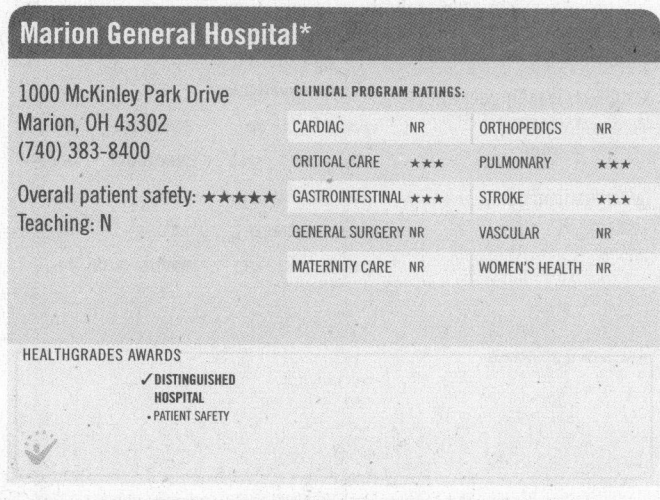

CLINICAL PROGRAM RATINGS:

CARDIAC	NR	ORTHOPEDICS	NR
CRITICAL CARE	★★★	PULMONARY	★★★
GASTROINTESTINAL	★★★	STROKE	★★★
GENERAL SURGERY	NR	VASCULAR	NR
MATERNITY CARE	NR	WOMEN'S HEALTH	NR

HEALTHGRADES AWARDS

✓ DISTINGUISHED HOSPITAL
- PATIENT SAFETY

Massillon Community Hospital

875 8th Street Northeast
Massillon, OH 44646
(330) 832-8761

Overall patient safety: ★★★
Teaching: N

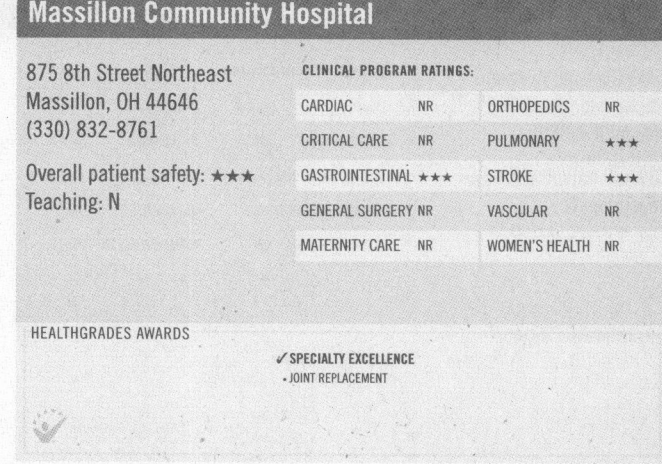

CLINICAL PROGRAM RATINGS:

CARDIAC	NR	ORTHOPEDICS	NR
CRITICAL CARE	NR	PULMONARY	★★★
GASTROINTESTINAL	★★★	STROKE	★★★
GENERAL SURGERY	NR	VASCULAR	NR
MATERNITY CARE	NR	WOMEN'S HEALTH	NR

HEALTHGRADES AWARDS

✓ SPECIALTY EXCELLENCE
- JOINT REPLACEMENT

Mary Rutan Hospital

205 Palmer Avenue
Bellefontaine, OH 43311
(937) 592-4015

Overall patient safety: ★★★
Teaching: Y

CLINICAL PROGRAM RATINGS:

CARDIAC	NR	ORTHOPEDICS	NR
CRITICAL CARE	NR	PULMONARY	★★★
GASTROINTESTINAL	NR	STROKE	★★★
GENERAL SURGERY	NR	VASCULAR	NR
MATERNITY CARE	NR	WOMEN'S HEALTH	NR

HEALTHGRADES AWARDS

McCullough-Hyde Memorial Hospital

110 North Poplar Street
Oxford, OH 45056
(513) 523-2111

Overall patient safety: ★★★
Teaching: N

CLINICAL PROGRAM RATINGS:

CARDIAC	NR	ORTHOPEDICS	NR
CRITICAL CARE	NR	PULMONARY	★★★
GASTROINTESTINAL	NR	STROKE	★
GENERAL SURGERY	NR	VASCULAR	NR
MATERNITY CARE	NR	WOMEN'S HEALTH	NR

HEALTHGRADES AWARDS

*This hospital reports its data to the federal government jointly with another hospital. Therefore the ratings and awards apply to multiple hospitals and this specific hospital may not provide all rated services.

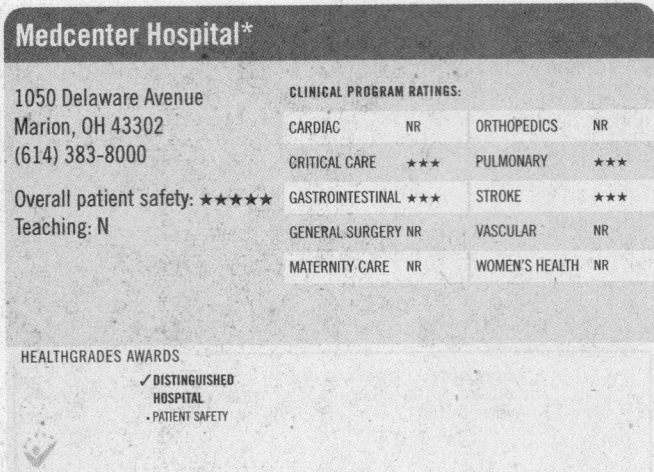

Medcenter Hospital*

1050 Delaware Avenue
Marion, OH 43302
(614) 383-8000

Overall patient safety: ★★★★★
Teaching: N

CLINICAL PROGRAM RATINGS:

CARDIAC	NR	ORTHOPEDICS	NR
CRITICAL CARE	★★★	PULMONARY	★★★
GASTROINTESTINAL	★★★	STROKE	★★★
GENERAL SURGERY	NR	VASCULAR	NR
MATERNITY CARE	NR	WOMEN'S HEALTH	NR

HEALTHGRADES AWARDS

✓ DISTINGUISHED HOSPITAL
- PATIENT SAFETY

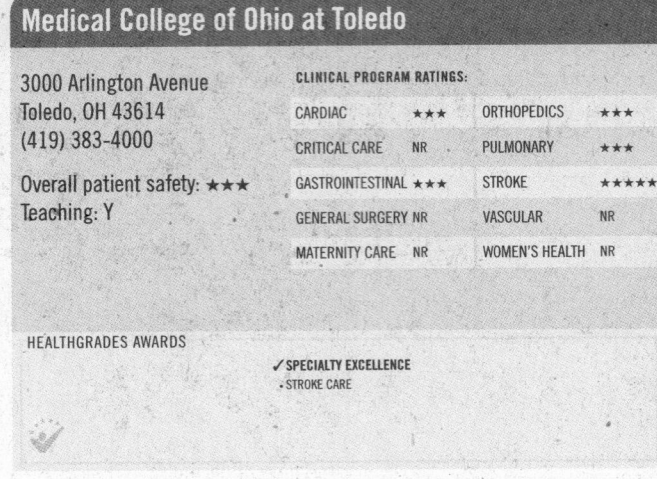

Medical College of Ohio at Toledo

3000 Arlington Avenue
Toledo, OH 43614
(419) 383-4000

Overall patient safety: ★★★
Teaching: Y

CLINICAL PROGRAM RATINGS:

CARDIAC	★★★	ORTHOPEDICS	★★★
CRITICAL CARE	NR	PULMONARY	★★★
GASTROINTESTINAL	★★★	STROKE	★★★★★
GENERAL SURGERY	NR	VASCULAR	NR
MATERNITY CARE	NR	WOMEN'S HEALTH	NR

HEALTHGRADES AWARDS

✓ SPECIALTY EXCELLENCE
- STROKE CARE

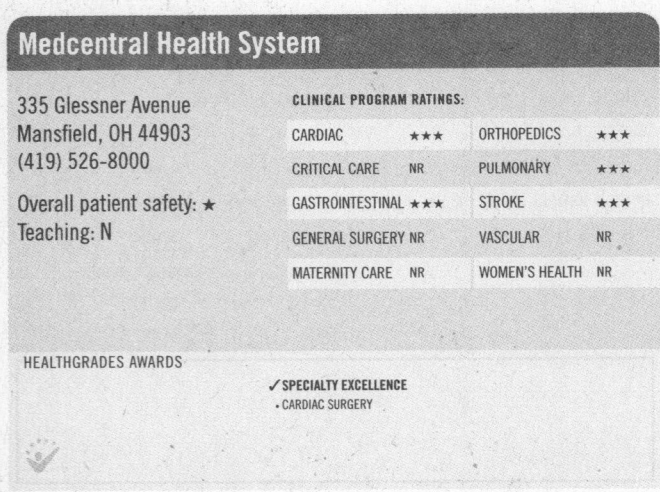

Medcentral Health System

335 Glessner Avenue
Mansfield, OH 44903
(419) 526-8000

Overall patient safety: ★
Teaching: N

CLINICAL PROGRAM RATINGS:

CARDIAC	★★★	ORTHOPEDICS	★★★
CRITICAL CARE	NR	PULMONARY	★★★
GASTROINTESTINAL	★★★	STROKE	★★★
GENERAL SURGERY	NR	VASCULAR	NR
MATERNITY CARE	NR	WOMEN'S HEALTH	NR

HEALTHGRADES AWARDS

✓ SPECIALTY EXCELLENCE
- CARDIAC SURGERY

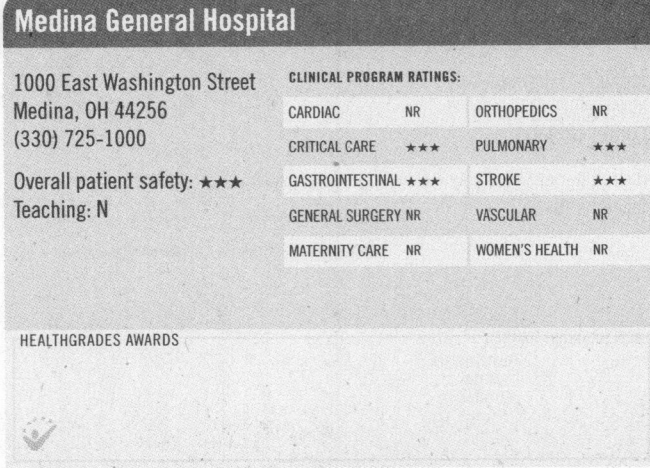

Medina General Hospital

1000 East Washington Street
Medina, OH 44256
(330) 725-1000

Overall patient safety: ★★★
Teaching: N

CLINICAL PROGRAM RATINGS:

CARDIAC	NR	ORTHOPEDICS	NR
CRITICAL CARE	★★★	PULMONARY	★★★
GASTROINTESTINAL	★★★	STROKE	★★★
GENERAL SURGERY	NR	VASCULAR	NR
MATERNITY CARE	NR	WOMEN'S HEALTH	NR

HEALTHGRADES AWARDS

Medcentral Health System Shelby Hospital

20 Morris Road
Shelby, OH 44875
(419) 342-5015

Overall patient safety: ★
Teaching: N

CLINICAL PROGRAM RATINGS:

CARDIAC	NR	ORTHOPEDICS	NR
CRITICAL CARE	NR	PULMONARY	★★★
GASTROINTESTINAL	NR	STROKE	NR
GENERAL SURGERY	NR	VASCULAR	NR
MATERNITY CARE	NR	WOMEN'S HEALTH	NR

HEALTHGRADES AWARDS

✓ SPECIALTY EXCELLENCE
- CARDIAC SURGERY

Memorial Hospital

715 South Taft Avenue
Fremont, OH 43420
(419) 332-7321

Overall patient safety: ★★★
Teaching: N

CLINICAL PROGRAM RATINGS:

CARDIAC	NR	ORTHOPEDICS	NR
CRITICAL CARE	NR	PULMONARY	★★★
GASTROINTESTINAL	NR	STROKE	★
GENERAL SURGERY	NR	VASCULAR	NR
MATERNITY CARE	NR	WOMEN'S HEALTH	NR

HEALTHGRADES AWARDS

KEY: ★★★★★ BEST   ★★★ AS EXPECTED   ★ POOR   NR NOT RATED BY HEALTHGRADES   For full definitions of ratings and awards, see Appendix.

Memorial Hospital of Union County

500 London Avenue
Marysville, OH 43040
(937) 644-6115

Overall patient safety: ★★★
Teaching: N

CLINICAL PROGRAM RATINGS:

CARDIAC	NR	ORTHOPEDICS	NR
CRITICAL CARE	NR	PULMONARY	★★★
GASTROINTESTINAL	NR	STROKE	★★★
GENERAL SURGERY	NR	VASCULAR	NR
MATERNITY CARE	NR	WOMEN'S HEALTH	NR

HEALTHGRADES AWARDS

Mercy Healthcare Center*

2200 Jefferson Avenue
Toledo, OH 43624
(419) 259-1500

Overall patient safety: ★★★★★
Teaching: Y

CLINICAL PROGRAM RATINGS:

CARDIAC	★★★	ORTHOPEDICS	★★★
CRITICAL CARE	NR	PULMONARY	★★★★★
GASTROINTESTINAL	★★★	STROKE	★★★
GENERAL SURGERY	NR	VASCULAR	★★★
MATERNITY CARE	NR	WOMEN'S HEALTH	NR

HEALTHGRADES AWARDS

✓ **DISTINGUISHED HOSPITAL**
· PATIENT SAFETY

✓ **SPECIALTY EXCELLENCE**
· PULMONARY CARE

Mercer County Joint Township Community

800 West Main Street
Coldwater, OH 45828
(419) 678-2341

Overall patient safety: ★
Teaching: N

CLINICAL PROGRAM RATINGS:

CARDIAC	NR	ORTHOPEDICS	NR
CRITICAL CARE	NR	PULMONARY	★★★
GASTROINTESTINAL	NR	STROKE	NR
GENERAL SURGERY	NR	VASCULAR	NR
MATERNITY CARE	NR	WOMEN'S HEALTH	NR

HEALTHGRADES AWARDS

Mercy Hospital—Anderson

7500 State Road
Anderson, OH 45255
(513) 624-4500

Overall patient safety: ★★★★★
Teaching: N

CLINICAL PROGRAM RATINGS:

CARDIAC	NR	ORTHOPEDICS	★★★
CRITICAL CARE	NR	PULMONARY	★★★
GASTROINTESTINAL	★★★	STROKE	★★★
GENERAL SURGERY	NR	VASCULAR	NR
MATERNITY CARE	NR	WOMEN'S HEALTH	NR

HEALTHGRADES AWARDS

✓ **DISTINGUISHED HOSPITAL**
· PATIENT SAFETY

Mercy Franciscan Hospital—Mount Airy

2446 Kipling Avenue
Cincinnati, OH 45239
(513) 853-5000

Overall patient safety: ★★★★★
Teaching: Y

CLINICAL PROGRAM RATINGS:

CARDIAC	NR	ORTHOPEDICS	★★★
CRITICAL CARE	NR	PULMONARY	★★★
GASTROINTESTINAL	★★★	STROKE	★★★
GENERAL SURGERY	NR	VASCULAR	NR
MATERNITY CARE	NR	WOMEN'S HEALTH	NR

HEALTHGRADES AWARDS

✓ **DISTINGUISHED HOSPITAL**
· PATIENT SAFETY

Mercy Hospital—Clermont

3000 Hospital Drive
Batavia, OH 45103
(513) 732-8200

Overall patient safety: ★★★
Teaching: N

CLINICAL PROGRAM RATINGS:

CARDIAC	NR	ORTHOPEDICS	NR
CRITICAL CARE	NR	PULMONARY	★★★
GASTROINTESTINAL	★★★	STROKE	★★★
GENERAL SURGERY	NR	VASCULAR	NR
MATERNITY CARE	NR	WOMEN'S HEALTH	NR

HEALTHGRADES AWARDS

*This hospital reports its data to the federal government jointly with another hospital. Therefore the ratings and awards apply to multiple hospitals and this specific hospital may not provide all rated services.

Mercy Hospital–Fairfield

3000 Mack Road
Fairfield, OH 45014
(513) 870-7000

Overall patient safety: ★★★
Teaching: N

CLINICAL PROGRAM RATINGS:

CARDIAC	★★★	ORTHOPEDICS	★★★
CRITICAL CARE	NR	PULMONARY	★★★
GASTROINTESTINAL	★★★	STROKE	★★★
GENERAL SURGERY	NR	VASCULAR	★★★
MATERNITY CARE	NR	WOMEN'S HEALTH	NR

HEALTHGRADES AWARDS

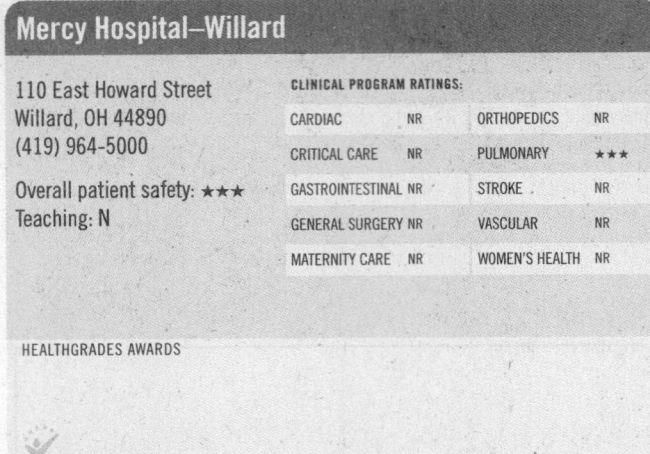

Mercy Hospital–Willard

110 East Howard Street
Willard, OH 44890
(419) 964-5000

Overall patient safety: ★★★
Teaching: N

CLINICAL PROGRAM RATINGS:

CARDIAC	NR	ORTHOPEDICS	NR
CRITICAL CARE	NR	PULMONARY	★★★
GASTROINTESTINAL	NR	STROKE	NR
GENERAL SURGERY	NR	VASCULAR	NR
MATERNITY CARE	NR	WOMEN'S HEALTH	NR

HEALTHGRADES AWARDS

Mercy Hospital–Tiffin Ohio

485 West Market Street
Tiffin, OH 44883
(419) 447-3130

Overall patient safety: ★★★★★
Teaching: N

CLINICAL PROGRAM RATINGS:

CARDIAC	NR	ORTHOPEDICS	NR
CRITICAL CARE	NR	PULMONARY	★★★
GASTROINTESTINAL	NR	STROKE	★★★
GENERAL SURGERY	NR	VASCULAR	NR
MATERNITY CARE	NR	WOMEN'S HEALTH	NR

HEALTHGRADES AWARDS

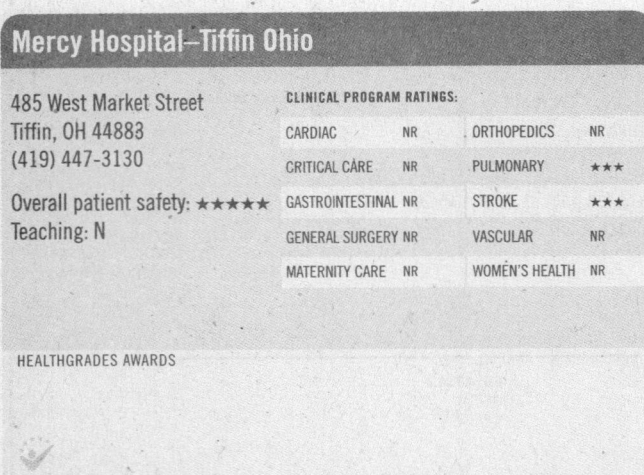

Mercy Medical Center

1320 Mercy Drive Northwest
Canton, OH 44708
(330) 489-1000

Overall patient safety: ★★★
Teaching: Y

CLINICAL PROGRAM RATINGS:

CARDIAC	★★★	ORTHOPEDICS	★★★
CRITICAL CARE	NR	PULMONARY	★★★
GASTROINTESTINAL	★★★	STROKE	★★★
GENERAL SURGERY	NR	VASCULAR	★★★
MATERNITY CARE	NR	WOMEN'S HEALTH	NR

HEALTHGRADES AWARDS

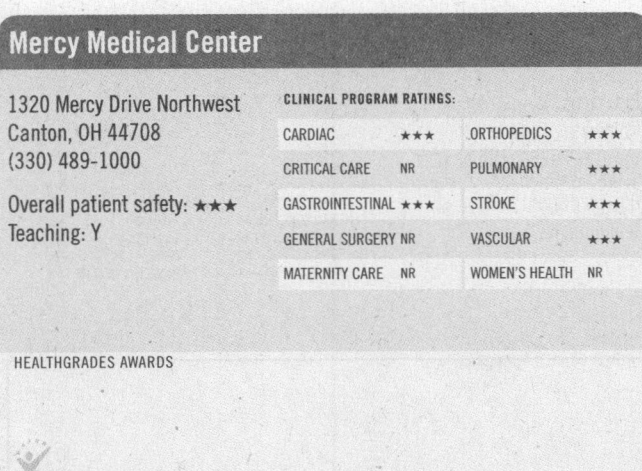

Mercy Hospital–Western Hills

3131 Queen City Avenue
Cincinnati, OH 45238
(513) 389-5000

Overall patient safety: ★★★★★
Teaching: N

CLINICAL PROGRAM RATINGS:

CARDIAC	NR	ORTHOPEDICS	★★★
CRITICAL CARE	NR	PULMONARY	★★★
GASTROINTESTINAL	★★★	STROKE	★★★
GENERAL SURGERY	NR	VASCULAR	NR
MATERNITY CARE	NR	WOMEN'S HEALTH	NR

HEALTHGRADES AWARDS

✓ DISTINGUISHED
HOSPITAL
- PATIENT SAFETY

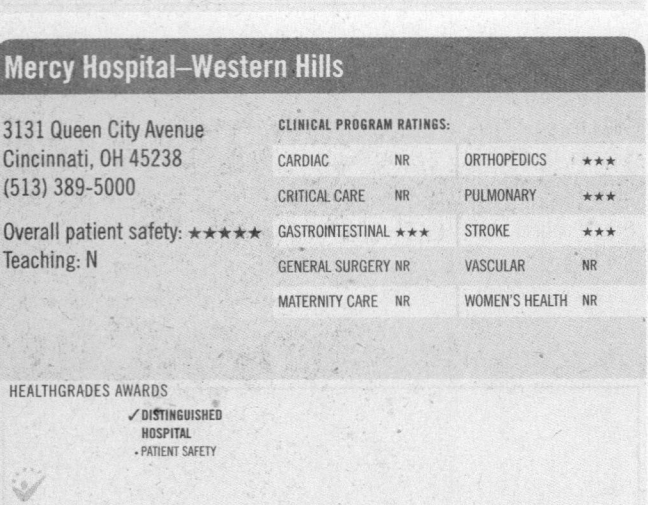

Mercy Medical Center of Springfield

1343 North Fountain Boulevard
Springfield, OH 45504
(937) 390-5000

Overall patient safety: ★★★★★
Teaching: N

CLINICAL PROGRAM RATINGS:

CARDIAC	★★★	ORTHOPEDICS	NR
CRITICAL CARE	NR	PULMONARY	★★★
GASTROINTESTINAL	★★★	STROKE	★★★
GENERAL SURGERY	NR	VASCULAR	★★★
MATERNITY CARE	NR	WOMEN'S HEALTH	NR

HEALTHGRADES AWARDS

✓ DISTINGUISHED
HOSPITAL
- PATIENT SAFETY

KEY: ★★★★★ BEST   ★★★ AS EXPECTED   ★ POOR   NR NOT RATED BY HEALTHGRADES   For full definitions of ratings and awards, see Appendix.

Mercy Memorial Hospital

904 Scioto Avenue
Urbana, OH 43078
(937) 653-5231

Overall patient safety: ★★★
Teaching: N

CLINICAL PROGRAM RATINGS:

CARDIAC	NR	ORTHOPEDICS	NR
CRITICAL CARE	NR	PULMONARY	★★★
GASTROINTESTINAL	NR	STROKE	★
GENERAL SURGERY	NR	VASCULAR	NR
MATERNITY CARE	NR	WOMEN'S HEALTH	NR

HEALTHGRADES AWARDS

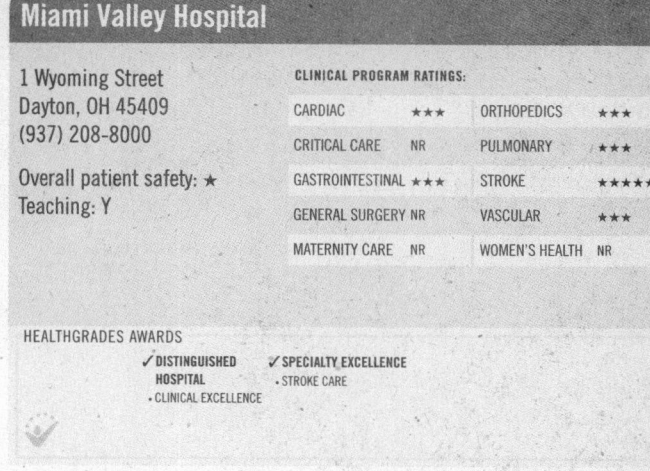

Miami Valley Hospital

1 Wyoming Street
Dayton, OH 45409
(937) 208-8000

Overall patient safety: ★
Teaching: Y

CLINICAL PROGRAM RATINGS:

CARDIAC	★★★	ORTHOPEDICS	★★★
CRITICAL CARE	NR	PULMONARY	★★★
GASTROINTESTINAL	★★★	STROKE	★★★★★
GENERAL SURGERY	NR	VASCULAR	★★★
MATERNITY CARE	NR	WOMEN'S HEALTH	NR

HEALTHGRADES AWARDS

✓ DISTINGUISHED HOSPITAL
• CLINICAL EXCELLENCE

✓ SPECIALTY EXCELLENCE
• STROKE CARE

Meridia Euclid Hospital

18901 Lake Shore Boulevard
Euclid, OH 44119
(216) 531-9000

Overall patient safety: ★★★
Teaching: N

CLINICAL PROGRAM RATINGS:

CARDIAC	NR	ORTHOPEDICS	★★★
CRITICAL CARE	★★★	PULMONARY	★★★
GASTROINTESTINAL	★★★	STROKE	★★★
GENERAL SURGERY	NR	VASCULAR	NR
MATERNITY CARE	NR	WOMEN'S HEALTH	NR

HEALTHGRADES AWARDS

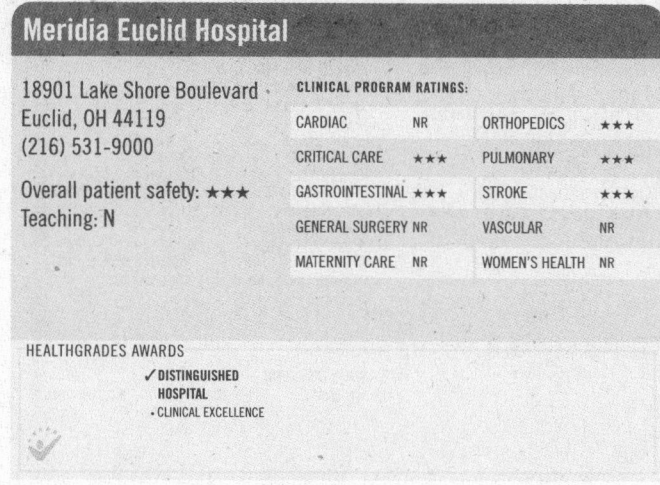

✓ DISTINGUISHED HOSPITAL
• CLINICAL EXCELLENCE

Middletown Regional Hospital

105 McKnight Drive
Middletown, OH 45044
(513) 424-2111

Overall patient safety: ★★★★★
Teaching: N

CLINICAL PROGRAM RATINGS:

CARDIAC	NR	ORTHOPEDICS	★★★
CRITICAL CARE	NR	PULMONARY	★★★
GASTROINTESTINAL	★★★	STROKE	★★★
GENERAL SURGERY	NR	VASCULAR	NR
MATERNITY CARE	NR	WOMEN'S HEALTH	NR

HEALTHGRADES AWARDS

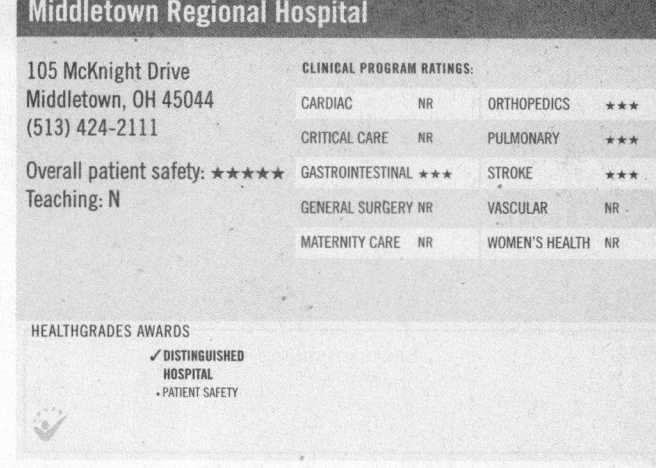

✓ DISTINGUISHED HOSPITAL
• PATIENT SAFETY

MetroHealth Medical Center

2500 MetroHealth Drive
Cleveland, OH 44109
(216) 778-7800

Overall patient safety: ★★★
Teaching: Y

CLINICAL PROGRAM RATINGS:

CARDIAC	★★★	ORTHOPEDICS	★★★
CRITICAL CARE	★★★	PULMONARY	★★★
GASTROINTESTINAL	NR	STROKE	★★★
GENERAL SURGERY	NR	VASCULAR	NR
MATERNITY CARE	NR	WOMEN'S HEALTH	NR

HEALTHGRADES AWARDS

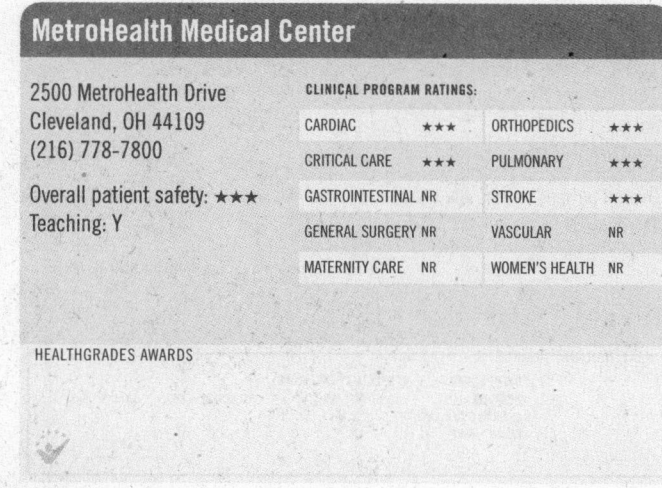

Mount Carmel Health

793 West State Street
Columbus, OH 43222
(614) 234-5000

Overall patient safety: ★★★
Teaching: Y

CLINICAL PROGRAM RATINGS:

CARDIAC	★★★	ORTHOPEDICS	★★★★★
CRITICAL CARE	★★★	PULMONARY	★★★
GASTROINTESTINAL	★★★	STROKE	★★★★★
GENERAL SURGERY	NR	VASCULAR	★★★
MATERNITY CARE	NR	WOMEN'S HEALTH	NR

HEALTHGRADES AWARDS

✓ SPECIALTY EXCELLENCE
• JOINT REPLACEMENT   • ORTHOPEDIC SURGERY   • STROKE CARE

Mount Carmel St. Ann's Hospital of Columbus

500 South Cleveland Avenue
Westerville, OH 43081
(614) 898-4000

Overall patient safety: ★★★
Teaching: Y

CLINICAL PROGRAM RATINGS:

CARDIAC	NR	ORTHOPEDICS	NR
CRITICAL CARE	★★★	PULMONARY	★★★
GASTROINTESTINAL	★★★	STROKE	★★★
GENERAL SURGERY	NR	VASCULAR	★★★
MATERNITY CARE	NR	WOMEN'S HEALTH	NR

HEALTHGRADES AWARDS

Ohio State University Hospital East

1492 East Broad Street
Columbus, OH 43205
(614) 257-3000

Overall patient safety: ★★★
Teaching: Y

CLINICAL PROGRAM RATINGS:

CARDIAC	NR	ORTHOPEDICS	★★★
CRITICAL CARE	★★★★★	PULMONARY	★★★★★
GASTROINTESTINAL	★★★	STROKE	★★★
GENERAL SURGERY	NR	VASCULAR	NR
MATERNITY CARE	NR	WOMEN'S HEALTH	NR

HEALTHGRADES AWARDS

✓ DISTINGUISHED HOSPITAL
• CLINICAL EXCELLENCE

✓ SPECIALTY EXCELLENCE
• CRITICAL CARE   • PULMONARY CARE

New Albany Surgical Hospital

7333 Smith's Mill Road
New Albany, OH 43054
(614) 775-6000

Overall patient safety: ★★★★★
Teaching: N

CLINICAL PROGRAM RATINGS:

CARDIAC	NR	ORTHOPEDICS	NR
CRITICAL CARE	NR	PULMONARY	NR
GASTROINTESTINAL	NR	STROKE	NR
GENERAL SURGERY	NR	VASCULAR	NR
MATERNITY CARE	NR	WOMEN'S HEALTH	NR

HEALTHGRADES AWARDS

✓ SPECIALTY EXCELLENCE
• JOINT REPLACEMENT

Ohio State University Hospitals

1375 Perry Street
Columbus, OH 43210
(614) 293-8000

Overall patient safety: ★
Teaching: Y

CLINICAL PROGRAM RATINGS:

CARDIAC	★	ORTHOPEDICS	NR
CRITICAL CARE	★★★★★	PULMONARY	★★★★★
GASTROINTESTINAL	★★★	STROKE	★★★
GENERAL SURGERY	NR	VASCULAR	★★★★★
MATERNITY CARE	NR	WOMEN'S HEALTH	NR

HEALTHGRADES AWARDS

✓ SPECIALTY EXCELLENCE
• CRITICAL CARE   • PULMONARY CARE   • VASCULAR SURGERY

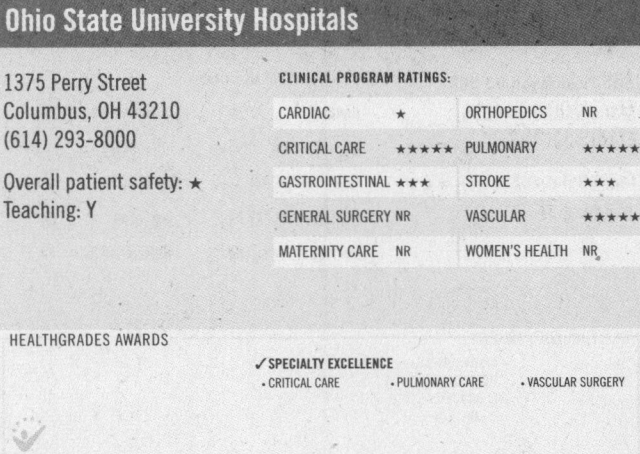

O. Bleness Memorial Hospital

55 Hospital Drive
Athens, OH 45701
(740) 593-5551

Overall patient safety: ★★★
Teaching: Y

CLINICAL PROGRAM RATINGS:

CARDIAC	NR	ORTHOPEDICS	NR
CRITICAL CARE	NR	PULMONARY	★★★
GASTROINTESTINAL	NR	STROKE	NR
GENERAL SURGERY	NR	VASCULAR	NR
MATERNITY CARE	NR	WOMEN'S HEALTH	NR

HEALTHGRADES AWARDS

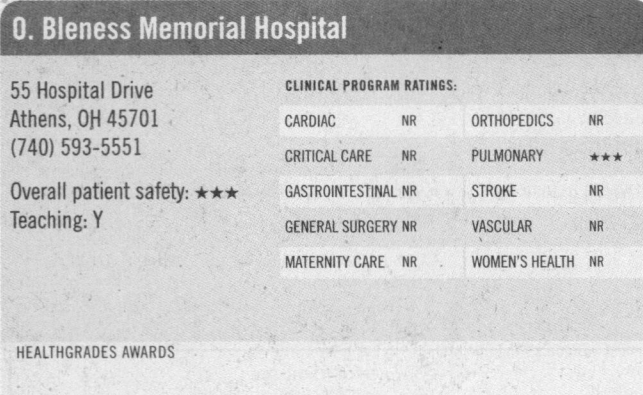

Parma Community General Hospital

7007 Powers Boulevard
Parma, OH 44129
(440) 743-4000

Overall patient safety: ★★★★★
Teaching: N

CLINICAL PROGRAM RATINGS:

CARDIAC	★★★	ORTHOPEDICS	NR
CRITICAL CARE	★★★	PULMONARY	★★★
GASTROINTESTINAL	★★★	STROKE	★★★★★
GENERAL SURGERY	NR	VASCULAR	★★★
MATERNITY CARE	NR	WOMEN'S HEALTH	NR

HEALTHGRADES AWARDS

✓ DISTINGUISHED HOSPITAL
• CLINICAL EXCELLENCE
• PATIENT SAFETY

✓ SPECIALTY EXCELLENCE
• CARDIAC CARE   • JOINT REPLACEMENT   • STROKE CARE

KEY: ★★★★★ BEST   ★★★ AS EXPECTED   ★ POOR   NR NOT RATED BY HEALTHGRADES   For full definitions of ratings and awards, see Appendix.

Paulding County Hospital

1035 West Wayne Street
Paulding, OH 45879
(419) 399-4080

Overall patient safety: ★★★
Teaching: N

CLINICAL PROGRAM RATINGS:

CARDIAC	NR	ORTHOPEDICS	NR
CRITICAL CARE	NR	PULMONARY	★★★
GASTROINTESTINAL	NR	STROKE	NR
GENERAL SURGERY	NR	VASCULAR	NR
MATERNITY CARE	NR	WOMEN'S HEALTH	NR

HEALTHGRADES AWARDS

Regency Hospital of Cincinnati

311 Straight Street, 4th Floor
Cincinnati, OH 45219
(513) 559-5957

Overall patient safety: ★★★★★
Teaching: N

CLINICAL PROGRAM RATINGS:

CARDIAC	NR	ORTHOPEDICS	★★★
CRITICAL CARE	NR	PULMONARY	★★★★★
GASTROINTESTINAL	★★★	STROKE	★★★
GENERAL SURGERY	NR	VASCULAR	NR
MATERNITY CARE	NR	WOMEN'S HEALTH	NR

HEALTHGRADES AWARDS

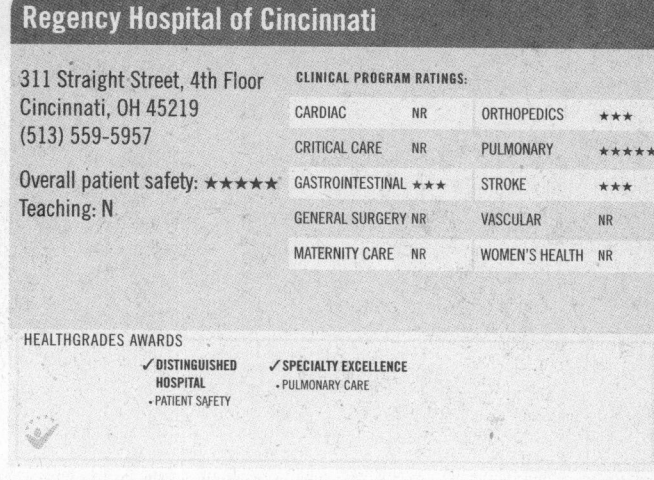
✓ DISTINGUISHED HOSPITAL
  • PATIENT SAFETY

✓ SPECIALTY EXCELLENCE
  • PULMONARY CARE

Peoples Hospital*

597 Park Avenue East
Mansfield, OH 44905
(419) 526-7300

Overall patient safety: ★★★
Teaching: N

CLINICAL PROGRAM RATINGS:

CARDIAC	NR	ORTHOPEDICS	NR
CRITICAL CARE	NR	PULMONARY	★★★
GASTROINTESTINAL	★★★	STROKE	★★★
GENERAL SURGERY	NR	VASCULAR	NR
MATERNITY CARE	NR	WOMEN'S HEALTH	NR

HEALTHGRADES AWARDS

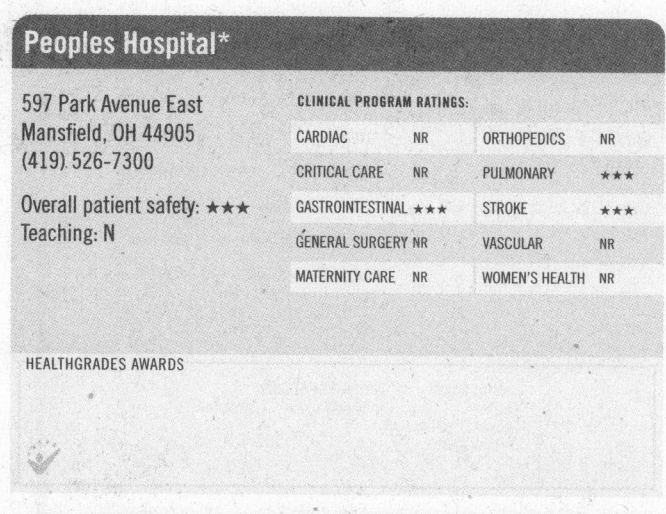

Riverside Methodist Hospital

3535 Olentangy River Road
Columbus, OH 43214
(614) 566-5000

Overall patient safety: ★★★★★
Teaching: Y

CLINICAL PROGRAM RATINGS:

CARDIAC	★★★	ORTHOPEDICS	★
CRITICAL CARE	★★★	PULMONARY	★★★
GASTROINTESTINAL	★★★	STROKE	★★★★★
GENERAL SURGERY	NR	VASCULAR	★★★
MATERNITY CARE	NR	WOMEN'S HEALTH	NR

HEALTHGRADES AWARDS

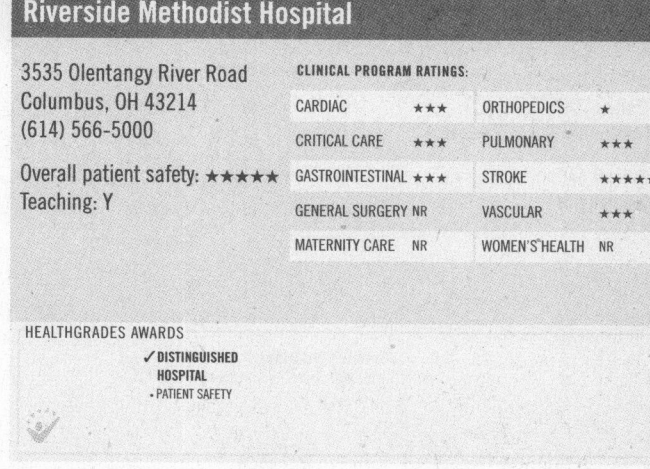
✓ DISTINGUISHED HOSPITAL
  • PATIENT SAFETY

Pike Community Hospital

100 Dawn Lane
Waverly, OH 45690
(740) 947-2186

Overall patient safety: NR
Teaching: N

CLINICAL PROGRAM RATINGS:

CARDIAC	NR	ORTHOPEDICS	NR
CRITICAL CARE	NR	PULMONARY	★
GASTROINTESTINAL	NR	STROKE	NR
GENERAL SURGERY	NR	VASCULAR	NR
MATERNITY CARE	NR	WOMEN'S HEALTH	NR

HEALTHGRADES AWARDS

Robinson Memorial Hospital

6847 North Chestnut Street
Ravenna, OH 44266
(330) 297-0811

Overall patient safety: ★★★
Teaching: Y

CLINICAL PROGRAM RATINGS:

CARDIAC	NR	ORTHOPEDICS	NR
CRITICAL CARE	★★★	PULMONARY	★★★
GASTROINTESTINAL	★★★	STROKE	★★★
GENERAL SURGERY	NR	VASCULAR	NR
MATERNITY CARE	NR	WOMEN'S HEALTH	NR

HEALTHGRADES AWARDS

*This hospital reports its data to the federal government jointly with another hospital. Therefore the ratings and awards apply to multiple hospitals and this specific hospital may not provide all rated services.

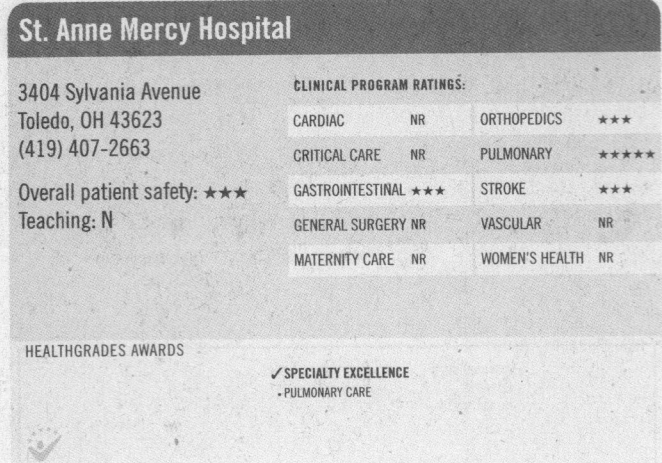

St. Anne Mercy Hospital

3404 Sylvania Avenue
Toledo, OH 43623
(419) 407-2663

Overall patient safety: ★★★
Teaching: N

CLINICAL PROGRAM RATINGS:

CARDIAC	NR	ORTHOPEDICS	★★★
CRITICAL CARE	NR	PULMONARY	★★★★★
GASTROINTESTINAL	★★★	STROKE	★★★
GENERAL SURGERY	NR	VASCULAR	NR
MATERNITY CARE	NR	WOMEN'S HEALTH	NR

HEALTHGRADES AWARDS

✓ SPECIALTY EXCELLENCE
· PULMONARY CARE

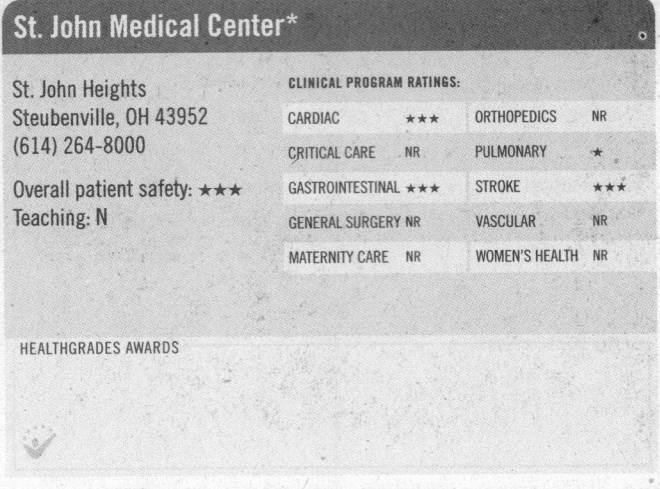

St. John Medical Center*

St. John Heights
Steubenville, OH 43952
(614) 264-8000

Overall patient safety: ★★★
Teaching: N

CLINICAL PROGRAM RATINGS:

CARDIAC	★★★	ORTHOPEDICS	NR
CRITICAL CARE	NR	PULMONARY	★
GASTROINTESTINAL	★★★	STROKE	★★★
GENERAL SURGERY	NR	VASCULAR	NR
MATERNITY CARE	NR	WOMEN'S HEALTH	NR

HEALTHGRADES AWARDS

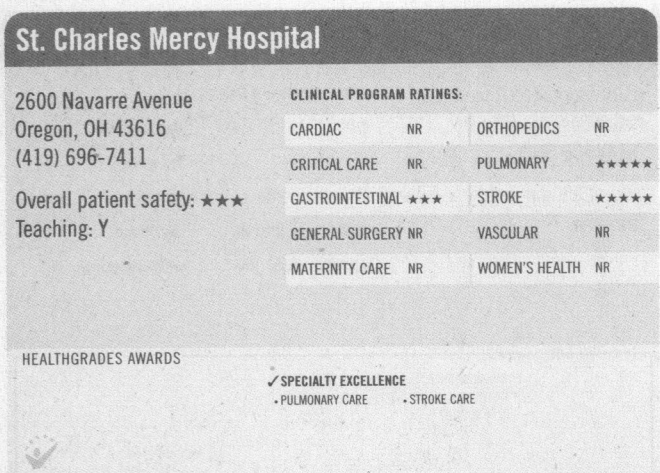

St. Charles Mercy Hospital

2600 Navarre Avenue
Oregon, OH 43616
(419) 696-7411

Overall patient safety: ★★★
Teaching: Y

CLINICAL PROGRAM RATINGS:

CARDIAC	NR	ORTHOPEDICS	NR
CRITICAL CARE	NR	PULMONARY	★★★★★
GASTROINTESTINAL	★★★	STROKE	★★★★★
GENERAL SURGERY	NR	VASCULAR	NR
MATERNITY CARE	NR	WOMEN'S HEALTH	NR

HEALTHGRADES AWARDS

✓ SPECIALTY EXCELLENCE
· PULMONARY CARE · STROKE CARE

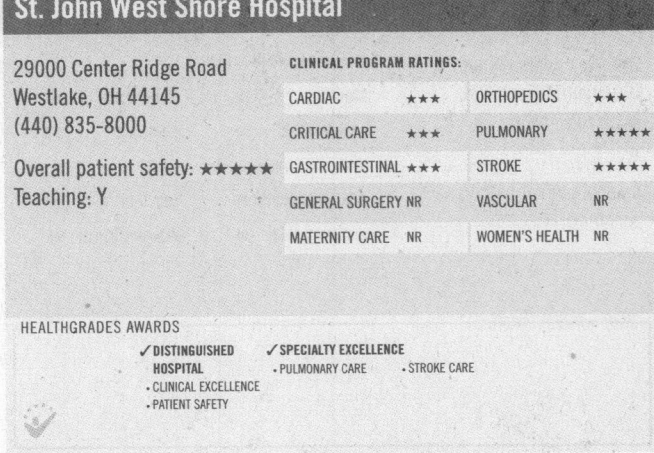

St. John West Shore Hospital

29000 Center Ridge Road
Westlake, OH 44145
(440) 835-8000

Overall patient safety: ★★★★★
Teaching: Y

CLINICAL PROGRAM RATINGS:

CARDIAC	★★★	ORTHOPEDICS	★★★
CRITICAL CARE	★★★	PULMONARY	★★★★★
GASTROINTESTINAL	★★★	STROKE	★★★★★
GENERAL SURGERY	NR	VASCULAR	NR
MATERNITY CARE	NR	WOMEN'S HEALTH	NR

HEALTHGRADES AWARDS

✓ DISTINGUISHED HOSPITAL
· CLINICAL EXCELLENCE
· PATIENT SAFETY

✓ SPECIALTY EXCELLENCE
· PULMONARY CARE · STROKE CARE

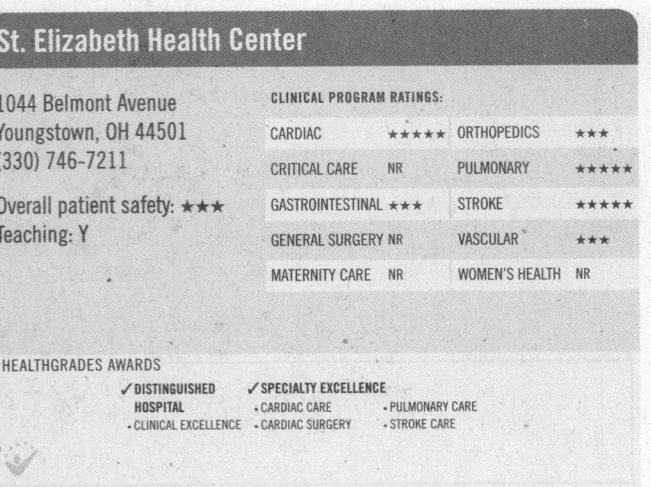

St. Elizabeth Health Center

1044 Belmont Avenue
Youngstown, OH 44501
(330) 746-7211

Overall patient safety: ★★★
Teaching: Y

CLINICAL PROGRAM RATINGS:

CARDIAC	★★★★★	ORTHOPEDICS	★★★
CRITICAL CARE	NR	PULMONARY	★★★★★
GASTROINTESTINAL	★★★	STROKE	★★★★★
GENERAL SURGERY	NR	VASCULAR	★★★
MATERNITY CARE	NR	WOMEN'S HEALTH	NR

HEALTHGRADES AWARDS

✓ DISTINGUISHED HOSPITAL
· CLINICAL EXCELLENCE

✓ SPECIALTY EXCELLENCE
· CARDIAC CARE
· CARDIAC SURGERY
· PULMONARY CARE
· STROKE CARE

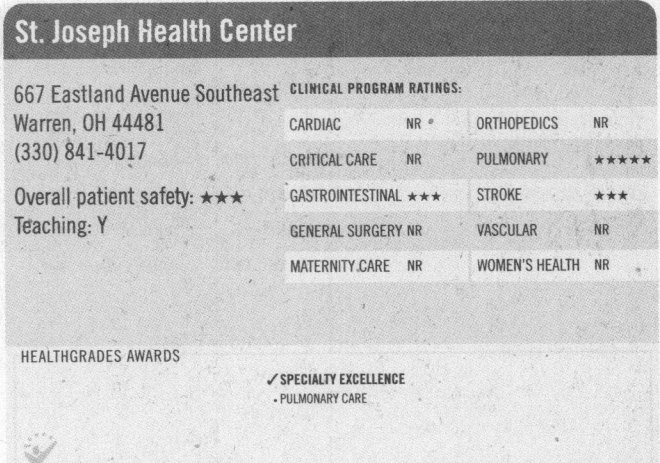

St. Joseph Health Center

667 Eastland Avenue Southeast
Warren, OH 44481
(330) 841-4017

Overall patient safety: ★★★
Teaching: Y

CLINICAL PROGRAM RATINGS:

CARDIAC	NR	ORTHOPEDICS	NR
CRITICAL CARE	NR	PULMONARY	★★★★★
GASTROINTESTINAL	★★★	STROKE	★★★
GENERAL SURGERY	NR	VASCULAR	NR
MATERNITY CARE	NR	WOMEN'S HEALTH	NR

HEALTHGRADES AWARDS

✓ SPECIALTY EXCELLENCE
· PULMONARY CARE

KEY: ★★★★★ BEST ★★★ AS EXPECTED ★ POOR NR NOT RATED BY HEALTHGRADES   For full definitions of ratings and awards, see Appendix.

St. Luke's Hospital

5901 Monclova Road
Maumee, OH 43537
(419) 893-5911

Overall patient safety: ★★★★★
Teaching: N

CLINICAL PROGRAM RATINGS:

CARDIAC	★★★	ORTHOPEDICS	★★★
CRITICAL CARE	NR	PULMONARY	★
GASTROINTESTINAL	★★★	STROKE	★★★
GENERAL SURGERY	NR	VASCULAR	NR
MATERNITY CARE	NR	WOMEN'S HEALTH	NR

HEALTHGRADES AWARDS

✓ **DISTINGUISHED HOSPITAL**
· PATIENT SAFETY

✓ **SPECIALTY EXCELLENCE**
· CARDIAC SURGERY

St. Vincent Mercy Medical Center*

2213 Cherry Street
Toledo, OH 43608
(419) 251-3232

Overall patient safety: ★★★★★
Teaching: Y

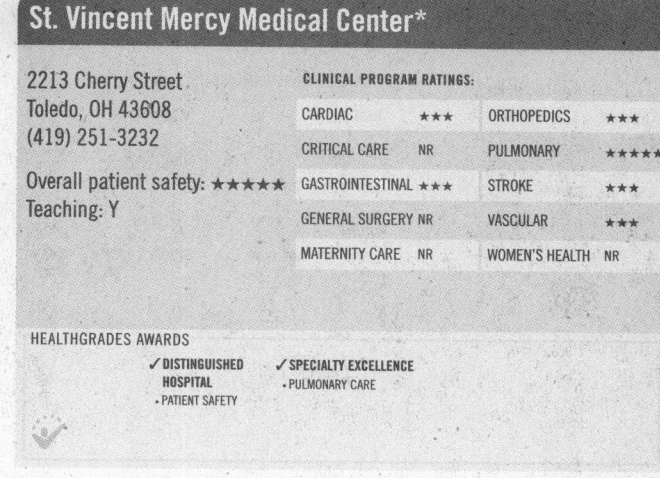

CLINICAL PROGRAM RATINGS:

CARDIAC	★★★	ORTHOPEDICS	★★★
CRITICAL CARE	NR	PULMONARY	★★★★★
GASTROINTESTINAL	★★★	STROKE	★★★
GENERAL SURGERY	NR	VASCULAR	★★★
MATERNITY CARE	NR	WOMEN'S HEALTH	NR

HEALTHGRADES AWARDS

✓ **DISTINGUISHED HOSPITAL**
· PATIENT SAFETY

✓ **SPECIALTY EXCELLENCE**
· PULMONARY CARE

St. Rita's Medical Center

730 West Market Street
6th Floor
Lima, OH 45801
(419) 227-3361

Overall patient safety: ★★★
Teaching: N

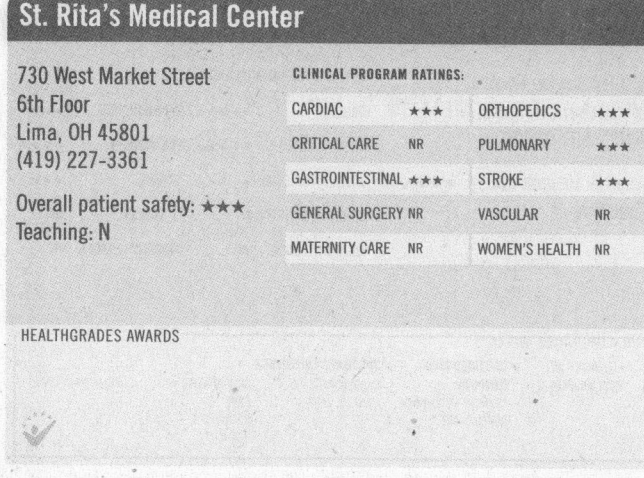

CLINICAL PROGRAM RATINGS:

CARDIAC	★★★	ORTHOPEDICS	★★★
CRITICAL CARE	NR	PULMONARY	★★★
GASTROINTESTINAL	★★★	STROKE	★★★
GENERAL SURGERY	NR	VASCULAR	NR
MATERNITY CARE	NR	WOMEN'S HEALTH	NR

HEALTHGRADES AWARDS

Salem Community Hospital

1995 East State Street
Salem, OH 44460
(330) 332-1551

Overall patient safety: ★★★
Teaching: N

CLINICAL PROGRAM RATINGS:

CARDIAC	NR	ORTHOPEDICS	★
CRITICAL CARE	NR	PULMONARY	★★★
GASTROINTESTINAL	NR	STROKE	★★★
GENERAL SURGERY	NR	VASCULAR	NR
MATERNITY CARE	NR	WOMEN'S HEALTH	NR

HEALTHGRADES AWARDS

St. Vincent Charity Hospital*

2351 East 22nd Street
Cleveland, OH 44115
(216) 861-6200

Overall patient safety: ★★★
Teaching: Y

CLINICAL PROGRAM RATINGS:

CARDIAC	★★★	ORTHOPEDICS	★★★
CRITICAL CARE	NR	PULMONARY	★★★★★
GASTROINTESTINAL	★★★	STROKE	★★★★★
GENERAL SURGERY	NR	VASCULAR	NR
MATERNITY CARE	NR	WOMEN'S HEALTH	NR

HEALTHGRADES AWARDS

✓ **DISTINGUISHED HOSPITAL**
· CLINICAL EXCELLENCE

✓ **SPECIALTY EXCELLENCE**
· PULMONARY CARE   · STROKE CARE

Samaritan Regional Health System*

1025 Center Street
Ashland, OH 44805
(419) 289-0491

Overall patient safety: ★★★
Teaching: N

CLINICAL PROGRAM RATINGS:

CARDIAC	NR	ORTHOPEDICS	NR
CRITICAL CARE	NR	PULMONARY	★★★
GASTROINTESTINAL	★★★	STROKE	★★★
GENERAL SURGERY	NR	VASCULAR	NR
MATERNITY CARE	NR	WOMEN'S HEALTH	NR

HEALTHGRADES AWARDS

*This hospital reports its data to the federal government jointly with another hospital. Therefore the ratings and awards apply to multiple hospitals and this specific hospital may not provide all rated services.

Selby General Hospital

1106 Colegate Drive
Marietta, OH 45750
(740) 568-2000

Overall patient safety: ★★★
Teaching: Y

CLINICAL PROGRAM RATINGS:

CARDIAC	NR	ORTHOPEDICS	NR
CRITICAL CARE	NR	PULMONARY	★★★
GASTROINTESTINAL	NR	STROKE	NR
GENERAL SURGERY	NR	VASCULAR	NR
MATERNITY CARE	NR	WOMEN'S HEALTH	NR

HEALTHGRADES AWARDS

Southern Ohio Medical Center

1805 27th Street
Portsmouth, OH 45662
(740) 356-5000

Overall patient safety: ★★★
Teaching: Y

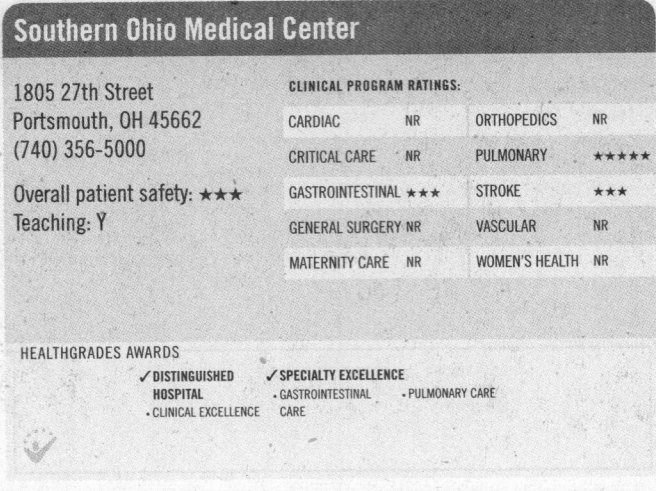

CLINICAL PROGRAM RATINGS:

CARDIAC	NR	ORTHOPEDICS	NR
CRITICAL CARE	NR	PULMONARY	★★★★★
GASTROINTESTINAL	★★★	STROKE	★★★
GENERAL SURGERY	NR	VASCULAR	NR
MATERNITY CARE	NR	WOMEN'S HEALTH	NR

HEALTHGRADES AWARDS

✓ DISTINGUISHED HOSPITAL
• CLINICAL EXCELLENCE

✓ SPECIALTY EXCELLENCE
• GASTROINTESTINAL CARE
• PULMONARY CARE

South Pointe Hospital

4110 Warrensville Center Road
Warrensville Heights, OH 44122
(216) 491-6000

Overall patient safety: ★★★
Teaching: Y

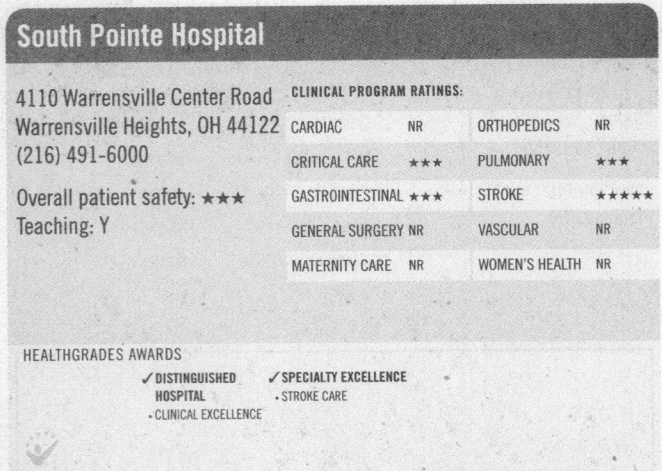

CLINICAL PROGRAM RATINGS:

CARDIAC	NR	ORTHOPEDICS	NR
CRITICAL CARE	★★★	PULMONARY	★★★
GASTROINTESTINAL	★★★	STROKE	★★★★★
GENERAL SURGERY	NR	VASCULAR	NR
MATERNITY CARE	NR	WOMEN'S HEALTH	NR

HEALTHGRADES AWARDS

✓ DISTINGUISHED HOSPITAL
• CLINICAL EXCELLENCE

✓ SPECIALTY EXCELLENCE
• STROKE CARE

Southwest General Health Center

18697 Bagley Road
Middleburg Heights, OH 44130
(440) 816-8000

Overall patient safety: ★★★★★
Teaching: Y

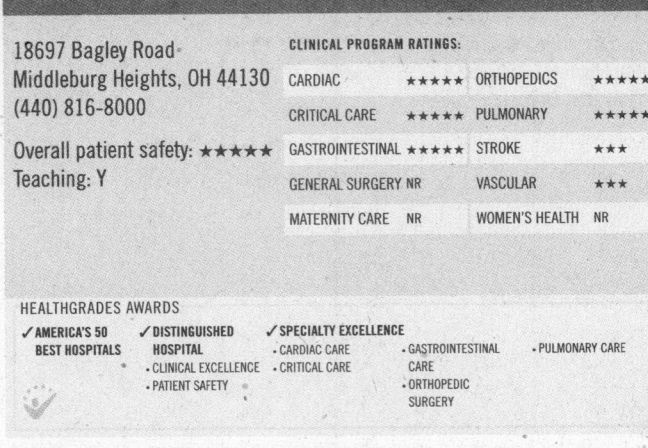

CLINICAL PROGRAM RATINGS:

CARDIAC	★★★★★	ORTHOPEDICS	★★★★★
CRITICAL CARE	★★★★★	PULMONARY	★★★★★
GASTROINTESTINAL	★★★★★	STROKE	★★★
GENERAL SURGERY	NR	VASCULAR	★★★
MATERNITY CARE	NR	WOMEN'S HEALTH	NR

HEALTHGRADES AWARDS

✓ AMERICA'S 50 BEST HOSPITALS

✓ DISTINGUISHED HOSPITAL
• CLINICAL EXCELLENCE
• PATIENT SAFETY

✓ SPECIALTY EXCELLENCE
• CARDIAC CARE
• CRITICAL CARE
• GASTROINTESTINAL CARE
• ORTHOPEDIC SURGERY
• PULMONARY CARE

Southeastern Ohio Regional Medical Center

1341 North Clark Street
Cambridge, OH 43725
(740) 439-3561

Overall patient safety: ★★★
Teaching: N

CLINICAL PROGRAM RATINGS:

CARDIAC	NR	ORTHOPEDICS	NR
CRITICAL CARE	NR	PULMONARY	★★★
GASTROINTESTINAL	★★★	STROKE	★★★
GENERAL SURGERY	NR	VASCULAR	NR
MATERNITY CARE	NR	WOMEN'S HEALTH	NR

HEALTHGRADES AWARDS

Summa Health Systems Hospitals

525 East Market Street
Akron, OH 44309
(330) 375-3000

Overall patient safety: ★★★
Teaching: Y

CLINICAL PROGRAM RATINGS:

CARDIAC	★★★	ORTHOPEDICS	★★★
CRITICAL CARE	★★★★★	PULMONARY	★★★★★
GASTROINTESTINAL	★★★	STROKE	★★★★★
GENERAL SURGERY	NR	VASCULAR	★★★
MATERNITY CARE	NR	WOMEN'S HEALTH	NR

HEALTHGRADES AWARDS

✓ AMERICA'S 50 BEST HOSPITALS

✓ DISTINGUISHED HOSPITAL
• CLINICAL EXCELLENCE

✓ SPECIALTY EXCELLENCE
• CRITICAL CARE
• PULMONARY CARE
• STROKE CARE

KEY: ★★★★★ BEST   ★★★ AS EXPECTED   ★ POOR   NR NOT RATED BY HEALTHGRADES   For full definitions of ratings and awards, see Appendix.

Toledo Hospital

2142 North Cove Boulevard
Toledo, OH 43606
(419) 291-4000

Overall patient safety: ★★★
Teaching: Y

CLINICAL PROGRAM RATINGS:

CARDIAC	★★★	ORTHOPEDICS	★★★
CRITICAL CARE	NR	PULMONARY	★★★
GASTROINTESTINAL	★★★	STROKE	★★★★★
GENERAL SURGERY	NR	VASCULAR	★★★
MATERNITY CARE	NR	WOMEN'S HEALTH	NR

HEALTHGRADES AWARDS

✓ SPECIALTY EXCELLENCE
· STROKE CARE

Twin City Hospital

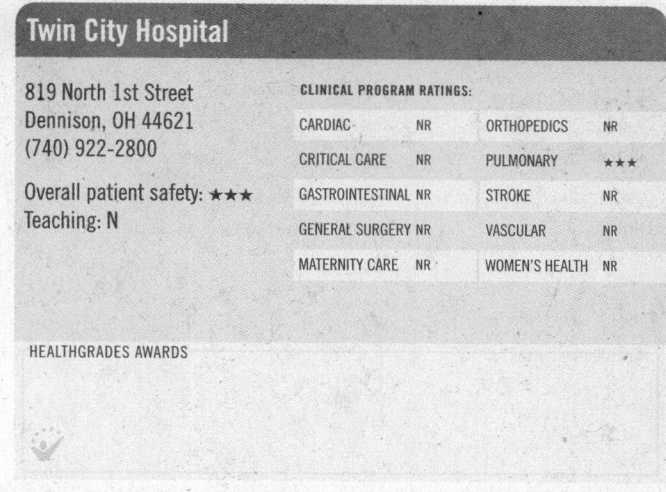

819 North 1st Street
Dennison, OH 44621
(740) 922-2800

Overall patient safety: ★★★
Teaching: N

CLINICAL PROGRAM RATINGS:

CARDIAC	NR	ORTHOPEDICS	NR
CRITICAL CARE	NR	PULMONARY	★★★
GASTROINTESTINAL	NR	STROKE	NR
GENERAL SURGERY	NR	VASCULAR	NR
MATERNITY CARE	NR	WOMEN'S HEALTH	NR

HEALTHGRADES AWARDS

Trinity Health System*

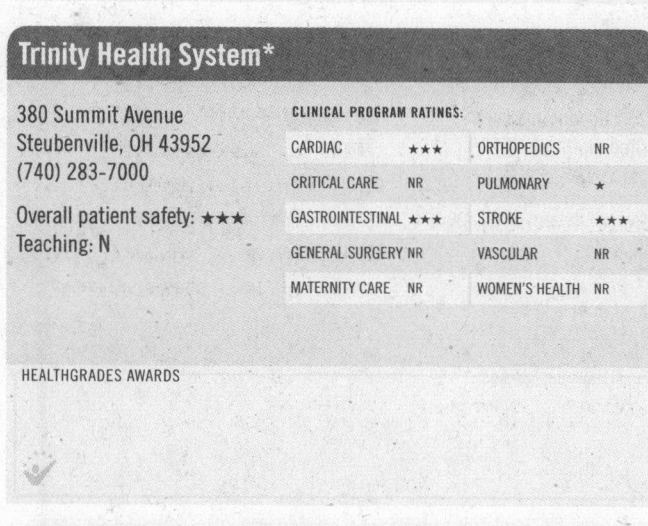

380 Summit Avenue
Steubenville, OH 43952
(740) 283-7000

Overall patient safety: ★★★
Teaching: N

CLINICAL PROGRAM RATINGS:

CARDIAC	★★★	ORTHOPEDICS	NR
CRITICAL CARE	NR	PULMONARY	★
GASTROINTESTINAL	★★★	STROKE	★★★
GENERAL SURGERY	NR	VASCULAR	NR
MATERNITY CARE	NR	WOMEN'S HEALTH	NR

HEALTHGRADES AWARDS

UHHS Bedford Medical Center

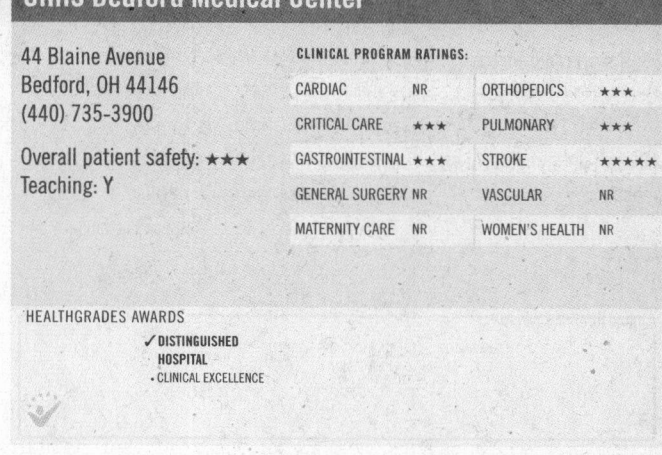

44 Blaine Avenue
Bedford, OH 44146
(440) 735-3900

Overall patient safety: ★★★
Teaching: Y

CLINICAL PROGRAM RATINGS:

CARDIAC	NR	ORTHOPEDICS	★★★
CRITICAL CARE	★★★	PULMONARY	★★★
GASTROINTESTINAL	★★★	STROKE	★★★★★
GENERAL SURGERY	NR	VASCULAR	NR
MATERNITY CARE	NR	WOMEN'S HEALTH	NR

HEALTHGRADES AWARDS

✓ DISTINGUISHED
  HOSPITAL
  · CLINICAL EXCELLENCE

Trumbull Memorial Hospital

1350 East Market Street
Warren, OH 44483
(330) 841-9011

Overall patient safety: ★★★
Teaching: N

CLINICAL PROGRAM RATINGS:

CARDIAC	★★★	ORTHOPEDICS	★★★
CRITICAL CARE	NR	PULMONARY	★★★★★
GASTROINTESTINAL	★★★	STROKE	★★★★★
GENERAL SURGERY	NR	VASCULAR	NR
MATERNITY CARE	NR	WOMEN'S HEALTH	NR

HEALTHGRADES AWARDS

✓ DISTINGUISHED   ✓ SPECIALTY EXCELLENCE
  HOSPITAL   · GASTROINTESTINAL   · PULMONARY CARE   · STROKE CARE
· CLINICAL EXCELLENCE   CARE

UHHS Brown Memorial Hospital

158 West Main Road
Conneaut, OH 44030
(440) 593-1131

Overall patient safety: ★★★
Teaching: N

CLINICAL PROGRAM RATINGS:

CARDIAC	NR	ORTHOPEDICS	NR
CRITICAL CARE	NR	PULMONARY	★★★
GASTROINTESTINAL	NR	STROKE	★★★
GENERAL SURGERY	NR	VASCULAR	NR
MATERNITY CARE	NR	WOMEN'S HEALTH	NR

HEALTHGRADES AWARDS

*This hospital reports its data to the federal government jointly with another hospital. Therefore the ratings and awards apply to multiple hospitals and this specific hospital may not provide all rated services.

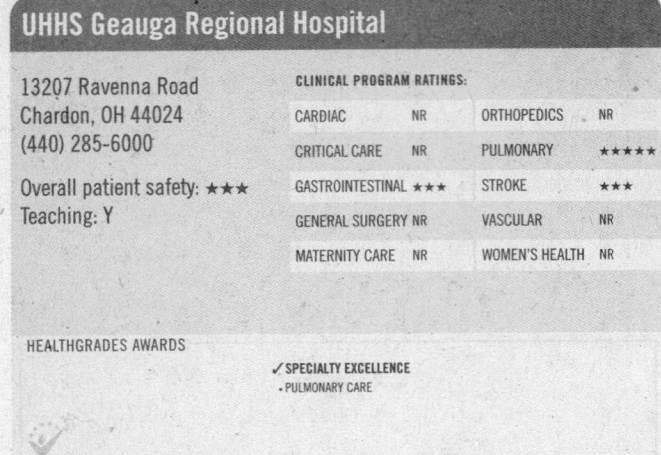

UHHS Geauga Regional Hospital

13207 Ravenna Road
Chardon, OH 44024
(440) 285-6000

Overall patient safety: ★★★
Teaching: Y

CLINICAL PROGRAM RATINGS:

CARDIAC	NR	ORTHOPEDICS	NR
CRITICAL CARE	NR	PULMONARY	★★★★★
GASTROINTESTINAL	★★★	STROKE	★★★
GENERAL SURGERY	NR	VASCULAR	NR
MATERNITY CARE	NR	WOMEN'S HEALTH	NR

HEALTHGRADES AWARDS

✓ SPECIALTY EXCELLENCE
• PULMONARY CARE

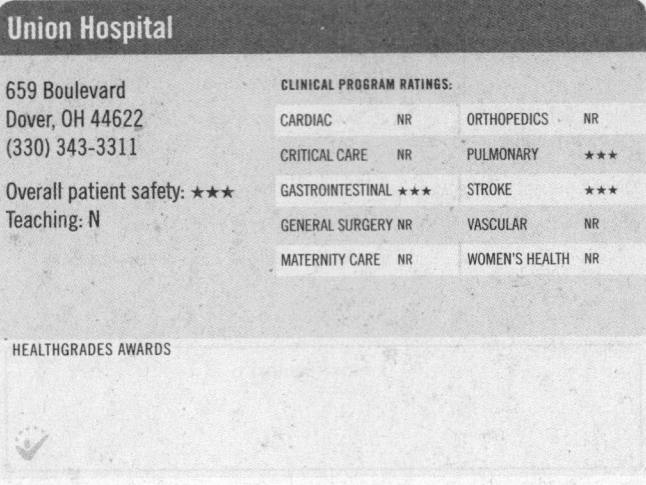

Union Hospital

659 Boulevard
Dover, OH 44622
(330) 343-3311

Overall patient safety: ★★★
Teaching: N

CLINICAL PROGRAM RATINGS:

CARDIAC	NR	ORTHOPEDICS	NR
CRITICAL CARE	NR	PULMONARY	★★★
GASTROINTESTINAL	★★★	STROKE	★★★
GENERAL SURGERY	NR	VASCULAR	NR
MATERNITY CARE	NR	WOMEN'S HEALTH	NR

HEALTHGRADES AWARDS

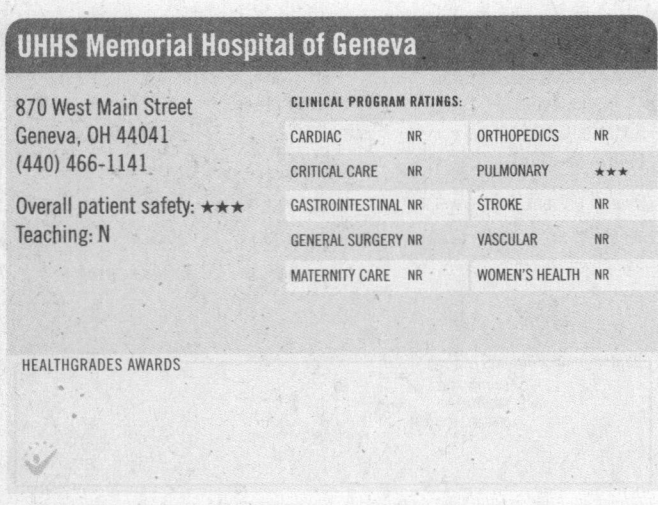

UHHS Memorial Hospital of Geneva

870 West Main Street
Geneva, OH 44041
(440) 466-1141

Overall patient safety: ★★★
Teaching: N

CLINICAL PROGRAM RATINGS:

CARDIAC	NR	ORTHOPEDICS	NR
CRITICAL CARE	NR	PULMONARY	★★★
GASTROINTESTINAL	NR	STROKE	NR
GENERAL SURGERY	NR	VASCULAR	NR
MATERNITY CARE	NR	WOMEN'S HEALTH	NR

HEALTHGRADES AWARDS

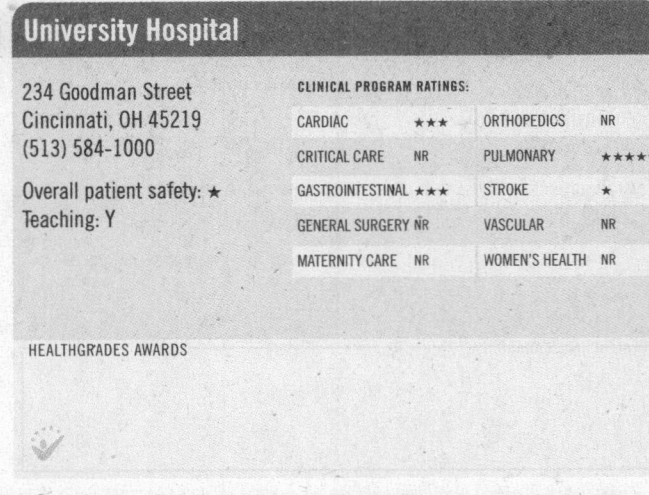

University Hospital

234 Goodman Street
Cincinnati, OH 45219
(513) 584-1000

Overall patient safety: ★
Teaching: Y

CLINICAL PROGRAM RATINGS:

CARDIAC	★★★	ORTHOPEDICS	NR
CRITICAL CARE	NR	PULMONARY	★★★★★
GASTROINTESTINAL	★★★	STROKE	★
GENERAL SURGERY	NR	VASCULAR	NR
MATERNITY CARE	NR	WOMEN'S HEALTH	NR

HEALTHGRADES AWARDS

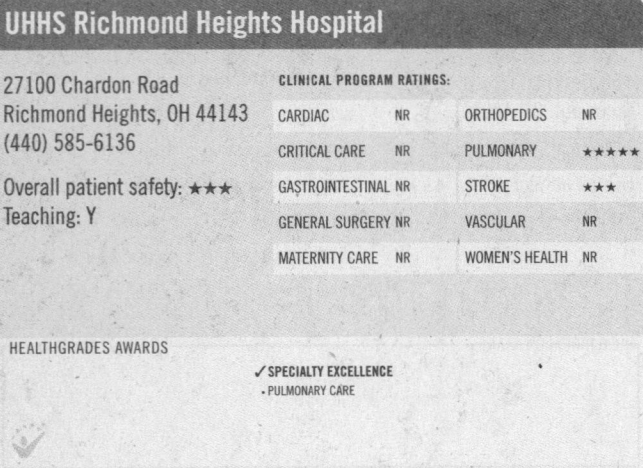

UHHS Richmond Heights Hospital

27100 Chardon Road
Richmond Heights, OH 44143
(440) 585-6136

Overall patient safety: ★★★
Teaching: Y

CLINICAL PROGRAM RATINGS:

CARDIAC	NR	ORTHOPEDICS	NR
CRITICAL CARE	NR	PULMONARY	★★★★★
GASTROINTESTINAL	NR	STROKE	★★★
GENERAL SURGERY	NR	VASCULAR	NR
MATERNITY CARE	NR	WOMEN'S HEALTH	NR

HEALTHGRADES AWARDS

✓ SPECIALTY EXCELLENCE
• PULMONARY CARE

University Hospitals Case Medical Center

11100 Euclid Avenue
Cleveland, OH 44106
(216) 844-1000

Overall patient safety: ★★★
Teaching: Y

CLINICAL PROGRAM RATINGS:

CARDIAC	★★★	ORTHOPEDICS	★★★
CRITICAL CARE	★★★	PULMONARY	★★★
GASTROINTESTINAL	★★★	STROKE	★★★★★
GENERAL SURGERY	NR	VASCULAR	★★★
MATERNITY CARE	NR	WOMEN'S HEALTH	NR

HEALTHGRADES AWARDS

KEY: ★★★★★ BEST   ★★★ AS EXPECTED   ★ POOR   NR NOT RATED BY HEALTHGRADES   For full definitions of ratings and awards, see Appendix.

Upper Valley Medical Center*

3130 North Dixie Highway
Troy, OH 45373
(937) 440-4000

Overall patient safety: ★
Teaching: N

CLINICAL PROGRAM RATINGS:

CARDIAC	NR	ORTHOPEDICS	NR
CRITICAL CARE	NR	PULMONARY	★★★
GASTROINTESTINAL	★★★	STROKE	★★★
GENERAL SURGERY	NR	VASCULAR	NR
MATERNITY CARE	NR	WOMEN'S HEALTH	NR

HEALTHGRADES AWARDS

Wadsworth Rittman Hospital

195 Wadsworth Road
Wadsworth, OH 44281
(330) 334-1504

Overall patient safety: ★★★
Teaching: N

CLINICAL PROGRAM RATINGS:

CARDIAC	NR	ORTHOPEDICS	NR
CRITICAL CARE	NR	PULMONARY	★★★
GASTROINTESTINAL	NR	STROKE	★★★
GENERAL SURGERY	NR	VASCULAR	NR
MATERNITY CARE	NR	WOMEN'S HEALTH	NR

HEALTHGRADES AWARDS

Upper Valley Medical Center*

624 Park Avenue
Piqua, OH 45356
(513) 778-6500

Overall patient safety: ★
Teaching: N

CLINICAL PROGRAM RATINGS:

CARDIAC	NR	ORTHOPEDICS	NR
CRITICAL CARE	NR	PULMONARY	★★★
GASTROINTESTINAL	★★★	STROKE	★★★
GENERAL SURGERY	NR	VASCULAR	NR
MATERNITY CARE	NR	WOMEN'S HEALTH	NR

HEALTHGRADES AWARDS

Wayne Hospital

835 Sweitzer Street
Greenville, OH 45331
(937) 548-1141

Overall patient safety: ★★★
Teaching: N

CLINICAL PROGRAM RATINGS:

CARDIAC	NR	ORTHOPEDICS	NR
CRITICAL CARE	NR	PULMONARY	★
GASTROINTESTINAL	★★★	STROKE	★
GENERAL SURGERY	NR	VASCULAR	NR
MATERNITY CARE	NR	WOMEN'S HEALTH	NR

HEALTHGRADES AWARDS

Van Wert County Hospital

1250 South Washington Street
Van Wert, OH 45891
(419) 238-2390

Overall patient safety: ★★★
Teaching: N

CLINICAL PROGRAM RATINGS:

CARDIAC	NR	ORTHOPEDICS	NR
CRITICAL CARE	NR	PULMONARY	★
GASTROINTESTINAL	NR	STROKE	★★★
GENERAL SURGERY	NR	VASCULAR	NR
MATERNITY CARE	NR	WOMEN'S HEALTH	NR

HEALTHGRADES AWARDS

Western Reserve Care System

500 Gypsy Lane
Youngstown, OH 44501
(330) 884-1000

Overall patient safety: ★★★
Teaching: Y

CLINICAL PROGRAM RATINGS:

CARDIAC	★★★	ORTHOPEDICS	★★★
CRITICAL CARE	★★★★★	PULMONARY	★★★
GASTROINTESTINAL	★★★	STROKE	★★★
GENERAL SURGERY	NR	VASCULAR	NR
MATERNITY CARE	NR	WOMEN'S HEALTH	NR

HEALTHGRADES AWARDS

✓ SPECIALTY EXCELLENCE
• CRITICAL CARE

*This hospital reports its data to the federal government jointly with another hospital. Therefore the ratings and awards apply to multiple hospitals and this specific hospital may not provide all rated services.

CHAPTER 6: HOSPITAL RATINGS BY CLINICAL SPECIALTY   **529**

Wilson Memorial Hospital

915 West Michigan Street
Sidney, OH 45365
(937) 498-2311

Overall patient safety: ★★★
Teaching: N

CLINICAL PROGRAM RATINGS:

CARDIAC	NR	ORTHOPEDICS	NR
CRITICAL CARE	NR	PULMONARY	★★★
GASTROINTESTINAL	NR	STROKE	NR
GENERAL SURGERY	NR	VASCULAR	NR
MATERNITY CARE	NR	WOMEN'S HEALTH	NR

HEALTHGRADES AWARDS

Wooster Community Hospital

1761 Beall Avenue
Wooster, OH 44691
(330) 263-8100

Overall patient safety: ★★★★★
Teaching: N

CLINICAL PROGRAM RATINGS:

CARDIAC	NR	ORTHOPEDICS	NR
CRITICAL CARE	NR	PULMONARY	★★★
GASTROINTESTINAL	★★★	STROKE	★★★
GENERAL SURGERY	NR	VASCULAR	NR
MATERNITY CARE	NR	WOMEN'S HEALTH	NR

HEALTHGRADES AWARDS

✓ DISTINGUISHED HOSPITAL
 - PATIENT SAFETY

✓ SPECIALTY EXCELLENCE
 - GASTROINTESTINAL CARE

Wood County Hospital

950 West Wooster Street
Bowling Green, OH 43402
(419) 354-8900

Overall patient safety: ★★★
Teaching: N

CLINICAL PROGRAM RATINGS:

CARDIAC	NR	ORTHOPEDICS	NR
CRITICAL CARE	NR	PULMONARY	★★★
GASTROINTESTINAL	NR	STROKE	★
GENERAL SURGERY	NR	VASCULAR	NR
MATERNITY CARE	NR	WOMEN'S HEALTH	NR

HEALTHGRADES AWARDS

Wyandot Memorial Hospital

885 North Sandusky Avenue
Upper Sandusky, OH 43351
(419) 294-4991

Overall patient safety: ★★★
Teaching: N

CLINICAL PROGRAM RATINGS:

CARDIAC	NR	ORTHOPEDICS	NR
CRITICAL CARE	NR	PULMONARY	★★★
GASTROINTESTINAL	NR	STROKE	★★★
GENERAL SURGERY	NR	VASCULAR	NR
MATERNITY CARE	NR	WOMEN'S HEALTH	NR

HEALTHGRADES AWARDS

OKLAHOMA HOSPITALS: RATINGS BY CLINICAL SPECIALTY

American Transitional Hospital

5501 North Portland Avenue
Oklahoma City, OK 73112
(405) 951-4017

Overall patient safety: ★★★
Teaching: Y

CLINICAL PROGRAM RATINGS:

CARDIAC	★★★	ORTHOPEDICS	NR
CRITICAL CARE	NR	PULMONARY	★★★
GASTROINTESTINAL	★★★	STROKE	★★★
GENERAL SURGERY	NR	VASCULAR	NR
MATERNITY CARE	NR	WOMEN'S HEALTH	NR

HEALTHGRADES AWARDS

American Transitional Hospital—Tulsa

744 West 9th Street
6th Floor
Tulsa, OK 74127
(918) 599-5665

Overall patient safety: ★
Teaching: Y

CLINICAL PROGRAM RATINGS:

CARDIAC	★★★	ORTHOPEDICS	NR
CRITICAL CARE	NR	PULMONARY	★★★
GASTROINTESTINAL	NR	STROKE	★
GENERAL SURGERY	NR	VASCULAR	NR
MATERNITY CARE	NR	WOMEN'S HEALTH	NR

HEALTHGRADES AWARDS

KEY: ★★★★★ BEST ★★★ AS EXPECTED ★ POOR NR NOT RATED BY HEALTHGRADES For full definitions of ratings and awards, see Appendix.

Arbuckle Memorial Hospital

2011 West Broadway
Sulphur, OK 73086
(580) 622-2161

Overall patient safety: NR
Teaching: N

CLINICAL PROGRAM RATINGS:

CARDIAC	NR	ORTHOPEDICS	NR
CRITICAL CARE	NR	PULMONARY	★
GASTROINTESTINAL	NR	STROKE	NR
GENERAL SURGERY	NR	VASCULAR	NR
MATERNITY CARE	NR	WOMEN'S HEALTH	NR

HEALTHGRADES AWARDS

Bone and Joint Hospital

1111 North Dewey Avenue
Oklahoma City, OK 73103
(405) 272-9671

Overall patient safety: ★★★★★
Teaching: Y

CLINICAL PROGRAM RATINGS:

CARDIAC	NR	ORTHOPEDICS	★★★
CRITICAL CARE	NR	PULMONARY	NR
GASTROINTESTINAL	NR	STROKE	NR
GENERAL SURGERY	NR	VASCULAR	NR
MATERNITY CARE	NR	WOMEN'S HEALTH	NR

HEALTHGRADES AWARDS

✓ SPECIALTY EXCELLENCE
  • JOINT REPLACEMENT

Ardmore Adventist Hospital*

1012 14th Northwest
Ardmore, OK 73401
(405) 223-4050

Overall patient safety: ★★★★★
Teaching: N

CLINICAL PROGRAM RATINGS:

CARDIAC	NR	ORTHOPEDICS	NR
CRITICAL CARE	NR	PULMONARY	★
GASTROINTESTINAL	★★★	STROKE	★★★
GENERAL SURGERY	NR	VASCULAR	NR
MATERNITY CARE	NR	WOMEN'S HEALTH	NR

HEALTHGRADES AWARDS

✓ DISTINGUISHED
  HOSPITAL
  • PATIENT SAFETY

Bristow Medical Center

700 West 7th Street
Bristow, OK 74010
(918) 367-2215

Overall patient safety: NR
Teaching: N

CLINICAL PROGRAM RATINGS:

CARDIAC	NR	ORTHOPEDICS	NR
CRITICAL CARE	NR	PULMONARY	★★★
GASTROINTESTINAL	NR	STROKE	NR
GENERAL SURGERY	NR	VASCULAR	NR
MATERNITY CARE	NR	WOMEN'S HEALTH	NR

HEALTHGRADES AWARDS

Atoka Memorial Hospital

1501 South Virginia Avenue
Atoka, OK 74525
(580) 889-3333

Overall patient safety: NR
Teaching: N

CLINICAL PROGRAM RATINGS:

CARDIAC	NR	ORTHOPEDICS	NR
CRITICAL CARE		PULMONARY	★★★
GASTROINTESTINAL	NR	STROKE	NR
GENERAL SURGERY	NR	VASCULAR	NR
MATERNITY CARE	NR	WOMEN'S HEALTH	NR

HEALTHGRADES AWARDS

Carl Albert Indian Health Facility

1001 North Country Club Road
Ada, OK 74820
(580) 436-3980

Overall patient safety: ★★★
Teaching: N

CLINICAL PROGRAM RATINGS:

CARDIAC	NR	ORTHOPEDICS	NR
CRITICAL CARE	NR	PULMONARY	★
GASTROINTESTINAL	NR	STROKE	NR
GENERAL SURGERY	NR	VASCULAR	NR
MATERNITY CARE	NR	WOMEN'S HEALTH	NR

HEALTHGRADES AWARDS

*This hospital reports its data to the federal government jointly with another hospital. Therefore the ratings and awards apply to multiple hospitals and this specific hospital may not provide all rated services.

OKLAHOMA HOSPITALS: RATINGS BY CLINICAL SPECIALTY

Carnegie Tri-County Municipal Hospital

102 North Broadway
Carnegie, OK 73015
(580) 654-1050

Overall patient safety: NR
Teaching: N

CLINICAL PROGRAM RATINGS:

CARDIAC	NR	ORTHOPEDICS	NR
CRITICAL CARE	NR	PULMONARY	★
GASTROINTESTINAL	NR	STROKE	NR
GENERAL SURGERY	NR	VASCULAR	NR
MATERNITY CARE	NR	WOMEN'S HEALTH	NR

HEALTHGRADES AWARDS

Claremore Indian Hospital

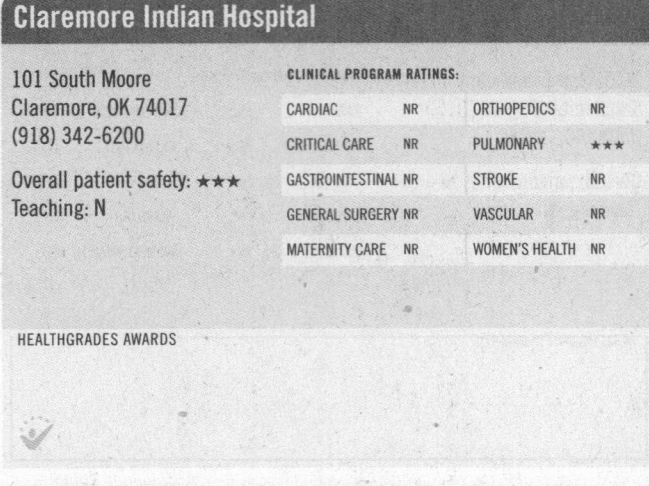

101 South Moore
Claremore, OK 74017
(918) 342-6200

Overall patient safety: ★★★
Teaching: N

CLINICAL PROGRAM RATINGS:

CARDIAC	NR	ORTHOPEDICS	NR
CRITICAL CARE	NR	PULMONARY	★★★
GASTROINTESTINAL	NR	STROKE	NR
GENERAL SURGERY	NR	VASCULAR	NR
MATERNITY CARE	NR	WOMEN'S HEALTH	NR

HEALTHGRADES AWARDS

Choctaw Memorial Hospital

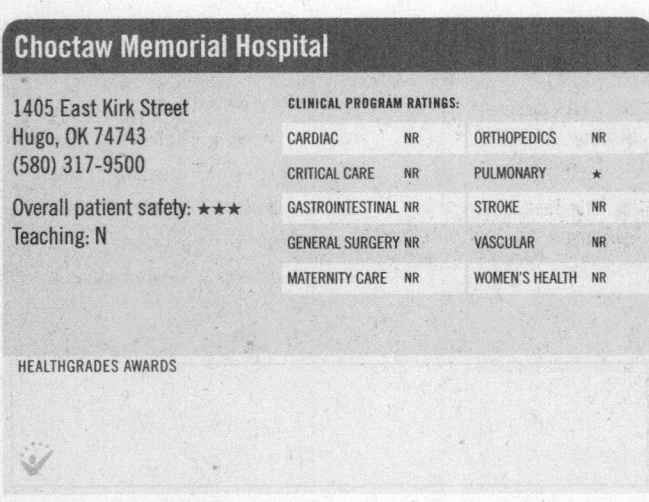

1405 East Kirk Street
Hugo, OK 74743
(580) 317-9500

Overall patient safety: ★★★
Teaching: N

CLINICAL PROGRAM RATINGS:

CARDIAC	NR	ORTHOPEDICS	NR
CRITICAL CARE	NR	PULMONARY	★
GASTROINTESTINAL	NR	STROKE	NR
GENERAL SURGERY	NR	VASCULAR	NR
MATERNITY CARE	NR	WOMEN'S HEALTH	NR

HEALTHGRADES AWARDS

Claremore Regional Hospital

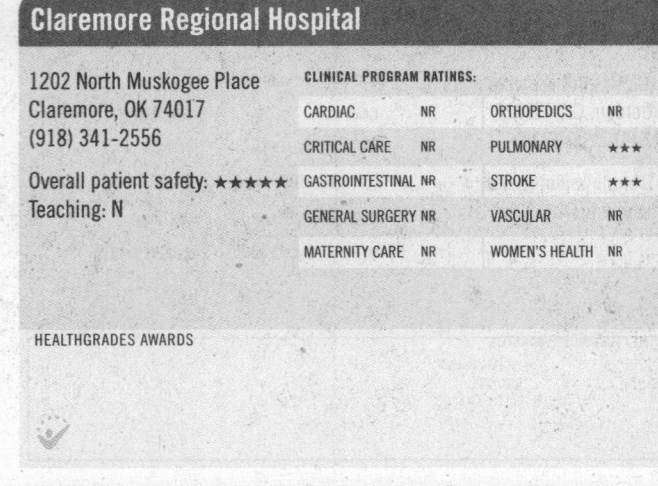

1202 North Muskogee Place
Claremore, OK 74017
(918) 341-2556

Overall patient safety: ★★★★★
Teaching: N

CLINICAL PROGRAM RATINGS:

CARDIAC	NR	ORTHOPEDICS	NR
CRITICAL CARE	NR	PULMONARY	★★★
GASTROINTESTINAL	NR	STROKE	★★★
GENERAL SURGERY	NR	VASCULAR	NR
MATERNITY CARE	NR	WOMEN'S HEALTH	NR

HEALTHGRADES AWARDS

Choctaw Nation Health Services Authority

1 Choctaw Way
Talihina, OK 74571
(918) 567-7000

Overall patient safety: ★★★
Teaching: N

CLINICAL PROGRAM RATINGS:

CARDIAC	NR	ORTHOPEDICS	NR
CRITICAL CARE	NR	PULMONARY	★★★
GASTROINTESTINAL	NR	STROKE	NR
GENERAL SURGERY	NR	VASCULAR	NR
MATERNITY CARE	NR	WOMEN'S HEALTH	NR

HEALTHGRADES AWARDS

Comanche County Memorial Hospital

3401 West Gore Boulevard
Lawton, OK 73505
(580) 355-8620

Overall patient safety: ★★★
Teaching: Y

CLINICAL PROGRAM RATINGS:

CARDIAC	★★★	ORTHOPEDICS	★★★
CRITICAL CARE	NR	PULMONARY	★★★
GASTROINTESTINAL	★★★	STROKE	★★★
GENERAL SURGERY	NR	VASCULAR	NR
MATERNITY CARE	NR	WOMEN'S HEALTH	NR

HEALTHGRADES AWARDS

KEY: ★★★★★ BEST ★★★ AS EXPECTED ★ POOR NR NOT RATED BY HEALTHGRADES   For full definitions of ratings and awards, see Appendix.

Community Hospital

3100 Southwest 89th Street
Oklahoma City, OK 73159
(405) 602-8100

Overall patient safety: ★★★
Teaching: N

CLINICAL PROGRAM RATINGS:

CARDIAC	NR	ORTHOPEDICS	NR
CRITICAL CARE	NR	PULMONARY	NR
GASTROINTESTINAL	NR	STROKE	NR
GENERAL SURGERY	NR	VASCULAR	NR
MATERNITY CARE	NR	WOMEN'S HEALTH	NR

HEALTHGRADES AWARDS

Creek Nation Community Hospital

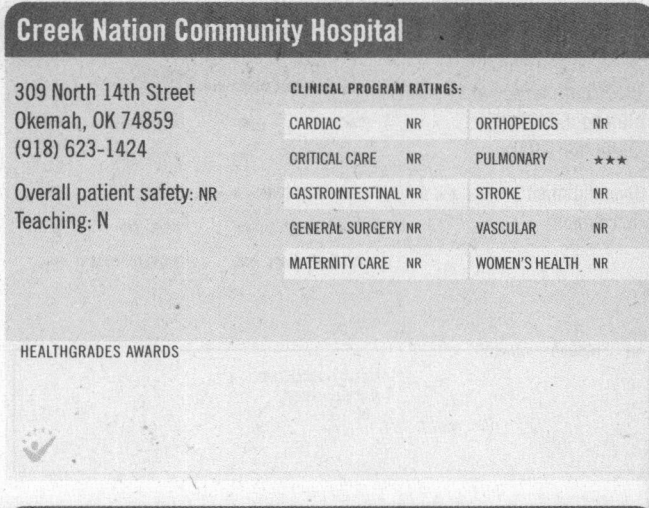

309 North 14th Street
Okemah, OK 74859
(918) 623-1424

Overall patient safety: NR
Teaching: N

CLINICAL PROGRAM RATINGS:

CARDIAC	NR	ORTHOPEDICS	NR
CRITICAL CARE	NR	PULMONARY	★★★
GASTROINTESTINAL	NR	STROKE	NR
GENERAL SURGERY	NR	VASCULAR	NR
MATERNITY CARE	NR	WOMEN'S HEALTH	NR

HEALTHGRADES AWARDS

Cordell Memorial Hospital

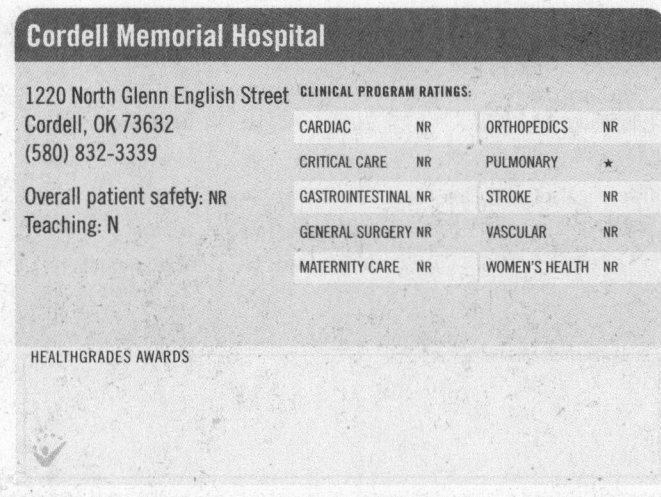

1220 North Glenn English Street
Cordell, OK 73632
(580) 832-3339

Overall patient safety: NR
Teaching: N

CLINICAL PROGRAM RATINGS:

CARDIAC	NR	ORTHOPEDICS	NR
CRITICAL CARE	NR	PULMONARY	★
GASTROINTESTINAL	NR	STROKE	NR
GENERAL SURGERY	NR	VASCULAR	NR
MATERNITY CARE	NR	WOMEN'S HEALTH	NR

HEALTHGRADES AWARDS

Cushing Regional Hospital

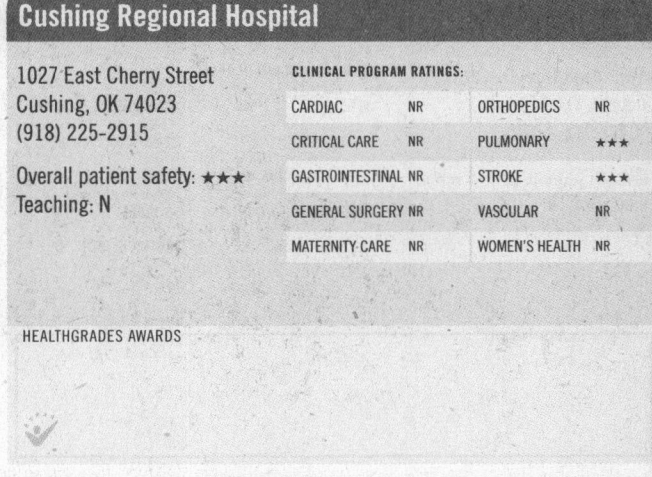

1027 East Cherry Street
Cushing, OK 74023
(918) 225-2915

Overall patient safety: ★★★
Teaching: N

CLINICAL PROGRAM RATINGS:

CARDIAC	NR	ORTHOPEDICS	NR
CRITICAL CARE	NR	PULMONARY	★★★
GASTROINTESTINAL	NR	STROKE	★★★
GENERAL SURGERY	NR	VASCULAR	NR
MATERNITY CARE	NR	WOMEN'S HEALTH	NR

HEALTHGRADES AWARDS

Craig General Hospital

735 North Foreman Street
Vinita, OK 74301
(918) 256-7551

Overall patient safety: ★★★
Teaching: N

CLINICAL PROGRAM RATINGS:

CARDIAC	NR	ORTHOPEDICS	NR
CRITICAL CARE	NR	PULMONARY	★★★
GASTROINTESTINAL	NR	STROKE	★
GENERAL SURGERY	NR	VASCULAR	NR
MATERNITY CARE	NR	WOMEN'S HEALTH	NR

HEALTHGRADES AWARDS

Deaconess Hospital

5501 North Portland Avenue
Oklahoma City, OK 73112
(405) 604-6000

Overall patient safety: ★★★
Teaching: Y

CLINICAL PROGRAM RATINGS:

CARDIAC	★★★	ORTHOPEDICS	NR
CRITICAL CARE	NR	PULMONARY	★★★
GASTROINTESTINAL	★★★	STROKE	★★★
GENERAL SURGERY	NR	VASCULAR	NR
MATERNITY CARE	NR	WOMEN'S HEALTH	NR

HEALTHGRADES AWARDS

Duncan Regional Hospital

1407 North Whisenant Drive
Duncan, OK 73534
(580) 252-5300

Overall patient safety: ★★★★★
Teaching: N

CLINICAL PROGRAM RATINGS:

CARDIAC	NR	ORTHOPEDICS	NR
CRITICAL CARE	NR	PULMONARY	★★★
GASTROINTESTINAL	★★★	STROKE	★★★
GENERAL SURGERY	NR	VASCULAR	NR
MATERNITY CARE	NR	WOMEN'S HEALTH	NR

HEALTHGRADES AWARDS

✓ SPECIALTY EXCELLENCE
· JOINT REPLACEMENT

Elkview General Hospital

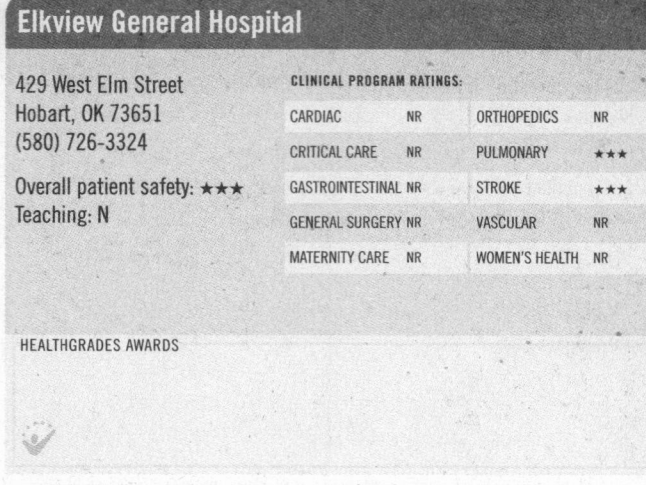

429 West Elm Street
Hobart, OK 73651
(580) 726-3324

Overall patient safety: ★★★
Teaching: N

CLINICAL PROGRAM RATINGS:

CARDIAC	NR	ORTHOPEDICS	NR
CRITICAL CARE	NR	PULMONARY	★★★
GASTROINTESTINAL	NR	STROKE	★★★
GENERAL SURGERY	NR	VASCULAR	NR
MATERNITY CARE	NR	WOMEN'S HEALTH	NR

HEALTHGRADES AWARDS

Eastern Oklahoma Medical Center

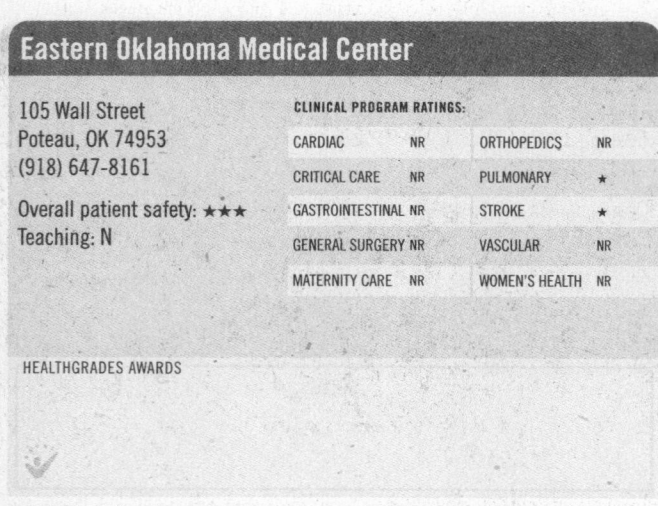

105 Wall Street
Poteau, OK 74953
(918) 647-8161

Overall patient safety: ★★★
Teaching: N

CLINICAL PROGRAM RATINGS:

CARDIAC	NR	ORTHOPEDICS	NR
CRITICAL CARE	NR	PULMONARY	★
GASTROINTESTINAL	NR	STROKE	★
GENERAL SURGERY	NR	VASCULAR	NR
MATERNITY CARE	NR	WOMEN'S HEALTH	NR

HEALTHGRADES AWARDS

Grady Memorial Hospital

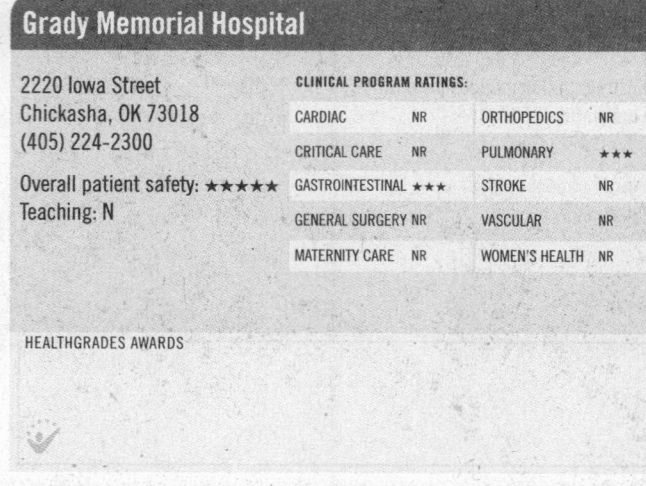

2220 Iowa Street
Chickasha, OK 73018
(405) 224-2300

Overall patient safety: ★★★★★
Teaching: N

CLINICAL PROGRAM RATINGS:

CARDIAC	NR	ORTHOPEDICS	NR
CRITICAL CARE	NR	PULMONARY	★★★
GASTROINTESTINAL	★★★	STROKE	NR
GENERAL SURGERY	NR	VASCULAR	NR
MATERNITY CARE	NR	WOMEN'S HEALTH	NR

HEALTHGRADES AWARDS

Edmond Medical Center

1 South Bryant Avenue
Edmond, OK 73034
(405) 341-6100

Overall patient safety: ★★★
Teaching: N

CLINICAL PROGRAM RATINGS:

CARDIAC	NR	ORTHOPEDICS	NR
CRITICAL CARE	NR	PULMONARY	★★★
GASTROINTESTINAL	★★★	STROKE	★★★
GENERAL SURGERY	NR	VASCULAR	NR
MATERNITY CARE	NR	WOMEN'S HEALTH	NR

HEALTHGRADES AWARDS

Great Plains Regional Medical Center

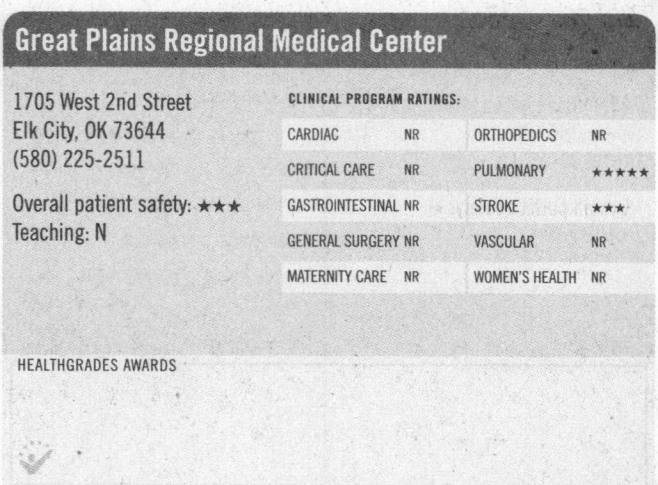

1705 West 2nd Street
Elk City, OK 73644
(580) 225-2511

Overall patient safety: ★★★
Teaching: N

CLINICAL PROGRAM RATINGS:

CARDIAC	NR	ORTHOPEDICS	NR
CRITICAL CARE	NR	PULMONARY	★★★★★
GASTROINTESTINAL	NR	STROKE	★★★
GENERAL SURGERY	NR	VASCULAR	NR
MATERNITY CARE	NR	WOMEN'S HEALTH	NR

HEALTHGRADES AWARDS

KEY: ★★★★★ BEST   ★★★ AS EXPECTED   ★ POOR   NR NOT RATED BY HEALTHGRADES   For full definitions of ratings and awards, see Appendix.

Haskell County Hospital

401 Northwest H Street
Stigler, OK 74462
(918) 967-4682

Overall patient safety: ★★★
Teaching: N

CLINICAL PROGRAM RATINGS:

CARDIAC	NR	ORTHOPEDICS	NR
CRITICAL CARE	NR	PULMONARY	★
GASTROINTESTINAL	NR	STROKE	★
GENERAL SURGERY	NR	VASCULAR	NR
MATERNITY CARE	NR	WOMEN'S HEALTH	NR

HEALTHGRADES AWARDS

Holdenville General Hospital

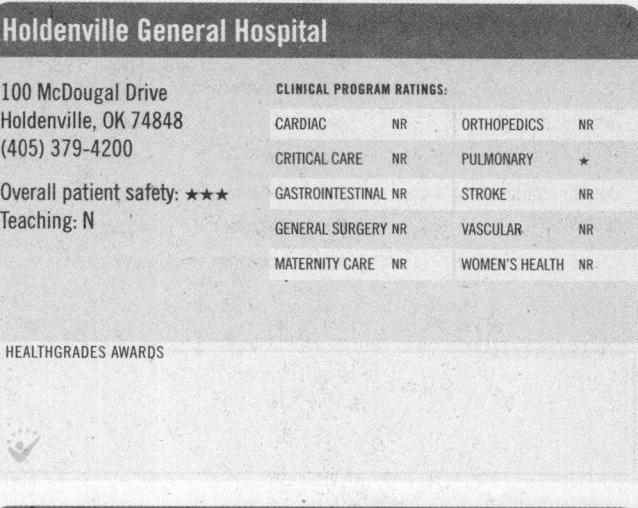

100 McDougal Drive
Holdenville, OK 74848
(405) 379-4200

Overall patient safety: ★★★
Teaching: N

CLINICAL PROGRAM RATINGS:

CARDIAC	NR	ORTHOPEDICS	NR
CRITICAL CARE	NR	PULMONARY	★
GASTROINTESTINAL	NR	STROKE	NR
GENERAL SURGERY	NR	VASCULAR	NR
MATERNITY CARE	NR	WOMEN'S HEALTH	NR

HEALTHGRADES AWARDS

Henryetta Medical Center

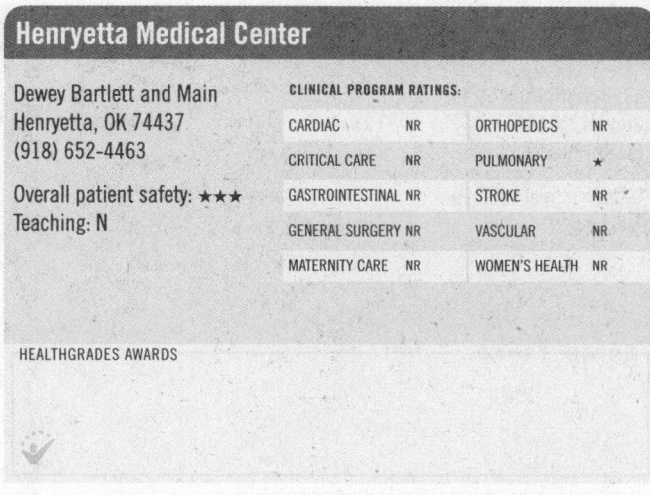

Dewey Bartlett and Main
Henryetta, OK 74437
(918) 652-4463

Overall patient safety: ★★★
Teaching: N

CLINICAL PROGRAM RATINGS:

CARDIAC	NR	ORTHOPEDICS	NR
CRITICAL CARE	NR	PULMONARY	★
GASTROINTESTINAL	NR	STROKE	NR
GENERAL SURGERY	NR	VASCULAR	NR
MATERNITY CARE	NR	WOMEN'S HEALTH	NR

HEALTHGRADES AWARDS

Integris Baptist Medical Center

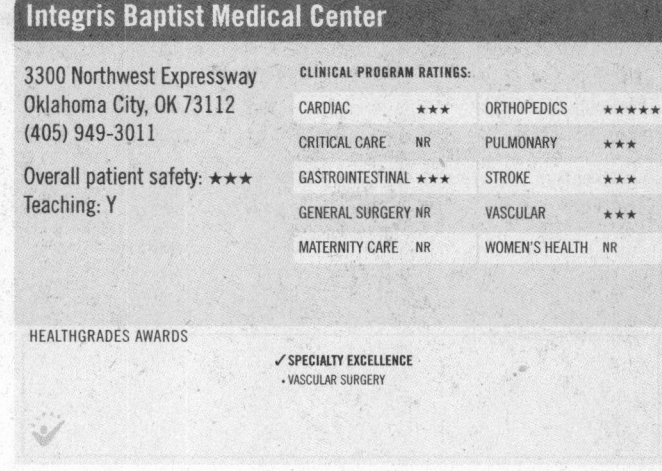

3300 Northwest Expressway
Oklahoma City, OK 73112
(405) 949-3011

Overall patient safety: ★★★
Teaching: Y

CLINICAL PROGRAM RATINGS:

CARDIAC	★★★	ORTHOPEDICS	★★★★★
CRITICAL CARE	NR	PULMONARY	★★★
GASTROINTESTINAL	★★★	STROKE	★★★
GENERAL SURGERY	NR	VASCULAR	★★★
MATERNITY CARE	NR	WOMEN'S HEALTH	NR

HEALTHGRADES AWARDS

✓ **SPECIALTY EXCELLENCE**
• VASCULAR SURGERY

Hillcrest Medical Center

1120 South Utica Avenue
Tulsa, OK 74104
(918) 579-1000

Overall patient safety: ★
Teaching: Y

CLINICAL PROGRAM RATINGS:

CARDIAC	★★★	ORTHOPEDICS	★★★
CRITICAL CARE	NR	PULMONARY	★★★
GASTROINTESTINAL	★★★	STROKE	★★★
GENERAL SURGERY	NR	VASCULAR	NR
MATERNITY CARE	NR	WOMEN'S HEALTH	NR

HEALTHGRADES AWARDS

Integris Baptist Regional Health Center

200 2nd Avenue Southwest
Miami, OK 74354
(918) 542-6611

Overall patient safety: ★★★
Teaching: N

CLINICAL PROGRAM RATINGS:

CARDIAC	NR	ORTHOPEDICS	NR
CRITICAL CARE	NR	PULMONARY	★★★
GASTROINTESTINAL	NR	STROKE	★★★
GENERAL SURGERY	NR	VASCULAR	NR
MATERNITY CARE	NR	WOMEN'S HEALTH	NR

HEALTHGRADES AWARDS

Integris Bass Baptist Health Center

600 South Monroe
Enid, OK 73701
(580) 233-2300

Overall patient safety: ★★★
Teaching: Y

CLINICAL PROGRAM RATINGS:

CARDIAC	★	ORTHOPEDICS	NR
CRITICAL CARE	NR	PULMONARY	★★★
GASTROINTESTINAL	NR	STROKE	★★★
GENERAL SURGERY	NR	VASCULAR	NR
MATERNITY CARE	NR	WOMEN'S HEALTH	NR

HEALTHGRADES AWARDS

Integris Clinton Regional Hospital

100 North 30th Street
Clinton, OK 73601
(580) 323-2363

Overall patient safety: ★★★
Teaching: N

CLINICAL PROGRAM RATINGS:

CARDIAC	NR	ORTHOPEDICS	NR
CRITICAL CARE	NR	PULMONARY	★★★★★
GASTROINTESTINAL	NR	STROKE	★★★
GENERAL SURGERY	NR	VASCULAR	NR
MATERNITY CARE	NR	WOMEN'S HEALTH	NR

HEALTHGRADES AWARDS

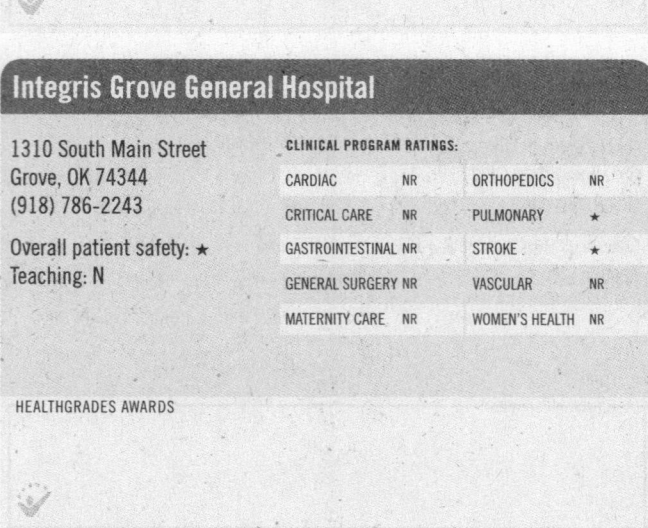

✓ SPECIALTY EXCELLENCE
- PULMONARY CARE

Integris Blackwell Regional Hospital

710 South 13th Street
Blackwell, OK 74631
(580) 363-2311

Overall patient safety: ★★★
Teaching: N

CLINICAL PROGRAM RATINGS:

CARDIAC	NR	ORTHOPEDICS	NR
CRITICAL CARE	NR	PULMONARY	★
GASTROINTESTINAL	NR	STROKE	★★★
GENERAL SURGERY	NR	VASCULAR	NR
MATERNITY CARE	NR	WOMEN'S HEALTH	NR

HEALTHGRADES AWARDS

Integris Grove General Hospital

1310 South Main Street
Grove, OK 74344
(918) 786-2243

Overall patient safety: ★
Teaching: N

CLINICAL PROGRAM RATINGS:

CARDIAC	NR	ORTHOPEDICS	NR
CRITICAL CARE	NR	PULMONARY	★
GASTROINTESTINAL	NR	STROKE	★
GENERAL SURGERY	NR	VASCULAR	NR
MATERNITY CARE	NR	WOMEN'S HEALTH	NR

HEALTHGRADES AWARDS

Integris Canadian Valley Regional Hospital

1201 Health Center Parkway
Yukon, OK 73099
(405) 717-7999

Overall patient safety: ★★★
Teaching: N

CLINICAL PROGRAM RATINGS:

CARDIAC	NR	ORTHOPEDICS	NR
CRITICAL CARE	NR	PULMONARY	★★★
GASTROINTESTINAL	NR	STROKE	★★★
GENERAL SURGERY	NR	VASCULAR	NR
MATERNITY CARE	NR	WOMEN'S HEALTH	NR

HEALTHGRADES AWARDS

Integris Marshall County Medical Center

1 Hospital Drive
Madill, OK 73446
(580) 795-3384

Overall patient safety: ★★★
Teaching: N

CLINICAL PROGRAM RATINGS:

CARDIAC	NR	ORTHOPEDICS	NR
CRITICAL CARE	NR	PULMONARY	★
GASTROINTESTINAL	NR	STROKE	NR
GENERAL SURGERY	NR	VASCULAR	NR
MATERNITY CARE	NR	WOMEN'S HEALTH	NR

HEALTHGRADES AWARDS

KEY: ★★★★★ BEST   ★★★ AS EXPECTED   ★ POOR   NR NOT RATED BY HEALTHGRADES   For full definitions of ratings and awards, see Appendix.

Integris Mayes County Medical Center

129 North Kentucky Street
Pryor, OK 74361
(918) 825-1600

Overall patient safety: ★★★
Teaching: N

CLINICAL PROGRAM RATINGS:

CARDIAC	NR	ORTHOPEDICS	NR
CRITICAL CARE	NR	PULMONARY	★★★
GASTROINTESTINAL	NR	STROKE	★★★
GENERAL SURGERY	NR	VASCULAR	NR
MATERNITY CARE	NR	WOMEN'S HEALTH	NR

HEALTHGRADES AWARDS

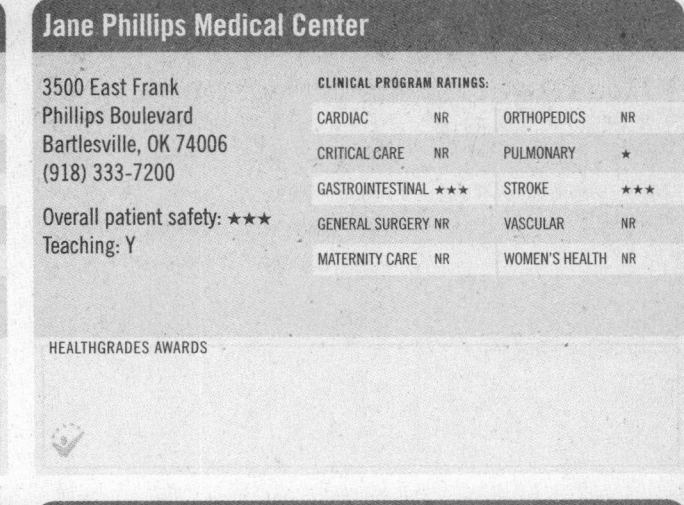

Jane Phillips Medical Center

3500 East Frank
Phillips Boulevard
Bartlesville, OK 74006
(918) 333-7200

Overall patient safety: ★★★
Teaching: Y

CLINICAL PROGRAM RATINGS:

CARDIAC	NR	ORTHOPEDICS	NR
CRITICAL CARE	NR	PULMONARY	★
GASTROINTESTINAL	★★★	STROKE	★★★
GENERAL SURGERY	NR	VASCULAR	NR
MATERNITY CARE	NR	WOMEN'S HEALTH	NR

HEALTHGRADES AWARDS

Integris Southwest Medical Center

4401 South Western
Oklahoma City, OK 73109
(405) 636-7000

Overall patient safety: ★★★
Teaching: Y

CLINICAL PROGRAM RATINGS:

CARDIAC	★★★	ORTHOPEDICS	★★★
CRITICAL CARE	NR	PULMONARY	★★★
GASTROINTESTINAL	★★★	STROKE	★★★
GENERAL SURGERY	NR	VASCULAR	NR
MATERNITY CARE	NR	WOMEN'S HEALTH	NR

HEALTHGRADES AWARDS

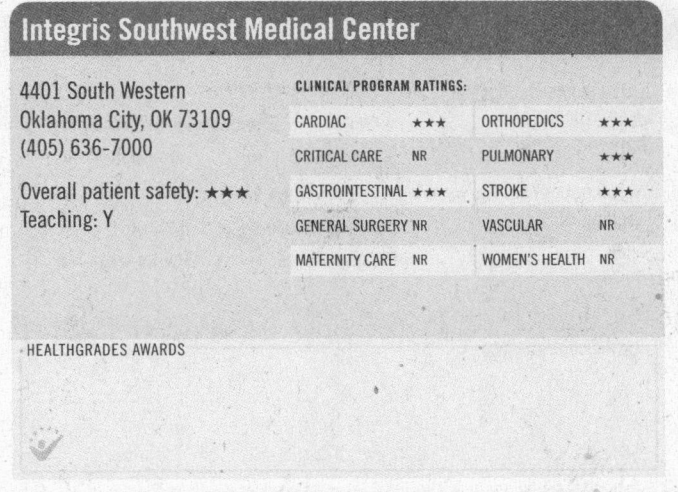

Johnston Memorial Hospital

1000 South Bryd
Tishomingo, OK 73460
(580) 371-2327

Overall patient safety: ★★★
Teaching: N

CLINICAL PROGRAM RATINGS:

CARDIAC	NR	ORTHOPEDICS	NR
CRITICAL CARE	NR	PULMONARY	★★★
GASTROINTESTINAL	NR	STROKE	NR
GENERAL SURGERY	NR	VASCULAR	NR
MATERNITY CARE	NR	WOMEN'S HEALTH	NR

HEALTHGRADES AWARDS

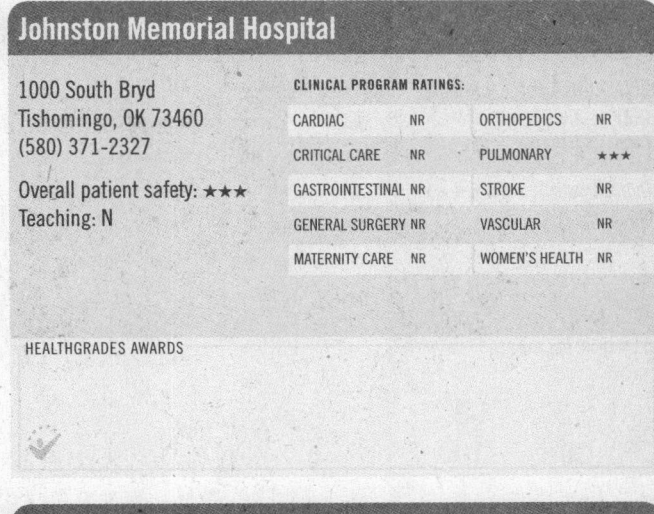

Jackson County Memorial Hospital

1200 East Pecan Street
Altus, OK 73521
(580) 482-4781

Overall patient safety: ★★★
Teaching: N

CLINICAL PROGRAM RATINGS:

CARDIAC	NR	ORTHOPEDICS	NR
CRITICAL CARE	NR	PULMONARY	★★★
GASTROINTESTINAL	NR	STROKE	★★★
GENERAL SURGERY	NR	VASCULAR	NR
MATERNITY CARE	NR	WOMEN'S HEALTH	NR

HEALTHGRADES AWARDS

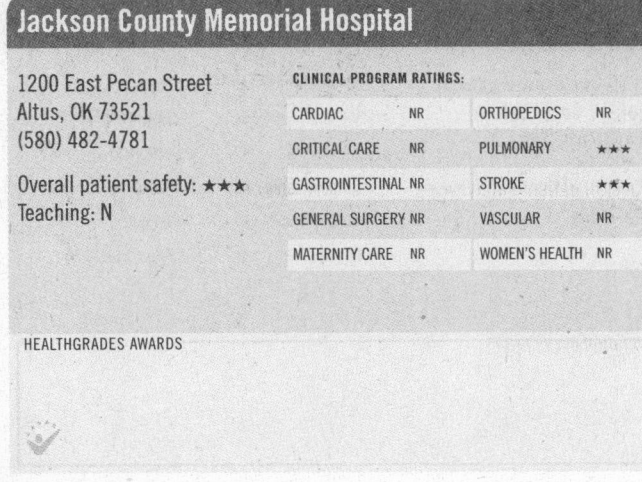

Kingfisher Regional Hospital

500 South 9th Street
Kingfisher, OK 73750
(405) 375-3141

Overall patient safety: ★★★
Teaching: N

CLINICAL PROGRAM RATINGS:

CARDIAC	NR	ORTHOPEDICS	NR
CRITICAL CARE	NR	PULMONARY	★
GASTROINTESTINAL	NR	STROKE	NR
GENERAL SURGERY	NR	VASCULAR	NR
MATERNITY CARE	NR	WOMEN'S HEALTH	NR

HEALTHGRADES AWARDS

Latimer County General Hospital

806 Highway 2 North
Wilburton, OK 74578
(918) 465-2391

Overall patient safety: NR
Teaching: N

CLINICAL PROGRAM RATINGS:

CARDIAC	NR	ORTHOPEDICS	NR
CRITICAL CARE	NR	PULMONARY	★★★
GASTROINTESTINAL	NR	STROKE	NR
GENERAL SURGERY	NR	VASCULAR	NR
MATERNITY CARE	NR	WOMEN'S HEALTH	NR

HEALTHGRADES AWARDS

McBride Clinic Orthopedic Hospital

9600 North Broadway Extension
Oklahoma City, OK 73114
(405) 478-1717

Overall patient safety: ★★★
Teaching: N

CLINICAL PROGRAM RATINGS:

CARDIAC	NR	ORTHOPEDICS	★★★★★
CRITICAL CARE	NR	PULMONARY	NR
GASTROINTESTINAL	NR	STROKE	NR
GENERAL SURGERY	NR	VASCULAR	NR
MATERNITY CARE	NR	WOMEN'S HEALTH	NR

HEALTHGRADES AWARDS

✓ SPECIALTY EXCELLENCE
• ORTHOPEDIC SURGERY

Logan Medical Center

200 South Academy Road
Guthrie, OK 73044
(405) 282-6700

Overall patient safety: ★★★
Teaching: N

CLINICAL PROGRAM RATINGS:

CARDIAC	NR	ORTHOPEDICS	NR
CRITICAL CARE	NR	PULMONARY	★★★
GASTROINTESTINAL	NR	STROKE	★★★
GENERAL SURGERY	NR	VASCULAR	NR
MATERNITY CARE	NR	WOMEN'S HEALTH	NR

HEALTHGRADES AWARDS

McCurtain Memorial Hospital

1301 Lincoln Road
Idabel, OK 74745
(580) 286-7623

Overall patient safety: ★★★
Teaching: N

CLINICAL PROGRAM RATINGS:

CARDIAC	NR	ORTHOPEDICS	NR
CRITICAL CARE	NR	PULMONARY	★
GASTROINTESTINAL	NR	STROKE	★★★
GENERAL SURGERY	NR	VASCULAR	NR
MATERNITY CARE	NR	WOMEN'S HEALTH	NR

HEALTHGRADES AWARDS

McAlester Regional Health Center

1 Clark Bass Boulevard
McAlester, OK 74501
(918) 426-1800

Overall patient safety: ★★★
Teaching: N

CLINICAL PROGRAM RATINGS:

CARDIAC	NR	ORTHOPEDICS	NR
CRITICAL CARE	NR	PULMONARY	★★★
GASTROINTESTINAL	★★★	STROKE	★★★
GENERAL SURGERY	NR	VASCULAR	NR
MATERNITY CARE	NR	WOMEN'S HEALTH	NR

HEALTHGRADES AWARDS

Medical Center of Southeastern Oklahoma

1800 University Boulevard
Durant, OK 74701
(580) 924-3080

Overall patient safety: ★★★
Teaching: Y

CLINICAL PROGRAM RATINGS:

CARDIAC	NR	ORTHOPEDICS	NR
CRITICAL CARE	NR	PULMONARY	★★★
GASTROINTESTINAL	NR	STROKE	★
GENERAL SURGERY	NR	VASCULAR	NR
MATERNITY CARE	NR	WOMEN'S HEALTH	NR

HEALTHGRADES AWARDS

KEY: ★★★★★ BEST ★★★ AS EXPECTED ★ POOR NR NOT RATED BY HEALTHGRADES For full definitions of ratings and awards, see Appendix.

Memorial Hospital and Physician Group

319 East Josephine Avenue
Frederick, OK 73542
(580) 335-7565

Overall patient safety: ★★★
Teaching: N

CLINICAL PROGRAM RATINGS:

CARDIAC	NR	ORTHOPEDICS	NR
CRITICAL CARE	NR	PULMONARY	★★★
GASTROINTESTINAL	NR	STROKE	★★★
GENERAL SURGERY	NR	VASCULAR	NR
MATERNITY CARE	NR	WOMEN'S HEALTH	NR

HEALTHGRADES AWARDS

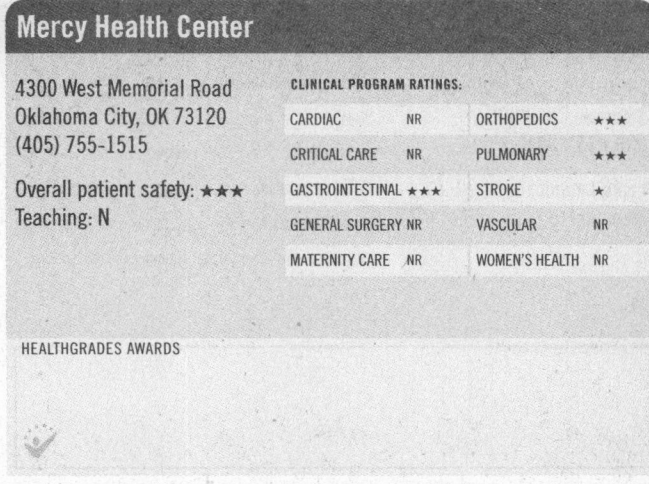

Mercy Health Center

4300 West Memorial Road
Oklahoma City, OK 73120
(405) 755-1515

Overall patient safety: ★★★
Teaching: N

CLINICAL PROGRAM RATINGS:

CARDIAC	NR	ORTHOPEDICS	★★★
CRITICAL CARE	NR	PULMONARY	★★★
GASTROINTESTINAL	★★★	STROKE	★
GENERAL SURGERY	NR	VASCULAR	NR
MATERNITY CARE	NR	WOMEN'S HEALTH	NR

HEALTHGRADES AWARDS

Memorial Hospital of Stilwell

1401 West Locust Street
Stilwell, OK 74960
(918) 696-3101

Overall patient safety: ★★★
Teaching: N

CLINICAL PROGRAM RATINGS:

CARDIAC	NR	ORTHOPEDICS	NR
CRITICAL CARE	NR	PULMONARY	★★★
GASTROINTESTINAL	NR	STROKE	NR
GENERAL SURGERY	NR	VASCULAR	NR
MATERNITY CARE	NR	WOMEN'S HEALTH	NR

HEALTHGRADES AWARDS

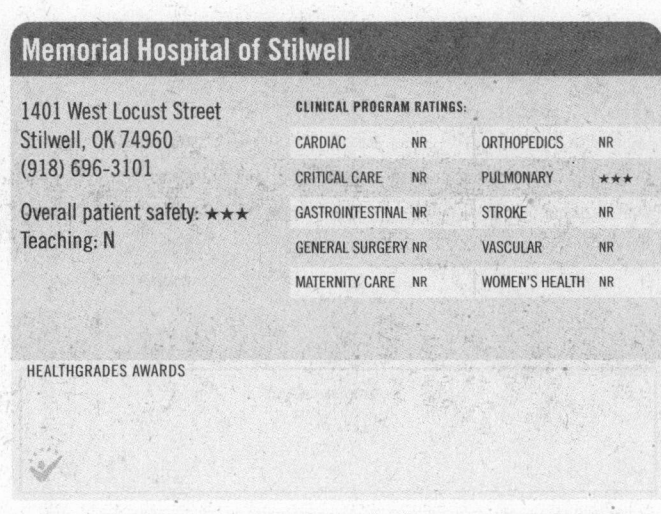

Mercy Memorial Health Center*

1011 14th Avenue Northwest
Ardmore, OK 73401
(580) 223-5400

Overall patient safety: ★★★★★
Teaching: N

CLINICAL PROGRAM RATINGS:

CARDIAC	NR	ORTHOPEDICS	NR
CRITICAL CARE	NR	PULMONARY	★
GASTROINTESTINAL	★★★	STROKE	★★★
GENERAL SURGERY	NR	VASCULAR	NR
MATERNITY CARE	NR	WOMEN'S HEALTH	NR

HEALTHGRADES AWARDS

✓ DISTINGUISHED
   HOSPITAL
 • PATIENT SAFETY

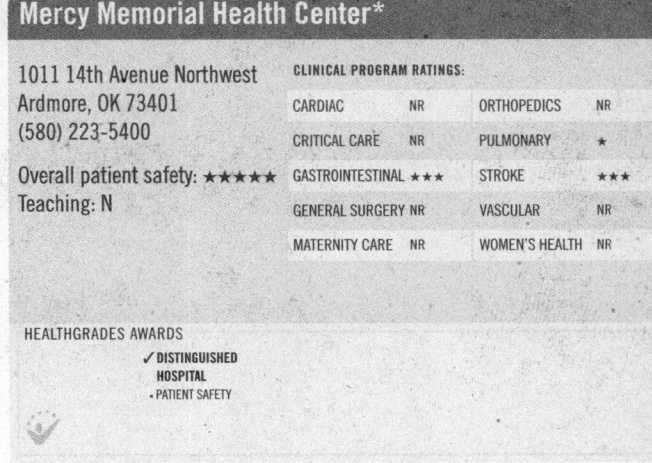

Memorial Hospital of Texas County

520 Medical Drive
Guymon, OK 73942
(580) 338-6515

Overall patient safety: ★★★
Teaching: N

CLINICAL PROGRAM RATINGS:

CARDIAC	NR	ORTHOPEDICS	NR
CRITICAL CARE	NR	PULMONARY	★★★
GASTROINTESTINAL	NR	STROKE	NR
GENERAL SURGERY	NR	VASCULAR	NR
MATERNITY CARE	NR	WOMEN'S HEALTH	NR

HEALTHGRADES AWARDS

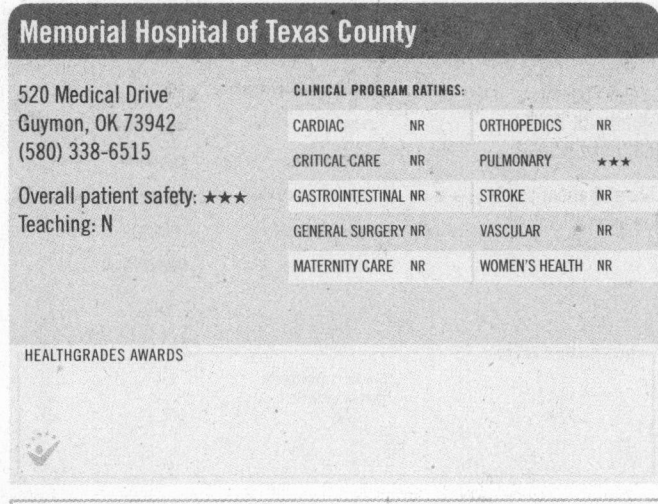

Midwest Regional Medical Center

2825 Parklawn Drive
Midwest City, OK 73110
(405) 610-4411

Overall patient safety: ★★★★★
Teaching: Y

CLINICAL PROGRAM RATINGS:

CARDIAC	★★★	ORTHOPEDICS	★★★★★
CRITICAL CARE	NR	PULMONARY	★★★
GASTROINTESTINAL	★★★	STROKE	★★★
GENERAL SURGERY	NR	VASCULAR	NR
MATERNITY CARE	NR	WOMEN'S HEALTH	NR

HEALTHGRADES AWARDS

✓ DISTINGUISHED   ✓ SPECIALTY EXCELLENCE
   HOSPITAL   • ORTHOPEDIC
 • PATIENT SAFETY   SURGERY

*This hospital reports its data to the federal government jointly with another hospital. Therefore the ratings and awards apply to multiple hospitals and this specific hospital may not provide all rated services.

Mission Hill Memorial Hospital*

1900 Gordon Cooper Drive
Shawnee, OK 74801
(405) 273-2240

Overall patient safety: ★★★
Teaching: N

CLINICAL PROGRAM RATINGS:

CARDIAC	NR	ORTHOPEDICS	NR
CRITICAL CARE	NR	PULMONARY	★
GASTROINTESTINAL	★★★	STROKE	★
GENERAL SURGERY	NR	VASCULAR	NR
MATERNITY CARE	NR	WOMEN'S HEALTH	NR

HEALTHGRADES AWARDS

Norman Regional Hospital

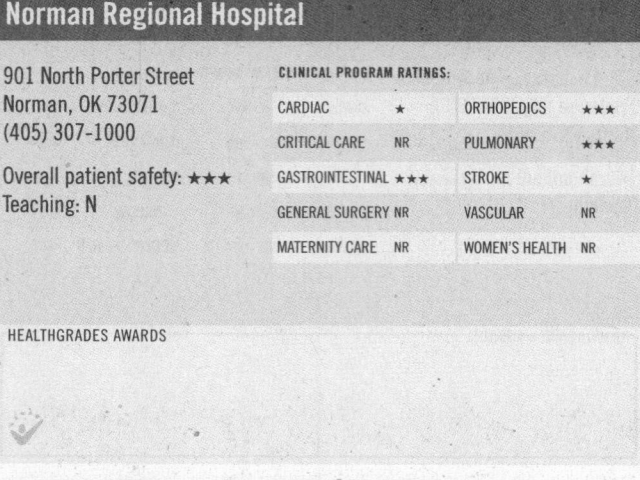

901 North Porter Street
Norman, OK 73071
(405) 307-1000

Overall patient safety: ★★★
Teaching: N

CLINICAL PROGRAM RATINGS:

CARDIAC	★	ORTHOPEDICS	★★★
CRITICAL CARE	NR	PULMONARY	★★★
GASTROINTESTINAL	★★★	STROKE	★
GENERAL SURGERY	NR	VASCULAR	NR
MATERNITY CARE	NR	WOMEN'S HEALTH	NR

HEALTHGRADES AWARDS

Muskogee Regional Medical Center

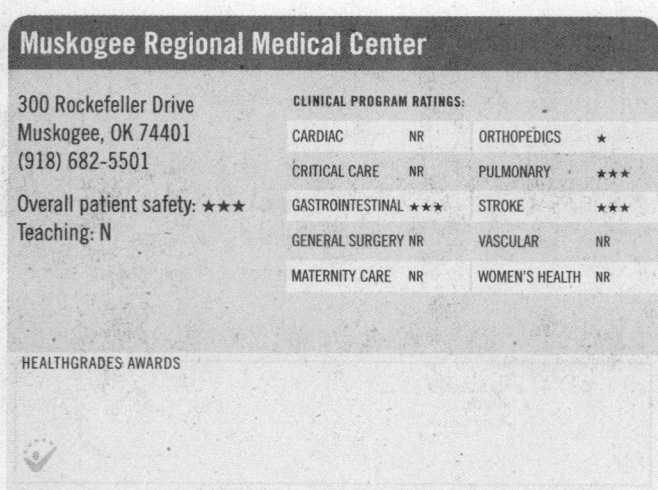

300 Rockefeller Drive
Muskogee, OK 74401
(918) 682-5501

Overall patient safety: ★★★
Teaching: N

CLINICAL PROGRAM RATINGS:

CARDIAC	NR	ORTHOPEDICS	★
CRITICAL CARE	NR	PULMONARY	★★★
GASTROINTESTINAL	★★★	STROKE	★★★
GENERAL SURGERY	NR	VASCULAR	NR
MATERNITY CARE	NR	WOMEN'S HEALTH	NR

HEALTHGRADES AWARDS

Oklahoma Heart Hospital

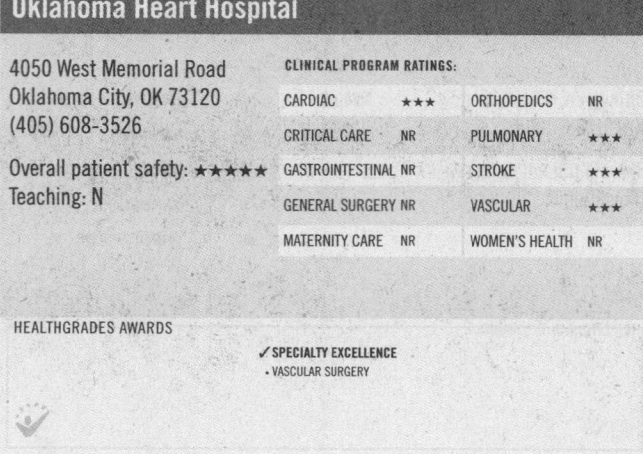

4050 West Memorial Road
Oklahoma City, OK 73120
(405) 608-3526

Overall patient safety: ★★★★★
Teaching: N

CLINICAL PROGRAM RATINGS:

CARDIAC	★★★	ORTHOPEDICS	NR
CRITICAL CARE	NR	PULMONARY	★★★
GASTROINTESTINAL	NR	STROKE	★★★
GENERAL SURGERY	NR	VASCULAR	★★★
MATERNITY CARE	NR	WOMEN'S HEALTH	NR

HEALTHGRADES AWARDS

✓ SPECIALTY EXCELLENCE
• VASCULAR SURGERY

Newman Memorial Hospital

905 South Main Street
Shattuck, OK 73858
(580) 938-2551

Overall patient safety: ★★★
Teaching: N

CLINICAL PROGRAM RATINGS:

CARDIAC	NR	ORTHOPEDICS	NR
CRITICAL CARE	NR	PULMONARY	★★★
GASTROINTESTINAL	NR	STROKE	NR
GENERAL SURGERY	NR	VASCULAR	NR
MATERNITY CARE	NR	WOMEN'S HEALTH	NR

HEALTHGRADES AWARDS

Oklahoma Surgical Hospital

2408 East 81st Street
Tulsa, OK 74137
(918) 477-5000

Overall patient safety: ★★★★★
Teaching: N

CLINICAL PROGRAM RATINGS:

CARDIAC	NR	ORTHOPEDICS	NR
CRITICAL CARE	NR	PULMONARY	NR
GASTROINTESTINAL	NR	STROKE	NR
GENERAL SURGERY	NR	VASCULAR	NR
MATERNITY CARE	NR	WOMEN'S HEALTH	NR

HEALTHGRADES AWARDS

✓ SPECIALTY EXCELLENCE
• JOINT REPLACEMENT

KEY: ★★★★★ BEST ★★★ AS EXPECTED ★ POOR NR NOT RATED BY HEALTHGRADES For full definitions of ratings and awards, see Appendix.

Oklahoma University Medical Center

700 Northeast 13th Street
Oklahoma City, OK 73104
(405) 271-5100

Overall patient safety: ★★★
Teaching: Y

CLINICAL PROGRAM RATINGS:

CARDIAC	★★★	ORTHOPEDICS	NR
CRITICAL CARE	NR	PULMONARY	★★★
GASTROINTESTINAL	NR	STROKE	★
GENERAL SURGERY	NR	VASCULAR	NR
MATERNITY CARE	NR	WOMEN'S HEALTH	NR

HEALTHGRADES AWARDS

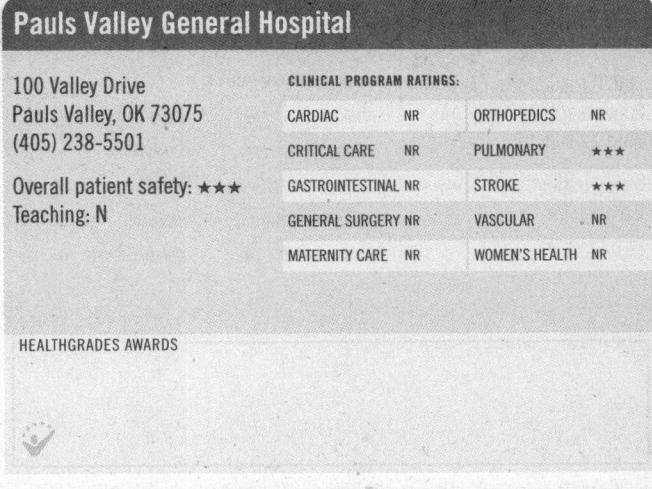

Pauls Valley General Hospital

100 Valley Drive
Pauls Valley, OK 73075
(405) 238-5501

Overall patient safety: ★★★
Teaching: N

CLINICAL PROGRAM RATINGS:

CARDIAC	NR	ORTHOPEDICS	NR
CRITICAL CARE	NR	PULMONARY	★★★
GASTROINTESTINAL	NR	STROKE	★★★
GENERAL SURGERY	NR	VASCULAR	NR
MATERNITY CARE	NR	WOMEN'S HEALTH	NR

HEALTHGRADES AWARDS

Okmulgee Memorial Hospital

1401 Morris Drive
Okmulgee, OK 74447
(918) 756-4233

Overall patient safety: ★
Teaching: N

CLINICAL PROGRAM RATINGS:

CARDIAC	NR	ORTHOPEDICS	NR
CRITICAL CARE	NR	PULMONARY	★
GASTROINTESTINAL	NR	STROKE	NR
GENERAL SURGERY	NR	VASCULAR	NR
MATERNITY CARE	NR	WOMEN'S HEALTH	NR

HEALTHGRADES AWARDS

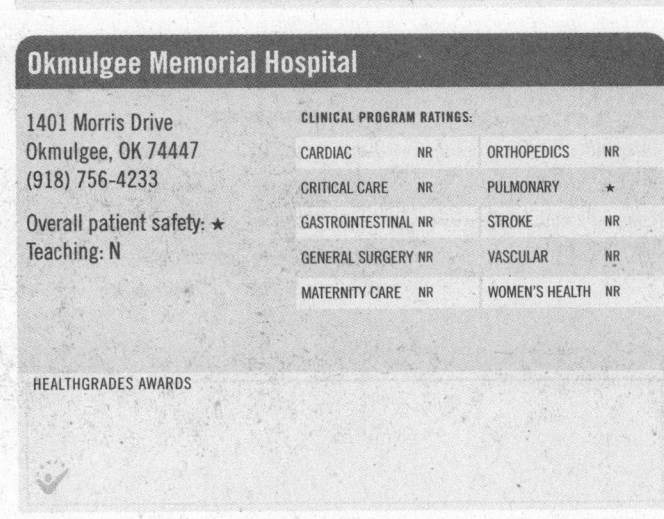

Pawnee Municipal Hospital

1212 4th Street
Pawnee, OK 74058
(918) 762-2577

Overall patient safety: ★★★
Teaching: N

CLINICAL PROGRAM RATINGS:

CARDIAC	NR	ORTHOPEDICS	NR
CRITICAL CARE	NR	PULMONARY	★★★
GASTROINTESTINAL	NR	STROKE	NR
GENERAL SURGERY	NR	VASCULAR	NR
MATERNITY CARE	NR	WOMEN'S HEALTH	NR

HEALTHGRADES AWARDS

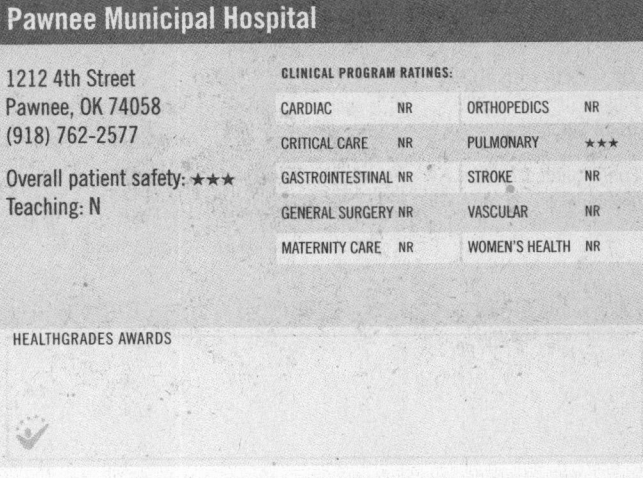

Parkview Hospital

2115 Parkview Drive
El Reno, OK 73036
(405) 262-2640

Overall patient safety: ★★★
Teaching: N

CLINICAL PROGRAM RATINGS:

CARDIAC	NR	ORTHOPEDICS	NR
CRITICAL CARE	NR	PULMONARY	★★★
GASTROINTESTINAL	NR	STROKE	★
GENERAL SURGERY	NR	VASCULAR	NR
MATERNITY CARE	NR	WOMEN'S HEALTH	NR

HEALTHGRADES AWARDS

Perry Memorial Hospital

501 14th Street
Perry, OK 73077
(580) 336-3541

Overall patient safety: ★★★
Teaching: N

CLINICAL PROGRAM RATINGS:

CARDIAC	NR	ORTHOPEDICS	NR
CRITICAL CARE	NR	PULMONARY	★★★
GASTROINTESTINAL	NR	STROKE	★★★
GENERAL SURGERY	NR	VASCULAR	NR
MATERNITY CARE	NR	WOMEN'S HEALTH	NR

HEALTHGRADES AWARDS

*This hospital reports its data to the federal government jointly with another hospital. Therefore the ratings and awards apply to multiple hospitals and this specific hospital may not provide all rated services.

Physicians' Hospital in Anadarko

1002 East Central Boulevard
Anadarko, OK 73005
(405) 247-2551

Overall patient safety: ★★★
Teaching: N

CLINICAL PROGRAM RATINGS:

CARDIAC	NR	ORTHOPEDICS	NR
CRITICAL CARE	NR	PULMONARY	★★★
GASTROINTESTINAL	NR	STROKE	NR
GENERAL SURGERY	NR	VASCULAR	NR
MATERNITY CARE	NR	WOMEN'S HEALTH	NR

HEALTHGRADES AWARDS

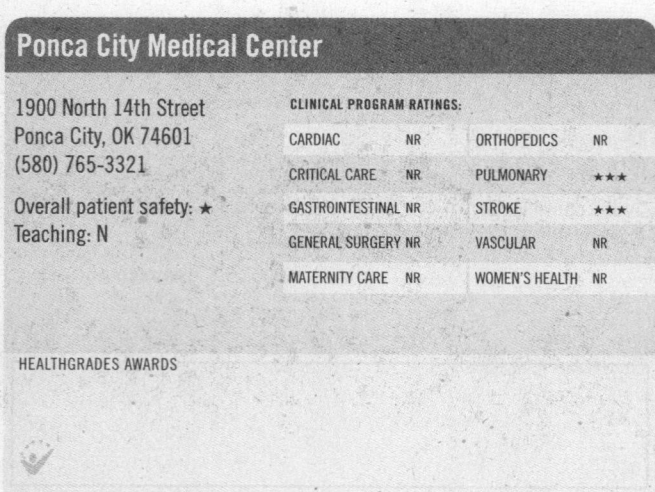

Pushmataha County—Town of Antlers Hospital Authority

510 East Main Street
Antlers, OK 74523
(580) 298-3341

Overall patient safety: ★★★
Teaching: N

CLINICAL PROGRAM RATINGS:

CARDIAC	NR	ORTHOPEDICS	NR
CRITICAL CARE	NR	PULMONARY	★★★
GASTROINTESTINAL	NR	STROKE	★★★
GENERAL SURGERY	NR	VASCULAR	NR
MATERNITY CARE	NR	WOMEN'S HEALTH	NR

HEALTHGRADES AWARDS

Ponca City Medical Center

1900 North 14th Street
Ponca City, OK 74601
(580) 765-3321

Overall patient safety: ★
Teaching: N

CLINICAL PROGRAM RATINGS:

CARDIAC	NR	ORTHOPEDICS	NR
CRITICAL CARE	NR	PULMONARY	★★★
GASTROINTESTINAL	NR	STROKE	★★★
GENERAL SURGERY	NR	VASCULAR	NR
MATERNITY CARE	NR	WOMEN'S HEALTH	NR

HEALTHGRADES AWARDS

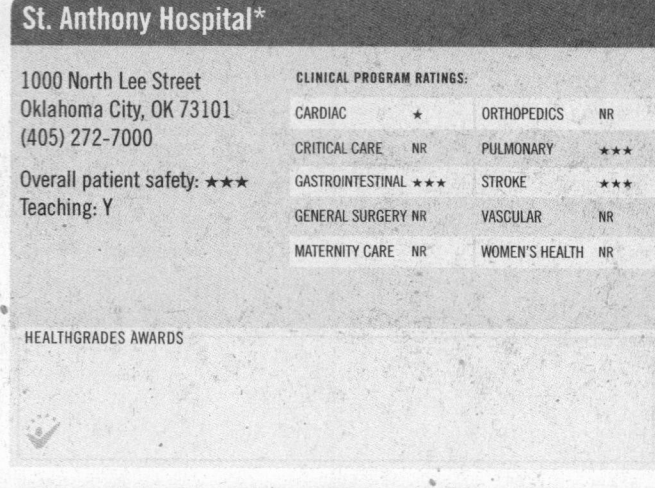

St. Anthony Hospital*

1000 North Lee Street
Oklahoma City, OK 73101
(405) 272-7000

Overall patient safety: ★★★
Teaching: Y

CLINICAL PROGRAM RATINGS:

CARDIAC	★	ORTHOPEDICS	NR
CRITICAL CARE	NR	PULMONARY	★★★
GASTROINTESTINAL	★★★	STROKE	★★★
GENERAL SURGERY	NR	VASCULAR	NR
MATERNITY CARE	NR	WOMEN'S HEALTH	NR

HEALTHGRADES AWARDS

Purcell Municipal Hospital

1500 North Green Avenue
Purcell, OK 73080
(405) 527-6524

Overall patient safety: ★★★
Teaching: N

CLINICAL PROGRAM RATINGS:

CARDIAC	NR	ORTHOPEDICS	NR
CRITICAL CARE	NR	PULMONARY	★★★
GASTROINTESTINAL	NR	STROKE	★
GENERAL SURGERY	NR	VASCULAR	NR
MATERNITY CARE	NR	WOMEN'S HEALTH	NR

HEALTHGRADES AWARDS

St. Francis Hospital

6161 South Yale Avenue
Tulsa, OK 74136
(918) 494-2200

Overall patient safety: ★
Teaching: Y

CLINICAL PROGRAM RATINGS:

CARDIAC	★	ORTHOPEDICS	★★★
CRITICAL CARE	NR	PULMONARY	★★★
GASTROINTESTINAL	★★★	STROKE	★★★
GENERAL SURGERY	NR	VASCULAR	★★★
MATERNITY CARE	NR	WOMEN'S HEALTH	NR

HEALTHGRADES AWARDS

KEY: ★★★★★ BEST   ★★★ AS EXPECTED   ★ POOR   NR NOT RATED BY HEALTHGRADES   For full definitions of ratings and awards, see Appendix.

St. Francis Hospital—Broken Arrow

3000 South Elm Place
Broken Arrow, OK 74012
(918) 455-3535

Overall patient safety: ★★★
Teaching: N

CLINICAL PROGRAM RATINGS:

CARDIAC	NR	ORTHOPEDICS	NR
CRITICAL CARE	NR	PULMONARY	★★★
GASTROINTESTINAL	NR	STROKE	★★★
GENERAL SURGERY	NR	VASCULAR	NR
MATERNITY CARE	NR	WOMEN'S HEALTH	NR

HEALTHGRADES AWARDS

St. Michael Hospital*

2129 Southwest 59th Street
Oklahoma City, OK 73119
(405) 685-6671

Overall patient safety: ★★★
Teaching: Y

CLINICAL PROGRAM RATINGS:

CARDIAC	★	ORTHOPEDICS	NR
CRITICAL CARE	NR	PULMONARY	★★★
GASTROINTESTINAL	★★★	STROKE	★★★
GENERAL SURGERY	NR	VASCULAR	NR
MATERNITY CARE	NR	WOMEN'S HEALTH	NR

HEALTHGRADES AWARDS

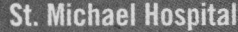

St. John Medical Center

1923 South Utica Avenue
Tulsa, OK 74104
(918) 744-2345

Overall patient safety: ★
Teaching: Y

CLINICAL PROGRAM RATINGS:

CARDIAC	★★★	ORTHOPEDICS	★★★
CRITICAL CARE	NR	PULMONARY	★
GASTROINTESTINAL	★★★	STROKE	★★★
GENERAL SURGERY	NR	VASCULAR	★★★
MATERNITY CARE	NR	WOMEN'S HEALTH	NR

HEALTHGRADES AWARDS

Seminole Medical Center

2401 Wrangler Boulevard
Seminole, OK 74868
(405) 303-4000

Overall patient safety: ★★★
Teaching: N

CLINICAL PROGRAM RATINGS:

CARDIAC	NR	ORTHOPEDICS	NR
CRITICAL CARE	NR	PULMONARY	★
GASTROINTESTINAL	NR	STROKE	NR
GENERAL SURGERY	NR	VASCULAR	NR
MATERNITY CARE	NR	WOMEN'S HEALTH	NR

HEALTHGRADES AWARDS

St. Mary's Regional Medical Center

305 South 5th Street
Enid, OK 73701
(580) 233-6100

Overall patient safety: ★★★
Teaching: N

CLINICAL PROGRAM RATINGS:

CARDIAC	★★★	ORTHOPEDICS	★★★
CRITICAL CARE	NR	PULMONARY	★★★
GASTROINTESTINAL	★★★	STROKE	★★★
GENERAL SURGERY	NR	VASCULAR	NR
MATERNITY CARE	NR	WOMEN'S HEALTH	NR

HEALTHGRADES AWARDS

Sequoyah Memorial Hospital

213 East Redwood
Sallisaw, OK 74955
(918) 774-1100

Overall patient safety: ★★★
Teaching: N

CLINICAL PROGRAM RATINGS:

CARDIAC	NR	ORTHOPEDICS	NR
CRITICAL CARE	NR	PULMONARY	★
GASTROINTESTINAL	NR	STROKE	★
GENERAL SURGERY	NR	VASCULAR	NR
MATERNITY CARE	NR	WOMEN'S HEALTH	NR

HEALTHGRADES AWARDS

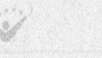

*This hospital reports its data to the federal government jointly with another hospital. Therefore the ratings and awards apply to multiple hospitals and this specific hospital may not provide all rated services.

Share Memorial Hospital

800 Share Drive
Alva, OK 73717
(580) 327-2800

Overall patient safety: ★★★
Teaching: N

CLINICAL PROGRAM RATINGS:

CARDIAC	NR	ORTHOPEDICS	NR
CRITICAL CARE	NR	PULMONARY	★
GASTROINTESTINAL	NR	STROKE	NR
GENERAL SURGERY	NR	VASCULAR	NR
MATERNITY CARE	NR	WOMEN'S HEALTH	NR

HEALTHGRADES AWARDS

Southwestern Memorial Hospital

215 North Kansas Street
Weatherford, OK 73096
(580) 772-5551

Overall patient safety: ★★★
Teaching: N

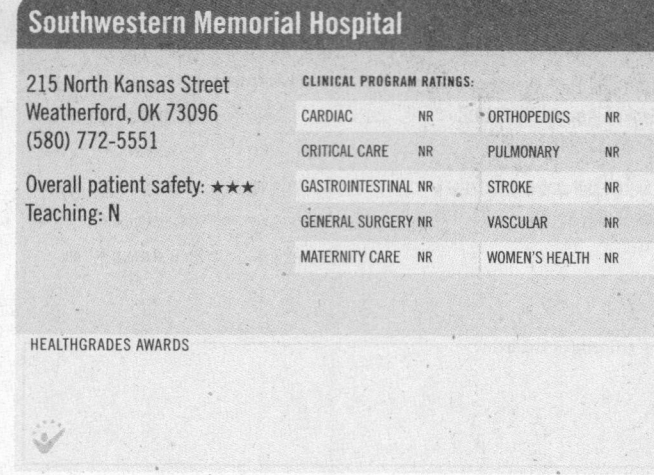

CLINICAL PROGRAM RATINGS:

CARDIAC	NR	ORTHOPEDICS	NR
CRITICAL CARE	NR	PULMONARY	NR
GASTROINTESTINAL	NR	STROKE	NR
GENERAL SURGERY	NR	VASCULAR	NR
MATERNITY CARE	NR	WOMEN'S HEALTH	NR

HEALTHGRADES AWARDS

SouthCrest Hospital

8801 South 101st East Avenue
Tulsa, OK 74133
(918) 294-4000

Overall patient safety: ★★★
Teaching: N

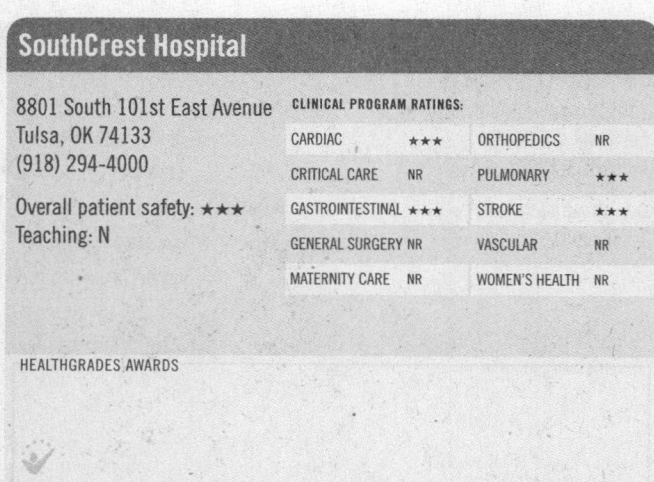

CLINICAL PROGRAM RATINGS:

CARDIAC	★★★	ORTHOPEDICS	NR
CRITICAL CARE	NR	PULMONARY	★★★
GASTROINTESTINAL	★★★	STROKE	★★★
GENERAL SURGERY	NR	VASCULAR	NR
MATERNITY CARE	NR	WOMEN'S HEALTH	NR

HEALTHGRADES AWARDS

Stillwater Medical Center

1323 West 6th Street
Stillwater, OK 74074
(405) 372-1480

Overall patient safety: ★★★
Teaching: N

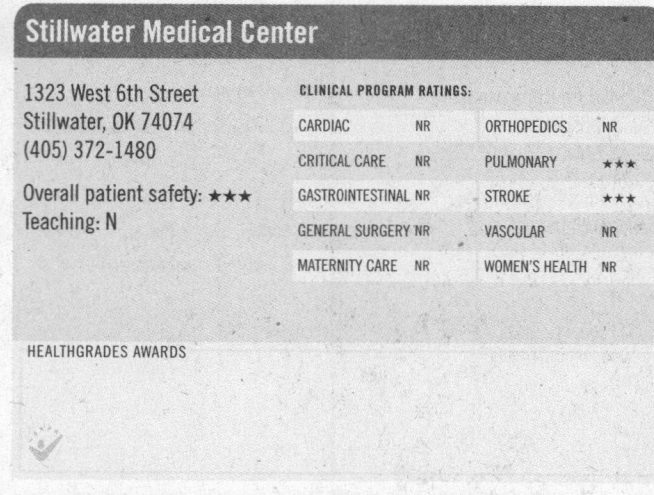

CLINICAL PROGRAM RATINGS:

CARDIAC	NR	ORTHOPEDICS	NR
CRITICAL CARE	NR	PULMONARY	★★★
GASTROINTESTINAL	NR	STROKE	★★★
GENERAL SURGERY	NR	VASCULAR	NR
MATERNITY CARE	NR	WOMEN'S HEALTH	NR

HEALTHGRADES AWARDS

Southwestern Medical Center

5602 Southwest Lee Boulevard
Lawton, OK 73505
(580) 531-4700

Overall patient safety: ★★★
Teaching: N

CLINICAL PROGRAM RATINGS:

CARDIAC	NR	ORTHOPEDICS	NR
CRITICAL CARE	NR	PULMONARY	★★★
GASTROINTESTINAL	NR	STROKE	★★★
GENERAL SURGERY	NR	VASCULAR	NR
MATERNITY CARE	NR	WOMEN'S HEALTH	NR

HEALTHGRADES AWARDS

Stroud Regional Medical Center

2308 Highway 66 West
Stroud, OK 74079
(918) 968-3571

Overall patient safety: ★★★
Teaching: N

CLINICAL PROGRAM RATINGS:

CARDIAC	NR	ORTHOPEDICS	NR
CRITICAL CARE	NR	PULMONARY	★★★
GASTROINTESTINAL	NR	STROKE	NR
GENERAL SURGERY	NR	VASCULAR	NR
MATERNITY CARE	NR	WOMEN'S HEALTH	NR

HEALTHGRADES AWARDS

KEY: ★★★★★ BEST   ★★★ AS EXPECTED   ★ POOR   NR NOT RATED BY HEALTHGRADES   For full definitions of ratings and awards, see Appendix.

Tahlequah City Hospital

1400 East Downing Street
Tahlequah, OK 74465
(918) 456-0641

Overall patient safety: ★★★
Teaching: N

CLINICAL PROGRAM RATINGS:

CARDIAC	NR	ORTHOPEDICS	NR
CRITICAL CARE	NR	PULMONARY	★
GASTROINTESTINAL	NR	STROKE	★
GENERAL SURGERY	NR	VASCULAR	NR
MATERNITY CARE	NR	WOMEN'S HEALTH	NR

HEALTHGRADES AWARDS

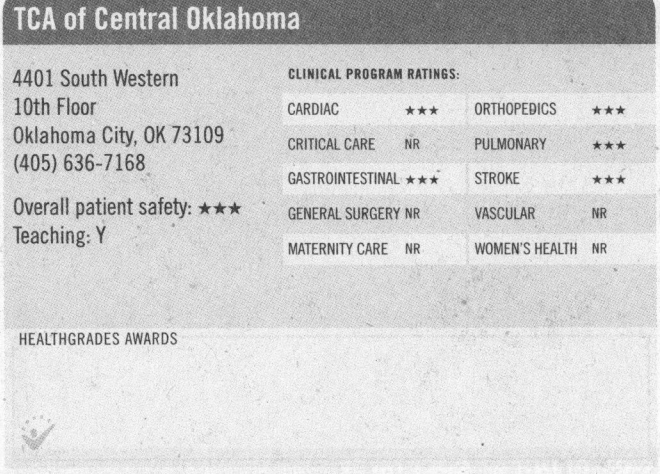

Unity Health Center*

1102 West Macarthur
Shawnee, OK 74804
(405) 273-2270

Overall patient safety: ★★★
Teaching: N

CLINICAL PROGRAM RATINGS:

CARDIAC	NR	ORTHOPEDICS	NR
CRITICAL CARE	NR	PULMONARY	★
GASTROINTESTINAL	★★★	STROKE	★
GENERAL SURGERY	NR	VASCULAR	NR
MATERNITY CARE	NR	WOMEN'S HEALTH	NR

HEALTHGRADES AWARDS

TCA of Central Oklahoma

4401 South Western
10th Floor
Oklahoma City, OK 73109
(405) 636-7168

Overall patient safety: ★★★
Teaching: Y

CLINICAL PROGRAM RATINGS:

CARDIAC	★★★	ORTHOPEDICS	★★★
CRITICAL CARE	NR	PULMONARY	★★★
GASTROINTESTINAL	★★★	STROKE	★★★
GENERAL SURGERY	NR	VASCULAR	NR
MATERNITY CARE	NR	WOMEN'S HEALTH	NR

HEALTHGRADES AWARDS

Valley View Regional Hospital

430 North Monta Vista
Ada, OK 74820
(580) 332-2323

Overall patient safety: ★★★
Teaching: N

CLINICAL PROGRAM RATINGS:

CARDIAC	NR	ORTHOPEDICS	NR
CRITICAL CARE	NR	PULMONARY	★★★
GASTROINTESTINAL	★★★	STROKE	★★★
GENERAL SURGERY	NR	VASCULAR	NR
MATERNITY CARE	NR	WOMEN'S HEALTH	NR

HEALTHGRADES AWARDS

Tulsa Regional Medical Center

744 West 9th Street
Tulsa, OK 74127
(918) 579-7974

Overall patient safety: ★
Teaching: Y

CLINICAL PROGRAM RATINGS:

CARDIAC	★★★	ORTHOPEDICS	NR
CRITICAL CARE	NR	PULMONARY	★★★
GASTROINTESTINAL	NR	STROKE	★
GENERAL SURGERY	NR	VASCULAR	NR
MATERNITY CARE	NR	WOMEN'S HEALTH	NR

HEALTHGRADES AWARDS

W. W. Hastings Indian Hospital

100 South Bliss Avenue
Tahlequah, OK 74464
(918) 458-3100

Overall patient safety: ★★★
Teaching: N

CLINICAL PROGRAM RATINGS:

CARDIAC	NR	ORTHOPEDICS	NR
CRITICAL CARE	NR	PULMONARY	★
GASTROINTESTINAL	NR	STROKE	NR
GENERAL SURGERY	NR	VASCULAR	NR
MATERNITY CARE	NR	WOMEN'S HEALTH	NR

HEALTHGRADES AWARDS

*This hospital reports its data to the federal government jointly with another hospital. Therefore the ratings and awards apply to multiple hospitals and this specific hospital may not provide all rated services.

OKLAHOMA HOSPITALS: RATINGS BY CLINICAL SPECIALTY

Wagoner Community Hospital

1200 West Cherokee
Wagoner, OK 74467
(918) 485-5514

Overall patient safety: ★★★
Teaching: N

CLINICAL PROGRAM RATINGS:

CARDIAC	NR	ORTHOPEDICS	NR
CRITICAL CARE	NR	PULMONARY	★★★
GASTROINTESTINAL	NR	STROKE	NR
GENERAL SURGERY	NR	VASCULAR	NR
MATERNITY CARE	NR	WOMEN'S HEALTH	NR

HEALTHGRADES AWARDS

Woodward Regional Hospital

900 17th Street
Woodward, OK 73801
(580) 256-5511

Overall patient safety: ★★★
Teaching: N

CLINICAL PROGRAM RATINGS:

CARDIAC	NR	ORTHOPEDICS	NR
CRITICAL CARE	NR	PULMONARY	★★★
GASTROINTESTINAL	NR	STROKE	★★★
GENERAL SURGERY	NR	VASCULAR	NR
MATERNITY CARE	NR	WOMEN'S HEALTH	NR

HEALTHGRADES AWARDS

Watonga Municipal Hospital

500 North Clarence
Nash Boulevard
Watonga, OK 73772
(580) 623-7211

Overall patient safety: NR
Teaching: N

CLINICAL PROGRAM RATINGS:

CARDIAC	NR	ORTHOPEDICS	NR
CRITICAL CARE	NR	PULMONARY	★
GASTROINTESTINAL	NR	STROKE	NR
GENERAL SURGERY	NR	VASCULAR	NR
MATERNITY CARE	NR	WOMEN'S HEALTH	NR

HEALTHGRADES AWARDS

OREGON HOSPITALS: RATINGS BY CLINICAL SPECIALTY

Adventist Medical Center

10123 Southeast
Market Street
Portland, OR 97216
(503) 257-2500

Overall patient safety: ★
Teaching: N

CLINICAL PROGRAM RATINGS:

CARDIAC	NR	ORTHOPEDICS	★★★
CRITICAL CARE	NR	PULMONARY	★
GASTROINTESTINAL	NR	STROKE	★
GENERAL SURGERY	★★★	VASCULAR	NR
MATERNITY CARE	★★★	WOMEN'S HEALTH	NR

HEALTHGRADES AWARDS

Ashland Community Hospital

280 Maple Street
Ashland, OR 97520
(541) 482-2441

Overall patient safety: ★★★
Teaching: N

CLINICAL PROGRAM RATINGS:

CARDIAC	NR	ORTHOPEDICS	★★★
CRITICAL CARE	NR	PULMONARY	★★★
GASTROINTESTINAL	NR	STROKE	★★★
GENERAL SURGERY	NR	VASCULAR	NR
MATERNITY CARE	★	WOMEN'S HEALTH	NR

HEALTHGRADES AWARDS

KEY: ★★★★★ BEST ★★★ AS EXPECTED ★ POOR NR NOT RATED BY HEALTHGRADES For full definitions of ratings and awards, see Appendix.

Bay Area Hospital

1775 Thompson Road
Coos Bay, OR 97420
(541) 269-8111

Overall patient safety: ★★★
Teaching: N

CLINICAL PROGRAM RATINGS:

CARDIAC	NR	ORTHOPEDICS	★★★
CRITICAL CARE	NR	PULMONARY	★★★
GASTROINTESTINAL	★★★	STROKE	★
GENERAL SURGERY	★★★	VASCULAR	NR
MATERNITY CARE	★★★	WOMEN'S HEALTH	NR

HEALTHGRADES AWARDS

Coquille Valley Hospital

940 East 5th Street
Coquille, OR 97423
(541) 396-3101

Overall patient safety: ★★★
Teaching: N

CLINICAL PROGRAM RATINGS:

CARDIAC	NR	ORTHOPEDICS	NR
CRITICAL CARE	NR	PULMONARY	NR
GASTROINTESTINAL	NR	STROKE	NR
GENERAL SURGERY	NR	VASCULAR	NR
MATERNITY CARE	★	WOMEN'S HEALTH	NR

HEALTHGRADES AWARDS

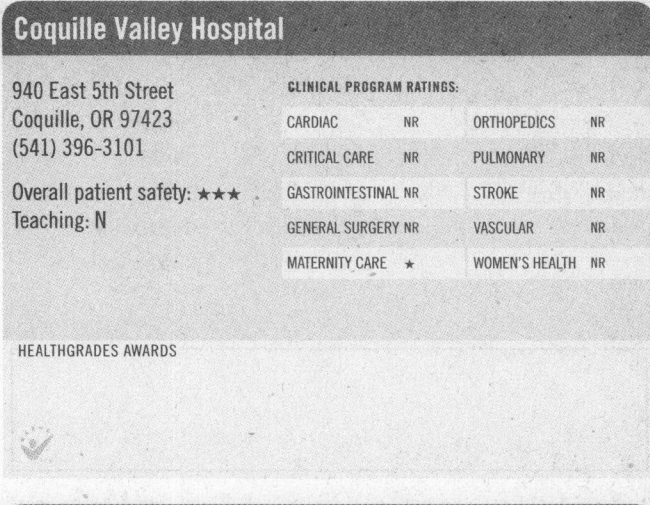

Blue Mountain Hospital District

170 Ford Road
John Day, OR 97845
(541) 575-1311

Overall patient safety: ★★★
Teaching: N

CLINICAL PROGRAM RATINGS:

CARDIAC	NR	ORTHOPEDICS	NR
CRITICAL CARE	NR	PULMONARY	★★★
GASTROINTESTINAL	NR	STROKE	NR
GENERAL SURGERY	NR	VASCULAR	NR
MATERNITY CARE	★	WOMEN'S HEALTH	NR

HEALTHGRADES AWARDS

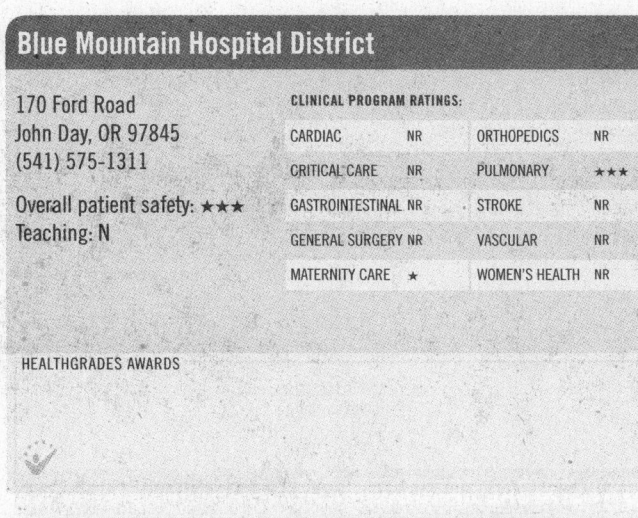

Good Samaritan Regional Medical Center

3600 Northwest
Samaritan Drive
Corvallis, OR 97330
(541) 768-5111

Overall patient safety: ★★★
Teaching: N

CLINICAL PROGRAM RATINGS:

CARDIAC	★★★	ORTHOPEDICS	★★★
CRITICAL CARE	NR	PULMONARY	★★★
GASTROINTESTINAL	★★★	STROKE	★★★
GENERAL SURGERY	★★★★★	VASCULAR	★★★
MATERNITY CARE	★	WOMEN'S HEALTH	★★★

HEALTHGRADES AWARDS

✓ SPECIALTY EXCELLENCE
• GENERAL SURGERY

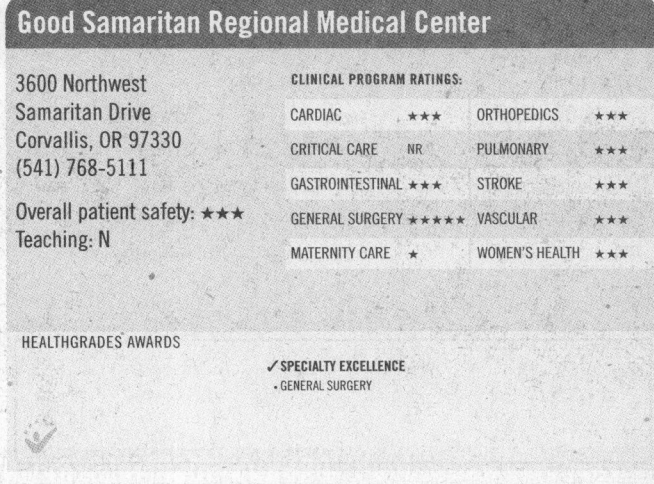

Columbia Memorial Hospital

2111 Exchange Street
Astoria, OR 97103
(503) 338-7505

Overall patient safety: ★
Teaching: N

CLINICAL PROGRAM RATINGS:

CARDIAC	NR	ORTHOPEDICS	NR
CRITICAL CARE	NR	PULMONARY	★
GASTROINTESTINAL	NR	STROKE	★
GENERAL SURGERY	★★★	VASCULAR	NR
MATERNITY CARE	★★★	WOMEN'S HEALTH	NR

HEALTHGRADES AWARDS

Good Shepherd Medical Center

610 Northwest 11th Street
Hermiston, OR 97838
(541) 667-3400

Overall patient safety: NR
Teaching: N

CLINICAL PROGRAM RATINGS:

CARDIAC	NR	ORTHOPEDICS	NR
CRITICAL CARE	NR	PULMONARY	★★★
GASTROINTESTINAL	NR	STROKE	★★★
GENERAL SURGERY	NR	VASCULAR	NR
MATERNITY CARE	NR	WOMEN'S HEALTH	NR

HEALTHGRADES AWARDS

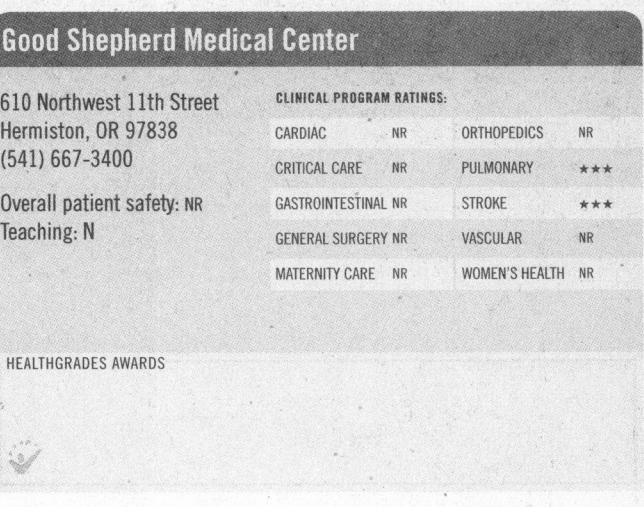

Grande Ronde Hospital

900 Sunset Drive
La Grande, OR 97850
(541) 963-8421

Overall patient safety: ★★★
Teaching: N

CLINICAL PROGRAM RATINGS:

CARDIAC	NR	ORTHOPEDICS	NR
CRITICAL CARE	NR	PULMONARY	★★★
GASTROINTESTINAL	NR	STROKE	★★★
GENERAL SURGERY	★★★	VASCULAR	NR
MATERNITY CARE	★	WOMEN'S HEALTH	NR

HEALTHGRADES AWARDS

Legacy Emanuel Hospital

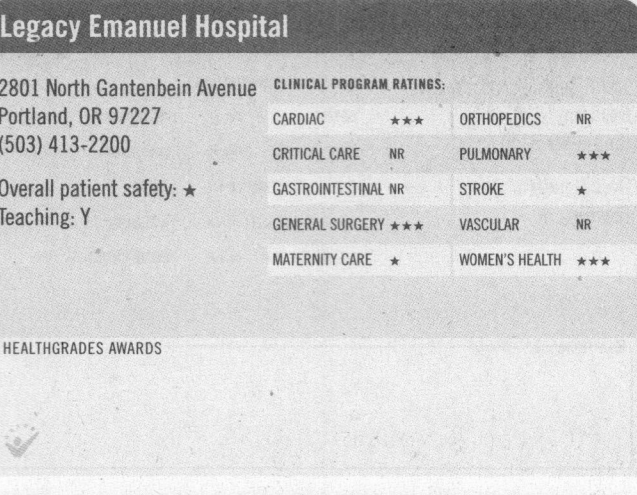

2801 North Gantenbein Avenue
Portland, OR 97227
(503) 413-2200

Overall patient safety: ★
Teaching: Y

CLINICAL PROGRAM RATINGS:

CARDIAC	★★★	ORTHOPEDICS	NR
CRITICAL CARE	NR	PULMONARY	★★★
GASTROINTESTINAL	NR	STROKE	★
GENERAL SURGERY	★★★	VASCULAR	NR
MATERNITY CARE	★	WOMEN'S HEALTH	★★★

HEALTHGRADES AWARDS

Holy Rosary Medical Center

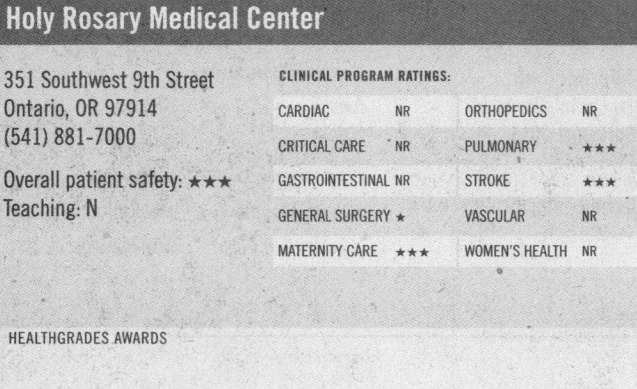

351 Southwest 9th Street
Ontario, OR 97914
(541) 881-7000

Overall patient safety: ★★★
Teaching: N

CLINICAL PROGRAM RATINGS:

CARDIAC	NR	ORTHOPEDICS	NR
CRITICAL CARE	NR	PULMONARY	★★★
GASTROINTESTINAL	NR	STROKE	★★★
GENERAL SURGERY	★	VASCULAR	NR
MATERNITY CARE	★★★	WOMEN'S HEALTH	NR

HEALTHGRADES AWARDS

Legacy Good Samaritan Hospital

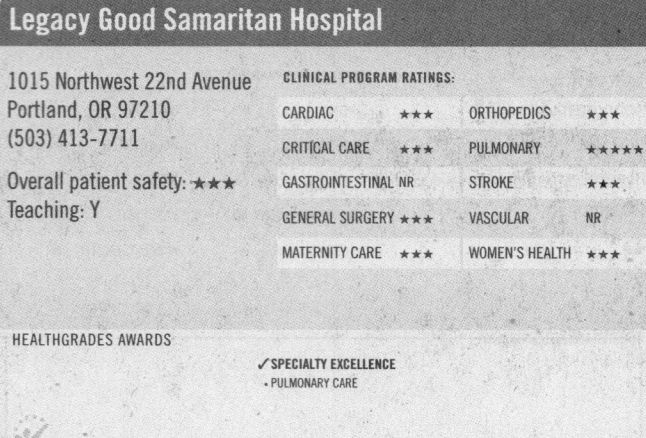

1015 Northwest 22nd Avenue
Portland, OR 97210
(503) 413-7711

Overall patient safety: ★★★
Teaching: Y

CLINICAL PROGRAM RATINGS:

CARDIAC	★★★	ORTHOPEDICS	★★★
CRITICAL CARE	★★★	PULMONARY	★★★★★
GASTROINTESTINAL	NR	STROKE	★★★
GENERAL SURGERY	★★★	VASCULAR	NR
MATERNITY CARE	★★★	WOMEN'S HEALTH	★★★

HEALTHGRADES AWARDS

✓ SPECIALTY EXCELLENCE
- PULMONARY CARE

Kaiser Sunnyside Medical Center

10180 Southeast
Sunnyside Road
Clackamas, OR 97015
(503) 652-2880

Overall patient safety: ★★★
Teaching: Y

CLINICAL PROGRAM RATINGS:

CARDIAC	NR	ORTHOPEDICS	NR
CRITICAL CARE	NR	PULMONARY	NR
GASTROINTESTINAL	NR	STROKE	★★★
GENERAL SURGERY	NR	VASCULAR	NR
MATERNITY CARE	★★★	WOMEN'S HEALTH	NR

HEALTHGRADES AWARDS

Legacy Meridian Park Hospital

19300 Southwest 65th Avenue
Tualatin, OR 97062
(503) 692-1212

Overall patient safety: ★★★
Teaching: N

CLINICAL PROGRAM RATINGS:

CARDIAC	NR	ORTHOPEDICS	★★★
CRITICAL CARE	NR	PULMONARY	★
GASTROINTESTINAL	★★★	STROKE	★
GENERAL SURGERY	★★★	VASCULAR	NR
MATERNITY CARE	★★★	WOMEN'S HEALTH	NR

HEALTHGRADES AWARDS

KEY: ★★★★★ BEST   ★★★ AS EXPECTED   ★ POOR   NR NOT RATED BY HEALTHGRADES   For full definitions of ratings and awards, see Appendix.

Legacy Mount Hood Medical Center

24800 Southeast Stark Street
Gresham, OR 97030
(503) 674-1122

Overall patient safety: ★
Teaching: N

CLINICAL PROGRAM RATINGS:

CARDIAC	NR	ORTHOPEDICS	NR
CRITICAL CARE	NR	PULMONARY	★
GASTROINTESTINAL	NR	STROKE	★★★
GENERAL SURGERY	★★★	VASCULAR	NR
MATERNITY CARE	★★★	WOMEN'S HEALTH	NR

HEALTHGRADES AWARDS

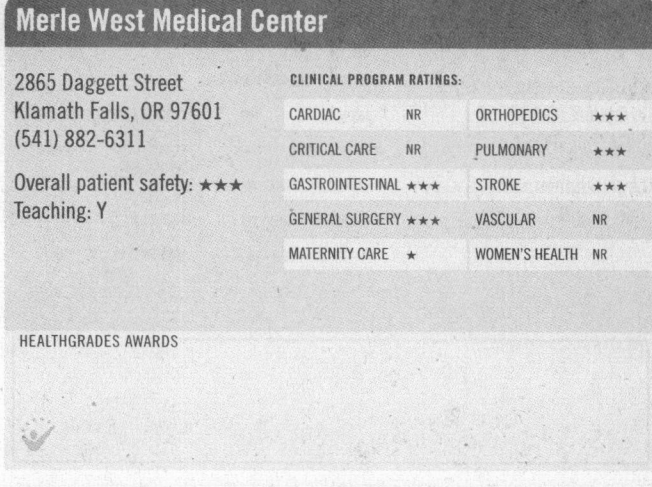

Merle West Medical Center

2865 Daggett Street
Klamath Falls, OR 97601
(541) 882-6311

Overall patient safety: ★★★
Teaching: Y

CLINICAL PROGRAM RATINGS:

CARDIAC	NR	ORTHOPEDICS	★★★
CRITICAL CARE	NR	PULMONARY	★★★
GASTROINTESTINAL	★★★	STROKE	★★★
GENERAL SURGERY	★★★	VASCULAR	NR
MATERNITY CARE	★	WOMEN'S HEALTH	NR

HEALTHGRADES AWARDS

McKenzie-Willamette Medical Center

1460 G Street
Springfield, OR 97477
(541) 726-4400

Overall patient safety: ★★★
Teaching: N

CLINICAL PROGRAM RATINGS:

CARDIAC	NR	ORTHOPEDICS	★★★
CRITICAL CARE	NR	PULMONARY	★★★
GASTROINTESTINAL	★★★	STROKE	★★★
GENERAL SURGERY	★★★	VASCULAR	NR
MATERNITY CARE	★★★	WOMEN'S HEALTH	NR

HEALTHGRADES AWARDS

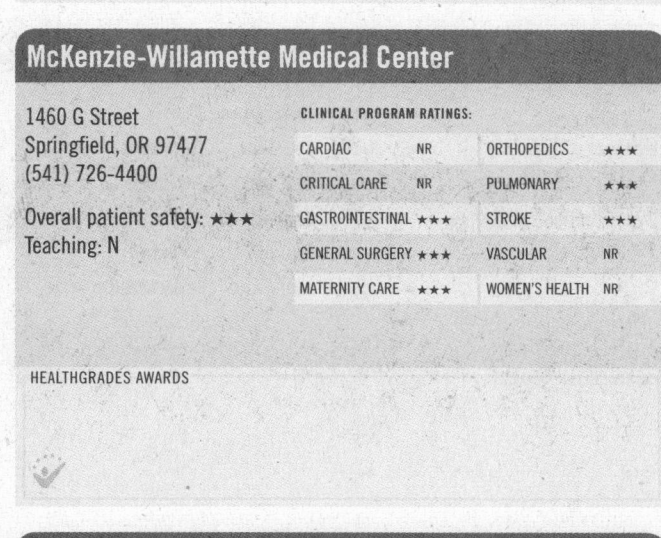

Mid-Columbia Medical Center

1700 East 19th Street
The Dalles, OR 97058
(541) 296-1111

Overall patient safety: ★
Teaching: N

CLINICAL PROGRAM RATINGS:

CARDIAC	NR	ORTHOPEDICS	NR
CRITICAL CARE	NR	PULMONARY	★★★
GASTROINTESTINAL	NR	STROKE	★★★
GENERAL SURGERY	★★★	VASCULAR	NR
MATERNITY CARE	★★★	WOMEN'S HEALTH	NR

HEALTHGRADES AWARDS

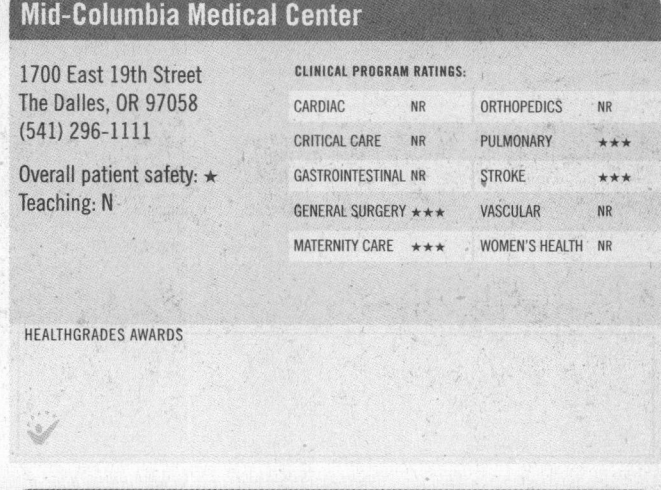

Mercy Medical Center

2700 Stewart Parkway
Roseburg, OR 97470
(541) 673-0611

Overall patient safety: ★★★
Teaching: N

CLINICAL PROGRAM RATINGS:

CARDIAC	NR	ORTHOPEDICS	★★★
CRITICAL CARE	★★★★★	PULMONARY	★★★★★
GASTROINTESTINAL	★★★	STROKE	★★★
GENERAL SURGERY	★★★	VASCULAR	NR
MATERNITY CARE	★★★★★	WOMEN'S HEALTH	NR

HEALTHGRADES AWARDS

✓ **DISTINGUISHED HOSPITAL**
· CLINICAL EXCELLENCE

✓ **SPECIALTY EXCELLENCE**
· CRITICAL CARE
· GASTROINTESTINAL CARE
· GENERAL SURGERY
· PULMONARY CARE

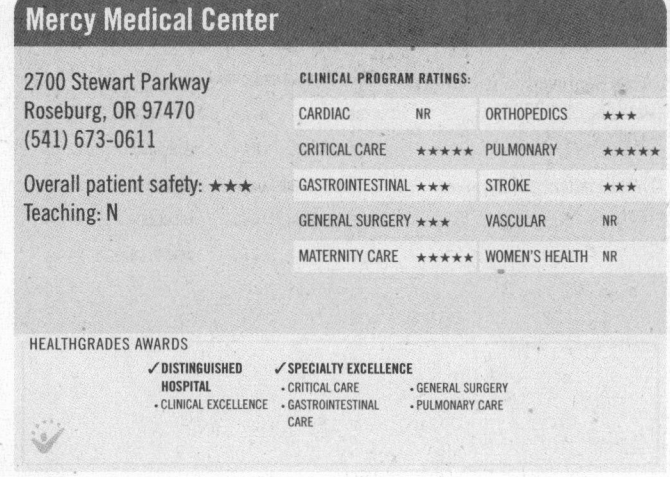

OHSU Hospital

3181 Southwest Sam
Jackson Park Road
Portland, OR 97239
(503) 494-8311

Overall patient safety: ★
Teaching: Y

CLINICAL PROGRAM RATINGS:

CARDIAC	★★★	ORTHOPEDICS	★
CRITICAL CARE	NR	PULMONARY	★★★
GASTROINTESTINAL	NR	STROKE	★★★★★
GENERAL SURGERY	★★★	VASCULAR	★★★
MATERNITY CARE	★	WOMEN'S HEALTH	★★★

HEALTHGRADES AWARDS

Pioneer Memorial Hospital

1201 Northeast Elm Street
Prineville, OR 97754
(541) 447-6254

Overall patient safety: ★★★
Teaching: N

CLINICAL PROGRAM RATINGS:

CARDIAC	NR	ORTHOPEDICS	NR
CRITICAL CARE	NR	PULMONARY	★★★
GASTROINTESTINAL	NR	STROKE	NR
GENERAL SURGERY	NR	VASCULAR	NR
MATERNITY CARE	★★★	WOMEN'S HEALTH	NR

HEALTHGRADES AWARDS

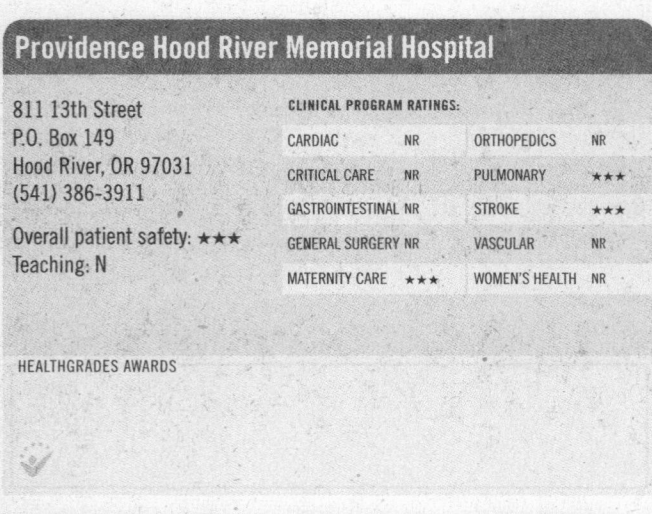

Providence Milwaukie Hospital

10150 Southeast 32nd Avenue
Milwaukie, OR 97222
(503) 513-8300

Overall patient safety: ★★★
Teaching: Y

CLINICAL PROGRAM RATINGS:

CARDIAC	NR	ORTHOPEDICS	NR
CRITICAL CARE	NR	PULMONARY	★★★
GASTROINTESTINAL	NR	STROKE	★★★
GENERAL SURGERY	NR	VASCULAR	NR
MATERNITY CARE	★★★	WOMEN'S HEALTH	NR

HEALTHGRADES AWARDS

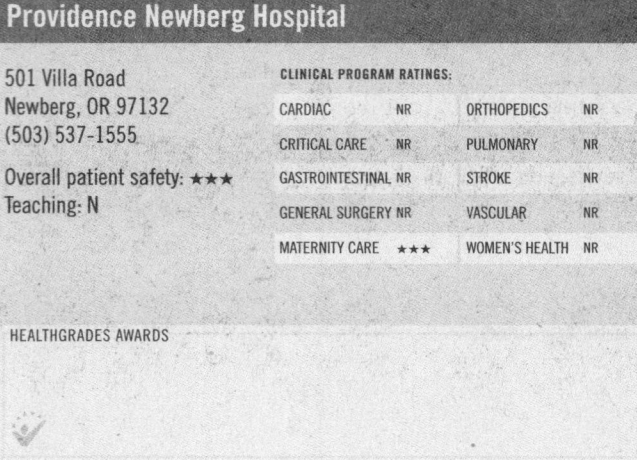

Providence Hood River Memorial Hospital

811 13th Street
P.O. Box 149
Hood River, OR 97031
(541) 386-3911

Overall patient safety: ★★★
Teaching: N

CLINICAL PROGRAM RATINGS:

CARDIAC	NR	ORTHOPEDICS	NR
CRITICAL CARE	NR	PULMONARY	★★★
GASTROINTESTINAL	NR	STROKE	★★★
GENERAL SURGERY	NR	VASCULAR	NR
MATERNITY CARE	★★★	WOMEN'S HEALTH	NR

HEALTHGRADES AWARDS

Providence Newberg Hospital

501 Villa Road
Newberg, OR 97132
(503) 537-1555

Overall patient safety: ★★★
Teaching: N

CLINICAL PROGRAM RATINGS:

CARDIAC	NR	ORTHOPEDICS	NR
CRITICAL CARE	NR	PULMONARY	NR
GASTROINTESTINAL	NR	STROKE	NR
GENERAL SURGERY	NR	VASCULAR	NR
MATERNITY CARE	★★★	WOMEN'S HEALTH	NR

HEALTHGRADES AWARDS

Providence Medford Medical Center

1111 Crater Lake Avenue
Medford, OR 97504
(541) 732-5000

Overall patient safety: ★★★★★
Teaching: N

CLINICAL PROGRAM RATINGS:

CARDIAC	NR	ORTHOPEDICS	NR
CRITICAL CARE	★★★	PULMONARY	★★★
GASTROINTESTINAL	★★★	STROKE	★
GENERAL SURGERY	★★★	VASCULAR	NR
MATERNITY CARE	★★★	WOMEN'S HEALTH	NR

HEALTHGRADES AWARDS
✓ DISTINGUISHED
  HOSPITAL
- PATIENT SAFETY

Providence Portland Medical Center

4805 Northeast Glisan Street
Portland, OR 97213
(503) 215-1111

Overall patient safety: ★★★
Teaching: Y

CLINICAL PROGRAM RATINGS:

CARDIAC	★★★	ORTHOPEDICS	★★★
CRITICAL CARE	★★★	PULMONARY	★★★
GASTROINTESTINAL	★★★	STROKE	★★★
GENERAL SURGERY	★★★	VASCULAR	★★★
MATERNITY CARE	★★★	WOMEN'S HEALTH	★★★

HEALTHGRADES AWARDS

KEY: ★★★★★ BEST   ★★★ AS EXPECTED   ★ POOR   NR NOT RATED BY HEALTHGRADES   For full definitions of ratings and awards, see Appendix.

Providence Seaside Hospital

725 South Wahanna Road
Seaside, OR 97138
(503) 717-7000

Overall patient safety: ★
Teaching: N

CLINICAL PROGRAM RATINGS:

CARDIAC	NR	ORTHOPEDICS	NR
CRITICAL CARE	NR	PULMONARY	★★★
GASTROINTESTINAL	NR	STROKE	★★★
GENERAL SURGERY	NR	VASCULAR	NR
MATERNITY CARE	★★★	WOMEN'S HEALTH	NR

HEALTHGRADES AWARDS

Sacred Heart Medical Center—University District

1255 Hilyard Street
Eugene, OR 97401
(541) 686-7300

Overall patient safety: ★★★
Teaching: N

CLINICAL PROGRAM RATINGS:

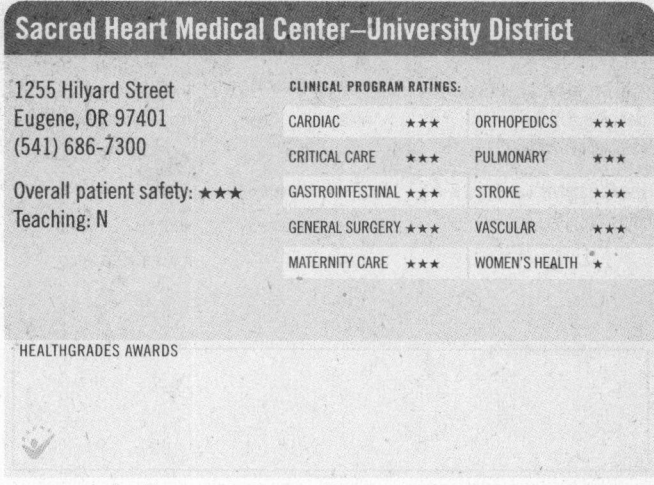

CARDIAC	★★★	ORTHOPEDICS	★★★
CRITICAL CARE	★★★	PULMONARY	★★★
GASTROINTESTINAL	★★★	STROKE	★★★
GENERAL SURGERY	★★★	VASCULAR	★★★
MATERNITY CARE	★★★	WOMEN'S HEALTH	★

HEALTHGRADES AWARDS

Providence St. Vincent Medical Center

9205 Southwest Barnes Road
Portland, OR 97225
(503) 216-1234

Overall patient safety: ★★★★★
Teaching: Y

CLINICAL PROGRAM RATINGS:

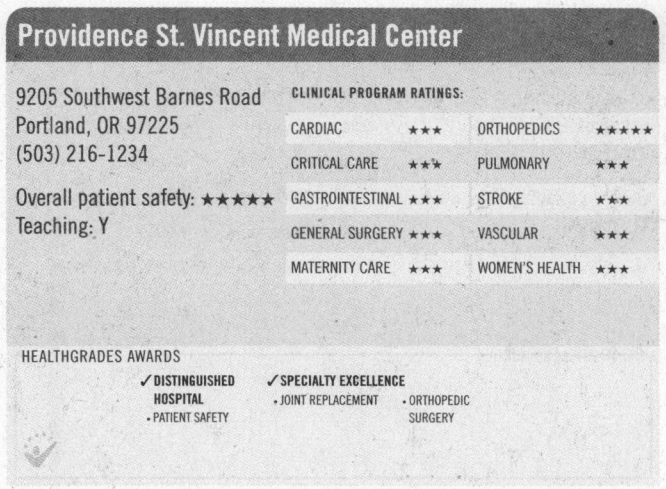

CARDIAC	★★★	ORTHOPEDICS	★★★★★
CRITICAL CARE	★★★	PULMONARY	★★★
GASTROINTESTINAL	★★★	STROKE	★★★
GENERAL SURGERY	★★★	VASCULAR	★★★
MATERNITY CARE	★★★	WOMEN'S HEALTH	★★★

HEALTHGRADES AWARDS

✓ DISTINGUISHED HOSPITAL
- PATIENT SAFETY

✓ SPECIALTY EXCELLENCE
- JOINT REPLACEMENT
- ORTHOPEDIC SURGERY

St. Anthony Hospital

1601 Southeast Court Avenue
Pendleton, OR 97801
(541) 276-5121

Overall patient safety: ★★★
Teaching: N

CLINICAL PROGRAM RATINGS:

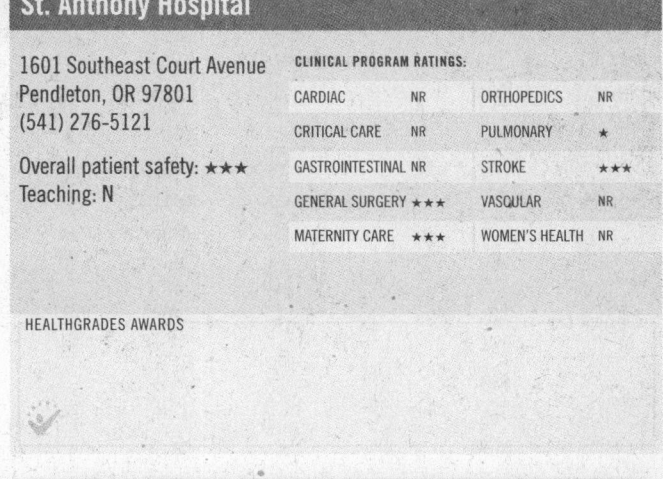

CARDIAC	NR	ORTHOPEDICS	NR
CRITICAL CARE	NR	PULMONARY	★
GASTROINTESTINAL	NR	STROKE	★★★
GENERAL SURGERY	★★★	VASCULAR	NR
MATERNITY CARE	★★★	WOMEN'S HEALTH	NR

HEALTHGRADES AWARDS

Rogue Valley Medical Center

2825 Barnett Road East
Medford, OR 97504
(541) 789-7000

Overall patient safety: ★★★★★
Teaching: N

CLINICAL PROGRAM RATINGS:

CARDIAC	★★★	ORTHOPEDICS	★★★
CRITICAL CARE	★★★	PULMONARY	★★★
GASTROINTESTINAL	★★★	STROKE	★★★
GENERAL SURGERY	★★★	VASCULAR	★★★
MATERNITY CARE	★★★	WOMEN'S HEALTH	★

HEALTHGRADES AWARDS

✓ DISTINGUISHED HOSPITAL
- PATIENT SAFETY

St. Charles Medical Center—Bend

2500 Northeast Neff Road
Bend, OR 97701
(541) 382-4321

Overall patient safety: ★★★
Teaching: Y

CLINICAL PROGRAM RATINGS:

CARDIAC	★★★	ORTHOPEDICS	★★★★★
CRITICAL CARE	NR	PULMONARY	★★★
GASTROINTESTINAL	★★★	STROKE	★★★
GENERAL SURGERY	★★★	VASCULAR	NR
MATERNITY CARE	★★★	WOMEN'S HEALTH	★★★

HEALTHGRADES AWARDS

✓ DISTINGUISHED HOSPITAL
- PATIENT SAFETY

St. Charles Medical Center--Redmond

1253 North Canal Boulevard
Redmond, OR 97756
(541) 548-8131

Overall patient safety: ★★★
Teaching: N

CLINICAL PROGRAM RATINGS:

CARDIAC	NR	ORTHOPEDICS	NR
CRITICAL CARE	NR	PULMONARY	★★★
GASTROINTESTINAL	NR	STROKE	★★★
GENERAL SURGERY	NR	VASCULAR	NR
MATERNITY CARE	★	WOMEN'S HEALTH	NR

HEALTHGRADES AWARDS

Samaritan Albany General Hospital

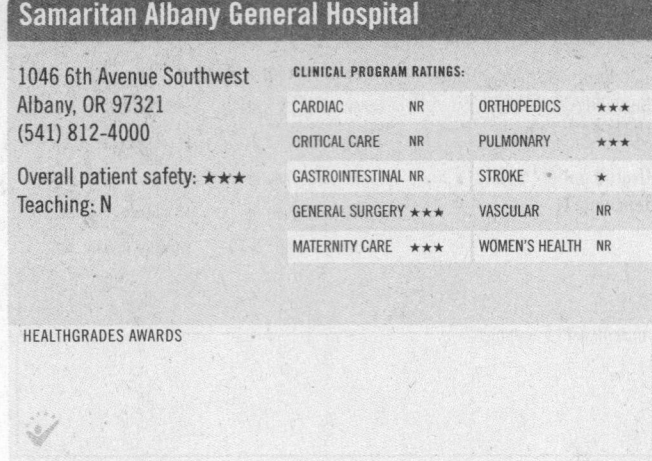

1046 6th Avenue Southwest
Albany, OR 97321
(541) 812-4000

Overall patient safety: ★★★
Teaching: N

CLINICAL PROGRAM RATINGS:

CARDIAC	NR	ORTHOPEDICS	★★★
CRITICAL CARE	NR	PULMONARY	★★★
GASTROINTESTINAL	NR	STROKE	★
GENERAL SURGERY	★★★	VASCULAR	NR
MATERNITY CARE	★★★	WOMEN'S HEALTH	NR

HEALTHGRADES AWARDS

St. Elizabeth Health Services

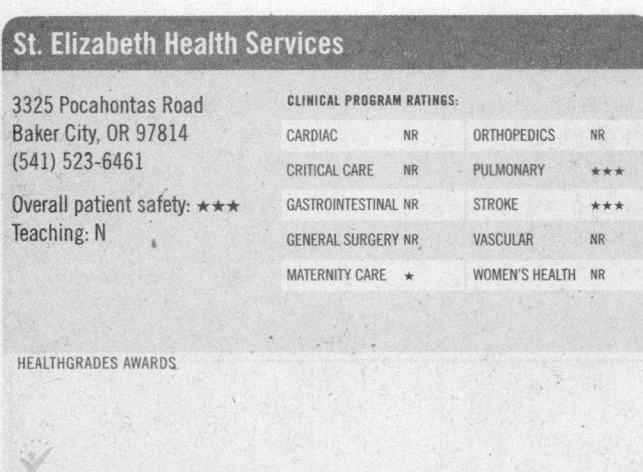

3325 Pocahontas Road
Baker City, OR 97814
(541) 523-6461

Overall patient safety: ★★★
Teaching: N

CLINICAL PROGRAM RATINGS:

CARDIAC	NR	ORTHOPEDICS	NR
CRITICAL CARE	NR	PULMONARY	★★★
GASTROINTESTINAL	NR	STROKE	★★★
GENERAL SURGERY	NR	VASCULAR	NR
MATERNITY CARE	★	WOMEN'S HEALTH	NR

HEALTHGRADES AWARDS

Samaritan Lebanon Community Hospital

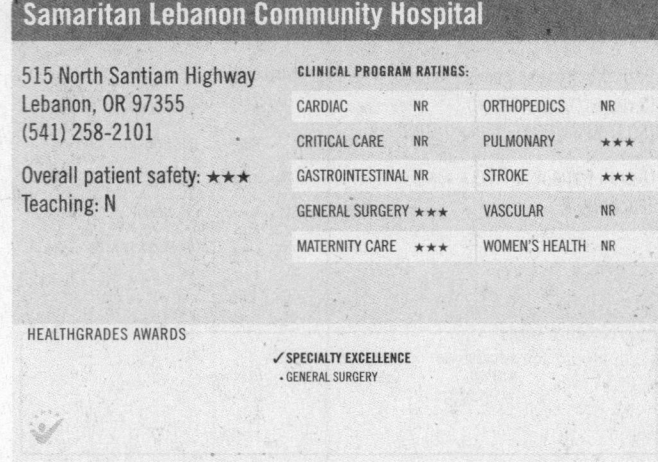

515 North Santiam Highway
Lebanon, OR 97355
(541) 258-2101

Overall patient safety: ★★★
Teaching: N

CLINICAL PROGRAM RATINGS:

CARDIAC	NR	ORTHOPEDICS	NR
CRITICAL CARE	NR	PULMONARY	★★★
GASTROINTESTINAL	NR	STROKE	★★★
GENERAL SURGERY	★★★	VASCULAR	NR
MATERNITY CARE	★★★	WOMEN'S HEALTH	NR

HEALTHGRADES AWARDS

✓ SPECIALTY EXCELLENCE
- GENERAL SURGERY

Salem Hospital

665 Winter Street Southeast
Salem, OR 97301
(503) 561-5200

Overall patient safety: ★★★
Teaching: N

CLINICAL PROGRAM RATINGS:

CARDIAC	★★★	ORTHOPEDICS	★★★
CRITICAL CARE	★	PULMONARY	★
GASTROINTESTINAL	★★★	STROKE	★★★
GENERAL SURGERY	★★★	VASCULAR	NR
MATERNITY CARE	★★★	WOMEN'S HEALTH	★

HEALTHGRADES AWARDS

Samaritan North Lincoln Hospital

3043 Northeast 28th Street
Lincoln City, OR 97367
(541) 994-3661

Overall patient safety: ★★★
Teaching: N

CLINICAL PROGRAM RATINGS:

CARDIAC	NR	ORTHOPEDICS	NR
CRITICAL CARE	NR	PULMONARY	★★★
GASTROINTESTINAL	NR	STROKE	★★★
GENERAL SURGERY	NR	VASCULAR	NR
MATERNITY CARE	★	WOMEN'S HEALTH	NR

HEALTHGRADES AWARDS

KEY: ★★★★★ BEST   ★★★ AS EXPECTED   ★ POOR   NR NOT RATED BY HEALTHGRADES   For full definitions of ratings and awards, see Appendix.

Samaritan Pacific Community Hospital

930 Southwest Abbey Street
Newport, OR 97365
(541) 265-2244

Overall patient safety: ★★★
Teaching: N

CLINICAL PROGRAM RATINGS:

CARDIAC	NR	ORTHOPEDICS	NR
CRITICAL CARE	NR	PULMONARY	★
GASTROINTESTINAL	NR	STROKE	★
GENERAL SURGERY	NR	VASCULAR	NR
MATERNITY CARE	★★★	WOMEN'S HEALTH	NR

HEALTHGRADES AWARDS

Three Rivers Community Hospital*

500 Southwest Ramsey Avenue
Grants Pass, OR 97527
(541) 472-7000

Overall patient safety: ★★★
Teaching: Y

CLINICAL PROGRAM RATINGS:

CARDIAC	NR	ORTHOPEDICS	NR
CRITICAL CARE	NR	PULMONARY	★★★
GASTROINTESTINAL	★★★	STROKE	★
GENERAL SURGERY	★★★	VASCULAR	NR
MATERNITY CARE	★	WOMEN'S HEALTH	NR

HEALTHGRADES AWARDS

Santiam Memorial Hospital

1401 North 10th Avenue
Stayton, OR 97383
(503) 769-2175

Overall patient safety: ★★★
Teaching: N

CLINICAL PROGRAM RATINGS:

CARDIAC	NR	ORTHOPEDICS	NR
CRITICAL CARE	NR	PULMONARY	★
GASTROINTESTINAL	NR	STROKE	NR
GENERAL SURGERY	NR	VASCULAR	NR
MATERNITY CARE	★★★	WOMEN'S HEALTH	NR

HEALTHGRADES AWARDS

Three Rivers Community Hospital Washington Output Ctr.*

1505 Northwest Washington
Boulevard
Grants Pass, OR 97526
(541) 479-7531

Overall patient safety: ★★★
Teaching: Y

CLINICAL PROGRAM RATINGS:

CARDIAC	NR	ORTHOPEDICS	NR
CRITICAL CARE	NR	PULMONARY	★★★
GASTROINTESTINAL	★★★	STROKE	★
GENERAL SURGERY	★★★	VASCULAR	NR
MATERNITY CARE	★	WOMEN'S HEALTH	NR

HEALTHGRADES AWARDS

Silverton Hospital

342 Fairview Street
Silverton, OR 97381
(503) 873-1500

Overall patient safety: ★★★
Teaching: N

CLINICAL PROGRAM RATINGS:

CARDIAC	NR	ORTHOPEDICS	NR
CRITICAL CARE	NR	PULMONARY	NR
GASTROINTESTINAL	NR	STROKE	★
GENERAL SURGERY	NR	VASCULAR	NR
MATERNITY CARE	★★★	WOMEN'S HEALTH	NR

HEALTHGRADES AWARDS

Tillamook County General Hospital

1000 3rd Street
Tillamook, OR 97141
(503) 815-2260

Overall patient safety: ★★★
Teaching: N

CLINICAL PROGRAM RATINGS:

CARDIAC	NR	ORTHOPEDICS	NR
CRITICAL CARE	NR	PULMONARY	★
GASTROINTESTINAL	NR	STROKE	★
GENERAL SURGERY	★★★	VASCULAR	NR
MATERNITY CARE	★★★	WOMEN'S HEALTH	NR

HEALTHGRADES AWARDS

*This hospital reports its data to the federal government jointly with another hospital. Therefore the ratings and awards apply to multiple hospitals and this specific hospital may not provide all rated services.

Tuality Community Hospital*

335 Southeast 8th Street
Hillsboro, OR 97123
(503) 681-1111

Overall patient safety: ★★★
Teaching: N

CLINICAL PROGRAM RATINGS:

CARDIAC	★★★	ORTHOPEDICS	★★★
CRITICAL CARE	NR	PULMONARY	★
GASTROINTESTINAL	NR	STROKE	★
GENERAL SURGERY	★★★	VASCULAR	NR
MATERNITY CARE	★★★	WOMEN'S HEALTH	★★★

HEALTHGRADES AWARDS

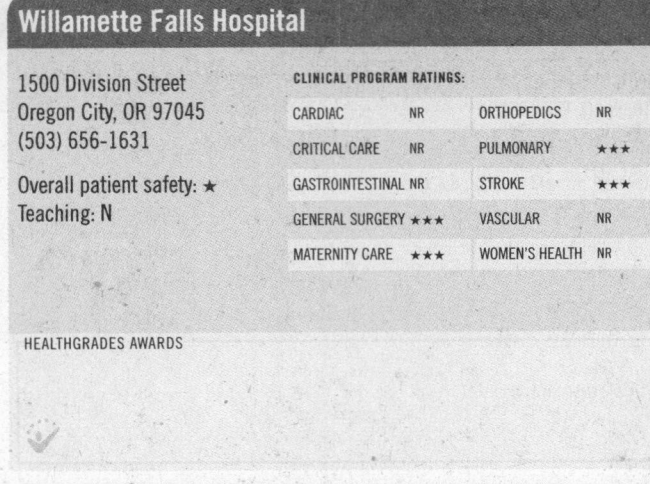

Willamette Falls Hospital

1500 Division Street
Oregon City, OR 97045
(503) 656-1631

Overall patient safety: ★
Teaching: N

CLINICAL PROGRAM RATINGS:

CARDIAC	NR	ORTHOPEDICS	NR
CRITICAL CARE	NR	PULMONARY	★★★
GASTROINTESTINAL	NR	STROKE	★★★
GENERAL SURGERY	★★★	VASCULAR	NR
MATERNITY CARE	★★★	WOMEN'S HEALTH	NR

HEALTHGRADES AWARDS

Tuality Forest Grove Hospital*

1809 Maple Street
Forest Grove, OR 97116
(503) 357-2173

Overall patient safety: ★★★
Teaching: N

CLINICAL PROGRAM RATINGS:

CARDIAC	★★★	ORTHOPEDICS	★★★
CRITICAL CARE	NR	PULMONARY	★
GASTROINTESTINAL	NR	STROKE	★
GENERAL SURGERY	★★★	VASCULAR	NR
MATERNITY CARE	★★★	WOMEN'S HEALTH	★★★

HEALTHGRADES AWARDS

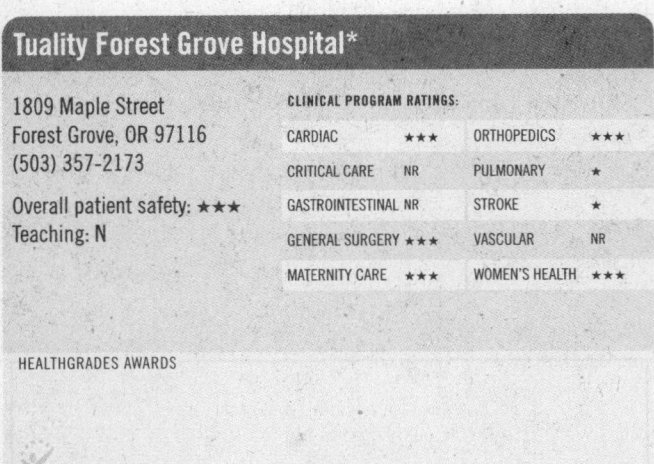

Willamette Valley Medical Center

2700 Southeast Stratus Avenue
McMinnville, OR 97128
(503) 472-6131

Overall patient safety: ★★★
Teaching: N

CLINICAL PROGRAM RATINGS:

CARDIAC	NR	ORTHOPEDICS	NR
CRITICAL CARE	NR	PULMONARY	★★★
GASTROINTESTINAL	NR	STROKE	★★★
GENERAL SURGERY	★★★	VASCULAR	NR
MATERNITY CARE	★★★	WOMEN'S HEALTH	NR

HEALTHGRADES AWARDS

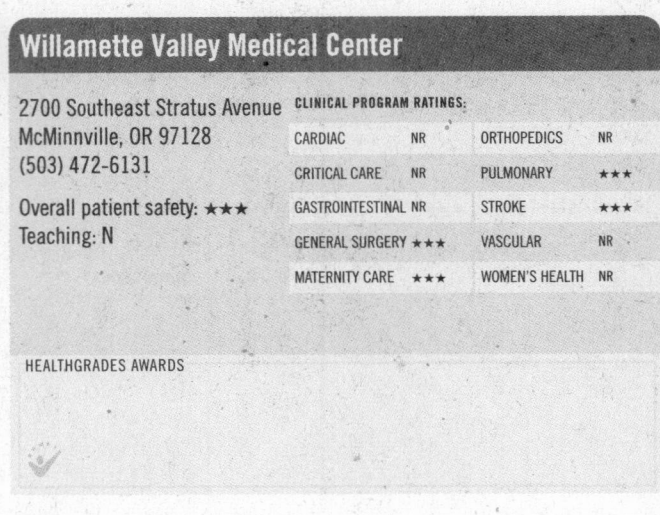

Wallowa Memorial Hospital

601 Medical Parkway
Enterprise, OR 97828
(541) 426-3111

Overall patient safety: ★★★
Teaching: N

CLINICAL PROGRAM RATINGS:

CARDIAC	NR	ORTHOPEDICS	NR
CRITICAL CARE	NR	PULMONARY	★★★
GASTROINTESTINAL	NR	STROKE	NR
GENERAL SURGERY	NR	VASCULAR	NR
MATERNITY CARE	★★★	WOMEN'S HEALTH	NR

HEALTHGRADES AWARDS

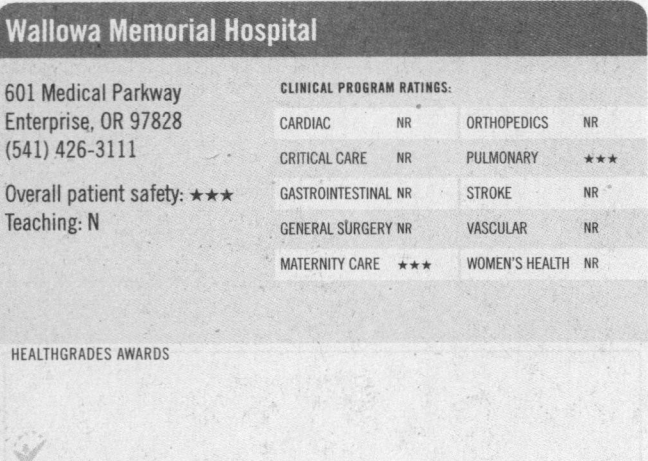

KEY: ★★★★★ BEST ★★★ AS EXPECTED ★ POOR NR NOT RATED BY HEALTHGRADES For full definitions of ratings and awards, see Appendix.

Abington Memorial Hospital

1200 Old York Road
Abington, PA 19001
(215) 481-2000

Overall patient safety: ★★★
Teaching: Y

CLINICAL PROGRAM RATINGS:			
CARDIAC	★★★	ORTHOPEDICS	★★★
CRITICAL CARE	NR	PULMONARY	★★★
GASTROINTESTINAL	★★★	STROKE	★★★
GENERAL SURGERY	★★★★★	VASCULAR	★★★
MATERNITY CARE	★★★	WOMEN'S HEALTH	★★★

HEALTHGRADES AWARDS

✓ SPECIALTY EXCELLENCE
· GASTROINTESTINAL   · GENERAL SURGERY
  CARE

Aliquippa Community Hospital

2500 Hospital Drive
Aliquippa, PA 15001
(724) 857-1212

Overall patient safety: ★★★
Teaching: N

CLINICAL PROGRAM RATINGS:			
CARDIAC	NR	ORTHOPEDICS	NR
CRITICAL CARE	NR	PULMONARY	★★★
GASTROINTESTINAL	NR	STROKE	NR
GENERAL SURGERY	NR	VASCULAR	NR
MATERNITY CARE	NR	WOMEN'S HEALTH	NR

HEALTHGRADES AWARDS

ACMH Hospital

1 Nolte Drive
Kittanning, PA 16201
(724) 543-8500

Overall patient safety: ★★★
Teaching: N

CLINICAL PROGRAM RATINGS:			
CARDIAC	NR	ORTHOPEDICS	NR
CRITICAL CARE	NR	PULMONARY	★
GASTROINTESTINAL	NR	STROKE	★
GENERAL SURGERY	★★★	VASCULAR	NR
MATERNITY CARE	★	WOMEN'S HEALTH	NR

HEALTHGRADES AWARDS

Alle Kiski Medical Center

1301 Carlisle Street
Natrona Heights, PA 15065
(724) 224-5100

Overall patient safety: ★★★
Teaching: N

CLINICAL PROGRAM RATINGS:			
CARDIAC	NR	ORTHOPEDICS	★★★
CRITICAL CARE	NR	PULMONARY	★★★★★
GASTROINTESTINAL	★★★	STROKE	★★★
GENERAL SURGERY	★★★	VASCULAR	NR
MATERNITY CARE	★★★	WOMEN'S HEALTH	NR

HEALTHGRADES AWARDS

✓ DISTINGUISHED   ✓ SPECIALTY EXCELLENCE
  HOSPITAL   · PULMONARY CARE
· CLINICAL EXCELLENCE

Albert Einstein Medical Center

5501 Old York Road
Philadelphia, PA 19141
(215) 456-7890

Overall patient safety: ★
Teaching: Y

CLINICAL PROGRAM RATINGS:			
CARDIAC	★★★	ORTHOPEDICS	★★★
CRITICAL CARE	NR	PULMONARY	★★★★★
GASTROINTESTINAL	★★★	STROKE	★★★
GENERAL SURGERY	★★★	VASCULAR	NR
MATERNITY CARE	★★★	WOMEN'S HEALTH	★★★

HEALTHGRADES AWARDS

Allegheny General Hospital*

320 East North Avenue
Pittsburgh, PA 15212
(412) 359-3131

Overall patient safety: ★★★
Teaching: Y

CLINICAL PROGRAM RATINGS:			
CARDIAC	★★★	ORTHOPEDICS	★★★
CRITICAL CARE	★★★	PULMONARY	★★★
GASTROINTESTINAL	★★★	STROKE	★★★★★
GENERAL SURGERY	★★★	VASCULAR	★★★
MATERNITY CARE	★★★	WOMEN'S HEALTH	★★★

HEALTHGRADES AWARDS

✓ SPECIALTY EXCELLENCE
· STROKE CARE

*This hospital reports its data to the federal government jointly with another hospital. Therefore the ratings and awards apply to multiple hospitals and this specific hospital may not provide all rated services.

Allegheny General Hospital—Suburban Campus*

100 South Jackson Avenue
Pittsburgh, PA 15202
(412) 734-6000

Overall patient safety: ★★★
Teaching: Y

CLINICAL PROGRAM RATINGS:

CARDIAC	★★★	ORTHOPEDICS	★★★
CRITICAL CARE	★★★	PULMONARY	★★★
GASTROINTESTINAL	★★★	STROKE	★★★★★
GENERAL SURGERY	★★★	VASCULAR	★★★
MATERNITY CARE	★★★	WOMEN'S HEALTH	★★★

HEALTHGRADES AWARDS

✓ SPECIALTY EXCELLENCE
• STROKE CARE

Berwick Hospital Center

701 East 16th Street
Berwick, PA 18603
(570) 759-5000

Overall patient safety: ★★★
Teaching: N

CLINICAL PROGRAM RATINGS:

CARDIAC	NR	ORTHOPEDICS	NR
CRITICAL CARE	NR	PULMONARY	★★★
GASTROINTESTINAL	NR	STROKE	★★★
GENERAL SURGERY	★★★★★	VASCULAR	NR
MATERNITY CARE	★★★	WOMEN'S HEALTH	NR

HEALTHGRADES AWARDS

✓ SPECIALTY EXCELLENCE
• GENERAL SURGERY

Altoona Hospital*

620 Howard Avenue
Altoona, PA 16601
(814) 889-2011

Overall patient safety: ★★★
Teaching: Y

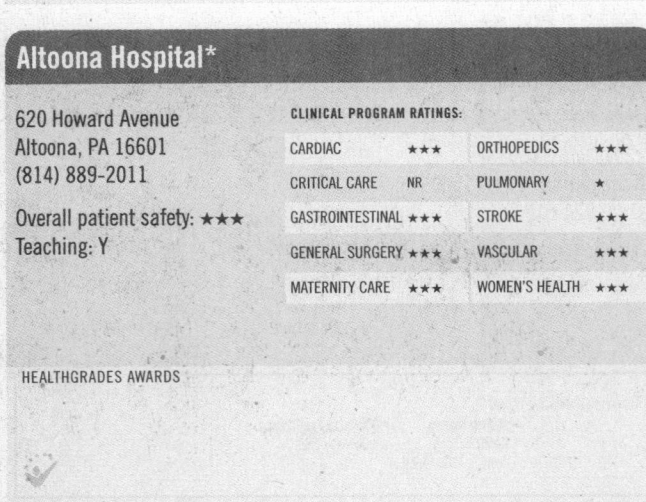

CLINICAL PROGRAM RATINGS:

CARDIAC	★★★	ORTHOPEDICS	★★★
CRITICAL CARE	NR	PULMONARY	★
GASTROINTESTINAL	★★★	STROKE	★★★
GENERAL SURGERY	★★★	VASCULAR	★★★
MATERNITY CARE	★★★	WOMEN'S HEALTH	★★★

HEALTHGRADES AWARDS

Bloomsburg Hospital

549 East Fair Street
Bloomsburg, PA 17815
(570) 387-2100

Overall patient safety: ★★★
Teaching: N

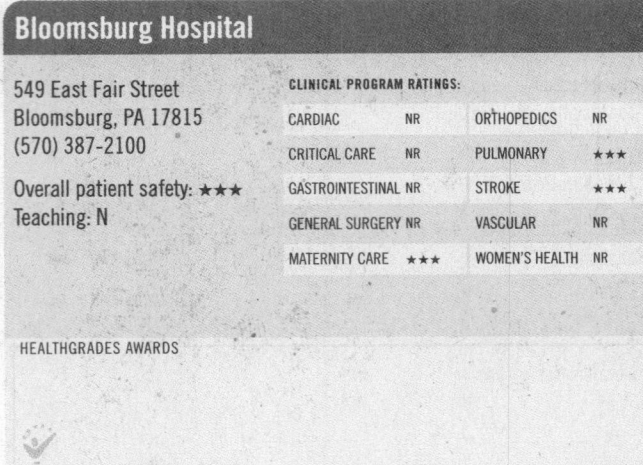

CLINICAL PROGRAM RATINGS:

CARDIAC	NR	ORTHOPEDICS	NR
CRITICAL CARE	NR	PULMONARY	★★★
GASTROINTESTINAL	NR	STROKE	★★★
GENERAL SURGERY	NR	VASCULAR	NR
MATERNITY CARE	★★★	WOMEN'S HEALTH	NR

HEALTHGRADES AWARDS

Barnes-Kasson County Hospital

400 Turnpike Street
Susquehanna, PA 18847
(570) 853-3135

Overall patient safety: ★★★
Teaching: N

CLINICAL PROGRAM RATINGS:

CARDIAC	NR	ORTHOPEDICS	NR
CRITICAL CARE	NR	PULMONARY	★★★
GASTROINTESTINAL	NR	STROKE	NR
GENERAL SURGERY	NR	VASCULAR	NR
MATERNITY CARE	★★★	WOMEN'S HEALTH	NR

HEALTHGRADES AWARDS

Bon Secours Mercy Hospital*

2500 7th Avenue
Altoona, PA 16602
(814) 944-1681

Overall patient safety: ★★★
Teaching: Y

CLINICAL PROGRAM RATINGS:

CARDIAC	★★★	ORTHOPEDICS	★★★
CRITICAL CARE	NR	PULMONARY	★
GASTROINTESTINAL	★★★	STROKE	★★★
GENERAL SURGERY	★★★	VASCULAR	★★★
MATERNITY CARE	★★★	WOMEN'S HEALTH	★★★

HEALTHGRADES AWARDS

KEY: ★★★★★ BEST   ★★★ AS EXPECTED   ★ POOR   NR NOT RATED BY HEALTHGRADES   For full definitions of ratings and awards, see Appendix.

Bradford Regional Medical Center

116 Interstate Parkway
Bradford, PA 16701
(814) 368-4143

Overall patient safety: ★★★
Teaching: N

CLINICAL PROGRAM RATINGS:

CARDIAC	NR	ORTHOPEDICS	NR
CRITICAL CARE	NR	PULMONARY	★
GASTROINTESTINAL	NR	STROKE	★★★
GENERAL SURGERY	NR	VASCULAR	NR
MATERNITY CARE	★★★	WOMEN'S HEALTH	NR

HEALTHGRADES AWARDS

Butler Memorial Hospital

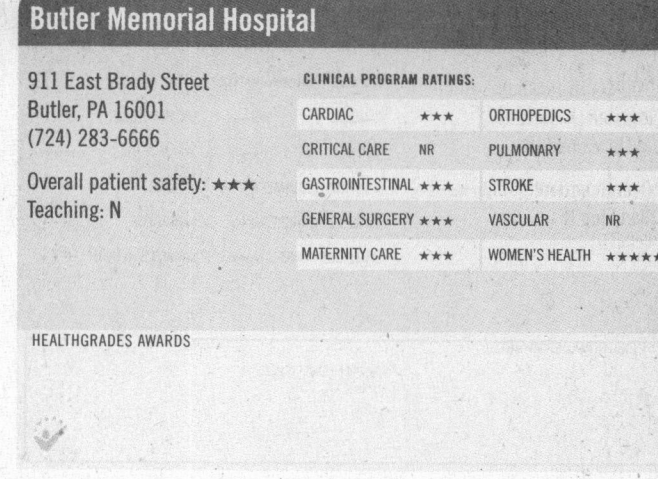

911 East Brady Street
Butler, PA 16001
(724) 283-6666

Overall patient safety: ★★★
Teaching: N

CLINICAL PROGRAM RATINGS:

CARDIAC	★★★	ORTHOPEDICS	★★★
CRITICAL CARE	NR	PULMONARY	★★★
GASTROINTESTINAL	★★★	STROKE	★★★
GENERAL SURGERY	★★★	VASCULAR	NR
MATERNITY CARE	★★★	WOMEN'S HEALTH	★★★★★

HEALTHGRADES AWARDS

Brandywine Hospital

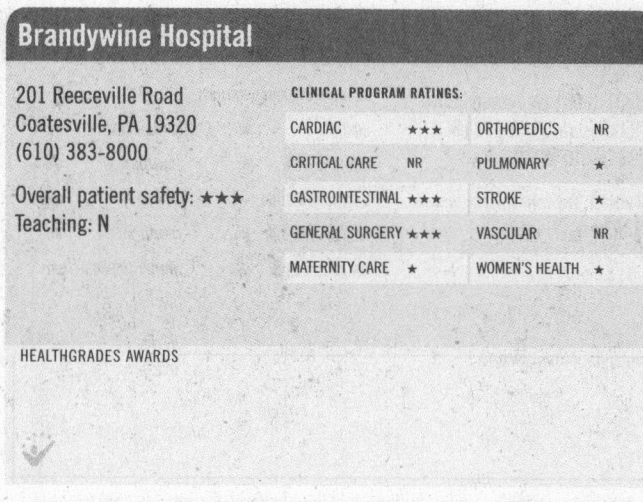

201 Reecceville Road
Coatesville, PA 19320
(610) 383-8000

Overall patient safety: ★★★
Teaching: N

CLINICAL PROGRAM RATINGS:

CARDIAC	★★★	ORTHOPEDICS	NR
CRITICAL CARE	NR	PULMONARY	★
GASTROINTESTINAL	★★★	STROKE	★
GENERAL SURGERY	★★★	VASCULAR	NR
MATERNITY CARE	★	WOMEN'S HEALTH	★

HEALTHGRADES AWARDS

Canonsburg General Hospital

100 Medical Boulevard
Canonsburg, PA 15317
(724) 745-6100

Overall patient safety: ★★★
Teaching: N

CLINICAL PROGRAM RATINGS:

CARDIAC	NR	ORTHOPEDICS	NR
CRITICAL CARE	NR	PULMONARY	★★★
GASTROINTESTINAL	NR	STROKE	★★★
GENERAL SURGERY	★★★	VASCULAR	NR
MATERNITY CARE	NR	WOMEN'S HEALTH	NR

HEALTHGRADES AWARDS

Brookville Hospital

100 Hospital Road
Brookville, PA 15825
(814) 849-1461

Overall patient safety: ★★★★★
Teaching: N

CLINICAL PROGRAM RATINGS:

CARDIAC	NR	ORTHOPEDICS	NR
CRITICAL CARE	NR	PULMONARY	★★★
GASTROINTESTINAL	NR	STROKE	★★★
GENERAL SURGERY	★★★	VASCULAR	NR
MATERNITY CARE	NR	WOMEN'S HEALTH	NR

HEALTHGRADES AWARDS

Carlisle Regional Medical Center

246 Parker Street
Carlisle, PA 17013
(717) 249-1212

Overall patient safety: ★★★
Teaching: N

CLINICAL PROGRAM RATINGS:

CARDIAC	NR	ORTHOPEDICS	★★★
CRITICAL CARE	NR	PULMONARY	★
GASTROINTESTINAL	★★★	STROKE	★
GENERAL SURGERY	★★★	VASCULAR	NR
MATERNITY CARE	★★★	WOMEN'S HEALTH	NR

HEALTHGRADES AWARDS

*This hospital reports its data to the federal government jointly with another hospital. Therefore the ratings and awards apply to multiple hospitals and this specific hospital may not provide all rated services.

Central Montgomery Medical Center

100 Medical Campus Drive
Lansdale, PA 19446
(215) 368-2100

Overall patient safety: ★★★
Teaching: N

CLINICAL PROGRAM RATINGS:

CARDIAC	NR	ORTHOPEDICS	NR
CRITICAL CARE	NR	PULMONARY	★★★
GASTROINTESTINAL	NR	STROKE	★★★
GENERAL SURGERY	★★★	VASCULAR	NR
MATERNITY CARE	★★★	WOMEN'S HEALTH	NR

HEALTHGRADES AWARDS

Chester County Hospital

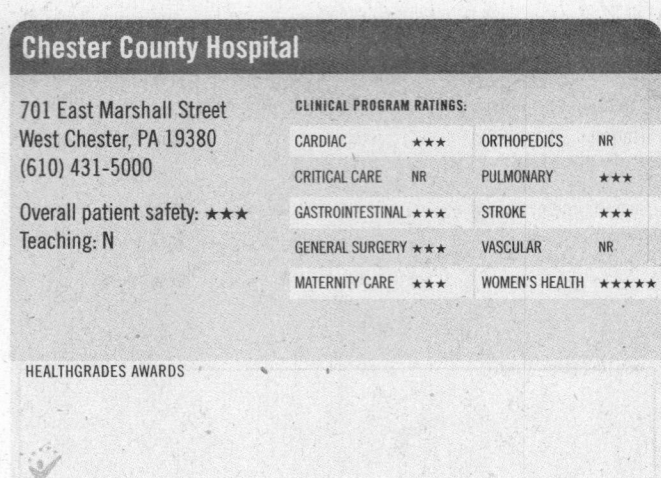

701 East Marshall Street
West Chester, PA 19380
(610) 431-5000

Overall patient safety: ★★★
Teaching: N

CLINICAL PROGRAM RATINGS:

CARDIAC	★★★	ORTHOPEDICS	NR
CRITICAL CARE	NR	PULMONARY	★★★
GASTROINTESTINAL	★★★	STROKE	★★★
GENERAL SURGERY	★★★	VASCULAR	NR
MATERNITY CARE	★★★	WOMEN'S HEALTH	★★★★★

HEALTHGRADES AWARDS

Chambersburg Hospital

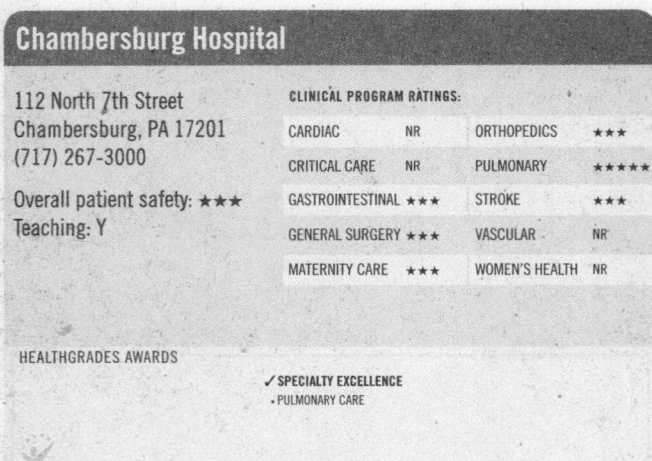

112 North 7th Street
Chambersburg, PA 17201
(717) 267-3000

Overall patient safety: ★★★
Teaching: Y

CLINICAL PROGRAM RATINGS:

CARDIAC	NR	ORTHOPEDICS	★★★
CRITICAL CARE	NR	PULMONARY	★★★★★
GASTROINTESTINAL	★★★	STROKE	★★★
GENERAL SURGERY	★★★	VASCULAR	NR
MATERNITY CARE	★★★	WOMEN'S HEALTH	NR

HEALTHGRADES AWARDS

✓ SPECIALTY EXCELLENCE
• PULMONARY CARE

Chestnut Hill Hospital

8835 Germantown Avenue
Philadelphia, PA 19118
(215) 248-8200

Overall patient safety: ★★★
Teaching: Y

CLINICAL PROGRAM RATINGS:

CARDIAC	NR	ORTHOPEDICS	NR
CRITICAL CARE	NR	PULMONARY	★★★
GASTROINTESTINAL	★★★	STROKE	★★★
GENERAL SURGERY	★★★	VASCULAR	NR
MATERNITY CARE	★★★	WOMEN'S HEALTH	NR

HEALTHGRADES AWARDS

Charles Cole Memorial Hospital

1001 East 2nd Street
Coudersport, PA 16915
(814) 274-9300

Overall patient safety: ★★★
Teaching: N

CLINICAL PROGRAM RATINGS:

CARDIAC	NR	ORTHOPEDICS	NR
CRITICAL CARE	NR	PULMONARY	★★★
GASTROINTESTINAL	NR	STROKE	★
GENERAL SURGERY	★★★	VASCULAR	NR
MATERNITY CARE	★★★	WOMEN'S HEALTH	NR

HEALTHGRADES AWARDS

Clarion Hospital

1 Hospital Drive
Clarion, PA 16214
(814) 226-9500

Overall patient safety: ★★★
Teaching: Y

CLINICAL PROGRAM RATINGS:

CARDIAC	NR	ORTHOPEDICS	NR
CRITICAL CARE	NR	PULMONARY	★
GASTROINTESTINAL	★★★	STROKE	★★★
GENERAL SURGERY	★★★	VASCULAR	NR
MATERNITY CARE	★	WOMEN'S HEALTH	NR

HEALTHGRADES AWARDS

KEY: ★★★★★ BEST ★★★ AS EXPECTED ★ POOR NR NOT RATED BY HEALTHGRADES For full definitions of ratings and awards, see Appendix.

Clearfield Hospital

809 Turnpike Avenue
Clearfield, PA 16830
(814) 765-5341

Overall patient safety: ★★★★★
Teaching: N

CLINICAL PROGRAM RATINGS:

CARDIAC	NR	ORTHOPEDICS	NR
CRITICAL CARE	NR	PULMONARY	★★★
GASTROINTESTINAL	★★★	STROKE	★★★
GENERAL SURGERY	★★★	VASCULAR	NR
MATERNITY CARE	★★★	WOMEN'S HEALTH	NR

HEALTHGRADES AWARDS

Conemaugh Valley Memorial Hospital

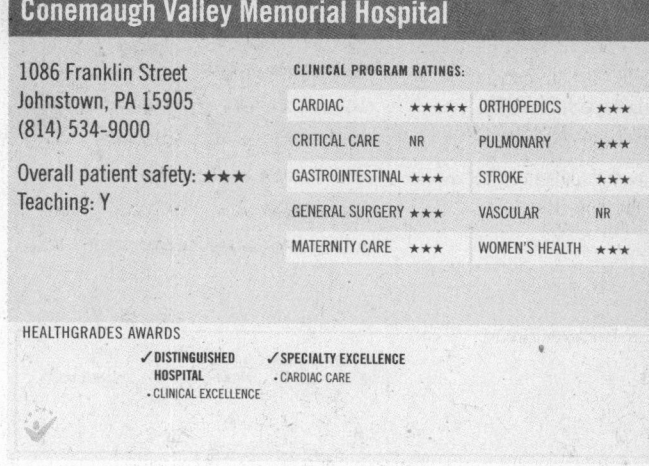

1086 Franklin Street
Johnstown, PA 15905
(814) 534-9000

Overall patient safety: ★★★
Teaching: Y

CLINICAL PROGRAM RATINGS:

CARDIAC	★★★★★	ORTHOPEDICS	★★★
CRITICAL CARE	NR	PULMONARY	★★★
GASTROINTESTINAL	★★★	STROKE	★★★
GENERAL SURGERY	★★★	VASCULAR	NR
MATERNITY CARE	★★★	WOMEN'S HEALTH	★★★

HEALTHGRADES AWARDS

✓ DISTINGUISHED
  HOSPITAL
  - CLINICAL EXCELLENCE

✓ SPECIALTY EXCELLENCE
  - CARDIAC CARE

Community Hospital

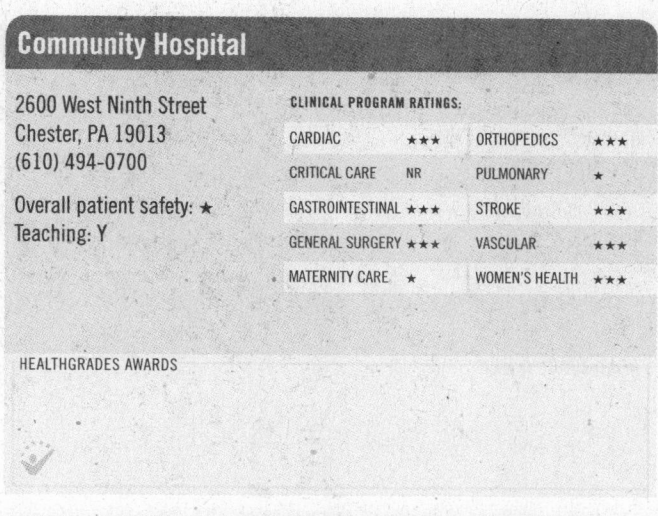

2600 West Ninth Street
Chester, PA 19013
(610) 494-0700

Overall patient safety: ★
Teaching: Y

CLINICAL PROGRAM RATINGS:

CARDIAC	★★★	ORTHOPEDICS	★★★
CRITICAL CARE	NR	PULMONARY	★
GASTROINTESTINAL	★★★	STROKE	★★★
GENERAL SURGERY	★★★	VASCULAR	★★★
MATERNITY CARE	★	WOMEN'S HEALTH	★★★

HEALTHGRADES AWARDS

Crozer-Chester Medical Center*

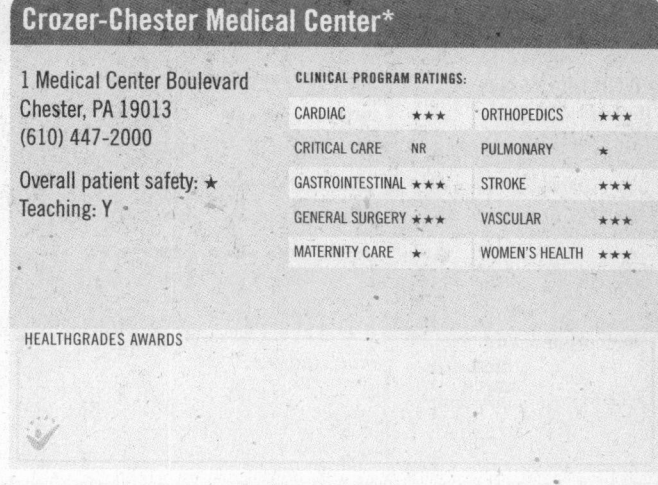

1 Medical Center Boulevard
Chester, PA 19013
(610) 447-2000

Overall patient safety: ★
Teaching: Y

CLINICAL PROGRAM RATINGS:

CARDIAC	★★★	ORTHOPEDICS	★★★
CRITICAL CARE	NR	PULMONARY	★
GASTROINTESTINAL	★★★	STROKE	★★★
GENERAL SURGERY	★★★	VASCULAR	★★★
MATERNITY CARE	★	WOMEN'S HEALTH	★★★

HEALTHGRADES AWARDS

Community Medical Center

1800 Mulberry Street
Scranton, PA 18501
(570) 969-8000

Overall patient safety: ★★★★★
Teaching: Y

CLINICAL PROGRAM RATINGS:

CARDIAC	★★★	ORTHOPEDICS	★★★
CRITICAL CARE	NR	PULMONARY	★★★
GASTROINTESTINAL	★★★	STROKE	★★★
GENERAL SURGERY	★★★	VASCULAR	NR
MATERNITY CARE	★★★★★	WOMEN'S HEALTH	★★★★★

HEALTHGRADES AWARDS

✓ DISTINGUISHED
  HOSPITAL
  - PATIENT SAFETY

✓ SPECIALTY EXCELLENCE
  - CARDIAC SURGERY   - WOMEN'S HEALTH

Delaware County Memorial Hospital

501 North Lansdowne Avenue
Drexel Hill, PA 19026
(610) 284-8100

Overall patient safety: ★★★
Teaching: Y

CLINICAL PROGRAM RATINGS:

CARDIAC	NR	ORTHOPEDICS	NR
CRITICAL CARE	NR	PULMONARY	★
GASTROINTESTINAL	★★★	STROKE	★★★
GENERAL SURGERY	★★★	VASCULAR	NR
MATERNITY CARE	★★★	WOMEN'S HEALTH	NR

HEALTHGRADES AWARDS

*This hospital reports its data to the federal government jointly with another hospital. Therefore the ratings and awards apply to multiple hospitals and this specific hospital may not provide all rated services.

Doylestown Hospital

595 West State Street
Doylestown, PA 18901
(215) 345-2200

Overall patient safety: ★★★
Teaching: N

CLINICAL PROGRAM RATINGS:

CARDIAC	★★★	ORTHOPEDICS	★★★
CRITICAL CARE	NR	PULMONARY	★
GASTROINTESTINAL	★★★	STROKE	★★★
GENERAL SURGERY	★★★	VASCULAR	NR
MATERNITY CARE	★★★★★	WOMEN'S HEALTH	★★★★★

HEALTHGRADES AWARDS

✓ SPECIALTY EXCELLENCE
· GENERAL SURGERY   · MATERNITY CARE   · WOMEN'S HEALTH

Elk Regional Health Center

763 Johnsonburg Road
St. Marys, PA 15857
(814) 788-8000

Overall patient safety: ★★★
Teaching: N

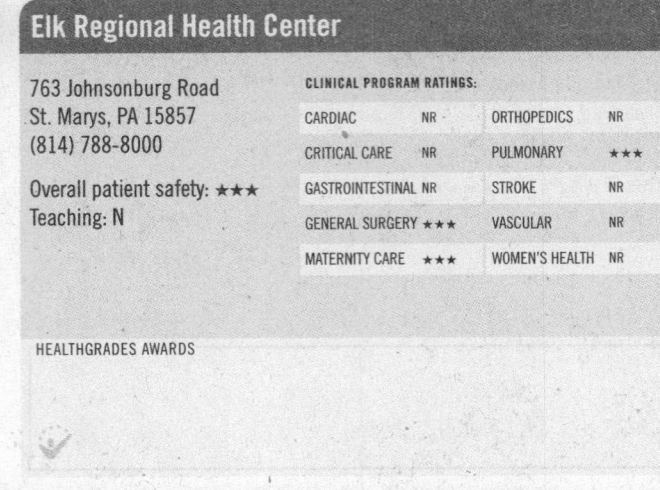

CLINICAL PROGRAM RATINGS:

CARDIAC	NR	ORTHOPEDICS	NR
CRITICAL CARE	NR	PULMONARY	★★★
GASTROINTESTINAL	NR	STROKE	NR
GENERAL SURGERY	★★★	VASCULAR	NR
MATERNITY CARE	★★★	WOMEN'S HEALTH	NR

HEALTHGRADES AWARDS

DuBois Regional Medical Center

100 Hospital Avenue
DuBois, PA 15801
(814) 371-2200

Overall patient safety: ★★★★★
Teaching: N

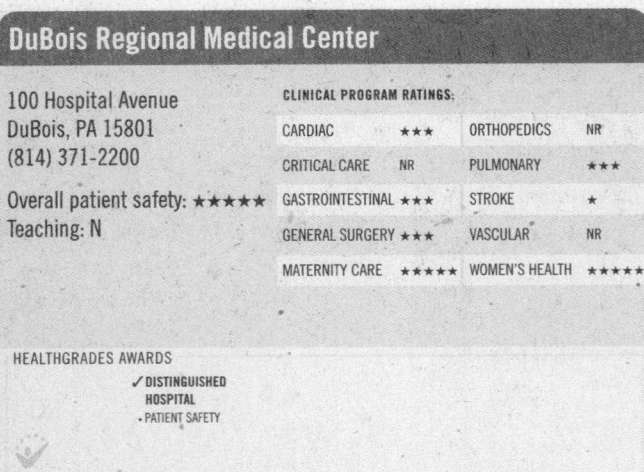

CLINICAL PROGRAM RATINGS:

CARDIAC	★★★	ORTHOPEDICS	NR
CRITICAL CARE	NR	PULMONARY	★★★
GASTROINTESTINAL	★★★	STROKE	★
GENERAL SURGERY	★★★	VASCULAR	NR
MATERNITY CARE	★★★★★	WOMEN'S HEALTH	★★★★★

HEALTHGRADES AWARDS

✓ DISTINGUISHED
HOSPITAL
· PATIENT SAFETY

Ellwood City Hospital

724 Pershing Street
Ellwood City, PA 16117
(724) 752-0081

Overall patient safety: ★★★
Teaching: N

CLINICAL PROGRAM RATINGS:

CARDIAC	NR	ORTHOPEDICS	NR
CRITICAL CARE	NR	PULMONARY	★
GASTROINTESTINAL	NR	STROKE	NR
GENERAL SURGERY	NR	VASCULAR	NR
MATERNITY CARE	★★★	WOMEN'S HEALTH	NR

HEALTHGRADES AWARDS

Easton Hospital

250 South 21st Street
Easton, PA 18042
(610) 250-4000

Overall patient safety: ★★★
Teaching: Y

CLINICAL PROGRAM RATINGS:

CARDIAC	★★★	ORTHOPEDICS	NR
CRITICAL CARE	NR	PULMONARY	★★★★★
GASTROINTESTINAL	★★★	STROKE	★★★
GENERAL SURGERY	★★★★★	VASCULAR	NR
MATERNITY CARE	★★★	WOMEN'S HEALTH	★★★

HEALTHGRADES AWARDS

✓ AMERICA'S 50   ✓ DISTINGUISHED   ✓ SPECIALTY EXCELLENCE
BEST HOSPITALS   HOSPITAL   · GASTROINTESTINAL   · GENERAL SURGERY   · PULMONARY CARE
                      · CLINICAL EXCELLENCE   CARE

Ephrata Community Hospital

169 Martin Avenue
Ephrata, PA 17522
(717) 733-0311

Overall patient safety: ★★★★★
Teaching: N

CLINICAL PROGRAM RATINGS:

CARDIAC	NR	ORTHOPEDICS	★★★
CRITICAL CARE	NR	PULMONARY	★★★★★
GASTROINTESTINAL	★★★	STROKE	★★★★★
GENERAL SURGERY	★★★	VASCULAR	NR
MATERNITY CARE	★	WOMEN'S HEALTH	NR

HEALTHGRADES AWARDS

✓ DISTINGUISHED   ✓ SPECIALTY EXCELLENCE
HOSPITAL   · GASTROINTESTINAL   · PULMONARY CARE
· PATIENT SAFETY   CARE

KEY: ★★★★★ BEST   ★★★ AS EXPECTED   ★ POOR   NR NOT RATED BY HEALTHGRADES   For full definitions of ratings and awards, see Appendix.

560   CHAPTER 6: HOSPITAL RATINGS BY CLINICAL SPECIALTY

Evangelical Community Hospital

1 Hospital Drive
Lewisburg, PA 17837
(570) 522-2000

Overall patient safety: ★★★
Teaching: N

CLINICAL PROGRAM RATINGS:

CARDIAC	NR	ORTHOPEDICS	★
CRITICAL CARE	NR	PULMONARY	★★★
GASTROINTESTINAL	★★★	STROKE	★★★
GENERAL SURGERY	★★★	VASCULAR	NR
MATERNITY CARE	★★★	WOMEN'S HEALTH	NR

HEALTHGRADES AWARDS

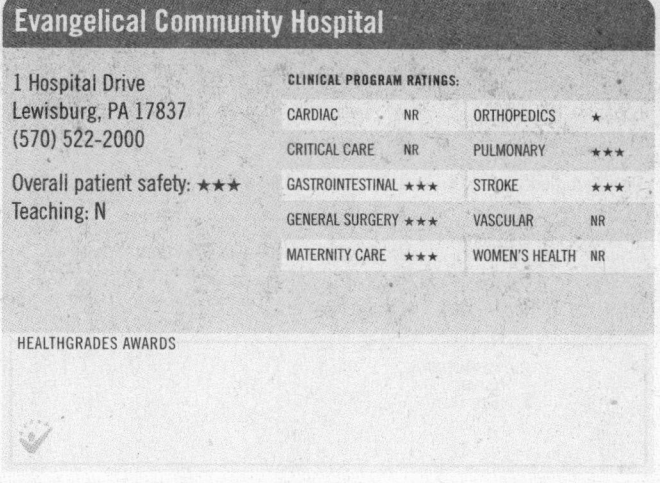

Fulton County Medical Center

216 South 1st Street
McConnellsburg, PA 17233
(717) 485-3155

Overall patient safety: ★★★
Teaching: N

CLINICAL PROGRAM RATINGS:

CARDIAC	NR	ORTHOPEDICS	NR
CRITICAL CARE	NR	PULMONARY	★★★
GASTROINTESTINAL	NR	STROKE	NR
GENERAL SURGERY	NR	VASCULAR	NR
MATERNITY CARE	NR	WOMEN'S HEALTH	NR

HEALTHGRADES AWARDS

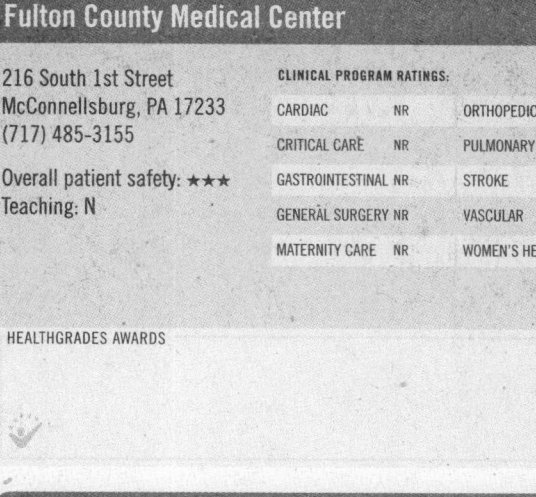

Frankford Hospital–Torresdale Campus

Knights and Red Lion Roads
Philadelphia, PA 19114
(215) 612-4000

Overall patient safety: ★★★
Teaching: Y

CLINICAL PROGRAM RATINGS:

CARDIAC	★★★	ORTHOPEDICS	NR
CRITICAL CARE	NR	PULMONARY	★★★
GASTROINTESTINAL	★★★	STROKE	★★★
GENERAL SURGERY	★★★	VASCULAR	NR
MATERNITY CARE	★★★	WOMEN'S HEALTH	★★★

HEALTHGRADES AWARDS

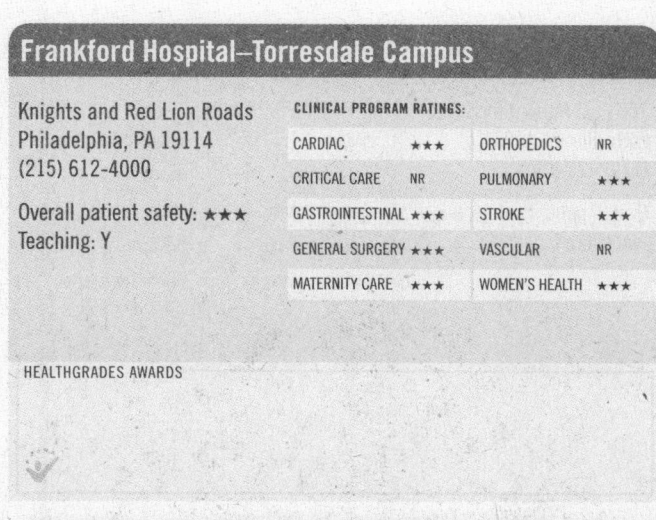

Geisinger Medical Center

100 North Academy Avenue
Danville, PA 17822
(570) 271-6211

Overall patient safety: ★★★
Teaching: Y

CLINICAL PROGRAM RATINGS:

CARDIAC	★★★	ORTHOPEDICS	★★★
CRITICAL CARE	NR	PULMONARY	★★★
GASTROINTESTINAL	★★★	STROKE	★★★
GENERAL SURGERY	★★★	VASCULAR	★★★
MATERNITY CARE	★	WOMEN'S HEALTH	★★★

HEALTHGRADES AWARDS

✓ SPECIALTY EXCELLENCE
· BARIATRIC SURGERY

Frick Hospital

508 South Church Street
Mt. Pleasant, PA 15666
(724) 547-1500

Overall patient safety: ★
Teaching: N

CLINICAL PROGRAM RATINGS:

CARDIAC	NR	ORTHOPEDICS	NR
CRITICAL CARE	NR	PULMONARY	★★★
GASTROINTESTINAL	NR	STROKE	★★★
GENERAL SURGERY	★★★	VASCULAR	NR
MATERNITY CARE	NR	WOMEN'S HEALTH	NR

HEALTHGRADES AWARDS

Geisinger South Wilkes-Barre

25 Church Street
Wilkes-Barre, PA 18765
(570) 826-3100

Overall patient safety: ★★★
Teaching: Y

CLINICAL PROGRAM RATINGS:

CARDIAC	★★★	ORTHOPEDICS	NR
CRITICAL CARE	NR	PULMONARY	★★★
GASTROINTESTINAL	★★★	STROKE	★★★★★
GENERAL SURGERY	★★★	VASCULAR	NR
MATERNITY CARE	★★★	WOMEN'S HEALTH	★★★★★

HEALTHGRADES AWARDS

✓ SPECIALTY EXCELLENCE
· STROKE CARE   · WOMEN'S HEALTH

Geisinger Wyoming Valley Medical Center

1000 East Mountain Boulevard
Wilkes-Barre, PA 18711
(570) 826-7300

Overall patient safety: ★★★
Teaching: Y

CLINICAL PROGRAM RATINGS:

CARDIAC	★★★	ORTHOPEDICS	NR
CRITICAL CARE	NR	PULMONARY	★★★
GASTROINTESTINAL	★★★	STROKE	★★★
GENERAL SURGERY	★★★	VASCULAR	NR
MATERNITY CARE	★★★	WOMEN'S HEALTH	★★★

HEALTHGRADES AWARDS

Good Samaritan Hospital

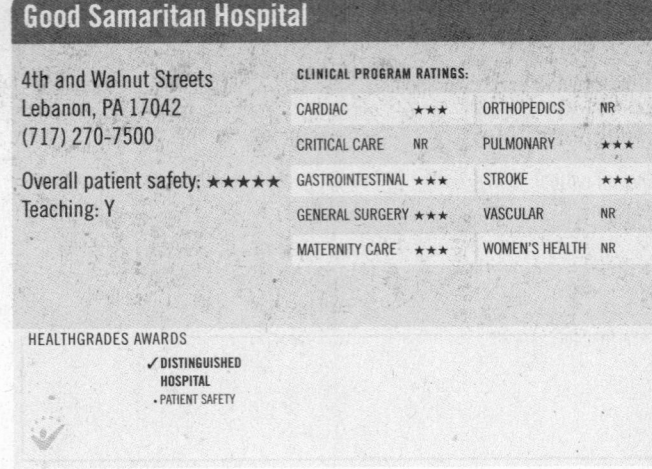

4th and Walnut Streets
Lebanon, PA 17042
(717) 270-7500

Overall patient safety: ★★★★★
Teaching: Y

CLINICAL PROGRAM RATINGS:

CARDIAC	★★★	ORTHOPEDICS	NR
CRITICAL CARE	NR	PULMONARY	★★★
GASTROINTESTINAL	★★★	STROKE	★★★
GENERAL SURGERY	★★★	VASCULAR	NR
MATERNITY CARE	★★★	WOMEN'S HEALTH	NR

HEALTHGRADES AWARDS
✓ DISTINGUISHED HOSPITAL
• PATIENT SAFETY

Gettysburg Hospital

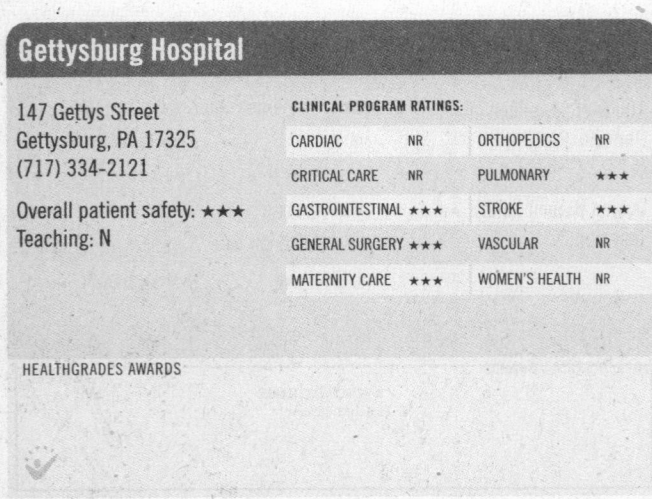

147 Gettys Street
Gettysburg, PA 17325
(717) 334-2121

Overall patient safety: ★★★
Teaching: N

CLINICAL PROGRAM RATINGS:

CARDIAC	NR	ORTHOPEDICS	NR
CRITICAL CARE	NR	PULMONARY	★★★
GASTROINTESTINAL	★★★	STROKE	★★★
GENERAL SURGERY	★★★	VASCULAR	NR
MATERNITY CARE	★★★	WOMEN'S HEALTH	NR

HEALTHGRADES AWARDS

Good Samaritan Regional Medical Center

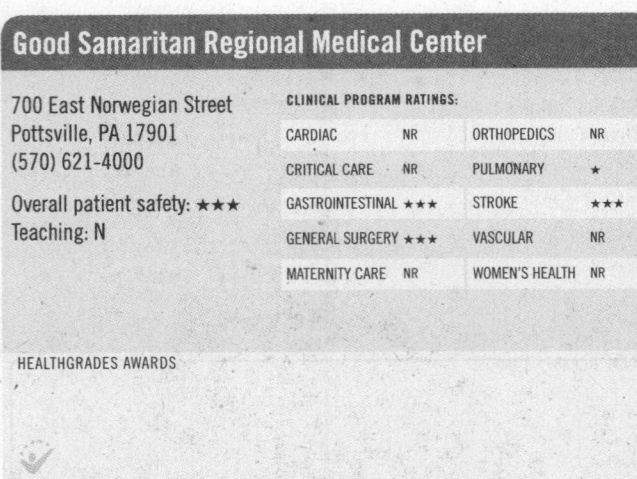

700 East Norwegian Street
Pottsville, PA 17901
(570) 621-4000

Overall patient safety: ★★★
Teaching: N

CLINICAL PROGRAM RATINGS:

CARDIAC	NR	ORTHOPEDICS	NR
CRITICAL CARE	NR	PULMONARY	★
GASTROINTESTINAL	★★★	STROKE	★★★
GENERAL SURGERY	★★★	VASCULAR	NR
MATERNITY CARE	NR	WOMEN'S HEALTH	NR

HEALTHGRADES AWARDS

Gnaden Huetten Memorial Hospital

211 North 12th Street
Lehighton, PA 18235
(610) 377-1300

Overall patient safety: ★★★
Teaching: N

CLINICAL PROGRAM RATINGS:

CARDIAC	NR	ORTHOPEDICS	NR
CRITICAL CARE	NR	PULMONARY	★★★
GASTROINTESTINAL	NR	STROKE	★★★
GENERAL SURGERY	★★★	VASCULAR	NR
MATERNITY CARE	★★★	WOMEN'S HEALTH	NR

HEALTHGRADES AWARDS

Graduate Hospital

1800 Lombard Street
Philadelphia, PA 19146
(215) 893-2000

Overall patient safety: ★★★
Teaching: Y

CLINICAL PROGRAM RATINGS:

CARDIAC	★★★	ORTHOPEDICS	NR
CRITICAL CARE	NR	PULMONARY	★★★
GASTROINTESTINAL	NR	STROKE	★★★
GENERAL SURGERY	NR	VASCULAR	NR
MATERNITY CARE	NR	WOMEN'S HEALTH	NR

HEALTHGRADES AWARDS

KEY: ★★★★★ BEST ★★★ AS EXPECTED ★ POOR NR NOT RATED BY HEALTHGRADES For full definitions of ratings and awards, see Appendix.

Grand View Hospital

700 Lawn Avenue
Sellersville, PA 18960
(215) 453-4000

Overall patient safety: ★★★
Teaching: N

CLINICAL PROGRAM RATINGS:

CARDIAC	NR	ORTHOPEDICS	NR
CRITICAL CARE	NR	PULMONARY	★★★
GASTROINTESTINAL	NR	STROKE	★★★
GENERAL SURGERY	★★★	VASCULAR	NR
MATERNITY CARE	★★★★★	WOMEN'S HEALTH	NR

HEALTHGRADES AWARDS

Hamot Medical Center

201 State Street
Erie, PA 16550
(814) 877-6000

Overall patient safety: ★★★
Teaching: Y

CLINICAL PROGRAM RATINGS:

CARDIAC	★★★★★	ORTHOPEDICS	★★★
CRITICAL CARE	NR	PULMONARY	★★★★★
GASTROINTESTINAL	★★★	STROKE	★★★★★
GENERAL SURGERY	★★★	VASCULAR	★★★
MATERNITY CARE	★★★	WOMEN'S HEALTH	★★★

HEALTHGRADES AWARDS

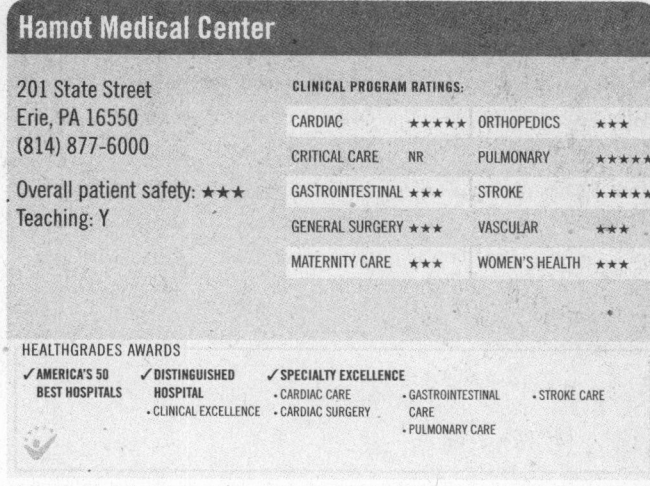

✓ AMERICA'S 50 BEST HOSPITALS
✓ DISTINGUISHED HOSPITAL
- CLINICAL EXCELLENCE
✓ SPECIALTY EXCELLENCE
- CARDIAC CARE
- CARDIAC SURGERY
- GASTROINTESTINAL CARE
- PULMONARY CARE
- STROKE CARE

Grove City Medical Center

631 North Broad
Street Extension
Grove City, PA 16127
(724) 450-7000

Overall patient safety: ★★★
Teaching: N

CLINICAL PROGRAM RATINGS:

CARDIAC	NR	ORTHOPEDICS	NR
CRITICAL CARE	NR	PULMONARY	★
GASTROINTESTINAL	NR	STROKE	★★★
GENERAL SURGERY	NR	VASCULAR	NR
MATERNITY CARE	★★★	WOMEN'S HEALTH	NR

HEALTHGRADES AWARDS

Hanover General Hospital

300 Highland Avenue
Hanover, PA 17331
(717) 637-3711

Overall patient safety: ★★★
Teaching: N

CLINICAL PROGRAM RATINGS:

CARDIAC	NR	ORTHOPEDICS	★★★★★
CRITICAL CARE	NR	PULMONARY	★
GASTROINTESTINAL	★★★	STROKE	★
GENERAL SURGERY	★★★	VASCULAR	NR
MATERNITY CARE	★★★★★	WOMEN'S HEALTH	NR

HEALTHGRADES AWARDS

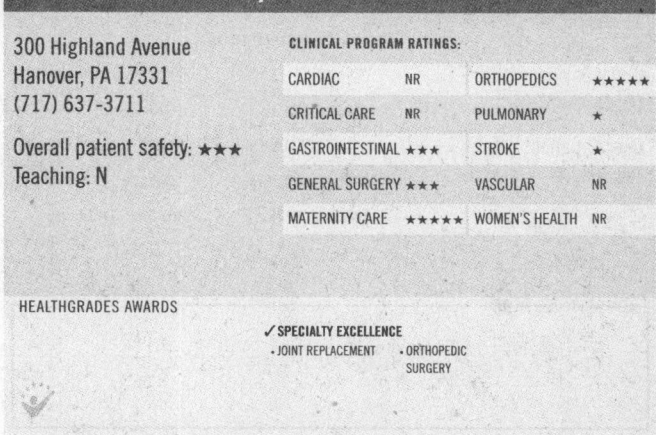

✓ SPECIALTY EXCELLENCE
- JOINT REPLACEMENT
- ORTHOPEDIC SURGERY

Hahnemann University Hospital*

230 North Broad Street
Philadelphia, PA 19102
(215) 762-7000

Overall patient safety: ★
Teaching: Y

CLINICAL PROGRAM RATINGS:

CARDIAC	★★★	ORTHOPEDICS	NR
CRITICAL CARE	NR	PULMONARY	★★★
GASTROINTESTINAL	NR	STROKE	★★★
GENERAL SURGERY	★★★	VASCULAR	NR
MATERNITY CARE	★★★	WOMEN'S HEALTH	★★★

HEALTHGRADES AWARDS

Hazleton General Hospital

700 East Broad Street
Hazleton, PA 18201
(570) 501-4000

Overall patient safety: ★★★
Teaching: Y

CLINICAL PROGRAM RATINGS:

CARDIAC	NR	ORTHOPEDICS	NR
CRITICAL CARE	NR	PULMONARY	★★★★★
GASTROINTESTINAL	★★★	STROKE	★★★
GENERAL SURGERY	★★★	VASCULAR	NR
MATERNITY CARE	★★★	WOMEN'S HEALTH	NR

HEALTHGRADES AWARDS

✓ SPECIALTY EXCELLENCE
- PULMONARY CARE

---

*This hospital reports its data to the federal government jointly with another hospital. Therefore the ratings and awards apply to multiple hospitals and this specific hospital may not provide all rated services.

Heart of Lancaster Regional Medical Center

1500 Highlands Drive
Lititz, PA 17543
(717) 397-3711

Overall patient safety: ★★★
Teaching: Y

CLINICAL PROGRAM RATINGS:

CARDIAC	NR	ORTHOPEDICS	NR
CRITICAL CARE	NR	PULMONARY	★★★
GASTROINTESTINAL	NR	STROKE	★
GENERAL SURGERY	★★★	VASCULAR	NR
MATERNITY CARE	★★★	WOMEN'S HEALTH	NR

HEALTHGRADES AWARDS

Holy Spirit Hospital

503 North 21st Street
Camp Hill, PA 17011
(717) 763-2100

Overall patient safety: ★★★
Teaching: Y

CLINICAL PROGRAM RATINGS:

CARDIAC	★★★	ORTHOPEDICS	★★★
CRITICAL CARE	NR	PULMONARY	★★★
GASTROINTESTINAL	★★★	STROKE	★★★
GENERAL SURGERY	★	VASCULAR	★★★
MATERNITY CARE	★★★	WOMEN'S HEALTH	★★★

HEALTHGRADES AWARDS

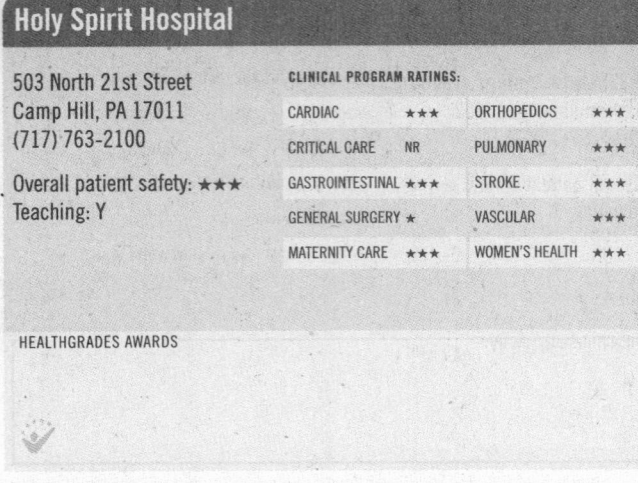

Highlands Hospital

401 East Murphy Avenue
Connellsville, PA 15425
(724) 628-1500

Overall patient safety: ★★★
Teaching: N

CLINICAL PROGRAM RATINGS:

CARDIAC	NR	ORTHOPEDICS	NR
CRITICAL CARE	NR	PULMONARY	★★★
GASTROINTESTINAL	NR	STROKE	NR
GENERAL SURGERY	NR	VASCULAR	NR
MATERNITY CARE	NR	WOMEN'S HEALTH	NR

HEALTHGRADES AWARDS

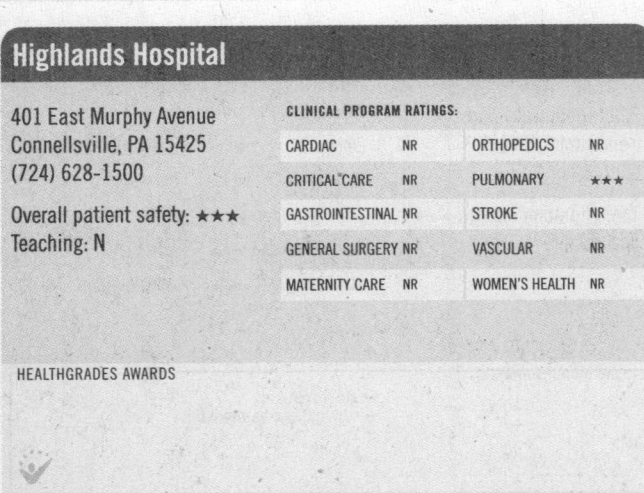

Hospital of the University of Pennsylvania

3400 Spruce Street
Philadelphia, PA 19104
(215) 662-4000

Overall patient safety: ★★★
Teaching: Y

CLINICAL PROGRAM RATINGS:

CARDIAC	★★★	ORTHOPEDICS	NR
CRITICAL CARE	NR	PULMONARY	★★★
GASTROINTESTINAL	★★★	STROKE	★★★
GENERAL SURGERY	★★★	VASCULAR	★★★
MATERNITY CARE	★	WOMEN'S HEALTH	★

HEALTHGRADES AWARDS

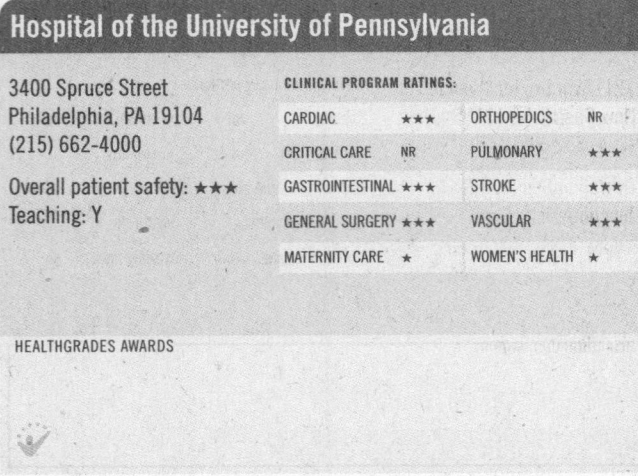

Holy Redeemer Hospital and Medical Center

1648 Huntington Pike
Meadowbrook, PA 19046
(215) 947-3000

Overall patient safety: ★★★
Teaching: Y

CLINICAL PROGRAM RATINGS:

CARDIAC	NR	ORTHOPEDICS	★★★
CRITICAL CARE	NR	PULMONARY	★★★
GASTROINTESTINAL	★★★	STROKE	★★★
GENERAL SURGERY	★★★	VASCULAR	NR
MATERNITY CARE	★★★	WOMEN'S HEALTH	NR

HEALTHGRADES AWARDS

Indiana Regional Medical Center

835 Hospital Road
Indiana, PA 15701
(724) 357-7000

Overall patient safety: ★★★★★
Teaching: N

CLINICAL PROGRAM RATINGS:

CARDIAC	NR	ORTHOPEDICS	NR
CRITICAL CARE	NR	PULMONARY	★★★
GASTROINTESTINAL	★★★	STROKE	★★★
GENERAL SURGERY	★★★	VASCULAR	NR
MATERNITY CARE	★★★★★	WOMEN'S HEALTH	NR

HEALTHGRADES AWARDS
✓ DISTINGUISHED HOSPITAL
- PATIENT SAFETY

KEY: ★★★★★ BEST ★★★ AS EXPECTED ★ POOR NR NOT RATED BY HEALTHGRADES For full definitions of ratings and awards, see Appendix.

J. C. Blair Memorial Hospital

1225 Warm Springs Avenue
Huntingdon, PA 16652
(814) 643-2290

Overall patient safety: ★★★
Teaching: N

CLINICAL PROGRAM RATINGS:

CARDIAC	NR	ORTHOPEDICS	NR
CRITICAL CARE	NR	PULMONARY	★★★
GASTROINTESTINAL	NR	STROKE	★
GENERAL SURGERY	★	VASCULAR	NR
MATERNITY CARE	★★★	WOMEN'S HEALTH	NR

HEALTHGRADES AWARDS

Jefferson Regional Medical Center

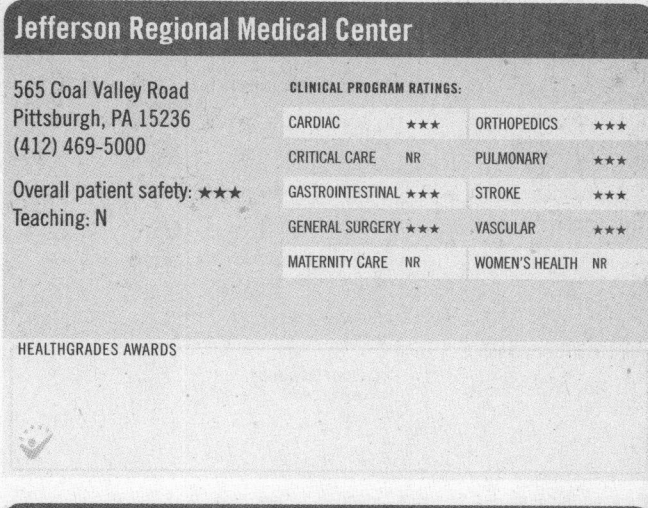

565 Coal Valley Road
Pittsburgh, PA 15236
(412) 469-5000

Overall patient safety: ★★★
Teaching: N

CLINICAL PROGRAM RATINGS:

CARDIAC	★★★	ORTHOPEDICS	★★★
CRITICAL CARE	NR	PULMONARY	★★★
GASTROINTESTINAL	★★★	STROKE	★★★
GENERAL SURGERY	★★★	VASCULAR	★★★
MATERNITY CARE	NR	WOMEN'S HEALTH	NR

HEALTHGRADES AWARDS

Jameson Memorial Hospital

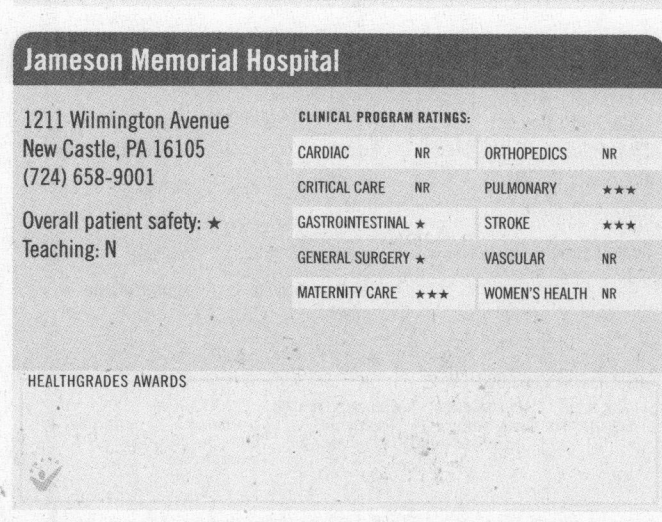

1211 Wilmington Avenue
New Castle, PA 16105
(724) 658-9001

Overall patient safety: ★
Teaching: N

CLINICAL PROGRAM RATINGS:

CARDIAC	NR	ORTHOPEDICS	NR
CRITICAL CARE	NR	PULMONARY	★★★
GASTROINTESTINAL	★	STROKE	★★★
GENERAL SURGERY	★	VASCULAR	NR
MATERNITY CARE	★★★	WOMEN'S HEALTH	NR

HEALTHGRADES AWARDS

Jennersville Regional Hospital

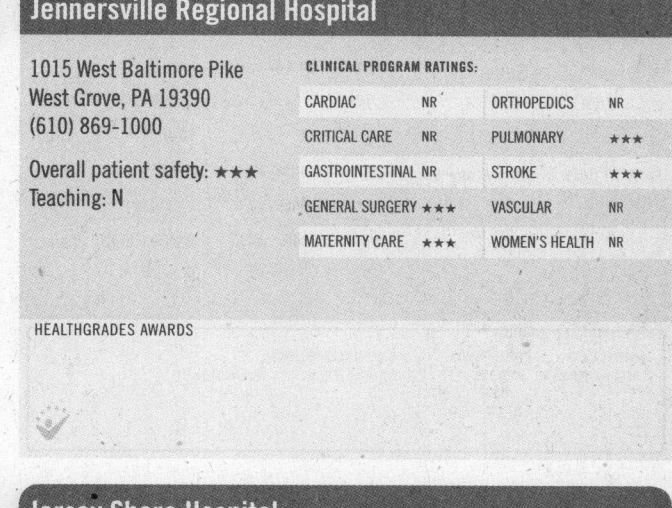

1015 West Baltimore Pike
West Grove, PA 19390
(610) 869-1000

Overall patient safety: ★★★
Teaching: N

CLINICAL PROGRAM RATINGS:

CARDIAC	NR	ORTHOPEDICS	NR
CRITICAL CARE	NR	PULMONARY	★★★
GASTROINTESTINAL	NR	STROKE	★★★
GENERAL SURGERY	★★★	VASCULAR	NR
MATERNITY CARE	★★★	WOMEN'S HEALTH	NR

HEALTHGRADES AWARDS

Jeanes Hospital

7600 Central Avenue
Philadelphia, PA 19111
(215) 728-2000

Overall patient safety: ★★★
Teaching: Y

CLINICAL PROGRAM RATINGS:

CARDIAC	NR	ORTHOPEDICS	NR
CRITICAL CARE	NR	PULMONARY	★★★
GASTROINTESTINAL	★★★	STROKE	★★★
GENERAL SURGERY	★★★	VASCULAR	NR
MATERNITY CARE	★★★	WOMEN'S HEALTH	NR

HEALTHGRADES AWARDS

Jersey Shore Hospital

1020 Thompson Street
Jersey Shore, PA 17740
(570) 398-0100

Overall patient safety: ★★★
Teaching: N

CLINICAL PROGRAM RATINGS:

CARDIAC	NR	ORTHOPEDICS	NR
CRITICAL CARE	NR	PULMONARY	★★★
GASTROINTESTINAL	NR	STROKE	★★★
GENERAL SURGERY	NR	VASCULAR	NR
MATERNITY CARE	NR	WOMEN'S HEALTH	NR

HEALTHGRADES AWARDS

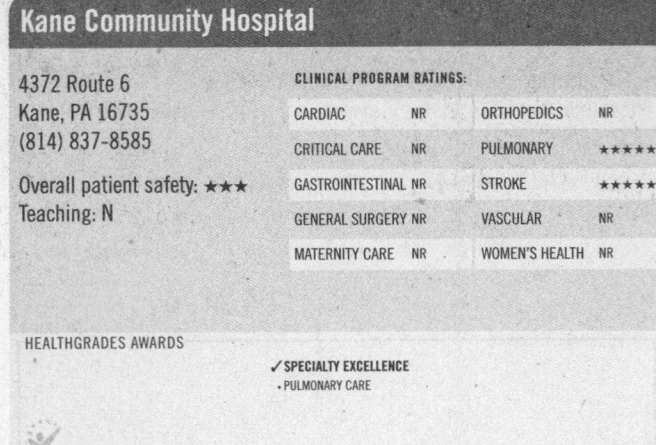

Kane Community Hospital

4372 Route 6
Kane, PA 16735
(814) 837-8585

Overall patient safety: ★★★
Teaching: N

CLINICAL PROGRAM RATINGS:

CARDIAC	NR	ORTHOPEDICS	NR
CRITICAL CARE	NR	PULMONARY	★★★★★
GASTROINTESTINAL	NR	STROKE	★★★★★
GENERAL SURGERY	NR	VASCULAR	NR
MATERNITY CARE	NR	WOMEN'S HEALTH	NR

HEALTHGRADES AWARDS

✓ SPECIALTY EXCELLENCE
· PULMONARY CARE

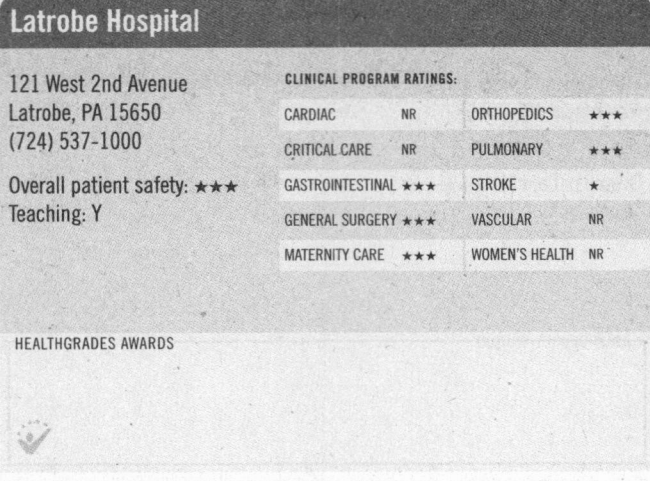

Latrobe Hospital

121 West 2nd Avenue
Latrobe, PA 15650
(724) 537-1000

Overall patient safety: ★★★
Teaching: Y

CLINICAL PROGRAM RATINGS:

CARDIAC	NR	ORTHOPEDICS	★★★
CRITICAL CARE	NR	PULMONARY	★★★
GASTROINTESTINAL	★★★	STROKE	★
GENERAL SURGERY	★★★	VASCULAR	NR
MATERNITY CARE	★★★	WOMEN'S HEALTH	NR

HEALTHGRADES AWARDS

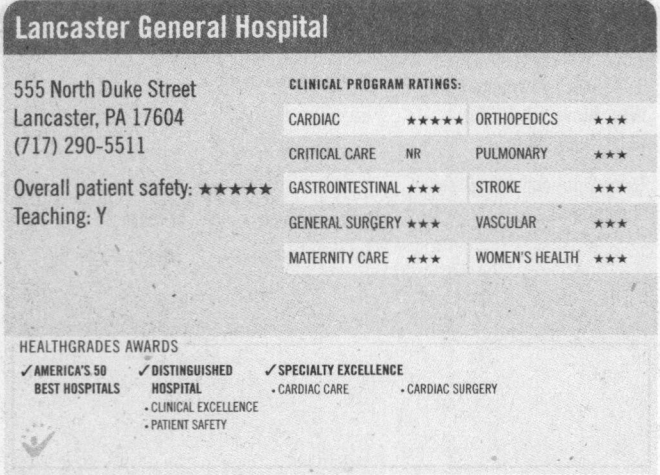

Lancaster General Hospital

555 North Duke Street
Lancaster, PA 17604
(717) 290-5511

Overall patient safety: ★★★★★
Teaching: Y

CLINICAL PROGRAM RATINGS:

CARDIAC	★★★★★	ORTHOPEDICS	★★★
CRITICAL CARE	NR	PULMONARY	★★★
GASTROINTESTINAL	★★★	STROKE	★★★
GENERAL SURGERY	★★★	VASCULAR	★★★
MATERNITY CARE	★★★	WOMEN'S HEALTH	★★★

HEALTHGRADES AWARDS

✓ AMERICA'S 50 BEST HOSPITALS

✓ DISTINGUISHED HOSPITAL
· CLINICAL EXCELLENCE
· PATIENT SAFETY

✓ SPECIALTY EXCELLENCE
· CARDIAC CARE
· CARDIAC SURGERY

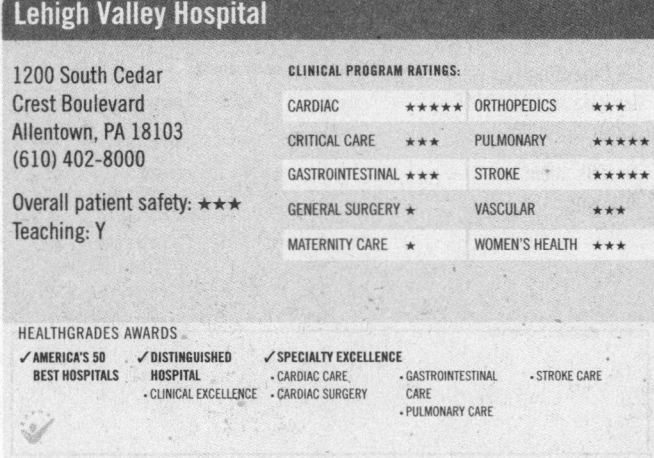

Lehigh Valley Hospital

1200 South Cedar
Crest Boulevard
Allentown, PA 18103
(610) 402-8000

Overall patient safety: ★★★
Teaching: Y

CLINICAL PROGRAM RATINGS:

CARDIAC	★★★★★	ORTHOPEDICS	★★★
CRITICAL CARE	★★★	PULMONARY	★★★★★
GASTROINTESTINAL	★★★	STROKE	★★★★★
GENERAL SURGERY	★	VASCULAR	★★★
MATERNITY CARE	★	WOMEN'S HEALTH	★★★

HEALTHGRADES AWARDS

✓ AMERICA'S 50 BEST HOSPITALS

✓ DISTINGUISHED HOSPITAL
· CLINICAL EXCELLENCE

✓ SPECIALTY EXCELLENCE
· CARDIAC CARE
· CARDIAC SURGERY
· GASTROINTESTINAL CARE
· PULMONARY CARE
· STROKE CARE

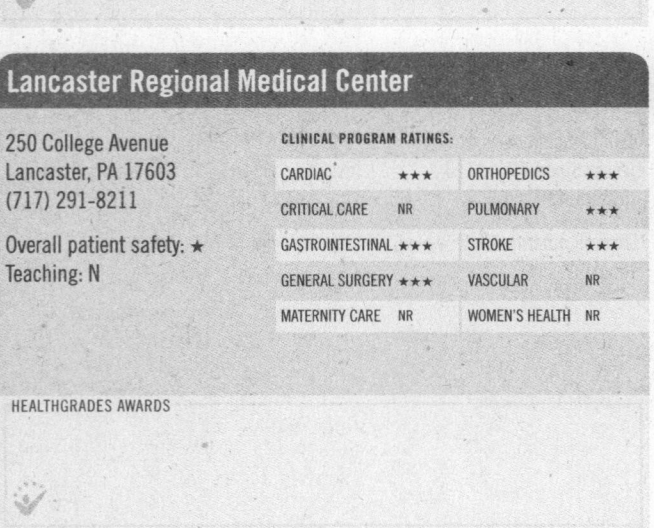

Lancaster Regional Medical Center

250 College Avenue
Lancaster, PA 17603
(717) 291-8211

Overall patient safety: ★
Teaching: N

CLINICAL PROGRAM RATINGS:

CARDIAC	★★★	ORTHOPEDICS	★★★
CRITICAL CARE	NR	PULMONARY	★★★
GASTROINTESTINAL	★★★	STROKE	★★★
GENERAL SURGERY	★★★	VASCULAR	NR
MATERNITY CARE	NR	WOMEN'S HEALTH	NR

HEALTHGRADES AWARDS

Lehigh Valley Hospital–Muhlenberg

2545 Schoenersville Road
Bethlehem, PA 18017
(610) 402-2200

Overall patient safety: ★★★
Teaching: Y

CLINICAL PROGRAM RATINGS:

CARDIAC	★★★	ORTHOPEDICS	★★★
CRITICAL CARE	★★★	PULMONARY	★★★★★
GASTROINTESTINAL	★★★	STROKE	★★★
GENERAL SURGERY	★★★	VASCULAR	NR
MATERNITY CARE	NR	WOMEN'S HEALTH	NR

HEALTHGRADES AWARDS

✓ DISTINGUISHED HOSPITAL
· CLINICAL EXCELLENCE

✓ SPECIALTY EXCELLENCE
· GASTROINTESTINAL CARE

KEY: ★★★★★ BEST   ★★★ AS EXPECTED   ★ POOR   NR NOT RATED BY HEALTHGRADES   For full definitions of ratings and awards, see Appendix.

Lewistown Hospital

400 Highland Avenue
Lewistown, PA 17044
(717) 248-5411

Overall patient safety: ★★★
Teaching: N

CLINICAL PROGRAM RATINGS:

CARDIAC	NR	ORTHOPEDICS	NR
CRITICAL CARE	NR	PULMONARY	★
GASTROINTESTINAL	★★★	STROKE	★
GENERAL SURGERY	★★★	VASCULAR	NR
MATERNITY CARE	★★★	WOMEN'S HEALTH	NR

HEALTHGRADES AWARDS

✓ SPECIALTY EXCELLENCE
· GENERAL SURGERY

Magee-Womens Hospital of the UPMC Health System

300 Halket Street
Pittsburgh, PA 15213
(412) 641-1000

Overall patient safety: ★★★
Teaching: Y

CLINICAL PROGRAM RATINGS:

CARDIAC	NR	ORTHOPEDICS	NR
CRITICAL CARE	NR	PULMONARY	NR
GASTROINTESTINAL	NR	STROKE	NR
GENERAL SURGERY	NR	VASCULAR	NR
MATERNITY CARE	★	WOMEN'S HEALTH	NR

HEALTHGRADES AWARDS

Lock Haven Hospital

24 Cree Drive
Lock Haven, PA 17745
(570) 893-5000

Overall patient safety: ★★★
Teaching: N

CLINICAL PROGRAM RATINGS:

CARDIAC	NR	ORTHOPEDICS	NR
CRITICAL CARE	NR	PULMONARY	★
GASTROINTESTINAL	NR	STROKE	★★★
GENERAL SURGERY	NR	VASCULAR	NR
MATERNITY CARE	★★★	WOMEN'S HEALTH	NR

HEALTHGRADES AWARDS

Main Line Hospitals—Bryn Mawr

130 South Bryn Mawr Avenue
Bryn Mawr, PA 19010
(610) 526-3000

Overall patient safety: ★★★
Teaching: Y

CLINICAL PROGRAM RATINGS:

CARDIAC	★★★	ORTHOPEDICS	★★★
CRITICAL CARE	NR	PULMONARY	★★★★★
GASTROINTESTINAL	★★★	STROKE	★★★★★
GENERAL SURGERY	★★★	VASCULAR	★★★
MATERNITY CARE	★★★	WOMEN'S HEALTH	★★★

HEALTHGRADES AWARDS

Lower Bucks Hospital

501 Bath Road
Bristol, PA 19007
(215) 785-9200

Overall patient safety: ★★★
Teaching: Y

CLINICAL PROGRAM RATINGS:

CARDIAC	★★★	ORTHOPEDICS	NR
CRITICAL CARE	NR	PULMONARY	★★★
GASTROINTESTINAL	NR	STROKE	★★★
GENERAL SURGERY	NR	VASCULAR	NR
MATERNITY CARE	★★★	WOMEN'S HEALTH	★

HEALTHGRADES AWARDS

Main Line Hospitals—Lankenau

100 Lancaster Avenue
Wynnewood, PA 19096
(610) 645-2000

Overall patient safety: ★★★
Teaching: Y

CLINICAL PROGRAM RATINGS:

CARDIAC	★★★★★	ORTHOPEDICS	★★★
CRITICAL CARE	NR	PULMONARY	★★★★★
GASTROINTESTINAL	★★★	STROKE	★★★
GENERAL SURGERY	★★★	VASCULAR	NR
MATERNITY CARE	★	WOMEN'S HEALTH	★★★

HEALTHGRADES AWARDS

✓ AMERICA'S 50 BEST HOSPITALS   ✓ DISTINGUISHED HOSPITAL
· CLINICAL EXCELLENCE   ✓ SPECIALTY EXCELLENCE
· CARDIAC CARE   · CARDIAC SURGERY   · PULMONARY CARE

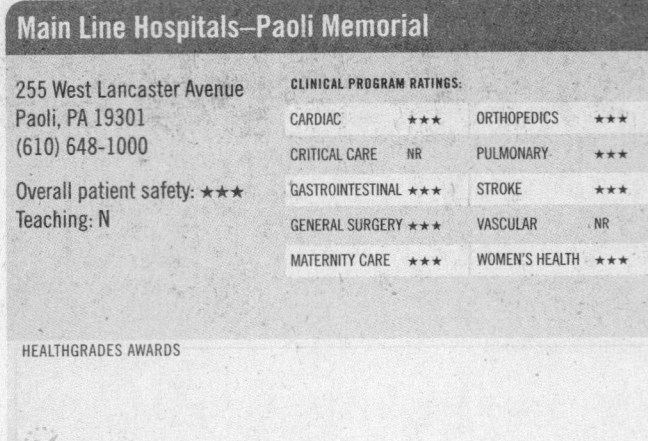

Main Line Hospitals—Paoli Memorial

255 West Lancaster Avenue
Paoli, PA 19301
(610) 648-1000

Overall patient safety: ★★★
Teaching: N

CLINICAL PROGRAM RATINGS:

CARDIAC	★★★	ORTHOPEDICS	★★★
CRITICAL CARE	NR	PULMONARY	★★★
GASTROINTESTINAL	★★★	STROKE	★★★
GENERAL SURGERY	★★★	VASCULAR	NR
MATERNITY CARE	★★★	WOMEN'S HEALTH	★★★

HEALTHGRADES AWARDS

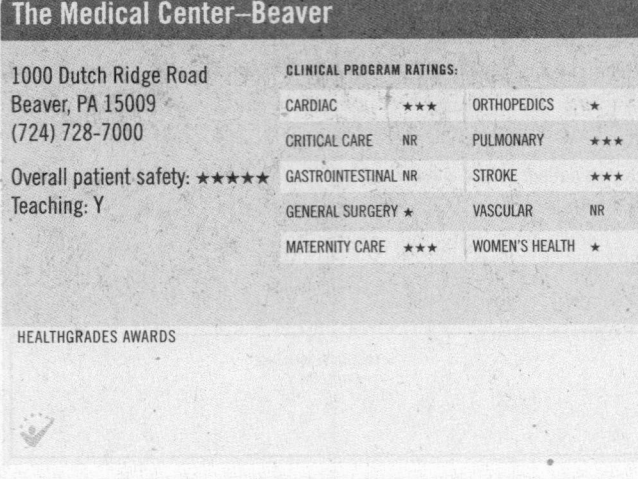

The Medical Center—Beaver

1000 Dutch Ridge Road
Beaver, PA 15009
(724) 728-7000

Overall patient safety: ★★★★★
Teaching: Y

CLINICAL PROGRAM RATINGS:

CARDIAC	★★★	ORTHOPEDICS	★
CRITICAL CARE	NR	PULMONARY	★★★
GASTROINTESTINAL	NR	STROKE	★★★
GENERAL SURGERY	★	VASCULAR	NR
MATERNITY CARE	★★★	WOMEN'S HEALTH	★

HEALTHGRADES AWARDS

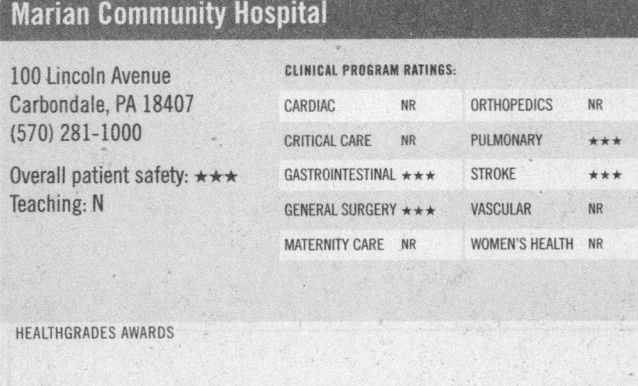

Marian Community Hospital

100 Lincoln Avenue
Carbondale, PA 18407
(570) 281-1000

Overall patient safety: ★★★
Teaching: N

CLINICAL PROGRAM RATINGS:

CARDIAC	NR	ORTHOPEDICS	NR
CRITICAL CARE	NR	PULMONARY	★★★
GASTROINTESTINAL	★★★	STROKE	★★★
GENERAL SURGERY	★★★	VASCULAR	NR
MATERNITY CARE	NR	WOMEN'S HEALTH	NR

HEALTHGRADES AWARDS

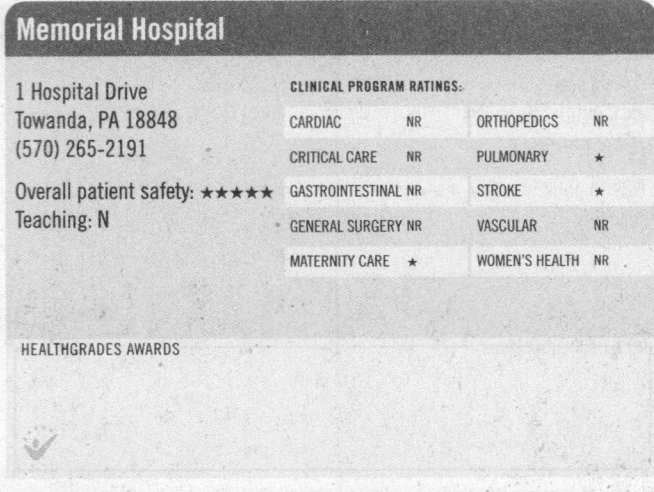

Memorial Hospital

1 Hospital Drive
Towanda, PA 18848
(570) 265-2191

Overall patient safety: ★★★★★
Teaching: N

CLINICAL PROGRAM RATINGS:

CARDIAC	NR	ORTHOPEDICS	NR
CRITICAL CARE	NR	PULMONARY	★
GASTROINTESTINAL	NR	STROKE	★
GENERAL SURGERY	NR	VASCULAR	NR
MATERNITY CARE	★	WOMEN'S HEALTH	NR

HEALTHGRADES AWARDS

Meadville Medical Center

751 Liberty Street
Meadville, PA 16335
(814) 333-5000

Overall patient safety: ★★★
Teaching: Y

CLINICAL PROGRAM RATINGS:

CARDIAC	NR	ORTHOPEDICS	NR
CRITICAL CARE	NR	PULMONARY	★★★
GASTROINTESTINAL	★★★	STROKE	★★★
GENERAL SURGERY	★★★	VASCULAR	NR
MATERNITY CARE	★★★	WOMEN'S HEALTH	NR

HEALTHGRADES AWARDS

Memorial Hospital

325 South Belmont Street
York, PA 17403
(717) 843-8623

Overall patient safety: ★★★
Teaching: Y

CLINICAL PROGRAM RATINGS:

CARDIAC	NR	ORTHOPEDICS	★★★
CRITICAL CARE	NR	PULMONARY	★★★
GASTROINTESTINAL	★★★	STROKE	★
GENERAL SURGERY	★	VASCULAR	NR
MATERNITY CARE	★★★	WOMEN'S HEALTH	NR

HEALTHGRADES AWARDS

PENNSYLVANIA HOSPITALS: RATINGS BY CLINICAL SPECIALTY

KEY: ★★★★★ BEST   ★★★ AS EXPECTED   ★ POOR   NR NOT RATED BY HEALTHGRADES   For full definitions of ratings and awards, see Appendix.

Mercy Fitzgerald Hospital

1500 Lansdowne Avenue
Darby, PA 19023
(610) 237-4000

Overall patient safety: ★
Teaching: Y

CLINICAL PROGRAM RATINGS:

CARDIAC	★★★	ORTHOPEDICS	NR
CRITICAL CARE	NR	PULMONARY	★★★
GASTROINTESTINAL	★★★	STROKE	★★★
GENERAL SURGERY	★★★	VASCULAR	NR
MATERNITY CARE	NR	WOMEN'S HEALTH	NR

HEALTHGRADES AWARDS

Mercy Jeannette Hospital

600 Jefferson Avenue
Jeannette, PA 15644
(724) 527-3551

Overall patient safety: ★★★
Teaching: N

CLINICAL PROGRAM RATINGS:

CARDIAC	NR	ORTHOPEDICS	NR
CRITICAL CARE	NR	PULMONARY	★★★
GASTROINTESTINAL	NR	STROKE	★★★
GENERAL SURGERY	★★★	VASCULAR	NR
MATERNITY CARE	★★★★★	WOMEN'S HEALTH	NR

HEALTHGRADES AWARDS

✓ SPECIALTY EXCELLENCE
- BARIATRIC SURGERY

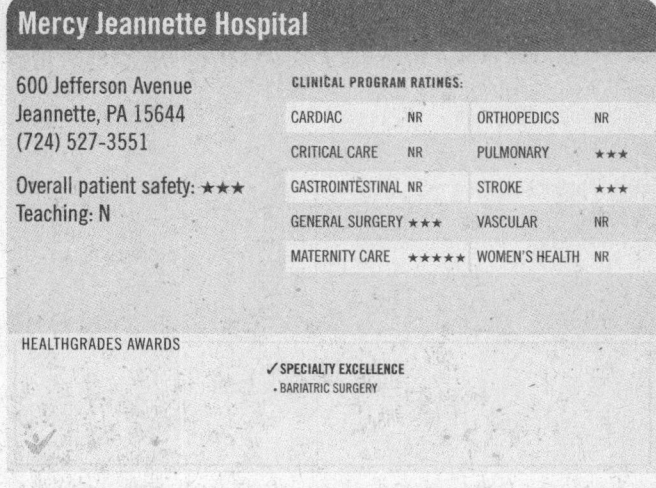

Mercy Hospital*

1400 Locust Street
Pittsburgh, PA 15219
(412) 232-8111

Overall patient safety: ★
Teaching: Y

CLINICAL PROGRAM RATINGS:

CARDIAC	★★★	ORTHOPEDICS	★★★
CRITICAL CARE	NR	PULMONARY	★★★★★
GASTROINTESTINAL	★★★	STROKE	★★★
GENERAL SURGERY	★	VASCULAR	★★★
MATERNITY CARE	★★★	WOMEN'S HEALTH	★

HEALTHGRADES AWARDS

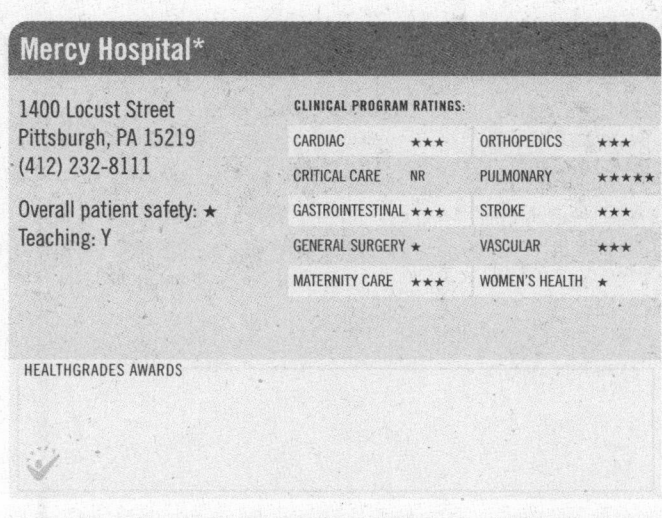

Mercy Providence Hospital*

1004 Arch Street
Pittsburgh, PA 15212
(412) 323-5600

Overall patient safety: ★
Teaching: Y

CLINICAL PROGRAM RATINGS:

CARDIAC	★★★	ORTHOPEDICS	★★★
CRITICAL CARE	NR	PULMONARY	★★★★★
GASTROINTESTINAL	★★★	STROKE	★★★
GENERAL SURGERY	★	VASCULAR	★★★
MATERNITY CARE	★★★	WOMEN'S HEALTH	★

HEALTHGRADES AWARDS

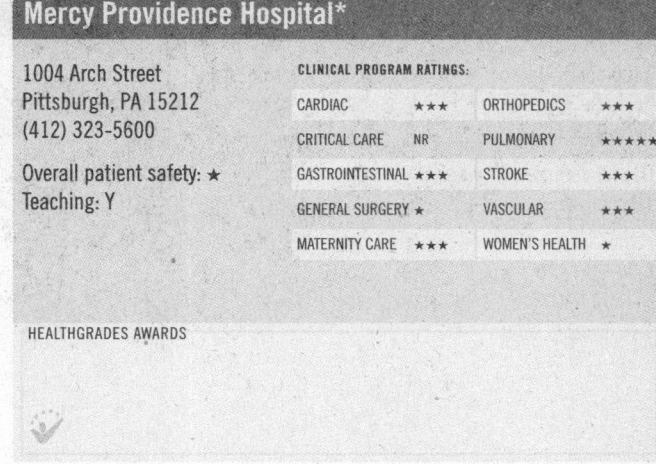

Mercy Hospital Scranton

746 Jefferson Avenue
Scranton, PA 18501
(570) 348-7100

Overall patient safety: ★★★★★
Teaching: Y

CLINICAL PROGRAM RATINGS:

CARDIAC	★★★	ORTHOPEDICS	NR
CRITICAL CARE	NR	PULMONARY	★★★
GASTROINTESTINAL	★★★	STROKE	★★★
GENERAL SURGERY	★★★	VASCULAR	NR
MATERNITY CARE	★★★	WOMEN'S HEALTH	★★★★★

HEALTHGRADES AWARDS

✓ AMERICA'S 50 BEST HOSPITALS
✓ DISTINGUISHED HOSPITAL
- CLINICAL EXCELLENCE
- PATIENT SAFETY
✓ SPECIALTY EXCELLENCE
- CARDIAC CARE
- WOMEN'S HEALTH

Mercy Suburban Hospital

2701 DeKalb Pike
Norristown, PA 19401
(610) 278-2000

Overall patient safety: ★
Teaching: Y

CLINICAL PROGRAM RATINGS:

CARDIAC	NR	ORTHOPEDICS	NR
CRITICAL CARE	NR	PULMONARY	★
GASTROINTESTINAL	NR	STROKE	★★★
GENERAL SURGERY	NR	VASCULAR	NR
MATERNITY CARE	★	WOMEN'S HEALTH	NR

HEALTHGRADES AWARDS

*This hospital reports its data to the federal government jointly with another hospital. Therefore the ratings and awards apply to multiple hospitals and this specific hospital may not provide all rated services.

Methodist Hospital*

2301 South Broad Street
Philadelphia, PA 19148
(215) 952-9000

Overall patient safety: ★
Teaching: Y

CLINICAL PROGRAM RATINGS:

CARDIAC	★★★	ORTHOPEDICS	★★★
CRITICAL CARE	NR	PULMONARY	★★★★★
GASTROINTESTINAL	★★★	STROKE	★★★
GENERAL SURGERY	★★★	VASCULAR	NR
MATERNITY CARE	★	WOMEN'S HEALTH	★★★

HEALTHGRADES AWARDS

✓ SPECIALTY EXCELLENCE
· PULMONARY CARE

Milton S. Hershey Medical Center

500 University Drive
Hershey, PA 17033
(717) 531-8521

Overall patient safety: ★
Teaching: Y

CLINICAL PROGRAM RATINGS:

CARDIAC	★★★	ORTHOPEDICS	★★★
CRITICAL CARE	NR	PULMONARY	★★★
GASTROINTESTINAL	★★★	STROKE	★★★★★
GENERAL SURGERY	★★★	VASCULAR	★★★
MATERNITY CARE	★	WOMEN'S HEALTH	★★★

HEALTHGRADES AWARDS

✓ SPECIALTY EXCELLENCE
· STROKE CARE

Mid-Valley Hospital

1400 South Main Street
Peckville, PA 18452
(570) 383-5600

Overall patient safety: ★★★
Teaching: N

CLINICAL PROGRAM RATINGS:

CARDIAC	NR	ORTHOPEDICS	NR
CRITICAL CARE	NR	PULMONARY	★★★
GASTROINTESTINAL	NR	STROKE	★★★
GENERAL SURGERY	NR	VASCULAR	NR
MATERNITY CARE	NR	WOMEN'S HEALTH	NR

HEALTHGRADES AWARDS

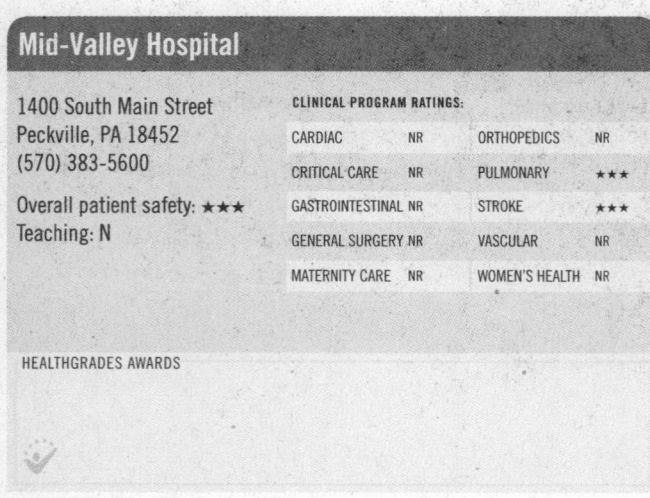

Miners Medical Center

290 Haida Avenue
Hastings, PA 16646
(814) 247-3100

Overall patient safety: ★★★
Teaching: N

CLINICAL PROGRAM RATINGS:

CARDIAC	NR	ORTHOPEDICS	NR
CRITICAL CARE	NR	PULMONARY	★★★
GASTROINTESTINAL	NR	STROKE	NR
GENERAL SURGERY	NR	VASCULAR	NR
MATERNITY CARE	NR	WOMEN'S HEALTH	NR

HEALTHGRADES AWARDS

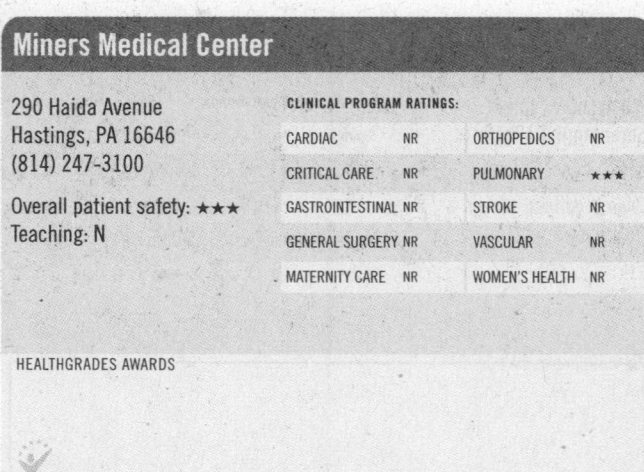

Millcreek Community Hospital

5515 Peach Street
Erie, PA 16509
(814) 864-4031

Overall patient safety: ★★★
Teaching: Y

CLINICAL PROGRAM RATINGS:

CARDIAC	NR	ORTHOPEDICS	NR
CRITICAL CARE	NR	PULMONARY	★
GASTROINTESTINAL	NR	STROKE	★★★
GENERAL SURGERY	NR	VASCULAR	NR
MATERNITY CARE	★★★	WOMEN'S HEALTH	NR

HEALTHGRADES AWARDS

Monongahela Valley Hospital

1163 Country Club Road
Monongahela, PA 15063
(724) 258-1000

Overall patient safety: ★★★
Teaching: N

CLINICAL PROGRAM RATINGS:

CARDIAC	NR	ORTHOPEDICS	NR
CRITICAL CARE	NR	PULMONARY	★★★
GASTROINTESTINAL	★★★	STROKE	★
GENERAL SURGERY	★★★	VASCULAR	NR
MATERNITY CARE	★★★	WOMEN'S HEALTH	NR

HEALTHGRADES AWARDS

KEY: ★★★★★ BEST   ★★★ AS EXPECTED   ★ POOR   NR NOT RATED BY HEALTHGRADES   For full definitions of ratings and awards, see Appendix.

Montgomery Hospital

1301 Powell Street
Norristown, PA 19401
(610) 270-2000

Overall patient safety: ★★★
Teaching: Y

CLINICAL PROGRAM RATINGS:

CARDIAC	NR	ORTHOPEDICS	NR
CRITICAL CARE	NR	PULMONARY	★
GASTROINTESTINAL	NR	STROKE	★
GENERAL SURGERY	★★★	VASCULAR	NR
MATERNITY CARE	★★★	WOMEN'S HEALTH	NR

HEALTHGRADES AWARDS

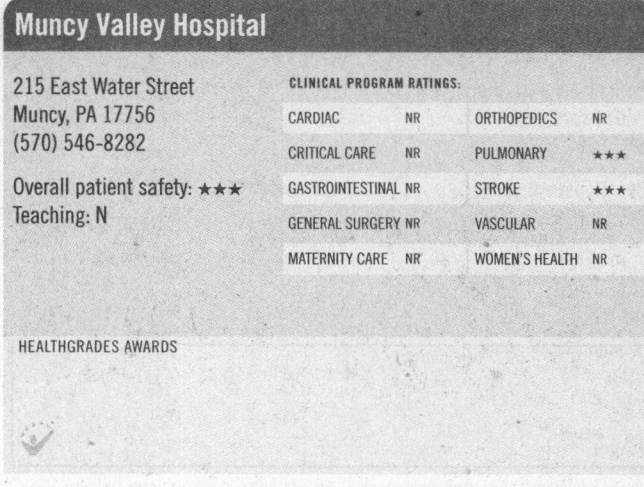

Muncy Valley Hospital

215 East Water Street
Muncy, PA 17756
(570) 546-8282

Overall patient safety: ★★★
Teaching: N

CLINICAL PROGRAM RATINGS:

CARDIAC	NR	ORTHOPEDICS	NR
CRITICAL CARE	NR	PULMONARY	★★★
GASTROINTESTINAL	NR	STROKE	★★★
GENERAL SURGERY	NR	VASCULAR	NR
MATERNITY CARE	NR	WOMEN'S HEALTH	NR

HEALTHGRADES AWARDS

Moses Taylor Hospital

700 Quincy Avenue
Scranton, PA 18510
(570) 340-2100

Overall patient safety: ★★★
Teaching: Y

CLINICAL PROGRAM RATINGS:

CARDIAC	NR	ORTHOPEDICS	NR
CRITICAL CARE	NR	PULMONARY	★★★
GASTROINTESTINAL	★★★	STROKE	★★★
GENERAL SURGERY	★★★	VASCULAR	NR
MATERNITY CARE	★★★	WOMEN'S HEALTH	NR

HEALTHGRADES AWARDS

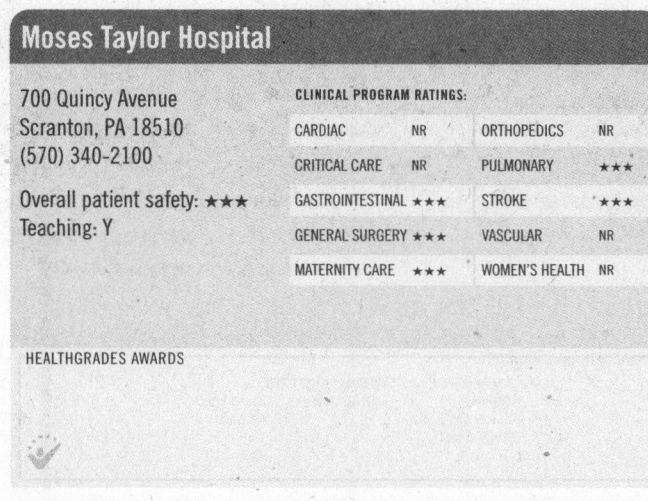

Nason Hospital

105 Nason Drive
Roaring Spring, PA 16673
(814) 224-2141

Overall patient safety: ★★★
Teaching: N

CLINICAL PROGRAM RATINGS:

CARDIAC	NR	ORTHOPEDICS	NR
CRITICAL CARE	NR	PULMONARY	★
GASTROINTESTINAL	NR	STROKE	★★★
GENERAL SURGERY	NR	VASCULAR	NR
MATERNITY CARE	★★★	WOMEN'S HEALTH	NR

HEALTHGRADES AWARDS

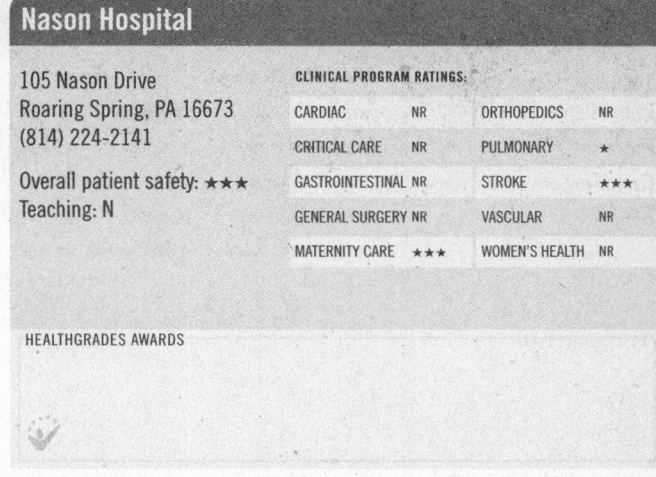

Mount Nittany Medical Center

1800 East Park Avenue
State College, PA 16803
(814) 231-7000

Overall patient safety: ★★★
Teaching: N

CLINICAL PROGRAM RATINGS:

CARDIAC	NR	ORTHOPEDICS	★★★
CRITICAL CARE	NR	PULMONARY	★★★
GASTROINTESTINAL	★★★	STROKE	★
GENERAL SURGERY	★★★	VASCULAR	NR
MATERNITY CARE	★★★	WOMEN'S HEALTH	NR

HEALTHGRADES AWARDS

Nazareth Hospital

2601 Holme Avenue
Philadelphia, PA 19152
(215) 335-6000

Overall patient safety: ★★★
Teaching: N

CLINICAL PROGRAM RATINGS:

CARDIAC	NR	ORTHOPEDICS	★★★
CRITICAL CARE	NR	PULMONARY	★★★
GASTROINTESTINAL	★★★	STROKE	★★★★★
GENERAL SURGERY	★★★	VASCULAR	NR
MATERNITY CARE	NR	WOMEN'S HEALTH	NR

HEALTHGRADES AWARDS

✓ SPECIALTY EXCELLENCE
· JOINT REPLACEMENT   · STROKE CARE

*This hospital reports its data to the federal government jointly with another hospital. Therefore the ratings and awards apply to multiple hospitals and this specific hospital may not provide all rated services.

North Philadelphia Health System*

16th Street and Girard Avenue
Philadelphia, PA 19122
(215) 787-2000

Overall patient safety: ★
Teaching: Y

CLINICAL PROGRAM RATINGS:

CARDIAC	NR	ORTHOPEDICS	NR
CRITICAL CARE	NR	PULMONARY	★★★
GASTROINTESTINAL	NR	STROKE	★
GENERAL SURGERY	NR	VASCULAR	NR
MATERNITY CARE	NR	WOMEN'S HEALTH	NR

HEALTHGRADES AWARDS

Palmerton Hospital

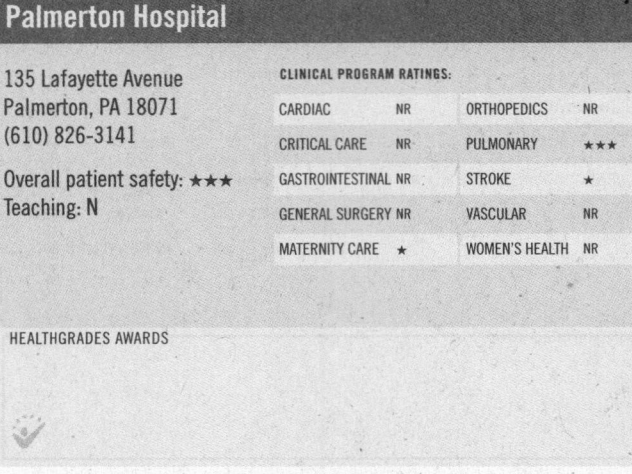

135 Lafayette Avenue
Palmerton, PA 18071
(610) 826-3141

Overall patient safety: ★★★
Teaching: N

CLINICAL PROGRAM RATINGS:

CARDIAC	NR	ORTHOPEDICS	NR
CRITICAL CARE	NR	PULMONARY	★★★
GASTROINTESTINAL	NR	STROKE	★
GENERAL SURGERY	NR	VASCULAR	NR
MATERNITY CARE	★	WOMEN'S HEALTH	NR

HEALTHGRADES AWARDS

Northeastern Hospital

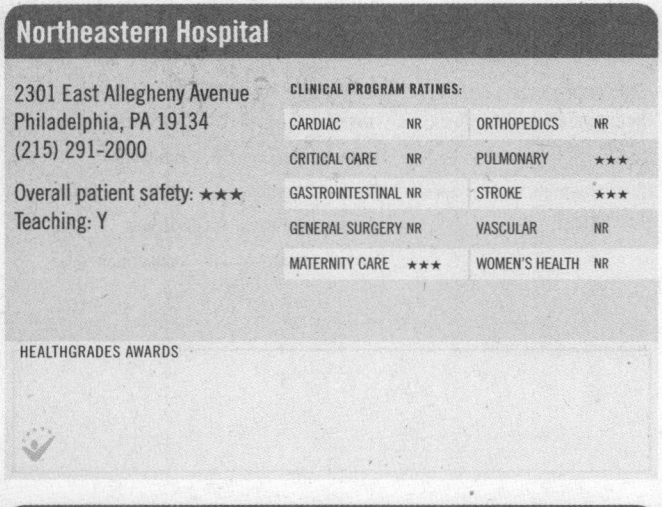

2301 East Allegheny Avenue
Philadelphia, PA 19134
(215) 291-2000

Overall patient safety: ★★★
Teaching: Y

CLINICAL PROGRAM RATINGS:

CARDIAC	NR	ORTHOPEDICS	NR
CRITICAL CARE	NR	PULMONARY	★★★
GASTROINTESTINAL	NR	STROKE	★★★
GENERAL SURGERY	NR	VASCULAR	NR
MATERNITY CARE	★★★	WOMEN'S HEALTH	NR

HEALTHGRADES AWARDS

Pennsylvania Hospital

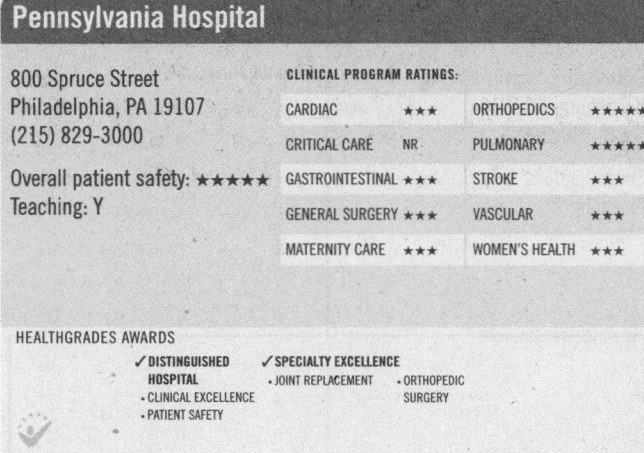

800 Spruce Street
Philadelphia, PA 19107
(215) 829-3000

Overall patient safety: ★★★★★
Teaching: Y

CLINICAL PROGRAM RATINGS:

CARDIAC	★★★	ORTHOPEDICS	★★★★★
CRITICAL CARE	NR	PULMONARY	★★★★★
GASTROINTESTINAL	★★★	STROKE	★★★
GENERAL SURGERY	★★★	VASCULAR	★★★
MATERNITY CARE	★★★	WOMEN'S HEALTH	★★★

HEALTHGRADES AWARDS

✓ **DISTINGUISHED HOSPITAL**
· CLINICAL EXCELLENCE
· PATIENT SAFETY

✓ **SPECIALTY EXCELLENCE**
· JOINT REPLACEMENT
· ORTHOPEDIC SURGERY

Ohio Valley General Hospital

25 Heckel Road
McKees Rocks, PA 15136
(412) 777-6161

Overall patient safety: ★★★★★
Teaching: N

CLINICAL PROGRAM RATINGS:

CARDIAC	NR	ORTHOPEDICS	NR
CRITICAL CARE	NR	PULMONARY	★
GASTROINTESTINAL	NR	STROKE	★★★
GENERAL SURGERY	NR	VASCULAR	NR
MATERNITY CARE	★★★	WOMEN'S HEALTH	NR

HEALTHGRADES AWARDS

Pennsylvania Presbyterian Medical Center

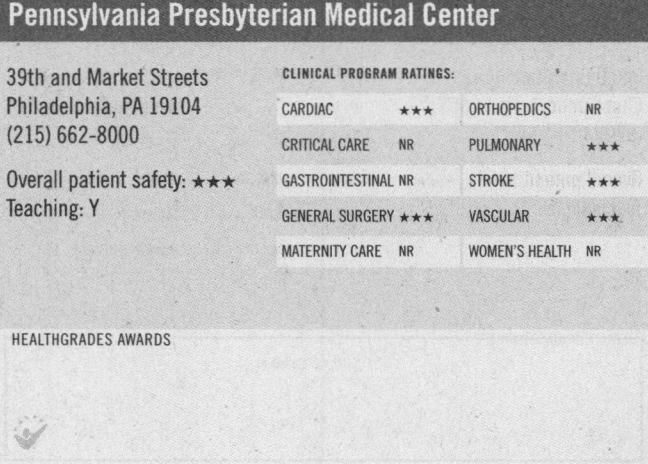

39th and Market Streets
Philadelphia, PA 19104
(215) 662-8000

Overall patient safety: ★★★
Teaching: Y

CLINICAL PROGRAM RATINGS:

CARDIAC	★★★	ORTHOPEDICS	NR
CRITICAL CARE	NR	PULMONARY	★★★
GASTROINTESTINAL	NR	STROKE	★★★
GENERAL SURGERY	★★★	VASCULAR	★★★
MATERNITY CARE	NR	WOMEN'S HEALTH	NR

HEALTHGRADES AWARDS

KEY: ★★★★★ BEST   ★★★ AS EXPECTED   ★ POOR   NR NOT RATED BY HEALTHGRADES   For full definitions of ratings and awards, see Appendix.

PENNSYLVANIA HOSPITALS: RATINGS BY CLINICAL SPECIALTY

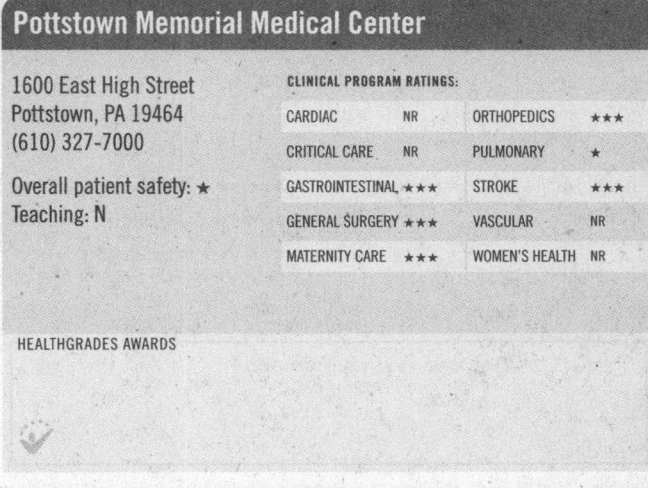

Phoenixville Hospital

140 Nutt Road
Phoenixville, PA 19460
(610) 983-1000

Overall patient safety: ★
Teaching: N

CLINICAL PROGRAM RATINGS:

CARDIAC	★★★	ORTHOPEDICS	NR
CRITICAL CARE	NR	PULMONARY	★★★
GASTROINTESTINAL	★	STROKE	★★★
GENERAL SURGERY	★	VASCULAR	NR
MATERNITY CARE	★★★	WOMEN'S HEALTH	★★★

HEALTHGRADES AWARDS

✓ SPECIALTY EXCELLENCE
- CARDIAC SURGERY

Pottstown Memorial Medical Center

1600 East High Street
Pottstown, PA 19464
(610) 327-7000

Overall patient safety: ★
Teaching: N

CLINICAL PROGRAM RATINGS:

CARDIAC	NR	ORTHOPEDICS	★★★
CRITICAL CARE	NR	PULMONARY	★
GASTROINTESTINAL	★★★	STROKE	★★★
GENERAL SURGERY	★★★	VASCULAR	NR
MATERNITY CARE	★★★	WOMEN'S HEALTH	NR

HEALTHGRADES AWARDS

Pinnacle Health System

111 South Front Street
Harrisburg, PA 17104
(717) 231-8200

Overall patient safety: ★★★★★
Teaching: Y

CLINICAL PROGRAM RATINGS:

CARDIAC	★★★	ORTHOPEDICS	★★★
CRITICAL CARE	NR	PULMONARY	★★★★★
GASTROINTESTINAL	★★★	STROKE	★★★★★
GENERAL SURGERY	★★★	VASCULAR	★★★
MATERNITY CARE	★★★	WOMEN'S HEALTH	★★★

HEALTHGRADES AWARDS

✓ DISTINGUISHED HOSPITAL
- CLINICAL EXCELLENCE
- PATIENT SAFETY

✓ SPECIALTY EXCELLENCE
- GASTROINTESTINAL CARE
- STROKE CARE

Pottsville Hospital and Warne Clinic

420 South Jackson Street
Pottsville, PA 17901
(570) 621-5000

Overall patient safety: ★★★
Teaching: N

CLINICAL PROGRAM RATINGS:

CARDIAC	NR	ORTHOPEDICS	NR
CRITICAL CARE	NR	PULMONARY	★
GASTROINTESTINAL	★★★	STROKE	★
GENERAL SURGERY	★★★	VASCULAR	NR
MATERNITY CARE	★★★★★	WOMEN'S HEALTH	NR

HEALTHGRADES AWARDS

✓ SPECIALTY EXCELLENCE
- MATERNITY CARE

Pocono Medical Center

206 East Brown Street
East Stroudsburg, PA 18301
(570) 421-4000

Overall patient safety: ★★★
Teaching: N

CLINICAL PROGRAM RATINGS:

CARDIAC	NR	ORTHOPEDICS	NR
CRITICAL CARE	NR	PULMONARY	★★★
GASTROINTESTINAL	★★★	STROKE	★★★★★
GENERAL SURGERY	★★★	VASCULAR	★★★
MATERNITY CARE	★	WOMEN'S HEALTH	NR

HEALTHGRADES AWARDS

✓ SPECIALTY EXCELLENCE
- STROKE CARE

Punxsutawney Area Hospital

81 Hilcrest Drive
Punxsutawney, PA 15767
(814) 938-1800

Overall patient safety: ★★★
Teaching: N

CLINICAL PROGRAM RATINGS:

CARDIAC	NR	ORTHOPEDICS	NR
CRITICAL CARE	NR	PULMONARY	★★★
GASTROINTESTINAL	NR	STROKE	NR
GENERAL SURGERY	★★★	VASCULAR	NR
MATERNITY CARE	★★★	WOMEN'S HEALTH	NR

HEALTHGRADES AWARDS

*This hospital reports its data to the federal government jointly with another hospital. Therefore the ratings and awards apply to multiple hospitals and this specific hospital may not provide all rated services.

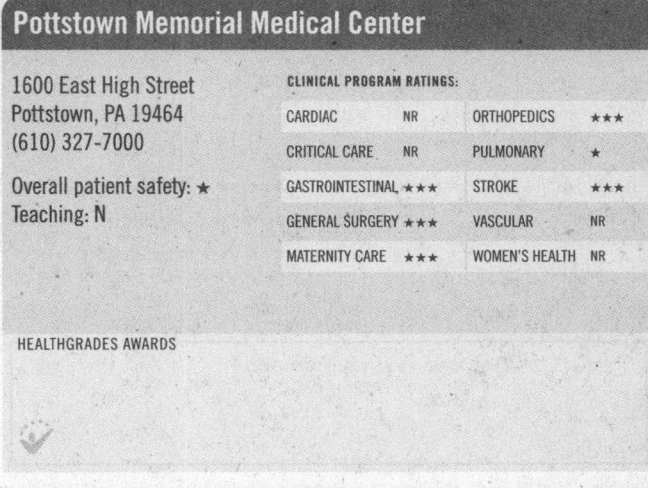

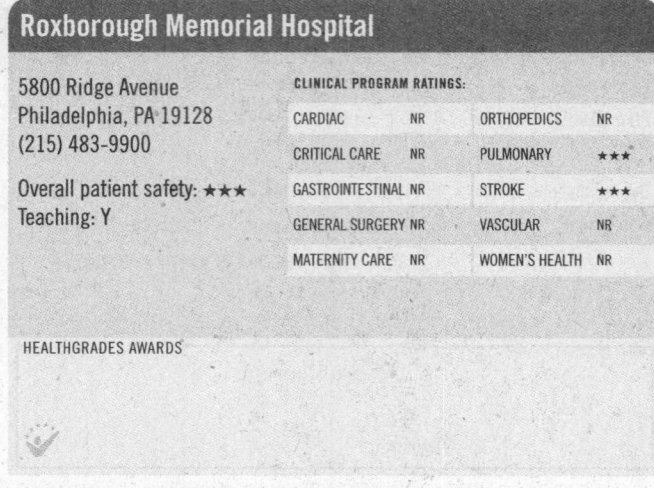

The Reading Hospital and Medical Center

6th Avenue and Spruce Street
West Reading, PA 19611
(610) 988-8000

Overall patient safety: ★★★★★
Teaching: Y

CLINICAL PROGRAM RATINGS:

CARDIAC	★★★	ORTHOPEDICS	★★★
CRITICAL CARE	NR	PULMONARY	★★★
GASTROINTESTINAL	★★★	STROKE	★★★★★
GENERAL SURGERY	★★★	VASCULAR	★★★
MATERNITY CARE	★★★	WOMEN'S HEALTH	★★★

HEALTHGRADES AWARDS

✓ DISTINGUISHED HOSPITAL
· PATIENT SAFETY

✓ SPECIALTY EXCELLENCE
· CARDIAC SURGERY   · STROKE CARE

Roxborough Memorial Hospital

5800 Ridge Avenue
Philadelphia, PA 19128
(215) 483-9900

Overall patient safety: ★★★
Teaching: Y

CLINICAL PROGRAM RATINGS:

CARDIAC	NR	ORTHOPEDICS	NR
CRITICAL CARE	NR	PULMONARY	★★★
GASTROINTESTINAL	NR	STROKE	★★★
GENERAL SURGERY	NR	VASCULAR	NR
MATERNITY CARE	NR	WOMEN'S HEALTH	NR

HEALTHGRADES AWARDS

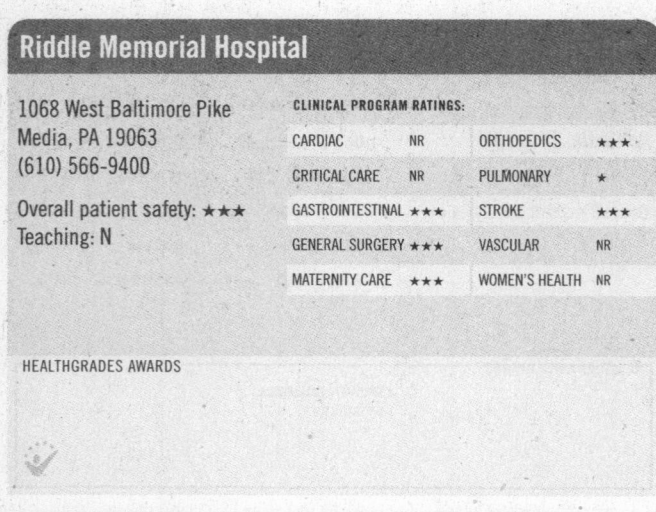

Riddle Memorial Hospital

1068 West Baltimore Pike
Media, PA 19063
(610) 566-9400

Overall patient safety: ★★★
Teaching: N

CLINICAL PROGRAM RATINGS:

CARDIAC	NR	ORTHOPEDICS	★★★
CRITICAL CARE	NR	PULMONARY	★
GASTROINTESTINAL	★★★	STROKE	★★★
GENERAL SURGERY	★★★	VASCULAR	NR
MATERNITY CARE	★★★	WOMEN'S HEALTH	NR

HEALTHGRADES AWARDS

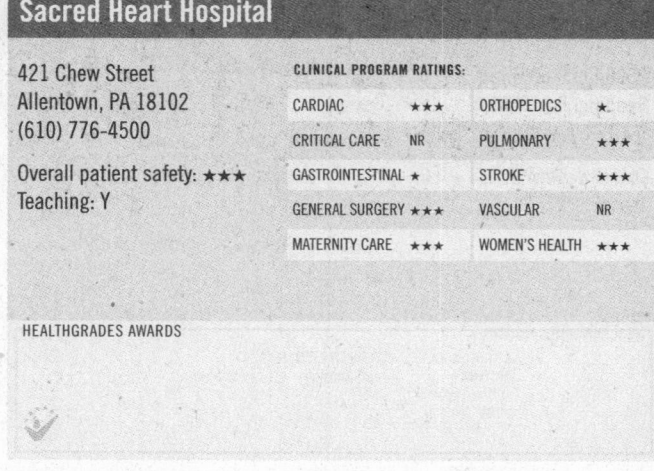

Sacred Heart Hospital

421 Chew Street
Allentown, PA 18102
(610) 776-4500

Overall patient safety: ★★★
Teaching: Y

CLINICAL PROGRAM RATINGS:

CARDIAC	★★★	ORTHOPEDICS	★
CRITICAL CARE	NR	PULMONARY	★★★
GASTROINTESTINAL	★	STROKE	★★★
GENERAL SURGERY	★★★	VASCULAR	NR
MATERNITY CARE	★★★	WOMEN'S HEALTH	★★★

HEALTHGRADES AWARDS

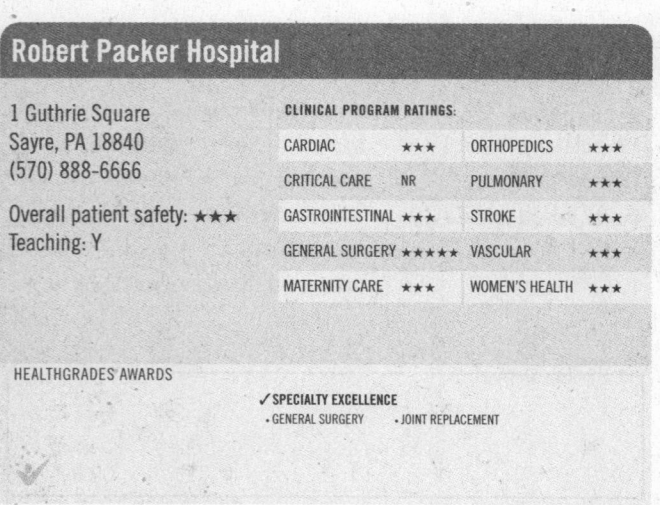

Robert Packer Hospital

1 Guthrie Square
Sayre, PA 18840
(570) 888-6666

Overall patient safety: ★★★
Teaching: Y

CLINICAL PROGRAM RATINGS:

CARDIAC	★★★	ORTHOPEDICS	★★★
CRITICAL CARE	NR	PULMONARY	★★★
GASTROINTESTINAL	★★★	STROKE	★★★
GENERAL SURGERY	★★★★★	VASCULAR	★★★
MATERNITY CARE	★★★	WOMEN'S HEALTH	★★★

HEALTHGRADES AWARDS

✓ SPECIALTY EXCELLENCE
· GENERAL SURGERY   · JOINT REPLACEMENT

St. Catherine Medical Center—Fountain Springs

101 Broad Street
Ashland, PA 17921
(570) 875-2000

Overall patient safety: NR
Teaching: N

CLINICAL PROGRAM RATINGS:

CARDIAC	NR	ORTHOPEDICS	NR
CRITICAL CARE	NR	PULMONARY	★
GASTROINTESTINAL	NR	STROKE	NR
GENERAL SURGERY	NR	VASCULAR	NR
MATERNITY CARE	NR	WOMEN'S HEALTH	NR

HEALTHGRADES AWARDS

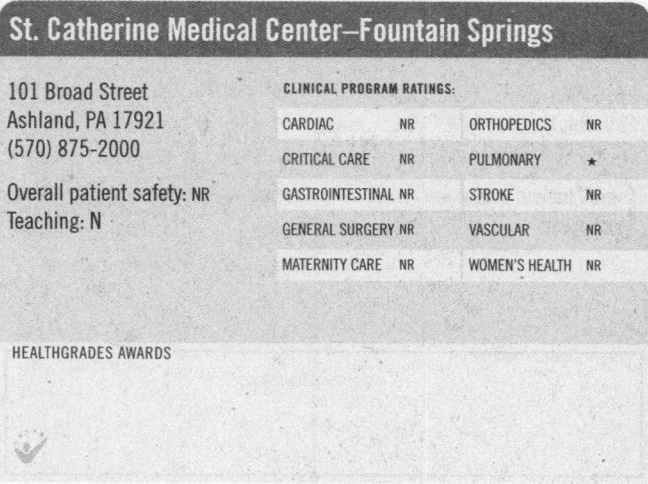

KEY: ★★★★★ BEST ★★★ AS EXPECTED ★ POOR NR NOT RATED BY HEALTHGRADES For full definitions of ratings and awards, see Appendix.

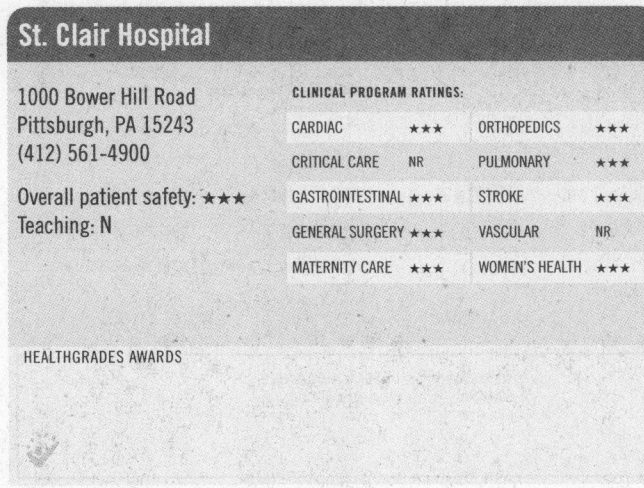

St. Clair Hospital

1000 Bower Hill Road
Pittsburgh, PA 15243
(412) 561-4900

Overall patient safety: ★★★
Teaching: N

CLINICAL PROGRAM RATINGS:

CARDIAC	★★★	ORTHOPEDICS	★★★
CRITICAL CARE	NR	PULMONARY	★★★
GASTROINTESTINAL	★★★	STROKE	★★★
GENERAL SURGERY	★★★	VASCULAR	NR
MATERNITY CARE	★★★	WOMEN'S HEALTH	★★★

HEALTHGRADES AWARDS

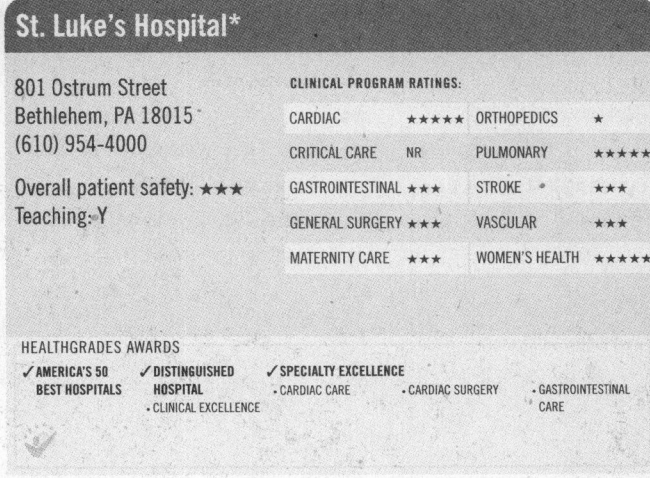

St. Luke's Hospital*

801 Ostrum Street
Bethlehem, PA 18015
(610) 954-4000

Overall patient safety: ★★★
Teaching: Y

CLINICAL PROGRAM RATINGS:

CARDIAC	★★★★★	ORTHOPEDICS	★
CRITICAL CARE	NR	PULMONARY	★★★★★
GASTROINTESTINAL	★★★	STROKE	★★★
GENERAL SURGERY	★★★	VASCULAR	★★★
MATERNITY CARE	★★★	WOMEN'S HEALTH	★★★★★

HEALTHGRADES AWARDS

✓ AMERICA'S 50 BEST HOSPITALS   ✓ DISTINGUISHED HOSPITAL   ✓ SPECIALTY EXCELLENCE
• CLINICAL EXCELLENCE   • CARDIAC CARE   • CARDIAC SURGERY   • GASTROINTESTINAL CARE

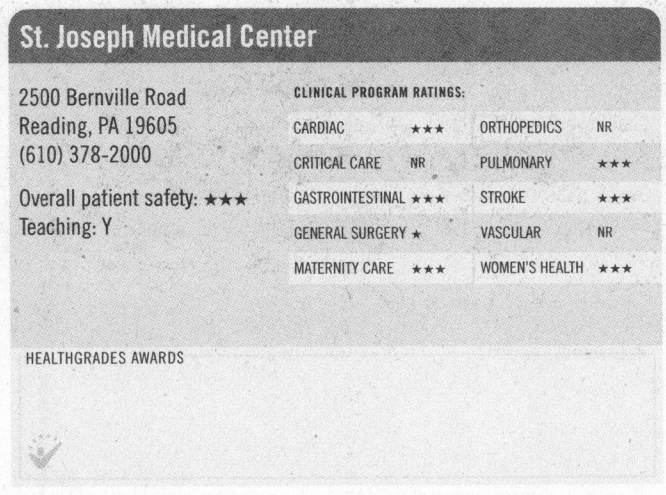

St. Joseph Medical Center

2500 Bernville Road
Reading, PA 19605
(610) 378-2000

Overall patient safety: ★★★
Teaching: Y

CLINICAL PROGRAM RATINGS:

CARDIAC	★★★	ORTHOPEDICS	NR
CRITICAL CARE	NR	PULMONARY	★★★
GASTROINTESTINAL	★★★	STROKE	★★★
GENERAL SURGERY	★	VASCULAR	NR
MATERNITY CARE	★★★	WOMEN'S HEALTH	★★★

HEALTHGRADES AWARDS

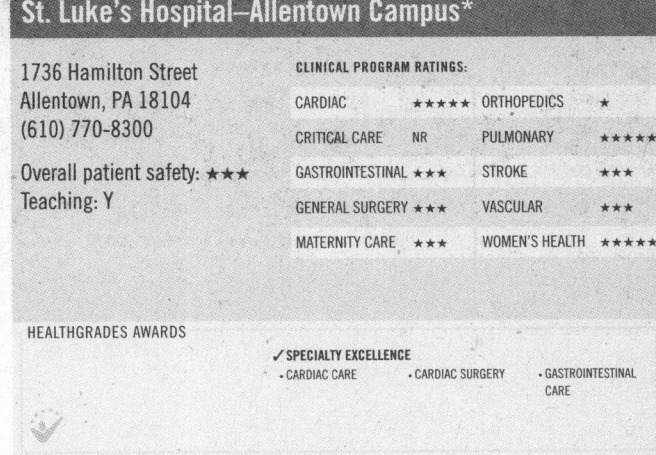

St. Luke's Hospital—Allentown Campus*

1736 Hamilton Street
Allentown, PA 18104
(610) 770-8300

Overall patient safety: ★★★
Teaching: Y

CLINICAL PROGRAM RATINGS:

CARDIAC	★★★★★	ORTHOPEDICS	★
CRITICAL CARE	NR	PULMONARY	★★★★★
GASTROINTESTINAL	★★★	STROKE	★★★
GENERAL SURGERY	★★★	VASCULAR	★★★
MATERNITY CARE	★★★	WOMEN'S HEALTH	★★★★★

HEALTHGRADES AWARDS

✓ SPECIALTY EXCELLENCE
• CARDIAC CARE   • CARDIAC SURGERY   • GASTROINTESTINAL CARE

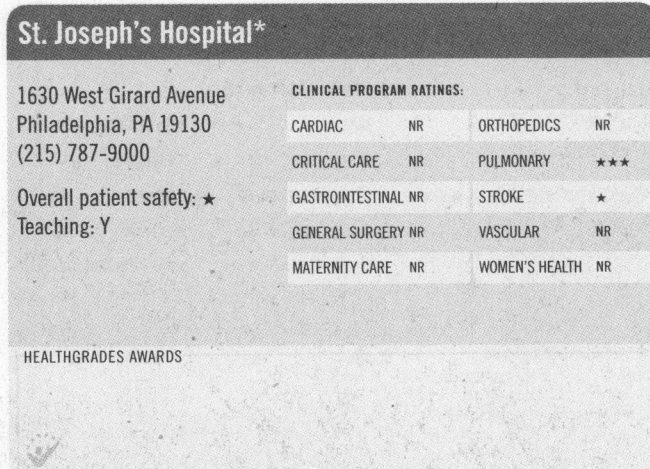

St. Joseph's Hospital*

1630 West Girard Avenue
Philadelphia, PA 19130
(215) 787-9000

Overall patient safety: ★
Teaching: Y

CLINICAL PROGRAM RATINGS:

CARDIAC	NR	ORTHOPEDICS	NR
CRITICAL CARE	NR	PULMONARY	★★★
GASTROINTESTINAL	NR	STROKE	★
GENERAL SURGERY	NR	VASCULAR	NR
MATERNITY CARE	NR	WOMEN'S HEALTH	NR

HEALTHGRADES AWARDS

St. Luke's Miners Memorial Hospital

360 West Ruddle Street
Coaldale, PA 18218
(570) 645-2131

Overall patient safety: ★★★
Teaching: N

CLINICAL PROGRAM RATINGS:

CARDIAC	NR	ORTHOPEDICS	NR
CRITICAL CARE	NR	PULMONARY	★★★★★
GASTROINTESTINAL	NR	STROKE	NR
GENERAL SURGERY	NR	VASCULAR	NR
MATERNITY CARE	NR	WOMEN'S HEALTH	NR

HEALTHGRADES AWARDS

*This hospital reports its data to the federal government jointly with another hospital. Therefore the ratings and awards apply to multiple hospitals and this specific hospital may not provide all rated services.

St. Luke's Quakertown Hospital

1021 Park Avenue
Quakertown, PA 18951
(215) 538-4500

Overall patient safety: ★★★
Teaching: N

CLINICAL PROGRAM RATINGS:

CARDIAC	NR	ORTHOPEDICS	★★★
CRITICAL CARE	NR	PULMONARY	★★★
GASTROINTESTINAL	NR	STROKE	★
GENERAL SURGERY	★★★	VASCULAR	NR
MATERNITY CARE	NR	WOMEN'S HEALTH	NR

HEALTHGRADES AWARDS

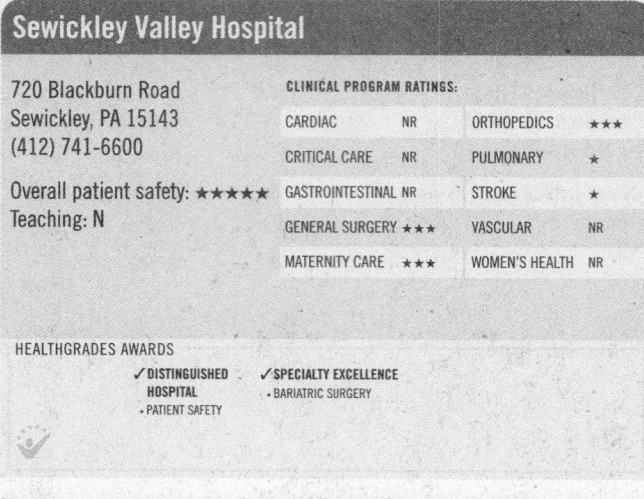

Sewickley Valley Hospital

720 Blackburn Road
Sewickley, PA 15143
(412) 741-6600

Overall patient safety: ★★★★★
Teaching: N

CLINICAL PROGRAM RATINGS:

CARDIAC	NR	ORTHOPEDICS	★★★
CRITICAL CARE	NR	PULMONARY	★
GASTROINTESTINAL	NR	STROKE	★
GENERAL SURGERY	★★★	VASCULAR	NR
MATERNITY CARE	★★★	WOMEN'S HEALTH	NR

HEALTHGRADES AWARDS

✓ DISTINGUISHED HOSPITAL
- PATIENT SAFETY

✓ SPECIALTY EXCELLENCE
- BARIATRIC SURGERY

St. Mary Medical Center

1201 Langhorne Newtown Road
Langhorne, PA 19047
(215) 710-2000

Overall patient safety: ★★★
Teaching: N

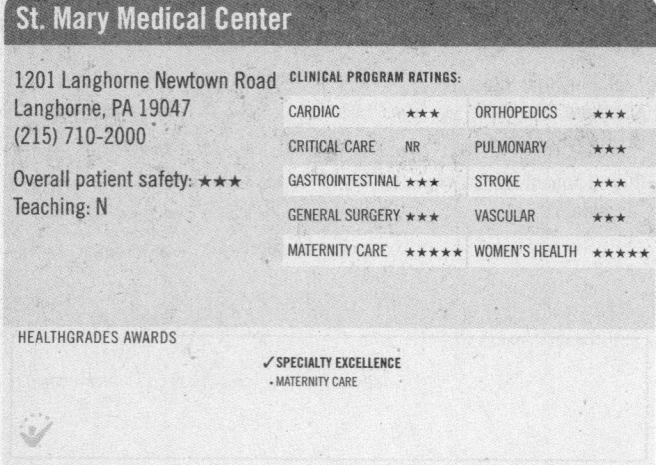

CLINICAL PROGRAM RATINGS:

CARDIAC	★★★	ORTHOPEDICS	★★★
CRITICAL CARE	NR	PULMONARY	★★★
GASTROINTESTINAL	★★★	STROKE	★★★
GENERAL SURGERY	★★★	VASCULAR	★★★
MATERNITY CARE	★★★★★	WOMEN'S HEALTH	★★★★★

HEALTHGRADES AWARDS

✓ SPECIALTY EXCELLENCE
- MATERNITY CARE

Shamokin Area Community Hospital

4200 Hospital Road
Coal Township, PA 17866
(570) 644-4200

Overall patient safety: ★★★
Teaching: N

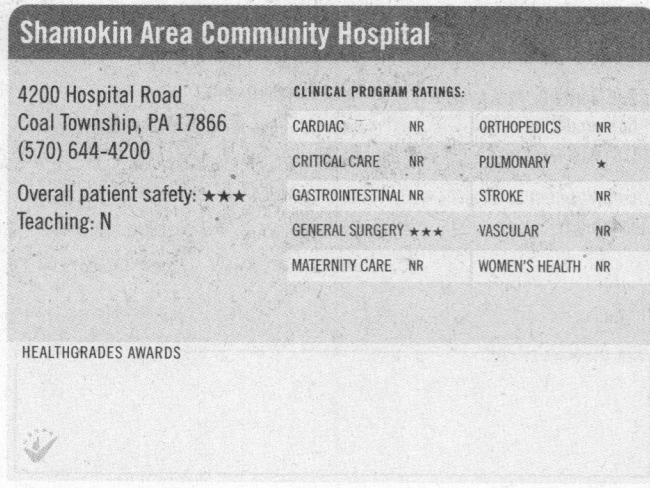

CLINICAL PROGRAM RATINGS:

CARDIAC	NR	ORTHOPEDICS	NR
CRITICAL CARE	NR	PULMONARY	★
GASTROINTESTINAL	NR	STROKE	NR
GENERAL SURGERY	★★★	VASCULAR	NR
MATERNITY CARE	NR	WOMEN'S HEALTH	NR

HEALTHGRADES AWARDS

St. Vincent Health Center

232 West 25th Street
Erie, PA 16544
(814) 452-5000

Overall patient safety: ★★★
Teaching: Y

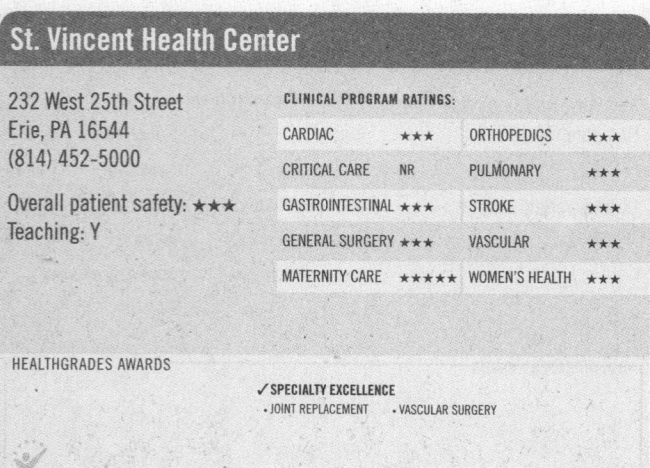

CLINICAL PROGRAM RATINGS:

CARDIAC	★★★	ORTHOPEDICS	★★★
CRITICAL CARE	NR	PULMONARY	★★★
GASTROINTESTINAL	★★★	STROKE	★★★
GENERAL SURGERY	★★★	VASCULAR	★★★
MATERNITY CARE	★★★★★	WOMEN'S HEALTH	★★★

HEALTHGRADES AWARDS

✓ SPECIALTY EXCELLENCE
- JOINT REPLACEMENT   - VASCULAR SURGERY

Sharon Regional Health System

740 East State Street
Sharon, PA 16146
(724) 983-3911

Overall patient safety: ★★★★★
Teaching: N

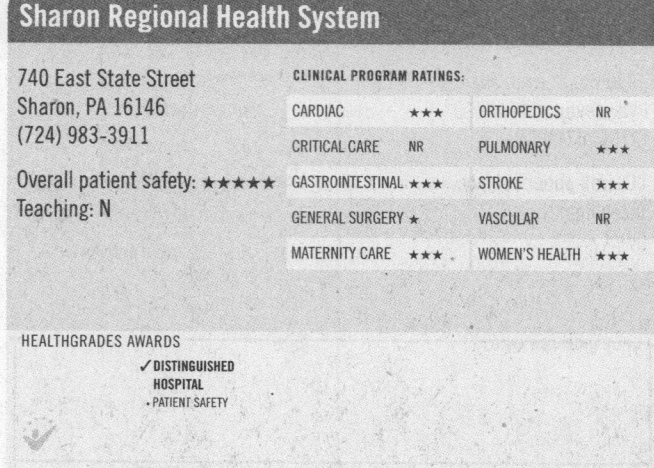

CLINICAL PROGRAM RATINGS:

CARDIAC	★★★	ORTHOPEDICS	NR
CRITICAL CARE	NR	PULMONARY	★★★
GASTROINTESTINAL	★★★	STROKE	★★★
GENERAL SURGERY	★	VASCULAR	NR
MATERNITY CARE	★★★	WOMEN'S HEALTH	★★★

HEALTHGRADES AWARDS

✓ DISTINGUISHED HOSPITAL
- PATIENT SAFETY

KEY: ★★★★★ BEST   ★★★ AS EXPECTED   ★ POOR   NR NOT RATED BY HEALTHGRADES   For full definitions of ratings and awards, see Appendix.

Soldiers and Sailors Memorial Hospital

32-36 Central Avenue
Wellsboro, PA 16901
(570) 723-7764

Overall patient safety: ★★★
Teaching: N

CLINICAL PROGRAM RATINGS:

CARDIAC	NR	ORTHOPEDICS	NR
CRITICAL CARE	NR	PULMONARY	★
GASTROINTESTINAL	NR	STROKE	★
GENERAL SURGERY	★★★	VASCULAR	NR
MATERNITY CARE	★★★	WOMEN'S HEALTH	NR

HEALTHGRADES AWARDS

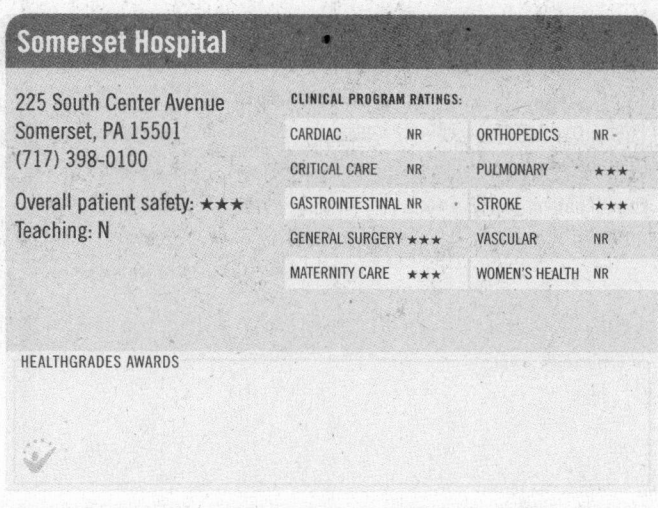

Springfield Hospital*

190 Sproul Road
Springfield, PA 19064
(215) 328-8700

Overall patient safety: ★
Teaching: Y

CLINICAL PROGRAM RATINGS:

CARDIAC	★★★	ORTHOPEDICS	★★★
CRITICAL CARE	NR	PULMONARY	★
GASTROINTESTINAL	★★★	STROKE	★★★
GENERAL SURGERY	★★★	VASCULAR	★★★
MATERNITY CARE	★	WOMEN'S HEALTH	★★★

HEALTHGRADES AWARDS

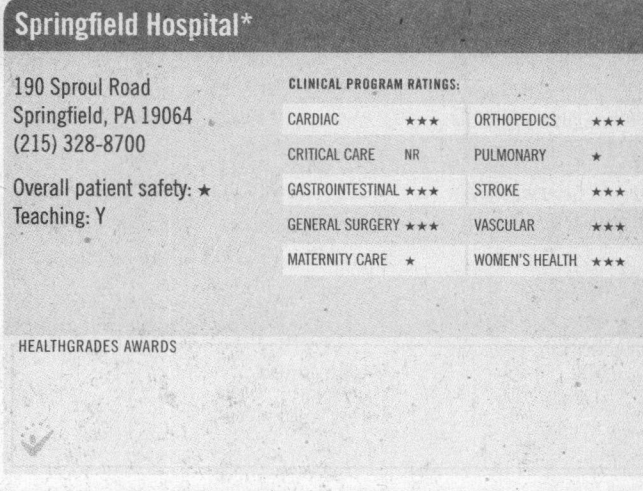

Somerset Hospital

225 South Center Avenue
Somerset, PA 15501
(717) 398-0100

Overall patient safety: ★★★
Teaching: N

CLINICAL PROGRAM RATINGS:

CARDIAC	NR	ORTHOPEDICS	NR
CRITICAL CARE	NR	PULMONARY	★★★
GASTROINTESTINAL	NR	STROKE	★★★
GENERAL SURGERY	★★★	VASCULAR	NR
MATERNITY CARE	★★★	WOMEN'S HEALTH	NR

HEALTHGRADES AWARDS

Sunbury Community Hospital

350 North 11th Street
Sunbury, PA 17801
(570) 286-3333

Overall patient safety: ★★★★★
Teaching: N

CLINICAL PROGRAM RATINGS:

CARDIAC	NR	ORTHOPEDICS	NR
CRITICAL CARE	NR	PULMONARY	★★★
GASTROINTESTINAL	NR	STROKE	★★★
GENERAL SURGERY	★★★	VASCULAR	NR
MATERNITY CARE	NR	WOMEN'S HEALTH	NR

HEALTHGRADES AWARDS

Southwest Regional Medical Center

350 Bonar Avenue
Waynesburg, PA 15370
(724) 627-3101

Overall patient safety: ★★★
Teaching: N

CLINICAL PROGRAM RATINGS:

CARDIAC	NR	ORTHOPEDICS	NR
CRITICAL CARE	NR	PULMONARY	★★★
GASTROINTESTINAL	NR	STROKE	★★★
GENERAL SURGERY	NR	VASCULAR	NR
MATERNITY CARE	NR	WOMEN'S HEALTH	NR

HEALTHGRADES AWARDS

Temple University Hospital

3401 North Broad Street
Philadelphia, PA 19140
(215) 707-2000

Overall patient safety: ★
Teaching: Y

CLINICAL PROGRAM RATINGS:

CARDIAC	★★★	ORTHOPEDICS	★★★
CRITICAL CARE	NR	PULMONARY	★★★
GASTROINTESTINAL	NR	STROKE	★★★
GENERAL SURGERY	NR	VASCULAR	NR
MATERNITY CARE	★	WOMEN'S HEALTH	★

HEALTHGRADES AWARDS

*This hospital reports its data to the federal government jointly with another hospital. Therefore the ratings and awards apply to multiple hospitals and this specific hospital may not provide all rated services.

Thomas Jefferson University Hospital*

111 South 11th Street
Philadelphia, PA 19107
(215) 955-6000

Overall patient safety: ★
Teaching: Y

CLINICAL PROGRAM RATINGS:

CARDIAC	★★★	ORTHOPEDICS	★★★
CRITICAL CARE	NR	PULMONARY	★★★★★
GASTROINTESTINAL	★★★	STROKE	★★★
GENERAL SURGERY	★★★	VASCULAR	NR
MATERNITY CARE	★	WOMEN'S HEALTH	★★★

HEALTHGRADES AWARDS

✓ SPECIALTY EXCELLENCE
- PULMONARY CARE

Tyler Memorial Hospital

880 SR 6 West
Tunkhannock, PA 18657
(570) 836-2161

Overall patient safety: ★★★
Teaching: N

CLINICAL PROGRAM RATINGS:

CARDIAC	NR	ORTHOPEDICS	NR
CRITICAL CARE	NR	PULMONARY	★★★
GASTROINTESTINAL	NR	STROKE	★★★
GENERAL SURGERY	NR	VASCULAR	NR
MATERNITY CARE	★★★	WOMEN'S HEALTH	NR

HEALTHGRADES AWARDS

Titusville Hospital

406 West Oak Street
Titusville, PA 16354
(814) 827-1851

Overall patient safety: ★★★
Teaching: N

CLINICAL PROGRAM RATINGS:

CARDIAC	NR	ORTHOPEDICS	NR
CRITICAL CARE	NR	PULMONARY	★★★
GASTROINTESTINAL	NR	STROKE	★★★
GENERAL SURGERY	★★★	VASCULAR	NR
MATERNITY CARE	★★★	WOMEN'S HEALTH	NR

HEALTHGRADES AWARDS

Tyrone Hospital

1 Hospital Drive
Tyrone, PA 16686
(814) 684-1255

Overall patient safety: ★★★
Teaching: N

CLINICAL PROGRAM RATINGS:

CARDIAC	NR	ORTHOPEDICS	NR
CRITICAL CARE	NR	PULMONARY	★★★
GASTROINTESTINAL	NR	STROKE	★★★
GENERAL SURGERY	NR	VASCULAR	NR
MATERNITY CARE	★★★	WOMEN'S HEALTH	NR

HEALTHGRADES AWARDS

Troy Community Hospital

100 John Street
Troy, PA 16947
(570) 297-2121

Overall patient safety: ★★★
Teaching: N

CLINICAL PROGRAM RATINGS:

CARDIAC	NR	ORTHOPEDICS	NR
CRITICAL CARE	NR	PULMONARY	★★★
GASTROINTESTINAL	NR	STROKE	NR
GENERAL SURGERY	NR	VASCULAR	NR
MATERNITY CARE	NR	WOMEN'S HEALTH	NR

HEALTHGRADES AWARDS

Uniontown Hospital

500 West Berkeley Street
Uniontown, PA 15401
(724) 430-5000

Overall patient safety: ★★★
Teaching: N

CLINICAL PROGRAM RATINGS:

CARDIAC	NR	ORTHOPEDICS	NR
CRITICAL CARE	NR	PULMONARY	★★★
GASTROINTESTINAL	★★★	STROKE	★★★
GENERAL SURGERY	★★★★★	VASOULAR	NR
MATERNITY CARE	★★★	WOMEN'S HEALTH	NR

HEALTHGRADES AWARDS

✓ SPECIALTY EXCELLENCE
- GASTROINTESTINAL   - GENERAL SURGERY
  CARE

KEY: ★★★★★ BEST   ★★★ AS EXPECTED   ★ POOR   NR NOT RATED BY HEALTHGRADES   For full definitions of ratings and awards, see Appendix.

University of Pittsburgh Medical Center–Bedford

10455 Lincoln Highway
Everett, PA 15537
(814) 623-6161

Overall patient safety: ★★★
Teaching: N

CLINICAL PROGRAM RATINGS:

CARDIAC	NR	ORTHOPEDICS	NR
CRITICAL CARE	NR	PULMONARY	★★★
GASTROINTESTINAL	NR	STROKE	★★★
GENERAL SURGERY	NR	VASCULAR	NR
MATERNITY CARE	★★★	WOMEN'S HEALTH	NR

HEALTHGRADES AWARDS

University of Pittsburgh Medical Center–Horizon

110 North Main Street
Greenville, PA 16125
(724) 588-2100

Overall patient safety: ★★★
Teaching: Y

CLINICAL PROGRAM RATINGS:

CARDIAC	NR	ORTHOPEDICS	NR
CRITICAL CARE	★★★	PULMONARY	★★★
GASTROINTESTINAL	★★★	STROKE	★★★
GENERAL SURGERY	★★★	VASCULAR	NR
MATERNITY CARE	★★★	WOMEN'S HEALTH	NR

HEALTHGRADES AWARDS

University of Pittsburgh Medical Center–Braddock

400 Holland Avenue
Braddock, PA 15104
(412) 636-5000

Overall patient safety: ★★★
Teaching: N

CLINICAL PROGRAM RATINGS:

CARDIAC	NR	ORTHOPEDICS	NR
CRITICAL CARE	NR	PULMONARY	★★★
GASTROINTESTINAL	NR	STROKE	★★★
GENERAL SURGERY	★★★	VASCULAR	NR
MATERNITY CARE	NR	WOMEN'S HEALTH	NR

HEALTHGRADES AWARDS

University of Pittsburgh Medical Center–Lee

320 Main Street
Johnstown, PA 15901
(814) 533-0123

Overall patient safety: ★★★
Teaching: Y

CLINICAL PROGRAM RATINGS:

CARDIAC	★★★★★	ORTHOPEDICS	★★★
CRITICAL CARE	NR	PULMONARY	★★★
GASTROINTESTINAL	★★★	STROKE	★★★
GENERAL SURGERY	★★★	VASCULAR	NR
MATERNITY CARE	★★★	WOMEN'S HEALTH	★★★

HEALTHGRADES AWARDS

✓ SPECIALTY EXCELLENCE
 - CARDIAC CARE

University of Pittsburgh Medical Center–Cranberry*

1 St. Francis Way
Cranberry Township, PA 16066
(724) 772-5300

Overall patient safety: ★★★★★
Teaching: N

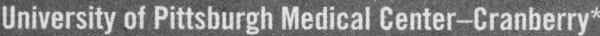

CLINICAL PROGRAM RATINGS:

CARDIAC	★★★	ORTHOPEDICS	★★★
CRITICAL CARE	★★★	PULMONARY	★★★
GASTROINTESTINAL	★★★	STROKE	★★★
GENERAL SURGERY	★	VASCULAR	NR
MATERNITY CARE	NR	WOMEN'S HEALTH	NR

HEALTHGRADES AWARDS

✓ DISTINGUISHED
 HOSPITAL
 - PATIENT SAFETY

University of Pittsburgh Medical Center–McKeesport

1500 5th Avenue
McKeesport, PA 15132
(412) 664-2000

Overall patient safety: ★★★
Teaching: Y

CLINICAL PROGRAM RATINGS:

CARDIAC	NR	ORTHOPEDICS	NR
CRITICAL CARE	★★★★★	PULMONARY	★★★★★
GASTROINTESTINAL	★★★	STROKE	★★★
GENERAL SURGERY	★★★	VASCULAR	NR
MATERNITY CARE	NR	WOMEN'S HEALTH	NR

HEALTHGRADES AWARDS

✓ SPECIALTY EXCELLENCE
 - CRITICAL CARE - PULMONARY CARE

*This hospital reports its data to the federal government jointly with another hospital. Therefore the ratings and awards apply to multiple hospitals and this specific hospital may not provide all rated services.

University of Pittsburgh Medical Center–Northwest*

100 Fairfield Drive
Seneca, PA 16346
(814) 676-7600

Overall patient safety: ★★★★★
Teaching: N

CLINICAL PROGRAM RATINGS:

CARDIAC	NR	ORTHOPEDICS	NR
CRITICAL CARE	★	PULMONARY	★★★
GASTROINTESTINAL	★★★	STROKE	★★★
GENERAL SURGERY	★★★	VASCULAR	NR
MATERNITY CARE	★★★	WOMEN'S HEALTH	NR

HEALTHGRADES AWARDS

✓ DISTINGUISHED HOSPITAL
• PATIENT SAFETY

University of Pittsburgh Medical Center–St. Margaret

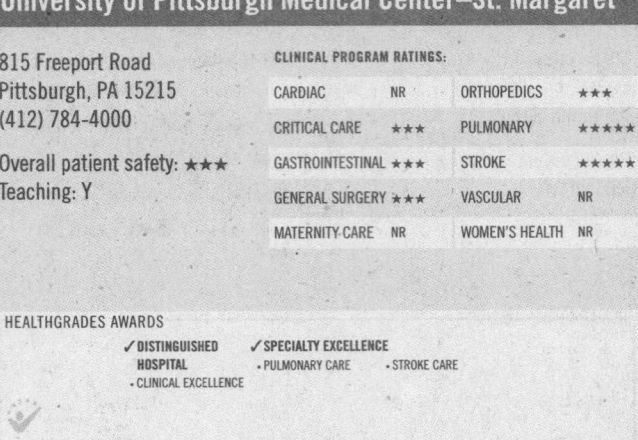

815 Freeport Road
Pittsburgh, PA 15215
(412) 784-4000

Overall patient safety: ★★★
Teaching: Y

CLINICAL PROGRAM RATINGS:

CARDIAC	NR	ORTHOPEDICS	★★★
CRITICAL CARE	★★★	PULMONARY	★★★★★
GASTROINTESTINAL	★★★	STROKE	★★★★★
GENERAL SURGERY	★★★	VASCULAR	NR
MATERNITY CARE	NR	WOMEN'S HEALTH	NR

HEALTHGRADES AWARDS

✓ DISTINGUISHED HOSPITAL
• CLINICAL EXCELLENCE

✓ SPECIALTY EXCELLENCE
• PULMONARY CARE   • STROKE CARE

University of Pittsburgh Medical Center–Passavant*

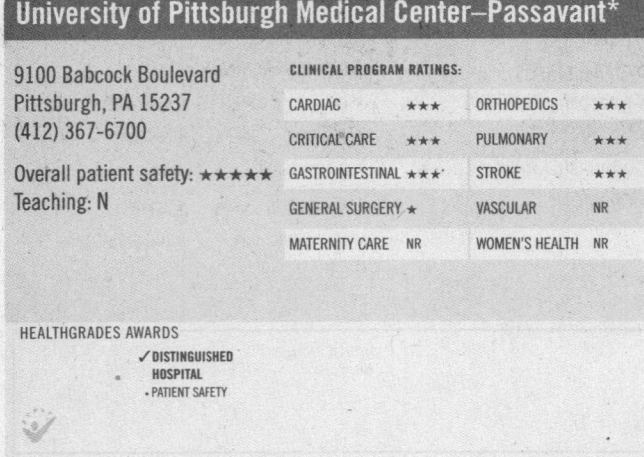

9100 Babcock Boulevard
Pittsburgh, PA 15237
(412) 367-6700

Overall patient safety: ★★★★★
Teaching: N

CLINICAL PROGRAM RATINGS:

CARDIAC	★★★	ORTHOPEDICS	★★★
CRITICAL CARE	★★★	PULMONARY	★★★
GASTROINTESTINAL	★★★	STROKE	★★★
GENERAL SURGERY	★	VASCULAR	NR
MATERNITY CARE	NR	WOMEN'S HEALTH	NR

HEALTHGRADES AWARDS

✓ DISTINGUISHED HOSPITAL
• PATIENT SAFETY

University of Pittsburgh Medical Center–Shadyside*

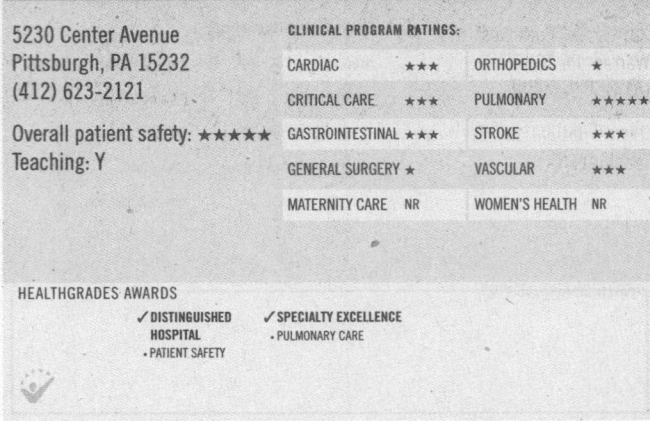

5230 Center Avenue
Pittsburgh, PA 15232
(412) 623-2121

Overall patient safety: ★★★★★
Teaching: Y

CLINICAL PROGRAM RATINGS:

CARDIAC	★★★	ORTHOPEDICS	★
CRITICAL CARE	★★★	PULMONARY	★★★★★
GASTROINTESTINAL	★★★	STROKE	★★★
GENERAL SURGERY	★	VASCULAR	★★★
MATERNITY CARE	NR	WOMEN'S HEALTH	NR

HEALTHGRADES AWARDS

✓ DISTINGUISHED HOSPITAL
• PATIENT SAFETY

✓ SPECIALTY EXCELLENCE
• PULMONARY CARE

University of Pittsburgh Med. Ctr.–Presbyterian Shadyside*

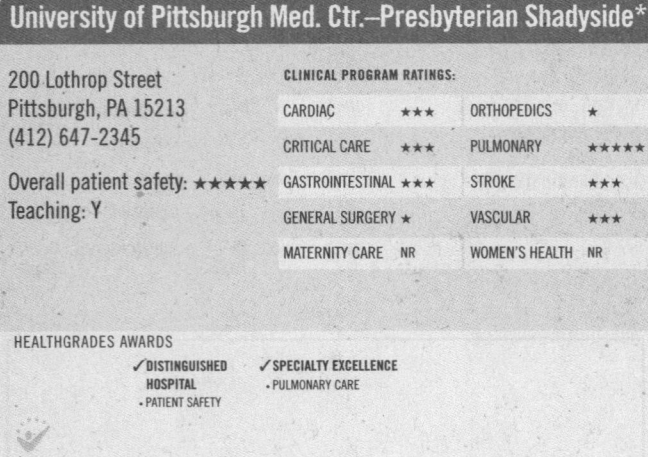

200 Lothrop Street
Pittsburgh, PA 15213
(412) 647-2345

Overall patient safety: ★★★★★
Teaching: Y

CLINICAL PROGRAM RATINGS:

CARDIAC	★★★	ORTHOPEDICS	★
CRITICAL CARE	★★★	PULMONARY	★★★★★
GASTROINTESTINAL	★★★	STROKE	★★★
GENERAL SURGERY	★	VASCULAR	★★★
MATERNITY CARE	NR	WOMEN'S HEALTH	NR

HEALTHGRADES AWARDS

✓ DISTINGUISHED HOSPITAL
• PATIENT SAFETY

✓ SPECIALTY EXCELLENCE
• PULMONARY CARE

University of Pittsburgh Medical Center–South Side

2000 Mary Street
Pittsburgh, PA 15203
(412) 488-5550

Overall patient safety: ★★★
Teaching: Y

CLINICAL PROGRAM RATINGS:

CARDIAC	NR	ORTHOPEDICS	NR
CRITICAL CARE	NR	PULMONARY	★★★
GASTROINTESTINAL	★★★	STROKE	★★★
GENERAL SURGERY	★★★	VASCULAR	NR
MATERNITY CARE	NR	WOMEN'S HEALTH	NR

HEALTHGRADES AWARDS

KEY: ★★★★★ BEST   ★★★ AS EXPECTED   ★ POOR   NR **NOT RATED BY HEALTHGRADES**   For full definitions of ratings and awards, see Appendix.

Warminster Hospital

225 Newtown Road
Warminster, PA 18974
(215) 441-6601

Overall patient safety: ★★★
Teaching: Y

CLINICAL PROGRAM RATINGS:

CARDIAC	NR	ORTHOPEDICS	NR
CRITICAL CARE	NR	PULMONARY	★★★
GASTROINTESTINAL	NR	STROKE	★★★
GENERAL SURGERY	NR	VASCULAR	NR
MATERNITY CARE	NR	WOMEN'S HEALTH	NR

HEALTHGRADES AWARDS

Wayne Memorial Hospital

601 Park Street
Honesdale, PA 18431
(570) 253-8100

Overall patient safety: ★★★
Teaching: N

CLINICAL PROGRAM RATINGS:

CARDIAC	NR	ORTHOPEDICS	NR
CRITICAL CARE	NR	PULMONARY	★★★
GASTROINTESTINAL	★★★	STROKE	★★★
GENERAL SURGERY	★★★	VASCULAR	NR
MATERNITY CARE	★★★	WOMEN'S HEALTH	NR

HEALTHGRADES AWARDS

Warren General Hospital

2 Crescent Park West
Warren, PA 16365
(814) 723-4973

Overall patient safety: ★★★
Teaching: N

CLINICAL PROGRAM RATINGS:

CARDIAC	NR	ORTHOPEDICS	NR
CRITICAL CARE	NR	PULMONARY	★★★
GASTROINTESTINAL	NR	STROKE	★★★
GENERAL SURGERY	NR	VASCULAR	NR
MATERNITY CARE	★	WOMEN'S HEALTH	NR

HEALTHGRADES AWARDS

Waynesboro Hospital

501 East Main Street
Waynesboro, PA 17268
(717) 765-4000

Overall patient safety: ★
Teaching: N

CLINICAL PROGRAM RATINGS:

CARDIAC	NR	ORTHOPEDICS	NR
CRITICAL CARE	NR	PULMONARY	★★★
GASTROINTESTINAL	★★★	STROKE	★★★
GENERAL SURGERY	★★★	VASCULAR	NR
MATERNITY CARE	★	WOMEN'S HEALTH	NR

HEALTHGRADES AWARDS

Washington Hospital

155 Wilson Avenue
Washington, PA 15301
(724) 225-7000

Overall patient safety: ★★★
Teaching: Y

CLINICAL PROGRAM RATINGS:

CARDIAC	★★★	ORTHOPEDICS	★★★★★
CRITICAL CARE	NR	PULMONARY	★
GASTROINTESTINAL	★★★	STROKE	★★★
GENERAL SURGERY	★★★	VASCULAR	NR
MATERNITY CARE	★★★★★	WOMEN'S HEALTH	★★★★★

HEALTHGRADES AWARDS

✓ SPECIALTY EXCELLENCE
- CARDIAC SURGERY
- JOINT REPLACEMENT
- ORTHOPEDIC SURGERY
- WOMEN'S HEALTH

Western Pennsylvania Hospital

4800 Friendship Avenue
Pittsburgh, PA 15224
(412) 578-5000

Overall patient safety: ★★★
Teaching: Y

CLINICAL PROGRAM RATINGS:

CARDIAC	★★★	ORTHOPEDICS	★★★
CRITICAL CARE	NR	PULMONARY	★★★
GASTROINTESTINAL	★★★	STROKE	★★★
GENERAL SURGERY	★★★	VASCULAR	★★★
MATERNITY CARE	★	WOMEN'S HEALTH	★

HEALTHGRADES AWARDS

✓ SPECIALTY EXCELLENCE
- BARIATRIC SURGERY
- JOINT REPLACEMENT

*This hospital reports its data to the federal government jointly with another hospital. Therefore the ratings and awards apply to multiple hospitals and this specific hospital may not provide all rated services.

Western Pennsylvania Hospital—Forbes Regional Campus

2570 Haymaker Road
Monroeville, PA 15146
(412) 858-2000

Overall patient safety: ★★★
Teaching: Y

CLINICAL PROGRAM RATINGS:

CARDIAC	NR	ORTHOPEDICS	NR
CRITICAL CARE	NR	PULMONARY	★★★
GASTROINTESTINAL	★★★	STROKE	★★★
GENERAL SURGERY	★★★	VASCULAR	NR
MATERNITY CARE	★★★	WOMEN'S HEALTH	NR

HEALTHGRADES AWARDS

Williamsport Hospital and Medical Center

777 Rural Avenue
Williamsport, PA 17701
(570) 321-1000

Overall patient safety: ★★★
Teaching: Y

CLINICAL PROGRAM RATINGS:

CARDIAC	★★★	ORTHOPEDICS	★★★
CRITICAL CARE	NR	PULMONARY	★★★
GASTROINTESTINAL	NR	STROKE	★★★
GENERAL SURGERY	★★★	VASCULAR	NR
MATERNITY CARE	★★★	WOMEN'S HEALTH	★

HEALTHGRADES AWARDS

Westmoreland Regional Hospital

532 West Pittsburgh Street
Greensburg, PA 15601
(724) 832-4000

Overall patient safety: ★★★
Teaching: N

CLINICAL PROGRAM RATINGS:

CARDIAC	★★★	ORTHOPEDICS	★★★
CRITICAL CARE	NR	PULMONARY	★★★
GASTROINTESTINAL	★★★	STROKE	★★★
GENERAL SURGERY	★★★	VASCULAR	NR
MATERNITY CARE	★★★★★	WOMEN'S HEALTH	★★★★★

HEALTHGRADES AWARDS

✓ SPECIALTY EXCELLENCE
• MATERNITY CARE

Windber Hospital

600 Somerset Avenue
Windber, PA 15963
(814) 467-3000

Overall patient safety: ★★★
Teaching: N

CLINICAL PROGRAM RATINGS:

CARDIAC	NR	ORTHOPEDICS	NR
CRITICAL CARE	NR	PULMONARY	★★★
GASTROINTESTINAL	NR	STROKE	★★★
GENERAL SURGERY	NR	VASCULAR	NR
MATERNITY CARE	★★★	WOMEN'S HEALTH	NR

HEALTHGRADES AWARDS

Wilkes-Barre General Hospital*

North River and Auburn Streets
Wilkes-Barre, PA 18764
(717) 829-8111

Overall patient safety: ★★★★★
Teaching: Y

CLINICAL PROGRAM RATINGS:

CARDIAC	★★★	ORTHOPEDICS	★★★
CRITICAL CARE	NR	PULMONARY	★★★
GASTROINTESTINAL	★★★	STROKE	★★★
GENERAL SURGERY	★★★	VASCULAR	★★★
MATERNITY CARE	★★★★★	WOMEN'S HEALTH	★★★

HEALTHGRADES AWARDS

✓ DISTINGUISHED HOSPITAL
• PATIENT SAFETY

✓ SPECIALTY EXCELLENCE
• MATERNITY CARE

WVHCS Hospital*

575 North River Street
Wilkes-Barre, PA 18764
(570) 829-8111

Overall patient safety: ★★★★★
Teaching: Y

CLINICAL PROGRAM RATINGS:

CARDIAC	★★★	ORTHOPEDICS	★★★
CRITICAL CARE	NR	PULMONARY	★★★
GASTROINTESTINAL	★★★	STROKE	★★★
GENERAL SURGERY	★★★	VASCULAR	★★★
MATERNITY CARE	★★★★★	WOMEN'S HEALTH	★★★

HEALTHGRADES AWARDS

✓ DISTINGUISHED HOSPITAL
• PATIENT SAFETY

✓ SPECIALTY EXCELLENCE
• MATERNITY CARE

KEY: ★★★★★ BEST   ★★★ AS EXPECTED   ★ POOR   NR NOT RATED BY HEALTHGRADES   For full definitions of ratings and awards, see Appendix.

York Hospital

1001 South George Street
York, PA 17405
(717) 851-2345

Overall patient safety: ★★★★★
Teaching: Y

CLINICAL PROGRAM RATINGS:

CARDIAC	★★★	ORTHOPEDICS	★★★★★
CRITICAL CARE	NR	PULMONARY	★★★
GASTROINTESTINAL	★★★	STROKE	★
GENERAL SURGERY	★★★★★	VASCULAR	★★★
MATERNITY CARE	★★★	WOMEN'S HEALTH	★★★

HEALTHGRADES AWARDS

✓ DISTINGUISHED HOSPITAL
- PATIENT SAFETY

✓ SPECIALTY EXCELLENCE
- GASTROINTESTINAL CARE
- GENERAL SURGERY
- ORTHOPEDIC SURGERY

RHODE ISLAND HOSPITALS: RATINGS BY CLINICAL SPECIALTY

John Fogarty Memorial Hospital*

Eddie Dowling Highway
Woonsocket, RI 02895
(401) 769-2200

Overall patient safety: ★★★
Teaching: N

CLINICAL PROGRAM RATINGS:

CARDIAC	NR	ORTHOPEDICS	NR
CRITICAL CARE	NR	PULMONARY	★★★
GASTROINTESTINAL	★★★	STROKE	★★★
GENERAL SURGERY	★★★	VASCULAR	NR
MATERNITY CARE	★★★	WOMEN'S HEALTH	NR

HEALTHGRADES AWARDS

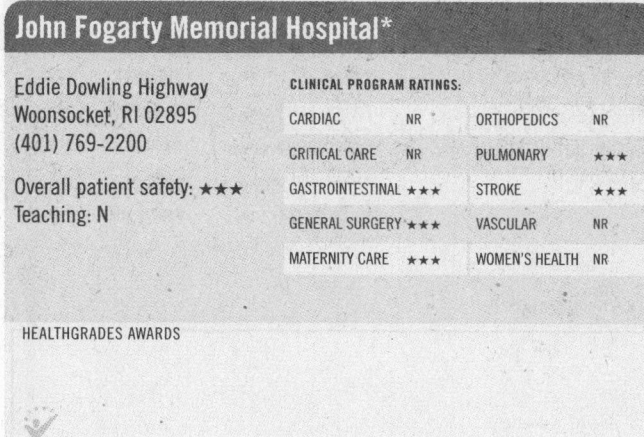

Landmark Medical Center*

115 Cass Avenue
Woonsocket, RI 02895
(401) 769-4100

Overall patient safety: ★★★
Teaching: N

CLINICAL PROGRAM RATINGS:

CARDIAC	NR	ORTHOPEDICS	NR
CRITICAL CARE	NR	PULMONARY	★★★
GASTROINTESTINAL	★★★	STROKE	★★★
GENERAL SURGERY	★★★	VASCULAR	NR
MATERNITY CARE	★★★	WOMEN'S HEALTH	NR

HEALTHGRADES AWARDS

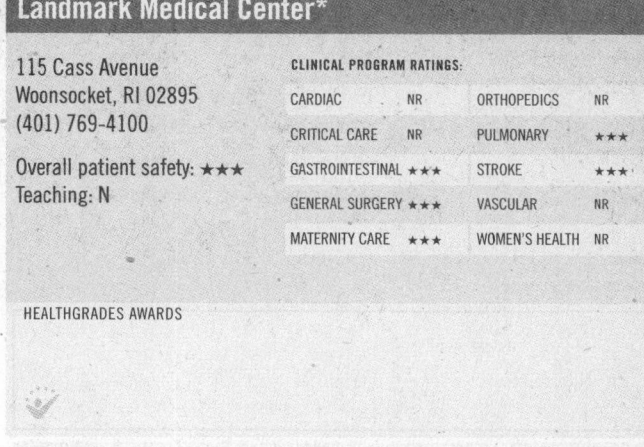

Kent County Memorial Hospital

455 Tollgate Road
Warwick, RI 02886
(401) 737-7000

Overall patient safety: ★★★
Teaching: N

CLINICAL PROGRAM RATINGS:

CARDIAC	NR	ORTHOPEDICS	★★★
CRITICAL CARE	NR	PULMONARY	★★★
GASTROINTESTINAL	★★★	STROKE	★
GENERAL SURGERY	★★★	VASCULAR	NR
MATERNITY CARE	★★★	WOMEN'S HEALTH	NR

HEALTHGRADES AWARDS

Memorial Hospital of Rhode Island

111 Brewster Street
Pawtucket, RI 02860
(401) 729-2000

Overall patient safety: ★★★
Teaching: Y

CLINICAL PROGRAM RATINGS:

CARDIAC	NR	ORTHOPEDICS	NR
CRITICAL CARE	NR	PULMONARY	★★★
GASTROINTESTINAL	★★★	STROKE	★★★★★
GENERAL SURGERY	★★★	VASCULAR	NR
MATERNITY CARE	★★★	WOMEN'S HEALTH	NR

HEALTHGRADES AWARDS

✓ SPECIALTY EXCELLENCE
- GASTROINTESTINAL CARE
- STROKE CARE

---

*This hospital reports its data to the federal government jointly with another hospital. Therefore the ratings and awards apply to multiple hospitals and this specific hospital may not provide all rated services.

Miriam Hospital

164 Summit Avenue
Providence, RI 02906
(401) 793-2500

Overall patient safety: ★★★
Teaching: Y

CLINICAL PROGRAM RATINGS:

CARDIAC	★★★	ORTHOPEDICS	★★★
CRITICAL CARE	NR	PULMONARY	★★★
GASTROINTESTINAL	★★★	STROKE	★★★
GENERAL SURGERY	★★★	VASCULAR	NR
MATERNITY CARE	NR	WOMEN'S HEALTH	NR

HEALTHGRADES AWARDS

Roger Williams Hospital

825 Chalkstone Avenue
Providence, RI 02908
(401) 456-2000

Overall patient safety: ★
Teaching: Y

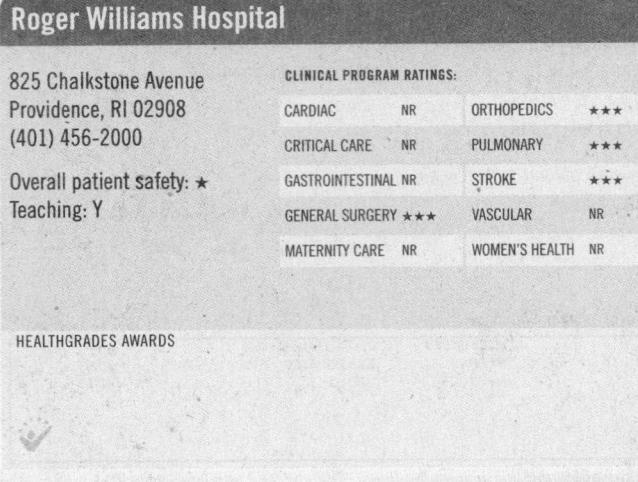

CLINICAL PROGRAM RATINGS:

CARDIAC	NR	ORTHOPEDICS	★★★
CRITICAL CARE	NR	PULMONARY	★★★
GASTROINTESTINAL	NR	STROKE	★★★
GENERAL SURGERY	★★★	VASCULAR	NR
MATERNITY CARE	NR	WOMEN'S HEALTH	NR

HEALTHGRADES AWARDS

Newport Hospital

11 Friendship Street
Newport, RI 02840
(401) 846-6400

Overall patient safety: ★★★★★
Teaching: N

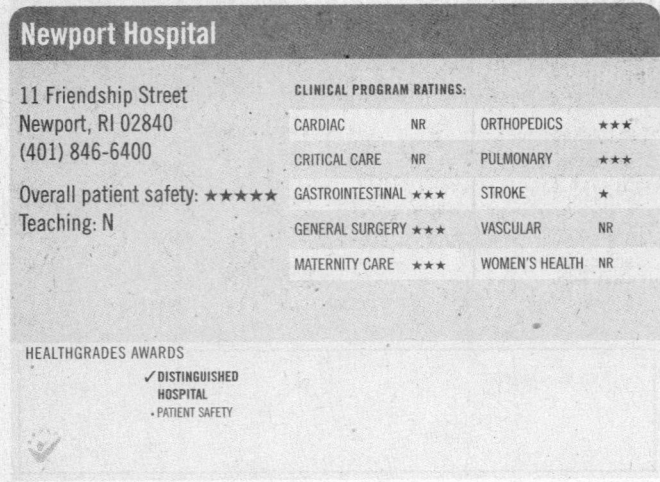

CLINICAL PROGRAM RATINGS:

CARDIAC	NR	ORTHOPEDICS	★★★
CRITICAL CARE	NR	PULMONARY	★★★
GASTROINTESTINAL	★★★	STROKE	★
GENERAL SURGERY	★★★	VASCULAR	NR
MATERNITY CARE	★★★	WOMEN'S HEALTH	NR

HEALTHGRADES AWARDS

✓ DISTINGUISHED
HOSPITAL
• PATIENT SAFETY

St. Joseph Health Services of Rhode Island

200 High Service Avenue
North Providence, RI 02904
(401) 456-3000

Overall patient safety: ★
Teaching: N

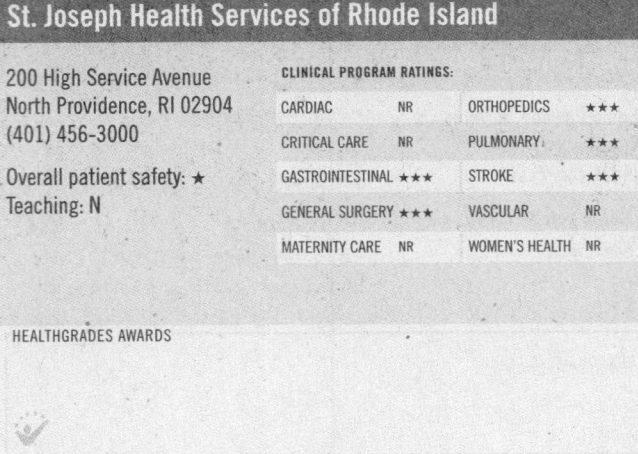

CLINICAL PROGRAM RATINGS:

CARDIAC	NR	ORTHOPEDICS	★★★
CRITICAL CARE	NR	PULMONARY	★★★
GASTROINTESTINAL	★★★	STROKE	★★★
GENERAL SURGERY	★★★	VASCULAR	NR
MATERNITY CARE	NR	WOMEN'S HEALTH	NR

HEALTHGRADES AWARDS

Rhode Island Hospital

593 Eddy Street
Providence, RI 02903
(401) 444-4000

Overall patient safety: ★★★
Teaching: Y

CLINICAL PROGRAM RATINGS:

CARDIAC	★★★★★	ORTHOPEDICS	★
CRITICAL CARE	NR	PULMONARY	★★★
GASTROINTESTINAL	★★★	STROKE	★★★
GENERAL SURGERY	★★★	VASCULAR	★
MATERNITY CARE	NR	WOMEN'S HEALTH	NR

HEALTHGRADES AWARDS

✓ SPECIALTY EXCELLENCE
• CARDIAC CARE

South County Hospital

100 Kenyon Avenue
Wakefield, RI 02879
(401) 782-8000

Overall patient safety: ★★★
Teaching: N

CLINICAL PROGRAM RATINGS:

CARDIAC	NR	ORTHOPEDICS	★★★
CRITICAL CARE	NR	PULMONARY	★★★
GASTROINTESTINAL	NR	STROKE	★★★
GENERAL SURGERY	★★★	VASCULAR	NR
MATERNITY CARE	★★★	WOMEN'S HEALTH	NR

HEALTHGRADES AWARDS

KEY: ★★★★★ BEST   ★★★ AS EXPECTED   ★ POOR   NR NOT RATED BY HEALTHGRADES   For full definitions of ratings and awards, see Appendix.

Westerly Hospital

25 Wells Street
Westerly, RI 02891
(401) 596-6000

Overall patient safety: ★★★
Teaching: N

CLINICAL PROGRAM RATINGS:

CARDIAC	NR	ORTHOPEDICS	NR
CRITICAL CARE	NR	PULMONARY	★★★
GASTROINTESTINAL	★★★	STROKE	★
GENERAL SURGERY	★	VASCULAR	NR
MATERNITY CARE	★★★	WOMEN'S HEALTH	NR

HEALTHGRADES AWARDS

SOUTH CAROLINA HOSPITALS: RATINGS BY CLINICAL SPECIALTY

Abbeville County Memorial Hospital

901 West Greenwood Street
Abbeville, SC 29620
(864) 366-3312

Overall patient safety: ★★★
Teaching: N

CLINICAL PROGRAM RATINGS:

CARDIAC	NR	ORTHOPEDICS	NR
CRITICAL CARE	NR	PULMONARY	★★★
GASTROINTESTINAL	NR	STROKE	★★★
GENERAL SURGERY	NR	VASCULAR	NR
MATERNITY CARE	NR	WOMEN'S HEALTH	NR

HEALTHGRADES AWARDS

Allen Bennett Memorial Hospital

313 Memorial Drive
Greer, SC 29650
(864) 848-8200

Overall patient safety: ★★★
Teaching: N

CLINICAL PROGRAM RATINGS:

CARDIAC	NR	ORTHOPEDICS	NR
CRITICAL CARE	NR	PULMONARY	★★★
GASTROINTESTINAL	★★★	STROKE	★★★
GENERAL SURGERY	NR	VASCULAR	NR
MATERNITY CARE	NR	WOMEN'S HEALTH	NR

HEALTHGRADES AWARDS

Aiken Regional Medical Center

302 University Parkway
Aiken, SC 29801
(803) 641-5600

Overall patient safety: ★
Teaching: N

CLINICAL PROGRAM RATINGS:

CARDIAC	★★★	ORTHOPEDICS	★★★
CRITICAL CARE	NR	PULMONARY	★★★
GASTROINTESTINAL	★★★	STROKE	★
GENERAL SURGERY	NR	VASCULAR	NR
MATERNITY CARE	NR	WOMEN'S HEALTH	NR

HEALTHGRADES AWARDS

Anmed Health

800 North Fant Street
Anderson, SC 29621
(864) 261-1000

Overall patient safety: ★★★★★
Teaching: Y

CLINICAL PROGRAM RATINGS:

CARDIAC	★★★	ORTHOPEDICS	★★★
CRITICAL CARE	★★★★★	PULMONARY	★★★★★
GASTROINTESTINAL	★★★	STROKE	★★★
GENERAL SURGERY	NR	VASCULAR	★★★
MATERNITY CARE	NR	WOMEN'S HEALTH	NR

HEALTHGRADES AWARDS

✓ DISTINGUISHED HOSPITAL
· CLINICAL EXCELLENCE
· PATIENT SAFETY

✓ SPECIALTY EXCELLENCE
· CARDIAC SURGERY · CRITICAL CARE · PULMONARY CARE

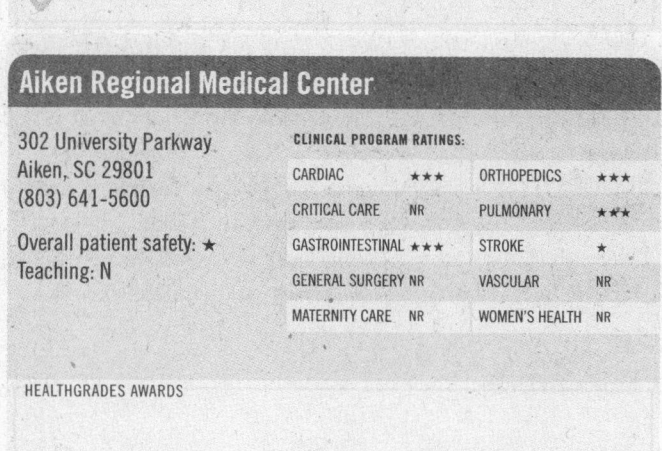

Bamberg County Memorial Hospital

509 North Street
Bamberg, SC 29003
(803) 245-4321

Overall patient safety: ★★★
Teaching: N

CLINICAL PROGRAM RATINGS:

CARDIAC	NR	ORTHOPEDICS	NR
CRITICAL CARE	NR	PULMONARY	★★★
GASTROINTESTINAL	NR	STROKE	NR
GENERAL SURGERY	NR	VASCULAR	NR
MATERNITY CARE	NR	WOMEN'S HEALTH	NR

HEALTHGRADES AWARDS

Bon Secours St. Francis Hospital

2095 Henry Tecklenburg Drive
Charleston, SC 29414
(843) 402-1000

Overall patient safety: ★
Teaching: N

CLINICAL PROGRAM RATINGS:

CARDIAC	NR	ORTHOPEDICS	NR
CRITICAL CARE	NR	PULMONARY	★★★
GASTROINTESTINAL	★★★	STROKE	★★★
GENERAL SURGERY	NR	VASCULAR	NR
MATERNITY CARE	NR	WOMEN'S HEALTH	NR

HEALTHGRADES AWARDS

Barnwell County Hospital

811 Reynolds Road
Barnwell, SC 29812
(803) 259-1000

Overall patient safety: ★★★
Teaching: N

CLINICAL PROGRAM RATINGS:

CARDIAC	NR	ORTHOPEDICS	NR
CRITICAL CARE	NR	PULMONARY	★★★
GASTROINTESTINAL	NR	STROKE	NR
GENERAL SURGERY	NR	VASCULAR	NR
MATERNITY CARE	NR	WOMEN'S HEALTH	NR

HEALTHGRADES AWARDS

Cannon Memorial Hospital

123 West G. Acker Drive
Pickens, SC 29671
(864) 878-4791

Overall patient safety: ★★★
Teaching: N

CLINICAL PROGRAM RATINGS:

CARDIAC	NR	ORTHOPEDICS	NR
CRITICAL CARE	NR	PULMONARY	★
GASTROINTESTINAL	NR	STROKE	★★★
GENERAL SURGERY	NR	VASCULAR	NR
MATERNITY CARE	NR	WOMEN'S HEALTH	NR

HEALTHGRADES AWARDS

Beaufort Memorial Hospital

955 Ribaut Road
Beaufort, SC 29902
(843) 522-5200

Overall patient safety: ★★★
Teaching: N

CLINICAL PROGRAM RATINGS:

CARDIAC	NR	ORTHOPEDICS	★★★★★
CRITICAL CARE	NR	PULMONARY	★★★
GASTROINTESTINAL	★★★	STROKE	★
GENERAL SURGERY	NR	VASCULAR	NR
MATERNITY CARE	NR	WOMEN'S HEALTH	NR

HEALTHGRADES AWARDS

✓ SPECIALTY EXCELLENCE
· ORTHOPEDIC
  SURGERY

Carolina Pines Regional Medical Center

1304 West Bobo
Newsom Highway
Hartsville, SC 29550
(843) 339-2100

Overall patient safety: ★★★
Teaching: N

CLINICAL PROGRAM RATINGS:

CARDIAC	NR	ORTHOPEDICS	NR
CRITICAL CARE	★★★	PULMONARY	★★★
GASTROINTESTINAL	★★★	STROKE	★
GENERAL SURGERY	NR	VASCULAR	NR
MATERNITY CARE	NR	WOMEN'S HEALTH	NR

HEALTHGRADES AWARDS

KEY: ★★★★★ BEST ★★★ AS EXPECTED ★ POOR NR NOT RATED BY HEALTHGRADES For full definitions of ratings and awards, see Appendix.

Carolinas Hospital System

805 Pamplico Highway
Box 100550
Florence, SC 29505
(843) 674-5000

Overall patient safety: ★★★
Teaching: N

CLINICAL PROGRAM RATINGS:

CARDIAC	★★★	ORTHOPEDICS	★★★
CRITICAL CARE	★★★	PULMONARY	★★★
GASTROINTESTINAL	★★★	STROKE	★★★
GENERAL SURGERY	NR	VASCULAR	★★★
MATERNITY CARE	NR	WOMEN'S HEALTH	NR

HEALTHGRADES AWARDS

Clarendon Memorial Hospital

10 Hospital Street
Manning, SC 29102
(803) 435-8463

Overall patient safety: ★★★
Teaching: N

CLINICAL PROGRAM RATINGS:

CARDIAC	NR	ORTHOPEDICS	NR
CRITICAL CARE	NR	PULMONARY	★★★
GASTROINTESTINAL	NR	STROKE	NR
GENERAL SURGERY	NR	VASCULAR	NR
MATERNITY CARE	NR	WOMEN'S HEALTH	NR

HEALTHGRADES AWARDS

Chester Regional Medical Center

1 Medical Park Drive
Chester, SC 29706
(803) 581-3151

Overall patient safety: ★
Teaching: N

CLINICAL PROGRAM RATINGS:

CARDIAC	NR	ORTHOPEDICS	NR
CRITICAL CARE	NR	PULMONARY	★★★
GASTROINTESTINAL	NR	STROKE	NR
GENERAL SURGERY	NR	VASCULAR	NR
MATERNITY CARE	NR	WOMEN'S HEALTH	NR

HEALTHGRADES AWARDS

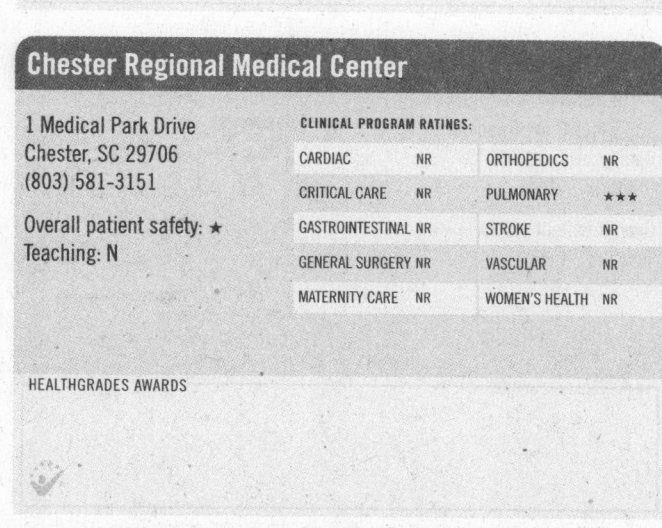

Coastal Carolina Medical Center

1000 Medical Center Drive
Hardeeville, SC 29927
(843) 784-8000

Overall patient safety: ★★★
Teaching: N

CLINICAL PROGRAM RATINGS:

CARDIAC	NR	ORTHOPEDICS	NR
CRITICAL CARE	NR	PULMONARY	★★★
GASTROINTESTINAL	NR	STROKE	NR
GENERAL SURGERY	NR	VASCULAR	NR
MATERNITY CARE	NR	WOMEN'S HEALTH	NR

HEALTHGRADES AWARDS

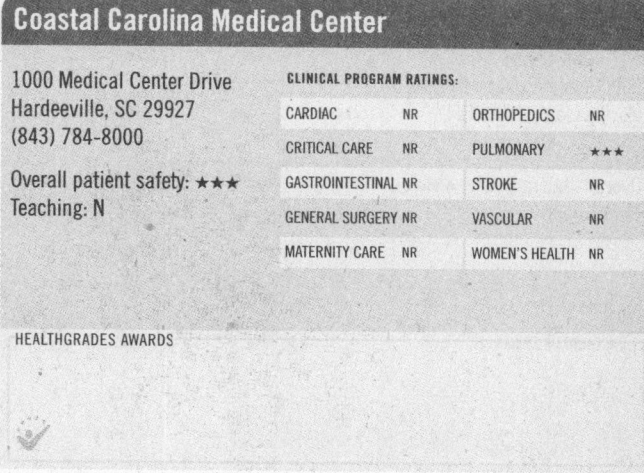

Chesterfield General Hospital

711 Chesterfield Highway
Cheraw, SC 29520
(843) 537-7881

Overall patient safety: ★★★
Teaching: N

CLINICAL PROGRAM RATINGS:

CARDIAC	NR	ORTHOPEDICS	NR
CRITICAL CARE	NR	PULMONARY	★★★
GASTROINTESTINAL	NR	STROKE	NR
GENERAL SURGERY	NR	VASCULAR	NR
MATERNITY CARE	NR	WOMEN'S HEALTH	NR

HEALTHGRADES AWARDS

Colleton Medical Center

501 Robertson Boulevard
Walterboro, SC 29488
(843) 549-2000

Overall patient safety: ★
Teaching: N

CLINICAL PROGRAM RATINGS:

CARDIAC	NR	ORTHOPEDICS	NR
CRITICAL CARE	★★★	PULMONARY	★★★
GASTROINTESTINAL	★★★	STROKE	★★★
GENERAL SURGERY	NR	VASCULAR	NR
MATERNITY CARE	NR	WOMEN'S HEALTH	NR

HEALTHGRADES AWARDS

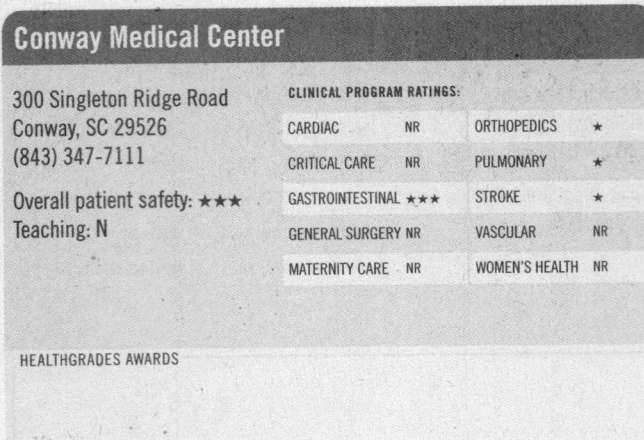

Conway Medical Center

300 Singleton Ridge Road
Conway, SC 29526
(843) 347-7111

Overall patient safety: ★★★
Teaching: N

CLINICAL PROGRAM RATINGS:

CARDIAC	NR	ORTHOPEDICS	★
CRITICAL CARE	NR	PULMONARY	★
GASTROINTESTINAL	★★★	STROKE	★
GENERAL SURGERY	NR	VASCULAR	NR
MATERNITY CARE	NR	WOMEN'S HEALTH	NR

HEALTHGRADES AWARDS

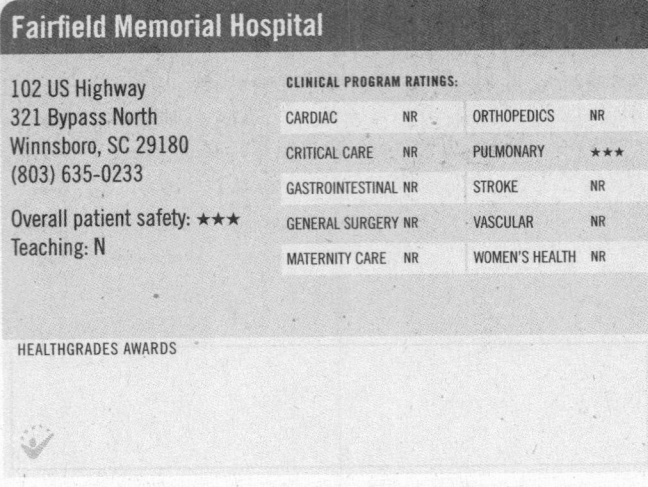

Fairfield Memorial Hospital

102 US Highway
321 Bypass North
Winnsboro, SC 29180
(803) 635-0233

Overall patient safety: ★★★
Teaching: N

CLINICAL PROGRAM RATINGS:

CARDIAC	NR	ORTHOPEDICS	NR
CRITICAL CARE	NR	PULMONARY	★★★
GASTROINTESTINAL	NR	STROKE	NR
GENERAL SURGERY	NR	VASCULAR	NR
MATERNITY CARE	NR	WOMEN'S HEALTH	NR

HEALTHGRADES AWARDS

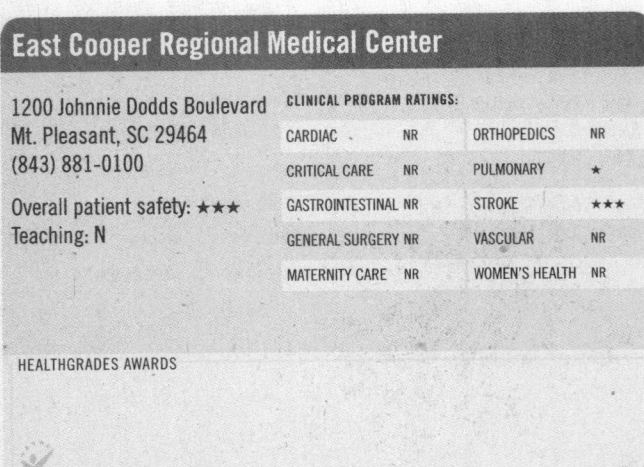

East Cooper Regional Medical Center

1200 Johnnie Dodds Boulevard
Mt. Pleasant, SC 29464
(843) 881-0100

Overall patient safety: ★★★
Teaching: N

CLINICAL PROGRAM RATINGS:

CARDIAC	NR	ORTHOPEDICS	NR
CRITICAL CARE	NR	PULMONARY	★
GASTROINTESTINAL	NR	STROKE	★★★
GENERAL SURGERY	NR	VASCULAR	NR
MATERNITY CARE	NR	WOMEN'S HEALTH	NR

HEALTHGRADES AWARDS

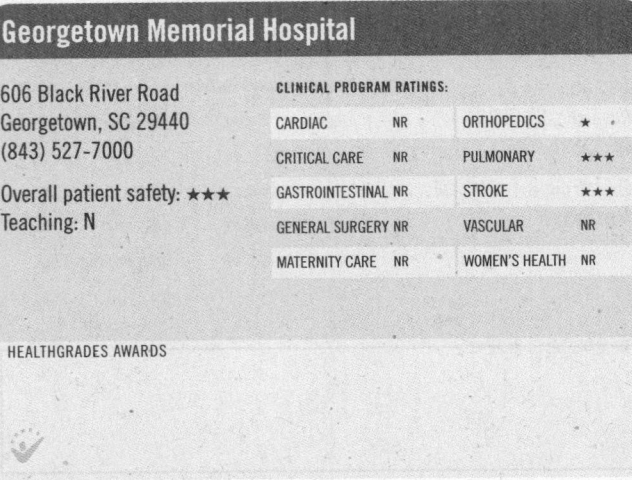

Georgetown Memorial Hospital

606 Black River Road
Georgetown, SC 29440
(843) 527-7000

Overall patient safety: ★★★
Teaching: N

CLINICAL PROGRAM RATINGS:

CARDIAC	NR	ORTHOPEDICS	★
CRITICAL CARE	NR	PULMONARY	★★★
GASTROINTESTINAL	NR	STROKE	★★★
GENERAL SURGERY	NR	VASCULAR	NR
MATERNITY CARE	NR	WOMEN'S HEALTH	NR

HEALTHGRADES AWARDS

Edgefield County Hospital

300 Ridge Medical Plaza
Edgefield, SC 29824
(803) 637-1150

Overall patient safety: NR
Teaching: N

CLINICAL PROGRAM RATINGS:

CARDIAC	NR	ORTHOPEDICS	NR
CRITICAL CARE	NR	PULMONARY	★★★
GASTROINTESTINAL	NR	STROKE	NR
GENERAL SURGERY	NR	VASCULAR	NR
MATERNITY CARE	NR	WOMEN'S HEALTH	NR

HEALTHGRADES AWARDS

Grand Strand Regional Medical Center

809 82nd Parkway
Myrtle Beach, SC 29572
(843) 692-1000

Overall patient safety: ★★★
Teaching: N

CLINICAL PROGRAM RATINGS:

CARDIAC	★★★	ORTHOPEDICS	★★★
CRITICAL CARE	★★★	PULMONARY	★★★
GASTROINTESTINAL	★★★	STROKE	★★★
GENERAL SURGERY	NR	VASCULAR	★★★
MATERNITY CARE	NR	WOMEN'S HEALTH	NR

HEALTHGRADES AWARDS

KEY: ★★★★★ BEST ★★★ AS EXPECTED ★ POOR NR NOT RATED BY HEALTHGRADES *For full definitions of ratings and awards, see Appendix.

Greenville Memorial Hospital

701 Grove Road
Greenville, SC 29605
(864) 455-7000

Overall patient safety: ★★★
Teaching: Y

CLINICAL PROGRAM RATINGS:

CARDIAC	★★★	ORTHOPEDICS	★★★
CRITICAL CARE	★★★	PULMONARY	★★★
GASTROINTESTINAL	★★★	STROKE	★★★
GENERAL SURGERY	NR	VASCULAR	★★★
MATERNITY CARE	NR	WOMEN'S HEALTH	NR

HEALTHGRADES AWARDS

Hilton Head Regional Medical Center

25 Hospital Center Boulevard
Hilton Head Island, SC 29926
(843) 681-6122

Overall patient safety: ★★★
Teaching: N

CLINICAL PROGRAM RATINGS:

CARDIAC	★★★	ORTHOPEDICS	NR
CRITICAL CARE	NR	PULMONARY	★★★
GASTROINTESTINAL	★★★	STROKE	★★★
GENERAL SURGERY	NR	VASCULAR	NR
MATERNITY CARE	NR	WOMEN'S HEALTH	NR

HEALTHGRADES AWARDS

Hampton Regional Medical Center

595 Carolina Avenue West
Varnville, SC 29944
(803) 943-2771

Overall patient safety: ★★★
Teaching: N

CLINICAL PROGRAM RATINGS:

CARDIAC	NR	ORTHOPEDICS	NR
CRITICAL CARE	NR	PULMONARY	★★★
GASTROINTESTINAL	NR	STROKE	NR
GENERAL SURGERY	NR	VASCULAR	NR
MATERNITY CARE	NR	WOMEN'S HEALTH	NR

HEALTHGRADES AWARDS

Kershaw County Medical Center

1315 Roberts Street
Camden, SC 29020
(803) 432-4311

Overall patient safety: ★★★★★
Teaching: N

CLINICAL PROGRAM RATINGS:

CARDIAC	NR	ORTHOPEDICS	NR
CRITICAL CARE	NR	PULMONARY	★★★
GASTROINTESTINAL	★★★	STROKE	★★★
GENERAL SURGERY	NR	VASCULAR	NR
MATERNITY CARE	NR	WOMEN'S HEALTH	NR

HEALTHGRADES AWARDS

Hillcrest Memorial Hospital

729 Southeast Main Street
Simpsonville, SC 29681
(864) 967-6100

Overall patient safety: ★★★
Teaching: N

CLINICAL PROGRAM RATINGS:

CARDIAC	NR	ORTHOPEDICS	NR
CRITICAL CARE	NR	PULMONARY	★★★
GASTROINTESTINAL	NR	STROKE	★★★
GENERAL SURGERY	NR	VASCULAR	NR
MATERNITY CARE	NR	WOMEN'S HEALTH	NR

HEALTHGRADES AWARDS

Laurens County Healthcare System

22725 Highway 76 East
Clinton, SC 29325
(864) 833-9100

Overall patient safety: ★★★
Teaching: N

CLINICAL PROGRAM RATINGS:

CARDIAC	NR	ORTHOPEDICS	NR
CRITICAL CARE	NR	PULMONARY	★
GASTROINTESTINAL	NR	STROKE	★★★
GENERAL SURGERY	NR	VASCULAR	NR
MATERNITY CARE	NR	WOMEN'S HEALTH	NR

HEALTHGRADES AWARDS

Lexington Medical Center

2720 Sunset Boulevard
West Columbia, SC 29169
(803) 791-2000

Overall patient safety: ★★★
Teaching: N

CLINICAL PROGRAM RATINGS:

CARDIAC	NR	ORTHOPEDICS	★★★
CRITICAL CARE	NR	PULMONARY	★
GASTROINTESTINAL	★★★	STROKE	★
GENERAL SURGERY	NR	VASCULAR	★★★
MATERNITY CARE	NR	WOMEN'S HEALTH	NR

HEALTHGRADES AWARDS

Marlboro Park Hospital

1138 Cheraw Highway
Bennettsville, SC 29512
(843) 479-2881

Overall patient safety: ★★★
Teaching: N

CLINICAL PROGRAM RATINGS:

CARDIAC	NR	ORTHOPEDICS	NR
CRITICAL CARE	NR	PULMONARY	★★★
GASTROINTESTINAL	NR	STROKE	NR
GENERAL SURGERY	NR	VASCULAR	NR
MATERNITY CARE	NR	WOMEN'S HEALTH	NR

HEALTHGRADES AWARDS

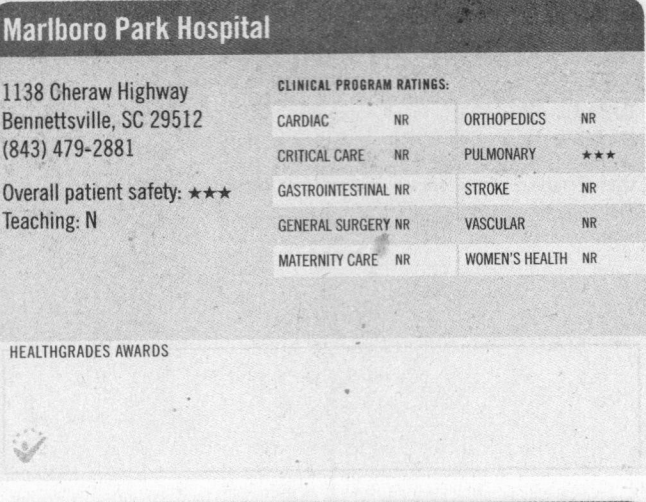

Loris Community Hospital

3655 Mitchell Street
Loris, SC 29569
(843) 716-7000

Overall patient safety: ★★★
Teaching: N

CLINICAL PROGRAM RATINGS:

CARDIAC	NR	ORTHOPEDICS	NR
CRITICAL CARE	NR	PULMONARY	★★★
GASTROINTESTINAL	NR	STROKE	★
GENERAL SURGERY	NR	VASCULAR	NR
MATERNITY CARE	NR	WOMEN'S HEALTH	NR

HEALTHGRADES AWARDS

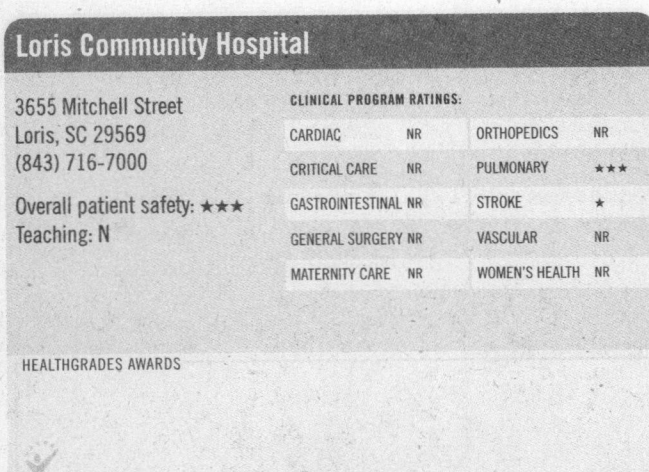

Mary Black Memorial Hospital

1700 Skylyn Drive
Spartanburg, SC 29307
(864) 573-3000

Overall patient safety: ★★★
Teaching: N

CLINICAL PROGRAM RATINGS:

CARDIAC	NR	ORTHOPEDICS	NR
CRITICAL CARE	NR	PULMONARY	★★★
GASTROINTESTINAL	★★★	STROKE	★
GENERAL SURGERY	NR	VASCULAR	★★★
MATERNITY CARE	NR	WOMEN'S HEALTH	NR

HEALTHGRADES AWARDS

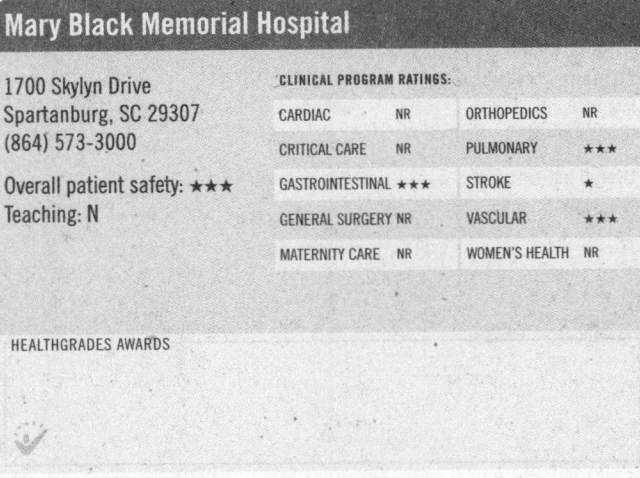

Marion County Medical Center

2829 East Highway 76
P.O. Box 1150
Marion, SC 29571
(843) 431-2000

Overall patient safety: ★★★
Teaching: N

CLINICAL PROGRAM RATINGS:

CARDIAC	NR	ORTHOPEDICS	NR
CRITICAL CARE	NR	PULMONARY	★★★
GASTROINTESTINAL	NR	STROKE	★★★
GENERAL SURGERY	NR	VASCULAR	NR
MATERNITY CARE	NR	WOMEN'S HEALTH	NR

HEALTHGRADES AWARDS

McLeod Medical Center–Darlington

701 Cashua Ferry Road
Darlington, SC 29532
(843) 395-1100

Overall patient safety: ★★★
Teaching: N

CLINICAL PROGRAM RATINGS:

CARDIAC	NR	ORTHOPEDICS	NR
CRITICAL CARE	NR	PULMONARY	★★★
GASTROINTESTINAL	NR	STROKE	★★★
GENERAL SURGERY	NR	VASCULAR	NR
MATERNITY CARE	NR	WOMEN'S HEALTH	NR

HEALTHGRADES AWARDS

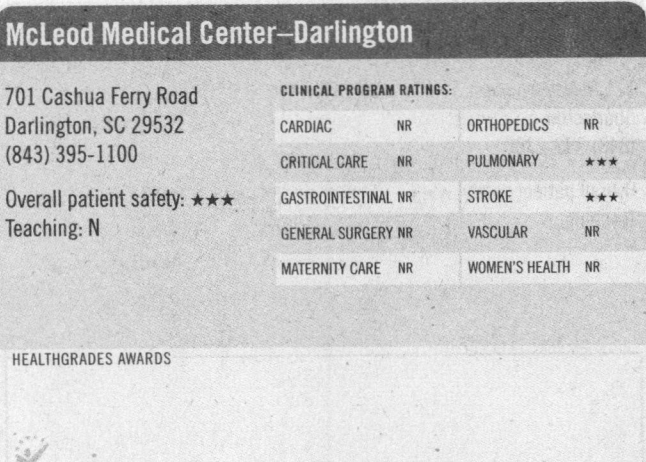

KEY: ★★★★★ BEST   ★★★ AS EXPECTED   ★ POOR   NR NOT RATED BY HEALTHGRADES   For full definitions of ratings and awards, see Appendix.

McLeod Medical Center—Dillon

301 East Jackson
Dillon, SC 29536
(843) 774-4111

Overall patient safety: ★★★
Teaching: N

CLINICAL PROGRAM RATINGS:

CARDIAC	NR	ORTHOPEDICS	NR
CRITICAL CARE	NR	PULMONARY	★★★
GASTROINTESTINAL	NR	STROKE	NR
GENERAL SURGERY	NR	VASCULAR	NR
MATERNITY CARE	NR	WOMEN'S HEALTH	NR

HEALTHGRADES AWARDS

Newberry County Memorial Hospital

2669 Kinard Street
Newberry, SC 29108
(803) 276-7570

Overall patient safety: ★★★
Teaching: N

CLINICAL PROGRAM RATINGS:

CARDIAC	NR	ORTHOPEDICS	NR
CRITICAL CARE	NR	PULMONARY	★
GASTROINTESTINAL	NR	STROKE	★★★
GENERAL SURGERY	NR	VASCULAR	NR
MATERNITY CARE	NR	WOMEN'S HEALTH	NR

HEALTHGRADES AWARDS

McLeod Regional Medical Center

555 East Cheves Street
Florence, SC 29506
(843) 777-2000

Overall patient safety: ★★★★★
Teaching: Y

CLINICAL PROGRAM RATINGS:

CARDIAC	★★★	ORTHOPEDICS	★★★
CRITICAL CARE	★★★	PULMONARY	★★★
GASTROINTESTINAL	★★★	STROKE	★★★
GENERAL SURGERY	NR	VASCULAR	NR
MATERNITY CARE	NR	WOMEN'S HEALTH	NR

HEALTHGRADES AWARDS

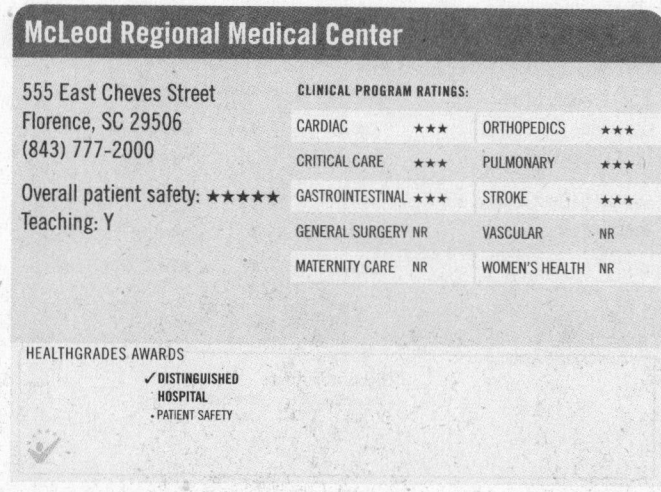

✓ DISTINGUISHED
   HOSPITAL
 • PATIENT SAFETY

Oconee Memorial Hospital

298 Memorial Drive
Seneca, SC 29672
(864) 882-3351

Overall patient safety: ★★★
Teaching: Y

CLINICAL PROGRAM RATINGS:

CARDIAC	NR	ORTHOPEDICS	NR
CRITICAL CARE	NR	PULMONARY	★★★★★
GASTROINTESTINAL	★★★	STROKE	★★★
GENERAL SURGERY	NR	VASCULAR	NR
MATERNITY CARE	NR	WOMEN'S HEALTH	NR

HEALTHGRADES AWARDS

Medical University Hospital

171 Ashley Avenue
Charleston, SC 29425
(843) 792-2300

Overall patient safety: ★★★
Teaching: Y

CLINICAL PROGRAM RATINGS:

CARDIAC	★★★	ORTHOPEDICS	★★★
CRITICAL CARE	★★★	PULMONARY	★★★
GASTROINTESTINAL	★★★	STROKE	★
GENERAL SURGERY	NR	VASCULAR	★★★
MATERNITY CARE	NR	WOMEN'S HEALTH	NR

HEALTHGRADES AWARDS

Palmetto Health Baptist

Taylor at Marion Street
Columbia, SC 29220
(803) 296-5010

Overall patient safety: ★★★
Teaching: N

CLINICAL PROGRAM RATINGS:

CARDIAC	NR	ORTHOPEDICS	★★★
CRITICAL CARE	★★★	PULMONARY	★★★
GASTROINTESTINAL	★★★	STROKE	★★★
GENERAL SURGERY	NR	VASCULAR	NR
MATERNITY CARE	NR	WOMEN'S HEALTH	NR

HEALTHGRADES AWARDS

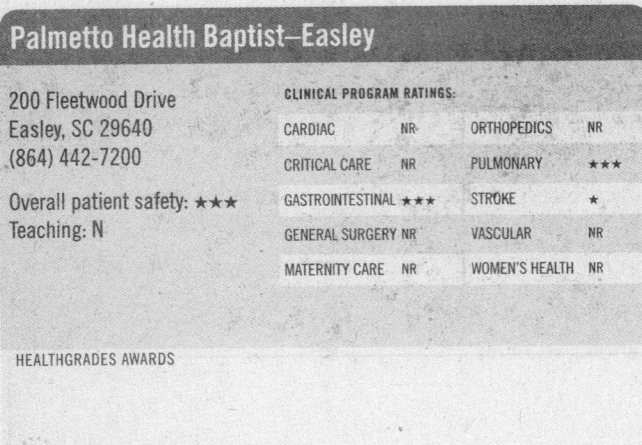

Palmetto Health Baptist—Easley

200 Fleetwood Drive
Easley, SC 29640
(864) 442-7200

Overall patient safety: ★★★
Teaching: N

CLINICAL PROGRAM RATINGS:

CARDIAC	NR	ORTHOPEDICS	NR
CRITICAL CARE	NR	PULMONARY	★★★
GASTROINTESTINAL	★★★	STROKE	★
GENERAL SURGERY	NR	VASCULAR	NR
MATERNITY CARE	NR	WOMEN'S HEALTH	NR

HEALTHGRADES AWARDS

Roper Hospital

316 Calhoun Street
Charleston, SC 29401
(843) 724-2000

Overall patient safety: ★★★
Teaching: N

CLINICAL PROGRAM RATINGS:

CARDIAC	★★★	ORTHOPEDICS	★
CRITICAL CARE	NR	PULMONARY	★★★
GASTROINTESTINAL	★★★	STROKE	★★★
GENERAL SURGERY	NR	VASCULAR	★★★
MATERNITY CARE	NR	WOMEN'S HEALTH	NR

HEALTHGRADES AWARDS

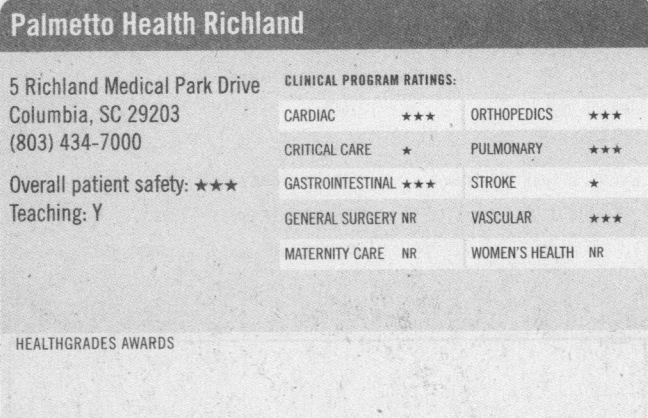

Palmetto Health Richland

5 Richland Medical Park Drive
Columbia, SC 29203
(803) 434-7000

Overall patient safety: ★★★
Teaching: Y

CLINICAL PROGRAM RATINGS:

CARDIAC	★★★	ORTHOPEDICS	★★★
CRITICAL CARE	★	PULMONARY	★★★
GASTROINTESTINAL	★★★	STROKE	★
GENERAL SURGERY	NR	VASCULAR	★★★
MATERNITY CARE	NR	WOMEN'S HEALTH	NR

HEALTHGRADES AWARDS

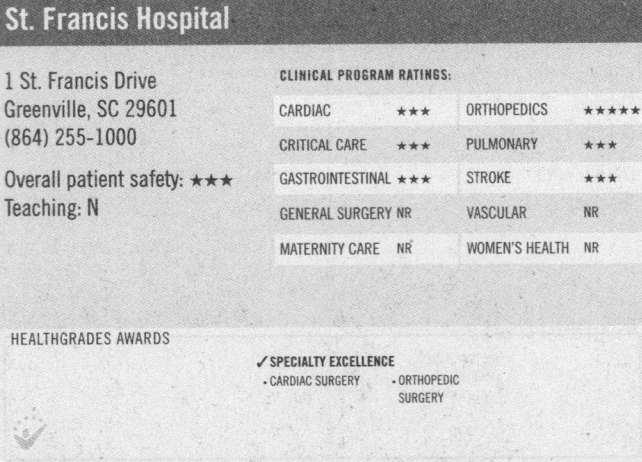

St. Francis Hospital

1 St. Francis Drive
Greenville, SC 29601
(864) 255-1000

Overall patient safety: ★★★
Teaching: N

CLINICAL PROGRAM RATINGS:

CARDIAC	★★★	ORTHOPEDICS	★★★★★
CRITICAL CARE	★★★	PULMONARY	★★★
GASTROINTESTINAL	★★★	STROKE	★★★
GENERAL SURGERY	NR	VASCULAR	NR
MATERNITY CARE	NR	WOMEN'S HEALTH	NR

HEALTHGRADES AWARDS

✓ SPECIALTY EXCELLENCE
- CARDIAC SURGERY
- ORTHOPEDIC SURGERY

Piedmont Medical Center

222 South Herlong Avenue
Rock Hill, SC 29732
(803) 329-1234

Overall patient safety: ★★★
Teaching: N

CLINICAL PROGRAM RATINGS:

CARDIAC	★★★	ORTHOPEDICS	★★★
CRITICAL CARE	★★★	PULMONARY	★★★★★
GASTROINTESTINAL	★	STROKE	★★★
GENERAL SURGERY	NR	VASCULAR	★★★
MATERNITY CARE	NR	WOMEN'S HEALTH	NR

HEALTHGRADES AWARDS

✓ SPECIALTY EXCELLENCE
- PULMONARY CARE

Self Regional Healthcare

1325 Spring Street
Greenwood, SC 29646
(864) 227-4111

Overall patient safety: ★★★
Teaching: Y

CLINICAL PROGRAM RATINGS:

CARDIAC	★★★	ORTHOPEDICS	★★★
CRITICAL CARE	★	PULMONARY	★★★
GASTROINTESTINAL	★★★	STROKE	★★★
GENERAL SURGERY	NR	VASCULAR	★★★
MATERNITY CARE	NR	WOMEN'S HEALTH	NR

HEALTHGRADES AWARDS

KEY: ★★★★★ BEST   ★★★ AS EXPECTED   ★ POOR   NR NOT RATED BY HEALTHGRADES   For full definitions of ratings and awards, see Appendix.

Sisters of Charity Providence Hospitals

2435 Forest Drive
Columbia, SC 29204
(803) 256-5300

Overall patient safety: ★★★
Teaching: N

CLINICAL PROGRAM RATINGS:

CARDIAC	★★★	ORTHOPEDICS	★★★
CRITICAL CARE	NR	PULMONARY	★★★
GASTROINTESTINAL	★★★	STROKE	★
GENERAL SURGERY	NR	VASCULAR	NR
MATERNITY CARE	NR	WOMEN'S HEALTH	NR

HEALTHGRADES AWARDS

Trident Medical Center

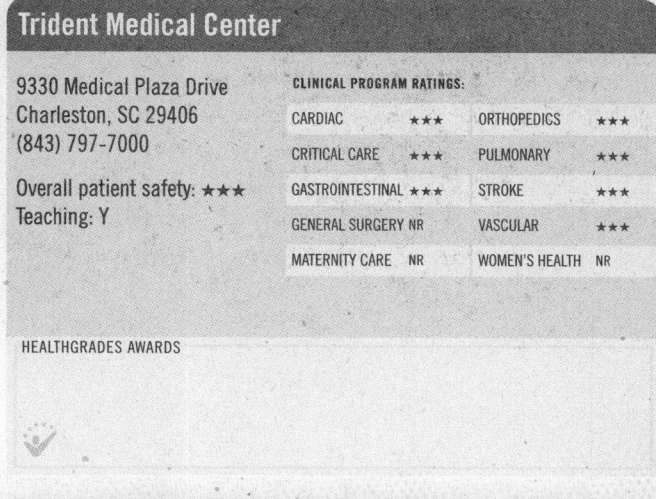

9330 Medical Plaza Drive
Charleston, SC 29406
(843) 797-7000

Overall patient safety: ★★★
Teaching: Y

CLINICAL PROGRAM RATINGS:

CARDIAC	★★★	ORTHOPEDICS	★★★
CRITICAL CARE	★★★	PULMONARY	★★★
GASTROINTESTINAL	★★★	STROKE	★★★
GENERAL SURGERY	NR	VASCULAR	★★★
MATERNITY CARE	NR	WOMEN'S HEALTH	NR

HEALTHGRADES AWARDS

Spartanburg Regional Medical Center

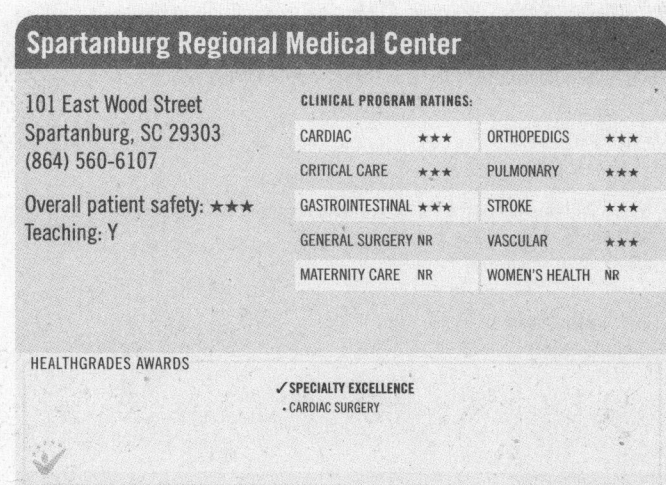

101 East Wood Street
Spartanburg, SC 29303
(864) 560-6107

Overall patient safety: ★★★
Teaching: Y

CLINICAL PROGRAM RATINGS:

CARDIAC	★★★	ORTHOPEDICS	★★★
CRITICAL CARE	★★★	PULMONARY	★★★
GASTROINTESTINAL	★★★	STROKE	★★★
GENERAL SURGERY	NR	VASCULAR	★★★
MATERNITY CARE	NR	WOMEN'S HEALTH	NR

HEALTHGRADES AWARDS

✓ SPECIALTY EXCELLENCE
· CARDIAC SURGERY

TRMC of Orangeburg and Calhoun

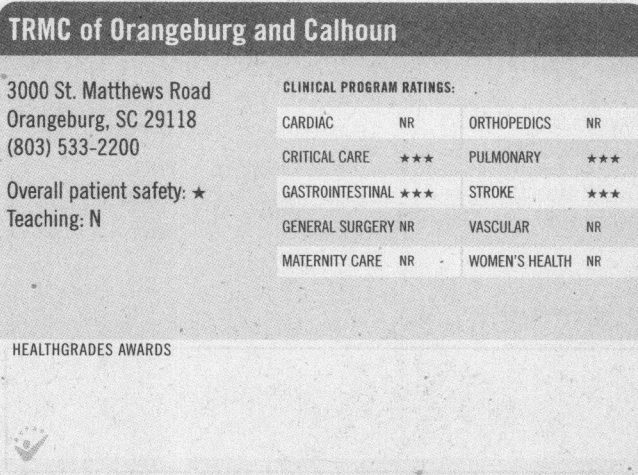

3000 St. Matthews Road
Orangeburg, SC 29118
(803) 533-2200

Overall patient safety: ★
Teaching: N

CLINICAL PROGRAM RATINGS:

CARDIAC	NR	ORTHOPEDICS	NR
CRITICAL CARE	★★★	PULMONARY	★★★
GASTROINTESTINAL	★★★	STROKE	★★★
GENERAL SURGERY	NR	VASCULAR	NR
MATERNITY CARE	NR	WOMEN'S HEALTH	NR

HEALTHGRADES AWARDS

Springs Memorial Hospital

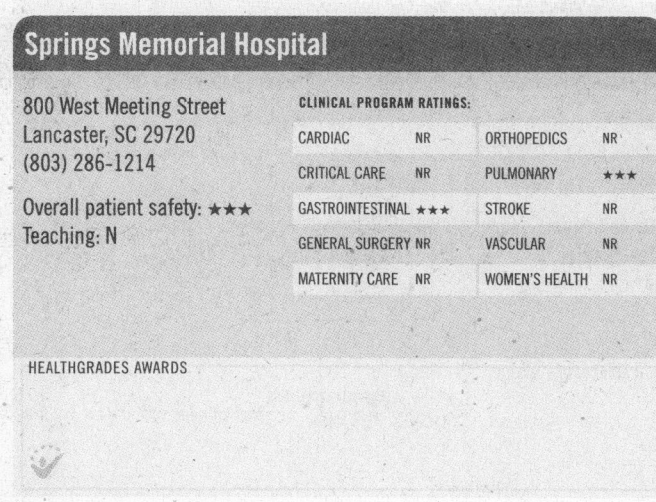

800 West Meeting Street
Lancaster, SC 29720
(803) 286-1214

Overall patient safety: ★★★
Teaching: N

CLINICAL PROGRAM RATINGS:

CARDIAC	NR	ORTHOPEDICS	NR
CRITICAL CARE	NR	PULMONARY	★★★
GASTROINTESTINAL	★★★	STROKE	NR
GENERAL SURGERY	NR	VASCULAR	NR
MATERNITY CARE	NR	WOMEN'S HEALTH	NR

HEALTHGRADES AWARDS

Tuomey Healthcare System

129 North Washington Street
Sumter, SC 29150
(803) 778-9000

Overall patient safety: ★★★★★
Teaching: N

CLINICAL PROGRAM RATINGS:

CARDIAC	NR	ORTHOPEDICS	NR
CRITICAL CARE	NR	PULMONARY	★★★
GASTROINTESTINAL	★★★	STROKE	★★★
GENERAL SURGERY	NR	VASCULAR	NR
MATERNITY CARE	NR	WOMEN'S HEALTH	NR

HEALTHGRADES AWARDS

✓ DISTINGUISHED
HOSPITAL
· PATIENT SAFETY

Upstate Carolina Medical Center

1530 North Limestone Street
Gaffney, SC 29340
(864) 487-4271

Overall patient safety: ★
Teaching: N

CLINICAL PROGRAM RATINGS:

CARDIAC	NR	ORTHOPEDICS	NR
CRITICAL CARE	NR	PULMONARY	★
GASTROINTESTINAL	★★★	STROKE	★
GENERAL SURGERY	NR	VASCULAR	NR
MATERNITY CARE	NR	WOMEN'S HEALTH	NR

HEALTHGRADES AWARDS

Wallace Thomson Hospital

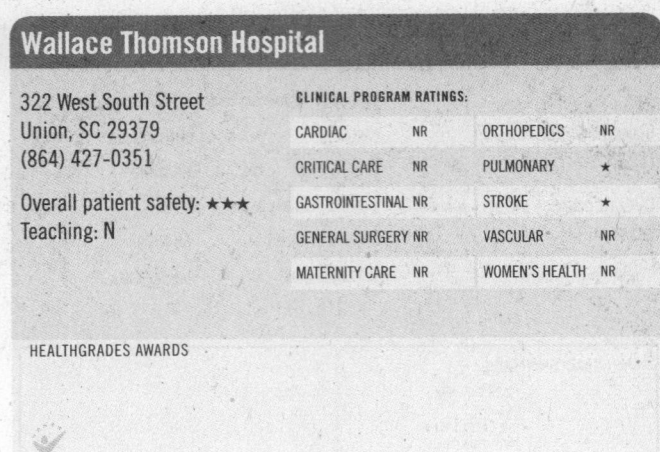

322 West South Street
Union, SC 29379
(864) 427-0351

Overall patient safety: ★★★
Teaching: N

CLINICAL PROGRAM RATINGS:

CARDIAC	NR	ORTHOPEDICS	NR
CRITICAL CARE	NR	PULMONARY	★
GASTROINTESTINAL	NR	STROKE	★
GENERAL SURGERY	NR	VASCULAR	NR
MATERNITY CARE	NR	WOMEN'S HEALTH	NR

HEALTHGRADES AWARDS

Waccamaw Community Hospital

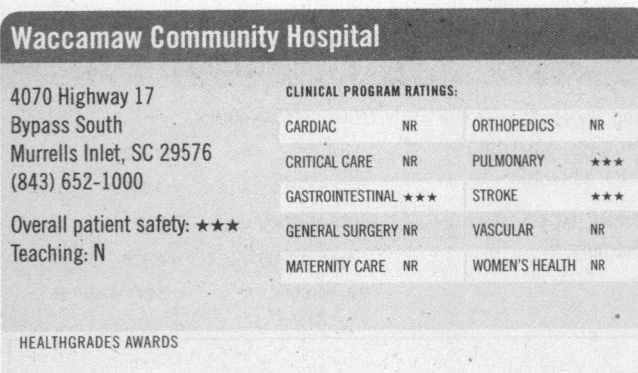

4070 Highway 17
Bypass South
Murrells Inlet, SC 29576
(843) 652-1000

Overall patient safety: ★★★
Teaching: N

CLINICAL PROGRAM RATINGS:

CARDIAC	NR	ORTHOPEDICS	NR
CRITICAL CARE	NR	PULMONARY	★★★
GASTROINTESTINAL	★★★	STROKE	★★★
GENERAL SURGERY	NR	VASCULAR	NR
MATERNITY CARE	NR	WOMEN'S HEALTH	NR

HEALTHGRADES AWARDS

Williamsburg Regional Hospital

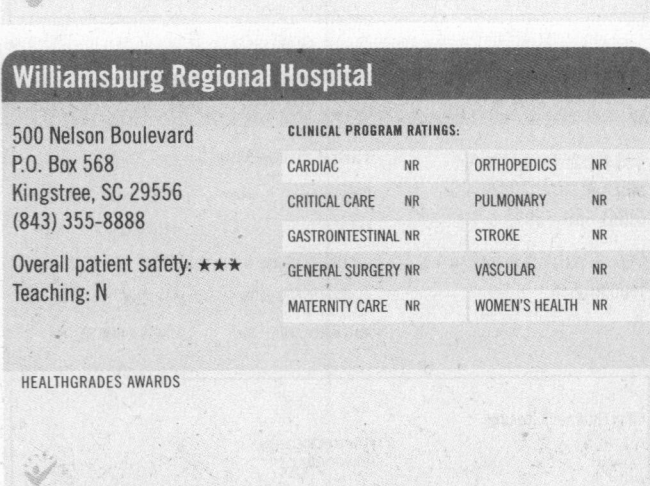

500 Nelson Boulevard
P.O. Box 568
Kingstree, SC 29556
(843) 355-8888

Overall patient safety: ★★★
Teaching: N

CLINICAL PROGRAM RATINGS:

CARDIAC	NR	ORTHOPEDICS	NR
CRITICAL CARE	NR	PULMONARY	NR
GASTROINTESTINAL	NR	STROKE	NR
GENERAL SURGERY	NR	VASCULAR	NR
MATERNITY CARE	NR	WOMEN'S HEALTH	NR

HEALTHGRADES AWARDS

SOUTH DAKOTA HOSPITALS: RATINGS BY CLINICAL SPECIALTY

Avera Gregory Healthcare Center

400 Park Avenue
Gregory, SD 57533
(605) 835-8394

Overall patient safety: ★★★
Teaching: N

CLINICAL PROGRAM RATINGS:

CARDIAC	NR	ORTHOPEDICS	NR
CRITICAL CARE	NR	PULMONARY	NR
GASTROINTESTINAL	NR	STROKE	NR
GENERAL SURGERY	NR	VASCULAR	NR
MATERNITY CARE	NR	WOMEN'S HEALTH	NR

HEALTHGRADES AWARDS

Avera Heart Hospital of South Dakota

4500 West 69th Street
Sioux Falls, SD 57108
(605) 977-7000

Overall patient safety: ★★★★★
Teaching: N

CLINICAL PROGRAM RATINGS:

CARDIAC	★★★★★	ORTHOPEDICS	NR
CRITICAL CARE	NR	PULMONARY	NR
GASTROINTESTINAL	NR	STROKE	NR
GENERAL SURGERY	NR	VASCULAR	★★★
MATERNITY CARE	NR	WOMEN'S HEALTH	NR

HEALTHGRADES AWARDS

✓ SPECIALTY EXCELLENCE
• CARDIAC CARE   • CARDIAC SURGERY

KEY: ★★★★★ BEST   ★★★ AS EXPECTED   ★ POOR   NR NOT RATED BY HEALTHGRADES   For full definitions of ratings and awards, see Appendix.

Avera McKennan Hospital and University Health Center

800 East 21st Street
Sioux Falls, SD 57117
(605) 322-8000

Overall patient safety: ★★★★★
Teaching: Y

CLINICAL PROGRAM RATINGS:

CARDIAC	NR	ORTHOPEDICS	★★★
CRITICAL CARE	NR	PULMONARY	★★★★★
GASTROINTESTINAL	★★★	STROKE	★★★★★
GENERAL SURGERY	NR	VASCULAR	NR
MATERNITY CARE	NR	WOMEN'S HEALTH	NR

HEALTHGRADES AWARDS

✓ DISTINGUISHED HOSPITAL
- CLINICAL EXCELLENCE
- PATIENT SAFETY

✓ SPECIALTY EXCELLENCE
- JOINT REPLACEMENT - STROKE CARE

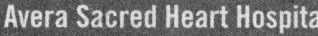

Avera St. Luke's*

305 South State Street
Aberdeen, SD 57401
(605) 622-5000

Overall patient safety: ★★★
Teaching: N

CLINICAL PROGRAM RATINGS:

CARDIAC	NR	ORTHOPEDICS	★★★
CRITICAL CARE	NR	PULMONARY	★★★
GASTROINTESTINAL	★★★	STROKE	★★★
GENERAL SURGERY	NR	VASCULAR	NR
MATERNITY CARE	NR	WOMEN'S HEALTH	NR

HEALTHGRADES AWARDS

Avera Queen of Peace

525 North Foster Street
Mitchell, SD 57301
(605) 995-2000

Overall patient safety: ★★★
Teaching: N

CLINICAL PROGRAM RATINGS:

CARDIAC	NR	ORTHOPEDICS	NR
CRITICAL CARE	NR	PULMONARY	★★★
GASTROINTESTINAL	NR	STROKE	★★★
GENERAL SURGERY	NR	VASCULAR	NR
MATERNITY CARE	NR	WOMEN'S HEALTH	NR

HEALTHGRADES AWARDS

Brookings Hospital

300 22nd Avenue
Brookings, SD 57006
(605) 696-9000

Overall patient safety: ★★★
Teaching: N

CLINICAL PROGRAM RATINGS:

CARDIAC	NR	ORTHOPEDICS	NR
CRITICAL CARE	NR	PULMONARY	★★★
GASTROINTESTINAL	NR	STROKE	★★★
GENERAL SURGERY	NR	VASCULAR	NR
MATERNITY CARE	NR	WOMEN'S HEALTH	NR

HEALTHGRADES AWARDS

Avera Sacred Heart Hospital

501 Summit Street
Yankton, SD 57078
(605) 668-8000

Overall patient safety: ★★★
Teaching: N

CLINICAL PROGRAM RATINGS:

CARDIAC	NR	ORTHOPEDICS	NR
CRITICAL CARE	NR	PULMONARY	★
GASTROINTESTINAL	NR	STROKE	★★★
GENERAL SURGERY	NR	VASCULAR	NR
MATERNITY CARE	NR	WOMEN'S HEALTH	NR

HEALTHGRADES AWARDS

Community Memorial Hospital

111 West 10th Avenue
Redfield, SD 57469
(605) 472-1110

Overall patient safety: NR
Teaching: N

CLINICAL PROGRAM RATINGS:

CARDIAC	NR	ORTHOPEDICS	NR
CRITICAL CARE	NR	PULMONARY	★★★
GASTROINTESTINAL	NR	STROKE	NR
GENERAL SURGERY	NR	VASCULAR	NR
MATERNITY CARE	NR	WOMEN'S HEALTH	NR

HEALTHGRADES AWARDS

*This hospital reports its data to the federal government jointly with another hospital. Therefore the ratings and awards apply to multiple hospitals and this specific hospital may not provide all rated services.

Dakota Midland Hospital*

1400 15th Avenue Northwest
Aberdeen, SD 57401
(605) 622-3300

Overall patient safety: ★★★
Teaching: N

CLINICAL PROGRAM RATINGS:

CARDIAC	NR	ORTHOPEDICS	★★★
CRITICAL CARE	NR	PULMONARY	★★★
GASTROINTESTINAL	★★★	STROKE	★★★
GENERAL SURGERY	NR	VASCULAR	NR
MATERNITY CARE	NR	WOMEN'S HEALTH	NR

HEALTHGRADES AWARDS

Madison Community Hospital

917 North Washington Avenue
Madison, SD 57042
(605) 256-6551

Overall patient safety: ★
Teaching: N

CLINICAL PROGRAM RATINGS:

CARDIAC	NR	ORTHOPEDICS	NR
CRITICAL CARE	NR	PULMONARY	★★★
GASTROINTESTINAL	NR	STROKE	★★★
GENERAL SURGERY	NR	VASCULAR	NR
MATERNITY CARE	NR	WOMEN'S HEALTH	NR

HEALTHGRADES AWARDS

Hand County Memorial Hospital

300 West 5th Street
Miller, SD 57362
(605) 853-2421

Overall patient safety: NR
Teaching: N

CLINICAL PROGRAM RATINGS:

CARDIAC	NR	ORTHOPEDICS	NR
CRITICAL CARE	NR	PULMONARY	★★★
GASTROINTESTINAL	NR	STROKE	NR
GENERAL SURGERY	NR	VASCULAR	NR
MATERNITY CARE	NR	WOMEN'S HEALTH	NR

HEALTHGRADES AWARDS

Mid-Dakota Medical Center

300 South Byron Boulevard
Chamberlain, SD 57325
(605) 234-5511

Overall patient safety: ★★★
Teaching: N

CLINICAL PROGRAM RATINGS:

CARDIAC	NR	ORTHOPEDICS	NR
CRITICAL CARE	NR	PULMONARY	★★★
GASTROINTESTINAL	NR	STROKE	NR
GENERAL SURGERY	NR	VASCULAR	NR
MATERNITY CARE	NR	WOMEN'S HEALTH	NR

HEALTHGRADES AWARDS

Huron Regional Medical Center

172 4th Street Southeast
Huron, SD 57350
(605) 353-6200

Overall patient safety: ★★★
Teaching: N

CLINICAL PROGRAM RATINGS:

CARDIAC	NR	ORTHOPEDICS	NR
CRITICAL CARE	NR	PULMONARY	NR
GASTROINTESTINAL	NR	STROKE	★★★
GENERAL SURGERY	NR	VASCULAR	NR
MATERNITY CARE	NR	WOMEN'S HEALTH	NR

HEALTHGRADES AWARDS

Milbank Area Hospital—Avera Health

901 East Virgil Avenue
Milbank, SD 57252
(605) 432-4538

Overall patient safety: ★★★
Teaching: N

CLINICAL PROGRAM RATINGS:

CARDIAC	NR	ORTHOPEDICS	NR
CRITICAL CARE	NR	PULMONARY	NR
GASTROINTESTINAL	NR	STROKE	★
GENERAL SURGERY	NR	VASCULAR	NR
MATERNITY CARE	NR	WOMEN'S HEALTH	NR

HEALTHGRADES AWARDS

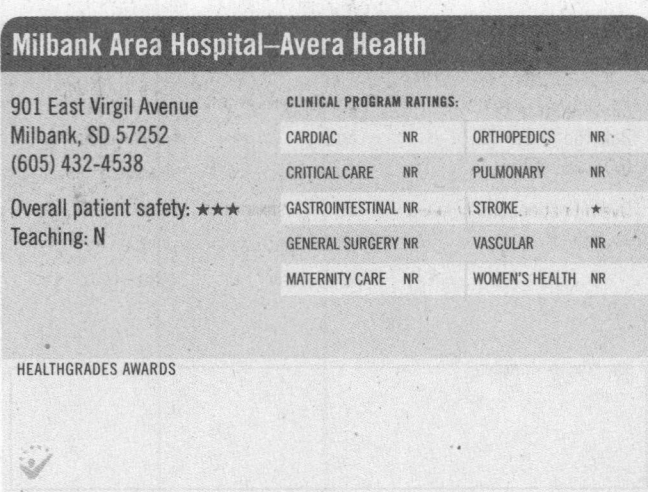

KEY: ★★★★★ **BEST**   ★★★ **AS EXPECTED**   ★ **POOR**   NR **NOT RATED BY HEALTHGRADES**   For full definitions of ratings and awards, see Appendix.

Mobridge Regional Hospital

1401 10th Avenue West
Mobridge, SD 57601
(605) 845-3692

Overall patient safety: ★★★
Teaching: N

CLINICAL PROGRAM RATINGS:

CARDIAC	NR	ORTHOPEDICS	NR
CRITICAL CARE	NR	PULMONARY	★
GASTROINTESTINAL	NR	STROKE	NR
GENERAL SURGERY	NR	VASCULAR	NR
MATERNITY CARE	NR	WOMEN'S HEALTH	NR

HEALTHGRADES AWARDS

Prairie Lakes Hospital and Care Center

400 10th Avenue Northwest
Watertown, SD 57201
(605) 882-7000

Overall patient safety: ★★★
Teaching: N

CLINICAL PROGRAM RATINGS:

CARDIAC	NR	ORTHOPEDICS	NR
CRITICAL CARE	NR	PULMONARY	★★★
GASTROINTESTINAL	★★★	STROKE	★
GENERAL SURGERY	NR	VASCULAR	NR
MATERNITY CARE	NR	WOMEN'S HEALTH	NR

HEALTHGRADES AWARDS

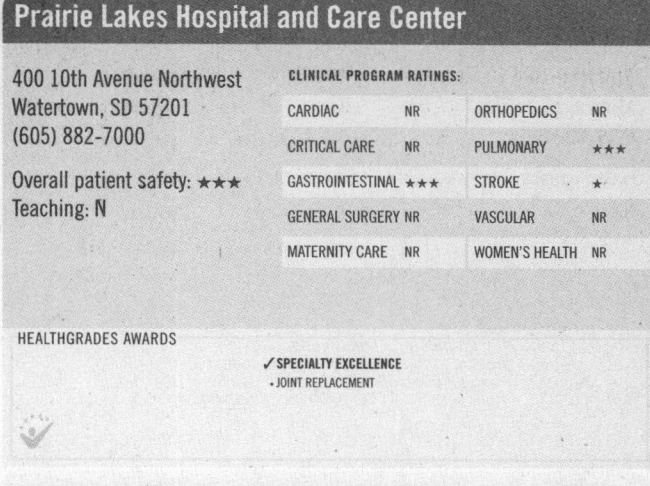

✓ SPECIALTY EXCELLENCE
· JOINT REPLACEMENT

Physicians Indian Hospital

111 Washington Avenue
Box 490
Wagner, SD 57380
(605) 384-3621

Overall patient safety: ★★★
Teaching: N

CLINICAL PROGRAM RATINGS:

CARDIAC	NR	ORTHOPEDICS	NR
CRITICAL CARE	NR	PULMONARY	★★★
GASTROINTESTINAL	NR	STROKE	NR
GENERAL SURGERY	NR	VASCULAR	NR
MATERNITY CARE	NR	WOMEN'S HEALTH	NR

HEALTHGRADES AWARDS

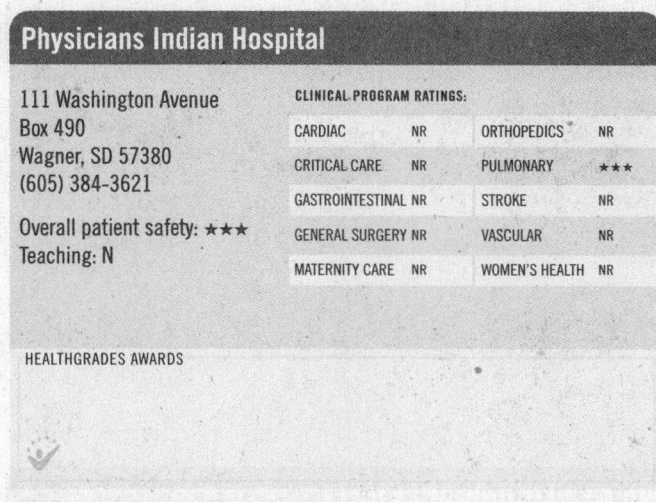

Rapid City Regional Hospital

353 Fairmont Boulevard
Rapid City, SD 57701
(605) 719-1000

Overall patient safety: ★★★
Teaching: Y

CLINICAL PROGRAM RATINGS:

CARDIAC	★★★	ORTHOPEDICS	★★★
CRITICAL CARE	NR	PULMONARY	★★★
GASTROINTESTINAL	★★★	STROKE	★
GENERAL SURGERY	NR	VASCULAR	★★★
MATERNITY CARE	NR	WOMEN'S HEALTH	NR

HEALTHGRADES AWARDS

Physicians Indian Hospital at Pine Ridge

East Highway 18
Pine Ridge, SD 57770
(605) 867-5131

Overall patient safety: ★★★
Teaching: N

CLINICAL PROGRAM RATINGS:

CARDIAC	NR	ORTHOPEDICS	NR
CRITICAL CARE	NR	PULMONARY	★★★
GASTROINTESTINAL	NR	STROKE	NR
GENERAL SURGERY	NR	VASCULAR	NR
MATERNITY CARE	NR	WOMEN'S HEALTH	NR

HEALTHGRADES AWARDS

St. Mary's Hospital

801 East Sioux Avenue
Pierre, SD 57501
(605) 224-3100

Overall patient safety: ★★★
Teaching: N

CLINICAL PROGRAM RATINGS:

CARDIAC	NR	ORTHOPEDICS	★★★
CRITICAL CARE	NR	PULMONARY	★★★
GASTROINTESTINAL	NR	STROKE	★★★
GENERAL SURGERY	NR	VASCULAR	NR
MATERNITY CARE	NR	WOMEN'S HEALTH	NR

HEALTHGRADES AWARDS

*This hospital reports its data to the federal government jointly with another hospital. Therefore the ratings and awards apply to multiple hospitals and this specific hospital may not provide all rated services.

Sanford USD Medical Center

1305 West 18th Street
Sioux Falls, SD 57117
(605) 333-1000

Overall patient safety: ★★★★★
Teaching: Y

CLINICAL PROGRAM RATINGS:

CARDIAC	★★★	ORTHOPEDICS	★★★★★
CRITICAL CARE	NR	PULMONARY	★★★
GASTROINTESTINAL	★★★	STROKE	★★★
GENERAL SURGERY	NR	VASCULAR	★★★
MATERNITY CARE	NR	WOMEN'S HEALTH	NR

HEALTHGRADES AWARDS

✓ DISTINGUISHED HOSPITAL
- CLINICAL EXCELLENCE
- PATIENT SAFETY

✓ SPECIALTY EXCELLENCE
- GASTROINTESTINAL CARE
- JOINT REPLACEMENT
- ORTHOPEDIC SURGERY
- VASCULAR SURGERY

Sturgis Regional Hospital

949 Harmon Street
Sturgis, SD 57785
(605) 347-2536

Overall patient safety: ★★★
Teaching: N

CLINICAL PROGRAM RATINGS:

CARDIAC	NR	ORTHOPEDICS	NR
CRITICAL CARE	NR	PULMONARY	★★★
GASTROINTESTINAL	NR	STROKE	NR
GENERAL SURGERY	NR	VASCULAR	NR
MATERNITY CARE	NR	WOMEN'S HEALTH	NR

HEALTHGRADES AWARDS

Spearfish Regional Hospital

1440 North Main Street
Spearfish, SD 57783
(605) 644-4000

Overall patient safety: ★★★
Teaching: N

CLINICAL PROGRAM RATINGS:

CARDIAC	NR	ORTHOPEDICS	NR
CRITICAL CARE	NR	PULMONARY	★★★
GASTROINTESTINAL	NR	STROKE	★★★
GENERAL SURGERY	NR	VASCULAR	NR
MATERNITY CARE	NR	WOMEN'S HEALTH	NR

HEALTHGRADES AWARDS

Winner Regional Healthcare Center

745 East 8th Street
Winner, SD 57580
(605) 842-7100

Overall patient safety: ★★★
Teaching: N

CLINICAL PROGRAM RATINGS:

CARDIAC	NR	ORTHOPEDICS	NR
CRITICAL CARE	NR	PULMONARY	★★★
GASTROINTESTINAL	NR	STROKE	NR
GENERAL SURGERY	NR	VASCULAR	NR
MATERNITY CARE	NR	WOMEN'S HEALTH	NR

HEALTHGRADES AWARDS

TENNESSEE HOSPITALS: RATINGS BY CLINICAL SPECIALTY

Athens Regional Medical Center

1114 West Madison Avenue
Athens, TN 37371
(423) 745-1411

Overall patient safety: ★★★
Teaching: N

CLINICAL PROGRAM RATINGS:

CARDIAC	NR	ORTHOPEDICS	NR
CRITICAL CARE	NR	PULMONARY	★
GASTROINTESTINAL	NR	STROKE	★
GENERAL SURGERY	NR	VASCULAR	NR
MATERNITY CARE	NR	WOMEN'S HEALTH	NR

HEALTHGRADES AWARDS

Baptist Hospital

2000 Church Street
Nashville, TN 37236
(615) 284-5555

Overall patient safety: ★★★
Teaching: Y

CLINICAL PROGRAM RATINGS:

CARDIAC	★★★	ORTHOPEDICS	★★★
CRITICAL CARE	★★★	PULMONARY	★★★★★
GASTROINTESTINAL	★★★	STROKE	★★★
GENERAL SURGERY	NR	VASCULAR	★★★
MATERNITY CARE	NR	WOMEN'S HEALTH	NR

HEALTHGRADES AWARDS

✓ SPECIALTY EXCELLENCE
- PULMONARY CARE

KEY: ★★★★★ BEST   ★★★ AS EXPECTED   ★ POOR   NR NOT RATED BY HEALTHGRADES   For full definitions of ratings and awards, see Appendix.

Baptist Hospital of Cocke County

435 2nd Street
Newport, TN 37821
(423) 625-2200

Overall patient safety: ★★★
Teaching: N

CLINICAL PROGRAM RATINGS:

CARDIAC	NR	ORTHOPEDICS	NR
CRITICAL CARE	NR	PULMONARY	★★★
GASTROINTESTINAL	NR	STROKE	★★★
GENERAL SURGERY	NR	VASCULAR	NR
MATERNITY CARE	NR	WOMEN'S HEALTH	NR

HEALTHGRADES AWARDS

Baptist Memorial Hospital

6019 Walnut Grove Road
Memphis, TN 38120
(901) 226-5000

Overall patient safety: ★★★
Teaching: Y

CLINICAL PROGRAM RATINGS:

CARDIAC	★★★	ORTHOPEDICS	★★★
CRITICAL CARE	★★★	PULMONARY	★★★
GASTROINTESTINAL	★★★★★	STROKE	★★★★★
GENERAL SURGERY	NR	VASCULAR	★★★
MATERNITY CARE	NR	WOMEN'S HEALTH	NR

HEALTHGRADES AWARDS

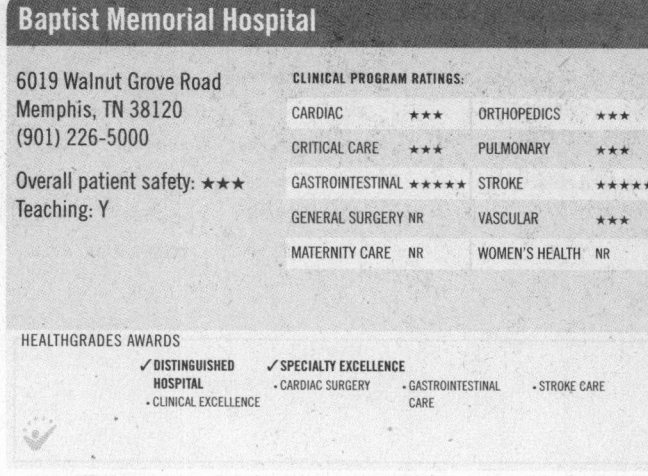

✓ DISTINGUISHED HOSPITAL
· CLINICAL EXCELLENCE

✓ SPECIALTY EXCELLENCE
· CARDIAC SURGERY   · GASTROINTESTINAL   · STROKE CARE
                      CARE

Baptist Hospital of East Tennessee

137 Blount Avenue Southeast
Knoxville, TN 37920
(865) 632-5011

Overall patient safety: ★
Teaching: N

CLINICAL PROGRAM RATINGS:

CARDIAC	★★★	ORTHOPEDICS	NR
CRITICAL CARE	★★★★★	PULMONARY	★★★★★
GASTROINTESTINAL	★★★	STROKE	★★★
GENERAL SURGERY	NR	VASCULAR	NR
MATERNITY CARE	NR	WOMEN'S HEALTH	NR

HEALTHGRADES AWARDS

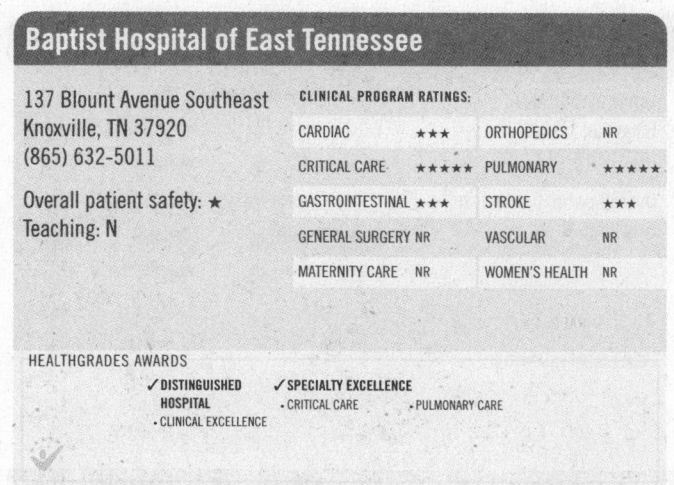

✓ DISTINGUISHED HOSPITAL
· CLINICAL EXCELLENCE

✓ SPECIALTY EXCELLENCE
· CRITICAL CARE   · PULMONARY CARE

Baptist Memorial Hospital—Collierville

1500 West Poplar Avenue
Collierville, TN 38017
(901) 861-9000

Overall patient safety: ★★★
Teaching: N

CLINICAL PROGRAM RATINGS:

CARDIAC	NR	ORTHOPEDICS	★★★
CRITICAL CARE	NR	PULMONARY	★★★
GASTROINTESTINAL	NR	STROKE	★★★
GENERAL SURGERY	NR	VASCULAR	NR
MATERNITY CARE	NR	WOMEN'S HEALTH	NR

HEALTHGRADES AWARDS

Baptist Hospital West

10820 Parkside Drive
Knoxville, TN 37922
(865) 218-7090

Overall patient safety: ★★★
Teaching: N

CLINICAL PROGRAM RATINGS:

CARDIAC	NR	ORTHOPEDICS	NR
CRITICAL CARE	NR	PULMONARY	★★★
GASTROINTESTINAL	NR	STROKE	★★★
GENERAL SURGERY	NR	VASCULAR	NR
MATERNITY CARE	NR	WOMEN'S HEALTH	NR

HEALTHGRADES AWARDS

Baptist Memorial Hospital—Huntingdon

631 R. B. Wilson Drive
Huntingdon, TN 38344
(731) 986-4461

Overall patient safety: ★★★
Teaching: N

CLINICAL PROGRAM RATINGS:

CARDIAC	NR	ORTHOPEDICS	NR
CRITICAL CARE	NR	PULMONARY	★
GASTROINTESTINAL	NR	STROKE	★
GENERAL SURGERY	NR	VASCULAR	NR
MATERNITY CARE	NR	WOMEN'S HEALTH	NR

HEALTHGRADES AWARDS

Baptist Memorial Hospital—Lauderdale

326 Asbury Avenue
Ripley, TN 38063
(731) 221-2200

Overall patient safety: ★★★
Teaching: N

CLINICAL PROGRAM RATINGS:

CARDIAC	NR	ORTHOPEDICS	NR
CRITICAL CARE	NR	PULMONARY	★★★
GASTROINTESTINAL	NR	STROKE	NR
GENERAL SURGERY	NR	VASCULAR	NR
MATERNITY CARE	NR	WOMEN'S HEALTH	NR

HEALTHGRADES AWARDS

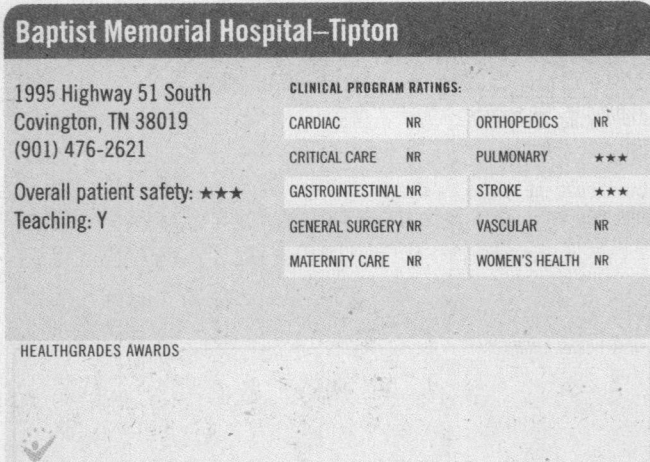

Bedford County Medical Center

845 Union Street
Shelbyville, TN 37160
(931) 685-5433

Overall patient safety: ★
Teaching: N

CLINICAL PROGRAM RATINGS:

CARDIAC	NR	ORTHOPEDICS	NR
CRITICAL CARE	NR	PULMONARY	★★★
GASTROINTESTINAL	NR	STROKE	★
GENERAL SURGERY	NR	VASCULAR	NR
MATERNITY CARE	NR	WOMEN'S HEALTH	NR

HEALTHGRADES AWARDS

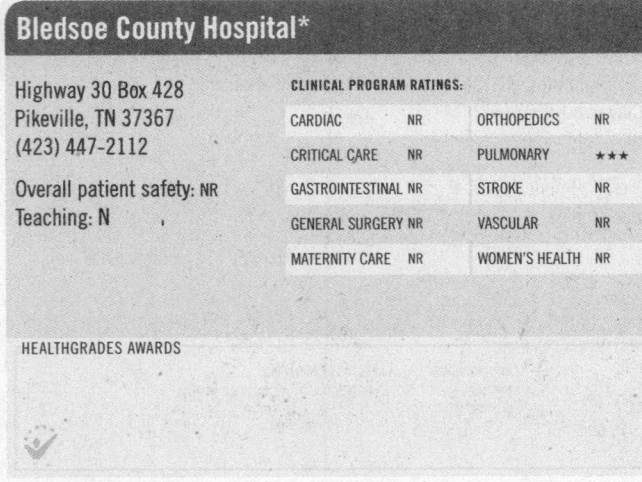

Baptist Memorial Hospital—Tipton

1995 Highway 51 South
Covington, TN 38019
(901) 476-2621

Overall patient safety: ★★★
Teaching: Y

CLINICAL PROGRAM RATINGS:

CARDIAC	NR	ORTHOPEDICS	NR
CRITICAL CARE	NR	PULMONARY	★★★
GASTROINTESTINAL	NR	STROKE	★★★
GENERAL SURGERY	NR	VASCULAR	NR
MATERNITY CARE	NR	WOMEN'S HEALTH	NR

HEALTHGRADES AWARDS

Bledsoe County Hospital*

Highway 30 Box 428
Pikeville, TN 37367
(423) 447-2112

Overall patient safety: NR
Teaching: N

CLINICAL PROGRAM RATINGS:

CARDIAC	NR	ORTHOPEDICS	NR
CRITICAL CARE	NR	PULMONARY	★★★
GASTROINTESTINAL	NR	STROKE	NR
GENERAL SURGERY	NR	VASCULAR	NR
MATERNITY CARE	NR	WOMEN'S HEALTH	NR

HEALTHGRADES AWARDS

Baptist Memorial Hospital—Union City

1201 Bishop Street
Union City, TN 38261
(731) 885-2410

Overall patient safety: ★★★
Teaching: N

CLINICAL PROGRAM RATINGS:

CARDIAC	NR	ORTHOPEDICS	NR
CRITICAL CARE	NR	PULMONARY	★
GASTROINTESTINAL	NR	STROKE	★
GENERAL SURGERY	NR	VASCULAR	NR
MATERNITY CARE	NR	WOMEN'S HEALTH	NR

HEALTHGRADES AWARDS

Blount Memorial Hospital

907 East Lamar
Alexander Parkway
Maryville, TN 37804
(865) 983-7211

Overall patient safety: ★
Teaching: N

CLINICAL PROGRAM RATINGS:

CARDIAC	NR	ORTHOPEDICS	★★★
CRITICAL CARE	★★★	PULMONARY	★★★
GASTROINTESTINAL	★★★	STROKE	★
GENERAL SURGERY	NR	VASCULAR	NR
MATERNITY CARE	NR	WOMEN'S HEALTH	NR

HEALTHGRADES AWARDS

KEY: ★★★★★ BEST   ★★★ AS EXPECTED   ★ POOR   NR NOT RATED BY HEALTHGRADES   For full definitions of ratings and awards, see Appendix.

Bolivar General Hospital

650 Nuckolls Road
Bolivar, TN 38008
(731) 658-3100

Overall patient safety: ★★★
Teaching: N

CLINICAL PROGRAM RATINGS:

CARDIAC	NR	ORTHOPEDICS	NR
CRITICAL CARE	NR	PULMONARY	★
GASTROINTESTINAL	NR	STROKE	NR
GENERAL SURGERY	NR	VASCULAR	NR
MATERNITY CARE	NR	WOMEN'S HEALTH	NR

HEALTHGRADES AWARDS

Carthage General Hospital

130 Lebanon Highway
Carthage, TN 37030
(615) 735-9815

Overall patient safety: ★★★
Teaching: N

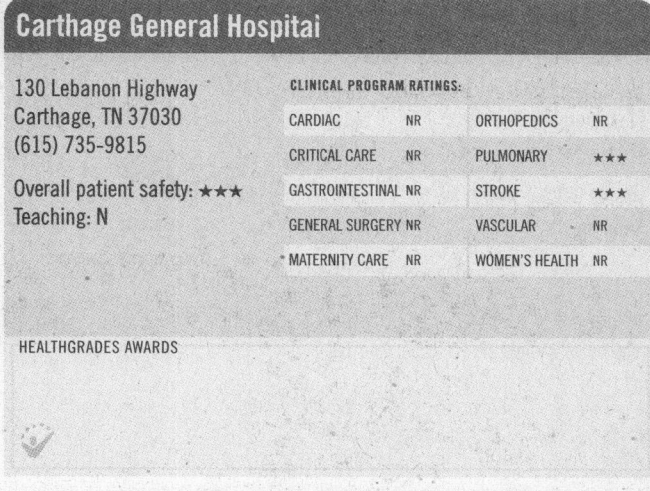

CLINICAL PROGRAM RATINGS:

CARDIAC	NR	ORTHOPEDICS	NR
CRITICAL CARE	NR	PULMONARY	★★★
GASTROINTESTINAL	NR	STROKE	★★★
GENERAL SURGERY	NR	VASCULAR	NR
MATERNITY CARE	NR	WOMEN'S HEALTH	NR

HEALTHGRADES AWARDS

Bradley Memorial Hospital

2305 Chambliss Avenue
Cleveland, TN 37311
(423) 559-6000

Overall patient safety: ★
Teaching: N

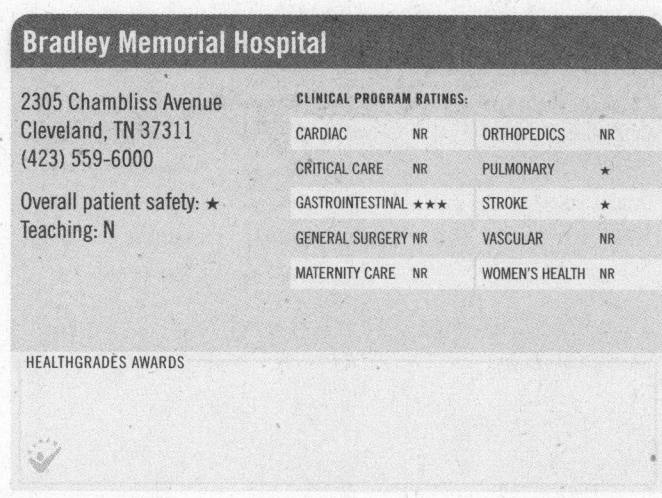

CLINICAL PROGRAM RATINGS:

CARDIAC	NR	ORTHOPEDICS	NR
CRITICAL CARE	NR	PULMONARY	★
GASTROINTESTINAL	★★★	STROKE	★
GENERAL SURGERY	NR	VASCULAR	NR
MATERNITY CARE	NR	WOMEN'S HEALTH	NR

HEALTHGRADES AWARDS

Centennial Medical Center

2300 Patterson Street
Nashville, TN 37203
(615) 342-1000

Overall patient safety: ★★★★★
Teaching: N

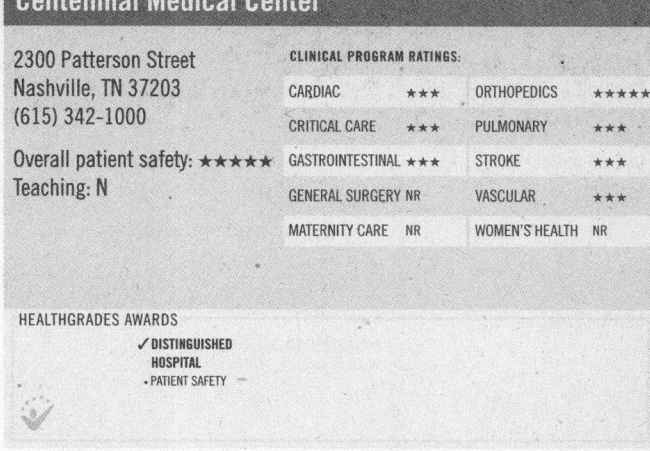

CLINICAL PROGRAM RATINGS:

CARDIAC	★★★	ORTHOPEDICS	★★★★★
CRITICAL CARE	★★★	PULMONARY	★★★
GASTROINTESTINAL	★★★	STROKE	★★★
GENERAL SURGERY	NR	VASCULAR	★★★
MATERNITY CARE	NR	WOMEN'S HEALTH	NR

HEALTHGRADES AWARDS

✓ DISTINGUISHED
HOSPITAL
- PATIENT SAFETY

Camden General Hospital

175 Hospital Drive
Camden, TN 38320
(731) 584-6135

Overall patient safety: NR
Teaching: N

CLINICAL PROGRAM RATINGS:

CARDIAC	NR	ORTHOPEDICS	NR
CRITICAL CARE	NR	PULMONARY	NR
GASTROINTESTINAL	NR	STROKE	NR
GENERAL SURGERY	NR	VASCULAR	NR
MATERNITY CARE	NR	WOMEN'S HEALTH	NR

HEALTHGRADES AWARDS

Claiborne County Hospital

1850 Old Knoxville Road
Tazewell, TN 37879
(423) 626-4211

Overall patient safety: ★★★
Teaching: N

CLINICAL PROGRAM RATINGS:

CARDIAC	NR	ORTHOPEDICS	NR
CRITICAL CARE	NR	PULMONARY	★★★
GASTROINTESTINAL	NR	STROKE	NR
GENERAL SURGERY	NR	VASCULAR	NR
MATERNITY CARE	NR	WOMEN'S HEALTH	NR

HEALTHGRADES AWARDS

---

*This hospital reports its data to the federal government jointly with another hospital. Therefore the ratings and awards apply to multiple hospitals and this specific hospital may not provide all rated services.

Cleveland Community Hospital

2800 Westside Drive Northwest
Cleveland, TN 37312
(423) 339-4100

Overall patient safety: ★★★
Teaching: N

CLINICAL PROGRAM RATINGS:

CARDIAC	NR	ORTHOPEDICS	NR
CRITICAL CARE	NR	PULMONARY	★★★
GASTROINTESTINAL	NR	STROKE	★★★
GENERAL SURGERY	NR	VASCULAR	NR
MATERNITY CARE	NR	WOMEN'S HEALTH	NR

HEALTHGRADES AWARDS

Crockett Hospital

1607 South Locust Avenue
Highway 43
Lawrenceburg, TN 38464
(931) 762-6571

Overall patient safety: ★★★
Teaching: N

CLINICAL PROGRAM RATINGS:

CARDIAC	NR	ORTHOPEDICS	NR
CRITICAL CARE	NR	PULMONARY	★★★
GASTROINTESTINAL	NR	STROKE	★★★
GENERAL SURGERY	NR	VASCULAR	NR
MATERNITY CARE	NR	WOMEN'S HEALTH	NR

HEALTHGRADES AWARDS

Cookeville Regional Medical Center

142 West 5th Street
Cookeville, TN 38501
(931) 528-2541

Overall patient safety: ★★★
Teaching: N

CLINICAL PROGRAM RATINGS:

CARDIAC	★★★	ORTHOPEDICS	★★★
CRITICAL CARE	NR	PULMONARY	★★★
GASTROINTESTINAL	★★★	STROKE	★
GENERAL SURGERY	NR	VASCULAR	★★★★★
MATERNITY CARE	NR	WOMEN'S HEALTH	NR

HEALTHGRADES AWARDS

✓ SPECIALTY EXCELLENCE
- VASCULAR SURGERY

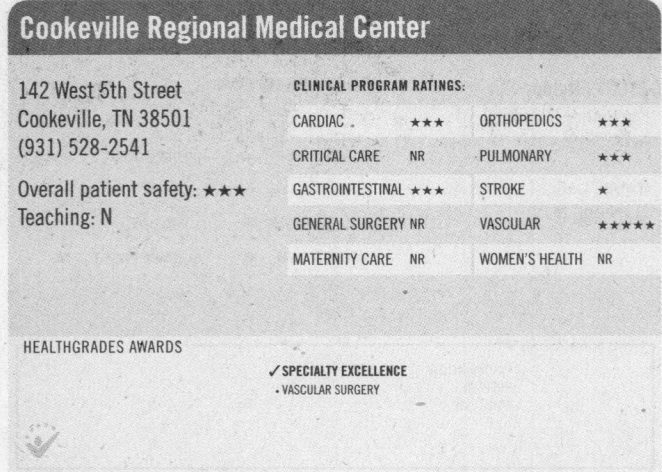

Cumberland Medical Center

421 South Main Street
Crossville, TN 38555
(931) 484-9511

Overall patient safety: ★★★
Teaching: N

CLINICAL PROGRAM RATINGS:

CARDIAC	NR	ORTHOPEDICS	NR
CRITICAL CARE	NR	PULMONARY	★★★
GASTROINTESTINAL	★★★	STROKE	★★★
GENERAL SURGERY	NR	VASCULAR	NR
MATERNITY CARE	NR	WOMEN'S HEALTH	NR

HEALTHGRADES AWARDS

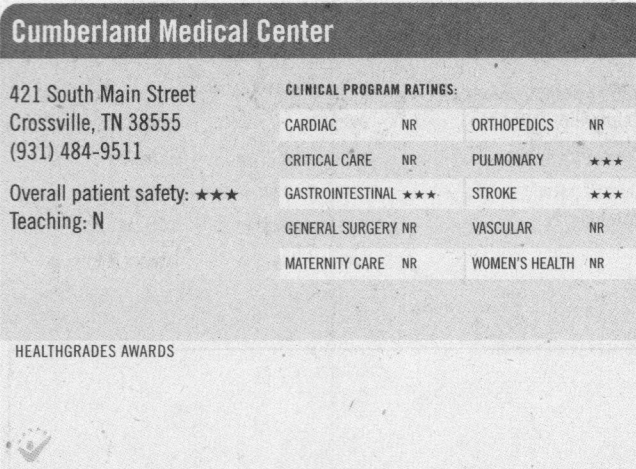

Copper Basin Medical Center

144 Medical Center Drive
P.O. Box 990
Copperhill, TN 37317
(423) 496-5511

Overall patient safety: ★★★
Teaching: N

CLINICAL PROGRAM RATINGS:

CARDIAC	NR	ORTHOPEDICS	NR
CRITICAL CARE	NR	PULMONARY	★★★
GASTROINTESTINAL	NR	STROKE	NR
GENERAL SURGERY	NR	VASCULAR	NR
MATERNITY CARE	NR	WOMEN'S HEALTH	NR

HEALTHGRADES AWARDS

Cumberland River Hospital

100 Old Jefferson Street
Celina, TN 38551
(931) 243-3581

Overall patient safety: ★★★
Teaching: N

CLINICAL PROGRAM RATINGS:

CARDIAC	NR	ORTHOPEDICS	NR
CRITICAL CARE	NR	PULMONARY	★★★★★
GASTROINTESTINAL	NR	STROKE	NR
GENERAL SURGERY	NR	VASCULAR	NR
MATERNITY CARE	NR	WOMEN'S HEALTH	NR

HEALTHGRADES AWARDS

✓ SPECIALTY EXCELLENCE
- PULMONARY CARE

KEY: ★★★★★ BEST   ★★★ AS EXPECTED   ★ POOR   NR NOT RATED BY HEALTHGRADES   For full definitions of ratings and awards, see Appendix.

Decatur County General Hospital

969 Tennessee Avenue South
Parsons, TN 38363
(731) 847-3031

Overall patient safety: ★★★
Teaching: N

CLINICAL PROGRAM RATINGS:

CARDIAC	NR	ORTHOPEDICS	NR
CRITICAL CARE	NR	PULMONARY	★
GASTROINTESTINAL	NR	STROKE	★★★
GENERAL SURGERY	NR	VASCULAR	NR
MATERNITY CARE	NR	WOMEN'S HEALTH	NR

HEALTHGRADES AWARDS

Dyersburg Regional Medical Center

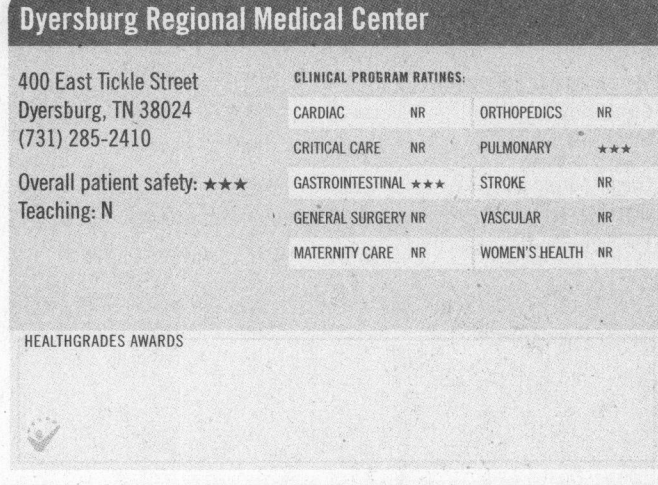

400 East Tickle Street
Dyersburg, TN 38024
(731) 285-2410

Overall patient safety: ★★★
Teaching: N

CLINICAL PROGRAM RATINGS:

CARDIAC	NR	ORTHOPEDICS	NR
CRITICAL CARE	NR	PULMONARY	★★★
GASTROINTESTINAL	★★★	STROKE	NR
GENERAL SURGERY	NR	VASCULAR	NR
MATERNITY CARE	NR	WOMEN'S HEALTH	NR

HEALTHGRADES AWARDS

Dekalb Hospital

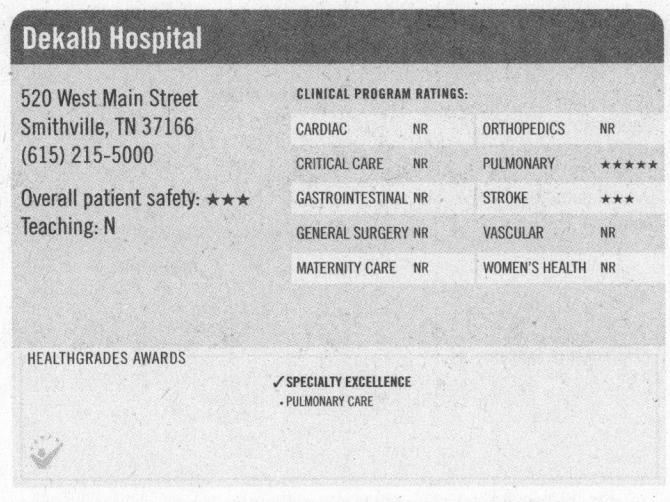

520 West Main Street
Smithville, TN 37166
(615) 215-5000

Overall patient safety: ★★★
Teaching: N

CLINICAL PROGRAM RATINGS:

CARDIAC	NR	ORTHOPEDICS	NR
CRITICAL CARE	NR	PULMONARY	★★★★★
GASTROINTESTINAL	NR	STROKE	★★★
GENERAL SURGERY	NR	VASCULAR	NR
MATERNITY CARE	NR	WOMEN'S HEALTH	NR

HEALTHGRADES AWARDS

✓ SPECIALTY EXCELLENCE
- PULMONARY CARE

Erlanger Bledsoe Hospital*

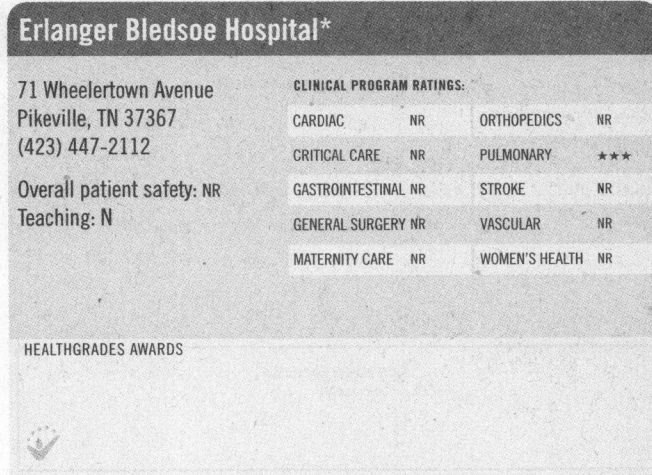

71 Wheelertown Avenue
Pikeville, TN 37367
(423) 447-2112

Overall patient safety: NR
Teaching: N

CLINICAL PROGRAM RATINGS:

CARDIAC	NR	ORTHOPEDICS	NR
CRITICAL CARE	NR	PULMONARY	★★★
GASTROINTESTINAL	NR	STROKE	NR
GENERAL SURGERY	NR	VASCULAR	NR
MATERNITY CARE	NR	WOMEN'S HEALTH	NR

HEALTHGRADES AWARDS

Delta Medical Center

3000 Getwell Road
Memphis, TN 38118
(901) 369-8100

Overall patient safety: ★★★
Teaching: N

CLINICAL PROGRAM RATINGS:

CARDIAC	NR	ORTHOPEDICS	NR
CRITICAL CARE	NR	PULMONARY	★★★
GASTROINTESTINAL	NR	STROKE	NR
GENERAL SURGERY	NR	VASCULAR	NR
MATERNITY CARE	NR	WOMEN'S HEALTH	NR

HEALTHGRADES AWARDS

Erlanger Medical Center*

975 East 3rd Street
Chattanooga, TN 37403
(423) 778-7000

Overall patient safety: ★★★
Teaching: Y

CLINICAL PROGRAM RATINGS:

CARDIAC	★★★	ORTHOPEDICS	★★★
CRITICAL CARE	★★★	PULMONARY	★★★
GASTROINTESTINAL	★★★	STROKE	★★★
GENERAL SURGERY	NR	VASCULAR	★★★
MATERNITY CARE	NR	WOMEN'S HEALTH	NR

HEALTHGRADES AWARDS

*This hospital reports its data to the federal government jointly with another hospital. Therefore the ratings and awards apply to multiple hospitals and this specific hospital may not provide all rated services.

Fort Loudoun Medical Center

550 Fort Loudoun Medical
Center Drive
Lenoir City, TN 37772
(865) 271-6000

Overall patient safety: ★★★
Teaching: N

CLINICAL PROGRAM RATINGS:

CARDIAC	NR	ORTHOPEDICS	NR
CRITICAL CARE	NR	PULMONARY	★★★
GASTROINTESTINAL	NR	STROKE	★★★
GENERAL SURGERY	NR	VASCULAR	NR
MATERNITY CARE	NR	WOMEN'S HEALTH	NR

HEALTHGRADES AWARDS

Gateway Medical Center

1771 Madison Street
Clarksville, TN 37043
(931) 552-6622

Overall patient safety: ★
Teaching: N

CLINICAL PROGRAM RATINGS:

CARDIAC	NR	ORTHOPEDICS	NR
CRITICAL CARE	NR	PULMONARY	★★★
GASTROINTESTINAL	★★★	STROKE	★★★
GENERAL SURGERY	NR	VASCULAR	NR
MATERNITY CARE	NR	WOMEN'S HEALTH	NR

HEALTHGRADES AWARDS

Fort Sanders Regional Medical Center

1901 Clinch Avenue Southwest
Knoxville, TN 37916
(865) 541-1111

Overall patient safety: ★
Teaching: N

CLINICAL PROGRAM RATINGS:

CARDIAC	★★★	ORTHOPEDICS	★
CRITICAL CARE	★★★★★	PULMONARY	★★★
GASTROINTESTINAL	★★★	STROKE	★★★
GENERAL SURGERY	NR	VASCULAR	NR
MATERNITY CARE	NR	WOMEN'S HEALTH	NR

HEALTHGRADES AWARDS

✓ SPECIALTY EXCELLENCE
• CRITICAL CARE

Germantown Community Hospital*

7691 Poplar Avenue
Germantown, TN 38138
(901) 516-6418

Overall patient safety: ★
Teaching: Y

CLINICAL PROGRAM RATINGS:

CARDIAC	★	ORTHOPEDICS	★★★★★
CRITICAL CARE	★★★	PULMONARY	★
GASTROINTESTINAL	★★★	STROKE	★★★
GENERAL SURGERY	NR	VASCULAR	★★★
MATERNITY CARE	NR	WOMEN'S HEALTH	NR

HEALTHGRADES AWARDS

✓ SPECIALTY EXCELLENCE
• JOINT REPLACEMENT • ORTHOPEDIC
SURGERY

Fort Sanders Sevier Medical Center

709 Middle Creek Road
Sevierville, TN 37862
(865) 429-6100

Overall patient safety: ★★★
Teaching: N

CLINICAL PROGRAM RATINGS:

CARDIAC	NR	ORTHOPEDICS	NR
CRITICAL CARE	NR	PULMONARY	★★★
GASTROINTESTINAL	NR	STROKE	★★★
GENERAL SURGERY	NR	VASCULAR	NR
MATERNITY CARE	NR	WOMEN'S HEALTH	NR

HEALTHGRADES AWARDS

Gibson General Hospital

200 Hospital Drive
Trenton, TN 38382
(731) 855-7900

Overall patient safety: ★★★
Teaching: N

CLINICAL PROGRAM RATINGS:

CARDIAC	NR	ORTHOPEDICS	NR
CRITICAL CARE	NR	PULMONARY	★
GASTROINTESTINAL	NR	STROKE	★
GENERAL SURGERY	NR	VASCULAR	NR
MATERNITY CARE	NR	WOMEN'S HEALTH	NR

HEALTHGRADES AWARDS

KEY: ★★★★★ BEST ★★★ AS EXPECTED ★ POOR NR NOT RATED BY HEALTHGRADES   For full definitions of ratings and awards, see Appendix.

Grandview Medical Center

1000 Highway 28
Jasper, TN 37347
(423) 837-9500

Overall patient safety: ★★★
Teaching: N

CLINICAL PROGRAM RATINGS:

CARDIAC	NR	ORTHOPEDICS	NR
CRITICAL CARE	NR	PULMONARY	★★★
GASTROINTESTINAL	NR	STROKE	NR
GENERAL SURGERY	NR	VASCULAR	NR
MATERNITY CARE	NR	WOMEN'S HEALTH	NR

HEALTHGRADES AWARDS

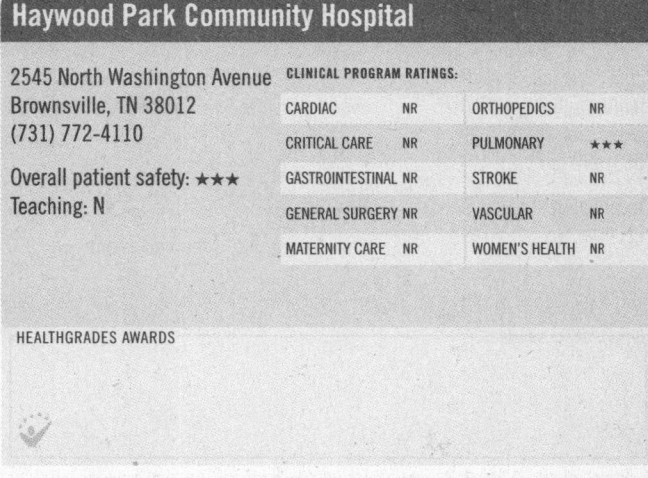

Haywood Park Community Hospital

2545 North Washington Avenue
Brownsville, TN 38012
(731) 772-4110

Overall patient safety: ★★★
Teaching: N

CLINICAL PROGRAM RATINGS:

CARDIAC	NR	ORTHOPEDICS	NR
CRITICAL CARE	NR	PULMONARY	★★★
GASTROINTESTINAL	NR	STROKE	NR
GENERAL SURGERY	NR	VASCULAR	NR
MATERNITY CARE	NR	WOMEN'S HEALTH	NR

HEALTHGRADES AWARDS

Hardin Medical Center

2006 Wayne Road
Savannah, TN 38372
(731) 926-8000

Overall patient safety: ★★★
Teaching: N

CLINICAL PROGRAM RATINGS:

CARDIAC	NR	ORTHOPEDICS	NR
CRITICAL CARE	NR	PULMONARY	★
GASTROINTESTINAL	NR	STROKE	★
GENERAL SURGERY	NR	VASCULAR	NR
MATERNITY CARE	NR	WOMEN'S HEALTH	NR

HEALTHGRADES AWARDS

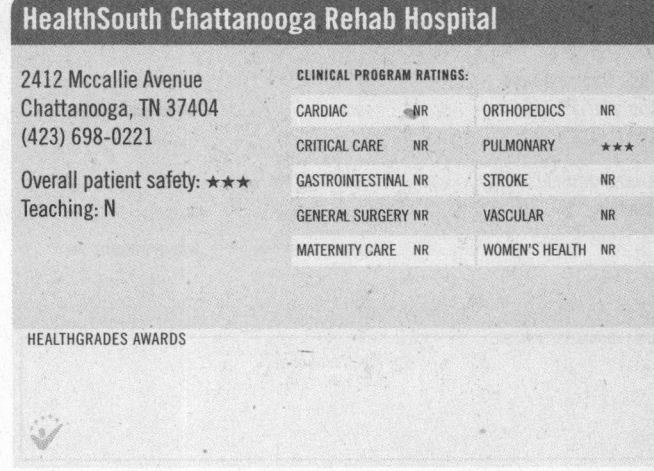

HealthSouth Chattanooga Rehab Hospital

2412 Mccallie Avenue
Chattanooga, TN 37404
(423) 698-0221

Overall patient safety: ★★★
Teaching: N

CLINICAL PROGRAM RATINGS:

CARDIAC	NR	ORTHOPEDICS	NR
CRITICAL CARE	NR	PULMONARY	★★★
GASTROINTESTINAL	NR	STROKE	NR
GENERAL SURGERY	NR	VASCULAR	NR
MATERNITY CARE	NR	WOMEN'S HEALTH	NR

HEALTHGRADES AWARDS

Harton Regional Medical Center

1801 North Jackson Street
Tullahoma, TN 37388
(931) 393-3000

Overall patient safety: ★★★
Teaching: N

CLINICAL PROGRAM RATINGS:

CARDIAC	NR	ORTHOPEDICS	NR
CRITICAL CARE	NR	PULMONARY	★
GASTROINTESTINAL	★	STROKE	★
GENERAL SURGERY	NR	VASCULAR	NR
MATERNITY CARE	NR	WOMEN'S HEALTH	NR

HEALTHGRADES AWARDS

Henderson County Community Hospital

200 West Church Street
Lexington, TN 38351
(731) 968-3646

Overall patient safety: ★★★
Teaching: N

CLINICAL PROGRAM RATINGS:

CARDIAC	NR	ORTHOPEDICS	NR
CRITICAL CARE	NR	PULMONARY	★
GASTROINTESTINAL	NR	STROKE	★
GENERAL SURGERY	NR	VASCULAR	NR
MATERNITY CARE	NR	WOMEN'S HEALTH	NR

HEALTHGRADES AWARDS

*This hospital reports its data to the federal government jointly with another hospital. Therefore the ratings and awards apply to multiple hospitals and this specific hospital may not provide all rated services.

Hendersonville Medical Center

355 New Shackle Island Road
Hendersonville, TN 37075
(615) 264-4000

Overall patient safety: ★★★
Teaching: N

CLINICAL PROGRAM RATINGS:

CARDIAC	NR	ORTHOPEDICS	NR
CRITICAL CARE	NR	PULMONARY	★★★
GASTROINTESTINAL	★★★	STROKE	★★★
GENERAL SURGERY	NR	VASCULAR	NR
MATERNITY CARE	NR	WOMEN'S HEALTH	NR

HEALTHGRADES AWARDS

Hillside Hospital

1265 East College Street
Pulaski, TN 38478
(931) 363-7531

Overall patient safety: ★★★
Teaching: N

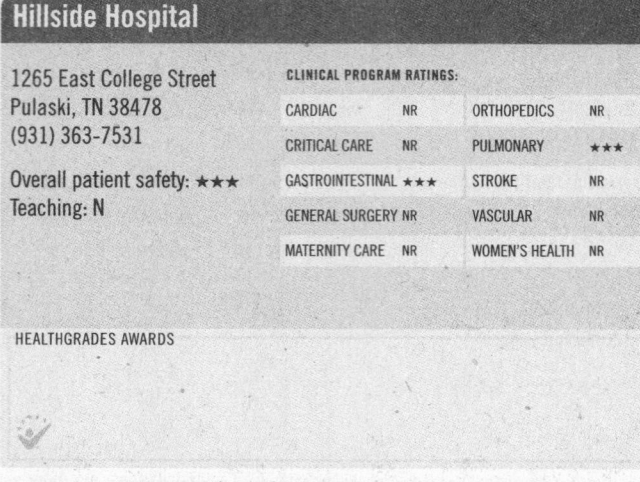

CLINICAL PROGRAM RATINGS:

CARDIAC	NR	ORTHOPEDICS	NR
CRITICAL CARE	NR	PULMONARY	★★★
GASTROINTESTINAL	★★★	STROKE	NR
GENERAL SURGERY	NR	VASCULAR	NR
MATERNITY CARE	NR	WOMEN'S HEALTH	NR

HEALTHGRADES AWARDS

Henry County Medical Center

301 Tyson Avenue
Paris, TN 38242
(731) 642-1220

Overall patient safety: ★★★
Teaching: N

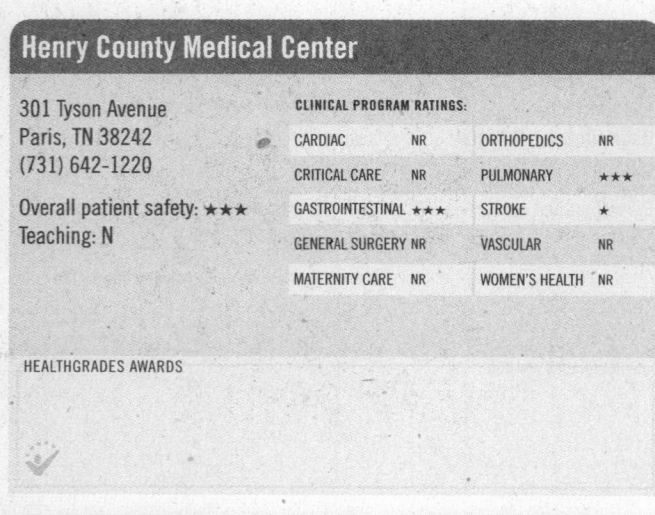

CLINICAL PROGRAM RATINGS:

CARDIAC	NR	ORTHOPEDICS	NR
CRITICAL CARE	NR	PULMONARY	★★★
GASTROINTESTINAL	★★★	STROKE	★
GENERAL SURGERY	NR	VASCULAR	NR
MATERNITY CARE	NR	WOMEN'S HEALTH	NR

HEALTHGRADES AWARDS

Horizon Medical Center

111 Highway 70 East
Dickson, TN 37055
(615) 446-0446

Overall patient safety: ★★★
Teaching: N

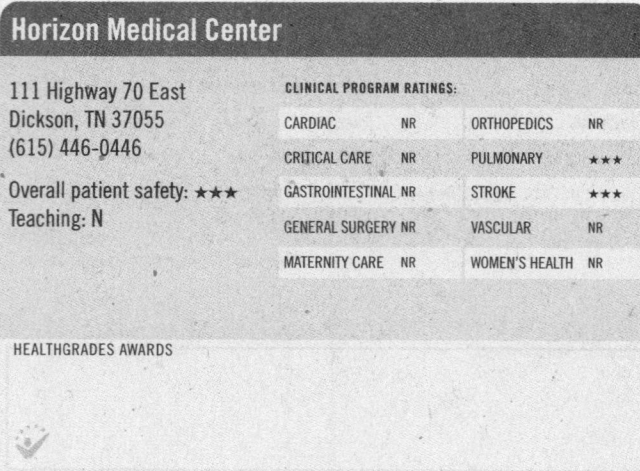

CLINICAL PROGRAM RATINGS:

CARDIAC	NR	ORTHOPEDICS	NR
CRITICAL CARE	NR	PULMONARY	★★★
GASTROINTESTINAL	NR	STROKE	★★★
GENERAL SURGERY	NR	VASCULAR	NR
MATERNITY CARE	NR	WOMEN'S HEALTH	NR

HEALTHGRADES AWARDS

Hickman Community Health Services

135 East Swan Street
Centerville, TN 37033
(931) 729-4271

Overall patient safety: NR
Teaching: N

CLINICAL PROGRAM RATINGS:

CARDIAC	NR	ORTHOPEDICS	NR
CRITICAL CARE	NR	PULMONARY	★★★
GASTROINTESTINAL	NR	STROKE	NR
GENERAL SURGERY	NR	VASCULAR	NR
MATERNITY CARE	NR	WOMEN'S HEALTH	NR

HEALTHGRADES AWARDS

Humboldt General Hospital

3525 Chere Carol Road
Humboldt, TN 38343
(731) 784-2321

Overall patient safety: ★★★
Teaching: N

CLINICAL PROGRAM RATINGS:

CARDIAC	NR	ORTHOPEDICS	NR
CRITICAL CARE	NR	PULMONARY	★
GASTROINTESTINAL	NR	STROKE	★
GENERAL SURGERY	NR	VASCULAR	NR
MATERNITY CARE	NR	WOMEN'S HEALTH	NR

HEALTHGRADES AWARDS

KEY: ★★★★★ BEST   ★★★ AS EXPECTED   ★ POOR   NR NOT RATED BY HEALTHGRADES   For full definitions of ratings and awards, see Appendix.

Indian Path Medical Center

2000 Brookside Drive
Kingsport, TN 37660
(423) 392-7000

Overall patient safety: ★★★
Teaching: Y

CLINICAL PROGRAM RATINGS:

CARDIAC	NR	ORTHOPEDICS	★★★
CRITICAL CARE	NR	PULMONARY	★
GASTROINTESTINAL	★★★	STROKE	★★★
GENERAL SURGERY	NR	VASCULAR	NR
MATERNITY CARE	NR	WOMEN'S HEALTH	NR

HEALTHGRADES AWARDS

Jellico Community Hospital

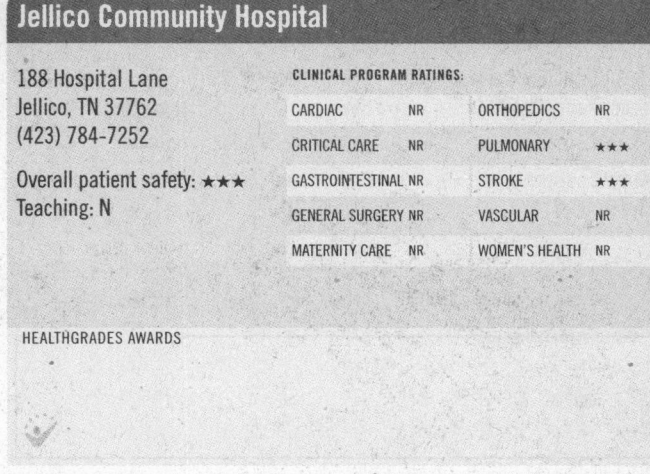

188 Hospital Lane
Jellico, TN 37762
(423) 784-7252

Overall patient safety: ★★★
Teaching: N

CLINICAL PROGRAM RATINGS:

CARDIAC	NR	ORTHOPEDICS	NR
CRITICAL CARE	NR	PULMONARY	★★★
GASTROINTESTINAL	NR	STROKE	★★★
GENERAL SURGERY	NR	VASCULAR	NR
MATERNITY CARE	NR	WOMEN'S HEALTH	NR

HEALTHGRADES AWARDS

Jackson-Madison County General Hospital

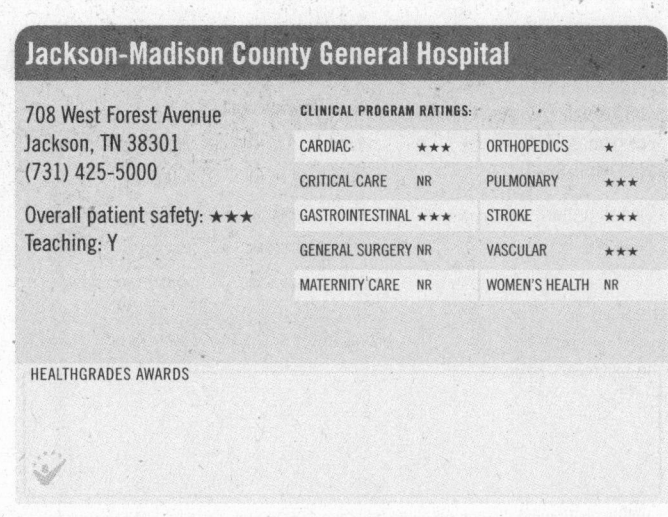

708 West Forest Avenue
Jackson, TN 38301
(731) 425-5000

Overall patient safety: ★★★
Teaching: Y

CLINICAL PROGRAM RATINGS:

CARDIAC	★★★	ORTHOPEDICS	★
CRITICAL CARE	NR	PULMONARY	★★★
GASTROINTESTINAL	★★★	STROKE	★★★
GENERAL SURGERY	NR	VASCULAR	★★★
MATERNITY CARE	NR	WOMEN'S HEALTH	NR

HEALTHGRADES AWARDS

Johnson City Medical Center

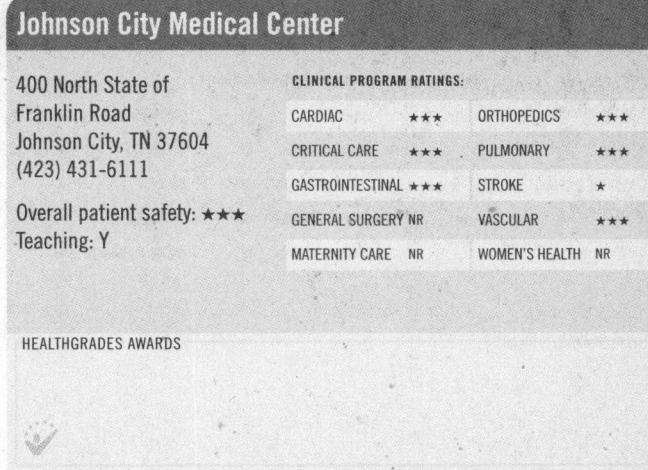

400 North State of
Franklin Road
Johnson City, TN 37604
(423) 431-6111

Overall patient safety: ★★★
Teaching: Y

CLINICAL PROGRAM RATINGS:

CARDIAC	★★★	ORTHOPEDICS	★★★
CRITICAL CARE	★★★	PULMONARY	★★★
GASTROINTESTINAL	★★★	STROKE	★
GENERAL SURGERY	NR	VASCULAR	★★★
MATERNITY CARE	NR	WOMEN'S HEALTH	NR

HEALTHGRADES AWARDS

Jamestown Regional Medical Center

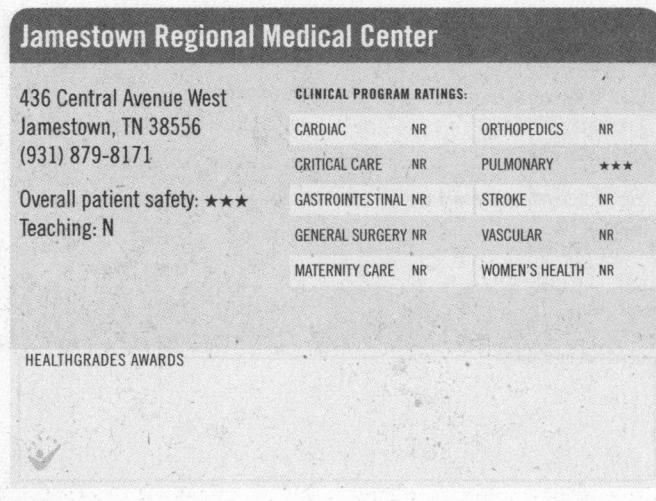

436 Central Avenue West
Jamestown, TN 38556
(931) 879-8171

Overall patient safety: ★★★
Teaching: N

CLINICAL PROGRAM RATINGS:

CARDIAC	NR	ORTHOPEDICS	NR
CRITICAL CARE	NR	PULMONARY	★★★
GASTROINTESTINAL	NR	STROKE	NR
GENERAL SURGERY	NR	VASCULAR	NR
MATERNITY CARE	NR	WOMEN'S HEALTH	NR

HEALTHGRADES AWARDS

Lakeway Regional Hospital

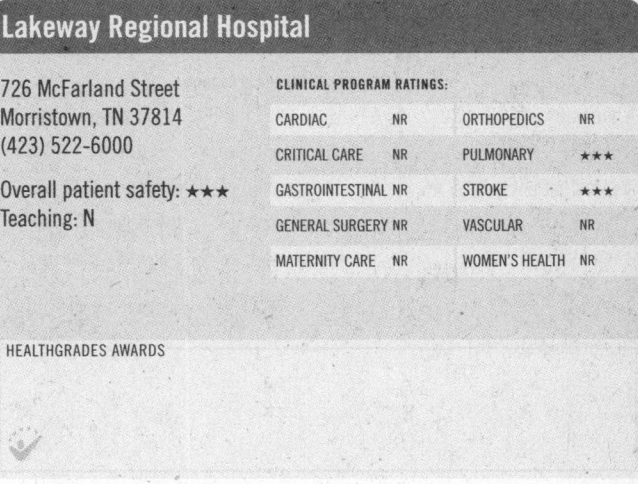

726 McFarland Street
Morristown, TN 37814
(423) 522-6000

Overall patient safety: ★★★
Teaching: N

CLINICAL PROGRAM RATINGS:

CARDIAC	NR	ORTHOPEDICS	NR
CRITICAL CARE	NR	PULMONARY	★★★
GASTROINTESTINAL	NR	STROKE	★★★
GENERAL SURGERY	NR	VASCULAR	NR
MATERNITY CARE	NR	WOMEN'S HEALTH	NR

HEALTHGRADES AWARDS

Laughlin Memorial Hospital

1420 Tusculum Boulevard
Greeneville, TN 37745
(423) 787-5000

Overall patient safety: ★★★
Teaching: N

CLINICAL PROGRAM RATINGS:

CARDIAC	NR	ORTHOPEDICS	NR
CRITICAL CARE	★★★	PULMONARY	★
GASTROINTESTINAL	NR	STROKE	★
GENERAL SURGERY	NR	VASCULAR	NR
MATERNITY CARE	NR	WOMEN'S HEALTH	NR

HEALTHGRADES AWARDS

Macon County General Hospital

204 Medical Drive
Lafayette, TN 37083
(615) 666-2147

Overall patient safety: NR
Teaching: N

CLINICAL PROGRAM RATINGS:

CARDIAC	NR	ORTHOPEDICS	NR
CRITICAL CARE	NR	PULMONARY	★★★
GASTROINTESTINAL	NR	STROKE	NR
GENERAL SURGERY	NR	VASCULAR	NR
MATERNITY CARE	NR	WOMEN'S HEALTH	NR

HEALTHGRADES AWARDS

Lincoln Medical Center

106 Medical Center Boulevard
Fayetteville, TN 37334
(931) 438-1100

Overall patient safety: ★★★
Teaching: N

CLINICAL PROGRAM RATINGS:

CARDIAC	NR	ORTHOPEDICS	NR
CRITICAL CARE	NR	PULMONARY	★★★
GASTROINTESTINAL	NR	STROKE	★★★
GENERAL SURGERY	NR	VASCULAR	NR
MATERNITY CARE	NR	WOMEN'S HEALTH	NR

HEALTHGRADES AWARDS

Marshall Medical Center

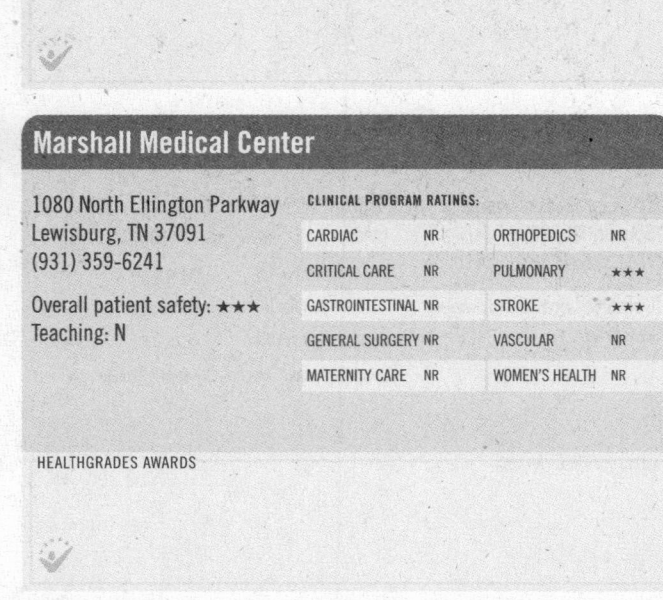

1080 North Ellington Parkway
Lewisburg, TN 37091
(931) 359-6241

Overall patient safety: ★★★
Teaching: N

CLINICAL PROGRAM RATINGS:

CARDIAC	NR	ORTHOPEDICS	NR
CRITICAL CARE	NR	PULMONARY	★★★
GASTROINTESTINAL	NR	STROKE	★★★
GENERAL SURGERY	NR	VASCULAR	NR
MATERNITY CARE	NR	WOMEN'S HEALTH	NR

HEALTHGRADES AWARDS

Livingston Regional Hospital

315 Oak Street
Livingston, TN 38570
(931) 823-5611

Overall patient safety: ★★★
Teaching: N

CLINICAL PROGRAM RATINGS:

CARDIAC	NR	ORTHOPEDICS	NR
CRITICAL CARE	NR	PULMONARY	★★★
GASTROINTESTINAL	NR	STROKE	★
GENERAL SURGERY	NR	VASCULAR	NR
MATERNITY CARE	NR	WOMEN'S HEALTH	NR

HEALTHGRADES AWARDS

Maury Regional Hospital

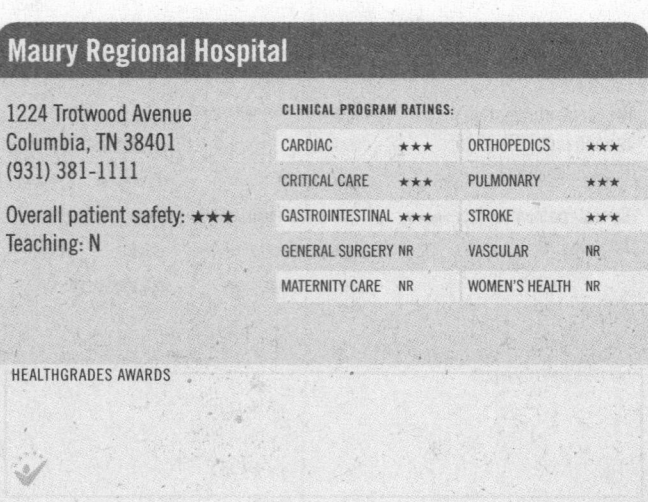

1224 Trotwood Avenue
Columbia, TN 38401
(931) 381-1111

Overall patient safety: ★★★
Teaching: N

CLINICAL PROGRAM RATINGS:

CARDIAC	★★★	ORTHOPEDICS	★★★
CRITICAL CARE	★★★	PULMONARY	★★★
GASTROINTESTINAL	★★★	STROKE	★★★
GENERAL SURGERY	NR	VASCULAR	NR
MATERNITY CARE	NR	WOMEN'S HEALTH	NR

HEALTHGRADES AWARDS

KEY: ★★★★★ BEST   ★★★ AS EXPECTED   ★ POOR   NR NOT RATED BY HEALTHGRADES   For full definitions of ratings and awards, see Appendix.

McKenzie Regional Hospital

161 Hospital Drive
McKenzie, TN 38201
(731) 352-9105

Overall patient safety: ★★★
Teaching: N

CLINICAL PROGRAM RATINGS:

CARDIAC	NR	ORTHOPEDICS	NR
CRITICAL CARE	NR	PULMONARY	★
GASTROINTESTINAL	NR	STROKE	★
GENERAL SURGERY	NR	VASCULAR	NR
MATERNITY CARE	NR	WOMEN'S HEALTH	NR

HEALTHGRADES AWARDS

Memorial Healthcare System

2525 DeSales Avenue
Chattanooga, TN 37404
(423) 495-2525

Overall patient safety: ★★★
Teaching: N

CLINICAL PROGRAM RATINGS:

CARDIAC	★★★	ORTHOPEDICS	★★★
CRITICAL CARE	★★★★★	PULMONARY	★★★★★
GASTROINTESTINAL	★★★★★	STROKE	★★★
GENERAL SURGERY	NR	VASCULAR	★★★
MATERNITY CARE	NR	WOMEN'S HEALTH	NR

HEALTHGRADES AWARDS

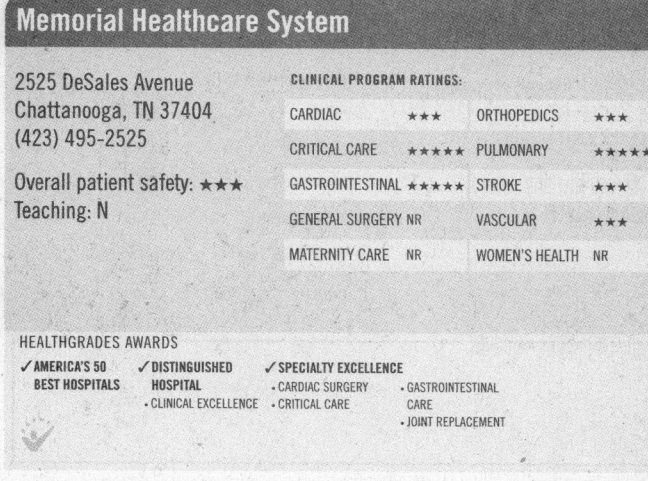

✓ AMERICA'S 50 BEST HOSPITALS   ✓ DISTINGUISHED HOSPITAL   ✓ SPECIALTY EXCELLENCE
- CLINICAL EXCELLENCE
- CARDIAC SURGERY
- CRITICAL CARE
- GASTROINTESTINAL CARE
- JOINT REPLACEMENT

McNairy Regional Hospital

705 East Poplar Avenue
Selmer, TN 38375
(731) 645-3221

Overall patient safety: ★★★
Teaching: N

CLINICAL PROGRAM RATINGS:

CARDIAC	NR	ORTHOPEDICS	NR
CRITICAL CARE	NR	PULMONARY	★
GASTROINTESTINAL	NR	STROKE	★★★
GENERAL SURGERY	NR	VASCULAR	NR
MATERNITY CARE	NR	WOMEN'S HEALTH	NR

HEALTHGRADES AWARDS

Methodist Healthcare Fayette Hospital

214 Lakeview Drive
Somerville, TN 38068
(901) 465-3594

Overall patient safety: ★★★
Teaching: N

CLINICAL PROGRAM RATINGS:

CARDIAC	NR	ORTHOPEDICS	NR
CRITICAL CARE	NR	PULMONARY	★
GASTROINTESTINAL	NR	STROKE	NR
GENERAL SURGERY	NR	VASCULAR	NR
MATERNITY CARE	NR	WOMEN'S HEALTH	NR

HEALTHGRADES AWARDS

Medical Center of Manchester

481 Interstate Drive
Manchester, TN 37355
(931) 728-6354

Overall patient safety: ★★★
Teaching: N

CLINICAL PROGRAM RATINGS:

CARDIAC	NR	ORTHOPEDICS	NR
CRITICAL CARE	NR	PULMONARY	★★★
GASTROINTESTINAL	NR	STROKE	NR
GENERAL SURGERY	NR	VASCULAR	NR
MATERNITY CARE	NR	WOMEN'S HEALTH	NR

HEALTHGRADES AWARDS

Methodist Healthcare Memphis Hospitals*

1265 Union Avenue
Memphis, TN 38104
(901) 726-7000

Overall patient safety: ★
Teaching: Y

CLINICAL PROGRAM RATINGS:

CARDIAC	★	ORTHOPEDICS	★★★★★
CRITICAL CARE	★★★	PULMONARY	★
GASTROINTESTINAL	★★★	STROKE	★★★
GENERAL SURGERY	NR	VASCULAR	★★★
MATERNITY CARE	NR	WOMEN'S HEALTH	NR

HEALTHGRADES AWARDS

✓ SPECIALTY EXCELLENCE
- JOINT REPLACEMENT
- ORTHOPEDIC SURGERY

*This hospital reports its data to the federal government jointly with another hospital. Therefore the ratings and awards apply to multiple hospitals and this specific hospital may not provide all rated services.

Methodist Medical Center of Oak Ridge

990 Oak Ridge Turnpike
Oak Ridge, TN 37831
(865) 481-1000

Overall patient safety: ★
Teaching: N

CLINICAL PROGRAM RATINGS:

CARDIAC	★★★	ORTHOPEDICS	★★★★★
CRITICAL CARE	★★★★★	PULMONARY	★★★
GASTROINTESTINAL	★★★	STROKE	★★★
GENERAL SURGERY	NR	VASCULAR	★★★
MATERNITY CARE	NR	WOMEN'S HEALTH	NR

HEALTHGRADES AWARDS

✓ SPECIALTY EXCELLENCE
• CRITICAL CARE   • JOINT REPLACEMENT   • ORTHOPEDIC SURGERY

Milan General Hospital

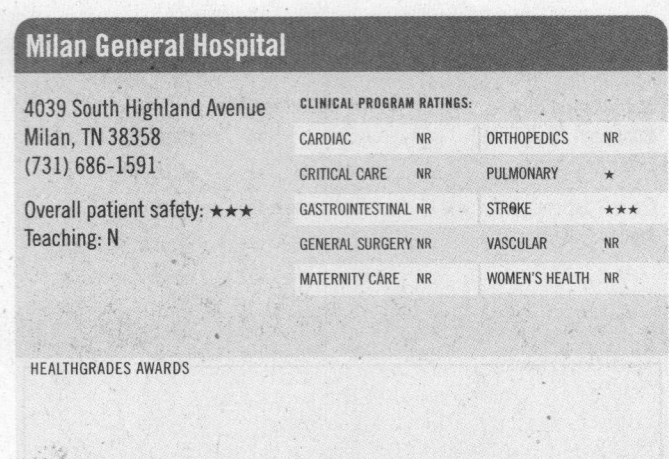

4039 South Highland Avenue
Milan, TN 38358
(731) 686-1591

Overall patient safety: ★★★
Teaching: N

CLINICAL PROGRAM RATINGS:

CARDIAC	NR	ORTHOPEDICS	NR
CRITICAL CARE	NR	PULMONARY	★
GASTROINTESTINAL	NR	STROKE	★★★
GENERAL SURGERY	NR	VASCULAR	NR
MATERNITY CARE	NR	WOMEN'S HEALTH	NR

HEALTHGRADES AWARDS

Metro Nashville General Hospital

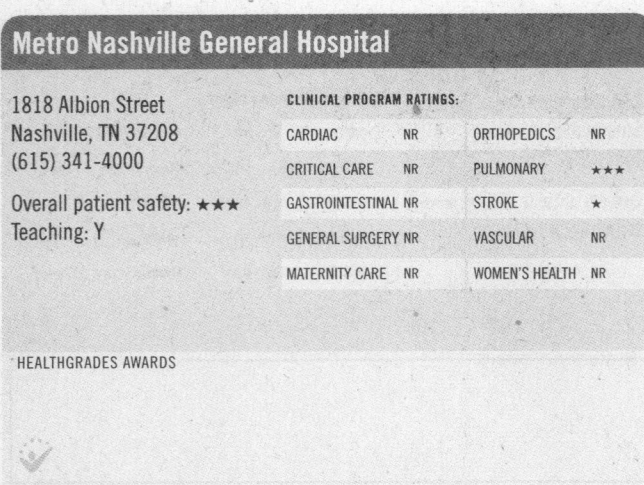

1818 Albion Street
Nashville, TN 37208
(615) 341-4000

Overall patient safety: ★★★
Teaching: Y

CLINICAL PROGRAM RATINGS:

CARDIAC	NR	ORTHOPEDICS	NR
CRITICAL CARE	NR	PULMONARY	★★★
GASTROINTESTINAL	NR	STROKE	★
GENERAL SURGERY	NR	VASCULAR	NR
MATERNITY CARE	NR	WOMEN'S HEALTH	NR

HEALTHGRADES AWARDS

Morristown-Hamblen Healthcare System

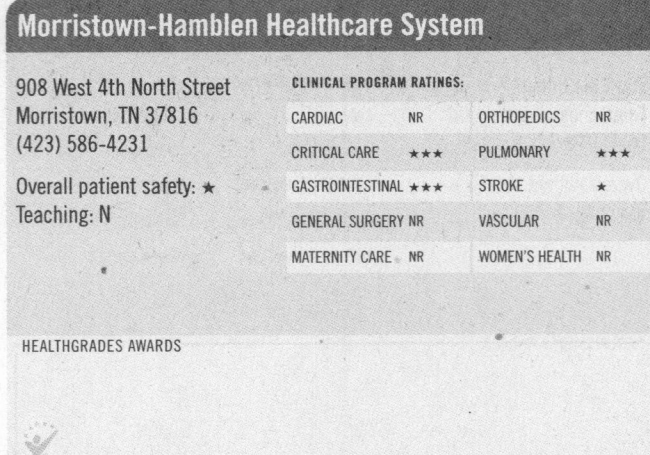

908 West 4th North Street
Morristown, TN 37816
(423) 586-4231

Overall patient safety: ★
Teaching: N

CLINICAL PROGRAM RATINGS:

CARDIAC	NR	ORTHOPEDICS	NR
CRITICAL CARE	★★★	PULMONARY	★★★
GASTROINTESTINAL	★★★	STROKE	★
GENERAL SURGERY	NR	VASCULAR	NR
MATERNITY CARE	NR	WOMEN'S HEALTH	NR

HEALTHGRADES AWARDS

Middle Tennessee Medical Center

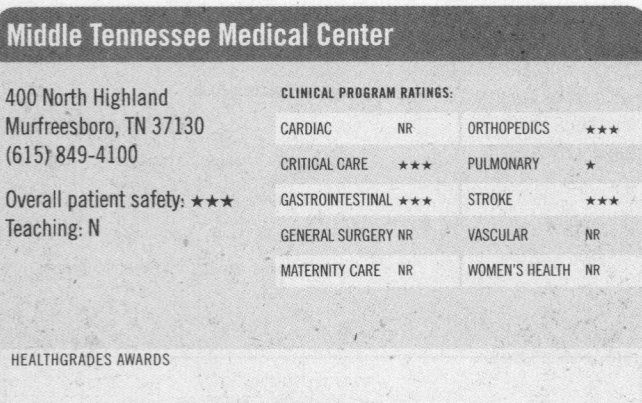

400 North Highland
Murfreesboro, TN 37130
(615) 849-4100

Overall patient safety: ★★★
Teaching: N

CLINICAL PROGRAM RATINGS:

CARDIAC	NR	ORTHOPEDICS	★★★
CRITICAL CARE	★★★	PULMONARY	★
GASTROINTESTINAL	★★★	STROKE	★★★
GENERAL SURGERY	NR	VASCULAR	NR
MATERNITY CARE	NR	WOMEN'S HEALTH	NR

HEALTHGRADES AWARDS

NorthCrest Medical Center

100 NorthCrest Drive
Springfield, TN 37172
(615) 384-2411

Overall patient safety: ★★★
Teaching: N

CLINICAL PROGRAM RATINGS:

CARDIAC	NR	ORTHOPEDICS	NR
CRITICAL CARE	★★★	PULMONARY	★★★
GASTROINTESTINAL	★★★	STROKE	★★★
GENERAL SURGERY	NR	VASCULAR	NR
MATERNITY CARE	NR	WOMEN'S HEALTH	NR

HEALTHGRADES AWARDS

KEY: ★★★★★ BEST   ★★★ AS EXPECTED   ★ POOR   NR NOT RATED BY HEALTHGRADES   For full definitions of ratings and awards, see Appendix.

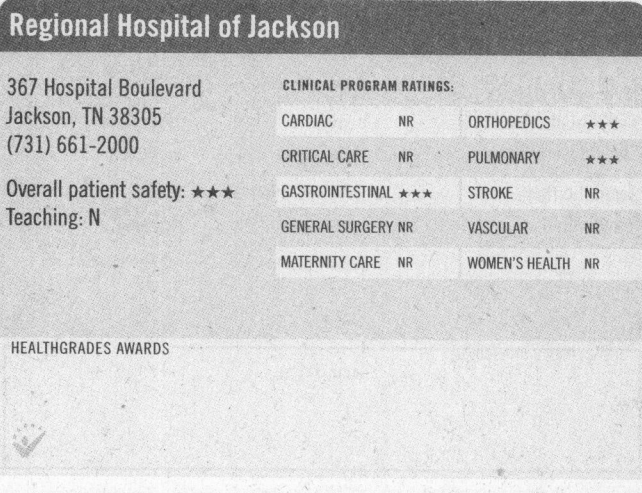

Northside Hospital

401 Princeton Road
Johnson City, TN 37601
(423) 854-5600

Overall patient safety: ★★★
Teaching: N

CLINICAL PROGRAM RATINGS:

CARDIAC	NR	ORTHOPEDICS	NR
CRITICAL CARE	NR	PULMONARY	★★★
GASTROINTESTINAL	NR	STROKE	NR
GENERAL SURGERY	NR	VASCULAR	NR
MATERNITY CARE	NR	WOMEN'S HEALTH	NR

HEALTHGRADES AWARDS

Regional Hospital of Jackson

367 Hospital Boulevard
Jackson, TN 38305
(731) 661-2000

Overall patient safety: ★★★
Teaching: N

CLINICAL PROGRAM RATINGS:

CARDIAC	NR	ORTHOPEDICS	★★★
CRITICAL CARE	NR	PULMONARY	★★★
GASTROINTESTINAL	★★★	STROKE	NR
GENERAL SURGERY	NR	VASCULAR	NR
MATERNITY CARE	NR	WOMEN'S HEALTH	NR

HEALTHGRADES AWARDS

Parkridge Medical Center

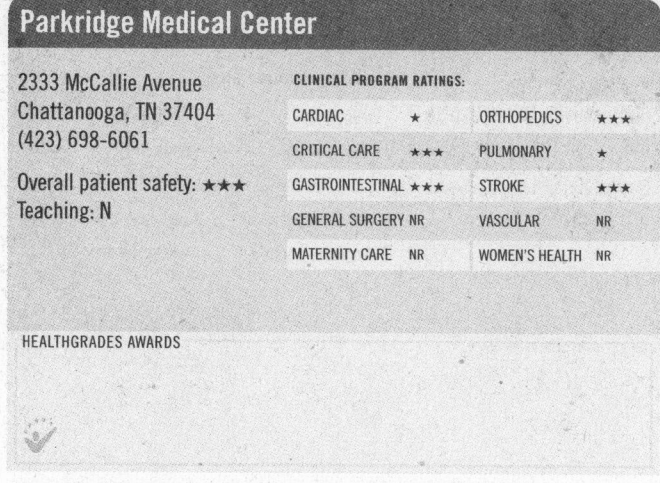

2333 McCallie Avenue
Chattanooga, TN 37404
(423) 698-6061

Overall patient safety: ★★★
Teaching: N

CLINICAL PROGRAM RATINGS:

CARDIAC	★	ORTHOPEDICS	★★★
CRITICAL CARE	★★★	PULMONARY	★
GASTROINTESTINAL	★★★	STROKE	★★★
GENERAL SURGERY	NR	VASCULAR	NR
MATERNITY CARE	NR	WOMEN'S HEALTH	NR

HEALTHGRADES AWARDS

Regional Medical Center at Memphis

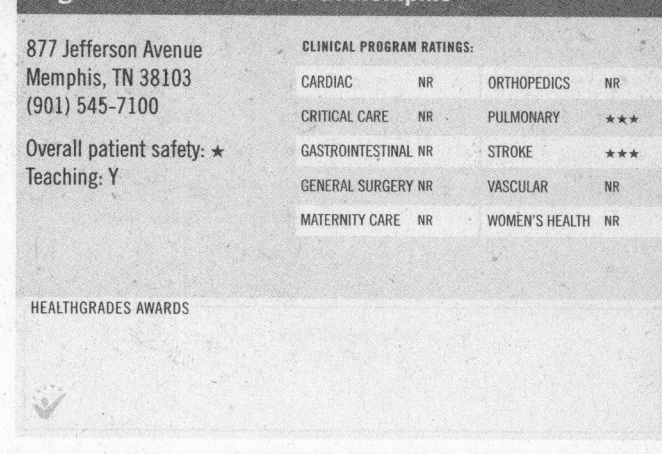

877 Jefferson Avenue
Memphis, TN 38103
(901) 545-7100

Overall patient safety: ★
Teaching: Y

CLINICAL PROGRAM RATINGS:

CARDIAC	NR	ORTHOPEDICS	NR
CRITICAL CARE	NR	PULMONARY	★★★
GASTROINTESTINAL	NR	STROKE	★★★
GENERAL SURGERY	NR	VASCULAR	NR
MATERNITY CARE	NR	WOMEN'S HEALTH	NR

HEALTHGRADES AWARDS

Parkwest Medical Center

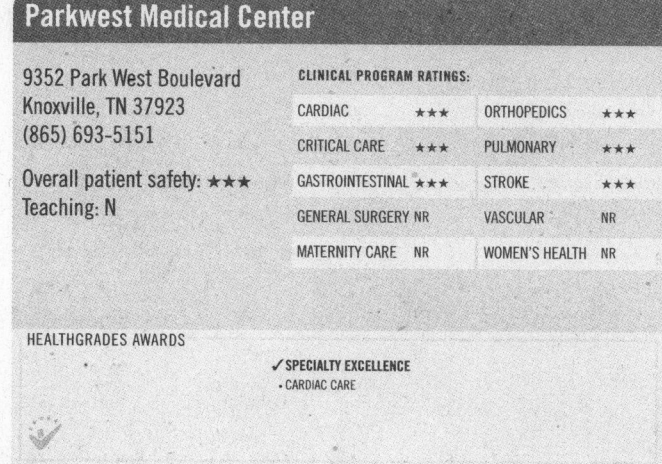

9352 Park West Boulevard
Knoxville, TN 37923
(865) 693-5151

Overall patient safety: ★★★
Teaching: N

CLINICAL PROGRAM RATINGS:

CARDIAC	★★★	ORTHOPEDICS	★★★
CRITICAL CARE	★★★	PULMONARY	★★★
GASTROINTESTINAL	★★★	STROKE	★★★
GENERAL SURGERY	NR	VASCULAR	NR
MATERNITY CARE	NR	WOMEN'S HEALTH	NR

HEALTHGRADES AWARDS

✓ SPECIALTY EXCELLENCE
· CARDIAC CARE

Rhea Medical Center

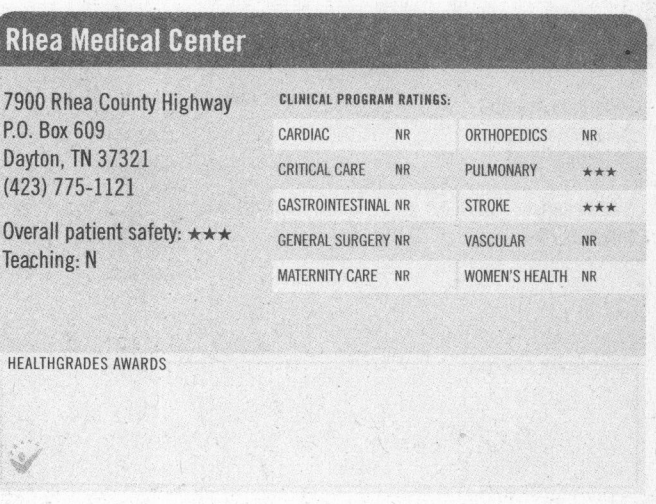

7900 Rhea County Highway
P.O. Box 609
Dayton, TN 37321
(423) 775-1121

Overall patient safety: ★★★
Teaching: N

CLINICAL PROGRAM RATINGS:

CARDIAC	NR	ORTHOPEDICS	NR
CRITICAL CARE	NR	PULMONARY	★★★
GASTROINTESTINAL	NR	STROKE	★★★
GENERAL SURGERY	NR	VASCULAR	NR
MATERNITY CARE	NR	WOMEN'S HEALTH	NR

HEALTHGRADES AWARDS

River Park Hospital

1559 Sparta Road
McMinnville, TN 37110
(931) 815-4000

Overall patient safety: ★★★
Teaching: N

CLINICAL PROGRAM RATINGS:

CARDIAC	NR	ORTHOPEDICS	NR
CRITICAL CARE	NR	PULMONARY	★★★
GASTROINTESTINAL	NR	STROKE	★★★
GENERAL SURGERY	NR	VASCULAR	NR
MATERNITY CARE	NR	WOMEN'S HEALTH	NR

HEALTHGRADES AWARDS

St. Francis Hospital—Bartlett

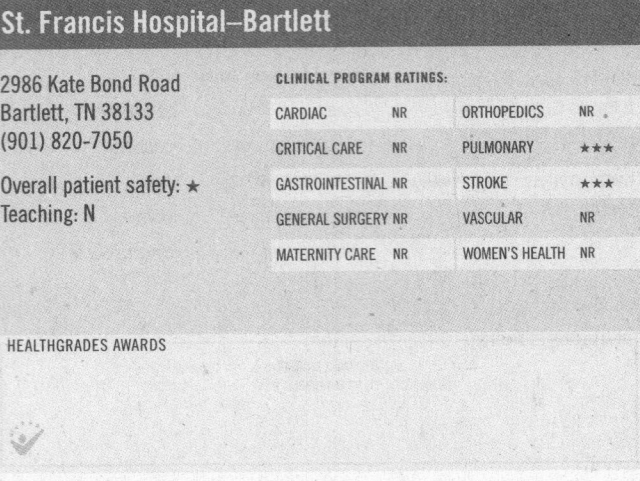

2986 Kate Bond Road
Bartlett, TN 38133
(901) 820-7050

Overall patient safety: ★
Teaching: N

CLINICAL PROGRAM RATINGS:

CARDIAC	NR	ORTHOPEDICS	NR
CRITICAL CARE	NR	PULMONARY	★★★
GASTROINTESTINAL	NR	STROKE	★★★
GENERAL SURGERY	NR	VASCULAR	NR
MATERNITY CARE	NR	WOMEN'S HEALTH	NR

HEALTHGRADES AWARDS

Roane Medical Center

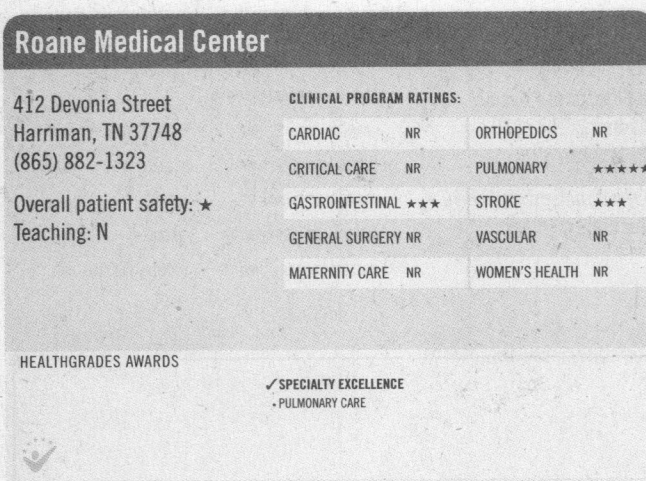

412 Devonia Street
Harriman, TN 37748
(865) 882-1323

Overall patient safety: ★
Teaching: N

CLINICAL PROGRAM RATINGS:

CARDIAC	NR	ORTHOPEDICS	NR
CRITICAL CARE	NR	PULMONARY	★★★★★
GASTROINTESTINAL	★★★	STROKE	★★★
GENERAL SURGERY	NR	VASCULAR	NR
MATERNITY CARE	NR	WOMEN'S HEALTH	NR

HEALTHGRADES AWARDS

✓ SPECIALTY EXCELLENCE
• PULMONARY CARE

St. Mary's Jefferson Memorial Hospital

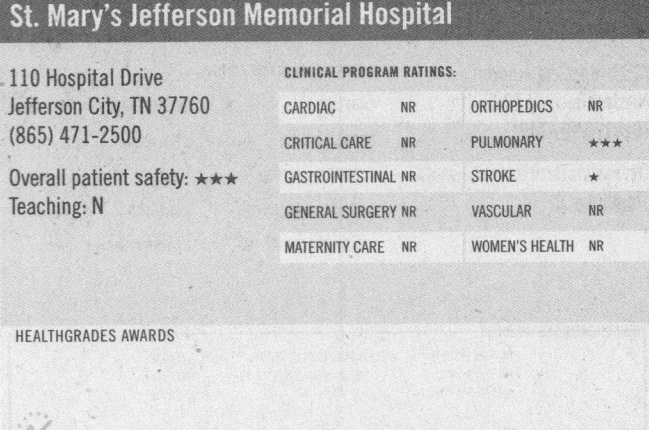

110 Hospital Drive
Jefferson City, TN 37760
(865) 471-2500

Overall patient safety: ★★★
Teaching: N

CLINICAL PROGRAM RATINGS:

CARDIAC	NR	ORTHOPEDICS	NR
CRITICAL CARE	NR	PULMONARY	★★★
GASTROINTESTINAL	NR	STROKE	★
GENERAL SURGERY	NR	VASCULAR	NR
MATERNITY CARE	NR	WOMEN'S HEALTH	NR

HEALTHGRADES AWARDS

St. Francis Hospital

5959 Park Avenue
Memphis, TN 38119
(901) 765-1000

Overall patient safety: ★
Teaching: Y

CLINICAL PROGRAM RATINGS:

CARDIAC	★★★	ORTHOPEDICS	★★★
CRITICAL CARE	★★★	PULMONARY	★
GASTROINTESTINAL	★★★	STROKE	★
GENERAL SURGERY	NR	VASCULAR	★★★
MATERNITY CARE	NR	WOMEN'S HEALTH	NR

HEALTHGRADES AWARDS

St. Mary's Medical Center

900 East Oak Hill Avenue
Knoxville, TN 37917
(865) 545-8000

Overall patient safety: ★★★
Teaching: N

CLINICAL PROGRAM RATINGS:

CARDIAC	★★★	ORTHOPEDICS	★★★★★
CRITICAL CARE	★★★	PULMONARY	★★★★★
GASTROINTESTINAL	★★★	STROKE	★
GENERAL SURGERY	NR	VASCULAR	NR
MATERNITY CARE	NR	WOMEN'S HEALTH	NR

HEALTHGRADES AWARDS

✓ SPECIALTY EXCELLENCE
• JOINT REPLACEMENT   • ORTHOPEDIC SURGERY   • PULMONARY CARE

KEY: ★★★★★ BEST   ★★★ AS EXPECTED   ★ POOR   NR NOT RATED BY HEALTHGRADES   For full definitions of ratings and awards, see Appendix.

St. Mary's Medical Center of Campbell County

923 East Central Avenue
La Follette, TN 37766
(423) 907-1200

Overall patient safety: ★★★★★
Teaching: N

CLINICAL PROGRAM RATINGS:

CARDIAC	NR	ORTHOPEDICS	NR
CRITICAL CARE	NR	PULMONARY	★★★★★
GASTROINTESTINAL	NR	STROKE	NR
GENERAL SURGERY	NR	VASCULAR	NR
MATERNITY CARE	NR	WOMEN'S HEALTH	NR

HEALTHGRADES AWARDS

✓ **SPECIALTY EXCELLENCE**
• PULMONARY CARE

Select Specialty Hospital—Tricities

1 Medical Park Boulevard
5th Floor
Bristol, TN 37620
(423) 968-1121

Overall patient safety: ★★★
Teaching: Y

CLINICAL PROGRAM RATINGS:

CARDIAC	★★★	ORTHOPEDICS	★
CRITICAL CARE	★★★	PULMONARY	★★★
GASTROINTESTINAL	★★★	STROKE	★★★
GENERAL SURGERY	NR	VASCULAR	NR
MATERNITY CARE	NR	WOMEN'S HEALTH	NR

HEALTHGRADES AWARDS

St. Thomas Hospital

4220 Harding Road
Nashville, TN 37205
(615) 222-2111

Overall patient safety: ★★★★★
Teaching: Y

CLINICAL PROGRAM RATINGS:

CARDIAC	★★★	ORTHOPEDICS	★★★★★
CRITICAL CARE	★★★	PULMONARY	★★★
GASTROINTESTINAL	★★★	STROKE	★
GENERAL SURGERY	NR	VASCULAR	★★★
MATERNITY CARE	NR	WOMEN'S HEALTH	NR

HEALTHGRADES AWARDS

✓ **DISTINGUISHED HOSPITAL**
• PATIENT SAFETY

✓ **SPECIALTY EXCELLENCE**
• VASCULAR SURGERY

Skyline Madison Campus

500 Hospital Drive
Madison, TN 37115
(615) 865-2373

Overall patient safety: ★★★
Teaching: N

CLINICAL PROGRAM RATINGS:

CARDIAC	NR	ORTHOPEDICS	NR
CRITICAL CARE	NR	PULMONARY	★★★★★
GASTROINTESTINAL	NR	STROKE	★★★
GENERAL SURGERY	NR	VASCULAR	NR
MATERNITY CARE	NR	WOMEN'S HEALTH	NR

HEALTHGRADES AWARDS

Scott County Hospital

18797 Alberta Street
Oneida, TN 37841
(423) 569-8521

Overall patient safety: ★★★
Teaching: N

CLINICAL PROGRAM RATINGS:

CARDIAC	NR	ORTHOPEDICS	NR
CRITICAL CARE	NR	PULMONARY	★★★
GASTROINTESTINAL	NR	STROKE	NR
GENERAL SURGERY	NR	VASCULAR	NR
MATERNITY CARE	NR	WOMEN'S HEALTH	NR

HEALTHGRADES AWARDS

Skyline Medical Center

3441 Dickerson Pike
Nashville, TN 37207
(615) 769-2000

Overall patient safety: ★★★
Teaching: N

CLINICAL PROGRAM RATINGS:

CARDIAC	NR	ORTHOPEDICS	★★★
CRITICAL CARE	★★★	PULMONARY	★★★
GASTROINTESTINAL	★★★	STROKE	★★★
GENERAL SURGERY	NR	VASCULAR	NR
MATERNITY CARE	NR	WOMEN'S HEALTH	NR

HEALTHGRADES AWARDS

Smith County Memorial Hospital

158 Hospital Drive
Carthage, TN 37030
(615) 735-1560

Overall patient safety: ★★★
Teaching: N

CLINICAL PROGRAM RATINGS:

CARDIAC	NR	ORTHOPEDICS	NR
CRITICAL CARE	NR	PULMONARY	★★★
GASTROINTESTINAL	NR	STROKE	★★★
GENERAL SURGERY	NR	VASCULAR	NR
MATERNITY CARE	NR	WOMEN'S HEALTH	NR

HEALTHGRADES AWARDS

Stonecrest Medical Center

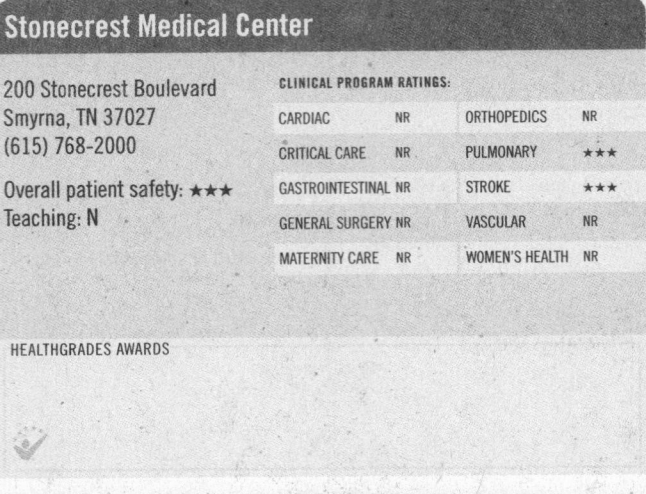

200 Stonecrest Boulevard
Smyrna, TN 37027
(615) 768-2000

Overall patient safety: ★★★
Teaching: N

CLINICAL PROGRAM RATINGS:

CARDIAC	NR	ORTHOPEDICS	NR
CRITICAL CARE	NR	PULMONARY	★★★
GASTROINTESTINAL	NR	STROKE	★★★
GENERAL SURGERY	NR	VASCULAR	NR
MATERNITY CARE	NR	WOMEN'S HEALTH	NR

HEALTHGRADES AWARDS

Southern Hills Medical Center

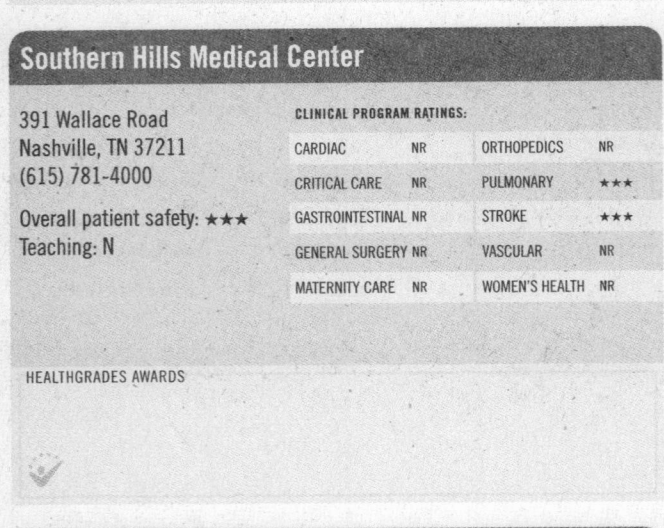

391 Wallace Road
Nashville, TN 37211
(615) 781-4000

Overall patient safety: ★★★
Teaching: N

CLINICAL PROGRAM RATINGS:

CARDIAC	NR	ORTHOPEDICS	NR
CRITICAL CARE	NR	PULMONARY	★★★
GASTROINTESTINAL	NR	STROKE	★★★
GENERAL SURGERY	NR	VASCULAR	NR
MATERNITY CARE	NR	WOMEN'S HEALTH	NR

HEALTHGRADES AWARDS

Stones River Hospital

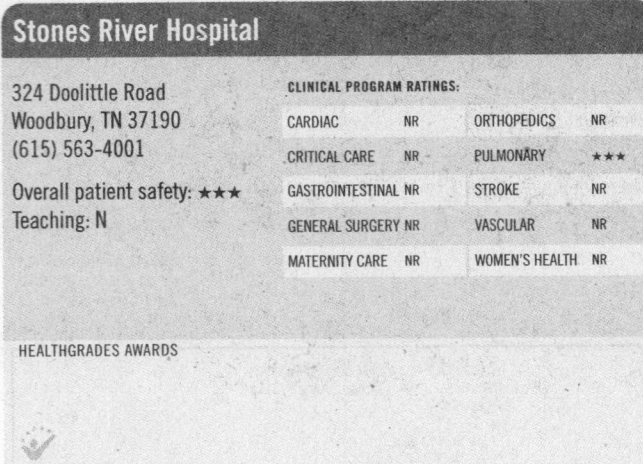

324 Doolittle Road
Woodbury, TN 37190
(615) 563-4001

Overall patient safety: ★★★
Teaching: N

CLINICAL PROGRAM RATINGS:

CARDIAC	NR	ORTHOPEDICS	NR
CRITICAL CARE	NR	PULMONARY	★★★
GASTROINTESTINAL	NR	STROKE	NR
GENERAL SURGERY	NR	VASCULAR	NR
MATERNITY CARE	NR	WOMEN'S HEALTH	NR

HEALTHGRADES AWARDS

Southern Tennessee Medical Center

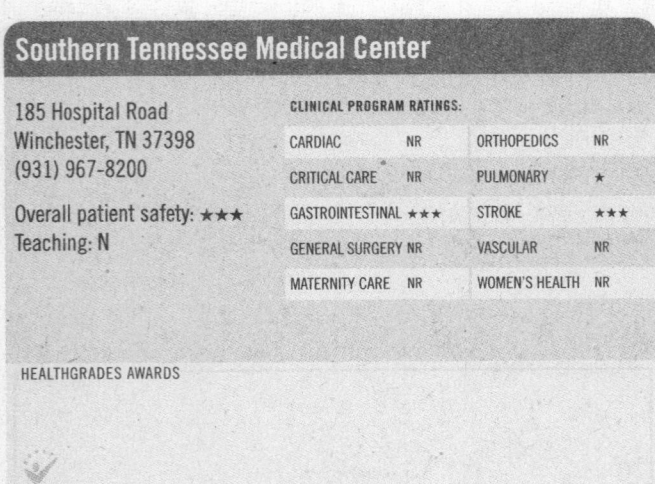

185 Hospital Road
Winchester, TN 37398
(931) 967-8200

Overall patient safety: ★★★
Teaching: N

CLINICAL PROGRAM RATINGS:

CARDIAC	NR	ORTHOPEDICS	NR
CRITICAL CARE	NR	PULMONARY	★
GASTROINTESTINAL	★★★	STROKE	★★★
GENERAL SURGERY	NR	VASCULAR	NR
MATERNITY CARE	NR	WOMEN'S HEALTH	NR

HEALTHGRADES AWARDS

Summit Medical Center

5655 Frist Boulevard
Hermitage, TN 37076
(615) 316-3000

Overall patient safety: ★
Teaching: N

CLINICAL PROGRAM RATINGS:

CARDIAC	NR	ORTHOPEDICS	★
CRITICAL CARE	NR	PULMONARY	★★★★★
GASTROINTESTINAL	★★★	STROKE	★
GENERAL SURGERY	NR	VASCULAR	NR
MATERNITY CARE	NR	WOMEN'S HEALTH	NR

HEALTHGRADES AWARDS

✓ SPECIALTY EXCELLENCE
- PULMONARY CARE

KEY: ★★★★★ BEST   ★★★ AS EXPECTED   ★ POOR   NR NOT RATED BY HEALTHGRADES   For full definitions of ratings and awards, see Appendix.

Sumner Regional Medical Center

555 Hartsville Pike
Gallatin, TN 37066
(615) 452-4210

Overall patient safety: ★
Teaching: N

CLINICAL PROGRAM RATINGS:

CARDIAC	NR	ORTHOPEDICS	NR
CRITICAL CARE	NR	PULMONARY	★★★
GASTROINTESTINAL	★★★	STROKE	★★★
GENERAL SURGERY	NR	VASCULAR	NR
MATERNITY CARE	NR	WOMEN'S HEALTH	NR

HEALTHGRADES AWARDS

Takoma Adventist Hospital

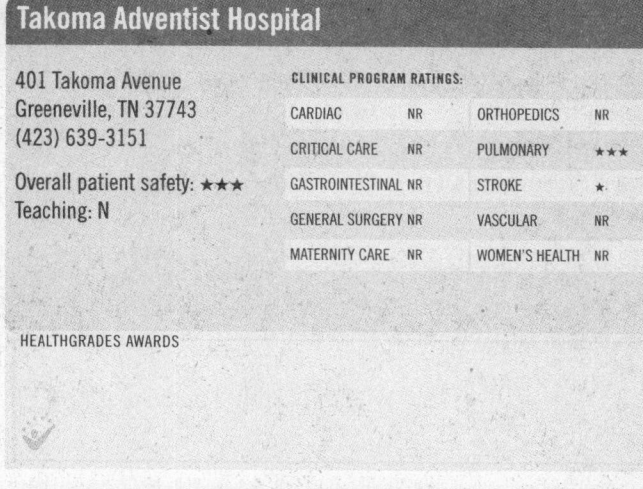

401 Takoma Avenue
Greeneville, TN 37743
(423) 639-3151

Overall patient safety: ★★★
Teaching: N

CLINICAL PROGRAM RATINGS:

CARDIAC	NR	ORTHOPEDICS	NR
CRITICAL CARE	NR	PULMONARY	★★★
GASTROINTESTINAL	NR	STROKE	★
GENERAL SURGERY	NR	VASCULAR	NR
MATERNITY CARE	NR	WOMEN'S HEALTH	NR

HEALTHGRADES AWARDS

Sweetwater Hospital Association

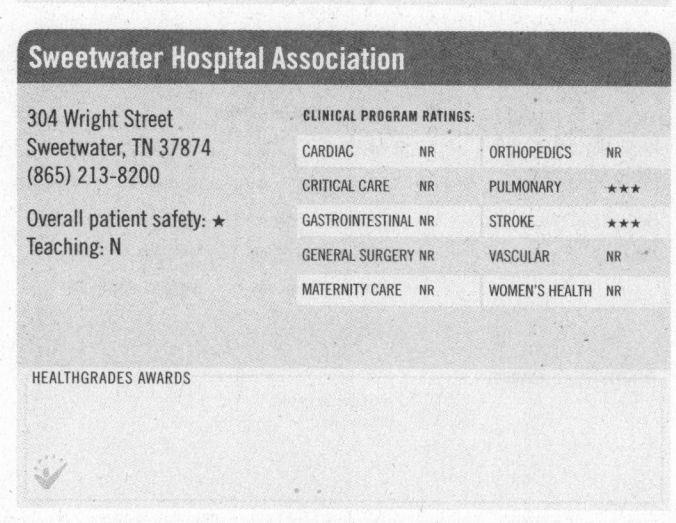

304 Wright Street
Sweetwater, TN 37874
(865) 213-8200

Overall patient safety: ★
Teaching: N

CLINICAL PROGRAM RATINGS:

CARDIAC	NR	ORTHOPEDICS	NR
CRITICAL CARE	NR	PULMONARY	★★★
GASTROINTESTINAL	NR	STROKE	★★★
GENERAL SURGERY	NR	VASCULAR	NR
MATERNITY CARE	NR	WOMEN'S HEALTH	NR

HEALTHGRADES AWARDS

Three Rivers Hospital

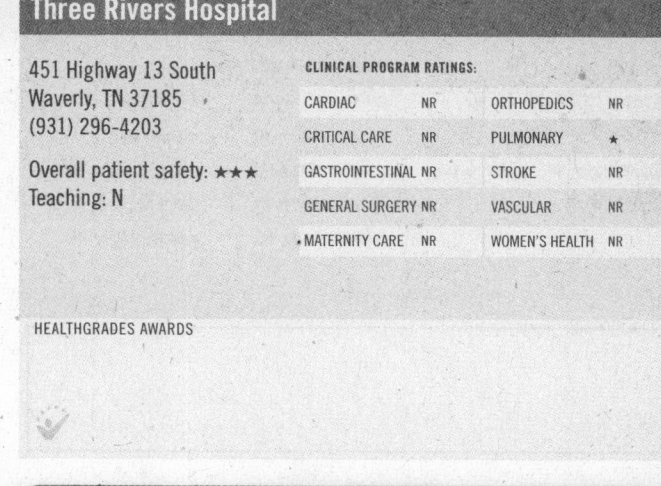

451 Highway 13 South
Waverly, TN 37185
(931) 296-4203

Overall patient safety: ★★★
Teaching: N

CLINICAL PROGRAM RATINGS:

CARDIAC	NR	ORTHOPEDICS	NR
CRITICAL CARE	NR	PULMONARY	★
GASTROINTESTINAL	NR	STROKE	NR
GENERAL SURGERY	NR	VASCULAR	NR
MATERNITY CARE	NR	WOMEN'S HEALTH	NR

HEALTHGRADES AWARDS

Sycamore Shoals Hospital

1501 West Elk Avenue
Elizabethton, TN 37643
(423) 542-1300

Overall patient safety: ★★★
Teaching: N

CLINICAL PROGRAM RATINGS:

CARDIAC	NR	ORTHOPEDICS	NR
CRITICAL CARE	NR	PULMONARY	★
GASTROINTESTINAL	★★★	STROKE	★
GENERAL SURGERY	NR	VASCULAR	NR
MATERNITY CARE	NR	WOMEN'S HEALTH	NR

HEALTHGRADES AWARDS

Trinity Hospital

302 East Main Street
Erin, TN 37061
(931) 289-4211

Overall patient safety: ★★★
Teaching: N

CLINICAL PROGRAM RATINGS:

CARDIAC	NR	ORTHOPEDICS	NR
CRITICAL CARE	NR	PULMONARY	★★★
GASTROINTESTINAL	NR	STROKE	★★★
GENERAL SURGERY	NR	VASCULAR	NR
MATERNITY CARE	NR	WOMEN'S HEALTH	NR

HEALTHGRADES AWARDS

Trousdale Medical Center

500 Church Street
Hartsville, TN 37074
(615) 374-2221

Overall patient safety: ★★★
Teaching: N

CLINICAL PROGRAM RATINGS:

CARDIAC	NR	ORTHOPEDICS	NR
CRITICAL CARE	NR	PULMONARY	★★★
GASTROINTESTINAL	NR	STROKE	NR
GENERAL SURGERY	NR	VASCULAR	NR
MATERNITY CARE	NR	WOMEN'S HEALTH	NR

HEALTHGRADES AWARDS

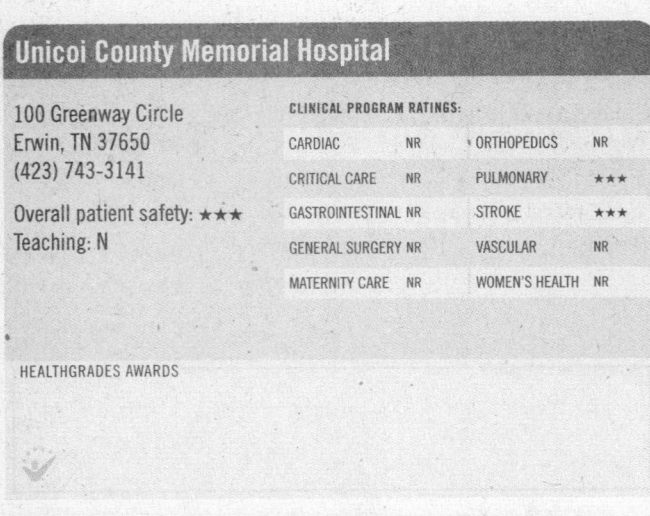

University Medical Center

1411 Baddour Parkway
Lebanon, TN 37087
(615) 444-8262

Overall patient safety: ★★★
Teaching: N

CLINICAL PROGRAM RATINGS:

CARDIAC	NR	ORTHOPEDICS	NR
CRITICAL CARE	NR	PULMONARY	★
GASTROINTESTINAL	★★★	STROKE	★★★
GENERAL SURGERY	NR	VASCULAR	NR
MATERNITY CARE	NR	WOMEN'S HEALTH	NR

HEALTHGRADES AWARDS

Unicoi County Memorial Hospital

100 Greenway Circle
Erwin, TN 37650
(423) 743-3141

Overall patient safety: ★★★
Teaching: N

CLINICAL PROGRAM RATINGS:

CARDIAC	NR	ORTHOPEDICS	NR
CRITICAL CARE	NR	PULMONARY	★★★
GASTROINTESTINAL	NR	STROKE	★★★
GENERAL SURGERY	NR	VASCULAR	NR
MATERNITY CARE	NR	WOMEN'S HEALTH	NR

HEALTHGRADES AWARDS

University of Tennessee Memorial Hospital

1924 Alcoa Highway
Knoxville, TN 37920
(865) 544-9000

Overall patient safety: ★
Teaching: Y

CLINICAL PROGRAM RATINGS:

CARDIAC	★★★	ORTHOPEDICS	★★★
CRITICAL CARE	★★★★★	PULMONARY	★★★★★
GASTROINTESTINAL	★★★	STROKE	★
GENERAL SURGERY	NR	VASCULAR	★★★
MATERNITY CARE	NR	WOMEN'S HEALTH	NR

HEALTHGRADES AWARDS

✓ SPECIALTY EXCELLENCE
· CRITICAL CARE

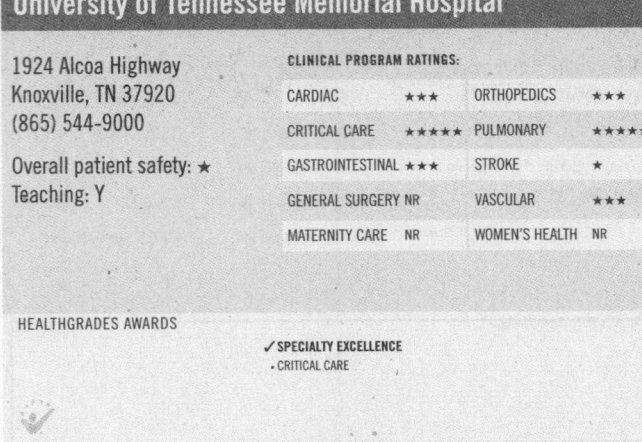

United Regional Medical Center

1001 McArthur Drive
Manchester, TN 37355
(931) 728-3586

Overall patient safety: ★★★
Teaching: N

CLINICAL PROGRAM RATINGS:

CARDIAC	NR	ORTHOPEDICS	NR
CRITICAL CARE	NR	PULMONARY	★★★
GASTROINTESTINAL	NR	STROKE	NR
GENERAL SURGERY	NR	VASCULAR	NR
MATERNITY CARE	NR	WOMEN'S HEALTH	NR

HEALTHGRADES AWARDS

Vanderbilt University Hospital

1660 21st Avenue South
Nashville, TN 37232
(615) 322-5000

Overall patient safety: ★★★
Teaching: Y

CLINICAL PROGRAM RATINGS:

CARDIAC	★★★	ORTHOPEDICS	★★★
CRITICAL CARE	★★★	PULMONARY	★★★
GASTROINTESTINAL	★★★	STROKE	★★★
GENERAL SURGERY	NR	VASCULAR	★★★
MATERNITY CARE	NR	WOMEN'S HEALTH	NR

HEALTHGRADES AWARDS

KEY: ★★★★★ BEST   ★★★ AS EXPECTED   ★ POOR   NR NOT RATED BY HEALTHGRADES   For full definitions of ratings and awards, see Appendix.

Volunteer Community Hospital

161 Mount Pelia Road
Martin, TN 38237
(731) 587-4261

Overall patient safety: ★★★
Teaching: N

CLINICAL PROGRAM RATINGS:

CARDIAC	NR	ORTHOPEDICS	NR
CRITICAL CARE	NR	PULMONARY	★★★
GASTROINTESTINAL	NR	STROKE	★★★
GENERAL SURGERY	NR	VASCULAR	NR
MATERNITY CARE	NR	WOMEN'S HEALTH	NR

HEALTHGRADES AWARDS

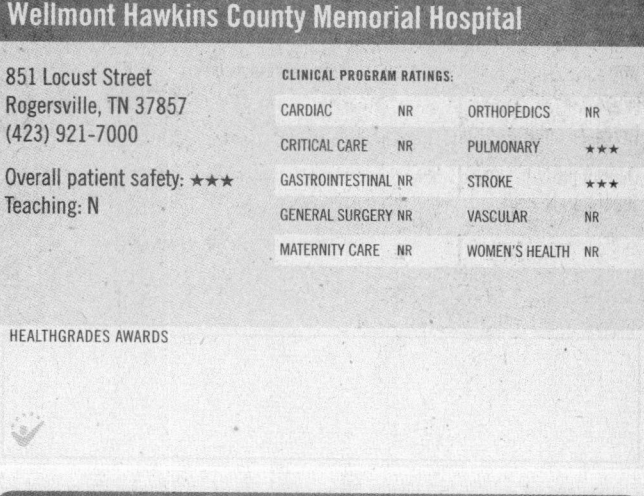

Wellmont Hawkins County Memorial Hospital

851 Locust Street
Rogersville, TN 37857
(423) 921-7000

Overall patient safety: ★★★
Teaching: N

CLINICAL PROGRAM RATINGS:

CARDIAC	NR	ORTHOPEDICS	NR
CRITICAL CARE	NR	PULMONARY	★★★
GASTROINTESTINAL	NR	STROKE	★★★
GENERAL SURGERY	NR	VASCULAR	NR
MATERNITY CARE	NR	WOMEN'S HEALTH	NR

HEALTHGRADES AWARDS

Wayne Medical Center

103 J V Mangubat Drive
Waynesboro, TN 38485
(931) 722-5411

Overall patient safety: NR
Teaching: N

CLINICAL PROGRAM RATINGS:

CARDIAC	NR	ORTHOPEDICS	NR
CRITICAL CARE	NR	PULMONARY	★★★
GASTROINTESTINAL	NR	STROKE	NR
GENERAL SURGERY	NR	VASCULAR	NR
MATERNITY CARE	NR	WOMEN'S HEALTH	NR

HEALTHGRADES AWARDS

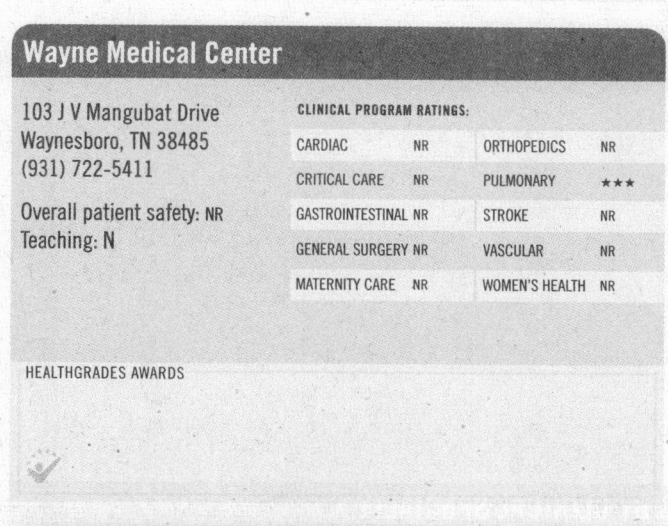

Wellmont Holston Valley Medical Center

130 West Ravine
Kingsport, TN 37660
(423) 224-4000

Overall patient safety: ★★★
Teaching: Y

CLINICAL PROGRAM RATINGS:

CARDIAC	★★★	ORTHOPEDICS	★★★
CRITICAL CARE	★★★	PULMONARY	★★★
GASTROINTESTINAL	★★★	STROKE	★★★
GENERAL SURGERY	NR	VASCULAR	★★★
MATERNITY CARE	NR	WOMEN'S HEALTH	NR

HEALTHGRADES AWARDS

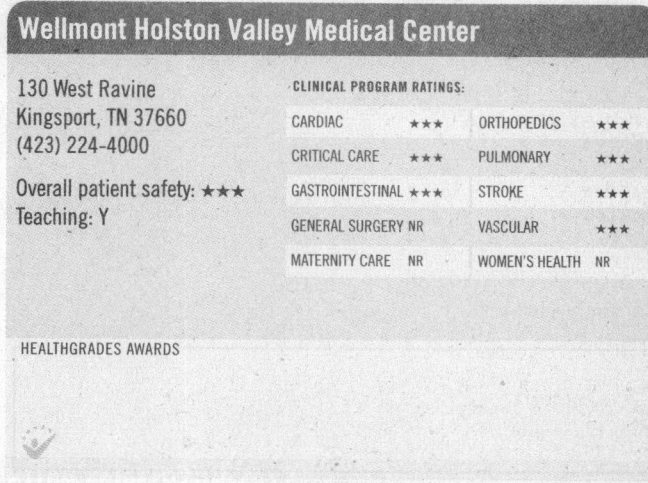

Wellmont Bristol Regional Medical Center

1 Medical Park Boulevard
Bristol, TN 37620
(423) 844-1121

Overall patient safety: ★★★
Teaching: Y

CLINICAL PROGRAM RATINGS:

CARDIAC	★★★	ORTHOPEDICS	★
CRITICAL CARE	★★★	PULMONARY	★★★
GASTROINTESTINAL	★★★	STROKE	★★★
GENERAL SURGERY	NR	VASCULAR	NR
MATERNITY CARE	NR	WOMEN'S HEALTH	NR

HEALTHGRADES AWARDS

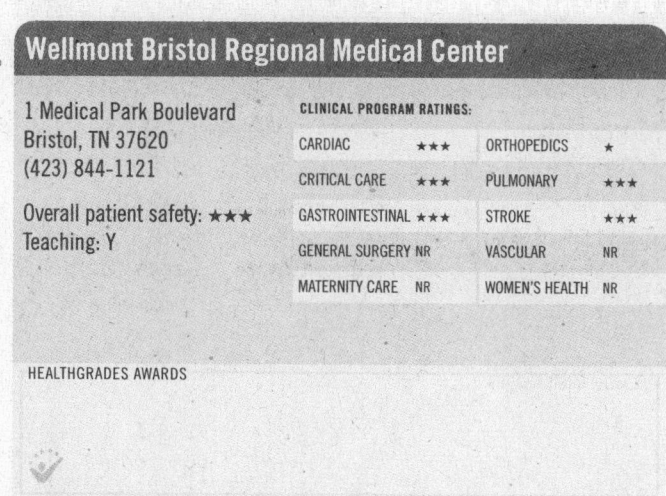

White County Community Hospital

401 Sewell Road
Sparta, TN 38583
(931) 738-9211

Overall patient safety: ★★★
Teaching: N

CLINICAL PROGRAM RATINGS:

CARDIAC	NR	ORTHOPEDICS	NR
CRITICAL CARE	NR	PULMONARY	★★★
GASTROINTESTINAL	NR	STROKE	★★★
GENERAL SURGERY	NR	VASCULAR	NR
MATERNITY CARE	NR	WOMEN'S HEALTH	NR

HEALTHGRADES AWARDS

Williamson Medical Center

2021 Carothers Road
Franklin, TN 37067
(615) 791-0500

Overall patient safety: ★★★
Teaching: N

CLINICAL PROGRAM RATINGS:

CARDIAC	NR	ORTHOPEDICS	★★★
CRITICAL CARE	NR	PULMONARY	★★★
GASTROINTESTINAL	NR	STROKE	★★★
GENERAL SURGERY	NR	VASCULAR	NR
MATERNITY CARE	NR	WOMEN'S HEALTH	NR

HEALTHGRADES AWARDS

Woods Memorial Hospital

886 Highway 411 North
Etowah, TN 37331
(423) 263-3600

Overall patient safety: ★★★
Teaching: N

CLINICAL PROGRAM RATINGS:

CARDIAC	NR	ORTHOPEDICS	NR
CRITICAL CARE	NR	PULMONARY	★
GASTROINTESTINAL	NR	STROKE	★
GENERAL SURGERY	NR	VASCULAR	NR
MATERNITY CARE	NR	WOMEN'S HEALTH	NR

HEALTHGRADES AWARDS

Women's East Pavilion*

1751 Gunbarrel Road
Chattanooga, TN 37421
(423) 954-8700

Overall patient safety: ★★★
Teaching: Y

CLINICAL PROGRAM RATINGS:

CARDIAC	★★★	ORTHOPEDICS	★★★
CRITICAL CARE	★★★	PULMONARY	★★★
GASTROINTESTINAL	★★★	STROKE	★★★
GENERAL SURGERY	NR	VASCULAR	★★★
MATERNITY CARE	NR	WOMEN'S HEALTH	NR

HEALTHGRADES AWARDS

TEXAS HOSPITALS: RATINGS BY CLINICAL SPECIALTY

Abilene Regional Medical Center

6250 Highway 83-84 at
Antilley Road
Abilene, TX 79606
(325) 695-9900

Overall patient safety: ★★★
Teaching: N

CLINICAL PROGRAM RATINGS:

CARDIAC	★★★	ORTHOPEDICS	★★★
CRITICAL CARE	NR	PULMONARY	★★★
GASTROINTESTINAL	★★★	STROKE	★★★
GENERAL SURGERY	★★★	VASCULAR	NR
MATERNITY CARE	★★★	WOMEN'S HEALTH	★

HEALTHGRADES AWARDS

✓ SPECIALTY EXCELLENCE
• CARDIAC SURGERY

Alliance Hospital

515 North Adams
Odessa, TX 79761
(432) 550-1903

Overall patient safety: ★★★
Teaching: N

CLINICAL PROGRAM RATINGS:

CARDIAC	★★★	ORTHOPEDICS	★★★
CRITICAL CARE	NR	PULMONARY	★★★
GASTROINTESTINAL	NR	STROKE	★★★
GENERAL SURGERY	NR	VASCULAR	NR
MATERNITY CARE	NR	WOMEN'S HEALTH	NR

HEALTHGRADES AWARDS

KEY: ★★★★★ BEST   ★★★ AS EXPECTED   ★ POOR   NR NOT RATED BY HEALTHGRADES   For full definitions of ratings and awards, see Appendix.

American Transitional Hospital–Houston W

8850 Long Point Road
6th Floor Tower
Houston, TX 77055
(713) 984-2273

Overall patient safety: ★★★
Teaching: N

CLINICAL PROGRAM RATINGS:

CARDIAC	★★★	ORTHOPEDICS	★★★
CRITICAL CARE	NR	PULMONARY	★★★★★
GASTROINTESTINAL	★★★	STROKE	★★★
GENERAL SURGERY	★★★	VASCULAR	NR
MATERNITY CARE	NR	WOMEN'S HEALTH	NR

HEALTHGRADES AWARDS

✓ SPECIALTY EXCELLENCE
• PULMONARY CARE

Arlington Memorial Hospital

800 West Randol Mill Road
Arlington, TX 76012
(817) 548-6100

Overall patient safety: ★
Teaching: N

CLINICAL PROGRAM RATINGS:

CARDIAC	★	ORTHOPEDICS	★★★
CRITICAL CARE	★★★	PULMONARY	★★★
GASTROINTESTINAL	★★★	STROKE	★★★
GENERAL SURGERY	★★★★★	VASCULAR	★★★
MATERNITY CARE	★★★	WOMEN'S HEALTH	★★★

HEALTHGRADES AWARDS

✓ SPECIALTY EXCELLENCE
• GASTROINTESTINAL   • GENERAL SURGERY
  CARE

Angleton-Danbury Medical Center

132 Hospital Drive
Angleton, TX 77515
(979) 849-7721

Overall patient safety: ★★★
Teaching: N

CLINICAL PROGRAM RATINGS:

CARDIAC	NR	ORTHOPEDICS	NR
CRITICAL CARE	NR	PULMONARY	★
GASTROINTESTINAL	NR	STROKE	NR
GENERAL SURGERY	★★★	VASCULAR	NR
MATERNITY CARE	★★★	WOMEN'S HEALTH	NR

HEALTHGRADES AWARDS

Atlanta Memorial Hospital

1007 South William Street
Atlanta, TX 75551
(903) 799-3000

Overall patient safety: ★★★
Teaching: N

CLINICAL PROGRAM RATINGS:

CARDIAC	NR	ORTHOPEDICS	NR
CRITICAL CARE	NR	PULMONARY	★★★
GASTROINTESTINAL	NR	STROKE	★★★
GENERAL SURGERY	NR	VASCULAR	NR
MATERNITY CARE	NR	WOMEN'S HEALTH	NR

HEALTHGRADES AWARDS

Anson General Hospital

101 Avenue J
Anson, TX 79501
(325) 823-3231

Overall patient safety: ★★★
Teaching: N

CLINICAL PROGRAM RATINGS:

CARDIAC	NR	ORTHOPEDICS	NR
CRITICAL CARE	NR	PULMONARY	★★★
GASTROINTESTINAL	NR	STROKE	NR
GENERAL SURGERY	NR	VASCULAR	NR
MATERNITY CARE	NR	WOMEN'S HEALTH	NR

HEALTHGRADES AWARDS

Baptist Health System*

111 Dallas Street
San Antonio, TX 78205
(210) 297-7000

Overall patient safety: ★★★
Teaching: N

CLINICAL PROGRAM RATINGS:

CARDIAC	★★★	ORTHOPEDICS	★★★
CRITICAL CARE	NR	PULMONARY	★★★
GASTROINTESTINAL	★★★	STROKE	★★★
GENERAL SURGERY	★★★	VASCULAR	★★★★★
MATERNITY CARE	★★★	WOMEN'S HEALTH	★★★

HEALTHGRADES AWARDS

✓ SPECIALTY EXCELLENCE
• VASCULAR SURGERY

*This hospital reports its data to the federal government jointly with another hospital. Therefore the ratings and awards apply to multiple hospitals and this specific hospital may not provide all rated services.

Baptist St. Anthony's Health System

1600 Wallace Boulevard
Amarillo, TX 79106
(806) 212-2000

Overall patient safety: ★★★★★
Teaching: Y

CLINICAL PROGRAM RATINGS:

CARDIAC	★★★	ORTHOPEDICS	★★★
CRITICAL CARE	NR	PULMONARY	★★★
GASTROINTESTINAL	★★★	STROKE	★★★
GENERAL SURGERY	★★★	VASCULAR	★★★
MATERNITY CARE	★★★	WOMEN'S HEALTH	★★★

HEALTHGRADES AWARDS

✓ DISTINGUISHED HOSPITAL
· PATIENT SAFETY

✓ SPECIALTY EXCELLENCE
· GENERAL SURGERY

Baylor Medical Center at Garland

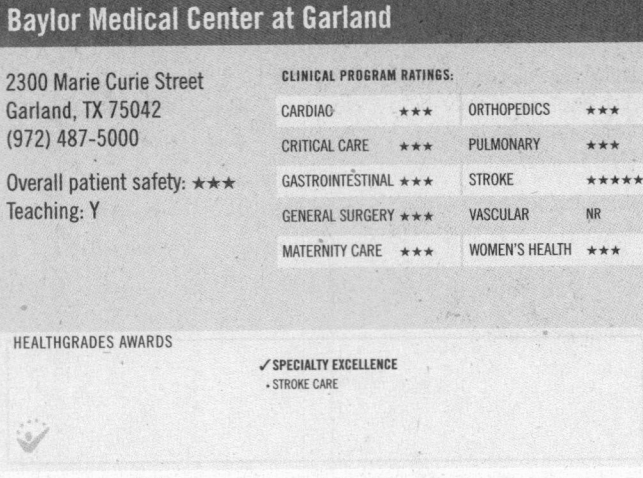

2300 Marie Curie Street
Garland, TX 75042
(972) 487-5000

Overall patient safety: ★★★
Teaching: Y

CLINICAL PROGRAM RATINGS:

CARDIAC	★★★	ORTHOPEDICS	★★★
CRITICAL CARE	★★★	PULMONARY	★★★
GASTROINTESTINAL	★★★	STROKE	★★★★★
GENERAL SURGERY	★★★	VASCULAR	NR
MATERNITY CARE	★★★	WOMEN'S HEALTH	★★★

HEALTHGRADES AWARDS

✓ SPECIALTY EXCELLENCE
· STROKE CARE

Baylor All Saints Medical Center at Fort Worth

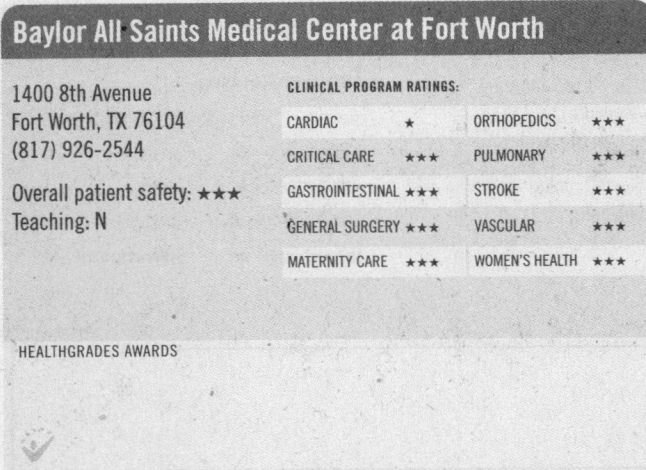

1400 8th Avenue
Fort Worth, TX 76104
(817) 926-2544

Overall patient safety: ★★★
Teaching: N

CLINICAL PROGRAM RATINGS:

CARDIAC	★	ORTHOPEDICS	★★★
CRITICAL CARE	★★★	PULMONARY	★★★
GASTROINTESTINAL	★★★	STROKE	★★★
GENERAL SURGERY	★★★	VASCULAR	★★★
MATERNITY CARE	★★★	WOMEN'S HEALTH	★★★

HEALTHGRADES AWARDS

Baylor Medical Center at Irving

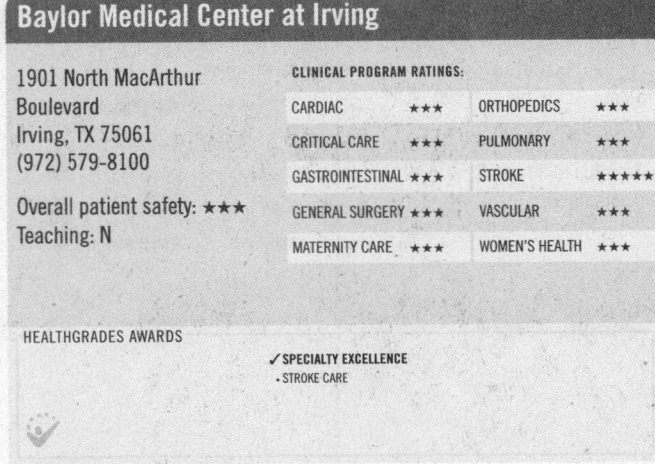

1901 North MacArthur Boulevard
Irving, TX 75061
(972) 579-8100

Overall patient safety: ★★★
Teaching: N

CLINICAL PROGRAM RATINGS:

CARDIAC	★★★	ORTHOPEDICS	★★★
CRITICAL CARE	★★★	PULMONARY	★★★
GASTROINTESTINAL	★★★	STROKE	★★★★★
GENERAL SURGERY	★★★	VASCULAR	★★★
MATERNITY CARE	★★★	WOMEN'S HEALTH	★★★

HEALTHGRADES AWARDS

✓ SPECIALTY EXCELLENCE
· STROKE CARE

Baylor Heart and Vascular Center

621 North Hall Street
Suite 150
Dallas, TX 75226
(214) 820-0600

Overall patient safety: ★★★★★
Teaching: Y

CLINICAL PROGRAM RATINGS:

CARDIAC	NR	ORTHOPEDICS	NR
CRITICAL CARE	NR	PULMONARY	NR
GASTROINTESTINAL	NR	STROKE	NR
GENERAL SURGERY	NR	VASCULAR	★★★
MATERNITY CARE	NR	WOMEN'S HEALTH	NR

HEALTHGRADES AWARDS

✓ SPECIALTY EXCELLENCE
· VASCULAR SURGERY

Baylor Medical Center at Waxahachie

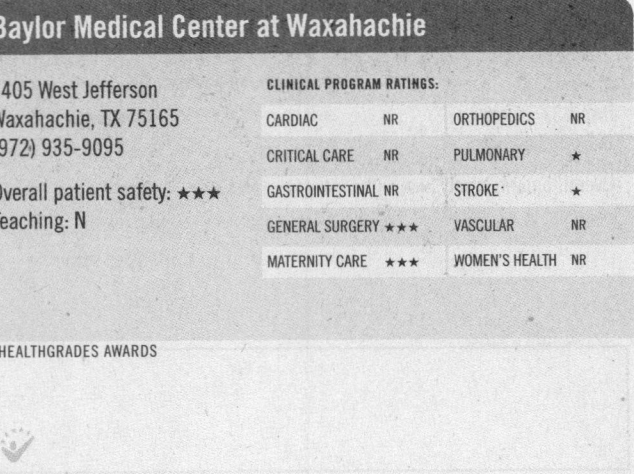

1405 West Jefferson
Waxahachie, TX 75165
(972) 935-9095

Overall patient safety: ★★★
Teaching: N

CLINICAL PROGRAM RATINGS:

CARDIAC	NR	ORTHOPEDICS	NR
CRITICAL CARE	NR	PULMONARY	★
GASTROINTESTINAL	NR	STROKE	★
GENERAL SURGERY	★★★	VASCULAR	NR
MATERNITY CARE	★★★	WOMEN'S HEALTH	NR

HEALTHGRADES AWARDS

KEY: ★★★★★ BEST ★★★ AS EXPECTED ★ POOR NR NOT RATED BY HEALTHGRADES For full definitions of ratings and awards, see Appendix.

Baylor Regional Medical Center at Grapevine

1650 West College Street
Grapevine, TX 76051
(817) 481-1588

Overall patient safety: ★★★
Teaching: N

CLINICAL PROGRAM RATINGS:

CARDIAC	★★★	ORTHOPEDICS	★★★
CRITICAL CARE	NR	PULMONARY	★★★
GASTROINTESTINAL	NR	STROKE	★★★
GENERAL SURGERY	★★★	VASCULAR	NR
MATERNITY CARE	★★★	WOMEN'S HEALTH	★★★

HEALTHGRADES AWARDS

Bayshore Medical Center in Pasadena*

4000 Spencer Highway
Pasadena, TX 77504
(713) 359-2000

Overall patient safety: ★★★
Teaching: N

CLINICAL PROGRAM RATINGS:

CARDIAC	★★★	ORTHOPEDICS	★★★★★
CRITICAL CARE	★★★	PULMONARY	★★★
GASTROINTESTINAL	★★★	STROKE	★★★
GENERAL SURGERY	★★★★★	VASCULAR	NR
MATERNITY CARE	★★★★★	WOMEN'S HEALTH	★★★

HEALTHGRADES AWARDS

✓ DISTINGUISHED HOSPITAL
 • CLINICAL EXCELLENCE

✓ SPECIALTY EXCELLENCE
 • GASTROINTESTINAL CARE
 • GENERAL SURGERY
 • MATERNITY CARE
 • ORTHOPEDIC SURGERY

Baylor Regional Medical Center at Plano

4700 Alliance Boulevard
Plano, TX 75093
(469) 814-2000

Overall patient safety: ★★★
Teaching: N

CLINICAL PROGRAM RATINGS:

CARDIAC	★★★	ORTHOPEDICS	NR
CRITICAL CARE	NR	PULMONARY	★★★
GASTROINTESTINAL	NR	STROKE	★★★
GENERAL SURGERY	★★★	VASCULAR	NR
MATERNITY CARE	NR	WOMEN'S HEALTH	NR

HEALTHGRADES AWARDS

Bellville General Hospital

44 North Cummings
Bellville, TX 77418
(979) 865-3141

Overall patient safety: ★★★
Teaching: N

CLINICAL PROGRAM RATINGS:

CARDIAC	NR	ORTHOPEDICS	NR
CRITICAL CARE	NR	PULMONARY	★
GASTROINTESTINAL	NR	STROKE	NR
GENERAL SURGERY	NR	VASCULAR	NR
MATERNITY CARE	NR	WOMEN'S HEALTH	NR

HEALTHGRADES AWARDS

Baylor University Medical Center

3500 Gaston Avenue
Dallas, TX 75246
(214) 820-0111

Overall patient safety: ★★★
Teaching: Y

CLINICAL PROGRAM RATINGS:

CARDIAC	★	ORTHOPEDICS	★★★
CRITICAL CARE	★★★	PULMONARY	★★★
GASTROINTESTINAL	★★★	STROKE	★★★★★
GENERAL SURGERY	★★★	VASCULAR	★★★
MATERNITY CARE	★★★	WOMEN'S HEALTH	★★★

HEALTHGRADES AWARDS

✓ SPECIALTY EXCELLENCE
 • GASTROINTESTINAL CARE
 • STROKE CARE

Big Bend Regional Medical Center

2600 Highway 118 North
Alpine, TX 79830
(432) 837-3447

Overall patient safety: ★★★
Teaching: N

CLINICAL PROGRAM RATINGS:

CARDIAC	NR	ORTHOPEDICS	NR
CRITICAL CARE	NR	PULMONARY	★★★
GASTROINTESTINAL	NR	STROKE	NR
GENERAL SURGERY	★★★	VASCULAR	NR
MATERNITY CARE	★★★	WOMEN'S HEALTH	NR

HEALTHGRADES AWARDS

*This hospital reports its data to the federal government jointly with another hospital. Therefore the ratings and awards apply to multiple hospitals and this specific hospital may not provide all rated services.

Bowie Memorial Hospital

705 East Greenwood Avenue
Bowie, TX 76230
(940) 872-1126

Overall patient safety: ★★★
Teaching: N

CLINICAL PROGRAM RATINGS:

CARDIAC	NR	ORTHOPEDICS	NR
CRITICAL CARE	NR	PULMONARY	★★★
GASTROINTESTINAL	NR	STROKE	★
GENERAL SURGERY	NR	VASCULAR	NR
MATERNITY CARE	NR	WOMEN'S HEALTH	NR

HEALTHGRADES AWARDS

Brownfield Regional Medical Center

705 East Felt Street
Brownfield, TX 79316
(806) 637-3551

Overall patient safety: ★★★
Teaching: N

CLINICAL PROGRAM RATINGS:

CARDIAC	NR	ORTHOPEDICS	NR
CRITICAL CARE	NR	PULMONARY	★★★
GASTROINTESTINAL	NR	STROKE	NR
GENERAL SURGERY	NR	VASCULAR	NR
MATERNITY CARE	★★★	WOMEN'S HEALTH	NR

HEALTHGRADES AWARDS

Brackenridge Hospital

601 East 15th Street
Austin, TX 78701
(512) 324-7000

Overall patient safety: ★★★
Teaching: Y

CLINICAL PROGRAM RATINGS:

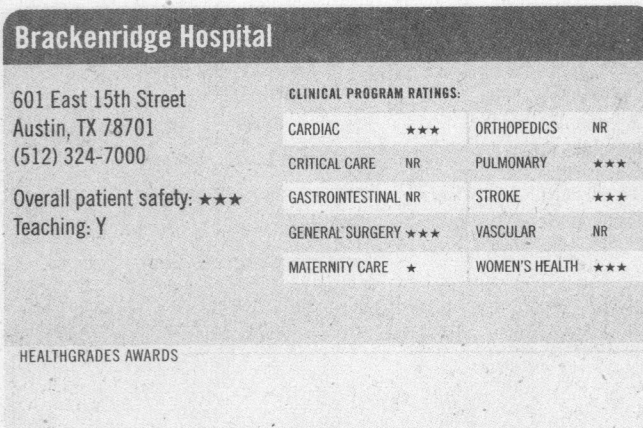

CARDIAC	★★★	ORTHOPEDICS	NR
CRITICAL CARE	NR	PULMONARY	★★★
GASTROINTESTINAL	NR	STROKE	★★★
GENERAL SURGERY	★★★	VASCULAR	NR
MATERNITY CARE	★	WOMEN'S HEALTH	★★★

HEALTHGRADES AWARDS

Brownwood Regional Medical Center

1501 Burnet Drive
Brownwood, TX 76801
(325) 646-8541

Overall patient safety: ★
Teaching: N

CLINICAL PROGRAM RATINGS:

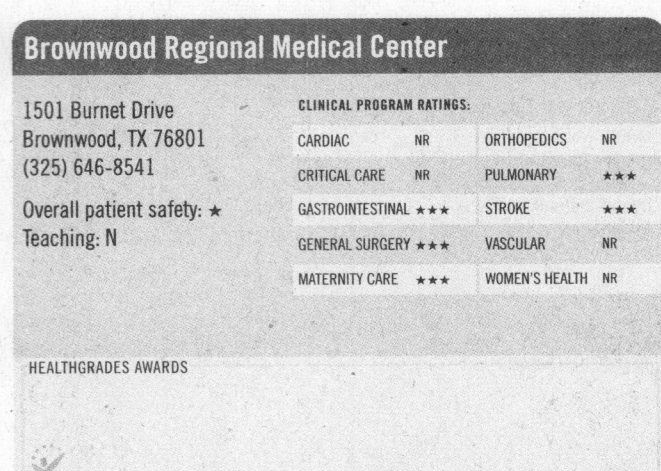

CARDIAC	NR	ORTHOPEDICS	NR
CRITICAL CARE	NR	PULMONARY	★★★
GASTROINTESTINAL	★★★	STROKE	★★★
GENERAL SURGERY	★★★	VASCULAR	NR
MATERNITY CARE	★★★	WOMEN'S HEALTH	NR

HEALTHGRADES AWARDS

Brazosport Regional Health System

100 Medical Drive
Lake Jackson, TX 77566
(979) 297-4411

Overall patient safety: ★
Teaching: N

CLINICAL PROGRAM RATINGS:

CARDIAC	NR	ORTHOPEDICS	NR
CRITICAL CARE	NR	PULMONARY	★★★
GASTROINTESTINAL	★★★	STROKE	★
GENERAL SURGERY	★★★	VASCULAR	NR
MATERNITY CARE	★★★	WOMEN'S HEALTH	NR

HEALTHGRADES AWARDS

Campbell Health System

713 East Anderson Street
Weatherford, TX 76086
(817) 596-8751

Overall patient safety: ★★★
Teaching: N

CLINICAL PROGRAM RATINGS:

CARDIAC	NR	ORTHOPEDICS	NR
CRITICAL CARE	NR	PULMONARY	★★★
GASTROINTESTINAL	★★★	STROKE	★★★
GENERAL SURGERY	★★★	VASCULAR	NR
MATERNITY CARE	★★★	WOMEN'S HEALTH	NR

HEALTHGRADES AWARDS

KEY: ★★★★★ BEST   ★★★ AS EXPECTED   ★ POOR   NR NOT RATED BY HEALTHGRADES   For full definitions of ratings and awards, see Appendix.

Centennial Medical Center

12505 Lebanon Road
Frisco, TX 75035
(972) 963-3333

Overall patient safety: ★★★
Teaching: N

CLINICAL PROGRAM RATINGS:

CARDIAC	NR	ORTHOPEDICS	NR
CRITICAL CARE	NR	PULMONARY	★★★
GASTROINTESTINAL	NR	STROKE	★★★
GENERAL SURGERY	NR	VASCULAR	NR
MATERNITY CARE	★★★	WOMEN'S HEALTH	NR

HEALTHGRADES AWARDS

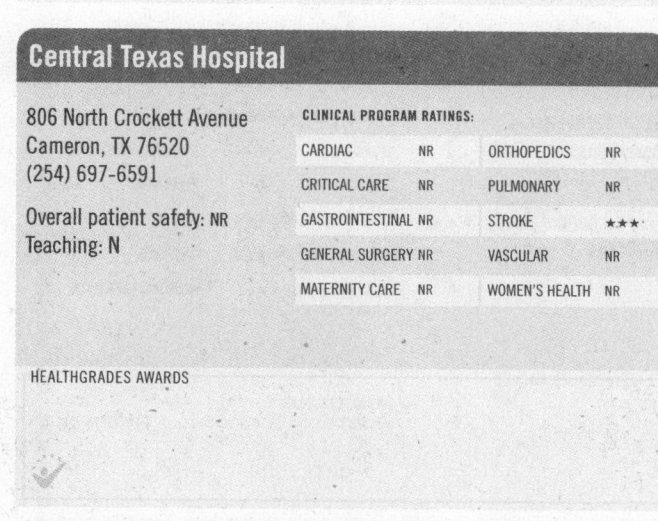

Charlton Methodist Hospital

3500 Wheatland Road
Dallas, TX 75237
(214) 947-7777

Overall patient safety: ★★★
Teaching: Y

CLINICAL PROGRAM RATINGS:

CARDIAC	NR	ORTHOPEDICS	★★★
CRITICAL CARE	★★★	PULMONARY	★★★
GASTROINTESTINAL	★★★	STROKE	★★★
GENERAL SURGERY	★★★	VASCULAR	NR
MATERNITY CARE	★★★★★	WOMEN'S HEALTH	NR

HEALTHGRADES AWARDS

✓ SPECIALTY EXCELLENCE
• MATERNITY CARE

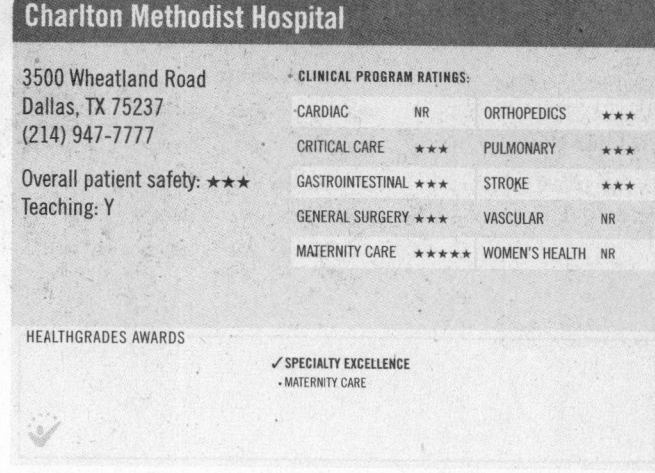

Central Texas Hospital

806 North Crockett Avenue
Cameron, TX 76520
(254) 697-6591

Overall patient safety: NR
Teaching: N

CLINICAL PROGRAM RATINGS:

CARDIAC	NR	ORTHOPEDICS	NR
CRITICAL CARE	NR	PULMONARY	NR
GASTROINTESTINAL	NR	STROKE	★★★
GENERAL SURGERY	NR	VASCULAR	NR
MATERNITY CARE	NR	WOMEN'S HEALTH	NR

HEALTHGRADES AWARDS

Childress Regional Medical Center

Highway 83 North
Childress, TX 79201
(940) 937-6371

Overall patient safety: ★★★
Teaching: Y

CLINICAL PROGRAM RATINGS:

CARDIAC	NR	ORTHOPEDICS	NR
CRITICAL CARE	NR	PULMONARY	★
GASTROINTESTINAL	NR	STROKE	NR
GENERAL SURGERY	NR	VASCULAR	NR
MATERNITY CARE	NR	WOMEN'S HEALTH	NR

HEALTHGRADES AWARDS

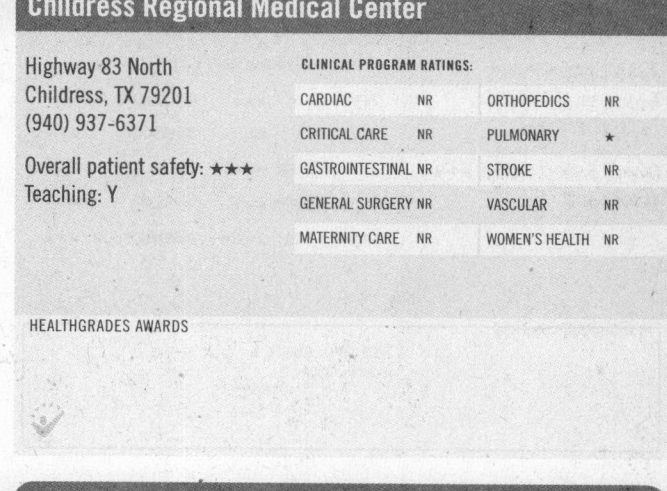

Central Texas Medical Center

1301 Wonder World Drive
San Marcos, TX 78666
(512) 753-3657

Overall patient safety: ★
Teaching: N

CLINICAL PROGRAM RATINGS:

CARDIAC	NR	ORTHOPEDICS	NR
CRITICAL CARE	NR	PULMONARY	★★★
GASTROINTESTINAL	★★★	STROKE	★★★
GENERAL SURGERY	★★★	VASCULAR	NR
MATERNITY CARE	★★★	WOMEN'S HEALTH	NR

HEALTHGRADES AWARDS

Christus Jasper Memorial Hospital

1275 Marvin Hancock Drive
Jasper, TX 75951
(409) 384-5461

Overall patient safety: ★★★
Teaching: N

CLINICAL PROGRAM RATINGS:

CARDIAC	NR	ORTHOPEDICS	NR
CRITICAL CARE	NR	PULMONARY	★★★
GASTROINTESTINAL	NR	STROKE	NR
GENERAL SURGERY	NR	VASCULAR	NR
MATERNITY CARE	★★★	WOMEN'S HEALTH	NR

HEALTHGRADES AWARDS

Christus St. Catherine Health and Wellness Center

701 South Fry Road
Katy, TX 77450
(281) 599-5700

Overall patient safety: ★★★
Teaching: N

CLINICAL PROGRAM RATINGS:

CARDIAC	NR	ORTHOPEDICS	NR
CRITICAL CARE	NR	PULMONARY	★★★★★
GASTROINTESTINAL	NR	STROKE	★★★
GENERAL SURGERY	★★★	VASCULAR	NR
MATERNITY CARE	★★★	WOMEN'S HEALTH	NR

HEALTHGRADES AWARDS

✓ SPECIALTY EXCELLENCE
· PULMONARY CARE

Christus St. Mary Hospital

3600 Gates Boulevard
Port Arthur, TX 77642
(409) 985-7431

Overall patient safety: ★★★
Teaching: N

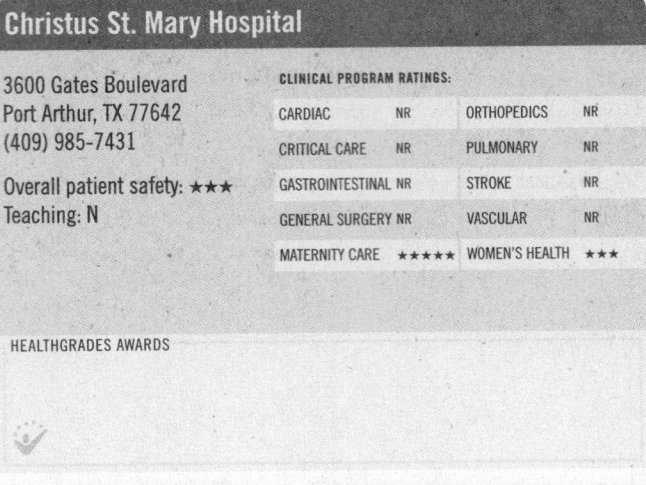

CLINICAL PROGRAM RATINGS:

CARDIAC	NR	ORTHOPEDICS	NR
CRITICAL CARE	NR	PULMONARY	NR
GASTROINTESTINAL	NR	STROKE	NR
GENERAL SURGERY	NR	VASCULAR	NR
MATERNITY CARE	★★★★★	WOMEN'S HEALTH	★★★

HEALTHGRADES AWARDS

Christus St. Elizabeth Hospital

2830 Calder Avenue
Beaumont, TX 77726
(409) 892-7171

Overall patient safety: ★★★
Teaching: N

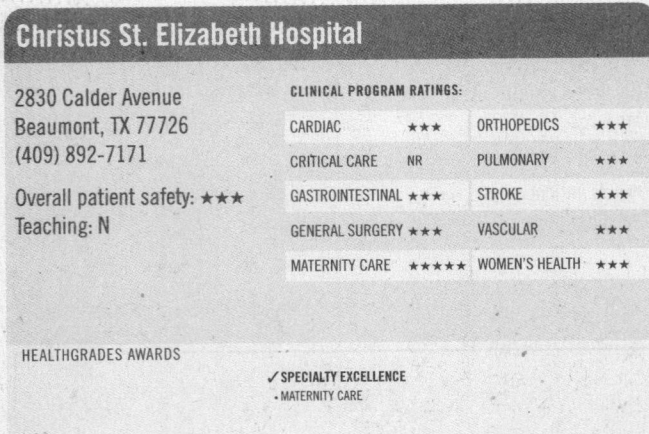

CLINICAL PROGRAM RATINGS:

CARDIAC	★★★	ORTHOPEDICS	★★★
CRITICAL CARE	NR	PULMONARY	★★★
GASTROINTESTINAL	★★★	STROKE	★★★
GENERAL SURGERY	★★★	VASCULAR	★★★
MATERNITY CARE	★★★★★	WOMEN'S HEALTH	★★★

HEALTHGRADES AWARDS

✓ SPECIALTY EXCELLENCE
· MATERNITY CARE

Christus St. Michael Health System

2600 St. Michael Drive
Texarkana, TX 75503
(903) 614-1000

Overall patient safety: ★★★
Teaching: Y

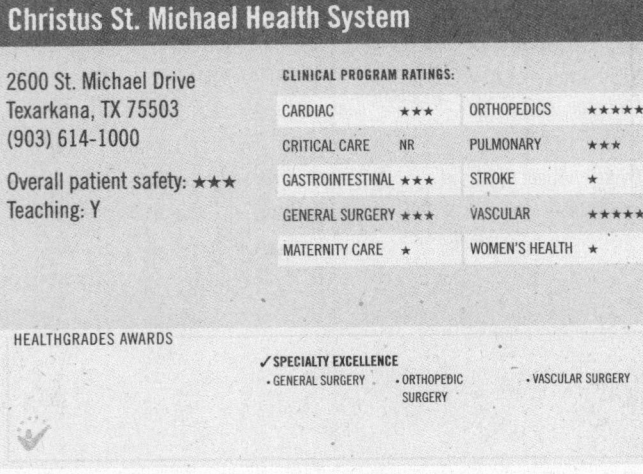

CLINICAL PROGRAM RATINGS:

CARDIAC	★★★	ORTHOPEDICS	★★★★★
CRITICAL CARE	NR	PULMONARY	★★★
GASTROINTESTINAL	★★★	STROKE	★
GENERAL SURGERY	★★★	VASCULAR	★★★★★
MATERNITY CARE	★	WOMEN'S HEALTH	★

HEALTHGRADES AWARDS

✓ SPECIALTY EXCELLENCE
· GENERAL SURGERY   · ORTHOPEDIC SURGERY   · VASCULAR SURGERY

Christus St. John Hospital

18300 St. John Drive
Houston, TX 77058
(281) 333-5503

Overall patient safety: ★★★
Teaching: N

CLINICAL PROGRAM RATINGS:

CARDIAC	NR	ORTHOPEDICS	★★★
CRITICAL CARE	NR	PULMONARY	★★★
GASTROINTESTINAL	NR	STROKE	★★★
GENERAL SURGERY	★★★	VASCULAR	NR
MATERNITY CARE	★★★★★	WOMEN'S HEALTH	NR

HEALTHGRADES AWARDS

Christus Santa Rosa Healthcare

333 North Santa Rosa Street
San Antonio, TX 78207
(210) 704-2011

Overall patient safety: ★★★
Teaching: Y

CLINICAL PROGRAM RATINGS:

CARDIAC	★★★	ORTHOPEDICS	NR
CRITICAL CARE	NR	PULMONARY	★★★★★
GASTROINTESTINAL	★★★	STROKE	★★★
GENERAL SURGERY	★★★	VASCULAR	NR
MATERNITY CARE	★★★	WOMEN'S HEALTH	★★★

HEALTHGRADES AWARDS

✓ DISTINGUISHED HOSPITAL   ✓ SPECIALTY EXCELLENCE
· CLINICAL EXCELLENCE   · JOINT REPLACEMENT   · PULMONARY CARE

KEY: ★★★★★ BEST   ★★★ AS EXPECTED   ★ POOR   NR NOT RATED BY HEALTHGRADES   For full definitions of ratings and awards, see Appendix.

Christus Spohn Hospital Corpus Christi—South*

5950 Saratoga Boulevard
Corpus Christi, TX 78414
(361) 985-5000

Overall patient safety: ★★★★★
Teaching: Y

CLINICAL PROGRAM RATINGS:

CARDIAC	★★★	ORTHOPEDICS	★★★
CRITICAL CARE	NR	PULMONARY	★★★★★
GASTROINTESTINAL	★★★	STROKE	★★★★★
GENERAL SURGERY	★★★	VASCULAR	NR
MATERNITY CARE	★★★★★	WOMEN'S HEALTH	★★★

HEALTHGRADES AWARDS

✓ DISTINGUISHED HOSPITAL
• PATIENT SAFETY

✓ SPECIALTY EXCELLENCE
• MATERNITY CARE   • PULMONARY CARE

Christus Spohn Hospital—Corpus Christi Memorial*

2606 Hospital Boulevard
Corpus Christi, TX 78405
(361) 902-4000

Overall patient safety: ★★★★★
Teaching: Y

CLINICAL PROGRAM RATINGS:

CARDIAC	★★★	ORTHOPEDICS	★★★
CRITICAL CARE	NR	PULMONARY	★★★★★
GASTROINTESTINAL	★★★	STROKE	★★★★★
GENERAL SURGERY	★★★	VASCULAR	NR
MATERNITY CARE	★★★★★	WOMEN'S HEALTH	★★★

HEALTHGRADES AWARDS

✓ DISTINGUISHED HOSPITAL
• CLINICAL EXCELLENCE
• PATIENT SAFETY

✓ SPECIALTY EXCELLENCE
• MATERNITY CARE   • PULMONARY CARE

Christus Spohn Hospital—Alice

2500 East Main Street
Alice, TX 78332
(361) 661-8000

Overall patient safety: ★★★★★
Teaching: N

CLINICAL PROGRAM RATINGS:

CARDIAC	NR	ORTHOPEDICS	NR
CRITICAL CARE	NR	PULMONARY	★★★★★
GASTROINTESTINAL	★★★★★	STROKE	★★★
GENERAL SURGERY	★★★	VASCULAR	NR
MATERNITY CARE	★★★	WOMEN'S HEALTH	NR

HEALTHGRADES AWARDS

✓ SPECIALTY EXCELLENCE
• GASTROINTESTINAL CARE   • GENERAL SURGERY   • PULMONARY CARE

Christus Spohn Hospital—Kleberg

1311 East General
Cavazos Boulevard
Kingsville, TX 78363
(361) 595-1661

Overall patient safety: ★★★
Teaching: N

CLINICAL PROGRAM RATINGS:

CARDIAC	NR	ORTHOPEDICS	NR
CRITICAL CARE	NR	PULMONARY	★★★
GASTROINTESTINAL	NR	STROKE	★★★
GENERAL SURGERY	★★★★★	VASCULAR	NR
MATERNITY CARE	★★★	WOMEN'S HEALTH	NR

HEALTHGRADES AWARDS

✓ SPECIALTY EXCELLENCE
• GENERAL SURGERY

Christus Spohn Hospital—Beeville

1500 East Houston Highway
Beeville, TX 78102
(361) 354-2000

Overall patient safety: ★★★
Teaching: N

CLINICAL PROGRAM RATINGS:

CARDIAC	NR	ORTHOPEDICS	NR
CRITICAL CARE	NR	PULMONARY	★★★
GASTROINTESTINAL	NR	STROKE	★★★
GENERAL SURGERY	NR	VASCULAR	NR
MATERNITY CARE	★★★	WOMEN'S HEALTH	NR

HEALTHGRADES AWARDS

Citizens Medical Center

2701 Hospital Drive
Victoria, TX 77901
(361) 573-9181

Overall patient safety: ★★★★★
Teaching: N

CLINICAL PROGRAM RATINGS:

CARDIAC	★★★	ORTHOPEDICS	★★★
CRITICAL CARE	NR	PULMONARY	★★★
GASTROINTESTINAL	★★★	STROKE	★★★
GENERAL SURGERY	★★★	VASCULAR	NR
MATERNITY CARE	★★★	WOMEN'S HEALTH	★★★

HEALTHGRADES AWARDS

✓ DISTINGUISHED HOSPITAL
• PATIENT SAFETY

✓ SPECIALTY EXCELLENCE
• BARIATRIC SURGERY   • JOINT REPLACEMENT

*This hospital reports its data to the federal government jointly with another hospital. Therefore the ratings and awards apply to multiple hospitals and this specific hospital may not provide all rated services.

TEXAS HOSPITALS: RATINGS BY CLINICAL SPECIALTY

Clay County Memorial Hospital

310 West South Street
Henrietta, TX 76365
(940) 538-5621

Overall patient safety: ★★★
Teaching: N

CLINICAL PROGRAM RATINGS:

CARDIAC	NR	ORTHOPEDICS	NR
CRITICAL CARE	NR	PULMONARY	★★★
GASTROINTESTINAL	NR	STROKE	★★★
GENERAL SURGERY	NR	VASCULAR	NR
MATERNITY CARE	NR	WOMEN'S HEALTH	NR

HEALTHGRADES AWARDS

Cleveland Regional Medical Center

300 East Crockett Street
Cleveland, TX 77327
(281) 593-1811

Overall patient safety: ★★★
Teaching: N

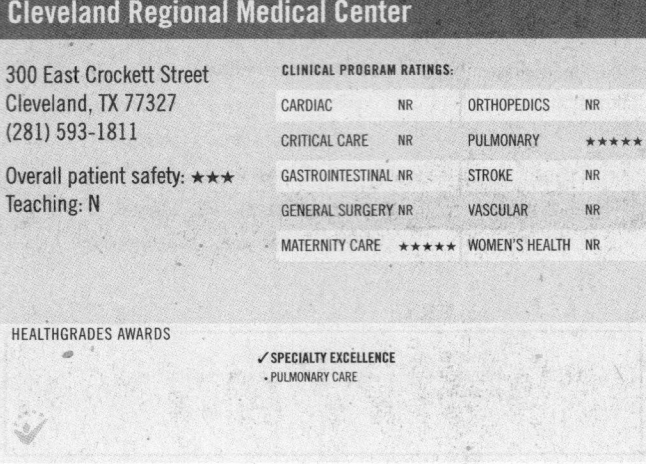

CLINICAL PROGRAM RATINGS:

CARDIAC	NR	ORTHOPEDICS	NR
CRITICAL CARE	NR	PULMONARY	★★★★★
GASTROINTESTINAL	NR	STROKE	NR
GENERAL SURGERY	NR	VASCULAR	NR
MATERNITY CARE	★★★★★	WOMEN'S HEALTH	NR

HEALTHGRADES AWARDS

✓ SPECIALTY EXCELLENCE
· PULMONARY CARE

Clear Lake Regional Medical Center

500 Medical Center Boulevard
Webster, TX 77598
(281) 332-2511

Overall patient safety: ★★★
Teaching: N

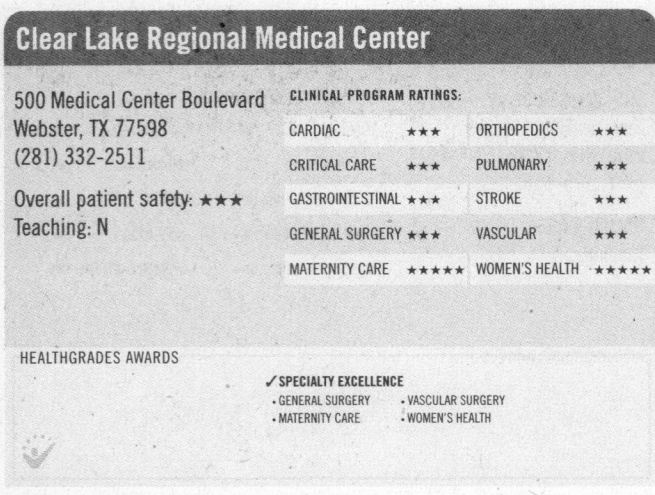

CLINICAL PROGRAM RATINGS:

CARDIAC	★★★	ORTHOPEDICS	★★★
CRITICAL CARE	★★★	PULMONARY	★★★
GASTROINTESTINAL	★★★	STROKE	★★★
GENERAL SURGERY	★★★	VASCULAR	★★★
MATERNITY CARE	★★★★★	WOMEN'S HEALTH	★★★★★

HEALTHGRADES AWARDS

✓ SPECIALTY EXCELLENCE
· GENERAL SURGERY   · VASCULAR SURGERY
· MATERNITY CARE   · WOMEN'S HEALTH

Coleman County Medical Center

310 South Pecos Street
Coleman, TX 76834
(325) 625-2135

Overall patient safety: ★★★
Teaching: N

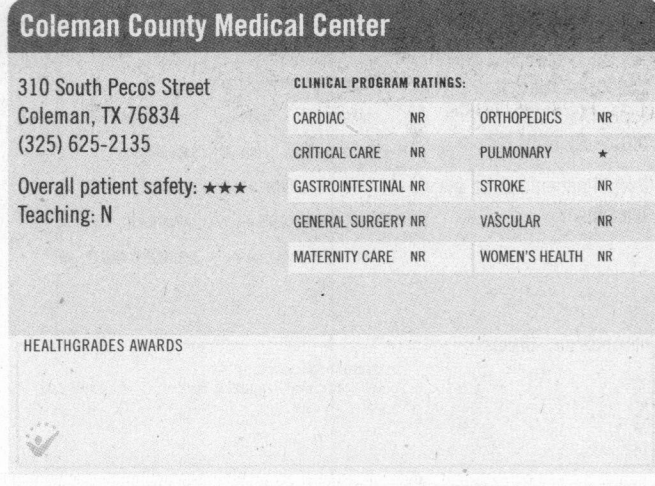

CLINICAL PROGRAM RATINGS:

CARDIAC	NR	ORTHOPEDICS	NR
CRITICAL CARE	NR	PULMONARY	★
GASTROINTESTINAL	NR	STROKE	NR
GENERAL SURGERY	NR	VASCULAR	NR
MATERNITY CARE	NR	WOMEN'S HEALTH	NR

HEALTHGRADES AWARDS

Clearview Hospital*

200 South County Road 1233
Box 4757
Midland, TX 79704
(915) 697-5200

Overall patient safety: ★★★
Teaching: Y

CLINICAL PROGRAM RATINGS:

CARDIAC	★★★	ORTHOPEDICS	★★★★★
CRITICAL CARE	NR	PULMONARY	★
GASTROINTESTINAL	★★★	STROKE	★
GENERAL SURGERY	★★★	VASCULAR	★★★
MATERNITY CARE	★★★	WOMEN'S HEALTH	★★★

HEALTHGRADES AWARDS

✓ SPECIALTY EXCELLENCE
· ORTHOPEDIC
  SURGERY

College Station Medical Center

1604 Rock Prairie Road
College Station, TX 77845
(979) 764-5100

Overall patient safety: ★★★
Teaching: Y

CLINICAL PROGRAM RATINGS:

CARDIAC	★★★	ORTHOPEDICS	NR
CRITICAL CARE	NR	PULMONARY	★★★
GASTROINTESTINAL	NR	STROKE	★★★
GENERAL SURGERY	★★★	VASCULAR	NR
MATERNITY CARE	★★★	WOMEN'S HEALTH	NR

HEALTHGRADES AWARDS

KEY: ★★★★★ BEST   ★★★ AS EXPECTED   ★ POOR   NR NOT RATED BY HEALTHGRADES   For full definitions of ratings and awards, see Appendix.

Columbus Community Hospital

110 Shult Drive
Columbus, TX 78934
(979) 732-2371

Overall patient safety: ★★★
Teaching: N

CLINICAL PROGRAM RATINGS:

CARDIAC	NR	ORTHOPEDICS	NR
CRITICAL CARE	NR	PULMONARY	★
GASTROINTESTINAL	NR	STROKE	★★★
GENERAL SURGERY	NR	VASCULAR	NR
MATERNITY CARE	NR	WOMEN'S HEALTH	NR

HEALTHGRADES AWARDS

Corpus Christi Medical Center

7101 South Padre Island Drive
Corpus Christi, TX 78412
(361) 761-1200

Overall patient safety: ★★★
Teaching: Y

CLINICAL PROGRAM RATINGS:

CARDIAC	★★★	ORTHOPEDICS	★★★
CRITICAL CARE	★★★	PULMONARY	★★★
GASTROINTESTINAL	★★★	STROKE	★★★
GENERAL SURGERY	★★★	VASCULAR	★★★
MATERNITY CARE	★★★★★	WOMEN'S HEALTH	★★★

HEALTHGRADES AWARDS

✓ SPECIALTY EXCELLENCE
- VASCULAR SURGERY   - MATERNITY CARE

Connally Memorial Medical Center

499 10th Street
Floresville, TX 78114
(830) 393-3122

Overall patient safety: ★★★
Teaching: N

CLINICAL PROGRAM RATINGS:

CARDIAC	NR	ORTHOPEDICS	NR
CRITICAL CARE	NR	PULMONARY	★★★
GASTROINTESTINAL	NR	STROKE	NR
GENERAL SURGERY	NR	VASCULAR	NR
MATERNITY CARE	NR	WOMEN'S HEALTH	NR

HEALTHGRADES AWARDS

Coryell Memorial Hospital

1507 West Main Street
Gatesville, TX 76528
(254) 865-8251

Overall patient safety: ★★★
Teaching: N

CLINICAL PROGRAM RATINGS:

CARDIAC	NR	ORTHOPEDICS	NR
CRITICAL CARE	NR	PULMONARY	★★★
GASTROINTESTINAL	NR	STROKE	NR
GENERAL SURGERY	NR	VASCULAR	NR
MATERNITY CARE	NR	WOMEN'S HEALTH	NR

HEALTHGRADES AWARDS

Conroe Regional Medical Center

504 Medical Center Boulevard
Conroe, TX 77304
(936) 539-1111

Overall patient safety: ★
Teaching: Y

CLINICAL PROGRAM RATINGS:

CARDIAC	★★★	ORTHOPEDICS	★★★
CRITICAL CARE	★★★	PULMONARY	★★★
GASTROINTESTINAL	★★★	STROKE	★
GENERAL SURGERY	★★★	VASCULAR	★★★
MATERNITY CARE	★★★	WOMEN'S HEALTH	★★★

HEALTHGRADES AWARDS

Covenant Hospital Levelland

1900 South College Avenue
Levelland, TX 79336
(806) 894-4963

Overall patient safety: ★★★
Teaching: N

CLINICAL PROGRAM RATINGS:

CARDIAC	NR	ORTHOPEDICS	NR
CRITICAL CARE	NR	PULMONARY	★★★
GASTROINTESTINAL	NR	STROKE	NR
GENERAL SURGERY	NR	VASCULAR	NR
MATERNITY CARE	★★★	WOMEN'S HEALTH	NR

HEALTHGRADES AWARDS

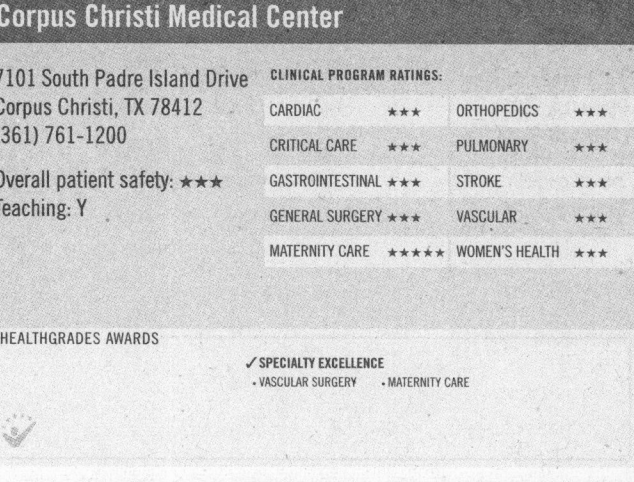

*This hospital reports its data to the federal government jointly with another hospital. Therefore the ratings and awards apply to multiple hospitals and this specific hospital may not provide all rated services.

Covenant Hospital Plainview

2601 Dimmitt Road
Plainview, TX 79072
(806) 296-5531

Overall patient safety: ★
Teaching: N

CLINICAL PROGRAM RATINGS:

CARDIAC	NR	ORTHOPEDICS	NR
CRITICAL CARE	NR	PULMONARY	★
GASTROINTESTINAL	NR	STROKE	★
GENERAL SURGERY	★★★	VASCULAR	NR
MATERNITY CARE	★★★	WOMEN'S HEALTH	NR

HEALTHGRADES AWARDS

Cuero Community Hospital

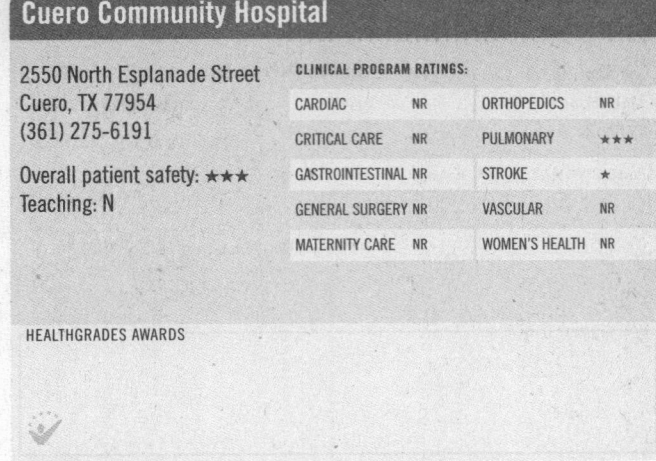

2550 North Esplanade Street
Cuero, TX 77954
(361) 275-6191

Overall patient safety: ★★★
Teaching: N

CLINICAL PROGRAM RATINGS:

CARDIAC	NR	ORTHOPEDICS	NR
CRITICAL CARE	NR	PULMONARY	★★★
GASTROINTESTINAL	NR	STROKE	★
GENERAL SURGERY	NR	VASCULAR	NR
MATERNITY CARE	NR	WOMEN'S HEALTH	NR

HEALTHGRADES AWARDS

Covenant Medical Center

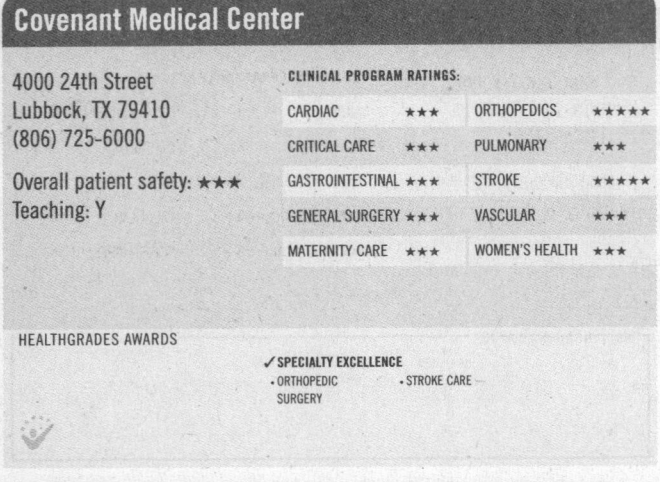

4000 24th Street
Lubbock, TX 79410
(806) 725-6000

Overall patient safety: ★★★
Teaching: Y

CLINICAL PROGRAM RATINGS:

CARDIAC	★★★	ORTHOPEDICS	★★★★★
CRITICAL CARE	★★★	PULMONARY	★★★
GASTROINTESTINAL	★★★	STROKE	★★★★★
GENERAL SURGERY	★★★	VASCULAR	★★★
MATERNITY CARE	★★★	WOMEN'S HEALTH	★★★

HEALTHGRADES AWARDS

✓ SPECIALTY EXCELLENCE
• ORTHOPEDIC   • STROKE CARE
  SURGERY

Cypress Fairbanks Medical Center

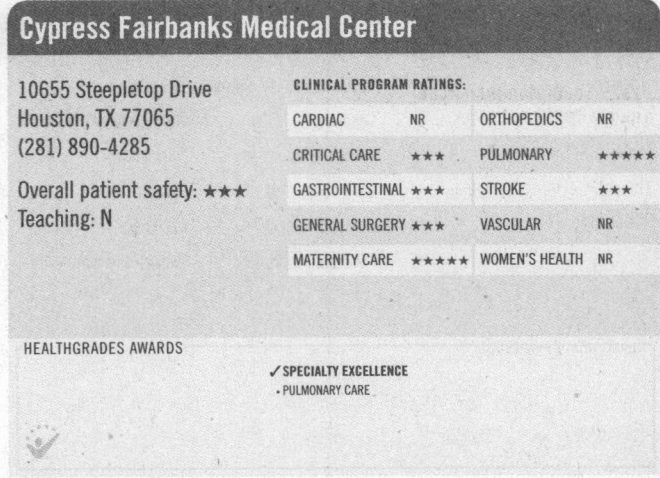

10655 Steepletop Drive
Houston, TX 77065
(281) 890-4285

Overall patient safety: ★★★
Teaching: N

CLINICAL PROGRAM RATINGS:

CARDIAC	NR	ORTHOPEDICS	NR
CRITICAL CARE	★★★	PULMONARY	★★★★★
GASTROINTESTINAL	★★★	STROKE	★★★
GENERAL SURGERY	★★★	VASCULAR	NR
MATERNITY CARE	★★★★★	WOMEN'S HEALTH	NR

HEALTHGRADES AWARDS

✓ SPECIALTY EXCELLENCE
• PULMONARY CARE

Crosbyton Clinic Hospital

710 West Main Street
Crosbyton, TX 79322
(806) 675-2382

Overall patient safety: NR
Teaching: N

CLINICAL PROGRAM RATINGS:

CARDIAC	NR	ORTHOPEDICS	NR
CRITICAL CARE	NR	PULMONARY	★★★
GASTROINTESTINAL	NR	STROKE	NR
GENERAL SURGERY	NR	VASCULAR	NR
MATERNITY CARE	NR	WOMEN'S HEALTH	NR

HEALTHGRADES AWARDS

D. M. Cogdell Memorial Hospital

1700 Cogdell Boulevard
Snyder, TX 79549
(325) 573-6374

Overall patient safety: ★★★
Teaching: N

CLINICAL PROGRAM RATINGS:

CARDIAC	NR	ORTHOPEDICS	NR
CRITICAL CARE	NR	PULMONARY	★★★
GASTROINTESTINAL	NR	STROKE	NR
GENERAL SURGERY	NR	VASCULAR	NR
MATERNITY CARE	NR	WOMEN'S HEALTH	NR

HEALTHGRADES AWARDS

KEY: ★★★★★ BEST   ★★★ AS EXPECTED   ★ POOR   NR NOT RATED BY HEALTHGRADES   For full definitions of ratings and awards, see Appendix.

Dallas Regional Medical Center–Galloway Campus

1011 North Galloway Avenue
Mesquite, TX 75149
(214) 320-7000

Overall patient safety: ★★★
Teaching: N

CLINICAL PROGRAM RATINGS:

CARDIAC	★★★	ORTHOPEDICS	NR
CRITICAL CARE	NR	PULMONARY	★★★
GASTROINTESTINAL	NR	STROKE	★★★
GENERAL SURGERY	★★★	VASCULAR	NR
MATERNITY CARE	★★★	WOMEN'S HEALTH	★★★

HEALTHGRADES AWARDS

Denton Regional Medical Center

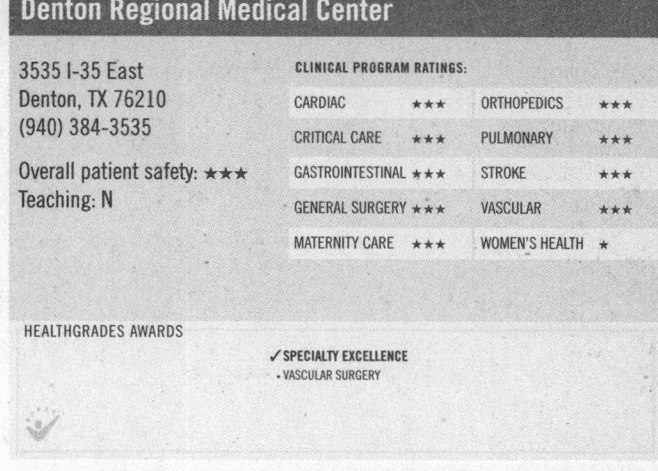

3535 I-35 East
Denton, TX 76210
(940) 384-3535

Overall patient safety: ★★★
Teaching: N

CLINICAL PROGRAM RATINGS:

CARDIAC	★★★	ORTHOPEDICS	★★★
CRITICAL CARE	★★★	PULMONARY	★★★
GASTROINTESTINAL	★★★	STROKE	★★★
GENERAL SURGERY	★★★	VASCULAR	★★★
MATERNITY CARE	★★★	WOMEN'S HEALTH	★

HEALTHGRADES AWARDS

✓ SPECIALTY EXCELLENCE
  · VASCULAR SURGERY

Dallas Southwest Medical Center*

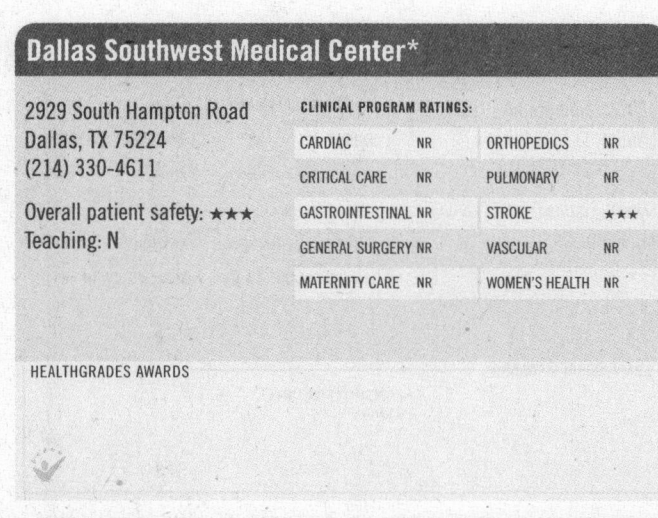

2929 South Hampton Road
Dallas, TX 75224
(214) 330-4611

Overall patient safety: ★★★
Teaching: N

CLINICAL PROGRAM RATINGS:

CARDIAC	NR	ORTHOPEDICS	NR
CRITICAL CARE	NR	PULMONARY	NR
GASTROINTESTINAL	NR	STROKE	★★★
GENERAL SURGERY	NR	VASCULAR	NR
MATERNITY CARE	NR	WOMEN'S HEALTH	NR

HEALTHGRADES AWARDS

Detar Hospital Navarro*

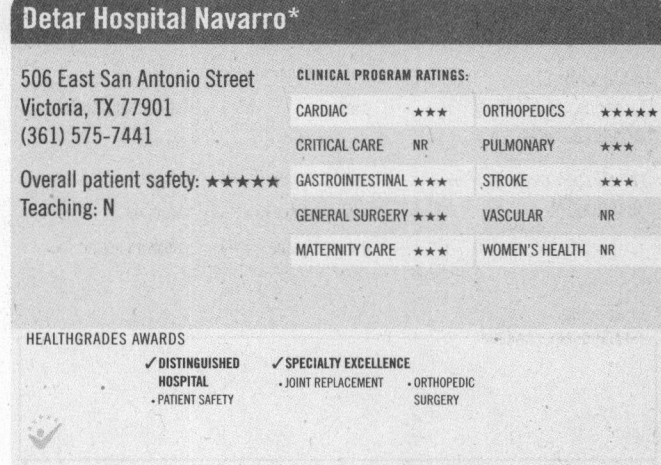

506 East San Antonio Street
Victoria, TX 77901
(361) 575-7441

Overall patient safety: ★★★★★
Teaching: N

CLINICAL PROGRAM RATINGS:

CARDIAC	★★★	ORTHOPEDICS	★★★★★
CRITICAL CARE	NR	PULMONARY	★★★
GASTROINTESTINAL	★★★	STROKE	★★★
GENERAL SURGERY	★★★	VASCULAR	NR
MATERNITY CARE	★★★	WOMEN'S HEALTH	NR

HEALTHGRADES AWARDS

✓ DISTINGUISHED HOSPITAL
  · PATIENT SAFETY

✓ SPECIALTY EXCELLENCE
  · JOINT REPLACEMENT   · ORTHOPEDIC SURGERY

Del Sol Medical Center

10301 Gateway West
El Paso, TX 79925
(915) 595-9000

Overall patient safety: ★
Teaching: N

CLINICAL PROGRAM RATINGS:

CARDIAC	★★★	ORTHOPEDICS	NR
CRITICAL CARE	★★★	PULMONARY	★★★
GASTROINTESTINAL	★★★	STROKE	★★★
GENERAL SURGERY	★★★★★	VASCULAR	NR
MATERNITY CARE	★★★★★	WOMEN'S HEALTH	★★★

HEALTHGRADES AWARDS

✓ SPECIALTY EXCELLENCE
  · GENERAL SURGERY

Detar Hospital North*

101 Medical Drive
Victoria, TX 77904
(361) 573-6100

Overall patient safety: ★★★★★
Teaching: N

CLINICAL PROGRAM RATINGS:

CARDIAC	★★★	ORTHOPEDICS	★★★★★
CRITICAL CARE	NR	PULMONARY	★★★
GASTROINTESTINAL	★★★	STROKE	★★★
GENERAL SURGERY	★★★	VASCULAR	NR
MATERNITY CARE	★★★	WOMEN'S HEALTH	NR

HEALTHGRADES AWARDS

✓ DISTINGUISHED HOSPITAL
  · PATIENT SAFETY

✓ SPECIALTY EXCELLENCE
  · JOINT REPLACEMENT   · ORTHOPEDIC SURGERY

---

*This hospital reports its data to the federal government jointly with another hospital. Therefore the ratings and awards apply to multiple hospitals and this specific hospital may not provide all rated services.

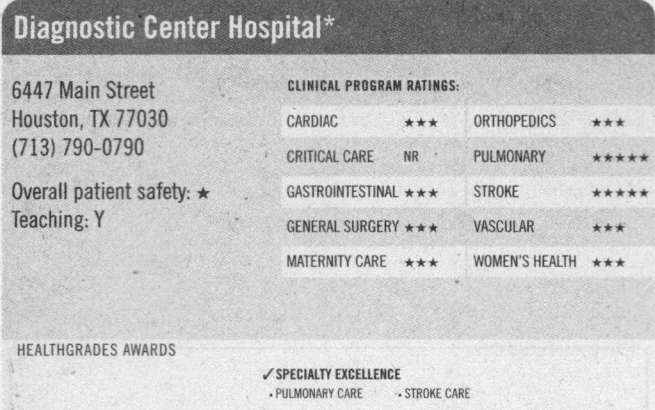

Diagnostic Center Hospital*

6447 Main Street
Houston, TX 77030
(713) 790-0790

Overall patient safety: ★
Teaching: Y

CLINICAL PROGRAM RATINGS:

CARDIAC	★★★	ORTHOPEDICS	★★★
CRITICAL CARE	NR	PULMONARY	★★★★★
GASTROINTESTINAL	★★★	STROKE	★★★★★
GENERAL SURGERY	★★★	VASCULAR	★★★
MATERNITY CARE	★★★	WOMEN'S HEALTH	★★★

HEALTHGRADES AWARDS

✓ SPECIALTY EXCELLENCE
• PULMONARY CARE   • STROKE CARE

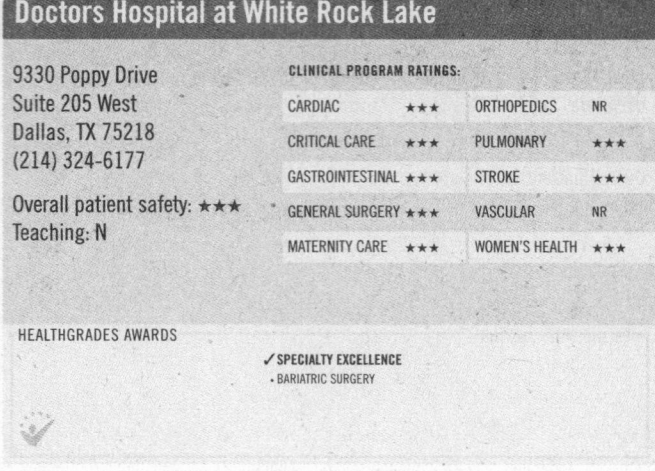

Doctors Hospital at White Rock Lake

9330 Poppy Drive
Suite 205 West
Dallas, TX 75218
(214) 324-6177

Overall patient safety: ★★★
Teaching: N

CLINICAL PROGRAM RATINGS:

CARDIAC	★★★	ORTHOPEDICS	NR
CRITICAL CARE	★★★	PULMONARY	★★★
GASTROINTESTINAL	★★★	STROKE	★★★
GENERAL SURGERY	★★★	VASCULAR	NR
MATERNITY CARE	★★★	WOMEN'S HEALTH	★★★

HEALTHGRADES AWARDS

✓ SPECIALTY EXCELLENCE
• BARIATRIC SURGERY

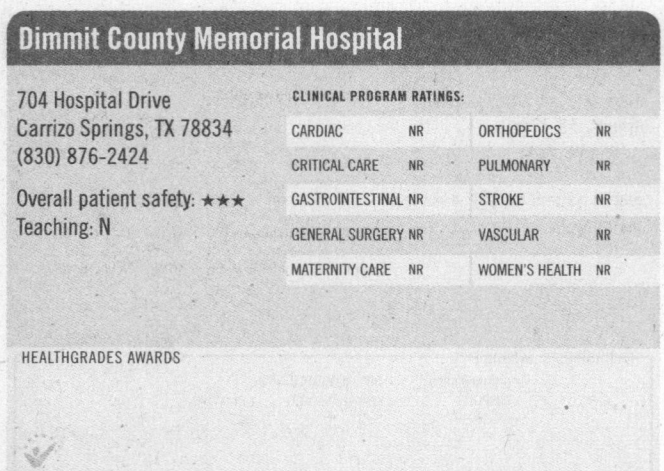

Dimmit County Memorial Hospital

704 Hospital Drive
Carrizo Springs, TX 78834
(830) 876-2424

Overall patient safety: ★★★
Teaching: N

CLINICAL PROGRAM RATINGS:

CARDIAC	NR	ORTHOPEDICS	NR
CRITICAL CARE	NR	PULMONARY	NR
GASTROINTESTINAL	NR	STROKE	NR
GENERAL SURGERY	NR	VASCULAR	NR
MATERNITY CARE	NR	WOMEN'S HEALTH	NR

HEALTHGRADES AWARDS

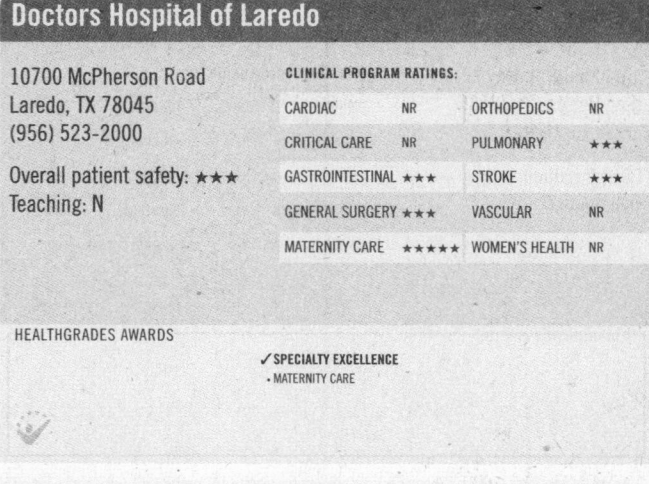

Doctors Hospital of Laredo

10700 McPherson Road
Laredo, TX 78045
(956) 523-2000

Overall patient safety: ★★★
Teaching: N

CLINICAL PROGRAM RATINGS:

CARDIAC	NR	ORTHOPEDICS	NR
CRITICAL CARE	NR	PULMONARY	★★★
GASTROINTESTINAL	★★★	STROKE	★★★
GENERAL SURGERY	★★★	VASCULAR	NR
MATERNITY CARE	★★★★★	WOMEN'S HEALTH	NR

HEALTHGRADES AWARDS

✓ SPECIALTY EXCELLENCE
• MATERNITY CARE

Doctors Hospital at Renaissance

5501 South McColl Road
Edinburg, TX 78539
(956) 666-7100

Overall patient safety: ★★★
Teaching: N

CLINICAL PROGRAM RATINGS:

CARDIAC	★★★	ORTHOPEDICS	★★★
CRITICAL CARE	NR	PULMONARY	★★★★★
GASTROINTESTINAL	★★★	STROKE	★★★★★
GENERAL SURGERY	★★★	VASCULAR	NR
MATERNITY CARE	NR	WOMEN'S HEALTH	NR

HEALTHGRADES AWARDS

✓ DISTINGUISHED   ✓ SPECIALTY EXCELLENCE
  HOSPITAL   • PULMONARY CARE
• CLINICAL EXCELLENCE

Doctors Hospital–Parkway*

233 West Parker Road
Houston, TX 77076
(281) 765-2600

Overall patient safety: ★
Teaching: N

CLINICAL PROGRAM RATINGS:

CARDIAC	NR	ORTHOPEDICS	NR
CRITICAL CARE	NR	PULMONARY	★★★
GASTROINTESTINAL	NR	STROKE	★★★
GENERAL SURGERY	NR	VASCULAR	NR
MATERNITY CARE	★★★	WOMEN'S HEALTH	NR

HEALTHGRADES AWARDS

KEY: ★★★★★ BEST   ★★★ AS EXPECTED   ★ POOR   NR NOT RATED BY HEALTHGRADES   For full definitions of ratings and awards, see Appendix.

Doctors Hospital—Tidwell*

510 West Tidwell Road
Houston, TX 77091
(281) 618-8500

Overall patient safety: ★
Teaching: N

CLINICAL PROGRAM RATINGS:

CARDIAC	NR	ORTHOPEDICS	NR
CRITICAL CARE	NR	PULMONARY	★★★
GASTROINTESTINAL	NR	STROKE	★★★
GENERAL SURGERY	NR	VASCULAR	NR
MATERNITY CARE	★★★	WOMEN'S HEALTH	NR

HEALTHGRADES AWARDS

East Texas Medical Center

1000 South Beckham Street
Tyler, TX 75701
(903) 597-0351

Overall patient safety: ★★★★★
Teaching: N

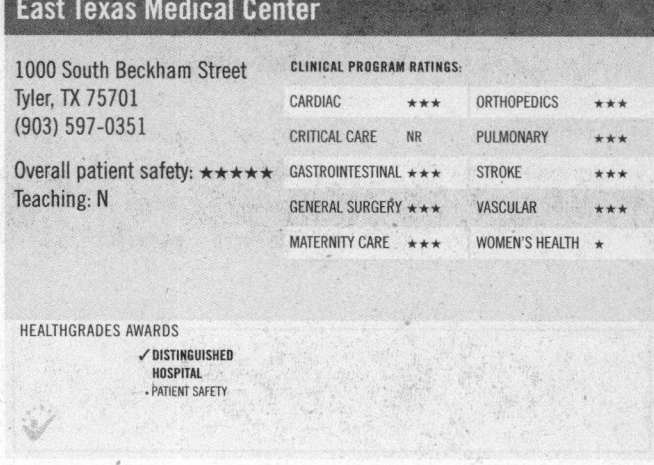

CLINICAL PROGRAM RATINGS:

CARDIAC	★★★	ORTHOPEDICS	★★★
CRITICAL CARE	NR	PULMONARY	★★★
GASTROINTESTINAL	★★★	STROKE	★★★
GENERAL SURGERY	★★★	VASCULAR	★★★
MATERNITY CARE	★★★	WOMEN'S HEALTH	★

HEALTHGRADES AWARDS

✓ DISTINGUISHED
HOSPITAL
· PATIENT SAFETY

Dolly Vinsant Memorial Hospital

400 East Highway 77
San Benito, TX 78586
(956) 399-1313

Overall patient safety: ★★★
Teaching: N

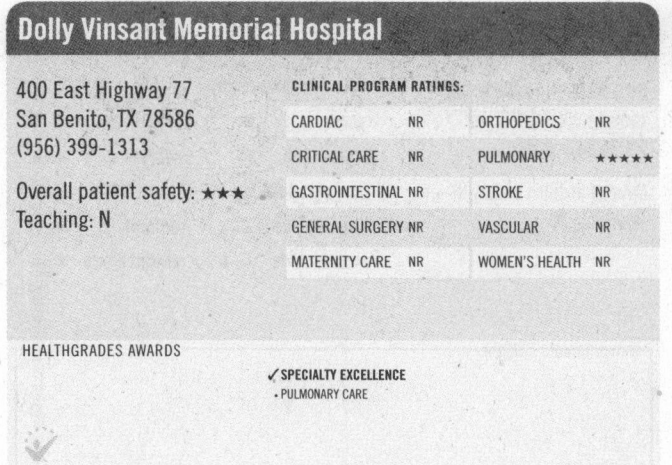

CLINICAL PROGRAM RATINGS:

CARDIAC	NR	ORTHOPEDICS	NR
CRITICAL CARE	NR	PULMONARY	★★★★★
GASTROINTESTINAL	NR	STROKE	NR
GENERAL SURGERY	NR	VASCULAR	NR
MATERNITY CARE	NR	WOMEN'S HEALTH	NR

HEALTHGRADES AWARDS

✓ SPECIALTY EXCELLENCE
· PULMONARY CARE

East Texas Medical Center—Athens

2000 South Palestine Street
Athens, TX 75751
(903) 676-1000

Overall patient safety: ★★★★★
Teaching: N

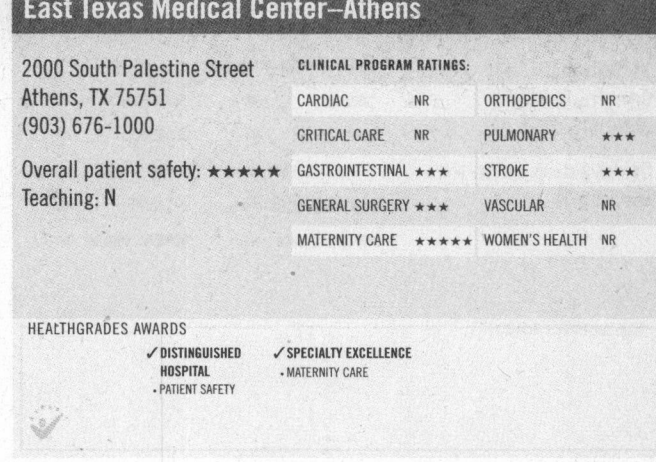

CLINICAL PROGRAM RATINGS:

CARDIAC	NR	ORTHOPEDICS	NR
CRITICAL CARE	NR	PULMONARY	★★★
GASTROINTESTINAL	★★★	STROKE	★★★
GENERAL SURGERY	★★★	VASCULAR	NR
MATERNITY CARE	★★★★★	WOMEN'S HEALTH	NR

HEALTHGRADES AWARDS

✓ DISTINGUISHED   ✓ SPECIALTY EXCELLENCE
HOSPITAL   · MATERNITY CARE
· PATIENT SAFETY

East Houston Regional Medical Center*

13111 East Freeway
Houston, TX 77015
(713) 393-2000

Overall patient safety: ★★★
Teaching: N

CLINICAL PROGRAM RATINGS:

CARDIAC	NR	ORTHOPEDICS	NR
CRITICAL CARE	NR	PULMONARY	★★★
GASTROINTESTINAL	★★★	STROKE	★★★★★
GENERAL SURGERY	★★★	VASCULAR	NR
MATERNITY CARE	★★★	WOMEN'S HEALTH	NR

HEALTHGRADES AWARDS

East Texas Medical Center—Carthage

409 West Cottage Road
Carthage, TX 75633
(903) 693-3841

Overall patient safety: ★★★
Teaching: N

CLINICAL PROGRAM RATINGS:

CARDIAC	NR	ORTHOPEDICS	NR
CRITICAL CARE	NR	PULMONARY	★★★
GASTROINTESTINAL	NR	STROKE	NR
GENERAL SURGERY	NR	VASCULAR	NR
MATERNITY CARE	★★★	WOMEN'S HEALTH	NR

HEALTHGRADES AWARDS

*This hospital reports its data to the federal government jointly with another hospital. Therefore the ratings and awards apply to multiple hospitals and this specific hospital may not provide all rated services.

East Texas Medical Center—Clarksville

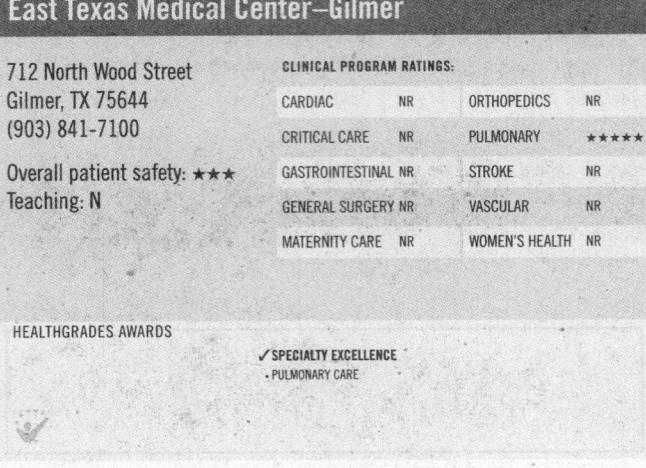

3000 Highway 82 West
Clarksville, TX 75426
(903) 427-3851

Overall patient safety: ★★★
Teaching: N

CLINICAL PROGRAM RATINGS:

CARDIAC	NR	ORTHOPEDICS	NR
CRITICAL CARE	NR	PULMONARY	★★★
GASTROINTESTINAL	NR	STROKE	★★★
GENERAL SURGERY	NR	VASCULAR	NR
MATERNITY CARE	NR	WOMEN'S HEALTH	NR

HEALTHGRADES AWARDS

East Texas Medical Center—Gilmer

712 North Wood Street
Gilmer, TX 75644
(903) 841-7100

Overall patient safety: ★★★
Teaching: N

CLINICAL PROGRAM RATINGS:

CARDIAC	NR	ORTHOPEDICS	NR
CRITICAL CARE	NR	PULMONARY	★★★★★
GASTROINTESTINAL	NR	STROKE	NR
GENERAL SURGERY	NR	VASCULAR	NR
MATERNITY CARE	NR	WOMEN'S HEALTH	NR

HEALTHGRADES AWARDS

✓ SPECIALTY EXCELLENCE
• PULMONARY CARE

East Texas Medical Center—Crockett

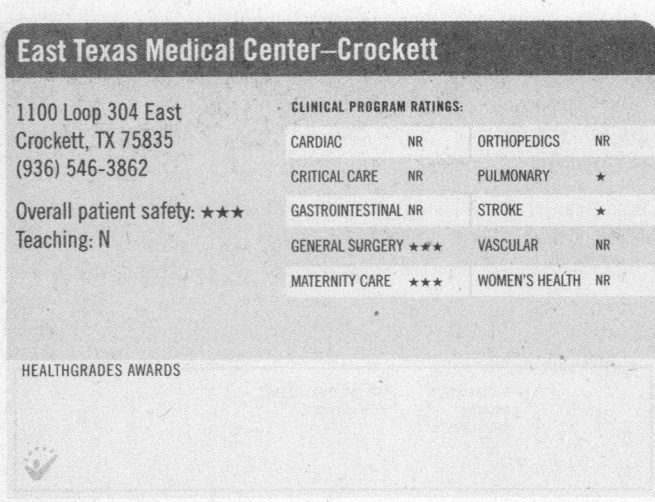

1100 Loop 304 East
Crockett, TX 75835
(936) 546-3862

Overall patient safety: ★★★
Teaching: N

CLINICAL PROGRAM RATINGS:

CARDIAC	NR	ORTHOPEDICS	NR
CRITICAL CARE	NR	PULMONARY	★
GASTROINTESTINAL	NR	STROKE	★
GENERAL SURGERY	★★★	VASCULAR	NR
MATERNITY CARE	★★★	WOMEN'S HEALTH	NR

HEALTHGRADES AWARDS

East Texas Medical Center—Jacksonville

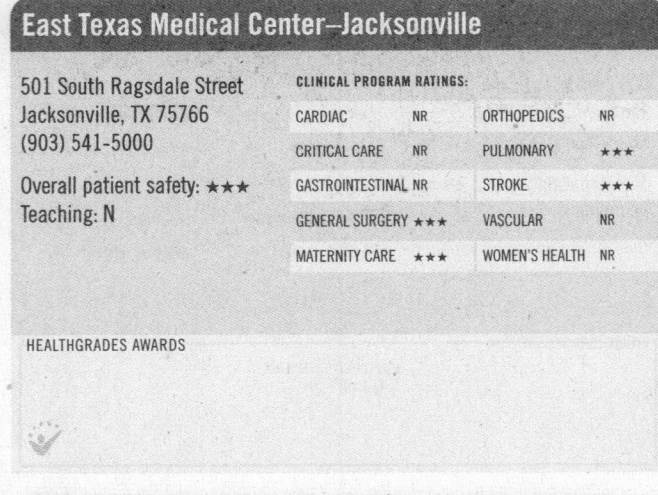

501 South Ragsdale Street
Jacksonville, TX 75766
(903) 541-5000

Overall patient safety: ★★★
Teaching: N

CLINICAL PROGRAM RATINGS:

CARDIAC	NR	ORTHOPEDICS	NR
CRITICAL CARE	NR	PULMONARY	★★★
GASTROINTESTINAL	NR	STROKE	★★★
GENERAL SURGERY	★★★	VASCULAR	NR
MATERNITY CARE	★★★	WOMEN'S HEALTH	NR

HEALTHGRADES AWARDS

East Texas Medical Center—Fairfield

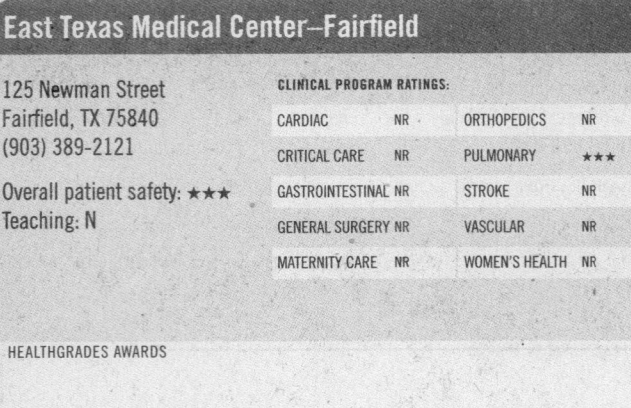

125 Newman Street
Fairfield, TX 75840
(903) 389-2121

Overall patient safety: ★★★
Teaching: N

CLINICAL PROGRAM RATINGS:

CARDIAC	NR	ORTHOPEDICS	NR
CRITICAL CARE	NR	PULMONARY	★★★
GASTROINTESTINAL	NR	STROKE	NR
GENERAL SURGERY	NR	VASCULAR	NR
MATERNITY CARE	NR	WOMEN'S HEALTH	NR

HEALTHGRADES AWARDS

East Texas Medical Center—Mt. Vernon

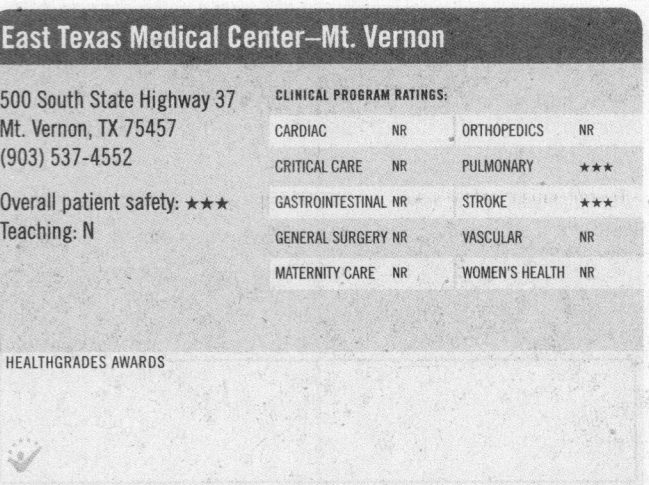

500 South State Highway 37
Mt. Vernon, TX 75457
(903) 537-4552

Overall patient safety: ★★★
Teaching: N

CLINICAL PROGRAM RATINGS:

CARDIAC	NR	ORTHOPEDICS	NR
CRITICAL CARE	NR	PULMONARY	★★★
GASTROINTESTINAL	NR	STROKE	★★★
GENERAL SURGERY	NR	VASCULAR	NR
MATERNITY CARE	NR	WOMEN'S HEALTH	NR

HEALTHGRADES AWARDS

KEY: ★★★★★ BEST   ★★★ AS EXPECTED   ★ POOR   NR NOT RATED BY HEALTHGRADES   For full definitions of ratings and awards, see Appendix.

East Texas Medical Center—Quitman

117 North Winnsboro Street
Quitman, TX 75783
(903) 763-6300

Overall patient safety: ★★★
Teaching: N

CLINICAL PROGRAM RATINGS:

CARDIAC	NR	ORTHOPEDICS	NR
CRITICAL CARE	NR	PULMONARY	★
GASTROINTESTINAL	NR	STROKE	NR
GENERAL SURGERY	NR	VASCULAR	NR
MATERNITY CARE	★★★	WOMEN'S HEALTH	NR

HEALTHGRADES AWARDS

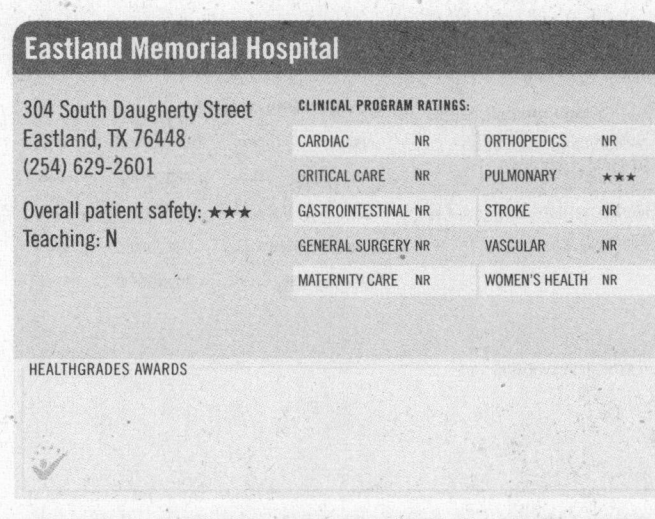

El Campo Memorial Hospital

303 Sandy Corner Road
El Campo, TX 77437
(979) 543-6251

Overall patient safety: ★★★
Teaching: N

CLINICAL PROGRAM RATINGS:

CARDIAC	NR	ORTHOPEDICS	NR
CRITICAL CARE	NR	PULMONARY	★★★
GASTROINTESTINAL	NR	STROKE	NR
GENERAL SURGERY	NR	VASCULAR	NR
MATERNITY CARE	NR	WOMEN'S HEALTH	NR

HEALTHGRADES AWARDS

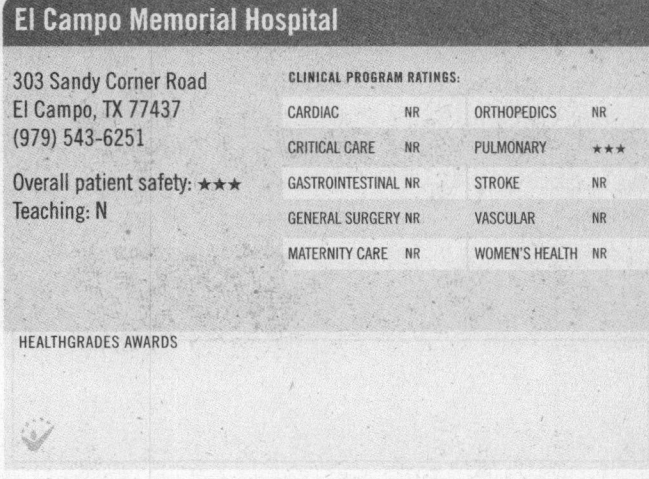

Eastland Memorial Hospital

304 South Daugherty Street
Eastland, TX 76448
(254) 629-2601

Overall patient safety: ★★★
Teaching: N

CLINICAL PROGRAM RATINGS:

CARDIAC	NR	ORTHOPEDICS	NR
CRITICAL CARE	NR	PULMONARY	★★★
GASTROINTESTINAL	NR	STROKE	NR
GENERAL SURGERY	NR	VASCULAR	NR
MATERNITY CARE	NR	WOMEN'S HEALTH	NR

HEALTHGRADES AWARDS

El Paso Specialty Hospital

1755 Curie Drive
Suite A
El Paso, TX 79902
(915) 544-3636

Overall patient safety: ★★★★★
Teaching: N

CLINICAL PROGRAM RATINGS:

CARDIAC	NR	ORTHOPEDICS	NR
CRITICAL CARE	NR	PULMONARY	NR
GASTROINTESTINAL	NR	STROKE	NR
GENERAL SURGERY	NR	VASCULAR	NR
MATERNITY CARE	NR	WOMEN'S HEALTH	NR

HEALTHGRADES AWARDS

✓ SPECIALTY EXCELLENCE
· JOINT REPLACEMENT

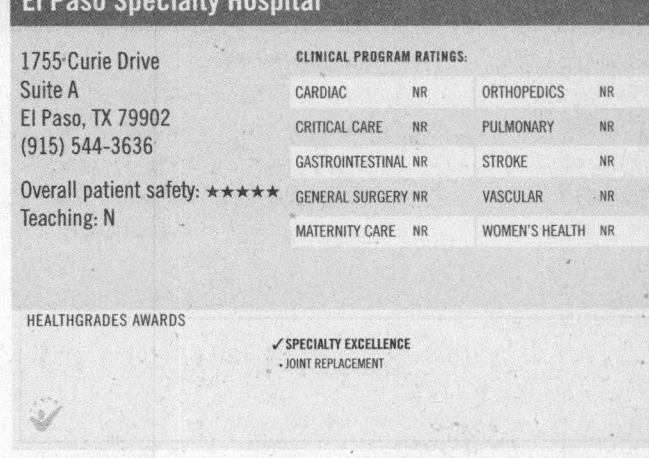

Edinburg Regional Medical Center

1102 West Trenton Road
Edinburg, TX 78539
(956) 388-6000

Overall patient safety: ★★★
Teaching: N

CLINICAL PROGRAM RATINGS:

CARDIAC	NR	ORTHOPEDICS	NR
CRITICAL CARE	NR	PULMONARY	★★★★★
GASTROINTESTINAL	NR	STROKE	NR
GENERAL SURGERY	★★★	VASCULAR	NR
MATERNITY CARE	NR	WOMEN'S HEALTH	NR

HEALTHGRADES AWARDS

✓ SPECIALTY EXCELLENCE
· PULMONARY CARE

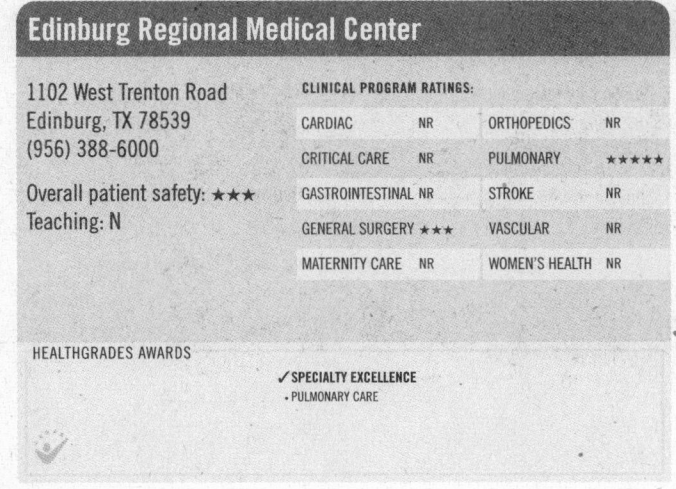

Electra Memorial Hospital

1207 South Bailey Street
Electra, TX 76360
(940) 495-3981

Overall patient safety: ★★★
Teaching: N

CLINICAL PROGRAM RATINGS:

CARDIAC	NR	ORTHOPEDICS	NR
CRITICAL CARE	NR	PULMONARY	★★★
GASTROINTESTINAL	NR	STROKE	NR
GENERAL SURGERY	NR	VASCULAR	NR
MATERNITY CARE	NR	WOMEN'S HEALTH	NR

HEALTHGRADES AWARDS

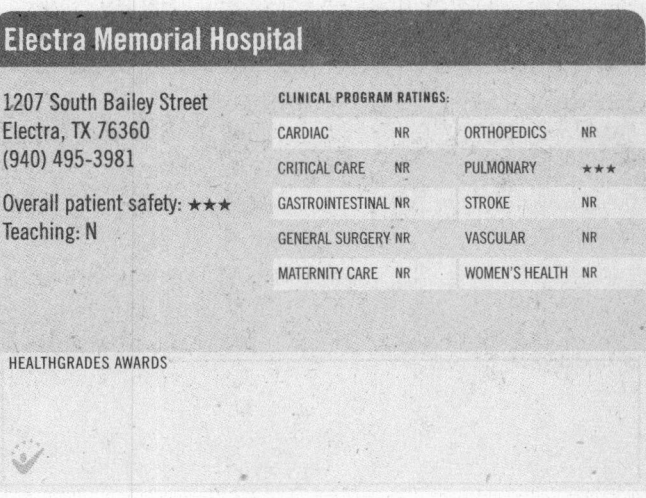

Ennis Regional Medical Center

2201 West Lampasas
Ennis, TX 75119
(972) 875-0900

Overall patient safety: ★★★
Teaching: N

CLINICAL PROGRAM RATINGS:

CARDIAC	NR	ORTHOPEDICS	NR
CRITICAL CARE	NR	PULMONARY	★★★
GASTROINTESTINAL	NR	STROKE	★
GENERAL SURGERY	NR	VASCULAR	NR
MATERNITY CARE	★★★	WOMEN'S HEALTH	NR

HEALTHGRADES AWARDS

Fort Duncan Medical Center

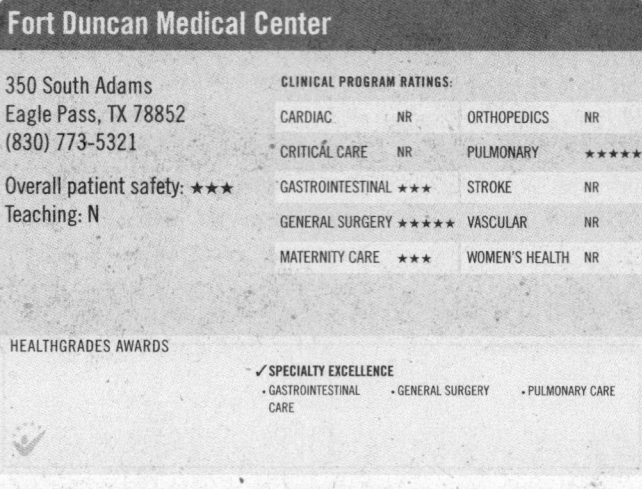

350 South Adams
Eagle Pass, TX 78852
(830) 773-5321

Overall patient safety: ★★★
Teaching: N

CLINICAL PROGRAM RATINGS:

CARDIAC	NR	ORTHOPEDICS	NR
CRITICAL CARE	NR	PULMONARY	★★★★★
GASTROINTESTINAL	★★★	STROKE	NR
GENERAL SURGERY	★★★★★	VASCULAR	NR
MATERNITY CARE	★★★	WOMEN'S HEALTH	NR

HEALTHGRADES AWARDS

✓ SPECIALTY EXCELLENCE
· GASTROINTESTINAL CARE   · GENERAL SURGERY   · PULMONARY CARE

ETMC Pittsburg

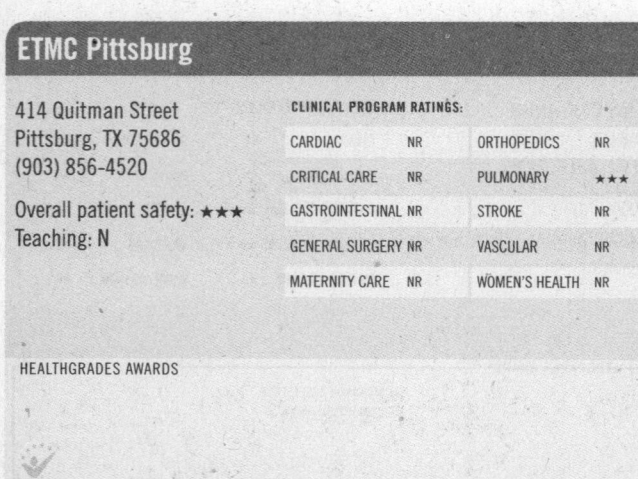

414 Quitman Street
Pittsburg, TX 75686
(903) 856-4520

Overall patient safety: ★★★
Teaching: N

CLINICAL PROGRAM RATINGS:

CARDIAC	NR	ORTHOPEDICS	NR
CRITICAL CARE	NR	PULMONARY	★★★
GASTROINTESTINAL	NR	STROKE	NR
GENERAL SURGERY	NR	VASCULAR	NR
MATERNITY CARE	NR	WOMEN'S HEALTH	NR

HEALTHGRADES AWARDS

Georgetown Hospital

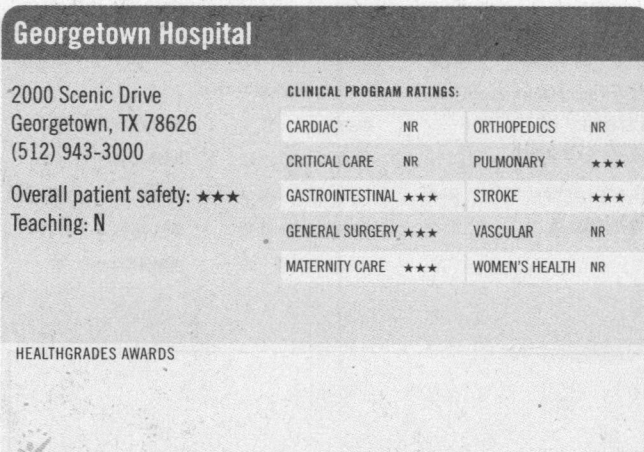

2000 Scenic Drive
Georgetown, TX 78626
(512) 943-3000

Overall patient safety: ★★★
Teaching: N

CLINICAL PROGRAM RATINGS:

CARDIAC	NR	ORTHOPEDICS	NR
CRITICAL CARE	NR	PULMONARY	★★★
GASTROINTESTINAL	★★★	STROKE	★★★
GENERAL SURGERY	★★★	VASCULAR	NR
MATERNITY CARE	★★★	WOMEN'S HEALTH	NR

HEALTHGRADES AWARDS

Falls Community Hospital and Clinic

322 Coleman Street
Marlin, TX 76661
(254) 803-3561

Overall patient safety: NR
Teaching: N

CLINICAL PROGRAM RATINGS:

CARDIAC	NR	ORTHOPEDICS	NR
CRITICAL CARE	NR	PULMONARY	★★★★★
GASTROINTESTINAL	NR	STROKE	NR
GENERAL SURGERY	NR	VASCULAR	NR
MATERNITY CARE	NR	WOMEN'S HEALTH	NR

HEALTHGRADES AWARDS

Golden Plains Community Hospital

200 South McGee Street
Borger, TX 79007
(806) 273-1100

Overall patient safety: ★★★
Teaching: N

CLINICAL PROGRAM RATINGS:

CARDIAC	NR	ORTHOPEDICS	NR
CRITICAL CARE	NR	PULMONARY	★★★
GASTROINTESTINAL	NR	STROKE	NR
GENERAL SURGERY	NR	VASCULAR	NR
MATERNITY CARE	NR	WOMEN'S HEALTH	NR

HEALTHGRADES AWARDS

KEY: ★★★★★ BEST   ★★★ AS EXPECTED   ★ POOR   NR NOT RATED BY HEALTHGRADES   For full definitions of ratings and awards, see Appendix.

Good Shepherd Medical Center*

700 East Marshall Avenue
Longview, TX 75601
(903) 315-2000

Overall patient safety: ★★★
Teaching: N

CLINICAL PROGRAM RATINGS:

CARDIAC	★★★	ORTHOPEDICS	★★★★★
CRITICAL CARE	NR	PULMONARY	★★★
GASTROINTESTINAL	★★★	STROKE	★★★★★
GENERAL SURGERY	★★★	VASCULAR	★★★
MATERNITY CARE	★★★	WOMEN'S HEALTH	★★★

HEALTHGRADES AWARDS

✓ SPECIALTY EXCELLENCE
• GENERAL SURGERY • ORTHOPEDIC SURGERY

Graham Regional Medical Center

1301 Montgomery Road
Graham, TX 76450
(940) 549-3400

Overall patient safety: ★★★
Teaching: N

CLINICAL PROGRAM RATINGS:

CARDIAC	NR	ORTHOPEDICS	NR
CRITICAL CARE	NR	PULMONARY	★★★
GASTROINTESTINAL	NR	STROKE	★★★
GENERAL SURGERY	NR	VASCULAR	NR
MATERNITY CARE	★★★	WOMEN'S HEALTH	NR

HEALTHGRADES AWARDS

Good Shepherd Medical Center--Linden

404 North Kaufman Street
Linden, TX 75563
(903) 756-5561

Overall patient safety: ★
Teaching: N

CLINICAL PROGRAM RATINGS:

CARDIAC	NR	ORTHOPEDICS	NR
CRITICAL CARE	NR	PULMONARY	★
GASTROINTESTINAL	NR	STROKE	★★★
GENERAL SURGERY	NR	VASCULAR	NR
MATERNITY CARE	★★★	WOMEN'S HEALTH	NR

HEALTHGRADES AWARDS

Guadalupe Valley Hospital

1215 East Court Street
Seguin, TX 78155
(830) 379-2411

Overall patient safety: ★
Teaching: N

CLINICAL PROGRAM RATINGS:

CARDIAC	NR	ORTHOPEDICS	NR
CRITICAL CARE	NR	PULMONARY	★
GASTROINTESTINAL	★★★	STROKE	★★★
GENERAL SURGERY	★★★	VASCULAR	NR
MATERNITY CARE	★	WOMEN'S HEALTH	NR

HEALTHGRADES AWARDS

Goodall Witcher Healthcare Foundation

101 South Avenue T
Clifton, TX 76634
(254) 675-8322

Overall patient safety: ★★★
Teaching: N

CLINICAL PROGRAM RATINGS:

CARDIAC	NR	ORTHOPEDICS	NR
CRITICAL CARE	NR	PULMONARY	★
GASTROINTESTINAL	NR	STROKE	★
GENERAL SURGERY	NR	VASCULAR	NR
MATERNITY CARE	NR	WOMEN'S HEALTH	NR

HEALTHGRADES AWARDS

Gulf Coast Medical Center

1400 Highway 59
Wharton, TX 77488
(979) 532-2500

Overall patient safety: ★
Teaching: N

CLINICAL PROGRAM RATINGS:

CARDIAC	NR	ORTHOPEDICS	NR
CRITICAL CARE	NR	PULMONARY	★★★
GASTROINTESTINAL	★★★	STROKE	★★★
GENERAL SURGERY	★★★	VASCULAR	NR
MATERNITY CARE	★★★	WOMEN'S HEALTH	NR

HEALTHGRADES AWARDS

*This hospital reports its data to the federal government jointly with another hospital. Therefore the ratings and awards apply to multiple hospitals and this specific hospital may not provide all rated services.

Hamilton General Hospital

400 North Brown Street
Hamilton, TX 76531
(254) 386-3151

Overall patient safety: ★★★
Teaching: N

CLINICAL PROGRAM RATINGS:

CARDIAC	NR	ORTHOPEDICS	NR
CRITICAL CARE	NR	PULMONARY	★★★
GASTROINTESTINAL	NR	STROKE	NR
GENERAL SURGERY	NR	VASCULAR	NR
MATERNITY CARE	NR	WOMEN'S HEALTH	NR

HEALTHGRADES AWARDS

Harris County Hospital District

2525 Holly Hall Street
Houston, TX 77054
(713) 566-6400

Overall patient safety: ★★★
Teaching: Y

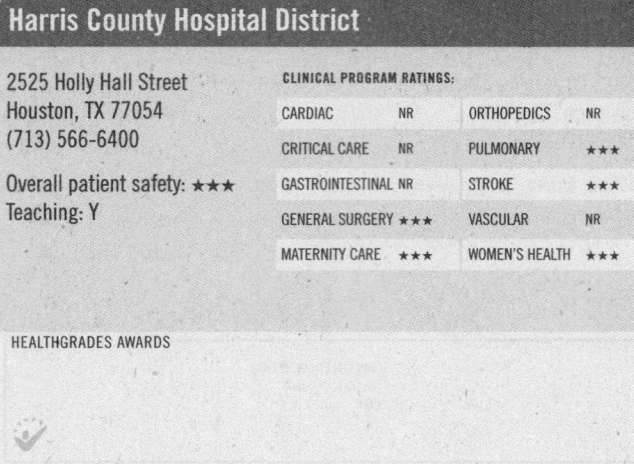

CLINICAL PROGRAM RATINGS:

CARDIAC	NR	ORTHOPEDICS	NR
CRITICAL CARE	NR	PULMONARY	★★★
GASTROINTESTINAL	NR	STROKE	★★★
GENERAL SURGERY	★★★	VASCULAR	NR
MATERNITY CARE	★★★	WOMEN'S HEALTH	★★★

HEALTHGRADES AWARDS

Hamlin Memorial Hospital

632 Northwest 2nd Street
Hamlin, TX 79520
(325) 576-3646

Overall patient safety: NR
Teaching: N

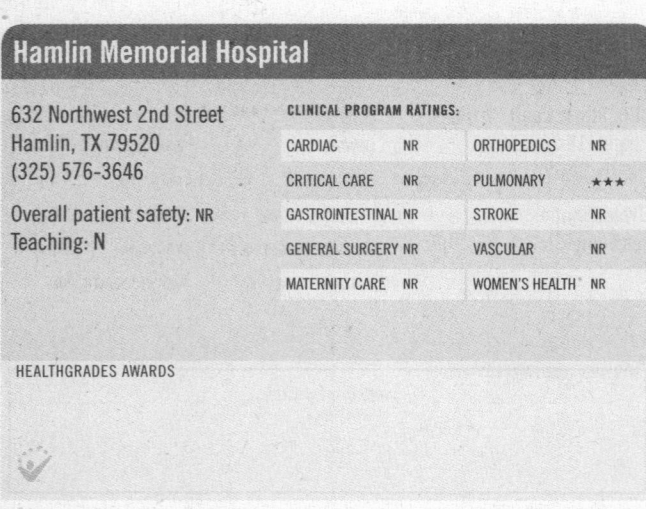

CLINICAL PROGRAM RATINGS:

CARDIAC	NR	ORTHOPEDICS	NR
CRITICAL CARE	NR	PULMONARY	★★★
GASTROINTESTINAL	NR	STROKE	NR
GENERAL SURGERY	NR	VASCULAR	NR
MATERNITY CARE	NR	WOMEN'S HEALTH	NR

HEALTHGRADES AWARDS

Harris Methodist Dublin*

205 North Patrick Street
Dublin, TX 76446
(817) 445-3322

Overall patient safety: ★★★
Teaching: N

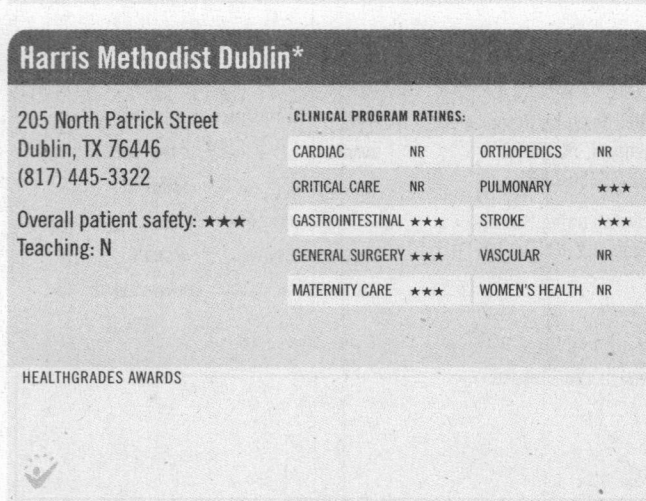

CLINICAL PROGRAM RATINGS:

CARDIAC	NR	ORTHOPEDICS	NR
CRITICAL CARE	NR	PULMONARY	★★★
GASTROINTESTINAL	★★★	STROKE	★★★
GENERAL SURGERY	★★★	VASCULAR	NR
MATERNITY CARE	★★★	WOMEN'S HEALTH	NR

HEALTHGRADES AWARDS

Harlingen Medical Center

5501 South Expressway 77
Harlingen, TX 78550
(956) 365-1000

Overall patient safety: ★★★★★
Teaching: N

CLINICAL PROGRAM RATINGS:

CARDIAC	★★★	ORTHOPEDICS	NR
CRITICAL CARE	NR	PULMONARY	★★★★★
GASTROINTESTINAL	★★★	STROKE	★★★
GENERAL SURGERY	★★★	VASCULAR	NR
MATERNITY CARE	★★★	WOMEN'S HEALTH	★★★★★

HEALTHGRADES AWARDS

✓DISTINGUISHED HOSPITAL
· CLINICAL EXCELLENCE
· PATIENT SAFETY

✓SPECIALTY EXCELLENCE
· CARDIAC CARE
· GASTROINTESTINAL CARE
· PULMONARY CARE

Harris Methodist Erath County*

411 North Belknap Street
Stephenville, TX 76401
(254) 965-1500

Overall patient safety: ★★★
Teaching: N

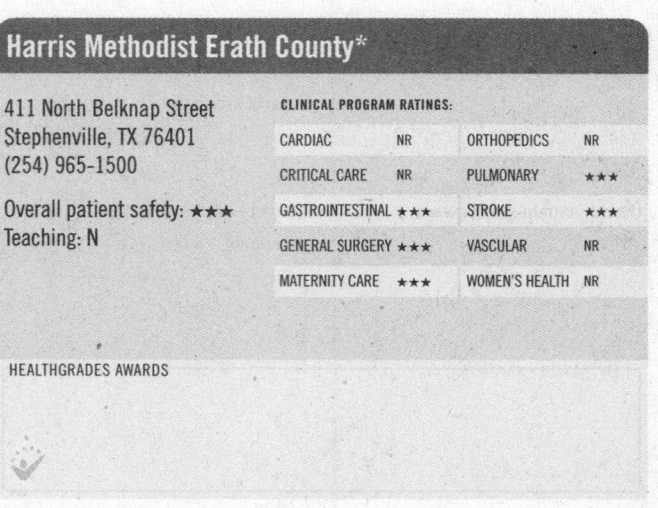

CLINICAL PROGRAM RATINGS:

CARDIAC	NR	ORTHOPEDICS	NR
CRITICAL CARE	NR	PULMONARY	★★★
GASTROINTESTINAL	★★★	STROKE	★★★
GENERAL SURGERY	★★★	VASCULAR	NR
MATERNITY CARE	★★★	WOMEN'S HEALTH	NR

HEALTHGRADES AWARDS

KEY: ★★★★★ BEST   ★★★ AS EXPECTED   ★ POOR   NR NOT RATED BY HEALTHGRADES   For full definitions of ratings and awards, see Appendix.

Harris Methodist Fort Worth

1301 Pennsylvania Avenue
Fort Worth, TX 76104
(817) 882-2000

Overall patient safety: ★★★★★
Teaching: Y

CLINICAL PROGRAM RATINGS:

CARDIAC	★★★	ORTHOPEDICS	★★★
CRITICAL CARE	★★★	PULMONARY	★★★★★
GASTROINTESTINAL	★★★	STROKE	★★★
GENERAL SURGERY	★★★	VASCULAR	★★★
MATERNITY CARE	★★★	WOMEN'S HEALTH	★★★

HEALTHGRADES AWARDS

✓ DISTINGUISHED HOSPITAL
  · PATIENT SAFETY

✓ SPECIALTY EXCELLENCE
  · GASTROINTESTINAL CARE

Healthsouth Medical Center

2124 Research Row
Dallas, TX 75235
(214) 904-6100

Overall patient safety: ★★★
Teaching: N

CLINICAL PROGRAM RATINGS:

CARDIAC	NR	ORTHOPEDICS	NR
CRITICAL CARE	NR	PULMONARY	★★★
GASTROINTESTINAL	NR	STROKE	NR
GENERAL SURGERY	NR	VASCULAR	NR
MATERNITY CARE	NR	WOMEN'S HEALTH	NR

HEALTHGRADES AWARDS

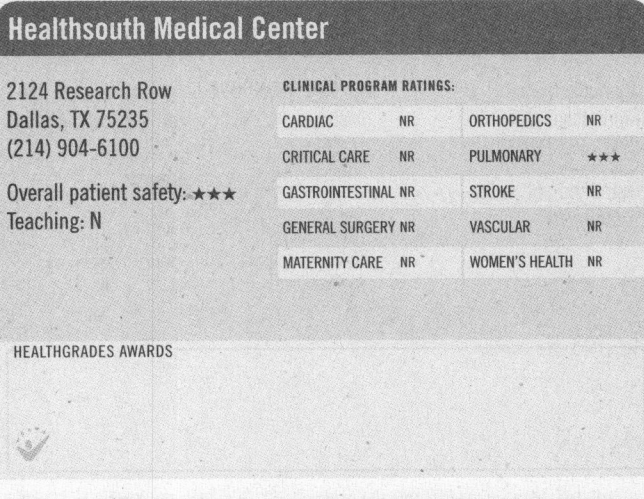

Harris Methodist HEB Hospital

1600 Hospital Parkway
Bedford, TX 76022
(817) 685-4000

Overall patient safety: ★★★
Teaching: N

CLINICAL PROGRAM RATINGS:

CARDIAC	★★★	ORTHOPEDICS	★★★
CRITICAL CARE	★★★	PULMONARY	★★★
GASTROINTESTINAL	★★★	STROKE	★★★
GENERAL SURGERY	★★★	VASCULAR	NR
MATERNITY CARE	★★★	WOMEN'S HEALTH	★★★

HEALTHGRADES AWARDS

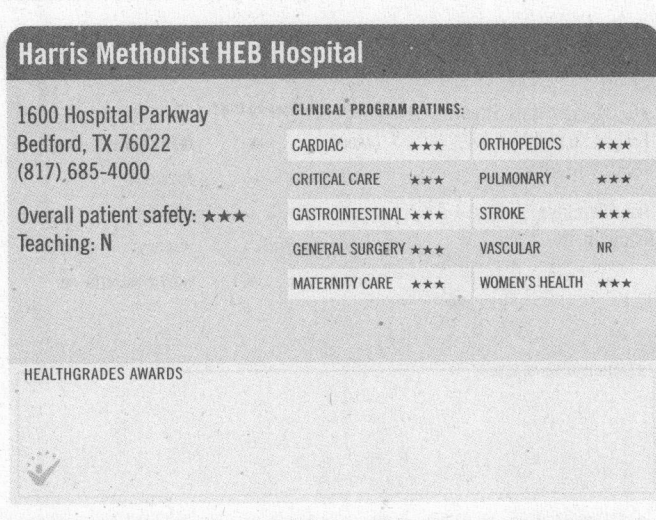

Heart Hospital of Austin

3801 North Lamar Boulevard
Austin, TX 78756
(512) 407-7000

Overall patient safety: ★★★★★
Teaching: N

CLINICAL PROGRAM RATINGS:

CARDIAC	★★★★★	ORTHOPEDICS	NR
CRITICAL CARE	NR	PULMONARY	★★★
GASTROINTESTINAL	NR	STROKE	NR
GENERAL SURGERY	NR	VASCULAR	★★★
MATERNITY CARE	NR	WOMEN'S HEALTH	NR

HEALTHGRADES AWARDS

✓ SPECIALTY EXCELLENCE
  · CARDIAC CARE   · CARDIAC SURGERY

Harris Methodist Southwest

6100 Harris Parkway
Fort Worth, TX 76132
(817) 346-5000

Overall patient safety: ★★★
Teaching: N

CLINICAL PROGRAM RATINGS:

CARDIAC	NR	ORTHOPEDICS	NR
CRITICAL CARE	NR	PULMONARY	★★★
GASTROINTESTINAL	★★★	STROKE	★★★
GENERAL SURGERY	★★★	VASCULAR	NR
MATERNITY CARE	★★★	WOMEN'S HEALTH	NR

HEALTHGRADES AWARDS

Heart of Texas Memorial Hospital

2008 Nine Road
Brady, TX 76825
(325) 597-2901

Overall patient safety: ★★★
Teaching: N

CLINICAL PROGRAM RATINGS:

CARDIAC	NR	ORTHOPEDICS	NR
CRITICAL CARE	NR	PULMONARY	★
GASTROINTESTINAL	NR	STROKE	NR
GENERAL SURGERY	NR	VASCULAR	NR
MATERNITY CARE	NR	WOMEN'S HEALTH	NR

HEALTHGRADES AWARDS

*This hospital reports its data to the federal government jointly with another hospital. Therefore the ratings and awards apply to multiple hospitals and this specific hospital may not provide all rated services.

Henderson Memorial Hospital

300 Wilson Street
Henderson, TX 75652
(903) 657-7541

Overall patient safety: ★★★
Teaching: N

CLINICAL PROGRAM RATINGS:

CARDIAC	NR	ORTHOPEDICS	NR
CRITICAL CARE	NR	PULMONARY	★★★
GASTROINTESTINAL	NR	STROKE	★★★
GENERAL SURGERY	NR	VASCULAR	NR
MATERNITY CARE	★★★★★	WOMEN'S HEALTH	NR

HEALTHGRADES AWARDS

Highland Medical Center

2412 50th Street
Lubbock, TX 79412
(806) 788-4100

Overall patient safety: ★★★
Teaching: N

CLINICAL PROGRAM RATINGS:

CARDIAC	NR	ORTHOPEDICS	NR
CRITICAL CARE	NR	PULMONARY	★★★
GASTROINTESTINAL	NR	STROKE	NR
GENERAL SURGERY	NR	VASCULAR	NR
MATERNITY CARE	★★★	WOMEN'S HEALTH	NR

HEALTHGRADES AWARDS

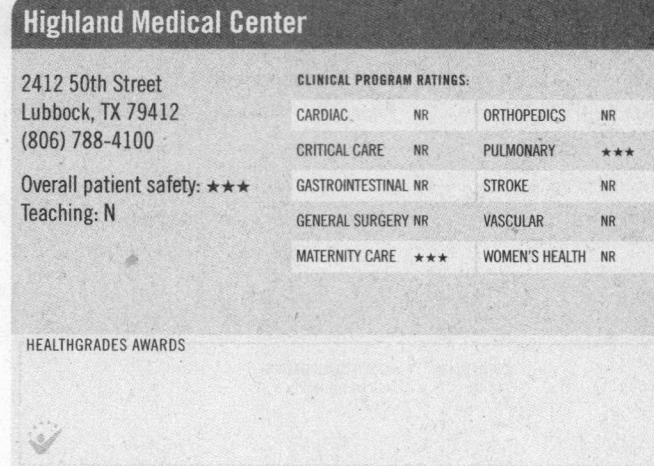

Hendrick Medical Center

1900 Pine Street
Abilene, TX 79601
(325) 670-2000

Overall patient safety: ★★★
Teaching: Y

CLINICAL PROGRAM RATINGS:

CARDIAC	★	ORTHOPEDICS	★★★
CRITICAL CARE	NR	PULMONARY	★★★
GASTROINTESTINAL	★	STROKE	★
GENERAL SURGERY	★★★	VASCULAR	NR
MATERNITY CARE	★★★	WOMEN'S HEALTH	★

HEALTHGRADES AWARDS

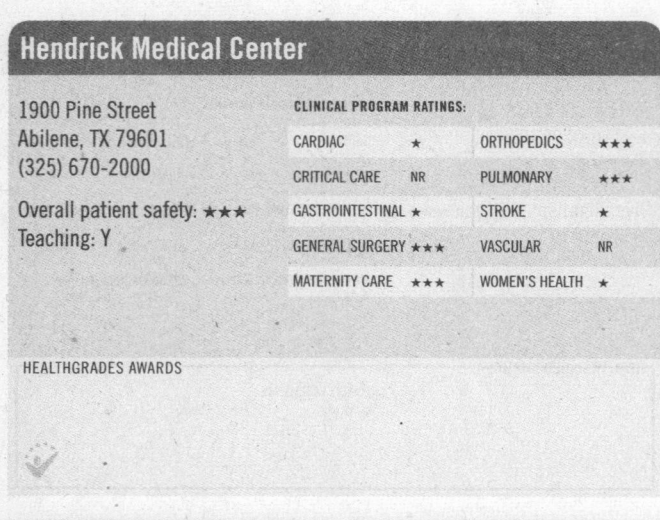

Hill Country Memorial Hospital

1020 South State Highway 16
Fredericksburg, TX 78624
(830) 997-4353

Overall patient safety: ★★★
Teaching: N

CLINICAL PROGRAM RATINGS:

CARDIAC	NR	ORTHOPEDICS	NR
CRITICAL CARE	NR	PULMONARY	★
GASTROINTESTINAL	★★★	STROKE	★
GENERAL SURGERY	NR	VASCULAR	NR
MATERNITY CARE	★	WOMEN'S HEALTH	NR

HEALTHGRADES AWARDS

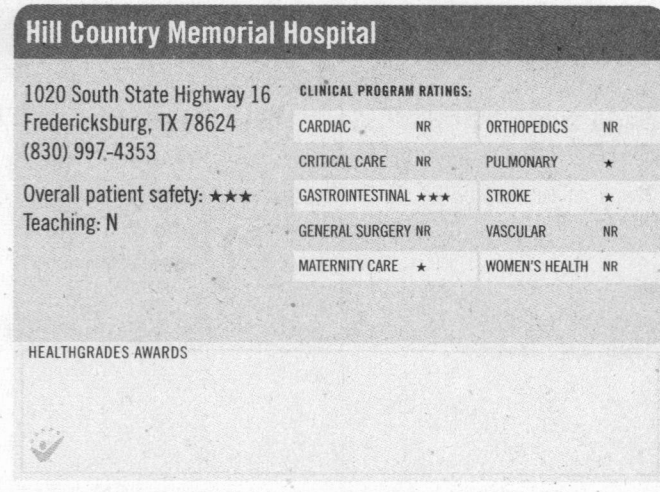

Hereford Regional Medical Center

801 East 3rd Street
Hereford, TX 79045
(806) 364-2141

Overall patient safety: ★★★
Teaching: N

CLINICAL PROGRAM RATINGS:

CARDIAC	NR	ORTHOPEDICS	NR
CRITICAL CARE	NR	PULMONARY	★
GASTROINTESTINAL	NR	STROKE	NR
GENERAL SURGERY	NR	VASCULAR	NR
MATERNITY CARE	NR	WOMEN'S HEALTH	NR

HEALTHGRADES AWARDS

Hill Regional Hospital

101 Circle Drive
Hillsboro, TX 76645
(254) 580-8500

Overall patient safety: ★★★
Teaching: N

CLINICAL PROGRAM RATINGS:

CARDIAC	NR	ORTHOPEDICS	NR
CRITICAL CARE	NR	PULMONARY	★★★
GASTROINTESTINAL	NR	STROKE	★★★
GENERAL SURGERY	★★★	VASCULAR	NR
MATERNITY CARE	★	WOMEN'S HEALTH	NR

HEALTHGRADES AWARDS

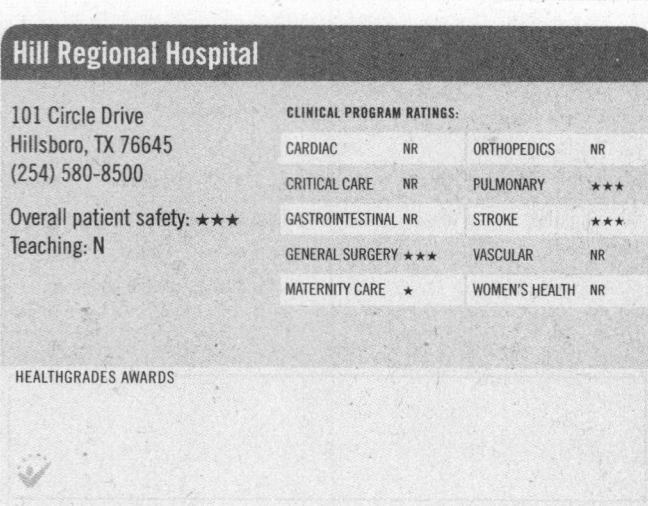

KEY: ★★★★★ BEST   ★★★ AS EXPECTED   ★ POOR   NR NOT RATED BY HEALTHGRADES   For full definitions of ratings and awards, see Appendix.

Hillcrest Baptist Medical Center

3000 Herring Avenue
Waco, TX 76708
(254) 202-2000

Overall patient safety: ★★★
Teaching: Y

CLINICAL PROGRAM RATINGS:

CARDIAC	★★★	ORTHOPEDICS	★★★★★
CRITICAL CARE	NR	PULMONARY	★★★
GASTROINTESTINAL	★★★	STROKE	★
GENERAL SURGERY	★★★	VASCULAR	NR
MATERNITY CARE	★★★	WOMEN'S HEALTH	★★★

HEALTHGRADES AWARDS

✓ SPECIALTY EXCELLENCE
- ORTHOPEDIC SURGERY

Houston Northwest Medical Center

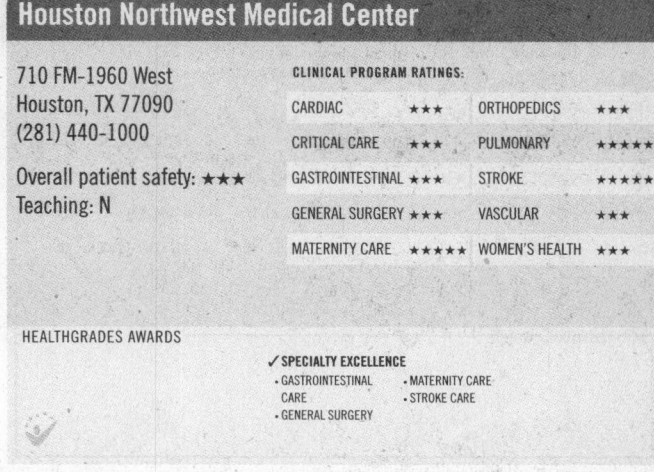

710 FM-1960 West
Houston, TX 77090
(281) 440-1000

Overall patient safety: ★★★
Teaching: N

CLINICAL PROGRAM RATINGS:

CARDIAC	★★★	ORTHOPEDICS	★★★
CRITICAL CARE	★★★	PULMONARY	★★★★★
GASTROINTESTINAL	★★★	STROKE	★★★★★
GENERAL SURGERY	★★★	VASCULAR	★★★
MATERNITY CARE	★★★★★	WOMEN'S HEALTH	★★★

HEALTHGRADES AWARDS

✓ SPECIALTY EXCELLENCE
- GASTROINTESTINAL CARE
- GENERAL SURGERY
- MATERNITY CARE
- STROKE CARE

Hopkins County Memorial Hospital

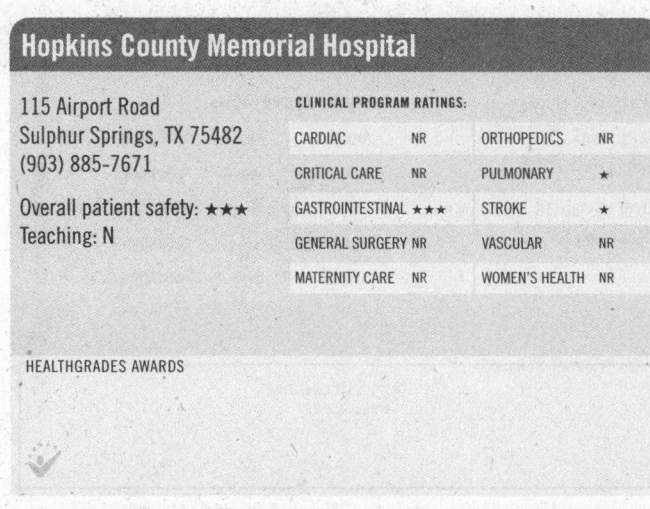

115 Airport Road
Sulphur Springs, TX 75482
(903) 885-7671

Overall patient safety: ★★★
Teaching: N

CLINICAL PROGRAM RATINGS:

CARDIAC	NR	ORTHOPEDICS	NR
CRITICAL CARE	NR	PULMONARY	★
GASTROINTESTINAL	★★★	STROKE	★
GENERAL SURGERY	NR	VASCULAR	NR
MATERNITY CARE	NR	WOMEN'S HEALTH	NR

HEALTHGRADES AWARDS

Huguley Memorial Medical Center

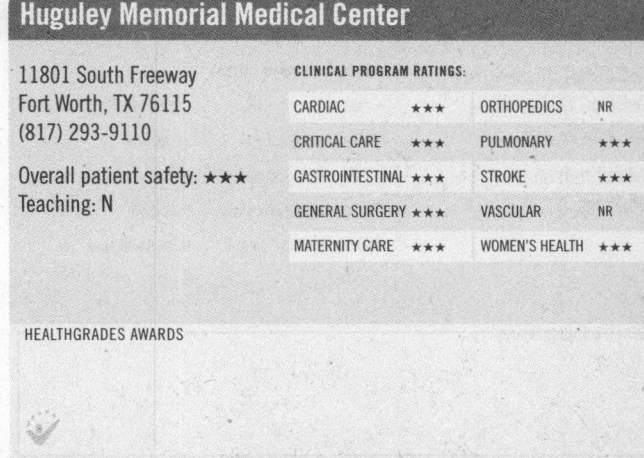

11801 South Freeway
Fort Worth, TX 76115
(817) 293-9110

Overall patient safety: ★★★
Teaching: N

CLINICAL PROGRAM RATINGS:

CARDIAC	★★★	ORTHOPEDICS	NR
CRITICAL CARE	★★★	PULMONARY	★★★
GASTROINTESTINAL	★★★	STROKE	★★★
GENERAL SURGERY	★★★	VASCULAR	NR
MATERNITY CARE	★★★	WOMEN'S HEALTH	★★★

HEALTHGRADES AWARDS

The Hospital at Westlake Medical Center

5656 Bee Caves Road
Suite M-302
Austin, TX 78746
(512) 327-0000

Overall patient safety: NR
Teaching: N

CLINICAL PROGRAM RATINGS:

CARDIAC	NR	ORTHOPEDICS	NR
CRITICAL CARE	NR	PULMONARY	NR
GASTROINTESTINAL	NR	STROKE	NR
GENERAL SURGERY	NR	VASCULAR	NR
MATERNITY CARE	NR	WOMEN'S HEALTH	NR

HEALTHGRADES AWARDS

Huntsville Memorial Hospital

110 Memorial Hospital Drive
Huntsville, TX 77340
(936) 291-3411

Overall patient safety: ★★★
Teaching: N

CLINICAL PROGRAM RATINGS:

CARDIAC	NR	ORTHOPEDICS	NR
CRITICAL CARE	NR	PULMONARY	★
GASTROINTESTINAL	NR	STROKE	★★★
GENERAL SURGERY	★	VASCULAR	NR
MATERNITY CARE	★★★	WOMEN'S HEALTH	NR

HEALTHGRADES AWARDS

Johns Community Hospital

205 Mallard Lane
Taylor, TX 76574
(512) 352-4215

Overall patient safety: ★★★
Teaching: N

CLINICAL PROGRAM RATINGS:

CARDIAC	NR	ORTHOPEDICS	NR
CRITICAL CARE	NR	PULMONARY	★★★
GASTROINTESTINAL	NR	STROKE	NR
GENERAL SURGERY	NR	VASCULAR	NR
MATERNITY CARE	NR	WOMEN'S HEALTH	NR

HEALTHGRADES AWARDS

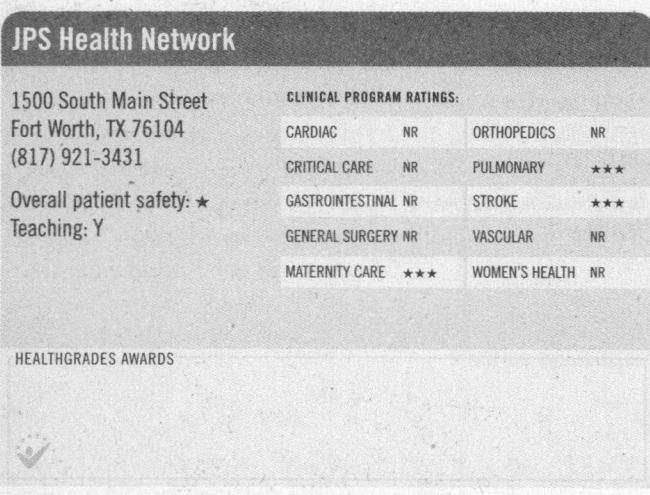

King's Daughters Hospital

1901 Southwest H. K.
Dodgen Loop
Temple, TX 76502
(254) 771-8600

Overall patient safety: ★★★
Teaching: N

CLINICAL PROGRAM RATINGS:

CARDIAC	NR	ORTHOPEDICS	NR.
CRITICAL CARE	NR	PULMONARY	★★★
GASTROINTESTINAL	NR	STROKE	★★★
GENERAL SURGERY	★★★	VASCULAR	NR
MATERNITY CARE	★★★	WOMEN'S HEALTH	NR

HEALTHGRADES AWARDS

JPS Health Network

1500 South Main Street
Fort Worth, TX 76104
(817) 921-3431

Overall patient safety: ★
Teaching: Y

CLINICAL PROGRAM RATINGS:

CARDIAC	NR	ORTHOPEDICS	NR
CRITICAL CARE	NR	PULMONARY	★★★
GASTROINTESTINAL	NR	STROKE	★★★
GENERAL SURGERY	NR	VASCULAR	NR
MATERNITY CARE	★★★	WOMEN'S HEALTH	NR

HEALTHGRADES AWARDS

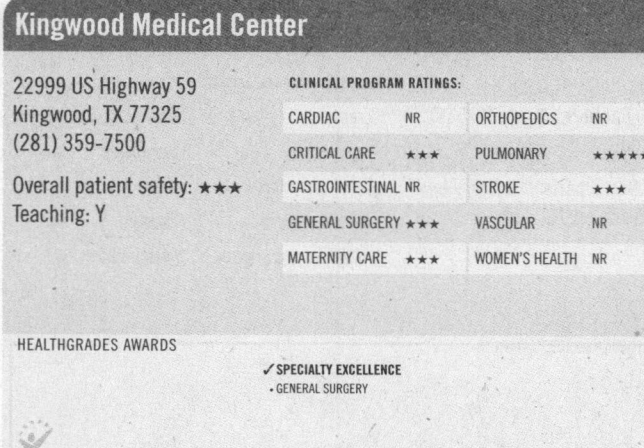

Kingwood Medical Center

22999 US Highway 59
Kingwood, TX 77325
(281) 359-7500

Overall patient safety: ★★★
Teaching: Y

CLINICAL PROGRAM RATINGS:

CARDIAC	NR	ORTHOPEDICS	NR
CRITICAL CARE	★★★	PULMONARY	★★★★★
GASTROINTESTINAL	NR	STROKE	★★★
GENERAL SURGERY	★★★	VASCULAR	NR
MATERNITY CARE	★★★	WOMEN'S HEALTH	NR

HEALTHGRADES AWARDS

✓ SPECIALTY EXCELLENCE
- GENERAL SURGERY

Kell West Regional Hospital

5402 Kell West Boulevard
Wichita Falls, TX 76310
(940) 692-5888

Overall patient safety: ★★★
Teaching: N

CLINICAL PROGRAM RATINGS:

CARDIAC	NR	ORTHOPEDICS	NR
CRITICAL CARE	NR	PULMONARY	★★★
GASTROINTESTINAL	NR	STROKE	NR
GENERAL SURGERY	NR	VASCULAR	NR
MATERNITY CARE	NR	WOMEN'S HEALTH	NR

HEALTHGRADES AWARDS

✓ SPECIALTY EXCELLENCE
- JOINT REPLACEMENT

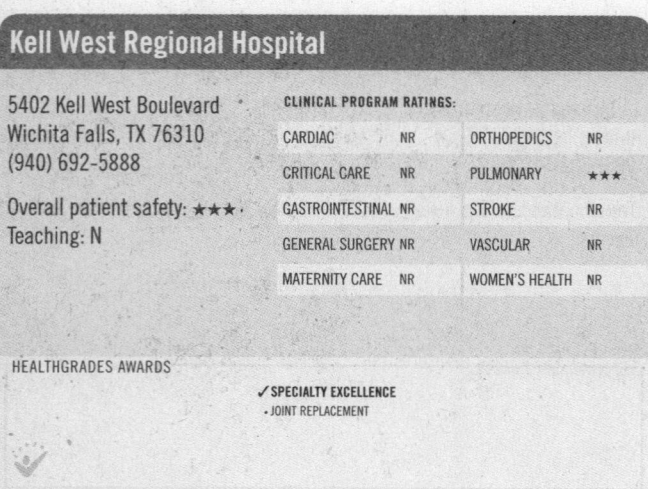

Knapp Medical Center

1401 East 8th Street
Weslaco, TX 78596
(956) 968-8567

Overall patient safety: ★★★
Teaching: N

CLINICAL PROGRAM RATINGS:

CARDIAC	NR	ORTHOPEDICS	NR
CRITICAL CARE	NR	PULMONARY	★★★★★
GASTROINTESTINAL	★★★	STROKE	★★★
GENERAL SURGERY	★★★	VASCULAR	NR
MATERNITY CARE	★★★	WOMEN'S HEALTH	NR

HEALTHGRADES AWARDS

✓ SPECIALTY EXCELLENCE
- GASTROINTESTINAL CARE
- PULMONARY CARE

KEY: ★★★★★ BEST   ★★★ AS EXPECTED   ★ POOR   NR NOT RATED BY HEALTHGRADES   For full definitions of ratings and awards, see Appendix.

Laird Memorial Hospital

1612 South Henderson
Boulevard
Kilgore, TX 75662
(903) 984-3505

Overall patient safety: ★★★
Teaching: N

CLINICAL PROGRAM RATINGS:

CARDIAC	NR	ORTHOPEDICS	NR
CRITICAL CARE	NR	PULMONARY	★★★
GASTROINTESTINAL	NR	STROKE	★★★
GENERAL SURGERY	★★★	VASCULAR	NR
MATERNITY CARE	★★★★★	WOMEN'S HEALTH	NR

HEALTHGRADES AWARDS

Lake Whitney Medical Center

200 North San Jacinto Street
Whitney, TX 76692
(254) 694-3165

Overall patient safety: NR
Teaching: N

CLINICAL PROGRAM RATINGS:

CARDIAC	NR	ORTHOPEDICS	NR
CRITICAL CARE	NR	PULMONARY	★★★★★
GASTROINTESTINAL	NR	STROKE	NR
GENERAL SURGERY	NR	VASCULAR	NR
MATERNITY CARE	NR	WOMEN'S HEALTH	NR

HEALTHGRADES AWARDS

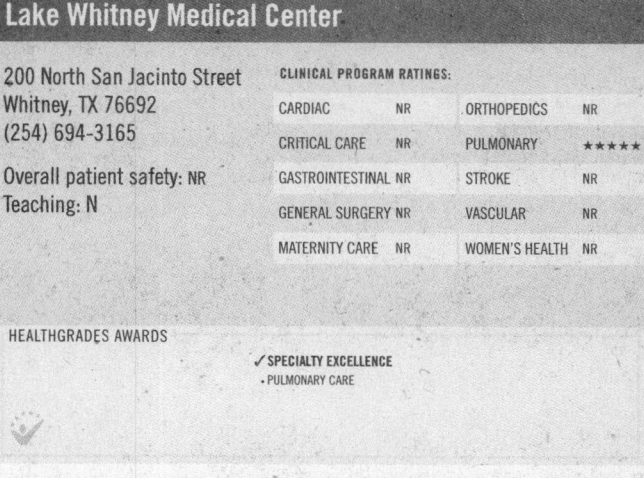

✓ SPECIALTY EXCELLENCE
 • PULMONARY CARE

Lake Granbury Medical Center

1310 Paluxy Road
Granbury, TX 76048
(817) 573-2683

Overall patient safety: ★★★
Teaching: N

CLINICAL PROGRAM RATINGS:

CARDIAC	NR	ORTHOPEDICS	NR
CRITICAL CARE	NR	PULMONARY	★★★
GASTROINTESTINAL	NR	STROKE	★★★
GENERAL SURGERY	★★★	VASCULAR	NR
MATERNITY CARE	★★★	WOMEN'S HEALTH	NR

HEALTHGRADES AWARDS

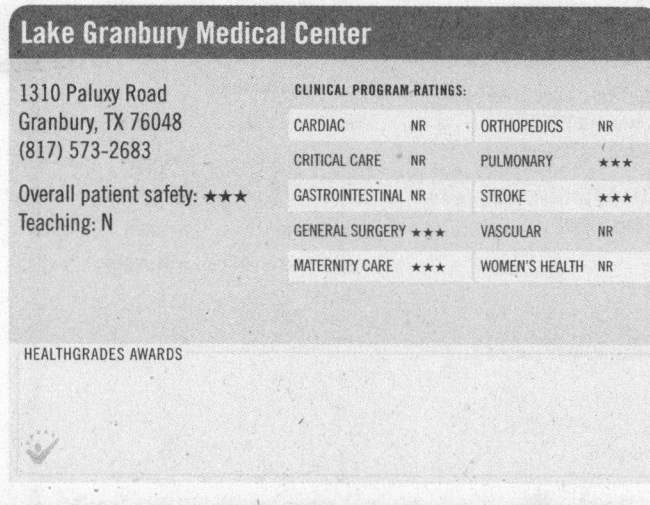

Lamb Healthcare Center

1500 South Sunset Avenue
Littlefield, TX 79339
(806) 385-6411

Overall patient safety: ★★★
Teaching: N

CLINICAL PROGRAM RATINGS:

CARDIAC	NR	ORTHOPEDICS	NR
CRITICAL CARE	NR	PULMONARY	★★★
GASTROINTESTINAL	NR	STROKE	NR
GENERAL SURGERY	NR	VASCULAR	NR
MATERNITY CARE	NR	WOMEN'S HEALTH	NR

HEALTHGRADES AWARDS

Lake Pointe Medical Center

6800 Scenic Drive
Rowlett, TX 75088
(972) 412-2273

Overall patient safety: ★
Teaching: N

CLINICAL PROGRAM RATINGS:

CARDIAC	NR	ORTHOPEDICS	NR
CRITICAL CARE	★★★	PULMONARY	★
GASTROINTESTINAL	★★★	STROKE	★★★
GENERAL SURGERY	★★★	VASCULAR	NR
MATERNITY CARE	★★★	WOMEN'S HEALTH	NR

HEALTHGRADES AWARDS

Laredo Medical Center

1700 East Saunders Street
Laredo, TX 78041
(956) 796-5000

Overall patient safety: ★★★
Teaching: N

CLINICAL PROGRAM RATINGS:

CARDIAC	★★★	ORTHOPEDICS	NR
CRITICAL CARE	NR	PULMONARY	★★★
GASTROINTESTINAL	★★★	STROKE	★★★★★
GENERAL SURGERY	★★★	VASCULAR	NR
MATERNITY CARE	★★★	WOMEN'S HEALTH	★★★

HEALTHGRADES AWARDS

✓ SPECIALTY EXCELLENCE
 • GASTROINTESTINAL   • STROKE CARE
   CARE

Las Colinas Medical Center

6800 North MacArthur
Boulevard
Irving, TX 75039
(972) 969-2000

Overall patient safety: ★★★
Teaching: N

CLINICAL PROGRAM RATINGS:

CARDIAC	NR	ORTHOPEDICS	NR
CRITICAL CARE	NR	PULMONARY	★★★
GASTROINTESTINAL	NR	STROKE	★★★
GENERAL SURGERY	NR	VASCULAR	NR
MATERNITY CARE	★★★	WOMEN'S HEALTH	NR

HEALTHGRADES AWARDS

Liberty Dayton Community Hospital

1353 North Travis Street
Liberty, TX 77575
(936) 336-7316

Overall patient safety: ★★★
Teaching: N

CLINICAL PROGRAM RATINGS:

CARDIAC	NR	ORTHOPEDICS	NR
CRITICAL CARE	NR	PULMONARY	★★★
GASTROINTESTINAL	NR	STROKE	NR
GENERAL SURGERY	NR	VASCULAR	NR
MATERNITY CARE	NR	WOMEN'S HEALTH	NR

HEALTHGRADES AWARDS

Las Palmas Medical Center

1801 North Oregon Street
El Paso, TX 79902
(915) 521-1200

Overall patient safety: ★
Teaching: N

CLINICAL PROGRAM RATINGS:

CARDIAC	★	ORTHOPEDICS	★★★
CRITICAL CARE	★★★	PULMONARY	★★★
GASTROINTESTINAL	★★★	STROKE	★★★★★
GENERAL SURGERY	★★★	VASCULAR	NR
MATERNITY CARE	★★★★★	WOMEN'S HEALTH	★★★

HEALTHGRADES AWARDS

✓ SPECIALTY EXCELLENCE
· JOINT REPLACEMENT   · MATERNITY CARE

Llano Memorial Healthcare System

200 West Ollie Street
Llano, TX 78643
(325) 247-5040

Overall patient safety: ★★★
Teaching: N

CLINICAL PROGRAM RATINGS:

CARDIAC	NR	ORTHOPEDICS	NR
CRITICAL CARE	NR	PULMONARY	★★★
GASTROINTESTINAL	NR	STROKE	★★★
GENERAL SURGERY	NR	VASCULAR	NR
MATERNITY CARE	★★★	WOMEN'S HEALTH	NR

HEALTHGRADES AWARDS

Lavaca Medical Center

1400 North Texana Street
Hallettsville, TX 77964
(361) 798-3671

Overall patient safety: NR
Teaching: N

CLINICAL PROGRAM RATINGS:

CARDIAC	NR	ORTHOPEDICS	NR
CRITICAL CARE	NR	PULMONARY	★★★
GASTROINTESTINAL	NR	STROKE	★★★
GENERAL SURGERY	NR	VASCULAR	NR
MATERNITY CARE	NR	WOMEN'S HEALTH	NR

HEALTHGRADES AWARDS

Longview Regional Medical Center

2901 North 4th Street
Longview, TX 75605
(903) 758-1818

Overall patient safety: ★
Teaching: N

CLINICAL PROGRAM RATINGS:

CARDIAC	★★★	ORTHOPEDICS	★★★
CRITICAL CARE	NR	PULMONARY	★★★★★
GASTROINTESTINAL	★★★	STROKE	★★★
GENERAL SURGERY	★★★	VASCULAR	NR
MATERNITY CARE	★★★	WOMEN'S HEALTH	★★★

HEALTHGRADES AWARDS

KEY: ★★★★★ BEST   ★★★ AS EXPECTED   ★ POOR   NR NOT RATED BY HEALTHGRADES   For full definitions of ratings and awards, see Appendix.

Lubbock Heart Hospital

4810 North Loop 289
Lubbock, TX 79416
(806) 687-7777

Overall patient safety: ★★★★★
Teaching: N

CLINICAL PROGRAM RATINGS:

CARDIAC	★★★	ORTHOPEDICS	NR
CRITICAL CARE	NR	PULMONARY	★★★
GASTROINTESTINAL	NR	STROKE	★★★
GENERAL SURGERY	NR	VASCULAR	★★★★★
MATERNITY CARE	NR	WOMEN'S HEALTH	NR

HEALTHGRADES AWARDS

✓ SPECIALTY EXCELLENCE
- CARDIAC CARE
- VASCULAR SURGERY

Matagorda General Hospital

1115 Avenue G
Bay City, TX 77414
(979) 245-6383

Overall patient safety: ★★★
Teaching: N

CLINICAL PROGRAM RATINGS:

CARDIAC	NR	ORTHOPEDICS	NR
CRITICAL CARE	NR	PULMONARY	★
GASTROINTESTINAL	NR	STROKE	★★★
GENERAL SURGERY	★★★	VASCULAR	NR
MATERNITY CARE	★	WOMEN'S HEALTH	NR

HEALTHGRADES AWARDS

Mainland Medical Center

6801 Emmett Lowry
Expressway
Texas City, TX 77591
(409) 938-5000

Overall patient safety: ★★★
Teaching: N

CLINICAL PROGRAM RATINGS:

CARDIAC	NR	ORTHOPEDICS	NR
CRITICAL CARE	NR	PULMONARY	★★★
GASTROINTESTINAL	★★★	STROKE	★★★
GENERAL SURGERY	★★★	VASCULAR	NR
MATERNITY CARE	★	WOMEN'S HEALTH	NR

HEALTHGRADES AWARDS

✓ SPECIALTY EXCELLENCE
- GASTROINTESTINAL
  CARE

McAllen Medical Center/Heart Hospital

301 West Expressway 83
McAllen, TX 78503
(956) 632-4000

Overall patient safety: ★★★
Teaching: Y

CLINICAL PROGRAM RATINGS:

CARDIAC	★★★★★	ORTHOPEDICS	NR
CRITICAL CARE	NR	PULMONARY	★★★★★
GASTROINTESTINAL	★★★	STROKE	★★★★★
GENERAL SURGERY	★★★	VASCULAR	NR
MATERNITY CARE	★★★	WOMEN'S HEALTH	★★★★★

HEALTHGRADES AWARDS

✓ DISTINGUISHED   ✓ SPECIALTY EXCELLENCE
  HOSPITAL
- CLINICAL EXCELLENCE
- CARDIAC CARE
- CARDIAC SURGERY
- PULMONARY CARE
- STROKE CARE
- WOMEN'S HEALTH

Marshall Regional Medical Center

811 South Washington Avenue
Marshall, TX 75670
(903) 927-6000

Overall patient safety: ★★★
Teaching: N

CLINICAL PROGRAM RATINGS:

CARDIAC	NR	ORTHOPEDICS	NR
CRITICAL CARE	NR	PULMONARY	★★★
GASTROINTESTINAL	NR	STROKE	★★★
GENERAL SURGERY	★★★	VASCULAR	NR
MATERNITY CARE	★★★★★	WOMEN'S HEALTH	NR

HEALTHGRADES AWARDS

✓ SPECIALTY EXCELLENCE
- MATERNITY CARE

McKenna Memorial Hospital

600 North Union Avenue
New Braunfels, TX 78130
(830) 606-9111

Overall patient safety: ★★★
Teaching: N

CLINICAL PROGRAM RATINGS:

CARDIAC	NR	ORTHOPEDICS	NR
CRITICAL CARE	NR	PULMONARY	★
GASTROINTESTINAL	★★★	STROKE	★★★
GENERAL SURGERY	★★★	VASCULAR	★★★
MATERNITY CARE	★★★	WOMEN'S HEALTH	NR

HEALTHGRADES AWARDS

✓ SPECIALTY EXCELLENCE
- JOINT REPLACEMENT

Medical Arts Hospital

1600 North Bryan Avenue
Lamesa, TX 79331
(806) 872-2183

Overall patient safety: ★★★
Teaching: N

CLINICAL PROGRAM RATINGS:

CARDIAC	NR	ORTHOPEDICS	NR
CRITICAL CARE	NR	PULMONARY	★★★
GASTROINTESTINAL	NR	STROKE	NR
GENERAL SURGERY	NR	VASCULAR	NR
MATERNITY CARE	NR	WOMEN'S HEALTH	NR

HEALTHGRADES AWARDS

Medical Center at Lancaster

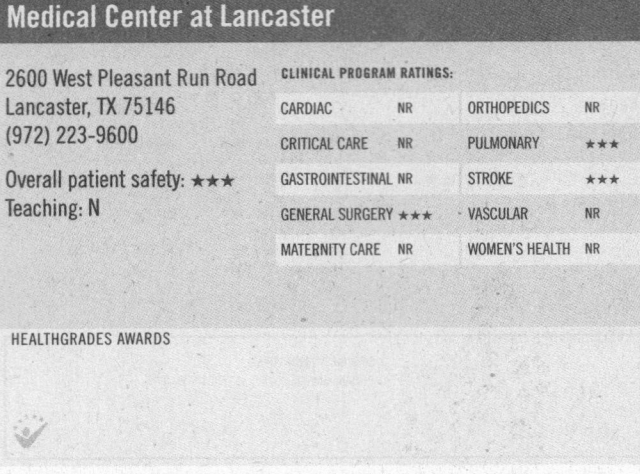

2600 West Pleasant Run Road
Lancaster, TX 75146
(972) 223-9600

Overall patient safety: ★★★
Teaching: N

CLINICAL PROGRAM RATINGS:

CARDIAC	NR	ORTHOPEDICS	NR
CRITICAL CARE	NR	PULMONARY	★★★
GASTROINTESTINAL	NR	STROKE	★★★
GENERAL SURGERY	★★★	VASCULAR	NR
MATERNITY CARE	NR	WOMEN'S HEALTH	NR

HEALTHGRADES AWARDS

Medical Centre Surgical Hospital

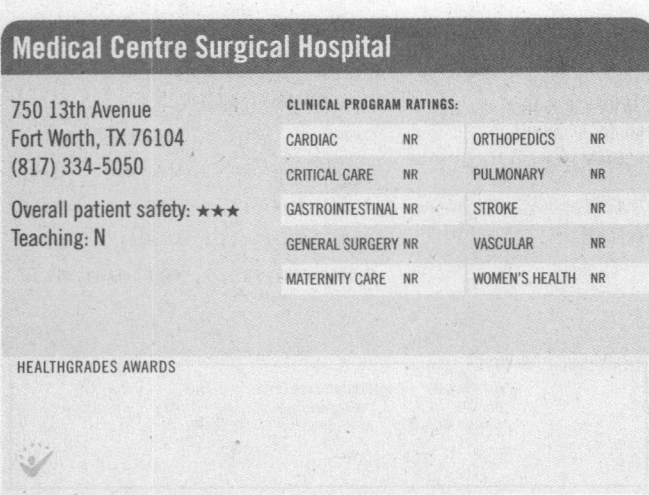

750 13th Avenue
Fort Worth, TX 76104
(817) 334-5050

Overall patient safety: ★★★
Teaching: N

CLINICAL PROGRAM RATINGS:

CARDIAC	NR	ORTHOPEDICS	NR
CRITICAL CARE	NR	PULMONARY	NR
GASTROINTESTINAL	NR	STROKE	NR
GENERAL SURGERY	NR	VASCULAR	NR
MATERNITY CARE	NR	WOMEN'S HEALTH	NR

HEALTHGRADES AWARDS

Medical Center Hospital

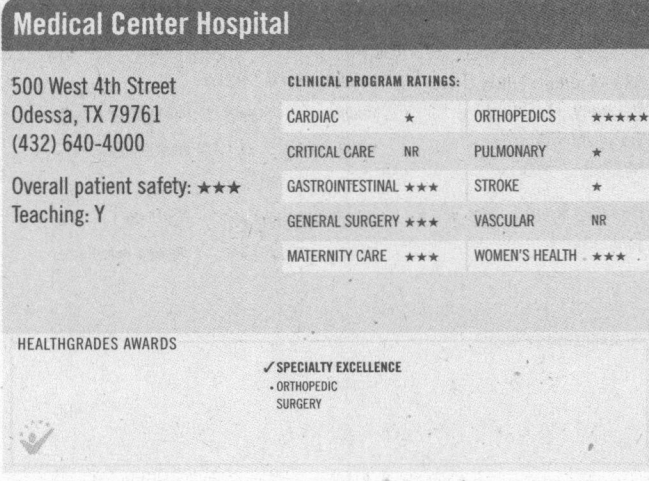

500 West 4th Street
Odessa, TX 79761
(432) 640-4000

Overall patient safety: ★★★
Teaching: Y

CLINICAL PROGRAM RATINGS:

CARDIAC	★	ORTHOPEDICS	★★★★★
CRITICAL CARE	NR	PULMONARY	★
GASTROINTESTINAL	★★★	STROKE	★
GENERAL SURGERY	★★★	VASCULAR	NR
MATERNITY CARE	★★★	WOMEN'S HEALTH	★★★

HEALTHGRADES AWARDS

✓ SPECIALTY EXCELLENCE
• ORTHOPEDIC SURGERY

Medical City Dallas Hospital

7777 Forest Lane
Dallas, TX 75230
(972) 661-7000

Overall patient safety: ★★★
Teaching: Y

CLINICAL PROGRAM RATINGS:

CARDIAC	★★★	ORTHOPEDICS	★★★
CRITICAL CARE	★	PULMONARY	★★★
GASTROINTESTINAL	★★★	STROKE	★★★
GENERAL SURGERY	★★★	VASCULAR	★★★
MATERNITY CARE	★★★	WOMEN'S HEALTH	★

HEALTHGRADES AWARDS

✓ SPECIALTY EXCELLENCE
• JOINT REPLACEMENT

Medical Center of Arlington

3301 Matlock Road
Arlington, TX 76015
(817) 465-3241

Overall patient safety: ★★★
Teaching: N

CLINICAL PROGRAM RATINGS:

CARDIAC	★★★	ORTHOPEDICS	NR
CRITICAL CARE	★★★	PULMONARY	★★★
GASTROINTESTINAL	★★★	STROKE	★★★★★
GENERAL SURGERY	★★★	VASCULAR	NR
MATERNITY CARE	★★★	WOMEN'S HEALTH	★★★

HEALTHGRADES AWARDS

✓ SPECIALTY EXCELLENCE
• STROKE CARE

KEY: ★★★★★ BEST   ★★★ AS EXPECTED   ★ POOR   NR NOT RATED BY HEALTHGRADES   For full definitions of ratings and awards, see Appendix.

Medical Center of Lewisville

500 West Main Street
Lewisville, TX 75057
(972) 420-1000

Overall patient safety: ★
Teaching: N

CLINICAL PROGRAM RATINGS:

CARDIAC	NR	ORTHOPEDICS	★★★
CRITICAL CARE	★★★	PULMONARY	★★★
GASTROINTESTINAL	★★★	STROKE	★★★
GENERAL SURGERY	★★★	VASCULAR	NR
MATERNITY CARE	★	WOMEN'S HEALTH	NR

HEALTHGRADES AWARDS

The Medical Center of Southeast Texas

3050 39th Street
Port Arthur, TX 77642
(409) 983-4951

Overall patient safety: ★★★
Teaching: N

CLINICAL PROGRAM RATINGS:

CARDIAC	★★★	ORTHOPEDICS	NR
CRITICAL CARE	NR	PULMONARY	★★★
GASTROINTESTINAL	NR	STROKE	★★★
GENERAL SURGERY	NR	VASCULAR	NR
MATERNITY CARE	★★★★★	WOMEN'S HEALTH	★★★

HEALTHGRADES AWARDS

✓ SPECIALTY EXCELLENCE
• MATERNITY CARE

Medical Center of McKinney*

4500 Medical Center Drive
McKinney, TX 75069
(972) 547-8000

Overall patient safety: ★★★
Teaching: N

CLINICAL PROGRAM RATINGS:

CARDIAC	★★★	ORTHOPEDICS	NR
CRITICAL CARE	★★★	PULMONARY	★★★
GASTROINTESTINAL	★★★	STROKE	★★★
GENERAL SURGERY	★★★	VASCULAR	NR
MATERNITY CARE	★★★	WOMEN'S HEALTH	NR

HEALTHGRADES AWARDS

Medina Community Hospital

3100 Avenue East
Hondo, TX 78861
(830) 741-4677

Overall patient safety: ★★★
Teaching: N

CLINICAL PROGRAM RATINGS:

CARDIAC	NR	ORTHOPEDICS	NR
CRITICAL CARE	NR	PULMONARY	★★★
GASTROINTESTINAL	NR	STROKE	NR
GENERAL SURGERY	NR	VASCULAR	NR
MATERNITY CARE	NR	WOMEN'S HEALTH	NR

HEALTHGRADES AWARDS

Medical Center of Plano

3901 West 15th Street
Plano, TX 75075
(972) 596-6800

Overall patient safety: ★★★
Teaching: N

CLINICAL PROGRAM RATINGS:

CARDIAC	★★★	ORTHOPEDICS	NR
CRITICAL CARE	★★★	PULMONARY	★★★
GASTROINTESTINAL	★★★	STROKE	★★★
GENERAL SURGERY	★★★	VASCULAR	NR
MATERNITY CARE	★★★	WOMEN'S HEALTH	★

HEALTHGRADES AWARDS

Memorial Acute Long Term Care Hospital

1201 Frank Street
Suite D-5
Lufkin, TX 75901
(409) 639-7975

Overall patient safety: ★★★
Teaching: N

CLINICAL PROGRAM RATINGS:

CARDIAC	★★★	ORTHOPEDICS	★★★★★
CRITICAL CARE	NR	PULMONARY	★★★
GASTROINTESTINAL	★★★	STROKE	★★★
GENERAL SURGERY	★★★	VASCULAR	NR
MATERNITY CARE	★★★★★	WOMEN'S HEALTH	★★★

HEALTHGRADES AWARDS

✓ SPECIALTY EXCELLENCE
• JOINT REPLACEMENT   • ORTHOPEDIC SURGERY

*This hospital reports its data to the federal government jointly with another hospital. Therefore the ratings and awards apply to multiple hospitals and this specific hospital may not provide all rated services.

Memorial Hermann Baptist Beaumont Hospital

3576 College Street
Beaumont, TX 77701
(409) 388-1411

Overall patient safety: ★★★
Teaching: N

CLINICAL PROGRAM RATINGS:

CARDIAC	★	ORTHOPEDICS	★★★★★
CRITICAL CARE	NR	PULMONARY	★
GASTROINTESTINAL	★★★	STROKE	★
GENERAL SURGERY	★★★	VASCULAR	NR
MATERNITY CARE	★★★	WOMEN'S HEALTH	★

HEALTHGRADES AWARDS

✓ SPECIALTY EXCELLENCE
· JOINT REPLACEMENT   · ORTHOPEDIC SURGERY

Memorial Hermann Katy Hospital

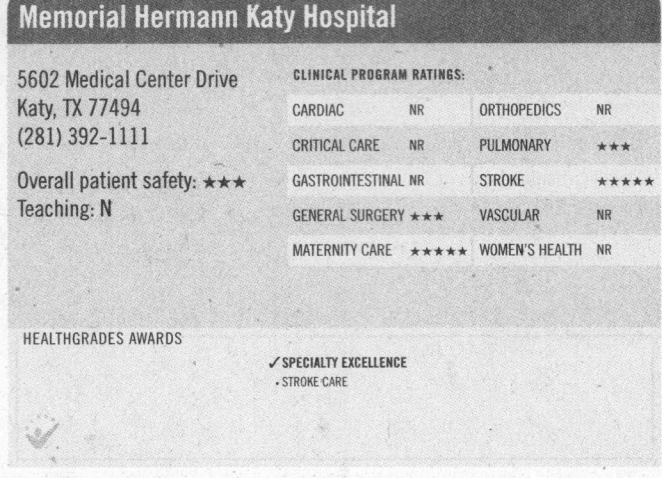

5602 Medical Center Drive
Katy, TX 77494
(281) 392-1111

Overall patient safety: ★★★
Teaching: N

CLINICAL PROGRAM RATINGS:

CARDIAC	NR	ORTHOPEDICS	NR
CRITICAL CARE	NR	PULMONARY	★★★
GASTROINTESTINAL	NR	STROKE	★★★★★
GENERAL SURGERY	★★★	VASCULAR	NR
MATERNITY CARE	★★★★★	WOMEN'S HEALTH	NR

HEALTHGRADES AWARDS

✓ SPECIALTY EXCELLENCE
· STROKE CARE

Memorial Hermann Baptist Orange Hospital

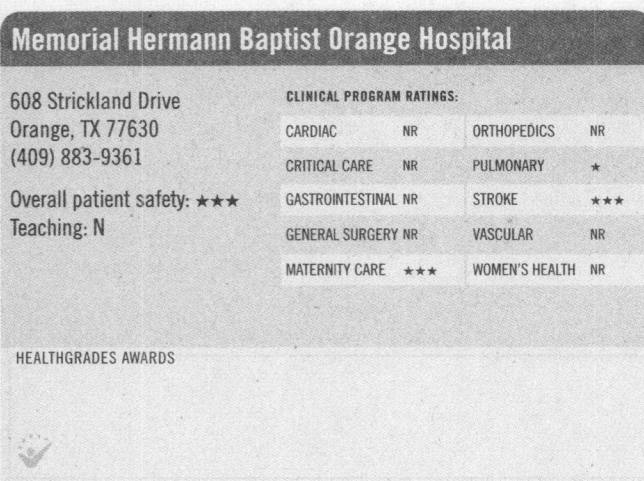

608 Strickland Drive
Orange, TX 77630
(409) 883-9361

Overall patient safety: ★★★
Teaching: N

CLINICAL PROGRAM RATINGS:

CARDIAC	NR	ORTHOPEDICS	NR
CRITICAL CARE	NR	PULMONARY	★
GASTROINTESTINAL	NR	STROKE	★★★
GENERAL SURGERY	NR	VASCULAR	NR
MATERNITY CARE	★★★	WOMEN'S HEALTH	NR

HEALTHGRADES AWARDS

Memorial Hermann Memorial City Medical Center

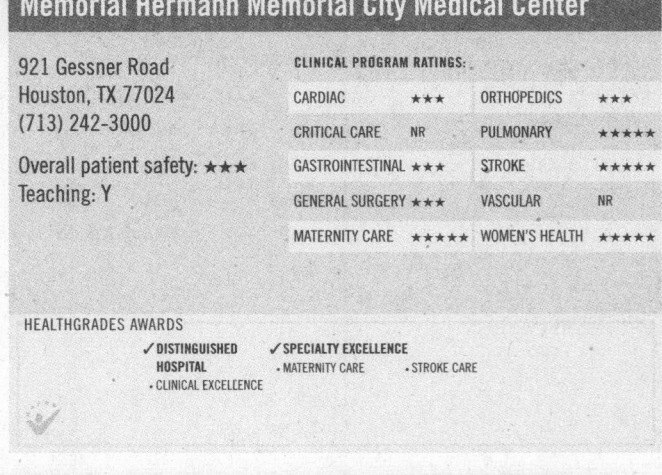

921 Gessner Road
Houston, TX 77024
(713) 242-3000

Overall patient safety: ★★★
Teaching: Y

CLINICAL PROGRAM RATINGS:

CARDIAC	★★★	ORTHOPEDICS	★★★
CRITICAL CARE	NR	PULMONARY	★★★★★
GASTROINTESTINAL	★★★	STROKE	★★★★★
GENERAL SURGERY	★★★	VASCULAR	NR
MATERNITY CARE	★★★★★	WOMEN'S HEALTH	★★★★★

HEALTHGRADES AWARDS

✓ DISTINGUISHED HOSPITAL   ✓ SPECIALTY EXCELLENCE
· CLINICAL EXCELLENCE   · MATERNITY CARE   · STROKE CARE

Memorial Hermann Fort Bend Hospital

3803 FM 1092
Missouri City, TX 77459
(281) 499-4800

Overall patient safety: ★★★
Teaching: N

CLINICAL PROGRAM RATINGS:

CARDIAC	NR	ORTHOPEDICS	NR
CRITICAL CARE	NR	PULMONARY	★★★★★
GASTROINTESTINAL	NR	STROKE	★★★★★
GENERAL SURGERY	NR	VASCULAR	NR
MATERNITY CARE	★★★	WOMEN'S HEALTH	NR

HEALTHGRADES AWARDS

Memorial Hermann Southwest Hospital

7600 Beechnut Street
Houston, TX 77074
(713) 867-2000

Overall patient safety: ★
Teaching: Y

CLINICAL PROGRAM RATINGS:

CARDIAC	★★★	ORTHOPEDICS	★★★
CRITICAL CARE	NR	PULMONARY	★★★★★
GASTROINTESTINAL	★★★	STROKE	★★★★★
GENERAL SURGERY	★★★★★	VASCULAR	★★★
MATERNITY CARE	★★★★★	WOMEN'S HEALTH	★★★★★

HEALTHGRADES AWARDS

✓ DISTINGUISHED HOSPITAL   ✓ SPECIALTY EXCELLENCE
· CLINICAL EXCELLENCE   · GASTROINTESTINAL CARE   · MATERNITY CARE   · STROKE CARE
· GENERAL SURGERY   · PULMONARY CARE   · WOMEN'S HEALTH
· JOINT REPLACEMENT

KEY: ★★★★★ BEST   ★★★ AS EXPECTED   ★ POOR   NR NOT RATED BY HEALTHGRADES   For full definitions of ratings and awards, see Appendix.

TEXAS HOSPITALS: RATINGS BY CLINICAL SPECIALTY

Memorial Hermann–Texas Medical Center

6411 Fannin Street
Houston, TX 77030
(713) 704-4000

Overall patient safety: ★
Teaching: Y

CLINICAL PROGRAM RATINGS:

CARDIAC	★★★	ORTHOPEDICS	★★★
CRITICAL CARE	NR	PULMONARY	★★★
GASTROINTESTINAL	★★★	STROKE	★★★
GENERAL SURGERY	★★★	VASCULAR	★★★
MATERNITY CARE	★	WOMEN'S HEALTH	★

HEALTHGRADES AWARDS

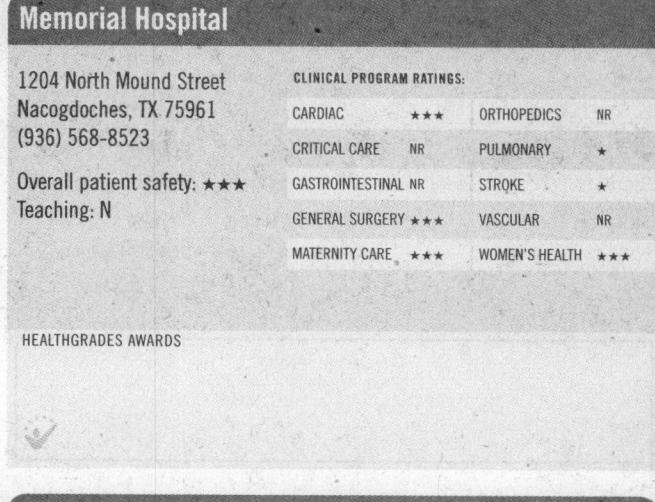

Memorial Hospital

1204 North Mound Street
Nacogdoches, TX 75961
(936) 568-8523

Overall patient safety: ★★★
Teaching: N

CLINICAL PROGRAM RATINGS:

CARDIAC	★★★	ORTHOPEDICS	NR
CRITICAL CARE	NR	PULMONARY	★
GASTROINTESTINAL	NR	STROKE	★
GENERAL SURGERY	★★★	VASCULAR	NR
MATERNITY CARE	★★★	WOMEN'S HEALTH	★★★

HEALTHGRADES AWARDS

Memorial Hospital

224 East 2nd Street
Dumas, TX 79029
(806) 935-7171

Overall patient safety: ★★★
Teaching: N

CLINICAL PROGRAM RATINGS:

CARDIAC	NR	ORTHOPEDICS	NR
CRITICAL CARE	NR	PULMONARY	★★★
GASTROINTESTINAL	NR	STROKE	NR
GENERAL SURGERY	NR	VASCULAR	NR
MATERNITY CARE	★★★	WOMEN'S HEALTH	NR

HEALTHGRADES AWARDS

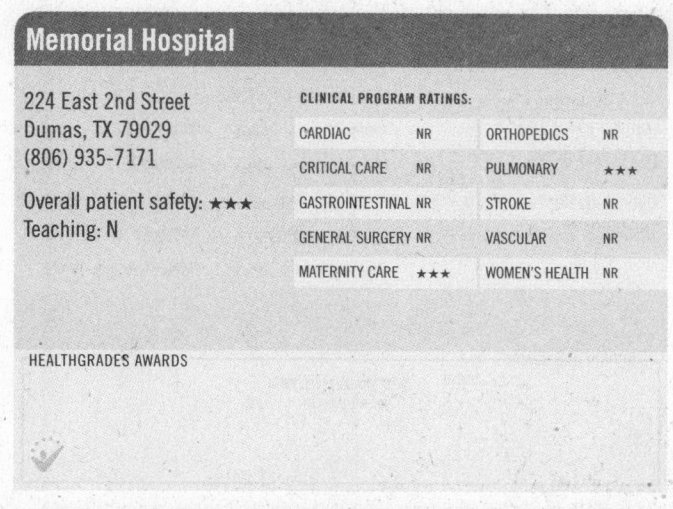

Memorial Hospital

209 Northwest 8th Street
Seminole, TX 79360
(432) 758-4854

Overall patient safety: ★★★
Teaching: N

CLINICAL PROGRAM RATINGS:

CARDIAC	NR	ORTHOPEDICS	NR
CRITICAL CARE	NR	PULMONARY	★★★
GASTROINTESTINAL	NR	STROKE	NR
GENERAL SURGERY	NR	VASCULAR	NR
MATERNITY CARE	NR	WOMEN'S HEALTH	NR

HEALTHGRADES AWARDS

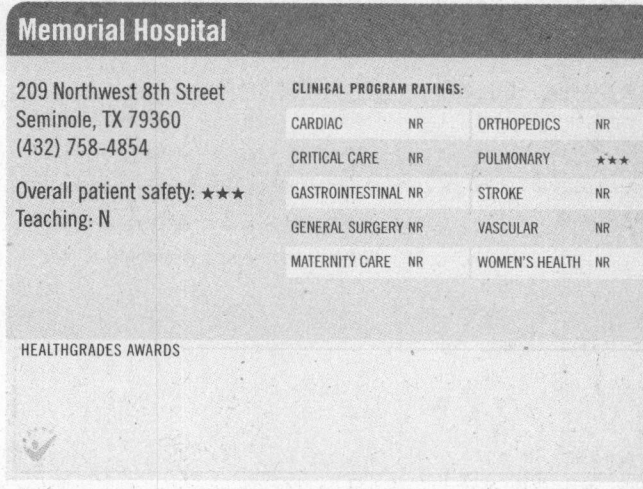

Memorial Hospital

1110 Sara Dewitt Drive
Gonzales, TX 78629
(830) 672-7581

Overall patient safety: ★★★
Teaching: N

CLINICAL PROGRAM RATINGS:

CARDIAC	NR	ORTHOPEDICS	NR
CRITICAL CARE	NR	PULMONARY	★
GASTROINTESTINAL	NR	STROKE	★★★
GENERAL SURGERY	NR	VASCULAR	NR
MATERNITY CARE	NR	WOMEN'S HEALTH	NR

HEALTHGRADES AWARDS

Memorial Medical Center

815 North Virginia Street
Port Lavaca, TX 77979
(361) 552-6713

Overall patient safety: ★★★
Teaching: N

CLINICAL PROGRAM RATINGS:

CARDIAC	NR	ORTHOPEDICS	NR
CRITICAL CARE	NR	PULMONARY	★
GASTROINTESTINAL	NR	STROKE	NR
GENERAL SURGERY	NR	VASCULAR	NR
MATERNITY CARE	NR	WOMEN'S HEALTH	NR

HEALTHGRADES AWARDS

Memorial Medical Center of East Texas

1201 Frank Street
Lufkin, TX 75904
(936) 634-8111

Overall patient safety: ★★★
Teaching: N

CLINICAL PROGRAM RATINGS:

CARDIAC	★★★	ORTHOPEDICS	★★★★★
CRITICAL CARE	NR	PULMONARY	★★★
GASTROINTESTINAL	★★★	STROKE	★★★
GENERAL SURGERY	★★★	VASCULAR	NR
MATERNITY CARE	★★★★★	WOMEN'S HEALTH	★★★

HEALTHGRADES AWARDS

✓ SPECIALTY EXCELLENCE
- JOINT REPLACEMENT   - ORTHOPEDIC SURGERY

Methodist Hospital*

7700 Floyd Curl Drive
San Antonio, TX 78229
(210) 575-4000

Overall patient safety: ★
Teaching: Y

CLINICAL PROGRAM RATINGS:

CARDIAC	★★★	ORTHOPEDICS	★★★
CRITICAL CARE	★★★	PULMONARY	★★★
GASTROINTESTINAL	★★★	STROKE	★★★
GENERAL SURGERY	★★★	VASCULAR	★★★
MATERNITY CARE	★★★★★	WOMEN'S HEALTH	★★★

HEALTHGRADES AWARDS

✓ SPECIALTY EXCELLENCE
- VASCULAR SURGERY

Memorial Medical Center–Livingston

1717 Highway 59 Bypass
Livingston, TX 77351
(936) 329-8700

Overall patient safety: ★★★
Teaching: N

CLINICAL PROGRAM RATINGS:

CARDIAC	NR	ORTHOPEDICS	NR
CRITICAL CARE	NR	PULMONARY	★★★
GASTROINTESTINAL	NR	STROKE	NR
GENERAL SURGERY	★	VASCULAR	NR
MATERNITY CARE	★★★	WOMEN'S HEALTH	NR

HEALTHGRADES AWARDS

Methodist Medical Center

1441 North Beckley Avenue
Dallas, TX 75203
(214) 947-8181

Overall patient safety: ★★★
Teaching: Y

CLINICAL PROGRAM RATINGS:

CARDIAC	★★★	ORTHOPEDICS	★★★
CRITICAL CARE	★★★	PULMONARY	★★★
GASTROINTESTINAL	★★★	STROKE	★★★★★
GENERAL SURGERY	★★★★★	VASCULAR	★★★
MATERNITY CARE	★★★	WOMEN'S HEALTH	★★★

HEALTHGRADES AWARDS

✓ SPECIALTY EXCELLENCE
- GENERAL SURGERY

Methodist Hospital*

6565 Fannin Street
Houston, TX 77030
(713) 790-3311

Overall patient safety: ★
Teaching: Y

CLINICAL PROGRAM RATINGS:

CARDIAC	★★★	ORTHOPEDICS	★★★
CRITICAL CARE	NR	PULMONARY	★★★★★
GASTROINTESTINAL	★★★	STROKE	★★★★★
GENERAL SURGERY	★★★	VASCULAR	★★★
MATERNITY CARE	★★★	WOMEN'S HEALTH	★★★

HEALTHGRADES AWARDS

✓ SPECIALTY EXCELLENCE
- PULMONARY CARE   - STROKE CARE

Methodist Specialty and Transplant Hospital*

8026 Floyd Curl Drive
San Antonio, TX 78229
(210) 575-0355

Overall patient safety: ★
Teaching: Y

CLINICAL PROGRAM RATINGS:

CARDIAC	★★★	ORTHOPEDICS	★★★
CRITICAL CARE	★★★	PULMONARY	★★★
GASTROINTESTINAL	★★★	STROKE	★★★
GENERAL SURGERY	★★★	VASCULAR	★★★
MATERNITY CARE	★★★★★	WOMEN'S HEALTH	★★★

HEALTHGRADES AWARDS

✓ SPECIALTY EXCELLENCE
- VASCULAR SURGERY

KEY: ★★★★★ BEST   ★★★ AS EXPECTED   ★ POOR   NR NOT RATED BY HEALTHGRADES   For full definitions of ratings and awards, see Appendix.

Methodist Sugar Land Hospital

16655 Southwest Freeway
Sugar Land, TX 77479
(281) 274-8000

Overall patient safety: ★★★
Teaching: N

CLINICAL PROGRAM RATINGS:

CARDIAC	NR	ORTHOPEDICS	NR
CRITICAL CARE	NR	PULMONARY	★★★
GASTROINTESTINAL	★★★	STROKE	NR
GENERAL SURGERY	★★★	VASCULAR	NR
MATERNITY CARE	★★★	WOMEN'S HEALTH	NR

HEALTHGRADES AWARDS

Metropolitan Methodist Hospital*

1310 McCullough
San Antonio, TX 78212
(210) 208-2200

Overall patient safety: ★
Teaching: Y

CLINICAL PROGRAM RATINGS:

CARDIAC	★★★	ORTHOPEDICS	★★★
CRITICAL CARE	★★★	PULMONARY	★★★
GASTROINTESTINAL	★★★	STROKE	★★★
GENERAL SURGERY	★★★	VASCULAR	★★★
MATERNITY CARE	★★★★★	WOMEN'S HEALTH	★★★

HEALTHGRADES AWARDS

✓ **SPECIALTY EXCELLENCE**
- VASCULAR SURGERY

Methodist Willowbrook Hospital

18220 Tomball Parkway
Houston, TX 77070
(281) 477-1000

Overall patient safety: ★★★
Teaching: N

CLINICAL PROGRAM RATINGS:

CARDIAC	NR	ORTHOPEDICS	★★★
CRITICAL CARE	NR	PULMONARY	★★★
GASTROINTESTINAL	NR	STROKE	★★★★★
GENERAL SURGERY	★★★	VASCULAR	NR
MATERNITY CARE	★★★	WOMEN'S HEALTH	NR

HEALTHGRADES AWARDS

Midland Memorial Hospital*

2200 West Illinois Avenue
Midland, TX 79701
(432) 685-1111

Overall patient safety: ★★★
Teaching: Y

CLINICAL PROGRAM RATINGS:

CARDIAC	★★★	ORTHOPEDICS	★★★★★
CRITICAL CARE	NR	PULMONARY	★
GASTROINTESTINAL	★★★	STROKE	★
GENERAL SURGERY	★★★	VASCULAR	★★★
MATERNITY CARE	★★★	WOMEN'S HEALTH	★★★

HEALTHGRADES AWARDS

✓ **SPECIALTY EXCELLENCE**
- ORTHOPEDIC SURGERY

Metroplex Hospital

2201 South Clear Creek Road
Killeen, TX 76542
(254) 526-7523

Overall patient safety: ★★★
Teaching: N

CLINICAL PROGRAM RATINGS:

CARDIAC	NR	ORTHOPEDICS	NR
CRITICAL CARE	NR	PULMONARY	★★★
GASTROINTESTINAL	NR	STROKE	★★★
GENERAL SURGERY	★★★	VASCULAR	NR
MATERNITY CARE	★★★	WOMEN'S HEALTH	NR

HEALTHGRADES AWARDS

Mission Regional Medical Center

900 South Bryan Road
Mission, TX 78572
(956) 580-9000

Overall patient safety: ★
Teaching: N

CLINICAL PROGRAM RATINGS:

CARDIAC	NR	ORTHOPEDICS	NR
CRITICAL CARE	NR	PULMONARY	★★★★★
GASTROINTESTINAL	★★★	STROKE	★★★
GENERAL SURGERY	★★★	VASCULAR	NR
MATERNITY CARE	★★★★★	WOMEN'S HEALTH	NR

HEALTHGRADES AWARDS

✓ **SPECIALTY EXCELLENCE**
- MATERNITY CARE   - PULMONARY CARE

*This hospital reports its data to the federal government jointly with another hospital. Therefore the ratings and awards apply to multiple hospitals and this specific hospital may not provide all rated services.

Mitchell County Hospital

997 West I-20
Colorado City, TX 79512
(325) 728-3431

Overall patient safety: ★★★
Teaching: N

CLINICAL PROGRAM RATINGS:

CARDIAC	NR	ORTHOPEDICS	NR
CRITICAL CARE	NR	PULMONARY	★
GASTROINTESTINAL	NR	STROKE	NR
GENERAL SURGERY	NR	VASCULAR	NR
MATERNITY CARE	NR	WOMEN'S HEALTH	NR

HEALTHGRADES AWARDS

Muleshoe Area Medical Center

708 South 1st Street
Muleshoe, TX 79347
(806) 272-4524

Overall patient safety: ★★★
Teaching: N

CLINICAL PROGRAM RATINGS:

CARDIAC	NR	ORTHOPEDICS	NR
CRITICAL CARE	NR	PULMONARY	★★★
GASTROINTESTINAL	NR	STROKE	NR
GENERAL SURGERY	NR	VASCULAR	NR
MATERNITY CARE	NR	WOMEN'S HEALTH	NR

HEALTHGRADES AWARDS

Mother Frances Hospital—Jacksonville

2026 South Jackson Street
Jacksonville, TX 75766
(903) 541-4500

Overall patient safety: ★★★
Teaching: N

CLINICAL PROGRAM RATINGS:

CARDIAC	NR	ORTHOPEDICS	NR
CRITICAL CARE	NR	PULMONARY	★★★
GASTROINTESTINAL	NR	STROKE	NR
GENERAL SURGERY	NR	VASCULAR	NR
MATERNITY CARE	NR	WOMEN'S HEALTH	NR

HEALTHGRADES AWARDS

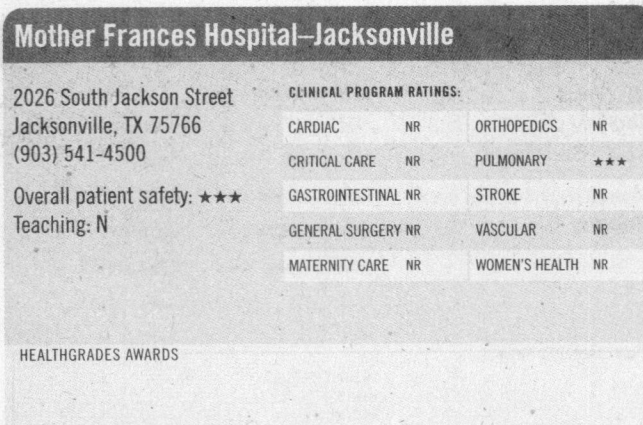

Nacogdoches Medical Center

4920 North East Stallings Drive
Nacogdoches, TX 75965
(936) 569-9481

Overall patient safety: ★★★
Teaching: N

CLINICAL PROGRAM RATINGS:

CARDIAC	★★★	ORTHOPEDICS	NR
CRITICAL CARE	★★★	PULMONARY	★
GASTROINTESTINAL	★★★	STROKE	★★★
GENERAL SURGERY	★★★	VASCULAR	NR
MATERNITY CARE	★	WOMEN'S HEALTH	★

HEALTHGRADES AWARDS

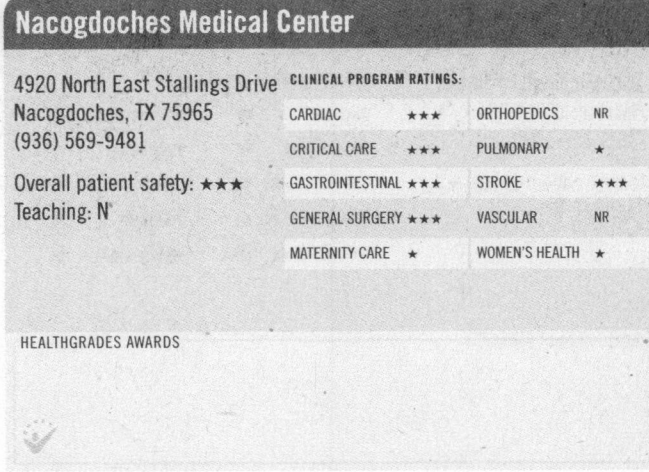

Mother Frances Hospital—Tyler

800 East Dawson Street
Tyler, TX 75701
(903) 593-8441

Overall patient safety: ★★★★★
Teaching: Y

CLINICAL PROGRAM RATINGS:

CARDIAC	★★★	ORTHOPEDICS	★★★
CRITICAL CARE	NR	PULMONARY	★★★
GASTROINTESTINAL	★★★	STROKE	★★★★★
GENERAL SURGERY	★★★★★	VASCULAR	★★★
MATERNITY CARE	★★★	WOMEN'S HEALTH	★★★

HEALTHGRADES AWARDS

✓ **DISTINGUISHED HOSPITAL** · PATIENT SAFETY

✓ **SPECIALTY EXCELLENCE** · GASTROINTESTINAL CARE · GENERAL SURGERY · STROKE CARE

Navarro Regional Hospital

3201 West Highway 22
Corsicana, TX 75110
(903) 654-6800

Overall patient safety: ★★★
Teaching: N

CLINICAL PROGRAM RATINGS:

CARDIAC	NR	ORTHOPEDICS	NR
CRITICAL CARE	NR	PULMONARY	★
GASTROINTESTINAL	NR	STROKE	★★★
GENERAL SURGERY	★★★	VASCULAR	NR
MATERNITY CARE	★	WOMEN'S HEALTH	NR

HEALTHGRADES AWARDS

KEY: ★★★★★ BEST   ★★★ AS EXPECTED   ★ POOR   NR NOT RATED BY HEALTHGRADES   For full definitions of ratings and awards, see Appendix.

Nix Health Care System

414 Navarro Street
San Antonio, TX 78205
(210) 271-1800

Overall patient safety: ★★★
Teaching: N

CLINICAL PROGRAM RATINGS:

CARDIAC	NR	ORTHOPEDICS	NR
CRITICAL CARE	NR	PULMONARY	★★★
GASTROINTESTINAL	NR	STROKE	★★★
GENERAL SURGERY	★★★	VASCULAR	NR
MATERNITY CARE	★★★	WOMEN'S HEALTH	NR

HEALTHGRADES AWARDS

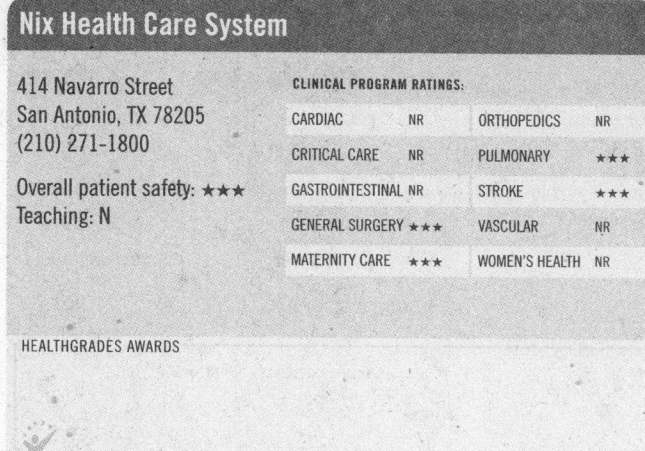

North Bay Hospital

1711 West Wheeler Avenue
Aransas Pass, TX 78336
(361) 758-8585

Overall patient safety: ★★★
Teaching: N

CLINICAL PROGRAM RATINGS:

CARDIAC	NR	ORTHOPEDICS	NR
CRITICAL CARE	NR	PULMONARY	★★★
GASTROINTESTINAL	NR	STROKE	★★★
GENERAL SURGERY	NR	VASCULAR	NR
MATERNITY CARE	NR	WOMEN'S HEALTH	NR

HEALTHGRADES AWARDS

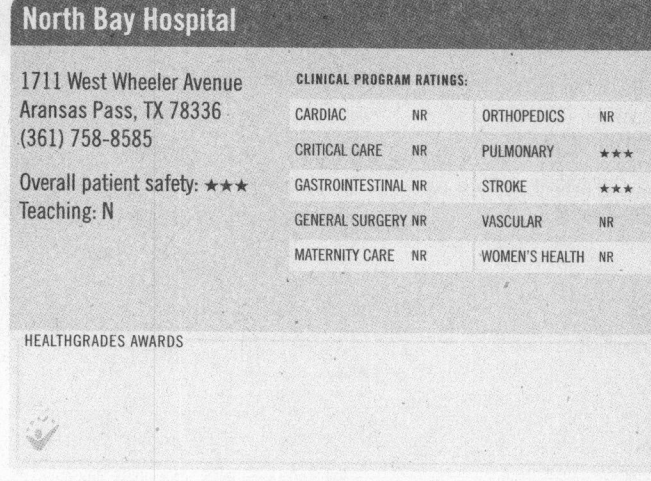

Nocona General Hospital

100 Park Road
Nocona, TX 76255
(940) 825-3235

Overall patient safety: ★★★
Teaching: N

CLINICAL PROGRAM RATINGS:

CARDIAC	NR	ORTHOPEDICS	NR
CRITICAL CARE	NR	PULMONARY	★★★
GASTROINTESTINAL	NR	STROKE	★
GENERAL SURGERY	NR	VASCULAR	NR
MATERNITY CARE	NR	WOMEN'S HEALTH	NR

HEALTHGRADES AWARDS

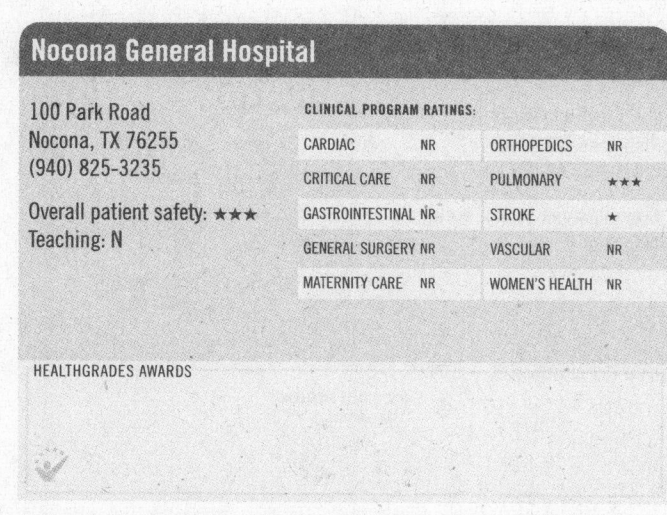

North Hills Hospital

4401 Booth Calloway Road
North Richland Hills, TX 76180
(817) 255-1000

Overall patient safety: ★★★
Teaching: N

CLINICAL PROGRAM RATINGS:

CARDIAC	★★★	ORTHOPEDICS	NR
CRITICAL CARE	★	PULMONARY	★★★
GASTROINTESTINAL	★★★	STROKE	★★★
GENERAL SURGERY	★★★	VASCULAR	NR
MATERNITY CARE	★★★	WOMEN'S HEALTH	★

HEALTHGRADES AWARDS

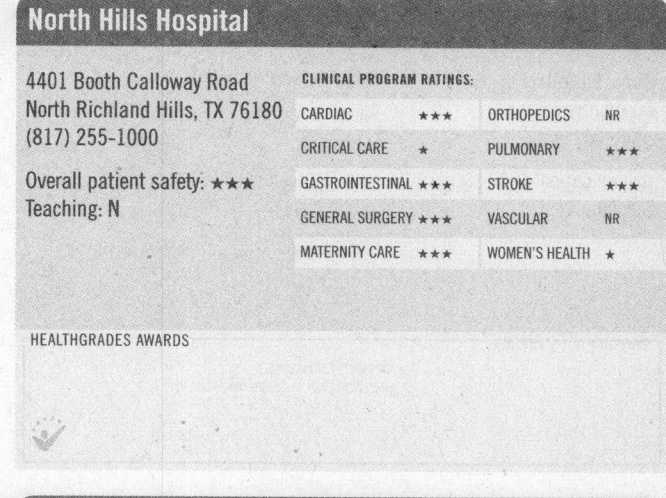

North Austin Medical Center

12221 Mopac Expressway North
Austin, TX 78758
(512) 901-1000

Overall patient safety: ★★★
Teaching: Y

CLINICAL PROGRAM RATINGS:

CARDIAC	★★★	ORTHOPEDICS	★★★
CRITICAL CARE	★★★	PULMONARY	★★★
GASTROINTESTINAL	★★★	STROKE	★★★
GENERAL SURGERY	★★★	VASCULAR	NR
MATERNITY CARE	★★★★★	WOMEN'S HEALTH	★★★

HEALTHGRADES AWARDS

✓ SPECIALTY EXCELLENCE
- MATERNITY CARE

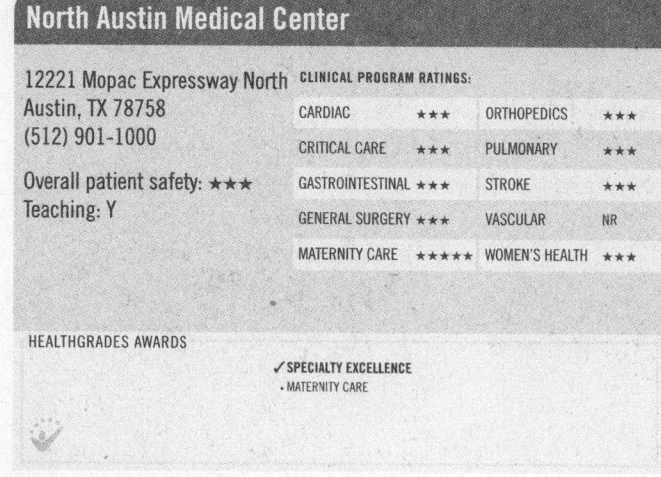

North Texas Medical Center

1900 Hospital Boulevard
Gainesville, TX 76240
(940) 665-1751

Overall patient safety: ★★★
Teaching: N

CLINICAL PROGRAM RATINGS:

CARDIAC	NR	ORTHOPEDICS	NR
CRITICAL CARE	NR	PULMONARY	★★★
GASTROINTESTINAL	NR	STROKE	★★★
GENERAL SURGERY	NR	VASCULAR	NR
MATERNITY CARE	NR	WOMEN'S HEALTH	NR

HEALTHGRADES AWARDS

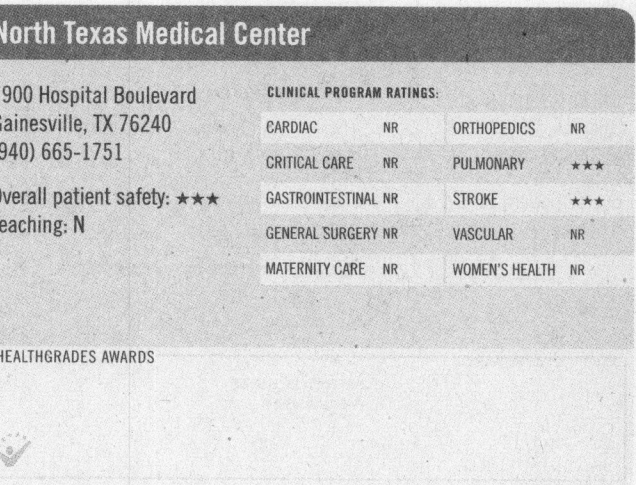

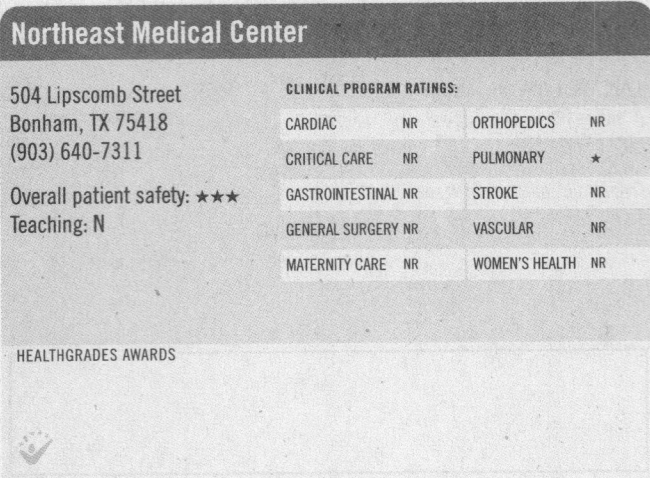

Northeast Medical Center

504 Lipscomb Street
Bonham, TX 75418
(903) 640-7311

Overall patient safety: ★★★
Teaching: N

CLINICAL PROGRAM RATINGS:

CARDIAC	NR	ORTHOPEDICS	NR
CRITICAL CARE	NR	PULMONARY	★
GASTROINTESTINAL	NR	STROKE	NR
GENERAL SURGERY	NR	VASCULAR	NR
MATERNITY CARE	NR	WOMEN'S HEALTH	NR

HEALTHGRADES AWARDS

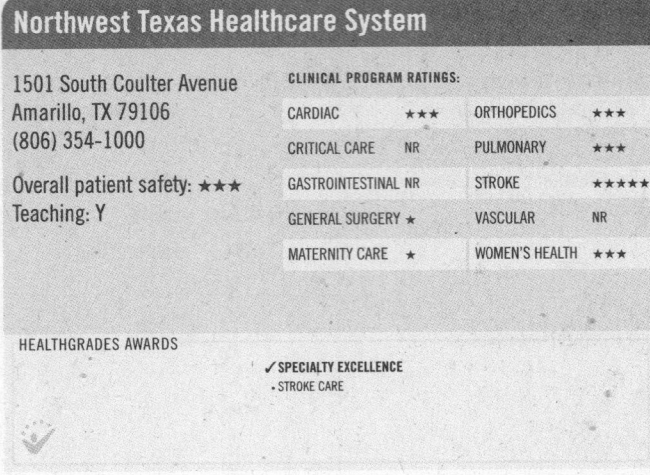

Northwest Texas Healthcare System

1501 South Coulter Avenue
Amarillo, TX 79106
(806) 354-1000

Overall patient safety: ★★★
Teaching: Y

CLINICAL PROGRAM RATINGS:

CARDIAC	★★★	ORTHOPEDICS	★★★
CRITICAL CARE	NR	PULMONARY	★★★
GASTROINTESTINAL	NR	STROKE	★★★★★
GENERAL SURGERY	★	VASCULAR	NR
MATERNITY CARE	★	WOMEN'S HEALTH	★★★

HEALTHGRADES AWARDS

✓ SPECIALTY EXCELLENCE
• STROKE CARE

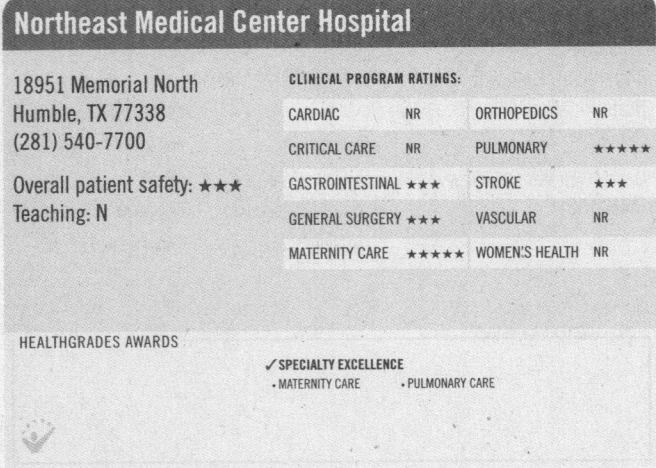

Northeast Medical Center Hospital

18951 Memorial North
Humble, TX 77338
(281) 540-7700

Overall patient safety: ★★★
Teaching: N

CLINICAL PROGRAM RATINGS:

CARDIAC	NR	ORTHOPEDICS	NR
CRITICAL CARE	NR	PULMONARY	★★★★★
GASTROINTESTINAL	★★★	STROKE	★★★
GENERAL SURGERY	★★★	VASCULAR	NR
MATERNITY CARE	★★★★★	WOMEN'S HEALTH	NR

HEALTHGRADES AWARDS

✓ SPECIALTY EXCELLENCE
• MATERNITY CARE   • PULMONARY CARE

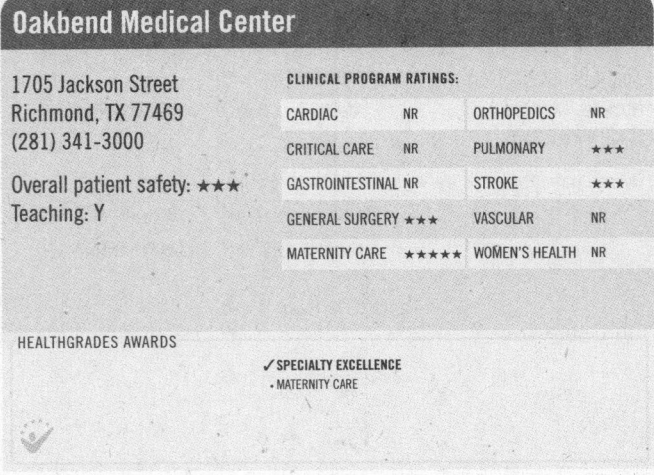

Oakbend Medical Center

1705 Jackson Street
Richmond, TX 77469
(281) 341-3000

Overall patient safety: ★★★
Teaching: Y

CLINICAL PROGRAM RATINGS:

CARDIAC	NR	ORTHOPEDICS	NR
CRITICAL CARE	NR	PULMONARY	★★★
GASTROINTESTINAL	NR	STROKE	★★★
GENERAL SURGERY	★★★	VASCULAR	NR
MATERNITY CARE	★★★★★	WOMEN'S HEALTH	NR

HEALTHGRADES AWARDS

✓ SPECIALTY EXCELLENCE
• MATERNITY CARE

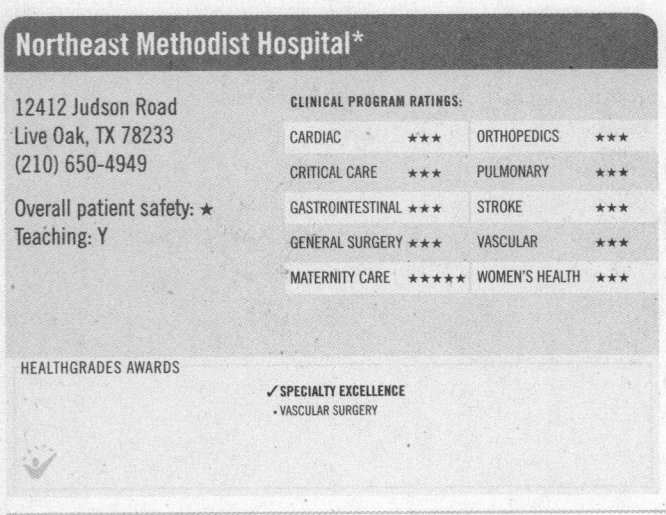

Northeast Methodist Hospital*

12412 Judson Road
Live Oak, TX 78233
(210) 650-4949

Overall patient safety: ★
Teaching: Y

CLINICAL PROGRAM RATINGS:

CARDIAC	★★★	ORTHOPEDICS	★★★
CRITICAL CARE	★★★	PULMONARY	★★★
GASTROINTESTINAL	★★★	STROKE	★★★
GENERAL SURGERY	★★★	VASCULAR	★★★
MATERNITY CARE	★★★★★	WOMEN'S HEALTH	★★★

HEALTHGRADES AWARDS

✓ SPECIALTY EXCELLENCE
• VASCULAR SURGERY

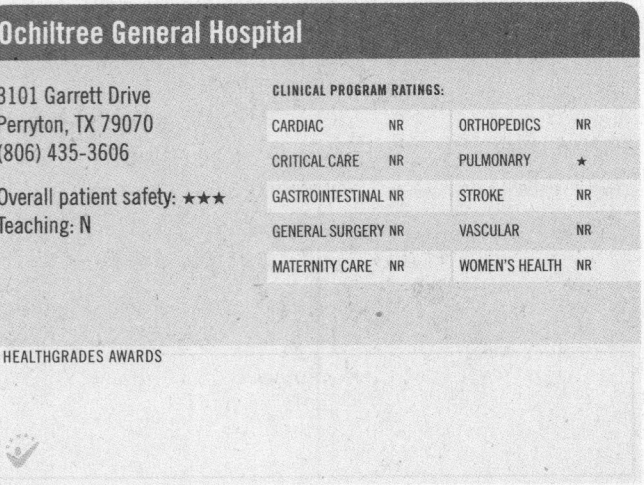

Ochiltree General Hospital

3101 Garrett Drive
Perryton, TX 79070
(806) 435-3606

Overall patient safety: ★★★
Teaching: N

CLINICAL PROGRAM RATINGS:

CARDIAC	NR	ORTHOPEDICS	NR
CRITICAL CARE	NR	PULMONARY	★
GASTROINTESTINAL	NR	STROKE	NR
GENERAL SURGERY	NR	VASCULAR	NR
MATERNITY CARE	NR	WOMEN'S HEALTH	NR

HEALTHGRADES AWARDS

KEY: ★★★★★ BEST   ★★★ AS EXPECTED   ★ POOR   NR NOT RATED BY HEALTHGRADES   For full definitions of ratings and awards, see Appendix.

Odessa Regional Medical Center

520 East 6th Street
Odessa, TX 79761
(432) 334-8200

Overall patient safety: ★★★
Teaching: N

CLINICAL PROGRAM RATINGS:

CARDIAC	NR	ORTHOPEDICS	NR
CRITICAL CARE	NR	PULMONARY	★★★
GASTROINTESTINAL	NR	STROKE	NR
GENERAL SURGERY	NR	VASCULAR	NR
MATERNITY CARE	★★★★★	WOMEN'S HEALTH	NR

HEALTHGRADES AWARDS

Palo Pinto General Hospital

400 Southwest 25th Avenue
Mineral Wells, TX 76067
(940) 325-7891

Overall patient safety: ★★★
Teaching: N

CLINICAL PROGRAM RATINGS:

CARDIAC	NR	ORTHOPEDICS	NR
CRITICAL CARE	NR	PULMONARY	★
GASTROINTESTINAL	NR	STROKE	★★★
GENERAL SURGERY	NR	VASCULAR	NR
MATERNITY CARE	★★★	WOMEN'S HEALTH	NR

HEALTHGRADES AWARDS

Otto Kaiser Memorial Hospital

3349 South Highway 181
Kenedy, TX 78119
(830) 583-3401

Overall patient safety: ★★★
Teaching: N

CLINICAL PROGRAM RATINGS:

CARDIAC	NR	ORTHOPEDICS	NR
CRITICAL CARE	NR	PULMONARY	★
GASTROINTESTINAL	NR	STROKE	NR
GENERAL SURGERY	NR	VASCULAR	NR
MATERNITY CARE	NR	WOMEN'S HEALTH	NR

HEALTHGRADES AWARDS

Pampa Regional Medical Center

1 Medical Plaza
Pampa, TX 79065
(806) 665-3721

Overall patient safety: ★★★
Teaching: N

CLINICAL PROGRAM RATINGS:

CARDIAC	NR	ORTHOPEDICS	NR
CRITICAL CARE	NR	PULMONARY	★★★
GASTROINTESTINAL	NR	STROKE	★★★
GENERAL SURGERY	NR	VASCULAR	NR
MATERNITY CARE	★	WOMEN'S HEALTH	NR

HEALTHGRADES AWARDS

Palestine Regional Medical Center

2900 South Loop 256
Palestine, TX 75801
(903) 731-1000

Overall patient safety: ★★★
Teaching: N

CLINICAL PROGRAM RATINGS:

CARDIAC	NR	ORTHOPEDICS	NR
CRITICAL CARE	NR	PULMONARY	★
GASTROINTESTINAL	★★★	STROKE	★
GENERAL SURGERY	★★★	VASCULAR	NR
MATERNITY CARE	★	WOMEN'S HEALTH	NR

HEALTHGRADES AWARDS

Paris Regional Medical Center

820 Clarksville Street
Paris, TX 75460
(903) 785-4521

Overall patient safety: ★★★
Teaching: N

CLINICAL PROGRAM RATINGS:

CARDIAC	★	ORTHOPEDICS	★★★
CRITICAL CARE	NR	PULMONARY	★
GASTROINTESTINAL	★★★	STROKE	★★★
GENERAL SURGERY	★★★	VASCULAR	NR
MATERNITY CARE	NR	WOMEN'S HEALTH	NR

HEALTHGRADES AWARDS

*This hospital reports its data to the federal government jointly with another hospital. Therefore the ratings and awards apply to multiple hospitals and this specific hospital may not provide all rated services.

Park Plaza Hospital and Medical Center

1313 Herman Drive
Houston, TX 77004
(713) 527-5000

Overall patient safety: ★
Teaching: Y

CLINICAL PROGRAM RATINGS:

CARDIAC	NR	ORTHOPEDICS	★★★
CRITICAL CARE	★★★	PULMONARY	★★★
GASTROINTESTINAL	★★★	STROKE	★★★
GENERAL SURGERY	★★★	VASCULAR	NR
MATERNITY CARE	★★★★★	WOMEN'S HEALTH	NR

HEALTHGRADES AWARDS

✓ SPECIALTY EXCELLENCE
· MATERNITY CARE

Pecos County Memorial Hospital

387 West Highway 10
Fort Stockton, TX 79735
(432) 336-2241

Overall patient safety: ★★★
Teaching: N

CLINICAL PROGRAM RATINGS:

CARDIAC	NR	ORTHOPEDICS	NR
CRITICAL CARE	NR	PULMONARY	★
GASTROINTESTINAL	NR	STROKE	NR
GENERAL SURGERY	NR	VASCULAR	NR
MATERNITY CARE	NR	WOMEN'S HEALTH	NR

HEALTHGRADES AWARDS

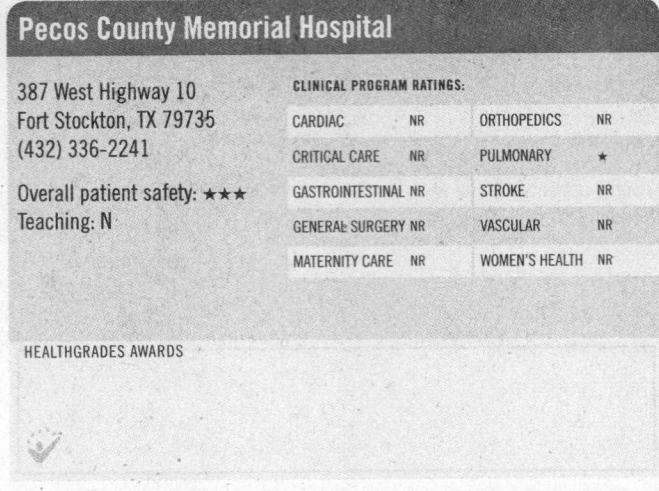

Parkland Health and Hospital System

5201 Harry Hines Boulevard
Dallas, TX 75235
(214) 590-8000

Overall patient safety: ★
Teaching: Y

CLINICAL PROGRAM RATINGS:

CARDIAC	NR	ORTHOPEDICS	NR
CRITICAL CARE	NR	PULMONARY	★★★
GASTROINTESTINAL	NR	STROKE	★★★
GENERAL SURGERY	★	VASCULAR	NR
MATERNITY CARE	★	WOMEN'S HEALTH	NR

HEALTHGRADES AWARDS

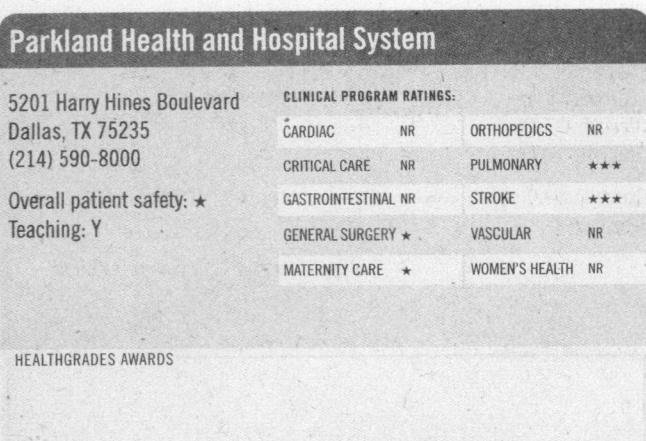

Permian Regional Medical Center

720 Hospital Drive
Andrews, TX 79714
(432) 523-2200

Overall patient safety: ★★★
Teaching: N

CLINICAL PROGRAM RATINGS:

CARDIAC	NR	ORTHOPEDICS	NR
CRITICAL CARE	NR	PULMONARY	★★★
GASTROINTESTINAL	NR	STROKE	NR
GENERAL SURGERY	NR	VASCULAR	NR
MATERNITY CARE	NR	WOMEN'S HEALTH	NR

HEALTHGRADES AWARDS

Parkview Regional Hospital

600 South Bonham Street
Mexia, TX 76667
(254) 562-5332

Overall patient safety: ★★★★★
Teaching: N

CLINICAL PROGRAM RATINGS:

CARDIAC	NR	ORTHOPEDICS	NR
CRITICAL CARE	NR	PULMONARY	★★★
GASTROINTESTINAL	NR	STROKE	★★★★★
GENERAL SURGERY	NR	VASCULAR	NR
MATERNITY CARE	NR	WOMEN'S HEALTH	NR

HEALTHGRADES AWARDS

✓ SPECIALTY EXCELLENCE
· STROKE CARE

Physicians Specialty Hospital of El Paso

1416 George Dieter
El Paso, TX 79936
(915) 598-4240

Overall patient safety: ★★★
Teaching: N

CLINICAL PROGRAM RATINGS:

CARDIAC	NR	ORTHOPEDICS	NR
CRITICAL CARE	NR	PULMONARY	★★★★★
GASTROINTESTINAL	NR	STROKE	NR
GENERAL SURGERY	NR	VASCULAR	NR
MATERNITY CARE	NR	WOMEN'S HEALTH	NR

HEALTHGRADES AWARDS

KEY: ★★★★★ BEST   ★★★ AS EXPECTED   ★ POOR   NR NOT RATED BY HEALTHGRADES   For full definitions of ratings and awards, see Appendix.

Plaza Medical Center of Fort Worth

900 Eighth Avenue
Fort Worth, TX 76104
(817) 336-2100

Overall patient safety: ★★★
Teaching: Y

CLINICAL PROGRAM RATINGS:

CARDIAC	★	ORTHOPEDICS	★★★
CRITICAL CARE	★★★	PULMONARY	★★★
GASTROINTESTINAL	★★★	STROKE	★★★
GENERAL SURGERY	★★★	VASCULAR	★★★
MATERNITY CARE	NR	WOMEN'S HEALTH	NR

HEALTHGRADES AWARDS

Presbyterian Hospital of Denton

207 North Bonnie Brae Street
Denton, TX 76201
(940) 898-7000

Overall patient safety: ★★★
Teaching: N

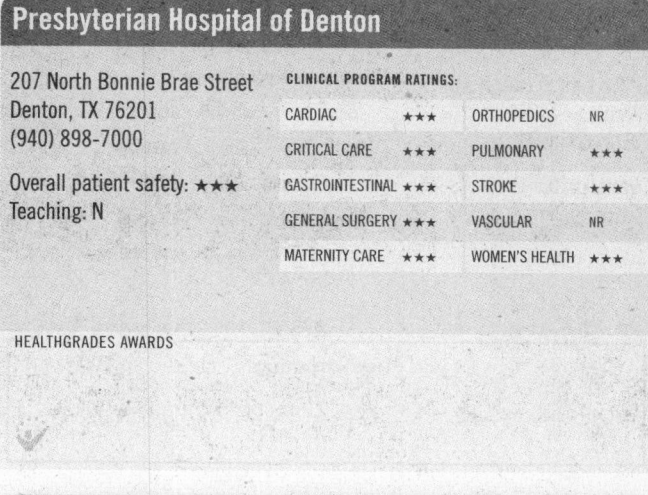

CLINICAL PROGRAM RATINGS:

CARDIAC	★★★	ORTHOPEDICS	NR
CRITICAL CARE	★★★	PULMONARY	★★★
GASTROINTESTINAL	★★★	STROKE	★★★
GENERAL SURGERY	★★★	VASCULAR	NR
MATERNITY CARE	★★★	WOMEN'S HEALTH	★★★

HEALTHGRADES AWARDS

Presbyterian Hospital of Allen

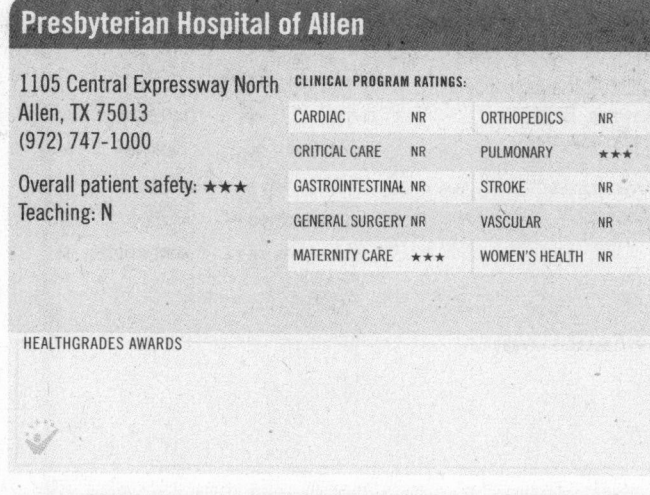

1105 Central Expressway North
Allen, TX 75013
(972) 747-1000

Overall patient safety: ★★★
Teaching: N

CLINICAL PROGRAM RATINGS:

CARDIAC	NR	ORTHOPEDICS	NR
CRITICAL CARE	NR	PULMONARY	★★★
GASTROINTESTINAL	NR	STROKE	NR
GENERAL SURGERY	NR	VASCULAR	NR
MATERNITY CARE	★★★	WOMEN'S HEALTH	NR

HEALTHGRADES AWARDS

Presbyterian Hospital of Greenville

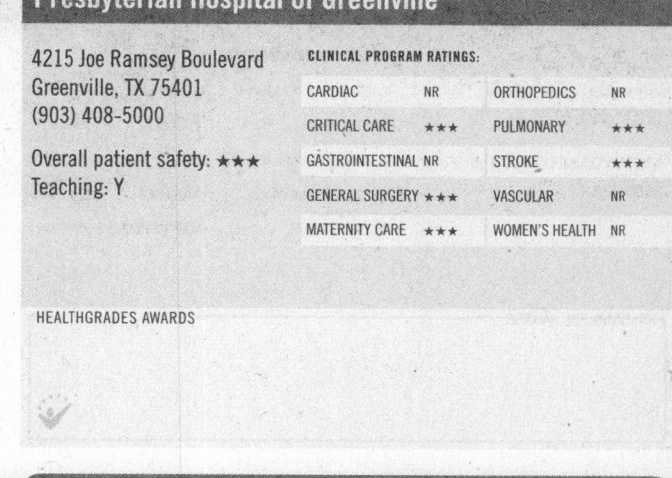

4215 Joe Ramsey Boulevard
Greenville, TX 75401
(903) 408-5000

Overall patient safety: ★★★
Teaching: Y

CLINICAL PROGRAM RATINGS:

CARDIAC	NR	ORTHOPEDICS	NR
CRITICAL CARE	★★★	PULMONARY	★★★
GASTROINTESTINAL	NR	STROKE	★★★
GENERAL SURGERY	★★★	VASCULAR	NR
MATERNITY CARE	★★★	WOMEN'S HEALTH	NR

HEALTHGRADES AWARDS

Presbyterian Hospital of Dallas

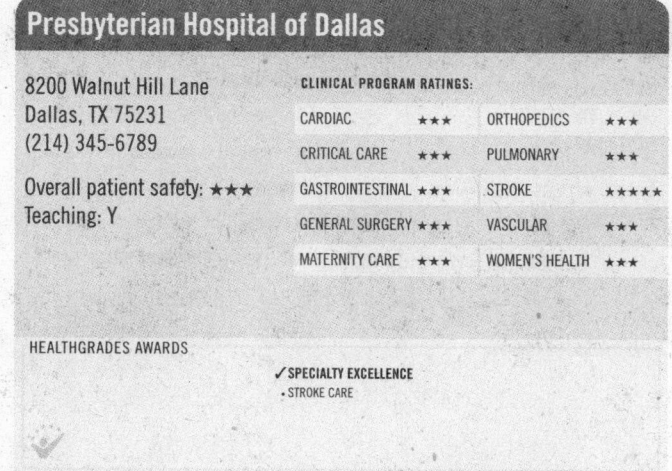

8200 Walnut Hill Lane
Dallas, TX 75231
(214) 345-6789

Overall patient safety: ★★★
Teaching: Y

CLINICAL PROGRAM RATINGS:

CARDIAC	★★★	ORTHOPEDICS	★★★
CRITICAL CARE	★★★	PULMONARY	★★★
GASTROINTESTINAL	★★★	STROKE	★★★★★
GENERAL SURGERY	★★★	VASCULAR	★★★
MATERNITY CARE	★★★	WOMEN'S HEALTH	★★★

HEALTHGRADES AWARDS

✓ SPECIALTY EXCELLENCE
• STROKE CARE

Presbyterian Hospital of Kaufman

850 Highway 243 West
Kaufman, TX 75142
(972) 932-7200

Overall patient safety: ★★★
Teaching: N

CLINICAL PROGRAM RATINGS:

CARDIAC	NR	ORTHOPEDICS	NR
CRITICAL CARE	NR	PULMONARY	★
GASTROINTESTINAL	NR	STROKE	★
GENERAL SURGERY	★★★	VASCULAR	NR
MATERNITY CARE	★★★	WOMEN'S HEALTH	NR

HEALTHGRADES AWARDS

Presbyterian Hospital of Plano

6200 West Parker Road
Plano, TX 75093
(972) 608-8000

Overall patient safety: ★★★
Teaching: N

CLINICAL PROGRAM RATINGS:

CARDIAC	★★★	ORTHOPEDICS	★★★★★
CRITICAL CARE	★★★	PULMONARY	★★★
GASTROINTESTINAL	★★★	STROKE	★★★
GENERAL SURGERY	★★★	VASCULAR	NR
MATERNITY CARE	★★★	WOMEN'S HEALTH	★★★

HEALTHGRADES AWARDS

✓ SPECIALTY EXCELLENCE
· JOINT REPLACEMENT · ORTHOPEDIC SURGERY

Providence Memorial Hospital

2001 North Oregon Street
El Paso, TX 79902
(915) 577-6011

Overall patient safety: ★
Teaching: Y

CLINICAL PROGRAM RATINGS:

CARDIAC	★★★	ORTHOPEDICS	★★★
CRITICAL CARE	★★★★★	PULMONARY	★★★
GASTROINTESTINAL	★★★	STROKE	★★★
GENERAL SURGERY	★★★	VASCULAR	NR
MATERNITY CARE	★★★★★	WOMEN'S HEALTH	★★★

HEALTHGRADES AWARDS

✓ SPECIALTY EXCELLENCE
· CRITICAL CARE · MATERNITY CARE

Presbyterian Hospital of Winnsboro

719 West Coke Road
Winnsboro, TX 75494
(903) 342-5227

Overall patient safety: ★★★★★
Teaching: N

CLINICAL PROGRAM RATINGS:

CARDIAC	NR	ORTHOPEDICS	NR
CRITICAL CARE	NR	PULMONARY	★★★
GASTROINTESTINAL	NR	STROKE	★
GENERAL SURGERY	NR	VASCULAR	NR
MATERNITY CARE	NR	WOMEN'S HEALTH	NR

HEALTHGRADES AWARDS

R. E. Thomason General Hospital

4815 Alameda Avenue
El Paso, TX 79905
(915) 544-1200

Overall patient safety: ★★★
Teaching: Y

CLINICAL PROGRAM RATINGS:

CARDIAC	NR	ORTHOPEDICS	NR
CRITICAL CARE	NR	PULMONARY	★★★
GASTROINTESTINAL	★★★	STROKE	★★★
GENERAL SURGERY	★★★	VASCULAR	NR
MATERNITY CARE	★★★	WOMEN'S HEALTH	NR

HEALTHGRADES AWARDS

Providence Healthcare Network

6901 Medical Parkway
Waco, TX 76712
(254) 751-4000

Overall patient safety: ★★★★★
Teaching: Y

CLINICAL PROGRAM RATINGS:

CARDIAC	★★★	ORTHOPEDICS	★★★★★
CRITICAL CARE	NR	PULMONARY	★★★
GASTROINTESTINAL	★★★	STROKE	★★★
GENERAL SURGERY	★★★	VASCULAR	★★★
MATERNITY CARE	★★★	WOMEN'S HEALTH	★★★

HEALTHGRADES AWARDS

✓ DISTINGUISHED HOSPITAL
· PATIENT SAFETY

✓ SPECIALTY EXCELLENCE
· JOINT REPLACEMENT · ORTHOPEDIC SURGERY

Reeves County Hospital District

2323 Texas Street
Pecos, TX 79772
(432) 447-3551

Overall patient safety: ★★★
Teaching: N

CLINICAL PROGRAM RATINGS:

CARDIAC	NR	ORTHOPEDICS	NR
CRITICAL CARE	NR	PULMONARY	★★★
GASTROINTESTINAL	NR	STROKE	NR
GENERAL SURGERY	NR	VASCULAR	NR
MATERNITY CARE	NR	WOMEN'S HEALTH	NR

HEALTHGRADES AWARDS

KEY: ★★★★★ BEST ★★★ AS EXPECTED ★ POOR NR NOT RATED BY HEALTHGRADES For full definitions of ratings and awards, see Appendix.

Renaissance Hospital

2807 Little York Road
Houston, TX 77093
(713) 697-2961

Overall patient safety: ★★★
Teaching: N

CLINICAL PROGRAM RATINGS:

CARDIAC	NR	ORTHOPEDICS	NR
CRITICAL CARE	NR	PULMONARY	★★★
GASTROINTESTINAL	NR	STROKE	NR
GENERAL SURGERY	NR	VASCULAR	NR
MATERNITY CARE	NR	WOMEN'S HEALTH	NR

HEALTHGRADES AWARDS

Renaissance Hospital—Terrell

1551 Highway 34 South
Terrell, TX 75160
(972) 563-7611

Overall patient safety: ★★★
Teaching: N

CLINICAL PROGRAM RATINGS:

CARDIAC	NR	ORTHOPEDICS	NR
CRITICAL CARE	NR	PULMONARY	★★★
GASTROINTESTINAL	NR	STROKE	★★★
GENERAL SURGERY	NR	VASCULAR	NR
MATERNITY CARE	★★★	WOMEN'S HEALTH	NR

HEALTHGRADES AWARDS

Renaissance Hospital

5500 39th Street
Groves, TX 77619
(409) 962-5733

Overall patient safety: ★★★
Teaching: Y

CLINICAL PROGRAM RATINGS:

CARDIAC	NR	ORTHOPEDICS	NR
CRITICAL CARE	NR	PULMONARY	★★★
GASTROINTESTINAL	NR	STROKE	★★★
GENERAL SURGERY	NR	VASCULAR	NR
MATERNITY CARE	NR	WOMEN'S HEALTH	NR

HEALTHGRADES AWARDS

RHD Memorial Medical Center

7 Medical Parkway
Dallas, TX 75234
(972) 247-1000

Overall patient safety: ★★★
Teaching: N

CLINICAL PROGRAM RATINGS:

CARDIAC	NR	ORTHOPEDICS	NR
CRITICAL CARE	NR	PULMONARY	★★★
GASTROINTESTINAL	NR	STROKE	★★★★★
GENERAL SURGERY	★★★	VASCULAR	NR
MATERNITY CARE	★	WOMEN'S HEALTH	NR

HEALTHGRADES AWARDS

✓ SPECIALTY EXCELLENCE
· BARIATRIC SURGERY   · STROKE CARE

Renaissance Hospital—Dallas*

2929 South Hampton Road
Dallas, TX 75224
(214) 623-4400

Overall patient safety: ★★★
Teaching: N

CLINICAL PROGRAM RATINGS:

CARDIAC	NR	ORTHOPEDICS	NR
CRITICAL CARE	NR	PULMONARY	NR
GASTROINTESTINAL	NR	STROKE	★★★
GENERAL SURGERY	NR	VASCULAR	NR
MATERNITY CARE	NR	WOMEN'S HEALTH	NR

HEALTHGRADES AWARDS

Richards Memorial Hospital

1700 Brazos
Rockdale, TX 76567
(512) 446-2513

Overall patient safety: ★★★
Teaching: N

CLINICAL PROGRAM RATINGS:

CARDIAC	NR	ORTHOPEDICS	NR
CRITICAL CARE	NR	PULMONARY	★★★
GASTROINTESTINAL	NR	STROKE	NR
GENERAL SURGERY	NR	VASCULAR	NR
MATERNITY CARE	NR	WOMEN'S HEALTH	NR

HEALTHGRADES AWARDS

*This hospital reports its data to the federal government jointly with another hospital. Therefore the ratings and awards apply to multiple hospitals and this specific hospital may not provide all rated services.

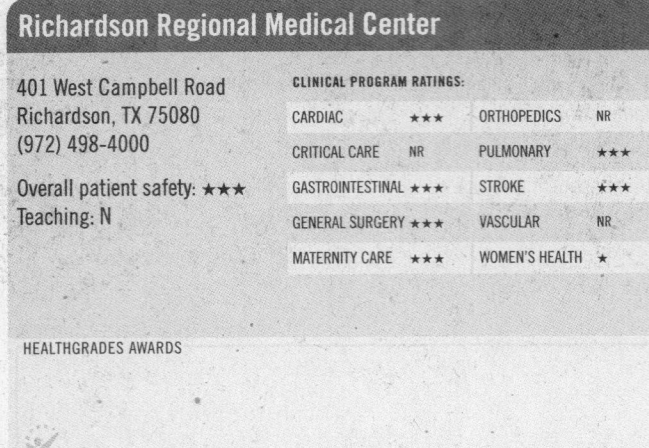

Richardson Regional Medical Center

401 West Campbell Road
Richardson, TX 75080
(972) 498-4000

Overall patient safety: ★★★
Teaching: N

CLINICAL PROGRAM RATINGS:

CARDIAC	★★★	ORTHOPEDICS	NR
CRITICAL CARE	NR	PULMONARY	★★★
GASTROINTESTINAL	★★★	STROKE	★★★
GENERAL SURGERY	★★★	VASCULAR	NR
MATERNITY CARE	★★★	WOMEN'S HEALTH	★

HEALTHGRADES AWARDS

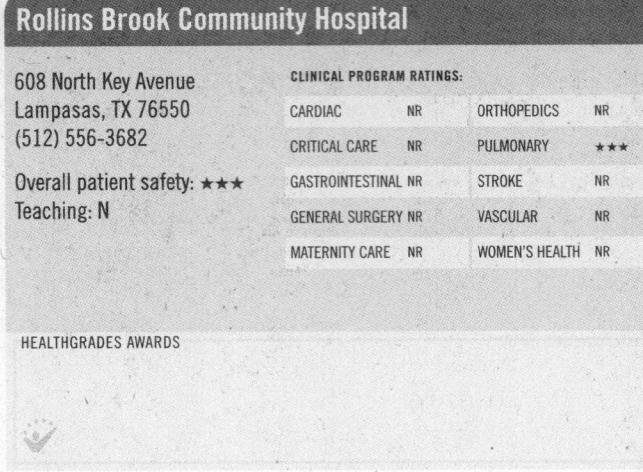

Rollins Brook Community Hospital

608 North Key Avenue
Lampasas, TX 76550
(512) 556-3682

Overall patient safety: ★★★
Teaching: N

CLINICAL PROGRAM RATINGS:

CARDIAC	NR	ORTHOPEDICS	NR
CRITICAL CARE	NR	PULMONARY	★★★
GASTROINTESTINAL	NR	STROKE	NR
GENERAL SURGERY	NR	VASCULAR	NR
MATERNITY CARE	NR	WOMEN'S HEALTH	NR

HEALTHGRADES AWARDS

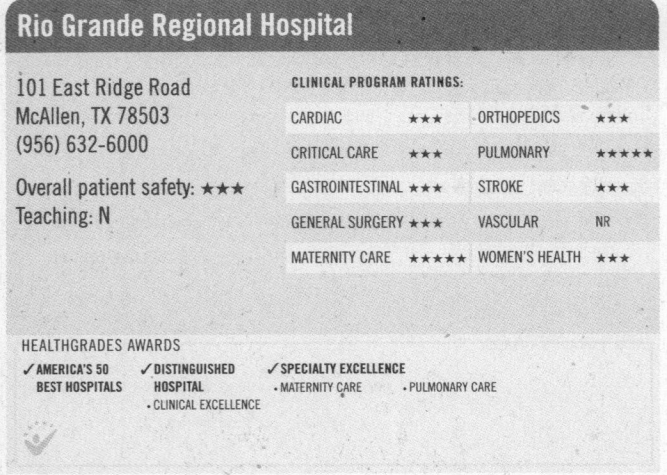

Rio Grande Regional Hospital

101 East Ridge Road
McAllen, TX 78503
(956) 632-6000

Overall patient safety: ★★★
Teaching: N

CLINICAL PROGRAM RATINGS:

CARDIAC	★★★	ORTHOPEDICS	★★★
CRITICAL CARE	★★★	PULMONARY	★★★★★
GASTROINTESTINAL	★★★	STROKE	★★★
GENERAL SURGERY	★★★	VASCULAR	NR
MATERNITY CARE	★★★★★	WOMEN'S HEALTH	★★★

HEALTHGRADES AWARDS

✓ AMERICA'S 50 BEST HOSPITALS   ✓ DISTINGUISHED HOSPITAL   ✓ SPECIALTY EXCELLENCE
• CLINICAL EXCELLENCE   • MATERNITY CARE   • PULMONARY CARE

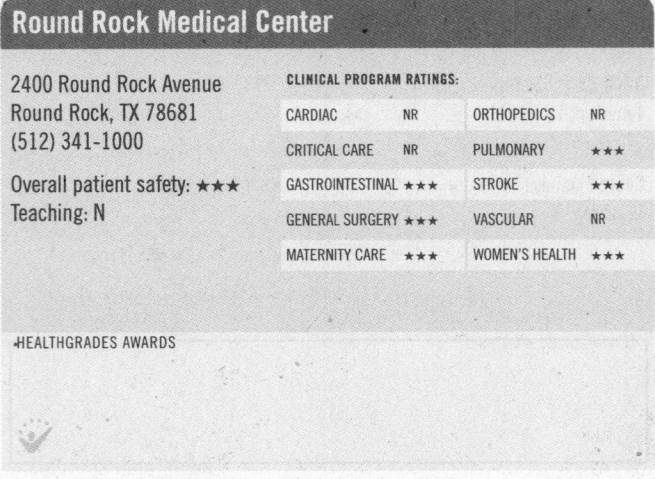

Round Rock Medical Center

2400 Round Rock Avenue
Round Rock, TX 78681
(512) 341-1000

Overall patient safety: ★★★
Teaching: N

CLINICAL PROGRAM RATINGS:

CARDIAC	NR	ORTHOPEDICS	NR
CRITICAL CARE	NR	PULMONARY	★★★
GASTROINTESTINAL	★★★	STROKE	★★★
GENERAL SURGERY	★★★	VASCULAR	NR
MATERNITY CARE	★★★	WOMEN'S HEALTH	★★★

HEALTHGRADES AWARDS

Rolling Plains Memorial Hospital

200 East Arizona Street
Sweetwater, TX 79556
(325) 235-1701

Overall patient safety: ★★★
Teaching: N

CLINICAL PROGRAM RATINGS:

CARDIAC	NR	ORTHOPEDICS	NR
CRITICAL CARE	NR	PULMONARY	★★★
GASTROINTESTINAL	NR	STROKE	★★★
GENERAL SURGERY	NR	VASCULAR	NR
MATERNITY CARE	NR	WOMEN'S HEALTH	NR

HEALTHGRADES AWARDS

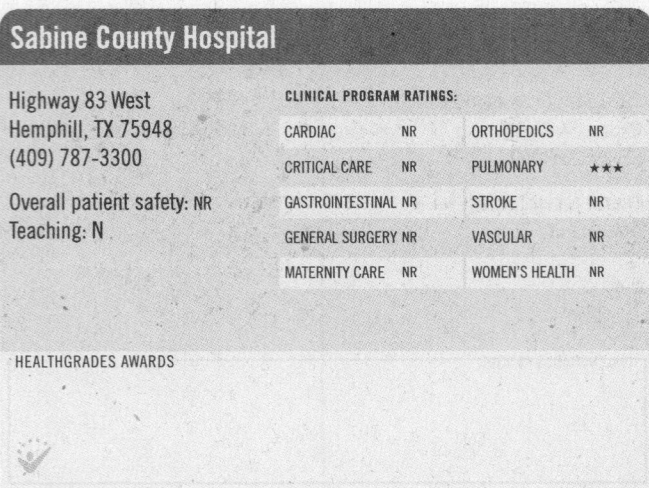

Sabine County Hospital

Highway 83 West
Hemphill, TX 75948
(409) 787-3300

Overall patient safety: NR
Teaching: N

CLINICAL PROGRAM RATINGS:

CARDIAC	NR	ORTHOPEDICS	NR
CRITICAL CARE	NR	PULMONARY	★★★
GASTROINTESTINAL	NR	STROKE	NR
GENERAL SURGERY	NR	VASCULAR	NR
MATERNITY CARE	NR	WOMEN'S HEALTH	NR

HEALTHGRADES AWARDS

KEY: ★★★★★ BEST   ★★★ AS EXPECTED   ★ POOR   NR NOT RATED BY HEALTHGRADES   For full definitions of ratings and awards, see Appendix.

St. David's Hospital

919 East 32nd Street
Austin, TX 78705
(512) 476-7111

Overall patient safety: ★★★
Teaching: Y

CLINICAL PROGRAM RATINGS:

CARDIAC	★★★	ORTHOPEDICS	★★★
CRITICAL CARE	★★★	PULMONARY	★★★★★
GASTROINTESTINAL	★★★	STROKE	★★★
GENERAL SURGERY	★★★	VASCULAR	NR
MATERNITY CARE	★★★★★	WOMEN'S HEALTH	★★★

HEALTHGRADES AWARDS

✓ DISTINGUISHED HOSPITAL
- CLINICAL EXCELLENCE

✓ SPECIALTY EXCELLENCE
- GENERAL SURGERY
- MATERNITY CARE

St. Luke's Baptist Hospital*

7930 Floyd Curl Drive
San Antonio, TX 78229
(210) 297-5000

Overall patient safety: ★★★
Teaching: N

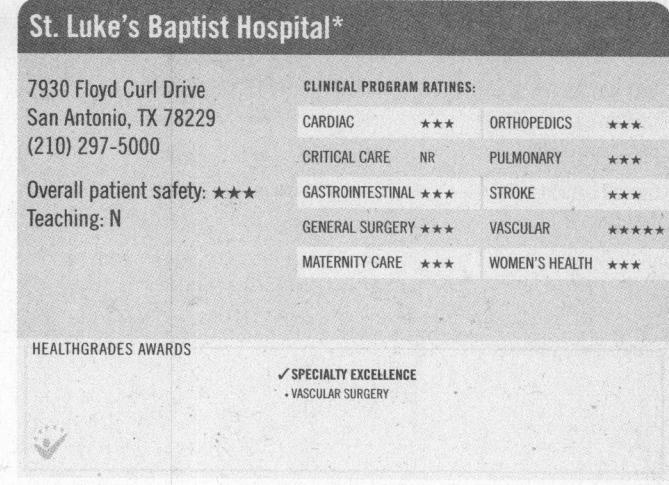

CLINICAL PROGRAM RATINGS:

CARDIAC	★★★	ORTHOPEDICS	★★★
CRITICAL CARE	NR	PULMONARY	★★★
GASTROINTESTINAL	★★★	STROKE	★★★
GENERAL SURGERY	★★★	VASCULAR	★★★★★
MATERNITY CARE	★★★	WOMEN'S HEALTH	★★★

HEALTHGRADES AWARDS

✓ SPECIALTY EXCELLENCE
- VASCULAR SURGERY

St. Joseph Medical Center

1401 Street Joseph Parkway
Houston, TX 77002
(713) 757-1000

Overall patient safety: ★
Teaching: Y

CLINICAL PROGRAM RATINGS:

CARDIAC	★★★	ORTHOPEDICS	★★★
CRITICAL CARE	NR	PULMONARY	★★★
GASTROINTESTINAL	★★★	STROKE	★★★
GENERAL SURGERY	★★★	VASCULAR	NR
MATERNITY CARE	★★★	WOMEN'S HEALTH	★★★

HEALTHGRADES AWARDS

St. Luke's Community Medical Center–The Woodlands

17200 St. Luke's Way
The Woodlands, TX 77384
(936) 266-4050

Overall patient safety: ★★★
Teaching: N

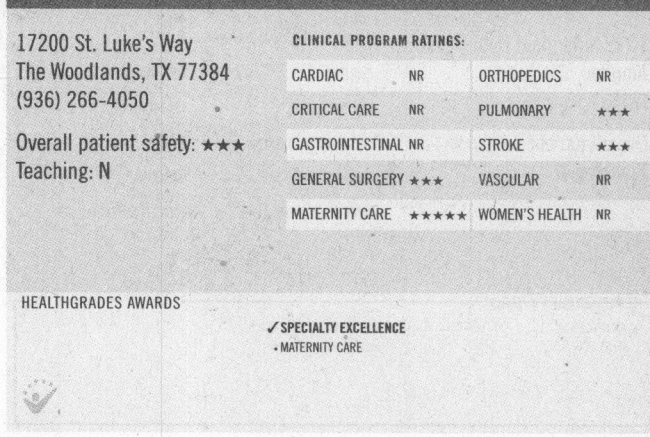

CLINICAL PROGRAM RATINGS:

CARDIAC	NR	ORTHOPEDICS	NR
CRITICAL CARE	NR	PULMONARY	★★★
GASTROINTESTINAL	NR	STROKE	★★★
GENERAL SURGERY	★★★	VASCULAR	NR
MATERNITY CARE	★★★★★	WOMEN'S HEALTH	NR

HEALTHGRADES AWARDS

✓ SPECIALTY EXCELLENCE
- MATERNITY CARE

St. Joseph Regional Health Center

2801 Franciscan Drive
Bryan, TX 77802
(979) 776-3777

Overall patient safety: ★★★
Teaching: Y

CLINICAL PROGRAM RATINGS:

CARDIAC	★★★	ORTHOPEDICS	★★★
CRITICAL CARE	NR	PULMONARY	★★★
GASTROINTESTINAL	★★★	STROKE	★★★
GENERAL SURGERY	★★★	VASCULAR	NR
MATERNITY CARE	★	WOMEN'S HEALTH	★

HEALTHGRADES AWARDS

St. Luke's Episcopal Hospital

6720 Bertner Avenue
Houston, TX 77030
(713) 785-8537

Overall patient safety: ★★★
Teaching: Y

CLINICAL PROGRAM RATINGS:

CARDIAC	★★★	ORTHOPEDICS	★★★
CRITICAL CARE	NR	PULMONARY	★★★★★
GASTROINTESTINAL	★★★	STROKE	★★★★★
GENERAL SURGERY	★★★	VASCULAR	★★★
MATERNITY CARE	★★★	WOMEN'S HEALTH	★★★

HEALTHGRADES AWARDS

✓ DISTINGUISHED HOSPITAL
- CLINICAL EXCELLENCE

✓ SPECIALTY EXCELLENCE
- GASTROINTESTINAL CARE
- PULMONARY CARE
- STROKE CARE
- VASCULAR SURGERY

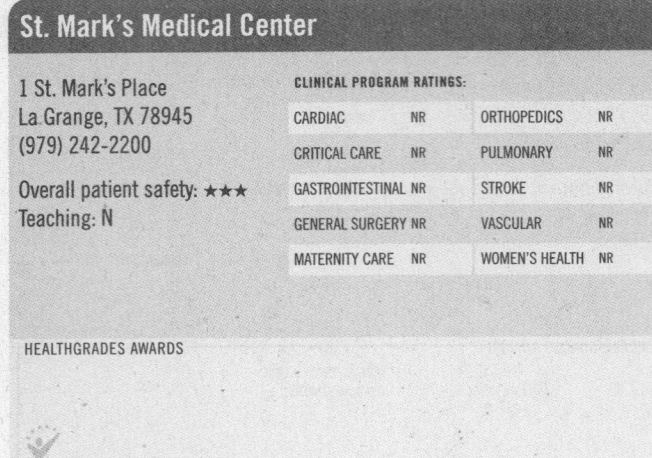

St. Mark's Medical Center

1 St. Mark's Place
La Grange, TX 78945
(979) 242-2200

Overall patient safety: ★★★
Teaching: N

CLINICAL PROGRAM RATINGS:

CARDIAC	NR	ORTHOPEDICS	NR
CRITICAL CARE	NR	PULMONARY	NR
GASTROINTESTINAL	NR	STROKE	NR
GENERAL SURGERY	NR	VASCULAR	NR
MATERNITY CARE	NR	WOMEN'S HEALTH	NR

HEALTHGRADES AWARDS

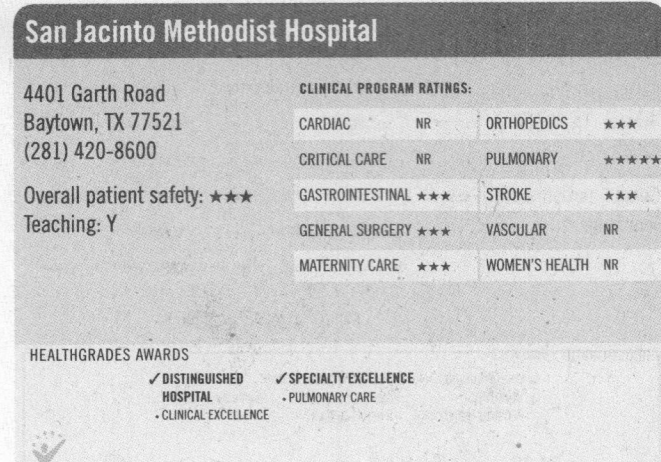

San Jacinto Methodist Hospital

4401 Garth Road
Baytown, TX 77521
(281) 420-8600

Overall patient safety: ★★★
Teaching: Y

CLINICAL PROGRAM RATINGS:

CARDIAC	NR	ORTHOPEDICS	★★★
CRITICAL CARE	NR	PULMONARY	★★★★★
GASTROINTESTINAL	★★★	STROKE	★★★
GENERAL SURGERY	★★★	VASCULAR	NR
MATERNITY CARE	★★★	WOMEN'S HEALTH	NR

HEALTHGRADES AWARDS

✓ DISTINGUISHED HOSPITAL
• CLINICAL EXCELLENCE

✓ SPECIALTY EXCELLENCE
• PULMONARY CARE

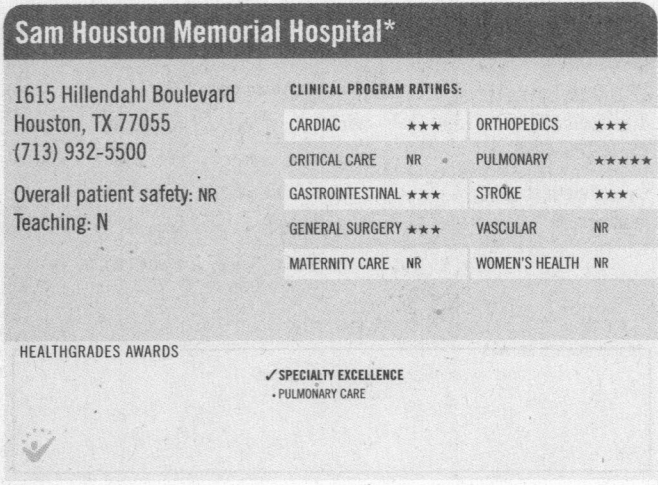

Sam Houston Memorial Hospital*

1615 Hillendahl Boulevard
Houston, TX 77055
(713) 932-5500

Overall patient safety: NR
Teaching: N

CLINICAL PROGRAM RATINGS:

CARDIAC	★★★	ORTHOPEDICS	★★★
CRITICAL CARE	NR	PULMONARY	★★★★★
GASTROINTESTINAL	★★★	STROKE	★★★
GENERAL SURGERY	★★★	VASCULAR	NR
MATERNITY CARE	NR	WOMEN'S HEALTH	NR

HEALTHGRADES AWARDS

✓ SPECIALTY EXCELLENCE
• PULMONARY CARE

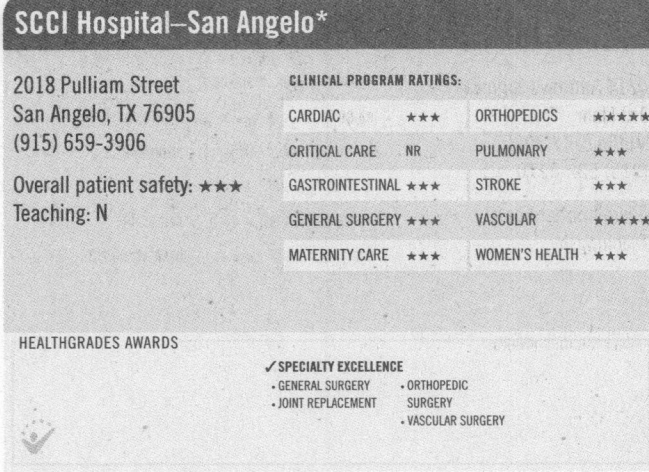

SCCI Hospital—San Angelo*

2018 Pulliam Street
San Angelo, TX 76905
(915) 659-3906

Overall patient safety: ★★★
Teaching: N

CLINICAL PROGRAM RATINGS:

CARDIAC	★★★	ORTHOPEDICS	★★★★★
CRITICAL CARE	NR	PULMONARY	★★★
GASTROINTESTINAL	★★★	STROKE	★★★
GENERAL SURGERY	★★★	VASCULAR	★★★★★
MATERNITY CARE	★★★	WOMEN'S HEALTH	★★★

HEALTHGRADES AWARDS

✓ SPECIALTY EXCELLENCE
• GENERAL SURGERY
• JOINT REPLACEMENT
• ORTHOPEDIC SURGERY
• VASCULAR SURGERY

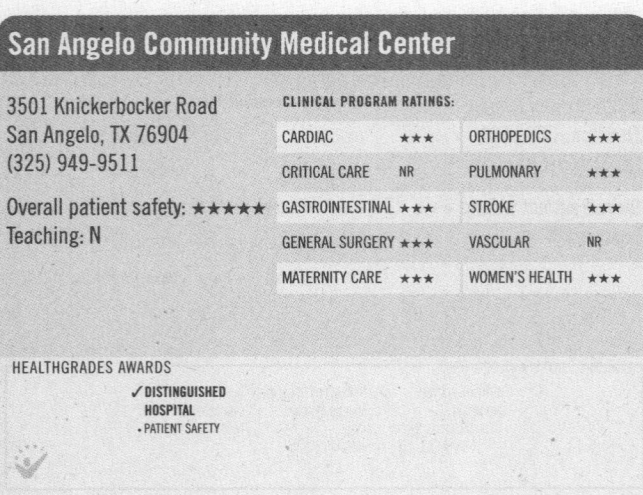

San Angelo Community Medical Center

3501 Knickerbocker Road
San Angelo, TX 76904
(325) 949-9511

Overall patient safety: ★★★★★
Teaching: N

CLINICAL PROGRAM RATINGS:

CARDIAC	★★★	ORTHOPEDICS	★★★
CRITICAL CARE	NR	PULMONARY	★★★
GASTROINTESTINAL	★★★	STROKE	★★★
GENERAL SURGERY	★★★	VASCULAR	NR
MATERNITY CARE	★★★	WOMEN'S HEALTH	★★★

HEALTHGRADES AWARDS

✓ DISTINGUISHED HOSPITAL
• PATIENT SAFETY

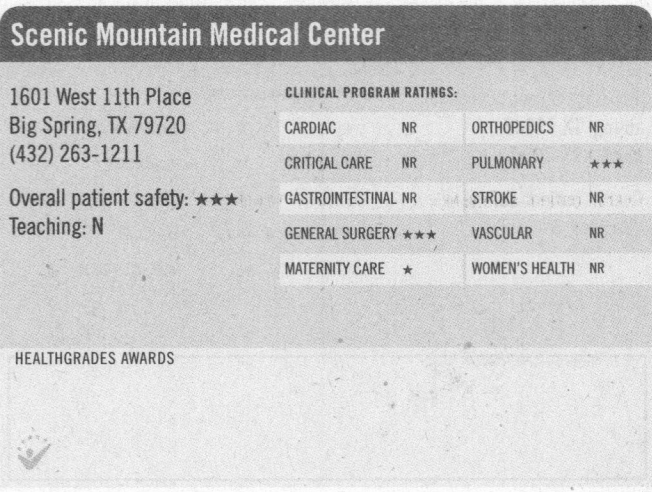

Scenic Mountain Medical Center

1601 West 11th Place
Big Spring, TX 79720
(432) 263-1211

Overall patient safety: ★★★
Teaching: N

CLINICAL PROGRAM RATINGS:

CARDIAC	NR	ORTHOPEDICS	NR
CRITICAL CARE	NR	PULMONARY	★★★
GASTROINTESTINAL	NR	STROKE	NR
GENERAL SURGERY	★★★	VASCULAR	NR
MATERNITY CARE	★	WOMEN'S HEALTH	NR

HEALTHGRADES AWARDS

KEY: ★★★★★ BEST ★★★ AS EXPECTED ★ POOR NR NOT RATED BY HEALTHGRADES   For full definitions of ratings and awards, see Appendix.

Scott and White Memorial Hospital

2401 South 31st Street
Temple, TX 76508
(254) 724-2111

Overall patient safety: ★★★★★
Teaching: Y

CLINICAL PROGRAM RATINGS:

CARDIAC	★★★	ORTHOPEDICS	★★★★★
CRITICAL CARE	NR	PULMONARY	★★★
GASTROINTESTINAL	★★★	STROKE	★★★
GENERAL SURGERY	★★★★★	VASCULAR	NR
MATERNITY CARE	★★★	WOMEN'S HEALTH	★★★

HEALTHGRADES AWARDS

✓ **DISTINGUISHED HOSPITAL**
- PATIENT SAFETY

✓ **SPECIALTY EXCELLENCE**
- BARIATRIC SURGERY
- GENERAL SURGERY
- JOINT REPLACEMENT
- ORTHOPEDIC SURGERY

Seton Highland Lakes

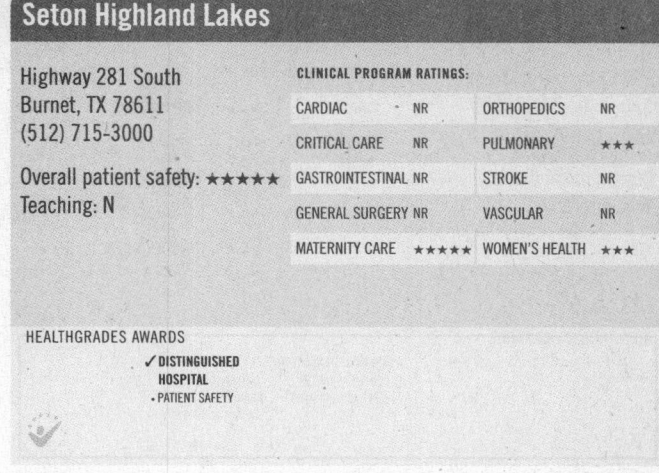

Highway 281 South
Burnet, TX 78611
(512) 715-3000

Overall patient safety: ★★★★★
Teaching: N

CLINICAL PROGRAM RATINGS:

CARDIAC	NR	ORTHOPEDICS	NR
CRITICAL CARE	NR	PULMONARY	★★★
GASTROINTESTINAL	NR	STROKE	NR
GENERAL SURGERY	NR	VASCULAR	NR
MATERNITY CARE	★★★★★	WOMEN'S HEALTH	★★★

HEALTHGRADES AWARDS

✓ **DISTINGUISHED HOSPITAL**
- PATIENT SAFETY

Sempercare Hospital of Midland

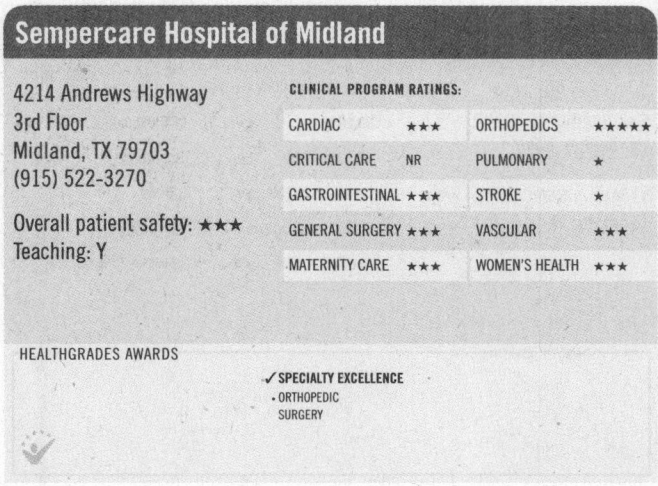

4214 Andrews Highway
3rd Floor
Midland, TX 79703
(915) 522-3270

Overall patient safety: ★★★
Teaching: Y

CLINICAL PROGRAM RATINGS:

CARDIAC	★★★	ORTHOPEDICS	★★★★★
CRITICAL CARE	NR	PULMONARY	★
GASTROINTESTINAL	★★★	STROKE	★
GENERAL SURGERY	★★★	VASCULAR	★★★
MATERNITY CARE	★★★	WOMEN'S HEALTH	★★★

HEALTHGRADES AWARDS

✓ **SPECIALTY EXCELLENCE**
- ORTHOPEDIC SURGERY

Seton Medical Center

1201 West 38th Street
Austin, TX 78705
(512) 324-1000

Overall patient safety: ★★★★★
Teaching: N

CLINICAL PROGRAM RATINGS:

CARDIAC	★★★	ORTHOPEDICS	★★★★★
CRITICAL CARE	NR	PULMONARY	★★★
GASTROINTESTINAL	★★★	STROKE	★★★
GENERAL SURGERY	NR	VASCULAR	★★★
MATERNITY CARE	★★★★★	WOMEN'S HEALTH	★★★

HEALTHGRADES AWARDS

✓ **DISTINGUISHED HOSPITAL**
- CLINICAL EXCELLENCE
- PATIENT SAFETY

✓ **SPECIALTY EXCELLENCE**
- JOINT REPLACEMENT
- ORTHOPEDIC SURGERY

Seton Edgar B. Davis Hospital

130 Hays Street
Luling, TX 78648
(830) 875-7000

Overall patient safety: NR
Teaching: N

CLINICAL PROGRAM RATINGS:

CARDIAC	NR	ORTHOPEDICS	NR
CRITICAL CARE	NR	PULMONARY	★★★
GASTROINTESTINAL	NR	STROKE	★★★★★
GENERAL SURGERY	NR	VASCULAR	NR
MATERNITY CARE	NR	WOMEN'S HEALTH	NR

HEALTHGRADES AWARDS

Seton Northwest Hospital

11113 Research Boulevard
Austin, TX 78759
(512) 324-6000

Overall patient safety: ★★★
Teaching: N

CLINICAL PROGRAM RATINGS:

CARDIAC	NR	ORTHOPEDICS	NR
CRITICAL CARE	NR	PULMONARY	★★★
GASTROINTESTINAL	NR	STROKE	★★★
GENERAL SURGERY	★★★	VASCULAR	NR
MATERNITY CARE	★★★	WOMEN'S HEALTH	NR

HEALTHGRADES AWARDS

*This hospital reports its data to the federal government jointly with another hospital. Therefore the ratings and awards apply to multiple hospitals and this specific hospital may not provide all rated services.

Shannon West Texas Medical Center*

120 East Harris Street
San Angelo, TX 76903
(325) 653-6741

Overall patient safety: ★★★
Teaching: N

CLINICAL PROGRAM RATINGS:

CARDIAC	★★★	ORTHOPEDICS	★★★★★
CRITICAL CARE	NR	PULMONARY	★★★
GASTROINTESTINAL	★★★	STROKE	★★★
GENERAL SURGERY	★★★	VASCULAR	★★★★★
MATERNITY CARE	★★★	WOMEN'S HEALTH	★★★

HEALTHGRADES AWARDS

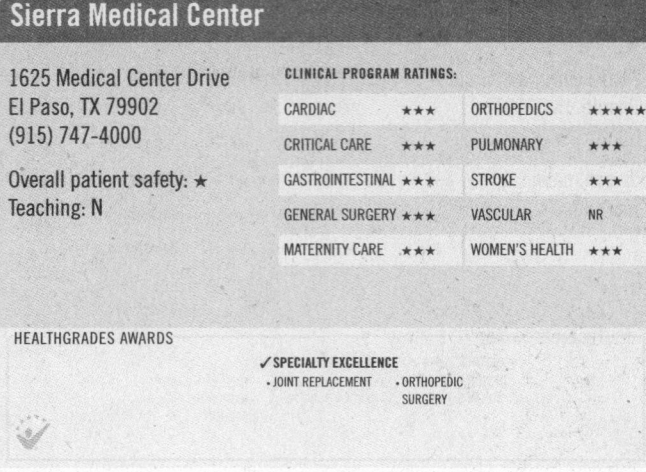

✓ SPECIALTY EXCELLENCE
• GENERAL SURGERY   • ORTHOPEDIC
• JOINT REPLACEMENT   SURGERY
                     • VASCULAR SURGERY

Sierra Medical Center

1625 Medical Center Drive
El Paso, TX 79902
(915) 747-4000

Overall patient safety: ★
Teaching: N

CLINICAL PROGRAM RATINGS:

CARDIAC	★★★	ORTHOPEDICS	★★★★★
CRITICAL CARE	★★★	PULMONARY	★★★
GASTROINTESTINAL	★★★	STROKE	★★★
GENERAL SURGERY	★★★	VASCULAR	NR
MATERNITY CARE	★★★	WOMEN'S HEALTH	★★★

HEALTHGRADES AWARDS

✓ SPECIALTY EXCELLENCE
• JOINT REPLACEMENT   • ORTHOPEDIC
                        SURGERY

Shelby Regional Medical Center

602 Hurst Street
Center, TX 75935
(936) 598-2781

Overall patient safety: ★★★
Teaching: N

CLINICAL PROGRAM RATINGS:

CARDIAC	NR	ORTHOPEDICS	NR
CRITICAL CARE	NR	PULMONARY	★
GASTROINTESTINAL	NR	STROKE	NR
GENERAL SURGERY	NR	VASCULAR	NR
MATERNITY CARE	★	WOMEN'S HEALTH	NR

HEALTHGRADES AWARDS

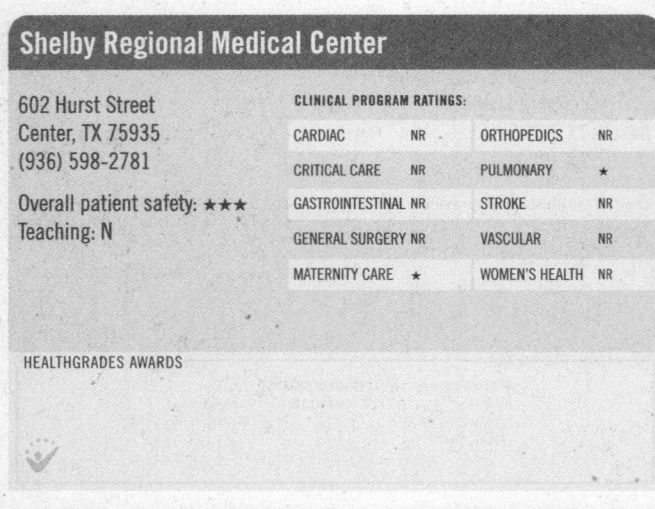

Smithville Regional Hospital

800 East Highway 71
Smithville, TX 78957
(512) 237-3214

Overall patient safety: ★★★
Teaching: N

CLINICAL PROGRAM RATINGS:

CARDIAC	NR	ORTHOPEDICS	NR
CRITICAL CARE	NR	PULMONARY	★★★
GASTROINTESTINAL	NR	STROKE	★
GENERAL SURGERY	NR	VASCULAR	NR
MATERNITY CARE	★★★	WOMEN'S HEALTH	NR

HEALTHGRADES AWARDS

Sid Peterson Memorial Hospital

710 Water Street
Kerrville, TX 78028
(830) 896-4200

Overall patient safety: ★★★
Teaching: N

CLINICAL PROGRAM RATINGS:

CARDIAC	NR	ORTHOPEDICS	NR
CRITICAL CARE	NR	PULMONARY	★
GASTROINTESTINAL	★★★	STROKE	★★★
GENERAL SURGERY	★★★	VASCULAR	NR
MATERNITY CARE	★★★	WOMEN'S HEALTH	NR

HEALTHGRADES AWARDS

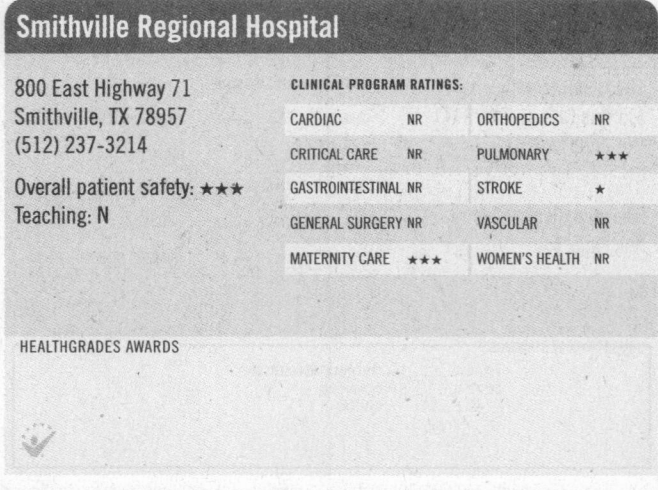

South Austin Hospital

901 West Ben White Boulevard
Austin, TX 78704
(512) 447-2211

Overall patient safety: ★★★★★
Teaching: N

CLINICAL PROGRAM RATINGS:

CARDIAC	★★★	ORTHOPEDICS	★★★
CRITICAL CARE	★★★	PULMONARY	★★★
GASTROINTESTINAL	★★★	STROKE	★★★
GENERAL SURGERY	★★★★★	VASCULAR	NR
MATERNITY CARE	★★★	WOMEN'S HEALTH	★★★★★

HEALTHGRADES AWARDS

✓ DISTINGUISHED   ✓ SPECIALTY EXCELLENCE
   HOSPITAL   • GASTROINTESTINAL   • GENERAL SURGERY
• PATIENT SAFETY   CARE

KEY: ★★★★★ BEST   ★★★ AS EXPECTED   ★ POOR   NR NOT RATED BY HEALTHGRADES   For full definitions of ratings and awards, see Appendix.

South Texas Regional Medical Center

Highway 97 East
Jourdanton, TX 78026
(830) 769-3515

Overall patient safety: ★★★
Teaching: N

CLINICAL PROGRAM RATINGS:

CARDIAC	NR	ORTHOPEDICS	NR
CRITICAL CARE	NR	PULMONARY	★★★★★
GASTROINTESTINAL	NR	STROKE	★★★
GENERAL SURGERY	★★★	VASCULAR	NR
MATERNITY CARE	★	WOMEN'S HEALTH	NR

HEALTHGRADES AWARDS

✓ SPECIALTY EXCELLENCE
· PULMONARY CARE

Southwestern General Hospital

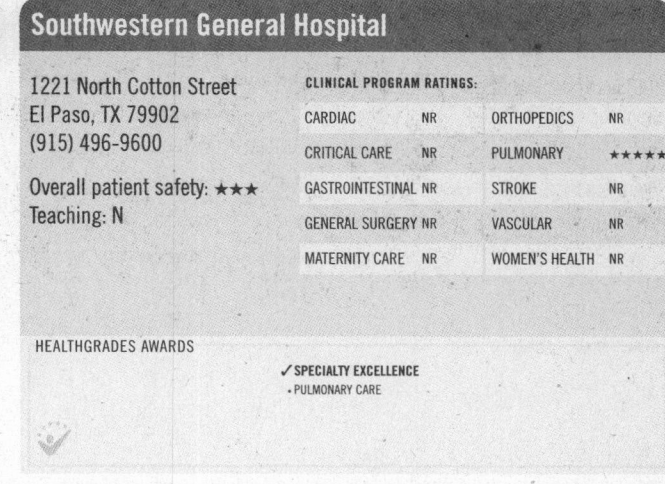

1221 North Cotton Street
El Paso, TX 79902
(915) 496-9600

Overall patient safety: ★★★
Teaching: N

CLINICAL PROGRAM RATINGS:

CARDIAC	NR	ORTHOPEDICS	NR
CRITICAL CARE	NR	PULMONARY	★★★★★
GASTROINTESTINAL	NR	STROKE	NR
GENERAL SURGERY	NR	VASCULAR	NR
MATERNITY CARE	NR	WOMEN'S HEALTH	NR

HEALTHGRADES AWARDS

✓ SPECIALTY EXCELLENCE
· PULMONARY CARE

Southside Health Center*

4626 Weber Road
Corpus Christi, TX 78411
(512) 854-2031

Overall patient safety: ★★★★★
Teaching: Y

CLINICAL PROGRAM RATINGS:

CARDIAC	★★★	ORTHOPEDICS	★★★
CRITICAL CARE	NR	PULMONARY	★★★★★
GASTROINTESTINAL	★★★	STROKE	★★★★★
GENERAL SURGERY	★★★	VASCULAR	NR
MATERNITY CARE	★★★★★	WOMEN'S HEALTH	★★★

HEALTHGRADES AWARDS

✓ DISTINGUISHED HOSPITAL
· PATIENT SAFETY

✓ SPECIALTY EXCELLENCE
· MATERNITY CARE   · PULMONARY CARE

Spring Branch Medical Center*

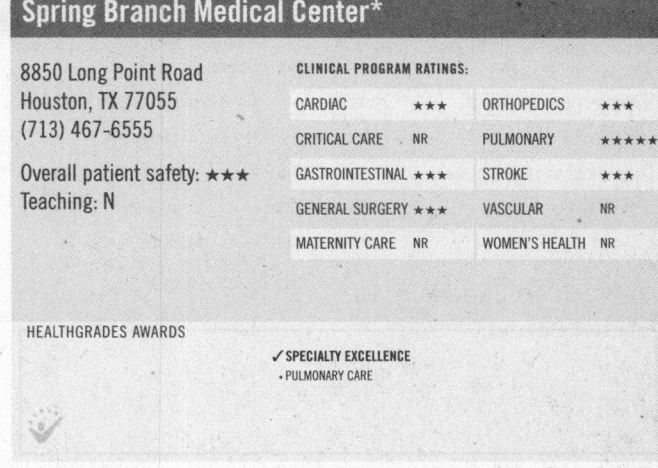

8850 Long Point Road
Houston, TX 77055
(713) 467-6555

Overall patient safety: ★★★
Teaching: N

CLINICAL PROGRAM RATINGS:

CARDIAC	★★★	ORTHOPEDICS	★★★
CRITICAL CARE	NR	PULMONARY	★★★★★
GASTROINTESTINAL	★★★	STROKE	★★★
GENERAL SURGERY	★★★	VASCULAR	NR
MATERNITY CARE	NR	WOMEN'S HEALTH	NR

HEALTHGRADES AWARDS

✓ SPECIALTY EXCELLENCE
· PULMONARY CARE

Southwest General Hospital

7400 Barlite Boulevard
San Antonio, TX 78224
(210) 921-2000

Overall patient safety: ★★★
Teaching: N

CLINICAL PROGRAM RATINGS:

CARDIAC	NR	ORTHOPEDICS	NR
CRITICAL CARE	NR	PULMONARY	★★★
GASTROINTESTINAL	NR	STROKE	★
GENERAL SURGERY	★★★	VASCULAR	NR
MATERNITY CARE	★★★★★	WOMEN'S HEALTH	NR

HEALTHGRADES AWARDS

✓ SPECIALTY EXCELLENCE
· MATERNITY CARE

Starr County Memorial Hospital

2573 Hospital Court
Rio Grande City, TX 78582
(956) 487-5561

Overall patient safety: ★★★
Teaching: N

CLINICAL PROGRAM RATINGS:

CARDIAC	NR	ORTHOPEDICS	NR
CRITICAL CARE	NR	PULMONARY	★★★
GASTROINTESTINAL	NR	STROKE	NR
GENERAL SURGERY	NR	VASCULAR	NR
MATERNITY CARE	★★★	WOMEN'S HEALTH	NR

HEALTHGRADES AWARDS

*This hospital reports its data to the federal government jointly with another hospital. Therefore the ratings and awards apply to multiple hospitals and this specific hospital may not provide all rated services.

Stephens Memorial Hospital

200 South Geneva Street
Breckenridge, TX 76424
(254) 559-2241

Overall patient safety: ★★★
Teaching: N

CLINICAL PROGRAM RATINGS:

CARDIAC	NR	ORTHOPEDICS	NR
CRITICAL CARE	NR	PULMONARY	★★★
GASTROINTESTINAL	NR	STROKE	NR
GENERAL SURGERY	NR	VASCULAR	NR
MATERNITY CARE	NR	WOMEN'S HEALTH	NR

HEALTHGRADES AWARDS

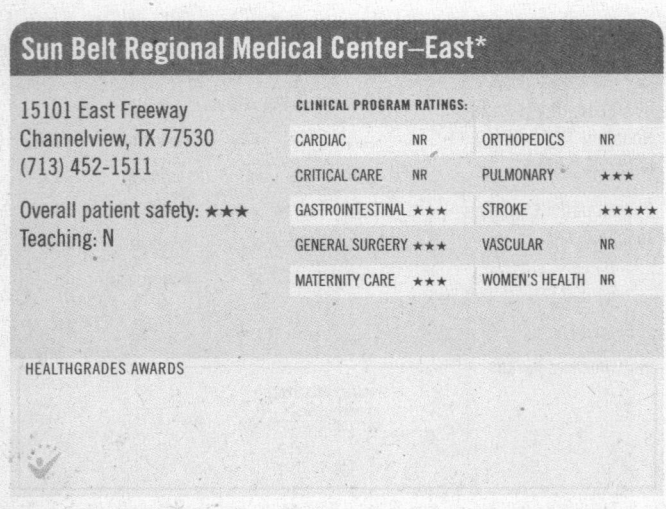

Texoma Medical Center

1000 Memorial Drive
Denison, TX 75020
(903) 416-4000

Overall patient safety: ★★★★★
Teaching: N

CLINICAL PROGRAM RATINGS:

CARDIAC	★★★	ORTHOPEDICS	★★★★★
CRITICAL CARE	★★★	PULMONARY	★★★
GASTROINTESTINAL	★★★	STROKE	★★★★★
GENERAL SURGERY	★★★	VASCULAR	NR
MATERNITY CARE	★★★	WOMEN'S HEALTH	★★★

HEALTHGRADES AWARDS

✓ **DISTINGUISHED HOSPITAL**
• PATIENT SAFETY

✓ **SPECIALTY EXCELLENCE**
• GASTROINTESTINAL CARE
• GENERAL SURGERY

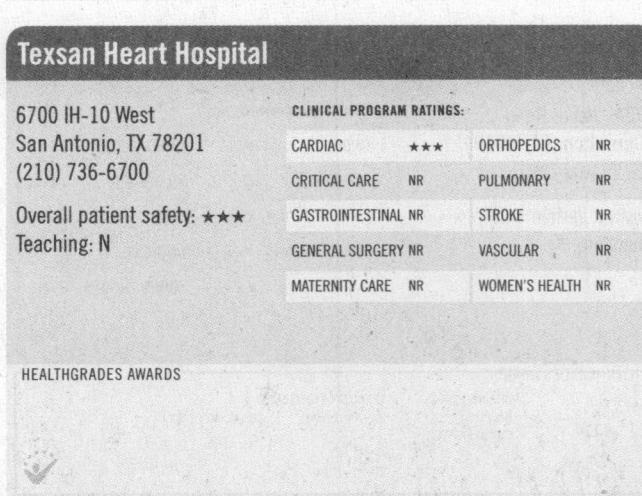

Sun Belt Regional Medical Center–East*

15101 East Freeway
Channelview, TX 77530
(713) 452-1511

Overall patient safety: ★★★
Teaching: N

CLINICAL PROGRAM RATINGS:

CARDIAC	NR	ORTHOPEDICS	NR
CRITICAL CARE	NR	PULMONARY	★★★
GASTROINTESTINAL	★★★	STROKE	★★★★★
GENERAL SURGERY	★★★	VASCULAR	NR
MATERNITY CARE	★★★	WOMEN'S HEALTH	NR

HEALTHGRADES AWARDS

Texsan Heart Hospital

6700 IH-10 West
San Antonio, TX 78201
(210) 736-6700

Overall patient safety: ★★★
Teaching: N

CLINICAL PROGRAM RATINGS:

CARDIAC	★★★	ORTHOPEDICS	NR
CRITICAL CARE	NR	PULMONARY	NR
GASTROINTESTINAL	NR	STROKE	NR
GENERAL SURGERY	NR	VASCULAR	NR
MATERNITY CARE	NR	WOMEN'S HEALTH	NR

HEALTHGRADES AWARDS

Texas Orthopedic Hospital

7401 South Main Street
Houston, TX 77030
(713) 799-8600

Overall patient safety: ★★★
Teaching: N

CLINICAL PROGRAM RATINGS:

CARDIAC	NR	ORTHOPEDICS	NR
CRITICAL CARE	NR	PULMONARY	NR
GASTROINTESTINAL	NR	STROKE	NR
GENERAL SURGERY	NR	VASCULAR	NR
MATERNITY CARE	NR	WOMEN'S HEALTH	NR

HEALTHGRADES AWARDS

✓ **SPECIALTY EXCELLENCE**
• JOINT REPLACEMENT

Titus County Memorial Hospital

2001 North Jefferson
Mt. Pleasant, TX 75455
(903) 577-6000

Overall patient safety: ★★★
Teaching: N

CLINICAL PROGRAM RATINGS:

CARDIAC	NR	ORTHOPEDICS	NR
CRITICAL CARE	NR	PULMONARY	★★★★★
GASTROINTESTINAL	NR	STROKE	★★★
GENERAL SURGERY	NR	VASCULAR	NR
MATERNITY CARE	★	WOMEN'S HEALTH	NR

HEALTHGRADES AWARDS

KEY: ★★★★★ BEST   ★★★ AS EXPECTED   ★ POOR   NR NOT RATED BY HEALTHGRADES   For full definitions of ratings and awards, see Appendix.

Tomball Regional Hospital

605 Holderrieth Boulevard
Tomball, TX 77375
(281) 351-1623

Overall patient safety: ★
Teaching: N

CLINICAL PROGRAM RATINGS:

CARDIAC	★★★	ORTHOPEDICS	★★★
CRITICAL CARE	NR	PULMONARY	★★★
GASTROINTESTINAL	★★★	STROKE	★★★★★
GENERAL SURGERY	★★★	VASCULAR	NR
MATERNITY CARE	★★★	WOMEN'S HEALTH	★★★

HEALTHGRADES AWARDS

✓ SPECIALTY EXCELLENCE
• STROKE CARE

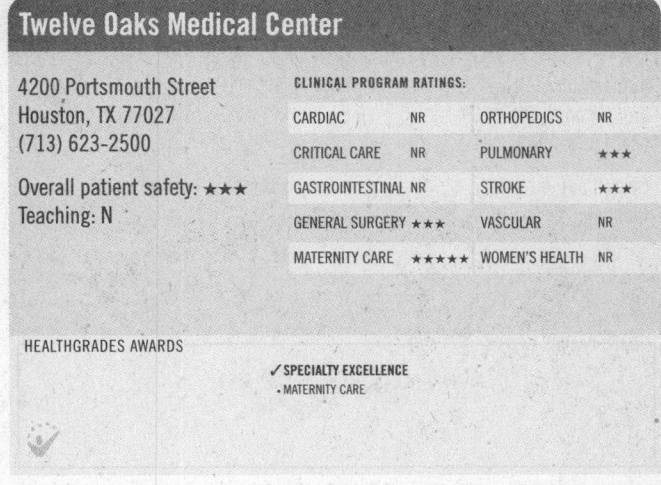

Twelve Oaks Medical Center

4200 Portsmouth Street
Houston, TX 77027
(713) 623-2500

Overall patient safety: ★★★
Teaching: N

CLINICAL PROGRAM RATINGS:

CARDIAC	NR	ORTHOPEDICS	NR
CRITICAL CARE	NR	PULMONARY	★★★
GASTROINTESTINAL	NR	STROKE	★★★
GENERAL SURGERY	★★★	VASCULAR	NR
MATERNITY CARE	★★★★★	WOMEN'S HEALTH	NR

HEALTHGRADES AWARDS

✓ SPECIALTY EXCELLENCE
• MATERNITY CARE

Trinity Medical Center

4343 North Josey Lane
Carrollton, TX 75010
(972) 492-1010

Overall patient safety: ★
Teaching: N

CLINICAL PROGRAM RATINGS:

CARDIAC	NR	ORTHOPEDICS	NR
CRITICAL CARE	NR	PULMONARY	★
GASTROINTESTINAL	NR	STROKE	★★★
GENERAL SURGERY	★★★	VASCULAR	NR
MATERNITY CARE	★★★	WOMEN'S HEALTH	NR

HEALTHGRADES AWARDS

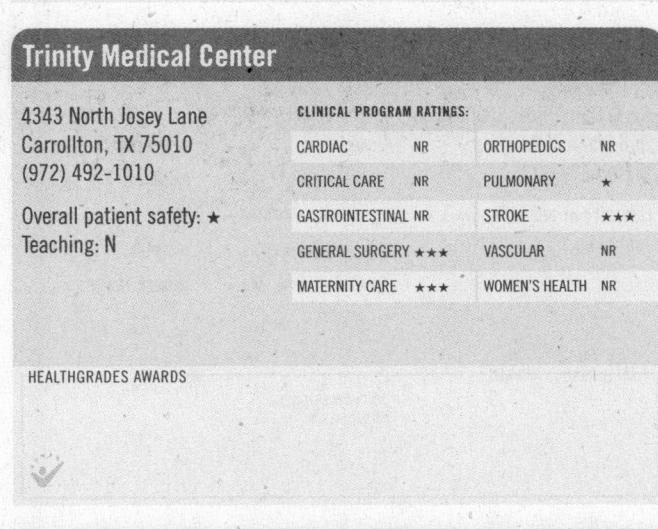

Tyler County Hospital

1100 West Bluff Street
Woodville, TX 75979
(409) 283-8141

Overall patient safety: ★★★
Teaching: N

CLINICAL PROGRAM RATINGS:

CARDIAC	NR	ORTHOPEDICS	NR
CRITICAL CARE	NR	PULMONARY	★
GASTROINTESTINAL	NR	STROKE	★
GENERAL SURGERY	NR	VASCULAR	NR
MATERNITY CARE	NR	WOMEN'S HEALTH	NR

HEALTHGRADES AWARDS

Trinity Medical Center

700 Medical Parkway
Brenham, TX 77833
(979) 836-6173

Overall patient safety: ★
Teaching: N

CLINICAL PROGRAM RATINGS:

CARDIAC	NR	ORTHOPEDICS	NR
CRITICAL CARE	NR	PULMONARY	★
GASTROINTESTINAL	NR	STROKE	★
GENERAL SURGERY	NR	VASCULAR	NR
MATERNITY CARE	NR	WOMEN'S HEALTH	NR

HEALTHGRADES AWARDS

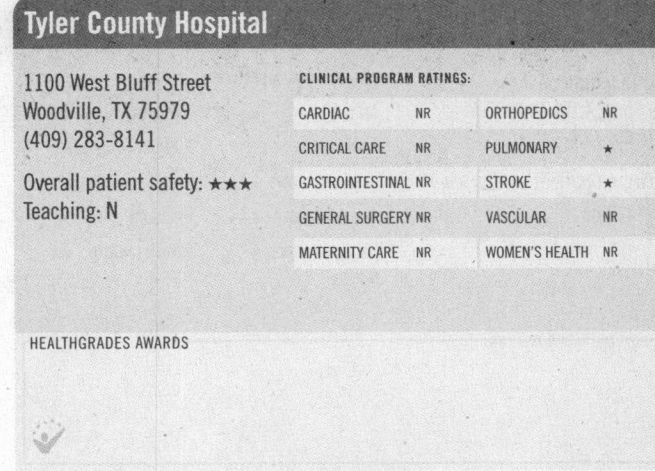

United Regional Health Care System

1600 10th Street
Wichita Falls, TX 76301
(940) 764-7000

Overall patient safety: ★★★★★
Teaching: Y

CLINICAL PROGRAM RATINGS:

CARDIAC	★★★	ORTHOPEDICS	★★★★★
CRITICAL CARE	NR	PULMONARY	★★★
GASTROINTESTINAL	★★★	STROKE	★★★
GENERAL SURGERY	★★★	VASCULAR	NR
MATERNITY CARE	★★★★★	WOMEN'S HEALTH	★★★

HEALTHGRADES AWARDS

✓ DISTINGUISHED HOSPITAL
• PATIENT SAFETY

✓ SPECIALTY EXCELLENCE
• BARIATRIC SURGERY   • ORTHOPEDIC SURGERY

*This hospital reports its data to the federal government jointly with another hospital. Therefore the ratings and awards apply to multiple hospitals and this specific hospital may not provide all rated services.

University Health System

4502 Medical Drive
San Antonio, TX 78229
(210) 358-4000

Overall patient safety: ★
Teaching: Y

CLINICAL PROGRAM RATINGS:

CARDIAC	★★★	ORTHOPEDICS	NR
CRITICAL CARE	NR	PULMONARY	★★★
GASTROINTESTINAL	NR	STROKE	★★★
GENERAL SURGERY	★★★	VASCULAR	NR
MATERNITY CARE	★★★	WOMEN'S HEALTH	★★★

HEALTHGRADES AWARDS

✓ SPECIALTY EXCELLENCE
• GENERAL SURGERY

University of Texas Medical Branch Galveston

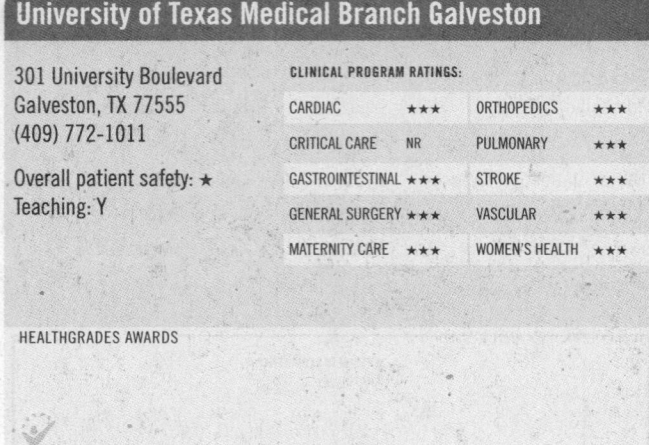

301 University Boulevard
Galveston, TX 77555
(409) 772-1011

Overall patient safety: ★
Teaching: Y

CLINICAL PROGRAM RATINGS:

CARDIAC	★★★	ORTHOPEDICS	★★★
CRITICAL CARE	NR	PULMONARY	★★★
GASTROINTESTINAL	★★★	STROKE	★★★
GENERAL SURGERY	★★★	VASCULAR	★★★
MATERNITY CARE	★★★	WOMEN'S HEALTH	★★★

HEALTHGRADES AWARDS

University Medical Center

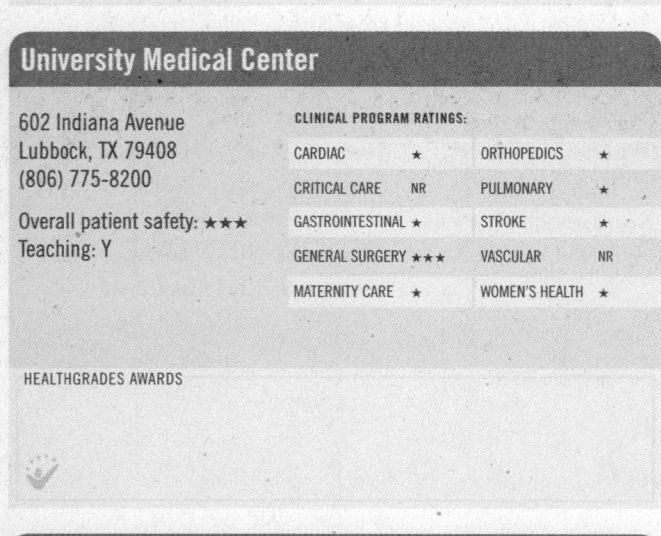

602 Indiana Avenue
Lubbock, TX 79408
(806) 775-8200

Overall patient safety: ★★★
Teaching: Y

CLINICAL PROGRAM RATINGS:

CARDIAC	★	ORTHOPEDICS	★
CRITICAL CARE	NR	PULMONARY	★
GASTROINTESTINAL	★	STROKE	★
GENERAL SURGERY	★★★	VASCULAR	NR
MATERNITY CARE	★	WOMEN'S HEALTH	★

HEALTHGRADES AWARDS

UT Southwestern Medical Center

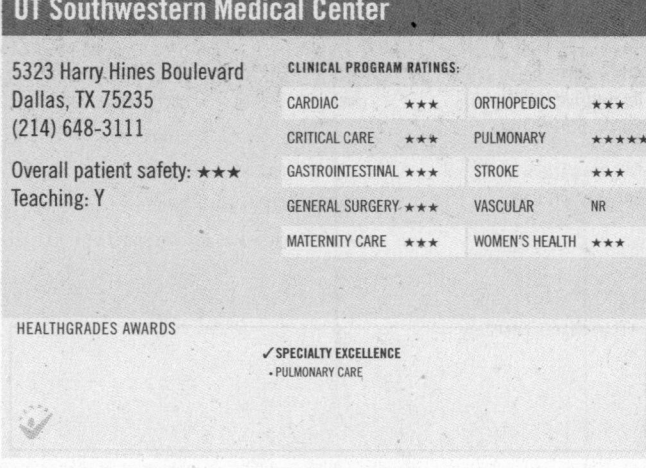

5323 Harry Hines Boulevard
Dallas, TX 75235
(214) 648-3111

Overall patient safety: ★★★
Teaching: Y

CLINICAL PROGRAM RATINGS:

CARDIAC	★★★	ORTHOPEDICS	★★★
CRITICAL CARE	★★★	PULMONARY	★★★★★
GASTROINTESTINAL	★★★	STROKE	★★★
GENERAL SURGERY	★★★	VASCULAR	NR
MATERNITY CARE	★★★	WOMEN'S HEALTH	★★★

HEALTHGRADES AWARDS

✓ SPECIALTY EXCELLENCE
• PULMONARY CARE

University of Texas Health Center at Tyler

11937 US Highway 271
Tyler, TX 75708
(903) 877-3451

Overall patient safety: ★★★
Teaching: Y

CLINICAL PROGRAM RATINGS:

CARDIAC	★★★	ORTHOPEDICS	NR
CRITICAL CARE	NR	PULMONARY	★★★
GASTROINTESTINAL	NR	STROKE	★★★★★
GENERAL SURGERY	NR	VASCULAR	NR
MATERNITY CARE	NR	WOMEN'S HEALTH	NR

HEALTHGRADES AWARDS

UT Southwestern Zale Lipshy Hospital

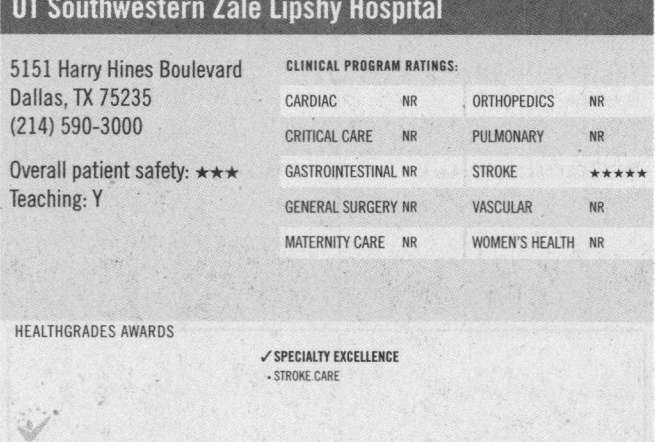

5151 Harry Hines Boulevard
Dallas, TX 75235
(214) 590-3000

Overall patient safety: ★★★
Teaching: Y

CLINICAL PROGRAM RATINGS:

CARDIAC	NR	ORTHOPEDICS	NR
CRITICAL CARE	NR	PULMONARY	NR
GASTROINTESTINAL	NR	STROKE	★★★★★
GENERAL SURGERY	NR	VASCULAR	NR
MATERNITY CARE	NR	WOMEN'S HEALTH	NR

HEALTHGRADES AWARDS

✓ SPECIALTY EXCELLENCE
• STROKE CARE

KEY: ★★★★★ BEST ★★★ AS EXPECTED ★ POOR NR NOT RATED BY HEALTHGRADES For full definitions of ratings and awards, see Appendix.

Uvalde Memorial Hospital

1025 Garner Field Road
Uvalde, TX 78801
(830) 278-6251

Overall patient safety: ★★★
Teaching: N

CLINICAL PROGRAM RATINGS:

CARDIAC	NR	ORTHOPEDICS	NR
CRITICAL CARE	NR	PULMONARY	★★★
GASTROINTESTINAL	NR	STROKE	NR
GENERAL SURGERY	NR	VASCULAR	NR
MATERNITY CARE	NR	WOMEN'S HEALTH	NR

HEALTHGRADES AWARDS

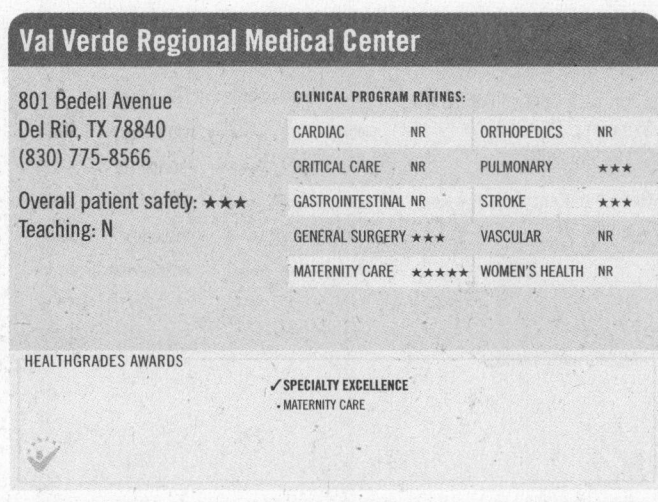

Valley Baptist Medical Center—Brownsville

1040 West Jefferson Street
Brownsville, TX 78520
(956) 544-1400

Overall patient safety: ★★★
Teaching: N

CLINICAL PROGRAM RATINGS:

CARDIAC	★★★	ORTHOPEDICS	NR
CRITICAL CARE	NR	PULMONARY	★★★★★
GASTROINTESTINAL	★★★	STROKE	★★★★★
GENERAL SURGERY	★★★★★	VASCULAR	NR
MATERNITY CARE	★★★	WOMEN'S HEALTH	★★★

HEALTHGRADES AWARDS

✓ SPECIALTY EXCELLENCE
• GENERAL SURGERY   • PULMONARY CARE   • STROKE CARE

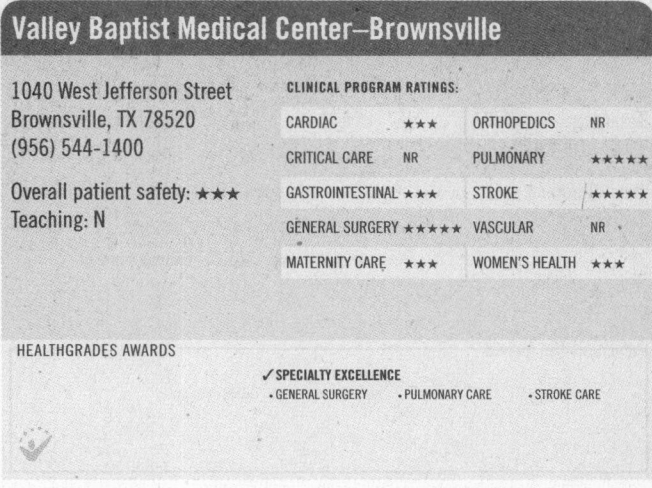

Val Verde Regional Medical Center

801 Bedell Avenue
Del Rio, TX 78840
(830) 775-8566

Overall patient safety: ★★★
Teaching: N

CLINICAL PROGRAM RATINGS:

CARDIAC	NR	ORTHOPEDICS	NR
CRITICAL CARE	NR	PULMONARY	★★★
GASTROINTESTINAL	NR	STROKE	★★★
GENERAL SURGERY	★★★	VASCULAR	NR
MATERNITY CARE	★★★★★	WOMEN'S HEALTH	NR

HEALTHGRADES AWARDS

✓ SPECIALTY EXCELLENCE
• MATERNITY CARE

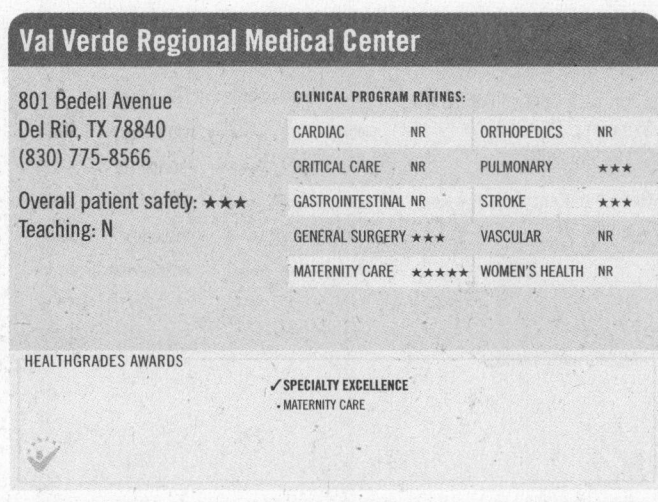

Valley Regional Medical Center

100 East Alton
Gloor Boulevard
Brownsville, TX 78526
(956) 350-7000

Overall patient safety: ★★★
Teaching: N

CLINICAL PROGRAM RATINGS:

CARDIAC	★★★	ORTHOPEDICS	NR
CRITICAL CARE	NR	PULMONARY	★★★
GASTROINTESTINAL	★★★	STROKE	★★★★★
GENERAL SURGERY	★★★★★	VASCULAR	NR
MATERNITY CARE	★★★	WOMEN'S HEALTH	★★★

HEALTHGRADES AWARDS

✓ DISTINGUISHED
HOSPITAL
• CLINICAL EXCELLENCE

✓ SPECIALTY EXCELLENCE
• GASTROINTESTINAL   • GENERAL SURGERY   • STROKE CARE
CARE

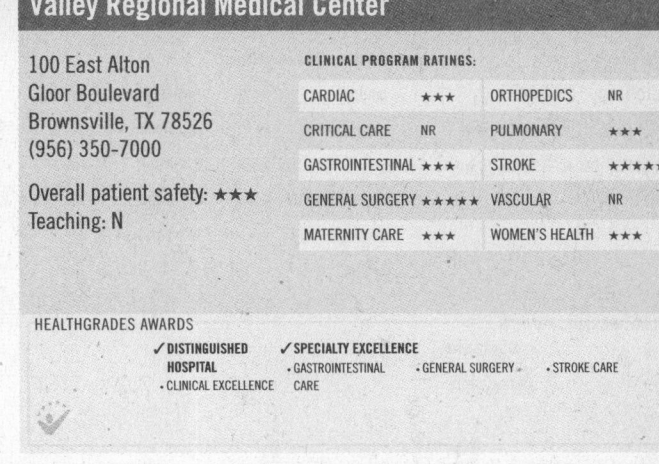

Valley Baptist Medical Center

2101 Pease Street
Harlingen, TX 78550
(956) 389-1100

Overall patient safety: ★★★
Teaching: Y

CLINICAL PROGRAM RATINGS:

CARDIAC	★★★	ORTHOPEDICS	★★★
CRITICAL CARE	NR	PULMONARY	★★★★★
GASTROINTESTINAL	★★★	STROKE	★★★★★
GENERAL SURGERY	★★★★★	VASCULAR	★★★
MATERNITY CARE	★★★	WOMEN'S HEALTH	★★★

HEALTHGRADES AWARDS

✓ DISTINGUISHED
HOSPITAL
• CLINICAL EXCELLENCE

✓ SPECIALTY EXCELLENCE
• CARDIAC SURGERY   • GENERAL SURGERY   • PULMONARY CARE
• GASTROINTESTINAL   • JOINT REPLACEMENT   • STROKE CARE
CARE

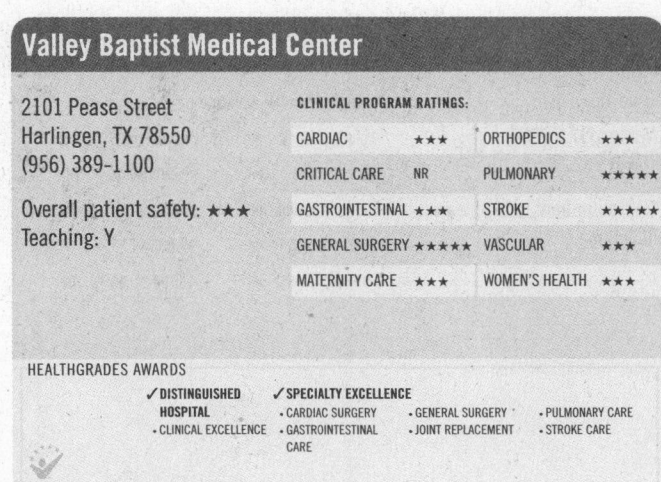

W. J. Mangold Memorial Hospital

320 North Main
Lockney, TX 79241
(806) 652-3373

Overall patient safety: NR
Teaching: N

CLINICAL PROGRAM RATINGS:

CARDIAC	NR	ORTHOPEDICS	NR
CRITICAL CARE	NR	PULMONARY	★★★
GASTROINTESTINAL	NR	STROKE	NR
GENERAL SURGERY	NR	VASCULAR	NR
MATERNITY CARE	NR	WOMEN'S HEALTH	NR

HEALTHGRADES AWARDS

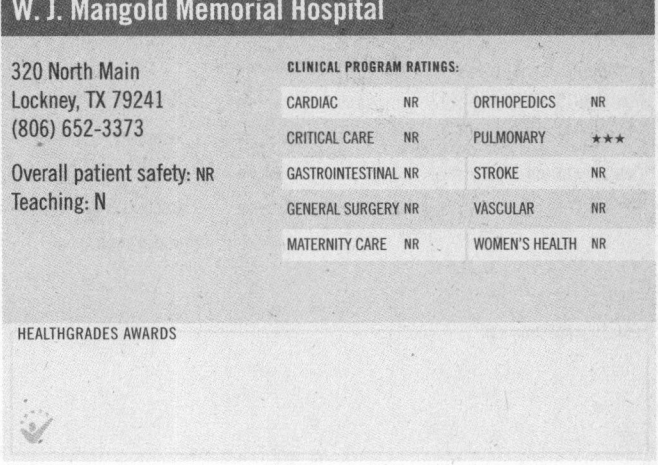

Wadley Regional Medical Center

1000 Pine Street
Texarkana, TX 75501
(903) 798-8000

Overall patient safety: ★★★
Teaching: Y

CLINICAL PROGRAM RATINGS:

CARDIAC	★★★	ORTHOPEDICS	★★★
CRITICAL CARE	NR	PULMONARY	★★★
GASTROINTESTINAL	★★★	STROKE	★★★
GENERAL SURGERY	★★★	VASCULAR	★★★★★
MATERNITY CARE	★★★	WOMEN'S HEALTH	★

HEALTHGRADES AWARDS

✓ SPECIALTY EXCELLENCE
- JOINT REPLACEMENT   - VASCULAR SURGERY

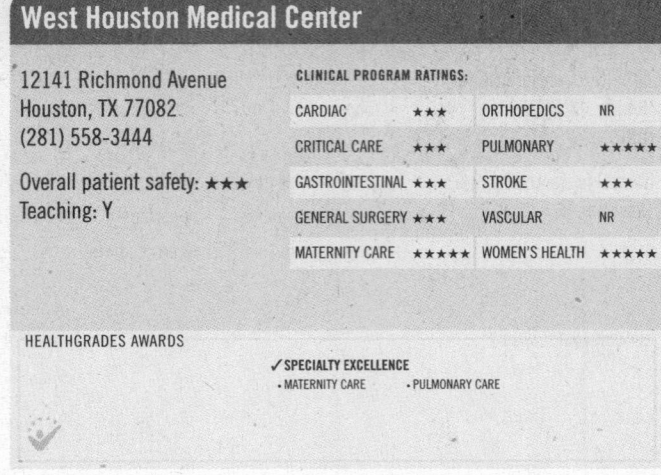

West Houston Medical Center

12141 Richmond Avenue
Houston, TX 77082
(281) 558-3444

Overall patient safety: ★★★
Teaching: Y

CLINICAL PROGRAM RATINGS:

CARDIAC	★★★	ORTHOPEDICS	NR
CRITICAL CARE	★★★	PULMONARY	★★★★★
GASTROINTESTINAL	★★★	STROKE	★★★
GENERAL SURGERY	★★★	VASCULAR	NR
MATERNITY CARE	★★★★★	WOMEN'S HEALTH	★★★★★

HEALTHGRADES AWARDS

✓ SPECIALTY EXCELLENCE
- MATERNITY CARE   - PULMONARY CARE

Walls Regional Hospital

201 Walls Drive
Cleburne, TX 76033
(817) 641-2551

Overall patient safety: ★★★★★
Teaching: N

CLINICAL PROGRAM RATINGS:

CARDIAC	NR	ORTHOPEDICS	NR
CRITICAL CARE	NR	PULMONARY	★★★
GASTROINTESTINAL	★★★	STROKE	★★★
GENERAL SURGERY	★★★	VASCULAR	NR
MATERNITY CARE	★★★	WOMEN'S HEALTH	NR

HEALTHGRADES AWARDS

✓ DISTINGUISHED HOSPITAL
- PATIENT SAFETY

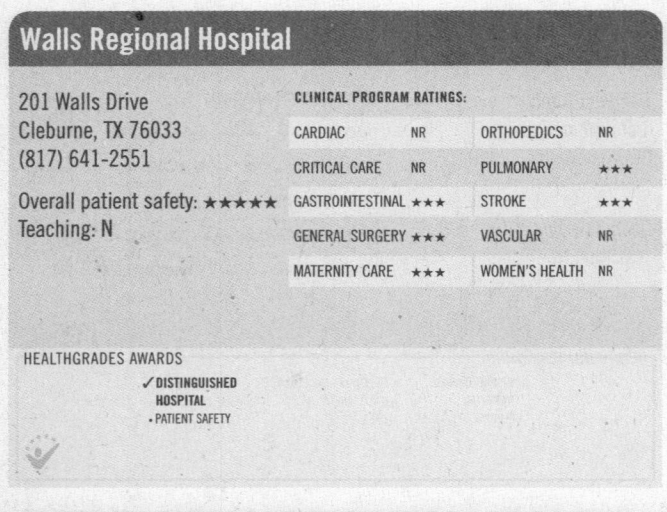

Westpark Medical Center*

130 South Central Expressway
McKinney, TX 75069
(214) 542-9382

Overall patient safety: ★★★
Teaching: N

CLINICAL PROGRAM RATINGS:

CARDIAC	★★★	ORTHOPEDICS	NR
CRITICAL CARE	★★★	PULMONARY	★★★
GASTROINTESTINAL	★★★	STROKE	★★★
GENERAL SURGERY	★★★	VASCULAR	NR
MATERNITY CARE	★★★	WOMEN'S HEALTH	NR

HEALTHGRADES AWARDS

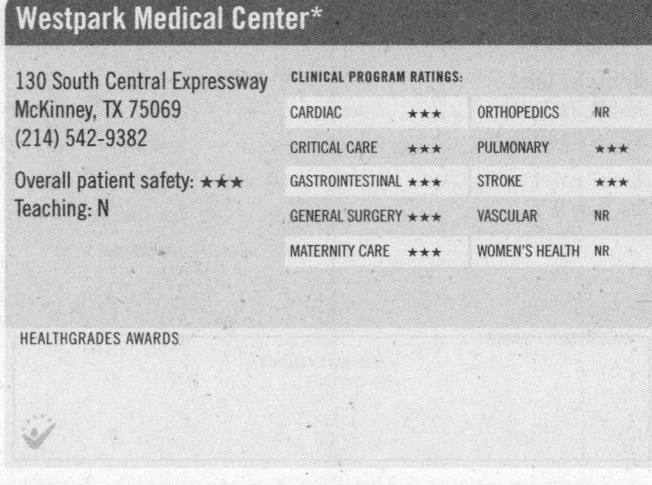

Ward Memorial Hospital

406 South Gary Street
Monahans, TX 79756
(432) 943-7537

Overall patient safety: NR
Teaching: N

CLINICAL PROGRAM RATINGS:

CARDIAC	NR	ORTHOPEDICS	NR
CRITICAL CARE	NR	PULMONARY	★★★
GASTROINTESTINAL	NR	STROKE	NR
GENERAL SURGERY	NR	VASCULAR	NR
MATERNITY CARE	NR	WOMEN'S HEALTH	NR

HEALTHGRADES AWARDS

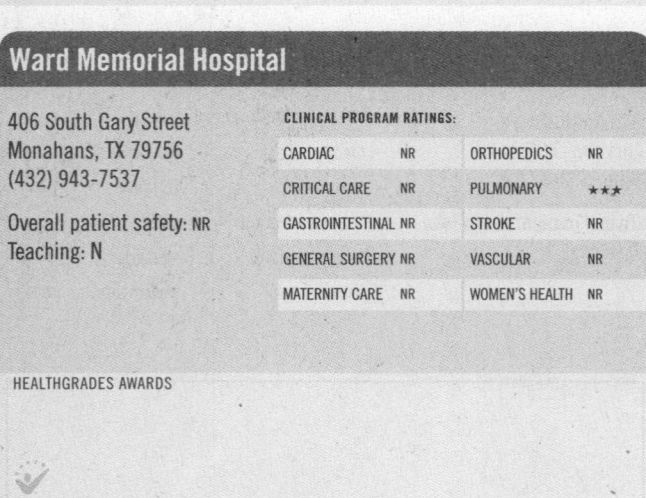

Wilbarger General Hospital

920 Hillcrest Drive
Vernon, TX 76384
(940) 552-9351

Overall patient safety: ★★★
Teaching: N

CLINICAL PROGRAM RATINGS:

CARDIAC	NR	ORTHOPEDICS	NR
CRITICAL CARE	NR	PULMONARY	★
GASTROINTESTINAL	NR	STROKE	NR
GENERAL SURGERY	NR	VASCULAR	NR
MATERNITY CARE	NR	WOMEN'S HEALTH	NR

HEALTHGRADES AWARDS

KEY: ★★★★★ BEST   ★★★ AS EXPECTED   ★ POOR   NR NOT RATED BY HEALTHGRADES   For full definitions of ratings and awards, see Appendix.

TEXAS HOSPITALS: RATINGS BY CLINICAL SPECIALTY

Wilson N. Jones Medical Center

500 North Highland Avenue
Sherman, TX 75092
(903) 870-4611

Overall patient safety: ★★★
Teaching: N

CLINICAL PROGRAM RATINGS:

CARDIAC	★★★	ORTHOPEDICS	★★★
CRITICAL CARE	★	PULMONARY	★
GASTROINTESTINAL	★★★	STROKE	★★★
GENERAL SURGERY	★★★	VASCULAR	NR
MATERNITY CARE	★★★	WOMEN'S HEALTH	★★★

HEALTHGRADES AWARDS

Woman's Hospital at Dallas Regional Medical Center

3500 Interstate 30
Mesquite, TX 75150
(972) 698-3300

Overall patient safety: ★★★
Teaching: N

CLINICAL PROGRAM RATINGS:

CARDIAC	NR	ORTHOPEDICS	NR
CRITICAL CARE	NR	PULMONARY	★★★
GASTROINTESTINAL	NR	STROKE	★★★
GENERAL SURGERY	★★★	VASCULAR	NR
MATERNITY CARE	★★★★★	WOMEN'S HEALTH	NR

HEALTHGRADES AWARDS

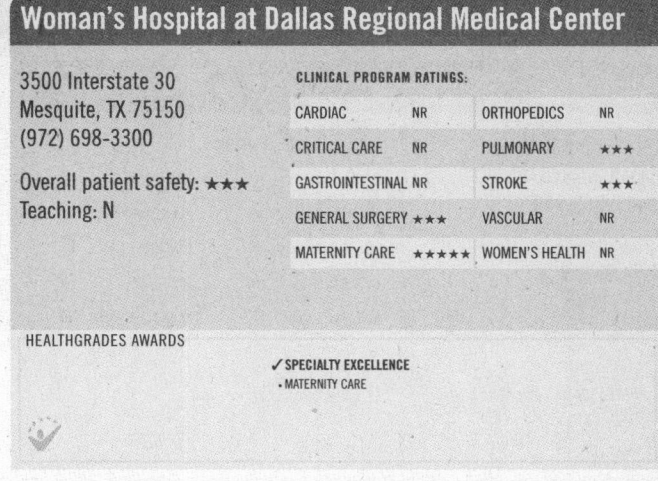

✓ SPECIALTY EXCELLENCE
• MATERNITY CARE

Winkler County Memorial Hospital

821 Jeffee Drive
Kermit, TX 79745
(432) 586-5864

Overall patient safety: NR
Teaching: N

CLINICAL PROGRAM RATINGS:

CARDIAC	NR	ORTHOPEDICS	NR
CRITICAL CARE	NR	PULMONARY	★★★
GASTROINTESTINAL	NR	STROKE	NR
GENERAL SURGERY	NR	VASCULAR	NR
MATERNITY CARE	NR	WOMEN'S HEALTH	NR

HEALTHGRADES AWARDS

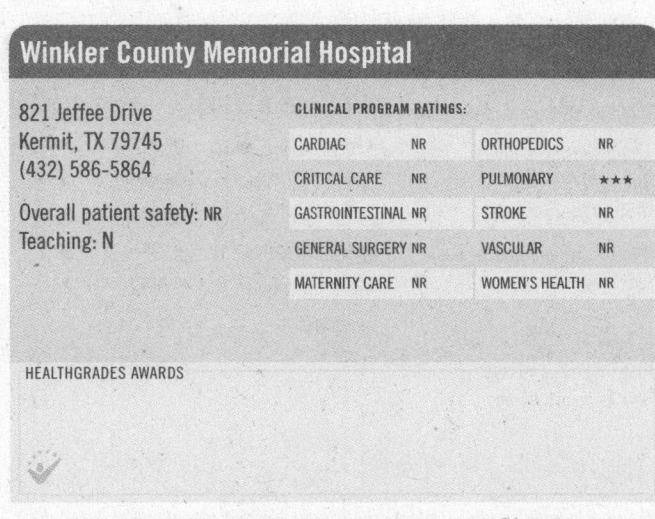

Woodland Heights Medical Center

505 South John Redditt Drive
Lufkin, TX 75904
(936) 634-8311

Overall patient safety: ★★★
Teaching: N

CLINICAL PROGRAM RATINGS:

CARDIAC	★★★	ORTHOPEDICS	NR
CRITICAL CARE	NR	PULMONARY	★★★★★
GASTROINTESTINAL	★★★	STROKE	★★★
GENERAL SURGERY	★★★	VASCULAR	NR
MATERNITY CARE	★★★	WOMEN'S HEALTH	NR

HEALTHGRADES AWARDS

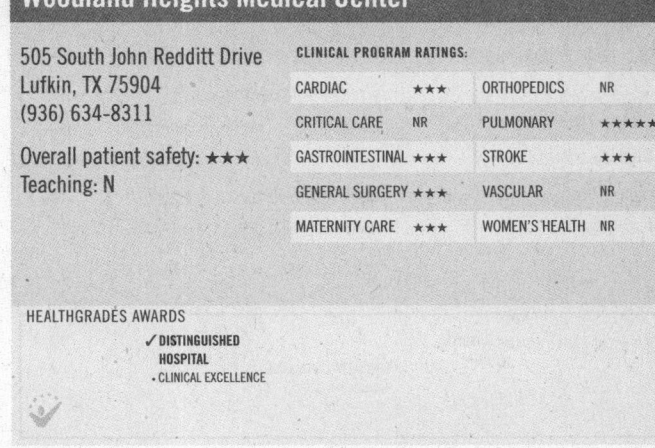

✓ DISTINGUISHED
   HOSPITAL
• CLINICAL EXCELLENCE

Wise Regional Health System

2000 FM 51 South
Decatur, TX 76234
(940) 627-5921

Overall patient safety: ★
Teaching: N

CLINICAL PROGRAM RATINGS:

CARDIAC	NR	ORTHOPEDICS	NR
CRITICAL CARE	NR	PULMONARY	★★★
GASTROINTESTINAL	NR	STROKE	★★★
GENERAL SURGERY	NR	VASCULAR	NR
MATERNITY CARE	NR	WOMEN'S HEALTH	NR

HEALTHGRADES AWARDS

Yoakum Community Hospital

1200 Carl Ramert Drive
Yoakum, TX 77995
(361) 293-2321

Overall patient safety: ★★★
Teaching: N

CLINICAL PROGRAM RATINGS:

CARDIAC	NR	ORTHOPEDICS	NR
CRITICAL CARE	NR	PULMONARY	★★★
GASTROINTESTINAL	NR	STROKE	★★★
GENERAL SURGERY	NR	VASCULAR	NR
MATERNITY CARE	★	WOMEN'S HEALTH	NR

HEALTHGRADES AWARDS

*This hospital reports its data to the federal government jointly with another hospital. Therefore the ratings and awards apply to multiple hospitals and this specific hospital may not provide all rated services.

Allen Memorial Hospital

719 West 400 North
Moab, UT 84532
(435) 259-7191

Overall patient safety: ★★★
Teaching: N

CLINICAL PROGRAM RATINGS:

CARDIAC	NR	ORTHOPEDICS	NR
CRITICAL CARE	NR	PULMONARY	★★★
GASTROINTESTINAL	NR	STROKE	NR
GENERAL SURGERY	NR	VASCULAR	NR
MATERNITY CARE	★	WOMEN'S HEALTH	NR

HEALTHGRADES AWARDS

Ashley Valley Medical Center

151 West 200 North
Vernal, UT 84078
(435) 789-3342

Overall patient safety: ★★★
Teaching: N

CLINICAL PROGRAM RATINGS:

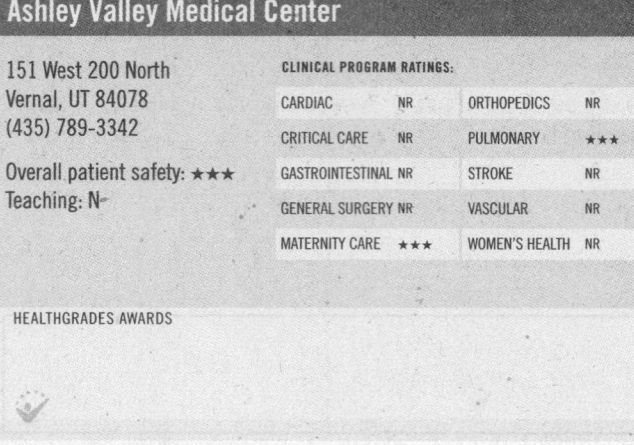

CARDIAC	NR	ORTHOPEDICS	NR
CRITICAL CARE	NR	PULMONARY	★★★
GASTROINTESTINAL	NR	STROKE	NR
GENERAL SURGERY	NR	VASCULAR	NR
MATERNITY CARE	★★★	WOMEN'S HEALTH	NR

HEALTHGRADES AWARDS

Alta View Hospital

9660 South 1300 East
Sandy, UT 84094
(801) 501-2600

Overall patient safety: ★★★
Teaching: N

CLINICAL PROGRAM RATINGS:

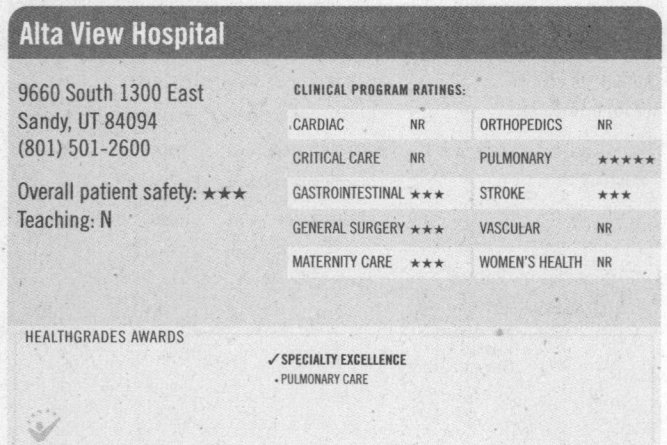

CARDIAC	NR	ORTHOPEDICS	NR
CRITICAL CARE	NR	PULMONARY	★★★★★
GASTROINTESTINAL	★★★	STROKE	★★★
GENERAL SURGERY	★★★	VASCULAR	NR
MATERNITY CARE	★★★	WOMEN'S HEALTH	NR

HEALTHGRADES AWARDS

✓ SPECIALTY EXCELLENCE
• PULMONARY CARE

Beaver Valley Hospital

1109 North 100 West
Beaver, UT 84713
(435) 438-7100

Overall patient safety: ★★★
Teaching: N

CLINICAL PROGRAM RATINGS:

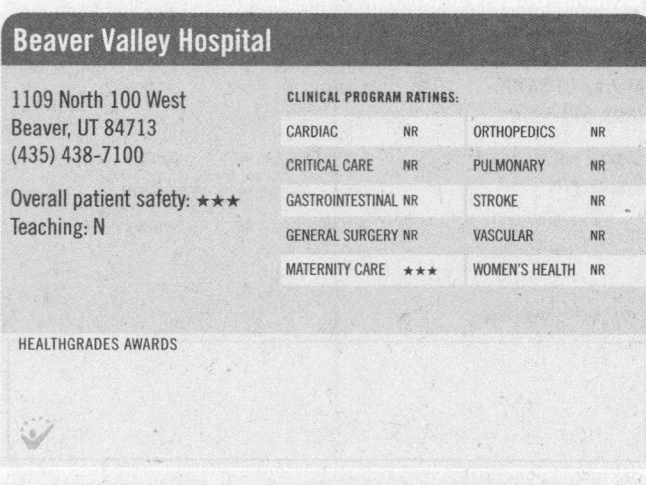

CARDIAC	NR	ORTHOPEDICS	NR
CRITICAL CARE	NR	PULMONARY	NR
GASTROINTESTINAL	NR	STROKE	NR
GENERAL SURGERY	NR	VASCULAR	NR
MATERNITY CARE	★★★	WOMEN'S HEALTH	NR

HEALTHGRADES AWARDS

American Fork Hospital

170 North 1100 East
American Fork, UT 84003
(801) 763-3300

Overall patient safety: ★★★
Teaching: N

CLINICAL PROGRAM RATINGS:

CARDIAC	NR	ORTHOPEDICS	NR
CRITICAL CARE	NR	PULMONARY	★★★
GASTROINTESTINAL	NR	STROKE	★★★
GENERAL SURGERY	★★★	VASCULAR	NR
MATERNITY CARE	★★★	WOMEN'S HEALTH	NR

HEALTHGRADES AWARDS

Brigham City Community Hospital

950 South Medical Drive
Brigham City, UT 84302
(435) 734-9471

Overall patient safety: ★★★
Teaching: N

CLINICAL PROGRAM RATINGS:

CARDIAC	NR	ORTHOPEDICS	NR
CRITICAL CARE	NR	PULMONARY	NR
GASTROINTESTINAL	NR	STROKE	★★★
GENERAL SURGERY	NR	VASCULAR	NR
MATERNITY CARE	★★★	WOMEN'S HEALTH	NR

HEALTHGRADES AWARDS

KEY: ★★★★★ BEST   ★★★ AS EXPECTED   ★ POOR   NR NOT RATED BY HEALTHGRADES   For full definitions of ratings and awards, see Appendix.

Castleview Hospital

300 North Hospital Drive
Price, UT 84501
(435) 637-4800

Overall patient safety: ★★★
Teaching: N

CLINICAL PROGRAM RATINGS:

CARDIAC	NR	ORTHOPEDICS	NR
CRITICAL CARE	NR	PULMONARY	★
GASTROINTESTINAL	NR	STROKE	★★★
GENERAL SURGERY	★★★	VASCULAR	NR
MATERNITY CARE	★★★	WOMEN'S HEALTH	NR

HEALTHGRADES AWARDS

Dixie Regional Medical Center

1380 East Medical Center Drive
St. George, UT 84790
(435) 634-4000

Overall patient safety: ★★★
Teaching: N

CLINICAL PROGRAM RATINGS:

CARDIAC	★★★	ORTHOPEDICS	★★★
CRITICAL CARE	NR	PULMONARY	★★★
GASTROINTESTINAL	★★★	STROKE	★★★
GENERAL SURGERY	★★★★★	VASCULAR	NR
MATERNITY CARE	★★★★★	WOMEN'S HEALTH	★★★

HEALTHGRADES AWARDS

✓ **SPECIALTY EXCELLENCE**
- GENERAL SURGERY   - MATERNITY CARE

Cottonwood Hospital

5770 South 300 East
Murray, UT 84107
(801) 314-5300

Overall patient safety: ★★★
Teaching: N

CLINICAL PROGRAM RATINGS:

CARDIAC	NR	ORTHOPEDICS	★
CRITICAL CARE	NR	PULMONARY	★★★
GASTROINTESTINAL	★★★	STROKE	★★★
GENERAL SURGERY	★★★	VASCULAR	NR
MATERNITY CARE	★★★★★	WOMEN'S HEALTH	NR

HEALTHGRADES AWARDS

Garfield Memorial Hospital

200 North 400 East
Panguitch, UT 84759
(435) 676-8811

Overall patient safety: ★★★
Teaching: N

CLINICAL PROGRAM RATINGS:

CARDIAC	NR	ORTHOPEDICS	NR
CRITICAL CARE	NR	PULMONARY	NR
GASTROINTESTINAL	NR	STROKE	NR
GENERAL SURGERY	NR	VASCULAR	NR
MATERNITY CARE	★	WOMEN'S HEALTH	NR

HEALTHGRADES AWARDS

Davis Hospital and Medical Center

1600 West Antelope Drive
Layton, UT 84041
(801) 825-9561

Overall patient safety: ★★★
Teaching: N

CLINICAL PROGRAM RATINGS:

CARDIAC	NR	ORTHOPEDICS	★★★
CRITICAL CARE	NR	PULMONARY	★
GASTROINTESTINAL	★★★	STROKE	★
GENERAL SURGERY	★★★	VASCULAR	NR
MATERNITY CARE	★★★	WOMEN'S HEALTH	NR

HEALTHGRADES AWARDS

Gunnison Valley Hospital

64 East 100 North
Gunnison, UT 84634
(435) 528-7246

Overall patient safety: ★★★
Teaching: N

CLINICAL PROGRAM RATINGS:

CARDIAC	NR	ORTHOPEDICS	NR
CRITICAL CARE	NR	PULMONARY	NR
GASTROINTESTINAL	NR	STROKE	NR
GENERAL SURGERY	NR	VASCULAR	NR
MATERNITY CARE	★★★	WOMEN'S HEALTH	NR

HEALTHGRADES AWARDS

Jordan Valley Hospital

3580 West 9000 South
West Jordan, UT 84088
(801) 561-8888

Overall patient safety: ★★★
Teaching: N

CLINICAL PROGRAM RATINGS:

CARDIAC	NR	ORTHOPEDICS	NR
CRITICAL CARE	NR	PULMONARY	★★★
GASTROINTESTINAL	NR	STROKE	★★★
GENERAL SURGERY	★	VASCULAR	NR
MATERNITY CARE	★★★	WOMEN'S HEALTH	NR

HEALTHGRADES AWARDS

LDS Hospital

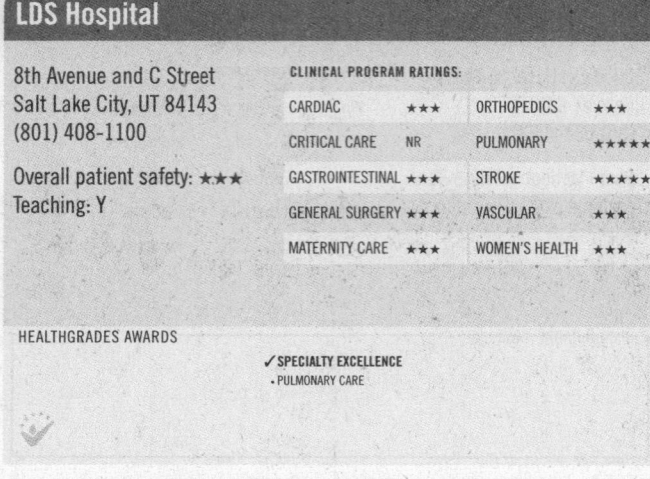

8th Avenue and C Street
Salt Lake City, UT 84143
(801) 408-1100

Overall patient safety: ★★★
Teaching: Y

CLINICAL PROGRAM RATINGS:

CARDIAC	★★★	ORTHOPEDICS	★★★
CRITICAL CARE	NR	PULMONARY	★★★★★
GASTROINTESTINAL	★★★	STROKE	★★★★★
GENERAL SURGERY	★★★	VASCULAR	★★★
MATERNITY CARE	★★★	WOMEN'S HEALTH	★★★

HEALTHGRADES AWARDS

✓ SPECIALTY EXCELLENCE
• PULMONARY CARE

Kane County Hospital

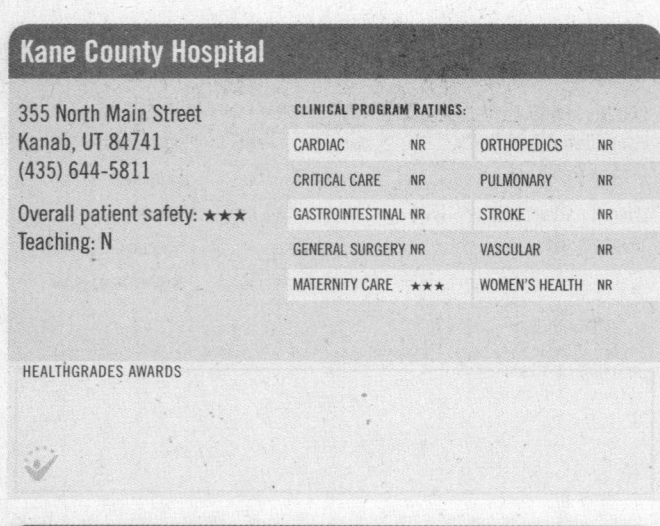

355 North Main Street
Kanab, UT 84741
(435) 644-5811

Overall patient safety: ★★★
Teaching: N

CLINICAL PROGRAM RATINGS:

CARDIAC	NR	ORTHOPEDICS	NR
CRITICAL CARE	NR	PULMONARY	NR
GASTROINTESTINAL	NR	STROKE	NR
GENERAL SURGERY	NR	VASCULAR	NR
MATERNITY CARE	★★★	WOMEN'S HEALTH	NR

HEALTHGRADES AWARDS

Logan Regional Hospital

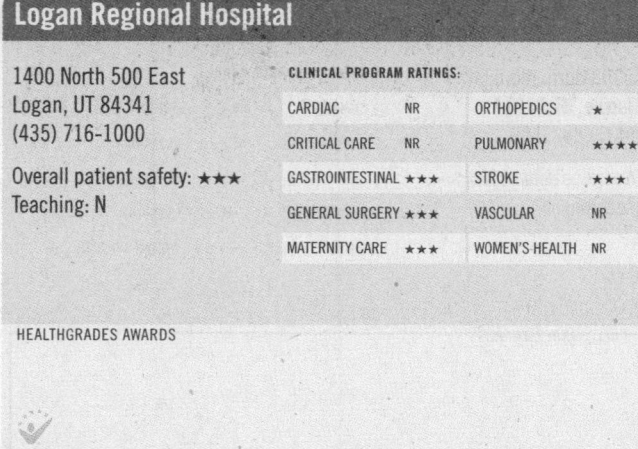

1400 North 500 East
Logan, UT 84341
(435) 716-1000

Overall patient safety: ★★★
Teaching: N

CLINICAL PROGRAM RATINGS:

CARDIAC	NR	ORTHOPEDICS	★
CRITICAL CARE	NR	PULMONARY	★★★★★
GASTROINTESTINAL	★★★	STROKE	★★★
GENERAL SURGERY	★★★	VASCULAR	NR
MATERNITY CARE	★★★	WOMEN'S HEALTH	NR

HEALTHGRADES AWARDS

Lakeview Hospital

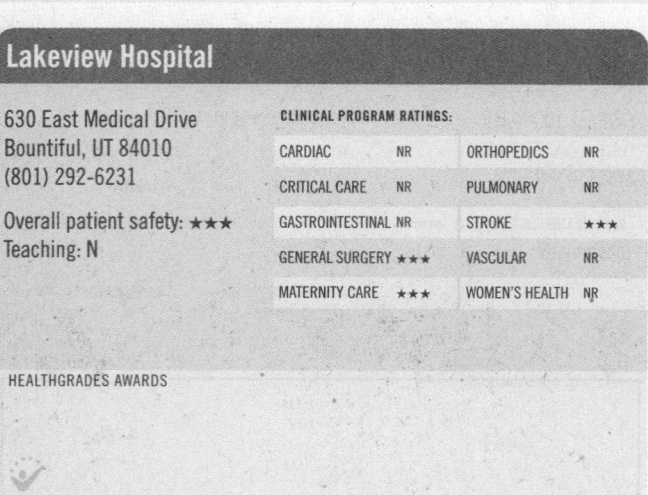

630 East Medical Drive
Bountiful, UT 84010
(801) 292-6231

Overall patient safety: ★★★
Teaching: N

CLINICAL PROGRAM RATINGS:

CARDIAC	NR	ORTHOPEDICS	NR
CRITICAL CARE	NR	PULMONARY	NR
GASTROINTESTINAL	NR	STROKE	★★★
GENERAL SURGERY	★★★	VASCULAR	NR
MATERNITY CARE	★★★	WOMEN'S HEALTH	NR

HEALTHGRADES AWARDS

McKay-Dee Hospital Center

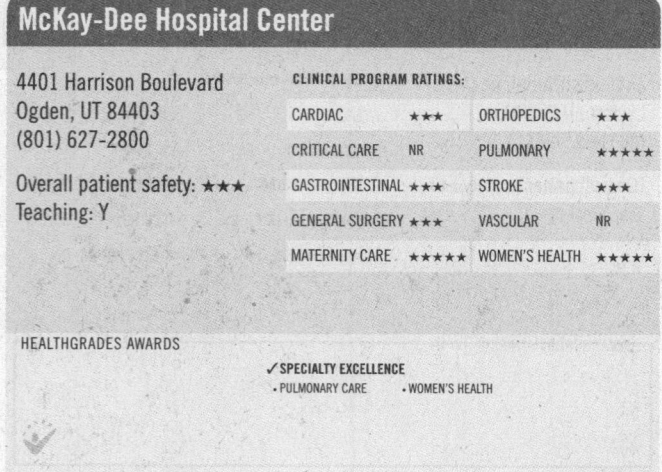

4401 Harrison Boulevard
Ogden, UT 84403
(801) 627-2800

Overall patient safety: ★★★
Teaching: Y

CLINICAL PROGRAM RATINGS:

CARDIAC	★★★	ORTHOPEDICS	★★★
CRITICAL CARE	NR	PULMONARY	★★★★★
GASTROINTESTINAL	★★★	STROKE	★★★
GENERAL SURGERY	★★★	VASCULAR	NR
MATERNITY CARE	★★★★★	WOMEN'S HEALTH	★★★★★

HEALTHGRADES AWARDS

✓ SPECIALTY EXCELLENCE
• PULMONARY CARE   • WOMEN'S HEALTH

KEY: ★★★★★ BEST   ★★★ AS EXPECTED   ★ POOR   NR NOT RATED BY HEALTHGRADES   For full definitions of ratings and awards, see Appendix.

Mountain View Hospital

1000 East 100 North
Payson, UT 84651
(801) 465-7000

Overall patient safety: ★★★
Teaching: N

CLINICAL PROGRAM RATINGS:

CARDIAC	NR	ORTHOPEDICS	★★★
CRITICAL CARE	NR	PULMONARY	★★★
GASTROINTESTINAL	NR	STROKE	★
GENERAL SURGERY	★★★	VASCULAR	NR
MATERNITY CARE	★★★	WOMEN'S HEALTH	NR

HEALTHGRADES AWARDS

Pioneer Valley Hospital

3460 South Pioneer Parkway
West Valley City, UT 84120
(801) 964-3100

Overall patient safety: ★★★
Teaching: N

CLINICAL PROGRAM RATINGS:

CARDIAC	NR	ORTHOPEDICS	NR
CRITICAL CARE	NR	PULMONARY	★★★
GASTROINTESTINAL	★★★	STROKE	★★★
GENERAL SURGERY	★★★	VASCULAR	NR
MATERNITY CARE	★★★	WOMEN'S HEALTH	NR

HEALTHGRADES AWARDS

Mountain West Medical Center

2055 North Main Street
Tooele, UT 84074
(435) 882-1697

Overall patient safety: ★★★
Teaching: N

CLINICAL PROGRAM RATINGS:

CARDIAC	NR	ORTHOPEDICS	NR
CRITICAL CARE	NR	PULMONARY	★★★
GASTROINTESTINAL	NR	STROKE	NR
GENERAL SURGERY	NR	VASCULAR	NR
MATERNITY CARE	★★★	WOMEN'S HEALTH	NR

HEALTHGRADES AWARDS

Salt Lake Regional Medical Center

1050 East South Temple
Salt Lake City, UT 84102
(801) 350-4111

Overall patient safety: ★★★
Teaching: Y

CLINICAL PROGRAM RATINGS:

CARDIAC	★★★	ORTHOPEDICS	NR
CRITICAL CARE	NR	PULMONARY	★★★★★
GASTROINTESTINAL	NR	STROKE	★★★
GENERAL SURGERY	★★★	VASCULAR	NR
MATERNITY CARE	★★★	WOMEN'S HEALTH	NR

HEALTHGRADES AWARDS

Ogden Regional Medical Center

5475 South 500 East
Ogden, UT 84405
(801) 479-2111

Overall patient safety: ★★★
Teaching: N

CLINICAL PROGRAM RATINGS:

CARDIAC	★★★	ORTHOPEDICS	NR
CRITICAL CARE	NR	PULMONARY	★★★
GASTROINTESTINAL	★★★	STROKE	★★★
GENERAL SURGERY	★★★	VASCULAR	NR
MATERNITY CARE	★★★★★	WOMEN'S HEALTH	★★★★★

HEALTHGRADES AWARDS

✓ SPECIALTY EXCELLENCE
· GENERAL SURGERY   · MATERNITY CARE   · WOMEN'S HEALTH

St. Mark's Hospital

1200 East 3900 South
Salt Lake City, UT 84124
(801) 268-7111

Overall patient safety: ★★★
Teaching: Y

CLINICAL PROGRAM RATINGS:

CARDIAC	★★★	ORTHOPEDICS	★★★
CRITICAL CARE	★★★★★	PULMONARY	★★★★★
GASTROINTESTINAL	★★★	STROKE	★★★
GENERAL SURGERY	★★★	VASCULAR	NR
MATERNITY CARE	★★★	WOMEN'S HEALTH	★★★

HEALTHGRADES AWARDS

✓ DISTINGUISHED HOSPITAL   ✓ SPECIALTY EXCELLENCE
· CLINICAL EXCELLENCE   · CRITICAL CARE   · JOINT REPLACEMENT   · PULMONARY CARE

Sevier Valley Medical Center

1100 North Main Street
Richfield, UT 84701
(435) 896-8271

Overall patient safety: ★★★
Teaching: N

CLINICAL PROGRAM RATINGS:

CARDIAC	NR	ORTHOPEDICS	NR
CRITICAL CARE	NR	PULMONARY	NR
GASTROINTESTINAL	NR	STROKE	NR
GENERAL SURGERY	★★★	VASCULAR	NR
MATERNITY CARE	★	WOMEN'S HEALTH	NR

HEALTHGRADES AWARDS

University of Utah Hospital

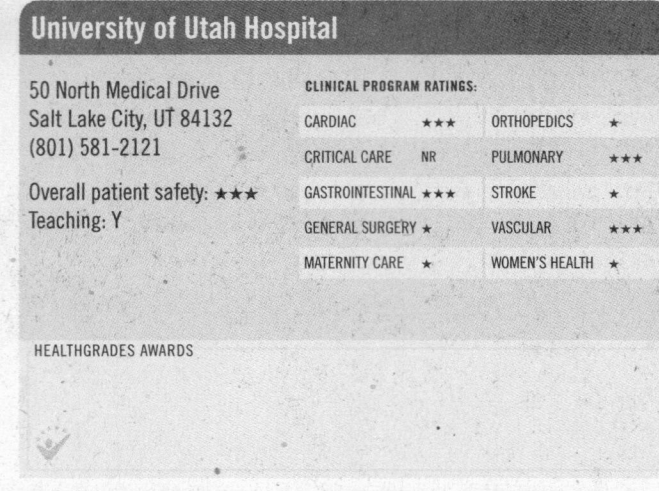

50 North Medical Drive
Salt Lake City, UT 84132
(801) 581-2121

Overall patient safety: ★★★
Teaching: Y

CLINICAL PROGRAM RATINGS:

CARDIAC	★★★	ORTHOPEDICS	★
CRITICAL CARE	NR	PULMONARY	★★★
GASTROINTESTINAL	★★★	STROKE	★
GENERAL SURGERY	★	VASCULAR	★★★
MATERNITY CARE	★	WOMEN'S HEALTH	★

HEALTHGRADES AWARDS

Timpanogos Regional Hospital

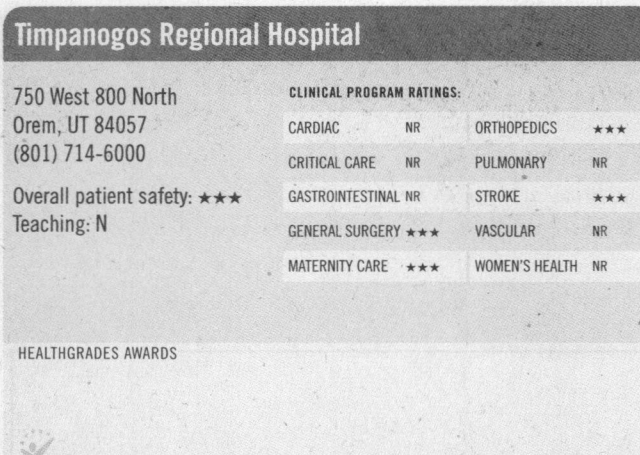

750 West 800 North
Orem, UT 84057
(801) 714-6000

Overall patient safety: ★★★
Teaching: N

CLINICAL PROGRAM RATINGS:

CARDIAC	NR	ORTHOPEDICS	★★★
CRITICAL CARE	NR	PULMONARY	NR
GASTROINTESTINAL	NR	STROKE	★★★
GENERAL SURGERY	★★★	VASCULAR	NR
MATERNITY CARE	★★★	WOMEN'S HEALTH	NR

HEALTHGRADES AWARDS

Utah Valley Regional Medical Center

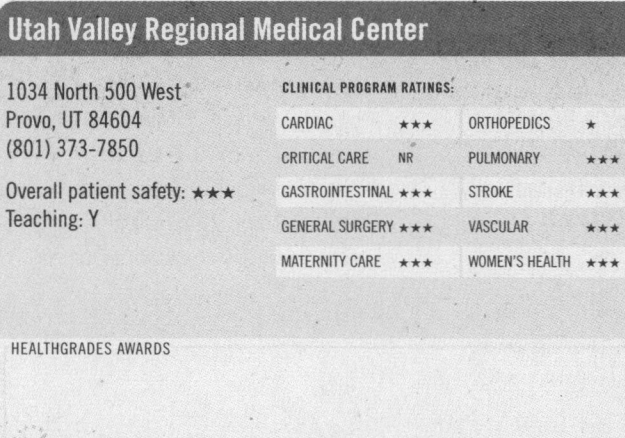

1034 North 500 West
Provo, UT 84604
(801) 373-7850

Overall patient safety: ★★★
Teaching: Y

CLINICAL PROGRAM RATINGS:

CARDIAC	★★★	ORTHOPEDICS	★
CRITICAL CARE	NR	PULMONARY	★★★
GASTROINTESTINAL	★★★	STROKE	★★★
GENERAL SURGERY	★★★	VASCULAR	★★★
MATERNITY CARE	★★★	WOMEN'S HEALTH	★★★

HEALTHGRADES AWARDS

Uintah Basin Medical Center

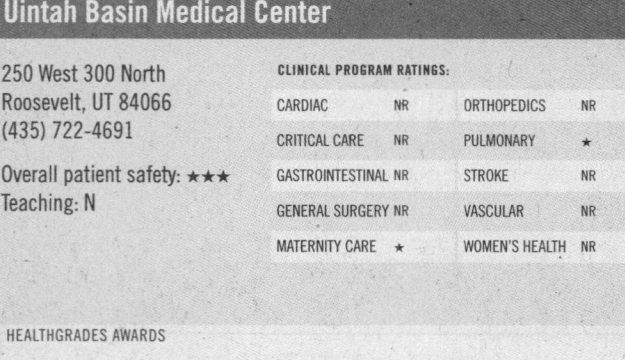

250 West 300 North
Roosevelt, UT 84066
(435) 722-4691

Overall patient safety: ★★★
Teaching: N

CLINICAL PROGRAM RATINGS:

CARDIAC	NR	ORTHOPEDICS	NR
CRITICAL CARE	NR	PULMONARY	★
GASTROINTESTINAL	NR	STROKE	NR
GENERAL SURGERY	NR	VASCULAR	NR
MATERNITY CARE	★	WOMEN'S HEALTH	NR

HEALTHGRADES AWARDS

Valley View Medical Center

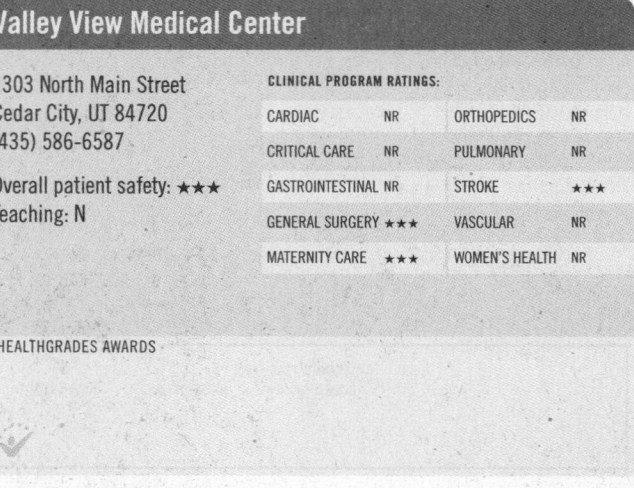

1303 North Main Street
Cedar City, UT 84720
(435) 586-6587

Overall patient safety: ★★★
Teaching: N

CLINICAL PROGRAM RATINGS:

CARDIAC	NR	ORTHOPEDICS	NR
CRITICAL CARE	NR	PULMONARY	NR
GASTROINTESTINAL	NR	STROKE	★★★
GENERAL SURGERY	★★★	VASCULAR	NR
MATERNITY CARE	★★★	WOMEN'S HEALTH	NR

HEALTHGRADES AWARDS

KEY: ★★★★★ BEST ★★★ AS EXPECTED ★ POOR NR NOT RATED BY HEALTHGRADES   For full definitions of ratings and awards, see Appendix.

Brattleboro Memorial Hospital

17 Belmont Avenue
Brattleboro, VT 05301
(802) 257-0341

Overall patient safety: ★★★
Teaching: N

CLINICAL PROGRAM RATINGS:

CARDIAC	NR	ORTHOPEDICS	NR
CRITICAL CARE	NR	PULMONARY	★
GASTROINTESTINAL	NR	STROKE	★★★
GENERAL SURGERY	NR	VASCULAR	NR
MATERNITY CARE	NR	WOMEN'S HEALTH	NR

HEALTHGRADES AWARDS

Gifford Medical Center

44 South Main Street
Randolph, VT 05060
(802) 728-4441

Overall patient safety: ★
Teaching: N

CLINICAL PROGRAM RATINGS:

CARDIAC	NR	ORTHOPEDICS	NR
CRITICAL CARE	NR	PULMONARY	★★★
GASTROINTESTINAL	NR	STROKE	NR
GENERAL SURGERY	NR	VASCULAR	NR
MATERNITY CARE	NR	WOMEN'S HEALTH	NR

HEALTHGRADES AWARDS

Central Vermont Medical Center

130 Fisher Road
Barre, VT 05641
(802) 371-4100

Overall patient safety: ★★★
Teaching: N

CLINICAL PROGRAM RATINGS:

CARDIAC	NR	ORTHOPEDICS	NR
CRITICAL CARE	NR	PULMONARY	★★★
GASTROINTESTINAL	NR	STROKE	★
GENERAL SURGERY	NR	VASCULAR	NR
MATERNITY CARE	NR	WOMEN'S HEALTH	NR

HEALTHGRADES AWARDS

North Country Hospital and Health Center

189 Prouty Drive
Newport, VT 05855
(802) 334-7331

Overall patient safety: ★★★
Teaching: N

CLINICAL PROGRAM RATINGS:

CARDIAC	NR	ORTHOPEDICS	NR
CRITICAL CARE	NR	PULMONARY	★★★★★
GASTROINTESTINAL	NR	STROKE	★★★
GENERAL SURGERY	NR	VASCULAR	NR
MATERNITY CARE	NR	WOMEN'S HEALTH	NR

HEALTHGRADES AWARDS

✓ SPECIALTY EXCELLENCE
• PULMONARY CARE

Fletcher Allen Hospital of Vermont

111 Colchester Avenue
Burlington, VT 05401
(802) 847-0000

Overall patient safety: ★★★
Teaching: Y

CLINICAL PROGRAM RATINGS:

CARDIAC	★★★	ORTHOPEDICS	★★★
CRITICAL CARE	NR	PULMONARY	★★★
GASTROINTESTINAL	★★★	STROKE	★★★★★
GENERAL SURGERY	NR	VASCULAR	★★★
MATERNITY CARE	NR	WOMEN'S HEALTH	NR

HEALTHGRADES AWARDS

✓ SPECIALTY EXCELLENCE
• STROKE CARE

Northeastern Vermont Regional Hospital

1315 Hospital Drive
St. Johnsbury, VT 05819
(802) 748-7400

Overall patient safety: ★★★★★
Teaching: N

CLINICAL PROGRAM RATINGS:

CARDIAC	NR	ORTHOPEDICS	NR
CRITICAL CARE	NR	PULMONARY	★
GASTROINTESTINAL	NR	STROKE	NR
GENERAL SURGERY	NR	VASCULAR	NR
MATERNITY CARE	NR	WOMEN'S HEALTH	NR

HEALTHGRADES AWARDS

VERMONT HOSPITALS: RATINGS BY CLINICAL SPECIALTY

Northwestern Medical Center

133 Fairfield Street
St. Albans, VT 05478
(802) 524-5911

Overall patient safety: ★★★
Teaching: N

CLINICAL PROGRAM RATINGS:

CARDIAC	NR	ORTHOPEDICS	NR
CRITICAL CARE	NR	PULMONARY	★
GASTROINTESTINAL	NR	STROKE	★★★
GENERAL SURGERY	NR	VASCULAR	NR
MATERNITY CARE	NR	WOMEN'S HEALTH	NR

HEALTHGRADES AWARDS

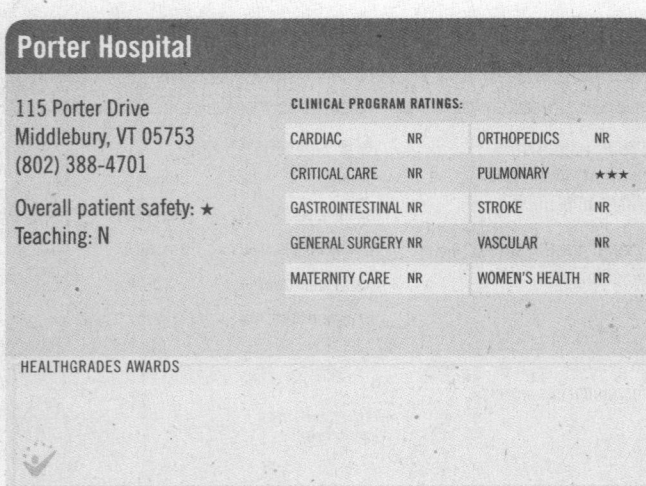

Southwestern Vermont Medical Center

100 Hospital Drive
Bennington, VT 05201
(802) 442-6361

Overall patient safety: ★★★
Teaching: N

CLINICAL PROGRAM RATINGS:

CARDIAC	NR	ORTHOPEDICS	★
CRITICAL CARE	NR	PULMONARY	★★★
GASTROINTESTINAL	★★★	STROKE	★★★
GENERAL SURGERY	NR	VASCULAR	NR
MATERNITY CARE	NR	WOMEN'S HEALTH	NR

HEALTHGRADES AWARDS

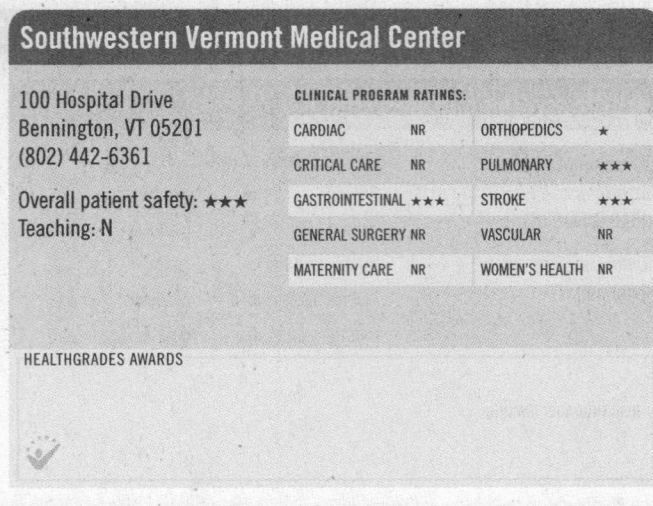

Porter Hospital

115 Porter Drive
Middlebury, VT 05753
(802) 388-4701

Overall patient safety: ★
Teaching: N

CLINICAL PROGRAM RATINGS:

CARDIAC	NR	ORTHOPEDICS	NR
CRITICAL CARE	NR	PULMONARY	★★★
GASTROINTESTINAL	NR	STROKE	NR
GENERAL SURGERY	NR	VASCULAR	NR
MATERNITY CARE	NR	WOMEN'S HEALTH	NR

HEALTHGRADES AWARDS

Springfield Hospital

P.O. Box 2003
Springfield, VT 05156
(802) 885-2151

Overall patient safety: NR
Teaching: N

CLINICAL PROGRAM RATINGS:

CARDIAC	NR	ORTHOPEDICS	NR
CRITICAL CARE	NR	PULMONARY	★
GASTROINTESTINAL	NR	STROKE	★
GENERAL SURGERY	NR	VASCULAR	NR
MATERNITY CARE	NR	WOMEN'S HEALTH	NR

HEALTHGRADES AWARDS

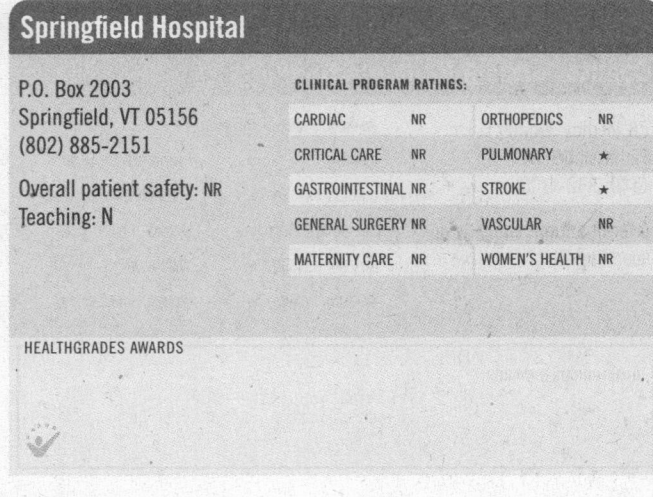

Rutland Regional Medical Center

160 Allen Street
Rutland, VT 05701
(802) 775-7111

Overall patient safety: ★★★
Teaching: N

CLINICAL PROGRAM RATINGS:

CARDIAC	NR	ORTHOPEDICS	★★★
CRITICAL CARE	NR	PULMONARY	★
GASTROINTESTINAL	★★★	STROKE	★
GENERAL SURGERY	NR	VASCULAR	NR
MATERNITY CARE	NR	WOMEN'S HEALTH	NR

HEALTHGRADES AWARDS

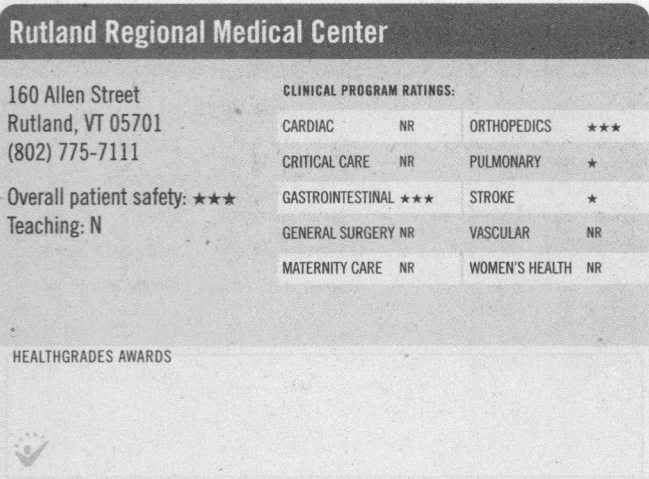

KEY: ★★★★★ BEST ★★★ AS EXPECTED ★ POOR NR NOT RATED BY HEALTHGRADES For full definitions of ratings and awards, see Appendix.

Alleghany Regional Hospital

1 Arh Lane
Low Moor, VA 24457
(540) 862-6011

Overall patient safety: ★★★
Teaching: N

CLINICAL PROGRAM RATINGS:

CARDIAC	NR	ORTHOPEDICS	NR
CRITICAL CARE	NR	PULMONARY	★★★
GASTROINTESTINAL	NR	STROKE	★
GENERAL SURGERY	★★★	VASCULAR	NR
MATERNITY CARE	NR	WOMEN'S HEALTH	NR

HEALTHGRADES AWARDS

Bedford Memorial Hospital

1613 Oakwood Street
Bedford, VA 24523
(540) 586-2441

Overall patient safety: ★★★
Teaching: N

CLINICAL PROGRAM RATINGS:

CARDIAC	NR	ORTHOPEDICS	NR
CRITICAL CARE	NR	PULMONARY	★★★
GASTROINTESTINAL	NR	STROKE	★
GENERAL SURGERY	NR	VASCULAR	NR
MATERNITY CARE	★★★	WOMEN'S HEALTH	NR

HEALTHGRADES AWARDS

Augusta Medical Center

78 Medical Center Drive
Fishersville, VA 22939
(540) 932-4000

Overall patient safety: ★★★
Teaching: N

CLINICAL PROGRAM RATINGS:

CARDIAC	NR	ORTHOPEDICS	★★★
CRITICAL CARE	NR	PULMONARY	★★★
GASTROINTESTINAL	★★★	STROKE	★★★
GENERAL SURGERY	★★★	VASCULAR	NR
MATERNITY CARE	★★★	WOMEN'S HEALTH	NR

HEALTHGRADES AWARDS

✓ SPECIALTY EXCELLENCE
• GENERAL SURGERY   • JOINT REPLACEMENT

Bon Secours DePaul Medical Center

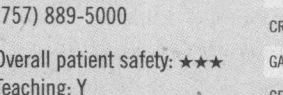

150 Kingsley Lane
Norfolk, VA 23505
(757) 889-5000

Overall patient safety: ★★★
Teaching: Y

CLINICAL PROGRAM RATINGS:

CARDIAC	NR	ORTHOPEDICS	★
CRITICAL CARE	★★★	PULMONARY	★★★
GASTROINTESTINAL	★★★	STROKE	★★★
GENERAL SURGERY	★	VASCULAR	★★★
MATERNITY CARE	★★★	WOMEN'S HEALTH	NR

HEALTHGRADES AWARDS

Bath County Community Hospital

Route 220 North and
Park Lane
Hot Springs, VA 24445
(540) 839-7000

Overall patient safety: NR
Teaching: N

CLINICAL PROGRAM RATINGS:

CARDIAC	NR	ORTHOPEDICS	NR
CRITICAL CARE	NR	PULMONARY	★★★
GASTROINTESTINAL	NR	STROKE	NR
GENERAL SURGERY	NR	VASCULAR	NR
MATERNITY CARE	NR	WOMEN'S HEALTH	NR

HEALTHGRADES AWARDS

Bon Secours Maryview Medical Center

3636 High Street
Portsmouth, VA 23707
(757) 398-2200

Overall patient safety: ★★★
Teaching: Y

CLINICAL PROGRAM RATINGS:

CARDIAC	NR	ORTHOPEDICS	★★★
CRITICAL CARE	★★★	PULMONARY	★★★
GASTROINTESTINAL	★★★	STROKE	★★★
GENERAL SURGERY	★★★	VASCULAR	NR
MATERNITY CARE	★★★	WOMEN'S HEALTH	NR

HEALTHGRADES AWARDS

✓ SPECIALTY EXCELLENCE
• BARIATRIC SURGERY

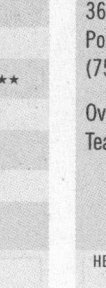

Bon Secours Memorial Regional Medical Center

8260 Atlee Road
Mechanicsville, VA 23116
(804) 764-6000

Overall patient safety: ★
Teaching: N

CLINICAL PROGRAM RATINGS:

CARDIAC	★★★	ORTHOPEDICS	★★★
CRITICAL CARE	★★★	PULMONARY	★★★★★
GASTROINTESTINAL	★★★	STROKE	★★★★★
GENERAL SURGERY	★★★	VASCULAR	★★★
MATERNITY CARE	★★★	WOMEN'S HEALTH	★★★

HEALTHGRADES AWARDS

✓DISTINGUISHED HOSPITAL
- CLINICAL EXCELLENCE

✓SPECIALTY EXCELLENCE
- CARDIAC CARE
- CARDIAC SURGERY
- PULMONARY CARE
- STROKE CARE

Bon Secours St. Mary's Hospital

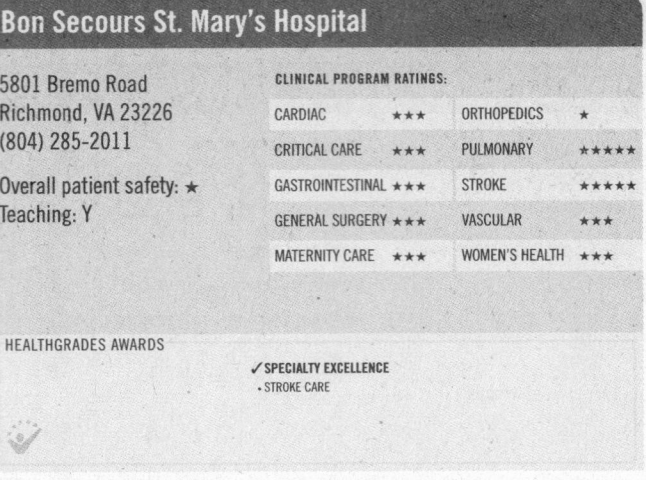

5801 Bremo Road
Richmond, VA 23226
(804) 285-2011

Overall patient safety: ★
Teaching: Y

CLINICAL PROGRAM RATINGS:

CARDIAC	★★★	ORTHOPEDICS	★
CRITICAL CARE	★★★	PULMONARY	★★★★★
GASTROINTESTINAL	★★★	STROKE	★★★★★
GENERAL SURGERY	★★★	VASCULAR	★★★
MATERNITY CARE	★★★	WOMEN'S HEALTH	★★★

HEALTHGRADES AWARDS

✓SPECIALTY EXCELLENCE
- STROKE CARE

Bon Secours Richmond Community Hospital

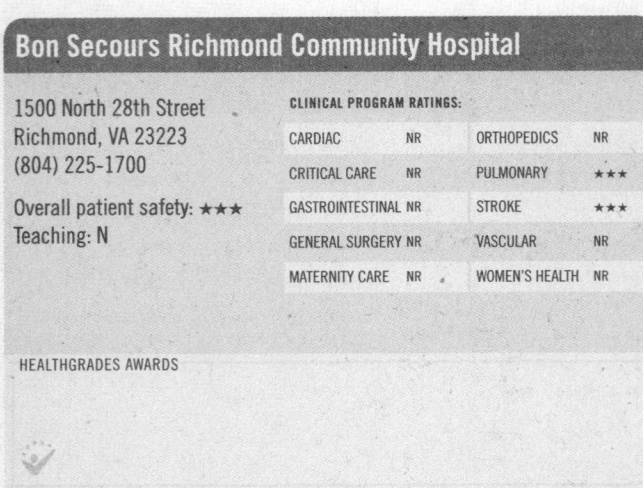

1500 North 28th Street
Richmond, VA 23223
(804) 225-1700

Overall patient safety: ★★★
Teaching: N

CLINICAL PROGRAM RATINGS:

CARDIAC	NR	ORTHOPEDICS	NR
CRITICAL CARE	NR	PULMONARY	★★★
GASTROINTESTINAL	NR	STROKE	★★★
GENERAL SURGERY	NR	VASCULAR	NR
MATERNITY CARE	NR	WOMEN'S HEALTH	NR

HEALTHGRADES AWARDS

Buchanan General Hospital*

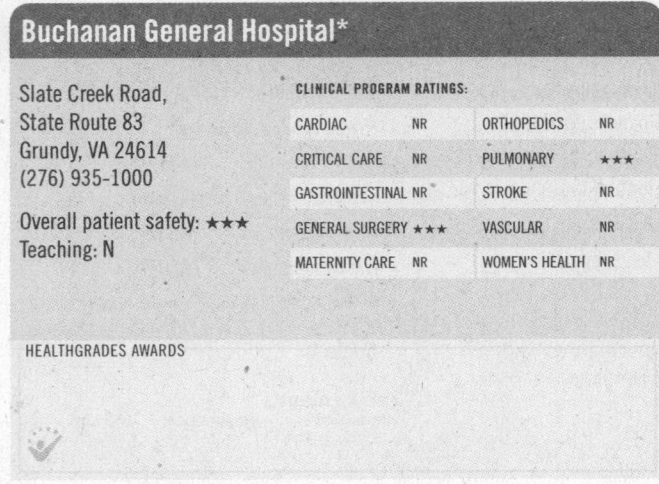

Slate Creek Road,
State Route 83
Grundy, VA 24614
(276) 935-1000

Overall patient safety: ★★★
Teaching: N

CLINICAL PROGRAM RATINGS:

CARDIAC	NR	ORTHOPEDICS	NR
CRITICAL CARE	NR	PULMONARY	★★★
GASTROINTESTINAL	NR	STROKE	NR
GENERAL SURGERY	★★★	VASCULAR	NR
MATERNITY CARE	NR	WOMEN'S HEALTH	NR

HEALTHGRADES AWARDS

Bon Secours St. Francis Medical Center

13700 St. Francis Boulevard
Midlothian, VA 23114
(804) 594-7404

Overall patient safety: ★★★
Teaching: N

CLINICAL PROGRAM RATINGS:

CARDIAC	NR	ORTHOPEDICS	NR
CRITICAL CARE	NR	PULMONARY	★★★
GASTROINTESTINAL	NR	STROKE	NR
GENERAL SURGERY	NR	VASCULAR	NR
MATERNITY CARE	★★★	WOMEN'S HEALTH	NR

HEALTHGRADES AWARDS

Carilion Franklin Memorial Hospital

180 Floyd Avenue
Rocky Mount, VA 24151
(540) 483-5277

Overall patient safety: ★★★
Teaching: N

CLINICAL PROGRAM RATINGS:

CARDIAC	NR	ORTHOPEDICS	NR
CRITICAL CARE	NR	PULMONARY	★★★
GASTROINTESTINAL	NR	STROKE	★★★
GENERAL SURGERY	★★★	VASCULAR	NR
MATERNITY CARE	★★★	WOMEN'S HEALTH	NR

HEALTHGRADES AWARDS

✓SPECIALTY EXCELLENCE
- GENERAL SURGERY

KEY: ★★★★★ BEST   ★★★ AS EXPECTED   ★ POOR   NR NOT RATED BY HEALTHGRADES   For full definitions of ratings and awards, see Appendix.

Carilion Giles Memorial Hospital

1 Taylor Avenue
Pearisburg, VA 24134
(540) 921-6000

Overall patient safety: ★★★
Teaching: N

CLINICAL PROGRAM RATINGS:

CARDIAC	NR	ORTHOPEDICS	NR
CRITICAL CARE	NR	PULMONARY	★★★
GASTROINTESTINAL	NR	STROKE	★★★
GENERAL SURGERY	NR	VASCULAR	NR
MATERNITY CARE	NR	WOMEN'S HEALTH	NR

HEALTHGRADES AWARDS

Centra Health*

3300 Rivermont Avenue
Lynchburg, VA 24503
(434) 947-4700

Overall patient safety: ★★★
Teaching: Y

CLINICAL PROGRAM RATINGS:

CARDIAC	★★★	ORTHOPEDICS	★★★★★
CRITICAL CARE	★★★	PULMONARY	★★★
GASTROINTESTINAL	★★★	STROKE	★★★
GENERAL SURGERY	★★★★★	VASCULAR	★★★
MATERNITY CARE	★★★	WOMEN'S HEALTH	★★★

HEALTHGRADES AWARDS

✓ DISTINGUISHED HOSPITAL
- CLINICAL EXCELLENCE

✓ SPECIALTY EXCELLENCE
- GASTROINTESTINAL CARE
- GENERAL SURGERY
- JOINT REPLACEMENT
- ORTHOPEDIC SURGERY

Carilion Medical Center

1906 Belleview Avenue
Roanoke, VA 24014
(540) 981-7000

Overall patient safety: ★★★
Teaching: Y

CLINICAL PROGRAM RATINGS:

CARDIAC	★★★	ORTHOPEDICS	★★★
CRITICAL CARE	★	PULMONARY	★★★
GASTROINTESTINAL	★★★	STROKE	★★★
GENERAL SURGERY	★★★	VASCULAR	★★★
MATERNITY CARE	★	WOMEN'S HEALTH	★

HEALTHGRADES AWARDS

✓ SPECIALTY EXCELLENCE
- VASCULAR SURGERY

Chesapeake General Hospital

736 Battlefield Boulevard North
Chesapeake, VA 23320
(757) 312-8121

Overall patient safety: ★★★
Teaching: N

CLINICAL PROGRAM RATINGS:

CARDIAC	NR	ORTHOPEDICS	★★★
CRITICAL CARE	★★★	PULMONARY	★★★★★
GASTROINTESTINAL	★★★	STROKE	★★★
GENERAL SURGERY	★★★	VASCULAR	NR
MATERNITY CARE	★★★	WOMEN'S HEALTH	NR

HEALTHGRADES AWARDS

✓ SPECIALTY EXCELLENCE
- PULMONARY CARE

Carilion New River Valley Medical Center

2900 Lamb Circle
Christiansburg, VA 24073
(540) 731-2000

Overall patient safety: ★★★
Teaching: N

CLINICAL PROGRAM RATINGS:

CARDIAC	NR	ORTHOPEDICS	NR
CRITICAL CARE	★★★	PULMONARY	★★★
GASTROINTESTINAL	★★★	STROKE	★★★
GENERAL SURGERY	★★★	VASCULAR	★★★
MATERNITY CARE	★★★	WOMEN'S HEALTH	NR

HEALTHGRADES AWARDS

CJW Medical Center--Chippenham Campus

7101 Jahnke Road
Richmond, VA 23225
(804) 320-3911

Overall patient safety: ★★★
Teaching: Y

CLINICAL PROGRAM RATINGS:

CARDIAC	★★★★★	ORTHOPEDICS	★★★
CRITICAL CARE	★★★	PULMONARY	★★★★★
GASTROINTESTINAL	★★★	STROKE	★★★
GENERAL SURGERY	★★★	VASCULAR	★★★
MATERNITY CARE	★★★	WOMEN'S HEALTH	★★★

HEALTHGRADES AWARDS

✓ AMERICA'S 50 BEST HOSPITALS

✓ DISTINGUISHED HOSPITAL
- CLINICAL EXCELLENCE

✓ SPECIALTY EXCELLENCE
- CARDIAC CARE
- CARDIAC SURGERY

---

*This hospital reports its data to the federal government jointly with another hospital. Therefore the ratings and awards apply to multiple hospitals and this specific hospital may not provide all rated services.

Clinch Valley Medical Center

2949 West Front Street
Richlands, VA 24641
(276) 596-6000

Overall patient safety: ★★★
Teaching: N

CLINICAL PROGRAM RATINGS:

CARDIAC	NR	ORTHOPEDICS	NR
CRITICAL CARE	NR	PULMONARY	★★★
GASTROINTESTINAL	NR	STROKE	★★★
GENERAL SURGERY	★★★	VASCULAR	NR
MATERNITY CARE	★★★	WOMEN'S HEALTH	NR

HEALTHGRADES AWARDS

Danville Regional Medical Center

142 South Main Street
Danville, VA 24541
(434) 799-2100

Overall patient safety: ★★★
Teaching: N

CLINICAL PROGRAM RATINGS:

CARDIAC	★★★	ORTHOPEDICS	★★★★★
CRITICAL CARE	★★★	PULMONARY	★★★★★
GASTROINTESTINAL	★★★	STROKE	★★★★★
GENERAL SURGERY	★★★★★	VASCULAR	NR
MATERNITY CARE	★★★	WOMEN'S HEALTH	★★★

HEALTHGRADES AWARDS

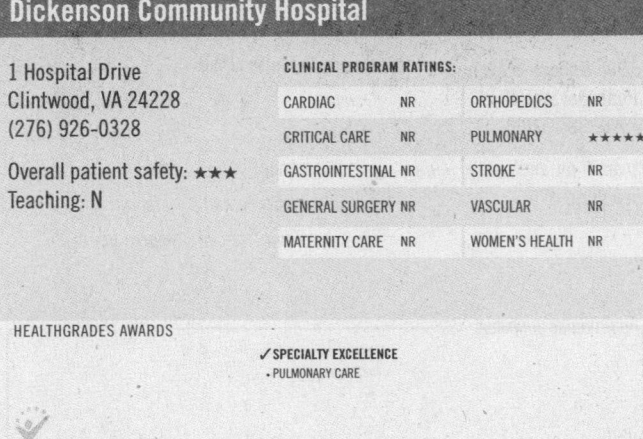

✓ SPECIALTY EXCELLENCE
- GENERAL SURGERY
- ORTHOPEDIC SURGERY
- PULMONARY CARE
- STROKE CARE

Community Memorial Healthcenter

125 Buena Vista Circle
South Hill, VA 23970
(434) 447-3151

Overall patient safety: ★★★
Teaching: N

CLINICAL PROGRAM RATINGS:

CARDIAC	NR	ORTHOPEDICS	NR
CRITICAL CARE	NR	PULMONARY	★★★
GASTROINTESTINAL	★★★	STROKE	★★★
GENERAL SURGERY	★★★	VASCULAR	NR
MATERNITY CARE	★★★	WOMEN'S HEALTH	NR

HEALTHGRADES AWARDS

Dickenson Community Hospital

1 Hospital Drive
Clintwood, VA 24228
(276) 926-0328

Overall patient safety: ★★★
Teaching: N

CLINICAL PROGRAM RATINGS:

CARDIAC	NR	ORTHOPEDICS	NR
CRITICAL CARE	NR	PULMONARY	★★★★★
GASTROINTESTINAL	NR	STROKE	NR
GENERAL SURGERY	NR	VASCULAR	NR
MATERNITY CARE	NR	WOMEN'S HEALTH	NR

HEALTHGRADES AWARDS

✓ SPECIALTY EXCELLENCE
- PULMONARY CARE

Culpeper Memorial Hospital

501 Sunset Lane
Culpeper, VA 22701
(540) 829-4100

Overall patient safety: ★★★
Teaching: N

CLINICAL PROGRAM RATINGS:

CARDIAC	NR	ORTHOPEDICS	★★★
CRITICAL CARE	NR	PULMONARY	★★★
GASTROINTESTINAL	NR	STROKE	★
GENERAL SURGERY	NR	VASCULAR	NR
MATERNITY CARE	★★★	WOMEN'S HEALTH	NR

HEALTHGRADES AWARDS

Fauquier Hospital

500 Hospital Drive
Warrenton, VA 20186
(540) 349-0550

Overall patient safety: ★★★
Teaching: N

CLINICAL PROGRAM RATINGS:

CARDIAC	NR	ORTHOPEDICS	★★★
CRITICAL CARE	NR	PULMONARY	★★★
GASTROINTESTINAL	★★★	STROKE	★
GENERAL SURGERY	★★★	VASCULAR	NR
MATERNITY CARE	★★★	WOMEN'S HEALTH	NR

HEALTHGRADES AWARDS

KEY: ★★★★★ BEST   ★★★ AS EXPECTED   ★ POOR   NR NOT RATED BY HEALTHGRADES   For full definitions of ratings and awards, see Appendix.

Grundy Hospital*

Main Street
Grundy, VA 24614
(703) 935-2111

Overall patient safety: ★★★
Teaching: N

CLINICAL PROGRAM RATINGS:

CARDIAC	NR	ORTHOPEDICS	NR
CRITICAL CARE	NR	PULMONARY	★★★
GASTROINTESTINAL	NR	STROKE	NR
GENERAL SURGERY	★★★	VASCULAR	NR
MATERNITY CARE	NR	WOMEN'S HEALTH	NR

HEALTHGRADES AWARDS

Henrico Doctors' Hospital—Parham*

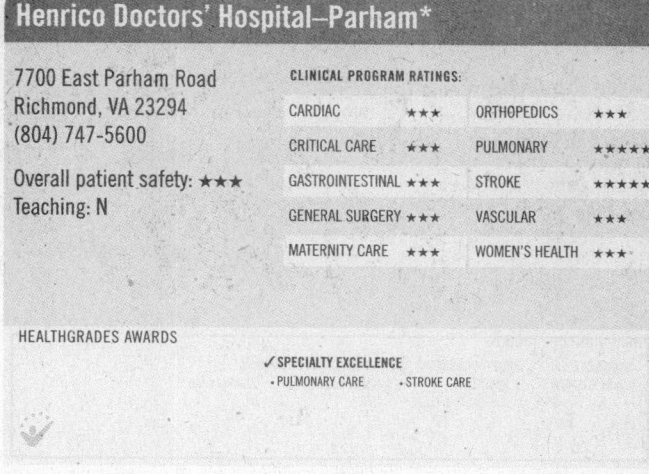

7700 East Parham Road
Richmond, VA 23294
(804) 747-5600

Overall patient safety: ★★★
Teaching: N

CLINICAL PROGRAM RATINGS:

CARDIAC	★★★	ORTHOPEDICS	★★★
CRITICAL CARE	★★★	PULMONARY	★★★★★
GASTROINTESTINAL	★★★	STROKE	★★★★★
GENERAL SURGERY	★★★	VASCULAR	★★★
MATERNITY CARE	★★★	WOMEN'S HEALTH	★★★

HEALTHGRADES AWARDS

✓ SPECIALTY EXCELLENCE
- PULMONARY CARE   - STROKE CARE

Halifax Regional Hospital

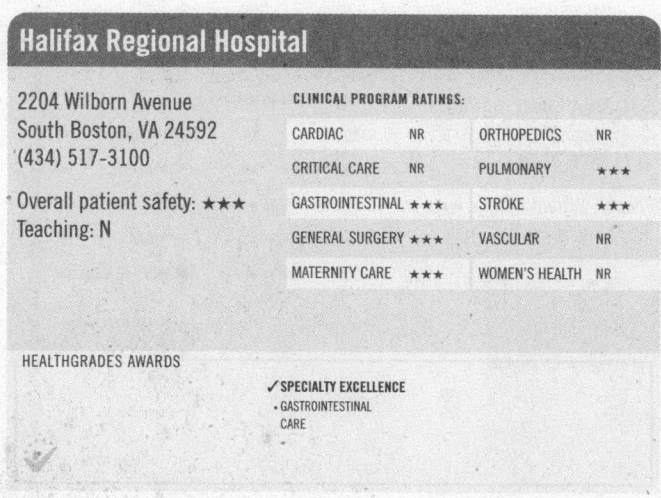

2204 Wilborn Avenue
South Boston, VA 24592
(434) 517-3100

Overall patient safety: ★★★
Teaching: N

CLINICAL PROGRAM RATINGS:

CARDIAC	NR	ORTHOPEDICS	NR
CRITICAL CARE	NR	PULMONARY	★★★
GASTROINTESTINAL	★★★	STROKE	★★★
GENERAL SURGERY	★★★	VASCULAR	NR
MATERNITY CARE	★★★	WOMEN'S HEALTH	NR

HEALTHGRADES AWARDS

✓ SPECIALTY EXCELLENCE
- GASTROINTESTINAL CARE

Inova Alexandria Hospital

4320 Seminary Road
Alexandria, VA 22304
(703) 504-3000

Overall patient safety: ★
Teaching: N

CLINICAL PROGRAM RATINGS:

CARDIAC	★★★	ORTHOPEDICS	★★★
CRITICAL CARE	★★★	PULMONARY	★★★★★
GASTROINTESTINAL	★★★	STROKE	★★★★★
GENERAL SURGERY	★★★	VASCULAR	★★★
MATERNITY CARE	★★★★★	WOMEN'S HEALTH	★★★★★

HEALTHGRADES AWARDS

✓ DISTINGUISHED HOSPITAL
- CLINICAL EXCELLENCE

✓ SPECIALTY EXCELLENCE
- GASTROINTESTINAL CARE   - PULMONARY CARE   - WOMEN'S HEALTH
- MATERNITY CARE   - STROKE CARE

Henrico Doctors' Hospital*

1602 Skipwith Road
Richmond, VA 23229
(804) 289-4500

Overall patient safety: ★★★
Teaching: N

CLINICAL PROGRAM RATINGS:

CARDIAC	★★★	ORTHOPEDICS	★★★
CRITICAL CARE	★★★	PULMONARY	★★★★★
GASTROINTESTINAL	★★★	STROKE	★★★★★
GENERAL SURGERY	★★★	VASCULAR	★★★
MATERNITY CARE	★★★	WOMEN'S HEALTH	★★★

HEALTHGRADES AWARDS

✓ AMERICA'S 50 BEST HOSPITALS

✓ DISTINGUISHED HOSPITAL
- CLINICAL EXCELLENCE

✓ SPECIALTY EXCELLENCE
- PULMONARY CARE   - STROKE CARE

Inova Fair Oaks Hospital

3600 Joseph Siewick Drive
Fairfax, VA 22033
(703) 391-3600

Overall patient safety: ★★★
Teaching: N

CLINICAL PROGRAM RATINGS:

CARDIAC	NR	ORTHOPEDICS	★★★
CRITICAL CARE	★★★	PULMONARY	★★★
GASTROINTESTINAL	★★★	STROKE	★★★
GENERAL SURGERY	★★★	VASCULAR	NR
MATERNITY CARE	★★★★★	WOMEN'S HEALTH	NR

HEALTHGRADES AWARDS

✓ SPECIALTY EXCELLENCE
- BARIATRIC SURGERY   - MATERNITY CARE

*This hospital reports its data to the federal government jointly with another hospital. Therefore the ratings and awards apply to multiple hospitals and this specific hospital may not provide all rated services.

CHAPTER 6: HOSPITAL RATINGS BY CLINICAL SPECIALTY   681

VIRGINIA HOSPITALS: RATINGS BY CLINICAL SPECIALTY

Inova Fairfax Hospital

3300 Gallows Road
Falls Church, VA 22042
(703) 698-1110

Overall patient safety: ★★★
Teaching: Y

CLINICAL PROGRAM RATINGS:

CARDIAC	★★★	ORTHOPEDICS	★★★
CRITICAL CARE	★★★	PULMONARY	★★★★★
GASTROINTESTINAL	★★★	STROKE	★★★★★
GENERAL SURGERY	★★★	VASCULAR	★★★
MATERNITY CARE	★★★	WOMEN'S HEALTH	★★★★★

HEALTHGRADES AWARDS

✓ AMERICA'S 50 BEST HOSPITALS ✓ DISTINGUISHED HOSPITAL · CLINICAL EXCELLENCE ✓ SPECIALTY EXCELLENCE · GASTROINTESTINAL CARE · STROKE CARE

John Randolph Medical Center

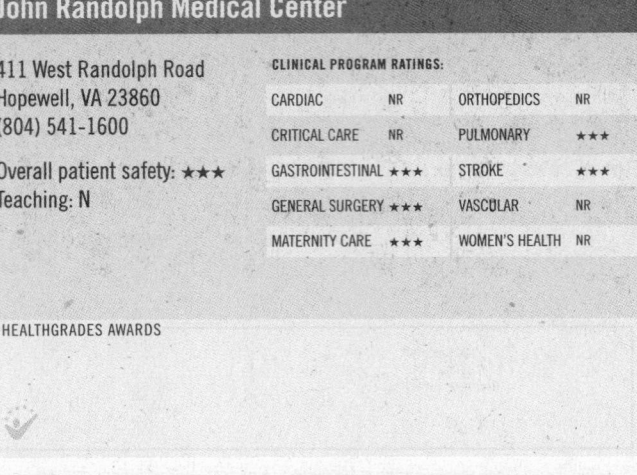

411 West Randolph Road
Hopewell, VA 23860
(804) 541-1600

Overall patient safety: ★★★
Teaching: N

CLINICAL PROGRAM RATINGS:

CARDIAC	NR	ORTHOPEDICS	NR
CRITICAL CARE	NR	PULMONARY	★★★
GASTROINTESTINAL	★★★	STROKE	★★★
GENERAL SURGERY	★★★	VASCULAR	NR
MATERNITY CARE	★★★	WOMEN'S HEALTH	NR

HEALTHGRADES AWARDS

Inova Loudoun Hospital

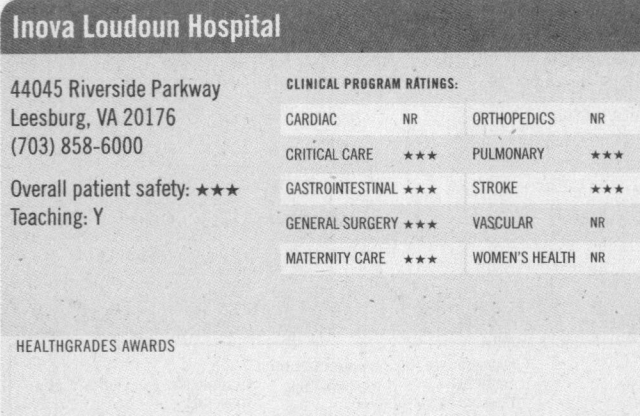

44045 Riverside Parkway
Leesburg, VA 20176
(703) 858-6000

Overall patient safety: ★★★
Teaching: Y

CLINICAL PROGRAM RATINGS:

CARDIAC	NR	ORTHOPEDICS	NR
CRITICAL CARE	★★★	PULMONARY	★★★
GASTROINTESTINAL	★★★	STROKE	★★★
GENERAL SURGERY	★★★	VASCULAR	NR
MATERNITY CARE	★★★	WOMEN'S HEALTH	NR

HEALTHGRADES AWARDS

Johnston Memorial Hospital

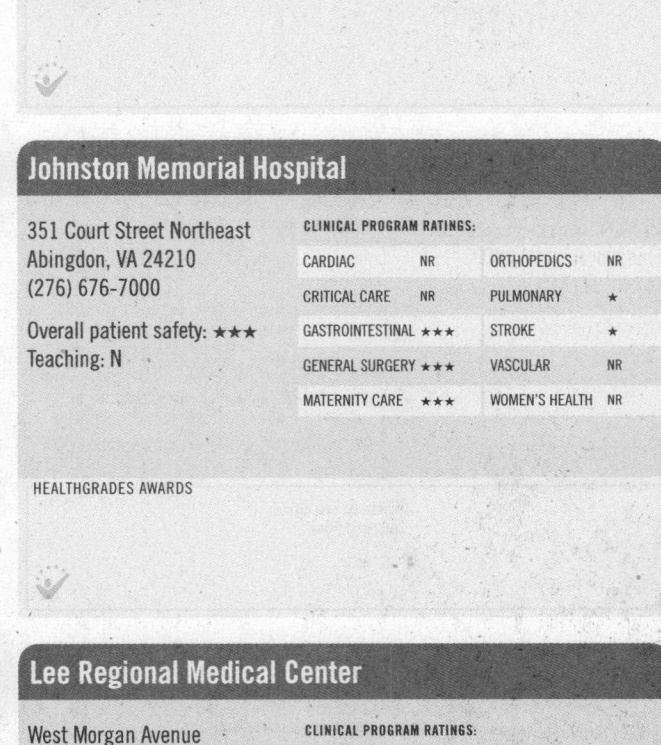

351 Court Street Northeast
Abingdon, VA 24210
(276) 676-7000

Overall patient safety: ★★★
Teaching: N

CLINICAL PROGRAM RATINGS:

CARDIAC	NR	ORTHOPEDICS	NR
CRITICAL CARE	NR	PULMONARY	★
GASTROINTESTINAL	★★★	STROKE	★
GENERAL SURGERY	★★★	VASCULAR	NR
MATERNITY CARE	★★★	WOMEN'S HEALTH	NR

HEALTHGRADES AWARDS

Inova Mount Vernon Hospital

2501 Parkers Lane
Alexandria, VA 22306
(703) 664-7000

Overall patient safety: ★★★
Teaching: N

CLINICAL PROGRAM RATINGS:

CARDIAC	NR	ORTHOPEDICS	★★★
CRITICAL CARE	★★★	PULMONARY	★
GASTROINTESTINAL	★★★	STROKE	★★★
GENERAL SURGERY	★	VASCULAR	NR
MATERNITY CARE	NR	WOMEN'S HEALTH	NR

HEALTHGRADES AWARDS

✓ SPECIALTY EXCELLENCE · JOINT REPLACEMENT

Lee Regional Medical Center

West Morgan Avenue
Pennington Gap, VA 24277
(276) 546-1440

Overall patient safety: ★
Teaching: N

CLINICAL PROGRAM RATINGS:

CARDIAC	NR	ORTHOPEDICS	NR
CRITICAL CARE	NR	PULMONARY	★★★
GASTROINTESTINAL	NR	STROKE	★★★
GENERAL SURGERY	NR	VASCULAR	NR
MATERNITY CARE	NR	WOMEN'S HEALTH	NR

HEALTHGRADES AWARDS

KEY: ★★★★★ BEST ★★★ AS EXPECTED ★ POOR NR NOT RATED BY HEALTHGRADES For full definitions of ratings and awards, see Appendix.

Lewis-Gale Medical Center

1900 Electric Road
Salem, VA 24153
(540) 776-4000

Overall patient safety: ★★★
Teaching: N

CLINICAL PROGRAM RATINGS:

CARDIAC	★★★	ORTHOPEDICS	★★★
CRITICAL CARE	★★★★★	PULMONARY	★★★
GASTROINTESTINAL	★★★	STROKE	★★★
GENERAL SURGERY	★★★	VASCULAR	NR
MATERNITY CARE	★★★	WOMEN'S HEALTH	★★★

HEALTHGRADES AWARDS

✓ **DISTINGUISHED HOSPITAL**
· CLINICAL EXCELLENCE

✓ **SPECIALTY EXCELLENCE**
· CRITICAL CARE

Mary Immaculate Hospital

2 Bernardine Drive
Newport News, VA 23602
(757) 886-6000

Overall patient safety: ★
Teaching: N

CLINICAL PROGRAM RATINGS:

CARDIAC	NR	ORTHOPEDICS	★★★★★
CRITICAL CARE	★★★	PULMONARY	★
GASTROINTESTINAL	★★★	STROKE	★★★
GENERAL SURGERY	★★★	VASCULAR	NR
MATERNITY CARE	★★★	WOMEN'S HEALTH	NR

HEALTHGRADES AWARDS

✓ **SPECIALTY EXCELLENCE**
· ORTHOPEDIC SURGERY

Lynchburg General Hospital*

1901 Tate Springs Road
Lynchburg, VA 24501
(434) 947-3000

Overall patient safety: ★★★
Teaching: Y

CLINICAL PROGRAM RATINGS:

CARDIAC	★★★	ORTHOPEDICS	★★★★★
CRITICAL CARE	★★★	PULMONARY	★★★
GASTROINTESTINAL	★★★	STROKE	★★★
GENERAL SURGERY	★★★★★	VASCULAR	★★★
MATERNITY CARE	★★★	WOMEN'S HEALTH	★★★

HEALTHGRADES AWARDS

✓ **SPECIALTY EXCELLENCE**
· GASTROINTESTINAL CARE
· GENERAL SURGERY
· JOINT REPLACEMENT
· ORTHOPEDIC SURGERY

Mary Washington Hospital

1001 Sam Perry Boulevard
Fredericksburg, VA 22401
(540) 899-1410

Overall patient safety: ★★★
Teaching: N

CLINICAL PROGRAM RATINGS:

CARDIAC	★★★	ORTHOPEDICS	★
CRITICAL CARE	★★★	PULMONARY	★★★★★
GASTROINTESTINAL	★★★	STROKE	★★★
GENERAL SURGERY	★★★	VASCULAR	★★★
MATERNITY CARE	★★★	WOMEN'S HEALTH	★★★

HEALTHGRADES AWARDS

✓ **SPECIALTY EXCELLENCE**
· PULMONARY CARE

Martha Jefferson Hospital

459 Locust Avenue
Charlottesville, VA 22902
(434) 982-7000

Overall patient safety: ★★★★★
Teaching: N

CLINICAL PROGRAM RATINGS:

CARDIAC	NR	ORTHOPEDICS	★
CRITICAL CARE	★★★	PULMONARY	★★★★★
GASTROINTESTINAL	★★★	STROKE	★★★
GENERAL SURGERY	★★★	VASCULAR	★★★
MATERNITY CARE	★★★	WOMEN'S HEALTH	NR

HEALTHGRADES AWARDS

✓ **DISTINGUISHED HOSPITAL**
· PATIENT SAFETY

Memorial Hospital of Martinsville and Henry County

320 Hospital Drive
Martinsville, VA 24112
(276) 666-7200

Overall patient safety: ★★★
Teaching: N

CLINICAL PROGRAM RATINGS:

CARDIAC	NR	ORTHOPEDICS	NR
CRITICAL CARE	NR	PULMONARY	★★★
GASTROINTESTINAL	★★★	STROKE	★
GENERAL SURGERY	★★★	VASCULAR	NR
MATERNITY CARE	★	WOMEN'S HEALTH	NR

HEALTHGRADES AWARDS

*This hospital reports its data to the federal government jointly with another hospital. Therefore the ratings and awards apply to multiple hospitals and this specific hospital may not provide all rated services.

Montgomery Regional Hospital

3700 South Main Street
Blacksburg, VA 24060
(540) 951-1111

Overall patient safety: ★★★
Teaching: N

CLINICAL PROGRAM RATINGS:

CARDIAC	NR	ORTHOPEDICS	NR
CRITICAL CARE	★★★	PULMONARY	★★★
GASTROINTESTINAL	NR	STROKE	★
GENERAL SURGERY	★★★	VASCULAR	NR
MATERNITY CARE	★★★	WOMEN'S HEALTH	NR

HEALTHGRADES AWARDS

Norton Community Hospital

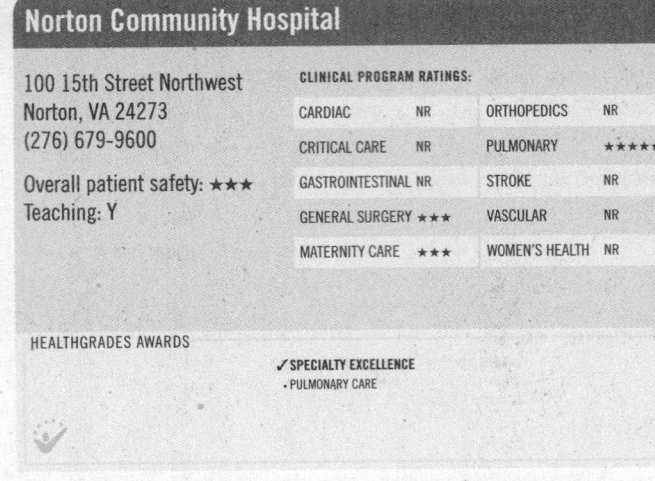

100 15th Street Northwest
Norton, VA 24273
(276) 679-9600

Overall patient safety: ★★★
Teaching: Y

CLINICAL PROGRAM RATINGS:

CARDIAC	NR	ORTHOPEDICS	NR
CRITICAL CARE	NR	PULMONARY	★★★★★
GASTROINTESTINAL	NR	STROKE	NR
GENERAL SURGERY	★★★	VASCULAR	NR
MATERNITY CARE	★★★	WOMEN'S HEALTH	NR

HEALTHGRADES AWARDS

✓ SPECIALTY EXCELLENCE
• PULMONARY CARE

Mountain View Regional Medical Center

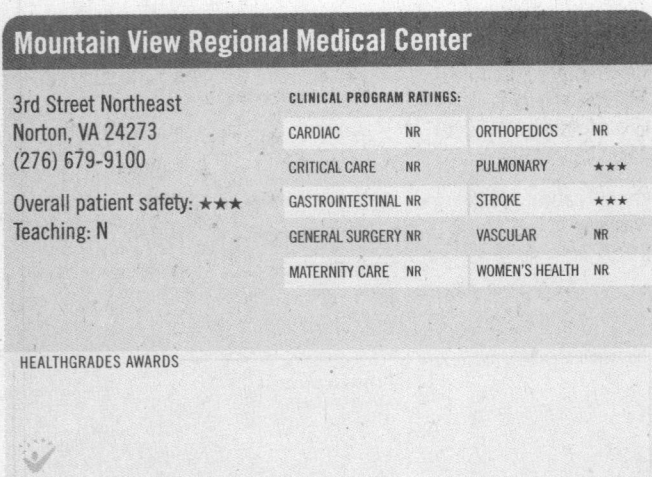

3rd Street Northeast
Norton, VA 24273
(276) 679-9100

Overall patient safety: ★★★
Teaching: N

CLINICAL PROGRAM RATINGS:

CARDIAC	NR	ORTHOPEDICS	NR
CRITICAL CARE	NR	PULMONARY	★★★
GASTROINTESTINAL	NR	STROKE	★★★
GENERAL SURGERY	NR	VASCULAR	NR
MATERNITY CARE	NR	WOMEN'S HEALTH	NR

HEALTHGRADES AWARDS

Obici Hospital

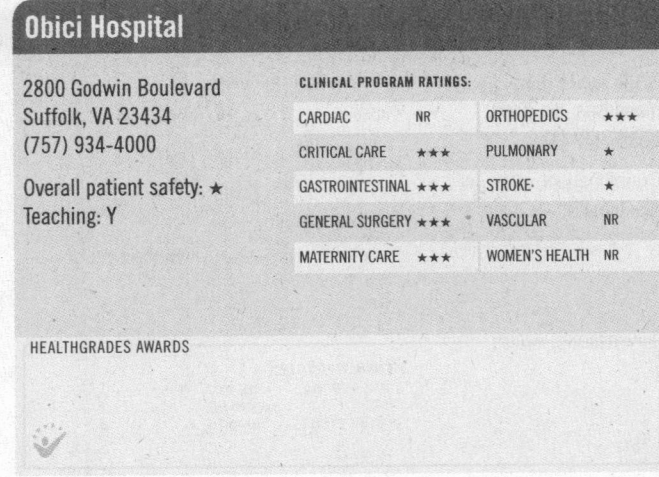

2800 Godwin Boulevard
Suffolk, VA 23434
(757) 934-4000

Overall patient safety: ★
Teaching: Y

CLINICAL PROGRAM RATINGS:

CARDIAC	NR	ORTHOPEDICS	★★★
CRITICAL CARE	★★★	PULMONARY	★
GASTROINTESTINAL	★★★	STROKE	★
GENERAL SURGERY	★★★	VASCULAR	NR
MATERNITY CARE	★★★	WOMEN'S HEALTH	NR

HEALTHGRADES AWARDS

Northern Virginia Community Hospital

601 South Carlin Springs Road
Arlington, VA 22204
(703) 671-1200

Overall patient safety: ★
Teaching: N

CLINICAL PROGRAM RATINGS:

CARDIAC	NR	ORTHOPEDICS	NR
CRITICAL CARE	NR	PULMONARY	NR
GASTROINTESTINAL	NR	STROKE	NR
GENERAL SURGERY	NR	VASCULAR	NR
MATERNITY CARE	NR	WOMEN'S HEALTH	NR

HEALTHGRADES AWARDS

Page Memorial Hospital

200 Memorial Drive
Luray, VA 22835
(540) 743-4561

Overall patient safety: ★★★
Teaching: N

CLINICAL PROGRAM RATINGS:

CARDIAC	NR	ORTHOPEDICS	NR
CRITICAL CARE	NR	PULMONARY	★★★
GASTROINTESTINAL	NR	STROKE	★★★★★
GENERAL SURGERY	NR	VASCULAR	NR
MATERNITY CARE	NR	WOMEN'S HEALTH	NR

HEALTHGRADES AWARDS

KEY: ★★★★★ BEST   ★★★ AS EXPECTED   ★ POOR   NR NOT RATED BY HEALTHGRADES   For full definitions of ratings and awards, see Appendix.

Potomac Hospital

2300 Opitz Boulevard
Woodbridge, VA 22191
(703) 670-1313

Overall patient safety: ★★★
Teaching: N

CLINICAL PROGRAM RATINGS:

CARDIAC	NR	ORTHOPEDICS	NR
CRITICAL CARE	★★★	PULMONARY	★★★
GASTROINTESTINAL	★★★	STROKE	★★★
GENERAL SURGERY	★★★	VASCULAR	NR
MATERNITY CARE	★★★	WOMEN'S HEALTH	NR

HEALTHGRADES AWARDS

✓ SPECIALTY EXCELLENCE
· BARIATRIC SURGERY · GASTROINTESTINAL · GENERAL SURGERY
 CARE

R. J. Reynolds Patrick County Memorial Hospital

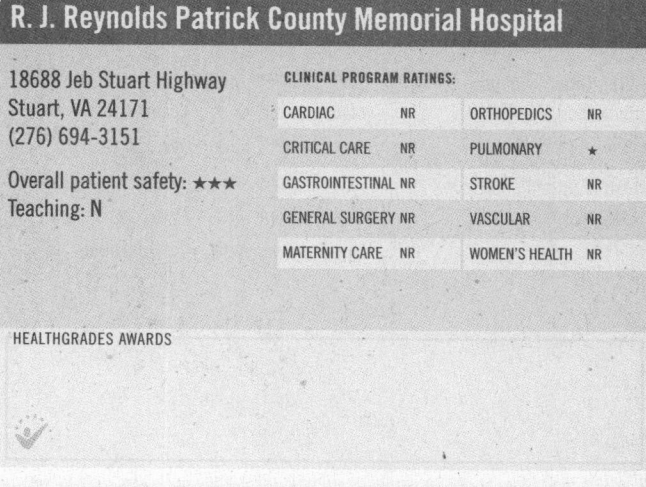

18688 Jeb Stuart Highway
Stuart, VA 24171
(276) 694-3151

Overall patient safety: ★★★
Teaching: N

CLINICAL PROGRAM RATINGS:

CARDIAC	NR	ORTHOPEDICS	NR
CRITICAL CARE	NR	PULMONARY	★
GASTROINTESTINAL	NR	STROKE	NR
GENERAL SURGERY	NR	VASCULAR	NR
MATERNITY CARE	NR	WOMEN'S HEALTH	NR

HEALTHGRADES AWARDS

Prince William Hospital

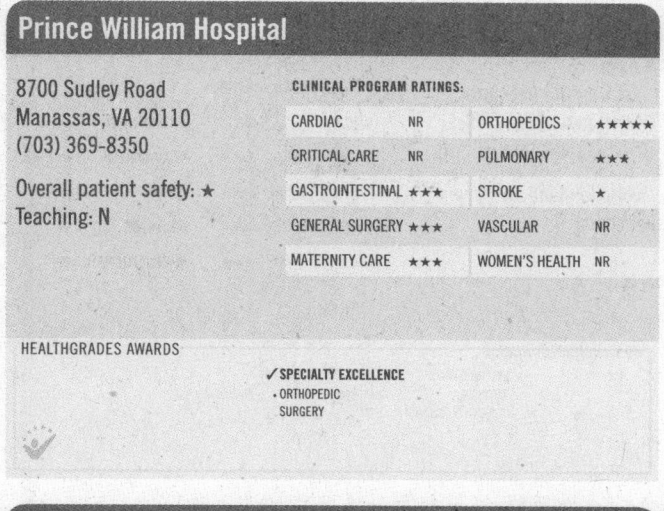

8700 Sudley Road
Manassas, VA 20110
(703) 369-8350

Overall patient safety: ★
Teaching: N

CLINICAL PROGRAM RATINGS:

CARDIAC	NR	ORTHOPEDICS	★★★★★
CRITICAL CARE	NR	PULMONARY	★★★
GASTROINTESTINAL	★★★	STROKE	★
GENERAL SURGERY	★★★	VASCULAR	NR
MATERNITY CARE	★★★	WOMEN'S HEALTH	NR

HEALTHGRADES AWARDS

✓ SPECIALTY EXCELLENCE
· ORTHOPEDIC
 SURGERY

Rappahannock General Hospital

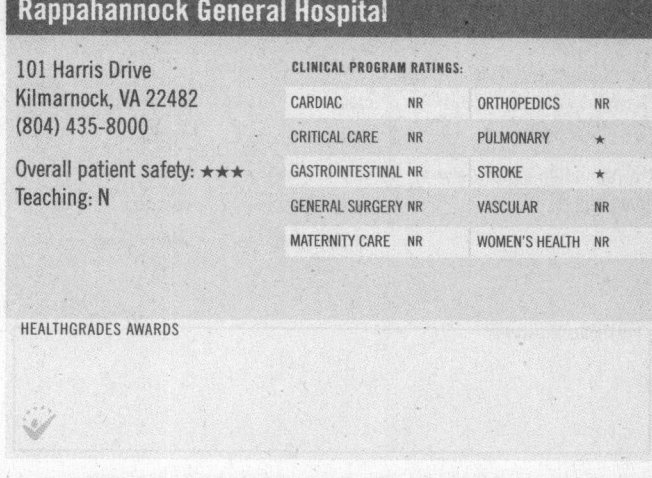

101 Harris Drive
Kilmarnock, VA 22482
(804) 435-8000

Overall patient safety: ★★★
Teaching: N

CLINICAL PROGRAM RATINGS:

CARDIAC	NR	ORTHOPEDICS	NR
CRITICAL CARE	NR	PULMONARY	★
GASTROINTESTINAL	NR	STROKE	★
GENERAL SURGERY	NR	VASCULAR	NR
MATERNITY CARE	NR	WOMEN'S HEALTH	NR

HEALTHGRADES AWARDS

Pulaski Community Hospital

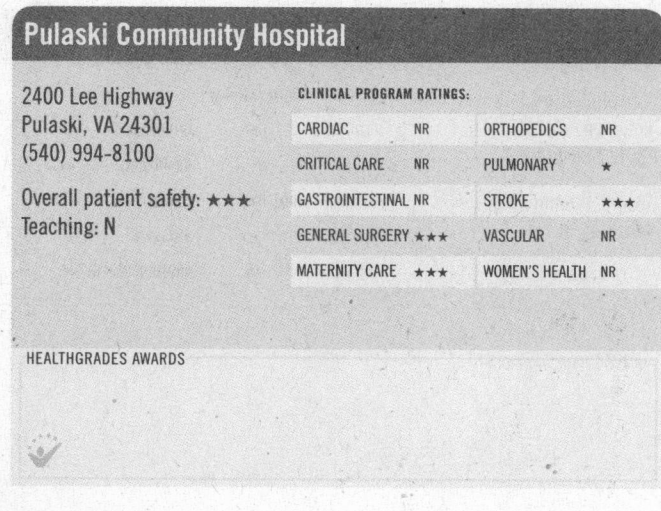

2400 Lee Highway
Pulaski, VA 24301
(540) 994-8100

Overall patient safety: ★★★
Teaching: N

CLINICAL PROGRAM RATINGS:

CARDIAC	NR	ORTHOPEDICS	NR
CRITICAL CARE	NR	PULMONARY	★
GASTROINTESTINAL	NR	STROKE	★★★
GENERAL SURGERY	★★★	VASCULAR	NR
MATERNITY CARE	★★★	WOMEN'S HEALTH	NR

HEALTHGRADES AWARDS

Reston Hospital Center

1850 Town Center Parkway
Reston, VA 20190
(703) 689-9000

Overall patient safety: ★★★
Teaching: N

CLINICAL PROGRAM RATINGS:

CARDIAC	NR	ORTHOPEDICS	★★★
CRITICAL CARE	★★★	PULMONARY	★
GASTROINTESTINAL	NR	STROKE	★★★
GENERAL SURGERY	★★★	VASCULAR	NR
MATERNITY CARE	★★★	WOMEN'S HEALTH	NR

HEALTHGRADES AWARDS

Retreat Hospital

2621 Grove Avenue
Richmond, VA 23220
(804) 254-5100

Overall patient safety: ★
Teaching: N

CLINICAL PROGRAM RATINGS:

CARDIAC	NR	ORTHOPEDICS	NR
CRITICAL CARE	NR	PULMONARY	★★★
GASTROINTESTINAL	NR	STROKE	★★★
GENERAL SURGERY	★★★	VASCULAR	NR
MATERNITY CARE	NR	WOMEN'S HEALTH	NR

HEALTHGRADES AWARDS

Riverside Walter Reed Hospital

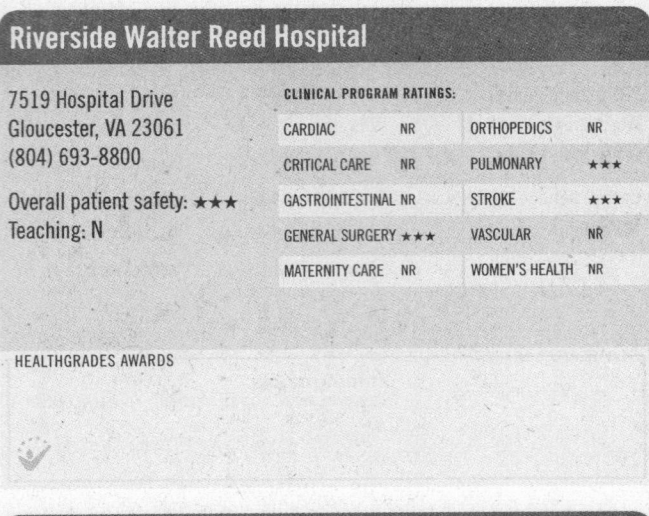

7519 Hospital Drive
Gloucester, VA 23061
(804) 693-8800

Overall patient safety: ★★★
Teaching: N

CLINICAL PROGRAM RATINGS:

CARDIAC	NR	ORTHOPEDICS	NR
CRITICAL CARE	NR	PULMONARY	★★★
GASTROINTESTINAL	NR	STROKE	★★★
GENERAL SURGERY	★★★	VASCULAR	NR
MATERNITY CARE	NR	WOMEN'S HEALTH	NR

HEALTHGRADES AWARDS

Riverside Regional Medical Center

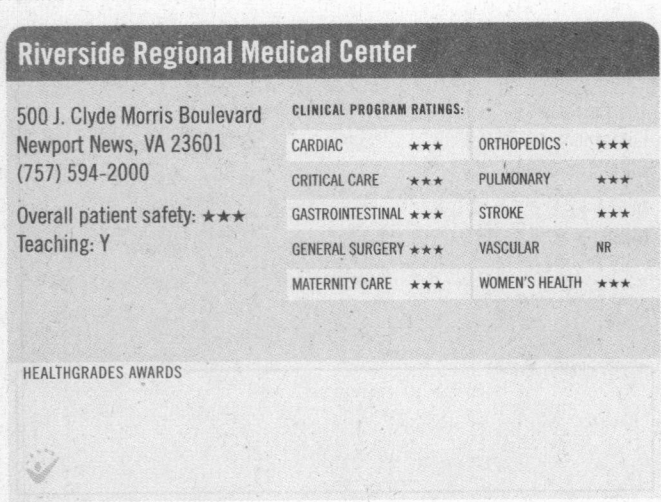

500 J. Clyde Morris Boulevard
Newport News, VA 23601
(757) 594-2000

Overall patient safety: ★★★
Teaching: Y

CLINICAL PROGRAM RATINGS:

CARDIAC	★★★	ORTHOPEDICS	★★★
CRITICAL CARE	★★★	PULMONARY	★★★
GASTROINTESTINAL	★★★	STROKE	★★★
GENERAL SURGERY	★★★	VASCULAR	NR
MATERNITY CARE	★★★	WOMEN'S HEALTH	★★★

HEALTHGRADES AWARDS

Rockingham Memorial Hospital

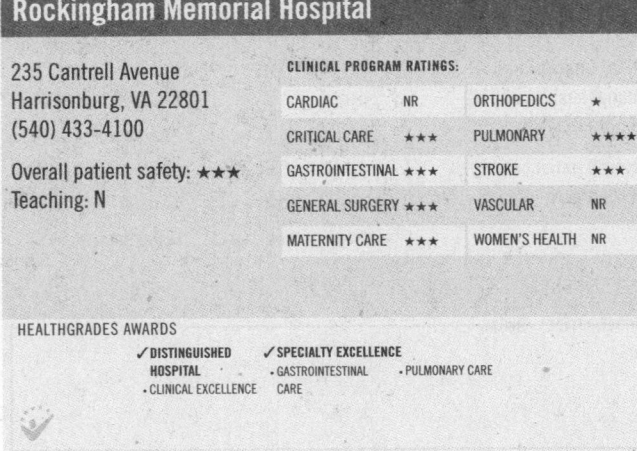

235 Cantrell Avenue
Harrisonburg, VA 22801
(540) 433-4100

Overall patient safety: ★★★
Teaching: N

CLINICAL PROGRAM RATINGS:

CARDIAC	NR	ORTHOPEDICS	★
CRITICAL CARE	★★★	PULMONARY	★★★★★
GASTROINTESTINAL	★★★	STROKE	★★★
GENERAL SURGERY	★★★	VASCULAR	NR
MATERNITY CARE	★★★	WOMEN'S HEALTH	NR

HEALTHGRADES AWARDS

✓ **DISTINGUISHED HOSPITAL**
• CLINICAL EXCELLENCE

✓ **SPECIALTY EXCELLENCE**
• GASTROINTESTINAL CARE
• PULMONARY CARE

Riverside Tappahannock Hospital

618 Hospital Road
Tappahannock, VA 22560
(804) 443-3311

Overall patient safety: ★★★
Teaching: N

CLINICAL PROGRAM RATINGS:

CARDIAC	NR	ORTHOPEDICS	NR
CRITICAL CARE	★★★	PULMONARY	★★★
GASTROINTESTINAL	NR	STROKE	NR
GENERAL SURGERY	NR	VASCULAR	NR
MATERNITY CARE	NR	WOMEN'S HEALTH	NR

HEALTHGRADES AWARDS

Russell County Medical Center

Carroll and Tate Streets
Lebanon, VA 24266
(276) 883-8000

Overall patient safety: ★
Teaching: N

CLINICAL PROGRAM RATINGS:

CARDIAC	NR	ORTHOPEDICS	NR
CRITICAL CARE	NR	PULMONARY	★
GASTROINTESTINAL	NR	STROKE	★
GENERAL SURGERY	★★★	VASCULAR	NR
MATERNITY CARE	NR	WOMEN'S HEALTH	NR

HEALTHGRADES AWARDS

KEY: ★★★★★ BEST ★★★ AS EXPECTED ★ POOR NR NOT RATED BY HEALTHGRADES For full definitions of ratings and awards, see Appendix.

Sentara Bayside Hospital

800 Independence Boulevard
Virginia Beach, VA 23455
(757) 363-6100

Overall patient safety: ★
Teaching: Y

CLINICAL PROGRAM RATINGS:

CARDIAC	NR	ORTHOPEDICS	NR
CRITICAL CARE	★★★	PULMONARY	★★★
GASTROINTESTINAL	★★★	STROKE	★★★
GENERAL SURGERY	★★★	VASCULAR	NR
MATERNITY CARE	NR	WOMEN'S HEALTH	NR

HEALTHGRADES AWARDS

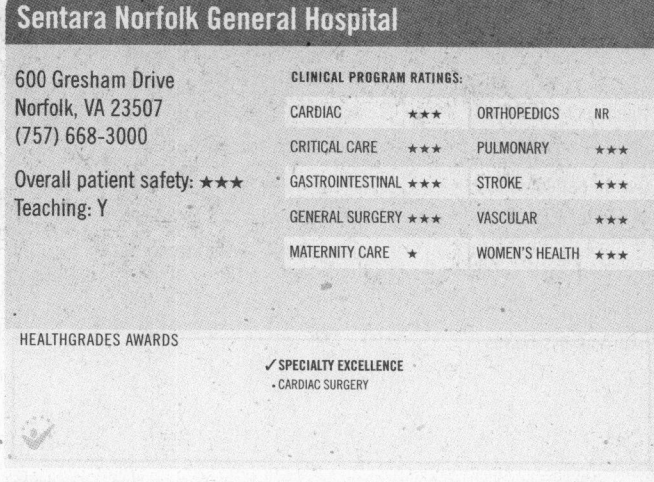

Sentara Norfolk General Hospital

600 Gresham Drive
Norfolk, VA 23507
(757) 668-3000

Overall patient safety: ★★★
Teaching: Y

CLINICAL PROGRAM RATINGS:

CARDIAC	★★★	ORTHOPEDICS	NR
CRITICAL CARE	★★★	PULMONARY	★★★
GASTROINTESTINAL	★★★	STROKE	★★★
GENERAL SURGERY	★★★	VASCULAR	★★★
MATERNITY CARE	★	WOMEN'S HEALTH	★★★

HEALTHGRADES AWARDS

✓ SPECIALTY EXCELLENCE
- CARDIAC SURGERY

Sentara Careplex Hospital

3000 Coliseum Drive
Hampton, VA 23666
(757) 727-7000

Overall patient safety: ★
Teaching: N

CLINICAL PROGRAM RATINGS:

CARDIAC	NR	ORTHOPEDICS	★★★
CRITICAL CARE	★★★★★	PULMONARY	★★★
GASTROINTESTINAL	★★★	STROKE	★★★
GENERAL SURGERY	★★★	VASCULAR	★★★
MATERNITY CARE	★★★	WOMEN'S HEALTH	NR

HEALTHGRADES AWARDS

✓ SPECIALTY EXCELLENCE
- BARIATRIC SURGERY   - CRITICAL CARE

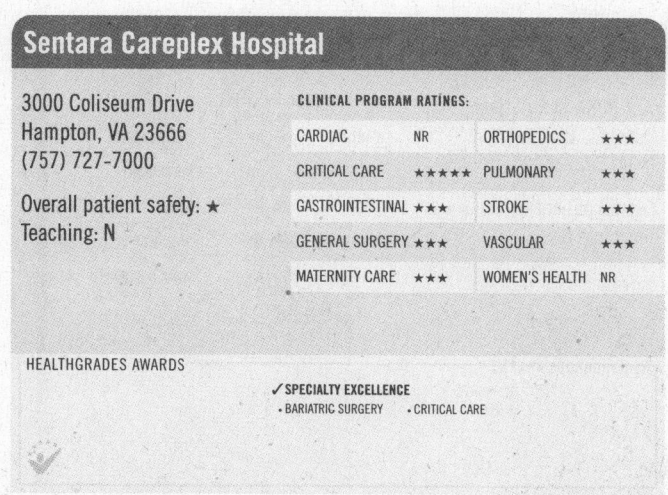

Sentara Virginia Beach General Hospital

1060 1st Colonial Road
Virginia Beach, VA 23454
(757) 395-8000

Overall patient safety: ★★★
Teaching: Y

CLINICAL PROGRAM RATINGS:

CARDIAC	★★★	ORTHOPEDICS	★
CRITICAL CARE	★★★★★	PULMONARY	★★★★★
GASTROINTESTINAL	★★★	STROKE	★★★★★
GENERAL SURGERY	★★★	VASCULAR	★★★
MATERNITY CARE	★★★	WOMEN'S HEALTH	★★★

HEALTHGRADES AWARDS

✓ DISTINGUISHED HOSPITAL
- CLINICAL EXCELLENCE

✓ SPECIALTY EXCELLENCE
- CARDIAC CARE   - GASTROINTESTINAL CARE   - STROKE CARE
- CRITICAL CARE   - PULMONARY CARE

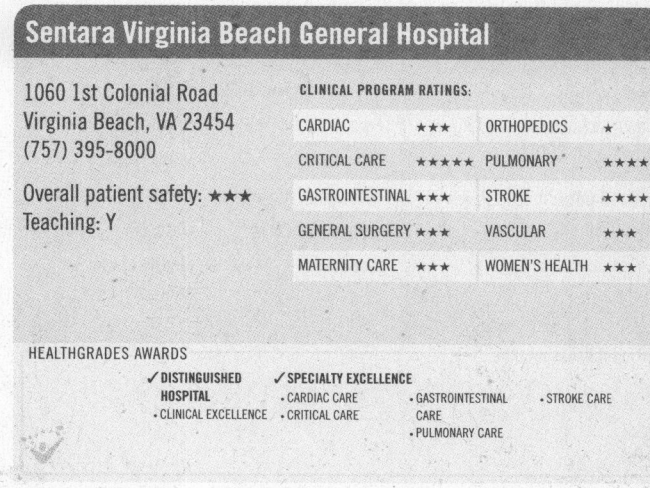

Sentara Leigh Hospital

830 Kempsville Road
Norfolk, VA 23502
(757) 466-6000

Overall patient safety: ★★★
Teaching: Y

CLINICAL PROGRAM RATINGS:

CARDIAC	NR	ORTHOPEDICS	★★★
CRITICAL CARE	★★★	PULMONARY	★★★★★
GASTROINTESTINAL	★★★	STROKE	★★★
GENERAL SURGERY	★	VASCULAR	NR
MATERNITY CARE	★★★★★	WOMEN'S HEALTH	NR

HEALTHGRADES AWARDS

✓ SPECIALTY EXCELLENCE
- BARIATRIC SURGERY   - MATERNITY CARE   - PULMONARY CARE

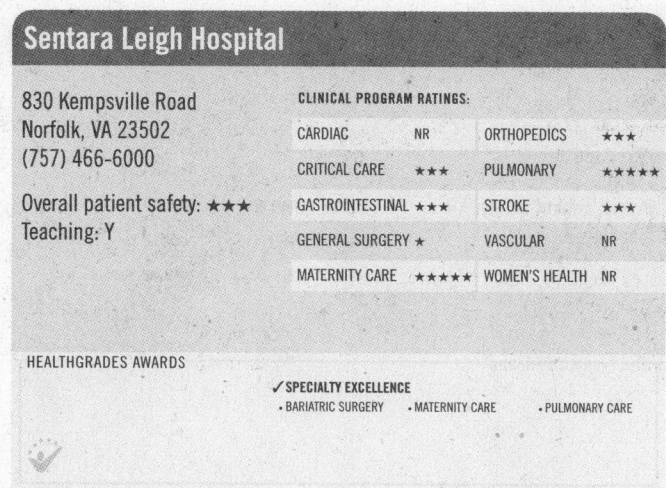

Sentara Williamsburg Regional Medical Center

100 Sentara Circle
Williamsburg, VA 23188
(757) 259-6000

Overall patient safety: ★★★
Teaching: N

CLINICAL PROGRAM RATINGS:

CARDIAC	NR	ORTHOPEDICS	★★★
CRITICAL CARE	★★★	PULMONARY	★★★
GASTROINTESTINAL	★★★	STROKE	★
GENERAL SURGERY	★★★	VASCULAR	NR
MATERNITY CARE	★★★	WOMEN'S HEALTH	NR

HEALTHGRADES AWARDS

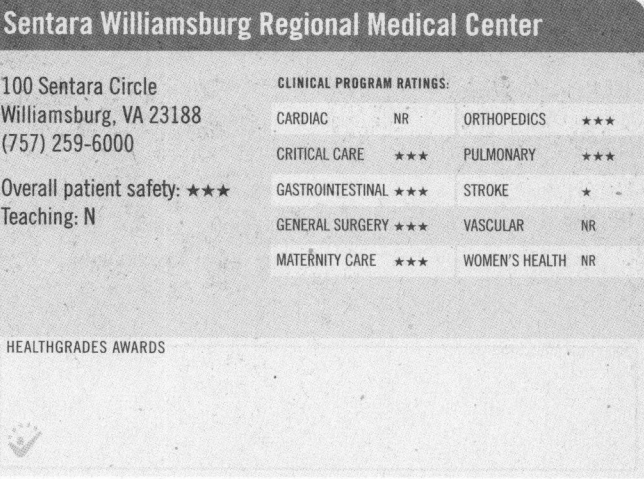

Shenandoah Memorial Hospital

759 South Main Street
Woodstock, VA 22664
(540) 459-1100

Overall patient safety: ★★★
Teaching: N

CLINICAL PROGRAM RATINGS:

CARDIAC	NR	ORTHOPEDICS	NR
CRITICAL CARE	NR	PULMONARY	★★★
GASTROINTESTINAL	NR	STROKE	NR
GENERAL SURGERY	NR	VASCULAR	NR
MATERNITY CARE	★★★	WOMEN'S HEALTH	NR

HEALTHGRADES AWARDS

Southampton Memorial Hospital

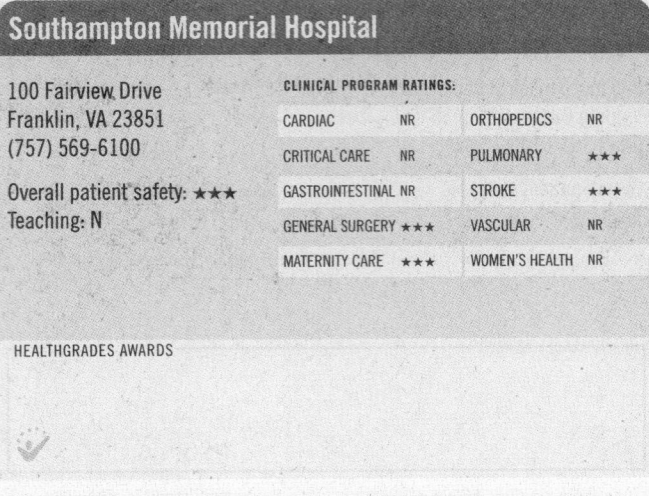

100 Fairview Drive
Franklin, VA 23851
(757) 569-6100

Overall patient safety: ★★★
Teaching: N

CLINICAL PROGRAM RATINGS:

CARDIAC	NR	ORTHOPEDICS	NR
CRITICAL CARE	NR	PULMONARY	★★★
GASTROINTESTINAL	NR	STROKE	★★★
GENERAL SURGERY	★★★	VASCULAR	NR
MATERNITY CARE	★★★	WOMEN'S HEALTH	NR

HEALTHGRADES AWARDS

Shore Memorial Hospital

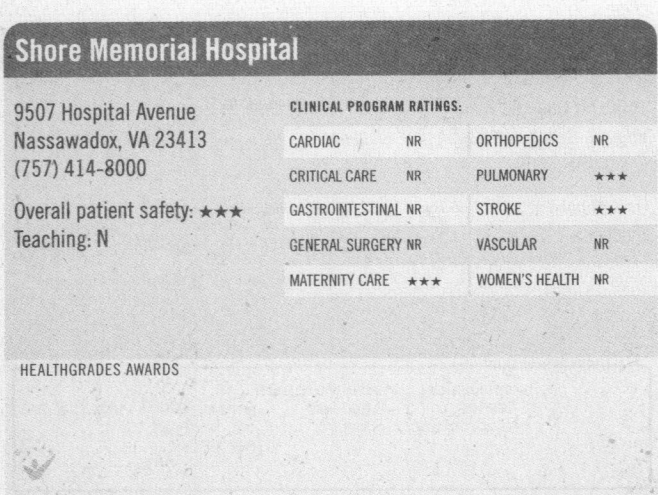

9507 Hospital Avenue
Nassawadox, VA 23413
(757) 414-8000

Overall patient safety: ★★★
Teaching: N

CLINICAL PROGRAM RATINGS:

CARDIAC	NR	ORTHOPEDICS	NR
CRITICAL CARE	NR	PULMONARY	★★★
GASTROINTESTINAL	NR	STROKE	★★★
GENERAL SURGERY	NR	VASCULAR	NR
MATERNITY CARE	★★★	WOMEN'S HEALTH	NR

HEALTHGRADES AWARDS

Southern Virginia Regional Medical Center

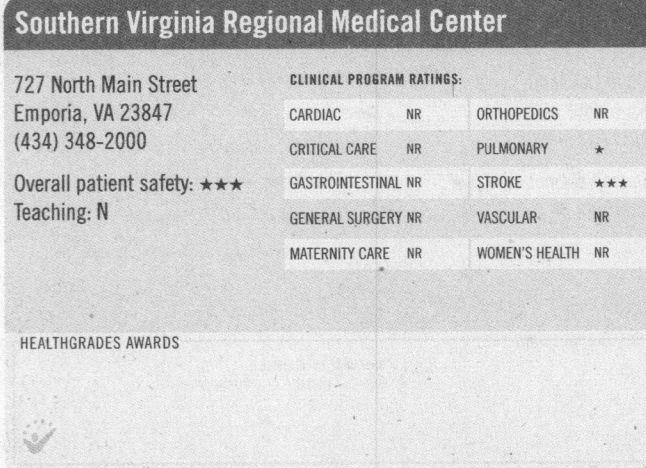

727 North Main Street
Emporia, VA 23847
(434) 348-2000

Overall patient safety: ★★★
Teaching: N

CLINICAL PROGRAM RATINGS:

CARDIAC	NR	ORTHOPEDICS	NR
CRITICAL CARE	NR	PULMONARY	★
GASTROINTESTINAL	NR	STROKE	★★★
GENERAL SURGERY	NR	VASCULAR	NR
MATERNITY CARE	NR	WOMEN'S HEALTH	NR

HEALTHGRADES AWARDS

Smyth County Community Hospital

565 Radio Hill Road
Marion, VA 24354
(276) 782-1234

Overall patient safety: ★
Teaching: N

CLINICAL PROGRAM RATINGS:

CARDIAC	NR	ORTHOPEDICS	NR
CRITICAL CARE	NR	PULMONARY	★
GASTROINTESTINAL	★★★	STROKE	★★★
GENERAL SURGERY	★★★	VASCULAR	NR
MATERNITY CARE	★★★	WOMEN'S HEALTH	NR

HEALTHGRADES AWARDS

Southside Community Hospital

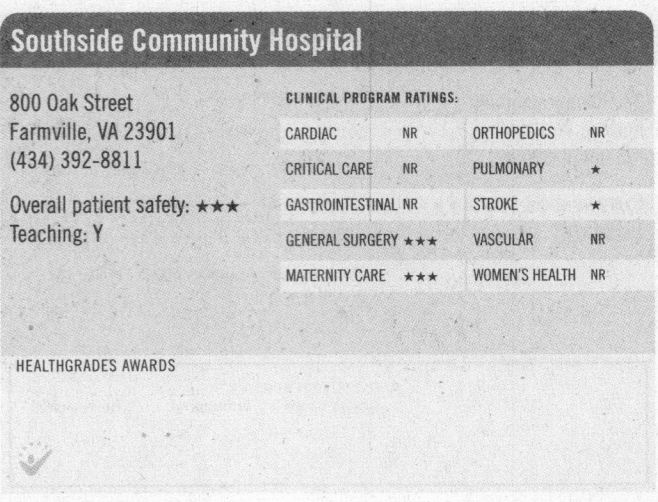

800 Oak Street
Farmville, VA 23901
(434) 392-8811

Overall patient safety: ★★★
Teaching: Y

CLINICAL PROGRAM RATINGS:

CARDIAC	NR	ORTHOPEDICS	NR
CRITICAL CARE	NR	PULMONARY	★
GASTROINTESTINAL	NR	STROKE	★
GENERAL SURGERY	★★★	VASCULAR	NR
MATERNITY CARE	★★★	WOMEN'S HEALTH	NR

HEALTHGRADES AWARDS

KEY: ★★★★★ BEST   ★★★ AS EXPECTED   ★ POOR   NR NOT RATED BY HEALTHGRADES   For full definitions of ratings and awards, see Appendix.

Southside Regional Medical Center

801 South Adams Street
Petersburg, VA 23803
(804) 862-5000

Overall patient safety: ★
Teaching: N

CLINICAL PROGRAM RATINGS:

CARDIAC	NR	ORTHOPEDICS	NR
CRITICAL CARE	★★★	PULMONARY	★★★
GASTROINTESTINAL	★★★	STROKE	★★★
GENERAL SURGERY	★★★	VASCULAR	NR
MATERNITY CARE	★★★	WOMEN'S HEALTH	NR

HEALTHGRADES AWARDS

Twin County Regional Hospital

200 Hospital Drive
Galax, VA 24333
(276) 236-8181

Overall patient safety: ★
Teaching: N

CLINICAL PROGRAM RATINGS:

CARDIAC	NR	ORTHOPEDICS	NR
CRITICAL CARE	NR	PULMONARY	★★★
GASTROINTESTINAL	★★★	STROKE	★
GENERAL SURGERY	★	VASCULAR	NR
MATERNITY CARE	★★★	WOMEN'S HEALTH	NR

HEALTHGRADES AWARDS

Stonewall Jackson Hospital

1 Health Circle
Lexington, VA 24450
(540) 458-3300

Overall patient safety: ★★★★★
Teaching: N

CLINICAL PROGRAM RATINGS:

CARDIAC	NR	ORTHOPEDICS	NR
CRITICAL CARE	NR	PULMONARY	★★★
GASTROINTESTINAL	NR	STROKE	★
GENERAL SURGERY	NR	VASCULAR	NR
MATERNITY CARE	★★★	WOMEN'S HEALTH	NR

HEALTHGRADES AWARDS

University of Virginia Hospital

Jefferson Parks Avenue
Charlottesville, VA 22908
(434) 924-0211

Overall patient safety: ★★★
Teaching: Y

CLINICAL PROGRAM RATINGS:

CARDIAC	★★★	ORTHOPEDICS	★
CRITICAL CARE	★★★	PULMONARY	★★★
GASTROINTESTINAL	★★★	STROKE	★★★
GENERAL SURGERY	★★★	VASCULAR	★★★
MATERNITY CARE	★★★	WOMEN'S HEALTH	★★★

HEALTHGRADES AWARDS

Tazewell Community Hospital

141 Ben Bolt Avenue
Tazewell, VA 24651
(276) 988-8700

Overall patient safety: ★★★
Teaching: N

CLINICAL PROGRAM RATINGS:

CARDIAC	NR	ORTHOPEDICS	NR
CRITICAL CARE	NR	PULMONARY	★
GASTROINTESTINAL	NR	STROKE	NR
GENERAL SURGERY	NR	VASCULAR	NR
MATERNITY CARE	NR	WOMEN'S HEALTH	NR

HEALTHGRADES AWARDS

Virginia Commonwealth University Health System

1250 East Marshall Street
Richmond, VA 23298
(804) 828-9000

Overall patient safety: ★
Teaching: Y

CLINICAL PROGRAM RATINGS:

CARDIAC	★★★	ORTHOPEDICS	★
CRITICAL CARE	★★★	PULMONARY	★★★
GASTROINTESTINAL	★★★	STROKE	★★★
GENERAL SURGERY	★★★	VASCULAR	NR
MATERNITY CARE	★	WOMEN'S HEALTH	★

HEALTHGRADES AWARDS

Virginia Hospital Center—Arlington

1701 North George Mason Drive
Arlington, VA 22205
(703) 558-5000

Overall patient safety: ★★★
Teaching: Y

CLINICAL PROGRAM RATINGS:

CARDIAC	★★★	ORTHOPEDICS	★★★
CRITICAL CARE	★★★	PULMONARY	★★★
GASTROINTESTINAL	★★★★★	STROKE	★★★
GENERAL SURGERY	★★★★★	VASCULAR	NR
MATERNITY CARE	★★★	WOMEN'S HEALTH	★

HEALTHGRADES AWARDS

✓ DISTINGUISHED HOSPITAL
- CLINICAL EXCELLENCE

✓ SPECIALTY EXCELLENCE
- GASTROINTESTINAL CARE
- GENERAL SURGERY

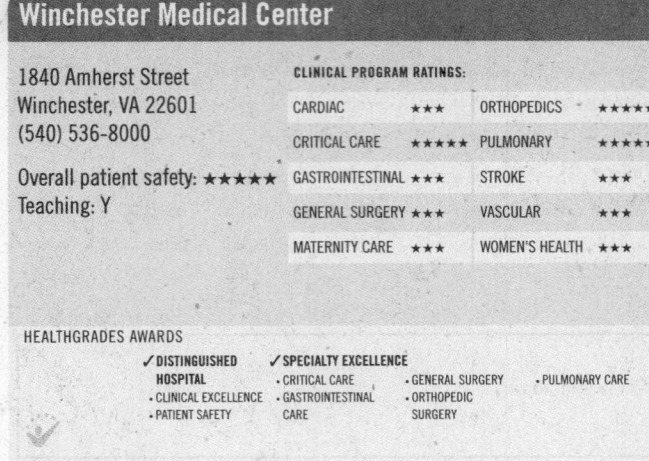

Winchester Medical Center

1840 Amherst Street
Winchester, VA 22601
(540) 536-8000

Overall patient safety: ★★★★★
Teaching: Y

CLINICAL PROGRAM RATINGS:

CARDIAC	★★★	ORTHOPEDICS	★★★★★
CRITICAL CARE	★★★★★	PULMONARY	★★★★★
GASTROINTESTINAL	★★★	STROKE	★★★
GENERAL SURGERY	★★★	VASCULAR	★★★
MATERNITY CARE	★★★	WOMEN'S HEALTH	★★★

HEALTHGRADES AWARDS

✓ DISTINGUISHED HOSPITAL
- CLINICAL EXCELLENCE
- PATIENT SAFETY

✓ SPECIALTY EXCELLENCE
- CRITICAL CARE
- GASTROINTESTINAL CARE
- GENERAL SURGERY
- ORTHOPEDIC SURGERY
- PULMONARY CARE

Warren Memorial Hospital

1000 Shenandoah Avenue
Front Royal, VA 22630
(540) 636-0300

Overall patient safety: ★★★
Teaching: Y

CLINICAL PROGRAM RATINGS:

CARDIAC	NR	ORTHOPEDICS	NR
CRITICAL CARE	NR	PULMONARY	★★★
GASTROINTESTINAL	NR	STROKE	★★★
GENERAL SURGERY	NR	VASCULAR	NR
MATERNITY CARE	★★★	WOMEN'S HEALTH	NR

HEALTHGRADES AWARDS

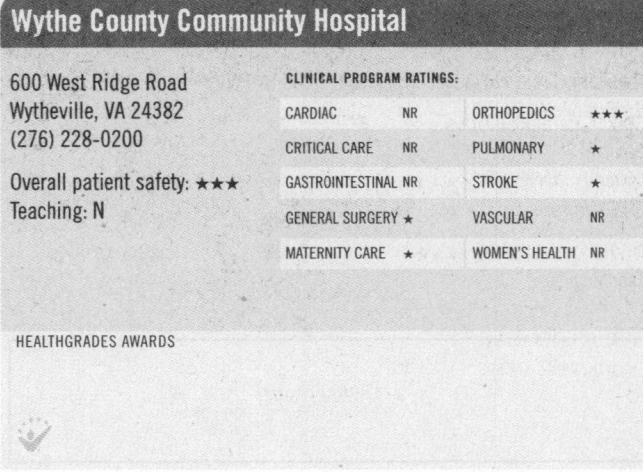

Wythe County Community Hospital

600 West Ridge Road
Wytheville, VA 24382
(276) 228-0200

Overall patient safety: ★★★
Teaching: N

CLINICAL PROGRAM RATINGS:

CARDIAC	NR	ORTHOPEDICS	★★★
CRITICAL CARE	NR	PULMONARY	★
GASTROINTESTINAL	NR	STROKE	★
GENERAL SURGERY	★	VASCULAR	NR
MATERNITY CARE	★	WOMEN'S HEALTH	NR

HEALTHGRADES AWARDS

Wellmont Lonesome Pine Hospital

1990 Holton Avenue East
Big Stone Gap, VA 24219
(276) 523-3111

Overall patient safety: ★
Teaching: N

CLINICAL PROGRAM RATINGS:

CARDIAC	NR	ORTHOPEDICS	NR
CRITICAL CARE	NR	PULMONARY	★★★
GASTROINTESTINAL	NR	STROKE	★★★
GENERAL SURGERY	NR	VASCULAR	NR
MATERNITY CARE	★★★	WOMEN'S HEALTH	NR

HEALTHGRADES AWARDS

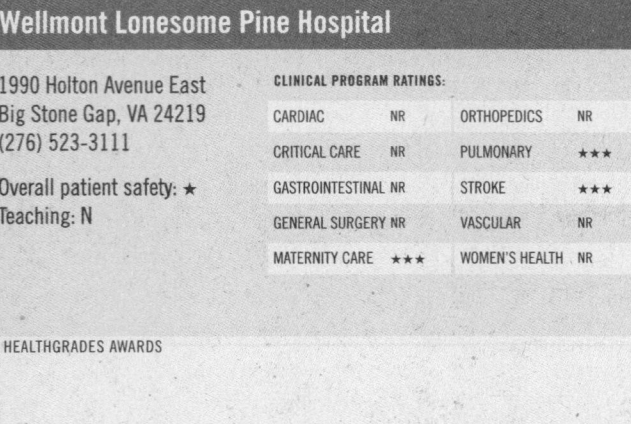

KEY: ★★★★★ BEST   ★★★ AS EXPECTED   ★ POOR   NR NOT RATED BY HEALTHGRADES   For full definitions of ratings and awards, see Appendix.

Auburn Regional Medical Center

202 North Division Street
Auburn, WA 98001
(253) 833-7711

Overall patient safety: ★
Teaching: N

CLINICAL PROGRAM RATINGS:

CARDIAC	NR	ORTHOPEDICS	★★★
CRITICAL CARE	NR	PULMONARY	★★★
GASTROINTESTINAL	★★★	STROKE	★★★
GENERAL SURGERY	★★★	VASCULAR	NR
MATERNITY CARE	★★★	WOMEN'S HEALTH	NR

HEALTHGRADES AWARDS

Central Washington Hospital

1201 South Miller Street
Wenatchee, WA 98801
(509) 662-1511

Overall patient safety: ★★★
Teaching: N

CLINICAL PROGRAM RATINGS:

CARDIAC	★★★	ORTHOPEDICS	★★★★★
CRITICAL CARE	★★★	PULMONARY	★★★
GASTROINTESTINAL	★★★	STROKE	★★★★★
GENERAL SURGERY	★★★★★	VASCULAR	★★★
MATERNITY CARE	★★★	WOMEN'S HEALTH	★★★

HEALTHGRADES AWARDS

✓ DISTINGUISHED HOSPITAL
• CLINICAL EXCELLENCE

✓ SPECIALTY EXCELLENCE
• GASTROINTESTINAL CARE
• GENERAL SURGERY
• STROKE CARE

Capital Medical Center

3900 Capital Mall Drive
Southwest
Olympia, WA 98502
(360) 754-5858

Overall patient safety: ★★★
Teaching: N

CLINICAL PROGRAM RATINGS:

CARDIAC	NR	ORTHOPEDICS	★★★★★
CRITICAL CARE	NR	PULMONARY	★★★
GASTROINTESTINAL	NR	STROKE	★★★
GENERAL SURGERY	★★★	VASCULAR	NR
MATERNITY CARE	★★★	WOMEN'S HEALTH	NR

HEALTHGRADES AWARDS

✓ SPECIALTY EXCELLENCE
• JOINT REPLACEMENT
• ORTHOPEDIC SURGERY

Coulee Community Hospital

411 Fortuyn Road
Grand Coulee, WA 99133
(509) 633-1753

Overall patient safety: ★★★
Teaching: N

CLINICAL PROGRAM RATINGS:

CARDIAC	NR	ORTHOPEDICS	NR
CRITICAL CARE	NR	PULMONARY	NR
GASTROINTESTINAL	NR	STROKE	NR
GENERAL SURGERY	NR	VASCULAR	NR
MATERNITY CARE	★★★	WOMEN'S HEALTH	NR

HEALTHGRADES AWARDS

Cascade Valley Hospital

330 South Stillaguamish
Avenue
Arlington, WA 98223
(360) 435-2133

Overall patient safety: ★★★
Teaching: N

CLINICAL PROGRAM RATINGS:

CARDIAC	NR	ORTHOPEDICS	NR
CRITICAL CARE	NR	PULMONARY	★★★
GASTROINTESTINAL	NR	STROKE	NR
GENERAL SURGERY	NR	VASCULAR	NR
MATERNITY CARE	★★★	WOMEN'S HEALTH	NR

HEALTHGRADES AWARDS

Deaconess Medical Center*

800 West 5th Avenue
Spokane, WA 99204
(509) 458-5800

Overall patient safety: ★★★
Teaching: Y

CLINICAL PROGRAM RATINGS:

CARDIAC	★★★	ORTHOPEDICS	★
CRITICAL CARE	NR	PULMONARY	★★★
GASTROINTESTINAL	★★★	STROKE	★★★
GENERAL SURGERY	★	VASCULAR	★★★
MATERNITY CARE	★	WOMEN'S HEALTH	★★★

HEALTHGRADES AWARDS

*This hospital reports its data to the federal government jointly with another hospital. Therefore the ratings and awards apply to multiple hospitals and this specific hospital may not provide all rated services.

Doctors Hospital of Tacoma*

737 Fawcett Avenue
Tacoma, WA 98405
(206) 627-8111

Overall patient safety: ★★★
Teaching: Y

CLINICAL PROGRAM RATINGS:

CARDIAC	★★★	ORTHOPEDICS	★★★
CRITICAL CARE	★★★	PULMONARY	★★★
GASTROINTESTINAL	★★★	STROKE	★★★
GENERAL SURGERY	★	VASCULAR	★★★
MATERNITY CARE	★	WOMEN'S HEALTH	★

HEALTHGRADES AWARDS

Good Samaritan Hospital and Rehabilitation Center

407 14th Avenue Southeast
Puyallup, WA 98372
(253) 697-4000

Overall patient safety: ★★★★★
Teaching: N

CLINICAL PROGRAM RATINGS:

CARDIAC	NR	ORTHOPEDICS	★★★
CRITICAL CARE	★★★	PULMONARY	★
GASTROINTESTINAL	★★★	STROKE	★★★
GENERAL SURGERY	★★★	VASCULAR	★★★
MATERNITY CARE	★★★★★	WOMEN'S HEALTH	NR

HEALTHGRADES AWARDS

✓ DISTINGUISHED HOSPITAL • PATIENT SAFETY

✓ SPECIALTY EXCELLENCE • GENERAL SURGERY • MATERNITY CARE

Enumclaw Community Hospital

1450 Battersby Avenue
Enumclaw, WA 98022
(360) 825-2505

Overall patient safety: ★★★
Teaching: N

CLINICAL PROGRAM RATINGS:

CARDIAC	NR	ORTHOPEDICS	NR
CRITICAL CARE	NR	PULMONARY	★
GASTROINTESTINAL	NR	STROKE	★★★
GENERAL SURGERY	NR	VASCULAR	NR
MATERNITY CARE	★★★	WOMEN'S HEALTH	NR

HEALTHGRADES AWARDS

Grays Harbor Community Hospital*

915 Anderson Drive
Aberdeen, WA 98520
(360) 537-5000

Overall patient safety: ★★★
Teaching: N

CLINICAL PROGRAM RATINGS:

CARDIAC	NR	ORTHOPEDICS	NR
CRITICAL CARE	NR	PULMONARY	★
GASTROINTESTINAL	★★★	STROKE	★
GENERAL SURGERY	★★★	VASCULAR	NR
MATERNITY CARE	★★★	WOMEN'S HEALTH	NR

HEALTHGRADES AWARDS

Evergreen Hospital Medical Center

12040 Northeast 128th Street
Kirkland, WA 98034
(425) 899-1000

Overall patient safety: ★★★
Teaching: N

CLINICAL PROGRAM RATINGS:

CARDIAC	NR	ORTHOPEDICS	★★★
CRITICAL CARE	NR	PULMONARY	★★★
GASTROINTESTINAL	★★★	STROKE	★★★
GENERAL SURGERY	★★★	VASCULAR	NR
MATERNITY CARE	★★★★★	WOMEN'S HEALTH	NR

HEALTHGRADES AWARDS

Group Health Eastside Hospital

2700 152nd Avenue Northeast
Redmond, WA 98052
(425) 883-5151

Overall patient safety: ★★★
Teaching: N

CLINICAL PROGRAM RATINGS:

CARDIAC	NR	ORTHOPEDICS	NR
CRITICAL CARE	NR	PULMONARY	NR
GASTROINTESTINAL	NR	STROKE	NR
GENERAL SURGERY	NR	VASCULAR	NR
MATERNITY CARE	★★★	WOMEN'S HEALTH	NR

HEALTHGRADES AWARDS

KEY: ★★★★★ **BEST** ★★★ **AS EXPECTED** ★ **POOR** NR **NOT RATED BY HEALTHGRADES** For full definitions of ratings and awards, see Appendix.

Harborview Medical Center

325 9th Avenue
Seattle, WA 98104
(206) 223-3000

Overall patient safety: ★
Teaching: Y

CLINICAL PROGRAM RATINGS:

CARDIAC	NR	ORTHOPEDICS	NR
CRITICAL CARE	NR	PULMONARY	★★★
GASTROINTESTINAL	NR	STROKE	★
GENERAL SURGERY	NR	VASCULAR	NR
MATERNITY CARE	NR	WOMEN'S HEALTH	NR

HEALTHGRADES AWARDS

Holy Family Hospital

5633 North Lidgerwood Street
Spokane, WA 99208
(509) 482-0111

Overall patient safety: ★★★★★
Teaching: N

CLINICAL PROGRAM RATINGS:

CARDIAC	NR	ORTHOPEDICS	★★★
CRITICAL CARE	★★★	PULMONARY	★★★
GASTROINTESTINAL	★★★	STROKE	★★★
GENERAL SURGERY	★★★	VASCULAR	NR
MATERNITY CARE	★★★	WOMEN'S HEALTH	NR

HEALTHGRADES AWARDS

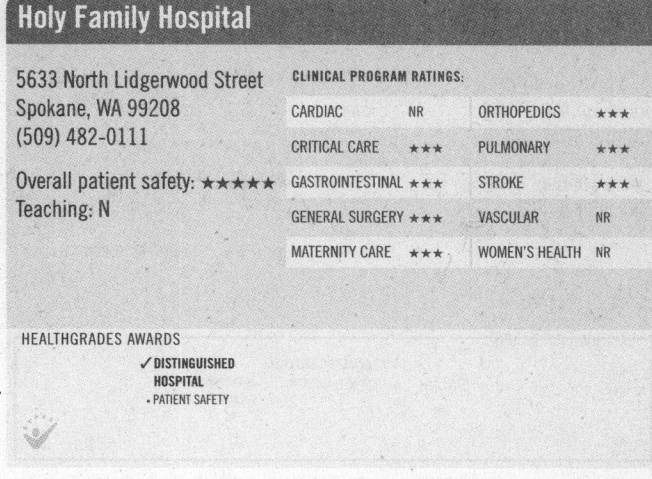

✓ DISTINGUISHED
  HOSPITAL
• PATIENT SAFETY

Harrison Medical Center

2520 Cherry Avenue
Bremerton, WA 98310
(360) 377-3911

Overall patient safety: ★
Teaching: N

CLINICAL PROGRAM RATINGS:

CARDIAC	★★★	ORTHOPEDICS	★★★
CRITICAL CARE	★★★	PULMONARY	★★★
GASTROINTESTINAL	★★★	STROKE	★
GENERAL SURGERY	★★★	VASCULAR	★★★
MATERNITY CARE	★★★	WOMEN'S HEALTH	★★★

HEALTHGRADES AWARDS

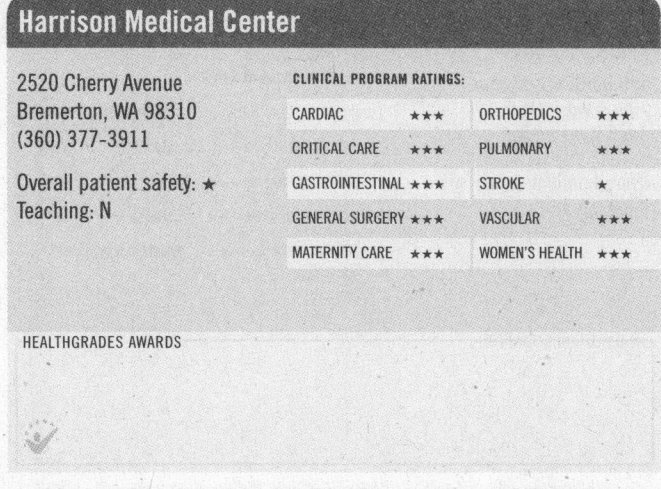

Island Hospital

1211 24th Street
Anacortes, WA 98221
(360) 299-1300

Overall patient safety: ★★★
Teaching: N

CLINICAL PROGRAM RATINGS:

CARDIAC	NR	ORTHOPEDICS	NR
CRITICAL CARE	NR	PULMONARY	★★★
GASTROINTESTINAL	NR	STROKE	★★★
GENERAL SURGERY	★★★	VASCULAR	NR
MATERNITY CARE	★★★	WOMEN'S HEALTH	NR

HEALTHGRADES AWARDS

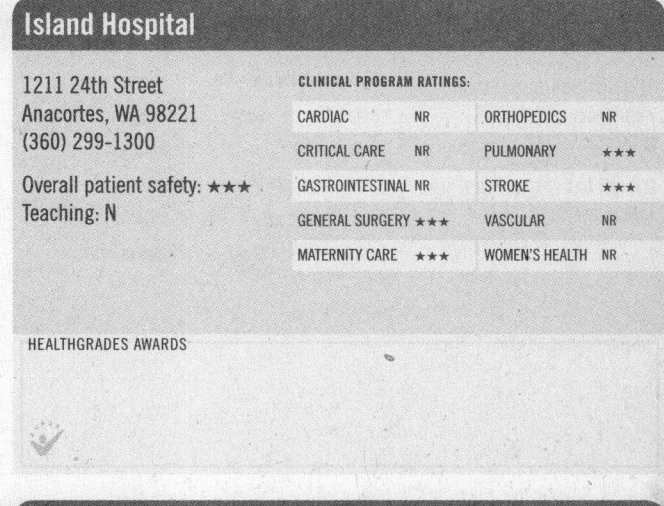

Highline Community Hospital

16251 Sylvester Road
Southwest
Burien, WA 98166
(206) 244-9970

Overall patient safety: ★★★
Teaching: N

CLINICAL PROGRAM RATINGS:

CARDIAC	NR	ORTHOPEDICS	★★★
CRITICAL CARE	NR	PULMONARY	★
GASTROINTESTINAL	NR	STROKE	★★★
GENERAL SURGERY	★★★	VASCULAR	NR
MATERNITY CARE	★★★	WOMEN'S HEALTH	NR

HEALTHGRADES AWARDS

Jefferson General Hospital

834 Sheridan Street
Port Townsend, WA 98368
(360) 385-2200

Overall patient safety: ★
Teaching: N

CLINICAL PROGRAM RATINGS:

CARDIAC	NR	ORTHOPEDICS	NR
CRITICAL CARE	NR	PULMONARY	★★★
GASTROINTESTINAL	NR	STROKE	★
GENERAL SURGERY	NR	VASCULAR	NR
MATERNITY CARE	★★★	WOMEN'S HEALTH	NR

HEALTHGRADES AWARDS

*This hospital reports its data to the federal government jointly with another hospital. Therefore the ratings and awards apply to multiple hospitals and this specific hospital may not provide all rated services.

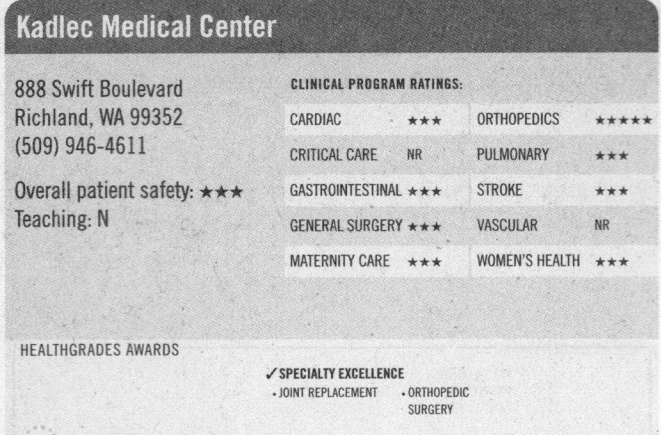

Kadlec Medical Center

888 Swift Boulevard
Richland, WA 99352
(509) 946-4611

Overall patient safety: ★★★
Teaching: N

CLINICAL PROGRAM RATINGS:

CARDIAC	★★★	ORTHOPEDICS	★★★★★
CRITICAL CARE	NR	PULMONARY	★★★
GASTROINTESTINAL	★★★	STROKE	★★★
GENERAL SURGERY	★★★	VASCULAR	NR
MATERNITY CARE	★★★	WOMEN'S HEALTH	★★★

HEALTHGRADES AWARDS

✓ SPECIALTY EXCELLENCE
• JOINT REPLACEMENT • ORTHOPEDIC SURGERY

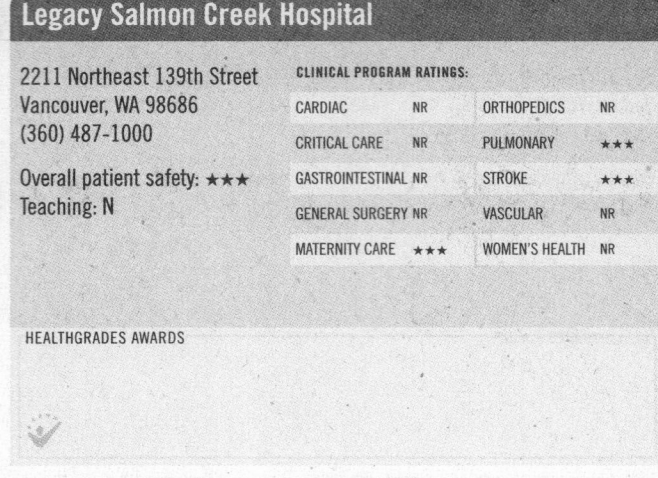

Legacy Salmon Creek Hospital

2211 Northeast 139th Street
Vancouver, WA 98686
(360) 487-1000

Overall patient safety: ★★★
Teaching: N

CLINICAL PROGRAM RATINGS:

CARDIAC	NR	ORTHOPEDICS	NR
CRITICAL CARE	NR	PULMONARY	★★★
GASTROINTESTINAL	NR	STROKE	★★★
GENERAL SURGERY	NR	VASCULAR	NR
MATERNITY CARE	★★★	WOMEN'S HEALTH	NR

HEALTHGRADES AWARDS

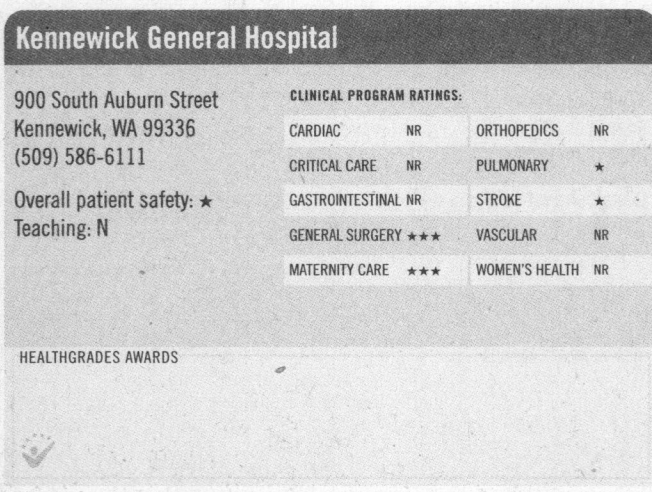

Kennewick General Hospital

900 South Auburn Street
Kennewick, WA 99336
(509) 586-6111

Overall patient safety: ★
Teaching: N

CLINICAL PROGRAM RATINGS:

CARDIAC	NR	ORTHOPEDICS	NR
CRITICAL CARE	NR	PULMONARY	★
GASTROINTESTINAL	NR	STROKE	★
GENERAL SURGERY	★★★	VASCULAR	NR
MATERNITY CARE	★★★	WOMEN'S HEALTH	NR

HEALTHGRADES AWARDS

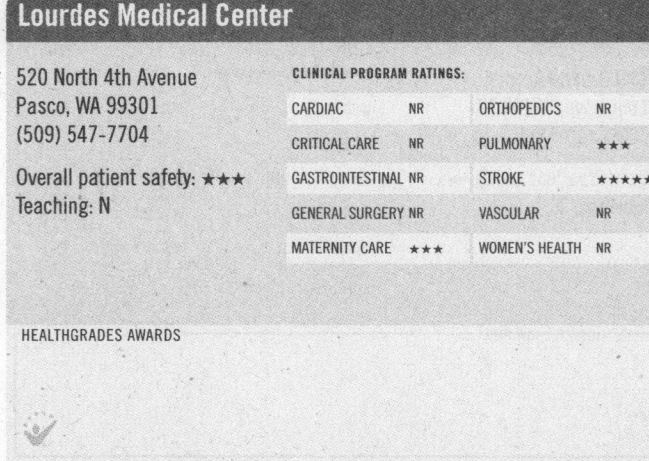

Lourdes Medical Center

520 North 4th Avenue
Pasco, WA 99301
(509) 547-7704

Overall patient safety: ★★★
Teaching: N

CLINICAL PROGRAM RATINGS:

CARDIAC	NR	ORTHOPEDICS	NR
CRITICAL CARE	NR	PULMONARY	★★★
GASTROINTESTINAL	NR	STROKE	★★★★★
GENERAL SURGERY	NR	VASCULAR	NR
MATERNITY CARE	★★★	WOMEN'S HEALTH	NR

HEALTHGRADES AWARDS

Kittitas Valley Community Hospital

603 South Chestnut Street
Ellensburg, WA 98926
(509) 962-9841

Overall patient safety: ★★★
Teaching: N

CLINICAL PROGRAM RATINGS:

CARDIAC	NR	ORTHOPEDICS	NR
CRITICAL CARE	NR	PULMONARY	★★★
GASTROINTESTINAL	NR	STROKE	★★★
GENERAL SURGERY	★★★	VASCULAR	NR
MATERNITY CARE	★	WOMEN'S HEALTH	NR

HEALTHGRADES AWARDS

Mason General Hospital

901 Mount View Drive
Shelton, WA 98584
(360) 426-1611

Overall patient safety: ★
Teaching: N

CLINICAL PROGRAM RATINGS:

CARDIAC	NR	ORTHOPEDICS	NR
CRITICAL CARE	NR	PULMONARY	★★★
GASTROINTESTINAL	NR	STROKE	★
GENERAL SURGERY	NR	VASCULAR	NR
MATERNITY CARE	★★★	WOMEN'S HEALTH	NR

HEALTHGRADES AWARDS

KEY: ★★★★★ BEST   ★★★ AS EXPECTED   ★ POOR   NR NOT RATED BY HEALTHGRADES   For full definitions of ratings and awards, see Appendix.

Mid-Valley Hospital

810 Jasmine Street
Omak, WA 98841
(509) 826-1760

Overall patient safety: ★
Teaching: N

CLINICAL PROGRAM RATINGS:

CARDIAC	NR	ORTHOPEDICS	NR
CRITICAL CARE	NR	PULMONARY	NR
GASTROINTESTINAL	NR	STROKE	NR
GENERAL SURGERY	NR	VASCULAR	NR
MATERNITY CARE	★★★	WOMEN'S HEALTH	NR

HEALTHGRADES AWARDS

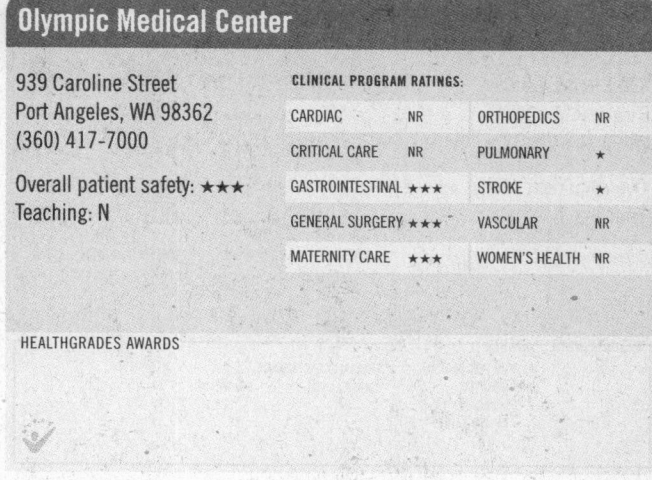

Olympic Medical Center

939 Caroline Street
Port Angeles, WA 98362
(360) 417-7000

Overall patient safety: ★★★
Teaching: N

CLINICAL PROGRAM RATINGS:

CARDIAC	NR	ORTHOPEDICS	NR
CRITICAL CARE	NR	PULMONARY	★
GASTROINTESTINAL	★★★	STROKE	★
GENERAL SURGERY	★★★	VASCULAR	NR
MATERNITY CARE	★★★	WOMEN'S HEALTH	NR

HEALTHGRADES AWARDS

Monticello Medical Center*

600 Broadway
Longview, WA 98632
(206) 423-5850

Overall patient safety: ★★★
Teaching: N

CLINICAL PROGRAM RATINGS:

CARDIAC	NR	ORTHOPEDICS	NR
CRITICAL CARE	NR	PULMONARY	★
GASTROINTESTINAL	★★★	STROKE	★★★
GENERAL SURGERY	★★★	VASCULAR	NR
MATERNITY CARE	★★★	WOMEN'S HEALTH	NR

HEALTHGRADES AWARDS

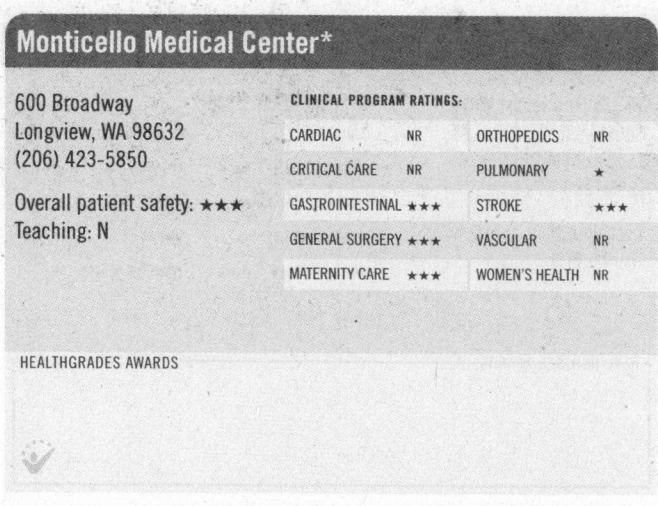

Overlake Hospital Medical Center

1035 116th Avenue Northeast
Bellevue, WA 98004
(425) 688-5000

Overall patient safety: ★★★
Teaching: Y

CLINICAL PROGRAM RATINGS:

CARDIAC	★★★	ORTHOPEDICS	★★★
CRITICAL CARE	NR	PULMONARY	★
GASTROINTESTINAL	★★★	STROKE	★★★
GENERAL SURGERY	★★★	VASCULAR	★★★
MATERNITY CARE	★★★★★	WOMEN'S HEALTH	★★★★★

HEALTHGRADES AWARDS

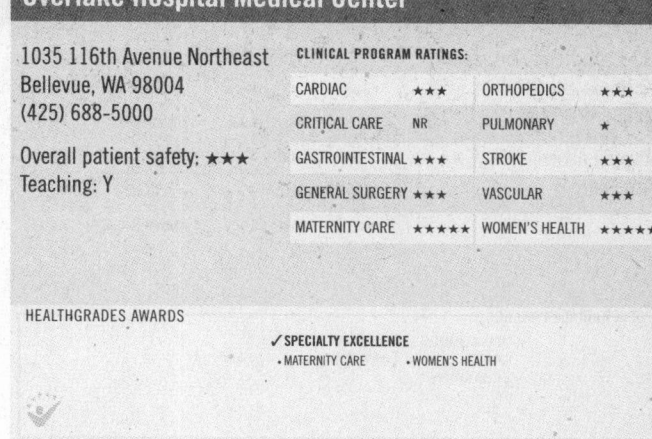

✓ SPECIALTY EXCELLENCE
• MATERNITY CARE   • WOMEN'S HEALTH

Northwest Hospital and Medical Center

1550 North 115th Street
Seattle, WA 98133
(206) 364-0500

Overall patient safety: ★★★★★
Teaching: N

CLINICAL PROGRAM RATINGS:

CARDIAC	★★★	ORTHOPEDICS	★★★
CRITICAL CARE	★★★	PULMONARY	★★★
GASTROINTESTINAL	★★★	STROKE	★★★★★
GENERAL SURGERY	★★★	VASCULAR	NR
MATERNITY CARE	★★★	WOMEN'S HEALTH	NR

HEALTHGRADES AWARDS

✓ DISTINGUISHED   ✓ SPECIALTY EXCELLENCE
   HOSPITAL   • STROKE CARE
   • PATIENT SAFETY

Providence Centralia Hospital

914 South Scheuber Road
Centralia, WA 98531
(360) 736-2803

Overall patient safety: ★
Teaching: N

CLINICAL PROGRAM RATINGS:

CARDIAC	NR	ORTHOPEDICS	★★★
CRITICAL CARE	NR	PULMONARY	★★★
GASTROINTESTINAL	NR	STROKE	★
GENERAL SURGERY	★★★	VASCULAR	NR
MATERNITY CARE	★	WOMEN'S HEALTH	NR

HEALTHGRADES AWARDS

*This hospital reports its data to the federal government jointly with another hospital. Therefore the ratings and awards apply to multiple hospitals and this specific hospital may not provide all rated services.

Providence Everett Medical Center–Colby Campus*

1321 Colby Avenue
Everett, WA 98201
(425) 261-2000

Overall patient safety: ★★★★★
Teaching: N

CLINICAL PROGRAM RATINGS:

CARDIAC	★★★	ORTHOPEDICS	★
CRITICAL CARE	★★★★★	PULMONARY	★★★★★
GASTROINTESTINAL	★★★	STROKE	★★★★★
GENERAL SURGERY	★★★	VASCULAR	★★★
MATERNITY CARE	★★★	WOMEN'S HEALTH	★★★

HEALTHGRADES AWARDS

✓ DISTINGUISHED HOSPITAL
- CLINICAL EXCELLENCE
- PATIENT SAFETY

✓ SPECIALTY EXCELLENCE
- CRITICAL CARE
- STROKE CARE

Sacred Heart Medical Center

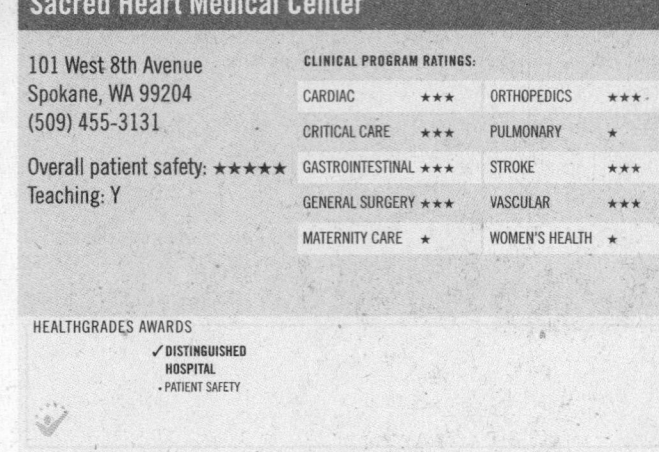

101 West 8th Avenue
Spokane, WA 99204
(509) 455-3131

Overall patient safety: ★★★★★
Teaching: Y

CLINICAL PROGRAM RATINGS:

CARDIAC	★★★	ORTHOPEDICS	★★★
CRITICAL CARE	★★★	PULMONARY	★
GASTROINTESTINAL	★★★	STROKE	★★★
GENERAL SURGERY	★★★	VASCULAR	★★★
MATERNITY CARE	★	WOMEN'S HEALTH	★

HEALTHGRADES AWARDS

✓ DISTINGUISHED HOSPITAL
- PATIENT SAFETY

Providence St. Peter Hospital

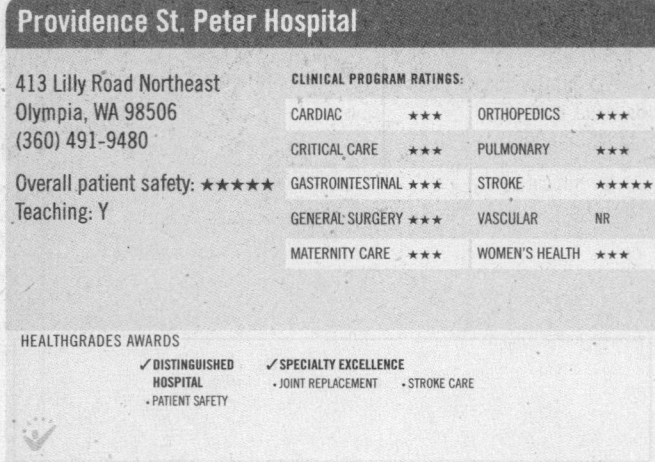

413 Lilly Road Northeast
Olympia, WA 98506
(360) 491-9480

Overall patient safety: ★★★★★
Teaching: Y

CLINICAL PROGRAM RATINGS:

CARDIAC	★★★	ORTHOPEDICS	★★★
CRITICAL CARE	★★★	PULMONARY	★★★
GASTROINTESTINAL	★★★	STROKE	★★★★★
GENERAL SURGERY	★★★	VASCULAR	NR
MATERNITY CARE	★★★	WOMEN'S HEALTH	★★★

HEALTHGRADES AWARDS

✓ DISTINGUISHED HOSPITAL
- PATIENT SAFETY

✓ SPECIALTY EXCELLENCE
- JOINT REPLACEMENT
- STROKE CARE

St. Clare Hospital

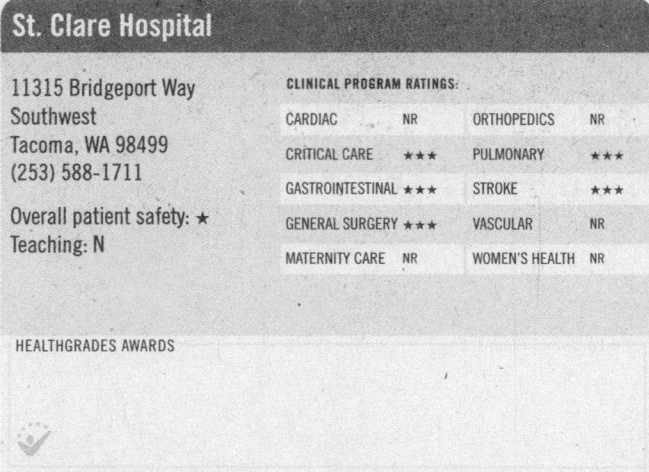

11315 Bridgeport Way
Southwest
Tacoma, WA 98499
(253) 588-1711

Overall patient safety: ★
Teaching: N

CLINICAL PROGRAM RATINGS:

CARDIAC	NR	ORTHOPEDICS	NR
CRITICAL CARE	★★★	PULMONARY	★★★
GASTROINTESTINAL	★★★	STROKE	★★★
GENERAL SURGERY	★★★	VASCULAR	NR
MATERNITY CARE	NR	WOMEN'S HEALTH	NR

HEALTHGRADES AWARDS

Pullman Memorial Hospital

1125 Northeast Washington
Avenue
Pullman, WA 99163
(509) 332-2541

Overall patient safety: ★★★
Teaching: N

CLINICAL PROGRAM RATINGS:

CARDIAC	NR	ORTHOPEDICS	NR
CRITICAL CARE	NR	PULMONARY	NR
GASTROINTESTINAL	NR	STROKE	NR
GENERAL SURGERY	NR	VASCULAR	NR
MATERNITY CARE	★	WOMEN'S HEALTH	NR

HEALTHGRADES AWARDS

St. Francis Community Hospital

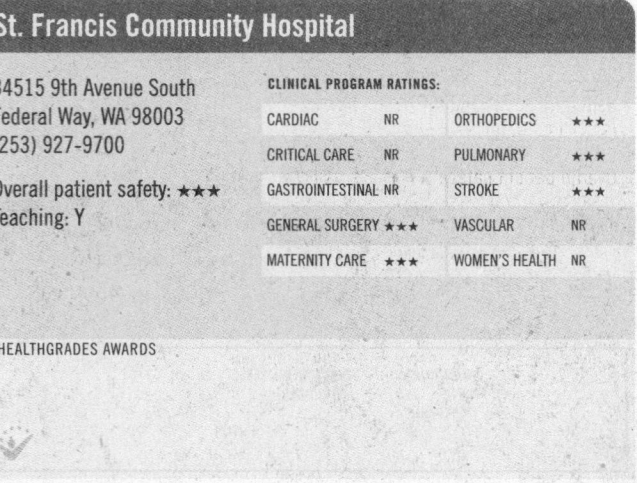

34515 9th Avenue South
Federal Way, WA 98003
(253) 927-9700

Overall patient safety: ★★★
Teaching: Y

CLINICAL PROGRAM RATINGS:

CARDIAC	NR	ORTHOPEDICS	★★★
CRITICAL CARE	NR	PULMONARY	★★★
GASTROINTESTINAL	NR	STROKE	★★★
GENERAL SURGERY	★★★	VASCULAR	NR
MATERNITY CARE	★★★	WOMEN'S HEALTH	NR

HEALTHGRADES AWARDS

KEY: ★★★★★ BEST ★★★ AS EXPECTED ★ POOR NR NOT RATED BY HEALTHGRADES For full definitions of ratings and awards, see Appendix.

St. John Medical Center Peacehealth*

1615 Delaware Street
Longview, WA 98632
(360) 414-2000

Overall patient safety: ★★★
Teaching: N

CLINICAL PROGRAM RATINGS:

CARDIAC	NR	ORTHOPEDICS	NR
CRITICAL CARE	NR	PULMONARY	★
GASTROINTESTINAL	★★★	STROKE	★★★
GENERAL SURGERY	★★★	VASCULAR	NR
MATERNITY CARE	★★★	WOMEN'S HEALTH	NR

HEALTHGRADES AWARDS

St. Joseph Medical Center

1717 South J Street
Tacoma, WA 98405
(253) 627-4101

Overall patient safety: ★★★
Teaching: N

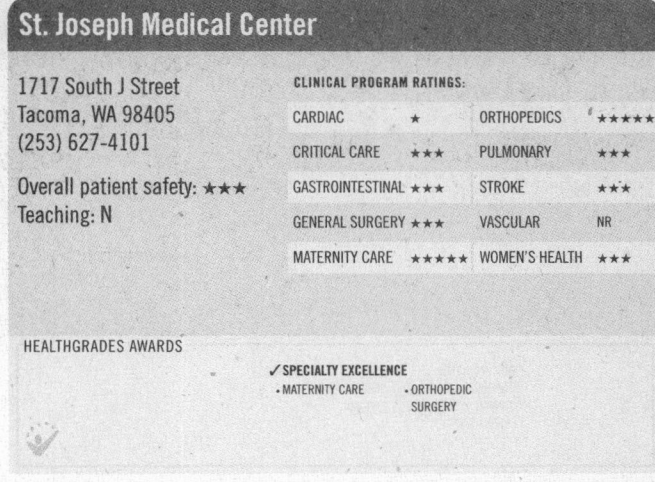

CLINICAL PROGRAM RATINGS:

CARDIAC	★	ORTHOPEDICS	★★★★★
CRITICAL CARE	★★★	PULMONARY	★★★
GASTROINTESTINAL	★★★	STROKE	★★★
GENERAL SURGERY	★★★	VASCULAR	NR
MATERNITY CARE	★★★★★	WOMEN'S HEALTH	★★★

HEALTHGRADES AWARDS

✓ SPECIALTY EXCELLENCE
- MATERNITY CARE   - ORTHOPEDIC SURGERY

St. Joseph Hospital*

1006 North H Street
Aberdeen, WA 98520
(206) 533-0450

Overall patient safety: ★★★
Teaching: N

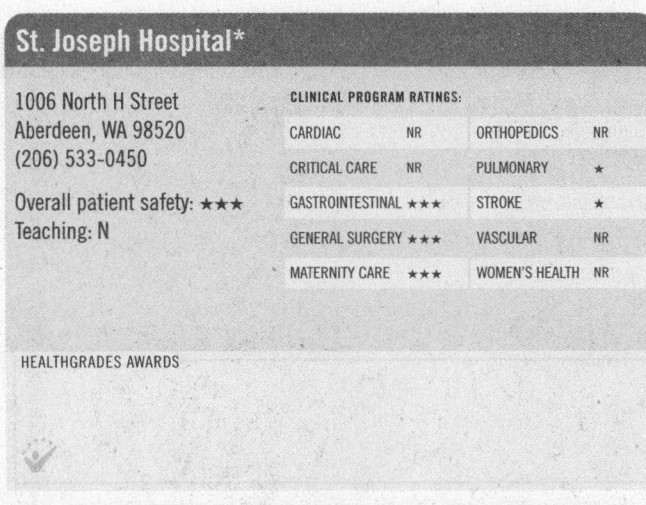

CLINICAL PROGRAM RATINGS:

CARDIAC	NR	ORTHOPEDICS	NR
CRITICAL CARE	NR	PULMONARY	★
GASTROINTESTINAL	★★★	STROKE	★
GENERAL SURGERY	★★★	VASCULAR	NR
MATERNITY CARE	★★★	WOMEN'S HEALTH	NR

HEALTHGRADES AWARDS

St. Joseph's Hospital of Chewelah

500 East Webster Avenue
Chewelah, WA 99109
(509) 935-8211

Overall patient safety: NR
Teaching: N

CLINICAL PROGRAM RATINGS:

CARDIAC	NR	ORTHOPEDICS	NR
CRITICAL CARE	NR	PULMONARY	★★★
GASTROINTESTINAL	NR	STROKE	NR
GENERAL SURGERY	NR	VASCULAR	NR
MATERNITY CARE	★	WOMEN'S HEALTH	NR

HEALTHGRADES AWARDS

St. Joseph Hospital*

2901 Squalicum Parkway
Bellingham, WA 98225
(360) 734-5400

Overall patient safety: ★★★
Teaching: N

CLINICAL PROGRAM RATINGS:

CARDIAC	★★★	ORTHOPEDICS	★★★
CRITICAL CARE	★★★	PULMONARY	★★★★★
GASTROINTESTINAL	★★★	STROKE	★★★
GENERAL SURGERY	★★★	VASCULAR	NR
MATERNITY CARE	★★★	WOMEN'S HEALTH	★★★

HEALTHGRADES AWARDS

✓ SPECIALTY EXCELLENCE
- PULMONARY CARE

St. Luke's Memorial Hospital*

S 711 Cowley
Spokane, WA 99210
(509) 838-4771

Overall patient safety: ★★★
Teaching: Y

CLINICAL PROGRAM RATINGS:

CARDIAC	★★★	ORTHOPEDICS	★
CRITICAL CARE	NR	PULMONARY	★★★
GASTROINTESTINAL	★★★	STROKE	★★★
GENERAL SURGERY	★	VASCULAR	★★★
MATERNITY CARE	★	WOMEN'S HEALTH	★★★

HEALTHGRADES AWARDS

*This hospital reports its data to the federal government jointly with another hospital. Therefore the ratings and awards apply to multiple hospitals and this specific hospital may not provide all rated services.

St. Mary Medical Center

401 West Poplar Street
Walla Walla, WA 99362
(509) 525-3320

Overall patient safety: ★★★★★
Teaching: N

CLINICAL PROGRAM RATINGS:

CARDIAC	NR	ORTHOPEDICS	★★★★★
CRITICAL CARE	NR	PULMONARY	★★★
GASTROINTESTINAL	★★★	STROKE	★★★
GENERAL SURGERY	★★★	VASCULAR	NR
MATERNITY CARE	★★★	WOMEN'S HEALTH	NR

HEALTHGRADES AWARDS

✓ DISTINGUISHED HOSPITAL
• CLINICAL EXCELLENCE
• PATIENT SAFETY

✓ SPECIALTY EXCELLENCE
• ORTHOPEDIC SURGERY

Stevens Hospital

21601 76th Avenue West
Edmonds, WA 98026
(425) 640-4000

Overall patient safety: ★★★
Teaching: N

CLINICAL PROGRAM RATINGS:

CARDIAC	NR	ORTHOPEDICS	NR
CRITICAL CARE	★★★	PULMONARY	★★★
GASTROINTESTINAL	NR	STROKE	★★★
GENERAL SURGERY	★★★	VASCULAR	NR
MATERNITY CARE	★★★	WOMEN'S HEALTH	NR

HEALTHGRADES AWARDS

Samaritan Hospital

801 East Wheeler Road
Moses Lake, WA 98837
(509) 765-5606

Overall patient safety: ★★★
Teaching: N

CLINICAL PROGRAM RATINGS:

CARDIAC	NR	ORTHOPEDICS	NR
CRITICAL CARE	NR	PULMONARY	★★★
GASTROINTESTINAL	NR	STROKE	★★★
GENERAL SURGERY	★★★	VASCULAR	NR
MATERNITY CARE	★	WOMEN'S HEALTH	NR

HEALTHGRADES AWARDS

Sunnyside Community Hospital*

1016 Tacoma Avenue
Sunnyside, WA 98944
(509) 837-1500

Overall patient safety: ★★★
Teaching: N

CLINICAL PROGRAM RATINGS:

CARDIAC	NR	ORTHOPEDICS	NR
CRITICAL CARE	NR	PULMONARY	★★★
GASTROINTESTINAL	NR	STROKE	NR
GENERAL SURGERY	NR	VASCULAR	NR
MATERNITY CARE	★	WOMEN'S HEALTH	NR

HEALTHGRADES AWARDS

Skagit Valley Hospital

1415 Kincaid Street
Mount Vernon, WA 98274
(360) 424-4111

Overall patient safety: ★
Teaching: N

CLINICAL PROGRAM RATINGS:

CARDIAC	NR	ORTHOPEDICS	★★★
CRITICAL CARE	NR	PULMONARY	★★★
GASTROINTESTINAL	★★★	STROKE	★
GENERAL SURGERY	★★★	VASCULAR	NR
MATERNITY CARE	★★★	WOMEN'S HEALTH	NR

HEALTHGRADES AWARDS

Southwest Washington Medical Center

400 Northeast Mother
Joseph Place
Vancouver, WA 98668
(360) 256-2000

Overall patient safety: ★★★
Teaching: Y

CLINICAL PROGRAM RATINGS:

CARDIAC	★★★	ORTHOPEDICS	★★★★★
CRITICAL CARE	★★★	PULMONARY	★★★
GASTROINTESTINAL	★★★	STROKE	★★★
GENERAL SURGERY	★★★	VASCULAR	NR
MATERNITY CARE	★★★	WOMEN'S HEALTH	★★★

HEALTHGRADES AWARDS

KEY: ★★★★★ BEST   ★★★ AS EXPECTED   ★ POOR   NR NOT RATED BY HEALTHGRADES   For full definitions of ratings and awards, see Appendix.

Swedish Medical Center–Ballard Campus*

5409 Barnes Avenue Northwest
Seattle, WA 98107
(206) 386-6000

Overall patient safety: ★★★
Teaching: Y

CLINICAL PROGRAM RATINGS:

CARDIAC	★	ORTHOPEDICS	★★★
CRITICAL CARE	★★★★★	PULMONARY	★★★★★
GASTROINTESTINAL	★★★	STROKE	★★★★★
GENERAL SURGERY	★★★	VASCULAR	★★★
MATERNITY CARE	★★★	WOMEN'S HEALTH	★★★

HEALTHGRADES AWARDS

✓ SPECIALTY EXCELLENCE
- CRITICAL CARE
- GASTROINTESTINAL CARE
- GENERAL SURGERY
- STROKE CARE

Tacoma General Allenmore Hospital*

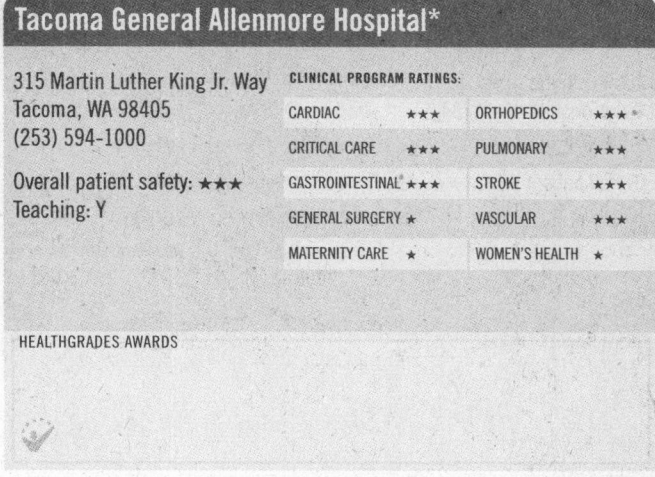

315 Martin Luther King Jr. Way
Tacoma, WA 98405
(253) 594-1000

Overall patient safety: ★★★
Teaching: Y

CLINICAL PROGRAM RATINGS:

CARDIAC	★★★	ORTHOPEDICS	★★★
CRITICAL CARE	★★★	PULMONARY	★★★
GASTROINTESTINAL	★★★	STROKE	★★★
GENERAL SURGERY	★	VASCULAR	★★★
MATERNITY CARE	★	WOMEN'S HEALTH	★

HEALTHGRADES AWARDS

Swedish Medical Center–Cherry Hills Campus

500 17th Avenue
Seattle, WA 98124
(206) 320-2000

Overall patient safety: ★★★
Teaching: Y

CLINICAL PROGRAM RATINGS:

CARDIAC	★★★	ORTHOPEDICS	★★★
CRITICAL CARE	★★★	PULMONARY	★★★
GASTROINTESTINAL	NR	STROKE	★★★★★
GENERAL SURGERY	NR	VASCULAR	★
MATERNITY CARE	NR	WOMEN'S HEALTH	NR

HEALTHGRADES AWARDS

✓ SPECIALTY EXCELLENCE
- STROKE CARE

Toppenish Community Hospital

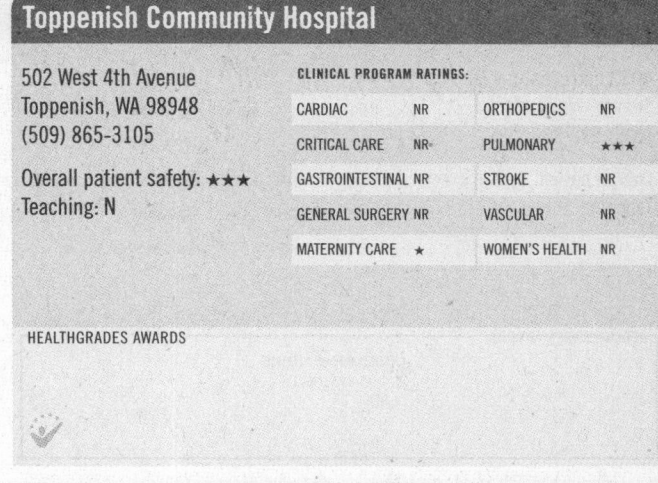

502 West 4th Avenue
Toppenish, WA 98948
(509) 865-3105

Overall patient safety: ★★★
Teaching: N

CLINICAL PROGRAM RATINGS:

CARDIAC	NR	ORTHOPEDICS	NR
CRITICAL CARE	NR	PULMONARY	★★★
GASTROINTESTINAL	NR	STROKE	NR
GENERAL SURGERY	NR	VASCULAR	NR
MATERNITY CARE	★	WOMEN'S HEALTH	NR

HEALTHGRADES AWARDS

Swedish Medical Center–First Hill*

747 Broadway
Seattle, WA 98122
(206) 386-6000

Overall patient safety: ★★★
Teaching: Y

CLINICAL PROGRAM RATINGS:

CARDIAC	★	ORTHOPEDICS	★★★
CRITICAL CARE	★★★★★	PULMONARY	★★★★★
GASTROINTESTINAL	★★★	STROKE	★★★★★
GENERAL SURGERY	★★★	VASCULAR	★★★
MATERNITY CARE	★★★	WOMEN'S HEALTH	★★★

HEALTHGRADES AWARDS

✓ SPECIALTY EXCELLENCE
- CRITICAL CARE
- GASTROINTESTINAL CARE
- GENERAL SURGERY
- STROKE CARE

Tri-State Memorial Hospital

1221 Highland Avenue
Clarkston, WA 99403
(509) 758-5511

Overall patient safety: ★★★
Teaching: N

CLINICAL PROGRAM RATINGS:

CARDIAC	NR	ORTHOPEDICS	NR
CRITICAL CARE	NR	PULMONARY	★★★
GASTROINTESTINAL	NR	STROKE	★★★
GENERAL SURGERY	★★★	VASCULAR	NR
MATERNITY CARE	NR	WOMEN'S HEALTH	NR

HEALTHGRADES AWARDS

✓ SPECIALTY EXCELLENCE
- JOINT REPLACEMENT

*This hospital reports its data to the federal government jointly with another hospital. Therefore the ratings and awards apply to multiple hospitals and this specific hospital may not provide all rated services.

United General Hospital

2000 Hospital Drive
Sedro Woolley, WA 98284
(360) 856-6021

Overall patient safety: ★★★
Teaching: N

CLINICAL PROGRAM RATINGS:

Program	Rating	Program	Rating
CARDIAC	NR	ORTHOPEDICS	NR
CRITICAL CARE	NR	PULMONARY	★
GASTROINTESTINAL	NR	STROKE	NR
GENERAL SURGERY	NR	VASCULAR	NR
MATERNITY CARE	NR	WOMEN'S HEALTH	NR

HEALTHGRADES AWARDS

Valley Hospital and Medical Center

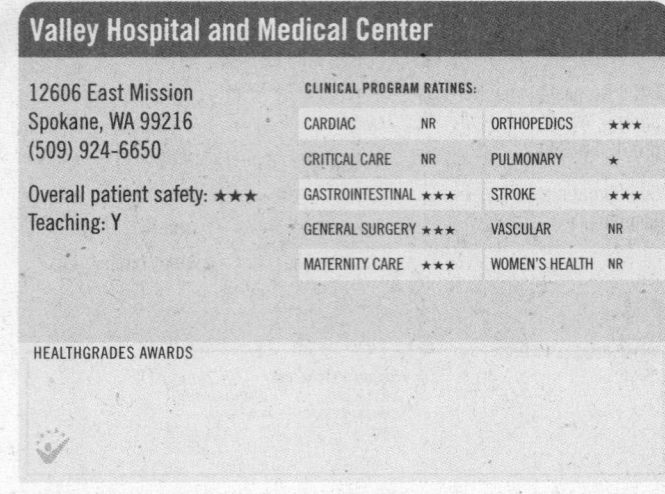

12606 East Mission
Spokane, WA 99216
(509) 924-6650

Overall patient safety: ★★★
Teaching: Y

CLINICAL PROGRAM RATINGS:

Program	Rating	Program	Rating
CARDIAC	NR	ORTHOPEDICS	★★★
CRITICAL CARE	NR	PULMONARY	★
GASTROINTESTINAL	★★★	STROKE	★★★
GENERAL SURGERY	★★★	VASCULAR	NR
MATERNITY CARE	★★★	WOMEN'S HEALTH	NR

HEALTHGRADES AWARDS

University of Washington Medical Center

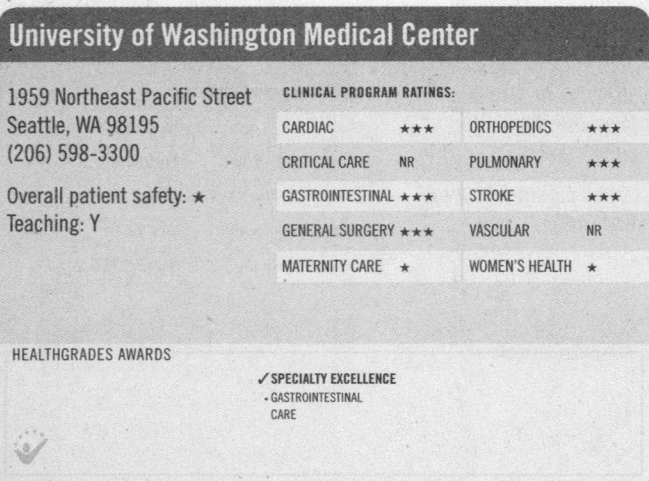

1959 Northeast Pacific Street
Seattle, WA 98195
(206) 598-3300

Overall patient safety: ★
Teaching: Y

CLINICAL PROGRAM RATINGS:

Program	Rating	Program	Rating
CARDIAC	★★★	ORTHOPEDICS	★★★
CRITICAL CARE	NR	PULMONARY	★★★
GASTROINTESTINAL	★★★	STROKE	★★★
GENERAL SURGERY	★★★	VASCULAR	NR
MATERNITY CARE	★	WOMEN'S HEALTH	★

HEALTHGRADES AWARDS

✓ SPECIALTY EXCELLENCE
· GASTROINTESTINAL CARE

Valley Medical Center

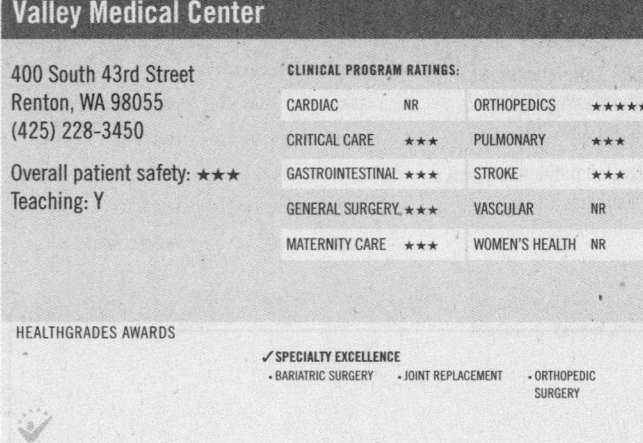

400 South 43rd Street
Renton, WA 98055
(425) 228-3450

Overall patient safety: ★★★
Teaching: Y

CLINICAL PROGRAM RATINGS:

Program	Rating	Program	Rating
CARDIAC	NR	ORTHOPEDICS	★★★★★
CRITICAL CARE	★★★	PULMONARY	★★★
GASTROINTESTINAL	★★★	STROKE	★★★
GENERAL SURGERY	★★★	VASCULAR	NR
MATERNITY CARE	★★★	WOMEN'S HEALTH	NR

HEALTHGRADES AWARDS

✓ SPECIALTY EXCELLENCE
· BARIATRIC SURGERY   · JOINT REPLACEMENT   · ORTHOPEDIC SURGERY

Valley General Hospital

14701 179 Avenue Southeast
Monroe, WA 98272
(360) 794-7497

Overall patient safety: ★★★
Teaching: N

CLINICAL PROGRAM RATINGS:

Program	Rating	Program	Rating
CARDIAC	NR	ORTHOPEDICS	NR
CRITICAL CARE	NR	PULMONARY	★★★
GASTROINTESTINAL	NR	STROKE	★★★
GENERAL SURGERY	NR	VASCULAR	NR
MATERNITY CARE	★★★	WOMEN'S HEALTH	NR

HEALTHGRADES AWARDS

Valley Memorial Hospital*

Tenth and Tacoma
Sunnyside, WA 98944
(509) 837-2101

Overall patient safety: ★★★
Teaching: N

CLINICAL PROGRAM RATINGS:

Program	Rating	Program	Rating
CARDIAC	NR	ORTHOPEDICS	NR
CRITICAL CARE	NR	PULMONARY	★★★
GASTROINTESTINAL	NR	STROKE	NR
GENERAL SURGERY	NR	VASCULAR	NR
MATERNITY CARE	★	WOMEN'S HEALTH	NR

HEALTHGRADES AWARDS

KEY: ★★★★★ BEST   ★★★ AS EXPECTED   ★ POOR   NR NOT RATED BY HEALTHGRADES   For full definitions of ratings and awards, see Appendix.

Virginia Mason Medical Center

1100 9th Avenue
Seattle, WA 98101
(206) 223-6600

Overall patient safety: ★★★
Teaching: Y

CLINICAL PROGRAM RATINGS:

CARDIAC	★★★	ORTHOPEDICS	★★★
CRITICAL CARE	NR	PULMONARY	★★★
GASTROINTESTINAL	★★★	STROKE	★★★
GENERAL SURGERY	★★★	VASCULAR	★★★
MATERNITY CARE	NR	WOMEN'S HEALTH	NR

HEALTHGRADES AWARDS

Whitman Hospital and Medical Center

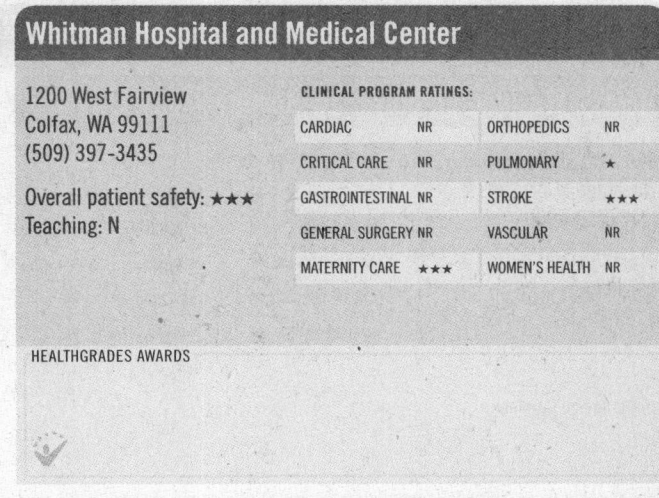

1200 West Fairview
Colfax, WA 99111
(509) 397-3435

Overall patient safety: ★★★
Teaching: N

CLINICAL PROGRAM RATINGS:

CARDIAC	NR	ORTHOPEDICS	NR
CRITICAL CARE	NR	PULMONARY	★
GASTROINTESTINAL	NR	STROKE	★★★
GENERAL SURGERY	NR	VASCULAR	NR
MATERNITY CARE	★★★	WOMEN'S HEALTH	NR

HEALTHGRADES AWARDS

Walla Walla General Hospital

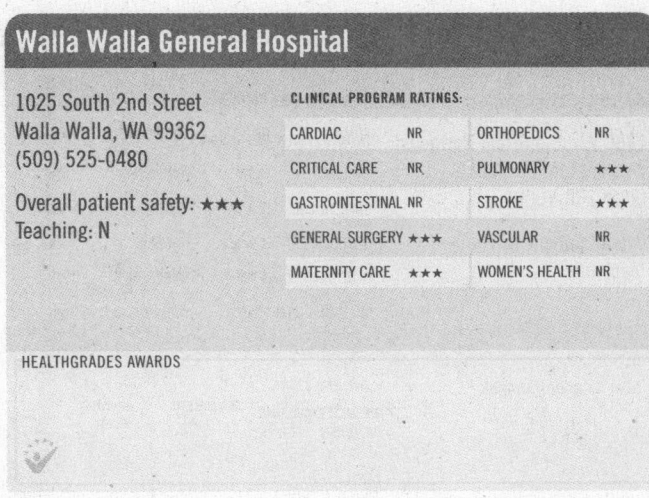

1025 South 2nd Street
Walla Walla, WA 99362
(509) 525-0480

Overall patient safety: ★★★
Teaching: N

CLINICAL PROGRAM RATINGS:

CARDIAC	NR	ORTHOPEDICS	NR
CRITICAL CARE	NR	PULMONARY	★★★
GASTROINTESTINAL	NR	STROKE	★★★
GENERAL SURGERY	★★★	VASCULAR	NR
MATERNITY CARE	★★★	WOMEN'S HEALTH	NR

HEALTHGRADES AWARDS

Yakima Regional Medical and Cardiac Center

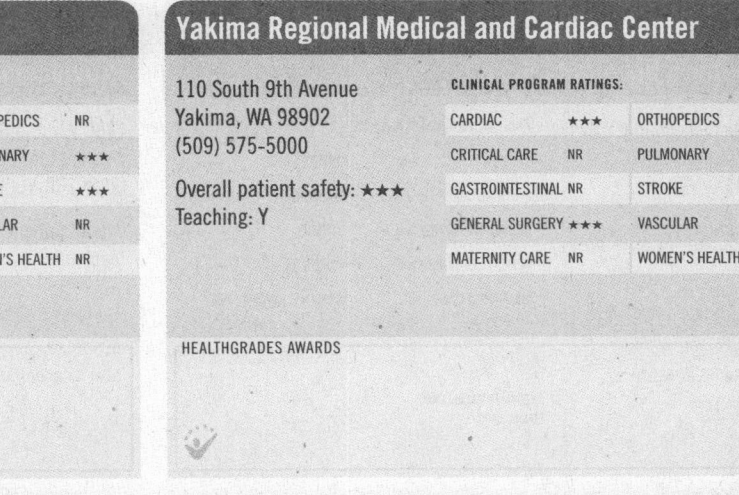

110 South 9th Avenue
Yakima, WA 98902
(509) 575-5000

Overall patient safety: ★★★
Teaching: Y

CLINICAL PROGRAM RATINGS:

CARDIAC	★★★	ORTHOPEDICS	NR
CRITICAL CARE	NR	PULMONARY	★★★
GASTROINTESTINAL	NR	STROKE	★★★
GENERAL SURGERY	★★★	VASCULAR	NR
MATERNITY CARE	NR	WOMEN'S HEALTH	NR

HEALTHGRADES AWARDS

Whidbey General Hospital

101 North Main Street
Coupeville, WA 98239
(360) 678-5151

Overall patient safety: ★
Teaching: N

CLINICAL PROGRAM RATINGS:

CARDIAC	NR	ORTHOPEDICS	NR
CRITICAL CARE	NR	PULMONARY	★★★
GASTROINTESTINAL	NR	STROKE	★
GENERAL SURGERY	★★★	VASCULAR	NR
MATERNITY CARE	★★★	WOMEN'S HEALTH	NR

HEALTHGRADES AWARDS

Yakima Valley Memorial Hospital

2811 Tieton Drive
Yakima, WA 98902
(509) 575-8000

Overall patient safety: ★★★
Teaching: Y

CLINICAL PROGRAM RATINGS:

CARDIAC	NR	ORTHOPEDICS	★★★
CRITICAL CARE	★★★	PULMONARY	★★★
GASTROINTESTINAL	★★★	STROKE	★
GENERAL SURGERY	★★★	VASCULAR	NR
MATERNITY CARE	★★★	WOMEN'S HEALTH	NR

HEALTHGRADES AWARDS

*This hospital reports its data to the federal government jointly with another hospital. Therefore the ratings and awards apply to multiple hospitals and this specific hospital may not provide all rated services.

WASHINGTON, DC HOSPITALS: RATINGS BY CLINICAL SPECIALTY

George Washington University Hospital

900 23rd Street Northwest
Washington, DC 20037
(202) 715-4000

Overall patient safety: ★
Teaching: Y

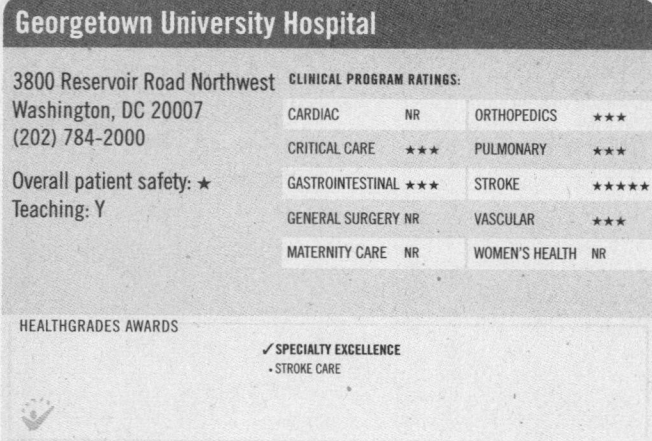

CLINICAL PROGRAM RATINGS:

CARDIAC	★★★	ORTHOPEDICS	★★★
CRITICAL CARE	NR	PULMONARY	★★★
GASTROINTESTINAL	NR	STROKE	★★★
GENERAL SURGERY	NR	VASCULAR	NR
MATERNITY CARE	NR	WOMEN'S HEALTH	NR

HEALTHGRADES AWARDS

Howard University Hospital

2041 Georgia Avenue Northwest
Washington, DC 20060
(202) 865-6100

Overall patient safety: ★
Teaching: Y

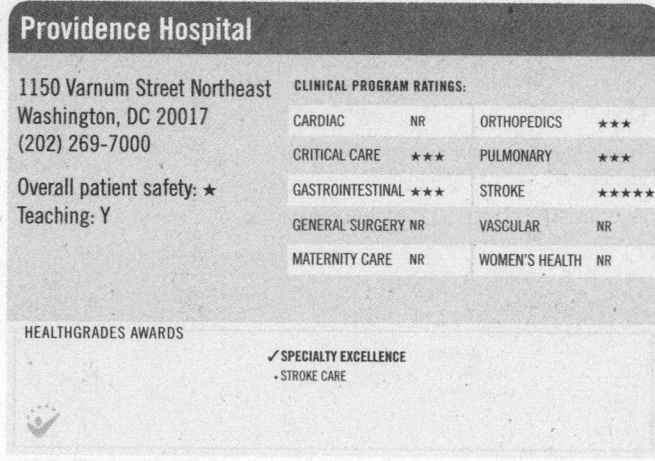

CLINICAL PROGRAM RATINGS:

CARDIAC	NR	ORTHOPEDICS	NR
CRITICAL CARE	★	PULMONARY	★★★
GASTROINTESTINAL	NR	STROKE	★★★★★
GENERAL SURGERY	NR	VASCULAR	NR
MATERNITY CARE	NR	WOMEN'S HEALTH	NR

HEALTHGRADES AWARDS

✓ SPECIALTY EXCELLENCE
• STROKE CARE

Georgetown University Hospital

3800 Reservoir Road Northwest
Washington, DC 20007
(202) 784-2000

Overall patient safety: ★
Teaching: Y

CLINICAL PROGRAM RATINGS:

CARDIAC	NR	ORTHOPEDICS	★★★
CRITICAL CARE	★★★	PULMONARY	★★★
GASTROINTESTINAL	★★★	STROKE	★★★★★
GENERAL SURGERY	NR	VASCULAR	★★★
MATERNITY CARE	NR	WOMEN'S HEALTH	NR

HEALTHGRADES AWARDS

✓ SPECIALTY EXCELLENCE
• STROKE CARE

Providence Hospital

1150 Varnum Street Northeast
Washington, DC 20017
(202) 269-7000

Overall patient safety: ★
Teaching: Y

CLINICAL PROGRAM RATINGS:

CARDIAC	NR	ORTHOPEDICS	★★★
CRITICAL CARE	★★★	PULMONARY	★★★
GASTROINTESTINAL	★★★	STROKE	★★★★★
GENERAL SURGERY	NR	VASCULAR	NR
MATERNITY CARE	NR	WOMEN'S HEALTH	NR

HEALTHGRADES AWARDS

✓ SPECIALTY EXCELLENCE
• STROKE CARE

Greater Southeast Community Hospital

1310 Southern Avenue
Southeast
Washington, DC 20032
(202) 574-6000

Overall patient safety: ★
Teaching: N

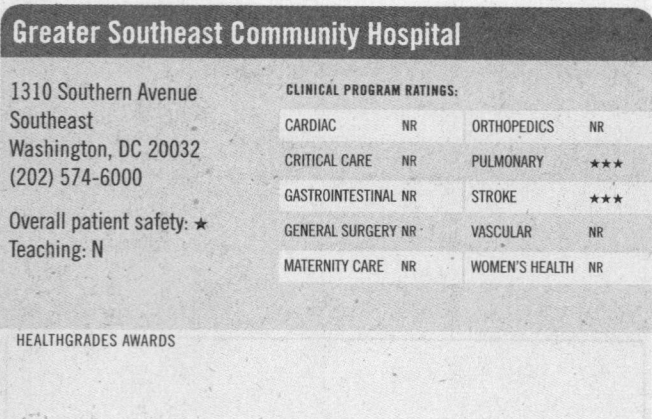

CLINICAL PROGRAM RATINGS:

CARDIAC	NR	ORTHOPEDICS	NR
CRITICAL CARE	NR	PULMONARY	★★★
GASTROINTESTINAL	NR	STROKE	★★★
GENERAL SURGERY	NR	VASCULAR	NR
MATERNITY CARE	NR	WOMEN'S HEALTH	NR

HEALTHGRADES AWARDS

Sibley Memorial Hospital

5255 Loughboro Road
Northwest
Washington, DC 20016
(202) 537-4000

Overall patient safety: ★★★
Teaching: Y

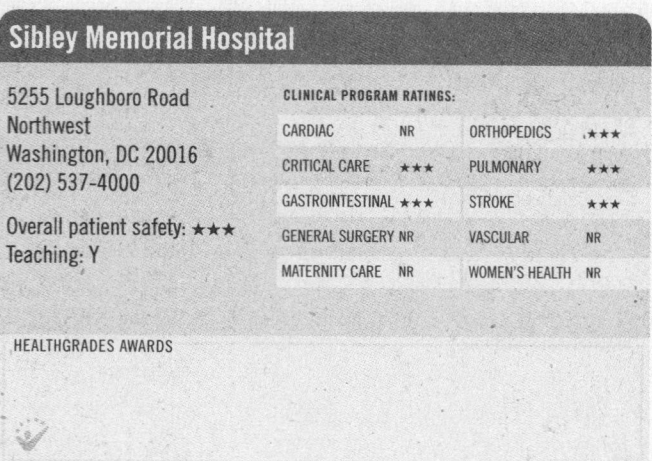

CLINICAL PROGRAM RATINGS:

CARDIAC	NR	ORTHOPEDICS	★★★
CRITICAL CARE	★★★	PULMONARY	★★★
GASTROINTESTINAL	★★★	STROKE	★★★
GENERAL SURGERY	NR	VASCULAR	NR
MATERNITY CARE	NR	WOMEN'S HEALTH	NR

HEALTHGRADES AWARDS

KEY: ★★★★★ BEST   ★★★ AS EXPECTED   ★ POOR   NR NOT RATED BY HEALTHGRADES   For full definitions of ratings and awards, see Appendix.

Washington Hospital Center

110 Irving Street Northwest
Washington, DC 20010
(202) 877-7000

Overall patient safety: ★
Teaching: Y

CLINICAL PROGRAM RATINGS:

CARDIAC	★★★	ORTHOPEDICS	★★★
CRITICAL CARE	★★★	PULMONARY	★★★★★
GASTROINTESTINAL	★★★	STROKE	★★★★★
GENERAL SURGERY	NR	VASCULAR	★★★
MATERNITY CARE	NR	WOMEN'S HEALTH	NR

HEALTHGRADES AWARDS

✓ **SPECIALTY EXCELLENCE**
- PULMONARY CARE   - STROKE CARE

WEST VIRGINIA HOSPITALS: RATINGS BY CLINICAL SPECIALTY

Beckley ARH Hospital

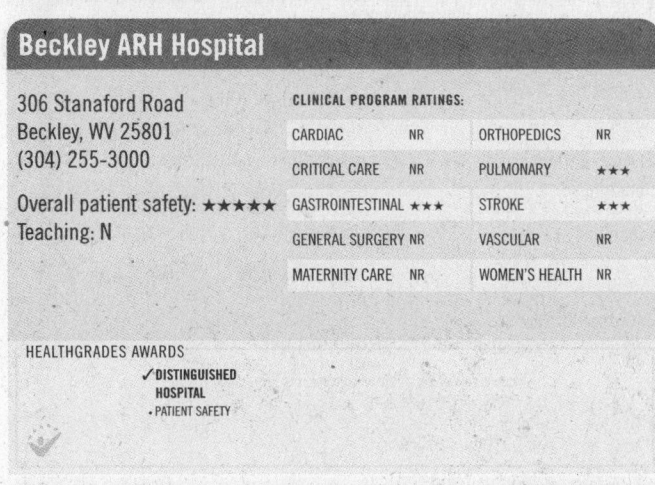

306 Stanaford Road
Beckley, WV 25801
(304) 255-3000

Overall patient safety: ★★★★★
Teaching: N

CLINICAL PROGRAM RATINGS:

CARDIAC	NR	ORTHOPEDICS	NR
CRITICAL CARE	NR	PULMONARY	★★★
GASTROINTESTINAL	★★★	STROKE	★★★
GENERAL SURGERY	NR	VASCULAR	NR
MATERNITY CARE	NR	WOMEN'S HEALTH	NR

HEALTHGRADES AWARDS

✓ **DISTINGUISHED HOSPITAL**
- PATIENT SAFETY

Boone Memorial Hospital

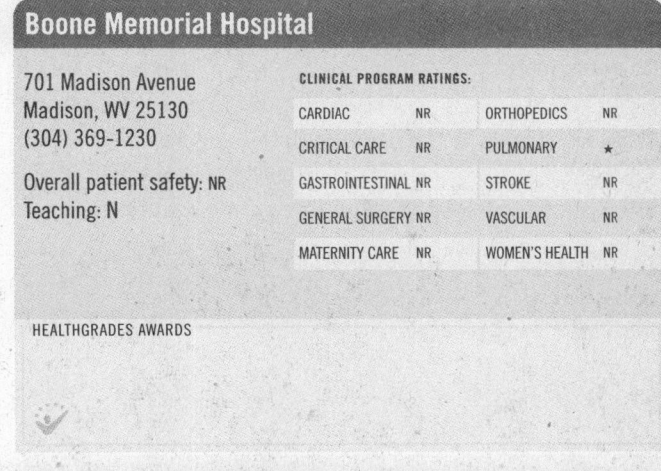

701 Madison Avenue
Madison, WV 25130
(304) 369-1230

Overall patient safety: NR
Teaching: N

CLINICAL PROGRAM RATINGS:

CARDIAC	NR	ORTHOPEDICS	NR
CRITICAL CARE	NR	PULMONARY	★
GASTROINTESTINAL	NR	STROKE	NR
GENERAL SURGERY	NR	VASCULAR	NR
MATERNITY CARE	NR	WOMEN'S HEALTH	NR

HEALTHGRADES AWARDS

Bluefield Regional Medical Center

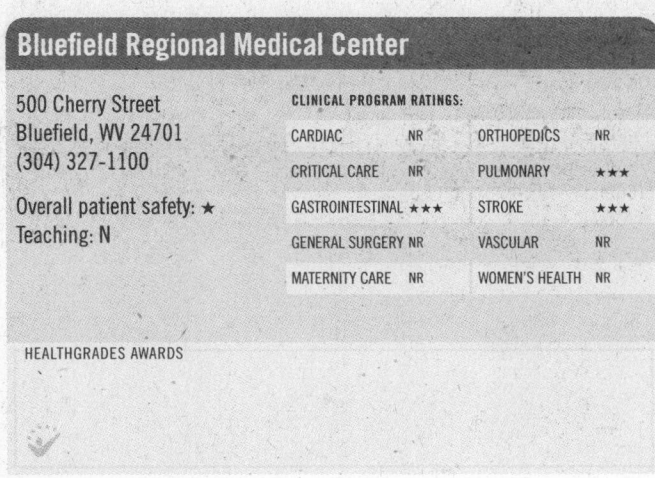

500 Cherry Street
Bluefield, WV 24701
(304) 327-1100

Overall patient safety: ★
Teaching: N

CLINICAL PROGRAM RATINGS:

CARDIAC	NR	ORTHOPEDICS	NR
CRITICAL CARE	NR	PULMONARY	★★★
GASTROINTESTINAL	★★★	STROKE	★★★
GENERAL SURGERY	NR	VASCULAR	NR
MATERNITY CARE	NR	WOMEN'S HEALTH	NR

HEALTHGRADES AWARDS

Braxton County Memorial Hospital

100 Hoylman Drive
Gassaway, WV 26624
(304) 364-5156

Overall patient safety: ★★★
Teaching: N

CLINICAL PROGRAM RATINGS:

CARDIAC	NR	ORTHOPEDICS	NR
CRITICAL CARE	NR	PULMONARY	★
GASTROINTESTINAL	NR	STROKE	★
GENERAL SURGERY	NR	VASCULAR	NR
MATERNITY CARE	NR	WOMEN'S HEALTH	NR

HEALTHGRADES AWARDS

Cabell-Huntington Hospital

1340 Hal Greer Boulevard
Huntington, WV 25701
(304) 526-2000

Overall patient safety: ★
Teaching: Y

CLINICAL PROGRAM RATINGS:

CARDIAC	NR	ORTHOPEDICS	★★★
CRITICAL CARE	NR	PULMONARY	★★★
GASTROINTESTINAL	NR	STROKE	★
GENERAL SURGERY	NR	VASCULAR	NR
MATERNITY CARE	NR	WOMEN'S HEALTH	NR

HEALTHGRADES AWARDS

✓ SPECIALTY EXCELLENCE
· JOINT REPLACEMENT

Camden Clark Memorial Hospital

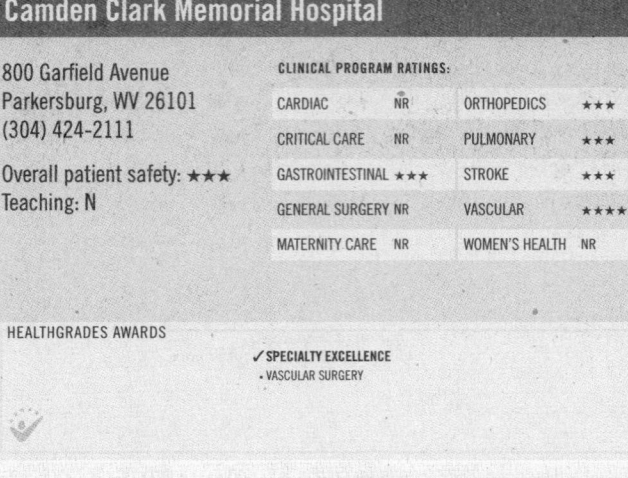

800 Garfield Avenue
Parkersburg, WV 26101
(304) 424-2111

Overall patient safety: ★★★
Teaching: N

CLINICAL PROGRAM RATINGS:

CARDIAC	NR	ORTHOPEDICS	★★★
CRITICAL CARE	NR	PULMONARY	★★★
GASTROINTESTINAL	★★★	STROKE	★★★
GENERAL SURGERY	NR	VASCULAR	★★★★★
MATERNITY CARE	NR	WOMEN'S HEALTH	NR

HEALTHGRADES AWARDS

✓ SPECIALTY EXCELLENCE
· VASCULAR SURGERY

Calhoun General Hospital County*

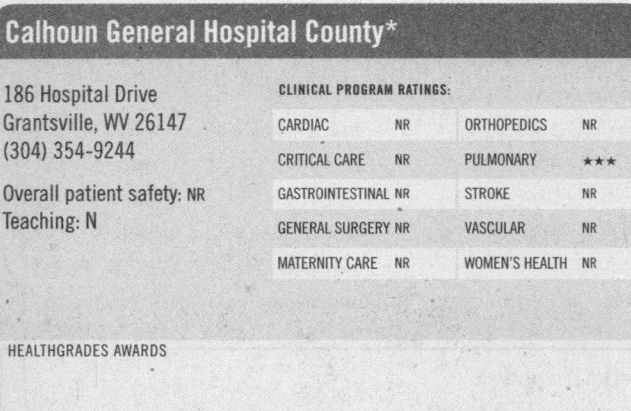

186 Hospital Drive
Grantsville, WV 26147
(304) 354-9244

Overall patient safety: NR
Teaching: N

CLINICAL PROGRAM RATINGS:

CARDIAC	NR	ORTHOPEDICS	NR
CRITICAL CARE	NR	PULMONARY	★★★
GASTROINTESTINAL	NR	STROKE	NR
GENERAL SURGERY	NR	VASCULAR	NR
MATERNITY CARE	NR	WOMEN'S HEALTH	NR

HEALTHGRADES AWARDS

Charleston Area Medical Center

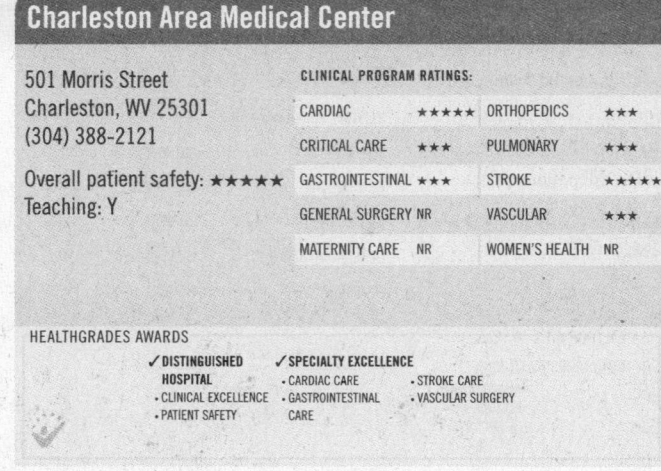

501 Morris Street
Charleston, WV 25301
(304) 388-2121

Overall patient safety: ★★★★★
Teaching: Y

CLINICAL PROGRAM RATINGS:

CARDIAC	★★★★★	ORTHOPEDICS	★★★
CRITICAL CARE	★★★	PULMONARY	★★★
GASTROINTESTINAL	★★★	STROKE	★★★★★
GENERAL SURGERY	NR	VASCULAR	★★★
MATERNITY CARE	NR	WOMEN'S HEALTH	NR

HEALTHGRADES AWARDS

✓ DISTINGUISHED HOSPITAL
· CLINICAL EXCELLENCE
· PATIENT SAFETY

✓ SPECIALTY EXCELLENCE
· CARDIAC CARE
· GASTROINTESTINAL CARE
· STROKE CARE
· VASCULAR SURGERY

CAMC Teays Valley Hospital

1400 Hospital Drive
Hurricane, WV 25526
(304) 757-1700

Overall patient safety: ★★★
Teaching: N

CLINICAL PROGRAM RATINGS:

CARDIAC	NR	ORTHOPEDICS	NR
CRITICAL CARE	NR	PULMONARY	★★★
GASTROINTESTINAL	NR	STROKE	★★★
GENERAL SURGERY	NR	VASCULAR	NR
MATERNITY CARE	NR	WOMEN'S HEALTH	NR

HEALTHGRADES AWARDS

City Hospital

Dry Run Road
Martinsburg, WV 25401
(304) 264-1000

Overall patient safety: ★★★
Teaching: Y

CLINICAL PROGRAM RATINGS:

CARDIAC	NR	ORTHOPEDICS	NR
CRITICAL CARE	NR	PULMONARY	★★★
GASTROINTESTINAL	NR	STROKE	★★★
GENERAL SURGERY	NR	VASCULAR	NR
MATERNITY CARE	NR	WOMEN'S HEALTH	NR

HEALTHGRADES AWARDS

KEY: ★★★★★ BEST   ★★★ AS EXPECTED   ★ POOR   NR NOT RATED BY HEALTHGRADES   For full definitions of ratings and awards, see Appendix.

Davis Memorial Hospital

Reed Street and
Gorman Avenue
Elkins, WV 26241
(304) 636-3300

Overall patient safety: ★★★★★
Teaching: N

CLINICAL PROGRAM RATINGS:

CARDIAC	NR	ORTHOPEDICS	NR
CRITICAL CARE	NR	PULMONARY	★★★
GASTROINTESTINAL	NR.	STROKE	★
GENERAL SURGERY	NR	VASCULAR	NR
MATERNITY CARE	NR	WOMEN'S HEALTH	NR

HEALTHGRADES AWARDS

✓ DISTINGUISHED   ✓ SPECIALTY EXCELLENCE
  HOSPITAL   • JOINT REPLACEMENT
• PATIENT SAFETY

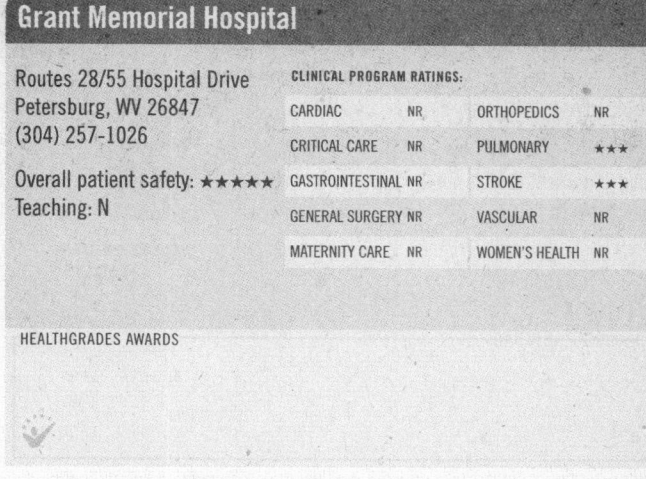

Grant Memorial Hospital

Routes 28/55 Hospital Drive
Petersburg, WV 26847
(304) 257-1026

Overall patient safety: ★★★★★
Teaching: N

CLINICAL PROGRAM RATINGS:

CARDIAC	NR	ORTHOPEDICS	NR
CRITICAL CARE	NR	PULMONARY	★★★
GASTROINTESTINAL	NR	STROKE	★★★
GENERAL SURGERY	NR	VASCULAR	NR
MATERNITY CARE	NR	WOMEN'S HEALTH	NR

HEALTHGRADES AWARDS

Fairmont General Hospital

1325 Locust Avenue
Fairmont, WV 26554
(304) 367-7100

Overall patient safety: ★★★
Teaching: N

CLINICAL PROGRAM RATINGS:

CARDIAC	NR	ORTHOPEDICS	NR
CRITICAL CARE	NR	PULMONARY	★★★
GASTROINTESTINAL	★★★	STROKE	★★★
GENERAL SURGERY	NR	VASCULAR	NR
MATERNITY CARE	NR	WOMEN'S HEALTH	NR

HEALTHGRADES AWARDS

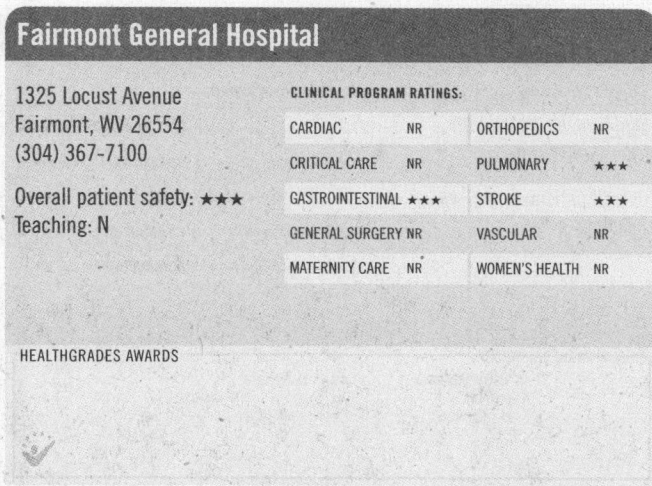

Greenbrier Valley Medical Center

202 Maplewood Avenue
Ronceverte, WV 24970
(304) 647-4411

Overall patient safety: ★★★★★
Teaching: Y

CLINICAL PROGRAM RATINGS:

CARDIAC	NR	ORTHOPEDICS	NR
CRITICAL CARE	NR	PULMONARY	★★★
GASTROINTESTINAL	★★★	STROKE	★★★
GENERAL SURGERY	NR	VASCULAR	NR
MATERNITY CARE	NR	WOMEN'S HEALTH	NR

HEALTHGRADES AWARDS

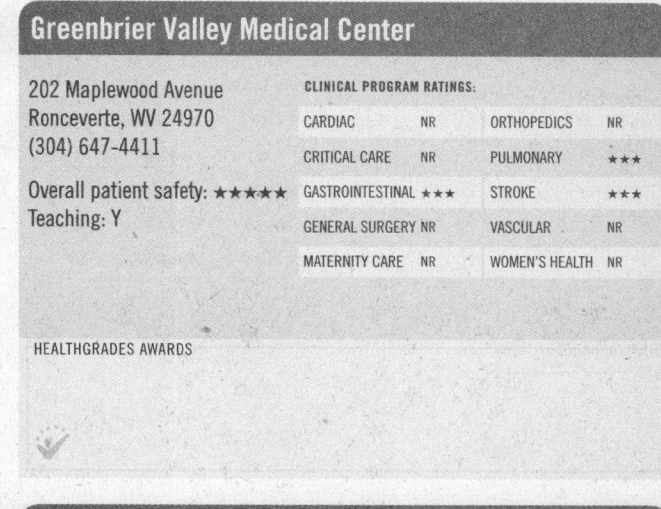

Grafton City Hospital

500 Market Street
Grafton, WV 26354
(304) 265-0400

Overall patient safety: ★★★
Teaching: N

CLINICAL PROGRAM RATINGS:

CARDIAC	NR	ORTHOPEDICS	NR
CRITICAL CARE	NR	PULMONARY	★
GASTROINTESTINAL	NR	STROKE	NR
GENERAL SURGERY	NR	VASCULAR	NR
MATERNITY CARE	NR	WOMEN'S HEALTH	NR

HEALTHGRADES AWARDS

Hampshire Memorial Hospital

549 Center Avenue
Romney, WV 26757
(304) 822-4561

Overall patient safety: ★★★
Teaching: N

CLINICAL PROGRAM RATINGS:

CARDIAC	NR	ORTHOPEDICS	NR
CRITICAL CARE	NR	PULMONARY	★★★
GASTROINTESTINAL	NR	STROKE	NR
GENERAL SURGERY	NR	VASCULAR	NR
MATERNITY CARE	NR	WOMEN'S HEALTH	NR

HEALTHGRADES AWARDS

*This hospital reports its data to the federal government jointly with another hospital. Therefore the ratings and awards apply to multiple hospitals and this specific hospital may not provide all rated services..

Jackson General Hospital

122 Pinnell Street
Ripley, WV 25271
(304) 372-2731

Overall patient safety: ★★★
Teaching: N

CLINICAL PROGRAM RATINGS:

CARDIAC	NR	ORTHOPEDICS	NR
CRITICAL CARE	NR	PULMONARY	★★★
GASTROINTESTINAL	NR	STROKE	★★★
GENERAL SURGERY	NR	VASCULAR	NR
MATERNITY CARE	NR	WOMEN'S HEALTH	NR

HEALTHGRADES AWARDS

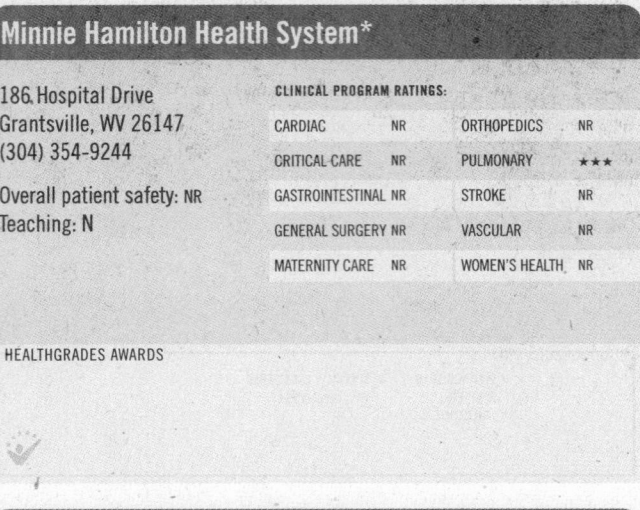

Minnie Hamilton Health System*

186 Hospital Drive
Grantsville, WV 26147
(304) 354-9244

Overall patient safety: NR
Teaching: N

CLINICAL PROGRAM RATINGS:

CARDIAC	NR	ORTHOPEDICS	NR
CRITICAL CARE	NR	PULMONARY	★★★
GASTROINTESTINAL	NR	STROKE	NR
GENERAL SURGERY	NR	VASCULAR	NR
MATERNITY CARE	NR	WOMEN'S HEALTH	NR

HEALTHGRADES AWARDS

Jefferson Memorial Hospital

300 South Preston Street
Ranson, WV 25438
(304) 728-1600

Overall patient safety: ★★★
Teaching: Y

CLINICAL PROGRAM RATINGS:

CARDIAC	NR	ORTHOPEDICS	NR
CRITICAL CARE	NR	PULMONARY	★
GASTROINTESTINAL	NR	STROKE	★★★
GENERAL SURGERY	NR	VASCULAR	NR
MATERNITY CARE	NR	WOMEN'S HEALTH	NR

HEALTHGRADES AWARDS

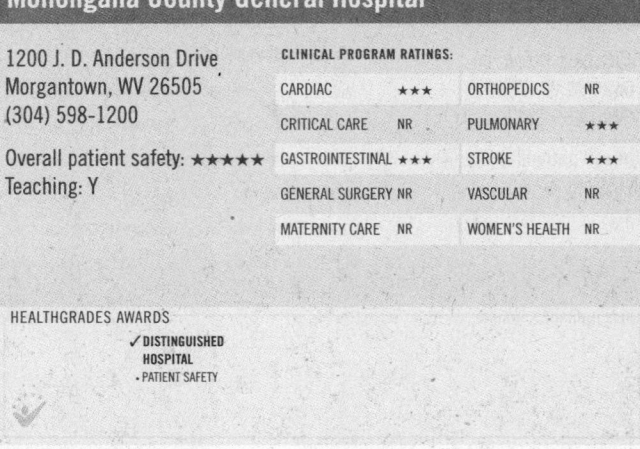

Monongalia County General Hospital

1200 J. D. Anderson Drive
Morgantown, WV 26505
(304) 598-1200

Overall patient safety: ★★★★★
Teaching: Y

CLINICAL PROGRAM RATINGS:

CARDIAC	★★★	ORTHOPEDICS	NR
CRITICAL CARE	NR	PULMONARY	★★★
GASTROINTESTINAL	★★★	STROKE	★★★
GENERAL SURGERY	NR	VASCULAR	NR
MATERNITY CARE	NR	WOMEN'S HEALTH	NR

HEALTHGRADES AWARDS

✓ DISTINGUISHED
  HOSPITAL
- PATIENT SAFETY

Logan Regional Medical Center

20 Hospital Drive
Logan, WV 25601
(304) 831-1350

Overall patient safety: ★★★
Teaching: N

CLINICAL PROGRAM RATINGS:

CARDIAC	NR	ORTHOPEDICS	NR
CRITICAL CARE	NR	PULMONARY	★★★
GASTROINTESTINAL	NR	STROKE	★★★
GENERAL SURGERY	NR	VASCULAR	NR
MATERNITY CARE	NR	WOMEN'S HEALTH	NR

HEALTHGRADES AWARDS

Montgomery General Hospital

401 6th Avenue
Montgomery, WV 25136
(304) 442-5151

Overall patient safety: ★★★
Teaching: N

CLINICAL PROGRAM RATINGS:

CARDIAC	NR	ORTHOPEDICS	NR
CRITICAL CARE	NR	PULMONARY	★★★
GASTROINTESTINAL	NR	STROKE	NR
GENERAL SURGERY	NR	VASCULAR	NR
MATERNITY CARE	NR	WOMEN'S HEALTH	NR

HEALTHGRADES AWARDS

KEY: ★★★★★ BEST   ★★★ AS EXPECTED   ★ POOR   NR NOT RATED BY HEALTHGRADES   For full definitions of ratings and awards, see Appendix.

Ohio Valley Medical Center

2000 Eoff Street
Wheeling, WV 26003
(304) 234-0123

Overall patient safety: ★
Teaching: Y

CLINICAL PROGRAM RATINGS:

CARDIAC	NR	ORTHOPEDICS	NR
CRITICAL CARE	NR	PULMONARY	★
GASTROINTESTINAL	NR	STROKE	★★★
GENERAL SURGERY	NR	VASCULAR	NR
MATERNITY CARE	NR	WOMEN'S HEALTH	NR

HEALTHGRADES AWARDS

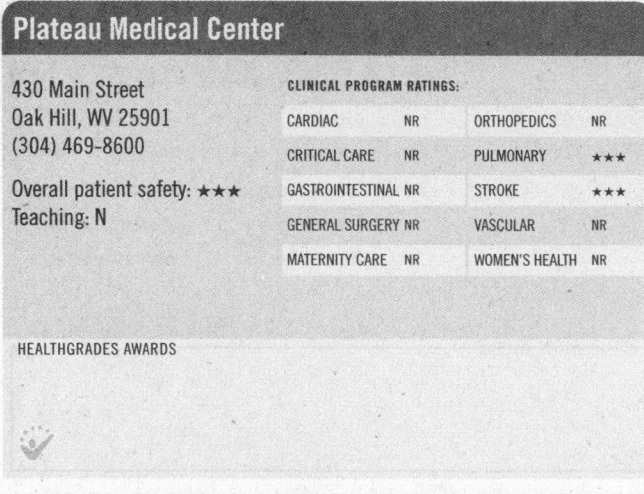

Pocahontas Memorial Hospital

Duncan Road
Buckeye, WV 24924
(304) 799-7400

Overall patient safety: ★★★
Teaching: N

CLINICAL PROGRAM RATINGS:

CARDIAC	NR	ORTHOPEDICS	NR
CRITICAL CARE	NR	PULMONARY	★
GASTROINTESTINAL	NR	STROKE	NR
GENERAL SURGERY	NR	VASCULAR	NR
MATERNITY CARE	NR	WOMEN'S HEALTH	NR

HEALTHGRADES AWARDS

Plateau Medical Center

430 Main Street
Oak Hill, WV 25901
(304) 469-8600

Overall patient safety: ★★★
Teaching: N

CLINICAL PROGRAM RATINGS:

CARDIAC	NR	ORTHOPEDICS	NR
CRITICAL CARE	NR	PULMONARY	★★★
GASTROINTESTINAL	NR	STROKE	★★★
GENERAL SURGERY	NR	VASCULAR	NR
MATERNITY CARE	NR	WOMEN'S HEALTH	NR

HEALTHGRADES AWARDS

Potomac Valley Hospital

167 South Mineral Street
Keyser, WV 26726
(304) 597-1100

Overall patient safety: ★★★
Teaching: N

CLINICAL PROGRAM RATINGS:

CARDIAC	NR	ORTHOPEDICS	NR
CRITICAL CARE	NR	PULMONARY	★★★
GASTROINTESTINAL	NR	STROKE	★
GENERAL SURGERY	NR	VASCULAR	NR
MATERNITY CARE	NR	WOMEN'S HEALTH	NR

HEALTHGRADES AWARDS

Pleasant Valley Hospital

2520 Valley Drive
Point Pleasant, WV 25550
(304) 675-4340

Overall patient safety: ★★★
Teaching: N

CLINICAL PROGRAM RATINGS:

CARDIAC	NR	ORTHOPEDICS	NR
CRITICAL CARE	NR	PULMONARY	★
GASTROINTESTINAL	NR	STROKE	★
GENERAL SURGERY	NR	VASCULAR	NR
MATERNITY CARE	NR	WOMEN'S HEALTH	NR

HEALTHGRADES AWARDS

Preston Memorial Hospital

300 South Price Street
Kingwood, WV 26537
(304) 329-1400

Overall patient safety: ★★★
Teaching: N

CLINICAL PROGRAM RATINGS:

CARDIAC	NR	ORTHOPEDICS	NR
CRITICAL CARE	NR	PULMONARY	★
GASTROINTESTINAL	NR	STROKE	NR
GENERAL SURGERY	NR	VASCULAR	NR
MATERNITY CARE	NR	WOMEN'S HEALTH	NR

HEALTHGRADES AWARDS

*This hospital reports its data to the federal government jointly with another hospital. Therefore the ratings and awards apply to multiple hospitals and this specific hospital may not provide all rated services.

Princeton Community Hospital

122 12th Street
Princeton, WV 24740
(304) 487-7000

Overall patient safety: ★★★
Teaching: N

CLINICAL PROGRAM RATINGS:

CARDIAC	NR	ORTHOPEDICS	★★★
CRITICAL CARE	NR	PULMONARY	★★★
GASTROINTESTINAL	★★★	STROKE	★★★
GENERAL SURGERY	NR	VASCULAR	NR
MATERNITY CARE	NR	WOMEN'S HEALTH	NR

HEALTHGRADES AWARDS

Richwood Area Community Hospital

75 Avenue B
Richwood, WV 26261
(304) 846-2573

Overall patient safety: NR
Teaching: N

CLINICAL PROGRAM RATINGS:

CARDIAC	NR	ORTHOPEDICS	NR
CRITICAL CARE	NR	PULMONARY	★★★
GASTROINTESTINAL	NR	STROKE	NR
GENERAL SURGERY	NR	VASCULAR	NR
MATERNITY CARE	NR	WOMEN'S HEALTH	NR

HEALTHGRADES AWARDS

Raleigh General Hospital

1710 Harper Road
Beckley, WV 25801
(304) 256-4100

Overall patient safety: ★★★
Teaching: N

CLINICAL PROGRAM RATINGS:

CARDIAC	NR	ORTHOPEDICS	NR
CRITICAL CARE	NR	PULMONARY	★★★
GASTROINTESTINAL	★★★	STROKE	★★★
GENERAL SURGERY	NR	VASCULAR	NR
MATERNITY CARE	NR	WOMEN'S HEALTH	NR

HEALTHGRADES AWARDS

Roane General Hospital

200 Hospital Drive
Spencer, WV 25276
(304) 927-4444

Overall patient safety: ★★★
Teaching: N

CLINICAL PROGRAM RATINGS:

CARDIAC	NR	ORTHOPEDICS	NR
CRITICAL CARE	NR	PULMONARY	★
GASTROINTESTINAL	NR	STROKE	NR
GENERAL SURGERY	NR	VASCULAR	NR
MATERNITY CARE	NR	WOMEN'S HEALTH	NR

HEALTHGRADES AWARDS

Reynolds Memorial Hospital

800 Wheeling Avenue
Glen Dale, WV 26038
(304) 845-3211

Overall patient safety: ★★★
Teaching: N

CLINICAL PROGRAM RATINGS:

CARDIAC	NR	ORTHOPEDICS	NR
CRITICAL CARE	NR	PULMONARY	★
GASTROINTESTINAL	NR	STROKE	★★★
GENERAL SURGERY	NR	VASCULAR	NR
MATERNITY CARE	NR	WOMEN'S HEALTH	NR

HEALTHGRADES AWARDS

St. Francis Hospital

333 Laidley Street
Charleston, WV 25301
(304) 347-6500

Overall patient safety: ★★★
Teaching: N

CLINICAL PROGRAM RATINGS:

CARDIAC	NR	ORTHOPEDICS	NR
CRITICAL CARE	NR	PULMONARY	★★★★★
GASTROINTESTINAL	★★★	STROKE	★★★
GENERAL SURGERY	NR	VASCULAR	NR
MATERNITY CARE	NR	WOMEN'S HEALTH	NR

HEALTHGRADES AWARDS

✓ SPECIALTY EXCELLENCE
 - PULMONARY CARE

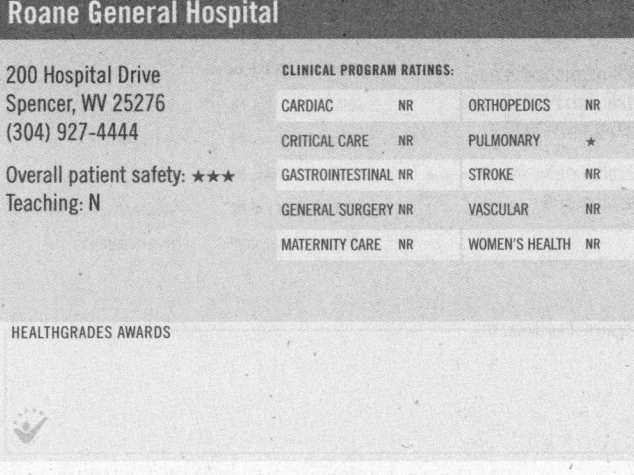

KEY: ★★★★★ BEST ★★★ AS EXPECTED ★ POOR NR NOT RATED BY HEALTHGRADES For full definitions of ratings and awards, see Appendix.

708 CHAPTER 6: HOSPITAL RATINGS BY CLINICAL SPECIALTY

St. Joseph Hospital

1 Amalia Drive
Buckhannon, WV 26201
(304) 473-2000

Overall patient safety: ★★★
Teaching: N

CLINICAL PROGRAM RATINGS:

CARDIAC	NR	ORTHOPEDICS	NR
CRITICAL CARE	NR	PULMONARY	★
GASTROINTESTINAL	NR	STROKE	★
GENERAL SURGERY	NR	VASCULAR	NR
MATERNITY CARE	NR	WOMEN'S HEALTH	NR

HEALTHGRADES AWARDS

Stonewall Jackson Memorial Hospital

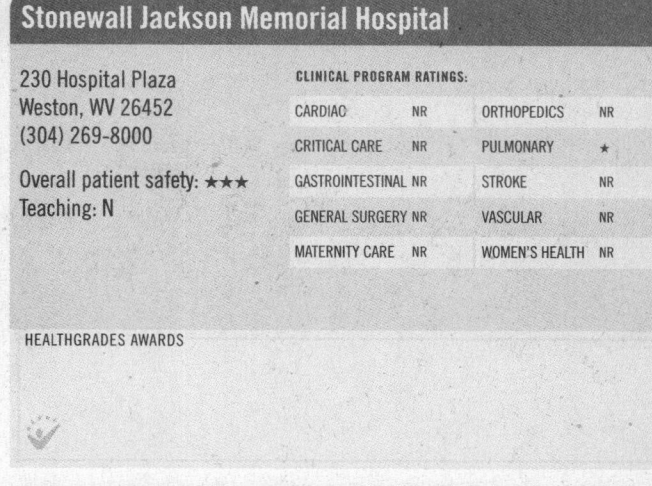

230 Hospital Plaza
Weston, WV 26452
(304) 269-8000

Overall patient safety: ★★★
Teaching: N

CLINICAL PROGRAM RATINGS:

CARDIAC	NR	ORTHOPEDICS	NR
CRITICAL CARE	NR	PULMONARY	★
GASTROINTESTINAL	NR	STROKE	NR
GENERAL SURGERY	NR	VASCULAR	NR
MATERNITY CARE	NR	WOMEN'S HEALTH	NR

HEALTHGRADES AWARDS

St. Joseph's Hospital

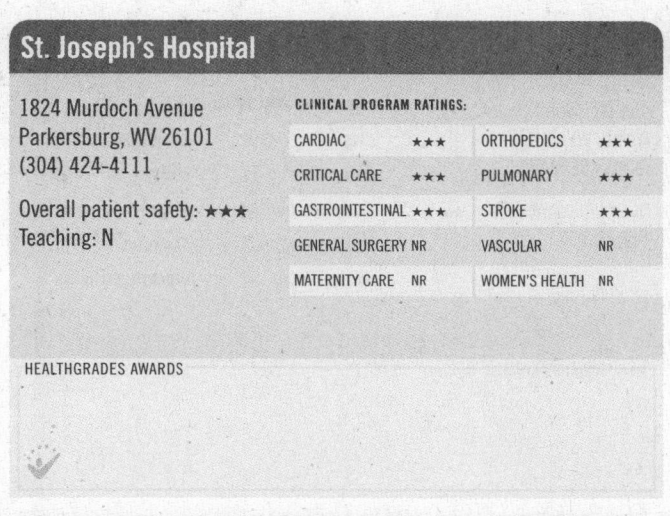

1824 Murdoch Avenue
Parkersburg, WV 26101
(304) 424-4111

Overall patient safety: ★★★
Teaching: N

CLINICAL PROGRAM RATINGS:

CARDIAC	★★★	ORTHOPEDICS	★★★
CRITICAL CARE	★★★	PULMONARY	★★★
GASTROINTESTINAL	★★★	STROKE	★★★
GENERAL SURGERY	NR	VASCULAR	NR
MATERNITY CARE	NR	WOMEN'S HEALTH	NR

HEALTHGRADES AWARDS

Summers County ARH Hospital

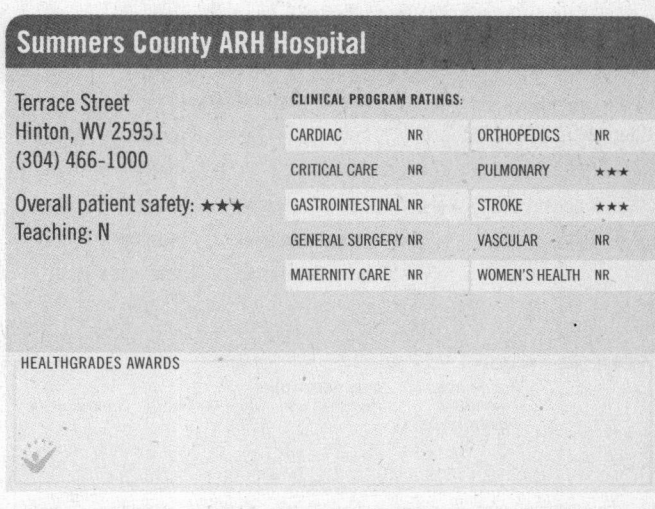

Terrace Street
Hinton, WV 25951
(304) 466-1000

Overall patient safety: ★★★
Teaching: N

CLINICAL PROGRAM RATINGS:

CARDIAC	NR	ORTHOPEDICS	NR
CRITICAL CARE	NR	PULMONARY	★★★
GASTROINTESTINAL	NR	STROKE	★★★
GENERAL SURGERY	NR	VASCULAR	NR
MATERNITY CARE	NR	WOMEN'S HEALTH	NR

HEALTHGRADES AWARDS

St. Mary's Medical Center

2900 1st Avenue
Huntington, WV 25702
(304) 526-1234

Overall patient safety: ★★★
Teaching: Y

CLINICAL PROGRAM RATINGS:

CARDIAC	★★★	ORTHOPEDICS	★★★
CRITICAL CARE	NR	PULMONARY	★★★
GASTROINTESTINAL	★★★	STROKE	★★★
GENERAL SURGERY	NR	VASCULAR	NR
MATERNITY CARE	NR	WOMEN'S HEALTH	NR

HEALTHGRADES AWARDS

Summersville Memorial Hospital

400 Fairview Heights Road
Summersville, WV 26651
(304) 872-2891

Overall patient safety: ★★★
Teaching: N

CLINICAL PROGRAM RATINGS:

CARDIAC	NR	ORTHOPEDICS	NR
CRITICAL CARE	NR	PULMONARY	★★★
GASTROINTESTINAL	NR	STROKE	★★★
GENERAL SURGERY	NR	VASCULAR	NR
MATERNITY CARE	NR	WOMEN'S HEALTH	NR

HEALTHGRADES AWARDS

Thomas Memorial Hospital

4605 MacCorkle Avenue
Southwest
South Charleston, WV 25309
(304) 766-3600

Overall patient safety: ★★★
Teaching: N

CLINICAL PROGRAM RATINGS:

CARDIAC	NR	ORTHOPEDICS	NR
CRITICAL CARE	NR	PULMONARY	★★★
GASTROINTESTINAL	★★★	STROKE	★★★
GENERAL SURGERY	NR	VASCULAR	NR
MATERNITY CARE	NR	WOMEN'S HEALTH	NR

HEALTHGRADES AWARDS

Weirton Medical Center

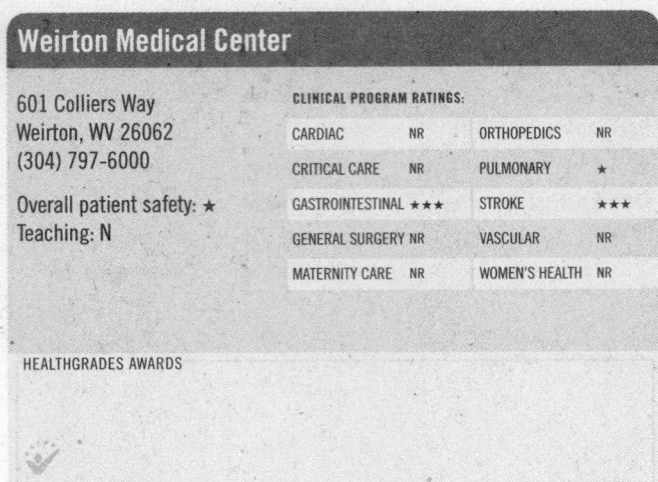

601 Colliers Way
Weirton, WV 26062
(304) 797-6000

Overall patient safety: ★
Teaching: N

CLINICAL PROGRAM RATINGS:

CARDIAC	NR	ORTHOPEDICS	NR
CRITICAL CARE	NR	PULMONARY	★
GASTROINTESTINAL	★★★	STROKE	★★★
GENERAL SURGERY	NR	VASCULAR	NR
MATERNITY CARE	NR	WOMEN'S HEALTH	NR

HEALTHGRADES AWARDS

United Hospital Center

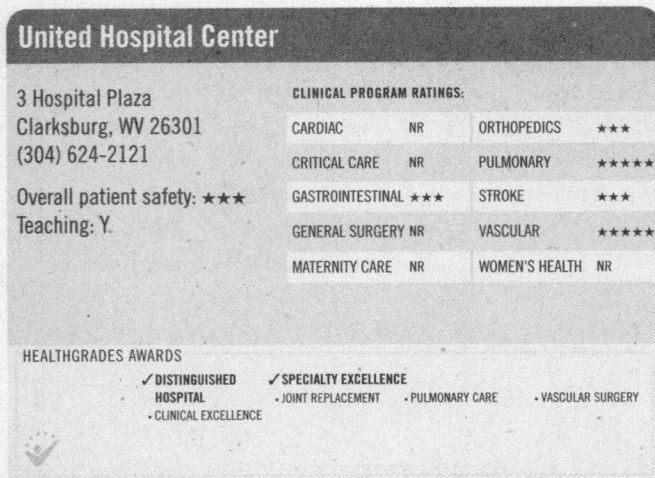

3 Hospital Plaza
Clarksburg, WV 26301
(304) 624-2121

Overall patient safety: ★★★
Teaching: Y

CLINICAL PROGRAM RATINGS:

CARDIAC	NR	ORTHOPEDICS	★★★
CRITICAL CARE	NR	PULMONARY	★★★★★
GASTROINTESTINAL	★★★	STROKE	★★★
GENERAL SURGERY	NR	VASCULAR	★★★★★
MATERNITY CARE	NR	WOMEN'S HEALTH	NR

HEALTHGRADES AWARDS

✓ **DISTINGUISHED HOSPITAL**
• CLINICAL EXCELLENCE

✓ **SPECIALTY EXCELLENCE**
• JOINT REPLACEMENT • PULMONARY CARE • VASCULAR SURGERY

Welch Community Hospital

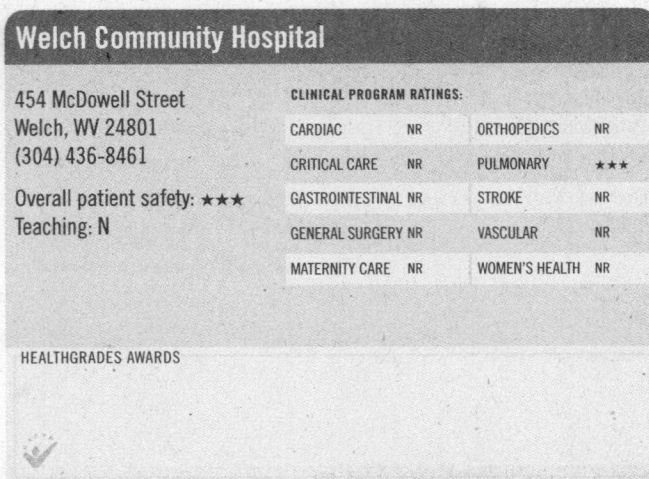

454 McDowell Street
Welch, WV 24801
(304) 436-8461

Overall patient safety: ★★★
Teaching: N

CLINICAL PROGRAM RATINGS:

CARDIAC	NR	ORTHOPEDICS	NR
CRITICAL CARE	NR	PULMONARY	★★★
GASTROINTESTINAL	NR	STROKE	NR
GENERAL SURGERY	NR	VASCULAR	NR
MATERNITY CARE	NR	WOMEN'S HEALTH	NR

HEALTHGRADES AWARDS

War Memorial Hospital

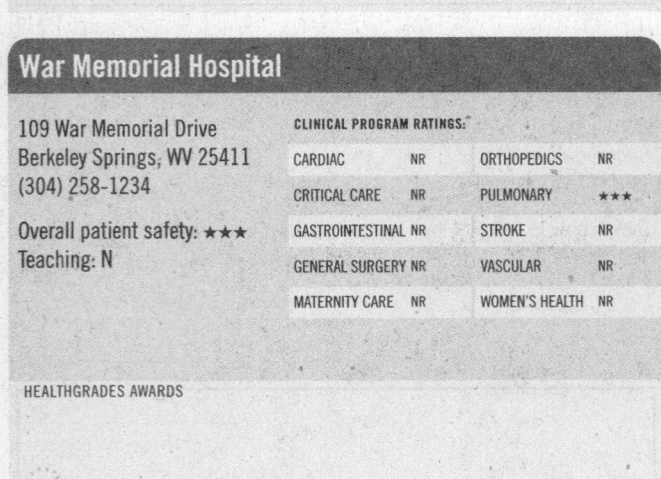

109 War Memorial Drive
Berkeley Springs, WV 25411
(304) 258-1234

Overall patient safety: ★★★
Teaching: N

CLINICAL PROGRAM RATINGS:

CARDIAC	NR	ORTHOPEDICS	NR
CRITICAL CARE	NR	PULMONARY	★★★
GASTROINTESTINAL	NR	STROKE	NR
GENERAL SURGERY	NR	VASCULAR	NR
MATERNITY CARE	NR	WOMEN'S HEALTH	NR

HEALTHGRADES AWARDS

West Virginia University Hospitals

1 Medical Center Drive
Morgantown, WV 26506
(304) 598-4000

Overall patient safety: ★★★
Teaching: Y

CLINICAL PROGRAM RATINGS:

CARDIAC	★★★	ORTHOPEDICS	★
CRITICAL CARE	★★★	PULMONARY	★★★
GASTROINTESTINAL	NR	STROKE	★
GENERAL SURGERY	NR	VASCULAR	NR
MATERNITY CARE	NR	WOMEN'S HEALTH	NR

HEALTHGRADES AWARDS

KEY: ★★★★★ **BEST** ★★★ **AS EXPECTED** ★ **POOR** NR **NOT RATED BY HEALTHGRADES** For full definitions of ratings and awards, see Appendix.

Wetzel County Hospital

3 East Benjamin Drive
New Martinsville, WV 26155
(304) 455-8000

Overall patient safety: ★★★
Teaching: N

CLINICAL PROGRAM RATINGS:

CARDIAC	NR	ORTHOPEDICS	NR
CRITICAL CARE	NR	PULMONARY	★★★
GASTROINTESTINAL	NR	STROKE	★★★
GENERAL SURGERY	NR	VASCULAR	NR
MATERNITY CARE	NR	WOMEN'S HEALTH	NR

HEALTHGRADES AWARDS

Williamson Memorial Hospital

859 Alderson Street
Williamson, WV 25661
(304) 235-2500

Overall patient safety: ★★★
Teaching: N

CLINICAL PROGRAM RATINGS:

CARDIAC	NR	ORTHOPEDICS	NR
CRITICAL CARE	NR	PULMONARY	★
GASTROINTESTINAL	NR	STROKE	★★★
GENERAL SURGERY	NR	VASCULAR	NR
MATERNITY CARE	NR	WOMEN'S HEALTH	NR

HEALTHGRADES AWARDS

Wheeling Hospital

1 Medical Park
Wheeling, WV 26003
(304) 243-3000

Overall patient safety: ★★★★★
Teaching: Y

CLINICAL PROGRAM RATINGS:

CARDIAC	★★★	ORTHOPEDICS	★★★★★
CRITICAL CARE	NR	PULMONARY	★
GASTROINTESTINAL	★★★	STROKE	★
GENERAL SURGERY	NR	VASCULAR	★★★
MATERNITY CARE	NR	WOMEN'S HEALTH	NR

HEALTHGRADES AWARDS

✓ SPECIALTY EXCELLENCE
• ORTHOPEDIC SURGERY

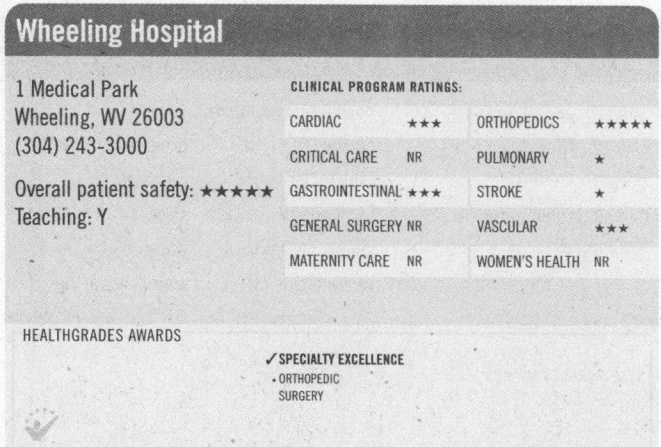

WISCONSIN HOSPITALS: RATINGS BY CLINICAL SPECIALTY

All Saints Medical Center–St. Mary's Campus*

3801 Spring Street
Racine, WI 53405
(262) 687-4011

Overall patient safety: ★★★
Teaching: Y

CLINICAL PROGRAM RATINGS:

CARDIAC	★★★	ORTHOPEDICS	★★★
CRITICAL CARE	★★★	PULMONARY	★★★
GASTROINTESTINAL	★★★	STROKE	★★★★★
GENERAL SURGERY	★★★	VASCULAR	NR
MATERNITY CARE	★★★	WOMEN'S HEALTH	★★★

HEALTHGRADES AWARDS

✓ SPECIALTY EXCELLENCE
• STROKE CARE

All Saints St. Luke's Hospital*

1320 Wisconsin Avenue
Racine, WI 53403
(262) 687-2011

Overall patient safety: ★★★
Teaching: Y

CLINICAL PROGRAM RATINGS:

CARDIAC	★★★	ORTHOPEDICS	★★★
CRITICAL CARE	★★★	PULMONARY	★★★
GASTROINTESTINAL	★★★	STROKE	★★★★★
GENERAL SURGERY	★★★	VASCULAR	NR
MATERNITY CARE	★★★	WOMEN'S HEALTH	★★★

HEALTHGRADES AWARDS

✓ SPECIALTY EXCELLENCE
• STROKE CARE

*This hospital reports its data to the federal government jointly with another hospital. Therefore the ratings and awards apply to multiple hospitals and this specific hospital may not provide all rated services.

Amery Regional Medical Center

225 Scholl Court
Amery, WI 54001
(715) 268-8000

Overall patient safety: ★★★
Teaching: N

CLINICAL PROGRAM RATINGS:

CARDIAC	NR	ORTHOPEDICS	NR
CRITICAL CARE	NR	PULMONARY	★
GASTROINTESTINAL	NR	STROKE	★★★
GENERAL SURGERY	NR	VASCULAR	NR
MATERNITY CARE	★	WOMEN'S HEALTH	NR

HEALTHGRADES AWARDS

Aurora Baycare Medical Center

2845 Greenbrier Road
Green Bay, WI 54311
(920) 288-8000

Overall patient safety: ★★★
Teaching: N

CLINICAL PROGRAM RATINGS:

CARDIAC	★★★	ORTHOPEDICS	★★★
CRITICAL CARE	NR	PULMONARY	★★★
GASTROINTESTINAL	★★★	STROKE	★★★★★
GENERAL SURGERY	★★★	VASCULAR	NR
MATERNITY CARE	★★★	WOMEN'S HEALTH	★★★★★

HEALTHGRADES AWARDS

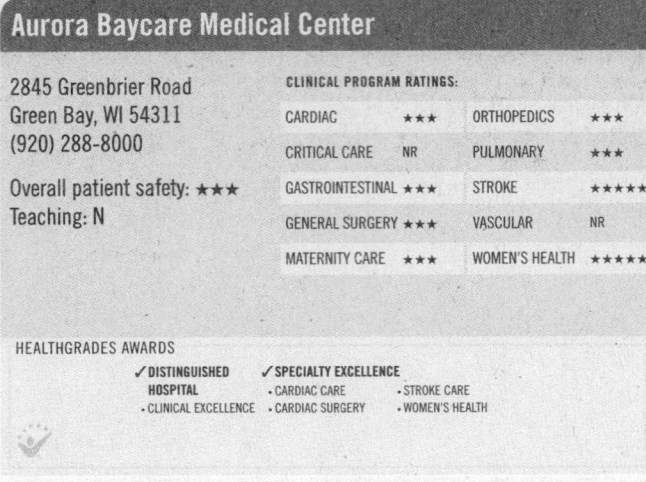

✓ DISTINGUISHED HOSPITAL
• CLINICAL EXCELLENCE

✓ SPECIALTY EXCELLENCE
• CARDIAC CARE
• CARDIAC SURGERY
• STROKE CARE
• WOMEN'S HEALTH

Appleton Medical Center

1818 North Meade Street
Appleton, WI 54911
(920) 731-4101

Overall patient safety: ★★★
Teaching: Y

CLINICAL PROGRAM RATINGS:

CARDIAC	★★★	ORTHOPEDICS	NR
CRITICAL CARE	★★★	PULMONARY	★★★
GASTROINTESTINAL	★★★	STROKE	★★★
GENERAL SURGERY	★★★	VASCULAR	★★★
MATERNITY CARE	★★★	WOMEN'S HEALTH	★★★

HEALTHGRADES AWARDS

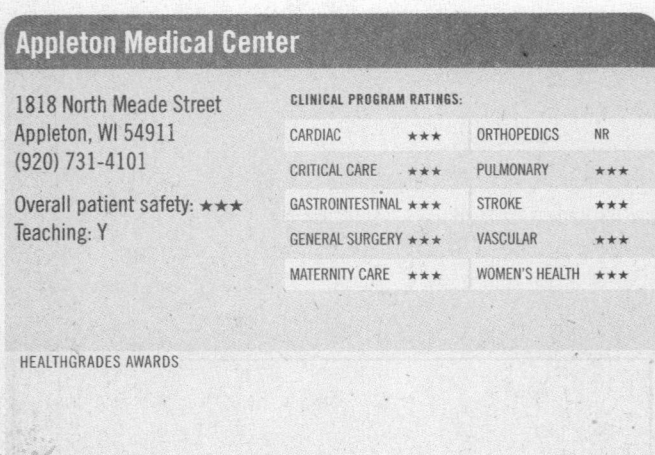

Aurora Lakeland Medical Center

3985 County Road North
Elkhorn, WI 53121
(262) 741-2000

Overall patient safety: ★
Teaching: N

CLINICAL PROGRAM RATINGS:

CARDIAC	NR	ORTHOPEDICS	NR
CRITICAL CARE	NR	PULMONARY	★
GASTROINTESTINAL	★★★	STROKE	NR
GENERAL SURGERY	★★★	VASCULAR	NR
MATERNITY CARE	★	WOMEN'S HEALTH	NR

HEALTHGRADES AWARDS

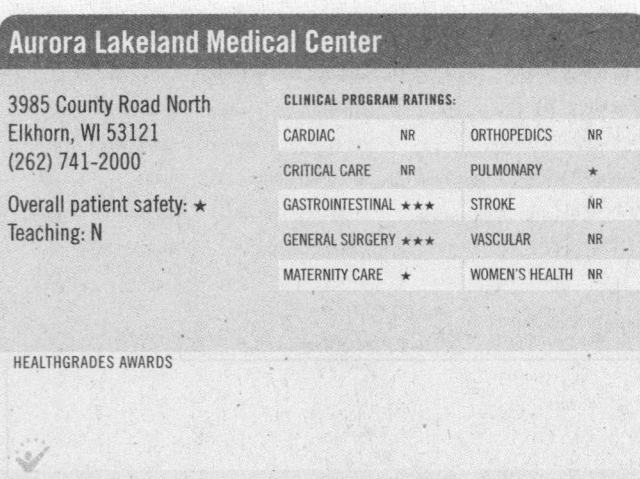

Aspirus Wausau Hospital

333 Pine Ridge Boulevard
Wausau, WI 54401
(715) 847-2121

Overall patient safety: ★★★★★
Teaching: Y

CLINICAL PROGRAM RATINGS:

CARDIAC	★★★★★	ORTHOPEDICS	★★★
CRITICAL CARE	★★★	PULMONARY	★★★★★
GASTROINTESTINAL	★★★	STROKE	★★★★★
GENERAL SURGERY	★★★	VASCULAR	★★★
MATERNITY CARE	★★★	WOMEN'S HEALTH	★★★

HEALTHGRADES AWARDS

✓ DISTINGUISHED HOSPITAL
• CLINICAL EXCELLENCE
• PATIENT SAFETY

✓ SPECIALTY EXCELLENCE
• CARDIAC CARE
• CARDIAC SURGERY
• GENERAL SURGERY
• PULMONARY CARE
• STROKE CARE

Aurora Medical Center—Kenosha

10400 75th Street
Kenosha, WI 53142
(262) 948-5600

Overall patient safety: ★
Teaching: N

CLINICAL PROGRAM RATINGS:

CARDIAC	NR	ORTHOPEDICS	NR
CRITICAL CARE	NR	PULMONARY	★★★
GASTROINTESTINAL	NR	STROKE	★
GENERAL SURGERY	★★★	VASCULAR	NR
MATERNITY CARE	★★★	WOMEN'S HEALTH	NR

HEALTHGRADES AWARDS

KEY: ★★★★★ BEST   ★★★ AS EXPECTED   ★ POOR   NR NOT RATED BY HEALTHGRADES   For full definitions of ratings and awards, see Appendix.

Aurora Medical Center—Manitowoc City

5000 Memorial Drive
Two Rivers, WI 54241
(920) 794-5000

Overall patient safety: ★★★
Teaching: N

CLINICAL PROGRAM RATINGS:

CARDIAC	NR	ORTHOPEDICS	NR
CRITICAL CARE	NR	PULMONARY	★★★
GASTROINTESTINAL	NR	STROKE	★★★
GENERAL SURGERY	★★★	VASCULAR	NR
MATERNITY CARE	★★★	WOMEN'S HEALTH	NR

HEALTHGRADES AWARDS

Aurora Sheboygan Memorial Medical Center

2629 North 7th Street
Sheboygan, WI 53083
(920) 451-5000

Overall patient safety: ★★★
Teaching: N

CLINICAL PROGRAM RATINGS:

CARDIAC	NR	ORTHOPEDICS	NR
CRITICAL CARE	★★★	PULMONARY	★
GASTROINTESTINAL	NR	STROKE	★
GENERAL SURGERY	★★★	VASCULAR	NR
MATERNITY CARE	★	WOMEN'S HEALTH	NR

HEALTHGRADES AWARDS

✓ SPECIALTY EXCELLENCE
- JOINT REPLACEMENT

Aurora Medical Center—Oshkosh

855 North Westhaven Drive
Oshkosh, WI 54904
(920) 456-6000

Overall patient safety: ★★★
Teaching: N

CLINICAL PROGRAM RATINGS:

CARDIAC	NR	ORTHOPEDICS	NR
CRITICAL CARE	NR	PULMONARY	★★★
GASTROINTESTINAL	NR	STROKE	★
GENERAL SURGERY	★★★	VASCULAR	NR
MATERNITY CARE	★	WOMEN'S HEALTH	NR

HEALTHGRADES AWARDS

Aurora Sinai Medical Center

945 North 12th Street
Milwaukee, WI 53233
(414) 219-2000

Overall patient safety: ★★★
Teaching: Y

CLINICAL PROGRAM RATINGS:

CARDIAC	★★★	ORTHOPEDICS	NR
CRITICAL CARE	NR	PULMONARY	★★★★★
GASTROINTESTINAL	NR	STROKE	★★★
GENERAL SURGERY	NR	VASCULAR	NR
MATERNITY CARE	★★★	WOMEN'S HEALTH	★★★

HEALTHGRADES AWARDS

✓ SPECIALTY EXCELLENCE
- PULMONARY CARE

Aurora Medical Center—Washington County

1032 East Sumner Street
Hartford, WI 53027
(262) 673-2300

Overall patient safety: ★★★
Teaching: N

CLINICAL PROGRAM RATINGS:

CARDIAC	NR	ORTHOPEDICS	NR
CRITICAL CARE	NR	PULMONARY	★★★
GASTROINTESTINAL	NR	STROKE	★★★
GENERAL SURGERY	★★★	VASCULAR	NR
MATERNITY CARE	★★★	WOMEN'S HEALTH	NR

HEALTHGRADES AWARDS

Aurora St. Luke's Medical Center*

2900 West Oklahoma Avenue
Milwaukee, WI 53215
(414) 649-6000

Overall patient safety: ★★★★★
Teaching: Y

CLINICAL PROGRAM RATINGS:

CARDIAC	★★★	ORTHOPEDICS	★
CRITICAL CARE	★★★★★	PULMONARY	★★★★★
GASTROINTESTINAL	★★★	STROKE	★★★★★
GENERAL SURGERY	★★★	VASCULAR	★
MATERNITY CARE	NR	WOMEN'S HEALTH	NR

HEALTHGRADES AWARDS

✓ DISTINGUISHED HOSPITAL
- CLINICAL EXCELLENCE
- PATIENT SAFETY

✓ SPECIALTY EXCELLENCE
- CRITICAL CARE
- PULMONARY CARE

*This hospital reports its data to the federal government jointly with another hospital. Therefore the ratings and awards apply to multiple hospitals and this specific hospital may not provide all rated services.

Baldwin Area Medical Center

730 10th Avenue
Baldwin, WI 54002
(715) 684-3311

Overall patient safety: ★★★
Teaching: N

CLINICAL PROGRAM RATINGS:

CARDIAC	NR	ORTHOPEDICS	NR
CRITICAL CARE	NR	PULMONARY	★
GASTROINTESTINAL	NR	STROKE	NR
GENERAL SURGERY	NR	VASCULAR	NR
MATERNITY CARE	★	WOMEN'S HEALTH	NR

HEALTHGRADES AWARDS

Beaver Dam Community Hospital

707 South University Avenue
Beaver Dam, WI 53916
(920) 887-7181

Overall patient safety: ★★★
Teaching: N

CLINICAL PROGRAM RATINGS:

CARDIAC	NR	ORTHOPEDICS	NR
CRITICAL CARE	NR	PULMONARY	★★★
GASTROINTESTINAL	NR	STROKE	★★★
GENERAL SURGERY	NR	VASCULAR	NR
MATERNITY CARE	★★★	WOMEN'S HEALTH	NR

HEALTHGRADES AWARDS

Barron Memorial Medical Center Mayo

1222 East Woodland Avenue
Barron, WI 54812
(715) 537-3186

Overall patient safety: ★★★
Teaching: N

CLINICAL PROGRAM RATINGS:

CARDIAC	NR	ORTHOPEDICS	NR
CRITICAL CARE	NR	PULMONARY	★★★
GASTROINTESTINAL	NR	STROKE	★
GENERAL SURGERY	NR	VASCULAR	NR
MATERNITY CARE	★★★	WOMEN'S HEALTH	NR

HEALTHGRADES AWARDS

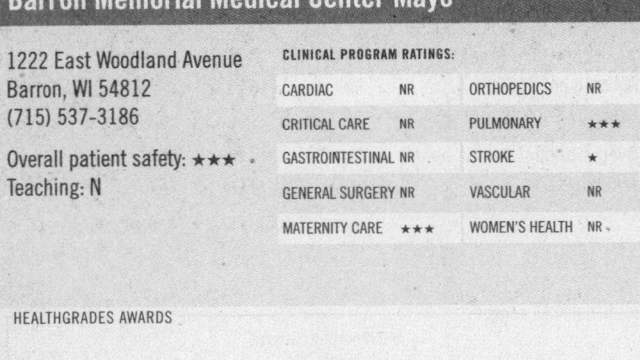

Bellin Memorial Hospital

744 South Webster Avenue
Green Bay, WI 54301
(920) 433-3500

Overall patient safety: ★★★★★
Teaching: N

CLINICAL PROGRAM RATINGS:

CARDIAC	★★★	ORTHOPEDICS	NR
CRITICAL CARE	NR	PULMONARY	★★★
GASTROINTESTINAL	★★★	STROKE	★★★
GENERAL SURGERY	★★★	VASCULAR	NR
MATERNITY CARE	★★★	WOMEN'S HEALTH	★★★

HEALTHGRADES AWARDS

✓ DISTINGUISHED
HOSPITAL
• PATIENT SAFETY

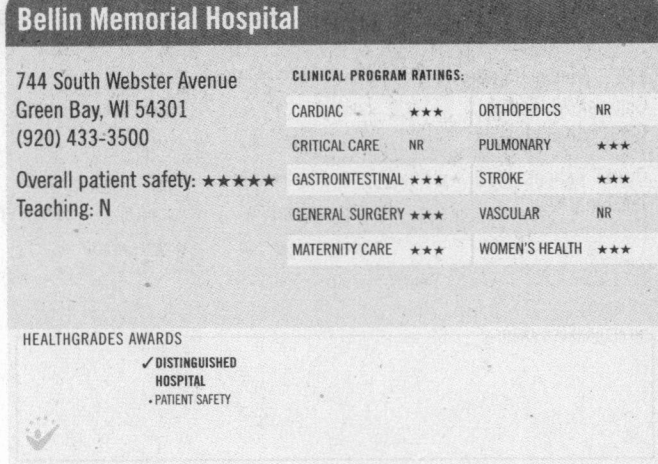

Bay Area Medical Center

3100 Shore Drive
Marinette, WI 54143
(715) 735-6621

Overall patient safety: ★★★★★
Teaching: N

CLINICAL PROGRAM RATINGS:

CARDIAC	NR	ORTHOPEDICS	NR
CRITICAL CARE	NR	PULMONARY	★★★
GASTROINTESTINAL	★★★	STROKE	★★★
GENERAL SURGERY	★★★	VASCULAR	NR
MATERNITY CARE	★★★	WOMEN'S HEALTH	NR

HEALTHGRADES AWARDS

✓ DISTINGUISHED
HOSPITAL
• PATIENT SAFETY

Beloit Memorial Hospital

1969 West Hart Road
Beloit, WI 53511
(608) 364-5011

Overall patient safety: ★★★
Teaching: N

CLINICAL PROGRAM RATINGS:

CARDIAC	NR	ORTHOPEDICS	NR
CRITICAL CARE	NR	PULMONARY	★
GASTROINTESTINAL	★★★	STROKE	★
GENERAL SURGERY	★★★	VASCULAR	NR
MATERNITY CARE	★★★	WOMEN'S HEALTH	NR

HEALTHGRADES AWARDS

KEY: ★★★★★ BEST   ★★★ AS EXPECTED   ★ POOR   NR NOT RATED BY HEALTHGRADES   For full definitions of ratings and awards, see Appendix.

Berlin Memorial Hospital

225 Memorial Drive
Berlin, WI 54923
(920) 361-1313

Overall patient safety: ★★★
Teaching: N

CLINICAL PROGRAM RATINGS:

CARDIAC	NR	ORTHOPEDICS	NR
CRITICAL CARE	NR	PULMONARY	★★★
GASTROINTESTINAL	NR	STROKE	★
GENERAL SURGERY	★★★	VASCULAR	NR
MATERNITY CARE	★	WOMEN'S HEALTH	NR

HEALTHGRADES AWARDS

✓ SPECIALTY EXCELLENCE
• JOINT REPLACEMENT

Burnett Medical Center

257 West St. George Avenue
Grantsburg, WI 54840
(715) 463-5353

Overall patient safety: ★★★
Teaching: N

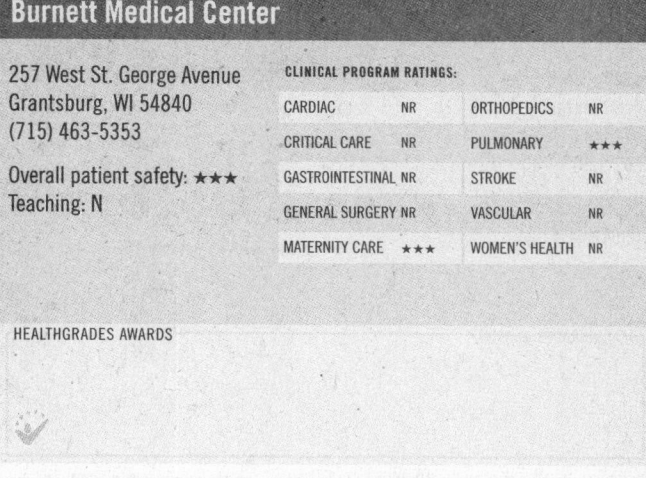

CLINICAL PROGRAM RATINGS:

CARDIAC	NR	ORTHOPEDICS	NR
CRITICAL CARE	NR	PULMONARY	★★★
GASTROINTESTINAL	NR	STROKE	NR
GENERAL SURGERY	NR	VASCULAR	NR
MATERNITY CARE	★★★	WOMEN'S HEALTH	NR

HEALTHGRADES AWARDS

Bloomer Medical Center

1501 Thompson Street
Bloomer, WI 54724
(715) 568-2000

Overall patient safety: ★★★
Teaching: N

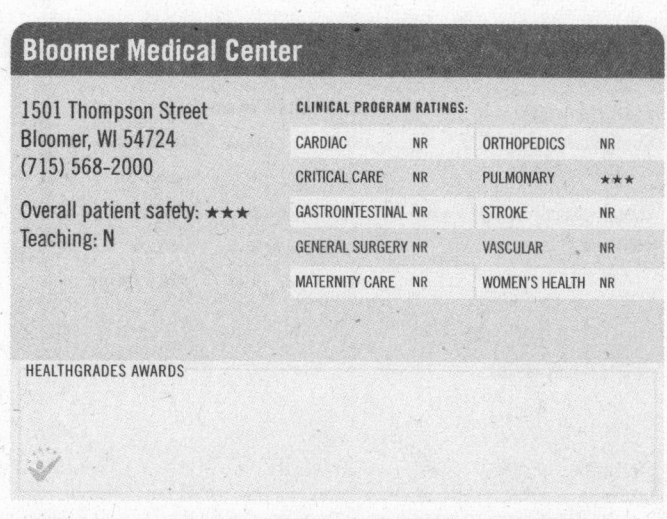

CLINICAL PROGRAM RATINGS:

CARDIAC	NR	ORTHOPEDICS	NR
CRITICAL CARE	NR	PULMONARY	★★★
GASTROINTESTINAL	NR	STROKE	NR
GENERAL SURGERY	NR	VASCULAR	NR
MATERNITY CARE	NR	WOMEN'S HEALTH	NR

HEALTHGRADES AWARDS

Chippewa Valley Hospital

1220 3rd Avenue West
Durand, WI 54736
(715) 672-4211

Overall patient safety: ★★★
Teaching: N

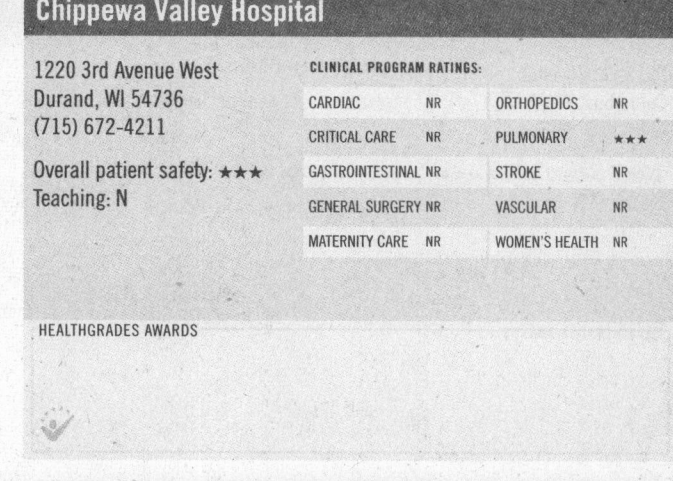

CLINICAL PROGRAM RATINGS:

CARDIAC	NR	ORTHOPEDICS	NR
CRITICAL CARE	NR	PULMONARY	★★★
GASTROINTESTINAL	NR	STROKE	NR
GENERAL SURGERY	NR	VASCULAR	NR
MATERNITY CARE	NR	WOMEN'S HEALTH	NR

HEALTHGRADES AWARDS

Boscobel Area Health Care

205 Parker Street
Boscobel, WI 53805
(608) 375-4112

Overall patient safety: ★★★
Teaching: N

CLINICAL PROGRAM RATINGS:

CARDIAC	NR	ORTHOPEDICS	NR
CRITICAL CARE	NR	PULMONARY	NR
GASTROINTESTINAL	NR	STROKE	NR
GENERAL SURGERY	NR	VASCULAR	NR
MATERNITY CARE	★★★	WOMEN'S HEALTH	NR

HEALTHGRADES AWARDS

Columbia St. Mary's Hospital Milwaukee

2323 North Lake Drive
Milwaukee, WI 53211
(414) 291-1000

Overall patient safety: ★★★
Teaching: Y

CLINICAL PROGRAM RATINGS:

CARDIAC	★★★	ORTHOPEDICS	★★★
CRITICAL CARE	★★★	PULMONARY	★★★
GASTROINTESTINAL	★★★	STROKE	★★★★★
GENERAL SURGERY	★★★	VASCULAR	NR
MATERNITY CARE	★★★	WOMEN'S HEALTH	★★★

HEALTHGRADES AWARDS

✓ SPECIALTY EXCELLENCE
• STROKE CARE

Columbia St. Mary's Hospital Ozaukee

13111 North Port
Washington Road
Mequon, WI 53097
(262) 243-7300

Overall patient safety: ★★★
Teaching: Y

CLINICAL PROGRAM RATINGS:

CARDIAC	★★★	ORTHOPEDICS	★★★
CRITICAL CARE	★★★	PULMONARY	★★★
GASTROINTESTINAL	★★★	STROKE	★★★
GENERAL SURGERY	★★★	VASCULAR	NR
MATERNITY CARE	★★★	WOMEN'S HEALTH	NR

HEALTHGRADES AWARDS

Community Memorial Hospital

855 South Main Street
Oconto Falls, WI 54154
(920) 846-3444

Overall patient safety: ★★★
Teaching: N

CLINICAL PROGRAM RATINGS:

CARDIAC	NR	ORTHOPEDICS	NR
CRITICAL CARE	NR	PULMONARY	★★★
GASTROINTESTINAL	NR	STROKE	★★★
GENERAL SURGERY	NR	VASCULAR	NR
MATERNITY CARE	★★★	WOMEN'S HEALTH	NR

HEALTHGRADES AWARDS

Columbus Community Hospital

1515 Park Avenue
Columbus, WI 53925
(920) 623-2200

Overall patient safety: ★★★
Teaching: N

CLINICAL PROGRAM RATINGS:

CARDIAC	NR	ORTHOPEDICS	NR
CRITICAL CARE	NR	PULMONARY	★★★
GASTROINTESTINAL	NR	STROKE	★★★
GENERAL SURGERY	NR	VASCULAR	NR
MATERNITY CARE	★★★	WOMEN'S HEALTH	NR

HEALTHGRADES AWARDS

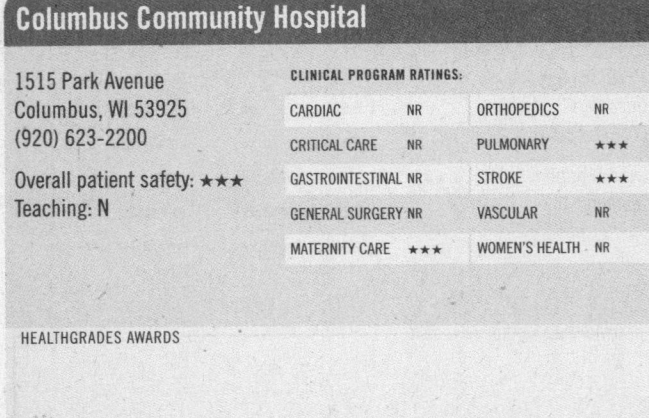

Cumberland Memorial Hospital

1110 7th Avenue
Cumberland, WI 54829
(715) 822-2741

Overall patient safety: ★★★
Teaching: N

CLINICAL PROGRAM RATINGS:

CARDIAC	NR	ORTHOPEDICS	NR
CRITICAL CARE	NR	PULMONARY	★
GASTROINTESTINAL	NR	STROKE	NR
GENERAL SURGERY	NR	VASCULAR	NR
MATERNITY CARE	★★★	WOMEN'S HEALTH	NR

HEALTHGRADES AWARDS

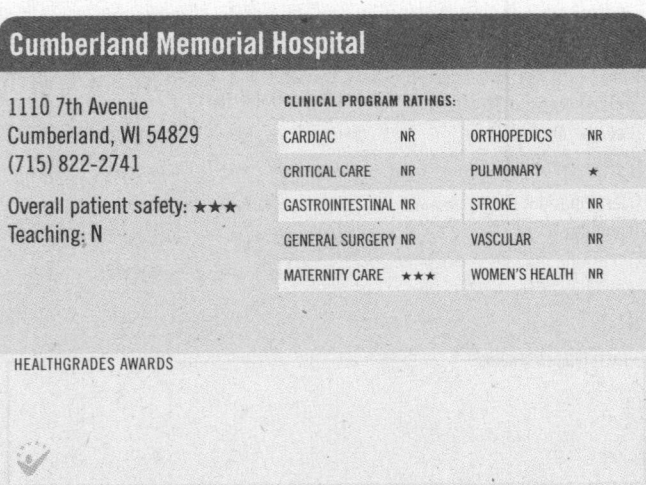

Community Memorial Hospital

West 180 N8085
Town Hall Road
Menomonee Falls, WI 53051
(262) 251-1000

Overall patient safety: ★★★
Teaching: N

CLINICAL PROGRAM RATINGS:

CARDIAC	★★★	ORTHOPEDICS	★★★
CRITICAL CARE	★★★	PULMONARY	★
GASTROINTESTINAL	★★★	STROKE	★
GENERAL SURGERY	★★★	VASCULAR	NR
MATERNITY CARE	★	WOMEN'S HEALTH	★

HEALTHGRADES AWARDS

Divine Savior Healthcare

2817 New Pinery Road
Portage, WI 53901
(608) 742-4131

Overall patient safety: ★
Teaching: N

CLINICAL PROGRAM RATINGS:

CARDIAC	NR	ORTHOPEDICS	NR
CRITICAL CARE	NR	PULMONARY	★★★
GASTROINTESTINAL	NR	STROKE	★
GENERAL SURGERY	★	VASCULAR	NR
MATERNITY CARE	★	WOMEN'S HEALTH	NR

HEALTHGRADES AWARDS

KEY: ★★★★★ **BEST**   ★★★ **AS EXPECTED**   ★ **POOR**   NR **NOT RATED BY HEALTHGRADES**   For full definitions of ratings and awards, see Appendix.

Door County Memorial Hospital

323 South 18th Avenue
Sturgeon Bay, WI 54235
(920) 743-5566

Overall patient safety: NR
Teaching: N

CLINICAL PROGRAM RATINGS:

CARDIAC	NR	ORTHOPEDICS	NR
CRITICAL CARE	NR	PULMONARY	★★★
GASTROINTESTINAL	NR	STROKE	★★★
GENERAL SURGERY	NR	VASCULAR	NR
MATERNITY CARE	NR	WOMEN'S HEALTH	NR

HEALTHGRADES AWARDS

Fort Healthcare

611 East Sherman Avenue
Fort Atkinson, WI 53538
(920) 568-5000

Overall patient safety: ★★★
Teaching: N

CLINICAL PROGRAM RATINGS:

CARDIAC	NR	ORTHOPEDICS	NR
CRITICAL CARE	NR	PULMONARY	★★★
GASTROINTESTINAL	NR	STROKE	★
GENERAL SURGERY	★★★	VASCULAR	NR
MATERNITY CARE	★★★	WOMEN'S HEALTH	NR

HEALTHGRADES AWARDS

Edgerton Hospital and Health Services

313 Stoughton Road
Edgerton, WI 53534
(608) 884-3441

Overall patient safety: ★★★
Teaching: N

CLINICAL PROGRAM RATINGS:

CARDIAC	NR	ORTHOPEDICS	NR
CRITICAL CARE	NR	PULMONARY	★★★
GASTROINTESTINAL	NR	STROKE	NR
GENERAL SURGERY	NR	VASCULAR	NR
MATERNITY CARE	NR	WOMEN'S HEALTH	NR

HEALTHGRADES AWARDS

Franciscan Skemp La Crosse Hospital

700 West Avenue South
La Crosse, WI 54601
(608) 785-0940

Overall patient safety: ★★★
Teaching: Y

CLINICAL PROGRAM RATINGS:

CARDIAC	NR	ORTHOPEDICS	★
CRITICAL CARE	NR	PULMONARY	★★★
GASTROINTESTINAL	★★★	STROKE	★
GENERAL SURGERY	★	VASCULAR	NR
MATERNITY CARE	★★★	WOMEN'S HEALTH	NR

HEALTHGRADES AWARDS

Flambeau Hospital

98 Sherry Avenue
Park Falls, WI 54552
(715) 762-7500

Overall patient safety: ★★★
Teaching: N

CLINICAL PROGRAM RATINGS:

CARDIAC	NR	ORTHOPEDICS	NR
CRITICAL CARE	NR	PULMONARY	★★★
GASTROINTESTINAL	NR	STROKE	★★★
GENERAL SURGERY	NR	VASCULAR	NR
MATERNITY CARE	★	WOMEN'S HEALTH	NR

HEALTHGRADES AWARDS

Franciscan Skemp Sparta Hospital

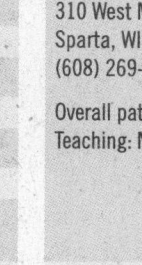

310 West Main Street
Sparta, WI 54656
(608) 269-2132

Overall patient safety: ★★★
Teaching: N

CLINICAL PROGRAM RATINGS:

CARDIAC	NR	ORTHOPEDICS	NR
CRITICAL CARE	NR	PULMONARY	NR
GASTROINTESTINAL	NR	STROKE	NR
GENERAL SURGERY	NR	VASCULAR	NR
MATERNITY CARE	★	WOMEN'S HEALTH	NR

HEALTHGRADES AWARDS

Frederic Municipal Hospital Association*

Highway 35 and United Way
Frederic, WI 54837
(715) 327-4201

Overall patient safety: ★★★
Teaching: N

CLINICAL PROGRAM RATINGS:

CARDIAC	NR	ORTHOPEDICS	NR
CRITICAL CARE	NR	PULMONARY	★★★
GASTROINTESTINAL	NR	STROKE	NR
GENERAL SURGERY	NR	VASCULAR	NR
MATERNITY CARE	★★★	WOMEN'S HEALTH	NR

HEALTHGRADES AWARDS

Grant Regional Health Center

507 South Monroe Street
Lancaster, WI 53813
(608) 723-2143

Overall patient safety: ★★★
Teaching: N

CLINICAL PROGRAM RATINGS:

CARDIAC	NR	ORTHOPEDICS	NR
CRITICAL CARE	NR	PULMONARY	★★★
GASTROINTESTINAL	NR	STROKE	★
GENERAL SURGERY	NR	VASCULAR	NR
MATERNITY CARE	★★★	WOMEN'S HEALTH	NR

HEALTHGRADES AWARDS

Froedtert Memorial Lutheran Hospital

9200 West Wisconsin Avenue
Milwaukee, WI 53226
(414) 805-3000

Overall patient safety: ★
Teaching: Y

CLINICAL PROGRAM RATINGS:

CARDIAC	★★★	ORTHOPEDICS	★★★
CRITICAL CARE	★★★	PULMONARY	★★★
GASTROINTESTINAL	★★★	STROKE	★★★
GENERAL SURGERY	★★★	VASCULAR	★★★
MATERNITY CARE	★★★	WOMEN'S HEALTH	★★★

HEALTHGRADES AWARDS

Gundersen Lutheran Medical Center

1900 South Avenue
La Crosse, WI 54601
(608) 782-7300

Overall patient safety: ★★★
Teaching: Y

CLINICAL PROGRAM RATINGS:

CARDIAC	★★★	ORTHOPEDICS	★★★
CRITICAL CARE	★★★★★	PULMONARY	★★★
GASTROINTESTINAL	★★★	STROKE	★★★
GENERAL SURGERY	★★★★★	VASCULAR	★★★
MATERNITY CARE	★	WOMEN'S HEALTH	★★★

HEALTHGRADES AWARDS

✓ DISTINGUISHED HOSPITAL
· CLINICAL EXCELLENCE

✓ SPECIALTY EXCELLENCE
· BARIATRIC SURGERY
· CRITICAL CARE
· GASTROINTESTINAL CARE
· GENERAL SURGERY
· JOINT REPLACEMENT

Good Samaritan Health Center

601 South Center Avenue
Merrill, WI 54452
(715) 536-5511

Overall patient safety: ★★★
Teaching: N

CLINICAL PROGRAM RATINGS:

CARDIAC	NR	ORTHOPEDICS	NR
CRITICAL CARE	NR	PULMONARY	★★★
GASTROINTESTINAL	NR	STROKE	★
GENERAL SURGERY	NR	VASCULAR	NR
MATERNITY CARE	★	WOMEN'S HEALTH	NR

HEALTHGRADES AWARDS

Hayward Area Memorial Hospital

11040 North State Road 77
Hayward, WI 54843
(715) 934-4321

Overall patient safety: ★★★
Teaching: N

CLINICAL PROGRAM RATINGS:

CARDIAC	NR	ORTHOPEDICS	NR
CRITICAL CARE	NR	PULMONARY	★★★
GASTROINTESTINAL	NR	STROKE	★★★
GENERAL SURGERY	★★★	VASCULAR	NR
MATERNITY CARE	★★★	WOMEN'S HEALTH	NR

HEALTHGRADES AWARDS

✓ SPECIALTY EXCELLENCE
· GENERAL SURGERY

KEY: ★★★★★ BEST   ★★★ AS EXPECTED   ★ POOR   NR NOT RATED BY HEALTHGRADES   For full definitions of ratings and awards, see Appendix.

Hess Memorial Hospital

1050 Division Street
Mauston, WI 53948
(608) 847-6161

Overall patient safety: ★★★
Teaching: N

CLINICAL PROGRAM RATINGS:

CARDIAC	NR	ORTHOPEDICS	NR
CRITICAL CARE	NR	PULMONARY	★★★
GASTROINTESTINAL	NR	STROKE	NR
GENERAL SURGERY	NR	VASCULAR	NR
MATERNITY CARE	★	WOMEN'S HEALTH	NR

HEALTHGRADES AWARDS

Howard Young Medical Center

240 Maple Street
Woodruff, WI 54568
(715) 356-8000

Overall patient safety: ★★★
Teaching: N

CLINICAL PROGRAM RATINGS:

CARDIAC	NR	ORTHOPEDICS	NR
CRITICAL CARE	NR	PULMONARY	★★★
GASTROINTESTINAL	★★★	STROKE	★★★
GENERAL SURGERY	★★★	VASCULAR	NR
MATERNITY CARE	★	WOMEN'S HEALTH	NR

HEALTHGRADES AWARDS

✓ SPECIALTY EXCELLENCE
• JOINT REPLACEMENT

Holy Family Hospital New Richmond

535 Hospital Road
New Richmond, WI 54017
(715) 246-2101

Overall patient safety: ★★★
Teaching: N

CLINICAL PROGRAM RATINGS:

CARDIAC	NR	ORTHOPEDICS	NR
CRITICAL CARE	NR	PULMONARY	★★★
GASTROINTESTINAL	NR	STROKE	★★★
GENERAL SURGERY	NR	VASCULAR	NR
MATERNITY CARE	★★★	WOMEN'S HEALTH	NR

HEALTHGRADES AWARDS

Hudson Hospital

405 Stageline Road
Hudson, WI 54016
(715) 531-6000

Overall patient safety: ★★★
Teaching: N

CLINICAL PROGRAM RATINGS:

CARDIAC	NR	ORTHOPEDICS	NR
CRITICAL CARE	NR	PULMONARY	NR
GASTROINTESTINAL	NR	STROKE	NR
GENERAL SURGERY	NR	VASCULAR	NR
MATERNITY CARE	★★★	WOMEN'S HEALTH	NR

HEALTHGRADES AWARDS

Holy Family Memorial*

2300 Western Avenue
Manitowoc, WI 54220
(920) 684-2011

Overall patient safety: ★★★
Teaching: N

CLINICAL PROGRAM RATINGS:

CARDIAC	NR	ORTHOPEDICS	NR
CRITICAL CARE	NR	PULMONARY	★★★
GASTROINTESTINAL	★★★	STROKE	★★★
GENERAL SURGERY	★★★	VASCULAR	NR
MATERNITY CARE	★	WOMEN'S HEALTH	NR

HEALTHGRADES AWARDS

✓ SPECIALTY EXCELLENCE
• GENERAL SURGERY

Indianhead Medical Center*

113 4th Avenue
Shell Lake, WI 54871
(715) 468-7833

Overall patient safety: ★★★
Teaching: N

CLINICAL PROGRAM RATINGS:

CARDIAC	NR	ORTHOPEDICS	NR
CRITICAL CARE	NR	PULMONARY	★★★
GASTROINTESTINAL	NR	STROKE	NR
GENERAL SURGERY	NR	VASCULAR	NR
MATERNITY CARE	★★★	WOMEN'S HEALTH	NR

HEALTHGRADES AWARDS

*This hospital reports its data to the federal government jointly with another hospital. Therefore the ratings and awards apply to multiple hospitals and this specific hospital may not provide all rated services.

Ladd Memorial Hospital

301 River Street
Osceola, WI 54020
(715) 294-2111

Overall patient safety: ★★★
Teaching: N

CLINICAL PROGRAM RATINGS:

CARDIAC	NR	ORTHOPEDICS	NR
CRITICAL CARE	NR	PULMONARY	NR
GASTROINTESTINAL	NR	STROKE	NR
GENERAL SURGERY	NR	VASCULAR	NR
MATERNITY CARE	★★★	WOMEN'S HEALTH	NR

HEALTHGRADES AWARDS

Langlade Memorial Hospital

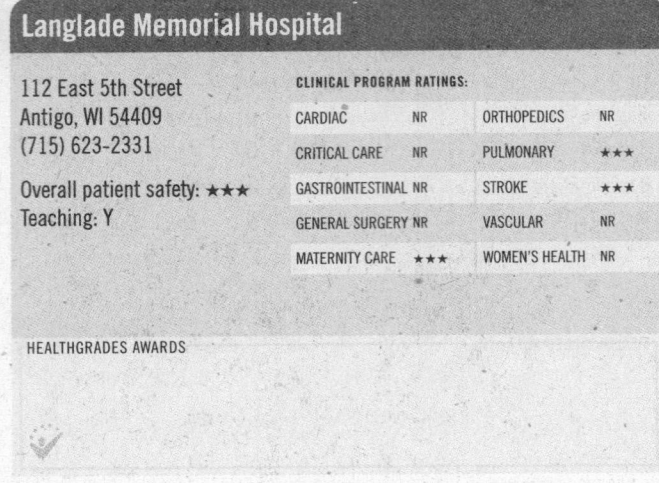

112 East 5th Street
Antigo, WI 54409
(715) 623-2331

Overall patient safety: ★★★
Teaching: Y

CLINICAL PROGRAM RATINGS:

CARDIAC	NR	ORTHOPEDICS	NR
CRITICAL CARE	NR	PULMONARY	★★★
GASTROINTESTINAL	NR	STROKE	★★★
GENERAL SURGERY	NR	VASCULAR	NR
MATERNITY CARE	★★★	WOMEN'S HEALTH	NR

HEALTHGRADES AWARDS

Lakeview Hospital*

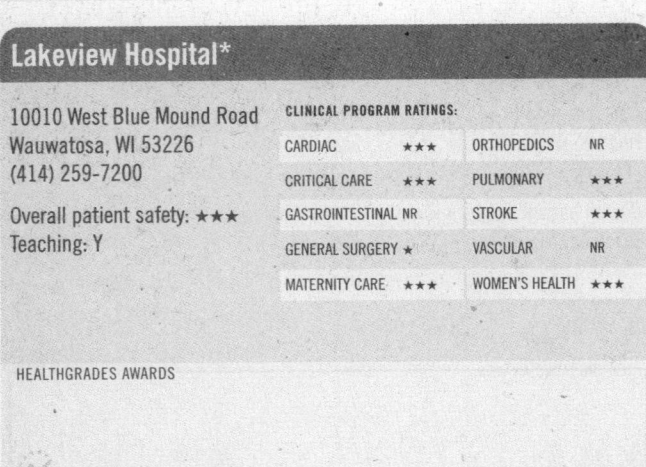

10010 West Blue Mound Road
Wauwatosa, WI 53226
(414) 259-7200

Overall patient safety: ★★★
Teaching: Y

CLINICAL PROGRAM RATINGS:

CARDIAC	★★★	ORTHOPEDICS	NR
CRITICAL CARE	★★★	PULMONARY	★★★
GASTROINTESTINAL	NR	STROKE	★★★
GENERAL SURGERY	★	VASCULAR	NR
MATERNITY CARE	★★★	WOMEN'S HEALTH	★★★

HEALTHGRADES AWARDS

Luther Hospital Mayo Health System

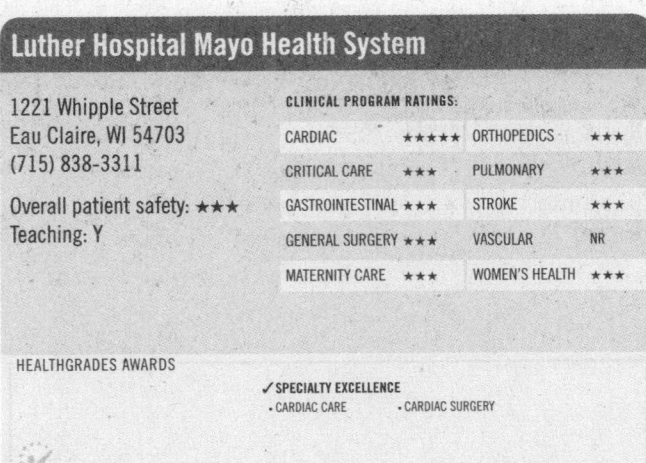

1221 Whipple Street
Eau Claire, WI 54703
(715) 838-3311

Overall patient safety: ★★★
Teaching: Y

CLINICAL PROGRAM RATINGS:

CARDIAC	★★★★★	ORTHOPEDICS	★★★
CRITICAL CARE	★★★	PULMONARY	★★★
GASTROINTESTINAL	★★★	STROKE	★★★
GENERAL SURGERY	★★★	VASCULAR	NR
MATERNITY CARE	★★★	WOMEN'S HEALTH	★★★

HEALTHGRADES AWARDS

✓ SPECIALTY EXCELLENCE
· CARDIAC CARE   · CARDIAC SURGERY

Lakeview Medical Center

1100 North Main Street
Rice Lake, WI 54868
(715) 234-1515

Overall patient safety: ★★★
Teaching: N

CLINICAL PROGRAM RATINGS:

CARDIAC	NR	ORTHOPEDICS	NR
CRITICAL CARE	NR	PULMONARY	★★★
GASTROINTESTINAL	NR	STROKE	★★★
GENERAL SURGERY	★★★	VASCULAR	NR
MATERNITY CARE	★	WOMEN'S HEALTH	NR

HEALTHGRADES AWARDS

✓ SPECIALTY EXCELLENCE
· JOINT REPLACEMENT

Memorial Health Center

135 South Gibson Street
Medford, WI 54451
(715) 748-8100

Overall patient safety: ★★★
Teaching: N

CLINICAL PROGRAM RATINGS:

CARDIAC	NR	ORTHOPEDICS	NR
CRITICAL CARE	NR	PULMONARY	★★★
GASTROINTESTINAL	NR	STROKE	★★★
GENERAL SURGERY	NR	VASCULAR	NR
MATERNITY CARE	★★★	WOMEN'S HEALTH	NR

HEALTHGRADES AWARDS

KEY: ★★★★★ BEST   ★★★ AS EXPECTED   ★ POOR   NR NOT RATED BY HEALTHGRADES   For full definitions of ratings and awards, see Appendix.

Memorial Hospital*

333 Reed Avenue
Manitowoc, WI 54220
(414) 682-7765

Overall patient safety: ★★★
Teaching: N

CLINICAL PROGRAM RATINGS:

CARDIAC	NR	ORTHOPEDICS	NR
CRITICAL CARE	NR	PULMONARY	★★★
GASTROINTESTINAL	★★★	STROKE	★★★
GENERAL SURGERY	★★★	VASCULAR	NR
MATERNITY CARE	★	WOMEN'S HEALTH	NR

HEALTHGRADES AWARDS

✓ SPECIALTY EXCELLENCE
• GENERAL SURGERY

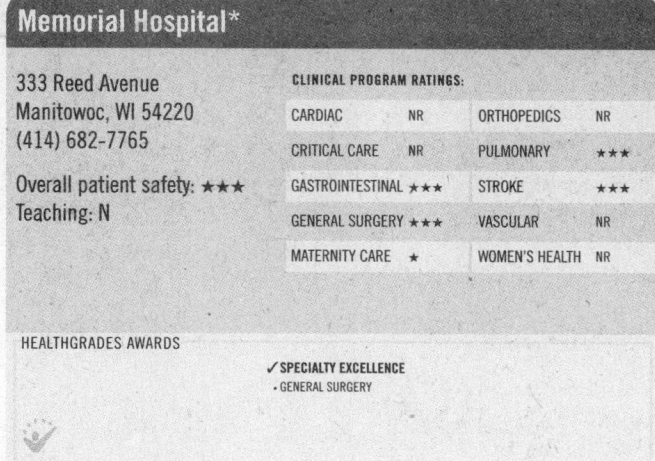

Memorial Medical Center

1615 Maple Lane
Ashland, WI 54806
(715) 682-4563

Overall patient safety: ★★★
Teaching: N

CLINICAL PROGRAM RATINGS:

CARDIAC	NR	ORTHOPEDICS	NR
CRITICAL CARE	NR	PULMONARY	★★★
GASTROINTESTINAL	NR	STROKE	★★★
GENERAL SURGERY	★★★	VASCULAR	NR
MATERNITY CARE	★★★	WOMEN'S HEALTH	NR

HEALTHGRADES AWARDS

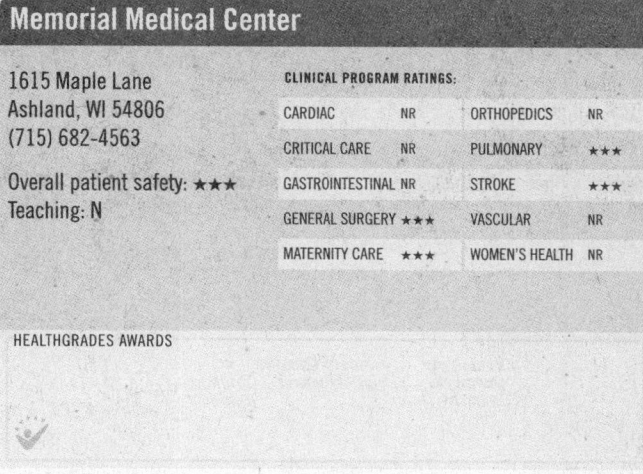

Memorial Hospital Burlington

252 McHenry Street
Burlington, WI 53105
(262) 767-6000

Overall patient safety: ★★★★★
Teaching: N

CLINICAL PROGRAM RATINGS:

CARDIAC	NR	ORTHOPEDICS	NR
CRITICAL CARE	NR	PULMONARY	★★★
GASTROINTESTINAL	★★★	STROKE	★★★
GENERAL SURGERY	★★★	VASCULAR	NR
MATERNITY CARE	★★★	WOMEN'S HEALTH	NR

HEALTHGRADES AWARDS

✓ DISTINGUISHED
HOSPITAL
• PATIENT SAFETY

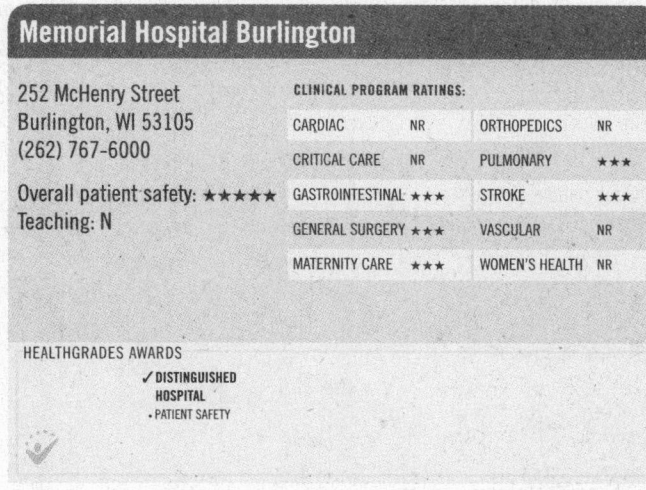

Memorial Medical Center

216 Sunset Place
Neillsville, WI 54456
(715) 743-3101

Overall patient safety: ★★★
Teaching: N

CLINICAL PROGRAM RATINGS:

CARDIAC	NR	ORTHOPEDICS	NR
CRITICAL CARE	NR	PULMONARY	★★★
GASTROINTESTINAL	NR	STROKE	NR
GENERAL SURGERY	NR	VASCULAR	NR
MATERNITY CARE	★★★	WOMEN'S HEALTH	NR

HEALTHGRADES AWARDS

Memorial Hospital Lafayette City

800 Clay Street
Darlington, WI 53530
(608) 776-4466

Overall patient safety: ★★★
Teaching: N

CLINICAL PROGRAM RATINGS:

CARDIAC	NR	ORTHOPEDICS	NR
CRITICAL CARE	NR	PULMONARY	★★★
GASTROINTESTINAL	NR	STROKE	NR
GENERAL SURGERY	NR	VASCULAR	NR
MATERNITY CARE	★★★	WOMEN'S HEALTH	NR

HEALTHGRADES AWARDS

Mercy Health System

1000 Mineral Point Avenue
Janesville, WI 53545
(608) 756-6000

Overall patient safety: ★★★
Teaching: Y

CLINICAL PROGRAM RATINGS:

CARDIAC	★★★	ORTHOPEDICS	★
CRITICAL CARE	★★★	PULMONARY	★★★
GASTROINTESTINAL	★★★	STROKE	★★★
GENERAL SURGERY	★★★	VASCULAR	NR
MATERNITY CARE	★★★	WOMEN'S HEALTH	★★★

HEALTHGRADES AWARDS

*This hospital reports its data to the federal government jointly with another hospital. Therefore the ratings and awards apply to multiple hospitals and this specific hospital may not provide all rated services.

Mercy Medical Center

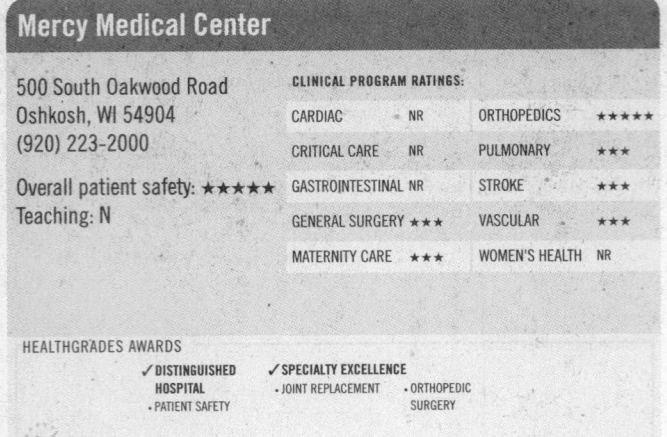

500 South Oakwood Road
Oshkosh, WI 54904
(920) 223-2000

Overall patient safety: ★★★★★
Teaching: N

CLINICAL PROGRAM RATINGS:

CARDIAC	NR	ORTHOPEDICS	★★★★★
CRITICAL CARE	NR	PULMONARY	★★★
GASTROINTESTINAL	NR	STROKE	★★★
GENERAL SURGERY	★★★	VASCULAR	★★★
MATERNITY CARE	★★★	WOMEN'S HEALTH	NR

HEALTHGRADES AWARDS

✓ DISTINGUISHED HOSPITAL
- PATIENT SAFETY

✓ SPECIALTY EXCELLENCE
- JOINT REPLACEMENT
- ORTHOPEDIC SURGERY

Moundview Memorial Hospital and Clinics

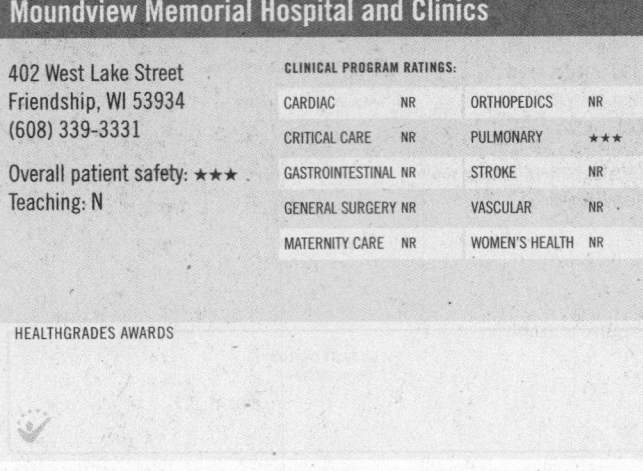

402 West Lake Street
Friendship, WI 53934
(608) 339-3331

Overall patient safety: ★★★
Teaching: N

CLINICAL PROGRAM RATINGS:

CARDIAC	NR	ORTHOPEDICS	NR
CRITICAL CARE	NR	PULMONARY	★★★
GASTROINTESTINAL	NR	STROKE	NR
GENERAL SURGERY	NR	VASCULAR	NR
MATERNITY CARE	NR	WOMEN'S HEALTH	NR

HEALTHGRADES AWARDS

Meriter Hospital*

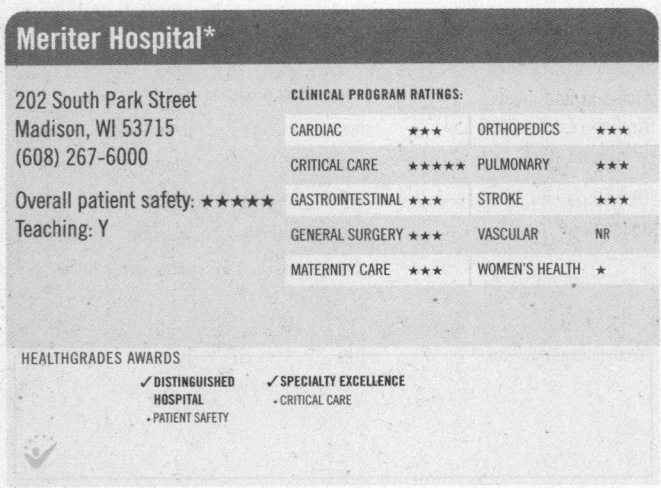

202 South Park Street
Madison, WI 53715
(608) 267-6000

Overall patient safety: ★★★★★
Teaching: Y

CLINICAL PROGRAM RATINGS:

CARDIAC	★★★	ORTHOPEDICS	★★★
CRITICAL CARE	★★★★★	PULMONARY	★★★
GASTROINTESTINAL	★★★	STROKE	★★★
GENERAL SURGERY	★★★	VASCULAR	NR
MATERNITY CARE	★★★	WOMEN'S HEALTH	★

HEALTHGRADES AWARDS

✓ DISTINGUISHED HOSPITAL
- PATIENT SAFETY

✓ SPECIALTY EXCELLENCE
- CRITICAL CARE

New London Family Medical Center

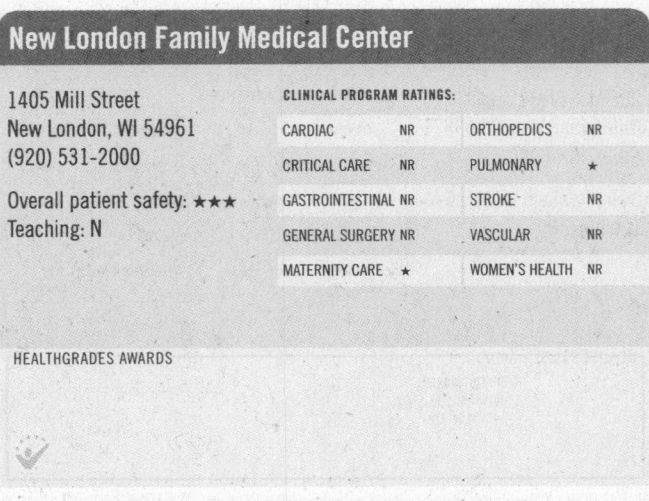

1405 Mill Street
New London, WI 54961
(920) 531-2000

Overall patient safety: ★★★
Teaching: N

CLINICAL PROGRAM RATINGS:

CARDIAC	NR	ORTHOPEDICS	NR
CRITICAL CARE	NR	PULMONARY	★
GASTROINTESTINAL	NR	STROKE	NR
GENERAL SURGERY	NR	VASCULAR	NR
MATERNITY CARE	★	WOMEN'S HEALTH	NR

HEALTHGRADES AWARDS

Monroe Clinic

515 22nd Avenue
Monroe, WI 53566
(608) 324-1000

Overall patient safety: ★★★
Teaching: Y

CLINICAL PROGRAM RATINGS:

CARDIAC	NR	ORTHOPEDICS	NR
CRITICAL CARE	NR	PULMONARY	★★★
GASTROINTESTINAL	★★★	STROKE	★★★
GENERAL SURGERY	★★★	VASCULAR	NR
MATERNITY CARE	★★★	WOMEN'S HEALTH	NR

HEALTHGRADES AWARDS

Oconomowoc Memorial Hospital

791 Summit Avenue
Oconomowoc, WI 53066
(262) 569-9400

Overall patient safety: ★★★
Teaching: N

CLINICAL PROGRAM RATINGS:

CARDIAC	NR	ORTHOPEDICS	NR
CRITICAL CARE	NR	PULMONARY	★★★★★
GASTROINTESTINAL	NR	STROKE	★★★
GENERAL SURGERY	★★★	VASCULAR	NR
MATERNITY CARE	★★★	WOMEN'S HEALTH	NR

HEALTHGRADES AWARDS

✓ SPECIALTY EXCELLENCE
- PULMONARY CARE

KEY: ★★★★★ BEST ★★★ AS EXPECTED ★ POOR NR NOT RATED BY HEALTHGRADES   For full definitions of ratings and awards, see Appendix.

Our Lady of Victory Hospital

1120 Pine Street
Stanley, WI 54768
(715) 644-5571

Overall patient safety: ★★★
Teaching: N

CLINICAL PROGRAM RATINGS:

CARDIAC	NR	ORTHOPEDICS	NR
CRITICAL CARE	NR	PULMONARY	★★★
GASTROINTESTINAL	NR	STROKE	NR
GENERAL SURGERY	NR	VASCULAR	NR
MATERNITY CARE	NR	WOMEN'S HEALTH	NR

HEALTHGRADES AWARDS

Reedsburg Area Medical Center

2000 North Dewey Avenue
Reedsburg, WI 53959
(608) 524-6487

Overall patient safety: ★★★
Teaching: N

CLINICAL PROGRAM RATINGS:

CARDIAC	NR	ORTHOPEDICS	NR
CRITICAL CARE	NR	PULMONARY	★★★
GASTROINTESTINAL	NR	STROKE	★★★
GENERAL SURGERY	NR	VASCULAR	NR
MATERNITY CARE	★	WOMEN'S HEALTH	NR

HEALTHGRADES AWARDS

Prairie Du Chien Memorial Hospital

705 East Taylor Street
Prairie Du Chien, WI 53821
(608) 357-2000

Overall patient safety: ★★★
Teaching: N

CLINICAL PROGRAM RATINGS:

CARDIAC	NR	ORTHOPEDICS	NR
CRITICAL CARE	NR	PULMONARY	★★★
GASTROINTESTINAL	NR	STROKE	★
GENERAL SURGERY	NR	VASCULAR	NR
MATERNITY CARE	★★★	WOMEN'S HEALTH	NR

HEALTHGRADES AWARDS

Richland Hospital

333 East 2nd Street
Richland Center, WI 53581
(608) 647-6321

Overall patient safety: ★★★★★
Teaching: N

CLINICAL PROGRAM RATINGS:

CARDIAC	NR	ORTHOPEDICS	NR
CRITICAL CARE	NR	PULMONARY	★★★
GASTROINTESTINAL	NR	STROKE	★★★
GENERAL SURGERY	NR	VASCULAR	NR
MATERNITY CARE	★	WOMEN'S HEALTH	NR

HEALTHGRADES AWARDS

Red Cedar Medical Center—Mayo Health System

2321 Stout Road
Menomonie, WI 54751
(715) 235-5531

Overall patient safety: ★★★
Teaching: N

CLINICAL PROGRAM RATINGS:

CARDIAC	NR	ORTHOPEDICS	NR
CRITICAL CARE	NR	PULMONARY	★★★
GASTROINTESTINAL	NR	STROKE	★★★
GENERAL SURGERY	NR	VASCULAR	NR
MATERNITY CARE	★★★	WOMEN'S HEALTH	NR

HEALTHGRADES AWARDS

River Falls Area Hospital

1629 East Division Street
River Falls, WI 54022
(715) 426-6155

Overall patient safety: ★★★
Teaching: N

CLINICAL PROGRAM RATINGS:

CARDIAC	NR	ORTHOPEDICS	NR
CRITICAL CARE	NR	PULMONARY	★
GASTROINTESTINAL	NR	STROKE	★★★
GENERAL SURGERY	NR	VASCULAR	NR
MATERNITY CARE	★★★	WOMEN'S HEALTH	NR

HEALTHGRADES AWARDS

*This hospital reports its data to the federal government jointly with another hospital. Therefore the ratings and awards apply to multiple hospitals and this specific hospital may not provide all rated services.

Riverside Medical Center

800 Riverside Drive
Waupaca, WI 54981
(715) 258-1000

Overall patient safety: ★★★
Teaching: N

CLINICAL PROGRAM RATINGS:

CARDIAC	NR	ORTHOPEDICS	NR
CRITICAL CARE	NR	PULMONARY	★
GASTROINTESTINAL	NR	STROKE	★★★
GENERAL SURGERY	★★★	VASCULAR	NR
MATERNITY CARE	★★★	WOMEN'S HEALTH	NR

HEALTHGRADES AWARDS

Sacred Heart Hospital

900 West Clairemont Avenue
Eau Claire, WI 54701
(715) 839-4121

Overall patient safety: ★★★
Teaching: Y

CLINICAL PROGRAM RATINGS:

CARDIAC	NR	ORTHOPEDICS	★★★
CRITICAL CARE	★★★	PULMONARY	★★★
GASTROINTESTINAL	★★★	STROKE	★★★
GENERAL SURGERY	★★★	VASCULAR	NR
MATERNITY CARE	★★★	WOMEN'S HEALTH	NR

HEALTHGRADES AWARDS

✓ SPECIALTY EXCELLENCE
- JOINT REPLACEMENT

Riverview Hospital

410 Dewey Street
Wisconsin Rapids, WI 54495
(715) 423-6060

Overall patient safety: ★★★★★
Teaching: N

CLINICAL PROGRAM RATINGS:

CARDIAC	NR	ORTHOPEDICS	NR
CRITICAL CARE	NR	PULMONARY	★★★
GASTROINTESTINAL	NR	STROKE	★
GENERAL SURGERY	★★★	VASCULAR	NR
MATERNITY CARE	★★★	WOMEN'S HEALTH	NR

HEALTHGRADES AWARDS

St. Agnes Hospital

430 East Division Street
Fond Du Lac, WI 54935
(920) 929-2300

Overall patient safety: ★★★
Teaching: N

CLINICAL PROGRAM RATINGS:

CARDIAC	★★★	ORTHOPEDICS	★★★
CRITICAL CARE	NR	PULMONARY	★★★
GASTROINTESTINAL	★★★	STROKE	★
GENERAL SURGERY	★★★	VASCULAR	NR
MATERNITY CARE	★★★	WOMEN'S HEALTH	NR

HEALTHGRADES AWARDS

Rusk County Memorial Hospital

900 College Avenue West
Ladysmith, WI 54848
(715) 532-5561

Overall patient safety: ★★★
Teaching: N

CLINICAL PROGRAM RATINGS:

CARDIAC	NR	ORTHOPEDICS	NR
CRITICAL CARE	NR	PULMONARY	★★★
GASTROINTESTINAL	NR	STROKE	★★★
GENERAL SURGERY	NR	VASCULAR	NR
MATERNITY CARE	★★★	WOMEN'S HEALTH	NR

HEALTHGRADES AWARDS

St. Clare Hospital Health Services

707 14th Street
Baraboo, WI 53913
(608) 356-1400

Overall patient safety: ★★★
Teaching: Y

CLINICAL PROGRAM RATINGS:

CARDIAC	NR	ORTHOPEDICS	NR
CRITICAL CARE	NR	PULMONARY	★★★
GASTROINTESTINAL	NR	STROKE	NR
GENERAL SURGERY	NR	VASCULAR	NR
MATERNITY CARE	★★★	WOMEN'S HEALTH	NR

HEALTHGRADES AWARDS

KEY: ★★★★★ BEST   ★★★ AS EXPECTED   ★ POOR   NR NOT RATED BY HEALTHGRADES   For full definitions of ratings and awards, see Appendix.

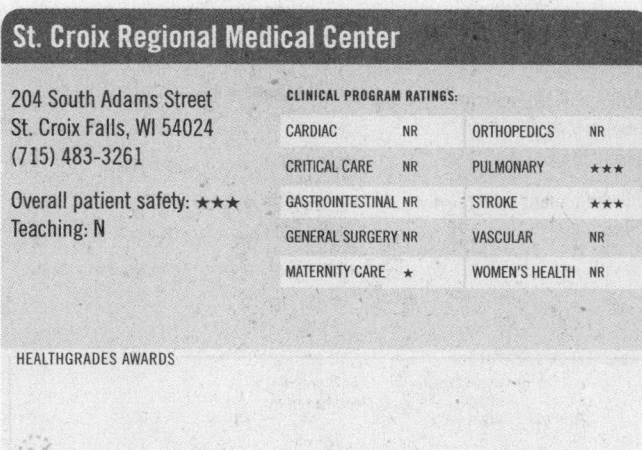

St. Croix Regional Medical Center

204 South Adams Street
St. Croix Falls, WI 54024
(715) 483-3261

Overall patient safety: ★★★
Teaching: N

CLINICAL PROGRAM RATINGS:

CARDIAC	NR	ORTHOPEDICS	NR
CRITICAL CARE	NR	PULMONARY	★★★
GASTROINTESTINAL	NR	STROKE	★★★
GENERAL SURGERY	NR	VASCULAR	NR
MATERNITY CARE	★	WOMEN'S HEALTH	NR

HEALTHGRADES AWARDS

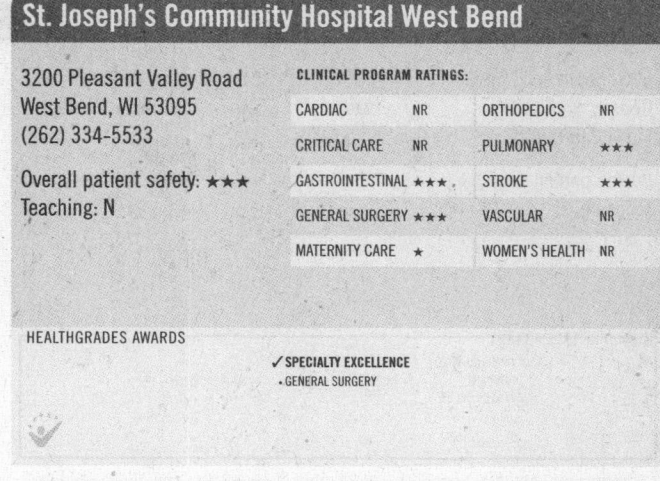

St. Joseph's Community Hospital West Bend

3200 Pleasant Valley Road
West Bend, WI 53095
(262) 334-5533

Overall patient safety: ★★★
Teaching: N

CLINICAL PROGRAM RATINGS:

CARDIAC	NR	ORTHOPEDICS	NR
CRITICAL CARE	NR	PULMONARY	★★★
GASTROINTESTINAL	★★★	STROKE	★★★
GENERAL SURGERY	★★★	VASCULAR	NR
MATERNITY CARE	★	WOMEN'S HEALTH	NR

HEALTHGRADES AWARDS

✓ **SPECIALTY EXCELLENCE**
• GENERAL SURGERY

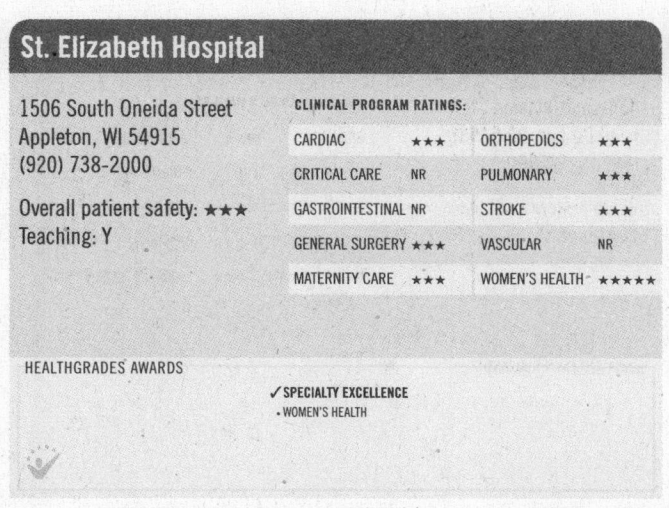

St. Elizabeth Hospital

1506 South Oneida Street
Appleton, WI 54915
(920) 738-2000

Overall patient safety: ★★★
Teaching: Y

CLINICAL PROGRAM RATINGS:

CARDIAC	★★★	ORTHOPEDICS	★★★
CRITICAL CARE	NR	PULMONARY	★★★
GASTROINTESTINAL	NR	STROKE	★★★
GENERAL SURGERY	★★★	VASCULAR	NR
MATERNITY CARE	★★★	WOMEN'S HEALTH	★★★★★

HEALTHGRADES AWARDS

✓ **SPECIALTY EXCELLENCE**
• WOMEN'S HEALTH

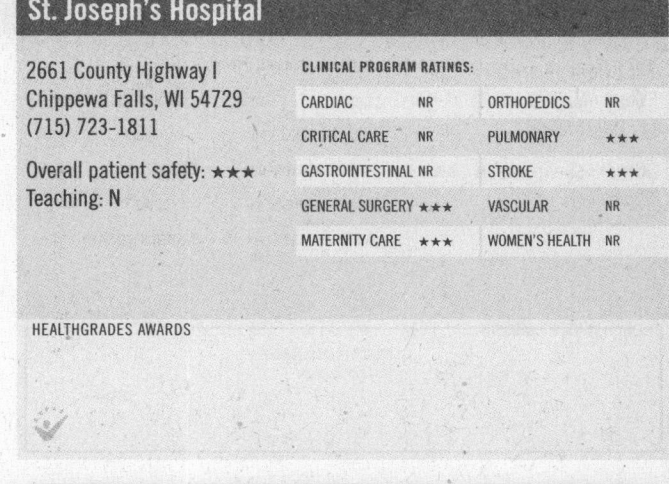

St. Joseph's Hospital

2661 County Highway I
Chippewa Falls, WI 54729
(715) 723-1811

Overall patient safety: ★★★
Teaching: N

CLINICAL PROGRAM RATINGS:

CARDIAC	NR	ORTHOPEDICS	NR
CRITICAL CARE	NR	PULMONARY	★★★
GASTROINTESTINAL	NR	STROKE	★★★
GENERAL SURGERY	★★★	VASCULAR	NR
MATERNITY CARE	★★★	WOMEN'S HEALTH	NR

HEALTHGRADES AWARDS

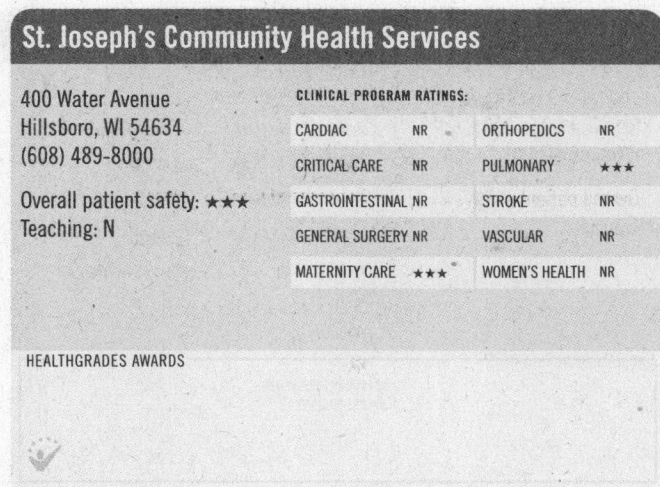

St. Joseph's Community Health Services

400 Water Avenue
Hillsboro, WI 54634
(608) 489-8000

Overall patient safety: ★★★
Teaching: N

CLINICAL PROGRAM RATINGS:

CARDIAC	NR	ORTHOPEDICS	NR
CRITICAL CARE	NR	PULMONARY	★★★
GASTROINTESTINAL	NR	STROKE	NR
GENERAL SURGERY	NR	VASCULAR	NR
MATERNITY CARE	★★★	WOMEN'S HEALTH	NR

HEALTHGRADES AWARDS

St. Joseph's Hospital

611 St. Joseph Avenue
Marshfield, WI 54449
(715) 387-1713

Overall patient safety: ★★★
Teaching: Y

CLINICAL PROGRAM RATINGS:

CARDIAC	★★★★★	ORTHOPEDICS	★★★
CRITICAL CARE	★★★	PULMONARY	★★★★★
GASTROINTESTINAL	★★★	STROKE	★★★★★
GENERAL SURGERY	★★★★★	VASCULAR	★★★
MATERNITY CARE	★	WOMEN'S HEALTH	★★★

HEALTHGRADES AWARDS

✓ **DISTINGUISHED HOSPITAL**
• CLINICAL EXCELLENCE

✓ **SPECIALTY EXCELLENCE**
• CARDIAC CARE
• GENERAL SURGERY
• PULMONARY CARE
• STROKE CARE

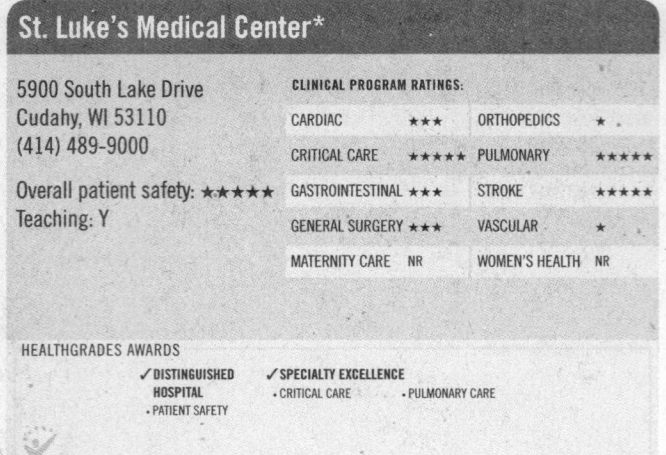

St. Luke's Medical Center*

5900 South Lake Drive
Cudahy, WI 53110
(414) 489-9000

Overall patient safety: ★★★★★
Teaching: Y

CLINICAL PROGRAM RATINGS:

CARDIAC	★★★	ORTHOPEDICS	★
CRITICAL CARE	★★★★★	PULMONARY	★★★★★
GASTROINTESTINAL	★★★	STROKE	★★★★★
GENERAL SURGERY	★★★	VASCULAR	★
MATERNITY CARE	NR	WOMEN'S HEALTH	NR

HEALTHGRADES AWARDS

✓ DISTINGUISHED HOSPITAL
 • PATIENT SAFETY

✓ SPECIALTY EXCELLENCE
 • CRITICAL CARE • PULMONARY CARE

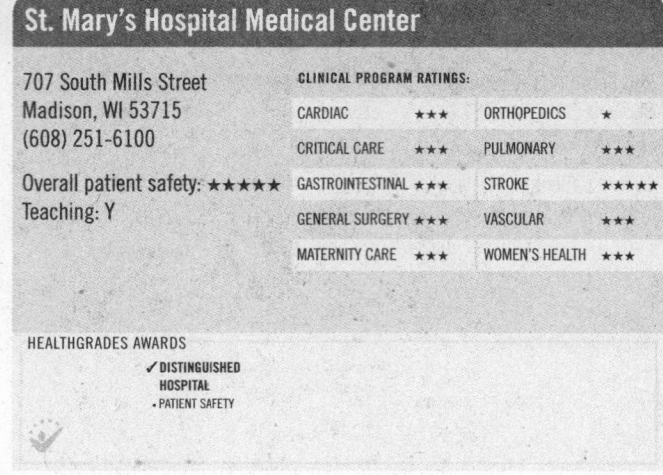

St. Mary's Hospital Medical Center

707 South Mills Street
Madison, WI 53715
(608) 251-6100

Overall patient safety: ★★★★★
Teaching: Y

CLINICAL PROGRAM RATINGS:

CARDIAC	★★★	ORTHOPEDICS	★
CRITICAL CARE	★★★	PULMONARY	★★★
GASTROINTESTINAL	★★★	STROKE	★★★★★
GENERAL SURGERY	★★★	VASCULAR	★★★
MATERNITY CARE	★★★	WOMEN'S HEALTH	★★★

HEALTHGRADES AWARDS

✓ DISTINGUISHED HOSPITAL
 • PATIENT SAFETY

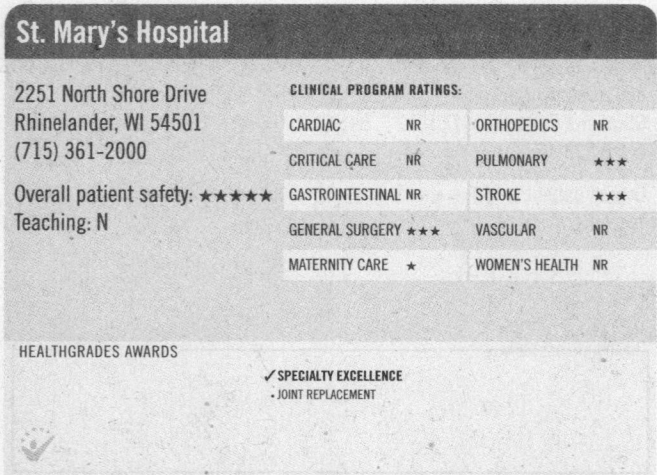

St. Mary's Hospital

2251 North Shore Drive
Rhinelander, WI 54501
(715) 361-2000

Overall patient safety: ★★★★★
Teaching: N

CLINICAL PROGRAM RATINGS:

CARDIAC	NR	ORTHOPEDICS	NR
CRITICAL CARE	NR	PULMONARY	★★★
GASTROINTESTINAL	NR	STROKE	★★★
GENERAL SURGERY	★★★	VASCULAR	NR
MATERNITY CARE	★	WOMEN'S HEALTH	NR

HEALTHGRADES AWARDS

✓ SPECIALTY EXCELLENCE
 • JOINT REPLACEMENT

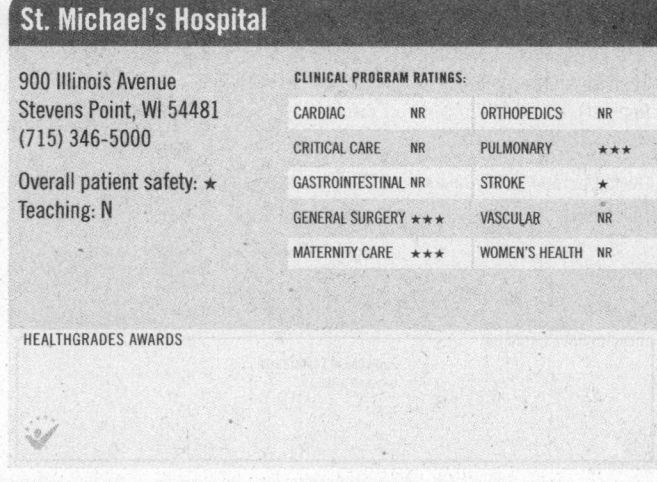

St. Michael's Hospital

900 Illinois Avenue
Stevens Point, WI 54481
(715) 346-5000

Overall patient safety: ★
Teaching: N

CLINICAL PROGRAM RATINGS:

CARDIAC	NR	ORTHOPEDICS	NR
CRITICAL CARE	NR	PULMONARY	★★★
GASTROINTESTINAL	NR	STROKE	★
GENERAL SURGERY	★★★	VASCULAR	NR
MATERNITY CARE	★★★	WOMEN'S HEALTH	NR

HEALTHGRADES AWARDS

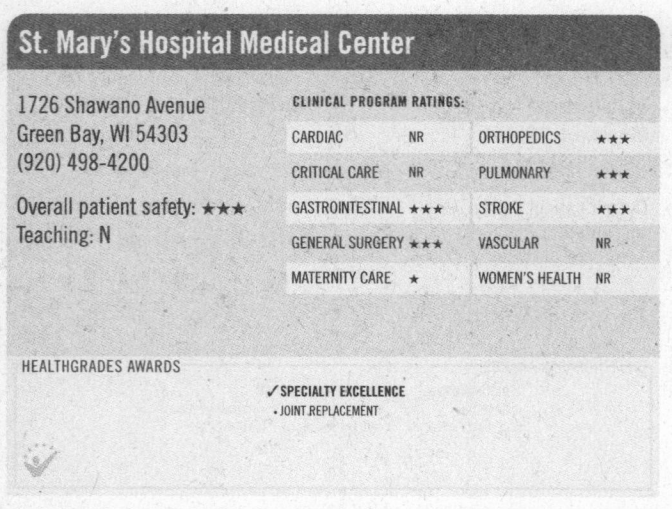

St. Mary's Hospital Medical Center

1726 Shawano Avenue
Green Bay, WI 54303
(920) 498-4200

Overall patient safety: ★★★
Teaching: N

CLINICAL PROGRAM RATINGS:

CARDIAC	NR	ORTHOPEDICS	★★★
CRITICAL CARE	NR	PULMONARY	★★★
GASTROINTESTINAL	★★★	STROKE	★★★
GENERAL SURGERY	★★★	VASCULAR	NR
MATERNITY CARE	★	WOMEN'S HEALTH	NR

HEALTHGRADES AWARDS

✓ SPECIALTY EXCELLENCE
 • JOINT REPLACEMENT

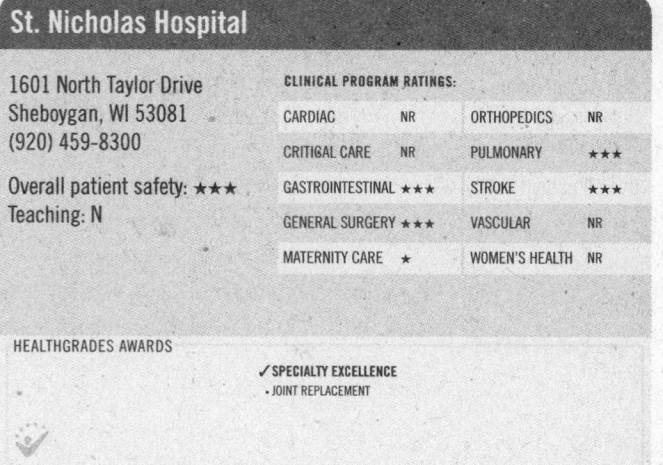

St. Nicholas Hospital

1601 North Taylor Drive
Sheboygan, WI 53081
(920) 459-8300

Overall patient safety: ★★★
Teaching: N

CLINICAL PROGRAM RATINGS:

CARDIAC	NR	ORTHOPEDICS	NR
CRITICAL CARE	NR	PULMONARY	★★★
GASTROINTESTINAL	★★★	STROKE	★★★
GENERAL SURGERY	★★★	VASCULAR	NR
MATERNITY CARE	★	WOMEN'S HEALTH	NR

HEALTHGRADES AWARDS

✓ SPECIALTY EXCELLENCE
 • JOINT REPLACEMENT

KEY: ★★★★★ BEST ★★★ AS EXPECTED ★ POOR NR NOT RATED BY HEALTHGRADES   For full definitions of ratings and awards, see Appendix.

St. Vincent Hospital

835 South Van Buren Street
Green Bay, WI 54301
(920) 433-0111

Overall patient safety: ★★★
Teaching: N

CLINICAL PROGRAM RATINGS:

CARDIAC	NR	ORTHOPEDICS	★★★
CRITICAL CARE	★★★	PULMONARY	★★★★★
GASTROINTESTINAL	★★★	STROKE	★★★
GENERAL SURGERY	★★★★★	VASCULAR	★★★
MATERNITY CARE	★★★	WOMEN'S HEALTH	NR

HEALTHGRADES AWARDS

✓ SPECIALTY EXCELLENCE
· GASTROINTESTINAL   · GENERAL SURGERY   · PULMONARY CARE
CARE

Southwest Health Center

1400 East Side Road
Platteville, WI 53818
(608) 342-4701

Overall patient safety: ★★★
Teaching: N

CLINICAL PROGRAM RATINGS:

CARDIAC	NR	ORTHOPEDICS	NR
CRITICAL CARE	NR	PULMONARY	★★★
GASTROINTESTINAL	NR	STROKE	★
GENERAL SURGERY	NR	VASCULAR	NR
MATERNITY CARE	★★★	WOMEN'S HEALTH	NR

HEALTHGRADES AWARDS

Sauk Prairie Memorial Hospital

80 1st Street
Prairie Du Sac, WI 53578
(608) 643-3311

Overall patient safety: ★★★
Teaching: Y

CLINICAL PROGRAM RATINGS:

CARDIAC	NR	ORTHOPEDICS	NR
CRITICAL CARE	NR	PULMONARY	★★★
GASTROINTESTINAL	NR	STROKE	★★★
GENERAL SURGERY	NR	VASCULAR	NR
MATERNITY CARE	★★★	WOMEN'S HEALTH	NR

HEALTHGRADES AWARDS

✓ SPECIALTY EXCELLENCE
· JOINT REPLACEMENT

Spooner Health System

819 Ash Street
Spooner, WI 54801
(715) 635-2111

Overall patient safety: ★★★
Teaching: N

CLINICAL PROGRAM RATINGS:

CARDIAC	NR	ORTHOPEDICS	NR
CRITICAL CARE	NR	PULMONARY	★★★
GASTROINTESTINAL	NR	STROKE	★★★
GENERAL SURGERY	NR	VASCULAR	NR
MATERNITY CARE	★★★	WOMEN'S HEALTH	NR

HEALTHGRADES AWARDS

Shawano Medical Center

309 North Bartlette Street
Shawano, WI 54166
(715) 526-2111

Overall patient safety: ★★★
Teaching: N

CLINICAL PROGRAM RATINGS:

CARDIAC	NR	ORTHOPEDICS	NR
CRITICAL CARE	NR	PULMONARY	★★★
GASTROINTESTINAL	NR	STROKE	★★★
GENERAL SURGERY	NR	VASCULAR	NR
MATERNITY CARE	★	WOMEN'S HEALTH	NR

HEALTHGRADES AWARDS

Theda Clark Medical Center

130 2nd Street
Neenah, WI 54956
(920) 729-3100

Overall patient safety: ★★★
Teaching: N

CLINICAL PROGRAM RATINGS:

CARDIAC	NR	ORTHOPEDICS	★★★
CRITICAL CARE	★★★	PULMONARY	★★★
GASTROINTESTINAL	★★★	STROKE	★★★
GENERAL SURGERY	★★★	VASCULAR	NR
MATERNITY CARE	★★★	WOMEN'S HEALTH	NR

HEALTHGRADES AWARDS

*This hospital reports its data to the federal government jointly with another hospital. Therefore the ratings and awards apply to multiple hospitals and this specific hospital may not provide all rated services.

Tomah Memorial Hospital

321 Butts Avenue
Tomah, WI 54660
(608) 372-2181

Overall patient safety: ★★★
Teaching: N

CLINICAL PROGRAM RATINGS:

CARDIAC	NR	ORTHOPEDICS	NR
CRITICAL CARE	NR	PULMONARY	★★★
GASTROINTESTINAL	NR	STROKE	★★★
GENERAL SURGERY	NR	VASCULAR	NR
MATERNITY CARE	★★★★★	WOMEN'S HEALTH	NR

HEALTHGRADES AWARDS

UW Health-UW Hospitals and Clinics

600 Highland Avenue
Madison, WI 53792
(608) 263-6400

Overall patient safety: ★★★
Teaching: Y

CLINICAL PROGRAM RATINGS:

CARDIAC	★★★	ORTHOPEDICS	★
CRITICAL CARE	★★★★★	PULMONARY	★★★★★
GASTROINTESTINAL	★★★	STROKE	★★★
GENERAL SURGERY	★★★	VASCULAR	★★★
MATERNITY CARE	NR	WOMEN'S HEALTH	NR

HEALTHGRADES AWARDS

✓ **DISTINGUISHED HOSPITAL**
· CLINICAL EXCELLENCE

✓ **SPECIALTY EXCELLENCE**
· CARDIAC SURGERY
· CRITICAL CARE
· GASTROINTESTINAL CARE
· PULMONARY CARE

United Hospital System

6308 8th Avenue
Kenosha, WI 53143
(262) 656-2011

Overall patient safety: ★★★
Teaching: N

CLINICAL PROGRAM RATINGS:

CARDIAC	★★★	ORTHOPEDICS	★★★
CRITICAL CARE	★	PULMONARY	★
GASTROINTESTINAL	★★★	STROKE	★
GENERAL SURGERY	★★★	VASCULAR	NR
MATERNITY CARE	★★★	WOMEN'S HEALTH	★

HEALTHGRADES AWARDS

✓ **SPECIALTY EXCELLENCE**
· CARDIAC SURGERY

Vernon Memorial Hospital

507 Main Street
Viroqua, WI 54665
(608) 637-2101

Overall patient safety: ★★★
Teaching: N

CLINICAL PROGRAM RATINGS:

CARDIAC	NR	ORTHOPEDICS	NR
CRITICAL CARE	NR	PULMONARY	NR
GASTROINTESTINAL	NR	STROKE	★★★
GENERAL SURGERY	NR	VASCULAR	NR
MATERNITY CARE	★★★	WOMEN'S HEALTH	NR

HEALTHGRADES AWARDS

Upland Hills Health

800 Compassion Way
Dodgeville, WI 53533
(608) 930-8000

Overall patient safety: ★★★
Teaching: N

CLINICAL PROGRAM RATINGS:

CARDIAC	NR	ORTHOPEDICS	NR
CRITICAL CARE	NR	PULMONARY	★★★
GASTROINTESTINAL	NR	STROKE	★★★
GENERAL SURGERY	NR	VASCULAR	NR
MATERNITY CARE	★★★	WOMEN'S HEALTH	NR

HEALTHGRADES AWARDS

Watertown Memorial Hospital

125 Hospital Drive
Watertown, WI 53098
(920) 261-4210

Overall patient safety: ★★★
Teaching: N

CLINICAL PROGRAM RATINGS:

CARDIAC	NR	ORTHOPEDICS	NR
CRITICAL CARE	NR	PULMONARY	★★★
GASTROINTESTINAL	NR	STROKE	★★★
GENERAL SURGERY	★★★	VASCULAR	NR
MATERNITY CARE	★★★	WOMEN'S HEALTH	NR

HEALTHGRADES AWARDS

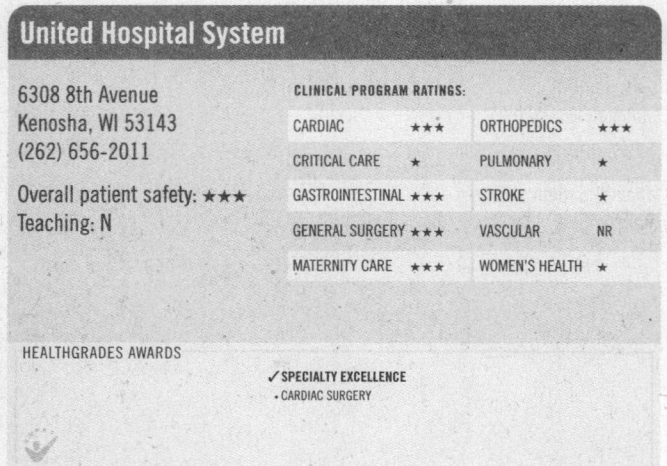
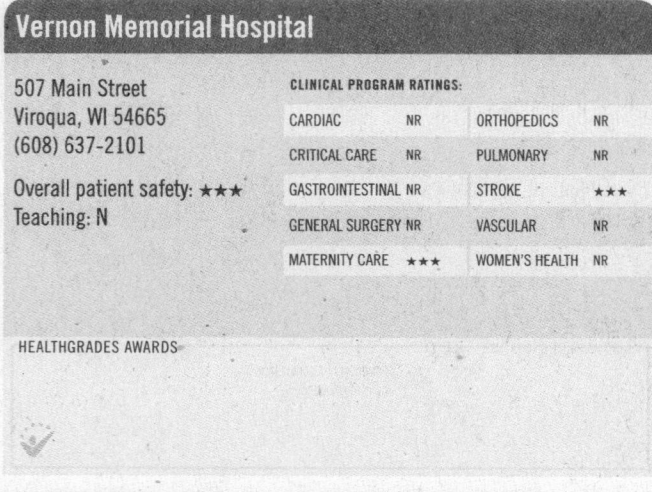
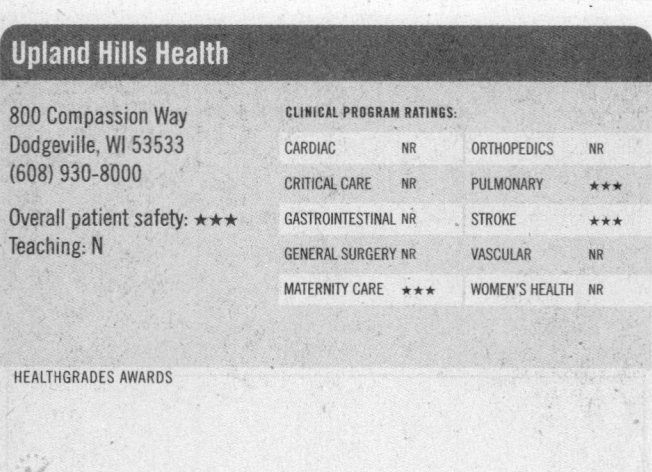

KEY: ★★★★★ BEST ★★★ AS EXPECTED ★ POOR NR NOT RATED BY HEALTHGRADES For full definitions of ratings and awards, see Appendix.

Waukesha Memorial Hospital

725 American Avenue
Waukesha, WI 53188
(262) 928-1000

Overall patient safety: ★★★★★
Teaching: Y

CLINICAL PROGRAM RATINGS:

CARDIAC	★★★	ORTHOPEDICS	★★★
CRITICAL CARE	★★★	PULMONARY	★★★
GASTROINTESTINAL	★★★	STROKE	★
GENERAL SURGERY	★★★	VASCULAR	★★★
MATERNITY CARE	★★★	WOMEN'S HEALTH	★★★★★

HEALTHGRADES AWARDS

✓ DISTINGUISHED HOSPITAL
- PATIENT SAFETY

✓ SPECIALTY EXCELLENCE
- CARDIAC CARE
- CARDIAC SURGERY
- WOMEN'S HEALTH

Wheaton Franciscan Healthcare—Elmbrook Memorial

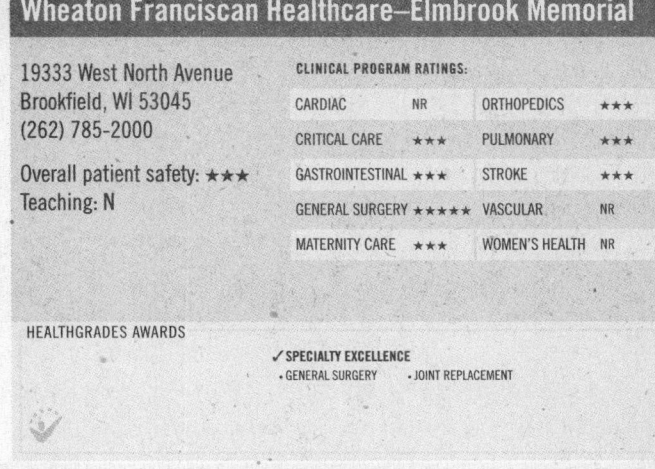

19333 West North Avenue
Brookfield, WI 53045
(262) 785-2000

Overall patient safety: ★★★
Teaching: N

CLINICAL PROGRAM RATINGS:

CARDIAC	NR	ORTHOPEDICS	★★★
CRITICAL CARE	★★★	PULMONARY	★★★
GASTROINTESTINAL	★★★	STROKE	★★★
GENERAL SURGERY	★★★★★	VASCULAR	NR
MATERNITY CARE	★★★	WOMEN'S HEALTH	NR

HEALTHGRADES AWARDS

✓ SPECIALTY EXCELLENCE
- GENERAL SURGERY
- JOINT REPLACEMENT

Waupun Memorial Hospital

620 West Brown Street
Waupun, WI 53963
(920) 324-5581

Overall patient safety: ★★★
Teaching: N

CLINICAL PROGRAM RATINGS:

CARDIAC	NR	ORTHOPEDICS	NR
CRITICAL CARE	NR	PULMONARY	★★★
GASTROINTESTINAL	NR	STROKE	★★★
GENERAL SURGERY	NR	VASCULAR	NR
MATERNITY CARE	★	WOMEN'S HEALTH	NR

HEALTHGRADES AWARDS

Wheaton Franciscan Healthcare—St. Francis

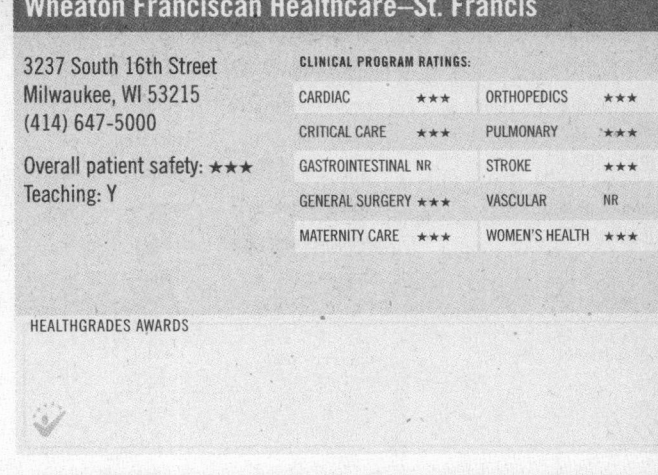

3237 South 16th Street
Milwaukee, WI 53215
(414) 647-5000

Overall patient safety: ★★★
Teaching: Y

CLINICAL PROGRAM RATINGS:

CARDIAC	★★★	ORTHOPEDICS	★★★
CRITICAL CARE	★★★	PULMONARY	★★★
GASTROINTESTINAL	NR	STROKE	★★★
GENERAL SURGERY	★★★	VASCULAR	NR
MATERNITY CARE	★★★	WOMEN'S HEALTH	★★★

HEALTHGRADES AWARDS

West Allis Memorial Hospital

8901 West Lincoln Avenue
West Allis, WI 53227
(414) 328-6000

Overall patient safety: ★★★★★
Teaching: Y

CLINICAL PROGRAM RATINGS:

CARDIAC	NR	ORTHOPEDICS	★★★
CRITICAL CARE	★★★★★	PULMONARY	★★★
GASTROINTESTINAL	★★★	STROKE	★★★★★
GENERAL SURGERY	★★★	VASCULAR	NR
MATERNITY CARE	★★★	WOMEN'S HEALTH	NR

HEALTHGRADES AWARDS

✓ DISTINGUISHED HOSPITAL
- CLINICAL EXCELLENCE
- PATIENT SAFETY

✓ SPECIALTY EXCELLENCE
- CRITICAL CARE
- GASTROINTESTINAL CARE
- STROKE CARE

Wheaton Franciscan Healthcare—St. Joseph*

5000 West Chambers Street
Milwaukee, WI 53210
(414) 447-2000

Overall patient safety: ★★★
Teaching: Y

CLINICAL PROGRAM RATINGS:

CARDIAC	★★★	ORTHOPEDICS	NR
CRITICAL CARE	★★★	PULMONARY	★★★
GASTROINTESTINAL	NR	STROKE	★★★
GENERAL SURGERY	★	VASCULAR	NR
MATERNITY CARE	★★★	WOMEN'S HEALTH	★★★

HEALTHGRADES AWARDS

*This hospital reports its data to the federal government jointly with another hospital. Therefore the ratings and awards apply to multiple hospitals and this specific hospital may not provide all rated services.

Wisconsin Heart Hospital

10000 West Blue Mound Road
Wauwatosa, WI 53226
(414) 778-7800

Overall patient safety: ★★★
Teaching: N

CLINICAL PROGRAM RATINGS:

CARDIAC	★★★	ORTHOPEDICS	NR
CRITICAL CARE	NR	PULMONARY	NR
GASTROINTESTINAL	NR	STROKE	NR
GENERAL SURGERY	NR	VASCULAR	NR
MATERNITY CARE	NR	WOMEN'S HEALTH	NR

HEALTHGRADES AWARDS

WYOMING HOSPITALS: RATINGS BY CLINICAL SPECIALTY

Campbell County Memorial Hospital

501 South Burma Avenue
Gillette, WY 82716
(307) 682-8811

Overall patient safety: ★
Teaching: N

CLINICAL PROGRAM RATINGS:

CARDIAC	NR	ORTHOPEDICS	NR
CRITICAL CARE	NR	PULMONARY	★★★
GASTROINTESTINAL	NR	STROKE	★★★
GENERAL SURGERY	NR	VASCULAR	NR
MATERNITY CARE	NR	WOMEN'S HEALTH	NR

HEALTHGRADES AWARDS

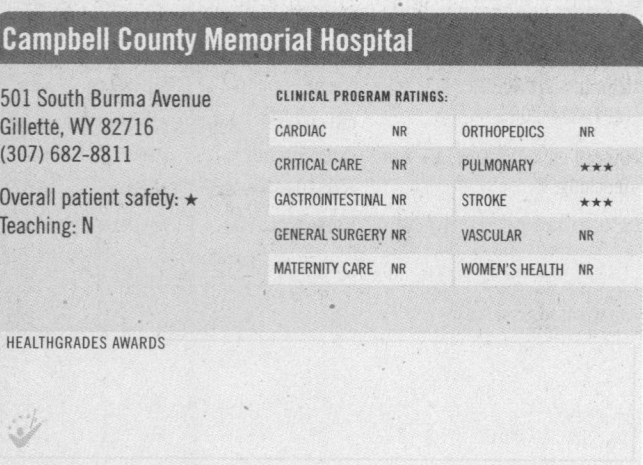

Community Hospital

2000 Campbell Drive
Torrington, WY 82240
(307) 532-4181

Overall patient safety: ★★★
Teaching: N

CLINICAL PROGRAM RATINGS:

CARDIAC	NR	ORTHOPEDICS	NR
CRITICAL CARE	NR	PULMONARY	★
GASTROINTESTINAL	NR	STROKE	NR
GENERAL SURGERY	NR	VASCULAR	NR
MATERNITY CARE	NR	WOMEN'S HEALTH	NR

HEALTHGRADES AWARDS

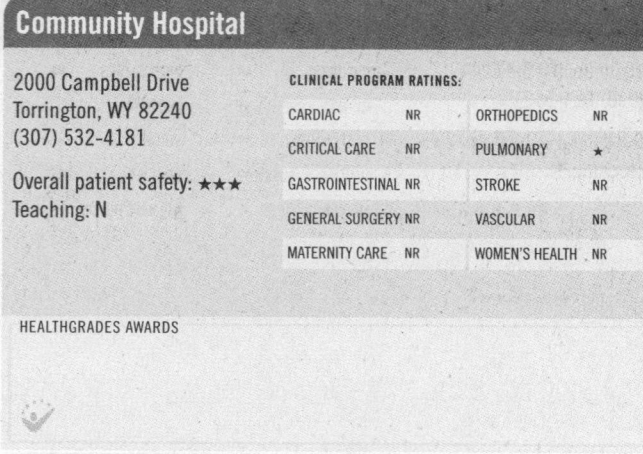

Cheyenne Regional Medical Center*

214 East 23rd Street
Cheyenne, WY 82001
(307) 634-2273

Overall patient safety: ★★★
Teaching: Y

CLINICAL PROGRAM RATINGS:

CARDIAC	★	ORTHOPEDICS	★★★
CRITICAL CARE	NR	PULMONARY	★
GASTROINTESTINAL	★★★	STROKE	★★★
GENERAL SURGERY	NR	VASCULAR	NR
MATERNITY CARE	NR	WOMEN'S HEALTH	NR

HEALTHGRADES AWARDS

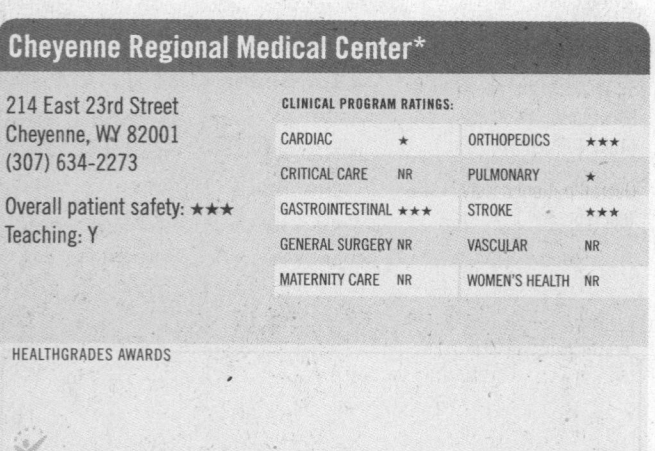

Depaul Hospital*

2600 East 18th Street
Cheyenne, WY 82001
(307) 632-6411

Overall patient safety: ★★★
Teaching: Y

CLINICAL PROGRAM RATINGS:

CARDIAC	★	ORTHOPEDICS	★★★
CRITICAL CARE	NR	PULMONARY	★
GASTROINTESTINAL	★★★	STROKE	★★★
GENERAL SURGERY	NR	VASCULAR	NR
MATERNITY CARE	NR	WOMEN'S HEALTH	NR

HEALTHGRADES AWARDS

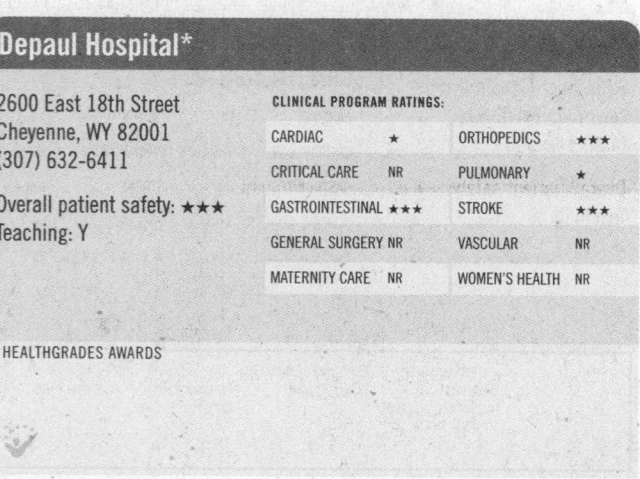

KEY: ★★★★★ BEST ★★★ AS EXPECTED ★ POOR NR NOT RATED BY HEALTHGRADES For full definitions of ratings and awards, see Appendix.

Evanston Regional Hospital

190 Arrowhead Drive
Evanston, WY 82930
(307) 789-3636

Overall patient safety: ★★★
Teaching: N

CLINICAL PROGRAM RATINGS:

CARDIAC	NR	ORTHOPEDICS	NR
CRITICAL CARE	NR	PULMONARY	★★★
GASTROINTESTINAL	NR	STROKE	NR
GENERAL SURGERY	NR	VASCULAR	NR
MATERNITY CARE	NR	WOMEN'S HEALTH	NR

HEALTHGRADES AWARDS

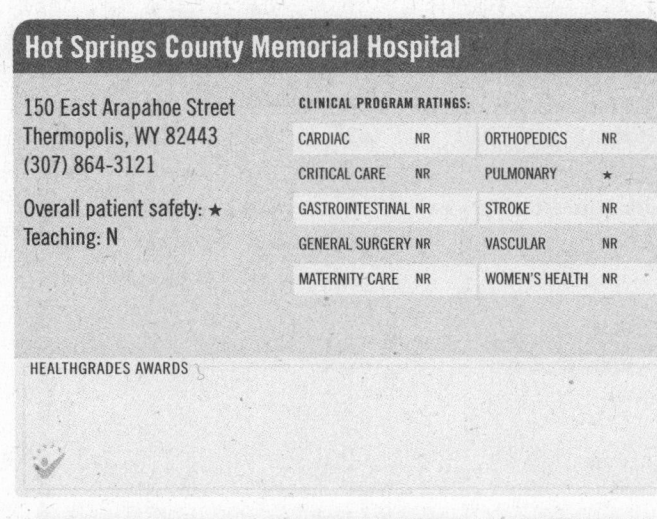

Lander Valley Medical Center

1320 Bishop Randall Drive
Lander, WY 82520
(307) 332-4420

Overall patient safety: ★★★
Teaching: N

CLINICAL PROGRAM RATINGS:

CARDIAC	NR	ORTHOPEDICS	NR
CRITICAL CARE	NR	PULMONARY	★★★
GASTROINTESTINAL	NR	STROKE	NR
GENERAL SURGERY	NR	VASCULAR	NR
MATERNITY CARE	NR	WOMEN'S HEALTH	NR

HEALTHGRADES AWARDS

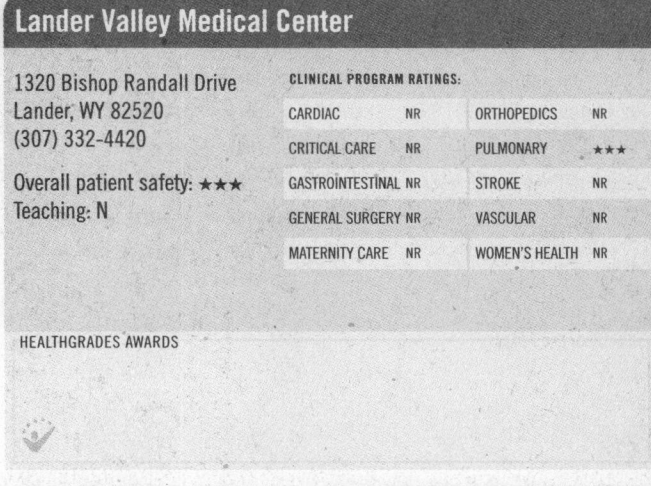

Hot Springs County Memorial Hospital

150 East Arapahoe Street
Thermopolis, WY 82443
(307) 864-3121

Overall patient safety: ★
Teaching: N

CLINICAL PROGRAM RATINGS:

CARDIAC	NR	ORTHOPEDICS	NR
CRITICAL CARE	NR	PULMONARY	★
GASTROINTESTINAL	NR	STROKE	NR
GENERAL SURGERY	NR	VASCULAR	NR
MATERNITY CARE	NR	WOMEN'S HEALTH	NR

HEALTHGRADES AWARDS

Memorial Hospital of Carbon County

2221 West Elm Street
Rawlins, WY 82301
(307) 324-2221

Overall patient safety: ★★★
Teaching: N

CLINICAL PROGRAM RATINGS:

CARDIAC	NR	ORTHOPEDICS	NR
CRITICAL CARE	NR	PULMONARY	★★★
GASTROINTESTINAL	NR	STROKE	NR
GENERAL SURGERY	NR	VASCULAR	NR
MATERNITY CARE	NR	WOMEN'S HEALTH	NR

HEALTHGRADES AWARDS

Ivinson Memorial Hospital

255 North 30th Street
Laramie, WY 82072
(307) 742-2141

Overall patient safety: ★★★
Teaching: N

CLINICAL PROGRAM RATINGS:

CARDIAC	NR	ORTHOPEDICS	★★★
CRITICAL CARE	NR	PULMONARY	★★★
GASTROINTESTINAL	NR	STROKE	★★★
GENERAL SURGERY	NR	VASCULAR	NR
MATERNITY CARE	NR	WOMEN'S HEALTH	NR

HEALTHGRADES AWARDS

Memorial Hospital of Sheridan County

1401 West 5th Street
Sheridan, WY 82801
(307) 672-1000

Overall patient safety: ★★★
Teaching: N

CLINICAL PROGRAM RATINGS:

CARDIAC	NR	ORTHOPEDICS	★★★
CRITICAL CARE	NR	PULMONARY	★
GASTROINTESTINAL	NR	STROKE	★
GENERAL SURGERY	NR	VASCULAR	NR
MATERNITY CARE	NR	WOMEN'S HEALTH	NR

HEALTHGRADES AWARDS

*This hospital reports its data to the federal government jointly with another hospital. Therefore the ratings and awards apply to multiple hospitals and this specific hospital may not provide all rated services.

Memorial Hospital Sweetwater County

1200 College Drive
Rock Springs, WY 82901
(307) 362-3711

Overall patient safety: ★★★
Teaching: N

CLINICAL PROGRAM RATINGS:

CARDIAC	NR	ORTHOPEDICS	NR
CRITICAL CARE	NR	PULMONARY	★★★
GASTROINTESTINAL	NR	STROKE	★
GENERAL SURGERY	NR	VASCULAR	NR
MATERNITY CARE	NR	WOMEN'S HEALTH	NR

HEALTHGRADES AWARDS

Riverton Memorial Hospital

2100 West Sunset Drive
Riverton, WY 82501
(307) 856-4161

Overall patient safety: ★★★
Teaching: N

CLINICAL PROGRAM RATINGS:

CARDIAC	NR	ORTHOPEDICS	NR
CRITICAL CARE	NR	PULMONARY	★★★
GASTROINTESTINAL	NR	STROKE	★★★
GENERAL SURGERY	NR	VASCULAR	NR
MATERNITY CARE	NR	WOMEN'S HEALTH	NR

HEALTHGRADES AWARDS

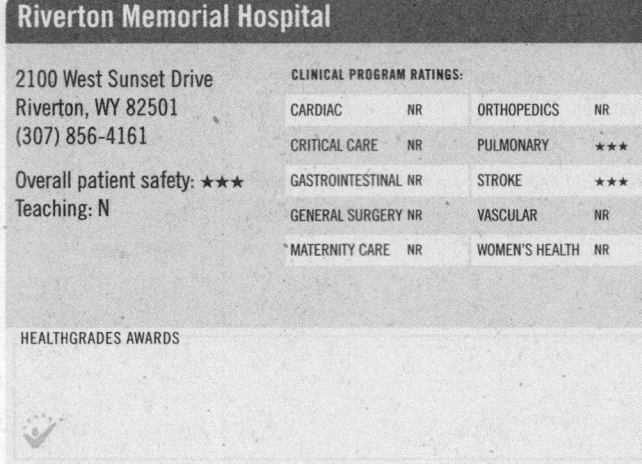

Platte County Memorial Hospital

201 14th Street
Wheatland, WY 82201
(307) 322-3636

Overall patient safety: ★★★
Teaching: N

CLINICAL PROGRAM RATINGS:

CARDIAC	NR	ORTHOPEDICS	NR
CRITICAL CARE	NR	PULMONARY	★★★
GASTROINTESTINAL	NR	STROKE	NR
GENERAL SURGERY	NR	VASCULAR	NR
MATERNITY CARE	NR	WOMEN'S HEALTH	NR

HEALTHGRADES AWARDS

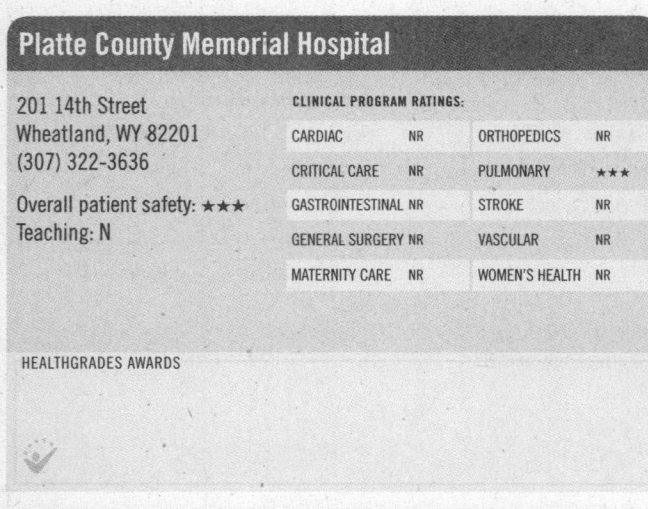

St. John's Medical Center

625 East Broadway
Jackson Hole, WY 83001
(307) 733-3636

Overall patient safety: ★★★
Teaching: N

CLINICAL PROGRAM RATINGS:

CARDIAC	NR	ORTHOPEDICS	NR
CRITICAL CARE	NR	PULMONARY	★★★
GASTROINTESTINAL	NR	STROKE	NR
GENERAL SURGERY	NR	VASCULAR	NR
MATERNITY CARE	NR	WOMEN'S HEALTH	NR

HEALTHGRADES AWARDS

Powell Valley Hospital

777 Avenue H
Powell, WY 82435
(307) 754-2267

Overall patient safety: ★★★
Teaching: N

CLINICAL PROGRAM RATINGS:

CARDIAC	NR	ORTHOPEDICS	NR
CRITICAL CARE	NR	PULMONARY	★★★
GASTROINTESTINAL	NR	STROKE	★★★
GENERAL SURGERY	NR	VASCULAR	NR
MATERNITY CARE	NR	WOMEN'S HEALTH	NR

HEALTHGRADES AWARDS

Washakie Medical Center

400 South 15th Street
Worland, WY 82401
(307) 347-3221

Overall patient safety: ★★★
Teaching: N

CLINICAL PROGRAM RATINGS:

CARDIAC	NR	ORTHOPEDICS	NR
CRITICAL CARE	NR	PULMONARY	★
GASTROINTESTINAL	NR	STROKE	NR
GENERAL SURGERY	NR	VASCULAR	NR
MATERNITY CARE	NR	WOMEN'S HEALTH	NR

HEALTHGRADES AWARDS

KEY: ★★★★★ BEST   ★★★ AS EXPECTED   ★ POOR   NR NOT RATED BY HEALTHGRADES   For full definitions of ratings and awards, see Appendix.

West Park Hospital District

707 Sheridan Avenue
Cody, WY 82414
(307) 527-7501

Overall patient safety: ★
Teaching: N

CLINICAL PROGRAM RATINGS:

CARDIAC	NR	ORTHOPEDICS	★
CRITICAL CARE	NR	PULMONARY	★★★★★
GASTROINTESTINAL	NR	STROKE	★★★
GENERAL SURGERY	NR	VASCULAR	NR
MATERNITY CARE	NR	WOMEN'S HEALTH	NR

HEALTHGRADES AWARDS

Wyoming Medical Center

1233 East 2nd Street
Casper, WY 82601
(307) 577-7201

Overall patient safety: ★★★
Teaching: Y

CLINICAL PROGRAM RATINGS:

CARDIAC	★★★	ORTHOPEDICS	★★★
CRITICAL CARE	NR	PULMONARY	★★★
GASTROINTESTINAL	★★★	STROKE	★★★
GENERAL SURGERY	NR	VASCULAR	NR
MATERNITY CARE	NR	WOMEN'S HEALTH	NR

HEALTHGRADES AWARDS

CHAPTER 7

FIVE STAR RATED HOSPITALS

FIVE STAR RATED HOSPITALS

In this chapter, you will find a listing of hospitals that HealthGrades has awarded with a five star rating. These "top hospitals" have passed through HealthGrades' rigorous screening process, and have demonstrated better results than their competitors by having lower mortality and complication rates over a three-year period.

All of the hospitals in this section are listed by state for easy reference, as location is frequently the first determining factor when choosing a hospital. After you have located a selection of hospitals that are conveniently located, you will be able to peruse the listing of clinical specialties in which each hospital excels, such as maternity or cardiac care. Once you have determined which five star rated hospital best suits your needs, you can find the hospital's contact information by referring to Chapter 6, titled "Hospital Ratings by Clinical Specialty."

Once you've selected the best hospital for your needs, you'll be ready to research the top physicians in their fields who might perform your procedure or provide any type of healthcare. To do so, turn to Chapter 9, titled "Top Doctors," for our listing of exemplary physicians.

BARIATRIC SURGERY

None

CARDIAC

ATRIAL FIBRILLATION

None

CORONARY INTERVENTIONAL PROCEDURES (ANGIOPLASTY/STENT)

Providence Hospital, Mobile

HEART ATTACK

None

HEART BYPASS SURGERY

Huntsville Hospital, Huntsville
Northeast Alabama Regional Medical Center, Anniston
University of Alabama Hospital, Birmingham

HEART FAILURE

DCH Regional Medical Center, Tuscaloosa
LTC Hospital of Tuscaloosa, Tuscaloosa

VALVE REPLACEMENT SURGERY

Huntsville Hospital, Huntsville
University of Alabama Hospital, Birmingham

CRITICAL CARE

DIABETIC ACIDOSIS AND COMA

Mobile Infirmary, Mobile

PULMONARY EMBOLISM

None

RESPIRATORY FAILURE

Chilton Medical Center, Clanton
DCH Regional Medical Center, Tuscaloosa
LTC Hospital of Tuscaloosa, Tuscaloosa
Walker Baptist Medical Center, Jasper

SEPSIS

Andalusia Regional Hospital, Andalusia
G. H. Lanier Memorial Hospital, Valley
Lawrence Medical Center, Moulton
Southwest Alabama Medical Center, Thomasville

GASTROINTESTINAL

BOWEL OBSTRUCTION

L. V. Stabler Memorial Hospital, Greenville
Walker Baptist Medical Center, Jasper

CHOLECYSTECTOMY

Andalusia Regional Hospital, Andalusia
Baptist Medical Center–Dekalb, Fort Payne
Baptist Medical Center–South, Montgomery
East Alabama Medical Center and Skilled Nursing Facility, Opelika
G. H. Lanier Memorial Hospital, Valley
Huntsville Hospital, Huntsville
Marshall Medical Center–North, Guntersville
Providence Hospital, Mobile
Troy Regional Medical Center, Troy
Wiregrass Medical Center, Geneva

GASTROINTESTINAL BLEED

DCH Regional Medical Center, Tuscaloosa
Lake Martin Community Hospital, Dadeville
LTC Hospital of Tuscaloosa, Tuscaloosa
South Baldwin Regional Medical Center, Foley

GASTROINTESTINAL SURGERIES AND PROCEDURES

None

PANCREATITIS

Springhill Medical Center, Mobile

GENERAL SURGERY

APPENDECTOMY

None

MATERNITY CARE

None

ORTHOPEDICS

BACK AND NECK SURGERY (EXCEPT SPINAL FUSION)

East Alabama Medical Center and Skilled Nursing Facility, Opelika
Jackson Hospital and Clinic, Montgomery
St. Vincent's–East, Birmingham

BACK AND NECK SURGERY (SPINAL FUSION)

Brookwood Medical Center, Birmingham
Carraway Methodist Medical Center, Birmingham
Gadsden Regional Medical Center, Gadsden
Jackson Hospital and Clinic, Montgomery
Mobile Infirmary, Mobile
St. Vincent's–East, Birmingham
University of Alabama Hospital, Birmingham
Walker Baptist Medical Center, Jasper

HIP FRACTURE REPAIR

Carraway Methodist Medical Center, Birmingham
Cullman Regional Medical Center, Cullman
East Alabama Medical Center and Skilled Nursing Facility, Opelika
Mobile Infirmary, Mobile
Northeast Alabama Regional Medical Center, Anniston
Riverview Regional Medical Center, Gadsden
St. Vincent's–Birmingham, Birmingham
Shoals Hospital, Muscle Shoals
Walker Baptist Medical Center, Jasper
Woodland Medical Center, Cullman

TOTAL HIP REPLACEMENT

None

TOTAL KNEE REPLACEMENT

Andalusia Regional Hospital, Andalusia
Brookwood Medical Center, Birmingham
Crestwood Medical Center, Huntsville
East Alabama Medical Center and Skilled Nursing Facility, Opelika
Huntsville Hospital, Huntsville
Jackson Hospital and Clinic, Montgomery
Providence Hospital, Mobile
St. Vincent's–Birmingham, Birmingham
Walker Baptist Medical Center, Jasper

PROSTATECTOMY

Andalusia Regional Hospital, Andalusia
Brookwood Medical Center, Birmingham
St. Vincent's–Birmingham, Birmingham

PULMONARY

CHRONIC OBSTRUCTIVE PULMONARY DISEASE (COPD)

Baptist Citizens, Talladega
DCH Regional Medical Center, Tuscaloosa
G. H. Lanier Memorial Hospital, Valley
LTC Hospital of Tuscaloosa, Tuscaloosa
Wiregrass Medical Center, Geneva

PNEUMONIA

DCH Regional Medical Center, Tuscaloosa
Flowers Hospital, Dothan
G. H. Lanier Memorial Hospital, Valley
Lawrence Medical Center, Moulton
LTC Hospital of Tuscaloosa, Tuscaloosa

Hospitals receiving a five star rating in a particular procedure have patient outcomes that put them among the best in the nation. For full definitions of ratings and awards, see Appendix.

STROKE

Coosa Valley Medical Center, Sylacauga
DCH Regional Medical Center, Tuscaloosa
Lawrence Medical Center, Moulton
LTC Hospital of Tuscaloosa, Tuscaloosa
Providence Hospital, Mobile
Riverview Regional Medical Center, Gadsden

VASCULAR

CAROTID SURGERY
Baptist Medical Center–South, Montgomery
Brookwood Medical Center, Birmingham

PERIPHERAL VASCULAR BYPASS
Gadsden Regional Medical Center, Gadsden
Mobile Infirmary, Mobile

RESECTION/REPLACEMENT OF ABDOMINAL AORTA
None

WOMEN'S HEALTH
None

ALASKA HOSPITALS: FIVE STAR RATED FACILITIES

BARIATRIC SURGERY
None

CARDIAC

ATRIAL FIBRILLATION
Providence Alaska Medical Center, Anchorage

CORONARY INTERVENTIONAL PROCEDURES (ANGIOPLASTY/STENT)
None

HEART ATTACK
None

HEART BYPASS SURGERY
Providence Alaska Medical Center, Anchorage

HEART FAILURE
None

VALVE REPLACEMENT SURGERY
Providence Alaska Medical Center, Anchorage

CRITICAL CARE

DIABETIC ACIDOSIS AND COMA
None

PULMONARY EMBOLISM
None

RESPIRATORY FAILURE
None

SEPSIS
Alaska Native Medical Center, Anchorage
Providence Alaska Medical Center, Anchorage

GASTROINTESTINAL

BOWEL OBSTRUCTION
None

CHOLECYSTECTOMY
Providence Alaska Medical Center, Anchorage

GASTROINTESTINAL BLEED
Providence Alaska Medical Center, Anchorage

GASTROINTESTINAL SURGERIES AND PROCEDURES
None

PANCREATITIS
None

GENERAL SURGERY

APPENDECTOMY
None

MATERNITY CARE
None

ORTHOPEDICS

BACK AND NECK SURGERY (EXCEPT SPINAL FUSION)
None

BACK AND NECK SURGERY (SPINAL FUSION)
None

HIP FRACTURE REPAIR
None

TOTAL HIP REPLACEMENT
None

TOTAL KNEE REPLACEMENT
None

PROSTATECTOMY
None

PULMONARY

CHRONIC OBSTRUCTIVE PULMONARY DISEASE (COPD)
None

PNEUMONIA
Providence Alaska Medical Center, Anchorage

STROKE
None

VASCULAR

CAROTID SURGERY
None

PERIPHERAL VASCULAR BYPASS
None

RESECTION/REPLACEMENT OF ABDOMINAL AORTA
None

WOMEN'S HEALTH
None

BARIATRIC SURGERY

Banner Good Samaritan Medical Center, Phoenix
Mayo Clinic Hospital, Phoenix
Scottsdale Healthcare—Shea, Scottsdale

CARDIAC

ATRIAL FIBRILLATION

Banner Baywood Heart Hospital, Mesa
Banner Good Samaritan Medical Center, Phoenix
Mayo Clinic Hospital, Phoenix
Tucson Heart Hospital, Tucson
Walter O. Boswell Memorial Hospital, Sun City

CORONARY INTERVENTIONAL PROCEDURES (ANGIOPLASTY/STENT)

Arizona Heart Hospital, Phoenix
Banner Thunderbird Medical Center, Glendale
Mayo Clinic Hospital, Phoenix

HEART ATTACK

Arizona Heart Hospital, Phoenix
Banner Baywood Heart Hospital, Mesa
Banner Baywood Medical Center, Mesa
Banner Thunderbird Medical Center, Glendale
Mayo Clinic Hospital, Phoenix
Northwest Medical Center, Tucson
Scottsdale Healthcare—Osborn, Scottsdale
Scottsdale Healthcare—Shea, Scottsdale
Tucson Heart Hospital, Tucson
University Medical Center, Tucson
West Valley Hospital, Goodyear

HEART BYPASS SURGERY

Banner Desert Medical Center, Mesa
Tucson Medical Center, Tucson

HEART FAILURE

Arizona Heart Hospital, Phoenix
Banner Baywood Heart Hospital, Mesa
Banner Baywood Medical Center, Mesa
Banner Estrella Medical Center, Phoenix
Banner Good Samaritan Medical Center, Phoenix
Banner Thunderbird Medical Center, Glendale
Casa Grande Regional Medical Center, Casa Grande
Chandler Regional Hospital, Chandler
Del E. Webb Memorial Hospital, Sun City West
John C. Lincoln Deer Valley Hospital, Phoenix
John C. Lincoln North Mountain Hospital, Phoenix
Mayo Clinic Hospital, Phoenix
Northwest Medical Center, Tucson
Paradise Valley Hospital, Phoenix

Payson Regional Medical Center, Payson
Scottsdale Healthcare—Osborn, Scottsdale
Scottsdale Healthcare—Shea, Scottsdale
Tempe St. Luke's Hospital, Tempe
Tucson Heart Hospital, Tucson
Walter O. Boswell Memorial Hospital, Sun City
Yuma Regional Medical Center, Yuma

VALVE REPLACEMENT SURGERY

Banner Good Samaritan Medical Center, Phoenix
Mayo Clinic Hospital, Phoenix
Walter O. Boswell Memorial Hospital, Sun City

CRITICAL CARE

DIABETIC ACIDOSIS AND COMA

Flagstaff Medical Center, Flagstaff
Yuma Regional Medical Center, Yuma

PULMONARY EMBOLISM

Walter O. Boswell Memorial Hospital, Sun City

RESPIRATORY FAILURE

Arrowhead Hospital, Glendale
Banner Baywood Medical Center, Mesa
Banner Thunderbird Medical Center, Glendale
Casa Grande Regional Medical Center, Casa Grande
John C. Lincoln Deer Valley Hospital, Phoenix
Maryvale Hospital, Phoenix
Payson Regional Medical Center, Payson
Scottsdale Healthcare—Shea, Scottsdale

SEPSIS

Arrowhead Hospital, Glendale
Banner Baywood Medical Center, Mesa
Banner Estrella Medical Center, Phoenix
Banner Good Samaritan Medical Center, Phoenix
Banner Thunderbird Medical Center, Glendale
Casa Grande Regional Medical Center, Casa Grande
Del E. Webb Memorial Hospital, Sun City West
Maryvale Hospital, Phoenix
Mayo Clinic Hospital, Phoenix
Northwest Medical Center, Tucson
Paradise Valley Hospital, Phoenix
Payson Regional Medical Center, Payson
Phoenix Memorial Hospital, Phoenix
St. Joseph's Hospital and Medical Center, Phoenix
Scottsdale Healthcare—Osborn, Scottsdale
Tucson Medical Center, Tucson
University Medical Center, Tucson
Walter O. Boswell Memorial Hospital, Sun City
West Valley Hospital, Goodyear

GASTROINTESTINAL

BOWEL OBSTRUCTION

Banner Baywood Medical Center, Mesa
Northwest Medical Center, Tucson
Tucson Medical Center, Tucson

CHOLECYSTECTOMY

Kingman Regional Medical Center, Kingman
Mayo Clinic Hospital, Phoenix
Tucson Medical Center, Tucson
Yavapai Regional Medical Center, Prescott

GASTROINTESTINAL BLEED

Banner Thunderbird Medical Center, Glendale
Del E. Webb Memorial Hospital, Sun City West
La Paz Regional Hospital, Parker
Maricopa Medical Center, Phoenix

GASTROINTESTINAL SURGERIES AND PROCEDURES

Chandler Regional Hospital, Chandler
Mayo Clinic Hospital, Phoenix
Northwest Medical Center, Tucson
Payson Regional Medical Center, Payson
St. Joseph's Hospital and Medical Center, Phoenix
Scottsdale Healthcare—Osborn, Scottsdale

PANCREATITIS

None

GENERAL SURGERY

APPENDECTOMY

Banner Baywood Medical Center, Mesa
Banner Mesa Medical Center, Mesa
Del E. Webb Memorial Hospital, Sun City West
Kingman Regional Medical Center, Kingman
Scottsdale Healthcare—Osborn, Scottsdale
Scottsdale Healthcare—Shea, Scottsdale
Yavapai Regional Medical Center, Prescott

MATERNITY CARE

Arrowhead Hospital, Glendale
Banner Baywood Medical Center, Mesa
Carondelet Holy Cross Hospital, Nogales
John C. Lincoln North Mountain Hospital, Phoenix
Paradise Valley Hospital, Phoenix
Scottsdale Healthcare—Osborn, Scottsdale
Verde Valley Medical Center, Cottonwood

ORTHOPEDICS

BACK AND NECK SURGERY (EXCEPT SPINAL FUSION)
Carondelet St. Joseph's Hospital and Health Center, Tucson
Mayo Clinic Hospital, Phoenix

BACK AND NECK SURGERY (SPINAL FUSION)
Flagstaff Medical Center, Flagstaff
Mayo Clinic Hospital, Phoenix

HIP FRACTURE REPAIR
Arrowhead Hospital, Glendale
Banner Baywood Medical Center, Mesa
Banner Estrella Medical Center, Phoenix
Havasu Regional Medical Center, Lake Havasu City
Northwest Medical Center, Tucson
Paradise Valley Hospital, Phoenix
Scottsdale Healthcare–Shea, Scottsdale
Tucson Medical Center, Tucson
Yavapai Regional Medical Center, Prescott

TOTAL HIP REPLACEMENT
Northwest Medical Center, Tucson
Northwest Medical Center–Oro Valley, Oro Valley
Scottsdale Healthcare–Osborn, Scottsdale
Walter O. Boswell Memorial Hospital, Sun City
Yavapai Regional Medical Center, Prescott

TOTAL KNEE REPLACEMENT
Casa Grande Regional Medical Center, Casa Grande
Scottsdale Healthcare–Osborn, Scottsdale
Yavapai Regional Medical Center, Prescott

PROSTATECTOMY
Mayo Clinic Hospital, Phoenix
Scottsdale Healthcare–Shea, Scottsdale
Tucson Medical Center, Tucson

PULMONARY

CHRONIC OBSTRUCTIVE PULMONARY DISEASE (COPD)
Arizona Heart Hospital, Phoenix
Banner Thunderbird Medical Center, Glendale
Del E. Webb Memorial Hospital, Sun City West
John C. Lincoln Deer Valley Hospital, Phoenix
La Paz Regional Hospital, Parker
Maricopa Medical Center, Phoenix

PNEUMONIA
Arizona Heart Hospital, Phoenix
Arrowhead Hospital, Glendale
Banner Baywood Heart Hospital, Mesa
Banner Baywood Medical Center, Mesa
Banner Good Samaritan Medical Center, Phoenix
Banner Mesa Medical Center, Mesa
Banner Thunderbird Medical Center, Glendale
Carondelet St. Mary's Hospital and Health Center, Tucson
Chandler Regional Hospital, Chandler
Del E. Webb Memorial Hospital, Sun City West
El Dorado Hospital, Tucson
John C. Lincoln Deer Valley Hospital, Phoenix
La Paz Regional Hospital, Parker
Maricopa Medical Center, Phoenix
Maryvale Hospital, Phoenix
Mayo Clinic Hospital, Phoenix
Navapache Regional Medical Center, Show Low
Northwest Medical Center, Tucson
Paradise Valley Hospital, Phoenix
Payson Regional Medical Center, Payson
Phoenix Baptist Hospital, Phoenix
St. Joseph's Hospital and Medical Center, Phoenix
St. Luke's Medical Center, Phoenix
St. Lukes Behaviorial Health Center, Phoenix
Scottsdale Healthcare–Osborn, Scottsdale
Scottsdale Healthcare–Shea, Scottsdale
Tempe St. Luke's Hospital, Tempe
Tucson Heart Hospital, Tucson
Tucson Medical Center, Tucson
University Medical Center, Tucson

University Physicians Healthcare Hospital at Kino, Tucson
Walter O. Boswell Memorial Hospital, Sun City
West Valley Hospital, Goodyear

STROKE
Arrowhead Hospital, Glendale
Banner Baywood Medical Center, Mesa
Banner Good Samaritan Medical Center, Phoenix
Banner Mesa Medical Center, Mesa
Banner Thunderbird Medical Center, Glendale
Carondelet St. Mary's Hospital and Health Center, Tucson
Del E. Webb Memorial Hospital, Sun City West
El Dorado Hospital, Tucson
Flagstaff Medical Center, Flagstaff
John C. Lincoln Deer Valley Hospital, Phoenix
Northwest Medical Center, Tucson
Phoenix Baptist Hospital, Phoenix
St. Joseph's Hospital and Medical Center, Phoenix
Scottsdale Healthcare–Osborn, Scottsdale
Tempe St. Luke's Hospital, Tempe
Tucson Heart Hospital, Tucson
Tucson Medical Center, Tucson
Walter O. Boswell Memorial Hospital, Sun City
Western Arizona Regional Medical Center, Bullhead City
Yuma Regional Medical Center, Yuma

VASCULAR

CAROTID SURGERY
Arizona Heart Hospital, Phoenix

PERIPHERAL VASCULAR BYPASS
Kingman Regional Medical Center, Kingman

RESECTION/REPLACEMENT OF ABDOMINAL AORTA
None

WOMEN'S HEALTH
Northwest Medical Center, Tucson
Scottsdale Healthcare–Osborn, Scottsdale
Yuma Regional Medical Center, Yuma

ARKANSAS HOSPITALS: FIVE STAR RATED FACILITIES

BARIATRIC SURGERY
None

CARDIAC

ATRIAL FIBRILLATION
None

CORONARY INTERVENTIONAL PROCEDURES (ANGIOPLASTY/STENT)
Arkansas Heart Hospital, Little Rock

HEART ATTACK
Arkansas Heart Hospital, Little Rock

HEART BYPASS SURGERY
None

HEART FAILURE
Arkansas Heart Hospital, Little Rock
Harris Hospital, Newport
St. Vincent Doctors Hospital, Little Rock
St. Vincent Infirmary Medical Center, Little Rock

VALVE REPLACEMENT SURGERY
None

CRITICAL CARE

DIABETIC ACIDOSIS AND COMA
None

PULMONARY EMBOLISM
St. Joseph's Mercy Health Center, Hot Springs

RESPIRATORY FAILURE
St. Edward Mercy Medical Center, Fort Smith
St. Joseph's Mercy Health Center, Hot Springs
St. Vincent Doctors Hospital, Little Rock
St. Vincent Infirmary Medical Center, Little Rock
Sparks Regional Medical Center, Fort Smith

SEPSIS
Medical Park Hospital, Hope
St. Joseph's Mercy Health Center, Hot Springs
St. Vincent Doctors Hospital, Little Rock
St. Vincent Infirmary Medical Center, Little Rock

GASTROINTESTINAL

BOWEL OBSTRUCTION
Sparks Regional Medical Center, Fort Smith

CHOLECYSTECTOMY
Arkansas Methodist Medical Center, Paragould
Chicot Memorial Hospital, Lake Village
Howard Memorial Hospital, Nashville
North Arkansas Regional Medical Center, Harrison
St. Vincent Doctors Hospital, Little Rock
St. Vincent Infirmary Medical Center, Little Rock
White County Medical Center—South Campus, Searcy

GASTROINTESTINAL BLEED
Baptist Health Medical Center—North Little Rock,
    North Little Rock

GASTROINTESTINAL SURGERIES
AND PROCEDURES
None

PANCREATITIS
None

GENERAL SURGERY

APPENDECTOMY
None

MATERNITY CARE

None

ORTHOPEDICS

BACK AND NECK SURGERY
(EXCEPT SPINAL FUSION)
Baptist Health Medical Center—Little Rock,
    Little Rock
Northwest Medical Center—Benton County,
    Bentonville
St. Joseph's Mercy Health Center, Hot Springs
St. Vincent Doctors Hospital, Little Rock
St. Vincent Infirmary Medical Center, Little Rock
St. Vincent Medical Center—North, Sherwood
UAMS Medical Center, Little Rock
White County Medical Center—North Campus, Searcy
White County Medical Center—South Campus, Searcy

BACK AND NECK SURGERY (SPINAL FUSION)
St. Bernards Medical Center, Jonesboro
St. Vincent Doctors Hospital, Little Rock
St. Vincent Infirmary Medical Center, Little Rock
St. Vincent Medical Center—North, Sherwood

HIP FRACTURE REPAIR
Arkansas Methodist Medical Center, Paragould
Medical Center—South Arkansas, El Dorado
Randolph County Medical Center, Pocahontas
St. Bernards Medical Center, Jonesboro
St. Joseph's Mercy Health Center, Hot Springs
St. Mary's Regional Medical Center, Russellville
Sparks Regional Medical Center, Fort Smith
White River Medical Center, Batesville

TOTAL HIP REPLACEMENT
St. Mary's Regional Medical Center, Russellville
St. Vincent Doctors Hospital, Little Rock
St. Vincent Infirmary Medical Center, Little Rock

TOTAL KNEE REPLACEMENT
Arkansas Methodist Medical Center, Paragould
Conway Regional Medical Center, Conway
Medical Center—South Arkansas, El Dorado
St. Mary's Regional Medical Center, Russellville
St. Vincent Doctors Hospital, Little Rock
St. Vincent Infirmary Medical Center, Little Rock
Sparks Regional Medical Center, Fort Smith

PROSTATECTOMY

St. Vincent Doctors Hospital, Little Rock
St. Vincent Infirmary Medical Center, Little Rock

PULMONARY

CHRONIC OBSTRUCTIVE PULMONARY DISEASE
(COPD)
Arkansas Heart Hospital, Little Rock
Jefferson Regional Medical Center, Pine Bluff
John Ed Chambers Memorial Hospital, Danville
St. Joseph's Mercy Health Center, Hot Springs
Sparks Regional Medical Center, Fort Smith

PNEUMONIA
Arkansas Heart Hospital, Little Rock
Harris Hospital, Newport
Little River Memorial Hospital, Ashdown
Medical Park Hospital, Hope
St. Joseph's Mercy Health Center, Hot Springs
St. Vincent Doctors Hospital, Little Rock
St. Vincent Infirmary Medical Center, Little Rock
Southwest Regional Medical Center, Little Rock
Sparks Regional Medical Center, Fort Smith

STROKE

None

VASCULAR

CAROTID SURGERY
Baptist Health Medical Center—Little Rock,
    Little Rock
Northwest Medical Center—Washington County,
    Springdale
St. Joseph's Mercy Health Center, Hot Springs

PERIPHERAL VASCULAR BYPASS
St. Vincent Doctors Hospital, Little Rock
St. Vincent Infirmary Medical Center, Little Rock

RESECTION/REPLACEMENT OF ABDOMINAL AORTA
None

WOMEN'S HEALTH

None

Hospitals receiving a five star rating in a particular procedure have patient outcomes that put them among the best in the nation. For full definitions of ratings and awards, see Appendix.

740   CHAPTER 7: FIVE STAR RATED HOSPITALS

BARIATRIC SURGERY

California Pacific Medical Center, San Francisco
Cedars-Sinai Medical Center, Los Angeles
Clovis Community Medical Center, Clovis
Community Memorial Hospital of San
    Buenaventura, Ventura
El Camino Hospital, Mountain View
Huntington Memorial Hospital, Pasadena
Methodist Hospital of Southern California, Arcadia
Mills Health Center, San Mateo
Mills Peninsula Health Services, Burlingame
Pacific Campus Hospital, San Francisco
Providence Saint Joseph Medical Center, Burbank
St. John's Regional Medical Center, Oxnard
San Joaquin Community Hospital, Bakersfield
Scripps Mercy Hospital, San Diego
Scripps Mercy Hospital—Chula Vista, Chula Vista
South Coast Medical Center, Laguna Beach
Southwest Healthcare System—Inland Valley
    Medical Center, Wildomar
Southwest Healthcare System—Rancho Springs
    Medical Center, Murrieta
Sutter General Hospital, Sacramento
Sutter Medical Center of Santa Rosa—Chanate,
    Santa Rosa

CARDIAC

ATRIAL FIBRILLATION

Alta Bates Summit—Summit Campus, Oakland
Little Company of Mary Hospital, Torrance
Mercy General Hospital, Sacramento
Saddleback Memorial Medical Center, Laguna Hills
Saddleback Memorial Medical Center—San
    Clemente, San Clemente

CORONARY INTERVENTIONAL PROCEDURES
(ANGIOPLASTY/STENT)

Downey Regional Medical Center, Downey
El Camino Hospital, Mountain View
Sequoia Hospital, Redwood City
Sharp Memorial Hospital, San Diego

HEART ATTACK

Citrus Valley Medical Center—IC Campus, Covina
Fresno Heart and Surgical Hospital, Fresno
John Muir Medical Center, Walnut Creek
LAC Olive View—UCLA Medical Center, Sylmar
St. John's Health Center, Santa Monica
St. John's Regional Medical Center, Oxnard
St. Joseph Hospital, Orange

St. Vincent Medical Center, Los Angeles
Temple Community Hospital, Los Angeles

HEART BYPASS SURGERY

Anaheim Memorial Hospital, Anaheim
Loma Linda University Medical Center, Loma Linda
Mercy General Hospital, Sacramento
Presbyterian Intercommunity Hospital, Whittier
St. John's Regional Medical Center, Oxnard
St. Joseph's Medical Center of Stockton, Stockton
White Memorial Medical Center, Los Angeles

HEART FAILURE

Alameda County Medical Center, San Leandro
Alameda Hospital, Alameda
Alhambra Hospital and Medical Center, Alhambra
Cedars-Sinai Medical Center, Los Angeles
Desert Valley Hospital, Victorville
Doctor's Hospital Medical Center of Montclair,
    Montclair
El Camino Hospital, Mountain View
Fountain Valley Regional Hospital and Medical
    Center, Fountain Valley
Garfield Medical Center, Monterey Park
Glendale Memorial Hospital and Health Center,
    Glendale
Hollywood Community Hospital, Hollywood
John Muir Medical Center, Walnut Creek
Menifee Valley Medical Center, Sun City
Moreno Valley Medical Center, Moreno Valley
Northridge Hospital Medical Center, Northridge
Pacific Alliance Medical Center, Los Angeles
Paradise Valley Hospital, National City
Pomona Valley Hospital Medical Center, Pomona
Providence Holy Cross Medical Center, Mission Hills
Queen of the Valley, Napa
Saddleback Memorial Medical Center, Laguna Hills
Saddleback Memorial Medical
    Center—San Clemente, San Clemente
St. John's Health Center, Santa Monica
Santa Monica—UCLA Medical Center, Santa Monica
Scripps Memorial Hospital—La Jolla, La Jolla
Scripps Mercy Hospital, San Diego
Scripps Mercy Hospital—Chula Vista, Chula Vista
Sierra Nevada Memorial Hospital, Grass Valley
Southwest Healthcare System—Inland Valley
    Medical Center, Wildomar
Southwest Healthcare System—Rancho Springs
    Medical Center, Murrieta
Sutter Auburn Faith Hospital, Auburn
Sutter Roseville Medical Center, Roseville

Tri-City Regional Medical Center, Hawaiian Gardens
White Memorial Medical Center, Los Angeles
Whittier Hospital, Whittier

VALVE REPLACEMENT SURGERY

Bakersfield Heart Hospital, Bakersfield
Cedars-Sinai Medical Center, Los Angeles
Fremont Medical Center, Yuba City
Hoag Memorial Hospital Presbyterian,
    Newport Beach
Marin General Hospital, Greenbrae
Rideout Memorial Hospital, Marysville
Sharp Memorial Hospital, San Diego
Sutter Medical Center of Santa Rosa—Chanate,
    Santa Rosa
Sutter Warrack Hospital, Santa Rosa
UCLA Medical Center, Los Angeles
USC University Hospital, Los Angeles

CRITICAL CARE

DIABETIC ACIDOSIS AND COMA

Glendale Adventist Medical Center, Glendale

PULMONARY EMBOLISM

Eisenhower Medical Center, Rancho Mirage
Mission Hospital Regional Medical Center,
    Mission Viejo
West Hills Medical Center, West Hills

RESPIRATORY FAILURE

Beverly Hospital, Montebello
Feather River Hospital, Paradise
Good Samaritan Hospital, Los Angeles
Greater El Monte Community Hospital,
    South El Monte
Hollywood Community Hospital, Hollywood
Hollywood Presbyterian Medical Center, Los Angeles
Huntington Beach Hospital, Huntington Beach
John Muir Medical Center, Walnut Creek
La Palma Intercommunity Hospital, La Palma
Long Beach Memorial Medical Center, Long Beach
Marshall Medical Center, Placerville
Monterey Park Hospital, Monterey Park
Ridgecrest Regional Hospital, Ridgecrest
St. Louise Regional Hospital, Gilroy
St. Mary Medical Center, Long Beach
San Antonio Community Hospital, Upland
San Gabriel Valley Medical Center, San Gabriel
Scripps Memorial Hospital—La Jolla, La Jolla
Scripps Mercy Hospital, San Diego
Scripps Mercy Hospital—Chula Vista, Chula Vista

Sutter Auburn Faith Hospital, Auburn
West Hills Medical Center, West Hills
Western Medical Center Hospital Anaheim, Anaheim
White Memorial Medical Center, Los Angeles

SEPSIS

Alhambra Hospital and Medical Center, Alhambra
Anaheim General Hospital, Anaheim
Anaheim Memorial Hospital, Anaheim
Brotman Medical Center, Culver City
Centinela Freeman Regional Medical
   Center–Memorial, Inglewood
Century City Doctors Hospital, Los Angeles
Chino Valley Medical Center, Chino
Citrus Valley Medical Center–IC Campus, Covina
Citrus Valley Medical Center–QV Campus,
   West Covina
City of Angels Medical Center, Los Angeles
Community Hospital of San Bernardino,
   San Bernardino
Doctor's Hospital Medical Center of Montclair,
   Montclair
East Valley Hospital Medical Center, Glendora
El Camino Hospital, Mountain View
Feather River Hospital, Paradise
Garfield Medical Center, Monterey Park
Glendale Adventist Medical Center, Glendale
Good Samaritan Hospital, Los Angeles
Greater El Monte Community Hospital,
   South El Monte
Henry Mayo Newhall Memorial Hospital, Valencia
Hollywood Community Hospital, Hollywood
Hollywood Presbyterian Medical Center, Los Angeles
Huntington Beach Hospital, Huntington Beach
John Muir Medical Center, Walnut Creek
Kaiser Foundation Hospital–South San Francisco,
   South San Francisco
Little Company of Mary Hospital, Torrance
Loma Linda University Medical Center, Loma Linda
Long Beach Memorial Medical Center, Long Beach
Los Angeles Community Hospital, Los Angeles
Los Angeles Metropolitan Medical Center,
   Los Angeles
Los Robles Regional Medical Center, Thousand Oaks
Marshall Medical Center, Placerville
Mendocino Coast District Hospital, Fort Bragg
Methodist Hospital of Southern California, Arcadia
Mills Health Center, San Mateo
Mills Peninsula Health Services, Burlingame
Northridge Hospital Medical Center, Northridge
Norwalk Community Hospital, Norwalk
Olympia Medical Center, Los Angeles

Orange Coast Memorial Medical Center,
   Fountain Valley
Pacific Alliance Medical Center, Los Angeles
Paradise Valley Hospital, National City
Petaluma Valley Hospital, Petaluma
Pomona Valley Hospital Medical Center, Pomona
Presbyterian Intercommunity Hospital, Whittier
Providence Holy Cross Medical Center, Mission Hills
Queen of the Valley, Napa
Regional Medical Center of San Jose, San Jose
Saddleback Memorial Medical Center, Laguna Hills
Saddleback Memorial Medical
   Center–San Clemente, San Clemente
St. Bernardine Medical Center, San Bernardino
St. Louise Regional Hospital, Gilroy
St. Mary Medical Center, Long Beach
San Antonio Community Hospital, Upland
San Gabriel Valley Medical Center, San Gabriel
Santa Clara Valley Medical Center, San Jose
Scripps Memorial Hospital–Encinitas, Encinitas
Scripps Memorial Hospital–La Jolla, La Jolla
Scripps Mercy Hospital, San Diego
Scripps Mercy Hospital–Chula Vista, Chula Vista
Sherman Oaks Hospital, Sherman Oaks
Sierra Nevada Memorial Hospital, Grass Valley
Simi Valley Hospital and Health Care Service,
   Simi Valley
Southwest Healthcare System–Inland Valley
   Medical Center, Wildomar
Southwest Healthcare System–Rancho Springs
   Medical Center, Murrieta
Sutter Davis Hospital, Davis
Sutter Lakeside Hospital, Lakeport
Temple Community Hospital, Los Angeles
Tri-City Regional Medical Center, Hawaiian Gardens
University of California–San Diego Medical
   Center, San Diego
West Anaheim Medical Center, Anaheim
West Hills Medical Center, West Hills
Western Medical Center Hospital Anaheim, Anaheim
Whittier Hospital, Whittier

GASTROINTESTINAL

BOWEL OBSTRUCTION

Cedars-Sinai Medical Center, Los Angeles
Desert Valley Hospital, Victorville
Dominican Hospital, Santa Cruz
Huntington Memorial Hospital, Pasadena
Mills Health Center, San Mateo
Mills Peninsula Health Services, Burlingame
Novato Community Hospital, Novato
Pacific Alliance Medical Center, Los Angeles

St. Helena Hospital, Deer Park
St. Joseph Hospital, Orange
St. Rose Hospital, Hayward
San Leandro Hospital, San Leandro
UCSF Medical Center, San Francisco

CHOLECYSTECTOMY

Arroyo Grande Community Hospital, Arroyo Grande
Community Hospital of the Monterey Peninsula,
   Monterey
Dominican Hospital, Santa Cruz
Eden Medical Center, Castro Valley
Eisenhower Medical Center, Rancho Mirage
Glendale Adventist Medical Center, Glendale
Glendale Memorial Hospital and Health Center,
   Glendale
Good Samaritan Hospital, San Jose
Lodi Memorial Hospital, Lodi
Pacific Alliance Medical Center, Los Angeles
St. Bernardine Medical Center, San Bernardino
St. Elizabeth Community Hospital, Red Bluff
Scripps Green Hospital, La Jolla
Sierra Vista Regional Medical Center,
   San Luis Obispo

GASTROINTESTINAL BLEED

Enloe Medical Center, Chico
Garfield Medical Center, Monterey Park
Good Samaritan Hospital, Los Angeles
Hoag Memorial Hospital Presbyterian, Newport Beach
Huntington Memorial Hospital, Pasadena
John Muir Medical Center, Walnut Creek
Marin General Hospital, Greenbrae
St. Elizabeth Community Hospital, Red Bluff
Salinas Valley Memorial Health Care System,
   Salinas
Scripps Memorial Hospital–La Jolla, La Jolla
Sutter Delta Medical Center, Antioch
White Memorial Medical Center, Los Angeles

GASTROINTESTINAL SURGERIES
AND PROCEDURES

Alvarado Hospital Medical Center, San Diego
Beverly Hospital, Montebello
Cedars-Sinai Medical Center, Los Angeles
Community Hospital of the Monterey Peninsula,
   Monterey
Eisenhower Medical Center, Rancho Mirage
Good Samaritan Hospital, Los Angeles
Henry Mayo Newhall Memorial Hospital, Valencia
John Muir Medical Center, Walnut Creek
Mills Health Center, San Mateo
Mills Peninsula Health Services, Burlingame

Hospitals receiving a five star rating in a particular procedure have patient outcomes that put them among the best in the nation. For full definitions of ratings and awards, see Appendix.

Mt. Diablo Hospital Medical Center, Concord
Orange Coast Memorial Medical Center,
  Fountain Valley
Presbyterian Intercommunity Hospital, Whittier
St. John's Health Center, Santa Monica
St. John's Pleasant Valley Hospital, Camarillo
San Leandro Hospital, San Leandro
Santa Barbara Cottage Hospital, Santa Barbara
Scripps Memorial Hospital–La Jolla, La Jolla
Simi Valley Hospital and Health Care Service,
  Simi Valley
Sutter Auburn Faith Hospital, Auburn

PANCREATITIS

Beverly Hospital, Montebello
The Cancer Center at Riverside Community
  Hospital, Riverside
Cedars-Sinai Medical Center, Los Angeles
Glendale Adventist Medical Center, Glendale
John Muir Medical Center, Walnut Creek
Pacific Alliance Medical Center, Los Angeles
Riverside Community Hospital, Riverside
Scripps Memorial Hospital–La Jolla, La Jolla
Sutter Roseville Medical Center, Roseville

GENERAL SURGERY

APPENDECTOMY

Alameda County Medical Center, San Leandro
Antelope Valley Hospital, Lancaster
Arrowhead Regional Medical Center, Colton
California Pacific Medical Center, San Francisco
Chino Valley Medical Center, Chino
Coastal Communities Hospital, Santa Ana
Corona Regional Medical Center, Corona
Dameron Hospital Association, Stockton
Doctor's Hospital Medical Center of Montclair,
  Montclair
Doctors Medical Center of Modesto, Modesto
Dominican Hospital, Santa Cruz
Fremont Medical Center, Yuba City
Garden Grove Hospital and Medical Center,
  Garden Grove
Garfield Medical Center, Monterey Park
Glendale Adventist Medical Center, Glendale
Good Samaritan Hospital, San Jose
Hoag Memorial Hospital Presbyterian,
  Newport Beach
Hollywood Presbyterian Medical Center,
  Los Angeles
Kaiser Foundation Hospital, Bellflower
Kaiser Foundation Hospital, Panorama City
Kaiser Santa Clara Medical Center, Santa Clara

LAC+USC Medical Center, Los Angeles
LAC Harbor-UCLA Medical Center, Torrance
Lakewood Regional Medical Center, Lakewood
Los Robles Regional Medical Center, Thousand Oaks
Marin General Hospital, Greenbrae
Mills Health Center, San Mateo
Mills Peninsula Health Services, Burlingame
Olympia Medical Center, Los Angeles
Pacific Campus Hospital, San Francisco
Pacifica Hospital of the Valley, Sun Valley
Placentia-Linda Hospital, Placentia
Pomona Valley Hospital Medical Center, Pomona
Rideout Memorial Hospital, Marysville
St. Joseph Hospital, Orange
San Dimas Community Hospital, San Dimas
San Francisco General Hospital, San Francisco
San Joaquin General Hospital, French Camp
San Mateo Medical Center, San Mateo
Santa Barbara Cottage Hospital, Santa Barbara
Southwest Healthcare System–Inland Valley
  Medical Center, Wildomar
Southwest Healthcare System–Rancho Springs
  Medical Center, Murrieta
Tulare District Hospital, Tulare
Twin Cities Community Hospital, Templeton
Washington Hospital Healthcare System, Fremont
Western Medical Center Santa Ana, Santa Ana

MATERNITY CARE

Anaheim General Hospital, Anaheim
Antelope Valley Hospital, Lancaster
Arrowhead Regional Medical Center, Colton
Chino Valley Medical Center, Chino
Citrus Valley Medical Center–QV Campus,
  West Covina
Community and Mission Hospital of Huntington
  Park, Huntington Park
Community Hospital of Los Gatos, Los Gatos
Dameron Hospital Association, Stockton
Doctor's Hospital Medical Center of Montclair,
  Montclair
Downey Regional Medical Center, Downey
East Los Angeles Doctors Hospital, Los Angeles
Emanuel Medical Center, Turlock
Encino-Tarzana Regional Medical Center–Tarzana
  Campus, Tarzana
Garden Grove Hospital and Medical Center,
  Garden Grove
Good Samaritan Hospital, Los Angeles
Greater El Monte Community Hospital,
  South El Monte

Grossmont Hospital, La Mesa
Huntington Memorial Hospital, Pasadena
Kaiser Foundation Hospital, Panorama City
Los Angeles Community Hospital, Los Angeles
Los Angeles Metropolitan Medical Center,
  Los Angeles
Mercy General Hospital, Sacramento
Monterey Park Hospital, Monterey Park
Northridge Hospital Medical Center, Northridge
Norwalk Community Hospital, Norwalk
O'Connor Hospital, San Jose
Pacific Alliance Medical Center, Los Angeles
Paradise Valley Hospital, National City
Parkview Community Hospital, Riverside
Pioneers Memorial Health Care District, Brawley
Pomerado Hospital, Poway
Pomona Valley Hospital Medical Center, Pomona
Providence Saint Joseph Medical Center, Burbank
Saint Agnes Medical Center, Fresno
St. Louise Regional Hospital, Gilroy
San Antonio Community Hospital, Upland
San Joaquin Community Hospital, Bakersfield
Santa Barbara Cottage Hospital, Santa Barbara
Scripps Memorial Hospital–La Jolla, La Jolla
Scripps Mercy Hospital, San Diego
Scripps Mercy Hospital–Chula Vista, Chula Vista
Sharp Chula Vista Medical Center, Chula Vista
South Coast Medical Center, Laguna Beach
Valley Presbyterian Hospital, Van Nuys
Verdugo Hills Hospital, Glendale
Victor Valley Community Hospital, Victorville
West Hills Medical Center, West Hills
Western Medical Center Hospital Anaheim,
  Anaheim
Whittier Hospital, Whittier

ORTHOPEDICS

BACK AND NECK SURGERY
(EXCEPT SPINAL FUSION)

Alvarado Hospital Medical Center, San Diego
Community Memorial Hospital of San
  Buenaventura, Ventura
Garfield Medical Center, Monterey Park
Hoag Memorial Hospital Presbyterian,
  Newport Beach
Los Robles Regional Medical Center, Thousand Oaks
Saddleback Memorial Medical Center, Laguna Hills
Saddleback Memorial Medical
  Center–San Clemente, San Clemente
Saint Agnes Medical Center, Fresno
Santa Barbara Cottage Hospital, Santa Barbara
Scripps Green Hospital, La Jolla

Southwest Healthcare System—Inland Valley Medical Center, Wildomar
Southwest Healthcare System—Rancho Springs Medical Center, Murrieta

BACK AND NECK SURGERY (SPINAL FUSION)

Alvarado Hospital Medical Center, San Diego
Community Memorial Hospital of San Buenaventura, Ventura
El Camino Hospital, Mountain View
St. Bernardine Medical Center, San Bernardino
Santa Barbara Cottage Hospital, Santa Barbara
Scripps Green Hospital, La Jolla
Stanford Hospital, Stanford
Sutter Roseville Medical Center, Roseville

HIP FRACTURE REPAIR

Arroyo Grande Community Hospital, Arroyo Grande
Brotman Medical Center, Culver City
Citrus Valley Medical Center—QV Campus, West Covina
Clovis Community Medical Center, Clovis
Community Hospital of Los Gatos, Los Gatos
Community Hospital of the Monterey Peninsula, Monterey
Community Memorial Hospital of San Buenaventura, Ventura
Community Regional Medical Center, Fresno
Desert Regional Medical Center, Palm Springs
East Valley Hospital Medical Center, Glendora
Eisenhower Medical Center, Rancho Mirage
Encino-Tarzana Regional Medical Center, Encino
Fountain Valley Regional Hospital and Medical Center, Fountain Valley
Garfield Medical Center, Monterey Park
Glendale Adventist Medical Center, Glendale
Glendale Memorial Hospital and Health Center, Glendale
Hemet Valley Medical Center, Hemet
Hoag Memorial Hospital Presbyterian, Newport Beach
Hollywood Presbyterian Medical Center, Los Angeles
John F. Kennedy Memorial Hospital, Indio
Kaweah Delta District Hospital, Visalia
LAC+USC Medical Center, Los Angeles
Lodi Memorial Hospital, Lodi
Lompoc Healthcare District, Lompoc
Menifee Valley Medical Center, Sun City
Mt. Diablo Hospital Medical Center, Concord
Olympia Medical Center, Los Angeles
Pomona Valley Hospital Medical Center, Pomona
St. Bernardine Medical Center, San Bernardino
St. Elizabeth Community Hospital, Red Bluff
St. Francis Medical Center, Lynwood

St. John's Pleasant Valley Hospital, Camarillo
St. Joseph Hospital, Eureka
St. Jude Medical Center, Fullerton
San Joaquin General Hospital, French Camp
Shasta Regional Medical Center, Redding
Sierra Vista Regional Medical Center, San Luis Obispo
Sutter General Hospital, Sacramento
Tulare District Hospital, Tulare
University Medical Center, Fresno
Whittier Hospital, Whittier

TOTAL HIP REPLACEMENT

California Pacific Medical Center, San Francisco
Cedars-Sinai Medical Center, Los Angeles
Centinela Freeman Regional Medical Center—Centinela, Inglewood
Clovis Community Medical Center, Clovis
Community Hospital of Los Gatos, Los Gatos
Community Hospital of the Monterey Peninsula, Monterey
Community Regional Medical Center, Fresno
Eisenhower Medical Center, Rancho Mirage
Emanuel Medical Center, Turlock
Encino-Tarzana Regional Medical Center, Encino
Feather River Hospital, Paradise
Goleta Valley Cottage Hospital, Santa Barbara
Good Samaritan Hospital, Los Angeles
Grossmont Hospital, La Mesa
Hoag Memorial Hospital Presbyterian, Newport Beach
Loma Linda University Medical Center, Loma Linda
Long Beach Memorial Medical Center, Long Beach
Mercy Medical Center Merced, Merced
Mercy Medical Center Redding, Redding
Methodist Hospital, Sacramento
O'Connor Hospital, San Jose
Pacific Campus Hospital, San Francisco
Saint Agnes Medical Center, Fresno
St. Bernardine Medical Center, San Bernardino
Saint Francis Memorial Hospital, San Francisco
St. Mary's Medical Center, San Francisco
Santa Barbara Cottage Hospital, Santa Barbara
Scripps Green Hospital, La Jolla
Shasta Regional Medical Center, Redding
Sierra Nevada Memorial Hospital, Grass Valley
Stanford Hospital, Stanford
Sutter General Hospital, Sacramento
Sutter Lakeside Hospital, Lakeport
Sutter Medical Center of Santa Rosa—Chanate, Santa Rosa
Sutter Warrack Hospital, Santa Rosa
Twin Cities Community Hospital, Templeton

University Medical Center, Fresno
Washington Hospital Healthcare System, Fremont

TOTAL KNEE REPLACEMENT

Arroyo Grande Community Hospital, Arroyo Grande
California Hospital Medical Center—Los Angeles, Los Angeles
California Pacific Medical Center, San Francisco
Centinela Freeman Regional Medical Center—Centinela, Inglewood
Community Hospital of the Monterey Peninsula, Monterey
Dameron Hospital Association, Stockton
Desert Regional Medical Center, Palm Springs
Dominican Hospital, Santa Cruz
Eisenhower Medical Center, Rancho Mirage
El Centro Regional Medical Center, El Centro
Emanuel Medical Center, Turlock
Encino-Tarzana Regional Medical Center, Encino
Fallbrook Hospital, Fallbrook
Feather River Hospital, Paradise
French Hospital Medical Center, San Luis Obispo
Glendale Memorial Hospital and Health Center, Glendale
Goleta Valley Cottage Hospital, Santa Barbara
Good Samaritan Hospital, Los Angeles
Healdsburg District Hospital, Healdsburg
Hoag Memorial Hospital Presbyterian, Newport Beach
John F. Kennedy Memorial Hospital, Indio
Kaweah Delta District Hospital, Visalia
Long Beach Memorial Medical Center, Long Beach
Mercy Medical Center Redding, Redding
Methodist Hospital, Sacramento
Pacific Campus Hospital, San Francisco
Palomar Medical Center, Escondido
Redlands Community Hospital, Redlands
Regional Medical Center of San Jose, San Jose
Saint Agnes Medical Center, Fresno
St. Bernardine Medical Center, San Bernardino
St. Elizabeth Community Hospital, Red Bluff
St. Joseph Hospital, Orange
Santa Barbara Cottage Hospital, Santa Barbara
Scripps Green Hospital, La Jolla
Sharp Coronado Hospital and Healthcare Center, Coronado
Sierra Nevada Memorial Hospital, Grass Valley
Sierra Vista Regional Medical Center, San Luis Obispo
Stanford Hospital, Stanford
Sutter General Hospital, Sacramento
Sutter Solano Medical Center, Vallejo
Washington Hospital Healthcare System, Fremont

Hospitals receiving a five star rating in a particular procedure have patient outcomes that put them among the best in the nation. For full definitions of ratings and awards, see Appendix.

PROSTATECTOMY

Eisenhower Medical Center, Rancho Mirage
Emanuel Medical Center, Turlock
Glendale Adventist Medical Center, Glendale
Hanford Community Medical Center, Hanford
Hoag Memorial Hospital Presbyterian,
    Newport Beach
Mercy Medical Center Merced, Merced
St. John's Regional Medical Center, Oxnard
Santa Monica–UCLA Medical Center,
    Santa Monica

PULMONARY

CHRONIC OBSTRUCTIVE PULMONARY DISEASE (COPD)

Alameda Hospital, Alameda
Beverly Hospital, Montebello
Citrus Valley Medical Center–IC Campus, Covina
Fountain Valley Regional Hospital and Medical
    Center, Fountain Valley
Glendale Memorial Hospital and Health Center,
    Glendale
Henry Mayo Newhall Memorial Hospital, Valencia
John Muir Medical Center, Walnut Creek
Kaiser Walnut Creek Medical Center, Walnut Creek
Los Angeles Community Hospital, Los Angeles
Marshall Medical Center, Placerville
Norwalk Community Hospital, Norwalk
Pacific Alliance Medical Center, Los Angeles
Paradise Valley Hospital, National City
Providence Holy Cross Medical Center,
    Mission Hills
St. Louise Regional Hospital, Gilroy
St. Vincent Medical Center, Los Angeles
San Gabriel Valley Medical Center, San Gabriel
Sierra Vista Regional Medical Center,
    San Luis Obispo
Stanford Hospital, Stanford
Tri-City Regional Medical Center, Hawaiian Gardens
West Anaheim Medical Center, Anaheim

PNEUMONIA

Alhambra Hospital and Medical Center, Alhambra
Alta Bates Summit–Summit Campus, Oakland
Anaheim Memorial Hospital, Anaheim
Barstow Community Hospital, Barstow
Bellflower Medical Center, Bellflower
Beverly Hospital, Montebello
Brotman Medical Center, Culver City
California Pacific Medical Center, San Francisco
Cedars-Sinai Medical Center, Los Angeles

Centinela Freeman Regional Medical Center–
    Memorial, Inglewood
Chino Valley Medical Center, Chino
Citrus Valley Medical Center–QV Campus,
    West Covina
Coast Plaza Doctors Hospital, Norwalk
Corona Regional Medical Center, Corona
Desert Valley Hospital, Victorville
Doctor's Hospital Medical Center of Montclair,
    Montclair
East Los Angeles Doctors Hospital, Los Angeles
El Camino Hospital, Mountain View
Fountain Valley Regional Hospital and Medical
    Center, Fountain Valley
Garfield Medical Center, Monterey Park
Glendale Memorial Hospital and Health Center,
    Glendale
Good Samaritan Hospital, Los Angeles
Greater El Monte Community Hospital,
    South El Monte
Hollywood Community Hospital, Hollywood
Hollywood Presbyterian Medical Center, Los Angeles
John Muir Medical Center, Walnut Creek
Los Angeles Metropolitan Medical Center, Los Angeles
Los Robles Regional Medical Center, Thousand Oaks
Marshall Medical Center, Placerville
Mercy General Hospital, Sacramento
Mills Health Center, San Mateo
Mills Peninsula Health Services, Burlingame
Mission Community Hospital–Panorama,
    Panorama City
Monterey Park Hospital, Monterey Park
Mt. Diablo Hospital Medical Center, Concord
Novato Community Hospital, Novato
Olympia Medical Center, Los Angeles
Orange Coast Memorial Medical Center,
    Fountain Valley
Oroville Hospital, Oroville
Pacific Alliance Medical Center, Los Angeles
Pacific Campus Hospital, San Francisco
Pacific Hospital of Long Beach, Long Beach
Paradise Valley Hospital, National City
Pomona Valley Hospital Medical Center, Pomona
Presbyterian Intercommunity Hospital, Whittier
Providence Holy Cross Medical Center, Mission Hills
Saddleback Memorial Medical Center, Laguna Hills
Saddleback Memorial Medical
    Center–San Clemente, San Clemente
St. John's Health Center, Santa Monica
St. Louise Regional Hospital, Gilroy
St. Luke's Hospital, San Francisco
St. Mary Medical Center, Long Beach

St. Mary's Medical Center, San Francisco
St. Rose Hospital, Hayward
St. Vincent Medical Center, Los Angeles
San Fernando Community Hospital, San Fernando
San Gabriel Valley Medical Center, San Gabriel
San Ramon Regional Medical Center, San Ramon
Santa Clara Valley Medical Center, San Jose
Santa Monica–UCLA Medical Center, Santa Monica
Scripps Memorial Hospital–Encinitas, Encinitas
Scripps Memorial Hospital–La Jolla, La Jolla
Scripps Mercy Hospital, San Diego
Scripps Mercy Hospital–Chula Vista, Chula Vista
Sharp Memorial Hospital, San Diego
Sierra Nevada Memorial Hospital, Grass Valley
Simi Valley Hospital and Health Care Service,
    Simi Valley
Sutter Auburn Faith Hospital, Auburn
Sutter General Hospital, Sacramento
Sutter Lakeside Hospital, Lakeport
Tri-City Regional Medical Center, Hawaiian Gardens
UCLA Medical Center, Los Angeles
UCSF Medical Center, San Francisco
University of California–San Diego Medical
    Center, San Diego
Valley Care Medical Center, Pleasanton
Valley Memorial Hospital, Livermore
West Hills Medical Center, West Hills
White Memorial Medical Center, Los Angeles
Whittier Hospital, Whittier

STROKE

Alhambra Hospital and Medical Center, Alhambra
Alta Bates Summit–Alta Bates Campus, Berkeley
Alta Bates Summit–Summit Campus, Oakland
Alvarado Hospital Medical Center, San Diego
Anaheim Memorial Hospital, Anaheim
Beverly Hospital, Montebello
Brotman Medical Center, Culver City
California Hospital Medical Center–Los Angeles,
    Los Angeles
California Pacific Medical Center–Davies
    Campus, San Francisco
Centinela Freeman Regional Medical Center–
    Centinela, Inglewood
Centinela Freeman Regional Medical Center–
    Memorial, Inglewood
Century City Doctors Hospital, Los Angeles
Chinese Hospital, San Francisco
Chino Valley Medical Center, Chino
Citrus Valley Medical Center–IC Campus, Covina
Citrus Valley Medical Center–QV Campus,
    West Covina

Community Hospital of San Bernardino, San Bernardino
Corona Regional Medical Center, Corona
Downey Regional Medical Center, Downey
Eden Medical Center, Castro Valley
Eisenhower Medical Center, Rancho Mirage
Encino-Tarzana Regional Medical Center—Tarzana Campus, Tarzana
Fountain Valley Regional Hospital and Medical Center, Fountain Valley
Garfield Medical Center, Monterey Park
Glendale Adventist Medical Center, Glendale
Glendale Memorial Hospital and Health Center, Glendale
Good Samaritan Hospital, Los Angeles
Henry Mayo Newhall Memorial Hospital, Valencia
Hoag Memorial Hospital Presbyterian, Newport Beach
Hollywood Presbyterian Medical Center, Los Angeles
Huntington Memorial Hospital, Pasadena
John Muir Medical Center, Walnut Creek
Kaiser San Francisco Medical Center, San Francisco
Long Beach Memorial Medical Center, Long Beach
Methodist Hospital of Southern California, Arcadia
Mills Health Center, San Mateo
Mills Peninsula Health Services, Burlingame
Monterey Park Hospital, Monterey Park
Mt. Diablo Hospital Medical Center, Concord
O'Connor Hospital, San Jose
Pacific Alliance Medical Center, Los Angeles
Petaluma Valley Hospital, Petaluma
Presbyterian Intercommunity Hospital, Whittier
Providence Holy Cross Medical Center, Mission Hills
Providence Saint Joseph Medical Center, Burbank
Saddleback Memorial Medical Center, Laguna Hills

Saddleback Memorial Medical Center—San Clemente, San Clemente
Saint Agnes Medical Center, Fresno
St. Francis Medical Center, Lynwood
Saint Francis Memorial Hospital, San Francisco
St. John's Pleasant Valley Hospital, Camarillo
St. Joseph Hospital, Orange
St. Jude Medical Center, Fullerton
St. Vincent Medical Center, Los Angeles
San Antonio Community Hospital, Upland
San Gabriel Valley Medical Center, San Gabriel
San Leandro Hospital, San Leandro
Scripps Memorial Hospital—Encinitas, Encinitas
Scripps Mercy Hospital, San Diego
Scripps Mercy Hospital—Chula Vista, Chula Vista
Sequoia Hospital, Redwood City
Sharp Chula Vista Medical Center, Chula Vista
Sharp Memorial Hospital, San Diego
Sherman Oaks Hospital, Sherman Oaks
Sierra Nevada Memorial Hospital, Grass Valley
Sutter Delta Medical Center, Antioch
Sutter Roseville Medical Center, Roseville
UCSF Medical Center, San Francisco
USC University Hospital, Los Angeles
West Anaheim Medical Center, Anaheim
White Memorial Medical Center, Los Angeles

VASCULAR

CAROTID SURGERY
Brotman Medical Center, Culver City
El Camino Hospital, Mountain View
French Hospital Medical Center, San Luis Obispo
Hoag Memorial Hospital Presbyterian, Newport Beach

Torrance Memorial Medical Center, Torrance
Tri-City Medical Center, Oceanside
UCSF Medical Center, San Francisco

PERIPHERAL VASCULAR BYPASS
San Leandro Hospital, San Leandro

RESECTION/REPLACEMENT OF ABDOMINAL AORTA
None

WOMEN'S HEALTH

Cedars-Sinai Medical Center, Los Angeles
Community Memorial Hospital of San Buenaventura, Ventura
Downey Regional Medical Center, Downey
El Camino Hospital, Mountain View
Encino-Tarzana Regional Medical Center—Tarzana Campus, Tarzana
Fountain Valley Regional Hospital and Medical Center, Fountain Valley
Garfield Medical Center, Monterey Park
Glendale Adventist Medical Center, Glendale
Glendale Memorial Hospital and Health Center, Glendale
Good Samaritan Hospital, Los Angeles
Huntington Memorial Hospital, Pasadena
Northridge Hospital Medical Center, Northridge
O'Connor Hospital, San Jose
Providence Holy Cross Medical Center, Mission Hills
Providence Saint Joseph Medical Center, Burbank
Saint Agnes Medical Center, Fresno
St. Mary Medical Center, Long Beach
Scripps Memorial Hospital—La Jolla, La Jolla
Sharp Chula Vista Medical Center, Chula Vista

COLORADO HOSPITALS: FIVE STAR RATED FACILITIES

BARIATRIC SURGERY
None

CARDIAC

ATRIAL FIBRILLATION
None

CORONARY INTERVENTIONAL PROCEDURES (ANGIOPLASTY/STENT)
Memorial Hospital, Colorado Springs
Poudre Valley Hospital, Fort Collins

HEART ATTACK
Centura Health—Penrose St. Francis Health Services, Colorado Springs
Centura Health—St. Anthony North Hospital, Westminster
Exempla Saint Joseph Hospital, Denver
Longmont United Hospital, Longmont
Memorial Hospital, Colorado Springs
North Colorado Medical Center, Greeley
Poudre Valley Hospital, Fort Collins
Southwest Memorial Hospital, Cortez
University of Colorado Hospital Authority, Aurora

HEART BYPASS SURGERY
Centura Health—St. Anthony Central Hospital, Denver
Memorial Hospital, Colorado Springs

HEART FAILURE
Centura Health—Parker Adventist Hospital, Parker
Centura Health—Penrose St. Francis Health Services, Colorado Springs
Centura Health—Porter Adventist Hospital, Denver
Exempla Lutheran Medical Center, Wheat Ridge
Exempla Saint Joseph Hospital, Denver

Hospitals receiving a five star rating in a particular procedure have patient outcomes that put them among the best in the nation. For full definitions of ratings and awards, see Appendix.

Longmont United Hospital, Longmont
Medical Center of Aurora, Aurora
North Colorado Medical Center, Greeley
North Suburban Medical Center, Thornton
Poudre Valley Hospital, Fort Collins
Prowers Medical Center, Lamar
Rose Medical Center, Denver
University of Colorado Hospital Authority, Aurora

VALVE REPLACEMENT SURGERY
None

CRITICAL CARE

DIABETIC ACIDOSIS AND COMA
Centura Health—Penrose St. Francis Health
    Services, Colorado Springs

PULMONARY EMBOLISM
Centura Health—Penrose St. Francis Health
    Services, Colorado Springs
Poudre Valley Hospital, Fort Collins
Rose Medical Center, Denver

RESPIRATORY FAILURE
Centura Health—Littleton Adventist Hospital,
    Littleton
Centura Health—Parker Adventist Hospital, Parker
Centura Health—Penrose St. Francis Health
    Services, Colorado Springs
Centura Health—Porter Adventist Hospital, Denver
Centura Health—St. Anthony Central Hospital,
    Denver
Medical Center of Aurora, Aurora
North Colorado Medical Center, Greeley
Presbyterian/St. Luke's Medical Center, Denver
Rose Medical Center, Denver

SEPSIS
Centura Health—Littleton Adventist Hospital,
    Littleton
Centura Health—Penrose St. Francis Health
    Services, Colorado Springs
Centura Health—Porter Adventist Hospital, Denver
Longmont United Hospital, Longmont
Medical Center of Aurora, Aurora
Memorial Hospital, Colorado Springs
North Colorado Medical Center, Greeley
Poudre Valley Hospital, Fort Collins
Presbyterian/St. Luke's Medical Center, Denver
Rose Medical Center, Denver

GASTROINTESTINAL

BOWEL OBSTRUCTION
Centura Health—Littleton Adventist Hospital,
    Littleton
Centura Health—Parker Adventist Hospital, Parker
Centura Health—St. Anthony Central Hospital,
    Denver
Community Hospital, Grand Junction
Exempla Saint Joseph Hospital, Denver
Rose Medical Center, Denver

CHOLECYSTECTOMY
Mercy Regional Medical Center, Durango
St. Mary's Hospital and Medical Center,
    Grand Junction
Sterling Regional Medical Center, Sterling

GASTROINTESTINAL BLEED
Centura Health—Penrose St. Francis Health
    Services, Colorado Springs
Centura Health—Porter Adventist Hospital, Denver
Medical Center of Aurora, Aurora
North Colorado Medical Center, Greeley
Poudre Valley Hospital, Fort Collins

GASTROINTESTINAL SURGERIES
AND PROCEDURES
Centura Health—Littleton Adventist Hospital,
    Littleton
Centura Health—Penrose St. Francis Health
    Services, Colorado Springs
Centura Health—Porter Adventist Hospital, Denver
Exempla Lutheran Medical Center, Wheat Ridge
Medical Center of Aurora, Aurora
Memorial Hospital, Colorado Springs
North Colorado Medical Center, Greeley
Poudre Valley Hospital, Fort Collins
Sky Ridge Medical Center, Lone Tree
Swedish Medical Center, Englewood

PANCREATITIS
North Colorado Medical Center, Greeley
Swedish Medical Center, Englewood

GENERAL SURGERY

APPENDECTOMY
None

MATERNITY CARE

None

ORTHOPEDICS

BACK AND NECK SURGERY
(EXCEPT SPINAL FUSION)
Poudre Valley Hospital, Fort Collins
St. Mary's Hospital and Medical Center,
    Grand Junction

BACK AND NECK SURGERY (SPINAL FUSION)
North Colorado Medical Center, Greeley
St. Mary's Hospital and Medical Center,
    Grand Junction

HIP FRACTURE REPAIR
Centura Health—St. Anthony Central Hospital,
    Denver
Centura Health—St. Thomas More Hospital,
    Canon City
Community Hospital, Grand Junction
McKee Medical Center, Loveland
Poudre Valley Hospital, Fort Collins
St. Joseph Hospital, Florence
St. Mary's Hospital and Medical Center,
    Grand Junction
Swedish Medical Center, Englewood

TOTAL HIP REPLACEMENT
Exempla Lutheran Medical Center, Wheat Ridge
Memorial Hospital, Colorado Springs
Poudre Valley Hospital, Fort Collins
Valley View Hospital Association,
    Glenwood Springs

TOTAL KNEE REPLACEMENT
Centura Health—St. Thomas More Hospital,
    Canon City
Community Hospital, Grand Junction
McKee Medical Center, Loveland
Memorial Hospital, Colorado Springs
Poudre Valley Hospital, Fort Collins
Presbyterian/St. Luke's Medical Center, Denver
St. Joseph Hospital, Florence
St. Mary's Hospital and Medical Center,
    Grand Junction

PROSTATECTOMY

Centura Health—Porter Adventist Hospital, Denver
Parkview Medical Center, Pueblo
Swedish Medical Center, Englewood

PULMONARY

CHRONIC OBSTRUCTIVE PULMONARY DISEASE (COPD)

Centura Health—St. Anthony North Hospital, Westminster
Centura Health—St. Thomas More Hospital, Canon City
Exempla Lutheran Medical Center, Wheat Ridge
North Colorado Medical Center, Greeley
Platte Valley Medical Center, Brighton
Rose Medical Center, Denver
St. Joseph Hospital, Florence
Swedish Medical Center, Englewood

PNEUMONIA

Centura Health—Littleton Adventist Hospital, Littleton
Centura Health—Penrose St. Francis Health Services, Colorado Springs
Centura Health—Porter Adventist Hospital, Denver
Centura Health—St. Anthony Central Hospital, Denver
Exempla Lutheran Medical Center, Wheat Ridge
Exempla Saint Joseph Hospital, Denver
Longmont United Hospital, Longmont
Medical Center of Aurora, Aurora
North Colorado Medical Center, Greeley
Poudre Valley Hospital, Fort Collins
Presbyterian/St. Luke's Medical Center, Denver
Rose Medical Center, Denver
University of Colorado Hospital Authority, Aurora

STROKE

Boulder Community Hospital, Boulder
Centura Health—Penrose St. Francis Health Services, Colorado Springs
Centura Health—Porter Adventist Hospital, Denver
Exempla Lutheran Medical Center, Wheat Ridge
Exempla Saint Joseph Hospital, Denver
North Colorado Medical Center, Greeley
Poudre Valley Hospital, Fort Collins
Presbyterian/St. Luke's Medical Center, Denver
Rose Medical Center, Denver
Swedish Medical Center, Englewood
University of Colorado Hospital Authority, Aurora

VASCULAR

CAROTID SURGERY
None

PERIPHERAL VASCULAR BYPASS
None

RESECTION/REPLACEMENT OF ABDOMINAL AORTA
Poudre Valley Hospital, Fort Collins

WOMEN'S HEALTH
None

CONNECTICUT HOSPITALS: FIVE STAR RATED FACILITIES

COLORADO / CONNECTICUT HOSPITALS: FIVE STAR RATED FACILITIES

BARIATRIC SURGERY

None

CARDIAC

ATRIAL FIBRILLATION
Danbury Hospital, Danbury
Manchester Memorial Hospital, Manchester
Middlesex Hospital, Middletown
Milford Hospital, Milford
Yale-New Haven Hospital, New Haven

CORONARY INTERVENTIONAL PROCEDURES (ANGIOPLASTY/STENT)
Hospital of St. Raphael, New Haven
St. Vincent's Medical Center, Bridgeport

HEART ATTACK
Danbury Hospital, Danbury
Griffin Hospital, Derby
Hospital of St. Raphael, New Haven
Middlesex Hospital, Middletown
Midstate Medical Center, Meriden
St. Vincent's Medical Center, Bridgeport
William W. Backus Hospital, Norwich
World War II Veterans Memorial Hospital, Meriden

HEART BYPASS SURGERY
Danbury Hospital, Danbury
St. Vincent's Medical Center, Bridgeport

HEART FAILURE
Danbury Hospital, Danbury
Griffin Hospital, Derby
Hospital of Central Connecticut—New Britain General, New Britain
Hospital of St. Raphael, New Haven
Middlesex Hospital, Middletown
Yale-New Haven Hospital, New Haven

VALVE REPLACEMENT SURGERY
Hospital of St. Raphael, New Haven
Yale-New Haven Hospital, New Haven

CRITICAL CARE

DIABETIC ACIDOSIS AND COMA
None

PULMONARY EMBOLISM
Danbury Hospital, Danbury
Middlesex Hospital, Middletown
St. Vincent's Medical Center, Bridgeport

RESPIRATORY FAILURE
Danbury Hospital, Danbury
Middlesex Hospital, Middletown
Rockville General Hospital, Vernon Rockville
Yale-New Haven Hospital, New Haven

SEPSIS
Danbury Hospital, Danbury
Hartford Hospital, Hartford
Middlesex Hospital, Middletown
Yale-New Haven Hospital, New Haven

GASTROINTESTINAL

BOWEL OBSTRUCTION
Middlesex Hospital, Middletown

CHOLECYSTECTOMY
Danbury Hospital, Danbury
Day Kimball Hospital, Putnam
Hartford Hospital, Hartford
Hospital of Central Connecticut—New Britain General, New Britain
Lawrence and Memorial Hospital, New London
St. Vincent's Medical Center, Bridgeport
William W. Backus Hospital, Norwich

GASTROINTESTINAL BLEED
Danbury Hospital, Danbury
Middlesex Hospital, Middletown
Sharon Hospital, Sharon
Stamford Hospital, Stamford
William W. Backus Hospital, Norwich

GASTROINTESTINAL SURGERIES AND PROCEDURES
Hartford Hospital, Hartford
Middlesex Hospital, Middletown
William W. Backus Hospital, Norwich

Hospitals receiving a five star rating in a particular procedure have patient outcomes that put them among the best in the nation. For full definitions of ratings and awards, see Appendix.

PANCREATITIS
Middlesex Hospital, Middletown

GENERAL SURGERY

APPENDECTOMY
None

MATERNITY CARE

None

ORTHOPEDICS

BACK AND NECK SURGERY (EXCEPT SPINAL FUSION)
Greenwich Hospital Association, Greenwich
Hartford Hospital, Hartford
Norwalk Hospital Association, Norwalk
St. Francis Hospital and Medical Center, Hartford
St. Mary's Hospital, Waterbury

BACK AND NECK SURGERY (SPINAL FUSION)
Hospital of Central Connecticut—New Britain General, New Britain
John Dempsey Hospital, Farmington
St. Francis Hospital and Medical Center, Hartford
St. Mary's Hospital, Waterbury
Stamford Hospital, Stamford

HIP FRACTURE REPAIR
Charlotte Hungerford Hospital, Torrington
Danbury Hospital, Danbury

Greenwich Hospital Association, Greenwich
Hartford Hospital, Hartford
Middlesex Hospital, Middletown
Midstate Medical Center, Meriden
Norwalk Hospital Association, Norwalk
William W. Backus Hospital, Norwich
World War II Veterans Memorial Hospital, Meriden

TOTAL HIP REPLACEMENT
Charlotte Hungerford Hospital, Torrington
Danbury Hospital, Danbury
Hartford Hospital, Hartford
Hospital of Central Connecticut—New Britain General, New Britain
Waterbury Hospital Health Center, Waterbury

TOTAL KNEE REPLACEMENT
Hartford Hospital, Hartford
St. Francis Hospital and Medical Center, Hartford
Waterbury Hospital Health Center, Waterbury

PROSTATECTOMY

Hartford Hospital, Hartford
Middlesex Hospital, Middletown

PULMONARY

CHRONIC OBSTRUCTIVE PULMONARY DISEASE (COPD)
Danbury Hospital, Danbury
Griffin Hospital, Derby

Middlesex Hospital, Middletown
William W. Backus Hospital, Norwich
Yale-New Haven Hospital, New Haven

PNEUMONIA
Danbury Hospital, Danbury
Griffin Hospital, Derby
Hospital of St. Raphael, New Haven
Manchester Memorial Hospital, Manchester
Middlesex Hospital, Middletown
Yale-New Haven Hospital, New Haven

STROKE

Danbury Hospital, Danbury
Norwalk Hospital Association, Norwalk

VASCULAR

CAROTID SURGERY
Middlesex Hospital, Middletown

PERIPHERAL VASCULAR BYPASS
None

RESECTION/REPLACEMENT OF ABDOMINAL AORTA
None

WOMEN'S HEALTH

None

DELAWARE HOSPITALS: FIVE STAR RATED FACILITIES

BARIATRIC SURGERY

None

CARDIAC

ATRIAL FIBRILLATION
None

CORONARY INTERVENTIONAL PROCEDURES (ANGIOPLASTY/STENT)
None

HEART ATTACK
Bayhealth Medical Center—Kent General Hospital, Dover
Bayhealth Medical Center—Milford Memorial Campus, Milford

HEART BYPASS SURGERY
None

HEART FAILURE
Bayhealth Medical Center—Kent General Hospital, Dover
Bayhealth Medical Center—Milford Memorial Campus, Milford
Beebe Medical Center, Lewes
Christiana Care Health System—Christiana Hospital, Newark
Wilmington Hospital, Wilmington

VALVE REPLACEMENT SURGERY
Bayhealth Medical Center—Kent General Hospital, Dover
Bayhealth Medical Center—Milford Memorial Campus, Milford

CRITICAL CARE

DIABETIC ACIDOSIS AND COMA
None

PULMONARY EMBOLISM
None

RESPIRATORY FAILURE
Bayhealth Medical Center—Kent General Hospital, Dover
Bayhealth Medical Center—Milford Memorial Campus, Milford
Christiana Care Health System—Christiana Hospital, Newark
Wilmington Hospital, Wilmington

SEPSIS
Christiana Care Health System—Christiana Hospital, Newark
Wilmington Hospital, Wilmington

GASTROINTESTINAL

BOWEL OBSTRUCTION
Christiana Care Health System—Christiana
 Hospital, Newark
Wilmington Hospital, Wilmington

CHOLECYSTECTOMY
St. Francis Hospital, Wilmington

GASTROINTESTINAL BLEED
None

GASTROINTESTINAL SURGERIES AND PROCEDURES
None

PANCREATITIS
None

GENERAL SURGERY

APPENDECTOMY
None

MATERNITY CARE
None

ORTHOPEDICS

BACK AND NECK SURGERY (EXCEPT SPINAL FUSION)
None

BACK AND NECK SURGERY (SPINAL FUSION)
None

HIP FRACTURE REPAIR
Beebe Medical Center, Lewes

TOTAL HIP REPLACEMENT
St. Francis Hospital, Wilmington

TOTAL KNEE REPLACEMENT
Beebe Medical Center, Lewes
St. Francis Hospital, Wilmington

PROSTATECTOMY
None

PULMONARY

CHRONIC OBSTRUCTIVE PULMONARY DISEASE (COPD)
Christiana Care Health System—Christiana
 Hospital, Newark

St. Francis Hospital, Wilmington
Wilmington Hospital, Wilmington

PNEUMONIA
Beebe Medical Center, Lewes
Christiana Care Health System—Christiana
 Hospital, Newark
Wilmington Hospital, Wilmington

STROKE
None

VASCULAR

CAROTID SURGERY
None

PERIPHERAL VASCULAR BYPASS
Beebe Medical Center, Lewes

RESECTION/REPLACEMENT OF ABDOMINAL AORTA
None

WOMEN'S HEALTH
None

FLORIDA HOSPITALS: FIVE STAR RATED FACILITIES

BARIATRIC SURGERY

Bay Medical Center, Panama City
Cedars Medical Center, Miami
Gulf Coast Medical Center, Panama City
Hialeah Hospital, Hialeah
Memorial Hospital—Jacksonville, Jacksonville
Memorial Hospital—Pembroke, Pembroke Pines
Mercy Hospital, Miami
Munroe Regional Medical Center, Ocala
Ocala Regional Medical Center, Ocala
Palmetto General Hospital, Hialeah
Pasco Regional Medical Center, Dade City
Santa Rosa Medical Center, Milton
Tallahassee Memorial Healthcare, Tallahassee
Town and Country Hospital, Tampa
University Hospital and Medical Center, Tamarac

CARDIAC

ATRIAL FIBRILLATION
Charlotte Regional Medical Center, Punta Gorda
Flagler Hospital, St. Augustine
Florida Hospital, Orlando
Holy Cross Hospital, Fort Lauderdale

JFK Medical Center, Atlantis
Palm Beach Gardens Medical Center,
 Palm Beach Gardens
Venice Regional Medical Center, Venice
Westside Regional Medical Center, Plantation

CORONARY INTERVENTIONAL PROCEDURES (ANGIOPLASTY/STENT)
Baptist Hospital Pensacola, Pensacola
Baptist Medical Center, Jacksonville
Blake Medical Center, Bradenton
Central Florida Regional Hospital, Sanford
Cleveland Clinic Hospital, Weston
Delray Medical Center, Delray Beach
Florida Hospital—Oceanside, Ormond Beach
Florida Hospital—Ormond Beach, Ormond Beach
Holmes Regional Medical Center, Melbourne
JFK Medical Center, Atlantis
Morton Plant Hospital, Clearwater
Munroe Regional Medical Center, Ocala
NCH Healthcare System, Naples
North Ridge Medical Center, Fort Lauderdale
Osceola Regional Medical Center, Kissimmee
Palm Beach Gardens Medical Center,
 Palm Beach Gardens

St. Vincent's Medical Center, Jacksonville
Sarasota Memorial Hospital, Sarasota
Wuesthoff Medical Center—Rockledge, Rockledge

HEART ATTACK
Bay Medical Center, Panama City
Bethesda Memorial Hospital, Boynton Beach
Blake Medical Center, Bradenton
Broward General Medical Center, Fort Lauderdale
Charlotte Regional Medical Center, Punta Gorda
Cleveland Clinic Hospital, Weston
Delray Medical Center, Delray Beach
Desoto Memorial Hospital, Arcadia
Englewood Community Hospital, Englewood
Fawcett Memorial Hospital, Port Charlotte
Flagler Hospital, St. Augustine
Florida Hospital—Deland, Deland
Florida Hospital—Flagler, Palm Coast
Florida Hospital—Oceanside, Ormond Beach
Florida Hospital—Ormond Beach, Ormond Beach
Florida Hospital—Waterman, Tavares
Florida Medical Center, Fort Lauderdale
Heart of Florida Regional Medical Center, Davenport
Hialeah Hospital, Hialeah
Holmes Regional Medical Center, Melbourne

Jackson North Medical Center, North Miami Beach
JFK Medical Center, Atlantis
Kendall Regional Medical Center, Miami
Lakewood Ranch Medical Center, Bradenton
Lawnwood Regional Medical Center and Heart
    Institute, Fort Pierce
Lee Memorial Hospital, Fort Myers
Manatee Memorial Hospital, Bradenton
Martin Memorial Medical Center, Stuart
Mease Healthcare Dunedin, Dunedin
Memorial Hospital—West, Pembroke Pines
Morton Plant Hospital, Clearwater
Morton Plant Mease Healthcare Countryside,
    Safety Harbor
NCH Healthcare System, Naples
North Ridge Medical Center, Fort Lauderdale
Ocala Regional Medical Center, Ocala
Palm Beach Gardens Medical Center,
    Palm Beach Gardens
Peace River Regional Medical Center, Port Charlotte
Raulerson Hospital, Okeechobee
St. Joseph's Hospital, Tampa
St. Joseph's Women's Hospital, Tampa
St. Luke's Hospital, Jacksonville
Sarasota Memorial Hospital, Sarasota
Sebastian River Medical Center, Sebastian
West Boca Medical Center, Boca Raton
Westside Regional Medical Center, Plantation

HEART BYPASS SURGERY

Charlotte Regional Medical Center, Punta Gorda
Delray Medical Center, Delray Beach
Flagler Hospital, St. Augustine
JFK Medical Center, Atlantis
NCH Healthcare System, Naples
Venice Regional Medical Center, Venice

HEART FAILURE

Alachua General Hospital, Gainesville
Baptist Hospital of Miami, Miami
Baptist Medical Center, Jacksonville
Bay Medical Center, Panama City
Bert Fish Medical Center, New Smyrna Beach
Bethesda Memorial Hospital, Boynton Beach
Blake Medical Center, Bradenton
Brandon Regional Hospital, Brandon
Brooksville Regional Hospital, Brooksville
Broward General Medical Center, Fort Lauderdale
Cape Coral Hospital, Cape Coral
Cedars Medical Center, Miami
Central Florida Regional Hospital, Sanford
Charlotte Regional Medical Center, Punta Gorda
Cleveland Clinic Hospital, Weston

Community Hospital, New Port Richey
Coral Springs Medical Center, Coral Springs
Delray Medical Center, Delray Beach
Fawcett Memorial Hospital, Port Charlotte
Flagler Hospital, St. Augustine
Florida Hospital, Orlando
Florida Hospital—Deland, Deland
Florida Hospital—Fish Memorial, Orange City
Florida Hospital—Heartland Medical Center, Sebring
Florida Hospital—Oceanside, Ormond Beach
Florida Hospital—Ormond Beach, Ormond Beach
Florida Hospital—Waterman, Tavares
Florida Medical Center, Fort Lauderdale
Good Samaritan Medical Center, West Palm Beach
Gulf Breeze Hospital, Gulf Breeze
Gulf Coast Medical Center, Panama City
Halifax Medical Center, Daytona Beach
Hollywood Medical Center, Hollywood
Holmes Regional Medical Center, Melbourne
Holy Cross Hospital, Fort Lauderdale
JFK Medical Center, Atlantis
Jupiter Medical Center, Jupiter
Kendall Regional Medical Center, Miami
Lakewood Ranch Medical Center, Bradenton
Largo Medical Center, Largo
Lawnwood Regional Medical Center and Heart
    Institute, Fort Pierce
Lee Memorial Hospital, Fort Myers
Mariners Hospital, Tavernier
Martin Memorial Medical Center, Stuart
Mease Healthcare Dunedin, Dunedin
Memorial Hospital—Jacksonville, Jacksonville
Memorial Hospital—Miramar, Miramar
Memorial Hospital—Pembroke, Pembroke Pines
Memorial Hospital—West, Pembroke Pines
Mercy Hospital, Miami
Morton Plant Mease Healthcare Countryside,
    Safety Harbor
Morton Plant North Bay Hospital, New Port Richey
Munroe Regional Medical Center, Ocala
NCH Healthcare System, Naples
North Broward Medical Center, Deerfield Beach
Northwest Medical Center, Margate
Ocala Regional Medical Center, Ocala
Orange Park Medical Center, Orange Park
Osceola Regional Medical Center, Kissimmee
Palm Beach Gardens Medical Center,
    Palm Beach Gardens
Palmetto General Hospital, Hialeah
Palms West Hospital, Loxahatchee
Pan American Hospital, Miami
Parrish Medical Center, Titusville

Peace River Regional Medical Center, Port Charlotte
Physicians Regional Medical Center, Naples
Raulerson Hospital, Okeechobee
Regional Medical Center—Bayonet Point, Hudson
St. Joseph's Hospital, Tampa
St. Joseph's Women's Hospital, Tampa
St. Lucie Medical Center, Port St. Lucie
St. Luke's Hospital, Jacksonville
St. Vincent's Medical Center, Jacksonville
Sarasota Memorial Hospital, Sarasota
Shands Hospital at the University of Florida,
    Gainesville
Shands Jacksonville, Jacksonville
South Bay Hospital, Sun City Center
South Florida Baptist Hospital, Plant City
South Lake Hospital, Clermont
University Hospital and Medical Center, Tamarac
The Villages Regional Hospital, The Villages
Wellington Regional Medical Center, Wellington
Westside Regional Medical Center, Plantation
Wuesthoff Medical Center—Rockledge, Rockledge

VALVE REPLACEMENT SURGERY

Charlotte Regional Medical Center, Punta Gorda
Delray Medical Center, Delray Beach
JFK Medical Center, Atlantis

CRITICAL CARE

DIABETIC ACIDOSIS AND COMA
Florida Hospital, Orlando

PULMONARY EMBOLISM
Baptist Hospital of Miami, Miami
Boca Raton Community Hospital, Boca Raton
Brandon Regional Hospital, Brandon
Flagler Hospital, St. Augustine
Florida Hospital—Waterman, Tavares
Good Samaritan Medical Center, West Palm Beach
Jupiter Medical Center, Jupiter
Leesburg Regional Medical Center, Leesburg
Martin Memorial Medical Center, Stuart
Ocala Regional Medical Center, Ocala
Palms of Pasadena Hospital, St. Petersburg
South Bay Hospital, Sun City Center
The Villages Regional Hospital, The Villages

RESPIRATORY FAILURE
Aventura Hospital and Medical Center, Aventura
Baptist Medical Center, Jacksonville
Bay Medical Center, Panama City
Bert Fish Medical Center, New Smyrna Beach
Bethesda Memorial Hospital, Boynton Beach
Boca Raton Community Hospital, Boca Raton

Brandon Regional Hospital, Brandon
Cedars Medical Center, Miami
Central Florida Regional Hospital, Sanford
Community Hospital, New Port Richey
Coral Gables Hospital, Coral Gables
Coral Springs Medical Center, Coral Springs
Delray Medical Center, Delray Beach
Doctors Hospital of Sarasota, Sarasota
Flagler Hospital, St. Augustine
Florida Hospital, Orlando
Florida Hospital—Deland, Deland
Florida Hospital—Fish Memorial, Orange City
Florida Hospital—Oceanside, Ormond Beach
Florida Hospital—Ormond Beach, Ormond Beach
Florida Hospital—Waterman, Tavares
Florida Medical Center, Fort Lauderdale
Good Samaritan Medical Center, West Palm Beach
Gulf Breeze Hospital, Gulf Breeze
Gulf Coast Medical Center, Panama City
Helen Ellis Memorial Hospital, Tarpon Springs
Hollywood Medical Center, Hollywood
JFK Medical Center, Atlantis
Jupiter Medical Center, Jupiter
Kendall Regional Medical Center, Miami
Lake City Medical Center, Lake City
Lawnwood Regional Medical Center and Heart
    Institute, Fort Pierce
Lee Memorial Hospital, Fort Myers
Martin Memorial Medical Center, Stuart
Memorial Hospital—Pembroke, Pembroke Pines
Memorial Hospital—West, Pembroke Pines
Memorial Regional Hospital, Hollywood
Mercy Hospital, Miami
Morton Plant North Bay Hospital, New Port Richey
Munroe Regional Medical Center, Ocala
North Broward Medical Center, Deerfield Beach
Northwest Medical Center, Margate
Ocala Regional Medical Center, Ocala
Palmetto General Hospital, Hialeah
Palms West Hospital, Loxahatchee
Peace River Regional Medical Center, Port Charlotte
Raulerson Hospital, Okeechobee
Regional Medical Center—Bayonet Point, Hudson
St. Joseph's Hospital, Tampa
St. Joseph's Women's Hospital, Tampa
Santa Rosa Medical Center, Milton
South Bay Hospital, Sun City Center
South Lake Hospital, Clermont
Southwest Florida Regional Medical Center,
    Fort Myers
University Hospital and Medical Center, Tamarac
Wellington Regional Medical Center, Wellington

Westside Regional Medical Center, Plantation
Winter Haven Hospital, Winter Haven
Wuesthoff Medical Center—Rockledge, Rockledge

SEPSIS

Aventura Hospital and Medical Center, Aventura
Baptist Medical Center, Jacksonville
Bay Medical Center, Panama City
Bert Fish Medical Center, New Smyrna Beach
Bethesda Memorial Hospital, Boynton Beach
Boca Raton Community Hospital, Boca Raton
Brandon Regional Hospital, Brandon
Brooksville Regional Hospital, Brooksville
Cedars Medical Center, Miami
Central Florida Regional Hospital, Sanford
Cleveland Clinic Hospital, Weston
Columbia Hospital, West Palm Beach
Coral Gables Hospital, Coral Gables
Coral Springs Medical Center, Coral Springs
Delray Medical Center, Delray Beach
Doctors Hospital, Coral Gables
Fawcett Memorial Hospital, Port Charlotte
Flagler Hospital, St. Augustine
Florida Hospital, Orlando
Florida Hospital—Deland, Deland
Florida Hospital—Fish Memorial, Orange City
Florida Hospital—Flagler, Palm Coast
Florida Hospital—Heartland Medical Center, Sebring
Florida Hospital—Oceanside, Ormond Beach
Florida Hospital—Ormond Beach, Ormond Beach
Florida Hospital—Waterman, Tavares
Florida Medical Center, Fort Lauderdale
Gulf Breeze Hospital, Gulf Breeze
Gulf Coast Medical Center, Panama City
Hialeah Hospital, Hialeah
Holy Cross Hospital, Fort Lauderdale
Jackson Hospital, Marianna
JFK Medical Center, Atlantis
Jupiter Medical Center, Jupiter
Kendall Regional Medical Center, Miami
Larkin Community Hospital, South Miami
Lawnwood Regional Medical Center and Heart
    Institute, Fort Pierce
Lee Memorial Hospital, Fort Myers
Martin Memorial Medical Center, Stuart
Memorial Hospital—Jacksonville, Jacksonville
Memorial Hospital—Miramar, Miramar
Memorial Hospital—Pembroke, Pembroke Pines
Memorial Hospital—West, Pembroke Pines
Memorial Regional Hospital, Hollywood
Morton Plant North Bay Hospital, New Port Richey
Munroe Regional Medical Center, Ocala
NCH Healthcare System, Naples

North Okaloosa Medical Center, Crestview
Northwest Medical Center, Margate
Oak Hill Hospital, Brooksville
Palms West Hospital, Loxahatchee
Parrish Medical Center, Titusville
Peace River Regional Medical Center, Port Charlotte
Physicians Regional Medical Center, Naples
Raulerson Hospital, Okeechobee
St. Anthony's Hospital, St. Petersburg
St. Joseph's Hospital, Tampa
St. Joseph's Women's Hospital, Tampa
St. Vincent's Medical Center, Jacksonville
Sarasota Memorial Hospital, Sarasota
South Florida Baptist Hospital, Plant City
South Lake Hospital, Clermont
University Hospital and Medical Center, Tamarac
The Villages Regional Hospital, The Villages
Wellington Regional Medical Center, Wellington
Westside Regional Medical Center, Plantation
Wuesthoff Medical Center—Rockledge, Rockledge

GASTROINTESTINAL

BOWEL OBSTRUCTION

Baptist Medical Center, Jacksonville
Cape Coral Hospital, Cape Coral
Community Hospital, New Port Richey
Doctors Hospital of Sarasota, Sarasota
Doctors Hospital, Coral Gables
Flagler Hospital, St. Augustine
Florida Hospital, Orlando
Florida Hospital—Heartland Medical Center, Sebring
Gulf Breeze Hospital, Gulf Breeze
Gulf Coast Medical Center, Panama City
Halifax Medical Center, Daytona Beach
JFK Medical Center, Atlantis
Lee Memorial Hospital, Fort Myers
Palm Beach Gardens Medical Center,
    Palm Beach Gardens
Peace River Regional Medical Center,
    Port Charlotte
Physicians Regional Medical Center, Naples
University Hospital and Medical Center, Tamarac
Westside Regional Medical Center, Plantation

CHOLECYSTECTOMY

Aventura Hospital and Medical Center, Aventura
Bay Medical Center, Panama City
Cape Coral Hospital, Cape Coral
Cedars Medical Center, Miami
Community Hospital, New Port Richey
Doctors' Memorial Hospital, Perry
Englewood Community Hospital, Englewood

Hospitals receiving a five star rating in a particular procedure have patient outcomes that put them among the best in the nation. For full definitions of ratings and awards, see Appendix.

Fawcett Memorial Hospital, Port Charlotte
Flagler Hospital, St. Augustine
Fort Walton Beach Medical Center,
  Fort Walton Beach
Gulf Coast Medical Center, Panama City
JFK Medical Center, Atlantis
Lake City Medical Center, Lake City
Lakeland Regional Medical Center, Lakeland
Largo Medical Center, Largo
Lawnwood Regional Medical Center and Heart
  Institute, Fort Pierce
Lehigh Regional Medical Center, Lehigh Acres
Morton Plant Hospital, Clearwater
North Florida Regional Medical Center, Gainesville
Ocala Regional Medical Center, Ocala
Pasco Regional Medical Center, Dade City
Peace River Regional Medical Center, Port Charlotte
St. Lucie Medical Center, Port St. Lucie
Santa Rosa Medical Center, Milton
Sebastian River Medical Center, Sebastian
South Bay Hospital, Sun City Center
South Lake Hospital, Clermont
Tallahassee Memorial Healthcare, Tallahassee
Twin Cities Hospital, Niceville
University Community Hospital at Carrollwood,
  Tampa
The Villages Regional Hospital, The Villages
Wuesthoff Medical Center—Rockledge, Rockledge

GASTROINTESTINAL BLEED

Alachua General Hospital, Gainesville
Bethesda Memorial Hospital, Boynton Beach
Boca Raton Community Hospital, Boca Raton
Cleveland Clinic Hospital, Weston
Community Hospital, New Port Richey
Delray Medical Center, Delray Beach
Fishermen's Hospital, Marathon
Flagler Hospital, St. Augustine
Florida Hospital—Deland, Deland
Florida Hospital—Fish Memorial, Orange City
Florida Hospital—Oceanside, Ormond Beach
Florida Hospital—Ormond Beach, Ormond Beach
Florida Medical Center, Fort Lauderdale
Good Samaritan Medical Center, West Palm Beach
Gulf Coast Medical Center, Panama City
Heart of Florida Regional Medical Center, Davenport
Holmes Regional Medical Center, Melbourne
JFK Medical Center, Atlantis
Jupiter Medical Center, Jupiter
Lucerne Medical Center, Orlando
Martin Memorial Medical Center, Stuart
Memorial Hospital—Pembroke, Pembroke Pines

Memorial Hospital—West, Pembroke Pines
Memorial Regional Hospital, Hollywood
Morton Plant Hospital, Clearwater
NCH Healthcare System, Naples
North Okaloosa Medical Center, Crestview
Orlando Regional Healthcare, Orlando
Palms of Pasadena Hospital, St. Petersburg
Peace River Regional Medical Center, Port Charlotte
Sarasota Memorial Hospital, Sarasota
Sebastian River Medical Center, Sebastian
Shands Hospital at the University of Florida,
  Gainesville
Westside Regional Medical Center, Plantation

GASTROINTESTINAL SURGERIES
AND PROCEDURES

Boca Raton Community Hospital, Boca Raton
Cleveland Clinic Hospital, Weston
Community Hospital, New Port Richey
Coral Springs Medical Center, Coral Springs
Delray Medical Center, Delray Beach
Fawcett Memorial Hospital, Port Charlotte
Flagler Hospital, St. Augustine
Florida Hospital, Orlando
Florida Hospital—Fish Memorial, Orange City
Florida Hospital—Oceanside, Ormond Beach
Florida Hospital—Ormond Beach, Ormond Beach
Florida Hospital—Waterman, Tavares
Good Samaritan Medical Center, West Palm Beach
Gulf Breeze Hospital, Gulf Breeze
Gulf Coast Medical Center, Panama City
Halifax Medical Center, Daytona Beach
Holmes Regional Medical Center, Melbourne
Holy Cross Hospital, Fort Lauderdale
JFK Medical Center, Atlantis
Lake City Medical Center, Lake City
Memorial Hospital—Tampa, Tampa
North Ridge Medical Center, Fort Lauderdale
Northwest Medical Center, Margate
Osceola Regional Medical Center, Kissimmee
Palms West Hospital, Loxahatchee
Parrish Medical Center, Titusville
Raulerson Hospital, Okeechobee
Regional Medical Center—Bayonet Point, Hudson
St. Joseph's Hospital, Tampa
St. Joseph's Women's Hospital, Tampa
St. Luke's Hospital, Jacksonville
Santa Rosa Medical Center, Milton
Shands Lake Shore, Lake City
University Hospital and Medical Center, Tamarac
Wellington Regional Medical Center, Wellington
Westside Regional Medical Center, Plantation

PANCREATITIS

Baptist Hospital Pensacola, Pensacola
Bethesda Memorial Hospital, Boynton Beach
Delray Medical Center, Delray Beach
Doctors Hospital, Coral Gables
Good Samaritan Medical Center, West Palm Beach
Lee Memorial Hospital, Fort Myers
NCH Healthcare System, Naples
St. Anthony's Hospital, St. Petersburg
Venice Regional Medical Center, Venice

GENERAL SURGERY

APPENDECTOMY

Baptist Hospital of Miami, Miami
Baptist Hospital Pensacola, Pensacola
Englewood Community Hospital, Englewood
Florida Hospital—Oceanside, Ormond Beach
Florida Hospital—Ormond Beach, Ormond Beach
Fort Walton Beach Medical Center, Fort Walton Beach
Gulf Coast Hospital, Fort Myers
Halifax Medical Center, Daytona Beach
Heart of Florida Regional Medical Center, Davenport
Indian River Medical Center, Vero Beach
JFK Medical Center, Atlantis
Jupiter Medical Center, Jupiter
Kendall Regional Medical Center, Miami
Lake City Medical Center, Lake City
Lakeland Regional Medical Center, Lakeland
Largo Medical Center, Largo
Lawnwood Regional Medical Center and Heart
  Institute, Fort Pierce
Memorial Hospital—Jacksonville, Jacksonville
Morton Plant Hospital, Clearwater
Morton Plant Mease Healthcare Countryside,
  Safety Harbor
North Florida Regional Medical Center, Gainesville
Northwest Medical Center, Margate
Oak Hill Hospital, Brooksville
Ocala Regional Medical Center, Ocala
Palm Springs General Hospital, Hialeah
Palms West Hospital, Loxahatchee
Pasco Regional Medical Center, Dade City
Regional Medical Center—Bayonet Point, Hudson
Sacred Heart Hospital at the Emerald Coast, Destin
St. Lucie Medical Center, Port St. Lucie
St. Petersburg General Hospital, St. Petersburg
Sebastian River Medical Center, Sebastian
South Lake Hospital, Clermont
Southwest Florida Regional Medical Center,
  Fort Myers
Tallahassee Memorial Healthcare, Tallahassee

Twin Cities Hospital, Niceville
University Hospital and Medical Center, Tamarac
The Villages Regional Hospital, The Villages

MATERNITY CARE

Baptist Hospital of Miami, Miami
Bartow Regional Medical Center, Bartow
Bethesda Memorial Hospital, Boynton Beach
Cape Coral Hospital, Cape Coral
Community Hospital, New Port Richey
Desoto Memorial Hospital, Arcadia
Florida Hospital, Orlando
Florida Keys Memorial Hospital, Key West
Gulf Coast Hospital, Fort Myers
Halifax Medical Center, Daytona Beach
Heart of Florida Regional Medical Center, Davenport
Helen Ellis Memorial Hospital, Tarpon Springs
Hialeah Hospital, Hialeah
Holy Cross Hospital, Fort Lauderdale
Jackson North Medical Center, North Miami Beach
Kendall Regional Medical Center, Miami
Lower Keys Medical Center, Key West
Manatee Memorial Hospital, Bradenton
Memorial Regional Hospital, Hollywood
Mercy Hospital, Miami
Miami Beach Community Hospital, Miami Beach
Mt. Sinai Medical Center, Miami Beach
Mt. Sinai Medical Center and Miami Heart Institute, Miami Beach
Munroe Regional Medical Center, Ocala
NCH Healthcare System, Naples
North Shore Medical Center, Miami
Northwest Medical Center, Margate
Orange Park Medical Center, Orange Park
Osceola Regional Medical Center, Kissimmee
Palmetto General Hospital, Hialeah
Palms West Hospital, Loxahatchee
Plantation General Hospital, Plantation
St. Petersburg General Hospital, St. Petersburg
Sarasota Memorial Hospital, Sarasota
South Miami Hospital, South Miami
Wellington Regional Medical Center, Wellington
West Boca Medical Center, Boca Raton
West Florida Hospital, Pensacola

ORTHOPEDICS

BACK AND NECK SURGERY (EXCEPT SPINAL FUSION)

Blake Medical Center, Bradenton
Capital Regional Medical Center, Tallahassee
Citrus Memorial Hospital, Inverness

Flagler Hospital, St. Augustine
Fort Walton Beach Medical Center, Fort Walton Beach
Good Samaritan Medical Center, West Palm Beach
Gulf Coast Hospital, Fort Myers
Gulf Coast Medical Center, Panama City
Halifax Medical Center, Daytona Beach
Indian River Medical Center, Vero Beach
Lee Memorial Hospital, Fort Myers
Lucerne Medical Center, Orlando
NCH Healthcare System, Naples
Ocala Regional Medical Center, Ocala
Orlando Regional Healthcare, Orlando
Physicians Regional Medical Center, Naples
Sarasota Memorial Hospital, Sarasota
Sebastian River Medical Center, Sebastian
Seven Rivers Regional Medical Center, Crystal River
South Bay Hospital, Sun City Center
Tallahassee Memorial Healthcare, Tallahassee
University Community Hospital, Tampa
Venice Regional Medical Center, Venice

BACK AND NECK SURGERY (SPINAL FUSION)

Aventura Hospital and Medical Center, Aventura
Bethesda Memorial Hospital, Boynton Beach
Citrus Memorial Hospital, Inverness
Flagler Hospital, St. Augustine
Fort Walton Beach Medical Center, Fort Walton Beach
Halifax Medical Center, Daytona Beach
Helen Ellis Memorial Hospital, Tarpon Springs
Holy Cross Hospital, Fort Lauderdale
Jupiter Medical Center, Jupiter
Lee Memorial Hospital, Fort Myers
Leesburg Regional Medical Center, Leesburg
Lucerne Medical Center, Orlando
NCH Healthcare System, Naples
Ocala Regional Medical Center, Ocala
Orlando Regional Healthcare, Orlando
Parrish Medical Center, Titusville
St. Lucie Medical Center, Port St. Lucie
Sarasota Memorial Hospital, Sarasota
Seven Rivers Regional Medical Center, Crystal River
South Bay Hospital, Sun City Center

HIP FRACTURE REPAIR

Aventura Hospital and Medical Center, Aventura
Baptist Hospital of Miami, Miami
Bay Medical Center, Panama City
Cape Coral Hospital, Cape Coral
Delray Medical Center, Delray Beach
Englewood Community Hospital, Englewood
Fawcett Memorial Hospital, Port Charlotte
Florida Hospital–Flagler, Palm Coast
Florida Hospital–Heartland Medical Center, Sebring

Florida Medical Center, Fort Lauderdale
Fort Walton Beach Medical Center, Fort Walton Beach
Gulf Breeze Hospital, Gulf Breeze
Halifax Medical Center, Daytona Beach
Helen Ellis Memorial Hospital, Tarpon Springs
Hialeah Hospital, Hialeah
Hollywood Medical Center, Hollywood
Holy Cross Hospital, Fort Lauderdale
JFK Medical Center, Atlantis
Jupiter Medical Center, Jupiter
Kendall Regional Medical Center, Miami
Lakeland Regional Medical Center, Lakeland
Largo Medical Center, Largo
Lawnwood Regional Medical Center and Heart Institute, Fort Pierce
Martin Memorial Medical Center, Stuart
Mercy Hospital, Miami
Morton Plant Mease Healthcare Countryside, Safety Harbor
North Broward Medical Center, Deerfield Beach
Northside Hospital, St. Petersburg
Oak Hill Hospital, Brooksville
Palm Beach Gardens Medical Center, Palm Beach Gardens
Palm Springs General Hospital, Hialeah
Parrish Medical Center, Titusville
Pasco Regional Medical Center, Dade City
Regional Medical Center–Bayonet Point, Hudson
St. Lucie Medical Center, Port St. Lucie
St. Mary's Medical Center, West Palm Beach
Seven Rivers Regional Medical Center, Crystal River
South Lake Hospital, Clermont
South Miami Hospital, South Miami
Sun Coast Hospital, Largo
Twin Cities Hospital, Niceville
University Community Hospital, Tampa
University Hospital and Medical Center, Tamarac
Westchester General Hospital, Miami
Wuesthoff Medical Center–Rockledge, Rockledge

TOTAL HIP REPLACEMENT

Citrus Memorial Hospital, Inverness
Delray Medical Center, Delray Beach
Englewood Community Hospital, Englewood
Florida Hospital, Orlando
Halifax Medical Center, Daytona Beach
Helen Ellis Memorial Hospital, Tarpon Springs
Holy Cross Hospital, Fort Lauderdale
Jupiter Medical Center, Jupiter
Lakeland Regional Medical Center, Lakeland
Largo Medical Center, Largo
Lee Memorial Hospital, Fort Myers

Hospitals receiving a five star rating in a particular procedure have patient outcomes that put them among the best in the nation. For full definitions of ratings and awards, see Appendix.

Martin Memorial Medical Center, Stuart
Palm Beach Gardens Medical Center,
    Palm Beach Gardens
St. Luke's Hospital, Jacksonville
South Bay Hospital, Sun City Center
Tallahassee Memorial Healthcare, Tallahassee

TOTAL KNEE REPLACEMENT

Alachua General Hospital, Gainesville
Cape Coral Hospital, Cape Coral
Charlotte Regional Medical Center, Punta Gorda
Citrus Memorial Hospital, Inverness
Flagler Hospital, St. Augustine
Fort Walton Beach Medical Center, Fort Walton Beach
Gulf Coast Hospital, Fort Myers
Halifax Medical Center, Daytona Beach
Heart of Florida Regional Medical Center, Davenport
Helen Ellis Memorial Hospital, Tarpon Springs
Holy Cross Hospital, Fort Lauderdale
Indian River Medical Center, Vero Beach
Jupiter Medical Center, Jupiter
Lakeland Regional Medical Center, Lakeland
Largo Medical Center, Largo
Manatee Memorial Hospital, Bradenton
Mercy Hospital, Miami
Morton Plant Mease Healthcare Countryside,
    Safety Harbor
Palmetto General Hospital, Hialeah
Palms of Pasadena Hospital, St. Petersburg
Pasco Regional Medical Center, Dade City
Physicians Regional Medical Center, Naples
St. Luke's Hospital, Jacksonville
Santa Rosa Medical Center, Milton
Seven Rivers Regional Medical Center, Crystal River
Shands Hospital at the University of Florida,
    Gainesville
South Miami Hospital, South Miami
Tallahassee Memorial Healthcare, Tallahassee
Twin Cities Hospital, Niceville
University Community Hospital, Tampa
Venice Regional Medical Center, Venice
West Florida Hospital, Pensacola

PROSTATECTOMY

Aventura Hospital and Medical Center, Aventura
Baptist Hospital of Miami, Miami
Boca Raton Community Hospital, Boca Raton
Coral Gables Hospital, Coral Gables
Flagler Hospital, St. Augustine
Fort Walton Beach Medical Center,
    Fort Walton Beach
Jupiter Medical Center, Jupiter

Munroe Regional Medical Center, Ocala
Oak Hill Hospital, Brooksville
Ocala Regional Medical Center, Ocala
St. Anthony's Hospital, St. Petersburg
St. Lucie Medical Center, Port St. Lucie
St. Luke's Hospital, Jacksonville
Seven Rivers Regional Medical Center,
    Crystal River
University Community Hospital, Tampa
Wuesthoff Medical Center–Melbourne, Melbourne
Wuesthoff Medical Center–Rockledge, Rockledge

PULMONARY

CHRONIC OBSTRUCTIVE PULMONARY DISEASE (COPD)

Baptist Medical Center, Jacksonville
Bethesda Memorial Hospital, Boynton Beach
Boca Raton Community Hospital, Boca Raton
Cedars Medical Center, Miami
Cleveland Clinic Hospital, Weston
Delray Medical Center, Delray Beach
Doctors Hospital, Coral Gables
Englewood Community Hospital, Englewood
Florida Hospital–Fish Memorial, Orange City
Florida Hospital–Waterman, Tavares
Florida Medical Center, Fort Lauderdale
Glades General Hospital, Belle Glade
Helen Ellis Memorial Hospital, Tarpon Springs
Jupiter Medical Center, Jupiter
Kendall Regional Medical Center, Miami
Lakeland Regional Medical Center, Lakeland
Lee Memorial Hospital, Fort Myers
Mease Healthcare Dunedin, Dunedin
Memorial Hospital–Pembroke, Pembroke Pines
Memorial Hospital–West, Pembroke Pines
Morton Plant Mease Healthcare Countryside,
    Safety Harbor
Munroe Regional Medical Center, Ocala
North Okaloosa Medical Center, Crestview
Ocala Regional Medical Center, Ocala
Orange Park Medical Center, Orange Park
Palm Beach Gardens Medical Center,
    Palm Beach Gardens
Raulerson Hospital, Okeechobee
Regional Medical Center–Bayonet Point, Hudson
St. Luke's Hospital, Jacksonville
St. Vincent's Medical Center, Jacksonville
Sarasota Memorial Hospital, Sarasota
Shands Lake Shore, Lake City
South Lake Hospital, Clermont
Southwest Florida Regional Medical Center,
    Fort Myers

Twin Cities Hospital, Niceville
Wuesthoff Medical Center–Rockledge, Rockledge

PNEUMONIA

Alachua General Hospital, Gainesville
Aventura Hospital and Medical Center, Aventura
Baptist Hospital of Miami, Miami
Baptist Medical Center, Jacksonville
Baptist Medical Center–Beaches, Jacksonville Beach
Bartow Regional Medical Center, Bartow
Bay Medical Center, Panama City
Bethesda Memorial Hospital, Boynton Beach
Boca Raton Community Hospital, Boca Raton
Brandon Regional Hospital, Brandon
Brooksville Regional Hospital, Brooksville
Broward General Medical Center, Fort Lauderdale
Cape Canaveral Hospital, Cocoa Beach
Cedars Medical Center, Miami
Central Florida Regional Hospital, Sanford
Charlotte Regional Medical Center, Punta Gorda
Cleveland Clinic Hospital, Weston
Community Hospital, New Port Richey
Coral Springs Medical Center, Coral Springs
Delray Medical Center, Delray Beach
Doctors Hospital of Sarasota, Sarasota
Doctors Hospital, Coral Gables
Fawcett Memorial Hospital, Port Charlotte
Flagler Hospital, St. Augustine
Florida Hospital, Orlando
Florida Hospital–Deland, Deland
Florida Hospital–Fish Memorial, Orange City
Florida Hospital–Heartland Medical Center, Sebring
Florida Hospital–Waterman, Tavares
Florida Medical Center, Fort Lauderdale
Glades General Hospital, Belle Glade
Good Samaritan Medical Center, West Palm Beach
Gulf Breeze Hospital, Gulf Breeze
Gulf Coast Hospital, Fort Myers
Gulf Coast Medical Center, Panama City
Health Central, Ocoee
Helen Ellis Memorial Hospital, Tarpon Springs
Hollywood Medical Center, Hollywood
Holmes Regional Medical Center, Melbourne
Holy Cross Hospital, Fort Lauderdale
Imperial Point Medical Center, Fort Lauderdale
JFK Medical Center, Atlantis
Jupiter Medical Center, Jupiter
Kendall Regional Medical Center, Miami
Lawnwood Regional Medical Center and Heart
    Institute, Fort Pierce
Lee Memorial Hospital, Fort Myers
Lucerne Medical Center, Orlando

Manatee Memorial Hospital, Bradenton
Martin Memorial Medical Center, Stuart
Mease Healthcare Dunedin, Dunedin
Memorial Hospital–Pembroke, Pembroke Pines
Memorial Hospital–Tampa, Tampa
Memorial Hospital–West, Pembroke Pines
Memorial Regional Hospital, Hollywood
Mercy Hospital, Miami
Morton Plant Hospital, Clearwater
Morton Plant Mease Healthcare Countryside,
  Safety Harbor
Morton Plant North Bay Hospital, New Port Richey
Munroe Regional Medical Center, Ocala
NCH Healthcare System, Naples
North Broward Medical Center, Deerfield Beach
North Okaloosa Medical Center, Crestview
Northside Hospital, St. Petersburg
Oak Hill Hospital, Brooksville
Ocala Regional Medical Center, Ocala
Orange Park Medical Center, Orange Park
Orlando Regional Healthcare, Orlando
Palm Beach Gardens Medical Center,
  Palm Beach Gardens
Palms West Hospital, Loxahatchee
Pan American Hospital, Miami
Parrish Medical Center, Titusville
Pasco Regional Medical Center, Dade City
Peace River Regional Medical Center, Port Charlotte
Raulerson Hospital, Okeechobee
St. Joseph's Hospital, Tampa
St. Joseph's Women's Hospital, Tampa
St. Petersburg General Hospital, St. Petersburg
St. Vincent's Medical Center, Jacksonville
Santa Rosa Medical Center, Milton
Sarasota Memorial Hospital, Sarasota
Shands Hospital at the University of Florida,
  Gainesville
Shands Lake Shore, Lake City
South Lake Hospital, Clermont
South Miami Hospital, South Miami
Southwest Florida Regional Medical Center,
  Fort Myers
University Community Hospital at Carrollwood,
  Tampa
University Hospital and Medical Center, Tamarac
The Villages Regional Hospital, The Villages
Wellington Regional Medical Center, Wellington
West Boca Medical Center, Boca Raton
Westside Regional Medical Center, Plantation
Wuesthoff Medical Center–Rockledge, Rockledge

STROKE

Aventura Hospital and Medical Center, Aventura
Baptist Hospital of Miami, Miami
Baptist Medical Center, Jacksonville
Bartow Regional Medical Center, Bartow
Bay Medical Center, Panama City
Bert Fish Medical Center, New Smyrna Beach
Bethesda Memorial Hospital, Boynton Beach
Boca Raton Community Hospital, Boca Raton
Brandon Regional Hospital, Brandon
Brooksville Regional Hospital, Brooksville
Cape Canaveral Hospital, Cocoa Beach
Cape Coral Hospital, Cape Coral
Cedars Medical Center, Miami
Central Florida Regional Hospital, Sanford
Community Hospital, New Port Richey
Coral Springs Medical Center, Coral Springs
Delray Medical Center, Delray Beach
Doctors Hospital of Sarasota, Sarasota
Englewood Community Hospital, Englewood
Fawcett Memorial Hospital, Port Charlotte
Flagler Hospital, St. Augustine
Florida Hospital, Orlando
Florida Hospital-Zephyrhills, Zephyrhills
Florida Hospital–Deland, Deland
Florida Hospital–Waterman, Tavares
Florida Medical Center, Fort Lauderdale
Good Samaritan Medical Center, West Palm Beach
Halifax Medical Center, Daytona Beach
Hialeah Hospital, Hialeah
Holmes Regional Medical Center, Melbourne
Holy Cross Hospital, Fort Lauderdale
JFK Medical Center, Atlantis
Jupiter Medical Center, Jupiter
Kendall Regional Medical Center, Miami
Lake City Medical Center, Lake City
Lakewood Ranch Medical Center, Bradenton
Lawnwood Regional Medical Center and Heart
  Institute, Fort Pierce
Lee Memorial Hospital, Fort Myers
Leesburg Regional Medical Center, Leesburg
Lucerne Medical Center, Orlando
Martin Memorial Medical Center, Stuart
Mease Healthcare Dunedin, Dunedin
Memorial Hospital–West, Pembroke Pines
Mercy Hospital, Miami
Miami Beach Community Hospital, Miami Beach
Morton Plant Mease Healthcare Countryside,
  Safety Harbor
Mt. Sinai Medical Center, Miami Beach

Mt. Sinai Medical Center and Miami Heart
  Institute, Miami Beach
Munroe Regional Medical Center, Ocala
North Broward Medical Center, Deerfield Beach
North Florida Regional Medical Center, Gainesville
Northwest Medical Center, Margate
Oak Hill Hospital, Brooksville
Ocala Regional Medical Center, Ocala
Orange Park Medical Center, Orange Park
Orlando Regional Healthcare, Orlando
Osceola Regional Medical Center, Kissimmee
Palm Beach Gardens Medical Center,
  Palm Beach Gardens
Palm Springs General Hospital, Hialeah
Palms West Hospital, Loxahatchee
Parrish Medical Center, Titusville
Pasco Regional Medical Center, Dade City
Raulerson Hospital, Okeechobee
Regional Medical Center–Bayonet Point, Hudson
Sacred Heart Hospital, Pensacola
St. Anthony's Hospital, St. Petersburg
St. Joseph's Hospital, Tampa
St. Joseph's Women's Hospital, Tampa
St. Lucie Medical Center, Port St. Lucie
St. Luke's Hospital, Jacksonville
St. Mary's Medical Center, West Palm Beach
St. Vincent's Medical Center, Jacksonville
Sarasota Memorial Hospital, Sarasota
Sebastian River Medical Center, Sebastian
Shands Lake Shore, Lake City
South Lake Hospital, Clermont
Southwest Florida Regional Medical Center,
  Fort Myers
University Hospital and Medical Center, Tamarac
Wellington Regional Medical Center, Wellington
Westchester General Hospital, Miami
Westside Regional Medical Center, Plantation

VASCULAR

CAROTID SURGERY

Aventura Hospital and Medical Center, Aventura
Bayfront Medical Center, St. Petersburg
Fawcett Memorial Hospital, Port Charlotte
Flagler Hospital, St. Augustine
Halifax Medical Center, Daytona Beach
Holmes Regional Medical Center, Melbourne
Indian River Medical Center, Vero Beach
Largo Medical Center, Largo
Martin Memorial Medical Center, Stuart
Memorial Hospital–Jacksonville, Jacksonville
North Florida Regional Medical Center, Gainesville

Hospitals receiving a five star rating in a particular procedure have patient outcomes that put them among the best in the nation. For full definitions of ratings and awards, see Appendix.

Ocala Regional Medical Center, Ocala
Orange Park Medical Center, Orange Park
Osceola Regional Medical Center, Kissimmee
Palm Beach Gardens Medical Center,
    Palm Beach Gardens

PERIPHERAL VASCULAR BYPASS

Baptist Hospital of Miami, Miami
Baptist Hospital Pensacola, Pensacola
Delray Medical Center, Delray Beach
Holmes Regional Medical Center, Melbourne
Largo Medical Center, Largo

Martin Memorial Medical Center, Stuart
Sacred Heart Hospital, Pensacola
Southwest Florida Regional Medical Center,
    Fort Myers

RESECTION/REPLACEMENT OF ABDOMINAL AORTA

Sacred Heart Hospital, Pensacola
Sarasota Memorial Hospital, Sarasota

WOMEN'S HEALTH

Baptist Hospital of Miami, Miami
Broward General Medical Center, Fort Lauderdale

Flagler Hospital, St. Augustine
Florida Hospital, Orlando
Florida Hospital—Oceanside, Ormond Beach
Florida Hospital—Ormond Beach, Ormond Beach
Halifax Medical Center, Daytona Beach
Holy Cross Hospital, Fort Lauderdale
Lee Memorial Hospital, Fort Myers
Munroe Regional Medical Center, Ocala
NCH Healthcare System, Naples
Osceola Regional Medical Center, Kissimmee
Sarasota Memorial Hospital, Sarasota
South Miami Hospital, South Miami

GEORGIA HOSPITALS: FIVE STAR RATED FACILITIES

BARIATRIC SURGERY

None

CARDIAC

ATRIAL FIBRILLATION
None

CORONARY INTERVENTIONAL PROCEDURES (ANGIOPLASTY/STENT)
Saint Joseph's Hospital of Atlanta, Atlanta

HEART ATTACK

Colquitt Regional Medical Center, Moultrie
Dekalb Medical Center, Decatur
Emory Crawford Long Hospital, Atlanta
Gwinnett Medical Center, Lawrenceville
John D. Archbold Memorial Hospital, Thomasville
Meadows Regional Medical Center, Vidalia
Piedmont Hospital, Atlanta
Saint Joseph's Hospital of Atlanta, Atlanta

HEART BYPASS SURGERY

Athens Regional Medical Center, Athens
Northeast Georgia Medical Center, Gainesville
Northeast Georgia Medical Center—Lanier Park
    Campus, Gainesville
Piedmont Hospital, Atlanta

HEART FAILURE

Atlanta Medical Center, Atlanta
Candler Hospital, Savannah
Colquitt Regional Medical Center, Moultrie
East Georgia Regional Medical Center, Statesboro
Elbert Memorial Hospital, Elberton
Emory Adventist Hospital, Smyrna
Emory Dunwoody Medical Center, Atlanta
Gwinnett Medical Center, Lawrenceville

Houston Medical Center, Warner Robins
Meadows Regional Medical Center, Vidalia
Memorial Health University Medical Center,
    Savannah
North Fulton Regional Hospital, Roswell
Northeast Georgia Medical Center, Gainesville
Northeast Georgia Medical Center—Lanier Park
    Campus, Gainesville
Piedmont Fayette Hospital, Fayetteville
Satilla Regional Medical Center, Waycross
South Fulton Medical Center, East Point
Wellstar Cobb Hospital, Austell
Wellstar Kennestone Hospital, Marietta

VALVE REPLACEMENT SURGERY

Northeast Georgia Medical Center, Gainesville
Northeast Georgia Medical Center—Lanier Park
    Campus, Gainesville

CRITICAL CARE

DIABETIC ACIDOSIS AND COMA
Candler Hospital, Savannah

PULMONARY EMBOLISM
Candler Hospital, Savannah
Memorial Health University Medical Center,
    Savannah
Northeast Georgia Medical Center, Gainesville
Northeast Georgia Medical Center—Lanier Park
    Campus, Gainesville
Oconee Regional Medical Center, Milledgeville

RESPIRATORY FAILURE
Candler Hospital, Savannah
East Georgia Regional Medical Center, Statesboro
Floyd Medical Center, Rome
Houston Medical Center, Warner Robins

North Fulton Regional Hospital, Roswell
Northside Hospital Forsyth, Cumming
Oconee Regional Medical Center, Milledgeville
Southern Regional Medical Center, Riverdale
Spalding Regional Medical Center, Griffin

SEPSIS

Candler Hospital, Savannah
Dekalb Medical Center, Decatur
Gwinnett Medical Center, Lawrenceville
Houston Medical Center, Warner Robins
Hutcheson Medical Center, Fort Oglethorpe
Memorial Health University Medical Center,
    Savannah
Northside Hospital Forsyth, Cumming
Oconee Regional Medical Center, Milledgeville
Perry General Hospital, Perry
St. Joseph's Hospital, Savannah
South Fulton Medical Center, East Point

GASTROINTESTINAL

BOWEL OBSTRUCTION

Candler Hospital, Savannah
Meadows Regional Medical Center, Vidalia
Northeast Georgia Medical Center, Gainesville
Northeast Georgia Medical Center—Lanier Park
    Campus, Gainesville
Piedmont Hospital, Atlanta

CHOLECYSTECTOMY

Coliseum Northside Hospital, Macon
Fannin Regional Hospital, Blue Ridge
Hamilton Medical Center, Dalton
Hart County Hospital, Hartwell
Memorial Hospital and Manor, Bainbridge
Perry General Hospital, Perry
Piedmont Hospital, Atlanta

Redmond Regional Medical Center, Rome
Saint Joseph's Hospital of Atlanta, Atlanta
Sempercare Hospital of Augusta, Augusta
University Hospital, Augusta
West Georgia Medical Center, Lagrange

GASTROINTESTINAL BLEED

Candler Hospital, Savannah
Houston Medical Center, Warner Robins
Meadows Regional Medical Center, Vidalia
Memorial Health University Medical Center,
  Savannah
Northside Hospital Cherokee, Canton
Saint Joseph's Hospital of Atlanta, Atlanta

GASTROINTESTINAL SURGERIES AND PROCEDURES

Candler Hospital, Savannah
Northeast Georgia Medical Center, Gainesville
Northeast Georgia Medical Center—Lanier Park
  Campus, Gainesville
Northside Hospital Forsyth, Cumming
Oconee Regional Medical Center, Milledgeville
Saint Joseph's Hospital of Atlanta, Atlanta
Southern Regional Medical Center, Riverdale

PANCREATITIS

Northeast Georgia Medical Center, Gainesville
Northeast Georgia Medical Center—Lanier Park
  Campus, Gainesville

GENERAL SURGERY

APPENDECTOMY

None

MATERNITY CARE

None

ORTHOPEDICS

BACK AND NECK SURGERY (EXCEPT SPINAL FUSION)

Henry Medical Center, Stockbridge
Redmond Regional Medical Center, Rome
Saint Joseph's Hospital of Atlanta, Atlanta
Sempercare Hospital of Augusta, Augusta
South Georgia Medical Center, Valdosta
University Hospital, Augusta

BACK AND NECK SURGERY (SPINAL FUSION)

Floyd Medical Center, Rome
Hughston Orthopedic Hospital, Columbus
John D. Archbold Memorial Hospital, Thomasville

Medical Center, Columbus
Memorial Health University Medical Center,
  Savannah
Northside Hospital, Atlanta
Piedmont Hospital, Atlanta
Redmond Regional Medical Center, Rome
St. Joseph's Hospital, Savannah
Saint Joseph's Hospital of Atlanta, Atlanta
South Georgia Medical Center, Valdosta
Tanner Medical Center—Carrollton, Carrollton

HIP FRACTURE REPAIR

Colquitt Regional Medical Center, Moultrie
Gordon Hospital, Calhoun
Gwinnett Medical Center, Lawrenceville
Hutcheson Medical Center, Fort Oglethorpe
McDuffie Regional Medical Center, Thomson
Medical Center, Columbus
North Fulton Regional Hospital, Roswell
Northeast Georgia Medical Center, Gainesville
Northeast Georgia Medical Center—Lanier Park
  Campus, Gainesville
Oconee Regional Medical Center, Milledgeville
Piedmont Fayette Hospital, Fayetteville
Redmond Regional Medical Center, Rome
St. Francis Hospital, Columbus
Saint Joseph's Hospital of Atlanta, Atlanta
South Fulton Medical Center, East Point
Southern Regional Medical Center, Riverdale
Tanner Medical Center—Carrollton, Carrollton
Tift Regional Medical Center, Tifton
Upson Regional Medical Center, Thomaston
Washington County Regional Medical Center,
  Sandersville
Wayne Memorial Hospital, Jesup
Wellstar Cobb Hospital, Austell
Wellstar Kennestone Hospital, Marietta
West Georgia Medical Center, Lagrange

TOTAL HIP REPLACEMENT

Dekalb Medical Center, Decatur
Hughston Orthopedic Hospital, Columbus
Piedmont Hospital, Atlanta
St. Joseph Hospital—Augusta, Augusta
Saint Joseph's Hospital of Atlanta, Atlanta
West Georgia Medical Center, Lagrange

TOTAL KNEE REPLACEMENT

Chestatee Regional Hospital, Dahlonega
Hughston Orthopedic Hospital, Columbus
Piedmont Fayette Hospital, Fayetteville
Piedmont Hospital, Atlanta
St. Joseph Hospital—Augusta, Augusta

Saint Joseph's Hospital of Atlanta, Atlanta
St. Mary's Hospital of Athens, Athens
Southeast Georgia Regional Medical Center,
  Brunswick
Upson Regional Medical Center, Thomaston
Wayne Memorial Hospital, Jesup

PROSTATECTOMY

Hamilton Medical Center, Dalton
Memorial Health University Medical Center,
  Savannah
Redmond Regional Medical Center, Rome
St. Joseph's Hospital, Savannah
Sempercare Hospital of Augusta, Augusta
Southern Regional Medical Center, Riverdale
University Hospital, Augusta
Wayne Memorial Hospital, Jesup
Wellstar Kennestone Hospital, Marietta

PULMONARY

CHRONIC OBSTRUCTIVE PULMONARY DISEASE (COPD)

Candler Hospital, Savannah
Colquitt Regional Medical Center, Moultrie
Emory University Hospital, Atlanta
Floyd Medical Center, Rome
Houston Medical Center, Warner Robins
Memorial Health University Medical Center,
  Savannah
Northeast Georgia Medical Center, Gainesville
Northeast Georgia Medical Center—Lanier Park
  Campus, Gainesville
Northside Hospital Forsyth, Cumming
Piedmont Fayette Hospital, Fayetteville
Saint Joseph's Hospital of Atlanta, Atlanta
Stephens County Hospital, Toccoa
Tanner Medical Center—Carrollton, Carrollton
Wheeler County Hospital, Glenwood

PNEUMONIA

Candler Hospital, Savannah
Emanuel County Hospital, Swainsboro
Emory Eastside Medical Center, Snellville
Gwinnett Medical Center, Lawrenceville
Habersham County Medical Center, Demorest
Houston Medical Center, Warner Robins
Memorial Health University Medical Center,
  Savannah
Northside Hospital Forsyth, Cumming
Perry General Hospital, Perry
Piedmont Fayette Hospital, Fayetteville

Piedmont Hospital, Atlanta
St. Joseph Hospital—Augusta, Augusta

STROKE

Colquitt Regional Medical Center, Moultrie
Crisp Regional Hospital, Cordele
Dekalb Medical Center, Decatur
Emory Adventist Hospital, Smyrna
Gwinnett Medical Center, Lawrenceville
Saint Joseph's Hospital of Atlanta, Atlanta
Wellstar Douglas Hospital, Douglasville

VASCULAR

CAROTID SURGERY

Coliseum Medical Center, Macon
Hamilton Medical Center, Dalton
Medical Center of Central Georgia, Macon
Redmond Regional Medical Center, Rome
St. Francis Hospital, Columbus
Saint Joseph's Hospital of Atlanta, Atlanta
Wellstar Kennestone Hospital, Marietta

PERIPHERAL VASCULAR BYPASS

Candler Hospital, Savannah

Saint Joseph's Hospital of Atlanta, Atlanta
South Fulton Medical Center, East Point
Wellstar Cobb Hospital, Austell

RESECTION/REPLACEMENT OF ABDOMINAL AORTA

Medical Center of Central Georgia, Macon
Redmond Regional Medical Center, Rome
Wellstar Cobb Hospital, Austell

WOMEN'S HEALTH

None

HAWAII HOSPITALS: FIVE STAR RATED FACILITIES

BARIATRIC SURGERY

None

CARDIAC

ATRIAL FIBRILLATION
None

CORONARY INTERVENTIONAL PROCEDURES (ANGIOPLASTY/STENT)
None

HEART ATTACK
None

HEART BYPASS SURGERY
None

HEART FAILURE
None

VALVE REPLACEMENT SURGERY
None

CRITICAL CARE

DIABETIC ACIDOSIS AND COMA
None

PULMONARY EMBOLISM
None

RESPIRATORY FAILURE
None

SEPSIS
Hawaii Medical Center—West, Ewa Beach
Kuakini Medical Center, Honolulu

GASTROINTESTINAL

BOWEL OBSTRUCTION
None

CHOLECYSTECTOMY
Hawaii Medical Center—East, Honolulu
Kapi'olani Medical Center at Pali Momi, Aiea
The Queen's Medical Center, Honolulu
Select Specialty Hospital, Honolulu
Straub Clinic and Hospital, Honolulu

GASTROINTESTINAL BLEED
None

GASTROINTESTINAL SURGERIES AND PROCEDURES
None

PANCREATITIS
None

GENERAL SURGERY

APPENDECTOMY
None

MATERNITY CARE

None

ORTHOPEDICS

BACK AND NECK SURGERY (EXCEPT SPINAL FUSION)
None

BACK AND NECK SURGERY (SPINAL FUSION)
None

HIP FRACTURE REPAIR
Kapi'olani Medical Center at Pali Momi, Aiea
The Queen's Medical Center, Honolulu
Select Specialty Hospital, Honolulu
Straub Clinic and Hospital, Honolulu
Wahiawa General Hospital, Wahiawa

TOTAL HIP REPLACEMENT
The Queen's Medical Center, Honolulu
Select Specialty Hospital, Honolulu

TOTAL KNEE REPLACEMENT
Kapi'olani Medical Center at Pali Momi, Aiea
Kuakini Medical Center, Honolulu

PROSTATECTOMY

None

PULMONARY

CHRONIC OBSTRUCTIVE PULMONARY DISEASE (COPD)
None

PNEUMONIA
None

STROKE

Hawaii Medical Center—West, Ewa Beach

VASCULAR

CAROTID SURGERY
None

PERIPHERAL VASCULAR BYPASS
The Queen's Medical Center, Honolulu
Select Specialty Hospital, Honolulu

RESECTION/REPLACEMENT OF ABDOMINAL AORTA
None

WOMEN'S HEALTH

None

BARIATRIC SURGERY
None

CARDIAC

ATRIAL FIBRILLATION
St. Alphonsus Regional Medical Center, Boise

CORONARY INTERVENTIONAL PROCEDURES
(ANGIOPLASTY/STENT)
None

HEART ATTACK
None

HEART BYPASS SURGERY
None

HEART FAILURE
None

VALVE REPLACEMENT SURGERY
St. Luke's Boise Medical Center, Boise

CRITICAL CARE

DIABETIC ACIDOSIS AND COMA
None

PULMONARY EMBOLISM
None

RESPIRATORY FAILURE
None

SEPSIS
None

GASTROINTESTINAL

BOWEL OBSTRUCTION
St. Luke's Boise Medical Center, Boise

CHOLECYSTECTOMY
None

GASTROINTESTINAL BLEED
None

GASTROINTESTINAL SURGERIES
AND PROCEDURES
None

PANCREATITIS
None

GENERAL SURGERY

APPENDECTOMY
None

MATERNITY CARE
None

ORTHOPEDICS

BACK AND NECK SURGERY
(EXCEPT SPINAL FUSION)
None

BACK AND NECK SURGERY (SPINAL FUSION)
None

HIP FRACTURE REPAIR
Bonner General Hospital, Sandpoint

TOTAL HIP REPLACEMENT
Portneuf Medical Center, Pocatello
St. Alphonsus Regional Medical Center, Boise

TOTAL KNEE REPLACEMENT
Gritman Medical Center, Moscow
St. Alphonsus Regional Medical Center, Boise
St. Joseph Regional Medical Center, Lewiston
St. Luke's Magic Valley Regional Medical Center,
   Twin Falls

PROSTATECTOMY
None

PULMONARY

CHRONIC OBSTRUCTIVE PULMONARY DISEASE
(COPD)
None

PNEUMONIA
None

STROKE
None

VASCULAR

CAROTID SURGERY
St. Luke's Boise Medical Center, Boise

PERIPHERAL VASCULAR BYPASS
None

RESECTION/REPLACEMENT OF ABDOMINAL AORTA
None

WOMEN'S HEALTH
None

BARIATRIC SURGERY

None

CARDIAC

ATRIAL FIBRILLATION
Alexian Brothers Medical Center, Elk Grove Village
Carle Foundation Hospital, Urbana
La Grange Memorial Hospital, La Grange
Little Company of Mary Hospital, Evergreen Park
Memorial Medical Center, Springfield

Northwest Community Hospital, Arlington Heights
St. James Hospital and Health Center,
   Chicago Heights
St. James Hospital and Health Center—Olympia
   Fields, Olympia Fields
University of Chicago Medical Center, Chicago

CORONARY INTERVENTIONAL PROCEDURES
(ANGIOPLASTY/STENT)

Advocate Good Samaritan Hospital, Downers Grove
Advocate Good Shepherd Hospital, Barrington

Alexian Brothers Medical Center, Elk Grove Village
Decatur Memorial Hospital, Decatur
Gateway Regional Medical Center, Granite City
Hinsdale Hospital, Hinsdale
Northwest Community Hospital, Arlington Heights
Our Lady of the Resurrection Medical Center, Chicago
Rush North Shore Medical Center, Skokie
St. John's Hospital, Springfield
Trinity Medical Center—7th Street Campus, Moline
Trinity Medical Center—West Campus, Rock Island
University of Chicago Medical Center, Chicago

Hospitals receiving a five star rating in a particular procedure have patient outcomes that put them among the best in the nation. For full definitions of ratings and awards, see Appendix.

HEART ATTACK

Advocate Good Shepherd Hospital, Barrington
Advocate Lutheran General Hospital, Park Ridge
Centegra Memorial Medical Center, Woodstock
Delnor Community Hospital, Geneva
Edward Hospital, Naperville
Evanston Northwestern Healthcare, Evanston
Highland Park Hospital, Highland Park
Ingalls Memorial Hospital, Harvey
La Grange Memorial Hospital, La Grange
Louis A. Weiss Memorial Hospital, Chicago
Mercy Hospital and Medical Center, Chicago
Morris Hospital and Healthcare Center, Morris
Northwest Community Hospital, Arlington Heights
Palos Community Hospital, Palos Heights
Provena Covenant Medical Center, Urbana
Provena St. Joseph Medical Center, Joliet
Resurrection Medical Center, Chicago
Rush North Shore Medical Center, Skokie
St. Alexius Medical Center, Hoffman Estates
St. Anthony Medical Center, Rockford
St. Francis Hospital and Health Center, Blue Island
Sherman Hospital, Elgin
Silver Cross Hospital, Joliet
Swedish Covenant Hospital, Chicago

HEART BYPASS SURGERY

Decatur Memorial Hospital, Decatur
MacNeal Hospital, Berwyn
Northwest Community Hospital, Arlington Heights
Northwestern Memorial Hospital, Chicago
Riverside Medical Center, Kankakee
St. Francis Hospital and Health Center, Blue Island
St. Joseph Hospital, Elgin
Swedish American Hospital, Rockford
Trinity Medical Center–7th Street Campus, Moline
Trinity Medical Center–West Campus, Rock Island

HEART FAILURE

Adventist Glenoaks, Glendale Heights
Advocate Bethany Hospital, Chicago
Advocate Christ Hospital and Medical Center,
  Oak Lawn
Advocate Good Samaritan Hospital, Downers Grove
Advocate Good Shepherd Hospital, Barrington
Advocate Illinois Masonic Medical Center, Chicago
Advocate Lutheran General Hospital, Park Ridge
Advocate South Suburban Hospital, Hazel Crest
Advocate Trinity Hospital, Chicago
Alexian Brothers Medical Center, Elk Grove Village
Carle Foundation Hospital, Urbana
Centegra Memorial Medical Center, Woodstock

Centegra Northern Illinois Medical Center, McHenry
Central Dupage Hospital, Winfield
Edward Hospital, Naperville
Evanston Northwestern Healthcare, Evanston
Highland Park Hospital, Highland Park
Hinsdale Hospital, Hinsdale
Illini Hospital, Silvis
Ingalls Memorial Hospital, Harvey
Iroquois Memorial Hospital, Watseka
Kenneth Hall Regional Hospital, East St. Louis
La Grange Memorial Hospital, La Grange
Loretto Hospital, Chicago
Loyola University Medical Center, Maywood
MacNeal Hospital, Berwyn
Mercy Hospital and Medical Center, Chicago
Michael Reese Hospital and Medical Center, Chicago
Northwest Community Hospital, Arlington Heights
Northwestern Memorial Hospital, Chicago
Oak Park Hospital, Oak Park
Palos Community Hospital, Palos Heights
Provena St. Joseph Medical Center, Joliet
Provident Hospital of Chicago, Chicago
Resurrection Medical Center, Chicago
Riverside Medical Center, Kankakee
Roseland Community Hospital, Chicago
Rush North Shore Medical Center, Skokie
Rush University Medical Center, Chicago
St. Alexius Medical Center, Hoffman Estates
St. Anthony Hospital, Chicago
St. Bernard Hospital, Chicago
St. Francis Hospital and Health Center, Blue Island
St. James Hospital and Health Center,
  Chicago Heights
St. James Hospital and Health Center–Olympia
  Fields, Olympia Fields
St. John's Hospital, Springfield
St. Joseph Hospital, Chicago
St. Joseph Hospital, Elgin
St. Mary and Elizabeth Medical Center–Division,
  Chicago
Sherman Hospital, Elgin
Thorek Memorial Hospital, Chicago
University of Chicago Medical Center, Chicago
West Suburban Hospital Medical Center, Oak Park
Westlake Community Hospital, Melrose Park

VALVE REPLACEMENT SURGERY

Alexian Brothers Medical Center, Elk Grove Village
Elmhurst Memorial Hospital, Elmhurst
Northwest Community Hospital, Arlington Heights
St. Francis Hospital and Health Center, Blue Island

CRITICAL CARE

DIABETIC ACIDOSIS AND COMA

Our Lady of the Resurrection Medical Center, Chicago

PULMONARY EMBOLISM

Advocate Good Samaritan Hospital, Downers Grove
Palos Community Hospital, Palos Heights
Resurrection Medical Center, Chicago
St. Alexius Medical Center, Hoffman Estates
Westlake Community Hospital, Melrose Park

RESPIRATORY FAILURE

Adventist Glenoaks, Glendale Heights
Advocate Christ Hospital and Medical Center,
  Oak Lawn
Advocate Good Shepherd Hospital, Barrington
Advocate South Suburban Hospital, Hazel Crest
Alexian Brothers Medical Center, Elk Grove Village
Delnor Community Hospital, Geneva
Evanston Northwestern Healthcare, Evanston
Highland Park Hospital, Highland Park
Holy Cross Hospital, Chicago
Ingalls Memorial Hospital, Harvey
Little Company of Mary Hospital, Evergreen Park
Louis A. Weiss Memorial Hospital, Chicago
Memorial Hospital, Belleville
Mercy Hospital and Medical Center, Chicago
Oak Park Hospital, Oak Park
Our Lady of the Resurrection Medical Center,
  Chicago
Palos Community Hospital, Palos Heights
Passavant Area Hospital, Jacksonville
Provena Mercy Center, Aurora
Resurrection Medical Center, Chicago
St. Alexius Medical Center, Hoffman Estates
St. Anthony's Health Center, Alton
St. Elizabeth Hospital, Belleville
St. Francis Hospital and Health Center, Blue Island
St. James Hospital and Health Center,
  Chicago Heights
St. James Hospital and Health Center–Olympia
  Fields, Olympia Fields
St. Joseph's Hospital, Alton
St. Mary's Hospital, Centralia
Sherman Hospital, Elgin
University of Chicago Medical Center, Chicago
Westlake Community Hospital, Melrose Park

SEPSIS

Adventist Glenoaks, Glendale Heights
Advocate Christ Hospital and Medical Center,
  Oak Lawn

Advocate Good Samaritan Hospital, Downers Grove
Advocate Trinity Hospital, Chicago
Alexian Brothers Medical Center, Elk Grove Village
Centegra Memorial Medical Center, Woodstock
Central Dupage Hospital, Winfield
Evanston Northwestern Healthcare, Evanston
Greenville Regional Hospital, Greenville
Heartland Regional Medical Center, Marion
Highland Park Hospital, Highland Park
Hinsdale Hospital, Hinsdale
Holy Cross Hospital, Chicago
Ingalls Memorial Hospital, Harvey
La Grange Memorial Hospital, La Grange
Lake Forest Hospital, Lake Forest
Little Company of Mary Hospital, Evergreen Park
Memorial Hospital, Belleville
Mercy Hospital and Medical Center, Chicago
Methodist Hospital of Chicago, Chicago
Northwest Community Hospital, Arlington Heights
Norwegian-American Hospital, Chicago
Our Lady of the Resurrection Medical Center, Chicago
Palos Community Hospital, Palos Heights
Provena Mercy Center, Aurora
Provena St. Joseph Medical Center, Joliet
Resurrection Medical Center, Chicago
Richland Memorial Hospital, Olney
Rush Copley Memorial Hospital, Aurora
Rush North Shore Medical Center, Skokie
St. Alexius Medical Center, Hoffman Estates
St. Elizabeth Hospital, Belleville
St. Francis Hospital and Health Center, Blue Island
St. James Hospital and Health Center,
    Chicago Heights
St. James Hospital and Health Center—Olympia
    Fields, Olympia Fields
St. Joseph Hospital, Chicago
St. Mary and Elizabeth Medical
    Center—Claremont, Chicago
Sherman Hospital, Elgin
Westlake Community Hospital, Melrose Park

GASTROINTESTINAL

BOWEL OBSTRUCTION
Advocate Lutheran General Hospital, Park Ridge
Alexian Brothers Medical Center, Elk Grove Village
Evanston Northwestern Healthcare, Evanston
Highland Park Hospital, Highland Park
Lake Forest Hospital, Lake Forest
Northwestern Memorial Hospital, Chicago
Oak Park Hospital, Oak Park
Palos Community Hospital, Palos Heights

Resurrection Medical Center, Chicago
Rush North Shore Medical Center, Skokie
Rush University Medical Center, Chicago
St. Alexius Medical Center, Hoffman Estates
St. Joseph's Hospital, Breese
St. Mary Medical Center, Galesburg
Valley West Community Hospital, Sandwich

CHOLECYSTECTOMY
Advocate Good Samaritan Hospital, Downers Grove
Advocate Good Shepherd Hospital, Barrington
Decatur Memorial Hospital, Decatur
Good Samaritan Regional Health Center,
    Mount Vernon
Graham Hospital Association, Canton
Hopedale Medical Complex, Hopedale
Ingalls Memorial Hospital, Harvey
Katherine Shaw Bethea Hospital, Dixon
Little Company of Mary Hospital, Evergreen Park
RHC St. Francis Hospital, Evanston
Trinity Medical Center—7th Street Campus, Moline
Trinity Medical Center—West Campus, Rock Island

GASTROINTESTINAL BLEED
Advocate Good Samaritan Hospital, Downers Grove
Advocate Good Shepherd Hospital, Barrington
Advocate Lutheran General Hospital, Park Ridge
Alexian Brothers Medical Center, Elk Grove Village
Edward Hospital, Naperville
Evanston Northwestern Healthcare, Evanston
Highland Park Hospital, Highland Park
Kishwaukee Community Hospital, DeKalb
La Grange Memorial Hospital, La Grange
Northwest Community Hospital, Arlington Heights
Our Lady of the Resurrection Medical Center, Chicago
Palos Community Hospital, Palos Heights
Rush North Shore Medical Center, Skokie
St. Alexius Medical Center, Hoffman Estates
St. Joseph Hospital, Chicago
West Suburban Hospital Medical Center, Oak Park

GASTROINTESTINAL SURGERIES
AND PROCEDURES
Advocate Lutheran General Hospital, Park Ridge
Alexian Brothers Medical Center, Elk Grove Village
Centegra Memorial Medical Center, Woodstock
Central Dupage Hospital, Winfield
Elmhurst Memorial Hospital, Elmhurst
Evanston Northwestern Healthcare, Evanston
Harrisburg Medical Center, Harrisburg
Highland Park Hospital, Highland Park
Illini Hospital, Silvis
Little Company of Mary Hospital, Evergreen Park

Mercy Hospital and Medical Center, Chicago
Northwest Community Hospital, Arlington Heights
Our Lady of the Resurrection Medical Center,
    Chicago
RHC St. Francis Hospital, Evanston
Rush North Shore Medical Center, Skokie
Sherman Hospital, Elgin
Swedish Covenant Hospital, Chicago
University of Chicago Medical Center, Chicago

PANCREATITIS
Carle Foundation Hospital, Urbana
La Grange Memorial Hospital, La Grange

GENERAL SURGERY

APPENDECTOMY
None

MATERNITY CARE

None

ORTHOPEDICS

BACK AND NECK SURGERY
(EXCEPT SPINAL FUSION)
Condell Medical Center, Libertyville
Decatur Memorial Hospital, Decatur
Kishwaukee Community Hospital, DeKalb
Northwest Community Hospital, Arlington Heights
Trinity Medical Center—7th Street Campus, Moline
Trinity Medical Center—West Campus, Rock Island

BACK AND NECK SURGERY (SPINAL FUSION)
Loyola University Medical Center, Maywood
Memorial Medical Center, Springfield
Rockford Memorial Hospital, Rockford
St. John's Hospital, Springfield
St. Joseph Medical Center, Bloomington

HIP FRACTURE REPAIR
Advocate Good Samaritan Hospital, Downers Grove
Advocate South Suburban Hospital, Hazel Crest
Advocate Trinity Hospital, Chicago
Blessing Hospital, Quincy
Bromenn Healthcare, Normal
Central Dupage Hospital, Winfield
Condell Medical Center, Libertyville
Illinois Valley Community Hospital, Peru
Ingalls Memorial Hospital, Harvey
Katherine Shaw Bethea Hospital, Dixon
Methodist Hospital of Chicago, Chicago
Methodist Medical Center of Illinois, Peoria
Passavant Area Hospital, Jacksonville

Hospitals receiving a five star rating in a particular procedure have patient outcomes that put them among the best in the nation. For full definitions of ratings and awards, see Appendix.

Provena St. Mary's Hospital, Kankakee
RHC St. Francis Hospital, Evanston
St. James Hospital and Health Center,
   Chicago Heights
St. James Hospital and Health Center—Olympia
   Fields, Olympia Fields
St. Joseph Hospital, Chicago
St. Mary Hospital, Quincy
Swedish Covenant Hospital, Chicago
Vista Medical Center—East, Waukegan
Westlake Community Hospital, Melrose Park

TOTAL HIP REPLACEMENT
Advocate South Suburban Hospital, Hazel Crest
Advocate Trinity Hospital, Chicago
Bromenn Healthcare, Normal
Illinois Valley Community Hospital, Peru
Little Company of Mary Hospital, Evergreen Park
Memorial Medical Center, Springfield
Morris Hospital and Healthcare Center, Morris
Northwestern Memorial Hospital, Chicago
Our Lady of the Resurrection Medical Center, Chicago
Passavant Area Hospital, Jacksonville
Rush University Medical Center, Chicago
St. James Hospital and Health Center,
   Chicago Heights
St. James Hospital and Health Center—Olympia
   Fields, Olympia Fields
Sarah Bush Lincoln Health Center, Mattoon

TOTAL KNEE REPLACEMENT
Advocate Lutheran General Hospital, Park Ridge
Delnor Community Hospital, Geneva
Evanston Northwestern Healthcare, Evanston
Galesburg Cottage Hospital, Galesburg
Highland Park Hospital, Highland Park
Illinois Valley Community Hospital, Peru
Illini Hospital, Silvis
McDonough District Hospital, Macomb
Memorial Hospital, Belleville
Memorial Medical Center, Springfield
Northwestern Memorial Hospital, Chicago
Oak Park Hospital, Oak Park
Provena Covenant Medical Center, Urbana
Provena St. Joseph Medical Center, Joliet
Provena St. Mary's Hospital, Kankakee
Riverside Medical Center, Kankakee
Rush North Shore Medical Center, Skokie
Rush University Medical Center, Chicago
St. Anthony Medical Center, Rockford
St. Mary's Hospital, Decatur
Sarah Bush Lincoln Health Center, Mattoon

PROSTATECTOMY
Bromenn Healthcare, Normal
Elmhurst Memorial Hospital, Elmhurst
Northwestern Memorial Hospital, Chicago
Our Lady of the Resurrection Medical Center,
   Chicago
Riverside Medical Center, Kankakee

PULMONARY
CHRONIC OBSTRUCTIVE PULMONARY DISEASE (COPD)
Advocate Bethany Hospital, Chicago
Advocate Christ Hospital and Medical Center,
   Oak Lawn
Advocate Good Samaritan Hospital, Downers Grove
Advocate Lutheran General Hospital, Park Ridge
Advocate Trinity Hospital, Chicago
Alexian Brothers Medical Center, Elk Grove Village
Centegra Memorial Medical Center, Woodstock
Centegra Northern Illinois Medical Center, McHenry
FHN Memorial Hospital, Freeport
Galesburg Cottage Hospital, Galesburg
Heartland Regional Medical Center, Marion
Ingalls Memorial Hospital, Harvey
Iroquois Memorial Hospital, Watseka
Mercy Hospital and Medical Center, Chicago
Palos Community Hospital, Palos Heights
Provena St. Joseph Medical Center, Joliet
Provena St. Mary's Hospital, Kankakee
Rockford Memorial Hospital, Rockford
Rush North Shore Medical Center, Skokie
St. Alexius Medical Center, Hoffman Estates
St. Anthony's Health Center, Alton
St. Anthony Hospital, Chicago
St. Bernard Hospital, Chicago
St. Francis Hospital and Health Center, Blue Island
St. Joseph Hospital, Elgin
St. Joseph's Hospital, Alton
South Shore Hospital, Chicago
University of Illinois Medical Center, Chicago
West Suburban Hospital Medical Center, Oak Park

PNEUMONIA
Adventist Glenoaks, Glendale Heights
Advocate Christ Hospital and Medical Center,
   Oak Lawn
Advocate Good Samaritan Hospital, Downers Grove
Advocate Good Shepherd Hospital, Barrington
Advocate Illinois Masonic Medical Center, Chicago
Advocate Trinity Hospital, Chicago
Alexian Brothers Medical Center, Elk Grove Village

Centegra Memorial Medical Center, Woodstock
Centegra Northern Illinois Medical Center, McHenry
Central Dupage Hospital, Winfield
Community Memorial Hospital, Staunton
Edward Hospital, Naperville
Evanston Northwestern Healthcare, Evanston
FHN Memorial Hospital, Freeport
Greenville Regional Hospital, Greenville
Highland Park Hospital, Highland Park
Hinsdale Hospital, Hinsdale
Holy Cross Hospital, Chicago
Ingalls Memorial Hospital, Harvey
La Grange Memorial Hospital, La Grange
Lake Forest Hospital, Lake Forest
Louis A. Weiss Memorial Hospital, Chicago
Mercy Hospital and Medical Center, Chicago
Methodist Hospital of Chicago, Chicago
Northwest Community Hospital, Arlington Heights
Norwegian-American Hospital, Chicago
Oak Park Hospital, Oak Park
Our Lady of the Resurrection Medical Center,
   Chicago
Palos Community Hospital, Palos Heights
Provena St. Joseph Medical Center, Joliet
RHC St. Francis Hospital, Evanston
Roseland Community Hospital, Chicago
Rush North Shore Medical Center, Skokie
Rush University Medical Center, Chicago
St. Alexius Medical Center, Hoffman Estates
St. Anthony Medical Center, Rockford
St. Bernard Hospital, Chicago
St. Francis Hospital and Health Center, Blue Island
St. James Hospital and Health Center,
   Chicago Heights
St. James Hospital and Health Center—Olympia
   Fields, Olympia Fields
St. Joseph Hospital, Chicago
St. Joseph Hospital, Elgin
Shelby Memorial Hospital, Shelbyville
Sherman Hospital, Elgin
Swedish Covenant Hospital, Chicago
Thorek Memorial Hospital, Chicago
University of Chicago Medical Center, Chicago
University of Illinois Medical Center, Chicago
Vista Medical Center—East, Waukegan
West Suburban Hospital Medical Center, Oak Park
Westlake Community Hospital, Melrose Park

STROKE
Adventist Glenoaks, Glendale Heights
Advocate Christ Hospital and Medical Center,
   Oak Lawn

Advocate Good Shepherd Hospital, Barrington
Advocate Lutheran General Hospital, Park Ridge
Alexian Brothers Medical Center, Elk Grove Village
Carle Foundation Hospital, Urbana
Centegra Memorial Medical Center, Woodstock
Central Dupage Hospital, Winfield
Condell Medical Center, Libertyville
Crossroads Community Hospital, Mount Vernon
Edward Hospital, Naperville
Eureka Community Hospital, Eureka
Evanston Northwestern Healthcare, Evanston
Highland Park Hospital, Highland Park
Hinsdale Hospital, Hinsdale
Holy Cross Hospital, Chicago
Ingalls Memorial Hospital, Harvey
Iroquois Memorial Hospital, Watseka
Lake Forest Hospital, Lake Forest
MacNeal Hospital, Berwyn
Memorial Hospital of Carbondale, Carbondale
Mercy Hospital and Medical Center, Chicago
Morris Hospital and Healthcare Center, Morris
Northwest Community Hospital, Arlington Heights
Northwestern Memorial Hospital, Chicago
Oak Park Hospital, Oak Park

Our Lady of the Resurrection Medical Center, Chicago
Palos Community Hospital, Palos Heights
Provena St. Joseph Medical Center, Joliet
Resurrection Medical Center, Chicago
Rockford Memorial Hospital, Rockford
Rush Copley Memorial Hospital, Aurora
Rush North Shore Medical Center, Skokie
Rush University Medical Center, Chicago
St. Alexius Medical Center, Hoffman Estates
St. Anthony Medical Center, Rockford
St. Francis Hospital and Health Center, Blue Island
St. James Hospital and Health Center,
    Chicago Heights
St. James Hospital and Health Center—Olympia
    Fields, Olympia Fields
St. Joseph Hospital, Chicago
St. Joseph Hospital, Elgin
St. Mary and Elizabeth Medical Center—
    Claremont, Chicago
Sarah Bush Lincoln Health Center, Mattoon
Swedish Covenant Hospital, Chicago
University of Chicago Medical Center, Chicago
University of Illinois Medical Center, Chicago
Westlake Community Hospital, Melrose Park

VASCULAR

CAROTID SURGERY
Bromenn Healthcare, Normal
Memorial Hospital of Carbondale, Carbondale
Our Lady of the Resurrection Medical Center, Chicago
St. John's Hospital, Springfield
Sarah Bush Lincoln Health Center, Mattoon
Trinity Medical Center—7th Street Campus, Moline
Trinity Medical Center—West Campus, Rock Island

PERIPHERAL VASCULAR BYPASS
Resurrection Medical Center, Chicago

RESECTION/REPLACEMENT OF ABDOMINAL AORTA
Advocate Lutheran General Hospital, Park Ridge
Alexian Brothers Medical Center, Elk Grove Village
Evanston Northwestern Healthcare, Evanston
Highland Park Hospital, Highland Park
Northwest Community Hospital, Arlington Heights

WOMEN'S HEALTH
None

INDIANA HOSPITALS: FIVE STAR RATED FACILITIES

BARIATRIC SURGERY
None

CARDIAC

ATRIAL FIBRILLATION
St. Vincent Heart Center of Indiana, Indianapolis

CORONARY INTERVENTIONAL PROCEDURES (ANGIOPLASTY/STENT)
Columbus Regional Hospital, Columbus
Lutheran Hospital of Indiana, Fort Wayne
St. Vincent Heart Center of Indiana, Indianapolis

HEART ATTACK
Clark Memorial Hospital, Jeffersonville
Community Hospital of Anderson
    and Madison County, Anderson
Daviess Community Hospital, Washington
Fayette Memorial Hospital, Connersville
Hancock Regional Hospital, Greenfield
Hendricks Regional Health, Danville
St. Catherine Hospital, East Chicago
St. Vincent Heart Center of Indiana, Indianapolis

HEART BYPASS SURGERY
Ball Memorial Hospital, Muncie
Community Hospital, Munster
St. Vincent Heart Center of Indiana, Indianapolis

HEART FAILURE
Clark Memorial Hospital, Jeffersonville
Community Hospital, Munster
Floyd Memorial Hospital and Health Services,
    New Albany
Howard Regional Health System, Kokomo
Laporte Hospital and Health Services, La Porte
St. Catherine Hospital, East Chicago
St. Francis Hospital and Health Center,
    Indianapolis
St. Margaret Mercy Healthcare Center, Dyer
St. Margaret Mercy Healthcare Center, Hammond
St. Vincent Hospital and Health Services,
    Indianapolis
St. Vincent Heart Center of Indiana, Indianapolis

VALVE REPLACEMENT SURGERY
Deaconess Hospital, Evansville

CRITICAL CARE

DIABETIC ACIDOSIS AND COMA
None

PULMONARY EMBOLISM
Community Hospitals Indianapolis, Indianapolis

RESPIRATORY FAILURE
Clark Memorial Hospital, Jeffersonville
Fayette Memorial Hospital, Connersville
Floyd Memorial Hospital and Health Services,
    New Albany
Memorial Hospital of Michigan City, Michigan City
Methodist Hospital Southlake, Merrillville
Methodist Hospital, Gary
St. Anthony Memorial Health Center, Michigan City
St. Elizabeth Medical Center, Lafayette
St. Francis Hospital and Health Center, Beech Grove
St. Joseph Hospital and Health Center, Kokomo
St. Vincent Hospital and Health Services,
    Indianapolis

SEPSIS
Clark Memorial Hospital, Jeffersonville
Community Hospital South, Indianapolis

Hospitals receiving a five star rating in a particular procedure have patient outcomes that put them among the best in the nation. For full definitions of ratings and awards, see Appendix.

Community Hospital, Munster
Community Hospitals Indianapolis, Indianapolis
Major Hospital, Shelbyville
Memorial Hospital of South Bend, South Bend
St. Elizabeth Medical Center, Lafayette
St. Francis Hospital and Health Center, Beech Grove
St. Margaret Mercy Healthcare Center, Hammond
St. Vincent Hospital and Health Services,
    Indianapolis
Schneck Medical Center, Seymour

GASTROINTESTINAL

BOWEL OBSTRUCTION
Columbus Regional Hospital, Columbus
St. Vincent Hospital and Health Services,
    Indianapolis

CHOLECYSTECTOMY
Clark Memorial Hospital, Jeffersonville
Community Hospital, Munster
Floyd Memorial Hospital and Health Services,
    New Albany
Good Samaritan Hospital, Vincennes
Henry County Memorial Hospital, New Castle
The King's Daughters' Hospital and Health
    Services, Madison
Memorial Hospital of South Bend, South Bend
Morgan Hospital and Medical Center, Martinsville
St. Joseph Regional Medical Center—South Bend,
    South Bend
St. Mary's Medical Center—Hobart, Hobart
Terre Haute Regional Hospital, Terre Haute

GASTROINTESTINAL BLEED
Community Hospital, Munster
Community Hospitals Indianapolis, Indianapolis
Dearborn County Hospital, Lawrenceburg
Good Samaritan Hospital, Vincennes
Major Hospital, Shelbyville

GASTROINTESTINAL SURGERIES
AND PROCEDURES
Community Hospitals Indianapolis, Indianapolis
Memorial Hospital of South Bend, South Bend
St. Francis Hospital and Health Center, Beech Grove
St. Vincent Hospital and Health Services,
    Indianapolis

PANCREATITIS
Columbus Regional Hospital, Columbus
Memorial Hospital of South Bend, South Bend

GENERAL SURGERY

APPENDECTOMY
None

MATERNITY CARE
None

ORTHOPEDICS

BACK AND NECK SURGERY
(EXCEPT SPINAL FUSION)
Columbus Regional Hospital, Columbus
Community Hospital, Munster
Indiana Orthopaedic Hospital, Indianapolis
Marion General Hospital, Marion
St. Francis Hospital and Health Center, Beech Grove
St. Joseph Regional Medical Center—South Bend,
    South Bend
Terre Haute Regional Hospital, Terre Haute

BACK AND NECK SURGERY (SPINAL FUSION)
Bloomington Hospital, Bloomington
Community Hospital, Munster
Indiana Orthopaedic Hospital, Indianapolis
Lutheran Hospital of Indiana, Fort Wayne
St. Joseph Regional Medical Center—South Bend,
    South Bend

HIP FRACTURE REPAIR
Ball Memorial Hospital, Muncie
Community Hospital of Anderson and Madison
    County, Anderson
Community Hospital, Munster
Daviess Community Hospital, Washington
Floyd Memorial Hospital and Health Services,
    New Albany
Good Samaritan Hospital, Vincennes
The King's Daughters' Hospital and Health
    Services, Madison
Laporte Hospital and Health Services, La Porte
Marion General Hospital, Marion
Memorial Hospital and Health Care Center, Jasper
Memorial Hospital of Michigan City, Michigan City
Methodist Hospital Southlake, Merrillville
Methodist Hospital, Gary
Parkview Hospital, Fort Wayne
St. Anthony Medical Center of Crown Point,
    Crown Point
St. Anthony Memorial Health Center, Michigan City
St. Catherine Hospital, East Chicago
St. Clare Medical Center, Crawfordsville

St. Francis Hospital and Health Center,
    Beech Grove
St. Joseph Hospital, Fort Wayne
St. Joseph Regional Medical
    Center—South Bend, South Bend
St. Margaret Mercy Healthcare Center, Dyer
St. Margaret Mercy Healthcare Center, Hammond
Witham Health Services, Lebanon

TOTAL HIP REPLACEMENT
Bluffton Regional Medical Center, Bluffton
Community Hospital, Munster
Indiana Orthopaedic Hospital, Indianapolis
Parkview Hospital, Fort Wayne
Porter, Valparaiso
St. Anthony Medical Center of Crown Point,
    Crown Point
St. Francis Hospital and Health Center, Beech
    Grove
St. Francis Hospital Mooresville, Mooresville
St. Joseph Regional Medical
    Center—South Bend, South Bend
St. Mary's Medical Center—Evansville, Evansville
Welborn Baptist Hospital, Evansville

TOTAL KNEE REPLACEMENT
Community Hospital, Munster
Good Samaritan Hospital, Vincennes
Indiana Orthopaedic Hospital, Indianapolis
Laporte Hospital and Health Services, La Porte
Porter, Valparaiso
St. Elizabeth Ann Seton Speciality Care, Carmel
St. Francis Hospital and Health Center,
    Beech Grove
St. Francis Hospital Mooresville, Mooresville
St. Joseph Regional Medical
    Center—South Bend, South Bend
St. Mary's Medical Center—Evansville, Evansville
St. Mary's Medical Center—Hobart, Hobart
St. Vincent Carmel Hospital, Carmel
Tipton Hospital, Tipton
Welborn Baptist Hospital, Evansville

PROSTATECTOMY
Community Hospital, Munster
The King's Daughters' Hospital and Health
    Services, Madison
Marion General Hospital, Marion
St. Anthony Medical Center of Crown Point,
    Crown Point

PULMONARY

CHRONIC OBSTRUCTIVE PULMONARY DISEASE (COPD)

Bluffton Regional Medical Center, Bluffton
Clarian Health Partners, Indianapolis
Clarian West Medical Center, Avon
Community Hospital of Anderson
    and Madison County, Anderson
Community Hospital, Munster
Dupont Hospital, Fort Wayne
Fayette Memorial Hospital, Connersville
Indiana University Medical Center, Indianapolis
Memorial Hospital of South Bend, South Bend
Methodist Hospital Southlake, Merrillville
Methodist Hospital, Gary
St. Catherine Hospital, East Chicago
Saint John's Health System, Anderson
St. Vincent Hospital and Health Services,
    Indianapolis
St. Vincent Mercy Hospital, Elwood
William N. Wishard Memorial Hospital,
    Indianapolis

PNEUMONIA

Ball Memorial Hospital, Muncie
Clark Memorial Hospital, Jeffersonville
Columbus Regional Hospital, Columbus
Community Hospital South, Indianapolis
Community Hospital, Munster
Deaconess Hospital, Evansville
Dearborn County Hospital, Lawrenceburg
Dupont Hospital, Fort Wayne
Floyd Memorial Hospital and Health Services,
    New Albany
Hancock Regional Hospital, Greenfield
Howard Regional Health System, Kokomo
Jay County Hospital, Portland
Laporte Hospital and Health Services, La Porte
Major Hospital, Shelbyville
St. Catherine Hospital, East Chicago
St. Francis Hospital and Health Center, Beech
    Grove
St. Mary's Medical Center—Hobart, Hobart
St. Vincent Hospital and Health Services,
    Indianapolis
St. Vincent Mercy Hospital, Elwood
William N. Wishard Memorial Hospital,
    Indianapolis
Witham Health Services, Lebanon

STROKE

Clarian Health Partners, Indianapolis
Community Hospitals Indianapolis, Indianapolis
Daviess Community Hospital, Washington
Howard Regional Health System, Kokomo
Indiana University Medical Center, Indianapolis
Methodist Hospital Southlake, Merrillville

Methodist Hospital, Gary
Reid Hospital and Health Care Services,
    Richmond
St. Francis Hospital and Health Center,
    Beech Grove
St. Joseph Regional Medical
    Center—South Bend, South Bend
St. Margaret Mercy Healthcare Center, Dyer
St. Vincent Hospital and Health Services,
    Indianapolis

VASCULAR

CAROTID SURGERY

Columbus Regional Hospital, Columbus
Community Hospital, Munster
Good Samaritan Hospital, Vincennes
Memorial Hospital of South Bend, South Bend
Porter, Valparaiso
St. Joseph Regional Medical
    Center—South Bend, South Bend

PERIPHERAL VASCULAR BYPASS

St. Mary's Medical Center—Hobart, Hobart

RESECTION/REPLACEMENT OF ABDOMINAL AORTA

None

WOMEN'S HEALTH

None

IOWA HOSPITALS: FIVE STAR RATED FACILITIES

BARIATRIC SURGERY

None

CARDIAC

ATRIAL FIBRILLATION

Covenant Medical Center, Waterloo

CORONARY INTERVENTIONAL PROCEDURES (ANGIOPLASTY/STENT)

Allen Memorial Hospital, Waterloo
Mercy Medical Center—North Iowa, Mason City
Mercy Medical Center—Sioux City, Sioux City

HEART ATTACK

Great River Medical Center, West Burlington
Grinnell Regional Medical Center, Grinnell
Henry County Health Center, Mount Pleasant
Mercy Medical Center—Des Moines, Des Moines
Mercy Medical Center—North Iowa, Mason City
Metropolitan Medical Center, Des Moines

Ottumwa Regional Health Center, Ottumwa
St. Luke's Hospital, Cedar Rapids

HEART BYPASS SURGERY

None

HEART FAILURE

Great River Medical Center, West Burlington
Grinnell Regional Medical Center, Grinnell
Keokuk Area Hospital, Keokuk
Mercy Medical Center—Des Moines, Des Moines
Metropolitan Medical Center, Des Moines
Ottumwa Regional Health Center, Ottumwa
St. Luke's Hospital, Cedar Rapids

VALVE REPLACEMENT SURGERY

None

CRITICAL CARE

DIABETIC ACIDOSIS AND COMA

None

PULMONARY EMBOLISM

None

RESPIRATORY FAILURE

Broadlawns Medical Center, Des Moines
Mercy Medical Center—Cedar Rapids, Cedar Rapids
Mercy Medical Center—Clinton, Clinton
Mercy Medical Center—Des Moines, Des Moines
Metropolitan Medical Center, Des Moines
Ottumwa Regional Health Center, Ottumwa
St. Luke's Hospital, Cedar Rapids

SEPSIS

Alegent Health Community Memorial Hospital,
    Missouri Valley
Buena Vista Regional Medical Center, Storm Lake
Mercy Medical Center—Cedar Rapids,
    Cedar Rapids
Mercy Medical Center—Clinton, Clinton
Mercy Medical Center—Des Moines, Des Moines
Mercy Medical Center—North Iowa, Mason City

Hospitals receiving a five star rating in a particular procedure have patient outcomes that put them among the best in the nation. For full definitions of ratings and awards, see Appendix.

Mercy Medical Center—Sioux City, Sioux City
Metropolitan Medical Center, Des Moines
Ottumwa Regional Health Center, Ottumwa
St. Luke's Hospital, Cedar Rapids

GASTROINTESTINAL

BOWEL OBSTRUCTION
St. Luke's Regional Medical Center, Sioux City

CHOLECYSTECTOMY
Iowa Methodist Medical Center, Des Moines
Mercy Medical Center—Dubuque, Dubuque
Mercy Medical Center—Sioux City, Sioux City

GASTROINTESTINAL BLEED
Mary Greeley Medical Center, Ames
Mercy Medical Center—Des Moines, Des Moines
Mercy Medical Center—Dubuque, Dubuque
Metropolitan Medical Center, Des Moines
Ottumwa Regional Health Center, Ottumwa

GASTROINTESTINAL SURGERIES AND PROCEDURES
None

PANCREATITIS
St. Luke's Hospital, Cedar Rapids

GENERAL SURGERY

APPENDECTOMY
Iowa Methodist Medical Center, Des Moines
Lakes Regional Healthcare, Spirit Lake
Mahaska County Hospital, Oskaloosa
Mary Greeley Medical Center, Ames
Mercy Medical Center—Dubuque, Dubuque
Mercy Medical Center—Sioux City, Sioux City
St. Luke's Hospital, Cedar Rapids

MATERNITY CARE

Mercy Medical Center—Des Moines, Des Moines
Metropolitan Medical Center, Des Moines

ORTHOPEDICS

BACK AND NECK SURGERY (EXCEPT SPINAL FUSION)
Genesis Medical Center—Davenport, Davenport
Iowa Methodist Medical Center, Des Moines

Jennie Edmundson Hospital, Council Bluffs
Mercy Medical Center—Cedar Rapids, Cedar Rapids
Mercy Medical Center—Sioux City, Sioux City

BACK AND NECK SURGERY (SPINAL FUSION)
Iowa Methodist Medical Center, Des Moines
Mercy Hospital—Iowa City, Iowa City
Mercy Medical Center—North Iowa, Mason City

HIP FRACTURE REPAIR
Alegent Health Mercy Hospital, Council Bluffs
Mercy Medical Center—Dubuque, Dubuque
Mercy Medical Center—Sioux City, Sioux City
St. Luke's Hospital, Cedar Rapids
Spencer Municipal Hospital, Spencer
Unity Hospital, Muscatine

TOTAL HIP REPLACEMENT
Jennie Edmundson Hospital, Council Bluffs
Mercy Medical Center—Des Moines, Des Moines
Mercy Medical Center—Dubuque, Dubuque
Mercy Medical Center—North Iowa, Mason City
Mercy Medical Center—Sioux City, Sioux City
Metropolitan Medical Center, Des Moines
Spencer Municipal Hospital, Spencer

TOTAL KNEE REPLACEMENT
Lakes Regional Healthcare, Spirit Lake
Mercy Hospital—Iowa City, Iowa City
Mercy Medical Center—North Iowa, Mason City
Mercy Medical Center—Sioux City, Sioux City
Spencer Municipal Hospital, Spencer
Trinity Medical Center—Terrace Park Campus, Bettendorf
Trinity Regional Medical Center, Fort Dodge

PROSTATECTOMY

St. Luke's Hospital, Cedar Rapids

PULMONARY

CHRONIC OBSTRUCTIVE PULMONARY DISEASE (COPD)
Mercy Medical Center—Des Moines, Des Moines
Metropolitan Medical Center, Des Moines

PNEUMONIA
Allen Memorial Hospital, Waterloo
Covenant Medical Center, Waterloo

Floyd County Memorial Hospital, Charles City
Great River Medical Center, West Burlington
Grinnell Regional Medical Center, Grinnell
Loring Hospital, Sac City
Mercy Medical Center—Cedar Rapids, Cedar Rapids
Mercy Medical Center—Clinton, Clinton
Mercy Medical Center—Des Moines, Des Moines
Mercy Medical Center—North Iowa, Mason City
Metropolitan Medical Center, Des Moines
Orange City Area Health System, Orange City
Ottumwa Regional Health Center, Ottumwa
St. Luke's Hospital, Cedar Rapids
St. Luke's Regional Medical Center, Sioux City
Virginia Gay Hospital, Vinton

STROKE

Mercy Medical Center—North Iowa, Mason City

VASCULAR

CAROTID SURGERY
Allen Memorial Hospital, Waterloo
Iowa Methodist Medical Center, Des Moines
Mary Greeley Medical Center, Ames
Mercy Medical Center—Dubuque, Dubuque
Mercy Medical Center—North Iowa, Mason City
Mercy Medical Center—Sioux City, Sioux City
St. Luke's Hospital, Cedar Rapids

PERIPHERAL VASCULAR BYPASS
Allen Memorial Hospital, Waterloo

RESECTION/REPLACEMENT OF ABDOMINAL AORTA
University of Iowa Hospital and Clinics, Iowa City

WOMEN'S HEALTH

Mercy Medical Center—Des Moines, Des Moines
Metropolitan Medical Center, Des Moines

BARIATRIC SURGERY

None

CARDIAC

ATRIAL FIBRILLATION

St. Joseph Medical Center, Wichita
Via Christi Regional Medical Center, Wichita

CORONARY INTERVENTIONAL PROCEDURES (ANGIOPLASTY/STENT)

None

HEART ATTACK

St. Francis Health Center, Topeka
St. Joseph Medical Center, Wichita
University of Kansas Hospital, Kansas City
Via Christi Regional Medical Center, Wichita

HEART BYPASS SURGERY

St. Joseph Medical Center, Wichita
Via Christi Regional Medical Center, Wichita

HEART FAILURE

Kansas Heart Hospital, Wichita
Newman Regional Health, Emporia
Newton Medical Center, Newton
Shawnee Mission Medical Center,
  Shawnee Mission

VALVE REPLACEMENT SURGERY

St. Joseph Medical Center, Wichita
Via Christi Regional Medical Center, Wichita

CRITICAL CARE

DIABETIC ACIDOSIS AND COMA

None

PULMONARY EMBOLISM

None

RESPIRATORY FAILURE

Coffeyville Regional Medical Center, Coffeyville
St. Joseph Medical Center, Wichita
Via Christi Regional Medical Center, Wichita

SEPSIS

Coffeyville Regional Medical Center, Coffeyville
Kingman Community Hospital, Kingman
University of Kansas Hospital, Kansas City

GASTROINTESTINAL

BOWEL OBSTRUCTION

Southwest Medical Center, Liberal

CHOLECYSTECTOMY

Select Specialty Hospital Wichita, Wichita
Wesley Medical Center, Wichita

GASTROINTESTINAL BLEED

None

GASTROINTESTINAL SURGERIES AND PROCEDURES

Lawrence Memorial Hospital, Lawrence
Olathe Medical Center, Olathe
Southwest Medical Center, Liberal

PANCREATITIS

Select Specialty Hospital Wichita, Wichita
Wesley Medical Center, Wichita

GENERAL SURGERY

APPENDECTOMY

None

MATERNITY CARE

None

ORTHOPEDICS

BACK AND NECK SURGERY (EXCEPT SPINAL FUSION)

Heartland Surgical Specialty Hospital,
  Overland Park
Providence Medical Center, Kansas City

BACK AND NECK SURGERY (SPINAL FUSION)

Heartland Surgical Specialty Hospital,
  Overland Park
Providence Medical Center, Kansas City
Select Specialty Hospital Wichita, Wichita
Wesley Medical Center, Wichita

HIP FRACTURE REPAIR

Newton Medical Center, Newton
Shawnee Mission Medical Center,
  Shawnee Mission

TOTAL HIP REPLACEMENT

Central Kansas Medical Center, Great Bend
Hays Medical Center, Hays
Stormont-Vail Healthcare, Topeka

TOTAL KNEE REPLACEMENT

Central Kansas Medical Center, Great Bend
Hays Medical Center, Hays
Mercy Hospital of Kansas Independence,
  Independence
Mercy Regional Health Center, Manhattan
Select Specialty Hospital Wichita, Wichita
Wesley Medical Center, Wichita

PROSTATECTOMY

St. Joseph Medical Center, Wichita
Select Specialty Hospital Wichita, Wichita
Via Christi Regional Medical Center, Wichita
Wesley Medical Center, Wichita

PULMONARY

CHRONIC OBSTRUCTIVE PULMONARY DISEASE (COPD)

Galichia Heart Hospital, Wichita
St. Joseph Medical Center, Wichita
Shawnee Mission Medical Center,
  Shawnee Mission
University of Kansas Hospital, Kansas City
Via Christi Regional Medical Center, Wichita

PNEUMONIA

Coffeyville Regional Medical Center, Coffeyville
Newman Regional Health, Emporia
Providence Medical Center, Kansas City
St. Francis Health Center, Topeka
St. John Hospital, Leavenworth
Stormont-Vail Healthcare, Topeka

STROKE

Mercy Health Center, Fort Scott
St. Francis Health Center, Topeka
St. Joseph Medical Center, Wichita
Shawnee Mission Medical Center,
  Shawnee Mission
Via Christi Regional Medical Center, Wichita

Hospitals receiving a five star rating in a particular procedure have patient outcomes that put them among the best in the nation. For full definitions of ratings and awards, see Appendix.

VASCULAR

CAROTID SURGERY
Kansas Heart Hospital, Wichita
Menorah Medical Center, Overland Park
St. Joseph Medical Center, Wichita

Select Specialty Hospital Wichita, Wichita
Via Christi Regional Medical Center, Wichita
Wesley Medical Center, Wichita

PERIPHERAL VASCULAR BYPASS
None

RESECTION/REPLACEMENT OF ABDOMINAL AORTA
None

WOMEN'S HEALTH
None

BARIATRIC SURGERY
None

CARDIAC

ATRIAL FIBRILLATION
None

CORONARY INTERVENTIONAL PROCEDURES (ANGIOPLASTY/STENT)
None

HEART ATTACK
Baptist Hospital East, Louisville
Cardinal Hill Specialty Hospital, Fort Thomas
Clark Regional Medical Center, Winchester
Jackson Purchase Medical Center, Mayfield
Jennie Stuart Medical Center, Hopkinsville
Jewish Hospital, Louisville
Marymount Medical Center, London
Norton Audubon Hospital, Louisville
Norton Hospital, Louisville
Norton Southwest Hospital, Louisville
Norton Suburban Hospital, Louisville
Our Lady of Bellefonte Hospital, Ashland
St. Elizabeth Medical Center—South, Edgewood
St. Joseph Hospital, Lexington
St. Luke Hospital East, Fort Thomas
St. Luke Hospital West, Florence
Sts. Mary and Elizabeth Hospital, Louisville
University of Louisville Hospital, Louisville

HEART BYPASS SURGERY
King's Daughters Medical Center, Ashland

HEART FAILURE
Baptist Hospital East, Louisville
Baptist Hospital Northeast, La Grange
Carroll County Hospital, Carrollton
Clark Regional Medical Center, Winchester
Ephraim McDowell Regional Medical Center, Danville
Jewish Hospital, Louisville
King's Daughters Medical Center, Ashland
Marymount Medical Center, London

Oak Tree Hospital at Baptist Hospital Northeast, La Grange
St. Elizabeth Medical Center—South, Edgewood
St. Luke Hospital West, Florence
Sts. Mary and Elizabeth Hospital, Louisville

VALVE REPLACEMENT SURGERY
Baptist Hospital East, Louisville
Medical Center, Bowling Green

CRITICAL CARE

DIABETIC ACIDOSIS AND COMA
None

PULMONARY EMBOLISM
Jewish Hospital, Louisville
Sts. Mary and Elizabeth Hospital, Louisville

RESPIRATORY FAILURE
ARH Regional Medical Center—Hazard, Hazard
Baptist Hospital East, Louisville
Baptist Regional Medical Center, Corbin
Cardinal Hill Specialty Hospital, Fort Thomas
Clark Regional Medical Center, Winchester
Greenview Regional Hospital, Bowling Green
Hardin Memorial Hospital, Elizabethtown
Jewish Hospital, Louisville
Kentucky River Medical Center, Jackson
King's Daughters Medical Center, Ashland
Mary Chiles Hospital, Mount Sterling
Marymount Medical Center, London
Medical Center, Bowling Green
Norton Audubon Hospital, Louisville
Norton Hospital, Louisville
Norton Southwest Hospital, Louisville
Norton Suburban Hospital, Louisville
Oak Tree Hospital at Baptist Regional Medical Center, Corbin
Our Lady of Bellefonte Hospital, Ashland
Pattie A. Clay Regional Medical Center, Richmond
Russell County Hospital, Russell Springs
St. Claire Medical Center, Morehead
St. Elizabeth Medical Center—South, Edgewood
St. Joseph Hospital, Lexington

St. Luke Hospital East, Fort Thomas
St. Luke Hospital West, Florence
Sts. Mary and Elizabeth Hospital, Louisville
Western Baptist Hospital, Paducah

SEPSIS
Baptist Hospital East, Louisville
Baptist Hospital Northeast, La Grange
Clark Regional Medical Center, Winchester
Hardin Memorial Hospital, Elizabethtown
Marymount Medical Center, London
Murray-Calloway County Hospital, Murray
Norton Audubon Hospital, Louisville
Norton Hospital, Louisville
Norton Southwest Hospital, Louisville
Norton Suburban Hospital, Louisville
Oak Tree Hospital at Baptist Hospital Northeast, La Grange
Our Lady of Bellefonte Hospital, Ashland
Owensboro Medical Health System, Owensboro
Owensboro Mercy Health System Ford, Owensboro
St. Elizabeth Medical Center—South, Edgewood
St. Joseph Hospital, Lexington
St. Luke Hospital West, Florence
Taylor Regional Hospital, Campbellsville

GASTROINTESTINAL

BOWEL OBSTRUCTION
Highlands Regional Medical Center, Prestonsburg
Jewish Hospital, Louisville
Sts. Mary and Elizabeth Hospital, Louisville

CHOLECYSTECTOMY
Ephraim McDowell Regional Medical Center, Danville
Hardin Memorial Hospital, Elizabethtown
Lake Cumberland Regional Hospital, Somerset
Meadowview Regional Medical Center, Maysville
Murray-Calloway County Hospital, Murray
Owensboro Medical Health System, Owensboro
Owensboro Mercy Health System Ford, Owensboro
Pikeville Medical Center, Pikeville
Pineville Community Hospital, Pineville
T. J. Samson Community Hospital, Glasgow

GASTROINTESTINAL BLEED
Central Baptist Hospital, Lexington
Jennie Stuart Medical Center, Hopkinsville
Norton Audubon Hospital, Louisville
Norton Hospital, Louisville
Norton Southwest Hospital, Louisville
Norton Suburban Hospital, Louisville

GASTROINTESTINAL SURGERIES AND PROCEDURES
Samaritan Hospital, Lexington
Select Specialty Hospital Lexington, Lexington

PANCREATITIS
None

GENERAL SURGERY

APPENDECTOMY
None

MATERNITY CARE

None

ORTHOPEDICS

BACK AND NECK SURGERY (EXCEPT SPINAL FUSION)
Lake Cumberland Regional Hospital, Somerset
Owensboro Medical Health System, Owensboro
Owensboro Mercy Health System Ford, Owensboro
St. Elizabeth Medical Center–South, Edgewood

BACK AND NECK SURGERY (SPINAL FUSION)
St. Joseph Hospital, Lexington

HIP FRACTURE REPAIR
Baptist Hospital East, Louisville
Baptist Regional Medical Center, Corbin
Flaget Memorial Hospital, Bardstown
Georgetown Community Hospital, Georgetown
Greenview Regional Hospital, Bowling Green
Hardin Memorial Hospital, Elizabethtown
Lake Cumberland Regional Hospital, Somerset
Medical Center, Bowling Green
Murray-Calloway County Hospital, Murray
Oak Tree Hospital at Baptist Regional
    Medical Center, Corbin
Pattie A. Clay Regional Medical Center, Richmond
Pikeville Medical Center, Pikeville

St. Elizabeth Medical Center–South, Edgewood
T. J. Samson Community Hospital, Glasgow

TOTAL HIP REPLACEMENT
Baptist Hospital East, Louisville
Greenview Regional Hospital, Bowling Green
Jackson Purchase Medical Center, Mayfield
Murray-Calloway County Hospital, Murray
Owensboro Medical Health System, Owensboro
Owensboro Mercy Health System Ford, Owensboro

TOTAL KNEE REPLACEMENT
Baptist Hospital East, Louisville
Greenview Regional Hospital, Bowling Green
Jackson Purchase Medical Center, Mayfield
Murray-Calloway County Hospital, Murray
Owensboro Medical Health System, Owensboro
Owensboro Mercy Health System Ford, Owensboro
St. Elizabeth Medical Center–South, Edgewood
T. J. Samson Community Hospital, Glasgow

PROSTATECTOMY

None

PULMONARY

CHRONIC OBSTRUCTIVE PULMONARY DISEASE (COPD)
Cardinal Hill Specialty Hospital, Fort Thomas
Ephraim McDowell Regional Medical Center,
    Danville
Frankfort Regional Medical Center, Frankfort
Jennie Stuart Medical Center, Hopkinsville
Jewish Hospital, Louisville
Kentucky River Medical Center, Jackson
King's Daughters Medical Center, Ashland
Mary Breckinridge Hospital, Hyden
Marymount Medical Center, London
Pattie A. Clay Regional Medical Center, Richmond
St. Elizabeth Medical Center–South, Edgewood
St. Joseph East, Lexington
St. Luke Hospital East, Fort Thomas
Sts. Mary and Elizabeth Hospital, Louisville
T. J. Samson Community Hospital, Glasgow
University of Louisville Hospital, Louisville

PNEUMONIA
ARH Regional Medical Center–Hazard, Hazard
Baptist Hospital East, Louisville

Baptist Hospital Northeast, La Grange
Cardinal Hill Specialty Hospital, Fort Thomas
Central Baptist Hospital, Lexington
Clark Regional Medical Center, Winchester
Hardin Memorial Hospital, Elizabethtown
Jewish Hospital, Louisville
Kentucky River Medical Center, Jackson
King's Daughters Medical Center, Ashland
Logan Memorial Hospital, Russellville
Marymount Medical Center, London
Norton Audubon Hospital, Louisville
Norton Hospital, Louisville
Norton Southwest Hospital, Louisville
Norton Suburban Hospital, Louisville
Oak Tree Hospital at Baptist Hospital Northeast,
    La Grange
Our Lady of Bellefonte Hospital, Ashland
Paul B. Hall Regional Medical Center, Paintsville
St. Claire Medical Center, Morehead
St. Elizabeth Medical Center–South, Edgewood
St. Luke Hospital East, Fort Thomas
Sts. Mary and Elizabeth Hospital, Louisville
Taylor Regional Hospital, Campbellsville

STROKE

Baptist Hospital Northeast, La Grange
Lourdes Hospital, Paducah
Oak Tree Hospital at Baptist Hospital Northeast,
    La Grange
St. Joseph Hospital, Lexington

VASCULAR

CAROTID SURGERY
Lourdes Hospital, Paducah
Medical Center, Bowling Green
Pattie A. Clay Regional Medical Center, Richmond

PERIPHERAL VASCULAR BYPASS
Medical Center, Bowling Green

RESECTION/REPLACEMENT OF ABDOMINAL AORTA
None

WOMEN'S HEALTH

None

Hospitals receiving a five star rating in a particular procedure have patient outcomes that put them among the best in the nation. For full definitions of ratings and awards, see Appendix.

BARIATRIC SURGERY

None

CARDIAC

ATRIAL FIBRILLATION

Willis Knighton Bossier Health Center, Bossier City
Willis Knighton Medical Center, Shreveport

CORONARY INTERVENTIONAL PROCEDURES (ANGIOPLASTY/STENT)

Heart Hospital of Lafayette, Lafayette
Southwest Medical Center, Lafayette

HEART ATTACK

Baton Rouge General Medical Center, Baton Rouge
Beauregard Memorial Hospital, Deridder
Jennings American Legion Hospital, Jennings
LSU Health Sciences Center–Shreveport, Shreveport

HEART BYPASS SURGERY

East Jefferson General Hospital, Metairie
St. Francis Medical Center, Monroe

HEART FAILURE

Christus Schumpert Health System, Shreveport
Citizens Medical Center, Columbia
Dauterive Hospital, New Iberia
Dubuis Hospital Continuing Care Shreveport, Shreveport
Iberia Medical Center, New Iberia
Louisiana Heart Hospital, Lacombe
Ochsner St. Anne General Hospital, Raceland
Southwest Medical Center, Lafayette
Ville Platte Medical Center, Ville Platte
Willis Knighton Bossier Health Center, Bossier City
Willis Knighton Medical Center, Shreveport

VALVE REPLACEMENT SURGERY

Louisiana Heart Hospital, Lacombe
Rapides Regional Medical Center, Alexandria

CRITICAL CARE

DIABETIC ACIDOSIS AND COMA

None

PULMONARY EMBOLISM

Glenwood Regional Medical Center, West Monroe

RESPIRATORY FAILURE

Baton Rouge General Medical Center, Baton Rouge
Glenwood Regional Medical Center, West Monroe

Willis Knighton Bossier Health Center, Bossier City
Willis Knighton Medical Center, Shreveport

SEPSIS

Baton Rouge General Medical Center, Baton Rouge
Byrd Regional Hospital, Leesville
Glenwood Regional Medical Center, West Monroe
Oakdale Community Hospital, Oakdale
Richland Parish Hospital Delhi, Delhi
Riverside Medical Center, Franklinton
St. Francis Medical Center, Monroe
Ville Platte Medical Center, Ville Platte
West Jefferson Medical Center, Marrero
Willis Knighton Bossier Health Center, Bossier City

GASTROINTESTINAL

BOWEL OBSTRUCTION

Rapides Regional Medical Center, Alexandria
Thibodaux Regional Medical Center, Thibodaux
Willis Knighton Medical Center, Shreveport

CHOLECYSTECTOMY

Iberia Medical Center, New Iberia
Lafayette General Medical Center, Lafayette
Our Lady of Lourdes Regional Medical Center, Lafayette
St. Brendan Rehab and Specialty Hospital, Lafayette
Thibodaux Regional Medical Center, Thibodaux
West Calcasieu Cameron Hospital, Sulphur

GASTROINTESTINAL BLEED

Byrd Regional Hospital, Leesville
Dauterive Hospital, New Iberia
Glenwood Regional Medical Center, West Monroe
Lake Charles Memorial Hospital, Lake Charles
Willis Knighton Bossier Health Center, Bossier City

GASTROINTESTINAL SURGERIES AND PROCEDURES

Christus St. Francis Cabrini Hospital, Alexandria
Lakeview Regional Medical Center, Covington
St. Francis Medical Center, Monroe

PANCREATITIS

None

GENERAL SURGERY

APPENDECTOMY

None

MATERNITY CARE

None

ORTHOPEDICS

BACK AND NECK SURGERY (EXCEPT SPINAL FUSION)

None

BACK AND NECK SURGERY (SPINAL FUSION)

Lafayette General Medical Center, Lafayette
Lake Charles Memorial Hospital, Lake Charles
Terrebonne General Hospital, Houma
Willis Knighton Medical Center, Shreveport

HIP FRACTURE REPAIR

Abbeville General Hospital, Abbeville
Christus St. Francis Cabrini Hospital, Alexandria
Glenwood Regional Medical Center, West Monroe
Lakeview Regional Medical Center, Covington
Lincoln General Hospital, Ruston
Our Lady of Lourdes Regional Medical Center, Lafayette
St. Brendan Rehab and Specialty Hospital, Lafayette
St. Francis Medical Center, Monroe
St. Francis North Hospital, Monroe
Slidell Memorial Hospital, Slidell

TOTAL HIP REPLACEMENT

Glenwood Regional Medical Center, West Monroe

TOTAL KNEE REPLACEMENT

Glenwood Regional Medical Center, West Monroe
Lafayette General Medical Center, Lafayette

PROSTATECTOMY

Iberia Medical Center, New Iberia
Lallie Kemp Medical Center, Independence
Ochsner Clinic Foundation, New Orleans

PULMONARY

CHRONIC OBSTRUCTIVE PULMONARY DISEASE (COPD)

Byrd Regional Hospital, Leesville
East Jefferson General Hospital, Metairie
Lincoln General Hospital, Ruston
Our Lady of the Lake Regional Medical Center, Baton Rouge
Willis Knighton Bossier Health Center, Bossier City
Willis Knighton Medical Center, Shreveport

PNEUMONIA

Christus Schumpert Health System, Shreveport
Christus St. Patrick Hospital, Lake Charles
Dubuis Hospital Continuing Care Shreveport, Shreveport
East Jefferson General Hospital, Metairie
Jennings American Legion Hospital, Jennings
Lady of the Sea General Hospital, Cut Off
Oakdale Community Hospital, Oakdale
Ochsner Clinic Foundation, New Orleans
Richland Parish Hospital Delhi, Delhi
Riverland Medical Center, Ferriday
St. Francis Medical Center, Monroe
Ville Platte Medical Center, Ville Platte

Willis Knighton Bossier Health Center, Bossier City
Willis Knighton Medical Center, Shreveport

STROKE

Columbia Jefferson Medical Center, Jefferson
Oakdale Community Hospital, Oakdale
St. Francis Medical Center, Monroe
Tulane University Hospital, New Orleans

VASCULAR

CAROTID SURGERY

Glenwood Regional Medical Center, West Monroe
Lafayette General Medical Center, Lafayette

Southwest Medical Center, Lafayette
Thibodaux Regional Medical Center, Thibodaux

PERIPHERAL VASCULAR BYPASS
None

RESECTION/REPLACEMENT OF ABDOMINAL AORTA
None

WOMEN'S HEALTH
None

MAINE HOSPITALS: FIVE STAR RATED FACILITIES

BARIATRIC SURGERY

None

CARDIAC

ATRIAL FIBRILLATION
None

CORONARY INTERVENTIONAL PROCEDURES (ANGIOPLASTY/STENT)
Brighton Medical Center, Portland
Maine Medical Center, Portland

HEART ATTACK
Kennebec Valley Medical Center, Augusta
Maine General Medical Center, Waterville
Mid Coast Hospital, Brunswick
Northern Maine Medical Center, Fort Kent

HEART BYPASS SURGERY
None

HEART FAILURE
Cary Medical Center, Caribou
Franklin Memorial Hospital, Farmington

VALVE REPLACEMENT SURGERY
None

CRITICAL CARE

DIABETIC ACIDOSIS AND COMA
None

PULMONARY EMBOLISM
None

RESPIRATORY FAILURE
Kennebec Valley Medical Center, Augusta
Maine General Medical Center, Waterville
Redington Fairview General Hospital, Skowhegan

SEPSIS
Inland Hospital, Waterville
Kennebec Valley Medical Center, Augusta
Maine General Medical Center, Waterville
Redington Fairview General Hospital, Skowhegan

GASTROINTESTINAL

BOWEL OBSTRUCTION
St. Joseph Hospital, Bangor

CHOLECYSTECTOMY
None

GASTROINTESTINAL BLEED
None

GASTROINTESTINAL SURGERIES AND PROCEDURES
None

PANCREATITIS
St. Joseph Hospital, Bangor

GENERAL SURGERY

APPENDECTOMY
Brighton Medical Center, Portland
Down East Community Hospital, Machias
Maine Medical Center, Portland
Mayo Regional Hospital, Dover Foxcroft
Waldo County General Hospital, Belfast

MATERNITY CARE
None

ORTHOPEDICS

BACK AND NECK SURGERY (EXCEPT SPINAL FUSION)
Mercy Hospital, Portland
Westbrook Community Hospital, Westbrook

BACK AND NECK SURGERY (SPINAL FUSION)
Mercy Hospital, Portland
Westbrook Community Hospital, Westbrook

HIP FRACTURE REPAIR
St. Joseph Hospital, Bangor

TOTAL HIP REPLACEMENT
Brighton Medical Center, Portland
Central Maine Medical Center, Lewiston
Eastern Maine Medical Center, Bangor
Maine Medical Center, Portland

TOTAL KNEE REPLACEMENT
Brighton Medical Center, Portland
Maine Medical Center, Portland
Southern Maine Medical Center, Biddeford

PROSTATECTOMY
None

PULMONARY

CHRONIC OBSTRUCTIVE PULMONARY DISEASE (COPD)
None

Hospitals receiving a five star rating in a particular procedure have patient outcomes that put them among the best in the nation. For full definitions of ratings and awards, see Appendix.

PNEUMONIA
Franklin Memorial Hospital, Farmington
Miles Memorial Hospital, Damariscotta

STROKE
None

BARIATRIC SURGERY
Johns Hopkins Bayview Medical Center, Baltimore
Shady Grove Adventist Hospital, Rockville

CARDIAC

ATRIAL FIBRILLATION
Harford Memorial Hospital, Havre De Grace
St. Mary's Hospital, Leonardtown
Washington County Hospital, Hagerstown

CORONARY INTERVENTIONAL PROCEDURES (ANGIOPLASTY/STENT)
Union Memorial Hospital, Baltimore

HEART ATTACK
Bon Secours Hospital, Baltimore
Civista Medical Center, La Plata
Franklin Square Hospital Center, Baltimore
Good Samaritan Hospital, Baltimore
Greater Baltimore Medical Center, Baltimore
Laurel Regional Hospital, Laurel
Mercy Medical Center, Baltimore
Northwest Hospital Center, Randallstown
Suburban Hospital, Bethesda

HEART BYPASS SURGERY
Sacred Heart Hospital, Cumberland

HEART FAILURE
Anne Arundel Medical Center, Annapolis
Atlantic General Hospital, Berlin
Baltimore Washington Medical Center, Glen Burnie
Bon Secours Hospital, Baltimore
Calvert Memorial Hospital, Prince Frederick
Carroll Hospital Center, Westminster
Civista Medical Center, La Plata
Franklin Square Hospital Center, Baltimore
Good Samaritan Hospital, Baltimore
Greater Baltimore Medical Center, Baltimore
Harbor Hospital, Baltimore
Holy Cross Hospital, Silver Spring
Howard County General Hospital, Columbia
Johns Hopkins Bayview Medical Center, Baltimore

Johns Hopkins Hospital, Baltimore
Laurel Regional Hospital, Laurel
Maryland General Hospital, Baltimore
Northwest Hospital Center, Randallstown
Prince George's Hospital Center, Cheverly
St. Joseph Medical Center, Towson
St. Mary's Hospital, Leonardtown
Suburban Hospital, Bethesda
Union Memorial Hospital, Baltimore
Upper Chesapeake Medical Center, Bel Air
Washington Adventist Hospital, Takoma Park
Washington County Hospital, Hagerstown

VALVE REPLACEMENT SURGERY
Sacred Heart Hospital, Cumberland
St. Joseph Medical Center, Towson

CRITICAL CARE

DIABETIC ACIDOSIS AND COMA
Johns Hopkins Bayview Medical Center, Baltimore
St. Agnes Hospital, Baltimore
St. Joseph Medical Center, Towson
Sinai Hospital of Baltimore, Baltimore

PULMONARY EMBOLISM
Frederick Memorial Hospital, Frederick
Greater Baltimore Medical Center, Baltimore
Howard County General Hospital, Columbia

RESPIRATORY FAILURE
Atlantic General Hospital, Berlin
Doctors Community Hospital, Lanham
Franklin Square Hospital Center, Baltimore
Greater Baltimore Medical Center, Baltimore
Howard County General Hospital, Columbia
Maryland General Hospital, Baltimore
Northwest Hospital Center, Randallstown
Suburban Hospital, Bethesda
Upper Chesapeake Medical Center, Bel Air

SEPSIS
Bon Secours Hospital, Baltimore
Civista Medical Center, La Plata

Doctors Community Hospital, Lanham
Franklin Square Hospital Center, Baltimore
Good Samaritan Hospital, Baltimore
Greater Baltimore Medical Center, Baltimore
Harbor Hospital, Baltimore
Howard County General Hospital, Columbia
Maryland General Hospital, Baltimore
Northwest Hospital Center, Randallstown
Peninsula Regional Medical Center, Salisbury
Sacred Heart Hospital, Cumberland
St. Joseph Medical Center, Towson
Shady Grove Adventist Hospital, Rockville
Suburban Hospital, Bethesda
Washington Adventist Hospital, Takoma Park

GASTROINTESTINAL

BOWEL OBSTRUCTION
Baltimore Washington Medical Center, Glen Burnie
Fort Washington Hospital, Fort Washington
Greater Baltimore Medical Center, Baltimore
St. Joseph Medical Center, Towson
Union Hospital of Cecil County, Elkton

CHOLECYSTECTOMY
Franklin Square Hospital Center, Baltimore

GASTROINTESTINAL BLEED
Baltimore Washington Medical Center, Glen Burnie
Calvert Memorial Hospital, Prince Frederick
Franklin Square Hospital Center, Baltimore
Holy Cross Hospital, Silver Spring
Johns Hopkins Bayview Medical Center, Baltimore
Laurel Regional Hospital, Laurel
Maryland General Hospital, Baltimore
Mercy Medical Center, Baltimore
St. Agnes Hospital, Baltimore
St. Joseph Medical Center, Towson
St. Mary's Hospital, Leonardtown
Shady Grove Adventist Hospital, Rockville
Suburban Hospital, Bethesda
Union Hospital of Cecil County, Elkton

VASCULAR

CAROTID SURGERY
Central Maine Medical Center, Lewiston

PERIPHERAL VASCULAR BYPASS
None

RESECTION/REPLACEMENT OF ABDOMINAL AORTA
None

WOMEN'S HEALTH
None

GASTROINTESTINAL SURGERIES AND PROCEDURES

Doctors Community Hospital, Lanham
Fort Washington Hospital, Fort Washington
Franklin Square Hospital Center, Baltimore
Greater Baltimore Medical Center, Baltimore
Mercy Medical Center, Baltimore
Sinai Hospital of Baltimore, Baltimore
Southern Maryland Hospital Center, Clinton
Suburban Hospital, Bethesda

PANCREATITIS

Good Samaritan Hospital, Baltimore
Greater Baltimore Medical Center, Baltimore
Sinai Hospital of Baltimore, Baltimore

GENERAL SURGERY

APPENDECTOMY

Baltimore Washington Medical Center, Glen Burnie
Upper Chesapeake Medical Center, Bel Air

MATERNITY CARE

Greater Baltimore Medical Center, Baltimore
Holy Cross Hospital, Silver Spring

ORTHOPEDICS

BACK AND NECK SURGERY (EXCEPT SPINAL FUSION)

Carroll Hospital Center, Westminster
Shady Grove Adventist Hospital, Rockville

BACK AND NECK SURGERY (SPINAL FUSION)

Baltimore Washington Medical Center, Glen Burnie
Prince George's Hospital Center, Cheverly

HIP FRACTURE REPAIR

Maryland General Hospital, Baltimore
Montgomery General Hospital, Olney
Peninsula Regional Medical Center, Salisbury

TOTAL HIP REPLACEMENT

None

TOTAL KNEE REPLACEMENT

Harford Memorial Hospital, Havre De Grace
Peninsula Regional Medical Center, Salisbury
Upper Chesapeake Medical Center, Bel Air
Washington County Hospital, Hagerstown

PROSTATECTOMY

Franklin Square Hospital Center, Baltimore
Peninsula Regional Medical Center, Salisbury

PULMONARY

CHRONIC OBSTRUCTIVE PULMONARY DISEASE (COPD)

Atlantic General Hospital, Berlin
Bon Secours Hospital, Baltimore
Calvert Memorial Hospital, Prince Frederick
Doctors Community Hospital, Lanham
Greater Baltimore Medical Center, Baltimore
Howard County General Hospital, Columbia
Johns Hopkins Bayview Medical Center, Baltimore
Northwest Hospital Center, Randallstown
St. Joseph Medical Center, Towson
St. Mary's Hospital, Leonardtown
Suburban Hospital, Bethesda
Union Hospital of Cecil County, Elkton
Upper Chesapeake Medical Center, Bel Air
Washington Adventist Hospital, Takoma Park

PNEUMONIA

Atlantic General Hospital, Berlin
Civista Medical Center, La Plata
Doctors Community Hospital, Lanham
Franklin Square Hospital Center, Baltimore
Good Samaritan Hospital, Baltimore
Greater Baltimore Medical Center, Baltimore
Harbor Hospital, Baltimore

Holy Cross Hospital, Silver Spring
Howard County General Hospital, Columbia
Johns Hopkins Bayview Medical Center, Baltimore
Maryland General Hospital, Baltimore
Mercy Medical Center, Baltimore
Northwest Hospital Center, Randallstown
St. Agnes Hospital, Baltimore
St. Joseph Medical Center, Towson
St. Mary's Hospital, Leonardtown
Shady Grove Adventist Hospital, Rockville
Southern Maryland Hospital Center, Clinton
Suburban Hospital, Bethesda
Union Hospital of Cecil County, Elkton
Washington Adventist Hospital, Takoma Park

STROKE

Anne Arundel Medical Center, Annapolis
Greater Baltimore Medical Center, Baltimore
Northwest Hospital Center, Randallstown
Prince George's Hospital Center, Cheverly
St. Joseph Medical Center, Towson
Suburban Hospital, Bethesda

VASCULAR

CAROTID SURGERY

Baltimore Washington Medical Center, Glen Burnie

PERIPHERAL VASCULAR BYPASS

Baltimore Washington Medical Center, Glen Burnie
Upper Chesapeake Medical Center, Bel Air

RESECTION/REPLACEMENT OF ABDOMINAL AORTA

None

WOMEN'S HEALTH

None

MASSACHUSETTS HOSPITALS: FIVE STAR RATED FACILITIES

BARIATRIC SURGERY

Newton-Wellesley Hospital, Newton
UMass Memorial Medical Center, Worcester
UMass Memorial Medical Center–Memorial
  Campus, Worcester
Winchester Hospital, Winchester

CARDIAC

ATRIAL FIBRILLATION

Atlanticare Medical Center–Union, Lynn

Berkshire Medical Center, Pittsfield
Hillcrest Hospital, Pittsfield
Mary and Arthur Clapham Hospital, Burlington
North Shore Medical Center, Salem

CORONARY INTERVENTIONAL PROCEDURES (ANGIOPLASTY/STENT)

Baystate Medical Center, Springfield
Cape Cod Hospital, Hyannis
Southcoast Hospitals Group–Charlton Memorial,
  Fall River

Southcoast Hospitals Group–St. Luke's Hospital,
  New Bedford
Southcoast Hospitals Group–Tobey Hospital,
  Wareham

HEART ATTACK

Baystate Franklin Medical Center, Greenfield
Baystate Mary Lane Hospital, Ware
Baystate Medical Center, Springfield
Berkshire Medical Center, Pittsfield
Cooley Dickinson Hospital, Northampton

Hospitals receiving a five star rating in a particular procedure have patient outcomes that put them among the best in the nation. For full definitions of ratings and awards, see Appendix.

Falmouth Hospital, Falmouth
HealthAlliance Hospital Burbank Campus,
  Fitchburg
HealthAlliance Hospital Leominster Campus,
  Leominster
Hillcrest Hospital, Pittsfield
Holyoke Medical Center, Holyoke
Milford Regional Medical Center, Milford
Milton Hospital, Milton
Morton Hospital and Medical Center, Taunton
North Adams Regional Hospital, North Adams

HEART BYPASS SURGERY

Baystate Medical Center, Springfield
Mount Auburn Hospital, Cambridge

HEART FAILURE

Atlanticare Medical Center–Union, Lynn
Baystate Franklin Medical Center, Greenfield
Beth Israel Deaconess Hospital–Needham, Needham
Caritas Carney Hospital, Dorchester
Falmouth Hospital, Falmouth
HealthAlliance Hospital Burbank Campus,
  Fitchburg
HealthAlliance Hospital Leominster Campus,
  Leominster
Morton Hospital and Medical Center, Taunton
Newton-Wellesley Hospital, Newton
Noble Hospital, Westfield
North Shore Medical Center, Salem
Southcoast Hospitals Group–Charlton Memorial,
  Fall River
Southcoast Hospitals Group–St. Luke's Hospital,
  New Bedford
Southcoast Hospitals Group–Tobey Hospital,
  Wareham

VALVE REPLACEMENT SURGERY

Atlanticare Medical Center–Union, Lynn
Baystate Medical Center, Springfield
Beth Israel Deaconess Medical Center, Boston
Mount Auburn Hospital, Cambridge
North Shore Medical Center, Salem

CRITICAL CARE

DIABETIC ACIDOSIS AND COMA
None

PULMONARY EMBOLISM
Caritas Good Samaritan Medical Center, Brockton

RESPIRATORY FAILURE
Atlanticare Medical Center–Union, Lynn
North Shore Medical Center, Salem

SEPSIS
HealthAlliance Hospital Burbank Campus,
  Fitchburg
HealthAlliance Hospital Leominster Campus,
  Leominster

GASTROINTESTINAL

BOWEL OBSTRUCTION
Baystate Medical Center, Springfield
Caritas Norwood Hospital, Norwood
Caritas Southwood Hospital, Norfolk
Emerson Hospital, Concord
Falmouth Hospital, Falmouth

CHOLECYSTECTOMY
Cape Cod Hospital, Hyannis
Caritas Norwood Hospital, Norwood
Caritas Southwood Hospital, Norfolk
Massachusetts General Hospital, Boston
Newton-Wellesley Hospital, Newton

GASTROINTESTINAL BLEED
Addison Gilbert Hospital, Gloucester
Berkshire Medical Center, Pittsfield
Beth Israel Deaconess Medical Center, Boston
Beverly Hospital, Beverly
Brigham and Women's Hospital, Boston
Cambridge Health Alliance, Cambridge
Cape Cod Hospital, Hyannis
Caritas Good Samaritan Medical Center, Brockton
HealthAlliance Hospital Burbank Campus,
  Fitchburg
HealthAlliance Hospital Leominster Campus,
  Leominster
Heritage Hospital, Somerville
Hillcrest Hospital, Pittsfield
Massachusetts General Hospital, Boston
Newton-Wellesley Hospital, Newton
Somerville Hospital, Somerville

GASTROINTESTINAL SURGERIES
AND PROCEDURES
Beth Israel Deaconess Medical Center, Boston
Newton-Wellesley Hospital, Newton

PANCREATITIS
Newton-Wellesley Hospital, Newton
Southcoast Hospitals Group–Charlton Memorial,
  Fall River
Southcoast Hospitals Group–St. Luke's Hospital,
  New Bedford
Southcoast Hospitals Group–Tobey Hospital,
  Wareham

GENERAL SURGERY

APPENDECTOMY
HealthAlliance Hospital Burbank Campus,
  Fitchburg
HealthAlliance Hospital Leominster Campus,
  Leominster
Newton-Wellesley Hospital, Newton
North Adams Regional Hospital, North Adams
St. Vincent Hospital, Worcester

MATERNITY CARE

Emerson Hospital, Concord
Hallmark Health, Medford
Melrose-Wakefield Hospital, Melrose
Mount Auburn Hospital, Cambridge
Newton-Wellesley Hospital, Newton
Southcoast Hospitals Group–Charlton Memorial,
  Fall River
Southcoast Hospitals Group–St. Luke's Hospital,
  New Bedford
Whidden Memorial Hospital, Everett

ORTHOPEDICS

BACK AND NECK SURGERY
(EXCEPT SPINAL FUSION)
Boston Medical Center, Boston
Caritas Holy Family Hospital and Medical Center,
  Methuen
Hallmark Health, Medford
Lawrence General Hospital, Lawrence
Malden Hospital, Malden
Melrose-Wakefield Hospital, Melrose
St. Vincent Hospital, Worcester
Whidden Memorial Hospital, Everett

BACK AND NECK SURGERY (SPINAL FUSION)
UMass Memorial Medical Center, Worcester
UMass Memorial Medical Center–Memorial
  Campus, Worcester

HIP FRACTURE REPAIR
None

TOTAL HIP REPLACEMENT
Jordan Hospital, Plymouth
Marlborough Hospital, Marlborough
New England Baptist Hospital, Boston

TOTAL KNEE REPLACEMENT
Cape Cod Hospital, Hyannis
Jordan Hospital, Plymouth
Massachusetts General Hospital, Boston
New England Baptist Hospital, Boston

PROSTATECTOMY

Atlanticare Medical Center—Union, Lynn
Cape Cod Hospital, Hyannis
Caritas Good Samaritan Medical Center, Brockton
Caritas Norwood Hospital, Norwood
Caritas Southwood Hospital, Norfolk
Massachusetts General Hospital, Boston
North Shore Medical Center, Salem

PULMONARY

CHRONIC OBSTRUCTIVE PULMONARY DISEASE (COPD)

Berkshire Medical Center, Pittsfield
Caritas Carney Hospital, Dorchester
Caritas St. Elizabeth's Medical Center, Boston
HealthAlliance Hospital Burbank Campus, Fitchburg
HealthAlliance Hospital Leominster Campus, Leominster
Hillcrest Hospital, Pittsfield
Mary and Arthur Clapham Hospital, Burlington
Milton Hospital, Milton
South Shore Hospital, South Weymouth

PNEUMONIA

Addison Gilbert Hospital, Gloucester
Atlanticare Medical Center—Union, Lynn
Beth Israel Deaconess Medical Center, Boston
Beverly Hospital, Beverly
Boston Medical Center, Boston
Brigham and Women's Hospital, Boston
HealthAlliance Hospital Burbank Campus, Fitchburg
HealthAlliance Hospital Leominster Campus, Leominster
Leonard Morse Hospital, Natick
MetroWest Medical Center, Framingham
Milford Regional Medical Center, Milford
Nashoba Valley Medical Center, Ayer
New England Baptist Hospital, Boston
Newton-Wellesley Hospital, Newton
North Shore Medical Center, Salem
South Shore Hospital, South Weymouth
Wing Memorial Hospital and Medical Center, Palmer

STROKE

Atlanticare Medical Center—Union, Lynn
Cape Cod Hospital, Hyannis
Emerson Hospital, Concord
HealthAlliance Hospital Burbank Campus, Fitchburg
HealthAlliance Hospital Leominster Campus, Leominster
Merrimack Valley Hospital, Haverhill
North Shore Medical Center, Salem

VASCULAR

CAROTID SURGERY

Baystate Medical Center, Springfield
Falmouth Hospital, Falmouth
Massachusetts General Hospital, Boston

PERIPHERAL VASCULAR BYPASS

None

RESECTION/REPLACEMENT OF ABDOMINAL AORTA

None

WOMEN'S HEALTH

None

MICHIGAN HOSPITALS: FIVE STAR RATED FACILITIES

BARIATRIC SURGERY

None

CARDIAC

ATRIAL FIBRILLATION

Beaumont Hospital—Royal Oak, Royal Oak
Beaumont Hospital—Troy, Troy
Huron Valley Sinai Hospital, Commerce Township
Lapeer Regional Medical Center, Lapeer
Oakwood Heritage Hospital, Taylor
St. Joseph Mercy Oakland, Pontiac

CORONARY INTERVENTIONAL PROCEDURES (ANGIOPLASTY/STENT)

Beaumont Hospital—Royal Oak, Royal Oak
Beaumont Hospital—Troy, Troy

HEART ATTACK

Beaumont Hospital—Grosse Pointe, Grosse Pointe
Beaumont Hospital—Royal Oak, Royal Oak
Beaumont Hospital—Troy, Troy
Community Hospital Foundation, Almont
Crittenton Hospital Medical Center, Rochester
Genesys Regional Medical Center, Grand Blanc
Gerber Memorial Health Services, Fremont
Hackley Hospital, Muskegon
Henry Ford Hospital, Detroit
Henry Ford Macomb Hospital, Clinton Township
Huron Valley Sinai Hospital, Commerce Township
Lapeer Regional Medical Center, Lapeer
Mecosta County Medical Center, Big Rapids
Mercy Hospital—Grayling, Grayling
Mercy Memorial Hospital, Monroe
Oakwood Annapolis Hospital, Wayne
Oakwood Southshore Medical Center, Trenton
Pennock Hospital, Hastings
Portage Health System, Hancock
Providence Hospital, Southfield
St. John Hospital and Medical Center, Detroit
St. John Oakland Hospital, Madison Heights
St. Mary's Health Care, Grand Rapids
Spectrum Health Hospitals, Grand Rapids
United Memorial Health Center, Greenville

HEART BYPASS SURGERY

Beaumont Hospital—Troy, Troy
Crittenton Hospital Medical Center, Rochester
Genesys Regional Medical Center, Grand Blanc
Providence Hospital, Southfield
St. Joseph Mercy Oakland, Pontiac
Spectrum Health Hospitals, Grand Rapids
University of Michigan Hospital, Ann Arbor

HEART FAILURE

Beaumont Hospital—Royal Oak, Royal Oak
Beaumont Hospital—Troy, Troy
Bronson Methodist Hospital, Kalamazoo
Central Michigan Community Hospital, Mount Pleasant
Cheboygan Memorial Hospital, Cheboygan
Community Hospital Foundation, Almont
Crittenton Hospital Medical Center, Rochester
Garden City Osteopathic Hospital, Garden City
Genesys Regional Medical Center, Grand Blanc
Harper University Hospital, Detroit
Henry Ford Hospital, Detroit
Henry Ford Macomb Hospital, Clinton Township
Henry Ford Wyandotte Hospital, Wyandotte
Huron Valley Sinai Hospital, Commerce Township
Hutzel Hospital, Detroit
Lapeer Regional Medical Center, Lapeer
Madison Community Hospital, Madison Heights
McLaren Regional Medical Center, Flint
Mercy Hospital—Grayling, Grayling

Hospitals receiving a five star rating in a particular procedure have patient outcomes that put them among the best in the nation. For full definitions of ratings and awards, see Appendix.

Mount Clemens Regional Medical Center,
    Mount Clemens
Oakwood Hospital and Medical Center–Dearborn,
    Dearborn
Oakwood Southshore Medical Center, Trenton
Providence Hospital, Southfield
St. John Detroit Riverview Hospital, Detroit
St. John Hospital and Medical Center, Detroit
St. John Macomb Hospital, Warren
St. John Oakland Hospital, Madison Heights
St. Joseph Mercy Hospital, Ypsilanti
St. Mary Mercy Hospital, Livonia
St. Mary's Health Care, Grand Rapids
Spectrum Health Hospitals, Grand Rapids
Standish Community Hospital, Standish
United Memorial Health Center, Greenville

VALVE REPLACEMENT SURGERY

Beaumont Hospital–Royal Oak, Royal Oak
Mercy General Health Partners, Muskegon
Munson Medical Center, Traverse City
Spectrum Health Hospitals, Grand Rapids

CRITICAL CARE

DIABETIC ACIDOSIS AND COMA

Beaumont Hospital–Royal Oak, Royal Oak
Detroit Receiving Hospital and University Health
    Center, Detroit
St. Joseph Mercy Hospital, Ypsilanti

PULMONARY EMBOLISM

Community Hospital Foundation, Almont
Henry Ford Macomb Hospital, Clinton Township
Metro Health Hospital, Wyoming
St. Mary Mercy Hospital, Livonia

RESPIRATORY FAILURE

Beaumont Hospital–Royal Oak, Royal Oak
Cheboygan Memorial Hospital, Cheboygan
Community Health Center of Branch County,
    Coldwater
Community Hospital Foundation, Almont
Covenant Medical Center, Saginaw
Dickinson County Healthcare System,
    Iron Mountain
Genesys Regional Medical Center, Grand Blanc
Hackley Hospital, Muskegon
Henry Ford Hospital, Detroit
Henry Ford Macomb Hospital, Clinton Township
Henry Ford Wyandotte Hospital, Wyandotte
McLaren Regional Medical Center, Flint
Mecosta County Medical Center, Big Rapids
Mercy General Health Partners, Muskegon

Mercy Hospital–Grayling, Grayling
Metro Health Hospital, Wyoming
Oakwood Heritage Hospital, Taylor
Oakwood Hospital and Medical Center–Dearborn,
    Dearborn
St. John Detroit Riverview Hospital, Detroit
St. John Oakland Hospital, Madison Heights
St. Mary Mercy Hospital, Livonia
St. Mary's Health Care, Grand Rapids
St. Mary's of Michigan Medical Center, Saginaw
Select Specialty Hospital–Saginaw, Saginaw
Sinai-Grace Hospital, Detroit
United Memorial Health Center, Greenville
Wa Foote Hospital, Jackson

SEPSIS

Bay Regional Medical Center, Bay City
Beaumont Hospital–Grosse Pointe, Grosse Pointe
Beaumont Hospital–Royal Oak, Royal Oak
Beaumont Hospital–Troy, Troy
Borgess Medical Center, Kalamazoo
Borgess Pipp Health Center, Plainwell
Cheboygan Memorial Hospital, Cheboygan
Community Hospital Foundation, Almont
Crittenton Hospital Medical Center, Rochester
Garden City Osteopathic Hospital, Garden City
Genesys Regional Medical Center, Grand Blanc
Gratiot Medical Center, Alma
Hackley Hospital, Muskegon
Henry Ford Bi-County Hospital, Warren
Henry Ford Hospital, Detroit
Henry Ford Macomb Hospital, Clinton Township
Henry Ford Wyandotte Hospital, Wyandotte
Holland Community Hospital, Holland
Hurley Medical Center, Flint
Huron Valley Sinai Hospital, Commerce Township
Lapeer Regional Medical Center, Lapeer
McLaren Regional Medical Center, Flint
Mercy Hospital–Cadillac, Cadillac
Mercy Hospital–Grayling, Grayling
Metro Health Hospital, Wyoming
MidMichigan Medical Center–Midland, Midland
Mount Clemens Regional Medical Center,
    Mount Clemens
Munson Medical Center, Traverse City
North Oakland Medical Center, Pontiac
Oakwood Annapolis Hospital, Wayne
Oakwood Heritage Hospital, Taylor
Oakwood Hospital and Medical Center–Dearborn,
    Dearborn
Oakwood Southshore Medical Center, Trenton
Otsego Memorial Hospital, Gaylord
Pennock Hospital, Hastings

POH Regional Medical Center, Pontiac
Port Huron Hospital, Port Huron
Providence Hospital, Southfield
St. John Detroit Riverview Hospital, Detroit
St. John Macomb Hospital, Warren
St. John Oakland Hospital, Madison Heights
St. Joseph Health System–Tawas, Tawas City
St. Joseph Mercy Oakland, Pontiac
St. Mary Mercy Hospital, Livonia
St. Mary's Health Care, Grand Rapids
Sinai-Grace Hospital, Detroit
United Memorial Health Center, Greenville
Zeeland Community Hospital, Zeeland

GASTROINTESTINAL

BOWEL OBSTRUCTION

Beaumont Hospital–Troy, Troy
Cheboygan Memorial Hospital, Cheboygan
Crittenton Hospital Medical Center, Rochester
Dickinson County Healthcare System,
    Iron Mountain
Genesys Regional Medical Center, Grand Blanc
Harper University Hospital, Detroit
Hutzel Hospital, Detroit
Lakeview Community Hospital, Paw Paw
Madison Community Hospital, Madison Heights
McLaren Regional Medical Center, Flint
Munson Medical Center, Traverse City
Providence Hospital, Southfield
St. John River District Hospital, East China
St. Mary's Health Care, Grand Rapids
Spectrum Health Hospitals, Grand Rapids

CHOLECYSTECTOMY

Battle Creek Health System, Battle Creek
Beaumont Hospital–Royal Oak, Royal Oak
Community Health Center of Branch County, Coldwater
Crittenton Hospital Medical Center, Rochester
Edward W. Sparrow Hospital Association, Lansing
Henry Ford Wyandotte Hospital, Wyandotte
Mercy Memorial Hospital, Monroe
Mount Clemens Regional Medical Center,
    Mount Clemens
Munson Medical Center, Traverse City
Northern Michigan Hospital, Petoskey
Oakwood Southshore Medical Center, Trenton
Providence Hospital, Southfield
Sinai-Grace Hospital, Detroit
West Branch Regional Medical Center, West Branch

GASTROINTESTINAL BLEED

Beaumont Hospital–Royal Oak, Royal Oak
Botsford Hospital, Farmington Hills

Community Hospital Foundation, Almont
Garden City Osteopathic Hospital, Garden City
Grand View Hospital, Ironwood
Harper University Hospital, Detroit
Henry Ford Bi-County Hospital, Warren
Henry Ford Macomb Hospital, Clinton Township
Hutzel Hospital, Detroit
Lapeer Regional Medical Center, Lapeer
Madison Community Hospital, Madison Heights
Mercy Hospital—Grayling, Grayling
Mount Clemens Regional Medical Center,
    Mount Clemens
Munson Medical Center, Traverse City
North Oakland Medical Center, Pontiac
Oakwood Annapolis Hospital, Wayne
Oakwood Heritage Hospital, Taylor
Oakwood Southshore Medical Center, Trenton
St. John Macomb Hospital, Warren
St. John Oakland Hospital, Madison Heights
St. Mary Mercy Hospital, Livonia
Spectrum Health Hospitals, Grand Rapids

GASTROINTESTINAL SURGERIES AND PROCEDURES

Beaumont Hospital—Royal Oak, Royal Oak
Crittenton Hospital Medical Center, Rochester
Hackley Hospital, Muskegon
Henry Ford Wyandotte Hospital, Wyandotte
Munson Medical Center, Traverse City
Oakwood Southshore Medical Center, Trenton
Port Huron Hospital, Port Huron
Providence Hospital, Southfield

PANCREATITIS

Community Hospital Foundation, Almont
Crittenton Hospital Medical Center, Rochester
Genesys Regional Medical Center, Grand Blanc
Henry Ford Hospital, Detroit
Henry Ford Macomb Hospital, Clinton Township
Huron Valley Sinai Hospital, Commerce Township

GENERAL SURGERY

APPENDECTOMY
None

MATERNITY CARE
None

ORTHOPEDICS

BACK AND NECK SURGERY (EXCEPT SPINAL FUSION)

Bay Regional Medical Center, Bay City

Beaumont Hospital—Royal Oak, Royal Oak
Covenant Medical Center, Saginaw
Garden City Osteopathic Hospital, Garden City
Hackley Hospital, Muskegon
Metro Health Hospital, Wyoming
Munson Medical Center, Traverse City
Northern Michigan Hospital, Petoskey
St. Mary's of Michigan Medical Center, Saginaw
Select Specialty Hospital—Saginaw, Saginaw

BACK AND NECK SURGERY (SPINAL FUSION)

Bay Regional Medical Center, Bay City
Beaumont Hospital—Royal Oak, Royal Oak
Beaumont Hospital—Troy, Troy
Borgess Medical Center, Kalamazoo
Borgess Pipp Health Center, Plainwell
Bronson Methodist Hospital, Kalamazoo
Covenant Medical Center, Saginaw
Genesys Regional Medical Center, Grand Blanc
Hackley Hospital, Muskegon
MidMichigan Medical Center—Midland, Midland
Munson Medical Center, Traverse City
Northern Michigan Hospital, Petoskey
St. John Macomb Hospital, Warren
St. Mary's of Michigan Medical Center, Saginaw
Select Specialty Hospital—Saginaw, Saginaw
Wa Foote Hospital, Jackson

HIP FRACTURE REPAIR

Battle Creek Health System, Battle Creek
Bay Regional Medical Center, Bay City
Beaumont Hospital—Grosse Pointe, Grosse Pointe
Beaumont Hospital—Royal Oak, Royal Oak
Beaumont Hospital—Troy, Troy
Borgess Medical Center, Kalamazoo
Borgess Pipp Health Center, Plainwell
Botsford Hospital, Farmington Hills
Cheboygan Memorial Hospital, Cheboygan
Crittenton Hospital Medical Center, Rochester
Garden City Osteopathic Hospital, Garden City
Genesys Regional Medical Center, Grand Blanc
Hackley Hospital, Muskegon
Henry Ford Wyandotte Hospital, Wyandotte
Herrick Memorial Hospital, Tecumseh
Huron Medical Center, Bad Axe
Mercy Hospital—Port Huron, Port Huron
Munson Medical Center, Traverse City
North Ottawa Community Hospital, Grand Haven
Oakwood Annapolis Hospital, Wayne
Oakwood Heritage Hospital, Taylor
Oakwood Hospital and Medical Center—Dearborn,
    Dearborn
Oakwood Southshore Medical Center, Trenton

St. John Macomb Hospital, Warren
St. John River District Hospital, East China
St. Mary Mercy Hospital, Livonia
St. Mary's of Michigan Medical Center, Saginaw

TOTAL HIP REPLACEMENT

Allegan General Hospital, Allegan
Beaumont Hospital—Royal Oak, Royal Oak
Borgess Medical Center, Kalamazoo
Borgess Pipp Health Center, Plainwell
Bronson Methodist Hospital, Kalamazoo
Covenant Medical Center, Saginaw
Garden City Osteopathic Hospital, Garden City
Huron Medical Center, Bad Axe
Ingham Regional Medical Center, Lansing
Marquette General Hospital, Marquette
Mecosta County Medical Center, Big Rapids
Mercy General Health Partners, Muskegon
MidMichigan Medical Center—Midland, Midland
Munson Medical Center, Traverse City
Oakwood Hospital and Medical Center—Dearborn,
    Dearborn
Oakwood Southshore Medical Center, Trenton
St. Joseph Mercy Oakland, Pontiac
Select Specialty Hospital—Saginaw, Saginaw
Spectrum Health Hospitals, Grand Rapids

TOTAL KNEE REPLACEMENT

Battle Creek Health System, Battle Creek
Bay Regional Medical Center, Bay City
Beaumont Hospital—Grosse Pointe, Grosse Pointe
Beaumont Hospital—Royal Oak, Royal Oak
Borgess Medical Center, Kalamazoo
Borgess Pipp Health Center, Plainwell
Bronson Methodist Hospital, Kalamazoo
Central Michigan Community Hospital,
    Mount Pleasant
Community Health Center of Branch County,
    Coldwater
Community Hospital—Watervliet, Watervliet
Covenant Medical Center, Saginaw
Garden City Osteopathic Hospital, Garden City
Henry Ford Wyandotte Hospital, Wyandotte
Herrick Memorial Hospital, Tecumseh
Huron Medical Center, Bad Axe
Ingham Regional Medical Center, Lansing
Lakeland Hospital—St. Joseph, St. Joseph
Lakeland Medical Center—Niles, Niles
Mecosta County Medical Center, Big Rapids
Memorial Medical Center of West Michigan,
    Ludington
Mercy General Health Partners, Muskegon
MidMichigan Medical Center—Midland, Midland

Munson Medical Center, Traverse City
North Ottawa Community Hospital, Grand Haven
Northern Michigan Hospital, Petoskey
Oaklawn Hospital, Marshall
Oakwood Heritage Hospital, Taylor
Oakwood Hospital and Medical Center—Dearborn,
    Dearborn
Otsego Memorial Hospital, Gaylord
St. Joseph Mercy Livingston Hospital, Howell
St. Joseph Mercy Oakland, Pontiac
Select Specialty Hospital—Saginaw, Saginaw
Sinai-Grace Hospital, Detroit
Spectrum Health Hospitals, Grand Rapids
Wa Foote Hospital, Jackson

PROSTATECTOMY

Beaumont Hospital—Royal Oak, Royal Oak
Bronson Methodist Hospital, Kalamazoo
Community Hospital Foundation, Almont
Hackley Hospital, Muskegon
Henry Ford Hospital, Detroit
Henry Ford Macomb Hospital, Clinton Township
Oakwood Annapolis Hospital, Wayne
St. Joseph Mercy Oakland, Pontiac
St. Mary Mercy Hospital, Livonia
Spectrum Health Hospitals, Grand Rapids

PULMONARY

CHRONIC OBSTRUCTIVE PULMONARY DISEASE (COPD)

Beaumont Hospital—Royal Oak, Royal Oak
Garden City Osteopathic Hospital, Garden City
Genesys Regional Medical Center, Grand Blanc
Henry Ford Hospital, Detroit
Henry Ford Wyandotte Hospital, Wyandotte
Mercy General Health Partners, Muskegon
Metro Health Hospital, Wyoming
Munson Medical Center, Traverse City
Oakwood Heritage Hospital, Taylor
Oakwood Hospital and Medical Center—Dearborn,
    Dearborn
Oakwood Southshore Medical Center, Trenton
St. John Detroit Riverview Hospital, Detroit
St. John Hospital and Medical Center, Detroit
St. John Macomb Hospital, Warren
St. Mary Mercy Hospital, Livonia

PNEUMONIA

Beaumont Hospital—Grosse Pointe, Grosse Pointe
Beaumont Hospital—Royal Oak, Royal Oak
Beaumont Hospital—Troy, Troy
Bronson Methodist Hospital, Kalamazoo

Cheboygan Memorial Hospital, Cheboygan
Community Hospital Foundation, Almont
Covenant Medical Center, Saginaw
Crittenton Hospital Medical Center, Rochester
Garden City Osteopathic Hospital, Garden City
Genesys Regional Medical Center, Grand Blanc
Gerber Memorial Health Services, Fremont
Gratiot Medical Center, Alma
Hackley Hospital, Muskegon
Henry Ford Hospital, Detroit
Henry Ford Macomb Hospital, Clinton Township
Huron Valley Sinai Hospital, Commerce Township
Lapeer Regional Medical Center, Lapeer
McLaren Regional Medical Center, Flint
Mercy Hospital—Grayling, Grayling
Metro Health Hospital, Wyoming
MidMichigan Medical Center—Clare, Clare
MidMichigan Medical Center—Gladwin, Gladwin
Mount Clemens Regional Medical Center,
    Mount Clemens
Munson Medical Center, Traverse City
Oakwood Annapolis Hospital, Wayne
Oakwood Heritage Hospital, Taylor
Oakwood Hospital and Medical Center—Dearborn,
    Dearborn
Oakwood Southshore Medical Center, Trenton
Otsego Memorial Hospital, Gaylord
POH Regional Medical Center, Pontiac
Port Huron Hospital, Port Huron
Providence Hospital, Southfield
St. John Detroit Riverview Hospital, Detroit
St. John Hospital and Medical Center, Detroit
St. John Macomb Hospital, Warren
St. John Oakland Hospital, Madison Heights
St. Joseph Mercy Oakland, Pontiac
St. Mary Mercy Hospital, Livonia
St. Mary's Health Care, Grand Rapids
St. Mary's of Michigan Medical Center, Saginaw
Select Specialty Hospital—Saginaw, Saginaw
Sinai-Grace Hospital, Detroit
Spectrum Health—Reed City Campus, Reed City
United Memorial Health Center, Greenville

STROKE

Beaumont Hospital—Grosse Pointe, Grosse Pointe
Beaumont Hospital—Royal Oak, Royal Oak
Beaumont Hospital—Troy, Troy
Borgess Medical Center, Kalamazoo
Borgess Pipp Health Center, Plainwell
Bronson Methodist Hospital, Kalamazoo
Chelsea Community Hospital, Chelsea
Community Hospital Foundation, Almont

Covenant Medical Center, Saginaw
Genesys Regional Medical Center, Grand Blanc
Harper University Hospital, Detroit
Henry Ford Bi-County Hospital, Warren
Henry Ford Hospital, Detroit
Henry Ford Macomb Hospital, Clinton Township
Herrick Memorial Hospital, Tecumseh
Holland Community Hospital, Holland
Hutzel Hospital, Detroit
Lapeer Regional Medical Center, Lapeer
Madison Community Hospital, Madison Heights
McLaren Regional Medical Center, Flint
Mount Clemens Regional Medical Center,
    Mount Clemens
Oakwood Heritage Hospital, Taylor
Oakwood Hospital and Medical Center—Dearborn,
    Dearborn
Portage Health System, Hancock
Providence Hospital, Southfield
St. John Hospital and Medical Center, Detroit
St. John Macomb Hospital, Warren
St. John Oakland Hospital, Madison Heights
St. Mary Mercy Hospital, Livonia
Select Specialty Hospital—Saginaw, Saginaw
Sinai-Grace Hospital, Detroit

VASCULAR

CAROTID SURGERY

Alpena Regional Medical Center, Alpena
Beaumont Hospital—Royal Oak, Royal Oak
Beaumont Hospital—Troy, Troy
Botsford Hospital, Farmington Hills
Ingham Regional Medical Center, Lansing
Mercy General Health Partners, Muskegon
Mercy Hospital—Port Huron, Port Huron
Mercy Memorial Hospital, Monroe
Northern Michigan Hospital, Petoskey
Port Huron Hospital, Port Huron
St. Mary Mercy Hospital, Livonia

PERIPHERAL VASCULAR BYPASS

Borgess Medical Center, Kalamazoo
Borgess Pipp Health Center, Plainwell
Ingham Regional Medical Center, Lansing
Munson Medical Center, Traverse City
Port Huron Hospital, Port Huron

RESECTION/REPLACEMENT OF ABDOMINAL AORTA

Bronson Methodist Hospital, Kalamazoo
Mercy General Health Partners, Muskegon

WOMEN'S HEALTH

None

BARIATRIC SURGERY

None

CARDIAC

ATRIAL FIBRILLATION

North Country Regional Hospital, Bemidji
St. Mary's Duluth Clinic, Duluth
St. Marys Hospital, Rochester
University of Minnesota Hospital and Clinic, Minneapolis
University of Minnesota Medical Center–Fairview, Minneapolis

CORONARY INTERVENTIONAL PROCEDURES (ANGIOPLASTY/STENT)

Fairview Southdale Hospital, Edina
Mercy Hospital, Coon Rapids
North Memorial Health Care, Robbinsdale

HEART ATTACK

Fairview Hospital Chisago Lakes, Chisago City
Fairview Lakes Health Services, Wyoming
Fairview Southdale Hospital, Edina
Methodist Hospital, Minneapolis
New Ulm Medical Center, New Ulm
Regions Hospital, St. Paul
Riverview Hospital, Crookston
Rush City Hospital, Rush City
St. Mary's Duluth Clinic, Duluth
St. Marys Hospital, Rochester
St. Mary's Regional Health Center, Detroit Lakes
United Hospitals, St. Paul
Unity Hospital, Fridley
Winona Community Memorial Hospital, Winona

HEART BYPASS SURGERY

North Memorial Health Care, Robbinsdale
St. Mary's Duluth Clinic, Duluth

HEART FAILURE

Abbott-Northwestern Hospital, Minneapolis
Austin Medical Center, Austin
Cambridge Medical Center, Cambridge
Clearwater Health Services, Bagley
Fairview Hospital Chisago Lakes, Chisago City
Fairview Lakes Health Services, Wyoming
Fairview Southdale Hospital, Edina
Hennepin County Medical Center, Minneapolis
Mercy Hospital, Coon Rapids
Methodist Hospital, Minneapolis

North Country Regional Hospital, Bemidji
Rush City Hospital, Rush City
St. Cloud Hospital, St. Cloud
St. Joseph's Hospital, St. Paul
St. Luke's Hospital, Duluth
St. Marys Hospital, Rochester
United Hospitals, St. Paul
Unity Hospital, Fridley

VALVE REPLACEMENT SURGERY

St. Cloud Hospital, St. Cloud

CRITICAL CARE

DIABETIC ACIDOSIS AND COMA

None

PULMONARY EMBOLISM

St. Marys Hospital, Rochester
Unity Hospital, Fridley

RESPIRATORY FAILURE

Fairview Southdale Hospital, Edina
Hutchinson Area Health Care, Hutchinson
Mercy Hospital, Coon Rapids
Methodist Hospital, Minneapolis
North Memorial Health Care, Robbinsdale
Regions Hospital, St. Paul
St. Luke's Hospital, Duluth
St. Mary's Duluth Clinic, Duluth
Unity Hospital, Fridley

SEPSIS

Abbott-Northwestern Hospital, Minneapolis
Douglas County Hospital, Alexandria
Fairview Southdale Hospital, Edina
Healtheast St. John's Hospital, Maplewood
Mercy Hospital, Coon Rapids
Methodist Hospital, Minneapolis
North Memorial Health Care, Robbinsdale
St. Joseph's Hospital, St. Paul
St. Luke's Hospital, Duluth
St. Mary's Duluth Clinic, Duluth
St. Marys Hospital, Rochester
Unity Hospital, Fridley
University of Minnesota Hospital and Clinic, Minneapolis
University of Minnesota Medical Center–Fairview, Minneapolis
Virginia Regional Medical Center, Virginia

GASTROINTESTINAL

BOWEL OBSTRUCTION

Abbott-Northwestern Hospital, Minneapolis
Austin Medical Center, Austin
Douglas County Hospital, Alexandria
Fairview Ridges Hospital, Burnsville
Hutchinson Area Health Care, Hutchinson
Mercy Hospital, Coon Rapids
Methodist Hospital, Minneapolis
North Country Regional Hospital, Bemidji
St. Cloud Hospital, St. Cloud
St. Joseph's Hospital, St. Paul
St. Marys Hospital, Rochester
United Hospitals, St. Paul

CHOLECYSTECTOMY

Chippewa County Hospital, Montevideo
Community Memorial Hospital, Cloquet
Lakeview Hospital, Stillwater
St. Mary's Regional Health Center, Detroit Lakes
University Medical Center–Mesabi, Hibbing

GASTROINTESTINAL BLEED

Austin Medical Center, Austin
Cambridge Medical Center, Cambridge
Methodist Hospital, Minneapolis
North Memorial Health Care, Robbinsdale
Regions Hospital, St. Paul
St. Cloud Hospital, St. Cloud
St. Francis Regional Medical Center, Shakopee
St. Joseph's Hospital, St. Paul
St. Marys Hospital, Rochester

GASTROINTESTINAL SURGERIES AND PROCEDURES

Methodist Hospital, Minneapolis
Rochester Methodist Hospital, Rochester
St. Luke's Hospital, Duluth
St. Marys Hospital, Rochester
Winona Community Memorial Hospital, Winona

PANCREATITIS

None

GENERAL SURGERY

APPENDECTOMY

None

MATERNITY CARE

None

Hospitals receiving a five star rating in a particular procedure have patient outcomes that put them among the best in the nation. For full definitions of ratings and awards, see Appendix.

ORTHOPEDICS

BACK AND NECK SURGERY (EXCEPT SPINAL FUSION)
Healtheast St. John's Hospital, Maplewood
Healtheast Woodwinds Hospital, Woodbury
Lakeview Hospital, Stillwater
St. Joseph's Hospital, St. Paul

BACK AND NECK SURGERY (SPINAL FUSION)
Healtheast Woodwinds Hospital, Woodbury
Lakeview Hospital, Stillwater
St. Cloud Hospital, St. Cloud
St. Luke's Hospital, Duluth

HIP FRACTURE REPAIR
Healtheast St. John's Hospital, Maplewood
Lakeview Hospital, Stillwater
Riverview Hospital, Crookston
St. Luke's Hospital, Duluth

TOTAL HIP REPLACEMENT
Healtheast St. John's Hospital, Maplewood
Healtheast Woodwinds Hospital, Woodbury
Lakeview Hospital, Stillwater
Rice Memorial Hospital, Willmar
St. Cloud Hospital, St. Cloud

TOTAL KNEE REPLACEMENT
Glencoe Regional Health Services, Glencoe
Healtheast Woodwinds Hospital, Woodbury
Lakeview Hospital, Stillwater
Pipestone County Medical Center Ashton Care Center, Pipestone
Rice Memorial Hospital, Willmar
St. Cloud Hospital, St. Cloud
St. Joseph's Hospital, St. Paul
St. Luke's Hospital, Duluth

PROSTATECTOMY
Healtheast St. John's Hospital, Maplewood
Rice Memorial Hospital, Willmar
St. Cloud Hospital, St. Cloud
St. Joseph's Hospital, St. Paul

PULMONARY

CHRONIC OBSTRUCTIVE PULMONARY DISEASE (COPD)
Fairview Southdale Hospital, Edina
Mercy Hospital, Coon Rapids
North Country Regional Hospital, Bemidji
St. Marys Hospital, Rochester
United Hospitals, St. Paul
University of Minnesota Hospital and Clinic, Minneapolis
University of Minnesota Medical Center—Fairview, Minneapolis

PNEUMONIA
Fairview Hospital Chisago Lakes, Chisago City
Fairview Lakes Health Services, Wyoming
Fairview Ridges Hospital, Burnsville
Fairview Southdale Hospital, Edina
Healtheast St. John's Hospital, Maplewood
Hennepin County Medical Center, Minneapolis
Mercy Hospital, Coon Rapids
Methodist Hospital, Minneapolis
Monticello-Big Lake Community Hospital, Monticello
North Memorial Health Care, Robbinsdale
Rochester Methodist Hospital, Rochester
Rush City Hospital, Rush City
St. Cloud Hospital, St. Cloud
St. Mary's Duluth Clinic, Duluth
St. Marys Hospital, Rochester

St. Peter Community Hospital, St. Peter
United Hospitals, St. Paul
Unity Hospital, Fridley

STROKE
Abbott-Northwestern Hospital, Minneapolis
Fairview Southdale Hospital, Edina
Healtheast St. John's Hospital, Maplewood
Mercy Hospital, Coon Rapids
Methodist Hospital, Minneapolis
North Memorial Health Care, Robbinsdale
St. Joseph's Hospital, St. Paul
St. Mary's Duluth Clinic, Duluth
University Medical Center—Mesabi, Hibbing
University of Minnesota Hospital and Clinic, Minneapolis
University of Minnesota Medical Center—Fairview, Minneapolis

VASCULAR

CAROTID SURGERY
None

PERIPHERAL VASCULAR BYPASS
None

RESECTION/REPLACEMENT OF ABDOMINAL AORTA
North Memorial Health Care, Robbinsdale

WOMEN'S HEALTH
None

MISSISSIPPI HOSPITALS: FIVE STAR RATED FACILITIES

BARIATRIC SURGERY
None

CARDIAC

ATRIAL FIBRILLATION
None

CORONARY INTERVENTIONAL PROCEDURES (ANGIOPLASTY/STENT)
None

HEART ATTACK
Parkview Regional Medical Center, Vicksburg
River Region Health System, Vicksburg

Trace Regional Hospital, Houston

HEART BYPASS SURGERY
None

HEART FAILURE
None

VALVE REPLACEMENT SURGERY
None

CRITICAL CARE

DIABETIC ACIDOSIS AND COMA
None

PULMONARY EMBOLISM
None

RESPIRATORY FAILURE
None

SEPSIS
None

GASTROINTESTINAL

BOWEL OBSTRUCTION
None

CHOLECYSTECTOMY

Baptist Memorial Hospital—Golden Triangle, Columbus
Delta Regional Medical Center, Greenville
George Regional Health System, Lucedale
Grenada Lake Medical Center, Grenada
Jeff Anderson Regional Medical Center, Meridian
King's Daughters Hospital—Greenville, Greenville
Mississippi Baptist Medical Center, Jackson
Natchez Community Hospital, Natchez
North Mississippi Medical Center, Tupelo
Parkview Regional Medical Center, Vicksburg
River Region Health System, Vicksburg

GASTROINTESTINAL BLEED

None

GASTROINTESTINAL SURGERIES AND PROCEDURES

Mississippi Baptist Medical Center, Jackson
St. Dominic-Jackson Memorial Hospital, Jackson
Singing River Hospital System, Pascagoula

PANCREATITIS

Mississippi Baptist Medical Center, Jackson

GENERAL SURGERY

APPENDECTOMY

None

MATERNITY CARE

None

ORTHOPEDICS

BACK AND NECK SURGERY (EXCEPT SPINAL FUSION)

Baptist Memorial Hospital—North Mississippi, Oxford
Mississippi Baptist Medical Center, Jackson
River Oaks Hospital, Jackson

BACK AND NECK SURGERY (SPINAL FUSION)

Baptist Memorial Hospital—Golden Triangle, Columbus
Forrest General Hospital, Hattiesburg
North Mississippi Medical Center, Tupelo
River Oaks Hospital, Jackson

HIP FRACTURE REPAIR

Forrest General Hospital, Hattiesburg
Gulf Coast Medical Center, Biloxi
Jeff Anderson Regional Medical Center, Meridian
Oktibbeha County Hospital, Starkville
Rush Foundation Hospital, Meridian

TOTAL HIP REPLACEMENT

Baptist Memorial Hospital—De Soto, Southaven
Gulf Coast Medical Center, Biloxi
River Oaks Hospital, Jackson

TOTAL KNEE REPLACEMENT

Baptist Memorial Hospital—Golden Triangle, Columbus
Garden Park Medical Center, Gulfport
Greenwood Leflore Hospital, Greenwood
Gulf Coast Medical Center, Biloxi
University of Mississippi Medical Center, Jackson
Wesley Medical Center, Hattiesburg

PROSTATECTOMY

Baptist Memorial Hospital—North Mississippi, Oxford
Greenwood Leflore Hospital, Greenwood
Mississippi Baptist Medical Center, Jackson

PULMONARY

CHRONIC OBSTRUCTIVE PULMONARY DISEASE (COPD)

None

PNEUMONIA

Trace Regional Hospital, Houston

STROKE

None

VASCULAR

CAROTID SURGERY

Forrest General Hospital, Hattiesburg
Memorial Hospital at Gulfport, Gulfport
Mississippi Baptist Medical Center, Jackson

PERIPHERAL VASCULAR BYPASS

Forrest General Hospital, Hattiesburg
Mississippi Baptist Medical Center, Jackson
North Mississippi Medical Center, Tupelo
Southwest Mississippi Regional Medical Center, McComb

RESECTION/REPLACEMENT OF ABDOMINAL AORTA

None

WOMEN'S HEALTH

None

MISSOURI HOSPITALS: FIVE STAR RATED FACILITIES

BARIATRIC SURGERY

None

CARDIAC

ATRIAL FIBRILLATION

St. Francis Medical Center, Cape Girardeau

CORONARY INTERVENTIONAL PROCEDURES (ANGIOPLASTY/STENT)

Barnes Hospital, St. Louis
Barnes-Jewish Hospital, St. Louis
St. Luke's Cancer Institute, Kansas City
Saint Luke's Hospital of Kansas City, Kansas City

HEART ATTACK

Missouri Baptist Medical Center, St. Louis
SSM St. Joseph Hospital West, Lake St. Louis
Texas County Memorial Hospital, Houston

HEART BYPASS SURGERY

Freeman Health System, Joplin

HEART FAILURE

Barnes Hospital, St. Louis
Barnes-Jewish Hospital, St. Louis
Christian Hospital Northeast, St. Louis
Missouri Baptist Medical Center, St. Louis
Missouri Southern Healthcare, Dexter
Ray County Memorial Hospital, Richmond
St. Joseph Medical Center, Kansas City

St. Louis University Hospital, St. Louis
St. Luke's Hospital, Chesterfield
Scotland County Memorial Hospital, Memphis
Skaggs Community Health Center, Branson
SSM DePaul Health Center, Bridgeton
SSM St. Joseph Hospital West, Lake St. Louis

VALVE REPLACEMENT SURGERY

Freeman Health System, Joplin
SSM St. Joseph Health Center, St. Charles
SSM St. Joseph Health Center—Wentzville, Wentzville

CRITICAL CARE

DIABETIC ACIDOSIS AND COMA

None

PULMONARY EMBOLISM
St. Luke's Hospital, Chesterfield
SSM St. Mary's Health Center, St. Louis

RESPIRATORY FAILURE
Audrain Medical Center, Mexico
Barnes Hospital, St. Louis
Barnes-Jewish Hospital, St. Louis
Hannibal Regional Hospital, Hannibal
Heartland Regional Medical Center, St. Joseph
Moberly Regional Medical Center, Moberly
Ray County Memorial Hospital, Richmond
St. Alexius Hospital, St. Louis
St. Anthony's Medical Center, St. Louis
St. John's Regional Medical Center, Joplin
Skaggs Community Health Center, Branson
South Point Hospital, St. Louis
SSM DePaul Health Center, Bridgeton
SSM St. Joseph Health Center, St. Charles
SSM St. Joseph Health Center—Wentzville,
   Wentzville
SSM St. Joseph Hospital West, Lake St. Louis
SSM St. Mary's Health Center, St. Louis

SEPSIS
Bonne Terre Hospital, Bonne Terre
Christian Hospital Northeast, St. Louis
Freeman Neosho Hospital, Neosho
Grim-Smith Hospital and Clinic, Kirksville
Moberly Regional Medical Center, Moberly
Northeast Regional Medical Center, Kirksville
Parkland Health Center, Farmington
St. John's Regional Medical Center, Joplin
Ste. Genevieve County Memorial Hospital,
   Sainte Genevieve
Skaggs Community Health Center, Branson
SSM DePaul Health Center, Bridgeton
SSM St. Joseph Health Center, St. Charles
SSM St. Joseph Health Center—Wentzville,
   Wentzville
SSM St. Joseph Hospital of Kirkwood, Kirkwood
SSM St. Joseph Hospital West, Lake St. Louis
SSM St. Mary's Health Center, St. Louis

GASTROINTESTINAL

BOWEL OBSTRUCTION
Baptist Lutheran Medical Center, Kansas City
Barnes Hospital, St. Louis
Barnes-Jewish Hospital, St. Louis

CHOLECYSTECTOMY
Boone Hospital Center, Columbia
Grim-Smith Hospital and Clinic, Kirksville

Northeast Regional Medical Center, Kirksville
Skaggs Community Health Center, Branson
SSM St. Joseph Health Center, St. Charles
SSM St. Joseph Health Center—Wentzville,
   Wentzville

GASTROINTESTINAL BLEED
Barnes Hospital, St. Louis
Barnes-Jewish Hospital, St. Louis
Barnes-Jewish St. Peters Hospital, St. Peters
Missouri Baptist Medical Center, St. Louis

GASTROINTESTINAL SURGERIES
AND PROCEDURES
Heartland Regional Medical Center, St. Joseph
SSM St. Joseph Hospital of Kirkwood, Kirkwood
SSM St. Mary's Health Center, St. Louis

PANCREATITIS
None

GENERAL SURGERY

APPENDECTOMY
None

MATERNITY CARE

None

ORTHOPEDICS

BACK AND NECK SURGERY
(EXCEPT SPINAL FUSION)
Heartland Regional Medical Center, St. Joseph
St. Joseph Medical Center, Kansas City
SSM St. Joseph Health Center, St. Charles
SSM St. Joseph Health Center—Wentzville,
   Wentzville

BACK AND NECK SURGERY (SPINAL FUSION)
Research Medical Center, Kansas City
St. Luke's Hospital, Chesterfield

HIP FRACTURE REPAIR
Audrain Medical Center, Mexico
Boone Hospital Center, Columbia
Cass Medical Center, Harrisonville
Golden Valley Memorial Hospital, Clinton
Grim-Smith Hospital and Clinic, Kirksville
Heartland Regional Medical Center, St. Joseph
Lafayette Regional Health Center, Lexington
Mineral Area Regional Medical Center, Farmington
Northeast Regional Medical Center, Kirksville
St. Alexius Hospital, St. Louis
St. Anthony's Medical Center, St. Louis
South Point Hospital, St. Louis

SSM St. Mary's Health Center, St. Louis
Western Missouri Medical Center, Warrensburg

TOTAL HIP REPLACEMENT
Audrain Medical Center, Mexico
Boone Hospital Center, Columbia
Centerpoint Medical Center, Independence
Columbia Regional Hospital, Columbia
Freeman Health System, Joplin
Heartland Regional Medical Center, St. Joseph
St. John's Regional Health Center, Springfield
St. John's Regional Medical Center, Joplin
SSM St. Mary's Health Center, St. Louis

TOTAL KNEE REPLACEMENT
Audrain Medical Center, Mexico
Barnes-Jewish West County Hospital, St. Louis
Boone Hospital Center, Columbia
Cass Medical Center, Harrisonville
Columbia Regional Hospital, Columbia
Des Peres Hospital, St. Louis
Golden Valley Memorial Hospital, Clinton
Heartland Regional Medical Center, St. Joseph
Lake Regional Health System, Osage Beach
St. John's Regional Health Center, Springfield
St. John's Regional Medical Center, Joplin
St. Joseph Medical Center, Kansas City
Western Missouri Medical Center, Warrensburg

PROSTATECTOMY

Barnes-Jewish West County Hospital, St. Louis
Boone Hospital Center, Columbia
University of Missouri Hospital and Clinics,
   Columbia

PULMONARY

CHRONIC OBSTRUCTIVE PULMONARY DISEASE
(COPD)
Audrain Medical Center, Mexico
Heartland Regional Medical Center, St. Joseph
Moberly Regional Medical Center, Moberly
Research Medical Center, Kansas City
St. Anthony's Medical Center, St. Louis
St. Joseph Medical Center, Kansas City
St. Luke's Hospital, Chesterfield
SSM DePaul Health Center, Bridgeton
Truman Medical Center—Hospital Hill, Kansas City

PNEUMONIA
Christian Hospital Northeast, St. Louis
Ellett Memorial Hospital, Appleton City
Freeman Neosho Hospital, Neosho
Heartland Regional Medical Center, St. Joseph

Jefferson Memorial Hospital, Crystal City
Liberty Hospital, Liberty
Missouri Baptist Medical Center, St. Louis
Missouri Southern Healthcare, Dexter
Moberly Regional Medical Center, Moberly
Northwest Medical Center, Albany
Ray County Memorial Hospital, Richmond
St. Anthony's Medical Center, St. Louis
St. John's Regional Medical Center, Joplin
St. Luke's Hospital, Chesterfield
Ste. Genevieve County Memorial Hospital,
    Sainte Genevieve
SSM DePaul Health Center, Bridgeton
SSM St. Joseph Health Center, St. Charles
SSM St. Joseph Health Center—Wentzville,
    Wentzville
SSM St. Joseph Hospital of Kirkwood, Kirkwood

SSM St. Mary's Health Center, St. Louis
Truman Medical Center—Hospital Hill, Kansas City
Twin Rivers Regional Medical Center, Kennett

STROKE

Christian Hospital Northeast, St. Louis
Liberty Hospital, Liberty
Missouri Baptist Medical Center, St. Louis
St. Joseph Medical Center, Kansas City
Skaggs Community Health Center, Branson
SSM DePaul Health Center, Bridgeton
SSM St. Mary's Health Center, St. Louis

VASCULAR

CAROTID SURGERY
Boone Hospital Center, Columbia
Centerpoint Medical Center, Independence

Lake Regional Health System, Osage Beach
Liberty Hospital, Liberty
Menorah Medical Center, Kansas City
Ozarks Medical Center, West Plains
St. Francis Medical Center, Cape Girardeau
St. Joseph Medical Center, Kansas City

PERIPHERAL VASCULAR BYPASS
Research Medical Center, Kansas City
Southeast Missouri Hospital, Cape Girardeau

RESECTION/REPLACEMENT OF ABDOMINAL AORTA
Boone Hospital Center, Columbia
St. Luke's Cancer Institute, Kansas City
Saint Luke's Hospital of Kansas City, Kansas City

WOMEN'S HEALTH

None

MONTANA HOSPITALS: FIVE STAR RATED FACILITIES

BARIATRIC SURGERY

None

CARDIAC

ATRIAL FIBRILLATION
Kalispell Regional Hospital, Kalispell

CORONARY INTERVENTIONAL PROCEDURES (ANGIOPLASTY/STENT)
None

HEART ATTACK
Missoula General Hospital, Missoula
St. Patrick Hospital and Health Sciences Center,
    Missoula

HEART BYPASS SURGERY
None

HEART FAILURE
Kalispell Regional Hospital, Kalispell

VALVE REPLACEMENT SURGERY
None

CRITICAL CARE

DIABETIC ACIDOSIS AND COMA
None

PULMONARY EMBOLISM
None

RESPIRATORY FAILURE
Benefis Healthcare, Great Falls

SEPSIS
Benefis Healthcare, Great Falls
Kalispell Regional Hospital, Kalispell

GASTROINTESTINAL

BOWEL OBSTRUCTION
St. Vincent Healthcare, Billings

CHOLECYSTECTOMY
Billings Clinic, Billings

GASTROINTESTINAL BLEED
None

GASTROINTESTINAL SURGERIES AND PROCEDURES
Benefis Healthcare, Great Falls

PANCREATITIS
None

GENERAL SURGERY

APPENDECTOMY
None

MATERNITY CARE

None

ORTHOPEDICS

BACK AND NECK SURGERY (EXCEPT SPINAL FUSION)
Billings Clinic, Billings

BACK AND NECK SURGERY (SPINAL FUSION)
None

HIP FRACTURE REPAIR
Benefis Healthcare, Great Falls
Billings Clinic, Billings

TOTAL HIP REPLACEMENT
Billings Clinic, Billings

TOTAL KNEE REPLACEMENT
Billings Clinic, Billings

PROSTATECTOMY

Billings Clinic, Billings

PULMONARY

CHRONIC OBSTRUCTIVE PULMONARY DISEASE (COPD)
None

PNEUMONIA
None

STROKE

Benefis Healthcare, Great Falls

Hospitals receiving a five star rating in a particular procedure have patient outcomes that put them among the best in the nation. For full definitions of ratings and awards, see Appendix.

VASCULAR

CAROTID SURGERY
Billings Clinic, Billings
St. Vincent Healthcare, Billings

PERIPHERAL VASCULAR BYPASS
Billings Clinic, Billings
St. Vincent Healthcare, Billings

RESECTION/REPLACEMENT OF ABDOMINAL AORTA
None

WOMEN'S HEALTH
None

NEBRASKA HOSPITALS: FIVE STAR RATED FACILITIES

BARIATRIC SURGERY

None

CARDIAC

ATRIAL FIBRILLATION
St. Francis Medical Center, Grand Island

CORONARY INTERVENTIONAL PROCEDURES (ANGIOPLASTY/STENT)
None

HEART ATTACK
None

HEART BYPASS SURGERY
Nebraska Heart Hospital, Lincoln
St. Elizabeth Regional Medical Center, Lincoln

HEART FAILURE
Nebraska Heart Hospital, Lincoln

VALVE REPLACEMENT SURGERY
None

CRITICAL CARE

DIABETIC ACIDOSIS AND COMA
None

PULMONARY EMBOLISM
None

RESPIRATORY FAILURE
None

SEPSIS
St. Elizabeth Regional Medical Center, Lincoln

GASTROINTESTINAL

BOWEL OBSTRUCTION
None

CHOLECYSTECTOMY
None

GASTROINTESTINAL BLEED
None

GASTROINTESTINAL SURGERIES AND PROCEDURES
Bryanlgh Medical Center, Lincoln
Bryanlgh Medical Center—West, Lincoln

PANCREATITIS
St. Francis Medical Center, Grand Island

GENERAL SURGERY

APPENDECTOMY
None

MATERNITY CARE

None

ORTHOPEDICS

BACK AND NECK SURGERY (EXCEPT SPINAL FUSION)
Regional West Medical Center, Scottsbluff
St. Elizabeth Regional Medical Center, Lincoln

BACK AND NECK SURGERY (SPINAL FUSION)
Alegent Health—Bergan Mercy Medical Center, Omaha
Alegent Health—Immanuel Medical Center, Omaha
Bryanlgh Medical Center, Lincoln
Bryanlgh Medical Center—West, Lincoln

HIP FRACTURE REPAIR
Alegent Health—Immanuel Medical Center, Omaha
Bryanlgh Medical Center, Lincoln
Bryanlgh Medical Center—West, Lincoln
Community Hospital, McCook
Great Plains Regional Medical Center, North Platte
Regional West Medical Center, Scottsbluff
St. Francis Medical Center, Grand Island

TOTAL HIP REPLACEMENT
Bryanlgh Medical Center, Lincoln
Bryanlgh Medical Center—West, Lincoln
Faith Regional Health Services, Norfolk
Great Plains Regional Medical Center, North Platte
Lutheran Community Hospital, Norfolk
Our Lady of Lourdes Hospital, Norfolk
Regional West Medical Center, Scottsbluff

TOTAL KNEE REPLACEMENT
Alegent Health—Bergan Mercy Medical Center, Omaha
Faith Regional Health Services, Norfolk
Good Samaritan Hospital, Kearney
Jefferson Community Health Center, Fairbury
Lutheran Community Hospital, Norfolk
Our Lady of Lourdes Hospital, Norfolk
Regional West Medical Center, Scottsbluff
St. Francis Memorial Hospital, West Point

PROSTATECTOMY

None

PULMONARY

CHRONIC OBSTRUCTIVE PULMONARY DISEASE (COPD)
None

PNEUMONIA
Alegent Health—Bergan Mercy Medical Center, Omaha
Bryanlgh Medical Center, Lincoln
Bryanlgh Medical Center—West, Lincoln
Jennie M. Melham Memorial Medical Center, Broken Bow

STROKE

Bryanlgh Medical Center, Lincoln
Bryanlgh Medical Center—West, Lincoln

VASCULAR

CAROTID SURGERY
Creighton University Medical Center, Omaha
Nebraska Heart Hospital, Lincoln

PERIPHERAL VASCULAR BYPASS
None

RESECTION/REPLACEMENT OF ABDOMINAL AORTA
None

WOMEN'S HEALTH

None

BARIATRIC SURGERY

Desert Springs Hospital, Las Vegas
North Vista Hospital, North Las Vegas
Renown Regional Medical Center, Reno
St. Rose Dominican Hospital, Henderson

CARDIAC

ATRIAL FIBRILLATION
St. Rose Dominican Hospital—Siena Campus, Henderson

CORONARY INTERVENTIONAL PROCEDURES (ANGIOPLASTY/STENT)
None

HEART ATTACK
None

HEART BYPASS SURGERY
None

HEART FAILURE
Sunrise Hospital and Medical Center, Las Vegas

VALVE REPLACEMENT SURGERY
St. Rose Dominican Hospital—Siena Campus, Henderson

CRITICAL CARE

DIABETIC ACIDOSIS AND COMA
None

PULMONARY EMBOLISM
None

RESPIRATORY FAILURE
Valley Hospital Medical Center, Las Vegas

SEPSIS
Northern Nevada Medical Center, Sparks
Renown Regional Medical Center, Reno
St. Rose Dominican Hospital, Henderson
Summerlin Hospital Medical Center, Las Vegas

GASTROINTESTINAL

BOWEL OBSTRUCTION
North Vista Hospital, North Las Vegas

CHOLECYSTECTOMY
None

GASTROINTESTINAL BLEED
Carson Tahoe Regional Medical Center, Carson City
St. Rose Dominican Hospital—Siena Campus, Henderson

GASTROINTESTINAL SURGERIES AND PROCEDURES
Carson Tahoe Regional Medical Center, Carson City
Southern Hills Hospital and Medical Center, Las Vegas
Summerlin Hospital Medical Center, Las Vegas

PANCREATITIS
None

GENERAL SURGERY

APPENDECTOMY
None

MATERNITY CARE

Mountainview Hospital, Las Vegas
North Vista Hospital, North Las Vegas
St. Mary's Regional Medical Center, Reno

ORTHOPEDICS

BACK AND NECK SURGERY (EXCEPT SPINAL FUSION)
Sunrise Hospital and Medical Center, Las Vegas

BACK AND NECK SURGERY (SPINAL FUSION)
Desert Springs Hospital, Las Vegas
Sunrise Hospital and Medical Center, Las Vegas

HIP FRACTURE REPAIR
North Vista Hospital, North Las Vegas
Valley Hospital Medical Center, Las Vegas

TOTAL HIP REPLACEMENT
None

TOTAL KNEE REPLACEMENT
North Vista Hospital, North Las Vegas

PROSTATECTOMY

None

PULMONARY

CHRONIC OBSTRUCTIVE PULMONARY DISEASE (COPD)
None

PNEUMONIA
Desert Springs Hospital, Las Vegas
North Vista Hospital, North Las Vegas
St. Rose Dominican Hospital—Siena Campus, Henderson
Sunrise Hospital and Medical Center, Las Vegas
Valley Hospital Medical Center, Las Vegas

STROKE

St. Rose Dominican Hospital—Siena Campus, Henderson
Southern Hills Hospital and Medical Center, Las Vegas
Sunrise Hospital and Medical Center, Las Vegas
UMC of Southern Nevada, Las Vegas
Valley Hospital Medical Center, Las Vegas

VASCULAR

CAROTID SURGERY
None

PERIPHERAL VASCULAR BYPASS
None

RESECTION/REPLACEMENT OF ABDOMINAL AORTA
None

WOMEN'S HEALTH

None

Hospitals receiving a five star rating in a particular procedure have patient outcomes that put them among the best in the nation. For full definitions of ratings and awards, see Appendix.

BARIATRIC SURGERY

None

CARDIAC

ATRIAL FIBRILLATION
Mary Hitchcock Memorial Hospital, Lebanon

CORONARY INTERVENTIONAL PROCEDURES (ANGIOPLASTY/STENT)
None

HEART ATTACK
Androscoggin Valley Hospital, Berlin
Cheshire Medical Center, Keene
Mary Hitchcock Memorial Hospital, Lebanon
Southern New Hampshire Medical Center, Nashua

HEART BYPASS SURGERY
None

HEART FAILURE
Mary Hitchcock Memorial Hospital, Lebanon
Valley Regional Hospital, Claremont

VALVE REPLACEMENT SURGERY
None

CRITICAL CARE

DIABETIC ACIDOSIS AND COMA
None

PULMONARY EMBOLISM
None

RESPIRATORY FAILURE
None

SEPSIS
None

GASTROINTESTINAL

BOWEL OBSTRUCTION
Mary Hitchcock Memorial Hospital, Lebanon

CHOLECYSTECTOMY
None

GASTROINTESTINAL BLEED
Mary Hitchcock Memorial Hospital, Lebanon
Portsmouth Regional Hospital, Portsmouth

GASTROINTESTINAL SURGERIES AND PROCEDURES
None

PANCREATITIS
None

GENERAL SURGERY

APPENDECTOMY
None

MATERNITY CARE

None

ORTHOPEDICS

BACK AND NECK SURGERY (EXCEPT SPINAL FUSION)
Concord Hospital, Concord

BACK AND NECK SURGERY (SPINAL FUSION)
None

HIP FRACTURE REPAIR
Franklin Regional Hospital, Franklin

TOTAL HIP REPLACEMENT
Cheshire Medical Center, Keene
Concord Hospital, Concord

TOTAL KNEE REPLACEMENT
Cheshire Medical Center, Keene
Concord Hospital, Concord
Mary Hitchcock Memorial Hospital, Lebanon

PROSTATECTOMY
None

PULMONARY

CHRONIC OBSTRUCTIVE PULMONARY DISEASE (COPD)
None

PNEUMONIA
Androscoggin Valley Hospital, Berlin
Mary Hitchcock Memorial Hospital, Lebanon
Weeks Medical Center, Lancaster

STROKE
Mary Hitchcock Memorial Hospital, Lebanon

VASCULAR

CAROTID SURGERY
Catholic Medical Center, Manchester

PERIPHERAL VASCULAR BYPASS
None

RESECTION/REPLACEMENT OF ABDOMINAL AORTA
None

WOMEN'S HEALTH
None

BARIATRIC SURGERY

Chilton Memorial Hospital, Pompton Plains
Hackensack University Medical Center, Hackensack
Morristown Memorial Hospital, Morristown
St. Barnabas Medical Center, Livingston
Somerset Medical Center, Somerville
South Jersey Healthcare Regional Medical Center, Vineland
UMDNJ-University Hospital, Newark

CARDIAC

ATRIAL FIBRILLATION
None

CORONARY INTERVENTIONAL PROCEDURES (ANGIOPLASTY/STENT)
Muhlenberg Regional Medical Center, Plainfield
St. Barnabas Medical Center, Livingston
Mountainside Hospital, Montclair

HEART ATTACK
Hackensack University Medical Center, Hackensack
St. Barnabas Medical Center, Livingston
Virtua Memorial Hospital—Burlington County, Mount Holly
Warren Hospital, Phillipsburg

HEART BYPASS SURGERY
Deborah Heart and Lung Center, Browns Mills
Hackensack University Medical Center, Hackensack
Jersey Shore University Medical Center, Neptune

HEART FAILURE

Clara Maass Medical Center, Belleville
Hackensack University Medical Center, Hackensack
Jersey Shore University Medical Center, Neptune
Monmouth Medical Center, Long Branch
Ocean Medical Center, Brick
Riverview Medical Center, Red Bank
Robert Wood Johnson University Hospital at
    Hamilton, Hamilton
St. Francis Medical Center, Trenton
Somerset Medical Center, Somerville
UMDNJ-University Hospital, Newark

VALVE REPLACEMENT SURGERY

Atlanticare Regional Medical Center, Atlantic City
Hackensack University Medical Center, Hackensack
St. Barnabas Medical Center, Livingston

CRITICAL CARE

DIABETIC ACIDOSIS AND COMA

St. Joseph's Wayne Hospital, Wayne

PULMONARY EMBOLISM

Community Medical Center, Toms River
Kimball Medical Center, Lakewood
Mountainside Hospital, Montclair
Underwood Memorial Hospital, Woodbury

RESPIRATORY FAILURE

Bayshore Community Hospital, Holmdel
Cape Regional Medical Center, Cape May Court
    House
Community Medical Center, Toms River
Hackensack University Medical Center,
    Hackensack
Robert Wood Johnson University Hospital at
    Hamilton, Hamilton

SEPSIS

Bayonne Hospital, Bayonne
Clara Maass Medical Center, Belleville
Hunterdon Medical Center, Flemington
JFK Medical Center, Edison
Monmouth Medical Center, Long Branch
Raritan Bay Medical Center, Perth Amboy
Robert Wood Johnson University Hospital at
    Hamilton, Hamilton
Warren Hospital, Phillipsburg

GASTROINTESTINAL

BOWEL OBSTRUCTION

Clara Maass Medical Center, Belleville
Southern Ocean County Hospital, Manahawkin

CHOLECYSTECTOMY

Hackensack University Medical Center, Hackensack
Memorial Hospital of Salem County, Salem
Robert Wood Johnson University Hospital at
    Hamilton, Hamilton

GASTROINTESTINAL BLEED

Centrastate Medical Center, Freehold
Robert Wood Johnson University Hospital at
    Hamilton, Hamilton
Somerset Medical Center, Somerville
Warren Hospital, Phillipsburg

GASTROINTESTINAL SURGERIES AND PROCEDURES

Centrastate Medical Center, Freehold
Clara Maass Medical Center, Belleville
Monmouth Medical Center, Long Branch
Raritan Bay Medical Center, Perth Amboy
Valley Hospital, Ridgewood
Warren Hospital, Phillipsburg

PANCREATITIS

Jersey Shore University Medical Center, Neptune
JFK Medical Center, Edison
Somerset Medical Center, Somerville
Southern Ocean County Hospital, Manahawkin

GENERAL SURGERY

APPENDECTOMY

Hackensack University Medical Center, Hackensack
Hunterdon Medical Center, Flemington
Monmouth Medical Center, Long Branch
Palisades Medical Center, North Bergen
Raritan Bay Medical Center, Perth Amboy
Robert Wood Johnson University Hospital at
    Hamilton, Hamilton
St. Joseph's Hospital and Medical Center, Paterson
Southern Ocean County Hospital, Manahawkin
University Medical Center at Princeton, Princeton

MATERNITY CARE

Centrastate Medical Center, Freehold
Christ Hospital, Jersey City
Columbus Hospital, Newark
Community Medical Center, Toms River
Englewood Hospital and Medical Center,
    Englewood
Hackettstown Community Hospital, Hackettstown
Holy Name Hospital, Teaneck
Kimball Medical Center, Lakewood
Meadowlands Hospital, Secaucus

Morristown Memorial Hospital, Morristown
Newark Beth Israel Medical Center, Newark
Palisades Medical Center, North Bergen
Riverside Hospital, Boonton
Riverview Medical Center, Red Bank
St. Barnabas Medical Center, Livingston
St. Clare's Hospital/Denville, Denville
St. James Hospital, Newark
St. Mary's Hospital, Passaic
University Medical Center at Princeton, Princeton
Valley Hospital, Ridgewood

ORTHOPEDICS

BACK AND NECK SURGERY (EXCEPT SPINAL FUSION)

Community Medical Center, Toms River
Hackensack University Medical Center,
    Hackensack
Somerset Medical Center, Somerville

BACK AND NECK SURGERY (SPINAL FUSION)

Morristown Memorial Hospital, Morristown

HIP FRACTURE REPAIR

Atlanticare Regional Medical Center, Atlantic City
Clara Maass Medical Center, Belleville
Community Medical Center, Toms River
Hackensack University Medical Center, Hackensack
Hunterdon Medical Center, Flemington
Kimball Medical Center, Lakewood
Morristown Memorial Hospital, Morristown
St. Joseph's Hospital and Medical Center, Paterson
Somerset Medical Center, Somerville

TOTAL HIP REPLACEMENT

Atlanticare Regional Medical Center, Atlantic City
Hackensack University Medical Center,
    Hackensack
Valley Hospital, Ridgewood

TOTAL KNEE REPLACEMENT

Clara Maass Medical Center, Belleville
Hoboken University Medical Center, Hoboken
St. Peter's University Hospital, New Brunswick
University Medical Center at Princeton, Princeton

PROSTATECTOMY

Hackensack University Medical Center,
    Hackensack
Newton Memorial Hospital, Newton
St. Mary's Hospital, Passaic
St. Peter's University Hospital, New Brunswick
Somerset Medical Center, Somerville

Hospitals receiving a five star rating in a particular procedure have patient outcomes that put them among the best in the nation. For full definitions of ratings and awards, see Appendix.

PULMONARY

CHRONIC OBSTRUCTIVE PULMONARY DISEASE (COPD)
Centrastate Medical Center, Freehold
Kimball Medical Center, Lakewood
Robert Wood Johnson University Hospital at Hamilton, Hamilton
Mountainside Hospital, Montclair

PNEUMONIA
Bayshore Community Hospital, Holmdel
Clara Maass Medical Center, Belleville
Community Medical Center, Toms River
Hunterdon Medical Center, Flemington
Kimball Medical Center, Lakewood
Memorial Hospital of Salem County, Salem
Monmouth Medical Center, Long Branch
Riverview Medical Center, Red Bank
Robert Wood Johnson University Hospital at Hamilton, Hamilton
St. Francis Medical Center, Trenton

STROKE
Capital Health System—Fuld Campus, Trenton
Centrastate Medical Center, Freehold
Chilton Memorial Hospital, Pompton Plains
Hackensack University Medical Center, Hackensack
JFK Medical Center, Edison
Monmouth Medical Center, Long Branch
Mountainside Hospital, Montclair
Muhlenberg Regional Medical Center, Plainfield
Robert Wood Johnson University Hospital at Hamilton, Hamilton
Robert Wood Johnson University Hospital—Rahway, Rahway
St. Francis Medical Center, Trenton
St. Mary's Hospital, Passaic

VASCULAR

CAROTID SURGERY
Kennedy Memorial Hospitals—Stratford, Stratford
Our Lady of Lourdes Medical Center, Camden

South Jersey Healthcare Regional Medical Center, Vineland
Underwood Memorial Hospital, Woodbury
Virtua West Jersey Hospital—Berlin, Berlin
Virtua West Jersey Hospital—Marlton, Marlton
Warren Hospital, Phillipsburg

PERIPHERAL VASCULAR BYPASS
Atlanticare Regional Medical Center, Atlantic City

RESECTION/REPLACEMENT OF ABDOMINAL AORTA
None

WOMEN'S HEALTH
Hackensack University Medical Center, Hackensack
Newark Beth Israel Medical Center, Newark
St. Barnabas Medical Center, Livingston
Valley Hospital, Ridgewood

NEW MEXICO HOSPITALS: FIVE STAR RATED FACILITIES

BARIATRIC SURGERY
None

CARDIAC

ATRIAL FIBRILLATION
Heart Hospital of New Mexico, Albuquerque

CORONARY INTERVENTIONAL PROCEDURES (ANGIOPLASTY/STENT)
St. Vincent Hospital, Santa Fe

HEART ATTACK
Carlsbad Medical Center, Carlsbad
Lovelace Medical Center—Gibson, Albuquerque
Mimbres Memorial Hospital, Deming

HEART BYPASS SURGERY
Mountainview Regional Medical Center, Las Cruces

HEART FAILURE
Española Hospital, Española

VALVE REPLACEMENT SURGERY
None

CRITICAL CARE

DIABETIC ACIDOSIS AND COMA
None

PULMONARY EMBOLISM
None

RESPIRATORY FAILURE
Lea Regional Hospital, Hobbs
Lovelace Medical Center—Downtown, Albuquerque
Lovelace Westside Hospital, Albuquerque
Lovelace Women's Hospital, Albuquerque

SEPSIS
Lea Regional Hospital, Hobbs
Miners' Colfax Medical Center, Raton

GASTROINTESTINAL

BOWEL OBSTRUCTION
None

CHOLECYSTECTOMY
Mimbres Memorial Hospital, Deming
Mountainview Regional Medical Center, Las Cruces

GASTROINTESTINAL BLEED
None

GASTROINTESTINAL SURGERIES AND PROCEDURES
Mountainview Regional Medical Center, Las Cruces

PANCREATITIS
None

GENERAL SURGERY

APPENDECTOMY
None

MATERNITY CARE
None

ORTHOPEDICS

BACK AND NECK SURGERY (EXCEPT SPINAL FUSION)
None

BACK AND NECK SURGERY (SPINAL FUSION)
None

HIP FRACTURE REPAIR
None

TOTAL HIP REPLACEMENT
Presbyterian Hospital, Albuquerque

TOTAL KNEE REPLACEMENT
Plains Regional Medical Center—Clovis, Clovis
Presbyterian Hospital, Albuquerque

PROSTATECTOMY

Lovelace Medical Center—Downtown, Albuquerque

PULMONARY

CHRONIC OBSTRUCTIVE PULMONARY DISEASE (COPD)

None

PNEUMONIA

Carlsbad Medical Center, Carlsbad
Lea Regional Hospital, Hobbs
Lovelace Women's Hospital, Albuquerque

STROKE

None

VASCULAR

CAROTID SURGERY

None

PERIPHERAL VASCULAR BYPASS

Mountainview Regional Medical Center, Las Cruces

RESECTION/REPLACEMENT OF ABDOMINAL AORTA

None

WOMEN'S HEALTH

None

NEW YORK HOSPITALS: FIVE STAR RATED FACILITIES

BARIATRIC SURGERY

Arnot Ogden Medical Center, Elmira
Bon Secours Community Hospital, Port Jervis
Brookdale Hospital Medical Center, Brooklyn
Children's Hospital Rehab Center, Utica
Faxton-Childrens Hospital, Utica
Faxton-St. Luke's Healthcare, Utica
Highland Hospital, Rochester
Lawrence Hospital Center, Bronxville
Mercy Medical Center, Rockville Centre
Mohawk Valley General Hospital, Ilion
New York University Medical Center—Tisch Hospital, New York
St. Catherine of Siena Hospital, Smithtown
St. Luke's Roosevelt Hospital, New York
Sisters of Charity Hospital, Buffalo
Southside Hospital, Bay Shore
Victory Memorial Hospital, Brooklyn
Westchester Medical Center, Valhalla

CARDIAC

ATRIAL FIBRILLATION

Rochester General Hospital, Rochester

CORONARY INTERVENTIONAL PROCEDURES (ANGIOPLASTY/STENT)

Champlain Valley Physicians Hospital Medical Center, Plattsburgh
Ellis Hospital, Schenectady
Lenox Hill Hospital, New York
Long Island Jewish Medical Center, New Hyde Park
Maimonides Medical Center, Brooklyn
Montefiore Medical Center, Bronx
Mount Sinai Hospital, New York
North Shore University Hospital Syosset, Syosset
North Shore University Hospital, Manhasset

Rochester General Hospital, Rochester
St. Joseph's Hospital Health Center, Syracuse
Staten Island University Hospital, Staten Island
United Health Services Hospitals, Binghamton
Westchester Medical Center, Valhalla

HEART ATTACK

Cayuga Medical Center at Ithaca, Ithaca
F. F. Thompson Hospital, Canandaigua
Northern Westchester Hospital, Mount Kisco
St. Clare's Hospital, Schenectady
St. Luke's Cornwall Hospital, Cornwall
Saratoga Hospital, Saratoga Springs
Unity Hospital, Rochester
Unity St. Mary's Campus, Rochester

HEART BYPASS SURGERY

Buffalo General Hospital—Kaleida Health, Buffalo
Degraff Memorial Hospital, North Tonawanda
Millard Fillmore Hospital, Buffalo
St. Joseph's Hospital Health Center, Syracuse
Stony Brook University Medical Center, Stony Brook
Vassar Brothers Medical Center, Poughkeepsie
Winthrop-University Hospital, Mineola

HEART FAILURE

Lenox Hill Hospital, New York
Maimonides Medical Center, Brooklyn
St. Luke's Cornwall Hospital, Cornwall
Saratoga Hospital, Saratoga Springs

VALVE REPLACEMENT SURGERY

Albany Medical CenterHospital, Albany
New York Presbyterian—Columbia, New York
New York-Presbyterian/Weill Cornell, New York
North Shore University Hospital Syosset, Syosset
North Shore University Hospital, Manhasset
St. Joseph's Hospital Health Center, Syracuse
Vassar Brothers Medical Center, Poughkeepsie

CRITICAL CARE

DIABETIC ACIDOSIS AND COMA

Maimonides Medical Center, Brooklyn
University Hospital SUNY Upstate Medical University, Syracuse

PULMONARY EMBOLISM

Mercy Hospital, Buffalo
Sound Shore Medical Center of Westchester, New Rochelle

RESPIRATORY FAILURE

Horton Memorial Hospital, Middletown
Maimonides Medical Center, Brooklyn
Mercy Hospital, Buffalo
Orange Regional Medical Center, Goshen
St. James Mercy Hospital, Hornell
St. Vincent's Hospital—Manhattan, New York

SEPSIS

Claxton-Hepburn Medical Center, Ogdensburg
Corning Hospital, Corning
Horton Memorial Hospital, Middletown
Mercy Hospital, Buffalo
Mount St. Mary's Hospital and Health Center, Lewiston
Nyack Hospital, Nyack
Orange Regional Medical Center, Goshen
St. Francis Hospital, Poughkeepsie
St. Luke's Cornwall Hospital, Cornwall
Wyckoff Heights Medical Center, Brooklyn

GASTROINTESTINAL

BOWEL OBSTRUCTION

Glens Falls Hospital, Glens Falls
St. James Mercy Hospital, Hornell

NEW MEXICO / NEW YORK HOSPITALS: FIVE STAR RATED FACILITIES

Hospitals receiving a five star rating in a particular procedure have patient outcomes that put them among the best in the nation. For full definitions of ratings and awards, see Appendix.

CHOLECYSTECTOMY

Champlain Valley Physicians Hospital Medical
  Center, Plattsburgh
Claxton-Hepburn Medical Center, Ogdensburg
Jacobi Medical Center, Bronx
John T. Mather Memorial Hospital of Port
  Jefferson, Port Jefferson
Kingsbrook Jewish Medical Center, Brooklyn
Lincoln Medical and Mental Health Center, Bronx
Mary Immaculate Hospital, Jamaica
New York Downtown Hospital, New York
Osteopathic Hospital Clinic of New York, Flushing
Parkway Hospital, Forest Hills
St. Francis Hospital—Roslyn, Roslyn
Victory Memorial Hospital, Brooklyn

GASTROINTESTINAL BLEED

St. Peter's Hospital, Albany

GASTROINTESTINAL SURGERIES AND PROCEDURES

Mount Sinai Hospital, New York

PANCREATITIS

None

GENERAL SURGERY

APPENDECTOMY

Bellevue Hospital Center, New York
Bronx-Lebanon Hospital Center, Bronx
Champlain Valley Physicians Hospital Medical
  Center, Plattsburgh
City Hospital Center at Elmhurst, Elmhurst
Coney Island Hospital, Brooklyn
Cortland Regional Medical Center, Cortland
Good Samaritan Hospital of Suffern, Suffern
John T. Mather Memorial Hospital of
  Port Jefferson, Port Jefferson
Long Island College Hospital, Brooklyn
Mary Immaculate Hospital, Jamaica
Mercy Medical Center, Rockville Centre
Mount St. Mary's Hospital and Health Center, Lewiston
New York Downtown Hospital, New York
New York Westchester Square Medical Center, Bronx
North Shore University Hospital Syosset, Syosset
North Shore University Hospital, Manhasset
Osteopathic Hospital Clinic of New York, Flushing
Peconic Bay Medical Center, Riverhead
Phelps Memorial Hospital Association,
  Sleepy Hollow
St. Catherine of Siena Hospital, Smithtown
St. Joseph Hospital of Cheektowaga New York,
  Cheektowaga

St. Luke's Cornwall Hospital, Cornwall
Southside Hospital, Bay Shore
Staten Island University Hospital, Staten Island
Woodhull Medical and Mental Health Center,
  Brooklyn
Wyckoff Heights Medical Center, Brooklyn
Wyoming County Community Hospital, Warsaw

MATERNITY CARE

Bayley Seton Hospital, Staten Island
Beth Israel Medical Center, New York
Bronx-Lebanon Hospital Center, Bronx
Cayuga Medical Center at Ithaca, Ithaca
Children's Hospital Rehab Center, Utica
Faxton-Childrens Hospital, Utica
Faxton-St. Luke's Healthcare, Utica
Flushing Hospital Medical Center, Flushing
Forest Hills Hospital, Forest Hills
Glens Falls Hospital, Glens Falls
Good Samaritan Hospital of Suffern, Suffern
Kings Highway Hospital, Brooklyn
Lenox Hill Hospital, New York
Maimonides Medical Center, Brooklyn
Mary Immaculate Hospital, Jamaica
Mercy Medical Center, Rockville Centre
Mohawk Valley General Hospital, Ilion
New York Downtown Hospital, New York
New York Hospital Medical Center of Queens,
  Flushing
Northern Dutchess Hospital, Rhinebeck
Nyack Hospital, Nyack
Osteopathic Hospital Clinic of New York, Flushing
Our Lady of Mercy Medical Center, Bronx
Plainview Hospital, Plainview
St. Catherine of Siena Hospital, Smithtown
St. Charles Hospital, Port Jefferson
St. John's Episcopal Hospital at South Shore,
  Far Rockaway
St. John's Riverside Hospital, Yonkers
St. Luke's Cornwall Hospital, Cornwall
St. Mary's Hospital, Amsterdam
St. Vincent's Hospital—Manhattan, New York
Sound Shore Medical Center of Westchester,
  New Rochelle
South Nassau Communities Hospital, Oceanside
Southampton Hospital, Southampton
Southside Hospital, Bay Shore
SVCMC—St. Vincent's Hospital Staten Island,
  Staten Island
White Plains Hospital Center, White Plains
Winthrop-University Hospital, Mineola
Yonkers General Hospital, Yonkers

ORTHOPEDICS

BACK AND NECK SURGERY (EXCEPT SPINAL FUSION)

Beth Israel Medical Center, New York
Community-General Hospital of Greater Syracuse,
  Syracuse
Ellis Hospital, Schenectady
Horton Memorial Hospital, Middletown
Kings Highway Hospital, Brooklyn
New York Presbyterian—Columbia, New York
New York-Presbyterian/Weill Cornell, New York
North Shore University Hospital Syosset, Syosset
North Shore University Hospital, Manhasset
Orange Regional Medical Center, Goshen
St. Luke's Cornwall Hospital, Cornwall
Strong Memorial Hospital, Rochester

BACK AND NECK SURGERY (SPINAL FUSION)

Beth Israel Medical Center, New York
Community-General Hospital of Greater Syracuse,
  Syracuse
Crouse Hospital, Syracuse
Ellis Hospital, Schenectady
Erie County Medical Center, Buffalo
Good Samaritan Hospital Medical Center, West Islip
Highland Hospital, Rochester
Hospital for Joint Diseases Orthopaedic Institute,
  New York
Kings Highway Hospital, Brooklyn
Lutheran Medical Center, Brooklyn
Maimonides Medical Center, Brooklyn
Mercy Medical Center, Rockville Centre
St. Joseph's Hospital Health Center, Syracuse
St. Luke's Roosevelt Hospital, New York
St. Peter's Hospital, Albany
Strong Memorial Hospital, Rochester

HIP FRACTURE REPAIR

Arnot Ogden Medical Center, Elmira
Auburn Memorial Hospital, Auburn
Beth Israel Medical Center, New York
Community-General Hospital of Greater Syracuse,
  Syracuse
Ellis Hospital, Schenectady
Kings Highway Hospital, Brooklyn
Kingston Hospital, Kingston
Leonard Hospital, Troy
Mercy Medical Center, Rockville Centre
New York Community Hospital of Brooklyn,
  Brooklyn
New York Westchester Square Medical Center,
  Bronx
North Shore University Hospital Syosset, Syosset

North Shore University Hospital, Manhasset
Oneida Healthcare Center, Oneida
St. Joseph's Hospital, Elmira
Seton Health System—St. Mary's Campus, Troy
Victory Memorial Hospital, Brooklyn

TOTAL HIP REPLACEMENT

Albany Medical CenterHospital, Albany
Arnot Ogden Medical Center, Elmira
Cayuga Medical Center at Ithaca, Ithaca
Claxton-Hepburn Medical Center, Ogdensburg
Community Memorial Hospital, Hamilton
Community-General Hospital of Greater Syracuse,
    Syracuse
Good Samaritan Hospital of Suffern, Suffern
Hospital for Special Surgery, New York
Kenmore Mercy Hospital, Kenmore
Leonard Hospital, Troy
Samaritan Medical Center, Watertown
Seton Health System—St. Mary's Campus, Troy

TOTAL KNEE REPLACEMENT

Albany Medical CenterHospital, Albany
Arnot Ogden Medical Center, Elmira
Auburn Memorial Hospital, Auburn
Beth Israel Medical Center, New York
Cayuga Medical Center at Ithaca, Ithaca
Community Memorial Hospital, Hamilton
Community-General Hospital of Greater Syracuse,
    Syracuse
Crouse Hospital, Syracuse
Ellis Hospital, Schenectady
Hospital for Special Surgery, New York
Kenmore Mercy Hospital, Kenmore
Kings Highway Hospital, Brooklyn
Kingsbrook Jewish Medical Center, Brooklyn
Mercy Medical Center, Rockville Centre
New York Hospital Medical Center of Queens,
    Flushing
Newark-Wayne Community Hospital, Newark
Northern Dutchess Hospital, Rhinebeck
St. Francis Hospital, Poughkeepsie

St. Joseph's Hospital Health Center, Syracuse
St. Luke's Cornwall Hospital, Cornwall
St. Peter's Hospital, Albany
Woman's Christian Association, Jamestown

PROSTATECTOMY

Auburn Memorial Hospital, Auburn
Clifton Springs Hospital and Clinic, Clifton Springs
Community-General Hospital of Greater Syracuse,
    Syracuse
Good Samaritan Hospital Medical Center,
    West Islip
Leonard Hospital, Troy
Mercy Medical Center, Rockville Centre
New York Community Hospital of Brooklyn,
    Brooklyn
Our Lady of Lourdes Memorial Hospital,
    Binghamton
Phelps Memorial Hospital Association,
    Sleepy Hollow
Rochester General Hospital, Rochester
St. Luke's Cornwall Hospital, Cornwall
Samaritan Medical Center, Watertown
Seton Health System—St. Mary's Campus, Troy
Strong Memorial Hospital, Rochester
Woman's Christian Association, Jamestown

PULMONARY

CHRONIC OBSTRUCTIVE PULMONARY DISEASE (COPD)

Jacobi Medical Center, Bronx
New York Presbyterian—Columbia, New York
New York-Presbyterian/Weill Cornell, New York
Our Lady of Lourdes Memorial Hospital, Binghamton
St. Clare's Hospital, Schenectady
St. James Mercy Hospital, Hornell

PNEUMONIA

Brooklyn Hospital Center at Downtown Campus,
    Brooklyn
Delaware Valley Hospital, Walton

Ellis Hospital, Schenectady
John T. Mather Memorial Hospital of Port
    Jefferson, Port Jefferson
Maimonides Medical Center, Brooklyn
St. Clare's Hospital, Schenectady
St. Luke's Cornwall Hospital, Cornwall
Sound Shore Medical Center of Westchester,
    New Rochelle
Unity Hospital, Rochester
Unity St. Mary's Campus, Rochester
Wyckoff Heights Medical Center, Brooklyn

STROKE

New York Methodist Hospital, Brooklyn
St. Anthony Community Hospital, Warwick
St. Francis Hospital—Roslyn, Roslyn
St. Vincent's Hospital—Manhattan, New York
Unity Hospital, Rochester
Unity St. Mary's Campus, Rochester

VASCULAR

CAROTID SURGERY

Mercy Medical Center, Rockville Centre
North Shore University Hospital Syosset, Syosset
North Shore University Hospital, Manhasset
St. Francis Hospital, Poughkeepsie
St. Francis Hospital—Roslyn, Roslyn
St. Luke's Cornwall Hospital, Cornwall
St. Peter's Hospital, Albany

PERIPHERAL VASCULAR BYPASS

Good Samaritan Hospital Medical Center, West Islip

RESECTION/REPLACEMENT OF ABDOMINAL AORTA

Good Samaritan Hospital Medical Center, West Islip

WOMEN'S HEALTH

Maimonides Medical Center, Brooklyn

NORTH CAROLINA HOSPITALS: FIVE STAR RATED FACILITIES

BARIATRIC SURGERY

Cape Fear Hospital, Wilmington
Cape Fear Valley Medical Center, Fayetteville
Carolinas Medical Center—NorthEast, Concord
Franklin Regional Medical Center, Louisburg
New Hanover Regional Medical Center, Wilmington
North Carolina Baptist Hospital, Winston-Salem
Presbyterian Hospital, Charlotte

CARDIAC

ATRIAL FIBRILLATION

Carolinas Medical Center—Union, Monroe
Haywood Regional Medical Center, Clyde
Lake Norman Regional Medical Center, Mooresville
University of North Carolina Hospital, Chapel Hill

CORONARY INTERVENTIONAL PROCEDURES (ANGIOPLASTY/STENT)

None

HEART ATTACK

Carolinas Medical Center—Union, Monroe
Lenoir Memorial Hospital, Kinston
Nash General Hospital, Rocky Mount
Randolph Hospital, Asheboro

Hospitals receiving a five star rating in a particular procedure have patient outcomes that put them among the best in the nation. For full definitions of ratings and awards, see Appendix.

Rex Hospital, Raleigh
Stanly Memorial Hospital, Albemarle

HEART BYPASS SURGERY
None

HEART FAILURE
Carolinas Medical Center–Union, Monroe
Franklin Regional Medical Center, Louisburg
Haywood Regional Medical Center, Clyde
Hugh Chatham Memorial Hospital, Elkin
Martin General Hospital, Williamston
Presbyterian Hospital Matthews, Matthews
Randolph Hospital, Asheboro
Roanoke Chowan Hospital, Ahoskie

VALVE REPLACEMENT SURGERY
Carolinas Medical Center–NorthEast, Concord
Duke University Hospital, Durham
Gaston Memorial Hospital, Gastonia

CRITICAL CARE

DIABETIC ACIDOSIS AND COMA
Cape Fear Valley Medical Center, Fayetteville

PULMONARY EMBOLISM
Mission Hospitals–Memorial Campus, Asheville
Presbyterian Hospital, Charlotte
Rex Hospital, Raleigh
Roanoke Chowan Hospital, Ahoskie
Rutherford Hospital, Rutherfordton
St. Joseph's Hospital, Asheville

RESPIRATORY FAILURE
Ashe Memorial Hospital, Jefferson
Cape Fear Valley Medical Center, Fayetteville
Carolinas Medical Center–Lincoln, Lincolnton
Carolinas Medical Center–Union, Monroe
Gaston Memorial Hospital, Gastonia
Harris Regional Hospital, Sylva
Haywood Regional Medical Center, Clyde
Hugh Chatham Memorial Hospital, Elkin
Murphy Medical Center, Murphy
Northern Hospital of Surry County, Mount Airy
Randolph Hospital, Asheboro
Rutherford Hospital, Rutherfordton
Stanly Memorial Hospital, Albemarle

SEPSIS
Anson Community Hospital, Wadesboro
Cape Fear Valley Medical Center, Fayetteville
Carolinas Medical Center–Union, Monroe
Gaston Memorial Hospital, Gastonia
Harris Regional Hospital, Sylva
Haywood Regional Medical Center, Clyde

Hugh Chatham Memorial Hospital, Elkin
Park Ridge Hospital, Fletcher
Randolph Hospital, Asheboro
Rex Hospital, Raleigh
Stanly Memorial Hospital, Albemarle

GASTROINTESTINAL

BOWEL OBSTRUCTION
Haywood Regional Medical Center, Clyde
Mission Hospitals–Memorial Campus, Asheville
Rex Hospital, Raleigh
St. Joseph's Hospital, Asheville

CHOLECYSTECTOMY
Albemarle Hospital Authority, Elizabeth City
Annie Penn Memorial Hospital, Reidsville
Carteret General Hospital, Morehead City
Duke Health Raleigh Hospital, Raleigh
FirstHealth Moore Regional Hospital, Pinehurst
Halifax Regional Medical Center, Roanoke Rapids
Hugh Chatham Memorial Hospital, Elkin
Moses H. Cone Memorial Hospital, Greensboro
Northern Hospital of Surry County, Mount Airy
Presbyterian Hospital Matthews, Matthews
Wesley Long Community Hospital, Greensboro

GASTROINTESTINAL BLEED
Brunswick Community Hospital, Supply
Haywood Regional Medical Center, Clyde
Mission Hospitals–Memorial Campus, Asheville
St. Joseph's Hospital, Asheville

GASTROINTESTINAL SURGERIES AND PROCEDURES
Gaston Memorial Hospital, Gastonia
Haywood Regional Medical Center, Clyde
Mission Hospitals–Memorial Campus, Asheville
Rex Hospital, Raleigh
St. Joseph's Hospital, Asheville

PANCREATITIS
Margaret R. Pardee Memorial Hospital, Hendersonville

GENERAL SURGERY

APPENDECTOMY
Annie Penn Memorial Hospital, Reidsville
Carolinas Medical Center–Union, Monroe
Carteret General Hospital, Morehead City
Chowan Hospital, Edenton
Duke Health Raleigh Hospital, Raleigh
FirstHealth Moore Regional Hospital, Pinehurst
Grace Hospital, Morganton

Granville Medical Center, Oxford
Halifax Regional Medical Center, Roanoke Rapids
Lenoir Memorial Hospital, Kinston
Moses H. Cone Memorial Hospital, Greensboro
Wesley Long Community Hospital, Greensboro

MATERNITY CARE

Carolinas Medical Center–Union, Monroe
Cleveland Regional Medical Center, Shelby
Durham Regional Hospital, Durham
Grace Hospital, Morganton
Heritage Hospital, Tarboro
Lexington Memorial Hospital, Lexington
Onslow Memorial Hospital, Jacksonville
Wakemed Cary Hospital, Cary

ORTHOPEDICS

BACK AND NECK SURGERY (EXCEPT SPINAL FUSION)
Catawba Valley Medical Center, Hickory
Forsyth Memorial Hospital, Winston-Salem
Gaston Memorial Hospital, Gastonia
Mission Hospitals–Memorial Campus, Asheville
Nash General Hospital, Rocky Mount
St. Joseph's Hospital, Asheville

BACK AND NECK SURGERY (SPINAL FUSION)
Annie Penn Memorial Hospital, Reidsville
Davis Regional Medical Center, Statesville
Forsyth Memorial Hospital, Winston-Salem
Gaston Memorial Hospital, Gastonia
Moses H. Cone Memorial Hospital, Greensboro
North Carolina Baptist Hospital, Winston-Salem
Wesley Long Community Hospital, Greensboro

HIP FRACTURE REPAIR
Alamance Regional Medical Center, Burlington
Albemarle Hospital Authority, Elizabeth City
Angel Medical Center, Franklin
Cape Fear Hospital, Wilmington
FirstHealth Moore Regional Hospital, Pinehurst
Forsyth Memorial Hospital, Winston-Salem
Halifax Regional Medical Center, Roanoke Rapids
Hugh Chatham Memorial Hospital, Elkin
Lenoir Memorial Hospital, Kinston
New Hanover Regional Medical Center, Wilmington
Presbyterian Orthopaedic Hospital, Charlotte
Southeastern Regional Medical Center, Lumberton

TOTAL HIP REPLACEMENT
Annie Penn Memorial Hospital, Reidsville
Brunswick Community Hospital, Supply
FirstHealth Moore Regional Hospital, Pinehurst

Forsyth Memorial Hospital, Winston-Salem
Margaret R. Pardee Memorial Hospital,
   Hendersonville
Moses H. Cone Memorial Hospital, Greensboro
Presbyterian Orthopaedic Hospital, Charlotte
Wesley Long Community Hospital, Greensboro
Wilson Medical Center, Wilson

TOTAL KNEE REPLACEMENT

Alamance Regional Medical Center, Burlington
Cape Fear Hospital, Wilmington
Chowan Hospital, Edenton
FirstHealth Moore Regional Hospital, Pinehurst
Forsyth Memorial Hospital, Winston-Salem
Margaret R. Pardee Memorial Hospital,
   Hendersonville
Mission Hospitals—Memorial Campus, Asheville
North Carolina Baptist Hospital, Winston-Salem
Nash General Hospital, Rocky Mount
New Hanover Regional Medical Center, Wilmington
Presbyterian Orthopaedic Hospital, Charlotte
Rowan Regional Medical Center, Salisbury
St. Joseph's Hospital, Asheville

PROSTATECTOMY

Annie Penn Memorial Hospital, Reidsville
Carolinas Medical Center—University, Charlotte

Moses H. Cone Memorial Hospital, Greensboro
Presbyterian Hospital, Charlotte
Wesley Long Community Hospital, Greensboro

PULMONARY

CHRONIC OBSTRUCTIVE PULMONARY DISEASE (COPD)

Alamance Regional Medical Center, Burlington
Carolinas Medical Center—Union, Monroe
Davis Regional Medical Center, Statesville
Mission Hospitals—Memorial Campus, Asheville
North Carolina Baptist Hospital, Winston-Salem
Pender Memorial Hospital, Burgaw
Randolph Hospital, Asheboro
Rutherford Hospital, Rutherfordton
St. Joseph's Hospital, Asheville

PNEUMONIA

Anson Community Hospital, Wadesboro
Cape Fear Valley Medical Center, Fayetteville
Carolinas Medical Center—Union, Monroe
Margaret R. Pardee Memorial Hospital,
   Hendersonville
Mission Hospitals—Memorial Campus, Asheville
North Carolina Baptist Hospital, Winston-Salem
Northern Hospital of Surry County, Mount Airy
Randolph Hospital, Asheboro

St. Joseph's Hospital, Asheville
University of North Carolina Hospital, Chapel Hill

STROKE

Angel Medical Center, Franklin
Duke University Hospital, Durham

VASCULAR

CAROTID SURGERY

FirstHealth Moore Regional Hospital, Pinehurst
North Carolina Baptist Hospital, Winston-Salem

PERIPHERAL VASCULAR BYPASS

Cape Fear Hospital, Wilmington
Cape Fear Valley Medical Center, Fayetteville
New Hanover Regional Medical Center, Wilmington

RESECTION/REPLACEMENT OF ABDOMINAL AORTA

Rex Hospital, Raleigh

WOMEN'S HEALTH

None

NORTH DAKOTA HOSPITALS: FIVE STAR RATED FACILITIES

BARIATRIC SURGERY

None

CARDIAC

ATRIAL FIBRILLATION
None

CORONARY INTERVENTIONAL PROCEDURES (ANGIOPLASTY/STENT)
St. Alexius Medical Center, Bismarck

HEART ATTACK
Altru Hospital, Grand Forks
St. Alexius Medical Center, Bismarck

HEART BYPASS SURGERY
Meritcare Health System, Fargo
St. Alexius Medical Center, Bismarck

HEART FAILURE
Medcenter One, Bismarck
Mercy Hospital of Valley City, Valley City
Mercy Medical Center, Williston

VALVE REPLACEMENT SURGERY
None

CRITICAL CARE

DIABETIC ACIDOSIS AND COMA
None

PULMONARY EMBOLISM
None

RESPIRATORY FAILURE
Medcenter One, Bismarck

SEPSIS
Altru Hospital, Grand Forks
Innovis Health, Fargo
Meritcare Health System, Fargo

GASTROINTESTINAL

BOWEL OBSTRUCTION
None

CHOLECYSTECTOMY
Altru Hospital, Grand Forks
St. Alexius Medical Center, Bismarck

GASTROINTESTINAL BLEED
None

GASTROINTESTINAL SURGERIES AND PROCEDURES
None

PANCREATITIS
None

GENERAL SURGERY

APPENDECTOMY
None

MATERNITY CARE

None

Hospitals receiving a five star rating in a particular procedure have patient outcomes that put them among the best in the nation. For full definitions of ratings and awards, see Appendix.

ORTHOPEDICS

BACK AND NECK SURGERY
(EXCEPT SPINAL FUSION)
Innovis Health, Fargo
Meritcare Health System, Fargo
St. Alexius Medical Center, Bismarck

BACK AND NECK SURGERY (SPINAL FUSION)
None

HIP FRACTURE REPAIR
Altru Hospital, Grand Forks

TOTAL HIP REPLACEMENT
St. Alexius Medical Center, Bismarck
Trinity Hospitals, Minot
Trinity Medical Center, Minot

TOTAL KNEE REPLACEMENT
Altru Hospital, Grand Forks
Medcenter One, Bismarck

Mercy Medical Center, Williston
St. Alexius Medical Center, Bismarck
Trinity Hospitals, Minot
Trinity Medical Center, Minot

PROSTATECTOMY

Altru Hospital, Grand Forks
Innovis Health, Fargo

PULMONARY

CHRONIC OBSTRUCTIVE PULMONARY DISEASE (COPD)
Innovis Health, Fargo
Medcenter One, Bismarck

PNEUMONIA
Innovis Health, Fargo
Mercy Hospital of Valley City, Valley City
Meritcare Health System, Fargo

St. Alexius Medical Center, Bismarck
St. Luke's Hospital, Crosby
West River Regional Medical Center, Hettinger

STROKE

None

VASCULAR

CAROTID SURGERY
None

PERIPHERAL VASCULAR BYPASS
None

RESECTION/REPLACEMENT OF ABDOMINAL AORTA
Medcenter One, Bismarck

WOMEN'S HEALTH

None

OHIO HOSPITALS: FIVE STAR RATED FACILITIES

BARIATRIC SURGERY

None

CARDIAC

ATRIAL FIBRILLATION
Adena Regional Medical Center, Chillicothe
Fort Hamilton Hughes Memorial Hospital, Hamilton
Kettering Medical Center, Kettering
Marietta Memorial Hospital, Marietta
Marymount Hospital, Garfield Heights
Mercy Healthcare Center, Toledo
Miami Valley Hospital, Dayton
Parma Community General Hospital, Parma
Robinson Memorial Hospital, Ravenna
St. John West Shore Hospital, Westlake
St. Vincent Mercy Medical Center, Toledo

CORONARY INTERVENTIONAL PROCEDURES (ANGIOPLASTY/STENT)
Akron General Medical Center, Akron
Christ Hospital, Cincinnati
Dayton Heart Hospital, Dayton
Fairfield Medical Center, Lancaster
Fairview Hospital, Cleveland
Jewish Hospital, Cincinnati
Lake Hospital System, Painesville
Parma Community General Hospital, Parma
Southwest General Health Center,
    Middleburg Heights

HEART ATTACK
Akron General Medical Center, Akron
Ashtabula County Medical Center, Ashtabula
Bethesda North Hospital, Cincinnati
Christ Hospital, Cincinnati
Cuyahoga Falls General Hospital, Cuyahoga Falls
Dayton Heart Hospital, Dayton
Fairfield Medical Center, Lancaster
Fairview Hospital, Cleveland
Firelands Regional Medical Center—Main Campus,
    Sandusky
Fort Hamilton Hughes Memorial Hospital, Hamilton
Good Samaritan Hospital, Cincinnati
Grandview Medical Center, Dayton
Hillcrest Hospital, Mayfield Heights
Jewish Hospital, Cincinnati
Lake Hospital System, Painesville
Mercy Memorial Hospital, Urbana
Meridia Euclid Hospital, Euclid
Miami Valley Hospital, Dayton
Ohio State University Hospital East, Columbus
Parma Community General Hospital, Parma
Robinson Memorial Hospital, Ravenna
St. Charles Mercy Hospital, Oregon
South Pointe Hospital, Warrensville Heights
Southwest General Health Center,
    Middleburg Heights
Summa Health Systems Hospitals, Akron
Toledo Hospital, Toledo

Trumbull Memorial Hospital, Warren
UHHS Bedford Medical Center, Bedford
Upper Valley Medical Center, Piqua
Upper Valley Medical Center, Troy
Wilson Memorial Hospital, Sidney

HEART BYPASS SURGERY
Aultman Hospital, Canton
Cleveland Clinic, Cleveland
Dayton Heart Hospital, Dayton
EMH Regional Medical Center, Elyria
Fairview Hospital, Cleveland
Hillcrest Hospital, Mayfield Heights
Lake Hospital System, Painesville
Medcentral Health System, Mansfield
St. Elizabeth Health Center, Youngstown
Summa Health Systems Hospitals, Akron

HEART FAILURE
Akron General Medical Center, Akron
Ashtabula County Medical Center, Ashtabula
Barberton Citizens Hospital, Barberton
Berger Hospital, Circleville
Bethesda North Hospital, Cincinnati
Brown County Hospital, Georgetown
Christ Hospital, Cincinnati
Cleveland Clinic, Cleveland
Community Health Partners of Ohio—West, Lorain
Dayton Heart Hospital, Dayton
Deaconess Hospital, Cincinnati

Emh Regional Medical Center, Elyria
Fairview Hospital, Cleveland
Fort Hamilton Hughes Memorial Hospital, Hamilton
Genesis Healthcare System, Zanesville
Good Samaritan Hospital, Cincinnati
Grandview Medical Center, Dayton
Hillcrest Hospital, Mayfield Heights
Huron Hospital, East Cleveland
Jewish Hospital, Cincinnati
Joint Township District Memorial Hospital,
    St. Marys
Kettering Medical Center, Kettering
Kettering Medical Center–Sycamore, Miamisburg
Lake Hospital System, Painesville
Lakewood Hospital, Lakewood
Licking Memorial Hospital, Newark
Lutheran Hospital, Cleveland
Marymount Hospital, Garfield Heights
Mercy Healthcare Center, Toledo
Mercy Hospital–Clermont, Batavia
Mercy Hospital–Western Hills, Cincinnati
Mercy Medical Center of Springfield, Springfield
Mercy Medical Center, Canton
Miami Valley Hospital, Dayton
Ohio State University Hospital East, Columbus
Parma Community General Hospital, Parma
Regency Hospital of Cincinnati, Cincinnati
St. Anne Mercy Hospital, Toledo
St. Charles Mercy Hospital, Oregon
St. John West Shore Hospital, Westlake
St. Vincent Charity Hospital, Cleveland
St. Vincent Mercy Medical Center, Toledo
South Pointe Hospital, Warrensville Heights
Southern Ohio Medical Center, Portsmouth
Southwest General Health Center,
    Middleburg Heights
Summa Health Systems Hospitals, Akron
Toledo Hospital, Toledo
UHHS Bedford Medical Center, Bedford
UHHS Memorial Hospital of Geneva, Geneva
UHHS Richmond Heights Hospital,
    Richmond Heights
University Hospital, Cincinnati
Western Reserve Care System, Youngstown
Wooster Community Hospital, Wooster

VALVE REPLACEMENT SURGERY
Akron General Medical Center, Akron
Aultman Hospital, Canton
Cleveland Clinic, Cleveland
Dayton Heart Hospital, Dayton
Fairview Hospital, Cleveland
Lake Hospital System, Painesville

Medcentral Health System, Mansfield
Parma Community General Hospital, Parma

CRITICAL CARE

DIABETIC ACIDOSIS AND COMA
Akron General Medical Center, Akron
Grandview Medical Center, Dayton
Summa Health Systems Hospitals, Akron

PULMONARY EMBOLISM
Akron General Medical Center, Akron
Bethesda North Hospital, Cincinnati
Christ Hospital, Cincinnati
Deaconess Hospital, Cincinnati
Good Samaritan Hospital, Dayton
Hillcrest Hospital, Mayfield Heights
Jewish Hospital, Cincinnati
Kettering Medical Center, Kettering
Kettering Medical Center–Sycamore, Miamisburg
Middletown Regional Hospital, Middletown
Regency Hospital of Cincinnati, Cincinnati
St. Charles Mercy Hospital, Oregon
Southwest General Health Center,
    Middleburg Heights
Summa Health Systems Hospitals, Akron

RESPIRATORY FAILURE
Adena Regional Medical Center, Chillicothe
Akron General Medical Center, Akron
Aultman Hospital, Canton
Barberton Citizens Hospital, Barberton
Bethesda North Hospital, Cincinnati
Brown County Hospital, Georgetown
Christ Hospital, Cincinnati
Community Health Partners of Ohio–West, Lorain
Deaconess Hospital, Cincinnati
Fairfield Medical Center, Lancaster
Fairview Hospital, Cleveland
Fort Hamilton Hughes Memorial Hospital, Hamilton
Good Samaritan Hospital, Cincinnati
Good Samaritan Hospital, Dayton
Grandview Medical Center, Dayton
Hillcrest Hospital, Mayfield Heights
Huron Hospital, East Cleveland
Jewish Hospital, Cincinnati
Kettering Medical Center, Kettering
Lakewood Hospital, Lakewood
Licking Memorial Hospital, Newark
Marymount Hospital, Garfield Heights
Medina General Hospital, Medina
Mercy Franciscan Hospital–Mount Airy, Cincinnati
Mercy Healthcare Center, Toledo
Mercy Hospital–Anderson, Anderson
Mercy Medical Center, Canton

Meridia Euclid Hospital, Euclid
Miami Valley Hospital, Dayton
Middletown Regional Hospital, Middletown
Ohio State University Hospital East, Columbus
Ohio State University Hospitals, Columbus
Parma Community General Hospital, Parma
Regency Hospital of Cincinnati, Cincinnati
Robinson Memorial Hospital, Ravenna
St. Charles Mercy Hospital, Oregon
St. Joseph Health Center, Warren
St. Vincent Mercy Medical Center, Toledo
South Pointe Hospital, Warrensville Heights
Southern Ohio Medical Center, Portsmouth
Southwest General Health Center,
    Middleburg Heights
Summa Health Systems Hospitals, Akron
Toledo Hospital, Toledo
UHHS Bedford Medical Center, Bedford
UHHS Memorial Hospital of Geneva, Geneva
Wooster Community Hospital, Wooster

SEPSIS
Akron General Medical Center, Akron
Ashtabula County Medical Center, Ashtabula
Aultman Hospital, Canton
Barberton Citizens Hospital, Barberton
Bethesda North Hospital, Cincinnati
Christ Hospital, Cincinnati
Community Health Partners of Ohio–West, Lorain
Community Hospital of Springfield and Clark
    County, Springfield
Deaconess Hospital, Cincinnati
Fort Hamilton Hughes Memorial Hospital, Hamilton
Genesis Healthcare System, Zanesville
Good Samaritan Hospital, Cincinnati
Good Samaritan Hospital, Dayton
Grandview Medical Center, Dayton
Hillcrest Hospital, Mayfield Heights
Jewish Hospital, Cincinnati
Kettering Medical Center, Kettering
Kettering Medical Center–Sycamore, Miamisburg
Lake Hospital System, Painesville
Lakewood Hospital, Lakewood
Licking Memorial Hospital, Newark
Marymount Hospital, Garfield Heights
Mercy Healthcare Center, Toledo
Mercy Hospital–Anderson, Anderson
Mercy Hospital–Fairfield, Fairfield
Mercy Hospital–Western Hills, Cincinnati
Meridia Euclid Hospital, Euclid
Miami Valley Hospital, Dayton
Middletown Regional Hospital, Middletown
Ohio State University Hospital East, Columbus
Ohio State University Hospitals, Columbus

Hospitals receiving a five star rating in a particular procedure have patient outcomes that put them among the best in the nation. For full definitions of ratings and awards, see Appendix.

Parma Community General Hospital, Parma
Regency Hospital of Cincinnati, Cincinnati
Riverside Methodist Hospital, Columbus
Robinson Memorial Hospital, Ravenna
St. Anne Mercy Hospital, Toledo
St. Charles Mercy Hospital, Oregon
St. Luke's Hospital, Maumee
St. Vincent Charity Hospital, Cleveland
St. Vincent Mercy Medical Center, Toledo
South Pointe Hospital, Warrensville Heights
Southeastern Ohio Regional Medical Center,
    Cambridge
Southern Ohio Medical Center, Portsmouth
Southwest General Health Center,
    Middleburg Heights
Summa Health Systems Hospitals, Akron
Toledo Hospital, Toledo
UHHS Bedford Medical Center, Bedford
UHHS Geauga Regional Hospital, Chardon
UHHS Memorial Hospital of Geneva, Geneva
UHHS Richmond Heights Hospital,
    Richmond Heights
Western Reserve Care System, Youngstown
Wooster Community Hospital, Wooster

GASTROINTESTINAL

BOWEL OBSTRUCTION
Christ Hospital, Cincinnati
Cleveland Clinic, Cleveland
Fort Hamilton Hughes Memorial Hospital, Hamilton
Good Samaritan Hospital, Cincinnati
Grandview Medical Center, Dayton
Huron Hospital, East Cleveland
Jewish Hospital, Cincinnati
Mercy Hospital—Clermont, Batavia
Riverside Methodist Hospital, Columbus
St. Elizabeth Health Center, Youngstown
St. Vincent Charity Hospital, Cleveland
Southwest General Health Center,
    Middleburg Heights
Upper Valley Medical Center, Piqua
Upper Valley Medical Center, Troy

CHOLECYSTECTOMY
Aultman Hospital, Canton
Barberton Citizens Hospital, Barberton
Barnesville Hospital Association, Barnesville
Bellevue Hospital, Bellevue
Community Hospital of Springfield and
    Clark County, Springfield
Community Hospital, Bryan
Fisher Titus Memorial Hospital, Norwalk
Flower Hospital, Sylvania

Fulton County Health Center, Wauseon
Marietta Memorial Hospital, Marietta
Mercy Hospital—Anderson, Anderson
Middletown Regional Hospital, Middletown
St. Anne Mercy Hospital, Toledo
St. John Medical Center, Steubenville
Southwest General Health Center,
    Middleburg Heights
Trinity Health System, Steubenville

GASTROINTESTINAL BLEED
Akron General Medical Center, Akron
Christ Hospital, Cincinnati
Fairview Hospital, Cleveland
Greene Memorial Hospital, Xenia
Huron Hospital, East Cleveland
Kettering Medical Center, Kettering
Kettering Medical Center—Sycamore, Miamisburg
Lake Hospital System, Painesville
Lakewood Hospital, Lakewood
Marymount Hospital, Garfield Heights
Medical College of Ohio at Toledo, Toledo
Miami Valley Hospital, Dayton
Ohio State University Hospitals, Columbus
South Pointe Hospital, Warrensville Heights
Southern Ohio Medical Center, Portsmouth
Southwest General Health Center,
    Middleburg Heights
Summa Health Systems Hospitals, Akron
Trumbull Memorial Hospital, Warren
University Hospital, Cincinnati
Western Reserve Care System, Youngstown
Wooster Community Hospital, Wooster

GASTROINTESTINAL SURGERIES
AND PROCEDURES
Aultman Hospital, Canton
Bethesda North Hospital, Cincinnati
Christ Hospital, Cincinnati
Cleveland Clinic, Cleveland
Community Health Partners of Ohio—West, Lorain
Genesis Healthcare System, Zanesville
Good Samaritan Hospital, Cincinnati
Hillcrest Hospital, Mayfield Heights
Huron Hospital, East Cleveland
Jewish Hospital, Cincinnati
Kettering Medical Center, Kettering
Lakewood Hospital, Lakewood
Mercy Hospital—Western Hills, Cincinnati
Mercy Medical Center, Canton
Parma Community General Hospital, Parma
St. Anns Hospital of Columbus, Westerville
St. Luke's Hospital, Maumee

Southwest General Health Center,
    Middleburg Heights
Trumbull Memorial Hospital, Warren

PANCREATITIS
Christ Hospital, Cincinnati
Cleveland Clinic, Cleveland
Marietta Memorial Hospital, Marietta
Mercy Hospital—Western Hills, Cincinnati
Ohio State University Hospital East, Columbus
St. Luke's Hospital, Maumee

GENERAL SURGERY

APPENDECTOMY
None

MATERNITY CARE

None

ORTHOPEDICS

BACK AND NECK SURGERY
(EXCEPT SPINAL FUSION)
Aultman Hospital, Canton
Emh Regional Medical Center, Elyria
Mercy Hospital—Anderson, Anderson
Miami Valley Hospital, Dayton
New Albany Surgical Hospital, New Albany
St. Luke's Hospital, Maumee
St. Vincent Charity Hospital, Cleveland

BACK AND NECK SURGERY (SPINAL FUSION)
Bethesda North Hospital, Cincinnati
Firelands Regional Medical Center—Main Campus,
    Sandusky
Mercy Hospital—Anderson, Anderson
Meridia Euclid Hospital, Euclid
New Albany Surgical Hospital, New Albany
Southwest General Health Center,
    Middleburg Heights

HIP FRACTURE REPAIR
Adena Regional Medical Center, Chillicothe
Barberton Citizens Hospital, Barberton
Bethesda North Hospital, Cincinnati
Community Hospital, Bryan
Fairfield Medical Center, Lancaster
Fort Hamilton Hughes Memorial Hospital, Hamilton
Good Samaritan Hospital, Dayton
Hillcrest Hospital, Mayfield Heights
Huron Hospital, East Cleveland
Jewish Hospital, Cincinnati
Joel Pomerene Memorial Hospital, Millersburg
Kettering Medical Center—Sycamore, Miamisburg

Knox Community Hospital, Mount Vernon
Massillon Community Hospital, Massillon
Medina General Hospital, Medina
Memorial Hospital, Fremont
Mercer County Joint Township Community, Coldwater
Middletown Regional Hospital, Middletown
Mount Carmel Health, Columbus
Ohio State University Hospitals, Columbus
Parma Community General Hospital, Parma
St. Elizabeth Health Center, Youngstown
St. John Medical Center, Steubenville
St. Joseph Health Center, Warren
Southwest General Health Center,
  Middleburg Heights
Summa Health Systems Hospitals, Akron
Trinity Health System, Steubenville
UHHS Bedford Medical Center, Bedford
University Hospitals Case Medical Center,
  Cleveland
Van Wert County Hospital, Van Wert
Western Reserve Care System, Youngstown
Wood County Hospital, Bowling Green

TOTAL HIP REPLACEMENT

Alliance Community Hospital, Alliance
Bethesda North Hospital, Cincinnati
Firelands Regional Medical Center–Main Campus,
  Sandusky
Fulton County Health Center, Wauseon
Good Samaritan Hospital, Dayton
Massillon Community Hospital, Massillon
Medina General Hospital, Medina
Mount Carmel Health, Columbus
New Albany Surgical Hospital, New Albany
Parma Community General Hospital, Parma

TOTAL KNEE REPLACEMENT

Adena Regional Medical Center, Chillicothe
Bellevue Hospital, Bellevue
Blanchard Valley Regional Health Center, Findlay
Community Hospital, Bryan
Good Samaritan Hospital, Dayton
Joel Pomerene Memorial Hospital, Millersburg
Kettering Medical Center–Sycamore, Miamisburg
Marietta Memorial Hospital, Marietta
Mary Rutan Hospital, Bellefontaine
Massillon Community Hospital, Massillon
Medcentral Health System Shelby Hospital, Shelby
Meridia Euclid Hospital, Euclid
Mount Carmel Health, Columbus
New Albany Surgical Hospital, New Albany
Parma Community General Hospital, Parma

St. Luke's Hospital, Maumee
Southwest General Health Center,
  Middleburg Heights

PROSTATECTOMY

Barberton Citizens Hospital, Barberton
Mount Carmel Health, Columbus
Mount Carmel St. Ann's Hospital of Columbus,
  Westerville
Southern Ohio Medical Center, Portsmouth

PULMONARY

CHRONIC OBSTRUCTIVE PULMONARY DISEASE (COPD)

Akron General Medical Center, Akron
Barberton Citizens Hospital, Barberton
Barnesville Hospital Association, Barnesville
Bethesda North Hospital, Cincinnati
Christ Hospital, Cincinnati
Cleveland Clinic, Cleveland
Community Health Partners of Ohio–West, Lorain
Cuyahoga Falls General Hospital, Cuyahoga Falls
Deaconess Hospital, Cincinnati
East Liverpool City Hospital, East Liverpool
Emh Regional Medical Center, Elyria
Fairview Hospital, Cleveland
Fort Hamilton Hughes Memorial Hospital, Hamilton
Good Samaritan Hospital, Dayton
Holzer Medical Center, Gallipolis
Huron Hospital, East Cleveland
Lake Hospital System, Painesville
Lakewood Hospital, Lakewood
Licking Memorial Hospital, Newark
Marymount Hospital, Garfield Heights
MetroHealth Medical Center, Cleveland
Ohio State University Hospital East, Columbus
Parma Community General Hospital, Parma
Regency Hospital of Cincinnati, Cincinnati
St. John West Shore Hospital, Westlake
Southern Ohio Medical Center, Portsmouth
Southwest General Health Center,
  Middleburg Heights
Summa Health Systems Hospitals, Akron
Trumbull Memorial Hospital, Warren
UHHS Geauga Regional Hospital, Chardon
UHHS Richmond Heights Hospital,
  Richmond Heights
University Hospital, Cincinnati
University Hospitals Case Medical Center,
  Cleveland

PNEUMONIA

Adena Regional Medical Center, Chillicothe
Akron General Medical Center, Akron
Allen Medical Center, Oberlin
Ashtabula County Medical Center, Ashtabula
Barberton Citizens Hospital, Barberton
Bethesda North Hospital, Cincinnati
Brown County Hospital, Georgetown
Christ Hospital, Cincinnati
Community Health Partners of Ohio–West, Lorain
Dayton Heart Hospital, Dayton
Deaconess Hospital, Cincinnati
Doctors Hospital Ohio Health, Columbus
Emh Regional Medical Center, Elyria
Fairview Hospital, Cleveland
Fort Hamilton Hughes Memorial Hospital, Hamilton
Genesis Healthcare System, Zanesville
Good Samaritan Hospital, Cincinnati
Good Samaritan Hospital, Dayton
Grandview Medical Center, Dayton
Hillcrest Hospital, Mayfield Heights
Jewish Hospital, Cincinnati
Joint Township District Memorial Hospital,
  St. Marys
Kettering Medical Center, Kettering
Kettering Medical Center–Sycamore, Miamisburg
Lake Hospital System, Painesville
Lakewood Hospital, Lakewood
Licking Memorial Hospital, Newark
Lutheran Hospital, Cleveland
Marymount Hospital, Garfield Heights
Medical College of Ohio at Toledo, Toledo
Mercy Hospital–Anderson, Anderson
Mercy Hospital–Fairfield, Fairfield
Mercy Hospital–Western Hills, Cincinnati
Mercy Medical Center, Canton
Miami Valley Hospital, Dayton
Mount Carmel Health, Columbus
Ohio State University Hospital East, Columbus
Ohio State University Hospitals, Columbus
Parma Community General Hospital, Parma
Regency Hospital of Cincinnati, Cincinnati
Robinson Memorial Hospital, Ravenna
St. Anne Mercy Hospital, Toledo
St. Charles Mercy Hospital, Oregon
St. Elizabeth Health Center, Youngstown
St. John West Shore Hospital, Westlake
St. Joseph Health Center, Warren
St. Vincent Charity Hospital, Cleveland
Southeastern Ohio Regional Medical Center,
  Cambridge

Hospitals receiving a five star rating in a particular procedure have patient outcomes that put them among the best in the nation. For full definitions of ratings and awards, see Appendix.

Southern Ohio Medical Center, Portsmouth
Southwest General Health Center,
   Middleburg Heights
Summa Health Systems Hospitals, Akron
Toledo Hospital, Toledo
Trumbull Memorial Hospital, Warren
UHHS Bedford Medical Center, Bedford
UHHS Geauga Regional Hospital, Chardon
UHHS Richmond Heights Hospital,
   Richmond Heights
Union Hospital, Dover
University Hospitals Case Medical Center,
   Cleveland
Upper Valley Medical Center, Piqua
Upper Valley Medical Center, Troy
Wadsworth Rittman Hospital, Wadsworth
Wooster Community Hospital, Wooster

STROKE

Akron General Medical Center, Akron
Ashtabula County Medical Center, Ashtabula
Barberton Citizens Hospital, Barberton
Bay Park Community Hospital, Oregon
Bethesda North Hospital, Cincinnati
Christ Hospital, Cincinnati
Cleveland Clinic, Cleveland
Clinton Memorial Hospital, Wilmington
Community Health Partners of Ohio—West, Lorain
Emh Regional Medical Center, Elyria
Fairview Hospital, Cleveland
Fort Hamilton Hughes Memorial Hospital, Hamilton
Genesis Healthcare System, Zanesville

Good Samaritan Hospital, Dayton
Grandview Medical Center, Dayton
Greene Memorial Hospital, Xenia
Hillcrest Hospital, Mayfield Heights
Hocking Valley Community Hospital, Logan
Jewish Hospital, Cincinnati
Joel Pomerene Memorial Hospital, Millersburg
Kettering Medical Center, Kettering
Lake Hospital System, Painesville
Lakewood Hospital, Lakewood
Licking Memorial Hospital, Newark
Marymount Hospital, Garfield Heights
Medical College of Ohio at Toledo, Toledo
Mercy Healthcare Center, Toledo
Mercy Hospital—Anderson, Anderson
Mercy Hospital—Western Hills, Cincinnati
Mercy Medical Center, Canton
Meridia Euclid Hospital, Euclid
Miami Valley Hospital, Dayton
Mount Carmel Health, Columbus
Parma Community General Hospital, Parma
Robinson Memorial Hospital, Ravenna
St. Anne Mercy Hospital, Toledo
St. Charles Mercy Hospital, Oregon
St. Elizabeth Health Center, Youngstown
St. John West Shore Hospital, Westlake
St. Vincent Charity Hospital, Cleveland
St. Vincent Mercy Medical Center, Toledo
South Pointe Hospital, Warrensville Heights
Southwest General Health Center,
   Middleburg Heights
Summa Health Systems Hospitals, Akron

Toledo Hospital, Toledo
UHHS Bedford Medical Center, Bedford
UHHS Geauga Regional Hospital, Chardon
University Hospitals Case Medical Center,
   Cleveland
Upper Valley Medical Center, Piqua
Upper Valley Medical Center, Troy

VASCULAR

CAROTID SURGERY

Alliance Community Hospital, Alliance
Aultman Hospital, Canton
Dayton Heart Hospital, Dayton
Emh Regional Medical Center, Elyria
Fairfield Medical Center, Lancaster
Firelands Regional Medical Center—Main Campus,
   Sandusky
Mercy Medical Center of Springfield, Springfield
Robinson Memorial Hospital, Ravenna
Southwest General Health Center,
   Middleburg Heights

PERIPHERAL VASCULAR BYPASS

Ohio State University Hospitals, Columbus

RESECTION/REPLACEMENT OF ABDOMINAL AORTA

Aultman Hospital, Canton
Cleveland Clinic, Cleveland
Ohio State University Hospitals, Columbus
Toledo Hospital, Toledo

WOMEN'S HEALTH

None

OKLAHOMA HOSPITALS: FIVE STAR RATED FACILITIES

BARIATRIC SURGERY

None

CARDIAC

ATRIAL FIBRILLATION

Integris Southwest Medical Center, Oklahoma City
TCA of Central Oklahoma, Oklahoma City

CORONARY INTERVENTIONAL PROCEDURES
(ANGIOPLASTY/STENT)

None

HEART ATTACK

Integris Baptist Regional Health Center, Miami

HEART BYPASS SURGERY

None

HEART FAILURE

Integris Baptist Medical Center, Oklahoma City
Integris Canadian Valley Regional Hospital, Yukon

VALVE REPLACEMENT SURGERY

None

CRITICAL CARE

DIABETIC ACIDOSIS AND COMA

American Transitional Hospital, Oklahoma City
Deaconess Hospital, Oklahoma City

PULMONARY EMBOLISM

None

RESPIRATORY FAILURE

St. Francis Hospital—Broken Arrow, Broken Arrow

SEPSIS

Duncan Regional Hospital, Duncan
Great Plains Regional Medical Center, Elk City

GASTROINTESTINAL

BOWEL OBSTRUCTION

American Transitional Hospital, Oklahoma City
Deaconess Hospital, Oklahoma City

CHOLECYSTECTOMY

Ardmore Adventist Hospital, Ardmore
Duncan Regional Hospital, Duncan
Grady Memorial Hospital, Chickasha
Integris Southwest Medical Center, Oklahoma City
Medical Center of Southeastern Oklahoma, Durant
Mercy Memorial Health Center, Ardmore
Midwest Regional Medical Center, Midwest City

Parkview Hospital, El Reno
SouthCrest Hospital, Tulsa
TCA of Central Oklahoma, Oklahoma City

GASTROINTESTINAL BLEED
None

GASTROINTESTINAL SURGERIES
AND PROCEDURES
None

PANCREATITIS
None

GENERAL SURGERY

APPENDECTOMY
None

MATERNITY CARE

None

ORTHOPEDICS

BACK AND NECK SURGERY
(EXCEPT SPINAL FUSION)
Comanche County Memorial Hospital, Lawton
Hillcrest Medical Center, Tulsa
McBride Clinic Orthopedic Hospital, Oklahoma City
Midwest Regional Medical Center, Midwest City

BACK AND NECK SURGERY (SPINAL FUSION)
Comanche County Memorial Hospital, Lawton
Oklahoma University Medical Center,
   Oklahoma City

HIP FRACTURE REPAIR
American Transitional Hospital, Oklahoma City

Ardmore Adventist Hospital, Ardmore
Deaconess Hospital, Oklahoma City
Duncan Regional Hospital, Duncan
Grady Memorial Hospital, Chickasha
Integris Baptist Medical Center, Oklahoma City
Integris Canadian Valley Regional Hospital, Yukon
Integris Southwest Medical Center, Oklahoma City
McBride Clinic Orthopedic Hospital, Oklahoma City
Mercy Memorial Health Center, Ardmore
Midwest Regional Medical Center, Midwest City
Norman Regional Hospital, Norman
St. Francis Hospital, Tulsa
Stillwater Medical Center, Stillwater
TCA of Central Oklahoma, Oklahoma City
Valley View Regional Hospital, Ada

TOTAL HIP REPLACEMENT
Bone and Joint Hospital, Oklahoma City
McAlester Regional Health Center, McAlester
Mercy Health Center, Oklahoma City
Oklahoma Surgical Hospital, Tulsa
St. John Medical Center, Tulsa

TOTAL KNEE REPLACEMENT
American Transitional Hospital, Oklahoma City
Bone and Joint Hospital, Oklahoma City
Deaconess Hospital, Oklahoma City
Duncan Regional Hospital, Duncan
Integris Baptist Medical Center, Oklahoma City
McBride Clinic Orthopedic Hospital, Oklahoma City
Oklahoma Surgical Hospital, Tulsa

PROSTATECTOMY

Ardmore Adventist Hospital, Ardmore
Integris Baptist Medical Center, Oklahoma City

Mercy Memorial Health Center, Ardmore
Norman Regional Hospital, Norman

PULMONARY

CHRONIC OBSTRUCTIVE PULMONARY DISEASE
(COPD)
Integris Southwest Medical Center, Oklahoma City
TCA of Central Oklahoma, Oklahoma City

PNEUMONIA
American Transitional Hospital—Tulsa, Tulsa
Great Plains Regional Medical Center, Elk City
Tulsa Regional Medical Center, Tulsa
Woodward Regional Hospital, Woodward

STROKE

None

VASCULAR

CAROTID SURGERY
Comanche County Memorial Hospital, Lawton
Integris Baptist Medical Center, Oklahoma City
Oklahoma Heart Hospital, Oklahoma City
St. Anthony Hospital, Oklahoma City
St. Michael Hospital, Oklahoma City

PERIPHERAL VASCULAR BYPASS
American Transitional Hospital—Tulsa, Tulsa
Tulsa Regional Medical Center, Tulsa

RESECTION/REPLACEMENT OF ABDOMINAL AORTA
St. Francis Hospital, Tulsa

WOMEN'S HEALTH

None

OREGON HOSPITALS: FIVE STAR RATED FACILITIES

BARIATRIC SURGERY

None

CARDIAC

ATRIAL FIBRILLATION
None

CORONARY INTERVENTIONAL PROCEDURES
(ANGIOPLASTY/STENT)
None

HEART ATTACK
Mercy Medical Center, Roseburg
Providence Medford Medical Center, Medford

Providence Milwaukie Hospital, Milwaukie
Providence Seaside Hospital, Seaside

HEART BYPASS SURGERY
None

HEART FAILURE
Mercy Medical Center, Roseburg

VALVE REPLACEMENT SURGERY
Legacy Emanuel Hospital, Portland

CRITICAL CARE

DIABETIC ACIDOSIS AND COMA
None

PULMONARY EMBOLISM
None

RESPIRATORY FAILURE
Holy Rosary Medical Center, Ontario
Mercy Medical Center, Roseburg

SEPSIS
Holy Rosary Medical Center, Ontario
McKenzie-Willamette Medical Center, Springfield
Mercy Medical Center, Roseburg
Providence Portland Medical Center, Portland

Hospitals receiving a five star rating in a particular procedure have patient outcomes that put them among the best in the nation. For full definitions of ratings and awards, see Appendix.

GASTROINTESTINAL

BOWEL OBSTRUCTION
None

CHOLECYSTECTOMY
Bay Area Hospital, Coos Bay
Good Samaritan Regional Medical Center,
  Corvallis
The Mid-Columbia Medical Center, Dalles
Sacred Heart Medical Center—University District,
  Eugene
Salem Hospital, Salem
Tillamook County General Hospital, Tillamook

GASTROINTESTINAL BLEED
St. Charles Medical Center—Bend, Bend

GASTROINTESTINAL SURGERIES
AND PROCEDURES
McKenzie-Willamette Medical Center, Springfield
Providence Medford Medical Center, Medford
Providence St. Vincent Medical Center, Portland
Rogue Valley Medical Center, Medford

PANCREATITIS
Mercy Medical Center, Roseburg

GENERAL SURGERY

APPENDECTOMY
Good Samaritan Regional Medical Center,
  Corvallis
Legacy Meridian Park Hospital, Tualatin
Legacy Mount Hood Medical Center, Gresham
Mercy Medical Center, Roseburg
Merle West Medical Center, Klamath Falls
Providence Portland Medical Center, Portland
Providence Seaside Hospital, Seaside
Samaritan Lebanon Community Hospital, Lebanon
Silverton Hospital, Silverton
Willamette Falls Hospital, Oregon City

MATERNITY CARE

Mercy Medical Center, Roseburg

ORTHOPEDICS

BACK AND NECK SURGERY
(EXCEPT SPINAL FUSION)
Legacy Good Samaritan Hospital, Portland
Mercy Medical Center, Roseburg
Providence St. Vincent Medical Center, Portland
Rogue Valley Medical Center, Medford
St. Charles Medical Center—Bend, Bend
Salem Hospital, Salem

BACK AND NECK SURGERY (SPINAL FUSION)
Adventist Medical Center, Portland
Bay Area Hospital, Coos Bay
Providence Medford Medical Center, Medford
Providence Portland Medical Center, Portland
St. Charles Medical Center—Bend, Bend

HIP FRACTURE REPAIR
Providence Milwaukie Hospital, Milwaukie
Providence Newberg Hospital, Newberg
Samaritan Lebanon Community Hospital, Lebanon

TOTAL HIP REPLACEMENT
Bay Area Hospital, Coos Bay
Providence St. Vincent Medical Center, Portland
Salem Hospital, Salem
Willamette Falls Hospital, Oregon City

TOTAL KNEE REPLACEMENT
Good Samaritan Regional Medical Center,
  Corvallis
The Mid-Columbia Medical Center, Dalles
Providence Hood River Memorial Hospital,
  Hood River
Providence Portland Medical Center, Portland
Providence St. Vincent Medical Center, Portland
Rogue Valley Medical Center, Medford

Sacred Heart Medical Center—University District,
  Eugene
St. Charles Medical Center—Bend, Bend

PROSTATECTOMY
Providence St. Vincent Medical Center, Portland

PULMONARY

CHRONIC OBSTRUCTIVE PULMONARY DISEASE
(COPD)
Holy Rosary Medical Center, Ontario
Legacy Good Samaritan Hospital, Portland

PNEUMONIA
Holy Rosary Medical Center, Ontario
Mercy Medical Center, Roseburg

STROKE
OHSU Hospital, Portland
St. Elizabeth Health Services, Baker City

VASCULAR

CAROTID SURGERY
Good Samaritan Regional Medical Center,
  Corvallis
OHSU Hospital, Portland
Providence St. Vincent Medical Center, Portland
Rogue Valley Medical Center, Medford

PERIPHERAL VASCULAR BYPASS
None

RESECTION/REPLACEMENT OF ABDOMINAL AORTA
None

WOMEN'S HEALTH
None

PENNSYLVANIA HOSPITALS: FIVE STAR RATED FACILITIES

BARIATRIC SURGERY

Geisinger Medical Center, Danville
Mercy Jeannette Hospital, Jeannette
Pennsylvania Hospital, Philadelphia
Pinnacle Health System, Harrisburg
Sewickley Valley Hospital, Sewickley
Western Pennsylvania Hospital, Pittsburgh
York Hospital, York

CARDIAC

ATRIAL FIBRILLATION
Mercy Hospital Scranton, Scranton
Methodist Hospital, Philadelphia
Pinnacle Health System, Harrisburg
St. Luke's Hospital, Bethlehem
St. Luke's Hospital—Allentown Campus, Allentown
Shamokin Area Community Hospital, Coal Township
Thomas Jefferson University Hospital, Philadelphia

CORONARY INTERVENTIONAL PROCEDURES
(ANGIOPLASTY/STENT)
Chambersburg Hospital, Chambersburg
Hamot Medical Center, Erie
Mercy Hospital Scranton, Scranton
St. Luke's Hospital, Bethlehem
St. Luke's Hospital—Allentown Campus, Allentown
York Hospital, York

HEART ATTACK

Community Medical Center, Scranton
Conemaugh Valley Memorial Hospital, Johnstown
Doylestown Hospital, Doylestown
Easton Hospital, Easton
Elk Regional Health Center, St. Marys
Gettysburg Hospital, Gettysburg
Hamot Medical Center, Erie
Lancaster General Hospital, Lancaster
Lehigh Valley Hospital, Allentown
Lehigh Valley Hospital—Muhlenberg, Bethlehem
Lewistown Hospital, Lewistown
Main Line Hospitals—Lankenau, Wynnewood
Mercy Hospital Scranton, Scranton
Mercy Hospital, Pittsburgh
Mercy Providence Hospital, Pittsburgh
Pinnacle Health System, Harrisburg
The Reading Hospital and Medical Center,
    West Reading
Robert Packer Hospital, Sayre
Sacred Heart Hospital, Allentown
St. Luke's Hospital, Bethlehem
St. Luke's Hospital—Allentown Campus, Allentown
Shamokin Area Community Hospital, Coal Township
Titusville Hospital, Titusville
University of Pittsburgh Medical
    Center—Lee, Johnstown
University of Pittsburgh Medical
    Center—McKeesport, McKeesport
University of Pittsburgh Medical
    Center—St. Margaret, Pittsburgh
University of Pittsburgh Medical
    Center—South Side, Pittsburgh
York Hospital, York

HEART BYPASS SURGERY

Butler Memorial Hospital, Butler
Community Medical Center, Scranton
Geisinger South Wilkes-Barre, Wilkes-Barre
Hamot Medical Center, Erie
Jefferson Regional Medical Center, Pittsburgh
Lancaster General Hospital, Lancaster
Main Line Hospitals—Lankenau, Wynnewood
Phoenixville Hospital, Phoenixville
The Reading Hospital and Medical Center,
    West Reading
St. Luke's Hospital, Bethlehem
St. Luke's Hospital—Allentown Campus, Allentown
Washington Hospital, Washington

HEART FAILURE

Abington Memorial Hospital, Abington
Alle Kiski Medical Center, Natrona Heights
Allegheny General Hospital, Pittsburgh
Allegheny General Hospital—Suburban Campus,
    Pittsburgh
Brandywine Hospital, Coatesville
Chambersburg Hospital, Chambersburg
Chestnut Hill Hospital, Philadelphia
Clearfield Hospital, Clearfield
Ephrata Community Hospital, Ephrata
Frankford Hospital—Torresdale Campus,
    Philadelphia
Geisinger South Wilkes-Barre, Wilkes-Barre
Hamot Medical Center, Erie
Holy Redeemer Hospital and Medical Center,
    Meadowbrook
Jeanes Hospital, Philadelphia
Jefferson Regional Medical Center, Pittsburgh
Lancaster General Hospital, Lancaster
Lehigh Valley Hospital, Allentown
Lehigh Valley Hospital—Muhlenberg, Bethlehem
Main Line Hospitals—Bryn Mawr, Bryn Mawr
Main Line Hospitals—Lankenau, Wynnewood
Mercy Fitzgerald Hospital, Darby
Mercy Hospital Scranton, Scranton
Nazareth Hospital, Philadelphia
Pennsylvania Hospital, Philadelphia
Robert Packer Hospital, Sayre
Sacred Heart Hospital, Allentown
St. Luke's Hospital, Bethlehem
St. Luke's Hospital—Allentown Campus, Allentown
University of Pittsburgh Medical
    Center—McKeesport, McKeesport
University of Pittsburgh Medical
    Center—St. Margaret, Pittsburgh
University of Pittsburgh Medical
    Center—Shadyside, Pittsburgh
University of Pittsburgh Medical Center—
    Presbyterian Shadyside, Pittsburgh
Warminster Hospital, Warminster
Western Pennsylvania Hospital, Pittsburgh

VALVE REPLACEMENT SURGERY

Conemaugh Valley Memorial Hospital, Johnstown
Geisinger South Wilkes-Barre, Wilkes-Barre
Lancaster General Hospital, Lancaster
Lehigh Valley Hospital, Allentown
Main Line Hospitals—Bryn Mawr, Bryn Mawr
Mercy Hospital Scranton, Scranton
University of Pittsburgh Medical
    Center—Lee, Johnstown
Washington Hospital, Washington
York Hospital, York

CRITICAL CARE

DIABETIC ACIDOSIS AND COMA

Albert Einstein Medical Center, Philadelphia
Mercy Hospital, Pittsburgh
Mercy Providence Hospital, Pittsburgh
University of Pittsburgh Medical
    Center—McKeesport, McKeesport

PULMONARY EMBOLISM

Chambersburg Hospital, Chambersburg
Chestnut Hill Hospital, Philadelphia
Easton Hospital, Easton
Hazleton General Hospital, Hazleton
Lancaster General Hospital, Lancaster
Pinnacle Health System, Harrisburg
University of Pittsburgh Medical Center—
    McKeesport, McKeesport

RESPIRATORY FAILURE

Alle Kiski Medical Center, Natrona Heights
Chestnut Hill Hospital, Philadelphia
Conemaugh Valley Memorial Hospital, Johnstown
Geisinger South Wilkes-Barre, Wilkes-Barre
Geisinger Wyoming Valley Medical Center,
    Wilkes-Barre
Gettysburg Hospital, Gettysburg
Hamot Medical Center, Erie
Hazleton General Hospital, Hazleton
Heart of Lancaster Regional Medical Center, Lititz
Lancaster Regional Medical Center, Lancaster
Mercy Hospital Scranton, Scranton
Montgomery Hospital, Norristown
Moses Taylor Hospital, Scranton
Pinnacle Health System, Harrisburg
St. Joseph Medical Center, Reading
University of Pittsburgh Medical
    Center—Lee, Johnstown
University of Pittsburgh Medical
    Center—McKeesport, McKeesport
University of Pittsburgh Medical
    Center—St. Margaret, Pittsburgh

SEPSIS

Alle Kiski Medical Center, Natrona Heights
Butler Memorial Hospital, Butler
Chestnut Hill Hospital, Philadelphia
Clearfield Hospital, Clearfield
Conemaugh Valley Memorial Hospital, Johnstown
Easton Hospital, Easton
Frick Hospital, Mt. Pleasant
Hamot Medical Center, Erie
Hazleton General Hospital, Hazleton
Kane Community Hospital, Kane

Hospitals receiving a five star rating in a particular procedure have patient outcomes that put them among the best in the nation. For full definitions of ratings and awards, see Appendix.

Lehigh Valley Hospital, Allentown
Pinnacle Health System, Harrisburg
Pocono Medical Center, East Stroudsburg
Robert Packer Hospital, Sayre
University of Pittsburgh Medical
Center—Lee, Johnstown
University of Pittsburgh Medical
Center—McKeesport, McKeesport
York Hospital, York

GASTROINTESTINAL

BOWEL OBSTRUCTION

Easton Hospital, Easton
Hamot Medical Center, Erie
Lancaster Regional Medical Center, Lancaster
Lehigh Valley Hospital—Muhlenberg, Bethlehem
Pinnacle Health System, Harrisburg
St. Luke's Hospital, Bethlehem
St. Luke's Hospital—Allentown Campus, Allentown
Uniontown Hospital, Uniontown

CHOLECYSTECTOMY

Abington Memorial Hospital, Abington
Berwick Hospital Center, Berwick
Brookville Hospital, Brookville
Lewistown Hospital, Lewistown
Robert Packer Hospital, Sayre
St. Luke's Quakertown Hospital, Quakertown
Uniontown Hospital, Uniontown
York Hospital, York

GASTROINTESTINAL BLEED

Abington Memorial Hospital, Abington
Community Medical Center, Scranton
Ephrata Community Hospital, Ephrata
Evangelical Community Hospital, Lewisburg
Geisinger Wyoming Valley Medical Center,
Wilkes-Barre
Hamot Medical Center, Erie
Indiana Regional Medical Center, Indiana
Lehigh Valley Hospital, Allentown
Lehigh Valley Hospital—Muhlenberg, Bethlehem
Main Line Hospitals—Bryn Mawr, Bryn Mawr
North Philadelphia Health System, Philadelphia
Pennsylvania Hospital, Philadelphia
Pinnacle Health System, Harrisburg
St. Joseph's Hospital, Philadelphia
University of Pittsburgh Medical
Center—McKeesport, McKeesport
Warminster Hospital, Warminster
Waynesboro Hospital, Waynesboro

GASTROINTESTINAL SURGERIES
AND PROCEDURES

Community Medical Center, Scranton
Easton Hospital, Easton
Ephrata Community Hospital, Ephrata
Geisinger Medical Center, Danville
Hamot Medical Center, Erie
Lehigh Valley Hospital, Allentown
Lehigh Valley Hospital—Muhlenberg, Bethlehem
Mercy Hospital Scranton, Scranton
St. Luke's Hospital, Bethlehem
St. Luke's Hospital—Allentown Campus, Allentown
University of Pittsburgh Medical
Center—St. Margaret, Pittsburgh
Western Pennsylvania Hospital—Forbes Regional
Campus, Monroeville
York Hospital, York

PANCREATITIS

Geisinger Medical Center, Danville
Lehigh Valley Hospital, Allentown
Methodist Hospital, Philadelphia
Thomas Jefferson University Hospital, Philadelphia
Wilkes-Barre General Hospital, Wilkes-Barre
WVHCS Hospital, Wilkes-Barre

GENERAL SURGERY

APPENDECTOMY

Abington Memorial Hospital, Abington
Berwick Hospital Center, Berwick
Canonsburg General Hospital, Canonsburg
Chester County Hospital, West Chester
Chestnut Hill Hospital, Philadelphia
Conemaugh Valley Memorial Hospital, Johnstown
Delaware County Memorial Hospital, Drexel Hill
Doylestown Hospital, Doylestown
Easton Hospital, Easton
Good Samaritan Regional Medical Center,
Pottsville
Jersey Shore Hospital, Jersey Shore
Lancaster General Hospital, Lancaster
Lewistown Hospital, Lewistown
Lock Haven Hospital, Lock Haven
Main Line Hospitals—Lankenau, Wynnewood
Main Line Hospitals—Paoli Memorial, Paoli
Mount Nittany Medical Center, State College
Pennsylvania Hospital, Philadelphia
Pottstown Memorial Medical Center, Pottstown
Pottsville Hospital and Warne Clinic, Pottsville
Riddle Memorial Hospital, Media
Robert Packer Hospital, Sayre
Uniontown Hospital, Uniontown
University of Pittsburgh Medical Center—Bedford,
Everett

University of Pittsburgh Medical Center—Lee,
Johnstown
Wayne Memorial Hospital, Honesdale
Western Pennsylvania Hospital—Forbes Regional
Campus, Monroeville
York Hospital, York

MATERNITY CARE

Community Medical Center, Scranton
Doylestown Hospital, Doylestown
DuBois Regional Medical Center, DuBois
Grand View Hospital, Sellersville
Hanover General Hospital, Hanover
Indiana Regional Medical Center, Indiana
Mercy Jeannette Hospital, Jeannette
Pottsville Hospital and Warne Clinic, Pottsville
St. Mary Medical Center, Langhorne
St. Vincent Health Center, Erie
Washington Hospital, Washington
Westmoreland Regional Hospital, Greensburg
Wilkes-Barre General Hospital, Wilkes-Barre
WVHCS Hospital, Wilkes-Barre

ORTHOPEDICS

BACK AND NECK SURGERY
(EXCEPT SPINAL FUSION)

Community Medical Center, Scranton
Doylestown Hospital, Doylestown
Lancaster General Hospital, Lancaster
Pennsylvania Hospital, Philadelphia
Williamsport Hospital and Medical Center,
Williamsport

BACK AND NECK SURGERY (SPINAL FUSION)

Hanover General Hospital, Hanover
Main Line Hospitals—Paoli Memorial, Paoli
Methodist Hospital, Philadelphia
Mount Nittany Medical Center, State College
Pennsylvania Hospital, Philadelphia
Robert Packer Hospital, Sayre
Sewickley Valley Hospital, Sewickley
Thomas Jefferson University Hospital, Philadelphia
Williamsport Hospital and Medical Center,
Williamsport

HIP FRACTURE REPAIR

Albert Einstein Medical Center, Philadelphia
Canonsburg General Hospital, Canonsburg
Carlisle Regional Medical Center, Carlisle
Chester County Hospital, West Chester
Clearfield Hospital, Clearfield
Conemaugh Valley Memorial Hospital, Johnstown
Delaware County Memorial Hospital, Drexel Hill

DuBois Regional Medical Center, DuBois
Grand View Hospital, Sellersville
Hanover General Hospital, Hanover
Indiana Regional Medical Center, Indiana
Jersey Shore Hospital, Jersey Shore
Main Line Hospitals—Lankenau, Wynnewood
Mercy Jeannette Hospital, Jeannette
Pottstown Memorial Medical Center, Pottstown
Sewickley Valley Hospital, Sewickley
Uniontown Hospital, Uniontown
University of Pittsburgh Medical Center—Lee,
  Johnstown
University of Pittsburgh Medical
  Center—McKeesport, McKeesport
Washington Hospital, Washington
Wayne Memorial Hospital, Honesdale
Western Pennsylvania Hospital—Forbes Regional
  Campus, Monroeville
Wilkes-Barre General Hospital, Wilkes-Barre
WVHCS Hospital, Wilkes-Barre
York Hospital, York

TOTAL HIP REPLACEMENT

Geisinger Medical Center, Danville
Good Samaritan Regional Medical Center, Pottsville
Hanover General Hospital, Hanover
Jefferson Regional Medical Center, Pittsburgh
Methodist Hospital, Philadelphia
Nazareth Hospital, Philadelphia
Pennsylvania Hospital, Philadelphia
Robert Packer Hospital, Sayre
St. Vincent Health Center, Erie
Thomas Jefferson University Hospital, Philadelphia
Washington Hospital, Washington
Western Pennsylvania Hospital, Pittsburgh
Westmoreland Regional Hospital, Greensburg
Wilkes-Barre General Hospital, Wilkes-Barre
WVHCS Hospital, Wilkes-Barre

TOTAL KNEE REPLACEMENT

Altoona Hospital, Altoona
Bon Secours Mercy Hospital, Altoona
Brookville Hospital, Brookville
Central Montgomery Medical Center, Lansdale
Chambersburg Hospital, Chambersburg
Conemaugh Valley Memorial Hospital, Johnstown
Delaware County Memorial Hospital, Drexel Hill
DuBois Regional Medical Center, DuBois
Geisinger Wyoming Valley Medical Center,
  Wilkes-Barre
Hanover General Hospital, Hanover
Magee-Womens Hospital of the UPMC
  Health System, Pittsburgh
Meadville Medical Center, Meadville
Memorial Hospital, Towanda

Mercy Hospital Scranton, Scranton
Milton S. Hershey Medical Center, Hershey
Mount Nittany Medical Center, State College
Nazareth Hospital, Philadelphia
Pennsylvania Hospital, Philadelphia
Pottsville Hospital and Warne Clinic, Pottsville
Punxsutawney Area Hospital, Punxsutawney
Robert Packer Hospital, Sayre
St. Vincent Health Center, Erie
St. Luke's Quakertown Hospital, Quakertown
Uniontown Hospital, Uniontown
University of Pittsburgh Medical Center—Bedford,
  Everett
University of Pittsburgh Medical Center—Lee,
  Johnstown
Washington Hospital, Washington
Western Pennsylvania Hospital, Pittsburgh
York Hospital, York

PROSTATECTOMY

Butler Memorial Hospital, Butler
Conemaugh Valley Memorial Hospital, Johnstown
Hospital of the University of Pennsylvania,
  Philadelphia
Jefferson Regional Medical Center, Pittsburgh
Pennsylvania Hospital, Philadelphia
Pennsylvania Presbyterian Medical Center,
  Philadelphia
University of Pittsburgh Medical Center—Bedford,
  Everett
University of Pittsburgh Medical Center—Lee,
  Johnstown

PULMONARY

CHRONIC OBSTRUCTIVE PULMONARY DISEASE (COPD)

Central Montgomery Medical Center, Lansdale
Chestnut Hill Hospital, Philadelphia
Community Medical Center, Scranton
Ephrata Community Hospital, Ephrata
Hamot Medical Center, Erie
Mid-Valley Hospital, Peckville
Pinnacle Health System, Harrisburg
St. Clair Hospital, Pittsburgh
University of Pittsburgh Medical
  Center—McKeesport, McKeesport
University of Pittsburgh Medical
  Center—St. Margaret, Pittsburgh
University of Pittsburgh Medical
  Center—Shadyside, Pittsburgh
University of Pittsburgh Medical Center—
  Presbyterian Shadyside, Pittsburgh

PNEUMONIA

Albert Einstein Medical Center, Philadelphia
Alle Kiski Medical Center, Natrona Heights
Easton Hospital, Easton
Ephrata Community Hospital, Ephrata
Hamot Medical Center, Erie
Hazleton General Hospital, Hazleton
Kane Community Hospital, Kane
Lancaster General Hospital, Lancaster
Lehigh Valley Hospital, Allentown
Lehigh Valley Hospital—Muhlenberg, Bethlehem
Main Line Hospitals—Bryn Mawr, Bryn Mawr
Main Line Hospitals—Lankenau, Wynnewood
Mercy Hospital Scranton, Scranton
Mercy Hospital, Pittsburgh
Mercy Providence Hospital, Pittsburgh
Methodist Hospital, Philadelphia
Mid-Valley Hospital, Peckville
Nazareth Hospital, Philadelphia
Pennsylvania Hospital, Philadelphia
Pocono Medical Center, East Stroudsburg
St. Luke's Hospital, Bethlehem
St. Luke's Hospital—Allentown Campus, Allentown
St. Luke's Quakertown Hospital, Quakertown
St. Luke's Miners Memorial Hospital, Coaldale
Thomas Jefferson University Hospital, Philadelphia
University of Pittsburgh Medical
  Center—McKeesport, McKeesport
University of Pittsburgh Medical
  Center—St. Margaret, Pittsburgh
University of Pittsburgh Medical
  Center—Shadyside, Pittsburgh
University of Pittsburgh Medical Center—
  Presbyterian Shadyside, Pittsburgh
Warminster Hospital, Warminster
Williamsport Hospital and Medical Center,
  Williamsport

STROKE

Abington Memorial Hospital, Abington
Central Montgomery Medical Center, Lansdale
Ephrata Community Hospital, Ephrata
Geisinger South Wilkes-Barre, Wilkes-Barre
Hamot Medical Center, Erie
Jefferson Regional Medical Center, Pittsburgh
Lancaster General Hospital, Lancaster
Lehigh Valley Hospital, Allentown
Lehigh Valley Hospital—Muhlenberg, Bethlehem
Main Line Hospitals—Bryn Mawr, Bryn Mawr
Main Line Hospitals—Lankenau, Wynnewood
Mercy Fitzgerald Hospital, Darby
Mercy Hospital Scranton, Scranton

Milton S. Hershey Medical Center, Hershey
Nazareth Hospital, Philadelphia
Pinnacle Health System, Harrisburg
The Reading Hospital and Medical Center,
    West Reading
University of Pittsburgh Medical Center–Horizon,
    Greenville
University of Pittsburgh Medical
    Center–St. Margaret, Pittsburgh

VASCULAR

CAROTID SURGERY

Allegheny General Hospital, Pittsburgh
Allegheny General Hospital–Suburban Campus,
    Pittsburgh
Brookville Hospital, Brookville

DuBois Regional Medical Center, DuBois
Pennsylvania Hospital, Philadelphia
Pocono Medical Center, East Stroudsburg
Robert Packer Hospital, Sayre
St. Vincent Health Center, Erie
Sewickley Valley Hospital, Sewickley

PERIPHERAL VASCULAR BYPASS

Albert Einstein Medical Center, Philadelphia
Carlisle Regional Medical Center, Carlisle
DuBois Regional Medical Center, DuBois
The Reading Hospital and Medical Center,
    West Reading

RESECTION/REPLACEMENT OF ABDOMINAL AORTA

University of Pittsburgh Medical
    Center–Shadyside, Pittsburgh

University of Pittsburgh Medical Center–
    Presbyterian Shadyside, Pittsburgh

WOMEN'S HEALTH

Butler Memorial Hospital, Butler
Chester County Hospital, West Chester
Community Medical Center, Scranton
Doylestown Hospital, Doylestown
DuBois Regional Medical Center, DuBois
Geisinger South Wilkes-Barre, Wilkes-Barre
Mercy Hospital Scranton, Scranton
St. Luke's Hospital, Bethlehem
St. Luke's Hospital–Allentown Campus, Allentown
St. Mary Medical Center, Langhorne
Washington Hospital, Washington
Westmoreland Regional Hospital, Greensburg

RHODE ISLAND HOSPITALS: FIVE STAR RATED FACILITIES

BARIATRIC SURGERY

None

CARDIAC

ATRIAL FIBRILLATION
None

CORONARY INTERVENTIONAL PROCEDURES (ANGIOPLASTY/STENT)
Rhode Island Hospital, Providence

HEART ATTACK
None

HEART BYPASS SURGERY
None

HEART FAILURE
Rhode Island Hospital, Providence

VALVE REPLACEMENT SURGERY
None

CRITICAL CARE

DIABETIC ACIDOSIS AND COMA
None

PULMONARY EMBOLISM
None

RESPIRATORY FAILURE
None

SEPSIS
None

GASTROINTESTINAL

BOWEL OBSTRUCTION
Memorial Hospital of Rhode Island, Pawtucket

CHOLECYSTECTOMY
None

GASTROINTESTINAL BLEED
None

GASTROINTESTINAL SURGERIES AND PROCEDURES
None

PANCREATITIS
None

GENERAL SURGERY

APPENDECTOMY
None

MATERNITY CARE

None

ORTHOPEDICS

BACK AND NECK SURGERY (EXCEPT SPINAL FUSION)
None

BACK AND NECK SURGERY (SPINAL FUSION)
Roger Williams Hospital, Providence
South County Hospital, Wakefield

HIP FRACTURE REPAIR
None

TOTAL HIP REPLACEMENT
None

TOTAL KNEE REPLACEMENT
None

PROSTATECTOMY

None

PULMONARY

CHRONIC OBSTRUCTIVE PULMONARY DISEASE (COPD)
None

PNEUMONIA
Rhode Island Hospital, Providence

STROKE

Memorial Hospital of Rhode Island, Pawtucket

VASCULAR

CAROTID SURGERY
None

PERIPHERAL VASCULAR BYPASS
None

RESECTION/REPLACEMENT OF ABDOMINAL AORTA
Kent County Memorial Hospital, Warwick

WOMEN'S HEALTH

None

BARIATRIC SURGERY

None

CARDIAC

ATRIAL FIBRILLATION
St. Francis Hospital, Greenville

CORONARY INTERVENTIONAL PROCEDURES (ANGIOPLASTY/STENT)
None

HEART ATTACK
Spartanburg Regional Medical Center, Spartanburg
Springs Memorial Hospital, Lancaster

HEART BYPASS SURGERY
Anmed Health, Anderson
Greenville Memorial Hospital, Greenville
St. Francis Hospital, Greenville
Spartanburg Regional Medical Center, Spartanburg

HEART FAILURE
Chesterfield General Hospital, Cheraw

VALVE REPLACEMENT SURGERY
Greenville Memorial Hospital, Greenville

CRITICAL CARE

DIABETIC ACIDOSIS AND COMA
None

PULMONARY EMBOLISM
Anmed Health, Anderson
Palmetto Health Baptist–Easley, Easley
Piedmont Medical Center, Rock Hill

RESPIRATORY FAILURE
Anmed Health, Anderson
Chester Regional Medical Center, Chester
Hillcrest Memorial Hospital, Simpsonville
McLeod Medical Center–Darlington, Darlington
McLeod Medical Center–Dillon, Dillon
Oconee Memorial Hospital, Seneca

SEPSIS
Anmed Health, Anderson
Hillcrest Memorial Hospital, Simpsonville
McLeod Medical Center–Darlington, Darlington
Oconee Memorial Hospital, Seneca

GASTROINTESTINAL

BOWEL OBSTRUCTION
None

CHOLECYSTECTOMY
Aiken Regional Medical Center, Aiken
Beaufort Memorial Hospital, Beaufort
Self Regional Healthcare, Greenwood
Trident Medical Center, Charleston
Tuomey Healthcare System, Sumter

GASTROINTESTINAL BLEED
None

GASTROINTESTINAL SURGERIES AND PROCEDURES
None

PANCREATITIS
Greenville Memorial Hospital, Greenville

GENERAL SURGERY

APPENDECTOMY
None

MATERNITY CARE

None

ORTHOPEDICS

BACK AND NECK SURGERY (EXCEPT SPINAL FUSION)
Beaufort Memorial Hospital, Beaufort
Medical University Hospital, Charleston
Self Regional Healthcare, Greenwood
Trident Medical Center, Charleston

BACK AND NECK SURGERY (SPINAL FUSION)
Beaufort Memorial Hospital, Beaufort
East Cooper Regional Medical Center, Mt. Pleasant
Self Regional Healthcare, Greenwood
Sisters of Charity Providence Hospitals, Columbia

HIP FRACTURE REPAIR
Allen Bennett Memorial Hospital, Greer
Anmed Health, Anderson
East Cooper Regional Medical Center, Mt. Pleasant
Hillcrest Memorial Hospital, Simpsonville
Laurens County Healthcare System, Clinton
Oconee Memorial Hospital, Seneca
Piedmont Medical Center, Rock Hill
St. Francis Hospital, Greenville
Springs Memorial Hospital, Lancaster
Tuomey Healthcare System, Sumter

TOTAL HIP REPLACEMENT
Lexington Medical Center, West Columbia
Loris Community Hospital, Loris
Oconee Memorial Hospital, Seneca
Palmetto Health Richland, Columbia
Sisters of Charity Providence Hospitals, Columbia
Spartanburg Regional Medical Center, Spartanburg

TOTAL KNEE REPLACEMENT
Beaufort Memorial Hospital, Beaufort
Cannon Memorial Hospital, Pickens
Palmetto Health Baptist–Easley, Easley
St. Francis Hospital, Greenville
Tuomey Healthcare System, Sumter

PROSTATECTOMY

Allen Bennett Memorial Hospital, Greer
Marion County Medical Center, Marion
Self Regional Healthcare, Greenwood

PULMONARY

CHRONIC OBSTRUCTIVE PULMONARY DISEASE (COPD)
Piedmont Medical Center, Rock Hill

PNEUMONIA
Abbeville County Memorial Hospital, Abbeville
Anmed Health, Anderson
Oconee Memorial Hospital, Seneca

STROKE

None

VASCULAR

CAROTID SURGERY
Conway Medical Center, Conway
Medical University Hospital, Charleston
Self Regional Healthcare, Greenwood
Spartanburg Regional Medical Center, Spartanburg

PERIPHERAL VASCULAR BYPASS
Anmed Health, Anderson

RESECTION/REPLACEMENT OF ABDOMINAL AORTA
Greenville Memorial Hospital, Greenville

WOMEN'S HEALTH

None

Hospitals receiving a five star rating in a particular procedure have patient outcomes that put them among the best in the nation. For full definitions of ratings and awards, see Appendix.

BARIATRIC SURGERY

None

CARDIAC

ATRIAL FIBRILLATION

Avera Heart Hospital of South Dakota, Sioux Falls

CORONARY INTERVENTIONAL PROCEDURES (ANGIOPLASTY/STENT)

Avera Heart Hospital of South Dakota, Sioux Falls

HEART ATTACK

Avera Heart Hospital of South Dakota, Sioux Falls
Sanford USD Medical Center, Sioux Falls

HEART BYPASS SURGERY

Avera Heart Hospital of South Dakota, Sioux Falls

HEART FAILURE

Avera Heart Hospital of South Dakota, Sioux Falls

VALVE REPLACEMENT SURGERY

Avera Heart Hospital of South Dakota, Sioux Falls
Sanford USD Medical Center, Sioux Falls

CRITICAL CARE

DIABETIC ACIDOSIS AND COMA

None

PULMONARY EMBOLISM

None

RESPIRATORY FAILURE

Avera McKennan Hospital and University
    Health Center, Sioux Falls
Sanford USD Medical Center, Sioux Falls

SEPSIS

Avera McKennan Hospital and University
    Health Center, Sioux Falls
Avera Queen of Peace, Mitchell
St. Mary's Hospital, Pierre

GASTROINTESTINAL

BOWEL OBSTRUCTION

Prairie Lakes Hospital and Care Center, Watertown

CHOLECYSTECTOMY

None

GASTROINTESTINAL BLEED

Sanford USD Medical Center, Sioux Falls

GASTROINTESTINAL SURGERIES AND PROCEDURES

Avera McKennan Hospital and University
    Health Center, Sioux Falls
Sanford USD Medical Center, Sioux Falls

PANCREATITIS

None

GENERAL SURGERY

APPENDECTOMY

None

MATERNITY CARE

None

ORTHOPEDICS

BACK AND NECK SURGERY (EXCEPT SPINAL FUSION)

Sanford USD Medical Center, Sioux Falls

BACK AND NECK SURGERY (SPINAL FUSION)

Sanford USD Medical Center, Sioux Falls

HIP FRACTURE REPAIR

Rapid City Regional Hospital, Rapid City

TOTAL HIP REPLACEMENT

Avera McKennan Hospital and University
    Health Center, Sioux Falls
Prairie Lakes Hospital and Care Center, Watertown
Sanford USD Medical Center, Sioux Falls

TOTAL KNEE REPLACEMENT

Avera McKennan Hospital and University
    Health Center, Sioux Falls
Prairie Lakes Hospital and Care Center, Watertown
Sanford USD Medical Center, Sioux Falls

PROSTATECTOMY

None

PULMONARY

CHRONIC OBSTRUCTIVE PULMONARY DISEASE (COPD)

None

PNEUMONIA

Avera Gregory Healthcare Center, Gregory
Avera McKennan Hospital and University
    Health Center, Sioux Falls
Hand County Memorial Hospital, Miller
St. Mary's Hospital, Pierre

STROKE

Avera McKennan Hospital and University
    Health Center, Sioux Falls

VASCULAR

CAROTID SURGERY

None

PERIPHERAL VASCULAR BYPASS

Sanford USD Medical Center, Sioux Falls

RESECTION/REPLACEMENT OF ABDOMINAL AORTA

Avera Heart Hospital of South Dakota, Sioux Falls
Sanford USD Medical Center, Sioux Falls

WOMEN'S HEALTH

None

BARIATRIC SURGERY

None

CARDIAC

ATRIAL FIBRILLATION

Baptist Hospital of East Tennessee, Knoxville
Blount Memorial Hospital, Maryville
Cumberland Medical Center, Crossville
Wellmont Holston Valley Medical Center, Kingsport

CORONARY INTERVENTIONAL PROCEDURES (ANGIOPLASTY/STENT)

Baptist Hospital, Nashville
Parkwest Medical Center, Knoxville

HEART ATTACK

Macon County General Hospital, Lafayette
Memorial Healthcare System, Chattanooga
Parkwest Medical Center, Knoxville
Skyline Medical Center, Nashville
Southern Tennessee Medical Center, Winchester

HEART BYPASS SURGERY

Baptist Memorial Hospital, Memphis

HEART FAILURE

Cumberland River Hospital, Celina
Memorial Healthcare System, Chattanooga
Parkwest Medical Center, Knoxville
Roane Medical Center, Harriman
United Regional Medical Center, Manchester
White County Community Hospital, Sparta

VALVE REPLACEMENT SURGERY

Memorial Healthcare System, Chattanooga

CRITICAL CARE

DIABETIC ACIDOSIS AND COMA

Erlanger Medical Center, Chattanooga
Wellmont Holston Valley Medical Center, Kingsport
Women's East Pavilion, Chattanooga

PULMONARY EMBOLISM

Baptist Memorial Hospital—Collierville, Collierville
Fort Sanders Regional Medical Center, Knoxville
Johnson City Medical Center, Johnson City
Parkwest Medical Center, Knoxville

RESPIRATORY FAILURE

Jamestown Regional Medical Center, Jamestown
Jellico Community Hospital, Jellico
Memorial Healthcare System, Chattanooga
Methodist Medical Center of Oak Ridge, Oak Ridge
NorthCrest Medical Center, Springfield
Parkridge Medical Center, Chattanooga
Scott County Hospital, Oneida
Takoma Adventist Hospital, Greeneville
Vanderbilt University Hospital, Nashville
Wellmont Hawkins County Memorial Hospital, Rogersville
Wellmont Holston Valley Medical Center, Kingsport

SEPSIS

Baptist Hospital of Cocke County, Newport
Baptist Hospital of East Tennessee, Knoxville
Centennial Medical Center, Nashville
Memorial Healthcare System, Chattanooga
Methodist Medical Center of Oak Ridge, Oak Ridge
Skyline Medical Center, Nashville
Takoma Adventist Hospital, Greeneville

GASTROINTESTINAL

BOWEL OBSTRUCTION

Memorial Healthcare System, Chattanooga

CHOLECYSTECTOMY

Baptist Memorial Hospital, Memphis
Cookeville Regional Medical Center, Cookeville
Hillside Hospital, Pulaski
Memorial Healthcare System, Chattanooga
River Park Hospital, McMinnville
St. Thomas Hospital, Nashville
Skyline Medical Center, Nashville
Sumner Regional Medical Center, Gallatin

GASTROINTESTINAL BLEED

Memorial Healthcare System, Chattanooga
St. Mary's Medical Center, Knoxville
Select Specialty Hospital—Tricities, Bristol
Volunteer Community Hospital, Martin
Wellmont Bristol Regional Medical Center, Bristol
Wellmont Holston Valley Medical Center, Kingsport

GASTROINTESTINAL SURGERIES AND PROCEDURES

Baptist Memorial Hospital, Memphis
Centennial Medical Center, Nashville
Memorial Healthcare System, Chattanooga
St. Francis Hospital, Memphis

PANCREATITIS

Centennial Medical Center, Nashville
Erlanger Medical Center, Chattanooga
Select Specialty Hospital—Tricities, Bristol

University of Tennessee Memorial Hospital, Knoxville
Wellmont Bristol Regional Medical Center, Bristol
Women's East Pavilion, Chattanooga

GENERAL SURGERY

APPENDECTOMY

None

MATERNITY CARE

None

ORTHOPEDICS

BACK AND NECK SURGERY (EXCEPT SPINAL FUSION)

Baptist Memorial Hospital, Memphis
Cookeville Regional Medical Center, Cookeville
Germantown Community Hospital, Germantown
Harton Regional Medical Center, Tullahoma
Methodist Healthcare Memphis Hospitals, Memphis
Regional Hospital of Jackson, Jackson
St. Thomas Hospital, Nashville
Skyline Medical Center, Nashville

BACK AND NECK SURGERY (SPINAL FUSION)

Baptist Hospital West, Knoxville
Centennial Medical Center, Nashville
Cookeville Regional Medical Center, Cookeville
Germantown Community Hospital, Germantown
Methodist Healthcare Memphis Hospitals, Memphis
Middle Tennessee Medical Center, Murfreesboro
St. Mary's Medical Center, Knoxville
St. Thomas Hospital, Nashville

HIP FRACTURE REPAIR

Baptist Hospital West, Knoxville
Blount Memorial Hospital, Maryville
Cumberland Medical Center, Crossville
Germantown Community Hospital, Germantown
Indian Path Medical Center, Kingsport
Maury Regional Hospital, Columbia
Methodist Healthcare Memphis Hospitals, Memphis
Methodist Medical Center of Oak Ridge, Oak Ridge
NorthCrest Medical Center, Springfield
Parkwest Medical Center, Knoxville
St. Mary's Medical Center, Knoxville
Sumner Regional Medical Center, Gallatin
Volunteer Community Hospital, Martin

Hospitals receiving a five star rating in a particular procedure have patient outcomes that put them among the best in the nation. For full definitions of ratings and awards, see Appendix.

TOTAL HIP REPLACEMENT

Cookeville Regional Medical Center, Cookeville
Germantown Community Hospital, Germantown
Memorial Healthcare System, Chattanooga
Methodist Healthcare Memphis Hospitals,
    Memphis
Methodist Medical Center of Oak Ridge, Oak Ridge
St. Mary's Medical Center, Knoxville

TOTAL KNEE REPLACEMENT

Baptist Hospital of East Tennessee, Knoxville
Baptist Hospital, Nashville
Centennial Medical Center, Nashville
Delta Medical Center, Memphis
Germantown Community Hospital, Germantown
Memorial Healthcare System, Chattanooga
Methodist Healthcare Memphis Hospitals,
    Memphis
Methodist Medical Center of Oak Ridge, Oak Ridge
St. Mary's Medical Center, Knoxville
St. Thomas Hospital, Nashville
Williamson Medical Center, Franklin

PROSTATECTOMY

Baptist Hospital of East Tennessee, Knoxville
Centennial Medical Center, Nashville
Crockett Hospital, Lawrenceburg
St. Thomas Hospital, Nashville
Vanderbilt University Hospital, Nashville
Williamson Medical Center, Franklin

PULMONARY

CHRONIC OBSTRUCTIVE PULMONARY DISEASE (COPD)

Baptist Hospital of East Tennessee, Knoxville
Cleveland Community Hospital, Cleveland

Cookeville Regional Medical Center, Cookeville
Haywood Park Community Hospital, Brownsville
Johnson City Medical Center, Johnson City
Medical Center of Manchester, Manchester
River Park Hospital, McMinnville
Roane Medical Center, Harriman
St. Mary's Medical Center of Campbell County,
    La Follette
St. Mary's Medical Center, Knoxville
Select Specialty Hospital—Tricities, Bristol
Skyline Madison Campus, Madison
University of Tennessee Memorial Hospital, Knoxville
Wellmont Bristol Regional Medical Center, Bristol
White County Community Hospital, Sparta

PNEUMONIA

Baptist Hospital, Nashville
Cumberland River Hospital, Celina
Dekalb Hospital, Smithville
Fort Loudoun Medical Center, Lenoir City
HealthSouth Chattanooga Rehab Hospital,
    Chattanooga
Horizon Medical Center, Dickson
Lakeway Regional Hospital, Morristown
Medical Center of Manchester, Manchester
Memorial Healthcare System, Chattanooga
Roane Medical Center, Harriman
St. Mary's Medical Center of Campbell County,
    La Follette
St. Mary's Medical Center, Knoxville
St. Thomas Hospital, Nashville
Smith County Memorial Hospital, Carthage
Summit Medical Center, Hermitage
Vanderbilt University Hospital, Nashville
Wellmont Holston Valley Medical Center, Kingsport

STROKE

Baptist Memorial Hospital, Memphis
Erlanger Medical Center, Chattanooga
Memorial Healthcare System, Chattanooga
Women's East Pavilion, Chattanooga

VASCULAR

CAROTID SURGERY

Baptist Memorial Hospital, Memphis
Blount Memorial Hospital, Maryville
Centennial Medical Center, Nashville
Cookeville Regional Medical Center, Cookeville
Johnson City Medical Center, Johnson City
Methodist Medical Center of Oak Ridge, Oak Ridge
St. Thomas Hospital, Nashville
Skyline Medical Center, Nashville
Williamson Medical Center, Franklin

PERIPHERAL VASCULAR BYPASS

Baptist Hospital, Nashville
Memorial Healthcare System, Chattanooga
Skyline Medical Center, Nashville

RESECTION/REPLACEMENT OF ABDOMINAL AORTA

Cookeville Regional Medical Center, Cookeville

WOMEN'S HEALTH

None

TEXAS HOSPITALS: FIVE STAR RATED FACILITIES

BARIATRIC SURGERY

American Transitional Hospital—Houston W,
    Houston
Citizens Medical Center, Victoria
College Station Medical Center, College Station
Cypress Fairbanks Medical Center, Houston
Doctors Hospital at White Rock Lake, Dallas
East Texas Medical Center, Tyler
Memorial Hermann—Texas Medical Center,
    Houston
Nix Health Care System, San Antonio
RHD Memorial Medical Center, Dallas
Scott and White Memorial Hospital, Temple

Spring Branch Medical Center, Houston
Twelve Oaks Medical Center, Houston
United Regional Health Care System, Wichita Falls
Valley Baptist Medical Center, Harlingen

CARDIAC

ATRIAL FIBRILLATION

Brownwood Regional Medical Center, Brownwood
Heart Hospital of Austin, Austin
Memorial Hermann Southwest Hospital, Houston
South Austin Hospital, Austin
United Regional Health Care System, Wichita Falls

CORONARY INTERVENTIONAL PROCEDURES (ANGIOPLASTY/STENT)

Baylor Heart and Vascular Center, Dallas
Harris Methodist HEB Hospital, Bedford
Heart Hospital of Austin, Austin
Lubbock Heart Hospital, Lubbock
Texsan Heart Hospital, San Antonio
University of Texas Medical Branch Galveston,
    Galveston

HEART ATTACK

Baptist Health System, San Antonio
Baptist St. Anthony's Health System, Amarillo

Baylor All Saints Medical Center at Fort Worth, Fort Worth
Coryell Memorial Hospital, Gatesville
Doctors Hospital—Parkway, Houston
Doctors Hospital—Tidwell, Houston
Edinburg Regional Medical Center, Edinburg
Fort Duncan Medical Center, Eagle Pass
Good Shepherd Medical Center, Longview
Harlingen Medical Center, Harlingen
Harris Methodist Dublin, Dublin
Harris Methodist Erath County, Stephenville
Heart Hospital of Austin, Austin
Lubbock Heart Hospital, Lubbock
Marshall Regional Medical Center, Marshall
Memorial Hermann Katy Hospital, Katy
Methodist Willowbrook Hospital, Houston
Northeast Medical Center, Bonham
Northwest Texas Healthcare System, Amarillo
Renaissance Hospital—Terrell, Terrell
St. Luke's Baptist Hospital, San Antonio
San Jacinto Methodist Hospital, Baytown
Seton Medical Center, Austin
South Austin Hospital, Austin
South Texas Regional Medical Center, Jourdanton
University of Texas Health Center at Tyler, Tyler
West Houston Medical Center, Houston

HEART BYPASS SURGERY

Abilene Regional Medical Center, Abilene
Harlingen Medical Center, Harlingen
Heart Hospital of Austin, Austin
McAllen Medical Center/Heart Hospital, McAllen

HEART FAILURE

Baylor Heart and Vascular Center, Dallas
Baylor Regional Medical Center at Grapevine, Grapevine
Baylor Regional Medical Center at Plano, Plano
Bayshore Medical Center in Pasadena, Pasadena
Christus Santa Rosa Healthcare, San Antonio
Christus Spohn Hospital Corpus Christi—South, Corpus Christi
Christus Spohn Hospital—Corpus Christi Memorial, Corpus Christi
Clear Lake Regional Medical Center, Webster
Connally Memorial Medical Center, Floresville
Conroe Regional Medical Center, Conroe
Doctors Hospital at Renaissance, Edinburg
East Texas Medical Center—Gilmer, Gilmer
Edinburg Regional Medical Center, Edinburg
El Campo Memorial Hospital, El Campo
Ennis Regional Medical Center, Ennis
Fort Duncan Medical Center, Eagle Pass

Good Shepherd Medical Center, Longview
Harlingen Medical Center, Harlingen
Harris Methodist Fort Worth, Fort Worth
Heart Hospital of Austin, Austin
Huguley Memorial Medical Center, Fort Worth
Lubbock Heart Hospital, Lubbock
Mainland Medical Center, Texas City
McAllen Medical Center/Heart Hospital, McAllen
Medical Center at Lancaster, Lancaster
Memorial Hermann Fort Bend Hospital, Missouri City
Memorial Hermann Katy Hospital, Katy
Memorial Hermann Southwest Hospital, Houston
Memorial Hermann—Texas Medical Center, Houston
Methodist Hospital, San Antonio
Methodist Specialty and Transplant Hospital, San Antonio
Methodist Sugar Land Hospital, Sugar Land
Metropolitan Methodist Hospital, San Antonio
Northeast Methodist Hospital, Live Oak
Northwest Texas Healthcare System, Amarillo
Oakbend Medical Center, Richmond
Pampa Regional Medical Center, Pampa
Renaissance Hospital—Terrell, Terrell
St. David's Hospital, Austin
San Jacinto Methodist Hospital, Baytown
South Austin Hospital, Austin
South Texas Regional Medical Center, Jourdanton
Southside Health Center, Corpus Christi
Southwest General Hospital, San Antonio
Texsan Heart Hospital, San Antonio
Tomball Regional Hospital, Tomball
University of Texas Medical Branch Galveston, Galveston
West Houston Medical Center, Houston

VALVE REPLACEMENT SURGERY
None

CRITICAL CARE

DIABETIC ACIDOSIS AND COMA
Memorial Hermann Southwest Hospital, Houston
Memorial Hermann—Texas Medical Center, Houston
Providence Memorial Hospital, El Paso

PULMONARY EMBOLISM
Baylor All Saints Medical Center at Fort Worth, Fort Worth
Baylor Medical Center at Irving, Irving
Detar Hospital Navarro, Victoria
Detar Hospital North, Victoria

RESPIRATORY FAILURE
American Transitional Hospital—Houston W, Houston
Baptist Health System, San Antonio
Baptist St. Anthony's Health System, Amarillo
Baylor University Medical Center, Dallas
Bayshore Medical Center in Pasadena, Pasadena
Central Texas Hospital, Cameron
Christus Santa Rosa Healthcare, San Antonio
Clear Lake Regional Medical Center, Webster
Clearview Hospital, Midland
Cypress Fairbanks Medical Center, Houston
Doctors Hospital—Parkway, Houston
Doctors Hospital—Tidwell, Houston
East Houston Regional Medical Center, Houston
East Texas Medical Center, Tyler
Edinburg Regional Medical Center, Edinburg
Good Shepherd Medical Center, Longview
Harris Methodist Fort Worth, Fort Worth
Houston Northwest Medical Center, Houston
Huguley Memorial Medical Center, Fort Worth
McKenna Memorial Hospital, New Braunfels
Medical Center at Lancaster, Lancaster
Medical Center of Arlington, Arlington
Memorial Acute Long Term Care Hospital, Lufkin
Memorial Hermann Fort Bend Hospital, Missouri City
Memorial Hermann Memorial City Medical Center, Houston
Memorial Hermann Southwest Hospital, Houston
Memorial Medical Center of East Texas, Lufkin
Methodist Sugar Land Hospital, Sugar Land
Midland Memorial Hospital, Midland
Northwest Texas Healthcare System, Amarillo
Oakbend Medical Center, Richmond
Pampa Regional Medical Center, Pampa
Presbyterian Hospital of Plano, Plano
Providence Healthcare Network, Waco
Renaissance Hospital—Terrell, Terrell
RHD Memorial Medical Center, Dallas
Rio Grande Regional Hospital, McAllen
St. Luke's Baptist Hospital, San Antonio
St. Luke's Episcopal Hospital, Houston
Sam Houston Memorial Hospital, Houston
San Jacinto Methodist Hospital, Baytown
Sempercare Hospital of Midland, Midland
Spring Branch Medical Center, Houston
Sun Belt Regional Medical Center—East, Channelview
Titus County Memorial Hospital, Mt. Pleasant
University of Texas Health Center at Tyler, Tyler
Woodland Heights Medical Center, Lufkin

Hospitals receiving a five star rating in a particular procedure have patient outcomes that put them among the best in the nation. For full definitions of ratings and awards, see Appendix.

SEPSIS

American Transitional Hospital—Houston W, Houston
Baptist Health System, San Antonio
Baptist St. Anthony's Health System, Amarillo
Baylor Medical Center at Irving, Irving
Baylor University Medical Center, Dallas
Bayshore Medical Center in Pasadena, Pasadena
Brackenridge Hospital, Austin
Christus Santa Rosa Healthcare, San Antonio
Christus Spohn Hospital Corpus Christi—South, Corpus Christi
Christus Spohn Hospital—Corpus Christi Memorial, Corpus Christi
Clear Lake Regional Medical Center, Webster
Connally Memorial Medical Center, Floresville
Cypress Fairbanks Medical Center, Houston
Dallas Southwest Medical Center, Dallas
Doctors Hospital at Renaissance, Edinburg
Doctors Hospital of Laredo, Laredo
Doctors Hospital—Parkway, Houston
Doctors Hospital—Tidwell, Houston
East Houston Regional Medical Center, Houston
Falls Community Hospital and Clinic, Marlin
Fort Duncan Medical Center, Eagle Pass
Good Shepherd Medical Center, Longview
Gulf Coast Medical Center, Wharton
Heart Hospital of Austin, Austin
Hill Regional Hospital, Hillsboro
Houston Northwest Medical Center, Houston
Laredo Medical Center, Laredo
Longview Regional Medical Center, Longview
Memorial Hermann Fort Bend Hospital, Missouri City
Memorial Hermann Katy Hospital, Katy
Memorial Hermann Memorial City Medical Center, Houston
Memorial Hermann Southwest Hospital, Houston
Methodist Sugar Land Hospital, Sugar Land
Mother Frances Hospital—Tyler, Tyler
Northeast Medical Center Hospital, Humble
Northwest Texas Healthcare System, Amarillo
Oakbend Medical Center, Richmond
Presbyterian Hospital of Plano, Plano
Renaissance Hospital—Dallas, Dallas
Renaissance Hospital—Terrell, Terrell
Rio Grande Regional Hospital, McAllen
St. David's Hospital, Austin
St. Luke's Baptist Hospital, San Antonio
St. Luke's Episcopal Hospital, Houston
Sam Houston Memorial Hospital, Houston
San Jacinto Methodist Hospital, Baytown
Seton Medical Center, Austin
South Austin Hospital, Austin
Southside Health Center, Corpus Christi
Spring Branch Medical Center, Houston
Sun Belt Regional Medical Center—East, Channelview
UT Southwestern Medical Center, Dallas
Valley Baptist Medical Center, Harlingen
West Houston Medical Center, Houston

GASTROINTESTINAL

BOWEL OBSTRUCTION

Arlington Memorial Hospital, Arlington
Baptist St. Anthony's Health System, Amarillo
Baylor Medical Center at Waxahachie, Waxahachie
Doctors Hospital at Renaissance, Edinburg
Mainland Medical Center, Texas City
Medical Center of Plano, Plano
Methodist Willowbrook Hospital, Houston
Mother Frances Hospital—Tyler, Tyler
Presbyterian Hospital of Plano, Plano
Seton Medical Center, Austin
Texoma Medical Center, Denison
UT Southwestern Medical Center, Dallas

CHOLECYSTECTOMY

American Transitional Hospital—Houston W, Houston
Arlington Memorial Hospital, Arlington
Bayshore Medical Center in Pasadena, Pasadena
Central Texas Medical Center, San Marcos
Christus St. Elizabeth Hospital, Beaumont
Christus St. Michael Health System, Texarkana
Christus Spohn Hospital—Alice, Alice
Christus Spohn Hospital—Kleberg, Kingsville
Citizens Medical Center, Victoria
Conroe Regional Medical Center, Conroe
Covenant Hospital Plainview, Plainview
Del Sol Medical Center, El Paso
Doctors Hospital of Laredo, Laredo
East Texas Medical Center, Tyler
East Texas Medical Center—Crockett, Crockett
Fort Duncan Medical Center, Eagle Pass
Georgetown Hospital, Georgetown
Harlingen Medical Center, Harlingen
Hillcrest Baptist Medical Center, Waco
Houston Northwest Medical Center, Houston
Knapp Medical Center, Weslaco
Marshall Regional Medical Center, Marshall
Medical Center Hospital, Odessa
Memorial Acute Long Term Care Hospital, Lufkin
Memorial Hermann Baptist Beaumont Hospital, Beaumont

Memorial Hermann Memorial City Medical Center, Houston
Memorial Hermann Southwest Hospital, Houston
Memorial Medical Center of East Texas, Lufkin
Methodist Medical Center, Dallas
Mother Frances Hospital—Tyler, Tyler
North Hills Hospital, North Richland Hills
Pampa Regional Medical Center, Pampa
Parkview Regional Hospital, Mexia
St. Luke's Community Medical Center—The Woodlands, The Woodlands
Sam Houston Memorial Hospital, Houston
SCCI Hospital—San Angelo, San Angelo
Scott and White Memorial Hospital, Temple
Shannon West Texas Medical Center, San Angelo
South Austin Hospital, Austin
Spring Branch Medical Center, Houston
Texoma Medical Center, Denison
Val Verde Regional Medical Center, Del Rio
Valley Baptist Medical Center, Harlingen
Valley Regional Medical Center, Brownsville
Wadley Regional Medical Center, Texarkana

GASTROINTESTINAL BLEED

Harris Methodist Fort Worth, Fort Worth
Kingwood Medical Center, Kingwood
Memorial Hermann Southwest Hospital, Houston
Methodist Hospital, San Antonio
Methodist Specialty and Transplant Hospital, San Antonio
Metropolitan Methodist Hospital, San Antonio
Northeast Medical Center Hospital, Humble
Northeast Methodist Hospital, Live Oak
Scott and White Memorial Hospital, Temple

GASTROINTESTINAL SURGERIES AND PROCEDURES

American Transitional Hospital—Houston W, Houston
Baylor Regional Medical Center at Grapevine, Grapevine
Baylor University Medical Center, Dallas
Campbell Health System, Weatherford
Christus Santa Rosa Healthcare, San Antonio
Christus Spohn Hospital—Alice, Alice
Harlingen Medical Center, Harlingen
Harris Methodist Fort Worth, Fort Worth
Houston Northwest Medical Center, Houston
Knapp Medical Center, Weslaco
Laredo Medical Center, Laredo
Mainland Medical Center, Texas City
McKenna Memorial Hospital, New Braunfels
Medical Center of McKinney, McKinney

Medical Center of Plano, Plano
Memorial Acute Long Term Care Hospital, Lufkin
Memorial Hermann Southwest Hospital, Houston
Memorial Medical Center of East Texas, Lufkin
Methodist Hospital, San Antonio
Methodist Specialty and Transplant Hospital, San Antonio
Metropolitan Methodist Hospital, San Antonio
Northeast Methodist Hospital, Live Oak
Providence Memorial Hospital, El Paso
Rolling Plains Memorial Hospital, Sweetwater
Round Rock Medical Center, Round Rock
Sam Houston Memorial Hospital, Houston
South Austin Hospital, Austin
Spring Branch Medical Center, Houston
Texoma Medical Center, Denison
United Regional Health Care System, Wichita Falls
Westpark Medical Center, McKinney

PANCREATITIS

Baylor All Saints Medical Center at Fort Worth, Fort Worth
Christus St. Michael Health System, Texarkana
Clearview Hospital, Midland
Cypress Fairbanks Medical Center, Houston
Harris Methodist Fort Worth, Fort Worth
Mainland Medical Center, Texas City
Midland Memorial Hospital, Midland
Northeast Medical Center Hospital, Humble
Sempercare Hospital of Midland, Midland

GENERAL SURGERY

APPENDECTOMY

Abilene Regional Medical Center, Abilene
Angleton-Danbury Medical Center, Angleton
Arlington Memorial Hospital, Arlington
Baptist St. Anthony's Health System, Amarillo
Baylor Regional Medical Center at Grapevine, Grapevine
Bayshore Medical Center in Pasadena, Pasadena
Big Bend Regional Medical Center, Alpine
Brazosport Regional Health System, Lake Jackson
Brownwood Regional Medical Center, Brownwood
Christus St. Michael Health System, Texarkana
Christus Spohn Hospital—Kleberg, Kingsville
Clear Lake Regional Medical Center, Webster
Clearview Hospital, Midland
Corpus Christi Medical Center, Corpus Christi
Del Sol Medical Center, El Paso
Fort Duncan Medical Center, Eagle Pass
Good Shepherd Medical Center, Longview
Harris County Hospital District, Houston

Kingwood Medical Center, Kingwood
Medical City Dallas Hospital, Dallas
Medical Center of Arlington, Arlington
Medical Center of Lewisville, Lewisville
Memorial Hermann Baptist Beaumont Hospital, Beaumont
Memorial Hermann Southwest Hospital, Houston
Methodist Medical Center, Dallas
Midland Memorial Hospital, Midland
Paris Regional Medical Center, Paris
Presbyterian Hospital of Winnsboro, Winnsboro
RHD Memorial Medical Center, Dallas
Round Rock Medical Center, Round Rock
St. David's Hospital, Austin
St. Joseph Regional Health Center, Bryan
SCCI Hospital—San Angelo, San Angelo
Scott and White Memorial Hospital, Temple
Sempercare Hospital of Midland, Midland
Seton Highland Lakes, Burnet
Seton Medical Center, Austin
Shannon West Texas Medical Center, San Angelo
Sierra Medical Center, El Paso
Smithville Regional Hospital, Smithville
South Austin Hospital, Austin
University Health System, San Antonio
Valley Baptist Medical Center, Harlingen
Valley Baptist Medical Center—Brownsville, Brownsville
Valley Regional Medical Center, Brownsville
Walls Regional Hospital, Cleburne
West Houston Medical Center, Houston

MATERNITY CARE

Bayshore Medical Center in Pasadena, Pasadena
Charlton Methodist Hospital, Dallas
Christus St. Elizabeth Hospital, Beaumont
Christus St. John Hospital, Houston
Christus St. Mary Hospital, Port Arthur
Christus Spohn Hospital Corpus Christi—South, Corpus Christi
Christus Spohn Hospital—Corpus Christi Memorial, Corpus Christi
Clear Lake Regional Medical Center, Webster
Cleveland Regional Medical Center, Cleveland
Corpus Christi Medical Center, Corpus Christi
Cypress Fairbanks Medical Center, Houston
Del Sol Medical Center, El Paso
Doctors Hospital of Laredo, Laredo
East Texas Medical Center—Athens, Athens
Henderson Memorial Hospital, Henderson
Houston Northwest Medical Center, Houston
Laird Memorial Hospital, Kilgore

Las Palmas Medical Center, El Paso
Marshall Regional Medical Center, Marshall
The Medical Center of Southeast Texas, Port Arthur
Memorial Acute Long Term Care Hosp, Lufkin
Memorial Hermann Katy Hospital, Katy
Memorial Hermann Memorial City Medical Center, Houston
Memorial Hermann Southwest Hospital, Houston
Memorial Medical Center of East Texas, Lufkin
Methodist Hospital, San Antonio
Methodist Specialty and Transplant Hospital, San Antonio
Metropolitan Methodist Hospital, San Antonio
Mission Regional Medical Center, Mission
North Austin Medical Center, Austin
Northeast Medical Center Hospital, Humble
Northeast Methodist Hospital, Live Oak
Oakbend Medical Center, Richmond
Odessa Regional Medical Center, Odessa
Park Plaza Hospital and Medical Center, Houston
Providence Memorial Hospital, El Paso
Rio Grande Regional Hospital, McAllen
St. David's Hospital, Austin
St. Luke's Community Medical Center—The Woodlands, The Woodlands
Seton Highland Lakes, Burnet
Seton Medical Center, Austin
Southside Health Center, Corpus Christi
Southwest General Hospital, San Antonio
Twelve Oaks Medical Center, Houston
United Regional Health Care System, Wichita Falls
Val Verde Regional Medical Center, Del Rio
West Houston Medical Center, Houston
Woman's Hospital at Dallas Regional Medical Center, Mesquite

ORTHOPEDICS

BACK AND NECK SURGERY
(EXCEPT SPINAL FUSION)

Arlington Memorial Hospital, Arlington
Baylor University Medical Center, Dallas
Bayshore Medical Center in Pasadena, Pasadena
Christus St. Elizabeth Hospital, Beaumont
Clearview Hospital, Midland
Detar Hospital Navarro, Victoria
Detar Hospital North, Victoria
Diagnostic Center Hospital, Houston
Good Shepherd Medical Center, Longview
Memorial Acute Long Term Care Hospital, Lufkin
Memorial Hermann Baptist Beaumont Hospital, Beaumont

Hospitals receiving a five star rating in a particular procedure have patient outcomes that put them among the best in the nation. For full definitions of ratings and awards, see Appendix.

Memorial Hermann Memorial City Medical Center, Houston
Memorial Medical Center of East Texas, Lufkin
Methodist Hospital, Houston
Midland Memorial Hospital, Midland
Presbyterian Hospital of Dallas, Dallas
Rio Grande Regional Hospital, McAllen
St. Joseph Regional Health Center, Bryan
San Jacinto Methodist Hospital, Baytown
SCCI Hospital—San Angelo, San Angelo
Sempercare Hospital of Midland, Midland
Seton Medical Center, Austin
Shannon West Texas Medical Center, San Angelo
Sierra Medical Center, El Paso
UT Southwestern Medical Center, Dallas

BACK AND NECK SURGERY (SPINAL FUSION)
Baptist St. Anthony's Health System, Amarillo
Baylor University Medical Center, Dallas
Bayshore Medical Center in Pasadena, Pasadena
Christus St. Elizabeth Hospital, Beaumont
Clearview Hospital, Midland
College Station Medical Center, College Station
Corpus Christi Medical Center, Corpus Christi
Detar Hospital Navarro, Victoria
Detar Hospital North, Victoria
Diagnostic Center Hospital, Houston
Doctors Hospital at Renaissance, Edinburg
Good Shepherd Medical Center, Longview
Harlingen Medical Center, Harlingen
Houston Northwest Medical Center, Houston
Memorial Hermann Baptist Beaumont Hospital, Beaumont
Methodist Hospital, Houston
Midland Memorial Hospital, Midland
Plaza Medical Center of Fort Worth, Fort Worth
Providence Healthcare Network, Waco
SCCI Hospital—San Angelo, San Angelo
Scott and White Memorial Hospital, Temple
Sempercare Hospital of Midland, Midland
Shannon West Texas Medical Center, San Angelo
Texas Orthopedic Hospital, Houston
Wadley Regional Medical Center, Texarkana

HIP FRACTURE REPAIR
Angleton-Danbury Medical Center, Angleton
Arlington Memorial Hospital, Arlington
Baptist Health System, San Antonio
Baptist St. Anthony's Health System, Amarillo
Baylor Medical Center at Garland, Garland
Bayshore Medical Center in Pasadena, Pasadena
Central Texas Medical Center, San Marcos
Christus St. Catherine Health and Wellness Center, Katy

Christus St. Michael Health System, Texarkana
Christus Santa Rosa Healthcare, San Antonio
Clear Lake Regional Medical Center, Webster
Clearview Hospital, Midland
Covenant Medical Center, Lubbock
Del Sol Medical Center, El Paso
Detar Hospital Navarro, Victoria
Detar Hospital North, Victoria
East Houston Regional Medical Center, Houston
East Texas Medical Center, Tyler
Ennis Regional Medical Center, Ennis
Georgetown Hospital, Georgetown
Good Shepherd Medical Center, Longview
Guadalupe Valley Hospital, Seguin
Harlingen Medical Center, Harlingen
Hill Country Memorial Hospital, Fredericksburg
Hillcrest Baptist Medical Center, Waco
Kell West Regional Hospital, Wichita Falls
Kingwood Medical Center, Kingwood
Lake Granbury Medical Center, Granbury
Matagorda General Hospital, Bay City
Medical Center Hospital, Odessa
Medical Center of Arlington, Arlington
Memorial Hermann Baptist Beaumont Hospital, Beaumont
Memorial Hermann Southwest Hospital, Houston
Metroplex Hospital, Killeen
Midland Memorial Hospital, Midland
North Austin Medical Center, Austin
Paris Regional Medical Center, Paris
Presbyterian Hospital of Denton, Denton
Presbyterian Hospital of Plano, Plano
Providence Healthcare Network, Waco
Providence Memorial Hospital, El Paso
St. David's Hospital, Austin
St. Luke's Baptist Hospital, San Antonio
St. Luke's Episcopal Hospital, Houston
Scott and White Memorial Hospital, Temple
Sempercare Hospital of Midland, Midland
Seton Medical Center, Austin
Sierra Medical Center, El Paso
Sun Belt Regional Medical Center—East, Channelview
Texoma Medical Center, Denison
Trinity Medical Center, Carrollton
United Regional Health Care System, Wichita Falls

TOTAL HIP REPLACEMENT
Clearview Hospital, Midland
Doctors Hospital at White Rock Lake, Dallas
El Paso Specialty Hospital, El Paso
Kell West Regional Hospital, Wichita Falls
Las Palmas Medical Center, El Paso

Memorial Hermann Baptist Beaumont Hospital, Beaumont
Midland Memorial Hospital, Midland
Presbyterian Hospital of Plano, Plano
Providence Healthcare Network, Waco
SCCI Hospital—San Angelo, San Angelo
Scott and White Memorial Hospital, Temple
Sempercare Hospital of Midland, Midland
Seton Medical Center, Austin
Shannon West Texas Medical Center, San Angelo
Texas Orthopedic Hospital, Houston
Valley Baptist Medical Center, Harlingen
Wadley Regional Medical Center, Texarkana
Walls Regional Hospital, Cleburne
Woodland Heights Medical Center, Lufkin

TOTAL KNEE REPLACEMENT
Christus St. Michael Health System, Texarkana
Christus Santa Rosa Healthcare, San Antonio
Citizens Medical Center, Victoria
Covenant Medical Center, Lubbock
Detar Hospital Navarro, Victoria
Detar Hospital North, Victoria
Doctors Hospital of Laredo, Laredo
El Paso Specialty Hospital, El Paso
Highland Medical Center, Lubbock
Hillcrest Baptist Medical Center, Waco
Kell West Regional Hospital, Wichita Falls
Laredo Medical Center, Laredo
Las Palmas Medical Center, El Paso
McKenna Memorial Hospital, New Braunfels
Medical City Dallas Hospital, Dallas
Medical Center Hospital, Odessa
Memorial Acute Long Term Care Hospital, Lufkin
Memorial Hermann Baptist Beaumont Hospital, Beaumont
Memorial Hermann Southwest Hospital, Houston
Memorial Medical Center of East Texas, Lufkin
Nix Health Care System, San Antonio
Presbyterian Hospital of Denton, Denton
Presbyterian Hospital of Plano, Plano
Providence Healthcare Network, Waco
St. Joseph Regional Health Center, Bryan
SCCI Hospital—San Angelo, San Angelo
Scott and White Memorial Hospital, Temple
Seton Medical Center, Austin
Shannon West Texas Medical Center, San Angelo
Sid Peterson Memorial Hospital, Kerrville
Sierra Medical Center, El Paso
Texas Orthopedic Hospital, Houston
Texoma Medical Center, Denison
United Regional Health Care System, Wichita Falls
Valley Baptist Medical Center, Harlingen

Valley Regional Medical Center, Brownsville
Wadley Regional Medical Center, Texarkana
Woman's Hospital at Dallas Regional Medical
    Center, Mesquite

PROSTATECTOMY

Baptist Health System, San Antonio
Baylor University Medical Center, Dallas
Christus St. Michael Health System, Texarkana
Good Shepherd Medical Center, Longview
Harris Methodist Dublin, Dublin
Harris Methodist Erath County, Stephenville
Harris Methodist Fort Worth, Fort Worth
The Hospital at Westlake Medical Center, Austin
Physicians Specialty Hospital of El Paso, El Paso
Providence Healthcare Network, Waco
Providence Memorial Hospital, El Paso
St. David's Hospital, Austin
St. Luke's Baptist Hospital, San Antonio
St. Luke's Episcopal Hospital, Houston
Scott and White Memorial Hospital, Temple
South Austin Hospital, Austin

PULMONARY

CHRONIC OBSTRUCTIVE PULMONARY DISEASE (COPD)

Abilene Regional Medical Center, Abilene
American Transitional Hospital—Houston W,
    Houston
Baylor Medical Center at Garland, Garland
Brackenridge Hospital, Austin
Christus Spohn Hospital Corpus Christi—South,
    Corpus Christi
Christus Spohn Hospital—Alice, Alice
Christus Spohn Hospital—Corpus Christi
    Memorial, Corpus Christi
Cleveland Regional Medical Center, Cleveland
Conroe Regional Medical Center, Conroe
Cypress Fairbanks Medical Center, Houston
Fort Duncan Medical Center, Eagle Pass
Harris County Hospital District, Houston
Henderson Memorial Hospital, Henderson
Hendrick Medical Center, Abilene
Knapp Medical Center, Weslaco
Memorial Acute Long Term Care Hospital, Lufkin
Memorial Hermann Katy Hospital, Katy
Memorial Hermann Southwest Hospital, Houston
Memorial Medical Center of East Texas, Lufkin
Mission Regional Medical Center, Mission
Mother Frances Hospital—Tyler, Tyler
North Hills Hospital, North Richland Hills

Northeast Medical Center Hospital, Humble
Northwest Texas Healthcare System, Amarillo
R. E. Thomason General Hospital, El Paso
Renaissance Hospital—Terrell, Terrell
Rio Grande Regional Hospital, McAllen
Rolling Plains Memorial Hospital, Sweetwater
St. Luke's Community Medical Center—The
    Woodlands, The Woodlands
St. Luke's Episcopal Hospital, Houston
Sam Houston Memorial Hospital, Houston
San Jacinto Methodist Hospital, Baytown
Smithville Regional Hospital, Smithville
South Texas Regional Medical Center, Jourdanton
Southside Health Center, Corpus Christi
Spring Branch Medical Center, Houston
Tomball Regional Hospital, Tomball
United Regional Health Care System, Wichita Falls
West Houston Medical Center, Houston

PNEUMONIA

American Transitional Hospital—Houston W,
    Houston
Baptist Health System, San Antonio
Baptist St. Anthony's Health System, Amarillo
Baylor All Saints Medical Center at Fort Worth,
    Fort Worth
Baylor Medical Center at Irving, Irving
Baylor Regional Medical Center at Grapevine,
    Grapevine
Bayshore Medical Center in Pasadena, Pasadena
Brazosport Regional Health System, Lake Jackson
Central Texas Medical Center, San Marcos
Christus St. Catherine Health and Wellness
    Center, Katy
Christus St. John Hospital, Houston
Christus Santa Rosa Healthcare, San Antonio
Clear Lake Regional Medical Center, Webster
Cleveland Regional Medical Center, Cleveland
Conroe Regional Medical Center, Conroe
Cypress Fairbanks Medical Center, Houston
Dallas Regional Medical Center—Galloway
    Campus, Mesquite
Doctors Hospital at Renaissance, Edinburg
Doctors Hospital—Parkway, Houston
Doctors Hospital—Tidwell, Houston
Dolly Vinsant Memorial Hospital, San Benito
East Houston Regional Medical Center, Houston
East Texas Medical Center—Gilmer, Gilmer
Edinburg Regional Medical Center, Edinburg
Electra Memorial Hospital, Electra
Falls Community Hospital and Clinic, Marlin
Fort Duncan Medical Center, Eagle Pass

Good Shepherd Medical Center, Longview
Harlingen Medical Center, Harlingen
Harris Methodist Dublin, Dublin
Harris Methodist Erath County, Stephenville
Harris Methodist Fort Worth, Fort Worth
Heart Hospital of Austin, Austin
Houston Northwest Medical Center, Houston
Huguley Memorial Medical Center, Fort Worth
Kingwood Medical Center, Kingwood
Knapp Medical Center, Weslaco
Lake Granbury Medical Center, Granbury
Lake Whitney Medical Center, Whitney
Las Palmas Medical Center, El Paso
Longview Regional Medical Center, Longview
McAllen Medical Center/Heart Hospital, McAllen
Medical Center at Lancaster, Lancaster
Memorial Hermann Fort Bend Hospital,
    Missouri City
Memorial Hermann Katy Hospital, Katy
Memorial Hermann Memorial City Medical Center,
    Houston
Memorial Hermann Southwest Hospital, Houston
Methodist Hospital, San Antonio
Methodist Specialty and Transplant Hospital,
    San Antonio
Methodist Willowbrook Hospital, Houston
Metropolitan Methodist Hospital, San Antonio
Mission Regional Medical Center, Mission
Northeast Medical Center Hospital, Humble
Northeast Methodist Hospital, Live Oak
Northwest Texas Healthcare System, Amarillo
Oakbend Medical Center, Richmond
Park Plaza Hospital and Medical Center, Houston
Physicians Specialty Hospital of El Paso, El Paso
Presbyterian Hospital of Greenville, Greenville
Renaissance Hospital, Groves
Rio Grande Regional Hospital, McAllen
Rolling Plains Memorial Hospital, Sweetwater
St. David's Hospital, Austin
St. Luke's Baptist Hospital, San Antonio
St. Luke's Episcopal Hospital, Houston
Sam Houston Memorial Hospital, Houston
San Jacinto Methodist Hospital, Baytown
Seton Northwest Hospital, Austin
Smithville Regional Hospital, Smithville
South Texas Regional Medical Center, Jourdanton
Southwestern General Hospital, El Paso
Spring Branch Medical Center, Houston
Sun Belt Regional Medical Center—East, Channelview
Titus County Memorial Hospital, Mt. Pleasant
UT Southwestern Medical Center, Dallas
UT Southwestern Zale Lipshy Hospital, Dallas

Hospitals receiving a five star rating in a particular procedure have patient outcomes that put them among the best in the nation. For full definitions of ratings and awards, see Appendix.

Valley Baptist Medical Center, Harlingen
W. J. Mangold Memorial Hospital, Lockney
Walls Regional Hospital, Cleburne
West Houston Medical Center, Houston
Woodland Heights Medical Center, Lufkin

STROKE

Baptist St. Anthony's Health System, Amarillo
Baylor All Saints Medical Center at Fort Worth, Fort Worth
Baylor Medical Center at Garland, Garland
Baylor Medical Center at Irving, Irving
Brackenridge Hospital, Austin
Charlton Methodist Hospital, Dallas
Clear Lake Regional Medical Center, Webster
Covenant Medical Center, Lubbock
Cypress Fairbanks Medical Center, Houston
Diagnostic Center Hospital, Houston
Doctors Hospital at Renaissance, Edinburg
East Houston Regional Medical Center, Houston
East Texas Medical Center, Tyler
Good Shepherd Medical Center, Longview
Harris Methodist Fort Worth, Fort Worth
Harris Methodist Southwest, Fort Worth
Houston Northwest Medical Center, Houston
Huguley Memorial Medical Center, Fort Worth
Laird Memorial Hospital, Kilgore
Laredo Medical Center, Laredo
Las Palmas Medical Center, El Paso
Longview Regional Medical Center, Longview
McAllen Medical Center/Heart Hospital, McAllen
Medical Center at Lancaster, Lancaster
Medical Center of Arlington, Arlington
Memorial Acute Long Term Care Hospital, Lufkin
Memorial Hermann Katy Hospital, Katy
Memorial Hermann Memorial City Medical Center, Houston
Memorial Hermann Southwest Hospital, Houston
Memorial Medical Center of East Texas, Lufkin
Methodist Hospital, Houston
Methodist Medical Center, Dallas
Methodist Willowbrook Hospital, Houston
Mother Frances Hospital—Tyler, Tyler
North Austin Medical Center, Austin
North Hills Hospital, North Richland Hills
Northwest Texas Healthcare System, Amarillo
Oakbend Medical Center, Richmond
Parkview Regional Hospital, Mexia
Plaza Medical Center of Fort Worth, Fort Worth
Presbyterian Hospital of Dallas, Dallas
Presbyterian Hospital of Denton, Denton

Providence Healthcare Network, Waco
St. David's Hospital, Austin
St. Joseph Medical Center, Houston
St. Luke's Community Medical Center—The Woodlands, The Woodlands
St. Luke's Episcopal Hospital, Houston
San Jacinto Methodist Hospital, Baytown
Scott and White Memorial Hospital, Temple
Sun Belt Regional Medical Center—East, Channelview
Titus County Memorial Hospital, Mt. Pleasant
University of Texas Health Center at Tyler, Tyler
UT Southwestern Zale Lipshy Hospital, Dallas
Valley Baptist Medical Center, Harlingen
Valley Baptist Medical Center—Brownsville, Brownsville

VASCULAR

CAROTID SURGERY

Arlington Memorial Hospital, Arlington
Baptist Health System, San Antonio
Baylor Heart and Vascular Center, Dallas
Christus St. Elizabeth Hospital, Beaumont
Christus St. Michael Health System, Texarkana
Christus Spohn Hospital Corpus Christi—South, Corpus Christi
Christus Spohn Hospital—Corpus Christi Memorial, Corpus Christi
Clear Lake Regional Medical Center, Webster
Conroe Regional Medical Center, Conroe
Corpus Christi Medical Center, Corpus Christi
Denton Regional Medical Center, Denton
Diagnostic Center Hospital, Houston
East Texas Medical Center, Tyler
Lubbock Heart Hospital, Lubbock
The Medical Center of Southeast Texas, Port Arthur
Memorial Hermann Baptist Beaumont Hospital, Beaumont
Methodist Hospital, Houston
Presbyterian Hospital of Dallas, Dallas
St. David's Hospital, Austin
St. Joseph Medical Center, Houston
St. Joseph Regional Health Center, Bryan
St. Luke's Baptist Hospital, San Antonio
St. Luke's Episcopal Hospital, Houston
SCCI Hospital—San Angelo, San Angelo
Scott and White Memorial Hospital, Temple
Shannon West Texas Medical Center, San Angelo
Sierra Medical Center, El Paso
Southside Health Center, Corpus Christi
Texoma Medical Center, Denison

United Regional Health Care System, Wichita Falls
University of Texas Health Center at Tyler, Tyler
UT Southwestern Zale Lipshy Hospital, Dallas
Valley Baptist Medical Center, Harlingen
Valley Regional Medical Center, Brownsville
Wadley Regional Medical Center, Texarkana
West Houston Medical Center, Houston
Woodland Heights Medical Center, Lufkin

PERIPHERAL VASCULAR BYPASS

Alliance Hospital, Odessa
American Transitional Hospital—Houston W, Houston
Baptist Health System, San Antonio
Christus St. Michael Health System, Texarkana
Christus Spohn Hospital Corpus Christi—South, Corpus Christi
Christus Spohn Hospital—Corpus Christi Memorial, Corpus Christi
Good Shepherd Medical Center, Longview
Lubbock Heart Hospital, Lubbock
Memorial Hermann Baptist Beaumont Hospital, Beaumont
Memorial Hermann Southwest Hospital, Houston
Methodist Hospital, San Antonio
Methodist Specialty and Transplant Hospital, San Antonio
Metropolitan Methodist Hospital, San Antonio
Northeast Methodist Hospital, Live Oak
Rio Grande Regional Hospital, McAllen
St. Joseph Regional Health Center, Bryan
St. Luke's Baptist Hospital, San Antonio
Sam Houston Memorial Hospital, Houston
SCCI Hospital—San Angelo, San Angelo
Shannon West Texas Medical Center, San Angelo
Southside Health Center, Corpus Christi
Spring Branch Medical Center, Houston
Wadley Regional Medical Center, Texarkana

RESECTION/REPLACEMENT OF ABDOMINAL AORTA

Memorial Hermann—Texas Medical Center, Houston

WOMEN'S HEALTH

Clear Lake Regional Medical Center, Webster
Harlingen Medical Center, Harlingen
McAllen Medical Center/Heart Hospital, McAllen
Memorial Hermann Memorial City Medical Center, Houston
Memorial Hermann Southwest Hospital, Houston
South Austin Hospital, Austin
West Houston Medical Center, Houston

BARIATRIC SURGERY

None

CARDIAC

ATRIAL FIBRILLATION

St. Mark's Hospital, Salt Lake City

CORONARY INTERVENTIONAL PROCEDURES (ANGIOPLASTY/STENT)

None

HEART ATTACK

None

HEART BYPASS SURGERY

None

HEART FAILURE

Ogden Regional Medical Center, Ogden
St. Mark's Hospital, Salt Lake City

VALVE REPLACEMENT SURGERY

None

CRITICAL CARE

DIABETIC ACIDOSIS AND COMA

LDS Hospital, Salt Lake City

PULMONARY EMBOLISM

Alta View Hospital, Sandy
St. Mark's Hospital, Salt Lake City

RESPIRATORY FAILURE

St. Mark's Hospital, Salt Lake City

SEPSIS

Alta View Hospital, Sandy
Castleview Hospital, Price
Cottonwood Hospital, Murray
Dixie Regional Medical Center, St. George
Mountain View Hospital, Payson
Mountain West Medical Center, Tooele

GASTROINTESTINAL

BOWEL OBSTRUCTION

Cottonwood Hospital, Murray
Dixie Regional Medical Center, St. George
LDS Hospital, Salt Lake City
Logan Regional Hospital, Logan
McKay-Dee Hospital Center, Ogden

CHOLECYSTECTOMY

None

GASTROINTESTINAL BLEED

Cottonwood Hospital, Murray
Mountain West Medical Center, Tooele
St. Mark's Hospital, Salt Lake City

GASTROINTESTINAL SURGERIES AND PROCEDURES

Davis Hospital and Medical Center, Layton
Salt Lake Regional Medical Center, Salt Lake City

PANCREATITIS

None

GENERAL SURGERY

APPENDECTOMY

Davis Hospital and Medical Center, Layton
Dixie Regional Medical Center, St. George
Ogden Regional Medical Center, Ogden
St. Mark's Hospital, Salt Lake City
Timpanogos Regional Hospital, Orem

MATERNITY CARE

Cottonwood Hospital, Murray
Dixie Regional Medical Center, St. George
McKay-Dee Hospital Center, Ogden
Ogden Regional Medical Center, Ogden

ORTHOPEDICS

BACK AND NECK SURGERY (EXCEPT SPINAL FUSION)

None

BACK AND NECK SURGERY (SPINAL FUSION)

None

HIP FRACTURE REPAIR

Davis Hospital and Medical Center, Layton
Ogden Regional Medical Center, Ogden
Valley View Medical Center, Cedar City

TOTAL HIP REPLACEMENT

Cottonwood Hospital, Murray
Davis Hospital and Medical Center, Layton
Lakeview Hospital, Bountiful
LDS Hospital, Salt Lake City
St. Mark's Hospital, Salt Lake City

TOTAL KNEE REPLACEMENT

St. Mark's Hospital, Salt Lake City
Valley View Medical Center, Cedar City

PROSTATECTOMY

None

PULMONARY

CHRONIC OBSTRUCTIVE PULMONARY DISEASE (COPD)

St. Mark's Hospital, Salt Lake City

PNEUMONIA

Alta View Hospital, Sandy
Cottonwood Hospital, Murray
LDS Hospital, Salt Lake City
Logan Regional Hospital, Logan
McKay-Dee Hospital Center, Ogden
Mountain West Medical Center, Tooele
St. Mark's Hospital, Salt Lake City
Salt Lake Regional Medical Center, Salt Lake City
University of Utah Hospital, Salt Lake City

STROKE

St. Mark's Hospital, Salt Lake City

VASCULAR

CAROTID SURGERY

None

PERIPHERAL VASCULAR BYPASS

None

RESECTION/REPLACEMENT OF ABDOMINAL AORTA

None

WOMEN'S HEALTH

McKay-Dee Hospital Center, Ogden
Ogden Regional Medical Center, Ogden

Hospitals receiving a five star rating in a particular procedure have patient outcomes that put them among the best in the nation. For full definitions of ratings and awards, see Appendix.

BARIATRIC SURGERY

None

CARDIAC

ATRIAL FIBRILLATION
None

CORONARY INTERVENTIONAL PROCEDURES
(ANGIOPLASTY/STENT)
None

HEART ATTACK
Northeastern Vermont Regional Hospital,
St. Johnsbury

HEART BYPASS SURGERY
None

HEART FAILURE
None

VALVE REPLACEMENT SURGERY
None

CRITICAL CARE

DIABETIC ACIDOSIS AND COMA
None

PULMONARY EMBOLISM
None

RESPIRATORY FAILURE
None

SEPSIS
None

GASTROINTESTINAL

BOWEL OBSTRUCTION
None

CHOLECYSTECTOMY
None

GASTROINTESTINAL BLEED
None

GASTROINTESTINAL SURGERIES
AND PROCEDURES
None

PANCREATITIS
None

GENERAL SURGERY

APPENDECTOMY
None

MATERNITY CARE

None

ORTHOPEDICS

BACK AND NECK SURGERY
(EXCEPT SPINAL FUSION)
None

BACK AND NECK SURGERY (SPINAL FUSION)
None

HIP FRACTURE REPAIR
None

TOTAL HIP REPLACEMENT
None

TOTAL KNEE REPLACEMENT
Rutland Regional Medical Center, Rutland

PROSTATECTOMY

Fletcher Allen Hospital of Vermont, Burlington

PULMONARY

CHRONIC OBSTRUCTIVE PULMONARY DISEASE
(COPD)
Central Vermont Medical Center, Barre
North Country Hospital and Health Center,
Newport

PNEUMONIA
Southwestern Vermont Medical Center, Bennington

STROKE

Fletcher Allen Hospital of Vermont, Burlington

VASCULAR

CAROTID SURGERY
None

PERIPHERAL VASCULAR BYPASS
None

RESECTION/REPLACEMENT OF ABDOMINAL AORTA
None

WOMEN'S HEALTH

None

BARIATRIC SURGERY

Bon Secours Maryview Medical Center, Portsmouth
Inova Fair Oaks Hospital, Fairfax
Inova Fairfax Hospital, Falls Church
Lewis-Gale Medical Center, Salem
Northern Virginia Community Hospital, Arlington
Potomac Hospital, Woodbridge
Russell County Medical Center, Lebanon
Sentara Careplex Hospital, Hampton
Sentara Leigh Hospital, Norfolk

CARDIAC

ATRIAL FIBRILLATION
None

CORONARY INTERVENTIONAL PROCEDURES
(ANGIOPLASTY/STENT)
Rockingham Memorial Hospital, Harrisonburg

HEART ATTACK
Augusta Medical Center, Fishersville
Bon Secours Memorial Regional Medical Center,
Mechanicsville
Halifax Regional Hospital, South Boston
Inova Fairfax Hospital, Falls Church

Prince William Hospital, Manassas
Riverside Regional Medical Center, Newport News
Winchester Medical Center, Winchester

HEART BYPASS SURGERY
Bon Secours Memorial Regional Medical Center,
Mechanicsville
CJW Medical Center—Chippenham Campus,
Richmond

HEART FAILURE
Bon Secours Memorial Regional Medical Center,
Mechanicsville
Carilion Giles Memorial Hospital, Pearisburg

CJW Medical Center–Chippenham Campus, Richmond
Danville Regional Medical Center, Danville
Norton Community Hospital, Norton
Rockingham Memorial Hospital, Harrisonburg
Sentara Virginia Beach General Hospital, Virginia Beach

VALVE REPLACEMENT SURGERY
Centra Health, Lynchburg
CJW Medical Center–Chippenham Campus, Richmond
Inova Fairfax Hospital, Falls Church
Lynchburg General Hospital, Lynchburg
Sentara Virginia Beach General Hospital, Virginia Beach

CRITICAL CARE

DIABETIC ACIDOSIS AND COMA
Inova Fairfax Hospital, Falls Church

PULMONARY EMBOLISM
CJW Medical Center–Chippenham Campus, Richmond
Henrico Doctors' Hospital, Richmond
Henrico Doctors' Hospital–Parham, Richmond
Sentara Virginia Beach General Hospital, Virginia Beach

RESPIRATORY FAILURE
Bon Secours Memorial Regional Medical Center, Mechanicsville
Bon Secours St. Mary's Hospital, Richmond
Chesapeake General Hospital, Chesapeake
Halifax Regional Hospital, South Boston
Inova Fair Oaks Hospital, Fairfax
Lewis-Gale Medical Center, Salem
Norton Community Hospital, Norton
Rockingham Memorial Hospital, Harrisonburg
Winchester Medical Center, Winchester

SEPSIS
Bon Secours Memorial Regional Medical Center, Mechanicsville
Bon Secours St. Mary's Hospital, Richmond
Centra Health, Lynchburg
Inova Fair Oaks Hospital, Fairfax
Inova Fairfax Hospital, Falls Church
Lewis-Gale Medical Center, Salem
Lynchburg General Hospital, Lynchburg
Mountain View Regional Medical Center, Norton
Rockingham Memorial Hospital, Harrisonburg
Sentara Virginia Beach General Hospital, Virginia Beach

Virginia Hospital Center–Arlington, Arlington
Winchester Medical Center, Winchester

GASTROINTESTINAL

BOWEL OBSTRUCTION
Danville Regional Medical Center, Danville
Norton Community Hospital, Norton
Potomac Hospital, Woodbridge
Sentara Virginia Beach General Hospital, Virginia Beach
Virginia Hospital Center–Arlington, Arlington

CHOLECYSTECTOMY
Carilion Franklin Memorial Hospital, Rocky Mount
Centra Health, Lynchburg
Clinch Valley Medical Center, Richlands
Halifax Regional Hospital, South Boston
Inova Loudoun Hospital, Leesburg
Lynchburg General Hospital, Lynchburg
Potomac Hospital, Woodbridge
Rappahannock General Hospital, Kilmarnock
Rockingham Memorial Hospital, Harrisonburg

GASTROINTESTINAL BLEED
Bon Secours Memorial Regional Medical Center, Mechanicsville
CJW Medical Center–Chippenham Campus, Richmond
Inova Fairfax Hospital, Falls Church
Lewis-Gale Medical Center, Salem
Mary Washington Hospital, Fredericksburg
Rockingham Memorial Hospital, Harrisonburg
Sentara Leigh Hospital, Norfolk
Wellmont Lonesome Pine Hospital, Big Stone Gap
Winchester Medical Center, Winchester

GASTROINTESTINAL SURGERIES AND PROCEDURES
Fauquier Hospital, Warrenton
Halifax Regional Hospital, South Boston
Henrico Doctors' Hospital, Richmond
Henrico Doctors' Hospital–Parham, Richmond
Inova Alexandria Hospital, Alexandria
Inova Fair Oaks Hospital, Fairfax
Inova Fairfax Hospital, Falls Church
Virginia Hospital Center–Arlington, Arlington
Winchester Medical Center, Winchester

PANCREATITIS
Sentara Virginia Beach General Hospital, Virginia Beach
Virginia Hospital Center–Arlington, Arlington

GENERAL SURGERY

APPENDECTOMY
Augusta Medical Center, Fishersville
Centra Health, Lynchburg
Culpeper Memorial Hospital, Culpeper
Danville Regional Medical Center, Danville
Inova Alexandria Hospital, Alexandria
Lewis-Gale Medical Center, Salem
Lynchburg General Hospital, Lynchburg
Russell County Medical Center, Lebanon
Virginia Hospital Center–Arlington, Arlington
Winchester Medical Center, Winchester

MATERNITY CARE
Inova Alexandria Hospital, Alexandria
Inova Fair Oaks Hospital, Fairfax
Sentara Leigh Hospital, Norfolk

ORTHOPEDICS

BACK AND NECK SURGERY (EXCEPT SPINAL FUSION)
Bon Secours DePaul Medical Center, Norfolk
Lewis-Gale Medical Center, Salem
Sentara Williamsburg Regional Medical Center, Williamsburg
Virginia Hospital Center–Arlington, Arlington

BACK AND NECK SURGERY (SPINAL FUSION)
Inova Fair Oaks Hospital, Fairfax
Inova Fairfax Hospital, Falls Church
Lewis-Gale Medical Center, Salem
Sentara Williamsburg Regional Medical Center, Williamsburg

HIP FRACTURE REPAIR
Centra Health, Lynchburg
Danville Regional Medical Center, Danville
Halifax Regional Hospital, South Boston
Lee Regional Medical Center, Pennington Gap
Lynchburg General Hospital, Lynchburg
Mary Immaculate Hospital, Newport News
Obici Hospital, Suffolk
Potomac Hospital, Woodbridge
Prince William Hospital, Manassas
Rappahannock General Hospital, Kilmarnock
Sentara Bayside Hospital, Virginia Beach
Virginia Hospital Center–Arlington, Arlington
Winchester Medical Center, Winchester

TOTAL HIP REPLACEMENT
Augusta Medical Center, Fishersville
Centra Health, Lynchburg

Hospitals receiving a five star rating in a particular procedure have patient outcomes that put them among the best in the nation. For full definitions of ratings and awards, see Appendix.

Henrico Doctors' Hospital, Richmond
Henrico Doctors' Hospital–Parham, Richmond
Inova Mount Vernon Hospital, Alexandria
Lynchburg General Hospital, Lynchburg
Wythe County Community Hospital, Wytheville

TOTAL KNEE REPLACEMENT

Augusta Medical Center, Fishersville
Centra Health, Lynchburg
Danville Regional Medical Center, Danville
Inova Mount Vernon Hospital, Alexandria
Lynchburg General Hospital, Lynchburg
Mary Immaculate Hospital, Newport News
Prince William Hospital, Manassas
Sentara Leigh Hospital, Norfolk
Winchester Medical Center, Winchester

PROSTATECTOMY

Inova Fairfax Hospital, Falls Church

PULMONARY

CHRONIC OBSTRUCTIVE PULMONARY DISEASE (COPD)

Bon Secours Memorial Regional Medical Center, Mechanicsville
Danville Regional Medical Center, Danville
Henrico Doctors' Hospital, Richmond
Henrico Doctors' Hospital–Parham, Richmond

Norton Community Hospital, Norton
Rockingham Memorial Hospital, Harrisonburg
Winchester Medical Center, Winchester

PNEUMONIA

Bon Secours Memorial Regional Medical Center, Mechanicsville
Bon Secours St. Mary's Hospital, Richmond
CJW Medical Center–Chippenham Campus, Richmond
Danville Regional Medical Center, Danville
Dickenson Community Hospital, Clintwood
Inova Alexandria Hospital, Alexandria
Inova Fairfax Hospital, Falls Church
Inova Loudoun Hospital, Leesburg
Martha Jefferson Hospital, Charlottesville
Norton Community Hospital, Norton
Prince William Hospital, Manassas
Riverside Tappahannock Hospital, Tappahannock
Rockingham Memorial Hospital, Harrisonburg
Sentara Virginia Beach General Hospital, Virginia Beach
Winchester Medical Center, Winchester

STROKE

Danville Regional Medical Center, Danville
Henrico Doctors' Hospital, Richmond
Henrico Doctors' Hospital–Parham, Richmond

Inova Fair Oaks Hospital, Fairfax
Inova Fairfax Hospital, Falls Church
Martha Jefferson Hospital, Charlottesville
Page Memorial Hospital, Luray
Virginia Hospital Center–Arlington, Arlington
Winchester Medical Center, Winchester

VASCULAR

CAROTID SURGERY

Carilion Medical Center, Roanoke
CJW Medical Center–Chippenham Campus, Richmond
Lewis-Gale Medical Center, Salem
Sentara Williamsburg Regional Medical Center, Williamsburg
University of Virginia Hospital, Charlottesville
Virginia Hospital Center–Arlington, Arlington
Winchester Medical Center, Winchester

PERIPHERAL VASCULAR BYPASS

None

RESECTION/REPLACEMENT OF ABDOMINAL AORTA

Inova Fairfax Hospital, Falls Church

WOMEN'S HEALTH

Inova Alexandria Hospital, Alexandria
Inova Fairfax Hospital, Falls Church

WASHINGTON HOSPITALS: FIVE STAR RATED FACILITIES

BARIATRIC SURGERY

Overlake Hospital Medical Center, Bellevue
St. Francis Community Hospital, Federal Way
Valley Medical Center, Renton
Virginia Mason Medical Center, Seattle

CARDIAC

ATRIAL FIBRILLATION

Virginia Mason Medical Center, Seattle

CORONARY INTERVENTIONAL PROCEDURES (ANGIOPLASTY/STENT)

None

HEART ATTACK

Evergreen Hospital Medical Center, Kirkland
Kittitas Valley Community Hospital, Ellensburg
Monticello Medical Center, Longview
Providence Everett Medical Center–Colby Campus, Everett

Sacred Heart Medical Center, Spokane
St. John Medical Center Peacehealth, Longview

HEART BYPASS SURGERY

None

HEART FAILURE

Evergreen Hospital Medical Center, Kirkland
Legacy Salmon Creek Hospital, Vancouver
Northwest Hospital and Medical Center, Seattle
Overlake Hospital Medical Center, Bellevue
Providence Everett Medical Center–Colby Campus, Everett
Valley Medical Center, Renton

VALVE REPLACEMENT SURGERY

Overlake Hospital Medical Center, Bellevue

CRITICAL CARE

DIABETIC ACIDOSIS AND COMA

None

PULMONARY EMBOLISM

Providence Everett Medical Center–Colby Campus, Everett

RESPIRATORY FAILURE

Auburn Regional Medical Center, Auburn
Providence Centralia Hospital, Centralia
Providence Everett Medical Center–Colby Campus, Everett
St. Mary Medical Center, Walla Walla
Yakima Valley Memorial Hospital, Yakima

SEPSIS

Evergreen Hospital Medical Center, Kirkland
Harrison Medical Center, Bremerton
Holy Family Hospital, Spokane
Kadlec Medical Center, Richland
Monticello Medical Center, Longview
Providence Centralia Hospital, Centralia
Providence Everett Medical Center–Colby Campus, Everett

Providence St. Peter Hospital, Olympia
St. John Medical Center Peacehealth, Longview
St. Joseph Hospital, Bellingham
Swedish Medical Center–Ballard Campus, Seattle
Swedish Medical Center–First Hill, Seattle

GASTROINTESTINAL

BOWEL OBSTRUCTION
Central Washington Hospital, Wenatchee
Evergreen Hospital Medical Center, Kirkland
Olympic Medical Center, Port Angeles
Virginia Mason Medical Center, Seattle

CHOLECYSTECTOMY
Harrison Medical Center, Bremerton
University of Washington Medical Center, Seattle
Valley Hospital and Medical Center, Spokane

GASTROINTESTINAL BLEED
Auburn Regional Medical Center, Auburn
Central Washington Hospital, Wenatchee
Doctors Hospital of Tacoma, Tacoma
Monticello Medical Center, Longview
Providence Everett Medical Center–Colby
  Campus, Everett
Providence St. Peter Hospital, Olympia
St. John Medical Center Peacehealth, Longview
St. Mary Medical Center, Walla Walla
Southwest Washington Medical Center, Vancouver
Tacoma General Allenmore Hospital, Tacoma

GASTROINTESTINAL SURGERIES
AND PROCEDURES
Central Washington Hospital, Wenatchee
Monticello Medical Center, Longview
St. Francis Community Hospital, Federal Way
St. John Medical Center Peacehealth, Longview
St. Joseph Hospital, Bellingham
St. Joseph Medical Center, Tacoma
Southwest Washington Medical Center, Vancouver
Swedish Medical Center–Ballard Campus, Seattle
Swedish Medical Center–First Hill, Seattle

PANCREATITIS
University of Washington Medical Center, Seattle

GENERAL SURGERY

APPENDECTOMY
Central Washington Hospital, Wenatchee
Good Samaritan Hospital and Rehabilitation
  Center, Puyallup
Providence Centralia Hospital, Centralia

Providence Everett Medical Center–Colby
  Campus, Everett
Providence St. Peter Hospital, Olympia
Swedish Medical Center–Ballard Campus, Seattle
Swedish Medical Center–First Hill, Seattle
Yakima Valley Memorial Hospital, Yakima

MATERNITY CARE

Evergreen Hospital Medical Center, Kirkland
Good Samaritan Hospital and Rehabilitation
  Center, Puyallup
Overlake Hospital Medical Center, Bellevue
St. Joseph Medical Center, Tacoma

ORTHOPEDICS

BACK AND NECK SURGERY
(EXCEPT SPINAL FUSION)
Central Washington Hospital, Wenatchee
Good Samaritan Hospital and Rehabilitation
  Center, Puyallup
Kadlec Medical Center, Richland
Northwest Hospital and Medical Center, Seattle
Overlake Hospital Medical Center, Bellevue
Sacred Heart Medical Center, Spokane
St. Joseph Medical Center, Tacoma
St. Mary Medical Center, Walla Walla
Southwest Washington Medical Center, Vancouver
Valley Hospital and Medical Center, Spokane
Valley Medical Center, Renton

BACK AND NECK SURGERY (SPINAL FUSION)
Capital Medical Center, Olympia
Central Washington Hospital, Wenatchee
Kadlec Medical Center, Richland
St. Mary Medical Center, Walla Walla
Southwest Washington Medical Center, Vancouver

HIP FRACTURE REPAIR
Capital Medical Center, Olympia
St. Clare Hospital, Tacoma
St. Francis Community Hospital, Federal Way
St. Joseph Medical Center, Tacoma
St. Mary Medical Center, Walla Walla
Valley Medical Center, Renton

TOTAL HIP REPLACEMENT
Capital Medical Center, Olympia
Good Samaritan Hospital and Rehabilitation
  Center, Puyallup
Kadlec Medical Center, Richland
Providence St. Peter Hospital, Olympia
Skagit Valley Hospital, Mount Vernon
Swedish Medical Center–Ballard Campus, Seattle

Swedish Medical Center–First Hill, Seattle
Tri-State Memorial Hospital, Clarkston
Valley Medical Center, Renton

TOTAL KNEE REPLACEMENT
Capital Medical Center, Olympia
Central Washington Hospital, Wenatchee
Kadlec Medical Center, Richland
Monticello Medical Center, Longview
Olympic Medical Center, Port Angeles
Overlake Hospital Medical Center, Bellevue
Providence St. Peter Hospital, Olympia
St. John Medical Center Peacehealth, Longview
St. Mary Medical Center, Walla Walla
Southwest Washington Medical Center, Vancouver
Tri-State Memorial Hospital, Clarkston
Valley Medical Center, Renton
Virginia Mason Medical Center, Seattle
Yakima Valley Memorial Hospital, Yakima

PROSTATECTOMY

Central Washington Hospital, Wenatchee
St. Mary Medical Center, Walla Walla
University of Washington Medical Center, Seattle

PULMONARY

CHRONIC OBSTRUCTIVE PULMONARY DISEASE
(COPD)
St. Joseph Hospital, Bellingham
Virginia Mason Medical Center, Seattle

PNEUMONIA
Auburn Regional Medical Center, Auburn
Doctors Hospital of Tacoma, Tacoma
Providence Everett Medical Center–Colby
  Campus, Everett
St. Francis Community Hospital, Federal Way
St. Joseph Hospital, Bellingham
Southwest Washington Medical Center, Vancouver
Swedish Medical Center–Ballard Campus, Seattle
Swedish Medical Center–Cherry Hills Campus,
  Seattle
Swedish Medical Center–First Hill, Seattle
Tacoma General Allenmore Hospital, Tacoma
Virginia Mason Medical Center, Seattle
Yakima Regional Medical and Cardiac Center,
  Yakima

STROKE

Central Washington Hospital, Wenatchee
Doctors Hospital of Tacoma, Tacoma
Evergreen Hospital Medical Center, Kirkland

Hospitals receiving a five star rating in a particular procedure have patient outcomes that put them among the best in the nation. For full definitions of ratings and awards, see Appendix.

Lourdes Medical Center, Pasco
Monticello Medical Center, Longview
Providence Everett Medical Center—Colby
   Campus, Everett
Providence St. Peter Hospital, Olympia
St. Francis Community Hospital, Federal Way
St. John Medical Center Peacehealth, Longview
Tacoma General Allenmore Hospital, Tacoma

VASCULAR

CAROTID SURGERY
Capital Medical Center, Olympia
Overlake Hospital Medical Center, Bellevue

PERIPHERAL VASCULAR BYPASS
None

RESECTION/REPLACEMENT OF ABDOMINAL AORTA
Central Washington Hospital, Wenatchee
Providence Everett Medical Center—Colby
   Campus, Everett

WOMEN'S HEALTH
Overlake Hospital Medical Center, Bellevue

WASHINGTON, DC HOSPITALS: FIVE STAR RATED FACILITIES

BARIATRIC SURGERY
None

CARDIAC

ATRIAL FIBRILLATION
None

CORONARY INTERVENTIONAL PROCEDURES
(ANGIOPLASTY/STENT)
None

HEART ATTACK
Sibley Memorial Hospital, Washington

HEART BYPASS SURGERY
None

HEART FAILURE
Washington Hospital Center, Washington

VALVE REPLACEMENT SURGERY
None

CRITICAL CARE

DIABETIC ACIDOSIS AND COMA
None

PULMONARY EMBOLISM
None

RESPIRATORY FAILURE
None

SEPSIS
None

GASTROINTESTINAL

BOWEL OBSTRUCTION
Georgetown University Hospital, Washington

CHOLECYSTECTOMY
None

GASTROINTESTINAL BLEED
None

GASTROINTESTINAL SURGERIES
AND PROCEDURES
Providence Hospital, Washington

PANCREATITIS
None

GENERAL SURGERY

APPENDECTOMY
None

MATERNITY CARE
None

ORTHOPEDICS

BACK AND NECK SURGERY
(EXCEPT SPINAL FUSION)
Sibley Memorial Hospital, Washington
Washington Hospital Center, Washington

BACK AND NECK SURGERY (SPINAL FUSION)
Washington Hospital Center, Washington

HIP FRACTURE REPAIR
None

TOTAL HIP REPLACEMENT
Sibley Memorial Hospital, Washington

TOTAL KNEE REPLACEMENT
None

PROSTATECTOMY
George Washington University Hospital,
   Washington
Georgetown University Hospital, Washington
Washington Hospital Center, Washington

PULMONARY

CHRONIC OBSTRUCTIVE PULMONARY DISEASE
(COPD)
None

PNEUMONIA
None

STROKE
Georgetown University Hospital, Washington
Howard University Hospital, Washington
Providence Hospital, Washington
Washington Hospital Center, Washington

VASCULAR

CAROTID SURGERY
None

PERIPHERAL VASCULAR BYPASS
None

RESECTION/REPLACEMENT OF ABDOMINAL AORTA
None

WOMEN'S HEALTH
None

BARIATRIC SURGERY

None

CARDIAC

ATRIAL FIBRILLATION
Monongalia County General Hospital, Morgantown

CORONARY INTERVENTIONAL PROCEDURES (ANGIOPLASTY/STENT)
Charleston Area Medical Center, Charleston

HEART ATTACK
Charleston Area Medical Center, Charleston
Greenbrier Valley Medical Center, Ronceverte

HEART BYPASS SURGERY
None

HEART FAILURE
Charleston Area Medical Center, Charleston
Potomac Valley Hospital, Keyser
St. Francis Hospital, Charleston
Thomas Memorial Hospital, South Charleston

VALVE REPLACEMENT SURGERY
None

CRITICAL CARE

DIABETIC ACIDOSIS AND COMA
None

PULMONARY EMBOLISM
United Hospital Center, Clarksburg

RESPIRATORY FAILURE
Davis Memorial Hospital, Elkins
Greenbrier Valley Medical Center, Ronceverte
Raleigh General Hospital, Beckley
Thomas Memorial Hospital, South Charleston
United Hospital Center, Clarksburg

SEPSIS
Greenbrier Valley Medical Center, Ronceverte
Potomac Valley Hospital, Keyser
Princeton Community Hospital, Princeton

GASTROINTESTINAL

BOWEL OBSTRUCTION
Raleigh General Hospital, Beckley

CHOLECYSTECTOMY
Cabell-Huntington Hospital, Huntington
Charleston Area Medical Center, Charleston
Davis Memorial Hospital, Elkins
Fairmont General Hospital, Fairmont
St. Francis Hospital, Charleston
Summersville Memorial Hospital, Summersville

GASTROINTESTINAL BLEED
Raleigh General Hospital, Beckley

GASTROINTESTINAL SURGERIES AND PROCEDURES
None

PANCREATITIS
Camden Clark Memorial Hospital, Parkersburg
Raleigh General Hospital, Beckley

GENERAL SURGERY

APPENDECTOMY
None

MATERNITY CARE

None

ORTHOPEDICS

BACK AND NECK SURGERY (EXCEPT SPINAL FUSION)
Princeton Community Hospital, Princeton
Wheeling Hospital, Wheeling

BACK AND NECK SURGERY (SPINAL FUSION)
None

HIP FRACTURE REPAIR
Camden Clark Memorial Hospital, Parkersburg
Charleston Area Medical Center, Charleston

TOTAL HIP REPLACEMENT
Cabell-Huntington Hospital, Huntington
Davis Memorial Hospital, Elkins

St. Joseph's Hospital, Parkersburg
United Hospital Center, Clarksburg

TOTAL KNEE REPLACEMENT
Cabell-Huntington Hospital, Huntington
Davis Memorial Hospital, Elkins
United Hospital Center, Clarksburg
Wheeling Hospital, Wheeling

PROSTATECTOMY

Davis Memorial Hospital, Elkins
Logan Regional Medical Center, Logan
St. Francis Hospital, Charleston

PULMONARY

CHRONIC OBSTRUCTIVE PULMONARY DISEASE (COPD)
United Hospital Center, Clarksburg

PNEUMONIA
Thomas Memorial Hospital, South Charleston
United Hospital Center, Clarksburg

STROKE

Charleston Area Medical Center, Charleston

VASCULAR

CAROTID SURGERY
Camden Clark Memorial Hospital, Parkersburg
Charleston Area Medical Center, Charleston
St. Francis Hospital, Charleston
Thomas Memorial Hospital, South Charleston
United Hospital Center, Clarksburg

PERIPHERAL VASCULAR BYPASS
Camden Clark Memorial Hospital, Parkersburg
United Hospital Center, Clarksburg

RESECTION/REPLACEMENT OF ABDOMINAL AORTA
None

WOMEN'S HEALTH

None

Hospitals receiving a five star rating in a particular procedure have patient outcomes that put them among the best in the nation. For full definitions of ratings and awards, see Appendix.

BARIATRIC SURGERY

Aurora Sinai Medical Center, Milwaukee
Froedtert Memorial Lutheran Hospital, Milwaukee
Gundersen Lutheran Medical Center, La Crosse

CARDIAC

ATRIAL FIBRILLATION

Appleton Medical Center, Appleton
Howard Young Medical Center, Woodruff
Waukesha Memorial Hospital, Waukesha
Wheaton Franciscan Healthcare—St. Francis,
    Milwaukee

CORONARY INTERVENTIONAL PROCEDURES
(ANGIOPLASTY/STENT)
None

HEART ATTACK

Aspirus Wausau Hospital, Wausau
Aurora Baycare Medical Center, Green Bay
Aurora Medical Center—Kenosha, Kenosha
Gundersen Lutheran Medical Center, La Crosse
Luther Hospital Mayo Health System, Eau Claire
St. Croix Regional Medical Center, St. Croix Falls
St. Joseph's Hospital, Marshfield

HEART BYPASS SURGERY

Aspirus Wausau Hospital, Wausau
Aurora Baycare Medical Center, Green Bay
Luther Hospital Mayo Health System, Eau Claire
United Hospital System, Kenosha
UW Health-UW Hospitals and Clinics, Madison

HEART FAILURE

Aurora Lakeland Medical Center, Elkhorn
Aurora St. Luke's Medical Center, Milwaukee
Aurora Sinai Medical Center, Milwaukee
Beaver Dam Community Hospital, Beaver Dam
Froedtert Memorial Lutheran Hospital, Milwaukee
Good Samaritan Health Center, Merrill
Gundersen Lutheran Medical Center, La Crosse
Monroe Clinic, Monroe
St. Joseph's Hospital, Marshfield
St. Luke's Medical Center, Cudahy
Waukesha Memorial Hospital, Waukesha
West Allis Memorial Hospital, West Allis

VALVE REPLACEMENT SURGERY

Columbia St. Mary's Hospital Milwaukee, Milwaukee
UW Health-UW Hospitals and Clinics, Madison
Waukesha Memorial Hospital, Waukesha

CRITICAL CARE

DIABETIC ACIDOSIS AND COMA

Gundersen Lutheran Medical Center, La Crosse

PULMONARY EMBOLISM

St. Mary's Hospital Medical Center, Green Bay
Theda Clark Medical Center, Neenah
Wheaton Franciscan Healthcare—St. Francis,
    Milwaukee

RESPIRATORY FAILURE

Aspirus Wausau Hospital, Wausau
Gundersen Lutheran Medical Center, La Crosse
Lakeview Hospital, Wauwatosa
West Allis Memorial Hospital, West Allis
Wheaton Franciscan Healthcare—Elmbrook
    Memorial, Brookfield
Wheaton Franciscan Healthcare—St. Francis,
    Milwaukee
Wheaton Franciscan Healthcare—St. Joseph,
    Milwaukee

SEPSIS

All Saints Medical Center—St. Mary's Campus, Racine
All Saints St. Luke's Hospital, Racine
Appleton Medical Center, Appleton
Aurora Baycare Medical Center, Green Bay
Aurora St. Luke's Medical Center, Milwaukee
Bellin Memorial Hospital, Green Bay
Columbia St. Mary's Hospital Ozaukee, Mequon
Froedtert Memorial Lutheran Hospital, Milwaukee
Gundersen Lutheran Medical Center, La Crosse
Lakeview Hospital, Wauwatosa
Mercy Medical Center, Oshkosh
Meriter Hospital, Madison
Oconomowoc Memorial Hospital, Oconomowoc
St. Joseph's Hospital, Chippewa Falls
St. Joseph's Hospital, Marshfield
St. Luke's Medical Center, Cudahy
Theda Clark Medical Center, Neenah
UW Health-UW Hospitals and Clinics, Madison
Waukesha Memorial Hospital, Waukesha
West Allis Memorial Hospital, West Allis
Wheaton Franciscan Healthcare—St. Francis,
    Milwaukee
Wheaton Franciscan Healthcare—St. Joseph,
    Milwaukee

GASTROINTESTINAL

BOWEL OBSTRUCTION

Aurora St. Luke's Medical Center, Milwaukee
Bellin Memorial Hospital, Green Bay
St. Joseph's Hospital, Chippewa Falls
St. Luke's Medical Center, Cudahy
St. Vincent Hospital, Green Bay
UW Health-UW Hospitals and Clinics, Madison

CHOLECYSTECTOMY

Aurora Sheboygan Memorial Medical Center,
    Sheboygan
Berlin Memorial Hospital, Berlin
Hayward Area Memorial Hospital, Hayward
Holy Family Memorial, Manitowoc
Memorial Hospital Burlington, Burlington
Memorial Hospital, Manitowoc
St. Mary's Hospital Medical Center, Green Bay
West Allis Memorial Hospital, West Allis
Wheaton Franciscan Healthcare—Elmbrook
    Memorial, Brookfield

GASTROINTESTINAL BLEED

Appleton Medical Center, Appleton
Aurora St. Luke's Medical Center, Milwaukee
Lakeview Medical Center, Rice Lake
St. Luke's Medical Center, Cudahy
Waukesha Memorial Hospital, Waukesha
Wheaton Franciscan Healthcare—St. Francis,
    Milwaukee

GASTROINTESTINAL SURGERIES
AND PROCEDURES

Bay Area Medical Center, Marinette
Fort Healthcare, Fort Atkinson
Gundersen Lutheran Medical Center, La Crosse
West Allis Memorial Hospital, West Allis
Wheaton Franciscan Healthcare—Elmbrook
    Memorial, Brookfield

PANCREATITIS

Theda Clark Medical Center, Neenah

GENERAL SURGERY

APPENDECTOMY

All Saints Medical Center—St. Mary's Campus, Racine
All Saints St. Luke's Hospital, Racine
Aspirus Wausau Hospital, Wausau
Barron Memorial Medical Center Mayo, Barron
Gundersen Lutheran Medical Center, La Crosse
Riverview Hospital, Wisconsin Rapids

Sacred Heart Hospital, Eau Claire
St. Joseph's Community Hospital West Bend, West Bend
St. Joseph's Hospital, Marshfield
St. Vincent Hospital, Green Bay
Wheaton Franciscan Healthcare—Elmbrook Memorial, Brookfield

MATERNITY CARE

Tomah Memorial Hospital, Tomah

ORTHOPEDICS

BACK AND NECK SURGERY (EXCEPT SPINAL FUSION)
Luther Hospital Mayo Health System, Eau Claire
Mercy Medical Center, Oshkosh

BACK AND NECK SURGERY (SPINAL FUSION)
Aurora Baycare Medical Center, Green Bay
Columbia St. Mary's Hospital Milwaukee, Milwaukee
Gundersen Lutheran Medical Center, La Crosse
Mercy Medical Center, Oshkosh
St. Joseph's Hospital, Marshfield
Waukesha Memorial Hospital, Waukesha

HIP FRACTURE REPAIR
Aurora Sheboygan Memorial Medical Center, Sheboygan
Berlin Memorial Hospital, Berlin
Columbia St. Mary's Hospital Milwaukee, Milwaukee
Gundersen Lutheran Medical Center, La Crosse
Monroe Clinic, Monroe
New London Family Medical Center, New London
St. Mary's Hospital, Rhinelander
West Allis Memorial Hospital, West Allis

TOTAL HIP REPLACEMENT
Aurora Sheboygan Memorial Medical Center, Sheboygan
Bay Area Medical Center, Marinette
Berlin Memorial Hospital, Berlin
Gundersen Lutheran Medical Center, La Crosse
Howard Young Medical Center, Woodruff
Lakeview Hospital, Wauwatosa
Lakeview Medical Center, Rice Lake
Mercy Medical Center, Oshkosh
Meriter Hospital, Madison
Sacred Heart Hospital, Eau Claire

St. Mary's Hospital, Rhinelander
St. Mary's Hospital Medical Center, Green Bay
St. Nicholas Hospital, Sheboygan
Sauk Prairie Memorial Hospital, Prairie Du Sac
Wheaton Franciscan Healthcare—Elmbrook Memorial, Brookfield
Wheaton Franciscan Healthcare—St. Joseph, Milwaukee

TOTAL KNEE REPLACEMENT
All Saints Medical Center—St. Mary's Campus, Racine
All Saints St. Luke's Hospital, Racine
Aurora Sheboygan Memorial Medical Center, Sheboygan
Berlin Memorial Hospital, Berlin
Gundersen Lutheran Medical Center, La Crosse
Holy Family Memorial, Manitowoc
Howard Young Medical Center, Woodruff
Lakeview Medical Center, Rice Lake
Memorial Hospital, Manitowoc
Mercy Medical Center, Oshkosh
Monroe Clinic, Monroe
Riverview Hospital, Wisconsin Rapids
Sacred Heart Hospital, Eau Claire
St. Joseph's Hospital, Marshfield
St. Mary's Hospital, Rhinelander
St. Mary's Hospital Medical Center, Green Bay
St. Nicholas Hospital, Sheboygan
Sauk Prairie Memorial Hospital, Prairie Du Sac
Vernon Memorial Hospital, Viroqua
Wheaton Franciscan Healthcare—Elmbrook Memorial, Brookfield

PROSTATECTOMY

Columbia St. Mary's Hospital Milwaukee, Milwaukee
St. Mary's Hospital Medical Center, Madison
West Allis Memorial Hospital, West Allis

PULMONARY

CHRONIC OBSTRUCTIVE PULMONARY DISEASE (COPD)
Aspirus Wausau Hospital, Wausau
Aurora St. Luke's Medical Center, Milwaukee
Aurora Sinai Medical Center, Milwaukee
St. Luke's Medical Center, Cudahy

PNEUMONIA
Aurora Baycare Medical Center, Green Bay
Aurora Sinai Medical Center, Milwaukee

Aurora St. Luke's Medical Center, Milwaukee
Door County Memorial Hospital, Sturgeon Bay
Froedtert Memorial Lutheran Hospital, Milwaukee
Oconomowoc Memorial Hospital, Oconomowoc
St. Elizabeth Hospital, Appleton
St. Joseph's Hospital, Marshfield
St. Luke's Medical Center, Cudahy
UW Health-UW Hospitals and Clinics, Madison
West Allis Memorial Hospital, West Allis

STROKE

All Saints Medical Center—St. Mary's Campus, Racine
All Saints St. Luke's Hospital, Racine
Appleton Medical Center, Appleton
Aspirus Wausau Hospital, Wausau
Aurora Baycare Medical Center, Green Bay
Columbia St. Mary's Hospital Milwaukee, Milwaukee
Lakeview Hospital, Wauwatosa
Oconomowoc Memorial Hospital, Oconomowoc
St. Joseph's Hospital, Marshfield
St. Mary's Hospital Medical Center, Madison
Shawano Medical Center, Shawano
Theda Clark Medical Center, Neenah
West Allis Memorial Hospital, West Allis
Wheaton Franciscan Healthcare—St. Francis, Milwaukee
Wheaton Franciscan Healthcare—St. Joseph, Milwaukee

VASCULAR

CAROTID SURGERY
Aspirus Wausau Hospital, Wausau
Memorial Hospital Burlington, Burlington
Meriter Hospital, Madison
Monroe Clinic, Monroe
St. Mary's Hospital Medical Center, Green Bay
United Hospital System, Kenosha

PERIPHERAL VASCULAR BYPASS
None

RESECTION/REPLACEMENT OF ABDOMINAL AORTA
None

WOMEN'S HEALTH

Aurora Baycare Medical Center, Green Bay
St. Elizabeth Hospital, Appleton
Waukesha Memorial Hospital, Waukesha

Hospitals receiving a five star rating in a particular procedure have patient outcomes that put them among the best in the nation. For full definitions of ratings and awards, see Appendix.

BARIATRIC SURGERY

None

CARDIAC

ATRIAL FIBRILLATION
None

CORONARY INTERVENTIONAL PROCEDURES
(ANGIOPLASTY/STENT)
None

HEART ATTACK
None

HEART BYPASS SURGERY
None

HEART FAILURE
None

VALVE REPLACEMENT SURGERY
None

CRITICAL CARE

DIABETIC ACIDOSIS AND COMA
None

PULMONARY EMBOLISM
None

RESPIRATORY FAILURE
None

SEPSIS
None

GASTROINTESTINAL

BOWEL OBSTRUCTION
Cheyenne Regional Medical Center, Cheyenne
Depaul Hospital, Cheyenne

CHOLECYSTECTOMY
None

GASTROINTESTINAL BLEED
None

GASTROINTESTINAL SURGERIES
AND PROCEDURES
None

PANCREATITIS
None

GENERAL SURGERY

APPENDECTOMY
None

MATERNITY CARE

None

ORTHOPEDICS

BACK AND NECK SURGERY
(EXCEPT SPINAL FUSION)
Wyoming Medical Center, Casper

BACK AND NECK SURGERY (SPINAL FUSION)
Powell Valley Hospital, Powell

HIP FRACTURE REPAIR
None

TOTAL HIP REPLACEMENT
Ivinson Memorial Hospital, Laramie

TOTAL KNEE REPLACEMENT
Lander Valley Medical Center, Lander

PROSTATECTOMY

None

PULMONARY

CHRONIC OBSTRUCTIVE PULMONARY DISEASE
(COPD)
None

PNEUMONIA
West Park Hospital District, Cody

STROKE

None

VASCULAR

CAROTID SURGERY
None

PERIPHERAL VASCULAR BYPASS
None

RESECTION/REPLACEMENT OF ABDOMINAL AORTA
None

WOMEN'S HEALTH

None

CHAPTER 8

HOSPITAL RATINGS BY PROCEDURE

HOSPITAL RATINGS BY PROCEDURE

This chapter works as an at-a-glance guide to all the HealthGrades star ratings for virtually every hospital in the country. You can look at the information in this section in two different ways:

First, you can locate and research your local hospital to learn about its star ratings across all thirty-one procedures and treatments. That will give you a good idea of the hospital's specific quality ratings across the board, covering everything from appendectomies to women's health. Don't be alarmed if your local hospital doesn't fare well across the board. Although some exceptional hospitals perform better than their competitors across nearly all service lines, most hospitals specialize in a few clinical areas such as cardiac surgery or orthopedics. So don't be surprised to see a hospital rated as five star in one area and to only have one or three stars in others.

The second way to view and use this section is to locate the particular procedure or treatment of interest to you listed at the top of each column, and then run your eyes down the column to see the ratings for each hospital in your state for that particular procedure. This is a great way to compare hospital quality if you already know your diagnosis or required procedure.

ALABAMA HOSPITALS: RATINGS BY PROCEDURE

	Appendectomy	Atrial Fibrillation	Back and Neck Surgery (except Spinal Fusion)	Back and Neck Surgery (Spinal Fusion)	Bariatric Surgery	Bowel Obstruction	Carotid Surgery	Cholecystectomy (Gall Bladder Removal)	Chronic Obstructive Pulmonary Disease (COPD)	Coronary Bypass Surgery	Coronary Interventional Procedures (Angioplasty/Stent)	Diabetic Acidosis a...
1. Andalusia Regional Hospital, Andalusia	NR	★★★	★★★	★★★	NR	★★★	NR	★★★★★	★★★	NR	NR	NR
2. Athens-Limestone Hospital, Athens	NR	★★★	NR	NR	NR	★★★	NR	★★★	★★★	NR	NR	★★★
3. Atmore Community Hospital, Atmore	NR	★★★	NR	NR	NR	NR	NR	NR	★★★	NR	NR	NR
4. Baptist Cherokee, Centre	NR	★★★	NR	NR	NR	★★★	NR	NR	★	NR	NR	NR
5. Baptist Citizens, Talladega	NR	★★★	NR	NR	★	NR	NR	★★★	★★★★★	NR	NR	★★★
6. Baptist Medical Center–Dekalb, Fort Payne	NR	★★★	NR	NR	NR	★★★	NR	★★★★★	★	NR	NR	NR
7. Baptist Medical Center–East, Montgomery	NR	★★★	NR	★★★	NR	★★★	★★★	★★★	★★★	NR	NR	NR
8. Baptist Medical Center–South, Montgomery	NR	★	★★★	★	NR	★★★	★★★★★	★★★★★	★★★	★	★★★	★★★
9. Baptist Princeton, Birmingham	NR	★	★	NR	NR	★★★	★★★	★	★★★	★★★	★	★★★
10. Baptist Shelby, Alabaster	NR	★	★	★★★	NR	★★★	★★★	★★★	★★★	★★★	★★★	★★★
11. Brookwood Medical Center, Birmingham	NR	★★★	★★★	★★★★★	NR	★★★	★★★★★	★★★	★★★	★	★★★	★★★
12. Bryan W. Whitfield Memorial Hospital, Demopolis	NR	★★★	NR	NR	NR	NR	NR	NR	★★★	NR	NR	★★★
13. Bullock County Hospital, Union Springs	NR	NR	NR	NR	NR	NR	NR	NR	★	NR	NR	NR
14. Carraway Methodist Medical Center, Birmingham	NR	★★★	★★★	★★★★★	NR	★★★	★★★	★	★★★	NR	★	★★★
15. Chilton Medical Center, Clanton	NR	NR	NR	NR	NR	NR	NR	NR	★★★	NR	NR	NR
16. Clay County Hospital, Ashland	NR	★	NR	NR	NR	NR	NR	NR	★★★	NR	NR	NR
17. Community Hospital, Tallassee	NR	★★★	NR	NR	NR	★★★	NR	NR	★★★	NR	NR	★★★
18. Coosa Valley Medical Center, Sylacauga	NR	★	NR	NR	NR	★	NR	★★★	★★★	NR	NR	★
19. Crenshaw Community Hospital, Luverne	NR	NR	NR	NR	NR	NR	NR	NR	NR	NR	NR	NR
20. Crestwood Medical Center, Huntsville	NR	★★★	★★★	★★★	NR	★★★	★★★	★★★	★★★	NR	★★★	NR
21. Cullman Regional Medical Center, Cullman	NR	★★★	★★★	★★★	NR	★★★	★★★	★★★	★★★	NR	NR	★
22. D. W. McMillan Memorial Hospital, Brewton	NR	★★★	NR	NR	NR	★	NR	★★★	★	NR	NR	★★★
23. Dale Medical Center, Ozark	NR	★★★	NR	NR	NR	★★★	NR	★	★★★	NR	NR	NR
24. DCH Regional Medical Center, Tuscaloosa	NR	★★★	★★★	★★★	NR	★★★	★	★★★★★	★★★	★★★	★★★	★★★
25. Decatur General Hospital, Decatur	NR	★★★	NR	NR	NR	★★★	★★★	★★★	★★★	★	★★★	★★★
26. East Alabama Med. Ctr. and Skilled Nursing Facility, Opelika	NR	★★★	★★★★★	NR	NR	★★★	★★★	★★★★★	★★★	★	★★★	★★★
27. Eliza Coffee Memorial Hospital, Florence	NR	★★★	★★★	★★★	NR	★★★	★★★	★★★	★★★	★	★★★	★★★
28. Elmore Community Hospital, Wetumpka	NR	NR	NR	NR	NR	NR	NR	NR	★★★	NR	NR	NR
29. Evergreen Medical Center, Evergreen	NR	★★★	NR	NR	NR	★★★	NR	★★★	★★★	NR	NR	NR
30. Fayette Medical Center, Fayette	NR	★★★	NR	NR	NR	NR	NR	★★★	★★★	NR	NR	NR
31. Flowers Hospital, Dothan	NR	★	★	★★★	NR	★★★	★★★	★	★★★	★★★	★★★	★★★
32. G. H. Lanier Memorial Hospital, Valley	NR	★★★	NR	NR	NR	★★★	NR	★★★★★	★★★★★	NR	NR	★★★
33. Gadsden Regional Medical Center, Gadsden	NR	★★★	★★★	★★★★★	NR	★★★	★★★	★★★	★	★★★	★	★★★
34. Hale County Hospital, Greensboro	NR	NR	NR	NR	NR	NR	NR	NR	★★★	NR	NR	NR
35. Hartselle Medical Center, Hartselle	NR	★★★	NR	NR	NR	★★★	NR	★★★	★★★	NR	NR	NR
36. Helen Keller Hospital, Sheffield	NR	★★★	★★★	NR	NR	★★★	NR	★★★	★★★	NR	NR	★★★
37. Huntsville Hospital, Huntsville	NR	★★★	★	★★★	NR	★★★	★★★	★★★★★	★	★★★★★	★★★	★
38. Jackson County Hospital, Scottsboro	NR	★★★	NR	NR	NR	★★★	NR	★	★★★	NR	NR	★★★
39. Jackson Hospital and Clinic, Montgomery	NR	★★★	★★★★★	★★★★★	NR	★	★★★	★★★	NR	★★★	★★★	★★★
40. Jackson Medical Center, Jackson	NR	★★★	NR	NR	NR	NR	NR	NR	★★★	NR	NR	NR
41. Jacksonville Medical Center, Jacksonville	NR	NR	NR	NR	NR	★★★	NR	NR	★★★	NR	NR	NR
42. L. V. Stabler Memorial Hospital, Greenville	NR	★★★	NR	NR	NR	★★★★★	NR	★★★	★★★	NR	NR	NR
43. Lake Martin Community Hospital, Dadeville	NR	NR	NR	NR	NR	NR	NR	NR	★★★	NR	NR	NR
44. Lakeland Community Hospital, Haleyville	NR	★★★	NR	NR	NR	★★★	NR	★★★	★	NR	NR	NR
45. Lakeview Community Hospital, Eufaula	NR	★★★	NR	NR	NR	NR	NR	★★★	NR	NR	NR	NR
46. Lawrence Medical Center, Moulton	NR	★★★	NR	NR	NR	★★★	NR	★★★	★★★	NR	NR	NR
47. LTC Hospital at Southeast Alabama Medical Ctr., Dothan	NR	★★★	★	★	NR	★★★	★★★	★★★	★★★	★★★	★★★	★★★
48. LTC Hospital of Tuscaloosa, Tuscaloosa	NR	★★★	★★★	★★★	NR	★★★	★	★★★	★★★★★	★★★	★★★	★★★
49. Marion Regional Medical Center, Hamilton	NR	NR	NR	NR	NR	NR	NR	NR	★★★	NR	NR	NR
50. Marshall Medical Center–North, Guntersville	NR	★★★	NR	NR	NR	★★★	NR	★★★★★	★★★	NR	NR	NR

KEY: ★★★★★ BEST   ★★★ AS EXPECTED   ★ POOR   NR NOT RATED BY HEALTHGRADES   For full definitions of ratings and awards, see Appendix.

Gastrointestinal Bleed	Gastrointestinal Surgeries and Procedures	Heart Attack	Heart Failure	Hip Fracture Repair	Maternity Care	Pancreatitis	Peripheral Vascular Bypass	Pneumonia	Prostatectomy	Pulmonary Embolism	Resection/Replacement of Abdominal Aorta	Respiratory Failure	Sepsis	Stroke	Total Hip Replacement	Total Knee Replacement	Valve Replacement	Women's Health
★★★	NR	NR	★★★	★★★	NR	★★★	NR	★★★	★★★★★	NR	NR	NR	★★★★★	★★★	★★★	★★★★★	NR	NR
★★★	★★★	★	★★★	★	NR	★★★	NR	★★★	★★★	NR	NR	★★★	★	★	NR	★★★	NR	NR
★★★	NR	NR	★★★	NR	NR	NR	NR	★★★	NR	NR	NR	★★★	★★★	NR	NR	NR	NR	NR
★★★	NR	NR	★	NR	NR	NR	NR	★	NR	★★★	NR	NR	NR	NR	NR	NR	NR	NR
★★★	NR	★★★	★★★	★★★	NR	NR	NR	★★★	★★★	NR	NR	★★★	★★★	★★★	NR	NR	NR	NR
★★★	★★★	★★★	★★★	★★★	NR	★★★	NR	★★★	★★★	NR	NR	★★★	★★★	★★★	NR	NR	NR	NR
★	★	★	★★★	★	NR	★★★	★★★	★★★	★★★	★★★	★★★	★	★	★	★★★	★★★	★★★	NR
★★★	★	★	★★★	★★★	NR	★★★	★★★	★★★	★★★	★★★	★★★	★★★	★	★★★	★	★	★★★	NR
★★★	★★★	★★★	★★★	★★★	NR	★★★	NR	★★★	★★★	★	NR	★★★	★★★	★	★★★	★★★	NR	NR
★	★★★	★	★★★	★★★	NR	★★★	★★★	★	★★★★★	★★★	NR	★★★	★	★★★	★★★	★★★★★	★	NR
★	NR	★	★	NR	NR	NR	NR	★	NR	NR	NR	NR	★★★	NR	NR	NR	NR	NR
★★★	NR	NR	★	NR	NR	NR	NR	★★★	NR	NR	NR	NR	NR	NR	NR	NR	NR	NR
★	★★★	★	★	★★★★★	NR	★	★★★	★★★	★★★	NR	NR	★	NR	NR	★★★	★	NR	NR
NR	NR	NR	★★★	NR	NR	NR	NR	★★★	NR	NR	NR	★★★★★	★★★	NR	NR	NR	NR	NR
★★★	NR	NR	★★★	NR	NR	NR	NR	★★★	NR	NR	NR	NR	★	★★★	NR	NR	NR	NR
★★★	NR	★★★	★	NR	NR	NR	NR	★	NR	NR	NR	★	★	NR	NR	NR	NR	NR
★★★	NR	★★★	★★★	★★★	NR	★★★	NR	★	NR	NR	NR	★★★	★★★	★★★★★	NR	★★★	NR	NR
★	NR	NR	★	NR	NR	NR	NR	★	NR	NR	NR	NR	★★★	NR	NR	NR	NR	NR
★★★	★★★	★★★	★	★★★	NR	★★★	★★★	★★★	★★★	★★★	NR	★★★	NR	★★★	★★★	★★★★★	NR	NR
★★★	★★★	★	★	★★★★★	NR	★	NR	★	★★★	★	NR	★★★	NR	★★★	★★★	★★★	NR	NR
★★★	★	NR	★★★	NR	NR	NR	NR	NR	NR	NR	NR	★	NR	NR	NR	NR	NR	NR
★★★	NR	★★★	★★★	★★★	NR	NR	NR	★★★	NR	NR	NR	★★★	★★★	★★★	NR	NR	NR	NR
★★★★★	★★★	★	★★★★★	★★★	NR	★★★	★★★	★★★★★	★★★	★★★	★★★	★★★★★	★★★	★★★★★	★★★	★	★★★	NR
★★★	★	★★★	★	★★★★★	NR	★★★	★★★	★	★★★	NR	NR	★	NR	★★★	★★★	★★★★★	★★★	NR
★★★	★	★	★★★	★	NR	★	NR	★★★	NR	★	NR	★★★	★★★	★	★★★	★★★	★	NR
★★★	★★★	NR	★★★	NR	NR	NR	NR	★	NR	NR	NR	NR	NR	★★★	NR	NR	NR	NR
★★★	★★★	NR	★★★	NR	NR	NR	NR	★★★	NR	NR	NR	NR	★	★★★	NR	NR	NR	NR
★★★	★★★	★	★	★	NR	★★★	NR	★★★★★	NR	★	★★★	★★★	NR	★★★	★★★	★★★	★★★	NR
★★★	★★★	★★★	★	NR	NR	NR	NR	★★★★★	NR	NR	NR	★★★	★★★★★	★	NR	NR	★★★	NR
★★★	★★★	★	★	★★★	NR	★★★	★★★★★	★★★	★★★	★★★	NR	★	★	★	★★★	NR	★★★	NR
NR	NR	NR	★★★	NR	NR	NR	NR	★	NR	NR	NR	NR	NR	NR	NR	NR	NR	NR
★★★	NR	★★★	★★★	NR	NR	NR	NR	★★★	NR	NR	NR	NR	NR	★★★	NR	NR	NR	NR
★★★	★	★★★	★★★	★★★	NR	★★★	NR	★	NR	★★★	NR	★	★	★	★★★	★★★★★	★★★★★	NR
★★★	NR	★	★★★	NR	NR	NR	NR	★	NR	NR	NR	★★★	NR	NR	NR	NR	NR	NR
★★★	★★★	★★★	★★★	★★★	NR	★	NR	★★★	★★★	★★★	NR	★	★★★	★	★★★	★★★★★	★★★	NR
★★★	NR	NR	★★★	NR	NR	NR	NR	★★★	NR	NR	NR	★★★	NR	NR	NR	NR	NR	NR
★★★	NR	★	★★★	NR	NR	NR	NR	★	★★★	NR	NR	★★★	★	NR	NR	NR	NR	NR
★★★	★★★	NR	★★★	NR	NR	NR	NR	★★★	NR	NR	NR	★★★	★★★	NR	NR	NR	NR	NR
★★★★★	NR	NR	★★★	NR	NR	NR	NR	★★★	NR	NR	NR	★★★	NR	NR	NR	NR	NR	NR
★★★	NR	★	★★★	NR	NR	NR	NR	★★★	NR	NR	NR	★★★	★★★	NR	NR	NR	NR	NR
★★★	NR	NR	★★★	NR	NR	NR	NR	★★★	NR	NR	NR	★★★	★	★★★	NR	NR	NR	NR
★★★	NR	★★★	★★★	NR	NR	NR	NR	★★★★★	NR	NR	NR	★★★★★	★★★★★	★★★	NR	NR	NR	NR
★★★	★★★	★★★	★★★	★★★	NR	★★★	★	★★★	★	★★★	★★★	★★★	★★★	★★★	★★★	★	★★★	NR
★★★★★	★★★	★★★	★★★★★	★★★	NR	★★★	★★★	★★★★★	★★★	★★★	★★★	★★★★★	★★★	★★★★★	★★★	★	★★★	NR
★★★	NR	NR	★★★	NR	NR	NR	NR	★★★	NR	NR	NR	NR	★★★	NR	NR	NR	NR	NR
★★★	★	NR	★	★★★	NR	★★★	NR	★	NR	NR	NR	★	★	★	NR	★★★	NR	NR

	Appendectomy	Atrial Fibrillation	Back and Neck Surgery (except Spinal Fusion)	Back and Neck Surgery (Spinal Fusion)	Bariatric Surgery	Bowel Obstruction	Carotid Surgery	Cholecystectomy (Gall Bladder Removal)	Chronic Obstructive Pulmonary Disease (COPD)	Coronary Bypass Surgery	Coronary Interventional Procedures (Angioplasty/Stent)	Diabetic Acidosis a...
51. Marshall Medical Center–South, Boaz	NR	★★★	NR	NR	NR	★★★	NR	★★★	★★★	NR	NR	★★★
52. Medical Center Enterprise, Enterprise	NR	★★★	NR	NR	NR	★★★	NR	★★★	★★★	NR	NR	★★★
53. Mizell Memorial Hospital, Opp	NR	★★★	NR	NR	NR	★★★	NR	★★★	★	NR	NR	NR
54. Mobile Infirmary, Mobile	NR	★★★	★★★	★★★★★	NR	★★★	★★★	★★★	★★★	★	★★★	★★★★★
55. Monroe County Hospital, Monroeville	NR	NR	NR	NR	NR	★★★	NR	★★★	★	NR	NR	NR
56. North Baldwin Infirmary, Bay Minette	NR	★★★	NR	NR	NR	NR	NR	NR	★★★	NR	NR	NR
57. Northeast Alabama Regional Medical Center, Anniston	NR	★★★	NR	NR	★	★	★★★	★★★	★★★	★★★★★	★	★
58. Northport Medical Center, Northport	NR	★★★	★★★	★★★	NR	★★★	NR	★★★	★★★	NR	NR	★★★
59. Northwest Medical Center, Russellville	NR	★★★	NR	NR	NR	★★★	NR	★★★	★★★	NR	NR	NR
60. Northwest Medical Center, Winfield	NR	★★★	NR	NR	NR	★★★	NR	★★★	★★★	NR	NR	NR
61. Parkway Medical Center Hospital, Decatur	NR	★★★	NR	NR	NR	★★★	NR	★★★	★★★	NR	NR	★★★
62. Pickens County Medical Center, Carrollton	NR	NR	NR	NR	NR	NR	NR	★★★	★★★	NR	NR	NR
63. Prattville Baptist Hospital, Prattville	NR	★★★	NR	NR	NR	★★★	NR	NR	★★★	NR	NR	NR
64. Providence Hospital, Mobile	NR	★★★	★★★	★★★	NR	★★★	★★★	★★★★★	★★★	★	★★★★★	★★★
65. Randolph Medical Center, Roanoke	NR	NR	NR	NR	NR	NR	NR	NR	★★★	NR	NR	NR
66. Red Bay Hospital, Red Bay	NR	NR	NR	NR	NR	NR	NR	NR	★★★	NR	NR	NR
67. Riverview Regional Medical Center, Gadsden	NR	★★★	★★★	NR	NR	★	★★★	★★★	NR	★★★	★★★	★★★
68. Russell Medical Center, Alexander City	NR	★★★	NR	NR	NR	★★★	NR	★	★★★	NR	★★★	NR
69. Russellville Hospital, Russellville	NR	★★★	NR	NR	NR	★★★	NR	★★★	★★★	NR	NR	NR
70. St. Vincent's–Birmingham, Birmingham	NR	★★★	★★★	★★★	NR	★★★	★★★	★★★	★★★	★★★	★★★	★
71. St. Vincent's–Blount, Oneonta	NR	★★★	NR	NR	NR	★★★	NR	NR	★★★	NR	NR	NR
72. St. Vincent's–East, Birmingham	NR	★★★	★★★★★	★★★★★	NR	★	★★★	★★★	★★★	NR	★★★	★
73. St. Vincent's–St. Clair, Pell City	NR	★★★	NR	NR	NR	★★★	NR	★★★	★★★	NR	NR	NR
74. Shoals Hospital, Muscle Shoals	NR	★★★	NR	NR	NR	★★★	NR	★★★	★★★	NR	NR	NR
75. South Baldwin Regional Medical Center, Foley	NR	★★★	NR	NR	NR	★★★	NR	★★★	★★★	NR	NR	NR
76. Southeast Alabama Medical Center, Dothan	NR	★★★	★	★	NR	★★★	★★★	★★★	★★★	★★★	★★★	★★★
77. Southwest Alabama Medical Center, Thomasville	NR	NR	NR	NR	NR	NR	NR	NR	★★★	NR	NR	★★★
78. Springhill Medical Center, Mobile	NR	★★★	★★★	★★★	NR	★★★	★★★	★★★	★★★	★	★★★	★★★
79. Stringfellow Memorial Hospital, Anniston	NR	★★★	NR	NR	NR	★★★	★★★	★★★	★★★	NR	★	★★★
80. Thomas Hospital, Fairhope	NR	★★★	★★★	★★★	NR	★★★	★★★	★★★	★★★	★★★	★★★	★★★
81. Trinity Medical Center, Birmingham	NR	★★★	★★★	★★★	NR	★★★	★★★	★	★★★	★★★	★★★	★★★
82. Troy Regional Medical Center, Troy	NR	★★★	NR	NR	NR	★★★	NR	★★★★★	★★★	NR	NR	★★★
83. University of Alabama Hospital, Birmingham	NR	★★★	★★★	★★★★★	NR	★	★★★	★★★	★	★★★★★	★	★★★
84. University of Alabama Medical West, Bessemer	NR	★★★	★★★	NR	NR	★★★	NR	★★★	★★★	NR	NR	★★★
85. University of South Alabama Medical Center, Mobile	NR	NR	NR	NR	NR	NR	NR	NR	NR	★	★★★	NR
86. University of South Alabama–Knollwood Hospital, Mobile	NR	NR	NR	NR	NR	NR	NR	★	NR	NR	NR	NR
87. Vaughan Regional Medical Center–Parkway Campus, Selma	NR	★	NR	NR	NR	★	NR	★★★	★★★	NR	NR	★★★
88. Walker Baptist Medical Center, Jasper	NR	★★★	★★★	★★★★★	NR	★★★★★	NR	★★★	★★★	NR	★★★	★★★
89. Wedowee Hospital, Wedowee	NR	NR	NR	NR	NR	NR	NR	NR	★★★	NR	NR	NR
90. Wiregrass Medical Center, Geneva	NR	★★★	NR	NR	NR	★★★	NR	★★★★★	★★★★★	NR	NR	NR
91. Woodland Medical Center, Cullman	NR	★★★	NR	NR	NR	★★★	NR	★★★	★★★	NR	NR	NR

KEY: ★★★★★ BEST   ★★★ AS EXPECTED   ★ POOR   NR NOT RATED BY HEALTHGRADES   For full definitions of ratings and awards, see Appendix.

Gastrointestinal Bleed	Gastrointestinal Surgeries and Procedures	Heart Attack	Heart Failure	Hip Fracture Repair	Maternity Care	Pancreatitis	Peripheral Vascular Bypass	Pneumonia	Prostatectomy	Pulmonary Embolism	Resection/Replacement of Abdominal Aorta	Respiratory Failure	Sepsis	Stroke	Total Hip Replacement	Total Knee Replacement	Valve Replacement	Women's Health
★★★	★★★	★	★	★★★	NR	★	NR	★	★★★	NR	NR	★	★	★	NR	NR	NR	NR
★★★	★★★	★	★	★★★	NR	NR	NR	★★★	NR	NR	NR	★	★	★★★	★	★	NR	NR
★★★	NR	NR	★	★	NR	NR	NR	★	NR	NR	NR	NR	★	★★★	NR	NR	NR	NR
★★★	★★★	★	★★★	★★★★★	NR	★	★★★★★	★★★	★★★	★★★	★★★	★★★	★★★	★	★★★	★★★	★★★	NR
★★★	NR	NR	★★★	NR	NR	NR	NR	★	NR	NR	NR	NR	★	NR	NR	NR	NR	NR
★	NR	NR	★	★★★	NR	NR	NR	★★★	NR	NR	NR	NR	★★★	NR	NR	NR	NR	NR
★	★★★	★	★★★	★★★★★	NR	★★★	NR	★★★	★	★★★	NR	★★★	★★★	★★★	★	★★★	NR	NR
★★★	★★★	NR	★★★	★★★	NR	NR	NR	★★★	NR	NR	NR	★★★	★★★	★★★	★★★	★★★	NR	NR
★	NR	★★★	★	★★★	NR	NR	NR	★★★	NR	NR	NR	★★★	★	★★★	NR	★★★	NR	NR
★★★	NR	★★★	★★★	★	NR	NR	NR	★★★	NR	NR	NR	★★★	★★★	★★★	NR	NR	NR	NR
★★★	NR	★	★★★	NR	NR	NR	NR	★★★	NR	NR	NR	★★★	★★★	★★★	NR	NR	NR	NR
★★★	NR	NR	★	NR	NR	NR	NR	★	NR	NR	NR	NR	★	NR	NR	NR	NR	NR
NR	NR	NR	★	NR	NR	NR	NR	★	NR	NR	NR	NR	★	NR	NR	NR	NR	NR
★★★	★★★	★	★★★	★★★★★	NR	★★★	★★★	★★★	★	★★★	NR	★	★★★	★★★★★	★★★	★★★	★★★	NR
★★★	★★★	★★★	★★★	★	NR	★★★	NR	★	NR	NR	NR	★★★	★	★★★	NR	★	NR	NR
★	NR	★★★	★	★★★	NR	NR	NR	★★★	NR	NR	NR	★★★	★	★★★	NR	★★★	NR	NR
★★★	★★★	★★★	★	★★★★★	NR	★★★	★★★	★★★	★★★★★	NR	★★★	★★★	★★★	★	★★★	★★★★★	NR	NR
★★★	NR	NR	★	NR	NR	NR	NR	★	NR	NR	NR	NR	★	★★★	NR	NR	NR	NR
★	★	★★★	★★★	★★★	NR	★	★★★	★	★★★	★	★★★	★	★	★	★★★	★★★	★★★	NR
★★★	NR	NR	★★★	NR	NR	NR	NR	★★★	NR	NR	NR	NR	★★★	NR	★	NR	NR	NR
★★★	NR	NR	★	★★★★★	NR	NR	NR	★	NR	NR	NR	★★★	★★★	NR	★★★	★★★	NR	NR
★★★★★	★★★	★★★	★★★	★★★	NR	★★★	NR	★★★	★★★	★★★	NR	★★★	★★★	★	NR	★★★	NR	NR
★★★	★★★	★★★	NR	★★★	NR	★★★	★	NR	NR	★★★	NR	★★★	★★★	NR	★	NR	★★★	NR
★★★	NR	NR	★★★	NR	NR	NR	NR	★★★	NR	NR	NR	NR	★★★★★	NR	NR	NR	NR	NR
★★★	★★★	★	★	★★★★★	NR	★★★	★★★	★★★	★★★	NR	★	NR	★★★	★	★★★	★★★	NR	NR
★★★	★★★	★★★	★★★	★★★	NR	★★★	★★★	★★★	★★★	NR	★★★	NR	★★★	★★★	NR	★★★	NR	NR
★★★	★★★	★★★	★★★	★★★	★★★	★★★	★★★	★★★	★★★	★	★★★	★★★	★★★	★★★	★★★	★★★	NR
★★★	★★★	NR	★★★	★	NR	NR	★★★	NR	★★★	★★★	★★★	NR	★	★★★	★★★	NR	NR
★★★	★★★	★★★	★★★	★	NR	★★★	★★★	★★★	★★★	★★★	★★★	★	★★★	★★★	NR	★★★★★	NR
★★★	NR	★★★	★★★	★★★	NR	NR	★	NR	★★★	NR	NR	★★★	NR	NR	NR	NR	NR	NR
★★★	NR	NR	★★★	★★★	NR	NR	★	NR	★★★	NR	NR	★	NR	NR	NR	NR	NR	NR
★★★	★	★★★	★	NR	NR	★★★	NR	★★★	★★★	★★★	NR	★★★	★	★	NR	NR	NR	NR
★	★★★	★★★	★★★	★★★★★	NR	★★★	NR	★★★	★★★	★★★	★★★★★	★★★	★	★★★	★★★★★	NR	NR
NR	NR	NR	★★★	NR	NR	NR	NR	★★★	NR	NR	NR	NR	NR	NR	NR	NR	NR	NR
★★★	NR	NR	NR	NR	NR	NR	NR	★★★	NR	NR	NR	NR	★	★	NR	NR	NR	NR
★	★★★	★	★	★★★★★	NR	★★★	NR	★	NR	NR	NR	★★★	★★★	NR	★★★	NR	NR

	Appendectomy	Atrial Fibrillation	Back and Neck Surgery (except Spinal Fusion)	Back and Neck Surgery (Spinal Fusion)	Bariatric Surgery	Bowel Obstruction	Carotid Surgery	Cholecystectomy (Gall Bladder Removal)	Chronic Obstructive Pulmonary Disease (COPD)	Coronary Bypass Surgery	Coronary Interventional Procedures (Angioplasty/Stent)	Diabetic Acidosis a
1. **Alaska Native Medical Center**, Anchorage	NR	★★★	NR	NR	NR	★★★	NR	★★★	★★★	NR	NR	NR	
2. **Alaska Regional Hospital**, Anchorage	NR	★★★	★	★★★	NR	★★★	★★★	NR	★★★	★★★	★★★	NR	
3. **Bartlett Regional Hospital**, Juneau	NR	NR	NR	NR	NR	★★★	NR	NR	★★★	NR	NR	NR	
4. **Central Peninsula General Hospital**, Soldotna	NR	★★★	NR	NR	NR	★	NR	★★★	★★★	NR	NR	NR	
5. **Fairbanks Memorial Hospital**, Fairbanks	NR	★★★	NR	NR	NR	★★★	NR	★★★	★★★	NR	NR	NR	
6. **Ketchikan General Hospital**, Ketchikan	NR	NR	NR	NR	NR	★★★	NR	NR	★★★	NR	NR	NR	
7. **Mat-Su Regional Medical Center**, Palmer	NR	★★★	NR	NR	NR	★★★	NR	★★★	★★★	NR	NR	NR	
8. **Mt. Edgecumbe Hospital**, Sitka	NR	★★★	NR	NR	NR	NR	NR	NR	★★★	NR	NR	NR	
9. **Providence Alaska Medical Center**, Anchorage	NR	★★★★★	★★★	★★★	NR	★★★	★★★	★★★★★	★★★	★★★★★	★★★	★★★	
10. **Yukon Kuskokwim Delta Regional Hospital**, Bethel	NR	NR	NR	NR	NR	NR	NR	NR	★★★	NR	NR	NR	

KEY: ★★★★★ **BEST** ★★★ **AS EXPECTED** ★ **POOR** NR **NOT RATED BY HEALTHGRADES** For full definitions of ratings and awards, see Appendix.

832 CHAPTER 8: HOSPITAL RATINGS BY PROCEDURE

ALASKA HOSPITALS: RATINGS BY PROCEDURE

Gastrointestinal Bleed	Gastrointestinal Surgeries and Procedures	Heart Attack	Heart Failure	Hip Fracture Repair	Maternity Care	Pancreatitis	Peripheral Vascular Bypass	Pneumonia	Prostatectomy	Pulmonary Embolism	Resection/Replacement of Abdominal Aorta	Respiratory Failure	Sepsis	Stroke	Total Hip Replacement	Total Knee Replacement	Valve Replacement	Women's Health
★★★	★★★	NR	★★★	★★★	NR	NR	NR	★★★	★	NR	NR	★★★	★★★★★	★	NR	★★★	NR	NR
★★★	★★★	★★★	★	★★★	NR	NR	NR	★★★	★★★	NR	NR	NR	★★★	★★★	★★★	★★★	★★★	NR
★★★	NR	NR	★★★	★★★	NR	NR	NR	★★★	NR	NR	NR	★★★	NR	NR	NR	★★★	NR	NR
★★★	NR	NR	★★★	★★★	NR	NR	NR	★★★	NR	NR	NR	★★★	NR	NR	NR	★★★	NR	NR
★★★	★★★	NR	★★★	★★★	NR	NR	NR	★★★	NR	NR	NR	★★★	★★★	★★★	★	★	NR	NR
NR	NR	NR	★★★	★★★	NR	NR	NR	★★★	NR	NR	NR	NR	NR	NR	NR	NR	NR	NR
★★★	★★★	★★★	★★★	★★★	NR	NR	NR	★★★	★★★	NR	NR	★★★	★★★	NR	★	NR	NR	NR
NR	NR	NR	NR	NR	NR	NR	NR	★★★	NR	NR	NR	NR	NR	NR	NR	NR	NR	NR
★★★★★	★★★	★	★★★	★★★	NR	★★★	NR	★★★★★	★	★★★	★	★★★	★★★★★	★	★★★	★★★	★★★★★	NR
NR	NR	NR	★★★	NR	NR	NR	NR	★★★	NR	NR	NR	NR	NR	NR	NR	NR	NR	NR

ARIZONA HOSPITALS: RATINGS BY PROCEDURE

Hospital	Appendectomy	Atrial Fibrillation	Back and Neck Surgery (except Spinal Fusion)	Back and Neck Surgery (Spinal Fusion)	Bariatric Surgery	Bowel Obstruction	Carotid Surgery	Cholecystectomy (Gall Bladder Removal)	Chronic Obstructive Pulmonary Disease (COPD)	Coronary Bypass Surgery	Coronary Interventional Procedures (Angioplasty/Stent)	Diabetic Acidosis and...
1. Arizona Heart Hospital, Phoenix	NR	★★★	NR	NR	NR	NR	★★★★★	NR	★★★★★	★★★	★★★★★	NR
2. Arrowhead Hospital, Glendale	★★★	★★★	NR	NR	NR	★★★	NR	★	★★★	NR	★★★	NR
3. Banner Baywood Heart Hospital, Mesa	NR	★★★★★	NR	NR	NR	NR	★★★	NR	★★★	★★★	★★★	NR
4. Banner Baywood Medical Center, Mesa	★★★★★	★★★	NR	NR	NR	★★★★★	NR	★	★★★	NR	NR	★★★
5. Banner Desert Medical Center, Mesa	★★★	★★★	★	★	NR	★★★	★	★	★★★	★★★★★	★★★	★★★
6. Banner Estrella Medical Center, Phoenix	★★★	★★★	NR	NR	NR	NR	NR	NR	★★★	NR	★★★	NR
7. Banner Good Samaritan Medical Center, Phoenix	★★★	★★★★★	★	★	★★★★★	★★★	★★★	★★★	★★★	★★★	★★★	★★★
8. Banner Mesa Medical Center, Mesa	★★★★★	★★★	NR	NR	NR	★★★	NR	★★★	★★★	NR	NR	★★★
9. Banner Thunderbird Medical Center, Glendale	★★★	★★★	★★★	NR	NR	★★★	★★★	★	★★★★★	★★★	★★★★★	★★★
10. Carondelet Holy Cross Hospital, Nogales	★★★	NR	NR	NR	NR	NR	NR	NR	★	NR	NR	NR
11. Carondelet St. Joseph's Hospital and Health Center, Tucson	★	★★★	★★★★★	NR	NR	★★★	★★★	★	★★★	NR	★★★	★★★
12. Carondelet St. Mary's Hospital and Health Center, Tucson	★★★	★★★	★★★	NR	NR	★★★	★★★	★	★★★	NR	★★★	★★★
13. Casa Grande Regional Medical Center, Casa Grande	★	★★★	NR	NR	NR	★★★	NR	★★★	★★★	NR	NR	★★★
14. Chandler Regional Hospital, Chandler	★	★★★	NR	NR	NR	★★★	★	★★★	★★★	★★★	★★★	★★★
15. Cobre Valley Community Hospital, Globe	★★★	★	NR	NR	NR	★★★	NR	NR	★★★	NR	NR	★
16. Del E. Webb Memorial Hospital, Sun City West	★★★★★	★★★	NR	NR	NR	★★★	★★★	★★★	★★★★★	NR	★★★	★★★
17. El Dorado Hospital, Tucson	★★★	★★★	★★★	★★★	NR	★★★	★★★	★★★	★★★	NR	★★★	NR
18. Flagstaff Medical Center, Flagstaff	★	★	★★★	★★★★★	★★★	★★★	★★★	★★★	★	★★★	★★★	★★★★★
19. Fort Defiance Indian Hospital, Fort Defiance	NR	NR	NR	NR	NR	NR	NR	NR	NR	NR	NR	★★★
20. Havasu Regional Medical Center, Lake Havasu City	★★★	★★★	★★★	★★★	NR	★★★	NR	★	★★★	NR	★★★	★★★
21. John C. Lincoln Deer Valley Hospital, Phoenix	★★★	★★★	NR	NR	NR	★★★	★	★	★★★★★	★★★	★★★	★★★
22. John C. Lincoln North Mountain Hospital, Phoenix	★★★	★★★	★★★	★★★	NR	★★★	★★★	★★★	★★★★★	★★★	★★★	★★★
23. Kingman Regional Medical Center, Kingman	★★★★★	★★★	NR	NR	NR	★★★	★	★★★	★★★★★	NR	★	★★★
24. La Paz Regional Hospital, Parker	★★★	★★★	NR	NR	NR	★★★	NR	★★★	★★★★★	NR	NR	★★★
25. Maricopa Medical Center, Phoenix	★	NR	NR	NR	NR	★★★	NR	NR	★★★★★	NR	★	★★★
26. Maryvale Hospital, Phoenix	★	NR	NR	NR	NR	★★★	NR	★★★	★★★	NR	★★★	NR
27. Mayo Clinic Hospital, Phoenix	★★★	★★★★★	★★★★★	★★★★★	★★★★★	★★★	★★★	★★★★★	★★★	★★★	★★★★★	NR
28. Mesa General Hospital, Mesa	★★★	★★★	NR	NR	NR	NR	★★★	NR	★★★	★★★	★★★	NR
29. Mt. Graham Regional Medical Center, Safford	★	★★★	NR	NR	NR	★	NR	★★★	★	NR	NR	NR
30. Navapache Regional Medical Center, Show Low	★★★	★★★	NR	NR	NR	★★★	NR	★★★	★★★	NR	★★★	NR
31. Northwest Medical Center, Tucson	★★★	★★★	★★★	★★★	★★★	★★★★★	★★★	★★★	★★★	★★★	★★★	★★★
32. Northwest Medical Center—Oro Valley, Oro Valley	★★★	★★★	NR	NR	NR	★★★	NR	★★★	★★★	NR	★★★	★★★
33. Paradise Valley Hospital, Phoenix	★★★	★	NR	NR	NR	★★★	★★★	★★★	★★★	NR	NR	NR
34. Payson Regional Medical Center, Payson	★★★	★★★	★★★	NR	NR	★★★	NR	★★★	★★★	NR	NR	NR
35. Phoenix Baptist Hospital, Phoenix	★	★★★	NR	NR	NR	★★★	★★★	★★★	★★★	★★★	★★★	NR
36. Phoenix Memorial Hospital, Phoenix	★	NR	NR	NR	★★★	NR	★★★	NR	★★★	NR	★★★	NR
37. St. Joseph's Hospital and Medical Center, Phoenix	★	★★★	★	★	NR	★★★	★★★	★	★★★	★★★	★★★	★★★
38. St. Luke's Medical Center, Phoenix	★★★	★★★	★★★	NR	★	NR	NR	NR	★★★	★★★	★	NR
39. St. Lukes Behaviorial Health Center, Phoenix	★★★	★★★	★★★	NR	NR	NR	NR	NR	★★★	NR	NR	NR
40. Scottsdale Healthcare—Osborn, Scottsdale	★★★★★	★★★	★★★	★★★	NR	★★★	★★★	★★★	★★★	★★★	NR	★★★
41. Scottsdale Healthcare—Shea, Scottsdale	★★★★★	★★★	★★★	★★★	★★★★★	★★★	★★★	★★★	★★★	★★★	★★★	★★★
42. Sierra Vista Regional Health Center, Sierra Vista	★★★	★★★	NR	NR	NR	★★★	NR	★★★	★★★	NR	NR	NR
43. Southeast Arizona Medical Center, Douglas	NR	NR	NR	NR	NR	NR	NR	NR	★★★	NR	NR	NR
44. Tempe St. Luke's Hospital, Tempe	★★★	★★★	NR	NR	★★★	★★★	NR	★★★	★★★	NR	NR	NR
45. Tucson Heart Hospital, Tucson	NR	★★★★★	NR	NR	NR	NR	★★★	NR	★★★	★★★	★★★	★★★
46. Tucson Medical Center, Tucson	★★★	★★★	★	★	NR	★★★★★	★	★★★★★	★★★	★★★★★	★	★★★
47. University Medical Center, Tucson	★	★★★	★★★	★	NR	★★★	★★★	★	★★★	★★★	★★★	★★★
48. University Physicians Healthcare Hospital at Kino, Tucson	★★★	NR	NR	NR	NR	NR	NR	NR	★★★	NR	NR	NR
49. Verde Valley Medical Center, Cottonwood	★★★	★★★	NR	NR	NR	★★★	NR	★★★	★★★	NR	★★★	★★★
50. Walter O. Boswell Memorial Hospital, Sun City	★★★	★★★★★	★★★	★★★	NR	★★★	★	★★★	★★★	★★★	★★★	★★★

KEY: ★★★★★ BEST ★★★ AS EXPECTED ★ POOR NR NOT RATED BY HEALTHGRADES For full definitions of ratings and awards, see Appendix.

Gastrointestinal Bleed	Gastrointestinal Surgeries and Procedures	Heart Attack	Heart Failure	Hip Fracture Repair	Maternity Care	Pancreatitis	Peripheral Vascular Bypass	Pneumonia	Prostatectomy	Pulmonary Embolism	Resection/Replacement of Abdominal Aorta	Respiratory Failure	Sepsis	Stroke	Total Hip Replacement	Total Knee Replacement	Valve Replacement	Women's Health
NR	NR	★★★★★	★★★★★	NR	NR	NR	★★★	★★★★★	NR	NR	★★★	★★★	NR	NR	NR	NR	★★★	NR
★★★	★★★	★★★	★★★	★★★★★	★★★★★	NR	NR	★★★★★	★★★	NR	NR	★★★★★	★★★★★	★★★★★	★★★	★★★	NR	NR
NR	NR	★★★★★	★★★★★	NR	NR	NR	★★★	★★★★★	NR	★★★	★★★	★★★	NR	★★★	NR	NR	★	NR
★★★	★★★	★★★★★	★★★★★	★★★★★	★★★★★	★★★	NR	★★★★★	★★★	★★★	NR	★★★★★	★★★★★	★★★★★	★★★	★★★	NR	NR
★★★	★★★	★★★	★★★	★★★	★★★	★★★	★★★	★★★	★	★★★	★★★	★★★	★★★	★★★	★★★	★	★★★	★★★
★★★	NR	★★★	★★★★★	★★★★★	★★★	NR	NR	★★★	NR	NR	NR	★★★★★	NR	★★★	★★★	NR	NR	NR
★★★	★★★	★★★	★★★★★	★★★	★★★	★★★	★★★★★	★	★★★	★★★	★★★	★★★	★★★★★	★★★★★	★	★	★★★★★	★★★
★★★	★★★	★★★	★★★	★★★	★★★	★★★	★★★★★	★★★	★★★	★★★	NR	★★★	★★★	★★★★★	★	★	NR	NR
★★★★★	★★★	★★★★★	★★★★★	★★★	★★★	★★★	★★★★★	★	★★★	★★★	★★★	★★★★★	★★★★★	★★★★★	★	★★★	★★★	★★★
NR	NR	NR	NR	NR	★★★★★	NR	NR	★★★	NR	NR	NR	NR	NR	NR	NR	NR	NR	NR
★★★	★	★★★	★★★	★★★	★★★	★★★	★★★	★★★	★★★	★★★	★★★	★	★★★	★★★	★★★	★★★	★★★	NR
★★★	★★★	★★★	★★★	★★★	NR	★★★	NR	★★★★★	★★★	★★★	NR	★★★	★★★	★★★★★	NR	★	NR	NR
★★★	★★★	★★★	★★★★★	★★★	★★★	★★★	NR	★★★	★★★	★★★	NR	★★★★★	★★★★★	★★★	★★★	★★★★★	NR	NR
★★★	★★★★★	★★★	★★★★★	★★★	★★★	★★★	NR	★★★★★	★★★	★★★	NR	★★★	★★★	★★★	★★★	NR	NR	★★★
★★★	NR	NR	★	★★★	★★★	NR	NR	★	NR	NR	NR	NR	NR	★	NR	NR	★★★	NR
★★★★★	★★★	★★★	★★★★★	★★★	★★★	NR	NR	★★★★★	★★★	NR	NR	★★★	★★★★★	★★★★★	★★★	★★★	NR	NR
★★★	★★★	★★★	★★★	NR	NR	★★★	NR	★★★★★	NR	NR	NR	★★★	★★★★★	★★★★★	NR	NR	NR	NR
★★★	★★★	★★★	★★★	★★★	★★★	★★★	NR	★★★	★★★	NR	★	★★★	★★★★★	★★★★★	★★★	NR	NR	★★★
NR	NR	NR	★	NR	NR	NR	NR	★★★	NR	NR	NR	NR	NR	NR	NR	NR	NR	NR
★★★	★★★	★★★	★★★	★★★★★	★★★	★★★	NR	★	★★★	★★★	NR	★	★	★★★	★★★	★	NR	NR
★★★	★★★	★★★	★★★★★	★	NR	★★★	NR	★★★★★	★★★	★★★	NR	★★★★★	★★★	★★★	★★★	NR	NR	NR
★★★	★★★	★★★	★★★★★	★★★	★★★★★	★★★	NR	★★★	★★★	★★★	NR	★★★	★★★★★	★★★	★★★	★★★	NR	★★★
★	★★★	★★★	★	★★★	★★★	★★★	★★★★★	★★★	★★★	★	NR	★★★	★★★	★★★	★★★	NR	NR	NR
★★★★★	NR	NR	★★★	NR	★★★★★	NR	NR	★★★★★	NR	NR	NR	NR	NR	NR	NR	NR	NR	NR
★★★★★	NR	★★★	★★★	★★★	★	NR	NR	★★★★★	NR	NR	★	NR	★★★	★★★	NR	NR	NR	NR
★★★	NR	★★★	★★★	NR	★★★	NR	NR	★★★★★	NR	NR	NR	★★★★★	★★★★★	★★★	★★★	NR	NR	NR
★★★	★★★★★	★★★★★	★★★★★	★★★	NR	★	★★★	★★★★★	★★★★★	★★★	★★★	★	★★★★★	★★★	★★★	★	★★★★★	NR
★★★	NR	★★★	NR	★★★	★★★	NR	★★★	★★★	★★★	NR	NR	★★★	★★★	★★★	NR	★★★	★★★	★★★
★★★	NR	★★★	★★★	★	NR	NR	NR	★★★	NR	NR	NR	★★★	★★★	★★★	★★★	★★★	NR	NR
★★★	★★★★★	★★★★★	★★★★★	★★★★★	NR	★	★★★★★	★★★★★	★★★	★★★	★★★	★★★★★	★★★★★	★★★★★	★★★	★★★	NR	★★★★★
★★★	★	★★★	★★★	NR	★★★	NR	NR	★★★	★★★	★★★	NR	★★★	★★★	★★★★★	★★★	NR	NR	NR
★★★	★★★	★★★	★★★★★	★★★★★	★★★★★	★★★	★★★	★★★★★	★★★	★★★	NR	★★★★★	★★★	★★★	★★★	★★★	NR	NR
★★★	★★★★★	NR	★★★★★	★★★	★★★	NR	NR	★★★★★	★★★	★★★	NR	★★★★★	★★★★★	★★★	★	★	NR	NR
★★★	★★★	★★★	★★★	★★★	NR	NR	★★★★★	★★★	NR	★★★	NR	★★★	★★★★★	★★★	★	NR	NR	★★★
★★★	NR	★★★	★★★	NR	★★★	NR	NR	★★★	NR	NR	NR	★★★	★★★★★	NR	NR	NR	NR	NR
★★★	★★★★★	★★★	★★★	★★★	★	NR	NR	★★★★★	★★★	★★★	NR	★★★★★	★★★★★	NR	★★★	★★★	★★★	★★★
★★★	NR	★★★	★★★	★★★	NR	NR	NR	★★★★★	NR	NR	NR	★★★	★★★	NR	★★★	★★★	NR	NR
★★★	★★★★★	★★★★★	★★★★★	★★★	★★★★★	★★★	★★★★★	★★★★★	★★★	★★★	★★★	★★★★★	★★★★★	★★★★★	★★★★★	★★★	★★★★★	★★★★★
★★★	★★★	★★★★★	★★★★★	★★★★★	★★★	★★★	NR	★★★★★	★★★★★	★★★	NR	★★★★★	★★★	★★★	★★★	★★★	★★★	★★★
★★★	★★★	★★★	★★★	★★★	★★★	★★★	NR	★★★	NR	★★★	NR	★★★	★★★	★★★	★★★	★	NR	NR
NR	NR	NR	★★★	NR	NR	NR	NR	★★★	NR	NR	NR	NR	NR	NR	NR	NR	NR	NR
★★★	NR	NR	★★★★★	★★★	NR	NR	NR	★★★★★	NR	NR	NR	★★★	★★★★★	NR	NR	NR	NR	NR
★★★	NR	★★★★★	★★★★★	NR	NR	NR	★★★	★★★★★	NR	★★★	★★★	NR	NR	NR	NR	★★★	NR	NR
★★★	★★★	★★★	★★★	★★★★★	★★★	★★★	NR	★★★★★	★★★★★	NR	NR	★★★★★	★★★★★	★★★	★★★	★★★	NR	★★★
★★★	★★★	★★★★★	★★★	★	★	NR	NR	★★★★★	★★★	★★★	★★★	★★★★★	★★★	★★★	★★★	★★★	★★★	★★★
NR	NR	NR	★★★	NR	NR	NR	NR	★★★★★	★★★	NR	NR	NR	NR	NR	NR	NR	NR	NR
★	★★★	★★★	★	★★★	★★★★★	★★★	★	★★★	★★★	★★★	NR	★★★	★★★	★★★	★★★	NR	NR	NR
★★★	★★★	★★★	★★★★★	★★★	NR	★★★	★★★	★★★★★	★★★	★★★★★	★★★	★★★	★★★★★	★★★★★	★★★★★	★★★	★★★★★	NR

	Appendectomy	Atrial Fibrillation	Back and Neck Surgery (except Spinal Fusion)	Back and Neck Surgery (Spinal Fusion)	Bariatric Surgery	Bowel Obstruction	Carotid Surgery	Cholecystectomy (Gall Bladder Removal)	Chronic Obstructive Pulmonary Disease (COPD)	Coronary Bypass Surgery	Coronary Interventional Procedures (Angioplasty/Stent)	Diabetic Acidosis and
51. **West Valley Hospital**, Goodyear	★	★★★	NR	NR	NR	NR	NR	NR	★★★	★★★	★★★	NR
52. **Western Arizona Regional Medical Center**, Bullhead City	★	★★★	NR	★	NR	★★★	★★★	★	★★★	NR	★★★	★★★
53. **Winslow Memorial Hospital**, Winslow	NR	NR	NR	NR	NR	NR	NR	NR	NR	NR	NR	NR
54. **Yavapai Regional Medical Center**, Prescott	★★★★★	★★★	NR	NR	NR	★★★	★★★	★★★★★	★★★	NR	★★★	★★★
55. **Yuma Regional Medical Center**, Yuma	★★★	★★★	★	★★★	NR	★★★	★	★★★	★★★	★★★	★★★	★★★★★

KEY: ★★★★★ BEST   ★★★ AS EXPECTED   ★ POOR   NR NOT RATED BY HEALTHGRADES   For full definitions of ratings and awards, see Appendix.

Gastrointestinal Bleed	Gastrointestinal Surgeries and Procedures	Heart Attack	Heart Failure	Hip Fracture Repair	Maternity Care	Pancreatitis	Peripheral Vascular Bypass	Pneumonia	Prostatectomy	Pulmonary Embolism	Resection/Replacement of Abdominal Aorta	Respiratory Failure	Sepsis	Stroke	Total Hip Replacement	Total Knee Replacement	Valve Replacement	Women's Health
★★★	NR	★★★★★	★★★	★★★	★★★	NR	NR	★★★★★	NR	NR	NR	★★★	★★★★★	★★★	NR	★★★	NR	NR
★★★	★★★	★★★	★★★	★★★	★★★	★★★	★★★	★★★	★	NR	★★★	★★★	★★★	★★★★★	★★★	★★★	NR	NR
NR	NR	NR	★★★	NR	★★★	NR	NR	★	NR	NR	NR	NR	NR	NR	NR	NR	NR	NR
★★★	★★★	★★★	★★★	★★★★★	★★★	★★★	★★★	★★★	★★★	★★★	NR	★★★	★★★	★★★	★★★★★	★★★★★	NR	NR
★★★	★★★	★★★	★★★★★	★★★	★★★	★★★	NR	★★★	★★★	★★★	NR	★★★	★★★	★★★★★	★	★★★	★★★	★★★★★

ARKANSAS HOSPITALS: RATINGS BY PROCEDURE

	Appendectomy	Atrial Fibrillation	Back and Neck Surgery (except Spinal Fusion)	Back and Neck Surgery (Spinal Fusion)	Bariatric Surgery	Bowel Obstruction	Carotid Surgery	Cholecystectomy (Gall Bladder Removal)	Chronic Obstructive Pulmonary Disease (COPD)	Coronary Bypass Surgery	Coronary Interventional Procedures (Angioplasty/Stent)	Diabetic Acidosis and
1. Arkansas Heart Hospital, Little Rock	NR	★★★	NR	NR	NR	NR	★★★	NR	★★★★★	★★★	★★★★★	NR
2. Arkansas Methodist Medical Center, Paragould	NR	★★★	NR	NR	NR	★★★	NR	★★★★★	★★★	NR	★★★	NR
3. Ashley County Medical Center, Crossett	NR	★★★	NR	NR	NR	★★★	NR	★	NR	NR	NR	NR
4. Baptist Health Medical Center–Arkadelphia, Arkadelphia	NR	★★★	NR	NR	NR	NR	NR	NR	★★★	NR	NR	NR
5. Baptist Health Medical Center–Heber Spings, Heber Springs	NR	NR	NR	NR	NR	★★★	NR	NR	★★★	NR	NR	NR
6. Baptist Health Medical Center–Little Rock, Little Rock	NR	★	★★★★★	★★★	NR	★★★	★★★★★	★	★	★	★★★	★★★
7. Baptist Health Medical Center–North Little Rock, North Little Rock	NR	★	★★★	★★★	NR	★★★	★	★	★	★★★	★★★	★★★
8. Baptist Memorial Hospital–Forrest City, Forrest City	NR	★★★	NR	NR	NR	★★★	NR	NR	★★★	NR	NR	NR
9. Baxter Regional Medical Center, Mountain Home	NR	★★★	NR	★	NR	★★★	★★★	★★★	★★★	★★★	★	★★★
10. Booneville Community Hospital, Booneville	NR	NR	NR	NR	NR	NR	NR	NR	★★★	NR	NR	
11. Bradley County Medical Center, Warren	NR	NR	NR	NR	NR	NR	NR	NR	NR	NR	NR	
12. Chicot Memorial Hospital, Lake Village	NR	NR	NR	NR	NR	★★★	NR	★★★★★	★	NR	NR	
13. Community Medical Center–Izard County, Calico Rock	NR	NR	NR	NR	NR	NR	NR	NR	NR	NR	NR	
14. Conway Regional Medical Center, Conway	NR	★	NR	NR	NR	★★★	★★★	★★★	★	★★★	★★★	★
15. Crittenden Regional Hospital, West Memphis	NR	★★★	NR	NR	NR	★	NR	★★★	★★★	NR	NR	
16. De Queen Medical Center, De Queen	NR	NR	NR	NR	NR	NR	NR	NR	★★★	NR	NR	
17. De Witt City Hospital, De Witt	NR	NR	NR	NR	NR	NR	NR	NR	★★★	NR	NR	
18. Delta Memorial Hospital Association, Dumas	NR	NR	NR	NR	NR	NR	NR	NR	NR	NR	NR	
19. Drew Memorial Hospital, Monticello	NR	★★★	NR	NR	NR	NR	NR	NR	★★★	NR	NR	
20. Fulton County Hospital, Salem	NR	NR	NR	NR	NR	NR	NR	NR	★	NR	NR	
21. Great River Medical Center, Blytheville	NR	NR	NR	NR	NR	★	NR	NR	★	NR	NR	
22. Harris Hospital, Newport	NR	NR	NR	NR	NR	★★★	NR	NR	★★★	NR	NR	
23. Helena Regional Medical Center, Helena	NR	★★★	NR	NR	NR	★★★	NR	NR	★★★	NR	★★★	
24. Hot Spring County Medical Center, Malvern	NR	★	NR	NR	NR	★★★	NR	NR	★★★	NR	NR	
25. Howard Memorial Hospital, Nashville	NR	★	NR	NR	NR	NR	NR	★★★★★	★★★	NR	NR	
26. Jefferson Regional Medical Center, Pine Bluff	NR	★★★	★★★	NR	NR	★★★	★★★	★★★	★★★★★	★★★	★★★	★★★
27. John Ed Chambers Memorial Hospital, Danville	NR	NR	NR	NR	NR	NR	NR	★★★★★	NR	NR	NR	
28. Johnson Regional Medical Center, Clarksville	NR	★★★	NR	NR	NR	★★★	NR	NR	★★★	NR	NR	
29. Little River Memorial Hospital, Ashdown	NR	NR	NR	NR	NR	NR	NR	NR	★★★	NR	NR	
30. Magnolia Hospital, Magnolia	NR	★★★	NR	NR	NR	★★★	NR	NR	★★★	NR	NR	
31. McGehee Desha County Hospital, McGehee	NR	NR	NR	NR	NR	NR	NR	NR	★	NR	NR	
32. Medical Center–South Arkansas, El Dorado	NR	★	NR	NR	NR	★★★	NR	★★★	★★★	NR	★★★	
33. Medical Park Hospital, Hope	NR	★★★	NR	NR	NR	★★★	NR	★★★	★★★	NR	NR	
34. Mena Medical Center, Mena	NR	★	NR	NR	NR	NR	NR	NR	★	NR	NR	
35. Mercy Hospital–Turner Memorial, Ozark	NR	★★★	NR	NR	NR	NR	NR	NR	★★★	NR	NR	
36. National Park Medical Center, Hot Springs	NR	★★★	★★★	NR	NR	★	★★★	★	★★★	★★★	★★★	
37. Nea Medical Center, Jonesboro	NR	★★★	★★★	★★★	NR	★★★	★★★	★★★	★★★	★★★	★★★	
38. North Arkansas Regional Medical Center, Harrison	NR	★★★	NR	NR	NR	★★★	NR	★★★★★	★★★	NR	NR	
39. Northwest Medical Center–Benton County, Bentonville	NR	★★★	★★★★★	★★★	NR	★★★	★★★	★★★	★★★	★★★	★★★	
40. Northwest Medical Center–Washington County, Springdale	NR	★★★	★★★	★★★	NR	★★★	★★★★★	★★★	★	★★★	★★★	
41. Ouachita County Medical Center, Camden	NR	★	NR	NR	NR	★	NR	★★★	★★★	NR	★★★	
42. Ozark Health, Clinton	NR	★	NR	NR	NR	NR	NR	NR	★★★	NR	NR	
43. Piggott Community Hospital, Piggott	NR	NR	NR	NR	NR	NR	NR	NR	★★★	NR	NR	
44. Pike County Memorial Hospital, Murfreesboro	NR	NR	NR	NR	NR	NR	NR	NR	★★★	NR	NR	
45. Randolph County Medical Center, Pocahontas	NR	NR	NR	NR	NR	NR	NR	NR	★★★	NR	NR	
46. Rebsamen Medical Center, Jacksonville	NR	★★★	NR	NR	NR	★★★	NR	★★★	★★★	NR	NR	
47. St. Anthony's Healthcare Center, Morrilton	NR	★★★	NR	NR	NR	★★★	NR	★★★	★★★	NR	NR	
48. St. Bernards Medical Center, Jonesboro	NR	★★★	★★★	★★★★★	NR	★	★★★	★★★	★★★	★★★	★	★★★
49. St. Edward Mercy Medical Center, Fort Smith	NR	★★★	★★★	★★★	NR	★★★	NR	★★★	★★★	★	★★★	★★★
50. St. John's Hospital–Berryville, Berryville	NR	★★★	NR	NR	NR	★★★	NR	NR	★★★	NR	NR	

KEY: ★★★★★ BEST   ★★★ AS EXPECTED   ★ POOR   NR NOT RATED BY HEALTHGRADES   For full definitions of ratings and awards, see Appendix.

Gastrointestinal Bleed	Gastrointestinal Surgeries and Procedures	Heart Attack	Heart Failure	Hip Fracture Repair	Maternity Care	Pancreatitis	Peripheral Vascular Bypass	Pneumonia	Prostatectomy	Pulmonary Embolism	Resection/Replacement of Abdominal Aorta	Respiratory Failure	Sepsis	Stroke	Total Hip Replacement	Total Knee Replacement	Valve Replacement	Women's Health
★★★	NR	★★★★★	★★★★★	NR	NR	NR	★★★	★★★★★	NR	★★★	NR	★★★	★★★	★	NR	NR	★★★	NR
★★★	★★★	★	★	★★★★★	NR	★★★	NR	★★★	★★★	NR	NR	★★★	★★★	★★★	NR	★★★★★	NR	NR
★	NR	NR	★	NR	NR	NR	NR	★	NR	NR	NR	NR	★	★★★	NR	NR	NR	NR
★★★	NR	NR	★	★★★	NR	NR	NR	★	NR	NR	NR	NR	★★★	NR	NR	NR	NR	NR
★★★	NR	NR	★★★	NR	NR	NR	NR	★★★	NR	NR	NR	NR	★★★	NR	NR	NR	NR	NR
★★★	★★★	★	★	★	NR	★★★	★★★	★★★	★	★★★	★★★	★	★★★	★★★	★★★	★	★★★	NR
★★★★★	★★★	★★★	★	★	NR	★★★	★★★	★★★	★	★★★	NR	★★★	★	★★★	★★★	★	★★★	NR
★★★	NR	NR	★	NR	NR	NR	NR	★	NR	NR	NR	★	★★★	NR	NR	NR	NR	NR
★★★	★★★	★★★	★★★	★★★	NR	★★★	★★★	★★★	NR	★★★	★★★	★	NR	★	★★★	★	NR	NR
NR	NR	NR	★★★	NR	NR	NR	NR	★★★	NR	NR	NR	NR	NR	NR	NR	NR	NR	NR
★★★	NR	NR	★	NR	NR	NR	NR	★★★	NR	NR	NR	NR	★★★	NR	NR	NR	NR	NR
★	NR	NR	★	NR	NR	NR	NR	★★★	NR	NR	NR	★	NR	NR	NR	NR	NR	NR
★★★	★	★	★	★★★	NR	★★★	★★★	★	★★★	★★★	NR	★	NR	★	★★★	★★★★★	NR	NR
★	NR	NR	★★★	★★★	NR	★	NR	★★★	NR	★★★	NR	★	★★★	NR	NR	NR	NR	NR
★★★	NR	NR	★★★	NR	NR	NR	NR	★★★	NR	NR	NR	NR	NR	NR	NR	NR	NR	NR
NR	NR	NR	★	NR	NR	NR	NR	★★★	NR	NR	★★★	NR	★	NR	NR	NR	NR	NR
NR	NR	NR	★★★	NR	NR	NR	NR	★★★	NR	NR	NR	NR	★★★	NR	NR	NR	NR	NR
★★★	NR	NR	★	NR	NR	NR	NR	★	NR	NR	NR	NR	★★★	NR	NR	NR	NR	NR
NR	NR	NR	★	NR	NR	NR	NR	★	NR	NR	NR	★	NR	NR	NR	NR	NR	NR
★★★	NR	★	★★★	NR	NR	NR	NR	★	NR	NR	NR	★	★★★	★	NR	NR	NR	NR
★★★	NR	★★★★★	NR	NR	NR	NR	★★★★★	NR	NR	NR	NR	★★★	NR	NR	NR	NR	NR	NR
★★★	NR	★★★	★★★	NR	★★★	NR	NR	★	NR	NR	NR	NR	★★★	★★★	NR	NR	NR	NR
★★★	NR	★★★	★	★	NR	NR	NR	★	NR	NR	NR	★★★	★★★	NR	NR	★★★	NR	NR
NR	NR	★★★	★★★	NR	NR	★★★	NR	★★★★★	NR	NR	NR	NR	★★★	NR	NR	NR	NR	NR
★★★	NR	NR	★	NR	NR	NR	NR	★	NR	NR	NR	★★★	★★★	★★★	NR	NR	NR	NR
★★★	NR	NR	★★★	NR	NR	NR	NR	★	NR	NR	NR	NR	NR	NR	NR	NR	NR	NR
★★★	★★★	★★★	★	★★★★★	NR	★★★	NR	★	NR	★★★	NR	★★★	★	★	★★★	★★★★★	NR	NR
★★★	NR	★★★	★★★	NR	NR	NR	NR	★★★★★	NR	NR	NR	★★★	★★★★★	★★★	NR	NR	NR	NR
★★★	NR	★	★	NR	NR	NR	NR	★	NR	NR	NR	NR	NR	NR	NR	NR	NR	NR
NR	NR	NR	★	NR	NR	NR	NR	★	NR	NR	NR	NR	NR	NR	NR	NR	NR	NR
★★★	★★★	★★★	★★★	★	NR	NR	★	★	★	NR	★	★★★	★	★	NR	★★★	★★★	NR
★	NR	★★★	★	★★★	NR	★★★	NR	★	NR	★	NR	★	★★★	★	★★★	NR	★★★	NR
★★★	★★★	★★★	★★★	★★★	NR	★★★	NR	★★★	★★★	★	NR	★★★	★★★	★★★	NR	★★★	★★★	NR
★★★	★	★★★	★	★★★	NR	★★★	NR	★★★	★★★	NR	NR	★★★	★★★	NR	★★★	★★★	★★★	NR
★	★★★	★	★★★	★★★	NR	★★★	★★★	★★★	★★★	NR	★★★	★	★★★	★	★	★	NR	NR
★★★	NR	★	★★★	NR	NR	NR	NR	★	★★★	NR	★★★	★	★★★	NR	NR	NR	NR	NR
★★★	NR	NR	★★★	NR	NR	NR	NR	★★★	NR	NR	NR	NR	NR	NR	NR	NR	NR	NR
★★★	NR	★★★	★	NR	NR	NR	NR	★★★	NR	NR	NR	★★★	★★★	NR	NR	NR	NR	NR
NR	NR	NR	★	NR	NR	NR	NR	★	NR	NR	NR	NR	NR	NR	NR	NR	NR	NR
★★★	NR	NR	★★★★★	NR	NR	NR	NR	★★★	NR	NR	NR	NR	NR	NR	NR	★★★	NR	NR
★★★	★	★	★★★	★★★	NR	NR	NR	★★★	NR	NR	NR	★★★	★★★	★★★	NR	★	NR	NR
★	NR	NR	★★★	NR	NR	NR	NR	★	NR	NR	NR	★★★	★★★	★★★	NR	NR	★★★	NR
★	★	★	★★★★★	NR	NR	★	★★★	NR	★★★	★	★★★	★★★	NR	NR	NR	★★★	NR	NR
★★★	★★★	★★★	★★★	★	NR	★★★	NR	★★★	★	★★★	★★★	★★★★★	★★★	★	★	★	★★★	NR
★★★	NR	★★★	★★★	NR	NR	NR	★★★	NR	NR	NR	★	★★★	NR	NR	NR	NR	NR	NR

	Appendectomy	Atrial Fibrillation	Back and Neck Surgery (except Spinal Fusion)	Back and Neck Surgery (Spinal Fusion)	Bariatric Surgery	Bowel Obstruction	Carotid Surgery	Cholecystectomy (Gall Bladder Removal)	Chronic Obstructive Pulmonary Disease (COPD)	Coronary Bypass Surgery	Coronary Interventional Procedures (Angioplasty/Stent)	Diabetic Acidosis and
51. St. Joseph's Mercy Health Center, Hot Springs	NR	★★★	★★★★★	★★★	NR	★★★	★★★★★	★★★	★★★★★	★★★	★	★★★
52. St. Mary Rogers Memorial Hospital, Rogers	NR	★★★	NR	NR	NR	★★★	★	★★★	★★★	★	★★★	★★★
53. St. Mary's Regional Medical Center, Russellville	NR	★	★★★	NR	NR	★	NR	★★★	★	NR	NR	NR
54. St. Vincent Doctors Hospital, Little Rock	NR	★★★	★★★★★	★★★★★	NR	★★★	★★★	★★★★★	★★★	★	★★★	★★★
55. St. Vincent Infirmary Medical Center, Little Rock	NR	★★★	★★★★★	★★★★★	NR	★★★	★★★	★★★★★	★★★	★	★★★	★★★
56. St. Vincent Medical Center—North, Sherwood	NR	★★★	★★★★★	★★★★★	NR	★★★	NR	NR	★★★	NR	NR	NR
57. Saline Memorial Hospital, Benton	NR	★★★	NR	NR	NR	★★★	NR	★★★	★★★	NR	NR	NR
58. Siloam Springs Memorial Hospital, Siloam Springs	NR	★★★	NR	NR	NR	★★★	NR	★★★	★★★	NR	NR	NR
59. SMC Regional Medical Center, Osceola	NR	NR	NR	NR	NR	NR	NR	NR	★★★	NR	NR	NR
60. Southwest Regional Medical Center, Little Rock	NR	★★★	NR	NR	NR	★★★	NR	NR	★★★	NR	NR	NR
61. Sparks Regional Medical Center, Fort Smith	NR	★	★★★	★	NR	★★★★★	★★★	★★★	★★★★★	★★★	★	★★★
62. Stone County Medical Center, Mountain View	NR	NR	NR	NR	NR	NR	NR	NR	★★★	NR	NR	NR
63. Stuttgart Regional Medical Center, Stuttgart	NR	★★★	NR	NR	NR	★★★	NR	NR	★	NR	NR	NR
64. Summit Medical Center, Van Buren	NR	NR	NR	NR	NR	★★★	NR	NR	★	NR	NR	NR
65. UAMS Medical Center, Little Rock	NR	★★★	★★★★★	★★★	NR	★	★★★	★★★	★★★	★★★	★★★	★★★
66. Washington Regional Medical Center at North Hills, Fayetteville	NR	★★★	★	★★★	NR	★	★★★	★★★	★★★	★	★★★	★★★
67. White County Medical Center—North Campus, Searcy	NR	★★★	★★★★★	★★★	NR	★★★	★★★	★★★	★★★	★	★★★	★★★
68. White County Medical Center—South Campus, Searcy	NR	★★★	★★★★★	★★★	NR	★★★	★★★	★★★★★	★★★	★	★★★	★★★
69. White River Medical Center, Batesville	NR	★★★	NR	NR	NR	★★★	★★★	★★★	★★★	NR	★★★	★★★

KEY: ★★★★★ BEST   ★★★ AS EXPECTED   ★ POOR   NR NOT RATED BY HEALTHGRADES   For full definitions of ratings and awards, see Appendix.

Gastrointestinal Bleed	Gastrointestinal Surgeries and Procedures	Heart Attack	Heart Failure	Hip Fracture Repair	Maternity Care	Pancreatitis	Peripheral Vascular Bypass	Pneumonia	Prostatectomy	Pulmonary Embolism	Resection/Replacement of Abdominal Aorta	Respiratory Failure	Sepsis	Stroke	Total Hip-Replacement	Total Knee Replacement	Valve Replacement	Women's Health
★★★	★★★	★	★★★	★★★★★	NR	★★★	NR	★★★★★	★★★	★★★★★	★★★	★★★★★	★★★★★	★★★	★★★	★★★	★★★	NR
★★★	★★★	★★★	★★★	★★★	NR	★★★	NR	★★★	★★★	★★★	NR	★★★	★★★	★	★	★★★	NR	NR
★	★★★	★★★	★	★★★★★	NR	★★★	NR	★	★★★	NR	NR	NR	★	★	★★★★★	★★★★★	NR	NR
★★★	★★★	★★★	★★★★★	★★★	NR	★★★	★★★★★	★★★★★	★★★★★	★★★	★★★	★★★★★	★★★★★	★★★	★★★★★	★★★★★	★★★	NR
★★★	★★★	★★★	★★★★★	★★★	NR	★★★	★★★★★	★★★★★	★★★★★	★★★	★★★	★★★★★	★★★★★	★★★	★★★★★	★★★★★	★★★	NR
★★★	NR	★★★	★	★★★	NR	NR	NR	★★★	NR	NR	NR	NR	★★★	★★★	NR	NR	NR	NR
★★★	★★★	★★★	★★★	★★★	NR	★★★	NR	★	NR	★★★	NR	★★★	★★★	★	★★★	★★★	NR	NR
★★★	★	★★★	★★★	★★★	NR	NR	NR	★	NR	NR	NR	★	★	★	NR	NR	NR	NR
NR	NR	NR	★	NR	NR	NR	NR	★	NR	NR	NR	NR	NR	★	NR	NR	NR	NR
★★★	NR	NR	★★★	NR	NR	NR	NR	★★★★★	NR	NR	NR	★★★	★★★	NR	★★★	★★★	NR	NR
★★★	★★★	★	★	★★★★★	NR	★★★	★★★	★★★★★	★★★	NR	★★★	★★★★★	★★★	★★★	★★★	★★★★★	★	NR
★★★	NR	NR	★★★	NR	NR	NR	NR	★★★	NR	NR	NR	★★★	★★★	NR	NR	★★★	NR	NR
★★★	NR	★★★	★★★	NR	NR	NR	NR	★★★	NR	NR	NR	★★★	★★★	★	NR	★★★	NR	NR
★★★	NR	★★★	★	★★★	NR	★★★	NR	★	★★★	NR	NR	NR	★	NR	NR	★★★	NR	NR
★★★	★★★	★★★	★	★★★	NR	NR	NR	★	★★★	★★★	★★★	NR	★	★	★★★	★★★	NR	NR
★	★★★	★★★	★	★	NR	★★★	★★★	★★★	★★★	★★★	★★★	★★★	★★★	★★★	★★★	★★★	★	NR
★★★	★★★	★	★	★★★	NR	★★★	NR	★★★	★	NR	NR	★★★	★	★★★	★	★★★	NR	NR
★	★	★	★	★★★	NR	★★★	NR	★★★	NR	★★★	NR	★★★	★★★	★★★	NR	★★★	NR	NR
★	★	★★★	★	★★★★★	NR	★	NR	★★★	★★★	★	NR	★★★	★	★★★	★★★	★★★	NR	NR

CALIFORNIA HOSPITALS: RATINGS BY PROCEDURE

Hospital	Appendectomy	Atrial Fibrillation	Back and Neck Surgery (except Spinal Fusion)	Back and Neck Surgery (Spinal Fusion)	Bariatric Surgery	Bowel Obstruction	Carotid Surgery	Cholecystectomy (Gall Bladder Removal)	Chronic Obstructive Pulmonary Disease (COPD)	Coronary Bypass Surgery	Coronary Interventional Procedures (Angioplasty/Stent)	Diabetic Acidosis and...
1. Alameda County Medical Center, San Leandro	★★★★★	NR	NR	NR	NR	NR	NR	NR	★★★	NR	NR	NR
2. Alameda Hospital, Alameda	★★★	★★★	NR	NR	NR	★★★	NR	NR	★★★★★	NR	NR	NR
3. Alhambra Hospital and Medical Center, Alhambra	NR	★★★	NR	NR	NR	★★★	NR	★★★	★★★	NR	NR	★★★
4. Alta Bates Summit—Alta Bates Campus, Berkeley	★	★★★	NR	NR	NR	★★★	★★★	★	★★★	NR	★	★★★
5. Alta Bates Summit—Summit Campus, Oakland	★★★	★★★★★	NR	NR	★	★	★★★	★★★	★★★	★★★	★★★	★★★
6. Alvarado Hospital Medical Center, San Diego	★★★	★★★	★★★★★	★★★★★	★★★	★★★	★★★	★★★	★★★	★★★	★★★	★★★
7. Anaheim General Hospital, Anaheim	★★★	NR	NR	NR	NR	★★★	NR	NR	★★★	NR	NR	NR
8. Anaheim Memorial Hospital, Anaheim	★★★	★★★	NR	NR	★★★	★★★	★★★	★★★	★★★★★	★★★	★★★	★★★
9. Antelope Valley Hospital, Lancaster	★★★★★	★★★	NR	NR	★★★	★★★	★★★	★★★	★★★	★★★	★★★	★★★
10. Arrowhead Regional Medical Center, Colton	★★★★★	★	NR	NR	NR	NR	NR	NR	★★★	NR	NR	★★★
11. Arroyo Grande Community Hospital, Arroyo Grande	★★★	★★★	NR	NR	★★★	★★★	★★★★★	★★★	NR	NR	★★★	
12. Bakersfield Heart Hospital, Bakersfield	NR	★★★	NR	NR	NR	★★★	★★★	NR	★★★	★	★★★	
13. Bakersfield Memorial Hospital, Bakersfield	★★★	★★★	★	★★★	NR	★★★	★★★	★	★★★	★★★	★★★	★★★
14. Banner Lassen Medical Center, Susanville	NR	NR	NR	NR	NR	NR	NR	NR	★★★	NR	NR	NR
15. Barstow Community Hospital, Barstow	★★★	★★★	NR	NR	NR	★★★	NR	★★★	★★★	NR	NR	★★★
16. Barton Memorial Hospital, South Lake Tahoe	★	★★★	NR	★★★	NR	★★★	NR	★	★★★	NR	NR	★★★
17. Bellflower Medical Center, Bellflower	★★★	★★★	NR	NR	★★★	NR	NR	NR	★★★	NR	NR	★★★
18. Beverly Hospital, Montebello	★★★	★★★	NR	NR	★★★	NR	★★★	★★★★★	★★★	★★★	★★★	
19. Brotman Medical Center, Culver City	NR	★★★	NR	NR	★★★	★★★★★	★	★	NR	★★★	★★★	
20. California Hospital Medical Center—Los Angeles, Los Angeles	★★★	★★★	NR	NR	★★★	NR	★★★	★★★	NR	NR	★★★	
21. California Pacific Medical Center, San Francisco	★★★★★	★★★	★★★	★★★	★★★★★	★★★	★★★	★	★★★	★★★	★★★	★★★
22. California Pacific Medical Center—Davies Campus, San Francisco	NR	★★★	★★★	NR	NR	NR	NR	★★★	★★★	NR	★★★	★★★
23. The Cancer Center at Riverside Community Hospital, Riverside	★★★	★★★	★	★★★	NR	★★★	★★★	★★★	★★★	★★★	★★★	★★★
24. Cedars-Sinai Medical Center, Los Angeles	★★★	★★★	★★★	★	★★★★★	★★★★★	★★★	★★★	★★★	★★★	★★★	★★★
25. Centinela Freeman Regional Med. Ctr.—Centinela, Inglewood	★★★	★★★	★★★	★★★	NR	★	★	★★★	★★★	★★★	★★★	
26. Centinela Freeman Regional Med. Ctr.—Marina, Marina Del Rey	★	★★★	★★★	NR	NR	★★★	NR	NR	★★★	NR	NR	NR
27. Centinela Freeman Regional Med. Ctr.—Memorial, Inglewood	★★★	★★★	NR	NR	★★★	★★★	NR	NR	★★★	NR	NR	★★★
28. Central Valley General Hospital, Hanford	★★★	NR	NR	NR	NR	NR	NR	NR	★	NR	NR	NR
29. Century City Doctors Hospital, Los Angeles	NR	NR	★	★	NR	NR	NR	NR	★★★	NR	NR	NR
30. Chapman Medical Center, Orange	NR	NR	NR	NR	★★★	★★★	NR	NR	★★★	NR	NR	NR
31. Chinese Hospital, San Francisco	★★★	★★★	NR	NR	★★★	NR	★★★	★★★	★★★	NR	NR	
32. Chino Valley Medical Center, Chino	★★★★★	★★★	NR	NR	★★★	NR	★★★	★★★	NR	NR	★★★	
33. Citrus Valley Medical Center—IC Campus, Covina	★★★	★★★	NR	NR	★★★	★★★	★★★★★	★★★	★★★	★★★		
34. Citrus Valley Medical Center—QV Campus, West Covina	★★★	★★★	★★★	★★★	NR	★★★	★★★	★★★	NR	NR	★	
35. City of Angels Medical Center, Los Angeles	NR	NR	NR	NR	NR	NR	NR	NR	★★★	NR	NR	
36. Clovis Community Medical Center, Clovis	★★★	★★★	NR	NR	★★★★★	★★★	NR	★★★	★	NR	NR	
37. Coast Plaza Doctors Hospital, Norwalk	★★★	NR	NR	NR	NR	NR	NR	★★★	★★★	NR	NR	★★★
38. Coastal Communities Hospital, Santa Ana	★★★★★	NR	NR	NR	NR	★★★	NR	★★★	★★★	NR	NR	NR
39. Colorado River Medical Center, Needles	NR	NR	NR	NR	NR	NR	NR	★★★	NR	NR	NR	
40. Colusa Regional Medical Center, Colusa	NR											
41. Community and Mission Hospital of Huntington Park, Huntington Park	★★★	NR	NR	NR	NR	NR	NR	★★★	★★★	NR	NR	★★★
42. Community Hospital of Gardena, Gardena	NR	NR	NR	NR	NR	NR	NR	★	NR	NR	NR	
43. Community Hospital of Long Beach, Long Beach	★★★	★★★	NR	NR	★	NR	NR	★★★	NR	NR	★★★	
44. Community Hospital of Los Gatos, Los Gatos	★★★	★★★	★★★	★	NR	★★★	NR	★★★	★★★	NR	NR	★★★
45. Community Hospital of the Monterey Peninsula, Monterey	★★★	★★★	★★★	★★★	★★★	★★★	★	★★★★★	★★★	NR	NR	★★★
46. Community Hospital of San Bernardino, San Bernardino	★★★	NR	NR	NR	★★★	NR	★★★	★★★	★★★	NR	NR	★★★
47. Community Memorial Hospital of San Buenaventura, Ventura	★★★	★★★	★★★★★	★★★★★	★★★★★	★	★★★	★★★	★★★	★★★	★★★	★★★
48. Community Regional Medical Center, Fresno	★★★	★★★	★★★	★★★	NR	★★★	★★★	★★★	★	★★★	NR	★★★
49. Contra Costa Regional Medical Center, Martinez	★	NR	NR	NR	★★★	NR	NR	★★★	★★★	NR	NR	NR
50. Corona Regional Medical Center, Corona	★★★★★	★★★	NR	NR	NR	★★★	NR	★★★	★★★	NR	NR	★★★

KEY: ★★★★★ BEST   ★★★ AS EXPECTED   ★ POOR   NR NOT RATED BY HEALTHGRADES   For full definitions of ratings and awards, see Appendix.

Gastrointestinal Bleed	Gastrointestinal Surgeries and Procedures	Heart Attack	Heart Failure	Hip Fracture Repair	Maternity Care	Pancreatitis	Peripheral Vascular Bypass	Pneumonia	Prostatectomy	Pulmonary Embolism	Resection/Replacement of Abdominal Aorta	Respiratory Failure	Sepsis	Stroke	Total Hip Replacement	Total Knee Replacement	Valve Replacement	Women's Health
★★★	NR	★★★	★★★★★	NR	★★★	NR	NR	★★★	NR	NR	NR	NR	★★★	★	NR	NR	NR	NR
★★★	NR	★★★	★★★★★	★★★	NR	NR	NR	★★★	NR	NR	NR	NR	★★★	★★★	NR	★★★	NR	NR
★★★	NR	★★★	★★★★★	★★★	NR	NR	NR	★★★★★	★★★	NR	NR	★★★	★★★	★★★★★	★★★★★	NR	NR	NR
★★★	★★★	★★★	★★★	★★★	★★★	★★★	NR	★★★	★★★	NR	NR	★★★	★★★	★★★★★	★	★	NR	NR
★★★	★★★★★	★★★	★★★	★★★	NR	★★★	★★★	★★★	★★★★★	★★★	★★★	★★★	★★★	★★★★★	★★★	★★★	★★★	NR
★★★	NR	NR	★★★	★★★★★	NR	★★★	★★★	★★★	★★★	NR	★★★	★★★	★★★★★	★★★	NR	NR	NR	NR
★★★	★★★	★★★	★★★	★	★★★	★★★	NR	★★★★★	★★★	NR	NR	★★★	★★★★★	★★★★★	★★★	★★★	★★★	★★★
★★★	★★★	★★★	★★★	★★★★★	★	NR	NR	★★★	★★★	★	NR	★★★	★★★	★★★	NR	★★★	NR	★★★
★★★	NR	★	★★★	★★★	★★★★★	NR	NR	★★★	NR	NR	NR	★★★	★	★	NR	NR	NR	NR
★★★	★★★	★★★	★★★	★★★★★	NR	NR	NR	★★★	★★★	★★★	NR	★	★	★★★	★★★	★★★★★	NR	NR
★★★	NR	★★★	★★★	NR	NR	NR	NR	★★★	NR	★★★	NR	★	★	★★★	★★★	NR	★★★★★	NR
★★★	★★★	★★★	★★★	★★★	★★★	★★★	NR	★	★★★	★★★	NR	★	★	★★★	★★★	★★★	★★★	★★★
★★★	NR	NR	★	NR	NR	NR	NR	★	NR	NR	NR	NR	★★★	NR	NR	NR	NR	NR
★★★	NR	NR	★★★	NR	★★★	NR	NR	★★★★★	★	NR	NR	★★★	★★★	★★★	NR	NR	NR	NR
★	★★★	NR	★★★	★★★	★★★	NR	NR	★★★	NR	NR	NR	★★★	★★★	★★★	★★★	NR	NR	NR
★★★	NR	NR	★★★	NR	★★★	NR	NR	★★★★★	★★★	NR	NR	NR	★★★	NR	NR	NR	NR	NR
★★★	★★★★★	★★★	★★★	★★★	★★★	★★★★★	★★★	★★★★★	★★★	NR	NR	★★★★★	★★★	★★★★★	NR	★★★	NR	NR
★★★	★★★	★★★	★★★	★★★★★	NR	★★★	★★★	★★★★★	NR	NR	NR	★★★	★★★★★	★★★★★	NR	★	NR	NR
★★★	NR	★★★	★★★	★★★	★★★	NR	NR	★★★	NR	NR	NR	★★★	★★★	★★★★★	★★★	★★★★★	NR	NR
★★★	★★★	★★★	★★★	★★★	★★★	★★★	★★★	★★★★★	★★★	★★★	★★★	★	★★★	★★★	★★★★★	★★★★★	★★★	★★★
★	NR	NR	★★★	★★★	NR	NR	NR	★★★	★★★	NR	NR	★★★	★★★★★	NR	NR	NR	NR	NR
★	★★★	★★★	★★★	★★★	★★★	★★★★★	NR	★★★	★★★	NR	NR	★★★	★★★	★★★	★★★	★★★	NR	★★★
★★★	★★★★★	★★★	★★★★★	★★★	★★★★★	NR	NR	★★★	★★★	★★★	NR	★★★	★★★	★★★★★	★	NR	★★★★★	★★★★★
★	★★★	★★★	★★★	★★★	★★★	★★★	★★★	★★★	NR	NR	NR	★★★	★★★	★★★★★	★★★★★	★★★★★	★	★★★
★★★	NR	★★★	★★★	★★★	NR	NR	NR	★★★	NR	NR	NR	★★★	★★★	★★★	NR	NR	NR	NR
★★★	NR	★	★★★	★★★	★★★	★★★	★★★	★★★★★	★★★	NR	NR	★★★	★★★★★	★★★★★	NR	NR	NR	NR
★★★	NR	NR	★★★	NR	★★★	NR	NR	★★★	NR	NR	NR	NR	★★★	NR	NR	NR	NR	NR
★★★	NR	NR	★★★	★★★	NR	NR	NR	★★★	NR	NR	NR	★★★★★	★★★★★	★★★	★	NR	NR	NR
★★★	NR	NR	★★★	★★★	NR	NR	NR	★★★	★★★	NR	NR	NR	★★★★★	NR	NR	NR	NR	NR
★	NR	★★★	★★★	★★★	★★★★★	★★★	NR	★★★★★	NR	NR	NR	★	★★★★★	★★★★★	NR	NR	NR	NR
★★★	★★★	★★★★★	★★★	★★★	NR	NR	NR	★★★	NR	NR	NR	★★★	★★★★★	★★★★★	NR	★★★	★★★	NR
★★★	★	★★★	★★★	★★★★★	★★★★★	NR	NR	★★★★★	★★★	NR	NR	★★★	★★★	★★★	★★★	★★★	NR	NR
★	NR	NR	★★★	NR	NR	NR	NR	★★★	NR	NR	NR	★★★★★	★★★	NR	NR	NR	NR	NR
★★★	★★★	★★★	★	★★★★★	★★★	★★★	NR	★	★★★	NR	NR	★	★	★★★★★	★★★	NR	NR	NR
★	NR	NR	★★★	NR	NR	NR	NR	★★★★★	NR	NR	NR	★★★	★	NR	NR	NR	NR	NR
★★★	NR	★★★	★★★	NR	★★★	NR	NR	★★★	NR	NR	NR	★★★	★★★	★★★	NR	NR	NR	NR
NR	NR	NR	NR	NR	★★★★★	NR	NR	★★★	NR	NR	NR	NR	NR	NR	NR	NR	NR	NR
★★★	NR	NR	★★★	NR	★★★	NR	NR	★★★	NR	NR	NR	★	NR	NR	NR	NR	NR	NR
★★★	NR	NR	★★★	NR	★★★★★	NR	NR	★★★	NR	NR	NR	NR	★★★	NR	NR	★★★	NR	NR
NR	NR	NR	★★★	NR	NR	NR	NR	★★★	NR	NR	NR	NR	NR	★★★	NR	★★★	NR	NR
★★★	NR	NR	★★★	★★★	★★★	NR	NR	★★★	NR	NR	NR	★★★	★	★★★	NR	NR	NR	NR
★	★★★	NR	★	★★★★★	★★★★★	NR	NR	★	★★★	NR	NR	★	★	★★★	★★★★★	★★★	NR	NR
★★★	★★★★★	★★★	★★★	★★★★★	★★★	★★★	NR	★★★	★	★★★	NR	★	★★★	★★★	★★★★★	★★★★★	NR	NR
★★★	NR	★★★	★★★	★★★	★★★	NR	NR	★★★	NR	NR	NR	★★★	★★★★★	★★★★★	NR	NR	NR	NR
★★★	★★★	★★★	★★★	★★★★★	★★★	NR	★★★	★★★	★★★	★	NR	★★★	★★★	★★★	★★★	★★★	★★★	★★★★★
★★★	★★★	★★★	★	★★★★★	★★★	★★★	★★★	★	★★★	★★★	★★★	★	★	★	★★★★★	★★★	★★★	★
★★★	NR	NR	★★★	★★★	★★★	NR	NR	★★★	NR	NR	NR	NR	NR	★★★	NR	NR	NR	NR
★★★	★★★	★★★	★★★	★★★	★★★	★★★	NR	★★★★★	★★★	NR	NR	★★★	★★★	★★★★★	NR	★★★	NR	NR

	Appendectomy	Atrial Fibrillation	Back and Neck Surgery (except Spinal Fusion)	Back and Neck Surgery (Spinal Fusion)	Bariatric Surgery	Bowel Obstruction	Carotid Surgery	Cholecystectomy (Gall Bladder Removal)	Chronic Obstructive Pulmonary Disease (COPD)	Coronary Bypass Surgery	Coronary Interventional Procedures (Angioplasty/Stent)	Diabetic Acidosis and…
51. Dameron Hospital Association, Stockton	★★★★★	★	★	★★★	NR	★★★	★★★	★★★	★★★	★★★	★★★	★
52. Delano Regional Medical Center, Delano	★	★★★	NR	NR	★★★	NR	NR	★★★	NR	NR	NR	★
53. Desert Regional Medical Center, Palm Springs	★★★	★★★	★★★	NR	★	★★★	★★★	★★★	★	★★★	★★★	★★★
54. Desert Valley Hospital, Victorville	★★★	★★★	NR	NR	NR	★★★★★	NR	★★★	★★★	NR	★★★	★★★
55. Doctor's Hospital Medical Center of Montclair, Montclair	★★★★★	NR	★★★	NR	NR	★★★	NR	NR	★★★	NR	NR	NR
56. Doctors Hospital of Manteca, Manteca	★★★	★★★	NR	NR	NR	★★★	NR	★★★	★★★	NR	★★★	★★★
57. Doctors Medical Center of Modesto, Modesto	★★★★★	★★★	★★★	★★★	NR	★★★	★★★	★	★★★	★★★	★★★	★★★
58. Doctors Medical Center–San Pablo/Pinole, San Pablo	★★★	★★★	★★★	★★★	NR	★★★	NR	★★★	★★★	★★★	★★★	★★★
59. Dominican Hospital, Santa Cruz	★★★★★	★★★	★★★	★★★	NR	★★★★★	★★★	★★★★★	★★★	★★★	★★★★★	★★★
60. Downey Regional Medical Center, Downey	★★★	★★★	★★★	NR	NR	★★★	NR	★★★	★★★	★★★	★★★★★	★★★
61. East Los Angeles Doctors Hospital, Los Angeles	★★★	NR	NR	NR	NR	NR	NR	NR	★★★	NR	NR	NR
62. East Valley Hospital Medical Center, Glendora	NR	NR	NR	NR	NR	NR	NR	NR	★★★	NR	NR	NR
63. Eden Medical Center, Castro Valley	★★★	★★★	★★★	NR	NR	★★★	★★★	★★★★★	★★★	NR	NR	★★★
64. Eisenhower Medical Center, Rancho Mirage	★★★	★★★	★★★	★★★	NR	★★★	★★★	★★★★★	★★★	★★★	★★★	★★★
65. El Camino Hospital, Mountain View	★★★	★★★	★★★	★★★★★	★★★★★	★★★	★★★★★	★★★	★★★	★★★	★★★★★	★★★
66. El Centro Regional Medical Center, El Centro	★★★	★★★	NR	★	NR	NR	NR	★★★	★★★	NR	NR	★★★
67. Emanuel Medical Center, Turlock	★★★	★★★	NR	NR	NR	★	NR	★★★	★★★	NR	NR	★★★
68. Encino-Tarzana Regional Medical Center, Encino	NR	★★★	NR	NR	NR	★★★	NR	NR	★★★	NR	NR	NR
69. Encino-Tarzana Regional Med. Ctr.–Tarzana Campus, Tarzana	★★★	★★★	★★★	NR	NR	★★★	★★★	★★★	★★★	★★★	★★★	★★★
70. Enloe Medical Center, Chico	★★★	★★★	★★★	★★★	★	★★★	★★★	★	★★★	★★★	★★★	★★★
71. Fairchild Medical Center, Yreka	★★★	★★★	NR	NR	NR	★★★	★★★	★★★	★★★	NR	NR	NR
72. Fallbrook Hospital, Fallbrook	★	★★★	NR	NR	★	NR	NR	★★★	★★★	NR	NR	NR
73. Feather River Hospital, Paradise	★★★	★★★	NR	NR	★★★	NR	★	★★★	★★★	NR	NR	NR
74. Foothill Presbyterian Hospital, Glendora	★★★	★★★	NR	NR	NR	★★★	NR	★★★	★★★	NR	NR	NR
75. Fountain Valley Regional Hospital and Med. Ctr., Fountain Valley	★★★	★★★	NR	★★★	★	★★★	★★★	★	★★★★★	★★★	★★★	★★★
76. Frank R. Howard Memorial Hospital, Willits	NR	NR	NR	NR	NR	NR	NR	NR	★★★	NR	NR	NR
77. Fremont Medical Center, Yuba City	★★★★★	★★★	NR	★★★	NR	★★★	★	★★★	★★★	★★★	★★★	★★★
78. French Hospital Medical Center, San Luis Obispo	★★★	★★★	NR	NR	NR	★★★	★★★★★	★★★	★★★	★★★	★★★	NR
79. Fresno Heart and Surgical Hospital, Fresno	NR	★★★	NR	NR	NR	NR	★★★	NR	NR	★★★	★★★	NR
80. Garden Grove Hospital and Medical Center, Garden Grove	★★★★★	★★★	NR	NR	NR	★★★	NR	★★★	★★★	NR	NR	★★★
81. Garfield Medical Center, Monterey Park	★★★★★	★★★	★★★★★	★★★	NR	★★★	NR	★★★	★★★	★★★	★★★	★★★
82. George L. Mee Memorial Hospital, King City	★★★	NR	NR	NR	NR	★★★	NR	NR	★★★	NR	NR	NR
83. Glendale Adventist Medical Center, Glendale	★★★★★	★	★★★	★★★	NR	★★★	★	★★★★★	★★★	★★★	★★★	★★★★★
84. Glendale Memorial Hospital and Health Center, Glendale	★★★	★★★	★★★	NR	NR	★	★★★	★★★★★	★★★★★	★★★	★★★	★★★
85. Goleta Valley Cottage Hospital, Santa Barbara	★★★	NR	NR	NR	NR	★★★	NR	NR	NR	NR	NR	NR
86. Good Samaritan Hospital, Bakersfield	NR	NR	NR	NR	NR	NR	NR	NR	NR	★★★	NR	NR
87. Good Samaritan Hospital, Los Angeles	★★★	★★★	★★★	★★★	NR	★★★	★★★	★★★	★★★	★★★	★★★	★★★
88. Good Samaritan Hospital, San Jose	★★★★★	★★★	★★★	★★★	★★★	★★★	★★★	★★★★★	★★★	★	★	★★★
89. Greater El Monte Community Hospital, South El Monte	★★★	★★★	NR	NR	NR	NR	NR	NR	★★★	NR	NR	NR
90. Grossmont Hospital, La Mesa	★★★	★	★★★	★★★	NR	★★★	★★★	★	★★★	★★★	★★★	★★★
91. Hanford Community Medical Center, Hanford	★★★	★★★	NR	NR	NR	★	NR	★★★	★	NR	NR	NR
92. Hazel Hawkins Memorial Hospital, Hollister	★★★	★★★	NR	NR	NR	★★★	NR	★★★	★	NR	NR	NR
93. Healdsburg District Hospital, Healdsburg	NR	NR	NR	NR	NR	NR	NR	NR	NR	NR	NR	NR
94. Hemet Valley Medical Center, Hemet	★★★	★★★	NR	NR	★	★	★★★	★	NR	NR	NR	★★★
95. Henry Mayo Newhall Memorial Hospital, Valencia	★★★	★★★	NR	NR	NR	★★★	NR	★	★★★★★	NR	NR	★★★
96. Hi-Desert Medical Center, Joshua Tree	★★★	★★★	NR	NR	NR	★★★	NR	NR	★★★	NR	NR	★★★
97. Hoag Memorial Hospital Presbyterian, Newport Beach	★★★★★	★★★	★★★★★	★★★	NR	★★★	★★★★★	★★★	★	★★★	★★★	★★★
98. Hollywood Community Hospital, Hollywood	NR	NR	NR	NR	NR	NR	NR	NR	★★★	NR	NR	NR
99. Hollywood Presbyterian Medical Center, Los Angeles	★★★★★	★★★	★★★	NR	NR	★★★	NR	★★★	★★★	NR	NR	★★★
100. Huntington Beach Hospital, Huntington Beach	★	★★★	NR	NR	★★★	★★★	NR	NR	★★★	NR	NR	NR

KEY: ★★★★★ BEST ★★★ AS EXPECTED ★ POOR NR NOT RATED BY HEALTHGRADES   For full definitions of ratings and awards, see Appendix.

Gastrointestinal Bleed	Gastrointestinal Surgeries and Procedures	Heart Attack	Heart Failure	Hip Fracture Repair	Maternity Care	Pancreatitis	Peripheral Vascular Bypass	Pneumonia	Prostatectomy	Pulmonary Embolism	Resection/Replacement of Abdominal Aorta	Respiratory Failure	Sepsis	Stroke	Total Hip Replacement	Total Knee Replacement	Valve Replacement	Women's Health
★★★	NR	★	★	★★★	★★★★★	NR	NR	★	NR	NR	NR	★★★	★	★	★★★	★★★★★	NR	★★★
★	★	★	★★★	★★★	★★★	★	NR	★	NR	NR	NR	★	★★★	NR	NR	★★★	NR	NR
★	★	★★★	★	★★★★★	★★★	★★★	NR	★★★	★★★	★★★	NR	★★★	★★★	★★★	★★★	★★★★★	★★★	★★★
★	NR	★★★	★★★★★	★★★	★★★	★★★	NR	★★★★★	★★★	NR	NR	★★★	★★★	★★★	NR	★	NR	NR
★★★	NR	★★★	★★★★★	NR	★★★★★	NR	NR	★★★★★	NR	NR	NR	★★★	★★★★★	★★★	NR	NR	NR	NR
★★★	★★★	★★★	★	★★★	★★★	★★★	★	★	★	★★★	★★★	★★★	★	★★★	NR	★★★	★★★	★★★
★★★	★★★	★★★	★★★	★	★★★	NR	NR	★	★★★	★★★	NR	★★★	★	★★★	NR	NR	★★★	★★★
★	★★★	★★★	★★★	★★★	★★★	NR	NR	★★★	★★★	NR	NR	★★★	★★★	★★★★★	NR	★	NR	★★★★★
★	NR	★★★	★★★	NR	★★★★★	NR	NR	★★★★★	NR	NR	NR	★★★	NR	NR	NR	NR	NR	NR
★★★	NR	★★★	★★★★★	★★★	★★★	NR	NR	★★★	NR	NR	NR	★★★	★★★★★	★★★	NR	NR	NR	NR
★★★	★★★	★★★	★★★	★★★	NR	NR	NR	★★★	NR	NR	NR	★★★	★★★	★★★	★★★	★★★	NR	NR
★★★	★★★★★	★★★	★★★	★★★★★	NR	NR	NR	★★★	★★★★★	★★★★★	★★★	★★★	★★★★★	★★★★★	★★★★★	★★★★★	★★★★★	NR
★★★	★★★	★★★	★★★★★	★	★★★	NR	★★★	★★★★★	★★★	★★★	★★★	★★★	★★★	★★★★★	★★★	★★★	★★★	★★★★★
★★★	★★★	★	★★★	★★★	★★★★★	NR	NR	★★★	★★★	NR	NR	★★★	★★★	★★★	NR	★★★★★	NR	NR
★	★	★★★	★	★★★★★	★	NR	★	★★★★★	NR	NR	NR	★★★	★	★	★★★★★	★★★★★	NR	NR
★★★	★★★	★★★	★	★★★★★	NR	NR	NR	★★★	NR	NR	NR	★★★	★★★	★★★★★	NR	NR	★★★	★★★★★
★★★	★★★	★★★	★★★	★★★	★★★★★	★★★	★★★	★★★	★	NR	★★★	★★★	★★★	★★★★★	NR	NR	★★★	★★★★★
★★★★★	★★★	★	★	★★★	★★★	★★★	★	★	★★★	★★★	★	★★★	★★★	★	★	★★★	★★★	★★★
★★★	★★★	NR	★	★★★	★★★	NR	NR	★★★	★★★	NR	NR	NR	★★★	★★★	NR	★★★	NR	NR
★★★	NR	NR	★★★	★★★	★★★	NR	NR	★★★	NR	NR	NR	★★★	★★★	★★★	★★★	★★★★★	NR	NR
★★★	★★★	★★★	★★★★★	★★★★★	★★★	NR	NR	★★★★★	★★★	NR	★★★	★★★	★★★★★	★★★	★	NR	NR	★★★★★
★★★	NR	NR	★★★	★★★	NR	NR	NR	★★★	NR	NR	NR	★★★	★	★★★	★★★	NR	NR	NR
★★★	★★★	★	★★★	★	★★★	★★★	NR	★★★	★★★	★★★	NR	★	★★★	★	★	★★★★★	★★★	NR
★★★	★	★★★	★★★	★★★	★★★	NR	NR	★★★	★★★	NR	NR	★★★	★★★	★★★	★★★	★★★★★	★★★	★★★
NR	NR	★★★★★	★★★	NR	NR	NR	★★★	NR	NR	NR	NR	NR	NR	NR	★★★	★★★	★★★	NR
★★★	NR	★★★	★★★	★★★	★★★★★	NR	NR	★★★	★★★	NR	NR	★★★	★★★	★★★	NR	NR	NR	NR
★★★★★	★★★	★★★	★★★★★	★★★★★	★★★	NR	NR	★★★★★	★★★	NR	NR	★★★	★★★★★	★★★★★	NR	★★★	★★★	★★★★★
★★★	NR	NR	★★★	NR	★★★	NR	NR	★★★	NR	NR	NR	NR	NR	NR	NR	NR	NR	NR
★★★	★★★	★★★	★★★	★★★	★★★★★	NR	★★★	★★★	★★★★★	★★★	NR	★★★	★★★★★	★★★★★	★★★	★★★	★★★	★★★★★
★★★	★★★	★★★	★★★★★	★★★★★	★★★	NR	NR	★★★★★	★★★	NR	NR	★★★	★★★	★★★★★	★★★	★★★★★	NR	★★★★★
NR	NR	NR	★	★★★	★★★	NR	NR	★★★	NR	NR	NR	NR	NR	★★★★★	★★★★★	NR	NR	NR
NR	NR	NR	★★★	NR	NR	NR	NR	★★★	NR	NR	NR	NR	NR	NR	NR	NR	NR	NR
★★★★★	★★★★★	★★★	★★★	★★★	★★★★★	★★★	★★★	★★★★★	★★★	NR	NR	★★★★★	★★★★★	★★★★★	★★★★★	★★★★★	★★★★★	★★★★★
★★★	★★★	★★★	★	★★★	★★★	NR	NR	★★★	★★★	★★★	NR	★★★	★★★	★	★★★	NR	★★★	★★★
★★★	NR	★★★	★★★	NR	★★★★★	NR	NR	★★★★★	★★★	NR	★★★★★	★★★	NR	NR	NR	★★★	NR	★★★
★★★	★★★	★	★	★★★	★★★★★	NR	NR	★★★	★★★	★★★	★	★	★★★	★★★★★	★★★	★★★	★★★	★★★
★★★	★★★	★★★	★★★	★★★	★★★	NR	★	★★★★★	NR	NR	★	★★★	★★★	★	★★★	★★★	★★★	★★★
★★★	NR	NR	★★★	★★★	★★★	NR	NR	★★★	NR	NR	NR	★★★	★★★	★	NR	★★★★★	NR	NR
NR	NR	NR	★★★	NR	NR	NR	NR	★★★	NR	NR	NR	NR	NR	★★★	★★★	★★★★★	NR	NR
★★★	★★★	★★★	★★★	★★★★★	★★★	NR	★	★★★	★★★	NR	★	★★★	★★★	★★★	NR	NR	NR	NR
★★★	★★★★★	★★★	★★★	★★★	★★★	NR	NR	★★★	★★★	★★★	★★★	★★★★★	★★★★★	★★★	★★★	★★★	★★★	★★★
★★★	NR	★★★	★★★	★	NR	NR	NR	★★★	★★★	NR	★★★	★★★	NR	★★★	NR	NR	NR	NR
★★★★★	NR	★★★	★★★★★	★★★★★	★★★	NR	NR	★★★	★★★	★★★	★★★	★★★★★	★★★★★	★★★★★	★★★	★★★★★	★★★★★	★★★
★★★	NR	★★★	★★★★★	NR	★★★	NR	NR	★★★★★	★★★	NR	★★★	★★★★★	★★★★★	★★★	NR	NR	NR	NR
★★★	NR	★★★	★★★	★★★	★★★	NR	NR	★★★★★	★	NR	★★★★★	★★★★★	★★★★★	★★★	★★★	NR	NR	NR
★★★	★★★	★★★	★★★	★★★	NR	NR	NR	★★★	NR	NR	NR	★★★★★	★★★★★	★★★	NR	NR	NR	NR

	Appendectomy	Atrial Fibrillation	Back and Neck Surgery (except Spinal Fusion)	Back and Neck Surgery (Spinal Fusion)	Bariatric Surgery	Bowel Obstruction	Carotid Surgery	Cholecystectomy (Gall Bladder Removal)	Chronic Obstructive Pulmonary Disease (COPD)	Coronary Bypass Surgery	Coronary Interventional Procedures (Angioplasty/Stent)	Diabetic Acidosis and
101. Huntington Memorial Hospital, Pasadena	***	***	***	***	*****	*****	***	***	***	NR	***	NR
102. Irvine Regional Hospital, Irvine	***	***	NR	*	NR	***	NR	***	***	NR	***	***
103. John F. Kennedy Memorial Hospital, Indio	***	***	*	NR	NR	***	***	***	*****	NR	***	***
104. John Muir Medical Center, Walnut Creek	***	***	*	*	NR	***	***	NR	***	NR	***	***
105. Kaiser Foundation Hospital, Bellflower	*****	NR	NR	NR	NR	NR	NR	NR	***	NR	NR	NR
106. Kaiser Foundation Hospital, Harbor City	***	NR	NR	NR	***	NR	NR	NR	NR	NR	NR	NR
107. Kaiser Foundation Hospital, Los Angeles	***	NR	NR	NR	NR	NR	NR	NR	***	NR	NR	NR
108. Kaiser Foundation Hospital, Panorama City	*****	NR	NR	NR	NR	NR	NR	NR	NR	NR	NR	NR
109. Kaiser Foundation Hospital, San Diego	***	NR	NR	NR	NR	NR	NR	NR	***	NR	NR	NR
110. Kaiser Foundation Hospital—Anaheim, Anaheim	***	NR	NR	NR	NR	NR	NR	NR	NR	NR	NR	NR
111. Kaiser Foundation Hospital—Fontana, Fontana	*	NR	NR	NR	NR	NR	NR	NR	NR	NR	NR	NR
112. Kaiser Foundation Hospital—Fremont/Hayward, Hayward	***	NR	NR	NR	NR	***	NR	NR	***	NR	NR	NR
113. Kaiser Foundation Hospital—Manteca, Manteca	NR	NR	NR	NR	NR	NR	NR	NR	***	NR	NR	NR
114. Kaiser Foundation Hospital—Oakland/Richmond, Oakland	***	***	NR	*	NR	***	NR	NR	***	NR	NR	*
115. Kaiser Foundation Hospital–South San Francisco, South San Francisco	***	NR	NR	NR	***	NR	NR	NR	***	NR	NR	NR
116. Kaiser Foundation Hospital—Vallejo, Vallejo	*	***	NR	NR	NR	***	NR	NR	***	NR	NR	NR
117. Kaiser Fresno Medical Center, Fresno	***	NR	NR	NR	***	NR	NR	NR	NR	NR	NR	NR
118. Kaiser Redwood City Medical Center, Redwood City	***	NR	NR	NR	NR	NR	NR	NR	NR	NR	NR	NR
119. Kaiser Sacramento Medical Center, Sacramento	***	***	***	NR	NR	*	***	***	*	NR	NR	NR
120. Kaiser San Francisco Medical Center, San Francisco	***	NR	NR	NR	NR	NR	NR	NR	***	NR	***	***
121. Kaiser San Rafael Medical Center, San Rafael	***	NR	NR	NR	NR	NR	NR	NR	***	NR	NR	NR
122. Kaiser Santa Clara Medical Center, Santa Clara	*****	***	NR	NR	NR	NR	NR	NR	***	NR	NR	NR
123. Kaiser Santa Teresa Community Hospital, San Jose	***	NR	NR	NR	NR	***	NR	NR	***	NR	NR	NR
124. Kaiser South Sacramento Medical Center, Sacramento	***	NR	NR	NR	NR	NR	NR	NR	***	NR	NR	NR
125. Kaiser Walnut Creek Medical Center, Walnut Creek	***	NR	NR	NR	NR	NR	NR	NR	*****	NR	NR	NR
126. Kaweah Delta District Hospital, Visalia	***	***	***	***	NR	*	***	*	*	***	***	***
127. Kern Medical Center, Bakersfield	*	NR	NR	NR	*	NR	NR	NR	NR	NR	NR	NR
128. Kern Valley Healthcare District, Lake Isabella	NR	NR	NR	NR	NR	NR	NR	NR	***	NR	NR	NR
129. La Palma Intercommunity Hospital, La Palma	***	***	NR	NR	NR	NR	***	***	***	NR	NR	NR
130. LAC+USC Medical Center, Los Angeles	*****	***	NR	NR	NR	NR	NR	***	NR	NR	***	NR
131. LAC Harbor-UCLA Medical Center, Torrance	*****	NR	NR	NR	NR	NR	NR	***	NR	NR	***	NR
132. LAC Martin Luther King Jr. Multi Service Ambulatory Care Ctr., Los Angeles	***	NR	NR	NR	NR	NR	NR	***	NR	NR	NR	***
133. LAC Olive View-UCLA Medical Center, Sylmar	***	NR	NR	NR	NR	NR	NR	***	NR	NR	NR	NR
134. Lakewood Regional Medical Center, Lakewood	*****	***	NR	NR	NR	***	NR	*	***	***	***	***
135. Lancaster Community Hospital, Lancaster	***	***	NR	NR	NR	*	***	*	***	NR	***	***
136. Little Company of Mary Hospital, Torrance	***	*****	***	***	NR	***	***	*	***	*	*	*
137. Little Company of Mary Hospital—San Pedro, San Pedro	***	***	NR	NR	NR	***	NR	NR	***	NR	NR	NR
138. Lodi Memorial Hospital, Lodi	***	*	NR	NR	NR	***	***	*****	*	NR	NR	***
139. Loma Linda University Medical Center, Loma Linda	***	***	*	***	NR	***	***	NR	***	*****	***	***
140. Lompoc Healthcare District, Lompoc	***	NR	NR	NR	NR	***	NR	NR	***	NR	NR	NR
141. Long Beach Memorial Medical Center, Long Beach	***	*	***	***	NR	***	***	***	***	***	***	***
142. Los Alamitos Medical Center, Los Alamitos	***	*	NR	***	NR	***	***	***	***	NR	***	***
143. Los Angeles Community Hospital, Los Angeles	NR	***	NR	NR	NR	NR	NR	***	*****	NR	NR	***
144. Los Angeles Metropolitan Medical Center, Los Angeles	NR	NR	NR	NR	NR	NR	NR	***	***	NR	NR	***
145. Los Robles Regional Medical Center, Thousand Oaks	*****	***	*****	***	NR	***	***	***	***	***	***	***
146. Mad River Community Hospital, Arcata	***	***	NR	NR	NR	***	NR	***	***	NR	NR	NR
147. Madera Community Hospital, Madera	***	*	NR	NR	***	*	NR	***	***	NR	NR	***
148. Marian Medical Center, Santa Maria	***	*	***	***	NR	*	***	***	***	***	***	***
149. Marin General Hospital, Greenbrae	*****	*	***	*	NR	***	***	***	***	***	***	***
150. Mark Twain St. Joseph's Hospital, San Andreas	NR	***	NR	NR	NR	***	NR	NR	*	NR	NR	NR

KEY: ★★★★★ BEST   ★★★ AS EXPECTED   ★ POOR   NR NOT RATED BY HEALTHGRADES   For full definitions of ratings and awards, see Appendix.

Gastrointestinal Bleed	Gastrointestinal Surgeries and Procedures	Heart Attack	Heart Failure	Hip Fracture Repair	Maternity Care	Pancreatitis	Peripheral Vascular Bypass	Pneumonia	Prostatectomy	Pulmonary Embolism	Resection/Replacement of Abdominal Aorta	Respiratory Failure	Sepsis	Stroke	Total Hip Replacement	Total Knee Replacement	Valve Replacement	Women's Health
★★★★★	★★★	★★★	★★★	★★★	★★★★★	★★★	★★★	★★★	★★★	★★★	NR	★	★★★	★★★★★	★★★	★★★	★★★	★★★★★
★★★	★★★	★★★	★★★	★★★	★★★	★★★	NR	★★★	NR	NR	NR	★★★	★★★	★★★	NR	★★★	NR	NR
★★★	★★★	★★★	★★★	★★★★★	★★★	★★★	NR	★★★	NR	NR	NR	★★★	★★★	★★★	★★★	★★★★★	NR	NR
★★★★★	★★★★★	★★★★★	★★★★★	★★★	★★★	★★★★★	★★★	★★★★★	★★★	★★★	NR	★★★★★	★★★★★	★★★★★	★★★	★★★	NR	NR
NR	NR	NR	★★★	NR	★★★	NR	NR	NR	NR	NR	NR	NR	★	NR	NR	NR	NR	NR
NR	NR	NR	★★★	NR	★★★	NR	NR	★★★	NR	NR	NR	NR	NR	NR	NR	NR	NR	NR
NR	NR	★★★	★★★	NR	★	NR	NR	★★★	NR	NR	NR	NR	NR	NR	NR	NR	NR	★★★
NR	NR	NR	★★★	NR	★★★★★	NR	NR	★★★	NR	NR	NR	★★★	NR	NR	NR	NR	NR	NR
★★★	NR	★★★	★★★	NR	★★★	NR	★	★★★	NR	NR	NR	NR	NR	★★★	NR	NR	NR	NR
NR	NR	NR	★★★	NR	★★★	NR	NR	★★★	NR	NR	NR	NR	NR	NR	NR	NR	NR	NR
★★★	NR	★★★	★★★	★★★	★	NR	NR	★★★	NR	NR	NR	★★★	★★★	★★★	NR	★★★	NR	NR
★	NR	★★★	★★★	NR	NR	NR	NR	★★★	NR	NR	NR	★★★★★	NR	NR	NR	NR	NR	NR
★★★	NR	★★★	★★★	★★★	★★★	NR	NR	★★★	NR	NR	NR	★★★	★★★	★★★	NR	★	NR	NR
NR	NR	NR	NR	NR	★★★	NR	NR	NR	NR	NR	NR	NR	NR	NR	NR	NR	NR	NR
NR	NR	NR	NR	NR	★★★	NR	NR	NR	NR	NR	NR	NR	NR	NR	NR	NR	NR	NR
★★★	NR	★★★	★	★	★	NR	NR	★★★	★	NR	NR	★	★	★★★	★★★	★★★	NR	NR
★★★	NR	★★★	★★★	★★★	★★★	NR	NR	★★★	NR	NR	NR	★★★	★★★★★	NR	NR	★★★	NR	★★★
NR	NR	NR	★★★	★★★	NR	NR	NR	★★★	NR	NR	NR	★★★	★★★	NR	NR	★★★	NR	NR
★★★	NR	NR	★★★	★	★	NR	NR	★★★	NR	NR	NR	★★★	★★★	NR	NR	★★★	NR	NR
★★★	NR	★★★	★★★	NR	NR	NR	NR	★★★	NR	NR	NR	★★★	NR	NR	★★★	★	NR	NR
NR	NR	NR	★★★	NR	★★★	NR	NR	★★★	NR	NR	NR	NR	NR	NR	NR	NR	NR	NR
★★★	NR	★★★	★★★	NR	★★★	NR	NR	★★★	NR	NR	NR	NR	NR	★★★	★★★	NR	NR	NR
★	★	★★★	★	★★★★★	★★★	★	NR	★	★★★	★★★	NR	★	★	★	★★★	★★★★★	★★★	★★★
NR	NR	NR	★★★	★★★	★★★	NR	NR	★★★	NR	NR	NR	NR	★★★	NR	NR	NR	NR	NR
NR	NR	NR	★★★	NR	NR	NR	NR	★★★	NR	NR	NR	NR	NR	NR	NR	NR	NR	NR
★★★	NR	★★★	★★★	★★★	★★★	★★★	NR	★★★	NR	NR	NR	★★★★★	★★★	★★★	NR	NR	NR	NR
★★★	NR	★★★	★★★	★★★★★	★★★	NR	NR	★★★	NR	NR	NR	★★★	★★★	NR	NR	★★★	NR	NR
NR	NR	★★★	★★★	NR	★	NR	NR	★★★	NR	NR	★★★	NR	★★★	NR	NR	NR	NR	NR
NR	NR	★★★	★★★	NR	★★★	NR	NR	★★★	NR	NR	NR	★★★	★★★	NR	NR	NR	NR	NR
NR	NR	★★★★★	★★★	NR	★	NR	NR	★★★	NR	NR	NR	★	NR	NR	NR	NR	NR	NR
★★★	NR	★★★	★★★	★★★	NR	NR	NR	★★★	NR	NR	NR	★★★	★	★★★	NR	★★★	NR	NR
★★★	★★★	★★★	★★★	★★★	NR	NR	NR	★★★	★★★	★★★	NR	★★★	★	★★★	★★★	★★★	NR	NR
★★★	★★★	★★★	★★★	★	★★★	★★★	NR	★★★	★★★	★★★	NR	★★★	★★★★★	★★★	★★★	★★★	★	★★★
★★★	★★★	★★★	★★★	★★★	★★★	★★★	NR	★★★	★★★	NR	NR	★★★	★★★	★★★	★	★★★	★★★	NR
★★★	★★★	★	★	★★★★★	★★★	NR	NR	★	★★★	★★★	NR	★	★★★	★	★★★	★★★	NR	NR
★★★	★★★	★★★	★★★	★★★	★	NR	★★★	★★★	★★★	★★★	★★★	★★★★★	★★★	★★★★★	★★★	★★★	★★★	★
★★★	★★★	NR	★	★★★★★	★★★	NR	NR	★	NR	NR	NR	NR	★	★★★	★★★	NR	NR	NR
★★★	★★★	★	★★★	★★★	NR	★★★	★★★	★★★	★★★	★★★	★★★	★★★★★	★★★★★	★★★★★	★★★★★	★★★★★	★★★	NR
★★★	★★★	★	★★★	★★★	★★★	NR	NR	★	★★★	★★★	NR	★★★	★★★	NR	NR	★★★	NR	NR
★★★	NR	NR	★★★	NR	★★★★★	★★★	NR	★★★	NR	NR	NR	★★★	★★★★★	NR	NR	★★★	NR	NR
★★★	NR	NR	★★★	NR	★★★★★	NR	NR	★★★★★	NR	NR	NR	★★★	★★★★★	NR	NR	NR	NR	NR
★	★	★★★	★★★	★★★	★★★	★★★	★★★	★★★★★	★★★	★★★	NR	★	★★★★★	★★★	★★★	NR	★★★	★★★
★★★	★★★	★	★★★	NR	★	NR	NR	★★★	NR	NR	NR	★★★	★	NR	NR	★★★	NR	NR
★★★	★★★	★★★	★	★	★★★	★★★	NR	★★★	NR	NR	NR	★★★	★★★	NR	NR	★★★	NR	★
★★★★★	★★★	★	★	★★★	★★★	★★★	NR	★★★	★★★	★★★	NR	★★★	NR	★★★	NR	★★★	★★★★★	NR
★	NR	★★★	★★★	NR	★★★	★★★	NR	★★★	NR	NR	NR	★★★	★	NR	NR	★★★	NR	NR

	Appendectomy	Atrial Fibrillation	Back and Neck Surgery (except Spinal Fusion)	Back and Neck Surgery (Spinal Fusion)	Bariatric Surgery	Bowel Obstruction	Carotid Surgery	Cholecystectomy (Gall Bladder Removal)	Chronic Obstructive Pulmonary Disease (COPD)	Coronary Bypass Surgery	Coronary Interventional Procedures (Angioplasty/Stent)	Diabetic Acidosis and
151. Marshall Medical Center, Placerville	★★★	★★★	★★★	NR	NR	★★★	★★★	★★★	★★★★★	NR	NR	★★★
152. Memorial Hospital of Gardena, Gardena	★★★	NR	NR	NR	NR	NR	NR	NR	★★★	NR	NR	NR
153. Memorial Hospital–Los Banos, Los Banos	★★★	NR	NR	NR	NR	★★★	NR	NR	★★★	NR	NR	NR
154. Memorial Medical Center, Modesto	★★★	★★★	★★★	NR	★★★	★★★	★★★	★★★	★★★	★★★	★★★	★★★
155. Mendocino Coast District Hospital, Fort Bragg	★★★	★★★	NR	NR	NR	★★★	NR	NR	★	NR	NR	★★★
156. Menifee Valley Medical Center, Sun City	★★★	★★★	NR	NR	NR	★★★	★★★	★★★	★★★	★★★★★	★★★	★★★
157. Mercy General Hospital, Sacramento	★★★	★★★★★	★★★	★★★	NR	★★★	★★★	★★★	★★★	★★★★★	★★★	★★★
158. Mercy Hospital of Folsom, Folsom	★★★	★★★	NR	NR	NR	★★★	NR	★	★★★	NR	NR	★★★
159. Mercy Hospital, Bakersfield	★	NR	★★★	★	★	★★★	NR	★	★★★	NR	NR	★★★
160. Mercy Medical Center Merced, Merced	★	★★★	NR	NR	NR	★★★	NR	★★★	★★★	NR	NR	NR
161. Mercy Medical Center Mt. Shasta, Mt. Shasta	NR	★★★	NR	NR	NR	★★★	NR	★★★	★★★	NR	NR	★★★
162. Mercy Medical Center Redding, Redding	★★★	★★★	★	★★★	NR	★★★	★★★	★★★	★★★	★★★	★★★	★★★
163. Mercy San Juan Medical Center, Carmichael	★	★★★	★★★	NR	★★★	★★★	★★★	★★★	★★★	★★★	★★★	★★★
164. Methodist Hospital of Southern California, Arcadia	★★★	★	★★★	NR	★★★★★	★★★	★★★	★★★	★★★	★★★	★★★	★★★
165. Methodist Hospital, Sacramento	★★★	★	NR	NR	NR	★★★	NR	★★★	★★★	NR	NR	★★★
166. Mills Health Center, San Mateo	★★★★★	★	★★★	★★★	★★★★★	★★★★★	★★★	★★★	★★★	★★★	★★★	★★★
167. Mills Peninsula Health Services, Burlingame	★★★★★	★	★★★	★★★	★★★★★	★★★★★	★★★	★★★	★★★	★★★	★★★	★★★
168. Mission Community Hospital–Panorama, Panorama City	★★★	★★★	NR	NR	NR	★★★	NR	★★★	★★★	NR	NR	★★★
169. Mission Hospital Regional Medical Center, Mission Viejo	★★★	★★★	★★★	★★★	NR	★★★	★★★	★★★	★★★	★★★	★★★	★★★
170. Monterey Park Hospital, Monterey Park	NR	★★★	NR	NR	NR	★★★	NR	★★★	★★★	NR	NR	★★★
171. Moreno Valley Medical Center, Moreno Valley	★	NR	NR	★★★	NR	★★★	NR	★★★	★★★	NR	NR	★★★
172. Motion Picture and Television Hospital, Woodland Hills	NR	★★★	NR	NR	NR	NR	NR	★	NR	NR	NR	NR
173. Mt. Diablo Hospital Medical Center, Concord	★★★	★★★	NR	★★★	★★★	★★★	★★★	★★★	★★★	★★★	★	★★★
174. Natividad Medical Center, Salinas	★★★	NR	NR	NR	NR	★★★	NR	NR	★★★	NR	NR	★★★
175. NorthBay Medical Center, Fairfield	★★★	★★★	NR	NR	NR	★★★	NR	★	★★★	NR	NR	★★★
176. NorthBay VacaValley Hospital, Vacaville	★★★	★	NR	NR	NR	★★★	NR	★	★★★	NR	NR	★★★
177. Northern Inyo Hospital, Bishop	NR	NR	NR	NR	NR	NR	NR	★	★★★	NR	NR	NR
178. Northridge Hospital Medical Center, Northridge	★★★	★★★	★★★	★★★	NR	★★★	★★★	★★★	★★★	★★★	★★★	★★★
179. Norwalk Community Hospital, Norwalk	NR	★★★	NR	NR	NR	NR	NR	★★★	★★★★★	NR	NR	★★★
180. Novato Community Hospital, Novato	★★★	★★★	NR	NR	NR	★★★★★	NR	NR	★	NR	NR	NR
181. O'Connor Hospital, San Jose	★★★	★★★	★★★	NR	NR	★★★	★★★	★★★	★	★	★★★	★★★
182. Oak Valley District Hospital, Oakdale	★★★	NR	NR	NR	NR	★	NR	NR	★	NR	NR	NR
183. Ojai Valley Community Hospital, Ojai	★★★	★★★	NR	NR	NR	NR	NR	NR	★★★	NR	NR	NR
184. Olympia Medical Center, Los Angeles	★★★★★	★★★	★★★	NR	NR	★★★	NR	NR	★★★	NR	NR	★★★
185. Orange Coast Memorial Medical Center, Fountain Valley	★★★	★★★	NR	NR	★★★	★★★	NR	★★★	★★★	NR	NR	★★★
186. Oroville Hospital, Oroville	★	★★★	NR	NR	NR	★★★	★★★	★	★★★	NR	NR	★★★
187. Pacific Alliance Medical Center, Los Angeles	NR	★★★	NR	NR	NR	★★★★★	NR	★★★★★	★★★★★	NR	NR	★★★
188. Pacific Campus Hospital, San Francisco	★★★★★	★★★	★★★	★★★	★★★★★	★★★	★★★	★	★★★	★★★	★★★	★★★
189. Pacific Hospital of Long Beach, Long Beach	★★★	NR	NR	NR	NR	NR	NR	NR	★★★	NR	NR	★★★
190. Pacifica Hospital of the Valley, Sun Valley	★★★★★	NR	NR	NR	NR	NR	NR	NR	★★★	NR	NR	★★★
191. Palm Drive Hospital, Sebastopol	★★★	NR	NR	NR	NR	★★★	NR	NR	NR	NR	NR	NR
192. Palo Verde Hospital, Blythe	★★★	★★★	NR	NR	NR	NR	NR	NR	★★★	NR	NR	★★★
193. Palomar Medical Center, Escondido	★★★	★★★	★★★	★★★	NR	★★★	★★★	★★★	★★★	★★★	★★★	★★★
194. Paradise Valley Hospital, National City	★★★	★★★	NR	NR	NR	★★★	★	★	★★★★★	NR	NR	★★★
195. Parkview Community Hospital, Riverside	★★★	★★★	NR	NR	NR	★★★	NR	★★★	★★★	NR	NR	NR
196. Petaluma Valley Hospital, Petaluma	★★★	★★★	NR	NR	NR	★★★	NR	★★★	★★★	NR	NR	NR
197. Pioneers Memorial Health Care District, Brawley	★	★★★	NR	NR	NR	★	NR	★★★	★★★	NR	NR	★★★
198. Placentia-Linda Hospital, Placentia	★★★★★	★★★	★★★	NR	NR	★★★	NR	★★★	★★★	NR	NR	★★★
199. Pomerado Hospital, Poway	★	★	NR	NR	★	★★★	NR	★★★	★★★	NR	NR	★★★
200. Pomona Valley Hospital Medical Center, Pomona	★★★★★	★★★	★★★	★★★	NR	★★★	NR	★★★	★★★	★★★	★★★	★★★

KEY: ★★★★★ BEST   ★★★ AS EXPECTED   ★ POOR   NR NOT RATED BY HEALTHGRADES   For full definitions of ratings and awards, see Appendix.

Gastrointestinal Bleed	Gastrointestinal Surgeries and Procedures	Heart Attack	Heart Failure	Hip Fracture Repair	Maternity Care	Pancreatitis	Peripheral Vascular Bypass	Pneumonia	Prostatectomy	Pulmonary Embolism	Resection/Replacement of Abdominal Aorta	Respiratory Failure	Sepsis	Stroke	Total Hip Replacement	Total Knee Replacement	Valve Replacement	Women's Health
★★★	★★★	★★★	★★★	★★★	★★★	★★★	NR	★★★★★	★★★	★★★	NR	★★★★★	★★★★★	★★★	★★★	★	NR	NR
★★★	NR	NR	★★★	★★★	★★★	NR	NR	★★★	NR	NR	NR	★★★	★★★	★★★	NR	NR	NR	NR
★★★	NR	NR	★★★	NR	★★★	NR	NR	★★★	NR	NR	NR	★★★	★	★★★	NR	NR	NR	NR
★	★★★	★	★★★	★★★	★★★	★★★	★★★	★	★★★	NR	NR	★★★	★★★	★	★★★	★★★	★★★	★★★
★★★	NR	NR	★★★	★★★	★★★	NR	NR	★★★	NR	NR	NR	★★★★★	★★★	NR	NR	★★★	NR	NR
★★★	★★★	★★★	★★★★★	★★★★★	NR	★★★	NR	★★★	NR	★★★	NR	★★★	★★★	★★★	NR	NR	NR	NR
★★★	★★★	★★★	★★★	★★★★★	★★★	★★★	NR	★★★★★	★★★	★★★	NR	★★★	★★★	★★★	★★★	★★★	★	★★★
★★★	NR	NR	★★★	★★★	★★★	NR	NR	★	NR	★★★	NR	★	NR	★★★	★	★★★	NR	NR
★★★	★★★	★	★	★★★	★★★	★★★	NR	★★★	★	NR	NR	★	NR	★★★	NR	★★★	NR	NR
★★★	★★★	★★★	★★★	★★★	★★★	★★★	NR	★★★	★★★★★	★★★	NR	★★★	★★★	★★★	★★★★★	★★★	NR	NR
★★★	NR	NR	★★★	★★★	NR	NR	NR	★★★	★★★	NR	NR	★★★	★★★	★★★	NR	NR	NR	NR
★	★	★★★	★	★★★	★★★	★	★★★	★	★	★	★★★	★★★	★	★	★★★★★	★★★★★	★★★	★
★★★	★★★	★★★	★★★	★★★	★★★	★	NR	★★★	★★★	★★★	NR	★★★	★	★★★	★★★	★★★	NR	★★★
★★★	★★★	★★★	★★★	★★★	★★★	NR	NR	★★★	★	NR	NR	★★★	★★★★★	★★★	★★★	★★★	NR	★★★
★★★	★★★	★	★★★	★★★	NR	NR	NR	★★★	NR	NR	NR	★	★★★	NR	★★★★★	★★★★★	NR	NR
★★★	★★★★★	★★★	★★★	★★★	★★★	★★★	★★★	★★★★★	★★★	★★★	★★★	★★★	★★★★★	★★★★★	★★★	★	★★★	NR
★★★	★★★★★	★★★	★★★	★★★	★★★	★★★	★★★	★★★★★	★★★	★★★	★★★	★★★	★★★★★	★★★★★	★★★	★★★	★★★	NR
★★★	NR	NR	★★★	★★★	NR	NR	NR	★★★★★	NR	NR	NR	★★★	★★★	★★★	NR	NR	NR	NR
★★★	★★★	★★★	★★★	★★★	★★★	★★★	NR	★★★	★★★	★★★★★	★★★	★★★	★★★	★★★	★★★	★	★★★	★★★
★★★	NR	★★★	★★★	★★★	★★★★★	NR	NR	★★★★★	★	NR	NR	★★★★★	★★★	★★★★★	NR	NR	NR	NR
★★★	NR	NR	★★★★★	NR	★★★	NR	NR	★★★	NR	NR	NR	★★★	NR	NR	NR	NR	NR	NR
★★★	NR	NR	★★★	NR	NR	NR	NR	★★★	NR	NR	NR	NR	NR	NR	NR	NR	NR	NR
★★★	★★★★★	★★★	★★★	★★★★★	NR	★★★	★★★	★★★★★	★★★	★★★	★★★	★★★	★★★★★	★★★	★★★	★★★	★★★	NR
★★★	NR	NR	★★★	NR	★	NR	NR	★	NR	NR	NR	NR	NR	NR	NR	NR	NR	NR
★★★	★★★	★★★	★★★	★★★	★★★	★★★	NR	★★★	NR	NR	NR	★★★	★	★★★	★★★	★★★	NR	NR
★★★	NR	★★★	★★★	★★★	NR	★★★	NR	★★★	NR	NR	NR	★	★★★	NR	NR	★★★	NR	NR
★★★	NR	NR	★	★★★	★	NR	NR	★	NR	NR	NR	★★★	★★★	NR	NR	★★★	NR	NR
★★★	★★★	★★★	★★★★★	★★★	★★★★★	★★★	NR	★★★	★★★	★★★	NR	★★★	★★★★★	★★★	★★★	★	NR	★★★★★
★★★	NR	NR	★★★	NR	★★★★★	★★★	NR	★★★	★★★	NR	NR	★★★	★★★★★	★★★	★★★	★★★	NR	NR
★★★	NR	★★★	★★★	★★★	NR	NR	NR	★★★★★	NR	NR	NR	★★★	★★★	★★★	★★★	★★★	NR	NR
★★★	★★★	★★★	★★★	★★★	★★★★★	★★★	★★★	★★★	★★★	★★★	★★★	★★★	★★★	★★★★★	★★★★★	★★★	NR	★★★★★
★★★	NR	NR	★	NR	★★★	NR	NR	★★★	NR	NR	NR	★★★	★	★	NR	★★★	NR	NR
★★★	NR	★★★	★★★	★★★	NR	NR	NR	★★★	NR	NR	NR	★★★	★★★	NR	NR	★★★	NR	NR
★★★	★★★	★★★	★★★	★★★	NR	★★★	NR	★★★★★	★★★	NR	NR	★★★	★★★★★	★★★	NR	NR	NR	NR
★★★	★★★★★	★★★	★★★	★★★	★★★	NR	NR	★★★★★	NR	NR	NR	★★★	★★★★★	★★★	NR	NR	NR	NR
★	★★★	★★★	★★★	★★★	★★★	★★★	NR	★★★★★	★	★★★	NR	★★★	★	★★★	★★★	★★★	NR	NR
★★★	NR	★★★	★★★★★	★★★	★★★★★	★★★★★	NR	★★★★★	NR	NR	NR	★★★★★	★★★★★	NR	NR	NR	NR	NR
★★★	★★★	★★★	★★★	★★★	★★★	★★★	★★★	★★★★★	★★★	★★★	★★★	★	★★★★★	★★★★★	★★★	★★★	★★★	★★★
★	NR	NR	★★★	NR	NR	NR	NR	★★★★★	NR	NR	NR	★★★★★	★★★	NR	NR	★	NR	NR
★★★	NR	NR	★	★★★	★★★	NR	NR	★	NR	NR	NR	★	★	★	★★★	★★★	NR	NR
★★★	NR	NR	★★★	★★★	NR	NR	NR	★★★	NR	NR	NR	★★★	★★★	★★★	★★★	★★★	NR	NR
★★★	NR	NR	★★★	NR	★★★	NR	NR	★★★	NR	NR	NR	NR	NR	NR	NR	NR	NR	NR
★★★	★★★	★★★	★★★	★★★	★★★	★★★	★★★	★★★	★★★	★★★	NR	★★★	NR	★★★	★★★	★★★★★	★	★★★
★★★	★★★	★★★	★★★★★	★★★	★★★★★	★★★	★★★	★★★★★	NR	NR	NR	★★★★★	★★★	NR	★★★	NR	NR	NR
★★★	NR	★★★	★	★★★	★★★★★	NR	NR	★★★	NR	★★★	NR	★	★★★	★★★	NR	NR	NR	NR
★★★	★★★	★★★	★★★	★★★	★★★	★★★	NR	★★★	★★★	NR	NR	★★★★★	★★★★★	★★★	★★★	NR	NR	NR
★★★	NR	★★★	★★★	★★★	★★★★★	NR	NR	★	NR	NR	NR	★★★	★★★	NR	★★★	★★★	NR	NR
★★★	NR	NR	★★★	★★★	NR	NR	NR	★★★	NR	NR	NR	★★★	★★★	★★★	NR	NR	NR	NR
★★★	★★★	★★★	★★★	★★★	★★★★★	NR	NR	★★★	★★★	★★★	NR	★★★	★★★	★★★	★★★★★	NR	NR	NR
★	★★★	★★★	★★★★★	★★★★★	★★★★★	★★★	NR	★★★★★	★	NR	NR	★★★	★★★★★	★★★	★★★	★★★	★★★	★★★

	Appendectomy	Atrial Fibrillation	Back and Neck Surgery (except Spinal Fusion)	Back and Neck Surgery (Spinal Fusion)	Bariatric Surgery	Bowel Obstruction	Carotid Surgery	Cholecystectomy (Gall Bladder Removal)	Chronic Obstructive Pulmonary Disease (COPD)	Coronary Bypass Surgery	Coronary Interventional Procedures (Angioplasty/Stent)	Diabetic Acidosis a...
201. Presbyterian Intercommunity Hospital, Whittier	★★★	★★★	★	★★★	NR	★★★	★★★	★★★	★★★	★★★★★	★★★	★★★
202. Providence Holy Cross Medical Center, Mission Hills	★★★	★★★	NR	NR	NR	★★★	★★★	★★★	★★★★★	★★★	★★★	★★★
203. Providence Saint Joseph Medical Center, Burbank	★★★	★★★	★★★	★	★★★★★	★★★	★	★★★	★★★	★★★	★★★	★★★
204. Queen of the Valley, Napa	★★★	★★★	★★★	NR	NR	★★★	★★★	★★★	★★★	★★★	★★★	NR
205. Redbud Community Hospital, Clearlake	NR	NR	NR	NR	NR	★★★	NR	★★★	★★★	NR	NR	NR
206. Redlands Community Hospital, Redlands	★★★	★★★	★★★	NR	NR	★★★	★★★	★	★★★	★★★	★★★	★★★
207. Redwood Memorial Hospital, Fortuna	NR	NR	NR	NR	NR	NR	NR	★★★	★★★	NR	NR	NR
208. Regional Medical Center of San Jose, San Jose	★★★	★	NR	NR	NR	★★★	★★★	★★★	★★★	★★★	★★★	★★★
209. Rideout Memorial Hospital, Marysville	★★★★★	★★★	NR	NR	NR	★★★	★	★★★	★★★	★★★	★★★	★★★
210. Ridgecrest Regional Hospital, Ridgecrest	★★★	★★★	NR	NR	NR	★★★	NR	★★★	★	NR	NR	NR
211. Riverside Community Hospital, Riverside	★★★	★★★	★	★★★	NR	★★★	★★★	★★★	★★★	★★★	★★★	★★★
212. Riverside County Regional Medical Center, Moreno Valley	★★★	★★★	NR	NR	NR	NR	NR	NR	★★★	NR	NR	NR
213. Saddleback Memorial Medical Center, Laguna Hills	★★★	★★★★★	★★★★★	★★★	NR	★★★	NR	★★★	★★★	★★★	★★★	★★★
214. Saddleback Memorial Med. Ctr.–San Clemente, San Clemente	★★★	★★★★★	★★★★★	★★★	NR	★★★	NR	★★★	★★★	★★★	★★★	★★★
215. Saint Agnes Medical Center, Fresno	★★★	★★★	★★★★★	★★★	★★★	★★★	★★★	★★★	NR	★	★★★	★★★
216. St. Bernardine Medical Center, San Bernardino	★★★	★★★	★★★	★★★★★	★	★	★★★	★★★★★	★★★	★	★	★
217. St. Elizabeth Community Hospital, Red Bluff	★★★	★★★	NR	NR	NR	★★★	NR	★★★★★	★★★	NR	NR	NR
218. St. Francis Medical Center, Lynwood	★★★	★	NR	NR	NR	★★★	NR	★★★	★★★	★★★	★★★	★★★
219. Saint Francis Memorial Hospital, San Francisco	★★★	★★★	★	★	NR	★★★	NR	★★★	★★★	NR	NR	NR
220. St. Helena Hospital, Deer Park	NR	★★★	★★★	★★★	NR	★★★★★	★★★	★★★	★★★	★	★★★	★★★
221. St. John's Health Center, Santa Monica	★★★	★★★	★★★	★★★	NR	★★★	★★★	★★★	★★★	★★★	★★★	★★★
222. St. John's Pleasant Valley Hospital, Camarillo	★★★	★★★	NR	NR	NR	★★★	NR	★	★★★	★★★	NR	NR
223. St. John's Regional Medical Center, Oxnard	★★★	★★★	★★★	★★★	★★★★★	★★★	★	★★★	★★★	★★★★★	★★★	★★★
224. St. Joseph Hospital, Eureka	★★★	★★★	★	★	NR	★	★★★	★★★	★★★	★★★	★★★	NR
225. St. Joseph Hospital, Orange	★★★★★	★★★	★	★★★	★	★★★★★	★★★	★★★	★★★	★★★	★★★	★★★
226. St. Joseph's Medical Center of Stockton, Stockton	★	★	★	★★★	NR	★★★	★★★	★	★★★	★★★★★	★★★	★★★
227. St. Jude Medical Center, Fullerton	★★★	★★★	★★★	★★★	NR	★★★	★★★	★★★	★★★	★★★	★★★	★★★
228. St. Louise Regional Hospital, Gilroy	★★★	★★★	NR	NR	NR	★★★	NR	★★★	★★★★★	NR	NR	NR
229. St. Luke's Hospital, San Francisco	★★★	★★★	★★★	NR	NR	★★★	NR	★★★	★★★	NR	NR	★★★
230. St. Mary Medical Center, Apple Valley	★	★★★	★★★	★★★	NR	★★★	★★★	★	★★★	★★★	★★★	★★★
231. St. Mary Medical Center, Long Beach	★★★	★★★	NR	NR	NR	★★★	★★★	NR	★★★	★★★	★★★	★★★
232. St. Mary's Medical Center, San Francisco	★★★	★★★	★	★★★	★★★	★★★	★	★★★	★★★	★★★	★★★	NR
233. St. Rose Hospital, Hayward	★★★	★★★	NR	NR	NR	★★★★★	NR	★★★	★★★	NR	NR	★★★
234. St. Vincent Medical Center, Los Angeles	★★★	★★★	★	★★★	NR	★★★	★★★	★	★★★★★	★★★	★★★	★★★
235. Salinas Valley Memorial Health Care System, Salinas	★★★	★★★	★★★	★★★	NR	★★★	★★★	★	★	★★★	★★★	★★★
236. San Antonio Community Hospital, Upland	★★★	★★★	★★★	★★★	NR	★★★	★	★	★★★	★★★	★★★	★★★
237. San Dimas Community Hospital, San Dimas	★★★★★	NR	NR	NR	NR	NR	NR	NR	NR	NR	NR	NR
238. San Fernando Community Hospital, San Fernando	★★★	★★★	NR	NR	NR	★★★	NR	★★★	★★★	NR	NR	NR
239. San Francisco General Hospital, San Francisco	★★★★★	★	NR	NR	NR	★★★	NR	★★★	★★★	NR	NR	★★★
240. San Gabriel Valley Medical Center, San Gabriel	★★★	★★★	NR	NR	NR	★★★	NR	★★★	★★★★★	NR	NR	★★★
241. San Gorgonio Memorial Hospital, Banning	★★★	★★★	NR	NR	NR	★★★	NR	NR	★★★	NR	NR	NR
242. San Joaquin Community Hospital, Bakersfield	★★★	★★★	NR	★★★	★★★★★	★★★	★	★	★★★	★★★	★★★	★★★
243. San Joaquin General Hospital, French Camp	★★★★★	NR	NR	NR	NR	★★★	NR	★★★	★★★	★★★	NR	★★★
244. San Leandro Hospital, San Leandro	★★★	★★★	NR	NR	NR	★★★★★	★★★	★★★	★★★	NR	NR	★★★
245. San Mateo Medical Center, San Mateo	★★★★★	NR	NR	NR	NR	★★★	NR	NR	★★★	NR	NR	★★★
246. San Ramon Regional Medical Center, San Ramon	★	★★★	★★★	★	NR	★★★	NR	★	★★★	★★★	★★★	★★★
247. Santa Barbara Cottage Hospital, Santa Barbara	★★★★★	★★★	★★★★★	★★★★★	★★★	★★★	★★★	★★★	★	★★★	★★★	★★★
248. Santa Clara Valley Medical Center, San Jose	★★★	★★★	NR	NR	NR	★★★	NR	★★★	★★★	NR	★★★	★★★
249. Santa Monica–UCLA Medical Center, Santa Monica	★★★	★★★	★	★★★	★★★	★★★	NR	NR	★★★	NR	★★★	★★★
250. Santa Rosa Memorial Hospital, Santa Rosa	★★★	★	★★★	★★★	NR	★	★★★	★★★	★★★	★	★★★	★★★

KEY: ★★★★★ BEST ★★★ AS EXPECTED ★ POOR NR NOT RATED BY HEALTHGRADES For full definitions of ratings and awards, see Appendix.

Gastrointestinal Bleed	Gastrointestinal Surgeries and Procedures	Heart Attack	Heart Failure	Hip Fracture Repair	Maternity Care	Pancreatitis	Peripheral Vascular Bypass	Pneumonia	Prostatectomy	Pulmonary Embolism	Resection/Replacement of Abdominal Aorta	Respiratory Failure	Sepsis	Stroke	Total Hip Replacement	Total Knee Replacement	Valve Replacement	Women's Health
★★★	★★★★★	★★★	★★★	★★★	★★★	★★★	NR	★★★★★	★★★	NR	NR	★★★	★★★★★	★★★★★	★★★	★★★	NR	★★★
★★★	★★★	★★★	★★★★★	★★★	★★★	★★★	NR	★★★★★	★★★	NR	NR	★★★	★★★★★	★★★★★	★★★	★★★	★	★★★★★
★★★	★★★	★★★	★★★	★★★	★★★★★	★★★	★★★	★★★	★	★★★	★★★	★★★	★★★	★★★★★	★★★	★★★	★★★	★★★★★
★★★	★★★	★★★	★★★★★	★★★	★★★	★★★	★★★	★★★	★	★★★	NR	★★★	★★★★★	★★★★★	★★★	★★★	★★★	★★★
★★★	NR	NR	★★★	★	★★★	NR	NR	★★★	★	NR	NR	★★★	★	★	NR	NR	NR	NR
★★★	NR	★	★★★	★★★	NR	NR	NR	★★★	NR	NR	NR	★★★	★★★	★	★★★	★★★	NR	NR
★★★	★★★	★★★	★★★	★	★★★	★★★	NR	★★★	★★★	NR	NR	★★★	★★★★★	★	NR	★★★	★★★★★	NR
★★★	★★★	★	★★★	★	★★★	★★★	NR	★★★	★★★	★★★	NR	★	★★★	★★★	★	★★★★★	★★★	
★	★★★	★★★	★★★	NR	★★★	NR	NR	★★★	NR	NR	NR	★★★★★	★★★	★★★	NR	NR	NR	★★★
★	★★★	★★★	★★★	★★★	★★★	★★★★★	NR	★★★	★★★	NR	NR	★	★★★	★★★	★★★	★★★	★★★	★★★
★★★	NR	NR	★★★	★★★	★★★	NR	NR	★★★	NR	NR	NR	NR	NR	NR	NR	NR	NR	NR
★★★	★★★	★★★	★★★★★	★★★	★★★	★★★	NR	★★★★★	★★★	★★★	NR	★★★	★★★★★	★★★★★	★★★	★	★★★	★★★
★★★	★★★	★★★	★★★★★	★★★	★★★	★★★	NR	★★★★★	★★★	★★★	NR	★★★	★★★	★★★★★	★★★	★	★★★	★★★
★★★	★★★	★★★	★	★★★	★★★★★	★★★	★★★	★★★	★★★	★★★	NR	★	★★★★★	★★★★★	★★★★★	★★★★★	★★★	★★★★★
★★★	★★★	★★★	★★★★★	★★★	★★★	NR	★★★	★★★	★	NR	NR	★★★	★★★★★	★★★	★★★★★	★★★★★	★★★	★★★
★★★★★	★★★	★★★	★★★★★	★★★	★★★	★★★	★	★★★	★★★	NR	NR	★★★	★★★	★★★	★★★★★	NR	NR	
★	NR	★★★	★★★	★★★★★	★★★	★	NR	★★★	★★★	NR	NR	★	★★★	★★★★★	NR	★★★	NR	★★★
★★★	NR	★★★	★★★	★★★	NR	NR	NR	★★★	NR	NR	NR	★★★	★	★★★★★	★★★★★	★★★	NR	NR
★★★	★★★	★★★	★★★	★★★	NR	★★★	★★★	★★★	★★★	NR	NR	★	★★★	★★★	★★★	★★★	★	★★★
★★★	★★★★★	★★★★★	★★★★★	★	★★★	★★★	★★★	★★★★★	★★★	★★★	NR	★★★	★★★	★★★	★★★	★★★	★★★	★★★
★★★	★★★★★	★★★	★★★★★	★★★	NR	NR	★★★	NR	NR	NR	★★★	★★★	★★★★★	★★★	★★★	★★★	★★★	
★★★	★★★	★★★	★★★	★★★	★★★	★★★	★★★★★	★★★	NR	NR	★★★	★★★	★★★	★★★	★★★	★★★	★★★	
★★★	★★★	★★★	★★★★★	★★★	★★★	★★★	★	★★★	NR	NR	★★★	★	★★★	★★★	★★★★★	★★★	★★★	
★★★	★★★	★★★★★	★★★	★★★	★★★	★★★	★	★★★	★★★	★★★	★★★	★★★★★	★★★	★★★★★	★★★	★★★★★	★★★	
★	★★★	★	★	NR	★★★	★★★	★★★	★★★	★★★	★	★★★	★	★	★★★	NR	NR	★★★	★★★
★★★	★★★	★★★	★★★	★★★★★	★★★	★★★	NR	★★★	★★★	★★★	NR	★★★	★★★	★★★★★	★★★	★★★	★★★	★★★
★★★	NR	★★★	★★★	★★★	★★★★★	NR	NR	★★★★★	NR	NR	NR	★★★★★	★★★★★	★★★	NR	★	★★★	NR
★★★	NR	★★★	★★★	★★★	★★★	NR	NR	★★★★★	★	NR	NR	★★★	★★★	★★★	★★★	★	NR	NR
★	NR	★★★	★★★	★★★	★★★	★★★	★★★	★★★	★★★	★★★	NR	★★★	★★★	★★★	★	★★★	★★★	★★★
★★★	NR	★★★	★★★	★★★	★★★	NR	NR	★★★★★	★★★	NR	NR	★★★★★	★★★★★	★★★	★★★	★★★	★★★	★★★★★
★★★	★★★	★★★	★★★	★★★	NR	★★★	NR	★★★★★	★★★	NR	NR	★★★	★★★	★★★	★★★★★	★★★	★★★	NR
★★★	★★★	★★★	★★★	★★★	★★★	★★★	NR	★★★★★	NR	NR	NR	★★★	★★★	★★★	NR	★★★	NR	NR
★★★	★★★	★★★	★★★	★	NR	★★★	★	★★★★★	★★★	NR	NR	★★★	★★★★★	NR	★	★★★	★★★	NR
★★★★★	★★★	★★★	★	★	★★★	★★★	★★★	★	★	★	★★★	★	★	★★★	★★★	★★★	★★★	★★★
★★★	★★★	★★★	★★★	★	★★★★★	★★★	NR	★★★	★★★	★★★	NR	★★★★★	★★★★★	★★★★★	★	★	NR	★★★
★★★	NR	★★★	★★★	★★★	★★★	NR	NR	★★★	NR	NR	NR	★★★	★★★	★★★	★★★	★★★	NR	★★★
★★★	NR	NR	★★★	★★★	NR	NR	NR	★★★★★	NR	NR	NR	★★★	★★★	★★★	NR	NR	NR	NR
★★★	NR	★★★	★★★	★	NR	NR	NR	★★★	NR	NR	NR	NR	★	★	NR	NR	NR	★★★
★★★	★★★	★★★	★★★	★★★	★★★	NR	NR	★★★★★	★★★	NR	NR	★★★★★	★★★★★	★★★★★	★★★	★★★	★★★	★★★
★★★	NR	★★★	★★★	★	★★★	NR	NR	★★★	NR	NR	NR	★	★★★	★★★	NR	★★★	NR	★★★
★★★	★★★	★★★	★★★	★★★	★★★★★	★★★	NR	★★★	★★★	NR	NR	★	★★★	★★★	★★★	★★★	NR	★★★
★★★	NR	★★★	★★★	★★★★★	★★★	NR	NR	★	NR	NR	NR	NR	NR	★	NR	★★★	NR	NR
★★★	★★★★★	★★★	★★★	★★★	NR	★★★	★★★★★	★★★	★★★	★★★	NR	★★★	★★★★★	★★★	★★★	★★★	NR	★★★
NR	NR	NR	★★★	NR	NR	NR	NR	★★★	★★★	NR	NR	★	NR	NR	NR	NR	NR	NR
★★★	★★★	★★★	★★★	★★★	NR	★★★	NR	★★★★★	★★★	★★★	NR	★★★	★★★	★	★★★	★★★	NR	★★★
★★★	★★★★★	★★★	★★★	★★★★★	★★★	★★★	★★★	★★★	★★★	★★★	NR	NR	★★★	★★★★★	★★★★★	★★★	★★★	
★★★	NR	★★★	★★★	★★★	★	NR	NR	★★★★★	NR	NR	NR	★★★	★★★★★	★★★	NR	NR	NR	NR
★★★	★	★★★	★★★★★	★★★	NR	NR	★★★★★	★★★★★	★	NR	NR	★★★	★★★	★★★	★★★	★★★	NR	NR
★★★	★★★	★★★	★	★	★★★	★★★	NR	★★★	★★★	★★★	★★★	★★★	★★★	★	★★★	★★★	★	★

CALIFORNIA HOSPITALS: RATINGS BY PROCEDURE

	Appendectomy	Atrial Fibrillation	Back and Neck Surgery (except Spinal Fusion)	Back and Neck Surgery (Spinal Fusion)	Bariatric Surgery	Bowel Obstruction	Carotid Surgery	Cholecystectomy (Gall Bladder Removal)	Chronic Obstructive Pulmonary Disease (COPD)	Coronary Bypass Surgery	Coronary Interventional Procedures (Angioplasty/Stent)	Diabetic Acidosis
251. Scripps Green Hospital, La Jolla	***	***	*****	*****	***	***	***	*****	***	*	***	NR
252. Scripps Memorial Hospital—Encinitas, Encinitas	***	***	*	***	NR	***	***	***	***	NR	***	NR
253. Scripps Memorial Hospital—La Jolla, La Jolla	***	***	***	***	***	***	*	*	***	***	***	***
254. Scripps Mercy Hospital, San Diego	***	***	***	***	*****	***	***	***	***	***	***	***
255. Scripps Mercy Hospital—Chula Vista, Chula Vista	***	***	***	***	*****	***	***	***	***	***	***	***
256. Selma Community Hospital, Selma	***	NR	NR	NR	NR	NR	NR	NR	NR	NR	NR	NR
257. Sequoia Hospital, Redwood City	***	***	***	NR	NR	***	***	***	***	***	*****	***
258. Seton Medical Center, Daly City	***	*	NR	*	NR	***	***	***	***	***	***	***
259. Sharp Chula Vista Medical Center, Chula Vista	***	***	***	***	NR	***	***	***	***	***	***	***
260. Sharp Coronado Hospital and Healthcare Center, Coronado	***	***	NR	NR	NR	***	NR	***	***	NR	NR	NR
261. Sharp Memorial Hospital, San Diego	***	*	*	*	***	***	***	***	***	***	*****	***
262. Shasta Regional Medical Center, Redding	***	*	***	***	*	***	***	***	*	***	*	***
263. Sherman Oaks Hospital, Sherman Oaks	NR	***	NR	NR	NR	***	NR	***	***	NR	NR	NR
264. Sierra Kings District Hospital, Reedley	NR	NR	NR	NR	NR	NR	NR	***	***	NR	NR	NR
265. Sierra Nevada Memorial Hospital, Grass Valley	*	***	NR	NR	***	***	*	***	***	NR	NR	NR
266. Sierra View District Hospital, Porterville	***	***	NR	NR	***	***	***	***	NR	NR	NR	***
267. Sierra Vista Regional Medical Center, San Luis Obispo	***	*	***	***		***	***	*****	*****	***	***	NR
268. Simi Valley Hospital and Health Care Service, Simi Valley	***	***	NR	NR	NR	***	***	***	***	NR	NR	***
269. Sonoma Valley Hospital, Sonoma	***	***	NR	NR	NR	***	NR	***	***	NR	NR	NR
270. Sonora Regional Medical Center, Sonora	*	***	*	***	NR	***	NR	*	***	NR	NR	NR
271. South Coast Medical Center, Laguna Beach	***	***	NR	NR	*****	***	NR	NR	***	NR	NR	NR
272. Southwest Healthcare System—Inland Valley Med. Ctr., Wildomar	*****	***	*****	***	*****	*	***	***	***	NR	NR	***
273. Southwest Healthcare System—Rancho Springs Med. Ctr., Murrieta	*****	***	*****	***	*****	*	***	***	***	NR	NR	***
274. Stanford Hospital, Stanford	*	***	***	*****	***	***	***	***	*****	***	***	***
275. Sutter Amador Hospital, Jackson	***	***	NR	NR	NR	***	NR	***	***	NR	NR	NR
276. Sutter Auburn Faith Hospital, Auburn	***	***	NR	NR	*	***	NR	***	***	NR	NR	NR
277. Sutter Coast Hospital, Crescent City	***	***	NR	NR	NR	***	NR	***	***	NR	NR	NR
278. Sutter Davis Hospital, Davis	***	NR	***	NR	NR	***	***	***	***	NR	NR	NR
279. Sutter Delta Medical Center, Antioch	*	***	NR	NR	NR	***	NR	***	***	NR	NR	***
280. Sutter General Hospital, Sacramento	***	***	***	***	*****	***	***	***	***	***	***	***
281. Sutter Lakeside Hospital, Lakeport	***	NR	NR	NR	NR	*	NR	***	***	NR	NR	NR
282. Sutter Maternity and Surgery Center, Santa Cruz	NR	NR	NR	NR	NR	NR	NR	NR	NR	NR	NR	NR
283. Sutter Med. Ctr. of Santa Rosa—Chanate, Santa Rosa	***	***	NR	NR	*****	***	NR	***	***	***	***	NR
284. Sutter Memorial Hospital, Sacramento	*	NR	NR	NR	NR	NR	NR	NR	NR	NR	NR	NR
285. Sutter Roseville Medical Center, Roseville	***	***	***	*****	***	***	***	***	***	NR	***	***
286. Sutter Solano Medical Center, Vallejo	***	***	NR	NR	NR	***	NR	***	*	NR	NR	***
287. Sutter Tracy Community Hospital, Tracy	***	***	NR	NR	NR	***	NR	***	***	NR	NR	***
288. Sutter Warrack Hospital, Santa Rosa	***	***	NR	NR	NR	***	NR	***	***	***	***	***
289. Tahoe Forest Hospital District, Truckee	*	***	NR	NR	NR	***	NR	***	***	NR	NR	NR
290. Temple Community Hospital, Los Angeles	NR	***	NR	NR	NR	***	NR	NR	***	NR	NR	NR
291. Torrance Memorial Medical Center, Torrance	***	***	***	***	*	***	*****	***	***	*	***	***
292. Tri-City Medical Center, Oceanside	***	***	***	***	NR	***	*****	*	***	***	***	***
293. Tri-City Regional Medical Center, Hawaiian Gardens	NR	NR	NR	NR	*	NR	NR	***	*****	NR	NR	NR
294. Tulare District Hospital, Tulare	*****	*	NR	NR	NR	***	NR	***	***	NR	NR	***
295. Twin Cities Community Hospital, Templeton	*****	***	***	NR	NR	***	NR	***	***	NR	NR	NR
296. UCLA Medical Center, Los Angeles	***	***	***	*	***	***	***	***	***	***	***	***
297. UCSF Medical Center, San Francisco	***	***	***	*	***	*****	*****	***	***	***	***	***
298. Ukiah Valley Medical Center, Ukiah	***	***	NR	NR	NR	***	NR	***	***	NR	NR	NR
299. University Medical Center, Fresno	***	***	***	***	NR	***	***	***	***	*	***	***
300. University of California—Davis Med. Ctr., Sacramento	*	***	***	***	NR	***	***	***	***	***	*	***

KEY: *** BEST   *** AS EXPECTED   * POOR   NR NOT RATED BY HEALTHGRADES**   For full definitions of ratings and awards, see Appendix.

Gastrointestinal Bleed	Gastrointestinal Surgeries and Procedures	Heart Attack	Heart Failure	Hip Fracture Repair	Maternity Care	Pancreatitis	Peripheral Vascular Bypass	Pneumonia	Prostatectomy	Pulmonary Embolism	Resection/Replacement of Abdominal Aorta	Respiratory Failure	Sepsis	Stroke	Total Hip Replacement	Total Knee Replacement	Valve Replacement	Women's Health
★★★	★★★	★★★	★★★	★★★	NR	NR	★★★	★★★	★★★	★★★	★★★	NR	★★★	★★★	★★★★★	★★★★★	★★★	NR
★★★	★★★	★★★	★★★	★★★	★	NR	NR	★★★★★	★★★	★★★	NR	★★★	★★★★★	★★★★★	★★★	★	NR	NR
★★★★★	★★★★★	★★★	★★★★★	★	★★★★★	★★★★★	★	★★★★★	★★★	★★★	★★★	★★★★★	★★★★★	★★★	★★★	★★★	★★★	★★★★★
★★★	★★★	★★★	★★★★★	★★★	★★★★★	★★★	NR	★★★★★	★★★	★★★	★★★	★★★★★	★★★★★	★★★★★	★★★	★★★	★★★	★★★
NR	NR	NR	NR	NR	★★★	NR	★★★	NR	★★★	NR	NR	NR	NR	NR	NR	NR	NR	NR
★★★	★★★	★★★	★★★	★★★	★★★	★★★	★★★	★★★	★★★	★★★	NR	★★★	★★★★★	★★★	★★★	★★★	NR	NR
★	★★★	★	★	★★★	★	★★★	NR	★★★	★★★	★★★	★	★★★	★★★	★★★	★★★	★★★	★	NR
★★★	★★★	★★★	★★★	★★★★★	★★★	★★★	NR	★★★	★★★	★★★	NR	★★★	★★★	★★★	★★★	★★★	NR	★★★★★
★★★	NR	NR	★★★	★★★	★★★	NR	NR	NR	★★★	NR	NR	NR	★★★	★	★★★	★★★★★	NR	NR
★★★	★★★	★★★	★★★	★★★	NR	★★★	NR	★★★★★	★★★	★★★	★★★	★★★	★	★★★★★	★★★	★★★	★★★★★	NR
★★★	★★★	★	★★★	★★★★★	NR	★★★	★★★	★	★★★	★★★	NR	★★★	★★★	★★★	★★★★★	★★★	NR	NR
★★★	NR	NR	★★★	NR	★★★	NR	NR	★★★	NR	NR	NR	NR	★	★★★	NR	★★★	NR	NR
★★★	★★★	★★★	★★★★★	★★★	★★★	★★★	NR	★★★★★	★★★	★★★	NR	★★★★★	★★★★★	★★★★★	★★★★★	★★★★★	NR	NR
★★★	★★★	★★★	★	★★★	★★★	★★★	NR	★	★★★	NR	NR	★	★★★	★	★★★	★★★	NR	NR
★★★	★★★	★★★	★★★	★★★★★	★★★	NR	NR	★★★	★★★	NR	NR	★	★★★	★★★	★★★	★★★★★	★★★	★
★★★	★★★★★	★	★★★	★★★	★★★	NR	NR	★★★★★	NR	NR	NR	★★★	★★★★★	★★★	NR	★★★	NR	NR
★★★	NR	★★★	★★★	★★★	★★★	NR	NR	★	NR	NR	NR	★★★	★	★	★★★	★★★	NR	NR
★★★	★★★	★★★	★★★	★	★★★	★★★	NR	★★★	NR	★★★	NR	★★★	★★★	★	★	★★★	NR	NR
★★★	★★★	NR	★★★	★★★	★★★★★	NR	NR	★★★	NR	NR	NR	★★★	★★★	★★★	★★★	★★★	NR	NR
★★★	★	★★★	★★★★★	★★★	★★★	NR	NR	★★★	★★★	★★★	NR	★★★	★★★★★	★★★	★★★	★★★	NR	NR
★★★	★	★★★	★★★★★	★★★	★★★	NR	NR	★★★	★★★	★★★	NR	★★★	★★★★★	★★★	★★★	★★★	NR	NR
★★★	★★★	★★★	★★★	★	NR	★★★	★★★	★★★	★★★	★★★	★★★	★	★★★	★★★	★★★★★	★★★★★	★	NR
★★★	NR	NR	★	★★★	★★★	NR	NR	★★★	★★★	NR	★	★	★	★★★	NR	★	NR	NR
★★★	★★★★★	★★★	★★★★★	★★★	★★★	NR	NR	★★★★★	★★★	NR	NR	★★★★★	★★★	★★★	★★★	★★★	NR	NR
★★★	NR	★★★	★★★	NR	★★★	NR	NR	★★★	NR	NR	NR	★★★	★★★	★★★	NR	★★★	NR	NR
★★★	NR	NR	★★★	★★★	★★★	NR	NR	★★★	NR	NR	NR	★★★	★★★★★	★★★	NR	★★★	NR	NR
★★★★★	★★★	★★★	★★★	★★★	★★★	★★★	NR	★★★	NR	NR	NR	★★★	★★★	★★★★★	NR	★★★	NR	NR
★★★	★★★	★★★	★	★★★★★	NR	★★★	★	★★★★★	★★★	★★★	★★★	★	★★★	★★★	★★★★★	★★★★★	★★★	NR
★★★	★★★	★★★	★★★	★★★	★★★	NR	NR	★★★★★	★★★	NR	★★★	★★★	★★★	★★★★★	★★★	★★★★★	★★★	NR
NR	NR	NR	NR	NR	★★★	NR	NR	NR	NR	NR	NR	NR	NR	★★★	★★★	NR	NR	NR
★★★	★★★	★★★	★★★	★★★	★★★	NR	NR	★★★	NR	NR	NR	★★★	★★★	★★★	★★★★★	★★★	★★★★★	NR
NR	NR	NR	NR	NR	★★★	NR	NR	NR	NR	NR	NR	NR	NR	NR	NR	NR	NR	★★★
★★★	★★★	★★★	★★★★★	★★★	★★★	★★★★★	NR	★★★	★★★	★★★	NR	★★★	★★★	★★★★★	★★★	★★★	NR	NR
★★★	★★★	★★★	★★★	★★★	NR	NR	★★★	★	NR	NR	NR	★★★	★★★	★★★	★★★	★★★★★	NR	NR
★★★	NR	★★★	★★★	★★★	NR	NR	★★★	NR	NR	NR	★★★	★★★	★★★	NR	★★★	★★★★★	NR	NR
★★★	NR	NR	★★★	★★★★★	★★★	NR	★★★	★★★	NR	NR	NR	★★★★★	★★★	NR	★★★	★★★	NR	NR
★★★	★★★	★	★★★	★★★	★★★	★★★	★	★★★	★★★	★★★	NR	★★★	★★★	★★★	★★★	★★★	★★★	★★★
★★★	★★★	★★★	★	★★★	★★★	★★★	NR	★★★	★★★	★★★	★	★★★	★★★	★★★	★★★	★	★	★
★★★	NR	NR	★★★★★	NR	NR	★★★	NR	★★★★★	★★★	NR	NR	★★★★★	NR	NR	NR	★★★	NR	NR
★★★	NR	★★★	★★★★★	★★★	★★★	NR	★	NR	NR	NR	NR	★★★	★★★	NR	★★★	NR	NR	★★★★★
★★★	★★★	★	★★★	★★★	★★★	★★★	★	★★★	★★★	NR	★★★	★★★	★★★	★	★★★★★	★★★	NR	NR
★★★	★★★	★★★	★★★	★	★★★	★★★	★★★★★	★★★	★★★	★★★	NR	★★★	★★★	★	★★★	NR	★★★★★	NR
★★★	★★★	★★★	★	★	★★★	★★★	★★★★★	★★★	★★★	★★★	★★★★★	★	★★★	★★★	★★★	NR	★★★	★★★
★★★	★★★	★★★	★★★	★★★	NR	NR	★★★	★★★	NR	NR	★★★	★★★	★	NR	★★★	NR	NR	NR
★★★	★★★	★★★	★	★★★★★	★★★	★★★	★★★	★★★	★★★	★	★	★★★★★	★★★	★★★	★★★	NR	NR	NR
★★★	★★★	★★★	★★★	★★★	★	★★★	NR	★★★	★	★★★	★★★	★★★	★	★★★	★★★	★★★	★	NR

	Appendectomy	Atrial Fibrillation	Back and Neck Surgery (except Spinal Fusion)	Back and Neck Surgery (Spinal Fusion)	Bariatric Surgery	Bowel Obstruction	Carotid Surgery	Cholecystectomy (Gall Bladder Removal)	Chronic Obstructive Pulmonary Disease (COPD)	Coronary Bypass Surgery	Coronary Interventional Procedures (Angioplasty/Stent)	Diabetic Acidosis and
301. University of California–Irvine Med. Ctr., Orange	★★★	★★★	★★★	★★★	★★★	★★★	★★★	★	★★★	★★★	★★★	NR
302. University of California–San Diego Med. Ctr., San Diego	★	★★★	★★★	★	NR	★★★	★★★	★★★	★★★	★★★	★★★	NR
303. USC University Hospital, Los Angeles	NR	NR	★	★	★★★	★★★	★★★	NR	NR	★★★	★★★	NR
304. Valley Care Medical Center, Pleasanton	★★★	★	★	★	★★★	★★★	★★★	★	★★★	NR	★★★	NR
305. Valley Memorial Hospital, Livermore	★★★	★	★	★	★★★	★★★	★★★	★	★★★	NR	★★★	NR
306. Valley Presbyterian Hospital, Van Nuys	★★★	★★★	★★★	NR	NR	★★★	NR	★★★	★★★	NR	★★★	★★★
307. Ventura County Medical Center, Ventura	★★★	NR	NR	NR	NR	★★★	NR	NR	★	NR	NR	NR
308. Verdugo Hills Hospital, Glendale	★★★	★★★	NR	NR	NR	★★★	NR	NR	★★★	NR	NR	NR
309. Victor Valley Community Hospital, Victorville	★★★	NR	NR	NR	NR	NR	NR	NR	★	NR	NR	NR
310. Washington Hospital Healthcare System, Fremont	★★★★★	★★★	★★★	★★★	NR	★★★	★★★	★★★	★	★★★	★★★	★★★
311. Watsonville Community Hospital, Watsonville	★★★	★★★	★★★	★★★	NR	★★★	NR	★★★	★★★	NR	NR	NR
312. West Anaheim Medical Center, Anaheim	★★★	★★★	NR	NR	NR	★★★	NR	★	★★★★★	★★★	★	★★★
313. West Hills Medical Center, West Hills	★	★★★	NR	NR	★★★	★★★	★★★	★★★	★★★	★	★★★	★★★
314. Western Medical Center Hospital Anaheim, Anaheim	★★★	NR	NR	NR	NR	NR	NR	NR	★★★	★★★	★★★	NR
315. Western Medical Center Santa Ana, Santa Ana	★★★★★	★★★	NR	NR	NR	★★★	★★★	★★★	★★★	★★★	★★★	NR
316. White Memorial Medical Center, Los Angeles	★★★	★★★	NR	NR	NR	★★★	NR	★★★	★★★	★★★★★	★★★	★★★
317. Whittier Hospital, Whittier	★★★	★★★	NR	NR	NR	★★★	NR	★★★	★★★	NR	NR	★★★
318. Woodland Memorial Hospital, Woodland	★★★	NR	NR	NR	NR	★★★	NR	★★★	★★★	NR	NR	NR

KEY: ★★★★★ BEST ★★★ AS EXPECTED ★ POOR NR NOT RATED BY HEALTHGRADES For full definitions of ratings and awards, see Appendix.

Gastrointestinal Bleed	Gastrointestinal Surgeries and Procedures	Heart Attack	Heart Failure	Hip Fracture Repair	Maternity Care	Pancreatitis	Peripheral Vascular Bypass	Pneumonia	Prostatectomy	Pulmonary Embolism	Resection/Replacement of Abdominal Aorta	Respiratory Failure	Sepsis	Stroke	Total Hip Replacement	Total Knee Replacement	Valve Replacement	Women's Health
★★★	★★★	★★★	★★★	★	★	★★★	NR	★★★	★★★	NR	NR	★★★	★★★★★	★	★★★	★★★	NR	NR
★★★	★★★	★★★	★★★	★★★	★	NR	★★★	★★★★★	★	★★★	NR	★★★	★★★★★	★	★★★	★	★★★	★
NR	★★★	★★★	★★★	★★★	NR	NR	★★★	★★★	NR	NR	★★★	NR	NR	★★★★★	★★★	★	★★★★★	NR
★★★	★★★	★★★	★	★	★★★	★★★	NR	★★★★★	★	★★★	NR	★★★	★	★★★	★★★	★★★	NR	NR
★★★	★★★	★★★	★★★	★	★★★	★★★	NR	★★★★★	★	★★★	NR	★★★	★★★	★★★	★★★	★★★	NR	NR
★★★	★★★	★★★	★★★	★★★	★★★★★	NR	NR	★★★	NR	NR	NR	★★★	★	★★★	★	★	NR	NR
★★★	NR	NR	★★★	NR	★	NR	NR	★★★	NR	NR	NR	NR	NR	★★★	NR	NR	NR	NR
★★★	NR	★★★	★★★	★★★	★★★★★	NR	NR	★★★	★★★	NR	NR	★	★★★	NR	★★★	★★★	★★★	NR
★	NR	★★★	★★★	★★★	★★★★★	NR	NR	★★★	★★★	NR	NR	★★★	★	★	NR	NR	NR	NR
★★★	★★★	★	★	★★★	★★★	★★★	NR	★★★	★★★	★	NR	★★★	★★★	★★★	★★★★★	★★★★★	★★★	★★★
★★★	★	★★★	★	★★★	★★★	NR	NR	★★★	★★★	NR	NR	★★★	★★★	★★★	★★★	★★★	NR	NR
★★★	NR	★★★	★★★	★★★	NR	★★★	NR	★★★	NR	NR	NR	★★★	★★★★★	★★★★★	NR	★	NR	NR
★★★	★★★	★★★	★★★	★★★	★★★★★	★★★	NR	★★★★★	★★★	★★★★★	NR	★★★★★	★★★★★	★	★★★	★★★	NR	NR
★★★	NR	★★★	★★★	NR	★★★★★	NR	NR	★★★	NR	NR	NR	★★★★★	★★★★★	★★★	NR	NR	NR	NR
★★★	★★★	★★★	★★★	★★★	★★★	NR	NR	★★★	NR	NR	NR	★★★	★★★	★★★	NR	NR	NR	★★★
★★★★★	NR	★★★	★★★★★	★★★	★	NR	★★★	★★★★★	NR	NR	NR	★★★★★	★★★	★★★★★	NR	★★★	NR	NR
★★★	NR	★★★	★★★★★	★★★★★	★★★★★	NR	NR	★★★★★	NR	NR	NR	★★★	★★★★★	★★★	NR	NR	NR	NR
★★★	NR	★★★	★★★	★★★	★★★	NR	NR	★	NR	NR	NR	★★★	★★★	★★★	★★★	★★★	NR	NR

COLORADO HOSPITALS: RATINGS BY PROCEDURE

Hospital	Appendectomy	Atrial Fibrillation	Back and Neck Surgery (except Spinal Fusion)	Back and Neck Surgery (Spinal Fusion)	Bariatric Surgery	Bowel Obstruction	Carotid Surgery	Cholecystectomy (Gall Bladder Removal)	Chronic Obstructive Pulmonary Disease (COPD)	Coronary Bypass Surgery	Coronary Interventional Procedures (Angioplasty/Stent)	Diabetic Acidosis and...
1. Arkansas Valley Regional Medical Center, La Junta	NR	★★★	NR	NR	NR	★★★	NR	★★★	★★★	NR	NR	NR
2. Aspen Valley Hospital, Aspen	NR	★★★	NR	★	NR	★★★	NR	★★★	★★★	NR	NR	NR
3. Boulder Community Hospital, Boulder	NR	★★★	★★★	★	NR	★★★	★	★★★	★★★	★★★	★★★	NR
4. Centura Health–Avista Adventist Hospital, Louisville	NR	★★★	★	NR	NR	★★★	NR	★★★	★★★	NR	NR	NR
5. Centura Health–Littleton Adventist Hospital, Littleton	NR	★★★	★	★★★	NR	★★★★★	NR	★★★	★★★	NR	★★★	NR
6. Centura Health–Parker Adventist Hospital, Parker	NR	★★★	★	NR	NR	★★★★★	NR	★★★	★★★	NR	★★★	NR
7. Centura Health–Penrose St. Francis Health Services, Colorado Springs	NR	★★★	★★★	★★★	NR	★★★	★★★	★	★★★	★★★	★★★	★★★★★
8. Centura Health–Porter Adventist Hospital, Denver	NR	★★★	★★★	★★★	NR	★★★	★★★	★	★★★	★★★	★★★	★★★
9. Centura Health–St. Anthony Central Hospital, Denver	NR	★★★	★★★	★★★	NR	★★★★★	★★★	★★★	★★★	★★★★★	★★★	★★★
10. Centura Health–St. Anthony North Hospital, Westminster	NR	★★★	NR	★★★	NR	★★★	NR	★★★	★★★★★	NR	★★★	★★★
11. Centura Health–St. Mary Corwin Medical Center, Pueblo	NR	★★★	★	★	NR	★★★	NR	★	★★★	★★★	★	★★★
12. Centura Health–St. Thomas More Hospital, Canon City	NR	★★★	NR	NR	NR	★★★	NR	★★★	★★★★★	NR	NR	NR
13. Colorado Plains Medical Center, Fort Morgan	NR	★★★	NR	NR	NR	★★★	NR	★★★	★★★	NR	NR	NR
14. Community Hospital, Grand Junction	NR	★★★	★★★	★★★	NR	★★★★★	NR	★★★	★★★	NR	NR	NR
15. Delta County Memorial Hospital, Delta	NR	★★★	NR	NR	NR	★★★	NR	★★★	★★★	NR	NR	NR
16. Denver Health Medical Center, Denver	NR	★★★	NR	NR	NR	★★★	NR	NR	★★★	NR	NR	★★★
17. Exempla Lutheran Medical Center, Wheat Ridge	NR	★★★	★★★	★★★	NR	★★★	★	★★★	★★★★★	★★★	★★★	★★★
18. Exempla Saint Joseph Hospital, Denver	NR	★★★	★★★	NR	NR	★★★★★	NR	★★★	★★★	★★★	★★★	★★★
19. Grand River Medical Center, Rifle	NR	NR	NR	NR	NR	NR	NR	NR	★★★	NR	NR	NR
20. Heart of the Rockies Regional Medical Center, Salida	NR	NR	NR	NR	NR	★★★	NR	NR	★★★	NR	NR	NR
21. Longmont United Hospital, Longmont	NR	★★★	★★★	★★★	NR	★★★	★★★	★★★	★★★	★★★	★★★	★★★
22. McKee Medical Center, Loveland	NR	★★★	★★★	★★★	NR	★★★	NR	★	★★★	NR	★★★	★★★
23. Medical Center of Aurora, Aurora	NR	★★★	★	★	NR	★★★	★★★	★	★★★	★★★	★★★	★★★
24. Memorial Hospital, Colorado Springs	NR	★★★	★	★	NR	★★★	★★★	★	★★★	★★★★★	★★★★★	★★★
25. Memorial Hospital, Craig	NR	NR	NR	NR	NR	NR	NR	NR	★★★	NR	NR	NR
26. Mercy Regional Medical Center, Durango	NR	★★★	NR	★★★	NR	★★★	★★★	★★★★★	★★★	NR	★	NR
27. Montrose Memorial Hospital, Montrose	NR	★★★	NR	NR	NR	★★★	★★★	★★★	★	NR	★★★	NR
28. Mt. San Rafael Hospital, Trinidad	NR	NR	NR	NR	NR	NR	NR	NR	★★★	NR	NR	NR
29. North Colorado Medical Center, Greeley	NR	★★★	★★★	★★★★★	NR	★★★	★★★	★★★	★★★★★	★★★	★★★	★★★
30. North Suburban Medical Center, Thornton	NR	★★★	NR	★★★	NR	★★★	NR	★★★	★★★	NR	★★★	NR
31. Parkview Medical Center, Pueblo	NR	★★★	★	★	NR	★★★	★★★	★	★★★	★★★	★	★★★
32. Platte Valley Medical Center, Brighton	NR	★★★	NR	NR	NR	★★★	NR	★★★	★★★★★	NR	NR	NR
33. Poudre Valley Hospital, Fort Collins	NR	★★★	★★★★★	★★★	NR	★★★	★★★	★★★	★★★	★★★	★★★★★	★★★
34. Presbyterian/St. Luke's Medical Center, Denver	NR	★★★	★	★★★	NR	★★★	★	★★★	★★★	★★★	★★★	★★★
35. Prowers Medical Center, Lamar	NR	★★★	NR	NR	NR	★★★	NR	NR	★★★	NR	NR	NR
36. Rose Medical Center, Denver	NR	★★★	★	★	NR	★★★★★	★★★	★★★	★★★★★	★	★★★	★★★
37. St. Joseph Hospital, Florence	NR	★★★	NR	NR	NR	★★★	NR	★★★	★★★★★	NR	NR	NR
38. St. Mary's Hospital and Medical Center, Grand Junction	NR	★★★	★★★★★	★★★★★	NR	★★★	★★★	★★★★★	★★★	★★★	NR	NR
39. San Luis Valley Regional Medical Center, Alamosa	NR	★★★	NR	NR	NR	★★★	NR	★★★	★★★	NR	NR	NR
40. Sky Ridge Medical Center, Lone Tree	NR	★★★	★★★	★	NR	★★★	NR	★	★★★	NR	★★★	NR
41. Southwest Memorial Hospital, Cortez	NR	★★★	NR	NR	NR	★★★	NR	★	★★★	NR	NR	NR
42. Spanish Peaks Regional Health Center, Walsenburg	NR	NR	NR	NR	NR	NR	NR	NR	★★★	NR	NR	NR
43. Sterling Regional Medical Center, Sterling	NR	★★★	★★★	NR	NR	★★★	NR	★★★★★	★	NR	NR	NR
44. Swedish Medical Center, Englewood	NR	★★★	★★★	★★★	NR	★★★	★★★	★★★	★★★★★	★★★	★★★	★★★
45. University of Colorado Hospital Authority, Aurora	NR	★★★	★★★	★★★	NR	★★★	★★★	★★★	★★★	★★★	★★★	★★★
46. Vail Valley Medical Center, Vail	NR	NR	★	★★★	NR	NR	NR	NR	NR	NR	NR	NR
47. Valley View Hospital Association, Glenwood Springs	NR	★★★	NR	NR	NR	★★★	NR	★★★	★★★	★★★	NR	NR
48. Yampa Valley Medical Center, Steamboat Springs	NR	NR	NR	NR	NR	NR	NR	NR	★★★	NR	NR	NR

KEY: ★★★★★ BEST   ★★★ AS EXPECTED   ★ POOR   NR NOT RATED BY HEALTHGRADES   For full definitions of ratings and awards, see Appendix.

Gastrointestinal Bleed	Gastrointestinal Surgeries and Procedures	Heart Attack	Heart Failure	Hip Fracture Repair	Maternity Care	Pancreatitis	Peripheral Vascular Bypass	Pneumonia	Prostatectomy	Pulmonary Embolism	Resection/Replacement of Abdominal Aorta	Respiratory Failure	Sepsis	Stroke	Total Hip Replacement	Total Knee Replacement	Valve Replacement	Women's Health
★	NR	NR	★★★	NR	NR	NR	NR	★★★	NR	NR	NR	★	★★★	★	NR	NR	NR	NR
NR	NR	NR	★★★	NR	NR	NR	NR	★★★	NR	NR	NR	NR	NR	NR	NR	NR	NR	NR
★★★	★★★	★★★	★★★	★★★	NR	★★★	NR	★★★	★	★★★	NR	★★★	★★★	★★★★★	★★★	★★★	★★★	NR
★★★	NR	NR	★★★	★★★	NR	NR	NR	★★★	★★★	NR	NR	NR	★★★	★★★	★★★	★★★	NR	NR
★★★	★★★★★	★★★	★★★	★★★	NR	NR	NR	★★★★★	NR	★★★	NR	★★★★★	★★★★★	★★★	★★★	★★★	NR	NR
★★★	NR	★	★★★★★	★★★	NR	NR	NR	★★★	NR	NR	NR	★★★★★	★★★	★★★	NR	NR	NR	NR
★★★★★	★★★★★	★★★★★	★★★★★	★★★	NR	★★★	NR	★★★★★	★★★	★★★★★	NR	★★★★★	★★★★★	★★★★★	★★★	★★★	★★★	NR
★★★★★	★★★★★	★★★	★★★★★	★★★	NR	★	NR	★★★★★	★★★★★	★★★	NR	★★★★★	★★★★★	★★★★★	★★★	★	★★★	NR
★★★	★★★	★★★	★★★	★★★★★	NR	★★★	NR	★★★★★	★★★	NR	NR	★★★★★	★★★	★★★	★★★	★★★	★★★	NR
★★★	★★★	★★★★★	★★★	★★★	NR	NR	NR	★★★	NR	★★★	NR	★★★	★★★	★★★	NR	★★★	NR	NR
★★★	★★★	★★★	★★★	★★★	NR	★★★	NR	★★★	★★★	★★★	NR	★★★	★★★	★★★	★★★	NR	NR	NR
★★★	★★★	NR	★★★	★★★★★	NR	NR	NR	★★★	NR	★★★	NR	★★★	★★★	★★★	★★★	★★★★★	NR	NR
★★★	★★★	NR	★★★	★★★	NR	NR	NR	★★★	NR	NR	NR	★★★	★★★	★★★	★★★	NR	NR	NR
★★★	★★★	NR	★★★	★★★★★	NR	NR	NR	★	★★★	NR	NR	★★★	★★★	★★★	NR	★★★★★	NR	NR
★★★	★★★	★★★	★★★	★★★	NR	NR	NR	★★★	★	★★★	NR	★★★	★★★	★★★	NR	★	NR	NR
★★★	NR	★★★	★★★	★★★	NR	NR	NR	★★★	★★★	NR	NR	★★★	★★★	NR	NR	★	NR	NR
★★★	★★★★★	★★★	★★★★★	★★★	NR	★★★	NR	★★★★★	★★★	★★★	★★★	★★★	★★★	★★★★★	★★★★★	★★★	★★★	NR
★★★	★★★	★★★★★	★★★★★	★★★	NR	NR	NR	★★★★★	NR	★★★	NR	★★★	★★★	★★★★★	NR	NR	NR	NR
NR	NR	NR	★★★	NR	NR	NR	NR	★★★	NR	NR	NR	NR	NR	NR	NR	NR	NR	NR
★	NR	NR	★	★★★	NR	NR	NR	★★★	NR	NR	NR	★★★	★★★	NR	NR	★★★	NR	NR
★★★	★★★	★★★★★	★★★★★	★★★	NR	★★★	NR	★★★★★	★	NR	NR	★★★	★★★★★	★★★	★★★	★	NR	NR
★★★	★★★	★★★	★★★	★★★★★	NR	★★★	NR	★★★	★	NR	NR	★★★	★★★	★★★	★★★★★	NR	★★★	NR
★★★★★	★★★★★	★★★	★★★★★	★	NR	NR	NR	★★★★★	★★★	NR	NR	★★★	★★★	★★★	★	★★★	NR	NR
★★★	★★★	★★★	★★★	★★★	NR	NR	★★★	★★★	★★★	★★★	NR	★★★	★★★	★★★	★★★★★	★★★★★	★★★	NR
NR	NR	NR	★	NR	NR	NR	NR	★★★	NR	★★★	NR	NR	NR	NR	NR	NR	NR	NR
★★★	★★★	★★★	★★★	★★★	NR	NR	NR	★★★	NR	★★★	NR	★★★	★	★★★	★★★	NR	NR	NR
★	★★★	★★★	★	★★★	NR	NR	NR	★★★	NR	★★★	NR	★★★	★	★★★	★★★	NR	NR	NR
★★★	NR	NR	★★★	NR	NR	NR	NR	★★★	NR	NR	NR	★★★	★★★	NR	NR	NR	NR	NR
★★★★★	★★★★★	★★★★★	★★★★★	★★★	NR	★★★★★	NR	★★★★★	★★★	★★★	★★★	★★★★★	★★★★★	★★★★★	★★★	★	★★★	NR
★★★	★★★	★★★	★★★★★	★	NR	NR	NR	★★★	★★★	★★★	NR	★★★	★★★	★★★	★	★★★	NR	NR
★★★	★★★	★★★	★★★	★★★	NR	★★★	★★★	★★★	★★★★★	★★★	NR	★★★	★★★	★★★	★★★	★★★	★★★	NR
★★★	NR	NR	★★★	★★★	NR	NR	NR	★★★	NR	NR	NR	NR	★★★	NR	NR	★★★	NR	NR
★★★★★	★★★★★	★★★★★	★★★★★	★★★★★	NR	★★★	★★★	★★★★★	★★★	★★★★★	★★★★★	★★★	★★★★★	★★★★★	★★★★★	★★★★★	★★★	NR
★★★	★★★	★★★	★★★	★★★	NR	NR	★★★	★★★★★	★★★	★★★	★★★	★★★★★	★★★★★	★★★★★	★★★	★★★★★	★★★	NR
★★★	NR	NR	★★★★★	NR	NR	NR	NR	★★★	NR	NR	NR	NR	★★★	NR	NR	NR	NR	NR
★★★	★★★	★★★	★★★★★	★★★	NR	NR	NR	★★★★★	★★★	★★★★★	NR	★★★★★	★★★★★	★★★★★	★★★	★★★	NR	NR
★★★	★★★	★★★	★★★	★★★★★	NR	NR	NR	★★★	★★★	★★★	NR	★★★	★★★	★★★	★★★	★★★★★	NR	NR
★★★	★★★	★★★	★★★	★★★★★	NR	★★★	★★★	★	★★★	★★★	★★★	★	★★★	★	★★★	★★★★★	★★★	NR
★★★	NR	★★★	★★★	★★★	NR	NR	NR	★★★	NR	NR	NR	★★★	★★★	NR	★★★	★★★★★	NR	NR
★★★	★★★★★	★★★	★★★	★★★	NR	★★★	NR	★★★	NR	★★★	NR	★★★	★★★	★★★	★★★	★★★	NR	NR
★★★	★★★	★★★★★	★★★	★	NR	NR	NR	★★★	NR	★★★	NR	★★★	★	★	★	NR	NR	NR
NR	NR	NR	★★★	NR	NR	NR	NR	★★★	NR	NR	NR	NR	NR	NR	NR	NR	NR	NR
★★★	★★★	NR	★★★	★★★	NR	NR	NR	★★★	NR	NR	NR	★	★★★	NR	★★★	NR	NR	NR
★★★	★★★★★	★★★	★★★	★★★★★	NR	★★★★★	NR	★★★	★★★★★	★★★	★★★	★★★	★★★	★★★★★	★★★	★	★★★	NR
★★★	★★★	★★★★★	★★★★★	★★★	NR	NR	NR	★★★★★	★★★	★★★	NR	★★★	★★★	★★★★★	★★★	★★★	★★★	NR
NR	NR	NR	★★★	★★★	NR	NR	NR	★★★	NR	NR	NR	NR	NR	NR	★★★	NR	NR	NR
★★★	NR	NR	★	★★★	NR	NR	NR	★★★	★★★	NR	NR	NR	★★★	★★★	★★★★★	★★★	NR	NR
NR	NR	NR	★★★	NR	NR	NR	NR	★★★	★★★	NR	NR	NR	NR	NR	★★★	★★★	NR	NR

CONNECTICUT HOSPITALS: RATINGS BY PROCEDURE

Hospital	Appendectomy	Atrial Fibrillation	Back and Neck Surgery (except Spinal Fusion)	Back and Neck Surgery (Spinal Fusion)	Bariatric Surgery	Bowel Obstruction	Carotid Surgery	Cholecystectomy (Gall Bladder Removal)	Chronic Obstructive Pulmonary Disease (COPD)	Coronary Bypass Surgery	Coronary Interventional Procedures (Angioplasty/Stent)	Diabetic Acidosis an...
1. Bradley Memorial Hospital and Health Center, Southington	NR	★★★	NR	NR	NR	★★★	NR	★★★	★	NR	NR	NR
2. Bridgeport Hospital, Bridgeport	NR	★★★	★★★	★★★	NR	★★★	★★★	★★★	★★★	★★★	★★★	★★★
3. Bristol Hospital, Bristol	NR	★★★	NR	NR	NR	★★★	NR	★★★	★	NR	NR	★★★
4. Charlotte Hungerford Hospital, Torrington	NR	★	NR	★★★	NR	★★★	NR	★★★	★	NR	NR	★★★
5. Danbury Hospital, Danbury	NR	★★★★★	★★★	★	NR	★★★	★★★	★★★★★	★★★★★	★★★★★	★★★	★★★
6. Day Kimball Hospital, Putnam	NR	★	NR	NR-	NR	★★★	NR	★★★★★	★★★	NR	NR	★★★
7. Greenwich Hospital Association, Greenwich	NR	★★★	★★★★★	★	NR	★★★	★★★	★★★	★★★	NR	NR	★★★
8. Griffin Hospital, Derby	NR	★★★	★★★	NR	NR	★	★★★	★★★	★★★★★	NR	NR	★★★
9. Hartford Hospital, Hartford	NR	★★★	★★★★★	★★★	NR	★★★	★★★	★★★★★	★★★	★★★	★★★	★★★
10. Hospital of Central Connecticut–New Britain General, New Britain	NR	★★★	★★★	★★★★★	NR	★★★	★	★★★★★	★★★	NR	NR	★★★
11. Hospital of St. Raphael, New Haven	NR	★★★	★	★	NR	★★★	★★★	★	★★★	★	★★★★★	★★★
12. John Dempsey Hospital, Farmington	NR	★★★	★★★	★★★★★	NR	★★★	★★★	★★★	★★★	★★★	★★★	NR
13. Johnson Memorial Hospital, Stafford Springs	NR	★★★	NR	NR	NR	★★★	★★★	★★★	★★★	NR	NR	NR
14. Lawrence and Memorial Hospital, New London	NR	★★★	★★★	★★★	NR	★★★	★★★	★★★★★	★	NR	NR	★★★
15. Manchester Memorial Hospital, Manchester	NR	★★★★★	NR	NR	NR	★★★	★★★	★★★	★★★	NR	NR	★★★
16. Middlesex Hospital, Middletown	NR	★★★★★	NR	★★★	NR	★★★★★	★★★★★	★★★	★★★★★	NR	NR	★★★
17. Midstate Medical Center, Meriden	NR	★★★	★	NR	NR	★★★	★★★	★★★	★★★	NR	NR	★★★
18. Milford Hospital, Milford	NR	★★★★★	NR	NR	NR	★★★	★	★★★	★★★	NR	NR	★★★
19. New Milford Hospital, New Milford	NR	★	NR	★	NR	★★★	NR	★★★	★★★	NR	NR	NR
20. Norwalk Hospital Association, Norwalk	NR	★★★	★★★★★	★★★	NR	★★★	★★★	★★★	★★★	NR	NR	★★★
21. Rockville General Hospital, Vernon Rockville	NR	★★★	NR	NR	NR	★★★	★★★	★★★	★★★	NR	NR	★★★
22. St. Francis Hospital and Medical Center, Hartford	NR	★★★	★★★★★	★★★★★	NR	★★★	★★★	★★★	★★★	★★★	★★★	★★★
23. St. Mary's Hospital, Waterbury	NR	★★★	★★★★★	★★★★★	NR	★★★	★	★★★	★★★	★★★	★	★★★
24. St. Vincent's Medical Center, Bridgeport	NR	★★★	★★★	★★★	NR	★★★	★★★	★★★★★	★★★	★★★★★	★★★★★	★★★
25. Sharon Hospital, Sharon	NR	★★★	NR	NR	NR	★★★	NR	NR	★★★	NR	NR	NR
26. Stamford Hospital, Stamford	NR	★★★	★★★	★★★★★	NR	★★★	★★★	★★★	★★★	NR	NR	★★★
27. Waterbury Hospital Health Center, Waterbury	NR	★★★	★★★	★★★	NR	★★★	★	★★★	★★★	★★★	★★★	★★★
28. William W. Backus Hospital, Norwich	NR	★★★	★★★	★	NR	★★★	★★★	★★★★★	★★★★★	NR	★	
29. Windham Community Memorial Hospital and Hatch Hospital, Willimantic	NR	★	NR	NR	NR	★★★	NR	★★★	★★★	NR	NR	★★★
30. World War II Veterans Memorial Hospital, Meriden	NR	★★★	★	NR	NR	★★★	★★★	★★★	★★★	NR	NR	★★★
31. Yale-New Haven Hospital, New Haven	NR	★★★★★	★	★★★	NR	★★★	★	★★★	★★★★★	★★★	★★★	★★★

KEY: ★★★★★ **BEST**   ★★★ **AS EXPECTED**   ★ **POOR**   NR **NOT RATED BY HEALTHGRADES**   For full definitions of ratings and awards, see Appendix.

Gastrointestinal Bleed	Gastrointestinal Surgeries and Procedures	Heart Attack	Heart Failure	Hip Fracture Repair	Maternity Care	Pancreatitis	Peripheral Vascular Bypass	Pneumonia	Prostatectomy	Pulmonary Embolism	Resection/Replacement of Abdominal Aorta	Respiratory Failure	Sepsis	Stroke	Total Hip Replacement	Total Knee Replacement	Valve Replacement	Women's Health
★★★	★★★	★★★	★★★	★	NR	NR	NR	★	NR	NR	NR	NR	★	★★★	NR	★	NR	NR
★★★	★★★	★★★	★★★	★★★	NR	★★★	NR	★★★	★★★	★★★	★★★	★★★	★	★★★	★★★	★	★★★	NR
★★★	★★★	★★★	★	★★★	NR	★★★	★★★	★	★★★	★★★	NR	★	★	★★★	★★★	★	NR	NR
★★★	★	★★★	★★★	★★★★★	NR	★★★	NR	★★★	★★★	★★★	NR	★	★★★	★★★	★★★★★	★★★	NR	NR
★★★★★	★★★	★★★★★	★★★★★	★★★★★	NR	★★★	★★★	★★★★★	★★★	★★★★★	★★★	★★★★★	★★★★★	★★★★★	★★★★★	★★★	★★★	NR
★★★	★★★	★★★	★★★	★★★	NR	★★★	NR	★	★★★	NR	NR	★★★	★	★	★★★	★★★	NR	NR
★★★	★★★	★★★	★★★	★★★★★	NR	★★★	NR	★	★★★	★★★	NR	★	★	★	★	★★★	NR	NR
★★★	★	★★★★★	★★★★★	★★★	NR	★★★	★★★	★★★★★	★★★	NR	NR	★★★	★★★	★★★	★★★	★★★	NR	NR
★★★	★★★★★	★★★	★★★	★★★★★	NR	★★★	★★★	★★★	★★★★★	★★★	★★★	★★★	★★★★★	★	★★★★★	★★★★★	★★★	NR
★★★	★★★	★★★	★★★★★	★	NR	★★★	★★★	★★★	★★★	★★★	★	★	★★★	★★★	★★★★★	★★★	NR	NR
★★★	★★★	★★★★★	★★★★★	★★★	NR	★★★	★	★★★★★	★	★★★	★★★	★★★	★★★	★★★	★★★	★★★	★★★★★	NR
★★★	★	★★★	★★★	★★★	NR	NR	NR	★★★	★★★	★★★	NR	★★★	★	★★★	★★★	★★★	★	NR
★★★	★★★	★	★★★	★★★	NR	NR	★★★	★	★★★	NR	NR	★★★	★	★★★	★★★	★	NR	NR
★★★	★★★	★★★	★★★	★★★	NR	★★★	★★★	★	★★★	★★★	★★★	★	★★★	★★★	★★★	★★★	NR	NR
★★★	★★★	★★★	★★★	★★★	NR	★★★	NR	★★★★★	★★★	★★★	NR	★★★	★★★	★★★	★★★	★★★	NR	NR
★★★★★	★★★★★	★★★★★	★★★★★	★★★★★	NR	★★★★★	★★★	★★★★★	★★★★★	★★★★★	★★★	★★★★★	★★★★★	★★★	★★★	★★★	NR	NR
★★★	★★★	★★★★★	★★★	★★★★★	NR	★★★	★★★	★★★	★★★	★★★	NR	★	★	★★★	★★★	★★★	NR	NR
★	★★★	★★★	★★★	★★★	NR	★★★	NR	★	NR	★★★	NR	★★★	★	★★★	★★★	★★★	NR	NR
★★★	★★★	★★★	★★★	★	NR	NR	NR	★★★	★★★	NR	NR	★	★★★	★★★	★	★	NR	NR
★★★	★★★	★★★	★★★	★★★★★	NR	★★★	★★★	★	★★★	★★★	NR	★	★★★	★★★★★	★★★	★★★	NR	NR
★★★	★★★	★★★	★	NR	NR	★★★	NR	★★★	★★★	NR	NR	★★★★★	★★★	★★★	NR	NR	NR	NR
★★★	★★★	★	★★★	★★★	NR	★	★★★	★★★	★★★	★★★	★★★	★★★	★★★	★★★	★★★★★	★★★	NR	NR
★★★	★★★	★★★	★	★★★	NR	★★★	★★★	★★★	★★★	★	NR	★★★	★★★	★★★	★★★	NR	NR	NR
★★★	★★★	★★★★★	★	★★★	NR	★★★	★★★	★★★	★★★★★	★★★	NR	★	★★★	★	NR	★★★	NR	NR
★★★★★	NR	★★★	★★★	★★★	NR	NR	NR	★★★	★★★	NR	NR	★★★	★★★	★★★	NR	★	NR	NR
★★★★★	★★★	★★★	★	★	NR	★★★	NR	★★★	★★★	★★★	NR	★★★	★	★★★	★★★	NR	NR	NR
★★★	★★★	★★★	★★★	★★★	NR	★★★	★★★	★★★	★★★	NR	★★★	★★★	★	★★★	★★★★★	★★★★★	NR	NR
★★★★★	★★★★★	★★★★★	★★★	★★★★★	NR	★★★	★★★	★★★	★★★	★★★	★	★★★	★★★	★★★	★★★	★★★	NR	NR
★★★	★★★	★★★	★★★	★	NR	★★★	NR	★★★	★★★	NR	NR	★★★	★	★	★★★	★	NR	NR
★★★	★★★	★★★★★	★★★	★★★★★	NR	★★★	★★★	★★★	★★★	NR	★	★	★★★	★★★	★★★	★★★	NR	NR
★★★	★★★	★★★	★★★★★	★★★	NR	★★★	★	★★★★★	★★★	★★★	★★★	★★★★★	★★★★★	★★★	★★★	★★★	★★★★★	NR

DELAWARE HOSPITALS: RATINGS BY PROCEDURE

	Appendectomy	Atrial Fibrillation	Back and Neck Surgery (except Spinal Fusion)	Back and Neck Surgery (Spinal Fusion)	Bariatric Surgery	Bowel Obstruction	Carotid Surgery	Cholecystectomy (Gall Bladder Removal)	Chronic Obstructive Pulmonary Disease (COPD)	Coronary Bypass Surgery	Coronary Interventional Procedures (Angioplasty/Stent)	Diabetic Acidosis and
1. Bayhealth Medical Center–Kent General Hospital, Dover	NR	★★★	★★★	★★★	NR	★	★	★	★★★	★★★	★★★	★★★
2. Bayhealth Medical Center–Milford Memorial Campus, Milford	NR	★★★	★★★	★★★	NR	★	★	★	★★★	★★★	★★★	★★★
3. Beebe Medical Center, Lewes	NR	★★★	★★★	★★★	NR	★★★	★★★	★★★	★★★	NR	NR	★★★
4. Christiana Care Health System–Christiana Hospital, Newark	NR	★★★	★★★	★★★	NR	★★★★★	★★★	★★★	★★★★★	★★★	★★★	★★★
5. Nanticoke Memorial Hospital, Seaford	NR	★★★	NR	NR	NR	★★★	NR	★★★	★★★	NR	NR	★★★
6. St. Francis Hospital, Wilmington	NR	★★★	NR	NR	NR	★★★	★★★	★★★★★	★★★★★	★★★	★	★★★
7. Wilmington Hospital, Wilmington	NR	★★★	★★★	★★★	NR	★★★★★	★★★	★★★	★★★★★	★★★	★★★	★★★

KEY: ★★★★★ BEST   ★★★ AS EXPECTED   ★ POOR   NR NOT RATED BY HEALTHGRADES   For full definitions of ratings and awards, see Appendix.

Gastrointestinal Bleed	Gastrointestinal Surgeries and Procedures	Heart Attack	Heart Failure	Hip Fracture Repair	Maternity Care	Pancreatitis	Peripheral Vascular Bypass	Pneumonia	Prostatectomy	Pulmonary Embolism	Resection/Replacement of Abdominal Aorta	Respiratory Failure	Sepsis	Stroke	Total Hip Replacement	Total Knee Replacement	Valve Replacement	Women's Health
★★★	★★★	★★★★★	★★★★★	★	NR	★★★	★★★	★★★	★	★★★	NR	★★★★★	★★★	★★★	★	★	★★★★★	NR
★★★	★★★	★★★★★	★★★★★	★	NR	★★★	★★★	★★★	★	★★★	NR	★★★★★	★★★	★★★	★	★	★★★★★	NR
★★★	★★★	★★★	★★★★★	★★★★★	NR	★★★	★★★★★	★★★★★	★★★	★★★	★★★	★★★	★★★	★★★	★★★	★★★★★	NR	NR
★★★	★★★	★	★★★★★	★★★	NR	★★★	★★★	★★★★★	★★★	★★★	★	★★★★★	★★★★★	★★★	★★★	★★★	★★★	NR
★★★	★★★	★	★★★	★★★	NR	★★★	NR	★★★	★★★	★★★	NR	★★★	★	★	NR	NR	NR	NR
★★★	★★★	★	★★★	★★★	NR	★★★	NR	★★★	★★★	★★★	NR	★★★	★★★	★★★	★★★★★	★★★★★	★★★	NR
★★★	★★★	★	★★★★★	★★★	NR	★★★	★★★	★★★★★	★★★	★★★	★	★★★★★	★★★★★	★★★	★★★	★★★	★★★	NR

FLORIDA HOSPITALS: RATINGS BY PROCEDURE

	Appendectomy	Atrial Fibrillation	Back and Neck Surgery (except Spinal Fusion)	Back and Neck Surgery (Spinal Fusion)	Bariatric Surgery	Bowel Obstruction	Carotid Surgery	Cholecystectomy (Gall Bladder Removal)	Chronic Obstructive Pulmonary Disease (COPD)	Coronary Bypass Surgery	Coronary Interventional Procedures (Angioplasty/Stent)	Diabetic Acidosis
1. Alachua General Hospital, Gainesville	★★★	★★★	★	★★★	★	★★★	★★★	★★★	★★★	★★★	★★★	★★★
2. Aventura Hospital and Medical Center, Aventura	★★★	★★★	NR	★★★★★	NR	★★★	★★★★★	★★★★★	★★★	★★★	★★★	★★★
3. Baptist Hospital of Miami, Miami	★★★★★	★★★	★★★	★★★	★	★★★	★★★	★★★	★★★	★★★	★★★	★★★
4. Baptist Hospital Pensacola, Pensacola	★★★★★	★★★	★★★	★★★	★★★	★	★★★	★	★★★	★★★	★★★★★	★★★
5. Baptist Medical Center, Jacksonville	★★★	★★★	★★★	★★★	NR	★★★★★	★★★	★★★	★★★★★	★★★	★★★★★	★★★
6. Baptist Medical Center—Beaches, Jacksonville Beach	★	★★★	NR	NR	NR	★★★	★★★	★	★★★	NR	NR	★★★
7. Baptist Medical Center—Nassau, Fernandina Beach	★★★	★★★	NR	NR	NR	★★★	NR	NR	★★★	NR	NR	NR
8. Bartow Regional Medical Center, Bartow	★★★	★	NR	NR	NR	★★★	NR	★★★	★★★	NR	NR	★★★
9. Bay Medical Center, Panama City	★★★	★★★	NR	★★★	★★★★★	★★★	★★★	★★★★★	★★★	★★★	★★★	★★★
10. Bayfront Medical Center, St. Petersburg	★★★	★★★	★★★	★★★	NR	★★★	★★★★★	★★★	★★★	★★★	★	★★★
11. Bert Fish Medical Center, New Smyrna Beach	★★★	★★★	NR	NR	NR	★	NR	★★★	★★★	NR	NR	★★★
12. Bethesda Memorial Hospital, Boynton Beach	★★★	★★★	★★★	★★★★★	★★★	★★★	★★★	★★★	★★★★★	NR	★★★	★★★
13. Blake Medical Center, Bradenton	★★★	★★★	★★★★★	★★★	NR	★★★	★★★	★★★	★★★	★★★	★★★★★	★★★
14. Boca Raton Community Hospital, Boca Raton	★	★★★	★	★★★	★★★	★★★	★★★	★★★	★★★★★	NR	★★★	★★★
15. Brandon Regional Hospital, Brandon	★★★	★★★	★★★	NR	NR	★★★	★★★	★★★	★★★	★★★	★★★	★★★
16. Brooksville Regional Hospital, Brooksville	★★★	★★★	NR	NR	NR	★★★	★★★	★★★	★★★	NR	★★★	★★★
17. Broward General Medical Center, Fort Lauderdale	★★★	★★★	★★★	NR	NR	★★★	NR	★★★	★★★	★★★	★★★	★★★
18. Campbellton Graceville Hospital, Graceville	NR	NR	NR	NR	NR	NR	NR	NR	★★★	NR	NR	NR
19. Cape Canaveral Hospital, Cocoa Beach	★★★	★	NR	NR	NR	★★★	★★★	★★★	★★★	NR	NR	★★★
20. Cape Coral Hospital, Cape Coral	★★★	★★★	★	★★★	NR	★★★★★	★★★	★★★★★	★★★	NR	NR	★★★
21. Capital Regional Medical Center, Tallahassee	★★★	★	★★★★★	★★★	★	★★★	★★★	★★★	★★★	★★★	★★★	★★★
22. Cedars Medical Center, Miami	★★★	★★★	NR	NR	★★★★★	★★★	★★★	★★★★★	★★★★★	★	NR	★★★
23. Central Florida Regional Hospital, Sanford	★★★	★★★	★★★★★	★★★	NR	★★★	★★★	★★★	★★★	★	NR	★★★
24. Charlotte Regional Medical Center, Punta Gorda	★★★	★★★★★	★★★	NR	NR	★★★	★★★	★★★	★★★	★★★★★	NR	★★★
25. Citrus Memorial Hospital, Inverness	★★★	★★★	★★★★★	★★★★★	NR	★★★	★★★	★★★	★★★	★★★	NR	★★★
26. Cleveland Clinic Hospital, Weston	★	★★★	★★★	★	★★★	★★★	★★★	★★★	★★★★★	★★★	★★★★★	NR
27. Columbia Hospital, West Palm Beach	★★★	★★★	NR	NR	NR	★★★	★★★	NR	★★★	★★★	NR	★★★
28. Community Hospital, New Port Richey	★★★	★★★	★★★	★★★	★	★★★★★	★★★	★★★★★	★★★	NR	NR	★★★
29. Coral Gables Hospital, Coral Gables	★★★	★★★	NR	NR	NR	★★★	NR	★★★	★★★	NR	NR	★★★
30. Coral Springs Medical Center, Coral Springs	★★★	★★★	NR	NR	★	★★★	NR	★★★	★★★	NR	NR	★★★
31. Delray Medical Center, Delray Beach	★	★★★	★★★	★★★	★★★	★★★	★★★	★★★	★★★★★	★★★★★	★★★★★	★★★
32. Desoto Memorial Hospital, Arcadia	★★★	★★★	NR	NR	NR	★★★	NR	NR	★★★	NR	NR	NR
33. Doctors Hospital, Coral Gables	★★★	★★★	NR	★	★★★	★★★★★	NR	★★★	★★★★★	NR	NR	★★★
34. Doctors Hospital of Sarasota, Sarasota	★★★	★★★	★★★	★★★	NR	★★★★★	★★★	★★★	★★★	★★★	NR	★★★
35. Doctors Memorial Hospital, Bonifay	NR	NR	NR	NR	NR	NR	NR	NR	★★★	NR	NR	NR
36. Doctors' Memorial Hospital, Perry	★★★	★	NR	NR	NR	★★★	NR	★★★★★	★★★	NR	NR	★★★
37. Edward White Hospital, St. Petersburg	★★★	★★★	NR	NR	NR	★★★	NR	★	★★★	NR	NR	★★★
38. Englewood Community Hospital, Englewood	★★★★★	★★★	NR	NR	NR	★★★	★★★	★★★★★	★★★★★	NR	NR	★★★
39. Fawcett Memorial Hospital, Port Charlotte	★★★	★★★	★★★	★★★	NR	★★★	★★★★★	★★★★★	★★★	NR	NR	★★★
40. Fishermen's Hospital, Marathon	★	NR	NR	NR	NR	★★★	NR	★	★★★	NR	NR	NR
41. Flagler Hospital, St. Augustine	★★★	★★★★★	★★★★★	★★★★★	NR	★★★★★	★★★★★	★★★★★	★★★	★★★★★	★★★	★★★
42. Florida Hospital, Orlando	★	★★★★★	★★★	★★★	★	★★★★★	★★★	★	★★★	★★★	★★★	★★★★★
43. Florida Hospital—Deland, Deland	★★★	★★★	NR	NR	NR	★★★	★★★	★★★	★★★	★★★	NR	★★★
44. Florida Hospital—Fish Memorial, Orange City	★★★	★★★	★★★	★★★	NR	★★★	★★★	★	★★★★★	NR	NR	★★★
45. Florida Hospital—Flagler, Palm Coast	★★★	★★★	NR	NR	NR	★★★	★★★	★★★	★	NR	NR	★★★
46. Florida Hospital—Heartland Medical Center, Sebring	★★★	★★★	★★★	NR	NR	★★★★★	★★★	★★★	★★★	NR	NR	★★★
47. Florida Hospital—Oceanside, Ormond Beach	★★★★★	★★★	NR	NR	NR	★★★	★★★	★★★	★★★	★★★	★★★★★	NR
48. Florida Hospital—Ormond Beach, Ormond Beach	★★★★★	★★★	NR	NR	NR	★★★	★★★	★★★	★★★	★★★	★★★★★	NR
49. Florida Hospital—Waterman, Tavares	★★★	★★★	★★★	★★★	NR	★★★	★★★	★	★★★★★	NR	NR	★★★
50. Florida Hospital—Zephyrhills, Zephyrhills	★★★	★★★	NR	NR	NR	★★★	★★★	★★★	★★★	NR	★★★	★★★

KEY: ★★★★★ BEST   ★★★ AS EXPECTED   ★ POOR   NR NOT RATED BY HEALTHGRADES   For full definitions of ratings and awards, see Appendix.

Gastrointestinal Bleed	Gastrointestinal Surgeries and Procedures	Heart Attack	Heart Failure	Hip Fracture Repair	Maternity Care	Pancreatitis	Peripheral Vascular Bypass	Pneumonia	Prostatectomy	Pulmonary Embolism	Resection/Replacement of Abdominal Aorta	Respiratory Failure	Sepsis	Stroke	Total Hip Replacement	Total Knee Replacement	Valve Replacement	Women's Health
★★★★★	★★★	★★★	★★★★★	★★★	★★★	★	★★★	★★★★★	★★★	★★★	★★★	★	★★★	★★★	★★★★★	★★★	★★★	★★★
★★★	★★★	★★★	★★★	★★★★★	NR	★★★	NR	★★★★★	★★★★★	★★★	NR	★★★★★	★★★★★	★★★★★	★★★	★★★	NR	NR
★★★	★	★★★	★★★★★	★★★★★	★★★★★	★★★	★★★★★	★★★★★	★★★★★	★★★★★	★★★	★★★	★★★	★★★★★	★★★	★	★★★	★★★★★
★★★	★★★	★★★	★★★	★★★	★	★★★★★	★★★★★	★★★	★★★	★★★	★★★	★★★	★★★	★★★	★★★	★★★	★★★	★★★
★★★	★★★	★★★	★★★★★	★	★★★	★★★	★★★	★★★★★	★	★★★	★★★	★★★★★	★★★★★	★★★★★	★	★	★★★	★★★
★★★	NR	★★★	★★★	★★★	★★★	NR	NR	★	NR	NR	NR	★★★	★★★	★★★	NR	NR	NR	NR
★★★	NR	NR	★★★	★★★	★★★★★	★★★	NR	★★★★★	★★★	NR	NR	★★★	★★★	★★★★★	NR	NR	NR	NR
★★★	★★★	★★★★★	★★★★★	★★★★★	★★★	★★★	★★★	★★★★★	★★★	★★★	NR	★★★★★	★★★★★	★★★★★	★★★	★★★	★★★	★★★
★★★	★★★	★★★	★★★	★★★	★★★	★★★	NR	★	★★★	★★★	★	★	★★★	★★★	★★★	★★★	NR	★★★
★	★★★	★★★	★★★★★	★★★	NR	★★★	NR	★★★	★★★	★★★	NR	★★★★★	★★★★★	★★★★★	★★★	★★★	NR	★★★
★★★★★	★★★	★★★★★	★★★★★	★★★	★★★★★	★★★★★	★★★	★★★★★	★★★	★★★	★★★	★★★★★	★★★★★	★★★★★	★★★	★★★	NR	★★★
★★★	★★★	★★★★★	★★★	NR	★★★	NR	★★★	★★★	★★★	★★★	★★★	★★★	★★★	★★★	★★★	NR	NR	NR
★★★★★	★★★★★	★★★	★★★	★★★	★★★	★★★	★★★	★★★★★	★★★★★	★★★★★	★★★	★★★★★	★★★★★	★★★★★	★★★	★★★	NR	NR
★★★	★★★	★★★	★★★★★	★★★	★★★	★★★	★★★★★	NR	★★★★★	★★★★★	★★★★★	★★★★★	★★★★★	★★★★★	★	★	★★★	★★★
★★★	★★★	★★★	★★★★★	★★★	NR	★★★	NR	★★★★★	★★★	★★★	NR	★★★★★	★★★★★	★★★★★	★★★	★★★	NR	NR
★★★	★★★	★★★★★	★★★★★	★★★	★★★	NR	NR	★★★★★	★★★	NR	NR	★★★	★★★	★★★	★★★	★	★★★	★★★★★
NR	NR	NR	★★★	NR	NR	NR	NR	★★★	NR	NR	NR	NR	NR	NR	NR	NR	NR	NR
★★★	★★★	★★★	★★★	★★★	★★★	NR	NR	★★★★★	★★★	★★★	NR	★★★★★	★★★★★	★★★	★★★	★★★	★★★	★★★
★★★	★★★	★★★	★★★★★	★★★★★	★★★★★	★★★	★★★	★★★	★★★	★★★	★★★	★★★★★	★★★★★	★★★★★	★★★	★★★	★★★★★	NR
★★★	★★★	★★★	★★★★★	★★★	★★★	NR	★★★	★★★	NR	★★★	★★★	★★★	★★★	★★★	★★★	NR	NR	★★★
★★★	★★★	★★★	★★★★★	★★★★★	NR	★★★	NR	★★★	★★★	★★★	NR	★★★★★	★★★	★★★	★★★	NR	★★★	★★★
★★★	★★★	★★★★★	★★★★★	★★★	NR	★★★	★	★★★	★★★	★★★	★★★	★★★	★★★★★	★★★★★	★★★★★	★★★	★★★	★★★
★★★★★	★★★★★	★★★★★	★★★★★	★★★	NR	★★★	NR	★★★★★	NR	★★★	NR	★★★	★★★★★	★★★	★	★★★	★★★	★★★
★★★	★★★	★★★	★★★	★★★	NR	NR	NR	★★★	NR	★★★	NR	★★★	★★★★★	★★★	NR	NR	NR	NR
★★★★★	★★★★★	★★★	★	★★★★★	★★★	NR	★★★★★	★★★	★★★	NR	★★★★★	★★★★★	★★★★★	★★★	★	NR	NR	NR
★★★	★★★	★★★	★★★	★★★	NR	NR	NR	★★★	★★★★★	★★★	NR	★★★★★	★★★	★★★	NR	★	NR	NR
★★★	★★★★★	★★★	★★★	★★★	★★★	NR	NR	★★★★★	★★★	★★★	NR	★★★★★	★★★	★★★★★	★★★	★★★	NR	NR
★★★★★	★★★★★	★★★★★	★★★★★	★★★	★★★	★★★	★★★	★★★★★	★★★★★	★★★★★	NR	★★★★★	★★★★★	★★★★★	★★★★★	★★★	★★★★★	NR
★★★	NR	★★★★★	★★★	NR	★★★★★	NR	NR	★★★	NR	NR	NR	★★★	★★★	NR	NR	NR	NR	NR
★★★	★★★	★	★★★	★★★	NR	★★★★★	NR	★★★★★	★★★	★★★	NR	★★★	★★★★★	★★★	★	★★★	NR	NR
★★★	★★★	★★★	★★★	★★★	NR	★★★	★★★	★★★★★	★★★	★★★	NR	★★★★★	★★★	★★★★★	★★★	★★★	NR	NR
NR	NR	★★★	★	NR	NR	NR	NR	★★★	NR	NR	NR	NR	NR	NR	NR	NR	NR	NR
★★★	NR	NR	★★★	NR	★★★	NR	NR	★★★	NR	NR	NR	★★★	NR	NR	NR	NR	NR	NR
★★★	★★★	★★★	★★★	★★★	NR	NR	NR	★★★	★★★	NR	NR	★★★	★★★	★★★	★★★	★	NR	NR
★★★	★★★	★★★★★	★★★	★★★★★	NR	★★★	NR	★★★	★★★	★★★	NR	★★★	★★★★★	★★★★★	★★★	NR	NR	NR
★★★	★★★★★	★★★★★	★★★★★	★★★★★	NR	★★★	NR	★★★★★	★★★	★★★	★★★	★★★	★★★★★	★★★★★	★★★	★★★	NR	NR
★★★★★	NR	NR	★★★	NR	NR	NR	NR	★★★	NR	NR	NR	★★★	★★★	NR	★★★	NR	NR	NR
★★★★★	★★★★★	★★★★★	★★★★★	★★★	★★★	★★★	★★★	★★★★★	★★★★★	★★★★★	NR	★★★★★	★★★★★	★★★★★	★★★	★★★★★	★★★	★★★★★
★★★	★★★★★	★★★	★★★★★	★★★	★★★★★	★★★	★	★★★★★	★★★	★★★	★★★	★★★★★	★★★★★	★★★★★	★★★★★	★★★	★★★	★★★★★
★★★★★	★★★	★★★★★	★★★★★	★★★	★★★	★★★	NR	★★★★★	NR	★★★	NR	★★★★★	★★★★★	★★★★★	★★★	★	NR	NR
★★★★★	★★★★★	★★★	★★★★★	★	NR	★★★	NR	★★★★★	NR	★★★	NR	★★★★★	★★★★★	★★★	★	★	NR	NR
★★★	★★★	★★★★★	★★★	★★★★★	NR	★★★	NR	★★★	★★★	★★★	NR	★★★	★★★★★	★★★	★★★	★★★	NR	NR
★★★	★★★	★★★	★★★★★	★★★★★	★★★	★★★	NR	★★★★★	★	★★★	NR	★★★	★★★★★	★★★	★★★	★★★	NR	NR
★★★★★	★★★★★	★★★★★	★★★★★	★★★	★★★	★★★	★★★	★★★	★★★	★★★	NR	★★★★★	★★★★★	★★★	★	★★★	★★★	★★★★★
★★★★★	★★★	★★★	★★★★★	★★★	★★★	★★★	★★★	★★★	★★★	★★★	NR	★★★★★	★★★★★	★★★	★	★★★	★★★	★★★★★
★★★	★★★★★	★★★★★	★★★★★	★★★	★★★	★★★	★★★★★	★★★	★★★	★★★★★	NR	★★★★★	★★★★★	★★★★★	★★★	★	NR	NR
★★★	★★★	★	★★★	★★★	★	★★★	★★★	★★★	★★★	★★★	★★★	★★★	★★★★★	★★★	★	NR	NR	

	Appendectomy	Atrial Fibrillation	Back and Neck Surgery (except Spinal Fusion)	Back and Neck Surgery (Spinal Fusion)	Bariatric Surgery	Bowel Obstruction	Carotid Surgery	Cholecystectomy (Gall Bladder Removal)	Chronic Obstructive Pulmonary Disease (COPD)	Coronary Bypass Surgery	Coronary Interventional Procedures (Angioplasty/Stent)	Diabetic Acidosis a...
51. Florida Keys Memorial Hospital, Key West	***	***	NR	NR	NR	***	NR	***	***	NR	NR	NR
52. Florida Medical Center, Fort Lauderdale	***	***	NR	NR	*	***	***	***	*****	***	***	***
53. Fort Walton Beach Medical Center, Fort Walton Beach	*****	***	*****	*****	***	***	***	*****	***	***	***	***
54. Glades General Hospital, Belle Glade	***	NR	NR	NR	NR	NR	NR	NR	*****	NR	NR	NR
55. Good Samaritan Medical Center, West Palm Beach	*	***	*****	NR	NR	***	***	***	***	NR	NR	***
56. Gulf Breeze Hospital, Gulf Breeze	***	***	NR	NR	NR	*****	***	***	***	NR	***	NR
57. Gulf Coast Hospital, Fort Myers	*****	***	*****	NR	NR	***	NR	***	***	NR	NR	NR
58. Gulf Coast Medical Center, Panama City	***	***	*****	***	*****	*****	NR	*****	***	NR	NR	***
59. Halifax Medical Center, Daytona Beach	*****	***	*****	*****	***	*****	*****	***	***	***	***	***
60. Health Central, Ocoee	***	***	NR	NR	NR	***	***	***	***	NR	NR	***
61. Healthmark Regional Medical Center, Defuniak Springs	***	NR	NR	NR	NR	***	NR	NR	***	NR	NR	NR
62. Heart of Florida Regional Medical Center, Davenport	*****	***	NR	***	NR	***	***	***	***	NR	NR	***
63. Helen Ellis Memorial Hospital, Tarpon Springs	***	***	***	*****	NR	***	***	***	*****	NR	NR	***
64. Hendry Regional Medical Center, Clewiston	NR	NR	NR	NR	NR	NR	NR	NR	***	NR	NR	NR
65. Hialeah Hospital, Hialeah	***	***	NR	NR	*****	***	NR	***	***	NR	NR	***
66. Highlands Regional Medical Center, Sebring	***	***	***	NR	NR	***	*	***	*	NR	NR	***
67. Hollywood Medical Center, Hollywood	***	***	NR	NR	NR	***	NR	NR	***	NR	NR	NR
68. Holmes Regional Medical Center, Melbourne	*	***	***	*	***	***	*****	***	***	***	*****	***
69. Holy Cross Hospital, Fort Lauderdale	***	*****	***	*****	***	***	***	***	***	***	***	***
70. Homestead Hospital, Homestead	***	***	NR	NR	NR	***	***	***	***	NR	NR	NR
71. Imperial Point Medical Center, Fort Lauderdale	*	***	NR	NR	NR	***	NR	*	***	NR	NR	NR
72. Indian River Medical Center, Vero Beach	*****	*	*****	***	***	***	*****	***	***	NR	NR	***
73. Jackson Health System, Miami	***	***	***	***	***	***	***	***	***	NR	***	***
74. Jackson Hospital, Marianna	***	***	NR	NR	NR	***	NR	***	***	NR	NR	NR
75. Jackson North Medical Center, North Miami Beach	*	*	NR	NR	NR	***	NR	***	***	NR	NR	***
76. Jackson South Community Hospital, Miami	***	***	***	***	***	***	***	***	***	*	***	***
77. Jay Hospital, Jay	NR	NR	NR	NR	*	NR	NR	NR	***	NR	NR	NR
78. JFK Medical Center, Atlantis	*****	*****	***	***	***	*****	***	*****	***	*****	*****	***
79. Jupiter Medical Center, Jupiter	*****	***	***	*****	*	***	***	***	*****	NR	NR	***
80. Kendall Regional Medical Center, Miami	*****	***	NR	NR	***	***	***	*****	***	***	***	***
81. Lake City Medical Center, Lake City	*****	*	NR	NR	***	NR	***	*****	***	NR	NR	NR
82. Lake Wales Medical Center, Lake Wales	***	***	NR	NR	*	***	***	***	***	NR	NR	***
83. Lakeland Regional Medical Center, Lakeland	*****	***	*	***	NR	***	***	*****	*****	*	***	***
84. Lakewood Ranch Medical Center, Bradenton	***	***	NR	NR	NR	***	***	NR	***	NR	NR	NR
85. Largo Medical Center, Largo	*****	***	***	***	NR	***	*****	*****	***	***	***	***
86. Larkin Community Hospital, South Miami	NR	***	NR	NR	NR	***	NR	***	***	NR	NR	NR
87. Lawnwood Regional Medical Center and Heart Institute, Fort Pierce	*****	***	NR	NR	NR	***	***	*****	***	***	***	***
88. Lee Memorial Hospital, Fort Myers	***	***	*****	*****	NR	*****	***	***	*****	***	***	***
89. Leesburg Regional Medical Center, Leesburg	***	***	***	*****	***	*	***	***	***	***	***	***
90. Lehigh Regional Medical Center, Lehigh Acres	***	***	NR	NR	NR	***	NR	*****	***	NR	NR	NR
91. Lower Keys Medical Center, Key West	***	***	NR	NR	NR	***	NR	***	***	NR	NR	NR
92. Lucerne Medical Center, Orlando	***	***	*****	*****	NR	***	***	***	***	*	*	***
93. Madison County Memorial Hospital, Madison	NR	NR	NR	NR	NR	NR	NR	NR	***	NR	NR	NR
94. Manatee Memorial Hospital, Bradenton	*	***	***	***	***	***	***	***	***	***	***	***
95. Mariners Hospital, Tavernier	***	***	NR	NR	NR	***	NR	***	***	NR	NR	***
96. Martin Memorial Medical Center, Stuart	***	***	***	***	NR	***	*****	***	***	NR	***	***
97. Mease Healthcare Dunedin, Dunedin	*	***	***	***	NR	***	***	***	*****	NR	NR	***
98. Memorial Hospital–Jacksonville, Jacksonville	*****	***	***	***	*****	***	*****	*****	***	***	***	***
99. Memorial Hospital–Miramar, Miramar	*	NR	NR	NR	NR	NR	NR	NR	***	NR	NR	NR
100. Memorial Hospital–Pembroke, Pembroke Pines	*	***	NR	NR	*****	***	NR	***	*****	NR	NR	***

KEY: ***** BEST   *** AS EXPECTED   * POOR   NR NOT RATED BY HEALTHGRADES   For full definitions of ratings and awards, see Appendix.

Gastrointestinal Bleed	Gastrointestinal Surgeries and Procedures	Heart Attack	Heart Failure	Hip Fracture Repair	Maternity Care	Pancreatitis	Peripheral Vascular Bypass	Pneumonia	Prostatectomy	Pulmonary Embolism	Resection/Replacement of Abdominal Aorta	Respiratory Failure	Sepsis	Stroke	Total Hip Replacement	Total Knee Replacement	Valve Replacement	Women's Health
★	★★★	NR	★★★	★★★	★★★★★	NR	NR	★★★	NR	NR	NR	NR	★	★★★	NR	★	NR	NR
★★★★★	★★★	★★★★★	★★★★★	★★★★★	NR	★★★	NR	★★★★★	NR	★★★	NR	★★★★★	★★★★★	★★★★★	NR	★★★	★★★	NR
★★★	★★★	★★★	★★★	★★★★★	★★★	★★★	★★★	★	★★★★★	★★★	★★★	★	★	★★★	★★★	★★★★★	NR	★★★
★★★	NR	NR	★★★	NR	★★★	NR	NR	★★★★★	NR	NR	NR	★★★	★★★	NR	NR	NR	NR	NR
★★★★★	★★★★★	★★★	★★★★★	★	★★★	★★★★★	NR	★★★★★	★★★	★★★★★	NR	★★★★★	★★★	★★★★★	★★★	★★★	NR	NR
★★★	★★★★★	★★★	★★★★★	★★★★★	NR	★★★	NR	★★★★★	NR	★★★	NR	★★★★★	★★★★★	★★★	★★★	★★★	NR	NR
★★★	NR	NR	★★★	★★★	★★★★★	NR	NR	★★★★★	NR	NR	NR	★★★	★★★	NR	★★★	★★★★★	NR	NR
★★★★★	★★★★★	NR	★★★★★	★★★	★★★	★★★	NR	★★★★★	★★★	★★★	NR	★★★★★	★★★★★	★★★	★	★	NR	NR
★★★	★★★★★	★★★	★★★★★	★★★	★★★★★	★★★	★★★	★★★	★★★	★★★	★★★	★★★	★★★	★★★★★	★★★★★	★★★★★	★★★	★★★★★
★★★	★★★	★★★	★★★	★★★	★★★	★★★	NR	★★★★★	★★★	★★★	NR	★★★	★★★	★★★	NR	★★★	NR	NR
★★★	NR	NR	★★★	NR	NR	NR	NR	★	NR	NR	NR	NR	NR	★★★	NR	NR	NR	NR
★★★★★	★★★	★★★★★	★★★	★★★	★★★★★	★★★	NR	★★★	★★★	★★★	NR	★	★★★	★★★	★★★	★★★★★	NR	NR
★★★	★★★	★★★	★★★★★	★★★★★	NR	NR	NR	★★★★★	NR	★★★	NR	★★★★★	NR	★★★★★	★★★★★	★★★★★	NR	NR
★★★	NR	★★★★★	★★★	★★★★★	★★★★★	NR	NR	★★★	NR	★★★	NR	★★★	★★★★★	★★★★★	NR	NR	NR	NR
★★★	★★★	★★★	★★★	★★★	★★★	★★★	NR	★	NR	★★★	NR	★★★	★★★	★★★	★★★	★	NR	NR
★★★	NR	★★★	★★★★★	★★★★★	NR	NR	NR	★★★★★	NR	NR	NR	★★★★★	★★★	★★★	★★★	★★★	NR	NR
★★★★★	★★★★★	★★★★★	★★★★★	★★★	★★★	★★★	★★★★★	★★★★★	★	★★★	★★★	★★★	★★★	★★★★★	★	★	★★★	★★★
★★★	★★★★★	★★★	★★★★★	★★★★★	★★★★★	★★★	★★★	★★★★★	★★★	★★★	★★★	★★★	★★★★★	★★★★★	★★★★★	★★★★★	★★★	★★★★★
★★★	NR	★★★	★★★	★★★	★★★	NR	NR	★★★	NR	NR	NR	★★★	★★★	★★★	NR	NR	NR	NR
★★★	★★★	★★★	★★★	★★★	NR	NR	NR	★★★★★	NR	NR	NR	★★★	★★★	NR	NR	★	NR	NR
★★★	★★★	★	★★★	★★★	★★★	★★★	★★★	★★★	★	★★★	★★★	★★★	★	★★★	★★★	★★★★★	NR	NR
★★★	★	★	★★★	★★★	★★★	NR	NR	★★★	★★★	★★★	NR	★	★★★	★★★	NR	★★★	★★★	★
★★★	NR	★★★	★	★★★	★★★	★★★	NR	★★★	★★★	★★★	NR	★★★	★★★	★★★	NR	★★★	NR	NR
★★★	NR	★★★★★	★★★	★★★★★	NR	NR	NR	★★★	NR	NR	NR	★★★	★★★	★★★	NR	NR	NR	NR
★★★	★	★	★★★	★★★	★★★	★★★	NR	★★★	★★★	★★★	NR	★	★	★★★	NR	NR	★★★	★
NR	NR	NR	★	NR	NR	NR	NR	★★★	NR	NR	NR	NR	★★★	★★★	NR	NR	NR	NR
★★★★★	★★★★★	★★★★★	★★★★★	★★★★★	NR	★★★	★★★	★★★★★	★★★	★★★	★★★	★★★★★	★★★★★	★★★★★	★★★	★★★	★★★★★	NR
★★★★★	★★★	★★★	★★★★★	★★★★★	★★★	★★★	NR	★★★★★	★★★★★	★★★★★	★★★	★★★★★	★★★★★	★★★★★	★★★★★	★★★★★	NR	NR
★★★	★★★	★★★★★	★★★★★	★★★★★	★★★★★	★★★	NR	★★★★★	★	★★★	NR	★★★★★	★★★★★	★★★★★	NR	★★★	★★★	★★★
★★★	NR	★★★	★★★	NR	★★★	★★★★★	NR	★★★	★★★	★★★	NR	★★★★★	★★★★★	★★★★★	NR	NR	NR	NR
★★★	NR	★★★	★★★★★	★★★	★	NR	NR	★★★	NR	★★★	NR	★★★	★★★	★★★	NR	NR	NR	NR
★★★	★★★	★	★★★	★★★★★	★★★★★	★★★	★★★	★★★	NR	★	★	★★★	★★★	★★★★★	★★★★★	★★★	NR	★★★
★★★	NR	★★★★★	★★★★★	★★★★★	NR	★★★	NR	NR	NR	NR	NR	★★★	★★★	★★★★★	NR	★★★	NR	NR
★★★	★★★	★	★★★★★	★★★★★	NR	★★★	★★★★★	★★★	★★★	★★★	★★★	★★★	★★★	★★★★★	★★★★★	★	NR	NR
★★★	NR	★★★	★★★	NR	NR	★★★	NR	★★★	★★★	NR	NR	★★★★★	★★★	NR	NR	★★★	★★★	★★★
★★★	★★★	★★★★★	★★★★★	★★★	★★★	NR	★★★★★	★★★★★	★★★	★★★	NR	★★★★★	★★★★★	★★★★★	NR	★★★	★★★	★★★
★★★	★★★	★★★★★	★★★★★	★★★	★★★	★★★★★	★★★	★★★★★	★★★	★★★	★★★	★★★★★	★★★★★	★★★★★	★★★	★★★	★★★	★★★★★
★	★★★	★★★	★★★	★★★	★★★	★★★	NR	★★★	★★★	★★★★★	★★★	★★★	★★★	★★★	★★★	★★★	★★★	★★★
★★★	★★★	★	★★★	★★★	NR	★★★	NR	★★★	NR	★★★	★★★	★★★	★★★	★★★	NR	★★★	NR	NR
★	★★★	NR	★★★	★★★	★★★★★	NR	NR	★★★	NR	NR	NR	★	★★★	NR	★	NR	NR	NR
★★★★★	★★★	★	★★★	★★★	★★★	★★★	NR	★★★★★	★★★	★★★	★★★	★★★	★★★★★	★★★	★	★	★	★★★
NR	NR	NR	★★★	NR	NR	NR	NR	★	NR	NR	NR	NR	★★★	NR	NR	NR	★★★	NR
★★★	★★★	★★★★★	★★★	★★★	★★★★★	★	★★★	★★★★★	★★★	★★★	★★★	★★★	★★★	★	★★★★★	★	★★★	★★★
★★★	NR	★★★	★★★★★	★★★	NR	NR	NR	★★★	NR	NR	NR	★★★	★★★	NR	★★★★★	★	NR	★★★
★★★★★	★★★	★★★	★★★★★	★★★★★	★★★	★★★	★★★★★	★★★★★	★★★	★★★★★	★★★	★★★★★	★★★★★	★★★★★	★★★★★	★★★	NR	NR
★★★	★	★★★★★	★★★★★	★★★	★★★	★★★	NR	★★★★★	NR	★★★	NR	★★★	★★★	★★★★★	★★★	★★★	NR	NR
★★★	★★★	★★★	★★★★★	★★★	★★★	★★★	★★★	★★★	★★★	★★★	★★★	★★★★★	★★★	★★★	★★★	★★★	★★★	★★★
★★★	NR	★★★	★★★★★	NR	★★★	NR	NR	★★★	NR	NR	NR	★★★★★	NR	NR	NR	NR	NR	NR
★★★★★	★★★	★★★	★★★★★	★★★	NR	NR	NR	★★★★★	NR	NR	NR	★★★★★	★★★★★	★★★	NR	NR	NR	NR

Hospital	Appendectomy	Atrial Fibrillation	Back and Neck Surgery (except Spinal Fusion)	Back and Neck Surgery (Spinal Fusion)	Bariatric Surgery	Bowel Obstruction	Carotid Surgery	Cholecystectomy (Gall Bladder Removal)	Chronic Obstructive Pulmonary Disease (COPD)	Coronary Bypass Surgery	Coronary Interventional Procedures (Angioplasty/Stent)	Diabetic Acidosis and
101. Memorial Hospital–Tampa, Tampa	★★★	★★★	NR	NR	NR	★★★	★★★	★★★	★★★	NR	NR	NR
102. Memorial Hospital–West, Pembroke Pines	★	★★★	NR	NR	NR	★★★	★★★	★	★★★★★	NR	NR	★★★
103. Memorial Regional Hospital, Hollywood	★★★	★★★	★★★	★★★	★	★★★	★★★	★	★★★	★★★	★★★	★★★
104. Mercy Hospital, Miami	★★★	★★★	★★★	★★★	★★★★★	★★★	★★★	★★★	★★★	★★★	★★★	★★★
105. Miami Beach Community Hospital, Miami Beach	★★★	★★★	★★★	★★★	★★★	★★★	★★★	★★★	★	★	★★★	★
106. Morton Plant Hospital, Clearwater	★★★★★	★★★	★★★	★★★	★★★	★★★	★★★	★★★★★	★	★	★★★★★	★★★
107. Morton Plant Mease Healthcare Countryside, Safety Harbor	★★★★★	★★★	★★★	★★★	★★★	★★★	★★★	★★★	★★★★★	NR	NR	★★★
108. Morton Plant North Bay Hospital, New Port Richey	★	★★★	NR	NR	NR	★★★	NR	★★★	★★★	NR	NR	★★★
109. Mt. Sinai Medical Center, Miami Beach	★★★	★★★	★★★	★★★	★★★	★★★	★★★	★★★	★	★★★	★★★	
110. Mt. Sinai Medical Center and Miami Heart Institute, Miami Beach	★★★	★★★	★★★	★★★	★★★	★★★	★★★	★★★	★	★★★	★★★	
111. Munroe Regional Medical Center, Ocala	★★★	★★★	★★★	★★★	★★★★★	★★★	★	★★★	★★★★★	★★★	★★★★★	★★★
112. NCH Healthcare System, Naples	★★★	★★★	★★★★★	★★★★★	NR	★★★	★	★★★	★★★	★★★★★	★★★★★	★★★
113. North Broward Medical Center, Deerfield Beach	★★★	★★★	★★★	NR	NR	★★★	★★★	★★★	★★★	NR	NR	★★★
114. North Florida Regional Medical Center, Gainesville	★★★★★	★★★	★★★	★★★	★★★	★★★	★★★★★	★★★★★	★★★	★	★★★	★★★
115. North Okaloosa Medical Center, Crestview	★★★	★★★	NR	★	NR	★★★	★★★	★★★	★★★★★	NR	NR	NR
116. North Ridge Medical Center, Fort Lauderdale	★★★	★★★	★★★	★★★	★	★★★	★	★★★	★★★	★★★	★★★★★	★★★
117. North Shore Medical Center, Miami	★★★	★★★	NR	NR	NR	★★★	NR	NR	★★★	NR	NR	★★★
118. Northside Hospital, St. Petersburg	★★★	★★★	★★★	NR	NR	★★★	★★★	★★★	★★★	★★★	★★★	★★★
119. Northwest Florida Community Hospital, Chipley	NR	NR	NR	NR	NR	NR	NR	NR	★★★	NR	NR	NR
120. Northwest Medical Center, Margate	★★★★★	★★★	NR	NR	★★★	★★★	★★★	★★★	★★★	NR	NR	★★★
121. Oak Hill Hospital, Brooksville	★★★★★	★★★	★★★	NR	NR	★★★	★★★	★★★	★★★	NR	NR	★★★
122. Ocala Regional Medical Center, Ocala	★★★★★	★★★	★★★★★	★★★★★	★★★★★	★★★	★★★★★	★★★	★★★★★	★★★	★★★	★★★
123. Orange Park Medical Center, Orange Park	★★★	★★★	★★★★★	★★★	NR	★★★	★★★★★	★★★	★★★	★	★★★	★★★
124. Orlando Regional Healthcare, Orlando	★★★	★★★	★★★★★	★★★★★	★★★	★★★	★★★	★★★	★★★	★	★★★	★★★
125. Osceola Regional Medical Center, Kissimmee	★★★	★★★	NR	NR	NR	★★★	★★★	★★★	★★★	★★★★★	★★★	★★★
126. Palm Beach Gardens Medical Center, Palm Beach Gardens	★★★	★★★★★	NR	NR	NR	★★★★★	★★★★★	★★★	★★★★★	★★★	★★★★★	★★★
127. Palm Springs General Hospital, Hialeah	★★★★★	★	NR	NR	NR	★★★	★★★	★★★	★★★	NR	NR	★★★
128. Palmetto General Hospital, Hialeah	★	★★★	NR	NR	★★★★★	★★★	★★★	★	★★★	★★★	NR	★★★
129. Palms of Pasadena Hospital, St. Petersburg	★	★★★	★★★	★★★	★	★★★	★★★	★	★★★	NR	NR	★★★
130. Palms West Hospital, Loxahatchee	★★★★★	★★★	NR	NR	★★★	★★★	★★★	★★★	★★★	NR	NR	★★★
131. Pan American Hospital, Miami	★★★	★	NR	NR	NR	★★★	NR	★★★	★★★	NR	NR	★★★
132. Parrish Medical Center, Titusville	★★★	★★★	NR	★★★★★	NR	★★★	★★★	★★★	★★★	NR	NR	★★★
133. Pasco Regional Medical Center, Dade City	★★★★★	★★★	NR	NR	★★★★★	★★★	NR	★★★★★	★★★	NR	NR	NR
134. Peace River Regional Medical Center, Port Charlotte	★★★	★★★	★★★	★★★	NR	★★★★★	★★★	★★★★★	★★★	NR	NR	★★★
135. Physicians Regional Medical Center, Naples	★★★	★★★	★★★★★	★★★	★	★★★★★	★	★★★	★★★	NR	NR	NR
136. Plantation General Hospital, Plantation	★★★	NR	NR	NR	★★★	NR	NR	NR	★★★	NR	NR	NR
137. Putnam Community Medical Center, Palatka	★★★	★★★	NR	NR	NR	★★★	★★★	★★★	★★★★★	NR	NR	★★★
138. Raulerson Hospital, Okeechobee	★★★	★★★	NR	NR	NR	★★★	NR	★★★	★★★★★	NR	★★★	★★★
139. Regional Medical Center—Bayonet Point, Hudson	★★★★★	★★★	★★★	★★★	★★★	★★★	★★★	★★★	★★★★★	★★★	★★★	★★★
140. Sacred Heart Hospital at the Emerald Coast, Destin	★★★★★	★★★	★★★	NR	NR	★★★	★★★	★★★	★★★	NR	NR	★★★
141. Sacred Heart Hospital, Pensacola	★★★	★★★	★★★	★★★	NR	★★★	★★★	★★★	★★★	★★★	★★★	★★★
142. St. Anthony's Hospital, St. Petersburg	★★★	★★★	★★★	NR	NR	★	★★★	★	★★★	★★★	★★★	★★★
143. St. Cloud Regional Medical Center, St. Cloud	NR	NR	NR	NR	NR	NR	NR	NR	★★★	NR	NR	NR
144. St. Joseph's Hospital, Tampa	★	★★★	★	★	★★★	★★★	★	★★★	★★★	★★★	★★★	★★★
145. St. Joseph's Women's Hospital, Tampa	★	★★★	★	★	★★★	★★★	★	★★★	★★★	★★★	★★★	★★★
146. St. Lucie Medical Center, Port St. Lucie	★★★★★	★★★	★★★	★★★★★	NR	★★★	★★★	★★★	★★★★★	★★★	NR	★★★
147. St. Luke's Hospital, Jacksonville	★★★	★★★	★★★	★	NR	★★★	★★★	★★★	★★★	★★★★★	★★★	★★★
148. St. Mary's Medical Center, West Palm Beach	★	★★★	★★★	★★★	NR	★★★	NR	NR	★★★	NR	NR	NR
149. St. Petersburg General Hospital, St. Petersburg	★★★★★	★★★	NR	NR	★	★★★	★★★	★★★	★★★	NR	NR	★★★
150. St. Vincent's Medical Center, Jacksonville	★	★★★	★★★	★	NR	★★★	★★★	★★★	★★★★★	★★★	★★★★★	★★★

KEY: ★★★★★ BEST ★★★ AS EXPECTED ★ POOR NR NOT RATED BY HEALTHGRADES For full definitions of ratings and awards, see Appendix.

Gastrointestinal Bleed	Gastrointestinal Surgeries and Procedures	Heart Attack	Heart Failure	Hip Fracture Repair	Maternity Care	Pancreatitis	Peripheral Vascular Bypass	Pneumonia	Prostatectomy	Pulmonary Embolism	Resection/Replacement of Abdominal Aorta	Respiratory Failure	Sepsis	Stroke	Total Hip Replacement	Total Knee Replacement	Valve Replacement	Women's Health
★★★	★★★★★	★	★★★	★★★	NR	★★★	NR	★★★★★	★★★	★	NR	★★★	★★★	★★★	★★★	★★★	NR	NR
★★★★★	★★★	★★★★★	★★★★★	★★★	★★★	★★★	NR	★★★★★	★★★	★★★	NR	★★★★★	★★★★★	★★★★★	NR	★★★	NR	NR
★★★★★	★★★	★★★	★★★	★	★★★★★	★★★	★★★	★★★★★	★★★	★★★	★	★★★★★	★★★★★	★★★	★★★	★★★	★	★★★
★★★	★★★	★★★	★★★★★	★★★★★	★★★★★	★★★	NR	★★★★★	★★★	★★★	NR	★★★★★	★★★	★★★★★	★★★	★★★★★	★★★	★★★
★★★	★★★	★	★★★	★★★	★★★★★	★★★	★★★	★★★	★★★	★★★	★★★	★★★	★	★★★★★	★★★	★★★	★★★	★★★
★★★★★	★★★	★★★★★	★★★	★	★★★	★★★	★★★	★★★★★	★★★	★★★	★★★	★★★	★	★★★	★★★	★★★	★★★	★★★
★★★	★★★	★★★★★	★★★★★	★★★★★	★★★	★★★	★★★	★★★★★	★★★	★★★	★★★	★★★	★★★	★★★★★	★★★	★★★★★	NR	NR
★★★	NR	★★★	★★★★★	★★★	NR	NR	NR	★★★★★	★★★	NR	NR	★★★★★	★★★★★	★★★	★★★	★	NR	NR
★★★	★★★	★	★★★	★★★	★★★★★	★★★	★★★	★★★	★★★	★★★	★★★	★★★	★	★★★★★	★★★	★★★	★★★	★★★
★★★	★★★	★	★★★	★★★	★★★★★	★★★	★★★	★★★	★★★	★★★	★★★	★★★	★	★★★★★	★★★	★★★	★★★	★★★★★
★★★★★	★	★★★★★	★★★★★	★★★	★★★★★	★★★	★★★	★★★	★★★	★★★	★★★	★★★	★★★	★★★	★★★	★★★	★★★	★★★★★
★★★	★★★	★★★	★★★	★★★★★	NR	★★★	NR	★★★★★	★★★	NR	NR	★★★★★	★★★	★★★★★	★★★	★★★	NR	NR
★★★	★★★	★	★★★	★★★	★★★	★★★	★★★	★★★	★★★	★★★	★★★	★★★	★★★	★★★★★	★★★	★★★	★★★	★★★
★★★★★	NR	★	★★★	★★★	★★★	★	★★★	★★★★★	★★★	★	★★★	★★★	★★★★★	★★★	NR	★	NR	NR
★★★	★★★★★	★★★★★	★★★	★★★	NR	★★★	NR	★★★	★★★	★★★	★★★	★★★	★★★	★★★★★	★★★	★★★	NR	NR
★★★	NR	★★★	★★★	★★★★★	NR	NR	NR	★★★	NR	★★★	★★★	★★★	★★★	★★★	NR	NR	★★★	NR
★★★	★★★	★★★	★★★	★★★★★	★★★	NR	NR	★★★★★	NR	★★★	★★★	★★★	★★★	★★★	★★★	★★★	★★★	★★★
NR	NR	NR	★	NR	NR	NR	NR	★	NR	NR	NR	NR	NR	NR	NR	NR	NR	NR
★★★	★★★★★	★★★	★★★★★	★★★	★★★★★	★★★	NR	★★★★★	★★★	★★★	NR	★★★★★	★★★★★	★★★★★	NR	★★★	NR	NR
★★★	★★★	★★★	★★★	★★★★★	NR	★★★	★★★	★★★★★	★★★★★	★★★	★★★	★★★★★	★★★★★	★★★	★★★	★★★	★★★	★★★
★★★	★★★	★★★	★★★	★★★	★★★	★★★	★★★	★★★★★	★★★★★	★★★★★	NR	★★★	★★★★★	★★★★★	★★★	★★★	★★★	★★★
★★★★★	★★★	★	★★★	★★★	★★★	★★★	★★★★★	★★★	★★★	★★★	NR	★★★	★★★★★	★★★★★	★★★	★	★	★★★
★★★	★★★★★	★★★	★★★	★★★	★★★	★★★	★★★	★★★	★★★	★★★	NR	★★★	★★★★★	★★★★★	★★★	★★★	★★★	★★★★★
★★★	★★★★★	★★★	★★★	★★★	★★★	★★★	★★★	★★★★★	★★★	★★★	NR	★★★	★★★★★	★★★★★	★★★★★	★★★	★★★	★★★
★★★	★★★	★	★★★	★★★★★	★★★	★★★	NR	★	★★★	★★★	NR	★★★★★	★	★★★★★	NR	★★★	NR	NR
★	★★★	★★★	★★★★★	★★★	★★★★★	★★★	NR	★★★	★★★	★★★	NR	★★★★★	★★★	★★★	NR	★★★★★	NR	NR
★★★★★	★★★	★★★	★★★	★★★	★★★	★★★	★	★★★	★★★	★★★★★	NR	★★★	★★★	★★★	★★★★★	★★★	NR	NR
★★★	★★★★★	★★★	★★★★★	★★★	★★★★★	★★★	★★★★★	NR	NR	NR	NR	★★★★★	★★★★★	★★★★★	NR	NR	NR	★★★
★★★	NR	★★★	★★★★★	★★★	NR	★★★	NR	★★★★★	★★★	★★★	NR	★★★	★★★	★★★	NR	NR	NR	NR
★★★	★★★★★	★★★	★★★	★★★★★	★★★	★★★	NR	★★★★★	★★★	★★★	NR	★★★★★	★★★★★	★★★★★	★★★	★	NR	NR
★★★	★★★	★	★★★	★★★★★	★★★	NR	NR	★★★★★	★★★	★★★	NR	★★★★★	★★★★★	★★★	★★★	★★★★★	★★★	★★★
★★★★★	★★★	★★★★★	★★★★★	★★★	★★★	★★★	NR	★★★★★	★★★★★	★★★	★★★	★★★★★	★★★★★	★★★	★★★	★★★	★★★	★★★
★★★	★★★	★★★	★★★★★	★★★	NR	★★★	★★★	★★★	★★★	★	★★★	★★★	★★★★★	★★★	★★★	★★★	★★★★★	NR
★★★	NR	NR	★★★	NR	★★★★★	NR	NR	★★★	NR	NR	NR	NR	★★★	★★★	NR	NR	NR	NR
★★★	★★★	★★★	★★★	★★★	★	★★★	NR	★★★	NR	★★★	NR	★★★	★★★	★★★	NR	★★★	NR	NR
★★★	★★★★★	★★★	★★★	★★★	NR	★★★	NR	★★★★★	★★★	★★★	NR	★★★★★	★★★★★	★★★★★	NR	★★★	NR	NR
★★★	★★★★★	★★★	★★★	NR	NR	★★★	NR	★★★	★★★	★★★	NR	★★★★★	★★★★★	★★★	NR	★★★	★★★	NR
★★★	NR	★★★	★★★	★★★	NR	NR	NR	★★★	NR	NR	NR	★★★	★★★	★★★	★★★	★★★	NR	NR
★★★	★★★	★★★	★★★	★★★	NR	★★★	★★★★★	★★★	★★★	★★★★★	★★★	★★★	★★★★★	★★★	★★★	★★★	★★★	★
★	★★★	★★★	★★★	★★★	NR	★★★★★	★★★	★★★	★★★★★	★★★	★★★	★★★	★★★★★	★★★★★	★★★	★★★	NR	NR
NR	NR	NR	★★★	NR	NR	NR	NR	★★★	NR	NR	NR	NR	★★★	★★★	NR	NR	NR	NR
★★★	★★★★★	★★★★★	★★★★★	★	★★★	★★★	★★★	★★★★★	★★★	★★★	★★★★★	★★★★★	★★★★★	★	★★★	★★★	★★★
★★★	★★★★★	★★★★★	★★★★★	★★★	★	★★★	★★★	★★★★★	★★★	★★★	★★★★★	★★★★★	★★★★★	★	★★★	★★★	★★★
★	★★★	★★★	★★★★★	★★★★★	★★★	★★★	NR	★★★	★★★★★	★★★	NR	★★★	★	★★★★★	NR	★★★	NR	NR
★★★	★★★★★	★★★★★	★★★★★	★★★	★	★★★	★★★	★★★	★★★★★	★★★	★★★	★★★	★★★★★	★★★★★	★★★	★★★	★★★	★★★
★★★	NR	★★★	★★★	★★★★★	★★★	NR	NR	★★★	NR	NR	★★★	★★★	★★★	★★★★★	NR	★★★	NR	NR
★★★	★★★	★★★	★★★	★★★	★★★★★	★★★	NR	★★★★★	NR	★★★	NR	★	★★★	★★★	★★★	NR	NR	NR
★★★	★★★	★★★	★★★	★★★	★★★	★★★	★★★	★★★★★	★	NR	★	★★★	★★★★★	★★★★★	★★★	★	★★★	★★★

	Appendectomy	Atrial Fibrillation	Back and Neck Surgery (except Spinal Fusion)	Back and Neck Surgery (Spinal Fusion)	Bariatric Surgery	Bowel Obstruction	Carotid Surgery	Cholecystectomy (Gall Bladder Removal)	Chronic Obstructive Pulmonary Disease (COPD)	Coronary Bypass Surgery	Coronary Interventional Procedures (Angioplasty/Stent)	Diabetic Acidosis and C...
151. Santa Rosa Medical Center, Milton	★★★	★★★	NR	NR	★★★★★	★★★	NR	★★★★★	★★★	NR	NR	NR
152. Sarasota Memorial Hospital, Sarasota	★	★★★	★★★★★	★★★★★	★	★★★	★★★	★★★	★★★★★	★★★	★★★★★	★★★
153. Sebastian River Medical Center, Sebastian	★★★★★	★★★	★★★★★	NR	NR	★★★	★★★	★★★★★	★★★	NR	NR	★★★
154. Seven Rivers Regional Medical Center, Crystal River	★★★	★★★	★★★★★	★★★★★	NR	★★★	★★★	★★★	★★★	NR	NR	★★★
155. Shands Hospital at the University of Florida, Gainesville	★★★	★★★	★	★★★	★	★★★	★★★	★★★	★★★	★★★	★★★	★★★
156. Shands Jacksonville, Jacksonville	★★★	★★★	★★★	NR	★★★	★★★	★★★	★★★	★★★	★	★	★★★
157. Shands Lake Shore, Lake City	★★★	★★★	NR	NR	NR	★★★	NR	★★★	★★★★★	NR	NR	NR
158. Shands Starke, Starke	NR	★★★	NR	NR	NR	NR	NR	★★★	★★★	NR	NR	NR
159. South Bay Hospital, Sun City Center	★★★	★★★	★★★★★	★★★★★	NR	★★★	★★★	★★★★★	★★★	NR	NR	★★★
160. South Beach Community Hospital, Miami Beach	★★★	NR	NR	NR	NR	NR	NR	★★★	★★★	NR	NR	NR
161. South Florida Baptist Hospital, Plant City	★	★	NR	NR	NR	★★★	★★★	★★★	★★★	NR	NR	NR
162. South Lake Hospital, Clermont	★★★★★	★★★	NR	NR	NR	★★★	NR	★★★★★	★★★★★	NR	NR	★★★
163. South Miami Hospital, South Miami	★★★	★	★	NR	★	★★★	★★★	★★★	★★★★★	★★★	★★★	★★★
164. Southwest Florida Regional Medical Center, Fort Myers	★★★★★	★★★	★	★★★	NR	★	★★★	★★★★★	★★★★★	★★★	★★★	★★★
165. Sun Coast Hospital, Largo	★★★	★★★	NR	NR	★★★	★★★	★★★	★★★	★	NR	NR	NR
166. Tallahassee Memorial Healthcare, Tallahassee	★★★★★	★★★	★★★★★	★★★	★★★★★	★	★★★	★★★★★	★★★	★★★	★★★	★★★
167. Tampa General Hospital, Tampa	★★★	★★★	★	★	★★★	★★★	★	★★★	★★★	★★★	★★★	★★★
168. Town and Country Hospital, Tampa	★★★	★★★	NR	★★★	★★★★★	★★★	NR	★★★	★★★	★★★	NR	NR
169. Trinity Community Hospital, Jasper	NR	NR	NR	NR	NR	NR	NR	★★★	★★★	NR	NR	NR
170. Twin Cities Hospital, Niceville	★★★★★	★★★	NR	NR	NR	★★★	NR	★★★★★	★★★★★	NR	NR	NR
171. University Community Hospital at Carrollwood, Tampa	★★★	★★★	★★★	★★★	NR	★	NR	★★★★★	★★★	NR	NR	★★★
172. University Community Hospital, Tampa	★★★	★★★	★★★★★	★★★	NR	★	★★★	★★★	★	★	★★★	★★★
173. University Hospital and Medical Center, Tamarac	★★★★★	★★★	NR	NR	★★★★★	★★★★★	★★★	★★★	★★★	★★★	★★★	★★★
174. Venice Regional Medical Center, Venice	★★★	★★★★★	★★★★★	★★★	NR	★★★	★★★	★★★	★★★	★★★★★	★★★	★★★
175. Villages Regional Hospital, The Villages	★★★★★	★★★	NR	NR	NR	★★★	★★★	★★★★★	★★★	NR	NR	★★★
176. Wellington Regional Medical Center, Wellington	★★★	★★★	NR	NR	★★★	★★★	NR	★	★★★	NR	NR	NR
177. West Boca Medical Center, Boca Raton	★	★★★	NR	NR	NR	★★★	NR	★	★★★	NR	NR	★★★
178. West Florida Hospital, Pensacola	★★★	★★★	★	★★★	★★★	★★★	★★★	★★★	★★★	★★★	★★★	★★★
179. Westchester General Hospital, Miami	★★★	★★★	NR	NR	NR	★★★	★	★★★	★★★	NR	NR	★★★
180. Westside Regional Medical Center, Plantation	★★★	★★★★★	NR	NR	NR	★★★★★	NR	★★★	★★★	★★★	★★★	★★★
181. Winter Haven Hospital, Winter Haven	★	★★★	★★★	★★★	★★★	★★★	★★★	★★★	★★★	★★★	★★★	★★★
182. Wuesthoff Medical Center—Melbourne, Melbourne	★	★★★	NR	NR	NR	★★★	★★★	★★★	★★★	NR	NR	NR
183. Wuesthoff Medical Center—Rockledge, Rockledge	★★★	★★★	★★★	★★★	NR	★★★	★★★	★★★★★	★★★★★	★★★	★★★★★	★★★

KEY: ★★★★★ BEST   ★★★ AS EXPECTED   ★ POOR   NR NOT RATED BY HEALTHGRADES   For full definitions of ratings and awards, see Appendix.

Gastrointestinal Bleed	Gastrointestinal Surgeries and Procedures	Heart Attack	Heart Failure	Hip Fracture Repair	Maternity Care	Pancreatitis	Peripheral Vascular Bypass	Pneumonia	Prostatectomy	Pulmonary Embolism	Resection/Replacement of Abdominal Aorta	Respiratory Failure	Sepsis	Stroke	Total Hip Replacement	Total Knee Replacement	Valve Replacement	Women's Health
★★★	★★★★★	★★★	★★★	★★★	★★★	★★★	NR	★★★★★	NR	NR	NR	★★★★★	★	★★★	NR	★★★★★	NR	NR
★★★★★	★★★	★★★★★	★★★★★	★★★	★★★★★	★★★	★★★	★★★★★	★★★	★★★	★★★★★	★★★	★★★★★	★★★★★	★	★★★	★★★	★★★★★
★★★★★	★★★	★★★★★	★★★	★★★	NR	★★★	NR	★★★	★★★	★★★	NR	★★★	★★★	★★★★★	★★★	★★★	NR	NR
★★★	★★★	★	★★★	★★★★★	★★★	★★★	NR	★	★★★★★	★★★	NR	★	★	★★★	★★★	★★★★★	NR	NR
★★★★★	★★★	★★★	★★★★★	★★★	★★★	★	★★★	★★★★★	★★★	★★★	★★★	★★★	★	★★★	★★★	★★★★★	★★★	★★★
★★★	★	★	★★★★★	★★★	★	★★★	★	★★★	NR	★	NR	★	★	★★★	★★★	★★★	NR	★
★★★	★★★★★	★★★	★★★	★★★	★★★	NR	NR	★★★★★	NR	NR	NR	★★★	★★★	★★★★★	NR	★★★	NR	NR
NR	NR	NR	★★★	NR	NR	NR	NR	★★★	NR	NR	NR	NR	★★★	NR	NR	NR	NR	NR
★★★	★★★	★★★	★★★★★	★★★	NR	★★★	NR	★★★	★★★	★★★★★	NR	★★★★★	★★★	★★★	★★★★★	★★★	NR	NR
NR	NR	NR	★★★	NR	NR	NR	NR	★★★	NR	NR	NR	★	NR	NR	NR	NR	NR	NR
★★★	★★★	★★★	★★★	★★★	NR	NR	★★★	★★★	NR	NR	★★★	★★★★★	★★★	★★★	★★★	NR	NR	NR
★★★	★★★	★★★	★★★★★	★★★★★	★★★	★★★	NR	★★★★★	NR	★★★	NR	★★★★★	★★★★★	★★★★★	★★★	★★★	NR	NR
★★★	★★★	★★★	★★★	★★★★★	★★★★★	★★★	NR	★★★★★	★★★	★★★	★★★	★★★	★★★	★★★	★★★★★	★★★	★★★	★★★★★
★★★	★★★	★★★	★★★	★★★	NR	★★★	★★★★★	★★★★★	★★★	★★★	★★★	★★★★★	★★★	★★★	★★★	★★★★★	★★★	NR
★★★	★★★	★★★	★★★	★★★★★	NR	NR	NR	★★★	NR	NR	NR	★	★	★★★	★★★	★★★	★★★	NR
★★★	★★★	★★★	★★★	★★★	★★★	★★★	★	★★★	★★★	★	★★★	★★★	★	★★★	★★★★★	★★★★★	★★★	★★★
★★★	★★★	★	★	★★★	★	★★★	★★★	★★★	★★★	★★★	★★★	★★★	★★★	★★★	★	★	★	★
★★★	★★★	★★★	★★★	★★★	NR	NR	NR	★★★	★★★	NR	NR	★★★	★★★	★★★	NR	★★★	NR	NR
NR	NR	NR	★★★	NR	NR	NR	NR	★★★	NR	NR	NR	NR	★★★	NR	NR	NR	NR	NR
★★★	★★★	NR	★★★	★★★★★	NR	NR	★★★	NR	NR	NR	★★★	★★★	★	NR	★★★★★	NR	NR	
★★★	★★★	★★★	★★★	★★★	NR	★★★	NR	★★★★★	★★★	★★★	★★★	★★★	★★★	★★★	★★★	NR	NR	
★★★	★★★	★	★★★	★★★★★	★★★	★★★	★★★	★★★	★★★★★	★★★	★★★	★★★	★	★★★	★★★	★★★★★	★★★	★★★
★★★	★★★	★★★	★★★★★	★★★	NR	★★★	★★★	★★★★★	★★★	★★★	★★★	★★★★★	★★★★★	★★★	★★★	★★★	★★★	★★★
★★★	★	★★★	★★★	NR	★★★★★	★	★★★	★★★	★★★	★★★	★★★	★★★	★★★	★★★	★★★	★★★★★	★★★	★★★
★★★	★★★	★★★	★★★★★	★★★	NR	★★★	NR	★★★★★	NR	★★★★★	NR	★★★	★★★★★	★★★	NR	NR	★★★	NR
★★★	★★★★★	★★★	★★★★★	★★★	★★★★★	★★★	NR	★★★★★	NR	NR	NR	★★★★★	★★★★★	★★★★★	★★★	★★★	★★★	NR
★★★	★★★	★★★★★	★★★	★★★	★★★★★	★★★	NR	★★★★★	★	★★★	NR	★★★	★★★	★★★	★★★	★★★	★★★	NR
★★★	★★★	★	★	★★★	★★★★★	★★★	★★★	★★★	★★★	★★★	★★★	★★★	★★★	★★★	★★★★★	★★★	★★★	★★★
★★★	NR	★★★	★	★★★★★	NR	★★★	NR	★★★	NR	NR	NR	★★★	★★★	★★★★★	NR	NR	★★★	NR
★★★★★	★★★★★	★★★★★	★★★★★	★★★	NR	★★★	NR	★★★★★	★	★★★	NR	★★★★★	★★★★★	★★★★★	★★★	★★★	★★★	★★★
★★★	★★★	★★★	★★★	★★★	★★★	★★★	★★★	★★★	★★★	★★★	★★★	★★★★★	★	★★★	★★★	★★★	★★★	★★★
★★★	★★★	★★★	★	★★★	★★★	NR	NR	★	★★★★★	★★★	NR	★★★	★★★	★★★	★★★	★★★	NR	NR
★★★	★★★	★★★	★★★★★	★★★★★	★★★	★★★	★★★	★★★★★	★★★★★	★★★	★★★	★★★★★	★★★★★	★★★	★★★	★	★★★	★★★

GEORGIA HOSPITALS: RATINGS BY PROCEDURE

Hospital	Appendectomy	Atrial Fibrillation	Back and Neck Surgery (except Spinal Fusion)	Back and Neck Surgery (Spinal Fusion)	Bariatric Surgery	Bowel Obstruction	Carotid Surgery	Cholecystectomy (Gall Bladder Removal)	Chronic Obstructive Pulmonary Disease (COPD)	Coronary Bypass Surgery	Coronary Interventional Procedures (Angioplasty/Stent)	Diabetic Acidosis and...
1. Appling Hospital, Baxley	NR	NR	NR	NR	NR	***	NR	NR	***	NR	NR	NR
2. Athens Regional Medical Center, Athens	NR	***	***	*	NR	***	***	***	***	*****	***	***
3. Atlanta Medical Center, Atlanta	NR	***	***	***	NR	*	***	NR	***	*	***	***
4. Bacon County Hospital, Alma	NR	NR	NR	NR	NR	NR	NR	NR	***	NR	NR	NR
5. Barrow Regional Medical Center, Winder	NR	NR	NR	NR	NR	NR	NR	NR	***	NR	NR	NR
6. Berrien County Hospital, Nashville	NR	NR	NR	NR	NR	NR	NR	NR	***	NR	NR	NR
7. BJC Medical Center, Commerce	NR	*	NR	NR	NR	***	NR	***	***	NR	NR	NR
8. Brooks County Hospital, Quitman	NR	NR	NR	NR	NR	NR	NR	NR	***	NR	NR	NR
9. Burke Medical Center, Waynesboro	NR	NR	NR	NR	NR	***	NR	NR	***	NR	NR	NR
10. Calhoun Memorial Hospital, Arlington	NR	NR	NR	NR	NR	NR	NR	NR	***	NR	NR	NR
11. Camden Medical Center, St. Marys	NR	NR	NR	NR	NR	***	NR	NR	***	NR	NR	NR
12. Candler County Hospital, Metter	NR	***	NR	NR	NR	***	NR	NR	***	NR	NR	NR
13. Candler Hospital, Savannah	NR	***	NR	NR	NR	*****	NR	***	*****	NR	NR	*****
14. Cartersville Medical Center, Cartersville	NR	***	***	***	NR	***	***	***	***	NR	NR	***
15. Chatuge Regional Hospital, Hiawassee	NR	NR	NR	NR	NR	NR	NR	NR	***	NR	NR	NR
16. Chestatee Regional Hospital, Dahlonega	NR	***	NR	NR	NR	***	NR	***	***	NR	NR	NR
17. Cobb Memorial Hospital, Royston	NR	NR	NR	NR	NR	***	NR	NR	*	NR	NR	NR
18. Coffee Regional Medical Center, Douglas	NR	***	NR	NR	NR	***	NR	***	***	NR	NR	NR
19. Coliseum Medical Center, Macon	NR	*	NR	***	NR	***	*****	***	***	***	***	***
20. Coliseum Northside Hospital, Macon	NR	***	NR	***	NR	***	*****	***	NR	NR	NR	NR
21. Colquitt Regional Medical Center, Moultrie	NR	***	NR	NR	NR	***	NR	***	*****	NR	NR	NR
22. Columbus Doctors Hospital, Columbus	NR	***	NR	NR	NR	***	NR	***	*	NR	NR	***
23. Crisp Regional Hospital, Cordele	NR	***	NR	NR	NR	***	NR	***	***	NR	NR	***
24. Dekalb Medical Center, Decatur	NR	***	***	NR	NR	*	***	***	***	NR	NR	***
25. Doctors Hospital, Augusta	NR	***	***	***	NR	***	***	***	*	NR	NR	***
26. Dodge County Hospital, Eastman	NR	NR	NR	NR	NR	NR	NR	NR	***	NR	NR	NR
27. Donalsonville Hospital, Donalsonville	NR	NR	NR	NR	NR	NR	NR	NR	***	NR	NR	NR
28. Dorminy Medical Center, Fitzgerald	NR	***	NR	NR	NR	***	NR	NR	*	NR	NR	NR
29. East Georgia Regional Medical Center, Statesboro	NR	***	NR	NR	NR	*	NR	*	***	NR	NR	***
30. Elbert Memorial Hospital, Elberton	NR	***	NR	NR	NR	***	NR	*	***	NR	NR	NR
31. Emanuel County Hospital, Swainsboro	NR	***	NR	NR	NR	***	NR	***	***	NR	NR	NR
32. Emory Adventist Hospital, Smyrna	NR	***	NR	NR	NR	***	NR	***	***	NR	NR	NR
33. Emory Crawford Long Hospital, Atlanta	NR	***	*	*	NR	***	***	*	***	***	***	*
34. Emory Dunwoody Medical Center, Atlanta	NR	NR	NR	NR	NR	*	NR	NR	***	NR	NR	NR
35. Emory Eastside Medical Center, Snellville	NR	***	***	NR	NR	***	***	***	***	NR	NR	***
36. Emory University Hospital, Atlanta	NR	***	***	*	NR	***	*	*	*****	***	*	***
37. Evans Memorial Hospital, Claxton	NR	***	NR	NR	NR	***	NR	***	***	NR	NR	NR
38. Fairview Park Hospital, Dublin	NR	***	NR	NR	NR	*	***	***	***	NR	***	***
39. Fannin Regional Hospital, Blue Ridge	NR	***	NR	NR	NR	***	NR	*****	***	NR	NR	NR
40. Flint River Hospital, Montezuma	NR	NR	NR	NR	NR	NR	NR	NR	***	NR	NR	NR
41. Floyd Medical Center, Rome	NR	***	***	*****	NR	***	NR	***	*****	NR	NR	***
42. Gordon Hospital, Calhoun	NR	***	NR	NR	NR	***	NR	***	***	NR	NR	NR
43. Grady General Hospital, Cairo	NR	***	NR	NR	NR	***	NR	NR	***	NR	NR	NR
44. Grady Memorial Hospital, Atlanta	NR	*	NR	NR	NR	*	NR	***	***	***	***	***
45. Gwinnett Medical Center, Lawrenceville	NR	***	***	***	NR	***	***	***	***	NR	NR	***
46. Habersham County Medical Center, Demorest	NR	***	NR	NR	NR	*	NR	***	***	NR	NR	NR
47. Hamilton Medical Center, Dalton	NR	*	***	NR	NR	***	*****	*****	***	NR	NR	***
48. Hart County Hospital, Hartwell	NR	NR	NR	NR	NR	***	NR	*****	***	NR	NR	NR
49. Henry Medical Center, Stockbridge	NR	***	*****	NR	NR	***	*	***	***	NR	NR	***
50. Houston Medical Center, Warner Robins	NR	***	NR	***	NR	***	NR	***	*****	NR	NR	***

KEY: ***** BEST *** AS EXPECTED * POOR NR NOT RATED BY HEALTHGRADES For full definitions of ratings and awards, see Appendix.

Gastrointestinal Bleed	Gastrointestinal Surgeries and Procedures	Heart Attack	Heart Failure	Hip Fracture Repair	Maternity Care	Pancreatitis	Peripheral Vascular Bypass	Pneumonia	Prostatectomy	Pulmonary Embolism	Resection/Replacement of Abdominal Aorta	Respiratory Failure	Sepsis	Stroke	Total Hip Replacement	Total Knee Replacement	Valve Replacement	Women's Health
★★★	NR	NR	★★★	NR	NR	NR	NR	★★★	NR	NR	NR	★	★	NR	NR	NR	NR	NR
★★★	★★★	★	★★★	★	NR	★★★	★★★	★★★	★★★	★★★	★★★	★★★	★★★	★★★	★★★	★	★	NR
★	★	★★★	★★★★★	★	NR	NR	NR	★★★	NR	NR	★	★★★	★★★	★★★	NR	★★★	NR	NR
★	NR	NR	★★★	NR	NR	NR	NR	★★★	NR	NR	NR	★	NR	NR	NR	NR	NR	NR
★★★	NR	NR	★★★	NR	NR	NR	NR	★★★	NR	NR	NR	NR	NR	NR	NR	NR	NR	NR
NR	NR	NR	★★★	NR	NR	NR	NR	★★★	NR	NR	NR	★★★	NR	★	NR	NR	NR	NR
★★★	NR	★★★	★★★	★	NR	NR	NR	★★★	NR	NR	NR	★★★	★★★	★★★	NR	NR	NR	NR
NR	NR	NR	★★★	NR	NR	NR	NR	★★★	NR	NR	NR	★★★	★★★	NR	NR	NR	NR	NR
★★★	NR	NR	★★★	NR	NR	NR	NR	★★★	NR	NR	NR	★	★★★	★★★	NR	NR	NR	NR
NR	NR	NR	★★★	NR	NR	NR	NR	★★★	NR	NR	NR	NR	NR	NR	NR	NR	NR	NR
★★★	NR	NR	★★★	NR	NR	NR	NR	★★★	NR	NR	NR	★★★	NR	NR	NR	NR	NR	NR
★★★	NR	NR	★	NR	NR	NR	NR	★	NR	NR	NR	★	NR	NR	NR	NR	NR	NR
★★★★★	★★★★★	★★★	★★★★★	NR	NR	★★★	★★★★★	★★★★★	★★★	★★★★★	NR	★★★★★	★★★★★	★★★	NR	NR	NR	NR
★★★	★★★	★★★	★★★	★★★	NR	★★★	★★★	★★★	NR	★★★	NR	★★★	★★★	★★★	★	★★★	NR	NR
★★★	NR	NR	★★★	NR	NR	NR	NR	★★★	NR	NR	NR	NR	NR	NR	NR	NR	NR	NR
★★★	NR	NR	★	NR	NR	NR	NR	★★★	NR	NR	NR	★★★	★★★	NR	NR	★★★★★	NR	NR
★★★	NR	★★★	★★★	★	NR	NR	NR	★★★	★	NR	NR	★★★	★★★	★★★	NR	NR	NR	NR
★★★	★★★	★★★	★★★	★★★	NR	★★★	NR	★★★	NR	★★★	NR	★★★	★★★	★★★	NR	★★★	NR	NR
★★★	★★★	★★★★★	★★★★★	★★★★★	NR	★★★	NR	★★★	NR	★★★	NR	★★★	★★★	★★★★★	NR	★★★	NR	NR
★★★	★★★	★★★	★★★	★	NR	★★★	NR	★★★	★★★	NR	NR	★★★	★★★	★★★★★	NR	★★★	NR	NR
★★★	NR	★★★	★★★	★★★	NR	★★★	NR	★★★	NR	NR	NR	★★★	★★★	★★★★★	NR	NR	NR	NR
★★★	★	★★★★★	★★★	★★★	NR	★★★	★★★	★★★	★★★	★★★	NR	★★★	★★★★★	★★★★★	★★★★★	★★★	NR	NR
★★★	★★★	★	★★★	★★★	NR	★★★	★★★	★★★	★★★	NR	NR	★★★	★★★	★★★	★★★	★★★	NR	NR
★★★	NR	NR	★	NR	NR	NR	NR	★	NR	NR	NR	★	★	NR	NR	NR	NR	NR
★★★	NR	NR	★★★	NR	NR	NR	NR	★★★	NR	NR	NR	NR	NR	NR	NR	NR	NR	NR
★★★	NR	NR	★	NR	NR	NR	NR	★★★	NR	NR	NR	★★★	NR	NR	NR	NR	NR	NR
★★★	★	★★★	★★★★★	★★★	NR	NR	NR	★★★	★	NR	★★★	★★★★★	★★★	★★★	NR	★★★	NR	NR
★	NR	★★★	★★★★★	NR	NR	NR	NR	★	NR	NR	NR	★★★	★★★	NR	NR	★★★	NR	NR
★★★	NR	NR	★★★	NR	NR	NR	NR	★★★★★	NR	NR	NR	★★★	NR	NR	NR	NR	NR	NR
★★★	NR	NR	★★★★★	★★★	NR	NR	NR	★★★	NR	NR	NR	★★★	★★★	★★★★★	★	★★★	NR	NR
★★★	★★★	★★★★★	★★★	★★★	NR	★★★	★★★	★★★	★	★★★	NR	★★★	★★★	★★★	★	★	★★★	NR
★★★	NR	NR	★★★★★	★★★	NR	NR	NR	★★★	NR	NR	NR	★★★	NR	NR	NR	NR	NR	NR
★★★	★★★	★★★	★★★	★★★	NR	★★★	NR	★★★	NR	★	NR	★★★	★★★	★★★	NR	★★★	NR	NR
★★★	★★★	NR	★★★	★★★	NR	★★★	NR	★	NR	NR	NR	★★★	NR	NR	★★★	NR	NR	NR
★	NR	NR	★	NR	NR	NR	NR	★★★	NR	NR	NR	★★★	NR	★★★	NR	NR	NR	NR
★★★	★★★	★	★	★★★	NR	★★★	NR	★★★	★★★	★★★	NR	★★★★★	★★★	★	★★★	★★★	NR	NR
★★★	★★★	★★★	★★★	★★★★★	NR	NR	NR	★★★	NR	NR	NR	★★★	★★★	★★★	NR	NR	NR	NR
★★★	NR	NR	★	NR	NR	NR	NR	★	NR	NR	NR	★★★	★★★	★★★	NR	NR	NR	NR
★★★	★	★★★	★★★	★★★	NR	★★★	NR	★★★	NR	★★★	NR	★★★	★★★	★	NR	NR	NR	NR
★★★	★★★	★★★★★	★★★★★	★★★	NR	★★★	NR	★★★★★	★★★	★★★	NR	★★★	★★★★★	★★★★★	★★★	★	NR	NR
★★★	★★★	★	★★★	★★★	NR	★★★	NR	★	★★★★★	★★★	NR	★	★★★	★★★	★★★	★★★	NR	NR
★	★	★	★	★	NR	NR	NR	★★★	NR	NR	NR	★	★★★	NR	NR	★	NR	NR
★	★★★	★★★	★★★	★★★	NR	★★★	NR	★★★	★★★	NR	NR	★	★★★	★★★	★★★	★★★	NR	NR
★★★★★	★★★	★★★	★★★★★	★	NR	★★★	NR	★★★★★	★	NR	★★★	NR	★★★★★	★★★★★	★★★	★	★	NR

	Appendectomy	Atrial Fibrillation	Back and Neck Surgery (except Spinal Fusion)	Back and Neck Surgery (Spinal Fusion)	Bariatric Surgery	Bowel Obstruction	Carotid Surgery	Cholecystectomy (Gall Bladder Removal)	Chronic Obstructive Pulmonary Disease (COPD)	Coronary Bypass Surgery	Coronary Interventional Procedures (Angioplasty/Stent)	Diabetic Acidosis an...
51. Hughston Orthopedic Hospital, Columbus	NR	NR	★★★	★★★★★	NR	NR	NR	NR	NR	NR	NR	NR
52. Hutcheson Medical Center, Fort Oglethorpe	NR	★★★	NR	NR	NR	★	★★★	★★★	★	NR	NR	★★★
53. Irwin County Hospital, Ocilla	NR	NR	NR	NR	NR	NR	NR	★★★	NR	NR	NR	NR
54. Jeff Davis Hospital, Hazlehurst	NR	★★★	NR	NR	NR	NR	NR	NR	★	NR	NR	NR
55. Jefferson Hospital, Louisville	NR	NR	NR	NR	NR	★★★	NR	NR	★★★	NR	NR	NR
56. John D. Archbold Memorial Hospital, Thomasville	NR	★★★	NR	★★★★★	NR	★★★	★★★	★★★	★	NR	NR	★★★
57. Louis Smith Memorial Hospital, Lakeland	NR	NR	NR	NR	NR	NR	NR	NR	★★★	NR	NR	NR
58. McDuffie Regional Medical Center, Thomson	NR	NR	NR	NR	NR	NR	NR	NR	★★★	NR	NR	NR
59. Meadows Regional Medical Center, Vidalia	NR	★★★	NR	NR	NR	★★★★★	NR	NR	★★★	NR	NR	NR
60. Medical College of Georgia Hospitals and Clinics, Augusta	NR	★★★	★★★	★★★	NR	★★★	NR	★★★	★★★	★★★	★★★	★★★
61. Medical Center of Central Georgia, Macon	NR	★★★	★★★	★★★	NR	★★★	★★★★★	★	★	★★★	★★★	★★★
62. Medical Center, Columbus	NR	★★★	★★★	★★★★★	NR	★★★	★★★	★★★	★★★	NR	★★★	★★★
63. Memorial Health University Medical Center, Savannah	NR	★★★	★★★	★★★★★	NR	★★★	★★★	★★★	★★★★★	★★★	NR	★★★
64. Memorial Hospital and Manor, Bainbridge	NR	★	NR	NR	NR	★★★	NR	★★★★★	★	NR	NR	NR
65. Memorial Hospital of Adel, Adel	NR	NR	NR	NR	NR	NR	NR	NR	★★★	NR	NR	NR
66. Miller County Hospital, Colquitt	NR	NR	NR	NR	NR	NR	NR	NR	NR	NR	NR	
67. Mitchell County Hospital, Camilla	NR	NR	NR	NR	NR	NR	NR	NR	NR	NR	NR	
68. Monroe County Hospital, Forsyth	NR	NR	NR	NR	NR	NR	NR	NR	★★★	NR	NR	
69. Mountain Lakes Medical Center, Clayton	NR	NR	NR	NR	NR	NR	NR	NR	★★★	NR	NR	
70. Murray Medical Center, Chatsworth	NR	NR	NR	NR	NR	NR	NR	NR	★★★	NR	NR	
71. Newton Medical Center, Covington	NR	★★★	NR	NR	NR	★★★	★★★	★★★	★	NR	NR	★★★
72. North Fulton Regional Hospital, Roswell	NR	★★★	★★★	★★★	NR	★★★	NR	★★★	★★★	NR	NR	★★★
73. North Georgia Medical Center, Ellijay	NR	NR	NR	NR	NR	★★★	NR	NR	★★★	NR	NR	NR
74. Northeast Georgia Medical Center, Gainesville	NR	★★★	★	★	NR	★★★★★	★★★	NR	★★★★★	★★★★★	★★★	★★★
75. Northeast Georgia Med. Ctr.–Lanier Park Campus, Gainesville	NR	★★★	★	★	NR	★★★★★	★★★	NR	★★★★★	★★★★★	★★★	★★★
76. Northside Hospital Cherokee, Canton	NR	★★★	NR	NR	NR	★★★	NR	★★★	★★★	NR	NR	★★★
77. Northside Hospital Forsyth, Cumming	NR	★★★	★★★	NR	NR	★★★	NR	★★★	★★★★★	NR	NR	★★★
78. Northside Hospital, Atlanta	NR	★	★★★	★★★★★	NR	★★★	NR	★★★	★★★	NR	NR	★★★
79. Oconee Regional Medical Center, Milledgeville	NR	★★★	NR	NR	NR	★★★	NR	★★★	★★★	NR	NR	★★★
80. Palmyra Medical Center, Albany	NR	★★★	NR	★★★	NR	★★★	NR	★★★	★★★	NR	NR	★★★
81. Peach Regional Medical Center, Fort Valley	NR	NR	NR	NR	NR	NR	NR	NR	NR	NR	NR	
82. Perry General Hospital, Perry	NR	★★★	NR	NR	NR	★★★	NR	★★★★★	★★★	NR	NR	
83. Phoebe Putney Memorial Hospital, Albany	NR	★★★	★★★	★★★	NR	★	★★★	★★★	★	★★★	★★★	★★★
84. Phoebe Worth Medical Center, Sylvester	NR	NR	NR	NR	NR	NR	NR	NR	★★★	NR	NR	NR
85. Piedmont Fayette Hospital, Fayetteville	NR	★★★	NR	NR	NR	★★★	★★★	★★★	★★★★★	NR	NR	★
86. Piedmont Hospital, Atlanta	NR	★★★	★★★	★★★★★	NR	★★★★★	★★★	★★★★★	★★★	★★★★★	★★★	★★★
87. Piedmont Mountainside Hospital, Jasper	NR	★★★	NR	NR	NR	★★★	NR	★★★	★★★	NR	NR	NR
88. Piedmont Newnan Hospital, Newnan	NR	★★★	NR	NR	NR	★★★	NR	★★★	★★★	NR	NR	★★★
89. Putnam General Hospital, Eatonton	NR	NR	NR	NR	NR	NR	NR	NR	★★★	NR	NR	NR
90. Redmond Regional Medical Center, Rome	NR	★	★★★★★	★★★★★	NR	★	★★★★★	★★★★★	★★★	★★★	★★★	★★★
91. Rockdale Medical Center, Conyers	NR	★★★	NR	★	NR	★★★	★★★	★	★★★	NR	NR	NR
92. Roosevelt Warm Springs Rehabilitation Hospital, Warm Springs	NR	NR	NR	NR	NR	NR	NR	NR	NR	NR	NR	NR
93. St. Francis Hospital, Columbus	NR	★	★★★	★★★	NR	★★★	★★★★★	★★★	★★★	★	★★★	★★★
94. St. Joseph Hospital–Augusta, Augusta	NR	★★★	NR	NR	NR	★★★	NR	★	★★★	NR	NR	NR
95. St. Joseph's Hospital, Savannah	NR	★★★	★★★	★★★★★	NR	★★★	★★★	★	★★★	★★★	★★★	★★★
96. Saint Joseph's Hospital of Atlanta, Atlanta	NR	★★★	★★★★★	★★★★★	NR	★★★	★★★★★	★★★	★★★★★	★★★	★★★★★	★★★
97. St. Mary's Hospital of Athens, Athens	NR	★★★	★★★	★★★	NR	★★★	★	★★★	★★★	NR	NR	NR
98. Satilla Regional Medical Center, Waycross	NR	★★★	★★★	NR	NR	★★★	NR	★★★	★★★	NR	NR	★★★
99. Screven County Hospital, Sylvania	NR	NR	NR	NR	NR	NR	NR	NR	★★★	NR	NR	NR
100. Sempercare Hospital of Augusta, Augusta	NR	★	★★★★★	★★★	NR	★★★	★★★	★★★★★	★	★★★	★★★	★★★

KEY: ★★★★★ BEST   ★★★ AS EXPECTED   ★ POOR   NR NOT RATED BY HEALTHGRADES   For full definitions of ratings and awards, see Appendix.

GEORGIA HOSPITALS: RATINGS BY PROCEDURE

Gastrointestinal Bleed	Gastrointestinal Surgeries and Procedures	Heart Attack	Heart Failure	Hip Fracture Repair	Maternity Care	Pancreatitis	Peripheral Vascular Bypass	Pneumonia	Prostatectomy	Pulmonary Embolism	Resection/Replacement of Abdominal Aorta	Respiratory Failure	Sepsis	Stroke	Total Hip Replacement	Total Knee Replacement	Valve Replacement	Women's Health
NR	NR	NR	NR	★★★	NR	NR	NR	NR	NR	NR	NR	NR	NR	NR	★★★★★	★★★★★	NR	NR
★★★	★★★	★★★	★	★★★★★	NR	★★★	NR	★★★	NR	★★★	NR	★★★	★★★★★	★★★	NR	★	NR	NR
NR	NR	NR	★★★	NR	NR	NR	NR	★★★	NR	NR	NR	NR	NR	NR	NR	NR	NR	NR
★★★	NR	NR	★★★	NR	NR	NR	NR	NR	NR	NR	NR	NR	NR	NR	NR	NR	NR	NR
★★★	NR	NR	★★★	NR	NR	NR	NR	★★★	NR	NR	NR	NR	★★★	NR	NR	NR	NR	NR
★★★	★	★★★★★	★	NR	★★★	NR	★	NR	★★★	NR	NR	NR	★★★	★★★	★★★	★★★	★★★	NR
NR	NR	NR	★★★	NR	NR	NR	NR	★★★	NR	NR	NR	NR	NR	NR	NR	★★★	NR	NR
★★★	NR	NR	★	NR	★★★★★	NR	NR	NR	★	NR	NR	NR	★	NR	★★★	NR	★★★	NR
★★★★★	★★★	★★★★★	★★★★★	★★★	NR	NR	NR	★★★	★	NR	NR	NR	★★★	★★★	NR	★★★	NR	NR
★★★	★★★	★★★	★★★	★	NR	★★★	★★★	★★★	NR	★★★	NR	★★★	★	NR	★★★	★★★	★★★	NR
★	★	★★★	★★★	★★★	NR	★★★	★★★	★★★	★★★	★	★★★★★	★	NR	★★★	★	★★★	★	★★★
★	★★★	★	★★★	★★★★★	NR	★★★	NR	★	★★★	★★★	NR	★	★	★★★	NR	★★★	NR	NR
★★★★★	★★★	★★★★★	★★★★★	★★★	NR	★★★	★★★	★★★★★	★★★★★	★★★★★	★★★	★★★	★★★★★	★★★	★	★	★★★	NR
★★★	NR	★★★	★★★	★★★	NR	NR	NR	★★★	NR	NR	NR	NR	★★★	NR	NR	★★★	NR	NR
★★★	NR	NR	★	NR	NR	NR	NR	★★★	NR	NR	NR	NR	★	NR	★★★	NR	NR	NR
★★★	NR	NR	★★★	NR	NR	NR	NR	★★★	NR	NR	NR	NR	NR	NR	NR	NR	NR	NR
NR	NR	NR	★★★	NR	NR	NR	NR	★	NR	NR	NR	NR	★★★	NR	NR	NR	NR	NR
★★★	NR	NR	★	NR	NR	NR	NR	★	NR	NR	NR	NR	★★★	★	NR	NR	NR	NR
NR	NR	NR	★★★	NR	NR	NR	NR	★★★	NR	NR	NR	NR	NR	NR	NR	NR	NR	NR
★★★	NR	NR	★★★	NR	NR	NR	NR	★★★	NR	NR	NR	★★★	★★★	★★★	NR	NR	NR	NR
★★★	★★★	★★★	★	★	NR	★★★	NR	★★★	NR	★★★	NR	★★★	★	★★★	★	★	NR	NR
★★★	★★★	★★★	★★★★★	★★★★★	NR	★★★	NR	★★★	★★★	★★★	NR	★★★★★	★★★	★★★	★★★	★★★	NR	NR
★★★	NR	NR	★★★	NR	NR	NR	NR	★★★	NR	NR	NR	NR	NR	NR	NR	NR	NR	NR
★★★	★★★★★	★★★	★★★★★	★★★★★	NR	★★★★★	★	★★★	★	★★★★★	★★★	★★★	★★★	★★★	★★★	★★★	★★★★★	NR
★★★	★★★★★	★★★	★★★★★	★★★★★	NR	★★★★★	★	★★★	★	★★★★★	★★★	★★★	★★★	★★★	★★★	★★★	★★★★★	NR
★★★★★	★★★	★	★★★	★	NR	NR	NR	★★★	NR	★★★	NR	★★★	★★★	★★★	NR	★★★	NR	NR
★★★	★★★★★	★★★	★★★	★★★	NR	★★★	NR	★★★★★	NR	★★★	NR	★★★★★	★★★★★	★★★	★★★	★	NR	NR
★★★	★★★	★★★	★★★	★★★	NR	NR	NR	★★★	★★★	★★★	NR	★	★	★★★	★	★★★	NR	NR
★★★	★★★★★	★★★	★★★	★★★	NR	★★★	NR	★★★	NR	★★★★★	NR	★★★★★	★★★★★	★★★	NR	★★★	NR	NR
★★★	★★★	NR	★★★	★★★	NR	★★★	NR	★★★	★★★	NR	NR	★★★	★★★	★★★	★★★	★★★	NR	NR
★★★	NR	NR	★★★	NR	NR	NR	NR	★★★	NR	NR	NR	NR	★★★	NR	NR	NR	NR	NR
★★★	NR	★★★	★★★	★★★	NR	NR	NR	★★★★★	NR	NR	NR	★★★	★★★★★	NR	NR	NR	NR	NR
★★★	★★★	★★★	★★★	★★★	NR	★★★	★★★	★★★	★★★	★	★★★	★	★★★	★	★★★	★★★	★★★	NR
NR	NR	NR	★	NR	NR	NR	NR	★★★	NR	NR	NR	NR	NR	NR	NR	NR	NR	NR
★★★	★★★	★★★	★★★★★	★★★★★	NR	★★★	NR	★★★★★	★★★	★★★	NR	★★★	★★★	★★★	★★★	★★★★★	NR	NR
★★★	★★★	★★★★★	★★★	★★★	NR	★★★	★★★	★★★★★	★★★	★★★	NR	★★★	★★★	★★★	★★★★★	★★★★★	★★★	NR
★	NR	NR	★★★	NR	NR	★★★	NR	★★★	NR	NR	NR	★★★	★★★	★★★	★	NR	★★★	NR
★★★	★★★	NR	★★★	★★★	NR	NR	NR	★★★	★★★	★★★	NR	NR	NR	NR	NR	NR	NR	NR
★★★	★★★	★	★	★★★★★	NR	★★★	★★★	★★★	★★★★★	★★★	★★★★★	★★★	★★★	★	★★★	★★★	★	NR
★★★	★★★	★★★	★★★	★	NR	★★★	NR	★★★	★★★	NR	★	★	★★★	★★★	★★★	★★★	NR	NR
NR	NR	NR	★★★	NR	NR	NR	NR	★★★	NR	NR	NR	NR	NR	NR	NR	NR	NR	NR
★★★	★★★	NR	★★★★★	★★★	NR	★	★★★	★★★	★★★	★★★	★★★	★★★	★★★	★★★	★★★	★★★	★★★	NR
★★★	★★★	NR	★★★	★★★	NR	★★★	NR	★★★★★	★★★	NR	NR	★★★	★★★	★★★	★★★★★	★★★★★	NR	NR
★★★	★	★★★	★★★	NR	NR	★★★	★★★	★★★	★★★★★	★★★	★★★	★★★	★★★★★	★	★★★	★★★	★★★	NR
★★★★★	★★★★★	★★★★★	★★★★★	NR	NR	★★★	★★★★★	★★★	★★★	★★★	★★★	★	★★★	★★★★★	★★★★★	★★★★★	★★★	NR
★	★★★	★★★	★★★	★	NR	★★★	NR	★★★	★★★	★★★	NR	★★★	★★★	★★★	★★★	★★★★★	NR	NR
★★★	★★★	★★★	★★★★★	★★★	NR	★★★	★★★	★★★	★★★	NR	★	★★★	★★★	★★★	★★★	★	NR	NR
NR	NR	NR	★★★	NR	NR	NR	NR	★★★	NR	NR	NR	NR	NR	NR	NR	NR	NR	NR
★	★★★	★	★	★★★	NR	★★★	★★★	★	★★★★★	★★★	★★★	★	★	★	★★★	★★★	★	NR

	Appendectomy	Atrial Fibrillation	Back and Neck Surgery (except Spinal Fusion)	Back and Neck Surgery (Spinal Fusion)	Bariatric Surgery	Bowel Obstruction	Carotid Surgery	Cholecystectomy (Gall Bladder Removal)	Chronic Obstructive Pulmonary Disease (COPD)	Coronary Bypass Surgery	Coronary Interventional Procedures (Angioplasty/Stent)	Diabetic Acidosis and...
101. Smith Northview Hospital, Valdosta	NR	NR	NR	NR	NR	★★★	NR	★	★★★	NR	NR	NR
102. South Fulton Medical Center, East Point	NR	★★★	NR	NR	NR	★	NR	★★★	★★★	NR	NR	★★★
103. South Georgia Medical Center, Valdosta	NR	★	★★★★★	★★★★★	NR	★★★	★★★	★★★	★★★	★	★★★	★
104. Southeast Georgia Regional Medical Center, Brunswick	NR	★	★★★	★★★	NR	★	★★★	★★★	★	NR	NR	★★★
105. Southern Regional Medical Center, Riverdale	NR	★★★	★★★	★	NR	★	★	★★★	★★★	NR	NR	★★★
106. Spalding Regional Medical Center, Griffin	NR	★★★	NR	NR	NR	★★★	★★★	★★★	★★★	NR	NR	★★★
107. Stephens County Hospital, Toccoa	NR	★★★	NR	NR	NR	★★★	NR	★★★	★★★★★	NR	NR	NR
108. Stewart Webster Hospital, Richland	NR	NR	NR	NR	NR	NR	NR	NR	★★★	NR	NR	NR
109. Tanner Medical Center–Carrollton, Carrollton	NR	★★★	NR	★★★★★	NR	★★★	NR	NR	★★★★★	NR	NR	★★★
110. Tanner Medical Center–Villa Rica, Villa Rica	NR	★★★	NR	NR	NR	★	NR	NR	★★★	NR	NR	NR
111. Tattnall Community Hospital, Reidsville	NR	NR	NR	NR	NR	NR	NR	NR	★★★	NR	NR	NR
112. Taylor Regional Hospital, Hawkinsville	NR	★★★	NR	NR	NR	★★★	NR	NR	★★★	NR	NR	NR
113. Tift Regional Medical Center, Tifton	NR	★★★	NR	★★★	NR	★★★	NR	★★★	★★★	NR	NR	NR
114. Union General Hospital, Blairsville	NR	★★★	NR	NR	NR	★★★	NR	★★★	★	NR	NR	NR
115. University Hospital, Augusta	NR	★	★★★★★	★★★	NR	★★★	★★★	★★★★★	★	★★★	★★★	★★★
116. Upson Regional Medical Center, Thomaston	NR	★★★	NR	NR	NR	★★★	NR	★★★	★★★	NR	NR	NR
117. Walton Regional Medical Center, Monroe	NR	★	NR	NR	NR	★★★	NR	★★★	★★★	NR	NR	NR
118. Warm Springs Medical Center, Warm Springs	NR	NR	NR	NR	NR	NR	NR	NR	★★★	NR	NR	NR
119. Washington County Regional Medical Center, Sandersville	NR	NR	NR	NR	NR	★★★	NR	NR	★★★	NR	NR	NR
120. Wayne Memorial Hospital, Jesup	NR	★★★	NR	NR	NR	★★★	NR	NR	★★★	NR	NR	NR
121. Wellstar Cobb Hospital, Austell	NR	★★★	★★★	★★★	NR	★★★	★★★	★★★	★★★	NR	NR	★★★
122. Wellstar Douglas Hospital, Douglasville	NR	★★★	NR	NR	NR	★★★	NR	★★★	★★★	NR	NR	NR
123. Wellstar Kennestone Hospital, Marietta	NR	★★★	★★★	★	NR	★	★★★★★	★★★	★★★	★★★	★★★	★★★
124. Wellstar Paulding Hospital, Dallas	NR	★	NR	NR	NR	NR	NR	NR	★★★	NR	NR	NR
125. West Georgia Medical Center, Lagrange	NR	★★★	NR	NR	NR	★★★	★★★	★★★★★	★★★	NR	NR	★★★
126. Wheeler County Hospital, Glenwood	NR	NR	NR	NR	NR	NR	NR	NR	★★★★★	NR	NR	NR
127. Wills Memorial Hospital, Washington	NR	★★★	NR	NR	NR	NR	NR	NR	★★★	NR	NR	NR

KEY: ★★★★★ BEST   ★★★ AS EXPECTED   ★ POOR   NR NOT RATED BY HEALTHGRADES   For full definitions of ratings and awards, see Appendix.

Gastrointestinal Bleed	Gastrointestinal Surgeries and Procedures	Heart Attack	Heart Failure	Hip Fracture Repair	Maternity Care	Pancreatitis	Peripheral Vascular Bypass	Pneumonia	Prostatectomy	Pulmonary Embolism	Resection/Replacement of Abdominal Aorta	Respiratory Failure	Sepsis	Stroke	Total Hip Replacement	Total Knee Replacement	Valve Replacement	Women's Health
★★★	NR	NR	★★★	NR	NR		★★★	NR	★★★	★★★	NR		★★★	NR	NR	★★★	NR	NR
★★★	★★★	★★★	★★★★★	★★★★★	NR	★★★	★★★★★	★★★	★★★	★★★	NR	★★★	★★★★★	★★★	NR	NR	NR	NR
★	★★★	★	★	★★★	NR	★★★	★★★	★	★★★	★★★	NR	★	★	★	★★★	★★★	NR	NR
★	★★★	★★★	★	★★★	NR	★★★	NR	★	★★★	★★★	NR	★	★★★	★★★	★★★	★★★★★	NR	
★★★	★★★★★	★	★★★	★★★★★	NR	★★★	NR	★★★	★★★★★	★★★	★★★	★★★★★	★★★	★★★	★★★	NR		
★★★	★★★	★	★★★	★★★	NR	★★★	NR	★★★	★★★	★★★	NR	★★★★★	★★★	★	★★★	★	NR	
NR	NR	NR	★★★	NR	NR	★	NR	NR	NR	NR	NR	NR	NR	NR	NR	NR		
★★★	★★★	★★★	★★★	★★★★★	NR	★★★	NR	★★★	★★★	★	NR	★	★	★★★	★★★	★★★	NR	
★★★	NR	NR	★★★	NR	NR	★★★	NR	NR	NR	NR	★★★	★	NR	NR	NR			
NR	NR	NR	★★★	NR	NR	★	NR	NR	NR	NR	NR	NR	NR	NR				
★★★	NR	★★★	★★★	★★★	NR	★	NR	NR	NR	★	★	★★★	★★★	★★★	NR			
★★★	★★★	★★★	★★★★★	NR	★★★	NR	★★★	★★★	★★★	NR	★★★	★	★	★	NR			
★★★	NR	★	★★★	★★★	NR	★★★	NR	NR	NR	★	★★★	★★★	NR					
★	★★★	★	★	★★★	NR	★★★	★★★	★	★★★★★	★★★	★★★	★	★	★	★★★	★★★	★	
★	★★★	★★★	★	★★★★★	NR	★★★	★★★	★	NR	★★★	★★★	★	NR	★★★★★	NR			
★★★	★★★	★★★	★	★★★	NR	★★★	★★★	NR	★	★★★	★★★	NR	NR					
NR	NR	NR	★★★	NR	NR	★★★	NR	NR	NR	NR	NR	NR						
★★★	NR	NR	★★★	★★★★★	NR	★	NR	NR	★★★	★★★	NR							
★★★	NR	★	★★★	★★★★★	NR	★★★	★★★★★	NR	★★★	★★★★★	NR							
★★★	★★★	★	★★★★★	★★★★★	NR	★★★	★★★★★	★★★	★★★	★★★	★★★★★	★	★★★	★★★	★	★★★	NR	
★★★	★★★	★★★	★★★	★★★	NR	★★★	NR	★★★	NR	★★★	★★★	★★★	★★★★★	NR	★★★	NR		
★★★	★★★	★★★	★★★★★	★★★★★	NR	★★★	NR	★★★	★★★★★	★★★	★★★	★★★	★	★	★★★	★★★	★★★	
★★★	NR	NR	★★★	★★★	NR	NR	★★★	NR	NR	NR	★★★	NR	NR					
★	★★★	★	★	★★★★★	NR	★★★	NR	★	NR	★★★	★★★	★★★	★★★	★★★★★	★★★			
NR	NR	NR	★★★	NR	NR	★★★	NR	NR	NR	NR	NR	NR						
★	NR	NR	★★★	NR	NR	★★★	NR	NR	NR	★★★	NR	NR	NR	NR				

HAWAII HOSPITALS: RATINGS BY PROCEDURE

	Appendectomy	Atrial Fibrillation	Back and Neck Surgery (except Spinal Fusion)	Back and Neck Surgery (Spinal Fusion)	Bariatric Surgery	Bowel Obstruction	Carotid Surgery	Cholecystectomy (Gall Bladder Removal)	Chronic Obstructive Pulmonary Disease (COPD)	Coronary Bypass Surgery	Coronary Interventional Procedures (Angioplasty/Stent)	Diabetic Acidosis an
1. Castle Medical Center, Kailua	NR	★	NR	NR	NR	★	NR	★★★	★★★	NR	★	★★★
2. Hawaii Medical Center–East, Honolulu	NR	★★★	NR	NR	NR	★	NR	★★★★★	★★★	★	★★★	★★★
3. Hawaii Medical Center–West, Ewa Beach	NR	★★★	NR	NR	NR	★★★	NR	★★★	★	NR	NR	★★★
4. Hilo Medical Center, Hilo	NR	★★★	NR	NR	NR	★★★	NR	★★★	★★★	NR	NR	NR
5. Kaiser Foundation Hospital, Honolulu	NR	★★★	NR	NR	NR	★★★	NR	NR	★★★	★★★	★★★	NR
6. Kapi'olani Medical Center at Pali Momi, Aiea	NR	★★★	NR	★★★	NR	★★★	NR	★★★★★	★	NR	NR	★★★
7. Kona Community Hospital, Kealakekua	NR	NR	NR	NR	NR	★★★	NR	NR	★	NR	NR	NR
8. Kuakini Medical Center, Honolulu	NR	★★★	★★★	NR	NR	★★★	NR	★★★	★★★	★	★★★	★★★
9. Maui Memorial Medical Center, Wailuku	NR	★★★	NR	NR	NR	★	NR	★★★	★	NR	NR	★★★
10. North Hawaii Community Hospital, Kamuela	NR	★★★	NR	NR	NR	★★★	NR	NR	★★★	NR	NR	NR
11. The Queen's Medical Center, Honolulu	NR	★	★★★	★★★	NR	★★★	★	★★★★★	★★★	★★★	★★★	★★★
12. Select Specialty Hospital, Honolulu	NR	★	★★★	★★★	NR	★★★	★	★★★★★	★★★	★★★	★★★	★★★
13. Straub Clinic and Hospital, Honolulu	NR	★★★	★★★	NR	NR	★★★	★★★	★★★★★	★	NR	★★★	NR
14. Wahiawa General Hospital, Wahiawa	NR	★★★	NR	NR	NR	★★★	NR	NR	★★★	NR	NR	NR
15. Wilcox Memorial Hospital, Lihue	NR	★★★	NR	NR	NR	★★★	NR	★★★	★★★	NR	NR	NR

KEY: ★★★★★ BEST   ★★★ AS EXPECTED   ★ POOR   NR NOT RATED BY HEALTHGRADES   For full definitions of ratings and awards, see Appendix.

Gastrointestinal Bleed	Gastrointestinal Surgeries and Procedures	Heart Attack	Heart Failure	Hip Fracture Repair	Maternity Care	Pancreatitis	Peripheral Vascular Bypass	Pneumonia	Prostatectomy	Pulmonary Embolism	Resection/Replacement of Abdominal Aorta	Respiratory Failure	Sepsis	Stroke	Total Hip Replacement	Total Knee Replacement	Valve Replacement	Women's Health
★★★	NR	★★★	★★★	★★★	NR	★★★	NR	★	NR	NR	NR	★	★★★	★	★★★	★★★	NR	NR
★★★	NR	★	★★★	★★★	NR	★	NR	★★★	NR	NR	NR	★★★	★	★★★	NR	★★★	★	NR
★★★	NR	★	★★★	★★★	NR	★★★	NR	★★★	NR	NR	NR	★★★	★★★★★	★★★★★	NR	NR	NR	NR
★★★	NR	★★★	★	★★★	NR	NR	NR	★	NR	NR	NR	★★★	★★★	NR	NR	NR	NR	NR
★★★	NR	★★★	★★★	★★★	NR	NR	NR	★★★	NR	NR	NR	★★★	★★★	NR	★★★	NR	NR	NR
★★★	★★★	★	★★★	★★★★★	NR	★★★	NR	★★★	★★★	NR	NR	★★★	★★★	★★★	★★★★★	NR	NR	NR
★	NR	NR	★	★★★	NR	NR	NR	★	NR	NR	NR	NR	★★★	NR	NR	NR	NR	NR
★★★	★★★	★★★	★★★	★★★	NR	★★★	NR	★★★	★★★	NR	NR	★★★	★★★★★	★★★	★★★	★★★★★	★★★	NR
★★★	★★★	★★★	★	★	NR	NR	NR	★	NR	NR	NR	★	★	NR	★	NR	NR	NR
★★★	NR	NR	★	NR	NR	NR	NR	★★★	NR	NR	NR	NR	NR	★	NR	NR	NR	NR
★★★	★★★	★★★	★★★	★★★★★	NR	★★★	★★★★★	★	★★★	★★★	★★★	★★★	★★★	★★★	★★★★★	★★★	★★★	NR
★★★	★★★	★★★	★★★	★★★★★	NR	★★★	★★★★★	★	★★★	★★★	★★★	★★★	★★★	★★★	★★★★★	★★★	★★★	NR
★★★	★★★	★★★	★★★	★★★★★	NR	★★★	★★★	★★★	★★★	★★★	★★★	★	★★★	★★★	★★★	★★★	★★★	NR
★★★	NR	★★★	★★★	★★★★★	NR	NR	NR	★★★	NR	NR	NR	★	★★★	★★★	★★★	★★★	NR	NR
★★★	NR	★★★	★★★	★★★	NR	NR	NR	★	NR	NR	NR	★	★	NR	★★★	NR	NR	NR

IDAHO HOSPITALS: RATINGS BY PROCEDURE

	Appendectomy	Atrial Fibrillation	Back and Neck Surgery (except Spinal Fusion)	Back and Neck Surgery (Spinal Fusion)	Bariatric Surgery	Bowel Obstruction	Carotid Surgery	Cholecystectomy (Gall Bladder Removal)	Chronic Obstructive Pulmonary Disease (COPD)	Coronary Bypass Surgery	Coronary Interventional Procedures (Angioplasty/Stent)	Diabetic Acidosis and Coma
1. Bear Lake Memorial Hospital, Montpelier	NR	NR	NR	NR	NR	★★★	NR	NR	★	NR	NR	NR
2. Bingham Memorial Hospital, Blackfoot	NR	★★★	NR	★★★	NR	★★★	NR	★★★	★★★	NR	NR	NR
3. Bonner General Hospital, Sandpoint	NR	★★★	NR	NR	NR	★★★	NR	★	★★★	NR	NR	NR
4. Cassia Regional Medical Center, Burley	NR	★★★	NR	NR	NR	★★★	NR	★	NR	NR	NR	NR
5. Eastern Idaho Regional Medical Center, Idaho Falls	NR	★★★	★	★	NR	★★★	★★★	★★★	★	★	★	★★★
6. Gritman Medical Center, Moscow	NR	NR	NR	NR	NR	★★★	NR	★★★	★★★	NR	NR	NR
7. Kootenai Medical Center, Coeur d'Alene	NR	★	★★★	★★★	NR	★	★★★	★	★	★★★	★★★	★★★
8. Madison Memorial Hospital, Rexburg	NR	★★★	NR	NR	NR	★★★	NR	★★★	★★★	NR	NR	NR
9. Mercy Medical Center, Nampa	NR	★★★	NR	NR	NR	★★★	NR	★★★	NR	NR	★★★	NR
10. Minidoka Memorial Hospital, Rupert	NR	NR	NR	NR	NR	NR	NR	NR	★	NR	NR	NR
11. Portneuf Medical Center, Pocatello	NR	★★★	★★★	★★★	NR	★★★	NR	★★★	★	★★★	★★★	★★★
12. St. Alphonsus Regional Medical Center, Boise	NR	★★★★★	★★★	★★★	NR	★★★	★★★	★	★★★	★	★★★	NR
13. St. Joseph Regional Medical Center, Lewiston	NR	★★★	★★★	★★★	NR	★★★	★★★	★★★	★★★	NR	NR	★★★
14. St. Luke's Boise Medical Center, Boise	NR	★★★	★★★	★★★	NR	★★★★★	★★★★★	★	★★★	★★★	★★★	★★★
15. St. Luke's Magic Valley Regional Medical Center, Twin Falls	NR	★★★	★★★	★★★	NR	★★★	★★★	★★★	★★★	NR	★★★	★★★
16. St. Luke's Wood River Medical Center, Ketchum	NR	NR	NR	★★★	NR	NR	NR	NR	NR	NR	NR	NR
17. West Valley Medical Center, Caldwell	NR	★	NR	NR	NR	★★★	NR	★★★	★★★	NR	NR	NR

KEY: ★★★★★ BEST   ★★★ AS EXPECTED   ★ POOR   NR NOT RATED BY HEALTHGRADES   For full definitions of ratings and awards, see Appendix.

Gastrointestinal Bleed	Gastrointestinal Surgeries and Procedures	Heart Attack	Heart Failure	Hip Fracture Repair	Maternity Care	Pancreatitis	Peripheral Vascular Bypass	Pneumonia	Prostatectomy	Pulmonary Embolism	Resection/Replacement of Abdominal Aorta	Respiratory Failure	Sepsis	Stroke	Total Hip Replacement	Total Knee Replacement	Valve Replacement	Women's Health
NR	NR	NR	★	NR	NR	NR	★	NR	NR	NR	NR	NR	NR	NR	NR	NR	NR	NR
NR	NR	NR	★★★	★	NR	NR	★★★	NR	NR	NR	NR	NR	NR	NR	NR	NR	NR	NR
★★★	NR	★★★	★	★★★★★	NR	NR	★★★	NR	NR	NR	NR	NR	★	★★★	★★★	NR	NR	NR
★★★	NR	NR	★★★	★★★	NR	NR	★★★	NR	NR	NR	NR	★★★	★★★	★★★	★★★	NR	NR	NR
★★★	★★★	★	★	★	NR	★★★	NR	★	★★★	★★★	NR	★★★	★★★	★	★★★	★	★	NR
★★★	★	★★★	★	★★★	NR	★	★★★	★★★	★★★	★★★	NR	★★★	★	★★★	★★★	★★★	NR	NR
★★★	★★★	NR	★★★	★★★	NR	★★★	NR	★★★	★★★	★★★	NR	NR	★★★	★★★	★★★	★★★	NR	NR
★★★	★★★	★★★	★★★	★★★	NR	★★★	★	★★★	★★★	★★★	NR	★	★★★	★★★	★★★	★★★	NR	NR
★	NR	NR	★★★	NR	NR	NR	★★★	NR	NR	NR	NR	NR	NR	★★★	NR	NR	NR	NR
★	★	★★★	★	★★★	NR	★	★★★	★★★	★	NR	NR	★★★	★★★	★★★	★★★★★	★★★	NR	NR
★★★	★★★	★★★	★★★	★★★	NR	★★★	★★★	★★★	★★★	NR	NR	★★★	★★★	★★★	★★★★★	★★★★★	★★★	NR
★★★	★★★	★★★	★★★	★★★	NR	★★★	★	★★★	★★★	NR	NR	★★★	★	★	★★★	★★★★★	NR	NR
★★★	★★★	★★★	★★★	★	NR	★★★	★★★	★	★★★	★★★	NR	★★★	★★★	★★★	★★★	★★★	★★★★★	NR
★★★	★★★	★	★★★	★★★	NR	★★★	★	★★★	★★★	NR	NR	★★★	★★★	★	★★★	★★★★★	NR	NR
NR	NR	NR	★★★	NR	NR	NR	★★★	NR	NR	NR	NR	NR	NR	★★★	NR	NR	NR	NR
★★★	★★★	★★★	★★★	★	NR	NR	★★★	★	NR	NR	★	★★★	★★★	★★★	★★★	NR	NR	NR

ILLINOIS HOSPITALS: RATINGS BY PROCEDURE

Hospital	Appendectomy	Atrial Fibrillation	Back and Neck Surgery (except Spinal Fusion)	Back and Neck Surgery (Spinal Fusion)	Bariatric Surgery	Bowel Obstruction	Carotid Surgery	Cholecystectomy (Gall Bladder Removal)	Chronic Obstructive Pulmonary Disease (COPD)	Coronary Bypass Surgery	Coronary Interventional Procedures (Angioplasty/Stent)	Diabetic Acidosis and
1. Abraham Lincoln Memorial Hospital, Lincoln	NR	★★★	NR	NR	NR	★★★	NR	NR	★★★	★★★	NR	NR
2. Adventist GlenOaks, Glendale Heights	NR	NR	NR	NR	NR	★★★	NR	NR	★★★	★★★	NR	NR
3. Advocate Bethany Hospital, Chicago	NR	NR	NR	NR	NR	NR	NR	NR	★★★★★	NR	★★★	NR
4. Advocate Christ Hospital and Medical Center, Oak Lawn	NR	★★★	★★★	★	NR	★★★	★★★	★★★	★★★★★	★★★	★★★	★★★
5. Advocate Good Samaritan Hospital, Downers Grove	NR	★★★	★★★	★★★	NR	★★★	★★★	★★★★★	★★★★★	★★★	★★★★★	★
6. Advocate Good Shepherd Hospital, Barrington	NR	★★★	★	★	NR	★★★	NR	★★★	★★★★★	★★★	★★★★★	★★★
7. Advocate Illinois Masonic Medical Center, Chicago	NR	★★★	★★★	NR	NR.	★★★	★	★★★	★★★	★★★	★★★	★★★
8. Advocate Lutheran General Hospital, Park Ridge	NR	★★★	★★★	★★★	NR	★★★★★	★★★	★★★	★★★★★	★★★	★★★	★★★
9. Advocate South Suburban Hospital, Hazel Crest	NR	★★★	★★★	★★★	NR	★★★	★★★	★★★	★★★	NR	★★★	★★★
10. Advocate Trinity Hospital, Chicago	NR	★★★	NR	NR	NR	★★★	NR	★★★	★★★★★	NR	★★★	NR
11. Alexian Brothers Medical Center, Elk Grove Village	NR	★★★★★	★	NR	NR	★★★★★	★★★	★★★	★★★★★	★★★	★★★★★	★★★
12. Alton Memorial Hospital, Alton	NR	★★★	NR	NR	NR	★★★	NR	★★★	★★★	NR	★★★	NR
13. Anderson Hospital, Maryville	NR	★★★	NR	NR	NR	★	★	★	★★★	NR	★★★	NR
14. Blessing Hospital, Quincy	NR	★★★	★	★★★	NR	★★★	★	★★★	★★★	★★★	★★★	★
15. BroMenn Healthcare, Normal	NR	★★★	★★★	★★★	NR	★★★	★★★★★	★★★	★★★	★★★	★★★	NR
16. Carle Foundation Hospital, Urbana	NR	★★★★★	★	★	NR	★★★	★★★	★★★	★★★	★★★	★★★	★
17. Carlinville Area Hospital, Carlinville	NR	NR	NR	NR	NR	NR	NR	NR	★★★	NR	NR	NR
18. Centegra Memorial Medical Center, Woodstock	NR	★★★	★★★	NR	NR	★★★	★★★	★★★	★★★★★	NR	NR	NR
19. Centegra Northern Illinois Medical Center, McHenry	NR	★★★	★★★	NR	NR	★★★	★★★	★★★	★★★★★	NR	★★★	★★★
20. Central DuPage Hospital, Winfield	NR	★★★	★★★	★★★	NR	★★★	★★★	★★★	★★★	★★★	★★★	★★★
21. CGH Medical Center, Sterling	NR	★★★	NR	NR	NR	★★★	★★★	★★★	★★★	NR	NR	★★★
22. Community Hospital of Ottawa, Ottawa	NR	★★★	NR	NR	NR	★	NR	★	★★★	NR	NR	NR
23. Community Memorial Hospital, Staunton	NR	NR	NR	NR	NR	NR	NR	NR	NR	NR	NR	NR
24. Condell Medical Center, Libertyville	NR	★★★	★★★★★	★	NR	★★★	★	★★★	★★★	★★★	★★★	★★★
25. Crawford Memorial Hospital, Robinson	NR	★★★	NR	NR	NR	★★★	NR	NR	★★★	NR	NR	NR
26. Crossroads Community Hospital, Mount Vernon	NR	★★★	NR	NR	NR	★★★	NR	★★★	★★★	NR	NR	NR
27. Decatur Memorial Hospital, Decatur	NR	★	★★★★★	★★★	NR	★★★	★★★	★★★★★	★	★★★★★	★★★★★	★★★
28. Delnor Community Hospital, Geneva	NR	★★★	★★★	★	NR	★★★	★★★	★★★	★	NR	★★★	★★★
29. Edward Hospital, Naperville	NR	★★★	★★★	★	NR	★★★	★★★	★★★	★★★	★★★	★★★	★★★
30. Elmhurst Memorial Hospital, Elmhurst	NR	★★★	★★★	★★★	NR	★★★	★★★	★★★	★★★	★★★	★★★	★★★
31. Eureka Community Hospital, Eureka	NR	NR	NR	NR	NR	NR	NR	NR	★★★	NR	NR	NR
32. Evanston Northwestern Healthcare, Evanston	NR	★★★	★	NR	NR	★★★★★	★★★	★	★★★	★★★	★★★	★★★
33. Fairfield Memorial Hospital, Fairfield	NR	★★★	NR	NR	NR	★★★	NR	★★★	★★★	NR	NR	NR
34. Fayette County Hospital, Vandalia	NR	★★★	NR	NR	NR	★	NR	NR	★★★	NR	NR	NR
35. Ferrell Hospital Community Foundations, Eldorado	NR	NR	NR	NR	NR	★★★	NR	★★★	★	NR	NR	NR
36. FHN Memorial Hospital, Freeport	NR	★★★	NR	NR	NR	★★★	NR	★★★	★★★★★	NR	★★★	NR
37. Franklin Hospital, Benton	NR	NR	NR	NR	NR	NR	NR	NR	★★★	NR	NR	NR
38. Galesburg Cottage Hospital, Galesburg	NR	★	NR	NR	NR	★★★	★★★	★★★	★★★★★	NR	★★★	NR
39. Gateway Regional Medical Center, Granite City	NR	★★★	NR	NR	NR	★	NR	★★★	★★★	NR	★★★★★	NR
40. Gibson Community Hospital, Gibson City	NR	NR	NR	NR	NR	★★★	NR	NR	★★★	NR	NR	NR
41. Good Samaritan Regional Health Center, Mount Vernon	NR	★★★	NR	NR	NR	★★★	★★★	★★★★★	★★★	★★★	★★★	★★★
42. Gottlieb Memorial Hospital, Melrose Park	NR	★★★	★★★	NR	NR	★★★	★	★★★	★★★	★★★	★★★	★★★
43. Graham Hospital Association, Canton	NR	★★★	NR	NR	NR	★★★	NR	★★★★★	★★★	NR	NR	NR
44. Greenville Regional Hospital, Greenville	NR	★★★	NR	NR.	NR	★★★	NR	NR	★★★	NR	NR	NR
45. Hamilton Memorial Hospital District, McLeansboro	NR	NR	NR	NR	NR	NR	NR	NR	★★★	NR	NR	NR
46. Hammond Henry Hospital, Geneseo	NR	NR	NR	NR	NR	★	NR	NR	★★★	NR	NR	NR
47. Hardin County General Hospital, Rosiclare	NR	NR	NR	NR	NR	NR	NR	NR	★★★	NR	NR	NR
48. Harrisburg Medical Center, Harrisburg	NR	★★★	NR	NR	NR	★★★	NR	★★★	★★★	NR	NR	NR
49. Heartland Regional Medical Center, Marion	NR	★★★	NR	NR	NR	★★★	NR	★★★	★★★★★	★★★	★★★	★
50. Herrin Hospital, Herrin	NR	★★★	NR	NR	NR	★★★	NR	★★★	★★★	NR	NR	★

KEY: ★★★★★ BEST ★★★ AS EXPECTED ★ POOR NR NOT RATED BY HEALTHGRADES For full definitions of ratings and awards, see Appendix.

Gastrointestinal Bleed	Gastrointestinal Surgeries and Procedures	Heart Attack	Heart Failure	Hip Fracture Repair	Maternity Care	Pancreatitis	Peripheral Vascular Bypass	Pneumonia	Prostatectomy	Pulmonary Embolism	Resection/Replacement of Abdominal Aorta	Respiratory Failure	Sepsis	Stroke	Total Hip Replacement	Total Knee Replacement	Valve Replacement	Women's Health
★★★	NR	NR	★★★	NR	NR	NR	NR	★★★	NR	NR	NR	NR	★★★	★★★	NR	★	NR	NR
★★★	NR	★★★	★★★★★	★★★	NR	NR	NR	★★★★★	NR	NR	NR	★★★★★	★★★★★	★★★★★	NR	★★★	NR	NR
★★★	NR	NR	★★★★★	NR	NR	NR	NR	★★★	NR	NR	NR	NR	★★★	★★★	NR	NR	NR	NR
★★★	★★★	★★★	★★★★★	★★★	NR	★★★	★★★	★★★★★	★★★	★★★	★	★★★★★	★★★★★	★★★★★	★	★★★	★★★	NR
★★★★★	★★★	★★★	★★★★★	★★★★★	NR	★★★	NR	★★★★★	★★★	★★★★★	★★★	★★★	★★★★★	★★★	★	★★★	★★★	NR
★★★★★	★★★	★★★★★	★★★★★	★★★	NR	★★★	NR	★★★★★	★★★	NR	NR	★★★★★	★★★	★★★★★	★	★	★★★	NR
★★★	★★★	★★★	★★★★★	★★★	NR	NR	★★★	★★★★★	★★★	NR	NR	★★★	★★★	★★★	★★★	★★★	NR	NR
★★★★★	★★★★★	★★★★★	★★★★★	★★★	NR	★★★	★★★	★★★	★★★	★★★	★★★★★	★★★	★★★	★★★	★★★	★★★★★	★★★	NR
★★★	★★★	★★★	★★★★★	★★★	NR	★★★	NR	★★★★★	★★★	★★★	NR	★★★	★★★	★★★	★★★★★	★★★	NR	NR
★★★	★★★	★★★	★★★★★	★★★★★	NR	★★★	NR	★★★★★	★★★	★★★	NR	★★★	★★★★★	★★★	★★★★★	★★★	NR	NR
★★★★★	★★★★★	★★★	★★★★★	★★★	NR	★★★	NR	★★★★★	★	★★★	★★★★★	★★★	★★★★★	★★★★★	★★★★★	★★★	★★★★★	NR
★★★	★★★	★★★	★★★	★★★	NR	★★★	NR	★★★	NR	★★★	NR	★★★	★★★	★★★	★★★	★★★	NR	NR
★★★	★	★★★	★★★	★	NR	★	NR	★★★	NR	★★★	NR	★★★	★★★	★★★	★	NR	NR	NR
★★★	★★★	★★★	★★★★★	NR	NR	★★★	★★★	★	NR	★★★	★★★	★	★★★	★★★	★★★	NR	★★★	NR
★★★	★★★	★★★	★	★★★★★	NR	★★★	NR	★	★★★★★	★★★	★★★	★★★	★	★★★	★★★★★	NR	★★★	NR
★★★	★★★	★★★	★★★★★	★★★	NR	★★★★★	★★★	★★★	★★★	★★★	★★★	★★★	★★★	★★★★★	★	★	★★★	NR
★★★	NR	★★★	★★★	NR	NR	NR	NR	NR	NR	NR	NR	★	★	★	NR	NR	NR	NR
★★★	★★★★★	★★★★★	★★★★★	★★★	NR	★★★	★★★	★★★★★	★★★	★★★	★★★	★★★	★★★★★	★★★★★	★★★	NR	★★★	NR
★★★	★★★	★★★	★★★★★	★★★	NR	★★★	★★★	★★★★★	★★★	★★★	★★★	★★★	★★★★★	★★★	★	★★★	★★★	NR
★★★	★★★	★	★	★★★	NR	★	NR	★★★	★	★★★	NR	★★★	★★★	★★★	NR	★★★	NR	NR
★★★	★	★★★	★★★	★★★	NR	NR	★	NR	★★★	★★★	★	NR	★	NR	★★★	★★★	★★★	NR
★★★	NR	★★★	★★★★★	NR	NR	NR	★★★	★★★	NR	NR	NR	★★★	★★★★★	★★★★★	NR	★★★	NR	NR
★★★	NR	★★★	★	★★★	NR	NR	NR	★	NR	NR	NR	★★★	★	NR	NR	★★★	NR	NR
★★★	NR	NR	★★★	★★★	NR	NR	NR	★★★	NR	NR	NR	★★★	NR	★★★★★	NR	★★★	NR	NR
★★★	★	★★★	★	★★★	NR	★★★	NR	★	★★★	★★★	★★★	★★★	★	NR	★★★	★★★	★★★	NR
★★★	★★★	★★★★★	★	★★★	NR	★★★	NR	★★★	★★★	★★★	NR	★★★★★	★★★	★★★	★	★★★★★	★★★	NR
★★★★★	★★★	★★★★★	★★★★★	★★★	NR	★★★	NR	★★★★★	★★★	★★★	★★★	★★★	★★★★★	★	★★★	★★★	NR
★★★	★★★★★	★★★	★★★	★★★	NR	★★★	★	★★★	★★★★★	★★★	★★★	★★★	★★★	★★★	★	★★★★★
★★★	NR	NR	★★★	NR	NR	NR	NR	★	NR	NR	NR	NR	★★★	★★★★★	NR	NR	NR	NR
★★★★★	★★★★★	★★★★★	★★★★★	★★★	NR	★★★	★★★	★★★★★	★★★	★★★	★★★★★	★★★★★	★★★★★	★★★	★★★★★	★★★	
★	NR	NR	★★★	NR	NR	NR	NR	★	NR	NR	NR	NR	NR	NR	NR	NR	NR	NR
★★★	NR	★★★	★★★	NR	NR	NR	NR	★★★	NR	NR	NR	★★★	★★★	NR	★★★	NR	NR
★★★	NR	★★★	★	NR	NR	NR	NR	★★★	NR	NR	NR	★★★	★★★	NR	NR	NR	NR
★★★	★★★	★★★	★★★	★	NR	★★★	NR	★★★★★	★★★	★★★	NR	★★★	★★★	★★★	★	★	NR
★★★	NR	NR	★★★	NR	NR	NR	NR	★★★	NR	NR	NR	★★★	★★★	NR	NR	NR	NR
★★★	★	★★★	★★★	★★★	NR	★★★	NR	★★★	★	★★★	NR	★	★★★	★	★★★	★★★★★	NR
★★★	NR	★	★	★★★	NR	★	NR	★	NR	★★★	NR	★★★	★★★	★★★	★★★	★★★	NR
★★★	NR	NR	★★★	★	NR	NR	NR	★★★	NR	NR	NR	NR	NR	NR	NR	NR	NR
★★★	★★★	★★★	★★★	★★★	NR	★★★	NR	★★★	★★★	★★★	NR	★	★★★	★★★	★	★	NR
★	★	★★★	★★★	★★★	NR	★	★★★	★★★	★★★	★★★	NR	★★★	★★★	★★★	★★★	★★★★★	★	NR
★	★	NR	★	★★★	NR	NR	NR	★★★	★★★	NR	NR	★★★	★★★	NR	★★★	★★★	NR
★★★	NR	NR	★★★	NR	NR	NR	NR	★★★★★	NR	NR	NR	★★★★★	NR	NR	NR	NR	NR
★★★	NR	NR	★★★	NR	NR	NR	NR	★★★	NR	NR	NR	NR	★★★	NR	NR	NR	NR
★	NR	NR	★	★★★	NR	NR	NR	★★★	NR	NR	NR	NR	NR	NR	NR	NR	NR
★★★	NR	★★★	NR	NR	NR	NR	NR	★★★	NR	NR	NR	NR	★★★	NR	NR	NR	NR
★★★	★★★★★	★★★	★	NR	NR	NR	NR	★	NR	NR	NR	★★★	NR	NR	★	NR	NR
★★★	★★★	★★★	★★★	★	NR	NR	NR	★★★	★★★	★★★	NR	★★★	★★★★★	★★★	★	NR	NR
★★★	NR	★★★	★	★	NR	★★★	NR	★★★	NR	NR	NR	★★★	★	★★★	★	NR	NR

Hospital	Appendectomy	Atrial Fibrillation	Back and Neck Surgery (except Spinal Fusion)	Back and Neck Surgery (Spinal Fusion)	Bariatric Surgery	Bowel Obstruction	Carotid Surgery	Cholecystectomy (Gall Bladder Removal)	Chronic Obstructive Pulmonary Disease (COPD)	Coronary Bypass Surgery	Coronary Interventional Procedures (Angioplasty/Stent)	Diabetic Acidosis an…
51. **Highland Park Hospital**, Highland Park	NR	★★★	★	★	NR	★★★★★	★★★	★	NR	★★★	★★★	★★★
52. **Hillsboro Area Hospital**, Hillsboro	NR	★★★	NR	NR	NR	NR	NR	NR	★	NR	NR	NR
53. **Hinsdale Hospital**, Hinsdale	NR	★★★	★★★	★★★	NR	★★★	★★★	★	★★★	★★★	★★★★★	★★★
54. **Holy Cross Hospital**, Chicago	NR	★★★	NR	NR	NR	★★★	NR	★★★	★★★	NR	NR	★★★
55. **Hopedale Medical Complex**, Hopedale	NR	NR	NR	NR	NR	★★★	NR	★★★★★	★★★	NR	NR	NR
56. **Illinois Valley Community Hospital**, Peru	NR	★★★	NR	NR	NR	★★★	NR	★★★	★	NR	NR	NR
57. **Illini Community Hospital**, Pittsfield	NR	★★★	NR	NR	NR	NR	NR	NR	★★★	NR	NR	NR
58. **Illini Hospital**, Silvis	NR	★★★	NR	NR	NR	★★★	NR	★★★	★★★	NR	★★★	NR
59. **Ingalls Memorial Hospital**, Harvey	NR	★★★	★★★	NR	NR	★★★	★	★★★★★	★★★★★	★★★	★★★	★★★
60. **Iroquois Memorial Hospital**, Watseka	NR	★★★	NR	NR	NR	★★★	NR	NR	★★★★★	NR	NR	NR
61. **Jackson Park Hospital Foundation**, Chicago	NR	NR	NR	NR	NR	★★★	NR	NR	★★★	NR	NR	★★★
62. **Jersey Community Hospital**, Jerseyville	NR	★★★	NR	NR	NR	★★★	NR	★★★	★★★	NR	NR	NR
63. **John H. Stroger Jr. Hospital**, Chicago	NR	★★★	NR	NR	NR	★	NR	NR	★★★	★★★	★★★	★★★
64. **Katherine Shaw Bethea Hospital**, Dixon	NR	★★★	NR	NR	NR	★	★★★	★★★★★	★★★	NR	NR	NR
65. **Kenneth Hall Regional Hospital**, East St. Louis	NR	NR	NR	NR	NR	NR	NR	NR	NR	NR	NR	NR
66. **Kewanee Hospital**, Kewanee	NR	★	NR	NR	NR	★★★	NR	★★★	★★★	NR	NR	NR
67. **Kishwaukee Community Hospital**, DeKalb	NR	★★★	★★★★★	NR	NR	★★★	NR	★★★	★★★	NR	NR	★★★
68. **La Grange Memorial Hospital**, La Grange	NR	★★★★★	★★★	NR	NR	★★★	★★★	★	★★★	★	★★★	★★★
69. **Lake Forest Hospital**, Lake Forest	NR	★★★	★★★	★★★	NR	★★★★★	NR	★★★	★★★	NR	★★★	NR
70. **Lawrence County Memorial Hospital**, Lawrenceville	NR	NR	NR	NR	NR	NR	NR	NR	★★★	NR	NR	NR
71. **Lincoln Park Hospital**, Chicago	NR	★★★	NR	NR	NR	★★★	NR	★★★	★★★	NR	★★★	NR
72. **Little Company of Mary Hospital**, Evergreen Park	NR	★★★★★	★★★	NR	NR	★★★	★★★	★★★★★	★★★	NR	NR	★★★
73. **Loretto Hospital**, Chicago	NR	NR	NR	NR	NR	★★★	NR	NR	★★★	NR	NR	★★★
74. **Louis A. Weiss Memorial Hospital**, Chicago	NR	★★★	NR	NR	NR	★★★	NR	★★★	★★★	★★★	★★★	★★★
75. **Loyola University Medical Center**, Maywood	NR	★★★	★★★	★★★★★	NR	★★★	★★★	★★★	★★★	★★★	★★★	★★★
76. **MacNeal Hospital**, Berwyn	NR	★★★	★★★	NR	NR	★★★	★★★	★★★	★★★	★★★★★	★★★	★★★
77. **Marshall Browning Hospital**, DuQuoin	NR	NR	NR	NR	NR	NR	NR	NR	★★★	NR	NR	NR
78. **Mason District Hospital**, Havana	NR	NR	NR	NR	NR	NR	NR	NR	★★★	NR	NR	NR
79. **Massac Memorial Hospital**, Metropolis	NR	NR	NR	NR	NR	★★★	NR	NR	★★★	NR	NR	NR
80. **McDonough District Hospital**, Macomb	NR	★★★	NR	NR	NR	★★★	★★★	★★★	★★★	NR	NR	NR
81. **Memorial Hospital of Carbondale**, Carbondale	NR	★★★	NR	★★★	NR	★★★	★★★★★	★★★	★★★	★★★	★★★	NR
82. **Memorial Hospital**, Belleville	NR	★★★	★★★	NR	NR	★★★	★	★★★	★	★★★	★★★	★★★
83. **Memorial Hospital**, Carthage	NR	NR	NR	NR	NR	NR	NR	NR	★★★	NR	NR	NR
84. **Memorial Hospital**, Chester	NR	★★★	NR	NR	NR	NR	NR	NR	★★★	NR	NR	NR
85. **Memorial Medical Center**, Springfield	NR	★★★★★	★★★	★★★★★	NR	★★★	★★★	★★★	★★★	★	★★★	★
86. **Mendota Community Hospital**, Mendota	NR	★★★	NR	NR	NR	★★★	NR	NR	★★★	NR	NR	NR
87. **Mercy Harvard Hospital**, Harvard	NR	NR	NR	NR	NR	NR	NR	NR	NR	NR	NR	NR
88. **Mercy Hospital and Medical Center**, Chicago	NR	★★★	NR	NR	NR	★★★	★★★	★★★	★★★★★	★★★	★★★	★★★
89. **Methodist Hospital of Chicago**, Chicago	NR	★★★	NR	NR	NR	★★★	NR	★★★	★★★	NR	★★★	NR
90. **Methodist Medical Center of Illinois**, Peoria	NR	★★★	★★★	★★★	NR	★★★	★★★	★	★★★	★★★	★★★	★★★
91. **Michael Reese Hospital and Medical Center**, Chicago	NR	★★★	NR	NR	NR	★★★	NR	★★★	★★★	NR	★★★	NR
92. **Midwestern Region Medical Center**, Zion	NR	NR	NR	NR	NR	NR	NR	★★★	★★★	NR	NR	NR
93. **Morris Hospital and Healthcare Center**, Morris	NR	★★★	NR	NR	NR	★★★	NR	★★★	★★★	NR	★★★	NR
94. **Mt. Sinai Hospital Medical Center**, Chicago	NR	★	NR	NR	NR	★★★	NR	NR	★★★	NR	NR	NR
95. **Northwest Community Hospital**, Arlington Heights	NR	★★★★★	★★★★★	★★★	NR	★★★	★★★	★★★	★★★	★★★★★	★★★★★	★★★★★
96. **Northwestern Memorial Hospital**, Chicago	NR	★★★	★★★	★★★	NR	★★★★★	★★★	★★★	★★★	★★★★★	★★★	★★★
97. **Norwegian-American Hospital**, Chicago	NR	NR	NR	NR	NR	★★★	NR	★	NR	★	NR	★★★
98. **Oak Forest Hospital**, Oak Forest	NR	NR	NR	NR	NR	NR	NR	NR	★★★	NR	NR	NR
99. **Oak Park Hospital**, Oak Park	NR	★★★	NR	NR	NR	★★★★★	★	★★★	★★★	NR	NR	★★★
100. **Our Lady of the Resurrection Medical Center**, Chicago	NR	★	NR	NR	NR	★★★	★★★★★	★★★	★★★	NR	★★★★★	★★★★★

KEY: ★★★★★ BEST   ★★★ AS EXPECTED   ★ POOR   NR NOT RATED BY HEALTHGRADES   For full definitions of ratings and awards, see Appendix.

Gastrointestinal Bleed	Gastrointestinal Surgeries and Procedures	Heart Attack	Heart Failure	Hip Fracture Repair	Maternity Care	Pancreatitis	Peripheral Vascular Bypass	Pneumonia	Prostatectomy	Pulmonary Embolism	Resection/Replacement of Abdominal Aorta	Respiratory Failure	Sepsis	Stroke	Total Hip Replacement	Total Knee Replacement	Valve Replacement	Women's Health
★★★★★	★★★★★	★★★★★	★★★★★	★★★	NR	★★★	★★★	★★★★★	★★★	★★★	★★★★★	★★★★★	★★★★★	★★★★★	★★★	★★★★★	★★★	NR
★★★	NR	NR	★	NR	NR	NR	NR	★	NR	NR	NR	NR	★★★	★★★	NR	NR	NR	NR
★★★	★★★	★★★	★★★★★	★★★	NR	★★★	NR	★★★★★	★	★★★	NR	★★★	★★★★★	★★★★★	★	★	★★★	NR
★★★	★★★	★★★	★★★	★★★	NR	★★★	NR	★★★★★	★★★	★★★	NR	★★★★★	★★★★★	★★★★★	★★★	★★★	NR	NR
★★★	NR	NR	★★★	NR	NR	NR	NR	★★★	★★★	NR	NR	NR	NR	NR	NR	NR	NR	NR
★★★	★★★	NR	★	★★★★★	NR	NR	NR	★★★	★★★	NR	NR	NR	NR	★	★★★★★	★★★★★	NR	NR
★★★	★★★★★	★	★★★★★	★★★	NR	★★★	NR	★★★	★★★	NR	NR	★★★	★★★	★★★	★★★	★★★★★	NR	NR
★★★	★★★	★★★★★	★★★	★★★★★	NR	NR	NR	★★★	★★★	NR	★★★★★	★★★★★	★★★★★	★★★★★	NR	NR	NR	NR
★★★	NR	★★★	★★★★★	NR	NR	NR	NR	★★★	★★★	NR	NR	★★★	★★★	★★★★★	NR	NR	NR	NR
★★★	NR	NR	★	NR	NR	NR	NR	★★★	★★★	NR	NR	★★★	★★★	★★★	NR	NR	NR	NR
★★★	★★★	NR	★★★	★	NR	NR	NR	★★★	★★★	NR	NR	★★★	★★★	★★★	NR	NR	NR	NR
★★★	★	★★★	★	★★★★★	NR	★★★	NR	★★★	★★★	NR	NR	★★★	★★★	★★★	★★★	★★★	★★★	NR
★★★	NR	NR	★★★★★	NR	NR	NR	NR	★★★	★★★	NR	NR	NR	NR	NR	NR	NR	NR	NR
★★★	NR	NR	★★★	★★★	NR	NR	NR	★	NR	NR	NR	★	NR	NR	NR	NR	NR	NR
★★★★★	★★★	★★★	★	NR	NR	NR	NR	★★★	NR	★★★	NR	★	★★★	★★★	★	★	NR	NR
★★★★★	★★★	★★★★★	★★★★★	★	NR	★★★★★	NR	★★★★★	★	★★★	NR	★★★	★★★★★	★★★	★	★	★★★	NR
★★★	★★★	★★★	★	★★★	NR	★★★	NR	★★★★★	★★★	★★★	NR	★★★★★	★★★★★	★★★	★	NR	NR	NR
★★★	NR	★	★★★	NR	NR	NR	NR	★★★	NR	NR	NR	NR	★★★	NR	NR	NR	NR	NR
★★★	NR	★★★	★★★	★★★	NR	NR	NR	★★★	★★★	NR	NR	NR	★★★	NR	NR	NR	NR	NR
★★★	★★★★★	★★★	★★★	★★★	NR	★★★	★★★	★★★	★★★	★★★	NR	★★★★★	★★★★★	★★★	★★★★★	★★★	NR	NR
★★★	NR	★	★★★★★	NR	NR	NR	NR	★★★	NR	NR	NR	★★★	★★★	NR	NR	NR	NR	NR
★★★	★★★	★★★★★	★★★	★	NR	NR	NR	★★★★★	NR	NR	NR	★★★★★	★★★	★★★	NR	NR	NR	NR
★★★	★★★	★★★	★★★★★	★★★	NR	★★★	★★★	★★★	★★★	★★★	★★★	★★★	★	★★★	★★★	★★★	★★★	NR
★★★	★★★	★★★	★★★★★	★	NR	★★★	NR	★★★	★★★	★★★	NR	★★★	★★★	★★★★★	★★★	★★★	★★★	NR
★★★	NR	NR	★	NR	NR	NR	NR	★★★	NR	NR	NR	NR	NR	★	NR	NR	NR	NR
NR	NR	NR	★	★★★	NR	NR	NR	★★★	NR	NR	NR	NR	NR	NR	NR	NR	NR	NR
NR	NR	NR	★★★	NR	NR	NR	NR	★★★	NR	NR	NR	★★★	NR	★★★	NR	NR	NR	NR
★	★★★	★	★	★★★	NR	★★★	NR	★★★	NR	NR	NR	NR	★	★★★	★★★	★★★★★	NR	NR
★★★	★★★	★★★	★★★	★★★	NR	★★★	★★★	★★★	★	★★★	NR	★★★	★★★	★★★★★	★	★★★	★★★	NR
★★★	★	★★★	★★★	★★★	NR	★★★	★★★	★★★	★★★	★★★	NR	★★★★★	★★★★★	★★★	★★★	★★★★★	★★★	NR
NR	NR	NR	★	NR	NR	NR	NR	★★★	NR	NR	NR	NR	NR	NR	NR	NR	NR	NR
★★★	NR	NR	★★★	NR	NR	NR	NR	★★★	NR	NR	NR	NR	★★★	NR	★★★	NR	NR	NR
★★★	★★★	★★★	★★★	★★★	NR	★★★	★★★	★★★	★★★	★★★	★	★	★★★	★★★★★	★★★★★	★★★	NR	NR
★★★	NR	★★★	★★★	★★★	NR	NR	NR	★★★	NR	NR	NR	★★★	★★★	NR	NR	★★★	NR	NR
★★★	NR	★★★	★★★	NR	NR	NR	NR	★★★	NR	NR	NR	★★★	★★★	NR	NR	NR	NR	NR
★★★	★★★★★	★★★★★	★★★★★	★★★	NR	NR	NR	★★★★★	★★★	★★★	★★★	★★★★★	★★★★★	★★★★★	★★★	★★★	NR	NR
★★★	NR	NR	★★★	★★★★★	NR	NR	NR	★★★★★	NR	NR	NR	★★★	★★★★★	NR	NR	NR	NR	NR
★★★	★★★	★★★	★★★	★★★★★	NR	★★★	NR	★★★	★	★★★	★	★★★	★★★	★★★	★★★	★★★	NR	NR
★★★	NR	★★★	★★★★★	★★★	NR	NR	NR	★★★	★★★	★★★	NR	★★★	★★★	NR	NR	NR	NR	NR
NR	NR	NR	★	NR	NR	NR	NR	★★★	NR	NR	NR	★	★★★	NR	NR	NR	NR	NR
★★★	★★★	★★★★★	★★★	★★★	NR	★★★	NR	★★★	★★★	NR	NR	★★★	★★★★★	★★★★★	★★★	NR	NR	NR
★★★	NR	★★★	★★★	★★★	NR	NR	NR	★★★	NR	NR	NR	★★★	★	★★★	NR	NR	NR	NR
★★★★★	★★★★★	★★★	★★★★★	★★★	NR	★★★	★★★	★★★★★	★	★★★	★★★★★	★★★★★	★★★★★	★	★	★★★★★	NR	NR
★★★	★★★	★	★★★★★	★★★	NR	★★★	★★★	★★★	★★★★★	★★★	★★★	★★★	★★★★★	★★★★★	★★★★★	★★★	NR	NR
★	NR	★★★	★★★	NR	NR	NR	NR	★★★★★	★★★	NR	★★★★★	★★★	★★★★★	★★★	NR	NR	NR	NR
NR	NR	NR	★★★	NR	NR	NR	NR	★★★	NR	NR	NR	★	NR	NR	NR	NR	NR	NR
★★★	★★★	★★★	★★★★★	★★★	NR	NR	NR	★★★★★	★	★★★	NR	★★★★★	★★★★★	★★★★★	★★★	★★★★★	NR	NR
★★★★★	★★★★★	★★★	★★★	★★★	NR	★★★	NR	★★★★★	★★★★★	★★★	NR	★★★★★	★★★★★	★★★★★	★★★★★	★★★	NR	NR

	Appendectomy	Atrial Fibrillation	Back and Neck Surgery (except Spinal Fusion)	Back and Neck Surgery (Spinal Fusion)	Bariatric Surgery	Bowel Obstruction	Carotid Surgery	Cholecystectomy (Gall Bladder Removal)	Chronic Obstructive Pulmonary Disease (COPD)	Coronary Bypass Surgery	Coronary Interventional Procedures (Angioplasty/Stent)	Diabetic Acidosis
101. Palos Community Hospital, Palos Heights	NR	★★★	★★★	★★★	NR	★★★★★	★★★	★★★	★★★★★	★★★	★★★	★★★
102. Pana Community Hospital, Pana	NR	NR	NR	NR	NR	NR	NR	NR	★★★	NR	NR	NR
103. Paris Community Hospital, Paris	NR	NR	NR	NR	★	NR	NR	NR	★★★	NR	NR	NR
104. Passavant Area Hospital, Jacksonville	NR	★★★	NR	NR	★	NR	★★★	★★★	★★★	NR	NR	NR
105. Pekin Memorial Hospital, Pekin	NR	★★★	NR	NR	★★★	★	★	★	★★★	NR	NR	★
106. Perry Memorial Hospital, Princeton	NR	★★★	NR	NR	★	NR	★★★	★★★	★★★	NR	NR	NR
107. Pinckneyville Community Hospital, Pinckneyville	NR	★	NR	NR	NR	NR	NR	NR	★★★	NR	NR	NR
108. Proctor Hospital, Peoria	NR	★★★	NR	NR	★★★	★★★	★★★	★★★	★★★	★★★	★★★	★
109. Provena Covenant Medical Center, Urbana	NR	★★★	NR	NR	★★★	★★★	★★★	★★★	★★★	★★★	★★★	★★★
110. Provena Mercy Center, Aurora	NR	★★★	NR	NR	★★★	★★★	★★★	★★★	★★★	★★★	★★★	★★★
111. Provena St. Joseph Medical Center, Joliet	NR	★★★	★★★	NR	★★★	★★★	★★★	★★★★★	★★★	NR	★★★	★★★
112. Provena St. Mary's Hospital, Kankakee	NR	★★★	NR	NR	★★★	★★★	★★★	★★★★★	NR	NR	★★★	★★★
113. Provena United Samaritans Medical Center–Logan, Danville	NR	★★★	NR	NR	★★★	★★★	★★★	★★★	★★★	NR	★★★	★★★
114. Provident Hospital of Chicago, Chicago	NR	★★★	NR	NR	NR	NR	NR	★★★	★★★	NR	★★★	★★★
115. Red Bud Regional Hospital, Red Bud	NR	NR	NR	NR	NR	NR	NR	★★★	★★★	NR	NR	NR
116. Resurrection Medical Center, Chicago	NR	★★★	★★★	★★★	NR	★★★★★	★★★	★★★	★★★	★★★	★★★	★★★
117. RHC St. Francis Hospital, Evanston	NR	★★★	★★★	★★★	NR	★★★	★★★	★★★★★	★★★	★★★	★★★	★★★
118. Richland Memorial Hospital, Olney	NR	★★★	NR	NR	NR	★★★	NR	★★★	★★★	NR	NR	NR
119. Riverside Medical Center, Kankakee	NR	★★★	★★★	NR	NR	★★★	★★★	★★★	★★★★★	★★★	★★★	★★★
120. Rochelle Community Hospital, Rochelle	NR	NR	NR	NR	NR	★★★	NR	★★★	★★★	NR	NR	NR
121. Rockford Memorial Hospital, Rockford	NR	★★★	★★★	★★★★★	NR	★★★	★★★	★★★	★★★★★	★★★	★★★	★★★
122. Roseland Community Hospital, Chicago	NR	NR	NR	NR	NR	★★★	NR	★★★	★★★	NR	NR	★★★
123. Rush Copley Memorial Hospital, Aurora	NR	★★★	NR	★★★	NR	★★★	★★★	★★★	★★★	★★★	★★★	★★★
124. Rush North Shore Medical Center, Skokie	NR	★★★	★★★	★★★	NR	★★★★★	★	★★★	★★★★★	★★★	★★★★★	★★★
125. Rush University Medical Center, Chicago	NR	★★★	★	★	NR	★★★★★	★★★	★★★	★★★	★★★	★★★	★★★
126. Sacred Heart Hospital, Chicago	NR	★★★	NR	NR	NR	NR	NR	★★★	NR	NR	NR	NR
127. St. Alexius Medical Center, Hoffman Estates	NR	★★★	★★★	NR	NR	★★★★★	★★★	★★★	★★★★★	NR	★★★	★★★
128. St. Anthony Hospital, Chicago	NR	★	NR	NR	NR	★★★	NR	★★★	★★★★★	NR	NR	★★★
129. St. Anthony Medical Center, Rockford	NR	★★★	★★★	★★★	NR	★★★	★★★	★★★	★★★	★★★	★★★	★★★
130. St. Anthony's Health Center, Alton	NR	★★★	★★★	NR	NR	★★★	★★★	★★★	★★★★★	NR	★★★	★★★
131. St. Anthony's Memorial Hospital, Effingham	NR	★★★	★★★	NR	NR	★★★	NR	★	★★★	NR	★★★	★★★
132. St. Bernard Hospital, Chicago	NR	NR	NR	NR	NR	★★★	NR	★★★★★	NR	NR	NR	★★★
133. St. Elizabeth Hospital, Belleville	NR	★★★	★	NR	NR	★★★	★★★	★	★★★	★★★	★★★	★★★
134. St. Francis Hospital, Litchfield	NR	★★★	NR	NR	NR	★	NR	NR	★★★	NR	NR	NR
135. St. Francis Hospital and Health Center, Blue Island	NR	★★★	NR	NR	NR	★★★	★★★	★★★	★★★★★	★★★★★	★★★	★★★
136. Saint Francis Medical Center, Peoria	NR	★★★	★★★	★★★	NR	★★★	★★★	★★★	★★★	★★★	★★★	★★★
137. Saint James Hospital, Pontiac	NR	★★★	NR	NR	NR	★★★	NR	NR	★★★	NR	NR	NR
138. St. James Hospital and Health Center, Chicago Heights	NR	★★★★★	★	★	NR	★	★★★	★	★★★	★★★★★	★★★	★★★
139. St. James Hospital and Health Ctr.–Olympia Fields, Olympia Fields	NR	★★★★★	★	★	NR	★	★★★	★	★★★	★★★★★	★★★	★★★
140. St. John's Hospital, Springfield	NR	★★★	★	★★★★★	NR	★	★★★★★	★	★★★	★	★★★★★	★★★
141. St. Joseph Hospital, Chicago	NR	★★★	★★★	NR	NR	★★★	★★★	★★★	★★★	★★★	★★★	★★★
142. St. Joseph Hospital, Elgin	NR	★★★	NR	NR	NR	★★★	★★★	★★★	★★★★★	★★★★★	★	NR
143. St. Joseph Medical Center, Bloomington	NR	★★★	★★★	★★★★★	NR	★★★	★★★	★★★	★★★	★★★	★★★	★★★
144. St. Joseph Memorial Hospital, Murphysboro	NR	NR	NR	NR	NR	★★★	NR	★★★	★	NR	NR	NR
145. St. Joseph's Hospital, Highland	NR	★★★	NR	NR	NR	★★★	NR	★★★	★★★	NR	★★★	NR
146. St. Joseph's Hospital, Alton	NR	★★★	★★★	NR	NR	★★★	★★★	★★★	★★★★★	NR	★★★	★★★
147. St. Joseph's Hospital, Breese	NR	★★★	NR	NR	NR	★★★★★	NR	★★★	★★★	NR	★★★	★★★
148. St. Margaret's Hospital, Spring Valley	NR	★★★	NR	NR	NR	★★★	NR	★★★	★★★	NR	NR	NR
149. St. Mary and Elizabeth Medical Center–Claremont, Chicago	NR	★	NR	NR	NR	★★★	NR	★★★	★★★	NR	NR	★★★
150. St. Mary and Elizabeth Medical Center–Division, Chicago	NR	★★★	NR	NR	NR	★★★	NR	★★★	★★★	★★★	★★★	★★★

KEY: ★★★★★ BEST ★★★ AS EXPECTED ★ POOR NR NOT RATED BY HEALTHGRADES For full definitions of ratings and awards, see Appendix.

Gastrointestinal Bleed	Gastrointestinal Surgeries and Procedures	Heart Attack	Heart Failure	Hip Fracture Repair	Maternity Care	Pancreatitis	Peripheral Vascular Bypass	Pneumonia	Prostatectomy	Pulmonary Embolism	Resection/Replacement of Abdominal Aorta	Respiratory Failure	Sepsis	Stroke	Total Hip Replacement	Total Knee Replacement	Valve Replacement	Women's Health
★★★★★	★★★	★★★★★	★★★★★	★★★	NR	★★★	NR	★★★★★	★★★	★★★★★	NR	★★★★★	★★★★★	★★★★★	★★★	★	NR	NR
NR	NR	NR	★★★	NR	NR	NR	NR	★	NR	NR	NR	NR	NR	★★★	NR	NR	NR	NR
★★★	NR	NR	★★★	NR	NR	NR	NR	★	NR	NR	NR	NR	NR	★	NR	NR	NR	NR
★	★★★	★★★	★	★★★★★	NR	★★★	NR	★★★	★★★	NR	NR	★★★★★	★★★	★★★	★★★★★	★★★	NR	NR
★★★	★★★	★★★	★★★	★★★	NR	★★★	NR	★	★	NR	NR	★★★	★★★	★	★★★	★★★	NR	NR
★★★	NR	★★★	★	★	NR	NR	NR	★★★	NR	NR	NR	★★★	★	NR	NR	NR	NR	NR
★★★	NR	NR	★★★	NR	NR	NR	NR	★★★	NR	NR	NR	NR	★	NR	NR	NR	NR	NR
★★★	★★★	★★★	★★★	★★★	NR	★★★	NR	★	★★★	★	NR	★	★	★★★	★★★	★★★	★★★	NR
★	★	★★★★★	★★★	★★★	NR	★★★	★★★	★★★	★★★	★★★	NR	★	★★★	★★★	★★★	★★★★★	★★★	NR
★★★	★★★	★★★	★★★	★★★	NR	★★★	NR	★★★	★★★	★★★	NR	★★★★★	★★★★★	★★★	★★★	★★★	★★★	NR
★★★	★★★	★★★★★	★★★★★	★★★	NR	★★★	★	★★★★★	★★★	★★★	★★★	★★★★★	★★★★★	★	★★★★★	★★★★★	★★★	NR
★	★★★	★★★	★★★	★★★★★	NR	★★★	NR	★★★	★★★	NR	NR	★★★	★	★★★	★★★	★★★★★	NR	NR
★★★	★★★	★★★	★★★	NR	NR	★★★	NR	★★★	NR	★★★	NR	★	★	★★★	★	NR	NR	NR
★★★	NR	★★★	★★★★★	NR	NR	NR	NR	★★★	NR	NR	NR	NR	★	NR	NR	NR	NR	NR
★★★	NR	NR	★	NR	NR	NR	NR	★★★	NR	NR	NR	NR	NR	★★★	NR	NR	NR	NR
★★★	★★★	★★★★★	★★★★★	★★★	NR	★★★	★★★★★	★★★	★★★	★★★★★	★★★	★★★★★	★★★★★	★★★★★	★★★	★★★	★★★	NR
★★★	★★★★★	★	★★★	★★★★★	NR	★★★	★	★★★★★	★★★	★★★	NR	★★★	★★★★★	★★★	★★★	★★★	★★★★★	NR
★★★	NR	★★★	★★★★★	★★★	NR	NR	NR	★★★	★	NR	NR	★★★	★★★★★	NR	NR	★	NR	NR
★★★	★★★	★	★★★	★★★	NR	★★★	NR	★★★	★★★	★★★	NR	★★★	★★★	★★★★★	★★★	★★★	★★★	NR
★★★	NR	NR	★★★★★	NR	NR	NR	NR	★★★★★	NR	NR	NR	NR	★★★	NR	NR	NR	NR	NR
★★★	★★★	★★★	★★★	NR	NR	NR	NR	★★★	NR	NR	NR	NR	★★★	★★★★★	★	★	NR	NR
★★★★★	★★★★★	★★★★★	★★★★★	★★★	NR	★★★	NR	★★★★★	★★★	★★★	★	★★★	★★★	★★★★★	★★★★★	★★★★★	★★★	NR
★★★	★★★	★★★	★★★★★	★	NR	★★★	★★★	★★★★★	★★★	★★★	★★★	★★★	★★★	★★★★★	★★★★★	★★★★★	★★★	NR
NR	NR	NR	★★★	NR	NR	NR	NR	★★★	NR	NR	NR	NR	NR	NR	NR	NR	NR	NR
★★★★★	★★★	★★★★★	★★★★★	★★★	NR	★★★	NR	★★★★★	★★★	★★★★★	NR	★★★★★	★★★★★	★★★★★	★★★	★★★	NR	NR
★★★	NR	NR	★★★★★	NR	NR	★★★	NR	★★★	NR	NR	NR	★★★	NR	NR	NR	NR	NR	NR
★★★	★★★	★★★★★	★★★	★★★	NR	★★★	NR	★★★★★	★★★	★★★	NR	★★★	★	★★★★★	★★★	★★★★★	★★★	NR
★★★	★★★	★★★	★★★	★★★	NR	NR	NR	★★★	NR	★★★	NR	★★★★★	★★★★★	★★★	★★★	★★★	★★★	NR
★★★	NR	★★★	★	★★★	NR	NR	NR	★	NR	NR	NR	★★★	★	NR	★★★	★★★	NR	NR
★★★	★★★	★★★★★	★★★★★	★★★	NR	★★★	★	★★★★★	★★★	★★★	★★★	★★★★★	★★★★★	★★★★★	★	★	★★★★★	NR
★	★	★★★	★★★	★	NR	★★★	★★★	★★★	★	★★★	★★★	★★★	★	★	★★★	★★★	★★★	NR
★	NR	NR	★	★	NR	NR	NR	★★★	NR	NR	NR	NR	★	NR	★	NR	NR	NR
★★★	★★★	★★★	★★★★★	★★★★★	NR	★★★	★★★	★★★★★	★★★	★★★	NR	★★★★★	★★★★★	★★★★★	★★★★★	★	★★★	NR
★★★	★★★	★★★	★★★★★	★★★★★	NR	★★★	★★★	★★★★★	★★★	★★★	NR	★★★★★	★★★★★	★★★★★	★★★★★	★	★★★	NR
★	★★★	★★★	★★★★★	★	NR	★★★	★★★	★	★★★	★★★	★★★	★★★	★★★	★★★	★★★	★★★	★★★	NR
★★★★★	★★★	★★★	★★★★★	★★★★★	NR	★★★	★★★	★★★★★	★★★	★★★	★★★	★★★★★	★★★★★	★★★★★	★★★	★★★	★★★	NR
★★★	★★★	★★★	★★★★★	★★★	NR	NR	NR	★★★★★	★★★	★★★	NR	★★★	★★★	★★★★★	★★★	NR	NR	NR
★	★	★★★	★★★	★★★	NR	★	NR	★★★	NR	★★★	★★★	★★★	★★★	★★★	★	★	★	NR
★	NR	NR	★★★	NR	NR	NR	NR	★★★	NR	NR	NR	NR	NR	★★★	NR	NR	NR	NR
★★★	NR	NR	★★★	★★★	NR	NR	NR	★	NR	NR	NR	★★★	★	NR	NR	NR	NR	NR
★★★	★★★	★★★	★★★	★★★	NR	NR	NR	★★★	NR	★★★	NR	★★★★★	★★★	★★★	★★★	★★★	NR	NR
★★★	NR	NR	★★★	★★★	NR	NR	NR	★★★	NR	NR	NR	★	★	NR	NR	NR	NR	NR
★★★	NR	NR	★★★	NR	NR	NR	NR	★	★	NR	NR	★	★★★	★	NR	★	NR	NR
★★★	NR	NR	★★★	★★★	NR	★★★	NR	★★★	★★★	NR	NR	★★★	★★★★★	★★★★★	NR	NR	NR	NR
★★★	★★★	★	★★★★★	★★★	NR	★★★	★★★	★★★	★★★	NR	NR	★★★	★★★	NR	NR	NR	NR	NR

	Appendectomy	Atrial Fibrillation	Back and Neck Surgery (except Spinal Fusion)	Back and Neck Surgery (Spinal Fusion)	Bariatric Surgery	Bowel Obstruction	Carotid Surgery	Cholecystectomy (Gall Bladder Removal)	Chronic Obstructive Pulmonary Disease (COPD)	Coronary Bypass Surgery	Coronary Interventional Procedures (Angioplasty/Stent)	Diabetic Acidosis and...
151. St. Mary Hospital, Quincy	NR	★★★	★	★★★	NR	★★★	★	★★★	★★★	★★★	★★★	★
152. St. Mary Medical Center, Galesburg	NR	★★★	NR	NR	NR	★★★★★	★	★★★	★★★	NR	NR	★★★
153. St. Mary's Hospital, Centralia	NR	★★★	NR	NR	NR	★★★	★★★	★★★	★★★	NR	NR	★★★
154. St. Mary's Hospital, Decatur	NR	★★★	NR	NR	NR	★★★	★★★	★★★	★★★	NR	NR	NR
155. St. Mary's Hospital, Streator	NR	★	NR	NR	NR	★★★	NR	★★★	★★★	NR	NR	NR
156. Salem Township Hospital, Salem	NR	NR	NR	NR	NR	★★★	NR	★★★	★★★	NR	NR	NR
157. Sarah Bush Lincoln Health Center, Mattoon	NR	★★★	★★★	NR	NR	★★★	★★★★★	★★★	★★★	NR	NR	★★★
158. Sarah D. Culbertson Memorial Hospital, Rushville	NR	NR	NR	NR	NR	NR	NR	NR	★★★	NR	NR	NR
159. Shelby Memorial Hospital, Shelbyville	NR	★★★	NR	NR	NR	NR	NR	NR	★★★	NR	NR	NR
160. Sherman Hospital, Elgin	NR	★★★	NR	NR	NR	★★★	★★★	★	★★★	★★★	★★★	★★★
161. Silver Cross Hospital, Joliet	NR	★★★	NR	NR	NR	★★★	★★★	★★★	★★★	NR	★★★	★★★
162. South Shore Hospital, Chicago	NR	★	NR	NR	NR	★★★	NR	NR	★★★★★	NR	NR	★★★
163. Sparta Community Hospital, Sparta	NR	★★★	NR	NR	NR	NR	NR	NR	★★★	NR	NR	NR
164. Swedish American Hospital, Rockford	NR	★★★	★	★★★	NR	★	★★★	★★★	★★★	★★★★★	★★★	★★★
165. Swedish Covenant Hospital, Chicago	NR	★★★	NR	NR	NR	★★★	★★★	★★★	★★★	★★★	★★★	★★★
166. Taylorville Memorial Hospital, Taylorville	NR	★★★	NR	NR	NR	★★★	NR	NR	★★★	NR	NR	NR
167. Thomas H. Boyd Memorial Hospital, Carrollton	NR	NR	NR	NR	NR	NR	NR	NR	★★★	NR	NR	NR
168. Thorek Memorial Hospital, Chicago	NR	NR	NR	NR	NR	★★★	NR	NR	★★★	NR	NR	NR
169. Touchette Regional Hospital, Centreville	NR	NR	NR	NR	NR	NR	NR	NR	★★★	NR	NR	NR
170. Trinity Medical Center—7th Street Campus, Moline	NR	★★★	★★★★★	★★★	NR	★★★	★★★★★	★★★★★	★★★	★★★★★	★★★★★	★★★
171. Trinity Medical Center—West Campus, Rock Island	NR	★★★	★★★★★	★★★	NR	★★★	★★★★★	★★★★★	★★★	★★★★★	★★★★★	★★★
172. Union County Hospital District, Anna	NR	NR	NR	NR	NR	NR	NR	NR	★★★	NR	NR	NR
173. University of Chicago Medical Center, Chicago	NR	★★★★★	★★★	★	NR	★★★	★★★	★★★	★★★	★	★★★★★	★★★
174. University of Illinois Medical Center, Chicago	NR	★★★	★★★	NR	NR	★★★	★★★	★★★	★★★★★	★	★★★	★★★
175. Valley West Community Hospital, Sandwich	NR	★★★	NR	NR	NR	★★★★★	NR	NR	★★★	NR	NR	NR
176. Vista Medical Center—East, Waukegan	NR	★★★	NR	NR	NR	★★★	NR	★★★	★★★	NR	★	★★★
177. Wabash General Hospital, Mount Carmel	NR	★★★	NR	NR	NR	NR	NR	NR	★★★	NR	NR	NR
178. West Suburban Hospital Medical Center, Oak Park	NR	★★★	NR	NR	NR	★★★	★★★	★★★	★★★★★	NR	★★★	★★★
179. Westlake Community Hospital, Melrose Park	NR	★★★	NR	NR	NR	★★★	★★★	★★★	★★★	★★★	★	★★★
180. White County Medical Center, Carmi	NR	NR	NR	NR	NR	NR	NR	NR	★★★	NR	NR	NR

KEY: ★★★★★ BEST ★★★ AS EXPECTED ★ POOR NR NOT RATED BY HEALTHGRADES For full definitions of ratings and awards, see Appendix.

Gastrointestinal Bleed	Gastrointestinal Surgeries and Procedures	Heart Attack	Heart Failure	Hip Fracture Repair	Maternity Care	Pancreatitis	Peripheral Vascular Bypass	Pneumonia	Prostatectomy	Pulmonary Embolism	Resection/Replacement of Abdominal Aorta	Respiratory Failure	Sepsis	Stroke	Total Hip Replacement	Total Knee Replacement	Valve Replacement	Women's Health
★★★	★★★	★★★	★★★	★★★★★	NR	★	★★★	★	★★★	★★★	★★★	★	★	★★★	★★★	★★★	★★★	NR
★★★	★★★	★★★	★★★	★★★	NR	NR	NR	★★★	NR	NR	NR	★	★	★★★	★★★	★★★	NR	NR
★★★	★★★	★★★	★★★	★★★	NR	★★★	NR	★★★	NR	★★★	NR	★★★★★	★★★	★★★	NR	★★★	NR	NR
★★★	★	★★★	★	★★★	NR	NR	NR	★★★	★★★	★★★	NR	★★★	★★★	★★★	★★★	★★★★★	NR	NR
★★★	★	★★★	★★★	★	NR	NR	NR	★★★	NR	NR	NR	NR	★★★	★	NR	★	NR	NR
★★★	NR	NR	★★★	NR	NR	NR	NR	★★★	NR	NR	NR	NR	★★★	NR	NR	NR	NR	NR
★★★	★★★	★★★	★★★	★★★	NR	★★★	NR	★★★	★★★	★★★	NR	★★★	★	★★★★★	★★★★★	★★★★★	NR	NR
NR	NR	NR	★★★	NR	NR	NR	NR	★★★	NR	NR	NR	NR	★★★	NR	NR	NR	NR	NR
★★★	NR	NR	★★★	NR	NR	NR	NR	★★★★★	NR	NR	NR	NR	★★★	★★★	NR	NR	NR	NR
★★★	★★★★★	★★★★★	★★★★★	★★★	NR	★★★	NR	★★★★★	★	★★★	★★★	★★★★★	★★★★★	★★★	★★★	★	★★★	NR
★★★	★★★	★★★★★	★★★	★★★	NR	★★★	★★★	★★★	★★★	★★★	NR	★★★	★★★	★★★	★★★	★★★	NR	NR
★★★	NR	★	★★★	NR	NR	★★★	NR	★★★	★★★	NR	NR	★★★	★★★	NR	NR	NR	NR	NR
★★★	NR	NR	★★★	NR	NR	NR	NR	★	NR	NR	NR	★★★	★★★	NR	NR	NR	NR	NR
★★★	★★★	★★★	★★★	★★★	NR	★★★	NR	★★★	★★★	★★★	★★★	★★★	★	★★★	★★★	★	NR	NR
★★★	★★★★★	★★★★★	★★★	★★★★★	NR	★★★	NR	★★★★★	★★★	★★★	NR	★★★	★★★	★★★★★	★★★	★★★	★★★	NR
★★★	NR	★★★	★★★	★★★	NR	NR	NR	★★★	NR	NR	NR	★★★	★★★	★★★	NR	NR	NR	NR
NR	NR	NR	★★★	NR	NR	NR	NR	★★★	NR	NR	NR	NR	NR	NR	NR	NR	NR	NR
★★★	NR	NR	★★★★★	NR	NR	NR	NR	★★★★★	NR	NR	NR	★★★	★★★	NR	NR	NR	NR	NR
NR	NR	NR	★★★	NR	NR	NR	NR	★	NR	NR	NR	NR	NR	NR	NR	NR	NR	NR
★★★	★★★	★★★	★★★	★	NR	★★★	★★★	★	★★★	★	★★★	★★★	★★★	★★★	★★★	★★★	★★★	NR
★★★	★★★	★★★	★★★	★	NR	★★★	★★★	★	★★★	★	★★★	★★★	★★★	★★★	★★★	★★★	★★★	NR
NR	NR	NR	★	NR	NR	NR	NR	★	NR	NR	NR	★★★	★	NR	★	NR	NR	NR
★★★	★★★★★	★★★	★★★★★	★★★	NR	★★★	NR	★★★★★	★★★	★★★	★★★	★★★★★	★★★	★★★★★	★★★	★★★	★★★	NR
★★★	★★★	★★★	★★★	★★★	NR	★★★	NR	★★★★★	★★★	★★★	NR	★★★	★★★	★★★★★	★★★	★★★	NR	NR
★★★	★★★	★★★	★★★	★	NR	★★★	NR	★★★	NR	★★★	NR	★★★	NR	★★★	NR	NR	NR	NR
★★★	★★★	★★★	★★★	★★★★★	NR	★★★	NR	★★★★★	★	NR	NR	★	★★★	★★★	★★★	★★★	NR	NR
NR	NR	NR	★★★	NR	NR	NR	NR	★★★	NR	NR	NR	★	★★★	NR	NR	NR	NR	NR
★★★★★	★★★	★★★	★★★★★	★★★	NR	★★★	★★★	★★★★★	★★★	★★★	NR	★★★	★★★	★★★	★★★	★★★	★★★	NR
★★★	NR	★★★	★★★★★	★★★★★	NR	NR	NR	★★★★★	★★★	★★★★★	NR	★★★★★	★★★★★	★★★★★	NR	★★★	NR	NR
NR	NR	NR	★★★	NR	NR	NR	NR	★★★	NR	NR	NR	NR	NR	NR	NR	NR	NR	NR

INDIANA HOSPITALS: RATINGS BY PROCEDURE

Hospital	Appendectomy	Atrial Fibrillation	Back and Neck Surgery (except Spinal Fusion)	Back and Neck Surgery (Spinal Fusion)	Bariatric Surgery	Bowel Obstruction	Carotid Surgery	Cholecystectomy (Gall Bladder Removal)	Chronic Obstructive Pulmonary Disease (COPD)	Coronary Bypass Surgery	Coronary Interventional Procedures (Angioplasty/Stent)	Diabetic Acidosis an...
1. Adams County Memorial Hospital, Decatur	NR	★★★	NR	NR	NR	★★★	NR	★★★	★★★	NR	NR	NR
2. Adams Memorial Hospital, Decatur	NR	★★★	NR	NR	NR	★★★	NR	★★★	★★★	NR	NR	
3. Ball Memorial Hospital, Muncie	NR	★★★	★★★	★★★	NR	★★★	★★★	★★★	★★★	★★★★★	★★★	★★★
4. Bedford Regional Medical Center, Bedford	NR	★★★	NR	NR	NR	★★★	NR	★★★	★★★	NR	NR	
5. Bloomington Hospital of Orange County, Paoli	NR	NR	NR	NR	NR	NR	NR	NR	★	NR	NR	
6. Bloomington Hospital, Bloomington	NR	★★★	★★★	★★★★★	NR	★★★	★★★	★	★★★	★★★	★★★	★★★
7. Bluffton Regional Medical Center, Bluffton	NR	★★★	NR	NR	NR	★★★	NR	★★★	★★★★★	NR	NR	
8. Cameron Memorial Community Hospital, Angola	NR	NR	NR	NR	NR	★★★	NR	NR	★★★	NR	NR	
9. Clarian Health Partners, Indianapolis	NR	★★★	★	NR	NR	★★★	★	NR	★★★★★	★★★	NR	★★★
10. Clarian West Medical Center, Avon	NR	★★★	NR	NR	NR	★★★	NR	NR	★★★★★	★★★	NR	★★★
11. Clark Memorial Hospital, Jeffersonville	NR	★★★	★	★★★	NR	★★★	★★★	★★★★★	★★★	NR	★★★	★★★
12. Columbus Regional Hospital, Columbus	NR	★★★	★★★★★	★★★	NR	★★★★★	★★★★★	★★★	★★★	★★★	★★★★★	★★★
13. Community Hospital of Anderson and Madison County, Anderson	NR	★★★	NR	NR	NR	★★★	★★★	★★★	★★★★★	NR	NR	★
14. Community Hospital of Bremen, Bremen	NR	NR	NR	NR	NR	★★★	NR	NR	★★★	NR	NR	
15. Community Hospital South, Indianapolis	NR	★★★	NR	NR	NR	★	★★★	NR	NR	NR	★★★	
16. Community Hospital, Munster	NR	★★★	★★★★★	★★★★★	NR	★★★	★★★★★	★★★★★	★★★★★	★★★★★	★★★	★★★
17. Community Hospitals Indianapolis, Indianapolis	NR	★★★	★★★	★★★	NR	★★★	★★★	★★★	★★★	NR	★★★	★★★
18. Daviess Community Hospital, Washington	NR	★★★	NR	NR	NR	★★★	NR	★★★	★★★	NR	NR	
19. Deaconess Hospital, Evansville	NR	★★★	★★★	★★★	NR	★★★	★★★	★	★★★	★★★	★★★	★★★
20. Dearborn County Hospital, Lawrenceburg	NR	★★★	NR	NR	NR	★★★	NR	★	★★★	NR	NR	
21. Decatur County Memorial Hospital, Greensburg	NR	★	NR	NR	NR	★★★	NR	NR	★★★	NR	NR	
22. DeKalb Memorial Hospital, Auburn	NR	★★★	NR	NR	NR	★★★	NR	NR	★★★	NR	NR	
23. Dukes Memorial Hospital, Peru	NR	★★★	NR	NR	NR	NR	NR	NR	★★★	NR	NR	
24. Dunn Memorial Hospital, Bedford	NR	★★★	NR	NR	NR	★★★	NR	★★★	★★★	NR	★★★	
25. Dupont Hospital, Fort Wayne	NR	NR	★★★	★★★	NR	★★★	NR	★	★★★★★	NR	NR	
26. Elkhart General Hospital, Elkhart	NR	★★★	★★★	★★★	NR	★★★	★★★	★★★	★	NR	★★★	★★★
27. Fayette Memorial Hospital, Connersville	NR	★★★	NR	NR	NR	★★★	NR	NR	★★★★★	NR	NR	
28. Floyd Memorial Hospital and Health Services, New Albany	NR	★★★	NR	NR	NR	★★★	★★★	★★★★★	★★★	NR	★★★	★★★
29. Gibson General Hospital, Princeton	NR	NR	NR	NR	NR	NR	NR	NR	★★★	NR	NR	
30. Good Samaritan Hospital, Vincennes	NR	★★★	NR	NR	NR	★★★	★★★★★	★★★★★	★	★★★	★	★★★
31. Goshen General Hospital, Goshen	NR	★★★	NR	NR	NR	★★★	★	★★★	★	NR	★★★	
32. Greene County General Hospital, Linton	NR	★	NR	NR	NR	NR	NR	NR	★★★	NR	NR	
33. Hancock Regional Hospital, Greenfield	NR	★★★	NR	NR	NR	★★★	NR	★★★	★★★	NR	NR	
34. Harrison County Hospital, Corydon	NR	NR	NR	NR	NR	★★★	NR	★	★★★	NR	NR	
35. Hendricks Regional Health, Danville	NR	★★★	NR	NR	NR	★★★	NR	★★★	★★★	NR	NR	★★★
36. Henry County Memorial Hospital, New Castle	NR	★★★	NR	NR	NR	★★★	NR	★★★★★	★	NR	NR	
37. Howard Regional Health System, Kokomo	NR	★★★	NR	★★★	NR	★★★	NR	★★★	★★★	NR	★★★	
38. Indiana Heart Hospital, Indianapolis	NR	★★★	NR	NR	NR	NR	★★★	NR	NR	★★★	★★★	
39. Indiana Orthopaedic Hospital, Indianapolis	NR	NR	★★★★★	★★★★★	NR	NR	NR	NR	NR	NR	NR	
40. Indiana University Medical Center, Indianapolis	NR	★★★	★	★	NR	★★★	★	★	★★★★★	★★★	★★★	★★★
41. Jasper County Hospital, Rensselaer	NR	★	NR	NR	NR	★★★	NR	NR	★	NR	NR	
42. Jay County Hospital, Portland	NR	★★★	NR	NR	NR	NR	NR	NR	★★★	NR	NR	
43. Johnson Memorial Hospital, Franklin	NR	★★★	NR	NR	NR	★★★	NR	★★★	★★★	NR	NR	
44. The King's Daughters' Hospital and Health Services, Madison	NR	★★★	NR	NR	NR	★★★	NR	★★★★★	★★★	NR	NR	★★★
45. Kosciusko Community Hospital, Warsaw	NR	★★★	NR	NR	NR	★★★	NR	★★★	★★★	NR	NR	
46. Lafayette Home Hospital, Lafayette	NR	★★★	★	★	NR	★★★	★★★	★	★★★	NR	NR	
47. Laporte Hospital and Health Services, La Porte	NR	★★★	NR	NR	NR	★★★	NR	★★★	★★★	★★★	★★★	
48. Lutheran Hospital of Indiana, Fort Wayne	NR	★★★	★★★	★★★★★	NR	★★★	NR	★★★	★★★	★★★	★★★★★	★★★
49. Major Hospital, Shelbyville	NR	★★★	NR	NR	NR	★★★	NR	★★★	★★★	★★★	NR	NR
50. Margaret Mary Community Hospital, Batesville	NR	★★★	NR	NR	NR	★★★	NR	NR	★★★	NR	NR	

KEY: ★★★★★ BEST   ★★★ AS EXPECTED   ★ POOR   NR NOT RATED BY HEALTHGRADES   For full definitions of ratings and awards, see Appendix.

Gastrointestinal Bleed	Gastrointestinal Surgeries and Procedures	Heart Attack	Heart Failure	Hip Fracture Repair	Maternity Care	Pancreatitis	Peripheral Vascular Bypass	Pneumonia	Prostatectomy	Pulmonary Embolism	Resection/Replacement of Abdominal Aorta	Respiratory Failure	Sepsis	Stroke	Total Hip Replacement	Total Knee Replacement	Valve Replacement	Women's Health
★	★★★	★★★	★★★	★★★	NR	NR	NR	★★★	NR	NR	NR	NR	★★★	★★★	NR	NR	NR	NR
★	★★★	★★★	★★★	★★★	NR	NR	NR	★★★	NR	NR	NR	NR	★★★	★★★	NR	NR	NR	NR
★★★	★★★	★★★	★★★	★★★★★	NR	★★★	★★★	★★★★★	★★★	★★★	★★★	★★★	★★★	★★★	★★★	★★★	★★★	NR
★★★	NR	★★★	★★★	★★★	NR	NR	NR	★★★	NR	NR	NR	★★★	★	★★★	NR	NR	NR	NR
NR	NR	NR	★	NR	NR	NR	NR	★	NR	NR	NR	NR	NR	★	NR	NR	NR	NR
★★★	★★★	★★★	★	★★★	NR	★★★	★★★	★★★	★	★	★★★	★	★	★★★	★★★	★★★	★	NR
★★★	★★★	★★★	★★★	★★★	NR	★★★	NR	★★★	★★★	NR	NR	★★★	★★★	★★★	★★★★★	★★★	NR	NR
★★★	NR	NR	★★★	NR	NR	NR	NR	★	NR	NR	NR	NR	NR	NR	NR	NR	NR	NR
★★★	★★★	★★★	★★★	★	NR	★★★	★★★	★★★	★★★	★★★	★★★	★★★	★★★	★★★★★	★	★	★★★	NR
★★★	NR	NR	★★★	★	NR	NR	NR	★★★	NR	NR	NR	★★★	★★★	★★★	NR	★★★	NR	NR
★★★	★★★	★★★★★	★★★★★	★	NR	★★★	NR	★★★★★	★★★	★★★	NR	★★★★★	★★★★★	★★★	★	★	NR	NR
★★★	★★★	★★★	★★★	★	NR	★★★★★	★★★	★★★★★	★	★★★	NR	★★★	★★★	★★★	★★★	★★★	NR	NR
★	★★★	★★★★★	★★★	★★★★★	NR	★★★	NR	★★★	★★★	★★★	NR	★	★★★	★★★	★★★	★★★	NR	NR
NR	NR	NR	★★★	NR	NR	NR	NR	★★★	NR	NR	NR	NR	NR	★★★	NR	NR	NR	NR
★★★	★★★	★★★	★★★	★	NR	★★★	★★★	★★★★★	★	★★★	NR	★★★	★★★★★	★★★	★★★	★	NR	NR
★★★★★	★★★	★★★	★★★★★	★★★★★	NR	★★★	★★★	★★★★★	★★★★★	★★★	★★★	★★★	★★★★★	★★★	★★★★★	★★★★★	★★★	NR
★★★★★	★★★★★	★★★	★★★	★★★	NR	★★★	NR	★★★	★★★	★★★★★	NR	★★★	★★★★★	★★★	★	★★★	NR	NR
★★★	NR	★★★★★	★★★	★★★★★	NR	★★★	NR	★★★	NR	★★★	NR	★★★	★★★	★★★★★	NR	★★★	NR	NR
★★★	★★★	★★★	★★★	★	NR	★★★	★★★	★★★★★	★★★	★★★	NR	★★★	★★★	★	★	NR	★★★★★	NR
★★★★★	★★★	★★★	★	★★★	NR	★★★	NR	★★★★★	★★★	★★★	NR	★★★	★★★	★★★	★★★	NR	NR	NR
★★★	NR	NR	★★★	★★★	NR	NR	NR	★★★	NR	NR	NR	★★★	★★★	★★★	★★★	★★★	NR	NR
★★★	NR	NR	★★★	★★★	NR	NR	NR	★★★	NR	NR	NR	★★★	★★★	NR	NR	NR	NR	NR
★★★	★★★	★	★★★	★★★	NR	NR	NR	★★★	NR	NR	NR	★★★	★	★★★	NR	NR	NR	NR
NR	NR	NR	★★★	★★★	NR	NR	NR	★★★★★	★★★	NR	NR	NR	NR	★★★	★★★	NR	NR	NR
★★★	★	★★★	★★★	★★★	NR	★★★	NR	★★★	★★★	★★★	NR	★★★	★★★	★★★	★★★	★★★	★★★	NR
★★★	NR	★★★★★	★★★	★★★	NR	NR	NR	★★★	NR	NR	NR	★★★★★	★★★	★★★	NR	★★★	NR	NR
★★★	★★★	★★★	★★★★★	★★★★★	NR	★★★	★★★	★★★★★	★★★	★★★	NR	★★★★★	★★★	★★★	★★★	★★★	NR	NR
NR	NR	NR	★★★	NR	NR	NR	NR	★★★	NR	NR	NR	NR	NR	★★★	NR	NR	NR	NR
★★★★★	★★★	★★★	★★★	★★★★★	NR	★★★	NR	★★★	★★★	★★★	NR	★★★	★	★★★	★★★	★★★★★	NR	NR
★★★	★★★	★★★	★	★	NR	★	NR	★	★★★	★★★	NR	★	★	★★★	★★★	★★★	NR	NR
★★★	NR	NR	★★★	NR	NR	NR	NR	★	NR	NR	NR	NR	★	NR	NR	NR	NR	NR
★★★	★★★	★★★★★	★★★	★★★	NR	NR	NR	★★★★★	★★★	NR	NR	★★★	★★★	★★★	★★★	★★★	NR	NR
★★★	NR	★	★★★	★	NR	NR	NR	★	NR	NR	NR	★★★	★	★★★	NR	★★★	NR	NR
★★★	★★★	★★★★★	★★★	★	NR	★★★	NR	★	NR	★★★	NR	★★★	★★★	★★★	★	★★★	NR	NR
★★★	★	NR	★★★	★★★	NR	★★★	NR	★	★★★	NR	NR	★★★	★★★	★	★★★	★★★	NR	NR
★★★	★★★	★★★	★★★★★	★★★	NR	★★★	NR	★★★★★	★★★	★★★	NR	★★★	★★★	★★★★★	NR	★★★	NR	NR
NR	NR	★★★	★★★	NR	NR	★★★	★★★	NR	NR	★★★	NR	NR	NR	NR	NR	★★★	NR	NR
NR	NR	NR	NR	NR	NR	NR	NR	NR	NR	NR	NR	NR	NR	★★★★★	★★★★★	NR	NR	NR
★★★	★★★	★★★	★★★	★	NR	★★★	★★★	★★★	★★★	★★★	★★★	★★★	★★★★★	★	★	★★★	NR	NR
★★★	NR	NR	★	★★★	NR	NR	NR	★	★★★	NR	NR	NR	NR	★★★	NR	NR	NR	NR
★★★	NR	NR	★★★	NR	NR	NR	NR	★★★★★	NR	NR	NR	NR	NR	NR	NR	NR	NR	NR
★★★	★★★	NR	★★★	★★★	NR	★★★	NR	★★★	NR	NR	NR	★★★	★★★	NR	★★★	★★★	NR	NR
★★★	★★★	★	★★★	★★★★★	NR	NR	NR	★★★	★★★★★	NR	NR	★★★	★★★	★★★	★★★	★★★	NR	NR
★★★	★★★	★★★	★★★	★★★	NR	★★★	NR	★★★	NR	NR	NR	★★★	★★★	★★★	★★★	★★★	NR	NR
★	★★★	★★★	★	★	NR	★★★	NR	★★★	★	★★★	NR	★★★	★	★★★	★	★	NR	NR
★	★★★	★★★	★★★★★	★★★★★	NR	NR	NR	★★★★★	★★★	★★★	NR	★★★	★★★	★★★	★★★	★★★★★	NR	NR
★★★	★	★★★	★★★	★★★	NR	★★★	★★★	★★★	★★★	★★★	★★★	★★★	★★★	★★★	★	★★★	NR	NR
★★★★★	NR	★★★	★★★	★★★	NR	★★★	NR	★★★★★	NR	NR	NR	★★★	★★★★★	★★★	NR	★★★	NR	NR
★★★	NR	NR	★★★	★★★	NR	NR	NR	★★★	NR	NR	NR	NR	NR	★★★	NR	★	NR	NR

	Appendectomy	Atrial Fibrillation	Back and Neck Surgery (except Spinal Fusion)	Back and Neck Surgery (Spinal Fusion)	Bariatric Surgery	Bowel Obstruction	Carotid Surgery	Cholecystectomy (Gall Bladder Removal)	Chronic Obstructive Pulmonary Disease (COPD)	Coronary Bypass Surgery	Coronary Interventional Procedures (Angioplasty/Stent)	Diabetic Acidosis and...
51. Marion General Hospital, Marion	NR	★★★	★★★★★	NR	NR	★★★	NR	★★★	★★★	NR	NR	★★★
52. Memorial Hospital and Health Care Center, Jasper	NR	★★★	NR	NR	NR	★★★	★★★	★★★	★★★	NR	★★★	NR
53. Memorial Hospital of Michigan City, Michigan City	NR	★	NR	★	NR	★★★	★★★	★★★	★★★	NR	★★★	★★★
54. Memorial Hospital of South Bend, South Bend	NR	★★★	★★★	★★★	NR	★★★	★★★★★	★★★★★	★★★★★	★★★	★★★	★★★
55. Memorial Hospital, Logansport	NR	★★★	★★★	NR	NR	★★★	NR	★★★	★★★	NR	★★★	NR
56. Methodist Hospital Southlake, Merrillville	NR	★	★	★★★	NR	★★★	★★★	★★★	★★★★★	★★★	★★★	★★★
57. Methodist Hospital, Gary	NR	★	★	NR	NR	★★★	★★★	★★★	★★★★★	★★★	★★★	★★★
58. Morgan Hospital and Medical Center, Martinsville	NR	★★★	NR	NR	NR	★★★	NR	★★★★★	★★★	NR	NR	NR
59. Parkview Hospital, Fort Wayne	NR	★	★	★★★	NR	★★★	★	★	★★★	NR	★★★	★★★
60. Parkview Huntington Hospital, Huntington	NR	★★★	NR	NR	NR	★★★	NR	NR	★★★	NR	NR	NR
61. Parkview Lagrange Hospital, Lagrange	NR	NR	NR	NR	NR	NR	NR	NR	★★★	NR	NR	NR
62. Parkview Noble Hospital, Kendallville	NR	★★★	NR	NR	NR	★★★	NR	NR	★★★	NR	NR	NR
63. Parkview Whitley Hospital, Columbia City	NR	★★★	NR	NR	NR	★★★	NR	★★★	★★★	NR	NR	NR
64. Perry County Memorial Hospital, Tell City	NR	★★★	NR	NR	NR	NR	NR	NR	★★★	NR	NR	NR
65. Porter, Valparaiso	NR	★★★	★★★	★	NR	★★★	★★★★★	★★★	★★★	★★★	★★★	★★★
66. Putnam County Hospital, Greencastle	NR	NR	NR	NR	NR	★★★	NR	★	★★★	NR	NR	NR
67. Reid Hospital and Health Care Services, Richmond	NR	★★★	NR	★★★	NR	★★★	★★★	★★★	★★★	★★★	★★★	★★★
68. Riverview Hospital, Noblesville	NR	★★★	NR	NR	NR	★	★★★	★	★★★	NR	★★★	NR
69. St. Anthony Medical Center of Crown Point, Crown Point	NR	★★★	★★★	NR	NR	★★★	★★★	★★★	★★★	★★★	★★★	★★★
70. St. Anthony Memorial Health Center, Michigan City	NR	★	NR	★	NR	★★★	★★★	★★★	★★★	NR	★★★	★★★
71. St. Catherine Hospital, East Chicago	NR	★★★	NR	NR	NR	★★★	★★★	★★★	★★★★★	★★★	★★★	★★★
72. St. Catherine Regional Hospital, Charlestown	NR	★★★	NR	NR	NR	NR	NR	NR	★★★	NR	NR	NR
73. St. Clare Medical Center, Crawfordsville	NR	★	NR	NR	NR	★★★	NR	★★★	★★★	NR	NR	NR
74. St. Elizabeth Ann Seton Hospital, Boonville	NR	NR	NR	NR	NR	NR	NR	NR	★★★	NR	NR	NR
75. St. Elizabeth Ann Seton Speciality Care, Carmel	NR	★★★	★★★	★★★	NR	★★★	NR	★★★	★★★	NR	NR	NR
76. St. Elizabeth Medical Center, Lafayette	NR	★★★	★★★	★★★	NR	★★★	★	★	★★★	★★★	★★★	★★★
77. St. Francis Hospital and Health Center, Beech Grove	NR	★★★	★★★★★	★★★	NR	★★★	★	★★★	★★★	★	★★★	★★★
78. St. Francis Hospital and Health Center, Indianapolis	NR	★★★	NR	NR	NR	NR	★★★	NR	NR	★★★	★★★	NR
79. St. Francis Hospital Mooresville, Mooresville	NR	NR	NR	NR	NR	NR	NR	NR	NR	NR	NR	NR
80. Saint John's Health System, Anderson	NR	★★★	NR	★★★	NR	★★★	★★★	★★★	★★★★★	NR	NR	★★★
81. St. Joseph Community Hospital, Mishawaka	NR	★	NR	NR	NR	★★★	★★★	★★★	★	NR	★★★	★★★
82. St. Joseph Hospital, Fort Wayne	NR	★	NR	★★★	NR	★★★	★	NR	★★★	★★★	★★★	★
83. St. Joseph Hospital and Health Center, Kokomo	NR	★★★	NR	★★★	NR	★★★	★★★	★	★★★	NR	NR	NR
84. St. Joseph Regional Medical Center, Plymouth	NR	★★★	NR	NR	NR	★★★	NR	★	★★★	NR	NR	NR
85. St. Joseph Regional Medical Center–South Bend, South Bend	NR	★★★	★★★★★	★★★★★	NR	★★★	★★★★★	★★★★★	★★★	★★★	★★★	★★★
86. St. Margaret Mercy Healthcare Center, Dyer	NR	★★★	★★★	★★★	NR	★★★	★	★★★	★★★	★★★	★★★	★★★
87. St. Margaret Mercy Healthcare Center, Hammond	NR	★★★	★★★	NR	NR	★★★	★★★	★★★	★★★	★★★	★★★	★★★
88. St. Mary's Medical Center–Evansville, Evansville	NR	★	★★★	★★★	NR	★★★	★★★	★★★	★★★	★★★	★★★	★★★
89. St. Mary's Medical Center–Hobart, Hobart	NR	★★★	★★★	★★★	NR	★★★	★★★	★★★★★	★★★	★★★	★★★	NR
90. St. Mary's Warrick, Boonville	NR	NR	NR	NR	NR	NR	NR	NR	★★★	NR	NR	NR
91. St. Vincent Carmel Hospital, Carmel	NR	★★★	★★★	NR	NR	★★★	NR	★★★	★★★	NR	NR	NR
92. St. Vincent Frankfort Hospital, Frankfort	NR	★★★	NR	NR	NR	★★★	NR	NR	★★★	★	NR	NR
93. St. Vincent Heart Center of Indiana, Indianapolis	NR	★★★★★	NR	NR	NR	NR	★	NR	★★★	★★★★★	★★★★★	NR
94. St. Vincent Hospital and Health Services, Indianapolis	NR	★★★	★	★★★	NR	★★★★★	★	★	★★★★★	★★★	★★★	★★★
95. St. Vincent Mercy Hospital, Elwood	NR	★★★	NR	NR	NR	★★★	★	NR	★★★★★	NR	NR	NR
96. Schneck Medical Center, Seymour	NR	★★★	NR	NR	NR	★★★	★	★★★	★★★	NR	NR	NR
97. Scott Memorial Hospital, Scottsburg	NR	★★★	NR	NR	NR	★★★	NR	★★★	★★★	NR	NR	NR
98. Starke Memorial Hospital, Knox	NR	NR	NR	NR	NR	NR	NR	NR	★★★	NR	NR	NR
99. Sullivan County Community Hospital, Sullivan	NR	★★★	NR	NR	NR	★	NR	NR	★★★	NR	NR	NR
100. Terre Haute Regional Hospital, Terre Haute	NR	★★★	★★★★★	NR	NR	★★★	★★★	★★★★★	★★★	★★★	★★★	★

KEY: ★★★★★ BEST   ★★★ AS EXPECTED   ★ POOR   NR NOT RATED BY HEALTHGRADES   For full definitions of ratings and awards, see Appendix.

Gastrointestinal Bleed	Gastrointestinal Surgeries and Procedures	Heart Attack	Heart Failure	Hip Fracture Repair	Maternity Care	Pancreatitis	Peripheral Vascular Bypass	Pneumonia	Prostatectomy	Pulmonary Embolism	Resection/Replacement of Abdominal Aorta	Respiratory Failure	Sepsis	Stroke	Total Hip Replacement	Total Knee Replacement	Valve Replacement	Women's Health
★★★	★★★	★★★	★★★	★★★★★	NR	★★★	NR	★	★★★★★	★★★	NR	★★★	★	★	★★★	★★★	NR	NR
★★★	★★★	★★★	★	★★★★★	NR	★★★	NR	★★★	NR	★★★	NR	★★★	★★★	★★★	★★★	★★★	NR	NR
★★★	★★★	★★★	★★★	★★★★★	NR	NR	NR	★★★	★★★	NR	NR	★★★★★	★★★	★★★	★★★	★★★	NR	NR
★★★	★★★★★	★★★	★★★	★★★	NR	★★★★★	★★★	★★★	★★★	★★★	★★★	★★★	★★★★★	★	★★★	★	★★★	NR
★	★★★	NR	★	★★★	NR	NR	NR	★★★	NR	NR	NR	NR	★	★★★	★★★	★★★	NR	NR
★★★	★★★	★★★	★★★	★★★★★	NR	★★★	★	★★★	★★★	★★★	NR	★★★★★	★★★	★★★★★	★★★	★★★	NR	NR
★★★	★★★	★★★	★★★	★★★★★	NR	★★★	★	★★★	★★★	★★★	NR	★★★★★	★★★	★★★★★	★★★	★★★	NR	NR
★★★	NR	NR	★★★	★★★	NR	★★★	NR	★★★	★★★	NR	NR	★★★	★★★	★	NR	NR	NR	NR
★★★	★★★	★	★	★★★★★	NR	★★★	★★★	★★★	★★★	★★★	NR	★★★	★★★	★★★	★★★★★	★★★	★★★	NR
★★★	NR	NR	★★★	★★★	NR	NR	NR	★★★	NR	NR	NR	NR	★★★	★★★	NR	★★★	NR	NR
NR	NR	NR	★★★	NR	NR	NR	NR	★	NR	NR	NR	NR	★	NR	NR	NR	NR	NR
★★★	NR	NR	★★★	★★★	NR	★★★	NR	★★★	NR	NR	NR	NR	★★★	NR	NR	NR	NR	NR
★★★	★★★	★★★	★★★	★★★	NR	NR	NR	★★★	NR	NR	NR	★★★	★★★	NR	NR	NR	NR	NR
★	NR	NR	★★★	NR	NR	NR	NR	★	NR	NR	NR	NR	★★★	NR	NR	NR	NR	NR
★★★	★★★	★★★	★★★	NR	NR	★★★	★★★	★★★	★★★	★★★	NR	★★★	★★★	★★★	★★★★★	★★★★★	★★★	NR
★★★	NR	NR	★	★★★	NR	NR	NR	★	NR	NR	NR	NR	★	NR	NR	NR	NR	NR
★	★★★	★★★	★★★	NR	NR	★★★	★★★	★★★	★★★	★★★	NR	★★★	★	★★★★★	★★★	★	NR	NR
★★★	★	★★★	★★★	★★★	NR	NR	NR	★	NR	★★★	NR	NR	★	★★★	★★★	★★★	NR	NR
★★★	★★★	★★★	★★★	★★★★★	NR	★★★	NR	★★★	★★★★★	★	NR	★★★	★★★	★★★	★★★	★★★	NR	NR
★★★	★★★	★★★	★★★	★★★★★	NR	★★★	NR	★★★	★★★	NR	NR	★★★★★	★★★	★★★	★★★	★★★	NR	NR
★★★	NR	★★★★★	★★★★★	★★★★★	NR	★★★	★★★	★★★★★	★★★	NR	NR	★★★	★★★	★★★	★★★	★★★	NR	NR
★★★	NR	NR	★★★	NR	NR	NR	NR	★★★	NR	NR	NR	NR	★★★	NR	NR	NR	NR	NR
★	★★★	NR	★	★★★★★	NR	NR	NR	★	NR	NR	NR	NR	★★★	★★★	★★★	★★★	NR	NR
★★★	NR	★★★	★★★	★★★	NR	NR	NR	★★★	NR	NR	NR	NR	NR	NR	NR	NR	NR	NR
★	★★★	NR	★	★★★	NR	NR	NR	★★★	NR	NR	NR	★★★	★★★	★★★	★★★	★★★★★	NR	NR
★★★	★★★	★★★	★★★	★★★	NR	★★★	★	★★★	NR	★★★	NR	★★★★★	★★★★★	★★★	★★★	★★★	★★★	NR
★★★	★★★★★	★★★	★★★	★★★★★	NR	★★★	★	★★★★★	★★★	NR	★★★	★★★★★	★★★★★	★★★★★	★★★★★	★★★★★	★★★	NR
NR	NR	★★★	★★★★★	NR	NR	NR	NR	★★★	NR	NR	NR	NR	NR	★★★	NR	NR	NR	NR
NR	★★★	NR	NR	NR	NR	NR	NR	NR	NR	NR	NR	NR	NR	★★★★★	★★★★★	NR	NR	NR
★★★	★★★	★★★	★★★	★★★	NR	★★★	★★★	★★★	★★★	NR	★★★	★★★	★★★	★★★	★★★	NR	NR
★★★	★★★	★★★	★★★	NR	NR	NR	★★★	★★★	★★★	NR	NR	★★★	★★★	NR	★★★	NR	NR
★★★	NR	★	★	★★★★★	NR	NR	★★★	★★★	NR	★★★	NR	★★★	★★★	★★★	★★★	NR	NR
★★★	★★★	★	★	★	NR	★★★	★★★	★★★	★★★	NR	★★★★★	★★★	★	NR	NR
★★★	★★★	★★★	★★★	★★★	NR	NR	NR	★★★	NR	NR	NR	★★★	★★★	★★★	★★★	★★★	NR	NR
★★★	★★★	★★★	★★★★★	NR	NR	★★★	NR	★★★	★★★	★	NR	★★★	★★★	★★★★★	★★★★★	★★★★★	★★★	NR
★★★	★★★	★★★	★★★★★	★★★★★	NR	NR	NR	★★★	★★★	NR	NR	★★★	★★★	★★★★★	NR	★★★	NR	NR
★★★	★★★	★★★	★★★★★	★★★★★	NR	★★★	★★★	★★★	★★★	NR	NR	★★★★★	★★★	★★★	★★★	★★★	★★★	NR
★★★	★★★	★★★	★★★	NR	NR	★★★	★★★	★★★	★★★	★★★	NR	★★★	★	★★★★★	★★★★★	★★★	NR	NR
★★★	NR	★★★	★★★	NR	NR	NR	NR	★★★	NR	NR	NR	NR	NR	NR	NR	NR	NR	NR
★	★★★	NR	★	★★★	NR	NR	NR	★★★	NR	NR	NR	★★★	★★★	★★★	★★★	★★★★★	NR	NR
★	NR	NR	★	★★★	NR	NR	NR	★★★	NR	NR	NR	NR	NR	★★★	NR	NR	NR	NR
NR	NR	★★★★★	★★★★★	NR	NR	NR	NR	★★★	NR	NR	NR	NR	NR	NR	NR	NR	★★★	NR
★★★	★★★★★	★★★	★★★★★	★★★	NR	★★★	★★★	★★★★★	★★★	★★★	★	★★★★★	★★★★★	★★★★★	★★★	★	★★★	NR
★★★	NR	NR	★★★	NR	NR	NR	NR	★★★★★	NR	NR	NR	NR	★★★	NR	NR	NR	NR	NR
★★★	★★★	★★★	★	★★★	NR	NR	NR	★★★	★★★	NR	NR	★★★	★★★★★	★	★★★	★★★	NR	NR
★★★	NR	★★★	★★★	NR	NR	NR	NR	★★★	NR	NR	NR	★★★	NR	★★★	★★★	NR	NR	NR
★★★	NR	NR	★	★★★	NR	NR	NR	★	NR	NR	NR	★	★★★	NR	NR	NR	NR	NR
★	NR	★★★	★★★	NR	NR	NR	NR	★★★	NR	NR	NR	★★★	★★★	NR	NR	NR	NR	NR
★	★★★	★★★	★★★	★★★	NR	★★★	NR	★★★	NR	★★★	NR	★	★★★	★★★	★	★★★	NR	NR

	Appendectomy	Atrial Fibrillation	Back and Neck Surgery (except Spinal Fusion)	Back and Neck Surgery (Spinal Fusion)	Bariatric Surgery	Bowel Obstruction	Carotid Surgery	Cholecystectomy (Gall Bladder Removal)	Chronic Obstructive Pulmonary Disease (COPD)	Coronary Bypass Surgery	Coronary Interventional Procedures (Angioplasty/Stent)	Diabetic Acidosis and...
101. **Tipton Hospital,** Tipton	NR	★★★	NR	NR	NR	NR	NR	★★★	NR	NR	NR	★★★
102. **Union Hospital,** Terre Haute	NR	★★★	★	NR	NR	★	★★★	★★★	★	★★★	★★★	★
103. **Wabash County Hospital,** Wabash	NR	NR	NR	NR	NR	★★★	NR	NR	★★★	NR	NR	NR
104. **Washington County Memorial Hospital,** Salem	NR	NR	NR	NR	NR	NR	NR	NR	★	NR	NR	NR
105. **Welborn Baptist Hospital,** Evansville	NR	★	★★★	★★★	NR	★★★	★★★	★★★	★★★	★★★	★★★	★★★
106. **West Central Community Hospital,** Clinton	NR	NR	NR	NR	NR	NR	NR	NR	★★★	NR	NR	★★★
107. **Westview Hospital,** Indianapolis	NR	★★★	NR	NR	NR	NR	NR	NR	★★★	NR	NR	NR
108. **White County Memorial Hospital,** Monticello	NR	★★★	NR	NR	NR	★	NR	NR	★	NR	NR	NR
109. **William N. Wishard Memorial Hospital,** Indianapolis	NR	★★★	NR	NR	NR	★	NR	NR	★★★★★	NR	★★★	★★★
110. **Witham Health Services,** Lebanon	NR	★★★	NR	NR	NR	★★★	NR	NR	★★★	NR	NR	NR
111. **Woodlawn Hospital,** Rochester	NR	NR	NR	NR	NR	NR	NR	NR	★	NR	NR	NR

KEY: ★★★★★ BEST   ★★★ AS EXPECTED   ★ POOR   NR NOT RATED BY HEALTHGRADES   For full definitions of ratings and awards, see Appendix.

Gastrointestinal Bleed	Gastrointestinal Surgeries and Procedures	Heart Attack	Heart Failure	Hip Fracture Repair	Maternity Care	Pancreatitis	Peripheral Vascular Bypass	Pneumonia	Prostatectomy	Pulmonary Embolism	Resection/Replacement of Abdominal Aorta	Respiratory Failure	Sepsis	Stroke	Total Hip Replacement	Total Knee Replacement	Valve Replacement	Women's Health
★★★	NR	NR	★	★★★	NR	NR	NR	★	NR	NR	NR	NR	★★★	★★★	NR	★★★★★	NR	NR
★	★	★★★	★★★	★★★	NR	★	★★★	★★★	★★★	★★★	NR	★	★	★	★★★	★★★	★★★	NR
★	NR	NR	★★★	★★★	NR	NR	NR	★★★	NR	NR	NR	NR	NR	★★★	NR	NR	NR	NR
★★★	NR	★	★★★	★★★	NR	NR	NR	★	NR	NR	NR	NR	NR	NR	NR	NR	NR	NR
★★★	★★★	★★★	★★★	★★★	NR	★★★	★★★	★★★	★★★	★★★	★★★	★	★★★	★★★★★	★★★★★	★★★	NR	
★★★	NR	★★★	★★★	★★★	NR	NR	NR	★★★	NR	NR	NR	★★★	★★★	NR	NR	NR	NR	NR
★★★	NR	NR	★★★	★	NR	NR	NR	★★★	NR	NR	NR	★★★	★★★	NR	NR	NR	NR	NR
★★★	NR	NR	★	NR	NR	NR	NR	★	NR	NR	NR	NR	★	NR	NR	NR	NR	NR
★★★	NR	★★★	★★★	★★★	NR	★★★	NR	★★★★★	NR	★	NR	★★★	★★★	★★★	NR	NR	NR	NR
★★★	NR	★★★	★★★	★★★★★	NR	NR	NR	★★★★★	NR	NR	NR	NR	★★★	NR	★★★	NR	NR	NR
★★★	NR	NR	★★★	★★★	NR	NR	NR	★★★	NR	NR	NR	NR	NR	NR	★★★	NR	NR	NR

IOWA HOSPITALS: RATINGS BY PROCEDURE

	Appendectomy	Atrial Fibrillation	Back and Neck Surgery (except Spinal Fusion)	Back and Neck Surgery (Spinal Fusion)	Bariatric Surgery	Bowel Obstruction	Carotid Surgery	Cholecystectomy (Gall Bladder Removal)	Chronic Obstructive Pulmonary Disease (COPD)	Coronary Bypass Surgery	Coronary Interventional Procedures (Angioplasty/Stent)	Diabetic Acidosis
1. Alegent Health Community Memorial Hospital, Missouri Valley	NR	NR	NR	NR	NR	NR	NR	★★★	NR	NR	NR	
2. Alegent Health Mercy Hospital, Council Bluffs	★★★	★★★	NR	★★★	★	★★★	★★★	★★★	★	NR	NR	NR
3. Allen Memorial Hospital, Waterloo	★★★	★★★	★★★	★★★	NR	★★★	★★★★★	★★★	★★★	★★★	★★★★★	★★★
4. Boone County Hospital, Boone	NR	★★★	NR	NR	★	★★★	NR	★★★	NR	NR	NR	
5. Broadlawns Medical Center, Des Moines	NR	NR	NR	NR	NR	NR	NR	★★★	NR	NR	NR	
6. Buchanan County Health Center, Independence	NR	NR	NR	NR	NR	NR	NR	★★★	NR	NR	NR	
7. Buena Vista Regional Medical Center, Storm Lake	NR	★★★	NR	NR	NR	★★★	NR	★	NR	NR	NR	
8. Burgess Health Center, Onawa	NR	★★★	NR	NR	NR	★★★	NR	★★★	NR	NR	NR	
9. Cass County Memorial Hospital, Atlantic	NR	★★★	NR	NR	NR	★★★	NR	★★★	NR	NR	NR	
10. Cherokee Regional Medical Center, Cherokee	NR	★★★	NR	NR	NR	★★★	NR	★	NR	NR	NR	
11. Clarinda Regional Health Center, Clarinda	NR	NR	NR	NR	NR	NR	NR	★★★	NR	NR	NR	
12. Clarke County Hospital, Osceola	NR	NR	NR	NR	NR	NR	NR	★★★	NR	NR	NR	
13. Covenant Medical Center, Waterloo	★★★	★★★★★	★★★	★★★	NR	★★★	★	★★★	★★★	NR	NR	★★★
14. Crawford County Memorial Hospital, Denison	★★★	NR	NR	NR	NR	NR	NR	★★★	NR	NR	NR	
15. Davis County Hospital, Bloomfield	NR	NR	NR	NR	NR	NR	NR	NR	NR	NR	NR	
16. Decatur County Hospital, Leon	NR	NR	NR	NR	NR	NR	NR	NR	NR	NR	NR	
17. Ellsworth Municipal Hospital, Iowa Falls	NR	★★★	NR	NR	NR	★★★	NR	★	NR	NR	NR	
18. Finley Hospital, Dubuque	★★★	★★★	★★★	NR	NR	★★★	★★★	★★★	★★★	NR	NR	★★★
19. Floyd County Memorial Hospital, Charles City	NR	★★★	NR	NR	NR	★★★	NR	★	NR	NR	NR	
20. Floyd Valley Hospital, Le Mars	★★★	NR	NR	NR	NR	★★★	NR	★★★	★★★	NR	NR	
21. Fort Madison Community Hospital, Fort Madison	★★★	★	NR	NR	NR	★	NR	★★★	NR	NR	NR	
22. Genesis Medical Center–Davenport, Davenport	★	★★★	★★★★★	★★★	★★★	★★★	★★★	★★★	★	★	★★★	★★★
23. Grape Community Hospital, Hamburg	NR	NR	NR	NR	NR	★★★	NR	★★★	NR	NR	NR	
24. Great River Medical Center, West Burlington	★	★★★	NR	NR	NR	★★★	★★★	★★★	★★★	NR	NR	★★★
25. Greater Community Hospital, Creston	★	★★★	NR	NR	NR	★★★	NR	★★★	★★★	NR	NR	
26. Greene County Medical Center, Jefferson	NR	NR	NR	NR	NR	★★★	NR	★★★	NR	NR	NR	
27. Grinnell Regional Medical Center, Grinnell	★	NR	NR	★	NR	★★★	NR	★	NR	★★★	NR	
28. Guthrie County Hospital, Guthrie Center	NR	NR	NR	NR	NR	NR	NR	NR	NR	NR	NR	
29. Hamilton County Public Hospital, Webster City	NR	★★★	NR	NR	NR	★★★	NR	★★★	NR	NR	NR	
30. Hancock County Memorial Hospital, Britt	NR	NR	NR	NR	NR	NR	NR	★★★	NR	NR	NR	
31. Henry County Health Center, Mount Pleasant	NR	★★★	NR	NR	NR	★★★	NR	★★★	NR	NR	NR	
32. Horn Memorial Hospital, Ida Grove	NR	NR	NR	NR	NR	★★★	NR	★★★	NR	NR	NR	
33. Iowa Lutheran Hospital, Des Moines	★★★	★★★	★★★	NR	NR	★★★	★★★	★★★	★★★	★★★	★★★	★★★
34. Iowa Methodist Medical Center, Des Moines	★★★★★	★★★	★★★★★	★★★★★	NR	★★★	★★★★★	★★★★★	★★★	★★★	★★★	★★★
35. Jackson County Regional Health Center, Maquoketa	NR	NR	NR	NR	NR	NR	NR	★★★	NR	NR	NR	
36. Jefferson County Hospital, Fairfield	NR	NR	NR	NR	NR	NR	NR	★★★	NR	NR	NR	
37. Jennie Edmundson Hospital, Council Bluffs	★★★	★★★	★★★★★	★★★	★	★★★	★★★	★	NR	NR	★★★	NR
38. Jones Regional Medical Center, Anamosa	NR	NR	NR	NR	NR	NR	NR	★★★	NR	NR	NR	
39. Keokuk Area Hospital, Keokuk	★	★★★	NR	NR	NR	★★★	NR	★★★	NR	NR	NR	
40. Knoxville Hospital and Clinics, Knoxville	NR	NR	NR	NR	NR	★★★	NR	★★★	NR	NR	NR	
41. Lakes Regional Healthcare, Spirit Lake	★★★★★	★★★	NR	NR	NR	★★★	NR	★★★	★	NR	NR	
42. Loring Hospital, Sac City	NR	NR	NR	NR	NR	★★★	NR	★★★	NR	NR	NR	
43. Lucas County Health Center, Chariton	NR	NR	NR	NR	NR	NR	NR	★★★	NR	NR	NR	
44. Madison County Memorial Hospital, Winterset	NR	NR	NR	NR	NR	★★★	NR	★	NR	NR	NR	
45. Mahaska County Hospital, Oskaloosa	★★★★★	★★★	NR	NR	NR	★★★	NR	★★★	NR	NR	NR	
46. Marshalltown Medical and Surgical Center, Marshalltown	★	★★★	NR	NR	NR	★★★	NR	★	★	NR	NR	
47. Mary Greeley Medical Center, Ames	★★★★★	★★★	★★★	★	★★★	★★★	★★★★★	★★★	★★★	NR	★★★	NR
48. Mercy Hospital of Franciscan Sisters–Oelwein, Oelwein	NR	NR	NR	NR	NR	NR	NR	★★★	NR	NR	NR	
49. Mercy Hospital–Iowa City, Iowa City	★★★	★★★	★★★	★★★★★	NR	★★★	★★★	★	NR	★★★	★★★	
50. Mercy Medical Center–Cedar Rapids, Cedar Rapids	★★★	★★★	★★★★★	★★★	★★★	★	★★★	★★★	★★★	NR	★★★	★

KEY: ★★★★★ BEST   ★★★ AS EXPECTED   ★ POOR   NR NOT RATED BY HEALTHGRADES   For full definitions of ratings and awards, see Appendix.

Gastrointestinal Bleed	Gastrointestinal Surgeries and Procedures	Heart Attack	Heart Failure	Hip Fracture Repair	Maternity Care	Pancreatitis	Peripheral Vascular Bypass	Pneumonia	Prostatectomy	Pulmonary Embolism	Resection/Replacement of Abdominal Aorta	Respiratory Failure	Sepsis	Stroke	Total Hip Replacement	Total Knee Replacement	Valve Replacement	Women's Health
★★★	NR	NR	★★★	NR	NR	NR	NR	★★★	NR	NR	NR	NR	★★★★★	★★★	NR	NR	NR	NR
★★★	★	★★★	★★★	★★★★★	★★★	★	NR	★★★	NR	NR	NR	★★★	★★★	★★★	★★★	★★★	NR	NR
★★★	★★★	★★★	★	★★★	NR	★★★	★★★★★	★★★★★	★★★	★	★★★	★	★★★	★★★	★★★	★	★★★	NR
★★★	NR	NR	★	★★★	★★★	NR	NR	★	NR	NR	NR	★	★	NR	NR	NR	NR	NR
NR	NR	NR	★★★	NR	★★★	NR	NR	NR	NR	NR	NR	★★★★★	NR	NR	NR	NR	NR	NR
NR	NR	NR	★★★	NR	★★★	NR	NR	★★★	NR	NR	NR	NR	NR	NR	NR	NR	NR	NR
★★★	NR	★★★	★★★	★	NR	NR	NR	★★★	★	NR	NR	★★★★★	★★★	NR	NR	NR	NR	NR
★	NR	★★★	★★★	★★★	★	NR	NR	★	NR	NR	NR	★★★	NR	NR	NR	NR	NR	NR
★★★	NR	NR	★★★	NR	NR	NR	NR	★★★	NR	NR	NR	NR	★★★	NR	NR	NR	NR	NR
★★★	NR	NR	★★★	NR	★★★	NR	NR	★★★	NR	NR	NR	NR	★★★	NR	NR	NR	NR	NR
★★★	NR	NR	★★★	NR	NR	NR	NR	★	NR	NR	NR	NR	NR	NR	NR	NR	NR	NR
NR	NR	NR	★	NR	NR	NR	NR	★★★	NR	NR	NR	NR	NR	NR	NR	NR	NR	NR
★★★	★★★	★★★	★★★	★★★	★★★	★★★	NR	★★★★★	★★★	★★★	NR	★★★	★★★	★★★	★★★	★★★	NR	NR
★★★	NR	NR	★★★	NR	★	NR	NR	★★★	NR	NR	NR	NR	★★★	NR	NR	NR	NR	NR
NR	NR	NR.	★	NR	★★★	NR	NR	★	NR	NR	NR	NR	★★★	NR	NR	NR	NR	NR
NR	NR	NR	★★★	NR	★	NR	NR	★★★	NR	NR	NR	NR	★★★	NR	NR	NR	NR	NR
★★★	NR	NR	★★★	NR	★	NR	NR	★	NR	NR	NR	★	★★★	NR	NR	NR	NR	NR
★★★	★★★	★★★	★★★	★★★	NR	★★★	NR	★★★	★★★	★★★	NR	★★★	★★★	★★★	★★★	★★★	NR	NR
★★★	NR	★★★	★★★	NR	★★★	NR	NR	★★★★★	NR	NR	NR	NR	★★★	★★★	NR	NR	NR	NR
★★★	NR	NR	★★★	NR	★★★	NR	NR	★★★	NR	NR	NR	NR	★★★	NR	★★★	NR	NR	NR
★★★	NR	★	★★★	★★★	NR	NR	NR	★★★	★★★	NR	NR	★★★	★★★	★★★	★★★	NR	NR	NR
★	★	★	★	★★★	★★★	★★★	★★★	★★★	★★★	★★★	★★★	★	★	★	★★★	★★★	★	★★★
NR	NR	NR	★★★	NR	NR	NR	NR	★★★	NR	NR	NR	NR	NR	NR	NR	NR	NR	NR
★★★	★★★	★★★★★	★★★★★	★★★	★	NR	NR	★★★★★	★★★	★★★	NR	★★★	★★★	★★★	★★★	★★★	NR	NR
★	NR	★★★	★	★	NR	★★★	NR	★	NR	NR	NR	★	NR	NR	NR	NR	NR	NR
★★★	NR	NR	★	NR	★★★	NR	NR	★	NR	NR	NR	NR	★★★	NR	NR	NR	NR	NR
★★★	★★★	★★★★★	★★★★★	★	★	NR	NR	★★★★★	NR	NR	NR	NR	★★★	★★★	★	NR	NR	NR
NR	NR	NR	★★★	NR	NR	NR	NR	★	NR	NR	NR	NR	★★★	NR	NR	NR	NR	NR
★★★	NR	NR	★★★	NR	★★★	NR	NR	★★★	NR	NR	NR	NR	NR	NR	NR	NR	NR	NR
NR	NR	NR	★★★	NR	NR	NR	NR	★★★	NR	NR	NR	NR	★★★	NR	NR	NR	NR	NR
★	NR	★★★★★	★★★	★★★	★★★	NR	NR	★★★	NR	NR	NR	NR	★★★	NR	★★★	NR	NR	NR
★★★	NR	NR	★★★	NR	NR	NR	NR	★★★	NR	NR	NR	NR	NR	NR	NR	NR	NR	NR
★★★	★★★	★	★★★	★★★	NR	★★★	NR	★★★	★★★	★★★	NR	★★★	★★★	★★★	★★★	★★★	★★★	NR
★★★	★★★	★★★	★★★	★★★	NR	★★★	★★★	★★★	★★★	★★★	★★★	★	★★★	★★★	★★★	★★★	★	NR
★	NR	NR	★	NR	★★★	NR	NR	★★★	NR	NR	NR	NR	★★★	NR	NR	NR	NR	NR
★★★	NR	NR	★	★	NR	NR	NR	★★★	NR	NR	NR	NR	★★★	NR	★	NR	NR	NR
★	★	★★★	★	★★★	★★★	NR	★	★★★	★★★	NR	NR	★	★	★★★★★	★★★	NR	NR	NR
NR	NR	NR	★★★	NR	NR	NR	NR	★★★	NR	NR	NR	NR	NR	NR	NR	NR	NR	NR
★★★	NR	★★★	★★★★★	NR	★	★★★	NR	★★★	NR	NR	NR	★★★	★★★	NR	NR	NR	NR	NR
★★★	NR	NR	★★★	NR	★	NR	NR	★★★	NR	NR	NR	NR	★★★	NR	NR	NR	NR	NR
★★★	NR	NR	★★★	★★★	★★★	NR	NR	★	NR	NR	NR	NR	★★★	★★★	★★★★★	NR	NR	NR
★★★	NR	NR	★★★	NR	★	NR	NR	★★★★★	NR	NR	NR	NR	★★★	NR	NR	NR	NR	NR
★★★	NR	NR	★★★	NR	★★★	NR	NR	★	NR	NR	NR	NR	NR	NR	NR	NR	NR	NR
★★★	NR	NR	★	NR	NR	NR	NR	★	NR	NR	NR	NR	★★★	NR	NR	NR	NR	NR
★★★	NR	NR	★★★	★★★	★★★	NR	NR	★★★	NR	NR	NR	NR	★	NR	★★★	NR	NR	NR
★★★	★★★	★★★	★★★	★	★	★★★	NR	★★★	NR	NR	★★★	★★★	★★★	★	★	NR	NR	NR
★★★★★	★★★	★★★	★★★	★	★★★	★★★	NR	★★★	★★★	★★★	NR	★	★★★	★★★	★★★	★★★	NR	NR
★★★	NR	NR	★★★	NR	NR	NR	NR	★★★	NR	NR	NR	NR	NR	NR	NR	NR	NR	NR
★	★★★	★★★	★	★★★	★★★	★★★	NR	★★★	★★★	★★★	★★★	★	★★★	★	★★★	★★★★★	★	★
★★★	★★★	★★★	★★★	★★★	★★★	★★★	★★★	★★★★★	★★★	★★★	★★★	★★★★★	★★★★★	★★★	★	★★★	NR	NR

	Appendectomy	Atrial Fibrillation	Back and Neck Surgery (except Spinal Fusion)	Back and Neck Surgery (Spinal Fusion)	Bariatric Surgery	Bowel Obstruction	Carotid Surgery	Cholecystectomy (Gall Bladder Removal)	Chronic Obstructive Pulmonary Disease (COPD)	Coronary Bypass Surgery	Coronary Interventional Procedures (Angioplasty/Stent)	Diabetic Acidosis an...
51. Mercy Medical Center–Centerville, Centerville	NR	NR	NR	NR	NR	★★★	NR	★★★	★	NR	★★★	NR
52. Mercy Medical Center–Clinton, Clinton	★★★	★★★	NR	NR	NR	★★★	★★★	★★★	★★★	NR	★★★	NR
53. Mercy Medical Center–Des Moines, Des Moines	★★★	★★★	★★★	★★★	★	★★★	★	★	★★★★★	★★★	★★★	★★★
54. Mercy Medical Center–Dubuque, Dubuque	★★★★★	★★★	★★★	★★★	NR	★★★	★★★★★	★★★★★	★★★	★★★	★	NR
55. Mercy Medical Center–North Iowa, Mason City	★★★	★★★	★★★	★★★★★	NR	★★★	★★★★★	★★★	★★★	★★★	★★★★★	★★★
56. Mercy Medical Center–Sioux City, Sioux City	★★★★★	★★★	★★★★★	★★★	★	★★★	★★★★★	★★★★★	★★★	★★★	★★★★★	★★★
57. Metropolitan Medical Center, Des Moines	★★★	★★★	★★★	★★★	★	★★★	★	★	★★★★★	★★★	★★★	★★★
58. Mitchell County Regional Health, Osage	NR	★★★	NR	NR	NR	NR	NR	★★★	NR	NR	NR	NR
59. Montgomery County Memorial Hospital, Red Oak	★	★★★	NR	NR	★	NR	NR	★★★	NR	NR	NR	NR
60. Northwest Iowa Health Center, Sheldon	NR	★★★	NR	NR	★★★	NR	NR	★★★	NR	NR	NR	NR
61. Orange City Area Health System, Orange City	NR	★★★	NR	NR	★★★	NR	NR	★★★	NR	NR	NR	NR
62. Osceola Community Hospital, Sibley	NR	NR	NR	NR	NR	NR	NR	NR	NR	NR	NR	NR
63. Ottumwa Regional Health Center, Ottumwa	★	★★★	NR	NR	NR	★★★	★	★★★	NR	NR	NR	NR
64. Palmer Lutheran Health Center, West Union	NR	NR	NR	NR	NR	NR	NR	★★★	NR	NR	NR	NR
65. Pella Regional Health Center, Pella	★★★	NR	NR	NR	NR	★★★	NR	★★★	NR	NR	NR	NR
66. Regional Health Services of Howard County, Cresco	NR	NR	NR	NR	NR	NR	NR	★★★	NR	NR	NR	NR
67. Regional Medical Center, Manchester	NR	NR	NR	NR	NR	NR	NR	★★★	NR	NR	NR	NR
68. Ringgold County Hospital, Mount Ayr	NR	NR	NR	NR	NR	NR	NR	★★★	NR	NR	NR	NR
69. St. Anthony Regional Hospital, Carroll	★	★★★	NR	NR	NR	★★★	NR	★★★	NR	NR	NR	NR
70. St. Luke's Hospital, Cedar Rapids	★★★★★	★★★	★★★	★★★	★★★	★★★	★★★★★	★★★	★★★	★★★	★★★	★★★
71. St. Luke's Regional Medical Center, Sioux City	★	★★★	★	★	NR	★★★★★	★★★	★★★	★★★	NR	★★★	★★★
72. Sartori Memorial Hospital, Cedar Falls	★★★	★★★	NR	NR	★★★	★★★	NR	★★★	★★★	NR	NR	NR
73. Shelby County Myrtue Memorial Hospital, Harlan	★★★	★★★	NR	NR	NR	★★★	NR	★★★	★★★	NR	NR	NR
74. Shenandoah Memorial Hospital, Shenandoah	NR	NR	NR	NR	NR	NR	NR	★★★	NR	NR	NR	NR
75. Skiff Medical Center, Newton	NR	★★★	NR	NR	NR	★★★	NR	★★★	NR	NR	NR	NR
76. Spencer Municipal Hospital, Spencer	★★★	★★★	NR	NR	NR	★★★	NR	★★★	★★★	NR	NR	NR
77. Stewart Memorial Community Hospital, Lake City	NR	NR	NR	NR	★★★	NR	NR	★★★	★★★	NR	NR	NR
78. Trinity Medical Center–Terrace Park Campus, Bettendorf	★★★	★★★	NR	NR	NR	★★★	★★★	★★★	★★★	NR	★★★	NR
79. Trinity Regional Medical Center, Fort Dodge	★	★★★	NR	★★★	★	★★★	★	★	★	★	★	★★★
80. Unity Hospital, Muscatine	★★★	★★★	NR	NR	NR	★★★	NR	★★★	★	NR	NR	NR
81. University of Iowa Hospital and Clinics, Iowa City	★	★★★	★★★	★	★★★	★★★	★	★★★	★	★★★	★★★	★★★
82. Van Buren County Hospital, Keosauqua	NR	★★★	NR	NR	NR	★★★	NR	★★★	NR	NR	NR	NR
83. Veterans Memorial, Waukon	NR	★★★	NR	NR	NR	★★★	NR	★★★	NR	NR	NR	NR
84. Virginia Gay Hospital, Vinton	NR	NR	NR	NR	NR	NR	NR	★★★	NR	NR	NR	NR
85. Washington County Hospital, Washington	★	★★★	NR	NR	NR	★★★	NR	★★★	NR	NR	NR	NR
86. Waverly Health Center, Waverly	NR	NR	NR	NR	NR	NR	NR	★★★	NR	NR	NR	NR
87. Wayne County Hospital, Corydon	NR	NR	NR	NR	NR	NR	NR	★★★	NR	NR	NR	NR
88. Winneshiek Medical Center, Decorah	NR	★★★	NR	NR	NR	★★★	NR	★★★	NR	NR	NR	NR
89. Wright Medical Center, Clarion	NR	NR	NR	NR	NR	NR	NR	★★★	NR	NR	NR	NR

KEY: ★★★★★ BEST   ★★★ AS EXPECTED   ★ POOR   NR NOT RATED BY HEALTHGRADES   For full definitions of ratings and awards, see Appendix.

Gastrointestinal Bleed	Gastrointestinal Surgeries and Procedures	Heart Attack	Heart Failure	Hip Fracture Repair	Maternity Care	Pancreatitis	Peripheral Vascular Bypass	Pneumonia	Prostatectomy	Pulmonary Embolism	Resection/Replacement of Abdominal Aorta	Respiratory Failure	Sepsis	Stroke	Total Hip Replacement	Total Knee Replacement	Valve Replacement	Women's Health
★★★	NR	★★★	★	★★★	★★★	NR	NR	★	NR	NR	NR	NR	NR	★	NR	NR	NR	NR
★★★	★★★	★★★	★★★	★★★	★★★	★★★	NR	★★★★★	NR	★★★	NR	★★★★★	★★★★★	★	★★★	★★★	NR	NR
★★★★★	★★★	★★★★★	★★★★★	★★★	★★★★★	★★★	★★★	★★★★★	★★★	★★★	★★★	★★★★★	★★★★★	★★★	★★★★★	★	★★★	★★★★★
★★★★★	★★★	★★★	★	★★★★★	★★★	★	★★★	★★★	★★★	★★★	★★★	★	★★★	★★★	★★★★★	★★★	★★★	★★★
★★★	★★★	★★★★★	★★★	★★★	★★★	★★★	NR	★★★★★	★★★	★★★	★★★	★★★	★★★★★	★★★★★	★★★★★	★★★★★	★★★★★	★★★
★	★★★	★★★	★★★	★★★★★	★★★	★★★	★★★	★★★	★★★	★★★	★★★	★	★★★★★	★★★	★★★★★	★★★★★	★★★	★★★
★★★★★	★★★	★★★★★	★★★★★	★★★	★★★★★	★★★	★★★	★★★★★	★★★	★★★	★★★	★★★★★	★★★★★	★★★	★★★★★	★	★★★	★★★★★
★★★	NR	NR	★★★	NR	★	NR	NR	★★★	NR	NR	NR	NR	NR	NR	NR	NR	NR	NR
★★★	NR	NR	★★★	NR	★★★	NR	NR	★★★	NR	NR	NR	NR	★★★	★★★	NR	NR	NR	NR
★★★	NR	NR	★★★	NR	NR	NR	NR	★★★	NR	NR	NR	NR	★	NR	NR	NR	NR	NR
★★★	NR	NR	★	NR	★★★	NR	NR	★★★★★	NR	NR	NR	NR	NR	NR	NR	NR	NR	NR
NR	NR	NR	★	NR	★★★	NR	NR	★	NR	NR	NR	NR	NR	NR	NR	NR	NR	NR
★★★★★	★★★	★★★★★	★★★★★	★★★	NR	NR	NR	★★★★★	NR	NR	NR	★★★★★	★★★★★	★★★	★	★★★	NR	NR
NR	NR	NR	★★★	NR	★★★	NR	NR	★★★	NR	NR	NR	NR	NR	NR	NR	NR	NR	NR
★★★	NR	NR	★★★	★★★	★	NR	NR	★★★	★★★	NR	NR	NR	★★★	★★★	NR	★★★	NR	NR
NR	NR	NR	★	NR	★★★	NR	NR	★	NR	NR	NR	NR	NR	NR	NR	NR	NR	NR
★★★	NR	NR	★★★	NR	★	NR	NR	★★★	NR	NR	NR	NR	NR	★★★	NR	NR	NR	NR
NR	NR	NR	★	NR	NR	NR	NR	★★★	NR	NR	NR	NR	NR	NR	NR	NR	NR	NR
★★★	NR	★★★	★★★	★	★★★	NR	NR	★	NR	NR	NR	NR	★★★	★★★	★★★	★★★	NR	NR
★★★	★★★	★★★★★	★★★★★	★★★★★	NR	★★★★★	★★★	★★★★★	★★★★★	★★★	★★★	★★★★★	★★★★★	★★★	★★★	★★★	★★★	NR
★★★	★★★	★★★	★★★	★★★	★★★	★★★	NR	★★★★★	★★★	★	NR	★★★	★★★	★★★	★★★	★	NR	NR
★	★★★	★★★	★★★	★★★	NR	NR	NR	★★★	NR	NR	NR	NR	★★★	★★★	NR	NR	NR	NR
★★★	NR	NR	★★★	NR	★	NR	NR	★★★	NR	NR	NR	NR	★★★	★★★	NR	NR	NR	NR
★	NR	NR	★★★	NR	★	NR	NR	★★★	NR	NR	NR	NR	NR	NR	NR	NR	NR	NR
★★★	NR	★★★	★★★	★★★	NR	NR	NR	★★★	NR	NR	NR	NR	★★★	NR	NR	★★★	NR	NR
★★★	NR	★★★	★	★★★★★	★	NR	NR	★★★	★★★	NR	NR	NR	★★★	★	★★★★★	★★★★★	NR	NR
★★★	NR	NR	★★★	★★★	★★★	NR	NR	★★★	NR	NR	NR	NR	NR	NR	NR	NR	NR	NR
★★★	★★★	★★★	★★★	★★★	NR	NR	NR	★★★	NR	NR	★	NR	★★★	★★★	★★★	★★★★★	NR	NR
★	★	★	★★★	★	NR	★★★	★★★	★	NR	★★★	NR	★	★	★	★★★	★★★★★	★★★	NR
★★★	★★★	NR	★	★★★	★★★★★	★	NR	★	NR	NR	NR	★	★	★	NR	★★★	NR	NR
★★★	★★★	★★★	★	★	★	★★★	NR	★	★★★	★★★	★★★★★	NR	★	★★★	★★★	★★★	★★★	★
★★★	NR	NR	★★★	NR	★	NR	NR	★★★	NR	NR	NR	NR	★★★	NR	NR	NR	NR	NR
★★★	NR	NR	★★★	★★★	★★★	NR	NR	★	NR	NR	NR	NR	★	NR	NR	NR	NR	NR
NR	NR	NR	★★★	NR	NR	NR	★★★★★	NR	NR	NR	NR	NR	NR	NR	NR	NR	NR	NR
★★★	NR	NR	★★★	NR	★★★	NR	NR	★★★	NR	NR	NR	NR	NR	NR	NR	NR	NR	NR
★★★	NR	NR	★★★	★★★	★★★	NR	NR	★★★	NR	NR	NR	NR	★	NR	NR	★★★	NR	NR
★★★	NR	★	NR	★★★	★★★	NR	NR	★	NR	NR	NR	NR	★	NR	NR	NR	NR	NR
★★★	NR	NR	★★★	★★★	★	NR	NR	★★★	NR	NR	NR	NR	★★★	★	NR	★★★	NR	NR
NR	NR	NR	★★★	NR	★★★	NR	NR	★★★	NR	NR	NR	NR	NR	NR	NR	★★★	NR

KANSAS HOSPITALS: RATINGS BY PROCEDURE

	Appendectomy	Atrial Fibrillation	Back and Neck Surgery (except Spinal Fusion)	Back and Neck Surgery (Spinal Fusion)	Bariatric Surgery	Bowel Obstruction	Carotid Surgery	Cholecystectomy (Gall Bladder Removal)	Chronic Obstructive Pulmonary Disease (COPD)	Coronary Bypass Surgery	Coronary Interventional Procedures (Angioplasty/Stent)	Diabetic Acidosis and
1. Allen County Hospital, Iola	NR	★★★	NR	NR	NR	★★★	NR	NR	★	NR	NR	NR
2. Atchison Hospital, Atchison	NR	★★★	NR	NR	NR	★	NR	NR	★★★	NR	NR	NR
3. Bob Wilson Memorial Hospital, Ulysses	NR	NR	NR	NR	NR	NR	NR	NR	★★★	NR	NR	NR
4. Central Kansas Medical Center, Great Bend	NR	★★★	NR	NR	NR	★	NR	★★★	★	NR	NR	NR
5. Clara Barton Hospital, Hoisington	NR	NR	NR	NR	NR	★★★	NR	NR	NR	NR	NR	NR
6. Coffey County Hospital, Burlington	NR	NR	NR	NR	NR	NR	NR	NR	★	NR	NR	NR
7. Coffeyville Regional Medical Center, Coffeyville	NR	★★★	NR	NR	NR	★★★	NR	★★★	★★★	NR	NR	NR
8. Community Hospital—Onaga, Onaga	NR	NR	NR	NR	NR	NR	NR	NR	★★★	NR	NR	NR
9. Community Memorial Healthcare, Marysville	NR	NR	NR	NR	NR	★★★	NR	NR	★	NR	NR	NR
10. Cushing Memorial Hospital, Leavenworth	NR	★★★	NR	NR	NR	★★★	NR	NR	★★★	NR	NR	NR
11. Fredonia Regional Hospital, Fredonia	NR	NR	NR	NR	NR	NR	NR	NR	★★★	NR	NR	NR
12. Galichia Heart Hospital, Wichita	NR	★★★	NR	NR	NR	NR	★★★	NR	★★★★★	★★★	★★★	NR
13. Geary Community Hospital, Junction City	NR	★★★	NR	NR	NR	★	NR	★	★★★	NR	NR	NR
14. Greenwood County Hospital, Eureka	NR	NR	NR	NR	NR	NR	NR	NR	★★★	NR	NR	NR
15. Harper Hospital District #5, Harper	NR	NR	NR	NR	NR	NR	NR	NR	★★★	NR	NR	NR
16. Hays Medical Center, Hays	NR	★★★	★★★	★★★	NR	★★★	★★★	★★★	★★★	★★★	★★★	NR
17. Heartland Surgical Specialty Hospital, Overland Park	NR	NR	★★★★★	★★★★★	NR	NR	NR	NR	NR	NR	NR	NR
18. Hiawatha Community Hospital, Hiawatha	NR	★★★	NR	NR	NR	NR	NR	NR	★★★	NR	NR	NR
19. Hospital District #1 of Crawford County, Girard	NR	NR	NR	NR	NR	NR	NR	NR	★★★	NR	NR	NR
20. Hospital District #1 of Rice County, Lyons	NR	NR	NR	NR	NR	NR	NR	NR	★★★	NR	NR	NR
21. Hutchinson Hospital, Hutchinson	NR	★★★	★	★	NR	★★★	★	★	★★★	★★★	★	★★★
22. Kansas Heart Hospital, Wichita	NR	★★★	NR	NR	NR	NR	★★★★★	NR	NR	★★★	★★★	NR
23. Kingman Community Hospital, Kingman	NR	NR	NR	NR	NR	★★★	NR	NR	★★★	NR	NR	NR
24. Labette Health, Parsons	NR	★★★	NR	NR	NR	★★★	NR	★	★★★	NR	NR	NR
25. Lawrence Memorial Hospital, Lawrence	NR	★★★	NR	NR	NR	★★★	★★★	★★★	★★★	NR	★★★	NR
26. Logan County Hospital, Oakley	NR	NR	NR	NR	NR	NR	NR	NR	★★★	NR	NR	NR
27. Meade District Hospital, Meade	NR	NR	NR	NR	NR	NR	NR	NR	★★★	NR	NR	NR
28. Medicine Lodge Memorial Hospital, Medicine Lodge	NR	★★★	NR	NR	NR	NR	NR	★	★★★	NR	NR	NR
29. Memorial Hospital, Abilene	NR	NR	NR	NR	NR	★★★	NR	NR	★★★	NR	NR	NR
30. Memorial Hospital, McPherson	NR	NR	NR	NR	NR	★★★	NR	NR	★★★	NR	NR	NR
31. Menorah Medical Center, Overland Park	NR	★★★	★★★	★★★	NR	★★★	★★★★★	★★★	★★★	★★★	★	NR
32. Mercy Health Center, Fort Scott	NR	★★★	NR	NR	NR	★	NR	★★★	★★★	NR	NR	NR
33. Mercy Hospital of Kansas Independence, Independence	NR	NR	NR	NR	NR	★★★	NR	NR	★★★	NR	NR	NR
34. Mercy Regional Health Center, Manhattan	NR	★★★	★★★	NR	NR	★★★	★★★	★★★	★	NR	NR	NR
35. Mitchell County Hospital Health Systems, Beloit	NR	NR	NR	NR	NR	★★★	NR	★★★	★★★	NR	NR	NR
36. Morris County Hospital, Council Grove	NR	NR	NR	NR	NR	NR	NR	NR	★★★	NR	NR	NR
37. Morton County Hospital, Elkhart	NR	NR	NR	NR	NR	★★★	NR	NR	★★★	NR	NR	NR
38. Mt. Carmel Regional Medical Center, Pittsburg	NR	★★★	NR	NR	NR	★★★	NR	★★★	★★★	NR	★★★	NR
39. Neosho Memorial Regional Medical Center, Chanute	NR	★★★	NR	NR	NR	★★★	NR	★★★	NR	NR	NR	NR
40. Newman Regional Health, Emporia	NR	★★★	NR	NR	NR	★★★	★	★★★	★	NR	NR	★★★
41. Newton Medical Center, Newton	NR	★★★	NR	NR	NR	★★★	NR	★★★	★★★	NR	NR	NR
42. Norton County Hospital, Norton	NR	NR	NR	NR	NR	NR	NR	NR	★	NR	NR	NR
43. Olathe Medical Center, Olathe	NR	★	★	★★★	NR	★★★	★★★	★	★	★★★	★★★	★
44. Ottawa County Health Center, Minneapolis	NR	NR	NR	NR	NR	NR	NR	NR	★★★	NR	NR	NR
45. Overland Park Regional Medical Center, Overland Park	NR	★★★	NR	★★★	NR	★★★	★★★	★	★★★	★★★	★★★	NR
46. Phillips County Hospital, Phillipsburg	NR	NR	NR	NR	NR	NR	NR	NR	★★★	NR	NR	NR
47. Pratt Regional Medical Center, Pratt	NR	★★★	NR	NR	NR	★★★	NR	NR	★	NR	NR	NR
48. Providence Medical Center, Kansas City	NR	★★★	★★★★★	★★★★★	NR	★★★	★★★	★★★	★★★	★★★	★★★	★★★
49. Ransom Memorial Hospital, Ottawa	NR	★★★	NR	NR	NR	★★★	NR	NR	★★★	NR	NR	NR
50. Republic County Hospital, Belleville	NR	NR	NR	NR	NR	NR	NR	NR	★★★	NR	NR	NR

KEY: ★★★★★ BEST   ★★★ AS EXPECTED   ★ POOR   NR NOT RATED BY HEALTHGRADES   For full definitions of ratings and awards, see Appendix.

Gastrointestinal Bleed	Gastrointestinal Surgeries and Procedures	Heart Attack	Heart Failure	Hip Fracture Repair	Maternity Care	Pancreatitis	Peripheral Vascular Bypass	Pneumonia	Prostatectomy	Pulmonary Embolism	Resection/Replacement of Abdominal Aorta	Respiratory Failure	Sepsis	Stroke	Total Hip Replacement	Total Knee Replacement	Valve Replacement	Women's Health
★	NR	NR	★★★	NR	NR	NR	NR	★	NR	NR	NR	NR	NR	★★★	NR	NR	NR	NR
★★★	NR	NR	★	NR	NR	NR	NR	★★★	NR	NR	NR	NR	★★★	NR	NR	★★★	NR	NR
NR	NR	NR	★★★	NR	NR	NR	NR	★★★	NR	NR	NR	NR	★★★	NR	NR	NR	NR	NR
★	★★★	★★★	★	★★★	NR	NR	NR	★★★	NR	NR	NR	NR	★★★	★★★	★★★★★	★★★★★	NR	NR
NR	NR	NR	★★★	NR	NR	NR	NR	★★★	NR	NR	NR	NR	NR	NR	NR	NR	NR	NR
★★★	NR	NR	★★★	NR	NR	NR	NR	★	NR	NR	NR	NR	★★★	NR	★	NR	NR	NR
★★★	NR	★★★	★★★	★	NR	NR	★★★★★	★	NR	NR	★★★★★	★★★★★	★★★	NR	NR	NR	NR	NR
★★★	NR	NR	★★★	NR	NR	NR	NR	★★★	NR	NR	NR	NR	★★★	NR	NR	NR	NR	NR
★★★	NR	NR	★★★	NR	NR	NR	NR	★★★	NR	NR	NR	NR	★★★	NR	NR	NR	NR	NR
★★★	NR	NR	★★★	★	NR	NR	NR	★★★	NR	NR	NR	NR	NR	NR	NR	NR	NR	NR
★★★	NR	NR	★★★	NR	NR	NR	NR	★★★	NR	NR	NR	NR	NR	NR	NR	NR	NR	NR
★★★	NR	★★★	★★★	NR	NR	NR	★★★	★★★	NR	NR	★★★	NR	NR	★★★	NR	★★★	★★★	NR
★★★	NR	NR	★★★	NR	NR	NR	NR	★	NR	★★★	NR	NR	★	NR	★	NR	★	NR
NR	NR	NR	★★★	NR	NR	NR	NR	★★★	NR	NR	NR	NR	NR	NR	NR	NR	NR	NR
NR	NR	NR	★★★	NR	NR	NR	NR	★★★	NR	NR	NR	NR	NR	NR	NR	NR	NR	NR
★★★	★★★	★★★	★★★	★★★	NR	★★★	NR	★★★	★★★	★★★	NR	★	★	★★★	★★★★★	★★★★★	★★★	NR
NR	NR	NR	NR	NR	NR	NR	NR	NR	NR	NR	NR	NR	NR	NR	NR	★★★	NR	NR
★★★	NR	NR	★	NR	NR	NR	NR	★★★	NR	NR	NR	NR	NR	NR	NR	NR	NR	NR
★★★	NR	NR	★★★	NR	NR	NR	NR	★★★	NR	NR	NR	NR	NR	NR	NR	NR	NR	NR
NR	NR	NR	★★★	NR	NR	NR	NR	★★★	NR	NR	NR	NR	NR	NR	NR	NR	NR	NR
★	★	★★★	★★★	★	NR	★★★	NR	★★★	★★★	★★★	★★★	★	★	★★★	★★★	★★★	★★★	NR
NR	NR	★★★	★★★★★	NR	NR	NR	★★★	NR	NR	NR	★★★	NR	NR	NR	NR	★★★	NR	NR
★★★	NR	NR	★★★	NR	NR	NR	NR	★★★	NR	NR	NR	★★★★★	NR	NR	NR	NR	NR	NR
★★★	NR	NR	★★★	★★★	NR	NR	NR	★★★	★★★	NR	NR	NR	★	NR	★★★	★★★	NR	NR
★★★	★★★★★	★★★	★★★	★	NR	★★★	NR	★★★	★★★	★★★	NR	★★★	★★★	★★★	NR	★★★	NR	NR
NR	NR	NR	★★★	NR	NR	NR	NR	★★★	NR	NR	NR	NR	NR	NR	NR	NR	NR	NR
NR	NR	NR	★	NR	NR	NR	NR	★★★	NR	NR	NR	NR	NR	NR	NR	★★★	NR	NR
NR	NR	NR	★★★	NR	NR	NR	NR	★★★	NR	NR	NR	NR	NR	NR	NR	★★★	NR	NR
NR	NR	NR	★★★	NR	NR	NR	NR	★★★	NR	NR	NR	NR	NR	★★★	NR	NR	NR	NR
★★★	NR	NR	★★★	NR	NR	NR	NR	★★★	NR	NR	NR	NR	★★★	★★★	NR	NR	NR	NR
★★★	★★★	★★★	★★★	★	NR	★★★	NR	★	★★★	★★★	★★★	★	★★★	★★★	★★★	★	NR	NR
★★★	NR	★★★	★	★★★	NR	NR	NR	★★★	NR	NR	★★★	★	★★★★★	NR	NR	NR	NR	NR
★★★	NR	NR	★★★	★★★	NR	NR	NR	★★★	NR	NR	NR	NR	★★★	NR	★★★★★	NR	NR	NR
★★★	★★★	★★★	★	NR	NR	NR	NR	★★★	★★★	NR	NR	NR	★★★	★★★	★★★	★★★★★	NR	NR
★★★	NR	NR	★★★	NR	NR	NR	NR	★★★	NR	NR	NR	★★★	★★★	★★★	NR	NR	NR	NR
★★★	NR	NR	★	NR	NR	NR	NR	★★★	NR	NR	NR	NR	NR	NR	NR	NR	NR	NR
★★★	NR	NR	★★★	NR	NR	NR	NR	★★★	NR	NR	NR	NR	NR	★★★	NR	NR	NR	NR
★	★★★	★★★	★	★★★	NR	NR	NR	★	★★★	NR	★★★	★★★	★★★	★★★	NR	★★★	NR	NR
★★★	NR	★	★	★	NR	NR	NR	★★★	NR	NR	NR	NR	★★★	★★★	★★★	★	NR	NR
★★★	★★★	★★★	★★★★★	★	NR	★	NR	★★★★★	NR	NR	NR	★★★	NR	★★★	★★★	★	NR	NR
★	★★★	★★★	★★★★★	★★★★★	NR	★★★	NR	★★★	★★★	NR	NR	★★★	★★★	★★★	★★★	NR	NR	NR
NR	NR	NR	★★★	NR	NR	NR	NR	★	NR	NR	NR	NR	NR	NR	NR	NR	NR	NR
★★★	★★★★★	★	★★★	★	NR	NR	★★★	★★★	★★★	NR	★	★★★	★★★	★★★	★★★	★	★★★	NR
NR	NR	NR	★★★	NR	NR	NR	NR	★	NR	NR	NR	NR	NR	NR	NR	NR	NR	NR
★★★	★★★	★★★	★★★	★★★	NR	NR	NR	★★★	★★★	NR	★★★	★★★	★★★	★★★	★★★	★★★	NR	NR
★★★	NR	NR	★★★	NR	NR	NR	NR	★★★	NR	NR	NR	NR	★★★	★★★	★★★	★★★	NR	NR
★	★★★	NR	★	NR	★★★	NR	NR	★★★	NR	NR	NR	NR	★★★	★★★	★★★	★★★	NR	NR
★★★	★★★	★★★	★★★	★★★	NR	★★★	★★★	★★★★★	★★★	★★★	NR	★★★	★★★	★★★	★★★	★★★	NR	NR
★★★	NR	NR	★★★	NR	NR	NR	★★★	★★★	NR	NR	NR	NR	★★★	★★★	NR	★★★	NR	NR
NR	NR	★★★	★	NR	NR	NR	NR	★★★	NR	NR	NR	NR	NR	★★★	NR	★★★	NR	NR

	Appendectomy	Atrial Fibrillation	Back and Neck Surgery (except Spinal Fusion)	Back and Neck Surgery (Spinal Fusion)	Bariatric Surgery	Bowel Obstruction	Carotid Surgery	Cholecystectomy (Gall Bladder Removal)	Chronic Obstructive Pulmonary Disease (COPD)	Coronary Bypass Surgery	Coronary Interventional Procedures (Angioplasty/Stent)	Diabetic Acidosis and C
51. St. Catherine Hospital, Garden City	NR	★★★	NR	NR	NR	★	NR	★★★	★	NR	NR	NR
52. St. Francis Health Center, Topeka	NR	★	★★★	★★★	NR	★★★	★★★	★★★	★★★	★★★	★★★	★★★
53. St. John Hospital, Leavenworth	NR	★★★	NR	NR	NR	★★★	NR	NR	★★★	NR	NR	NR
54. St. Johns Regional Health Center, Salina	NR	★★★	★	★★★	NR	★	★★★	★★★	★	★	★★★	★
55. St. Joseph Medical Center, Wichita	NR	★★★★★	★★★	★★★	NR	★★★	★★★★★	★★★	★★★★★	★★★★★	★★★	★★★
56. St. Luke's South Hospital, Overland Park	NR	★★★	NR	★★★	NR	★★★	NR	★★★	★★★	★★★	★★★	NR
57. Salina Regional Health Center, Salina	NR	★★★	★	★★★	NR	★	★★★	★★★	★	★	★★★	NR
58. Scott County Hospital, Scott City	NR	★★★	NR	NR	NR	NR	NR	NR	★	NR	NR	NR
59. Select Specialty Hospital Wichita, Wichita	NR	★★★	★★★	★★★★★	NR	★★★	★★★★★	★★★★★	★★★	★★★	★★★	★★★
60. Shawnee Mission Medical Center, Shawnee Mission	NR	★★★	★★★	★★★	NR	★★★	★★★	★★★	★★★★★	★★★	★★★	★★★
61. Smith County Memorial Hospital, Smith Center	NR	NR	NR	NR	NR	NR	NR	★	NR	NR	NR	NR
62. South Central Kansas Regional Medical Center, Arkansas City	NR	★★★	NR	NR	NR	★★★	NR	★★★	★★★	NR	★★★	NR
63. Southwest Medical Center, Liberal	NR	★★★	NR	NR	NR	★★★★★	NR	★★★	★	NR	NR	NR
64. Stormont-Vail Healthcare, Topeka	NR	★★★	★★★	★★★	NR	★★★	★★★	★★★	★★★	★	★★★	★★★
65. Sumner Regional Medical Center, Wellington	NR	NR	NR	NR	NR	NR	NR	★★★	NR	NR	NR	NR
66. Susan B. Allen Memorial Hospital, El Dorado	NR	★★★	NR	NR	NR	★	NR	★★★	★★★	NR	NR	NR
67. Trego County Lemke Memorial Hospital, WaKeeney	NR	NR	NR	NR	NR	NR	NR	★★★	NR	NR	NR	NR
68. University of Kansas Hospital, Kansas City	NR	★	★	★★★	NR	★★★	★★★	★★★	★★★★★	★★★	★★★	★★★
69. Via Christi Regional Medical Center, Wichita	NR	★★★★★	★★★	★★★	NR	★★★	★★★★★	★★★	★★★★★	★★★★★	★★★	★★★
70. Wesley Medical Center, Wichita	NR	★★★	★★★	★★★★★	NR	★★★	★★★★★	★★★★★	★★★	★★★	★★★	★★★
71. Western Plains Medical Complex, Dodge City	NR	★★★	NR	NR	NR	★★★	NR	★★★	★★★	NR	★★★	NR
72. William Newton Hospital, Winfield	NR	★★★	NR	NR	NR	★★★	NR	NR	★★★	NR	NR	NR

KEY: ★★★★★ BEST ★★★ AS EXPECTED ★ POOR NR NOT RATED BY HEALTHGRADES For full definitions of ratings and awards, see Appendix.

Gastrointestinal Bleed	Gastrointestinal Surgeries and Procedures	Heart Attack	Heart Failure	Hip Fracture Repair	Maternity Care	Pancreatitis	Peripheral Vascular Bypass	Pneumonia	Prostatectomy	Pulmonary Embolism	Resection/Replacement of Abdominal Aorta	Respiratory Failure	Sepsis	Stroke	Total Hip Replacement	Total Knee Replacement	Valve Replacement	Women's Health
★	★	NR	★	★★★	NR	NR	NR	★	★★★	NR	NR	NR	★	★★★	★	★★★	NR	NR
★★★	★★★	★★★★★	★★★	★★★	NR	★★★	★	★★★★★	★	★★★	★★★	★★★	★★★	★★★★★	★★★	★★★	★★★	NR
★★★	NR	NR	★★★	★★★	NR	NR	NR	★★★★★	NR	NR	NR	NR	★	★★★	NR	NR	NR	NR
★★★	★★★	★★★	★★★	★	NR	★★★	★★★	★	★★★	★★★	★★★	★	★★★	★	★★★	★★★	★★★	NR
★	★★★	★★★★★	★★★	★★★	NR	★★★	★★★	★★★	★★★★★	★★★	★★★	★★★★★	★★★	★★★★★	★★★	★★★	★★★★★	NR
★★★	★★★	★	★★★	★	NR	★★★	NR	★★★	NR	NR	NR	★★★	★★★	★★★	★★★	★	NR	NR
★★★	★★★	★★★	★★★	★	NR	★★★	★★★	★	★★★	★★★	★★★	★	★★★	★	★★★	★★★	★★★	NR
NR	NR	NR	★★★	NR	NR	NR	NR	★★★	NR	NR	NR	NR	NR	NR	NR	NR	NR	NR
★★★	★★★	★★★	★	★★★	NR	★★★★★	★★★	★	★★★★★	★	★★★	★★★	★	★★★	★★★	★★★★★	★★★	NR
★★★	★★★	★★★	★★★★★	★★★★★	NR	★★★	★★★	★★★	★★★	★★★	NR	★★★	★★★	★★★★★	★★★	★	★★★	NR
NR	NR	NR	★★★	NR	NR	NR	NR	★	NR	NR	NR	NR	NR	NR	NR	NR	NR	NR
★★★	NR	NR	★★★	★★★	NR	NR	NR	★★★	NR	NR	NR	★★★	★★★	NR	★★★	NR	NR	NR
★	★★★★★	★★★	★	★	NR	NR	NR	★	NR	NR	NR	★★★	NR	★	NR	★	NR	NR
★★★	★★★	★★★	★★★	★★★	NR	★★★	NR	★★★★★	★	★★★	★★★	★	★★★	★★★★★	★★★	★★★	NR	NR
★★★	NR	NR	★★★	NR	NR	NR	NR	★★★	NR	NR	NR	NR	NR	★★★	NR	NR	NR	NR
★★★	NR	★★★	★	★★★	NR	NR	NR	★★★	★★★	NR	NR	★	★★★	NR	★★★	NR	NR	NR
★★★	NR	NR	★★★	NR	NR	NR	NR	★★★	NR	NR	NR	NR	NR	★★★	NR	NR	NR	NR
★★★	★★★	★★★★★	★★★	★	NR	★★★	★★★	★★★	★★★	★★★	★★★	★	★★★★★	★★★	★★★	★	★★★	NR
★	★★★	★★★★★	★★★	★★★	NR	★★★	★★★	★★★	★★★★★	★★★	★★★	★★★★★	★★★	★★★★★	★★★	★★★	★★★★★	NR
★★★	★★★	★★★	★	★★★	NR	★★★★★	★★★	★	★★★★★	★	★★★	★★★	★	★★★	★★★	★★★★★	★★★	NR
★★★	NR	★★★	★★★	★★★	NR	NR	NR	★★★	NR	NR	NR	★★★	★★★	★★★	★★★	★★★	NR	NR
★★★	★★★	NR	★★★	NR	NR	NR	NR	★★★	NR	NR	NR	★★★	★★★	NR	NR	NR	NR	NR

KENTUCKY HOSPITALS: RATINGS BY PROCEDURE

Hospital	Appendectomy	Atrial Fibrillation	Back and Neck Surgery (except Spinal Fusion)	Back and Neck Surgery (Spinal Fusion)	Bariatric Surgery	Bowel Obstruction	Carotid Surgery	Cholecystectomy (Gall Bladder Removal)	Chronic Obstructive Pulmonary Disease (COPD)	Coronary Bypass Surgery	Coronary Interventional Procedures (Angioplasty/Stent)	Diabetic Acidosis an...
1. ARH Regional Medical Center–Hazard, Hazard	NR	★★★	NR	NR	NR	★★★	NR	★★★	★★★	NR	★★★	★★★
2. Baptist Hospital East, Louisville	NR	★★★	★★★	★	NR	★★★	★★★	★★★	★★★	★★★	★★★	★★★
3. Baptist Hospital Northeast, La Grange	NR	★★★	NR	NR	NR	★★★	NR	★★★	★★★	NR	NR	NR
4. Baptist Regional Medical Center, Corbin	NR	★★★	NR	NR	NR	★★★	★	★★★	★★★	NR	NR	★★★
5. Berea Hospital, Berea	NR	★★★	NR	NR	NR	★★★	NR	NR	★★★	★★★	NR	NR
6. Bluegrass Community Hospital, Versailles	NR	NR	NR	NR	NR	NR	NR	NR	NR	★★★	NR	NR
7. Bourbon Community Hospital, Paris	NR	★★★	NR	NR	NR	★★★	NR	★★★	★★★	NR	NR	NR
8. Caldwell County Hospital, Princeton	NR	NR	NR	NR	★	NR	NR	NR	★★★	NR	NR	NR
9. Cardinal Hill Specialty Hospital, Fort Thomas	NR	★★★	NR	NR	NR	★★★	★	★	★★★★★	NR	NR	★★★
10. Carroll County Hospital, Carrollton	NR	NR	NR	NR	NR	NR	NR	NR	★★★	NR	NR	NR
11. Caverna Memorial Hospital, Horse Cave	NR	NR	NR	NR	NR	NR	NR	NR	★★★	NR	NR	NR
12. Central Baptist Hospital, Lexington	NR	★★★	★	★★★	NR	★★★	NR	★★★	★★★	★★★	★★★	★★★
13. Clark Regional Medical Center, Winchester	NR	★★★	NR	NR	NR	★★★	NR	★★★	★★★	NR	NR	NR
14. Clinton County Hospital, Albany	NR	★★★	NR	NR	NR	★★★	NR	★★★	★★★	NR	NR	NR
15. Crittenden Health Systems, Marion	NR	NR	NR	NR	NR	★★★	NR	★★★	★★★	NR	NR	NR
16. Cumberland County Hospital, Burkesville	NR	★★★	NR	NR	NR	NR	NR	NR	★★★	NR	NR	NR
17. Ephraim McDowell Regional Medical Center, Danville	NR	★★★	NR	NR	NR	★★★	NR	★★★★★	★★★★★	NR	NR	NR
18. Flaget Memorial Hospital, Bardstown	NR	★★★	NR	NR	NR	★★★	NR	NR	★★★	NR	NR	NR
19. Fleming County Hospital, Flemingsburg	NR	★★★	NR	NR	NR	★★★	NR	NR	★★★	NR	NR	NR
20. Fort Logan Hospital, Stanford	NR	NR	NR	NR	NR	NR	NR	NR	★★★	NR	NR	NR
21. Frankfort Regional Medical Center, Frankfort	NR	★★★	NR	NR	NR	★★★	NR	★★★	★★★★★	NR	NR	NR
22. Georgetown Community Hospital, Georgetown	NR	NR	NR	NR	NR	★★★	NR	★★★	★★★	NR	NR	NR
23. Greenview Regional Hospital, Bowling Green	NR	★★★	★★★	★★★	NR	★★★	NR	★★★	★★★	NR	NR	NR
24. Hardin Memorial Hospital, Elizabethtown	NR	★★★	NR	NR	NR	★★★	★★★	★★★★★	★★★	★	★★★	★★★
25. Harlan ARH Hospital, Harlan	NR	★★★	NR	NR	NR	★★★	NR	NR	★★★	NR	NR	NR
26. Harrison Memorial Hospital, Cynthiana	NR	★★★	NR	NR	NR	★★★	NR	NR	★★★	NR	NR	NR
27. Highlands Regional Medical Center, Prestonsburg	NR	★	NR	NR	NR	★★★★★	NR	★★★	★★★	NR	NR	★★★
28. Jackson Purchase Medical Center, Mayfield	NR	★★★	★★★	★★★	NR	★★★	NR	★★★	★★★	NR	NR	NR
29. James B. Haggin Memorial Hospital, Harrodsburg	NR	NR	NR	NR	NR	NR	NR	NR	★★★	NR	NR	NR
30. Jenkins Community Hospital, Jenkins	NR	NR	NR	NR	NR	NR	NR	NR	★★★	NR	NR	NR
31. Jennie Stuart Medical Center, Hopkinsville	NR	★★★	NR	NR	NR	★★★	★★★	★★★	★★★★★	NR	NR	★★★
32. Jewish Hospital, Louisville	NR	★★★	★	★	NR	★★★★★	★	★★★	★★★★★	★★★	★★★	★★★
33. Jewish Hospital–Shelbyville, Shelbyville	NR	★	NR	NR	NR	★	NR	★★★	★★★	NR	NR	NR
34. Kentucky River Medical Center, Jackson	NR	★★★	NR	NR	NR	NR	NR	NR	★★★★★	NR	NR	★★★
35. King's Daughters Medical Center, Ashland	NR	★	★★★	★★★	NR	★★★	★★★	★★★	★★★★★	★★★★★	★★★	★★★
36. Knox County Hospital, Barbourville	NR	★★★	NR	NR	NR	NR	NR	NR	★★★	NR	NR	NR
37. Lake Cumberland Regional Hospital, Somerset	NR	★★★	★★★★★	★★★	NR	★★★	★★★	★★★★★	★★★	★★★	★★★	★★★
38. Livingston Hospital and Healthcare, Salem	NR	★★★	NR	NR	NR	★★★	NR	NR	★★★	NR	NR	NR
39. Logan Memorial Hospital, Russellville	NR	NR	NR	NR	NR	NR	NR	NR	★★★	NR	NR	NR
40. Lourdes Hospital, Paducah	NR	★	NR	NR	NR	★★★	★★★★★	★★★	★★★	★★★	★★★	★★★
41. Manchester Memorial Hospital, Manchester	NR	NR	NR	NR	NR	NR	NR	★★★	★★★	NR	NR	NR
42. Marcum and Wallace Memorial Hospital, Irvine	NR	NR	NR	NR	NR	NR	NR	NR	★★★	NR	NR	NR
43. Marshall County Hospital, Benton	NR	NR	NR	NR	NR	★★★	NR	NR	★★★	NR	NR	NR
44. Mary Breckinridge Hospital, Hyden	NR	NR	NR	NR	NR	NR	NR	NR	★★★★★	NR	NR	NR
45. Mary Chiles Hospital, Mount Sterling	NR	★★★	NR	NR	NR	NR	NR	NR	★★★	NR	NR	NR
46. Marymount Medical Center, London	NR	★★★	NR	NR	NR	★★★	NR	★★★	★★★★★	NR	★★★	NR
47. McDowell ARH Hospital, McDowell	NR	NR	NR	NR	NR	NR	NR	NR	★★★	NR	NR	NR
48. Meadowview Regional Medical Center, Maysville	NR	★★★	NR	NR	NR	★★★	NR	★★★★★	★★★	NR	NR	NR
49. Medical Center, Bowling Green	NR	★★★	★★★	★★★	NR	★★★	★★★★★	★★★	★★★	★★★	★★★	★★★
50. Medical Center at Franklin, Franklin	NR	NR	NR	NR	NR	NR	NR	NR	★★★	NR	NR	NR

KEY: ★★★★★ BEST ★★★ AS EXPECTED ★ POOR NR NOT RATED BY HEALTHGRADES For full definitions of ratings and awards, see Appendix.

Gastrointestinal Bleed	Gastrointestinal Surgeries and Procedures	Heart Attack	Heart Failure	Hip Fracture Repair	Maternity Care	Pancreatitis	Peripheral Vascular Bypass	Pneumonia	Prostatectomy	Pulmonary Embolism	Resection/Replacement of Abdominal Aorta	Respiratory Failure	Sepsis	Stroke	Total Hip Replacement	Total Knee Replacement	Valve Replacement	Women's Health
★★★	★★★	★	★★★	★★★	NR	★★★	NR	★★★★★	★★★	★	NR	★★★★★	★★★	★★★	NR	★★★	★★★	NR
★★★	★★★	★★★★★	★★★★★	★★★★★	NR	★★★	★★★	★★★★★	★★★	★★★	★★★	★★★★★	★★★★★	★	★★★★★	★★★★★	★★★★★	NR
★★★	NR	★★★	★★★★★	★★★	NR	NR	NR	★★★★★	NR	NR	NR	★★★	★★★★★	★★★★★	★★★	★★★	NR	NR
★	★	★★★	★★★	★★★★★	NR	★★★	NR	★★★	NR	NR	NR	★★★★★	★★★	★★★	★★★	★★★	NR	NR
★★★	NR	NR	★★★	★★★	NR	NR	NR	★★★	NR	NR	NR	NR	★★★	★★★	NR	NR	NR	NR
★★★	NR	NR	★★★	NR	NR	NR	NR	★★★	NR	NR	NR	★★★	NR	NR	NR	NR	NR	NR
★★★	NR	NR	★★★	NR	NR	NR	NR	★★★	NR	NR	NR	★★★	NR	NR	NR	NR	NR	NR
★★★	NR	NR	★	NR	NR	NR	NR	★	NR	NR	NR	NR	NR	★	NR	NR	NR	NR
★★★	★★★	★★★★★	★★★	★	NR	★★★	NR	★★★★★	★	NR	★★★	NR	★★★★★	★★★	NR	★★★	NR	NR
★★★	NR	NR	★★★	★★★★★	NR	NR	NR	★★★	NR	NR	NR	NR	NR	NR	NR	NR	NR	NR
★★★	NR	NR	★★★	NR	NR	NR	NR	★	NR	NR	NR	NR	NR	★★★	NR	NR	NR	NR
★★★★★	★★★	★★★	★★★	★★★	NR	★★★	★★★	★★★★★	★★★	★★★	★★★	★★★	★★★	★★★	★	★	★★★	NR
★★★	NR	★★★★★	★★★★★	★★★	NR	NR	NR	★★★★★	★★★	NR	★★★★★	★★★★★	NR	NR	NR	NR	NR	NR
NR	NR	NR	★	NR	NR	NR	NR	★	NR	NR	NR	NR	NR	★	NR	NR	NR	NR
★	NR	★★★	★★★	NR	NR	NR	NR	★★★	NR	NR	NR	★★★	★★★	★★★	NR	NR	NR	NR
NR	NR	NR	★★★	NR	NR	NR	NR	★	NR	NR	NR	NR	NR	NR	NR	NR	NR	NR
★★★	★	★★★	★★★★★	★★★	NR	★★★	NR	★★★	★★★	★★★	NR	★★★	★★★	★★★	★★★	★★★	NR	NR
★★★	NR	★★★	★★★	★★★★★	NR	NR	NR	★★★	NR	NR	NR	★	★★★	★★★	★★★	NR	NR	NR
★★★	NR	★	★★★	★★★	NR	NR	NR	★★★	NR	NR	NR	★★★	★★★	★★★	NR	NR	NR	NR
NR	NR	NR	★★★	NR	NR	NR	NR	★★★	NR	NR	NR	NR	★	NR	NR	NR	NR	NR
★	★	★★★	★★★	★★★	NR	★★★	NR	★★★	★★★	★★★	NR	★	★	★★★	★★★	★	NR	NR
★★★	NR	NR	★★★	★★★★★	NR	NR	NR	★★★	NR	NR	NR	NR	★★★	NR	NR	NR	NR	NR
★★★	★★★	★★★	★★★	★★★	NR	★★★	NR	★★★	★★★	NR	★★★★★	★★★	★★★	★★★★★	★★★★★	NR	NR	NR
★★★	★★★	★	★★★	★★★	NR	★★★	NR	★★★★★	★★★	★★★	★	★★★★★	★★★★★	★	★★★	★★★	NR	NR
★★★	NR	★★★	★★★	★★★	NR	★★★	NR	★★★	NR	NR	NR	★★★	★★★	NR	NR	NR	NR	NR
★★★	NR	★★★	★★★	★★★	NR	NR	NR	★	NR	NR	NR	NR	★★★	NR	NR	NR	NR	NR
★★★	NR	★★★	★★★	★★★	NR	★	NR	★	NR	★★★	NR	★	★	NR	NR	NR	NR	NR
★★★	NR	★★★★★	★★★	★★★	NR	★★★	NR	★★★	NR	NR	NR	★★★	★	★★★	★★★★★	★★★★★	NR	NR
★★★	NR	NR	★	NR	NR	NR	NR	★	NR	NR	NR	NR	NR	NR	NR	NR	NR	NR
NR	NR	NR	★★★	NR	NR	NR	NR	★★★	NR	NR	NR	NR	NR	NR	NR	NR	NR	NR
★★★★★	★★★	★★★★★	★★★	★★★	NR	★★★	NR	★★★	★★★	NR	★★★	★★★	★★★	★★★	★★★	★★★	NR	NR
★★★	★★★	★★★★★	★★★★★	★★★	NR	★★★	★★★	★★★★★	★★★	★★★★★	★★★	★★★★★	★★★	★★★	★★★	★★★	★★★	NR
★★★	★★★	★★★	★★★	★★★	NR	NR	NR	★★★	NR	NR	NR	★★★	★	★	★★★	★★★	NR	NR
★★★	NR	★★★	★★★	NR	NR	NR	NR	★★★★★	NR	NR	NR	★★★★★	★★★	NR	NR	NR	NR	NR
★★★	★★★	★★★	★★★★★	★★★	NR	★★★	★★★	★★★★★	★★★	★★★	★	★★★★★	★★★	★	★★★	★	★★★	NR
★★★	NR	★★★	★★★	NR	NR	NR	NR	★★★	NR	NR	★	★★★	NR	NR	NR	NR	NR	NR
★★★	★	★★★	★	★★★★★	NR	★★★	★★★	★	NR	★★★	★★★	NR	★★★	★★★	★★★	★★★	NR	NR
★	NR	NR	★	NR	NR	NR	NR	★★★	NR	NR	NR	NR	NR	NR	NR	NR	NR	NR
★★★	NR	NR	★★★	NR	NR	★★★	NR	★★★★★	NR	NR	NR	★★★	NR	NR	NR	NR	NR	NR
★★★	★★★	★★★	★★★	★★★	NR	★★★	★★★	★★★	NR	★★★	NR	★★★	★★★	★★★★★	★★★	★★★	★	NR
★★★	NR	★★★	★★★	NR	NR	NR	NR	★★★	NR	NR	NR	★★★★★	★★★	NR	NR	NR	NR	NR
NR	NR	NR	★★★	NR	NR	NR	NR	★★★	NR	NR	NR	NR	NR	NR	NR	NR	NR	NR
★★★	NR	★★★	★★★	NR	NR	NR	NR	★	NR	NR	NR	NR	★★★	NR	NR	NR	NR	NR
NR	NR	NR	★★★	NR	NR	NR	NR	★★★	NR	NR	NR	NR	NR	NR	NR	NR	NR	NR
★★★	NR	★★★	★★★	★★★	NR	NR	NR	★★★	NR	NR	NR	★★★★★	★★★	NR	★★★	NR	NR	NR
★★★	★★★	★★★★★	★★★	★	NR	★★★	NR	★★★★★	NR	NR	★★★★★	★★★★★	★★★	NR	★★★	NR	NR	NR
NR	NR	★★★	NR	NR	NR	NR	NR	★★★	NR	NR	NR	★★★	NR	NR	NR	★★★	NR	NR
★★★	NR	★★★	★★★	NR	NR	★★★	★★★	★★★	★★★	NR	NR	★★★	★★★	★★★	★★★	★★★	NR	NR
★★★	★	★★★	★★★	★★★★★	NR	★★★	★★★★★	★	★★★	★★★	★★★	★★★★★	★★★	★	★★★	★★★	★★★★★	NR
NR	NR	NR	★	NR	NR	NR	NR	★★★	NR	NR	NR	NR	NR	NR	NR	NR	NR	NR

	Appendectomy	Atrial Fibrillation	Back and Neck Surgery (except Spinal Fusion)	Back and Neck Surgery (Spinal Fusion)	Bariatric Surgery	Bowel Obstruction	Carotid Surgery	Cholecystectomy (Gall Bladder Removal)	Chronic Obstructive Pulmonary Disease (COPD)	Coronary Bypass Surgery	Coronary Interventional Procedures (Angioplasty/Stent)	Diabetic Acidosis an...
51. The Medical Center at Scottsville, Scottsville	NR	NR	NR	NR	NR	NR	NR	NR	★★★	NR	NR	NR
52. Methodist Hospital Union County, Morganfield	NR	NR	NR	NR	NR	NR	NR	NR	★★★	NR	NR	NR
53. Methodist Hospital, Henderson	NR	★★★	NR	NR	NR	★★★	NR	★★★	★★★	NR	NR	★★★
54. Middlesboro ARH Hospital, Middlesboro	NR	★★★	NR	NR	NR	★★★	NR	NR	★★★	NR	NR	NR
55. Monroe County Medical Center, Tompkinsville	NR	NR	NR	NR	NR	NR	NR	NR	★	NR	NR	NR
56. Muhlenberg Community Hospital, Greenville	NR	★★★	NR	NR	NR	★★★	NR	★★★	★★★	NR	NR	NR
57. Murray-Calloway County Hospital, Murray	NR	★★★	NR	NR	NR	★★★	★★★	★★★★★	★★★	NR	NR	★★★
58. New Horizons Health Systems, Owenton	NR	NR	NR	NR	NR	NR	NR	NR	★★★	NR	NR	NR
59. Norton Audubon Hospital, Louisville	NR	★★★	★★★	★	NR	★★★	★★★	★★★	★★★	★★★	★★★	★★★
60. Norton Hospital, Louisville	NR	★★★	★★★	★	NR	★★★	★★★	★★★	★★★	★★★	★★★	★★★
61. Norton Southwest Hospital, Louisville	NR	★★★	★★★	★	NR	★★★	★★★	★★★	★★★	★★★	★★★	★★★
62. Norton Suburban Hospital, Louisville	NR	★★★	★★★	★	NR	★★★	★★★	★★★	★★★	★★★	★★★	★★★
63. Oak Tree Hospital at Baptist Hospital Northeast, La Grange	NR	★★★	NR	NR	NR	★★★	NR	★★★	★★★	NR	NR	NR
64. Oak Tree Hospital at Baptist Regional Medical Center, Corbin	NR	★★★	NR	NR	NR	★★★	NR	★	★★★	NR	NR	★★★
65. Ohio County Hospital, Hartford	NR	★★★	NR	NR	NR	NR	NR	NR	★★★	NR	NR	NR
66. Our Lady of Bellefonte Hospital, Ashland	NR	★★★	NR	NR	NR	★★★	★	★★★	★★★	NR	NR	★★★
67. Our Lady of the Way, Martin	NR	NR	NR	NR	NR	NR	NR	NR	★★★	NR	NR	NR
68. Owensboro Medical Health System, Owensboro	NR	★	★★★★★	★★★	NR	★★★	★★★	★★★★★	★★★	★★★	★★★	★★★
69. Owensboro Mercy Health System Ford, Owensboro	NR	★	★★★★★	★★★	NR	★★★	★★★	★★★★★	★★★	★★★	★★★	★★★
70. Parkway Regional Hospital, Fulton	NR	★★★	NR	NR	NR	NR	NR	★★★	★	NR	NR	NR
71. Pattie A. Clay Regional Medical Center, Richmond	NR	★★★	NR	NR	NR	★★★	★★★★★	★★★	★★★★★	NR	NR	NR
72. Paul B. Hall Regional Medical Center, Paintsville	NR	NR	NR	NR	NR	★★★	NR	★★★	★★★	NR	NR	NR
73. Pikeville Medical Center, Pikeville	NR	★★★	NR	NR	NR	★★★	★★★	★★★★★	★★★	★	★★★	★★★
74. Pineville Community Hospital, Pineville	NR	★★★	NR	NR	NR	★★★	★★★	★★★★★	★★★	NR	NR	NR
75. Regional Medical Center, Madisonville	NR	★★★	★	NR	NR	★★★	★★★	★★★	★★★	★★★	★★★	★★★
76. Rockcastle Hospital Respiratory Care Center, Mount Vernon	NR	★★★	NR	NR	NR	NR	NR	NR	★★★	NR	NR	NR
77. Russell County Hospital, Russell Springs	NR	★★★	NR	NR	NR	★★★	NR	NR	★★★	NR	NR	NR
78. St. Claire Medical Center, Morehead	NR	★★★	NR	NR	NR	★★★	★	★★★	★★★	NR	NR	NR
79. St. Elizabeth Medical Center–South, Edgewood	NR	★★★	★★★★★	NR	NR	★★★	★★★	★★★	★★★★★	★★★	★★★	★★★
80. St. Joseph East, Lexington	NR	★★★	★★★	NR	NR	★★★	NR	★★★	★★★★★	NR	★	NR
81. St. Joseph Hospital, Lexington	NR	★★★	★	★★★★★	NR	★★★	★★★	★★★	★★★	★★★	★★★	★★★
82. St. Luke Hospital East, Fort Thomas	NR	★★★	NR	NR	NR	★★★	★	★	★★★★★	NR	NR	★★★
83. St. Luke Hospital West, Florence	NR	★★★	NR	NR	NR	★★★	★★★	★	★★★	NR	NR	★★★
84. Sts. Mary and Elizabeth Hospital, Louisville	NR	★★★	★	★	NR	★★★★★	★	★★★	★★★★★	★★★	★★★	★★★
85. Samaritan Hospital, Lexington	NR	★★★	NR	NR	NR	★★★	NR	★★★	★★★	NR	NR	NR
86. Select Specialty Hospital Lexington, Lexington	NR	★★★	NR	NR	NR	★★★	NR	★★★	★★★	NR	NR	NR
87. Spring View Hospital, Lebanon	NR	★★★	NR	NR	NR	NR	NR	★	★★★	NR	NR	NR
88. T. J. Samson Community Hospital, Glasgow	NR	★★★	NR	NR	NR	★	★★★	★★★★★	★★★	NR	NR	★★★
89. Taylor Regional Hospital, Campbellsville	NR	★★★	NR	NR	NR	★★★	NR	★	★★★	NR	NR	NR
90. Three Rivers Medical Center, Louisa	NR	★★★	NR	NR	NR	★★★	NR	NR	★★★	NR	NR	NR
91. Trigg County Hospital, Cadiz	NR	NR	NR	NR	NR	NR	NR	NR	★★★	NR	NR	NR
92. Twin Lakes Regional Medical Center, Leitchfield	NR	★★★	NR	NR	NR	★★★	NR	★★★	★★★	NR	NR	★★★
93. University of Kentucky Hospital, Lexington	NR	★	★★★	★★★	NR	★★★	★	★	★★★	★★★	★	★★★
94. University of Louisville Hospital, Louisville	NR	★★★	NR	NR	NR	NR	NR	NR	★★★★★	NR	★★★	NR
95. Wayne County Hospital, Monticello	NR	NR	NR	NR	NR	NR	NR	NR	★★★	NR	NR	NR
96. Western Baptist Hospital, Paducah	NR	★★★	★	★★★	NR	★★★	★★★	★	★★★	★	★★★	★★★
97. Westlake Regional Hospital, Columbia	NR	★★★	NR	NR	NR	NR	NR	NR	★★★	NR	NR	NR
98. Whitesburg ARH Hospital, Whitesburg	NR	★★★	NR	NR	NR	★★★	NR	★	★	NR	NR	NR
99. Williamson ARH Hospital, South Williamson	NR	★	NR	NR	NR	★★★	NR	★★★	★★★	NR	NR	★★★

KEY: ★★★★★ BEST   ★★★ AS EXPECTED   ★ POOR   NR NOT RATED BY HEALTHGRADES   For full definitions of ratings and awards, see Appendix.

Gastrointestinal Bleed	Gastrointestinal Surgeries and Procedures	Heart Attack	Heart Failure	Hip Fracture Repair	Maternity Care	Pancreatitis	Peripheral Vascular Bypass	Pneumonia	Prostatectomy	Pulmonary Embolism	Resection/Replacement of Abdominal Aorta	Respiratory Failure	Sepsis	Stroke	Total Hip Replacement	Total Knee Replacement	Valve Replacement	Women's Health
NR	NR	NR	★★★	NR	NR	NR	NR	★★★	NR	NR	NR	NR	NR	NR	NR	NR	NR	NR
★★★	NR	NR	★★★	NR	NR	NR	NR	★	NR	NR	NR	NR	NR	NR	NR	NR	NR	NR
★★★	★	★★★	★★★	★★★	NR	NR	NR	★★★	★★★	NR	NR	★★★	★★★	★★★	NR	★★★	NR	NR
★★★	NR	NR	★	★	NR	NR	NR	★	NR	NR	NR	★	★★★	NR	NR	NR	NR	NR
★★★	NR	NR	★★★	NR	NR	NR	NR	★	NR	NR	NR	NR	★★★	NR	NR	NR	NR	NR
★★★	★★★	NR	★	NR	NR	★★★	NR	★★★	NR	NR	NR	★★★	★★★	NR	NR	NR	NR	NR
★★★	★	★★★	★	★★★★★	NR	★★★	NR	★	NR	NR	NR	★★★	★★★★★	★	★★★★★	★★★★★	NR	NR
NR	NR	NR	★★★	NR	NR	NR	NR	★★★	NR	NR	NR	NR	NR	NR	NR	NR	NR	NR
★★★★★	★★★	★★★★★	★★★	★★★	NR	★★★	★★★	★★★★★	★★★	★★★	★★★	★★★★★	★★★★★	★★★	★	★★★	★★★	NR
★★★★★	★★★	★★★★★	★★★	★★★	NR	★★★	★★★	★★★★★	★★★	★★★	★★★	★★★★★	★★★★★	★★★	★	★★★	★★★	NR
★★★★★	★★★	★★★★★	★★★	★★★	NR	★★★	★★★	★★★★★	★★★	★★★	★★★	★★★★★	★★★★★	★★★	★	★★★	★★★	NR
★★★★★	★★★	★★★★★	★★★	★★★	NR	★★★	★★★	★★★★★	★★★	★★★	★★★	★★★★★	★★★★★	★★★	★	★★★	★★★	NR
★★★	NR	★★★	★★★★★	★★★	NR	NR	NR	★★★★★	NR	NR	NR	★★★	★★★★★	★★★★★	★★★	★★★	NR	NR
★	★	★★★	★★★	★★★★★	NR	★★★	NR	★★★	NR	NR	NR	★★★★★	★★★	★★★	★★★	★★★	NR	NR
★★★	NR	NR	★★★	NR	NR	NR	NR	★★★	NR	NR	NR	★★★	★★★	NR	NR	NR	NR	NR
★★★	★★★	NR	★★★	★★★	NR	NR	NR	★★★	★★★	NR	NR	★★★★★	★★★★★	★★★	★★★	★★★	★★★	NR
NR	NR	NR	★★★	NR	NR	NR	NR	★★★	NR	NR	NR	NR	NR	NR	NR	NR	NR	NR
★★★	★★★	★★★	★	★★★	NR	★★★	NR	★★★	★	NR	NR	★★★	★★★★★	★	★★★★★	★★★★★	NR	NR
★★★	★★★	★★★	★	★★★	NR	★★★	★★★	★★★	★	NR	★	★★★	★★★★★	★	★★★★★	★★★★★	NR	NR
★	NR	NR	★★★	NR	NR	NR	NR	★★★	NR	NR	NR	NR	★★★	★★★	NR	NR	NR	NR
★★★	NR	★★★	★★★	NR	NR	★★★	NR	★★★	NR	NR	NR	★★★★★	★★★	NR	★	★★★	NR	NR
★★★	NR	NR	★★★	NR	NR	NR	NR	★★★★★	NR	NR	NR	★★★	★★★	NR	NR	NR	NR	NR
★★★	NR	★	★	★★★★★	NR	NR	NR	★★★	★★★	★★★	NR	★★★	★★★	★★★	★★★	★★★	★	NR
★★★	NR	★★★	★★★	NR	NR	NR	NR	★★★	NR	NR	NR	★★★	★	★	NR	NR	NR	NR
★★★	★	★★★	★	★	NR	★★★	NR	★★★	★	NR	NR	★★★	★★★	★★★	★★★	★	NR	NR
★★★	NR	★★★	★	NR	NR	NR	NR	★	NR	NR	NR	NR	NR	NR	NR	NR	NR	NR
★	NR	★★★	★★★	NR	NR	NR	NR	★★★	NR	NR	NR	★★★★★	NR	★★★	NR	NR	NR	NR
★★★	★★★	★★★	★★★	★★★	NR	★★★	NR	★★★★★	★	NR	NR	★★★★★	★★★	★★★	NR	NR	NR	NR
★★★	★★★	★★★★★	★★★★★	★★★★★	NR	★★★	★★★	★★★★★	★★★	★★★	★★★	★★★★★	★★★★★	★★★	★★★	★★★★★	★★★	NR
★★★	★★★	★★★	★	★★★	NR	★	NR	★★★	NR	★★★	NR	★★★	★	★★★	★★★	★★★	NR	NR
★★★	★★★	★★★★★	★★★	★★★	NR	★	NR	★★★	★★★	★★★	★★★	★★★★★	★★★★★	★★★★★	★★★	★★★	★★★	NR
★★★	★★★	★★★★★	★★★	★	NR	★★★	NR	★★★★★	★	NR	★★★	★★★★★	★★★	★★★	NR	★★★	NR	NR
★★★	★★★	★★★★★	★★★★★	★	NR	NR	NR	★★★	★★★	★★★	NR	★★★★★	★★★★★	★★★	NR	NR	NR	NR
★★★	★★★	★★★★★	★★★★★	★★★	NR	★★★	★★★	★★★★★	★★★	★★★★★	★★★	★★★★★	★★★	★★★	★★★	★★★	★★★	NR
★★★	★★★★★	NR	★★★	★★★	NR	NR	NR	★★★	★★★	NR	★★★	NR	★★★	★★★	★★★	★★★	NR	NR
★★★	★★★★★	NR	★★★	★★★	NR	NR	NR	★★★	★★★	NR	★★★	NR	★★★	★★★	★★★	★★★	NR	NR
★★★	NR	★★★	★★★	★★★	NR	NR	NR	★★★	NR	NR	NR	★★★	NR	NR	NR	★	NR	NR
★★★	★★★	★★★	★★★	★★★★★	NR	★★★	NR	★★★	★★★	★★★	NR	★★★	★★★	★★★	★★★	★★★★★	NR	NR
★★★	★★★	★	★★★	★★★	NR	NR	NR	★★★★★	NR	NR	NR	★★★	★★★★★	NR	NR	NR	NR	NR
★	NR	NR	★	NR	NR	★★★	NR	★	NR	NR	NR	★★★	NR	NR	NR	★★★	NR	NR
★★★	NR	NR	★★★	NR	NR	NR	NR	★★★	NR	NR	NR	NR	NR	NR	NR	NR	NR	NR
★	★★★	★★★	★★★	★★★	NR	NR	NR	★★★	★	NR	NR	★	NR	★★★	NR	★★★	NR	NR
★★★	★★★	★	★★★	★	NR	★★★	★★★	★	★★★	★	★★★	★	★★★	NR	★	★★★	NR	NR
★★★	★★★	★★★★★	★★★	★	NR	NR	NR	★★★	NR	NR	NR	★★★	NR	NR	NR	NR	NR	NR
★★★	NR	NR	★	NR	NR	NR	NR	★★★	NR	NR	NR	NR	NR	NR	NR	NR	NR	NR
★★★	★★★	★	★	NR	NR	★★★	★★★	★★★	★	NR	★★★	★★★	★★★★★	★★★	★	★★★	★★★	NR
★★★	NR	NR	★★★	NR	NR	NR	NR	★★★	NR	NR	NR	★★★	NR	NR	NR	NR	NR	NR
★★★	NR	NR	★★★	NR	NR	★★★	NR	★★★	NR	NR	NR	★	★	★★★	NR	NR	NR	NR
★★★	NR	★★★	★★★	NR	NR	NR	NR	★	NR	NR	NR	★★★	★★★	★★★	NR	NR	NR	NR

LOUISIANA HOSPITALS: RATINGS BY PROCEDURE

	Appendectomy	Atrial Fibrillation	Back and Neck Surgery (except Spinal Fusion)	Back and Neck Surgery (Spinal Fusion)	Bariatric Surgery	Bowel Obstruction	Carotid Surgery	Cholecystectomy (Gall Bladder Removal)	Chronic Obstructive Pulmonary Disease (COPD)	Coronary Bypass Surgery	Coronary Interventional Procedures (Angioplasty/Stent)	Diabetic Acidosis an...
1. Abbeville General Hospital, Abbeville	NR	★★★	NR	NR	NR	★	NR	★★★	★★★	NR	★★★	NR
2. Abrom Kaplan Memorial Hospital, Kaplan	NR	NR	NR	NR	NR	NR	NR	NR	★★★	NR	NR	NR
3. Acadian Medical Center, Eunice	NR	★★★	NR	NR	NR	★★★	NR	NR	★★★	NR	NR	NR
4. Allen Parish Hospital, Kinder	NR	NR	NR	NR	NR	NR	NR	NR	★★★	NR	NR	NR
5. American Legion Hospital, Crowley	NR	★★★	NR	NR	NR	★★★	NR	★★★	★	NR	NR	★★★
6. Avoyelles Hospital, Marksville	NR	★★★	NR	NR	NR	★★★	NR	NR	★★★	NR	NR	NR
7. Baton Rouge General Medical Center, Baton Rouge	NR	★★★	NR	NR	NR	★★★	★	★★★	★★★	★★★	★★★	★★★
8. Beauregard Memorial Hospital, Deridder	NR	★★★	NR	NR	NR	★★★	NR	NR	★★★	NR	NR	★
9. Bunkie General Hospital, Bunkie	NR	NR	NR	NR	NR	NR	NR	NR	★★★	NR	NR	NR
10. Byrd Regional Hospital, Leesville	NR	★★★	NR	NR	NR	★★★	NR	NR	★★★★★	NR	NR	★★★
11. Caldwell Memorial Hospital, Columbia	NR	NR	NR	NR	NR	NR	NR	NR	★★★	NR	NR	NR
12. Christus Coushatta Health Care Center, Coushatta	NR	NR	NR	NR	NR	NR	NR	NR	★★★	NR	NR	NR
13. Christus Coushatta Health Care, Coushatta	NR	NR	NR	NR	NR	NR	NR	NR	★★★	NR	NR	NR
14. Christus St. Francis Cabrini Hospital, Alexandria	NR	★★★	★★★	★★★	NR	★★★	★★★	★★★	★★★	★★★	★★★	★★★
15. Christus St. Patrick Hospital, Lake Charles	NR	★★★	★★★	★★★	NR	★★★	★★★	★★★	★★★	★★★	★★★	★★★
16. Christus Schumpert Health System, Shreveport	NR	★★★	★	★★★	NR	★★★	★	★	★★★	★★★	★★★	★★★
17. Citizens Medical Center, Columbia	NR	NR	NR	NR	NR	NR	NR	NR	★★★	NR	NR	NR
18. Columbia Jefferson Medical Center, Jefferson	NR	★★★	NR	NR	NR	★★★	★★★	NR	★★★	NR	★★★	NR
19. Dauterive Hospital, New Iberia	NR	★★★	NR	NR	NR	★★★	★★★	★★★	★★★	NR	★★★	NR
20. Desoto Regional Health System, Mansfield	NR	★★★	NR	NR	NR	★★★	NR	★★★	★★★	NR	NR	NR
21. Doctors' Hospital of Opelousas, Opelousas	NR	★★★	NR	NR	NR	★★★	NR	★	★★★	NR	★	★★★
22. Doctors' Hospital of Shreveport, Shreveport	NR	★★★	NR	NR	★	★★★	NR	NR	★★★	NR	NR	NR
23. Dubuis Hospital Continuing Care Shreveport, Shreveport	NR	★★★	★	★★★	NR	★★★	NR	★	★★★	★★★	★★★	★★★
24. E. A. Conway Medical Center, Monroe	NR	★★★	NR	NR	NR	NR	NR	★	★★★	NR	NR	NR
25. East Jefferson General Hospital, Metairie	NR	★★★	★★★	★★★	NR	★★★	★★★	★★★	★★★★★	★★★★★	★★★	★★★
26. Franklin Foundation Hospital, Franklin	NR	NR	NR	NR	NR	NR	NR	NR	★★★	NR	NR	NR
27. Franklin Medical Center, Winnsboro	NR	★	NR	NR	NR	★	NR	★★★	★★★	NR	NR	NR
28. Glenwood Regional Medical Center, West Monroe	NR	★★★	★	NR	NR	★★★	★★★★★	★★★	★★★	★★★	★★★	★★★
29. Hardtner Medical Center, Olla	NR	NR	NR	NR	NR	NR	NR	NR	★★★	NR	NR	NR
30. Heart Hospital of Lafayette, Lafayette	NR	★★★	NR	NR	NR	NR	★★★	NR	NR	★★★	★★★★★	NR
31. Homer Memorial Hospital, Homer	NR	NR	NR	NR	NR	★★★	NR	NR	★★★	NR	NR	NR
32. Iberia Medical Center, New Iberia	NR	★★★	NR	NR	NR	★★★	★★★	★★★★★	★★★	NR	★★★	★
33. Jackson Parish Hospital, Jonesboro	NR	NR	NR	NR	NR	NR	NR	NR	★★★	NR	NR	NR
34. Jennings American Legion Hospital, Jennings	NR	★	NR	NR	NR	★	NR	★★★	★★★	NR	NR	★★★
35. Lady of the Sea General Hospital, Cut Off	NR	NR	NR	NR	NR	NR	NR	NR	★★★	NR	NR	NR
36. Lafayette General Medical Center, Lafayette	NR	★★★	★★★	★★★★★	NR	★★★	★★★★★	★★★★★	★★★	★	★★★	★
37. Lake Charles Memorial Hospital, Lake Charles	NR	★★★	★	★★★★★	NR	★	★	★★★	★★★	★★★	★★★	★★★
38. Lakeview Regional Medical Center, Covington	NR	★★★	NR	NR	NR	★★★	★★★	★★★	★★★	★★★	★	NR
39. Lallie Kemp Medical Center, Independence	NR	NR	NR	NR	NR	NR	NR	NR	NR	NR	NR	NR
40. Lane Memorial Hospital, Zachary	NR	★★★	NR	NR	NR	★★★	NR	NR	★	NR	NR	★★★
41. Lasalle General Hospital, Jena	NR	NR	NR	NR	NR	★★★	NR	NR	★★★	NR	NR	NR
42. Leonard J Chabert Medical Center, Houma	NR	NR	NR	NR	NR	NR	NR	NR	★	NR	NR	NR
43. Lincoln General Hospital, Ruston	NR	★★★	NR	NR	NR	★★★	NR	★★★	★★★★★	NR	★★★	★
44. Louisiana Heart Hospital, Lacombe	NR	★★★	NR	★★★	NR	NR	★★★	NR	★★★	★★★	★★★	★★★
45. LSU Health Sciences Center–Shreveport, Shreveport	NR	★★★	★	★	NR	NR	NR	★★★	★★★	★★★	★★★	★★★
46. Madison Parish Hospital, Tallulah	NR	NR	NR	NR	NR	NR	NR	NR	★★★	NR	NR	NR
47. Minden Medical Center, Minden	NR	★★★	NR	NR	NR	★★★	NR	★	★★★	NR	★★★	★★★
48. Morehouse General Hospital, Bastrop	NR	★★★	NR	NR	NR	★★★	NR	★	★★★	NR	NR	NR
49. Natchitoches Regional Medical Center, Natchitoches	NR	★	NR	NR	NR	★	NR	★★★	★★★	NR	★★★	NR
50. North Caddo Medical Center, Vivian	NR	★★★	NR	NR	NR	NR	NR	NR	★★★	NR	NR	NR

KEY: ★★★★★ BEST ★★★ AS EXPECTED ★ POOR NR NOT RATED BY HEALTHGRADES For full definitions of ratings and awards, see Appendix.

Gastrointestinal Bleed	Gastrointestinal Surgeries and Procedures	Heart Attack	Heart Failure	Hip Fracture Repair	Maternity Care	Pancreatitis	Peripheral Vascular Bypass	Pneumonia	Prostatectomy	Pulmonary Embolism	Resection/Replacement of Abdominal Aorta	Respiratory Failure	Sepsis	Stroke	Total Hip Replacement	Total Knee Replacement	Valve Replacement	Women's Health
★★★	NR	★	★	★★★★★	NR	NR	NR	★★★	NR	NR	NR	NR	NR	★★★	NR	★★★	NR	NR
NR	NR	NR	★★★	NR	NR	NR	NR	★★★	NR	NR	NR	NR	NR	NR	NR	NR	NR	NR
★	NR	NR	★★★	NR	NR	NR	NR	★	NR	NR	NR	NR	★★★	NR	NR	NR	NR	NR
NR	NR	NR	★★★	NR	NR	NR	NR	★★★	NR	NR	NR	NR	★★★	NR	NR	NR	NR	NR
★★★	★★★	NR	★	★★★	NR	NR	NR	★	NR	NR	NR	★	★★★	NR	★★★	NR	NR	NR
★★★	NR	NR	★	NR	NR	NR	NR	★★★	NR	NR	NR	★★★	★★★	NR	NR	NR	NR	NR
★★★	★★★	★★★★★	★★★	★★★	NR	★★★	★★★	★★★	★★★	★★★	NR	★★★★★	★★★★★	★★★	★	★	★★★	NR
★★★	NR	★★★★★	★★★	★★★	NR	★★★	NR	★★★	NR	NR	NR	★	NR	★★★	NR	NR	NR	NR
NR	NR	NR	★★★	NR	NR	NR	NR	★★★	NR	NR	NR	NR	NR	NR	NR	NR	NR	NR
★★★★★	NR	★★★	★★★	★★★	NR	NR	NR	★★★	NR	NR	NR	★★★	★★★★★	★	NR	★★★	NR	NR
NR	NR	NR	★★★	NR	NR	NR	NR	★★★	NR	NR	NR	NR	NR	NR	NR	NR	NR	NR
★★★	NR	NR	★★★	NR	NR	NR	NR	★★★	NR	NR	NR	★★★	★★★	NR	NR	NR	NR	NR
★★★	NR	NR	★★★	NR	NR	NR	NR	★★★	NR	NR	NR	★★★	★★★	NR	NR	NR	NR	NR
★★★	★★★★★	★★★	★	★★★★★	NR	★★★	NR	★★★	★★★	★★★	★★★	★★★	★★★	★★★	★★★	★★★	★★★	★★★
★	★★★	★★★	★★★	★★★	NR	★★★	★★★★★	★★★	★★★	★★★	NR	★★★	★★★	★★★	★★★	★★★	★★★	★★★
★★★	★★★	★★★	★★★★★	★	NR	★★★	★	★★★★★	★★★	★★★	★★★	★★★	★★★	★★★	★	★	★	NR
NR	NR	NR	★★★★★	NR	NR	NR	NR	★★★	NR	NR	NR	★★★	★★★	NR	NR	NR	NR	NR
★★★	NR	★★★	★★★	★★★	NR	NR	NR	★★★	★★★	NR	NR	★★★	★★★★★	NR	NR	NR	NR	NR
★★★★★	NR	★★★	★★★★★	NR	NR	NR	NR	★★★	★★★	NR	NR	★★★	★	NR	NR	★★★	NR	NR
★★★	NR	NR	★★★	NR	NR	NR	NR	★★★	NR	NR	NR	★★★	★★★	NR	NR	NR	NR	NR
★★★	NR	★	★★★	★	NR	NR	NR	★★★	★	NR	NR	★★★	★	NR	NR	★	NR	NR
★★★	★★★	★★★	NR	NR	NR	NR	NR	★★★	NR	NR	NR	★	NR	★★★	NR	★★★	NR	NR
★★★	★★★	★★★	★★★★★	★	NR	★★★	★	★★★★★	★★★	★★★	★★★	★★★	★★★	★★★	★	★	★	NR
★★★	★★★	★★★	★★★	NR	NR	NR	NR	★★★	NR	NR	NR	NR	★★★	★★★	NR	NR	NR	NR
★★★	★★★	★★★	★★★	★★★	NR	★★★	★★★	★★★★★	★★★	★★★	NR	★	★★★	★★★	★★★	★★★	★★★	NR
★★★	NR	NR	★★★	NR	NR	NR	NR	★★★	NR	NR	NR	★	NR	NR	NR	NR	NR	NR
★	NR	★	★	NR	NR	NR	NR	★	NR	NR	NR	★	NR	NR	NR	NR	NR	NR
★★★★★	★★★	★★★	★★★	★★★★★	NR	★★★	NR	★★★	★★★	★★★★★	NR	★★★★★	★★★★★	★★★	★★★★★	★★★★★	★★★	NR
NR	NR	NR	★★★	NR	NR	NR	NR	★★★	NR	NR	NR	NR	NR	NR	NR	NR	NR	NR
NR	NR	★★★	★★★	NR	NR	NR	NR	NR	NR	NR	NR	NR	NR	NR	NR	NR	★★★	NR
★★★	NR	★	★	NR	NR	NR	NR	★★★	NR	NR	NR	★	NR	★★★	NR	NR	NR	NR
★★★	★★★	★★★	★★★★★	★★★	NR	★	NR	★★★	★★★★★	NR	NR	★★★	★★★	★	★★★	★★★	NR	NR
NR	NR	NR	★	NR	NR	NR	NR	★★★	NR	NR	NR	NR	★	NR	NR	NR	NR	NR
★★★	★★★	★★★★★	★	★	NR	NR	NR	★★★★★	NR	NR	NR	★	NR	★★★	NR	★	NR	NR
★★★	NR	★★★	★★★	NR	NR	NR	NR	★★★★★	NR	NR	NR	NR	★	NR	NR	NR	NR	NR
★★★	★★★	★	★★★	★★★	NR	★★★	★★★	★★★	★★★	★★★	NR	★★★	★★★	★★★	★★★	★★★★★	★	NR
★★★★★	★★★	★★★	★	★★★	NR	★★★	NR	★★★	★★★	★★★	NR	★★★	★★★	★★★	★★★	★★★	NR	NR
★★★	★★★★★	★	★★★	★★★★★	NR	★★★	NR	★	★★★	★	NR	★	NR	★★★	NR	★★★	NR	NR
NR	NR	NR	★★★	NR	NR	NR	NR	★★★★★	NR	NR	NR	NR	NR	NR	NR	NR	NR	NR
★	★★★	★★★	★★★	★★★	NR	NR	NR	★★★	NR	NR	NR	★★★	★	★★★	NR	NR	NR	NR
★★★	NR	★★★	★★★	NR	NR	NR	NR	★★★	NR	NR	NR	NR	★★★	NR	NR	NR	NR	NR
★	NR	★★★	★	NR	NR	NR	NR	★★★	NR	NR	NR	NR	NR	NR	NR	NR	NR	NR
★	★	★	★★★	★★★★★	NR	★	NR	★	NR	★	NR	★★★	★	★★★	NR	NR	NR	NR
★★★	NR	★★★	★★★★★	NR	NR	NR	NR	★★★	NR	NR	NR	★★★	★★★	NR	NR	★★★★★	NR	NR
★★★	★★★	★★★★★	★★★	★★★	NR	NR	NR	★	★★★	NR	NR	★★★	★★★	★	NR	NR	NR	NR
NR	NR	NR	★	NR	NR	NR	NR	★★★	NR	NR	NR	NR	NR	NR	NR	NR	NR	NR
★★★	NR	★	★	NR	NR	NR	NR	★★★	NR	NR	NR	★★★	★	NR	NR	★★★	NR	NR
★★★	NR	★	★	NR	NR	NR	NR	★	NR	NR	NR	NR	★	NR	NR	★★★	NR	NR
★★★	NR	★★★	★★★	★★★	NR	NR	NR	★★★	NR	NR	NR	★★★	★★★	NR	NR	★★★	NR	NR
★★★	NR	NR	★★★	NR	NR	NR	NR	★★★	NR	NR	NR	NR	NR	NR	NR	NR	NR	NR

	Appendectomy	Atrial Fibrillation	Back and Neck Surgery (except Spinal Fusion)	Back and Neck Surgery (Spinal Fusion)	Bariatric Surgery	Bowel Obstruction	Carotid Surgery	Cholecystectomy (Gall Bladder Removal)	Chronic Obstructive Pulmonary Disease (COPD)	Coronary Bypass Surgery	Coronary Interventional Procedures (Angioplasty/Stent)	Diabetic Acidosis an...
51. **North Oaks Medical Center North Campus,** Hammond	NR	***	NR	NR	NR	***	***	***	***	***	***	***
52. **North Oaks Medical Center,** Hammond	NR	***	NR	NR	NR	***	***	***	***	***	***	***
53. **Northshore Regional Medical Center,** Slidell	NR	***	***	NR	NR	***	***	***	***	***	***	NR
54. **Oakdale Community Hospital,** Oakdale	NR	NR	NR	NR	NR	***	NR	NR	***	NR	NR	NR
55. **Ochsner Clinic Foundation,** New Orleans	NR	***	***	***	NR	***	***	***	***	***	***	***
56. **Ochsner Medical Center–Baton Rouge,** Baton Rouge	NR	***	NR	NR	NR	*	NR	***	***	NR	***	***
57. **Ochsner Medical Center–Kenner,** Kenner	NR	***	NR	NR	NR	***	NR	NR	***	***	*	***
58. **Ochsner Medical Center–Westbank,** Gretna	NR	NR	NR	NR	NR	***	NR	NR	***	NR	NR	NR
59. **Ochsner St. Anne General Hospital,** Raceland	NR	NR	NR	NR	NR	***	NR	NR	***	NR	NR	NR
60. **Opelousas General Health System,** Opelousas	NR	***	***	***	NR	***	***	***	***	NR	***	***
61. **Our Lady of Lourdes Regional Medical Center,** Lafayette	NR	***	***	***	NR	*	***	*****	*	*	***	***
62. **Our Lady of the Lake Regional Medical Center,** Baton Rouge	NR	*	***	*	NR	*	***	*	*****	***	***	***
63. **Pointe Coupee General Hospital,** New Roads	NR	NR	NR	NR	NR	NR	NR	NR	***	NR	NR	NR
64. **Rapides Regional Medical Center,** Alexandria	NR	***	*	***	NR	*****	***	***	***	***	***	***
65. **Richardson Medical Center,** Rayville	NR	***	NR	NR	NR	***	NR	NR	***	NR	NR	*
66. **Richland Parish Hospital Delhi,** Delhi	NR	NR	NR	NR	NR	NR	NR	NR	***	NR	NR	NR
67. **River Parishes Hospital,** La Place	NR	***	NR	NR	NR	*	NR	*	***	NR	NR	NR
68. **River West Medical Center,** Plaquemine	NR	***	NR	NR	NR	***	NR	NR	***	NR	NR	NR
69. **Riverbend Rehab Hospital,** Columbia	NR	NR	NR	NR	NR	NR	NR	NR	***	NR	NR	NR
70. **Riverland Medical Center,** Ferriday	NR	NR	NR	NR	NR	NR	NR	NR	***	NR	NR	***
71. **Riverside Medical Center,** Franklinton	NR	NR	NR	NR	NR	NR	NR	NR	***	NR	NR	NR
72. **Sabine Medical Center,** Many	NR	***	NR	NR	NR	***	NR	NR	***	NR	NR	NR
73. **St. Brendan Rehab and Specialty Hospital,** Lafayette	NR	***	***	***	NR	*	***	*****	*	*	***	***
74. **St. Charles Parish Hospital,** Luling	NR	NR	NR	NR	NR	NR	NR	NR	***	NR	NR	NR
75. **St. Elizabeth Hospital,** Gonzales	NR	NR	NR	NR	NR	***	NR	***	***	NR	NR	***
76. **St. Francis Medical Center,** Monroe	NR	***	***	***	NR	***	***	***	***	*****	***	***
77. **St. Francis North Hospital,** Monroe	NR	*	NR	NR	NR	***	NR	***	***	*	***	*
78. **St. Helena Parish Hospital,** Greensburg	NR	NR	NR	NR	NR	NR	NR	NR	***	NR	NR	NR
79. **St. James Parish Hospital,** Lutcher	NR	NR	NR	NR	NR	NR	NR	NR	NR	NR	NR	NR
80. **St. Martin Hospital,** Breaux Bridge	NR	NR	NR	NR	NR	NR	NR	NR	***	NR	NR	NR
81. **St. Tammany Parish Hospital,** Covington	NR	***	***	NR	NR	***	***	***	***	***	***	***
82. **Savoy Medical Center,** Mamou	NR	***	NR	NR	NR	***	NR	***	***	NR	NR	NR
83. **Slidell Memorial Hospital,** Slidell	NR	***	***	NR	NR	***	***	***	***	***	***	***
84. **Southwest Medical Center,** Lafayette	NR	***	NR	NR	NR	***	*****	***	***	***	*****	NR
85. **Springhill Medical Center,** Springhill	NR	***	NR	NR	NR	***	NR	NR	*	NR	NR	NR
86. **Teche Regional Medical Center,** Morgan City	NR	*	NR	NR	NR	*	NR	*	***	NR	NR	NR
87. **Terrebonne General Hospital,** Houma	NR	***	***	*****	NR	***	***	***	***	***	***	***
88. **Thibodaux Regional Medical Center,** Thibodaux	NR	***	NR	NR	NR	*****	*****	*****	***	***	***	***
89. **Touro Infirmary,** New Orleans	NR	***	NR	***	NR	***	***	***	***	*	***	***
90. **Tulane University Hospital,** New Orleans	NR	***	NR	NR	NR	***	***	NR	***	NR	***	***
91. **Union General Hospital,** Farmerville	NR	NR	NR	NR	NR	NR	NR	NR	***	NR	NR	NR
92. **Ville Platte Medical Center,** Ville Platte	NR	***	NR	NR	NR	***	NR	***	***	NR	NR	NR
93. **Washington St. Tammany Parish Medical Center,** Bogalusa	NR	***	NR	NR	NR	***	NR	***	***	NR	NR	NR
94. **West Calcasieu Cameron Hospital,** Sulphur	NR	***	NR	NR	NR	***	NR	*****	***	NR	***	NR
95. **West Carroll Memorial Hospital,** Oak Grove	NR	NR	NR	NR	NR	NR	NR	NR	***	NR	NR	NR
96. **West Jefferson Medical Center,** Marrero	NR	***	NR	***	NR	***	***	***	***	***	*	***
97. **Willis Knighton Bossier Health Center,** Bossier City	NR	*****	***	NR	NR	***	*	***	*****	*	***	***
98. **Willis Knighton Medical Center,** Shreveport	NR	*****	***	*****	NR	*****	***	***	*****	***	***	*
99. **Winn Parish Medical Center,** Winnfield	NR	***	NR	NR	NR	*	NR	NR	*	NR	NR	NR

KEY: ***** **BEST** *** **AS EXPECTED** * **POOR** NR **NOT RATED BY HEALTHGRADES** For full definitions of ratings and awards, see Appendix.

Gastrointestinal Bleed	Gastrointestinal Surgeries and Procedures	Heart Attack	Heart Failure	Hip Fracture Repair	Maternity Care	Pancreatitis	Peripheral Vascular Bypass	Pneumonia	Prostatectomy	Pulmonary Embolism	Resection/Replacement of Abdominal Aorta	Respiratory Failure	Sepsis	Stroke	Total Hip Replacement	Total Knee Replacement	Valve Replacement	Women's Health
★★★	★★★	★★★	★★★	★★★	NR	★★★	★★★	★	★★★	★★★	★★★	★	★★★	★★★	★★★	★★★	NR	NR
★★★	★★★	★★★	★★★	★★★	NR	★★★	★★★	★	★★★	★★★	★★★	★	★	★★★	★★★	★★★	★★★	NR
★★★	NR	★★★	★★★	★★★	NR	NR	NR	★★★	★★★	NR	NR	NR	★★★	★★★	NR	★★★	NR	NR
★★★	NR	NR	★★★	NR	NR	NR	NR	★★★★★	NR	NR	NR	NR	★★★★★	★★★★★	NR	NR	NR	NR
★★★	★★★	★★★	★★★	★	NR	★★★	NR	★★★★★	★★★★★	★★★	★★★	★★★	★★★	★★★	★★★	★	★★★	NR
★★★	NR	★	★★★	★★★	NR	NR	NR	★★★	NR	NR	NR	★★★	★★★	★★★	NR	NR	NR	NR
★★★	NR	★	★★★	NR	NR	NR	NR	★★★	NR	NR	NR	★★★	★	NR	NR	NR	NR	NR
★★★	NR	★★★	★★★	★★★	NR	NR	NR	★★★	NR	NR	NR	★★★	★	★★★	NR	★★★	NR	NR
★	NR	NR	★★★★★	★★★	NR	NR	NR	★★★	NR	NR	NR	★★★	★★★	NR	NR	NR	NR	NR
★★★	★★★	★★★	★★★	★★★	NR	★★★	NR	★★★	★	★★★	NR	★★★	★	★★★	★★★	★★★	NR	NR
★★★	★★★	★	★	★★★★★	NR	★	NR	★★★	★★★	★	NR	★	★★★	★★★	★★★	★	NR	NR
★★★	★	★★★	★	★	NR	★★★	★	★★★	★★★	★★★	★★★	★	★★★	★★★	★★★	★	★★★	NR
NR	NR	NR	★★★	NR	NR	NR	NR	★★★	NR	NR	NR	NR	NR	NR	NR	NR	NR	NR
★★★	★★★	★★★	★★★	★★★	NR	★★★	★★★	★★★	★★★	★★★	★★★	★★★	★★★	★★★	★★★	★★★	★★★	★★★★★
★	NR	★	★★★	NR	NR	NR	NR	★	NR	NR	NR	★	★★★	NR	NR	NR	NR	NR
★★★	NR	NR	★★★	NR	NR	NR	NR	★★★★★	NR	NR	NR	★★★★★	NR	NR	NR	NR	NR	NR
★	NR	★★★	★★★	NR	NR	NR	NR	★	NR	NR	NR	★★★	★	★★★	NR	★	NR	NR
★	NR	★★★	★★★	NR	NR	NR	NR	★★★	NR	NR	NR	★	★★★	NR	NR	NR	NR	NR
NR	NR	NR	★★★	NR	NR	NR	NR	★★★	NR	NR	NR	NR	NR	NR	NR	NR	NR	NR
★★★	NR	★★★	★★★	NR	NR	NR	NR	★★★★★	NR	NR	NR	★★★	★★★	NR	NR	NR	NR	NR
★★★	NR	★★★	★★★	NR	NR	NR	NR	★★★	NR	NR	NR	★★★★★	★★★	NR	NR	NR	NR	NR
★★★	NR	★★★	★★★	NR	NR	NR	NR	★★★	NR	NR	NR	★★★	★★★	NR	NR	NR	NR	NR
★★★	★★★	★	★	★★★★★	NR	★	NR	★★★	★★★	★	NR	★★★	★★★	★★★	★★★	★	★	NR
★★★	★★★	★★★	NR	NR	NR	NR	NR	★★★	NR	NR	NR	★★★	★★★	NR	NR	NR	NR	NR
★★★	★★★	★★★	★★★	★★★★★	NR	★★★	NR	★★★	NR	NR	NR	★★★	★★★	NR	NR	★★★	NR	NR
★★★	NR	★★★	★★★★★	★★★	NR	NR	★★★	★★★	NR	NR	★★★	★★★	★★★	★★★	NR	★★★	★★★	NR
★★★	NR	NR	★★★	NR	NR	NR	NR	★★★	NR	NR	NR	★★★	NR	NR	NR	★★★	NR	NR
★★★	NR	★	★★★	★★★	NR	NR	NR	★★★	NR	NR	NR	★★★	★	★★★	NR	★★★	NR	NR
★★★	★★★	★★★	★★★	★★★	NR	★★★	NR	★★★	★★★	★★★	★★★	★★★	★	★★★	★★★	★★★	★★★	NR
★★★	★★★	★★★	★	★★★	NR	★★★	NR	★★★	★★★	★★★	NR	★★★	★	★★★	NR	★★★	NR	NR
★	★★★	★★★	★★★	★	NR	NR	NR	★★★	★	★★★	NR	★★★	★★★	★★★	★★★	NR	NR	NR
★★★	NR	★★★	★★★	★★★	NR	NR	NR	★★★	★★★	NR	NR	NR	★★★	★★★★★	NR	NR	NR	NR
NR	NR	NR	★★★	NR	NR	NR	NR	★★★	NR	NR	NR	NR	NR	NR	NR	NR	NR	NR
★★★	★★★	NR	★★★★★	NR	NR	NR	NR	★★★★★	★★★	NR	NR	★★★	★★★★★	★★★	NR	NR	NR	NR
★★★	NR	★	★★★	NR	NR	NR	NR	★★★	NR	NR	NR	★★★	★	NR	NR	NR	NR	NR
★★★	★★★	★★★	★★★	★★★	NR	NR	NR	★★★	★	NR	NR	★★★	★★★	NR	NR	★★★	NR	NR
NR	NR	NR	★★★	NR	NR	NR	NR	★★★	NR	NR	NR	★★★	NR	NR	NR	NR	NR	NR
★★★	★★★	★★★	★★★	★★★	NR	★★★	NR	★★★	NR	NR	NR	★★★	★★★★★	★★★	★	★★★	NR	NR
★★★★★	★★★	★★★	★★★★★	★	NR	★★★	NR	★★★★★	★★★	★★★	NR	★★★★★	★★★★★	★★★	★★★	★	NR	NR
★★★	★★★	★★★★★	★★★	NR	NR	★★★	★★★	★★★★★	★★★	★★★	★★★	★★★★★	★★★	★★★	★★★	★★★	★★★	NR
★★★	NR	NR	★★★	NR	NR	NR	NR	★★★	NR	NR	NR	★	NR	NR	NR	NR	NR	NR

MAINE HOSPITALS: RATINGS BY PROCEDURE

Hospital	Appendectomy	Atrial Fibrillation	Back and Neck Surgery (except Spinal Fusion)	Back and Neck Surgery (Spinal Fusion)	Bariatric Surgery	Bowel Obstruction	Carotid Surgery	Cholecystectomy (Gall Bladder Removal)	Chronic Obstructive Pulmonary Disease (COPD)	Coronary Bypass Surgery	Coronary Interventional Procedures (Angioplasty/Stent)	Diabetic Acidosis and C...
1. Aroostook Medical Center, Presque Isle	★★★	★★★	NR	NR	NR	★★★	NR	★★★	★★★	NR	NR	★★★
2. Blue Hill Memorial Hospital, Blue Hill	NR	★★★	NR	NR	NR	NR	NR	★★★	NR	NR	NR	
3. Bridgton Hospital, Bridgton	★★★	★★★	NR	NR	NR	★★★	NR	★★★	★★★	NR	NR	
4. Brighton Medical Center, Portland	★★★★★	★★★	★★★	★★★	★★★	★★★	★★★	★★★	★★★	★★★	★★★★★	★★★
5. Calais Regional Hospital, Calais	NR	★★★	NR	NR	NR	NR	NR	★★★	★★★	NR	NR	
6. Cary Medical Center, Caribou	★★★	★★★	NR	NR	NR	★★★	★★★	★★★	★★★	NR	NR	
7. Central Maine Medical Center, Lewiston	★★★	★★★	★★★	★★★	★	★★★	★★★★★	★★★	★★★	★★★	★★★	★★★
8. Down East Community Hospital, Machias	★★★★★	★★★	NR	NR	NR	★★★	NR	★★★	★★★	NR	NR	
9. Eastern Maine Medical Center, Bangor	★★★	★★★	★★★	★★★	★★★	★★★	★★★	★★★	★★★	★★★	★★★	★★★
10. Franklin Memorial Hospital, Farmington	★	★★★	NR	NR	NR	★★★	NR	★★★	★★★	NR	NR	
11. Henrietta D Goodall Hospital, Sanford	★★★	NR	NR	NR	NR	★	NR	★★★	★★★	NR	NR	
12. Houlton Regional Hospital, Houlton	NR	★★★	NR	NR	NR	★★★	NR	★★★	★★★	NR	NR	
13. Inland Hospital, Waterville	★★★	★★★	★★★	NR	NR	★★★	NR	NR	★★★	NR	NR	
14. Kennebec Valley Medical Center, Augusta	★★★	★★★	★★★	NR	★	★★★	★	★★★	★★★	NR	NR	★★★
15. Maine Coast Memorial Hospital, Ellsworth	★★★	★	NR	NR	NR	★★★	NR	★★★	★★★	NR	NR	
16. Maine General Medical Center, Waterville	★★★	★★★	★★★	NR	★	★★★	★	★★★	★★★	NR	NR	★★★
17. Maine Medical Center, Portland	★★★★★	★★★	★★★	★★★	★★★	★★★	★★★	★★★	★★★	★★★	★★★★★	★★★
18. Mayo Regional Hospital, Dover Foxcroft	★★★★★	NR	NR	NR	NR	★★★	NR	NR	★★★	NR	NR	
19. Mercy Hospital, Portland	★★★	★★★	★★★★★	★★★★★	NR	★★★	★★★	★★★	★★★	NR	NR	★★★
20. Mid Coast Hospital, Brunswick	★	★★★	NR	NR	NR	★★★	NR	★★★	★★★	NR	NR	
21. Miles Memorial Hospital, Damariscotta	NR	★★★	NR	NR	NR	★★★	NR	★★★	★★★	NR	NR	
22. Millinocket Regional Hospital, Millinocket	NR	★★★	NR	NR	NR	NR	NR	★★★	★★★	NR	NR	
23. Mount Desert Island Hospital, Bar Harbor	★★★	★★★	NR	NR	NR	★★★	NR	★★★	★★★	NR	NR	
24. Northern Maine Medical Center, Fort Kent	★★★	★★★	NR	NR	NR	NR	NR	★★★	★★★	NR	NR	
25. Parkview Adventist Medical Center, Brunswick	★	★★★	NR	NR	NR	★★★	NR	★★★	★★★	NR	NR	
26. Penobscot Bay Medical Center, Rockport	★	★	NR	NR	NR	★★★	NR	★★★	★	NR	NR	
27. Penobscot Valley Hospital, Lincoln	NR	★★★	NR	NR	NR	NR	NR	★★★	★★★	NR	NR	
28. Redington Fairview General Hospital, Skowhegan	NR	★★★	NR	NR	NR	★★★	NR	★	★★★	NR	NR	
29. Rumford Hospital, Rumford	NR	★★★	NR	NR	NR	★★★	NR	NR	★★★	NR	NR	
30. St. Andrews Hospital, Boothbay Harbor	NR	NR	NR	NR	NR	NR	NR	NR	★★★	NR	NR	
31. St. Joseph Hospital, Bangor	★★★	★★★	NR	NR	NR	★★★★★	NR	★★★	★★★	NR	NR	
32. St. Mary's Regional Medical Center, Lewiston	★	★★★	★★★	★★★	NR	★	★	★	★★★	NR	NR	
33. Sebasticook Valley Hospital, Pittsfield	NR	★★★	NR	NR	NR	★★★	NR	NR	★★★	NR	NR	
34. Southern Maine Medical Center, Biddeford	★★★	★★★	NR	NR	★	★	NR	★★★	★	NR	NR	★★★
35. Stephens Memorial Hospital, Norway	★	★★★	NR	NR	NR	★★★	NR	★	★★★	NR	NR	
36. Waldo County General Hospital, Belfast	★★★★★	★★★	NR	NR	NR	★★★	NR	NR	★★★	NR	NR	
37. Westbrook Community Hospital, Westbrook	★★★	★★★	★★★★★	★★★★★	NR	★★★	★★★	★★★	★★★	NR	NR	★★★
38. York Hospital, York	★★★	★★★	NR	NR	NR	★★★	NR	★★★	★	NR	★★★	NR

KEY: ★★★★★ BEST   ★★★ AS EXPECTED   ★ POOR   NR NOT RATED BY HEALTHGRADES   For full definitions of ratings and awards, see Appendix.

Gastrointestinal Bleed	Gastrointestinal Surgeries and Procedures	Heart Attack	Heart Failure	Hip Fracture Repair	Maternity Care	Pancreatitis	Peripheral Vascular Bypass	Pneumonia	Prostatectomy	Pulmonary Embolism	Resection/Replacement of Abdominal Aorta	Respiratory Failure	Sepsis	Stroke	Total Hip Replacement	Total Knee Replacement	Valve Replacement	Women's Health
★★★	★	★★★	★★★	★★★	★	NR	NR	★★★	★★★	NR	NR	NR	★★★	★★★	★★★	★★★	NR	NR
★★★	NR	★★★	★	NR	★	NR	NR	★★★	NR	NR	NR	NR	★★★	NR	NR	NR	NR	NR
NR	NR	NR	★★★	NR	★★★	NR	NR	★★★	NR	NR	NR	NR	★★★	NR	NR	NR	NR	NR
★★★	★★★	★★★	★	★★★	★	★★★	★	★★★	★★★	★★★	★★★	★	★★★	★★★	★★★★★	★★★★★	★★★	★
★★★	NR	★★★	★★★	★★★	★	NR	NR	★★★	NR	NR	NR	★★★	★★★	★	NR	NR	NR	NR
★★★	NR	★★★	★★★★★	NR	★	NR	NR	★★★	★	NR	NR	★★★	★★★	★★★	NR	★	NR	NR
★★★	★	★★★	★★★	★	★★★	★★★	★★★	★★★	★★★	★	NR	★★★	★★★	★	★★★★★	★	★★★	★★★
★★★	NR	★★★	★★★	NR	★	NR	NR	★★★	NR	NR	NR	NR	NR	NR	NR	NR	NR	NR
★★★	★★★	★★★	★★★	★	★★★	★★★	★★★	★★★	★★★	★★★	★★★	★	★	★★★	★★★★★	★★★	★★★	★★★
★★★	NR	★★★	★★★★★	★	★★★	NR	NR	★★★★★	NR	NR	NR	★★★	★★★	★★★	NR	★	NR	NR
★	NR	★★★	★★★	★	★★★	NR	NR	★★★	NR	NR	NR	★★★	★★★	★	NR	★★★	NR	NR
★★★	NR	★★★	★★★	★★★	★★★	NR	NR	★★★	NR	NR	NR	NR	NR	★★★	NR	NR	NR	NR
★★★	NR	★★★	★★★	★★★	★★★	NR	NR	★★★	NR	NR	NR	★★★	★★★★★	★★★	NR	★★★	NR	NR
★★★	★★★	★★★★★	★★★	★	★★★	★★★	★★★	★★★	★★★	★★★	NR	★★★★★	★★★★★	★	★	NR	NR	NR
★★★	★★★	★★★	★★★	★★★	★	★★★	★★★	★★★	★★★	NR	NR	★★★	★	NR	★★★	★★★	NR	NR
★★★	★★★	★★★★★	★★★	★	★★★	★★★	★★★	★★★	★★★	NR	NR	★★★★★	★★★★★	★	NR	★	NR	NR
★★★	★★★	★★★	★	★★★	★	★★★	★	★★★	★★★	★★★	★★★	★	★★★	NR	★★★★★	★★★★★	★★★	★
★★★	NR	★★★	★★★	★★★	★★★	NR	★	★★★	★★★	★★★	★★★	★	★★★	★	NR	★★★	NR	NR
★★★	★★★	★★★	★	★★★	★★★	★★★	★★★	★★★	★★★	★★★	★★★	★	★★★	★	NR	★★★	NR	NR
★★★	★★★	NR	★★★	★★★	NR	NR	NR	★★★★★	NR	NR	NR	★★★	★★★	NR	★	NR	NR	NR
★★★	NR	NR	★	★★★	NR	NR	NR	★★★	NR	NR	NR	NR	NR	NR	NR	★★★	NR	NR
★★★	NR	NR	★★★	NR	★★★	NR	NR	★★★	NR	NR	NR	NR	NR	NR	NR	NR	NR	NR
★★★	NR	★★★★★	★★★	NR	★	NR	NR	★★★	NR	NR	NR	★	★★★	NR	NR	NR	NR	NR
★★★	NR	★★★	★★★	★	★	NR	NR	★★★	★	NR	NR	★★★	★★★	★	★	★	NR	NR
★★★	★★★	★	NR	★★★	NR	NR	NR	★★★	NR	NR	NR	★★★★★	★★★★★	★★★	NR	NR	NR	NR
★★★	NR	★★★	NR	★★★	NR	NR	NR	★★★	NR	NR	NR	NR	NR	★★★	NR	NR	NR	NR
NR	NR	NR	★★★	NR	NR	NR	NR	★★★	NR	NR	NR	NR	NR	NR	NR	NR	NR	NR
★★★	★★★	★★★	★★★	★★★★★	NR	★★★★★	NR	★★★	★★★	NR	NR	★★★	★★★	NR	★★★	★★★	NR	NR
★★★	★★★	★★★	★★★	★★★	★★★	NR	NR	★★★	★★★	NR	NR	★★★	★★★	★★★	★★★	★	NR	NR
★★★	NR	★★★	★★★	NR	NR	NR	NR	★★★	NR	NR	NR	NR	★★★	NR	NR	NR	NR	NR
★	★★★	★★★	★★★	★	★★★	★	NR	★	★★★	NR	NR	★	★	NR	★★★	★★★★★	NR	NR
★★★	★★★	★★★	★	★	★	NR	NR	★	NR	NR	NR	★★★	★★★	★★★	★★★	★★★	NR	NR
★★★	NR	★★★	★★★	★★★	★★★	NR	NR	★	★	NR	NR	★★★	★	★	NR	NR	NR	NR
★★★	★★★	★★★	★	★★★	★★★	★★★	★★★	★★★	★★★	★★★	★	★★★	★	★★★	★★★	★★★	NR	NR
★★★	★★★	★	★	★★★	★★★	★★★	NR	★	NR	NR	NR	★	★★★	★	★★★	★★★	NR	NR

MARYLAND HOSPITALS: RATINGS BY PROCEDURE

	Appendectomy	Atrial Fibrillation	Back and Neck Surgery (except Spinal Fusion)	Back and Neck Surgery (Spinal Fusion)	Bariatric Surgery	Bowel Obstruction	Carotid Surgery	Cholecystectomy (Gall Bladder Removal)	Chronic Obstructive Pulmonary Disease (COPD)	Coronary Bypass Surgery	Coronary Interventional Procedures (Angioplasty/Stent)	Diabetic Acidosis and
1. Anne Arundel Medical Center, Annapolis	★	★★★	★★★	★	NR	★★★	★★★	★	★	NR	★★★	★★★
2. Atlantic General Hospital, Berlin	★	★★★	NR	NR	NR	★★★	NR	★	★★★★★	NR	NR	★★★
3. Baltimore Washington Medical Center, Glen Burnie	★★★★★	★★★	★★★	★★★★★	NR	★★★★★	★★★★★	★★★	★★★	NR	★★★	★★★
4. Bon Secours Hospital, Baltimore	★★★	★★★	NR	NR	NR	★★★	NR	★★★	★★★★★	NR	NR	★
5. Calvert Memorial Hospital, Prince Frederick	★★★	★★★	★★★	NR	NR	★★★	★★★	★★★	★★★★★	NR	NR	★★★
6. Carroll Hospital Center, Westminster	★★★	★★★	★★★★★	NR	NR	★★★	★★★	★★★	★★★	NR	NR	★★★
7. Chester River Hospital Center, Chestertown	★★★	★★★	NR	NR	NR	★★★	★	★	★★★	NR	NR	★★★
8. Civista Medical Center, La Plata	★★★	★★★	NR	NR	NR	★★★	NR	★★★	★★★	NR	NR	★★★
9. Doctors Community Hospital, Lanham	★	★★★	★	NR	NR	★★★	★	★★★	★★★★★	NR	NR	★★★
10. Fort Washington Hospital, Fort Washington	★★★	★★★	NR	NR	NR	★★★★★	NR	★★★	★★★	NR	NR	★★★
11. Franklin Square Hospital Center, Baltimore	★★★	★★★	★★★	★★★	★★★	★★★	★★★	★★★★★	★★★	NR	★★★	★★★
12. Frederick Memorial Hospital, Frederick	★	★★★	★★★	★★★	NR	★★★	★	★★★	★★★	NR	★★★	★★★
13. Garrett County Memorial Hospital, Oakland	★★★	★★★	NR	NR	NR	★★★	NR	★★★	★★★	NR	NR	
14. Good Samaritan Hospital, Baltimore	★	★★★	★★★	★	NR	★★★	★★★	★★★	★★★	NR	NR	★★★
15. Greater Baltimore Medical Center, Baltimore	★★★	★★★	★★★	★	★★★	★★★★★	★★★	★★★	★★★★★	NR	NR	★★★
16. Harbor Hospital, Baltimore	★	★★★	★★★	★★★	NR	★★★	★★★	★★★	★★★	NR	NR	★★★
17. Harford Memorial Hospital, Havre De Grace	★★★	★★★★★	NR	NR	★	★★★	NR	★★★	★★★	NR	NR	★★★
18. Holy Cross Hospital, Silver Spring	★	★★★	★★★	★★★	★★★	★★★	★★★	★	★★★	NR	NR	★★★
19. Howard County General Hospital, Columbia	★	★★★	★	★	NR	★★★	★	★	★★★★★	NR	NR	★★★
20. Johns Hopkins Bayview Medical Center, Baltimore	★	★★★	★★★	★	★★★★★	★★★	★	★	★★★★★	NR	NR	★★★★★
21. Johns Hopkins Hospital, Baltimore	★	★★★	★★★	★	NR	★★★	★★★	★★★	★★★	★★★	★	★★★
22. Laurel Regional Hospital, Laurel	★★★	★★★	NR	NR	NR	★★★	NR	★	★★★	NR	NR	★★★
23. Maryland General Hospital, Baltimore	★	★★★	NR	NR	NR	★★★	NR	★★★	★★★	NR	NR	★★★
24. McCready Memorial Hospital, Crisfield	NR	NR	NR	NR	NR	★★★	NR	NR	★★★	NR	NR	NR
25. Memorial Hospital and Med. Ctr.—Cumberland, Cumberland	★	★	NR	NR	NR	★★★	★★★	★★★	★	NR	NR	★★★
26. Memorial Hospital at Easton, Easton	★★★	★★★	★	NR	NR	★★★	★	★★★	★★★	NR	NR	★
27. Mercy Medical Center, Baltimore	★	★★★	★	★★★	NR	★★★	★	★★★	★★★	NR	NR	★★★
28. Montgomery General Hospital, Olney	★	★★★	★★★	★★★	NR	★★★	NR	★★★	★★★	NR	NR	★★★
29. Northwest Hospital Center, Randallstown	★	★★★	NR	★★★	NR	★★★	★	★★★	★★★★★	NR	NR	★★★
30. Peninsula Regional Medical Center, Salisbury	★	★★★	★★★	★★★	★★★	★★★	★★★	★★★	★★★	★	★★★	★★★
31. Prince George's Hospital Center, Cheverly	★★★	★★★	★★★	★★★★★	NR	★★★	★★★	★★★	★★★	★	★★★	★★★
32. Sacred Heart Hospital, Cumberland	★	★★★	★★★	NR	NR	★★★	★★★	★	★★★	★★★★★	★★★	★★★
33. St. Agnes Hospital, Baltimore	★	★★★	★★★	★★★	★★★	★★★	★	★	★★★	NR	★★★	★★★★★
34. St. Joseph Medical Center, Towson	★	★★★	★	★	★	★★★★★	★★★	★	★★★★★	★★★	★	★★★★★
35. St. Mary's Hospital, Leonardtown	★★★	★★★★★	NR	NR	NR	★★★	NR	★★★	★★★★★	NR	NR	★★★
36. Shady Grove Adventist Hospital, Rockville	★	★★★	★★★★★	★	★★★★★	★★★	★	★	★★★	NR	★★★	★★★
37. Sinai Hospital of Baltimore, Baltimore	★★★	★★★	★★★	★	★★★	★★★	★★★	★★★	★★★	★★★	★★★	★★★★★
38. Southern Maryland Hospital Center, Clinton	★	★★★	★★★	NR	NR	★	★★★	★★★	★★★	NR	★★★	★★★
39. Suburban Hospital, Bethesda	★	★★★	★★★	★★★	NR	★★★	★	★★★	★★★	NR	★★★	★★★
40. Union Hospital of Cecil County, Elkton	★★★	★★★	NR	NR	NR	★★★★★	NR	★★★	★★★	NR	NR	★★★
41. Union Memorial Hospital, Baltimore	★★★	★★★	★★★	★★★	★★★	★★★	★★★	★★★	★★★	★★★	★★★★★	★★★
42. University of Maryland Medical Center, Baltimore	★	★★★	★★★	★	★	★★★	★★★	★★★	★★★	★★★	★★★	★★★
43. Upper Chesapeake Medical Center, Bel Air	★★★★★	★★★	★★★	★★★	NR	★★★	★★★	★★★	★★★★★	NR	NR	★★★
44. Washington Adventist Hospital, Takoma Park	★	★★★	NR	NR	NR	★★★	★★★	★★★	★★★★★	★	★★★	★★★
45. Washington County Hospital, Hagerstown	★★★	★★★★★	★★★	★★★	NR	★★★	★★★	★	★★★	NR	NR	★★★

KEY: ★★★★★ BEST   ★★★ AS EXPECTED   ★ POOR   NR NOT RATED BY HEALTHGRADES   For full definitions of ratings and awards, see Appendix.

Gastrointestinal Bleed	Gastrointestinal Surgeries and Procedures	Heart Attack	Heart Failure	Hip Fracture Repair	Maternity Care	Pancreatitis	Peripheral Vascular Bypass	Pneumonia	Prostatectomy	Pulmonary Embolism	Resection/Replacement of Abdominal Aorta	Respiratory Failure	Sepsis	Stroke	Total Hip Replacement	Total Knee Replacement	Valve Replacement	Women's Health
★★★	★★★	★★★	★★★★★	★	★★★	★★★	★★★	★★★	★★★	★★★	★★★	★★★	★★★★★	★★★	★	NR	NR	
★★★	★★★	★★★	★★★★★	★	NR	★★★	NR	★★★★★	NR	NR	NR	★★★★★	★★★	★★★	★	★	NR	NR
★★★★★	★★★	★★★	★★★★★	★★★	NR	★★★	★★★★★	★★★	★★★	★★★	★★★	★★★	★★★	★★★	★	NR	NR	
★★★	★★★	★★★★★	★★★★★	★★★	NR	★★★	NR	★★★	★	NR	NR	★★★	★★★★★	★★★	NR	★	NR	
★★★★★	★★★	★★★	★★★★★	★	★★★	★★★	NR	★★★	NR	★★★	NR	★	★★★	★★★	★	★	NR	
★★★	★★★	★★★	★★★★★	★★★	★★★	★★★	★	★★★	★★★	★★★	★★★	★★★	★★★	★★★	★	NR	NR	
★★★	★★★	★★★	★★★	★	★	★★★	NR	★★★	NR	NR	NR	★★★	★	★	★	★	NR	
★★★	★★★	★★★★★	★★★★★	★★★	★★★	★★★	★★★	★★★★★	★★★	NR	NR	★★★	★★★★★	★★★	★★★	★	NR	
★★★	★★★★★	★	★★★	★★★	NR	★★★	★★★	★★★★★	★★★	★★★	NR	★★★★★	★★★	★★★	★★★	★★★	NR	
★★★	★★★★★	★★★	★★★	NR	NR	NR	NR	★★★	★★★	NR	NR	★★★	★★★	★★★	NR	★★★	NR	
★★★★★	★★★★★	★★★★★	★★★★★	★	★★★	★★★	★★★	★★★★★	★★★★★	★★★	NR	★★★★★	★★★★★	★★★	★★★	★★★	NR	
★★★	★★★	★★★	★★★	★	★★★	★★★	★★★	★★★	★★★	NR	★★★★★	★★★	★★★	★★★	★★★	★	NR	
★★★	NR	★★★	★★★	NR	NR	★★★★★	NR	★★★★★	★	NR	NR	★	★	★★★	★	NR	NR	
★★★	★★★	★★★	★★★★★	★	NR	★★★★★	★★★★★	★★★★★	★★★	NR	NR	★★★	★★★	★★★	★	NR	NR	
★★★	★★★★★	★★★★★	★★★★★	★★★	★★★★★	★★★★★	★★★★★	★★★	★★★★★	★★★	★★★	★★★★★	★★★★★	★★★	★	NR	NR	
★★★	★★★	★★★	★★★★★	★★★	★★★	★★★	★	★★★★★	★★★	★★★	NR	★★★	★★★	★★★	★	NR	NR	
★★★	★★★	★★★	★★★★★	NR	NR	★★★	★	★★★	★★★	★★★	NR	★★★	★★★	★★★	★★★★★	NR	NR	
★★★★★	★★★	★★★	★★★★★	★	★★★★★	★★★	★★★	★★★	★★★	★★★	NR	★★★	★★★	★★★	★	NR	NR	
★★★	★★★	★★★	★★★	★★★	★★★	NR	★★★	★★★★★	★	★★★★★	NR	★★★★★	★★★	★★★	★	NR	NR	
★★★★★	★★★	★★★	★★★	★★★	★★★	★★★	★	★★★★★	★	★★★	NR	★	★	★★★	★	★	NR	
★★★	★★★	★	★★★★★	★	★	★★★	NR	★★★	★★★	★★★	★★★	★★★	★	★★★	NR	★★★	★	★★★
★★★★★	★	★★★	★★★★★	★★★	★★★	★★★	NR	★★★	NR	NR	NR	★★★★★	★★★	★★★	NR	★★★	★	NR
★★★★★	★★★	NR	★★★★★	★★★★★	★	NR	★★★	★★★★★	★★★	NR	NR	★★★★★	★★★	★★★	NR	★★★	★	NR
★★★	NR	NR	★★★	NR	★★★	NR	★★★	★★★	★★★	NR	NR	★★★	★★★	NR	NR	NR	NR	
★★★	★★★	★★★	★★★	★	★★★	★★★	NR	★★★	NR	★★★	NR	★	★★★	★★★	★	NR	★★★	
★★★	★★★	★★★	★★★	★	★★★	★★★	★	★★★	★	★★★	NR	★★★	★	★★★	★★★	★★★	NR	
★★★★★	★★★★★	★★★★★	★★★	★★★	★★★	★★★	★★★	★★★★★	★★★	★★★	★★★	★★★	★★★	★★★	★★★	★★★	NR	
★★★	★★★	★★★	★★★	★	★★★★★	★★★	★★★	★★★	★★★	★★★	NR	★★★	★★★	★	★★★	★★★	NR	
★★★	★★★	★★★★★	★★★★★	★★★	NR	★★★	NR	★★★★★	★	★★★	NR	★★★★★	★★★★★	★	★	NR	NR	
★★★	★★★	★	★★★	★★★★★	★★★	★★★	★	★★★	★★★★★	★★★	★★★	★★★	★★★★★	★★★	★	★★★★★	★	★★★
★★★	★★★	★★★	★★★★★	★★★	★★★	NR	★★★	★★★	NR	★★★	NR	★	★★★	★★★★★	NR	★★★	NR	★★★
★★★	★★★	★★★	★★★	NR	NR	★★★	NR	★★★	★	★★★	★★★	★★★	★★★★★	★★★	NR	NR	★★★★★	NR
★★★★★	★★★	★★★	★★★	★	★★★	★★★	★★★	★★★★★	★★★	★★★	★	★	★★★	NR	★★★	★★★	NR	
★★★★★	★★★	★★★	★★★★★	★	★★★	★★★	★★★	★★★★★	★	★★★	★★★	★★★	★★★★★	★★★★★	★★★	★★★	★★★★★	★★★
★★★★★	★★★	★★★	★★★★★	★★★	★★★	★★★	NR	★★★★★	NR	★★★	NR	★★★	★★★	★★★	★	★	NR	
★★★★★	★★★	★	★★★	★★★	★★★	★★★	★★★	★★★★★	★★★	NR	★★★	★★★★★	★★★	★★★	★★★	NR	NR	
★★★	★★★★★	★★★	★★★	★	★★★	★★★★★	★★★	★★★	★★★	NR	★★★	★★★	★★★	★★★	★★★	★	★★★	
★★★	★★★★★	★★★	★★★	★★★	★★★	★	★★★★★	NR	★★★	NR	★★★	★★★	★★★	★★★	NR	NR	NR	
★★★★★	★★★★★	★★★★★	★★★★★	★★★	NR	★★★	★★★★★	★★★	★★★	★★★★★	★★★★★	★★★★★	★★★	★	★★★	NR	NR	
★★★★★	★★★	★★★	★★★	★★★	★★★	NR	★★★★★	NR	★★★	NR	★★★	★★★	★★★	★	★★★	NR	NR	
★	★★★	★★★	★★★★★	★★★	NR	★★★	★★★	★★★	★★★	★★★	★★★	★	★★★	★★★	★★★	★★★	NR	
★★★	★★★	★	★★★	★★★	★	★★★	★★★	★★★	NR	★★★	★★★	★★★	★	NR	NR	★★★	★	NR
★★★	★★★	★★★	★★★★★	★★★	★★★	★★★★★	★★★	★★★	★★★	NR	★★★★★	★★★	★★★	NR	★★★	★★★★★	NR	NR
★★★	★★★	★★★	★★★★★	★★★	★★★	★★★	★★★	★★★★★	★★★	★★★	NR	★★★	★★★★★	★★★	★★★	★	★	★★★
★★★	★★★	★★★	★★★★★	★★★	★★★	★★★	★★★	★★★	★★★	★★★	NR	★★★	★★★★★	★★★	★★★	★★★★★	NR	NR

MASSACHUSETTS HOSPITALS: RATINGS BY PROCEDURE

	Appendectomy	Atrial Fibrillation	Back and Neck Surgery (except Spinal Fusion)	Back and Neck Surgery (Spinal Fusion)	Bariatric Surgery	Bowel Obstruction	Carotid Surgery	Cholecystectomy (Gall Bladder Removal)	Chronic Obstructive Pulmonary Disease (COPD)	Coronary Bypass Surgery	Coronary Interventional Procedures (Angioplasty/Sten)	Diabetic Acidosis
1. Addison Gilbert Hospital, Gloucester	***	***	NR	NR	NR	***	*	***	***	NR	NR	***
2. Anna Jaques Hospital, Newburyport	***	***	NR	NR	NR	***	NR	***	***	NR	NR	***
3. Athol Memorial Hospital, Athol	NR	NR	NR	NR	NR	***	NR	NR	***	NR	NR	NR
4. Atlanticare Medical Center—Union, Lynn	*	*****	***	***	***	***	***	***	***	***	***	***
5. Baystate Franklin Medical Center, Greenfield	***	***	NR	NR	NR	***	NR	***	***	NR	NR	***
6. Baystate Mary Lane Hospital, Ware	***	***	NR	NR	NR	NR	NR	***	***	NR	NR	NR
7. Baystate Medical Center, Springfield	***	***	***	***	***	*****	*****	***	***	*****	*****	***
8. Berkshire Medical Center, Pittsfield	***	*****	NR	NR	NR	***	***	***	*****	NR	NR	*
9. Beth Israel Deaconess Hospital—Needham, Needham	***	***	NR	NR	NR	***	NR	***	***	NR	NR	***
10. Beth Israel Deaconess Medical Center, Boston	***	***	*	*	***	***	***	*	***	***	***	***
11. Beverly Hospital, Beverly	***	***	NR	NR	NR	***	*	***	***	NR	NR	***
12. Boston Medical Center, Boston	***	***	*****	***	*	***	***	***	***	***	***	***
13. Brigham and Women's Hospital, Boston	*	***	***	*	***	***	*	*	***	***	***	***
14. Brockton Hospital, Brockton	***	***	NR	NR	NR	***	***	***	***	NR	NR	***
15. Cambridge Health Alliance, Cambridge	***	***	NR	NR	NR	***	***	***	***	NR	NR	***
16. Cape Cod Hospital, Hyannis	***	***	***	***	NR	***	***	*****	***	***	*****	***
17. Caritas Carney Hospital, Dorchester	*	***	***	*	NR	***	***	***	*****	NR	NR	***
18. Caritas Good Samaritan Medical Center, Brockton	***	***	NR	NR	NR	***	*	***	***	NR	NR	***
19. Caritas Holy Family Hospital and Medical Center, Methuen	***	***	*****	NR	NR	***	***	***	***	NR	NR	***
20. Caritas Norwood Hospital, Norwood	*	***	***	NR	NR	*****	***	*****	***	NR	NR	***
21. Caritas St. Elizabeth's Medical Center, Boston	***	***	***	NR	***	***	***	***	*****	*	***	***
22. Caritas Southwood Hospital, Norfolk	*	***	***	NR	NR	*****	***	*****	***	NR	NR	***
23. Cooley Dickinson Hospital, Northampton	***	***	NR	***	NR	***	NR	***	*	NR	NR	***
24. Emerson Hospital, Concord	*	***	***	NR	NR	*****	NR	***	***	NR	NR	***
25. Falmouth Hospital, Falmouth	*	***	NR	NR	NR	*****	*****	***	***	NR	NR	NR
26. Faulkner Hospital, Boston	*	***	***	NR	*	***	NR	*	***	NR	NR	***
27. Hallmark Health, Medford	*	***	*****	NR	*	***	***	***	***	NR	NR	***
28. Harrington Memorial Hospital, Southbridge	***	***	NR	NR	NR	***	NR	NR	***	NR	NR	NR
29. HealthAlliance Hospital Burbank Campus, Fitchburg	*****	***	NR	NR	NR	***	***	NR	*****	NR	NR	NR
30. HealthAlliance Hospital Leominster Campus, Leominster	*****	***	NR	NR	NR	***	***	NR	*****	NR	NR	NR
31. Heritage Hospital, Somerville	***	***	NR	NR	NR	***	***	*	***	NR	NR	***
32. Heywood Hospital, Gardner	***	***	NR	NR	NR	***	NR	NR	***	NR	NR	NR
33. Hillcrest Hospital, Pittsfield	***	*****	***	NR	NR	***	***	***	*****	NR	NR	*
34. Holyoke Medical Center, Holyoke	***	***	***	NR	NR	***	***	***	***	NR	NR	***
35. Jordan Hospital, Plymouth	***	***	***	NR	NR	***	NR	***	***	NR	NR	***
36. Lawrence General Hospital, Lawrence	***	***	*****	NR	NR	***	***	***	***	NR	NR	***
37. Leonard Morse Hospital, Natick	***	***	***	***	NR	***	***	*	***	NR	NR	***
38. Lowell General Hospital, Lowell	*	***	***	NR	NR	*	***	***	***	NR	NR	***
39. Malden Hospital, Malden	*	***	*****	NR	*	***	***	***	***	NR	NR	***
40. Marlborough Hospital, Marlborough	***	***	NR	NR	NR	***	NR	NR	***	NR	NR	NR
41. Mary and Arthur Clapham Hospital, Burlington	***	*****	***	***	***	***	***	***	***	*****	***	***
42. Massachusetts General Hospital, Boston	***	***	*	*	***	***	***	*****	*****	***	***	***
43. Melrose-Wakefield Hospital, Melrose	*	***	*****	NR	*	***	***	***	***	NR	NR	***
44. Mercy Medical Center, Springfield	***	***	*	***	NR	***	***	***	***	NR	NR	***
45. Merrimack Valley Hospital, Haverhill	***	***	NR	NR	NR	***	NR	***	***	NR	NR	NR
46. MetroWest Medical Center, Framingham	***	***	***	***	NR	***	***	***	***	NR	NR	***
47. Milford Regional Medical Center, Milford	*	***	***	NR	NR	***	*	***	***	NR	NR	***
48. Milton Hospital, Milton	***	*	*	NR	NR	***	NR	***	*****	NR	NR	***
49. Morton Hospital and Medical Center, Taunton	***	***	NR	NR	***	***	NR	***	***	NR	NR	***
50. Mount Auburn Hospital, Cambridge	***	***	***	NR	NR	***	***	***	***	*****	***	***

KEY: ***** BEST *** AS EXPECTED * POOR NR NOT RATED BY HEALTHGRADES For full definitions of ratings and awards, see Appendix.

Gastrointestinal Bleed	Gastrointestinal Surgeries and Procedures	Heart Attack	Heart Failure	Hip Fracture Repair	Maternity Care	Pancreatitis	Peripheral Vascular Bypass	Pneumonia	Prostatectomy	Pulmonary Embolism	Resection/Replacement of Abdominal Aorta	Respiratory Failure	Sepsis	Stroke	Total Hip Replacement	Total Knee Replacement	Valve Replacement	Women's Health
★★★★★	★★★	★★★	★★★	★	★★★	★★★	NR	★★★★★	★★★	★★★	NR	★★★	★★★	★★★	★	★	NR	NR
★★★	★★★	★★★	★★★	★	★★★	NR	NR	★★★	★	NR	NR	★★★	★	★★★	★★★	★★★	NR	NR
★★★	NR	★★★	★★★	NR	NR	NR	NR	★★★	NR	NR	NR	NR	NR	NR	NR	NR	NR	NR
★★★	★★★	★★★	★★★★★	★★★	★★★	★★★	★★★	★★★★★	★★★★★	★★★	★★★	★★★★★	★★★	★★★★★	★	★★★	★★★★★	★★★
★★★	NR	★★★★★	★★★★★	★★★	★★★	NR	NR	★★★	NR	NR	NR	★	★★★	★★★	NR	NR	NR	NR
★★★	NR	★★★★★	★★★	★★★	★	NR	NR	★★★	NR	NR	NR	★★★	★★★	★★★	NR	NR	NR	NR
★★★	★★★	★★★★★	★★★	★	★★★	★★★	★★★	★★★	★★★	★★★	★★★	★★★	★	★	★★★	★★★	★★★★★	★★★
★★★★★	★★★	★★★★★	★★★	★	★★★	★★★	★	★★★	★	★★★	NR	★★★	★★★	★★★	★★★	★★★	★★★★★	NR
★★★	NR	★★★	★★★★★	★★★	NR	NR	NR	★★★	★★★	NR	NR	★★★	★★★	NR	★★★	★★★	NR	NR
★★★★★	★★★★★	★★★	★★★	★	★★★	★★★	★★★	★★★★★	★★★	★★★	★★★	★★★	★★★	★★★	★★★	★	★★★★★	★★★
★★★★★	★★★	★★★	★★★	★	★★★	★★★	NR	★★★★★	★★★	★★★	NR	★★★	★★★	★★★	★	★	NR	NR
★★★	★★★	★★★	★★★	★	★	★★★	★★★	★★★★★	★★★	★	★★★	★★★	★★★	★★★	★★★	★★★	★★★	★
★★★★★	★★★	★★★	★★★	★	★★★	★	★★★★★	★★★	★★★	★★★	NR	★★★	★	★★★	★★★	★★★	★★★	★★★
★★★	★	★★★	★	★★★	NR	NR	★★★	★★★	★★★	NR	NR	★★★	★	★★★	★★★	★★★	★★★	NR
★★★★★	★★★	★★★	★★★	★	★★★	★★★	★★★	★★★	★	NR	NR	★	★★★	NR	★	NR	NR	NR
★★★★★	★	★★★	★★★	★★★	★★★	★★★	★★★	★★★★★	★★★	★★★	NR	★	★★★	★★★★★	★★★	★★★★★	★★★	★★★
★★★	★★★	★★★	★★★★★	★	NR	NR	★★★	★★★	★★★	NR	NR	★★★	★★★	★	★★★	★	NR	NR
★★★★★	★★★	★★★	★	★	★★★	★★★	★	★★★★★	★★★★★	NR	★	★★★	★★★	★	★★★	★★★	NR	NR
★★★	★★★	★	★★★	★★★	★★★	★★★	★	★★★	★★★	NR	★	★★★	★	★★★	★★★	★★★	NR	NR
★★★	★★★	★	★	★	★★★	★	★★★	★★★★★	★★★	NR	★	★★★	★★★	★★★	★★★	NR	NR	NR
★	★	★★★	★★★	★	★★★	★★★	★★★	★★★	★★★	NR	★★★	★★★	★★★	★★★	★★★	★★★	★★★	★
★★★	★★★	★★★	★	★★★	★	NR	★★★	★★★	★★★	NR	★	★★★	★★★	★★★	★★★	NR	NR	NR
★★★	★★★	★★★★★	★★★	★★★	★★★	★★★	★★★	★★★	★★★	NR	★	★★★	★	★★★	★★★	★★★	NR	NR
★★★	★★★	★★★	★	★	★★★	NR	★★★	★★★	★★★	NR	NR	★	★★★★★	★★★	★★★	NR	NR	NR
★★★	★★★	★★★★★	★★★★★	★	★★★	★★★	★	★★★	★★★	NR	★★★	★★★	★★★	★	★★★	NR	NR	NR
★★★	★★★	★★★	★★★	★	NR	★★★	NR	★	★★★	★★★	NR	★	★★★	★★★	★	NR	NR	NR
★★★	★★★	★★★	★★★	★	★★★★★	★★★	★	★★★	★	★★★	NR	★	★	★★★	★★★	★	NR	NR
★★★	NR	★★★	★	★★★	★★★	NR	NR	★★★	NR	NR	NR	★	★★★	★	NR	★★★	NR	NR
★★★★★	★★★	★★★★★	★★★★★	★★★	★★★	NR	NR	★★★★★	★★★	NR	NR	★★★	★★★★★	★★★★★	★	★	NR	NR
★★★★★	★★★	★★★★★	★★★★★	★★★	★★★	NR	NR	★★★★★	★★★	NR	NR	★★★	★★★★★	★★★★★	★	★	NR	NR
★★★★★	★★★	★★★	★★★	★	★★★	★★★	NR	★★★	★★★	★	NR	★★★	★	★★★	NR	★	NR	NR
★★★	NR	★★★	★★★	★★★	★★★	NR	NR	★	NR	NR	NR	★	★★★	★★★	NR	★★★	NR	NR
★★★★★	★★★	★★★★★	★★★	★	★★★	★★★	★	★★★	★	★★★	NR	★★★	★★★	★★★	★★★	★★★	NR	NR
★★★	★★★	★★★★★	★★★	★★★	★★★	★★★	★★★	★★★	NR	★★★	NR	★★★	★★★	★★★	★★★	★★★	NR	NR
★★★	★★★	★★★	★★★	★★★	★★★	NR	★	★★★	★★★	NR	★	★	★★★	★★★★★	★★★★★	NR	NR	NR
★★★	★★★	★	★	★★★	★★★	★	★★★	★	★★★	NR	★	★	★★★	★★★	★★★	NR	NR	NR
★★★	★★★	★	★★★	★★★	★★★	★★★	★★★★★	★★★	★★★	★★★	★	★	★★★	★	★★★	NR	NR	NR
★★★	★	★★★	★★★	★	★★★	NR	★★★	★★★	NR	NR	★★★	★	★	★★★	★★★	★	NR	NR
★★★	★★★	★★★	★	★★★★★	★★★	★★★	★	★★★	NR	NR	NR	★★★	★	★★★	★★★	NR	NR	NR
★★★	NR	★★★	★★★	NR	NR	★★★	★★★	★★★	NR	★★★	★★★	★★★	★★★★★	★★★	NR	NR	NR	NR
★★★	★★★	★★★	★★★	★★★	NR	★★★	★	★★★	★★★	★★★	★★★	★	★	★	★★★	★★★	NR	NR
★★★★★	★★★	★★★	★	★	★★★	★★★	★	★★★	★★★★★	★	★★★	★★★	★	★	★★★	★★★★★	★★★	★★★
★★★	★★★	★★★	★★★	★	★★★★★	★★★	★	★★★	★	★★★	NR	★	★	★★★	★★★	★	NR	NR
★★★	★	★★★	★	★	★★★	★★★	★★★	★★★	★★★	★★★	NR	★	★	★★★	★	★	NR	NR
★★★	★	★★★	★	★★★	NR	NR	NR	★★★	★★★	NR	★	★★★	★★★★★	★★★	★★★	NR	NR	NR
★★★	★★★	★	★★★	★★★	★★★	NR	★★★	★★★★★	★★★	★★★	★★★	★★★	★	★★★	★★★	NR	NR	NR
★★★	★★★	★★★	★	★★★	NR	NR	★★★	★★★★★	★★★	★★★	NR	★★★	★	★★★	★★★	NR	NR	NR
★★★	★★★	★★★★★	★★★	★★★	NR	★★★	NR	★★★	NR	NR	NR	NR	★★★	★★★	★★★	NR	NR	NR
★★★	★★★	★★★★★	★★★★★	★	★★★	NR	NR	★★★	★★★	NR	★★★	★★★	★★★	★★★	NR	NR	NR	NR
★	★	★★★	★	★	★★★★★	★★★	★★★	★	★★★	★	NR	★★★	★★★	★	★★★	★★★★★	★★★

	Appendectomy	Atrial Fibrillation	Back and Neck Surgery (except Spinal Fusion)	Back and Neck Surgery (Spinal Fusion)	Bariatric Surgery	Bowel Obstruction	Carotid Surgery	Cholecystectomy (Gall Bladder Removal)	Chronic Obstructive Pulmonary Disease (COPD)	Coronary Bypass Surgery	Coronary Interventional Procedures (Angioplasty/Stent)	Diabetic Acidosis
51. Nashoba Valley Medical Center, Ayer	★★★	★★★	NR	NR	NR	★★★	NR	★★★	★★★	NR	NR	NR
52. New England Baptist Hospital, Boston	★	★★★	★	★	NR	★★★	NR	★★★	★★★	NR	NR	NR
53. Newton-Wellesley Hospital, Newton	★★★★★	★★★	★★★	NR	★★★★★	★★★	★★★	★★★★★	★★★	NR	NR	★★★
54. Noble Hospital, Westfield	★★★	★★★	NR	NR	NR	★★★	NR	★	★★★	NR	NR	NR
55. North Adams Regional Hospital, North Adams	★★★★★	★★★	NR	NR	NR	★★★	★	★★★	★★★	NR	NR	NR
56. North Shore Medical Center, Salem	★	★★★★★	★★★	★★★	★★★	★★★	★★★	★★★	★★★	★★★	★★★	★★★
57. Providence Hospital, Holyoke	★★★	★★★	★	★★★	★★★	★★★	★★★	★★★	★★★	NR	NR	★★★
58. Quincy Medical Center, Quincy	★	★★★	NR	NR	NR	★★★	NR	★★★	★★★	NR	NR	★★★
59. St. Anne's Hospital Corporation, Fall River	★	★★★	NR	NR	NR	★★★	NR	★	★★★	NR	NR	★★★
60. St. Vincent Hospital, Worcester	★★★★★	★★★	★★★★★	NR	★★★	★★★	★★★	★	★★★	★★★	★★★	★★★
61. Saints Medical Center, Lowell	★★★	★★★	★★★	NR	★★★	★★★	★★★	★★★	★★★	NR	★★★	★★★
62. Somerville Hospital, Somerville	★★★	★★★	NR	NR	★★★	★★★	★★★	★	★★★	NR	★★★	★★★
63. South Shore Hospital, South Weymouth	★	★★★	★★★	★★★	NR	★★★	★★★	★★★★★	NR	★★★	★★★	★★★
64. Southcoast Hospitals Group—Charlton Memorial, Fall River	★★★	★	★★★	★★★	★★★	★★★	★★★	★★★	★	★★★	★★★★★	★★★
65. Southcoast Hospitals Group—St. Luke's Hospital, New Bedford	★★★	★	★★★	★★★	★★★	★★★	★★★	★★★	★	★★★	★★★★★	★★★
66. Southcoast Hospitals Group—Tobey Hospital, Wareham	NR	★	★★★	★★★	NR	★★★	★★★	★★★	★	★★★	★★★★★	★★★
67. Sturdy Memorial Hospital, Attleboro	★	★★★	NR	NR	NR	★	★★★	★★★	★★★	NR	NR	★★★
68. Tufts-New England Medical Center, Boston	★★★	★★★	★★★	★★★	★★★	★★★	★★★	★★★	★★★	★★★	★★★	★★★
69. UMass Memorial Medical Center, Worcester	★★★	★★★	★★★	★★★★★	★★★★★	★★★	★★★	★★★	★★★	★★★	★★★	★★★
70. UMass Memorial Medical Center—Memorial Campus, Worcester	★★★	★★★	★★★	★★★★★	★★★★★	★★★	★★★	★★★	★★★	★★★	★★★	★★★
71. Whidden Memorial Hospital, Everett	★	★★★	★★★★★	NR	★	★★★	★★★	★★★	★★★	NR	NR	★★★
72. Winchester Hospital, Winchester	★	★★★	NR	NR	★★★★★	★★★	★★★	★	★★★	NR	NR	★★★
73. Wing Memorial Hospital and Medical Center, Palmer	★★★	★★★	NR	NR	NR	★★★	NR	NR	★★★	NR	NR	NR

KEY: ★★★★★ BEST   ★★★ AS EXPECTED   ★ POOR   NR NOT RATED BY HEALTHGRADES   For full definitions of ratings and awards, see Appendix.

Gastrointestinal Bleed	Gastrointestinal Surgeries and Procedures	Heart Attack	Heart Failure	Hip Fracture Repair	Maternity Care	Pancreatitis	Peripheral Vascular Bypass	Pneumonia	Prostatectomy	Pulmonary Embolism	Resection/Replacement of Abdominal Aorta	Respiratory Failure	Sepsis	Stroke	Total Hip Replacement	Total Knee Replacement	Valve Replacement	Women's Health
★★★	★★★	★★★	★★★	★★★	NR	★★★	NR	★★★★★	NR	NR	NR	NR	NR	NR	NR	★★★	NR	NR
★★★	★★★	NR	★★★	★	NR	NR	NR	★★★★★	★★★	NR	NR	NR	★★★	NR	★★★★★	★★★★★	NR	NR
★★★★★	★★★★★	★★★	★★★★★	★★★	★★★★★	★★★★★	NR	★★★★★	★★★	★★★	NR	★★★	★★★	★★★	★★★	★★★	NR	NR
★	★★★	★★★	★★★★★	★	NR	★★★	NR	★★★	NR	NR	NR	★★★	★★★	★★★	NR	★	NR	NR
★★★	★★★	★★★★★	★★★	★★★	★★★	NR	NR	★	NR	NR	NR	★★★	★	★★★	★★★	★★★	NR	NR
★★★	★★★	★★★	★★★★★	★★★	★★★	★★★	★★★	★★★★★	★★★★★	★★★	★★★	★★★★★	★★★	★★★★★	★	★★★	★★★★★	★★★
★★★	★	★★★	★	★	★★★	★★★	★★★	★★★	★★★	★★★	NR	★	★★★	★	★	★★★	NR	NR
★★★	★	★★★	★★★	★★★	NR	NR	NR	★★★	★★★	NR	★	★★★	★	★★★	★	★★★	NR	NR
★★★	★★★	★★★	★★★	★★★	NR	★★★	NR	★★★	★★★	★★★	NR	★★★	★	★★★	NR	★	NR	NR
★	★★★	★	★★★	★★★	★★★	★★★	NR	★★★	★★★	★	★★★	★	★★★	★★★	★★★	★★★	★★★	★★★
★★★	★	★★★	★★★	★	★★★	★★★	NR	★	★★★	★★★	★	★★★	★	★	★★★	★★★	NR	NR
★★★★★	★★★	★★★	★★★	★	★★★	★★★	NR	★★★	★★★	★	NR	★★★	★	★★★	★	★★★	NR	NR
★★★	★★★	★★★	★★★	★★★	★★★	★★★	★	★★★★★	★★★	★★★	★★★	★★★	★★★	★	★★★	★	★★★	★★★
★★★	★	★	★★★★★	★	★★★★★	★★★★★	★	★	★★★	★★★	★★★	★★★	★	★	★	★	★★★	★★★
★★★	★★★	★	★★★★★	★	★★★★★	★★★★★	★	★	★★★	★★★	★★★	★★★	★	★	★	★	★★★	★★★
★★★	★★★	★	★★★★★	★	NR	★★★★★	★	★	★★★	★★★	★★★	★★★	★	★	★	★	★★★	NR
★★★	★	★	★★★	★	★★★	★	NR	★★★	★	NR	NR	★★★	★	★★★	★	★	NR	NR
★★★	★★★	★★★	★★★	★★★	★	★★★	★★★	★	★★★	★★★	★★★	★★★	★	★★★	★	★★★	★★★	★★★
★★★	★	★	★★★	★	★★★	★★★	★	★★★	★★★	★★★	★★★	★★★	★	★★★	★★★	★★★	★★★	★★★
★★★	★	★	★★★	★	★★★	★★★	★	★★★	★★★	★★★	★★★	★★★	★	★★★	★★★	★★★	★★★	★★★
★★★	★★★	★★★	★★★	★	★★★★★	★★★	★	★★★	★	★★★	NR	★	★	★★★	★★★	★	NR	NR
★★★	★★★	★★★	★★★	★★★	★★★	★★★	★★★	★★★	★★★	★★★	NR	★★★	★	★★★	★★★	NR	NR	NR
★★★	NR	★★★	★★★	★	NR	★★★	NR	★★★★★	NR	NR	NR	★★★	★★★	★★★	NR	NR	NR	NR

MICHIGAN HOSPITALS: RATINGS BY PROCEDURE

	Appendectomy	Atrial Fibrillation	Back and Neck Surgery (except Spinal Fusion)	Back and Neck Surgery (Spinal Fusion)	Bariatric Surgery	Bowel Obstruction	Carotid Surgery	Cholecystectomy (Gall Bladder Removal)	Chronic Obstructive Pulmonary Disease (COPD)	Coronary Bypass Surgery	Coronary Interventional Procedures (Angioplasty/Stent)	Diabetic Acidosis a...
1. Allegan General Hospital, Allegan	NR	★★★	NR	NR	NR	★★★	NR	NR	★★★	NR	NR	NR
2. Alpena Regional Medical Center, Alpena	NR	★★★	NR	NR	NR	★	★★★★★	★★★	★★★	NR	NR	NR
3. Battle Creek Health System, Battle Creek	NR	★★★	★★★	★★★	NR	★★★	★★★	★★★★★	★★★	NR	★★★	★★★
4. Bay Regional Medical Center, Bay City	NR	★	★★★★★	★★★★★	NR	★★★	★★★	★★★	★	★★★	★	★★★
5. Beaumont Hospital—Grosse Pointe, Grosse Pointe	NR	★★★	★★★	★★★	NR	★★★	★★★	★★★	★★★	★★★	NR	★★★
6. Beaumont Hospital—Royal Oak, Royal Oak	NR	★★★★★	★★★★★	★★★★★	NR	★★★	★★★★★	★★★★★	★★★★★	★	★★★★★	★★★★★
7. Beaumont Hospital—Troy, Troy	NR	★★★★★	★★★	★★★★★	NR	★★★★★	★★★★★	★★★	★★★	★★★★★	★★★★★	★★★
8. Bell Memorial Hospital, Ishpeming	NR	★★★	NR	NR	NR	NR	NR	NR	★★★	NR	NR	NR
9. Borgess Medical Center, Kalamazoo	NR	★★★	★★★	★★★★★	NR	★★★	★★★	★★★	★★★	★★★	★★★	★★★
10. Borgess Pipp Health Center, Plainwell	NR	★★★	★★★	★★★★★	NR	★★★	★★★	★★★	★★★	★★★	★★★	★★★
11. Borgess-Lee Memorial Hospital, Dowagiac	NR	NR	NR	NR	NR	★★★	NR	NR	★★★	NR	NR	NR
12. Botsford Hospital, Farmington Hills	NR	★	★★★	★★★	NR	★★★	★★★★★	★	★★★	NR	NR	★★★
13. Bronson Methodist Hospital, Kalamazoo	NR	★★★	★★★	★★★★★	NR	★★★	★★★	★	★★★	★★★	★★★	★★★
14. Caro Community Hospital, Caro	NR	NR	NR	NR	NR	NR	NR	NR	★★★	NR	NR	NR
15. Carson City Hospital, Carson City	NR	★★★	NR	NR	NR	NR	NR	NR	★★★	NR	NR	NR
16. Central Michigan Community Hospital, Mount Pleasant	NR	★★★	NR	NR	NR	★★★	★★★	★★★	★★★	NR	NR	NR
17. Charlevoix Area Hospital, Charlevoix	NR	NR	NR	NR	NR	★★★	NR	NR	★★★	NR	NR	NR
18. Cheboygan Memorial Hospital, Cheboygan	NR	★	NR	NR	NR	★★★★★	NR	★★★	★★★	NR	NR	NR
19. Chelsea Community Hospital, Chelsea	NR	★★★	NR	★★★	NR	★★★	NR	★★★	★★★	NR	NR	NR
20. Chippewa County War Memorial Hospital, Sault Sainte Marie	NR	★★★	NR	NR	NR	★★★	NR	NR	★★★	NR	NR	NR
21. Clinton Memorial Hospital, St. Johns	NR	★★★	NR	NR	NR	★★★	NR	NR	★★★	NR	NR	NR
22. Community Health Center of Branch County, Coldwater	NR	★★★	★★★	NR	NR	★★★	NR	★★★★★	★★★	NR	NR	★
23. Community Hospital Foundation, Almont	NR	★★★	★★★	★★★	NR	★★★	★★★	★★★	★★★	★★★	★★★	★★★
24. Community Hospital—Watervliet, Watervliet	NR	★★★	NR	NR	NR	★★★	NR	NR	★★★	NR	NR	NR
25. Covenant Medical Center, Saginaw	NR	★★★	★★★★★	★★★★★	NR	★★★	★★★	★★★	★★★	★	★★★	★★★
26. Crittenton Hospital Medical Center, Rochester	NR	★★★	★★★	★★★	NR	★★★★★	★★★	★★★★★	★★★	★★★★★	★★★	★★★
27. Crystal Falls Community Hospital, Crystal Falls	NR	★★★	NR	NR	NR	★★★	NR	NR	★★★	NR	NR	NR
28. Detroit Rec Hospital and University Health Center, Detroit	NR	★★★	NR	NR	NR	★★★	NR	★★★	★★★	NR	★★★	★★★★★
29. Dickinson County Healthcare System, Iron Mountain	NR	★★★	NR	NR	NR	★★★★★	NR	★	★★★	NR	NR	NR
30. Eaton Rapids Medical Center, Eaton Rapids	NR	NR	NR	NR	NR	★★★	NR	NR	★★★	NR	NR	NR
31. Edward W. Sparrow Hospital Association, Lansing	NR	★★★	★★★	★★★	NR	★★★	★★★	★★★★★	★★★	★★★	★★★	★★★
32. Emma L. Bixby Medical Center, Adrian	NR	★★★	NR	NR	NR	★★★	NR	★★★	★★★	NR	NR	NR
33. Garden City Osteopathic Hospital, Garden City	NR	★★★	★★★★★	NR	NR	★★★	★	★★★	★★★★★	NR	NR	★★★
34. Genesys Regional Medical Center, Grand Blanc	NR	★★★	★★★	★★★★★	NR	★★★★★	★★★	★★★	★★★★★	★★★★★	★★★	★★★
35. Gerber Memorial Health Services, Fremont	NR	★★★	NR	NR	NR	★★★	NR	★★★	★	NR	NR	NR
36. Grand View Hospital, Ironwood	NR	★★★	NR	NR	NR	★★★	NR	★★★	★★★	NR	NR	NR
37. Gratiot Medical Center, Alma	NR	★★★	NR	NR	NR	★★★	★★★	★★★	★★★	NR	NR	NR
38. Hackley Hospital, Muskegon	NR	★★★	★★★★★	★★★★★	NR	★★★	★★★	★★★	★★★	NR	NR	NR
39. Harper University Hospital, Detroit	NR	★★★	★★★	★★★	NR	★★★★★	★	★★★	★★★	★★★	★★★	★★★
40. Hayes Green Beach Memorial Hospital, Charlotte	NR	★★★	NR	NR	NR	★★★	NR	★★★	★★★	NR	NR	NR
41. Helen Newberry Joy Hospital, Newberry	NR	NR	NR	NR	NR	NR	NR	NR	★	NR	NR	NR
42. Henry Ford Bi-County Hospital, Warren	NR	★★★	NR	NR	NR	★★★	★★★	★★★	★★★	NR	NR	★★★
43. Henry Ford Hospital, Detroit	NR	★★★	★★★	★	NR	★★★	★★★	★★★	★★★★★	★★★	★★★	★★★
44. Henry Ford Macomb Hospital, Clinton Township	NR	★★★	★★★	★★★	NR	★★★	★★★	★★★	★★★	★★★	★★★	★★★
45. Henry Ford Wyandotte Hospital, Wyandotte	NR	★★★	★★★	★★★	NR	★	★	★★★★★	★★★★★	NR	NR	★★★
46. Herrick Memorial Hospital, Tecumseh	NR	★★★	NR	NR	NR	★★★	NR	★★★	★★★	NR	NR	NR
47. Hills and Dales General Hospital, Cass City	NR	NR	NR	NR	NR	NR	NR	★★★	NR	NR	NR	NR
48. Hillsdale Community Health Center, Hillsdale	NR	★★★	NR	NR	NR	★★★	★★★	★★★	★★★	NR	NR	NR
49. Holland Community Hospital, Holland	NR	★★★	★★★	★★★	NR	★★★	NR	★★★	★★★	NR	NR	★★★
50. Hurley Medical Center, Flint	NR	★	NR	NR	NR	★★★	★	★★★	★★★	NR	NR	★★★

KEY: ★★★★★ BEST ★★★ AS EXPECTED ★ POOR NR NOT RATED BY HEALTHGRADES For full definitions of ratings and awards, see Appendix.

Gastrointestinal Bleed	Gastrointestinal Surgeries and Procedures	Heart Attack	Heart Failure	Hip Fracture Repair	Maternity Care	Pancreatitis	Peripheral Vascular Bypass	Pneumonia	Prostatectomy	Pulmonary Embolism	Resection/Replacement of Abdominal Aorta	Respiratory Failure	Sepsis	Stroke	Total Hip Replacement	Total Knee Replacement	Valve Replacement	Women's Health
★★★	NR	NR	★★★	★★★	NR	NR	NR	★★★	NR	★★★	NR	★★★	★★★	★★★	★★★★★	★★★	NR	NR
★★★	★★★	★★★	★	★★★	NR	NR	NR	★★★	★	★★★	NR	★★★	★★★	★★★	★	★	NR	NR
★	★★★	★★★	★★★	★★★★★	NR	★★★	★★★	★★★	★★★	★★★	★★★	★	★★★	★	★★★	★★★★★	NR	NR
★★★	★★★	★★★	★★★	★★★★★	NR	★★★	★★★	★★★	★★★	★★★	NR	★★★	★★★★★	★	★★★	★★★★★	★★★	NR
★★★	★★★	★★★★★	★★★	★★★★★	NR	★★★	★★★	★★★★★	★★★	★★★	★	★★★	★★★★★	★★★★★	★★★	★★★★★	NR	NR
★★★★★	★★★★★	★★★★★	★★★★★	★★★★★	NR	★★★	★★★	★★★★★	★★★★★	★★★	★★★	★★★★★	★★★★★	★★★★★	★★★★★	★★★★★	★★★★★	NR
★★★	★★★	★★★	★★★	★★★★★	NR	★★★	★★★	★★★★★	★★★	★★★	★★★	★★★★★	★★★★★	★★★	★★★	★★★	★★★	NR
★★★	NR	★★★	★	★★★	NR	NR	NR	★★★	NR	★★★	NR	★★★	★★★	★	NR	NR	NR	NR
★★★	★★★	★★★	★★★	★★★★★	NR	★★★	★★★	★★★	★★★	★★★	NR	★★★★★	★★★★★	★★★★★	★★★	★★★	★★★	NR
★★★	★★★	★★★	★★★	★★★	NR	★★★	★★★★★	★★★	★★★	★★★	NR	★★★★★	★★★★★	★★★★★	★★★★★	★★★★★	★★★	NR
★★★	NR	★★★	★★★	NR	NR	NR	NR	★★★	NR	NR	NR	★★★	★★★	NR	★★★	NR	NR	NR
★★★★★	★	★	★★★	★★★★★	NR	★★★	★★★	★★★	★★★	NR	★	★★★	★★★	★★★	★★★	★★★	NR	NR
★★★	★★★	★★★	★★★★★	★★★	NR	★★★	NR	★★★★★	★★★	★★★★★	★★★	★★★	★★★★★	★★★★★	★★★★★	★★★★★	★★★	NR
NR	NR	NR	★★★	NR	NR	NR	NR	★★★	NR	NR	NR	NR	NR	NR	NR	NR	NR	NR
★★★	NR	★★★	★★★	★★★	NR	NR	NR	★★★	NR	NR	NR	★	★★★	★★★	NR	★★★	NR	NR
★★★	★★★	★★★	★★★★★	★★★	NR	★★★	NR	★	★★★	NR	NR	★★★	★★★	★★★	★★★	★★★★★	NR	NR
★★★	★★★	NR	★★★	★★★	NR	NR	NR	★★★	★★★	NR	NR	★★★	★★★	★★★	NR	★★★	NR	NR
★★★	★★★	★★★	★★★★★	★★★★★	NR	★★★	NR	★★★★★	★★★	NR	NR	★★★★★	★★★★★	★★★	NR	★★★	NR	NR
★★★	NR	★★★	★★★	★★★	NR	NR	NR	★★★	★★★	NR	NR	★	★★★★★	★★★	★★★	★★★	NR	NR
★★★	★★★	★★★	★	★★★	NR	NR	NR	★★★	NR	NR	NR	★	★	★★★	★★★	★★★★★	NR	NR
★★★	NR	NR	★★★	NR	NR	NR	NR	★★★	NR	NR	NR	★★★	★	★	★★★	★★★	NR	NR
★★★	★★★	★	★★★	★★★	NR	NR	NR	★★★	NR	NR	NR	★★★★★	★★★	★	★★★	★★★★★	NR	NR
★★★★★	★★★	★★★★★	★★★★★	★★★	NR	★★★★★	NR	★★★★★	★★★★★	★★★★★	★★★	★★★★★	★★★★★	★★★★★	★★★	★★★	★★★	NR
★★★	NR	NR	★★★	★★★	NR	NR	NR	★★★	NR	NR	NR	NR	NR	★★★	NR	NR	NR	NR
★★★	★★★	★★★	★★★	★★★	NR	★★★	★★★	★★★★★	★★★	★★★	★★★	★★★★★	★★★	★★★★★	★★★★★	★★★★★	★★★	NR
★★★	★★★★★	★★★★★	★★★★★	★★★★★	NR	★★★★★	NR	★★★★★	★★★	★★★	NR	★★★	★★★★★	★★★	★★★	★★★	NR	NR
★★★	NR	NR	★★★	NR	NR	NR	NR	★★★	NR	NR	NR	NR	★★★	NR	NR	NR	NR	NR
★★★	★★★	★★★	★★★	★★★	NR	★	NR	★★★	NR	★★★	NR	★	★★★	★★★	NR	NR	NR	NR
★★★	★★★	★★★	★★★	★★★	NR	★	NR	★★★	NR	NR	NR	★★★★★	★★★	★	★★★	★	NR	NR
★★★	NR	NR	★★★	NR	NR	NR	NR	★★★	NR	NR	NR	NR	★★★	NR	NR	NR	NR	NR
★★★	★★★	★★★	★★★	★★★	NR	★★★	★★★	★★★	★★★	★★★	NR	★	★★★	★★★	★★★	★★★	★★★	NR
★★★	★★★	★★★	★★★	★★★	NR	NR	NR	★★★	★★★	NR	NR	★★★	★★★	★★★	★★★	★★★	NR	NR
★★★★★	★★★	★★★	★★★★★	★★★★★	NR	★★★	NR	★★★★★	★★★	★★★	NR	★★★	★★★★★	★★★	★★★★★	★★★★★	NR	NR
★★★	★★★	★★★★★	★★★★★	★★★★★	NR	★★★★★	★★★	★★★★★	★	★★★	★★★	★★★★★	★★★★★	★★★★★	★★★	★★★	★★★	NR
★★★	NR	★★★★★	★★★	★★★	NR	★★★	NR	★★★★★	NR	NR	NR	★★★	★★★	★★★	★★★	★★★	NR	NR
★★★★★	NR	★★★	★★★	★★★	NR	NR	NR	★★★	NR	NR	NR	NR	★★★	NR	★★★	★★★	NR	NR
★★★	★★★	★★★	★★★	★★★	NR	★★★	NR	★★★★★	★★★	NR	NR	★★★	★★★★★	★★★	★★★	★★★	NR	NR
★★★	★★★★★	★★★★★	★★★	★★★★★	NR	★★★	NR	★★★★★	★★★★★	★★★	NR	★★★★★	★★★	★★★	★★★	★★★	NR	NR
★★★★★	★★★	★	★★★★★	NR	NR	★★★	★	★★★	★★★	★★★	★	★★★★★	★★★	★★★★★	★★★	★★★	NR	NR
★★★	NR	NR	★★★	NR	NR	NR	NR	★★★	NR	NR	NR	★★★	★★★	NR	NR	★★★	NR	NR
★★★	NR	NR	★★★	★★★	NR	NR	NR	★★★	NR	NR	NR	NR	NR	NR	NR	NR	NR	NR
★★★★★	★★★	★	★★★	★	NR	★★★	NR	★★★	NR	NR	NR	★★★	★★★★★	★★★★★	★	★★★	NR	NR
★★★	★★★	★★★★★	★★★★★	★	NR	★★★★★	★★★	★★★★★	★★★★★	★★★	★★★	★★★★★	★★★★★	★★★★★	★★★	★★★	★	NR
★★★★★	★★★	★★★★★	★★★★★	★★★	NR	★★★★★	★★★	★★★★★	★★★★★	★★★★★	★★★	★★★★★	★★★★★	★★★★★	★★★	★★★	★★★★★	NR
★★★	★★★★★	★★★	★★★★★	★★★★★	NR	★★★	★★★	★★★	★★★	★★★	NR	★★★★★	★★★★★	★★★	★★★	★★★	★★★★★	NR
★★★	NR	★★★	★★★	★★★★★	NR	NR	NR	★★★	★★★	★★★	NR	★★★★★	★★★	★★★	★★★	★★★	NR	NR
★★★	NR	NR	★	NR	NR	NR	NR	★★★	NR	NR	NR	★★★	★★★	★★★	NR	NR	NR	NR
★	★★★	★★★	★★★	★★★	NR	NR	NR	★★★	★★★	★★★	NR	★★★	★★★★★	★★★★★	★★★	★★★	NR	NR
★★★	★★★	★★★	★★★	★	NR	★★★	NR	★★★	★★★	★★★	NR	★★★	★★★★★	★★★★★	★★★	★★★	NR	NR
★★★	★★★	★	★★★	★★★	NR	★★★	NR	★★★	★★★	★	NR	★★★	★★★★★	★★★	★★★	★★★	NR	NR

	Appendectomy	Atrial Fibrillation	Back and Neck Surgery (except Spinal Fusion)	Back and Neck Surgery (Spinal Fusion)	Bariatric Surgery	Bowel Obstruction	Carotid Surgery	Cholecystectomy (Gall Bladder Removal)	Chronic Obstructive Pulmonary Disease (COPD)	Coronary Bypass Surgery	Coronary Interventional Procedures (Angioplasty/Stent)	Diabetic Acidosis an...
51. Huron Medical Center, Bad Axe	NR	★★★	NR	NR	NR	★★★	★★★	NR	★★★	NR	NR	NR
52. Huron Valley Sinai Hospital, Commerce Township	NR	★★★★★	★★★	NR	NR	★★★	★★★	★	★★★	NR	NR	★★★
53. Hutzel Hospital, Detroit	NR	★★★	★★★	★★★	NR	★★★★★	★	★★★	★★★	★	★★★	★★★
54. Ingham Regional Medical Center, Lansing	NR	★★★	★★★	★★★	NR	★★★	★★★★★	★★★	★★★	★★★	★★★	★★★
55. Ionia County Memorial Hospital, Ionia	NR	NR	NR	NR	NR	★★★	NR	★	NR	NR	NR	NR
56. Iron County Community Hospital, Iron River	NR	★★★	NR	NR	NR	★★★	NR	★★★	★★★	NR	NR	NR
57. Keweenaw Memorial Medical Center, Laurium	NR	★	NR	NR	NR	★★★	NR	★★★	★★★	NR	NR	NR
58. Lakeland Hospital—St. Joseph, St. Joseph	NR	★★★	★★★	NR	NR	★★★	★★★	★★★	★★★	★★★	★★★	★★★
59. Lakeland Medical Center—Niles, Niles	NR	★★★	★★★	NR	NR	★★★	★★★	★★★	★★★	★★★	★★★	NR
60. Lakeview Community Hospital, Paw Paw	NR	★★★	NR	NR	NR	★★★★★	NR	NR	★★★	NR	NR	NR
61. Lapeer Regional Medical Center, Lapeer	NR	★★★★★	NR	NR	NR	★★★	NR	★★★	★★★	NR	NR	NR
62. Madison Community Hospital, Madison Heights	NR	★★★	★★★	★★★	NR	★★★★★	★	★★★	★★★	★	★★★	★★★
63. Marlette Community Hospital, Marlette	NR	NR	NR	NR	NR	★★★	NR	NR	★★★	NR	NR	NR
64. Marquette General Hospital, Marquette	NR	★★★	★★★	★★★	NR	★★★	★★★	★★★	NR	★★★	★★★	NR
65. McKenzie Memorial Hospital, Sandusky	NR	NR	NR	NR	NR	NR	NR	NR	★★★	NR	NR	NR
66. McLaren Regional Medical Center, Flint	NR	★★★	★★★	★★★	NR	★★★★★	★★★	★★★	★★★	★	★★★	★★★
67. Mecosta County Medical Center, Big Rapids	NR	★★★	NR	NR	NR	★★★	NR	★★★	★★★	NR	NR	NR
68. Memorial Healthcare Center, Owosso	NR	★★★	NR	NR	NR	★★★	★★★	★★★	★★★	NR	NR	NR
69. Memorial Medical Center of West Michigan, Ludington	NR	★★★	NR	NR	NR	★★★	★★★	★	★★★	NR	NR	NR
70. Mercy General Health Partners, Muskegon	NR	★★★	★★★	★★★	NR	★★★	★★★★★	★★★	★★★★★	★★★	★★★	★
71. Mercy Hospital—Cadillac, Cadillac	NR	★★★	NR	NR	NR	★★★	NR	★	★★★	NR	NR	★★★
72. Mercy Hospital—Grayling, Grayling	NR	★★★	NR	NR	NR	★★★	NR	★★★	★★★	NR	NR	★★★
73. Mercy Hospital—Port Huron, Port Huron	NR	★★★	NR	NR	NR	★★★	★★★★★	★★★	★★★	NR	NR	★★★
74. Mercy Memorial Hospital, Monroe	NR	★★★	NR	NR	NR	★★★	★★★★★	★★★★★	★★★	NR	NR	★★★
75. Metro Health Hospital, Wyoming	NR	★★★	★★★★★	★★★	NR	★★★	★★★	★★★	★★★★★	NR	NR	★★★
76. MidMichigan Medical Center—Clare, Clare	NR	★★★	NR	NR	NR	★★★	NR	★★★	★★★	NR	NR	NR
77. MidMichigan Medical Center—Gladwin, Gladwin	NR	★★★	NR	NR	NR	★★★	NR	NR	★★★	NR	NR	NR
78. MidMichigan Medical Center—Midland, Midland	NR	★★★	★★★	★★★★★	NR	★★★	★★★	★★★	★★★	NR	NR	★★★
79. Morenci Area Hospital, Morenci	NR	★★★	NR	NR	NR	★★★	NR	★★★	★★★	NR	NR	NR
80. Mount Clemens Regional Medical Center, Mount Clemens	NR	★★★	★★★	★★★	NR	★★★	★★★	★★★★★	★★★	★★★	★★★	★★★
81. Munson Medical Center, Traverse City	NR	★★★	★★★★★	★★★★★	NR	★★★★★	★★★	★★★★★	★★★★★	★★★	★★★	★★★
82. North Oakland Medical Center, Pontiac	NR	★★★	NR	★★★	NR	★★★	★	★	★★★	NR	NR	★★★
83. North Ottawa Community Hospital, Grand Haven	NR	★	NR	NR	NR	★★★	NR	★★★	★★★	NR	NR	NR
84. Northern Michigan Hospital, Petoskey	NR	★★★	★★★★★	★★★★★	NR	★★★	★★★★★	★★★★★	★★★	★★★	★	★★★
85. Oaklawn Hospital, Marshall	NR	★★★	NR	NR	NR	★★★	★★★	★★★	★★★	NR	NR	NR
86. Oakwood Annapolis Hospital, Wayne	NR	★★★	NR	NR	NR	★★★	★	★★★	★★★	NR	NR	★★★
87. Oakwood Heritage Hospital, Taylor	NR	★★★★★	NR	NR	NR	★★★	★	★★★	★★★★★	NR	NR	★★★
88. Oakwood Hospital and Medical Center—Dearborn, Dearborn	NR	★★★	★★★	★★★	NR	★★★	★	★★★	★★★★★	★★★	★★★	★★★
89. Oakwood Southshore Medical Center, Trenton	NR	★★★	NR	NR	NR	★★★	★★★	★★★★★	★★★	NR	NR	★★★
90. Otsego Memorial Hospital, Gaylord	NR	★★★	NR	NR	NR	★★★	NR	★★★	★★★	NR	NR	NR
91. Pennock Hospital, Hastings	NR	★★★	NR	NR	NR	★★★	NR	★★★	★★★	★	NR	NR
92. POH Regional Medical Center, Pontiac	NR	★★★	NR	NR	NR	★★★	NR	★★★	★★★	NR	NR	★★★
93. Port Huron Hospital, Port Huron	NR	★★★	★★★	★★★	NR	★★★	★★★★★	★★★	★★★	★★★	★★★	★★★
94. Portage Health System, Hancock	NR	★★★	NR	NR	NR	★★★	NR	★★★	★★★	NR	NR	NR
95. Providence Hospital, Southfield	NR	★★★	★★★	★★★	NR	★★★★★	★★★	★★★★★	★★★	★★★★★	★★★	★★★
96. St. Francis Hospital, Escanaba	NR	★★★	NR	NR	NR	★★★	★★★	★★★	★★★	NR	NR	NR
97. St. John Detroit Riverview Hospital, Detroit	NR	★	NR	NR	NR	★★★	★★★	★★★★★	NR	NR	NR	★★★
98. St. John Hospital and Medical Center, Detroit	NR	★★★	★★★	★★★	NR	★★★	★★★	★★★	★★★★★	★★★	★★★	★★★
99. St. John Macomb Hospital, Warren	NR	★★★	NR	★★★★★	NR	★★★	★★★	★★★	★★★★★	★★★	★★★	★★★
100. St. John Oakland Hospital, Madison Heights	NR	★	NR	NR	NR	★★★	★★★	★★★	★★★	NR	NR	★★★

KEY: ★★★★★ BEST ★★★ AS EXPECTED ★ POOR NR NOT RATED BY HEALTHGRADES For full definitions of ratings and awards, see Appendix.

Gastrointestinal Bleed	Gastrointestinal Surgeries and Procedures	Heart Attack	Heart Failure	Hip Fracture Repair	Maternity Care	Pancreatitis	Peripheral Vascular Bypass	Pneumonia	Prostatectomy	Pulmonary Embolism	Resection/Replacement of Abdominal Aorta	Respiratory Failure	Sepsis	Stroke	Total Hip Replacement	Total Knee Replacement	Valve Replacement	Women's Health
★★★	NR	NR	★★★	★★★★★	NR	NR	NR	★★★	NR	NR	NR	NR	NR	★★★	★★★★★	★★★★★	NR	NR
★★★	★★★	★★★★★	★★★★★	★★★	NR	★★★★★	NR	★★★★★	★★★	★★★	NR	★★★	★★★★★	★★★	★★★	★	NR	NR
★★★★★	★★★	★	★★★★★	NR	NR	★★★	★	★★★	★★★	★★★	★	★★★	★★★	★★★★★	★★★	★★★	★★★	NR
★★★	★★★	★★★	★★★	★★★	NR	★★★	★★★★★	★★★	★★★	★★★	★★★	★★★	★★★	★	★★★★★	★★★★★	★★★	NR
★★★	NR	NR	★	NR	NR	NR	NR	★★★	NR	NR	NR	NR	NR	★★★	NR	NR	NR	NR
★★★	NR	★★★	★	NR	NR	NR	NR	★★★	NR	NR	NR	NR	★★★	★★★	NR	★	NR	NR
★★★	★★★	★	★★★	★★★	NR	★★★	★★★	★★★	★★★	★★★	NR	★★★	★★★	★★★	★★★	★★★★★	★★★	NR
★★★	★★★	★	★★★	★★★	NR	★★★	★★★	★★★	★★★	★★★	NR	★★★	★★★	★★★	★★★	★★★★★	★★★	NR
★★★	NR	★★★	★★★	★★★	NR	NR	NR	★★★	NR	NR	NR	★★★	NR	NR	NR	NR	NR	NR
★★★★★	★★★	★★★★★	★★★★★	★★★	NR	NR	NR	★★★★★	★★★	★★★	NR	★★★	★★★★★	★★★★★	★★★	★★★	NR	NR
★★★★★	★★★	★	★★★★★	NR	NR	★★★	★	★★★	★★★	★★★	★	★★★	★★★	★★★★★	★★★	★★★	★★★	NR
★★★	NR	NR	★★★	NR	NR	NR	NR	★★★	NR	NR	NR	NR	NR	NR	NR	NR	NR	NR
★★★	★★★	★★★	★★★	★★★	NR	★★★	★★★	★★★	★★★	★★★	NR	★★★	★★★	★★★★★	★★★	★★★★★	★★★	NR
★★★	NR	NR	★	NR	NR	NR	NR	★★★	NR	NR	NR	NR	NR	NR	NR	NR	NR	NR
★★★	★★★	★★★	★★★★★	★★★	NR	★★★	★★★	★★★★★	★★★	★★★	★★★	★★★★★	★★★★★	★★★★★	★★★	★★★	★	NR
★★★	NR	★★★★★	★★★	★★★	NR	NR	NR	★★★	NR	NR	NR	★★★★★	★★★	★★★	★★★★★	★★★★★	NR	NR
★★★	★★★	★	★★★	★★★	NR	★★★	NR	★★★	★★★	NR	NR	★	★★★	★★★	★★★	★★★	NR	NR
★★★	★★★	★	★★★	★★★	NR	★★★	NR	★★★	★★★	NR	NR	★★★	★★★	★★★	★★★	★★★★★	NR	NR
★★★	★★★	★★★	★★★	★★★	NR	★	★★★	★★★	★★★	★★★	★★★★★	★★★★★	★★★★★	★	★★★★★	★★★★★	★★★★★	NR
★★★	★★★	★★★	★★★	★★★	NR	NR	NR	★★★	★★★	NR	NR	★★★	★★★★★	★★★	★★★	★★★	NR	NR
★★★★★	★★★	★★★	★★★★★	★	NR	★★★	NR	★★★★★	NR	NR	★★★★★	★★★★★	★★★	NR	★	NR	NR	NR
★★★	★	★★★	★★★	★★★★★	NR	★★★	★★★	★★★	★★★	NR	NR	★★★★★	★★★	★★★	★★★	★★★	NR	NR
★★★	★★★	★★★	★★★	NR	NR	★★★	NR	★★★★★	NR	★★★	★★★	★★★★★	★★★	★★★	NR	NR	NR	NR
★★★	NR	NR	★★★	NR	NR	NR	NR	★★★★★	NR	NR	NR	NR	★★★	NR	NR	NR	NR	NR
★★★	★★★	★★★	★★★	★★★	NR	NR	NR	★★★	★★★	★★★	NR	★★★	★★★	★★★★★	★★★★★	★★★★★	NR	NR
★★★	★★★	★★★	★★★	★★★	NR	NR	NR	★★★	★★★	NR	NR	★★★	★★★	★★★	★★★	★★★	NR	NR
★★★★★	★★★	★★★	★★★★★	★★★	NR	★★★	★★★	★★★	★★★	★★★	NR	★	★★★★★	★★★★★	★★★	★★★	★★★	NR
★★★★★	★★★★★	★★★	★★★★★	NR	NR	★★★	★★★★★	★★★★★	★★★★★	★★★	★★★	★★★	★★★★★	★★★	★★★★★	★★★★★	★★★★★	NR
★★★★★	★★★	★★★	★★★	NR	NR	★★★	NR	★★★	NR	NR	★★★	★★★★★	★★★	NR	★★★	★★★★★	NR	NR
★★★	★★★	★★★	★★★★★	★★★★★	NR	NR	NR	★	★★★	NR	NR	★★★★★	★★★★★	★★★★★	★★★★★	★★★★★	★★★	NR
★★★	★★★	★★★	★★★	★★★	NR	★★★	★★★	★	★★★	★★★	★	★★★	★★★	★★★	★★★	★★★★★	★	NR
★★★	★★★	NR	★★★	★★★	NR	★★★	NR	★★★	★★★	NR	NR	★★★	★★★	★★★	★★★	★★★★★	NR	NR
★★★★★	★★★	★★★★★	★★★	★★★★★	NR	★★★	NR	★★★★★	★★★★★	★★★	NR	★★★	★★★★★	★★★	★★★	★★★	NR	NR
★★★★★	NR	★★★	★★★	★★★★★	NR	★★★	NR	★★★★★	NR	NR	★★★★★	★★★★★	★★★★★	★★★	★★★★★	★★★	NR	NR
★★★	★★★	★★★	★★★★★	★★★★★	NR	★★★	★★★	★★★★★	★★★	★★★	★	★★★★★	★★★★★	★★★★★	★★★★★	★★★★★	★★★	NR
★★★★★	★★★★★	★★★★★	★★★★★	★★★★★	NR	★★★	NR	★★★★★	★★★	★★★	NR	★★★★★	★★★★★	★★★★★	★★★★★	★★★★★	NR	NR
★★★	NR	NR	★★★	★★★	NR	NR	NR	★★★★★	NR	NR	NR	★★★★★	★★★	★★★	★★★★★	NR	NR	NR
★★★	★★★	★★★★★	★	★★★	NR	★★★	NR	★★★	NR	★★★	NR	NR	★★★★★	★★★	★★★	★★★	NR	NR
★★★	NR	★★★	★★★	★★★	NR	NR	NR	★★★★★	NR	NR	NR	★★★	★★★★★	★★★	★★★	★★★	NR	NR
★★★	★★★★★	★★★	★★★	★★★	NR	★★★	★★★★★	★★★★★	★★★	★★★	NR	★★★	★★★★★	★★★	★★★	★★★	★★★	NR
★★★	NR	★★★★★	★★★	★★★	NR	NR	NR	★★★	NR	NR	NR	NR	★★★★★	NR	★★★	NR	NR	NR
★★★	★★★★★	★★★★★	★★★★★	★★★	NR	★★★	★★★	★★★★★	★★★	★★★	★★★	★★★	★★★★★	★★★★★	★★★	★★★	★★★	NR
★★★	★★★	★★★	★★★	★	NR	★★★	NR	★★★	NR	NR	NR	★★★	★★★	★	★	NR	NR	NR
★★★	★★★	★★★	★★★★★	NR	NR	★★★	NR	★★★★★	★★★	NR	NR	★★★★★	★★★★★	★★★	NR	★	NR	NR
★★★	★★★	★★★★★	★★★★★	★★★	NR	★★★	★★★	★★★★★	★★★	★★★	★	★★★	★★★	★★★★★	★★★	★★★	★★★	NR
★★★	★★★	★★★	★★★★★	★★★★★	NR	★★★	NR	★★★★★	★★★	★★★	NR	★★★★★	★★★★★	★★★★★	★★★	★★★	★★★	NR
★★★★★	★★★	★★★	★★★★★	★★★★★	NR	★★★	NR	★★★★★	★★★	NR	★★★	★★★★★	★★★★★	★★★★★	★★★	★★★	★★★	NR
★★★★★	★★★	★★★★★	★★★★★	★★★	NR	★★★	NR	★★★★★	NR	NR	NR	★★★★★	★★★★★	★★★★★	★★★	★★★	NR	NR

	Appendectomy	Atrial Fibrillation	Back and Neck Surgery (except Spinal Fusion)	Back and Neck Surgery (Spinal Fusion)	Bariatric Surgery	Bowel Obstruction	Carotid Surgery	Cholecystectomy (Gall Bladder Removal)	Chronic Obstructive Pulmonary Disease (COPD)	Coronary Bypass Surgery	Coronary Interventional Procedures (Angioplasty/Stent)	Diabetic Acidosis an...
101. St. John River District Hospital, East China	NR	★	NR	NR	NR	★★★★★	NR	★★★	★★★	NR	NR	NR
102. St. Joseph Health System—Tawas, Tawas City	NR	★★★	NR	NR	NR	★★★	NR	★★★	★★★	NR	NR	NR
103. St. Joseph Mercy Hospital, Ypsilanti	NR	★★★	★	★	NR	★★★	★★★	★★★	★★★	★★★	★★★	★★★★★
104. St. Joseph Mercy Livingston Hospital, Howell	NR	★★★	NR	NR	NR	★★★	NR	★	★★★	NR	NR	NR
105. St. Joseph Mercy Oakland, Pontiac	NR	★★★★★	★★★	★★★	NR	★★★	★★★	★★★	★★★	★★★★★	★★★	★★★
106. St. Joseph Mercy Saline Hospital, Saline	NR	★★★	NR	NR	NR	★★★	NR	NR	★	NR	NR	NR
107. St. Mary Mercy Hospital, Livonia	NR	★★★	★★★	★★★	NR	★★★	★★★★★	★★★	★★★★★	NR	★★★	★★★
108. St. Mary's Health Care, Grand Rapids	NR	★	★★★	★	NR	★★★★★	★	★★★	★★★	★★★	NR	NR
109. St. Mary's of Michigan Medical Center, Saginaw	NR	★	★★★★★	★★★★★	NR	★★★	★	★★★	★	★★★	★	★★★
110. Select Specialty Hospital—Saginaw, Saginaw	NR	★★★	★★★★★	★★★★★	NR	★★★	★★★	★★★	★★★	★	★★★	★★★
111. Sheridan Community Hospital, Sheridan	NR	NR	NR	NR	NR	NR	NR	NR	★★★	NR	NR	NR
112. Sinai-Grace Hospital, Detroit	NR	★★★	NR	NR	NR	★★★	★★★	★★★★★	★★★	★★★	★★★	★★★
113. South Haven Community Hospital, South Haven	NR	★	NR	NR	NR	NR	NR	NR	★★★	NR	NR	NR
114. Spectrum Health Hospitals, Grand Rapids	NR	★★★	★★★	★★★	NR	★★★★★	★★★	★★★	★★★	★★★★★	★★★	★★★
115. Spectrum Health—Reed City Campus, Reed City	NR	★★★	NR	NR	NR	★★★	NR	★★★	★★★	NR	NR	NR
116. Standish Community Hospital, Standish	NR	NR	NR	NR	NR	★★★	NR	★★★	★★★	NR	NR	NR
117. Sturgis Hospital, Sturgis	NR	★★★	NR	NR	NR	★★★	★★★	★★★	★★★	NR	NR	NR
118. Three Rivers Health, Three Rivers	NR	★★★	NR	NR	NR	★★★	NR	★★★	★★★	NR	NR	NR
119. United Memorial Health Center, Greenville	NR	★★★	NR	NR	NR	★★★	NR	★★★	★★★	NR	NR	NR
120. University of Michigan Hospital, Ann Arbor	NR	★★★	★	★	NR	★★★	★★★	★	★★★	★★★★★	★★★	★★★
121. Wa Foote Hospital, Jackson	NR	★★★	★★★	★★★★★	NR	★	★★★	★★★	★★★	NR	NR	★★★
122. West Branch Regional Medical Center, West Branch	NR	★★★	NR	NR	NR	★	NR	★★★★★	★	NR	NR	NR
123. West Shore Hospital, Manistee	NR	★	NR	NR	NR	★★★	★★★	★★★	★★★	NR	NR	NR
124. Zeeland Community Hospital, Zeeland	NR	★★★	NR	NR	NR	★★★	NR	★★★	★★★	NR	NR	NR

KEY: ★★★★★ BEST   ★★★ AS EXPECTED   ★ POOR   NR NOT RATED BY HEALTHGRADES   For full definitions of ratings and awards, see Appendix.

Gastrointestinal Bleed	Gastrointestinal Surgeries and Procedures	Heart Attack	Heart Failure	Hip Fracture Repair	Maternity Care	Pancreatitis	Peripheral Vascular Bypass	Pneumonia	Prostatectomy	Pulmonary Embolism	Resection/Replacement of Abdominal Aorta	Respiratory Failure	Sepsis	Stroke	Total Hip Replacement	Total Knee Replacement	Valve Replacement	Women's Health
★★★	★★★	★★★	★★★	★★★★★	NR	NR	NR	★★★	NR	NR	NR	★★★	★★★	★★★	NR	★★★	NR	NR
★★★	★★★	★★★	★★★	★	NR	NR	NR	★	★★★	NR	NR	NR	★★★★★	★★★	★★★	★	NR	NR
★★★	★★★	★★★	★★★★★	★	NR	★★★	★★★	★★★	★★★	★★★	★★★	★	★	★★★	★★★	★	★★★	NR
★★★	★★★	★★★	★★★	★★★	NR	★★★	NR	★★★	NR	★	NR	★★★	★★★	★	★★★	★★★★★	NR	NR
★★★	★★★	★★★	★★★	★★★	NR	★★★	★★★	★★★★★	★★★★★	★★★	★★★	★★★	★★★★★	★★★	★★★★★	★★★★★	★★★	NR
NR	NR	NR	★★★	★★★	NR	NR	NR	★★★	NR	NR	NR	NR	NR	★★★	NR	★★★	NR	NR
★★★★★	★★★	★★★	★★★★★	★★★★★	NR	★★★	★★★	★★★★★	★★★★★	★★★★★	NR	★★★★★	★★★★★	★★★★★	★★★	★★★	NR	NR
★★★	★★★	★★★★★	★★★★★	★	NR	★★★	NR	★★★★★	★	★★★	NR	★★★★★	★★★★★	★★★	★	★	NR	NR
★★★	★★★	★	★★★	★★★★★	NR	★★★	★★★	★★★★★	★★★	★★★	★★★	★★★★★	★★★	★★★	★★★	★★★	★★★	NR
★★★	★★★	★★★	★★★	★★★	NR	★★★	★★★	★★★★★	★★★	★★★	★★★	★★★★★	★★★	★★★★★	★★★★★	★★★★★	★★★	NR
NR	NR	NR	★★★	NR	NR	NR	NR	★★★	NR	NR	NR	NR	NR	NR	NR	NR	NR	NR
★★★	★★★	★★★	★★★	★★★	NR	★★★	★★★	★★★★★	★★★	★★★	NR	★★★★★	★★★★★	★★★★★	★	★★★★★	NR	NR
NR	NR	NR	★★★	★	NR	NR	NR	★★★	NR	NR	NR	NR	NR	NR	NR	★★★	NR	NR
★★★★★	★★★	★★★★★	★★★★★	★★★	NR	★	★★★	★★★	★★★★★	★★★	★★★	★	NR	NR	★★★★★	★★★★★	★★★★★	NR
★★★	NR	★★★	★★★	NR	NR	NR	NR	★★★★★	NR	NR	NR	NR	NR	NR	NR	NR	NR	NR
★★★	NR	NR	★★★★★	NR	NR	NR	NR	★★★	NR	NR	NR	★★★	★★★	NR	NR	NR	NR	NR
★★★	NR	★★★	★	★★★	NR	NR	NR	★	★★★	NR	NR	★★★	★★★	★★★	★★★	NR	NR	NR
★★★	NR	NR	★★★	NR	NR	NR	NR	★★★	NR	NR	NR	★★★	NR	NR	NR	NR	NR	NR
★★★	★★★	★★★★★	★★★★★	★	NR	NR	NR	★★★★★	NR	NR	NR	★★★★★	★★★★★	★★★	NR	★	NR	NR
★★★	★	★★★	★★★	★	NR	★★★	★★★	★★★	★★★	★★★	★★★	★	★	★★★	★	★★★	★★★	NR
★★★	★	★	★★★	★★★	NR	★★★	★★★	★	★★★	★★★	NR	★★★★★	★★★	★★★	★★★	★★★★★	NR	NR
★	★	★★★	★	★★★	NR	NR	NR	★	NR	NR	NR	NR	★★★	★★★	★★★	★★★	NR	NR
★★★	★★★	NR	★	★★★	NR	NR	NR	★★★	NR	NR	NR	★	NR	★	NR	★★★	NR	NR
★★★	NR	NR	★★★	★★★	NR	★★★	NR	★★★	NR	NR	NR	★★★★★	★★★	★★★	NR	★★★	NR	NR

MINNESOTA HOSPITALS: RATINGS BY PROCEDURE

	Appendectomy	Atrial Fibrillation	Back and Neck Surgery (except Spinal Fusion)	Back and Neck Surgery (Spinal Fusion)	Bariatric Surgery	Bowel Obstruction	Carotid Surgery	Cholecystectomy (Gall Bladder Removal)	Chronic Obstructive Pulmonary Disease (COPD)	Coronary Bypass Surgery	Coronary Interventional Procedures (Angioplasty/Stent)	Diabetic Acidosis an...
1. Abbott-Northwestern Hospital, Minneapolis	NR	★★★	★	★	NR	★★★★★	★★★	★★★	★★★	★★★	★★★	★★★
2. Albert Lea Medical Center–Mayo Health System, Albert Lea	NR	★★★	NR	NR	NR	★★★	NR	★★★	★★★	NR	NR	NR
3. Austin Medical Center, Austin	NR	★★★	NR	NR	NR	★★★★★	NR	★	★★★	NR	NR	NR
4. Avera Marshall Regional Medical Center, Marshall	NR	NR	NR	NR	NR	★★★	NR	NR	★★★	NR	NR	NR
5. Buffalo Hospital, Buffalo	NR	★★★	NR	NR	NR	★★★	NR	NR	★★★	NR	NR	NR
6. Cambridge Medical Center, Cambridge	NR	★★★	NR	NR	NR	★★★	NR	★★★	★★★	NR	NR	NR
7. Chippewa County Hospital, Montevideo	NR	★★★	NR	NR	NR	★★★	NR	★★★★★	★	NR	NR	NR
8. Clearwater Health Services, Bagley	NR	NR	NR	NR	NR	NR	NR	NR	★★★	NR	NR	NR
9. Community Memorial Hospital, Cloquet	NR	★★★	NR	NR	NR	★★★	NR	★★★★★	★	NR	NR	NR
10. Cuyuna Regional Medical Center, Crosby	NR	★★★	NR	NR	NR	★★★	NR	NR	★★★	NR	NR	NR
11. Douglas County Hospital, Alexandria	NR	★★★	★★★	★	NR	★★★★★	NR	★★★	★★★	NR	NR	NR
12. Ely Bloomenson Community Hospital, Ely	NR	NR	NR	NR	NR	NR	NR	NR	★★★	NR	NR	NR
13. Fairmont Medical Center, Fairmont	NR	★★★	★★★	NR	NR	★★★	NR	★	★★★	NR	NR	NR
14. Fairview Hospital Chisago Lakes, Chisago City	NR	★★★	NR	NR	NR	★★★	NR	★★★	★★★	NR	NR	NR
15. Fairview Lakes Health Services, Wyoming	NR	★★★	NR	NR	NR	★★★	NR	★★★	★★★	NR	NR	NR
16. Fairview Northland Regional Hospital, Princeton	NR	★★★	NR	NR	NR	★★★	NR	★★★	★★★	NR	NR	NR
17. Fairview Red Wing Hospital, Red Wing	NR	★★★	★★★	NR	NR	★★★	NR	★★★	★★★	NR	NR	NR
18. Fairview Ridges Hospital, Burnsville	NR	★★★	NR	NR	NR	★★★★★	NR	★	★★★	NR	NR	★★★
19. Fairview Southdale Hospital, Edina	NR	★★★	★★★	★	NR	★★★	★★★	★★★	★★★★★	★★★	★★★★★	★★★
20. Falls Memorial Hospital, International Falls	NR	NR	NR	NR	NR	★★★	NR	NR	★★★	NR	NR	NR
21. First Care Medical Services, Fosston	NR	NR	NR	NR	NR	NR	NR	NR	★★★	NR	NR	NR
22. Glacial Ridge Hospital, Glenwood	NR	★★★	NR	NR	NR	NR	NR	NR	★★★	NR	NR	NR
23. Glencoe Regional Health Services, Glencoe	NR	★★★	NR	NR	NR	NR	NR	NR	★★★	NR	NR	NR
24. Grand Itasca Clinic and Hospital, Grand Rapids	NR	★★★	NR	NR	NR	★★★	NR	★	★★★	NR	NR	NR
25. Healtheast St. John's Hospital, Maplewood	NR	★★★	★★★★★	★★★	NR	★★★	★★★	★★★	★★★	NR	NR	★★★
26. Healtheast Woodwinds Hospital, Woodbury	NR	★★★	★★★★★	★★★★★	NR	★★★	NR	★★★	★★★	NR	NR	NR
27. Hennepin County Medical Center, Minneapolis	NR	★★★	NR	NR	NR	★★★	NR	★★★	★★★	NR	★★★	★★★
28. Hutchinson Area Health Care, Hutchinson	NR	★★★	NR	NR	NR	★★★★★	NR	★★★	★★★	NR	NR	NR
29. Immanuel St. Joseph's–Mayo Health System, Mankato	NR	★★★	★★★	★	NR	★	NR	★★★	★	NR	★★★	★★★
30. Kanabec Hospital, Mora	NR	★★★	NR	NR	NR	NR	NR	NR	★★★	NR	NR	NR
31. Lake Region Healthcare Corporation, Fergus Falls	NR	★★★	NR	NR	NR	★★★	★	★	★★★	NR	NR	NR
32. Lakeview Hospital, Stillwater	NR	★★★	★★★★★	★★★★★	NR	★★★	NR	★★★★★	★★★	NR	NR	NR
33. Lakewood Health System, Staples	NR	★★★	NR	NR	NR	NR	NR	NR	★★★	NR	NR	NR
34. Luverne Community Hospital, Luverne	NR	★★★	NR	NR	NR	NR	NR	NR	★★★	NR	NR	NR
35. Madison Hospital, Madison	NR	NR	NR	NR	NR	★★★	NR	NR	NR	NR	NR	NR
36. Meeker County Memorial Hospital, Litchfield	NR	★★★	NR	NR	NR	★★★	NR	NR	★★★	NR	NR	NR
37. Melrose Area Hospital Centracare, Melrose	NR	★★★	NR	NR	NR	NR	NR	NR	★	NR	NR	NR
38. Mercy Hospital and Health Care Center, Moose Lake	NR	★★★	NR	NR	NR	★	NR	NR	★	NR	NR	NR
39. Mercy Hospital, Coon Rapids	NR	★★★	★★★	★★★	NR	★★★★★	★★★	★★★	★★★★★	★★★	★★★★★	★★★
40. Methodist Hospital, Minneapolis	NR	★★★	★	★	NR	★★★★★	★	★★★	★★★	★★★	★★★	★★★
41. Mille Lacs Health System, Onamia	NR	NR	NR	NR	NR	NR	NR	NR	★★★	NR	NR	NR
42. Monticello-Big Lake Community Hospital, Monticello	NR	NR	NR	NR	NR	★★★	NR	NR	★★★	NR	NR	NR
43. Municipal Hospital and Granite Manor, Granite Falls	NR	NR	NR	NR	NR	NR	NR	NR	★★★	NR	NR	NR
44. Murray County Memorial Hospital, Slayton	NR	★★★	NR	NR	NR	NR	NR	NR	★★★	NR	NR	NR
45. New Ulm Medical Center, New Ulm	NR	★★★	NR	NR	NR	★★★	NR	★★★	★★★	NR	NR	NR
46. North Country Regional Hospital, Bemidji	NR	★★★★★	NR	NR	NR	★★★★★	★★★	★	★★★★★	NR	NR	NR
47. North Memorial Health Care, Robbinsdale	NR	★★★	★★★	★★★	NR	★★★	★★★	★★★	★★★	★★★★★	★★★★★	★★★
48. Northfield Hospital, Northfield	NR	★★★	NR	NR	NR	★★★	NR	★★★	★★★	NR	NR	NR
49. Northwest Medical Center, Thief River Falls	NR	NR	NR	NR	NR	★★★	NR	NR	★★★	NR	NR	NR
50. Olmsted Medical Center, Rochester	NR	NR	NR	NR	NR	NR	NR	NR	★★★	NR	NR	NR

KEY: ★★★★★ BEST   ★★★ AS EXPECTED   ★ POOR   NR NOT RATED BY HEALTHGRADES   For full definitions of ratings and awards, see Appendix.

Gastrointestinal Bleed	Gastrointestinal Surgeries and Procedures	Heart Attack	Heart Failure	Hip Fracture Repair	Maternity Care	Pancreatitis	Peripheral Vascular Bypass	Pneumonia	Prostatectomy	Pulmonary Embolism	Resection/Replacement of Abdominal Aorta	Respiratory Failure	Sepsis	Stroke	Total Hip Replacement	Total Knee Replacement	Valve Replacement	Women's Health
★★★	★★★	★★★	★★★★★	★	NR	★★★	★★★	★★★	★★★	★★★	★★★	★★★	★★★★★	★★★★★	★	★	★★★	NR
★★★	★★★	★★★	★	★★★	NR	NR	NR	★★★	★★★	NR	NR	★	★★★	★★★	★	★	NR	NR
★★★★★	★★★	★★★	★★★★★	★	NR	NR	NR	★★★	★★★	NR	NR	★★★	★★★	★★★	★	★	NR	NR
★★★	NR	NR	★★★	NR	NR	NR	NR	★★★	NR	NR	NR	NR	NR	★	NR	★★★	NR	NR
★★★	NR	NR	★★★	★	NR	NR	NR	★★★	NR	NR	NR	★★★	★★★	★★★	★★★	★★★	NR	NR
★★★★★	NR	NR	★★★★★	★★★	NR	NR	NR	★★★	NR	NR	NR	★★★	★★★	★	★	NR	NR	NR
NR	NR	NR	★★★★★	NR	NR	NR	NR	★★★	NR	NR	NR	NR	NR	NR	NR	NR	NR	NR
★★★	NR	★★★	★★★	NR	NR	NR	NR	★★★	NR	NR	NR	NR	★	NR	NR	★★★	NR	NR
★★★	NR	NR	★★★	NR	NR	NR	NR	★★★	NR	NR	NR	NR	★★★	★★★	★★★	★★★	NR	NR
★★★	★★★	NR	★★★	★★★	NR	★★★	NR	★★★	★★★	NR	NR	★★★	★★★★★	★	★★★	★★★	NR	NR
NR	NR	NR	★★★	NR	NR	NR	NR	★★★	NR	NR	NR	NR	NR	NR	NR	NR	NR	NR
★★★	NR	★★★	★★★	★	NR	NR	NR	★	NR	NR	NR	NR	★★★	★★★	★	★	NR	NR
★★★	NR	★★★★★	★★★★★	★★★	NR	★★★	NR	★★★★★	NR	★★★	NR	★★★	★★★	★★★	★★★	★★★	NR	NR
★★★	NR	★★★★★	★★★★★	★★★	NR	★★★	NR	★★★★★	NR	★★★	NR	★★★	★★★	★★★	★★★	★★★	NR	NR
★★★	NR	★★★	★★★	★	NR	NR	NR	★★★	NR	NR	NR	★★★	★★★	★★★	★	★	NR	NR
★★★	NR	NR	★★★	★	NR	NR	NR	★★★	NR	NR	NR	★★★	★★★	★★★	★★★	★	NR	NR
★★★	★★★	★★★	★★★	★★★	NR	★★★	NR	★★★★★	NR	★★★	NR	★★★	★★★	★★★	★★★	★★★	NR	NR
★★★	★★★	★★★★★	★★★★★	★★★	NR	★★★	★★★	★★★★★	★★★	★★★	★★★	★★★★★	★★★★★	★★★★★	★★★	★★★	★★★	NR
★★★	NR	NR	★★★	NR	NR	NR	NR	★★★	NR	NR	NR	NR	★★★	★★★	NR	NR	NR	NR
NR	NR	NR	★★★	NR	NR	NR	NR	★★★	NR	NR	NR	NR	NR	★★★	NR	NR	NR	NR
NR	NR	NR	★★★	NR	NR	NR	NR	★★★	NR	NR	NR	NR	NR	NR	NR	NR	NR	NR
★★★	NR	NR	★	NR	NR	NR	NR	★★★	NR	NR	NR	NR	NR	NR	NR	★★★★★	NR	NR
★★★	★★★	★★★	★★★	★★★	NR	NR	NR	★★★	NR	NR	NR	★★★	★★★	★★★	★	NR	★	NR
★★★	★★★	★★★	★★★	★★★	NR	★★★	★★★	★★★★★	★★★★★	★★★	NR	★★★	★★★★★	★★★★★	★★★★★	★★★	NR	NR
★★★	NR	★★★	★★★★★	★	NR	★★★	NR	★★★★★	NR	★★★	★★★	★	★★★	★★★	★★★★★	★★★★★	NR	NR
★★★	★★★	NR	★★★	★	NR	NR	NR	★★★	NR	NR	NR	★★★★★	★★★	★★★	★	NR	★★★	NR
★★★	★★★	★★★	★	★	NR	★★★	NR	★★★	NR	★★★	NR	★	★★★	★★★	★★★	★★★	★★★	NR
★★★	NR	NR	★	NR	NR	NR	NR	★★★	NR	NR	NR	NR	★★★	NR	NR	★★★	NR	NR
★★★	★★★	★★★	★★★	★	NR	★★★	NR	★★★	NR	NR	NR	NR	★★★	★	★★★	★★★	NR	NR
★★★	★★★	★★★	★★★	★★★★★	NR	NR	NR	★★★	NR	NR	NR	NR	★★★	★★★	★★★★★	★★★★★	NR	NR
NR	NR	NR	★	NR	NR	NR	NR	★★★	NR	NR	NR	NR	NR	NR	NR	NR	NR	NR
★	NR	NR	★	NR	NR	NR	NR	★★★	NR	NR	NR	NR	★★★	★★★	NR	NR	NR	NR
NR	NR	NR	★★★	NR	NR	NR	NR	★★★	NR	NR	NR	NR	NR	NR	NR	NR	NR	NR
★★★	NR	NR	★★★	★	NR	NR	NR	★★★	NR	NR	NR	NR	★	NR	NR	NR	NR	NR
NR	NR	NR	★★★	NR	NR	NR	NR	★★★	NR	NR	NR	NR	NR	NR	NR	NR	NR	NR
★★★	NR	NR	★★★	NR	NR	NR	NR	★★★	NR	NR	NR	NR	NR	★★★	NR	NR	NR	NR
★★★	★★★	★★★	★★★★★	★	NR	★★★	★★★	★★★★★	★★★	★★★	★★★	★★★★★	★★★★★	★★★★★	★★★	★★★	★★★	NR
★★★★★	★★★★★	★★★★★	★★★★★	★	NR	★★★	★★★	★★★★★	★★★	★★★	★★★	★★★★★	★★★★★	★★★★★	★	★★★	★★★	NR
NR	NR	NR	★★★	NR	NR	NR	NR	★★★	NR	NR	NR	NR	NR	NR	NR	NR	NR	NR
★★★	NR	NR	★★★	★★★	NR	NR	NR	★★★★★	NR	NR	NR	NR	★★★	NR	NR	NR	NR	NR
★★★	NR	NR	★★★	NR	NR	NR	NR	★★★	NR	NR	NR	NR	NR	★★★	NR	NR	NR	NR
NR	NR	NR	★★★	NR	NR	NR	NR	★	NR	NR	NR	NR	NR	NR	NR	★★★	NR	NR
★★★	NR	★★★★★	★★★	★	NR	NR	NR	★★★	NR	NR	NR	NR	★★★	★★★	★	★	NR	NR
★★★	★★★	★★★	★★★★★	★★★	NR	NR	NR	★★★	★★★	NR	NR	★★★	★★★	★	★★★	★★★	NR	NR
★★★★★	★★★	★★★	★★★	★★★	NR	★★★	★★★	★★★★★	★	★★★	★★★★★	★★★★★	★★★★★	★★★★★	★★★	★	★★★	NR
★	NR	★★★	★★★	★	NR	NR	NR	★★★	★★★	NR	NR	NR	NR	NR	★★★	★	NR	NR
★★★	NR	★★★	★★★	NR	NR	NR	NR	★★★	NR	NR	NR	NR	★★★	★	★★★	★★★	NR	NR
★★★	NR	NR	★★★	NR	NR	NR	NR	★★★	NR	NR	NR	NR	NR	NR	NR	★★★	NR	NR

	Appendectomy	Atrial Fibrillation	Back and Neck Surgery (except Spinal Fusion)	Back and Neck Surgery (Spinal Fusion)	Bariatric Surgery	Bowel Obstruction	Carotid Surgery	Cholecystectomy (Gall Bladder Removal)	Chronic Obstructive Pulmonary Disease (COPD)	Coronary Bypass Surgery	Coronary Interventional Procedures (Angioplasty/Sten)	Diabetic Acidosis
51. Owatonna Hospital, Owatonna	NR	★★★	NR	NR	NR	★★★	NR	NR	★	NR	NR	NR
52. Paynesville Area Health Care System, Paynesville	NR	NR	NR	NR	NR	NR	NR	★★★	NR	NR	NR	NR
53. Perham Memorial Hospital and Home, Perham	NR	NR	NR	NR	NR	NR	NR	★★★	NR	NR	NR	NR
54. Pine Medical Center, Sandstone	NR	NR	NR	NR	NR	NR	NR	★★★	NR	NR	NR	NR
55. Pipestone County Medical Center Ashton Care Center, Pipestone	NR	NR	NR	NR	NR	NR	NR	NR	NR	NR	NR	NR
56. Queen of Peace Hospital, New Prague	NR	★★★	NR	NR	NR	★★★	NR	★★★	NR	NR	NR	NR
57. Redwood Area Hospital, Redwood Falls	NR	NR	NR	NR	NR	NR	NR	★★★	NR	NR	NR	NR
58. Regina Medical Center, Hastings	NR	★★★	NR	NR	NR	★★★	NR	★★★	NR	NR	NR	NR
59. Regions Hospital, St. Paul	NR	★★★	★★★	★★★	NR	★★★	★	★★★	★★★	★★★	★★★	★★★
60. Rice County District One Hospital, Faribault	NR	★★★	NR	NR	NR	★★★	NR	★★★	NR	NR	NR	NR
61. Rice Memorial Hospital, Willmar	NR	★★★	NR	NR	NR	★★★	★★★	★★★	★★★	NR	NR	NR
62. Ridgeview Medical Center, Waconia	NR	★	★★★	NR	NR	★★★	NR	★★★	★	NR	NR	NR
63. Riverview Hospital, Crookston	NR	NR	NR	NR	★	NR	NR	★★★	NR	NR	NR	NR
64. Rochester Methodist Hospital, Rochester	NR	NR	NR	NR	NR	★★★	NR	★★★	★	NR	★★★	NR
65. Roseau Area Hospital and Homes, Roseau	NR	NR	NR	NR	NR	NR	NR	★★★	NR	NR	NR	NR
66. Rush City Hospital, Rush City	NR	★★★	NR	NR	NR	★★★	NR	★★★	NR	NR	NR	NR
67. St. Cloud Hospital, St. Cloud	NR	★★★	★★★	★★★★★	NR	★★★★★	★★★	★★★	★★★	★★★	★★★	★★★
68. St. Elizabeth Medical Center, Wabasha	NR	★★★	NR	NR	NR	★★★	NR	NR	★★★	NR	NR	NR
69. St. Francis Medical Center, Breckenridge	NR	★★★	NR	NR	NR	★★★	NR	NR	★★★	NR	NR	NR
70. St. Francis Regional Medical Center, Shakopee	NR	★★★	NR	NR	NR	★★★	NR	★	★★★	NR	NR	NR
71. St. Gabriel's Hospital, Little Falls	NR	NR	NR	NR	NR	★★★	NR	★★★	★★★	NR	NR	NR
72. St. James Health Services, St. James	NR	NR	NR	NR	NR	NR	NR	★★★	NR	NR	NR	NR
73. St. Joseph's Hospital, St. Paul	NR	★★★	★★★★★	★★★	NR	★★★★★	★★★	★★★	★★★	★★★	★★★	★★★
74. St. Josephs Area Health Services, Park Rapids	NR	★★★	NR	NR	NR	★★★	NR	★★★	★★★	NR	NR	NR
75. St. Joseph's Medical Center, Brainerd	NR	★★★	NR	NR	NR	★★★	NR	★★★	★	NR	★★★	NR
76. St. Luke's Hospital, Duluth	NR	★★★	★★★	★★★★★	NR	★★★	★★★	★★★	★★★	★★★	★★★	NR
77. St. Mary's Duluth Clinic, Duluth	NR	★★★★★	★★★	★★★	NR	★★★	NR	★★★	★★★	★★★★★	★★★	★★★
78. St. Marys Hospital, Rochester	NR	★★★★★	★	★	NR	★★★★★	★	★	★★★★★	★★★	★★★	★★★
79. St. Mary's Regional Health Center, Detroit Lakes	NR	★★★	NR	NR	NR	★★★	NR	★★★★★	★★★	NR	NR	NR
80. St. Michael's Hospital and Nursing Home, Sauk Centre	NR	NR	NR	NR	NR	NR	NR	★★★	NR	NR	NR	NR
81. St. Peter Community Hospital, St. Peter	NR	NR	NR	NR	NR	NR	NR	★★★	NR	NR	NR	NR
82. Sioux Valley Canby Campus, Canby	NR	NR	NR	NR	NR	NR	NR	★★★	NR	NR	NR	NR
83. Stevens Community Medical Center, Morris	NR	★★★	NR	NR	NR	★★★	NR	NR	★★★	NR	NR	NR
84. Swift County Benson Hospital, Benson	NR	NR	NR	NR	NR	NR	NR	NR	NR	NR	NR	NR
85. Tracy Area Medical Services, Tracy	NR	NR	NR	NR	NR	NR	NR	★★★	NR	NR	NR	NR
86. Tri-County Hospital, Wadena	NR	★★★	NR	NR	NR	★★★	NR	★★★	★★★	NR	NR	NR
87. United Hospital District, Blue Earth	NR	NR	NR	NR	NR	NR	NR	★★★	NR	NR	NR	NR
88. United Hospitals, St. Paul	NR	★★★	★★★	★★★	NR	★★★★★	★★★	★★★	★★★★★	★★★	★★★	★★★
89. Unity Hospital, Fridley	NR	★★★	★	★	NR	★★★	★★★	★★★	★★★	NR	NR	★★★
90. University Medical Center—Mesabi, Hibbing	NR	★★★	NR	NR	NR	★★★	NR	★★★★★	★★★	NR	NR	★★★
91. University of Minnesota Hospital and Clinic, Minneapolis	NR	★★★★★	★	★	NR	★★★	NR	★★★	★★★★★	★★★	★	NR
92. University of Minnesota Med. Ctr.—Fairview, Minneapolis	NR	★★★★★	★	★	NR	★★★	NR	★★★	★★★★★	★★★	★	NR
93. Virginia Regional Medical Center, Virginia	NR	★★★	NR	NR	NR	★★★	NR	★★★	★★★	NR	NR	NR
94. Windom Area Hospital, Windom	NR	NR	NR	NR	NR	NR	NR	★★★	NR	NR	NR	NR
95. Winona Community Memorial Hospital, Winona	NR	★★★	NR	NR	NR	★★★	NR	★★★	★★★	NR	NR	NR
96. Worthington Regional Hospital, Worthington	NR	★★★	NR	NR	NR	★★★	NR	★★★	NR	NR	NR	NR

KEY: ★★★★★ BEST   ★★★ AS EXPECTED   ★ POOR   NR NOT RATED BY HEALTHGRADES   For full definitions of ratings and awards, see Appendix.

Gastrointestinal Bleed	Gastrointestinal Surgeries and Procedures	Heart Attack	Heart Failure	Hip Fracture Repair	Maternity Care	Pancreatitis	Peripheral Vascular Bypass	Pneumonia	Prostatectomy	Pulmonary Embolism	Resection/Replacement of Abdominal Aorta	Respiratory Failure	Sepsis	Stroke	Total Hip Replacement	Total Knee Replacement	Valve Replacement	Women's Health
★★★	NR	★★★	★★★	★★★	NR	NR	NR	★★★	NR	NR	NR	NR	★★★	★★★	★★★	★	NR	NR
NR	NR	NR	★	NR	NR	NR	NR	★	NR	NR	NR	NR	NR	★★★	NR	★★★	NR	NR
★★★	NR	NR	★	NR	NR	NR	NR	★★★	NR	NR	NR	NR	NR	NR	NR	NR	NR	NR
NR	NR	NR	★★★	NR	NR	NR	NR	★★★	NR	NR	NR	NR	NR	NR	NR	NR	NR	NR
★★★	NR	NR	★	NR	NR	NR	NR	★★★	NR	NR	NR	NR	NR	★★★	NR	★★★★★	NR	NR
★★★	NR	★★★	★	★★★	NR	NR	NR	★★★	NR	NR	NR	NR	NR	★★★	★★★	★★★	NR	NR
NR	NR	NR	★★★	NR	NR	NR	NR	★	NR	NR	NR	NR	NR	★	NR	NR	NR	NR
★★★	NR	NR	★★★	★★★	NR	NR	NR	★★★	★★★	NR	NR	NR	★★★	★★★	★★★	★	NR	NR
★★★★★	★★★	★★★★★	★★★	★	NR	★★★	NR	★★★	★★★	★★★	★★★	★★★★★	★★★	★★★	★★★	★	★★★	NR
★★★	NR	NR	★★★	★	NR	NR	NR	★★★	NR	NR	NR	★★★	★	★	★★★	NR	NR	NR
★★★	★	★★★	★★★	★★★	NR	NR	NR	★	★★★★★	NR	NR	NR	★	★★★	★★★★★	★★★★★	NR	NR
★★★	★★★	★★★	★★★	★★★	NR	★★★	NR	★★★	★★★	★★★	NR	★	★★★	★★★	★★★	NR	NR	NR
★★★	NR	★★★★★	★★★	★★★★★	NR	NR	NR	★	NR	NR	NR	★	NR	NR	NR	NR	NR	NR
★★★	★★★★★	NR	★★★	NR	NR	NR	NR	★★★★★	★★★	★★★	NR	★★★	NR	★	NR	NR	NR	NR
NR	NR	NR	★	NR	NR	NR	NR	★★★	NR	NR	NR	NR	NR	NR	NR	NR	NR	NR
★★★	NR	★★★★★	★★★★★	★★★	NR	★★★	NR	★★★★★	NR	★★★	NR	★★★	★★★	★★★	★★★	★★★	NR	NR
★★★★★	★★★	★★★	★★★★★	★★★	NR	★★★	★★★	★★★★★	★★★★★	★★★	★★★	★★★	★★★	★★★	★★★★★	★★★★★	★★★★★	NR
★★★	NR	NR	★★★	NR	NR	NR	NR	★★★	NR	NR	NR	NR	NR	NR	NR	NR	NR	NR
★★★	NR	NR	★	NR	NR	NR	NR	★★★	NR	NR	NR	NR	★★★	NR	NR	NR	NR	NR
★★★★★	★★★	NR	★★★	★	NR	NR	NR	★★★	NR	NR	NR	★★★	★★★	★★★	★	★★★	NR	NR
★★★	NR	NR	★	★★★	NR	NR	NR	★★★	NR	NR	NR	★★★	★★★	★	★★★	NR	NR	NR
NR	NR	NR	★★★	NR	NR	NR	NR	★★★	NR	NR	NR	NR	NR	NR	NR	NR	NR	NR
★★★★★	★★★	★★★	★★★	NR	NR	★★★	NR	★★★★★	★★★	★★★	★★★	★★★	★★★★★	★★★	★★★★★	★★★	NR	NR
★★★	★★★	★★★	★	NR	NR	★★★	NR	★★★	NR	NR	NR	★★★	★★★	NR	NR	NR	NR	NR
★★★	NR	★★★	★★★	★★★	NR	★★★	NR	★★★	★★★	★★★	NR	★★★	★★★	★★★	★★★	★★★	NR	NR
★★★	★★★★★	★★★	★★★★★	★★★★★	NR	★★★	NR	★★★	★★★	★★★	★★★	★★★★★	★★★★★	★★★	★★★	★★★★★	★	NR
★★★	★	★★★★★	★★★	★	NR	★★★	★	★★★★★	★★★	★★★	NR	★★★★★	★★★★★	★★★★★	★	★	★★★	NR
★★★★★	★★★★★	★★★★★	★★★★★	★	NR	★★★	★	★★★★★	★★★	★★★★★	★★★	★★★	★★★★★	★★★	★	★	★★★	NR
★★★	NR	★★★★★	★★★	★★★	NR	NR	NR	★	NR	NR	NR	NR	NR	★	NR	★★★	★★★	NR
NR	NR	NR	★★★	NR	NR	NR	NR	★★★	NR	NR	NR	NR	NR	NR	NR	NR	NR	NR
NR	NR	NR	★★★	NR	NR	NR	NR	★★★★★	NR	NR	NR	NR	NR	NR	NR	NR	NR	NR
NR	NR	NR	★★★	NR	NR	NR	NR	★★★	NR	NR	NR	NR	NR	NR	NR	NR	NR	NR
★★★	NR	NR	★★★	NR	NR	NR	NR	★★★	NR	NR	NR	NR	NR	NR	NR	NR	NR	NR
NR	NR	NR	★★★	NR	NR	NR	NR	★★★	NR	NR	NR	NR	NR	★★★	NR	NR	NR	NR
NR	NR	NR	★★★	NR	NR	NR	NR	★★★	NR	NR	NR	NR	NR	NR	NR	NR	NR	NR
★★★	NR	NR	★★★	★★★	NR	NR	NR	★★★	NR	NR	NR	NR	NR	★★★	NR	NR	NR	NR
NR	NR	NR	★★★	★★★	NR	NR	NR	★	NR	NR	NR	NR	NR	NR	★★★	★★★	NR	NR
★★★	★★★	★★★★★	★★★★★	★	NR	NR	★★★	★★★	★★★★★	★★★	★★★	★★★	★★★	★★★	★★★	★★★	★	★★★
★★★	★★★	★★★★★	★★★★★	★★★	NR	★★★	NR	★★★★★	★★★	★★★★★	NR	★★★★★	★★★★★	★★★	★	★	★★★	NR
★	★★★	★★★	★★★	★★★	NR	★	NR	★★★	★★★	NR	NR	★★★	★★★	★★★★★	★★★	★★★	NR	NR
★★★	★★★	★★★	★★★	★	NR	★★★	NR	★★★	★★★	★★★	NR	★★★	★★★★★	★★★★★	★	★	★★★	NR
★★★	★★★	★★★	★★★	★	NR	★★★	NR	★★★	★★★	★★★	NR	★★★	★★★★★	★★★★★	★	★	★★★	NR
★★★	★	★★★	★★★	★	NR	NR	NR	★★★	★★★	NR	NR	★★★	★★★★★	★★★	NR	NR	★★★	NR
★★★	NR	NR	★★★	NR	NR	NR	NR	★★★	NR	NR	NR	NR	NR	★	NR	NR	NR	NR
★★★	★★★★★	★★★★★	★★★	★★★	NR	NR	NR	★★★	NR	NR	NR	★★★	★★★	★★★	NR	NR	NR	NR
★★★	NR	NR	★★★	★	NR	NR	NR	★★★	NR	NR	NR	NR	NR	NR	NR	★★★	NR	NR

MISSISSIPPI HOSPITALS: RATINGS BY PROCEDURE

Hospital	Appendectomy	Atrial Fibrillation	Back and Neck Surgery (except Spinal Fusion)	Back and Neck Surgery (Spinal Fusion)	Bariatric Surgery	Bowel Obstruction	Carotid Surgery	Cholecystectomy (Gall Bladder Removal)	Chronic Obstructive Pulmonary Disease (COPD)	Coronary Bypass Surgery	Coronary Interventional Procedures (Angioplasty/Stent)	Diabetic Acidosis a...
1. Baptist Memorial Hospital—Booneville, Booneville	NR	★★★	NR	NR	NR	★★★	NR	★	★★★	NR	NR	NR
2. Baptist Memorial Hospital—De Soto, Southaven	NR	★★★	★★★	NR	★★★	★★★	★★★	★★★	★★★	★★★	★★★	★★★
3. Baptist Memorial Hospital—Golden Triangle, Columbus	NR	★★★	★★★	★★★★★	★★★	★★★	★★★★★	★	★★★	★★★	★	NR
4. Baptist Memorial Hospital—North Mississippi, Oxford	NR	★★★	★★★★★	NR	★	★★★	★★★	★	★★★	★★★	★	NR
5. Baptist Memorial Hospital—Union County, New Albany	NR	★★★	NR	NR	★★★	NR	★★★	★★★	★★★	NR	NR	NR
6. Batesville Specialty Hospital, Batesville	NR	NR	NR	NR	NR	NR	NR	★★★	NR	NR	NR	NR
7. Beacham Memorial, Magnolia	NR	★★★	NR	NR	NR	NR	NR	★★★	NR	NR	NR	NR
8. Biloxi Regional Medical Center, Biloxi	NR	★★★	★	★★★	NR	★★★	NR	★★★	★★★	NR	★★★	NR
9. Bolivar Medical Center, Cleveland	NR	★	NR	NR	NR	★★★	NR	★★★	★★★	NR	★★★	NR
10. Central Mississippi Medical Center, Jackson	NR	★★★	★★★	NR	NR	★★★	★★★	★★★	NR	★★★	★★★	★
11. Clay County Medical Center, West Point	NR	NR	NR	NR	NR	★★★	NR	★★★	★★★	NR	NR	NR
12. Covington County Hospital, Collins	NR	NR	NR	NR	NR	NR	NR	★★★	★★★	NR	NR	NR
13. Delta Regional Medical Center, Greenville	NR	★★★	NR	NR	★	★	★★★★★	★★★	★★★	★★★	★★★	★★★
14. Field Memorial Community Hospital, Centreville	NR	NR	NR	NR	NR	NR	NR	★★★	NR	NR	NR	NR
15. Forrest General Hospital, Hattiesburg	NR	★★★	★★★	★★★★★	NR	★★★	★★★★★	★★★	★★★	★★★	★★★	★
16. Franklin County Memorial Hospital, Meadville	NR	NR	NR	NR	NR	NR	NR	★★★	NR	NR	NR	NR
17. Garden Park Medical Center, Gulfport	NR	★★★	★★★	★★★	NR	★★★	NR	★★★	★★★	NR	NR	NR
18. George Regional Health System, Lucedale	NR	★★★	NR	NR	NR	★★★	NR	★★★★★	★★★	NR	NR	NR
19. Gilmore Memorial Hospital, Amory	NR	★★★	NR	NR	NR	★★★	NR	★★★	★	NR	NR	NR
20. Greenwood Leflore Hospital, Greenwood	NR	★★★	NR	NR	NR	★★★	NR	★★★	★★★	NR	NR	★★★
21. Grenada Lake Medical Center, Grenada	NR	★	NR	NR	NR	★	NR	★★★★★	★	NR	NR	NR
22. Gulf Coast Medical Center, Biloxi	NR	★	★★★	NR	NR	★★★	NR	NR	★★★	NR	NR	NR
23. H. C. Watkins Memorial Hospital, Quitman	NR	NR	NR	NR	NR	NR	NR	NR	★★★	NR	NR	NR
24. Hancock Medical Center, Bay St. Louis	NR	★★★	NR	NR	NR	★★★	NR	NR	★★★	★★★	NR	NR
25. Hardy Wilson Memorial Hospital, Hazlehurst	NR	NR	NR	NR	NR	NR	NR	NR	★	NR	NR	NR
26. Highland Community Hospital, Picayune	NR	★	NR	NR	NR	★★★	NR	NR	★★★	NR	NR	NR
27. Humphreys County Memorial Hospital, Belzoni	NR	NR	NR	NR	NR	NR	NR	NR	★★★	NR	NR	NR
28. Jeff Anderson Regional Medical Center, Meridian	NR	★	★★★	NR	NR	★	★★★	★★★★★	★★★	★	★★★	★
29. Jefferson Davis Community Hospital, Prentiss	NR	NR	NR	NR	NR	NR	NR	NR	★★★	NR	NR	NR
30. King's Daughters Medical Center—Brookhaven, Brookhaven	NR	★	NR	NR	NR	★★★	NR	★★★	★★★	NR	NR	★★★
31. King's Daughters Hospital, Yazoo City	NR	NR	NR	NR	NR	NR	NR	NR	★★★	NR	NR	NR
32. King's Daughters Hospital—Greenville, Greenville	NR	★★★	NR	NR	NR	★	★	★★★★★	★★★	★★★	★★★	★★★
33. Lackey Memorial Hospital, Forest	NR	NR	NR	NR	NR	NR	NR	NR	★★★	NR	NR	NR
34. Laird Hospital, Union	NR	NR	NR	NR	NR	NR	NR	NR	★★★	NR	NR	NR
35. Lawrence County Hospital, Monticello	NR	NR	NR	NR	NR	NR	NR	NR	★★★	NR	NR	NR
36. Leake County Memorial Hospital, Carthage	NR	NR	NR	NR	NR	NR	NR	NR	★★★	NR	NR	NR
37. Madison Regional Medical Center, Canton	NR	NR	NR	NR	NR	NR	NR	NR	★★★	NR	NR	NR
38. Magee General Hospital, Magee	NR	NR	NR	NR	NR	★★★	NR	NR	★★★	NR	NR	NR
39. Magnolia Regional Health Center, Corinth	NR	★★★	NR	NR	NR	★	NR	★★★	★★★	NR	★★★	★★★
40. Marion General Hospital, Columbia	NR	★	NR	NR	NR	★★★	NR	NR	★★★	NR	NR	★★★
41. Memorial Hospital at Gulfport, Gulfport	NR	★★★	★★★	NR	NR	★★★	★★★★★	★★★	★★★	★★★	★	★★★
42. Mississippi Baptist Medical Center, Jackson	NR	★	★★★★★	NR	NR	★★★	★★★★★	★★★★★	★★★	★★★	★★★	★★★
43. Montfort Jones Memorial Hospital, Kosciusko	NR	★	NR	NR	NR	★★★	NR	NR	★	NR	NR	★
44. Natchez Community Hospital, Natchez	NR	★★★	NR	NR	NR	★	NR	★★★★★	★	NR	NR	★★★
45. Natchez Regional Medical Center, Natchez	NR	★	NR	NR	NR	★★★	NR	★	★	NR	NR	NR
46. Neshoba County General Hospital, Philadelphia	NR	NR	NR	NR	NR	NR	NR	NR	★★★	NR	NR	NR
47. Newton Regional Hospital, Newton	NR	NR	NR	NR	NR	NR	NR	NR	★★★	NR	NR	NR
48. North Mississippi Medical Center, Tupelo	NR	★	★★★	★★★★★	NR	★	★★★	★★★★★	★★★	★★★	★★★	★★★
49. North Oak Regional Medical Center, Senatobia	NR	NR	NR	NR	NR	NR	NR	NR	★★★	NR	NR	★★★
50. North Sunflower Medical Center, Ruleville	NR	NR	NR	NR	NR	NR	NR	NR	★★★	NR	NR	NR

KEY: ★★★★★ BEST   ★★★ AS EXPECTED   ★ POOR   NR NOT RATED BY HEALTHGRADES   For full definitions of ratings and awards, see Appendix.

Gastrointestinal Bleed	Gastrointestinal Surgeries and Procedures	Heart Attack	Heart Failure	Hip Fracture Repair	Maternity Care	Pancreatitis	Peripheral Vascular Bypass	Pneumonia	Prostatectomy	Pulmonary Embolism	Resection/Replacement of Abdominal Aorta	Respiratory Failure	Sepsis	Stroke	Total Hip Replacement	Total Knee Replacement	Valve Replacement	Women's Health
★★★	NR	NR	★★★	NR	NR	NR	NR	★★★	NR	NR	NR	★★★	★	★	NR	NR	NR	NR
★★★	★★★	★★★	★★★	★★★	NR	★★★	NR	★★★	NR	★★★	NR	★★★	★★★	★★★	★★★★★	★★★	NR	NR
★★★	★★★	★	★	★★★	NR	★	NR	★	★★★	★	NR	★	★	★	★★★	★★★★★	NR	NR
★	★★★	★★★	★	★★★	NR	★	★★★	★	★★★★★	★★★	NR	★	★★★	★	★★★	★★★	NR	NR
★★★	NR	★★★	★	★★★	NR	NR	NR	★	NR	NR	NR	NR	★★★	★★★	NR	★★★	NR	NR
★★★	NR	NR	★★★	NR	NR	NR	NR	★★★	NR	NR	NR	★	NR	NR	NR	NR	NR	NR
NR	NR	NR	★	NR	NR	NR	NR	★	NR	NR	NR	NR	★★★	NR	NR	NR	NR	NR
★	★	NR	★	★★★	NR	NR	NR	★★★	★★★	NR	NR	★	★	★	NR	★★★	NR	NR
★★★	NR	★★★	★	★★★	NR	NR	NR	★	NR	NR	NR	★★★	★	★★★	NR	NR	NR	NR
★★★	★★★	★	★★★	★★★	NR	★★★	NR	★★★	★★★	★★★	NR	★★★	★	★★★	★★★	NR	NR	NR
★★★	NR	NR	★	★★★	NR	NR	NR	★	NR	NR	NR	★★★	★★★	★★★	NR	NR	NR	NR
★	NR	NR	★	NR	NR	NR	NR	★	NR	NR	NR	NR	NR	NR	NR	NR	NR	NR
★	★	★	★	★★★	NR	★	NR	★	★	★★★	NR	★	★	★	★★★	★★★	NR	NR
★★★	NR	NR	★★★	NR	NR	NR	NR	★★★	NR	NR	NR	NR	★★★	NR	NR	NR	NR	NR
★★★	★★★	NR	★	★★★★★	NR	★★★	★★★★★	★	★★★	★★★	★	★★★	★	★★★	★★★	★★★	★★★	NR
NR	NR	NR	★★★	NR	NR	NR	NR	★★★	NR	NR	NR	NR	NR	NR	NR	NR	NR	NR
★	NR	NR	★	★★★	NR	NR	NR	★	NR	NR	NR	★	★	★★★	★	★★★★★	NR	NR
★★★	★	★★★	★	NR	NR	NR	NR	★★★	NR	NR	NR	NR	★	★	NR	NR	NR	NR
★★★	★★★	★★★	★★★	NR	NR	NR	NR	★★★	NR	NR	NR	NR	★	★★★	NR	NR	NR	NR
★★★	★★★	★★★	★	★★★	NR	★★★	NR	★	★★★★★	NR	NR	★★★	★	NR	NR	★★★★★	NR	NR
★	NR	★★★	★	★★★	NR	NR	NR	★	NR	NR	NR	★	★	NR	NR	NR	NR	NR
★★★	NR	NR	★★★	★★★★★	NR	NR	NR	★★★	NR	NR	NR	NR	★★★	★★★★★	★★★★★	NR	NR	NR
NR	NR	NR	NR	NR	NR	NR	NR	★★★	NR	NR	NR	NR	NR	NR	NR	NR	NR	NR
★★★	NR	NR	★	NR	NR	NR	NR	★★★	NR	NR	NR	★★★	NR	NR	NR	NR	NR	NR
★★★	NR	NR	★	NR	NR	NR	NR	★	NR	NR	NR	★★★	NR	NR	NR	NR	NR	NR
★	NR	NR	★★★	★★★	NR	NR	NR	★★★	NR	NR	NR	★	NR	★	NR	NR	NR	NR
NR	NR	NR	★★★	NR	NR	NR	NR	★	NR	NR	NR	NR	NR	★	NR	NR	NR	NR
★★★	★★★	★	★	★★★★★	NR	★★★	NR	★	★★★	★★★	★★★	★★★	★★★	★★★	★★★	★★★	★★★	NR
NR	NR	NR	★★★	NR	NR	NR	NR	★	NR	NR	NR	NR	NR	NR	NR	NR	NR	NR
★★★	NR	★★★	★	★★★	NR	NR	NR	★★★	★★★	★★★	NR	NR	★	NR	★★★	NR	NR	NR
★★★	NR	NR	★★★	NR	NR	NR	NR	★★★	NR	NR	NR	NR	★★★	NR	NR	NR	NR	NR
★	★	★	★	★★★	NR	★	NR	★	★	★★★	NR	★	★	★★★	★★★	NR	NR	NR
NR	NR	NR	★	NR	NR	NR	NR	★★★	NR	NR	NR	NR	NR	NR	NR	NR	NR	NR
NR	NR	NR	★★★	NR	NR	NR	NR	★★★	NR	NR	NR	NR	NR	NR	NR	NR	NR	NR
NR	NR	NR	★★★	NR	NR	NR	NR	★★★	NR	NR	NR	NR	NR	NR	NR	NR	NR	NR
NR	NR	NR	★	NR	NR	NR	NR	★★★	NR	NR	NR	NR	★★★	NR	NR	NR	NR	NR
★★★	NR	★★★	★★★	NR	NR	NR	NR	★	NR	NR	NR	★★★	NR	NR	NR	NR	NR	NR
★	NR	NR	★★★	NR	NR	NR	NR	★	NR	NR	NR	NR	NR	NR	NR	NR	NR	NR
★★★	★★★	★	★	★★★	NR	★★★	NR	★	NR	★★★	NR	★★★	★	★	★★★	★★★	NR	NR
★★★	NR	★★★	★	NR	NR	NR	NR	★	NR	NR	NR	★	NR	NR	NR	NR	NR	NR
★★★	★★★	★	★	★★★	NR	★★★	★★★	★	★★★	★★★	★★★	★	★	★	★★★	★★★	★★★	NR
★★★	★★★★★	★★★	★★★	★★★	NR	★★★★★	★★★★★	★★★	★★★★★	★★★	★★★	★★★	★	★	★★★	★★★	★★★	NR
★★★	NR	NR	★	NR	NR	NR	NR	★	NR	NR	NR	★★★	★	NR	NR	NR	NR	NR
★	NR	★★★	★	★★★	NR	NR	NR	★	NR	NR	NR	★	NR	NR	★	★★★	NR	NR
★	NR	★★★	★	★★★	NR	NR	NR	★	NR	NR	NR	★	★	★★★	★★★	★★★	★★★	NR
★★★	NR	NR	★★★	NR	NR	NR	NR	★	NR	NR	NR	★★★	★★★	NR	NR	NR	NR	NR
NR	NR	NR	★★★	NR	NR	NR	NR	★	NR	NR	NR	NR	NR	NR	NR	NR	NR	NR
★	★★★	★	★	★★★	NR	★★★	★★★★★	★	★★★	★★★	★★★	★	★	★	★	★★★	★★★	NR
★★★	NR	NR	★★★	NR	NR	NR	NR	★★★	NR	NR	NR	NR	NR	NR	NR	NR	NR	NR
NR	NR	NR	★	NR	NR	NR	NR	★★★	NR	NR	NR	NR	★	NR	NR	NR	NR	NR

	Appendectomy	Atrial Fibrillation	Back and Neck Surgery (except Spinal Fusion)	Back and Neck Surgery (Spinal Fusion)	Bariatric Surgery	Bowel Obstruction	Carotid Surgery	Cholecystectomy (Gall Bladder Removal)	Chronic Obstructive Pulmonary Disease (COPD)	Coronary Bypass Surgery	Coronary Interventional Procedures (Angioplasty/Stent)	Diabetic Acidosis and
51. Northwest Mississippi Regional Med. Ctr., Clarksdale	NR	★★★	NR	NR	NR	★★★	NR	★★★	★★★	NR	NR	★★★
52. Noxubee General Critical Access Hospital, Macon	NR	NR	NR	NR	NR	NR	NR	NR	★★★	NR	NR	NR
53. Oktibbeha County Hospital, Starkville	NR	NR	NR	NR	NR	★★★	NR	NR	★★★	NR	NR	NR
54. Parkview Regional Medical Center, Vicksburg	NR	★★★	NR	NR	NR	★★★	★★★	★★★★★	★★★	★	★★★	★★★
55. Rankin Medical Center, Brandon	NR	★	NR	NR	NR	★★★	NR	★★★	★★★	NR	NR	★★★
56. Riley Hospital, Meridian	NR	★★★	NR	NR	NR	★★★	NR	★★★	★★★	NR	★★★	★★★
57. River Oaks Hospital, Jackson	NR	★★★	★★★★★	★★★★★	NR	★★★	NR	★	★★★	NR	NR	★★★
58. River Region Health System, Vicksburg	NR	★★★	NR	NR	NR	★★★	★★★	★★★★★	★★★	★	★★★	★★★
59. Rush Foundation Hospital, Meridian	NR	★★★	★★★	NR	NR	★	★★★	★★★	★★★	★	★★★	★★★
60. St. Dominic-Jackson Memorial Hospital, Jackson	NR	★★★	★	★★★	NR	★★★	★★★	★	★★★	★★★	★★★	★★★
61. Simpson General Hospital, Mendenhall	NR	NR	NR	NR	NR	NR	NR	NR	★	NR	NR	NR
62. Singing River Hospital System, Pascagoula	NR	★★★	★★★	★★★	NR	★★★	★	★★★	★★★	★★★	★★★	★★★
63. South Central Regional Medical Center, Laurel	NR	★★★	NR	NR	NR	★★★	★★★	★★★	★	NR	NR	★★★
64. South Sunflower County Hospital, Indianola	NR	NR	NR	NR	NR	NR	NR	NR	★★★	NR	NR	NR
65. Southwest Mississippi Regional Medical Center, McComb	NR	★★★	NR	NR	NR	★	★★★	★★★	★★★	★★★	NR	★★★
66. Stone County Hospital, Wiggins	NR	NR	NR	NR	NR	NR	NR	NR	★★★	NR	NR	NR
67. Tippah County Hospital, Ripley	NR	NR	NR	NR	NR	★★★	NR	NR	★★★	NR	NR	NR
68. Tishomingo Health Services, Iuka	NR	★★★	NR	NR	NR	NR	NR	NR	★★★	NR	NR	NR
69. Trace Regional Hospital, Houston	NR	NR	NR	NR	NR	NR	NR	NR	★★★	NR	NR	NR
70. Tri-Lakes Medical Center, Batesville	NR	NR	NR	NR	NR	NR	NR	NR	★★★	NR	NR	NR
71. Tyler Holmes Memorial Hospital, Winona	NR	NR	NR	NR	NR	NR	NR	NR	★★★	NR	NR	NR
72. University Hospital and Clinics—Holmes County, Lexington	NR	NR	NR	NR	NR	NR	NR	NR	★★★	NR	NR	NR
73. University of Mississippi Medical Center, Jackson	NR	★	★★★	★★★	NR	★	★★★	★★★	★★★	★	★★★	NR
74. Walthall County General Hospital, Tylertown	NR	NR	NR	NR	NR	NR	NR	NR	★★★	NR	NR	NR
75. Wayne General Hospital, Waynesboro	NR	NR	NR	NR	★★★	NR	NR	NR	★★★	NR	★	NR
76. Webster General Hospital, Eupora	NR	NR	NR	NR	NR	NR	NR	NR	★	NR	NR	NR
77. Wesley Medical Center, Hattiesburg	NR	★	★	★★★	NR	★★★	★★★	★★★	★	★★★	★	★★★
78. Winston Medical Center, Louisville	NR	NR	NR	NR	NR	NR	NR	NR	★★★	NR	NR	NR
79. Yalobusha General Hospital, Water Valley	NR	NR	NR	NR	NR	NR	NR	NR	★★★	NR	NR	NR

KEY: ★★★★★ BEST   ★★★ AS EXPECTED   ★ POOR   NR NOT RATED BY HEALTHGRADES   For full definitions of ratings and awards, see Appendix.

Gastrointestinal Bleed	Gastrointestinal Surgeries and Procedures	Heart Attack	Heart Failure	Hip Fracture Repair	Maternity Care	Pancreatitis	Peripheral Vascular Bypass	Pneumonia	Prostatectomy	Pulmonary Embolism	Resection/Replacement of Abdominal Aorta	Respiratory Failure	Sepsis	Stroke	Total Hip Replacement	Total Knee Replacement	Valve Replacement	Women's Health
★★★	NR	★	★	★★★	NR	★★★	NR	★★★	NR	NR	NR	★★★	★	★★★	NR	NR	NR	NR
NR	NR	NR	★★★	NR	NR	NR	NR	★★★	NR	NR	NR	NR	★★★	NR	NR	NR	NR	NR
★	NR	★★★	★	★★★★★	NR	NR	NR	★	NR	NR	NR	NR	★★★	★★★	NR	★★★	NR	NR
★	★★★	★★★★★	★	★★★	NR	★	NR	★	★★★	★	NR	★★★	★	★★★	★	★★★	NR	NR
★	NR	NR	★	★★★	NR	NR	NR	★	NR	NR	NR	★★★	★	★★★	NR	NR	NR	NR
★★★	★	★	★	★	NR	★★★	NR	★	NR	NR	NR	★★★	★	★★★	NR	NR	NR	NR
★★★	★★★	★★★	★★★	★	NR	★	NR	★★★	NR	NR	NR	★★★	★	★★★	★★★★★	★★★	NR	NR
★	★★★	★★★★★	★	★★★	NR	★	NR	★	★★★	★	NR	★★★	★	★★★	★	★★★	NR	NR
★★★	★	★	★★★	★★★★★	NR	★★★	NR	★	★★★	★★★	NR	★	★	★★★	★★★	★★★	NR	NR
★	★★★★★	★★★	★★★	★	NR	★	★★★	★★★	★	★★★	★★★	★★★	★	★★★	★	★	★★★	NR
NR	NR	NR	★	NR	NR	NR	★	NR	NR	NR	NR	NR	NR	NR	NR	NR	NR	NR
★	★★★★★	★	★	★★★	NR	★★★	★★★	★	★★★	★★★	NR	★★★	★	★	★★★	★★★	★	NR
★★★	★★★	★★★	★	★	NR	★★★	NR	★	★★★	★★★	NR	★	★★★	★★★	★	★	NR	NR
★★★	NR	★★★	★	NR	NR	NR	NR	★	NR	NR	NR	NR	NR	NR	NR	NR	NR	NR
★	★	★★★	NR	★★★	NR	★	★★★★★	★	★★★	NR	NR	★	★	NR	★	★★★	NR	NR
NR	NR	NR	NR	NR	NR	NR	★	NR	NR	NR	NR	NR	NR	NR	NR	NR	NR	NR
★★★	NR	NR	NR	NR	NR	NR	NR	★★★	NR	NR	NR	NR	★	NR	NR	NR	NR	NR
★★★	NR	NR	★	NR	NR	NR	NR	★★★	NR	NR	★★★	NR	★★★	NR	NR	NR	NR	NR
NR	NR	★★★★★	★★★	NR	NR	★★★	NR	★★★★★	NR	NR	NR	NR	★★★	NR	NR	NR	NR	NR
★★★	NR	NR	★★★	NR	NR	NR	NR	★★★	NR	NR	NR	NR	★	NR	NR	NR	NR	NR
★★★	NR	NR	★★★	NR	NR	NR	NR	★★★	NR	NR	NR	NR	NR	NR	★★★	NR	NR	NR
NR	NR	NR	★★★	NR	NR	NR	★	NR	NR	NR	NR	NR	★	NR	NR	NR	NR	NR
★	★	★	★★★	★★★	NR	NR	NR	★★★	NR	NR	★★★	★	★★★	★★★	★★★★★	NR	NR	NR
NR	NR	NR	★★★	NR	NR	NR	★	NR	NR	NR	NR	NR	★★★	★★★	NR	NR	NR	NR
★	NR	★	NR	NR	NR	NR	★	NR	NR	NR	NR	★	NR	NR	NR	NR	NR	NR
★★★	NR	NR	★	NR	NR	NR	★★★	NR	NR	NR	NR	★	★★★	NR	NR	NR	NR	NR
★★★	★	★★★	★	★★★	NR	★★★	★★★	★	★	NR	NR	★★★	★	★★★	★★★	★★★★★	★	NR
NR	NR	NR	★	NR	NR	NR	★	NR	NR	NR	NR	NR	★	NR	NR	NR	NR	NR
NR	NR	NR	★★★	NR	NR	NR	★	NR	NR	NR	NR	NR	NR	NR	NR	NR	NR	NR

MISSOURI HOSPITALS: RATINGS BY PROCEDURE

Hospital	Appendectomy	Atrial Fibrillation	Back and Neck Surgery (except Spinal Fusion)	Back and Neck Surgery (Spinal Fusion)	Bariatric Surgery	Bowel Obstruction	Carotid Surgery	Cholecystectomy (Gall Bladder Removal)	Chronic Obstructive Pulmonary Disease (COPD)	Coronary Bypass Surgery	Coronary Interventional Procedures (Angioplasty/Stent)	Diabetic Acidosis and Coma
1. Advanced Healthcare Medical Center, Ellington	NR	NR	NR	NR	NR	NR	NR	NR	NR	NR	NR	
2. Audrain Medical Center, Mexico	NR	★★★	NR	NR	NR	★★★	NR	★★★	★★★★★	NR	★★★	NR
3. Baptist Lutheran Medical Center, Kansas City	NR	★★★	NR	NR	NR	★★★★★	NR	★★★	★★★	NR	★★★	NR
4. Barnes Hospital, St. Louis	NR	★★★	★	★★★	NR	★★★★★	★★★	★★★	★★★	★★★	★★★★★	★★★
5. Barnes-Jewish Hospital, St. Louis	NR	★★★	★	★★★	NR	★★★★★	★★★	★★★	★★★	★★★	★★★★★	★★★
6. Barnes-Jewish St. Peters Hospital, St. Peters	NR	★★★	NR	★	NR	★★★	NR	★★★	★★★	NR	★★★	NR
7. Barnes-Jewish West County Hospital, St. Louis	NR	★★★	★★★	NR	NR	★★★	NR	★	★★★	NR	NR	NR
8. Barton County Memorial Hospital, Lamar	NR	★★★	NR	NR	NR	★★★	NR	★★★	★★★	NR	NR	NR
9. Bates County Memorial Hospital, Butler	NR	★★★	NR	NR	NR	★★★	NR	★★★	★★★	NR	NR	NR
10. Bonne Terre Hospital, Bonne Terre	NR	★★★	NR	NR	NR	★★★	NR	★	★★★	NR	★★★	NR
11. Boone Hospital Center, Columbia	NR	★★★	★★★	★★★	NR	★★★	★★★★★	★★★★★	★★★	★★★	★★★	★★★
12. Bothwell Regional Health Center, Sedalia	NR	★★★	NR	NR	NR	★★★	★★★	★★★	★★★	NR	★	
13. Callaway Community Hospital, Fulton	NR	★★★	NR	NR	NR	NR	NR	NR	★★★	NR	NR	
14. Cameron Regional Medical Center, Cameron	NR	★	NR	NR	NR	★★★	NR	★	★★★	NR	NR	
15. Capital Region Medical Center, Jefferson City	NR	★★★	★★★	★★★	NR	★★★	★★★	★★★	★★★	★★★	★★★	★★★
16. Carroll County Memorial Hospital, Carrollton	NR	NR	NR	NR	NR	NR	NR	NR	★★★	NR	NR	
17. Cass Medical Center, Harrisonville	NR	★★★	NR	NR	NR	★★★	NR	★★★	★★★	NR	NR	
18. Cedar County Memorial Hospital, El Dorado Springs	NR	NR	NR	NR	NR	NR	NR	NR	★★★	NR	NR	
19. Centerpoint Medical Center, Independence	NR	★	★★★	★★★	NR	★	★★★★★	★	★★★	★★★	★★★	★★★
20. Christian Hospital Northeast, St. Louis	NR	★★★	★	★	NR	★★★	★	★★★	★★★	★	★★★	★★★
21. Citizens Memorial Hospital, Bolivar	NR	★★★	NR	NR	NR	★★★	NR	★★★	★★★	NR	NR	
22. Columbia Regional Hospital, Columbia	NR	★★★	★★★	★	NR	★★★	NR	★★★	★★★	NR	★★★	NR
23. Community Hospital Association, Fairfax	NR	NR	NR	NR	NR	NR	NR	★	★★★	NR	NR	
24. Cooper County Memorial Hospital, Boonville	NR	NR	NR	NR	NR	NR	NR	NR	★★★	NR	NR	
25. Cox Medical Center, Springfield	NR	★★★	★	★	NR	★★★	★	★★★	★★★	★	★★★	★★★
26. Cox Monett Hospital, Monett	NR	NR	NR	NR	NR	★★★	NR	NR	★★★	NR	NR	
27. Des Peres Hospital, St. Louis	NR	★★★	★★★	★★★	NR	★★★	★★★	★★★	★★★	★★★	★★★	★★★
28. Ellett Memorial Hospital, Appleton City	NR	NR	NR	NR	NR	NR	NR	★	★★★	NR	NR	
29. Excelsior Springs Medical Center, Excelsior Springs	NR	NR	NR	NR	NR	NR	NR	NR	★★★	NR	NR	
30. Fitzgibbon Memorial Hospital, Marshall	NR	★★★	NR	NR	NR	★★★	NR	★★★	★★★	NR	NR	
31. Forest Park Community Hospital, St. Louis	NR	★★★	NR	NR	NR	★★★	NR	★★★	★★★	★	★★★	★
32. Freeman Health System, Joplin	NR	★★★	★★★	★★★	NR	★★★	★★★	★★★	★	★★★★★	★★★	★★★
33. Freeman Neosho Hospital, Neosho	NR	★★★	NR	NR	NR	★★★	NR	★	★★★	NR	NR	
34. Golden Valley Memorial Hospital, Clinton	NR	★★★	NR	NR	NR	★★★	NR	★★★	★★★	NR	NR	
35. Grim-Smith Hospital and Clinic, Kirksville	NR	★★★	NR	NR	NR	★★★	★★★	★★★★★	★★★	NR	NR	
36. Hannibal Regional Hospital, Hannibal	NR	★★★	★★★	NR	NR	★	★	★★★	★★★	NR	NR	
37. Heartland Regional Medical Center, St. Joseph	NR	★★★	★★★★★	NR	NR	★★★	★★★	★	★★★★★	★★★	★★★	★★★
38. Hermann Area District Hospital, Hermann	NR	NR	NR	NR	NR	NR	NR	★★★	★★★	NR	NR	
39. Jefferson Memorial Hospital, Crystal City	NR	★★★	NR	NR	NR	★★★	NR	★★★	★★★	★★★	NR	★★★
40. Lafayette Regional Health Center, Lexington	NR	★	NR	NR	NR	NR	NR	NR	★★★	NR	NR	
41. Lake Regional Health System, Osage Beach	NR	★★★	NR	NR	NR	★★★	★★★★★	★★★	★	★★★	★★★	NR
42. Lee's Summit Medical Center, Lee's Summit	NR	★★★	NR	NR	NR	★★★	★★★	★★★	★★★	NR	NR	
43. Liberty Hospital, Liberty	NR	★★★	★	NR	NR	★★★	★★★★★	★★★	★★★	NR	★★★	
44. Lincoln County Medical Center, Troy	NR	NR	NR	NR	NR	NR	NR	NR	★★★	NR	NR	
45. Macon County Samaritan Memorial Hospital, Macon	NR	NR	NR	NR	NR	NR	NR	NR	★★★	NR	NR	
46. Madison Medical Center, Fredericktown	NR	NR	NR	NR	NR	NR	NR	NR	★★★	NR	NR	
47. McCune-Brooks Hospital, Carthage	NR	NR	NR	NR	NR	★★★	NR	NR	★★★	NR	NR	
48. Menorah Medical Center, Kansas City	NR	★★★	★★★	★★★	NR	★★★	★★★★★	★★★	★★★	★★★	★	
49. Mineral Area Regional Medical Center, Farmington	NR	★★★	NR	NR	NR	★★★	NR	★★★	★★★	NR	NR	
50. Missouri Baptist Hospital Sullivan, Sullivan	NR	★★★	NR	NR	NR	★	NR	★★★	★	NR	NR	

KEY: ★★★★★ BEST   ★★★ AS EXPECTED   ★ POOR   NR NOT RATED BY HEALTHGRADES   For full definitions of ratings and awards, see Appendix.

Gastrointestinal Bleed	Gastrointestinal Surgeries and Procedures	Heart Attack	Heart Failure	Hip Fracture Repair	Maternity Care	Pancreatitis	Peripheral Vascular Bypass	Pneumonia	Prostatectomy	Pulmonary Embolism	Resection/Replacement of Abdominal Aorta	Respiratory Failure	Sepsis	Stroke	Total Hip Replacement	Total Knee Replacement	Valve Replacement	Women's Health
NR	NR	NR	★★★	NR	NR	NR	NR	★★★	NR	NR	NR	NR	NR	NR	NR	NR	NR	NR
★★★	★	★★★	★★★	★★★★★	NR	NR	NR	★★★	★★★	★★★	NR	★★★★★	★★★	★★★	★★★★★	★★★★★	NR	NR
★★★	NR	★★★	★★★	★★★	NR	NR	NR	★★★	★★★	NR	NR	★★★	★★★	★★★	★★★	★★★	NR	NR
★★★★★	★★★	★★★	★★★★★	★	NR	★★★	★	★★★	★★★	★★★	★★★	★★★★★	★	★★★	★★★	★★★	★★★	NR
★★★★★	★★★	★★★	★★★★★	★	NR	★★★	★	★★★	★★★	★★★	★★★	★★★★★	★	★★★	★★★	★★★	★★★	NR
★★★★★	★★★	★	★★★	★★★	NR	★★★	NR	★★★	★★★	NR	NR	★★★	★★★	★★★	★★★	★★★★★	NR	NR
★★★	NR	NR	★★★	★★★	NR	NR	NR	★★★	★★★★★	NR	NR	NR	NR	NR	★★★	★★★★★	NR	NR
★★★	NR	NR	★★★	NR	NR	NR	NR	★★★	NR	NR	NR	★★★	★★★	NR	NR	NR	NR	NR
★★★	NR	★★★	★★★	★★★	NR	NR	NR	★★★	NR	NR	NR	★★★	★★★	NR	★	NR	NR	NR
★★★	NR	★★★	★★★	★	NR	NR	NR	★★★	★	NR	NR	★★★	★★★★★	★★★	NR	★	NR	NR
★★★	★★★	★★★	★	★★★★★	NR	★	★★★	★★★	★★★★★	★★★	★★★★★	★	★★★	★	★★★★★	★★★★★	★★★	NR
★	★★★	★	★★★	★	NR	★★★	NR	★	★★★	NR	NR	★★★	★★★	★★★	★★★	★★★	★★★	NR
★★★	NR	NR	★★★	★★★	NR	NR	NR	★★★	NR	NR	NR	NR	★	NR	NR	NR	NR	NR
★	NR	NR	★	★★★	NR	NR	NR	★	NR	NR	NR	NR	NR	★★★	NR	★★★	NR	NR
★	★	★★★	★	★	NR	★	★★★	★★★	★★★	★★★	NR	★★★	★	★★★	★★★	★★★	★	NR
NR	NR	NR	★	NR	NR	NR	NR	★★★	NR	NR	NR	NR	NR	★★★	NR	NR	NR	NR
★★★	NR	NR	★★★	★★★★★	NR	NR	NR	★	NR	NR	NR	NR	NR	NR	NR	★★★★★	NR	NR
★★★	NR	NR	★★★	NR	NR	NR	NR	★	NR	NR	NR	NR	NR	NR	NR	NR	NR	NR
★	★	★	★★★	★★★	NR	★	NR	★	NR	NR	NR	★	★★★	★★★	★★★★★	★★★	NR	NR
★★★	★★★	★★★	★★★★★	★★★	NR	★★★	NR	★★★★★	★★★	★★★	NR	★★★	★★★★★	★★★★★	★★★	★★★	★	NR
★★★	★	★	★	★★★	NR	NR	NR	★★★	NR	NR	NR	★★★	★★★	★★★	★★★	★★★	NR	NR
★★★	NR	NR	★★★	★★★	NR	NR	NR	★★★	★★★	NR	NR	★★★	★★★	★★★★★	★★★★★	NR	NR	NR
NR	NR	NR	★★★	NR	NR	NR	NR	★★★	NR	NR	NR	★★★	NR	NR	NR	NR	NR	NR
★★★	NR	NR	★★★	★★★	NR	NR	NR	★	NR	NR	NR	★★★	★★★	NR	NR	NR	NR	NR
★★★	★★★	★★★	★	★	NR	★	NR	★★★	★	NR	★★★	★	★★★	★	NR	NR	★★★	NR
★★★	NR	NR	★	★★★	NR	NR	NR	★	NR	NR	NR	★★★	NR	★★★	NR	★★★	NR	NR
★	★★★	★★★	★★★	★★★	NR	NR	NR	★★★	NR	NR	NR	★	★	★★★	★★★★★	★★★	NR	NR
NR	NR	NR	★★★	NR	NR	NR	NR	★★★★★	NR	NR	NR	NR	NR	NR	NR	NR	NR	NR
NR	NR	NR	★★★	NR	NR	NR	NR	★★★	NR	NR	NR	NR	NR	NR	NR	NR	NR	NR
★★★	NR	NR	★★★	★★★	NR	★★★	NR	★★★	NR	NR	NR	★★★	★★★	★★★	★★★	★★★	NR	NR
★★★	★★★	★★★	★★★	★★★	NR	★★★	NR	★★★	★★★	★	★★★	★★★	★★★	★★★	★★★★★	★★★	★★★★★	NR
★★★	★★★	★★★	★★★	★★★	NR	NR	NR	★★★★★	NR	NR	NR	★★★★★	NR	★★★	NR	★★★★★	NR	NR
★★★	★★★	★	★★★	★★★★★	NR	★★★	NR	★★★	NR	NR	NR	★★★	★★★★★	★★★	NR	★★★★★	NR	NR
★★★	★	★	★★★	★	NR	NR	NR	★★★	★★★	★★★	NR	★★★★★	★	★★★	★★★	★★★	NR	NR
★★★	★★★★★	★★★	★★★★★	NR	NR	★★★	★★★	★★★★★	★★★	★★★	★★★	★★★★★	★★★	★★★	★★★★★	★★★★★	★★★	NR
NR	NR	NR	★★★	NR	NR	NR	NR	★★★	NR	NR	NR	NR	NR	NR	NR	NR	NR	NR
★★★	★★★	★★★	★★★	★★★	NR	NR	NR	★★★★★	NR	NR	NR	★★★	NR	★★★	★★★	NR	★	NR
★	NR	NR	★★★	★★★★★	NR	NR	NR	★★★	NR	NR	NR	NR	★★★	NR	NR	NR	NR	NR
★	★	★★★	★★★	★★★	NR	★★★	NR	★	★	★★★	NR	★	★★★	★★★	★★★	★★★★★	NR	NR
★★★	★★★	★	★★★	★	NR	★★★	NR	★★★	NR	NR	NR	★	★	★★★	★★★	★	NR	NR
★★★	★	★★★	★★★	★	NR	★	NR	★★★★★	★★★	★★★	★	★★★	★	★★★★★	★★★	★	NR	NR
★★★	NR	NR	★	★★★	NR	NR	NR	★★★	NR	NR	NR	NR	★★★	NR	★★★	NR	★★★	NR
NR	NR	NR	★★★	★★★	NR	NR	NR	★★★	NR	NR	NR	NR	NR	NR	NR	★★★	NR	NR
NR	NR	NR	★★★	NR	NR	NR	NR	★★★	NR	NR	NR	NR	NR	NR	NR	★★★	NR	NR
★★★	NR	★★★	★★★	NR	NR	NR	NR	★★★	NR	NR	NR	★★★	NR	★★★	★★★	NR	NR	NR
★★★	★★★	★★★	★★★	★	NR	★★★	NR	★	★★★	★★★	★★★	★	★★★	★★★	★★★	NR	NR	NR
★★★	NR	★★★	★	★★★★★	NR	NR	NR	★	NR	NR	NR	★	★	★★★	NR	★★★	NR	NR
★★★	NR	★★★	★	NR	NR	NR	NR	★★★	NR	NR	NR	★★★	★	★	NR	NR	NR	NR

Hospital	Appendectomy	Atrial Fibrillation	Back and Neck Surgery (except Spinal Fusion)	Back and Neck Surgery (Spinal Fusion)	Bariatric Surgery	Bowel Obstruction	Carotid Surgery	Cholecystectomy (Gall Bladder Removal)	Chronic Obstructive Pulmonary Disease (COPD)	Coronary Bypass Surgery	Coronary Interventional Procedures (Angioplasty/Stent)	Diabetic Acidosis and…
51. Missouri Baptist Medical Center, St. Louis	NR	★★★	★	★★★	NR	★★★	★	★	★★★	★★★	★★★	★★★
52. Missouri Delta Medical Center, Sikeston	NR	★★★	NR	NR	NR	★★★	NR	★	★	NR	NR	★
53. Missouri Southern Healthcare, Dexter	NR	★★★	NR	NR	NR	★★★	NR	NR	★★★	NR	NR	NR
54. Moberly Regional Medical Center, Moberly	NR	★★★	NR	NR	NR	★★★	NR	NR	★★★★★	NR	NR	NR
55. Nevada Regional Medical Center, Nevada	NR	★★★	NR	NR	NR	★★★	NR	NR	★★★	NR	NR	NR
56. North Kansas City Hospital, North Kansas City	NR	★★★	★★★	★★★	NR	★★★	★	★★★	★★★	★★★	★	★★★
57. Northeast Regional Medical Center, Kirksville	NR	★★★	NR	NR	NR	★★★	★★★	★★★★★	★★★	NR	NR	NR
58. Northwest Medical Center, Albany	NR	★★★	NR	NR	NR	NR	NR	NR	★★★	NR	NR	NR
59. Ozarks Community Hospital—Springfield, Springfield	NR	NR	NR	NR	NR	NR	NR	★	NR	NR	NR	NR
60. Ozarks Medical Center, West Plains	NR	★★★	NR	NR	★	★★★★★	★★★	★★★	NR	★	NR	
61. Parkland Health Center, Farmington	NR	★★★	NR	NR	NR	★★★	NR	★	★★★	NR	NR	★★★
62. Pemiscot Memorial Hospital, Hayti	NR	★	NR	NR	NR	★	NR	NR	★★★	NR	NR	★★★
63. Perry County Memorial Hospital, Perryville	NR	NR	NR	NR	NR	NR	NR	NR	NR	NR	NR	NR
64. Pershing Memorial Hospital, Brookfield	NR	NR	NR	NR	NR	NR	NR	NR	★★★	NR	NR	NR
65. Phelps County Regional Medical Center, Rolla	NR	★★★	NR	NR	NR	★★★	NR	★★★	★★★	NR	NR	★★★
66. Pike County Memorial Hospital, Louisiana	NR	NR	NR	NR	NR	NR	NR	NR	★★★	NR	NR	NR
67. Poplar Bluff Regional Medical Center, Poplar Bluff	NR	★★★	NR	NR	★	★★★	★★★	★	★	NR	★★★	★★★
68. Ray County Memorial Hospital, Richmond	NR	NR	NR	NR	NR	★★★	NR	NR	★★★	NR	NR	NR
69. Research Belton Hospital, Belton	NR	NR	NR	NR	NR	★★★	NR	NR	★★★	NR	NR	NR
70. Research Medical Center, Kansas City	NR	★	★★★	★★★★★	NR	★★★	★★★	★★★	★★★★★	★★★	★★★	★★★
71. Ripley County Memorial Hospital, Doniphan	NR	★★★	NR	NR	NR	★★★	NR	NR	★★★	NR	NR	NR
72. Sac-Osage Hospital, Osceola	NR	★★★	NR	NR	NR	★★★	NR	NR	NR	NR	NR	★★★
73. St. Alexius Hospital, St. Louis	NR	★★★	NR	NR	NR	★★★	NR	NR	NR	NR	NR	★★★
74. St. Anthony's Medical Center, St. Louis	NR	★★★	★★★	★	NR	★★★	★	★★★	★★★★★	NR	★★★	★★★
75. St. Francis Hospital, Maryville	NR	★★★	NR	NR	NR	★★★	NR	NR	NR	NR	NR	★★★
76. St. Francis Medical Center, Cape Girardeau	NR	★★★★★	★★★	★★★	NR	★★★	★★★★★	★★★	★★★	★	★★★	★★★
77. St. John's Hospital—Aurora, Aurora	NR	★★★	NR	NR	NR	NR	NR	NR	★★★	NR	NR	★★★
78. St. John's Hospital—Lebanon, Lebanon	NR	★★★	NR	NR	NR	★★★	NR	NR	★★★	NR	NR	★★★
79. St. John's Mercy Hospital, Washington	NR	★★★	NR	NR	NR	★★★	★★★	★★★	★★★	NR	NR	★★★
80. St. John's Mercy Medical Center, St. Louis	NR	★★★	★★★	★★★	NR	★★★	★★★	★★★	★★★	★★★	★★★	★★★
81. St. John's Regional Health Center, Springfield	NR	★★★	★★★	★	NR	★★★	★★★	★★★	★★★	★★★	★	★★★
82. St. John's Regional Medical Center, Joplin	NR	★★★	★★★	★	NR	★★★	★★★	★★★	★★★	★	★★★	★★★
83. St. Joseph Medical Center, Kansas City	NR	★★★	★★★★★	★★★	NR	★★★	★★★★★	★★★	★★★★★	★★★	★★★	★★★
84. St. Louis University Hospital, St. Louis	NR	★★★	★★★	★★★	★	★★★	NR	★★★	★★★	★★★	★	★★★
85. St. Luke's Cancer Institute, Kansas City	NR	★★★	★★★	★	NR	★★★	★★★	★★★	★★★	★★★	★★★★★	★★★
86. St. Luke's Hospital, Chesterfield	NR	★★★	★★★	★★★★★	NR	★★★	★★★	★★★	★★★★★	★★★	★★★	★★★
87. Saint Luke's Hospital of Kansas City, Kansas City	NR	★★★	★★★	★	NR	★★★	★★★	★★★	★★★	★★★	★★★★★	★★★
88. St. Luke's Northland Hospital, Kansas City	NR	★★★	NR	NR	NR	★★★	NR	★	★★★	NR	NR	NR
89. St. Mary's Health Center, Jefferson City	NR	★	NR	★★★	NR	★★★	★★★	★★★	★★★	★★★	★★★	★★★
90. St. Mary's Medical Center, Blue Springs	NR	★★★	NR	NR	NR	★★★	★★★	★★★	★	NR	NR	★★★
91. Ste. Genevieve County Memorial Hospital, Ste. Genevieve	NR	NR	NR	NR	NR	NR	NR	NR	★★★	NR	NR	NR
92. Scotland County Memorial Hospital, Memphis	NR	NR	NR	NR	NR	NR	NR	NR	★★★	NR	NR	NR
93. Skaggs Community Health Center, Branson	NR	★★★	NR	NR	NR	★★★	★★★	★★★★★	★★★	NR	★★★	★★★
94. South Point Hospital, St. Louis	NR	★★★	NR	NR	NR	★★★	NR	NR	★★★	NR	NR	★★★
95. Southeast Missouri Hospital, Cape Girardeau	NR	★★★	★★★	★	NR	★★★	★★★	★★★	★★★	★★★	★★★	★★★
96. SSM DePaul Health Center, Bridgeton	NR	★★★	★★★	★★★	NR	★★★	★★★	★★★	★★★★★	★★★	★★★	★★★
97. SSM St. Joseph Health Center, St. Charles	NR	★★★	★★★★★	NR	NR	★★★	★★★	★★★★★	★★★	★★★	★★★	★★★
98. SSM St. Joseph Health Center—Wentzville, Wentzville	NR	★★★	★★★★★	NR	NR	★★★	★★★	★★★★★	★★★	★★★	★★★	★★★
99. SSM St. Joseph Hospital of Kirkwood, Kirkwood	NR	★★★	NR	NR	NR	★★★	★★★	★★★	★★★	NR	★★★	★★★
100. SSM St. Joseph Hospital West, Lake St. Louis	NR	★★★	NR	NR	NR	★★★	NR	★★★	★★★	NR	NR	NR

KEY: ★★★★★ BEST   ★★★ AS EXPECTED   ★ POOR   NR NOT RATED BY HEALTHGRADES   For full definitions of ratings and awards, see Appendix.

Gastrointestinal Bleed	Gastrointestinal Surgeries and Procedures	Heart Attack	Heart Failure	Hip Fracture Repair	Maternity Care	Pancreatitis	Peripheral Vascular Bypass	Pneumonia	Prostatectomy	Pulmonary Embolism	Resection/Replacement of Abdominal Aorta	Respiratory Failure	Sepsis	Stroke	Total Hip Replacement	Total Knee Replacement	Valve Replacement	Women's Health
★★★★★	★★★	★★★★★	★★★★★	★	NR	★★★	NR	★★★	★★★	★★★★★	★	★★★	NR	★★★	NR	★	★★★	NR
★★★	★★★	★	★★★	★★★	NR	NR	NR	★★★	NR	★★★★★	NR	NR	★★★	★★★	★★★	NR	NR	NR
★★★	NR	★★★	★★★★★	NR	NR	NR	NR	★★★★★	NR	NR	NR	★★★★★	★★★★★	★★★	NR	NR	NR	NR
★★★	NR	NR	★★★	NR	NR	NR	NR	★★★	NR	NR	NR	★	★★★	★	NR	★★★	NR	NR
★★★	★★★	★	★★★	★	NR	★★★	NR	★★★	★	★★★	★★★	★★★	★★★	★★★	★	★	★	NR
★★★	★	★★★	★★★	★★★★★	NR	★★★	NR	★★★	★★★	NR	NR	★★★★★	★★★★★	★★★	NR	★★★	★★★	NR
NR	NR	NR	★★★	NR	NR	NR	NR	★★★★★	NR	NR	NR	NR	NR	NR	NR	NR	NR	NR
★★★	NR	NR	★	NR	NR	NR	NR	★	NR	NR	NR	NR	★★★	★★★	NR	NR	NR	NR
★★★	★★★	★★★	★★★	★★★	NR	★★★	NR	★★★	NR	★★★	NR	★★★	★★★	★★★	NR	★	NR	NR
★★★	NR	★★★	★★★	★	NR	NR	NR	★★★	★	NR	NR	★★★	★★★★★	★★★	NR	★	NR	NR
★★★	NR	NR	★★★	NR	NR	NR	NR	★★★	NR	NR	NR	NR	★★★	★★★	NR	NR	NR	NR
★★★	NR	NR	★★★	NR	NR	NR	NR	★★★	NR	NR	NR	NR	NR	NR	★★★	NR	NR	NR
NR	NR	NR	★★★	NR	NR	NR	NR	★★★	NR	NR	NR	NR	NR	NR	NR	NR	NR	NR
★	★★★	★★★	★	★★★	NR	★★★	NR	★	★★★	NR	★★★	★	★	★★★	★★★	NR	NR	NR
★★★	NR	NR	★★★	NR	NR	NR	NR	★★★	NR	NR	NR	NR	★★★	NR	NR	NR	NR	NR
★	★	★	★	★★★	NR	★	★★★	★	★★★	★	NR	★	★	★	★★★	★★★	NR	NR
★★★	NR	NR	★★★★★	NR	NR	NR	NR	★★★★★	NR	NR	NR	★★★★★	NR	NR	NR	NR	NR	NR
★★★	NR	NR	★★★	★★★	NR	NR	NR	★★★	NR	NR	NR	NR	NR	NR	NR	NR	★★★	NR
★★★	★★★	★★★	★★★	★★★	NR	★★★	★★★★★	★★★	★★★	★	★★★	★★★	★★★	★★★	★★★	★★★	★★★	NR
★★★	NR	NR	★	NR	NR	NR	NR	★★★	NR	NR	NR	NR	NR	NR	NR	NR	NR	NR
★★★	NR	NR	★	NR	NR	NR	NR	★	NR	NR	NR	NR	★★★	★	NR	NR	NR	NR
★★★	NR	★★★	★	★★★★★	NR	NR	NR	★★★	★★★	NR	NR	★★★★★	★★★	★	NR	NR	★★★	NR
★★★	★★★	★	★★★	★★★★★	NR	★	★★★	★★★★★	★★★	★★★	★★★	★★★★★	★★★	★★★	★★★	★★★	★★★	NR
★★★	NR	NR	★★★	★★★	NR	NR	NR	★	NR	NR	NR	NR	NR	★★★	NR	★★★	NR	NR
★★★	★★★	★★★	★	★★★	NR	★★★	★★★	★★★	★★★	★★★	★★★	★★★	★	★	★★★	★★★	★★★	NR
★★★	NR	NR	★★★	NR	NR	NR	NR	★★★	NR	NR	NR	NR	★★★	NR	NR	NR	NR	NR
★★★	NR	★	★	★	NR	★★★	NR	★	NR	NR	NR	★	★	★★★	★★★	★★★	NR	NR
★★★	★★★	★★★	★★★	★★★	NR	NR	NR	★★★	NR	★★★	NR	★★★	★★★	★★★	★★★	★	NR	NR
★★★	★★★	★★★	★★★	★	NR	★★★	★★★	★★★	★★★	★★★	★★★	★★★	★★★	★★★	★★★	★★★	★★★	NR
★★★	★★★	★	★	★★★	NR	★	★	★★★	★★★	★★★	★★★	★	★★★	★	★★★★★	★★★★★	★	NR
★★★	★★★	★	★	★★★	NR	★	★★★	★★★★★	★★★	★★★	★★★	★★★★★	★★★★★	★	★★★★★	★★★★★	★★★	NR
★★★	★★★	★★★	★★★★★	★★★	NR	★★★	★★★	★★★	★★★	★★★	★★★	★★★	★★★	★★★	★★★	★★★★★	★	NR
★★★	★★★	★★★	★★★★★	★★★	NR	★★★	NR	★★★	NR	★★★	★★★	★★★	★★★	★★★	★★★	★★★	NR	NR
★★★	★★★	★★★	★★★	★★★	NR	★★★	★	★★★	★★★	★★★	★★★★★	★	★★★	★★★	★★★	★★★	★★★	NR
★★★	★★★	★★★	★★★★★	★★★	NR	★★★	★	★★★★★	★★★	★★★★★	★	★★★	★★★	★★★	★★★	★★★	★★★	NR
★★★	★★★	★★★	★★★	★★★	NR	★★★	★	★★★	★★★	★★★★★	★	★★★	★★★	★★★	★★★	★★★	★★★	NR
★★★	★★★	★★★	★★★	★	NR	NR	NR	★★★	NR	★★★	NR	★★★	★★★	NR	★	★	NR	NR
★★★	★★★	★★★	★★★	★	NR	★★★	NR	★★★	★★★	★★★	NR	★★★	★★★	NR	NR	NR	NR	NR
★★★	★★★	★★★	★	★	NR	★★★	NR	★★★	★★★	★★★	NR	★	★★★	★★★	★★★	NR	NR	NR
★★★	NR	NR	★★★	NR	NR	NR	NR	★★★★★	NR	NR	NR	NR	★★★★★	NR	NR	NR	NR	NR
NR	NR	NR	★★★★★	NR	NR	NR	NR	★★★	NR	NR	NR	NR	NR	NR	NR	NR	NR	NR
★★★	★	★★★	★★★★★	★★★	NR	NR	NR	★★★	★★★	★★★	NR	★★★★★	★★★★★	★★★★★	NR	★★★	★★★	NR
★★★	NR	★★★	★	★★★★★	NR	NR	NR	★★★	★★★	NR	NR	★★★★★	★★★	★	NR	NR	★★★	NR
★★★	★★★	★	★★★	★★★	NR	★★★	★★★★★	★★★	★★★	★★★	★★★	★★★	★★★	★★★	★★★	★★★	★★★	NR
★★★	★★★	★★★★★	★★★	★★★	NR	★★★	★★★★★	★★★	★★★	★★★	★★★★★	★★★★★	★★★★★	★★★	★★★	★★★	★★★	NR
★★★	★★★	★★★	★★★	★★★	NR	★★★	★★★★★	★★★	★★★	★★★	★★★★★	★★★	★★★	★★★	★★★	★★★	★★★★★	NR
★★★	★★★	★★★	★★★	★★★	NR	NR	★★★	★★★	★★★	★★★	★★★	★★★	★★★	★★★	★★★	★★★	★★★★★	NR
★★★	★★★★★	★★★	★★★	★★★	NR	★★★	★★★★★	★★★	★★★	★★★	★★★	★★★	★★★★★	★★★	★★★	★★★★★	★★★	NR
★★★	★★★	★★★★★	★★★★★	★★★	NR	★★★	NR	★★★	NR	★★★	NR	★★★★★	★★★★★	★★★	★	★★★	NR	NR

	Appendectomy	Atrial Fibrillation	Back and Neck Surgery (except Spinal Fusion)	Back and Neck Surgery (Spinal Fusion)	Bariatric Surgery	Bowel Obstruction	Carotid Surgery	Cholecystectomy (Gall Bladder Removal)	Chronic Obstructive Pulmonary Disease (COPD)	Coronary Bypass Surgery	Coronary Interventional Procedures (Angioplasty/Stent)	Diabetic Acidosis an...
101. **SSM St. Mary's Health Center,** St. Louis	NR	★★★	★★★	★★★	NR	★★★	★★★	★★★	★	★★★	★★★	★
102. **Texas County Memorial Hospital,** Houston	NR	★★★	NR	NR	NR	★★★	NR	★★★	★★★	NR	NR	NR
103. **Truman Medical Center–Hospital Hill,** Kansas City	NR	★★★	NR	NR	NR	NR	NR	NR	★★★★★	NR	NR	★★★
104. **Truman Medical Center–Lakewood,** Kansas City	NR	NR	NR	NR	NR	NR	NR	NR	★★★	NR	NR	NR
105. **Twin Rivers Regional Medical Center,** Kennett	NR	★★★	NR	NR	NR	★	NR	NR	★★★	NR	NR	NR
106. **University of Missouri Hospital and Clinics,** Columbia	NR	★★★	NR	NR	NR	★★★	★★★	★★★	★★★	★★★	★★★	NR
107. **Washington County Memorial Hospital,** Potosi	NR	NR	NR	NR	NR	NR	NR	NR	★★★	NR	NR	NR
108. **Western Missouri Medical Center,** Warrensburg	NR	★★★	NR	NR	NR	★★★	NR	NR	★★★	NR	NR	NR
109. **Whispering Oaks Hospital,** Jefferson City	NR	★	NR	★★★	NR	★★★	★★★	★★★	★★★	★★★	★★★	★★★

KEY: ★★★★★ BEST   ★★★ AS EXPECTED   ★ POOR   NR NOT RATED BY HEALTHGRADES   For full definitions of ratings and awards, see Appendix.

Gastrointestinal Bleed	Gastrointestinal Surgeries and Procedures	Heart Attack	Heart Failure	Hip Fracture Repair	Maternity Care	Pancreatitis	Peripheral Vascular Bypass	Pneumonia	Prostatectomy	Pulmonary Embolism	Resection/Replacement of Abdominal Aorta	Respiratory Failure	Sepsis	Stroke	Total Hip Replacement	Total Knee Replacement	Valve Replacement	Women's Health
★★★	★★★★★	★★★	★★★	★★★★★	NR	★★★	★★★	★★★★★	★★★	★★★★★	★★★	★★★★★	★★★★★	★★★★★	★★★★★	★★★	★★★	NR
★★★	NR	★★★★★	★★★	NR	NR	NR	NR	★★★	NR	NR	NR	★★★	★★★	★★★	NR	NR	NR	NR
★★★	★	★★★	★★★	NR	NR	NR	NR	★★★★★	★★★	NR	NR	★★★	NR	★	NR	NR	NR	NR
NR	NR	NR	★★★	NR	NR	NR	NR	★★★	NR	NR	NR	NR	NR	NR	★★★	NR	NR	NR
★★★	NR	★★★	★★★	★★★	NR	NR	NR	★★★★★	NR	NR	NR	★★★	★★★	★	NR	NR	NR	NR
★★★	★	★	★★★	★★★	NR	★★★	NR	★★★	★★★★★	★★★	★	★	★★★	NR	NR	★★★	NR	NR
NR	NR	NR	★	NR	NR	NR	NR	★★★	NR	NR	NR	NR	NR	NR	NR	NR	NR	NR
★	★★★	★★★	★★★	★★★★★	NR	★★★	NR	★★★	NR	NR	NR	★	★★★	★★★	★★★★★	NR	NR	NR
★★★	★★★	★★★	★	★	NR	★★★	NR	★★★	★★★	★★★	NR	★★★	★★★	★★★	★★★	★★★	NR	NR

MONTANA HOSPITALS: RATINGS BY PROCEDURE

Hospital	Appendectomy	Atrial Fibrillation	Back and Neck Surgery (except Spinal Fusion)	Back and Neck Surgery (Spinal Fusion)	Bariatric Surgery	Bowel Obstruction	Carotid Surgery	Cholecystectomy (Gall Bladder Removal)	Chronic Obstructive Pulmonary Disease (COPD)	Coronary Bypass Surgery	Coronary Interventional Procedures (Angioplasty/Stent)	Diabetic Acidosis [a]
1. Benefis Healthcare, Great Falls	NR	★★★	★★★	★★★	NR	★★★	★★★	★★★	★★★	★★★	★★★	★★★
2. Billings Clinic, Billings	NR	★★★	★★★★★	★★★	NR	★★★	★★★★★	★★★★★	★★★	★★★	★★★	★★★
3. Bozeman Deaconess Hospital, Bozeman	NR	★★★	NR	★★★	NR	★	NR	★★★	★★★	NR	★★★	NR
4. Central Montana Medical Center, Lewistown	NR	★★★	NR	NR	NR	★★★	NR	NR	★★★	NR	NR	NR
5. Community Hospital of Anaconda, Anaconda	NR	★★★	NR	NR	NR	NR	NR	★	NR	NR	NR	NR
6. Community Medical Center, Missoula	NR	★★★	★★★	★★★	NR	★★★	★★★	★★★	★★★	NR	★★★	NR
7. Holy Rosary Healthcare, Miles City	NR	NR	NR	NR	NR	★★★	NR	★★★	★	NR	NR	NR
8. Kalispell Regional Hospital, Kalispell	NR	★★★★★	★	★★★	NR	★★★	★★★	★★★	★★★	★★★	★★★	NR
9. Marcus Daly Memorial Hospital, Hamilton	NR	★★★	NR	NR	NR	★★★	NR	NR	★★★	NR	NR	NR
10. Missoula General Hospital, Missoula	NR	★★★	★★★	★★★	NR	★★★	★★★	★★★	★	★★★	★★★	★★★
11. North Valley Hospital, Whitefish	NR	★★★	NR	NR	NR	★★★	NR	NR	★★★	NR	NR	NR
12. Northern Montana Hospital, Havre	NR	★★★	NR	NR	NR	★★★	NR	NR	★★★	NR	NR	★★★
13. PHS Indian Hospital–Browning, Browning	NR	NR	NR	NR	NR	NR	NR	NR	★★★	NR	NR	NR
14. St. James Healthcare, Butte	NR	★★★	★	★★★	NR	★★★	NR	★★★	★	NR	★	★
15. St. Patrick Hospital and Health Sciences Center, Missoula	NR	★★★	★★★	★★★	NR	★★★	★★★	★★★	★	★★★	★★★	★★★
16. St. Peter's Hospital, Helena	NR	★★★	★★★	NR	NR	★★★	★	★	★	NR	★	NR
17. St. Vincent Healthcare, Billings	NR	★★★	★★★	★	NR	★★★★★	★★★★★	★★★	★★★	★★★	★★★	★★★
18. Sidney Health Center, Sidney	NR	NR	NR	NR	NR	NR	NR	NR	★★★	NR	NR	NR

KEY: ★★★★★ BEST   ★★★ AS EXPECTED   ★ POOR   NR NOT RATED BY HEALTHGRADES   For full definitions of ratings and awards, see Appendix.

Gastrointestinal Bleed	Gastrointestinal Surgeries and Procedures	Heart Attack	Heart Failure	Hip Fracture Repair	Maternity Care	Pancreatitis	Peripheral Vascular Bypass	Pneumonia	Prostatectomy	Pulmonary Embolism	Resection/Replacement of Abdominal Aorta	Respiratory Failure	Sepsis	Stroke	Total Hip Replacement	Total Knee Replacement	Valve Replacement	Women's Health
★★★	★★★★★	★★★	★★★	★★★★★	NR	★★★	NR	★★★	★★★	★★★	★★★	★★★★★	★★★★★	★★★★★	★★★	★★★	★★★	NR
★★★	★★★	★★★	★★★	★★★★★	NR	★★★	★★★★★	★★★	★★★★★	★★★	★★★	★	★★★	★★★	★★★★★	★★★★★	★★★	NR
★★★	★★★	★★★	★★★	★★★	NR	★★★	NR	★★★	NR	★★★	NR	NR	★	★	★★★	★★★	NR	NR
★★★	NR	★★★	★★★	★★★	NR	NR	NR	★★★	NR	NR	NR	NR	NR	★★★	NR	NR	NR	NR
★★★	NR	NR	★★★	NR	NR	NR	★	NR	NR	NR	NR	NR	NR	NR	NR	NR	NR	NR
★★★	★★★	★★★	★★★	★	NR	★★★	NR	★★★	★★★	★★★	NR	★	★★★	★★★	★★★	★★★	NR	NR
★★★	NR	NR	★★★	★★★	NR	NR	NR	★★★	NR	NR	NR	NR	NR	★★★	★★★	NR	NR	NR
★★★	★★★	★★★	★★★★★	★★★	NR	★★★	NR	★★★	★★★	★★★	NR	★★★	★★★★★	★★★	★★★	★★★	NR	NR
★★★	NR	NR	★★★	★★★	NR	NR	NR	★★★	NR	NR	NR	NR	NR	★★★	NR	★	NR	NR
★★★	★★★	★★★★★	★★★	★★★	NR	★★★	★★★	★	★★★	★	★★★	★★★	★	★	★★★	★★★	★★★	NR
NR	NR	★★★	★★★	★★★	NR	NR	NR	★★★	NR	NR	NR	NR	★★★	★★★	NR	★★★	NR	NR
★★★	NR	NR	★★★	★	NR	NR	NR	★★★	NR	NR	NR	NR	NR	★	NR	★	NR	NR
NR	NR	NR	★	NR	NR	NR	NR	★★★	NR	NR	NR	NR	NR	NR	NR	NR	NR	NR
★★★	★★★	★	★	★	NR	NR	NR	★★★	★★★	NR	NR	★	NR	★★★	★★★	★★★	NR	NR
★★★	★★★	★★★★★	★★★	★★★	NR	★★★	★★★	★	★★★	★	NR	★★★	★★★	★	★★★	★★★	★★★	NR
★★★	★★★	★★★	★★★	★★★	NR	★★★	NR	★	★	NR	NR	NR	★	★★★	★	★	NR	NR
★★★	★★★	★★★	★★★	★	NR	★★★	★★★★★	★★★	★★★	★★★	★★★	★★★	★★★	★★★	★★★	★★★	★★★	NR
NR	NR	NR	★★★	★★★	NR	NR	NR	★★★	NR	NR	NR	NR	NR	★★★	NR	★★★	NR	NR

NEBRASKA HOSPITALS: RATINGS BY PROCEDURE

Hospital	Appendectomy	Atrial Fibrillation	Back and Neck Surgery (except Spinal Fusion)	Back and Neck Surgery (Spinal Fusion)	Bariatric Surgery	Bowel Obstruction	Carotid Surgery	Cholecystectomy (Gall Bladder Removal)	Chronic Obstructive Pulmonary Disease (COPD)	Coronary Bypass Surgery	Coronary Interventional Procedures (Angioplasty/Stent)	Diabetic Acidosis an...
1. Alegent Health–Bergan Mercy Medical Center, Omaha	NR	★★★	★★★	★★★★★	NR	★★★	★★★	★★★	★★★	★★★	★★★	
2. Alegent Health–Immanuel Medical Center, Omaha	NR	★★★	★★★	★★★★★	NR	★★★	★★★	★★★	★★★	★★★	★★★	
3. Alegent Health–Lakeside Hospital, Omaha	NR	★★★	NR	NR	NR	★★★	NR	NR	★★★	NR	★★★	
4. Alegent Health–Midlands Community Hospital, Papillion	NR	★★★	NR	NR	★	NR	NR	★★★	★★★	NR	★★★	
5. Avera St. Anthony's Hospital, Oneill	NR	★★★	NR	NR	NR	★★★	NR	NR	★	NR	NR	
6. Beatrice Community Hospital and Health Center, Beatrice	NR	NR	NR	NR	NR	★★★	NR	NR	★★★	NR	NR	
7. Boone County Health Center, Albion	NR	NR	NR	NR	NR	NR	NR	NR	★★★	NR	NR	
8. Box Butte General Hospital, Alliance	NR	★★★	NR	NR	NR	NR	NR	NR	★★★	NR	NR	
9. Brodstone Memorial Nuckolls County Hospital, Superior	NR	★★★	NR	NR	NR	NR	NR	NR	★★★	NR	NR	
10. Bryanlgh Medical Center, Lincoln	NR	★★★	★★★	★★★★★	NR	★★★	★★★	★★★	★★★	★★★	★★★	
11. Bryanlgh Medical Center–West, Lincoln	NR	★★★	★★★	★★★★★	NR	★★★	★★★	★★★	★★★	★★★	★★★	
12. Butler County Health Care Center, David City	NR	NR	NR	NR	NR	NR	NR	NR	★★★	NR	NR	
13. Chase County Community Hospital, Imperial	NR	NR	NR	NR	NR	NR	NR	NR	★★★	NR	NR	
14. Clarkson Bishop Memorial Hospital, Omaha	NR	★★★	★★★	★★★	★	★★★	★★★	NR	★★★	★★★	★★★	
15. Columbus Community Hospital, Columbus	NR	★★★	NR	NR	★	NR	NR	★★★	★	NR	NR	
16. Community Hospital, McCook	NR	★★★	NR	NR	NR	★★★	NR	NR	★★★	NR	NR	
17. Community Medical Center, Falls City	NR	NR	NR	NR	NR	NR	NR	NR	★	NR	NR	
18. Creighton University Medical Center, Omaha	NR	★★★	★	NR	★	★★★★★	★	★★★	★★★	★★★	★★★	
19. Faith Regional Health Services, Norfolk	NR	★★★	NR	★★★	NR	★★★	★★★	★★★	★★★	★★★	★★★	
20. Fremont Area Medical Center, Fremont	NR	★★★	NR	NR	NR	★★★	★★★	★★★	★	NR	★★★	
21. Good Samaritan Hospital, Kearney	NR	★★★	★★★	★★★	NR	★	★★★	★★★	NR	★★★	★	
22. Great Plains Regional Medical Center, North Platte	NR	★★★	NR	NR	★	NR	NR	★★★	★★★	NR	NR	
23. Howard County Community Hospital, St. Paul	NR	NR	NR	NR	NR	★★★	NR	NR	★★★	NR	NR	
24. Jefferson Community Health Center, Fairbury	NR	NR	NR	NR	NR	NR	NR	NR	★★★	NR	NR	
25. Jennie M. Melham Memorial Medical Center, Broken Bow	NR	★	NR	NR	NR	★★★	NR	NR	★★★	NR	NR	
26. Lutheran Community Hospital, Norfolk	NR	★★★	NR	★★★	NR	★★★	★★★	★★★	★★★	★★★	★★★	
27. Mary Lanning Memorial Hospital, Hastings	NR	★★★	★	NR	NR	★★★	★★★	★	★★★	NR	★★★	
28. Memorial Community Hospital, Blair	NR	★★★	NR	NR	NR	★★★	NR	NR	★★★	NR	NR	
29. Memorial Health Care Systems, Seward	NR	★★★	NR	NR	★	NR	NR	NR	NR	NR	NR	
30. Memorial Hospital, Aurora	NR	NR	NR	NR	NR	NR	NR	NR	★	NR	NR	
31. Nebraska Heart Hospital, Lincoln	NR	★★★	NR	NR	NR	NR	★★★★★	NR	NR	★★★★★	★★★	
32. Nebraska Medical Center, Omaha	NR	★★★	★★★	★★★	★	★★★	★★★	★	★★★	★★★	★★★	
33. Nebraska Methodist Hospital, Omaha	NR	★	★	★★★	NR	★★★	★★★	★	★★★	★★★	★★★	
34. Osmond General Hospital, Osmond	NR	NR	NR	NR	NR	NR	NR	NR	NR	NR	NR	
35. Our Lady of Lourdes Hospital, Norfolk	NR	★★★	NR	★★★	NR	★★★	★★★	★★★	★★★	★★★	★★★	
36. Pender Community Hospital, Pender	NR	NR	NR	NR	NR	NR	NR	NR	NR	NR	NR	
37. Phelps Memorial Health Center, Holdrege	NR	★★★	NR	NR	NR	★★★	NR	NR	★	NR	NR	
38. Providence Medical Center, Wayne	NR	NR	NR	NR	NR	NR	NR	NR	★★★	NR	NR	
39. Regional West Medical Center, Scottsbluff	NR	★★★	★★★★★	NR	NR	★★★	★★★	★★★	★★★	NR	★★★	
40. St. Elizabeth Regional Medical Center, Lincoln	NR	★	★★★★★	★★★	NR	★★★	★★★	★	★★★	★★★★★	★★★	
41. St. Francis Medical Center, Grand Island	NR	★★★★★	NR	NR	NR	★★★	NR	★★★	★★★	NR	★★★	
42. St. Francis Memorial Hospital, West Point	NR	NR	NR	NR	NR	★★★	NR	NR	★★★	NR	NR	
43. Saunders Medical Center, Wahoo	NR	NR	NR	NR	NR	NR	NR	NR	★★★	NR	NR	
44. Tri-County Area Hospital District, Lexington	NR	NR	NR	NR	NR	★★★	NR	NR	★★★	NR	NR	
45. York General Hospital, York	NR	★★★	NR	NR	NR	★★★	NR	NR	★	NR	NR	

KEY: ★★★★★ BEST   ★★★ AS EXPECTED   ★ POOR   NR NOT RATED BY HEALTHGRADES   For full definitions of ratings and awards, see Appendix.

Gastrointestinal Bleed	Gastrointestinal Surgeries and Procedures	Heart Attack	Heart Failure	Hip Fracture Repair	Maternity Care	Pancreatitis	Peripheral Vascular Bypass	Pneumonia	Prostatectomy	Pulmonary Embolism	Resection/Replacement of Abdominal Aorta	Respiratory Failure	Sepsis	Stroke	Total Hip Replacement	Total Knee Replacement	Valve Replacement	Women's Health
★★★	★★★	★★★	★★★	★★★	NR	★	★★★	★★★★★	★★★	★★★	★★★	★★★	★★★	★★★	★★★	★★★★★	★★★	NR
★★★	★★★	★★★	★★★	★★★★★	NR	★★★	NR	★★★	★★★	★★★	NR	★	★★★	★★★	★★★	★★★	★★★	NR
★★★	NR	★★★	★★★	★★★	NR	NR	NR	★★★	NR	NR	NR	NR	★★★	★★★	NR	NR	NR	NR
★	★★★	★	★★★	★★★	NR	★★★	NR	★	NR	★★★	NR	★	★★★	★	NR	★★★	NR	NR
★★★	NR	NR	★★★	NR	NR	NR	NR	★	NR	NR	NR	NR	NR	★	NR	NR	NR	NR
★★★	NR	NR	★★★	★★★	NR	NR	NR	★★★	NR	NR	NR	NR	NR	★★★	NR	★★★	NR	NR
NR	NR	NR	★★★	NR	NR	NR	NR	★★★	NR	NR	NR	NR	NR	★★★	NR	NR	NR	NR
★★★	NR	NR	★★★	NR	NR	NR	NR	★★★	NR	NR	NR	NR	NR	★	NR	NR	NR	NR
★★★	★★★★★	★★★	★★★	★★★★★	NR	★	★★★	★★★★★	★★★	★★★	★★★	★★★	★★★	★★★	★★★★★	★★★★★	★★★	NR
★★★	★★★★★	★★★	★★★	★★★★★	NR	★	★★★	★★★★★	★★★	★★★	★★★	★★★	★★★	★★★★★	★★★★★	★★★	★★★	NR
NR	NR	NR	★	NR	NR	NR	NR	★★★	NR	NR	NR	NR	NR	NR	NR	NR	NR	NR
NR	NR	NR	★★★	NR	NR	NR	NR	★★★	NR	NR	NR	NR	NR	NR	NR	NR	NR	NR
★★★	★	★	★★★	★★★	NR	★★★	★★★	★	★★★	★★★	★	★	★	★★★	★	★★★	★★★	NR
★★★	★	★	★	★★★	NR	★★★	NR	★	NR	NR	NR	★★★	NR	★	★★★	★★★	NR	NR
★★★	NR	NR	★	★★★★★	NR	NR	NR	★	NR	NR	NR	NR	NR	★	★★★	★★★	NR	NR
★★★	NR	NR	★★★	NR	NR	NR	NR	★★★	NR	NR	NR	NR	NR	★★★	NR	NR	NR	NR
★	★	★★★	★★★	★	NR	NR	NR	★★★	★★★	★★★	NR	★	★★★	★★★	NR	★★★	★★★	NR
★★★	★★★	★	★	★★★	NR	★★★	NR	★	★★★	★★★	NR	★	★★★	★★★★★	★★★★★	NR	NR	NR
★★★	★	★★★	★★★	★★★	NR	★★★	NR	★★★	NR	★★★	★★★	★	★★★	★★★	★★★	NR	NR	NR
★★★	★	★	★	★★★	NR	★★★	NR	★	★★★	NR	★★★	★★★	★	★★★	★★★	★★★★★	★★★	NR
NR	NR	★	NR	NR	NR	NR	NR	★★★	NR	NR	NR	NR	NR	NR	NR	NR	NR	NR
NR	NR	NR	★★★	NR	NR	NR	NR	★★★	NR	NR	NR	NR	NR	★★★★★	NR	NR	NR	NR
★★★	NR	NR	★★★	NR	NR	NR	NR	★★★★★	NR	NR	NR	NR	NR	NR	NR	NR	NR	NR
★★★	★★★	★	★	★★★	NR	★★★	NR	★	★★★	★★★	NR	★	★★★	★★★	★★★★★	★★★★★	NR	NR
★★★	★★★	★	★★★	★	NR	★★★	NR	★★★	★★★	★	NR	★	★★★	★★★	★	★	NR	NR
NR	NR	NR	★★★	NR	NR	NR	NR	★	NR	NR	NR	NR	NR	★★★	NR	NR	NR	NR
★★★	NR	NR	★	NR	NR	NR	NR	★	NR	NR	NR	NR	NR	★★★	NR	NR	NR	NR
NR	NR	★	NR	NR	NR	NR	NR	★★★	NR	NR	NR	NR	NR	NR	NR	NR	NR	NR
NR	NR	★★★	★★★★★	NR	NR	NR	★★★	NR	NR	NR	★★★	NR	NR	NR	NR	NR	★★★	NR
★★★	★	★	★★★	★★★	NR	★★★	★★★	★	★★★	★★★	★	★	★	★★★	★	★★★	★★★	NR
★★★	★	★★★	★★★	★	NR	★★★	★★★	★★★	★	★★★	★★★	★	★★★	★★★	★	★	★	NR
NR	NR	NR	★★★	NR	NR	NR	NR	★★★	NR	NR	NR	NR	NR	★★★	NR	NR	NR	NR
★★★	★★★	★	★	★★★	NR	★★★	NR	★	★★★	★★★	NR	★	★★★	★★★	★★★★★	★★★★★	NR	NR
★★★	NR	NR	★	NR	NR	NR	NR	★★★	NR	NR	NR	NR	NR	★★★	NR	NR	NR	NR
★★★	NR	NR	★★★	★★★	NR	NR	NR	★	NR	NR	NR	NR	NR	NR	NR	★★★	NR	NR
★★★	NR	NR	★★★	NR	NR	NR	NR	★★★	NR	NR	NR	NR	NR	NR	NR	NR	NR	NR
★★★	★	★★★	★★★	★★★★★	NR	★	NR	★	★★★	★★★	NR	★★★	★★★	★★★	★★★★★	★★★★★	NR	NR
★★★	★★★	★★★	★	★	NR	★★★	NR	★★★	★★★	★★★	NR	★	★★★★★	★	★★★	★★★	★★★	NR
★★★	★★★	★★★	★★★	★★★★★	NR	★★★★★	★★★	★★★	★★★	★★★	NR	★★★	★★★	★★★	★★★	★★★	NR	NR
★★★	NR	NR	★	NR	NR	NR	NR	★★★	NR	NR	NR	NR	NR	★	NR	★★★★★	NR	NR
NR	NR	NR	★★★	NR	NR	NR	NR	★★★	NR	NR	NR	NR	NR	NR	NR	NR	NR	NR
★★★	NR	NR	★	NR	NR	NR	NR	★★★	NR	NR	NR	NR	NR	★★★	NR	★★★	NR	NR
★★★	NR	NR	★★★	★★★	NR	NR	NR	★★★	NR	NR	NR	NR	NR	NR	NR	★★★	NR	NR

NEVADA HOSPITALS: RATINGS BY PROCEDURE

	Appendectomy	Atrial Fibrillation	Back and Neck Surgery (except Spinal Fusion)	Back and Neck Surgery (Spinal Fusion)	Bariatric Surgery	Bowel Obstruction	Carotid Surgery	Cholecystectomy (Gall Bladder Removal)	Chronic Obstructive Pulmonary Disease (COPD)	Coronary Bypass Surgery	Coronary Interventional Procedures (Angioplasty/Stent)	Diabetic Acidosis and...
1. Carson Tahoe Regional Medical Center, Carson City	★★★	★★★	★★★	★★★	★★★	★★★	★	★	★★★	NR	★★★	★★★
2. Churchill Community Hospital, Fallon	★	★	NR	NR	NR	★	NR	NR	★★★	NR	NR	NR
3. Desert Springs Hospital, Las Vegas	★★★	★★★	★★★	★★★★★	★★★★★	★★★	★★★	★★★	★★★	★	★★★	★★★
4. Mesa View Regional Hospital, Mesquite	NR	NR	NR	NR	NR	NR	NR	NR	★★★	NR	NR	NR
5. Mountainview Hospital, Las Vegas	★★★	★	★	★★★	★★★	★★★	★★★	★★★	★★★	★	★	★
6. North Vista Hospital, North Las Vegas	★★★	★★★	NR	NR	★★★★★	★★★★★	NR	NR	★★★	NR	NR	NR
7. Northeastern Nevada Regional Hospital, Elko	★★★	★★★	NR	NR	★★★	NR		★★★	★★★	NR	NR	NR
8. Northern Nevada Medical Center, Sparks	★	★★★	NR	★	NR	★★★	★★★	★	★★★	NR	NR	NR
9. Renown Regional Medical Center, Reno	★★★	★★★	★	★	★★★★★	★★★	★★★	★	★★★	★★★	★	★★★
10. Renown South Meadows Medical Center, Reno	★★★	★★★	NR	NR	★★★	★★★	NR	NR	★★★	NR	NR	
11. St. Mary's Regional Medical Center, Reno	★	★★★	★★★	★★★	★★★	★★★	★★★	★	★★★	★★★	★★★	NR
12. St. Rose Dominican Hospital, Henderson	★★★	★★★	NR	NR	★★★★★	★★★	NR	★★★	★★★	NR	★★★	
13. St. Rose Dominican Hospital–Siena Campus, Henderson	★	★★★★★	★★★	★★★	NR	★★★	★	★★★	★★★	★★★	★★★	★★★
14. Southern Hills Hospital and Medical Center, Las Vegas	★	★★★	NR	NR	NR	★★★	NR	★★★	★★★	NR	NR	NR
15. Spring Valley Hospital, Las Vegas	★★★	★★★	NR	NR	NR	★★★	NR	★★★	★★★	NR	NR	
16. Summerlin Hospital Medical Center, Las Vegas	★★★	★★★	NR	NR	★★★	★★★	★★★	★★★	★★★	NR	★★★	★★★
17. Sunrise Hospital and Medical Center, Las Vegas	★★★	★★★	★★★★★	★★★★★	NR	★	★★★	★	★★★	★★★	★★★	★★★
18. UMC of Southern Nevada, Las Vegas	★	★	★★★	★★★	NR	★★★	NR	★★★	★★★	★	★★★	★★★
19. Valley Hospital Medical Center, Las Vegas	★★★	★★★	★★★	★★★	★★★	★★★	★★★	★★★	★★★	★★★	★★★	★★★

KEY: ★★★★★ **BEST**   ★★★ **AS EXPECTED**   ★ **POOR**   NR **NOT RATED BY HEALTHGRADES**   For full definitions of ratings and awards, see Appendix.

Gastrointestinal Bleed	Gastrointestinal Surgeries and Procedures	Heart Attack	Heart Failure	Hip Fracture Repair	Maternity Care	Pancreatitis	Peripheral Vascular Bypass	Pneumonia	Prostatectomy	Pulmonary Embolism	Resection/Replacement of Abdominal Aorta	Respiratory Failure	Sepsis	Stroke	Total Hip Replacement	Total Knee Replacement	Valve Replacement	Women's Health
★★★★★	★★★★★	★★★	★★★	★	★★★	★★★	NR	★★★	★★★	★★★	NR	★★★	★★★	★	★	★	NR	NR
★★★	NR	NR	★★★	NR	★★★	NR	NR	★★★	NR	NR	NR	NR	NR	★	NR	NR	NR	NR
★★★	★★★	★	★★★	★★★	NR	★★★	★★★	★★★★★	★★★	★★★	NR	★★★	★★★	★★★	NR	NR	★★★	NR
NR	NR	NR	★★★	★★★	★★★	NR	NR	★★★	NR	NR	NR	NR	NR	NR	NR	★★★	NR	NR
★★★	★	★	★★★	★★★	★★★★★	★★★	NR	★★★	★★★	★★★	NR	★	★★★	★★★	★★★	★★★	NR	★★★
★★★	NR	★★★	★★★	★★★★★	★★★★★	NR	NR	★★★★★	NR	NR	NR	★★★	★★★	★★★	★★★	★★★★★	NR	NR
★★★	NR	NR	★★★	★	★★★	NR	NR	★	NR	NR	NR	★★★	★★★	★	NR	★	NR	NR
★★★	★★★	★★★	★★★	★★★	NR	NR	★★★	★★★	NR	NR	★★★	★★★★★	★★★	★★★	★★★	NR	NR	NR
★★★	★★★	★★★	★	★	★★★	★	★★★	★★★	★★★	★★★	★	★★★★★	★★★	★★★	★★★	★	NR	★★★
★★★	NR	NR	★★★	NR	NR	NR	NR	★★★	NR	NR	NR	★★★	★★★	NR	NR	★★★	NR	NR
★	★★★	★★★	★★★	★★★	★★★★★	★★★	★★★	★	NR	★★★	NR	★	★★★	★	★★★	★★★	★★★	★★★
★★★	★★★	★★★	★★★	★★★	★	★★★	NR	★★★	NR	★★★	NR	★★★	★★★★★	★★★	★★★	★★★	NR	NR
★★★★★	★★★	★★★	★★★	★★★	★★★	NR	★★★★★	★★★	★★★	NR	★★★	★★★★★	★★★	★	NR	★★★★★	★★★	
★★★	★★★★★	★★★	★★★	★	NR	NR	NR	★★★	NR	NR	NR	★★★	★★★	★★★★★	NR	★★★	NR	NR
★★★	★★★	★★★	★★★	★★★	NR	NR	NR	★★★	NR	NR	NR	★★★	★★★	★★★	★★★	★	NR	NR
★★★	★★★★★	★★★	★★★	★★★	★★★	NR	★★★	★	★★★	NR	★★★	★★★★★	★★★	★	★★★	NR	NR	
★★★	★★★★★	★★★	★★★★★	★★★	★★★	★★★	NR	★★★	★	★★★	★★★	★★★	★★★	★★★★★	★	★	★★★	★★★
★★★	★★★	★	★★★	★★★	★★★	NR	NR	★★★	NR	NR	★★★	★★★	★★★★★	★★★	★★★	★★★	★★★	
★★★	★★★	★★★	★★★	★★★★★	★★★	★	★★★	★★★★★	★★★	★★★	NR	★★★★★	★★★	★★★★★	★★★	★★★	★★★	★★★

NEW HAMPSHIRE HOSPITALS: RATINGS BY PROCEDURE

Hospital	Appendectomy	Atrial Fibrillation	Back and Neck Surgery (except Spinal Fusion)	Back and Neck Surgery (Spinal Fusion)	Bariatric Surgery	Bowel Obstruction	Carotid Surgery	Cholecystectomy (Gall Bladder Removal)	Chronic Obstructive Pulmonary Disease (COPD)	Coronary Bypass Surgery	Coronary Interventional Procedures (Angioplasty/Stent)	Diabetic Acidosis and
1. Alice Peck Day Memorial Hospital, Lebanon	NR	NR	★★★	★★★	NR	NR	NR	NR	NR	NR	NR	NR
2. Androscoggin Valley Hospital, Berlin	NR	★★★	NR	NR	NR	★★★	NR	NR	★★★	NR	NR	NR
3. Catholic Medical Center, Manchester	NR	★	★★★	★★★	NR	★★★	★★★★★	★★★	★★★	★	★★★	★★★
4. Cheshire Medical Center, Keene	NR	★★★	NR	NR	NR	★★★	NR	★★★	★	NR	NR	NR
5. Concord Hospital, Concord	NR	★★★	★★★★★	★★★	NR	★★★	★★★	★★★	★	★	★	★
6. Cottage Hospital, Woodsville	NR	★★★	NR	NR	NR	NR	NR	NR	★★★	NR	NR	NR
7. Elliot Hospital, Manchester	NR	★★★	★★★	★★★	NR	★★★	★	★	★★★	NR	★★★	NR
8. Exeter Hospital, Exeter	NR	★★★	NR	NR	NR	★★★	★★★	★★★	★★★	NR	★★★	★
9. Franklin Regional Hospital, Franklin	NR	★	NR	NR	NR	NR	NR	NR	★★★	NR	NR	NR
10. Frisbie Memorial Hospital, Rochester	NR	★★★	NR	NR	NR	★★★	NR	NR	★★★	NR	NR	NR
11. Huggins Hospital, Wolfeboro	NR	★★★	NR	NR	NR	★★★	NR	NR	★★★	NR	NR	NR
12. Lakes Region General Hospital, Laconia	NR	★★★	★★★	★★★	NR	★★★	★	★	★	NR	NR	NR
13. Littleton Regional Hospital, Littleton	NR	★	NR	NR	NR	NR	NR	NR	★★★	NR	NR	NR
14. Mary Hitchcock Memorial Hospital, Lebanon	NR	★★★★★	★★★	★★★	NR	★★★★★	★★★	★★★	★★★	★★★	★	★★★
15. Memorial Hospital, North Conway	NR	★★★	NR	NR	NR	NR	NR	★★★	NR	NR	NR	
16. Monadnock Community Hospital, Peterborough	NR	★	NR	NR	NR	★★★	NR	NR	★★★	NR	NR	NR
17. Parkland Medical Center, Derry	NR	★	NR	NR	NR	★★★	NR	NR	★★★	NR	NR	NR
18. Portsmouth Regional Hospital, Portsmouth	NR	★★★	★★★	NR	NR	★★★	★★★	★★★	★★★	★★★	★★★	NR
19. St. Joseph Hospital, Nashua	NR	★	NR	NR	NR	★★★	★★★	★★★	★★★	NR	NR	NR
20. Southern New Hampshire Medical Center, Nashua	NR	★★★	NR	NR	NR	★★★	NR	★★★	★★★	NR	NR	NR
21. Speare Memorial Hospital, Plymouth	NR	NR	NR	NR	NR	★★★	NR	NR	★	NR	NR	NR
22. Valley Regional Hospital, Claremont	NR	★★★	NR	NR	NR	NR	NR	NR	★★★	NR	NR	NR
23. Weeks Medical Center, Lancaster	NR	★	NR	NR	NR	NR	NR	NR	★	NR	NR	NR
24. Wentworth-Douglass Hospital, Dover	NR	★★★	★★★	★★★	NR	★★★	★★★	★★★	★★★	NR	★★★	★★★

KEY: ★★★★★ BEST   ★★★ AS EXPECTED   ★ POOR   NR NOT RATED BY HEALTHGRADES   For full definitions of ratings and awards, see Appendix.

	Gastrointestinal Bleed	Gastrointestinal Surgeries and Procedures	Heart Attack	Heart Failure	Hip Fracture Repair	Maternity Care	Pancreatitis	Peripheral Vascular Bypass	Pneumonia	Prostatectomy	Pulmonary Embolism	Resection/Replacement of Abdominal Aorta	Respiratory Failure	Sepsis	Stroke	Total Hip Replacement	Total Knee Replacement	Valve Replacement	Women's Health
	NR	NR	NR	NR	NR	NR	NR	★★★	NR	NR	NR	NR	NR	NR	NR	NR	★★★	NR	NR
	★★★	NR	★★★★★	★★★	★★★	NR	NR	NR	★★★★★	NR	NR	NR	NR	★★★	★★★	NR	★★★	NR	NR
	★★★	★★★	★	★	★★★	NR	★★★	★★★	★	★★★	★	★★★	★	★★★	★	★★★	★★★	★	NR
	★★★	★	★★★★★	★	★★★	NR	★★★	NR	★	NR	NR	NR	★	★	★★★★★	★★★★★	NR	NR	NR
	★	★★★	★★★	★★★	★★★	NR	★★★	NR	★★★	NR	★	NR	★★★	★★★	★★★★★	★★★★★	★★★	NR	NR
	★★★	NR	NR	★★★	★★★	NR	NR	NR	★	NR	NR	NR	★★★	★	NR	★★★	NR	NR	NR
	★★★	★★★	★★★	★	★	NR	★★★	★★★	★	★★★	★★★	NR	★★★	★	★★★	★	NR	NR	NR
	★★★	★★★	★★★	★★★	★	NR	★★★	★	★★★	★★★	★★★	NR	★★★	★	★★★	★★★	NR	NR	NR
	★★★	NR	★★★	★	★★★★★	NR	NR	NR	★★★	NR	NR	NR	★★★	★★★	NR	NR	NR	NR	NR
	★★★	NR	★★★	★★★	★	NR	★★★	NR	★	NR	NR	NR	★★★	★★★	★★★	NR	★	NR	NR
	★★★	★★★	★★★	★★★	★★★	NR	NR	NR	★★★	NR	NR	NR	★★★	★★★	NR	★★★	NR	NR	NR
	★★★	★★★	★	★	★★★	NR	★★★	★★★	★	NR	★★★	★	★	★★★	★★★	★★★	★★★	NR	NR
	★★★	NR	NR	★★★	★★★	NR	NR	NR	★★★	NR	NR	NR	★★★	NR	★★★	NR	★★★	NR	NR
	★★★★★	★★★	★★★★★	★★★★★	★★★	NR	★★★	★★★	★★★★★	★★★	★★★	★★★	★★★	★★★★★	★★★	★★★★★	★★★★★	★★★	
	★★★	NR	NR	★★★	★★★	NR	NR	NR	★★★	NR	NR	NR	NR	★★★	NR	★★★	NR	★★★	NR
	★★★	NR	★★★	★★★	★	NR	NR	NR	★★★	NR	NR	NR	★★★	★★★	★★★	★★★	★★★	NR	
	★★★	★★★	★★★	★★★	★	NR	NR	NR	★★★	NR	NR	★★★	★★★	★★★	★★★	★★★	NR	NR	
	★★★★★	★★★	★★★	★	★	NR	★	NR	★★★	★★★	NR	NR	★	★	★	★★★	★	★★★	
	★★★	★★★	★★★	★	★★★	NR	NR	NR	★	★	★★★	NR	★★★	★★★	★	★★★	NR	NR	
	★★★	★★★	★★★★★	★★★	★	NR	★★★	NR	★★★	★★★	NR	★★★	★★★	★★★	★	★	NR	NR	
	★★★	NR	★★★	★	★	NR	NR	NR	★★★	NR	NR	NR	★★★	★★★	NR	NR	NR	NR	
	★★★	NR	★★★	★★★★★	★	NR	NR	NR	★★★	NR	NR	NR	★★★	★★★	NR	★★★	NR	NR	
	★★★	NR	★★★	★★★	NR	NR	NR	NR	★★★★★	NR	NR	NR	★★★	NR	★★★	NR	NR	NR	
	★★★	★★★	★★★	★★★	NR	NR	★★★	★★★	NR	★★★	★★★	★★★	★★★	★★★	★★★	★	NR	NR	

NEW JERSEY HOSPITALS: RATINGS BY PROCEDURE

Hospital	Appendectomy	Atrial Fibrillation	Back and Neck Surgery (except Spinal Fusion)	Back and Neck Surgery (Spinal Fusion)	Bariatric Surgery	Bowel Obstruction	Carotid Surgery	Cholecystectomy (Gall Bladder Removal)	Chronic Obstructive Pulmonary Disease (COPD)	Coronary Bypass Surgery	Coronary Interventional Procedures (Angioplasty/Stent)	Diabetic Acidosis &
1. Atlanticare Regional Medical Center, Atlantic City	★★★	★★★	★★★	NR	★★★	★★★	★★★	★★★	★	★★★	★★★	★★★
2. Barnert Hospital, Paterson	★★★	★	NR	NR	★	★★★	NR	NR	★★★	NR	NR	★★★
3. Bayonne Hospital, Bayonne	★	★★★	NR	NR	NR	★★★	NR	★★★	★★★	NR		★★★
4. Bayshore Community Hospital, Holmdel	★★★	★★★	NR	NR	NR	★★★	★★★	★★★	★★★	NR		★★★
5. Bergen Regional Medical Center, Paramus	NR	NR	NR	NR	NR	NR	NR	NR	★★★	NR		NR
6. Cape Regional Medical Center, Cape May Court House	★★★	★★★	NR	NR	NR	★	★★★	★	★★★	NR		★★★
7. Capital Health System—Fuld Campus, Trenton	★	★★★	★★★	NR		★★★	★	★★★	★★★	NR		★★★
8. Capital Health System—Mercer Campus, Trenton	★★★	★★★	★	NR	★	★★★	★★★	★	★★★	NR		★★★
9. Centrastate Medical Center, Freehold	★★★	★★★	NR	NR	★	★★★	★★★	★	★★★★★	★★★		★★★
10. Chilton Memorial Hospital, Pompton Plains	★★★	★★★	★★★	NR	★★★★★	★★★	★★★	★	★★★	NR		★★★
11. Christ Hospital, Jersey City	★★★	★★★	NR	NR	★	★★★	★	★	★★★	NR		★★★
12. Clara Maass Medical Center, Belleville	★★★	★★★	NR	NR	★★★★★	★★★	★★★	★★★	★★★	NR		★★★
13. Columbus Hospital, Newark	★★★	★★★	NR	NR	NR	★★★	NR	★★★	★★★	NR		★★★
14. Community Medical Center, Toms River	★★★	★★★	★★★★★	★★★	NR	★★★	★★★	★★★	★★★	NR	★★★	★★★
15. Cooper University Hospital, Camden	★★★	★★★	NR	★★★	★	★★★	★★★	★	★★★	★		★★★
16. Deborah Heart and Lung Center, Browns Mills	NR	★★★	NR	NR	NR	★★★	NR	★★★	★★★★★	★★★	NR	
17. East Orange General Hospital, East Orange	NR	★	NR	NR	NR	★	NR	★★★	★★★	NR	NR	★
18. Englewood Hospital and Medical Center, Englewood	★★★	★	★★★	★★★	★	★★★	★	★★★	★★★	★★★	★★★	★★★
19. Greenville Hospital, Jersey City	★★★	NR	NR	NR	NR	★★★	NR	NR	★★★	NR		★★★
20. Hackensack University Medical Center, Hackensack	★★★★★	★★★	★★★★★	★★★	★★★★★	★★★	★★★	★★★★★	★★★	★★★★★		★★★
21. Hackettstown Community Hospital, Hackettstown	★★★	★★★	NR	NR	NR	★★★	NR	★★★	★★★	NR		★★★
22. Hoboken University Medical Center, Hoboken	★	★★★	NR	NR	NR	★★★	NR	★★★	★	NR		★★★
23. Holy Name Hospital, Teaneck	★★★	★★★	★★★	★★★	★	★★★	★★★	★★★	★★★	NR		★★★
24. Hunterdon Medical Center, Flemington	★★★★★	★★★	★★★	NR	NR	★★★	★★★	★★★	★★★	NR		★★★
25. Jersey City Medical Center, Jersey City	★★★	★★★	NR	NR	NR	★	NR	NR	★★★	★		★★★
26. Jersey Shore University Medical Center, Neptune	★★★	★★★	★★★	★★★	NR	★★★	★★★	★	★★★	★★★★★	★★★	★★★
27. JFK Medical Center, Edison	★	★★★	★★★	★	NR	★★★	★★★	★	★★★	★★★		★★★
28. Kennedy Memorial Hospitals—Stratford, Stratford	★★★	★★★	NR	NR	NR	★★★	★★★★★	★★★	★★★	★★★		★★★
29. Kessler Memorial Hospital, Hammonton	★★★	★★★	NR	NR	NR	★★★	NR	★	★★★	★★★		★★★
30. Kimball Medical Center, Lakewood	★★★	★★★	NR	NR	NR	★★★	★★★	★★★	★★★★★	NR		★★★
31. Lourdes Medical Center of Burlington County, Willingboro	★★★	★★★	NR	NR	★	★★★	NR	★★★	★★★	NR		★★★
32. Meadowlands Hospital, Secaucus	★★★	★	NR	NR	NR	★★★	NR	★★★	★	NR		★★★
33. Memorial Hospital of Salem County, Salem	★★★	★★★	NR	NR	NR	★★★	★★★	★★★★★	★★★	NR		★★★
34. Monmouth Medical Center, Long Branch	★★★★★	★★★	★★★	★★★	★	★★★	★	★	★★★	NR		★★★
35. Morristown Memorial Hospital, Morristown	★★★	★	★★★	★★★★★	★★★★★	★	★★★	★★★	★★★	★★★	★★★	★★★
36. Mountainside Hospital, Montclair	★★★	★★★	NR	NR	★★★	★★★	★	★	★★★★★	NR	★★★★★	★★★
37. Muhlenberg Regional Medical Center, Plainfield	★★★	★★★	NR	NR	NR	★★★	★★★	★	★★★	NR	★★★★★	★★★
38. Newark Beth Israel Medical Center, Newark	★★★	★★★	NR	NR	★	★★★	★★★	★★★	★★★	★★★	★★★	★★★
39. Newton Memorial Hospital, Newton	★★★	★★★	NR	NR	★	NR	NR	★★★	★★★	NR		★★★
40. Ocean Medical Center, Brick	★	★★★	★★★	★	NR	★★★	★★★	★★★	★★★	NR		★★★
41. Our Lady of Lourdes Medical Center, Camden	★★★	★★★	NR	NR	★★★	★★★	★★★★★	★★★	★★★	★★★		★★★
42. Overlook Hospital, Summit	★	★★★	★	★★★	★	★★★	★★★	★	★	NR		★★★
43. Palisades Medical Center, North Bergen	★★★★★	★	NR	NR	NR	★	NR	★★★	★★★	NR		★★★
44. Pascack Valley Hospital, Westwood	★★★	★★★	★★★	NR	★★★	★★★	★★★	★★★	★★★	NR		★★★
45. Raritan Bay Medical Center, Perth Amboy	★★★★★	★★★	NR	NR	NR	★★★	★★★	★★★	★	★★★		★★★
46. Riverside Hospital, Boonton	★★★	★★★	★★★	★★★	★	★★★	★★★	★★★	★★★	★		★★★
47. Riverview Medical Center, Red Bank	★	★★★	★★★	★★★	NR	★★★	★	★	★★★	NR		★★★
48. Robert Wood Johnson University Hospital at Hamilton, Hamilton	★★★★★	★★★	★★★	NR	NR	★★★	★★★	★★★★★	★★★★★	NR	★★★	★★★
49. Robert Wood Johnson University Hospital—Rahway, Rahway	★★★	★	NR	NR	NR	★★★	★★★	★★★	★★★	NR	NR	★★★
50. St. Barnabas Medical Center, Livingston	★★★	★★★	★★★	★★★	★★★★★	★★★	★★★	★	★★★	★★★	★★★★★	★★★

KEY: ★★★★★ BEST ★★★ AS EXPECTED ★ POOR NR NOT RATED BY HEALTHGRADES For full definitions of ratings and awards, see Appendix.

Gastrointestinal Bleed	Gastrointestinal Surgeries and Procedures	Heart Attack	Heart Failure	Hip Fracture Repair	Maternity Care	Pancreatitis	Peripheral Vascular Bypass	Pneumonia	Prostatectomy	Pulmonary Embolism	Resection/Replacement of Abdominal Aorta	Respiratory Failure	Sepsis	Stroke	Total Hip Replacement	Total Knee Replacement	Valve Replacement	Women's Health
***	*	***	***	*****	***	*		*****	***	***	***	NR	***	***	***	*****	***	*****
***	NR	NR	***	NR	***	NR	NR	***	NR	NR	NR	***	***	***	NR	NR	NR	NR
***	***	*	***	***	***	***	NR	***	***	***	NR	***	*****	***	NR	*	NR	NR
***	***	***	***	***	NR	***	NR	*****	***	***	NR	*****	***	***	***	***	NR	NR
***	NR	***	*	NR	NR	NR	NR	*	NR	NR	NR	NR	*	NR	NR	NR	NR	NR
*	*	*	***	***	***	***	NR	***	***	***	NR	*****	***	***	*	***	NR	NR
***	***	***	***	***	NR	NR	NR	***	***	***	NR	***	***	*****	***	***	NR	NR
***	***	***	***	***	***	NR	***	***	NR	***	NR	***	*	***	*	*	NR	NR
*****	*****	***	*	*****	***	***	***	*	***	***	***	***	*****	***	*	NR	NR	NR
***	***	***	***	***	***	***	*	***	***	***	NR	***	***	***	*	***	NR	NR
***	***	*	*	*	*****	***	*	***	***	***	NR	***	*	***	NR	***	NR	NR
***	*****	***	*****	*****	***	***	*****	***	***	NR	***	*****	***	***	*****	NR	NR	NR
***	*	***	***	*****	***	***	***	***	NR	***	NR	*	***	***	NR	NR	NR	NR
***	***	***	*****	***	***	***	*****	***	*****	NR	*****	***	***	***	***	NR	NR	NR
***	***	***	***	*	***	***	*	***	NR	NR	***	*	*	***	***	***	***	*
NR	NR	***	***	NR	NR	NR	NR	NR	NR	NR	***	NR	NR	NR	NR	NR	***	NR
***	NR	***	***	NR	*	NR	NR	***	*	***	NR	***	***	***	NR	NR	NR	NR
***	***	***	***	*	*****	***	*	***	***	***	***	***	***	***	***	***	***	***
***	***	***	***	NR	NR	NR	NR	***	NR	***	NR	***	*	***	NR	NR	NR	NR
***	***	*****	*****	*****	***	***	*	***	*****	***	***	*****	***	*****	*****	***	*****	*****
***	***	***	***	*****	***	NR	***	NR	NR	NR	***	***	***	*	***	NR	NR	NR
***	***	*	***	***	***	***	*	***	NR	***	***	***	NR	*****	NR	NR	NR	NR
***	***	***	***	*****	***	***	***	***	***	*	***	***	***	***	***	NR	NR	NR
***	NR	*	***	***	***	NR	NR	***	NR	NR	NR	***	***	*	NR	NR	NR	NR
***	*	***	*****	***	***	*****	***	***	***	***	*	*	***	***	*	***	***	***
***	***	***	***	*	***	*****	*	***	*	***	***	***	*****	*****	*	*	NR	NR
***	*	***	***	***	***	*	***	***	***	***	NR	***	*	***	***	*	NR	NR
***	NR	***	***	*	NR	***	NR	***	NR	NR	NR	***	NR	***	NR	NR	NR	NR
***	*	***	***	*****	*****	***	NR	*****	NR	*****	NR	***	***	***	NR	***	NR	NR
***	***	***	***	***	***	***	NR	***	***	NR	NR	***	*	*	NR	***	NR	NR
***	NR	NR	*	***	*****	NR	NR	*	NR	NR	NR	*	*	*	NR	NR	NR	NR
***	***	***	***	***	***	***	NR	*****	***	***	NR	***	***	***	NR	*	NR	NR
***	*****	***	*****	***	***	***	***	*****	***	***	NR	*****	*****	***	***	NR	NR	NR
***	***	***	*	*****	*****	***	*	***	***	***	***	*	*	***	***	***	***	***
***	***	***	***	***	***	***	***	***	***	*****	NR	***	*	*****	*	*	NR	NR
***	***	***	***	*****	***	***	***	***	***	***	***	***	***	NR	***	*	NR	*****
***	***	***	***	NR	NR	***	*****	*	NR	***	***	***	***	***	***	*	NR	NR
***	***	***	*****	***	***	***	***	***	***	***	***	***	*	***	***	***	***	*
***	***	*	***	*	*	***	***	*	***	***	***	***	***	*	*	*	NR	NR
***	***	*	*	***	*****	***	NR	***	***	NR	***	***	*****	***	***	***	NR	NR
***	***	*	***	***	***	NR	***	***	***	***	***	***	***	***	***	***	NR	NR
***	*****	***	***	***	*****	***	*	***	NR	***	*	***	*****	***	***	*	NR	NR
***	***	***	***	*****	***	*	***	*	***	NR	NR	***	***	***	*	*	NR	NR
*****	***	***	***	***	***	*	***	*****	***	***	***	*****	*****	***	*****	*****	***	NR
*	***	***	***	NR	***	***	***	***	***	NR	NR	*	*****	***	*****	***	NR	NR
***	***	*****	***	*	*****	*****	***	***	***	***	***	***	***	***	***	*****	*****

	Appendectomy	Atrial Fibrillation	Back and Neck Surgery (except Spinal Fusion)	Back and Neck Surgery (Spinal Fusion)	Bariatric Surgery	Bowel Obstruction	Carotid Surgery	Cholecystectomy (Gall Bladder Removal)	Chronic Obstructive Pulmonary Disease (COPD)	Coronary Bypass Surgery	Coronary Interventional Procedures (Angioplasty/Stent)	Diabetic Acidosis
51. St. Clare's Hospital/Denville, Denville	★★★	★★★	★★★	★★★	★	★	★★★	★★★	★	NR	★	★★★
52. St. Clare's Hospital/Sussex, Sussex	NR	★★★	NR	NR	NR	★★★	NR	NR	★	NR	NR	NR
53. St. Francis Medical Center, Trenton	★★★	★★★	★★★	NR	★	★★★	★	★★★	★★★	★★★	★★★	★★★
54. St. James Hospital, Newark	★★★	★★★	NR	NR	NR	★★★	NR	★★★	★★★	NR	NR	★★★
55. St. Joseph's Hospital and Medical Center, Paterson	★★★★★	★	★★★	★★★	NR	★★★	★★★	★★★	★★★	★★★	★	★★★
56. St. Joseph's Wayne Hospital, Wayne	★★★	★★★	NR	NR	★	★★★	★★★	★★★	★★★	NR	NR	★★★★★
57. St. Mary's Hospital, Passaic	★★★	★★★	NR	NR	★	★★★	★★★	★	★★★	★★★	★	
58. St. Michael's Medical Center, Newark	★★★	★	NR	NR	NR	★★★	★★★	★	★★★	★★★	★	★★★
59. St. Peter's University Hospital, New Brunswick	★★★	★★★	★★★	★★★	NR	★★★	★★★	★★★	★★★	NR		★
60. Shore Memorial Hospital, Somers Point	★	★★★	★★★	★★★	NR	★	★	★	★★★	NR	NR	★★★
61. Somerset Medical Center, Somerville	★★★	★★★	★★★★★	★★★	★★★★★	★★★	★★★	★★★	★	NR	★★★	★★★
62. South Jersey Healthcare Regional Medical Center, Vineland	★★★	★★★	★★★	NR	★★★★★	★★★	★★★★★	★★★	★	NR	NR	★
63. South Jersey Hospital—Elmer Division, Elmer	★★★	★	★★★	NR		★★★	NR	★★★	★★★	NR	NR	★★★
64. Southern Ocean County Hospital, Manahawkin	★★★★★	★★★	NR	NR	NR	★★★★★	★★★	★★★	★★★	NR	NR	★★★
65. Trinitas Hospital—Williamson, Elizabeth	★★★	★★★	NR	NR	★★★	★	★★★	★★★	★★★	NR	NR	★★★
66. UMDNJ-University Hospital, Newark	★★★	★★★	★★★	★★★	★★★★★	★★★	NR	NR	★★★	★★★	★★★	★
67. Underwood Memorial Hospital, Woodbury	★★★	★★★	NR	NR	NR	★★★	★★★★★	★★★	★	NR	NR	★
68. Union Hospital, Union	★★★	★★★	★★★	NR	NR	★	NR	★	★	NR	NR	★★★
69. University Medical Center at Princeton, Princeton	★★★★★	★★★	★★★	★★★	★	★★★	★★★	★★★	★	NR	NR	★★★
70. Valley Hospital, Ridgewood	★	★★★	★★★	★★★	★★★	★★★	★	★★★	★★★	★★★	★★★	★★★
71. Virtua Memorial Hospital—Burlington County, Mount Holly	★★★	★★★	★★★	★	★	★★★	★★★	★★★	★	NR	NR	★
72. Virtua West Jersey Hospital—Berlin, Berlin	★★★	★★★	★	★★★	NR	★	★★★★★	★	★★★	NR	NR	★★★
73. Virtua West Jersey Hospital—Marlton, Marlton	★★★	★★★	★	★★★	NR	★	★★★★★	★	★★★	NR	NR	★★★
74. Warren Hospital, Phillipsburg	★★★	★★★	★	NR	NR	★★★	★★★★★	★★★	★	NR	NR	★★★

KEY: ★★★★★ BEST   ★★★ AS EXPECTED   ★ POOR   NR NOT RATED BY HEALTHGRADES   For full definitions of ratings and awards, see Appendix.

Gastrointestinal Bleed	Gastrointestinal Surgeries and Procedures	Heart Attack	Heart Failure	Hip Fracture Repair	Maternity Care	Pancreatitis	Peripheral Vascular Bypass	Pneumonia	Prostatectomy	Pulmonary Embolism	Resection/Replacement of Abdominal Aorta	Respiratory Failure	Sepsis	Stroke	Total Hip Replacement	Total Knee Replacement	Valve Replacement	Women's Health
★★★	★★★	★	★	★★★	★★★★★	★	★★★	★	★★★	★★★		★	★	★★★	★★★	★	NR	NR
★	NR	NR	★	NR	NR	NR	NR	★★★	NR	NR	NR	NR	★★★	★	NR	NR	NR	NR
★★★	★★★	★★★	★★★★★	★★★	NR	NR	NR	★★★★★	★★★	NR	NR	★★★	★	★★★★★	NR	NR	★★★	NR
★	NR	★★★	★★★	NR	★★★★★	NR	NR	★★★	NR	NR	NR	★★★	★	★★★	NR	NR	★★★	NR
★★★	★	★	★★★	★★★★★	★★★	★★★	★★★	★★★	★★★	★★★	★★★	★	★★★	★★★	★★★	★★★	★★★	★★★
★	★★★	★	★★★	★★★	NR	★★★	NR	★	★★★	★★★	NR	★★★	★★★	★★★	★★★	★★★	★★★	NR
★	★★★	★	★	★★★★★	★★★	★★★	★★★	★★★★★	★★★	NR	★	★	★★★★★	★★★	★★★	★★★	★★★	NR
★★★	NR	★	★★★	★★★	★★★	NR	NR	★★★	NR	NR	NR	★	★	★★★	★★★	★★★	★★★	NR
★★★	★★★	★★★	★★★	★★★	★★★	★★★	★★★	★★★★★	★★★	★★★	★	★★★	★★★	★★★	★★★	★★★★★	NR	NR
★★★	★★★	★★★	★★★	★★★	★★★	★★★	★★★	★★★	★★★	★★★	NR	★	★	★★★	★	★★★	★★★	NR
★★★★★	★★★	★★★	★★★★★	★★★★★	★★★	★★★★★	★★★	★★★★★	★★★	★★★	★	★★★	★	★★★	★★★	★★★	NR	NR
★★★	★	★	★★★	★★★	★★★	★	★★★	★	★★★	★	NR	★	★	★★★	★★★	★★★	NR	NR
★★★	★★★	★★★	★★★	★★★	NR	NR	★★★	★★★	NR	NR	NR	★★★	★★★	★	★★★	★★★	NR	NR
★	★★★	★★★	★★★	★★★	★★★	★★★★★	NR	★★★	★★★	NR	NR	★★★	★★★	★	★★★	★★★	NR	NR
★	★	★	★★★	★★★	★★★	★★★	★	★★★	★	★★★	NR	★	★	★★★	NR	NR	NR	★
★★★	NR	★	★★★★★	★★★	★★★	NR	NR	★★★	NR	NR	NR	★★★	★★★	★★★	NR	NR	NR	★
★★★	★★★	★★★	★★★	★	★★★	★★★	★★★	★★★	★★★	★★★★★	★★★	★	★★★	★★★	★	NR	NR	NR
★	★	★★★	★★★	★	NR	★★★	NR	★	★	NR	NR	★	★★★	★★★	★★★	★★★	NR	NR
★★★	★★★	★★★	★	★	★★★★★	★★★	★★★	★★★	★★★	★★★	★★★	★	★★★	★★★	★★★	★★★★★	NR	NR
★★★	★★★★★	★★★	★★★	★★★	★★★★★	★	★	★★★	★★★	★★★	★★★	★★★	★★★	★★★	★★★★★	★★★	★★★	★★★★★
★★★	★	★★★★★	★★★	★	★★★	★	★★★	★★★	★★★	★★★	NR	★	★★★	★★★	★★★	★★★	NR	NR
★	★★★	★★★	★	★★★	★★★	★★★	★★★	★★★	★	★★★	NR	★	★★★	★★★	★★★	★★★	NR	NR
★	★★★	★★★	★	★★★	★★★	★★★	★★★	★	★	★★★	NR	★	★★★	★★★	★★★	★★★	NR	NR
★★★★★	★★★★★	★★★★★	★★★	★★★	★★★	★★★	NR	★★★	★★★	★★★	NR	★	★★★★★	★★★	★★★	★★★	NR	NR

NEW MEXICO HOSPITALS: RATINGS BY PROCEDURE

Hospital	Appendectomy	Atrial Fibrillation	Back and Neck Surgery (except Spinal Fusion)	Back and Neck Surgery (Spinal Fusion)	Bariatric Surgery	Bowel Obstruction	Carotid Surgery	Cholecystectomy (Gall Bladder Removal)	Chronic Obstructive Pulmonary Disease (COPD)	Coronary Bypass Surgery	Coronary Interventional Procedures (Angioplasty/Stent)	Diabetic Acidosis a
1. Alta Vista Regional Hospital, Las Vegas	NR	★★★	NR	NR	NR	★★★	NR	NR	★★★	NR	NR	NR
2. Artesia General Hospital, Artesia	NR	NR	NR	NR	NR	NR	NR	NR	★★★	NR	NR	NR
3. Carlsbad Medical Center, Carlsbad	NR	★★★	NR	NR	NR	★★★	NR	★	★★★	NR	NR	NR
4. Cibola General Hospital, Grants	NR	NR	NR	NR	NR	NR	NR	NR	★★★	NR	NR	NR
5. Dr. Dan C. Trigg Memorial Hospital, Tucumcari	NR	NR	NR	NR	NR	★★★	NR	NR	★★★	NR	NR	NR
6. Eastern New Mexico Medical Center, Roswell	NR	★★★	★★★	★★★	NR	★★★	★★★	★★★	★★★	NR	NR	NR
7. Española Hospital, Española	NR	NR	NR	NR	NR	★★★	NR	★★★	★★★	NR	NR	NR
8. Gallup Indian Medical Center, Gallup	NR	NR	NR	NR	NR	★★★	NR	NR	NR	NR	NR	NR
9. Gerald Champion Regional Medical Center, Alamogordo	NR	★★★	NR	★★★	NR	★	NR	★★★	★	NR	NR	NR
10. Gila Regional Medical Center, Silver City	NR	★★★	NR	NR	NR	★★★	NR	★★★	★★★	NR	NR	NR
11. Heart Hospital of New Mexico, Albuquerque	NR	★★★★★	NR	NR	NR	NR	★★★	NR	★★★	★★★	★★★	NR
12. Holy Cross Hospital, Taos	NR	★★★	NR	NR	NR	★★★	NR	NR	★★★	NR	NR	NR
13. Lea Regional Hospital, Hobbs	NR	NR	NR	NR	NR	★★★	NR	★★★	★★★	NR	NR	NR
14. Los Alamos Medical Center, Los Alamos	NR	NR	NR	NR	NR	NR	NR	NR	NR	NR	NR	NR
15. Lovelace Medical Center—Downtown, Albuquerque	NR	NR	★★★	★★★	NR	★★★	NR	★★★	★★★	NR	NR	★★★
16. Lovelace Medical Center—Gibson, Albuquerque	NR	★★★	★★★	NR	NR	★★★	NR	★★★	★★★	NR	★★★	NR
17. Lovelace Westside Hospital, Albuquerque	NR	NR	NR	NR	NR	NR	NR	NR	★★★	NR	NR	NR
18. Lovelace Women's Hospital, Albuquerque	NR	NR	★★★	NR	NR	NR	NR	NR	★★★	NR	NR	NR
19. Memorial Medical Center, Las Cruces	NR	★	NR	NR	NR	★★★	★★★	★★★	★	★★★	★★★	★★★
20. Mimbres Memorial Hospital, Deming	NR	★★★	NR	NR	NR	★★★	NR	★★★★★	★★★	NR	NR	NR
21. Miners' Colfax Medical Center, Raton	NR	NR	NR	NR	NR	★★★	NR	NR	★★★	NR	NR	NR
22. Mountainview Regional Medical Center, Las Cruces	NR	★★★	★★★	NR	NR	★★★	★★★	★★★★★	★★★	★★★★★	★★★	NR
23. Nor Lea General Hospital, Lovington	NR	NR	NR	NR	NR	NR	NR	NR	★★★	NR	NR	NR
24. Northern Navajo Physicians Indian Hospital, Shiprock	NR	NR	NR	NR	NR	★★★	NR	NR	NR	NR	★	NR
25. Plains Regional Medical Center—Clovis, Clovis	NR	★★★	NR	NR	NR	★★★	NR	NR	★★★	NR	★★★	NR
26. Presbyterian Hospital, Albuquerque	NR	★	★★★	★★★	NR	★★★	★★★	★	★	★★★	★★★	★★★
27. Presbyterian Kaseman Hospital, Albuquerque	NR	NR	NR	NR	NR	★★★	NR	NR	★	NR	NR	NR
28. Rehoboth McKinley Christian Health Services, Gallup	NR	★★★	NR	NR	NR	★★★	NR	★★★	★★★	NR	NR	NR
29. St. Vincent Hospital, Santa Fe	NR	★	★★★	★★★	NR	★★★	★★★	★★★	★★★	NR	★★★★★	★★★
30. San Juan Regional Medical Center, Farmington	NR	★★★	★★★	★★★	NR	★★★	NR	★★★	★★★	NR	★★★	NR
31. Sierra Vista Hospital, Truth Or Consequences	NR	NR	NR	NR	NR	NR	NR	NR	★★★	NR	NR	NR
32. Union County General Hospital, Clayton	NR	NR	NR	NR	NR	NR	NR	NR	★★★	NR	NR	NR
33. University of New Mexico Hospital, Albuquerque	NR	★★★	★★★	★	NR	★★★	NR	★★★	★★★	★	★★★	★★★

KEY: ★★★★★ BEST   ★★★ AS EXPECTED   ★ POOR   NR NOT RATED BY HEALTHGRADES   For full definitions of ratings and awards, see Appendix.

Gastrointestinal Bleed	Gastrointestinal Surgeries and Procedures	Heart Attack	Heart Failure	Hip Fracture Repair	Maternity Care	Pancreatitis	Peripheral Vascular Bypass	Pneumonia	Prostatectomy	Pulmonary Embolism	Resection/Replacement of Abdominal Aorta	Respiratory Failure	Sepsis	Stroke	Total Hip Replacement	Total Knee Replacement	Valve Replacement	Women's Health
★★★	NR	NR	★★★	★	NR	NR	NR	★	★	NR	NR	NR	★	★	NR	★★★	NR	NR
★★★	NR	NR	★★★	NR	NR	NR	NR	★★★	NR	NR	NR	NR	NR	★★★	NR	NR	NR	NR
★★★	★★★	★★★★★	★★★	★★★	NR	★★★	NR	★★★★★	★★★	NR	NR	★★★	★★★	★★★	★	★★★	NR	NR
NR	NR	NR	★★★	NR	NR	NR	NR	★★★	NR	NR	NR	NR	NR	NR	NR	NR	NR	NR
★★★	NR	NR	★	NR	NR	NR	NR	★★★	NR	NR	NR	NR	NR	NR	NR	NR	NR	NR
★	★★★	★★★	★★★	★★★	NR	★★★	NR	★★★	★★★	NR	NR	★★★	★★★	★★★	★★★	★★★	NR	NR
★★★	NR	NR	★★★★★	★★★	NR	NR	NR	★★★	NR	NR	NR	★★★	NR	NR	NR	NR	NR	NR
★	NR	NR	★★★	NR	NR	NR	NR	★	NR	NR	NR	NR	NR	NR	NR	NR	NR	NR
★★★	★★★	★	★	★★★	NR	★	NR	★	★★★	NR	NR	★	★★★	★	★	NR	★	NR
NR	NR	★★★	★★★	NR	NR	NR	★★★	★★★	NR	★★★	★★★	★★★	★★★	NR	NR	NR	★★★	NR
★★★	NR	NR	★★★	★★★	NR	NR	NR	★★★	★★★	NR	NR	NR	★★★	NR	NR	★	NR	NR
★★★	NR	NR	★★★	★★★	NR	NR	NR	★★★★★	★	NR	NR	★★★★★	★★★★★	NR	NR	★★★	NR	NR
★★★	NR	NR	★★★	★	NR	NR	NR	★	★★★	NR	NR	NR	NR	NR	NR	★★★	NR	NR
★★★	★★★	NR	★★★	★★★	NR	★★★	NR	★★★	★★★★★	★★★	NR	★★★★★	★★★	★★★	★★★	★★★	★★★	NR
★★★	★★★	★★★★★	★	★★★	NR	NR	NR	★	NR	NR	NR	★★★	★★★	★★★	★★★	★★★	NR	NR
★★★	NR	NR	★★★	★★★	NR	NR	NR	★★★★★	NR	NR	NR	★★★★★	★★★	NR	NR	★★★	NR	NR
★★★	★★★	★★★	★★★	★★★	NR	★★★	NR	★★★	★★★	★★★	★	NR	★★★	★★★	★★★	★★★	NR	NR
★	NR	★★★★★	★★★	NR	NR	NR	★★★	NR	NR	NR	NR	NR	★★★	★★★	NR	NR	NR	NR
★★★	NR	★★★	★★★	★★★	NR	NR	NR	★★★	NR	NR	NR	★★★★★	★★★	NR	NR	NR	★★★	NR
★★★	★★★★★	★★★	★★★	★★★	NR	★★★	NR	★★★★★	★★★	★	NR	★★★	★★★	★★★	★★★	★★★	★★★	NR
NR	NR	NR	★★★	NR	NR	NR	NR	★★★	NR	NR	NR	NR	NR	NR	NR	NR	NR	NR
★★★	NR	NR	★★★	★★★	NR	NR	NR	★	NR	NR	NR	NR	NR	NR	NR	NR	NR	NR
★★★	★★★	NR	★★★	★★★	NR	NR	NR	★	★★★	NR	NR	★	NR	★★★	★★★	★★★★★	NR	NR
★★★	★★★	★★★	★	★★★	NR	★★★	NR	★★★	★★★	★★★	★★★	★	★★★	★★★	★★★★★	★★★★★	★★★	NR
NR	NR	NR	★★★	NR	NR	NR	NR	★★★	NR	NR	NR	NR	NR	NR	NR	NR	NR	NR
★★★	NR	NR	★★★	★★★	NR	NR	NR	★★★	NR	NR	NR	★★★	★★★	★	NR	NR	NR	NR
★★★	★★★	★★★	★★★	★	NR	★★★	NR	★★★	★★★	★★★	NR	★	★★★	★	★★★	★★★	NR	NR
★★★	★★★	★★★	★	★	NR	★★★	NR	★★★	★★★	★★★	NR	★★★	★★★	★★★	★★★	★★★	NR	NR
NR	NR	NR	★★★	NR	NR	NR	NR	★★★	NR	NR	NR	NR	NR	NR	NR	NR	NR	NR
NR	NR	NR	★★★	NR	NR	NR	NR	★	NR	NR	NR	NR	NR	NR	NR	NR	NR	NR
★★★	★★★	★★★	★★★	★★★	NR	★★★	NR	★	★★★	NR	NR	★	★★★	★★★	★★★	NR	NR	NR

NEW YORK HOSPITALS: RATINGS BY PROCEDURE

	Appendectomy	Atrial Fibrillation	Back and Neck Surgery (except Spinal Fusion)	Back and Neck Surgery (Spinal Fusion)	Bariatric Surgery	Bowel Obstruction	Carotid Surgery	Cholecystectomy (Gall Bladder Removal)	Chronic Obstructive Pulmonary Disease (COPD)	Coronary Bypass Surgery	Coronary Interventional Procedures (Angioplasty/Stent)	Diabetic Acidosis a…
1. Adirondack Medical Center, Saranac Lake	***	***	NR	NR	***	***	***	***	***	NR	NR	***
2. Albany Medical Center Hospital, Albany	***	***	***	***	*	***	***	***	***	***	***	*
3. Albany Memorial Hospital, Albany	***	*	***	***	NR	***	***	*	***	NR	NR	***
4. Albert Lindley Lee Memorial Hospital, Fulton	*	***	NR	NR	NR	***	NR	*	*	NR	NR	***
5. Alice Hyde Medical Center, Malone	***	***	NR	NR	NR	***	NR	*	***	NR	NR	NR
6. Arnot Ogden Medical Center, Elmira	***	***	***	***	*****	***	***	***	***	***	***	***
7. Auburn Memorial Hospital, Auburn	***	***	NR	NR	*	***	NR	***	***	NR	NR	***
8. Aurelia Osborn Fox Memorial Hospital, Oneonta	***	***	NR	NR	NR	***	***	***	***	NR	NR	***
9. Bassett Hospital of Schoharie County, Cobleskill	NR	***	NR	NR	NR	NR	NR	NR	***	NR	NR	***
10. Bayley Seton Hospital, Staten Island	***	*	NR	NR	*	***	***	***	***	NR	NR	***
11. Bellevue Hospital Center, New York	*****	***	NR	NR	NR	***	***	***	***	***	***	***
12. Benedictine Hospital, Kingston	***	***	NR	NR	NR	***	***	***	***	NR	NR	***
13. Bertrand Chaffee Hospital, Springville	***	***	NR	NR	NR	NR	NR	***	***	NR	NR	NR
14. Beth Israel Medical Center, New York	***	*	*****	*****	***	*	***	***	***	***	NR	***
15. Bon Secours Community Hospital, Port Jervis	***	***	NR	NR	*****	***	NR	***	***	NR	NR	***
16. Bronx-Lebanon Hospital Center, Bronx	*****	***	NR	NR	NR	***	NR	*	***	NR	NR	***
17. Brookdale Hospital Medical Center, Brooklyn	***	***	NR	NR	*****	*	NR	***	*	NR	NR	***
18. Brookhaven Memorial Hospital Medical Center, Patchogue	*	***	*	*	NR	***	NR	*	***	NR	NR	***
19. Brooklyn Hospital Center at Downtown Campus, Brooklyn	***	***	NR	NR	***	***	NR	***	***	NR	NR	***
20. Brooks Memorial Hospital, Dunkirk	***	***	NR	NR	*	***	NR	NR	***	NR	NR	***
21. Buffalo General Hospital–Kaleida Health, Buffalo	***	***	***	***	***	***	***	***	*	*****	***	***
22. Cabrini Medical Center, New York	***	*	NR	NR	NR	***	NR	***	***	NR	NR	***
23. Canton-Potsdam Hospital, Potsdam	*	***	NR	NR	NR	***	NR	NR	***	NR	NR	***
24. Carthage Area Hospital, Carthage	***	***	NR	NR	NR	*	NR	NR	***	NR	NR	***
25. Catskill Regional Medical Center, Harris	***	***	NR	NR	NR	***	NR	***	***	NR	NR	***
26. Cayuga Medical Center at Ithaca, Ithaca	***	***	***	NR	***	***	***	***	***	NR	NR	***
27. Champlain Valley Physicians Hospital Medical Center, Plattsburgh	*****	*	NR	NR	NR	***	***	*****	***	***	*****	***
28. Chenango Memorial Hospital, Norwich	*	***	NR	NR	NR	***	NR	NR	*	NR	NR	***
29. Children's Hospital Rehab Center, Utica	***	*	*	***	*****	***	***	***	NR	NR	NR	***
30. City Hospital Center at Elmhurst, Elmhurst	*****	***	NR	NR	NR	***	NR	NR	***	NR	NR	***
31. Claxton-Hepburn Medical Center, Ogdensburg	***	***	NR	NR	*	***	NR	*****	***	NR	NR	***
32. Clifton Springs Hospital and Clinic, Clifton Springs	***	***	NR	NR	NR	*	NR	***	***	NR	NR	***
33. Columbia Memorial Hospital, Hudson	***	***	NR	NR	*	***	***	***	***	NR	NR	*
34. Community Hospital at Dobbs Ferry, Dobbs Ferry	***	***	NR	NR	*	***	NR	NR	***	NR	NR	***
35. Community Memorial Hospital, Hamilton	***	***	***	NR	NR	***	NR	NR	***	NR	NR	***
36. Community-General Hospital of Greater Syracuse, Syracuse	***	***	*****	*****	NR	***	***	***	*	NR	NR	***
37. Coney Island Hospital, Brooklyn	*****	***	NR	NR	*	*	NR	***	*	NR	NR	***
38. Corning Hospital, Corning	***	***	NR	NR	NR	***	NR	***	***	NR	NR	***
39. Cortland Regional Medical Center, Cortland	*****	***	NR	NR	NR	***	NR	***	***	NR	NR	***
40. Crouse Hospital, Syracuse	***	*	***	*****	NR	***	***	***	***	NR	***	***
41. Degraff Memorial Hospital, North Tonawanda	***	***	***	***	***	***	***	***	*	*****	***	***
42. Delaware Valley Hospital, Walton	NR	NR	NR	NR	NR	NR	NR	NR	***	NR	NR	NR
43. Eastern Long Island Hospital, Greenport	***	***	NR	NR	NR	***	NR	***	***	NR	NR	***
44. Edward John Noble Hospital of Gouverneur, Gouverneur	NR	NR	NR	NR	NR	NR	NR	NR	***	NR	NR	NR
45. Elizabethtown Community Hospital, Elizabethtown	NR	NR	NR	NR	NR	NR	NR	NR	*	NR	NR	NR
46. Ellis Hospital, Schenectady	***	***	*****	*****	***	***	***	***	***	*****	***	***
47. Erie County Medical Center, Buffalo	***	***	*****	*****	NR	***	***	***	***	***	***	***
48. F. F. Thompson Hospital, Canandaigua	***	***	NR	NR	NR	***	***	***	***	NR	NR	***
49. Faxton-Childrens Hospital, Utica	***	*	*	***	*****	***	***	***	***	NR	NR	***
50. Faxton-St. Luke's Healthcare, Utica	***	*	*	***	*****	***	***	***	*	NR	NR	***

KEY: ***** BEST   *** AS EXPECTED   * POOR   NR NOT RATED BY HEALTHGRADES   For full definitions of ratings and awards, see Appendix.

Gastrointestinal Bleed	Gastrointestinal Surgeries and Procedures	Heart Attack	Heart Failure	Hip Fracture Repair	Maternity Care	Pancreatitis	Peripheral Vascular Bypass	Pneumonia	Prostatectomy	Pulmonary Embolism	Resection/Replacement of Abdominal Aorta	Respiratory Failure	Sepsis	Stroke	Total Hip Replacement	Total Knee Replacement	Valve Replacement	Women's Health
***	***	***	*	*	***	NR	NR	*	***	NR	NR	NR	***	*	*	***	NR	NR
***	***	***	***	***	***	***	***	***	***	***	***	*	***	*	*****	*****	*****	***
***	***	***	*	*	NR	***	***	***	NR	NR	NR	*	***	***	*	*	NR	NR
***	***	*	***	***	NR	*	NR	***	NR	NR	NR	***	*	***	NR	NR	NR	NR
***	***	*	*	*	***	NR	NR	*	*	NR	NR	***	***	***	*	NR	NR	NR
***	***	***	*	*****	***	***	NR	***	***	***	NR	***	*	*	*****	*****	***	***
***	***	***	*	*****	***	***	NR	*	*****	NR	NR	*	*	*	***	*****	NR	NR
***	***	***	*	***	NR	***	NR	***	***	NR	NR	***	***	***	***	***	NR	NR
***	NR	NR	***	NR	***	NR	NR	***	NR	NR	NR	NR	***	*	NR	NR	NR	NR
*	***	***	***	***	*****	***	NR	*	***	NR	NR	***	*	***	NR	***	NR	NR
***	NR	***	***	*	*	NR	NR	***	NR	NR	NR	***	*	***	NR	NR	NR	*
***	***	***	***	***	***	***	***	***	***	***	NR	***	***	***	***	***	NR	NR
***	NR	***	***	NR	NR	NR	*	NR	NR	NR	NR	*	***	*	NR	NR	NR	NR
***	***	***	***	*****	*****	***	***	***	***	***	NR	***	***	***	***	*****	***	***
*	*	*	*	*	***	NR	NR	*	NR	NR	NR	***	***	***	NR	NR	NR	NR
***	*	***	***	NR	*****	NR	NR	*	NR	NR	NR	***	***	***	NR	NR	NR	NR
*	***	*	*	***	*	NR	NR	***	***	***	NR	*	*	*	NR	NR	NR	NR
***	***	*	***	***	***	*	NR	***	***	***	NR	***	***	*	***	NR	NR	NR
***	***	***	*	***	***	NR	NR	*****	***	***	NR	*	***	***	***	NR	NR	NR
***	NR	***	*	*	***	NR	NR	*	NR	NR	NR	NR	***	*	***	NR	NR	NR
***	***	***	***	***	***	***	NR	*	***	***	***	*	***	*	***	***	***	***
***	*	***	***	NR	*	***	NR	***	***	NR	NR	***	***	***	NR	***	NR	NR
***	***	***	***	***	***	NR	NR	*	NR	NR	NR	*	***	***	NR	***	NR	NR
***	NR	***	***	NR	***	NR	NR	*	NR	NR	NR	NR	***	*	***	NR	NR	NR
***	***	*****	***	***	*****	***	NR	***	***	***	NR	*	***	*	*****	*****	NR	NR
***	***	*	*	***	***	***	NR	*	***	NR	NR	***	***	*	***	***	NR	NR
***	***	***	*	***	NR	NR	***	NR	***	NR	NR	*	***	***	NR	***	NR	NR
*	*	***	***	***	*****	***	NR	*	***	***	NR	***	*	*	NR	***	NR	NR
***	NR	*	*	***	*	NR	NR	***	NR	NR	NR	NR	***	*	NR	NR	NR	NR
***	***	***	***	*	***	NR	NR	*	NR	NR	NR	NR	*****	***	*****	***	NR	NR
***	***	*	***	*	NR	NR	NR	*	*****	NR	NR	NR	***	***	***	NR	NR	NR
***	***	*	***	***	*	***	NR	***	*	NR	NR	*	***	***	NR	*	NR	NR
***	NR	***	***	*	NR	NR	NR	*	NR	NR	NR	NR	***	***	NR	NR	NR	NR
***	NR	***	***	***	***	NR	NR	*	NR	NR	NR	NR	***	*****	*****	NR	NR	NR
***	***	***	*	*****	***	***	***	*	*****	***	NR	*	***	*	*****	*****	NR	NR
***	*	***	***	***	***	***	NR	***	NR	***	NR	*	*	*	NR	NR	NR	NR
*	NR	***	***	***	***	NR	***	***	NR	***	*****	***	*	***	***	NR	NR	NR
***	*	***	*	***	NR	NR	NR	***	NR	NR	NR	*	***	***	***	NR	NR	NR
***	***	*	***	***	***	***	*	*	***	***	***	*	***	*	***	*	***	***
***	NR	***	***	NR	NR	NR	*****	NR	NR	NR	NR	NR	NR	NR	NR	NR	NR	NR
***	NR	***	***	***	NR	NR	***	NR	NR	NR	NR	***	***	NR	NR	NR	NR	NR
NR	NR	NR	***	NR	*	NR	*	NR	NR	NR	NR	NR	***	NR	NR	NR	NR	NR
NR	NR	NR	***	NR	NR	NR	***	NR	NR	NR	NR	NR	NR	NR	NR	NR	NR	NR
***	***	***	***	*****	NR	***	***	*****	***	***	***	***	***	***	***	*****	***	NR
***	*	***	***	***	NR	NR	*	NR	***	NR	*	*	*	***	***	***	NR	NR
***	***	*****	***	***	***	NR	NR	***	***	NR	NR	***	***	***	***	***	NR	NR
*	*	*	*	***	*****	***	NR	*	*	***	***	*	*	*	***	NR	NR	NR
*	*	*	*	***	*****	***	NR	*	*	***	***	*	*	*	***	NR	NR	NR

	Appendectomy	Atrial Fibrillation	Back and Neck Surgery (except Spinal Fusion)	Back and Neck Surgery (Spinal Fusion)	Bariatric Surgery	Bowel Obstruction	Carotid Surgery	Cholecystectomy (Gall Bladder Removal)	Chronic Obstructive Pulmonary Disease (COPD)	Coronary Bypass Surgery	Coronary Interventional Procedures (Angioplasty/Stent)	Diabetic Acidosis an...
51. Flushing Hospital Medical Center, Flushing	★★★	★★★	NR	NR	NR	★	NR	★★★	★	NR	NR	★★★
52. Forest Hills Hospital, Forest Hills	★★★	★	NR	NR	★★★	★★★	NR	★★★	★★★	NR	NR	★★★
53. Franklin Hospital, Valley Stream	★★★	★★★	NR	NR	★★★	★	NR	★★★	★	NR	NR	★★★
54. Geneva General Hospital, Geneva	★★★	★★★	★★★	NR	NR	★★★	★★★	NR	★★★	NR	NR	★★★
55. Glen Cove Hospital, Glen Cove	★★★	★★★	★★★	NR	NR	★★★	NR	★★★	★	NR	NR	★★★
56. Glens Falls Hospital, Glens Falls	★★★	★★★	★★★	NR	NR	★★★★★	★★★	★★★	★★★	NR	★★★	★★★
57. Good Samaritan Hospital Medical Center, West Islip	★★★	★★★	★★★	★★★★★	★★★	★★★	★★★	★★★	★	NR	★★★	★★★
58. Good Samaritan Hospital of Suffern, Suffern	★★★★★	★★★	★★★	NR	★★★	★★★	★★★	★★★	★★★	NR	★★★	★★★
59. Harlem Hospital Center, New York	★★★	★★★	NR	NR	NR	★	NR	NR	★★★	NR	NR	★
60. Highland Hospital, Rochester	★★★	★★★	★★★	★★★★★	★★★★★	★★★	NR	★	★★★	NR	NR	★★★
61. Horton Memorial Hospital, Middletown	★★★	★★★	★★★★★	NR	NR	★★★	NR	★★★	★	NR	NR	★★★
62. Hospital for Joint Diseases Orthopaedic Institute, New York	NR	NR	★★★	★★★★★	NR	NR	NR	NR	NR	NR	NR	NR
63. Hospital for Special Surgery, New York	NR	NR	★★★	★★★	NR	NR	NR	NR	NR	NR	NR	NR
64. Hudson Valley Hospital Center, Cortlandt Manor	★	★★★	NR	NR	NR	★★★	★	NR	★★★	NR	NR	★★★
65. Huntington Hospital, Huntington	★	★	★★★	★★★	NR	★★★	★★★	★★★	★	NR	NR	★★★
66. Inter-Community Memorial Hospital at Newfane, Newfane	★★★	★★★	NR	NR	NR	★★★	NR	NR	★★★	NR	NR	NR
67. Interfaith Medical Center, Brooklyn	★★★	NR	NR	NR	NR	★	NR	NR	★★★	NR	NR	★★★
68. Ira Davenport Memorial Hospital, Bath	★★★	★★★	NR	NR	NR	★★★	NR	NR	★★★	NR	NR	NR
69. Jacobi Medical Center, Bronx	★★★	★★★	NR	NR	★★★	★★★	NR	★★★★★	★★★★★	NR	NR	★★★
70. Jamaica Hospital Medical Center, Jamaica	★★★	★	NR	NR	NR	★	NR	★★★	★★★	NR	NR	★★★
71. John T. Mather Memorial Hospital of Port Jefferson, Port Jefferson	★★★★★	★★★	NR	NR	★★★	★★★	★★★	★★★★★	★★★	NR	NR	★
72. Jones Memorial Hospital, Wellsville	★★★	★★★	NR	NR	NR	★★★	NR	NR	★★★	NR	NR	NR
73. Kenmore Mercy Hospital, Kenmore	★★★	★	★★★	★★★	NR	★★★	NR	★★★	★	NR	NR	★★★
74. Kings County Hospital Center, Brooklyn	★★★	★★★	NR	NR	NR	★★★	NR	★★★	★★★	NR	NR	★★★
75. Kings Highway Hospital, Brooklyn	★★★	★	★★★★★	★★★★★	★★★	★	★★★	★★★	NR	★★★	★★★	★★★
76. Kingsbrook Jewish Medical Center, Brooklyn	★★★	★★★	NR	NR	NR	★	NR	★★★★★	★★★	NR	NR	★
77. Kingston Hospital, Kingston	★★★	★	NR	NR	NR	★★★	★★★	★★★	★★★	NR	NR	★★★
78. Lake Shore Hospital, Irving	★★★	★	NR	NR	NR	★★★	NR	NR	★	NR	NR	NR
79. Lakeside Memorial Hospital, Brockport	★★★	★★★	NR	NR	NR	★★★	NR	NR	★★★	NR	NR	NR
80. Lawrence Hospital Center, Bronxville	★★★	★★★	NR	NR	★★★★★	★★★	NR	★★★	NR	NR	NR	★★★
81. Lenox Hill Hospital, New York	★★★	★★★	★★★	★	★★★	★★★	★★★	★	★	★★★	★★★★★	★★★
82. Leonard Hospital, Troy	★★★	★★★	NR	★	NR	★★★	★★★	★★★	★★★	NR	NR	★
83. Lewis County General Hospital, Lowville	★	★	NR	NR	NR	★★★	NR	★★★	★★★	NR	NR	NR
84. Lincoln Medical and Mental Health Center, Bronx	★★★	★★★	NR	NR	NR	★★★	NR	★★★★★	★★★	NR	NR	★★★
85. Little Falls Hospital, Little Falls	NR	★★★	NR	NR	NR	★★★	NR	NR	★	NR	NR	NR
86. Lockport Memorial Hospital, Lockport	★★★	★★★	NR	NR	★★★	★	NR	★★★	★★★	NR	NR	NR
87. Long Beach Medical Center, Long Beach	★★★	★★★	NR	NR	NR	★	NR	★★★	★★★	NR	NR	★
88. Long Island College Hospital, Brooklyn	★★★★★	★	NR	NR	★★★	★★★	NR	★★★	★★★	NR	NR	★★★
89. Long Island Jewish Medical Center, New Hyde Park	★★★	★★★	★★★	★★★	★★★	★★★	★	★★★	NR	★★★	★★★★★	★
90. Lutheran Medical Center, Brooklyn	★★★	★★★	★★★	★★★★★	★★★	★★★	★★★	★★★	NR	NR	NR	★★★
91. Maimonides Medical Center, Brooklyn	★★★	★★★	NR	★★★★★	★★★	★★★	★	★	★	★	★★★★★	★★★★★
92. Mary Immaculate Hospital, Jamaica	★★★★★	★	NR	NR	NR	★	NR	★★★★★	★★★	NR	NR	★★★
93. Mary Imogene Bassett Hospital, Cooperstown	★★★	★★★	★★★	NR	★	★★★	★★★	★★★	★★★	★★★	★★★	★★★
94. Massena Memorial Hospital, Massena	★★★	★★★	NR	NR	NR	★★★	NR	★★★	★★★	NR	NR	★★★
95. Medina Memorial Hospital, Medina	★	NR	NR	NR	NR	★★★	NR	★★★	★★★	NR	NR	NR
96. Mercy Hospital, Buffalo	★★★	★	★★★	★★★	NR	★★★	NR	★★★	★★★	★★★	★★★	★★★
97. Mercy Medical Center, Rockville Centre	★★★★★	★★★	NR	★★★★★	★★★	★	★★★★★	★	NR	NR	NR	★★★
98. Metropolitan Hospital Center, New York	★★★	★★★	NR	NR	NR	★★★	NR	★★★	★★★	NR	NR	★★★
99. Millard Fillmore Hospital, Buffalo	★★★	★★★	★★★	★★★	★★★	★★★	★★★	★★★	★	★★★★★	★★★	★★★
100. Mohawk Valley General Hospital, Ilion	★★★	★	★	★★★	★★★★★	★★★	★★★	★★★	★	NR	NR	★★★

KEY: ★★★★★ BEST   ★★★ AS EXPECTED   ★ POOR   NR NOT RATED BY HEALTHGRADES   For full definitions of ratings and awards, see Appendix.

Gastrointestinal Bleed	Gastrointestinal Surgeries and Procedures	Heart Attack	Heart Failure	Hip Fracture Repair	Maternity Care	Pancreatitis	Peripheral Vascular Bypass	Pneumonia	Prostatectomy	Pulmonary Embolism	Resection/Replacement of Abdominal Aorta	Respiratory Failure	Sepsis	Stroke	Total Hip Replacement	Total Knee Replacement	Valve Replacement	Women's Health
★	★★★	★	★	★	★★★★★	NR	NR	★	NR	NR	NR	★★★	★	★	NR	NR	NR	NR
★★★	★★★	★	★★★	★★★	★★★★★	NR	NR	★★★	★★★	NR	NR	★★★	★	★	NR	★★★	NR	NR
★★★	★★★	★★★	★	★★★	★★★	★★★	NR	★	NR	★★★	NR	★	★	★★★	NR	★★★	NR	NR
★★★	★★★	★★★	★	★★★	NR	★★★	NR	★★★	NR	NR	NR	★★★	★★★	★★★	★	★★★	NR	NR
★★★	★★★	★★★	★	★	★★★★★	★★★	★	★	★★★	★★★	NR	★★★	★★★	★★★	★★★	★	NR	NR
★	★★★	★★★	★	★★★	★★★	★★★	★★★★★	★	★★★★★	★★★	★★★★★	★	★	★★★	★★★	★★★	NR	NR
★★★	★★★	★★★	★	★★★	★★★★★	★★★	★★★	★★★	★★★	★	★★★	★★★	★★★	★★★	★★★★★	★	NR	NR
★★★	NR	★	★★★	NR	★	NR	NR	★★★	NR	NR	NR	★	★	★	NR	NR	NR	NR
★	★	★★★	★★★	★★★	★	★★★	NR	★	★★★	★★★	NR	★	★	★★★	★★★	★★★	NR	NR
★	★★★	★★★	★★★	★★★	★★★	★★★	NR	★★★	★★★	★★★	NR	★★★★★	★★★★★	★★★	★★★	★	NR	NR
NR	NR	NR	NR	★★★	NR	NR	NR	NR	NR	NR	NR	NR	NR	NR	★★★	★★★	NR	NR
NR	NR	NR	NR	★★★	NR	NR	NR	NR	NR	NR	NR	NR	NR	NR	★★★★★	★★★★★	NR	NR
★	★★★	★★★	★	★★★	★★★	★★★	★★★	★★★	★	★★★	NR	★★★	★	★★★	★★★	★★★	NR	NR
★★★	★★★	★★★	★★★	★★★	★★★	★★★	★★★	★★★	★★★	★★★	NR	★	★★★	★★★	★★★	★★★	NR	NR
★★★	NR	★★★	★	NR	★★★	NR	NR	★	NR	NR	NR	NR	★	NR	NR	NR	NR	NR
★★★	NR	NR	★	NR	★★★	NR	NR	★	NR	NR	NR	★	★★★	★	NR	NR	NR	NR
★	NR	NR	★	★★★	★	NR	NR	★★★	NR	NR	NR	★★★	★★★	NR	NR	NR	NR	NR
★★★	NR	★★★	★★★	★	★	NR	NR	★★★	★★★	NR	NR	★★★	NR	★	★★★	NR	NR	NR
★	★	★	★	★★★	★★★	★★★	NR	★★★	NR	★★★	NR	★★★	★	★★★	NR	NR	NR	NR
★★★	★★★	★	★★★	★★★	NR	★★★	★★★	★★★★★	★★★	★★★	★★★	★★★	★	★	NR	NR	NR	NR
★	NR	★★★	★★★	★	★★★	★★★	NR	NR	★	NR	NR	★★★	★★★	★	NR	★★★	NR	NR
★★★	★★★	★★★	★	NR	★	★★★	NR	★	★★★	★★★	NR	★	★	★★★★★	★★★★★	NR	NR	NR
★	NR	★★★	★★★	★★★	★★★	★★★	NR	★★★	NR	NR	NR	★	★	★	NR	NR	NR	NR
★★★	★★★	★★★	★★★	★★★★★	★★★★★	★★★	★★★	★★★	★★★	★★★	NR	NR	★★★	★★★	★★★★★	★★★	★★★	
★★★	NR	★	★★★	NR	NR	NR	NR	★★★	★★★	NR	NR	★★★	★★★	★★★	NR	★★★★★	NR	NR
★★★	★★★	★	★★★	★★★★★	★★★	★★★	NR	★★★	★★★	NR	NR	★	★	★	★★★	★★★	NR	NR
★★★	NR	★★★	★	★★★	NR	NR	NR	★	NR	NR	NR	NR	NR	★★★	NR	★★★	NR	NR
★★★	NR	★★★	★	NR	★★★	NR	NR	★	NR	NR	NR	★★★	★★★	NR	NR	NR	NR	NR
★★★	★★★	★★★	★	★	★★★	NR	NR	★★★	★★★	NR	NR	★	★	★★★	★★★	★	NR	NR
★★★	★★★	★★★	★★★★★	★	★★★★★	★★★	★	★★★	★	★★★	★★★	★	★★★	★★★	★★★	★★★	★★★	★★★
★★★	★★★	★★★	★★★	★★★★★	★★★	★★★	NR	★★★	★★★★★	NR	NR	★★★	★★★	★★★★★	★★★	★★★★★	★★★	NR
★★★	NR	NR	★	NR	★	NR	NR	★★★	NR	NR	NR	NR	★★★	★★★	NR	★★★	NR	NR
★	★	★★★	★★★	★★★	★	★★★	★★★	NR	★★★	NR	NR	★	★★★	NR	NR	NR	NR	NR
★★★	NR	NR	★★★	NR	NR	NR	NR	★★★	NR	NR	NR	NR	NR	NR	NR	NR	NR	NR
★	NR	★★★	★	★★★	★★★	NR	NR	★	NR	NR	NR	★	★★★	★★★	NR	NR	NR	NR
★	NR	★	★★★	NR	★★★	NR	NR	★	★★★	NR	NR	★	★	★★★	NR	NR	NR	NR
★	★★★	★	★★★	★★★	★★★	★★★	NR	★	★★★	★	NR	★	★	★★★	★	NR	NR	NR
★	★	★★★	★	★★★	★★★	★★★	★	★★★	★★★	★★★	★	★★★	★	★	★★★	NR	NR	★★★
★★★	★	★★★	★	★★★	★★★	★★★	NR	★★★	★★★	NR	★★★	★★★	★★★	★	★★★	★★★	NR	★★★
★★★	★	★★★	★★★★★	★★★	★★★★★	★★★	★	★★★★★	★★★	★★★	★	★★★★★	★★★	★★★	★	★★★	★★★	★★★★★
★	★★★	★	★	★★★	★★★★★	★★★	★★★	★	★★★	★	NR	★	★	★	NR	★	NR	NR
★★★	★★★	★★★	★	★★★	★	★★★	★★★	★★★	★★★	★★★	★★★	★★★	★★★	★	★	★★★	★★★	★
★	NR	★★★	★★★	★	★★★	NR	NR	★	NR	NR	NR	★	★	NR	★★★	★★★	NR	NR
★★★	NR	★★★	★★★	★★★	★★★	NR	NR	★	NR	NR	NR	NR	★	NR	NR	NR	NR	NR
★★★	★★★	★★★	★	★★★	★★★	★★★	★★★	★★★	★★★★★	NR	★★★★★	★★★★★	★	★	★	NR	★★★	
★★★	★★★	★	★	★★★★★	★★★★★	★	★★★	★★★	★★★★★	★★★	★	★	★★★	★★★	★★★★★	NR	NR	★★★
★	NR	★★★	★★★	NR	★★★	NR	NR	★★★	★★★	NR	★★★	★	★	★★★	NR	NR	NR	NR
★★★	★★★	★	★★★	★★★	★★★	★★★	★	★	★★★	★★★	★★★	★	★★★	★	★★★	★★★	★★★	
★	★	★	★	★★★	★★★★★	★★★	NR	★	★	★★★	★★★	★	★	★	★	★★★	NR	NR

	Appendectomy	Atrial Fibrillation	Back and Neck Surgery (except Spinal Fusion)	Back and Neck Surgery (Spinal Fusion)	Bariatric Surgery	Bowel Obstruction	Carotid Surgery	Cholecystectomy (Gall Bladder Removal)	Chronic Obstructive Pulmonary Disease (COPD)	Coronary Bypass Surgery	Coronary Interventional Procedures (Angioplasty/Stent)	Diabetic Acidosis a...
101. Montefiore Medical Center, Bronx	★	★★★	★★★	★★★	★★★	★★★	★	★	★	★★★	★★★★★	★★★
102. Mount St. Mary's Hospital and Health Center, Lewiston	★★★★★	★	★★★	NR	NR	★★★	★★★	★★★	★	NR	NR	★★★
103. Mount Sinai Hospital, New York	★	★★★	★★★	★★★	★★★	★★★	★	★	★★★	★★★	★★★★★	★★★
104. Mount Vernon Hospital, Mount Vernon	★	★★★	NR	NR	NR	★	NR	NR	★★★	NR	NR	★★★
105. Nassau University Medical Center, East Meadow	★★★	★★★	NR	NR	★★★	★	NR	NR	★★★	NR	NR	★
106. Nathan Littauer Hospital, Gloversville	★★★	★★★	NR	NR	NR	★★★	NR	★★★	★	NR	NR	★★★
107. New Island Hospital, Bethpage	★★★	★★★	NR	NR	NR	★★★	NR	★★★	★★★	NR	NR	★★★
108. New York Community Hospital of Brooklyn, Brooklyn	★★★	★★★	NR	NR	NR	★★★	NR	★★★	★	NR	NR	★★★
109. New York Downtown Hospital, New York	★★★★★	★★★	NR	NR	NR	★★★	NR	★★★★★	★★★	NR	NR	★
110. New York Hospital Medical Center of Queens, Flushing	★★★	★★★	NR	NR	★★★	★★★	★★★	★★★	★★★	★★★	★	★★★
111. New York Methodist Hospital, Brooklyn	★★★	★★★	★★★	NR	★	★★★	★★★	★★★	★★★	★★★	★★★	★
112. New York Presbyterian—Columbia, New York	★	★★★	★★★★★	★★★	★★★	★★★	★★★	★★★	★★★★★	★★★	★★★	★★★
113. New York University Medical Center—Tisch Hospital, New York	★★★	★★★	★★★	★	★★★★★	★★★	★	★	★★★	★★★	★★★	★★★
114. New York Westchester Square Medical Center, Bronx	★★★★★	★	NR	NR	NR	★★★	★★★	★★★	★	NR	NR	★★★
115. New York-Presbyterian/Weill Cornell, New York	★	★★★	★★★★★	★★★	★★★	★★★	★★★	★★★	★★★★★	★★★	★★★	★★★
116. Newark-Wayne Community Hospital, Newark	★★★	★★★	NR	NR	NR	★★★	NR	★★★	★★★	NR	NR	NR
117. Niagara Falls Memorial Medical Center, Niagara Falls	★	★	NR	NR	★★★	★★★	★★★	NR	★	NR	NR	★★★
118. Nicholas H. Noyes Memorial Hospital, Dansville	★★★	★★★	NR	NR	NR	★★★	NR	★★★	★★★	NR	NR	NR
119. North Central Bronx Hospital, Bronx	★★★	NR	NR	NR	NR	NR	NR	★★★	★★★	NR	NR	★★★
120. North General Hospital, New York	NR	★★★	NR	NR	★★★	★★★	NR	★★★	★★★	NR	NR	★★★
121. North Shore University Hospital Syosset, Syosset	★★★★★	★★★	★★★★★	★★★	★★★	★★★	★★★★★	★★★	★★★	★★★	★★★★★	★★★
122. North Shore University Hospital, Manhasset	★★★★★	★★★	★★★★★	★★★	★★★	★★★	★★★★★	★★★	★★★	★★★	★★★★★	★★★
123. Northern Dutchess Hospital, Rhinebeck	★	★★★	NR	NR	NR	★★★	NR	★★★	★	NR	NR	NR
124. Northern Westchester Hospital, Mount Kisco	★	★★★	★	★★★	NR	★★★	★★★	★★★	★★★	NR	NR	★★★
125. Nyack Hospital, Nyack	★★★	★★★	NR	NR	NR	★★★	★★★	★★★	★★★	NR	NR	★
126. Olean General Hospital, Olean	★★★	★★★	NR	NR	NR	★	★★★	★★★	★	NR	NR	★★★
127. Oneida Healthcare Center, Oneida	★	★★★	NR	NR	NR	★★★	NR	★★★	★	NR	NR	NR
128. Orange Regional Medical Center, Goshen	★★★	★★★	★★★★★	NR	NR	★★★	★	★★★	★	NR	NR	★★★
129. Osteopathic Hospital Clinic of New York, Flushing	★★★★★	★	NR	NR	NR	★	NR	★★★★★	★★★	NR	NR	★★★
130. Oswego Hospital, Oswego	★★★	★★★	NR	NR	NR	★★★	NR	★	★★★	NR	NR	★★★
131. Our Lady of Lourdes Memorial Hospital, Binghamton	★★★	★★★	★★★	★★★	NR	★★★	★★★	★★★	★★★★★	NR	NR	★★★
132. Our Lady of Mercy Medical Center, Bronx	★★★	★★★	NR	NR	NR	★★★	NR	★★★	★★★	★★★	NR	★★★
133. Parkway Hospital, Forest Hills	★★★	★★★	NR	NR	NR	★★★	NR	★★★★★	★	NR	NR	★★★
134. Peconic Bay Medical Center, Riverhead	★★★★★	★★★	NR	NR	★★★	★	★★★	★★★	★★★	NR	NR	★★★
135. Peninsula Hospital Center, Far Rockaway	★★★	★★★	NR	NR	★★★	★★★	NR	★★★	★	NR	NR	★★★
136. Phelps Memorial Hospital Association, Sleepy Hollow	★★★★★	★★★	★★★	NR	★★★	★★★	NR	★★★	★★★	NR	NR	★
137. Plainview Hospital, Plainview	★	★	NR	NR	★★★	★★★	★★★	★★★	★★★	NR	NR	★★★
138. Putnam Hospital Center, Carmel	★★★	★★★	NR	NR	★	★	★★★	★★★	★★★	NR	NR	★★★
139. Queens Hospital Center, Jamaica	★★★	★★★	NR	NR	NR	★★★	NR	★★★	★★★	NR	NR	★★★
140. Rochester General Hospital, Rochester	★★★	★★★★★	★★★	★	★★★	★★★	★★★	★	★★★	★★★	★★★★★	★★★
141. Rome Memorial Hospital, Rome	★★★	★	NR	NR	NR	★★★	★★★	★★★	★	NR	NR	★★★
142. St. Anthony Community Hospital, Warwick	★★★	★	NR	NR	NR	★★★	NR	★	★★★	NR	NR	NR
143. St. Barnabas Hospital, Bronx	★★★	★★★	NR	NR	NR	★★★	NR	★	★★★	NR	NR	★★★
144. St. Catherine of Siena Hospital, Smithtown	★★★★★	★★★	★★★	★★★	★★★★★	★	★★★	★★★	★★★	NR	NR	★★★
145. St. Charles Hospital, Port Jefferson	★★★	★	★★★	NR	NR	★★★	NR	★★★	★★★	NR	NR	★★★
146. St. Clare's Hospital, Schenectady	★	★★★	NR	NR	NR	★★★	NR	★	★★★★★	NR	NR	★★★
147. St. Elizabeth Medical Center, Utica	★★★	★★★	★	★	★★★	★★★	★	★	★★★	★★★	★★★	★★★
148. St. Francis Hospital, Poughkeepsie	★★★	★	★★★	★★★	NR	★★★	★★★★★	★★★	★	NR	NR	★★★
149. St. Francis Hospital—Roslyn, Roslyn	★★★	★★★	NR	NR	NR	★★★	★★★★★	★★★★★	★	★★★	★★★	★
150. St. James Mercy Hospital, Hornell	★	★★★	NR	NR	NR	★★★★★	NR	NR	★★★★★	NR	NR	NR

KEY: ★★★★★ **BEST**   ★★★ **AS EXPECTED**   ★ **POOR**   NR **NOT RATED BY HEALTHGRADES**   For full definitions of ratings and awards, see Appendix.

Gastrointestinal Bleed	Gastrointestinal Surgeries and Procedures	Heart Attack	Heart Failure	Hip Fracture Repair	Maternity Care	Pancreatitis	Peripheral Vascular Bypass	Pneumonia	Prostatectomy	Pulmonary Embolism	Resection/Replacement of Abdominal Aorta	Respiratory Failure	Sepsis	Stroke	Total Hip Replacement	Total Knee Replacement	Valve Replacement	Women's Health
★	★★★	★★★	★	★	★★★	★★★	★	★★★	★★★	★★★	★	★	★	★	★	★	★★★	★
★★★	★★★	★★★	★	★★★	★★★	NR	NR	★★★	NR	NR	NR	★★★	★★★★★	★★★	★★★	★★★	NR	NR
★★★	★★★★★	★	★	★★★	★	★★★	★	★★★	★★★	★★★	★★★	★	★	★★★	★★★	★★★	★★★	★★★
★★★	NR	★★★	★★★	★★★	NR	NR	NR	★★★	★	NR	NR	★★★	NR	★	NR	NR	NR	NR
★	NR	★	★	★★★	★★★	NR	NR	★★★	NR	★★★	NR	★	★	★	NR	NR	NR	NR
★	★★★	★★★	★	★	★★★	NR	NR	★★★	NR	★★★	NR	★★★	★	★★★	★★★	★★★	NR	NR
★★★	★★★	★	★	★★★	NR	★★★	NR	★★★	★★★	NR	NR	★	★★★	★★★	★★★	★★★	NR	NR
★★★	★★★	★★★	★	★★★★★	NR	★	NR	★	★★★★★	NR	NR	★★★	★	★★★	NR	NR	NR	NR
★★★	NR	★★★	★	★★★	★★★★★	★★★	NR	★	NR	NR	NR	★★★	★	★★★	NR	NR	NR	NR
★	★★★	★★★	★	★	★★★★★	★★★	★★★	★	★★★	★★★	NR	★	★★★	★★★	★★★★★	★★★	★★★	★★★
★★★	★	★	★★★	★★★	★★★	★★★	★★★	★	★	★	NR	★	★★★★★	★★★	★	★★★	★★★	★★★
★★★	★★★	★★★	★★★	★	★★★	★★★	★★★	★★★	★★★	★	★★★	★★★	★★★	★★★	★★★	★	★★★★★	★★★
★★★	★	★	★★★	★	★★★	★	★	★★★	★	★★★	★★★	★★★	★★★	★★★	★★★	★	NR	★★★
★★★	★★★	★★★	★	★★★★★	NR	★★★	★★★	★	★★★	NR	NR	★★★	★	★★★	NR	★★★	NR	NR
★★★	★★★	★★★	★	★★★	★	★★★	★★★	★★★	★★★	★	NR	★★★	★★★	★★★	★	★★★★★	★★★	
★	NR	★★★	★	★★★	★★★	NR	NR	★	★	NR	NR	★	★★★	★★★	NR	★★★★★	NR	NR
★★★	★★★	★★★	★	★★★	★★★	NR	NR	★	NR	NR	NR	★★★	★	NR	NR	NR	NR	
★★★	★	★★★	★	★★★	★	NR	NR	★★★	NR	NR	NR	★★★	★	★★★	★★★	★★★	NR	NR
★★★	NR	NR	★★★	NR	★★★	NR	NR	★★★	NR	NR	NR	NR	★	NR	NR	NR	NR	
★	NR	★	★★★	NR	NR	NR	NR	★★★	NR	NR	NR	★★★	★	★★★	NR	NR	NR	NR
★★★	★★★	★★★	★	★★★★★	★★★	★★★	★★★	★	★★★	★★★	★★★	★	★	★	★★★	★★★	★★★★★	★★★
★★★	★★★	★★★	★	★★★★★	★★★	★★★	★★★	★	★★★	★★★	★★★	★	★	★	★★★	★★★	★★★★★	★★★
★★★	NR	★	★★★	★★★	★★★★★	★★★	NR	★	NR	NR	NR	★★★	★★★	★★★	★★★	★★★★★	NR	NR
★★★	★	★★★★★	★★★	★★★	★★★	★★★	NR	★	★★★	★★★	NR	★	★★★	★★★	★★★	★★★	NR	NR
★★★	★	★★★	★★★	★★★	★★★★★	★★★	★★★	★★★	★★★	★★★	★★★	★	★★★★★	★★★	NR	NR	NR	NR
★	★	★	★★★	★★★	★★★	NR	★	★★★	★★★	NR	★	★★★	★★★	★	NR	NR		
★★★	★★★	★	★	★★★★★	★★★	NR	NR	★	★★★	NR	NR	★★★	★	NR	★★★	NR	NR	
★	★★★	★★★	★★★	★★★	★★★	★★★	NR	★★★	★	★★★	NR	★★★★★	★★★★★	★★★	★★★	★	NR	NR
★	★★★	★★★	★	★★★	★★★★★	★★★	★★★	★	★★★	★	NR	★	NR	NR	NR	NR		
★★★	★★★	★	★	★★★	★★★	★★★	NR	★	NR	NR	NR	★	★	★★★	NR	★★★	NR	NR
★★★	★★★	★★★	★★★	★★★	★★★	★	★★★	★★★★★	★★★	★★★	★★★	★★★	★★★	★★★	★★★	NR	NR	
★★★	★★★	★	★★★	★★★★★	★★★	★★★	★	★★★	★★★	NR	NR	★	★★★	NR	NR			
★★★	★	★	★★★	★★★	★★★	★★★	★	★★★	NR	NR	NR	★★★	★★★	★★★	NR	NR		
★★★	★★★	★★★	★★★	★	★★★	★★★	★	★★★	NR	NR	NR	★★★	★★★	★★★	NR	NR		
★★★	★	★	★★★	★★★	NR	★★★	★	NR	NR	NR	★★★	★★★	★★★	NR	NR			
★	★★★	★★★	★	★★★	★★★	★	★★★	★	★★★★★	NR	NR	★★★	★★★	★★★	★★★	NR		
★	★★★	★★★	★	★★★	★★★★★	★★★	★★★	★	★★★	★★★	NR	NR	★★★	★★★	★★★	NR		
★★★	★★★	★★★	★★★	★★★	★★★	NR	★★★	★★★	NR	NR	★★★	★	★★★	★★★				
★★★	NR	NR	★★★	NR	★★★	★	★★★	NR	NR	NR	★★★	★★★	★★★	NR				
★★★	★	★★★	★★★	★★★	★★★	★★★	★★★	★★★	★★★★★	★★★	★★★	★★★	★★★	★★★	★★★	★★★	★★★	★★★
★	★★★	★	★★★	★★★	★	★★★	NR	★	NR	NR	NR	★	★	★★★	★★★	NR		
★★★	NR	★★★	★★★	★★★	NR	NR	★★★	NR	NR	NR	★★★	★★★★★	NR	NR	NR			
★★★	NR	★	★★★	★	★★★	★★★	NR	★★★	NR	NR	★★★	★	★★★	NR	NR			
★★★	★★★	★★★	★★★	★★★	★★★★★	★★★	NR	★	★★★	★★★	NR	★	★	★★★	★	NR		
★★★	NR	NR	★	★★★	★★★★★	NR	NR	★★★	NR	NR	NR	★★★	★★★	★★★	★★★	NR		
★★★	★★★	★★★★★	★	★	★★★	★★★	NR	★★★★★	NR	★★★	NR	★★★	★★★	★★★	★★★	★	NR	
★★★	★★★	★	★	★	NR	★★★	NR	★★★	NR	★★★	NR	★★★	★★★	★	★	★★★	★	
★★★	★★★	★★★	★	★★★	NR	★★★	NR	★★★	★★★	NR	NR	★★★	★★★★★	★	★★★	★★★★★	NR	
★	★★★	★	★	★★★	NR	★★★	★★★	★★★	★★★	★★★	★★★	★	★	★★★★★	★★★	★★★	★★★	
★★★	NR	★★★	★★★	★★★	★★★	NR	NR	★★★	NR	NR	NR	★★★★★	★★★	★	NR	NR	NR	NR

Hospital	Appendectomy	Atrial Fibrillation	Back and Neck Surgery (except Spinal Fusion)	Back and Neck Surgery (Spinal Fusion)	Bariatric Surgery	Bowel Obstruction	Carotid Surgery	Cholecystectomy (Gall Bladder Removal)	Chronic Obstructive Pulmonary Disease (COPD)	Coronary Bypass Surgery	Coronary Interventional Procedures (Angioplasty/Stent)	Diabetic Acidosis
151. St. John's Episcopal Hospital at South Shore, Far Rockaway	★★★	★	NR	NR	NR	★	NR	★	★	NR	NR	★★★
152. St. John's Riverside Hospital, Yonkers	★★★	★★★	NR	NR	NR	★★★	★	★★★	★★★	NR	NR	★★★
153. St. Joseph Hospital of Cheektowaga New York, Cheektowaga	★★★★★	★	★★★	NR	NR	★★★	★	★★★	★	NR	NR	★★★
154. St. Joseph's Hospital Health Center, Syracuse	★	★★★	★★★	★★★★★	NR	★★★	★★★	★★★	★★★	★★★★★	★★★★★	★★★
155. St. Joseph's Hospital Yonkers, Yonkers	★	★★★	NR	NR	★★★	★★★	NR	★	★★★	NR	NR	★
156. St. Joseph's Hospital, Elmira	★★★	★★★	NR	NR	NR	★★★	NR	★★★	★★★	NR	NR	★★★
157. St. Luke's Cornwall Hospital, Cornwall	★★★★★	★★★	★★★★★	NR	NR	★★★	★★★★★	★★★	★★★	NR	NR	★★★
158. St. Luke's Roosevelt Hospital, New York	★	★★★	★★★	★★★★★	★★★★★	★★★	★★★	★	★★★	★★★	★★★	★★★
159. St. Mary's Hospital, Amsterdam	★★★	★★★	NR	NR	NR	★	NR	★★★	★★★	NR	NR	★★★
160. St. Peter's Hospital, Albany	★★★	★	★★★	★★★★★	★	★★★	★★★★★	★	★★★	★★★	★★★	★★★
161. St. Vincent's Hospital–Manhattan, New York	★★★	★★★	★★★	★★★	★	★★★	★★★	★★★	★★★	★★★	★★★	★★★
162. Samaritan Hospital, Troy	★★★	★★★	NR	NR	NR	★★★	★★★	★★★	★★★	NR	NR	★★★
163. Samaritan Medical Center, Watertown	★★★	★	NR	NR	NR	★★★	NR	★★★	★★★	NR	NR	★★★
164. Saratoga Hospital, Saratoga Springs	★	★★★	NR	NR	NR	★	NR	★	★★★	NR	NR	★
165. Schuyler Hospital, Montour Falls	NR	NR	NR	NR	NR	★★★	NR	NR	★★★	NR	NR	NR
166. Seton Health System–St. Mary's Campus, Troy	★★★	★★★	NR	★	NR	★★★	★★★	★★★	★★★	NR	NR	★
167. Sisters of Charity Hospital, Buffalo	★★★	★★★	★★★	★★★	★★★★★	★★★	★★★	★★★	★★★	NR	NR	★★★
168. Soldiers and Sailors Memorial Hospital of Yates, Penn Yan	NR	NR	NR	NR	NR	NR	NR	NR	★★★	★★★	NR	NR
169. Sound Shore Medical Center of Westchester, New Rochelle	★★★	★★★	NR	★★★	★★★	★★★	NR	★★★	★★★	NR	NR	★★★
170. South Nassau Communities Hospital, Oceanside	★	★	★★★	NR	★★★	★	★★★	★	★★★	NR	NR	★★★
171. Southampton Hospital, Southampton	★★★	★★★	NR	NR	★★★	★★★	★★★	★★★	★★★	NR	NR	NR
172. Southside Hospital, Bay Shore	★★★★★	★★★	NR	NR	★★★★★	★★★	★	★★★	★★★	NR	★★★	★★★
173. Staten Island University Hospital, Staten Island	★★★★★	★★★	NR	NR	★	★★★	★★★	★	★★★	★★★	★★★★★	★★★
174. Stony Brook University Medical Center, Stony Brook	★★★	★★★	★	★★★	★★★	★★★	★	★★★	★★★	★★★★★	★★★	★
175. Strong Memorial Hospital, Rochester	★★★	★★★	★★★★★	★★★★★	★★★	★★★	★★★	★★★	★★★	★★★	★★★	★★★
176. SVCMC–St. Vincent's Hospital Staten Island, Staten Island	★★★	★	NR	NR	NR	★	★★★	★★★	★★★	NR	NR	★★★
177. Taylor Brown Memorial Hospital (Closed), Waterloo	★★★	★★★	★★★	NR	NR	★★★	NR	★★★	★★★	NR	NR	★★★
178. TLC Health Network, Gowanda	★★★	★	NR	NR	NR	★★★	NR	NR	★	NR	NR	★★★
179. United Health Services Hospitals, Binghamton	★★★	★★★	★	★★★	★★★	★★★	★	★★★	★★★	★★★	★★★★★	★
180. United Memorial Medical Center, Batavia	★★★	★★★	NR	NR	NR	★★★	★	★★★	★★★	NR	NR	NR
181. Unity Hospital, Rochester	★★★	★★★	NR	★★★	★★★	★★★	★★★	★★★	★★★	NR	NR	★★★
182. Unity St. Mary's Campus, Rochester	★★★	★★★	NR	★★★	★★★	★★★	★★★	★★★	★★★	NR	NR	★★★
183. University Hospital of Brooklyn–Downstate, Brooklyn	★★★	★★★	NR	NR	NR	★★★	NR	NR	★★★	★★★	★★★	★★★
184. University Hospital SUNY Upstate Medical University, Syracuse	★	★	★	★★★	★	★★★	★★★	★	★★★	★★★	★★★	★★★★★
185. Vassar Brothers Medical Center, Poughkeepsie	★	★★★	★★★	NR	NR	★★★	★★★	★★★	★	★★★★★	★★★	★★★
186. Victory Memorial Hospital, Brooklyn	★★★	★★★	NR	NR	★★★★★	★	NR	★★★★★	★	NR	NR	★★★
187. Westchester Medical Center, Valhalla	★★★	★★★	NR	★★★	★★★★★	★	★★★	★	★★★	★★★	★★★★★	★★★
188. Westfield Memorial Hospital, Westfield	NR	NR	NR	NR	NR	★★★	NR	NR	★★★	NR	NR	NR
189. White Plains Hospital Center, White Plains	★	★★★	★★★	★★★	★	★★★	★★★	★★★	★★★	NR	NR	★★★
190. Winthrop-University Hospital, Mineola	★★★	★★★	★★★	★	★★★	★★★	★★★	★	★★★★★	★★★	★★★	★★★
191. Woman's Christian Association, Jamestown	★★★	★★★	★★★	NR	NR	★★★	NR	★★★	★★★	NR	NR	★★★
192. Woodhull Medical and Mental Health Center, Brooklyn	★★★★★	★★★	NR	NR	NR	NR	NR	NR	★★★	NR	NR	★★★
193. Wyckoff Heights Medical Center, Brooklyn	★★★★★	★★★	NR	NR	★	NR	NR	★★★	★	NR	NR	★★★
194. Wyoming County Community Hospital, Warsaw	★★★★★	★★★	NR	NR	★	NR	NR	★★★	★★★	NR	NR	NR
195. Yonkers General Hospital, Yonkers	★★★	★★★	NR	NR	★★★	★	★★★	★★★	★★★	NR	NR	★★★

KEY: ★★★★★ BEST   ★★★ AS EXPECTED   ★ POOR   NR NOT RATED BY HEALTHGRADES   For full definitions of ratings and awards, see Appendix.

Gastrointestinal Bleed	Gastrointestinal Surgeries and Procedures	Heart Attack	Heart Failure	Hip Fracture Repair	Maternity Care	Pancreatitis	Peripheral Vascular Bypass	Pneumonia	Prostatectomy	Pulmonary Embolism	Resection/Replacement of Abdominal Aorta	Respiratory Failure	Sepsis	Stroke	Total Hip Replacement	Total Knee Replacement	Valve Replacement	Women's Health
★	★	★	★	★★★	★★★★★	NR	NR	★	★	NR	NR	★★★	★	★★★	NR	NR	NR	NR
★★★	★★★	★★★	★★★	★	★★★★★	★★★	★★★	★★★	★★★	NR	NR	★★★	★	★★★	★	★	NR	NR
★	★★★	★	★★★	★★★	NR	NR	NR	★	★★★	★★★	NR	★★★	★★★	★	★★★	★★★	NR	NR
★★★	★★★	★★★	★	★	★★★	★	★★★	★	★★★	★★★	★★★	★★★	★	★★★	★★★	★★★★★	★★★★★	★★★
★	★	★★★	★★★	★★★	NR	NR	★★★	★	★★★	NR	NR	★	★	NR	NR	NR	NR	NR
★★★	★	★★★	★	★★★★★	NR	★★★	★	★★★	★★★	★★★	NR	★★★	★★★	★	★★★	★★★	NR	NR
★★★	★★★	★★★★★	★★★★★	★★★	★★★★★	★★★	NR	★★★★★	★★★★★	★★★	NR	★★★	★★★★★	★	★★★	★★★★★	NR	NR
★★★	★★★	★	★★★	★	★★★	★★★	★	★	★★★	★	★★★	★★★	★	★★★	★★★	★★★	★★★	★
★★★	★	★	★★★	★★★	★★★★★	★	NR	★	★★★	★	NR	★★★	★	★★★	★★★	NR	★★★	NR
★★★★★	★★★	★★★	★★★	★★★	★★★	★★★	★	★★★	★★★	★	★★★	★★★	★	★★★	★★★	★★★★★	★★★	★★★
★	★★★	★★★	★	★★★	★★★	★	NR	★★★	★★★	NR	NR	★	★★★	★★★	★	★★★	NR	NR
★★★	★★★	★★★	★	★★★	★★★	★	NR	★	★★★★★	★★★	NR	★★★	★	★	★★★★★	★★★	NR	NR
★★★	★★★	★★★★★	★★★★★	★	NR	NR	NR	★★★	★★★	★★★	NR	★★★	★	★★★	★★★	NR	NR	NR
★★★	NR	★★★	★★★	NR	NR	NR	★★★	NR	NR	NR	NR	NR	NR	NR	NR	NR	NR	NR
★★★	★★★	★★★	★★★	★★★★★	★★★	★★★	NR	★★★	★★★★★	NR	★★★	★★★	★★★	★★★	★★★	★★★	NR	NR
★★★	★★★	★★★	★★★	★	★★★	★★★	★	★★★	★	NR	★★★	★★★	★★★	★★★	NR	NR	NR	NR
★★★	NR	★★★	★★★	NR	★	NR	NR	★★★	NR	NR	★★★	★★★	★★★	★★★	NR	NR	NR	NR
★★★	★★★	★★★	★★★	★★★★★	NR	★★★	★★★★★	★★★	★★★★★	NR	★★★	★★★	★★★	★★★	★	NR	NR	NR
★	★	★★★	★	★	★★★★★	★★★	★	NR	★	★★★	NR	★★★	★	★★★	★	NR	NR	NR
★★★	★★★	★★★	★★★	★★★★★	NR	★★★	NR	★	★★★	★	NR	★★★	★★★	★★★	NR	NR	NR	NR
★	★★★	★	★★★	★★★	★★★	★★★	★★★	★	★★★	★★★	★★★	★★★	★	★★★	★★★	★★★	★★★	★★★
★★★	★★★	★★★	★★★	★★★	★★★	★★★	★	★★★	★★★	★★★	★	★	★★★	★★★	★	★	★★★	★★★
★★★	★★★	★	★	★★★	★★★	★	NR	★	★★★★★	★★★	★	★	★	★	NR	★★★	★★★	★
★	★★★	★★★	★★★	★★★	★★★★★	★★★	NR	★	★★★	NR	NR	★★★	★	★★★	★	NR	★★★	NR
★★★	★★★	★★★	★	★★★	★★★	NR	NR	★★★	NR	NR	NR	★★★	★★★	★★★	★	NR	NR	NR
★★★	NR	★★★	★	★★★	NR	NR	NR	★	NR	NR	NR	★★★	★★★	★★★	NR	NR	NR	NR
★	★★★	★★★	★★★	★	★★★	★★★	★★★	★	★★★	★★★	★★★	★★★	★	★★★	★★★	★★★	★★★	★★★
★★★	NR	★★★	★	★★★	★★★	NR	NR	★	NR	★	NR	★★★	★★★	★	★★★	★★★	NR	NR
★★★	★★★	★★★★★	★★★	★★★	★★★	★★★	NR	★★★★★	NR	★★★	NR	★★★	★★★	★★★★★	★	★	NR	NR
★★★	★★★	★★★★★	★★★	★★★	★★★	NR	NR	★★★★★	NR	★★★	NR	★★★	★★★	★★★★★	★	★	NR	NR
★	★	★	★★★	NR	★★★	NR	NR	★★★	★★★	NR	NR	★★★	★★★	★	NR	★★★	NR	★★★
★★★	★★★	★	★★★	★★★	NR	★★★	NR	★★★	★★★	★	NR	★	★	★★★	★	★★★	★★★	★★★
★★★	★★★	★★★	★★★	★★★	★★★	★★★	★★★	★	★★★	★★★	★★★	★★★	★★★	★	NR	NR	★★★★★	★★★
★	★	★	★	★★★★★	★★★	★★★	★	★★★	NR	NR	★	★	★	NR	NR	NR	NR	NR
★	★★★	★★★	★	★	★	★	★★★	★	★★★	★	★★★	★	★★★	★★★	★★★	★★★	★★★	★★★
★★★	NR	NR	★★★	NR	★★★	NR	NR	★	NR	NR	NR	NR	NR	NR	NR	NR	NR	NR
★★★	★★★	★★★	★★★	★	★★★★★	★★★	★	★★★	★★★	★★★	NR	★★★	★	★★★	★★★	★	NR	NR
★★★	★★★	★★★	★★★	★	★★★★★	★★★	★	★★★	★★★	★★★	NR	★★★	★★★	★★★	★★★	★★★	★★★	★★★
★★★	★	★	★★★	★★★	★★★	★★★	NR	★	★★★★★	★★★	NR	★★★	★★★	★★★	★★★	★★★★★	NR	NR
★★★	NR	★★★	★★★	★★★	★★★	NR	NR	★★★	NR	NR	NR	★★★	★★★	★★★	NR	NR	NR	NR
★★★	★★★	★★★	★★★	★★★	★★★	NR	NR	★★★★★	★★★	NR	NR	★★★	★★★★★	★★★	NR	★★★	NR	NR
★★★	NR	★	★	★★★	★★★	NR	NR	★★★	NR	NR	NR	★★★	★★★	NR	NR	NR	NR	NR
★★★	★★★	★	★★★	★	★★★★★	★★★	★★★	★★★	★★★	NR	NR	★★★	★	★★★	★	★	NR	NR

NORTH CAROLINA HOSPITALS: RATINGS BY PROCEDURE

Hospital	Appendectomy	Atrial Fibrillation	Back and Neck Surgery (except Spinal Fusion)	Back and Neck Surgery (Spinal Fusion)	Bariatric Surgery	Bowel Obstruction	Carotid Surgery	Cholecystectomy (Gall Bladder Removal)	Chronic Obstructive Pulmonary Disease (COPD)	Coronary Bypass Surgery	Coronary Interventional Procedures (Angioplasty/Stent)	Diabetic Acidosis an...
1. Alamance Regional Medical Center, Burlington	★★★	★★★	NR	★★★	NR	★★★	★★★	★★★	★★★★★	NR	★★★	★★★
2. Albemarle Hospital Authority, Elizabeth City	★★★	★★★	★	NR	NR	★	★★★	★★★★★	★★★	NR	NR	★★★
3. Angel Medical Center, Franklin	NR	★★★	NR	NR	NR	★★★	NR	★★★	★★★	NR	NR	NR
4. Annie Penn Memorial Hospital, Reidsville	★★★★★	★	★★★	★★★★★	★★★	★	★★★	★★★★★	★	★★★	★★★	★★★
5. Anson Community Hospital, Wadesboro	NR	NR	NR	NR	NR	NR	NR	NR	★★★	NR	NR	NR
6. Ashe Memorial Hospital, Jefferson	★★★	★★★	NR	NR	NR	★★★	NR	★★★	★★★	NR	NR	NR
7. Beaufort County Hospital, Washington	★★★	★★★	NR	NR	NR	★★★	★★★	★★★	★	NR	NR	NR
8. Betsy Johnson Memorial Hospital, Dunn	★★★	★★★	NR	NR	NR	★	NR	★★★	★★★	NR	NR	★★★
9. Bladen County Hospital, Elizabethtown	NR	NR	NR	NR	NR	NR	NR	★★★	★★★	NR	NR	NR
10. Brunswick Community Hospital, Supply	★★★	★★★	NR	NR	★★★	★★★	★★★	★★★	★★★	NR	NR	★★★
11. Caldwell Memorial Hospital, Lenoir	★★★	★★★	NR	NR	★★★	NR	★★★	★★★	★★★	NR	NR	NR
12. Cape Fear Hospital, Wilmington	★★★	★★★	★★★	★★★	★★★★★	★★★	★	★★★	★★★	★★★	★	★★★
13. Cape Fear Valley Medical Center, Fayetteville	★★★	★★★	★★★	★★★	★★★★★	★★★	★★★	★★★	★★★	★	★★★	★★★★★
14. Carolinas Medical Center, Charlotte	★	★	★	★★★	★★★	★★★	★★★	★	★★★	★★★	★★★	★★★
15. Carolinas Medical Center–Lincoln, Lincolnton	★★★	★★★	NR	NR	★★★	★★★	★★★	★★★	★★★	NR	NR	★★★
16. Carolinas Medical Center–Mercy, Charlotte	★	★★★	NR	NR	NR	★★★	★★★	★★★	★★★	★★★	★★★	★★★
17. Carolinas Medical Center–NorthEast, Concord	★★★	★★★	★	★	★★★★★	★★★	★★★	★★★	★★★	★★★	★★★	★★★
18. Carolinas Medical Center–Union, Monroe	★★★★★	★★★★★	NR	NR	★★★	★★★	★★★	★★★	★★★★★	NR	★★★	★★★
19. Carolinas Medical Center–University, Charlotte	★★★	★★★	NR	NR	★★★	★★★	NR	★★★	★★★	★★★	NR	NR
20. Carteret General Hospital, Morehead City	★★★★★	★★★	NR	NR	★★★	★	★★★	★★★★★	★	NR	NR	★★★
21. Catawba Valley Medical Center, Hickory	★★★	★★★	★★★★★	★★★	★★★	★★★	★★★	★★★	★★★	NR	★★★	★★★
22. Central Carolina Hospital, Sanford	★★★	★★★	NR	NR	NR	★★★	★★★	★★★	★	NR	NR	★★★
23. Charles A. Cannon Jr. Memorial Hospital, Linville	★★★	★	NR	NR	★★★	NR	★★★	★★★	★★★	NR	NR	NR
24. Chowan Hospital, Edenton	★★★★★	★★★	NR	NR	NR	★★★	★★★	★★★	★★★	NR	NR	NR
25. Cleveland Regional Medical Center, Shelby	★★★	★★★	NR	NR	★★★	★	★★★	★★★	★★★	NR	NR	★★★
26. Columbus County Hospital, Whiteville	★★★	★★★	NR	NR	★	★★★	★★★	★★★	★★★	NR	NR	★★★
27. Craven Regional Medical Center, New Bern	★★★	★★★	★★★	★★★	★	★★★	★	★★★	★★★	★★★	★	★★★
28. Davis Regional Medical Center, Statesville	★★★	★★★	NR	★★★★★	★★★	NR	★★★	★★★★★	NR	NR	★★★	★★★
29. Duke Health Raleigh Hospital, Raleigh	★★★★★	★★★	★★★	★★★	★★★	NR	★★★	★★★★★	★★★	NR	NR	NR
30. Duke University Hospital, Durham	★	★★★	★★★	★	NR	★★★	★★★	★	★★★	★★★	★★★	★★★
31. Duplin General Hospital, Kenansville	★	★★★	NR	NR	★★★	NR	NR	★★★	★★★	NR	NR	★★★
32. Durham Regional Hospital, Durham	★★★	★★★	★	★★★	★	★★★	★★★	★★★	★★★	★★★	★★★	★★★
33. FirstHealth Moore Regional Hospital, Pinehurst	★★★★★	★★★	★★★	★★★	★★★	★	★★★★★	★★★★★	★★★	★★★	★★★	★★★
34. FirstHealth Richmond Memorial Hospital, Rockingham	★	★	NR	NR	★★★	NR	★★★	★★★	★★★	NR	NR	★★★
35. Forsyth Memorial Hospital, Winston-Salem	★★★	★	★★★★★	★★★★★	★	★	★★★	★★★	★	★★★	★	★★★
36. Franklin Regional Medical Center, Louisburg	★★★	★★★	NR	NR	★★★★★	★★★	NR	★★★	★★★	NR	NR	NR
37. Frye Regional Medical Center, Hickory	★★★	★★★	★★★	★★★	★	★	★★★	★★★	★	★★★	★★★	★★★
38. Gaston Memorial Hospital, Gastonia	★	★★★	★★★★★	★★★★★	★★★	★	★★★	★★★	★★★	★★★	★★★	★★★
39. Good Hope Hospital, Erwin	NR	NR	NR	NR	NR	NR	NR	★★★	NR	NR	NR	NR
40. Grace Hospital, Morganton	★★★★★	★★★	NR	NR	★★★	NR	★★★	★★★	★★★	NR	NR	★★★
41. Granville Medical Center, Oxford	★★★★★	★	NR	NR	★★★	NR	★★★	★★★	NR	NR	NR	NR
42. Halifax Regional Medical Center, Roanoke Rapids	★★★★★	★★★	NR	NR	★	NR	★★★★★	★★★	NR	NR	NR	★★★
43. Harris Regional Hospital, Sylva	★	★★★	NR	NR	★★★	NR	★★★	★★★	NR	NR	NR	NR
44. Haywood Regional Medical Center, Clyde	★★★	★★★★★	★★★	★★★	★★★★★	NR	★★★	★★★	NR	NR	NR	★★★
45. Heritage Hospital, Tarboro	★	★★★	NR	★★★	★★★	NR	★★★	★★★	NR	NR	NR	NR
46. High Point Regional Hospital, High Point	★★★	★★★	NR	★	★★★	★	★	★★★	★★★	★★★	★★★	★★★
47. Hugh Chatham Memorial Hospital, Elkin	★★★	★★★	NR	NR	★★★	NR	★★★★★	★★★	NR	NR	NR	★★★
48. Iredell Memorial Hospital, Statesville	★★★	★★★	NR	★★★	★★★	★★★	★★★	★★★	NR	NR	NR	★★★
49. J. Arthur Dosher Memorial Hospital, Southport	★★★	★★★	NR	NR	★★★	NR	★★★	★★★	★	NR	NR	NR
50. Johnston Memorial Hospital, Smithfield	★★★	★★★	NR	NR	NR	★★★	★★★	★★★	★	NR	NR	★★★

KEY: ★★★★★ BEST   ★★★ AS EXPECTED   ★ POOR   NR NOT RATED BY HEALTHGRADES   For full definitions of ratings and awards, see Appendix.

Gastrointestinal Bleed	Gastrointestinal Surgeries and Procedures	Heart Attack	Heart Failure	Hip Fracture Repair	Maternity Care	Pancreatitis	Peripheral Vascular Bypass	Pneumonia	Prostatectomy	Pulmonary Embolism	Resection/Replacement of Abdominal Aorta	Respiratory Failure	Sepsis	Stroke	Total Hip Replacement	Total Knee Replacement	Valve Replacement	Women's Health
★★★	★★★	★	★★★	★★★★★	★★★	★★★	NR	★★★	★★★	★★★	NR	★	★	★	★★★	★★★★★	NR	NR
★	★	★★★	★★★	★★★★★	★	★★★	NR	★	★★★	★	NR	★	★	★	★★★	★★★	NR	NR
★★★	NR	★★★	★★★	★★★★★	★★★	NR	NR	★	NR	NR	NR	NR	★★★	★★★★★	★★★	★★★	NR	NR
★	★★★	★	★	★★★	★★★	★★★	★★★	★	★★★★★	★★★	★★★	★	★	★	★★★★★	★★★	★★★	★★★
★	NR	NR	★★★	NR	NR	NR	NR	★★★★★	NR	NR	NR	★★★	★★★★★	★★★	NR	NR	NR	NR
★	NR	★	★★★	★	★	NR	NR	★★★	NR	NR	NR	★★★★★	★★★	★	NR	NR	NR	NR
★★★	★★★	★★★	★	★★★	★★★	NR	NR	★★★	★★★	NR	NR	★	★	NR	★★★	★★★	NR	NR
★★★	★	★★★	★★★	★	★★★	★★★	NR	★★★	★	NR	NR	★★★	★★★	★★★	NR	★★★	NR	NR
NR	NR	NR	★★★	NR	★★★	★★★	NR	★	NR	NR	NR	★	NR	NR	NR	NR	NR	NR
★★★★★	★★★	NR	★	★★★	★★★	★★★	NR	★★★	NR	★★★	NR	★★★	★★★	★	★★★★★	★	NR	NR
★★★	★★★	★★★	★★★	★	★★★	★★★	NR	★★★	NR	★★★	NR	★★★	★	★★★	★	★	NR	NR
★★★	★	★	★	★★★★★	★★★	★★★	★★★★★	★★★	★★★	★★★	★★★	★	★★★	★★★	★★★	★★★★★	★	★★★
★	★★★	★★★	★★★	★★★	★★★	★★★	★★★★★	★★★★★	★★★	★★★	★★★	★★★★★	★★★★★	★★★	★★★	★★★	★★★	★★★
★★★	★★★	★★★	★★★	★★★	★	★★★	★	★★★	★★★	★	★★★	★	★	★★★	★★★	★★★	★	★
★★★	NR	★	★★★	★★★	★★★	NR	NR	★★★	NR	NR	NR	★★★★★	★★★	★	NR	NR	NR	NR
★★★	★★★	★★★	★★★	★★★	★★★	NR	NR	★★★	★★★	★★★	NR	★★★	★	★★★	★★★	★★★	★	★★★
★★★	★★★	★★★	★★★	★	★★★	★★★	★★★	★	★★★	★★★	★★★	★	★	★★★	★★★	★	★★★★★	★★★
★★★	★★★	★★★★★	★★★★★	★★★	★★★★★	★★★	NR	★★★★★	★	★★★	NR	★★★★★	★★★★★	★★★	★★★	★★★	NR	NR
★★★	★★★	★★★	★★★	★★★	★★★	NR	NR	★★★	★★★★★	★★★	NR	★★★	★	★★★	★★★	★	NR	NR
★	★	★★★	★★★	★★★	★	★	NR	★	★★★	★	NR	NR	★	★★★	★★★	★★★	NR	NR
★★★	★★★	★★★	★★★	★★★	★★★	★★★	★★★	★★★	★★★	NR	★★★	★★★	★★★	★★★	★★★	★★★	NR	NR
★	★	★★★	★★★	★★★	★	★★★	NR	★	★	★★★	NR	★★★	★	★★★	NR	NR	NR	NR
★★★	NR	NR	★★★	NR	★	NR	NR	★	NR	NR	NR	★★★	★★★	★★★	NR	NR	NR	NR
★★★	NR	NR	★★★	★★★	★★★	NR	NR	★★★	NR	NR	NR	★★★	★	★★★	NR	★★★★★	NR	NR
★★★	★★★	★★★	★★★	★★★★★	★	NR	NR	★★★	★★★	★★★	NR	★★★	★	★★★	★★★	NR	NR	NR
★	★★★	NR	★★★	★★★	★★★	★	★★★	★	★★★	NR	NR	★★★	★	★★★	NR	★	NR	NR
★★★	★	★	★	★★★	★★★	★★★	★★★	★	★	★★★	★★★	★	★	★★★	★★★	★★★	★★★	★★★
★★★	★	NR	★★★	★★★	★★★	NR	NR	★★★	★★★	NR	NR	★★★	★	★★★	★★★	★★★	NR	NR
★★★	★★★	★★★	★	★★★	★★★	NR	NR	★★★	★★★	NR	NR	★	★	★★★	★★★	★★★	NR	NR
★★★	★★★	★★★	★★★	★	★	★★★	★	★★★	★	★★★	★★★	★	★★★★★	★	★★★	★★★★★	★★★	★
★★★	NR	★★★	★★★★★	★★★	NR	NR	NR	★	NR	NR	NR	★★★	★	NR	NR	★★★	NR	NR
★	★★★	★★★	★★★	★★★	★★★	★★★	NR	★	★★★	★★★	★★★	★★★	★	★★★	★★★	★★★	★★★	★★★
★★★	★★★★★	★★★	★★★	★★★	★★★	★★★	NR	★★★	★★★	★★★	★★★	★★★★★	★★★★★	★★★	★★★	★★★	★★★★★	★★★
★★★	NR	NR	★★★	NR	NR	NR	NR	★	NR	NR	NR	NR	NR	NR	NR	NR	NR	NR
★★★	★★★	★★★	★	★★★	★★★★★	★★★	NR	★★★	★★★	NR	NR	★★★	★★★	★★★	★★★	★★★	NR	NR
★★★	NR	★★★	★★★	★★★	★★★	NR	NR	★	NR	NR	NR	★★★	★	★★★	★★★	★★★	NR	NR
★★★	★★★	★	★★★	★★★★★	★	★★★	NR	★	★★★	★★★	NR	★★★	★	★	★★★	★★★	NR	NR
★★★	NR	★★★	★★★	★★★	★	NR	NR	★★★	NR	NR	NR	★★★★★	★★★★★	★★★	★★★	★★★	NR	NR
★★★★★	★★★★★	★★★	★★★★★	★★★	★★★	★★★	NR	★★★	★	NR	★★★	NR	★★★★★	★★★★★	★★★	★★★	★	NR
★★★	NR	★★★	★★★	★★★	★★★★★	★	NR	★★★	NR	NR	NR	★★★	★★★	★★★	NR	★★★	NR	NR
★★★	★★★	★★★	★★★	★★★	★★★	★★★	NR	★★★	★★★	★	★★★	★	★	★★★	★★★	★★★	★★★	★★★
★★★	NR	★★★	★★★★★	★★★★★	★★★	NR	NR	★★★	★★★	★★★	NR	★★★★★	★★★★★	★★★	★★★	★★★	NR	NR
★	★★★	★★★	★★★	★★★	★★★	★★★	NR	★	★	NR	NR	★	★	★★★	★★★	★★★	NR	NR
★★★	NR	NR	★★★	★★★	NR	NR	NR	★	NR	NR	NR	NR	★	★★★	NR	★★★	NR	NR
★	★★★	★	★★★	★	★★★	★★★	★	★	★★★	NR	NR	★	★★★	★★★	★★★	★	NR	NR

Hospital	Appendectomy	Atrial Fibrillation	Back and Neck Surgery (except Spinal Fusion)	Back and Neck Surgery (Spinal Fusion)	Bariatric Surgery	Bowel Obstruction	Carotid Surgery	Cholecystectomy (Gall Bladder Removal)	Chronic Obstructive Pulmonary Disease (COPD)	Coronary Bypass Surgery	Coronary Interventional Procedures (Angioplasty/Stent)	Diabetic Acidosis and
51. Kings Mountain Hospital, Kings Mountain	***	***	NR	NR	NR	***	NR	***	***	NR	NR	***
52. Lake Norman Regional Medical Center, Mooresville	***	*****	NR	NR	NR	*	NR	***	***	NR	NR	***
53. Lenoir Memorial Hospital, Kinston	*****	*	NR	NR	NR	*	***	***	*	NR	NR	***
54. Lexington Memorial Hospital, Lexington	***	***	NR	NR	NR	***	NR	NR	***	NR	NR	NR
55. Margaret R. Pardee Memorial Hospital, Hendersonville	*	***	NR	NR	NR	***	***	***	***	NR	NR	***
56. Maria Parham Hospital, Henderson	***	***	NR	NR	NR	*	NR	***	*	NR	NR	***
57. Martin General Hospital, Williamston	***	***	NR	NR	NR	***	NR	***	***	NR	NR	***
58. McDowell Hospital, Marion	***	***	NR	NR	NR	***	NR	***	***	NR	NR	NR
59. Medical Park Hospital, Winston-Salem	*	NR	NR	NR	NR	NR	NR	***	NR	NR	NR	NR
60. Mission Hospitals—Memorial Campus, Asheville	*	***	*****	*	***	*****	***	***	*****	***	***	***
61. Morehead Memorial Hospital, Eden	***	***	NR	NR	NR	***	NR	***	***	NR	NR	***
62. Moses H. Cone Memorial Hospital, Greensboro	*****	*	***	*****	***	NR	***	*****	***	***	***	***
63. Murphy Medical Center, Murphy	*	***	NR	NR	NR	***	NR	*	***	NR	NR	NR
64. North Carolina Baptist Hospital, Winston-Salem	***	***	***	*****	*****	***	*****	***	*****	*	***	***
65. Nash General Hospital, Rocky Mount	***	*	*****	***	NR	***	***	***	***	NR	NR	***
66. New Hanover Regional Medical Center, Wilmington	***	***	***	***	*****	***	*	***	***	***	*	***
67. Northern Hospital of Surry County, Mount Airy	***	***	NR	NR	NR	***	NR	*****	***	NR	NR	NR
68. Onslow Memorial Hospital, Jacksonville	***	***	NR	NR	NR	***	NR	***	***	NR	NR	***
69. Park Ridge Hospital, Fletcher	***	***	*	*	*	***	NR	***	***	***	NR	NR
70. Pender Memorial Hospital, Burgaw	NR	***	NR	NR	NR	***	NR	*****	NR	NR	NR	NR
71. Person Memorial Hospital, Roxboro	*	***	NR	NR	NR	*	NR	***	*	NR	NR	NR
72. Pitt County Memorial Hospital, Greenville	*	*	NR	***	*	***	***	***	*	***	***	*
73. Presbyterian Hospital Huntersville, Huntersville	***	***	NR	NR	NR	***	NR	***	***	NR	NR	NR
74. Presbyterian Hospital Matthews, Matthews	***	***	NR	NR	NR	***	NR	*****	***	NR	NR	***
75. Presbyterian Hospital, Charlotte	***	***	*	***	*****	***	***	***	*	***	***	***
76. Presbyterian Orthopaedic Hospital, Charlotte	NR	NR	*	***	NR	NR	NR	NR	NR	NR	NR	NR
77. Pungo District Hospital, Belhaven	NR	***	NR	NR	NR	NR	NR	***	NR	NR	NR	NR
78. Randolph Hospital, Asheboro	*	***	NR	NR	NR	***	NR	*	*****	NR	NR	NR
79. Rex Hospital, Raleigh	***	***	*	*	*	*****	***	***	***	***	***	***
80. Roanoke Chowan Hospital, Ahoskie	***	***	NR	NR	NR	***	NR	***	***	NR	NR	***
81. Rowan Regional Medical Center, Salisbury	*	***	*	***	NR	***	NR	***	***	NR	NR	***
82. Rutherford Hospital, Rutherfordton	*	***	NR	NR	NR	***	NR	***	*****	NR	NR	***
83. St. Joseph's Hospital, Asheville	*	***	*****	*	NR	*****	***	***	*****	***	***	***
84. St. Luke's Hospital, Columbus	***	***	NR	NR	NR	***	NR	***	***	NR	NR	NR
85. Sampson Regional Medical Center, Clinton	*	***	NR	NR	NR	***	NR	***	***	NR	NR	***
86. Sandhills Regional Medical Center, Hamlet	***	***	NR	NR	NR	***	***	***	*	NR	NR	***
87. Scotland Memorial Hospital, Laurinburg	***	***	NR	NR	NR	***	NR	NR	***	NR	NR	***
88. Southeastern Regional Medical Center, Lumberton	***	*	*	NR	NR	*	***	*	***	NR	NR	***
89. Spruce Pine Community Hospital, Spruce Pine	NR	***	NR	NR	NR	***	NR	***	***	NR	NR	NR
90. Stanly Memorial Hospital, Albemarle	***	***	NR	NR	NR	***	NR	***	***	NR	NR	NR
91. Stokes-Reynolds Memorial Hospital, Danbury	NR	NR	NR	NR	NR	NR	NR	***	***	NR	NR	NR
92. Swain County Hospital, Bryson City	NR	***	NR	NR	NR	NR	NR	***	***	NR	NR	NR
93. Thomasville Medical Center, Thomasville	***	***	NR	NR	NR	***	*	***	*	NR	NR	***
94. Transylvania Community Hospital, Brevard	*	***	NR	NR	NR	***	NR	***	***	NR	NR	NR
95. University of North Carolina Hospital, Chapel Hill	*	*****	NR	***	*	***	***	*	***	***	***	***
96. Valdese General Hospital, Valdese	***	***	NR	NR	NR	***	***	***	***	NR	NR	NR
97. Wakemed Cary Hospital, Cary	*	***	NR	NR	NR	***	NR	***	***	NR	NR	***
98. Wakemed—Raleigh Campus, Raleigh	*	***	***	*	NR	***	***	***	***	***	***	***
99. Washington County Hospital, Plymouth	NR	NR	NR	NR	NR	NR	NR	***	***	NR	NR	NR
100. Watauga Medical Center, Boone	***	***	NR	NR	NR	***	NR	*	***	NR	NR	NR

KEY: ***** BEST   *** AS EXPECTED   * POOR   NR NOT RATED BY HEALTHGRADES   For full definitions of ratings and awards, see Appendix.

Gastrointestinal Bleed	Gastrointestinal Surgeries and Procedures	Heart Attack	Heart Failure	Hip Fracture Repair	Maternity Care	Pancreatitis	Peripheral Vascular Bypass	Pneumonia	Prostatectomy	Pulmonary Embolism	Resection/Replacement of Abdominal Aorta	Respiratory Failure	Sepsis	Stroke	Total Hip Replacement	Total Knee Replacement	Valve Replacement	Women's Health
★★★	NR	NR	★★★	NR	NR	NR	NR	★★★	NR	NR	NR	★★★	★★★	★★★	NR	NR	NR	NR
★★★	★★★	★★★	★★★	★	★★★	★★★	NR	★★★	★★★	★★★	NR	★★★	★	★	★	★	NR	NR
★	★	★★★★★	★★★	★★★★★	★★★	★★★	★★★	★	★★★	★	NR	★★★	★★★	★	★	★	NR	NR
★	NR	★★★	★★★	★★★	★★★★★	★★★	NR	★	NR	★★★	NR	★	★	★★★	★★★	★★★	NR	NR
★★★	★★★	★★★	★★★	★★★	★★★	★★★★★	★★★	★★★★★	NR	★★★	NR	★★★	★★★	★★★	★★★★★	★★★★★	NR	NR
★	★	★★★	★★★	★★★	★	★★★	NR	★	★★★	★★★	NR	NR	★	★	NR	★	NR	NR
★★★	NR	★★★	★★★★★	NR	★★★	★	NR	★★★	NR	NR	NR	★★★	★★★	★★★	NR	NR	NR	NR
★	NR	★★★	★	★★★	★	NR	NR	★★★	NR	NR	NR	★★★	★★★	★★★	NR	NR	NR	NR
NR	★★★	NR	NR	NR	NR	NR	NR	NR	★★★	NR	NR	NR	NR	NR	NR	NR	NR	NR
★★★★★	★★★★★	★★★	★★★	★★★	★	★★★	★★★	★★★★★	★★★	★★★★★	★★★	★★★	★★★	★★★	★★★	★★★★★	★★★	★★★
★★★	NR	★	★★★	★	★★★	★★★	NR	★★★	★★★	★★★	NR	★★★	★	★	NR	NR	NR	NR
★	★★★	★	★	★★★	★★★	★★★	★★★	★	★★★★★	★★★	★★★	★	★	★	★★★★★	★★★	★★★	★★★
★	NR	★★★	★★★	★★★	★	NR	NR	★★★	NR	NR	NR	★★★★★	★★★	★★★	NR	NR	NR	NR
★★★	★	★	★★★	★	NR	★★★	★★★	★★★★★	★★★	★★★	★★★	★★★	★★★	★★★	★★★	★★★	★★★★★	★
★★★	★★★	★★★★★	★★★	★★★	★★★	★★★	NR	★★★	★★★	★★★	NR	★★★	★★★	★★★	★★★	★★★★★	NR	NR
★★★	★	★	★★★	★★★★★	★★★	★★★	★★★★★	★★★	★★★	★★★	★	★★★	★★★	★★★	★★★★★	★	NR	★★★
★★★	★★★	★★★	★★★	★★★	NR	★★★	NR	★★★★★	★★★	★★★	NR	★★★★★	★★★	★★★	NR	★	NR	NR
★★★	★★★	★	★★★	★★★★★	★★★	NR	★	★★★	NR	NR	NR	★★★	★	★	NR	★	NR	NR
★★★	NR	★★★	★★★	★★★	★★★	NR	NR	★★★	★★★	NR	NR	★★★	★★★★★	★★★	★★★	★★★	NR	NR
★	NR	NR	★	NR	NR	NR	NR	★★★	NR	NR	NR	NR	NR	NR	NR	NR	NR	NR
★★★	★★★	NR	★	★★★	★★★	★★★	NR	★	NR	NR	NR	NR	★	NR	NR	★★★	NR	NR
★★★	★	★	★	★	★★★	★	★★★	★	★★★	★	★★★	★	★	★	★	★	★	★
★★★	NR	NR	★★★	★★★	★★★	NR	NR	★★★	NR	NR	NR	★	★★★	★★★	NR	NR	NR	NR
★★★	★★★	★★★	★★★★★	★★★	★	★★★	NR	★★★	NR	★★★	NR	★★★	★★★	★★★	NR	NR	NR	NR
★★★	★★★	★★★	★	NR	★	★★★	★★★	★	★★★★★	★★★★★	★★★	★★★	★	NR	NR	★	NR	★
NR	NR	NR	NR	★★★★★	NR	NR	NR	NR	NR	NR	NR	NR	NR	NR	★★★★★	★★★★★	NR	NR
★★★	NR	NR	★★★	NR	NR	NR	NR	★★★	NR	NR	NR	NR	NR	NR	NR	NR	NR	NR
★★★	★★★	★★★★★	★★★★★	★	★★★	★	NR	★★★★★	★	★★★	NR	★★★★★	★★★★★	★★★	NR	★	NR	NR
★★★	★★★★★	★★★★★	★★★	★	★★★	★★★	★★★	★★★	★★★	★★★★★	★★★★★	★★★	★★★★★	★★★	★	NR	★★★	NR
★★★	★★★	NR	★★★★★	★★★	★★★	NR	NR	★★★	★	NR	NR	★★★★★	★★★	★★★	NR	NR	NR	NR
★★★	★	★★★	★★★	★★★	★	★★★	NR	★★★	★★★	★★★	NR	★★★★★	★	★★★	★★★	★★★★★	NR	NR
★★★	★★★	★★★	★★★	★★★	★★★	★★★	NR	★★★	NR	NR	NR	★★★★★	★★★	★★★	★★★	★★★	NR	NR
★★★★★	★★★★★	★★★	★★★	★★★	NR	★★★	★★★	★★★★★	★★★	★★★★★	★★★	★★★	★★★	★★★	★★★★★	★★★	NR	NR
★	★★★	★★★	★★★	★	★★★	★★★	NR	★	★★★	NR	NR	NR	NR	★★★	NR	★	NR	NR
★	★★★	★★★	★	★★★	★★★	★★★	NR	★	★★★	★★★	NR	NR	★	★★★	NR	★★★	NR	NR
★★★	NR	NR	★★★	NR	NR	NR	NR	★	NR	★	NR	NR	★	★	NR	NR	NR	NR
★★★	★★★	★★★	★★★	★★★	★★★	★★★	NR	★	★	★★★	NR	★★★	★★★	★	★★★	★★★	NR	NR
★★★	★★★	NR	★★★	★★★★★	★★★	★★★	NR	★	NR	★	NR	★★★	★★★	NR	★★★	★★★	NR	NR
★★★	★★★	NR	★★★	★	NR	NR	NR	★★★	NR	NR	NR	★★★★★	★★★	NR	★★★	★★★	NR	NR
★★★	★★★	★★★★★	★★★	★★★	★★★	★★★	NR	★★★	★★★	★★★	NR	★★★★★	★★★★★	★	NR	★★★	NR	NR
NR	NR	NR	★★★	NR	NR	NR	NR	★★★	NR	NR	NR	NR	NR	NR	NR	NR	NR	NR
NR	NR	NR	★★★	NR	NR	NR	NR	★★★	NR	NR	NR	NR	★★★	NR	NR	NR	NR	NR
★	★★★	★★★	★★★	★★★	★★★	NR	NR	★	★★★	NR	NR	★★★	★	NR	NR	NR	NR	NR
★★★	★	★	★★★	★	★	★★★	NR	★	★★★	NR	NR	★	★	NR	NR	★★★	NR	NR
★★★	★★★	★★★	★	★	★★★	★	★★★★★	★	★★★	★★★	★★★	★	★	★★★	★★★	★	★	★
★★★	★★★	★★★	★★★	NR	★★★	NR	★★★	★★★	★★★	★★★	NR	★★★	★★★	★★★	★★★	★★★	★	★
★★★	★★★	★	★	★★★★★	★	NR	NR	★	★	★★★	NR	★★★	★★★	★★★	★★★	★★★	NR	NR
★	★	★	★★★	★	★★★	★★★	★★★	★	★★★	★	NR	★	★★★	★	★	★★★	★★★	★★★
NR	NR	★★★	★★★	NR	NR	NR	NR	★★★	NR	NR	NR	NR	NR	NR	NR	NR	NR	NR
★★★	★★★	★★★	★	★	★★★	★★★	NR	★	★★★	★	NR	★	★	★	★	★	NR	NR

	Appendectomy	Atrial Fibrillation	Back and Neck Surgery (except Spinal Fusion)	Back and Neck Surgery (Spinal Fusion)	Bariatric Surgery	Bowel Obstruction	Carotid Surgery	Cholecystectomy (Gall Bladder Removal)	Chronic Obstructive Pulmonary Disease (COPD)	Coronary Bypass Surgery	Coronary Interventional Procedures (Angioplasty/Stent)	Diabetic Acidosis and
101. Wayne Memorial Hospital, Goldsboro	★★★	★	★★★	★★★	NR	★	★★★	★★★	★	NR	NR	★★★	
102. Wesley Long Community Hospital, Greensboro	★★★★★	★	★★★	★★★★★	★★★	★	★★★	★★★★★	★	★★★	★★★	★★★	
103. Wilkes Regional Medical Center, North Wilkesboro	★★★	★★★	NR	NR	NR	★★★	NR	★★★	★★★	NR	NR	NR	
104. Wilson Medical Center, Wilson	★★★	★	NR	NR	NR	★★★	NR	★★★	★★★	NR	NR	★	

KEY: ★★★★★ **BEST**   ★★★ **AS EXPECTED**   ★ **POOR**   NR **NOT RATED BY HEALTHGRADES**   For full definitions of ratings and awards, see Appendix.

Gastrointestinal Bleed	Gastrointestinal Surgeries and Procedures	Heart Attack	Heart Failure	Hip Fracture Repair	Maternity Care	Pancreatitis	Peripheral Vascular Bypass	Pneumonia	Prostatectomy	Pulmonary Embolism	Resection/Replacement of Abdominal Aorta	Respiratory Failure	Sepsis	Stroke	Total Hip Replacement	Total Knee Replacement	Valve Replacement	Women's Health
★★★	★★★	★★★	★	★★★	★★★	★★★	NR	★	★★★	★★★	NR	★	★	★	★★★	★★★	NR	NR
★	★★★	★	★	★★★	★★★	★★★	★★★	★★★★★	★★★	★★★	★	★	★	★	★★★★★	★★★	★★★	★★★
★	NR	★★★	★★★	★★★	★★★	NR	NR	★	★★★	NR	NR	★★★	★	★	NR	★	NR	NR
★	★★★	★	★	★★★	★★★	★★★	NR	★	★★★	★★★	NR	★★★	★	★	★★★★★	★★★	NR	NR

NORTH DAKOTA HOSPITALS: RATINGS BY PROCEDURE

	Appendectomy	Atrial Fibrillation	Back and Neck Surgery (except Spinal Fusion)	Back and Neck Surgery (Spinal Fusion)	Bariatric Surgery	Bowel Obstruction	Carotid Surgery	Cholecystectomy (Gall Bladder Removal)	Chronic Obstructive Pulmonary Disease (COPD)	Coronary Bypass Surgery	Coronary Interventional Procedures (Angioplasty/Stent)	Diabetic Acidosis and...
1. **Altru Hospital,** Grand Forks	NR	★★★	★★★	NR	NR	★★★	★★★	★★★★★	★★★	★★★	★★★	★★★
2. **Carrington Health Center,** Carrington	NR	★★★	NR	NR	NR	NR	NR	NR	★★★	NR	NR	NR
3. **Heart of America Medical Center,** Rugby	NR	★★★	NR	NR	NR	NR	NR	NR	★★★	NR	NR	NR
4. **Innovis Health,** Fargo	NR	★	★★★★★	★★★	NR	★★★	★★★	★★★	★★★★★	★★★	★★★	NR
5. **Jamestown Hospital,** Jamestown	NR	★★★	NR	NR	NR	★★★	NR	★★★	★★★	NR	NR	NR
6. **Medcenter One,** Bismarck	NR	★★★	★	★	NR	★	★★★	★★★	★★★★★	★★★	★★★	★
7. **Mercy Hospital of Valley City,** Valley City	NR	NR	NR	NR	NR	NR	NR	NR	★★★	NR	NR	NR
8. **Mercy Hospital,** Devils Lake	NR	★★★	NR	NR	NR	★★★	NR	★★★	★★★	NR	NR	NR
9. **Mercy Medical Center,** Williston	NR	★	NR	NR	NR	★★★	NR	★★★	★★★	NR	NR	NR
10. **Meritcare Health System,** Fargo	NR	★★★	★★★★★	★	NR	★★★	★★★	★★★	★★★	★★★★★	★★★	★★★
11. **Oakes Community Hospital,** Oakes	NR	NR	NR	NR	NR	NR	NR	NR	★★★	NR	NR	NR
12. **Pembina County Memorial Hospital,** Cavalier	NR	NR	NR	NR	NR	NR	NR	NR	★★★	NR	NR	NR
13. PHS Indian Hospital at Belcourt-Quentin N. Burdick Memorial, Belcourt	NR	NR	NR	NR	NR	NR	NR	NR	★★★	NR	NR	NR
14. **St. Alexius Medical Center,** Bismarck	NR	★★★	★★★★★	★★★	NR	★★★	★	★★★★★	★★★	★★★★★	★★★★★	NR
15. **St. Aloisius Medical Center,** Harvey	NR	NR	NR	NR	NR	NR	NR	NR	★★★	NR	NR	NR
16. **St. Joseph's Hospital and Health Center,** Dickinson	NR	★★★	NR	NR	NR	★★★	NR	★★★	★★★	NR	NR	NR
17. **St. Luke's Hospital,** Crosby	NR	NR	NR	NR	NR	NR	NR	NR	★★★	NR	NR	NR
18. **Tioga Medical Center,** Tioga	NR	NR	NR	NR	NR	NR	NR	NR	★★★	NR	NR	NR
19. **Trinity Hospitals,** Minot	NR	★★★	NR	NR	NR	★★★	★★★	★★★	★	★★★	★★★	★★★
20. **Trinity Medical Center,** Minot	NR	★★★	NR	NR	NR	★★★	★★★	★★★	★	★★★	★★★	★★★
21. **West River Regional Medical Center,** Hettinger	NR	★★★	NR	NR	NR	★★★	NR	NR	★★★	NR	NR	NR

KEY: ★★★★★ BEST ★★★ AS EXPECTED ★ POOR NR NOT RATED BY HEALTHGRADES For full definitions of ratings and awards, see Appendix.

Gastrointestinal Bleed	Gastrointestinal Surgeries and Procedures	Heart Attack	Heart Failure	Hip Fracture Repair	Maternity Care	Pancreatitis	Peripheral Vascular Bypass	Pneumonia	Prostatectomy	Pulmonary Embolism	Resection/Replacement of Abdominal Aorta	Respiratory Failure	Sepsis	Stroke	Total Hip Replacement	Total Knee Replacement	Valve Replacement	Women's Health
★★★	★	★★★★★	★★★	★★★★★	NR	★★★		★★★	★★★★★	★★★	★★★	★★★	★★★★★	★★★	★★★	★★★★★	★★★	NR
★★★	NR	NR	★★★	NR	NR	NR		★★★	NR	NR	NR	NR	NR	NR	NR	NR	NR	NR
★★★	NR	NR	★★★	NR	NR	NR		★★★	NR	NR	NR	NR	NR	★★★	NR	NR	NR	NR
★★★	★★★	★★★	★★★	★★★	NR	★★★	★★★	★★★★★	★★★★★	★★★	★★★	★★★	★★★★★	★★★	★★★	★★★	★	NR
★★★	★★★	★★★	★★★	★★★	NR	NR		★★★	NR	NR	NR	NR	★★★	NR	NR	★★★	NR	NR
★★★	★★★	★★★	★★★★★	★★★	NR	★★★	★★★	★★★	★★★	★	★★★★★	★★★★★	★★★	★	★★★	★★★★★	★★★	
★★★	NR	★★★	★★★★★	NR	NR	NR		★★★★★	NR	NR	NR	NR	★★★	NR	NR	NR	NR	
★★★	NR	★★★	★★★	NR	NR	NR		★★★	NR	NR	NR	NR	★★★	NR	NR	NR	NR	
★★★	★★★	NR	★★★★★	★★★	NR	NR		★★★	★★★	NR	NR	NR	★★★	NR	★★★	★★★★★	NR	
★★★	★★★	★★★	★★★	★	NR	★★★	★★★	★★★	★★★	★		★★★	★★★★★	★	★★★	★	★★★	
★★★	NR	NR	★★★	NR	NR	NR		★★★	NR	NR	NR	NR	NR	NR	NR	NR	NR	
NR	NR	NR	★	NR	NR	NR		★★★	NR	NR	NR	NR	NR	NR	NR	NR	NR	
NR	NR	NR	★★★	NR	NR	NR		★★★	NR	NR	NR	NR	NR	NR	NR	NR	NR	
★★★	★★★	★★★★★	★★★	★★★	NR	★★★		★★★★★	★★★	★★★	★★★	★★★	★★★	★★★	★★★★★	★★★★★	NR	
NR	NR	NR	★★★	NR	NR	NR		★★★	NR	NR	NR	NR	NR	NR	NR	NR	NR	
★★★	NR	★★★	★★★	★	NR	NR		★★★	NR	★★★	NR	★★★	★★★	★★★	★★★	★★★	NR	
NR	NR	NR	★★★	NR	NR	NR		★★★★★	NR	NR	NR	NR	NR	NR	NR	NR	NR	
NR	NR	NR	★★★	NR	NR	NR		★★★	NR	NR	NR	NR	NR	NR	NR	NR	NR	
★★★	★	★★★	★★★	★★★	NR	★★★		★★★	★★★	★★★	NR	★★★	★★★	★	★★★★★	★★★★★	★★★	
★★★	★	★★★	★★★	★★★	NR	★★★		★★★	★★★	★★★	NR	★★★	★★★	★	★★★★★	★★★★★	★★★	
★★★	NR	★★★	★★★	NR	NR	NR		★★★★★	NR	★★★	NR	NR	★★★	NR	NR	NR	NR	

OHIO HOSPITALS: RATINGS BY PROCEDURE

Hospital	Appendectomy	Atrial Fibrillation	Back and Neck Surgery (except Spinal Fusion)	Back and Neck Surgery (Spinal Fusion)	Bariatric Surgery	Bowel Obstruction	Carotid Surgery	Cholecystectomy (Gall Bladder Removal)	Chronic Obstructive Pulmonary Disease (COPD)	Coronary Bypass Surgery	Coronary Interventional Procedures (Angioplasty/Stent)	Diabetic Acidosis and
1. Adams County Regional Medical Center, Seaman	NR	★★★	NR	NR	NR	NR	NR	NR	★★★	NR	NR	
2. Adena Regional Medical Center, Chillicothe	NR	★★★★★	NR	NR	NR	★★★	★★★	★★★	★★★	NR	★★★	★★★
3. Akron General Medical Center, Akron	NR	★★★	★	★	NR	★★★	★★★	★★★	★★★★★	★★★	★★★★★	★★★★★
4. Allen Medical Center, Oberlin	NR	NR	NR	NR	NR	★	NR	NR	★★★	NR	NR	
5. Alliance Community Hospital, Alliance	NR	★★★	NR	NR	NR	★★★	★★★★★	★★★	★★★	NR	★★★	
6. Ashtabula County Medical Center, Ashtabula	NR	★★★	NR	NR	NR	★★★	★★★	★★★	★★★	NR	★★★	
7. Aultman Hospital, Canton	NR	★★★	★★★★★	★★★	NR	★★★	★★★★★	★★★★★	★★★	★★★★★	★★★	★★★
8. Barberton Citizens Hospital, Barberton	NR	★★★	NR	NR	NR	★★★	★★★	★★★★★	★★★★★	NR	★★★	★★★
9. Barnesville Hospital Association, Barnesville	NR	★★★	NR	NR	NR	NR	NR	★★★★★	★★★★★	NR	NR	
10. Bay Park Community Hospital, Oregon	NR	★★★	NR	NR	NR	★★★	★★★	★★★	★★★	NR	NR	
11. Bellevue Hospital, Bellevue	NR	★★★	NR	NR	NR	★★★	NR	★★★★★	★★★	NR	NR	
12. Belmont Community Hospital, Bellaire	NR	★	NR	NR	NR	★★★	NR	NR	★★★	NR	NR	
13. Berger Hospital, Circleville	NR	★★★	NR	NR	NR	★★★	★★★	NR	★★★	NR	NR	
14. Bethesda North Hospital, Cincinnati	NR	★★★	★★★	★★★★★	NR	★★★	★	★★★	★★★★★	★★★	★★★	★★★
15. Blanchard Valley Regional Health Center, Findlay	NR	★★★	★★★	★★★	NR	★	★★★	★★★	★★★	★★★	★★★	★★★
16. Brown County Hospital, Georgetown	NR	★★★	NR	NR	NR	★★★	NR	NR	★★★	NR	NR	
17. Christ Hospital, Cincinnati	NR	★★★	★	★★★	NR	★★★★★	★★★	★★★	★★★★★	★★★	★★★★★	★★★
18. Cleveland Clinic, Cleveland	NR	★★★	★	★	NR	★★★★★	★★★	★★★	★★★★★	★★★★★	★★★	★★★
19. Clinton Memorial Hospital, Wilmington	NR	★★★	NR	NR	NR	★★★	★★★	★	★★★	NR	NR	
20. Community Health Partners of Ohio—West, Lorain	NR	★★★	★★★	★★★	NR	★★★	★★★	★★★	★★★★★	★★★	★★★	★★★
21. Community Hospital of Springfield and Clark County, Springfield	NR	★★★	NR	NR	NR	★★★	★★★	★★★★★	★★★	★★★	★★★	★★★
22. Community Hospital, Bryan	NR	★★★	NR	NR	NR	★★★	NR	★★★★★	★★★	NR	★★★	
23. Community Memorial Hospital, Hicksville	NR	NR	NR	NR	NR	NR	NR	NR	★	NR	NR	
24. Coshocton County Memorial Hospital, Coshocton	NR	★★★	NR	NR	NR	★★★	NR	★★★	★	NR	NR	★★★
25. Cuyahoga Falls General Hospital, Cuyahoga Falls	NR	★★★	NR	NR	NR	★★★	★★★	★★★	★★★★★	NR	NR	
26. Dayton Heart Hospital, Dayton	NR	★★★	NR	NR	NR	NR	★★★★★	NR	★★★	★★★★★	★★★★★	NR
27. Deaconess Hospital, Cincinnati	NR	★★★	★★★	★★★	NR	★★★	NR	★★★	★★★★★	NR	★★★	★★★
28. Defiance Regional Medical Center, Defiance	NR	★★★	NR	NR	NR	★★★	NR	★★★	★★★	NR	NR	
29. Doctors Hospital of Nelsonville, Nelsonville	NR	NR	NR	NR	NR	NR	NR	NR	★★★	NR	NR	
30. Doctors Hospital of Stark County, Massillon	NR	★★★	★★★	NR	NR	★	★★★	★★★	★★★	★★★	★	NR
31. Doctors Hospital Ohio Health, Columbus	NR	★	NR	NR	NR	★★★	★★★	★★★	★★★	★★★	★★★	★★★
32. Dunlap Memorial Hospital, Orrville	NR	NR	NR	NR	NR	NR	NR	NR	★★★	NR	NR	
33. East Liverpool City Hospital, East Liverpool	NR	★★★	NR	NR	NR	★★★	NR	★	★★★★★	NR	★	
34. East Ohio Regional Hospital, Martins Ferry	NR	★	NR	NR	NR	★★★	★★★	★★★	★★★	NR	★★★	
35. Emh Regional Medical Center, Elyria	NR	★★★	★★★★★	NR	NR	★★★	★★★★★	★★★	★★★★★	★★★★★	★★★	★★★
36. Fairfield Medical Center, Lancaster	NR	★★★	★★★	NR	NR	★★★	★★★★★	★★★	★★★	★★★	★★★★★	★★★
37. Fairview Hospital, Cleveland	NR	★★★	★★★	NR	NR	★★★	★★★	★★★	★★★★★	★★★★★	★★★★★	★★★
38. Fayette County Memorial Hospital, Washington Court House	NR	NR	NR	NR	NR	★★★	NR	NR	★★★	NR	NR	
39. Firelands Regional Medical Center—Main Campus, Sandusky	NR	★★★	NR	★★★★★	NR	★★★★★	★★★	★★★	★★★	★★★	★★★	★★★
40. Fisher Titus Memorial Hospital, Norwalk	NR	★★★	NR	NR	NR	★★★	NR	★★★★★	★★★	NR	★★★	
41. Flower Hospital, Sylvania	NR	★★★	NR	NR	NR	★★★	★★★	★★★★★	★★★	NR	★★★	
42. Fort Hamilton Hughes Memorial Hospital, Hamilton	NR	★★★★★	NR	NR	NR	★★★★★	★★★	★★★	★★★★★	★★★	NR	★★★
43. Fostoria Community Hospital, Fostoria	NR	★★★	NR	NR	NR	★★★	NR	★★★	★★★	NR	NR	
44. Fulton County Health Center, Wauseon	NR	★★★	NR	NR	NR	★★★	NR	★★★★★	★★★	NR	NR	
45. Galion Community Hospital, Galion	NR	★★★	NR	NR	NR	★★★	NR	NR	★★★	NR	NR	
46. Genesis Healthcare System, Zanesville	NR	★★★	★★★	NR	NR	★★★	★	★	★★★	★★★	★★★	★★★
47. Good Samaritan Hospital, Cincinnati	NR	★★★	★★★	★★★	NR	★★★★★	★★★	★★★	★★★	★★★	★★★	★★★
48. Good Samaritan Hospital, Dayton	NR	★★★	★★★	★★★	NR	★★★	★★★	★★★	★★★★★	★★★	★★★	★★★
49. Grady Memorial Hospital, Delaware	NR	★★★	NR	NR	NR	★★★	NR	NR	★★★	NR	NR	
50. Grandview Medical Center, Dayton	NR	★★★	★★★	★★★	NR	★★★★★	★★★	★★★	★★★	★★★	★★★	★★★★★

KEY: ★★★★★ BEST   ★★★ AS EXPECTED   ★ POOR   NR NOT RATED BY HEALTHGRADES   For full definitions of ratings and awards, see Appendix.

Gastrointestinal Bleed	Gastrointestinal Surgeries and Procedures	Heart Attack	Heart Failure	Hip Fracture Repair	Maternity Care	Pancreatitis	Peripheral Vascular Bypass	Pneumonia	Prostatectomy	Pulmonary Embolism	Resection/Replacement of Abdominal Aorta	Respiratory Failure	Sepsis	Stroke	Total Hip Replacement	Total Knee Replacement	Valve Replacement	Women's Health
★★★	NR	NR	★	NR	NR	NR	NR	★★★	NR	NR	NR	NR	★★★	★★★	NR	NR	NR	NR
★★★	★★★	★★★	★	★★★★★	NR	★★★	★★★	★★★★★	★	★★★	NR	★★★★★	★★★	★	★★★	★★★★★	NR	NR
★★★★★	★★★	★★★★★	★★★★★	★★★	NR	★★★	★★★	★★★★★	★★★	★★★★★	★★★	★★★★★	★★★★★	★★★★★	★	★	★★★★★	NR
★★★	NR	NR	★★★	★★★	NR	NR	NR	★★★★★	NR	NR	NR	NR	NR	★★★	NR	NR	NR	NR
★★★	★★★	★★★	★★★	★★★	NR	★★★	NR	★★★	NR	NR	NR	★★★	★★★	★★★	★★★★★	★★★	NR	NR
★★★	★★★★★	★★★★★	★★★★★	★	NR	★★★	NR	★★★★★	NR	★★★	NR	★★★	★★★★★	★★★★★	★★★	★★★	NR	NR
★★★	★★★★★	★★★	★★★	★★★	NR	★★★	★★★	★★★	★★★	★★★	★★★★★	★★★★★	★★★★★	★★★	★★★	★★★	★★★★★	NR
★★★	★★★	★★★	★★★★★	★★★★★	NR	★★★	NR	★★★★★	★★★★★	NR	NR	★★★	★★★	★	NR	★★★	NR	NR
★★★	NR	★★★	★★★	★★★	NR	NR	NR	★★★	NR	NR	NR	NR	★★★	★★★★★	NR	NR	NR	NR
★★★	★★★	NR	★★★	★★★	NR	NR	NR	★★★	NR	NR	NR	NR	★★★	★★★	NR	★★★	NR	NR
★★★	NR	NR	★★★	★★★	NR	NR	NR	★★★	NR	NR	NR	NR	NR	★★★	NR	★★★★★	NR	NR
★★★	NR	★★★	★★★	NR	NR	NR	NR	★★★	NR	NR	NR	NR	NR	★★★	NR	NR	NR	NR
★★★	★★★★★	★★★	★★★★★	★★★★★	NR	★★★	NR	★★★★★	★★★	★★★★★	NR	★★★★★	★★★	★★★	★★★	★★★★★	NR	NR
★★★	★★★	★★★	★	NR	NR	★★★	NR	★★★	★★★	NR	NR	★	★★★	★★★	NR	NR	★★★★★	NR
★★★	NR	NR	★★★★★	★	NR	NR	NR	★★★★★	NR	NR	NR	★★★★★	★★★	★★★	NR	NR	NR	NR
★★★★★	★★★★★	★★★★★	★★★★★	★★★★★	NR	★★★★★	★★★	★★★★★	★★★	★★★★★	★★★	★★★★★	★★★★★	★★★★★	★★★	★	★★★	NR
★★★	★★★★★	★★★	★★★★★	★★★	NR	★★★★★	★	★★★	★★★	★★★★★	NR	★★★	★★★	★★★★★	★	★	NR	★★★★★
★★★	★★★★★	★★★	★	NR	NR	★★★	NR	★★★	★	NR	NR	★★★	★★★	★★★★★	★	NR	NR	NR
★★★	★★★★★	★★★	★★★★★	★★★	NR	★★★	NR	★★★★★	★	NR	NR	★★★★★	★★★★★	★★★★★	★★★	NR	★★★	NR
★★★	★	★★★	★★★	★★★	NR	NR	NR	★★★	★★★	NR	NR	★★★	★★★★★	★★★	★	★★★	NR	NR
★★★	★★★	★★★	★★★★★	NR	NR	NR	NR	★★★	NR	NR	NR	★	★★★	★★★	★★★	★★★★★	NR	NR
NR	NR	NR	★★★	NR	NR	NR	NR	★★★	NR	NR	NR	NR	NR	NR	NR	NR	NR	NR
★★★	★	★★★	★★★	★★★	NR	★★★	NR	★	NR	NR	NR	★★★	★★★	★	NR	NR	NR	NR
★	★★★	★★★★★	★★★	★★★	NR	★★★	NR	★★★	NR	NR	NR	★★★	★★★	★★★	NR	★★★	NR	NR
NR	NR	★★★★★	★★★★★	NR	NR	NR	★★★	★★★★★	NR	NR	NR	★★★	NR	NR	NR	NR	★★★★★	NR
★★★	★★★	★★★	★★★★★	★★★	NR	★★★	NR	★★★★★	NR	★★★★★	NR	★★★★★	★★★★★	★★★	★★★	★★★	NR	NR
★★★	★★★	★★★	★	★★★	NR	★★★	NR	★★★	NR	NR	NR	NR	★★★	★	NR	★	NR	NR
★★★	NR	NR	★	NR	NR	NR	NR	★★★	NR	NR	NR	NR	★★★	★★★	NR	NR	NR	NR
★★★	★★★	★★★	★★★	★★★	NR	NR	NR	★★★	NR	NR	NR	★★★	★★★	★★★	★★★	★★★	NR	NR
★★★	★	★★★	★★★	★	NR	NR	NR	★★★★★	NR	NR	NR	★★★	★★★	★★★	NR	★★★	★★★	NR
NR	NR	NR	★★★	NR	NR	NR	NR	★★★	NR	NR	NR	★★★	★★★	NR	NR	NR	NR	NR
★★★	★★★	★★★	★★★	★★★	NR	★★★	NR	★★★	★	NR	NR	★★★	★	★★★	★	★★★	NR	NR
★★★	NR	★★★	★★★	★★★	NR	NR	NR	★	★★★	NR	NR	★	★★★	★★★	★	★★★	NR	NR
★★★	★★★	★★★	★★★★★	★★★	NR	★★★	★★★	★★★★★	★★★	★★★	★★★	★★★	★★★	★★★★★	★★★	★★★	★★★	NR
★★★	★	★★★★★	★★★	★★★★★	NR	★★★	★★★	★★★	★★★	★★★	NR	★★★★★	★	★	★★★	★★★	★★★	NR
★★★★★	★★★	★★★★★	★★★★★	★★★	NR	★★★	★★★	★★★★★	★★★	★★★	NR	★★★★★	★★★	★★★★★	★	★	★★★★★	NR
★★★	NR	NR	★★★	NR	NR	NR	NR	★★★	NR	NR	NR	★	NR	NR	NR	NR	NR	NR
★★★	★★★	★★★★★	★★★	★★★	NR	★★★	★	★★★	★★★	NR	★★★	★★★	★★★	★★★	★★★★★	★★★	NR	NR
★★★	★★★	★★★	★★★	★★★	NR	NR	NR	★★★	★★★	NR	NR	★★★	★	★★★	★★★	NR	NR	NR
★★★	★	★★★	★★★	★★★	NR	★	NR	★★★	NR	★★★	NR	★★★	★★★	★★★	★	★	NR	NR
★★★	★★★	★★★★★	★★★★★	★★★★★	NR	★★★	★★★	★★★★★	★★★	NR	NR	★★★★★	★★★★★	★★★★★	NR	★★★	NR	NR
★★★	NR	NR	★	★★★	NR	NR	NR	★★★	NR	NR	NR	NR	NR	★★★	NR	★★★	NR	NR
★★★	★★★	★★★	★★★	★★★	NR	NR	NR	★	NR	NR	NR	NR	NR	★★★	★★★★★	★★★	NR	NR
★★★	NR	NR	★★★	NR	NR	NR	NR	★★★	NR	NR	NR	NR	★	★★★	NR	★★★	NR	NR
★★★	★★★★★	★★★	★★★★★	★★★	NR	★★★	★★★	★★★★★	★★★	★★★	NR	★★★★★	★★★★★	★★★★★	★★★	★	★★★	NR
★★★	★★★★★	★★★★★	★★★★★	★★★	NR	★★★	★	★★★★★	★★★	★★★	NR	★★★	★★★	★★★★★	★★★	★★★	NR	NR
★★★	★★★	★★★	★★★	★★★	NR	NR	NR	★★★	★★★	NR	NR	★★★★★	★★★★★	★★★★★	★★★★★	★★★★★	★★★	NR
★	★★★	★★★	★★★	★	NR	NR	NR	★★★	★★★	NR	NR	★★★	★	★★★	NR	★★★	NR	NR
★★★	★★★	★★★★★	★★★★★	★★★	NR	★★★	★★★	★★★★★	★	★★★	NR	★★★★★	★★★★★	★★★★★	★★★	★	NR	NR

	Appendectomy	Atrial Fibrillation	Back and Neck Surgery (except Spinal Fusion)	Back and Neck Surgery (Spinal Fusion)	Bariatric Surgery	Bowel Obstruction	Carotid Surgery	Cholecystectomy (Gall Bladder Removal)	Chronic Obstructive Pulmonary Disease (COPD)	Coronary Bypass Surgery	Coronary Interventional Procedures (Angioplasty/Stent)	Diabetic Acidosis and...
51. Grant Medical Center, Columbus	NR	★★★	★	★	NR	★★★	★★★	★	★★★	★★★	★★★	★★★
52. Greene Memorial Hospital, Xenia	NR	★★★	NR	NR	NR	★★★	NR	★★★	★★★	NR	NR	NR
53. Greenfield Area Medical Center, Greenfield	NR	NR	NR	NR	NR	NR	NR	NR	★★★	NR	NR	NR
54. H. B. Magruder Memorial Hospital, Port Clinton	NR	★★★	NR	NR	NR	★★★	NR	★★★	★★★	NR	NR	NR
55. Hardin Memorial Hospital, Kenton	NR	★★★	NR	NR	NR	★★★	NR	★	NR	NR	NR	NR
56. Harrison Community Hospital, Cadiz	NR	NR	NR	NR	NR	NR	NR	NR	★★★	NR	NR	NR
57. Henry County Hospital, Napoleon	NR	★★★	NR	NR	NR	★★★	NR	★	NR	NR	NR	NR
58. Highland District Hospital, Hillsboro	NR	★★★	NR	NR	NR	★★★	NR	★★★	★★★	NR	NR	NR
59. Hillcrest Hospital, Mayfield Heights	NR	★★★	★★★	★	NR	★★★	★	★	★★★	★★★★★	★★★	★★★
60. Hocking Valley Community Hospital, Logan	NR	NR	NR	NR	NR	★★★	NR	★★★	★★★	NR	NR	NR
61. Holzer Medical Center, Gallipolis	NR	★★★	NR	NR	NR	★★★	★★★	★★★	★★★★★	★★★	★★★	★★★
62. Hospital for Orthopaedic and Specialty Service, Amherst	NR	NR	NR	NR	NR	NR	NR	NR	★★★	NR	NR	NR
63. Huron Hospital, East Cleveland	NR	NR	NR	NR	NR	★★★★★	NR	NR	★★★★★	NR	NR	★★★
64. Jewish Hospital, Cincinnati	NR	★★★	★	NR	NR	★★★★★	★★★	★★★	★★★	★★★	★★★★★	★★★
65. Joel Pomerene Memorial Hospital, Millersburg	NR	★★★	NR	NR	NR	★★★	NR	★★★	★	NR	NR	NR
66. Joint Township District Memorial Hospital, St. Marys	NR	★★★	NR	NR	NR	★★★	NR	★★★	★★★	NR	NR	NR
67. Kettering Medical Center, Kettering	NR	★★★★★	★	★★★	NR	★★★	★★★	★★★	★★★	★★★	★★★	★★★
68. Kettering Medical Center–Sycamore, Miamisburg	NR	★★★	NR	NR	NR	★★★	NR	★★★	★★★	NR	★★★	★★★
69. Kettering-Mohican Area Medical Center, Loudonville	NR	★★★	NR	NR	NR	★★★	NR	★	★★★	NR	NR	NR
70. Knox Community Hospital, Mount Vernon	NR	★★★	NR	NR	NR	★★★	NR	★★★	★★★	NR	NR	NR
71. Lake Hospital System, Painesville	NR	★★★	★	★★★	NR	★★★	★★★	★	★★★★★	★★★★★	★★★★★	★★★
72. Lakewood Hospital, Lakewood	NR	★★★	★	NR	NR	★★★	★★★	★★★	★★★★★	★★★	★★★	★★★
73. Licking Memorial Hospital, Newark	NR	★★★	NR	NR	NR	★★★	★★★	★★★	★★★★★	NR	NR	★★★
74. Lima Memorial Health System, Lima	NR	★★★	★★★	NR	NR	★★★	★★★	★★★	★★★	★★★	★★★	★★★
75. Lutheran Hospital, Cleveland	NR	★★★	★★★	★	NR	★★★	NR	★★★	★★★	★★★	NR	NR
76. Madison County Hospital, London	NR	NR	NR	NR	NR	★★★	NR	NR	★★★	NR	NR	NR
77. Marietta Memorial Hospital, Marietta	NR	★★★★★	NR	★★★	NR	★★★	★★★	★★★★★	★★★	NR	NR	★★★
78. Marion General Hospital, Marion	NR	★★★	NR	NR	NR	★★★	★	★★★	★★★	NR	★★★	★★★
79. Mary Rutan Hospital, Bellefontaine	NR	★	NR	NR	NR	★★★	NR	★★★	★★★	NR	NR	NR
80. Marymount Hospital, Garfield Heights	NR	★★★★★	NR	NR	NR	★★★	★★★	★★★	★★★★★	NR	NR	★★★
81. Massillon Community Hospital, Massillon	NR	★★★	NR	NR	NR	★★★	NR	★★★	★★★	NR	NR	★★★
82. McCullough-Hyde Memorial Hospital, Oxford	NR	★★★	NR	NR	NR	★★★	NR	★	★★★	NR	NR	NR
83. Medcenter Hospital, Marion	NR	★★★	NR	NR	NR	★★★	★	★★★	★★★	NR	★★★	★★★
84. Medcentral Health System Shelby Hospital, Shelby	NR	NR	NR	NR	NR	NR	NR	NR	★★★	NR	NR	NR
85. Medcentral Health System, Mansfield	NR	★	★	★★★	NR	★★★	★★★	★★★	★★★	★★★★★	★★★	★★★
86. Medical College of Ohio at Toledo, Toledo	NR	★★★	★★★	★★★	NR	★	★★★	★★★	★★★	★★★	★★★	★★★
87. Medina General Hospital, Medina	NR	★★★	NR	NR	NR	★	NR	★★★	★★★	NR	NR	★★★
88. Memorial Hospital of Union County, Marysville	NR	★★★	NR	NR	NR	★★★	NR	★★★	★★★	NR	NR	NR
89. Memorial Hospital, Fremont	NR	★★★	NR	NR	NR	★★★	NR	★★★	★★★	NR	NR	NR
90. Mercer County Joint Township Community, Coldwater	NR	★★★	NR	NR	NR	★★★	NR	★★★	★★★	NR	NR	NR
91. Mercy Franciscan Hospital–Mount Airy, Cincinnati	NR	★★★	NR	★★★	NR	★★★	★★★	★★★	★★★	NR	NR	★★★
92. Mercy Healthcare Center, Toledo	NR	★★★★★	★★★	★★★	NR	★★★	★	★★★	★★★	★★★	★★★	★★★
93. Mercy Hospital–Anderson, Anderson	NR	★★★	★★★★★	★★★★★	NR	★★★	★	★★★★★	★★★	NR	★★★	★★★
94. Mercy Hospital–Clermont, Batavia	NR	★★★	NR	NR	NR	★★★★★	NR	★★★	★★★	NR	NR	NR
95. Mercy Hospital–Fairfield, Fairfield	NR	★★★	★★★	★★★	NR	★★★	★★★	★★★	★★★	★★★	★★★	★★★
96. Mercy Hospital–Tiffin Ohio, Tiffin	NR	★★★	NR	NR	NR	★★★	NR	★★★	★★★	NR	NR	NR
97. Mercy Hospital–Western Hills, Cincinnati	NR	★★★	★	NR	★★★	NR	★★★	★★★	★★★	★★★	NR	★★★
98. Mercy Hospital–Willard, Willard	NR	NR	NR	NR	NR	★★★	NR	NR	★★★	NR	NR	NR
99. Mercy Medical Center of Springfield, Springfield	NR	★★★	NR	NR	NR	★★★	★★★★★	★★★	★★★	NR	★★★	★★★
100. Mercy Medical Center, Canton	NR	★★★	★	★★★	NR	★★★	★★★	★★★	★★★	★★★	★★★	★★★

KEY: ★★★★★ BEST   ★★★ AS EXPECTED   ★ POOR   NR NOT RATED BY HEALTHGRADES   For full definitions of ratings and awards, see Appendix.

Gastrointestinal Bleed	Gastrointestinal Surgeries and Procedures	Heart Attack	Heart Failure	Hip Fracture Repair	Maternity Care	Pancreatitis	Peripheral Vascular Bypass	Pneumonia	Prostatectomy	Pulmonary Embolism	Resection/Replacement of Abdominal Aorta	Respiratory Failure	Sepsis	Stroke	Total Hip Replacement	Total Knee Replacement	Valve Replacement	Women's Health
★★★	★★★	★★★	★★★	★	NR	★★★	★★★	★★★	★★★	★★★	NR	★★★	★★★	★★★	★	★	★★★	NR
★★★★★	★★★	★★★	★★★	★★★	NR	★★★	NR	★★★	NR	★★★	NR	★★★	★★★	★★★★★	NR	★★★	NR	NR
NR	NR	NR	★★★	NR	NR	NR	NR	★★★	NR	NR	NR	NR	NR	NR	NR	NR	NR	NR
★★★	NR	★★★	★★★	★★★	NR	NR	NR	★★★	NR	NR	NR	NR	NR	★★★	NR	★★★	NR	NR
★★★	NR	★★★	★★★	★★★	NR	NR	NR	★★★	NR	NR	NR	★★★	★	NR	NR	NR	NR	NR
NR	NR	NR	★★★	NR	NR	NR	NR	★★★	NR	NR	NR	★★★	★★★	NR	NR	NR	NR	NR
★★★	NR	NR	★★★	NR	NR	NR	NR	★	NR	NR	NR	NR	NR	NR	NR	★★★	NR	NR
★★★	NR	NR	★★★	NR	NR	NR	NR	★	NR	NR	NR	★	★★★	NR	NR	NR	NR	NR
★★★	★★★★★	★★★★★	★★★★★	★★★★★	NR	★★★	★★★	★★★★★	★★★	★★★★★	★★★	★★★★★	★★★★★	★★★★★	★★★	★★★	★★★	NR
★★★	NR	★★★	★★★	★	NR	NR	NR	★★★	NR	NR	NR	★★★	NR	★★★★★	NR	★	NR	NR
★★★	★★★	★★★	★★★	NR	NR	★★★	NR	★★★	★★★	★★★	NR	★★★	★	NR	★★★	★★★	NR	NR
NR	NR	NR	★★★	NR	NR	NR	NR	NR	NR	NR	NR	NR	NR	★★★	★★★	NR	NR	NR
★★★★★	★★★★★	★★★	★★★★★	★★★★★	NR	★★★	★★★	★★★★★	★★★	★★★★★	NR	★★★★★	★★★★★	★★★	NR	★★★	NR	NR
★★★	★★★★★	★★★★★	★★★★★	★★★★★	NR	★★★	★★★	★★★★★	★★★	★★★★★	★★★	★★★★★	★★★★★	★★★★★	★	★	★★★	NR
★★★★★	★★★	★★★	★★★★★	★★★	NR	★★★	NR	★★★★★	★★★	★★★★★	NR	★★★	★★★★★	★★★	★★★	★★★★★	NR	NR
★★★★★	★★★	★★★	★★★★★	★★★	NR	★★★	NR	★★★★★	★★★	★★★★★	NR	★★★	★★★★★	★★★	★★★	★★★★★	NR	NR
★★★	★★★	★	★★★	★★★	NR	★★★	NR	★★★	★	NR	NR	★★★	★★★	★★★	★	★	NR	NR
★★★	★★★	★★★	★★★	★★★★★	NR	★★★	NR	★★★	★★★	NR	NR	★★★	★★★	★★★	★★★	★★★	NR	NR
★★★★★	★★★	★★★★★	★★★★★	★★★	NR	★★★	★★★	★★★★★	★	★★★	★★★	★★★	★★★★★	★★★★★	★	★★★	★★★★★	NR
★★★★★	★★★★★	★★★	★★★★★	★★★	NR	★★★	NR	★★★★★	★★★	★★★	NR	★★★★★	★★★★★	★★★★★	★★★	★★★	NR	NR
★★★	★★★	★★★	★★★★★	★★★	NR	★★★	NR	★★★★★	★★★	★★★	NR	★★★★★	★★★★★	★★★★★	★	★★★	NR	NR
★	★★★	★★★	★★★	★★★	NR	★★★	★★★	★★★	NR	★★★	★★★	★	★★★	★★★	★★★	★★★	★★★	NR
★★★	NR	★★★	★★★★★	★★★	NR	★★★	NR	★★★★★	★★★	NR	NR	★★★	★★★	★★★	★	★★★	NR	NR
★★★	NR	★★★	★★★	★	NR	NR	NR	★	NR	NR	NR	NR	★★★	NR	NR	NR	NR	NR
★★★	★★★	★★★	★★★	★★★	NR	★★★★★	NR	★★★	NR	★★★	NR	★★★	★	★★★	★★★	★★★★★	NR	NR
★★★	★	★★★	★★★	★★★	NR	★★★	NR	★★★	★★★	★★★	NR	★	★★★	★★★	★★★	★★★	NR	NR
★★★	NR	★★★	★★★	★★★	NR	NR	NR	★★★	NR	NR	NR	NR	★★★	★★★	★★★	★★★★★	NR	NR
★★★★★	★★★	★★★	★★★★★	★★★	NR	★★★	★	★★★★★	★★★	★★★	NR	★★★★★	★★★★★	★★★★★	★★★	★★★	NR	NR
★	★★★	★★★	★★★	★★★★★	NR	★★★	NR	★★★	NR	NR	NR	★★★	★★★	★★★	★★★★★	★★★★★	NR	NR
★★★	★★★	NR	★★★	★★★	NR	NR	NR	★★★	NR	NR	NR	★★★	★★★	★★★	★★★	NR	NR	NR
★★★	★	★★★	★★★	★★★	NR	★★★	NR	★★★	★★★	★★★	NR	★	★★★	★★★	★★★	★★★	NR	NR
NR	NR	NR	★★★	NR	NR	NR	NR	★★★	NR	NR	NR	NR	NR	NR	★★★	★★★★★	NR	NR
★★★	★★★	★★★	★★★	★★★	NR	★★★	NR	★★★	★★★	★	★★★	★★★	★	★★★	★★★	★★★	★★★★★	NR
★★★★★	★★★	★★★	★★★	★★★	NR	★★★	NR	★★★★★	★	★★★	★★★	★★★	★★★	★★★★★	★★★	★	NR	NR
★★★	★★★	★★★	★★★	★★★★★	NR	★★★	NR	★★★	★★★	★★★	NR	★★★★★	★★★	★★★★★	★★★	★★★	NR	NR
★★★	NR	NR	★★★	★★★	NR	NR	NR	★★★	NR	NR	NR	★★★	★★★	★★★	★	NR	NR	NR
★★★	★★★	NR	★★★	★★★★★	NR	NR	NR	★★★	NR	NR	NR	★★★	★★★	★★★	★	NR	NR	NR
★★★	NR	NR	★★★	★★★★★	NR	NR	NR	★★★	NR	NR	NR	NR	NR	★★★	★★★	NR	NR	NR
★★★	★★★	★★★	★★★★★	★★★	NR	★★★	NR	★★★	★	★★★	★★★	★★★★★	★★★★★	★★★★★	★	★★★	★★★	NR
★★★	★★★	★★★	★★★	★★★	NR	★★★	NR	★★★★★	★★★	★★★	★★★	★★★★★	★★★★★	★★★★★	★★★	★★★	★★★	NR
★★★	★★★	★★★	★★★	★	NR	★★★	NR	★★★★★	★	★★★	★★★	★★★	★★★	★★★	★★★	★★★	★★★	NR
★★★	NR	★★★	★★★	NR	NR	NR	NR	★★★★★	★	★★★	NR	★★★	★★★	★★★	★★★	★★★	NR	NR
★★★	★★★★★	★★★	★★★	NR	NR	★★★★★	NR	★★★★★	★★★	★★★	NR	★★★	★★★★★	★★★★★	★	★	NR	NR
NR	NR	NR	★★★	★★★	NR	NR	NR	★★★	NR	NR	NR	NR	NR	NR	NR	NR	NR	NR
★★★	★★★	★★★	★★★★★	★	NR	★★★	★★★	★★★	★★★	★★★	★★★	★★★	★★★	★★★	★	★★★	★★★	NR
★★★	★★★★★	★★★	★★★★★	★★★	NR	★★★	★★★	★★★★★	★★★	★★★	★★★	★★★★★	★★★	★★★★★	★★★	★★★	★★★	NR

	Appendectomy	Atrial Fibrillation	Back and Neck Surgery (except Spinal Fusion)	Back and Neck Surgery (Spinal Fusion)	Bariatric Surgery	Bowel Obstruction	Carotid Surgery	Cholecystectomy (Gall Bladder Removal)	Chronic Obstructive Pulmonary Disease (COPD)	Coronary Bypass Surgery	Coronary Interventional Procedures (Angioplasty/Stent)	Diabetic Acidosis and
101. Mercy Memorial Hospital, Urbana	NR	★★★	NR	NR	NR	★★★	NR	NR	★	NR	NR	NR
102. Meridia Euclid Hospital, Euclid	NR	★★★	★★★	★★★★★	NR	★★★	NR	★★★	★★★	NR	NR	★★★
103. MetroHealth Medical Center, Cleveland	NR	★	★	★★★	NR	★★★	★★★	★	★★★★★	★★★	★★★	★★★
104. Miami Valley Hospital, Dayton	NR	★★★★★	★★★★★	★★★	NR	★★★	★	★★★	★★★	★★★	★★★	★★★
105. Middletown Regional Hospital, Middletown	NR	★	★★★	★	NR	★★★	NR	★★★★★	★★★	NR	NR	★
106. Mount Carmel Health, Columbus	NR	★★★	★★★	★★★	NR	★★★	★★★	★★★	★★★	★★★	★★★	★★★
107. New Albany Surgical Hospital, New Albany	NR	NR	★★★★★	★★★★★	NR	NR	NR	NR	NR	NR	NR	NR
108. O. Bleness Memorial Hospital, Athens	NR	★★★	NR	NR	NR	★★★	NR	NR	★★★	NR	NR	NR
109. Ohio State University Hospital East, Columbus	NR	★★★	NR	★★★	NR	★★★	★★★	★★★	★★★★★	NR	★★★	★★★
110. Ohio State University Hospitals, Columbus	NR	★★★	★★★	★★★	NR	★★★	★★★	★★★	★★★	★★★	★	★★★
111. Parma Community General Hospital, Parma	NR	★★★★★	NR	NR	NR	★★★	★	★★★	★★★★★	★★★	★★★★★	★★★
112. Paulding County Hospital, Paulding	NR	NR	NR	NR	NR	NR	NR	NR	★★★	NR	NR	NR
113. Peoples Hospital, Mansfield	NR	★★★	NR	NR	NR	★★★	NR	★	★★★	NR	NR	NR
114. Pike Community Hospital, Waverly	NR	★★★	NR	NR	NR	NR	NR	NR	★★★	NR	NR	NR
115. Regency Hospital of Cincinnati, Cincinnati	NR	★★★	★★★	★★★	NR	★★★	NR	★★★	★★★★★	NR	★★★	★★★
116. Riverside Methodist Hospital, Columbus	NR	★★★	★	★	NR	★★★★★	★★★	★	★★★	★★★	★★★	★★★
117. Robinson Memorial Hospital, Ravenna	NR	★★★★★	NR	NR	NR	★★★	★★★★★	★★★	★★★	NR	NR	★★★
118. St. Anne Mercy Hospital, Toledo	NR	★★★	★★★	NR	NR	★★★	★★★	★★★★★	★★★	NR	NR	NR
119. St. Anns Hospital of Columbus, Westerville	NR	★★★	★★★	NR	NR	★★★	★★★	★★★	★★★	NR	NR	★★★
120. St. Charles Mercy Hospital, Oregon	NR	★★★	NR	NR	NR	★★★	★	★	★★★	NR	NR	★★★
121. St. Elizabeth Health Center, Youngstown	NR	★★★	★★★	★★★	NR	★★★★★	★★★	★★★	★★★	★★★★★	★★★	★★★
122. St. John Medical Center, Steubenville	NR	★★★	NR	NR	NR	★★★	★★★	★★★★★	★★★	★★★	★★★	★
123. St. John West Shore Hospital, Westlake	NR	★★★★★	★★★	NR	NR	★★★	★	★★★	★★★★★	★	★★★	★★★
124. St. Joseph Health Center, Warren	NR	★★★	NR	NR	NR	★★★	★★★	★★★	★★★	NR	NR	★★★
125. St. Luke's Hospital, Maumee	NR	★★★	★★★★★	★★★	NR	★★★	★★★	★★★	★	★★★	★★★	★★★
126. St. Rita's Medical Center, Lima	NR	★★★	★★★	★★★	NR	★★★	★	★★★	★★★	★★★	★★★	★
127. St. Vincent Charity Hospital, Cleveland	NR	★★★	★★★★★	★★★	NR	★★★★★	★★★	★★★	★★★	★★★	★★★	★★★
128. St. Vincent Mercy Medical Center, Toledo	NR	★★★★★	★★★	★★★	NR	★★★	★	★★★	★★★	★★★	★★★	★★★
129. Salem Community Hospital, Salem	NR	★★★	★	NR	NR	★★★	★★★	★★★	★★★	NR	NR	★
130. Samaritan Regional Health System, Ashland	NR	★★★	NR	NR	NR	★★★	NR	★	★★★	NR	NR	NR
131. Selby General Hospital, Marietta	NR	★★★	NR	NR	NR	NR	NR	NR	★★★	NR	NR	NR
132. South Pointe Hospital, Warrensville Heights	NR	★	NR	NR	NR	★★★	★★★	★★★	★	NR	NR	★★★
133. Southeastern Ohio Regional Medical Center, Cambridge	NR	★	NR	NR	NR	★★★	★	★★★	★★★	NR	NR	★★★
134. Southern Ohio Medical Center, Portsmouth	NR	★★★	NR	NR	NR	★★★	★★★	★★★	★★★★★	NR	NR	★★★
135. Southwest General Health Center, Middleburg Heights	NR	★★★	★★★	★★★★★	NR	★★★★★	★★★★★	★★★★★	★★★★★	★★★	★★★★★	★★★
136. Summa Health Systems Hospitals, Akron	NR	★	★★★	★	NR	★★★	★★★	★★★	★★★★★	★★★★★	★★★	★★★★★
137. Toledo Hospital, Toledo	NR	★★★	★	★★★	NR	★★★	★★★	★★★	★★★	★★★	★★★	★★★
138. Trinity Health System, Steubenville	NR	★★★	NR	NR	NR	★★★	★★★	★★★★★	★★★	★★★	★	
139. Trumbull Memorial Hospital, Warren	NR	★★★	★★★	NR	NR	★★★	★★★	★★★	★★★★★	★★★	★★★	★★★
140. Twin City Hospital, Dennison	NR	NR	NR	NR	NR	NR	NR	NR	★★★	NR	NR	NR
141. UHHS Bedford Medical Center, Bedford	NR	★★★	★	NR	NR	★★★	★★★	★★★	★★★	NR	NR	★★★
142. UHHS Brown Memorial Hospital, Conneaut	NR	★★★	NR	NR	NR	NR	NR	★	★★★	NR	NR	NR
143. UHHS Geauga Regional Hospital, Chardon	NR	★★★	NR	NR	NR	★★★	★★★	★★★	★★★★★	NR	NR	NR
144. UHHS Memorial Hospital of Geneva, Geneva	NR	★★★	NR	NR	NR	★★★	NR	NR	★★★	NR	NR	NR
145. UHHS Richmond Heights Hospital, Richmond Heights	NR	★★★	NR	NR	NR	★★★	NR	★★★	★★★★★	NR	NR	★★★
146. Union Hospital, Dover	NR	★	NR	NR	NR	★★★	★	★★★	★★★	NR	NR	★★★
147. University Hospital, Cincinnati	NR	★★★	★★★	★	NR	★★★	★★★	★★★	★★★★★	★★★	★★★	★★★
148. University Hospitals Case Medical Center, Cleveland	NR	★★★	★	★	NR	★★★	★★★	★★★	★★★★★	★★★	★★★	★★★
149. Upper Valley Medical Center, Piqua	NR	★★★	NR	NR	NR	★★★★★	★★★	★	★★★	NR	NR	★★★
150. Upper Valley Medical Center, Troy	NR	★★★	NR	NR	NR	★★★★★	★★★	★	★★★	NR	NR	★★★

KEY: ★★★★★ BEST   ★★★ AS EXPECTED   ★ POOR   NR NOT RATED BY HEALTHGRADES   For full definitions of ratings and awards, see Appendix.

Gastrointestinal Bleed	Gastrointestinal Surgeries and Procedures	Heart Attack	Heart Failure	Hip Fracture Repair	Maternity Care	Pancreatitis	Peripheral Vascular Bypass	Pneumonia	Prostatectomy	Pulmonary Embolism	Resection/Replacement of Abdominal Aorta	Respiratory Failure	Sepsis	Stroke	Total Hip Replacement	Total Knee Replacement	Valve Replacement	Women's Health
NR	NR	★★★★★	★★★	★★★	NR	NR	NR	★★★	NR	★★★	NR	★★★	★★★	★	NR	NR	NR	NR
★★★	★★★	★★★★★	★★★	★★★	NR	★★★	NR	★★★	★★★	★★★	NR	★★★★★	★★★★★	★★★★★	★★★	★★★★★	NR	NR
★★★	★	★★★	★★★	★	NR	NR	★★★	★★★	NR	★★★	NR	★	★★★	★	★★★	★★★	NR	NR
★★★★★	★★★	★★★★★	★★★★★	★★★	NR	★★★	★★★	★★★★★	★★★	★★★	★★★	★★★★★	★★★★★	★★★★★	★★★	★★★	★★★	NR
★★★	★★★	★★★	★	★★★★★	NR	★★★	★★★	★★★★★	★★★★★	NR	★★★	★★★	★★★	★★★★★	★★★★★	★★★★★	★★★	NR
NR	NR	NR	NR	NR	NR	NR	NR	NR	NR	NR	NR	NR	NR	NR	★★★★★	★★★★★	NR	NR
★★★	NR	★	★	★★★	NR	NR	NR	★★★	NR	NR	NR	NR	NR	NR	NR	NR	NR	NR
★★★	★★★	★★★★★	★★★★★	★★★	NR	★★★★★	★★★	★★★★★	NR	★★★	NR	★★★★★	★★★★★	★★★	★	★	NR	NR
★★★★★	★	★	★★★	★★★★★	NR	★★★	★★★	★★★★★	★★★★★	NR	★★★	★★★★★	★★★★★	★★★★★	★★★	NR	★	NR
★★★	★★★★★	★★★	★★★	★★★★★	NR	★★★	★★★	★★★★★	★★★	★★★	★★★	★★★★★	★★★★★	★★★★★	★★★★★	★★★★★	★★★★★	NR
NR	NR	NR	★	NR	NR	NR	NR	★★★	NR	NR	NR	NR	NR	NR	NR	NR	NR	NR
★★★	★★★	★	★★★	★★★	NR	NR	NR	★★★	★	NR	NR	NR	★★★	★	★	NR	★★★	NR
★★★	NR	NR	★★★	NR	NR	NR	NR	★	NR	NR	NR	NR	NR	NR	NR	NR	NR	NR
★★★	★★★	★★★	★★★★★	★★★	NR	★★★	★★★	★★★	NR	★★★★★	NR	★★★★★	★★★	★★★	★★★	★★★	NR	NR
★★★	★★★	★★★	★★★	★	NR	★★★	★★★	★★★	★★★	★	★★★	★	★★★★★	★★★	★	★	★★★	NR
★★★	★★★	★★★	★★★	★★★	NR	★★★	★★★	★★★★★	NR	★★★	NR	★★★	★★★★★	★★★	★★★★★	★	NR	NR
★★★	★★★★★	★★★	★★★	★★★	NR	★★★	NR	★★★	★★★★★	★★★	NR	★★★	★★★	★★★	★★★	★★★	NR	NR
★★★	★★★	★★★	★★★	★★★	NR	★★★	NR	★★★★★	NR	★★★★★	NR	★★★	★★★★★	★★★	★	★	★★★	NR
★★★	★★★	★★★	★★★★★	★★★	NR	★★★	★★★	★★★★★	★	★★★	★★★	★★★	★★★★★	★★★	★★★	★★★	★★★	NR
★★★	★★★	★★★	★★★★★	NR	NR	★★★	★★★	★★★★★	★	★★★	NR	★★★	★★★	★★★	★★★	★★★	NR	NR
★	NR	★★★	★★★★★	NR	NR	★★★	★★★	★★★★★	NR	★★★	★★★	★★★	★★★	★★★	NR	★	NR	NR
★	★★★★★	★★★	★★★	★★★	NR	★★★★★	NR	★★★	★★★	★★★	NR	★★★	★★★★★	★★★	★★★★★	★★★	NR	NR
★★★	★★★	★★★	★★★	★★★	NR	★★★	★	★★★	★★★	★★★	NR	★★★	★	★★★	★★★	★★★	NR	NR
★★★	★★★	★★★	★★★★★	★★★	NR	★★★	★★★	★★★★★	★★★	NR	NR	★★★	★★★★★	★★★★★	★★★	★★★	NR	NR
★★★	★★★	★★★	★★★	★★★	NR	NR	NR	★★★	★	★★★	NR	★	★★★	★★★	★	★	NR	NR
★★★	★★★	★	★★★	★★★	NR	★★★	NR	★★★	★	NR	NR	★★★	★★★	★★★	★	NR	NR	NR
★	★	NR	★★★	NR	NR	NR	NR	★★★	NR	NR	NR	NR	NR	NR	★★★	★★★	NR	NR
★★★★★	★★★	★★★★★	★★★★★	★★★	NR	★★★	★★★	★★★	★★★	★★★	NR	★★★★★	★★★★★	★★★★★	★★★	★★★	NR	NR
★★★	★★★	★★★	★★★	★★★	NR	★★★	NR	★★★★★	NR	★★★	NR	★★★	★★★★★	★★★	NR	★★★	NR	NR
★★★★★	★★★	★★★	★★★★★	★★★	NR	★★★	NR	★★★★★	★★★★★	★★★	NR	★★★★★	★★★★★	★★★	★★★	★	NR	NR
★★★★★	★★★★★	★★★★★	★★★★★	★★★★★	NR	★★★	★★★	★★★★★	★★★	★★★★★	★★★	★★★★★	★★★★★	★★★★★	★★★	★★★★★	★★★	NR
★★★★★	★★★	★★★★★	★★★★★	★★★★★	NR	★★★	★★★	★★★★★	★★★	★★★★★	★★★	★★★★★	★★★★★	★★★★★	★★★	★★★	★	NR
★★★	★★★	★★★★★	★★★★★	★★★	NR	★★★	★★★	★★★★★	★★★	★★★	★★★★★	★★★★★	★★★★★	★★★★★	★★★	★★★	NR	NR
★★★	★★★	★★★	★★★	★★★★★	NR	★★★	★★★	★	NR	NR	★★★	★	★★★	★★★	★★★	NR	NR	NR
★★★★★	★★★★★	★★★	★★★	★★★	NR	★★★	NR	★★★★★	NR	NR	★	★★★	★★★	★★★	NR	NR	NR	NR
NR	NR	NR	★★★	NR	NR	NR	NR	★★★	NR	NR	NR	NR	NR	NR	NR	NR	NR	NR
★★★	★★★	★★★★★	★★★★★	★★★★★	NR	★★★	★★★	★★★★★	★★★	★★★	NR	★★★★★	★★★★★	★★★	★★★	★★★	NR	NR
★★★	NR	NR	★★★	★★★	NR	★★★	NR	★★★	NR	NR	NR	★★★	★★★	★★★	★★★	NR	NR	NR
★★★	★★★	★★★	★★★	★★★	NR	★★★	★★★	★★★★★	★	NR	NR	★★★	★★★	★★★	★★★	NR	NR	NR
★★★	NR	NR	★★★★★	★★★	NR	★★★	NR	★★★	NR	NR	NR	★★★★★	★★★★★	NR	★★★	NR	NR	NR
★★★	★★★	★★★	★★★★★	★★★	NR	★★★	NR	★★★★★	NR	NR	NR	★★★	★★★★★	★★★	NR	★★★	NR	NR
★★★★★	★★★	★	★★★★★	★	NR	★★★	NR	★★★	NR	★	NR	★★★	★★★	★	NR	★★★	NR	NR
★★★	★★★	★★★	★★★	★★★★★	NR	★★★	★★★	★★★★★	★★★	★★★	NR	★★★	★★★	★★★★★	★★★★★	★	NR	NR
★★★	★★★	★★★★★	★★★	★★★	NR	★★★	NR	★★★★★	★	★	NR	★★★	★★★	★★★★★	★★★	★	NR	NR

	Appendectomy	Atrial Fibrillation	Back and Neck Surgery (except Spinal Fusion)	Back and Neck Surgery (Spinal Fusion)	Bariatric Surgery	Bowel Obstruction	Carotid Surgery	Cholecystectomy (Gall Bladder Removal)	Chronic Obstructive Pulmonary Disease (COPD)	Coronary Bypass Surgery	Coronary Interventional Procedures (Angioplasty/Stent)	Diabetic Acidosis and
151. Van Wert County Hospital, Van Wert	NR	★★★	NR	NR	NR	★★★	NR	NR	★★★	NR	NR	NR	
152. Wadsworth Rittman Hospital, Wadsworth	NR	★★★	NR	NR	NR	★★★	NR	★★★	★★★	NR	NR	NR	
153. Wayne Hospital, Greenville	NR	★★★	NR	NR	NR	★★★	NR	★★★	★★★	NR	NR	NR	
154. Western Reserve Care System, Youngstown	NR	★★★	★★★	★★★	NR	★★★	★	★★★	★★★	★★★	★★★	★★★	
155. Wilson Memorial Hospital, Sidney	NR	★★★	NR	NR	NR	★★★	NR	★★★	★★★	NR	NR	NR	
156. Wood County Hospital, Bowling Green	NR	★★★	NR	NR	NR	★★★	NR	★★★	★★★	NR	NR	NR	
157. Wooster Community Hospital, Wooster	NR	★★★	NR	NR	NR	★★★	★★★	★★★	★★★	NR	NR	NR	
158. Wyandot Memorial Hospital, Upper Sandusky	NR	NR	NR	NR	NR	★★★	NR	NR	★★★	NR	NR	NR	

KEY: ★★★★★ BEST   ★★★ AS EXPECTED   ★ POOR   NR NOT RATED BY HEALTHGRADES   For full definitions of ratings and awards, see Appendix.

Gastrointestinal Bleed	Gastrointestinal Surgeries and Procedures	Heart Attack	Heart Failure	Hip Fracture Repair	Maternity Care	Pancreatitis	Peripheral Vascular Bypass	Pneumonia	Prostatectomy	Pulmonary Embolism	Resection/Replacement of Abdominal Aorta	Respiratory Failure	Sepsis	Stroke	Total Hip Replacement	Total Knee Replacement	Valve Replacement	Women's Health
★★★	NR	★★★	★★★	★★★★★	NR	NR	NR	★	NR	NR	NR	NR	★★★	★★★	★★★	★★★	NR	NR
★★★	★★★	★★★	★★★	★★★	NR	NR	NR	★★★★★	★★★	NR	NR	NR	★★★	★★★	NR	★★★	NR	NR
★★★	★★★	★★★	★	★★★	NR	★★★	NR	★	NR	NR	NR	NR	★★★	★	NR	★★★	NR	NR
★★★★★	★★★	★★★	★★★★★	★★★★★	NR	★★★	★★★	★★★	NR	★★★	NR	★★★	★★★★★	★★★	★★★	★★★	★★★	NR
★★★	NR	★★★★★	★★★	★★★	NR	★★★	NR	★★★	NR	NR	NR	★★★	★★★	NR	★	★★★	NR	NR
★★★	NR	★★★	★★★	★★★★★	NR	NR	NR	★	NR	NR	NR	NR	★★★	★★★	★★★	★★★	NR	NR
★★★★★	★★★	★★★	★★★★★	★★★	NR	★★★	NR	★★★★★	★★★	★★★	NR	★★★★★	★★★★★	★★★	★★★	★★★	NR	NR
★★★	NR	NR	★★★	★★★	NR	NR	NR	★★★	NR	NR	NR	NR	★★★	NR	★★★	NR	NR	

OKLAHOMA HOSPITALS: RATINGS BY PROCEDURE

	Appendectomy	Atrial Fibrillation	Back and Neck Surgery (except Spinal Fusion)	Back and Neck Surgery (Spinal Fusion)	Bariatric Surgery	Bowel Obstruction	Carotid Surgery	Cholecystectomy (Gall Bladder Removal)	Chronic Obstructive Pulmonary Disease (COPD)	Coronary Bypass Surgery	Coronary Interventional Procedures (Angioplasty/Stent)	Diabetic Acidosis an...
1. American Transitional Hospital, Oklahoma City	NR	***	NR	NR	NR	*****	***	***	***	***	***	*****
2. American Transitional Hospital–Tulsa, Tulsa	NR	*	NR	NR	NR	***	***	*	***	***	***	***
3. Arbuckle Memorial Hospital, Sulphur	NR	NR	NR	NR	NR	***	NR	NR	***	NR	***	NR
4. Ardmore Adventist Hospital, Ardmore	NR	***	NR	NR	NR	***	*	*****	*	NR	***	***
5. Atoka Memorial Hospital, Atoka	NR	***	NR	NR	NR	NR	NR	NR	***	NR	NR	NR
6. Bone and Joint Hospital, Oklahoma City	NR	NR	NR	***	NR	NR	NR	NR	NR	NR	NR	NR
7. Bristow Medical Center, Bristow	NR	NR	NR	NR	NR	NR	NR	NR	***	NR	NR	NR
8. Carl Albert Indian Health Facility, Ada	NR	NR	NR	NR	NR	NR	NR	NR	***	NR	NR	NR
9. Carnegie Tri-County Municipal Hospital, Carnegie	NR	NR	NR	NR	NR	NR	NR	NR	***	NR	NR	NR
10. Choctaw Memorial Hospital, Hugo	NR	NR	NR	NR	NR	***	NR	NR	*	NR	NR	NR
11. Choctaw Nation Health Services Authority, Talihina	NR	NR	NR	NR	NR	NR	NR	NR	***	NR	NR	NR
12. Claremore Indian Hospital, Claremore	NR	NR	NR	NR	NR	NR	NR	NR	***	NR	NR	NR
13. Claremore Regional Hospital, Claremore	NR	***	NR	NR	NR	***	NR	***	***	NR	NR	NR
14. Comanche County Memorial Hospital, Lawton	NR	***	*****	*****	NR	***	*****	***	***	***	***	***
15. Community Hospital, Oklahoma City	NR	NR	***	***	NR	NR	NR	NR	NR	NR	NR	NR
16. Cordell Memorial Hospital, Cordell	NR	NR	NR	NR	NR	NR	NR	NR	*	NR	NR	NR
17. Craig General Hospital, Vinita	NR	***	NR	NR	NR	NR	NR	NR	*	NR	NR	NR
18. Creek Nation Community Hospital, Okemah	NR	NR	NR	NR	NR	NR	NR	NR	***	NR	NR	NR
19. Cushing Regional Hospital, Cushing	NR	***	NR	NR	NR	***	NR	NR	***	NR	NR	NR
20. Deaconess Hospital, Oklahoma City	NR	***	NR	NR	NR	*****	***	***	***	***	***	*****
21. Duncan Regional Hospital, Duncan	NR	***	NR	NR	NR	***	***	*****	***	NR	NR	NR
22. Eastern Oklahoma Medical Center, Poteau	NR	***	NR	NR	NR	***	NR	NR	***	NR	NR	NR
23. Edmond Medical Center, Edmond	NR	***	NR	NR	NR	***	NR	***	***	NR	***	NR
24. Elkview General Hospital, Hobart	NR	NR	NR	NR	NR	***	NR	NR	***	NR	NR	NR
25. Grady Memorial Hospital, Chickasha	NR	***	NR	NR	NR	***	NR	*****	***	NR	NR	NR
26. Great Plains Regional Medical Center, Elk City	NR	***	NR	NR	NR	*	NR	***	***	NR	NR	NR
27. Haskell County Hospital, Stigler	NR	NR	NR	NR	NR	NR	NR	NR	***	NR	NR	NR
28. Henryetta Medical Center, Henryetta	NR	NR	***	NR	NR	NR	NR	NR	***	NR	NR	NR
29. Hillcrest Medical Center, Tulsa	NR	***	*****	***	NR	***	*	***	***	***	***	***
30. Holdenville General Hospital, Holdenville	NR	NR	NR	NR	NR	NR	NR	NR	***	NR	NR	NR
31. Integris Baptist Medical Center, Oklahoma City	NR	***	***	***	NR	*	*****	***	***	***	*	***
32. Integris Baptist Regional Health Center, Miami	NR	***	NR	NR	NR	*	NR	***	***	NR	NR	NR
33. Integris Bass Baptist Health Center, Enid	NR	***	NR	NR	NR	***	***	***	***	*	*	NR
34. Integris Blackwell Regional Hospital, Blackwell	NR	NR	NR	NR	NR	***	NR	*	NR	NR	NR	NR
35. Integris Canadian Valley Regional Hospital, Yukon	NR	***	NR	NR	NR	*	NR	***	***	NR	NR	NR
36. Integris Clinton Regional Hospital, Clinton	NR	***	NR	NR	NR	***	NR	***	***	NR	NR	NR
37. Integris Grove General Hospital, Grove	NR	***	NR	NR	NR	*	NR	***	*	NR	***	NR
38. Integris Marshall County Medical Center, Madill	NR	***	NR	NR	NR	*	NR	NR	***	NR	NR	NR
39. Integris Mayes County Medical Center, Pryor	NR	NR	NR	NR	NR	***	NR	NR	***	NR	NR	NR
40. Integris Southwest Medical Center, Oklahoma City	NR	*****	NR	***	NR	***	***	*****	*****	*	***	***
41. Jackson County Memorial Hospital, Altus	NR	***	NR	NR	NR	*	***	***	***	NR	NR	***
42. Jane Phillips Medical Center, Bartlesville	NR	***	NR	NR	NR	***	*	***	***	NR	***	NR
43. Johnston Memorial Hospital, Tishomingo	NR	NR	NR	NR	NR	NR	NR	NR	***	NR	NR	NR
44. Kingfisher Regional Hospital, Kingfisher	NR	***	NR	NR	NR	NR	NR	NR	*	NR	NR	NR
45. Latimer County General Hospital, Wilburton	NR	NR	NR	NR	NR	NR	NR	NR	***	NR	NR	NR
46. Logan Medical Center, Guthrie	NR	NR	NR	NR	NR	***	NR	NR	***	NR	NR	NR
47. McAlester Regional Health Center, McAlester	NR	***	NR	NR	NR	*	NR	***	***	NR	NR	***
48. McBride Clinic Orthopedic Hospital, Oklahoma City	NR	NR	*****	NR	NR	NR	NR	NR	NR	NR	NR	NR
49. McCurtain Memorial Hospital, Idabel	NR	***	NR	NR	NR	*	NR	NR	***	NR	NR	NR
50. Medical Center of Southeastern Oklahoma, Durant	NR	***	NR	NR	NR	***	***	*****	***	NR	NR	***

KEY: ***** BEST *** AS EXPECTED * POOR NR NOT RATED BY HEALTHGRADES For full definitions of ratings and awards, see Appendix.

Gastrointestinal Bleed	Gastrointestinal Surgeries and Procedures	Heart Attack	Heart Failure	Hip Fracture Repair	Maternity Care	Pancreatitis	Peripheral Vascular Bypass	Pneumonia	Prostatectomy	Pulmonary Embolism	Resection/Replacement of Abdominal Aorta	Respiratory Failure	Sepsis	Stroke	Total Hip Replacement	Total Knee Replacement	Valve Replacement	Women's Health
★★★	★★★	★★★	★★★	★★★★★	NR	★★★	NR	★★★	★★★	★★★	NR	★★★	★★★	★★★	★★★	★★★★★	★★★	NR
★★★	★★★	★	★★★	★★★	NR	NR	★★★★★	★★★★★	NR	NR	NR	★★★	★★★	★	NR	★	NR	NR
★★★	NR	NR	★	NR	NR	NR	NR	★	NR	NR	NR	NR	NR	NR	NR	NR	NR	NR
★	★★★	★	★★★	★★★★★	NR	★★★	NR	★	★★★★★	NR	NR	★	★	★★★	★★★	★	NR	NR
NR	NR	NR	★	NR	NR	NR	NR	★★★	NR	NR	NR	NR	NR	NR	NR	NR	NR	NR
NR	NR	NR	NR	★★★	NR	NR	NR	NR	NR	NR	NR	NR	NR	NR	★★★★★	★★★★★	NR	NR
NR	NR	NR	★★★	NR	NR	NR	NR	★★★	NR	NR	NR	NR	NR	NR	NR	NR	NR	NR
NR	NR	NR	★★★	NR	NR	NR	NR	★	NR	NR	NR	NR	NR	NR	NR	NR	NR	NR
NR	NR	NR	★	NR	NR	NR	NR	★	NR	NR	NR	NR	NR	NR	NR	NR	NR	NR
★★★	NR	NR	★	NR	NR	NR	NR	★	NR	NR	NR	★★★	NR	NR	NR	NR	NR	NR
NR	NR	NR	★★★	NR	NR	NR	NR	★★★	NR	NR	NR	NR	NR	NR	NR	NR	NR	NR
NR	NR	NR	★★★	NR	NR	NR	NR	★★★	NR	NR	NR	NR	NR	NR	NR	NR	NR	NR
★★★	NR	★★★	★	★★★	NR	★★★	NR	★★★	★★★	NR	NR	★★★	★★★	NR	★	NR	NR	NR
★	★★★	★	★★★	★★★	NR	★★★	NR	★★★	★★★	★★★	★★★	★★★	★	★★★	★★★	★★★	★	NR
NR	NR	NR	NR	NR	NR	NR	NR	NR	NR	NR	NR	NR	NR	NR	NR	NR	★★★	NR
NR	NR	NR	★★★	NR	NR	NR	NR	★★★	NR	NR	NR	NR	NR	NR	NR	NR	NR	NR
★★★	NR	NR	★★★	NR	NR	NR	NR	★★★	NR	NR	NR	NR	★	NR	NR	NR	NR	NR
NR	NR	NR	NR	NR	NR	NR	NR	★★★	NR	NR	NR	NR	NR	NR	NR	NR	NR	NR
★★★	NR	NR	★★★	★★★	NR	★	NR	★★★	NR	NR	NR	★	NR	★★★	★★★	★	NR	NR
★★★	★★★	★★★	★★★	★★★★★	NR	★★★	NR	★★★	★★★	★★★	NR	★★★	★★★	★★★	★★★	★★★★★	★★★	NR
★★★	★★★	★★★	★★★	★★★★★	NR	★★★	NR	★★★	★★★	★★★	NR	★★★	★★★★★	★★★	★★★	★★★★★	★★★	NR
★	NR	★★★	★★★	NR	NR	NR	NR	★	NR	NR	NR	★	★	★	NR	NR	NR	NR
★★★	★★★	★★★	★★★	★★★	NR	★★★	NR	★★★	★★★	★★★	NR	★★★	★★★	★★★	★★★	NR	★★★	NR
★★★	NR	★★★	★★★	NR	NR	NR	NR	★★★	NR	NR	NR	★	★	★★★	NR	NR	NR	NR
★★★	★★★	NR	★★★	★★★★★	NR	★★★	NR	★★★	NR	NR	NR	★★★	★★★	NR	NR	★★★	NR	NR
★★★	NR	★★★	★★★	★	NR	NR	NR	★★★★★	★★★	NR	NR	★★★	★★★★★	★★★	★★★	★	NR	NR
NR	NR	★★★	★	NR	NR	NR	NR	★	NR	NR	NR	NR	★	NR	★★★	NR	NR	NR
★★★	NR	NR	★★★	★★★	NR	NR	NR	★	NR	NR	NR	★★★	NR	NR	NR	NR	NR	NR
★★★	★★★	★★★	★★★	★★★	NR	★★★	★★★	★★★	★★★	★★★	NR	★	★★★	★★★	★★★	★★★	★★★	NR
★★★	NR	NR	★	NR	NR	NR	NR	★	NR	NR	NR	NR	★★★	NR	NR	NR	NR	NR
★★★	★★★	★★★	★★★★★	★★★★★	NR	★★★	★★★	★★★	★★★★★	★★★	★★★	★★★	★★★	★★★	★★★	★★★★★	★★★	NR
★★★	NR	★★★★★	★★★	★★★	NR	NR	NR	★★★	NR	NR	NR	★★★	★★★	★★★	NR	★★★	NR	NR
★	★★★	★★★	★★★	★★★	NR	NR	NR	★★★	★★★	NR	NR	★★★	★★★	★★★	NR	★★★	★★★	NR
★★★	NR	NR	★★★	NR	NR	NR	NR	★	NR	NR	NR	★★★	★★★	NR	NR	NR	NR	NR
★★★	NR	NR	★★★★★	★★★★★	NR	NR	NR	★★★	NR	NR	NR	★★★	★★★	★★★	NR	NR	NR	NR
★★★	NR	NR	★★★	NR	NR	NR	NR	★★★	NR	NR	NR	★★★	★★★	★★★	NR	NR	NR	NR
★★★	NR	★★★	★★★	★★★	NR	★★★	NR	★	NR	NR	NR	★	★★★	★★★	★★★	NR	NR	NR
★★★	NR	NR	★	NR	NR	NR	NR	★★★	NR	NR	NR	NR	NR	NR	NR	NR	NR	NR
★★★	NR	NR	NR	NR	NR	NR	NR	★★★	NR	NR	NR	★★★	★★★	NR	NR	NR	NR	NR
★★★	★★★	★★★	★★★	★★★★★	NR	★★★	NR	★	★★★	★	NR	★	★	★★★	★★★	★★★	NR	NR
★★★	★★★	★	★★★	★	NR	NR	NR	★★★	★	NR	NR	★	★	★★★	★	★	★★★	NR
★★★	★★★	★	NR	★★★	NR	★★★	NR	★★★	★★★	★★★	NR	★	★★★	★★★	★★★	★	NR	NR
NR	NR	NR	★★★	NR	NR	NR	NR	★★★	NR	NR	NR	NR	NR	NR	NR	NR	NR	NR
★★★	NR	★	★	NR	NR	NR	NR	★	NR	NR	NR	NR	NR	NR	NR	NR	NR	NR
★★★	NR	NR	★	NR	NR	NR	NR	★★★	NR	NR	NR	NR	NR	NR	NR	NR	NR	NR
★★★	NR	★★★	★★★	NR	NR	NR	NR	★★★	NR	NR	NR	NR	★★★	NR	NR	NR	NR	NR
★★★	★	NR	★	★★★	NR	★★★	NR	★	★	NR	NR	★★★	★★★	NR	★★★★★	★★★	NR	NR
NR	NR	NR	NR	★★★★★	NR	NR	NR	NR	NR	NR	NR	NR	★★★	NR	★★★	★★★★★	NR	NR
★★★	NR	★★★	★★★	NR	NR	NR	NR	★	NR	NR	NR	★★★	★★★	NR	NR	NR	NR	NR
★★★	★	★★★	★★★	★★★	NR	NR	NR	★★★	NR	NR	NR	★	★	NR	NR	NR	NR	NR

	Appendectomy	Atrial Fibrillation	Back and Neck Surgery (except Spinal Fusion)	Back and Neck Surgery (Spinal Fusion)	Bariatric Surgery	Bowel Obstruction	Carotid Surgery	Cholecystectomy (Gall Bladder Removal)	Chronic Obstructive Pulmonary Disease (COPD)	Coronary Bypass Surgery	Coronary Interventional Procedures (Angioplasty/Stent)	Diabetic Acidosis
51. Memorial Hospital and Physician Group, Frederick	NR	NR	NR	NR	NR	NR	NR	NR	★★★	NR	NR	NR
52. Memorial Hospital of Stilwell, Stilwell	NR	NR	NR	NR	NR	NR	NR	NR	★★★	NR	NR	NR
53. Memorial Hospital of Texas County, Guymon	NR	NR	NR	NR	NR	NR	NR	NR	★★★	NR	NR	NR
54. Mercy Health Center, Oklahoma City	NR	★	★★★	★★★	NR	★★★	★★★	★	★★★	NR	NR	★★★
55. Mercy Memorial Health Center, Ardmore	NR	★★★	NR	NR	NR	★★★	★	★★★★★	★	NR	★★★	★★★
56. Midwest Regional Medical Center, Midwest City	NR	★★★	★★★★★	★★★	NR	★★★	★★★	★★★★★	★★★	★★★	★★★	★
57. Mission Hill Memorial Hospital, Shawnee	NR	★★★	NR	NR	NR	★★★	NR	★★★	★★★	NR	★★★	★★★
58. Muskogee Regional Medical Center, Muskogee	NR	★★★	★★★	NR	NR	★★★	NR	★★★	★★★	NR	NR	★★★
59. Newman Memorial Hospital, Shattuck	NR	NR	NR	NR	NR	★★★	NR	★★★	★★★	NR	NR	NR
60. Norman Regional Hospital, Norman	NR	★	★	★★★	NR	★	★★★	★★★	★★★	★	★	★★★
61. Oklahoma Heart Hospital, Oklahoma City	NR	★★★	NR	NR	NR	NR	★★★★★	NR	★★★	★	★★★	NR
62. Oklahoma Surgical Hospital, Tulsa	NR	NR	★★★	NR	NR	NR	NR	NR	NR	NR	NR	NR
63. Oklahoma University Medical Center, Oklahoma City	NR	★★★	★★★	★★★★★	NR	★★★	★★★	NR	★★★	★	★★★	★★★
64. Okmulgee Memorial Hospital, Okmulgee	NR	NR	NR	NR	NR	NR	NR	NR	★★★	NR	NR	NR
65. Parkview Hospital, El Reno	NR	NR	NR	NR	NR	★	NR	★★★★★	★★★	NR	NR	NR
66. Pauls Valley General Hospital, Pauls Valley	NR	★★★	NR	NR	NR	★★★	NR	★★★	★★★	NR	NR	NR
67. Pawnee Municipal Hospital, Pawnee	NR	NR	NR	NR	NR	NR	NR	NR	★★★	NR	NR	NR
68. Perry Memorial Hospital, Perry	NR	NR	NR	NR	NR	NR	NR	NR	★★★	NR	NR	NR
69. Physicians' Hospital in Anadarko, Anadarko	NR	NR	NR	NR	NR	NR	NR	NR	★★★	NR	NR	NR
70. Ponca City Medical Center, Ponca City	NR	★	NR	NR	★★★	NR	★★★	★★★	★★★	NR	NR	★★★
71. Purcell Municipal Hospital, Purcell	NR	★★★	NR	NR	NR	★★★	NR	★★★	★★★	NR	NR	NR
72. Pushmataha County–Town of Antlers Hospital Authority, Antlers	NR	★	NR	NR	NR	★★★	NR	★★★	★★★	NR	NR	NR
73. St. Anthony Hospital, Oklahoma City	NR	★★★	NR	★★★	NR	★★★	★★★★★	★★★	★★★	★★★	★	★★★
74. St. Francis Hospital, Tulsa	NR	★★★	★★★	★★★	NR	★★★	★★★	★★★	★★★	★	★★★	★★★
75. St. Francis Hospital–Broken Arrow, Broken Arrow	NR	NR	NR	NR	NR	★★★	NR	★★★	★★★	NR	NR	NR
76. St. John Medical Center, Tulsa	NR	★★★	★	★	NR	★★★	★★★	★★★	★★★	★★★	★★★	★★★
77. St. Mary's Regional Medical Center, Enid	NR	★★★	★	★★★	NR	★★★	★★★	★★★	★★★	★	★★★	NR
78. St. Michael Hospital, Oklahoma City	NR	★★★	NR	★★★	NR	★★★	★★★★★	★★★	★★★	★★★	★	★★★
79. Seminole Medical Center, Seminole	NR	NR	NR	NR	NR	★★★	NR	★★★	★★★	NR	NR	NR
80. Sequoyah Memorial Hospital, Sallisaw	NR	NR	NR	NR	NR	NR	NR	★	NR	NR	NR	NR
81. Share Memorial Hospital, Alva	NR	NR	NR	NR	NR	NR	NR	★	NR	NR	NR	NR
82. SouthCrest Hospital, Tulsa	NR	★★★	★★★	★	NR	★★★	★★★	★★★★★	★★★	★★★	★★★	★★★
83. Southwestern Medical Center, Lawton	NR	★★★	★★★	★	NR	★★★	NR	★★★	★★★	NR	NR	★★★
84. Southwestern Memorial Hospital, Weatherford	NR	NR	NR	NR	NR	★★★	NR	NR	NR	NR	NR	NR
85. Stillwater Medical Center, Stillwater	NR	★★★	NR	NR	NR	★★★	NR	★	★★★	NR	NR	NR
86. Stroud Regional Medical Center, Stroud	NR	NR	NR	NR	NR	NR	NR	NR	★★★	NR	NR	NR
87. Tahlequah City Hospital, Tahlequah	NR	★★★	NR	NR	NR	★	★★★	★★★	★★★	NR	★★★	NR
88. TCA of Central Oklahoma, Oklahoma City	NR	★★★★★	NR	★★★	NR	★★★	★★★	★★★★★	★★★★★	★	★★★	★★★
89. Tulsa Regional Medical Center, Tulsa	NR	★	NR	NR	NR	★★★	★★★	★	★★★	★★★	★★★	★★★
90. Unity Health Center, Shawnee	NR	★★★	NR	NR	NR	★★★	NR	★★★	★★★	NR	NR	NR
91. Valley View Regional Hospital, Ada	NR	★★★	NR	NR	NR	★★★	NR	★★★	★	NR	NR	★★★
92. W. W. Hastings Indian Hospital, Tahlequah	NR	★★★	NR	NR	NR	NR	NR	NR	★★★	NR	NR	NR
93. Wagoner Community Hospital, Wagoner	NR	NR	NR	NR	NR	NR	NR	NR	★★★	NR	NR	NR
94. Watonga Municipal Hospital, Watonga	NR	NR	NR	NR	NR	NR	NR	NR	★★★	NR	NR	NR
95. Woodward Regional Hospital, Woodward	NR	★	NR	NR	NR	★	NR	★	★★★	NR	NR	NR

KEY: ★★★★★ BEST   ★★★ AS EXPECTED   ★ POOR   NR NOT RATED BY HEALTHGRADES   For full definitions of ratings and awards, see Appendix.

Gastrointestinal Bleed	Gastrointestinal Surgeries and Procedures	Heart Attack	Heart Failure	Hip Fracture Repair	Maternity Care	Pancreatitis	Peripheral Vascular Bypass	Pneumonia	Prostatectomy	Pulmonary Embolism	Resection/Replacement of Abdominal Aorta	Respiratory Failure	Sepsis	Stroke	Total Hip Replacement	Total Knee Replacement	Valve Replacement	Women's Health
NR	NR	NR	★★★	NR	NR	NR	NR	★★★	NR	NR	NR	NR	★★★	★★★	NR	NR	NR	NR
NR	NR	NR	★★★	NR	NR	NR	NR	★	NR	NR	NR	NR	★★★	NR	NR	NR	NR	NR
★★★	NR	NR	★★★	NR	NR	NR	NR	★★★	NR	NR	NR	NR	NR	NR	NR	NR	NR	NR
★★★	★★★	★★★	★	★★★	NR	★★★	NR	★	★★★	★	NR	★★★	★★★	★	★★★★★	★★★	NR	NR
★	★★★	★	★★★	★★★★★	NR	★★★	NR	★	★★★★★	NR	NR	★	★	★★★	★★★	★	NR	NR
★★★	★★★	★★★	★★★	★★★★★	NR	★★★	★★★	★★★	★★★	★★★	NR	★★★	★★★	★★★	★★★	★★★	★★★	NR
★	★	★★★	★★★	★★★	NR	★★★	NR	★★★	NR	★★★	NR	★	★	★★★	★★★	★★★	★★★	NR
★★★	★★★	★★★	★★★	★	NR	★★★	NR	★★★	★★★	★★★	NR	★★★	★★★	★★★	★	★	NR	NR
★★★	NR	NR	★★★	NR	NR	NR	NR	★★★	NR	NR	NR	NR	NR	NR	NR	NR	NR	NR
★★★	★	★	★	★★★★★	NR	★★★	★★★	★	★★★★★	★★★	NR	★	★	★	★★★	★★★	★★★	NR
NR	NR	★★★	★★★	NR	NR	NR	★★★	★★★	NR	★★★	★★★	★	NR	★★★	NR	NR	★★★	NR
NR	NR	NR	NR	NR	NR	NR	NR	NR	NR	NR	NR	NR	NR	NR	★★★★★	★★★★★	NR	NR
★	★	★★★	★★★	★★★	NR	★★★	NR	★★★	★★★	NR	NR	★	★	★	NR	★★★	★★★	NR
★★★	NR	NR	★★★	★★★	NR	NR	NR	★	NR	★★★	NR	NR	NR	NR	NR	NR	NR	NR
★★★	★★★	★★★	★★★	NR	NR	★★★	NR	★★★	NR	NR	NR	NR	★★★	★★★	NR	NR	NR	NR
★★★	NR	★★★	★★★	NR	NR	NR	NR	★★★	NR	NR	NR	NR	★★★	★★★	NR	NR	NR	NR
★★★	NR	★★★	★★★	NR	NR	NR	NR	★★★	NR	NR	NR	NR	★★★	★★★	NR	NR	NR	NR
NR	NR	NR	★★★	NR	NR	NR	NR	★	NR	NR	NR	NR	NR	NR	NR	NR	NR	NR
★	★★★	★★★	★★★	★★★	NR	NR	NR	★★★	★	NR	★★★	★	★★★	★★★	NR	★	NR	NR
★	NR	NR	★★★	NR	NR	NR	NR	★★★	NR	NR	NR	NR	★★★	★	NR	NR	NR	NR
★★★	NR	NR	★	NR	NR	NR	NR	★	NR	NR	NR	NR	NR	★★★	NR	NR	NR	NR
★★★	★★★	★	★★★	★	NR	★★★	★★★	★★★	★★★	★★★	NR	★	★★★	★★★	NR	★	★★★	NR
★★★	★★★	★	★★★★★	★★★	NR	★	NR	★★★	NR	★	★★★★★	★★★	★★★	★★★	★★★	★★★	★	NR
★★★	NR	NR	★★★	★★★	NR	NR	NR	★★★	NR	NR	NR	★★★★★	★★★	★★★	★★★	★	NR	NR
★★★	★★★	★	★★★	★★★	NR	★	★★★	★	★★★	★★★	★★★	★	★	★★★	★★★★★	★★★	★★★	NR
★	★★★	★★★	★★★	★★★	NR	★★★	NR	★★★	★★★	NR	★★★	★★★	★★★	★★★	★★★	NR	NR	NR
★★★	★★★	★	★★★	★	NR	★★★	★★★	★★★	★★★	★★★	NR	★	★★★	★★★	NR	★	★★★	NR
★★★	NR	NR	★	NR	NR	NR	NR	★	NR	NR	NR	NR	NR	NR	NR	NR	NR	NR
NR	NR	NR	★	NR	NR	NR	NR	★	NR	NR	NR	NR	NR	★	NR	NR	NR	NR
★★★	NR	NR	★★★	NR	NR	NR	NR	★	NR	NR	NR	NR	NR	NR	NR	NR	NR	NR
★★★	★★★	★★★	★★★	★★★	NR	NR	NR	★★★	★★★	NR	NR	★★★	★★★	★★★	NR	NR	★★★	NR
★	★★★	★	★★★	★★★	NR	NR	NR	★★★	★★★	NR	NR	★	★★★	NR	NR	★★★	NR	NR
★★★	NR	NR	★★★	NR	NR	NR	NR	★	NR	NR	NR	NR	NR	NR	NR	NR	NR	NR
★★★	★★★	★★★	★	★★★★★	NR	NR	NR	★★★	★★★	NR	★★★	★★★	★★★	★	NR	★★★	NR	NR
NR	NR	NR	★★★	NR	NR	NR	NR	★★★	NR	NR	NR	NR	NR	NR	NR	NR	NR	NR
★★★	★★★	★★★	★★★	★★★	NR	NR	NR	★	NR	NR	NR	★★★	★★★	NR	★★★	NR	NR	NR
★★★	★★★	★★★	★★★	★★★★★	NR	★★★	NR	★	★★★	★	NR	★	★	★★★	★★★	★★★	NR	NR
★★★	★★★	★	★★★	★★★	NR	NR	★★★★★	★★★★★	NR	NR	★★★	★★★	★	NR	★	NR	NR	NR
★	★	★★★	★★★	★★★	NR	★★★	NR	★★★	NR	NR	★	★★★	★★★	★★★	NR	NR	NR	NR
★	★	★★★	★★★	★★★★★	NR	★★★	NR	★★★	★★★	NR	★	★	★★★	NR	★★★	NR	NR	NR
NR	NR	NR	★★★	NR	NR	NR	NR	★	NR	NR	NR	NR	NR	NR	NR	NR	NR	NR
★★★	NR	NR	★★★	NR	NR	NR	NR	★★★	NR	NR	NR	NR	NR	NR	NR	NR	NR	NR
NR	NR	NR	★★★	NR	NR	NR	NR	★	NR	NR	NR	NR	NR	NR	NR	NR	NR	NR
★	★	NR	★★★	★	NR	NR	NR	★★★★★	★	NR	NR	NR	★★★	★★★	NR	★	NR	NR

Hospital	Appendectomy	Atrial Fibrillation	Back and Neck Surgery (except Spinal Fusion)	Back and Neck Surgery (Spinal Fusion)	Bariatric Surgery	Bowel Obstruction	Carotid Surgery	Cholecystectomy (Gall Bladder Removal)	Chronic Obstructive Pulmonary Disease (COPD)	Coronary Bypass Surgery	Coronary Interventional Procedures (Angioplasty/Ste...	Diabetic Acidosi...
1. Adventist Medical Center, Portland	***	***	***	*****	***	***	***	***	***	NR	***	NR
2. Ashland Community Hospital, Ashland	***	*	***	***	NR	***	NR	NR	***	NR	NR	NR
3. Bay Area Hospital, Coos Bay	***	***	***	*****	***	*	***	*****	*	NR	*	
4. Blue Mountain Hospital District, John Day	NR	NR	NR	NR	NR	NR	NR	NR	***	NR	NR	NR
5. Columbia Memorial Hospital, Astoria	***	***	NR	NR	NR	***	NR	***	***	NR	NR	NR
6. Coquille Valley Hospital, Coquille	NR	NR	NR	NR	NR	NR	NR	NR	NR	NR	NR	
7. Good Samaritan Regional Medical Center, Corvallis	*****	***	***	***	***	***	*****	*****	***	***	***	
8. Good Shepherd Medical Center, Hermiston	NR	NR	NR	NR	NR	*	NR	NR	***	NR	NR	
9. Grande Ronde Hospital, La Grande	***	***	NR	NR	NR	***	NR	***	***	NR	NR	
10. Holy Rosary Medical Center, Ontario	*	***	NR	NR	NR	***	NR	*	*****	NR	NR	
11. Kaiser Sunnyside Medical Center, Clackamas	*	NR	NR	*	NR	NR	NR	NR	NR	NR	NR	
12. Legacy Emanuel Hospital, Portland	***	***	***	***	NR	***	***	***	***	***	***	
13. Legacy Good Samaritan Hospital, Portland	***	***	*****	NR	***	***	*	***	*****	*	***	***
14. Legacy Meridian Park Hospital, Tualatin	*****	***	***	***	NR	***	***	***	***	NR	***	NR
15. Legacy Mount Hood Medical Center, Gresham	*****	*	***	NR	NR	***	NR	***	***	NR	NR	
16. McKenzie-Willamette Medical Center, Springfield	***	***	***	***	NR	***	*	***	***	NR	NR	***
17. Mercy Medical Center, Roseburg	*****	***	*****	***	NR	***	***	***	***	NR	NR	***
18. Merle West Medical Center, Klamath Falls	*****	***	***	***	***	***	***	***	***	***	***	NR
19. Mid-Columbia Medical Center, The Dalles	***	***	NR	NR	NR	***	***	*****	***	NR	NR	
20. OHSU Hospital, Portland	*	***	*	*	*	***	*****	***	***	*	***	NR
21. Pioneer Memorial Hospital, Prineville	NR	***	NR	NR	NR	***	NR	NR	***	NR	NR	
22. Providence Hood River Memorial Hospital, Hood River	***	***	NR	NR	NR	***	NR	***	***	NR	NR	
23. Providence Medford Medical Center, Medford	*	***	***	*****	NR	***	***	***	***	NR	***	
24. Providence Milwaukie Hospital, Milwaukie	*	***	NR	NR	NR	***	NR	***	***	NR	NR	
25. Providence Newberg Hospital, Newberg	***	NR	NR	NR	NR	NR	NR	NR	***	NR	NR	
26. Providence Portland Medical Center, Portland	*****	***	***	*****	NR	***	***	*	***	***	***	***
27. Providence St. Vincent Medical Center, Portland	***	***	*****	***	NR	***	*****	***	***	***	***	***
28. Providence Seaside Hospital, Seaside	*****	***	NR	NR	NR	NR	NR	***	***	NR	NR	
29. Rogue Valley Medical Center, Medford	***	***	*****	***	NR	***	*****	***	***	***	***	***
30. Sacred Heart Medical Center—University District, Eugene	***	***	***	***	NR	***	***	*****	***	***	***	***
31. St. Anthony Hospital, Pendleton	***	***	NR	NR	NR	***	NR	*	***	NR	NR	NR
32. St. Charles Medical Center—Bend, Bend	***	***	*****	*****	*	***	***	***	***	***	***	***
33. St. Charles Medical Center—Redmond, Redmond	***	***	NR	NR	NR	***	NR	***	***	NR	NR	
34. St. Elizabeth Health Services, Baker City	***	NR	NR	NR	NR	***	NR	***	***	NR	NR	
35. Salem Hospital, Salem	***	*	*****	***	NR	***	***	*****	***	***	***	***
36. Samaritan Albany General Hospital, Albany	***	***	***	NR	NR	***	***	***	***	NR	NR	NR
37. Samaritan Lebanon Community Hospital, Lebanon	*****	***	NR	NR	NR	***	NR	***	*	NR	NR	
38. Samaritan North Lincoln Hospital, Lincoln City	***	***	NR	NR	NR	***	NR	NR	*	NR	NR	
39. Samaritan Pacific Community Hospital, Newport	NR	***	NR	NR	NR	***	NR	NR	*	NR	NR	
40. Santiam Memorial Hospital, Stayton	***	NR	NR	NR	NR	NR	NR	***	***	NR	NR	
41. Silverton Hospital, Silverton	*****	NR	NR	NR	NR	***	NR	NR	***	NR	NR	
42. Three Rivers Community Hospital, Grants Pass	***	***	NR	NR	NR	***	***	***	***	NR	NR	***
43. Three Rivers Community Hospital Washington Output Ctr., Grants Pass	***	***	NR	NR	NR	***	***	***	***	NR	NR	***
44. Tillamook County General Hospital, Tillamook	***	***	NR	NR	NR	***	NR	*****	***	NR	NR	
45. Tuality Community Hospital, Hillsboro	***	***	***	*	NR	*	NR	***	***	***	***	NR
46. Tuality Forest Grove Hospital, Forest Grove	***	***	***	*	NR	***	NR	***	***	***	***	NR
47. Wallowa Memorial Hospital, Enterprise	NR	***	NR	NR	NR	***	NR	***	***	NR	NR	
48. Willamette Falls Hospital, Oregon City	*****	***	NR	NR	NR	***	NR	*	***	NR	NR	
49. Willamette Valley Medical Center, McMinnville	***	***	NR	NR	NR	***	***	***	***	NR	NR	

KEY: ***** BEST   *** AS EXPECTED   * POOR   NR NOT RATED BY HEALTHGRADES   For full definitions of ratings and awards, see Appendix.

Gastrointestinal Bleed	Gastrointestinal Surgeries and Procedures	Heart Attack	Heart Failure	Hip Fracture Repair	Maternity Care	Pancreatitis	Peripheral Vascular Bypass	Pneumonia	Prostatectomy	Pulmonary Embolism	Resection/Replacement of Abdominal Aorta	Respiratory Failure	Sepsis	Stroke	Total Hip Replacement	Total Knee Replacement	Valve Replacement	Women's Health
★	★★★	★	★	★	★★★	NR	NR	★	★★★	★★★		★	★★★	★	★★★	★	NR	NR
★★★	NR	NR	★★★	★★★	★	NR	NR	★★★	NR	NR		NR	NR	★★★	★	★	NR	NR
★★★	★★★	★★★	★	★★★	★★★	★	★★★	★	★★★	★★★		★	★★★	★	★★★★★	★★★	NR	NR
NR	NR	NR	NR	NR	★	NR	NR	★★★	NR	NR		NR	NR	NR	NR	NR	NR	NR
★★★	NR	NR	★★★	★★★	★★★	NR	NR	★	NR	NR		NR	★★★	★	NR	NR	NR	NR
NR	NR	NR	★★★	NR	★	NR	NR	★	NR	NR		NR	NR	NR	NR	NR	NR	NR
★★★	★★★	★★★	★★★	★★★	★	★★★	★★★	★★★	★★★	★★★	★	★	★★★	★★★	★★★	★★★★★	★★★	★★★
★★★	NR	NR	★★★	★★★	★★★	NR	NR	★★★	NR	NR		NR	★★★	★★★	★★★	★★★	NR	NR
★★★	NR	NR	★★★	NR	★★★	NR	NR	★★★	NR	NR		NR	★★★	NR	NR	NR	NR	NR
★★★	★★★	★★★	★★★	★★★	★	NR	★★★★★	NR	★★★	NR	★★★★★	★★★★★	★★★	★★★	NR	NR	NR	NR
★★★	NR	★★★	★★★	NR	★★★	NR	NR	★★★	NR	NR		NR	★★★	NR	NR	NR	NR	NR
★★★	★★★	★	★★★	★★★	★	NR	★	★★★	★	NR		★	★★★	NR	NR	★★★★★	★★★	NR
★★★	★★★	★★★	★★★	★★★	★★★	NR	★★★	★★★	★	NR	★★★	★★★	★★★	★★★	★★★	★★★	★★★	★★★
★★★	★★★	★★★	★	★★★	★★★	★★★	★	NR	★★★	★★★		★★★	★★★	★★★	★★★	NR	NR	NR
★★★	★★★★★	★★★	★★★	★★★	★★★	★★★	NR	★★★	★	NR		★★★	★★★★★	★★★	★★★	★★★	NR	NR
★★★	★★★	★★★★★	★★★★★	★★★	★★★★★	★★★★★	NR	★★★★★	★★★	★★★		★★★★★	★★★★★	★★★	★★★	★★★	NR	NR
★★★	★★★	★★★	★	★	★★★	NR	★★★	★	★★★	★★★		★	★★★	★★★	★★★	★★★	NR	NR
★★★	★★★	★★★	★★★	★★★	★★★	NR	NR	★★★	★★★	NR		NR	★★★	★★★	★★★	★★★★★	NR	★★★
★★★	★★★	★★★	★★★	★	★	NR	★	★★★	★★★	NR	★★★	★★★	★★★	★★★★★	★	★	★★★	★★★
★★★	NR	NR	★★★	★	★★★	NR	NR	★★★	NR	NR		NR	NR	★★★	NR	NR	NR	NR
★★★	NR	NR	★★★	★★★	★★★	NR	NR	★★★	NR	NR		NR	★★★	★★★	★★★	★★★★★	NR	NR
★★★	★★★★★	★★★★★	★★★	★★★	★★★	★★★	★★★	★★★	★★★	★★★		★★★	★★★	★	NR	★★★	NR	NR
★★★	NR	★★★★★	★★★	★★★★★	★★★	NR	NR	★★★	NR	NR		NR	★	★★★	NR	NR	NR	NR
NR	NR	NR	★★★	★★★★★	★★★	NR	NR	★★★	NR	NR		NR	NR	★★★	★★★	NR	NR	NR
★★★	★	★★★	★★★	★	★★★	★★★	★★★	★★★	★★★	★★★	★★★	★★★	★★★★★	★★★	★★★	★★★★★	★★★	★★★
★★★	★★★★★	★★★	★★★	★★★	★★★	★★★	★★★	★★★	★★★★★	★★★	★★★	★	★★★	★★★	★★★★★	★★★★★	★★★	★★★
★★★	NR	★★★★★	★★★	★★★	★★★	NR	NR	★★★	NR	NR		NR	NR	★★★	NR	NR	NR	NR
★★★	★★★★★	★★★	★★★	★★★	★★★	★★★	★★★	★★★	★★★	★★★		★★★	★★★	★	★★★	★★★★★	★★★	★
★	★★★	★★★	★	★★★	★★★	★★★	★	★★★	★★★	★★★		★★★	★★★	★	★★★	★★★★★	★	★
★★★	NR	★	★★★	★	★★★	NR	NR	★	NR	NR		NR	★★★	★	★	★	NR	NR
★★★★★	★★★	★★★	★★★	★★★	★★★	★★★	NR	★★★	★★★	★★★		★★★	★★★	★★★	★★★	★★★★★	★★★	★★★
★★★	★★★	★★★	★★★	★★★	★	NR	NR	★★★	NR	NR		NR	★★★	★★★	★★★	★★★	NR	NR
★★★	NR	★★★	★	★★★	★	NR	NR	★★★	NR	NR		NR	NR	★★★★★	★★★	★★★	NR	NR
★★★	★★★	★★★	★★★	★★★	★★★	★★★	NR	★	★★★	★★★	★★★	★	★	★★★	★★★★★	★★★	★★★	★
★★★	★★★	★★★	★	★★★	★★★	NR	NR	★★★	★★★	NR		★★★	★★★	★★★	★★★	★★★	NR	NR
★	★★★	★★★	★★★	★★★★★	★★★	NR	NR	★★★	NR	NR		NR	★	★	NR	NR	NR	NR
★	NR	★★★	NR	NR	★	NR	NR	★★★	NR	NR		NR	★★★	NR	★★★	NR	NR	NR
★★★	NR	★★★	★★★	★★★	★	NR	NR	★★★	NR	NR		NR	★★★	★	★	★★★	NR	NR
★★★	NR	NR	★★★	NR	★★★	NR	NR	★	NR	NR		NR	NR	NR	NR	NR	NR	NR
★★★	NR	★★★	★★★	★★★	★★★	NR	NR	★	NR	NR		NR	★★★	★★★	NR	NR	NR	NR
★★★	★★★	★★★	★	★★★	★	★★★	NR	★★★	★★★	★★★		★★★	★★★	★★★	★	★★★	NR	NR
★★★	★★★	★★★	★	★	★★★	NR	★★★	★★★	★★★	★★★		★★★	★★★	★★★	★	★★★	NR	NR
★★★	★	NR	★★★	★★★	★★★	NR	NR	★★★	NR	NR		NR	★★★	★★★	★	★★★	NR	NR
★★★	★	★★★	★	★★★	★★★	NR	NR	★★★	★★★	NR		★★★	NR	★★★	★★★	★	NR	★★★
★★★	★	★★★	★★★	★★★	★★★	NR	NR	★★★	★★★	NR		NR	NR	★★★	NR	NR	NR	★★★
NR	NR	NR	★★★	NR	★★★	NR	NR	★	NR	NR		NR	NR	NR	NR	NR	NR	NR
★★★	★	★★★	★★★	★★★	★	NR	NR	★★★	NR	NR		NR	★★★	★★★	★★★★★	★★★	NR	NR
★★★	★★★	★★★	★★★	★	★★★	NR	NR	★★★	★	NR		NR	★★★	★★★	★★★	★★★	NR	NR

PENNSYLVANIA HOSPITALS: RATINGS BY PROCEDURE

Hospital	Appendectomy	Atrial Fibrillation	Back and Neck Surgery (except Spinal Fusion)	Back and Neck Surgery (Spinal Fusion)	Bariatric Surgery	Bowel Obstruction	Carotid Surgery	Cholecystectomy (Gall Bladder Removal)	Chronic Obstructive Pulmonary Disease (COPD)	Coronary Bypass Surgery	Coronary Interventional Procedures (Angioplasty/Stent)	Diabetic Acidosis a...
1. Abington Memorial Hospital, Abington	★★★★★	★★★	★★★	★★★	NR	★★★	★★★	★★★★★	★★★	★★★	★	★★★
2. ACMH Hospital, Kittanning	★★★	★	NR	NR	NR	★★★	NR	★★★	★	NR	NR	★★★
3. Albert Einstein Medical Center, Philadelphia	★★★	★	NR	★★★	★★★	★★★	★★★	★★★	★★★	★★★	★★★	★★★★★
4. Aliquippa Community Hospital, Aliquippa	NR	NR	NR	NR	★	NR	NR	NR	★★★	NR	NR	NR
5. Alle Kiski Medical Center, Natrona Heights	★	★★★	★★★	★★★	★★★	★★★	★★★	★★★	★★★	NR	NR	★★★
6. Allegheny General Hospital, Pittsburgh	★★★	★★★	★★★	★★★	★★★	★★★	★★★★★	★★★	★★★	★★★	★★★	★★★
7. Allegheny General Hospital–Suburban Campus, Pittsburgh	★★★	★★★	★★★	★★★	★★★	★★★	★★★★★	★★★	★★★	★★★	★★★	★★★
8. Altoona Hospital, Altoona	★★★	★★★	★★★	★★★	★★★	★	★★★	★★★	★	★★★	★★★	★★★
9. Barnes-Kasson County Hospital, Susquehanna	NR	★★★	NR	NR	NR	★	NR	NR	★★★	NR	NR	NR
10. Berwick Hospital Center, Berwick	★★★★★	★★★	NR	NR	NR	★★★	NR	★★★★★	★★★	NR	NR	NR
11. Bloomsburg Hospital, Bloomsburg	★★★	★★★	NR	NR	NR	★★★	NR	NR	★★★	NR	NR	NR
12. Bon Secours Mercy Hospital, Altoona	★★★	★★★	★★★	★★★	★★★	★	★★★	★★★	★	★★★	★★★	★★★
13. Bradford Regional Medical Center, Bradford	★	★★★	NR	NR	NR	★★★	★★★	NR	★★★	NR	NR	★★★
14. Brandywine Hospital, Coatesville	★	★★★	NR	NR	NR	★★★	★★★	★★★	★	★★★	★★★	★★★
15. Brookville Hospital, Brookville	★★★	★★★	NR	NR	NR	★★★	★★★★★	★★★★★	★★★	NR	NR	NR
16. Butler Memorial Hospital, Butler	★★★	★★★	★	NR	★	★★★	★★★	★★★	★★★	★★★★★	★★★	★★★
17. Canonsburg General Hospital, Canonsburg	★★★★★	★★★	NR	NR	NR	★★★	NR	★★★	★★★	NR	NR	NR
18. Carlisle Regional Medical Center, Carlisle	★★★	★★★	★★★	NR	NR	★★★	★★★	★★★	★	NR	NR	★★★
19. Central Montgomery Medical Center, Lansdale	★★★	★★★	NR	NR	NR	★★★	NR	★	★★★★★	NR	NR	NR
20. Chambersburg Hospital, Chambersburg	★	★★★	★	★★★	NR	★★★	★	★★★	★★★	NR	★★★★★	★★★
21. Charles Cole Memorial Hospital, Coudersport	★★★	★★★	NR	NR	NR	★★★	NR	★★★	★★★	NR	NR	NR
22. Chester County Hospital, West Chester	★★★★★	★★★	NR	NR	NR	★★★	★★★	★★★	★★★	★★★	★★★	★★★
23. Chestnut Hill Hospital, Philadelphia	★★★★★	★★★	NR	NR	NR	★★★	★★★	★★★★★	★★★	NR	NR	★★★
24. Clarion Hospital, Clarion	★★★	★★★	NR	NR	NR	★★★	NR	★★★	★★★	NR	NR	★★★
25. Clearfield Hospital, Clearfield	★★★	★★★	NR	NR	NR	★★★	NR	★★★	★★★	NR	NR	★★★
26. Community Hospital, Chester	★★★	★	★★★	NR	★★★	★	★★★	★	★	★★★	★★★	★★★
27. Community Medical Center, Scranton	★★★	★★★	★★★★★	★★★	★★★	★★★	★	★	★★★★★	★★★★★	★★★	★★★
28. Conemaugh Valley Memorial Hospital, Johnstown	★★★★★	★★★	★	★★★	★★★	★★★	★	★★★	★★★	★★★	★★★	★
29. Crozer-Chester Medical Center, Chester	★★★	★	★★★	NR	★★★	★	★★★	★	★	★★★	★★★	★★★
30. Delaware County Memorial Hospital, Drexel Hill	★★★★★	★★★	NR	NR	NR	★★★	★★★	★★★	★	NR	NR	★★★
31. Doylestown Hospital, Doylestown	★★★★★	★★★	★★★★★	NR	★★★	★★★	★	★★★	★	★★★	★★★	★★★
32. DuBois Regional Medical Center, DuBois	★★★	★★★	NR	NR	NR	★★★	★★★★★	★★★	★★★	★★★	★★★	★★★
33. Easton Hospital, Easton	★★★★★	★★★	NR	NR	★★★	★★★★★	★★★	★★★	★★★	★★★	★★★	★★★
34. Elk Regional Health Center, St. Marys	★★★	★★★	NR	NR	NR	★★★	NR	★★★	★★★	NR	NR	★★★
35. Ellwood City Hospital, Ellwood City	★★★	★★★	NR	NR	NR	★★★	NR	NR	★★★	NR	NR	NR
36. Ephrata Community Hospital, Ephrata	★	★★★	★★★	★★★	NR	★★★	★★★	★★★★★	★★★	NR	NR	★★★
37. Evangelical Community Hospital, Lewisburg	★★★	★★★	★★★	★★★	NR	★★★	★★★	★★★	★★★	NR	NR	★★★
38. Frankford Hospital–Torresdale Campus, Philadelphia	★★★	★★★	NR	NR	★	★★★	NR	★★★	★★★	★★★	★★★	★★★
39. Frick Hospital, Mt. Pleasant	★★★	★★★	NR	NR	NR	★★★	★★★	★★★	★★★	NR	NR	★★★
40. Fulton County Medical Center, McConnellsburg	NR	★★★	NR	NR	NR	NR	NR	NR	★★★	NR	NR	NR
41. Geisinger Medical Center, Danville	★★★	★★★	★★★	★	★★★★★	★★★	★★★	★★★	★★★	★★★	★★★	★★★
42. Geisinger South Wilkes-Barre, Wilkes-Barre	★★★	★★★	NR	NR	★	★★★	★	★★★	★★★	★★★★★	★★★	★★★
43. Geisinger Wyoming Valley Medical Center, Wilkes-Barre	★★★	★★★	NR	NR	★★★	★★★	★★★	★★★	★★★	★★★	★★★	★★★
44. Gettysburg Hospital, Gettysburg	★★★	★★★	NR	NR	NR	★★★	NR	★★★	★★★	NR	NR	★★★
45. Gnaden Huetten Memorial Hospital, Lehighton	★★★	★★★	NR	NR	NR	★★★	NR	★★★	★	NR	NR	★★★
46. Good Samaritan Hospital, Lebanon	★★★	★★★	NR	NR	NR	★★★	★★★	★★★	★★★	★★★	★★★	★★★
47. Good Samaritan Regional Medical Center, Pottsville	★★★★★	★★★	NR	NR	★	★★★	★★★	★	NR	NR	★★★	★★★
48. Graduate Hospital, Philadelphia	★★★	★	NR	NR	NR	★★★	NR	NR	★	★★★	★★★	★★★
49. Grand View Hospital, Sellersville	★	★★★	NR	NR	NR	★★★	★★★	★	★★★	NR	NR	★★★
50. Grove City Medical Center, Grove City	★★★	★★★	NR	NR	NR	★	NR	NR	★★★	NR	NR	NR

KEY: ★★★★★ BEST ★★★ AS EXPECTED ★ POOR NR NOT RATED BY HEALTHGRADES For full definitions of ratings and awards, see Appendix.

Gastrointestinal Bleed	Gastrointestinal Surgeries and Procedures	Heart Attack	Heart Failure	Hip Fracture Repair	Maternity Care	Pancreatitis	Peripheral Vascular Bypass	Pneumonia	Prostatectomy	Pulmonary Embolism	Resection/Replacement of Abdominal Aorta	Respiratory Failure	Sepsis	Stroke	Total Hip Replacement	Total Knee Replacement	Valve Replacement	Women's Health
★★★★★	★★★	★★★	★★★★★	★★★	★★★	★★★	★★★	★★★	★★★	★★★	★★★	★★★	★★★	★★★★★	★★★	★★★	★★★	★★★
★★★	★★★	★★★	★	★★★	★	NR	NR	★	★★★	NR	NR	NR	★	★	★★★	★★★	NR	NR
★★★	★★★	★★★	★★★	★★★★★	★★★	★★★	★★★★★	★★★★★	★★★	★★★	NR	★★★	★	★★★	★★★	★★★	NR	★★★
★★★	NR	NR	★★★	NR	NR	NR	NR	★★★	NR	NR	NR	NR	NR	NR	NR	NR	NR	NR
★★★	★★★	★★★	★★★★★	★★★	★★★	★★★	★★★	★★★	★★★	★★★	★★★★★	★★★★★	★★★	★★★	★★★	★★★	★★★	NR
★★★	★★★	★★★	★★★★★	★★★	★★★	★★★	★★★	★★★	★★★	★★★	★★★	★★★	★★★	★★★	★★★	★	★★★	★★★
★★★	★	★	★	★★★	★★★	★★★	★★★	★★★	★★★	★	★★★	★	★	★★★	★★★	★★★★★	★★★	★★★
★★★	NR	NR	★★★	NR	★★★	NR	NR	★★★	NR	NR	NR	NR	NR	NR	NR	NR	NR	NR
★★★	NR	★★★	★	★★★	★★★	NR	NR	★★★	NR	NR	NR	★	★★★	★★★	NR	NR	NR	NR
★★★	NR	★★★	★	★★★	★★★	NR	NR	★★★	NR	NR	NR	★★★	★★★	★★★	★★★	★★★	NR	NR
★★★	★	★	★	★★★	★★★	★★★	★★★	★★★	★★★	★	★★★	★	★	★★★	★★★	★★★★★	★★★	★★★
★★★	★★★	★★★	★★★	★★★	★★★	NR	★	★★★	NR	★★★	NR	★★★	★★★	★	★	NR	NR	NR
★★★	★★★	★★★	★★★★★	★★★	★	★★★	NR	★	NR	★★★	NR	★★★	★	★★★	NR	★★★★★	NR	NR
★★★	★★★	★★★	★★★	★★★	NR	★★★	★★★	★★★	★★★	NR	★★★	★★★	★★★	★★★	★★★	★★★★★	NR	NR
★★★	★★★	★★★	★★★	★★★	★★★	★	★★★	★★★	★★★★★	★★★	★★★	★★★	★★★★★	★★★	★★★	★★★	★★★	★★★★★
★★★	★★★	★	★★★	★★★	NR	★★★	★★★★★	★★★	NR	NR	★★★	★★★	★★★	★★★	★★★	★★★	★★★	★★★
★★★	★★★	★	★	★★★★★	★★★	NR	NR	★★★★★	★★★	NR	★	★★★	★★★	★★★	★★★	★★★	★★★	★★★★★
★★★	★★★	★★★	★★★★★	★★★	★★★	NR	NR	★★★	★	NR	★★★★★	★★★	★★★	★★★	★★★	★★★	★★★	★★★
★★★	★★★	★★★	★	★★★	★★★	NR	NR	★★★	NR	★★★	NR	★★★	★★★	★★★	★	★★★	★★★	★★★
★★★	★★★	★★★	★★★	★★★	★★★	★★★	★★★	★★★	★★★	★★★	★★★★★	★★★	★★★	★★★	★★★	★★★	★★★	★★★★★
★★★	★★★	★★★	★★★	★★★	★★★	NR	★★★	★★★	★★★★★	★★★	★★★	★★★	★★★	★★★	★★★	★★★	NR	★★★
★★★	★★★	★	★★★★★	★★★	★★★	NR	NR	★★★	NR	★★★	NR	★★★	★★★★★	★★★	★★★	NR	NR	NR
★★★	★	★★★	★★★	★★★	★	★★★	★★★	★★★	★★★	★★★	★★★	★	★	★★★	★★★	★	★★★	★★★
★★★★★	★★★★★	★★★★★	★★★	★★★	★★★★★	★★★	★★★	★★★	NR	★★★	NR	★★★	★★★	★★★	★★★	★★★	★★★	★★★★★
★	★★★	★★★★★	★★★	★★★★★	★★★	★★★	NR	★★★	★★★★★	★★★	★★★	★★★★★	★★★	★★★	★★★	★★★★★	★★★★★	★★★
★★★	★	★★★	★★★	★★★	★	★★★	★★★	★★★	★★★	★★★	★★★	★	★★★	★★★	★★★	★★★	★★★	★★★
★★★	★★★	★★★	★★★	★★★★★	★★★	★★★	NR	★	★★★	★★★	NR	NR	★	★★★	★★★	★★★★★	NR	NR
★★★	★★★	★★★★★	★★★	★★★	★★★★★	NR	★★★	★★★	★★★	★★★	NR	★★★	★★★	★★★	★★★	★★★	★★★	★★★★★
★★★	★	★★★	★★★	★★★★★	★★★★★	NR	★★★	★★★	★★★	★★★	NR	★★★	★★★	★★★	★★★★★	★★★	★★★★★	★★★★★
★★★	★★★★★	★★★★★	★★★	★★★	★★★	NR	★★★	★★★★★	★★★	★★★★★	NR	★★★	★★★★★	★★★	★★★	★	★★★	★★★
★★★	NR	★★★★★	★★★	★★★	★★★	NR	NR	★★★	★★★	NR	NR	★★★	★★★	NR	★★★	★★★	NR	NR
★★★	NR	NR	★★★	★★★	★★★	NR	NR	★★★	NR	NR	NR	NR	★	NR	NR	★★★	NR	NR
★★★★★	★★★★★	★★★	★★★★★	★★★	★	★★★	★★★	★★★★★	★	★★★	★★★	★★★	★★★★★	★	★	NR	NR	NR
★★★★★	★★★	★★★	★★★	★	★★★	★★★	NR	★★★	★★★	★★★	★★★	★★★	★★★	★	NR	NR	NR	NR
★★★	★★★	★★★	★★★★★	★	★★★	★★★	★★★	★★★	★★★	★★★	★	★★★	★★★	★	★★★	★★★	★★★	★★★
★★★	NR	★★★	★★★	★★★	NR	NR	NR	★★★	NR	NR	NR	★★★★★	★★★	NR	★★★	★★★	NR	NR
★★★	NR	NR	★★★	NR	NR	NR	NR	★★★	NR	NR	NR	NR	NR	NR	NR	NR	NR	NR
★★★	★★★★★	★★★	★★★	★★★	★	★★★★★	★★★	★★★	★★★	★★★	★★★	★★★	★★★	★★★	★★★★★	★★★	★★★	★★★
★★★	★	★★★	★★★★★	★★★	★★★	★★★	NR	★★★	NR	★★★	★★★★★	★	★★★★★	★	★★★	★★★★★	★★★★★	★★★★★
★★★★★	★★★	★★★	★★★	★★★	★★★	NR	NR	★★★	NR	NR	★★★★★	★★★	★★★	★★★	★★★★★	★★★	★★★	★★★
★★★	★★★	★★★★★	★★★	★★★	★★★	NR	NR	★★★	NR	★★★	★★★★★	★★★	★★★	★★★	★★★	NR	NR	NR
★★★	★★★	★★★	★★★	★★★	NR	NR	NR	★★★	NR	NR	NR	★★★	★	NR	★★★	★★★	NR	NR
★★★	★	★★★	★	★	★★★	★★★	NR	★	★	★★★	NR	★	★	★★★	★	★★★	NR	NR
★★★	★	★	★★★	NR	★★★	★★★	★★★	★★★	★★★	NR	★★★	★	★	★★★★★	★★★	★★★	NR	NR
★★★	NR	★★★	★★★	NR	NR	★★★	★★★	★★★	NR	NR	★★★	★★★	★★★	NR	★★★	★★★	NR	NR
★★★	★★★	★★★	★★★	★★★★★	★★★★★	NR	NR	★★★	★★★	★★★	NR	★★★	★★★	★★★	★★★	★★★	NR	NR
★★★	NR	NR	★★★	★★★	★★★	NR	★	★★★	NR	NR	NR	NR	★★★	NR	★	NR	NR	NR

Hospital	Appendectomy	Atrial Fibrillation	Back and Neck Surgery (except Spinal Fusion)	Back and Neck Surgery (Spinal Fusion)	Bariatric Surgery	Bowel Obstruction	Carotid Surgery	Cholecystectomy (Gall Bladder Removal)	Chronic Obstructive Pulmonary Disease (COPD)	Coronary Bypass Surgery	Coronary Interventional Procedures (Angioplasty/Stent)	Diabetic Acidosis a...
51. Hahnemann University Hospital, Philadelphia	***	***	NR	NR	***	***	***	***	***	*	***	***
52. Hamot Medical Center, Erie	***	***	*	***	*	*****	***	***	*****	*****	*****	***
53. Hanover General Hospital, Hanover	***	***	***	*****	NR	***	***	***	*	NR	NR	NR
54. Hazleton General Hospital, Hazleton	***	***	NR	NR	*	***	*	*	***	NR	NR	***
55. Heart of Lancaster Regional Medical Center, Lititz	***	***	NR	NR	NR	***	NR	***	***	NR	NR	***
56. Highlands Hospital, Connellsville	***	***	NR	NR	***	***	NR	NR	***	NR	NR	***
57. Holy Redeemer Hospital and Medical Center, Meadowbrook	***	***	***	NR	***	***	***	***	***	NR	***	***
58. Holy Spirit Hospital, Camp Hill	*	***	***	***	NR	***	***	***	***	***	***	***
59. Hospital of the University of Pennsylvania, Philadelphia	*	***	*	*	***	***	***	***	***	***	*	***
60. Indiana Regional Medical Center, Indiana	***	***	NR	NR	NR	***	***	***	***	NR	NR	***
61. J. C. Blair Memorial Hospital, Huntingdon	*	***	NR	NR	NR	***	*	***	***	NR	NR	***
62. Jameson Memorial Hospital, New Castle	*	***	NR	NR	NR	***	*	***	***	NR	***	***
63. Jeanes Hospital, Philadelphia	*	***	NR	NR	NR	***	***	***	***	NR	***	***
64. Jefferson Regional Medical Center, Pittsburgh	*	***	***	***	NR	***	***	***	***	*****	***	***
65. Jennersville Regional Hospital, West Grove	***	***	NR	NR	NR	***	NR	***	***	NR	NR	NR
66. Jersey Shore Hospital, Jersey Shore	*****	***	NR	NR	NR	***	NR	***	***	NR	NR	NR
67. Kane Community Hospital, Kane	NR	***	NR	NR	*	***	NR	***	***	NR	NR	NR
68. Lancaster General Hospital, Lancaster	*****	***	*****	***	NR	***	***	***	***	*****	***	***
69. Lancaster Regional Medical Center, Lancaster	***	***	***	***	*****	***	*	***	***	***	***	***
70. Latrobe Hospital, Latrobe	***	***	***	***	NR	***	***	***	***	NR	NR	***
71. Lehigh Valley Hospital, Allentown	*	***	*	***	***	***	*	*	***	***	***	***
72. Lehigh Valley Hospital–Muhlenberg, Bethlehem	*	***	***	NR	*****	***	***	***	***	***	***	***
73. Lewistown Hospital, Lewistown	*****	***	NR	NR	NR	***	***	*****	***	NR	NR	***
74. Lock Haven Hospital, Lock Haven	*****	***	NR	NR	NR	***	NR	NR	*	NR	NR	NR
75. Lower Bucks Hospital, Bristol	***	***	NR	NR	NR	***	***	***	***	***	***	***
76. Magee-Womens Hospital of the UPMC Health System, Pittsburgh	***	NR	NR	NR	***	NR	NR	NR	***	NR	NR	NR
77. Main Line Hospitals–Bryn Mawr, Bryn Mawr	***	***	***	NR	NR	***	***	***	***	***	***	***
78. Main Line Hospitals–Lankenau, Wynnewood	*****	***	***	NR	NR	***	***	***	***	*****	***	***
79. Main Line Hospitals–Paoli Memorial, Paoli	*****	***	***	*****	NR	***	***	***	***	***	***	***
80. Marian Community Hospital, Carbondale	***	*	NR	NR	NR	***	***	***	***	NR	NR	*
81. Meadville Medical Center, Meadville	***	***	NR	NR	NR	*	NR	***	*	NR	NR	***
82. The Medical Center–Beaver, Beaver	*	***	***	***	NR	***	***	*	***	***	***	***
83. Memorial Hospital, Towanda	***	*	NR	NR	NR	***	NR	NR	***	NR	NR	NR
84. Memorial Hospital, York	***	***	***	NR	NR	*	NR	*	***	NR	NR	***
85. Mercy Fitzgerald Hospital, Darby	***	*	NR	NR	NR	***	*	***	***	***	***	***
86. Mercy Hospital Scranton, Scranton	***	*****	NR	NR	NR	***	***	***	***	***	*****	***
87. Mercy Hospital, Pittsburgh	*	***	*	***	NR	***	***	*	***	***	*	*****
88. Mercy Jeannette Hospital, Jeannette	***	***	NR	NR	*****	***	NR	***	***	NR	NR	NR
89. Mercy Providence Hospital, Pittsburgh	*	***	*	***	NR	***	***	*	***	***	NR	*****
90. Mercy Suburban Hospital, Norristown	***	***	NR	NR	NR	***	NR	NR	*	NR	NR	***
91. Methodist Hospital, Philadelphia	***	*****	***	*****	NR	***	***	***	***	NR	***	***
92. Mid-Valley Hospital, Peckville	NR	***	*	NR	NR	NR	NR	***	*****	NR	NR	NR
93. Millcreek Community Hospital, Erie	***	***	NR	NR	NR	***	NR	NR	***	NR	NR	NR
94. Milton S. Hershey Medical Center, Hershey	*	***	*	*	*	***	***	***	***	***	***	***
95. Miners Medical Center, Hastings	NR	NR	NR	NR	NR	***	NR	NR	***	NR	NR	NR
96. Monongahela Valley Hospital, Monongahela	***	***	NR	NR	NR	***	***	***	***	***	***	***
97. Montgomery Hospital, Norristown	***	***	NR	NR	NR	***	NR	***	***	***	NR	***
98. Moses Taylor Hospital, Scranton	***	***	NR	NR	NR	***	NR	***	***	NR	NR	***
99. Mount Nittany Medical Center, State College	*****	***	***	*****	NR	*	***	***	***	NR	NR	***
100. Muncy Valley Hospital, Muncy	NR	***	NR	NR	NR	NR	NR	***	NR	NR	NR

KEY: ***** BEST   *** AS EXPECTED   * POOR   NR NOT RATED BY HEALTHGRADES   For full definitions of ratings and awards, see Appendix.

Gastrointestinal Bleed	Gastrointestinal Surgeries and Procedures	Heart Attack	Heart Failure	Hip Fracture Repair	Maternity Care	Pancreatitis	Peripheral Vascular Bypass	Pneumonia	Prostatectomy	Pulmonary Embolism	Resection/Replacement of Abdominal Aorta	Respiratory Failure	Sepsis	Stroke	Total Hip Replacement	Total Knee Replacement	Valve Replacement	Women's Health
★★★	★★★	★★★	★★★	★	★★★	NR	NR	★★★	NR	NR	NR	★★★	★	★★★	NR	★	★	★★★
★★★★★	★★★★★	★★★★★	★★★★★	★★★	★★★	★★★	★★★	★★★★★	★★★	★★★	★★★	★★★★★	★★★★★	★★★★★	★★★	★★★	★★★	★★★
★★★	★★★	★★★	★	★★★★★	★★★★★	★	NR	★	NR	★★★	NR	★	★★★	★	★★★★★	★★★★★	NR	NR
★★★	★★★	★★★	★★★	★★★	★★★	★★★	NR	★★★★★	★★★	★★★★★	NR	★★★★★	★★★★★	★★★	NR	NR	NR	NR
★★★	★★★	★★★	★★★	★★★	★★★	NR	NR	★★★	★★★	NR	NR	★★★★★	★★★	★★★	NR	★★★	NR	NR
★★★	NR	NR	★★★	★★★	NR	NR	NR	★★★	NR	NR	NR	★★★	★★★	NR	NR	NR	NR	NR
★★★	★★★	★★★	★★★★★	★★★	★★★	★★★	★★★	★★★	★★★	★★★	NR	★★★	★	★★★	★★★	★★★	NR	★★★
★★★	★	★★★	★	★★★	★★★	★★★	★★★	★★★	★★★	★★★	★★★	★	★★★	★	★★★	★★★	★★★	★★★
★★★	★★★	★★★	★★★	★	★	★★★	★	★★★	★★★★★	★★★	★★★	★★★	★★★	★★★	★★★	NR	★	★
★★★★★	★★★	★★★	★★★	★★★★★	★★★★★	★★★	NR	★★★	NR	★★★	NR	★★★	★★★	★★★	★★★	★★★	NR	NR
★★★	★★★	★★★	★★★	NR	★★★	NR	NR	★★★	NR	NR	NR	★★★	★★★	★	NR	NR	NR	NR
★	★	★★★	★★★	★	★★★	★★★	NR	★★★	★★★	★★★	NR	★	★★★	★★★	★	★	NR	NR
★★★	★★★	★★★	★★★★★	★★★	★★★	★★★	★★★	★★★	NR	NR	NR	★	★★★	★★★	★★★	★★★	NR	NR
★★★	NR	NR	★★★	★★★	★★★	NR	NR	★★★	★★★	NR	NR	★★★	★	★★★	NR	★★★	NR	NR
★★★	NR	★★★	★★★	★★★★★	NR	NR	NR	★★★	NR	NR	NR	NR	★★★	NR	NR	★★★	NR	NR
★★★	NR	★★★	★★★	★★★	NR	NR	NR	★★★★★	NR	NR	NR	★★★	★★★★★	★★★	NR	NR	NR	NR
★★★	★★★	★★★★★	★★★★★	★★★	★★★	★★★	★★★	★★★★★	★★★	★★★★★	★★★	★★★	★★★	★★★★★	★★★	★	★★★★★	★★★
★★★	★★★	★★★	★★★	★★★	NR	★★★	★	★★★	★★★	★★★	NR	★★★★★	★★★	★★★	★	★★★	★	★★★
★★★	★	★★★	★★★	★★★	★★★	★★★	NR	★★★	NR	★★★	NR	★★★	★★★	★★★	★★★	★★★	NR	★★★
★★★★★	★★★★★	★★★	★★★★★	★	★★★★★	★	★★★★★	★★★	★★★	★★★	★	★★★★★	★★★★★	★★★★★	★★★	★★★	★★★★★	★★★
★★★★★	★★★★★	★★★	★★★	NR	★★★	NR	★★★	★★★★★	★★★	★★★	NR	★★★	★★★★★	★★★	★	★★★	★★★	NR
★★★	★★★	★★★	★★★	★★★	NR	NR	NR	★★★	★★★	NR	NR	★★★	★★★	★★★	NR	★★★	NR	NR
★★★	★	★★★	★	NR	★★★	NR	NR	★★★	NR	NR	NR	★★★	★★★	★★★	NR	NR	NR	★
NR	NR	NR	NR	★	NR	NR	NR	NR	NR	NR	NR	NR	NR	NR	★★★	★★★★★	NR	NR
★★★★★	★★★	★★★	★★★★★	★★★	★★★	★★★	★★★★★	★★★	★★★	★★★	★★★	★★★	★★★★★	★★★	★★★★★	★★★	★★★★★	★★★
★★★	★★★	★★★★★	★★★★★	★★★★★	★	★★★	NR	★★★★★	★★★	★★★	★★★	★★★★★	★★★	★★★★★	★★★	★	★★★	★★★
★★★	★★★	★★★	★★★	★★★	★★★	NR	NR	★★★	NR	★	★★★	★★★	★★★	★★★	★★★	★★★	★	★★★
★★★	★	★★★	★★★	★★★	NR	★★★	NR	★★★	★★★	★★★	★	★★★	★★★	★★★	★★★	★★★	NR	NR
★★★	★★★	★	★★★	★	★★★	NR	NR	★★★	★★★	★	NR	★★★	★★★	★	★★★	★★★★★	NR	NR
★	NR	NR	★	NR	★★★	NR	NR	★	NR	NR	NR	★★★	★★★	NR	★★★★★	NR	NR	NR
★★★	★★★	★★★	★★★	★★★	★★★	★★★	NR	★★★	★★★	★★★	NR	★★★	★★★	★	★★★	★★★	NR	NR
★★★	★	★★★	★★★★★	★★★	NR	★★★	NR	★★★	★★★	★	NR	★	★★★	★★★★★	NR	★★★	NR	NR
★★★	★★★★★	★★★★★	★★★★★	★★★	★★★	NR	★★★★★	★★★	★★★	★	★★★★★	★★★	★★★★★	★★★	★★★★★	★★★★★	★★★★★
★★★	★★★	★★★★★	★★★	★★★	★★★	★★★	★★★	★★★★★	★★★	★★★	★★★	★★★	★	★★★	★	★★★	★
★★★	★★★	★★★	★★★	★★★★★	★★★★★	NR	NR	★★★	★	NR	NR	★★★	★★★	★	NR	NR	NR	NR
★★★	★★★	★★★★★	★★★	★★★	★★★	★★★	★★★	★★★★★	★★★	NR	★★★	★★★	★	★★★	★★★	★	NR
★★★	NR	★★★	★★★	★★★	★	NR	NR	★★★	NR	NR	★★★	★★★	★★★	NR	★★★	NR	NR
★★★	★	★★★	★★★	★★★	★	★★★★★	NR	★★★★★	★★★	★	★★★	★★★	★★★	★★★★★	★★★	★★★	★★★
★★★	NR	★★★	★★★	★★★	NR	NR	NR	★★★★★	NR	NR	NR	★★★	★★★	★★★	NR	NR	NR	NR
★	NR	NR	★★★	★★★	★★★	NR	NR	★	NR	NR	NR	NR	NR	★★★	NR	NR	NR	NR
★★★	★★★	★★★	★★★	★★★	★	★★★	★	★★★	★★★	★★★	★★★	★★★	★★★	★★★★★	★★★	★★★★★	★★★	★★★
★★★	NR	★★★	★★★	★★★	NR	NR	NR	★★★	NR	NR	NR	★★★	★★★	NR	NR	NR	NR	NR
★	★★★	★★★	★★★	★★★	★★★	★★★	NR	★★★	★★★	NR	NR	★★★	★	★★★	★★★	★★★	★★★	★★★
★★★	NR	★	★★★	★★★	NR	★	NR	★★★	NR	NR	NR	★★★★★	★	★	★★★	★★★	★★★	NR
★★★	★★★	★★★	★★★	★★★	★★★	★★★	NR	★★★	NR	NR	★★★	★★★★★	★★★	★★★	★★★	★★★	NR	NR
★★★	★★★	★★★	★	★★★	★★★	★★★	★	★★★	★★★	★★★	★	★★★	★	★★★	★★★	★★★★★	NR	NR
★★★	NR	★★★	★★★	NR	NR	NR	NR	★★★	NR	NR	NR	NR	NR	★★★	NR	NR	NR	NR

Hospital	Appendectomy	Atrial Fibrillation	Back and Neck Surgery (except Spinal Fusion)	Back and Neck Surgery (Spinal Fusion)	Bariatric Surgery	Bowel Obstruction	Carotid Surgery	Cholecystectomy (Gall Bladder Removal)	Chronic Obstructive Pulmonary Disease (COPD)	Coronary Bypass Surgery	Coronary Interventional Procedures (Angioplasty/Stent)	Diabetic Acidosis an...
101. **Nason Hospital**, Roaring Spring	★★★	★★★	NR	NR	★★★	★★★	NR	★★★	★★★	NR	NR	
102. **Nazareth Hospital**, Philadelphia	★★★	★★★	★★★	NR	NR	★★★	NR	★★★	★★★	NR	NR	★★★
103. **North Philadelphia Health System**, Philadelphia	NR	NR	NR	NR	NR	NR	NR	★★★	NR	NR	★★★	
104. **Northeastern Hospital**, Philadelphia	★★★	★★★	NR	NR	NR	★★★	NR	★★★	★★★	NR	NR	★★★
105. **Ohio Valley General Hospital**, McKees Rocks	★★★	★★★	NR	NR	★	★★★	NR	★★★	★★★	NR	NR	★★★
106. **Palmerton Hospital**, Palmerton	NR	★★★	NR	NR	NR	★★★	★★★	★★★	★★★	NR	NR	★★★
107. **Pennsylvania Hospital**, Philadelphia	★★★★★	★★★	★★★★★	★★★★★	★★★★★	★★★	★★★★★	★★★	★★★	★★★	★★★	★★★
108. **Pennsylvania Presbyterian Medical Center**, Philadelphia	★★★	★★★	NR	NR	★★★	★★★	NR	★★★	★★★	★★★	★★★	★★★
109. **Phoenixville Hospital**, Phoenixville	★★★	★★★	NR	NR	★	★★★	★	★★★	★★★★★	★★★	★	
110. **Pinnacle Health System**, Harrisburg	★	★★★★★	★★★	★★★	★★★★★	★★★★★	★★★	★★★★★	★★★★★	★★★	★★★	
111. **Pocono Medical Center**, East Stroudsburg	★★★	★★★	NR	NR	NR	★★★	★★★	★★★	★★★	★★★	NR	★★★
112. **Pottstown Memorial Medical Center**, Pottstown	★★★★★	★★★	★	NR	NR	★★★	NR	★★★	★★★	NR	NR	★★★
113. **Pottsville Hospital and Warne Clinic**, Pottsville	★★★★★	★★★	NR	NR	NR	★	NR	★★★	★	NR	NR	★★★
114. **Punxsutawney Area Hospital**, Punxsutawney	★★★	★★★	NR	NR	NR	★★★	NR	★★★	★★★	NR	NR	NR
115. **The Reading Hospital and Medical Center**, West Reading	★★★	★★★	NR	★	★★★	★★★	★★★	★★★	★★★	★★★★★	★★★	★★★
116. **Riddle Memorial Hospital**, Media	★★★★★	★★★	★★★	NR	★★★	★★★	NR	★★★	★★★	NR	NR	★
117. **Robert Packer Hospital**, Sayre	★★★★★	★★★	★★★	★★★★★	★★★	★★★★★	★★★★★	★★★	★★★	★★★	★★★	★★★
118. **Roxborough Memorial Hospital**, Philadelphia	★★★	★★★	NR	NR	★★★	NR	NR	★★★	NR	NR	NR	★★★
119. **Sacred Heart Hospital**, Allentown	★★★	★★★	★	NR	★★★	★★★	★	★★★	★★★	★★★	★★★	★★★
120. **St. Catherine Medical Center—Fountain Springs**, Ashland	NR	NR	NR	NR	★★★	NR	NR	★★★	NR	NR	NR	
121. **St. Clair Hospital**, Pittsburgh	★	★★★	★★★	★★★	★★★	★★★	★★★	★★★★★	★★★	★★★	★★★	★★★
122. **St. Joseph Medical Center**, Reading	★★★	★★★	NR	NR	★★★	★	★	★★★	★★★	★★★	★★★	★★★
123. **St. Joseph's Hospital**, Philadelphia	NR	NR	NR	NR	NR	NR	NR	★★★	NR	NR	★★★	
124. **St. Luke's Hospital**, Bethlehem	★★★	★★★★★	★★★	★	★★★★★	★★★	★★★	★★★	★★★	★★★★★	★★★★★	★★★
125. **St. Luke's Hospital—Allentown Campus**, Allentown	★★★	★★★★★	★	★	★	★★★★★	★★★	★★★	★★★	★★★★★	★★★★★	★★★
126. **St. Luke's Miners Memorial Hospital**, Coaldale	★★★	★★★	NR	NR	★★★	NR	NR	★★★	NR	NR	NR	
127. **St. Luke's Quakertown Hospital**, Quakertown	★★★	★★★	★★★	NR	★★★	NR	NR	★★★★★	★★★	NR	NR	
128. **St. Mary Medical Center**, Langhorne	★★★	★★★	★★★	NR	★★★	★★★	★★★	★★★	★★★	★★★	★★★	★★★
129. **St. Vincent Health Center**, Erie	★★★	★★★	★★★	NR	★★★	★★★★★	★★★	★★★	★★★	★★★	★★★	★★★
130. **Sewickley Valley Hospital**, Sewickley	★★★	★★★	★★★	★★★★★	★★★★★	★★★	★★★★★	★★★	★	NR	NR	
131. **Shamokin Area Community Hospital**, Coal Township	★★★	★★★★★	NR	NR	★★★	NR	★★★	★★★	NR	NR	★★★	
132. **Sharon Regional Health System**, Sharon	★	★★★	NR	NR	★	★★★	★★★	★★★	★★★	★★★	★★★	★★★
133. **Soldiers and Sailors Memorial Hospital**, Wellsboro	★★★	★★★	NR	NR	★★★	NR	★★★	★	NR	NR	NR	
134. **Somerset Hospital**, Somerset	★★★	★★★	NR	NR	★★★	NR	★★★	★★★	NR	NR	★★★	
135. **Southwest Regional Medical Center**, Waynesburg	★★★	★★★	NR	NR	★★★	NR	NR	★★★	NR	NR	NR	
136. **Springfield Hospital**, Springfield	★★★	★	★★★	NR	★★★	★	★★★	★	★	★★★	★★★	★★★
137. **Sunbury Community Hospital**, Sunbury	★★★	★★★	NR	NR	★★★	NR	NR	★★★	★★★	NR	NR	★★★
138. **Temple University Hospital**, Philadelphia	★	★★★	★	★★★	★★★	★★★	NR	NR	★★★	★★★	★★★	★★★
139. **Thomas Jefferson University Hospital**, Philadelphia	★★★	★★★★★	★★★	★★★★★	★★★	★★★	★★★	★★★	★★★	★★★	★★★	★★★
140. **Titusville Hospital**, Titusville	★★★	★★★	NR	NR	★★★	NR	★★★	★★★	NR	NR	NR	
141. **Troy Community Hospital**, Troy	NR	NR	NR	NR	NR	NR	NR	★★★	NR	NR	NR	
142. **Tyler Memorial Hospital**, Tunkhannock	★★★	★★★	NR	NR	NR	★★★	NR	★★★	NR	NR	NR	
143. **Tyrone Hospital**, Tyrone	NR	NR	NR	NR	NR	NR	NR	★★★	NR	NR	NR	
144. **Uniontown Hospital**, Uniontown	★★★★★	★★★	NR	NR	NR	★★★★★	★★★	★★★	★★★★★	NR	★★★	★★★
145. **University of Pittsburgh Med. Ctr.–Bedford**, Everett	★★★★★	★★★	NR	NR	NR	★★★	NR	★★★	★★★	NR	NR	★★★
146. **University of Pittsburgh Med. Ctr.–Braddock**, Braddock	★★★	★★★	NR	NR	NR	★★★	NR	★★★	★★★	NR	NR	
147. **University of Pittsburgh Med. Ctr.–Horizon**, Greenville	★★★	★★★	NR	NR	★	★★★	★★★	★	★★★	NR	NR	★★★
148. **University of Pittsburgh Med. Ctr.–Lee**, Johnstown	★★★★★	★★★	★	NR	★★★	★★★	NR	★★★	★★★	NR	NR	
149. **University of Pittsburgh Med. Ctr.–McKeesport**, McKeesport	★★★	★★★	NR	NR	★★★	★	NR	★★★★★	★★★	NR	NR	★
150. **University of Pittsburgh Med. Ctr.–Passavant**, Pittsburgh	★	★★★	★★★	★★★	★★★	★★★	★	★★★	★★★	★★★	★★★	

KEY: ★★★★★ BEST   ★★★ AS EXPECTED   ★ POOR   NR NOT RATED BY HEALTHGRADES   For full definitions of ratings and awards, see Appendix.

Gastrointestinal Bleed	Gastrointestinal Surgeries and Procedures	Heart Attack	Heart Failure	Hip Fracture Repair	Maternity Care	Pancreatitis	Peripheral Vascular Bypass	Pneumonia	Prostatectomy	Pulmonary Embolism	Resection/Replacement of Abdominal Aorta	Respiratory Failure	Sepsis	Stroke	Total Hip Replacement	Total Knee Replacement	Valve Replacement	Women's Health
★★★	NR	NR	★	★★★	★★★	NR	NR	★	NR	NR	NR	NR	NR	★★★	NR	★★★	NR	NR
★★★	★★★	★★★	★★★★★	★★★	NR	★★★	NR	★★★★★	NR	★★★	NR	★★★	★★★	★★★★★	★★★★★	★★★★★	NR	NR
★★★★★	NR	★★★	★★★	NR	NR	★★★	NR	★★★	NR	NR	NR	★★★	★★★	★★★	NR	NR	NR	NR
★★★	NR	★★★	★★★	★★★	★★★	NR	NR	★★★	NR	NR	NR	★★★	★★★	★★★	NR	★★★	NR	NR
★★★	NR	★★★	★★★	★★★	★★★	NR	NR	★★★	NR	NR	NR	★	★★★	★★★	NR	★★★	NR	NR
★★★	★★★	★★★	★★★	★★★	★	NR	NR	★★★	NR	NR	NR	★	★	NR	NR	★★★	NR	NR
★★★★★	★★★	★★★	★★★★★	★★★	★★★	★★★	★★★	★★★★★	★★★★★	NR	★★★	★★★	★★★	★★★	★★★★★	★★★★★	★★★	★★★
★★★	★★★	★★★	★★★	★	NR	NR	★★★	★★★	★★★★★	★★★	★★★	★★★	★	★★★	★★★	★★★	★★★	NR
★★★	★	★★★	★★★	★	★★★	★★★	★★★	★★★	NR	★★★	NR	★★★	★★★	★★★	NR	★★★	NR	★★★
★★★★★	★★★	★★★★★	★★★	★★★	★★★	★★★	★	★★★	★★★	★★★★★	★★★	★★★★★	★★★★★	★★★★★	★★★	★	★★★	★★★
★★★	★★★	★★★	★★★	★★★	★	★★★	★★★	★★★★★	★★★	★★★	★★★	★★★	★★★★★	★★★	★★★	★	NR	NR
★	★	★★★	★	★★★★★	★★★	★★★	NR	★	★★★	★★★	NR	★	★★★	★★★	★★★	★★★	NR	NR
★	★★★	★	★	★★★	★★★★★	★★★	★★★	★	★★★	★	NR	★★★	★★★	★	★★★	★★★★★	NR	NR
★★★	NR	★	★	★★★	★★★	NR	NR	★★★	NR	NR	NR	★★★	★★★	NR	NR	★★★★★	NR	NR
★★★	★★★	★★★★★	★★★	★★★	★★★	★★★	★★★★★	★★★	★★★	★★★	★★★	★★★	★★★	★★★★★	★★★	★★★	★★★	★★★
★★★	★★★	★★★	★★★	★★★	★★★	★★★	NR	★	★★★	★★★	★★★	★	★	★★★	★★★	★★★	NR	★★★
★★★	★★★	★★★★★	★★★★★	★★★	★★★	★★★	★★★	★★★	★★★	★★★	★★★	★★★★★	★★★	★★★★★	★★★★★	★★★	★★★	★★★
★★★	NR	★★★	★★★	★★★	NR	NR	NR	★★★	NR	NR	NR	★★★	★★★	★★★	NR	NR	NR	NR
★★★	★	★★★★★	★★★★★	★	★★★	★★★	NR	★★★	★★★	NR	NR	★★★	★	★	★★★	★★★	★★★	★★★
★★★	NR	★★★	★★★	★★★	NR	NR	NR	★★★	NR	NR	NR	★★★	★★★	NR	NR	NR	NR	NR
★★★	★★★	★★★	★★★	★★★	★★★	NR	★★★	★★★	★★★	★★★	NR	★★★	★★★	★★★	★★★	★★★	★★★	★★★
★★★	★★★	★★★	★★★	★	★★★	★★★	★	★★★	★★★	★★★	NR	★★★★★	★★★	★★★	★	★	★	★★★
★★★★★	NR	★★★	★★★	NR	NR	★★★	NR	★★★	NR	NR	NR	★★★	★★★	★★★	NR	NR	NR	NR
★★★	★★★★★	★★★★★	★★★★★	★★★	★★★	★★★	NR	★★★★★	★★★	★★★	★★★	★★★	★★★	★★★	★	★★★	★★★★★	★★★★★
★★★	★★★★★	★★★★★	★★★	★★★	★★★	★★★	NR	★★★★★	★★★	★★★	★★★	★★★	★★★	★★★	★	★★★	★★★★★	★★★★★
★★★	NR	★★★	★★★	★★★	NR	NR	NR	★★★★★	NR	NR	NR	★★★	NR	NR	★★★	NR	NR	NR
★★★	NR	★★★	★★★	★★★	NR	NR	NR	★★★★★	NR	NR	NR	★★★	★★★	★	★★★	★★★★★	NR	NR
★	★★★	★★★	★★★	★★★★★	★★★	★★★	★★★	★★★	★★★	★★★	★★★	★	★★★	★★★	★★★	★★★	★★★★★
★★★	★★★	★	★★★	★★★★★	★★★	NR	★★★	★★★	NR	NR	★★★	★★★	★	★★★★★	★★★★★	★★★	NR
★	NR	★★★★★	★★★	★★★	NR	★★★	NR	★★★	★★★	★★★	NR	★★★	★★★	NR	★★★	★★★	NR	NR
★★★	★	★★★	★★★	★	★★★	★★★	NR	★★★	★★★	★★★	★	★★★	★★★	★	★★★	★★★	NR	★★★
★★★	★★★	★★★	★★★	★★★	★★★	NR	★	★★★	★★★	NR	NR	★★★	★★★	NR	★★★	★★★	NR	NR
★★★	NR	★	★★★	★★★	★★★	NR	NR	★★★	NR	NR	NR	★★★	★★★	★★★	NR	NR	NR	NR
★★★	NR	★★★	★★★	★★★	NR	NR	NR	★★★	NR	NR	NR	★★★	★★★	★★★	NR	NR	NR	NR
★★★	★	★★★	★★★	★★★	★	★★★	★★★	★★★	★★★	★★★	★	★	★★★	★★★	★	★★★	★★★
★★★	NR	★★★	★★★	★★★	NR	NR	★★★	★★★	NR	NR	NR	★★★	★★★	★★★	★★★	NR	★★★	★★★
★★★	★	★	★★★	★★★	★★★	NR	★★★	★★★	★★★	NR	★★★	★★★	★★★	★★★	★★★	★★★	★
★★★	NR	★★★	★★★	★★★	★	★★★★★	NR	★★★★★	★	★★★	★★★	★★★	★★★	★★★★★	★★★	★★★	★★★
★★★	NR	★★★★★	★★★	★★★	★★★	NR	NR	★★★	★★★	NR	NR	NR	NR	★★★	★★★	NR	NR
★★★	NR	NR	★★★	NR	NR	NR	NR	★★★	NR	NR	NR	NR	NR	★★★	NR	NR	NR
★★★	NR	NR	★★★	NR	★★★	NR	NR	★★★	NR	NR	NR	★	★★★	NR	NR	NR	NR
NR	NR	★★★	★★★	★★★	★★★	NR	NR	★★★	NR	NR	NR	NR	★★★	NR	NR	NR	NR
★★★	★★★	★★★	★★★	★★★★★	★★★	★★★	NR	★	★★★	★★★	NR	★	★★★	★★★	★★★★★	NR	NR
★★★	★★★	★★★	★★★	★★★	★★★	NR	★★★	★★★★★	NR	NR	NR	NR	★★★	★★★	★★★★★	NR	NR
★★★	★★★	★★★	★★★	★★★	NR	NR	NR	★★★	NR	NR	★★★	★★★	★★★	NR	NR	NR	NR
★★★	★★★	★★★	★★★	★★★	★★★	NR	★★★	★★★	★★★	NR	★★★	★★★	★★★★★	★★★	★	NR	NR
★	★★★	★★★★★	★★★	★★★★★	★★★	★★★	★★★	★★★★★	★★★	★★★	★★★★★	★★★★★	★★★	★★★	★★★★★	★★★★★	★★★
★★★★★	★★★	★★★★★	★★★★★	★★★★★	NR	★★★	★★★	★★★★★	★★★	★★★★★	NR	★★★★★	★★★★★	★★★	NR	★★★	NR
★★★	★★★	★★★	★★★	★★★	NR	★★★	★★★	★★★	★	★★★	NR	★★★	★★★	★★★	★★★	★	★★★	NR

Hospital	Appendectomy	Atrial Fibrillation	Back and Neck Surgery (except Spinal Fusion)	Back and Neck Surgery (Spinal Fusion)	Bariatric Surgery	Bowel Obstruction	Carotid Surgery	Cholecystectomy (Gall Bladder Removal)	Chronic Obstructive Pulmonary Disease (COPD)	Coronary Bypass Surgery	Coronary Interventional Procedures (Angioplasty/Stent)	Diabetic Acidosis a...
151. University of Pittsburgh Med. Ctr.–St. Margaret, Pittsburgh	★	★★★	★★★	★	★★★	★★★	★★★	★★★	★★★★★	NR	NR	★★★
152. University of Pittsburgh Med. Ctr.–Shadyside, Pittsburgh	★	★★★	★	★	★★★	★★★	★	★	★★★★★	★★★	★★★	★★★
153. University of Pittsburgh Med. Ctr.–South Side, Pittsburgh	★★★	★★★	NR	NR	NR	★★★	NR	★★★	★★★	NR	NR	NR
154. University of Pittsburgh Med. Ctr.–Presbyterian Shadyside, Pittsburgh	★	★★★	★	★	★★★	★★★	★	★	★★★★★	★★★	★★★	★★★
155. University of Pittsburgh Med. Ctr.–Cranberry, Cranberry Township	★	★★★	★★★	★★★	NR	★★★	★★★	★	★★★	★★★	★★★	★★★
156. University of Pittsburgh Med. Ctr.–Northwest, Seneca	★★★	★	NR	NR	NR	★★★	★★★	★★★	★★★	NR	NR	★★★
157. Warminster Hospital, Warminster	★★★	★★★	NR	NR	NR	★	NR	NR	★★★	NR	NR	★
158. Warren General Hospital, Warren	★★★	★★★	NR	NR	NR	★	NR	NR	★★★	NR	NR	NR
159. Washington Hospital, Washington	★★★	★★★	★★★	★★★	NR	★★★	★★★	★★★	★★★	★★★★★	★★★	★★★
160. Wayne Memorial Hospital, Honesdale	★★★★★	★★★	NR	NR	NR	★★★	NR	★★★	★★★	NR	NR	NR
161. Waynesboro Hospital, Waynesboro	★★★	★★★	NR	NR	NR	★★★	NR	★★★	★★★	NR	NR	NR
162. Western Pennsylvania Hospital–Forbes Regional Campus, Monroeville	★★★★★	★★★	NR	NR	NR	★★★	★★★	★★★	★★★	NR	NR	★★★
163. Western Pennsylvania Hospital, Pittsburgh	★★★	★★★	★★★	★★★	★★★★★	★★★	★★★	★★★	★★★	★★★	★★★	★★★
164. Westmoreland Regional Hospital, Greensburg	★★★	★★★	★	NR	NR	★★★	★★★	★★★	★★★	★★★	★★★	★★★
165. Wilkes-Barre General Hospital, Wilkes-Barre	★	★★★	★	NR	NR	★★★	★★★	★★★	★★★	★★★	★★★	★★★
166. Williamsport Hospital and Medical Center, Williamsport	★★★	★★★	★★★★★	★★★★★	NR	★★★	★★★	★★★	★★★	★★★	★★★	★★★
167. Windber Hospital, Windber	★★★	NR	NR	NR	NR	NR	NR	★★★	NR	NR	NR	
168. WVHCS Hospital, Wilkes-Barre	★	★★★	★	NR	NR	★★★	★★★	★★★	★★★	★★★	★★★	★★★
169. York Hospital, York	★★★★★	★★★	★★★	★★★	★★★★★	★★★	★★★	★★★★★	★★★	★★★	★★★★★	★★★

KEY: ★★★★★ BEST   ★★★ AS EXPECTED   ★ POOR   NR NOT RATED BY HEALTHGRADES   For full definitions of ratings and awards, see Appendix.

Gastrointestinal Bleed	Gastrointestinal Surgeries and Procedures	Heart Attack	Heart Failure	Hip Fracture Repair	Maternity Care	Pancreatitis	Peripheral Vascular Bypass	Pneumonia	Prostatectomy	Pulmonary Embolism	Resection/Replacement of Abdominal Aorta	Respiratory Failure	Sepsis	Stroke	Total Hip Replacement	Total Knee Replacement	Valve Replacement	Women's Health
★★★	★★★★★	★★★★★	★★★★★	★★★	NR	★★★	★★★	★★★★★	★★★	★★★	NR	★★★★★	★★★	★★★★★	★★★	★★★	NR	NR
★★★	★★★	★★★	★★★★★	★	NR	★★★	★	★★★★★	★★★	★★★	★★★★★	★★★	★★★	★★★	★	★★★	★	NR
★★★	★★★	★★★★★	★★★	★★★	NR	★★★	NR	★★★	NR	NR	NR	★	★★★	★★★	NR	★★★	NR	NR
★★★	★★★	★★★	★★★★★	★	NR	★★★	★	★★★★★	★★★	★★★	★★★★★	★★★	★★★	★★★	★	★★★	★	NR
★★★	★★★	★★★	★★★	★★★	NR	★★★	★★★	★★★	★	★★★	NR	★★★	★★★	★★★	★★★	★	★★★	NR
★★★★★	NR	★★★	★★★★★	★★★	NR	NR	NR	★★★★★	NR	NR	NR	★★★	★★★	★★★	NR	★★★	NR	NR
★★★	★	★★★	★★★	★★★	★	NR	NR	★★★	NR	NR	NR	★★★	★★★	★★★	★★★	★★★	NR	NR
★★★	★	★★★	★★★	★★★★★	★★★★★	★★★	NR	★	★★★	★★★	NR	★★★	★	★★★	★★★★★	★★★★★	★★★★★	★★★★★
★★★	★★★	★★★	★★★	★★★★★	★★★	★★★	NR	★★★	NR	NR	NR	★★★	★★★	★★★	NR	★★★	NR	NR
★★★★★	★	★★★	★★★	★★★	★	★★★	NR	★★★	NR	★★★	NR	★★★	★★★	★★★	NR	★★★	NR	NR
★★★	★★★★★	★★★	★★★	★★★★★	★★★	★★★	NR	★★★	★★★	★★★	NR	★★★	★★★	★★★	★★★	★★★	NR	NR
★★★	★★★	★★★	★★★★★	★★★	★	★★★	★★★	★★★	★★★	★★★	★★★	★★★	★	★★★	★★★★★	★★★★★	★★★	★
★★★	★★★	★★★	★★★	★★★	★★★★★	★★★	NR	★★★	★★★	★★★	NR	★★★	★	★★★	★★★★★	★★★	★★★	★★★★★
★★★	★★★	★★★	★★★	★★★★★	★★★★★	★★★★★	★★★	★★★	★★★	★★★	★★★	★	★★★	★★★	★★★★★	★★★	★★★	★★★
★★★	★★★	★★★	★★★	★★★	★★★	NR	★★★	★★★★★	★★★	★★★	NR	★★★	★★★	★★★	★★★	★★★	★★★	★
★★★	NR	★★★	★★★	★★★	NR	NR	★★★	NR	NR	NR	★★★	★★★	★★★	NR	NR	NR	NR	NR
★★★	★★★	★★★	★★★	★★★★★	★★★★★	★★★★★	★★★	★★★	★★★	★★★	★	★★★	★★★	★★★★★	★★★	★★★	★★★	★★★
★★★	★★★★★	★★★★★	★★★	★★★★★	★★★★★	★★★	★★★	★★★	★★★	★★★	★	★★★★★	★	★★★	★★★★★	★★★★★	★★★	

RHODE ISLAND HOSPITALS: RATINGS BY PROCEDURE

Hospital	Appendectomy	Atrial Fibrillation	Back and Neck Surgery (except Spinal Fusion)	Back and Neck Surgery (Spinal Fusion)	Bariatric Surgery	Bowel Obstruction	Carotid Surgery	Cholecystectomy (Gall Bladder Removal)	Chronic Obstructive Pulmonary Disease (COPD)	Coronary Bypass Surgery	Coronary Interventional Procedures (Angioplasty/Stent)	Diabetic Acidosis
1. John Fogarty Memorial Hospital, Woonsocket	★★★	★★★	NR	NR	NR	★★★	★★★	★★★	★★★	NR	★	★★★
2. Kent County Memorial Hospital, Warwick	★★★	★★★	★★★	NR	NR	★★★	★	★★★	★	NR	NR	★★★
3. Landmark Medical Center, Woonsocket	★★★	★★★	NR	NR	NR	★★★	★★★	★★★	★★★	NR	★	★★★
4. Memorial Hospital of Rhode Island, Pawtucket	★★★	★★★	NR	NR	NR	★★★★★	★★★	★★★	★★★	NR	NR	★★★
5. Miriam Hospital, Providence	★★★	★★★	★★★	★★★	NR	★★★	★★★	★★★	★	★★★	★★★	★★★
6. Newport Hospital, Newport	★	★★★	★★★	NR	NR	★★★	★	★★★	★★★	NR	NR	NR
7. Rhode Island Hospital, Providence	★★★	★★★	★	★★★	★★★	★★★	★	★	★★★	★★★	★★★★★	★★★
8. Roger Williams Hospital, Providence	★★★	★★★	NR	★★★★★	★★★	★★★	NR	★	★★★	NR	NR	★
9. St. Joseph Health Services of Rhode Island, North Providence	★★★	★★★	★★★	★★★	NR	★★★	★★★	★★★	★★★	NR	NR	★★★
10. South County Hospital, Wakefield	★★★	★★★	NR	★★★★★	NR	★★★	★★★	★	★	NR	NR	NR
11. Westerly Hospital, Westerly	★	★★★	NR	NR	NR	★★★	NR	★	★★★	NR	NR	NR

KEY: ★★★★★ BEST   ★★★ AS EXPECTED   ★ POOR   NR NOT RATED BY HEALTHGRADES   For full definitions of ratings and awards, see Appendix.

Gastrointestinal Bleed	Gastrointestinal Surgeries and Procedures	Heart Attack	Heart Failure	Hip Fracture Repair	Maternity Care	Pancreatitis	Peripheral Vascular Bypass	Pneumonia	Prostatectomy	Pulmonary Embolism	Resection/Replacement of Abdominal Aorta	Respiratory Failure	Sepsis	Stroke	Total Hip Replacement	Total Knee Replacement	Valve Replacement	Women's Health
★★★	★★★	★★★	★	★	★★★	★★★	NR	★★★	NR	NR	NR	★★★	★★★	★★★	NR	★	NR	NR
★★★	★★★	★★★	★★★	★★★	★★★	★★★	NR	★★★	★★★	★★★	★★★★★	★★★	★★★	★★★	★★★	★★★	NR	NR
★★★	★★★	★★★	★	★	★★★	★★★	NR	★★★	NR	NR	NR	★★★	★★★	★★★	NR	★	NR	NR
★★★	★★★	★★★	★★★	★	★★★	★★★	NR	★★★	★★★	★★★	NR	★★★	★★★	★★★★★	NR	★	NR	NR
★★★	★	★★★	★★★	★★★	NR	★★★	NR	★★★	★★★	★★★	★★★	★	★	★★★	★★★	★★★	★	NR
★	★★★	★	★	★★★	★★★	★★★	NR	★★★	NR	★★★	NR	★	★★★	★	★★★	★★★	NR	NR
★★★	★★★	★★★	★★★★★	★	NR	★★★	★	★★★★★	★	★★★	★★★	★	★★★	★	★	★★★	★★★	NR
★★★	★★★	★★★	★★★	★	NR	NR	NR	★★★	NR	NR	NR	★	★	★★★	★★★	★	NR	NR
★★★	★★★	★★★	★	★★★	NR	★	NR	★★★	★★★	NR	NR	★★★	★	★★★	★★★	★★★	NR	NR
★★★	★★★	★★★	★★★	★	★★★	NR	NR	★★★	★★★	NR	NR	NR	★★★	★★★	★★★	★★★	NR	NR
★★★	★★★	★★★	★★★	★	★★★	★	NR	★★★	★	NR	NR	★★★	★★★	★	★★★	★★★	NR	NR

SOUTH CAROLINA HOSPITALS: RATINGS BY PROCEDURE

Hospital	Appendectomy	Atrial Fibrillation	Back and Neck Surgery (except Spinal Fusion)	Back and Neck Surgery (Spinal Fusion)	Bariatric Surgery	Bowel Obstruction	Carotid Surgery	Cholecystectomy (Gall Bladder Removal)	Chronic Obstructive Pulmonary Disease (COPD)	Coronary Bypass Surgery	Coronary Interventional Procedures (Angioplasty/Stent)	Diabetic Acidosis
1. Abbeville County Memorial Hospital, Abbeville	NR	***	NR	NR	NR	NR	NR	NR	***	NR	NR	NR
2. Aiken Regional Medical Center, Aiken	NR	*	***	***	NR	*	***	*****	***	***	***	*
3. Allen Bennett Memorial Hospital, Greer	NR	***	NR	NR	NR	***	NR	***	***	NR	NR	***
4. Anmed Health, Anderson	NR	***	***	***	NR	***	***	***	***	*****	*	***
5. Bamberg County Memorial Hospital, Bamberg	NR	NR	NR	NR	NR	NR	NR	NR	***	NR	NR	NR
6. Barnwell County Hospital, Barnwell	NR	NR	NR	NR	NR	NR	NR	NR	***	NR	NR	NR
7. Beaufort Memorial Hospital, Beaufort	NR	***	*****	*****	NR	***	***	*****	***	NR	NR	***
8. Bon Secours St. Francis Hospital, Charleston	NR	*	***	***	NR	***	NR	*	***	NR	NR	***
9. Cannon Memorial Hospital, Pickens	NR	***	NR	NR	NR	***	NR	***	***	NR	NR	NR
10. Carolina Pines Regional Medical Center, Hartsville	NR	***	NR	NR	NR	***	NR	***	***	NR	NR	***
11. Carolinas Hospital System, Florence	NR	***	***	***	NR	*	***	***	*	***	***	***
12. Chester Regional Medical Center, Chester	NR	***	NR	NR	NR	***	NR	NR	***	NR	NR	NR
13. Chesterfield General Hospital, Cheraw	NR	***	NR	NR	NR	*	NR	***	***	NR	NR	NR
14. Clarendon Memorial Hospital, Manning	NR	NR	NR	NR	NR	***	NR	NR	***	NR	NR	NR
15. Coastal Carolina Medical Center, Hardeeville	NR	NR	NR	NR	NR	NR	NR	NR	***	NR	NR	NR
16. Colleton Medical Center, Walterboro	NR	***	NR	NR	NR	*	NR	***	*	NR	NR	***
17. Conway Medical Center, Conway	NR	***	NR	***	NR	*	*****	***	***	NR	NR	***
18. East Cooper Regional Medical Center, Mt. Pleasant	NR	***	***	*****	NR	***	NR	***	***	NR	NR	*
19. Edgefield County Hospital, Edgefield	NR	NR	NR	NR	NR	***	NR	NR	***	NR	NR	NR
20. Fairfield Memorial Hospital, Winnsboro	NR	NR	NR	NR	NR	NR	NR	NR	***	NR	NR	NR
21. Georgetown Memorial Hospital, Georgetown	NR	***	NR	*	NR	***	***	***	*	NR	***	***
22. Grand Strand Regional Medical Center, Myrtle Beach	NR	***	***	***	NR	***	***	***	***	***	***	***
23. Greenville Memorial Hospital, Greenville	NR	*	*	*	NR	***	***	*	***	*****	***	***
24. Hampton Regional Medical Center, Varnville	NR	NR	NR	NR	NR	NR	NR	***	***	NR	NR	NR
25. Hillcrest Memorial Hospital, Simpsonville	NR	NR	NR	NR	NR	NR	NR	NR	***	NR	NR	NR
26. Hilton Head Regional Medical Center, Hilton Head Island	NR	***	NR	NR	NR	***	***	***	***	***	***	***
27. Kershaw County Medical Center, Camden	NR	***	NR	NR	NR	***	***	***	***	NR	NR	***
28. Laurens County Healthcare System, Clinton	NR	*	NR	NR	NR	NR	NR	*	***	NR	NR	***
29. Lexington Medical Center, West Columbia	NR	*	*	***	NR	*	***	***	*	NR	NR	***
30. Loris Community Hospital, Loris	NR	*	NR	NR	NR	***	NR	***	***	NR	NR	***
31. Marion County Medical Center, Marion	NR	***	NR	NR	NR	***	NR	***	***	NR	NR	***
32. Marlboro Park Hospital, Bennettsville	NR	NR	NR	NR	NR	NR	NR	***	***	NR	NR	NR
33. Mary Black Memorial Hospital, Spartanburg	NR	***	NR	NR	NR	***	***	***	***	NR	NR	***
34. McLeod Medical Center–Darlington, Darlington	NR	NR	NR	NR	NR	NR	NR	***	***	NR	NR	NR
35. McLeod Medical Center–Dillon, Dillon	NR	***	NR	NR	NR	***	NR	***	***	NR	NR	NR
36. McLeod Regional Medical Center, Florence	NR	***	***	*	NR	***	***	***	***	***	***	***
37. Medical University Hospital, Charleston	NR	***	*****	***	NR	*	*****	***	***	***	***	***
38. Newberry County Memorial Hospital, Newberry	NR	***	NR	NR	NR	***	NR	***	*	NR	NR	NR
39. Oconee Memorial Hospital, Seneca	NR	***	NR	NR	NR	***	NR	***	***	NR	NR	***
40. Palmetto Health Baptist, Columbia	NR	***	***	*	NR	***	***	***	*	NR	NR	***
41. Palmetto Health Baptist–Easley, Easley	NR	***	NR	NR	NR	***	NR	***	***	NR	NR	***
42. Palmetto Health Richland, Columbia	NR	*	***	*	NR	***	***	***	*	*	***	*
43. Piedmont Medical Center, Rock Hill	NR	*	*	***	NR	*	***	***	*****	*	***	***
44. Roper Hospital, Charleston	NR	***	*	***	NR	***	***	*	***	***	***	***
45. St. Francis Hospital, Greenville	NR	*****	***	***	NR	***	***	***	***	*****	*	***
46. Self Regional Healthcare, Greenwood	NR	*	*****	*****	NR	*	*****	*****	*	***	***	*
47. Sisters of Charity Providence Hospitals, Columbia	NR	***	***	*****	NR	***	***	***	***	NR	NR	***
48. Spartanburg Regional Medical Center, Spartanburg	NR	***	***	***	NR	***	*****	***	***	*****	***	***
49. Springs Memorial Hospital, Lancaster	NR	*	NR	NR	NR	*	NR	***	***	NR	NR	***
50. Trident Medical Center, Charleston	NR	*	*****	***	NR	***	***	*****	***	*	***	***

KEY: ***** BEST   *** AS EXPECTED   * POOR   NR NOT RATED BY HEALTHGRADES   For full definitions of ratings and awards, see Appendix.

Gastrointestinal Bleed	Gastrointestinal Surgeries and Procedures	Heart Attack	Heart Failure	Hip Fracture Repair	Maternity Care	Pancreatitis	Peripheral Vascular Bypass	Pneumonia	Prostatectomy	Pulmonary Embolism	Resection/Replacement of Abdominal Aorta	Respiratory Failure	Sepsis	Stroke	Total Hip Replacement	Total Knee Replacement	Valve Replacement	Women's Health
★★★	NR	NR	★★★	★★★	NR	NR	NR	★★★★★	NR	NR	NR	NR	★	★★★	NR	NR	NR	NR
★★★	★★★	★★★	★	★	NR	★	★★★	★	★★★	NR	NR	★★★	★★★	★★★	★★★	★★★	★★★	NR
★★★	★★★	NR	★	★★★★★	NR	★★★	NR	★★★	★★★★★	NR	NR	★	★	NR	★★★	NR	★★★	NR
★★★	★★★	★	★★★	★★★★★	NR	★★★	★★★★★	★★★★★	★★★	★★★★★	★★★	★★★★★	★★★★★	★★★	★★★	★	★★★	NR
★★★	NR	NR	★★★	NR	NR	NR	NR	★★★	NR	NR	NR	NR	★★★	NR	NR	NR	NR	NR
★★★	NR	NR	★★★	NR	NR	NR	NR	★★★	NR	NR	NR	NR	NR	NR	NR	NR	NR	NR
★★★	★★★	★	★★★	★★★	NR	★★★	NR	★★★	★★★	★★★	NR	★★★	★★★	★	NR	★★★	★★★★★	NR
★★★	★★★	★★★	★★★	★★★	NR	★★★	NR	★★★	★★★	★★★	NR	★★★	★★★	★★★	NR	★	NR	NR
★★★	NR	★★★	★	NR	NR	NR	NR	★	NR	NR	NR	NR	★★★	★	NR	★	★★★★★	NR
★★★	★	★★★	★★★	★★★	NR	★★★	NR	★	NR	★★★	NR	★★★	★	NR	★	★★★	NR	NR
★	★	★★★	★★★	★	NR	★★★	★	★★★	★★★	★	★★★	★★★	★	★	★★★	★★★	NR	NR
★★★	NR	NR	★★★	NR	NR	NR	NR	★★★	NR	NR	NR	★★★★★	★★★	NR	NR	NR	NR	NR
★★★	NR	NR	★★★★★	NR	NR	NR	NR	★★★	NR	NR	NR	★★★	★★★	NR	NR	NR	NR	NR
★★★	NR	★★★	★	NR	NR	NR	NR	★	NR	NR	NR	NR	★★★	NR	NR	NR	NR	NR
★★★	NR	NR	★★★	NR	NR	NR	NR	★★★	NR	NR	NR	NR	NR	NR	NR	NR	NR	NR
★★★	★★★	★★★	★★★	★★★	NR	★★★	NR	★★★	NR	★★★	NR	★★★	★★★	★★★	★★★	★★★	NR	NR
★	★	★★★	★	★	NR	★★★	★★★	★	★★★	★★★	NR	★	★★★	★	★	★	NR	NR
★	★★★	NR	★	★★★★★	NR	NR	NR	★	NR	NR	NR	★★★	★★★	★★★	NR	NR	NR	NR
★	NR	NR	★★★	NR	NR	NR	NR	★★★	NR	NR	NR	NR	NR	NR	NR	NR	NR	NR
★★★	NR	NR	★★★	NR	NR	NR	NR	★★★	NR	NR	NR	NR	NR	NR	NR	NR	NR	NR
★★★	★	★★★	★★★	★	NR	NR	NR	★	★★★	★★★	NR	★	★	★	★	★	NR	NR
★★★	★★★	★★★	★	★★★	NR	★★★	★★★	★★★	★★★	★★★	★★★	★★★	★★★	★	★★★	★	★★★	NR
★★★	★★★	★★★	★	★★★	NR	★★★★★	★★★	★★★	★	★★★	★★★★★	★★★	★	★	★★★	★★★	★★★★★	NR
★★★	NR	NR	★★★	NR	NR	NR	NR	★★★	NR	NR	NR	★★★	NR	NR	NR	NR	NR	NR
★★★	★★★	★★★	★★★	★★★★★	NR	NR	NR	★★★	NR	NR	NR	★★★★★	★★★★★	★★★	NR	★	NR	NR
★★★	★★★	★★★	★★★	★★★	NR	★★★	NR	★★★	★	NR	NR	★★★	★	★★★	★★★	★★★	NR	NR
★★★	★	★★★	★★★	★★★	NR	★★★	NR	★★★	NR	NR	NR	★★★	★	★★★	NR	★★★	NR	NR
★	NR	★★★	★	★★★★★	NR	★★★	NR	★	NR	NR	NR	★★★	★	★★★	NR	★★★	NR	NR
★	★	★	★	★★★	NR	★★★	★★★	★	★★★	★	★	★	★	★	★★★★★	★★★	NR	NR
★★★	★★★	★	★	★★★	NR	NR	NR	★	★★★	NR	★	★	★	★	★★★★★	★★★	NR	NR
★★★	NR	★	★★★	★★★	NR	★★★	NR	★	★★★★★	NR	NR	NR	★★★	★★★	NR	★	★★★	NR
★★★	NR	NR	★★★	NR	NR	NR	NR	★★★	NR	NR	NR	★★★	NR	NR	NR	NR	NR	NR
★★★	★★★	★★★	★★★	★★★	NR	★	★★★	★★★	★★★	★★★	★★★	★★★	★★★	NR	★★★	★★★	★★★	NR
★★★	NR	NR	★★★	NR	NR	NR	NR	★★★	NR	NR	NR	★★★★★	★★★★★	★★★	NR	NR	NR	NR
★★★	★★★	★★★	★★★	★★★	NR	★	NR	★★★	★★★	★★★	NR	★★★	★	★	★★★	★	★	NR
★★★	★★★	★★★	★★★	★★★	NR	★★★	★★★	★★★	★★★	★★★	NR	★★★	★★★	★★★	★★★	★★★	★★★	NR
★	NR	NR	★★★	★★★	NR	NR	NR	★	NR	NR	NR	NR	★	NR	NR	★★★	NR	NR
★★★	★★★	★★★	★★★	★★★★★	NR	★★★	NR	★★★★★	★	★★★	NR	★★★★★	★★★	★★★★★	★★★	★★★★★	★★★	NR
★★★	★★★	★★★	★★★	★	NR	★★★	NR	★	★★★	★★★	NR	★	★★★	★★★	★★★	★★★	★★★	NR
★★★	★★★	★	★	★★★	NR	★★★	NR	★★★	NR	★★★★★	NR	★★★	★★★	NR	NR	★★★★★	NR	NR
★	★	★★★	★	★★★	NR	★★★	★★★	★	NR	★★★	★★★	★	★	NR	★★★★★	★★★	★	NR
★	★	★	★★★	★★★★★	NR	★★★	★★★	★★★	★★★	★★★★★	★★★	★	★	NR	★★★	★★★	★★★	NR
★★★	★★★	★★★	★★★	★	NR	★★★	★★★	★★★	★★★	★★★	★★★	★	★★★	★★★	★	★	★★★	NR
★★★	★★★	★★★	★★★	★★★★★	NR	★★★	NR	★★★	★★★	★	NR	★	★★★	★★★	★★★	★★★★★	★★★	NR
★★★	★★★	★★★	★	★★★	NR	★	★★★	★★★	★★★★★	★★★	★★★	★	★★★	★★★	★★★	★★★	NR	NR
★★★	★	★	★	★★★	NR	★★★	NR	★	NR	★★★	★★★	★	★	NR	★★★★★	★★★	★★★	NR
★★★	★★★	★★★★★	★	★★★	NR	★★★	★	★	★	★★★	★★★	★★★	★★★	NR	★★★★★	★★★	★★★	NR
★★★	★★★	★★★★★	★	★★★★★	NR	★★★	NR	★★★	★★★	NR	NR	★★★	★★★	NR	NR	★★★	NR	NR
★	★★★	★	★	★★★	NR	★★★	★★★	★★★	★★★	★★★	★★★	★★★	★	★	★★★	★★★	★★★	NR

	Appendectomy	Atrial Fibrillation	Back and Neck Surgery (except Spinal Fusion)	Back and Neck Surgery (Spinal Fusion)	Bariatric Surgery	Bowel Obstruction	Carotid Surgery	Cholecystectomy (Gall Bladder Removal)	Chronic Obstructive Pulmonary Disease (COPD)	Coronary Bypass Surgery	Coronary Interventional Procedures (Angioplasty/Stent)	Diabetic Acidosis and
51. **TRMC of Orangeburg and Calhoun**, Orangeburg	NR	★★★	NR	NR	NR	★	★★★	★★★	★	NR	NR	★
52. **Tuomey Healthcare System**, Sumter	NR	★★★	NR	NR	NR	★★★	NR	★★★★★	★★★	NR	NR	★★★
53. **Upstate Carolina Medical Center**, Gaffney	NR	★★★	NR	NR	NR	★	NR	★★★	★	NR	NR	★★★
54. **Waccamaw Community Hospital**, Murrells Inlet	NR	★★★	NR	NR	NR	★★★	★★★	★★★	★★★	NR	NR	★★★
55. **Wallace Thomson Hospital**, Union	NR	★★★	NR	NR	NR	★	NR	★	★	NR	NR	★★★
56. **Williamsburg Regional Hospital**, Kingstree	NR	NR	NR	NR	NR	NR	NR	NR	NR	NR	NR	NR

KEY: ★★★★★ **BEST** ★★★ **AS EXPECTED** ★ **POOR** NR **NOT RATED BY HEALTHGRADES** For full definitions of ratings and awards, see Appendix.

Gastrointestinal Bleed	Gastrointestinal Surgeries and Procedures	Heart Attack	Heart Failure	Hip Fracture Repair	Maternity Care	Pancreatitis	Peripheral Vascular Bypass	Pneumonia	Prostatectomy	Pulmonary Embolism	Resection/Replacement of Abdominal Aorta	Respiratory Failure	Sepsis	Stroke	Total Hip Replacement	Total Knee Replacement	Valve Replacement	Women's Health
★	★★★	★★★	★	★★★	NR	★★★	NR	★	★★★	★★★	NR	★★★	★	★	NR	★★★	NR	NR
★★★	★★★	★★★	★	★★★★★	NR	★★★	NR	★	★★★	★★★	NR	★★★	★	★	★★★	★★★★★	NR	NR
★	★	★★★	★	★	NR	★★★	NR	★	★★★	NR	NR	★★★	★★★	★	NR	★★★	NR	NR
★★★	★★★	★★★	★★★	★	NR	★★★	NR	★★★	★★★	★★★	NR	★	★★★	★★★	★★★	★	NR	NR
★★★	NR	★	★	★	NR	★★★	NR	★	NR	★★★	NR	NR	★	★	NR	★	NR	NR
★★★	NR	NR	★★★	NR	NR	NR	NR	★	NR	NR	NR	NR	NR	NR	NR	NR	NR	NR

SOUTH DAKOTA HOSPITALS: RATINGS BY PROCEDURE

Hospital	Appendectomy	Atrial Fibrillation	Back and Neck Surgery (except Spinal Fusion)	Back and Neck Surgery (Spinal Fusion)	Bariatric Surgery	Bowel Obstruction	Carotid Surgery	Cholecystectomy (Gall Bladder Removal)	Chronic Obstructive Pulmonary Disease (COPD)	Coronary Bypass Surgery	Coronary Interventional Procedures (Angioplasty/Stent)	Diabetic Acidosis and C...
1. Avera Gregory Healthcare Center, Gregory	NR	NR	NR	NR	NR	NR	NR	NR	NR	NR	NR	
2. Avera Heart Hospital of South Dakota, Sioux Falls	NR	★★★★★	NR	NR	NR	NR	★★★	NR	NR	★★★★★	★★★★★	NR
3. Avera McKennan Hospital and University Health Center, Sioux Falls	NR	★★★	★★★	★★★	NR	★★★	★★★	★★★	★★★	NR	★★★	★★★
4. Avera Queen of Peace, Mitchell	NR	★★★	NR	NR	NR	★★★	NR	★★★	★★★	NR	NR	NR
5. Avera Sacred Heart Hospital, Yankton	NR	★★★	NR	NR	NR	★★★	★	★★★	★★★	NR	NR	NR
6. Avera St. Luke's, Aberdeen	NR	★★★	★★★	★★★	NR	★★★	★★★	★	★★★	NR	NR	NR
7. Brookings Hospital, Brookings	NR	NR	NR	NR	NR	★★★	NR	NR	★★★	NR	NR	NR
8. Community Memorial Hospital, Redfield	NR	NR	NR	NR	NR	NR	NR	NR	★★★	NR	NR	NR
9. Dakota Midland Hospital, Aberdeen	NR	★★★	★★★	★★★	NR	★★★	★★★	★	★★★	NR	NR	NR
10. Hand County Memorial Hospital, Miller	NR	NR	NR	NR	NR	NR	NR	NR	★★★	NR	NR	NR
11. Huron Regional Medical Center, Huron	NR	NR	NR	NR	NR	★★★	NR	NR	NR	NR	NR	NR
12. Madison Community Hospital, Madison	NR	NR	NR	NR	NR	NR	NR	NR	★★★	NR	NR	NR
13. Mid-Dakota Medical Center, Chamberlain	NR	NR	NR	NR	NR	NR	NR	NR	★★★	NR	NR	NR
14. Milbank Area Hospital—Avera Health, Milbank	NR	NR	NR	NR	NR	NR	NR	NR	NR	NR	NR	NR
15. Mobridge Regional Hospital, Mobridge	NR	NR	NR	NR	NR	NR	NR	★	NR	NR	NR	NR
16. Physicians Indian Hospital at Pine Ridge, Pine Ridge	NR	NR	NR	NR	NR	NR	NR	★★★	NR	NR	NR	NR
17. Physicians Indian Hospital, Wagner	NR	NR	NR	NR	NR	NR	NR	★★★	NR	NR	NR	NR
18. Prairie Lakes Hospital and Care Center, Watertown	NR	★★★	NR	NR	NR	★★★★★	NR	★★★	★★★	NR	NR	NR
19. Rapid City Regional Hospital, Rapid City	NR	★★★	★★★	★★★	NR	★★★	★	★★★	★	★	★★★	★★★
20. St. Mary's Hospital, Pierre	NR	★★★	★★★	NR	NR	★★★	NR	★★★	★★★	NR	NR	★★★
21. Sanford USD Medical Center, Sioux Falls	NR	★★★	★★★★★	★★★★★	NR	★★★	★★★	★★★	★★★	★★★	★★★	★★★
22. Spearfish Regional Hospital, Spearfish	NR	★★★	NR	NR	NR	★★★	NR	★★★	★	NR	NR	NR
23. Sturgis Regional Hospital, Sturgis	NR	NR	NR	NR	NR	NR	NR	★★★	NR	NR	NR	NR
24. Winner Regional Healthcare Center, Winner	NR	NR	NR	NR	NR	NR	NR	★★★	NR	NR	NR	NR

KEY: ★★★★★ BEST ★★★ AS EXPECTED ★ POOR NR NOT RATED BY HEALTHGRADES For full definitions of ratings and awards, see Appendix.

Gastrointestinal Bleed	Gastrointestinal Surgeries and Procedures	Heart Attack	Heart Failure	Hip Fracture Repair	Maternity Care	Pancreatitis	Peripheral Vascular Bypass	Pneumonia	Prostatectomy	Pulmonary Embolism	Resection/Replacement of Abdominal Aorta	Respiratory Failure	Sepsis	Stroke	Total Hip Replacement	Total Knee Replacement	Valve Replacement	Women's Health
★★★	NR	NR	★★★	NR	NR	NR	NR	★★★★★	NR	NR	NR	NR	NR	NR	NR	NR	NR	NR
NR	NR	★★★★★	★★★★★	NR	NR	NR	★★★	★★★	NR	★★★	★★★★★	NR	NR	NR	NR	NR	★★★★★	NR
★★★	★★★★★	★★★	★★★	★★★	NR	★★★	NR	★★★★★	★★★	★★★	NR	★★★★★	★★★★★	★★★★★	★★★★★	★★★★★	NR	NR
★★★	★★★	★★★	★★★	★★★	NR	NR	NR	★★★	★★★	NR	NR	★★★★★	★★★	★	★	NR	NR	NR
★★★	★★★	★★★	★	★★★	NR	★★★	NR	★★★	★	★★★	NR	★	★	★★★	★★★	★★★	NR	NR
★★★	NR	★★★	★	★★★	NR	NR	NR	★	NR	NR	NR	★★★	★★★	NR	NR	NR	NR	NR
NR	NR	NR	★★★	NR	NR	NR	NR	★★★	NR	NR	NR	NR	NR	NR	NR	NR	NR	NR
★★★	★★★	★★★	★	★★★	NR	★★★	NR	★★★	★	★★★	NR	★	★	★★★	★★★	★★★	NR	NR
NR	NR	NR	★★★	NR	NR	NR	NR	★★★★★	NR	NR	NR	NR	NR	NR	NR	NR	NR	NR
★★★	NR	★★★	★	★★★	NR	NR	NR	★★★	NR	NR	NR	★	NR	★★★	★★★	★★★	NR	NR
★★★	NR	NR	NR	NR	NR	NR	NR	★★★	NR	NR	NR	NR	NR	★★★	NR	NR	NR	NR
NR	NR	NR	★★★	NR	NR	NR	NR	★★★	NR	NR	NR	NR	NR	NR	NR	NR	NR	NR
NR	NR	NR	★★★	NR	NR	NR	NR	★	NR	NR	NR	★	NR	NR	NR	NR	NR	NR
★★★	NR	NR	★	NR	NR	NR	NR	★★★	NR	NR	NR	NR	NR	NR	NR	NR	NR	NR
NR	NR	NR	★★★	NR	NR	NR	NR	★★★	NR	NR	NR	NR	NR	NR	NR	NR	NR	NR
NR	NR	NR	★★★	NR	NR	NR	NR	★★★	NR	NR	NR	NR	NR	NR	NR	NR	NR	NR
★★★	★★★	★★★	★★★	★★★	NR	★★★	NR	★★★	★★★	NR	NR	★	★★★	★★★★★	★★★★★	NR	NR	NR
★	★★★	★★★	★★★	★★★★★	NR	★★★	★★★	★	★★★	★★★	★★★	★	★★★	★	★★★	★★★	★★★	NR
★★★	NR	NR	★	★★★	NR	NR	NR	★★★★★	NR	NR	NR	★★★★★	★★★	★★★	★★★	NR	NR	NR
★★★★★	★★★★★	★★★★★	★★★	★★★	NR	★★★	★★★★★	★★★	★	★★★	★★★★★	★★★★★	★	★★★	★★★★★	★★★★★	★★★★★	NR
★★★	NR	NR	★	★★★	NR	NR	NR	★★★	NR	NR	NR	★★★	★★★	★★★	NR	NR	NR	NR
★★★	NR	★★★	NR	NR	NR	NR	NR	★★★	NR	NR	NR	NR	NR	★★★	NR	NR	NR	NR
★★★	NR	NR	★	★★★	NR	NR	NR	★★★	NR	NR	NR	NR	NR	NR	NR	NR	NR	NR

TENNESSEE HOSPITALS: RATINGS BY PROCEDURE

	Appendectomy	Atrial Fibrillation	Back and Neck Surgery (except Spinal Fusion)	Back and Neck Surgery (Spinal Fusion)	Bariatric Surgery	Bowel Obstruction	Carotid Surgery	Cholecystectomy (Gall Bladder Removal)	Chronic Obstructive Pulmonary Disease (COPD)	Coronary Bypass Surgery	Coronary Interventional Procedures (Angioplasty/Stent)	Diabetic Acidosis and...
1. Athens Regional Medical Center, Athens	NR	★★★	NR	NR	NR	★★★	NR	★★★	★	NR	NR	NR
2. Baptist Hospital of Cocke County, Newport	NR	NR	NR	NR	NR	NR	NR	NR	★★★	NR	NR	NR
3. Baptist Hospital of East Tennessee, Knoxville	NR	★★★★★	NR	NR	NR	★★★	★★★	★★★	★★★★★	★★★	★★★	★★★
4. Baptist Hospital West, Knoxville	NR	★★★	★★★	★★★★★	NR	★★★	★★★	★★★	★	NR	★	NR
5. Baptist Hospital, Nashville	NR	★★★	★★★	★	NR	★★★	★★★	★★★	★★★	★★★	★★★★★	★★★
6. Baptist Memorial Hospital, Memphis	NR	★★★	★★★★★	★★★	NR	★★★	★★★★★	★★★★★	★	★★★★★	★	★★★
7. Baptist Memorial Hospital–Collierville, Collierville	NR	★	★	★★★	NR	★★★	NR	NR	★★★	NR	NR	NR
8. Baptist Memorial Hospital–Huntingdon, Huntingdon	NR	NR	NR	NR	NR	★	NR	NR	★★★	NR	NR	NR
9. Baptist Memorial Hospital–Lauderdale, Ripley	NR	NR	NR	NR	NR	NR	NR	NR	★★★	NR	NR	NR
10. Baptist Memorial Hospital–Tipton, Covington	NR	NR	NR	NR	NR	NR	NR	NR	★★★	NR	NR	NR
11. Baptist Memorial Hospital–Union City, Union City	NR	★★★	NR	NR	NR	★★★	NR	★★★	★★★	NR	NR	NR
12. Bedford County Medical Center, Shelbyville	NR	★★★	NR	NR	NR	★★★	★★★	NR	★★★	NR	NR	NR
13. Bledsoe County Hospital, Pikeville	NR	NR	NR	NR	NR	NR	NR	NR	★★★	NR	NR	NR
14. Blount Memorial Hospital, Maryville	NR	★★★★★	★★★	NR	NR	★★★	★★★★★	★★★	★★★	NR	★★★	★★★
15. Bolivar General Hospital, Bolivar	NR	NR	NR	NR	NR	NR	NR	NR	★	NR	NR	NR
16. Bradley Memorial Hospital, Cleveland	NR	★	NR	NR	NR	★★★	★★★	★★★	★★★	NR	NR	NR
17. Camden General Hospital, Camden	NR	NR	NR	NR	NR	NR	NR	NR	★★★	NR	NR	NR
18. Carthage General Hospital, Carthage	NR	NR	NR	NR	NR	NR	NR	NR	★★★	NR	NR	NR
19. Centennial Medical Center, Nashville	NR	★★★	★★★	★★★★★	NR	★★★	★★★★★	★★★	★★★	★★★	★★★	★
20. Claiborne County Hospital, Tazewell	NR	★★★	NR	NR	NR	★★★	NR	★★★	★★★	NR	NR	NR
21. Cleveland Community Hospital, Cleveland	NR	★★★	NR	NR	NR	★★★	NR	★	★★★	★★★★★	NR	NR
22. Cookeville Regional Medical Center, Cookeville	NR	★★★	★★★★★	★★★★★	NR	★★★	★★★★★	★★★★★	★★★★★	★★★	★★★	★★★
23. Copper Basin Medical Center, Copperhill	NR	NR	NR	NR	NR	NR	NR	NR	NR	NR	NR	NR
24. Crockett Hospital, Lawrenceburg	NR	★★★	NR	NR	NR	NR	NR	★★★	★★★	NR	NR	NR
25. Cumberland Medical Center, Crossville	NR	★★★★★	NR	NR	NR	★★★	NR	★★★	★★★	NR	★	NR
26. Cumberland River Hospital, Celina	NR	NR	NR	NR	NR	★★★	NR	NR	★★★	NR	NR	NR
27. Decatur County General Hospital, Parsons	NR	NR	NR	NR	NR	★★★	NR	NR	NR	NR	NR	NR
28. Dekalb Hospital, Smithville	NR	NR	NR	NR	NR	NR	NR	NR	★★★	NR	NR	NR
29. Delta Medical Center, Memphis	NR	NR	NR	NR	NR	NR	NR	NR	★	NR	NR	NR
30. Dyersburg Regional Medical Center, Dyersburg	NR	★★★	NR	NR	NR	★★★	NR	★★★	★★★	NR	NR	★★★
31. Erlanger Bledsoe Hospital, Pikeville	NR	NR	NR	NR	NR	NR	NR	NR	★★★	NR	NR	NR
32. Erlanger Medical Center, Chattanooga	NR	★★★	★★★	★★★	NR	★★★	★★★	★★★	★★★	★	★★★	★★★★★
33. Fort Loudoun Medical Center, Lenoir City	NR	NR	NR	NR	NR	NR	NR	NR	★★★	NR	NR	NR
34. Fort Sanders Regional Medical Center, Knoxville	NR	★★★	★	★	NR	★★★	★★★	★★★	★★★	★★★	★	★★★
35. Fort Sanders Sevier Medical Center, Sevierville	NR	★★★	NR	NR	NR	★	NR	★★★	★★★	NR	NR	NR
36. Gateway Medical Center, Clarksville	NR	★★★	NR	NR	NR	★★★	★★★	★	★★★	NR	★★★	★★★
37. Germantown Community Hospital, Germantown	NR	★	★★★★★	★★★★★	NR	★	★★★	★★★	★	★	★★★	★★★
38. Gibson General Hospital, Trenton	NR	NR	NR	NR	NR	★★★	NR	NR	★	NR	NR	NR
39. Grandview Medical Center, Jasper	NR	NR	NR	NR	NR	★★★	NR	NR	★★★	NR	NR	NR
40. Hardin Medical Center, Savannah	NR	NR	NR	NR	NR	★★★	NR	NR	★★★	NR	NR	NR
41. Harton Regional Medical Center, Tullahoma	NR	★★★	★★★★★	★★★	NR	★	★★★	★	★★★	NR	★★★	★★★
42. Haywood Park Community Hospital, Brownsville	NR	NR	NR	NR	NR	NR	NR	★★★★★	NR	NR	NR	NR
43. HealthSouth Chattanooga Rehab Hospital, Chattanooga	NR	NR	NR	NR	NR	NR	NR	★★★	NR	NR	NR	NR
44. Henderson County Community Hospital, Lexington	NR	NR	NR	NR	NR	★★★	NR	★	NR	NR	NR	NR
45. Hendersonville Medical Center, Hendersonville	NR	★★★	NR	NR	NR	★★★	★	★★★	★★★	NR	★★★	NR
46. Henry County Medical Center, Paris	NR	★	NR	NR	NR	★★★	★	★★★	★★★	NR	NR	NR
47. Hickman Community Health Services, Centerville	NR	NR	NR	NR	NR	NR	NR	NR	★★★	NR	NR	NR
48. Hillside Hospital, Pulaski	NR	★	NR	NR	NR	★★★	NR	★★★★★	★★★	NR	NR	NR
49. Horizon Medical Center, Dickson	NR	★★★	NR	NR	NR	★★★	NR	★★★	★★★	NR	★★★	NR
50. Humboldt General Hospital, Humboldt	NR	NR	NR	NR	NR	NR	NR	NR	★★★	NR	NR	NR

KEY: ★★★★★ BEST   ★★★ AS EXPECTED   ★ POOR   NR NOT RATED BY HEALTHGRADES   For full definitions of ratings and awards, see Appendix.

Gastrointestinal Bleed	Gastrointestinal Surgeries and Procedures	Heart Attack	Heart Failure	Hip Fracture Repair	Maternity Care	Pancreatitis	Peripheral Vascular Bypass	Pneumonia	Prostatectomy	Pulmonary Embolism	Resection/Replacement of Abdominal Aorta	Respiratory Failure	Sepsis	Stroke	Total Hip Replacement	Total Knee Replacement	Valve Replacement	Women's Health
★★★	NR	★★★	★	★★★	NR	NR	NR	★	NR	NR	NR	★★★	★	★	NR	NR	NR	NR
★★★	NR	★★★	★★★	NR	NR	NR	NR	★★★	NR	NR	NR	★★★	★★★★★	★★★	NR	NR	NR	NR
★★★	★★★	★★★	★★★	★★★	NR	★★★	NR	★★★	★★★★★	★★★	★	★★★	★★★★★	★	NR	★★★★★	★★★	NR
★★★	★★★	★★★	★★★	★★★★★	NR	NR	NR	★★★	NR	NR	NR	★★★	★★★	★★★	NR	★★★	NR	NR
★★★	★★★	★★★	★★★	★★★	NR	★★★	★★★★★	★★★★★	★★★	NR	★★★	★★★	★★★	★★★	★★★	★★★★★	★★★	NR
★★★	★★★★★	★	★	★★★	NR	★★★	★★★	★★★	★★★	NR	★★★	★★★	★★★	★★★★★	★★★	★★★	★★★	NR
★★★	NR	★	★★★	★★★	NR	★★★	NR	★★★	★★★	NR	★★★★★	NR	★★★	★★★	★★★	★★★	NR	NR
★★★	NR	★★★	★★★	★★★	NR	NR	NR	★★★	NR	NR	NR	★★★	★★★	NR	NR	NR	NR	NR
NR	NR	NR	★★★	NR	NR	NR	NR	★★★	NR	NR	NR	★★★	NR	NR	NR	NR	NR	NR
★★★	NR	★★★	★★★	NR	NR	NR	NR	★★★	★★★	NR	NR	NR	★★★	★	NR	NR	NR	NR
★	NR	★	★	★	NR	★	NR	★	NR	★	NR	★	★	★	NR	★★★	NR	NR
★★★	NR	NR	★	★★★	NR	NR	NR	★	NR	NR	NR	★	★★★	★★★	NR	NR	NR	NR
NR	NR	NR	★	NR	NR	NR	NR	★★★	NR	NR	NR	NR	NR	★★★	NR	NR	NR	NR
★★★	★★★	★★★	★★★	★★★★★	NR	★★★	NR	★★★	★★★	★★★	NR	★	NR	★	★★★	★★★	NR	NR
NR	★★★	NR	★	NR	NR	NR	NR	★	NR	NR	NR	NR	★★★	NR	NR	NR	NR	NR
★★★	★★★	★	★★★	★★★	NR	★★★	NR	★	★★★	★★★	NR	★	NR	★	★★★	★★★	NR	NR
NR	NR	NR	★	★	NR	NR	NR	★	NR	NR	NR	★	★★★	NR	NR	NR	NR	NR
★★★	NR	NR	★★★	NR	NR	NR	NR	★★★	NR	NR	NR	★★★	★★★	NR	NR	NR	NR	NR
★★★	★★★★★	★	★★★	★★★	NR	★★★★★	★★★	★★★	★★★★★	★★★	★★★	★★★	★★★★★	★★★	★★★	★★★★★	★★★	NR
★★★	NR	★★★	★★★	★	NR	★★★	NR	★★★	NR	NR	NR	★★★	★★★	NR	NR	NR	NR	NR
★★★	NR	★★★	★★★	★★★	NR	NR	NR	★★★	NR	NR	NR	★★★	★★★	★★★	NR	★	NR	NR
★★★	★	★★★	★★★	★★★	NR	★★★	★★★	★★★	★★★	★★★★★	NR	★★★	★	★★★★★	★★★	★★★	★★★	NR
NR	NR	NR	★★★★★	NR	NR	NR	NR	★★★★★	NR	NR	NR	NR	NR	NR	NR	NR	NR	NR
NR	NR	NR	★	NR	NR	NR	NR	★	NR	NR	NR	NR	★★★	★★★	NR	NR	NR	NR
★★★	NR	NR	★	★★★	NR	NR	NR	★★★★★	NR	NR	NR	★★★	NR	★	NR	★	NR	NR
★	NR	NR	★★★	NR	NR	NR	NR	★	NR	NR	NR	★	NR	NR	NR	★★★★★	NR	NR
★★★	★★★	★★★	★★★	★★★	NR	★★★	NR	★★★	NR	NR	NR	★★★	★	NR	NR	NR	NR	NR
NR	NR	NR	★	NR	NR	NR	NR	★★★	NR	NR	NR	NR	NR	NR	NR	NR	NR	NR
★★★	★★★	★★★	★★★	★★★	NR	★★★★★	★★★	★★★	★★★	★★★	★★★	★★★	★★★	★★★★★	★★★	★★★	★★★	NR
★★★	NR	★★★	★★★	NR	NR	NR	NR	★★★★★	NR	NR	NR	★★★	★★★	★★★	NR	NR	NR	NR
★★★	★★★	★★★	★★★	★★★	NR	★	NR	★	★★★	★★★★★	NR	★★★	★★★	★★★	NR	★	NR	NR
★★★	★★★	★★★	★	★★★	NR	NR	NR	★★★	NR	NR	NR	NR	NR	★★★	NR	★★★	NR	NR
★★★	★	★	★★★	★★★	NR	★★★	NR	★★★	★★★	★	NR	★	★	★★★	★★★	★★★	NR	NR
★★★	★	★	★	★★★★★	NR	★★★	★★★	★	★★★	★★★	★★★	★	★	★	★★★★★	★★★★★	★★★	NR
★	NR	NR	★	NR	NR	NR	NR	★	NR	NR	NR	NR	★	NR	NR	NR	NR	NR
★★★	NR	NR	★★★	★★★	NR	NR	NR	★★★	NR	NR	NR	★★★	NR	NR	NR	NR	NR	NR
★★★	NR	NR	★	★★★	NR	NR	NR	★	NR	NR	NR	★	★	NR	NR	NR	NR	NR
★★★	★	★★★	★	★★★	NR	★★★	NR	★	★★★	★★★	NR	★★★	★	NR	NR	★★★	NR	NR
NR	NR	NR	★★★	NR	NR	NR	NR	★	NR	NR	NR	NR	NR	NR	NR	NR	NR	NR
NR	NR	NR	★★★	NR	NR	NR	NR	★★★★★	NR	NR	NR	NR	NR	NR	NR	NR	NR	NR
★★★	NR	NR	★	NR	NR	NR	NR	★	NR	NR	NR	★	NR	NR	NR	NR	NR	NR
★★★	★★★	★★★	★★★	★★★	NR	★★★	NR	★★★	NR	★	NR	★★★	★★★	★★★	NR	★	NR	NR
★	★	★★★	★	★★★	NR	★★★	NR	★	★★★	NR	NR	★★★	★	NR	★	★★★	NR	NR
NR	NR	NR	★★★	NR	NR	NR	NR	★★★	NR	NR	NR	NR	NR	NR	NR	NR	NR	NR
★★★	★★★	★★★	★★★	★★★	NR	★★★	NR	★★★	NR	NR	NR	★★★	★★★	NR	NR	NR	NR	NR
★★★	★★★	★★★	★★★	★★★	NR	NR	NR	★★★★★	NR	NR	NR	★★★	★★★	★★★	NR	★★★	NR	NR
★★★	NR	NR	★	NR	NR	NR	NR	★	NR	NR	NR	★	NR	★	NR	NR	NR	NR

	Appendectomy	Atrial Fibrillation	Back and Neck Surgery (except Spinal Fusion)	Back and Neck Surgery (Spinal Fusion)	Bariatric Surgery	Bowel Obstruction	Carotid Surgery	Cholecystectomy (Gall Bladder Removal)	Chronic Obstructive Pulmonary Disease (COPD)	Coronary Bypass Surgery	Coronary Interventional Procedures (Angioplasty/Stent)	Diabetic Acidosis a...
51. Indian Path Medical Center, Kingsport	NR	★★★	★★★	NR	NR	★★★	NR	★★★	★★★	NR	NR	NR
52. Jackson-Madison County General Hospital, Jackson	NR	★★★	★	★	NR	★★★	★	★	★★★	★★★	★★★	★★★
53. Jamestown Regional Medical Center, Jamestown	NR	★★★	NR	NR	NR	★★★	NR	★★★	★★★	NR	NR	
54. Jellico Community Hospital, Jellico	NR	NR	NR	NR	NR	NR	NR	★★★	NR	NR	NR	
55. Johnson City Medical Center, Johnson City	NR	★	★★★	★★★	NR	★	★★★★★	★★★	★★★★★	★★★	★★★	★★★
56. Lakeway Regional Hospital, Morristown	NR	★★★	NR	NR	NR	★★★	NR	★★★	★★★	NR	NR	★★★
57. Laughlin Memorial Hospital, Greeneville	NR	★★★	NR	NR	NR	★★★	★★★	★★★	★	NR	NR	★★★
58. Lincoln Medical Center, Fayetteville	NR	NR	NR	NR	NR	★★★	NR	★★★	★★★	NR	NR	★★★
59. Livingston Regional Hospital, Livingston	NR	★★★	NR	NR	NR	★★★	NR	★★★	★★★	NR	NR	
60. Macon County General Hospital, Lafayette	NR	NR	NR	NR	NR	NR	NR	★★★	NR	NR	NR	
61. Marshall Medical Center, Lewisburg	NR	NR	NR	NR	NR	NR	NR	★★★	NR	NR	NR	
62. Maury Regional Hospital, Columbia	NR	★★★	NR	★★★	NR	★★★	★★★	★★★	★★★	★★★	★★★	★★★
63. McKenzie Regional Hospital, McKenzie	NR	NR	NR	NR	NR	★★★	NR	★★★	★★★	NR	NR	
64. McNairy Regional Hospital, Selmer	NR	NR	NR	NR	NR	★★★	NR	★★★	★★★	NR	NR	
65. Medical Center of Manchester, Manchester	NR	NR	NR	NR	NR	NR	NR	★★★★★	NR	NR		
66. Memorial Healthcare System, Chattanooga	NR	★★★	★★★	★★★	NR	★★★★★	★★★	★★★★★	★★★	★★★	★★★	★★★
67. Methodist Healthcare Fayette Hospital, Somerville	NR	NR	NR	NR	NR	NR	NR	★★★	NR	NR		
68. Methodist Healthcare Memphis Hospitals, Memphis	NR	★	★★★★★	★★★★★	NR	★	★★★	★★★	★	★	★★★	★★★
69. Methodist Medical Center of Oak Ridge, Oak Ridge	NR	★★★	★★★	★★★	NR	★★★	★★★★★	★★★	★★★	★★★	★	★★★
70. Metro Nashville General Hospital, Nashville	NR	NR	NR	NR	NR	NR	NR	★★★	★★★	NR	NR	
71. Middle Tennessee Medical Center, Murfreesboro	NR	★★★	★★★	★★★★★	NR	★	★★★	★★★	★★★	NR	NR	★★★
72. Milan General Hospital, Milan	NR	NR	NR	NR	NR	★★★	NR	NR	★	NR	NR	
73. Morristown-Hamblen Healthcare System, Morristown	NR	★★★	NR	NR	NR	★★★	★★★	★★★	★★★	NR	★★★	★★★
74. NorthCrest Medical Center, Springfield	NR	★★★	NR	NR	NR	★★★	NR	★★★	★★★	NR	★★★	★★★
75. Northside Hospital, Johnson City	NR	NR	NR	NR	NR	NR	NR	★★★	★★★	NR	NR	
76. Parkridge Medical Center, Chattanooga	NR	★★★	NR	★★★	NR	★	★★★	★★★	★★★	★	★	★★★
77. Parkwest Medical Center, Knoxville	NR	★★★	★★★	★★★	NR	★★★	★★★	★★★	★★★	★★★	★★★★★	★★★
78. Regional Hospital of Jackson, Jackson	NR	★	★★★★★	NR	NR	★★★	★	★★★	★★★	NR	★★★	NR
79. Regional Medical Center at Memphis, Memphis	NR	NR	NR	NR	NR	★★★	NR	NR	★★★	NR	NR	
80. Rhea Medical Center, Dayton	NR	NR	NR	NR	NR	★★★	NR	NR	★★★	NR	NR	
81. River Park Hospital, McMinnville	NR	★★★	NR	NR	NR	★★★	NR	★★★★★	★★★★★	NR	NR	
82. Roane Medical Center, Harriman	NR	★	NR	NR	NR	★★★	NR	★★★	★★★★★	NR	NR	★★★
83. St. Francis Hospital, Memphis	NR	★★★	★	★★★	NR	★	★★★	★★★	★	★★★	★★★	★★★
84. St. Francis Hospital–Bartlett, Bartlett	NR	NR	NR	NR	NR	★★★	NR	NR	★★★	NR	NR	
85. St. Mary's Jefferson Memorial Hospital, Jefferson City	NR	★★★	NR	NR	NR	★★★	NR	★★★	★★★	NR	NR	
86. St. Mary's Medical Center of Campbell County, La Follette	NR	★★★	NR	NR	NR	NR	NR	NR	★★★★★	NR	NR	
87. St. Mary's Medical Center, Knoxville	NR	★★★	★★★	★★★★★	NR	★★★	★★★	★★★	★★★★★	★★★	★★★	★★★
88. St. Thomas Hospital, Nashville	NR	★★★	★★★★★	★★★★★	NR	★★★	★★★★★	★★★★★	★	★★★	★★★	★★★
89. Scott County Hospital, Oneida	NR	★★★	NR	NR	NR	NR	NR	★★★	★★★	NR	NR	
90. Select Specialty Hospital–Tricities, Bristol	NR	★★★	★★★	★	NR	★	★★★	★★★	★★★★★	★★★	★★★	★★★
91. Skyline Madison Campus, Madison	NR	★★★	NR	NR	NR	★★★	NR	★★★	★★★★★	NR	NR	★★★
92. Skyline Medical Center, Nashville	NR	★★★	★★★★★	★★★	NR	★★★	★★★★★	★★★★★	★★★	NR	★★★	★★★
93. Smith County Memorial Hospital, Carthage	NR	NR	NR	NR	NR	★★★	NR	★★★	★★★	NR	NR	
94. Southern Hills Medical Center, Nashville	NR	★★★	NR	★★★	NR	★	★★★	★★★	★★★	NR	★★★	★★★
95. Southern Tennessee Medical Center, Winchester	NR	★★★	NR	NR	NR	★★★	NR	★★★	★★★	★	NR	★★★
96. Stonecrest Medical Center, Smyrna	NR	NR	NR	NR	NR	★★★	NR	★★★	★★★	NR	NR	★★★
97. Stones River Hospital, Woodbury	NR	NR	NR	NR	NR	NR	NR	★★★	★★★	NR	NR	
98. Summit Medical Center, Hermitage	NR	★★★	★	★	NR	★★★	★	★★★	★★★	NR	★★★	★★★
99. Sumner Regional Medical Center, Gallatin	NR	★★★	NR	NR	NR	★★★	NR	★★★★★	★★★	NR	NR	
100. Sweetwater Hospital Association, Sweetwater	NR	NR	NR	NR	NR	★★★	NR	★★★	★★★	NR	NR	

KEY: ★★★★★ BEST   ★★★ AS EXPECTED   ★ POOR   NR NOT RATED BY HEALTHGRADES   For full definitions of ratings and awards, see Appendix.

Gastrointestinal Bleed	Gastrointestinal Surgeries and Procedures	Heart Attack	Heart Failure	Hip Fracture Repair	Maternity Care	Pancreatitis	Peripheral Vascular Bypass	Pneumonia	Prostatectomy	Pulmonary Embolism	Resection/Replacement of Abdominal Aorta	Respiratory Failure	Sepsis	Stroke	Total Hip Replacement	Total Knee Replacement	Valve Replacement	Women's Health
★★★	★★★	★★★	★★★	★★★★★	NR	★★★	NR	★★★	★★★	NR	NR	★★★	★★★	★★★	★★★	★★★	NR	NR
★★★	★★★	★	★	★	NR	★★★	★★★	★	★	★★★	★★★	★★★	★★★	★★★	★	★	★★★	NR
★★★	NR	★★★	★★★	NR	NR	NR	NR	★★★	NR	NR	NR	★★★★★	★	NR	NR	NR	NR	NR
★★★	NR	★★★	★★★	NR	NR	NR	NR	★★★	NR	NR	NR	★★★★★	★★★	NR	NR	NR	NR	NR
★★★	★	★	★	★★★	NR	★	★★★	★	★★★	★★★★★	★★★	★	★	★	★★★	★★★	★★★	NR
★★★	NR	★★★	★★★	★	NR	★★★	NR	★★★★★	★★★	NR	NR	★★★	★	★★★	★★★	★★★	★★★	NR
★	NR	★	★	★★★	NR	★★★	NR	★	NR	★	NR	★★★	★★★	★	★	★★★	★★★	NR
★★★	NR	★★★	★	★★★	NR	★★★	NR	★★★	NR	NR	NR	★★★	NR	★	NR	NR	NR	NR
NR	NR	★★★★★	★★★	★★★	NR	NR	NR	★★★	NR	NR	NR	NR	NR	★★★	NR	NR	NR	NR
★★★	NR	NR	★★★	★★★	NR	NR	NR	★★★	NR	NR	NR	NR	NR	★★★	NR	NR	NR	NR
★★★	★★★	★★★	★★★	★★★★★	NR	★★★	NR	★★★	★★★	★★★	NR	★★★	★	★★★	★★★	★★★	★★★	NR
★	NR	★★★	★	★★★	NR	★★★	NR	★★★	NR	NR	NR	★	★	★★★	NR	NR	NR	NR
★★★	NR	NR	★★★	NR	NR	★	NR	★★★★★	NR	NR	NR	NR	NR	NR	NR	NR	NR	NR
★★★★★	★★★★★	★★★★★	★★★★★	★★★	NR	★★★	★★★★★	★★★★★	★★★	★★★	★★★	★★★★★	★★★★★	★★★★★	★★★★★	★★★★★	★★★★★	NR
NR	NR	NR	★	NR	NR	NR	★	NR	NR	NR	NR	NR	★★★	NR	NR	NR	NR	NR
★★★	NR	★	★	★★★★★	NR	★★★	★★★	★	★★★	★★★	★★★	★	★	★	★★★★★	★★★★★	★★★	NR
★★★	★	★★★	★★★	★★★★★	NR	★★★	★★★	★★★	★★★	★★★	★★★	★★★★★	★★★★★	★★★	★★★★★	★★★★★	★	NR
NR	NR	NR	★★★	NR	NR	NR	NR	★	NR	NR	NR	NR	★	NR	NR	NR	NR	NR
★	★★★	★	★	★★★	NR	★★★	★★★	★	★★★	★★★	NR	★★★	★	★★★	★★★	NR	NR	NR
★	★	NR	★★★	NR	NR	★★★	NR	★	NR	NR	NR	NR	★★★	NR	NR	NR	NR	NR
★★★	★★★	★	★★★	★★★	NR	★★★	NR	★★★	★★★	★★★	NR	★★★	NR	★★★	★	NR	NR	NR
★	★★★	★★★	★★★	★★★★★	NR	★★★	NR	★★★	NR	★★★	NR	★★★★★	NR	★★★	★★★	NR	NR	NR
NR	NR	NR	★★★	NR	NR	NR	NR	★	NR	NR	NR	★	NR	NR	NR	NR	NR	NR
★	★★★	★	★★★	★★★	NR	★★★	NR	★	★★★	★	NR	★★★★★	★★★	★★★	★★★	★★★	★★★	NR
★★★	★★★	★★★★★	★★★★★	★★★★★	NR	★★★	NR	★★★	★★★	★★★★★	★★★	★★★	★	★★★	★★★	★★★	★★★	NR
★★★	★★★	★	★★★	★★★	NR	★★★	NR	★★★	NR	★★★	NR	★★★	★★★	NR	★★★	★★★	NR	NR
★★★	NR	NR	★★★	★	NR	NR	NR	★★★	NR	NR	NR	★★★	★	★★★	NR	NR	NR	NR
★★★	NR	NR	★★★	NR	NR	NR	NR	★★★	NR	NR	NR	NR	NR	★★★	NR	NR	NR	NR
★★★	NR	★★★	★★★	★★★	NR	NR	NR	★	NR	★★★	NR	★	★★★	★	★★★	★★★	NR	NR
★★★	★★★	★★★	★★★★★	★	NR	★★★	NR	★★★★★	NR	NR	NR	★★★	★★★	★★★	NR	NR	NR	NR
★	★★★★★	★	★	★★★	NR	★★★	★★★	★	★★★	★★★	★★★	★	★	★	★★★	★★★	★★★	NR
★★★	NR	NR	★★★	★★★	NR	NR	NR	★★★	NR	NR	NR	★★★	★★★	★★★	NR	NR	NR	NR
★★★	NR	★★★	★★★	★★★	NR	NR	NR	★★★	NR	★★★	NR	★	★★★	★★★	NR	★★★	NR	NR
★★★	NR	★★★	★★★	NR	NR	★★★	NR	★★★★★	NR	NR	NR	★★★	★★★	NR	NR	NR	NR	NR
★★★★★	★★★	★★★	★★★	★★★★★	NR	★★★	NR	★★★★★	★★★	★★★	★★★	★★★	★	★★★★★	★★★★★	★★★	NR	NR
★★★	★★★	★★★	★★★	★★★	NR	★★★	★★★	★★★★★	★★★★★	★★★	★★★	★★★	NR	★★★	★★★★★	★★★	NR	NR
★★★	NR	NR	★★★	★★★	NR	NR	NR	★	NR	NR	NR	★★★★★	★★★	NR	NR	NR	NR	NR
★★★★★	★★★	★★★	★★★	★	NR	★★★★★	NR	★★★	NR	★★★	★★★	★	★★★	★★★	★	★	NR	NR
★★★	NR	NR	★★★	★★★	NR	NR	NR	★★★	NR	NR	NR	★★★	★★★	★★★	NR	★★★	NR	NR
★★★	★★★	★★★★★	★★★	★★★	NR	★★★	★★★★★	★★★	★★★	NR	★★★	★★★★★	★★★	★★★	★★★	NR	NR	NR
★★★	NR	NR	★★★	NR	NR	NR	NR	★★★★★	NR	NR	NR	NR	NR	★★★	NR	NR	NR	NR
★★★	NR	★	★★★	★★★	NR	NR	NR	★★★	★★★	NR	NR	★★★	★★★	★★★	NR	NR	NR	NR
★★★	★	★★★★★	★★★	★★★	NR	★★★	NR	★	NR	NR	NR	★★★	★	★★★	NR	★★★	NR	NR
NR	NR	★	NR	NR	NR	NR	NR	★★★	NR	NR	NR	★★★	NR	★★★	NR	NR	NR	NR
★★★	★★★	★★★	★★★	★	NR	★★★	NR	★★★★★	★★★	NR	NR	★★★	★	★★★	NR	★★★	NR	NR
★★★	★★★	★★★	★★★	★★★★★	NR	★★★	NR	★★★	★★★	★★★	NR	★★★	NR	★★★	NR	★★★	NR	NR
★★★	NR	★★★	★★★	★★★	NR	NR	NR	★★★	NR	NR	NR	★★★	★	★★★	NR	NR	NR	NR

	Appendectomy	Atrial Fibrillation	Back and Neck Surgery (except Spinal Fusion)	Back and Neck Surgery (Spinal Fusion)	Bariatric Surgery	Bowel Obstruction	Carotid Surgery	Cholecystectomy (Gall Bladder Removal)	Chronic Obstructive Pulmonary Disease (COPD)	Coronary Bypass Surgery	Coronary Interventional Procedures (Angioplasty/Stent)	Diabetic Acidosis an...
101. **Sycamore Shoals Hospital,** Elizabethton	NR	★★★	NR	NR	NR	★★★	NR	★★★	★★★	NR	NR	NR
102. **Takoma Adventist Hospital,** Greeneville	NR	★★★	NR	NR	NR	★★★	NR	★★★	★★★	NR	NR	NR
103. **Three Rivers Hospital,** Waverly	NR	NR	NR	NR	NR	NR	NR	NR	★★★	NR	NR	NR
104. **Trinity Hospital,** Erin	NR	★★★	NR	NR	NR	★★★	NR	NR	★★★	NR	NR	NR
105. **Trousdale Medical Center,** Hartsville	NR	NR	NR	NR	NR	NR	NR	NR	★★★	NR	NR	NR
106. **Unicoi County Memorial Hospital,** Erwin	NR	NR	NR	NR	NR	★★★	NR	NR	★★★	NR	NR	NR
107. **United Regional Medical Center,** Manchester	NR	NR	NR	NR	NR	NR	NR	NR	★★★	NR	NR	NR
108. **University Medical Center,** Lebanon	NR	★	NR	NR	NR	★★★	★★★	★★★	★	NR	NR	NR
109. **University of Tennessee Memorial Hospital,** Knoxville	NR	★★★	★★★	★★★	NR	★	★★★	★★★	★★★★★	★★★	★	★★★
110. **Vanderbilt University Hospital,** Nashville	NR	★★★	★★★	★★★	NR	★★★	★★★	★★★	★★★	★★★	★★★	★★★
111. **Volunteer Community Hospital,** Martin	NR	★★★	NR	NR	NR	★★★	NR	★★★	★★★	NR	NR	NR
112. **Wayne Medical Center,** Waynesboro	NR	NR	NR	NR	NR	NR	NR	NR	★	NR	NR	NR
113. **Wellmont Bristol Regional Medical Center,** Bristol	NR	★★★	★★★	★	NR	★	★★★	★★★	★★★★★	★★★	★★★	★★★
114. **Wellmont Hawkins County Memorial Hospital,** Rogersville	NR	★★★	NR	NR	NR	NR	NR	NR	★★★	NR	NR	NR
115. **Wellmont Holston Valley Medical Center,** Kingsport	NR	★★★★★	★★★	★	NR	★★★	★★★	★★★	★★★	★★★	★★★	★★★★★
116. **White County Community Hospital,** Sparta	NR	★★★	NR	NR	NR	★★★	NR	NR	★★★★★	NR	NR	NR
117. **Williamson Medical Center,** Franklin	NR	★★★	★★★	★★★	NR	★★★	★★★★★	★★★	★★★	NR	★★★	NR
118. **Women's East Pavilion,** Chattanooga	NR	★★★	★★★	★★★	NR	★★★	★★★	★★★	★★★	★	★★★	★★★★★
119. **Woods Memorial Hospital,** Etowah	NR	★★★	NR	NR	NR	★★★	NR	★★★	★	NR	NR	NR

KEY: ★★★★★ **BEST**   ★★★ **AS EXPECTED**   ★ **POOR**   NR **NOT RATED BY HEALTHGRADES**   For full definitions of ratings and awards, see Appendix.

Gastrointestinal Bleed	Gastrointestinal Surgeries and Procedures	Heart Attack	Heart Failure	Hip Fracture Repair	Maternity Care	Pancreatitis	Peripheral Vascular Bypass	Pneumonia	Prostatectomy	Pulmonary Embolism	Resection/Replacement of Abdominal Aorta	Respiratory Failure	Sepsis	Stroke	Total Hip Replacement	Total Knee Replacement	Valve Replacement	Women's Health
★★★	★★★	★★★	★★★	★★★	NR	★★★	NR	★	NR	NR	NR	★	NR	★	NR	NR	NR	NR
★★★	NR	★★★	★★★	★	NR	★	NR	★★★	NR	NR	NR	★★★★★	★★★★★	★★★	NR	★	NR	NR
NR	NR	NR	★	NR	NR	NR	NR	★	NR	NR	NR	NR	NR	NR	NR	NR	NR	NR
★★★	NR	NR	★★★	NR	NR	NR	NR	★★★	NR	NR	NR	★★★	★★★	NR	NR	NR	NR	NR
NR	NR	NR	★★★	NR	NR	NR	NR	★★★	NR	NR	NR	NR	NR	NR	NR	NR	NR	NR
★★★	NR	NR	★★★	★★★	NR	NR	NR	★★★	NR	NR	NR	★★★	NR	NR	NR	NR	NR	NR
NR	NR	NR	★★★★★	NR	NR	NR	NR	★★★	NR	NR	NR	NR	NR	NR	NR	NR	NR	NR
★	★★★	★★★	★★★	★★★	NR	★★★	NR	★	★★★	NR	★★★	★	★★★	★★★	★★★	★★★	NR	NR
★★★	★	★★★	★★★	★★★	NR	★★★★★	★★★	★★★	★★★	★★★	★★★	★	★★★	★	★★★	★	★★★	NR
★★★	★★★	★★★	★	★	NR	★★★	★★★	★★★★★	★★★★★	★★★	★★★	★★★★★	★★★	★★★	★★★	★★★	★★★	NR
★★★★★	NR	★★★	★★★	★★★★★	NR	NR	NR	★★★	NR	NR	NR	★	★	★★★	NR	NR	NR	NR
NR	NR	NR	★★★	NR	NR	NR	NR	★★★	NR	NR	NR	NR	★★★	NR	NR	NR	NR	NR
★★★★★	★★★	NR	★	NR	NR	★★★★★	NR	★★★	NR	★★★	★★★	★	★★★	★★★	★	★	NR	NR
★★★	★★★	NR	★★★	NR	NR	NR	NR	★★★	NR	NR	NR	★★★★★	★★★	★★★	NR	NR	NR	NR
★★★★★	★★★	★★★	★★★	★	NR	★★★	★	★★★★★	★	★★★	★★★	★★★★★	★★★	★★★	★★★	★★★	★★★	NR
★★★	NR	★★★	★★★★★	★★★	NR	NR	NR	★★★	NR	NR	NR	★★★	★★★	NR	NR	NR	NR	NR
★	★★★	★★★	★★★	★★★	NR	NR	NR	★★★	★★★★★	★★★	★★★	★★★	★	★★★	★★★	★★★★★	NR	NR
★★★	★★★	★★★	★★★	★★★	NR	★★★★★	★★★	★★★	★★★	★★★	★★★	★★★	★★★★★	★★★	★★★	★★★	★★★	NR
★	NR	NR	★★★	★★★	NR	NR	NR	★	NR	NR	NR	★	★	NR	NR	NR	NR	NR

TEXAS HOSPITALS: RATINGS BY PROCEDURE

Hospital	Appendectomy	Atrial Fibrillation	Back and Neck Surgery (except Spinal Fusion)	Back and Neck Surgery (Spinal Fusion)	Bariatric Surgery	Bowel Obstruction	Carotid Surgery	Cholecystectomy (Gall Bladder Removal)	Chronic Obstructive Pulmonary Disease (COPD)	Coronary Bypass Surgery	Coronary Interventional Procedures (Angioplasty/Stent)	Diabetic Acidosis an...
1. Abilene Regional Medical Center, Abilene	*****	***	NR	***	***	***	***	***	*****	*****	*	NR
2. Alliance Hospital, Odessa	NR	***	NR	***	NR	***	***	***	***	***	***	NR
3. American Transitional Hospital—Houston W, Houston	***	***	***	NR	*****	***	***	*****	*****	***	***	***
4. Angleton-Danbury Medical Center, Angleton	*****	NR	NR	NR	NR	*	NR	***	***	NR	NR	NR
5. Anson General Hospital, Anson	NR	NR	NR	NR	NR	NR	NR	NR	***	NR	NR	NR
6. Arlington Memorial Hospital, Arlington	*****	***	*****	***	NR	*****	*****	*****	***	*	*	***
7. Atlanta Memorial Hospital, Atlanta	NR	***	NR	NR	NR	***	NR	***	***	NR	NR	NR
8. Baptist Health System, San Antonio	***	***	***	***	NR	***	*****	***	***	***	***	***
9. Baptist St. Anthony's Health System, Amarillo	*****	***	***	*****	NR	*****	***	***	***	***	***	***
10. Baylor All Saints Medical Center at Fort Worth, Fort Worth	***	***	***	***	NR	***	***	***	***	*	*	***
11. Baylor Heart and Vascular Center, Dallas	NR	***	NR	NR	NR	NR	*****	NR	NR	NR	*****	NR
12. Baylor Medical Center at Garland, Garland	***	***	***	***	NR	***	***	***	*****	***	***	***
13. Baylor Medical Center at Irving, Irving	***	***	***	***	NR	***	***	***	***	***	***	***
14. Baylor Medical Center at Waxahachie, Waxahachie	***	***	NR	NR	***	*****	NR	***	***	NR	NR	***
15. Baylor Regional Medical Center at Grapevine, Grapevine	*****	***	***	***	NR	***	***	***	***	***	***	***
16. Baylor Regional Medical Center at Plano, Plano	***	***	NR	***	NR	***	***	***	***	***	***	***
17. Baylor University Medical Center, Dallas	***	*	*****	*****	*	***	***	***	***	*	***	***
18. Bayshore Medical Center in Pasadena, Pasadena	*****	***	*****	*****	***	***	***	*****	***	***	***	***
19. Bellville General Hospital, Bellville	NR	NR	NR	NR	NR	NR	NR	NR	***	NR	NR	NR
20. Big Bend Regional Medical Center, Alpine	*****	NR	NR	NR	NR	***	NR	***	***	NR	NR	NR
21. Bowie Memorial Hospital, Bowie	NR	***	NR	NR	NR	NR	NR	NR	***	NR	NR	NR
22. Brackenridge Hospital, Austin	***	***	***	*	NR	***	***	***	*****	***	***	***
23. Brazosport Regional Health System, Lake Jackson	*****	*	NR	NR	NR	***	NR	***	***	NR	NR	***
24. Brownfield Regional Medical Center, Brownfield	NR	NR	NR	NR	NR	NR	NR	NR	***	NR	NR	NR
25. Brownwood Regional Medical Center, Brownwood	*****	*****	NR	NR	NR	***	NR	***	***	NR	NR	***
26. Campbell Health System, Weatherford	***	***	NR	NR	NR	***	NR	***	***	***	NR	***
27. Centennial Medical Center, Frisco	***	NR	NR	NR	NR	NR	NR	***	***	***	NR	NR
28. Central Texas Hospital, Cameron	NR	NR	NR	NR	NR	NR	NR	***	***	NR	NR	NR
29. Central Texas Medical Center, San Marcos	***	***	NR	NR	***	NR	*****	***	***	NR	***	NR
30. Charlton Methodist Hospital, Dallas	*	***	***	NR	***	***	***	***	***	NR	***	***
31. Childress Regional Medical Center, Childress	NR	NR	NR	NR	NR	NR	NR	NR	*	NR	NR	NR
32. Christus Jasper Memorial Hospital, Jasper	***	***	NR	NR	NR	*	NR	NR	***	NR	NR	NR
33. Christus St. Catherine Health and Wellness Center, Katy	***	***	NR	NR	NR	*	NR	***	***	NR	NR	NR
34. Christus St. Elizabeth Hospital, Beaumont	***	***	*****	*****	NR	***	*****	*****	*	***	***	***
35. Christus St. John Hospital, Houston	***	***	***	***	NR	***	NR	***	NR	***	***	***
36. Christus St. Mary Hospital, Port Arthur	***	NR	NR	NR	NR	NR	NR	***	***	NR	NR	NR
37. Christus St. Michael Health System, Texarkana	*****	***	***	***	NR	*	*****	*****	***	***	***	***
38. Christus Santa Rosa Healthcare, San Antonio	***	***	NR	NR	NR	***	NR	***	***	***	***	***
39. Christus Spohn Hospital Corpus Christi—South, Corpus Christi	***	***	***	***	NR	***	*****	*****	***	*****	***	***
40. Christus Spohn Hospital—Alice, Alice	***	***	NR	NR	NR	***	NR	*****	*****	NR	NR	***
41. Christus Spohn Hospital—Beeville, Beeville	***	***	NR	NR	NR	***	NR	NR	***	NR	NR	***
42. Christus Spohn Hospital—Corpus Christi Memorial, Corpus Christi	***	***	***	***	NR	***	*****	***	*****	***	***	***
43. Christus Spohn Hospital—Kleberg, Kingsville	*****	***	NR	NR	NR	***	NR	*****	***	NR	NR	***
44. Citizens Medical Center, Victoria	***	***	NR	***	*****	***	***	*****	***	***	***	***
45. Clay County Memorial Hospital, Henrietta	NR	NR	NR	NR	NR	NR	NR	NR	***	NR	NR	NR
46. Clear Lake Regional Medical Center, Webster	*****	***	***	***	NR	***	*****	***	***	***	***	***
47. Clearview Hospital, Midland	*****	***	*****	*****	NR	***	***	***	*	*	***	***
48. Cleveland Regional Medical Center, Cleveland	NR	***	NR	NR	NR	***	NR	NR	*****	NR	NR	***
49. Coleman County Medical Center, Coleman	NR	NR	NR	NR	NR	NR	NR	NR	***	NR	NR	NR
50. College Station Medical Center, College Station	***	*	***	*****	*****	***	***	***	***	***	***	NR

KEY: ***** BEST   *** AS EXPECTED   * POOR   NR NOT RATED BY HEALTHGRADES   For full definitions of ratings and awards, see Appendix.

Gastrointestinal Bleed	Gastrointestinal Surgeries and Procedures	Heart Attack	Heart Failure	Hip Fracture Repair	Maternity Care	Pancreatitis	Peripheral Vascular Bypass	Pneumonia	Prostatectomy	Pulmonary Embolism	Resection/Replacement of Abdominal Aorta	Respiratory Failure	Sepsis	Stroke	Total Hip Replacement	Total Knee Replacement	Valve Replacement	Women's Health
★	★★★	★★★	★★★	★★★	★★★	★★★	★★★	★	★★★	★★★	NR	★★★	★★★	★★★	★★★	★★★	★★★	★
NR	NR	★★★	★★★	★★★	NR	NR	★★★★★	★★★	NR	NR	NR	NR	NR	★★★	★★★	★★★	★★★	NR
★★★	★★★★★	★★★	★★★	★★★	NR	★★★	★★★★★	★★★★★	★★★	NR	NR	★★★★★	★★★★★	★★★	★★★	★★★	NR	NR
★★★	NR	★★★	★	★★★★★	★★★	NR	NR	★★★	★★★	NR	NR	★★★	NR	NR	NR	NR	★★★	NR
NR	NR	NR	★★★	NR	NR	NR	NR	★★★	NR	NR	NR	★★★	NR	NR	NR	NR	NR	NR
★★★	★★★	★	★	★★★★★	★★★	★★★	★★★	★★★	NR	★★★	★★★	★	★	★★★	★★★	★★★	NR	★★★
★★★	NR	★★★	NR	NR	NR	NR	NR	★	NR	NR	NR	★★★	★	★★★	NR	NR	NR	NR
★	★★★	★★★★★	★★★	★★★★★	★★★	★★★	★★★★★	★★★	★★★★★	★★★★★	★★★	★★★	★★★★★	★★★	★★★	★★★	★★★	★★★
★★★	★★★	★★★	★★★	★★★	★★★	★★★	★★★★★	★★★	★★★	★★★	★★★	★★★★★	★★★★★	★★★★★	★★★★★	★★★	★	★★★
★★★	★★★	★★★★★	★★★★★	★★★	★★★	★★★★★	★★★	★★★	★★★	★★★	★★★★★	★★★	★★★	★★★★★	★★★	★★★	★★★	★★★
NR	NR	★★★	★★★★★	NR	NR	NR	★★★	NR	NR	NR	NR	★★★	NR	NR	NR	NR	NR	NR
★★★	★★★	★★★	★★★	★★★★★	★★★	★★★	NR	★★★	★★★	★★★	NR	★★★	★★★	★★★★★	★★★	★	★★★	★★★
★★★	★★★	★★★	★★★	★★★	★★★	★★★	★★★★★	★★★	★★★	NR	★★★★★	★★★	★★★	★★★	★★★	★★★	★★★	★★★
★★★	★★★	★★★★★	★	★★★	★★★	★★★	★	★★★	★★★	★★★★★	★★★	★★★	★★★	★★★	★	★★★	★★★	★★★
★★★	★★★	★★★★★	★★★	★★★★★	★★★★★	★★★★★	★★★	★★★	NR	★★★	NR	★★★	★★★	★★★	★★★	★★★	★★★	★★★
★★★	★★★★★	★★★	★★★	★★★	★★★	★★★	NR	★★★	★★★	★★★	★	★★★★★	★★★★★	★★★	★★★	★★★	★★★	★★★
★★★	NR	NR	★	NR	NR	NR	NR	★	NR	NR	NR	NR	NR	NR	NR	NR	NR	NR
★★★	NR	NR	★	NR	★★★	NR	NR	★★★	NR	NR	NR	★★★	NR	NR	NR	NR	NR	NR
★★★	NR	★★★	★	NR	NR	★★★	NR	★★★	NR	NR	NR	★★★	★★★	NR	NR	NR	NR	NR
★★★	NR	★★★	★★★	★★★	★	NR	NR	★★★	NR	NR	NR	★★★	★★★★★	★★★★★	NR	NR	NR	★★★
★★★	★★★	★★★	★★★	★★★	★★★	NR	★★★★★	★★★	NR	NR	NR	★★★★★	★★★	★★★	★★★	★★★	NR	NR
NR	NR	NR	★★★	★★★	NR	NR	NR	★★★	NR	NR	NR	NR	NR	NR	NR	NR	NR	NR
★★★	★★★	★	★★★	★★★	★★★	★★★	★★★	★★★	NR	NR	NR	★★★	★	★★★	★	★★★	★★★	NR
★	★★★★★	★★★	★★★	★★★	★★★	★★★	NR	★★★	NR	NR	NR	★	★★★	★★★	★★★	★★★	★★★	NR
★★★	NR	★★★	★★★	★★★	★★★	NR	NR	★★★	NR	NR	NR	★★★	★★★	NR	NR	NR	NR	NR
NR	NR	NR	NR	NR	NR	NR	NR	NR	NR	NR	NR	★★★★★	★	★★★	NR	NR	NR	NR
★★★	★★★	★★★	★★★	★★★★★	★★★	★★★	NR	★★★★★	★★★	NR	NR	★	★★★	NR	NR	NR	★★★	NR
★★★	★	★★★	★★★	★★★	★★★★★	★★★	NR	★★★	★★★	★★★	NR	★★★	★★★	★★★★★	★★★	★★★	NR	NR
★★★	NR	NR	★	★★★	NR	NR	★	NR	NR	NR	NR	NR	NR	NR	★★★	NR	NR	NR
★★★	NR	NR	★★★	★	★★★	★	NR	★★★	NR	NR	NR	★	NR	NR	NR	NR	NR	NR
★★★	NR	★★★	★★★	★★★★★	★★★	★★★	NR	★★★★★	NR	NR	NR	★★★	★★★	★★★	NR	★★★	NR	NR
★★★	★	★★★	★	★★★	★★★★★	★★★	★★★	★★★	★★★	★★★	NR	★★★	★★★	★★★	★★★	★★★	★★★	★★★
★★★	★★★	★	★★★	★★★	★★★★★	NR	★★★	★★★★★	NR	NR	NR	★★★	★★★	★★★	★	★★★	★★★	★★★
NR	NR	NR	NR	NR	★★★★★	NR	NR	NR	NR	NR	NR	NR	NR	NR	NR	NR	NR	★★★
★	★★★	★	★★★	★★★★★	★	★★★★★	★★★★★	★	★★★★★	★★★	★★★	★★★	★	★	★★★	★★★★★	★★★	★
★★★	★★★★★	★★★	★★★★★	★★★★★	★★★	★★★	★★★	★★★★★	★★★	★★★	NR	★★★★★	★★★★★	★★★	★★★	★★★★★	NR	NR
★	★★★	★★★	★★★	★★★	★★★	★★★	NR	★★★	★★★	★★★	NR	★★★	★★★	★★★	★★★	NR	★★★	★★★
★★★	★★★★★	★★★	★★★	★★★	★★★	★★★	NR	★★★	NR	NR	NR	★★★	★★★	★★★	★★★	★★★	NR	NR
★★★	NR	★★★	★★★	★★★	★★★	NR	NR	NR	NR	NR	NR	★★★	★★★	★★★	NR	NR	NR	NR
★	★★★	★★★	★★★	★★★	★★★★★	★★★	★★★★★	★★★	★★★	★★★	NR	★★★	★★★	★★★	★	★★★	★★★	★★★
★★★	NR	NR	★	NR	★★★	★★★	NR	★	NR	NR	NR	★★★	★★★	NR	NR	NR	NR	★★★
★★★	★★★	★	★★★	NR	★★★	★★★	NR	★★★	NR	NR	NR	★★★	★	★★★	★★★★★	★★★	NR	★★★
NR	NR	NR	★	NR	NR	NR	NR	★★★	NR	NR	NR	★★★	★★★	★★★	NR	NR	NR	NR
★★★	★★★	★★★	★★★★★	★★★★★	★★★★★	★★★★★	NR	★★★★★	★★★	NR	★★★	★★★	★★★	★★★★★	★★★★★	★★★	★★★	★★★★★
★★★	★★★	★★★	★★★★★	★★★	★★★★★	★★★★★	NR	★★★	★★★	★★★	NR	★★★★★	★★★★★	★★★★★	★★★	★★★	★★★	★★★
★★★	NR	★★★	★★★	NR	★★★★★	NR	NR	★★★★★	NR	NR	NR	★★★	NR	NR	NR	NR	★★★	NR
NR	NR	NR	★	NR	NR	NR	NR	★	NR	NR	NR	NR	NR	NR	NR	NR	NR	NR
★★★	★★★	★★★	★★★	★★★	★★★	NR	NR	★★★	NR	NR	NR	★★★	★★★	★★★	★★★	NR	★★★	NR

	Appendectomy	Atrial Fibrillation	Back and Neck Surgery (except Spinal Fusion)	Back and Neck Surgery (Spinal Fusion)	Bariatric Surgery	Bowel Obstruction	Carotid Surgery	Cholecystectomy (Gall Bladder Removal)	Chronic Obstructive Pulmonary Disease (COPD)	Coronary Bypass Surgery	Coronary Interventional Procedures (Angioplasty/Stent)	Diabetic Acidosis and
51. Columbus Community Hospital, Columbus	NR	NR	NR	NR	NR	★★★	NR	★★★	★	NR	NR	NR
52. Connally Memorial Medical Center, Floresville	NR	NR	NR	NR	NR	★★★	NR	NR	★★★	NR	NR	NR
53. Conroe Regional Medical Center, Conroe	★★★	★★★	★★★	NR	NR	★★★	★★★★★	★★★★★	★★★★★	★★★	★★★	★★★
54. Corpus Christi Medical Center, Corpus Christi	★★★★★	★★★	★★★	★★★★★	NR	★★★	★★★★★	★★★	★★★	★★★	★★★	★★★
55. Coryell Memorial Hospital, Gatesville	★★★	★★★	NR	NR	NR	NR	NR	NR	★★★	NR	NR	NR
56. Covenant Hospital Levelland, Levelland	NR	NR	NR	NR	NR	NR	NR	★	NR	NR	NR	NR
57. Covenant Hospital Plainview, Plainview	★★★	★★★	NR	NR	NR	★★★	NR	★★★★★	★	NR	NR	NR
58. Covenant Medical Center, Lubbock	★★★	★	★★★	★★★	★★★	★★★	★★★	★★★	★★★	★★★	★	★★★
59. Crosbyton Clinic Hospital, Crosbyton	NR	NR	NR	NR	NR	★★★	NR	NR	NR	NR	NR	NR
60. Cuero Community Hospital, Cuero	NR	★★★	NR	NR	NR	★★★	NR	NR	NR	NR	NR	★★★
61. Cypress Fairbanks Medical Center, Houston	★	★★★	NR	NR	★★★★★	★★★	NR	★★★	★★★★★	NR	★★★	★★★
62. D. M. Cogdell Memorial Hospital, Snyder	NR	NR	NR	NR	NR	★★★	NR	★★★	NR	NR	NR	NR
63. Dallas Regional Medical Center–Galloway Campus, Mesquite	★★★	★★★	NR	NR	NR	★★★	★	★★★	★★★	★★★	★	★★★
64. Dallas Southwest Medical Center, Dallas	★★★	NR	NR	NR	NR	★★★	NR	★★★	★★★	NR	NR	NR
65. Del Sol Medical Center, El Paso	★★★★★	★★★	NR	NR	★★★	★	NR	★★★★★	NR	★	★★★	★★★
66. Denton Regional Medical Center, Denton	★★★	★	★★★	★	★★★	★★★	★★★★★	★★★	★★★	★★★	★★★	★★★
67. Detar Hospital Navarro, Victoria	★★★	★★★	★★★★★	★★★★★	NR	★★★	★★★	★★★	★★★	★	★★★	★★★
68. Detar Hospital North, Victoria	★★★	★★★	★★★★★	★★★★★	NR	★★★	★★★	★★★	★★★	★	★★★	★★★
69. Diagnostic Center Hospital, Houston	★★★	★★★	★★★★★	★★★★★	★★★	★★★	★★★★★	★★★	★★★	★★★	★★★	★★★
70. Dimmit County Memorial Hospital, Carrizo Springs	NR	NR	NR	NR	NR	★★★	NR	NR	NR	NR	NR	NR
71. Doctors Hospital at Renaissance, Edinburg	★★★	★★★	★★★	★★★★★	★	★★★★★	★★★	★★★	★★★	★★★	★★★	★★★
72. Doctors Hospital at White Rock Lake, Dallas	★★★	★★★	NR	NR	★★★★★	★★★	★★★	★★★	★★★	★★★	★★★	★★★
73. Doctors Hospital of Laredo, Laredo	★★★	NR	NR	NR	NR	★★★	★★★	★★★★★	★★★	NR	NR	★
74. Doctors Hospital–Parkway, Houston	★★★	★★★	NR	NR	NR	★★★	NR	★★★	★★★	NR	NR	★★★
75. Doctors Hospital–Tidwell, Houston	★★★	★★★	NR	NR	NR	★★★	NR	★★★	★	NR	NR	★★★
76. Dolly Vinsant Memorial Hospital, San Benito	NR	NR	NR	NR	NR	NR	NR	NR	★★★	NR	NR	NR
77. East Houston Regional Medical Center, Houston	★★★	★★★	NR	NR	NR	★★★	NR	★★★	★★★	NR	NR	★★★
78. East Texas Medical Center, Tyler	★★★	★★★	★★★	★★★	★★★★★	★★★	★★★★★	★★★★★	★★★	★★★	★★★	★★★
79. East Texas Medical Center–Athens, Athens	★★★	★★★	NR	NR	NR	★★★	★★★	★★★	★★★	NR	NR	
80. East Texas Medical Center–Carthage, Carthage	NR	★★★	NR	NR	NR	★★★	NR	NR	★★★	NR	NR	NR
81. East Texas Medical Center–Clarksville, Clarksville	NR	NR	NR	NR	NR	★★★	NR	NR	★★★	NR	NR	NR
82. East Texas Medical Center–Crockett, Crockett	★★★	★★★	NR	NR	NR	★★★	NR	★★★★★	★★★	NR	NR	NR
83. East Texas Medical Center–Fairfield, Fairfield	NR	NR	NR	NR	NR	★★★	NR	NR	★★★	NR	NR	NR
84. East Texas Medical Center–Gilmer, Gilmer	NR	NR	NR	NR	NR	NR	NR	NR	★★★	NR	NR	NR
85. East Texas Medical Center–Jacksonville, Jacksonville	★★★	★★★	NR	NR	NR	★★★	NR	★★★	★★★	NR	NR	NR
86. East Texas Medical Center–Mt. Vernon, Mt. Vernon	NR	NR	NR	NR	NR	NR	NR	NR	★	NR	NR	NR
87. East Texas Medical Center–Quitman, Quitman	★★★	NR	NR	NR	NR	★★★	NR	NR	★	NR	NR	NR
88. Eastland Memorial Hospital, Eastland	NR	★★★	NR	NR	NR	★★★	NR	★★★	★	NR	NR	NR
89. Edinburg Regional Medical Center, Edinburg	★★★	★★★	NR	NR	NR	★★★	NR	★★★	★★★	NR	NR	★
90. El Campo Memorial Hospital, El Campo	NR	NR	NR	NR	NR	NR	NR	NR	★★★	NR	NR	NR
91. El Paso Specialty Hospital, El Paso	NR	NR	★★★	NR	NR	NR	NR	NR	NR	NR	NR	NR
92. Electra Memorial Hospital, Electra	NR	NR	NR	NR	NR	NR	NR	NR	★★★	NR	NR	NR
93. Ennis Regional Medical Center, Ennis	★★★	★★★	NR	NR	NR	★★★	NR	NR	★★★	NR	NR	NR
94. ETMC Pittsburg, Pittsburg	NR	NR	NR	NR	NR	★★★	NR	NR	★★★	NR	NR	NR
95. Falls Community Hospital and Clinic, Marlin	NR	NR	NR	NR	NR	NR	NR	★★★	★★★	NR	NR	NR
96. Fort Duncan Medical Center, Eagle Pass	★★★★★	★	NR	NR	NR	★★★	NR	★★★★★	★★★★★	NR	NR	★★★
97. Georgetown Hospital, Georgetown	★★★	★★★	NR	NR	NR	★★★	NR	★★★★★	★★★	NR	NR	NR
98. Golden Plains Community Hospital, Borger	NR	NR	NR	NR	NR	NR	NR	NR	★★★	NR	NR	NR
99. Good Shepherd Medical Center–Linden, Linden	NR	NR	NR	NR	NR	NR	NR	NR	★	NR	NR	NR
100. Good Shepherd Medical Center, Longview	★★★★★	★★★	★★★★★	★★★★★	NR	★★★	★★★	★★★	★★★	★	★★★	★★★

KEY: ★★★★★ BEST   ★★★ AS EXPECTED   ★ POOR   NR NOT RATED BY HEALTHGRADES   For full definitions of ratings and awards, see Appendix.

Gastrointestinal Bleed	Gastrointestinal Surgeries and Procedures	Heart Attack	Heart Failure	Hip Fracture Repair	Maternity Care	Pancreatitis	Peripheral Vascular Bypass	Pneumonia	Prostatectomy	Pulmonary Embolism	Resection/Replacement of Abdominal Aorta	Respiratory Failure	Sepsis	Stroke	Total Hip Replacement	Total Knee Replacement	Valve Replacement	Women's Health
★	NR	NR	★★★	★★★	NR	NR	NR	★★★	NR	NR	NR	NR	★★★	★★★	NR	★★★	NR	NR
★★★	NR	★★★	★★★★★	★★★	NR	NR	NR	★★★	NR	NR	NR	NR	★★★★★	NR	NR	NR	NR	NR
★★★	★★★	★★★	★★★★★	★	★★★	★★★	★★★	★★★★★	★★★	★★★	★★★	★★★	★★★	★★★	★★★	★★★	★★★	★★★
★★★	★★★	★★★	★★★	★★★	★★★★★	★★★	★★★	★★★	★★★	★★★	★★★	★★★	★★★	★★★	★★★	★★★	★★★	★★★
★★★	NR	★★★★★	★★★	NR	NR	NR	NR	★★★	NR	NR	NR	NR	★★★	NR	NR	NR	NR	NR
★★★	NR	NR	★	NR	★★★	NR	NR	★★★	NR	NR	NR	NR	NR	NR	NR	NR	NR	NR
★★★	★	NR	★	★★★	★★★	NR	NR	★	NR	NR	NR	NR	★★★	★★★	NR	★★★	NR	NR
★★★	★★★	★★★	★★★	★★★★★	★★★	★	★★★	★★★	★★★	★★★	★★★	★★★	★★★	★★★★★	★★★	★★★★★	★★★	★★★
NR	NR	NR	★	NR	NR	NR	NR	★★★	NR	NR	NR	NR	★★★	NR	NR	NR	NR	NR
★★★	NR	★	★	NR	NR	NR	NR	★	NR	★★★	NR	NR	★	★	NR	NR	NR	NR
★★★	★★★	★★★	★★★	★★★	★★★★★	★★★★★	NR	★★★★★	★★★	★★★	NR	★★★★★	★★★★★	★★★★★	NR	NR	NR	NR
★★★	NR	NR	★★★	NR	NR	NR	NR	★	NR	NR	NR	NR	NR	NR	NR	NR	NR	NR
★★★	NR	★★★	★★★	★★★	★★★	★★★	NR	★★★★★	NR	NR	NR	NR	★★★	★★★	NR	NR	NR	★★★
★★★	NR	NR	★★★	NR	NR	NR	NR	★★★	NR	NR	NR	NR	★★★★★	NR	NR	NR	NR	★★★
★★★	★★★	★	★★★	★★★★★	★★★★★	★★★	NR	★★★	★★★	★★★	NR	★★★	★★★	★★★	NR	★★★	NR	★★★
★★★	★★★	★★★	★	★★★	★★★	★★★	★★★	★	NR	★★★	★★★	★★★	★	★★★	★★★	★★★	★★★	★
★	★★★	★	★★★	★★★	★★★	★★★	NR	★★★	★★★	★★★★★	NR	★★★	★★★	★★★	★★★	★★★★★	NR	
★	★★★	★	★★★	★★★	★★★	★★★	NR	★★★	★★★	★★★★★	NR	★★★	★★★	★★★	★★★	★★★★★	NR	
★★★	★★★	★★★	★★★	★★★	★★★	★★★	NR	★★★	★★★	★★★	★★★	★★★	★★★	★★★★★	★★★	★★★	★★★	★★★
NR	NR	NR	★	NR	NR	NR	NR	★	NR	NR	NR	NR	★	NR	NR	NR	NR	NR
★★★	★★★	★★★	★★★★★	★★★	NR	★★★	★★★	★★★★★	★★★	NR	NR	★★★★★	★★★★★	★★★	★★★	NR	★★★	NR
★★★	★★★	★★★	★★★	NR	★★★	NR	NR	★★★	★★★	NR	NR	★★★	★★★	★★★★★	★	NR	NR	★★★
★	★★★	★★★	★★★	★★★★★	★	NR	NR	★★★	NR	NR	NR	NR	NR	NR	NR	★★★★★	NR	NR
★★★	★★★	★★★	★★★	NR	★★★	NR	NR	★★★★★	NR	NR	NR	★★★★★	★★★★★	NR	NR	NR	NR	NR
★★★	NR	★★★★★	★★★	★★★	★★★	NR	NR	★★★★★	NR	NR	NR	★★★★★	★★★★★	NR	NR	NR	NR	NR
NR	NR	NR	★★★	NR	NR	NR	NR	★★★★★	NR	NR	NR	NR	NR	NR	NR	NR	NR	NR
★★★	★★★	★★★	★★★	★★★★★	★★★	★★★	NR	★★★★★	NR	NR	NR	★★★★★	★★★★★	★★★★★	★★★	NR	NR	NR
★★★	★★★	★★★	★★★★★	★★★	★★★	★★★	★★★	★★★	★★★	★★★	★★★	★★★★★	★★★	★★★★★	★★★	★★★	★★★	★
★	★★★	★★★	★★★	★	★★★★★	★★★	NR	★★★	★★★	NR	NR	★★★	NR	★★★	★★★	★	NR	NR
★★★	NR	NR	★★★	NR	★★★	NR	NR	★★★	NR	NR	NR	★★★	NR	NR	NR	NR	NR	NR
★★★	NR	NR	★	NR	NR	NR	NR	★★★	NR	NR	NR	★	NR	★★★	NR	NR	NR	NR
★★★	NR	★★★	★	NR	★★★	NR	NR	★	NR	NR	NR	★	★	NR	NR	NR	NR	NR
NR	NR	NR	★★★	NR	NR	NR	NR	★★★	NR	NR	NR	NR	NR	NR	NR	NR	NR	NR
★★★	NR	NR	★★★★★	NR	NR	NR	NR	★★★★★	NR	NR	NR	NR	★★★	NR	NR	NR	NR	NR
★★★	NR	★	★★★	★★★	★★★	NR	NR	★★★	NR	NR	NR	★★★	★	★★★	NR	★	NR	NR
NR	NR	NR	★★★	NR	NR	NR	NR	★★★	NR	NR	NR	NR	★★★	NR	NR	NR	NR	NR
NR	NR	★	★	★★★	★★★	NR	NR	★	NR	NR	NR	NR	NR	NR	NR	NR	NR	NR
★	NR	NR	★	NR	NR	NR	NR	★	NR	NR	NR	★★★	NR	NR	NR	NR	NR	NR
★★★	NR	★★★★★	★★★★★	★★★	NR	★★★	NR	★★★★★	NR	NR	★★★★★	★★★	NR	NR	NR	NR	NR	NR
★★★	NR	NR	★★★★★	NR	NR	NR	NR	★★★	NR	NR	NR	★★★	NR	NR	NR	NR	NR	NR
NR	NR	NR	NR	NR	NR	NR	NR	NR	NR	NR	NR	NR	★★★★★	★★★★★	NR	NR	NR	NR
NR	NR	NR	★★★	NR	NR	NR	NR	★★★★★	NR	NR	NR	NR	NR	NR	NR	NR	NR	NR
★★★	NR	NR	★★★★★	★★★★★	★★★	NR	NR	★★★	NR	NR	NR	★★★	★★★	NR	NR	NR	NR	NR
NR	NR	NR	★★★	NR	NR	NR	NR	★★★	NR	NR	NR	NR	NR	NR	NR	NR	NR	NR
★★★	NR	NR	★★★	NR	NR	NR	NR	★★★★★	NR	NR	NR	★★★★★	NR	NR	NR	NR	NR	NR
★★★	★★★	★★★★★	★★★★★	★★★	★★★	★★★	NR	★★★★★	NR	NR	★★★	★★★★★	NR	NR	NR	NR	NR	NR
★★★	★★★	★★★	★★★	★★★★★	★★★	★★★	NR	★	NR	NR	NR	★★★	★★★	★★★	★★★	★★★	NR	NR
NR	NR	NR	★★★	NR	NR	NR	NR	★	NR	NR	NR	★★★	NR	NR	NR	NR	NR	NR
NR	NR	NR	★★★	NR	★★★	NR	NR	★★★	NR	NR	NR	★★★	★★★	NR	NR	NR	NR	NR
★★★	★★★	★★★★★	★★★★★	★★★★★	★★★	★★★	★★★★★	★★★★★	★★★★★	★★★	★★★	★★★★★	★★★★★	★★★★★	★★★	★★★	★	★★★

	Appendectomy	Atrial Fibrillation	Back and Neck Surgery (except Spinal Fusion)	Back and Neck Surgery (Spinal Fusion)	Bariatric Surgery	Bowel Obstruction	Carotid Surgery	Cholecystectomy (Gall Bladder Removal)	Chronic Obstructive Pulmonary Disease (COPD)	Coronary Bypass Surgery	Coronary Interventional Procedures (Angioplasty/Stent)	Diabetic Acidosis and...
101. Goodall Witcher Healthcare Foundation, Clifton	NR	***	NR	NR	NR	*	NR	NR	*	NR	NR	NR
102. Graham Regional Medical Center, Graham	NR	***	NR	NR	NR	***	NR	NR	***	NR	NR	NR
103. Guadalupe Valley Hospital, Seguin	***	*	NR	NR	***	***	NR	*	***	NR	NR	***
104. Gulf Coast Medical Center, Wharton	***	***	NR	NR	NR	***	NR	***	***	NR	NR	NR
105. Hamilton General Hospital, Hamilton	NR	***	NR	NR	NR	***	NR	NR	***	NR	NR	NR
106. Hamlin Memorial Hospital, Hamlin	NR	NR	NR	NR	NR	NR	NR	NR	***	NR	NR	NR
107. Harlingen Medical Center, Harlingen	***	***	***	*****	NR	***	***	*****	***	*****	***	***
108. Harris County Hospital District, Houston	*****	***	NR	NR	NR	***	NR	***	*****	NR	***	***
109. Harris Methodist Dublin, Dublin	***	***	NR	NR	NR	***	NR	***	***	NR	NR	NR
110. Harris Methodist Erath County, Stephenville	***	***	NR	NR	NR	***	NR	***	***	NR	NR	NR
111. Harris Methodist Fort Worth, Fort Worth	***	***	***	***	NR	***	***	***	***	*	*	***
112. Harris Methodist HEB Hospital, Bedford	***	***	***	***	NR	***	***	***	***	***	*****	***
113. Harris Methodist Southwest, Fort Worth	***	***	NR	NR	NR	***	NR	*	***	NR	NR	NR
114. Healthsouth Medical Center, Dallas	NR	NR	NR	NR	NR	NR	NR	***	NR	NR	NR	NR
115. Heart Hospital of Austin, Austin	NR	*****	NR	NR	NR	NR	***	NR	***	*****	*****	NR
116. Heart of Texas Memorial Hospital, Brady	NR	NR	NR	NR	NR	NR	NR	NR	***	NR	NR	NR
117. Henderson Memorial Hospital, Henderson	*	***	NR	NR	NR	***	NR	NR	*****	NR	NR	NR
118. Hendrick Medical Center, Abilene	***	*	***	***	NR	***	***	***	*****	***	*	***
119. Hereford Regional Medical Center, Hereford	NR	NR	NR	NR	NR	NR	NR	NR	***	NR	NR	NR
120. Highland Medical Center, Lubbock	NR	NR	NR	NR	NR	NR	NR	NR	***	NR	NR	NR
121. Hill Country Memorial Hospital, Fredericksburg	NR	***	NR	NR	NR	***	NR	***	*	NR	NR	NR
122. Hill Regional Hospital, Hillsboro	*	***	NR	NR	NR	***	NR	***	*	NR	NR	NR
123. Hillcrest Baptist Medical Center, Waco	***	***	***	***	NR	***	***	*****	***	***	***	***
124. Hopkins County Memorial Hospital, Sulphur Springs	NR	***	NR	NR	*	NR	NR	***	***	NR	NR	NR
125. The Hospital at Westlake Medical Center, Austin	NR	NR	NR	NR	NR	NR	NR	NR	NR	NR	***	NR
126. Houston Northwest Medical Center, Houston	***	***	***	*****	***	***	***	*****	***	*	***	***
127. Huguley Memorial Medical Center, Fort Worth	***	***	NR	NR	NR	***	***	***	***	*	***	***
128. Huntsville Memorial Hospital, Huntsville	*	***	NR	NR	NR	***	NR	*	*	NR	NR	NR
129. Johns Community Hospital, Taylor	NR	NR	NR	NR	NR	***	NR	NR	***	NR	NR	NR
130. JPS Health Network, Fort Worth	***	***	NR	NR	NR	*	***	NR	***	NR	***	***
131. Kell West Regional Hospital, Wichita Falls	NR	NR	NR	NR	NR	***	NR	NR	***	NR	NR	NR
132. King's Daughters Hospital, Temple	***	***	NR	NR	NR	***	***	***	***	NR	NR	***
133. Kingwood Medical Center, Kingwood	*****	***	NR	NR	NR	***	NR	***	***	NR	NR	***
134. Knapp Medical Center, Weslaco	***	***	NR	NR	***	***	NR	*****	*****	NR	NR	***
135. Laird Memorial Hospital, Kilgore	*	NR	NR	NR	NR	***	NR	***	***	NR	NR	NR
136. Lake Granbury Medical Center, Granbury	*	***	NR	NR	NR	***	NR	***	***	NR	NR	NR
137. Lake Pointe Medical Center, Rowlett	***	***	NR	NR	***	***	NR	***	***	NR	NR	***
138. Lake Whitney Medical Center, Whitney	NR	NR	NR	NR	NR	NR	NR	NR	***	NR	NR	NR
139. Lamb Healthcare Center, Littlefield	NR	NR	NR	NR	NR	NR	NR	NR	NR	NR	NR	NR
140. Laredo Medical Center, Laredo	***	***	NR	***	NR	***	***	***	***	*	***	***
141. Las Colinas Medical Center, Irving	***	***	NR	NR	NR	***	NR	***	***	NR	***	***
142. Las Palmas Medical Center, El Paso	***	***	***	***	NR	***	NR	***	***	*	***	***
143. Lavaca Medical Center, Hallettsville	NR	***	NR	NR	NR	NR	NR	NR	NR	NR	NR	NR
144. Liberty Dayton Community Hospital, Liberty	NR	NR	NR	NR	NR	NR	NR	***	NR	NR	NR	NR
145. Llano Memorial Healthcare System, Llano	NR	***	NR	NR	NR	***	NR	***	***	NR	NR	NR
146. Longview Regional Medical Center, Longview	***	***	***	***	NR	***	***	*	***	*	***	***
147. Lubbock Heart Hospital, Lubbock	NR	*	NR	NR	NR	NR	*****	***	***	***	*****	NR
148. Mainland Medical Center, Texas City	***	***	NR	NR	NR	*****	***	***	***	NR	NR	***
149. Marshall Regional Medical Center, Marshall	***	***	NR	NR	NR	***	NR	*****	***	NR	NR	***
150. Matagorda General Hospital, Bay City	***	***	NR	NR	NR	***	NR	***	*	NR	NR	NR

KEY: ***** BEST · *** AS EXPECTED · * POOR · NR NOT RATED BY HEALTHGRADES For full definitions of ratings and awards, see Appendix.

Gastrointestinal Bleed	Gastrointestinal Surgeries and Procedures	Heart Attack	Heart Failure	Hip Fracture Repair	Maternity Care	Pancreatitis	Peripheral Vascular Bypass	Pneumonia	Prostatectomy	Pulmonary Embolism	Resection/Replacement of Abdominal Aorta	Respiratory Failure	Sepsis	Stroke	Total Hip Replacement	Total Knee Replacement	Valve Replacement	Women's Health
***	NR	***	*	NR	NR	NR	NR	*	NR	NR	NR	NR	***	***	NR	NR	NR	NR
***	NR	NR	*	NR	***	NR	NR	***	NR	NR	NR	NR	***	***	NR	NR	NR	NR
***	***	***	***	*****	*	***	NR	*	***	NR	NR	*	*	***	***	***	NR	NR
***	***	*	***	***	***	***	NR	***	*	NR	NR	***	*****	***	NR	***	NR	NR
***	NR	NR	***	NR	NR	NR	NR	***	NR	NR	NR	NR	*	NR	NR	NR	NR	NR
NR	NR	NR	***	NR	NR	NR	NR	***	NR	NR	NR	NR	***	NR	NR	NR	NR	NR
*	*****	*****	*****	*****	***	***	NR	*****	NR	***	NR	***	***	***	NR	***	NR	*****
***	***	***	***	***	***	NR	NR	*	NR	NR	NR	*	*	***	NR	NR	NR	***
*	***	*****	***	***	NR	***	NR	*****	*****	NR	NR	***	***	***	***	***	NR	NR
*	***	*****	***	***	NR	***	NR	*****	*****	NR	NR	***	***	***	***	***	NR	NR
*****	*****	***	*****	***	*****	***	*****	*****	***	***	*****	***	*****	***	***	***	***	***
***	***	***	***	***	***	***	***	***	***	***	NR	***	***	***	***	*	NR	***
***	***	***	***	*	***	***	NR	***	***	***	NR	***	***	*****	***	***	NR	NR
NR	NR	NR	***	NR	NR	NR	NR	***	NR	NR	NR	NR	NR	NR	NR	NR	NR	NR
***	NR	*****	*****	NR	NR	NR	***	*****	NR	NR	***	***	*****	NR	NR	NR	***	NR
NR	NR	NR	*	NR	NR	NR	NR	*	NR	NR	NR	NR	NR	NR	NR	NR	NR	NR
***	NR	NR	***	***	*****	NR	NR	***	NR	NR	NR	***	***	***	***	*	NR	NR
***	***	*	*	***	***	*	NR	***	***	***	NR	*	***	***	***	*	***	*
*	NR	NR	*	NR	NR	NR	NR	*	NR	NR	NR	NR	NR	NR	NR	NR	NR	NR
NR	NR	NR	***	***	***	NR	NR	***	NR	NR	NR	NR	NR	***	***	*****	NR	NR
***	***	***	***	*****	*	***	NR	***	***	NR	NR	***	***	*	***	***	NR	NR
***	NR	*	***	NR	*	NR	NR	***	NR	NR	NR	***	*****	***	***	NR	NR	NR
***	***	***	***	*****	***	***	NR	***	***	***	NR	***	***	***	***	*****	NR	***
***	***	***	*	***	***	NR	NR	***	***	NR	NR	***	***	***	*	NR	NR	NR
NR	NR	NR	NR	NR	NR	NR	NR	*****	NR	NR	NR	NR	NR	NR	NR	***	NR	NR
***	*****	***	***	*****	***	***	NR	*****	*	***	*	*****	*****	*****	***	***	NR	***
***	***	*	***	*****	***	***	NR	*****	***	***	NR	*****	*****	*****	***	***	NR	***
***	NR	*	***	***	***	NR	NR	*	***	NR	NR	***	***	*	***	***	NR	NR
NR	NR	NR	***	NR	NR	NR	NR	***	NR	NR	NR	NR	NR	NR	NR	NR	NR	NR
***	***	***	*	***	***	NR	NR	***	NR	NR	NR	***	***	***	NR	***	NR	NR
***	***	NR	***	*****	NR	NR	NR	***	***	NR	NR	NR	NR	NR	*****	*****	NR	NR
***	***	***	***	***	***	NR	NR	*	NR	NR	NR	NR	***	NR	***	NR	NR	NR
*****	NR	***	*****	*****	***	***	NR	*****	***	***	NR	***	***	***	NR	***	NR	NR
***	*****	*	***	***	***	***	NR	*****	***	***	NR	***	***	***	NR	***	NR	NR
***	NR	NR	***	***	*****	NR	NR	***	NR	NR	NR	*	*****	NR	NR	NR	NR	NR
***	NR	NR	***	*****	***	NR	NR	*****	NR	NR	NR	***	***	***	NR	*	NR	NR
***	***	NR	***	***	***	NR	NR	*	NR	***	NR	***	***	***	NR	***	NR	NR
NR	NR	NR	***	NR	NR	NR	NR	*****	NR	NR	NR	NR	NR	NR	NR	NR	NR	NR
NR	NR	NR	***	NR	NR	NR	NR	***	NR	NR	NR	NR	NR	NR	NR	NR	NR	NR
***	*****	*	***	***	***	NR	***	***	***	NR	NR	***	*****	*****	NR	*****	NR	***
***	NR	NR	***	***	***	NR	NR	***	***	NR	NR	***	***	***	NR	*	NR	NR
***	***	*	***	***	*****	***	***	*****	***	***	NR	***	***	*****	*****	*****	NR	***
***	NR	NR	***	NR	NR	NR	NR	***	NR	NR	NR	***	***	***	NR	NR	NR	NR
NR	NR	NR	***	NR	NR	NR	NR	***	NR	NR	NR	NR	NR	NR	NR	NR	NR	NR
***	NR	***	***	NR	***	NR	NR	***	NR	NR	NR	NR	***	NR	NR	NR	NR	NR
***	***	***	***	***	***	***	NR	*****	***	***	NR	***	*****	*****	***	***	NR	***
***	NR	*****	*****	NR	NR	*****	***	NR	***	NR	NR	***	***	***	NR	NR	***	NR
***	*****	***	*****	***	*	*****	NR	***	***	NR	NR	***	*****	***	***	***	NR	NR
***	***	*****	***	***	*****	NR	NR	***	NR	NR	NR	***	***	***	NR	***	NR	NR
***	NR	***	***	*****	*	NR	NR	***	NR	NR	NR	NR	NR	***	NR	NR	NR	NR

	Appendectomy	Atrial Fibrillation	Back and Neck Surgery (except Spinal Fusion)	Back and Neck Surgery (Spinal Fusion)	Bariatric Surgery	Bowel Obstruction	Carotid Surgery	Cholecystectomy (Gall Bladder Removal)	Chronic Obstructive Pulmonary Disease (COPD)	Coronary Bypass Surgery	Coronary Interventional Procedures (Angioplasty/Stent)	Diabetic Acidosis
151. McAllen Medical Center/Heart Hospital, McAllen	***	***	***	*	*	*	***	***	***	*****	***	***
152. McKenna Memorial Hospital, New Braunfels	***	***	NR	NR	NR	***	***	***	***	NR	NR	***
153. Medical Arts Hospital, Lamesa	NR	***	NR	NR	NR	NR	NR	NR	***	NR	NR	NR
154. Medical Centre Surgical Hospital, Fort Worth	NR	NR	***	***	NR	NR	NR	NR	NR	NR	NR	NR
155. Medical City Dallas Hospital, Dallas	*****	*	***	***	*	***	***	***	***	***	***	***
156. Medical Center at Lancaster, Lancaster	***	***	NR	NR	***	*	NR	***	***	NR	NR	***
157. Medical Center Hospital, Odessa	***	***	***	***	***	***	***	*****	***	*	***	***
158. Medical Center of Arlington, Arlington	*****	*	NR	NR	***	*	NR	*	***	***	*	***
159. Medical Center of Lewisville, Lewisville	*****	***	***	NR	NR	*	NR	***	***	NR	*	***
160. Medical Center of McKinney, McKinney	***	***	NR	NR	***	***	***	***	***	***	***	***
161. Medical Center of Plano, Plano	***	*	***	*	NR	*****	***	***	***	***	***	***
162. The Medical Center of Southeast Texas, Port Arthur	***	***	NR	NR	***	*****	NR	***	***	***	***	NR
163. Medina Community Hospital, Hondo	NR	NR	NR	NR	NR	NR	NR	***	NR	NR	NR	NR
164. Memorial Acute Long Term Care Hospital, Lufkin	***	***	*****	NR	***	***	***	*****	*****	*	***	***
165. Memorial Hermann Baptist Beaumont Hospital, Beaumont	*****	***	*****	*****	NR	*	***	*****	*****	*	NR	NR
166. Memorial Hermann Baptist Orange Hospital, Orange	***	***	NR	NR	NR	***	***	***	***	NR	NR	NR
167. Memorial Hermann Fort Bend Hospital, Missouri City	*	NR	NR	NR	NR	***	***	***	***	NR	NR	NR
168. Memorial Hermann Katy Hospital, Katy	***	***	NR	NR	NR	***	***	***	*****	NR	NR	NR
169. Memorial Hermann Memorial City Medical Center, Houston	***	***	*****	***	***	***	***	*****	***	***	***	***
170. Memorial Hermann Southwest Hospital, Houston	*****	*****	***	*	***	***	***	*****	*****	*	***	*****
171. Memorial Hermann–Texas Medical Center, Houston	***	*	***	***	*****	***	***	***	***	***	***	*****
172. Memorial Hospital, Dumas	NR	NR	NR	NR	NR	***	NR	***	***	NR	NR	NR
173. Memorial Hospital, Gonzales	NR	NR	NR	NR	NR	***	NR	***	***	NR	NR	NR
174. Memorial Hospital, Nacogdoches	***	***	NR	NR	NR	***	***	***	*	NR	***	***
175. Memorial Hospital, Seminole	NR	NR	NR	NR	NR	NR	NR	***	***	NR	NR	NR
176. Memorial Medical Center of East Texas, Lufkin	***	***	*****	NR	***	***	***	*****	*****	*	***	***
177. Memorial Medical Center, Port Lavaca	NR	***	NR	NR	NR	***	NR	***	***	NR	NR	NR
178. Memorial Medical Center–Livingston, Livingston	*	***	NR	NR	NR	***	NR	*	***	NR	NR	NR
179. Methodist Hospital, Houston	***	***	*****	*****	***	***	*****	***	***	***	***	***
180. Methodist Hospital, San Antonio	***	***	***	***	***	***	***	*	***	*	***	***
181. Methodist Medical Center, Dallas	*****	***	***	***	***	***	***	*****	***	***	***	***
182. Methodist Specialty and Transplant Hospital, San Antonio	***	***	***	***	***	***	***	*	***	*	***	***
183. Methodist Sugar Land Hospital, Sugar Land	*	***	NR	NR	NR	***	***	***	***	NR	NR	NR
184. Methodist Willowbrook Hospital, Houston	***	***	NR	***	NR	*****	NR	***	***	NR	NR	NR
185. Metroplex Hospital, Killeen	***	***	NR	NR	NR	*	***	***	***	NR	NR	***
186. Metropolitan Methodist Hospital, San Antonio	***	***	***	***	***	***	***	*	***	NR	***	***
187. Midland Memorial Hospital, Midland	*****	***	*****	*****	NR	***	***	***	***	*	***	***
188. Mission Regional Medical Center, Mission	***	*	NR	NR	NR	***	***	***	*****	NR	***	*
189. Mitchell County Hospital, Colorado City	NR	NR	NR	NR	NR	NR	NR	NR	*	NR	NR	NR
190. Mother Frances Hospital–Jacksonville, Jacksonville	NR	***	NR	NR	NR	***	NR	***	***	NR	NR	NR
191. Mother Frances Hospital–Tyler, Tyler	***	***	*	***	*	*****	***	*****	*****	***	***	***
192. Muleshoe Area Medical Center, Muleshoe	NR	NR	NR	NR	NR	NR	NR	***	***	NR	NR	NR
193. Nacogdoches Medical Center, Nacogdoches	***	***	***	***	***	***	***	***	*	***	***	***
194. Navarro Regional Hospital, Corsicana	*	***	NR	NR	NR	***	NR	***	*	NR	NR	***
195. Nix Health Care System, San Antonio	***	***	NR	NR	*****	***	***	***	***	NR	***	***
196. Nocona General Hospital, Nocona	NR	***	NR	NR	NR	***	NR	*	NR	NR	NR	NR
197. North Austin Medical Center, Austin	***	***	***	***	NR	***	***	***	***	***	***	***
198. North Bay Hospital, Aransas Pass	***	NR	NR	NR	NR	***	***	***	***	NR	NR	NR
199. North Hills Hospital, North Richland Hills	***	***	NR	NR	*	***	***	*****	*****	***	***	***
200. North Texas Medical Center, Gainesville	NR	***	NR	NR	NR	***	*	***	***	NR	NR	NR

KEY: ***** BEST   *** AS EXPECTED   * POOR   NR NOT RATED BY HEALTHGRADES   For full definitions of ratings and awards, see Appendix.

Gastrointestinal Bleed	Gastrointestinal Surgeries and Procedures	Heart Attack	Heart Failure	Hip Fracture Repair	Maternity Care	Pancreatitis	Peripheral Vascular Bypass	Pneumonia	Prostatectomy	Pulmonary Embolism	Resection/Replacement of Abdominal Aorta	Respiratory Failure	Sepsis	Stroke	Total Hip Replacement	Total Knee Replacement	Valve Replacement	Women's Health
★★★	★★★	★★★	★★★★★	★★★	★★★	★★★	★★★	★★★★★	NR	★★★	NR	★★★	★★★	★★★★★	NR	★★★	★★★	★★★★★
★★★	★★★★★	★★★	★★★	★★★	★★★	★★★	★★★	★★★	★	★★★	★★★	★★★★★	★★★	★★★	★★★	★★★★★	NR	NR
NR	NR	NR	★★★	NR	NR	NR	NR	★★★	NR	NR	NR	NR	NR	NR	NR	NR	NR	NR
NR	NR	NR	NR	NR	NR	NR	NR	NR	NR	NR	NR	NR	NR	NR	NR	★★★	NR	NR
★★★	★★★	★★★	★	★★★	★★★	★	★★★	★★★	★★★	★	★★★	★★★	★	★	★★★	★★★★★	★★★	★
★★★	NR	NR	★★★★★	★★★	NR	NR	NR	★★★★★	NR	NR	NR	★★★★★	★★★	★★★★★	★★★	NR	NR	NR
★★★	★★★	★★★	★★★	★★★★★	★★★	★★★	★★★	★★★	★★★	★★★	NR	★★★	★★★	★★★	★★★	★★★★★	NR	★★★
★★★	★★★	★	★★★	★★★★★	★★★	★★★	★★★	★★★	NR	★	NR	★★★★★	★★★	★★★★★	★★★	★★★	★★★	★★★
★★★	★★★★★	★★★	★★★	★	★★★	★★★	★★★	★★★	★★★	★★★	NR	★★★	★★★	★★★	★★★	★★★	NR	★★★
★★★	★★★★★	★	★★★	★★★	★★★	★★★	★★★	★★★	★★★	★★★	NR	★★★	★★★	★★★	★★★	NR	★	★
★★★	NR	★★★	★★★	★★★	★★★★★	★	★★★	★★★	NR	NR	NR	★	★★★	★★★	★★★	★★★	★★★	★★★
NR	NR	NR	★	NR	NR	NR	★★★	★★★	NR	NR	NR	NR	NR	NR	NR	NR	NR	NR
★★★	★★★★★	★★★	★	★★★	★★★★★	★★★	★★★	★	★★★	★★★	NR	★★★★★	★★★	★★★★★	★★★★★	★★★★★	NR	★★★
★★★	★	★	★	★★★★★	★★★	★★★	★★★★★	★★★	★★★	★★★	NR	★	★★★	★★★	★★★★★	★★★★★	★★★	★
★★★	★★★	★★★	★★★	NR	★★★	NR	NR	★★★	NR	★★★	NR	★	★★★	★★★	★★★	★	★★★	★★★
★★★	NR	NR	★★★★★	★★★	NR	NR	NR	★★★★★	NR	NR	NR	★★★★★	★★★★★	★★★	NR	★	★★★	NR
★★★	★★★	★★★★★	★★★★★	★★★	★★★★★	NR	NR	★★★★★	NR	★★★	NR	★★★	★★★★★	★★★★★	★★★	★	★★★	★★★
★★★	★★★	★★★	★★★	★★★	★★★★★	NR	NR	★★★★★	★★★	★★★	NR	★★★★★	★★★	★★★	★★★	★	★★★	★★★★★
★★★★★	★★★★★	★★★	★★★	★★★★★	★★★	★★★★★	★★★★★	★★★★★	★★★	★★★	★★★	★★★★★	★★★★★	★★★★★	★★★	★★★★★	★	★★★★★
★★★	★★★★★	★★★	★★★★★	★	★★★	★★★	★★★	★★★	★★★	★★★	NR	★★★★★	★★★	★★★	★★★	★	★	★
★★★	NR	NR	★★★	★★★	★★★	NR	NR	★★★	NR	NR	NR	NR	NR	★★★	NR	★★★	NR	NR
★★★	NR	★	★★★	NR	NR	NR	★	NR	NR	NR	NR	NR	★★★	NR	NR	NR	NR	NR
★★★	★★★	★★★	★★★	★★★	NR	NR	★	NR	NR	NR	NR	★	★	★	NR	★★★	NR	★★★
NR	NR	NR	★★★	NR	NR	NR	NR	★★★	NR	NR	NR	NR	NR	NR	NR	NR	NR	NR
★★★	★★★★★	★★★	★	★★★	★★★★★	★★★	★	★★★	★★★	NR	NR	★★★★★	★	★★★★★	★★★	★★★★★	NR	★★★
★★★	NR	★	★★★	NR	NR	NR	★	NR	NR	NR	NR	NR	NR	NR	NR	NR	NR	NR
★★★	NR	NR	★★★	★★★	★★★	NR	NR	★★★	NR	NR	NR	NR	NR	★★★	NR	★★★	NR	NR
★★★	★★★	★★★	★★★	★★★	★★★	★★★	★★★	★★★	★★★	★★★	★★★	★★★	★★★	★★★★★	★★★	★★★	★★★	★★★
★★★★★	★★★★★	★★★	★★★★★	★★★	★★★★★	★★★	★★★★★	★★★★★	★	★★★	★★★	★★★	★★★	★★★	★★★	★★★	★★★	★★★
★★★	★★★	★★★	★★★	★★★	★★★	★★★	★★★	NR	★★★	★★★	★★★	★★★	★★★	★★★★★	★★★	★★★	★★★	★★★
★★★★★	★★★★★	★★★	★★★	★★★★★	★★★	★★★★★	★★★★★	★	★★★	★★★	★★★	★★★	★★★	★★★	★★★	★★★	★★★	★★★
★★★	★	★★★	★★★★★	★★★	★★★	★★★	★★★	NR	NR	NR	NR	★★★★★	★★★★★	NR	NR	★★★	★★★	NR
★★★	★★★	★★★★★	★★★	★★★	★★★	NR	★★★	★★★★★	NR	NR	NR	★★★	★★★	★★★★★	★★★	★★★	★★★	NR
★★★	NR	★★★	★	★★★★★	★★★	NR	★★★	★★★	NR	NR	NR	★★★	★	★★★	NR	★★★	★★★	NR
★★★★★	★★★★★	★★★	★★★★★	★★★	★★★★★	★★★	★★★★★	★★★★★	★	★★★	★★★	★★★	★★★	★★★	★★★	★★★	★★★	★★★
★★★	★★★	★★★	★★★	★★★★★	★★★	★★★★★	★★★	★★★	★★★	★★★	NR	★★★★★	★★★	★★★	★★★★★	★★★	★★★	★★★
★★★	★★★	★★★	★★★	★★★	★★★★★	★★★	★★★★★	NR	★★★	★★★	NR	★★★	★★★	★★★	★★★	★★★	★★★	★★★
NR	NR	NR	★★★	NR	NR	NR	NR	★	NR	NR	NR	NR	NR	NR	NR	NR	NR	NR
★★★	NR	NR	★★★	NR	NR	NR	NR	★★★	NR	NR	NR	NR	NR	NR	NR	★★★	NR	NR
★★★	★★★	★★★	★★★	★★★	★★★	★★★	★★★	★★★	★★★	★★★	★★★	★★★★★	★★★★★	★★★	★	★★★	★★★	★★★
★★★	NR	NR	★	NR	NR	NR	NR	★★★	NR	NR	NR	NR	NR	NR	NR	★★★	NR	NR
★	★★★	★	★	★★★	★	★★★	★	NR	★	NR	★★★	★★★	★★★	NR	★★★	★★★	★★★	★
★★★	★★★	★	★	★★★	★	NR	★★★	★★★	★★★	NR	★★★	★★★	★	★★★	NR	★★★	NR	NR
★★★	★★★	★★★	★★★	★★★	★★★	★★★	★★★	★★★	NR	★★★	★★★	★★★	★★★	★★★	★★★★★	NR	NR	NR
★★★	NR	NR	★★★	NR	NR	NR	NR	★★★	NR	NR	NR	★	★	NR	NR	NR	NR	NR
★	★★★	★★★	★★★	★★★★★	★★★★★	NR	★★★	★★★	★★★	★★★	NR	★★★	★★★	★★★★★	★★★	★★★	★★★	★★★
★★★	NR	NR	★★★	NR	NR	NR	NR	★★★	NR	NR	NR	NR	★★★	NR	NR	NR	NR	NR
★★★	★★★	★★★	★★★	★★★	NR	NR	★★★	★★★	NR	NR	NR	★★★	★★★★★	★★★	★★★	★★★	NR	NR
★★★	NR	★	★★★	★★★	NR	NR	NR	★	NR	NR	NR	NR	★★★	★★★	NR	★★★	NR	★

	Appendectomy	Atrial Fibrillation	Back and Neck Surgery (except Spinal Fusion)	Back and Neck Surgery (Spinal Fusion)	Bariatric Surgery	Bowel Obstruction	Carotid Surgery	Cholecystectomy (Gall Bladder Removal)	Chronic Obstructive Pulmonary Disease (COPD)	Coronary Bypass Surgery	Coronary Interventional Procedures (Angioplasty/Stent)	Diabetic Acidosis
201. Northeast Medical Center Hospital, Humble	★★★	★★★	NR	NR	NR	★★★	★	★★★	★★★★★	NR	NR	★★★
202. Northeast Medical Center, Bonham	NR	NR	NR	NR	NR	★★★	NR	NR	★	NR	NR	
203. Northeast Methodist Hospital, Live Oak	★★★	★★★	★★★	★★★	★★★	★★★	★★★	★	★★★	★	★★★	★★★
204. Northwest Texas Healthcare System, Amarillo	★	★★★	★	★	★★★	★★★	★★★	★	★★★★★	★★★	★★★	★★★
205. Oakbend Medical Center, Richmond	★★★	★★★	NR	NR	NR	★★★	NR	★★★	★★★	NR	★★★	
206. Ochiltree General Hospital, Perryton	NR	NR	NR	NR	NR	NR	NR	★★★	NR	NR		
207. Odessa Regional Medical Center, Odessa	★★★	NR	NR	NR	NR	★★★	NR	★★★	★★★	NR	★★★	
208. Otto Kaiser Memorial Hospital, Kenedy	NR	NR	NR	NR	NR	NR	NR	★★★	NR	NR		
209. Palestine Regional Medical Center, Palestine	★★★	★★★	NR	NR	★★★	★★★	NR	★★★	★★★	NR	★★★	
210. Palo Pinto General Hospital, Mineral Wells	NR	★★★	NR	NR	NR	★★★	★	★★★	★★★	NR	★★★	
211. Pampa Regional Medical Center, Pampa	NR	★★★	NR	NR	NR	★★★	NR	★★★★★	★★★	NR	★★★	
212. Paris Regional Medical Center, Paris	★★★★★	★★★	★★★	NR	★★★	★★★	★★★	★★★	★★★	★	★	★
213. Park Plaza Hospital and Medical Center, Houston	★	★★★	★★★	NR	★★★	★★★	★★★	★★★	★★★	★	★★★	
214. Parkland Health and Hospital System, Dallas	★	★★★	NR	NR	★★★	★	NR	★	★★★	★★★	★★★	
215. Parkview Regional Hospital, Mexia	NR	★★★	NR	NR	NR	★★★	NR	★★★★★	★★★	NR	NR	
216. Pecos County Memorial Hospital, Fort Stockton	NR	NR	NR	NR	★★★	NR	NR	★	NR	NR		
217. Permian Regional Medical Center, Andrews	NR	NR	NR	NR	NR	NR	NR	★★★	NR	NR		
218. Physicians Specialty Hospital of El Paso, El Paso	NR	★★★	NR	★★★	NR	★★★	NR	★★★	★★★	NR	★★★	NR
219. Plaza Medical Center of Fort Worth, Fort Worth	★★★	★★★	★★★	★★★★★	★★★	★	★★★	★★★	★★★	★★★	★	★★★
220. Presbyterian Hospital of Allen, Allen	★★★	NR	NR	NR	NR	NR	NR	★★★	NR	NR	NR	
221. Presbyterian Hospital of Dallas, Dallas	★★★	★★★	★★★★★	★★★	★★★	★★★	★★★★★	★	★★★	★★★	★	★★★
222. Presbyterian Hospital of Denton, Denton	★★★	★★★	NR	NR	★★★	★★★	★★★	★★★	★★★	★	★★★	★★★
223. Presbyterian Hospital of Greenville, Greenville	★★★	★★★	NR	NR	★	NR	★★★	★★★	★★★	NR	★★★	
224. Presbyterian Hospital of Kaufman, Kaufman	★	★★★	NR	NR	★	NR	★★★	★★★	★★★	NR	NR	
225. Presbyterian Hospital of Plano, Plano	★★★	★★★	★★★	★★★	★★★	★★★★★	★★★	★★★	★★★	★★★	★★★	★★★
226. Presbyterian Hospital of Winnsboro, Winnsboro	★★★★★	NR	NR	NR	NR	★★★	NR	★	NR	NR	NR	
227. Providence Healthcare Network, Waco	★★★	★★★	★★★	★★★★★	NR	★★★	★★★	★★★	★★★	★★★	★	★★★
228. Providence Memorial Hospital, El Paso	★★★	★★★	★★★	★★★	★★★	★★★	★★★	★★★	★★★	★	★	★★★★★
229. R. E. Thomason General Hospital, El Paso	★★★	★★★	NR	NR	NR	★	NR	★★★	★★★★★	NR	NR	★★★
230. Reeves County Hospital District, Pecos	NR	NR	NR	NR	NR	NR	NR	★★★	NR	NR		
231. Renaissance Hospital, Groves	NR	NR	NR	NR	★	NR	NR	★★★	NR	NR		
232. Renaissance Hospital, Houston	NR	NR	NR	NR	★★★	NR	NR	★★★	NR	NR		
233. Renaissance Hospital–Dallas, Dallas	★★★	NR	NR	NR	NR	NR	NR	NR	NR	★★★	NR	
234. Renaissance Hospital–Terrell, Terrell	★★★	★★★	NR	NR	NR	★★★	NR	★★★★★	NR	NR		
235. RHD Memorial Medical Center, Dallas	★★★★★	★★★	NR	NR	★★★★★	★	★★★	★★★	★★★	NR	★★★	NR
236. Richards Memorial Hospital, Rockdale	NR	NR	NR	NR	NR	NR	NR	★★★	★★★	NR	NR	
237. Richardson Regional Medical Center, Richardson	★	★★★	★★★	★★★	★★★	★★★	★★★	★★★	★★★	★★★	★★★	★★★
238. Rio Grande Regional Hospital, McAllen	★	★★★	★★★★★	NR	★★★	★★★	★★★	★★★	★★★★★	★★★	★★★	★★★
239. Rolling Plains Memorial Hospital, Sweetwater	NR	NR	NR	NR	NR	★★★	NR	★★★★★	NR	NR	NR	
240. Rollins Brook Community Hospital, Lampasas	NR	NR	NR	NR	NR	NR	NR	★★★	★★★	NR	NR	
241. Round Rock Medical Center, Round Rock	★★★★★	★★★	NR	NR	NR	★★★	NR	★★★	★★★	NR	NR	
242. Sabine County Hospital, Hemphill	NR	NR	NR	NR	NR	NR	NR	★	NR	NR		
243. St. David's Hospital, Austin	★★★★★	★★★	★★★	★★★	★★★	★★★	★★★★★	★★★	★★★	★★★	★★★	★★★
244. St. Joseph Medical Center, Houston	★★★	★★★	★★★	★★★	NR	★★★	★★★★★	★★★	★★★	★★★	★★★	★
245. St. Joseph Regional Health Center, Bryan	★★★★★	★★★	★★★★★	★★★	NR	★★★	★★★★★	★★★	★★★	★★★	★★★	★★★
246. St. Luke's Baptist Hospital, San Antonio	★★★	★★★	★★★	★★★	NR	★★★	★★★★★	★★★	★★★	★★★	★★★	★★★
247. St. Luke's Community Med. Ctr.–The Woodlands, The Woodlands	★★★	★★★	NR	NR	NR	★★★	NR	★★★★★	★★★★★	★★★	NR	
248. St. Luke's Episcopal Hospital, Houston	★★★	★★★	★★★	★★★	★★★	★★★	★★★★★	★★★	★★★★★	★★★	★★★	★★★
249. St. Mark's Medical Center, La Grange	NR	NR	NR	NR	NR	NR	NR	NR	NR	NR		
250. Sam Houston Memorial Hospital, Houston	★★★	★★★	★★★	NR	NR	★★★	★★★	★★★★★	★★★★★	★★★	★★★	★★★

KEY: ★★★★★ BEST ★★★ AS EXPECTED ★ POOR NR NOT RATED BY HEALTHGRADES For full definitions of ratings and awards, see Appendix.

Gastrointestinal Bleed	Gastrointestinal Surgeries and Procedures	Heart Attack	Heart Failure	Hip Fracture Repair	Maternity Care	Pancreatitis	Peripheral Vascular Bypass	Pneumonia	Prostatectomy	Pulmonary Embolism	Resection/Replacement of Abdominal Aorta	Respiratory Failure	Sepsis	Stroke	Total Hip Replacement	Total Knee Replacement	Valve Replacement	Women's Health
★★★★★	★★★	★	★★★	★★★	★★★★★	★★★★★	★★★	★★★★★	★★★	★★★	NR	★★★	★★★★★	★★★	★★★	★	NR	NR
★★★	NR	★★★★★	★★★	NR	NR	NR	NR	★★★	NR	NR	NR	NR	★★★	NR	★★★	NR	NR	NR
★★★★★	★★★★★	★★★	★★★★★	★★★	★★★★★	★★★	★★★★★	★★★★★	★	★★★	★★★	★★★	★★★	★★★	★★★	★★★	★★★	★★★
★★★	★★★	★★★★★	★★★★★	★★★	★	NR	★★★	★★★★★	NR	★★★	NR	★★★★★	★★★★★	★★★★★	★★★	★★★	★★★	★★★
★★★	NR	★★★	★★★★★	★★★	★★★★★	★★★	NR	★★★★★	NR	NR	NR	★★★★★	★★★★★	★★★★★	★★★	★★★	NR	NR
NR	NR	NR	★	NR	NR	NR	NR	★	NR	NR	NR	NR	NR	NR	NR	NR	NR	NR
NR	NR	NR	★★★	NR	★★★★★	NR	NR	★★★	NR	NR	NR	NR	NR	NR	NR	NR	NR	NR
NR	NR	NR	★	NR	NR	NR	NR	★★★	NR	NR	NR	NR	NR	NR	NR	NR	NR	NR
★★★	★★★	★	★★★	★★★	★	★★★	NR	★★★	NR	★	NR	★★★	★★★	★★★	★★★	★★★	NR	NR
★★★	NR	★	★	★★★	★★★	NR	NR	★	NR	★	NR	★★★	★★★	★★★	★★★	★★★	NR	NR
★	NR	NR	★★★★★	★★★	★	NR	NR	★★★	★★★	NR	NR	★★★★★	★★★	★★★	★★★	★	NR	NR
★★★	★★★	★	★★★	★★★★★	NR	★★★	★★★	★★★	★★★	★	NR	★★★	★	★	★★★	★★★	★★★	NR
★★★	★★★	★★★	★★★	★	★★★	★★★	★★★	★★★★★	★★★	NR	NR	★★★	★★★	★★★	★★★	★★★	★★★	NR
★★★	NR	★★★	★★★	NR	NR	★★★	NR	★★★	NR	NR	NR	★★★	★★★	★★★★★	NR	NR	★★★	NR
NR	NR	NR	★★★	NR	NR	NR	NR	★★★	NR	NR	NR	NR	NR	NR	NR	NR	NR	NR
★★★	NR	NR	★	NR	NR	NR	NR	★★★	NR	NR	NR	NR	NR	NR	NR	NR	NR	NR
★★★	NR	★★★	★★★	NR	NR	NR	NR	★★★★★	★★★★★	NR	NR	NR	★★★	★★★	NR	★★★	NR	NR
★★★	★★★	★★★	★★★	★	★★★	★★★	★★★	★★★	★★★	★★★	★★★	★★★	★★★★★	★	★	★★★	★★★	★★★
★★★	★★★	★★★	★★★★★	★★★	★★★	NR	★★★	★★★	★★★	★★★	NR	★★★	★★★★★	★★★	★★★★★	★★★	★★★	★★★
★★★	NR	★★★	★★★	★	NR	★★★	★★★★★	★★★★★	NR	NR	NR	★★★	★★★	★	NR	★★★	NR	NR
★★★	NR	★★★	★★★	★	NR	★	★★★	NR	NR	★	NR	★★★	★★★	★★★	★★★	NR	NR	NR
★★★	★★★	★★★	★★★	★★★	★★★	★★★	★★★	★★★	★★★	★★★★★	★★★★★	★★★	★★★★★	★★★★★	★★★★★	★★★★★	★★★	★★★
NR	NR	NR	★★★	NR	NR	NR	NR	★★★	NR	NR	NR	NR	★★★	★	NR	NR	NR	NR
★★★	★★★	★★★	★★★	★★★★★	★★★	★★★	★★★	★★★	★★★★★	★★★	★★★	★★★★★	★★★	★★★★★	★★★★★	★★★★★	★★★	★★★
★★★	★★★★★	★★★	★★★	★★★★★	★★★★★	★	★★★	★★★	★★★★★	★★★	NR	★★★	★	★★★	★★★	★★★	★	★★★
★★★	★	★★★	★★★	★★★	★★★	★★★	NR	★★★	★★★	NR	NR	★★★	★★★	★★★	NR	★★★	NR	NR
★★★	NR	NR	★★★	NR	NR	NR	NR	★	NR	NR	NR	NR	NR	NR	NR	NR	NR	NR
★★★	NR	NR	★★★	NR	NR	NR	NR	★★★★★	NR	NR	NR	NR	★★★	★★★	NR	NR	NR	NR
NR	NR	NR	★★★	NR	NR	NR	NR	★★★	NR	NR	NR	NR	NR	NR	NR	NR	NR	NR
★★★	NR	NR	★★★	NR	NR	NR	NR	★★★	NR	NR	NR	NR	★★★★★	★★★	NR	NR	NR	NR
★★★	NR	★★★★★	★★★★★	★★★	★★★	★★★	NR	★★★	NR	NR	NR	★★★★★	★★★★★	★★★	NR	NR	NR	NR
★★★	NR	★★★	★★★	★★★	★	NR	NR	★★★	★★★	NR	NR	★★★★★	★★★	NR	NR	★★★	NR	NR
NR	NR	NR	★★★	NR	NR	NR	NR	★★★	NR	NR	NR	NR	★★★	NR	NR	NR	NR	NR
★★★	★★★	★★★	★★★	★★★	★★★	★★★	NR	★★★	NR	NR	NR	★★★	★	★★★	NR	★	NR	★
★★★	★★★	★★★	★★★	★★★	★★★★★	★★★	★★★★★	★★★★★	★★★	★★★	NR	★★★★★	★★★	★★★	★★★	★★★	NR	★★★
★★★	★★★★★	NR	★★★	NR	NR	NR	★★★★★	★★★	NR	NR	NR	NR	★★★	★★★	NR	NR	NR	★★★
★★★	NR	NR	★★★	NR	NR	NR	NR	★★★	NR	NR	NR	NR	NR	NR	NR	NR	NR	NR
★★★	★★★★★	★★★	★★★	★★★	★★★	★★★	NR	★★★	★★★	★★★	NR	★★★	★★★	★★★	★★★	★★★	NR	★★★
NR	NR	NR	★★★	NR	NR	NR	NR	★★★	NR	NR	NR	NR	NR	NR	NR	NR	NR	NR
★★★	★★★	★★★	★★★★★	★★★★★	★★★★★	★★★	NR	★★★★★	★★★★★	★★★	NR	★★★	★★★★★	★★★★★	★★★	★★★	★★★	★★★
★★★	★★★	★★★	★★★	★★★	★★★	★★★	★★★	★★★	NR	NR	NR	★★★	★★★★★	★★★★★	★★★	★★★	★★★★★	★★★
★★★	NR	★	★★★	★★★	★	NR	★★★★★	★★★	★	★★★	NR	★★★	★★★	★	★★★	★★★★★	★★★	★
★	★★★	★★★★★	★★★	★★★★★	★★★	★★★	★★★★★	★★★	★	★★★	★★★	★★★★★	★★★★★	★★★	★★★	★★★	NR	★★★
★★★	NR	★★★	★★★	★★★	★★★★★	NR	★★★	★★★	★★★	NR	NR	★★★★★	★★★	★★★	★★★	★★★	NR	★★★
★★★	★★★	NR	★★★	★★★	★★★	★★★	★★★	★★★★★	★★★	★★★	NR	★★★★★	★★★★★	★★★★★	★★★	★	NR	★★★
★★★	NR	NR	★★★	★★★	NR	★★★	★★★	★★★	NR	NR	NR	★★★	★★★	NR	NR	NR	NR	NR
★★★	★★★★★	★★★	★★★	★★★	NR	★★★	★★★★★	★★★★★	★★★	NR	NR	★★★★★	★★★★★	★★★	★★★	★★★	NR	NR

	Appendectomy	Atrial Fibrillation	Back and Neck Surgery (except Spinal Fusion)	Back and Neck Surgery (Spinal Fusion)	Bariatric Surgery	Bowel Obstruction	Carotid Surgery	Cholecystectomy (Gall Bladder Removal)	Chronic Obstructive Pulmonary Disease (COPD)	Coronary Bypass Surgery	Coronary Interventional Procedures (Angioplasty/Stent)	Diabetic Acidosis a
251. San Angelo Community Medical Center, San Angelo	★	★★★	★★★	NR	NR	★★★	NR	★★★	★★★	★★★	★★★	
252. San Jacinto Methodist Hospital, Baytown	★★★	★★★	★★★★★	NR	NR	★★★	★	★★★	★★★★★	NR	★★★	★★★
253. SCCI Hospital–San Angelo, San Angelo	★★★★★	★★★	★★★★★	★★★★★	NR	★	★★★★★	★★★★★	★★★	★★★	★★★	
254. Scenic Mountain Medical Center, Big Spring	★★★	★★★	NR	NR	NR	★★★	NR	★★★	★★★	NR	★★★	
255. Scott and White Memorial Hospital, Temple	★★★★★	★★★	★★★	★★★★★	★★★★★	★★★	★★★★★	★★★★★	★★★	★★★	★★★	
256. Sempercare Hospital of Midland, Midland	★★★★★	★★★	★★★★★	★★★★★	NR	★★★	★★★	★★★	★	★	★★★	★★★
257. Seton Edgar B. Davis Hospital, Luling	NR	★★★	NR	NR	NR	★★★	NR	★★★	★★★	NR	★★★	
258. Seton Highland Lakes, Burnet	★★★★★	★★★	NR	NR	NR	★★★	★★★	★★★	★★★	NR	NR	
259. Seton Medical Center, Austin	★★★★★	★★★	★★★★★	★★★	★★★	★★★★★	★★★	★★★	★★★	★★★	★★★	
260. Seton Northwest Hospital, Austin	★★★	★	NR	NR	NR	★★★	NR	★★★	★★★	NR	NR	
261. Shannon West Texas Medical Center, San Angelo	★★★★★	★★★	★★★★★	★★★★★	NR	★	★★★★★	★★★★★	★★★	★★★	★★★	
262. Shelby Regional Medical Center, Center	NR	NR	NR	NR	NR	NR	NR	NR	★★★	NR	NR	
263. Sid Peterson Memorial Hospital, Kerrville	★	★★★	NR	NR	★★★	★★★	★★★	★	★★★	NR	NR	
264. Sierra Medical Center, El Paso	★★★★★	★★★	★★★★★	★★★	NR	★★★	★★★★★	★★★	★★★	★	★★★	★★★
265. Smithville Regional Hospital, Smithville	★★★★★	★★★	NR	NR	NR	★★★	NR	★★★	★★★★★	NR	NR	
266. South Austin Hospital, Austin	★★★★★	★★★★★	★★★	★★★	NR	★★★	★★★	★★★★★	★★★	★★★	★★★	★★★
267. South Texas Regional Medical Center, Jourdanton	★★★	★★★	NR	NR	NR	★★★	NR	★★★	★★★★★	NR	NR	
268. Southside Health Center, Corpus Christi	★★★	★★★	★★★	★★★	NR	★★★	★★★★★	★★★	★★★★★	★★★	★★★	★★★
269. Southwest General Hospital, San Antonio	★★★	★★★	NR	NR	★★★	★★★	NR	★★★	★★★	NR	★★★	
270. Southwestern General Hospital, El Paso	NR	NR	NR	NR	NR	NR	NR	★★★	NR	NR	NR	
271. Spring Branch Medical Center, Houston	★★★	★★★	★★★	NR	★★★★★	★★★	★★★	★★★★★	★★★★★	★★★	★★★	★★★
272. Starr County Memorial Hospital, Rio Grande City	NR	NR	NR	NR	NR	NR	NR	NR	★★★	NR	★★★	
273. Stephens Memorial Hospital, Breckenridge	NR	★★★	NR	NR	NR	NR	NR	NR	★★★	NR	NR	
274. Sun Belt Regional Medical Center–East, Channelview	★★★	★★★	NR	NR	NR	★★★	NR	★★★	★★★	NR	★★★	
275. Texas Orthopedic Hospital, Houston	NR	NR	★★★	★★★★★	NR	NR	NR	NR	NR	NR	NR	
276. Texoma Medical Center, Denison	★★★	★★★	★★★	★★★	NR	★★★★★	★★★★★	★★★★★	★★★	★★★	★★★	★★★
277. Texsan Heart Hospital, San Antonio	NR	★★★	NR	NR	NR	★★★	NR	NR	★	★★★★★	NR	
278. Titus County Memorial Hospital, Mt. Pleasant	NR	★★★	NR	NR	NR	★★★	NR	★★★	★★★	NR	NR	
279. Tomball Regional Hospital, Tomball	★★★	★★★	★★★	NR	NR	★★★	★★★	★★★	★★★★★	★★★	★	★★★
280. Trinity Medical Center, Brenham	NR	★★★	NR	NR	NR	★★★	NR	★★★	★★★	NR	NR	
281. Trinity Medical Center, Carrollton	★★★	★★★	NR	NR	★	★★★	NR	★★★	★★★	NR	NR	
282. Twelve Oaks Medical Center, Houston	★	★★★	★★★	★★★	★★★★★	★★★	NR	★★★	★★★	NR	★★★	
283. Tyler County Hospital, Woodville	NR	★★★	NR	NR	NR	★★★	NR	NR	★	NR	NR	
284. United Regional Health Care System, Wichita Falls	★★★	★★★★★	★★★	★★★	★★★★★	★★★	★★★★★	★★★	★★★★★	★★★	★★★	★★★
285. University Health System, San Antonio	★★★★★	★★★	NR	NR	★★★	★★★	NR	★★★	★★★	★★★	★	★★★
286. University Medical Center, Lubbock	★★★	★	★★★	★	★★★	★	★★★	★★★	★★★	★	★★★	★
287. University of Texas Health Center at Tyler, Tyler	NR	★★★	NR	NR	NR	★★★	★★★★★	★★★	★★★	★★★	★★★	NR
288. University of Texas Medical Branch Galveston, Galveston	★★★	★★★	★★★	★★★	★★★	★★★	★★★	★★★	★★★	★★★	★★★	
289. UT Southwestern Medical Center, Dallas	★★★	★★★	★★★★★	★★★★★	NR	★★★	★★★★★	★★★★★	★★★	★	★★★	
290. UT Southwestern Zale Lipshy Hospital, Dallas	NR	★★★	★★★	★★★	★★★	★★★	★★★	★★★★★	NR	NR	NR	
291. Uvalde Memorial Hospital, Uvalde	NR	★★★	NR	NR	NR	★★★	NR	★★★	★★★	NR	★★★	
292. Val Verde Regional Medical Center, Del Rio	★★★	★★★	NR	NR	NR	★★★	★★★	★★★★★	★★★	NR	★★★	
293. Valley Baptist Medical Center, Harlingen	★★★★★	★★★	★★★	★★★	★★★★★	★★★	★★★★★	★★★★★	★★★	★★★	★★★	★★★
294. Valley Baptist Medical Center–Brownsville, Brownsville	★★★★★	★★★	NR	NR	NR	★★★	NR	★★★	★★★	★★★	★★★	★
295. Valley Regional Medical Center, Brownsville	★★★★★	★★★	NR	★★★	★★★	★★★	NR	★★★★★	★★★★★	★★★	★★★	★★★
296. W. J. Mangold Memorial Hospital, Lockney	NR	NR	NR	NR	NR	NR	NR	NR	★★★	NR	NR	
297. Wadley Regional Medical Center, Texarkana	★★★	★★★	★★★	★★★★★	NR	★★★	★★★★★	★★★★★	★★★	★★★	★	
298. Walls Regional Hospital, Cleburne	★★★★★	★★★	NR	NR	NR	★★★	NR	★★★	★★★	NR	★★★	
299. Ward Memorial Hospital, Monahans	NR	NR	NR	NR	NR	NR	NR	★★★	NR	NR	NR	
300. West Houston Medical Center, Houston	★★★★★	★★★	NR	NR	NR	★★★	★★★★★	★★★★★	★★★	★★★	★★★	

KEY: ★★★★★ BEST ★★★ AS EXPECTED ★ POOR NR NOT RATED BY HEALTHGRADES For full definitions of ratings and awards, see Appendix.

Gastrointestinal Bleed	Gastrointestinal Surgeries and Procedures	Heart Attack	Heart Failure	Hip Fracture Repair	Maternity Care	Pancreatitis	Peripheral Vascular Bypass	Pneumonia	Prostatectomy	Pulmonary Embolism	Resection/Replacement of Abdominal Aorta	Respiratory Failure	Sepsis	Stroke	Total Hip Replacement	Total Knee Replacement	Valve Replacement	Women's Health
★★★	★	★★★	★★★	★★★	★★★	★★★	NR	★★★	★★★	NR	NR	NR	★	★★★	★★★	★★★	NR	★★★
★★★	★★★	★★★★★	★★★★★	★★★	★★★	★★★	NR	★★★★★	★★★	★★★	NR	★★★★★	★★★★★	★★★★★	★★★	★	NR	NR
★	★★★	★★★	★★★	★★★	★★★	★★★	★★★★★	★★★	★★★	★★★	★★★	★★★	★	★★★	★★★★★	★★★★★	★★★	★★★
★★★	NR	★★★	★★★	★★★	★	NR	NR	★★★	★★★	NR	NR	★	★★★	NR	NR	★	NR	NR
★★★★★	★★★	★★★	★★★	★★★★★	★★★	★★★	NR	★★★	★★★★★	★★★	★★★	★★★	★★★	★★★★★	★★★★★	★★★★★	★	★★★
★★★	★★★	★★★	★★★	★★★★★	★★★	★★★★★	★★★	★★★	★★★	★★★	★★★	★★★★★	★★★	★★★	★★★★★	★★★	NR	★★★
NR	NR	NR	★	NR	NR	NR	NR	★★★	NR	NR	NR	NR	NR	★★★	NR	NR	NR	NR
★★★	★★★	NR	★★★	NR	★★★★★	NR	NR	★★★	NR	NR	NR	NR	★★★	NR	NR	NR	NR	★★★
★★★	★★★	★★★★★	★★★	★★★★★	★★★★★	★★★	★★★	★★★	NR	★★★	★★★	★★★	★★★★★	NR	★★★★★	★★★★★	★★★	★★★
★★★	NR	★★★	★★★	★★★	★★★	★★★	NR	★★★★★	NR	NR	NR	★★★	★★★	★★★	NR	★★★	NR	NR
★	★★★	★★★	★★★	★★★	★★★	★★★	★★★★★	★★★	★★★	★★★	★★★	★★★	★	★★★	★★★★★	★★★	★★★	NR
★	NR	NR	★	NR	★	NR	NR	★	NR	NR	NR	NR	NR	NR	NR	NR	NR	NR
★★★	★★★	★★★	★	★★★	★★★	★★★	NR	★	★★★	★★★	★★★	★	★★★	★★★	★★★★★	NR	NR	NR
★★★	★★★	★★★	★★★	★★★★★	★★★	★★★	NR	★★★	★★★	★★★	★★★	★★★	★★★	★★★	★★★★★	★★★	NR	★★★
★★★	NR	NR	★★★	★★★	★★★	★★★	NR	★★★★★	NR	NR	NR	★★★	★★★	NR	NR	NR	NR	NR
★★★	★★★★★	★★★★★	★★★★★	★★★	★★★	★★★	NR	★★★	★★★★★	★★★	★★★	★	★★★★★	★	★★★	★★★	★★★	★★★★★
★★★	NR	★★★★★	★★★★★	★	NR	NR	NR	★★★★★	NR	NR	NR	★	★★★	★★★	NR	★★★	NR	NR
★	★★★	★★★	★★★★★	★★★	★★★★★	★★★	★★★★★	★★★	★★★	★★★	NR	★★★	★★★★★	★★★	★★★	★	★★★	★★★
★★★	NR	★★★	★★★★★	★★★	★★★★★	★★★	NR	★★★	★★★	NR	NR	★★★	★★★	★	NR	★★★	NR	NR
NR	NR	NR	★★★	NR	NR	NR	NR	★★★★★	NR	NR	NR	NR	NR	NR	NR	NR	NR	NR
★★★	★★★★★	★★★	★★★	★★★	NR	★★★	★★★★★	★★★	★★★	NR	★★★★★	★★★★★	★★★	★★★	★★★	★★★★★	NR	★★★
★★★	NR	★★★	★	NR	★★★	NR	NR	★★★	NR	NR	NR	NR	★	NR	NR	NR	NR	NR
★★★	NR	NR	★	NR	NR	NR	NR	★★★	NR	NR	NR	NR	NR	NR	NR	NR	NR	NR
★★★	★★★	★★★	★★★	NR	★★★	★★★	NR	★★★	NR	NR	NR	★★★★★	★★★★★	★★★★★	NR	NR	NR	NR
NR	NR	NR	NR	NR	NR	NR	NR	NR	NR	NR	NR	NR	NR	★★★★★	★★★★★	NR	NR	NR
★★★	★★★★★	★★★	★★★	NR	★★★	★★★	NR	★	★★★	★★★	★★★	★★★	★★★	★★★	★★★★★	NR	★★★	
NR	★★★	★★★	★★★★★	NR	NR	NR	NR	★★★	NR	NR	NR	★★★	★★★	★★★	NR	★★★		
★★★	★★★	★★★	★★★	★	NR	NR	NR	★★★★★	NR	NR	NR	★★★★★	★★★	★★★	NR	★	NR	NR
★★★	★★★	★★★★★	★★★	★★★	★★★	★★★	NR	★★★	★★★	★★★	NR	★★★	★★★	★	★★★	NR	★★★	
★★★	NR	★★★	★	★★★	NR	NR	NR	★	NR	NR	NR	★	★★★	★★★	NR	★★★	NR	NR
★★★	★★★	★★★	★★★★★	★★★	★★★	NR	NR	★★★	NR	NR	NR	★	★★★	★★★	NR	★	NR	★★★
★★★	NR	★★★	★★★	★★★	★★★★★	NR	NR	★★★	NR	NR	NR	★★★	★★★	NR	★★★	NR	NR	
★★★	NR	NR	★	NR	NR	NR	NR	★	NR	NR	NR	★	★★★	★	NR	NR	NR	NR
★★★	★★★★★	★★★	★★★	★★★★★	★★★★★	★★★	NR	★★★	★★★	★★★	★★★	★★★	★★★	★★★	★★★	★★★★★	★	★★★
★★★	★★★	★	★★★	★★★	★★★	NR	★★★	★★★	★★★	NR	NR	NR	★★★	NR	★★★	★★★	★★★	
★	★	★	★★★	★	★	★★★	NR	★	★★★	NR	NR	★★★	★★★	★	★★★	★	NR	★
★★★	★★★	★★★★★	NR	NR	★★★	★★★	NR	★★★	NR	NR	★★★★★	★★★	★★★★★	NR	NR	NR	NR	
★★★	★★★	★★★	★★★★★	★★★	★★★	★★★	★★★	★★★	NR	★★★	★★★	★★★	★	★★★	★	NR	★★★	
★★★	★★★	★	★★★	★★★	★★★	NR	★★★★★	NR	★★★	NR	★★★★★	★★★	★★★	★★★	NR	★★★	★★★	
★★★	★★★	NR	★★★	NR	NR	NR	NR	★★★★★	★★★	NR	NR	NR	★★★★★	★★★	★★★	NR	★★★	
★★★	NR	★	★★★	★★★	NR	NR	NR	★★★	NR	NR	NR	★★★	NR	NR	★	NR	NR	
★★★	★★★	★★★	★★★	★★★	★★★★★	NR	NR	★★★	★	NR	NR	★	★	★	NR	★★★	NR	NR
★★★	★★★	★★★	★★★	★★★	★★★	★★★	NR	★★★	★★★	★★★	★★★	★★★★★	★★★★★	★★★★★	★★★★★	★	★★★	
★	★★★	★★★	★★★	★★★	★★★	★★★	NR	★★★	NR	NR	NR	★★★	★★★	★★★★★	NR	★★★	★★★	
★★★	★★★	★★★	★★★	★★★	★★★	★★★	NR	★★★	★★★	NR	NR	★★★	★★★	★★★★★	NR	★★★	NR	NR
NR	NR	NR	★★★	NR	NR	NR	NR	★★★★★	NR	NR	NR	NR	NR	NR	NR	NR	NR	NR
★	★★★	★★★	★	★★★	★★★	★	★★★★★	★	★★★	★★★	★★★	★★★	★★★	★★★★★	★★★★★	NR	★	
★★★	★★★	★★★	★★★	★★★	★★★	★★★	NR	★★★★★	★★★	NR	NR	★★★	★★★	★★★★★	★★★	NR	NR	
NR	NR	NR	★★★	NR	NR	NR	NR	★★★	NR	NR	NR	NR	NR	NR	NR	NR	NR	NR
★★★	★★★	★★★★★	★★★★★	★★★	★★★★★	★★★	★★★	★★★★★	NR	★★★	NR	★★★	★★★★★	★★★	NR	★★★	NR	★★★★★

	Appendectomy	Atrial Fibrillation	Back and Neck Surgery (except Spinal Fusion)	Back and Neck Surgery (Spinal Fusion)	Bariatric Surgery	Bowel Obstruction	Carotid Surgery	Cholecystectomy (Gall Bladder Removal)	Chronic Obstructive Pulmonary Disease (COPD)	Coronary Bypass Surgery	Coronary Interventional Procedures (Angioplasty/Stent)	Diabetic Acidosis a
301. Westpark Medical Center, McKinney	★★★	★★★	NR	NR	NR	★★★	★★★	★★★	★★★	★★★	★★★	★★★	
302. Wilbarger General Hospital, Vernon	NR	NR	NR	NR	NR	★	NR	★★★	★★★	NR	NR	NR	
303. Wilson N. Jones Medical Center, Sherman	★★★	★	★★★	★★★	NR	★★★	★★★	★★★	★★★	★★★	★★★	★★★	
304. Winkler County Memorial Hospital, Kermit	NR	NR	NR	NR	NR	NR	NR	NR	★★★	NR	NR	NR	
305. Wise Regional Health System, Decatur	NR	★★★	NR	NR	NR	★★★	★★★	★★★	★★★	NR	NR	NR	
306. Woman's Hospital at Dallas Regional Medical Center, Mesquite	★★★	NR	NR	NR	★★★	★★★	NR	★★★	★★★	NR	NR	★★★	
307. Woodland Heights Medical Center, Lufkin	★★★	★★★	NR	NR	NR	★★★	★★★★★	★★★	★★★	★★★	★★★	★★★	
308. Yoakum Community Hospital, Yoakum	NR	★★★	NR	NR	NR	NR	NR	NR	★★★	NR	NR	NR	

KEY: ★★★★★ BEST   ★★★ AS EXPECTED   ★ POOR   NR NOT RATED BY HEALTHGRADES   For full definitions of ratings and awards, see Appendix.

Gastrointestinal Bleed	Gastrointestinal Surgeries and Procedures	Heart Attack	Heart Failure	Hip Fracture Repair	Maternity Care	Pancreatitis	Peripheral Vascular Bypass	Pneumonia	Prostatectomy	Pulmonary Embolism	Resection/Replacement of Abdominal Aorta	Respiratory Failure	Sepsis	Stroke	Total Hip Replacement	Total Knee Replacement	Valve Replacement	Women's Health
★★★	★★★★★	★★★	★★★	★	★★★	★★★	NR	★★★	★★★	★★★	NR	★★★	★★★	★★★	★	★★★	NR	NR
★	NR	NR	★★★	NR	NR	NR	★	NR	NR	NR	NR	NR	NR	★★★	★	NR	NR	NR
★	★	★	★	★★★	★★★	★★★	NR	★	★★★	★★★	NR	★	★	★★★	★★★	★★★	NR	★★★
NR	NR	NR	★★★	NR	NR	NR	NR	★★★	NR	NR	NR	NR	NR	NR	NR	NR	NR	NR
★★★	★★★	NR	★★★	★	NR	NR	NR	★★★	NR	NR	NR	★★★	★	★★★	NR	★	NR	NR
★★★	NR	★	★	★★★	★★★★★	NR	NR	★★★	NR	NR	★	★	★★★	★★★	★★★★★	NR	NR	NR
★★★	★★★	★★★	★★★	★★★	★★★	★★★	NR	★★★★★	★★★	★★★	★★★★★	★	★★★	★★★★★	★★★	NR	NR	NR
★★★	NR	NR	★★★	★	NR	NR	NR	★★★	NR	NR	NR	★	★★★	NR	NR	NR	NR	NR

UTAH HOSPITALS: RATINGS BY PROCEDURE

Hospital	Appendectomy	Atrial Fibrillation	Back and Neck Surgery (except Spinal Fusion)	Back and Neck Surgery (Spinal Fusion)	Bariatric Surgery	Bowel Obstruction	Carotid Surgery	Cholecystectomy (Gall Bladder Removal)	Chronic Obstructive Pulmonary Disease (COPD)	Coronary Bypass Surgery	Coronary Interventional Procedures (Angioplasty/Stent)	Diabetic Acidosis an...
1. Allen Memorial Hospital, Moab	NR	NR	NR	NR	NR	NR	NR	★★★	NR	NR	NR	
2. Alta View Hospital, Sandy	★★★	★★★	NR	NR	NR	★★★	NR	★	★★★	NR	NR	
3. American Fork Hospital, American Fork	★★★	★★★	NR	NR	NR	★★★	NR	★	★★★	NR	NR	
4. Ashley Valley Medical Center, Vernal	★★★	NR	NR	NR	NR	NR	NR	NR	★★★	NR	NR	
5. Beaver Valley Hospital, Beaver	NR	NR	NR	NR	NR	NR	NR	NR	NR	NR	NR	
6. Brigham City Community Hospital, Brigham City	★★★	NR	NR	NR	NR	NR	★★★	NR	★★★	NR	NR	
7. Castleview Hospital, Price	★★★	NR	NR	NR	NR	★★★	NR	★★★	★★★	NR	NR	
8. Cottonwood Hospital, Murray	★★★	★★★	★★★	★★★	★	★★★★★	NR	★	★★★	NR	★★★	★★★
9. Davis Hospital and Medical Center, Layton	★★★★★	★	★★★	NR	NR	★★★	NR	★★★	★	NR	★★★	
10. Dixie Regional Medical Center, St. George	★★★★★	★★★	★★★	★★★	★★★	★★★★★	★★★	★★★	★★★	★★★	★★★	★★★
11. Garfield Memorial Hospital, Panguitch	NR	NR	NR	NR	NR	NR	NR	NR	NR	NR	NR	
12. Gunnison Valley Hospital, Gunnison	NR	NR	NR	NR	NR	NR	NR	NR	NR	NR	NR	
13. Jordan Valley Hospital, West Jordan	★	NR	NR	NR	NR	★★★	NR	★	★★★	NR	NR	
14. Kane County Hospital, Kanab	NR	NR	NR	NR	NR	NR	NR	NR	NR	NR	NR	
15. Lakeview Hospital, Bountiful	★★★	★★★	NR	NR	NR	★★★	NR	★★★	NR	NR	★★★	
16. LDS Hospital, Salt Lake City	★★★	★★★	★★★	★★★	NR	★★★★★	★★★	★★★	★★★	★	★★★	★★★★★
17. Logan Regional Hospital, Logan	★	★★★	NR	★★★	NR	★★★★★	NR	★★★	★★★	NR	NR	
18. McKay-Dee Hospital Center, Ogden	★★★	★★★	★★★	★★★	NR	★★★★★	★	★	★★★	★★★	★★★	★★★
19. Mountain View Hospital, Payson	★★★	★★★	★★★	NR	★★★	★★★	NR	★★★	★★★	NR	★★★	
20. Mountain West Medical Center, Tooele	★★★	★★★	NR	NR	NR	★★★	NR	NR	★★★	NR	NR	
21. Ogden Regional Medical Center, Ogden	★★★★★	★★★	NR	NR	NR	★★★	NR	★★★	★★★	★★★	★★★	
22. Pioneer Valley Hospital, West Valley City	★★★	★★★	NR	NR	★★★	★★★	NR	★★★	★★★	NR	★★★	
23. St. Mark's Hospital, Salt Lake City	★★★★★	★★★★★	★★★	★★★	★★★	★★★	★★★	★★★	★★★★★	★★★	★	★★★
24. Salt Lake Regional Medical Center, Salt Lake City	★★★	★★★	★★★	★★★	★	★★★	★	★★★	★★★	★★★	★★★	
25. Sevier Valley Medical Center, Richfield	★★★	NR	NR	NR	NR	★★★	NR	★★★	NR	NR	NR	
26. Timpanogos Regional Hospital, Orem	★★★★★	★★★	★★★	★★★	NR	★★★	NR	★★★	NR	NR	★★★	
27. Uintah Basin Medical Center, Roosevelt	★★★	NR	NR	NR	NR	★★★	NR	NR	★	NR	NR	
28. University of Utah Hospital, Salt Lake City	★	★★★	★	★	NR	★★★	★★★	★	★★★	★★★	★★★	
29. Utah Valley Regional Medical Center, Provo	★	★★★	★★★	★★★	NR	★★★	★★★	★	★★★	★★★	★★★	
30. Valley View Medical Center, Cedar City	★★★	NR	NR	NR	NR	★★★	NR	★★★	NR	NR	NR	

KEY: ★★★★★ BEST   ★★★ AS EXPECTED   ★ POOR   NR NOT RATED BY HEALTHGRADES   For full definitions of ratings and awards, see Appendix.

Gastrointestinal Bleed	Gastrointestinal Surgeries and Procedures	Heart Attack	Heart Failure	Hip Fracture Repair	Maternity Care	Pancreatitis	Peripheral Vascular Bypass	Pneumonia	Prostatectomy	Pulmonary Embolism	Resection/Replacement of Abdominal Aorta	Respiratory Failure	Sepsis	Stroke	Total Hip Replacement	Total Knee Replacement	Valve Replacement	Women's Health
NR	NR	NR	★★★	NR	★	NR	NR	★★★	NR	NR	NR	NR	NR	NR	NR	NR	NR	NR
★★★	★★★	NR	★★★	★	★★★	★★★	NR	★★★★★	★	★★★★★	NR	★★★	★★★★★	★★★	★★★	★	NR	NR
★★★	NR	NR	★★★	★	★★★	★★★	NR	★★★	★★★	★★★	NR	NR	★★★	★★★	★★★	★★★	NR	NR
★★★	NR	NR	★★★	★★★	★★★	NR	NR	★★★	NR	NR	NR	NR	NR	NR	NR	NR	NR	NR
★★★	NR	NR	NR	★★★	★★★	NR	NR	★	NR	NR	NR	NR	NR	★★★	NR	★★★	NR	NR
★★★	NR	NR	★	★★★	★★★	NR	NR	★	NR	NR	NR	NR	★★★★★	★★★	★★★	★	NR	NR
★★★★★	★★★	★★★	★★★	★	★★★★★	★★★	NR	★★★★★	★★★	★★★	NR	★★★	★★★★★	★★★	★★★★★	★	NR	NR
★	★★★★★	★★★	★	★★★★★	★★★	★★★	NR	★★★	★	★★★	NR	★★★	★★★	★★★	★★★★★	★★★	NR	NR
★★★	★★★	★★★	★★★	★	★★★★★	★★★	NR	★★★	★★★	★★★	NR	★★★	★★★★★	★★★	★★★	★★★	★★★	★★★
NR	NR	NR	★★★	★	NR	NR	NR	★★★	NR	NR	NR	NR	NR	NR	NR	NR	NR	NR
NR	NR	NR	★★★	NR	★★★	NR	NR	★★★	NR	NR	NR	NR	NR	NR	NR	NR	NR	NR
★★★	NR	NR	★★★	★	★★★	NR	NR	★★★	NR	NR	NR	★★★	★★★	★★★	NR	★	NR	NR
NR	NR	NR	★★★	NR	★★★	NR	NR	★★★	NR	NR	NR	NR	NR	NR	NR	NR	NR	NR
★★★	★	★★★	★★★	★★★	★★★	NR	NR	★★★	★★★	★★★	NR	★★★	★★★	★★★	★★★★★	★★★	NR	NR
★★★	★★★	★★★	★★★	★★★	★★★	★★★	★★★	★★★★★	★★★	★★★	★★★	★★★	★★★	★★★	★★★★★	★★★	★★★	★★★
★★★	★★★	★★★	★★★	★	★★★	★★★	NR	★★★★★	★	★★★	NR	★★★	★★★	★★★	★	★	NR	NR
★★★	★★★	★★★	★★★	★★★	★★★★★	★★★	NR	★★★★★	★	★★★	NR	★★★	★★★	★★★	★★★	★★★	★★★	★★★★★
★★★	★★★	★★★	★★★	★	★★★	NR	NR	★★★	★★★	NR	NR	★★★	★★★★★	★	★★★	★★★	★★★	★★★
★★★★★	NR	NR	★★★	★★★	★★★	NR	NR	★★★★★	NR	NR	NR	★★★	★★★★★	NR	NR	★	NR	NR
★★★	★★★	★★★	★★★★★	★★★★★	★★★★★	★★★	NR	★★★	★	★★★	NR	★★★	★★★	★★★	★★★	★★★	NR	★★★★★
★★★	★★★	★★★	★★★	★★★	★★★	NR	NR	★★★	NR	★★★	NR	★★★	★★★	★★★	NR	★★★	NR	NR
★★★★★	★★★	★★★	★★★★★	★★★	★★★	NR	NR	★★★★★	★★★	★★★★★	★★★	★★★★★	★★★	★★★★★	★★★★★	★★★★★	★★★	★★★
★★★	★★★★★	★★★	★★★	★★★	★★★	NR	NR	★★★★★	★★★	NR	NR	★★★	★★★	★★★	NR	NR	★★★	★★★
★★★	NR	NR	★★★	NR	★	NR	NR	★★★	NR	NR	NR	NR	NR	NR	NR	NR	★★★	NR
★★★	NR	★★★	★★★	★	★★★	NR	NR	★★★	NR	★★★	NR	★★★	★	★	★	★★★	NR	NR
★	NR	NR	★	★★★	★	NR	NR	★	NR	NR	NR	NR	NR	NR	NR	★★★	NR	NR
★★★	★★★	★★★	★★★	★	★	★★★	★	★★★★★	★	★★★	★★★	★	★★★	★	★★★	★★★	★★★	★
★★★	★	★★★	★★★	★	★★★	★★★	★★★	★★★	★	★★★	★★★	★★★	★★★	★	★	★★★	★★★	★★★
★★★	★★★	NR	★★★	★★★★★	★★★	NR	NR	★★★	NR	NR	NR	NR	NR	★★★	★★★	★★★★★	NR	NR

VERMONT HOSPITALS: RATINGS BY PROCEDURE

	Appendectomy	Atrial Fibrillation	Back and Neck Surgery (except Spinal Fusion)	Back and Neck Surgery (Spinal Fusion)	Bariatric Surgery	Bowel Obstruction	Carotid Surgery	Cholecystectomy (Gall Bladder Removal)	Chronic Obstructive Pulmonary Disease (COPD)	Coronary Bypass Surgery	Coronary Interventional Procedures (Angioplasty/Stent)	Diabetic Acidosis a[...]
1. **Brattleboro Memorial Hospital,** Brattleboro	NR	★★★	NR	NR	NR	★★★	NR	NR	★★★	NR	NR	
2. **Central Vermont Medical Center,** Barre	NR	★★★	NR	NR	NR	★★★	NR	★★★	★★★★★	NR	NR	NR
3. **Fletcher Allen Hospital of Vermont,** Burlington	NR	★★★	★	★★★	NR	★★★	★★★	★★★	★★★	★★★	★★★	★
4. **Gifford Medical Center,** Randolph	NR	★★★	NR	NR	NR	NR	NR	NR	★★★	NR	NR	NR
5. **North Country Hospital and Health Center,** Newport	NR	★	NR	NR	NR	★★★	NR	NR	★★★★★	NR		
6. **Northeastern Vermont Regional Hospital,** St. Johnsbury	NR	★★★	NR	NR	NR	★★★	NR	NR	★	NR		
7. **Northwestern Medical Center,** St. Albans	NR	★★★	NR	NR	NR	★★★	NR	NR	★	NR		
8. **Porter Hospital,** Middlebury	NR	★	NR	NR	NR	★★★	NR	NR	★★★	NR		
9. **Rutland Regional Medical Center,** Rutland	NR	★	★★★	NR	NR	★	NR	★★★	★	NR	NR	
10. **Southwestern Vermont Medical Center,** Bennington	NR	★★★	★★★	★	NR	★★★	NR	★★★	★★★	NR	NR	
11. **Springfield Hospital,** Springfield	NR	★	NR	NR	NR	★★★	NR	NR	★★★	NR	NR	

KEY: ★★★★★ BEST   ★★★ AS EXPECTED   ★ POOR   NR NOT RATED BY HEALTHGRADES   For full definitions of ratings and awards, see Appendix.

Gastrointestinal Bleed	Gastrointestinal Surgeries and Procedures	Heart Attack	Heart Failure	Hip Fracture Repair	Maternity Care	Pancreatitis	Peripheral Vascular Bypass	Pneumonia	Prostatectomy	Pulmonary Embolism	Resection/Replacement of Abdominal Aorta	Respiratory Failure	Sepsis	Stroke	Total Hip Replacement	Total Knee Replacement	Valve Replacement	Women's Health
★★★	NR	★★★	★★★	★★★	NR	NR	NR	★	★★★	NR	NR	NR	★	★★★	★★★	★★★	NR	NR
★★★	★★★	★★★	★	★	NR	NR	NR	★★★	★★★	NR	NR	NR	★★★	★	★	★	NR	NR
★	★★★	★	★	★	NR	★★★	★★★	★★★	★★★★★	★★★	★★★	★	★★★	★★★★★	★★★	★★★	★	NR
★★★	NR	★★★	★★★	NR	NR	NR	NR	★★★	NR	NR	NR	NR	NR	NR	NR	NR	NR	NR
★★★	NR	★★★	★★★	NR	NR	NR	NR	★★★	NR	NR	NR	★★★	★★★	★★★	NR	NR	NR	NR
★★★	NR	★★★★★	★	★★★	NR	NR	NR	★★★	NR	NR	NR	NR	NR	NR	★★★	★	NR	NR
★★★	NR	★★★	★	★★★	NR	★	NR	NR	NR	NR	NR	★	NR	★★★	★★★	★★★	NR	NR
★	NR	NR	★★★	★★★	NR	NR	NR	★★★	NR	NR	NR	NR	NR	★★★	★★★	★	NR	NR
★★★	★★★	★★★	★	★★★	NR	★	NR	★★★	★★★	NR	★	★★★	★★★	★★★	★★★★★	NR	NR	NR
★★★	★★★	★★★	★★★	★	NR	★	NR	★★★★★	NR	NR	NR	★	★★★	★★★	★★★	★★★	NR	NR
★★★	NR	★★★	★★★	★★★	NR	NR	NR	★	NR	NR	NR	★★★	★	★	★★★	★★★	NR	NR

VIRGINIA HOSPITALS: RATINGS BY PROCEDURE

Hospital	Appendectomy	Atrial Fibrillation	Back and Neck Surgery (except Spinal Fusion)	Back and Neck Surgery (Spinal Fusion)	Bariatric Surgery	Bowel Obstruction	Carotid Surgery	Cholecystectomy (Gall Bladder Removal)	Chronic Obstructive Pulmonary Disease (COPD)	Coronary Bypass Surgery	Coronary Interventional Procedures (Angioplasty/Stent)	Diabetic Acidosis [a]
1. Alleghany Regional Hospital, Low Moor	★★★	★★★	NR	NR	★	★	NR	★★★	★★★	NR	NR	★
2. Augusta Medical Center, Fishersville	★★★★★	★★★	★★★	NR	NR	★★★	★★★	★★★	★★★	NR	NR	★★★
3. Bath County Community Hospital, Hot Springs	NR	NR	NR	NR	NR	NR	NR	★★★	★★★	NR		NR
4. Bedford Memorial Hospital, Bedford	★★★	★★★	NR	NR	NR	★★★	NR	NR	★★★	NR	NR	
5. Bon Secours DePaul Medical Center, Norfolk	★	★★★	★★★★★	★★★	NR	★★★	★★★	★	★★★	NR	★	★★★
6. Bon Secours Maryview Medical Center, Portsmouth	★★★	★★★	★★★	★★★	★★★★★	★★★	★★★	★★★	★★★	NR	★★★	★★★
7. Bon Secours Memorial Regional Medical Center, Mechanicsville	★★★	★★★	★★★	★	NR	★★★	★★★	★★★	★★★★★	★★★★★	★★★	★
8. Bon Secours Richmond Community Hospital, Richmond	NR	NR	NR	NR	NR	NR	NR	★★★	★★★	NR	NR	NR
9. Bon Secours St. Francis Medical Center, Midlothian	NR	NR	★	NR	NR	NR	NR	★★★	★★★	NR	NR	NR
10. Bon Secours St. Mary's Hospital, Richmond	★★★	★★★	★	★★★	★	★★★	★★★	★	★★★	★★★	NR	★★★
11. Buchanan General Hospital, Grundy	★★★	★★★	NR	NR	NR	★★★	NR	★★★	★★★	NR	NR	★★★
12. Carilion Franklin Memorial Hospital, Rocky Mount	★★★	★★★	NR	NR	NR	★★★	NR	★★★★★	★★★	NR	NR	★★★
13. Carilion Giles Memorial Hospital, Pearisburg	NR	★★★	NR	NR	NR	★★★	NR	★★★	★★★	NR	NR	★★★
14. Carilion Medical Center, Roanoke	★★★	★★★	★★★	★★★	★★★	★★★★★	★★★	★★★	★★★	★★★	NR	★★★
15. Carilion New River Valley Medical Center, Christiansburg	★★★	★★★	NR	NR	NR	★★★	★★★	★★★	★★★	NR	NR	★★★
16. Centra Health, Lynchburg	★★★★★	★★★	★★★	★★★	NR	★★★	★★★	★★★★★	★★★	★★★	★★★	★★★
17. Chesapeake General Hospital, Chesapeake	★★★	★★★	★★★	★	★★★	★★★	★★★	★★★	★★★	NR	★★★	★★★
18. CJW Medical Center–Chippenham Campus, Richmond	★★★	★★★	★	★	★★★	★★★★★	★★★	★★★	★★★★★	★★★	★★★	★★★
19. Clinch Valley Medical Center, Richlands	★★★	★★★	NR	NR	★	NR	★★★★★	★★★	★★★	NR	NR	★★★
20. Community Memorial Healthcenter, South Hill	★★★	★★★	NR	NR	★	NR	★★★	★★★	★★★	NR	NR	★★★
21. Culpeper Memorial Hospital, Culpeper	★★★★★	★★★	★★★	NR	NR	★★★	NR	★★★	★★★	NR	NR	NR
22. Danville Regional Medical Center, Danville	★★★★★	★★★	★★★	★★★	★★★★★	★★★	★★★	★★★★★	★	★★★	★★★	★★★
23. Dickenson Community Hospital, Clintwood	NR	NR	NR	NR	NR	NR	NR	★★★	★★★	NR	NR	NR
24. Fauquier Hospital, Warrenton	★★★	★★★	★★★	★★★	NR	★★★	★★★	★★★	★★★	NR	NR	★★★
25. Grundy Hospital, Grundy	★★★	★★★	NR	NR	NR	★★★	NR	★★★	★★★	NR	NR	★★★
26. Halifax Regional Hospital, South Boston	★★★	★★★	NR	NR	NR	★★★	NR	★★★★★	★★★	NR	NR	★★★
27. Henrico Doctors' Hospital, Richmond	★	★★★	★★★	★★★	★★★	★★★	★★★	★★★	★★★★★	★★★	★★★	★★★
28. Henrico Doctors' Hospital–Parham, Richmond	★	★★★	★★★	★★★	★★★	★★★	★★★	★★★	★★★★★	★★★	★★★	★★★
29. Inova Alexandria Hospital, Alexandria	★★★★★	★★★	★★★	★★★	NR	★★★	★★★	★★★	★★★	★★★	★★★	★★★
30. Inova Fair Oaks Hospital, Fairfax	★★★	★★★	★★★	★★★★★	★★★★★	★★★	★★★	★★★	★	NR	NR	★★★
31. Inova Fairfax Hospital, Falls Church	★★★	★★★	★★★	★★★★★	★★★★★	★★★	★★★	★★★	★★★	★★★	★★★	★★★★★
32. Inova Loudoun Hospital, Leesburg	★★★	★★★	NR	NR	NR	★★★	NR	★★★★★	★★★	NR	NR	★★★
33. Inova Mount Vernon Hospital, Alexandria	★	★★★	★★★	NR	NR	★★★	NR	★	★★★	NR	NR	★★★
34. John Randolph Medical Center, Hopewell	★★★	★	NR	NR	NR	★★★	NR	★★★	★★★	NR	NR	★★★
35. Johnston Memorial Hospital, Abingdon	★★★	★	NR	NR	NR	★★★	★★★	★★★	★	NR	NR	NR
36. Lee Regional Medical Center, Pennington Gap	NR	★★★	NR	NR	NR	★★★	NR	NR	★	NR	NR	★★★
37. Lewis-Gale Medical Center, Salem	★★★★★	★★★	★★★★★	★★★★★	★★★★★	★★★	★★★★★	★★★	★★★	★★★	★★★	★★★
38. Lynchburg General Hospital, Lynchburg	★★★★★	★★★	★★★	★★★	NR	★★★	★★★	★★★★★	★★★	★★★	★★★	★★★
39. Martha Jefferson Hospital, Charlottesville	★★★	★★★	★	NR	NR	★★★	★★★	★★★	★★★	NR	★★★	★★★
40. Mary Immaculate Hospital, Newport News	★★★	★★★	★★★	★★★	NR	★★★	NR	★★★	★★★	NR	NR	★★★
41. Mary Washington Hospital, Fredericksburg	★★★	★★★	★★★	★★★	NR	★★★	★★★	★★★	★★★	★★★	★★★	★★★
42. Memorial Hospital of Martinsville and Henry County, Martinsville	★★★	★	NR	NR	★	★★★	★★★	★★★	★★★	NR	NR	★★★
43. Montgomery Regional Hospital, Blacksburg	★★★	★★★	NR	NR	NR	★★★	NR	★★★	★★★	NR	NR	★★★
44. Mountain View Regional Medical Center, Norton	★★★	★★★	NR	NR	NR	NR	NR	NR	★★★	NR	NR	NR
45. Northern Virginia Community Hospital, Arlington	★★★	NR	NR	NR	★★★★★	NR	★★★	NR	NR	NR	NR	NR
46. Norton Community Hospital, Norton	★★★	★★★	NR	NR	NR	★★★★★	NR	★★★	★★★	NR	★★★★★	★★★
47. Obici Hospital, Suffolk	★★★	★★★	★★★	★★★	NR	★★★	★★★	★★★	★★★	NR	★★★	★
48. Page Memorial Hospital, Luray	NR	NR	NR	NR	NR	NR	NR	★★★	★★★	NR	NR	NR
49. Potomac Hospital, Woodbridge	★★★	★★★	NR	NR	★★★★★	★★★★★	NR	★★★★★	★★★	NR	NR	★★★
50. Prince William Hospital, Manassas	★★★	★★★	★★★	NR	NR	★★★	NR	★★★	★	NR	NR	NR

KEY: ★★★★★ BEST   ★★★ AS EXPECTED   ★ POOR   NR NOT RATED BY HEALTHGRADES   For full definitions of ratings and awards, see Appendix.

Gastrointestinal Bleed	Gastrointestinal Surgeries and Procedures	Heart Attack	Heart Failure	Hip Fracture Repair	Maternity Care	Pancreatitis	Peripheral Vascular Bypass	Pneumonia	Prostatectomy	Pulmonary Embolism	Resection/Replacement of Abdominal Aorta	Respiratory Failure	Sepsis	Stroke	Total Hip Replacement	Total Knee Replacement	Valve Replacement	Women's Health
★★★	NR	★★★	★★★	★★★	NR	★★★	★★★	★	NR	NR	NR	★★★	★	★	★★★	★★★	NR	NR
★★★	★★★	★★★★★	★★★	★★★	★★★	★★★	NR	★★★	★★★	★★★	NR	★★★	★★★	★★★	★★★★★	★★★★★	NR	NR
NR	NR	NR	★★★	NR	NR	NR	NR	★	NR	NR	NR	NR	NR	NR	NR	NR	NR	NR
★	NR	★★★	★★★	NR	★★★	NR	NR	★	NR	NR	NR	NR	★	★	NR	NR	NR	NR
★★★	★★★	★★★	★★★	★	★★★	★★★	★	★★★	NR	★★★	★★★	★★★	★★★	★★★	★	★	NR	NR
★★★	★★★	★★★	★	★★★	★★★	★★★	★★★	★★★	★★★	★★★	NR	★	★★★	★★★	★★★	★★★	NR	NR
★★★★★	★★★	★★★★★	★★★★★	★★★	★★★	★★★	★★★	★★★★★	★★★	★★★	★★★	★★★★★	★★★★★	★★★	★★★	★	★★★	★★★
★	NR	NR	★★★	NR	NR	NR	NR	★★★	NR	NR	NR	★★★	★★★	NR	NR	NR	NR	NR
★★★	NR	NR	★★★	NR	★★★	NR	NR	★★★	NR	★★★	NR	★★★	★★★	NR	★	★★★	NR	NR
★★★	★★★	★★★	★★★	★	★★★	★★★	★	★★★★★	★★★	★★★	★★★	★★★★★	★★★★★	★	★	★★★	★★★	★★★
★★★	NR	★	★★★	★	NR	★★★	NR	★★★	NR	★★★	★★★	NR	★	NR	NR	NR	NR	NR
★★★	NR	★★★	★★★	NR	★★★	NR	NR	★★★	NR	★★★	NR	NR	★	NR	★★★	NR	NR	NR
★★★	NR	NR	★★★★★	NR	NR	NR	NR	★★★	NR	NR	NR	★★★	NR	★★★	NR	NR	NR	NR
★★★	★	★★★	★★★	★★★	NR	★★★	★★★	★	★★★	★★★	★★★	NR	★	★★★	★★★	★★★	NR	★
★★★	★★★	★★★	★★★	★	★★★	★★★	★★★	★★★	★	★★★	★★★	NR	★★★	★	★★★	★★★	NR	NR
★★★	★★★	★★★	★★★★★	★★★	★★★	★★★	★★★	★★★	★★★	★	★★★	★★★★★	★★★	★★★★★	★★★★★	★★★★★	★★★	NR
★★★	★★★	★	★★★	NR	★★★	★★★	NR	★★★	NR	★★★★★	★★★	★★★	★★★	★	★★★	NR	NR
★★★★★	★	★★★	★★★★★	★★★	★★★	NR	★★★	★★★★★	★★★	★★★★★	NR	★★★	★	★	★★★★★	★★★	★★★★★	★★★
★★★	NR	★★★	★★★	★★★	★★★	NR	NR	★★★	NR	NR	NR	★★★	★★★	NR	★	★★★	NR	NR
★	★★★	★★★	★★★	★★★	★★★	NR	★★★	NR	★★★	NR	★	★★★	NR	NR	NR	NR	NR
★★★	NR	★★★	★★★	★★★	★★★	NR	★★★	NR	NR	★★★	★★★	★	NR	★	★★★	NR	NR
★★★	★	★	★★★★★	★★★★★	★★★	NR	★★★★★	★★★	★★★	NR	★★★	★	★★★★★	★★★	★★★★★	★	NR	NR
NR	NR	NR	★★★	NR	NR	NR	★★★★★	NR	NR	NR	NR	NR	★	★★★	NR	NR	NR	NR
★★★	★★★★★	★★★	★★★	★★★	★★★	★★★	★★★	★	★★★	NR	★★★	★★★	★	★★★	★★★	NR	NR
★★★	NR	★	★★★	★	NR	NR	★★★	NR	★★★	NR	★★★	★	NR	★★★	NR	NR	NR
★★★	★★★★★	★★★★★	★★★	★★★★★	★★★	★★★	NR	★★★	NR	★★★	NR	★★★★★	★★★	★★★	NR	★★★	NR
★	★★★★★	★★★	★★★	★★★	★★★	★★★	★★★	★★★	★★★	★★★★★	★★★	★★★	★★★	★★★★★	★★★★★	★★★	★★★	★★★
★	★★★★★	★★★	★★★	★★★	★★★	★★★	★★★	★★★	★★★	★★★★★	★★★	★★★	★★★	★★★★★	★★★★★	★★★	★★★	★★★
★★★	★★★★★	★★★	★★★	★★★	★★★	★★★	★★★	★★★★★	★★★	★★★	★★★	★★★	★★★	★★★	★★★	★★★	★★★	★★★★★
★★★	★★★★★	★★★	★★★	★★★	★★★★★	★★★	NR	★★★	★★★	★★★	NR	★★★★★	★★★★★	★★★★★	★★★	★★★	NR	NR
★★★★★	★★★★★	★★★★★	★★★	★★★	★★★	★★★	NR	★★★★★	★★★★★	★★★	★★★★★	★★★	★★★★★	★★★★★	★★★	★★★	★★★★★	★★★★★
★★★	★★★	★★★	★★★	★★★	★★★	★★★	NR	★★★★★	★★★	★★★	NR	★★★	★★★	★	★★★	★★★	NR	NR
★★★	★	★★★	★★★	★★★	NR	★★★	NR	★	NR	★★★	NR	★★★	★★★	★★★	★★★★★	★★★★★	NR	NR
★★★	★★★	★★★	★★★	★★★	★★★	★★★	NR	★★★	NR	NR	NR	★★★	★★★	★★★	NR	★	NR	NR
★	★	★★★	★	★★★	★★★	★★★	NR	★	NR	★★★	NR	★	★	★	★★★	★★★	NR	NR
★	NR	★★★	★	★★★★★	NR	NR	NR	★★★	NR	NR	NR	★★★	★	★	NR	NR	NR	NR
★★★★★	★★★	★★★	★★★	★★★	★★★	★★★	NR	★★★	★★★	★★★	NR	★★★★★	★★★★★	★★★	★★★	★★★	★★★	★★★
★★★	★★★	★★★	★★★	★★★★★	★★★	★★★	★★★	★★★	★★★	★★★	★	★★★	★★★★★	★★★	★★★★★	★★★★★	★★★★★	★★★
★★★	★★★	★★★	★	★★★	★★★	★★★	★★★★★	★	★★★	★★★	★★★	★★★	★★★★★	★	★	NR	NR
★	★★★	★★★	★★★★★	★★★	★★★	★★★	★	NR	★★★	★★★	★★★	★★★	★★★	★★★★★	NR	NR
★★★★★	★★★	★	★★★	★	★★★	★★★	★★★	★★★	★★★	★★★	★	★★★	★★★	★★★	★★★	★★★
★	★	★	★	★	★	★★★	NR	★	★	★	NR	★	★	★	★★★	★	NR	NR
★★★	★	★★★	★	★	★★★	★★★	NR	★★★	NR	★★★	★★★	★	★	★★★	★★★	NR	NR
★★★	NR	★★★	★	NR	NR	NR	NR	★★★	NR	NR	NR	★★★	★★★★★	★★★	NR	★★★	NR
NR	NR	NR	NR	NR	NR	NR	NR	NR	NR	NR	NR	NR	NR	NR	NR	NR	NR	NR
★★★	NR	★★★	★★★★★	★★★	★★★	NR	★★★★★	NR	★★★	NR	★★★★★	★★★	NR	★★★	★★★	NR	NR
★★★	★	★★★	★	★★★★★	★★★	★★★	★★★	★	★★★	★★★	★	★★★	★	★★★	★★★	★★★	NR
NR	NR	★★★	★★★	NR	NR	NR	★★★	NR	NR	NR	NR	★★★★★	NR	NR	NR	NR
★★★	★★★	★★★	★★★	★★★★★	★★★	★★★	★★★	★★★	★★★	NR	★★★	★★★	★★★	★★★	★★★	NR	NR
★★★	★	★★★★★	★★★	★★★★★	★★★	★★★	NR	★★★★★	★★★	★★★	NR	★★★	★	★★★	★★★	★★★★★	NR	NR

	Appendectomy	Atrial Fibrillation	Back and Neck Surgery (except Spinal Fusion)	Back and Neck Surgery (Spinal Fusion)	Bariatric Surgery	Bowel Obstruction	Carotid Surgery	Cholecystectomy (Gall Bladder Removal)	Chronic Obstructive Pulmonary Disease (COPD)	Coronary Bypass Surgery	Coronary Interventional Procedures (Angioplasty/Stent)	Diabetic Acidosis a...
51. Pulaski Community Hospital, Pulaski	★	★	NR	NR	NR	★★★	NR	★★★	★★★	NR	NR	NR
52. R. J. Reynolds Patrick County Memorial Hospital, Stuart	NR	NR	NR	NR	NR	NR	NR	NR	★	NR	NR	NR
53. Rappahannock General Hospital, Kilmarnock	NR	★★★	NR	NR	NR	★	NR	★★★★★	★	NR	NR	★★★
54. Reston Hospital Center, Reston	★★★	★★★	NR	★★★	NR	★★★	NR	★	★★★	NR	NR	★★★
55. Retreat Hospital, Richmond	★★★	★★★	NR	NR	★	★★★	★★★	★★★	★★★	NR	NR	NR
56. Riverside Regional Medical Center, Newport News	★★★	★★★	★★★	★★★	NR	★	★★★	★★★	★★★	★★★	★★★	★★★
57. Riverside Tappahannock Hospital, Tappahannock	★★★	★★★	NR	NR	NR	★★★	NR	NR	★★★	NR	NR	★★★
58. Riverside Walter Reed Hospital, Gloucester	★★★	★	NR	NR	NR	★★★	NR	★★★	★★★	NR	NR	★★★
59. Rockingham Memorial Hospital, Harrisonburg	★★★	★★★	★★★	★	NR	★★★	★★★	★★★★★	★★★★★	NR	★★★★★	★★★
60. Russell County Medical Center, Lebanon	★★★★★	★★★	NR	NR	★★★★★	★	NR	★★★	★★★	NR	NR	NR
61. Sentara Bayside Hospital, Virginia Beach	★★★	★★★	NR	NR	NR	★★★	NR	★★★	★★★	NR	★★★	★★★
62. Sentara Careplex Hospital, Hampton	★★★	★★★	★	★★★	★★★★★	★★★	★★★	★★★	★★★	NR	★★★	★★★
63. Sentara Leigh Hospital, Norfolk	★	★★★	★★★	★★★	★★★★★	★★★	NR	★	★★★	NR	★★★	★★★
64. Sentara Norfolk General Hospital, Norfolk	★	★★★	★★★	★★★	★★★	★★★	★★★	★★★	★★★	★★★	★★★	★★★
65. Sentara Virginia Beach General Hospital, Virginia Beach	★★★	★★★	★	★	★★★	★★★★★	★★★	★★★	★★★	★★★	★★★	★★★
66. Sentara Williamsburg Regional Medical Center, Williamsburg	★	★★★	★★★★★	★★★★★	NR	★★★	★★★★★	★★★	★★★	NR	★★★	★★★
67. Shenandoah Memorial Hospital, Woodstock	★★★	★	NR	NR	NR	★★★	NR	NR	★★★	NR	NR	NR
68. Shore Memorial Hospital, Nassawadox	★★★	★★★	NR	NR	NR	★★★	NR	NR	★★★	NR	★	
69. Smyth County Community Hospital, Marion	★★★	★★★	NR	NR	NR	★★★	NR	★	★	NR	NR	NR
70. Southampton Memorial Hospital, Franklin	★	★★★	NR	NR	NR	★★★	NR	★★★	★★★	NR	NR	NR
71. Southern Virginia Regional Medical Center, Emporia	★	★	NR	NR	NR	★★★	NR	NR	★★★	NR	NR	★★★
72. Southside Community Hospital, Farmville	★★★	★★★	NR	NR	NR	★★★	NR	★★★	★★★	NR	NR	★★★
73. Southside Regional Medical Center, Petersburg	★★★	★	NR	NR	NR	★	NR	★★★	★	NR	★★★	★★★
74. Stonewall Jackson Hospital, Lexington	NR	★★★	NR	NR	NR	★★★	NR	★★★	★★★	NR	NR	NR
75. Tazewell Community Hospital, Tazewell	NR	NR	NR	NR	NR	★★★	NR	★★★	★★★	NR	NR	NR
76. Twin County Regional Hospital, Galax	★	★★★	NR	NR	★	★★★	NR	★	★★★	NR	NR	★★★
77. University of Virginia Hospital, Charlottesville	★★★	★★★	★	★★★	★	★★★	★★★★★	★★★	★★★	★★★	★★★	★★★
78. Virginia Commonwealth University Health System, Richmond	★★★	★★★	★★★	★	★	★★★	★★★	★★★	★★★	★★★	★★★	★★★
79. Virginia Hospital Center–Arlington, Arlington	★★★★★	★★★	★★★★★	★★★	NR	★★★★★	★★★★★	★★★	★★★	★★★	★★★	★★★
80. Warren Memorial Hospital, Front Royal	★★★	★★★	NR	NR	NR	★★★	NR	NR	★★★	NR	NR	NR
81. Wellmont Lonesome Pine Hospital, Big Stone Gap	★★★	★★★	NR	NR	NR	★★★	NR	NR	★★★	NR	NR	NR
82. Winchester Medical Center, Winchester	★★★★★	★★★	★★★	★★★	NR	★★★	★★★★★	★★★	★★★★★	★★★	★★★	★★★
83. Wythe County Community Hospital, Wytheville	★	★★★	★	★★★	NR	★★★	NR	★	★	NR	NR	NR

KEY: ★★★★★ BEST ★★★ AS EXPECTED ★ POOR NR NOT RATED BY HEALTHGRADES For full definitions of ratings and awards, see Appendix.

Gastrointestinal Bleed	Gastrointestinal Surgeries and Procedures	Heart Attack	Heart Failure	Hip Fracture Repair	Maternity Care	Pancreatitis	Peripheral Vascular Bypass	Pneumonia	Prostatectomy	Pulmonary Embolism	Resection/Replacement of Abdominal Aorta	Respiratory Failure	Sepsis	Stroke	Total Hip Replacement	Total Knee Replacement	Valve Replacement	Women's Health
★★★	NR	★★★	★★★	★★★	★★★	NR	NR	★	NR	NR	NR	★★★	★	★★★	NR	★★★	NR	NR
★★★	NR	NR	★★★	NR	NR	NR	NR	★	NR	NR	NR	NR	★	NR	NR	NR	NR	NR
★	NR	★★★	★	★★★★★	NR	NR	NR	★	NR	NR	NR	NR	★★★	★	★★★	★★★	NR	NR
★★★	★★★	★★★	★★★	★★★	★★★	NR	NR	★★★	NR	★★★	NR	★★★	★★★	★★★	★★★	★★★	NR	NR
★★★	★★★	★★★	★★★	★★★	NR	NR	★★★	★★★	★	NR	NR	★★★	★★★	★★★	NR	★★★	NR	NR
★★★	★★★	★★★★★	★★★	★★★	★★★	★★★	★★★	★★★	★★★	★★★	★	NR	★★★	★★★	★★★	★★★	★★★	★★★
★★★	NR	★★★	★★★	★★★	NR	NR	★★★★★	★★★	NR	NR	★	NR	★★★	NR	NR	★★★	NR	NR
★★★	★★★	★★★	★	★★★	NR	NR	★	★★★	NR	★★★	★	NR	★★★	NR	★	NR	NR	NR
★★★★★	★★★	★★★	★★★★★	★	★★★	★★★	★★★	★★★★★	★★★	NR	★★★★★	★★★★★	★★★	★	★	★	NR	NR
★	NR	NR	★	★	★★★	NR	★	★	NR	NR	NR	★★★	★	★	NR	NR	NR	NR
★★★	★★★	★★★	★★★	★★★★★	NR	★	NR	★★★	NR	★★★	NR	★	★★★	★★★	★	★★★	NR	NR
★	★★★	★★★	★★★	★★★	★★★	★★★	★★★	★★★	★★★	★★★	★★★	★★★	★	★★★	★★★	★★★	NR	NR
★★★★★	★★★	★★★	★	★★★	★★★★★	★	NR	★★★	★★★	★★★	NR	★	★	★★★	★★★	★★★★★	NR	NR
★★★	★★★	★★★	★★★★★	★★★	★★★	★★★★★	★★★	★★★★★	★★★	★★★	★★★	★★★	★★★★★	★★★	★	NR	★★★★★	★★★
★★★	★★★	★★★	★★★	★★★	★★★	★★★	NR	★★★	★★★	★★★	★★★	★★★	★★★	★	★★★	★★★	★★★	NR
★★★	NR	NR	★	★	★★★	NR	★	★★★	★★★	NR	NR	NR	★	NR	NR	★	NR	NR
★★★	NR	★★★	★★★	★★★	★★★	NR	★	NR	NR	NR	NR	★★★	★★★	★★★	NR	NR	NR	NR
★★★	★★★	★★★	★	★	★★★	★★★	NR	★	NR	NR	NR	★★★	NR	NR	★★★	NR	★★★	NR
★★★	NR	★★★	★★★	NR	NR	NR	★	NR	NR	NR	NR	★★★	★★★	★	NR	NR	NR	NR
★	NR	★★★	★★★	★★★	★★★	NR	★	NR	★★★	NR	NR	★★★	★★★	★	★★★	NR	NR	NR
★★★	NR	★	★★★	NR	NR	NR	★	NR	NR	NR	NR	★★★	NR	★★★	★	NR	NR	NR
★★★	★	★	★	★	★★★	★★★	NR	★★★	NR	★★★	NR	★★★	★★★	★	★	★★★	★★★	NR
★★★	★	★★★	★★★	★★★	★★★	★★★	★★★	★★★	★★★	★★★	★★★	★	★★★	★	★	★★★	★★★	NR
★★★	★	★★★	★	★	★	NR	★★★	★	★★★	★★★	★★★	★★★	★	★★★	★	★★★	★	NR
★★★	★★★★★	★★★	★★★	★★★★★	★★★	★★★★★	★★★	★★★	★★★	★★★	★	★★★★★	★★★★★	★★★	★★★	★★★	★	NR
★★★	NR	★★★	★★★	★★★	★★★	NR	NR	★	NR	NR	NR	★★★	★★★	★★★	NR	NR	NR	NR
★★★★★	NR	★★★	★★★	★★★	★★★	NR	NR	★★★	NR	NR	NR	★★★	★★★	★★★	NR	NR	NR	NR
★★★★★	★★★★★	★★★★★	★★★	★★★★★	★★★	★★★	★★★	★★★★★	★★★	★★★	★★★	★★★★★	★★★★★	★★★★★	★★★	★★★★★	★★★	★★★
★★★	NR	★★★	★	★★★	★	NR	NR	★	NR	NR	NR	NR	★	★★★★★	★	NR	NR	NR

WASHINGTON HOSPITALS: RATINGS BY PROCEDURE

Hospital	Appendectomy	Atrial Fibrillation	Back and Neck Surgery (except Spinal Fusion)	Back and Neck Surgery (Spinal Fusion)	Bariatric Surgery	Bowel Obstruction	Carotid Surgery	Cholecystectomy (Gall Bladder Removal)	Chronic Obstructive Pulmonary Disease (COPD)	Coronary Bypass Surgery	Coronary Interventional Procedures (Angioplasty/Stent)	Diabetic Acidosis and...
1. Auburn Regional Medical Center, Auburn	★★★	★★★	★★★	★	NR	★★★	★★★	★	★★★	NR	★★★	NR
2. Capital Medical Center, Olympia	★★★	★★★	NR	★★★★★	★	★★★	★★★★★	★★★	★★★	NR	★★★	NR
3. Cascade Valley Hospital, Arlington	★★★	NR	NR	NR	NR	★★★	NR	NR	★★★	NR	NR	NR
4. Central Washington Hospital, Wenatchee	★★★★★	★★★	★★★★★	★★★★★	NR	★★★★★	★★★	★★★	★	★★★	★★★	★★★
5. Coulee Community Hospital, Grand Coulee	NR	NR	NR	NR	NR	NR	NR	NR	★★★	NR	NR	NR
6. Deaconess Medical Center, Spokane	★	★★★	★	★	NR	★★★	★★★	★★★	★★★	★★★	★★★	★★★
7. Doctors Hospital of Tacoma, Tacoma	★	★★★	★★★	★	NR	★★★	★★★	★	★★★	★★★	★	★★★
8. Enumclaw Community Hospital, Enumclaw	★★★	NR	NR	NR	NR	★★★	NR	NR	★★★	NR	NR	NR
9. Evergreen Hospital Medical Center, Kirkland	★★★	★★★	★★★	★★★	★	★★★★★	★★★	★★★	★★★	NR	★★★	NR
10. Good Samaritan Hospital and Rehabilitation Center, Puyallup	★★★★★	★★★	★★★★★	★★★	★★★	★★★	★★★	★★★	★	NR	★	★★★
11. Grays Harbor Community Hospital, Aberdeen	★★★	★★★	NR	NR	NR	★★★	NR	★★★	★★★	★	NR	NR
12. Group Health Eastside Hospital, Redmond	★★★	NR	NR	NR	★★★	NR	NR	NR	NR	NR	NR	NR
13. Harborview Medical Center, Seattle	★	★★★	★	★	NR	★★★	★★★	NR	★★★	NR	★★★	NR
14. Harrison Medical Center, Bremerton	★	★★★	★	★	NR	★	★★★	★★★★★	★★★	★★★	★★★	★★★
15. Highline Community Hospital, Burien	★★★	★★★	★	NR	NR	★★★	★★★	★	★	NR	★	NR
16. Holy Family Hospital, Spokane	★	★★★	★★★	★★★	NR	★★★	★★★	★★★	★★★	NR	★★★	★★★
17. Island Hospital, Anacortes	★★★	★	NR	NR	NR	★★★	NR	★★★	★★★	NR	NR	NR
18. Jefferson General Hospital, Port Townsend	★★★	★★★	NR	NR	NR	★★★	NR	NR	★★★	NR	NR	NR
19. Kadlec Medical Center, Richland	★★★	★★★	★★★★★	★★★★★	NR	★★★	★★★	★★★	★★★	★	★★★	NR
20. Kennewick General Hospital, Kennewick	★★★	★★★	NR	NR	★★★	★★★	★	★★★	★★★	NR	NR	NR
21. Kittitas Valley Community Hospital, Ellensburg	★★★	NR	NR	NR	NR	★★★	NR	★★★	★★★	NR	NR	NR
22. Legacy Salmon Creek Hospital, Vancouver	NR	★★★	NR	NR	NR	★	NR	NR	★★★	NR	★★★	NR
23. Lourdes Medical Center, Pasco	★★★	★★★	NR	NR	NR	★★★	NR	★★★	★★★	NR	★★★	NR
24. Mason General Hospital, Shelton	★★★	★★★	NR	NR	NR	★★★	NR	NR	★★★	NR	NR	NR
25. Mid-Valley Hospital, Omak	★★★	★★★	NR	NR	NR	★★★	NR	★★★	NR	NR	NR	NR
26. Monticello Medical Center, Longview	★★★	★★★	NR	NR	NR	★★★	★★★	★★★	★★★	NR	NR	NR
27. Northwest Hospital and Medical Center, Seattle	★★★	★★★	★★★★★	★★★	NR	★★★	★★★	★	★★★	★★★	★★★	★★★
28. Olympic Medical Center, Port Angeles	★★★	★★★	NR	NR	NR	★★★★★	NR	★	★	NR	NR	★★★
29. Overlake Hospital Medical Center, Bellevue	★★★	★★★	★★★★★	★★★	★★★★★	★★★	★★★★★	★★★	★★★	★★★	★★★	NR
30. Providence Centralia Hospital, Centralia	★★★★★	★★★	★★★	NR	NR	★★★	★★★	★★★	★★★	NR	NR	NR
31. Providence Everett Medical Center—Colby Campus, Everett	★★★★★	★★★	★★★	★★★	NR	★★★	★★★	★★★	★★★	★★★	★★★	★★★
32. Providence St. Peter Hospital, Olympia	★★★★★	★★★	★	NR	NR	★★★	★★★	★★★	★★★	★★★	★	★★★
33. Pullman Memorial Hospital, Pullman	★★★	NR	NR	NR	NR	★★★	NR	NR	NR	NR	NR	NR
34. Sacred Heart Medical Center, Spokane	★★★	★★★	★★★★★	★★★	★	★★★	★★★	★★★	★	★★★	★★★	★★★
35. St. Clare Hospital, Tacoma	★★★	★★★	NR	NR	NR	★★★	★★★	★	★★★	NR	NR	★★★
36. St. Francis Community Hospital, Federal Way	★★★	★	★★★	NR	★★★★★	★★★	★★★	★★★	★★★	NR	★★★	NR
37. St. John Medical Center Peacehealth, Longview	★★★	★★★	NR	NR	NR	★★★	★★★	★★★	★★★	★★★	NR	NR
38. St. Joseph Hospital, Aberdeen	★★★	★★★	NR	NR	NR	★★★	NR	★★★	★	NR	NR	NR
39. St. Joseph Hospital, Bellingham	★★★	★★★	★	★★★	★★★	★★★	★	★★★★★	★★★	★★★	★★★	★★★
40. St. Joseph Medical Center, Tacoma	★★★	★★★	★★★★★	★★★	★★★	★★★	★★★	★★★	★★★	★★★	★★★	★★★
41. St. Joseph's Hospital of Chewelah, Chewelah	NR	NR	NR	NR	NR	NR	NR	NR	NR	NR	NR	NR
42. St. Luke's Memorial Hospital, Spokane	★	★★★	★	★	NR	★★★	★★★	★	★★★	★★★	★★★	★★★
43. St. Mary Medical Center, Walla Walla	★★★	★★★	★★★★★	★★★★★	NR	★★★	★★★	★★★	★★★	★★★	★★★	★★★
44. Samaritan Hospital, Moses Lake	★★★	★★★	NR	NR	NR	★★★	NR	★★★	★★★	NR	NR	NR
45. Skagit Valley Hospital, Mount Vernon	★★★	★★★	★★★	★★★	NR	★★★	★★★	★★★	★★★	NR	★★★	NR
46. Southwest Washington Medical Center, Vancouver	★★★	★★★	★★★★★	★★★★★	★★★	★★★	★★★	★★★	★★★	★	★★★	★★★
47. Stevens Hospital, Edmonds	★★★	★★★	NR	NR	★★★	★★★	★★★	★★★	★★★	NR	★	★★★
48. Sunnyside Community Hospital, Sunnyside	★★★	NR	NR	NR	NR	★★★	NR	NR	★★★	NR	NR	NR
49. Swedish Medical Center—Ballard Campus, Seattle	★★★★★	★★★	★	★★★	★	★★★	★★★	★★★	★★★	★	★	★★★
50. Swedish Medical Center—Cherry Hills Campus, Seattle	★★★	★★★	★★★	★★★	NR	★★★	★★★	NR	★★★	★★★	★★★	★★★

KEY: ★★★★★ BEST ★★★ AS EXPECTED ★ POOR NR NOT RATED BY HEALTHGRADES For full definitions of ratings and awards, see Appendix.

Gastrointestinal Bleed	Gastrointestinal Surgeries and Procedures	Heart Attack	Heart Failure	Hip Fracture Repair	Maternity Care	Pancreatitis	Peripheral Vascular Bypass	Pneumonia	Prostatectomy	Pulmonary Embolism	Resection/Replacement of Abdominal Aorta	Respiratory Failure	Sepsis	Stroke	Total Hip Replacement	Total Knee Replacement	Valve Replacement	Women's Health
★★★★★	★★★	★★★	★★★	★★★	★★★	★★★	NR	★★★★★	★★★	★★★	NR	★★★★★	★★★	★★★	★★★	★★★	NR	NR
★★★	★★★	★★★	★★★	★★★★★	★★★	NR	★★★	★★★	★★★	NR	NR	★★★	★★★	★	★★★★★	★★★★★	NR	NR
★★★	NR	★★★	★★★	★★★	★★★	NR	NR	★★★	NR	NR	NR	NR	NR	NR	NR	NR	NR	NR
★★★★★	★★★★★	★★★	★★★	★★★	★★★	★★★	★★★	★★★	★★★★★	★★★	★★★★★	★★★	★★★	★★★★★	★★★	★★★★★	★★★	★★★
NR	NR	NR	★★★	NR	★★★	NR	NR	★★★	NR	NR	NR	NR	NR	NR	NR	NR	NR	NR
★★★	★★★	★★★	★★★	★	★	★★★	★	★★★	★	★★★	★★★	★★★	★★★	★★★	★★★	★★★	★★★	★★★
★★★★★	★★★	★★★	★★★	★★★	★	★★★	★★★	★★★★★	★★★	★★★	★★★	★	★★★	★★★★★	★★★	★★★	★★★	★
★★★	NR	NR	★★★	★★★	★★★	NR	★	NR	NR	NR	NR	NR	★★★	NR	★★★	NR	★★★	NR
★★★	★★★	★★★★★	★★★★★	★★★	★★★★★	★★★	★★★	★★★	★	★★★	NR	★★★	★★★★★	★★★★★	★★★	★★★★★	★★★	NR
★★★	★★★	★	★	★★★	★★★★★	★★★	★★★	★★★	★★★	★★★	NR	★★★	★★★	★★★	★★★★★	★★★	NR	NR
★★★	★★★	★★★	★★★	★★★	★★★	★★★	NR	★★★	NR	★★★	NR	★★★	★	★	★★★	★	NR	NR
NR	NR	NR	NR	NR	★★★	NR	NR	NR	NR	NR	NR	NR	NR	NR	NR	NR	NR	NR
★★★	★★★	★	★★★	★	NR	NR	NR	★★★	NR	★★★	NR	★★★	★★★	★★★	★	NR	NR	NR
★★★	★★★	★★★	★★★	★★★	★★★	★★★	★★★	★★★	★★★	★★★	★	★★★★★	★★★	★★★	★★★	★★★	★★★	★★★
★★★	★	★	★	★★★	★★★	NR	★★★	★★★	★★★	★★★	NR	★	★★★	★★★	★★★	★★★	NR	NR
★★★	★★★	★★★	★	★★★	★★★	★★★	NR	★★★	★★★	★	NR	★★★	★★★★★	★★★	★★★	★★★	NR	NR
★★★	NR	★★★	★	★	★★★	NR	NR	★	NR	NR	NR	★★★	NR	★★★	★★★	★★★	NR	NR
★★★	★★★	★★★	★★★	★★★	★★★	★★★	★★★	★★★	★★★	★★★	★★★	★	★★★★★	★★★	★★★★★	★★★★★	★★★	★★★
★★★	★★★	★★★	★★★	★★★	★★★	NR	★	NR	NR	★	NR	★★★	★★★	NR	★	NR	NR	NR
★★★	NR	★★★★★	★★★	★★★	★★★	NR	★	★★★	NR	NR	NR	★★★	★★★★★	★★★	NR	NR	NR	NR
★★★	NR	★★★	★★★	★★★	★★★	NR	★	NR	NR	NR	NR	NR	★★★★★	★★★	NR	NR	NR	NR
★★★	★	★★★	★★★	★★★	★★★	NR	NR	★★★	NR	NR	NR	NR	★★★	★★★	★★★	★★★	NR	NR
★★★	NR	NR	★★★	★★★	★★★	NR	★	NR	NR	NR	NR	NR	★★★	★★★	★★★	NR	NR	NR
★★★★★	★★★★★	★★★★★	★★★	★★★	★★★	★★★	NR	★★★	★	NR	NR	★★★	★★★★★	★★★★★	★★★	★★★★★	NR	NR
★★★	★★★	★	★★★★★	★★★	★★★	NR	★★★	★★★	★★★	★★★	★★★	★★★	★★★	★★★	★★★	★	NR	NR
★★★	★★★	★★★	★	★	★★★	★★★	NR	★	★	★★★	NR	★★★	★	★	★	★★★★★	NR	NR
★★★	★★★	★★★	★★★★★	★	★★★★★	★★★	★★★	★★★	★★★	★★★	★★★	★★★	★★★	★★★	★★★★★	★★★★★	★★★★★	★★★★★
★★★	★	★★★	★★★	★★★	★	NR	NR	★★★	★★★	NR	★★★	★★★★★	★★★★★	★★★	★★★	★★★	NR	NR
★★★★★	★★★	★★★★★	★★★★★	★★★	★★★	★★★	★★★	★★★★★	★★★	★★★★★	★★★★★	★★★★★	★★★★★	★★★★★	★	★	★★★	★★★
★★★★★	★★★	★★★	★★★	★★★	★★★	★★★	★★★	★★★	★★★	★★★	NR	★★★	★★★★★	★★★★★	★★★★★	★★★★★	★★★	★★★
★★★	NR	NR	★★★	NR	★	NR	NR	★★★	NR	NR	NR	NR	NR	★★★	★★★	NR	NR	NR
★★★	★★★	★★★★★	★★★	★	★	★★★	★★★	★	★★★	★★★	★★★	★	★★★	★★★	★	★★★	★★★	★
★★★	★★★	★	★	★★★★★	NR	★★★	★★★	★★★	★★★	NR	★★★	★★★	★★★	★★★	★★★	NR	NR	NR
★★★	★★★★★	★★★	★★★	★★★★★	★★★	NR	NR	★★★★★	NR	★★★	NR	★★★	★★★	★★★★★	★★★	★★★	NR	NR
★★★★★	★★★★★	★★★★★	★★★	★★★	★★★	★★★	NR	★★★	★	NR	NR	★★★	★★★★★	★★★★★	★★★	★★★★★	★★★	NR
★★★	★★★	★★★	★★★	★★★	★★★	★★★	NR	★★★	NR	★★★	NR	★★★	★	★★★	★	NR	NR	NR
★★★	★★★★★	★★★	★★★	★★★	★★★	★★★	NR	★★★★★	★★★	NR	★★★	★★★	★★★	★★★	★★★★★	★★★	★★★	★★★
★★★	★★★★★	★	★★★	★★★★★	★★★★★	★★★	★★★	★★★	★★★	NR	★	★★★	★★★	★★★	★★★	★	★★★	★★★
NR	NR	NR	★★★	NR	★	NR	NR	★★★	NR	NR	NR	NR	NR	NR	NR	NR	NR	NR
★★★	★★★	★★★	★★★	★	★	★★★	★	★★★	★	★★★	★★★	★★★	★★★	★★★	★★★	★★★	★★★	★★★
★★★★★	★★★	★★★	★★★	★★★★★	★★★	★★★	NR	★★★	★★★★★	NR	NR	★★★★★	★★★	★★★	★★★	★★★★★	★★★	NR
★★★	★★★	★★★	★★★	★	★	NR	NR	★★★	NR	NR	NR	★	★★★	★★★	★	NR	NR
★★★	★★★	★★★	★★★	★★★	★★★	NR	NR	★★★	★	NR	★	★★★	★★★	★★★★★	NR	NR	NR
★★★★★	★★★★★	★★★	★	★★★	★★★	★★★	NR	★★★★★	★★★	NR	★★★	★★★	★★★	★★★★★	★★★	★★★	★★★
★★★	★★★	★	★★★	★★★	★★★	NR	NR	★★★	NR	NR	★★★	★★★	★★★	★★★	NR	NR	NR
★★★	NR	NR	★★★	★★★	★	NR	NR	★★★	★★★	NR•	NR	NR	NR	NR	NR	NR	NR
★★★	★★★★★	★★★	★★★	★★★	★★★	★★★	★★★	★★★★★	★★★	★★★	★★★★★	★★★★★	★★★★★	★★★	★★★★★	★	★★★
★	★★★	★★★	★★★	★★★	NR	NR	★	★★★★★	NR	★★★	★	★★★	★★★	★★★	★★★	★	NR

	Appendectomy	Atrial Fibrillation	Back and Neck Surgery (except Spinal Fusion)	Back and Neck Surgery (Spinal Fusion)	Bariatric Surgery	Bowel Obstruction	Carotid Surgery	Cholecystectomy (Gall Bladder Removal)	Chronic Obstructive Pulmonary Disease (COPD)	Coronary Bypass Surgery	Coronary Interventional Procedures (Angioplasty/Stent)	Diabetic Acidosis and
51. Swedish Medical Center–First Hill, Seattle	★★★★★	★★★	★	★★★	★	★★★	★★★	★★★	★★★	★	★	★★★
52. Tacoma General Allenmore Hospital, Tacoma	★	★★★	★★★	★	NR	★★★	★★★	★	★★★	★★★	★	★★★
53. Toppenish Community Hospital, Toppenish	★★★	NR	NR	NR	NR	NR	NR	NR	★★★	NR	NR	NR
54. Tri-State Memorial Hospital, Clarkston	★★★	★★★	NR	NR	NR	★★★	NR	★★★	★★★	NR	NR	NR
55. United General Hospital, Sedro Woolley	NR	NR	NR	NR	NR	NR	NR	NR	★★★	NR	NR	NR
56. University of Washington Medical Center, Seattle	★★★	★★★	★★★	★★★	★	★★★	★★★	★★★★★	★★★	★★★	★	NR
57. Valley General Hospital, Monroe	★★★	★★★	★★★	NR	NR	★★★	NR	★★★	★★★	NR	NR	NR
58. Valley Hospital and Medical Center, Spokane	★★★	★★★	★★★★★	NR	NR	★★★	NR	★★★★★	★	NR	NR	NR
59. Valley Medical Center, Renton	★★★	★★★	★★★★★	★★★	★★★★★	★★★	★★★	★★★	★★★	NR	★★★	★★★
60. Valley Memorial Hospital, Sunnyside	★★★	NR	NR	NR	NR	★★★	NR	NR	★★★	★	NR	NR
61. Virginia Mason Medical Center, Seattle	★★★	★★★★★	★	★★★	★★★★★	★★★★★	★★★	★★★	★★★★★	★★★	★★★	NR
62. Walla Walla General Hospital, Walla Walla	★★★	★★★	NR	NR	NR	★★★	★★★	★★★	★★★	NR	NR	NR
63. Whidbey General Hospital, Coupeville	★★★	★★★	NR	NR	NR	★★★	NR	★★★	★	NR	NR	NR
64. Whitman Hospital and Medical Center, Colfax	NR	NR	NR	NR	NR	NR	NR	★★★	★★★	NR	NR	NR
65. Yakima Regional Medical and Cardiac Center, Yakima	★★★	★★★	★	★	NR	★★★	★★★	★★★	★★★	★	★★★	NR
66. Yakima Valley Memorial Hospital, Yakima	★★★★★	★★★	★★★	NR	NR	★★★	★★★	★★★	★★★	NR	★★★	★★★

KEY: ★★★★★ BEST   ★★★ AS EXPECTED   ★ POOR   NR NOT RATED BY HEALTHGRADES   For full definitions of ratings and awards, see Appendix.

Gastrointestinal Bleed	Gastrointestinal Surgeries and Procedures	Heart Attack	Heart Failure	Hip Fracture Repair	Maternity Care	Pancreatitis	Peripheral Vascular Bypass	Pneumonia	Prostatectomy	Pulmonary Embolism	Resection/Replacement of Abdominal Aorta	Respiratory Failure	Sepsis	Stroke	Total Hip Replacement	Total Knee Replacement	Valve Replacement	Women's Health
★★★	★★★★★	★★★	★★★	★★★	★★★	★★★	★★★	★★★★★	★★★	★★★	★★★	★★★	★★★★★	★★★	★★★★★	★★★	★	★★★
★★★★★	★★★	★★★	★★★	★★★	★	★★★	★★★	★★★★★	★★★	★★★	★★★	★	★★★	★★★★★	★★★	★★★	★★★	★
NR	NR	NR	★★★	NR	★	NR	NR	★★★	NR	NR	NR	NR	NR	NR	NR	NR	NR	NR
★★★	★★★	NR	★★★	★★★	NR	NR	NR	★	★★★	NR	NR	NR	★★★	★★★	★★★★★	★★★★★	NR	NR
★★★	NR	NR	★★★	NR	NR	NR	NR	★★★	NR	NR	NR	NR	NR	NR	NR	NR	NR	NR
★★★	★★★	★	★★★	★★★	★	★★★★★	NR	★★★	★★★★★	★★★	NR	★★★	★★★	★★★	★★★	★★★	★★★	★
NR	NR	NR	★★★	★★★	★★★	NR	NR	★★★	NR	NR	NR	NR	NR	★★★	NR	NR	NR	NR
★	★★★	★★★	★★★	★	★★★	★★★	NR	★★★	★★★	★★★	NR	★★★	★★★	★	★	★	NR	NR
★★★	★★★	★★★	★★★★★	★★★★★	★★★	★★★	NR	★★★	★★★	★★★	★★★	★★★	★★★	★★★	★★★★★	★★★★★	NR	NR
★★★	NR	NR	★★★	★★★	★	NR	NR	★★★	★★★	NR	NR	NR	NR	NR	NR	NR	NR	NR
★★★	★★★	★★★	★★★	★★★	NR	★★★	★	★★★★★	★★★	★★★	★★★	★	★★★	★★★	★★★★★	★★★		
★★★	★★★	★★★	★★★	★★★	★★★	NR	★★★	★★★	NR	NR	★★★	★★★	★★★	★★★	★★★	★★★	NR	NR
★★★	★★★	★★★	★★★	★★★	★★★	NR	NR	★★★	★★★	NR	NR	★	★★★	NR	NR	NR	NR	
NR	NR	NR	★	NR	★★★	NR	NR	★★★	NR	NR	NR	NR	NR	★★★	NR	★★★	NR	NR
★★★	NR	★★★	★★★	★★★	NR	NR	★★★★★	★★★	NR	NR	★★★	★★★	NR	NR	★★★	NR	★★★	NR
★★★	★★★	★★★	★★★	★	★★★	★★★	NR	★★★	★★★	★★★	NR	★★★★★	★★★	★	★★★	★★★★★	NR	NR

WASHINGTON, DC HOSPITALS: RATINGS BY PROCEDURE

	Appendectomy	Atrial Fibrillation	Back and Neck Surgery (except Spinal Fusion)	Back and Neck Surgery (Spinal Fusion)	Bariatric Surgery	Bowel Obstruction	Carotid Surgery	Cholecystectomy (Gall Bladder Removal)	Chronic Obstructive Pulmonary Disease (COPD)	Coronary Bypass Surgery	Coronary Interventional Procedures (Angioplasty/Stent)	Diabetic Acidosis and
1. George Washington University Hospital, Washington	NR	★★★	★★★	★★★	NR	★★★	NR	★★★	★	★	★★★	★★★
2. Georgetown University Hospital, Washington	NR	★★★	★★★	★	NR	★★★★★	★★★	★★★	★★★	NR	NR	★★★
3. Greater Southeast Community Hospital, Washington	NR	★★★	NR	NR	NR	★★★	NR	NR	★★★	NR	NR	★★★
4. Howard University Hospital, Washington	NR	★	NR	NR	NR	★★★	NR	NR	★	NR	★★★	★
5. Providence Hospital, Washington	NR	★★★	★★★	NR	NR	★★★	NR	★	★★★	NR	★★★	★★★
6. Sibley Memorial Hospital, Washington	NR	★★★	★★★★★	★	NR	★★★	★★★	★	★★★	NR	NR	★★★
7. Washington Hospital Center, Washington	NR	★★★	★★★★★	★★★★★	NR	★★★	★★★	★★★	★★★	★	★★★	★★★

KEY: ★★★★★ BEST   ★★★ AS EXPECTED   ★ POOR   NR NOT RATED BY HEALTHGRADES   For full definitions of ratings and awards, see Appendix.

Gastrointestinal Bleed	Gastrointestinal Surgeries and Procedures	Heart Attack	Heart Failure	Hip Fracture Repair	Maternity Care	Pancreatitis	Peripheral Vascular Bypass	Pneumonia	Prostatectomy	Pulmonary Embolism	Resection/Replacement of Abdominal Aorta	Respiratory Failure	Sepsis	Stroke	Total Hip Replacement	Total Knee Replacement	Valve Replacement	Women's Health
★★★	★★★	★★★	★★★	★★★	NR	NR	NR	★★★	★★★★★	★★★	NR	NR	★	★★★	★★★	★★★	★	NR
★★★	★★★	★★★	★★★	★★★	NR	★★★	★★★	★★★	★★★★★	★★★	★★★	★★★	★★★	★★★★★	★★★	★★★	NR	NR
★★★	NR	★★★	★★★	NR	NR	★★★	NR	★★★	★★★	NR	NR	★★★	★	★★★	NR	NR	NR	NR
★	★	★★★	★★★	★★★	NR	★★★	NR	★★★	★★★	★★★	NR	★	★	★★★★★	NR	NR	NR	NR
★★★	★★★★★	★★★	★★★	★★★	NR	★	★★★	★★★	★★★	★★★	NR	★★★	★★★	★★★★★	★★★	★★★	NR	NR
★★★	★★★	★★★★★	★★★	★★★	NR	★★★	NR	★★★	★★★	★★★	NR	★	★★★	★★★	★★★★★	★★★	NR	NR
★★★	★★★	★	★★★★★	★★★	NR	★★★	★★★	★★★	★★★★★	★★★	★	★★★	★★★	★★★★★	★★★	★★★	★	NR

WEST VIRGINIA HOSPITALS: RATINGS BY PROCEDURE

Hospital	Appendectomy	Atrial Fibrillation	Back and Neck Surgery (except Spinal Fusion)	Back and Neck Surgery (Spinal Fusion)	Bariatric Surgery	Bowel Obstruction	Carotid Surgery	Cholecystectomy (Gall Bladder Removal)	Chronic Obstructive Pulmonary Disease (COPD)	Coronary Bypass Surgery	Coronary Interventional Procedures (Angioplasty/Stent)	Diabetic Acidosis a...
1. Beckley ARH Hospital, Beckley	NR	★	NR	NR	NR	★★★	NR	★★★	★★★	NR	NR	★★★
2. Bluefield Regional Medical Center, Bluefield	NR	★★★	NR	NR	NR	★★★	NR	★★★	★★★	NR	NR	★★★
3. Boone Memorial Hospital, Madison	NR	NR	NR	NR	NR	NR	NR	NR	★★★	NR	NR	NR
4. Braxton County Memorial Hospital, Gassaway	NR	★	NR	NR	NR	NR	NR	NR	★★★	NR	NR	NR
5. Cabell-Huntington Hospital, Huntington	NR	★	★★★	NR	NR	★	★★★	★★★★★	★★★	NR	NR	★★★
6. Calhoun General Hospital County, Grantsville	NR	NR	NR	NR	NR	NR	NR	★★★	★★★	NR	NR	NR
7. CAMC Teays Valley Hospital, Hurricane	NR	★★★	NR	NR	NR	★★★	NR	★★★	★★★	NR	NR	★★★
8. Camden Clark Memorial Hospital, Parkersburg	NR	★★★	★	★★★	NR	★	★★★★★	★★★	★★★	NR	NR	★★★
9. Charleston Area Medical Center, Charleston	NR	★★★	★★★	★★★	NR	★★★	★★★★★	★★★★★	★★★	★★★	★★★★★	★★★
10. City Hospital, Martinsburg	NR	★★★	NR	NR	NR	★★★	NR	★★★	★★★	NR	NR	★★★
11. Davis Memorial Hospital, Elkins	NR	★★★	NR	NR	NR	★★★	NR	★★★★★	★★★	NR	NR	NR
12. Fairmont General Hospital, Fairmont	NR	★★★	NR	NR	NR	★★★	★★★	★★★★★	★★★	NR	NR	★★★
13. Grafton City Hospital, Grafton	NR	NR	NR	NR	NR	NR	NR	NR	★★★	NR	NR	NR
14. Grant Memorial Hospital, Petersburg	NR	★★★	NR	NR	NR	★★★	NR	NR	★★★	NR	NR	NR
15. Greenbrier Valley Medical Center, Ronceverte	NR	★	NR	NR	NR	★★★	NR	★★★	★★★	NR	NR	★★★
16. Hampshire Memorial Hospital, Romney	NR	NR	NR	NR	NR	NR	NR	NR	★★★	NR	NR	NR
17. Jackson General Hospital, Ripley	NR	★★★	NR	NR	NR	★★★	NR	NR	★★★	NR	NR	NR
18. Jefferson Memorial Hospital, Ranson	NR	★★★	NR	NR	NR	★★★	NR	★	NR	NR	NR	NR
19. Logan Regional Medical Center, Logan	NR	★★★	NR	NR	NR	★★★	NR	★★★	★★★	NR	NR	★★★
20. Minnie Hamilton Health System, Grantsville	NR	NR	NR	NR	NR	NR	NR	NR	★★★	NR	NR	NR
21. Monongalia County General Hospital, Morgantown	NR	★★★★★	NR	NR	NR	★★★	★	★★★	★	★★★	★★★	★
22. Montgomery General Hospital, Montgomery	NR	★★★	NR	NR	NR	NR	NR	NR	★★★	NR	NR	NR
23. Ohio Valley Medical Center, Wheeling	NR	★★★	NR	NR	NR	★★★	★★★	★	★	NR	NR	★★★
24. Plateau Medical Center, Oak Hill	NR	★★★	NR	NR	NR	★★★	NR	NR	★★★	NR	NR	NR
25. Pleasant Valley Hospital, Point Pleasant	NR	★★★	NR	NR	NR	★	NR	★★★	★	NR	NR	★★★
26. Pocahontas Memorial Hospital, Buckeye	NR	NR	NR	NR	NR	NR	NR	NR	★★★	NR	NR	NR
27. Potomac Valley Hospital, Keyser	NR	★★★	NR	NR	NR	NR	NR	NR	★★★	NR	NR	NR
28. Preston Memorial Hospital, Kingwood	NR	NR	NR	NR	NR	NR	NR	NR	★★★	NR	NR	NR
29. Princeton Community Hospital, Princeton	NR	★★★	★★★★★	NR	NR	★★★	NR	★★★	★★★	NR	NR	★★★
30. Raleigh General Hospital, Beckley	NR	★★★	NR	NR	NR	★★★★★	★★★	★★★	★	NR	NR	★★★
31. Reynolds Memorial Hospital, Glen Dale	NR	★	NR	NR	NR	★★★	★★★	★★★	★★★	NR	NR	NR
32. Richwood Area Community Hospital, Richwood	NR	NR	NR	NR	NR	NR	NR	NR	★★★	NR	NR	NR
33. Roane General Hospital, Spencer	NR	NR	NR	NR	NR	NR	NR	NR	★★★	NR	NR	NR
34. St. Francis Hospital, Charleston	NR	★★★	NR	NR	NR	★★★	★★★★★	★★★★★	★★★	NR	★	NR
35. St. Joseph Hospital, Buckhannon	NR	★★★	NR	NR	NR	★★★	NR	★★★	★★★	NR	NR	★★★
36. St. Joseph's Hospital, Parkersburg	NR	★★★	★★★	★★★	NR	★★★	★★★	★★★	★★★	★★★	★	★★★
37. St. Mary's Medical Center, Huntington	NR	★★★	★★★	★★★	NR	★★★	★★★	★★★	★★★	★★★	★	★★★
38. Stonewall Jackson Memorial Hospital, Weston	NR	★	NR	NR	NR	★★★	NR	★★★	★★★	NR	NR	NR
39. Summers County ARH Hospital, Hinton	NR	NR	NR	NR	NR	NR	NR	NR	★★★	NR	NR	NR
40. Summersville Memorial Hospital, Summersville	NR	★★★	NR	NR	NR	★	NR	★★★★★	★★★	NR	NR	NR
41. Thomas Memorial Hospital, South Charleston	NR	★★★	NR	NR	NR	★★★	★★★★★	★★★	★★★	NR	NR	★★★
42. United Hospital Center, Clarksburg	NR	★★★	★★★	NR	NR	★★★	★★★★★	★★★	★★★★★	NR	★★★	★★★
43. War Memorial Hospital, Berkeley Springs	NR	NR	NR	NR	NR	NR	NR	NR	★★★	NR	NR	NR
44. Weirton Medical Center, Weirton	NR	★★★	NR	NR	NR	★★★	★	★★★	★★★	NR	★★★	★★★
45. Welch Community Hospital, Welch	NR	NR	NR	NR	NR	NR	NR	NR	★★★	NR	NR	NR
46. West Virginia University Hospitals, Morgantown	NR	★★★	★	★	NR	★★★	★★★	NR	★★★	★★★	★★★	★★★
47. Wetzel County Hospital, New Martinsville	NR	★★★	NR	NR	NR	★★★	NR	NR	★★★	NR	NR	NR
48. Wheeling Hospital, Wheeling	NR	★★★	★★★★★	NR	NR	★★★	★★★	★★★	★★★	★★★	★★★	★★★
49. Williamson Memorial Hospital, Williamson	NR	★★★	NR	NR	NR	NR	NR	NR	★	NR	NR	★★★

KEY: ★★★★★ BEST ★★★ AS EXPECTED ★ POOR NR NOT RATED BY HEALTHGRADES   For full definitions of ratings and awards, see Appendix.

WEST VIRGINIA HOSPITALS: RATINGS BY PROCEDURE

Gastrointestinal Bleed	Gastrointestinal Surgeries and Procedures	Heart Attack	Heart Failure	Hip Fracture Repair	Maternity Care	Pancreatitis	Peripheral Vascular Bypass	Pneumonia	Prostatectomy	Pulmonary Embolism	Resection/Replacement of Abdominal Aorta	Respiratory Failure	Sepsis	Stroke	Total Hip Replacement	Total Knee Replacement	Valve Replacement	Women's Health
★★★	★★★	★★★	★★★	★★★	NR	★★★	NR	★★★	★★★	NR	NR	★	★	★★★	NR	NR	NR	NR
★★★	★★★	★★★	★★★	★★★	NR	★★★	NR	★★★	NR	★★★	NR	★★★	★★★	★	★★★	★	NR	NR
NR	NR	NR	★★★	NR	NR	NR	NR	★	NR	NR	NR	NR	NR	NR	NR	NR	NR	NR
NR	NR	★★★	★	NR	NR	NR	NR	★★★	NR	NR	NR	NR	★★★	★★★	NR	NR	NR	NR
★★★	★★★	★	★	★★★	NR	NR	NR	★★★	NR	★★★	NR	★★★	★★★	★	★★★★★	★★★★★	NR	NR
NR	NR	NR	★★★	NR	NR	NR	NR	★★★	NR	NR	NR	NR	NR	NR	NR	NR	NR	NR
★★★	★★★	★★★	★★★	★★★	NR	NR	NR	★	NR	NR	NR	★★★	★★★	★★★	NR	★★★	NR	NR
★★★	★	★★★	★★★	★★★★★	NR	★★★★★	★★★★★	★★★	★	★	★★★	★★★	★★★	★★★	★★★	★★★	NR	NR
★★★	★★★	★★★★★	★★★★★	★★★★★	NR	★★★	★★★	★★★	★★★	★★★	★★★	★★★	★★★	★★★★★	★★★	★★★	★★★	NR
★★★	★★★	★	★	★★★	NR	NR	NR	★★★	★★★	NR	NR	★	★	★★★	★★★	★★★	NR	NR
★★★	NR	★★★	★★★	★★★	NR	★	NR	★★★	★★★★★	NR	NR	★★★★★	★★★	★	★★★★★	★★★★★	NR	NR
★★★	★★★	★★★	★★★	★★★	NR	★★★	NR	★★★	★★★	NR	NR	★	★	★★★	★★★	★★★	NR	NR
NR	NR	NR	★	NR	NR	NR	NR	★	NR	NR	NR	NR	NR	★★★	NR	NR	NR	NR
★★★	NR	NR	★★★	NR	NR	NR	NR	★★★	NR	NR	NR	NR	NR	★	NR	NR	NR	NR
★★★	★★★	★★★★★	★★★	★★★	NR	★	NR	★★★	★★★	NR	NR	★★★★★	★★★★★	NR	NR	NR	NR	NR
NR	NR	NR	★★★	NR	NR	NR	NR	★★★	NR	NR	NR	NR	NR	NR	NR	NR	NR	NR
★★★	NR	★★★	★★★	NR	NR	NR	NR	★★★	NR	NR	NR	★	★	★★★	NR	NR	NR	NR
★	NR	★★★	★	NR	NR	NR	NR	★	NR	NR	NR	NR	NR	★★★	NR	NR	NR	NR
★★★	NR	★★★	★★★	★★★	NR	★	NR	★★★	★★★★★	NR	NR	★★★	★★★	★	NR	NR	NR	NR
NR	NR	NR	★★★	NR	NR	NR	NR	★	NR	NR	NR	NR	NR	NR	NR	NR	NR	NR
★★★	★★★	★	★	NR	NR	★★★	NR	★★★	★★★	★★★	NR	★★★	★★★	★★★	★★★	★	★★★	NR
★★★	NR	NR	★	NR	NR	NR	NR	★★★	NR	NR	NR	★★★	★★★	NR	NR	NR	NR	NR
★	★★★	★★★	★★★	★	NR	NR	NR	★	★★★	NR	NR	★★★	NR	NR	NR	NR	NR	NR
★★★	★★★	★★★	★★★	NR	NR	★★★	NR	★★★	NR	NR	NR	★★★	★★★	NR	NR	NR	NR	NR
★★★	NR	★	★	★	NR	NR	NR	★	★★★	NR	NR	NR	★	★★★	NR	★★★	NR	NR
NR	NR	NR	★	NR	NR	NR	NR	★	NR	NR	NR	NR	NR	NR	NR	NR	NR	NR
★★★	NR	NR	★★★★★	NR	NR	★★★	NR	★★★	NR	NR	NR	★★★	★★★★★	★★★	NR	NR	NR	NR
★	NR	★★★	★	NR	NR	NR	NR	★	NR	NR	NR	NR	NR	NR	NR	NR	NR	NR
★★★	★★★	★★★	★★★	★★★	NR	★★★	NR	★★★	★	★★★	NR	★★★	★★★★★	★	★	NR	NR	NR
★★★★★	★★★	★★★	★★★	★★★	NR	★★★★★	NR	★★★	★★★	★★★	NR	★★★★★	★★★	★★★	★★★	★	NR	NR
★★★	NR	★	★	★★★	NR	★★★	NR	★	★★★	NR	NR	NR	NR	★	NR	★★★	NR	NR
NR	NR	NR	★★★	NR	NR	NR	NR	★★★	NR	NR	NR	NR	NR	NR	NR	NR	NR	NR
★	NR	NR	★	NR	NR	NR	NR	★	NR	NR	NR	NR	NR	NR	NR	NR	NR	NR
★★★	★★★	★	★★★★★	★★★	NR	★★★	NR	★★★	★★★★★	NR	NR	★★★	★★★	★★★	★★★	★★★	NR	NR
★★★	NR	★★★	★	★	NR	NR	NR	★	NR	NR	NR	NR	NR	★	NR	★★★	NR	NR
★★★	★	★★★	★★★	★★★	NR	★★★	NR	★★★	★★★	★★★	NR	★★★	★	★★★	★★★★★	★★★	NR	NR
★★★	★★★	★★★	★★★	★★★	NR	★★★	NR	★	★	★★★	★★★	★	★★★	★★★	★★★	★★★	★★★	NR
★★★	NR	★	★★★	★★★	NR	NR	NR	★	★★★	NR	NR	★	★	NR	NR	NR	NR	NR
★★★	NR	NR	★★★	NR	NR	NR	NR	★★★	NR	NR	NR	★★★	★★★	NR	NR	NR	NR	NR
★★★	NR	★	★★★	★★★	NR	NR	NR	★★★	NR	NR	NR	★★★	★★★	NR	★★★	NR	NR	NR
★★★	★	★★★	★★★★★	★★★	NR	★★★	NR	★★★★★	★★★	NR	NR	★★★★★	★	★★★	★★★	★★★	NR	NR
★★★	★★★	★★★	★★★	★★★	NR	★★★	★★★★★	★★★★★	★	★★★★★	★★★	★★★★★	★★★	★★★	★★★★★	★★★★★	NR	NR
NR	NR	NR	★★★	NR	NR	NR	NR	★	NR	NR	NR	NR	NR	NR	NR	NR	NR	NR
★★★	★	★	★★★	★★★	NR	★★★	NR	★★★	NR	NR	NR	★★★	★★★	NR	★★★	NR	NR	NR
★★★	NR	NR	★★★	★★★	NR	NR	NR	★★★	NR	NR	NR	★	NR	NR	NR	NR	NR	NR
★★★	NR	★	★★★	★	NR	★★★	NR	★★★	★★★	★	★★★	★★★	★★★	NR	★	★★★	★★★	NR
★★★	NR	★★★	★	NR	NR	NR	NR	★	NR	NR	★★★	★★★	★★★	NR	NR	NR	NR	NR
★★★	★★★	★	★	★★★	NR	★★★	NR	★★★	NR	★★★	★	★★★	NR	★	★★★	★★★★★	★★★	NR
★★★	NR	NR	NR	★★★	NR	NR	NR	★★★	NR	NR	NR	★★★	★★★	NR	NR	NR	NR	NR

WISCONSIN HOSPITALS: RATINGS BY PROCEDURE

Hospital	Appendectomy	Atrial Fibrillation	Back and Neck Surgery (except Spinal Fusion)	Back and Neck Surgery (Spinal Fusion)	Bariatric Surgery	Bowel Obstruction	Carotid Surgery	Cholecystectomy (Gall Bladder Removal)	Chronic Obstructive Pulmonary Disease (COPD)	Coronary Bypass Surgery	Coronary Interventional Procedures (Angioplasty/Stent)	Diabetic Acidosis an...
1. All Saints Medical Center–St. Mary's Campus, Racine	★★★★★	★★★	★	★	★★★	★★★	★★★	★★★	★★★	★★★	★★★	★
2. All Saints St. Luke's Hospital, Racine	★★★★★	★★★	★	★	★★★	★★★	★★★	★★★	★★★	★★★	★★★	★
3. Amery Regional Medical Center, Amery	★★★	★★★	NR	NR	NR	★★★	NR	NR	★	NR	NR	NR
4. Appleton Medical Center, Appleton	★★★	★★★★★	NR	NR	NR	★★★	★★★	★★★	★★★	★★★	★	★★★
5. Aspirus Wausau Hospital, Wausau	★★★★★	★★★	★★★	★★★	★★★	★★★	★★★★★	★★★	★★★★★	★★★★★	★★★	★★★
6. Aurora Baycare Medical Center, Green Bay	★★★	★★★	★★★	★★★★★	★★★	★★★	★	★★★	★★★	★★★★★	★★★	NR
7. Aurora Lakeland Medical Center, Elkhorn	★★★	★★★	NR	NR	NR	★★★	NR	★★★	★	NR	NR	NR
8. Aurora Medical Center–Kenosha, Kenosha	★★★	★★★	NR	NR	NR	★★★	NR	★★★	★★★	NR	NR	NR
9. Aurora Medical Center–Manitowoc City, Two Rivers	★★★	★★★	NR	NR	NR	★★★	NR	★★★	★★★	NR	★★★	NR
10. Aurora Medical Center–Oshkosh, Oshkosh	★★★	★★★	NR	NR	NR	★★★	NR	★★★	★★★	NR	★★★	NR
11. Aurora Medical Center–Washington County, Hartford	★★★	★★★	NR	NR	NR	★★★	NR	★★★	★★★	NR	★★★	NR
12. Aurora Sheboygan Memorial Medical Center, Sheboygan	★★★	★★★	NR	NR	NR	★★★	NR	★★★★★	★★★	NR	★	NR
13. Aurora Sinai Medical Center, Milwaukee	★	★★★	NR	NR	★★★★★	★★★	NR	★★★★★	★★★	★★★	★★★	★★★
14. Aurora St. Luke's Medical Center, Milwaukee	★	★★★	★	★★★	★	★★★★★	★	★★★★★	★★★★★	★★★	★★★	★★★
15. Baldwin Area Medical Center, Baldwin	★★★	NR	NR	NR	NR	NR	NR	NR	★★★	NR	NR	NR
16. Barron Memorial Medical Center Mayo, Barron	★★★★★	NR	NR	NR	NR	NR	NR	NR	★★★	NR	NR	NR
17. Bay Area Medical Center, Marinette	★★★	★★★	NR	NR	NR	★★★	★	★★★	★★★	NR	NR	NR
18. Beaver Dam Community Hospital, Beaver Dam	★	★★★	NR	NR	NR	★★★	NR	★★★	★★★	NR	NR	NR
19. Bellin Memorial Hospital, Green Bay	★	★★★	NR	NR	★★★	★★★★★	★	★★★	★★★	★★★	★★★	NR
20. Beloit Memorial Hospital, Beloit	★	★★★	NR	NR	NR	★★★	NR	★★★	★	NR	★★★	★★★
21. Berlin Memorial Hospital, Berlin	★	★★★	NR	NR	NR	★★★	NR	★★★★★	★	NR	NR	NR
22. Bloomer Medical Center, Bloomer	NR	NR	NR	NR	NR	NR	NR	NR	★★★	NR	NR	NR
23. Boscobel Area Health Care, Boscobel	NR	NR	NR	NR	NR	NR	NR	NR	NR	NR	NR	NR
24. Burnett Medical Center, Grantsburg	NR	NR	NR	NR	NR	NR	NR	NR	★★★	NR	NR	NR
25. Chippewa Valley Hospital, Durand	NR	NR	NR	NR	NR	NR	NR	NR	★★★	NR	NR	NR
26. Columbia St. Mary's Hospital Milwaukee, Milwaukee	★★★	★★★	★	★★★★★	NR	★★★	★★★	★★★	★★★	★★★	★★★	★★★
27. Columbia St. Mary's Hospital Ozaukee, Mequon	★★★	★★★	★★★	★★★	NR	★★★	NR	★★★	★★★	★★★	★★★	★★★
28. Columbus Community Hospital, Columbus	NR	★★★	NR	NR	NR	NR	NR	NR	★★★	NR	NR	NR
29. Community Memorial Hospital, Menomonee Falls	★★★	★★★	★★★	★★★	★★★	★★★	★★★	★★★	★	★★★	★★★	★★★
30. Community Memorial Hospital, Oconto Falls	NR	★★★	NR	★★★	NR	★★★	NR	★★★	★★★	NR	NR	NR
31. Cumberland Memorial Hospital, Cumberland	NR	NR	NR	NR	NR	NR	NR	★	NR	NR	NR	NR
32. Divine Savior Healthcare, Portage	★★★	★★★	NR	NR	NR	★	NR	★	★★★	NR	NR	NR
33. Door County Memorial Hospital, Sturgeon Bay	NR	★★★	NR	NR	NR	★★★	NR	★★★	★★★	NR	NR	NR
34. Edgerton Hospital and Health Services, Edgerton	NR	NR	NR	NR	NR	NR	NR	NR	★★★	NR	NR	NR
35. Flambeau Hospital, Park Falls	NR	★★★	NR	NR	NR	NR	NR	NR	★★★	NR	NR	NR
36. Fort Healthcare, Fort Atkinson	★★★	★★★	NR	NR	NR	★★★	NR	★	★★★	NR	NR	NR
37. Franciscan Skemp La Crosse Hospital, La Crosse	★★★	★★★	★★★	★★★	NR	★	★	★	★★★	NR	★★★	NR
38. Franciscan Skemp Sparta Hospital, Sparta	★★★	NR	NR	NR	NR	NR	NR	NR	NR	NR	NR	NR
39. Frederic Municipal Hospital Association, Frederic	NR	NR	NR	NR	NR	NR	NR	NR	★★★	NR	NR	NR
40. Froedtert Memorial Lutheran Hospital, Milwaukee	★★★	★★★	★★★	★★★	★★★★★	★★★	★	★★★	★★★	★★★	NR	★★★
41. Good Samaritan Health Center, Merrill	★	★★★	NR	NR	NR	★★★	NR	★★★	★★★	NR	NR	NR
42. Grant Regional Health Center, Lancaster	NR	★★★	NR	NR	NR	NR	NR	NR	★★★	NR	NR	NR
43. Gundersen Lutheran Medical Center, La Crosse	★★★★★	★★★	★	★★★★★	★★★★★	★★★	★★★	★★★	★★★	★★★	★★★	★★★★★
44. Hayward Area Memorial Hospital, Hayward	★★★	★★★	NR	NR	NR	★★★	NR	★★★★★	★★★	NR	NR	NR
45. Hess Memorial Hospital, Mauston	★★★	★★★	NR	NR	NR	★★★	NR	★★★	★	NR	NR	★★★
46. Holy Family Hospital New Richmond, New Richmond	★★★	NR	NR	NR	NR	★★★	NR	★★★	★★★	NR	NR	NR
47. Holy Family Memorial, Manitowoc	★★★	★★★	NR	NR	NR	★★★	NR	★★★★★	★★★	★★★	★★★	NR
48. Howard Young Medical Center, Woodruff	★★★	★★★★★	NR	NR	★	★★★	★★★	NR	★★★	NR	NR	NR
49. Hudson Hospital, Hudson	★★★	NR	NR	NR	NR	NR	NR	NR	NR	NR	NR	NR
50. Indianhead Medical Center, Shell Lake	NR	NR	NR	NR	NR	NR	NR	NR	★★★	NR	NR	NR

KEY: ★★★★★ BEST ★★★ AS EXPECTED ★ POOR NR NOT RATED BY HEALTHGRADES For full definitions of ratings and awards, see Appendix.

Gastrointestinal Bleed	Gastrointestinal Surgeries and Procedures	Heart Attack	Heart Failure	Hip Fracture Repair	Maternity Care	Pancreatitis	Peripheral Vascular Bypass	Pneumonia	Prostatectomy	Pulmonary Embolism	Resection/Replacement of Abdominal Aorta	Respiratory Failure	Sepsis	Stroke	Total Hip Replacement	Total Knee Replacement	Valve Replacement	Women's Health
★★★	★★★	★★★	★★★	★	★★★	★★★	★★★	★★★	★★★	★★★	NR	★★★	★★★★★	★★★★★	★★★	★★★★★	NR	★★★
★★★	★★★	★★★	★★★	NR	★★★	★★★	★★★	★★★	★★★	★★★	NR	★★★	★★★★★	★★★★★	★★★	★★★★★	NR	★★★
★★★	NR	★★★	★	NR	★	NR	NR	★★★	NR	NR	NR	NR	NR	★★★	NR	★	NR	NR
★★★★★	★★★	★★★	★★★	★★★	★★★	★★★	★★★	★★★	★★★	★★★	★★★	★★★	★★★★★	★★★★★	★★★	★★★	★	★★★
★★★	★★★	★★★★★	★★★	★	★★★	★★★	★★★	★★★	★★★	★★★	NR	★★★	★★★★★	★★★★★	★★★	★★★	★★★	★★★
★★★	★★★	★★★★★	★★★	★★★	★★★	★★★	NR	★★★★★	★★★	NR	NR	★★★	★★★★★	★★★★★	★★★	★★★	★★★	★★★★★
★★★	★★★	★★★	★★★★★	★★★	★	★★★	NR	★★★	NR	★★★	NR	★★★	★	NR	★★★	★	NR	NR
★★★	★	★★★★★	★★★	★	NR	NR	NR	★★★	NR	NR	NR	★★★	★	NR	★★★	★★★	NR	NR
★★★	★★★	★★★	★★★	NR	★★★	NR	NR	★★★	NR	NR	NR	★★★	★★★	★★★	★★★	NR	NR	NR
★★★	★★★	★★★	★★★	★★★	★	NR	NR	★★★	NR	NR	NR	★★★	★★★	★★★	NR	★★★	NR	NR
★★★	★★★	★★★	★★★	NR	NR	NR	NR	★★★	NR	NR	NR	★★★	★★★	★★★	★★★	★★★	NR	NR
★	★★★	★★★	★	★★★★★	★	NR	NR	★	★★★	★★★	NR	★★★	★★★	★★★	★★★★★	★★★★★	NR	NR
★★★	★★★	★★★	★★★★★	★★★	★★★	NR	NR	★★★★★	NR	NR	NR	★★★	★★★	★★★	★	★★★	NR	★★★
★★★★★	★★★	★★★	★★★★★	★	NR	★★★	★	★★★★★	★	★★★	★★★	★★★	★★★★★	★★★	★	★★★	★★★	NR
★★★	NR	NR	★★★	NR	★	NR	NR	★★★	NR	NR	NR	NR	NR	NR	NR	★★★	NR	NR
★★★	NR	★★★	★★★	NR	★★★	NR	NR	★★★	NR	NR	NR	NR	NR	★	NR	NR	NR	NR
★★★	★★★★★	★★★	★★★	★★★	★★★	★★★	NR	★★★	★	★★★	NR	★★★	★★★	★★★	★★★★★	★★★	NR	NR
★★★	★★★	★★★	★★★★★	★★★	★★★	NR	NR	★★★	★★★	NR	NR	★★★	★★★	★★★	★★★	★★★	NR	NR
★★★	★★★	★★★	★★★	★	★★★	★★★	★★★	★★★	★★★	★★★	NR	★★★	★★★★★	★★★	★★★	★★★	★★★	★★★
★	★★★	★★★	★	★	★★★	★★★	NR	★	★	NR	NR	★	★	★	★	★	NR	NR
★★★	★★★	★	★★★	★★★★★	★	NR	NR	★★★	NR	NR	NR	★★★	★★★	★★★★★	★★★★★	NR	NR	NR
NR	NR	NR	★★★	NR	NR	NR	NR	★★★	NR	NR	NR	NR	NR	NR	NR	NR	NR	NR
★	NR	NR	★	NR	★★★	NR	NR	★	NR	NR	NR	NR	NR	NR	NR	NR	NR	NR
★★★	NR	NR	★	NR	★★★	NR	NR	★	NR	NR	NR	NR	NR	NR	NR	NR	NR	NR
NR	NR	NR	★★★	NR	★★★	NR	NR	★★★	NR	NR	NR	NR	NR	NR	NR	NR	NR	NR
★★★	★★★	★★★	★★★	★★★★★	★★★	★★★	★★★	★★★	★★★★★	★★★	NR	★★★	★★★	★★★★★	★★★	★★★	★★★★★	★★★
★★★	★★★	★	★	★★★	★★★	★★★	NR	★★★	★★★	★★★	NR	★	★★★★★	★★★	★★★	★★★	NR	NR
★	NR	★★★	★★★	★★★	★★★	NR	NR	★★★	NR	NR	NR	★★★	★★★	★★★	★★★	★★★	NR	NR
★★★	★★★	★★★	★★★	★★★	★	★★★	★★★	★	★★★	★★★	NR	★★★	★	★	★★★	★★★	★★★	★
★★★	NR	★★★	★★★	NR	★★★	NR	NR	★★★	NR	NR	NR	★★★	★★★	NR	★★★	NR	NR	NR
NR	NR	NR	★★★	NR	★★★	NR	NR	★★★	NR	NR	NR	NR	NR	NR	NR	NR	NR	NR
★★★	★★★	NR	★	★	★	NR	NR	★★★	NR	NR	NR	★★★	★	NR	★★★	NR	NR	NR
★★★	★★★	★★★	★★★	★★★	NR	NR	NR	★★★★★	★★★	★★★	NR	★★★	★★★	NR	★★★	NR	NR	NR
★★★	NR	NR	★★★	NR	NR	NR	NR	★★★	NR	NR	NR	NR	NR	NR	NR	NR	NR	NR
★★★	NR	NR	★★★	★	NR	NR	NR	★	NR	NR	NR	NR	★★★	NR	NR	NR	NR	NR
★★★	★★★★★	★★★	★	★	★★★	★★★	NR	★	★	★★★	NR	★★★	★★★	★★★	★★★	★★★	NR	NR
★★★	★	★★★	★★★	NR	★★★	★★★	NR	★	★★★	★★★	NR	★★★	★	★	★	★	NR	NR
NR	NR	NR	★★★	NR	★	NR	NR	★★★	NR	NR	NR	★★★	NR	NR	NR	NR	NR	NR
NR	NR	NR	★★★	NR	★★★	NR	NR	★★★	NR	NR	NR	NR	NR	NR	NR	NR	NR	NR
★★★	★★★	★★★	★★★★★	★	★★★	★★★	★★★	★★★★★	★★★	★★★	★★★	★★★	★★★★★	★★★	★★★	★★★★	★★★	★★★
★★★	NR	NR	★★★★★	★	★	NR	NR	★	NR	NR	NR	NR	★	NR	★	NR	NR	NR
★★★	NR	NR	★★★	★★★	NR	NR	NR	★★★	NR	NR	NR	★★★	NR	★★★	NR	NR	NR	NR
★★★	★★★★★	★★★★★	★★★★★	★★★★★	★	★★★	★★★	★★★	★★★	★★★	★★★	★★★★★	★★★★★	★★★	★★★★★	★★★★★	★★★	★★★
★★★	NR	NR	★★★	NR	★★★	NR	NR	★★★	NR	NR	NR	★★★	NR	★★★	NR	NR	NR	NR
★★★	NR	NR	★★★	★★★	NR	NR	NR	★★★	NR	NR	NR	★★★	NR	★★★	NR	★★★	NR	NR
★★★	NR	NR	★★★	★★★	★★★	NR	NR	★★★	NR	NR	NR	★★★	NR	★★★	NR	★★★	NR	NR
★★★	★★★	★★★	★	★★★	★	★★★	NR	★★★	★	★★★	★★★	★★★	★★★	★★★	★★★★★	NR	NR	NR
★★★	★★★	NR	★★★	★★★	★	★★★	NR	★★★	★★★	★★★	NR	★★★	★★★★★	★★★	NR	NR	NR	NR
NR	★★★	★★★	★★★	★★★	NR	NR	NR	★★★	NR	NR	NR	NR	NR	NR	NR	★★★	NR	NR
NR	NR	NR	★	NR	★★★	NR	NR	★★★	NR	NR	NR	NR	NR	NR	NR	NR	NR	NR

Hospital	Appendectomy	Atrial Fibrillation	Back and Neck Surgery (except Spinal Fusion)	Back and Neck Surgery (Spinal Fusion)	Bariatric Surgery	Bowel Obstruction	Carotid Surgery	Cholecystectomy (Gall Bladder Removal)	Chronic Obstructive Pulmonary Disease (COPD)	Coronary Bypass Surgery	Coronary Interventional Procedures (Angioplasty/Stent)	Diabetic Acidosis a...
51. Ladd Memorial Hospital, Osceola	NR	NR	NR	NR	NR	NR	NR	***	***	NR	NR	
52. Lakeview Hospital, Wauwatosa	*	***	NR	NR	NR	*	***	***	***	***	*	***
53. Lakeview Medical Center, Rice Lake	***	***	NR	NR	NR	***	NR	***	***	NR	NR	NR
54. Langlade Memorial Hospital, Antigo	***	***	NR	NR	NR	***	NR	***	***	NR	NR	NR
55. Luther Hospital Mayo Health System, Eau Claire	***	***	*****	***	NR	***	***	***	***	*****	***	***
56. Memorial Health Center, Medford	***	***	NR	NR	NR	***	NR	***	***	NR	NR	NR
57. Memorial Hospital Burlington, Burlington	***	***	NR	NR	NR	***	*****	*****	***	NR	NR	***
58. Memorial Hospital Lafayette City, Darlington	NR	NR	NR	NR	NR	NR	NR	***	***	NR	NR	
59. Memorial Hospital, Manitowoc	***	***	NR	NR	NR	***	NR	*****	***	NR	***	
60. Memorial Medical Center, Ashland	***	***	NR	NR	NR	***	NR	*	***	NR	***	
61. Memorial Medical Center, Neillsville	***	NR	NR	NR	NR	***	NR	***	***	NR	NR	
62. Mercy Health System, Janesville	*	***	***	NR	NR	***	***	***	***	***	***	***
63. Mercy Medical Center, Oshkosh	***	***	*****	*****	NR	***	***	***	***	NR	***	
64. Meriter Hospital, Madison	***	***	*	*	***	***	*****	***	***	***	***	***
65. Monroe Clinic, Monroe	***	***	NR	NR	NR	***	*****	***	***	NR		
66. Moundview Memorial Hospital and Clinics, Friendship	NR	NR	NR	NR	NR	NR	NR	NR	***	NR		
67. New London Family Medical Center, New London	***	NR	NR	NR	NR	NR	NR	NR	*	NR		
68. Oconomowoc Memorial Hospital, Oconomowoc	***	***	NR	NR	NR	***	***	*	***	NR	***	
69. Our Lady of Victory Hospital, Stanley	NR	NR	NR	NR	NR	NR	NR	*	NR			
70. Prairie Du Chien Memorial Hospital, Prairie Du Chien	***	***	NR	NR	NR	NR	NR	***	***	NR		
71. Red Cedar Medical Center–Mayo Health System, Menomonie	*	***	NR	NR	NR	***	NR	***	***	NR		
72. Reedsburg Area Medical Center, Reedsburg	***	***	NR	NR	NR	***	NR	***	***	NR		
73. Richland Hospital, Richland Center	NR	***	NR	NR	NR	NR	NR	***	***	NR		
74. River Falls Area Hospital, River Falls	***	***	NR	NR	NR	NR	***	***	***	NR		
75. Riverside Medical Center, Waupaca	***	***	NR	NR	NR	***	NR	***	***	NR		
76. Riverview Hospital, Wisconsin Rapids	*****	***	NR	NR	NR	***	NR	***	***	NR		
77. Rusk County Memorial Hospital, Ladysmith	***	***	NR	NR	NR	NR	NR	***	***	NR		
78. Sacred Heart Hospital, Eau Claire	*****	***	***	*	***	***	***	***	***	NR	***	***
79. St. Agnes Hospital, Fond Du Lac	***	***	***	NR	NR	***	***	***	***	***	***	
80. St. Clare Hospital Health Services, Baraboo	***	***	NR	NR	NR	***	NR	***	***	NR		
81. St. Croix Regional Medical Center, St. Croix Falls	***	***	NR	NR	NR	***	NR	***	***	NR		
82. St. Elizabeth Hospital, Appleton	***	***	***	NR	NR	***	***	***	***	***	***	
83. St. Joseph's Community Health Services, Hillsboro	NR	NR	NR	NR	NR	NR	NR	***	***	NR		
84. St. Joseph's Community Hospital West Bend, West Bend	*****	***	NR	NR	NR	***	***	***	***	NR		
85. St. Joseph's Hospital, Chippewa Falls	***	NR	NR	NR	NR	*****	NR	***	***	NR	NR	
86. St. Joseph's Hospital, Marshfield	*****	***	***	*****	***	***	***	***	***	***	***	***
87. St. Luke's Medical Center, Cudahy	*	***	*	***	*	*****	*	*	*****	***	***	***
88. St. Mary's Hospital, Rhinelander	***	***	NR	NR	NR	***	***	***	***	NR		
89. St. Mary's Hospital Medical Center, Green Bay	***	***	***	***	NR	***	*****	*****	***	***	*	
90. St. Mary's Hospital Medical Center, Madison	***	***	*	***	***	***	***	***	***	***	***	***
91. St. Michael's Hospital, Stevens Point	***	***	NR	NR	NR	***	***	***	***	NR		
92. St. Nicholas Hospital, Sheboygan	***	***	NR	NR	NR	***	***	***	***	NR		
93. St. Vincent Hospital, Green Bay	*****	***	***	***	*	*****	*	***	***	NR		
94. Sauk Prairie Memorial Hospital, Prairie Du Sac	***	***	NR	NR	NR	***	NR	NR	*	***		
95. Shawano Medical Center, Shawano	***	***	NR	NR	NR	***	NR	***	***	NR		
96. Southwest Health Center, Platteville	***	***	NR	NR	***	***	NR	***	***	NR		
97. Spooner Health System, Spooner	NR	NR	NR	NR	NR	NR	NR	NR	***	NR		
98. Theda Clark Medical Center, Neenah	***	***	***	***	***	***	***	***	***	***	***	***
99. Tomah Memorial Hospital, Tomah	***	NR	NR	NR	NR	NR	NR	***	***	NR		
100. United Hospital System, Kenosha	***	***	***	***	***	*	*****	***	*	*****	***	*

KEY: *** BEST   *** AS EXPECTED   * POOR   NR NOT RATED BY HEALTHGRADES**   For full definitions of ratings and awards, see Appendix.

Gastrointestinal Bleed	Gastrointestinal Surgeries and Procedures	Heart Attack	Heart Failure	Hip Fracture Repair	Maternity Care	Pancreatitis	Peripheral Vascular Bypass	Pneumonia	Prostatectomy	Pulmonary Embolism	Resection/Replacement of Abdominal Aorta	Respiratory Failure	Sepsis	Stroke	Total Hip Replacement	Total Knee Replacement	Valve Replacement	Women's Health
NR	NR	NR	★★★	NR	★★★	NR	NR	★★★	NR	NR	NR	NR	NR	NR	NR	★★★	NR	NR
★★★	★	★★★	★★★	★★★	★★★	NR	NR	★★★	★★★	★★★	★★★	★★★★★	★★★★★	★★★★★	★★★★★	★★★	★★★	★★★
★★★★★	★★★	★★★	★★★	★★★	★	NR	NR	★★★	NR	NR	NR	★★★	★★★	★★★	★★★★★	★★★★★	NR	NR
★★★	NR	NR	★★★	★★★	★★★	NR	NR	★★★	NR	NR	NR	NR	★★★	★★★	NR	★★★	NR	NR
★★★	★★★	★★★★★	★★★	★	★★★	★★★	★★★	★★★	★★★	★★★	NR	★★★	★★★	★	★★★	★	★★★	★★★
★★★	NR	NR	★★★	NR	★★★	NR	NR	★★★	NR	NR	NR	NR	★★★	★★★	NR	NR	NR	NR
★★★	★★★	★★★	★★★	★★★	★★★	★★★	★★★	★★★	NR	NR	NR	NR	★★★	★★★	NR	★★★	NR	NR
NR	NR	NR	★★★	NR	★★★	NR	NR	★★★	NR	NR	NR	NR	NR	NR	NR	★★★	NR	NR
★★★	★★★	★★★	★	★★★	★	NR	★★★	★★★	★	NR	★★★	NR	★★★	★★★	NR	★★★★★	NR	NR
★★★	NR	★★★	★★★	★★★	★★★	NR	NR	★	★★★	NR	NR	NR	★★★	★	★★★	★★★	NR	NR
NR	NR	NR	★	NR	★★★	NR	NR	★★★	NR	NR	NR	NR	NR	NR	NR	NR	NR	NR
★	★★★	★★★	★★★	★	★★★	★★★	NR	★	★★★	★★★	NR	★	★★★	★★★	NR	★	NR	★★★
★★★	★★★	★★★	★★★	★★★	★★★	NR	★★★	★★★	★★★	★★★	★★★	NR	★★★★★	NR	★★★★★	★★★★★	★★★	NR
★★★	★★★	★★★	★★★	★★★	★★★	★★★	★★★	★★★	★★★	★★★	NR	★	★★★	★★★	★★★★★	★★★	★★★	★
★★★	★★★	★★★	★★★★★	★★★★★	★★★	★★★	★★★	★★★	★★★	★★★	NR	★★★	★★★	★★★	★★★	★★★★★	NR	NR
NR	NR	NR	★★★	NR	NR	NR	NR	★★★	NR	NR	NR	NR	NR	★★★	NR	NR	NR	NR
★★★	NR	★★★	★★★	★★★★★	★	NR	NR	★	NR	NR	NR	NR	NR	NR	NR	★★★	NR	NR
★★★	★★★	★★★	★★★	★	★★★	NR	★★★★★	★★★	★★★	NR	NR	NR	★★★★★	★★★★★	★★★	★	NR	NR
NR	NR	NR	★★★	NR	NR	NR	NR	★★★	NR	NR	NR	NR	NR	NR	NR	NR	NR	NR
★★★	NR	NR	★★★	NR	NR	NR	NR	★★★	NR	NR	NR	NR	★★★	★★★	NR	NR	NR	NR
★★★	NR	NR	★★★	NR	NR	NR	NR	★★★	NR	NR	NR	NR	★★★	★★★	NR	★★★	NR	NR
★★★	NR	NR	★★★	★★★	★	NR	NR	★★★	NR	NR	NR	NR	★	NR	NR	★★★	NR	NR
★★★	NR	★	★★★	★	NR	NR	NR	★★★	NR	NR	NR	NR	★★★	NR	NR	★★★	NR	NR
★★★	NR	★	★★★	★	★★★	NR	NR	★	NR	NR	NR	NR	★★★	NR	NR	★★★	NR	NR
★	NR	★★★	★	★★★	★★★	NR	NR	★	NR	NR	NR	NR	★	★★★	NR	NR	NR	NR
★★★	★★★	★★★	★★★	★★★	★★★	NR	NR	★★★	★★★	NR	NR	NR	★	★	★★★	★★★★★	NR	NR
NR	NR	NR	★★★	NR	★★★	NR	NR	★★★	NR	NR	NR	NR	★★★	NR	NR	NR	NR	NR
★★★	★★★	★	★	★★★	★★★	★	★★★	★★★	★★★	★★★	NR	★	★★★	NR	★★★★★	★★★★★	NR	NR
★	★★★	★★★	★	★★★	★★★	★	NR	★	★★★	★	NR	★	★★★	★★★	★★★	★★★	★★★	NR
★★★	★★★	★★★	★★★	★★★	★★★	★★★	NR	NR	NR	NR	★★★	★★★	NR	★	★	NR	NR	NR
★★★	NR	★★★★★	★★★	★★★	★	NR	NR	★★★	NR	NR	NR	★★★	★★★	★★★	★★★	★★★	NR	NR
★★★	★★★	★★★	★★★	★	★★★	NR	★★★★★	★★★	★	★★★	NR	★★★	★★★	★★★	★★★	★★★	★★★	★★★★★
NR	NR	NR	★★★	NR	★★★	NR	NR	★★★	NR	NR	NR	NR	★★★	★★★	NR	NR	NR	NR
★★★	★★★	★★★	★★★	★★★	★	★★★	NR	★	★★★	★★★	NR	★★★	★★★	NR	★	★★★	NR	NR
★★★	NR	★★★	★★★	★★★	★★★	NR	NR	★★★	★★★	NR	NR	★★★	★★★★★	★★★	★★★	★★★	NR	NR
★★★	★	★★★★★	★★★★★	★★★	★	★★★	★★★	★★★★★	★★★	★★★	★★★	★★★	★★★★★	★★★★★	★★★	★★★★★	★★★	★★★
★★★★★	★★★	★★★	★★★★★	★	NR	★★★	★	★★★★★	★	★★★	★★★	NR	★★★★★	★★★	★	★★★	★★★	NR
★★★	★★★	★★★	★	★★★★★	★	NR	NR	★★★	★★★	NR	NR	★	★★★	★★★★★	★★★★★	NR	NR	NR
★★★	★★★	★	★★★	★★★	★	★★★	NR	★★★	★★★★★	NR	NR	★★★	★★★★★	★★★★★	NR	NR	NR	NR
★★★	★★★	★★★	★★★	★	★★★	★★★	★★★	★★★	★★★★★	★★★	★★★	★★★	★★★★★	★	★★★	★★★	★★★	★★★
★★★	★★★	★★★	★★★	★	★★★	NR	NR	★★★	★★★	NR	NR	★★★	★★★	★	★	★★★	NR	NR
★★★	★★★	★★★	★★★	★★★	★	NR	★★★	★★★	★★★	NR	NR	★★★	★★★	★★★★★	★★★★★	★★★	NR	NR
★★★	★★★	★★★	★	★★★	★★★	★★★	★★★	★★★	★★★	★★★	★★★	★★★	★★★	★	★★★	★★★	NR	NR
★★★	NR	NR	★★★	★★★	★★★	NR	NR	★★★	NR	NR	NR	★★★	★★★	★★★★★	★★★★★	★★★	NR	NR
★★★	NR	★★★	★	NR	★	NR	NR	★★★	NR	NR	NR	★★★	★★★★★	NR	NR	NR	NR	NR
★★★	NR	NR	★★★	NR	★★★	NR	NR	★★★	NR	NR	NR	NR	★	NR	NR	NR	NR	NR
★★★	NR	★★★	NR	NR	★★★	NR	NR	★★★	NR	NR	NR	NR	NR	NR	NR	NR	NR	NR
★★★	★★★	★★★	★★★	NR	★★★★★	NR	★★★	★★★	★★★	★★★★★	NR	★★★	★★★★★	NR	★★★	★★★	NR	NR
NR	NR	★★★	★	NR	★★★★★	NR	NR	★★★	NR	NR	NR	NR	★	NR	NR	NR	NR	NR
★★★	★★★	★★★	★	★★★	★★★	★★★	★★★	★	★★★	NR	NR	★	★	NR	★★★	★★★	★★★	★

	Appendectomy	Atrial Fibrillation	Back and Neck Surgery (except Spinal Fusion)	Back and Neck Surgery (Spinal Fusion)	Bariatric Surgery	Bowel Obstruction	Carotid Surgery	Cholecystectomy (Gall Bladder Removal)	Chronic Obstructive Pulmonary Disease (COPD)	Coronary Bypass Surgery	Coronary Interventional Procedures (Angioplasty/Stent)	Diabetic Acidosis and
101. **Upland Hills Health,** Dodgeville	NR	NR	NR	NR	★★★	★★★	NR	★★★	NR	★★★	NR	NR
102. **UW Health–UW Hospitals and Clinics,** Madison	★★★	★★★	★★★	★★★	★★★	★★★★★	★★★	★★★	★★★	★★★★★	★★★	★★★
103. **Vernon Memorial Hospital,** Viroqua	★★★	NR	NR	NR	NR	NR	NR	NR	NR	NR	NR	NR
104. **Watertown Memorial Hospital,** Watertown	★★★	★★★	NR	NR	NR	★★★	NR	★★★	★★★	NR	NR	NR
105. **Waukesha Memorial Hospital,** Waukesha	★★★	★★★★★	★★★	★★★★★	NR	★★★	★★★	★★★	★★★	★★★	★★★	★★★
106. **Waupun Memorial Hospital,** Waupun	★	NR	NR	NR	NR	NR	NR	★★★	★★★	NR	NR	NR
107. **West Allis Memorial Hospital,** West Allis	★★★	★★★	★★★	★★★	NR	★★★	★★★	★★★★★	★★★	NR	NR	★★★
108. **Wheaton Franciscan Healthcare–Elmbrook Memorial,** Brookfield	★★★★★	★★★	★★★	★★★	★★★	★★★	★★★	★★★★★	★★★	NR	NR	★★★
109. **Wheaton Franciscan Healthcare–St. Francis,** Milwaukee	★★★	★★★★★	★★★	NR	★★★	★★★	★★★	★★★	★★★	★★★	★★★	★★★
110. **Wheaton Franciscan Healthcare–St. Joseph,** Milwaukee	★	★★★	NR	NR	NR	★	★★★	★★★	★★★	★★★	★	★★★
111. **Wisconsin Heart Hospital,** Wauwatosa	NR	★★★	NR	NR	NR	NR	★★★	NR	NR	★★★	★★★	NR

KEY: ★★★★★ BEST   ★★★ AS EXPECTED   ★ POOR   NR NOT RATED BY HEALTHGRADES   For full definitions of ratings and awards, see Appendix.

Gastrointestinal Bleed	Gastrointestinal Surgeries and Procedures	Heart Attack	Heart Failure	Hip Fracture Repair	Maternity Care	Pancreatitis	Peripheral Vascular Bypass	Pneumonia	Prostatectomy	Pulmonary Embolism	Resection/Replacement of Abdominal Aorta	Respiratory Failure	Sepsis	Stroke	Total Hip Replacement	Total Knee Replacement	Valve Replacement	Women's Health
★★★	NR	NR	★	★	★★★	NR	NR	★★★	NR	NR	NR	NR	NR	★★★	NR	NR	NR	NR
★★★	★★★	★★★	★★★	★	NR	★★★	★★★	★★★★★	★★★	★★★	★★★	★★★	★★★★★	★★★	★★★	★	★★★★★	NR
★★★	NR	NR	★	NR	★★★	NR	NR	★★★	NR	NR	NR	NR	★★★	★★★	★★★	★★★★★	NR	NR
★★★	★★★	★★★	★★★	★	★★★	NR	NR	★★★	NR	★★★	NR	NR	★★★	★★★	★★★	★★★	NR	NR
★★★★★	★★★	★★★	★★★★★	★★★	★★★	★★★	★★★	★★★	★★★	★★★	★★★	★★★	★★★★★	★★★	★★★	★	★★★★★	★★★★★
★	NR	NR	★★★	★★★	★	NR	NR	★★★	NR	NR	NR	NR	★★★	NR	★★★	NR	NR	NR
★★★	★★★★★	★★★	★★★★★	★★★★★	★★★	★★★	★★★	★★★★★	★★★★★	★★★	NR	★★★★★	★★★★★	★★★★★	★★★	★★★	NR	NR
★★★	★★★★★	★★★	★★★	★★★	★★★	★	★★★	★	★★★	★★★	NR	★★★★★	★★★	★★★	★★★★★	★★★★★	NR	NR
★★★★★	★★★	★★★	★★★	★★★	★★★	NR	★★★	★★★	★★★	★★★★★	NR	★★★★★	★★★★★	★★★★★	★★★	★★★	NR	★★★
★★★	★	★★★	★★★	★★★	★★★	NR	NR	★★★	★★★	★★★	★★★	★★★★★	★★★★★	★★★★★	★★★★★	★★★	★★★	★★★
NR	NR	★★★	★★★	NR	NR	NR	NR	NR	NR	NR	NR	NR	NR	NR	NR	NR	★★★	NR

WYOMING HOSPITALS: RATINGS BY PROCEDURE

Hospital	Appendectomy	Atrial Fibrillation	Back and Neck Surgery (except Spinal Fusion)	Back and Neck Surgery (Spinal Fusion)	Bariatric Surgery	Bowel Obstruction	Carotid Surgery	Cholecystectomy (Gall Bladder Removal)	Chronic Obstructive Pulmonary Disease (COPD)	Coronary Bypass Surgery	Coronary Interventional Procedures (Angioplasty/Stent)	Diabetic Acidosis and...
1. Campbell County Memorial Hospital, Gillette	NR	★	NR	NR	NR	★★★	NR	★★★	NR	NR	★★★	
2. Cheyenne Regional Medical Center, Cheyenne	NR	★★★	★★★	★★★	NR	★★★★★	★★★	★	★★★	★	★	★★★
3. Community Hospital, Torrington	NR	NR	NR	NR	NR	★★★	NR	★	NR	NR	NR	
4. Depaul Hospital, Cheyenne	NR	★★★	★★★	★★★	NR	★★★★★	★★★	★	★★★	★	★	★★★
5. Evanston Regional Hospital, Evanston	NR	NR	NR	NR	NR	NR	NR	★★★	NR	NR	NR	
6. Hot Springs County Memorial Hospital, Thermopolis	NR	NR	NR	NR	NR	NR	NR	★	NR	NR	NR	
7. Ivinson Memorial Hospital, Laramie	NR	★★★	★★★	NR	NR	★★★	NR	★★★	NR	NR	NR	
8. Lander Valley Medical Center, Lander	NR	NR	NR	NR	NR	★★★	NR	★★★	NR	NR	NR	
9. Memorial Hospital of Carbon County, Rawlins	NR	NR	NR	NR	NR	★★★	NR	★★★	NR	NR	NR	
10. Memorial Hospital of Sheridan County, Sheridan	NR	★	★★★	NR	NR	★★★	★★★	★	NR	NR	NR	
11. Memorial Hospital Sweetwater County, Rock Springs	NR	★★★	NR	NR	NR	★★★	NR	★★★	NR	NR	NR	
12. Platte County Memorial Hospital, Wheatland	NR	NR	NR	NR	NR	NR	NR	★★★	NR	NR	NR	
13. Powell Valley Hospital, Powell	NR	NR	NR	★★★★★	NR	NR	NR	★★★	NR	NR	NR	
14. Riverton Memorial Hospital, Riverton	NR	★★★	NR	NR	NR	★★★	NR	★★★	NR	NR	NR	
15. St. John's Medical Center, Jackson Hole	NR	★★★	NR	NR	NR	★★★	★	★★★	NR	NR	NR	
16. Washakie Medical Center, Worland	NR	NR	NR	NR	NR	★★★	NR	★	NR	NR	NR	
17. West Park Hospital District, Cody	NR	★★★	★★★	★★★	NR	NR	NR	★★★	NR	NR	NR	
18. Wyoming Medical Center, Casper	NR	★★★	★★★★★	★★★	NR	★★★	★★★	★★★	★★★	★	★★★	NR

KEY: ★★★★★ BEST   ★★★ AS EXPECTED   ★ POOR   NR NOT RATED BY HEALTHGRADES   For full definitions of ratings and awards, see Appendix.

Gastrointestinal Bleed	Gastrointestinal Surgeries and Procedures	Heart Attack	Heart Failure	Hip Fracture Repair	Maternity Care	Pancreatitis	Peripheral Vascular Bypass	Pneumonia	Prostatectomy	Pulmonary Embolism	Resection/Replacement of Abdominal Aorta	Respiratory Failure	Sepsis	Stroke	Total Hip Replacement	Total Knee Replacement	Valve Replacement	Women's Health
★★★	NR	NR	★★★	★★★	NR	NR	NR	★★★	NR	NR	NR	★★★	NR	★★★	NR	★★★	NR	NR
★★★	★★★	★	★★★	★★★	NR	★★★	NR	★	★	★★★	NR	★★★	★★★	★★★	★	★★★	★★★	NR
★	NR	NR	★	NR	NR	NR	NR	★	NR	NR	NR	NR	NR	NR	NR	NR	NR	NR
★★★	★★★	★	★★★	★★★	NR	★★★	NR	★	★	★★★	NR	★★★	★★★	★★★	★	★★★	★★★	NR
NR	NR	NR	★★★	★★★	NR	NR	NR	★★★	NR	NR	NR	NR	NR	NR	NR	NR	NR	NR
★★★	NR	NR	★★★	NR	NR	NR	NR	★★★	NR	NR	NR	NR	NR	NR	NR	NR	NR	NR
★★★	NR	NR	★★★	★★★	NR	NR	NR	★★★	★★★	★★★	NR	NR	NR	★★★	★★★★★	★★★	NR	NR
★★★	NR	NR	★★★	★★★	NR	NR	NR	★★★	NR	NR	NR	NR	NR	NR	★★★	★★★★★	NR	NR
★★★	NR	NR	★	NR	NR	NR	NR	★★★	NR	NR	NR	NR	NR	NR	NR	NR	NR	NR
★★★	NR	NR	★★★	★★★	NR	NR	NR	★	★★★	NR	NR	★	★	★★★	★★★	NR	NR	NR
★★★	NR	NR	★★★	★	NR	NR	NR	★★★	★	★★★	NR	NR	★	NR	NR	NR	NR	NR
NR	NR	NR	★★★	NR	NR	NR	NR	★★★	NR	NR	NR	NR	NR	NR	NR	NR	NR	NR
★★★	NR	NR	★	NR	NR	NR	NR	★★★	NR	NR	NR	NR	★★★	NR	NR	NR	NR	NR
★★★	NR	NR	★★★	★★★	NR	NR	NR	★★★	NR	NR	NR	NR	★★★	NR	NR	NR	NR	NR
★★★	NR	NR	★★★	★	NR	NR	NR	★★★	★★★	NR	NR	NR	NR	NR	NR	★	NR	NR
★★★	NR	NR	★★★	NR	NR	NR	NR	★	NR	NR	NR	NR	NR	NR	NR	NR	NR	NR
★★★	NR	NR	★★★	★	NR	NR	NR	★★★★★	NR	NR	NR	NR	★★★	★	★	NR	NR	NR
★★★	★★★	★★★	★★★	★★★	NR	★	NR	★★★	★★★	★★★	NR	★★★	★	★★★	★★★	★★★	★★★	NR

CHAPTER 9

HEALTHGRADES TOP DOCTORS

HEALTHGRADES TOP DOCTORS

This section will help guide you to physicians who treat patients at hospitals that rate among the best in the nation in their particular specialties, such as cardiac care.

In the Top Doctors section you will find, listed by state, physicians who treat patients at hospitals HealthGrades has found to be among the top 10 percent in the nation for specific procedures and diagnosis. For example, if you know that you or a loved one need a stent placed in your heart to open a clogged artery, and you live in or near Rochester, New York, you may want to contact Dr. Martha Jones who practices at Unity Health System Park Ridge.

The lists of top doctors in this section reflect the first time that outstanding physicians across the country have been identified based on objective data derived from clinical results. It is this method of gathering information that sets HealthGrades' Top Doctors lists apart. While popular magazines and local reports use word of mouth and subjective surveys to gather their information, HealthGrades mines hospital reports for indisputable facts about patient outcomes.

ALABAMA TOP DOCTORS

CARDIAC SURGERY

Richard Clay, Huntsville Hospital, Huntsville
Evan Cohen, Huntsville Hospital, Huntsville
Charles Newton, Huntsville Hospital, Huntsville
Thomas Washburn Jr., Huntsville Hospital,
Huntsville

NEUROLOGY

Dinesh Bhambvani, Riverview Regional Medical
Center, Gadsden
John Just, Riverview Regional Medical Center,
Gadsden

ORTHOPEDIC SURGERY

Gary Russell, Walker Baptist Medical Center, Jasper
Kendall Vague, Walker Baptist Medical Center, Jasper
Erich Wouters, Walker Baptist Medical Center, Jasper

SPINE SURGERY

Mark Prevost, Walker Baptist Medical Center, Jasper

ARIZONA TOP DOCTORS

GENERAL SURGERY

Katie Artz, Tucson Medical Center, Tucson
Charles Atkinson, Tucson Medical Center, Tucson
James Balserak, Tucson Medical Center, Tucson
Kelly Favre, Tucson Medical Center, Tucson
Thomas Harmon, Tucson Medical Center, Tucson
James Herde, Tucson Medical Center, Tucson
Mark Kartchner, Tucson Medical Center, Tucson
Sitara Kommareddi, Tucson Medical Center, Tucson
Michael Lavor, Tucson Medical Center, Tucson
Daniel McCabe, Tucson Medical Center, Tucson
Michael Probstfeld, Tucson Medical Center, Tucson
U. Roeder, Tucson Medical Center, Tucson
Jolyon Schilling, Tucson Medical Center, Tucson
Patrick Smith, Tucson Medical Center, Tucson
Shawn Stevenson, Tucson Medical Center, Tucson
Mordechai Twena, Tucson Medical Center, Tucson

NEUROLOGY

Niteen Andalkar, Tucson Medical Center, Tucson

L. Anderson, Tucson Medical Center, Tucson
Hillel Baldwin, Tucson Medical Center, Tucson
Diana Benenati, Tucson Medical Center, Tucson
Arlo Brakel, Tucson Medical Center, Tucson
Joseph Christiano, Tucson Medical Center, Tucson
Jack Dunn, Tucson Medical Center, Tucson
John Iskandar, Tucson Medical Center, Tucson
Todd Levine, Banner Good Samaritan Medical
Center, Phoenix
William Lujan, Tucson Medical Center, Tucson
Thomas Norton, Tucson Medical Center, Tucson
Abhay Sanan, Tucson Medical Center, Tucson
Kurt Schroeder, Tucson Medical Center, Tucson
Eric Sipos, Tucson Medical Center, Tucson
Harry Tamm, Banner Good Samaritan Medical
Center, Phoenix
Matthew Wilson, Tucson Medical Center, Tucson

OBSTETRICS/GYNECOLOGY

Damian Bass, Arrowhead Hospital, Glendale
Rebecca Branaman, Arrowhead Hospital, Glendale

Carmen Brown, Arrowhead Hospital, Glendale
Mary-Helene Brown, Arrowhead Hospital, Glendale
William Castro, Arrowhead Hospital, Glendale
David Chisholm, Arrowhead Hospital, Glendale
Charles Clinch, Arrowhead Hospital, Glendale
Marvin Erickson, Arrowhead Hospital, Glendale
Bradley Folkestad, Arrowhead Hospital, Glendale
Scott Gulinson, Arrowhead Hospital, Glendale
Daniel Hu, Arrowhead Hospital, Glendale
Dawn Jenkins, Arrowhead Hospital, Glendale
Patrick Kennedy, Arrowhead Hospital, Glendale
Gary Kersten, Arrowhead Hospital, Glendale
Paul McKernan, Arrowhead Hospital, Glendale
Christopher Nahm, Arrowhead Hospital, Glendale
Charles Plimpton, Arrowhead Hospital, Glendale
Robert Saretsky, Arrowhead Hospital, Glendale
Allan Sawyer, Arrowhead Hospital, Glendale
Hetalkumar Shah, Arrowhead Hospital, Glendale
Frank Simchak, Arrowhead Hospital, Glendale
Padma Tummala, Arrowhead Hospital, Glendale

ARKANSAS TOP DOCTORS

ORTHOPEDIC SURGERY

Bruce Smith, St. Joseph's Mercy Health Center,
Hot Springs
Jason Brandt, Surgical Hospital of Jonesboro,
Jonesboro
D'Orsay Bryant, Medical Center–South Arkansas,
El Dorado
Edward Cooper, Surgical Hospital of Jonesboro,
Jonesboro
Dwayne Daniels, Medical Center–South Arkansas,
El Dorado
Thomas Day, Surgical Hospital of Jonesboro,
Jonesboro
Lawrence Dodd, St. Joseph's Mercy Health Center,
Hot Springs

Kenneth Gati, Medical Center–South Arkansas,
El Dorado
Greg Massanelli, Medical Center–South Arkansas,
El Dorado
Robert Olive, St. Joseph's Mercy Health Center,
Hot Springs
Kevin Rudder, St. Joseph's Mercy Health Center,
Hot Springs
James Schrantz, Surgical Hospital of Jonesboro,
Jonesboro
Henry Stroope, Surgical Hospital of Jonesboro,
Jonesboro
Christopher Young, St. Joseph's Mercy Health
Center, Hot Springs
Michael Young, St. Joseph's Mercy Health Center,
Hot Springs

SPINE SURGERY

Lawrence Dodd, St. Joseph's Mercy Health Center,
Hot Springs
Robert Olive, St. Joseph's Mercy Health Center,
Hot Springs
Kevin Rudder, St. Joseph's Mercy Health Center,
Hot Springs
Bruce Smith, St. Joseph's Mercy Health Center,
Hot Springs
Christopher Young, St. Joseph's Mercy Health
Center, Hot Springs
Michael Young, St. Joseph's Mercy Health Center,
Hot Springs

Top doctors are those that practice at hospitals that are rated in the top 10% in the nation for that clinical program area. For more information on how top doctors were selected, see Appendix.

CARDIAC SURGERY

Robert Adamson, Sharp Memorial Hospital, San Diego
Sam Baradarian, Sharp Memorial Hospital, San Diego
Joseph Chammas, Sharp Memorial Hospital, San Diego
Walter Dembitsky, Sharp Memorial Hospital, San Diego
Isam Felahy, St. Joseph's Medical Center of Stockton, Stockton
Keith Korver, Sutter Medical Center of Santa Rosa—Chanate, Santa Rosa
Jerome McDonald, St. Joseph's Medical Center of Stockton, Stockton
James Morrissey, St. Joseph's Medical Center of Stockton, Stockton

CARDIOLOGY

Edward Anderson, Sequoia Hospital, Redwood City
Benjamin Ansell, UCLA Medical Center, Los Angeles
Bruce Benedick, Sequoia Hospital, Redwood City
Noel Boyle, UCLA Medical Center, Los Angeles
Luis Castro, Sequoia Hospital, Redwood City
David Cesario, UCLA Medical Center, Los Angeles
John Child, UCLA Medical Center, Los Angeles
Jesse Currier, UCLA Medical Center, Los Angeles
Linda Demer, UCLA Medical Center, Los Angeles
Gregory Engel, Sequoia Hospital, Redwood City
Alan Fogelman, UCLA Medical Center, Los Angeles
Gregg Fonarow, UCLA Medical Center, Los Angeles
Osamu Fujimura, UCLA Medical Center, Los Angeles
Vincent Gaudiani, Sequoia Hospital, Redwood City
Joshua Goldhaber, UCLA Medical Center, Los Angeles
Peter Guzy, UCLA Medical Center, Los Angeles
Antoine Hage, UCLA Medical Center, Los Angeles
Michele Hamilton, UCLA Medical Center, Los Angeles
Adam Harmon, Sequoia Hospital, Redwood City
Tomoaki Hinohara, Sequoia Hospital, Redwood City
Henry Honda, UCLA Medical Center, Los Angeles
Jon Kobashigawa, UCLA Medical Center, Los Angeles
Janine Krivokapich, UCLA Medical Center, Los Angeles
Mary Larson, Sequoia Hospital, Redwood City
Andrew Lee, Sequoia Hospital, Redwood City
Michael Lee, UCLA Medical Center, Los Angeles
William MacLellan, UCLA Medical Center, Los Angeles
Bruce McAuley, Sequoia Hospital, Redwood City
Jaime Moriguchi, UCLA Medical Center, Los Angeles
Barbara Natterson, UCLA Medical Center, Los Angeles

Jignesh Patel, UCLA Medical Center, Los Angeles
William Reed, Sequoia Hospital, Redwood City
Michael Ruder, Sequoia Hospital, Redwood City
Donald St. Claire, Sequoia Hospital, Redwood City
Dennis Sheehan, Sequoia Hospital, Redwood City
Kalyanam Shivkumar, UCLA Medical Center, Los Angeles
John Simpson, Sequoia Hospital, Redwood City
Nellis Smith, Sequoia Hospital, Redwood City
Jan Tillisch, UCLA Medical Center, Los Angeles
Jonathan Tobis, UCLA Medical Center, Los Angeles
Helga Van Herle, UCLA Medical Center, Los Angeles
Conrad Vial, Sequoia Hospital, Redwood City
Andrew Watson, UCLA Medical Center, Los Angeles
Karol Watson, UCLA Medical Center, Los Angeles
James Weiss, UCLA Medical Center, Los Angeles
Roger Winkle, Sequoia Hospital, Redwood City
Lawrence Yeatman, UCLA Medical Center, Los Angeles

GASTROINTESTINAL

Gary Annunziata, Eisenhower Medical Center, Rancho Mirage
Ho Bae, Good Samaritan Hospital, Los Angeles
Carl Blau, Encino-Tarzana Regional Medical Center—Tarzana Campus, Tarzana
Hartley Cohen, Good Samaritan Hospital, Los Angeles
Noel Curry, Eisenhower Medical Center, Rancho Mirage
Caroline Diamant, Scripps Memorial Hospital—La Jolla, La Jolla
Anh Duong, Eisenhower Medical Center, Rancho Mirage
Richard Garrett, Encino-Tarzana Regional Medical Center—Tarzana Campus, Tarzana
Sheldon Getzug, Encino-Tarzana Regional Medical Center—Tarzana Campus, Tarzana
Robert Goldklang, Scripps Memorial Hospital—La Jolla, La Jolla
Maurice Gourdji, Encino-Tarzana Regional Medical Center—Tarzana Campus, Tarzana
Kenneth Hepps, Encino-Tarzana Regional Medical Center—Tarzana Campus, Tarzana
Lucien Jacobs, Encino-Tarzana Regional Medical Center—Tarzana Campus, Tarzana
Piyush Kumar, Scripps Memorial Hospital—La Jolla, La Jolla
Martin Lee, Good Samaritan Hospital, Los Angeles
Heinz Lenz, Scripps Memorial Hospital—La Jolla, La Jolla

Ariel Malamud, Encino-Tarzana Regional Medical Center—Tarzana Campus, Tarzana
Frank Mayer, Scripps Memorial Hospital—La Jolla, La Jolla
Otto Nebel, Scripps Memorial Hospital—La Jolla, La Jolla
Edward Paredez, Scripps Memorial Hospital—La Jolla, La Jolla
Vijayalakshmi Pratha, Scripps Memorial Hospital—La Jolla, La Jolla
Farshid Rahbar, Encino-Tarzana Regional Medical Center—Tarzana Campus, Tarzana
Simon Ritchken, Scripps Memorial Hospital—La Jolla, La Jolla
Donald Ritt, Scripps Memorial Hospital—La Jolla, La Jolla
David Roseman, Scripps Memorial Hospital—La Jolla, La Jolla
Shahid Sial, Good Samaritan Hospital, Los Angeles
Mordo Suchov, Encino-Tarzana Regional Medical Center—Tarzana Campus, Tarzana
Carlton Thomas, Eisenhower Medical Center, Rancho Mirage
Anthony Tornay, Eisenhower Medical Center, Rancho Mirage
Neil War Hirschenbein, Scripps Memorial Hospital—La Jolla, La Jolla

NEUROLOGY

David Alexander, Centinela Freeman Regional Medical Center—Memorial, Inglewood
Lancelot Alexander, Encino-Tarzana Regional Medical Center—Tarzana Campus, Tarzana
Arthur An, Methodist Hospital of Southern California, Arcadia
Isaac Bakst, Scripps Memorial Hospital—La Jolla, La Jolla
Sanjay Banerji, Good Samaritan Hospital, Los Angeles
Brian Beck, St. Jude Medical Center, Fullerton
Andrew Blumenfeld, Scripps Memorial Hospital—La Jolla, La Jolla
Andrew Brasch, Oroville Hospital, Oroville
Ellyn Bush, Sequoia Hospital, Redwood City
Kulreet Chaudhary, Scripps Memorial Hospital—La Jolla, La Jolla
George Chow, Encino-Tarzana Regional Medical Center—Tarzana Campus, Tarzana
Deepak Chugh, Encino-Tarzana Regional Medical Center—Tarzana Campus, Tarzana

CALIFORNIA TOP DOCTORS

Anthony Ciabarra, St. Jude Medical Center, Fullerton

Frederick De La Vega, Scripps Memorial Hospital—La Jolla, La Jolla

John Dietz, Encino-Tarzana Regional Medical Center—Tarzana Campus, Tarzana

Gary Duckwiler, UCLA Medical Center, Los Angeles

Fredric Edelman, Encino-Tarzana Regional Medical Center—Tarzana Campus, Tarzana

Thomas Ela, St. Jude Medical Center, Fullerton

Fares Elghazi, Citrus Valley Medical Center—IC Campus, Covina

Fares Elghazi, Citrus Valley Medical Center—QV Campus, West Covina

King Engel, Good Samaritan Hospital, Los Angeles

Shahin Etebar, Eisenhower Medical Center, Rancho Mirage

Tony Feuerman, Encino-Tarzana Regional Medical Center—Tarzana Campus, Tarzana

Jack Florin, St. Jude Medical Center, Fullerton

Vincent Fortanasce, Methodist Hospital of Southern California, Arcadia

John Frazee, UCLA Medical Center, Los Angeles

Benjamin Frishberg, Scripps Memorial Hospital—La Jolla, La Jolla

Andrew Geleris, Citrus Valley Medical Center—IC Campus, Covina

Andrew Geleris, Citrus Valley Medical Center—QV Campus, West Covina

Charles Glatstein, Citrus Valley Medical Center—IC Campus, Covina

Charles Glatstein, Citrus Valley Medical Center—QV Campus, West Covina

Nestor Gonzalez, UCLA Medical Center, Los Angeles

Ronald Greenwald, Sequoia Hospital, Redwood City

Randall Hawkins, Sharp Memorial Hospital, San Diego

Jeremy Hogan, Sharp Memorial Hospital, San Diego

William Hornstein, St. Mary Medical Center, Long Beach

Patrick Huott, Sharp Memorial Hospital, San Diego

Charles Imbus, Methodist Hospital of Southern California, Arcadia

Reza Jahan, UCLA Medical Center, Los Angeles

Fatima Janjua, Methodist Hospital of Southern California, Arcadia

Cleotilde Jose, Brotman Medical Center, Culver City

Surjit Kahlon, Methodist Hospital of Southern California, Arcadia

David Kheradyar, Centinela Freeman Regional Medical Center—Memorial, Inglewood

Naira Kocharian, Scripps Memorial Hospital—La Jolla, La Jolla

Kevin Kolostyak, Scripps Memorial Hospital—La Jolla, La Jolla

Arthur Kowell, Encino-Tarzana Regional Medical Center—Tarzana Campus, Tarzana

Mukhtair Kundi, Citrus Valley Medical Center—IC Campus, Covina

Muktair Kundi, Citrus Valley Medical Center—QV Campus, West Covina

Todd Lanman, Encino-Tarzana Regional Medical Center—Tarzana Campus, Tarzana

Timothy Lee, St. Mary Medical Center, Long Beach

Jonathan Licht, Sharp Memorial Hospital, San Diego

David Liebeskind, UCLA Medical Center, Los Angeles

Farhad Limonadi, Eisenhower Medical Center, Rancho Mirage

Frank Lin, Methodist Hospital of Southern California, Arcadia

June-Chih Liu, Methodist Hospital of Southern California, Arcadia

Michael Lobatz, Scripps Memorial Hospital—La Jolla, La Jolla

Peter Lorber, Good Samaritan Hospital, Los Angeles

Neil Martin, UCLA Medical Center, Los Angeles

James McFeely, Alta Bates Summit—Alta Bates Campus, Berkeley

Chad Miller, UCLA Medical Center, Los Angeles

Yafa Minazad, Methodist Hospital of Southern California, Arcadia

Robert Moon, St. Jude Medical Center, Fullerton

Kenneth Nazari, Centinela Freeman Regional Medical Center—Memorial, Inglewood

Richard Nusser, Alta Bates Summit—Alta Bates Campus, Berkeley

Richard Nusser, Alta Bates Summit—Summit Campus, Oakland

Robert Pavy, Sequoia Hospital, Redwood City

Erik Perkins, Sharp Memorial Hospital, San Diego

Meril Platzer, Encino-Tarzana Regional Medical Center—Tarzana Campus, Tarzana

Jeffrey Randall, Alta Bates Summit—Alta Bates Campus, Berkeley

Jeffrey Randall, Alta Bates Summit—Summit Campus, Oakland

Singh Ravinder, Brotman Medical Center, Culver City

Scott Riedler, Sharp Memorial Hospital, San Diego

Jack Rose, Pacific Campus Hospital, San Francisco

Bradley Rosenberg, Citrus Valley Medical Center—IC Campus, Covina

Bradley Rosenberg, Citrus Valley Medical Center—QV Campus, West Covina

Jay Rosenberg, Scripps Memorial Hospital—La Jolla, La Jolla

Johanna Rosenthal, St. Jude Medical Center, Fullerton

Peter Rossi, UCLA Medical Center, Los Angeles

Nancy Sajben, Scripps Memorial Hospital—La Jolla, La Jolla

Mark Saleh, Sequoia Hospital, Redwood City

Ayman Salem, Encino-Tarzana Regional Medical Center—Tarzana Campus, Tarzana

Jeffrey Saver, UCLA Medical Center, Los Angeles

Alfred Shen, Eisenhower Medical Center, Rancho Mirage

Richard Shubin, Methodist Hospital of Southern California, Arcadia

Dee Silver, Scripps Memorial Hospital—La Jolla, La Jolla

Kurt Slater, Methodist Hospital of Southern California, Arcadia

Sidney Starkman, UCLA Medical Center, Los Angeles

Shuichi Suzuki, Methodist Hospital of Southern California, Arcadia

Michael Tan, Methodist Hospital of Southern California, Arcadia

Satoshi Tateshima, UCLA Medical Center, Los Angeles

Jeffrey Thomas, Pacific Campus Hospital, San Francisco

David Tong, Pacific Campus Hospital, San Francisco

Guven Uzun, Brotman Medical Center, Culver City

Paul Vespa, UCLA Medical Center, Los Angeles

Kenneth Villa, Sharp Memorial Hospital, San Diego

Fernando Vinuela, UCLA Medical Center, Los Angeles

Stephen Waldman, St. Jude Medical Center, Fullerton

J. Wilson, Sequoia Hospital, Redwood City

Kenneth Wogensen, Methodist Hospital of Southern California, Arcadia

Qun Xu, St. Jude Medical Center, Fullerton

Sasan Yadegar, Encino-Tarzana Regional Medical Center—Tarzana Campus, Tarzana

Rosabel Young, Brotman Medical Center, Culver City

OBSTETRICS/GYNECOLOGY

Alex Abbassi, Encino-Tarzana Regional Medical Center—Tarzana Campus, Tarzana

Luis Acosta, Pioneers Memorial Health Care District, Brawley

Mohammad Ahmadinia, Victor Valley Community Hospital, Victorville

Eugene Albright, Parkview Community Hospital, Riverside

Mark Alwan, San Antonio Community Hospital, Upland

Todd Andrews, San Joaquin Community Hospital, Bakersfield

Robert Armada, San Antonio Community Hospital, Upland

Vijay Arora, Victor Valley Community Hospital, Victorville

Sahag Arslanian, Encino-Tarzana Regional Medical Center—Tarzana Campus, Tarzana

Azizeh Asgaripour, Encino-Tarzana Regional Medical Center—Tarzana Campus, Tarzana

Patrick Baggot, Greater El Monte Community Hospital, South El Monte

Vera Barile, Scripps Memorial Hospital—La Jolla, La Jolla

Viet Be, Garden Grove Hospital and Medical Center, Garden Grove

Michael Beaumont, Scripps Memorial Hospital—La Jolla, La Jolla

Carlos Beharie, Greater El Monte Community Hospital, South El Monte

Michael Berman, Garden Grove Hospital and Medical Center, Garden Grove

Wendy Brewster, Garden Grove Hospital and Medical Center, Garden Grove

Bijan Broukhim, Encino-Tarzana Regional Medical Center—Tarzana Campus, Tarzana

Darcy Bryan, Parkview Community Hospital, Riverside

Wendy Buchi, Scripps Memorial Hospital—La Jolla, La Jolla

Catherine Buerchner, Scripps Memorial Hospital—La Jolla, La Jolla

Seth Bulow, Scripps Memorial Hospital—La Jolla, La Jolla

Herman Carstens, Parkview Community Hospital, Riverside

Eric Chan, Greater El Monte Community Hospital, South El Monte

Daniel Channell, San Antonio Community Hospital, Upland

Edward Chen, Greater El Monte Community Hospital, South El Monte

Steve Cheung, Victor Valley Community Hospital, Victorville

Lisa Chong, San Antonio Community Hospital, Upland

Teresa Claus, Encino-Tarzana Regional Medical Center—Tarzana Campus, Tarzana

Gerilyn Cross, Scripps Memorial Hospital—La Jolla, La Jolla

Bijan Daneshgar, Encino-Tarzana Regional Medical Center—Tarzana Campus, Tarzana

Greggory De Vore, Encino-Tarzana Regional Medical Center—Tarzana Campus, Tarzana

Stephen DiMarzo, Scripps Memorial Hospital—La Jolla, La Jolla

Jonathan Dunn, Scripps Memorial Hospital—La Jolla, La Jolla

Mark Dwight, Good Samaritan Hospital, Los Angeles

Thomas Easter, San Antonio Community Hospital, Upland

Charles Edwards, Scripps Memorial Hospital—La Jolla, La Jolla

Donald Ehman, Pioneers Memorial Health Care District, Brawley

Scott Eisenkop, Encino-Tarzana Regional Medical Center—Tarzana Campus, Tarzana

Vivian Ellis, Scripps Memorial Hospital—La Jolla, La Jolla

Allen Entin, Encino-Tarzana Regional Medical Center—Tarzana Campus, Tarzana

Amin Fawwaz, Garden Grove Hospital and Medical Center, Garden Grove

Deng Fong, San Joaquin Community Hospital, Bakersfield

Mehrdad Forghani-Arani, Garden Grove Hospital and Medical Center, Garden Grove

Valerie Gafori, Scripps Memorial Hospital—La Jolla, La Jolla

Antonio Garcia, San Joaquin Community Hospital, Bakersfield

Richard Godt, San Antonio Community Hospital, Upland

Laurie Greenberg, Scripps Memorial Hospital—La Jolla, La Jolla

Amal Guha, Victor Valley Community Hospital, Victorville

Keerti Gurushanthaiah, Scripps Memorial Hospital—La Jolla, La Jolla

David Hagen, Pioneers Memorial Health Care District, Brawley

Ali Hamzeh, Garden Grove Hospital and Medical Center, Garden Grove

Kelly Harkey, Scripps Memorial Hospital—La Jolla, La Jolla

Jason Helliwell, San Joaquin Community Hospital, Bakersfield

Delroy Hewling, Greater El Monte Community Hospital, South El Monte

Allison Hill, Good Samaritan Hospital, Los Angeles

Linda Hillebrand, San Antonio Community Hospital, Upland

Umaima Jamaluddin, San Joaquin Community Hospital, Bakersfield

Hong-An Jan, Garden Grove Hospital and Medical Center, Garden Grove

Franklin Johnson, San Antonio Community Hospital, Upland

Ruslana Kadze, Encino-Tarzana Regional Medical Center—Tarzana Campus, Tarzana

Tanaz Kahen, Encino-Tarzana Regional Medical Center—Tarzana Campus, Tarzana

Farhat Kahn, Garden Grove Hospital and Medical Center, Garden Grove

Joseph Kahn, Garden Grove Hospital and Medical Center, Garden Grove

Siniva Kaneen, San Joaquin Community Hospital, Bakersfield

Behnam Kashanchi, Encino-Tarzana Regional Medical Center—Tarzana Campus, Tarzana

Katrina Kelly, Scripps Memorial Hospital—La Jolla, La Jolla

David Kim, Good Samaritan Hospital, Los Angeles

Hyung Kim, Garden Grove Hospital and Medical Center, Garden Grove

Jae Kim, Garden Grove Hospital and Medical Center, Garden Grove

Charles Kimelman, Encino-Tarzana Regional Medical Center—Tarzana Campus, Tarzana

John King, Parkview Community Hospital, Riverside

Lu-Wei King, Victor Valley Community Hospital, Victorville

Frederick Kohn, Encino-Tarzana Regional Medical Center—Tarzana Campus, Tarzana

Julius Kpaduwa, Greater El Monte Community Hospital, South El Monte

Witoon Krailas, Garden Grove Hospital and Medical Center, Garden Grove

Kestiutis Kuraitis, Pioneers Memorial Health Care District, Brawley

Mel Kurtulus, Scripps Memorial Hospital—La Jolla, La Jolla

Miguel Lascano, San Joaquin Community Hospital, Bakersfield

Rafik Latif, Encino-Tarzana Regional Medical Center—Tarzana Campus, Tarzana

Thuan Le, Parkview Community Hospital, Riverside

Karen Lee, Scripps Memorial Hospital—La Jolla, La Jolla

Kirstin Lee, Scripps Memorial Hospital—La Jolla, La Jolla

Patricia Lee, San Antonio Community Hospital, Upland

Sang Lee, Good Samaritan Hospital, Los Angeles

Thomas Lee, San Antonio Community Hospital, Upland

Kiat Lim, Scripps Memorial Hospital—La Jolla, La Jolla

Long-Dei Liu, Garden Grove Hospital and Medical Center, Garden Grove

Brent Livingston, Scripps Memorial Hospital—La Jolla, La Jolla

Elva Lopez, San Joaquin Community Hospital, Bakersfield

Kamran Malek, Encino-Tarzana Regional Medical Center—Tarzana Campus, Tarzana

Walter Marcus, Parkview Community Hospital, Riverside

Catharine Marshall, Scripps Memorial Hospital—La Jolla, La Jolla

Edward Matuga, Parkview Community Hospital, Riverside

Kevin McNeely, Scripps Memorial Hospital—La Jolla, La Jolla

Philipp Melendez, San Joaquin Community Hospital, Bakersfield

Jum Min, San Joaquin Community Hospital, Bakersfield

Dale Mitchell, Scripps Memorial Hospital—La Jolla, La Jolla

Victor Moneke, Victor Valley Community Hospital, Victorville

Bradley Monk, Garden Grove Hospital and Medical Center, Garden Grove

Renee Nelson, Scripps Memorial Hospital—La Jolla, La Jolla

Annmarie Nguyen, Garden Grove Hospital and Medical Center, Garden Grove

Nicole Nguyen, Scripps Memorial Hospital—La Jolla, La Jolla

Phu Nguyen, Garden Grove Hospital and Medical Center, Garden Grove

Alonso Ojeda, Parkview Community Hospital, Riverside

John Owens, San Joaquin Community Hospital, Bakersfield

Arthur Park, San Joaquin Community Hospital, Bakersfield

Min Park, Good Samaritan Hospital, Los Angeles

Dilipkumar Patel, Greater El Monte Community Hospital, South El Monte

Leonard Perez, San Joaquin Community Hospital, Bakersfield

Rebecca Perlow, Encino-Tarzana Regional Medical Center—Tarzana Campus, Tarzana

Stephen Pine, Encino-Tarzana Regional Medical Center—Tarzana Campus, Tarzana

Om Prakash, Victor Valley Community Hospital, Victorville

Michael Price, Pioneers Memorial Health Care District, Brawley

Mansoor Radpavar, Garden Grove Hospital and Medical Center, Garden Grove

Rebecca Rivera, San Joaquin Community Hospital, Bakersfield

William Rivera-Ortiz, Victor Valley Community Hospital, Victorville

Darryl Rodrigues, San Antonio Community Hospital, Upland

Rodney Root, San Joaquin Community Hospital, Bakersfield

Peter Rubenstein, Encino-Tarzana Regional Medical Center—Tarzana Campus, Tarzana

Joie Russo, Encino-Tarzana Regional Medical Center—Tarzana Campus, Tarzana

Tracy Ruymann, Scripps Memorial Hospital—La Jolla, La Jolla

Rodolfo Saenz, Parkview Community Hospital, Riverside

Norma Salceda, Encino-Tarzana Regional Medical Center—Tarzana Campus, Tarzana

Ronald Salzetti, Scripps Memorial Hospital—La Jolla, La Jolla

Richard Sand, Encino-Tarzana Regional Medical Center—Tarzana Campus, Tarzana

Cary Shakespeare, San Joaquin Community Hospital, Bakersfield

Rahul Sharma, San Joaquin Community Hospital, Bakersfield

Taaly Silberstein, Encino-Tarzana Regional Medical Center—Tarzana Campus, Tarzana

Allan Silver, Scripps Memorial Hospital—La Jolla, La Jolla

Elizabeth Silverman, Scripps Memorial Hospital—La Jolla, La Jolla

Christopher Smale, San Joaquin Community Hospital, Bakersfield

Gail Sowa, Scripps Memorial Hospital—La Jolla, La Jolla

Vasanthi Srinivas, San Joaquin Community Hospital, Bakersfield

Shanta Srivastava, San Antonio Community Hospital, Upland

Urvashi Sura, San Antonio Community Hospital, Upland

Krishnansu Tewari, Garden Grove Hospital and Medical Center, Garden Grove

Sherry Thomas, Encino-Tarzana Regional Medical Center—Tarzana Campus, Tarzana

Kevin Tieu, Garden Grove Hospital and Medical Center, Garden Grove

Kamran Torbati, Encino-Tarzana Regional Medical Center—Tarzana Campus, Tarzana

Thanh-Mai Trinh, Garden Grove Hospital and Medical Center, Garden Grove

Hiep Truong, Garden Grove Hospital and Medical Center, Garden Grove

Upland Women's Medical Group, San Antonio Community Hospital, Upland

Viruch Vachirakorntong, Victor Valley Community Hospital, Victorville

Monica Valenzuela-Gamm, San Antonio Community Hospital, Upland

Antero Velez, Encino-Tarzana Regional Medical Center—Tarzana Campus, Tarzana

Daniel Villarosa, Victor Valley Community Hospital, Victorville

Cau Vo, Garden Grove Hospital and Medical Center, Garden Grove

Toni Vu, San Antonio Community Hospital, Upland

Sherylann Wade, Victor Valley Community Hospital, Victorville

Armi Walker, San Joaquin Community Hospital, Bakersfield

Peter Wang, Garden Grove Hospital and Medical Center, Garden Grove

Linda Warren, San Joaquin Community Hospital, Bakersfield

Paul White, Victor Valley Community Hospital, Victorville

Christopher Winkle, Garden Grove Hospital and Medical Center, Garden Grove

Diana Wong, Encino-Tarzana Regional Medical Center—Tarzana Campus, Tarzana

Stanley Yang, San Antonio Community Hospital, Upland

Hung-Chou Yen, Garden Grove Hospital and Medical Center, Garden Grove

Elvin Yeo, Parkview Community Hospital, Riverside

ORTHOPEDIC SURGERY

Jack Akmakjian, St. Bernardine Medical Center, San Bernardino

Lawrence Albinski, St. Bernardine Medical Center, San Bernardino

David Anderson, St. Bernardine Medical Center, San Bernardino

James Bell, Desert Regional Medical Center, Palm Springs

Richard Biama, St. Bernardine Medical Center, San Bernardino

William Bugbee, Scripps Green Hospital, La Jolla

Paul Burton, St. Bernardine Medical Center, San Bernardino

Gurbir Chhabra, St. Bernardine Medical Center, San Bernardino

Loretta Chou, Stanford Hospital, Stanford

Steven Copp, Scripps Green Hospital, La Jolla

Michael Crane, St. Bernardine Medical Center, San Bernardino

Javier Descalzi, St. Bernardine Medical Center, San Bernardino

Thomas Donaldson, St. Bernardine Medical Center, San Bernardino

David Doty, St. Bernardine Medical Center, San Bernardino

David Duffner, Desert Regional Medical Center, Palm Springs

Eugene Emembolu, St. Bernardine Medical Center, San Bernardino

Kace Ezzet, Scripps Green Hospital, La Jolla

Gary Fanton, Stanford Hospital, Stanford

David Friscia, Eisenhower Medical Center, Rancho Mirage

Ronny Ghazal, St. Bernardine Medical Center, San Bernardino

Paramjeet Gill, Fresno Surgical Hospital, Fresno

Barry Grames, St. Bernardine Medical Center, San Bernardino

Mary Hurley, St. Bernardine Medical Center, San Bernardino

Imran Khan, St. Bernardine Medical Center, San Bernardino

Donald Kim, St. Bernardine Medical Center, San Bernardino

Amy Ladd, Stanford Hospital, Stanford

Edward Lembert, Fresno Surgical Hospital, Fresno

Paul Liu, St. Bernardine Medical Center, San Bernardino

William Maloney, Stanford Hospital, Stanford

James Matiko, St. Bernardine Medical Center, San Bernardino

Peter McGann, Fresno Surgical Hospital, Fresno

Clifford Merkel, St. Bernardine Medical Center, San Bernardino

David Mohler, Stanford Hospital, Stanford

Robert Murphy, Eisenhower Medical Center, Rancho Mirage

Stephen O'Connell, Eisenhower Medical Center, Rancho Mirage

Michael Oberto, Fresno Surgical Hospital, Fresno

Sean Rassman, St. Bernardine Medical Center, San Bernardino

Douglas Roger, Desert Regional Medical Center, Palm Springs

Adam Rosen, Scripps Green Hospital, La Jolla

Lawrence Serif, Desert Regional Medical Center, Palm Springs

Raj Sinha, Eisenhower Medical Center, Rancho Mirage

Peter Sofia, St. Bernardine Medical Center, San Bernardino

Louis Stabile, Desert Regional Medical Center, Palm Springs

John Velyvis, Eisenhower Medical Center, Rancho Mirage

Lawrence Walker, St. Bernardine Medical Center, San Bernardino

Richard Walker, Scripps Green Hospital, La Jolla

Bryan Wiley, St. Bernardine Medical Center, San Bernardino

Bruce Witmer, Fresno Surgical Hospital, Fresno

David Wood, St. Bernardine Medical Center, San Bernardino

SPINE SURGERY

Todd Alamin, Stanford Hospital, Stanford

Darren Bergey, St. Bernardine Medical Center, San Bernardino

James Bruffey, Scripps Green Hospital, La Jolla

Eugene Carragee, Stanford Hospital, Stanford

Ivan Cheng, Stanford Hospital, Stanford

Shahin Etebar, Eisenhower Medical Center, Rancho Mirage

Gail Hopkins, St. Bernardine Medical Center, San Bernardino

John Steinmann, St. Bernardine Medical Center, San Bernardino

Amir Tahernia, Eisenhower Medical Center, Rancho Mirage

Roger Thorne, Scripps Green Hospital, La Jolla

Christopher Uchiyama, Scripps Green Hospital, La Jolla

Gurvinder Uppal, St. Bernardine Medical Center, San Bernardino

COLORADO TOP DOCTORS

CARDIOLOGY

Burt Fowler, Memorial Hospital, Colorado Springs

Bryan Mahan, Memorial Hospital, Colorado Springs

NEUROLOGY

Robert Breeze, University of Colorado Hospital Authority, Aurora

Kerry Brega, University of Colorado Hospital Authority, Aurora

David Kumpe, University of Colorado Hospital Authority, Aurora

Robert Neumann, University of Colorado Hospital Authority, Aurora

CONNECTICUT TOP DOCTORS

GASTROINTESTINAL

Abera Abay, William W. Backus Hospital, Norwich

Tonya Hall, William W. Backus Hospital, Norwich

Ashan Manohar, William W. Backus Hospital, Norwich

You Sang, William W. Backus Hospital, Norwich

Kolala Sridhar, William W. Backus Hospital, Norwich

NEUROLOGY

Neil Culligan, Danbury Hospital, Danbury

John Murphy, Danbury Hospital, Danbury

ORTHOPEDIC SURGERY

Michael Aron, St. Francis Hospital and Medical Center, Hartford

Paul Beauvais, Waterbury Hospital Health Center, Waterbury

Steven Bond, St. Francis Hospital and Medical Center, Hartford

David Burstein, St. Francis Hospital and Medical Center, Hartford

William Flynn, Waterbury Hospital Health Center, Waterbury

Top doctors are those that practice at hospitals that are rated in the top 10% in the nation for that clinical program area. For more information on how top doctors were selected, see Appendix.

Andrew Gabow, St. Francis Hospital and Medical Center, Hartford

John Grady-Benson, St. Francis Hospital and Medical Center, Hartford

Robert Green, St. Francis Hospital and Medical Center, Hartford

Clinton Jambor, St. Francis Hospital and Medical Center, Hartford

Michael Joyce, St. Francis Hospital and Medical Center, Hartford

Michael Kaplan, Waterbury Hospital Health Center, Waterbury

John Keggi, Waterbury Hospital Health Center, Waterbury

Kristaps Keggi, Waterbury Hospital Health Center, Waterbury

Robert Kennon, Waterbury Hospital Health Center, Waterbury

Jay Kimmel, St. Francis Hospital and Medical Center, Hartford

David Kruger, St. Francis Hospital and Medical Center, Hartford

Courtland Lewis, St. Francis Hospital and Medical Center, Hartford

Todd Mailly, St. Francis Hospital and Medical Center, Hartford

John Mara, St. Francis Hospital and Medical Center, Hartford

Robert McCallister, St. Francis Hospital and Medical Center, Hartford

Paul Murray, St. Francis Hospital and Medical Center, Hartford

John O'Brien, St. Francis Hospital and Medical Center, Hartford

Eric Olson, Waterbury Hospital Health Center, Waterbury

Steven Schutzer, St. Francis Hospital and Medical Center, Hartford

Steven Selden, St. Francis Hospital and Medical Center, Hartford

Anthony Spinella, St. Francis Hospital and Medical Center, Hartford

Thomas Stevens, St. Francis Hospital and Medical Center, Hartford

Brett Wasserlauf, St. Francis Hospital and Medical Center, Hartford

Aris Yannopoulos, St. Francis Hospital and Medical Center, Hartford

Gordon Zimmerman, St. Francis Hospital and Medical Center, Hartford

SPINE SURGERY

Stephen Calderon, St. Francis Hospital and Medical Center, Hartford

Bruce Chozick, St. Francis Hospital and Medical Center, Hartford

Stephen Lange, St. Francis Hospital and Medical Center, Hartford

Howard Lantner, St. Francis Hospital and Medical Center, Hartford

FLORIDA TOP DOCTORS

CARDIAC SURGERY

George Abernathy, Venice Regional Medical Center, Venice

Victor Baga, Venice Regional Medical Center, Venice

William Corin, Venice Regional Medical Center, Venice

Mateo Dayo, Venice Regional Medical Center, Venice

Lawrence Elliott, Venice Regional Medical Center, Venice

Jonathan Fong, Venice Regional Medical Center, Venice

Ki Hassler, Venice Regional Medical Center, Venice

Heart and Vascular Center of Venice, Venice Regional Medical Center, Venice

Heart Institute of Venice, Venice Regional Medical Center, Venice

South County Heart Center, Venice Regional Medical Center, Venice

Barry Weckesser, Venice Regional Medical Center, Venice

William Woolverton, Venice Regional Medical Center, Venice

CARDIOLOGY

Edgar Abovich, Palm Beach Gardens Medical Center, Palm Beach Garden

Shakoor Arain, Lawnwood Regional Medical Center and Heart Institute, Fort Pierce

Haresh Asnani, Palm Beach Gardens Medical Center, Palm Beach Garden

David Axline, NCH Healthcare System, Naples

Brian Beaver, Palm Beach Gardens Medical Center, Palm Beach Garden

Ricardo Bedoya, Palm Beach Gardens Medical Center, Palm Beach Garden

Francis Boucek, NCH Healthcare System, Naples

Gabriel Breuer, Palm Beach Gardens Medical Center, Palm Beach Garden

James Buonavolonta, NCH Healthcare System, Naples

Randall Buss, NCH Healthcare System, Naples

Joseph Califano, NCH Healthcare System, Naples

Jorge Castriz, Palm Beach Gardens Medical Center, Palm Beach Garden

Prasad Chalasani, Lawnwood Regional Medical Center and Heart Institute, Fort Pierce

Charles Cousar, Baptist Medical Center, Jacksonville

Edgar Covarrubias, Palm Beach Gardens Medical Center, Palm Beach Garden

Chauncey Crandall, Palm Beach Gardens Medical Center, Palm Beach Garden

Paul Dillahunt, Baptist Medical Center, Jacksonville

Salvatore DiLoreto, Baptist Medical Center, Jacksonville

Walther Evenhuis, NCH Healthcare System, Naples

Paul Farrell, Baptist Medical Center, Jacksonville

Jeffrey Fenster, Palm Beach Gardens Medical Center, Palm Beach Garden

Michael Flynn, NCH Healthcare System, Naples

Jean Foucauld, Palm Beach Gardens Medical Center, Palm Beach Garden

George Gamouras, NCH Healthcare System, Naples

Bruce Gelinas, NCH Healthcare System, Naples

Burton Greenberg, Palm Beach Gardens Medical Center, Palm Beach Garden

Zannos Grekos, NCH Healthcare System, Naples

Sinan Gursoy, NCH Healthcare System, Naples

Holly Hancock, Baptist Medical Center, Jacksonville

Dennis Hanney, Palm Beach Gardens Medical Center, Palm Beach Garden

David Hassel, Baptist Medical Center, Jacksonville

John Hildreth, Palm Beach Gardens Medical Center, Palm Beach Garden

Brian Hummel, NCH Healthcare System, Naples

Yves Janin, Palm Beach Gardens Medical Center, Palm Beach Garden

Venu Jasti, Lawnwood Regional Medical Center and Heart Institute, Fort Pierce

Julian Javier, NCH Healthcare System, Naples

Steven Kessel, Palm Beach Gardens Medical Center, Palm Beach Garden

Predrag Knez, Palm Beach Gardens Medical Center, Palm Beach Garden

Steve Lebhar, NCH Healthcare System, Naples

Ronald Levine, NCH Healthcare System, Naples

Anthony Lewis, Lawnwood Regional Medical Center and Heart Institute, Fort Pierce

Marc Litt, Baptist Medical Center, Jacksonville

Zbigniew Litwinczuk, Palm Beach Gardens Medical Center, Palm Beach Garden

Gonzalo Loveday, Palm Beach Gardens Medical Center, Palm Beach Garden

Joshua Luce, Palm Beach Gardens Medical Center, Palm Beach Garden

Malvinder Makhni, Lawnwood Regional Medical Center and Heart Institute, Fort Pierce

Ziad Marjieh, Lawnwood Regional Medical Center and Heart Institute, Fort Pierce

Pedro Martinezclark, Palm Beach Gardens Medical Center, Palm Beach Garden

Michael Metke, NCH Healthcare System, Naples

Keith Meyer, Palm Beach Gardens Medical Center, Palm Beach Garden

Jyoti Mohanty, Palm Beach Gardens Medical Center, Palm Beach Garden

Edward Mostel, Palm Beach Gardens Medical Center, Palm Beach Garden

Tobia Palma, Palm Beach Gardens Medical Center, Palm Beach Garden

Robert Pascotto, NCH Healthcare System, Naples

Simie Platt, Palm Beach Gardens Medical Center, Palm Beach Garden

Kenneth Plunkitt, NCH Healthcare System, Naples

Richard Prewitt, NCH Healthcare System, Naples

Richard Price, Palm Beach Gardens Medical Center, Palm Beach Garden

Pamela Rama, Baptist Medical Center, Jacksonville

Kamalakar Rao, Lawnwood Regional Medical Center and Heart Institute, Fort Pierce

Ahmad Rashid, Lawnwood Regional Medical Center and Heart Institute, Fort Pierce

Michael Ravitsky, Palm Beach Gardens Medical Center, Palm Beach Garden

Mohammad Riaz, Lawnwood Regional Medical Center and Heart Institute, Fort Pierce

Tracey Roth, NCH Healthcare System, Naples

Carlo Santos-Ocampo, NCH Healthcare System, Naples

Joel Schrank, Baptist Medical Center, Jacksonville

Scot Schultz, NCH Healthcare System, Naples

Htwe Sein, Palm Beach Gardens Medical Center, Palm Beach Garden

Abdul Shadani, Lawnwood Regional Medical Center and Heart Institute, Fort Pierce

Neerav Shah, Palm Beach Gardens Medical Center, Palm Beach Garden

Babar Shareef, Lawnwood Regional Medical Center and Heart Institute, Fort Pierce

Girish Shroff, Baptist Medical Center, Jacksonville

Jane Silverstein, NCH Healthcare System, Naples

Mark Sims, Palm Beach Gardens Medical Center, Palm Beach Garden

Herman Spilker, NCH Healthcare System, Naples

Dennis Stapleton, NCH Healthcare System, Naples

Russell Stapleton, Baptist Medical Center, Jacksonville

Michael Stein, Palm Beach Gardens Medical Center, Palm Beach Garden

Robert Still, Baptist Medical Center, Jacksonville

David Stone, NCH Healthcare System, Naples

David Stroh, Baptist Medical Center, Jacksonville

Robert Tobar, Lawnwood Regional Medical Center and Heart Institute, Fort Pierce

Agustin Vargas, Palm Beach Gardens Medical Center, Palm Beach Garden

James Varnell, Palm Beach Gardens Medical Center, Palm Beach Garden

Amarnath Vedere, Palm Beach Gardens Medical Center, Palm Beach Garden

Augusto Villa, Palm Beach Gardens Medical Center, Palm Beach Garden

Craig Vogel, Palm Beach Gardens Medical Center, Palm Beach Garden

Randy Wainwright, Baptist Medical Center, Jacksonville

Steven Warshall, Palm Beach Gardens Medical Center, Palm Beach Garden

Arthur Yount, Palm Beach Gardens Medical Center, Palm Beach Garden

GASTROINTESTINAL

Ballapuran Adhinarayanan, Fawcett Memorial Hospital, Port Charlotte

James Amontree, Fawcett Memorial Hospital, Port Charlotte

John Chang, Raulerson Hospital, Okeechobee

David DePutron, Sebastian River Medical Center, Sebastian

Richard Dubno, Boca Raton Community Hospital, Boca Raton

Mitchell Duterte, Lake City Medical Center, Lake City

Jesse Eisenman, Good Samaritan Medical Center, West Palm Beach

Todd Eisner, Boca Raton Community Hospital, Boca Raton

Glenn Englander, Good Samaritan Medical Center, West Palm Beach

Mohammad Faisal, Lake City Medical Center, Lake City

Jeffrey Garelick, Good Samaritan Medical Center, West Palm Beach

Kenneth Haas, Raulerson Hospital, Okeechobee

Mohammad Idrees, Sebastian River Medical Center, Sebastian

Sovi Joseph, Fawcett Memorial Hospital, Port Charlotte

Steven Krumholz, Good Samaritan Medical Center, West Palm Beach

Alec Lui, Sebastian River Medical Center, Sebastian

Moideen Moopen, Fawcett Memorial Hospital, Port Charlotte

Denis Murphy, Good Samaritan Medical Center, West Palm Beach

Sidney Neimark, Good Samaritan Medical Center, West Palm Beach

Vito Proscia, Boca Raton Community Hospital, Boca Raton

Robert Raymond, Good Samaritan Medical Center, West Palm Beach

Ricardo Rosado, Lake City Medical Center, Lake City

Salvatore Senzatimore, Good Samaritan Medical Center, West Palm Beach

Hadi Shalhoub, Sebastian River Medical Center, Sebastian

Rizwana Thanawala, Lake City Medical Center, Lake City

Jeffrey Wenger, Good Samaritan Medical Center, West Palm Beach

GENERAL SURGERY

Sohrab Afshari, Memorial Hospital—Jacksonville, Jacksonville

Sam Bala, Pasco Regional Medical Center, Dade City

Alexander Balko, Largo Medical Center, Largo

Faramarz Behzadi, Memorial Hospital—Jacksonville, Jacksonville

Stephen Butler, Lakeland Regional Medical Center, Lakeland

Jim Cather, Lakeland Regional Medical Center, Lakeland

Paul Citrin, Pasco Regional Medical Center, Dade City

Ian Concilio, St. Lucie Medical Center, Port St. Lucie

John DePeri, Memorial Hospital—Jacksonville, Jacksonville

Richard DiCicco, Pasco Regional Medical Center, Dade City

Elisabeth Dupont, Lakeland Regional Medical Center, Lakeland

David Evans, Lakeland Regional Medical Center, Lakeland

Richard Fansler, Largo Medical Center, Largo

Larry Feinman, Largo Medical Center, Largo

Edwin Gonzalez, Lake City Medical Center, Lake City

Lee Grossbard, Pasco Regional Medical Center, Dade City

Kenneth Hagan, Memorial Hospital–Jacksonville, Jacksonville

John Hower, Lakeland Regional Medical Center, Lakeland

P. Krishnaraj, Pasco Regional Medical Center, Dade City

Adam Kurtin, St. Lucie Medical Center, Port St. Lucie

Edward Murphy, Sebastian River Medical Center, Sebastian

Michael Nerney, Largo Medical Center, Largo

Derek Paul, Sebastian River Medical Center, Sebastian

Lourdes Pelaez, Lake City Medical Center, Lake City

Ashok Roychoudhury, Memorial Hospital–Jacksonville, Jacksonville

Hadi Shalhoub, Sebastian River Medical Center, Sebastian

Alex Soler, Lake City Medical Center, Lake City

Nanjappa Subramanian, St. Lucie Medical Center, Port St. Lucie

NEUROLOGY

Darshan Aggarwal, Lawnwood Regional Medical Center and Heart Institute, Fort Pierce

Pedro Albanes, Hialeah Hospital, Hialeah

Peter Aldana, Lawnwood Regional Medical Center and Heart Institute, Fort Pierce

Richard Bailyn, Boca Raton Community Hospital, Boca Raton

Scott Blumenthal, Boca Raton Community Hospital, Boca Raton

Mark Brody, Bethesda Memorial Hospital, Boynton Beach

Paul Calise, Holy Cross Hospital, Fort Lauderdale

Delvis Celdran, Lawnwood Regional Medical Center and Heart Institute, Fort Pierce

James Cimera, Holy Cross Hospital, Fort Lauderdale

John Cintron, Kendall Regional Medical Center, Miami

Morton Corin, Palmetto General Hospital, Hialeah

Brian Costell, Kendall Regional Medical Center, Miami

Jonathan Cross, Mt. Sinai Medical Center, Miami Beach

Gilberto Cruz, Hialeah Hospital, Hialeah

Gilberto Cruz, Palmetto General Hospital, Hialeah

Mohan Deochand, Palmetto General Hospital, Hialeah

George Diaz, Mt. Sinai Medical Center, Miami Beach

Willis Dickens, Holy Cross Hospital, Fort Lauderdale

Ranjan Duara, Mt. Sinai Medical Center, Miami Beach

Joseph Durozel, Kendall Regional Medical Center, Miami

Joseph Durozel, Palmetto General Hospital, Hialeah

Waden Emery, Holy Cross Hospital, Fort Lauderdale

Oscar Farronay, Bethesda Memorial Hospital, Boynton Beach

Marc Feinberg, Boca Raton Community Hospital, Boca Raton

Paul Flaten, Holy Cross Hospital, Fort Lauderdale

Harold Friend, Boca Raton Community Hospital, Boca Raton

Ricardo Garcia-Rivera, Kendall Regional Medical Center, Miami

Gabriella Gerstle, Bethesda Memorial Hospital, Boynton Beach

Mark Goldberg, Hialeah Hospital, Hialeah

Mark Goldberg, Palmetto General Hospital, Hialeah

Anwar Gonzalez, Palmetto General Hospital, Hialeah

Thomas Hammond, Holy Cross Hospital, Fort Lauderdale

Jonathan Harris, Holy Cross Hospital, Fort Lauderdale

Frederick J Boltz, Boca Raton Community Hospital, Boca Raton

Edward Kaplan, Boca Raton Community Hospital, Boca Raton

Roy Katzin, Boca Raton Community Hospital, Boca Raton

Manley Kilgore, Baptist Medical Center, Jacksonville

Andrew Kovacs, Mt. Sinai Medical Center, Miami Beach

Philip Krampat, Holy Cross Hospital, Fort Lauderdale

Howard Kreger, Mt. Sinai Medical Center, Miami Beach

Hector Lalama, Hialeah Hospital, Hialeah

Rosendo Lopez-Jorge, Kendall Regional Medical Center, Miami

Antonio Mesa, Kendall Regional Medical Center, Miami

J. Michael Cochran, Boca Raton Community Hospital, Boca Raton

R. Montejo, Lawnwood Regional Medical Center and Heart Institute, Fort Pierce

Fernando Norona, Boca Raton Community Hospital, Boca Raton

Sean Orr, Baptist Medical Center, Jacksonville

Lekhraj Patel, Boca Raton Community Hospital, Boca Raton

Michael Paul, Lawnwood Regional Medical Center and Heart Institute, Fort Pierce

Scott Pearlman, Holy Cross Hospital, Fort Lauderdale

Jose Pozo, Lawnwood Regional Medical Center and Heart Institute, Fort Pierce

Marisa Prego-Lopez, Holy Cross Hospital, Fort Lauderdale

Carlos Sanchez, Hialeah Hospital, Hialeah

Robert Schiftan, Boca Raton Community Hospital, Boca Raton

Gregory Sengstock, Baptist Medical Center, Jacksonville

Maya Stambolisky, Cape Canaveral Hospital, Cocoa Beach

Alyssa Sussman, Bethesda Memorial Hospital, Boynton Beach

Marc Swerdloff, Holy Cross Hospital, Fort Lauderdale

Seth Tarras, Holy Cross Hospital, Fort Lauderdale

Harish Thaker, Holy Cross Hospital, Fort Lauderdale

Pedro Tirado, Bethesda Memorial Hospital, Boynton Beach

Herbert Todd, Holy Cross Hospital, Fort Lauderdale

Gonzalo Yanez, Hialeah Hospital, Hialeah

Gonzalo Yanez, Palmetto General Hospital, Hialeah

Basil Yates, Hialeah Hospital, Hialeah

OBSTETRICS/GYNECOLOGY

Jose Abreu, Palmetto General Hospital, Hialeah

Ghea Adeboyejo, Holy Cross Hospital, Fort Lauderdale

Miguel Albert, Hialeah Hospital, Hialeah

Rachel Bernstein, Holy Cross Hospital, Fort Lauderdale

Mauricio Bitran, Mt. Sinai Medical Center, Miami Beach

Leonardo Blachar, Mt. Sinai Medical Center, Miami Beach

Emilio Blanco, Hialeah Hospital, Hialeah

Emilio Blanco, Palmetto General Hospital, Hialeah

Frederick Bloom, Hialeah Hospital, Hialeah

France Bourget, Holy Cross Hospital, Fort Lauderdale

Elias Caltenco, Manatee Memorial Hospital, Bradenton

Patricia Calvo, Holy Cross Hospital, Fort Lauderdale

Phillip Caruso, Holy Cross Hospital, Fort Lauderdale

Celestino Castellon, Hialeah Hospital, Hialeah

Celestino Castellon, Palmetto General Hospital, Hialeah

Channing Coe, Holy Cross Hospital, Fort Lauderdale

Rochelle David, West Florida Hospital, Pensacola

Top doctors are those that practice at hospitals that are rated in the top 10% in the nation for that clinical program area. For more information on how top doctors were selected, see Appendix.

Armando De La Torre, Hialeah Hospital, Hialeah
Alberto Dominguez-Bali, Hialeah Hospital, Hialeah
Elham Elzind, Holy Cross Hospital, Fort Lauderdale
Elizabeth Etkin-Kramer, Mt. Sinai Medical Center, Miami Beach
Hector Fernandez, Palmetto General Hospital, Hialeah
Ramon Ferra, Mt. Sinai Medical Center, Miami Beach
Hugo Ferrara, Palmetto General Hospital, Hialeah
Jose Ferreira, Palmetto General Hospital, Hialeah
Roberto Fojo, Palmetto General Hospital, Hialeah
Richard Friefeld, Palmetto General Hospital, Hialeah
Miguel Gonzalez, Holy Cross Hospital, Fort Lauderdale
Rolando Gonzalez, Palmetto General Hospital, Hialeah
Raul Gonzalez-Napoles, Palmetto General Hospital, Hialeah
Jennifer Harper, Holy Cross Hospital, Fort Lauderdale
Ramon Hechavarria, Hialeah Hospital, Hialeah
William Joyner, Holy Cross Hospital, Fort Lauderdale
Nasim Kahn, West Florida Hospital, Pensacola
Eduardo Lavado, Hialeah Hospital, Hialeah
Eduardo Lavado, Palmetto General Hospital, Hialeah
John Lee, West Florida Hospital, Pensacola
Michele LeMay-Pace, Manatee Memorial Hospital, Bradenton
Moises Lichtinger, Holy Cross Hospital, Fort Lauderdale
Tomas Marimon, Hialeah Hospital, Hialeah
Jorge Martin, Palmetto General Hospital, Hialeah
Miguel Martinez, Palmetto General Hospital, Hialeah
Jose Matta, Manatee Memorial Hospital, Bradenton
David Mehta, West Florida Hospital, Pensacola
Luis Mendez, Palmetto General Hospital, Hialeah
Eric Mudafort, Manatee Memorial Hospital, Bradenton

Barbara Noel, Holy Cross Hospital, Fort Lauderdale
Edgardo Penabad, Hialeah Hospital, Hialeah
Manuel Penalver, Palmetto General Hospital, Hialeah
Jorge Perez, Hialeah Hospital, Hialeah
Paul Pietro, Palmetto General Hospital, Hialeah
I. Ramirez, Palmetto General Hospital, Hialeah
Wilfredo Rivera, Manatee Memorial Hospital, Bradenton
Emery Salom, Palmetto General Hospital, Hialeah
Helen Salsbury, Palmetto General Hospital, Hialeah
Lanalee Sam, Holy Cross Hospital, Fort Lauderdale
Laurie Scott, Palmetto General Hospital, Hialeah
Chatoor Singh, Holy Cross Hospital, Fort Lauderdale
R. Stuart, West Florida Hospital, Pensacola
Carlos Szajnert, Hialeah Hospital, Hialeah
Jacob Tangir, Palmetto General Hospital, Hialeah
Tracey Thomas-Doyle, West Florida Hospital, Pensacola
Lisa Tucker, West Florida Hospital, Pensacola
Francisco Tudela, Hialeah Hospital, Hialeah
Ronald Tuttelman, Holy Cross Hospital, Fort Lauderdale
Carlos Vazquez, Manatee Memorial Hospital, Bradenton
Raymond Whitted, Palmetto General Hospital, Hialeah

ORTHOPEDIC SURGERY

Richard Abdo, Largo Medical Center, Largo
Vladimir Alexander, Largo Medical Center, Largo
Jose Amundaray, Largo Medical Center, Largo
Andrew Beharrie, Largo Medical Center, Largo
Robert Biscup, Holy Cross Hospital, Fort Lauderdale
Kalman Blumberg, Holy Cross Hospital, Fort Lauderdale
Jeffrey Cantor, Holy Cross Hospital, Fort Lauderdale
Robert Catanzaro, Holy Cross Hospital, Fort Lauderdale
Philip Christ, Largo Medical Center, Largo

Lloyd Cope, Holy Cross Hospital, Fort Lauderdale
Derek Farr, Holy Cross Hospital, Fort Lauderdale
Brian Fingado, Holy Cross Hospital, Fort Lauderdale
David Gilbert, Holy Cross Hospital, Fort Lauderdale
Richard Giovanelli, Holy Cross Hospital, Fort Lauderdale
Ronald Hayter, Largo Medical Center, Largo
Gordon Hill, Holy Cross Hospital, Fort Lauderdale
Jóse Jackson, Holy Cross Hospital, Fort Lauderdale
Daniel Kanell, Holy Cross Hospital, Fort Lauderdale
Kevin Kessler, Holy Cross Hospital, Fort Lauderdale
William Leone, Holy Cross Hospital, Fort Lauderdale
Jonathan Levy, Holy Cross Hospital, Fort Lauderdale
Paul Meli, Holy Cross Hospital, Fort Lauderdale
Robert Mills, Holy Cross Hospital, Fort Lauderdale
George Morris, Largo Medical Center, Largo
William Near, Largo Medical Center, Largo
Michael Reilly, Holy Cross Hospital, Fort Lauderdale
Martin Roche, Holy Cross Hospital, Fort Lauderdale
Alan Routman, Holy Cross Hospital, Fort Lauderdale
Anthony Schiuma, Holy Cross Hospital, Fort Lauderdale
Mitchell Seavey, Holy Cross Hospital, Fort Lauderdale
Edward Williams, Holy Cross Hospital, Fort Lauderdale
Erol Yoldas, Holy Cross Hospital, Fort Lauderdale

SPINE SURGERY

Robert Donnelly, Largo Medical Center, Largo
Gordon Holen, Largo Medical Center, Largo
Ahmad Namatbakhsh, Largo Medical Center, Largo

VASCULAR SURGERY

Alexander Balko, Largo Medical Center, Largo
Larry Feinman, Largo Medical Center, Largo
Yves Gabriel, Largo Medical Center, Largo
Michael Nerney, Largo Medical Center, Largo

GEORGIA TOP DOCTORS

CARDIAC SURGERY

Ulfur Gudjonsson, Athens Regional Medical Center, Athens
Christopher Gullett, Athens Regional Medical Center, Athens
Vincent Maffei, Athens Regional Medical Center, Athens

GASTROENTEROLOGY

Gastroenterology Atlanta, LLC, Saint Joseph's Hospital of Atlanta, Atlanta
Gastroenterology Consultants, PC, Saint Joseph's Hospital of Atlanta, Atlanta
Gastroenterology of Northeast Georgia PC, Saint Joseph's Hospital of Atlanta, Atlanta

Metro Atlanta Gastroenterology, LLC, Saint Joseph's Hospital of Atlanta, Atlanta
Northeast Gastroenterology Associates, Saint Joseph's Hospital of Atlanta, Atlanta

Top doctors are those that practice at hospitals that are rated in the top 10% in the nation for that clinical program area. For more information on how top doctors were selected, see Appendix.

GASTROINTESTINAL

Agnes Han, Saint Joseph's Hospital of Atlanta, Atlanta

Claudia Kretzschmar, Athens Regional Medical Center, Athens

Ranjit Mathew, Athens Regional Medical Center, Athens

Lee Oberman, Saint Joseph's Hospital of Atlanta, Atlanta

Mario Ravry, Saint Joseph's Hospital of Atlanta, Atlanta

Christopher Sarzen, Saint Joseph's Hospital of Atlanta, Atlanta

Gregory Smith, Athens Regional Medical Center, Athens

J. West, Athens Regional Medical Center, Athens

Stephen Wilde, Athens Regional Medical Center, Athens

GENERAL SURGERY

William Ayers, West Georgia Medical Center, Lagrange
Brad Bowyer, West Georgia Medical Center, Lagrange
John Coggins, West Georgia Medical Center, Lagrange
Louellen Gurley, West Georgia Medical Center, Lagrange

Grant Major, West Georgia Medical Center, Lagrange
C. Major, Jr., West Georgia Medical Center, Lagrange
Madhav Naik, West Georgia Medical Center, Lagrange
William Turton, West Georgia Medical Center, Lagrange

NEUROLOGY

Robert Bashuk, Wellstar Cobb Hospital, Austell

Jeffrey Charpentier, Wellstar Cobb Hospital, Austell
Gary Kaplan, Wellstar Cobb Hospital, Austell
Mohammad Kukaswadia, Wellstar Cobb Hospital, Austell
Sandy McGaffigan, Wellstar Cobb Hospital, Austell
Gary Miller, Wellstar Cobb Hospital, Austell
Preethi Natarajan, Wellstar Cobb Hospital, Austell
Marvin Rachelefsky, Wellstar Cobb Hospital, Austell
William Tung, Wellstar Cobb Hospital, Austell
Daniel Zdonczyk, Wellstar Cobb Hospital, Austell

ORTHOPEDIC SURGERY

Atlanta Orthopaedic Specialist, PC, Saint Joseph's Hospital of Atlanta, Atlanta

Atlanta Spine Institute, Saint Joseph's Hospital of Atlanta, Atlanta

Atlanta Sports Medicine and Orthopaedic Center, Saint Joseph's Hospital of Atlanta, Atlanta

Andrew Bishop, Saint Joseph's Hospital of Atlanta, Atlanta

Capital City Orthopedics and Sports Medicine, Saint Joseph's Hospital of Atlanta, Atlanta

The Center for Orthopaedics and Sports Medicine, Saint Joseph's Hospital of Atlanta, Atlanta

Edward Crossland, St. Joseph Hospital—Augusta, Augusta

Dominion Orthopaedics and Sports Medicine, Saint Joseph's Hospital of Atlanta, Atlanta

Craig Kerins, St. Joseph Hospital—Augusta, Augusta

Kingloff Othopaedics, PC, Saint Joseph's Hospital of Atlanta, Atlanta

Thomas Myers, Saint Joseph's Hospital of Atlanta, Atlanta

Eugene Pendleton, Saint Joseph's Hospital of Atlanta, Atlanta

Resurgens Orthopaedics, Saint Joseph's Hospital of Atlanta, Atlanta

Spectrum Neurological Specialist, PC, Saint Joseph's Hospital of Atlanta, Atlanta

Paul Spiegl, Saint Joseph's Hospital of Atlanta, Atlanta

Warner Wood, Saint Joseph's Hospital of Atlanta, Atlanta

SPINE SURGERY

Tariq Javed, Saint Joseph's Hospital of Atlanta, Atlanta

VASCULAR SURGERY

Arun Chervu, Wellstar Cobb Hospital, Austell
Hector Dourron, Wellstar Cobb Hospital, Austell
Georgia Heart and Vascular Center, Medical Center of Central Georgia, Macon
Georgia Vascular Clinic, PA, Saint Joseph's Hospital of Atlanta, Atlanta
David Hafner, Wellstar Cobb Hospital, Austell
Gary Jacobson, Wellstar Cobb Hospital, Austell
John Jones, Wellstar Cobb Hospital, Austell
Charles Lewinstein, Wellstar Cobb Hospital, Austell
Steven Oweida, Wellstar Cobb Hospital, Austell
Jeffrey Reilly, Wellstar Cobb Hospital, Austell
Shariq Sayeed, Wellstar Cobb Hospital, Austell
Brooks Whitney, Wellstar Cobb Hospital, Austell
Jeffrey Winter, Wellstar Cobb Hospital, Austell
Charles Wyble, Wellstar Cobb Hospital, Austell
Joseph Zarge, Wellstar Cobb Hospital, Austell

ILLINOIS TOP DOCTORS

CARDIAC SURGERY

Rudolph Altergott, Trinity Medical Center—West Campus, Rock Island
Juan Bonilla, Trinity Medical Center—West Campus, Rock Island
David Cziperle, Trinity Medical Center—West Campus, Rock Island
Bryan Foy, Trinity Medical Center—West Campus, Rock Island
John Grieco, Trinity Medical Center—West Campus, Rock Island
Frank Lutrin, Trinity Medical Center—West Campus, Rock Island

Jeffrey Veluz, Trinity Medical Center—West Campus, Rock Island

CARDIOLOGY

Abas Amiry, Advocate Good Shepherd Hospital, Barrington
Michael Bresticker, Advocate Good Shepherd Hospital, Barrington
Vincent Bufalino, Advocate Good Shepherd Hospital, Barrington
George Christy, Advocate Good Shepherd Hospital, Barrington
Michael Fortsas, Advocate Good Shepherd Hospital, Barrington

Paul Gordon, Advocate Good Shepherd Hospital, Barrington
William Gries, Advocate Good Shepherd Hospital, Barrington
Raymond Helms, Advocate Good Shepherd Hospital, Barrington
Robert Hendel, Advocate Good Shepherd Hospital, Barrington
George Hodakowski, Advocate Good Shepherd Hospital, Barrington
Mehran Jabbarzadeh, Advocate Good Shepherd Hospital, Barrington
Sunil Kadakia, Advocate Good Shepherd Hospital, Barrington

GEORGIA / ILLINOIS TOP DOCTORS

Top doctors are those that practice at hospitals that are rated in the top 10% in the nation for that clinical program area. For more information on how top doctors were selected, see Appendix.

Raymond Kawasaki, Advocate Good Shepherd Hospital, Barrington

Anil Khemani, Advocate Good Shepherd Hospital, Barrington

Thomas Leskovac, Advocate Good Shepherd Hospital, Barrington

Authur Nazarian, Advocate Good Shepherd Hospital, Barrington

Daniel Orozco, St. Joseph Hospital, Chicago

Palatine Heart Center, Advocate Good Shepherd Hospital, Barrington

Patroklos Pappas, Advocate Good Shepherd Hospital, Barrington

Jack Pinto, Advocate Good Shepherd Hospital, Barrington

Paresh Rawal, Advocate Good Shepherd Hospital, Barrington

Joel Robbins, Advocate Good Shepherd Hospital, Barrington

Raja Sharma, Advocate Good Shepherd Hospital, Barrington

Alan Shepard, St. Joseph Hospital, Chicago

Hilliard Slavick, St. Joseph Hospital, Chicago

Irina Staicu, Advocate Good Shepherd Hospital, Barrington

Antone Tatooles, Advocate Good Shepherd Hospital, Barrington

Douglas Tomasian, Advocate Good Shepherd Hospital, Barrington

Russell Tonkovic, Advocate Good Shepherd Hospital, Barrington

Timothy Votapka, Advocate Good Shepherd Hospital, Barrington

GASTROINTESTINAL

Jagbir Ahuja, Advocate Good Shepherd Hospital, Barrington

Andrew Albert, Advocate Good Shepherd Hospital, Barrington

George Atia, Advocate Good Shepherd Hospital, Barrington

Dona Bartelt, Advocate Good Shepherd Hospital, Barrington

Mohammad Bawani, Advocate Good Shepherd Hospital, Barrington

Manish Bhuva, Advocate Good Shepherd Hospital, Barrington

Christopher Boutin, Elmhurst Memorial Hospital, Elmhurst

Dale Coy, Advocate Good Shepherd Hospital, Barrington

David Gerard, Elmhurst Memorial Hospital, Elmhurst

Dafna Gordon, Advocate Good Shepherd Hospital, Barrington

Stephen Grill, Elmhurst Memorial Hospital, Elmhurst

Shahid Ilahi, Advocate Good Shepherd Hospital, Barrington

Mary Kane, Advocate Good Shepherd Hospital, Barrington

Deepak Khurana, Advocate Good Shepherd Hospital, Barrington

Joseph Lagattuta, Elmhurst Memorial Hospital, Elmhurst

Michael McKenna, Elmhurst Memorial Hospital, Elmhurst

Kyoko Misawa, Advocate Good Shepherd Hospital, Barrington

George Morgan, Elmhurst Memorial Hospital, Elmhurst

Philip Nagel, Advocate Good Shepherd Hospital, Barrington

Phithao Nguyen, Advocate Good Shepherd Hospital, Barrington

Arun Ohri, Elmhurst Memorial Hospital, Elmhurst

Paul Parekh, Elmhurst Memorial Hospital, Elmhurst

Manfred Raiser, Elmhurst Memorial Hospital, Elmhurst

David Rzepczynski, Elmhurst Memorial Hospital, Elmhurst

Elizabeth Sack, Elmhurst Memorial Hospital, Elmhurst

Mohamed Sait, Elmhurst Memorial Hospital, Elmhurst

Amit Shah, Advocate Good Shepherd Hospital, Barrington

Matthew Smith, Elmhurst Memorial Hospital, Elmhurst

Anita Spiess, Advocate Good Shepherd Hospital, Barrington

George Stathopoulos, Elmhurst Memorial Hospital, Elmhurst

Gerard Sublette, Elmhurst Memorial Hospital, Elmhurst

George Zahrebelski, Advocate Good Shepherd Hospital, Barrington

NEUROLOGY

Ziauddin Ahmed, Our Lady of the Resurrection Medical Center, Chicago

Barry Bikshorn, St. Alexius Medical Center, Hoffman Estates

Ralph Cabin, Our Lady of the Resurrection Medical Center, Chicago

Prasad Chappidi, Our Lady of the Resurrection Medical Center, Chicago

Godwin D'Souza, Our Lady of the Resurrection Medical Center, Chicago

Mohammed Hussain, Our Lady of the Resurrection Medical Center, Chicago

Sanford Sherman, St. Alexius Medical Center, Hoffman Estates

ORTHOPEDIC SURGERY

Daniel Adair, Memorial Medical Center, Springfield

D. Allan, Memorial Medical Center, Springfield

Kevin Baumer, Memorial Hospital, Belleville

Tomasz Borowiecki, Memorial Medical Center, Springfield

Rodney Herrin, Memorial Medical Center, Springfield

Diane Hillard-Sembel, Memorial Medical Center, Springfield

Steven Horner, Memorial Hospital, Belleville

Aaron Humphreys, Memorial Medical Center, Springfield

Leo Ludwig, Memorial Medical Center, Springfield

David Mack, Memorial Medical Center, Springfield

Peter Meier, Illinois Valley Community Hospital, Peru

Robert Mitchell, Illinois Valley Community Hospital, Peru

Barry Mulshine, Memorial Medical Center, Springfield

David Olysav, Memorial Medical Center, Springfield

Stephen Pineda, Memorial Medical Center, Springfield

Ronald Romanelli, Memorial Medical Center, Springfield

Jeffrey Schopp, Memorial Medical Center, Springfield

Karolyn Senica, Memorial Medical Center, Springfield

Gregory Simmons, Memorial Hospital, Belleville

Michael Watson, Memorial Medical Center, Springfield

Donald Weimer, Memorial Hospital, Belleville

VASCULAR SURGERY

Afzal Abdullah, Trinity Medical Center—West Campus, Rock Island

John Klosak, Trinity Medical Center—West Campus, Rock Island

ILLINOIS TOP DOCTORS

CARDIAC SURGERY

Michael Koelsch, Ball Memorial Hospital, Muncie

GENERAL SURGERY

Stuart Coleman, Floyd Memorial Hospital and
Health Services, New Albany

David Dresner, Floyd Memorial Hospital and
Health Services, New Albany

William Garner, Floyd Memorial Hospital and
Health Services, New Albany

Kathryn Hutchens, Floyd Memorial Hospital and
Health Services, New Albany

Julie Hutchinson, Floyd Memorial Hospital and
Health Services, New Albany

Abdul Jabbar, Floyd Memorial Hospital and Health
Services, New Albany

Ashley Lankford, Floyd Memorial Hospital and
Health Services, New Albany

James McCullough, Floyd Memorial Hospital and
Health Services, New Albany

Huey Nguyen, Floyd Memorial Hospital and Health
Services, New Albany

James Strobel, Floyd Memorial Hospital and
Health Services, New Albany

NEUROLOGY

Steven James, St. Francis Hospital and Health
Center, Beech Grove

ORTHOPEDIC SURGERY

Christopher Balint, St. Joseph Regional Medical
Center–South Bend, South Bend

David Bankoff, St. Joseph Regional Medical
Center–South Bend, South Bend

Michael Berend, St. Francis Hospital Mooresville,
Mooresville

Center for Orthopedic Surgery and Sports
Medicine, St. Francis Hospital and Health
Center, Beech Grove

Robert Clayton, Indiana Orthopaedic Hospital,
Indianapolis

Robert Clemency, St. Joseph Regional Medical
Center–South Bend, South Bend

James Cole, St. Francis Hospital and Health
Center, Beech Grove

Robert Cravens, Indiana Orthopaedic Hospital,
Indianapolis

Henry Deleeuw, St. Joseph Regional Medical
Center–South Bend, South Bend

Daniel Edwards, Marion General Hospital, Marion

Philip Faris, St. Francis Hospital Mooresville,
Mooresville

Frederick Ferlic, St. Joseph Regional Medical
Center–South Bend, South Bend

Randolph Ferlic, St. Joseph Regional Medical
Center–South Bend, South Bend

David Fisher, Indiana Orthopaedic Hospital,
Indianapolis

Vincent Fragomeni, Indiana Orthopaedic Hospital,
Indianapolis

Karsten Fryburg, St. Francis Hospital and Health
Center, Beech Grove

Jamie Gottlieb, St. Joseph Regional Medical
Center–South Bend, South Bend

Howard Halstead, St. Joseph Regional Medical
Center–South Bend, South Bend

Earl Heller, St. Joseph Regional Medical
Center–South Bend, South Bend

Edward Hellman, Indiana Orthopaedic Hospital,
Indianapolis

Timothy Hupfer, Indiana Orthopaedic Hospital,
Indianapolis

Anthony Jabre, St. Francis Hospital and Health
Center, Beech Grove

Robert Jackson, Marion General Hospital, Marion

E. Keating, St. Francis Hospital Mooresville,
Mooresville

Charles Kershner, Marion General Hospital, Marion

Henry Kim, St. Joseph Regional Medical
Center–South Bend, South Bend

Frank Kolisek, Indiana Orthopaedic Hospital,
Indianapolis

Frank Kolisek, St. Francis Hospital and Health
Center, Beech Grove

David Levin, St. Francis Hospital and Health
Center, Beech Grove

Dean Maar, Indiana Orthopaedic Hospital,
Indianapolis

John Mahon, St. Joseph Regional Medical
Center–South Bend, South Bend

Robert Malinzak, St. Francis Hospital Mooresville,
Mooresville

John Meding, St. Francis Hospital Mooresville,
Mooresville

Adelbert Mencias, St. Joseph Regional Medical
Center–South Bend, South Bend

Stephen Mitros, St. Joseph Regional Medical
Center–South Bend, South Bend

Eric Monesmith, Indiana Orthopaedic Hospital,
Indianapolis

Eric Monesmith, St. Francis Hospital and
Health Center, Beech Grove

Neurosurgical Associates of St. Francis,
St. Francis Hospital and Health Center,
Beech Grove

Ortho Indy, St. Francis Hospital and Health Center,
Beech Grove

Salil Rajmaira, Marion General Hospital, Marion

Joseph Riina, St. Francis Hospital and Health
Center, Beech Grove

William Roper, Marion General Hospital, Marion

William Rozzi, St. Joseph Regional Medical
Center–South Bend, South Bend

D. Scheid, Indiana Orthopaedic Hospital,
Indianapolis

Thomas Trainer, Indiana Orthopaedic Hospital,
Indianapolis

Timothy Williams, St. Francis Hospital and Health
Center, Beech Grove

Thomas Woo, Indiana Orthopaedic Hospital,
Indianapolis

Jeffrey Yergler, St. Joseph Regional Medical
Center–South Bend, South Bend

Michael Yergler, St. Joseph Regional Medical
Center–South Bend, South Bend

Willard Yergler, St. Joseph Regional Medical
Center–South Bend, South Bend

SPINE SURGERY

John Peters, St. Francis Hospital and Health
Center, Beech Grove

GENERAL SURGERY

Gerald Baker, Iowa Methodist Medical Center, Des Moines
Daniel Kollmorgen, Iowa Methodist Medical Center, Des Moines
Michael Mohan, Iowa Methodist Medical Center, Des Moines

ORTHOPEDIC SURGERY

Timothy Gibbons, Mercy Medical Center–North Iowa, Mason City
Darron Jones, Mercy Medical Center–North Iowa, Mason City
Eric Nelson, Mercy Medical Center–North Iowa, Mason City
Eric Potthoff, Mercy Medical Center–North Iowa, Mason City
Michael Scherb, Mercy Medical Center–North Iowa, Mason City

VASCULAR SURGERY

E. Otoadese, Allen Memorial Hospital, Waterloo

NEUROLOGY

Arthur Allen, Shawnee Mission Medical Center, Shawnee Mission
Kimberly Cochran, Shawnee Mission Medical Center, Shawnee Mission
Gordon Kelley, Shawnee Mission Medical Center, Shawnee Mission
Michael Ryan, Shawnee Mission Medical Center, Shawnee Mission
Robert Satake, Shawnee Mission Medical Center, Shawnee Mission
John Seeley, Shawnee Mission Medical Center, Shawnee Mission

ORTHOPEDIC SURGERY

Richard Baker, Mercy Regional Health Center, Manhattan
Cris Barnthouse, Kansas City Orthopaedic Institute, Leawood
Jon Browne, Kansas City Orthopaedic Institute, Leawood
Bruce Buhr, Kansas Surgery and Recovery Center, Wichita
Scott Cook, Kansas City Orthopaedic Institute, Leawood
Robert Cusick, Kansas Surgery and Recovery Center, Wichita
John Fanning, Kansas Surgery and Recovery Center, Wichita

Shane Fejfar, Mercy Regional Health Center, Manhattan
Robert Gardiner, Kansas City Orthopaedic Institute, Leawood
Danny Gurba, Kansas City Orthopaedic Institute, Leawood
David Gwyn, Kansas Surgery and Recovery Center, Wichita
Phillip Hagan, Kansas Surgery and Recovery Center, Wichita
Bernard Hearon, Kansas Surgery and Recovery Center, Wichita
Daniel Hinkin, Mercy Regional Health Center, Manhattan
Peter Hodges, Mercy Regional Health Center, Manhattan
Allan Holiday, Mercy Regional Health Center, Manhattan
Kenneth Jansson, Kansas Surgery and Recovery Center, Wichita
William Jones, Mercy Regional Health Center, Manhattan
James Joseph, Kansas Surgery and Recovery Center, Wichita
Michelle Klaumann, Kansas Surgery and Recovery Center, Wichita
James McAtee, Mercy Regional Health Center, Manhattan

David McQueen, Kansas Surgery and Recovery Center, Wichita
Harry Morris, Kansas Surgery and Recovery Center, Wichita
Alan Moskowitz, Kansas Surgery and Recovery Center, Wichita
Bryce Palmgren, Mercy Regional Health Center, Manhattan
Paul Pappademos, Kansas Surgery and Recovery Center, Wichita
Daniel Prohaska, Kansas Surgery and Recovery Center, Wichita
Mark Rasmussen, Kansas City Orthopaedic Institute, Leawood
T. J. Rasmussen, Kansas City Orthopaedic Institute, Leawood
John Schurman, Kansas Surgery and Recovery Center, Wichita
Andrew Scott, Kansas City Orthopaedic Institute, Leawood
Naomi Shields, Kansas Surgery and Recovery Center, Wichita
Thomas Shriwise, Kansas City Orthopaedic Institute, Leawood
Daniel Stechschulte, Kansas City Orthopaedic Institute, Leawood
Camden Whitaker, Kansas Surgery and Recovery Center, Wichita

CARDIAC SURGERY

W. Carter, Medical Center, Bowling Green
Paul Moore, Medical Center, Bowling Green

GASTROINTESTINAL

M. Beebe, Central Baptist Hospital, Lexington

Adalberto Castellanos, Central Baptist Hospital, Lexington
Nathan Massey, Central Baptist Hospital, Lexington
James Pezzi, Central Baptist Hospital, Lexington
Stephen Schindler, Central Baptist Hospital, Lexington

NEUROLOGY

James Bean, Central Baptist Hospital, Lexington
William Brooks, Central Baptist Hospital, Lexington
Tim Coleman, Central Baptist Hospital, Lexington
David Kelly, Central Baptist Hospital, Lexington
Steven Kiefer, Central Baptist Hospital, Lexington
Brett Scott, Central Baptist Hospital, Lexington

Top doctors are those that practice at hospitals that are rated in the top 10% in the nation for that clinical program area. For more information on how top doctors were selected, see Appendix.

ORTHOPEDIC SURGERY

Gordon Air, St. Elizabeth Medical Center–South, Edgewood

John Bever, St. Elizabeth Medical Center–South, Edgewood

James Bilbo, St. Elizabeth Medical Center–South, Edgewood

Raymond Charette, Jackson Purchase Medical Center, Mayfield

Thomas Due, St. Elizabeth Medical Center–South, Edgewood

Nicholas Gates, St. Elizabeth Medical Center–South, Edgewood

Michael Grefer, St. Elizabeth Medical Center–South, Edgewood

Matthew Grunkemeyer, St. Elizabeth Medical Center–South, Edgewood

Samer Hasan, St. Elizabeth Medical Center–South, Edgewood

Forest Heis, St. Elizabeth Medical Center–South, Edgewood

Richard Hoblitzell, St. Elizabeth Medical Center–South, Edgewood

Bruce Holladay, St. Elizabeth Medical Center–South, Edgewood

John Larkin, St. Elizabeth Medical Center–South, Edgewood

Brion Moran, St. Elizabeth Medical Center–South, Edgewood

Michael O'Brien, St. Elizabeth Medical Center–South, Edgewood

VASCULAR SURGERY

Don Brown, Medical Center, Bowling Green

Michael Byrne, Medical Center, Bowling Green

LOUISIANA TOP DOCTORS

GASTROINTESTINAL

Stephen Duplechain, Thibodaux Regional Medical Center, Thibodaux

Charles Monier, Thibodaux Regional Medical Center, Thibodaux

Pasam Rao, Thibodaux Regional Medical Center, Thibodaux

NEUROLOGY

Vipul Shelat, St. Francis Medical Center, Monroe

VASCULAR SURGERY

David Allie, Southwest Medical Center, Lafayette

Antoine Keller, Southwest Medical Center, Lafayette

Mitchell Lirtzman, Southwest Medical Center, Lafayette

Charles Wyatt, Southwest Medical Center, Lafayette

MAINE TOP DOCTORS

NEUROLOGY

Marvin Eisengart, Inland Hospital, Waterville

Jennifer Yanoschak, Inland Hospital, Waterville

MARYLAND TOP DOCTORS

CARDIOLOGY

Mark Nelson, Sacred Heart Hospital, Cumberland

GASTROINTESTINAL

Thomas Abernathy, Jr., Baltimore Washington Medical Center, Glen Burnie

Bernardino Alonso, Baltimore Washington Medical Center, Glen Burnie

Michael Blume, Good Samaritan Hospital, Baltimore

Lester Bowser, Baltimore Washington Medical Center, Glen Burnie

Gelsimo Cruz, Baltimore Washington Medical Center, Glen Burnie

Sudhir Dutta, Sinai Hospital of Baltimore, Baltimore

Michael Epstein, Baltimore Washington Medical Center, Glen Burnie

David Fishbein, Baltimore Washington Medical Center, Glen Burnie

Steven Fleisher, Baltimore Washington Medical Center, Glen Burnie

Todd Heller, Baltimore Washington Medical Center, Glen Burnie

Gerald Hofkin, Baltimore Washington Medical Center, Glen Burnie

Niraj Jani, Sinai Hospital of Baltimore, Baltimore

Lubna Khan, Baltimore Washington Medical Center, Glen Burnie

Mukul Khandelwal, Baltimore Washington Medical Center, Glen Burnie

Charles King, Baltimore Washington Medical Center, Glen Burnie

George Kurian, Baltimore Washington Medical Center, Glen Burnie

Nii Lamptey-Mills, Baltimore Washington Medical Center, Glen Burnie

Loc Le, Baltimore Washington Medical Center, Glen Burnie

Alif Manejwala, Baltimore Washington Medical Center, Glen Burnie

Lawrence Mills, Good Samaritan Hospital, Baltimore

Jose Nepomuceno, Baltimore Washington Medical Center, Glen Burnie

Sivakolunt Pathmanathan, Baltimore Washington Medical Center, Glen Burnie

Michael Siuta, Baltimore Washington Medical Center, Glen Burnie

Top doctors are those that practice at hospitals that are rated in the top 10% in the nation for that clinical program area. For more information on how top doctors were selected, see Appendix.

Mahmood Solaiman, Baltimore Washington Medical Center, Glen Burnie

Lila Tarmin, Baltimore Washington Medical Center, Glen Burnie

Ernest Tsao, Baltimore Washington Medical Center, Glen Burnie

Edward Wolf, Baltimore Washington Medical Center, Glen Burnie

Edward Zimmerman, Baltimore Washington Medical Center, Glen Burnie

GENERAL SURGERY

Nabil Badro, Baltimore Washington Medical Center, Glen Burnie

Tsion Berhane, Baltimore Washington Medical Center, Glen Burnie

Dave Choi, Baltimore Washington Medical Center, Glen Burnie

Cynthia Drogula, Baltimore Washington Medical Center, Glen Burnie

Terrance Fullum, Baltimore Washington Medical Center, Glen Burnie

Sang Han, Baltimore Washington Medical Center, Glen Burnie

Craig Louisy, Baltimore Washington Medical Center, Glen Burnie

Cornelious Musara, Baltimore Washington Medical Center, Glen Burnie

Ashwin Nanavati, Baltimore Washington Medical Center, Glen Burnie

Anthony Raneri, Baltimore Washington Medical Center, Glen Burnie

John Roth, Baltimore Washington Medical Center, Glen Burnie

Samer Saiedy, Baltimore Washington Medical Center, Glen Burnie

Geoffrey Saunders, Baltimore Washington Medical Center, Glen Burnie

Pio Valle, Baltimore Washington Medical Center, Glen Burnie

Barry Wells, Baltimore Washington Medical Center, Glen Burnie

Samana Zulu, Baltimore Washington Medical Center, Glen Burnie

NEUROLOGY

Gurdeep Ahluwalia, Sinai Hospital of Baltimore, Baltimore

Nechama Bernhardt, Good Samaritan Hospital, Baltimore

Perry Foreman, Sinai Hospital of Baltimore, Baltimore

Majid Fotuhi, Sinai Hospital of Baltimore, Baltimore

Braeme Glaun, Sinai Hospital of Baltimore, Baltimore

Adrian Goldszmidt, Sinai Hospital of Baltimore, Baltimore

Bruce Rabin, Sinai Hospital of Baltimore, Baltimore

Saurabh Sinha, Sinai Hospital of Baltimore, Baltimore

Richard Taylor, Good Samaritan Hospital, Baltimore

Howard Weiss, Sinai Hospital of Baltimore, Baltimore

Michael Williams, Sinai Hospital of Baltimore, Baltimore

Robin Wilson, Sinai Hospital of Baltimore, Baltimore

VASCULAR SURGERY

Nabil Badro, Baltimore Washington Medical Center, Glen Burnie

Marshall Benjamin, Baltimore Washington Medical Center, Glen Burnie

Steven Busuttil, Baltimore Washington Medical Center, Glen Burnie

Dave Choi, Baltimore Washington Medical Center, Glen Burnie

Michael Curi, Baltimore Washington Medical Center, Glen Burnie

William Flinn, Baltimore Washington Medical Center, Glen Burnie

Sang Han, Baltimore Washington Medical Center, Glen Burnie

Michael Lilly, Baltimore Washington Medical Center, Glen Burnie

David Neschis, Baltimore Washington Medical Center, Glen Burnie

MASSACHUSETTS TOP DOCTORS

NEUROLOGY

David Crowley, North Shore Medical Center, Salem

Essex Neurological Associates, North Shore Medical Center, Salem

Andrew Leader-Cramer, North Shore Medical Center, Salem

Sanford Levy, North Shore Medical Center, Salem

Anna Litvak, North Shore Medical Center, Salem

Edgar Robertson, North Shore Medical Center, Salem

ORTHOPEDIC SURGERY

Peter Anas, New England Baptist Hospital, Boston

Benjamin Bierbaum, New England Baptist Hospital, Boston

James Bono, New England Baptist Hospital, Boston

Wolfgang Fitz, New England Baptist Hospital, Boston

Michael Mason, New England Baptist Hospital, Boston

David Mattingly, New England Baptist Hospital, Boston

Robert Miegel, New England Baptist Hospital, Boston

Douglas Patch, New England Baptist Hospital, Boston

Robert Patz, New England Baptist Hospital, Boston

Donald Reilly, New England Baptist Hospital, Boston

Arnold Scheller, New England Baptist Hospital, Boston

Richard Scott, New England Baptist Hospital, Boston

John Siliski, New England Baptist Hospital, Boston

Carl Talmo, New England Baptist Hospital, Boston

Geoffrey Van Flandern, New England Baptist Hospital, Boston

Daniel Ward, New England Baptist Hospital, Boston

CARDIAC SURGERY

Demetrios Apostolou, Providence Hospital, Southfield

Ingida Asfaw, Providence Hospital, Southfield

Joseph Bassett, Providence Hospital, Southfield

Gary Goodman, Providence Hospital, Southfield

Michael Lee, Providence Hospital, Southfield

Chris Liakonis, Providence Hospital, Southfield

Michael Parish, Providence Hospital, Southfield

Philip Robinson, Providence Hospital, Southfield

Marc Sakwa, Providence Hospital, Southfield

Nicholas Tepe, Providence Hospital, Southfield

CARDIOLOGY

Inderjit Aggarwal, Crittenton Hospital Medical Center, Rochester

Samer Kazziha, Crittenton Hospital Medical Center, Rochester

David Langholz, Spectrum Health Hospitals, Grand Rapids

Zakwan Mahjoub, Crittenton Hospital Medical Center, Rochester

Richard McNamara, Spectrum Health Hospitals, Grand Rapids

Divakar Pai, Crittenton Hospital Medical Center, Rochester

A. Shahbandar, Crittenton Hospital Medical Center, Rochester

Ronald Stewart, Crittenton Hospital Medical Center, Rochester

Alan Woelfel, Spectrum Health Hospitals, Grand Rapids

David Wohns, Spectrum Health Hospitals, Grand Rapids

GASTROINTESTINAL

Sami Akkary, Providence Hospital, Southfield

Kim Almodovar, Crittenton Hospital Medical Center, Rochester

Edward Clay, Harper University Hospital, Detroit

Mark DeVore, Providence Hospital, Southfield

Ravi Dhar, Harper University Hospital, Detroit

Murray Ehrinpreis, Harper University Hospital, Detroit

Prince Eubanks, Harper University Hospital, Detroit

Julia Greer, Providence Hospital, Southfield

Gregory Haynes, Harper University Hospital, Detroit

Marc Herschfus, Providence Hospital, Southfield

Herschel Jackson, Harper University Hospital, Detroit

Hershel Jackson, Providence Hospital, Southfield

Randall Jacobs, Providence Hospital, Southfield

Joseph Kinzie, Harper University Hospital, Detroit

Luis Maas, Providence Hospital, Southfield

Satish Maryala, Harper University Hospital, Detroit

Elizabeth May, Harper University Hospital, Detroit

Milton Mutchnick, Harper University Hospital, Detroit

Rene Peleman, Harper University Hospital, Detroit

Michael Piper, Providence Hospital, Southfield

Shivkumar Prabhu, Harper University Hospital, Detroit

Firdous Siddiqui, Harper University Hospital, Detroit

Sudarshan Singal, Harper University Hospital, Detroit

Freddy Sosa, Providence Hospital, Southfield

Laurence Stawick, Providence Hospital, Southfield

Ghiath Tayeb, Crittenton Hospital Medical Center, Rochester

Anthony Williams, Harper University Hospital, Detroit

NEUROLOGY

Amer Aboukasm, Beaumont Hospital–Grosse Pointe, Grosse Pointe

Gyula Acsadi, Beaumont Hospital–Grosse Pointe, Grosse Pointe

Steven Beall, Beaumont Hospital–Grosse Pointe, Grosse Pointe

Ronald Bennett, Beaumont Hospital–Grosse Pointe, Grosse Pointe

Norman Burns, Providence Hospital, Southfield

Tessy C. Jenkins, Beaumont Hospital–Grosse Pointe, Grosse Pointe

Seemant Chaturvedi, Harper University Hospital, Detroit

Abelardo Contreras, Sinai-Grace Hospital, Detroit

William Coplin, Harper University Hospital, Detroit

Paul Cullis, Beaumont Hospital–Grosse Pointe, Grosse Pointe

Sarih Dalati, Beaumont Hospital–Grosse Pointe, Grosse Pointe

Chandrakant Desai, Sinai-Grace Hospital, Detroit

Fernando Diaz, Providence Hospital, Southfield

Mitchell Elkiss, Providence Hospital, Southfield

Richard Fessler, Providence Hospital, Southfield

David Gaston, Sinai-Grace Hospital, Detroit

Thomas Giancarlo, Beaumont Hospital–Grosse Pointe, Grosse Pointe

Neil Gilbert, Providence Hospital, Southfield

Ramesh Gopalaswamy, Beaumont Hospital–Grosse Pointe, Grosse Pointe

Tessy Jenkins, Sinai-Grace Hospital, Detroit

Mark Kachadurian, Providence Hospital, Southfield

Brian Kirschner, Providence Hospital, Southfield

Bruce Kole, Providence Hospital, Southfield

Lawrence Konst, Beaumont Hospital–Grosse Pointe, Grosse Pointe

Jacqueline Kraus, Providence Hospital, Southfield

Benjamin Krpichak, Beaumont Hospital–Grosse Pointe, Grosse Pointe

Boris Leheta, Beaumont Hospital–Grosse Pointe, Grosse Pointe

Alicia Lumley, Beaumont Hospital–Grosse Pointe, Grosse Pointe

Ramesh Madhavan, Harper University Hospital, Detroit

Tracey Morson, Beaumont Hospital–Grosse Pointe, Grosse Pointe

Shyam Moudgil, Beaumont Hospital–Grosse Pointe, Grosse Pointe

Gregory Norris, Harper University Hospital, Detroit

Thomas O'Neil, St. John Macomb Hospital, Warren

Daniel Pieper, Providence Hospital, Southfield

Haranath Policherla, Beaumont Hospital–Grosse Pointe, Grosse Pointe

Kumar Rajamani, Harper University Hospital, Detroit

Chakrapani Ranganathan, St. John Macomb Hospital, Warren

Leonard Sahn, Sinai-Grace Hospital, Detroit

Sunitha Santhakumar, Harper University Hospital, Detroit

Manaf Seidarabi, Beaumont Hospital–Grosse Pointe, Grosse Pointe

Vaqar Siddiqui, Beaumont Hospital–Grosse Pointe, Grosse Pointe

Bruce Silverman, Providence Hospital, Southfield

Mark Silverman, Providence Hospital, Southfield

Teck-Mun Soo, Providence Hospital, Southfield

Yi Suleiman, Beaumont Hospital–Grosse Pointe, Grosse Pointe

Renee Van Stavern, Harper University Hospital, Detroit

Matthew Voci, Beaumont Hospital–Grosse Pointe, Grosse Pointe

Andrew Xavier, Harper University Hospital, Detroit

Top doctors are those that practice at hospitals that are rated in the top 10% in the nation for that clinical program area. For more information on how top doctors were selected, see Appendix.

ORTHOPEDIC SURGERY

Joeseph Walkiewicz, Garden City Osteopathic Hospital, Garden City

Jeffrey Anhalt, Mercy General Health Partners, Muskegon

William Athens, Oakwood Hospital and Medical Center–Dearborn, Dearborn

Michael Austin, Ingham Regional Medical Center, Lansing

Michael Baghdoian, Oakwood Hospital and Medical Center–Dearborn, Dearborn

Branislav Behan, Bay Regional Medical Center, Bay City

James Bookout, Beaumont Hospital–Grosse Pointe, Grosse Pointe

Jeffrey Carroll, Beaumont Hospital–Grosse Pointe, Grosse Pointe

Kenneth Cervone, Beaumont Hospital–Grosse Pointe, Grosse Pointe

Terrence Cherwin, Bay Regional Medical Center, Bay City

David Christ, Bronson Methodist Hospital, Kalamazoo

Kelly Coffey, Ingham Regional Medical Center, Lansing

Jerome Conrad, Mecosta County Medical Center, Big Rapids

Kevin Crawford, Oakwood Hospital and Medical Center–Dearborn, Dearborn

Steven Cusick, Beaumont Hospital–Grosse Pointe, Grosse Pointe

Mark Davis, Ingham Regional Medical Center, Lansing

Michael Demers, Beaumont Hospital–Grosse Pointe, Grosse Pointe

David Detrisac, Ingham Regional Medical Center, Lansing

James Dietz, Beaumont Hospital–Grosse Pointe, Grosse Pointe

Douglas Dietzel, Ingham Regional Medical Center, Lansing

Julie Dodds, Ingham Regional Medical Center, Lansing

Steven Drayer, Ingham Regional Medical Center, Lansing

Paul Drouillard, Garden City Osteopathic Hospital, Garden City

Christopher Eyke, Mercy General Health Partners, Muskegon

Meredith Fabing, Ingham Regional Medical Center, Lansing

Alfred Faulkner, Oakwood Hospital and Medical Center–Dearborn, Dearborn

Daniel Fett, Mercy General Health Partners, Muskegon

Joseph Finch, Oakwood Hospital and Medical Center–Dearborn, Dearborn

John Flood, Ingham Regional Medical Center, Lansing

Scott Free, Bronson Methodist Hospital, Kalamazoo

Donald Garver, Beaumont Hospital–Grosse Pointe, Grosse Pointe

Floyd Goodman, Ingham Regional Medical Center, Lansing

Yousif Hamati, Mercy General Health Partners, Muskegon

Todd Harburn, Ingham Regional Medical Center, Lansing

Julie Henry, Beaumont Hospital–Grosse Pointe, Grosse Pointe

Kenneth Highhouse, Bronson Methodist Hospital, Kalamazoo

Robert Highhouse, Bronson Methodist Hospital, Kalamazoo

Erich Hornbach, Ingham Regional Medical Center, Lansing

Gregory Housner, Oakwood Hospital and Medical Center–Dearborn, Dearborn

Kevin Howard, Ingham Regional Medical Center, Lansing

Ronald Irwin, Bay Regional Medical Center, Bay City

Edward Jeffries, Beaumont Hospital–Grosse Pointe, Grosse Pointe

Michael Kosinski, Beaumont Hospital–Grosse Pointe, Grosse Pointe

Christopher Lee, Beaumont Hospital–Grosse Pointe, Grosse Pointe

Terrence Lock, Beaumont Hospital–Grosse Pointe, Grosse Pointe

William Martin, Bay Regional Medical Center, Bay City

Brian McCardel, Ingham Regional Medical Center, Lansing

Michael McDermott, Ingham Regional Medical Center, Lansing

Rodney McFarland, Bay Regional Medical Center, Bay City

Robert Meehan, Oakwood Hospital and Medical Center–Dearborn, Dearborn

David Mendelson, St. John Macomb Hospital, Warren

Jeffery Mendelson, St. John Macomb Hospital, Warren

J. Mesko, Ingham Regional Medical Center, Lansing

David Michael, Ingham Regional Medical Center, Lansing

Michigan Orthopaedics and Sports Medicine, Spectrum Health Hospitals, Grand Rapids

Daniel Middleton, Bay Regional Medical Center, Bay City

Marc Milia, Oakwood Hospital and Medical Center–Dearborn, Dearborn

Glenn Minster, Beaumont Hospital–Grosse Pointe, Grosse Pointe

Scott Monson, Beaumont Hospital–Grosse Pointe, Grosse Pointe

Lawrence Morawa, Oakwood Hospital and Medical Center–Dearborn, Dearborn

Kenneth Morrison, Ingham Regional Medical Center, Lansing

Mark Moulton, Mercy General Health Partners, Muskegon

Richard Moulton, Mercy General Health Partners, Muskegon

Lawrence Mysliwiec, Ingham Regional Medical Center, Lansing

Sam Nasser, Beaumont Hospital–Grosse Pointe, Grosse Pointe

Mark Noffsinger, Bronson Methodist Hospital, Kalamazoo

Daniel Olenchak, Oakwood Hospital and Medical Center–Dearborn, Dearborn

Orthopaedic and Spinal Associates, Spectrum Health Hospitals, Grand Rapids

Richard Perry, Beaumont Hospital–Grosse Pointe, Grosse Pointe

Douglas Plagens, Oakwood Hospital and Medical Center–Dearborn, Dearborn

John Putz, Ingham Regional Medical Center, Lansing

Sudhir Rao, Mecosta County Medical Center, Big Rapids

Todd Ream, Bronson Methodist Hospital, Kalamazoo

Jeffrey Recknagel, Mercy General Health Partners, Muskegon

Bernard Roehr, Bronson Methodist Hospital, Kalamazoo

Bruce Rowe, Bronson Methodist Hospital, Kalamazoo

Mark Russell, Ingham Regional Medical Center, Lansing

John Sauchak, Ingham Regional Medical Center, Lansing

Robert Schneeberger, Mercy General Health Partners, Muskegon

Nicholas Schoch, Beaumont Hospital–Grosse Pointe, Grosse Pointe

Andrew Schorfhaar, Ingham Regional Medical Center, Lansing

Paul Schreck, Beaumont Hospital–Grosse Pointe, Grosse Pointe

Michael Shingles, Ingham Regional Medical Center, Lansing

David Shneider, Ingham Regional Medical Center, Lansing

Kanwaldeep Sidhu, Beaumont Hospital–Grosse Pointe, Grosse Pointe

Eric Silberg, Oakwood Hospital and Medical Center–Dearborn, Dearborn

Craig Silverton, Beaumont Hospital–Grosse Pointe, Grosse Pointe

Edward Sladek, Ingham Regional Medical Center, Lansing

Angelo Sorce, Oakwood Hospital and Medical Center–Dearborn, Dearborn

Kevin Sprague, Oakwood Hospital and Medical Center–Dearborn, Dearborn

Kenneth Stephens, Ingham Regional Medical Center, Lansing

Patrick Stephens, Beaumont Hospital–Grosse Pointe, Grosse Pointe

Mark Stewart, Bay Regional Medical Center, Bay City

J. Suleiman, Oakwood Hospital and Medical Center–Dearborn, Dearborn

Michael Swords, Ingham Regional Medical Center, Lansing

Charles Taunt, Ingham Regional Medical Center, Lansing

Aleksander Tosic, Mecosta County Medical Center, Big Rapids

Robert Travis, Oakwood Hospital and Medical Center–Dearborn, Dearborn

William Uggen, Bronson Methodist Hospital, Kalamazoo

Gregory Uitvlugt, Ingham Regional Medical Center, Lansing

Jeffrey Waldrop, Oakwood Hospital and Medical Center–Dearborn, Dearborn

Kenton Waterbrook, Ingham Regional Medical Center, Lansing

Michael Winkelpleck, Ingham Regional Medical Center, Lansing

Jeffrey Zacharias, Beaumont Hospital–Grosse Pointe, Grosse Pointe

Abbas Zand, Ingham Regional Medical Center, Lansing

Christopher Zingas, Beaumont Hospital–Grosse Pointe, Grosse Pointe

SPINE SURGERY

W. Athens, Oakwood Hospital and Medical Center–Dearborn, Dearborn

Srinivaschari Chakravarthi, Bay Regional Medical Center, Bay City

Roderick Claybrooks, Oakwood Hospital and Medical Center–Dearborn, Dearborn

Daniel Elskens, Beaumont Hospital–Grosse Pointe, Grosse Pointe

Randy Gehring, Beaumont Hospital–Grosse Pointe, Grosse Pointe

Mark Goldberger, Beaumont Hospital–Grosse Pointe, Grosse Pointe

Ravindra Goyal, Bay Regional Medical Center, Bay City

Devon Hoover, Beaumont Hospital–Grosse Pointe, Grosse Pointe

Louis Jacobs, Garden City Osteopathic Hospital, Garden City

Martin Kornblum, St. John Macomb Hospital, Warren

Daniel Michael, Beaumont Hospital–Grosse Pointe, Grosse Pointe

Manouchehr Nikpour, Beaumont Hospital–Grosse Pointe, Grosse Pointe

Anita North, Bay Regional Medical Center, Bay City

Rick Olson, St. John Macomb Hospital, Warren

Nilesh Patel, Oakwood Hospital and Medical Center–Dearborn, Dearborn

Siva Sriharan, Bay Regional Medical Center, Bay City

John Zinkel, Beaumont Hospital–Grosse Pointe, Grosse Pointe

VASCULAR SURGERY

Fred Brown, Mercy General Health Partners, Muskegon

Kurt Carter, Ingham Regional Medical Center, Lansing

Alonso Collar, Ingham Regional Medical Center, Lansing

Joseph Cotroneo, Ingham Regional Medical Center, Lansing

Andrew Duda, Ingham Regional Medical Center, Lansing

Victor Erzurum, Ingham Regional Medical Center, Lansing

Divyakant Gandhi, Ingham Regional Medical Center, Lansing

Anthony Holden, Ingham Regional Medical Center, Lansing

Gregory Landis, Ingham Regional Medical Center, Lansing

Lawrence Mallon, Mercy General Health Partners, Muskegon

Craig McBrayer, Mercy General Health Partners, Muskegon

Gary Roth, Ingham Regional Medical Center, Lansing

Vance Smith, Mercy General Health Partners, Muskegon

James Zito, Ingham Regional Medical Center, Lansing

MINNESOTA TOP DOCTORS

CARDIOLOGY

Greg Anderson, Fairview Southdale Hospital, Edina

Richard Aplin, St. Cloud Hospital, St. Cloud

Richard Backes, St. Cloud Hospital, St. Cloud

Stephen Battista, Fairview Southdale Hospital, Edina

David Benditt, St. Cloud Hospital, St. Cloud

Ann Dunnigan, St. Cloud Hospital, St. Cloud

Jacob Dutcher, St. Cloud Hospital, St. Cloud

Bernard Erickson, St. Cloud Hospital, St. Cloud

Mark Johnson, St. Cloud Hospital, St. Cloud

Richard Jolkovsky, St. Cloud Hospital, St. Cloud

David Laxson, Fairview Southdale Hospital, Edina

Keith Lurie, St. Cloud Hospital, St. Cloud

Brian Mahoney, United Hospitals, St. Paul

John Mahowald, St. Cloud Hospital, St. Cloud

Edward Martin, St. Cloud Hospital, St. Cloud

Mark Martone, St. Cloud Hospital, St. Cloud

Simón Milstein, St. Cloud Hospital, St. Cloud

Joe Nguyen, St. Cloud Hospital, St. Cloud

Jamie Pelzel, St. Cloud Hospital, St. Cloud

Peter Rusterholz, United Hospitals, St. Paul

Wade Schmidt, St. Cloud Hospital, St. Cloud

Timothy Schuchard, St. Cloud Hospital, St. Cloud

Mark Solfelt, Fairview Southdale Hospital, Edina

Michael Thurmes, Fairview Southdale Hospital, Edina

Daniel Tiede, St. Cloud Hospital, St. Cloud

Mevan Wijetunga, St. Cloud Hospital, St. Cloud

Howard Zimring, St. Cloud Hospital, St. Cloud

Top doctors are those that practice at hospitals that are rated in the top 10% in the nation for that clinical program area. For more information on how top doctors were selected, see Appendix.

GASTROINTESTINAL

Waldo Avello, St. Luke's Hospital, Duluth
Javier DeLaGarza, St. Luke's Hospital, Duluth

NEUROLOGY

Janiece Aldinger, Fairview Southdale Hospital,
Edina
Bruce Idelkope, Fairview Southdale Hospital, Edina
Michael Madison, Fairview Southdale Hospital, Edina

ORTHOPEDIC SURGERY

John Geiser, St. Cloud Hospital, St. Cloud
Eric Green, St. Cloud Hospital, St. Cloud
Patrick Hall, St. Luke's Hospital, Duluth
Chad Holien, St. Cloud Hospital, St. Cloud
David Kaus, St. Cloud Hospital, St. Cloud
Steven Mulawka, St. Cloud Hospital, St. Cloud
Michael Murphy, St. Cloud Hospital, St. Cloud
Joseph Nessler, St. Cloud Hospital, St. Cloud

Kim Schaap, St. Cloud Hospital, St. Cloud
Andrew Staiger, St. Cloud Hospital, St. Cloud
St. Cloud Orthopedic Associates, St. Cloud
Hospital, St. Cloud
Christopher Widstrom, St. Cloud Hospital, St. Cloud
Joel Zamzow, St. Luke's Hospital, Duluth

SPINE SURGERY

Stefan Konasiewicz, St. Luke's Hospital, Duluth

MISSISSIPPI TOP DOCTORS

ORTHOPEDIC SURGERY

Dudley Burwell, Gulf Coast Medical Center, Biloxi
David Clause, Gulf Coast Medical Center, Biloxi
Theodore Jordan, Gulf Coast Medical Center, Biloxi
James Thriffley, Gulf Coast Medical Center, Biloxi

SPINE SURGERY

Terry Smith, Gulf Coast Medical Center, Biloxi

VASCULAR SURGERY

Charles Omara, Mississippi Baptist Medical
Center, Jackson

Seshadri Raju, Mississippi Baptist Medical
Center, Jackson
Victor Weiss, Mississippi Baptist Medical Center,
Jackson

MISSOURI TOP DOCTORS

CARDIAC SURGERY

Randy Brown, Southeast Missouri Hospital,
Cape Girardeau
William Ogle, Southeast Missouri Hospital,
Cape Girardeau
Michael Phillips, Freeman Health System, Joplin
Darryl Ramsey, Southeast Missouri Hospital,
Cape Girardeau
Raymond Vetsch, Freeman Health System, Joplin

CARDIOLOGY

Richard Bach, Barnes-Jewish Hospital, St. Louis
Ben Barzilai, Barnes-Jewish Hospital, St. Louis
Michael Beardslee, Barnes-Jewish Hospital,
St. Louis
Joseph Billadello, Barnes-Jewish Hospital, St. Louis
Alan Braverman, Barnes-Jewish Hospital, St. Louis
Angela Brown, Barnes-Jewish Hospital, St. Louis
Jane Chen, Barnes-Jewish Hospital, St. Louis
Gregory Ewald, Barnes-Jewish Hospital, St. Louis
Mitchell Faddis, Barnes-Jewish Hospital, St. Louis
Edward Geltman, Barnes-Jewish Hospital,
St. Louis
Marye Gleva, Barnes-Jewish Hospital, St. Louis
Sudhir Jain, Barnes-Jewish Hospital, St. Louis
Andrew Kates, Barnes-Jewish Hospital, St. Louis
Robert Kleiger, Barnes-Jewish Hospital, St. Louis
Ronald Krone, Barnes-Jewish Hospital, St. Louis

Howard Kurz, Barnes-Jewish Hospital, St. Louis
John Lasala, Barnes-Jewish Hospital, St. Louis
Bruce Lindsay, Barnes-Jewish Hospital, St. Louis
Philip Ludbrook, Barnes-Jewish Hospital, St. Louis
Majesh Makan, Barnes-Jewish Hospital, St. Louis
Keith Mankowitz, Barnes-Jewish Hospital, St. Louis
Scott Nordlicht, Barnes-Jewish Hospital, St. Louis
Julio Perez, Barnes-Jewish Hospital, St. Louis
Craig Reiss, Barnes-Jewish Hospital, St. Louis
Michael Rich, Barnes-Jewish Hospital, St. Louis
Ibrahim Saeed, Barnes-Jewish Hospital, St. Louis
David Schwartz, Barnes-Jewish Hospital, St. Louis
Lynne Seacord, Barnes-Jewish Hospital, St. Louis
Jasvindar Singh, Barnes-Jewish Hospital, St. Louis
Timothy Smith, Barnes-Jewish Hospital, St. Louis
Joshua Stolker, Barnes-Jewish Hospital, St. Louis
Alan Weiss, Barnes-Jewish Hospital, St. Louis

GASTROINTESTINAL

Martin Altman, SSM St. Joseph Health Center,
St. Charles
Riad Azar, Barnes-Jewish Hospital, St. Louis
Bhaskar Banerjee, Barnes-Jewish Hospital,
St. Louis
Matthew Ciorba, Barnes-Jewish Hospital, St. Louis
Jeffery Crippin, Barnes-Jewish Hospital, St. Louis
Robert Cusworth, SSM St. Joseph Health Center,
St. Charles

Nicholas Davidson, Barnes-Jewish Hospital,
St. Louis
Dayna Early, Barnes-Jewish Hospital, St. Louis
Steven Edmundowicz, Barnes-Jewish Hospital,
St. Louis
Sreeni Jonnalagadda, Barnes-Jewish Hospital,
St. Louis
Kevin Korenblat, Barnes-Jewish Hospital, St. Louis
Mauricio Lisker-Melman, Barnes-Jewish Hospital,
St. Louis
Marin Marcu, SSM St. Joseph Health Center,
St. Charles
Rodney Newberry, Barnes-Jewish Hospital, St. Louis
Chandra Prakash, Barnes-Jewish Hospital,
St. Louis
Deborah Rubin, Barnes-Jewish Hospital, St. Louis
Gregory Sayuk, Barnes-Jewish Hospital, St. Louis
William Stenson, Barnes-Jewish Hospital, St. Louis
Christian Stone, Barnes-Jewish Hospital, St. Louis
Shelby Sullivan, Barnes-Jewish Hospital, St. Louis
Sandeep Tripathy, Barnes-Jewish Hospital,
St. Louis
Gary Zuckerman, Barnes-Jewish Hospital, St. Louis

NEUROLOGY

Diane Cornelison, Skaggs Community Health
Center, Branson
Donald Hopewell, Skaggs Community Health
Center, Branson

MINNESOTA / MISSISSIPPI / MISSOURI TOP DOCTORS

Mouhammed Kabbani, Skaggs Community Health
Center, Branson

Robert Margolis, Christian Hospital Northeast,
St. Louis

ORTHOPEDIC SURGERY

Thomas Aleto, Columbia Regional Hospital,
Columbia

B. Bal, Columbia Regional Hospital, Columbia

Peter Buchert, Columbia Regional Hospital,
Columbia

David Hockman, Columbia Regional Hospital,
Columbia

William Humphreys, Heartland Regional Medical
Center, St. Joseph

John Olson, Heartland Regional Medical Center,
St. Joseph

Brent Peterson, Heartland Regional Medical
Center, St. Joseph

Bruce Smith, Heartland Regional Medical Center,
St. Joseph

Daniel Smith, Heartland Regional Medical Center,
St. Joseph

VASCULAR SURGERY

Edward Bender, St. Francis Medical Center,
Cape Girardeau

R. New, St. Francis Medical Center,
Cape Girardeau

John Wiggans, St. Francis Medical Center,
Cape Girardeau

MONTANA TOP DOCTORS

CARDIOLOGY

Matt Maxwell, St. Patrick Hospital and Health
Sciences Center, Missoula

Stephen Tahta, St. Patrick Hospital and Health
Sciences Center, Missoula

ORTHOPEDIC SURGERY

Whitney Robinson, Billings Clinic, Billings

Robert Schultz, Billings Clinic, Billings

VASCULAR SURGERY

John Davis, Billings Clinic, Billings

Tim Dernbach, Billings Clinic, Billings

Barry Winton, Billings Clinic, Billings

NEBRASKA TOP DOCTORS

ORTHOPEDIC SURGERY

George Emodi, Alegent Health–Immanuel Medical
Center, Omaha

Mark Franco, Alegent Health–Immanuel Medical
Center, Omaha

Mark Pitner, Alegent Health–Immanuel Medical
Center, Omaha

Paul Watson, Alegent Health–Immanuel Medical
Center, Omaha

SPINE SURGERY

Timothy Burd, Alegent Health–Immanuel Medical
Center, Omaha

Jonathan Fuller, Alegent Health–Immanuel
Medical Center, Omaha

Michael Longley, Alegent Health–Immanuel
Medical Center, Omaha

John McClellan, Alegent Health–Immanuel
Medical Center, Omaha

Eric Phillips, Alegent Health–Immanuel Medical
Center, Omaha

H. Woodward, Alegent Health–Immanuel Medical
Center, Omaha

NEW HAMPSHIRE TOP DOCTORS

ORTHOPEDIC SURGERY

Wade Penny, Cheshire Medical Center, Keene

Anthony Presutti, Cheshire Medical Center, Keene

NEW JERSEY TOP DOCTORS

CARDIAC SURGERY

Lynn McGrath, Deborah Heart and Lung Center,
Browns Mills

Authur Ng, Deborah Heart and Lung Center,
Browns Mills

CARDIOLOGY

Kourosh Asgarian, Hackensack University Medical
Center, Hackensack

Fred Aueron, St. Barnabas Medical Center,
Livingston

Paul Burns, St. Barnabas Medical Center,
Livingston

John Ciccone, St. Barnabas Medical Center,
Livingston

Jeffrey Doskow, St. Barnabas Medical Center,
Livingston

Elie Elmann, Hackensack University Medical
Center, Hackensack

Deborah Friedman, St. Barnabas Medical Center,
Livingston

Jeffrey Gold, St. Barnabas Medical Center, Livingston

Mark Goldberg, St. Barnabas Medical Center, Livingston

Bruce Haik, St. Barnabas Medical Center, Livingston

James Hefferan, St. Barnabas Medical Center, Livingston

Ravindra Karanam, St. Barnabas Medical Center, Livingston

Constantine Kashnikow, St. Barnabas Medical Center, Livingston

Kenneth Miller, St. Barnabas Medical Center, Livingston

Peter Praeger, Hackensack University Medical Center, Hackensack

Brooke Ritvo, St. Barnabas Medical Center, Livingston

Marc Roelke, St. Barnabas Medical Center, Livingston

Gary Rogal, St. Barnabas Medical Center, Livingston

Fred Sardari, St. Barnabas Medical Center, Livingston

Roy Sauberman, St. Barnabas Medical Center, Livingston

Craig Saunders, St. Barnabas Medical Center, Livingston

Jacqueline Schwanwede, St. Barnabas Medical Center, Livingston

Susan Simandl, St. Barnabas Medical Center, Livingston

Eric Somberg, Hackensack University Medical Center, Hackensack

Sabino Torre, St. Barnabas Medical Center, Livingston

Paul Wangenheim, St. Barnabas Medical Center, Livingston

GASTROINTESTINAL

Joel Goldfarb, Holy Name Hospital, Teaneck
Barry Herman, Warren Hospital, Phillipsburg
Thomas Kantor, Warren Hospital, Phillipsburg
Chatargy Kaza, Warren Hospital, Phillipsburg
Manoj Mittal, Warren Hospital, Phillipsburg
Shanker Mukherjee, Warren Hospital, Phillipsburg
Vincent Rigoglioso, Holy Name Hospital, Teaneck
Michael Schmidt, Holy Name Hospital, Teaneck
Michael Sciarra, Holy Name Hospital, Teaneck

GENERAL SURGERY

John Bello, Hunterdon Medical Center, Flemington
Joseph Bello, Hunterdon Medical Center, Flemington

Douglas Benson, Hackensack University Medical Center, Hackensack

Stephen Pereira, Hackensack University Medical Center, Hackensack

NEUROLOGY

Charles Asta, Holy Name Hospital, Teaneck
Haidy Behman, Raritan Bay Medical Center, Perth Amboy

Eliot Chodosh, Chilton Memorial Hospital, Pompton Plains

Lyle Dennis, Hackensack University Medical Center, Hackensack

Damon Fellman, Holy Name Hospital, Teaneck
Frank Gazzillo, Chilton Memorial Hospital, Pompton Plains

Dev Gupta, Hackensack University Medical Center, Hackensack

Mark Haas, Holy Name Hospital, Teaneck
Annmarie Mascellino, Chilton Memorial Hospital, Pompton Plains

Terence McAlarney, Centrastate Medical Center, Freehold

Jennifer Monck, Chilton Memorial Hospital, Pompton Plains

Eyad Nayal, Chilton Memorial Hospital, Pompton Plains

John Nogueira, Holy Name Hospital, Teaneck
Farooq Rehman, Raritan Bay Medical Center, Perth Amboy

David Van Slooten, Holy Name Hospital, Teaneck
Robert Wagner, Chilton Memorial Hospital, Pompton Plains

OBSTETRICS/GYNECOLOGY

Melissa Ackerman, University Medical Center at Princeton, Princeton

Hina Ahmad, University Medical Center at Princeton, Princeton

Tatiana Ambarus, Newark Beth Israel Medical Center, Newark

Patrick Anderson, Newark Beth Israel Medical Center, Newark

Trissa Baden, University Medical Center at Princeton, Princeton

Roy Baldomero, Newark Beth Israel Medical Center, Newark

Debra Baseman, University Medical Center at Princeton, Princeton

Julio Caban, Newark Beth Israel Medical Center, Newark

Wendy Cervi, Newark Beth Israel Medical Center, Newark

Jeffrey Chait, University Medical Center at Princeton, Princeton

Gerald Ciciola, St. Barnabas Medical Center, Livingston

Shilpa Clott, University Medical Center at Princeton, Princeton

David Corley, University Medical Center at Princeton, Princeton

Seth Derman, University Medical Center at Princeton, Princeton

Christina DiVenti, University Medical Center at Princeton, Princeton

Richard Fain, St. Barnabas Medical Center, Livingston

Alan Friedman, University Medical Center at Princeton, Princeton

Eugene Gamburg, University Medical Center at Princeton, Princeton

Martin Gimovsky, Newark Beth Israel Medical Center, Newark

Shefali Goyal, University Medical Center at Princeton, Princeton

Jeffrey Gross, University Medical Center at Princeton, Princeton

Lanniece Hall, University Medical Center at Princeton, Princeton

Emad Hashemi, Newark Beth Israel Medical Center, Newark

Jeffrey Hofman, University Medical Center at Princeton, Princeton

Joseph Ivan, Newark Beth Israel Medical Center, Newark

Lillian Kaminsky, University Medical Center at Princeton, Princeton

Daria Klachko, St. Barnabas Medical Center, Livingston

Karen Koscica, Newark Beth Israel Medical Center, Newark

Luc Lemmerling, University Medical Center at Princeton, Princeton

Lawrence Lippert, University Medical Center at Princeton, Princeton

Sam Locatelli, Newark Beth Israel Medical Center, Newark

Robert Martin, University Medical Center at Princeton, Princeton

Robert Mayson, Centrastate Medical Center, Freehold

Richard Miller, St. Barnabas Medical Center, Livingston

Munir Nazir, Newark Beth Israel Medical Center, Newark

Vrunda Patel, University Medical Center at Princeton, Princeton

Alison Petraske, University Medical Center at Princeton, Princeton

Bruce Pierce, University Medical Center at Princeton, Princeton

Antonia Pinney, Newark Beth Israel Medical Center, Newark

Michael Pitter, Newark Beth Israel Medical Center, Newark

Joseph Polcaro, Newark Beth Israel Medical Center, Newark

Asha Proctor, University Medical Center at Princeton, Princeton

Alectis Santiago, University Medical Center at Princeton, Princeton

Bani Sarma, University Medical Center at Princeton, Princeton

Khalid Sawaged, Newark Beth Israel Medical Center, Newark

Elizabeth Scheff, University Medical Center at Princeton, Princeton

William Scorza, University Medical Center at Princeton, Princeton

Daniel Shapiro, University Medical Center at Princeton, Princeton

Glenn Sherman, University Medical Center at Princeton, Princeton

Anna Shoshilos, Newark Beth Israel Medical Center, Newark

Leon Smith, St. Barnabas Medical Center, Livingston

John Smulian, University Medical Center at Princeton, Princeton

George Taliadouros, University Medical Center at Princeton, Princeton

Kenneth Treadwell, Newark Beth Israel Medical Center, Newark

Kenneth Ung, University Medical Center at Princeton, Princeton

Joseph Vaydovsky, Newark Beth Israel Medical Center, Newark

Susan Warchaizer, University Medical Center at Princeton, Princeton

Krya Williams, University Medical Center at Princeton, Princeton

NEW MEXICO TOP DOCTORS

ORTHOPEDIC SURGERY

Franklin Guttmann, Presbyterian Hospital, Albuquerque

Sean Hassinger, Presbyterian Hospital, Albuquerque

NEW YORK TOP DOCTORS

CARDIOLOGY

Kara Bennorth, Westchester Medical Center, Valhalla

Israel Berkowitz, Lenox Hill Hospital, Manhattan

Ira Blaufarb, Lenox Hill Hospital, Manhattan

George Brief, Lenox Hill Hospital, Manhattan

Richard Charney, Westchester Medical Center, Valhalla

Saulat Chaudhry, Westchester Medical Center, Valhalla

Giovanni Ciuffo, Lenox Hill Hospital, Manhattan

Howard Cohen, Lenox Hill Hospital, Manhattan

Martin Cohen, Westchester Medical Center, Valhalla

Albert DeLuca, Westchester Medical Center, Valhalla

Alvaro Dominguez, Lenox Hill Hospital, Manhattan

Nicholas Dubois, Lenox Hill Hospital, Manhattan

Arlen Fleisher, Westchester Medical Center, Valhalla

William Frumkin, Lenox Hill Hospital, Manhattan

Kirk Garratt, Lenox Hill Hospital, Manhattan

Lynne Glasser, Lenox Hill Hospital, Manhattan

Simon Gorwara, Vassar Brothers Medical Center, Poughkeepsie

Stephen Green, North Shore University Hospital, Manhasset

Ahmad Hadid, Westchester Medical Center, Valhalla

Lawrence Hecker, Lenox Hill Hospital, Manhattan

Craig Hjemdahl-Monsen, Westchester Medical Center, Valhalla

Donna Ingram, Lenox Hill Hospital, Manhattan

Sriram Iyer, Lenox Hill Hospital, Manhattan

Mumtazuddin Jafar, Vassar Brothers Medical Center, Poughkeepsie

Kumar Kalapatapu, Westchester Medical Center, Valhalla

Ram Kalapatapu, Westchester Medical Center, Valhalla

Dina Katz, Westchester Medical Center, Valhalla

Stanley Katz, North Shore University Hospital, Manhasset

Richard Kay, Westchester Medical Center, Valhalla

Rocco Lafaro, Westchester Medical Center, Valhalla

Marie-Noelle Langan, Lenox Hill Hospital, Manhattan

Steven Lansman, Westchester Medical Center, Valhalla

Alexander Lee, North Shore University Hospital, Manhasset

Didier Loulmet, Lenox Hill Hospital, Manhattan

David Mackinnon, Lenox Hill Hospital, Manhattan

Ramin Malekan, Westchester Medical Center, Valhalla

Donna Marchant, North Shore University Hospital, Manhasset

Nino Marino, Lenox Hill Hospital, Manhattan

John McClung, Westchester Medical Center, Valhalla

David Messinger, Westchester Medical Center, Valhalla

Dayan Naik, Westchester Medical Center, Valhalla

Sanjay Naik, Westchester Medical Center, Valhalla

Marc Nolan, Lenox Hill Hospital, Manhattan

Daniel O'Dea, Vassar Brothers Medical Center, Poughkeepsie

Lawrence Ong, North Shore University Hospital, Manhasset

Manish Parikh, Lenox Hill Hospital, Manhattan

Nirav Patel, Lenox Hill Hospital, Manhattan

Robert Pilchik, Westchester Medical Center, Valhalla

Anthony Pucillo, Westchester Medical Center, Valhalla

Joseph Puma, Lenox Hill Hospital, Manhattan

Carl Reimers, Lenox Hill Hospital, Manhattan

Jae Ro, Westchester Medical Center, Valhalla

Paul Romanello, Lenox Hill Hospital, Manhattan

Warren Rosenblum, Westchester Medical Center, Valhalla

Gary Roubin, Lenox Hill Hospital, Manhattan

Carlos Ruiz, Lenox Hill Hospital, Manhattan

Mohan Sarabu, Vassar Brothers Medical Center, Poughkeepsie

Paul Saunders, Westchester Medical Center, Valhalla

Mark Schiffer, Lenox Hill Hospital, Manhattan

William Schwartz, Lenox Hill Hospital, Manhattan

Bonnie Seecharran, Westchester Medical Center, Valhalla

David Seinfeld, Lenox Hill Hospital, Manhattan

Suvro Sett, Westchester Medical Center, Valhalla

Rony Shimony, Lenox Hill Hospital, Manhattan

Inderpal Singh, Westchester Medical Center, Valhalla

Alan Slater, Westchester Medical Center, Valhalla

Carmine Sorbera, Westchester Medical Center, Valhalla

David Spielvogel, Westchester Medical Center, Valhalla

Suzanne Steinbaum, Lenox Hill Hospital, Manhattan

Valavanur Subramanian, Lenox Hill Hospital, Manhattan

Howard Tarkin, Westchester Medical Center, Valhalla

Jack Tighe, Westchester Medical Center, Valhalla

Ronald Wallach, Westchester Medical Center, Valhalla

Melvin Weiss, Westchester Medical Center, Valhalla

Peter Zakow, Vassar Brothers Medical Center, Poughkeepsie

Robert Zaloom, Lenox Hill Hospital, Manhattan

GENERAL SURGERY

Kishore Agrawal, Staten Island University Hospital, Staten Island

Lawrence Bodenstein, Staten Island University Hospital, Staten Island

Vinod Bopaiah, Staten Island University Hospital, Staten Island

Steven Brandeis, New York Downtown Hospital, New York

Michael Castellano, Staten Island University Hospital, Staten Island

Edwin Chang, Staten Island University Hospital, Staten Island

Charles Choy, Staten Island University Hospital, Staten Island

Gene Coppa, Staten Island University Hospital, Staten Island

Jerome Finkelstein, Staten Island University Hospital, Staten Island

Asaf Gave, Staten Island University Hospital, Staten Island

Ellen Hagopian, New York Downtown Hospital, New York

Shaw-Fu Hwang, New York Downtown Hospital, New York

Alan J Cherofsky, Staten Island University Hospital, Staten Island

Armen Kasabian, Staten Island University Hospital, Staten Island

Nachum Katlowitz, Staten Island University Hospital, Staten Island

Helen Kim, Staten Island University Hospital, Staten Island

Anthony Kopatsis, Staten Island University Hospital, Staten Island

Sam Kwauk, New York Downtown Hospital, New York

Frederick L. H. Sabido, Staten Island University Hospital, Staten Island

Har Lau, Phelps Memorial Hospital Association, Sleepy Hollow

Heather McMullen, Staten Island University Hospital, Staten Island

Frank Michael Rosell, Staten Island University Hospital, Staten Island

Jeffrey Nicastro, Staten Island University Hospital, Staten Island

Murlidhar Pahuja, Staten Island University Hospital, Staten Island

Thomas Panetta, Staten Island University Hospital, Staten Island

Marc Plawker, Staten Island University Hospital, Staten Island

Adley Raboy, Staten Island University Hospital, Staten Island

Robert Raniolo, Phelps Memorial Hospital Association, Sleepy Hollow

Ronald Scott Krantz, Staten Island University Hospital, Staten Island

Joel Sherman, Staten Island University Hospital, Staten Island

John Shiau, Staten Island University Hospital, Staten Island

Robert Silich, Staten Island University Hospital, Staten Island

Donald Summers, New York Downtown Hospital, New York

Stephen W. Hornyak, Staten Island University Hospital, Staten Island

NEUROLOGY

Donald Aberfeld, St. Vincent's Hospital–Manhattan, New York

Barbara Allis, Huntington Hospital, Huntington

Cary Buckner, New York Methodist Hospital, Brooklyn

Michael Bykofsky, St. Vincent's Hospital–Manhattan, New York

Christine Crisafulli, St. Vincent's Hospital–Manhattan, New York

Andrew Dawson, New York Methodist Hospital, Brooklyn

Alexandra Degenhardt, New York Methodist Hospital, Brooklyn

David Duncan, St. Vincent's Hospital–Manhattan, New York

Albert Favate, St. Vincent's Hospital–Manhattan, New York

Irving Fish, St. Vincent's Hospital–Manhattan, New York

Anthony Geraci, St. Vincent's Hospital–Manhattan, New York

Anne Kleiman, St. Vincent's Hospital–Manhattan, New York

Josiane LaJoie, St. Vincent's Hospital–Manhattan, New York

Claude Macaluso, St. Vincent's Hospital–Manhattan, New York

Paul Magda, St. Vincent's Hospital–Manhattan, New York

Anthony Maniscalco, St. Vincent's Hospital–Manhattan, New York

Carolyn Martin, St. Vincent's Hospital–Manhattan, New York

Daniel Miles, St. Vincent's Hospital–Manhattan, New York

Joseph Moreira, St. Vincent's Hospital–Manhattan, New York

Paul Mullin, St. Vincent's Hospital–Manhattan, New York

Shahin Nouri, New York Methodist Hospital, Brooklyn

Shalini Patcha, Huntington Hospital, Huntington

Nityananda Podder, St. Vincent's Hospital–Manhattan, New York

Max Rudansky, Huntington Hospital, Huntington

Miran Salgado, New York Methodist Hospital, Brooklyn

Howard Sander, St. Vincent's Hospital—Manhattan, New York

Marlon Seliger, St. Vincent's Hospital—Manhattan, New York

Musarat Shareeff, Huntington Hospital, Huntington

Keith Siller, New York University Medical Center—Tisch Hospital, New York

Josh Torgovnick, St. Vincent's Hospital—Manhattan, New York

Harold Weinberg, New York University Medical Center—Tisch Hospital, New York

John Wells, St. Vincent's Hospital—Manhattan, New York

David Younger, St. Vincent's Hospital—Manhattan, New York

Bruce Zablow, St. Vincent's Hospital—Manhattan, New York

OBSTETRICS/GYNECOLOGY

Vito Alamia, Southampton Hospital, Southampton
Dacarla Albright, Lenox Hill Hospital, Manhattan
Michael Arato, St. Charles Hospital, Port Jefferson
Theodore Blaszczyk, St. Charles Hospital, Port Jefferson
Damiano Buffa, St. Charles Hospital, Port Jefferson
Irving Buterman, Lenox Hill Hospital, Manhattan
Lyndon Chang, Lenox Hill Hospital, Manhattan
Louise Collins, Southampton Hospital, Southampton
Ramon Diaz, Southampton Hospital, Southampton
Michael Divon, Lenox Hill Hospital, Manhattan
Lance Edwards, St. Charles Hospital, Port Jefferson
Thomas Erhart, St. Charles Hospital, Port Jefferson
Tracey Fein, Lenox Hill Hospital, Manhattan
Asaf Ferber, Lenox Hill Hospital, Manhattan
Anthony Giammarino, St. Charles Hospital, Port Jefferson
Theodore Goldberg, St. Charles Hospital, Port Jefferson
John Hunt, Southampton Hospital, Southampton
Lisa Johnson, Lenox Hill Hospital, Manhattan
Edmund Kaplan, Lenox Hill Hospital, Manhattan
Harry Karamitsos, Lenox Hill Hospital, Manhattan
Robert Kramer, St. Charles Hospital, Port Jefferson
Mindy Kwan, Lenox Hill Hospital, Manhattan
Sarah Lazar, Southampton Hospital, Southampton
Douglas Lee, St. Charles Hospital, Port Jefferson
Samuel Levin, Lenox Hill Hospital, Manhattan
Paul Lograno, St. Charles Hospital, Port Jefferson

Philip Makowski, St. Charles Hospital, Port Jefferson
Janice Marks, Lenox Hill Hospital, Manhattan
Jennifer Marshak, St. Charles Hospital, Port Jefferson
Jeffery Mazlin, Lenox Hill Hospital, Manhattan
Ketly Michel, Lenox Hill Hospital, Manhattan
Karl-Heinz Moehlen, Lenox Hill Hospital, Manhattan
Jerry Ninia, St. Charles Hospital, Port Jefferson
Allen Ott, Southampton Hospital, Southampton
Ben Pascario, Lenox Hill Hospital, Manhattan
Dreux Patton, St. Charles Hospital, Port Jefferson
G. Peters, St. Charles Hospital, Port Jefferson
John Petraco, St. Charles Hospital, Port Jefferson
Michael Plakogiannis, Lenox Hill Hospital, Manhattan
Elizabeth Poynor, Lenox Hill Hospital, Manhattan
Samuel Rafalin, Lenox Hill Hospital, Manhattan
Amy Richter, St. Charles Hospital, Port Jefferson
Mary Rivera-Casamento, Lenox Hill Hospital, Manhattan
Florence Rolston, Southampton Hospital, Southampton
Adam Romoff, Lenox Hill Hospital, Manhattan
Steven Ross, St. Charles Hospital, Port Jefferson
Gerardo SanRoman, St. Charles Hospital, Port Jefferson
Gustavo SanRoman, St. Charles Hospital, Port Jefferson
Albert Sassoon, Lenox Hill Hospital, Manhattan
Geri Schmitt, Southampton Hospital, Southampton
Pedro Segarra, Lenox Hill Hospital, Manhattan
Mindy Shaffran, St. Charles Hospital, Port Jefferson
Howard Shaw, Lenox Hill Hospital, Manhattan
Dennis Strittmatter, St. Charles Hospital, Port Jefferson
Saul Stromer, Lenox Hill Hospital, Manhattan
Michael Strongin, Lenox Hill Hospital, Manhattan
Sylvia Tufano, St. Charles Hospital, Port Jefferson
Jennine Varhola, Southampton Hospital, Southampton
Jaqueline Worth, Lenox Hill Hospital, Manhattan
Jennifer Wu, Lenox Hill Hospital, Manhattan
Inga Zilberstein, Lenox Hill Hospital, Manhattan

ORTHOPEDIC SURGERY

Steven Arsht, Beth Israel Medical Center, New York
Stanley Asnis, North Shore University Hospital, Manhasset
Mansoor Beg, North Shore University Hospital, Manhasset

Steven Beldner, Beth Israel Medical Center, New York
Catherine Compito, Beth Israel Medical Center, New York
Salvatore Corso, North Shore University Hospital, Manhasset
Frances Cuomo, Beth Israel Medical Center, New York
Michael Cushner, Beth Israel Medical Center, New York
Richard D'Agostino, North Shore University Hospital, Manhasset
Martin Dolan, North Shore University Hospital, Manhasset
Excelsior Group, Kenmore Mercy Hospital, Kenmore
William Facibene, North Shore University Hospital, Manhasset
Ivan Fernandez-Madrid, Beth Israel Medical Center, New York
Jonathan Gordon, Beth Israel Medical Center, New York
Ivan Gowan, Community Memorial Hospital, Hamilton
Robert Haar, Beth Israel Medical Center, New York
Steven Harwin, Beth Israel Medical Center, New York
Stuart Hershon, North Shore University Hospital, Manhasset
Christopher Hubbard, Beth Israel Medical Center, New York
Joint Reconstruction Orthopedics, Kenmore Mercy Hospital, Kenmore
Alan Kadison, North Shore University Hospital, Manhasset
Donald Kastenbaum, Beth Israel Medical Center, New York
Samuel Kenan, North Shore University Hospital, Manhasset
Matthew Kilgo, North Shore University Hospital, Manhasset
Lewis Lane, North Shore University Hospital, Manhasset
Howard Levy, Beth Israel Medical Center, New York
Stanley Liebowitz, Beth Israel Medical Center, New York
Jerry Lubliner, Beth Israel Medical Center, New York
Joeseph Mannino, Community Memorial Hospital, Hamilton
Peter McCann, Beth Israel Medical Center, New York
Raymond Meeks, Community Memorial Hospital, Hamilton
Charles Melone, Beth Israel Medical Center, New York

Top doctors are those that practice at hospitals that are rated in the top 10% in the nation for that clinical program area. For more information on how top doctors were selected, see Appendix.

Kenji Miyasaka, Beth Israel Medical Center, New York

Hamid Mostafavi, North Shore University Hospital, Manhasset

Ron Noy, Beth Israel Medical Center, New York

Debra Parisi, Beth Israel Medical Center, New York

Kevin Plancher, Beth Israel Medical Center, New York

Daniel Polatsch, Beth Israel Medical Center, New York

John Ricci, North Shore University Hospital, Manhasset

Jeffrey Richmond, North Shore University Hospital, Manhasset

Marcus Romanowski, Kenmore Mercy Hospital, Kenmore

Jacob Rozbruch, Beth Israel Medical Center, New York

Stephen Rycyna, Kenmore Mercy Hospital, Kenmore

Thomas Scilaris, Beth Israel Medical Center, New York

Bruce Seideman, North Shore University Hospital, Manhasset

Nicholas Sgaglione, North Shore University Hospital, Manhasset

Jeffrey Shapiro, North Shore University Hospital, Manhasset

Peter Shields, Kenmore Mercy Hospital, Kenmore

Sheldon Simon, Beth Israel Medical Center, New York

James Slough, Kenmore Mercy Hospital, Kenmore

Peter Stein, North Shore University Hospital, Manhasset

Baruch Toledano, North Shore University Hospital, Manhasset

Michael Trepeta, North Shore University Hospital, Manhasset

David Tuckman, North Shore University Hospital, Manhasset

Andrew Turtel, Beth Israel Medical Center, New York

Max Tyorkin, Beth Israel Medical Center, New York

Paul Yerys, North Shore University Hospital, Manhasset

Michael Zahn, Community Memorial Hospital, Hamilton

Robert Ziets, Beth Israel Medical Center, New York

SPINE SURGERY

John Bania, North Shore University Hospital, Manhasset

Matthew Bank, North Shore University Hospital, Manhasset

Marvin Base, North Shore University Hospital, Manhasset

Steven Blau, North Shore University Hospital, Manhasset

Paolo Bolognese, North Shore University Hospital, Manhasset

Andrew Casden, Beth Israel Medical Center, New York

Saima Chaudhry, North Shore University Hospital, Manhasset

Mark Eisenberg, North Shore University Hospital, Manhasset

Itzhak Haimovic, North Shore University Hospital, Manhasset

Peter Hollis, North Shore University Hospital, Manhasset

Salvatore Insinga, North Shore University Hospital, Manhasset

Richard Johnson, North Shore University Hospital, Manhasset

Stuart Kahn, Beth Israel Medical Center, New York

Paul Kuflik, Beth Israel Medical Center, New York

Alexander Lee, Beth Israel Medical Center, New York

Michael Lefkowitz, North Shore University Hospital, Manhasset

Mitchell Levine, North Shore University Hospital, Manhasset

Thomas Mauri, North Shore University Hospital, Manhasset

Alan Mechanic, North Shore University Hospital, Manhasset

Thomas Milhorat, North Shore University Hospital, Manhasset

Alon Mogilner, North Shore University Hospital, Manhasset

John Morrison, North Shore University Hospital, Manhasset

Michael Neuwirth, Beth Israel Medical Center, New York

Dennis Ostrovskly, North Shore University Hospital, Manhasset

Michael Overby, North Shore University Hospital, Manhasset

John Platz, North Shore University Hospital, Manhasset

Rajesh Raina, North Shore University Hospital, Manhasset

Laura Schoenberg, North Shore University Hospital, Manhasset

Suhail Shah, North Shore University Hospital, Manhasset

Vikas Varma, North Shore University Hospital, Manhasset

NORTH CAROLINA TOP DOCTORS

GASTROINTESTINAL

Filiberto Colon, Haywood Regional Medical Center, Clyde

Harry Lipham, Haywood Regional Medical Center, Clyde

Alfred Mina, Haywood Regional Medical Center, Clyde

Henry Nathan, Haywood Regional Medical Center, Clyde

Benjamin Phillips, Haywood Regional Medical Center, Clyde

Eric Reitz, Haywood Regional Medical Center, Clyde

Bennie Sharpton, Haywood Regional Medical Center, Clyde

GENERAL SURGERY

D. Covington, Duke Health Raleigh Hospital, Raleigh

Joel Dragelin, Duke Health Raleigh Hospital, Raleigh

Kirk Faust, Duke Health Raleigh Hospital, Raleigh

Peter Ng, Duke Health Raleigh Hospital, Raleigh

Yale Podnos, Duke Health Raleigh Hospital, Raleigh

David Powell, Duke Health Raleigh Hospital, Raleigh

Jerry Stirman, Duke Health Raleigh Hospital, Raleigh

NEUROLOGY

Larry Goldstein, Duke University Hospital, Durham

Daniel Laskowitz, Duke University Hospital, Durham

OBSTETRICS/GYNECOLOGY

Martin Allen, Lexington Memorial Hospital, Lexington

Tiffeny Carroll, Lexington Memorial Hospital, Lexington

Samuel Harris, Lexington Memorial Hospital, Lexington

Lloyd Lohr, Lexington Memorial Hospital, Lexington

Joseph Niner, Lexington Memorial Hospital, Lexington

Piedmont Women's Healthcare, Lexington Memorial Hospital, Lexington

Women's Center of Lexington, Lexington Memorial Hospital, Lexington

ORTHOPEDIC SURGERY

Mark Brenner, FirstHealth Moore Regional Hospital, Pinehurst

Werner Brooks, Margaret R. Pardee Memorial Hospital, Hendersonville

Neil Conti, FirstHealth Moore Regional Hospital, Pinehurst

Amal Das, Margaret R. Pardee Memorial Hospital, Hendersonville

Jason Guevara, FirstHealth Moore Regional Hospital, Pinehurst

Suzanne Hall, Margaret R. Pardee Memorial Hospital, Hendersonville

Edward Lilly, Margaret R. Pardee Memorial Hospital, Hendersonville

David Mackel, Margaret R. Pardee Memorial Hospital, Hendersonville

John Moore, FirstHealth Moore Regional Hospital, Pinehurst

David Napoli, Margaret R. Pardee Memorial Hospital, Hendersonville

Ward Oakley, FirstHealth Moore Regional Hospital, Pinehurst

SPINE SURGERY

Henry Moyle, FirstHealth Moore Regional Hospital, Pinehurst

James Rice, FirstHealth Moore Regional Hospital, Pinehurst

Malcolm Shupeck, FirstHealth Moore Regional Hospital, Pinehurst

---

NORTH DAKOTA TOP DOCTORS

CARDIAC SURGERY

Michael Booth, St. Alexius Medical Center, Bismarck

Michael Brown, St. Alexius Medical Center, Bismarck

Jim Burdine, Meritcare Health System, Fargo

Ajit Damle, Meritcare Health System, Fargo

Roxanne Newman, Meritcare Health System, Fargo

Edward Williams, St. Alexius Medical Center, Bismarck

CARDIOLOGY

Stan Diede, St. Alexius Medical Center, Bismarck

Norman Eshoo, St. Alexius Medical Center, Bismarck

Sanathana Murthy, St. Alexius Medical Center, Bismarck

Robert Oatfield, St. Alexius Medical Center, Bismarck

Jose Wiley, St. Alexius Medical Center, Bismarck

John Windsor, St. Alexius Medical Center, Bismarck

GASTROINTESTINAL

William Altringer, St. Alexius Medical Center, Bismarck

Steven Johnson, St. Alexius Medical Center, Bismarck

Mustafa Kathawala, St. Alexius Medical Center, Bismarck

Gaylord Kavlie, St. Alexius Medical Center, Bismarck

Atam Mehdiratta, St. Alexius Medical Center, Bismarck

Michael Schmit, St. Alexius Medical Center, Bismarck

ORTHOPEDIC SURGERY

Timothy Bopp, St. Alexius Medical Center, Bismarck

Joseph Carlson, St. Alexius Medical Center, Bismarck

Charles Dahl, St. Alexius Medical Center, Bismarck

Mark Hart, St. Alexius Medical Center, Bismarck

David Larsen, St. Alexius Medical Center, Bismarck

Troy Pierce, St. Alexius Medical Center, Bismarck

OHIO TOP DOCTORS

CARDIAC SURGERY

David Brown, Medcentral Health System, Mansfield

Antonios Chryssos, Aultman Hospital, Canton

Fraser Keith, Medcentral Health System, Mansfield

Roberto Novoa, Aultman Hospital, Canton

Aqeel Sandhu, Aultman Hospital, Canton

Stephen Sanofsky, Aultman Hospital, Canton

Mark Tawil, Aultman Hospital, Canton

CARDIOLOGY

Donald Cho, Southwest General Health Center, Middleburg Heights

Michael Deucher, Southwest General Health Center, Middleburg Heights

Bartolomeo Giannattasio, Southwest General Health Center, Middleburg Heights

Michael Hughes, Akron General Medical Center, Akron

Marc Schrode, Southwest General Health Center, Middleburg Heights

Trilok Sharma, Southwest General Health Center, Middleburg Heights

Qarab Syed, Southwest General Health Center, Middleburg Heights

Touraj Taghizadeh, Southwest General Health Center, Middleburg Heights

S. Tobias, Akron General Medical Center, Akron

Sabino Velloze, Southwest General Health Center, Middleburg Heights

GASTROINTESTINAL

Sangeeta Agrawal, Kettering Medical Center, Kettering

Bikrem Ansil, Kettering Medical Center, Kettering

Christopher Barde, Kettering Medical Center, Kettering

Gregory Beck, Kettering Medical Center, Kettering

Nitin Davessar, Southwest General Health Center, Middleburg Heights

Steven Dellon, Kettering Medical Center, Kettering

Malay Dey, Kettering Medical Center, Kettering

Rupa Fritz, Kettering Medical Center, Kettering

Robert Gaylor, Kettering Medical Center, Kettering

Michael Gorsky, Kettering Medical Center, Kettering

Piush Gupta, Kettering Medical Center, Kettering

Richard Houston, Kettering Medical Center, Kettering

Vincent Jabour, Wooster Community Hospital, Wooster

Rajkamal Jit, Kettering Medical Center, Kettering

Javad Kardan, Kettering Medical Center, Kettering

Aaron Knoll, Kettering Medical Center, Kettering

Donald Lutter, Kettering Medical Center, Kettering

Suresh Mahajan, Southwest General Health Center, Middleburg Heights

Walter Maimon, Kettering Medical Center, Kettering

John Maxwell, Akron General Medical Center, Akron

Rajeev Mehta, Kettering Medical Center, Kettering

Mark Modic, Southwest General Health Center, Middleburg Heights

James Murphy, Wooster Community Hospital, Wooster

David Novick, Kettering Medical Center, Kettering
Nagaraja Oruganti, Kettering Medical Center, Kettering
Teressa Patrick, Kettering Medical Center, Kettering
Narayan Pedanna, Kettering Medical Center, Kettering
Lakshmaiah Pola, Southwest General Health Center, Middleburg Heights
Marios Pouagare, Kettering Medical Center, Kettering
Carlos Ricotti, Trumbull Memorial Hospital, Warren
David Romeo, Kettering Medical Center, Kettering
Giti Rostami, Kettering Medical Center, Kettering
Jonathan Saxe, Kettering Medical Center, Kettering
Martin Shill, Akron General Medical Center, Akron
Lisa Stone, Kettering Medical Center, Kettering
Ali Syed, Kettering Medical Center, Kettering
Niaz Usman, Kettering Medical Center, Kettering
Larry Weprin, Kettering Medical Center, Kettering
Christopher Wille, Kettering Medical Center, Kettering
Adel Youssef, Trumbull Memorial Hospital, Warren

NEUROLOGY

James Auberle, Toledo Hospital, Toledo
Faizan Hafeez, Medical College of Ohio at Toledo, Toledo
Kewal Mahajan, St. Charles Mercy Hospital, Oregon
Michael Nagel, Toledo Hospital, Toledo

Ravi Narra, St. Charles Mercy Hospital, Oregon
Robert Richardson, St. Vincent Charity Hospital, Cleveland
James Sander, Toledo Hospital, Toledo
Howard Schecht, Toledo Hospital, Toledo
Gretchen Tietjen, Medical College of Ohio at Toledo, Toledo
Peter Zangara, Toledo Hospital, Toledo

ORTHOPEDIC SURGERY

Abi Afonja, Southwest General Health Center, Middleburg Heights
Stephen Autry, Bethesda North Hospital, Cincinnati
Michael Banks, Southwest General Health Center, Middleburg Heights
John Briggs, Mount Carmel Health, Columbus
Robert Durbin, Mount Carmel Health, Columbus
Richard Gittinger, Southwest General Health Center, Middleburg Heights
Jerold Gurley, Southwest General Health Center, Middleburg Heights
Stephen Kolodzik, Mount Carmel Health, Columbus
Karl Kumler, Mount Carmel Health, Columbus
Larry Lika, Southwest General Health Center, Middleburg Heights
Mark Panigutti, Southwest General Health Center, Middleburg Heights

Joel Politi, Mount Carmel Health, Columbus
Dirk Pruis, Bethesda North Hospital, Cincinnati
Joseph Scarcella, Southwest General Health Center, Middleburg Heights

SPINE SURGERY

Johnathan Borden, Bethesda North Hospital, Cincinnati
Donald Rohl, Mount Carmel Health, Columbus
Paul Schwetschenau, Bethesda North Hospital, Cincinnati
Derek Snook, Mount Carmel Health, Columbus
Won Song, Mount Carmel Health, Columbus
Daryl Sybert, Mount Carmel Health, Columbus
Larry Todd, Mount Carmel Health, Columbus

VASCULAR SURGERY

Mohan Das, Ohio State University Hospitals, Columbus
William Smead, Ohio State University Hospitals, Columbus
Jean Starr, Ohio State University Hospitals, Columbus
Patrick Vaccaro, Ohio State University Hospitals, Columbus
Blair Vermilion, Ohio State University Hospitals, Columbus

OKLAHOMA TOP DOCTORS

ORTHOPEDIC SURGERY

Dennis Bond, Midwest Regional Medical Center, Midwest City
Rory Dunham, Midwest Regional Medical Center, Midwest City
Joel Frazier, Midwest Regional Medical Center, Midwest City
Bret Frey, Midwest Regional Medical Center, Midwest City
Robert Gunderson, Midwest Regional Medical Center, Midwest City
Joseph Hayhurst, Midwest Regional Medical Center, Midwest City

Daron Hitt, Midwest Regional Medical Center, Midwest City
Christopher Jordan, Midwest Regional Medical Center, Midwest City
George Matook, Midwest Regional Medical Center, Midwest City
Jeffery Meyer, Midwest Regional Medical Center, Midwest City
Stephen Mihalsky, Midwest Regional Medical Center, Midwest City
L. Olsen, Midwest Regional Medical Center, Midwest City

Robert Thompson, Midwest Regional Medical Center, Midwest City
Quang Tu, Midwest Regional Medical Center, Midwest City

SPINE SURGERY

J. Duncan, Comanche County Memorial Hospital, Lawton
Mark Duncan, Comanche County Memorial Hospital, Lawton
Stephen Ofori, Comanche County Memorial Hospital, Lawton

OREGON TOP DOCTORS

ORTHOPEDIC SURGERY

Paul Duwelius, Providence St. Vincent Medical Center, Portland
Hans Moller, Providence St. Vincent Medical Center, Portland

CARDIAC SURGERY

Brian Mott, Community Medical Center, Scranton

Russell Stahl, Community Medical Center, Scranton

CARDIOLOGY

Krishna Bhat, Conemaugh Valley Memorial Hospital, Johnstown

Thomas Cardellino, Conemaugh Valley Memorial Hospital, Johnstown

Rajsekhar Devineni, Conemaugh Valley Memorial Hospital, Johnstown

Virender Dhawer, Conemaugh Valley Memorial Hospital, Johnstown

Samir Hadeed, Conemaugh Valley Memorial Hospital, Johnstown

K. M. Hussain, Conemaugh Valley Memorial Hospital, Johnstown

Savas Mavridis, Conemaugh Valley Memorial Hospital, Johnstown

Mohan Mital, Conemaugh Valley Memorial Hospital, Johnstown

Jude Mugerwa, Conemaugh Valley Memorial Hospital, Johnstown

Cyril Nathaniel, Conemaugh Valley Memorial Hospital, Johnstown

Charles Oschwald, Conemaugh Valley Memorial Hospital, Johnstown

William Smeal, Conemaugh Valley Memorial Hospital, Johnstown

Robert Stenberg, Conemaugh Valley Memorial Hospital, Johnstown

James Tretter, Conemaugh Valley Memorial Hospital, Johnstown

Lear Von Koch, Mercy Hospital Scranton, Scranton

Rod Wall, Conemaugh Valley Memorial Hospital, Johnstown

GASTROINTESTINAL

Jeffrey Berman, Abington Memorial Hospital, Abington

Myhanh Bosse, Abington Memorial Hospital, Abington

Joseph Bruno, Abington Memorial Hospital, Abington

Martin Chatzinoff, Abington Memorial Hospital, Abington

Marta Dabezies, Abington Memorial Hospital, Abington

Cesar de la Torre, Abington Memorial Hospital, Abington

Eric Goosenberg, Abington Memorial Hospital, Abington

Harvey Guttmann, Abington Memorial Hospital, Abington

Barry Herman, Easton Hospital, Easton

William Ives, Ephrata Community Hospital, Ephrata

Stephen Kaufman, Abington Memorial Hospital, Abington

Chatargy Kaza, Easton Hospital, Easton

Steven Leskowitz, Abington Memorial Hospital, Abington

Stuart Lubinski, Abington Memorial Hospital, Abington

Manoj Mittal, Easton Hospital, Easton

Shanker Mukherjee, Easton Hospital, Easton

Anne Saris, Abington Memorial Hospital, Abington

Ellen Shaw, Abington Memorial Hospital, Abington

Robert Stein, Abington Memorial Hospital, Abington

Jonathan Sternlieb, Abington Memorial Hospital, Abington

Lindsley Van der Veer, Easton Hospital, Easton

GENERAL SURGERY

Donna Angotti, Abington Memorial Hospital, Abington

Robert Bloch, Easton Hospital, Easton

Fernando Bonanni, Abington Memorial Hospital, Abington

Victor Dy, Easton Hospital, Easton

Steven Fassler, Abington Memorial Hospital, Abington

Arthur Frankel, Abington Memorial Hospital, Abington

Ala Frey, Abington Memorial Hospital, Abington

Barry Glaser, Abington Memorial Hospital, Abington

Harsh Grewal, Abington Memorial Hospital, Abington

Steven Harper, Abington Memorial Hospital, Abington

Robert Josloff, Abington Memorial Hospital, Abington

Robert Jubelirer, Abington Memorial Hospital, Abington

Jeffrey Kolff, Abington Memorial Hospital, Abington

James Koren, Easton Hospital, Easton

John Kukora, Abington Memorial Hospital, Abington

James McClurken, Abington Memorial Hospital, Abington

William Meyers, Abington Memorial Hospital, Abington

James Moore, Abington Memorial Hospital, Abington

Joseph Nejman, Abington Memorial Hospital, Abington

Seth Newman, Abington Memorial Hospital, Abington

Michael Nussbaum, Abington Memorial Hospital, Abington

Diane Opatt, Abington Memorial Hospital, Abington

Ho Pak, Abington Memorial Hospital, Abington

Richard Parsons, Abington Memorial Hospital, Abington

Christopher Pezzi, Abington Memorial Hospital, Abington

Bhoompally Reddy, Easton Hospital, Easton

Chand Rohatgi, Easton Hospital, Easton

Robert Schmutzler, Abington Memorial Hospital, Abington

Theodore Sullivan, Abington Memorial Hospital, Abington

William Weintraub, Abington Memorial Hospital, Abington

James Yuschak, Abington Memorial Hospital, Abington

D. Zelbey, Abington Memorial Hospital, Abington

NEUROLOGY

Giriwarlal Gupta, Pocono Medical Center, East Stroudsburg

Alex Perez, Pocono Medical Center, East Stroudsburg

OBSTETRICS/GYNECOLOGY

Comprehensive Women's Health Services A Woman's Care, Pottsville Hospital and Warne Clinic, Pottsville

Timothy Grube, Pottsville Hospital and Warne Clinic, Pottsville

Ilene Katz-Weizer, Pottsville Hospital and Warne Clinic, Pottsville

David Krewson, Pottsville Hospital and Warne Clinic, Pottsville

J. Lee, Pottsville Hospital and Warne Clinic, Pottsville

Myron Levine, Pottsville Hospital and Warne Clinic, Pottsville

James Xenophon, Pottsville Hospital and Warne Clinic, Pottsville

Top doctors are those that practice at hospitals that are rated in the top 10% in the nation for that clinical program area. For more information on how top doctors were selected, see Appendix.

Robert Zimmerman, Pottsville Hospital and Warne Clinic, Pottsville

ORTHOPEDIC SURGERY

Arthur Bartolozzi, Pennsylvania Hospital, Philadelphia
Robert Bischoff, Hanover General Hospital, Hanover
Robert Booth, Pennsylvania Hospital, Philadelphia

Samuel D'Agata, Hanover General Hospital, Hanover
James Ellison, Hanover General Hospital, Hanover
Francis Kilkelly, Hanover General Hospital, Hanover
Thomas Raley Jr., Hanover General Hospital, Hanover

SPINE SURGERY

Richard Balderston, Pennsylvania Hospital, Philadelphia
Francis Kilkelly, Hanover General Hospital, Hanover
Scott Rushton, Pennsylvania Hospital, Philadelphia

VASCULAR SURGERY

Carl Lauer, St. Vincent Health Center, Erie

RHODE ISLAND TOP DOCTORS

GASTROINTESTINAL

Alyn Adrain, Memorial Hospital of Rhode Island, Pawtucket
Evan Cohen, Memorial Hospital of Rhode Island, Pawtucket
Neil Greenspan, Memorial Hospital of Rhode Island, Pawtucket
Brett Kalmowitz, Memorial Hospital of Rhode Island, Pawtucket
Herbert Rakatansky, Memorial Hospital of Rhode Island, Pawtucket

David Schreiber, Memorial Hospital of Rhode Island, Pawtucket
Samir Shah, Memorial Hospital of Rhode Island, Pawtucket
Jeremy Spector, Memorial Hospital of Rhode Island, Pawtucket

NEUROLOGY

Motasem Al-Yacoub, Memorial Hospital of Rhode Island, Pawtucket

Joseph Centofanti, Memorial Hospital of Rhode Island, Pawtucket
Richard Cervone, Memorial Hospital of Rhode Island, Pawtucket
Mason Gaspar, Memorial Hospital of Rhode Island, Pawtucket
Michelle Mellion, Memorial Hospital of Rhode Island, Pawtucket

SOUTH CAROLINA TOP DOCTORS

CARDIAC SURGERY

Michael Bucci, St. Francis Hospital, Greenville
Christie Mina, St. Francis Hospital, Greenville

ORTHOPEDIC SURGERY

Arnold Batson, St. Francis Hospital, Greenville
Thomas Baumgarten, St. Francis Hospital, Greenville
Edward Blocker, Beaufort Memorial Hospital, Beaufort
Mark Dean, Beaufort Memorial Hospital, Beaufort
William DeVault, St. Francis Hospital, Greenville
James Jennings, St. Francis Hospital, Greenville

W. Jernigan, St. Francis Hospital, Greenville
H. Jones, Beaufort Memorial Hospital, Beaufort
Chris Kavolus, St. Francis Hospital, Greenville
Daniel Lee, St. Francis Hospital, Greenville
Silas Lucas, St. Francis Hospital, Greenville
Ralph Moore, Beaufort Memorial Hospital, Beaufort
Michael O'Boyle, St. Francis Hospital, Greenville
Thomas Pace, St. Francis Hospital, Greenville
John Paylor, St. Francis Hospital, Greenville
Allen Posta, St. Francis Hospital, Greenville
Stephen Ridgeway, St. Francis Hospital, Greenville
John Rowell, St. Francis Hospital, Greenville

Ralph Salzer, Beaufort Memorial Hospital, Beaufort
Leland Stoddard, Beaufort Memorial Hospital, Beaufort
Michael Tollison, St. Francis Hospital, Greenville
John Vann, St. Francis Hospital, Greenville
Christopher VanPelt, St. Francis Hospital, Greenville

SPINE SURGERY

Jeffery Reuben, Beaufort Memorial Hospital, Beaufort
Scott Strohmeyer, Beaufort Memorial Hospital, Beaufort

SOUTH DAKOTA TOP DOCTORS

CARDIOLOGY

Mark Fox, Avera Heart Hospital of South Dakota, Sioux Falls
Carol Miles, Avera Heart Hospital of South Dakota, Sioux Falls
O. Opheim, Avera Heart Hospital of South Dakota, Sioux Falls
Harlan Payne, Avera Heart Hospital of South Dakota, Sioux Falls

Michael Puumala, Avera Heart Hospital of South Dakota, Sioux Falls
William Rossing, Avera Heart Hospital of South Dakota, Sioux Falls
Daniel Tynan, Avera Heart Hospital of South Dakota, Sioux Falls
Lisa Viola, Avera Heart Hospital of South Dakota, Sioux Falls
Todd Zimprich, Avera Heart Hospital of South Dakota, Sioux Falls

NEUROLOGY

Carol Miles, Avera McKennan Hospital and University Health Center, Sioux Falls
O. Opheim, Avera McKennan Hospital and University Health Center, Sioux Falls
Harlan Payne, Avera McKennan Hospital and University Health Center, Sioux Falls
William Rossing, Avera McKennan Hospital and University Health Center, Sioux Falls

Lisa Viola, Avera McKennan Hospital and University Health Center, Sioux Falls
Todd Zimprich, Avera McKennan Hospital and University Health Center, Sioux Falls

ORTHOPEDIC SURGERY

James MacDougall, Dakota Plains Surgical Center, Aberdeen
James Mantone, Dakota Plains Surgical Center, Aberdeen
Chester Mayo, Dakota Plains Surgical Center, Aberdeen

Matthew Reynen, Dakota Plains Surgical Center, Aberdeen
Gerald Rieber, Prairie Lakes Hospital and Care Center, Watertown
Michael Vener, Prairie Lakes Hospital and Care Center, Watertown

TENNESSEE TOP DOCTORS

CARDIAC SURGERY

Larry Burke, Baptist Memorial Hospital, Memphis
Russell Carter, Baptist Memorial Hospital, Memphis
Jerry Gooch, Baptist Memorial Hospital, Memphis
Harold Head, Memorial Healthcare System, Chattanooga
James Headrick, Memorial Healthcare System, Chattanooga
Patricio Ilabaca, Baptist Memorial Hospital, Memphis
Stephen Martin, Memorial Healthcare System, Chattanooga
Richard Morrison, Memorial Healthcare System, Chattanooga
E. Robbins, Baptist Memorial Hospital, Memphis
Bradley Wolf, Baptist Memorial Hospital, Memphis
Rodney Wolf, Baptist Memorial Hospital, Memphis
James Zellner, Memorial Healthcare System, Chattanooga

GASTROENTEROLOGY

University Surgical Associates Group, Memorial Healthcare System, Chattanooga

GASTROINTESTINAL

Coleman Arnold, Memorial Healthcare System, Chattanooga
Matthew Bagamery, Memorial Healthcare System, Chattanooga
Robert Barnett, Memorial Healthcare System, Chattanooga
Sumeet Bhushan, Memorial Healthcare System, Chattanooga
Paul Bierman, Baptist Memorial Hospital, Memphis
Chad Charapata, Memorial Healthcare System, Chattanooga
William Cockerham, Memorial Healthcare System, Chattanooga

David Collins, Memorial Healthcare System, Chattanooga
Kenneth Fields, Baptist Memorial Hospital, Memphis
Michael Goodman, Memorial Healthcare System, Chattanooga
John Gwin, Memorial Healthcare System, Chattanooga
Donald Hetzel, Memorial Healthcare System, Chattanooga
Marshall Horton, Memorial Healthcare System, Chattanooga
Isaac Jalfon, Baptist Memorial Hospital, Memphis
Richard Jennings III, Memorial Healthcare System, Chattanooga
Steven Kennedy, Memorial Healthcare System, Chattanooga
Martin Krecker, Memorial Healthcare System, Chattanooga
Roger Land, Memorial Healthcare System, Chattanooga
Myron Lewis, Baptist Memorial Hospital, Memphis
Gerald Lieberman, Baptist Memorial Hospital, Memphis
Donald Mackler, Memorial Healthcare System, Chattanooga
James Manton, Memorial Healthcare System, Chattanooga
Michael Mena, Memorial Healthcare System, Chattanooga
Richard Moore, Memorial Healthcare System, Chattanooga
Henry Paik, Memorial Healthcare System, Chattanooga
Ih-Koo Park, Memorial Healthcare System, Chattanooga
Manisha Patel, Memorial Healthcare System, Chattanooga
Jay Philippose, Memorial Healthcare System, Chattanooga
Charles Portera, Memorial Healthcare System, Chattanooga

Andrew Rittenberry, Memorial Healthcare System, Chattanooga
Walter Rose, Memorial Healthcare System, Chattanooga
Richard Sadowitz, Memorial Healthcare System, Chattanooga
Colleen Schmitt, Memorial Healthcare System, Chattanooga
Alan Shikoh, Memorial Healthcare System, Chattanooga
Edwin Shuck, Memorial Healthcare System, Chattanooga
Larry Shuster, Memorial Healthcare System, Chattanooga
John Stanley, Memorial Healthcare System, Chattanooga
Alvaro Valle, Memorial Healthcare System, Chattanooga
Douglas Vanderbilt, Memorial Healthcare System, Chattanooga
John Whitworth, Baptist Memorial Hospital, Memphis
Lawrence Wruble, Baptist Memorial Hospital, Memphis
Munford Yates, Memorial Healthcare System, Chattanooga

NEUROLOGY

Feiyu Chen, Baptist Memorial Hospital, Memphis
Michael Deshazo, Baptist Memorial Hospital, Memphis
Elias Giraldo, Baptist Memorial Hospital, Memphis
Michael Levin, Baptist Memorial Hospital, Memphis
Daniel Menkes, Baptist Memorial Hospital, Memphis
Moacir Schnapp, Baptist Memorial Hospital, Memphis
Lance Wright, Baptist Memorial Hospital, Memphis

Top doctors are those that practice at hospitals that are rated in the top 10% in the nation for that clinical program area. For more information on how top doctors were selected, see Appendix.

ORTHOPEDIC SURGERY

Paul Apyan, Memorial Healthcare System, Chattanooga

William Ballard, Memorial Healthcare System, Chattanooga

Todd Bell, Memorial Healthcare System, Chattanooga

Thomas Brown, Memorial Healthcare System, Chattanooga

William Bruce, Memorial Healthcare System, Chattanooga

Channappa Chandra, Memorial Healthcare System, Chattanooga

Eric Clarke, Memorial Healthcare System, Chattanooga

Thomas Currey, Memorial Healthcare System, Chattanooga

Richard Donaldson, Memorial Healthcare System, Chattanooga

Mark Freeman, Memorial Healthcare System, Chattanooga

William Hartley, Memorial Healthcare System, Chattanooga

Dale Ingram, Memorial Healthcare System, Chattanooga

Robert Mastey, Memorial Healthcare System, Chattanooga

William Matthews, Memorial Healthcare System, Chattanooga

John Nash, Memorial Healthcare System, Chattanooga

Alan Odom, Memorial Healthcare System, Chattanooga

Martin Redish, Memorial Healthcare System, Chattanooga

Chad Smalley, Memorial Healthcare System, Chattanooga

Neil Spitalny, Memorial Healthcare System, Chattanooga

Mark Sumida, Memorial Healthcare System, Chattanooga

W. Tew, Memorial Healthcare System, Chattanooga

VASCULAR SURGERY

Gerald Chapman, Cookeville Regional Medical Center, Cookeville

Scott Copeland, Cookeville Regional Medical Center, Cookeville

Brian Gerndt, Cookeville Regional Medical Center, Cookeville

Jeffrey McCarter, Cookeville Regional Medical Center, Cookeville

R. Wilson, Cookeville Regional Medical Center, Cookeville

TEXAS TOP DOCTORS

CARDIAC SURGERY

Lawrence Breitkreutz, Abilene Regional Medical Center, Abilene

David Carlson, Abilene Regional Medical Center, Abilene

Scott Crocker, Abilene Regional Medical Center, Abilene

GASTROINTESTINAL

Rajeshwar Abrol, Houston Northwest Medical Center, Houston

Darshan Anandu, Houston Northwest Medical Center, Houston

S. Badiga, Knapp Medical Center, Weslaco

Scott Becker, South Austin Hospital, Austin

Arturo Bravo, Knapp Medical Center, Weslaco

Sheela Chandra, Houston Northwest Medical Center, Houston

Lynn Copeland, Houston Northwest Medical Center, Houston

Edgar Cruz, Knapp Medical Center, Weslaco

Ali Dural, Houston Northwest Medical Center, Houston

Ben Echols, Houston Northwest Medical Center, Houston

Sandra Esquivel, Knapp Medical Center, Weslaco

Sohaib Faruqi, Houston Northwest Medical Center, Houston

David Folkers, South Austin Hospital, Austin

Jean-Pierre Forage, South Austin Hospital, Austin

Harish Gagneja, South Austin Hospital, Austin

Anna Gonzalez, Houston Northwest Medical Center, Houston

Rodolfo Guerrero, Knapp Medical Center, Weslaco

Maninder Guram, Houston Northwest Medical Center, Houston

Howard Hamat, Houston Northwest Medical Center, Houston

Chia-Wen Hsu, South Austin Hospital, Austin

Ayub Hussain, Houston Northwest Medical Center, Houston

Venodhar Julapalli, Houston Northwest Medical Center, Houston

S. A. Khan, Houston Northwest Medical Center, Houston

Udayini Kodali, Houston Northwest Medical Center, Houston

Eduardo Kofman, Valley Regional Medical Center, Brownsville

Beverly Lewis, Mainland Medical Center, Texas City

Gurinder Luthra, Houston Northwest Medical Center, Houston

Oscar Maldonado, Valley Regional Medical Center, Brownsville

Stephen Marcum, Mainland Medical Center, Texas City

Ilyas Memon, Houston Northwest Medical Center, Houston

Ravi Moparty, Houston Northwest Medical Center, Houston

Swaminathan Muralikrishna, Mainland Medical Center, Texas City

Ranga Nathan, Houston Northwest Medical Center, Houston

Ahmad Pacha, Houston Northwest Medical Center, Houston

Hari Pokala, Houston Northwest Medical Center, Houston

Carlos Ponce, Valley Regional Medical Center, Brownsville

Roberto Ponce, Valley Regional Medical Center, Brownsville

Guru Reddy, Houston Northwest Medical Center, Houston

Dan Rice, South Austin Hospital, Austin

Diane Robinson, Mainland Medical Center, Texas City

Ricardo Solis, South Austin Hospital, Austin

Kalyanam Subramanyam, Mainland Medical Center, Texas City

Douglas Thurman, Houston Northwest Medical Center, Houston

Steven Ugbarugba, Houston Northwest Medical Center, Houston

Stephen Utts, South Austin Hospital, Austin

Duc Vuong, Mainland Medical Center, Texas City

Abraham Winkelstein, Houston Northwest Medical Center, Houston

GENERAL SURGERY

Juliane Bingener-Casey, University Health System, San Antonio

Damian Chaupin, Houston Northwest Medical Center, Houston

Felix Cherico, St. David's Hospital, Austin

Peter Ching, St. David's Hospital, Austin

Peter Ching, South Austin Hospital, Austin

Stephen Clark, St. David's Hospital, Austin

Collom and Carney Clinic Association, Christus St. Michael Health System, Texarkana

Byron Cook, Good Shepherd Medical Center, Longview

Alfonso Cordoba, Houston Northwest Medical Center, Houston

Michael Corneille, University Health System, San Antonio

Daniel Dent, University Health System, San Antonio

Patrick Dillawn, St. David's Hospital, Austin

Richard Ehlers, Clear Lake Regional Medical Center, Webster

Alex Esquivel, South Austin Hospital, Austin

Steven Fass, South Austin Hospital, Austin

Tim Faulkenberry, St. David's Hospital, Austin

Anthony Fillmore, Baptist St. Anthony's Health System, Amarillo

Richard Fleming, St. David's Hospital, Austin

David Folkers, South Austin Hospital, Austin

Sashidhar Ganta, St. David's Hospital, Austin

David Gelber, Clear Lake Regional Medical Center, Webster

Philip Greger, Houston Northwest Medical Center, Houston

C. Hearn, Clear Lake Regional Medical Center, Webster

Matt Holcomb, Good Shepherd Medical Center, Longview

Jose Iglesias, Houston Northwest Medical Center, Houston

Kent Johnson, Houston Northwest Medical Center, Houston

Morton Kahlenberg, University Health System, San Antonio

Dean Kocay, South Austin Hospital, Austin

David Langley, Baptist St. Anthony's Health System, Amarillo

Michael Lary, Baptist St. Anthony's Health System, Amarillo

Philip Leggett, Houston Northwest Medical Center, Houston

Peter Lopez, University Health System, San Antonio

Rafael Lugo, Clear Lake Regional Medical Center, Webster

J. Mack, Good Shepherd Medical Center, Longview

Robert Markus, South Austin Hospital, Austin

Nancy Marquez, St. David's Hospital, Austin

William Mayer, St. David's Hospital, Austin

John McKinley, Baptist St. Anthony's Health System, Amarillo

Daniel Merritt, Good Shepherd Medical Center, Longview

Allen Milewicz, Clear Lake Regional Medical Center, Webster

Enrique Moncada, Valley Regional Medical Center, Brownsville

John Myers, University Health System, San Antonio

Cesar Nahas, Clear Lake Regional Medical Center, Webster

J. Neilson, Baptist St. Anthony's Health System, Amarillo

Khoa Nguyen, Houston Northwest Medical Center, Houston

Taylor Pickett, Houston Northwest Medical Center, Houston

Precision Surgery, Christus St. Michael Health System, Texarkana

Juan Rodriguez, Valley Regional Medical Center, Brownsville

Hector Salcedo-Dovi, Valley Regional Medical Center, Brownsville

Wayne Schwesinger, University Health System, San Antonio

H. Shin, St. David's Hospital, Austin

H. Shin, South Austin Hospital, Austin

Kenneth Sirinek, University Health System, San Antonio

Floyd Smith, St. David's Hospital, Austin

Brad Snyder, Houston Northwest Medical Center, Houston

Gustavo Stern, Valley Regional Medical Center, Brownsville

Ronald Stewart, University Health System, San Antonio

Surgery Associates of Texarkana, Christus St. Michael Health System, Texarkana

Phillip Sutton, Houston Northwest Medical Center, Houston

Dexter Turnquest, Houston Northwest Medical Center, Houston

Kent Van Sickle, University Health System, San Antonio

Texarkana Gastroenterology Consultants, P.A., Christus St. Michael Health System, Texarkana

Todd Waltrip, Good Shepherd Medical Center, Longview

John Winston, University Health System, San Antonio

Steven Wolf, University Health System, San Antonio

Eduardo Wolffe, Clear Lake Regional Medical Center, Webster

In Yo, Clear Lake Regional Medical Center, Webster

NEUROLOGY

Luis Gaitan, Valley Regional Medical Center, Brownsville

Robert Lozano, Valley Regional Medical Center, Brownsville

OBSTETRICS/GYNECOLOGY

Dennis Abbas, Woman's Hospital at Dallas Regional Medical Center, Mesquite

Lillian Abbott, Clear Lake Regional Medical Center, Webster

Anu Adeyemi, Woman's Hospital at Dallas Regional Medical Center, Mesquite

Carlos Almaguer, Rio Grande Regional Hospital, McAllen

James Biddle, Rio Grande Regional Hospital, McAllen

Bryan Blonder, Oakbend Medical Center, Richmond

Roberta Braun, St. David's Hospital, Austin

Cheryl Butler, St. David's Hospital, Austin

Salvador Cardenas, Rio Grande Regional Hospital, McAllen

Kimberly Carter, St. David's Hospital, Austin

R. Chouteau, St. David's Hospital, Austin

Linda Chung, Clear Lake Regional Medical Center, Webster

Sami Constantine, Woman's Hospital at Dallas Regional Medical Center, Mesquite

Cesar Coronado, Rio Grande Regional Hospital, McAllen

Shannon Crowe, Oakbend Medical Center, Richmond

Robert Crumb, St. David's Hospital, Austin

Deya Dafashy, Clear Lake Regional Medical Center, Webster

Hearther Daley, Rio Grande Regional Hospital, McAllen

Alecia Davis-Townsend, Clear Lake Regional Medical Center, Webster

Noble Doss, St. David's Hospital, Austin

Alberto Duran, Rio Grande Regional Hospital, McAllen

Steven Edmondson, Clear Lake Regional Medical Center, Webster

Diane Evering-Simms, Marshall Regional Medical Center, Marshall

Jose Fernandez, Rio Grande Regional Hospital, McAllen

Beth Files, Clear Lake Regional Medical Center, Webster

Joi Findley-Smith, Clear Lake Regional Medical Center, Webster

John Fitzwater, St. David's Hospital, Austin

Janet Frost, Woman's Hospital at Dallas Regional Medical Center, Mesquite

Charles Gaskin, Marshall Regional Medical Center, Marshall

Aurther Gore, St. David's Hospital, Austin

J. Grant, Woman's Hospital at Dallas Regional Medical Center, Mesquite

John Cuerra, Rio Grande Regional Hospital, McAllen

Stephen Guilliams, West Houston Medical Center, Houston

Glenford Guy, Rio Grande Regional Hospital, McAllen

Melissa Guzman-Winn, St. David's Hospital, Austin

Jeff Hagen, St. David's Hospital, Austin

Jacobo Hohenstein, Rio Grande Regional Hospital, McAllen

Angela Houghton, Clear Lake Regional Medical Center, Webster

Otohiel Huertas, Woman's Hospital at Dallas Regional Medical Center, Mesquite

Felix Hull, St. David's Hospital, Austin

Jeanie Huynh, West Houston Medical Center, Houston

Li-Min Hwang, Clear Lake Regional Medical Center, Webster

LaTasha Jarrett, Woman's Hospital at Dallas Regional Medical Center, Mesquite

Danielle Jimenez-Flores, Rio Grande Regional Hospital, McAllen

Gholam Kiani-Khozani, Rio Grande Regional Hospital, McAllen

Geffrey Klein, Clear Lake Regional Medical Center, Webster

Mary Klenz, Rio Grande Regional Hospital, McAllen

Stephanie Kodack, St. David's Hospital, Austin

Matti Korhonen, West Houston Medical Center, Houston

Erwin Korman, Clear Lake Regional Medical Center, Webster

Terrence Kuhlmann, St. David's Hospital, Austin

Ramiro Leal, Rio Grande Regional Hospital, McAllen

Peter Lotze, Clear Lake Regional Medical Center, Webster

Mikeal Love, St. David's Hospital, Austin

Anna Lozano, St. David's Hospital, Austin

Rodolfo Lozano, Rio Grande Regional Hospital, McAllen

Michael Magliolo, Clear Lake Regional Medical Center, Webster

Jewell Malick, Woman's Hospital at Dallas Regional Medical Center, Mesquite

C. McCathran, Marshall Regional Medical Center, Marshall

Orsel McGhee, Woman's Hospital at Dallas Regional Medical Center, Mesquite

Douglas McIntyre, St. David's Hospital, Austin

Cynthia Mingea, St. David's Hospital, Austin

Jorge Miranda, Rio Grande Regional Hospital, McAllen

Mary Mirto, St. David's Hospital, Austin

Brian Monks, St. David's Hospital, Austin

Guillermo Montanez, Rio Grande Regional Hospital, McAllen

Namitha Nagaraj, Rio Grande Regional Hospital, McAllen

Virginia Nisbet, Clear Lake Regional Medical Center, Webster

John O'Connor IV, Rio Grande Regional Hospital, McAllen

Mahendra Patel, Woman's Hospital at Dallas Regional Medical Center, Mesquite

Ricky Paul, Marshall Regional Medical Center, Marshall

Claude Perkins, Rio Grande Regional Hospital, McAllen

Michael Petitt, Clear Lake Regional Medical Center, Webster

Mary Poag, Clear Lake Regional Medical Center, Webster

Clive Polon, St. David's Hospital, Austin

Carol Poole, Woman's Hospital at Dallas Regional Medical Center, Mesquite

Bradley Price, St. David's Hospital, Austin

Roberto Prieto-Harris, Rio Grande Regional Hospital, McAllen

Nagamani Rao, Clear Lake Regional Medical Center, Webster

Maureen Ribail, Woman's Hospital at Dallas Regional Medical Center, Mesquite

Juan Rivera, Rio Grande Regional Hospital, McAllen

Magdy Rizk, West Houston Medical Center, Houston

Eduardo Robles-Emanuelli, Rio Grande Regional Hospital, McAllen

Edgar Rodriguez, Rio Grande Regional Hospital, McAllen

Maria Rodriguez de Lima, Rio Grande Regional Hospital, McAllen

Amber Salas, Marshall Regional Medical Center, Marshall

Kiran Shah, Clear Lake Regional Medical Center, Webster

Clayton Shaw, Woman's Hospital at Dallas Regional Medical Center, Mesquite

Rose Simani, Woman's Hospital at Dallas Regional Medical Center, Mesquite

Lenora Smith, St. David's Hospital, Austin

Robert Sorin, St. David's Hospital, Austin

Shraddha Talati, Woman's Hospital at Dallas Regional Medical Center, Mesquite

Marwan Tamim, Woman's Hospital at Dallas Regional Medical Center, Mesquite

Bassem Tawadrous, Clear Lake Regional Medical Center, Webster

Peggy Taylor, Clear Lake Regional Medical Center, Webster

Roosevelt Taylor, Woman's Hospital at Dallas Regional Medical Center, Mesquite

Alejandro Tey, Rio Grande Regional Hospital, McAllen

Reena Tharappel-Jacob, Clear Lake Regional Medical Center, Webster

Emilio Torres, St. David's Hospital, Austin

Steven Trostel, Woman's Hospital at Dallas Regional Medical Center, Mesquite

Rod Turner, Clear Lake Regional Medical Center, Webster

Luis Usuga, Woman's Hospital at Dallas Regional Medical Center, Mesquite

Francoise Vandaele, Clear Lake Regional Medical Center, Webster

Efraim Vela, Rio Grande Regional Hospital, McAllen

Christiaan Webb, Rio Grande Regional Hospital, McAllen

Christopher Wilson, St. David's Hospital, Austin

Wayne Wilson, Rio Grande Regional Hospital, McAllen

Douglas Wohlfahrt, West Houston Medical Center, Houston

Michael Yang, Woman's Hospital at Dallas Regional Medical Center, Mesquite

Jeffrey Youngkin, St. David's Hospital, Austin

Hugo Zapata, Rio Grande Regional Hospital, McAllen

ORTHOPEDIC SURGERY

Michael Andreo, Seton Medical Center, Austin

Austin Brain and Spine, Seton Medical Center, Austin

Robert Bell, Austin Surgical Hospital, Austin

Robert Bell, El Paso Specialty Hospital, El Paso
Shelby Carter, Seton Medical Center, Austin
Central Texas Spine Institute, Seton Medical Center, Austin
Collom and Carney Clinic Association, Christus St. Michael Health System, Texarkana
Don Davis, Seton Medical Center, Austin
John Dean, Midland Memorial Hospital, Midland
Franklin Dzida, Medical Center Hospital, Odessa
Jonathan Fontenot, Good Shepherd Medical Center, Longview
Orlando Garza, Medical Center Hospital, Odessa
John Genung, Seton Medical Center, Austin
Timothy Gueramy, Seton Medical Center, Austin
Malone Hill, Seton Medical Center, Austin
Terren Klein, Austin Surgical Hospital, Austin
Terren Klein, El Paso Specialty Hospital, El Paso
Stephen Littlejohn, Good Shepherd Medical Center, Longview
Michael Loeb, Seton Medical Center, Austin
Medical Park Orthopedic Clinic Association, Seton Medical Center, Austin
The Orthopaedic Group, Seton Medical Center, Austin
Orthopedic Specialists of Texarkana, P.L.L.C., Christus St. Michael Health System, Texarkana
William Parker, Seton Medical Center, Austin

Johan Penninck, Austin Surgical Hospital, Austin
David Power, Midland Memorial Hospital, Midland
Kenneth Reesor, Good Shepherd Medical Center, Longview
W. Schultz, Seton Medical Center, Austin
Jack Seaquist, Seton Medical Center, Austin
Eric Sides, Austin Surgical Hospital, Austin
Eric Sides, El Paso Specialty Hospital, El Paso
Spine and Rehabilitation Center, Seton Medical Center, Austin
Jordan Stanley, Good Shepherd Medical Center, Longview
Thomas Taylor, Good Shepherd Medical Center, Longview
Richard Westbrook, Austin Surgical Hospital, Austin
Richard Westbrook, El Paso Specialty Hospital, El Paso
Archie Whittemore, Seton Medical Center, Austin

SPINE SURGERY

Randall Dryer, Seton Medical Center, Austin
Matthew Geck, Seton Medical Center, Austin
Matthew Hummell, Seton Medical Center, Austin
Craig Kemper, Seton Medical Center, Austin
Jason Lowenstein, Seton Medical Center, Austin
Okay Onan, Seton Medical Center, Austin

James Smith, Seton Medical Center, Austin
John Stokes, Seton Medical Center, Austin
William Taylor, Seton Medical Center, Austin
George Tipton, Seton Medical Center, Austin
Viet Tran, Seton Medical Center, Austin
Hari Tumu, Seton Medical Center, Austin
Kurt Von Rueden, Seton Medical Center, Austin
Ronald Wilson, Seton Medical Center, Austin

VASCULAR SURGERY

Bill Chang, Clear Lake Regional Medical Center, Webster
Collom and Carney Clinic Association, Christus St. Michael Health System, Texarkana
Robert Connaughton, Denton Regional Medical Center, Denton
Carlos Cruz, Denton Regional Medical Center, Denton
Christos Katsigiannis, Clear Lake Regional Medical Center, Webster
Gordon Martin, Clear Lake Regional Medical Center, Webster
Cesar Nahas, Clear Lake Regional Medical Center, Webster
Precision Surgery, Christus St. Michael Health System, Texarkana
Surgery Associates of Texarkana, Christus St. Michael Health System, Texarkana

---

UTAH TOP DOCTORS

GENERAL SURGERY

Richard Alder, Ogden Regional Medical Center, Ogden
Steven Carabine, Ogden Regional Medical Center, Ogden
Sheila Garvey, Ogden Regional Medical Center, Ogden
Edward Jordan, Ogden Regional Medical Center, Ogden
John Miller, Dixie Regional Medical Center, St. George
Brad Myers, Dixie Regional Medical Center, St. George
J. Speakman, Dixie Regional Medical Center, St. George
Karen Tormey, Dixie Regional Medical Center, St. George
Gregory Watson, Dixie Regional Medical Center, St. George
Robert Whipple, Ogden Regional Medical Center, Ogden
Bruce Williams, Dixie Regional Medical Center, St. George
Richard Wintch, Dixie Regional Medical Center, St. George

OBSTETRICS/GYNECOLOGY

Jon Ahlstrom, Ogden Regional Medical Center, Ogden
Craig Astle, Dixie Regional Medical Center, St. George
Brady Benham, Dixie Regional Medical Center, St. George
Grant Carter, Dixie Regional Medical Center, St. George
Robert Chalmers, Dixie Regional Medical Center, St. George
Joan Eggert, Dixie Regional Medical Center, St. George
Robert Fagnant, Dixie Regional Medical Center, St. George
Albert Hartman, Ogden Regional Medical Center, Ogden
Darren Housel, Ogden Regional Medical Center, Ogden
Tracy Kvarfordt, Dixie Regional Medical Center, St. George

Chad Lunt, Dixie Regional Medical Center, St. George
Rodney Marriott, Ogden Regional Medical Center, Ogden
Jed Naisbitt, Ogden Regional Medical Center, Ogden
Richard Ott, Dixie Regional Medical Center, St. George
Jeffrey Rogers, Dixie Regional Medical Center, St. George
Larry Smithing, Ogden Regional Medical Center, Ogden
Joy Welsh, Dixie Regional Medical Center, St. George
Tracy Winward, Dixie Regional Medical Center, St. George

ORTHOPEDIC SURGERY

Michael Bourne, St. Mark's Hospital, Salt Lake City
David Curtis, St. Mark's Hospital, Salt Lake City
Robert Hansen, St. Mark's Hospital, Salt Lake City
E. Mariani, St. Mark's Hospital, Salt Lake City
Peter Novak, St. Mark's Hospital, Salt Lake City

CARDIAC SURGERY

Hormoz Azar, Sentara Norfolk General Hospital, Norfolk

Lenox Baker, Sentara Norfolk General Hospital, Norfolk

Wayne Derkac, Sentara Norfolk General Hospital, Norfolk

Kirk Fleischer, Sentara Norfolk General Hospital, Norfolk

Michael McGrath, Sentara Norfolk General Hospital, Norfolk

Joseph Newton, Sentara Norfolk General Hospital, Norfolk

Jeffrey Rich, Sentara Norfolk General Hospital, Norfolk

Scott Ross, Sentara Norfolk General Hospital, Norfolk

GENERAL SURGERY

David Caulkins, Augusta Medical Center, Fishersville

Douglas McKibbin, Augusta Medical Center, Fishersville

W. McKibbin, Augusta Medical Center, Fishersville

Joseph Ranzini, Augusta Medical Center, Fishersville

NEUROLOGY

Yamini Chennu, Henrico Doctors' Hospital, Richmond

Ken Ng, Henrico Doctors' Hospital, Richmond

John O'Bannon, Henrico Doctors' Hospital, Richmond

Alan Schulman, Henrico Doctors' Hospital, Richmond

Stephen Thurston, Henrico Doctors' Hospital, Richmond

ORTHOPEDIC SURGERY

Keith Albertson, Prince William Hospital, Manassas

Augusta Orthopedic Associates:, Augusta Medical Center, Fishersville

Kenneth Boatright, Augusta Medical Center, Fishersville

David Burgess, Augusta Medical Center, Fishersville

Ramon Esteban, Augusta Medical Center, Fishersville

Gabriel Gluck, Prince William Hospital, Manassas

George Godette, Augusta Medical Center, Fishersville

Lee Hereford, Augusta Medical Center, Fishersville

Christopher Highfill, Prince William Hospital, Manassas

W. Hosick, Prince William Hospital, Manassas

Subir Jossan, Prince William Hospital, Manassas

John Kim, Prince William Hospital, Manassas

Orthopedic Associates, Ltd., Augusta Medical Center, Fishersville

Jack Otteni, Augusta Medical Center, Fishersville

Kevin Peltier, Prince William Hospital, Manassas

Thomas Pereles, Augusta Medical Center, Fishersville

Matthew Pollard, Augusta Medical Center, Fishersville

SPINE SURGERY

James Melisi, Prince William Hospital, Manassas

Faisal Siddiqui, Prince William Hospital, Manassas

VASCULAR SURGERY

James Callis, Carilion Medical Center, Roanoke

Jesse Davidson, Carilion Medical Center, Roanoke

James Drougas, Carilion Medical Center, Roanoke

William H'Doubler, Carilion Medical Center, Roanoke

Stephen Hill, Carilion Medical Center, Roanoke

NEUROLOGY

Hojoong (Mike) Kim, Swedish Medical Center—Cherry Hills Campus, Seattle

Hojoong (Mike) Kim, Swedish Medical Center—First Hill, Seattle

Peter Balousek, Northwest Hospital and Medical Center, Seattle

William Berg, Swedish Medical Center—Cherry Hills Campus, Seattle

William Berg, Swedish Medical Center—First Hill, Seattle

Todd Czartoski, Swedish Medical Center—Cherry Hills Campus, Seattle

Todd Czartoski, Swedish Medical Center—First Hill, Seattle

Michael Doherty, Swedish Medical Center—Cherry Hills Campus, Seattle

Michael Doherty, Swedish Medical Center—First Hill, Seattle

Victor Erlich, Northwest Hospital and Medical Center, Seattle

James Gordon, Northwest Hospital and Medical Center, Seattle

Ryder Gwinn, Northwest Hospital and Medical Center, Seattle

Aaron Heide, Swedish Medical Center—First Hill, Seattle

Aaron Heide, Swedish Medical Center—Cherry Hills Campus, Seattle

Diana Herring, Northwest Hospital and Medical Center, Seattle

Stephen Houston, Northwest Hospital and Medical Center, Seattle

Marc Kirschner, Northwest Hospital and Medical Center, Seattle

Steve Klein, Northwest Hospital and Medical Center, Seattle

Jon Kooiker, Providence St. Peter Hospital, Olympia

Bjorn Krane, Northwest Hospital and Medical Center, Seattle

Daniel Lazar, Northwest Hospital and Medical Center, Seattle

William Likosky, Swedish Medical Center—Cherry Hills Campus, Seattle

William Likosky, Swedish Medical Center—First Hill, Seattle

Richard Marks, Northwest Hospital and Medical Center, Seattle

Marc Mayberg, Northwest Hospital and Medical Center, Seattle

James McDowell, Providence St. Peter Hospital, Olympia

David Newell, Northwest Hospital and Medical Center, Seattle

James Raisis, Northwest Hospital and Medical Center, Seattle

Stanley Schiff, Northwest Hospital and Medical Center, Seattle

Nancy Schuman, Northwest Hospital and Medical Center, Seattle

Sheila Smith, Swedish Medical Center—Cherry Hills Campus, Seattle

Sheila Smith, Swedish Medical Center—First Hill, Seattle

Christopher Smythies, Northwest Hospital and Medical Center, Seattle

Jayashree Srinivasan, Northwest Hospital and Medical Center, Seattle

Timothy Steege, Northwest Hospital and Medical Center, Seattle

Gary Stobbe, Swedish Medical Center–Cherry Hills Campus, Seattle

Gary Stobbe, Swedish Medical Center–First Hill, Seattle

Jacob Young, Northwest Hospital and Medical Center, Seattle

Ronald Young, Northwest Hospital and Medical Center, Seattle

OBSTETRICS/GYNECOLOGY

James Haines, Overlake Hospital Medical Center, Bellevue

Michael Lawler, Overlake Hospital Medical Center, Bellevue

ORTHOPEDIC SURGERY

L. Agtarap, Providence St. Peter Hospital, Olympia

Steven Boyea, Tri-State Memorial Hospital, Clarkston

Clyde Carpenter, Providence St. Peter Hospital, Olympia

Gregory Dietrich, Tri-State Memorial Hospital, Clarkston

Patrick Halpin, Capital Medical Center, Olympia

Patrick Halpin, Providence St. Peter Hospital, Olympia

Regan Hansen, Tri-State Memorial Hospital, Clarkston

Thomas Helpenstell, Providence St. Peter Hospital, Olympia

Richard Henderson, St. Mary Medical Center, Walla Walla

Ghalib Husseini, Providence St. Peter Hospital, Olympia

Orie Kaltenbaugh, Tri-State Memorial Hospital, Clarkston

Marvin Kym, Tri-State Memorial Hospital, Clarkston

Kenneth Partlow, Providence St. Peter Hospital, Olympia

William Peterson, Providence St. Peter Hospital, Olympia

Dennis Smith, Providence St. Peter Hospital, Olympia

Stephen Snow, Capital Medical Center, Olympia

Stephen Snow, Providence St. Peter Hospital, Olympia

Kirk Willard, St. Mary Medical Center, Walla Walla

P. Wood, Providence St. Peter Hospital, Olympia

Jerome Zechmann, Capital Medical Center, Olympia

Jerome Zechmann, Providence St. Peter Hospital, Olympia

SPINE SURGERY

Perry Camp, St. Mary Medical Center, Walla Walla

Clyde Carpenter, Capital Medical Center, Olympia

Guy Gehling, St. Mary Medical Center, Walla Walla

WEST VIRGINIA TOP DOCTORS

ORTHOPEDIC SURGERY

Ali Oliashirazi, Cabell-Huntington Hospital, Huntington

WISCONSIN TOP DOCTORS

CARDIAC SURGERY

Christopher Stone, United Hospital System, Kenosha

GASTROINTESTINAL

Roland Christian, St. Vincent Hospital, Green Bay

Peter Dzwonkowski, St. Vincent Hospital, Green Bay

Mark Laukka, St. Vincent Hospital, Green Bay

Mitchell Manthey, St. Vincent Hospital, Green Bay

Patrick Pfau, UW Health-UW Hospitals and Clinics, Madison

Mark Reichelderfer, UW Health-UW Hospitals and Clinics, Madison

Peter Stanko, St. Vincent Hospital, Green Bay

GENERAL SURGERY

James Kemmerling, St. Vincent Hospital, Green Bay

Patrick Kiefer, St. Vincent Hospital, Green Bay

Richard McNutt, St. Vincent Hospital, Green Bay

Paul Reckard, St. Vincent Hospital, Green Bay

Charles Saletta, St. Vincent Hospital, Green Bay

David Satchell, Holy Family Memorial, Manitowoc

Alan Sbar, Holy Family Memorial, Manitowoc

NEUROLOGY

Ofer Zikel, All Saints Medical Center–St. Mary's Campus, Racine

ORTHOPEDIC SURGERY

Roger Branham, Lakeview Medical Center, Rice Lake

John Cragg, Lakeview Medical Center, Rice Lake

James Dyreby, St. Mary's Hospital, Rhinelander

Thomas Florack, St. Mary's Hospital Medical Center, Green Bay

James Hinckley, St. Mary's Hospital Medical Center, Green Bay

Bryan Larson, Lakeview Medical Center, Rice Lake

Daniel Lochmann, Lakeview Medical Center, Rice Lake

Kent Lowry, St. Mary's Hospital, Rhinelander

Rolf Lulloff, St. Mary's Hospital Medical Center, Green Bay

Michael O'Reilly, St. Mary's Hospital Medical Center, Green Bay

William Padgett, St. Mary's Hospital, Rhinelander

Mark Schick, St. Mary's Hospital Medical Center, Green Bay

Daniel Tvedten, St. Mary's Hospital, Rhinelander

Donald Wackwitz, St. Mary's Hospital Medical Center, Green Bay

APPENDIX

INTRODUCTION

The *HealthGrades Guide to America's Hospitals and Doctors* methodology provides clinical quality information about America's hospitals. This guide provides information about the following regarding HealthGrades' methodology:

- Data Sources
- Clinical Specialty Ratings
- Star Ratings
- Patient Safety
- Awards
- Data Model Limitations

DATA SOURCES

HealthGrades quality ratings are derived from the following data sources:

- Medicare inpatient data purchased from the Centers for Medicare and Medicaid Services (MedPAR database) based on hospitalized Medicare patients for 2004 through 2006.
- Inpatient data for maternity care, women's health, bariatric surgery, and appendectomy provided by 19 states that provided this all-payer data (AZ, CA, FL, IA, MA, MD, ME, NC, NJ, NV, NY, OR, PA, RI, TX, UT, VA, WA, and WI) for 2003 through 2005.

CLINICAL SPECIALTY RATINGS FOR SERVICE AREAS

To help consumers evaluate and compare hospital performance, HealthGrades analyzed patient outcome data for virtually every hospital in the country. HealthGrades analyzed and assigned quality ratings to ten different clinical specialties. The rating of each clinical specialty area is a combined rating of one or more medical issues (e.g., heart attack, heart failure, and coronary bypass surgery). The following descriptions show how Health-Grades calculated each of the ten clinical specialty ratings.

Ten Identified Clinical Specialties

- Cardiac Care
- Critical Care
- Gastrointestinal Care
- General Surgery
- Maternity Care
- Orthopedic Surgery
- Pulmonary Care
- Stroke Care
- Vascular Surgery
- Women's Health

CARDIAC CARE

The Cardiac Care clinical specialty rating is based on:

- Coronary bypass surgery
- Valve replacement surgery
- Coronary interventional procedures (PTCA/angioplasty, stent, atherectomy)
- Heart attack
- Heart failure
- Atrial fibrillation

We first determine the star ratings for each of these procedures/ diagnoses by evenly weighting their individual mortality ratings (in-hospital mortality, in-hospital +1 month mortality, and in-hospital +6 month mortality). The Cardiac Care clinical specialty rating is then determined by evenly weighting the cardiac surgical star rating (coronary bypass surgery and valve replacement surgery), the medical star rating (heart attack, heart failure, and atrial fibrillation), and the rating for coronary interventional procedures. To receive a rating in this clinical specialty, a hospital had to provide coronary bypass surgery and have star ratings in four of the five other medical issues based on MedPAR data.

CRITICAL CARE

The Critical Care clinical specialty rating is based on:

- Diabetic acidosis and coma
- Sepsis
- Pulmonary embolism
- Respiratory failure
- Leapfrog's ICU specialist staffing

We first calculate the average star ratings for sepsis, pulmonary embolism, and respiratory failure for in-hospital mortality, in-hospital +1 month mortality, and in-hospital +6 month mortality; and the average star rating for diabetic acidosis and coma for in-hospital mortality and +1 month mortality. We then convert Leapfrog's ICU specialist staffing to a numeric value. The Critical Care clinical specialty rating is based on an average of these star ratings and values. To receive a rating in this clinical specialty, a hospital had to have star ratings in all four critical care areas based on MedPAR data, plus have a rating in Leapfrog's criteria for ICU specialist staffing. Leapfrog is an organization dedicated to reducing preventable mistakes in hospitals. Leapfrog promotes the use of physicians trained in critical care medicine in hospital ICUs. Hospitals that utilize these physicians in their ICUs qualify for the Critical Care specialty rating.

GASTROINTESTINAL CARE
The Gastrointestinal Care clinical specialty rating is based on:
- Gastrointestinal bleed
- Bowel obstruction
- Pancreatitis
- Gastrointestinal surgeries and procedures
- Cholecystectomy

We first calculate the average star ratings for gastrointestinal bleed, bowel obstruction, pancreatitis, and gastrointestinal surgeries and procedures for in-hospital mortality, in-hospital +1 month mortality, and in-hospital +6 month mortality. The Gastrointestinal Care clinical specialty rating is based on an average of these ratings, along with the cholecystectomy rating. To receive a rating in this clinical specialty, a hospital had to have star ratings in all five medical issues based on MedPAR data.

GENERAL SURGERY
The General Surgery clinical specialty rating is based on:
- Appendectomy
- Bowel obstruction
- Cholecystectomy

We first calculate the average star rating for bowel obstruction for in-hospital mortality, in-hospital +1 mortality, and in-hospital +6 month mortality. The General Surgery clinical specialty rating is based on the average star rating for bowel obstruction and the star ratings for appendectomy and cholecystectomy. To be rated, a hospital must be located in one of the nineteen all-payer states that provide appendectomy data, and the hospital must have star ratings in all three medical issues (that is, a state rating for appendectomy and MedPAR-based ratings for bowel obstruction and cholecystectomy).

ORTHOPEDIC SURGERY
The Orthopedic Surgery clinical specialty rating is based on:
- Total knee replacement
- Total hip replacement
- Hip fracture repair

- Back and neck surgery (except spinal fusion)
- Back and neck surgery (spinal fusion)

We first calculate star ratings for these procedures based on complication rates. The Orthopedic Surgery clinical specialty rating is based on a star average for these procedures. To receive a rating in this clinical specialty, a hospital had to have star ratings for four of the five medical issues based on MedPAR data and those four must include total knee replacement, total hip replacement, and hip fracture repair.

PULMONARY CARE
The Pulmonary clinical specialty rating is based on:
- Chronic obstructive pulmonary disease (COPD)
- Pneumonia

We first calculate the average star ratings for these medical issues by evenly weighting the individual mortality star ratings. For pneumonia we calculate in-hospital mortality, in-hospital +1 month mortality, and in-hospital +6 month mortality. For COPD we calculate in-hospital mortality and +6 month mortality. The Pulmonary Care clinical specialty rating is based on an average of the average star ratings. To receive a rating in this clinical specialty, a hospital had to have star ratings for both medical issues based on MedPAR data.

STROKE CARE
The Stroke clinical specialty rating is based on one medical issue: stroke. To receive a rating in this clinical specialty, a hospital had to have a transfer-out rate of less than 10 percent in the most recent year used (2005 for all-payer, 2006 for Medicare). The Stroke clinical specialty rating is based on the average of in-hospital mortality, in-hospital +1 month mortality, and in-hospital +6 month mortality.

VASCULAR SURGERY
The Vascular clinical specialty rating is based on:
- Resection/replacement of abdominal aorta
- Carotid surgery
- Peripheral vascular bypass

We first calculate the overall star ratings for resection/replacement of abdominal aorta by averaging the in-hospital mortality, in-hospital +1 month mortality, and in-hospital +6 month mortality. The Vascular Surgery clinical specialty rating is based on the average of the overall resection/replacement of abdominal aorta rating, plus carotid surgery and peripheral vascular bypass. To receive a rating in this clinical specialty, a hospital had to have star ratings for all three medical issues based on MedPAR data.

STAR RATINGS METHODOLOGIES FOR CLINICAL PROCEDURES AND DIAGNOSES

In addition to clinical specialty ratings which combine several procedures and diagnosis, HealthGrades also evaluates hospitals on individual procedures and diagnoses. For these ratings Health-Grades rates hospitals using the following methodologies:
- HealthGrades' proprietary risk-adjustment methodology
- Programmatic evaluations (maternity care and women's health)

HEALTHGRADES' PROPRIETARY RISK-ADJUSTMENT METHODOLOGY

When rating hospitals, there is a need to perform risk-adjustment. Risk adjustment is important because in healthcare, patients differ from one another with respect to their health status, demographics, and type of procedure performed. Risk factors include gender, age, specific procedure performed, and current health conditions such as hypertension, diabetes, and congestive heart failure. The risk-adjustment methodology HealthGrades uses takes these factors into consideration to make fair and accurate comparisons of hospitals based on the types of patients treated.

For 29 medical issues, the risk adjustment is based on a proprietary HealthGrades methodology. Developing ratings involved two steps. First, the **predicted** value for a specific outcome was estimated. Second, the predicted outcome was compared to the **actual** outcome. HealthGrades further determines if the difference between the predicted outcome and the actual outcome is statistically significant.

The twenty-nine medical issues using HealthGrades' risk-adjustment methodology are:

- Appendectomy
- Atrial fibrillation
- Back and neck surgery (except spinal fusion)
- Back and neck surgery (spinal fusion)
- Bariatric surgery
- Bowel obstruction
- Carotid surgery
- Cholecystectomy
- Chronic obstructive pulmonary disease
- Coronary bypass surgery
- Coronary interventional procedures
- Diabetic acidosis and coma
- Gastrointestinal bleed
- Gastrointestinal surgeries and procedures
- Heart attack
- Heart failure
- Hip fracture repair
- Pancreatitis
- Peripheral vascular bypass
- Pneumonia
- Prostatectomy
- Pulmonary embolism
- Resection/replacement of abdominal aorta
- Respiratory failure
- Sepsis
- Stroke
- Total hip replacement
- Total knee replacement
- Valve replacement surgery

HOW HEALTHGRADES RATES HOSPITALS

For each hospital, HealthGrades rated different procedures or diagnoses using risk-adjustment methodologies (except maternity care and women's health). Each of the procedures or diagnoses is rated in one or more categories:
- Survival
- Recovery
- Avoiding Complications

Survival and Recovery ratings are based on mortality outcomes while Avoiding Complications is based on complication outcomes.

HealthGrades risk-adjusts the data to ensure a fair comparison between hospitals. Each hospital receives one of the following ratings for each medical issue:

★★★★★ Best
★★★ As Expected
★ Poor

HOW HEALTHGRADES RATES HOSPITALS IN MATERNITY CARE

HealthGrades analyzes the following four factors for each hospital:
- Volume of vaginal and cesarean section (C-section) single live-born deliveries
- Maternal complication rate for single live-born deliveries for women undergoing vaginal or C-section delivery
- Maternal complication rate among women undergoing "patient-choice" or non-clinically indicated C-sections
- Newborn mortality rate stratified into nine birth weight categories

For each of the above factors except volume, hospitals are ranked separately based on whether or not they have a new-born ICU. The presence of a newborn ICU is defined as being an intermediate or intensive care unit for newborn care. Typically, intermediate care or intensive care newborn units allow for the care of premature infants, infants requiring mechanical ventilation or neonatal surgery, infants with congenital heart disease or malformations requiring immediate evaluations and monitoring, and/or infants with low birth weight.

The four factors were weighted using predetermined weights based on consensus from a physician panel. Each factor's score is multiplied by its weight and then summed to create an overall score for each hospital.

Based upon each hospital's overall score, HealthGrades applies the following star ratings for maternity care:

★★★★★ **Best** Top 15% of all hospitals within 19 states

★★★ **As Expected** Middle 70% of all hospitals within 19 states

★ **Poor** Bottom 15% of all hospitals within 19 states

HOW HEALTHGRADES RATES HOSPITALS IN WOMEN'S HEALTH

The Women's Health rating is based on several medical issues important to women, including maternity care and cardiac/stroke mortality outcomes for women. Hospitals had to have an overall rating from each area to be considered. Maternity care ratings are based on four factors related to deliveries and newborn care (methodology described above). For cardiac and stroke mortality for women, HealthGrades analyzes the following for female patients:

- Coronary bypass surgery
- Valve replacement surgery
- Coronary interventional procedures (PTCA/angioplasty, stent, atherectomy)
- Heart attack
- Heart failure
- Stroke

The maternity care percentile score is added to the cardiac/stroke percentile score to create a women's health score for each hospital. Hospitals are sorted with star ratings assigned in three tier levels.

The following star rating system is applied to the women's health score:

★★★★★ **Best** Top 15% of all hospitals within 19 states

★★★ **As Expected** Middle 70% of all hospitals within 19 states

★ **Poor** Bottom 15% of all hospitals within 19 states

PATIENT SAFETY

To help consumers evaluate and compare hospital performance, HealthGrades analyzes patient data for virtually every hospital in the country to determine patient safety outcomes.

HealthGrades uses Medicare inpatient data from the MedPAR database (purchased from the Centers for Medicare and Medicaid Services; 2003 through 2005 data) and Patient Safety Indicator software (QI Windows Software, Version 3.0a) from the Agency for Healthcare Research and Quality (AHRQ) to analyze the following 13 patient safety indicators (PSI):

- Prevention of death in procedures where mortality is usually very low
- Lack of pressure sores or bedsores acquired in the hospital
- Ability to diagnose and treat in time
- Absence of foreign body left in during procedure
- Avoidance of collapsed lung due to a procedure or surgery in or around the chest
- Lack of infections acquired at the hospital
- Absence of hip fracture after surgery
- Avoidance of excessive bruising or bleeding as a consequence of a procedure or surgery
- Adequate organ function and electrolyte and fluid balance after surgery
- Avoidance of respiratory failure following surgery
- Lack of deep blood clots in the lungs or legs after surgery
- Avoidance of severe infection following surgery
- Lack of surgical wound site breakdown

INDIVIDUAL PATIENT SAFETY INDICATOR RATING

For each PSI, HealthGrades then determines if the hospital's performance in each PSI was Best, Average, or Poor.

★★★★★ **Best**

★★★ **Average**

★ **Poor**

AWARDS SECTION

AMERICA'S 50 BEST HOSPITALS AWARD METHODOLOGY

Out of 5,000 hospitals in the nation, only fifty are recognized each year as HealthGrades' America's 50 Best Hospitals.

As with all HealthGrades awards, America's 50 Best are based on risk-adjusted mortality and complication rates. To receive a place on the HealthGrades America's 50 Best Hospitals list, the facilities must have patient outcomes that are in the top five percent in the nation the most consecutive times over the last five years, reflecting quality that is consistent across procedures and treatments and over time.

HealthGrades' America's 50 Best Hospitals Award recognizes hospitals for consistent excellence by identifying those hospitals that have received HealthGrades' Distinguished Hospital Award for Clinical Excellence (DHA-CE) designation for the most consecutive years. (For more information about the DHA-CE award see below.)

The list of hospitals contains well-known facilities, such as Cedars Sinai in Los Angeles, Mayo Clinic in Minnesota and the Cleveland Clinic. But it also contains hospitals without national reputations whose patients have superior outcomes compared with their peers across the country.

HealthGrades' America's 50 Best Hospitals list is announced each February.

DISTINGUISHED HOSPITAL AWARD—CLINICAL EXCELLENCE™ METHODOLOGY

Hospitals with overall clinical excellence in the top 5 percent in the nation are recognized with HealthGrades' Distinguished Hospital Award for Clinical Excellence.

HealthGrades evaluates clinical quality at all hospitals nationwide across twenty-eight procedures and diagnoses in clinical specialties such as cardiac surgery, cardiology, orthopedic surgery, vascular surgery, neurosciences, pulmonary care, and gastroenterology. Performance is statistically aggregated to create a hospital-wide evaluation of quality based on risk-adjusted mortality and complication rates.

HealthGrades' Distinguished Hospital Awards for Clinical Excellence are announced each January along with HealthGrades' annual Hospital Quality and Clinical Excellence study. For the Distinguished Hospital Award for Clinical Excellence, hospitals were segregated into two groups: teaching and non-teaching. To be considered for the Distinguished Hospital Award for Clinical Excellence (DHA-CE), a hospital had to have had in-hospital mortality or complication ratings in at least 20 of the 28 HealthGrades ratings using MedPAR data.

SPECIALTY EXCELLENCE AWARD™ METHODOLOGY
Introduction

HealthGrades recognizes hospitals performing in the top 10 percent in clinical excellence in each of thirteen specialty care areas.

The HealthGrades' Specialty Excellence Awards are announced each year in the following categories: bariatric surgery, cardiac, cardiac surgery, coronary intervention, critical care, gastrointestinal, gastrointestinal surgery, general surgery, joint replacement, maternity care, orthopedic, pulmonary, spine surgery, stroke, vascular, and women's health.

HealthGrades ratings of procedures and diagnoses are performed annually and released each October along with HealthGrades' annual Hospital Quality in America study. For more details on the methodology for each category, please see the "Star Ratings Methodologies" section on page 1084.

DISTINGUISHED HOSPITAL AWARD—PATIENT SAFETY™ METHODOLOGY (2003–2005 MEDPAR DATA)
Introduction

To help consumers evaluate and compare hospital patient safety performance, HealthGrades analyzes patient outcome data for virtually every hospital in the country. HealthGrades uses MedPAR file data from the Centers for Medicare and Medicaid Services (CMS) which contains the inpatient records for Medicare patients. The steps listed below are those taken to determine the recipients of the Distinguished Hospital Award for Patient Safety by creating an overall patient safety score for each hospital.

This methodology includes the following patient safety indicators (use the same descriptions as above):

- Prevention of death in procedures where mortality is usually very low
- Lack of pressure sores or bedsores acquired in the hospital
- Ability to diagnose and treat in time
- Absence of foreign body left in during procedure
- Avoidance of collapsed lung due to a procedure or surgery in or around the chest
- Lack of infections acquired at the hospital
- Absence of hip fracture after surgery
- Avoidance of excessive bruising or bleeding as a consequence of a procedure or surgery
- Adequate organ function and electrolyte and fluid balance after surgery

- Avoidance of respiratory failure following surgery
- Lack of deep blood clots in the lungs or legs after surgery
- Avoidance of severe infection following surgery
- Lack of surgical wound site breakdown

To determine a hospital's overall patient safety rating, their individual performance in each PSI are rolled up to an overall rating. Their overall score is then classified as:

★★★★★ **Best**
  ★★★ **Average**
    ★ **Poor**

Hospitals that are performing in the top 5 percent in the nation overall are awarded the HealthGrades Distinguished Hospital Award for Patient Safety.

LIMITATIONS OF THE DATA MODELS

It must be understood that while these models may be valuable in identifying hospitals that perform better than others, one should not use this information alone to determine the quality of care provided at each hospital. The models are limited by the following factors:

- Cases may have been coded incorrectly or incompletely by the hospital.
- The models can only account for risk factors that are coded into the billing data. Therefore, if a particular risk factor was not coded into the billing data (such as a patient's socioeconomic status and health behavior) then it was not accounted for with these models.
- Although HealthGrades has taken steps to carefully compile these data, no techniques are infallible; and therefore, some information may be missing, outdated, or incorrect.

Please note that if more than one hospital reported to CMS under a single provider ID, HealthGrades analyzed patient safety data for those hospitals as a single unit. Throughout this book, therefore, "hospital" refers to one hospital or a group of hospitals reporting under a single provider ID.

HEALTHGRADES TOP DOCTORS METHODOLOGY

INTRODUCTION

HealthGrades' lists of top doctors represent the first time that doctors have been identified across the nation based on patient outcomes at their hospitals. Lists of doctors published elsewhere have been created based on subjective measures, chiefly surveys of patients or other physicians. By contrast, doctors in this book were only eligible for inclusion if the hospitals at which they practice have objective mortality and complication rates in their area of specialty that are below the national average.

To identify the nation's top doctors, HealthGrades started by analyzing risk-adjusted patient outcomes for the nation's nearly five thousand non-federal hospitals. Those hospitals with outcomes in the top 10 percent in the nation for the nine medical specialties listed below were selected:

Cardiology, cardiac surgery, gastrointestinal care, general surgery, orthopedic surgery, spine surgery, stroke care (which includes neurology), vascular surgery, and maternity care.

Within each of these clinical specialty areas, HealthGrades identified specific treatments and diagnosis and measured risk-adjusted mortality and complication rates to assess the quality of each program.

HOW HOSPITALS WERE SELECTED

Every year HealthGrades analyzes more than forty million Medicare patient records from nearly five thousand hospitals nationwide. All hospitals with sufficient patient volumes are analyzed and rated based on risk-adjusted clinical outcomes. Hospitals cannot opt in or out of the rating process. The data used in the analysis primarily comes from the government's MedPAR database, purchased from the Centers for Medicare & Medicaid Services, which is part of the U.S. Department of Health and Human Services. The Medicare records analyzed for this book were based upon hospitalized patients for years 2004 through 2006. Inpatient data for two of the categories of medical care, maternity care and appendectomy, were gathered from the nineteen states which report all-payer data (AZ, CA, FL, IA, MA, MD, ME, NC, NJ, NV, NY, OR, PA, RI, TX, UT, VA, WA, and WI) for years 2004 through 2006.

HealthGrades risk-adjusted the mortality and complication rates for the nine specialty areas listed above to account for differences in the health and age of the patients. Researchers then identified those hospitals with risk-adjusted patient outcomes in the top 10 percent in the nation for each specialty.

COLLECTION OF PHYSICIAN NAMES

HealthGrades requested from each top-performing hospital the names of the physicians who provide inpatient care to patients within the specialty areas in which they ranked top 10 percent in the nation. Hospitals were encouraged to provide the names of physicians treating the highest volume of patients. HealthGrades accepted up to thirty physicians or physician group practice names. The physician and physician group practice information was matched against the HealthGrades physician database, and screened for state medical board sanction and disciplinary actions. Physicians with major sanctions or disciplinary actions were removed.

SPECIALTY AREAS FOR SELECTION OF TOP DOCTORS

HealthGrades' top doctors were identified in the following areas:

CARDIOLOGY

In the field of cardiology, the non-interventional area of cardiac care, HealthGrades lists doctors who primarily treat the following diagnosis or perform the following procedures:
- Heart attack
- Heart failure
- Atrial fibrillation
- Coronary interventional procedures (PTCA/angioplasty, stent, atherectomy)

CARDIAC SURGERY

The two most common surgeries performed by cardiac surgeons are:
- Coronary bypass surgery
- Valve replacement surgery

GASTROENTEROLOGY

Doctors who practice gastroenterology treat the following types of conditions. However, general surgeons often perform gastrointestinal surgeries such as appendectomy or treating a gastrointestinal bleed:
- Gastrointestinal bleed
- Bowel obstruction
- Pancreatitis
- Gastrointestinal surgeries and procedures
- Cholecystectomy

GENERAL SURGERY

General surgeons perform many types of surgeries. For the purposes of HealthGrades' book, hospitals were asked to provide the names of surgeons who primarily perform the following:
- Appendectomy
- Bowel obstruction
- Cholecystectomy

ORTHOPEDIC SURGERY

Orthopedic surgeons typically specialize in either joint surgery, including knee and hip surgery, or certain types of back and neck surgery, which can include spinal fusion. HealthGrades asked top orthopedic programs to supply the names of surgeons who perform the following:
- Total knee replacement
- Total hip replacement
- Hip fracture repair
- Back and neck surgery (except spinal fusion)
- Back and neck surgery (spinal fusion)

STROKE

There are several types of physicians who treat patients who come to a hospital with the diagnosis of stroke. HealthGrades asked hospitals to provide physicians treating stroke who specialize in the following:
- Neurology

VASCULAR SURGERY

Vascular surgeons primarily focus on the following procedures:
- Resection/replacement of abdominal aorta
- Carotid surgery
- Peripheral vascular bypass

A

Abbeville County Memorial Hospital (Abbeville SC), 585

Abbeville General Hospital (Abbeville LA), 303

Abbott-Northwestern Hospital (Minneapolis MN), 367

Abilene Regional Medical Center (Abilene TX), 618

Abington Memorial Hospital (Abington PA), 555

Abraham Lincoln Memorial Hospital (Lincoln IL), 211

Abrom Kaplan Memorial Hospital (Kaplan LA), 303

Acadian Medical Center (Eunice LA), 303

ACMH Hospital (Kittanning PA), 555

Adams Memorial Hospital (Decatur IN), 241

Adams County Memorial Hospital (Decatur IN), 241

Adams County Regional Medical Center (Seaman OH), 504

Addison Gilbert Hospital (Gloucester MA), 334

Adena Regional Medical Center (Chillicothe OH), 504

Adirondack Medical Center (Saranac Lake NY), 450

Advance Directive, 22–23

Advanced Healthcare Medical Center (Ellington MO), 396

Adventist Glenoaks (Glendale Heights IL), 211

Adventist Medical Center (Portland OR), 546

Advocate Bethany Hospital (Chicago IL), 211

Advocate Christ Hospital and Medical Center (Oak Lawn IL), 211

Advocate Good Samaritan Hospital (Downers Grove IL), 211

Advocate Good Shepherd Hospital (Barrington IL), 211

Advocate Illinois Masonic Medical Center (Chicago IL), 212

Advocate Lutheran General Hospital (Park Ridge IL), 212

Advocate South Suburban Hospital (Hazel Crest IL), 212

Advocate Trinity Hospital (Chicago IL), 212

advocates. *See* patient advocates

Aiken Regional Medical Center (Aiken SC), 585

Akron General Medical Center (Akron OH), 504

Alabama

   five star rated facilities, 736–37

   hospitals, 48–63

   procedure, hospital ratings by, 828–31

   top doctors, 1044

Alachua General Hospital (Gainesville FL), 153

Alamance Regional Medical Center (Burlington NC), 483

Alameda County Medical Center (San Leandro CA), 85

Alameda Hospital (Alameda CA), 85

Alaska

   five star rated facilities, 737

   hospitals, 63–64

   procedure, hospital ratings by, 832–33

Alaska Native Medical Center (Anchorage AK), 63

Alaska Regional Hospital (Anchorage AK), 63

Albany Medical Center Hospital (Albany NY), 450

Albany Memorial Hospital (Albany NY), 451

Albemarle Hospital Authority (Elizabeth City NC), 483

Albert Einstein Medical Center (Philadelphia PA), 555

Albert Lea Medical Center—Mayo Health System (Albert Lea MN), 367

Albert Lindley Lee Memorial Hospital (Fulton NY), 451

Albuquerque, New Mexico, 446, 447, 449, 450

Alegent Health—Bergan Mercy Medical Center (Omaha NE), 417

Alegent Health Community Memorial Hospital (Missouri Valley IA), 259

Alegent Health—Immanuel Medical Center (Omaha NE), 417

Alegent Health—Lakeside Hospital (Omaha NE), 418

Alegent Health Mercy Hospital (Council Bluffs IA), 259

Alegent Health—Midlands Community Hospital (Papillion NE), 418

Alexian Brothers Medical Center (Elk Grove Village IL), 212

Alhambra Hospital and Medical Center (Alhambra CA), 86

Alice Hyde Medical Center (Malone NY), 451

Alice Peck Day Memorial Hospital (Lebanon NH), 428

Aliquippa Community Hospital (Aliquippa PA), 555

All Saints Medical Center—St. Mary's Campus (Racine WI), 711

All Saints St. Luke's Hospital (Racine WI), 711

Alle Kiski Medical Center (Natrona Heights PA), 555

Allegan General Hospital (Allegan MI), 346

Alleghany Regional Hospital (Low Moor VA), 677

Allegheny General Hospital (Pittsburgh PA), 555

Allegheny General Hospital—Suburban Campus (Pittsburgh PA), 556

Allen Bennett Memorial Hospital (Greer SC), 585

Allen County Hospital (Iola KS), 274

Allen Medical Center (Oberlin OH), 504

Allen Memorial Hospital (Moab UT), 670

Allen Memorial Hospital (Waterloo IA), 260

Allen Parish Hospital (Kinder LA), 303

Alliance Community Hospital (Alliance OH), 505

Alliance Hospital (Odessa TX), 618

Alpena Regional Medical Center (Alpena MI), 346

Alta Bates Summit—Alta Bates Campus (Berkeley CA), 86

Alta Bates Summit—Summit Campus (Oakland CA), 86

Alta View Hospital (Sandy UT), 670

Alta Vista Regional Hospital (Las Vegas NM), 445

Alton Memorial Hospital (Alton IL), 212

Altoona Hospital (Altoona PA), 556

Altru Hospital (Grand Forks ND), 500

Alvarado Hospital Medical Center (San Diego CA), 86

American Fork Hospital (American Fork UT), 670

American Legion Hospital (Crowley LA), 304

American Transitional Hospital—Houston W (Houston TX), 619

American Transitional Hospital (Oklahoma City OK), 530

American Transitional Hospital—Tulsa (Tulsa OK), 530

Amery Regional Medical Center (Amery WI), 712

Anaheim, California, 86, 103, 137

Anaheim General Hospital (Anaheim CA), 86

Anaheim Memorial Hospital (Anaheim CA), 86

Andalusia Regional Hospital (Andalusia AL), 48

Anderson Hospital (Maryville IL), 213

Androscoggin Valley Hospital (Berlin NH), 428

anesthesia, general, 45

anesthesiologists, 40

Angel Medical Center (Franklin NC), 483

angioplasty, 42–43

Angleton-Danbury Medical Center (Angleton TX), 619

Anmed Health (Anderson SC), 585

Anna Jacques Hospital (Newburyport MA), 334

Anne Arundel Medical Center (Annapolis MD), 326

Annie Penn Memorial Hospital (Reidsville NC), 483

Anson Community Hospital (Wadesboro NC), 484

Anson General Hospital (Anson TX), 619

Antelope Valley Hospital (Lancaster CA), 87

antibiotics, 8

Appleton Medical Center (Appleton WI), 712

Appling Hospital (Baxley GA), 184

Arbuckle Memorial Hospital (Sulphur OK), 531

Ardmore Adventist Hospital (Ardmore OK), 531

ARH Regional Medical Center—Hazard (Hazard KY), 286

Arizona

   five star rated facilities, 738–39

   hospitals, 65–73

   procedure, hospital ratings by, 834–37

   top doctors, 1044

Arizona Heart Hospital (Phoenix AZ), 65

Arkansas

   five star rated facilities, 739–40

   hospitals, 74–85

   procedure, hospital ratings by, 838–41

   top doctors, 1044

Arkansas Heart Hospital (Little Rock AR), 74

Arkansas Methodist Medical Center (Paragould AR), 74

Arkansas Valley Regional Medical Center (La Junta CO), 138

Arnot Ogden Medical Center (Elmira NY), 451

Aroostook Medical Center (Presque Isle ME), 320

Arrowhead Hospital (Glendale AZ), 65

Arrowhead Regional Medical Center (Colton CA), 87

Arroyo Grande Community Hospital (Arroyo Grande CA), 87

Artesia General Hospital (Artesia NM), 445

Ashe Memorial Hospital (Jefferson NC), 484

Ashland Community Hospital (Ashland OR), 546

Ashley County Medical Center (Crossett AR), 74

Ashley Valley Medical Center (Vernal UT), 670

Ashtabula County Medical Center (Ashtabula OH), 505

asking questions. *See* questions, asking

Aspen Valley Hospital (Aspen CO), 138

Aspirus Wausau Hospital (Wausau WI), 712

assertive, being, 33

Atchison Hospital (Atchison KS), 274

Athens-Limestone Hospital (Athens AL), 48

Athens Regional Medical Center (Athens GA), 184

Athens Regional Medical Center (Athens TN), 598

Athol Memorial Hospital (Athol MA), 334

Atlanta, Georgia, 184, 189, 191, 196, 198, 199

Atlanta Medical Center (Atlanta GA), 184

Please note that all individual hospital listings provide page numbers for Chapter 6 (Hospital Ratings by Clinical Specialty) only. All other hospital listings can be found under their state listing.

Atlanta Memorial Hospital (Atlanta TX), 619
Atlantic General Hospital (Berlin MD), 326
Atlanticare Medical Center—Union (Lynn MA), 334
Atlanticare Regional Medical Center (Atlantic City NJ), 432
Atmore Community Hospital (Atmore AL), 48
Atoka Memorial Hospital (Atoka OK), 531
Auburn Memorial Hospital (Auburn NY), 451
Auburn Regional Medical Center (Auburn WA), 691
Audrain Medical Center (Mexico MO), 396
Augusta, Georgia, 188, 193, 199, 200, 203
Augusta Medical Center (Fishersville VA), 677
Aultman Hospital (Canton OH), 505
Aurelia Osborn Fox Memorial Hospital (Oneonta NY), 451
Aurora Baycare Medical Center (Green Bay WI), 712
Aurora Lakeland Medical Center (Elkhorn WI), 712
Aurora Medical Center—Kenosha (Kenosha WI), 712
Aurora Medical Center—Manitowoc City
    (Two Rivers WI), 713
Aurora Medical Center—Oshkosh (Oshkosh WI), 713
Aurora Medical Center—Washington County
    (Hartford WI), 713
Aurora Sheboygan Memorial Medical Center
    (Sheboygan WI), 713
Aurora Sinai Medical Center (Milwaukee WI), 713
Aurora St. Luke's Medical Center (Milwaukee WI), 713
Austin, Texas, 622, 637, 639, 651, 659, 661, 662
Austin Medical Center (Austin MN), 367
Aventura Hospital and Medical Center (Aventura FL), 153
Avera Gregory Healthcare Center (Gregory SD), 594
Avera Heart Hospital of South Dakota (Sioux Falls SD), 594
Avera Marshall Regional Medical Center (Marshall MN), 367
Avera McKennan Hospital and University Health Center
    (Sioux Falls SD), 595
Avera Queen of Peace (Mitchell SD), 595
Avera Sacred Heart Hospital (Yankton SD), 595
Avera St. Anthony's Hospital (Oneill NE), 418
Avera St. Luke's (Aberdeen SD), 595
Avoyelles Hospital (Marksville LA), 304

B
background checks, 6–8
Bacon County Hospital (Alma GA), 184
bacterial illnesses, 8
Bakersfield, California, 87, 99, 106, 111, 125
Bakersfield Heart Hospital (Bakersfield CA), 87
Bakersfield Memorial Hospital (Bakersfield CA), 87
Baldwin Area Medical Center (Baldwin WI), 714
Ball Memorial Hospital (Muncie IN), 241
Baltimore, Maryland, 326, 328, 330, 331, 332, 333
Baltimore Washington Medical Center (Glen Burnie MD), 326
Bamberg County Memorial Hospital (Bamberg SC), 586
Banner Baywood Heart Hospital (Mesa AZ), 65
Banner Baywood Medical Center (Mesa AZ), 65
Banner Desert Medical Center (Mesa AZ), 65
Banner Estrella Medical Center (Phoenix AZ), 65
Banner Good Samaritan Medical Center (Phoenix AZ), 66
Banner Lassen Medical Center (Susanville CA), 87
Banner Thunderbird Medical Center (Glendale AZ), 66

Baptist Cherokee (Centre AL), 48
Baptist Citizens (Talladega AL), 48
Baptist Health Medical Center—Arkadelphia
    (Arkadelphia AR), 74
Baptist Health Medical Center—Heber Springs
    (Heber Springs AR), 74
Baptist Health Medical Center—Little Rock
    (Little Rock AR), 74
Baptist Health Medical Center—North Little Rock
    (North Little Rock AR), 75
Baptist Health System (San Antonio TX), 619
Baptist Hospital (Nashville TN), 598
Baptist Hospital of Cocke County (Newport TN), 599
Baptist Hospital East (Louisville KY), 286
Baptist Hospital of East Tennessee (Knoxville TN), 599
Baptist Hospital of Miami (Miami FL), 153
Baptist Hospital Northeast (LaGrange KY), 287
Baptist Hospital Pensacola (Pensacola FL), 153
Baptist Hospital West (Knoxville TN), 599
Baptist Lutheran Medical Center (Kansas City MO), 396
Baptist Medical Center (Jacksonville FL), 154
Baptist Medical Center—Beaches
    (Jacksonville Beach FL), 154
Baptist Medical Center—Dekalb (Fort Payne AL), 48
Baptist Medical Center—East (Montgomery AL), 49
Baptist Medical Center—Nassau (Fernandina Beach FL),
    154
Baptist Medical Center—South (Montgomery AL), 49
Baptist Memorial Hospital (Memphis TN), 599
Baptist Memorial Hospital—Booneville (Booneville MS), 383
Baptist Memorial Hospital—Collierville (Collierville TN), 599
Baptist Memorial Hospital—De Soto (Southhaven MS), 383
Baptist Memorial Hospital—Forrest City (Forrest City AR),
    75
Baptist Memorial Hospital—Golden Triangle
    (Columbus MS), 383
Baptist Memorial Hospital—Huntingdon (Huntingdon TN),
    599
Baptist Memorial Hospital—Lauderdale (Ripley TN), 600
Baptist Memorial Hospital—North Mississippi
    (Oxford MS), 383
Baptist Memorial Hospital—Tipton (Covington TN), 600
Baptist Memorial Hospital—Union City (Union City TN), 600
Baptist Memorial Hospital—Union County
    (New Albany MS), 383
Baptist Princeton (Birmingham AL), 49
Baptist Regional Medical Center (Corbin KY), 287
Baptist Shelby (Alabaster AL), 49
Baptist St. Anthony's Health System (Amarillo TX), 620
Barberton Citizens Hospital (Barberton OH), 505
bare metal stents (BMS), 42
Barnert Hospital (Paterson NJ), 432
Barnes Hospital (St. Louis MO), 396
Barnes-Jewish Hospital (St. Louis MO), 397
Barnes-Jewish St. Peters Hospital (St. Peters MO), 397
Barnes-Jewish West County Hospital (St. Louis MO), 397
Barnes-Kasson County Hospital (Susquehanna PA), 556
Barnesville Hospital Association (Barnesville OH), 505

Barnwell County Hospital (Barnwell SC), 586
Barron Memorial Medical Center Mayo (Barron WI), 714
Barrow Regional Medical Center (Winder GA), 184
Barstow Community Hospital (Barstow CA), 88
Bartlett Regional Hospital (Juneau AK), 63
Barton County Memorial Hospital (Lamar MO), 397
Barton Memorial Hospital (South Lake Tahoe CA), 88
Bartow Regional Medical Center (Bartow FL), 154
Bassett Hospital of Schoharie County (Cobleskill NY), 452
Bates County Memorial Hospital (Butler MO), 397
Batesville Specialty Hospital (Batesville MS), 383
Bath County Community Hospital (Hot Springs VA), 677
Baton Rouge General Medical Center (Baton Rouge LA), 304
Battle Creek Health System (Battle Creek MI), 346
Baxter Regional Medical Center (Mountain Home AR), 75
Bay Area Hospital (Coos Bay OR), 547
Bay Area Medical Center (Marinette WI), 714
Bay Medical Center (Panama City FL), 154
Bay Park Community Hospital (Oregon OH), 505
Bay Regional Medical Center (Bay City MI), 346
Bayfront Medical Center (St. Petersburg FL), 154
Bayhealth Medical Center—Kent General Hospital
    (Dover DE), 152
Bayhealth Medical Center—Milford Memorial Campus
    (Milford DE), 152
Bayley Seton Hospital (Staten Island NY), 452
Baylor All Saints Medical Center at Fort Worth
    (Fort Worth TX), 620
Baylor Heart and Vascular Center (Dallas TX), 620
Baylor Medical Center at Garland (Garland TX), 620
Baylor Medical Center at Irving (Irving TX), 620
Baylor Medical Center at Waxahachie (Waxahachie TX), 620
Baylor Regional Medical Center at Grapevine
    (Grapevine TX), 621
Baylor Regional Medical Center at Plano (Plano TX), 621
Baylor University Medical Center (Dallas TX), 621
Bayonne Hospital (Bayonne NJ), 433
Bayshore Community Hospital (Holmdel NJ), 433
Bayshore Medical Center in Pasadena (Pasadena TX), 621
Baystate Franklin Medical Center (Greenfield MA), 334
Baystate Mary Lane Hospital (Ware MA), 334
Baystate Medical Center (Springfield MA), 335
Beacham Memorial (Magnolia MS), 384
Bear Lake Memorial Hospital (Montpelier ID), 208
Beatrice Community Hospital and Health Center
    (Beatrice NE), 418
Beaufort County Hospital (Washington NC), 484
Beaufort Memorial Hospital (Beaufort SC), 586
Beaumont Hospital—Grosse Pointe (Grosse Pointe MI), 347
Beaumont Hospital—Royal Oak (Royal Oak MI), 347
Beaumont Hospital—Troy (Troy MI), 347
Beauregard Memorial Hospital (Deridder LA), 304
Beaver Dam Community Hospital (Beaver Dam WI), 714
Beaver Valley Hospital (Beaver UT), 670
Beckley ARH Hospital (Beckley WV), 703
Bedford County Medical Center (Shelbyville TN), 600
Bedford Memorial Hospital (Bedford VA), 677
Bedford Regional Medical Center (Bedford IN), 241

Beebe Medical Center (Lewes DE), 152
Bell Memorial Hospital (Ishpeming MI), 347
Bellevue Hospital (Bellevue OH), 506
Bellevue Hospital Center (New York NY), 452
Bellflower Medical Center (Bellflower CA), 88
Bellin Memorial Hospital (Green Bay WI), 714
Bellville General Hospital (Bellville TX), 621
Belmont Community Hospital (Bellaire OH), 506
Beloit Memorial Hospital (Beloit WI), 714
Benedictine Hospital (Kingston NY), 452
Benefits Healthcare (Great Falls MT), 414
Berea Hospital (Berea KY), 287
Bergen Regional Medical Center (Paramus NJ), 433
Berger Hospital (Circleville OH), 506
Berkshire Medical Center (Pittsfield MA), 335
Berlin Memorial Hospital (Berlin WI), 715
Berrien County Hospital (Nashville GA), 184
Bert Fish Medical Center (New Smyrna Beach FL), 155
Bertrand Chaffee Hospital (Springville NY), 452
Berwick Hospital Center (Berwick PA), 556
beta blockers, 43
Beth Israel Deaconess Hospital—Needham
    (Needham MA), 335
Beth Israel Deaconess Medical Center (Boston MA), 335
Beth Israel Medical Center (New York NY), 452
Bethesda Memorial Hospital (Boynton Beach FL), 155
Bethesda North Hospital (Cincinnati OH), 506
Betsy Johnson Memorial Hospital (Dunn NC), 484
Beverly Hospital (Beverly MA), 335
Beverly Hospital (Montebello CA), 88
Big Bend Regional Medical Center (Alpine TX), 621
Billings Clinic (Billings MT), 414
Biloxi Regional Medical Center (Biloxi MS), 384
Bingham Memorial Hospital (Blackfoot ID), 208
Birmingham, Alabama, 49, 50, 59, 61
birth, giving, 40–42
BJC Medical Center (Commerce GA), 185
Bladen County Hospital (Elizabethtown NC), 484
Blake Medical Center (Bradenton FL), 155
Blanchard Valley Regional Medical Center (Findlay OH), 506
Bledsoe County Hospital (Pikeville TN), 600
Blessing Hospital (Quincy IL), 213
Bloomer Medical Center (Bloomer WI), 715
Bloomington Hospital (Bloomington IN), 241
Bloomington Hospital of Orange County (Paoli IN), 241
Bloomsburg Hospital (Bloomsburg PA), 556
Blount Memorial Hospital (Maryville TN), 600
Blue Hill Memorial Hospital (Blue Hill ME), 320
Blue Mountain Hospital District (John Day OR), 547
Bluefield Regional Medical Center (Bluefield WV), 703
Bluegrass Community Hospital (Versailles KY), 287
Bluffton Regional Medical Center (Bluffton IN), 242
BMS (bare metal stents), 42
board certification, 7
Bob Wilson Memorial Hospital (Ulysses KS), 275
Boca Raton Community Hospital (Boca Raton FL), 155
Bolivar General Hospital (Bolivar TN), 601
Bolivar Medical Center (Cleveland MS), 384

Bon Secours Community Hospital (Port Jervis NY), 453
Bon Secours DePaul Medical Center (Norfolk VA), 677
Bon Secours Hospital (Baltimore MD), 326
Bon Secours Maryview Medical Center (Portsmouth VA), 677
Bon Secours Memorial Regional Medical Center
    (Mechanicsville VA), 678
Bon Secours Mercy Hospital (Altoona PA), 556
Bon Secours Richmond Community Hospital
    (Richmond VA), 678
Bon Secours St. Francis Hospital (Charleston SC), 586
Bon Secours St. Francis Medical Center (Midlothian VA), 678
Bon Secours St. Mary's Hospital (Richmond VA), 678
Bone and Joint Hospital (Oklahoma City OK), 531
Bonne Terre Hospital (Bonne Terre MO), 397
Bonner General Hospital (Sandpoint ID), 208
Boone County Health Center (Albion NE), 418
Boone County Hospital (Boone IA), 260
Boone Hospital Center (Columbia MO), 398
Boone Memorial Hospital (Madison WV), 703
Booneville Community Hospital (Booneville AR), 75
boredom, avoiding, 36
Borgess Medical Center (Kalamazoo MI), 347
Borgess Pipp Health Center (Plainwell MI), 347
Borgess-Lee Memorial Hospital (Dowagiac MI), 348
Boscobel Area Health Care (Boscobel WI), 715
Boston, Massachusetts, 335, 336, 337, 338, 340, 342, 345
Boston Medical Center (Boston MA), 335
Bothwell Regional Health Center (Sedalia MO), 398
Botsford Hospital (Farmington Hills MI), 348
Boulder Community Hospital (Boulder CO), 139
Bourbon Community Hospital (Paris KY), 287
Bowie Memorial Hospital (Bowie TX), 622
Box Butte General Hospital (Alliance NE), 418
Bozeman Deaconess Hospital (Bozeman MT), 415
Brackenridge Hospital (Austin TX), 622
Bradford Regional Medical Center (Bradford PA), 557
Bradley County Medical Center (Warren AR), 75
Bradley Memorial Hospital (Cleveland TN), 601
Bradley Memorial Hospital and Health Center
    (Southington CT), 146
Brandon Regional Hospital (Brandon FL), 155
Brandywine Hospital (Coatesville PA), 557
Brattleboro Memorial Hospital (Brattleboro VT), 675
Braxton County Memorial Hospital (Gassaway WV), 703
Brazosport Regional Health System (Lake Jackson TX), 622
breaking up with your doctor, 12, 35
Bridgeport Hospital (Bridgeport CT), 146
Bridgton Hospital (Bridgton ME), 320
Brigham and Women's Hospital (Boston MA), 336
Brigham City Community Hospital (Brigham City UT), 670
Brighton Medical Center (Portland ME), 320
Bristol Hospital (Bristol CT), 147
Bristow Medical Center (Bristow OK), 531
Broadlawns Medical Center (Des Moines IA), 260
Brockton Hospital (Brockton MA), 336
Brodstone Memorial Nuckolls County Hospital
    (Superior NE), 419
Bromenn Healthcare (Normal IL), 213

Bronson Methodist Hospital (Kalamazoo MI), 348
Bronx, New York, 453, 462, 464, 467, 469, 470, 472, 474
Bronx-Lebanon Hospital Center (Bronx NY), 453
Brookdale Hospital Medical Center (Brooklyn NY), 453
Brookhaven Memorial Hospital Medical Center
    (Patchogue NY), 453
Brookings Hospital (Brookings SD), 595
Brooklyn, New York, 453, 456, 461, 462, 463, 465, 468,
    469, 481, 482
Brooklyn Hospital Center at Downtown Campus
    (Brooklyn NY), 453
Brooks County Hospital (Quitman GA), 185
Brooks Memorial Hospital (Dunkirk NY), 453
Brooksville Regional Hospital (Brooksville FL), 155
Brookville Hospital (Brookville PA), 557
Brookwood Medical Center (Birmingham AL), 49
Brotman Medical Center (Culver City CA), 88
Broward General Medical Center (Fort Lauderdale FL), 156
Brown County Hospital (Georgetown OH), 506
Brownfield Regional Medical Center (Brownfield TX), 622
Brownwood Regional Medical Center (Brownwood TX), 622
Brunswick Community Hospital (Supply NC), 484
Bryan W. Whitfield Memorial Hospital (Demopolis AL), 49
Bryanlgh Medical Center (Lincoln NE), 419
Bryanlgh Medical Center—West (Lincoln NE), 419
Buchanan County Health Center (Independence IA), 260
Buchanan General Hospital (Grundy VA), 678
Buena Vista Regional Medical Center (Storm Lake IA), 260
Buffalo, New York, 454, 458, 466, 467, 478
Buffalo General Hospital—Kaleida Health (Buffalo NY), 454
Buffalo Hospital (Buffalo MN), 367
Bullock County Hospital (Union Springs AL), 50
Bunkie General Hospital (Bunkie LA), 304
Burgess Health Center (Onawa IA), 260
Burke Medical Center (Waynesboro GA), 185
Burnett Medical Center (Grantsburg WI), 715
Butler County Health Care Center (David City NE), 419
Butler Memorial Hospital (Butler PA), 557
Byrd Regional Hospital (Leesville LA), 304

C

Cabell-Huntington Hospital (Huntington WV), 704
Cabrini Medical Center (New York NY), 454
Calais Regional Hospital (Calais ME), 320
Caldwell County Hospital (Princeton KY), 287
Caldwell Memorial Hospital (Columbia LA), 305
Caldwell Memorial Hospital (Lenoir NC), 485
Calhoun General Hospital County (Grantsville WV), 704
Calhoun Memorial Hospital (Arlington GA), 185
California
    five star rated facilities, 741–46
    hospitals, 85–138
    nurse-patient ratio in, 28
    procedure, hospital ratings by, 842–55
    top doctors, 1045–49
California Hospital Medical Center—Los Angeles
    (Los Angeles CA), 88
California Pacific Medical Center (San Francisco CA), 89

California Pacific Medical Center—Davies Campus (San Francisco CA), 89
Callaway Community Hospital (Fulton MO), 398
Calvert Memorial Hospital (Prince Frederick MD), 327
Cambridge Health Alliance (Cambridge MA), 336
Cambridge Medical Center (Cambridge MN), 367
CAMC Teays Valley Hospital (Hurricane WV), 704
Camden Clark Memorial Hospital (Parkersburg WV), 704
Camden General Hospital (Camden TN), 601
Camden Medical Center (St. Marys GA), 185
Cameron Memorial Community Hospital (Angola IN), 242
Cameron Regional Medical Center (Cameron MO), 398
Campbell County Memorial Hospital (Gillette WY), 730
Campbell Health System (Weatherford TX), 622
Campbellton Graceville Hospital (Graceville FL), 156
Cancer Center at Riverside Community Hospital, The (Riverside CA), 89
Candler County Hospital (Metter GA), 185
Candler Hospital (Savannah GA), 186
Cannon Memorial Hospital (Pickens SC), 586
Canonsburg General Hospital (Canonsburg PA), 557
Canton-Potsdam Hospital (Potsdam NY), 454
Cape Canaveral Hospital (Cocoa Beach FL), 156
Cape Cod Hospital (Hyannis MA), 336
Cape Coral Hospital (Cape Coral FL), 156
Cape Fear Hospital (Wilmington NC), 485
Cape Fear Valley Medical Center (Fayetteville NC), 485
Cape Regional Medical Center (Cape May Court House NJ), 433
Capital Health System—Fuld Campus (Trenton NJ), 433
Capital Health System—Mercer Campus (Trenton NJ), 433
Capital Medical Center (Olympia WA), 691
Capital Region Medical Center (Jefferson City MO), 398
Capital Regional Medical Center (Tallahassee FL), 156
cardiac procedure, getting a, 42–44
Cardinal Hill Specialty Hospital (Fort Thomas KY), 288
cardiologists, 42
Carilion Franklin Memorial Hospital (Rocky Mount VA), 678
Carilion Giles Memorial Hospital (Pearisburg VA), 679
Carilion Medical Center (Roanoke VA), 679
Carilion New River Valley Medical Center (Christiansburg VA), 679
Caritas Carney Hospital (Dorchester MA), 336
Caritas Good Samaritan Medical Center (Brockton MA), 336
Caritas Holy Family Hospital and Medical Center (Methuen MA), 337
Caritas Norwood Hospital (Norwood MA), 337
Caritas Southwood Hospital (Norfolk MA), 337
Caritas St. Elizabeth's Medical Center (Boston MA), 337
Carl Albert Indian Health Facility (Ada OK), 531
Carle Foundation Hospital (Urbana IL), 213
Carlinville Area Hospital (Carlinville IL), 213
Carlisle Regional Medical Center (Carlisle PA), 557
Carlsbad Medical Center (Carlsbad NM), 445
Carnegie Tri-County Municipal Hospital (Carnegie OK), 532
Caro Community Hospital (Caro MI), 348
Carolina Pines Regional Medical Center (Hartsville SC), 586
Carolinas Hospital System (Florence SC), 587

Carolinas Medical Center (Charlotte NC), 485
Carolinas Medical Center—Lincoln (Lincolnton NC), 485
Carolinas Medical Center—Mercy (Charlotte NC), 485
Carolinas Medical Center—NorthEast (Concord NC), 486
Carolinas Medical Center—Union (Monroe NC), 486
Carolinas Medical Center—University (Charlotte NC), 486
Carondelet Holy Cross Hospital (Nogales AZ), 66
Carondelet St. Joseph's Hospital and Health Center (Tucson AZ), 66
Carondelet St. Mary's Hospital and Health Center (Tucson AZ), 66
Carraway Methodist Medical Center (Birmingham AL), 50
Carrington Health Center (Carrington ND), 500
Carroll County Hospital (Carrollton KY), 288
Carroll County Memorial Hospital (Carrollton MO), 398
Carroll Hospital Center (Westminster MD), 327
Carson City Hospital (Carson City MI), 348
Carson Tahoe Regional Medical Center (Carson City NV), 425
Carteret General Hospital (Morehead City NC), 486
Cartersville Medical Center (Cartersville GA), 186
Carthage Area Hospital (Carthage NY), 454
Carthage General Hospital (Carthage TN), 601
Cary Medical Center (Caribou ME), 320
Casa Grande Regional Medical Center (Casa Grande AZ), 66
Cascade Valley Hospital (Arlington WA), 691
Cass County Memorial Hospital (Atlantic IA), 261
Cass Medical Center (Harrisonville MO), 399
Cassia Regional Medical Center (Burley ID), 208
Castle Medical Center (Kailua HI), 205
Castleview Hospital (Price UT), 671
Catawba Valley Medical Center (Hickory NC), 486
catheters, 35
Catholic Medical Center (Manchester NH), 429
Catskill Regional Medical Center (Harris NY), 454
Caverna Memorial Hospital (Horse Cave KY), 288
Cayuga Medical Center at Ithaca (Ithaca NY), 454
Cedar County Memorial Hospital (El Dorado Springs MO), 399
Cedars Medical Center (Miami FL), 156
Cedars-Sinai Medical Center (Los Angeles CA), 89
Centegra Memorial Medical Center (Woodstock IL), 213
Centegra Northern Illinois Medical Center (McHenry IL), 214
Centennial Medical Center (Frisco TX), 623
Centennial Medical Center (Nashville TN), 601
Centerpoint Medical Center (Independence MO), 399
Centers for Disease Control, 25
Centinela Freeman Regional Medical Center—Centinela (Inglewood CA), 89
Centinela Freeman Regional Medical Center—Marina (Marina Del Rey CA), 89
Centinela Freeman Regional Medical Center—Memorial (Inglewood CA), 90
Centra Health (Lynchburg VA), 679
Central Baptist Hospital (Lexington KY), 288
Central Carolina Hospital (Sanford NC), 486
Central Dupage Hospital (Winfield IL), 214
Central Florida Regional Hospital (Sanford FL), 157
Central Kansas Medical Center (Great Bend KS), 275
Central Maine Medical Center (Lewiston ME), 321

Central Michigan Community Hospital (Mount Pleasant MI), 348
Central Mississippi Medical Center (Jackson MS), 384
Central Montana Medical Center (Lewistown MT), 415
Central Montgomery Medical Center (Lansdale PA), 558
Central Peninsula General Hospital (Soldotna AK), 63
Central Texas Hospital (Cameron TX), 623
Central Texas Medical Center (San Marcos TX), 623
Central Valley General Hospital (Hanford CA), 90
Central Vermont Medical Center (Barre VT), 675
Central Washington Hospital (Wenatchee WA), 691
Centrastate Medical Center (Freehold NJ), 434
Centura Health—Avista Adventist Hospital (Louisville CO), 139
Centura Health—Littleton Adventist Hospital (Littleton CO), 139
Centura Health—Parker Adventist Hospital (Parker CO), 139
Centura Health—Penrose St. Francis Health Services (Colorado Springs CO), 139
Centura Health—Porter Adventist Hospital (Denver CO), 139
Centura Health—St. Anthony Central Hospital (Denver CO), 140
Centura Health—St. Anthony North Hospital (Westminster CO), 140
Centura Health—St. Mary Corwin Medical Center (Pueblo CO), 140
Centura Health—St. Thomas More Hospital (Canon City CO), 140
Century City Doctors Hospital (Los Angeles CA), 90
Cesarean section, 40–41
CGH Medical Center (Sterling IL), 214
Chambersburg Hospital (Chambersburg PA), 558
Champlain Valley Physicians Hospital Medical Center (Plattsburgh NY), 455
Chandler Regional Hospital (Chandler AZ), 67
Chapman Medical Center (Orange CA), 90
charge nurse, 28
Charles A. Cannon Jr. Memorial Hospital (Linville NC), 487
Charles Cole Memorial Hospital (Coudersport PA), 558
Charleston Area Medical Center (Charleston WV), 704
Charlevoix Area Hospital (Charlevoix MI), 349
Charlotte, North Carolina, 485, 486, 495
Charlotte Hungerford Hospital (Torrington CT), 147
Charlotte Regional Medical Center (Punta Gorda FL), 157
Charlton Methodist Hospital (Dallas TX), 623
Chase County Community Hospital (Imperial NE), 419
Chatuge Regional Hospital (Hiawassee GA), 186
Cheboygan Memorial Hospital (Cheboygan MI), 349
Chelsea Community Hospital (Chelsea MI), 349
Chenango Memorial Hospital (Norwich NY), 455
Cherokee Regional Medical Center (Cherokee IA), 261
Chesapeake General Hospital (Chesapeake VA), 679
Cheshire Medical Center (Keene NH), 429
Chestatee Regional Hospital (Dahlonega GA), 186
Chester County Hospital (West Chester PA), 558
Chester Regional Medical Center (Chester SC), 587
Chester River Hospital Center (Chestertown MD), 327
Chesterfield General Hospital (Cheraw SC), 587

Chestnut Hill Hospital (Philadelphia PA), 558
Cheyenne Regional Medical Center (Cheyenne WY), 730
Chicago, Illinois, 211, 212, 219, 221, 222, 223, 225–27,
    229–32, 234, 235, 237, 238, 239
Chicot Memorial Hospital (Lake Village AR), 75
Children's Hospital Rehab Center (Utica NY), 455
Childress Regional Medical Center (Childress TX), 623
Chilton Medical Center (Clanton AL), 50
Chilton Memorial Hospital (Pompton Plains NJ), 434
Chinese Hospital (San Francisco CA), 90
Chino Valley Medical Center (Chino CA), 90
Chippewa County Hospital (Montevideo MN), 368
Chippewa County War Memorial Hospital
    (Sault Ste. Marie MI), 349
Chippewa Valley Hospital (Durand WI), 715
Choctaw Memorial Hospital (Hugo OK), 532
Choctaw Nation Health Services Authority (Talihina OK), 532
Chowan Hospital (Edenton NC), 487
Christ Hospital (Cincinnati OH), 507
Christ Hospital (Jersey City NJ), 434
Christian Hospital Northeast (St. Louis MO), 399
Christiana Care Health System—Christiana Hospital
    (Newark DE), 152
Christus Coushatta Health Care (Coushatta LA), 305
Christus Coushatta Health Care Center (Coushatta LA), 305
Christus Jasper Memorial Hospital (Jasper TX), 623
Christus Santa Rosa Healthcare (San Antonio TX), 624
Christus Schumpert Health System (Shreveport LA), 305
Christus Spohn Hospital—Alice (Alice TX), 625
Christus Spohn Hospital—Beeville (Beeville TX), 625
Christus Spohn Hospital Corpus Christi—South
    (Corpus Christi TX), 625
Christus Spohn Hospital—Kleberg (Kingsville TX), 625
Christus St. Catherine Health and Wellness Center
    (Katy TX), 624
Christus St. Elizabeth Hospital (Beaumont TX), 624
Christus St. Francis Cabrini Hospital (Alexandria LA), 305
Christus St. John Hospital (Houston TX), 624
Christus St. Mary Hospital (Port Arthur TX), 624
Christus St. Michael Health System (Texarkana TX), 624
Christus St. Patrick Hospital (Lake Charles LA), 305
Churchill Community Hospital (Fallon NV), 425
Cibola General Hospital (Grants NM), 445
Cincinnati, Ohio, 506, 507, 508, 512, 514, 519, 520, 523,
    528
Citizens Medical Center (Columbia LA), 306
Citizens Medical Center (Victoria TX), 625
Citizens Memorial Hospital (Bolivar MO), 399
Citrus Memorial Hospital (Inverness FL), 157
Citrus Valley Medical Center—IC Campus (Covina CA), 91
Citrus Valley Medical Center—QV Campus
    (West Covina CA), 91
City Hospital (Martinsburg WV), 704
City Hospital Center at Elmhurst (Elmhurst NY), 455
City of Angels Medical Center (Los Angeles CA), 91
Civista Medical Center (La Plata MD), 327
CJW Medical Center—Chippenham Campus
    (Richmond VA), 679

Claiborne County Hospital (Tazewell TN), 601
Clara Barton Hospital (Hoisington KS), 275
Clara Maass Medical Center (Belleville NJ), 434
Claremore Indian Hospital (Claremore OK), 532
Claremore Regional Hospital (Claremore OK), 532
Clarendon Memorial Hospital (Manning SC), 587
Clarian Health Partners (Indianapolis IN), 242
Clarian West Medical Center (Avon IN), 242
Clarinda Regional Health Center (Clarinda IA), 261
Clarion Hospital (Clarion PA), 558
Clark Memorial Hospital (Jeffersonville IN), 242
Clark Regional Medical Center (Winchester KY), 288
Clarke County Hospital (Osceola IA), 261
Clarkson Bishop Memorial Hospital (Omaha NE), 419
Claxton-Hepburn Medical Center (Ogdensburg NY), 455
Clay County Hospital (Ashland AL), 50
Clay County Medical Center (West Point MS), 384
Clay County Memorial Hospital (Henrietta TX), 626
Clear Lake Regional Medical Center (Webster TX), 626
Clearfield Hospital (Clearfield PA), 559
Clearview Hospital (Midland TX), 626
Clearwater Health Services (Bagley MN), 368
Cleveland, Ohio, 507, 510, 516, 521, 525, 528
Cleveland Clinic (Cleveland OH), 507
Cleveland Clinic Hospital (Weston FL), 157
Cleveland Community Hospital (Cleveland TN), 602
Cleveland Regional Medical Center (Cleveland TX), 626
Cleveland Regional Medical Center (Shelby NC), 487
Clifton Springs Hospital and Clinic (Clifton Springs NY), 455
Clinch Valley Medical Center (Richlands VA), 680
clinical excellence, xiv
clinical specialty, xiii, xiv, 47, 48
Clinton County Hospital (Albany KY), 288
Clinton Memorial Hospital (St. Johns MI), 349
Clinton Memorial Hospital (Wilmington OH), 507
clopidogrel (Plavix), 43
Clovis Community Medical Center (Clovis CA), 91
Coast Plaza Doctors Hospital (Norwalk CA), 91
Coastal Carolina Medical Center (Hardeeville SC), 587
Coastal Communities Hospital (Santa Ana CA), 91
Cobb Memorial Hospital (Royston GA), 186
Cobre Valley Community Hospital (Globe AZ), 67
Coffee Regional Medical Center (Douglas GA), 186
Coffey County Hospital (Burlington KS), 275
Coffeyville Regional Medical Center (Coffeyville KS), 275
Coleman County Medical Center (Coleman TX), 626
Coliseum Medical Center (Macon GA), 187
Coliseum Northside Hospital (Macon GA), 187
College Station Medical Center (College Station TX), 626
Colleton Medical Center (Walterboro SC), 587
Colorado
    five star rated facilities, 746–48
    hospitals, 138–46
    procedure, hospital ratings by, 856–57
    top doctors, 1049
Colorado Plains Medical Center (Fort Morgan CO), 140
Colorado River Medical Center (Needles CA), 92
Colquitt Regional Medical Center (Moultrie GA), 187

Columbia Hospital (West Palm Beach FL), 157
Columbia Jefferson Medical Center (Jefferson LA), 306
Columbia Memorial Hospital (Astoria OR), 547
Columbia Memorial Hospital (Hudson NY), 456
Columbia Regional Hospital (Columbia MO), 399
Columbia St. Mary's Hospital Milwaukee (Milwaukee WI), 715
Columbia St. Mary's Hospital Ozaukee (Mequon WI), 716
Columbus, Ohio, 509, 512, 521, 522, 523
Columbus Community Hospital (Columbus NE), 420
Columbus Community Hospital (Columbus TX), 627
Columbus Community Hospital (Columbus WI), 716
Columbus County Hospital (Whiteville NC), 487
Columbus Doctors Hospital (Columbus GA), 187
Columbus Hospital (Newark NJ), 434
Columbus Regional Hospital (Columbus IN), 242
Colusa Regional Medical Center (Colusa CA), 92
Comanche County Memorial Hospital (Lawton OK), 532
Community and Mission Hospital of Huntington Park
    (Huntington Park CA), 92
Community Health Center of Branch County
    (Coldwater MI), 349
Community Health Partners of Ohio—West (Lorain OH), 507
Community-General Hospital of Greater Syracuse
    (Syracuse NY), 456
Community Hospital (Bryan OH), 507
Community Hospital (Chester PA), 559
Community Hospital (Grand Junction CO), 140
Community Hospital (McCook NE), 420
Community Hospital (Munster IN), 243
Community Hospital (New Port Richey FL), 157
Community Hospital (Oklahoma City OK), 533
Community Hospital (Tallassee AL), 50
Community Hospital (Torrington WY), 730
Community Hospital Association (Fairfax MO), 400
Community Hospital of Anaconda (Anaconda MT), 415
Community Hospital of Anderson and Madison County
    (Anderson IN), 243
Community Hospital of Bremen (Bremen IN), 243
Community Hospital at Dobbs Ferry (Dobbs Ferry NY), 456
Community Hospital Foundation (Almont MI), 350
Community Hospital of Gardena (Gardena CA), 92
Community Hospital of Long Beach (Long Beach CA), 92
Community Hospital of Los Gatos (Los Gatos CA), 92
Community Hospital of the Monterey Peninsula
    (Monterey CA), 93
Community Hospital—Onaga (Onaga KS), 275
Community Hospital of Ottawa (Ottawa IL), 214
Community Hospital of San Bernardino
    (San Bernardino CA), 93
Community Hospital South (Indianapolis IN), 243
Community Hospital of Springfield and Clark County
    (Springfield OH), 507
Community Hospital—Watervliet (Watervliet MI), 350
Community Hospitals Indianapolis (Indianapolis IN), 243
Community Medical Center (Falls City NE), 420
Community Medical Center (Missoula MT), 415
Community Medical Center (Scranton PA), 559
Community Medical Center (Toms River NJ), 434

Community Medical Center—Izard County
    (Calico Rock AR), 76
Community Memorial Healthcare (Marysville KS), 276
Community Memorial Healthcenter (South Hill VA), 680
Community Memorial Hospital (Cloquet MN), 368
Community Memorial Hospital (Hamilton NY), 456
Community Memorial Hospital (Hicksville OH), 508
Community Memorial Hospital (Menomonee Falls WI), 716
Community Memorial Hospital (Oconto Falls WI), 716
Community Memorial Hospital (Redfield SD), 595
Community Memorial Hospital (Staunton IL), 214
Community Memorial Hospital of San Buenaventura
    (Ventura CA), 93
Community Regional Medical Center (Fresno CA), 93
complications, 15, 16, 18, 42, 44, 45, xiii
Concord Hospital (Concord NH), 429
Condell Medical Center (Libertyville IL), 214
Conemaugh Valley Memorial Hospital (Johnstown PA), 559
Coney Island Hospital (Brooklyn NY), 456
Connally Memorial Medical Center (Floresville TX), 627
Connecticut
    five star rated facilities, 748–49
    hospitals, 146–51
    procedure, hospital ratings by, 858–59
    top doctors, 1049–50
Conroe Regional Medical Center (Conroe TX), 627
consumer, patient as, 2
Contra Costa Regional Medical Center (Martinez CA), 93
Conway Medical Center (Conway SC), 588
Conway Regional Medical Center (Conway AR), 76
Cookeville Regional Medical Center (Cookeville TN), 602
Cooley Dickinson Hospital (Northampton MA), 337
Cooper County Memorial Hospital (Boonville MO), 400
Cooper University Hospital (Camden NJ), 435
Coosa Valley Medical Center (Sylacauga AL), 50
Copper Basin Medical Center (Copperhill TN), 602
Coquille Valley Hospital (Coquille OR), 547
Coral Gables Hospital (Coral Gables FL), 158
Coral Springs Medical Center (Coral Springs FL), 158
Cordell Memorial Hospital (Cordell OK), 533
Corning Hospital (Corning NY), 456
Corona Regional Medical Center (Corona CA), 93
coronary heart disease, 42
Corpus Christi Medical Center (Corpus Christi TX), 627
Cortland Regional Medical Center (Cortland NY), 457
Coshocton County Memorial Hospital (Coshocton OH), 508
Cottage Hospital (Woodsville NH), 429
Cottonwood Hospital (Murray UT), 671
Coulee Community Hospital (Grand Coulee WA), 691
Covenant Hospital Levelland (Levelland TX), 627
Covenant Hospital Plainview (Plainview TX), 628
Covenant Medical Center (Lubbock TX), 628
Covenant Medical Center (Saginaw MI), 350
Covenant Medical Center (Waterloo IA), 261
Covington County Hospital (Collins MS), 384
Cox Medical Center (Springfield MO), 400
Cox Monett Hospital (Monett MO), 400
Coryell Memorial Hospital (Gatesville TX), 627

Craig General Hospital (Vinita OK), 533
Craven Regional Medical Center (New Bern NC), 487
Crawford County Memorial Hospital (Denison IA), 261
Crawford Memorial Hospital (Robinson IL), 215
Creek Nation Community Hospital (Okemah OK), 533
Creighton University Medical Center (Omaha NE), 420
Crenshaw Community Hospital (Luverne AL), 51
Crestwood Medical Center (Huntsville AL), 51
Crisp Regional Hospital (Cordele GA), 187
Crittenden Health Systems (Marion KY), 289
Crittenden Regional Hospital (West Memphis AR), 76
Crittenton Hospital Medical Center (Rochester MI), 350
Crockett Hospital (Lawrenceburg TN), 602
Crosbyton Clinic Hospital (Crosbyton TX), 628
Crossroads Community Hospital (Mount Vernon IL), 215
Crouse Hospital (Syracuse NY), 457
Crozer-Chester Medical Center (Chester PA), 559
Crystal Falls Community Hospital (Crystal Falls MI), 350
Cuero Community Hospital (Cuero TX), 628
Cullman Regional Medical Center (Cullman AL), 51
Culpeper Memorial Hospital (Culpeper VA), 680
Cumberland County Hospital (Burkesville KY), 289
Cumberland Medical Center (Crossville TN), 602
Cumberland Memorial Hospital (Cumberland WI), 716
Cumberland River Hospital (Celina TN), 602
Cushing Memorial Hospital (Leavenworth KS), 276
Cushing Regional Hospital (Cushing OK), 533
Cuyahoga Falls General Hospital (Cuyahoga Falls OH), 508
Cuyuna Regional Medical Center (Crosby MN), 368
Cypress Fairbanks Medical Center (Houston TX), 628

D

D. M. Cogdell Memorial Hospital (Snyder TX), 628
D. W. McMillan Memorial Hospital (Brewton AL), 51
Dakota Midland Hospital (Aberdeen SD), 596
Dale Medical Center (Ozark AL), 51
Dallas, Texas, 620, 621, 623, 629, 630, 637, 644, 648, 654,
    655, 657, 666
Dallas Regional Medical Center—Galloway Campus
    (Mesquite TX), 629
Dallas Southwest Medical Center (Dallas TX), 629
Dameron Hospital Association (Stockton CA), 94
Danbury Hospital (Danbury CT), 147
Danville Regional Medical Center (Danville VA), 680
Dauterive Hospital (New Iberia LA), 306
Daviess Community Hospital (Washington IN), 243
Davis County Hospital (Bloomfield IA), 262
Davis Memorial Hospital (Elkins WV), 705
Davis Memorial Hospital and Medical Center (Layton UT),
    671
Davis Regional Medical Center (Statesville NC), 487
Day Kimball Hospital (Putnam CT), 147
Dayton Heart Hospital (Dayton OH), 508
DCH Regional Medical Center (Tuscaloosa AL), 51
De Queen Medical Center (De Queen AR), 76
De Witt City Hospital (De Witt AR), 76
Deaconess Hospital (Cincinnati OH), 508
Deaconess Hospital (Evansville IN), 244

Deaconess Hospital (Oklahoma City OK), 533
Deaconess Medical Center (Spokane WA), 691
Dearborn County Hospital (Lawrenceburg IN), 244
Deborah Heart and Lung Center (Browns Mills NJ), 435
Decatur County General Hospital (Parsons TN), 603
Decatur County Hospital (Leon IA), 262
Decatur County Memorial Hospital (Greensburg IN), 244
Decatur General Hospital (Decatur AL), 52
Decatur Memorial Hospital (Decatur IL), 215
Defiance Regional Medical Center (Defiance OH), 508
Degraff Memorial Hospital (North Tonawanda NY), 457
Dekalb Hospital (Smithville TN), 603
Dekalb Medical Center (Decatur GA), 187
DeKalb Memorial Hospital (Auburn IN), 244
Del E. Webb Memorial Hospital (Sun City West AZ), 67
Del Sol Medical Center (El Paso TX), 629
Delano Regional Medical Center (Delano CA), 94
Delaware
    five star rated facilities, 749–50
    hospitals, 152–53
    procedure, hospital ratings by, 860–61
Delaware County Memorial Hospital (Drexel Hill PA), 559
Delaware Valley Hospital (Walton NY), 457
Delnor Community Hospital (Geneva IL), 215
Delray Medical Center (Delray Beach FL), 158
Delta County Memorial Hospital (Delta CO), 141
Delta Medical Center (Memphis TN), 603
Delta Memorial Hospital Association (Dumas AR), 76
Delta Regional Medical Center (Greenville MS), 385
Denver, Colorado, 139, 140, 141, 144
Denver Health Medical Center (Denver CO), 141
Depaul Hospital (Cheyenne WY), 730
DES (drug-eluting stents), 42, 43
Des Moines, Iowa, 260, 265, 268, 269
Des Peres Hospital (St. Louis MO), 400
Desert Regional Medical Center (Palm Springs CA), 94
Desert Springs Hospital (Las Vegas NV), 425
Desert Valley Hospital (Victorville CA), 94
Desoto Memorial Hospital (Arcadia FL), 158
Desoto Regional Health System (Mansfield LA), 306
Detar Hospital Navarro (Victoria TX), 629
Detar Hospital North (Victoria TX), 629
Detroit, Michigan, 350, 352, 353, 355, 362, 364
Detroit Receiving Hospital and University Health Center
    (Detroit MI), 350
diagnosis(-es), 4, 5, 8, 10–12, 15, 17, 26, 27, 36, 42
Diagnostic Center Hospital (Houston TX), 630
diagnostic tests, 35, 36
Dickenson Community Hospital (Clintwood VA), 680
Dickinson County Healthcare System (Iron Mountain MI), 351
Dimmit County Memorial Hospital (Carrizo Springs TX), 630
Divine Savior Healthcare (Portage WI), 716
Dixie Regional Medical Center (St. George UT), 671
doctor(s) (physicians)
    being comfortable with your, 4–6
    being proactive when searching for a, 2–4
    board-certified, 7
    breaking up with your, 12, 35

Please note that all individual hospital listings provide page numbers for Chapter 6 (Hospital Ratings by Clinical Specialty) only. All other hospital listings can be found under their state listing.

checking the background of, 6–8
choosing a, 2–12
first visit with your new, 10
hand washing by, 34
in the hospital, 27
interacting with, 32–36
interviewing, 9–11
and malpractice claims, 7, 8
and MDs vs. DOs, 8
and medical myths, 8
referrals from, 11
and search for a top hospital, 15–16
trusting your, 2, 10, 12, 15, 35
Dr. Dan C. Trigg Memorial Hospital (Tucumcari NM), 445
Doctors Community Hospital (Lanham MD), 327
Doctors Hospital (Augusta GA), 188
Doctors Hospital (Coral Gables FL), 158
Doctors Hospital of Laredo (Laredo TX), 630
Doctors Hospital of Manteca (Manteca CA), 94
Doctor's Hospital Medical Center of Montclair
    (Montclair CA), 94
Doctors Hospital of Nelsonville (Nelsonville OH), 509
Doctors Hospital Ohio Health (Columbus OH), 509
Doctors' Hospital of Opelousas (Opelousas LA), 306
Doctors Hospital—Parkway (Houston TX), 630
Doctors Hospital at Renaissance (Edinburg TX), 630
Doctors Hospital of Sarasota (Sarasota FL), 158
Doctors' Hospital of Shreveport (Shreveport LA), 306
Doctors Hospital of Stark County (Massillon OH), 509
Doctors Hospital of Tacoma (Tacoma WA), 692
Doctors Hospital—Tidwell (Houston TX), 631
Doctors Hospital at White Rock Lake (Dallas TX), 630
Doctors Medical Center of Modesto (Modesto CA), 95
Doctors Medical Center—San Pablo/Pinole
    (San Pablo CA), 95
Doctors Memorial Hospital (Bonifay FL), 159
Doctors' Memorial Hospital (Perry FL), 159
documentation, preparing, 22
Dodge County Hospital (Eastman GA), 188
Dolly Vinsant Memorial Hospital (San Benito TX), 631
Dominican Hospital (Santa Cruz CA), 95
Donalsonville Hospital (Donalsonville GA), 188
Door County Memorial Hospital (Sturgeon Bay WI), 717
Dorminy Medical Center (Fitzgerald GA), 188
DOs, 8
Douglas County Hospital (Alexandria MN), 368
Down East Community Hospital (Machias ME), 321
Downey Regional Medical Center (Downey CA), 95
Doylestown Hospital (Doylestown PA), 560
DPOA. See Durable Power of Attorney
Drew Memorial Hospital (Monticello AR), 77
drug-eluting stents (DES), 42, 43
DuBois Regional Medical Center (DuBois PA), 560
Dubuis Hospital Continuing Care Shreveport
    (Shreveport LA), 307
Duke Health Raleigh Hospital (Raleigh NC), 488
Duke University Hospital (Durham NC), 488
Dukes Memorial Hospital (Peru IN), 244

Duncan Regional Hospital (Duncan OK), 534
Dunlap Memorial Hospital (Orrville OH), 509
Dunn Memorial Hospital (Bedford IN), 244
Duplin General Hospital (Kenansville NC), 488
Dupont Hospital (Fort Wayne IN), 245
Durable Power of Attorney (DPOA), 22–23, 37
Durham Regional Hospital (Durham NC), 488
Dyersburg Regional Medical Center (Dyersburg TN), 603

E
E. A. Conway Medical Center (Monroe LA), 307
East Alabama Medical Center and Skilled Nursing Facility
    (Opelika AL), 52
East Cooper Regional Medical Center (Mt. Pleasant SC), 588
East Georgia Regional Medical Center (Statesboro GA), 188
East Houston Regional Medical Center (Houston TX), 631
East Jefferson General Hospital (Metairie LA), 307
East Liverpool City Hospital (East Liverpool OH), 509
East Los Angeles Doctors Hospital (Los Angeles CA), 95
East Ohio Regional Hospital (Martins Ferry OH), 509
East Orange General Hospital (East Orange NJ), 435
East Texas Medical Center (Tyler TX), 631
East Texas Medical Center—Athens (Athens TX), 631
East Texas Medical Center—Carthage (Carthage TX), 631
East Texas Medical Center—Clarksville (Clarksville TX), 632
East Texas Medical Center—Crockett (Crockett TX), 632
East Texas Medical Center—Fairfield (Fairfield TX), 632
East Texas Medical Center—Gilmer (Gilmer TX), 632
East Texas Medical Center—Jacksonville
    (Jacksonville TX), 632
East Texas Medical Center—Mt. Vernon (Mt. Vernon TX), 632
East Texas Medical Center—Quitman (Quitman TX), 633
East Valley Hospital Medical Center (Glendora CA), 95
Eastern Idaho Regional Medical Center (Idaho Falls ID), 208
Eastern Long Island Hospital (Greenport NY), 457
Eastern Maine Medical Center (Bangor ME), 321
Eastern New Mexico Medical Center (Roswell NM), 445
Eastern Oklahoma Medical Center (Poteau OK), 534
Eastland Memorial Hospital (Eastland TX), 633
Easton Hospital (Easton PA), 560
Eaton Rapids Medical Center (Eaton Rapids MI), 351
Eden Medical Center (Castro Valley CA), 96
Edgefield County Hospital (Edgefield SC), 588
Edgerton Hospital and Health Services (Edgerton WI), 717
Edinburg Regional Medical Center (Edinburg TX), 633
Edmond Medical Center (Edmond OK), 534
Edward Hospital (Naperville IL), 215
Edward John Noble Hospital of Gouverneur
    (Gouverneur NY), 457
Edward W. Sparrow Hospital Association (Lansing MI), 351
Edward White Hospital (St. Petersburg FL), 159
EEG. See electroencephalography
Eisenhower Medical Center (Rancho Mirage CA), 96
El Camino Hospital (Mountain View CA), 96
El Campo Memorial Hospital (El Campo TX), 633
El Centro Regional Medical Center (El Centro CA), 96
El Dorado Hospital (Tucson AZ), 67
El Paso, Texas, 629, 633, 642, 654, 656, 662, 663

El Paso Specialty Hospital (El Paso TX), 633
Elbert Memorial Hospital (Elberton GA), 188
Electra Memorial Hospital (Electra TX), 633
electroencephalography (EEG), 22
Eliza Coffee Memorial Hospital (Florence AL), 52
Elizabethtown Community Hospital (Elizabethtown NY), 458
Elk Regional Health Center (St. Marys PA), 560
Elkhart General Hospital (Elkhart IN), 245
Elkview General Hospital (Hobart OK), 534
Ellett Memorial Hospital (Appleton City MO), 400
Elliot Hospital (Manchester NH), 429
Ellis Hospital (Schenectady NY), 458
Ellsworth Municipal Hospital (Iowa Falls IA), 262
Ellwood City Hospital (Ellwood City PA), 560
Elmhurst Memorial Hospital (Elmhurst IL), 215
Elmore Community Hospital (Wetumpka AL), 52
Ely Bloomenson Community Hospital (Ely MN), 368
Emanuel County Hospital (Swainsboro GA), 189
Emanuel Medical Center (Turlock CA), 96
emergency room (ER), 23–27
    checking in to the, 24
    and "divert" status, 24
    exams in, 25–26
    and getting admitted, 26–27
    wait times in, 24–25
Emerson Hospital (Concord MA), 337
Emh Regional Medical Center (Elyria OH), 510
Emma L. Bixby Medical Center (Adrian MI), 351
Emory Adventist Hospital (Smyrna GA), 189
Emory Crawford Long Hospital (Atlanta GA), 189
Emory Dunwoody Medical Center (Atlanta GA), 189
Emory Eastside Medical Center (Snellville GA), 189
Emory University Hospital (Atlanta GA), 189
Encino-Tarzana Regional Medical Center (Encino CA), 96
Encino-Tarzana Regional Medical Center—Tarzana
    Campus (Tarzana CA), 97
Englewood Community Hospital (Englewood FL), 159
Englewood Hospital and Medical Center (Englewood NJ), 435
Enloe Medical Center (Chico CA), 97
Ennis Regional Medical Center (Ennis TX), 634
Enumclaw Community Hospital (Enumclaw WA), 692
Ephraim McDowell Regional Medical Center
    (Danville KY), 289
Ephrata Community Hospital (Ephrata PA), 560
epidurals, 40, 41, 45
ER. See emergency room
Erie County Medical Center (Buffalo NY), 458
Erlanger Bledsoe Hospital (Pikeville TN), 603
Erlanger Medical Center (Chattanooga TN), 603
errors, 15, 18, 28, 32, 37
errors, medical. See medical errors
Española Hospital (Española NM), 446
ETMC Pittsburg (Pittsburg TX), 634
Eureka Community Hospital (Eureka IL), 216
Evangelical Community Hospital (Lewisburg PA), 561
Evans Memorial Hospital (Claxton GA), 190
Evanston Northwestern Healthcare (Evanston IL), 216
Evanston Regional Hospital (Evanston WY), 731

Please note that all individual hospital listings provide page numbers for Chapter 6 (Hospital Ratings by Clinical Specialty) only. All other hospital listings can be found under their state listing.

Evergreen Hospital Medical Center (Kirkland WA), 692
Evergreen Medical Center (Evergreen AL), 52
exams, ER, 25–26
Excelsior Springs Medical Center (Excelsior Springs MO), 401
Exempla Lutheran Medical Center (Wheat Ridge CO), 141
Exempla Saint Joseph Hospital (Denver CO), 141
Exeter Hospital (Exeter NH), 429

F

F. F. Thompson Hospital (Canandaigua NY), 458
Fairbanks Memorial Hospital (Fairbanks AK), 64
Fairchild Medical Center (Yreka CA), 97
Fairfield Medical Center (Lancaster OH), 510
Fairfield Memorial Hospital (Fairfield IL), 216
Fairfield Memorial Hospital (Winnsboro SC), 588
Fairmont General Hospital (Fairmont WV), 705
Fairmont Medical Center (Fairmont MN), 369
Fairview Hospital (Cleveland OH), 510
Fairview Hospital Chisago Lakes (Chisago City MN), 369
Fairview Lakes Health Services (Wyoming MN), 369
Fairview Northland Regional Hospital (Princeton MN), 369
Fairview Park Hospital (Dublin GA), 190
Fairview Red Wing Hospital (Red Wing MN), 369
Fairview Ridges Hospital (Burnsville MN), 369
Fairview Southdale Hospital (Edina MN), 370
Faith Regional Health Services (Norfolk NE), 420
Fallbrook Hospital (Fallbrook CA), 97
Falls Community Hospital and Clinic (Marlin TX), 634
Falls Memorial Hospital (International Falls MN), 370
Falmouth Hospital (Falmouth MA), 338
Fannin Regional Hospital (Blue Ridge GA), 190
Faulkner Hospital (Boston MA), 338
Fauquier Hospital (Warrenton VA), 680
Fawcett Memorial Hospital (Port Charlotte FL), 159
Faxton-Childrens Hospital (Utica NY), 458
Faxton-St. Luke's Healthcare (Utica NY), 458
Fayette County Hospital (Vandalia IL), 216
Fayette County Memorial Hospital
    (Washington Court House OH), 510
Fayette Medical Center (Fayette AL), 52
Fayette Memorial Hospital (Connersville IN), 245
Feather River Hospital (Paradise CA), 97
fellows, 28
Ferrell Hospital Community Foundations (Eldorado IL), 216
FHN Memorial Hospital (Freeport IL), 216
Field Memorial Community Hospital (Centreville MS), 385
Finley Hospital (Dubuque IA), 262
Firelands Regional Medical Center—Main Campus
    (Sandusky OH), 510
First Care Medical Services (Fosston MN), 370
FirstHealth Moore Regional Hospital (Pinehurst NC), 488
FirstHealth Richmond Memorial Hospital
    (Rockingham NC), 488
Fisher Titus Memorial Hospital (Norwalk OH), 510
Fishermen's Hospital (Marathon FL), 159
Fitzgibbon Memorial Hospital (Marshall MO), 401
five star ratings, xiii, xiv, 16, 17
Flaget Memorial Hospital (Bardstown KY), 289

Flagler Hospital (St. Augustine FL), 160
Flagstaff Medical Center (Flagstaff AZ), 67
Flambeau Hospital (Park Falls WI), 717
Fleming County Hospital (Flemingsburg KY), 289
Fletcher Allen Hospital of Vermont (Burlington VT), 675
Flint River Hospital (Montezuma GA), 190
Florida
    five star rated facilities, 750–57
    hospitals, 153–83
    procedure, hospital ratings by, 862–69
    top doctors, 1050–53
Florida Hospital (Orlando FL), 160
Florida Hospital—Deland (Deland FL), 160
Florida Hospital—Fish Memorial (Orange City FL), 160
Florida Hospital—Flagler (Palm Coast FL), 160
Florida Hospital—Heartland Medical Center
    (Sebring FL), 160
Florida Hospital—Oceanside (Ormond Beach FL), 161
Florida Hospital—Ormond Beach (Ormond Beach FL), 161
Florida Hospital—Waterman (Tavares FL), 161
Florida Hospital—Zephyrhills (Zephyrhills FL), 161
Florida Keys Memorial Hospital (Key West FL), 161
Florida Medical Center (Fort Lauderdale FL), 161
Flower Hospital (Sylvania OH), 511
Flowers Hospital (Dothan AL), 53
Floyd County Memorial Hospital (Charles City IA), 262
Floyd Medical Center (Rome GA), 190
Floyd Memorial Hospital and Health Services
    (New Albany IN), 245
Floyd Valley Hospital (Le Mars IA), 262
Flushing Hospital Medical Center (Flushing NY), 459
Foothill Presbyterian Hospital (Glendora CA), 97
Forest Hills Hospital (Forest Hills NY), 459
Forest Park Community Hospital (St. Louis MO), 401
Forrest General Hospital (Hattiesburg MS), 385
Forsyth Memorial Hospital (Winston-Salem NC), 489
Fort Defiance Indian Hospital (Fort Defiance AZ), 67
Fort Duncan Medical Center (Eagle Pass TX), 634
Fort Hamilton Hughes Memorial Hospital (Hamilton OH), 511
Fort Healthcare (Fort Atkinson WI), 717
Fort Lauderdale, Florida, 156, 161, 164, 165, 172
Fort Logan Hospital (Stanford KY), 289
Fort Loudoun Medical Center (Lenoir City TN), 604
Fort Madison Community Hospital (Fort Madison IA), 263
Fort Sanders Regional Medical Center (Knoxville TN), 604
Fort Sanders Sevier Medical Center (Sevierville TN), 604
Fort Walton Beach Medical Center (Fort Walton Beach FL),
    162
Fort Washington Hospital (Fort Washington MD), 327
Fort Worth, Texas, 620, 637, 639, 640, 644, 655
Fostoria Community Hospital (Fostoria OH), 511
Fountain Valley Regional Hospital and Medical Center
    (Fountain Valley CA), 98
Franciscan Skemp La Crosse Hospital (La Crosse WI), 717
Franciscan Skemp Sparta Hospital (Sparta WI), 717
Frank R. Howard Memorial Hospital (Willits CA), 98
Frankford Hospital—Torresdale Campus
    (Philadelphia PA), 561

Frankfort Regional Medical Center (Frankfort KY), 290
Franklin County Memorial Hospital (Meadville MS), 385
Franklin Foundation Hospital (Franklin LA), 307
Franklin Hospital (Benton IL), 217
Franklin Hospital (Valley Stream NY), 459
Franklin Medical Center (Winnsboro LA), 307
Franklin Memorial Hospital (Farmington ME), 321
Franklin Regional Hospital (Franklin NH), 430
Franklin Regional Medical Center (Louisburg NC), 489
Franklin Square Hospital Center (Baltimore MD), 328
Frederic Municipal Hospital Association (Frederic WI), 718
Frederick Memorial Hospital (Frederick MD), 328
Fredonia Regional Hospital (Fredonia KS), 276
Freeman Health System (Joplin MO), 401
Freeman Neosho Hospital (Neosho MO), 401
Fremont Area Medical Center (Fremont NE), 420
Fremont Medical Center (Yuba City CA), 98
French Hospital Medical Center (San Luis Obispo CA), 98
Fresno, California, 93, 98, 105, 121, 135
Fresno Heart and Surgical Hospital (Fresno CA), 98
Frick Hospital (Mt. Pleasant PA), 561
Frisbie Memorial Hospital (Rochester NH), 430
Froedtert Memorial Lutheran Hospital (Milwaukee WI), 718
Frye Regional Medical Center (Hickory NC), 489
Fulton County Health Center (Wauseon OH), 511
Fulton County Hospital (Salem AR), 77
Fulton County Medical Center (McConnellsburg PA), 561

G

G. H. Lanier Memorial Hospital (Valley AL), 53
Gadsden Regional Medical Center (Gadsden AL), 53
Galesburg Cottage Hospital (Galesburg IL), 217
Galichia Heart Hospital (Wichita KS), 276
Galion Community Hospital (Galion OH), 511
Gallup Indian Medical Center (Gallup NM), 446
Garden City Osteopathic Hospital (Garden City MI), 351
Garden Grove Hospital and Medical Center
    (Garden Grove CA), 98
Garden Park Medical Center (Gulfport MS), 385
Garfield Medical Center (Monterey Park CA), 99
Garfield Memorial Hospital (Panguitch UT), 671
Garrett County Memorial Hospital (Oakland MD), 328
Gaston Memorial Hospital (Gastonia NC), 489
Gateway Medical Center (Clarksville TN), 604
Gateway Regional Medical Center (Granite City IL), 217
Geary Community Hospital (Junction City KS), 276
Geisinger Medical Center (Danville PA), 561
Geisinger South Wilkes-Barre (Wilkes-Barre PA), 561
Geisinger Wyoming Valley Medical Center
    (Wilkes-Barre PA), 562
general anesthesia, 45
Genesis Healthcare System (Zanesville OH), 511
Genesis Medical Center—Davenport (Davenport IA), 263
Genesys Regional Medical Center (Grand Blanc MI), 351
Geneva General Hospital (Geneva NY), 459
George L. Mee Memorial Hospital (King City CA), 99
George Regional Health System (Lucedale MS), 385
George Washington University Hospital (Washington DC), 702

Please note that all individual hospital listings provide page numbers for Chapter 6 (Hospital Ratings by Clinical Specialty) only. All other hospital listings can be found under their state listing.

Georgetown Community Hospital (Georgetown KY), 290
Georgetown Hospital (Georgetown TX), 634
Georgetown Memorial Hospital (Georgetown SC), 588
Georgetown University Hospital (Washington DC), 702
Georgia
    five star rated facilities, 757–59
    hospitals, 184–205
    procedure, hospital ratings by, 870–75
    top doctors, 1053–54
Gerald Champion Regional Medical Center
    (Alamogordo NM), 446
Gerber Memorial Health Services (Fremont MI), 352
Germantown Community Hospital (Germantown TN), 604
Gettysburg Hospital (Gettysburg PA), 562
Gibson Community Hospital (Gibson City IL), 217
Gibson General Hospital (Princeton IN), 245
Gibson General Hospital (Trenton TN), 604
Gifford Medical Center (Randolph VT), 675
Gila Regional Medical Center (Silver City NM), 446
Gilmore Memorial Hospital (Amory MS), 386
Glacial Ridge Hospital (Glenwood MN), 370
Glades General Hospital (Belle Glade FL), 162
Glen Cove Hospital (Glen Cove NY), 459
Glencoe Regional Health Services (Glencoe MN), 370
Glendale Adventist Medical Center (Glendale CA), 99
Glendale Memorial Hospital and Health Center
    (Glendale CA), 99
Glens Falls Hospital (Glens Falls NY), 459
Glenwood Regional Medical Center (West Monroe LA), 307
Gnaden Huetten Memorial Hospital (Lehighton PA), 562
goal for the day, 34
Golden Plains Community Hospital (Borger TX), 634
Golden Valley Memorial Hospital (Clinton MO), 401
Goleta Valley Cottage Hospital (Santa Barbara CA), 99
Good Hope Hospital (Erwin NC), 489
Good Samaritan Health Center (Merrill WI), 718
Good Samaritan Hospital (Bakersfield CA), 99
Good Samaritan Hospital (Baltimore MD), 328
Good Samaritan Hospital (Cincinnati OH), 512
Good Samaritan Hospital (Dayton OH), 512
Good Samaritan Hospital (Kearney NE), 421
Good Samaritan Hospital (Lebanon PA), 562
Good Samaritan Hospital (Los Angeles CA), 100
Good Samaritan Hospital (San Jose CA), 100
Good Samaritan Hospital (Vincennes IN), 245
Good Samaritan Hospital and Rehabilitation Center
    (Puyallup WA), 692
Good Samaritan Hospital Medical Center (West Islip NY), 460
Good Samaritan Hospital of Suffern (Suffern NY), 460
Good Samaritan Medical Center (West Palm Beach FL), 162
Good Samaritan Regional Health Center
    (Mount Vernon IL), 217
Good Samaritan Regional Medical Center (Corvallis OR), 547
Good Samaritan Regional Medical Center (Pottsville PA), 562
Good Shepherd Medical Center (Hermiston OR), 547
Good Shepherd Medical Center (Longview TX), 635
Good Shepherd Medical Center—Linden (Linden TX), 635
Goodall Witcher Healthcare Foundation (Clifton TX), 635

Gordon Hospital (Calhoun GA), 190
Goshen General Hospital (Goshen IN), 246
Gottlieb Memorial Hospital (Melrose Park IL), 217
Grace Hospital (Morganton NC), 489
Graduate Hospital (Philadelphia PA), 562
Grady General Hospital (Cairo GA), 191
Grady Memorial Hospital (Atlanta GA), 191
Grady Memorial Hospital (Chickasha OK), 534
Grady Memorial Hospital (Delaware OH), 512
Grafton City Hospital (Grafton WV), 705
Graham Hospital Association (Canton IL), 218
Graham Regional Medical Center (Graham TX), 635
Grand Itasca Clinic and Hospital (Grand Rapids MN), 370
Grand River Medical Center (Rifle CO), 141
Grand Strand Regional Medical Center (Myrtle Beach SC),
    588
Grand View Hospital (Ironwood MI), 352
Grand View Hospital (Sellersville PA), 563
Grande Ronde Hospital (La Grande OR), 548
Grandview Medical Center (Dayton OH), 512
Grandview Medical Center (Jasper TN), 605
Grant Medical Center (Columbus OH), 512
Grant Memorial Hospital (Petersburg WV), 705
Grant Regional Health Center (Lancaster WI), 718
Granville Medical Center (Oxford NC), 490
Grape Community Hospital (Hamburg IA), 263
Gratiot Medical Center (Alma MI), 352
Grays Harbor Community Hospital (Aberdeen WA), 692
Great Plains Regional Medical Center (Elk City OK), 534
Great Plains Regional Medical Center (North Platte NE), 421
Great River Medical Center (Blytheville AR), 77
Great River Medical Center (West Burlington IA), 263
Greater Baltimore Medical Center (Baltimore MD), 328
Greater Community Hospital (Creston IA), 263
Greater El Monte Community Hospital (South El Monte CA),
    100
Greater Southeast Community Hospital (Washington DC),
    702
Greenbrier Valley Medical Center (Ronceverte WV), 705
Greene County General Hospital (Linton IN), 246
Greene County Medical Center (Jefferson IA), 263
Greene Memorial Hospital (Xenia OH), 512
Greenfield Area Medical Center (Greenfield OH), 513
Greenview Regional Hospital (Bowling Green KY), 290
Greenville Hospital (Jersey City NJ), 435
Greenville Memorial Hospital (Greenville SC), 589
Greenville Regional Hospital (Greenville IL), 218
Greenwich Hospital Association (Greenwich CT), 147
Greenwood County Hospital (Eureka KS), 276
Greenwood Leflore Hospital (Greenwood MS), 386
Grenada Lake Medical Center (Grenada MS), 386
Griffin Hospital (Derby CT), 147
Grim-Smith Hospital and Clinic (Kirksville MO), 402
Grinnell Regional Medical Center (Grinnell IA), 264
Gritman Medical Center (Moscow ID), 208
Grossmont Hospital (La Mesa CA), 100
Group Health Eastside Hospital (Redmond WA), 692
Grove City Medical Center (Grove City PA), 563

Grundy Hospital (Grundy VA), 681
Guadalupe Valley Hospital (Seguin TX), 635
Gulf Breeze Hospital (Gulf Breeze FL), 162
Gulf Coast Hospital (Fort Myers FL), 162
Gulf Coast Medical Center (Biloxi MS), 386
Gulf Coast Medical Center (Panama City FL), 162
Gulf Coast Medical Center (Wharton TX), 635
Gundersen Lutheran Medical Center (La Crosse WI), 718
Gunnison Valley Hospital (Gunnison UT), 671
Guthrie County Hospital (Guthrie Center IA), 264
Gwinnett Medical Center (Lawrenceville GA), 191

H
H. B. Magruder Memorial Hospital (Port Clinton OH), 513
H. C. Watkins Memorial Hospital (Quitman MS), 386
Habersham County Medical Center (Demorest GA), 191
Hackensack University Medical Center (Hackensack NJ),
    435
Hackettstown Community Hospital (Hackettstown NJ), 436
Hackley Hospital (Muskegon MI), 352
Hahnemann University Hospital (Philadelphia PA), 563
Hale County Hospital (Greensboro AL), 53
Halifax Medical Center (Daytona Beach FL), 163
Halifax Regional Hospital (South Boston VA), 681
Halifax Regional Medical Center (Roanoke Rapids NC), 490
Hallmark Health (Medford MA), 338
Hamilton County Public Hospital (Webster City IA), 264
Hamilton General Hospital (Hamilton TX), 636
Hamilton Medical Center (Dalton GA), 191
Hamilton Memorial Hospital District (McLeansboro IL), 218
Hamlin Memorial Hospital (Hamlin TX), 636
Hammond Henry Hospital (Geneseo IL), 218
Hamot Medical Center (Erie PA), 563
Hampshire Memorial Hospital (Romney WV), 705
Hampton Regional Medical Center (Varnville SC), 589
Hancock County Memorial Hospital (Britt IA), 264
Hancock Medical Center (Bay St. Louis MS), 386
Hancock Regional Hospital (Greenfield IN), 246
Hand County Memorial Hospital (Miller SD), 596
hand washing, 34, 35
Hanford Community Medical Center (Hanford CA), 100
Hannibal Regional Hospital (Hannibal MO), 402
Hanover General Hospital (Hanover PA), 563
Harbor Hospital (Baltimore MD), 328
Harborview Medical Center (Seattle WA), 693
Hardin County General Hospital (Rosiclare IL), 218
Hardin Medical Center (Savannah TN), 605
Hardin Memorial Hospital (Elizabethtown KY), 290
Hardin Memorial Hospital (Kenton OH), 513
Hardtner Medical Center (Olla LA), 308
Hardy Wilson Memorial Hospital (Hazlehurst MS), 387
Harford Memorial Hospital (Havre De Grace MD), 329
Harlan ARH Hospital (Harlan KY), 290
Harlem Hospital Center (New York NY), 460
Harlingen Medical Center (Harlingen TX), 636
Harper Hospital District #5 (Harper KS), 277
Harper University Hospital (Detroit MI), 352
Harrington Memorial Hospital (Southbridge MA), 338

Harris County Hospital District (Houston TX), 636
Harris Hospital (Newport AR), 77
Harris Methodist Dublin (Dublin TX), 636
Harris Methodist Erath County (Stephenville TX), 636
Harris Methodist Fort Worth (Fort Worth TX), 637
Harris Methodist HEB Hospital (Bedford TX), 637
Harris Methodist Southwest (Fort Worth TX), 637
Harris Regional Hospital (Sylva NC), 490
Harrisburg Medical Center (Harrisburg IL), 218
Harrison Community Hospital (Cadiz OH), 513
Harrison County Hospital (Corydon IN), 246
Harrison Medical Center (Bremerton WA), 693
Harrison Memorial Hospital (Cynthiana KY), 290
Hart County Hospital (Hartwell GA), 191
Hartford Hospital (Hartford CT), 148
Harton Regional Medical Center (Tullahoma TN), 605
Hartselle Medical Center (Hartselle AL), 53
Haskell County Hospital (Stigler OK), 535
Havasu Regional Medical Center (Lake Havasu City AZ), 68
Hawaii
    five star rated facilities, 759
    hospitals, 205–7
    procedure, hospital ratings by, 876–77
Hawaii Medical Center—East (Honolulu HI), 205
Hawaii Medical Center—West (Ewa Beach HI), 205
Hayes Green Beach Memorial Hospital (Charlotte MI), 352
Hays Medical Center (Hays KS), 277
Hayward Area Memorial Hospital (Hayward WI), 718
Haywood Park Community Hospital (Brownsville TN), 605
Haywood Regional Medical Center (Clyde NC), 490
Hazel Hawkins Memorial Hospital (Hollister CA), 100
Hazleton General Hospital (Hazleton PA), 563
Healdsburg District Hospital (Healdsburg CA), 101
Health Central (Ocoee FL), 163
HealthAlliance Hospital Burbank Campus (Fitchburg MA),
    338
HealthAlliance Hospital Leominster Campus
    (Leominster MA), 338
Healtheast St. John's Hospital (Maplewood MN), 371
Healtheast Woodwinds Hospital (Woodbury MN), 371
HealthGrades, x–xv , 14, 16, 32
HealthGrades.com, 25
Healthmark Regional Medical Center
    (Defuniak Springs FL), 163
HealthSouth Chattanooga Rehab Hospital
    (Chattanooga TN), 605
Healthsouth Medical Center (Dallas TX), 637
Heart Hospital of Austin (Austin TX), 637
Heart Hospital of Lafayette (Lafayette LA), 308
Heart Hospital of New Mexico (Albuquerque NM), 446
Heart of America Medical Center (Rugby ND), 501
Heart of Florida Regional Medical Center (Davenport FL), 163
Heart of Lancaster Regional Medical Center (Lititz PA), 564
Heart of the Rockies Regional Medical Center
    (Salida CO), 141
Heart of Texas Memorial Hospital (Brady TX), 637
Heartland Regional Medical Center (Marion IL), 219
Heartland Regional Medical Center (St. Joseph MO), 402

Heartland Surgical Specialty Hospital (Overland Park KS),
    277
Helen Ellis Memorial Hospital (Tarpon Springs FL), 163
Helen Keller Hospital (Sheffield AL), 53
Helen Newberry Joy Hospital (Newberry MI), 353
Helena Regional Medical Center (Helena AR), 77
Hemet Valley Medical Center (Hemet CA), 101
Henderson County Community Hospital (Lexington TN), 605
Henderson Memorial Hospital (Henderson TX), 638
Hendersonville Medical Center (Hendersonville TN), 606
Hendrick Medical Center (Abilene TX), 638
Hendricks Regional Health (Danville IN), 246
Hendry Regional Medical Center (Clewiston FL), 163
Hennepin County Medical Center (Minneapolis MN), 371
Henrico Doctors' Hospital (Richmond VA), 681
Henrico Doctors' Hospital—Parham (Richmond VA), 681
Henrietta D. Goodall Hospital (Sanford ME), 321
Henry County Health Center (Mount Pleasant IA), 264
Henry County Hospital (Napoleon OH), 513
Henry County Medical Center (Paris TN), 606
Henry County Memorial Hospital (New Castle IN), 246
Henry Ford Bi-County Hospital (Warren MI), 353
Henry Ford Hospital (Detroit MI), 353
Henry Ford Macomb Hospital (Clinton Township MI), 353
Henry Ford Wyandotte Hospital (Wyandotte MI), 353
Henry Mayo Newhall Memorial Hospital (Valencia CA), 101
Henry Medical Center (Stockbridge GA), 192
Henryetta Medical Center (Henryetta OK), 535
Hereford Regional Medical Center (Hereford TX), 638
Heritage Hospital (Somerville MA), 339
Heritage Hospital (Tarboro NC), 490
Hermann Area District Hospital (Hermann MO), 402
Herrick Memorial Hospital (Tecumseh MI), 353
Herrin Hospital (Herrin IL), 219
Hess Memorial Hospital (Mauston WI), 719
Heywood Hospital (Gardner MA), 339
Hialeah Hospital (Hialeah FL), 164
Hiawatha Community Hospital (Hiawatha KS), 277
Hickman Community Health Services (Centerville TN), 606
Hi-Desert Medical Center (Joshua Tree CA), 101
High Point Regional Hospital (High Point NC), 490
Highland Community Hospital (Picayune MS), 387
Highland District Hospital (Hillsboro OH), 513
Highland Hospital (Rochester NY), 460
Highland Medical Center (Lubbock TX), 638
Highland Park Hospital (Highland Park IL), 219
Highlands Hospital (Connellsville PA), 564
Highlands Regional Medical Center (Prestonsburg KY), 291
Highlands Regional Medical Center (Sebring FL), 164
Highline Community Hospital (Burien WA), 693
Hill Country Memorial Hospital (Fredericksburg TX), 638
Hill Regional Hospital (Hillsboro TX), 638
Hillcrest Baptist Medical Center (Waco TX), 639
Hillcrest Hospital (Mayfield Heights OH), 514
Hillcrest Hospital (Pittsfield MA), 339
Hillcrest Medical Center (Tulsa OK), 535
Hillcrest Memorial Hospital (Simpsonville SC), 589
Hills and Dales General Hospital (Cass City MI), 354

Hillsboro Area Hospital (Hillsboro IL), 219
Hillsdale Community Health Center (Hillsdale MI), 354
Hillside Hospital (Pulaski TN), 606
Hilo Medical Center (Hilo HI), 205
Hilton Head Regional Medical Center
    (Hilton Head Island SC), 589
Hinsdale Hospital (Hinsdale IL), 219
hip replacement surgery, 44–45
Hoag Memorial Hospital Presbyterian (Newport Beach CA),
    101
Hoboken University Medical Center (Hoboken NJ), 436
Hocking Valley Community Hospital (Logan OH), 514
Holdenville General Hospital (Holdenville OK), 535
Holland Community Hospital (Holland MI), 354
Hollywood Community Hospital (Hollywood CA), 101
Hollywood Medical Center (Hollywood FL), 164
Hollywood Presbyterian Medical Center (Los Angeles CA), 102
Holmes Regional Medical Center (Melbourne FL), 164
Holy Cross Hospital (Chicago IL), 219
Holy Cross Hospital (Fort Lauderdale FL), 164
Holy Cross Hospital (Silver Spring MD), 329
Holy Cross Hospital (Taos NM), 446
Holy Family Hospital (Spokane WA), 693
Holy Family Hospital New Richmond (New Richmond WI), 719
Holy Family Memorial (Manitowoc WI), 719
Holy Name Hospital (Teaneck NJ), 436
Holy Redeemer Hospital and Medical Center
    (Meadowbrook PA), 564
Holy Rosary Healthcare (Miles City MT), 415
Holy Rosary Medical Center (Ontario OR), 548
Holy Spirit Hospital (Camp Hill PA), 564
Holyoke Medical Center (Holyoke MA), 339
Holzer Medical Center (Gallipolis OH), 514
Homer Memorial Hospital (Homer LA), 308
Homestead Hospital (Homestead FL), 164
Honolulu, Hawaii, 205, 206, 207
Hopedale Medical Complex (Hopedale IL), 220
Hopkins County Memorial Hospital (Sulphur Springs TX), 639
Horizon Medical Center (Dickson TN), 606
Horn Memorial Hospital (Ida Grove IA), 264
Horton Memorial Hospital (Middletown NY), 460
hospital(s)
    assessing, 16–18
    choosing a, 14–18
    doctor-recommended, 15–16
    emergency room of, 23–26
    getting admitted to the, 26–27
    length of stay in, 15
    nonprofit, 15
    personnel at, 27–29
    plan and goal for the day when in, 34
    preparing for a stay at the, 20–29
    reputation of, 15, 16
    scheduled stays at the, 21–23
    teaching vs. non-teaching, 27–28
    touring, 18
Hospital of Central Connecticut—New Britain General
    (New Britain CT), 148

Please note that all individual hospital listings provide page numbers for Chapter 6 (Hospital Ratings by Clinical Specialty) only. All other hospital listings can be found under their state listing.

INDEX

Hospital District #1 of Crawford County (Girard KS), 277

Hospital District #1 of Rice County (Lyons KS), 277

Hospital for Joint Diseases Orthopaedic Institute
(New York NY), 460

Hospital for Orthopaedic and Specialty Service
(Amherst OH), 514

Hospital for Special Surgery (New York NY), 461

Hospital of St. Raphael (New Haven CT), 148

Hospital of the University of Pennsylvania
(Philadelphia PA), 564

Hospital at Westlake Medical Center, The (Austin TX), 639

Hot Spring County Medical Center (Malvern AR), 77

Hot Springs County Memorial Hospital (Thermopolis WY),
731

Houlton Regional Hospital (Houlton ME), 321

Houston, Texas, 619, 624, 628, 630, 631, 636, 639,
646, 647, 648, 649, 654, 657, 659, 660, 663, 664,
665, 668

Houston Medical Center (Warner Robins GA), 192

Houston Northwest Medical Center (Houston TX), 639

Howard County Community Hospital (St. Paul NE), 421

Howard County General Hospital (Columbia MD), 329

Howard Memorial Hospital (Nashville AR), 78

Howard Regional Health System (Kokomo IN), 247

Howard University Hospital (Washington DC), 702

Howard Young Medical Center (Woodruff WI), 719

Hudson Hospital (Hudson WI), 719

Hudson Valley Hospital Center (Cortlandt Manor NY), 461

Huggins Hospital (Wolfeboro NH), 430

Hugh Chatham Memorial Hospital (Elkin NC), 491

Hughston Orthopedic Hospital (Columbus GA), 192

Huguley Memorial Medical Center (Fort Worth TX), 639

Humboldt General Hospital (Humboldt TN), 606

Humphreys County Memorial Hospital (Belzoni MS), 387

Hunterdon Medical Center (Flemington NJ), 436

Huntington Beach Hospital (Huntington Beach CA), 102

Huntington Hospital (Huntington NY), 461

Huntington Memorial Hospital (Pasadena CA), 102

Huntsville Hospital (Huntsville AL), 54

Huntsville Memorial Hospital (Huntsville TX), 639

Hurley Medical Center (Flint MI), 354

Huron Hospital (East Cleveland OH), 514

Huron Medical Center (Bad Axe MI), 354

Huron Regional Medical Center (Huron SD), 596

Huron Valley Sinai Hospital (Commerce Township MI), 354

Hutcheson Medical Center (Fort Oglethorpe GA), 192

Hutchinson Area Health Care (Hutchinson MN), 371

Hutchinson Hospital (Hutchinson KS), 278

Hutzel Hospital (Detroit MI), 355

I

Iberia Medical Center (New Iberia LA), 308

Idaho
five star rated facilities, 760
hospitals, 208–10
procedure, hospital ratings by, 878–79

Illini Community Hospital (Pittsfield IL), 220

Illini Hospital (Silvis IL), 220

Illinois
five star rated facilities, 760–64
hospitals, 211–40
procedure, hospital ratings by, 880–87
top doctors, 1054–55

Illinois Valley Community Hospital (Peru IL), 220

Immanuel St. Joseph's—Mayo Health System
(Mankato MN), 371

Imperial Point Medical Center (Fort Lauderdale FL), 165

Indian Path Medical Center (Kingsport TN), 607

Indian River Medical Center (Vero Beach FL), 165

Indiana
five star rated facilities, 764–66
hospitals, 241–59
procedure, hospital ratings by, 888–93
top doctors, 1056

Indiana Heart Hospital (Indianapolis IN), 247

Indiana Orthopaedic Hospital (Indianapolis IN), 247

Indiana Regional Medical Center (Indiana PA), 564

Indiana University Medical Center (Indianapolis IN), 247

Indianapolis, Indiana, 242, 243, 247, 253, 256, 258, 259

Indianhead Medical Center (Shell Lake WI), 719

Ingalls Memorial Hospital (Harvey IL), 220

Ingham Regional Medical Center (Lansing MI), 355

Inland Hospital (Waterville ME), 322

Innovis Health (Fargo ND), 501

Inova Alexandria Hospital (Alexandria VA), 681

Inova Fair Oaks Hospital (Fairfax VA), 681

Inova Fairfax Hospital (Falls Church VA), 682

Inova Loudoun Hospital (Leesburg VA), 682

Inova Mount Vernon Hospital (Alexandria VA), 682

Integris Baptist Medical Center (Oklahoma City OK), 535

Integris Baptist Regional Health Center (Miami OK), 535

Integris Bass Baptist Health Center (Enid OK), 536

Integris Blackwell Regional Hospital (Blackwell OK), 536

Integris Canadian Valley Regional Hospital (Yukon OK), 536

Integris Clinton Regional Hospital (Clinton OK), 536

Integris Grove General Hospital (Grove OK), 536

Integris Marshall County Medical Center (Madill OK), 536

Integris Mayes County Medical Center (Pryor OK), 537

Integris Southwest Medical Center (Oklahoma City OK), 537

Inter-Community Memorial Hospital at Newfane
(Newfane NY), 461

Interfaith Medical Center (Brooklyn NY), 461

interviewing your doctor, 9–11

Ionia County Memorial Hospital (Ionia MI), 355

Iowa
five star rated facilities, 766–67
hospitals, 259–74
procedure, hospital ratings by, 894–97
top doctors, 1057

Iowa Lutheran Hospital (Des Moines IA), 265

Iowa Methodist Medical Center (Des Moines IA), 265

Ira Davenport Memorial Hospital (Bath NY), 461

Iredell Memorial Hospital (Statesville NC), 491

Iron County Community Hospital (Iron River MI), 355

Iroquois Memorial Hospital (Watseka IL), 220

Irvine Regional Hospital (Irvine CA), 102

Irwin County Hospital (Ocilla GA), 192

Island Hospital (Anacortes WA), 693

Ivinson Memorial Hospital (Laramie WY), 731

IVs, asking about, 34–35

J

J. Arthur Dosher Memorial Hospital (Southport NC), 491

J. C. Blair Memorial Hospital (Huntingdon PA), 565

Jackson, Mississippi, 384, 389, 392, 395

Jackson County Hospital (Scottsboro AL), 54

Jackson County Memorial Hospital (Altus OK), 537

Jackson County Regional Health Center (Maquoketa IA), 265

Jackson General Hospital (Ripley WV), 706

Jackson Health System (Miami FL), 165

Jackson Hospital (Marianna FL), 165

Jackson Hospital and Clinic (Montgomery AL), 54

Jackson Medical Center (Jackson AL), 54

Jackson North Medical Center (North Miami Beach FL), 165

Jackson Parish Hospital (Jonesboro LA), 308

Jackson Park Hospital Foundation (Chicago IL), 221

Jackson Purchase Medical Center (Mayfield KY), 291

Jackson South Community Hospital (Miami FL), 165

Jackson-Madison County General Hospital (Jackson TN), 607

Jacksonville, Florida, 154, 169, 177, 178, 179

Jacksonville Medical Center (Jacksonville AL), 54

Jacobi Medical Center (Bronx NY), 462

Jamaica Hospital Medical Center (Jamaica NY), 462

James B. Haggin Memorial Hospital (Harrodsburg KY), 291

Jameson Memorial Hospital (New Castle PA), 565

Jamestown Hospital (Jamestown ND), 501

Jamestown Regional Medical Center (Jamestown TN), 607

Jane Phillips Medical Center (Bartlesville OK), 537

Jasper County Hospital (Rensselaer IN), 247

Jay County Hospital (Portland IN), 247

Jay Hospital (Jay FL), 166

Jeanes Hospital (Philadelphia PA), 565

Jeff Anderson Regional Medical Center (Meridian MS), 387

Jeff Davis Hospital (Hazlehurst GA), 192

Jefferson Community Health Center (Fairbury NE), 421

Jefferson County Hospital (Fairfield IA), 265

Jefferson Davis Community Hospital (Prentiss MS), 387

Jefferson General Hospital (Port Townsend WA), 693

Jefferson Hospital (Louisville GA), 193

Jefferson Memorial Hospital (Crystal City MO), 402

Jefferson Memorial Hospital (Ranson WV), 706

Jefferson Regional Medical Center (Pine Bluff AR), 78

Jefferson Regional Medical Center (Pittsburgh PA), 565

Jellico Community Hospital (Jellico TN), 607

Jenkins Community Hospital (Jenkins KY), 291

Jennersville Regional Hospital (West Grove PA), 565

Jennie Edmundson Hospital (Council Bluffs IA), 265

Jennie M. Melham Memorial Medical Center
(Broken Bow NE), 421

Jennie Stuart Medical Center (Hopkinsville KY), 291

Jennings American Legion Hospital (Jennings LA), 308

Jersey City Medical Center (Jersey City NJ), 436

Jersey Community Hospital (Jerseyville IL), 221

Jersey Shore Hospital (Jersey Shore PA), 565

Please note that all individual hospital listings provide page numbers for Chapter 6 (Hospital Ratings by Clinical Specialty) only. All other hospital listings can be found under their state listing.

Jersey Shore University Medical Center (Neptune NJ), 436
Jewish Hospital (Cincinnati OH), 514
Jewish Hospital (Louisville KY), 291
Jewish Hospital—Shelbyville (Shelbyville KY), 292
JFK Medical Center (Atlantis FL), 166
JFK Medical Center (Edison NJ), 437
Joel Pomerene Memorial Hospital (Millersburg OH), 515
John C. Lincoln Deer Valley Hospital (Phoenix AZ), 68
John C. Lincoln North Mountain Hospital (Phoenix AZ), 68
John D. Archbold Memorial Hospital (Thomasville GA), 193
John Dempsey Hospital (Farmington CT), 148
John Ed Chambers Memorial Hospital (Danville AR), 78
John F. Kennedy Memorial Hospital (Indio CA), 102
John Fogarty Memorial Hospital (Woonsocket RI), 583
John H. Stroger Jr. Hospital (Chicago IL), 221
John Muir Medical Center (Walnut Creek CA), 102
John Randolph Medical Center (Hopewell VA), 682
John T. Mather Memorial Hospital of Port Jefferson
    (Port Jefferson NY), 462
Johns Community Hospital (Taylor TX), 640
Johns Hopkins Bayview Medical Center (Baltimore MD), 329
Johns Hopkins Hospital (Baltimore MD), 329
Johnson City Medical Center (Johnson City TN), 607
Johnson Memorial Hospital (Franklin IN), 248
Johnson Memorial Hospital (Stafford Springs CT), 148
Johnson Regional Medical Center (Clarksville AR), 78
Johnston Memorial Hospital (Abingdon VA), 682
Johnston Memorial Hospital (Smithfield NC), 491
Johnston Memorial Hospital (Tishomingo OK), 537
Joint Township District Memorial Hospital (St. Marys OH), 515
Jones Memorial Hospital (Wellsville NY), 462
Jones Regional Medical Center (Anamosa IA), 265
Jordan Hospital (Plymouth MA), 339
Jordan Valley Hospital (West Jordan UT), 672
JPS Health Network (Fort Worth TX), 640
Jupiter Medical Center (Jupiter FL), 166

K

Kadlec Medical Center (Richland WA), 694
Kaiser Foundation Hospital (Bellflower CA), 103
Kaiser Foundation Hospital (Harbor City CA), 103
Kaiser Foundation Hospital (Honolulu HI), 206
Kaiser Foundation Hospital (Los Angeles CA), 103
Kaiser Foundation Hospital (Panorama City CA), 103
Kaiser Foundation Hospital (San Diego CA), 103
Kaiser Foundation Hospital—Anaheim (Anaheim CA), 103
Kaiser Foundation Hospital—Fontana (Fontana CA), 104
Kaiser Foundation Hospital—Fremont/Hayward
    (Hayward CA), 104
Kaiser Foundation Hospital—Manteca (Manteca CA), 104
Kaiser Foundation Hospital—Oakland/Richmond
    (Oakland CA), 104
Kaiser Foundation Hospital—South San Francisco
    (South San Francisco CA), 104
Kaiser Foundation Hospital—Vallejo (Vallejo CA), 104
Kaiser Fresno Medical Center (Fresno CA), 105
Kaiser Redwood City Medical Center (Redwood City CA), 105
Kaiser Sacramento Medical Center (Sacramento CA), 105

Kaiser San Francisco Medical Center (San Francisco CA), 105
Kaiser San Rafael Medical Center (San Rafael CA), 105
Kaiser Santa Clara Medical Center (Santa Clara CA), 105
Kaiser Santa Teresa Community Hospital (San Jose CA), 106
Kaiser South Sacramento Medical Center
    (Sacramento CA), 106
Kaiser Sunnyside Medical Center (Clackamas OR), 548
Kaiser Walnut Creek Medical Center (Walnut Creek CA), 106
Kalispell Regional Hospital (Kalispell MT), 415
Kanabec Hospital (Mora MN), 371
Kane Community Hospital (Kane PA), 566
Kane County Hospital (Kanab UT), 672
Kansas
    five star rated facilities, 768–69
    hospitals, 274–86
    procedure, hospital ratings by, 898–901
    top doctors, 1057
Kansas City, Missouri, 396, 404, 407, 410, 413
Kansas Heart Hospital (Wichita KS), 278
Kapi'olani Medical Center at Pali Momi (Aiea HI), 206
Katherine Shaw Bethea Hospital (Dixon IL), 221
Kaweah Delta District Hospital (Visalia CA), 106
Kell West Regional Hospital (Wichita Falls TX), 640
Kendall Regional Medical Center (Miami FL), 166
Kenmore Mercy Hospital (Kenmore NY), 462
Kennebec Valley Medical Center (Augusta ME), 322
Kennedy Memorial Hospitals—Stratford (Stratford NJ), 437
Kenneth Hall Regional Hospital (East St. Louis IL), 221
Kennewick General Hospital (Kennewick WA), 694
Kent County Memorial Hospital (Warwick RI), 583
Kentucky
    five star rated facilities, 769–70
    hospitals, 286–303
    procedure, hospital ratings by, 902–5
    top doctors, 1057–58
Kentucky River Medical Center (Jackson KY), 292
Keokuk Area Hospital (Keokuk IA), 266
Kern Medical Center (Bakersfield CA), 106
Kern Valley Healthcare District (Lake Isabella CA), 106
Kershaw County Medical Center (Camden SC), 589
Kessler Memorial Hospital (Hammonton NJ), 437
Ketchikan General Hospital (Ketchikan AK), 64
Kettering Medical Center (Kettering OH), 515
Kettering Medical Center—Sycamore (Miamisburg OH), 515
Kettering-Mohican Area Medical Center (Loudonville OH),
    515
Kewanee Hospital (Kewanee IL), 221
Keweenaw Memorial Medical Center (Laurium MI), 355
Kimball Medical Center (Lakewood NJ), 437
Kingfisher Regional Hospital (Kingfisher OK), 537
Kingman Community Hospital (Kingman KS), 278
Kingman Regional Medical Center (Kingman AZ), 68
Kings County Hospital Center (Brooklyn NY), 462
King's Daughters Hospital (Temple TX), 640
King's Daughters Hospital (Yazoo City MS), 388
King's Daughters' Hospital and Health Services, The
    (Madison IN), 248
King's Daughters Hospital—Greenville (Greenville MS), 388

King's Daughters Medical Center (Ashland KY), 292
King's Daughters Medical Center—Brookhaven
    (Brookhaven MS), 387
Kings Highway Hospital (Brooklyn NY), 463
Kings Mountain Hospital (Kings Mountain NC), 491
Kingsbrook Jewish Medical Center (Brooklyn NY), 463
Kingston Hospital (Kingston NY), 463
Kingwood Medical Center (Kingwood TX), 640
Kishwaukee Community Hospital (DeKalb IL), 222
Kittitas Valley Community Hospital (Ellensburg WA), 694
Knapp Medical Center (Weslaco TX), 640
knee replacement surgery, 44–45
Knox Community Hospital (Mount Vernon OH), 515
Knox County Hospital (Barbourville KY), 292
Knoxville, Tennessee, 599, 611, 612, 616
Knoxville Hospital and Clinics (Knoxville IA), 266
Kona Community Hospital (Kealakekua HI), 206
Kootenai Medical Center (Coeur d'Alene ID), 209
Kosciusko Community Hospital (Warsaw IN), 248
Kuakini Medical Center (Honolulu HI), 206

L

L. V. Stabler Memorial Hospital (Greenville AL), 54
La Grange Memorial Hospital (La Grange IL), 222
La Palma Intercommunity Hospital (La Palma CA), 107
La Paz Regional Hospital (Parker AZ), 68
Labette Health (Parsons KS), 278
LAC Harbor-UCLA Medical Center (Torrance CA), 107
LAC Martin Luther King Jr. Multi Service Ambulatory Care
    Ctr. (Los Angeles CA), 107
LAC Olive View-UCLA Medical Center (Sylmar CA), 107
LAC+USC Medical Center (Los Angeles CA), 107
Lackey Memorial Hospital (Forest MS), 388
Ladd Memorial Hospital (Osceola WI), 720
Lady of the Sea General Hospital (Cut Off LA), 309
Lafayette, Louisiana, 308, 309, 313, 315, 317
Lafayette General Medical Center (Lafayette LA), 309
Lafayette Home Hospital (Lafayette IN), 248
Lafayette Regional Health Center (Lexington MO), 402
Laird Hospital (Union MS), 388
Laird Memorial Hospital (Kilgore TX), 641
Lake Charles Memorial Hospital (Lake Charles LA), 309
Lake City Medical Center (Lake City FL), 166
Lake Cumberland Regional Hospital (Somerset KY), 292
Lake Forest Hospital (Lake Forest IL), 222
Lake Granbury Medical Center (Granbury TX), 641
Lake Hospital System (Painesville OH), 516
Lake Martin Community Hospital (Dadeville AL), 55
Lake Norman Regional Medical Center (Mooresville NC), 491
Lake Pointe Medical Center (Rowlett TX), 641
Lake Region Healthcare Corporation (Fergus Falls MN), 372
Lake Regional Health System (Osage Beach MO), 403
Lake Shore Hospital (Irving NY), 463
Lake Wales Medical Center (Lake Wales FL), 166
Lake Whitney Medical Center (Whitney TX), 641
Lakeland Community Hospital (Haleyville AL), 55
Lakeland Hospital—St. Joseph (St. Joseph MI), 355
Lakeland Medical Center—Niles (Niles MI), 356

Please note that all individual hospital listings provide page numbers for Chapter 6 (Hospital Ratings by Clinical Specialty) only. All other hospital listings can be found under their state listing.

Lakeland Regional Medical Center (Lakeland FL), 167
Lakes Region General Hospital (Laconia NH), 430
Lakes Regional Healthcare (Spirit Lake IA), 266
Lakeside Memorial Hospital (Brockport NY), 463
Lakeview Community Hospital (Eufaula AL), 55
Lakeview Community Hospital (Paw Paw MI), 356
Lakeview Hospital (Bountiful UT), 672
Lakeview Hospital (Stillwater MN), 372
Lakeview Hospital (Wauwatosa WI), 720
Lakeview Medical Center (Rice Lake WI), 720
Lakeview Regional Medical Center (Covington LA), 309
Lakeway Regional Hospital (Morristown TN), 607
Lakewood Health System (Staples MN), 372
Lakewood Hospital (Lakewood OH), 516
Lakewood Ranch Medical Center (Bradenton FL), 167
Lakewood Regional Medical Center (Lakewood CA), 107
Lallie Kemp Medical Center (Independence LA), 309
Lamb Healthcare Center (Littlefield TX), 641
Lancaster Community Hospital (Lancaster CA), 108
Lancaster General Hospital (Lancaster PA), 566
Lancaster Regional Medical Center (Lancaster PA), 566
Lander Valley Medical Center (Lander WY), 731
Landmark Medical Center (Woonsocket RI), 583
Lane Memorial Hospital (Zachary LA), 309
Langlade Memorial Hospital (Antigo WI), 720
Lapeer Regional Medical Center (Lapeer MI), 356
Laporte Hospital and Health Services (La Porte IN), 248
Laredo Medical Center (Laredo TX), 641
Largo Medical Center (Largo FL), 167
Larkin Community Hospital (South Miami FL), 167
Las Colinas Medical Center (Irving TX), 642
Las Palmas Medical Center (El Paso TX), 642
Las Vegas, Nevada, 425, 426, 427, 428
Lasalle General Hospital (Jena LA), 310
Latimer County General Hospital (Wilburton OK), 538
Latrobe Hospital (Latrobe PA), 566
Laughlin Memorial Hospital (Greeneville TN), 608
Laurel Regional Hospital (Laurel MD), 329
Laurens County Healthcare System (Clinton SC), 589
Lavaca Medical Center (Hallettsville TX), 642
Lawnwood Regional Medical Center and Heart Institute
    (Fort Pierce FL), 167
Lawrence and Memorial Hospital (New London CT), 148
Lawrence County Hospital (Monticello MS), 388
Lawrence County Memorial Hospital (Lawrenceville IL), 222
Lawrence General Hospital (Lawrence MA), 339
Lawrence Hospital Center (Bronxville NY), 463
Lawrence Medical Center (Moulton AL), 55
Lawrence Memorial Hospital (Lawrence KS), 278
LDS Hospital (Salt Lake City UT), 672
Lea Regional Hospital (Hobbs NM), 447
Leake County Memorial Hospital (Carthage MS), 388
Lee Memorial Hospital (Fort Myers FL), 167
Lee Regional Medical Center (Pennington Gap VA), 682
Lee's Summit Medical Center (Lee's Summit MO), 403
Leesburg Regional Medical Center (Leesburg FL), 168
Legacy Emanuel Hospital (Portland OR), 548
Legacy Good Samaritan Hospital (Portland OR), 548

Legacy Meridian Park Hospital (Tualatin OR), 548
Legacy Mount Hood Medical Center (Gresham OR), 549
Legacy Salmon Creek Hospital (Vancouver WA), 694
Lehigh Regional Medical Center (Lehigh Acres FL), 168
Lehigh Valley Hospital (Allentown PA), 566
Lehigh Valley Hospital—Muhlenberg (Bethlehem PA), 566
Lenoir Memorial Hospital (Kinston NC), 492
Lenox Hill Hospital (New York NY), 464
Leonard Hospital (Troy NY), 464
Leonard J. Chabert Medical Center (Houma LA), 310
Leonard Morse Hospital (Natick MA), 340
Lewis County General Hospital (Lowville NY), 464
Lewis-Gale Medical Center (Salem VA), 683
Lewistown Hospital (Lewistown PA), 567
Lexington, Kentucky, 288, 299, 300, 302
Lexington Medical Center (West Columbia SC), 590
Lexington Memorial Hospital (Lexington NC), 492
Liberty Dayton Community Hospital (Liberty TX), 642
Liberty Hospital (Liberty MO), 403
licensed practical nurses (LPNs), 28
Licking Memorial Hospital (Newark OH), 516
Lima Memorial Health System (Lima OH), 516
Lincoln County Medical Center (Troy MO), 403
Lincoln Medical and Mental Health Center (Bronx NY), 464
Lincoln Medical Center (Fayetteville TN), 608
Lincoln General Hospital (Ruston LA), 310
Lincoln Park Hospital (Chicago IL), 222
Little Rock Arkansas, 74, 82, 83, 84
Little Company of Mary Hospital (Evergreen Park IL), 222
Little Company of Mary Hospital (Torrance CA), 108
Little Company of Mary Hospital—San Pedro
    (San Pedro CA), 108
Little Falls Hospital (Little Falls NY), 464
Little River Memorial Hospital (Ashdown AR), 78
Littleton Regional Hospital (Littleton NH), 430
living will, 22–23
Livingston Hospital and Healthcare (Salem KY), 292
Livingston Regional Hospital (Livingston TN), 608
Llano Memorial Healthcare System (Llano TX), 642
Lock Haven Hospital (Lock Haven PA), 567
Lockport Memorial Hospital (Lockport NY), 464
Lodi Memorial Hospital (Lodi CA), 108
Logan County Hospital (Oakley KS), 278
Logan Medical Center (Guthrie OK), 538
Logan Memorial Hospital (Russellville KY), 293
Logan Regional Hospital (Logan UT), 672
Logan Regional Medical Center (Logan WV), 706
Loma Linda University Medical Center (Loma Linda CA), 108
Lompoc Healthcare District (Lompoc CA), 108
Long Beach Medical Center (Long Beach NY), 465
Long Beach Memorial Medical Center (Long Beach CA), 109
Long Island College Hospital (Brooklyn NY), 465
Long Island Jewish Medical Center (New Hyde Park NY), 465
Longmont United Hospital (Longmont CO), 142
Longview Regional Medical Center (Longview TX), 642
Loretto Hospital (Chicago IL), 223
Loring Hospital (Sac City IA), 266
Loris Community Hospital (Loris SC), 590

Los Alamitos Medical Center (Los Alamitos CA), 109
Los Alamos Medical Center (Los Alamos NM), 447
Los Angeles, California, 88, 89, 90, 91, 95, 100, 102, 103,
    107, 109, 116, 124, 133, 134, 136, 138
Los Angeles Community Hospital (Los Angeles CA), 109
Los Angeles Metropolitan Medical Center (Los Angeles CA),
    109
Los Robles Regional Medical Center (Thousand Oaks CA),
    109
Louis A. Weiss Memorial Hospital (Chicago IL), 223
Louis Smith Memorial Hospital (Lakeland GA), 193
Louisiana
    five star rated facilities, 771–72
    hospitals, 303–19
    procedure, hospital ratings by, 906–9
    top doctors, 1058
Louisiana Heart Hospital (Lacombe LA), 310
Louisville, Kentucky, 286, 291, 296, 300, 302
Lourdes Hospital (Paducah KY), 293
Lourdes Medical Center (Pasco WA), 694
Lourdes Medical Center of Burlington County
    (Willingboro NJ), 437
Lovelace Medical Center—Downtown (Albuquerque NM),
    447
Lovelace Medical Center—Gibson (Albuquerque NM), 447
Lovelace Westside Hospital (Albuquerque NM), 447
Lovelace Women's Hospital (Albuquerque NM), 447
Lowell General Hospital (Lowell MA), 340
Lower Bucks Hospital (Bristol PA), 567
Lower Keys Medical Center (Key West FL), 168
Loyola University Medical Center (Maywood IL), 223
LPNs (licensed practical nurses), 28
LSU Health Sciences Center—Shreveport (Shreveport LA),
    310
LTC Hospital at Southeast Alabama Medical Center
    (Dothan AL), 55
LTC Hospital of Tuscaloosa (Tuscaloosa AL), 55
Lubbock Heart Hospital (Lubbock TX), 643
Lucas County Health Center (Chariton IA), 266
Lucerne Medical Center (Orlando FL), 168
Luther Hospital Mayo Health System (Eau Claire WI), 720
Lutheran Community Hospital (Norfolk NE), 421
Lutheran Hospital (Cleveland OH), 516
Lutheran Hospital of Indiana (Fort Wayne IN), 248
Lutheran Medical Center (Brooklyn NY), 465
Luverne Community Hospital (Luverne MN), 372
Lynchburg General Hospital (Lynchburg VA), 683

M

MacNeal Hospital (Berwyn IL), 223
Macon County General Hospital (Lafayette TN), 608
Macon County Samaritan Memorial Hospital (Macon MO),
    403
Mad River Community Hospital (Arcata CA), 109
Madera Community Hospital (Madera CA), 110
Madison Community Hospital (Madison Heights MI), 356
Madison Community Hospital (Madison SD), 596
Madison County Hospital (London OH), 516

Please note that all individual hospital listings provide page numbers for Chapter 6 (Hospital Ratings by Clinical Specialty) only. All other hospital listings can be found under their state listing.

Madison County Memorial Hospital (Madison FL), 168
Madison County Memorial Hospital (Winterset IA), 266
Madison Hospital (Madison MN), 372
Madison Medical Center (Fredericktown MO), 403
Madison Memorial Hospital (Rexburg ID), 209
Madison Parish Hospital (Tallulah LA), 310
Madison Regional Medical Center (Canton MS), 389
Magee General Hospital (Magee MS), 389
Magee-Womens Hospital of the UPMC Health System
  (Pittsburgh PA), 567
Magnolia Hospital (Magnolia AR), 78
Magnolia Regional Health Center (Corinth MS), 389
Mahaska County Hospital (Oskaloosa IA), 267
Maimonides Medical Center (Brooklyn NY), 465
Main Line Hospitals—Bryn Mawr (Bryn Mawr PA), 567
Main Line Hospitals—Lankenau (Wynnewood PA), 567
Main Line Hospitals—Paoli Memorial (Paoli PA), 568
Maine
  five star rated facilities, 772–73
  hospitals, 320–26
  procedure, hospital ratings by, 910–11
  top doctors, 1058
Maine Coast Memorial Hospital (Ellsworth ME), 322
Maine General Medical Center (Waterville ME), 322
Maine Medical Center (Portland ME), 322
Mainland Medical Center (Texas City TX), 643
Major Hospital (Shelbyville IN), 249
Malden Hospital (Malden MA), 340
malpractice claims, 7, 8
Manatee Memorial Hospital (Bradenton FL), 168
Manchester Memorial Hospital (Manchester CT), 149
Manchester Memorial Hospital (Manchester KY), 293
Marcum and Wallace Memorial Hospital (Irvine KY), 293
Marcus Daly Memorial Hospital (Hamilton MT), 416
Margaret Mary Community Hospital (Batesville IN), 249
Margaret R. Pardee Memorial Hospital
  (Hendersonville NC), 492
Maria Parham Hospital (Henderson NC), 492
Marian Community Hospital (Carbondale PA), 568
Marian Medical Center (Santa Maria CA), 110
Maricopa Medical Center (Phoenix AZ), 68
Marietta Memorial Hospital (Marietta OH), 517
Marin General Hospital (Greenbrae CA), 110
Mariners Hospital (Tavernier FL), 169
Marion County Medical Center (Marion SC), 590
Marion General Hospital (Columbia MS), 389
Marion General Hospital (Marion IN), 249
Marion General Hospital (Marion OH), 517
Marion Regional Medical Center (Hamilton AL), 56
Mark Twain St. Joseph's Hospital (San Andreas CA), 110
Marlboro Park Hospital (Bennettsville SC), 590
Marlborough Hospital (Marlborough MA), 340
Marlette Community Hospital (Marlette MI), 356
Marquette General Hospital (Marquette MI), 356
Marshall County Hospital (Benton KY), 293
Marshall Medical Center (Lewisburg TN), 608
Marshall Medical Center (Placerville CA), 110
Marshall Medical Center—North (Guntersville AL), 56

Marshall Medical Center—South (Boaz AL), 56
Marshall Regional Medical Center (Marshall TX), 643
Marshalltown Medical and Surgical Center
  (Marshalltown IA), 267
Martha Jefferson Hospital (Charlottesville VA), 683
Martin General Hospital (Williamston NC), 492
Martin Memorial Medical Center (Stuart FL), 169
Mary and Arthur Clapham Hospital (Burlington MA), 340
Mary Black Memorial Hospital (Spartanburg SC), 590
Mary Breckinridge Hospital (Hyden KY), 293
Mary Chiles Hospital (Mount Sterling KY), 294
Mary Greeley Medical Center (Ames IA), 267
Mary Hitchcock Memorial Hospital (Lebanon NH), 430
Mary Immaculate Hospital (Jamaica NY), 465
Mary Immaculate Hospital (Newport News VA), 683
Mary Imogene Bassett Hospital (Cooperstown NY), 466
Mary Lanning Memorial Hospital (Hastings NE), 422
Mary Rutan Hospital (Bellefontaine OH), 517
Mary Washington Hospital (Fredericksburg VA), 683
Maryland
  five star rated facilities, 773–74
  hospitals, 326–33
  procedure, hospital ratings by, 912–13
  top doctors, 1058–59
Maryland General Hospital (Baltimore MD), 330
Marymount Hospital (Garfield Heights OH), 517
Marymount Medical Center (London KY), 294
Maryvale Hospital (Phoenix AZ), 69
Mason General Hospital (Shelton WA), 694
Mason District Hospital (Havana IL), 223
Massac Memorial Hospital (Metropolis IL), 224
Massachusetts
  five star rated facilities, 774–76
  hospitals, 334–46
  procedure, hospital ratings by, 914–17
  top doctors, 1059
Massachusetts General Hospital (Boston MA), 340
Massena Memorial Hospital (Massena NY), 466
Massillon Community Hospital (Massillon OH), 517
Matagorda General Hospital (Bay City TX), 643
Mat-Su Regional Medical Center (Palmer AK), 64
Maui Memorial Medical Center (Wailuku HI), 206
Maury Regional Hospital (Columbia TN), 608
Mayo Clinic Hospital (Phoenix AZ), 69
Mayo Regional Hospital (Dover Foxcroft ME), 322
McAlester Regional Health Center (McAlester OK), 538
McAllen Medical Center/Heart Hospital (McAllen TX), 643
McBride Clinic Orthopedic Hospital (Oklahoma City OK), 538
McCready Memorial Hospital (Crisfield MD), 330
McCullough-Hyde Memorial Hospital (Oxford OH), 517
McCune-Brooks Hospital (Carthage MO), 404
McCurtain Memorial Hospital (Idabel OK), 538
McDonough District Hospital (Macomb IL), 224
McDowell ARH Hospital (McDowell KY), 294
McDowell Hospital (Marion NC), 492
McDuffie Regional Medical Center (Thomson GA), 193
McGehee Desha County Hospital (McGehee AR), 79
McKay-Dee Hospital Center (Ogden UT), 672

McKee Medical Center (Loveland CO), 142
McKenna Memorial Hospital (New Braunfels TX), 643
McKenzie Memorial Hospital (Sandusky MI), 357
McKenzie Regional Hospital (McKenzie TN), 609
McKenzie-Willamette Medical Center (Springfield OR), 549
McLaren Regional Medical Center (Flint MI), 357
McLeod Medical Center—Darlington (Darlington SC), 590
McLeod Medical Center—Dillon (Dillon SC), 591
McLeod Regional Medical Center (Florence SC), 591
McNairy Regional Hospital (Selmer TN), 609
MDs, 8
Meade District Hospital (Meade KS), 279
Meadowlands Hospital (Secaucus NJ), 437
Meadows Regional Medical Center (Vidalia GA), 193
Meadowview Regional Medical Center (Maysville KY), 294
Meadville Medical Center (Meadville PA), 568
Mease Healthcare Dunedin (Dunedin FL), 169
Mecosta County Medical Center (Big Rapids MI), 357
Medcenter Hospital (Marion OH), 518
Medcenter One (Bismarck ND), 501
Medcentral Health System (Mansfield OH), 518
Medcentral Health System Shelby Hospital (Shelby OH), 518
Medical Arts Hospital (Lamesa TX), 644
Medical Center (Bowling Green KY), 294
Medical Center (Columbus GA), 194
Medical Center of Arlington (Arlington TX), 644
Medical Center of Aurora (Aurora CO), 142
Medical Center—Beaver (Beaver PA), 568
Medical Center of Central Georgia (Macon GA), 194
Medical Center Enterprise (Enterprise AL), 56
Medical Center at Franklin (Franklin KY), 294
Medical Center Hospital (Odessa TX), 644
Medical Center at Lancaster (Lancaster TX), 644
Medical Center of Lewisville (Lewisville TX), 645
Medical Center of Manchester (Manchester TN), 609
Medical Center of McKinney (McKinney TX), 645
Medical Center of Plano (Plano TX), 645
Medical Center at Scottsville, The (Scottsville KY), 295
Medical Center—South Arkansas (El Dorado AR), 79
Medical Center of Southeast Texas, The (Port Arthur TX), 645
Medical Center of Southeastern Oklahoma (Durant OK), 538
Medical Centre Surgical Hospital (Fort Worth TX), 644
Medical City Dallas Hospital (Dallas TX), 644
Medical College of Georgia Hospitals and Clinics
  (Augusta GA), 193
Medical College of Ohio at Toledo (Toledo OH), 518
medical errors, 32, 37
  deaths from, 32
  protecting yourself and your loved ones from, 32–37
  tips for avoiding, 35
Medical Park Hospital (Hope AR), 79
Medical Park Hospital (Winston-Salem NC), 493
medical students, 27, 28
Medical University Hospital (Charleston SC), 591
medications
  asking questions about, 34
  deaths related to, 32
  prices for, 43–44

Please note that all individual hospital listings provide page numbers for Chapter 6 (Hospital Ratings by Clinical Specialty) only. All other hospital listings can be found under their state listing.

Medicine Lodge Memorial Hospital (Medicine Lodge KS), 279

Medina Community Hospital (Hondo TX), 645

Medina General Hospital (Medina OH), 518

Medina Memorial Hospital (Medina NY), 466

Meeker County Memorial Hospital (Litchfield MN), 372

Melrose Area Hospital Centracare (Melrose MN), 373

Melrose-Wakefield Hospital (Melrose MA), 341

Memorial Acute Long Term Care Hospital (Lufkin TX), 645

Memorial Community Hospital (Blair NE), 422

Memorial Health Care Systems (Seward NE), 422

Memorial Health Center (Medford WI), 720

Memorial Health University Medical Center (Savannah GA), 194

Memorial Healthcare Center (Owosso MI), 357

Memorial Healthcare System (Chattanooga TN), 609

Memorial Hermann Baptist Beaumont Hospital (Beaumont TX), 646

Memorial Hermann Baptist Orange Hospital (Orange TX), 646

Memorial Hermann Fort Bend Hospital (Missouri City TX), 646

Memorial Hermann Katy Hospital (Katy TX), 646

Memorial Hermann Memorial City Medical Center (Houston TX), 646

Memorial Hermann Southwest Hospital (Houston TX), 646

Memorial Hermann—Texas Medical Center (Houston TX), 647

Memorial Hospital (Abilene KS), 279

Memorial Hospital (Aurora NE), 422

Memorial Hospital (Belleville IL), 224

Memorial Hospital (Carthage IL), 224

Memorial Hospital (Chester IL), 224

Memorial Hospital (Colorado Springs CO), 142

Memorial Hospital (Craig CO), 142

Memorial Hospital (Dumas TX), 647

Memorial Hospital (Fremont OH), 518

Memorial Hospital (Gonzales TX), 647

Memorial Hospital (Logansport IN), 249

Memorial Hospital (Manitowoc WI), 721

Memorial Hospital (McPherson KS), 279

Memorial Hospital (Nacogdoches TX), 647

Memorial Hospital (North Conway NH), 431

Memorial Hospital (Seminole TX), 647

Memorial Hospital (Towanda PA), 568

Memorial Hospital (York PA), 568

Memorial Hospital and Health Care Center (Jasper IN), 249

Memorial Hospital and Manor (Bainbridge GA), 194

Memorial Hospital and Medical Center—Cumberland (Cumberland MD), 330

Memorial Hospital and Physician Group (Frederick OK), 539

Memorial Hospital of Adel (Adel GA), 194

Memorial Hospital at Easton (Easton MD), 330

Memorial Hospital Burlington (Burlington WI), 721

Memorial Hospital of Carbon County (Rawlins WY), 731

Memorial Hospital of Carbondale (Carbondale IL), 224

Memorial Hospital of Gardena (Gardena CA), 110

Memorial Hospital at Gulfport (Gulfport MS), 389

Memorial Hospital—Jacksonville (Jacksonville FL), 169

Memorial Hospital Lafayette City (Darlington WI), 721

Memorial Hospital—Los Banos (Los Banos CA), 111

Memorial Hospital of Martinsville and Henry County (Martinsville VA), 683

Memorial Hospital of Michgan City (Michigan City IN), 249

Memorial Hospital—Miramar (Miramar FL), 169

Memorial Hospital—Pembroke (Pembroke Pines FL), 169

Memorial Hospital of Rhode Island (Pawtucket RI), 583

Memorial Hospital of Salem County (Salem NJ), 438

Memorial Hospital of Sheridan County (Sheridan WY), 731

Memorial Hospital of South Bend (South Bend IN), 250

Memorial Hospital of Stilwell (Stilwell OK), 539

Memorial Hospital Sweetwater County (Rock Springs WY), 732

Memorial Hospital—Tampa (Tampa FL), 170

Memorial Hospital of Texas County (Guymon OK), 539

Memorial Hospital of Union County (Marysville OH), 519

Memorial Hospital—West (Pembroke Pines FL), 170

Memorial Medical Center (Ashland WI), 721

Memorial Medical Center (Las Cruces NM), 448

Memorial Medical Center (Modesto CA), 111

Memorial Medical Center (Neillsville WI), 721

Memorial Medical Center (Port Lavaca TX), 647

Memorial Medical Center (Springfield IL), 225

Memorial Medical Center of East Texas (Lufkin TX), 648

Memorial Medical Center—Livingston (Livingston TX), 648

Memorial Medical Center of West Michigan (Ludington MI), 357

Memorial Regional Hospital (Hollywood FL), 170

Mena Medical Center (Mena AR), 79

Mendocino Coast District Hospital (Fort Bragg CA), 111

Mendota Community Hospital (Mendota IL), 225

Menifee Valley Medical Center (Sun City CA), 111

Menorah Medical Center (Kansas City MO), 404

Menorah Medical Center (Overland Park KS), 279

Mercer County Joint Township Community (Coldwater OH), 519

Mercy Fitzgerald Hospital (Darby PA), 569

Mercy Franciscan Hospital—Mount Airy (Cincinnati OH), 519

Mercy General Health Partners (Muskegon MI), 357

Mercy General Hospital (Sacramento CA), 111

Mercy Harvard Hospital (Harvard IL), 225

Mercy Health Center (Fort Scott KS), 279

Mercy Health Center (Oklahoma City OK), 539

Mercy Health System (Janesville WI), 721

Mercy Healthcare Center (Toledo OH), 519

Mercy Hospital (Bakersfield CA), 111

Mercy Hospital (Buffalo NY), 466

Mercy Hospital (Coon Rapids MN), 373

Mercy Hospital (Devils Lake ND), 501

Mercy Hospital (Miami FL), 170

Mercy Hospital (Pittsburgh PA), 569

Mercy Hospital (Portland ME), 323

Mercy Hospital and Health Care Center (Moose Lake MN), 373

Mercy Hospital and Medical Center (Chicago IL), 225

Mercy Hospital—Anderson (Anderson OH), 519

Mercy Hospital—Cadillac (Cadillac MI), 358

Mercy Hospital—Clermont (Batavia OH), 519

Mercy Hospital—Fairfield (Fairfield OH), 520

Mercy Hospital of Folsom (Folsom CA), 112

Mercy Hospital of Franciscan Sisters—Oelwein (Oelwein IA), 267

Mercy Hospital—Grayling (Grayling MI), 358

Mercy Hospital—Iowa City (Iowa City IA), 267

Mercy Hospital of Kansas Independence (Independence KS), 280

Mercy Hospital—Port Huron (Port Huron MI), 358

Mercy Hospital Scranton (Scranton PA), 569

Mercy Hospital—Tiffin Ohio (Tiffin OH), 520

Mercy Hospital—Turner Memorial (Ozark AR), 79

Mercy Hospital of Valley City (Valley City ND), 501

Mercy Hospital—Western Hills (Cincinnati OH), 520

Mercy Hospital—Willard (Willard OH), 520

Mercy Jeannette Hospital (Jeannette PA), 569

Mercy Medical Center (Baltimore MD), 330

Mercy Medical Center (Canton OH), 520

Mercy Medical Center (Nampa ID), 209

Mercy Medical Center (Oshkosh WI), 722

Mercy Medical Center (Rockville Centre NY), 466

Mercy Medical Center (Roseburg OR), 549

Mercy Medical Center (Springfield MA), 341

Mercy Medical Center (Williston ND), 502

Mercy Medical Center—Cedar Rapids (Cedar Rapids IA), 267

Mercy Medical Center—Centerville (Centerville IA), 268

Mercy Medical Center—Clinton (Clinton IA), 268

Mercy Medical Center—Des Moines (Des Moines IA), 268

Mercy Medical Center—Dubuque (Dubuque IA), 268

Mercy Medical Center Merced (Merced CA), 112

Mercy Medical Center Mt. Shasta (Mt. Shasta CA), 112

Mercy Medical Center—North Iowa (Mason City IA), 268

Mercy Medical Center of Springfield (Springfield OH), 520

Mercy Medical Center Redding (Redding CA), 112

Mercy Medical Center—Sioux City (Sioux City IA), 268

Mercy Memorial Health Center (Ardmore OK), 539

Mercy Memorial Hospital (Monroe MI), 358

Mercy Memorial Hospital (Urbana OH), 521

Mercy Providence Hospital (Pittsburgh PA), 569

Mercy Regional Health Center (Manhattan KS), 280

Mercy Regional Medical Center (Durango CO), 142

Mercy San Juan Medical Center (Carmichael CA), 112

Mercy Suburban Hospital (Norristown PA), 569

Meridia Euclid Hospital (Euclid OH), 521

Meritcare Health System (Fargo ND), 502

Meriter Hospital (Madison WI), 722

Merle West Medical Center (Klamath Falls OR), 549

Merrimack Valley Hospital (Haverhill MA), 341

Mesa General Hospital (Mesa AZ), 69

Mesa View Regional Hospital (Mesquite NV), 425

Methodist Healthcare Fayette Hospital (Somerville TN), 609

Methodist Healthcare Memphis Hospitals (Memphis TN), 609

Methodist Hospital (Gary IN), 250

Methodist Hospital (Henderson KY), 295

Methodist Hospital (Houston TX), 648

Methodist Hospital (Minneapolis MN), 373
Methodist Hospital (Philadelphia PA), 570
Methodist Hospital (Sacramento CA), 112
Methodist Hospital (San Antonio TX), 648
Methodist Hospital of Chicago (Chicago IL), 225
Methodist Hospital of Southern California (Arcadia CA), 113
Methodist Hospital Southlake (Merrillville IN), 250
Methodist Hospital Union County (Morganfield KY), 295
Methodist Medical Center (Dallas TX), 648
Methodist Medical Center of Illinois (Peoria IL), 225
Methodist Medical Center of Oak Ridge (Oak Ridge TN), 610
Methodist Specialty and Transplant Hospital
    (San Antonio TX), 648
Methodist Sugar Land Hospital (Sugar Land TX), 649
Methodist Willowbrook Hospital (Houston TX), 649
Metro Health Hospital (Wyoming MI), 358
Metro Nashville General Hospital (Nashville TN), 610
MetroHealth Medical Center (Cleveland OH), 521
Metroplex Hospital (Killeen TX), 649
Metropolitan Hospital Center (New York NY), 466
Metropolitan Medical Center (Des Moines IA), 269
Metropolitan Methodist Hospital (San Antonio TX), 649
MetroWest Medical Center (Framingham MA), 341
Miami, Florida, 153, 156, 165, 166, 170, 172, 175, 183
Miami Beach Community Hospital (Miami Beach FL), 170
Miami Valley Hospital (Dayton OH), 521
Michael Reese Hospital and Medical Center (Chicago IL),
    226
Michigan
    five star rated facilities, 776–79
    hospitals, 346–66
    procedure, hospital ratings by, 918–23
    top doctors, 1060–62
Mid Coast Hospital (Brunswick ME), 323
Mid-Columbia Medical Center (The Dalles OR), 549
Mid-Dakota Medical Center (Chamberlain SD), 596
Middle Tennessee Medical Center (Murfreesboro TN), 610
Middlesboro ARH Hospital (Middlesboro KY), 295
Middlesex Hospital (Middletown CT), 149
Middletown Regional Hospital (Middletown OH), 521
Midland Memorial Hospital (Midland TX), 649
MidMichigan Medical Center—Clare (Clare MI), 358
MidMichigan Medical Center—Gladwin (Gladwin MI), 359
MidMichigan Medical Center—Midland (Midland MI), 359
Midstate Medical Center (Meriden CT), 149
Mid-Valley Hospital (Omak WA), 695
Mid-Valley Hospital (Peckville PA), 570
Midwest Regional Medical Center (Midwest City OK), 539
Midwestern Region Medical Center (Zion IL), 226
midwives, 40
Milan General Hospital (Milan TN), 610
Milbank Area Hospital—Avera Health (Milbank SD), 596
Miles Memorial Hospital (Damariscotta ME), 323
Milford Hospital (Milford CT), 149
Milford Regional Medical Center (Milford MA), 341
Millard Fillmore Hospital (Buffalo NY), 467
Millcreek Community Hospital (Erie PA), 570
Mille Lacs Health System (Onamia MN), 373

Miller County Hospital (Colquitt GA), 194
Millinocket Regional Hospital (Millinocket ME), 323
Mills Health Center (San Mateo CA), 113
Mills Peninsula Health Services (Burlingame CA), 113
Milton Hospital (Milton MA), 341
Milton S. Hershey Medical Center (Hershey PA), 570
Milwaukee, Wisconsin, 713, 715, 718, 729
Mimbres Memorial Hospital (Deming NM), 448
Minden Medical Center (Minden LA), 311
Mineral Area Regional Medical Center (Farmington MO), 404
Miners' Colfax Medical Center (Raton NM), 448
Miners Medical Center (Hastings PA), 570
Minidoka Memorial Hospital (Rupert ID), 209
Minneapolis, Minnesota, 367, 371, 373, 382
Minnesota
    five star rated facilities, 780–81
    hospitals, 367–82
    procedure, hospital ratings by, 924–27
    top doctors, 1062–63
Minnie Hamilton Health System (Grantsville WV), 706
Miriam Hospital (Providence RI), 584
Mission Community Hospital—Panorama
    (Panorama City CA), 113
Mission Hill Memorial Hospital (Shawnee OK), 540
Mission Hospital Regional Medical Center
    (Mission Viejo CA), 113
Mission Hospitals—Memorial Campus (Asheville NC), 493
Mission Regional Medical Center (Mission TX), 649
Mississippi
    five star rated facilities, 781–82
    hospitals, 383–96
    procedure, hospital ratings by, 928–31
    top doctors, 1063
Mississippi Baptist Medical Center (Jackson MS), 389
Missoula General Hospital (Missoula MT), 416
Missouri
    five star rated facilities, 782–84
    hospitals, 396–414
    procedure, hospital ratings by, 932–37
    top doctors, 1063–64
Missouri Baptist Hospital Sullivan (Sullivan MO), 404
Missouri Baptist Medical Center (St. Louis MO), 404
Missouri Delta Medical Center (Sikeston MO), 404
Missouri Southern Healthcare (Dexter MO), 405
mistakes, medical. See medical errors
Mitchell County Hospital (Camilla GA), 195
Mitchell County Hospital (Colorado City TX), 650
Mitchell County Hospital Health Systems (Beloit KS), 280
Mitchell County Regional Health (Osage IA), 269
Mizell Memorial Hospital (Opp AL), 56
Moberly Regional Medical Center (Moberly MO), 405
Mobile, Alabama, 56, 58, 60, 62
Mobile Infirmary (Mobile AL), 56
Mobridge Regional Hospital (Mobridge SD), 597
Mohawk Valley General Hospital (Ilion NY), 467
Monadnock Community Hospital (Peterborough NH), 431
Monmouth Medical Center (Long Branch NJ), 438
Monongahela Valley Hospital (Monongahela PA), 570

Monongalia County General Hospital (Morgantown WV), 706
Monroe Clinic (Monroe WI), 722
Monroe County Hospital (Forsyth GA), 195
Monroe County Hospital (Monroeville AL), 57
Monroe County Medical Center (Tompkinsville KY), 295
Montana
    five star rated facilities, 784–85
    hospitals, 414–17
    procedure, hospital ratings by, 938–39
    top doctors, 1064
Montefiore Medical Center (Bronx NY), 467
Monterey Park Hospital (Monterey Park CA), 113
Montfort Jones Memorial Hospital (Kosciusko MS), 390
Montgomery County Memorial Hospital (Red Oak IA), 269
Montgomery General Hospital (Montgomery WV), 706
Montgomery General Hospital (Olney MD), 330
Montgomery Hospital (Norristown PA), 571
Montgomery Regional Hospital (Blacksburg VA), 684
Monticello Medical Center (Longview WA), 695
Monticello-Big Lake Community Hospital (Monticello MN),
    373
Montrose Memorial Hospital (Montrose CO), 143
Morehead Memorial Hospital (Eden NC), 493
Morehouse General Hospital (Bastrop LA), 311
Morenci Area Hospital (Morenci MI), 359
Moreno Valley Medical Center (Moreno Valley CA), 114
Morgan Hospital and Medical Center (Martinsville IN), 250
Morris County Hospital (Council Grove KS), 280
Morris Hospital and Healthcare Center (Morris IL), 226
Morristown Memorial Hospital (Morristown NJ), 438
Morristown-Hamblen Healthcare System (Morristown TN),
    610
Morton County Hospital (Elkhart KS), 280
Morton Hospital and Medical Center (Taunton MA), 342
Morton Plant Hospital (Clearwater FL), 170
Morton Plant Mease Healthcare Countryside
    (Safety Harbor FL), 171
Morton Plant North Bay Hospital (New Port Richey FL), 171
Moses H. Cone Memorial Hospital (Greensboro NC), 493
Moses Taylor Hospital (Scranton PA), 571
Mother Frances Hospital—Jacksonville (Jacksonville TX),
    650
Mother Frances Hospital—Tyler (Tyler TX), 650
Motion Picture and Television Hospital
    (Woodland Hills CA), 114
Moundview Memorial Hospital and Clinics
    (Friendship WI), 722
Mount Auburn Hospital (Cambridge MA), 342
Mount Carmel Health (Columbus OH), 521
Mt. Carmel Regional Medical Center (Pittsburg KS), 280
Mount Carmel St. Ann's Hospital of Columbus
    (Westerville OH), 522
Mount Clemens Regional Medical Center
    (Mount Clemens MI), 359
Mount Desert Island Hospital (Bar Harbor ME), 323
Mt. Diablo Hospital Medical Center (Concord CA), 114
Mt. Edgecumbe Hospital (Sitka AK), 64
Mt. Graham Regional Medical Center (Safford AZ), 69

Please note that all individual hospital listings provide page numbers for Chapter 6 (Hospital Ratings by Clinical Specialty) only. All other hospital listings can be found under their state listing.

Mount Nittany Medical Center (State College PA), 571

Mt. San Rafael Hospital (Trinidad CO), 143

Mount Sinai Hospital (New York NY), 467

Mt. Sinai Hospital Medical Center (Chicago IL), 226

Mt. Sinai Medical Center (Miami Beach FL), 171

Mt. Sinai Medical Center and Miami Heart Institute (Miami Beach FL), 171

Mount St. Mary's Hospital and Health Center (Lewiston NY), 467

Mount Vernon Hospital (Mount Vernon NY), 467

Mountain Lakes Medical Center (Clayton GA), 195

Mountain View Hospital (Payson UT), 673

Mountain View Regional Medical Center (Norton VA), 684

Mountain West Medical Center (Tooele UT), 673

Mountainside Hospital (Montclair NJ), 438

Mountainview Hospital (Las Vegas NV), 426

Mountainview Regional Medical Center (Las Cruces NM), 448

Muhlenberg Community Hospital (Greenville KY), 295

Muhlenberg Regional Medical Center (Plainfield NJ), 438

Muleshoe Area Medical Center (Muleshoe TX), 650

Muncy Valley Hospital (Muncy PA), 571

Municipal Hospital and Granite Manor (Granite Falls MN), 374

Munroe Regional Medical Center (Ocala FL), 171

Munson Medical Center (Traverse City MI), 359

Murphy Medical Center (Murphy NC), 493

Murray County Memorial Hospital (Slayton MN), 374

Murray Medical Center (Chatsworth GA), 195

Murray-Calloway County Hospital (Murray KY), 296

Muskogee Regional Medical Center (Muskogee OK), 540

N

Nacogdoches Medical Center (Nacogdoches TX), 650

Nanticoke Memorial Hospital (Seaford DE), 152

Nash General Hospital (Rocky Mount NC), 493

Nashoba Valley Medical Center (Ayer MA), 342

Nashville, Tennessee, 598, 601, 610, 613, 614, 616

Nason Hospital (Roaring Spring PA), 571

Nassau University Medical Center (East Meadow NY), 468

Natchez Community Hospital (Natchez MS), 390

Natchez Regional Medical Center (Natchez MS), 390

Natchitoches Regional Medical Center (Natchitoches LA), 311

Nathan Littauer Hospital (Gloversville NY), 468

National Park Medical Center (Hot Springs AR), 79

Natividad Medical Center (Salinas CA), 114

Navapache Regional Medical Center (Show Low AZ), 69

Navarro Regional Hospital (Corsicana TX), 650

Nazareth Hospital (Philadelphia PA), 571

NCH Healthcare System (Naples FL), 171

Nea Medical Center (Jonesboro AR), 80

Nebraska
    five star rated facilities, 785
    hospitals, 417–25
    procedure, hospital ratings by, 940–41
    top doctors, 1064

Nebraska Heart Hospital (Lincoln NE), 422

Nebraska Medical Center (Omaha NE), 422

Nebraska Methodist Hospital (Omaha NE), 423

Neosho Memorial Regional Medical Center (Chanute KS), 281

Neshoba County General Hospital (Philadelphia MS), 390

Nevada
    five star rated facilities, 786
    hospitals, 425–28
    procedure, hospital ratings by, 942–43

Nevada Regional Medical Center (Nevada MO), 405

New Albany Surgical Hospital (New Albany OH), 522

New England Baptist Hospital (Boston MA), 342

New Hampshire
    five star rated facilities, 787
    hospitals, 428–32
    procedure, hospital ratings by, 944–45
    top doctors, 1064

New Hanover Regional Medical Center (Wilmington NC), 494

New Horizons Health Systems (Owenton KY), 296

New Island Hospital (Bethpage NY), 468

New Jersey
    five star rated facilities, 787–89
    hospitals, 432–44
    procedure, hospital ratings by, 946–49
    top doctors, 1064–66

New London Family Medical Center (New London WI), 722

New Mexico
    five star rated facilities, 789–90
    hospitals, 445–50
    procedure, hospital ratings by, 950–51
    top doctors, 1066

New Milford Hospital (New Milford CT), 149

New Ulm Medical Center (New Ulm MN), 374

New York
    five star rated facilities, 790–92
    hospitals, 450–83
    procedure, hospital ratings by, 952–59
    top doctors, 1066–69

New York, New York, 452, 454, 460, 461, 464, 466, 467, 468, 469, 470, 476, 477

New York Community Hospital of Brooklyn (Brooklyn NY), 468

New York Downtown Hospital (New York NY), 468

New York Hospital Medical Center of Queens (Flushing NY), 468

New York Methodist Hospital (Brooklyn NY), 469

New York Presbyterian—Columbia (New York NY), 469

New York University Medical Center—Tisch Hospital (New York NY), 469

New York Westchester Square Medical Center (Bronx NY), 469

New York-Presbyterian/Weill Cornell (New York NY), 469

Newark, New Jersey, 434, 438, 441, 442, 443

Newark Beth Israel Medical Center (Newark NJ), 438

Newark-Wayne Community Hospital (Newark NY), 469

Newberry County Memorial Hospital (Newberry SC), 591

Newman Memorial Hospital (Shattuck OK), 540

Newman Regional Health (Emporia KS), 281

Newport Hospital (Newport RI), 584

Newton Medical Center (Covington GA), 195

Newton Medical Center (Newton KS), 281

Newton Memorial Hospital (Newton NJ), 439

Newton Regional Hospital (Newton MS), 390

Newton-Wellesley Hospital (Newton MA), 342

Niagara Falls Memorial Medical Center (Niagara Falls NY), 470

Nicholas H. Noyes Memorial Hospital (Dansville NY), 470

Nix Health Care System (San Antonio TX), 651

Noble Hospital (Westfield MA), 342

Nocona General Hospital (Nocona TX), 651

nonprofit hospitals, 15

Nor Lea General Hospital (Lovington NM), 448

Norman Regional Hospital (Norman OK), 540

North Adams Regional Hospital (North Adams MA), 343

North Arkansas Regional Medical Center (Harrison AR), 80

North Austin Medical Center (Austin TX), 651

North Baldwin Infirmary (Bay Minette AL), 57

North Bay Hospital (Aransas Pass TX), 651

North Broward Medical Center (Deerfield Beach FL), 172

North Caddo Medical Center (Vivian LA), 311

North Carolina
    five star rated facilities, 792–94
    hospitals, 483–500
    procedure, hospital ratings by, 960–65
    top doctors, 1069–70

North Carolina Baptist Hospital (Winston-Salem NC), 494

North Central Bronx Hospital (Bronx NY), 470

North Colorado Medical Center (Greeley CO), 143

North Country Hospital and Health Center (Newport VT), 675

North Country Regional Hospital (Bemidji MN), 374

North Dakota
    five star rated facilities, 794–95
    hospitals, 500–504
    procedure, hospital ratings by, 966–67
    top doctors, 1070

North Florida Regional Medical Center (Gainesville FL), 172

North Fulton Regional Hospital (Roswell GA), 195

North General Hospital (New York NY), 470

North Georgia Medical Center (Ellijay GA), 196

North Hawaii Community Hospital (Kamuela HI), 206

North Hills Hospital (North Richland Hills TX), 651

North Kansas City Hospital (North Kansas City MO), 405

North Memorial Health Care (Robbinsdale MN), 374

North Mississippi Medical Center (Tupelo MS), 390

North Oak Regional Medical Center (Senatobia MS), 391

North Oakland Medical Center (Pontiac MI), 359

North Oaks Medical Center (Hammond LA), 311

North Oaks Medical Center North Campus (Hammond LA), 311

North Okaloosa Medical Center (Crestview FL), 172

North Ottawa Community Hospital (Grand Haven MI), 360

North Philadelphia Health System (Philadelphia PA), 572

North Ridge Medical Center (Fort Lauderdale FL), 172

North Shore Medical Center (Miami FL), 172

North Shore Medical Center (Salem MA), 343

North Shore University Hospital (Manhasset NY), 470

North Shore University Hospital Syosset (Syosset NY), 470

North Suburban Medical Center (Thornton CO), 143

North Sunflower Medical Center (Ruleville MS), 391

North Texas Medical Center (Gainesville TX), 651
North Valley Hospital (Whitefish MT), 416
North Vista Hospital (North Las Vegas NV), 426
NorthBay Medical Center (Fairfield CA), 114
NorthBay VacaValley Hospital (Vacaville CA), 114
NorthCrest Medical Center (Springfield TN), 610
Northeast Alabama Regional Medical Center
    (Anniston AL), 57
Northeast Georgia Medical Center (Gainesville GA), 196
Northeast Georgia Medical Center—Lanier Park Campus
    (Gainesville GA), 196
Northeast Medical Center (Bonham TX), 652
Northeast Medical Center Hospital (Humble TX), 652
Northeast Methodist Hospital (Live Oak TX), 652
Northeast Regional Medical Center (Kirksville MO), 405
Northeastern Hospital (Philadelphia PA), 572
Northeastern Nevada Regional Hospital (Elko NV), 426
Northeastern Vermont Regional Hospital
    (St. Johnsbury VT), 675
Northern Dutchess Hospital (Rhinebeck NY), 471
Northern Hospital of Surry County (Mount Airy NC), 494
Northern Inyo Hospital (Bishop CA), 115
Northern Maine Medical Center (Fort Kent ME), 323
Northern Michigan Hospital (Petoskey MI), 360
Northern Montana Hospital (Havre MT), 416
Northern Navajo Physicians Indian Hospital
    (Shiprock NM), 448
Northern Nevada Medical Center (Sparks NV), 426
Northern Virginia Community Hospital (Arlington VA), 684
Northern Westchester Hospital (Mount Kisco NY), 471
Northfield Hospital (Northfield MN), 374
Northport Medical Center (Northport AL), 57
Northridge Hospital Medical Center (Northridge CA), 115
Northshore Regional Medical Center (Slidell LA), 312
Northside Hospital (Atlanta GA), 196
Northside Hospital (Johnson City TN), 611
Northside Hospital (St. Petersburg FL), 172
Northside Hospital Cherokee (Canton GA), 196
Northside Hospital Forsyth (Cumming GA), 196
Northwest Community Hospital (Arlington Heights IL), 226
Northwest Florida Community Hospital (Chipley FL), 173
Northwest Hospital and Medical Center (Seattle WA), 695
Northwest Hospital Center (Randallstown MD), 331
Northwest Iowa Health Center (Sheldon IA), 269
Northwest Medical Center (Albany MO), 405
Northwest Medical Center (Margate FL), 173
Northwest Medical Center (Russellville AL), 57
Northwest Medical Center (Thief River Falls MN), 375
Northwest Medical Center (Tucson AZ), 69
Northwest Medical Center (Winfield AL), 57
Northwest Medical Center—Benton County
    (Bentonville AR), 80
Northwest Medical Center—Oro Valley (Oro Valley AZ), 70
Northwest Medical Center—Washington County
    (Springdale AR), 80
Northwest Mississippi Regional Medical Center
    (Clarksdale MS), 391
Northwest Texas Healthcare System (Amarillo TX), 652

Northwestern Medical Center (St. Albans VT), 676
Northwestern Memorial Hospital (Chicago IL), 226
Norton Audubon Hospital (Louisville KY), 296
Norton Community Hospital (Norton VA), 684
Norton County Hospital (Norton KS), 281
Norton Hospital (Louisville KY), 296
Norton Southwest Hospital (Louisville KY), 296
Norton Suburban Hospital (Louisville KY), 296
Norwalk Community Hospital (Norwalk CA), 115
Norwalk Hospital Association (Norwalk CT), 149
Norwegian-American Hospital (Chicago IL), 227
Novato Community Hospital (Novato CA), 115
Noxubee General Critical Access Hospital (Macon MS), 391
nurses, 28–29
    talking with, 33
Nyack Hospital (Nyack NY), 471

O
O. Bleness Memorial Hospital (Athens OH), 522
Oak Forest Hospital (Oak Forest IL), 227
Oak Hill Hospital (Brooksville FL), 173
Oak Park Hospital (Oak Park IL), 227
Oak Tree Hospital at Baptist Hospital Northeast
    (La Grange KY), 297
Oak Tree Hospital at Baptist Regional Medical Center
    (Corbin KY), 297
Oak Valley District Hospital (Oakdale CA), 115
Oakbend Medical Center (Richmond TX), 652
Oakdale Community Hospital (Oakdale LA), 312
Oakes Community Hospital (Oakes ND), 502
Oaklawn Hospital (Marshall MI), 360
Oakwood Annapolis Hospital (Wayne MI), 360
Oakwood Heritage Hospital (Taylor MI), 360
Oakwood Hospital and Medical Center—Dearborn
    (Dearborn MI), 360
Oakwood Southsore Medical Center (Trenton MI), 361
Obici Hospital (Suffolk VA), 684
obstetricians, 40
Ocala Regional Medical Center (Ocala FL), 173
Ocean Medical Center (Brick NJ), 439
Ochiltree General Hospital (Perryton TX), 652
Ochsner Clinic Foundation (New Orleans LA), 312
Ochsner Medical Center—Baton Rouge (Baton Rouge LA),
    312
Ochsner Medical Center—Kenner (Kenner LA), 312
Ochsner Medical Center—Westbank (Gretna LA), 312
Ochsner St. Anne General Hospital (Raceland LA), 313
Oconee Memorial Hospital (Seneca SC), 591
Oconee Regional Medical Center (Milledgeville GA), 197
O'Connor Hospital (San Jose CA), 115
Oconomowoc Memorial Hospital (Oconomowoc WI), 722
Odessa Regional Medical Center (Odessa TX), 653
Ogden Regional Medical Center (Ogden UT), 673
Ohio
    five star rated facilities, 795–99
    hospitals, 504–30
    procedure, hospital ratings by, 968–75
    top doctors, 1070–71

Ohio County Hospital (Hartford KY), 297
Ohio State University Hospital East (Columbus OH), 522
Ohio State University Hospitals (Columbus OH), 522
Ohio Valley General Hospital (McKees Rocks PA), 572
Ohio Valley Medical Center (Wheeling WV), 707
OHSU Hospital (Portland OR), 549
Ojai Valley Community Hospital (Ojai CA), 116
Oklahoma
    five star rated facilities, 799–800
    hospitals, 530–46
    procedure, hospital ratings by, 976–79
    top doctors, 1071
Oklahoma City, Oklahoma, 530, 531, 533, 535, 537, 538,
    539, 540, 541, 542, 543, 545
Oklahoma Heart Hospital (Oklahoma City OK), 540
Oklahoma Surgical Hospital (Tulsa OK), 540
Oklahoma University Medical Center (Oklahoma City OK),
    541
Okmulgee Memorial Hospital (Okmulgee OK), 541
Oktibbeha County Hospital (Starkville MS), 391
Olathe Medical Center (Olathe KS), 281
Olean General Hospital (Olean NY), 471
Olmsted Medical Center (Rochester MN), 375
Olympia Medical Center (Los Angeles CA), 116
Olympic Medical Center (Port Angeles WA), 695
Omaha, Nebraska, 417, 418, 419, 420, 422, 423
on site visits, making, 18
one star ratings, xiii, xiv, 16
Oneida Healthcare Center (Oneida NY), 471
Onslow Memorial Hospital (Jacksonville NC), 494
Opelousas General Health System (Opelousas LA), 313
Orange City Area Health System (Orange City IA), 269
Orange Coast Memorial Medical Center
    (Fountain Valley CA), 116
Orange Park Medical Center (Orange Park FL), 173
Orange Regional Medical Center (Goshen NY), 471
Oregon
    five star rated facilities, 800–801
    hospitals, 546–54
    procedure, hospital ratings by, 980–81
    top doctors, 1071
Orlando Regional Healthcare (Orlando FL), 173
Oroville Hospital (Oroville CA), 116
orthopedic surgeons, 44
Osceola Community Hospital (Sibley IA), 269
Osceola Regional Medical Center (Kissimmee FL), 174
Osmond General Hospital (Osmond NE), 423
Osteopathic Hospital Clinic of New York (Flushing NY), 472
Oswego Hospital (Owsego NY), 472
Otsego Memorial Hospital (Gaylord MI), 361
Ottawa County Health Center (Minneapolis KS), 281
Otto Kaiser Memorial Hospital (Kenedy TX), 653
Ottumwa Regional Health Center (Ottumwa IA), 270
Ouachita County Medical Center (Camden AR), 80
Our Lady of Bellefonte Hospital (Ashland KY), 297
Our Lady of the Lake Regional Medical Center
    (Baton Rouge LA), 313
Our Lady of Lourdes Hospital (Norfolk NE), 423

Please note that all individual hospital listings provide page numbers for Chapter 6 (Hospital Ratings by Clinical Specialty) only. All other hospital listings can be found under their state listing.

Our Lady of Lourdes Medical Center (Camden NJ), 439
Our Lady of Lourdes Memorial Hospital (Binghamton NY), 472
Our Lady of Lourdes Regional Medical Center (Lafayette LA), 313
Our Lady of Mercy Medical Center (Bronx NY), 472
Our Lady of the Resurrection Medical Center (Chicago IL), 227
Our Lady of Victory Hospital (Stanley WI), 723
Our Lady of the Way (Martin KY), 297
outcomes, ix, xi–xiv, 16, 20, 25, 33, 44
Overlake Hospital Medical Center (Bellevue WA), 695
Overland Park Regional Medical Center (Overland Park KS), 282
Overlook Hospital (Summit NJ), 439
Owatonna Hospital (Owatonna MN), 375
Owensboro Medical Health System (Owensboro KY), 297
Owensboro Mercy Health System Ford (Owensboro KY), 298
Ozark Health (Clinton AR), 80
Ozarks Community Hospital—Springfield (Springfield MO), 406
Ozarks Medical Center (West Plains MO), 406

P

Pacific Alliance Medical Center (Los Angeles CA), 116
Pacific Campus Hospital (San Francisco CA), 116
Pacific Hospital of Long Beach (Long Beach CA), 117
Pacifica Hospital of the Valley (Sun Valley CA), 117
Page Memorial Hospital (Luray VA), 684
Palestine Regional Medical Center (Palestine TX), 653
Palisades Medical Center (North Bergen NJ), 439
Palm Beach Gardens Medical Center (Palm Beach Gardens FL), 174
Palm Drive Hospital (Sebastopol CA), 117
Palmer Lutheran Health Center (West Union IA), 270
Palmerton Hospital (Palmerton PA), 572
Palmetto General Hospital (Hialeah FL), 174
Palmetto Health Baptist (Columbia SC), 591
Palmetto Health Baptist—Easley (Easley SC), 592
Palmetto Health Richland (Columbia SC), 592
Palm Springs General Hospital (Hialeah FL), 174
Palms of Pasadena Hospital (St. Petersburg FL), 174
Palms West Hospital (Loxahatchee FL), 174
Palmyra Medical Center (Albany GA), 197
Palo Pinto General Hospital (Mineral Wells TX), 653
Palo Verde Hospital (Blythe CA), 117
Palomar Medical Center (Escondido CA), 117
Palos Community Hospital (Palos Heights IL), 227
Pampa Regional Medical Center (Pampa TX), 653
Pan American Hospital (Miami FL), 175
Pana Community Hospital (Pana IL), 227
Paradise Valley Hospital (National City CA), 117
Paradise Valley Hospital (Phoenix AZ), 70
Paris Community Hospital (Paris IL), 228
Paris Regional Medical Center (Paris TX), 653
Park Plaza Hospital and Medical Center (Houston TX), 654
Park Ridge Hospital (Fletcher NC), 494
Parkland Health and Hospital System (Dallas TX), 654

Parkland Health Center (Farmington MO), 406
Parkland Medical Center (Derry NH), 431
Parkridge Medical Center (Chattanooga TN), 611
Parkview Adventist Medical Center (Brunswick ME), 324
Parkview Community Hospital (Riverside CA), 118
Parkview Hospital (El Reno OK), 541
Parkview Hospital (Fort Wayne IN), 250
Parkview Huntington Hospital (Huntington IN), 250
Parkview Lagrange Hospital (Lagrange IN), 251
Parkview Medical Center (Pueblo CO), 143
Parkview Noble Hospital (Kendallville IN), 251
Parkview Regional Hospital (Mexia TX), 654
Parkview Regional Medical Center (Vicksburg MS), 391
Parkview Whitley Hospital (Columbia City IN), 251
Parkway Hospital (Forest Hills NY), 472
Parkway Medical Center Hospital (Decatur AL), 58
Parkway Regional Hospital (Fulton KY), 298
Parkwest Medical Center (Knoxville TN), 611
Parma Community General Hospital (Parma OH), 522
Parrish Medical Center (Titusville FL), 175
Pascack Valley Hospital (Westwood NJ), 439
Pasco Regional Medical Center (Dade City FL), 175
Passavant Area Hospital (Jacksonville IL), 228
patient advocates, 20, 21–22, 35, 36–37
patient outcomes, xii–xiv
patient safety, 25, 28, 32, 47, 48
Pattie A. Clay Regional Medical Center (Richmond KY), 298
Paul B. Hall Regional Medical Center (Paintsville KY), 298
Paulding County Hospital (Paulding OH), 523
Pauls Valley General Hospital (Pauls Valley OK), 541
Pawnee Municipal Hospital (Pawnee OK), 541
Paynesville Area Health Care System (Paynesville MN), 375
Payson Regional Medical Center (Payson AZ), 70
Peace River Regional Medical Center (Port Charlotte FL), 175
Peach Regional Medical Center (Fort Valley GA), 197
Peconic Bay Medical Center (Riverhead NY), 472
Pecos County Memorial Hospital (Fort Stockton TX), 654
Pekin Memorial Hospital (Pekin IL), 228
Pella Regional Health Center (Pella IA), 270
Pembina County Memorial Hospital (Cavalier ND), 502
Pemiscot Memorial Hospital (Hayti MO), 406
Pender Community Hospital (Pender NE), 423
Pender Memorial Hospital (Burgaw NC), 494
Peninsula Hospital Center (Far Rockaway NY), 473
Peninsula Regional Medical Center (Salisbury MD), 331
Pennock Hospital (Hastings MI), 361
Pennsylvania
   five star rated facilities, 801–5
   hospitals, 555–83
   procedure, hospital ratings by, 982–89
   top doctors, 1072–73
Pennsylvania Hospital (Philadelphia PA), 572
Pennsylvania Presbyterian Medical Center (Philadelphia PA), 572
Penobscot Bay Medical Center (Rockport ME), 324
Penobscot Valley Hospital (Lincoln ME), 324
Peoples Hospital (Mansfield OH), 523
Perham Memorial Hospital and Home (Perham MN), 375

Permian Regional Medical Center (Andrews TX), 654
Perry County Memorial Hospital (Perryville MO), 406
Perry County Memorial Hospital (Tell City IN), 251
Perry General Hospital (Perry GA), 197
Perry Memorial Hospital (Perry OK), 541
Perry Memorial Hospital (Princeton IL), 228
Pershing Memorial Hospital (Brookfield MO), 406
Person Memorial Hospital (Roxboro NC), 495
Petaluma Valley Hospital (Petaluma CA), 118
Phelps County Regional Medical Center (Rolla MO), 407
Phelps Memorial Health Center (Holdrege NE), 423
Phelps Memorial Hospital Association (Sleepy Hollow NY), 473
Philadelphia, Pennsylvania, 555, 558, 561, 562, 563, 564, 565, 570, 571, 572, 574, 575, 577, 578
Phillips County Hospital (Phillipsburg KS), 282
Phoebe Putney Memorial Hospital (Albany GA), 197
Phoebe Worth Medical Center (Sylvester GA), 197
Phoenix, Arizona, 65, 66, 68, 69, 70, 71
Phoenix Baptist Hospital (Phoenix AZ), 70
Phoenix Memorial Hospital (Phoenix AZ), 70
Phoenixville Hospital (Phoenixville PA), 573
PHS Indian Hospital at Belcourt-Quentin N. Burdick Memorial (Belcourt ND), 502
PHS Indian Hospital—Browning (Browning MT), 416
physicians. See doctor(s)
Physicians' Hospital in Anadarko (Anadarko OK), 542
Physicians Indian Hospital (Wagner SD), 597
Physicians Indian Hospital at Pine Ridge (Pine Ridge SD), 597
Physicians Regional Medical Center (Naples FL), 175
Physicians Specialty Hospital of El Paso (El Paso TX), 654
Pickens County Medical Center (Carrollton AL), 58
Piedmont Fayette Hospital (Fayetteville GA), 198
Piedmont Hospital (Atlanta GA), 198
Piedmont Medical Center (Rock Hill SC), 592
Piedmont Mountainside Hospital (Jasper GA), 198
Piedmont Newnan Hospital (Newnan GA), 198
Piggott Community Hospital (Piggott AR), 81
Pike Community Hospital (Waverly OH), 523
Pike County Memorial Hospital (Louisiana MO), 407
Pike County Memorial Hospital (Murfreesboro AR), 81
Pikeville Medical Center (Pikeville KY), 298
Pinckneyville Community Hospital (Pinckneyville IL), 228
Pine Medical Center (Sandstone MN), 375
Pineville Community Hospital (Pineville KY), 298
Pinnacle Health System (Harrisburg PA), 573
Pioneer Memorial Hospital (Prineville OR), 550
Pioneer Valley Hospital (West Valley City UT), 673
Pioneers Memorial Health Care District (Brawley CA), 118
Pipestone County Medical Center Ashton Care Center (Pipestone MN), 376
Pitt County Memorial Hospital (Greenville NC), 495
Pittsburgh, Pennsylvania, 555, 556, 565, 567, 569, 575, 580, 581
Placentia-Linda Hospital (Placentia CA), 118
Plains Regional Medical Center—Clovis (Clovis NM), 449
Plainview Hospital (Plainview NY), 473

Please note that all individual hospital listings provide page numbers for Chapter 6 (Hospital Ratings by Clinical Specialty) only. All other hospital listings can be found under their state listing.

plan for the day, 34, 35

Plantation General Hospital (Plantation FL), 175

Plateau Medical Center (Oak Hill WV), 707

Platte County Memorial Hospital (Wheatland WY), 732

Platte Valley Medical Center (Brighton CO), 143

Plavix (clopidogrel), 43

Plaza Medical Center of Fort Worth (Fort Worth TX), 655

Pleasant Valley Hospital (Point Pleasant WV), 707

Pocahontas Memorial Hospital (Buckeye WV), 707

Pocono Medical Center (East Stroudsburg PA), 573

POH Regional Medical Center (Pontiac MI), 361

Pointe Coupee General Hospital (New Roads LA), 313

Pomerado Hospital (Poway CA), 118

Pomona Valley Hospital Medical Center (Pomona CA), 118

Ponca City Medical Center (Ponca City OK), 542

Poplar Bluff Regional Medical Center (Poplar Bluff MO), 407

Port Huron Hospital (Port Huron MI), 361

Portage Health System (Hancock MI), 361

Porter (Valparaiso IN), 251

Porter Hospital (Middlebury VT), 676

Portland, Oregon, 546, 548, 549, 550, 551

Portneuf Medical Center (Pocatello ID), 209

Portsmouth Regional Hospital (Portsmouth NH), 431

Potomac Hospital (Woodbridge VA), 685

Potomac Valley Hospital (Keyser WV), 707

Pottstown Memorial Medical Center (Pottstown PA), 573

Pottsville Hospital and Warne Clinic (Pottsville PA), 573

Poudre Valley Hospital (Fort Collins CO), 144

Powell Valley Hospital (Powell WY), 732

Prairie Du Chien Memorial Hospital (Prairie Du Chien WI), 723

Prairie Lakes Hospital and Care Center (Watertown SD), 597

Pratt Regional Medical Center (Pratt KS), 282

Prattville Baptist Hospital (Prattville AL), 58

Presbyterian Hospital (Albuquerque NM), 449

Presbyterian Hospital (Charlotte NC), 495

Presbyterian Hospital of Allen (Allen TX), 655

Presbyterian Hospital of Dallas (Dallas TX), 655

Presbyterian Hospital of Denton (Denton TX), 655

Presbyterian Hospital of Greenville (Greenville TX), 655

Presbyterian Hospital Huntersville (Huntersville NC), 495

Presbyterian Hospital of Kaufman (Kaufman TX), 655

Presbyterian Hospital Matthews (Matthews NC), 495

Presbyterian Hospital of Plano (Plano TX), 656

Presbyterian Hospital of Winnsboro (Winnsboro TX), 656

Presbyterian Intercommunity Hospital (Whittier CA), 119

Presbyterian Kaseman Hospital (Albuquerque NM), 449

Presbyterian Orthopaedic Hospital (Charlotte NC), 495

Presbyterian/St. Luke's Medical Center (Denver CO), 144

prescriptions, 8, 43–44

Preston Memorial Hospital (Kingwood WV), 707

Prince George's Hospital Center (Cheverly MD), 331

Prince William Hospital (Manassas VA), 685

Princeton Community Hospital (Princeton WV), 708

privacy laws, 37

procedures, ix, xi, xiii–xv, 14–17, 27, 28, 33–35, 40, 42, 45

Proctor Hospital (Peoria IL), 228

Provena Covenant Medical Center (Urbana IL), 229

Provena Mercy Center (Aurora IL), 229

Provena St. Joseph Medical Center (Joliet IL), 229

Provena St. Mary's Hospital (Kankakee IL), 229

Provena United Samaritans Medical Center—Logan (Danville IL), 229

Providence Alaska Medical Center (Anchorage AK), 64

Providence Centralia Hospital (Centralia WA), 695

Providence Everett Medical Center—Colby Campus (Everett WA), 696

Providence Healthcare Network (Waco TX), 656

Providence Holy Cross Medical Center (Mission Hills CA), 119

Providence Hood River Memorial Hospital (Hood River OR), 550

Providence Hospital (Holyoke MA), 343

Providence Hospital (Mobile AL), 58

Providence Hospital (Southfield MI), 362

Providence Hospital (Washington DC), 702

Providence Medford Medical Center (Medford OR), 550

Providence Medical Center (Kansas City KS), 282

Providence Medical Center (Wayne NE), 423

Providence Memorial Hospital (El Paso TX), 656

Providence Milwaukie Hospital (Milwaukie OR), 550

Providence Newberg Hospital (Newberg OR), 550

Providence Portland Medical Center (Portland OR), 550

Providence Saint Joseph Medical Center (Burbank CA), 119

Providence St. Peter Hospital (Olympia WA), 696

Providence St. Vincent Medical Center (Portland OR), 551

Providence Seaside Hospital (Seaside OR), 551

Provident Hospital of Chicago (Chicago IL), 229

Prowers Medical Center (Lamar CO), 144

Pulaski Community Hospital (Pulaski VA), 685

Pullman Memorial Hospital (Pullman WA), 696

Pungo District Hospital (Belhaven NC), 496

Punxsutawney Area Hospital (Punxsutawney PA), 573

Purcell Municipal Hospital (Purcell OK), 542

Pushmataha County—Town of Antlers Hospital Authority (Antlers OK), 542

Putnam Community Medical Center (Palatka FL), 176

Putnam County Hospital (Greencastle IN), 251

Putnam General Hospital (Eatonton GA), 198

Putnam Hospital Center (Carmel NY), 473

Q

quality, x–xii, xiv, xv, 2, 4, 6–8, 11, 12, 14–18, 25, 32, 47

Queen of Peace Hospital (New Prague MN), 376

Queen of the Valley (Napa CA), 119

Queens Hospital Center (Jamaica NY), 473

Queen's Medical Center, The (Honolulu HI), 207

questions, asking

    and avoiding medical errors, 32–36

    before getting a cardiac procedure, 42–44

    before getting your knee or hip replaced, 44–45

    before giving birth for the first time, 40–42

Quincy Medical Center (Quincy MA), 343

R

R. E. Thomason General Hospital (El Paso TX), 656

R. J. Reynolds Patrick County Memorial Hospital (Stuart VA), 685

Raleigh General Hospital (Beckley WV), 708

Randolph County Medical Center (Pocahontas AR), 81

Randolph Hospital (Asheboro NC), 496

Randolph Medical Center (Roanoke AL), 58

Rankin Medical Center (Brandon MS), 392

Ransom Memorial Hospital (Ottawa KS), 282

Rapid City Regional Hospital (Rapid City SD), 597

Rapides Regional Medical Center (Alexandria LA), 313

Rappahannock General Hospital (Kilmarnock VA), 685

Raritan Bay Medical Center (Perth Amboy NJ), 440

ratings, xii–xiv, 16, 47

Raulerson Hospital (Okeechobee FL), 176

Ray County Memorial Hospital (Richmond MO), 407

Reading Hospital and Medical Center, The (West Reading PA), 574

Rebsamen Medical Center (Jacksonville AR), 81

Red Bay Hospital (Red Bay AL), 58

Red Bud Regional Hospital (Red Bud IL), 230

Red Cedar Medical Center—Mayo Health System (Menomonie WI), 723

Redbud Community Hospital (Clearlake CA), 119

Redington Fairview General Hospital (Skowhegan ME), 324

Redlands Community Hospital (Redlands CA), 119

Redmond Regional Medical Center (Rome GA), 198

Redwood Area Hospital (Redwood Falls MN), 376

Redwood Memorial Hospital (Fortuna CA), 120

Reedsburg Area Medical Center (Reedsburg WI), 723

Reeves County Hospital District (Pecos TX), 656

referrals, 11

Regency Hospital of Cincinnati (Cincinnati OH), 523

Regina Medical Center (Hastings MN), 376

Regional Health Services of Howard County (Cresco IA), 270

Regional Hospital of Jackson (Jackson TN), 611

Regional Medical Center (Madisonville KY), 299

Regional Medical Center (Manchester IA), 270

Regional Medical Center—Bayonet Point (Hudson FL), 176

Regional Medical Center at Memphis (Memphis TN), 611

Regional Medical Center of San Jose (San Jose CA), 120

Regional West Medical Center (Scottsbluff NE), 424

Regions Hospital (St. Paul MN), 376

registered nurses (RNs), 28

Rehoboth McKinley Christian Health Services (Gallup NM), 449

Reid Hospital and Health Care Services (Richmond IN), 252

Renaissance Hospital (Groves TX), 657

Renaissance Hospital (Houston TX), 657

Renaissance Hospital—Dallas (Dallas TX), 657

Renaissance Hospital—Terrell (Terrell TX), 657

Renown Regional Medical Center (Reno NV), 426

Renown South Meadows Medical Center (Reno NV), 426

Republic County Hospital (Belleville KS), 282

Research Belton Hospital (Belton MO), 407

Research Medical Center (Kansas City MO), 407

residents, 28

Reston Hospital Center (Reston VA), 685

Resurrection Medical Center (Chicago IL), 230

Retreat Hospital (Richmond VA), 685

Rex Hospital (Raleigh NC), 496

Please note that all individual hospital listings provide page numbers for Chapter 6 (Hospital Ratings by Clinical Specialty) only. All other hospital listings can be found under their state listing.

1108 INDEX

Reynolds Memorial Hospital (Glen Dale WV), 708
RHC St. Francis Hospital (Evanston IL), 230
RHD Memorial Medical Center (Dallas TX), 657
Rhea Medical Center (Dayton TN), 611
Rhode Island
   five star rated facilities, 805
   hospitals, 583–85
   procedure, hospital ratings by, 990–91
   top doctors, 1073
Rhode Island Hospital (Providence RI), 584
Rice County District One Hospital (Faribault MN), 376
Rice Memorial Hospital (Willmar MN), 377
Richards Memorial Hospital (Rockdale TX), 657
Richardson Medical Center (Rayville LA), 314
Richardson Regional Medical Center (Richardson TX), 658
Richland Hospital (Richland Center WI), 723
Richland Memorial Hospital (Olney IL), 230
Richland Parish Hospital Delhi (Delhi LA), 314
Richmond, Virginia, 678, 679, 681, 685, 689
Richwood Area Community Hospital (Richwood WV), 708
Riddle Memorial Hospital (Media PA), 574
Rideout Memorial Hospital (Marysville CA), 120
Ridgecrest Regional Hospital (Ridgecrest CA), 120
Ridgeview Medical Center (Waconia MN), 377
Riley Hospital (Meridian MS), 392
Ringgold County Hospital (Mount Ayr IA), 270
Rio Grande Regional Hospital (McAllen TX), 658
Ripley County Memorial Hospital (Doniphan MO), 408
River Falls Area Hospital (River Falls WI), 723
River Oaks Hospital (Jackson MS), 392
River Parishes Hospital (La Place LA), 314
River Park Hospital (McMinnville TN), 612
River Region Health System (Vicksburg MS), 392
River West Medical Center (Plaquemine LA), 314
Riverbend Rehab Hospital (Columbia LA), 314
Riverland Medical Center (Ferriday LA), 314
Riverside Community Hospital (Riverside CA), 120
Riverside County Regional Medical Center
   (Moreno Valley CA), 120
Riverside Hospital (Boonton NJ), 440
Riverside Medical Center (Franklinton LA), 315
Riverside Medical Center (Kankakee IL), 230
Riverside Medical Center (Waupaca WI), 724
Riverside Methodist Hospital (Columbus OH), 523
Riverside Regional Medical Center (Newport News VA), 685
Riverside Tappahannock Hospital (Tappahannock VA), 685
Riverside Water Reed Hospital (Gloucester VA), 685
Riverton Memorial Hospital (Riverton WY), 732
Riverview Hospital (Crookston MN), 377
Riverview Hospital (Noblesville IN), 252
Riverview Hospital (Wisconsin Rapids WI), 724
Riverview Medical Center (Red Bank NJ), 440
Riverview Regional Medical Center (Gadsden AL), 59
RNs. See registered nurses
Roane General Hospital (Spencer WV), 708
Roane Medical Center (Harriman TN), 612
Roanoke Chowan Hospital (Ahoskie NC), 496
Robert Packer Hospital (Sayre PA), 574

Robert Wood Johnson University Hospital at Hamilton
   (Hamilton NJ), 440
Robert Wood Johnson University Hospital—Rahway
   (Rahway NJ), 440
Robinson Memorial Hospital (Ravenna OH), 523
Rochelle Community Hospital (Rochelle IL), 230
Rochester, New York, 460, 473, 479, 480
Rochester General Hospital (Rochester NY), 473
Rochester Methodist Hospital (Rochester MN), 377
Rockcastle Hospital Respiratory Care Center
   (Mount Vernon KY), 299
Rockdale Medical Center (Conyers GA), 199
Rockford Memorial Hospital (Rockford IL), 231
Rockingham Memorial Hospital (Harrisonburg VA), 685
Rockville General Hospital (Vernon Rockville CT), 150
Roger Williams Hospital (Providence RI), 584
Rogue Valley Medical Center (Medford OR), 551
Rolling Plains Memorial Hospital (Sweetwater TX), 658
Rollins Brook Community Hospital (Lampasas TX), 658
Rome Memorial Hospital (Rome NY), 474
Roosevelt Warm Springs Rehabilitation Hospital
   (Warm Springs GA), 199
Roper Hospital (Charleston SC), 592
Rose Medical Center (Denver CO), 144
Roseau Area Hospital and Homes (Roseau MN), 377
Roseland Community Hospital (Chicago IL), 231
Round Rock Medical Center (Round Rock TX), 658
Rowan Regional Medical Center (Salisbury NC), 496
Roxborough Memorial Hospital (Philadelphia PA), 574
Rumford Hospital (Rumford ME), 324
Rush City Hospital (Rush City MN), 377
Rush Copley Memorial Hospital (Aurora IL), 231
Rush Foundation Hospital (Meridian MS), 392
Rush North Shore Medical Center (Skokie IL), 231
Rush University Medical Center (Chicago IL), 231
Rusk County Memorial Hospital (Ladysmith WI), 724
Russell County Hospital (Russell Springs KY), 299
Russell County Medical Center (Lebanon VA), 685
Russell Medical Center (Alexander City AL), 59
Russellville Hospital (Russellville AL), 59
Rutherford Hospital (Rutherfordton NC), 496
Rutland Regional Medical Center (Rutland VT), 676

S
Sabine County Hospital (Hemphill TX), 658
Sabine Medical Center (Many LA), 315
Sac-Osage Hospital (Osceola MO), 408
Sacramento, California, 105, 106, 111, 112, 132, 135
Sacred Heart Hospital (Allentown PA), 574
Sacred Heart Hospital (Chicago IL), 231
Sacred Heart Hospital (Cumberland MD), 331
Sacred Heart Hospital (Eau Claire WI), 724
Sacred Heart Hospital (Pensacola FL), 176
Sacred Heart Hospital at the Emerald Coast (Destin FL),
   176
Sacred Heart Medical Center (Spokane WA), 696
Sacred Heart Medical Center—University District
   (Eugene OR), 551

Saddleback Memorial Medical Center (Laguna Hills CA), 121
Saddleback Memorial Medical Center—San Clemente
   (San Clemente CA), 121
St. Agnes Hospital (Baltimore MD), 331
St. Agnes Hospital (Fond Du Lac WI), 724
Saint Agnes Medical Center (Fresno CA), 121
St. Alexius Hospital (St. Louis MO), 408
St. Alexius Medical Center (Bismarck ND), 502
St. Alexius Medical Center (Hoffman Estates IL), 232
St. Alosius Medical Center (Harvey ND), 503
St. Alphonsus Regional Medical Center (Boise ID), 209
St. Andrews Hospital (Boothbay Harbor ME), 324
St. Anne Mercy Hospital (Toledo OH), 524
St. Anne's Hospital Corporation (Fall River MA), 343
St. Anthony Community Hospital (Warwick NY), 474
St. Anthony Hospital (Chicago IL), 232
St. Anthony Hospital (Oklahoma City OK), 542
St. Anthony Hospital (Pendleton OR), 551
St. Anthony Medical Center (Rockford IL), 232
St. Anthony Medical Center of Crown Point
   (Crown Point IN), 252
St. Anthony Memorial Health Center (Michigan City IN), 252
St. Anthony Regional Hospital (Carroll IA), 271
St. Anthony's Health Center (Alton IL), 232
St. Anthony's Healthcare Center (Morrilton AR), 81
St. Anthony's Hospital (St. Petersburg FL), 176
St. Anthony's Medical Center (St. Louis MO), 408
St. Anthony's Memorial Hospital (Effingham IL), 232
St. Barnabas Hospital (Bronx NY), 474
St. Barnabas Medical Center (Livingston NJ), 440
St. Bernard Hospital (Chicago IL), 232
St. Bernardine Medical Center (San Bernardino CA), 121
St. Bernards Medical Center (Jonesboro AR), 81
St. Brendan Rehab and Specialty Hospital (Lafayette LA),
   315
St. Catherine Hospital (East Chicago IN), 252
St. Catherine Hospital (Garden City KS), 283
St. Catherine Medical Center—Fountain Springs
   (Ashland PA), 574
St. Catherine Regional Hospital (Charlestown IN), 252
St. Catherine of Siena Hospital (Smithtown NY), 474
St. Charles Hospital (Port Jefferson NY), 474
St. Charles Medical Center—Bend (Bend OR), 551
St. Charles Medical Center—Redmond (Redmond OR), 552
St. Charles Mercy Hospital (Oregon OH), 524
St. Charles Parish Hospital (Luling LA), 315
St. Clair Hospital (Pittsburgh PA), 575
St. Claire Medical Center (Morehead KY), 299
St. Clare Hospital (Tacoma WA), 696
St. Clare Hospital Health Services (Baraboo WI), 724
St. Clare Medical Center (Crawfordsville IN), 253
St. Clare's Hospital (Schenectady NY), 474
St. Clare's Hospital/Denville (Denville NJ), 441
St. Clare's Hospital/Sussex (Sussex NJ), 441
St. Cloud Hospital (St. Cloud MN), 378
St. Cloud Regional Medical Center (St. Cloud FL), 177
St. Croix Regional Medical Center (St. Croix Falls WI), 725
St. David's Hospital (Austin TX), 659

Please note that all individual hospital listings provide page numbers for Chapter 6 (Hospital Ratings by Clinical Specialty) only. All other hospital listings can be found under their state listing.

St. Dominic-Jackson Memorial Hospital (Jackson MS), 392
St. Edward Mercy Medical Center (Fort Smith AR), 82
St. Elizabeth Ann Seton Hospital (Boonville IN), 253
St. Elizabeth Ann Seton Specialty Care (Carmel IN), 253
St. Elizabeth Community Hospital (Red Bluff CA), 121
St. Elizabeth Health Center (Youngstown OH), 524
St. Elizabeth Health Services (Baker City OR), 552
St. Elizabeth Hospital (Appleton WI), 725
St. Elizabeth Hospital (Belleville IL), 233
St. Elizabeth Hospital (Gonzales LA), 315
St. Elizabeth Medical Center (Lafayette IN), 253
St. Elizabeth Medical Center (Utica NY), 475
St. Elizabeth Medical Center (Wabasha MN), 378
St. Elizabeth Medical Center—South (Edgewood KY), 299
St. Elizabeth Regional Medical Center (Lincoln NE), 424
St. Francis Community Hospital (Federal Way WA), 696
St. Francis Health Center (Topeka KS), 283
St. Francis Hospital (Charleston WV), 708
St. Francis Hospital (Columbus GA), 199
St. Francis Hospital (Escanaba MI), 362
St. Francis Hospital (Greenville SC), 592
St. Francis Hospital (Litchfield IL), 233
St. Francis Hospital (Maryville MO), 408
St. Francis Hospital (Memphis TN), 612
St. Francis Hospital (Poughkeepsie NY), 475
St. Francis Hospital (Tulsa OK), 542
St. Francis Hospital (Wilmington DE), 152
St. Francis Hospital and Health Center (Beech Grove IN), 253
St. Francis Hospital and Health Center (Blue Island IL), 233
St. Francis Hospital and Health Center (Indianapolis IN), 253
St. Francis Hospital and Medical Center (Hartford CT), 150
St. Francis Hospital—Bartlett (Bartlett TN), 612
St. Francis Hospital—Broken Arrow (Broken Arrow OK), 543
St. Francis Hospital Mooresville (Mooresville IN), 254
St. Francis Hospital—Roslyn (Roslyn NY), 475
St. Francis Medical Center (Breckenridge MN), 378
St. Francis Medical Center (Cape Girardeau MO), 408
St. Francis Medical Center (Grand Island NE), 424
St. Francis Medical Center (Lynwood CA), 121
St. Francis Medical Center (Monroe LA), 315
Saint Francis Medical Center (Peoria IL), 233
St. Francis Medical Center (Trenton NJ), 441
Saint Francis Memorial Hospital (San Francisco CA), 122
St. Francis Memorial Hospital (West Point NE), 424
St. Francis North Hospital (Monroe LA), 316
St. Francis Regional Medical Center (Shakopee MN), 378
St. Gabriel's Hospital (Little Falls MN), 378
St. Helena Hospital (Deer Park CA), 122
St. Helena Parish Hospital (Greensburg LA), 316
St. James Health Services (St. James MN), 378
St. James Healthcare (Butte MT), 416
St. James Hospital (Newark NJ), 441
Saint James Hospital (Pontiac IL), 233
St. James Hospital and Health Center (Chicago Heights IL), 233
St. James Hospital and Health Center—Olympia Fields (Olympia Fields IL), 234

St. James Mercy Hospital (Hornell NY), 475
St. James Parish Hospital (Lutcher LA), 316
St. John Detroit Riverview Hospital (Detroit MI), 362
St. John Hospital (Leavenworth KS), 283
St. John Hospital and Medical Center (Detroit MI), 362
St. John Macomb Hospital (Warren MI), 362
St. John Medical Center (Steubenville OH), 524
St. John Medical Center (Tulsa OK), 543
St. John Medical Center Peacehealth (Longview WA), 697
St. John Oakland Hospital (Madison Heights MI), 362
St. John River District Hospital (East China MI), 363
St. John West Shore Hospital (Westlake OH), 524
St. John's Episcopal Hospital at South Shore (Far Rockaway NY), 475
St. John's Health Center (Santa Monica CA), 122
Saint John's Health System (Anderson IN), 254
St. John's Hospital (Springfield IL), 234
St. John's Hospital—Aurora (Aurora MO), 409
St. John's Hospital—Berryville (Berryville AR), 82
St. John's Hospital—Lebanon (Lebanon MO), 409
St. John's Medical Center (Jackson Hole WY), 732
St. John's Mercy Hospital (Washington MO), 409
St. John's Mercy Medical Center (St. Louis MO), 409
St. John's Pleasant Valley Hospital (Camarillo CA), 122
St. Johns Regional Health Center (Salina KS), 283
St. John's Regional Health Center (Springfield MO), 409
St. John's Regional Medical Center (Joplin MO), 409
St. John's Regional Medical Center (Oxnard CA), 122
St. John's Riverside Hospital (Yonkers NY), 475
St. Joseph Community Hospital (Mishawaka IN), 254
St. Joseph East (Lexington KY), 299
St. Joseph Health Center (Warren OH), 524
St. Joseph Health Services of Rhode Island (North Providence RI), 584
St. Joseph Health System—Tawas (Tawas City MI), 363
St. Joseph Hospital (Aberdeen WA), 697
St. Joseph Hospital (Bangor ME), 325
St. Joseph Hospital (Bellingham WA), 697
St. Joseph Hospital (Buckhannon WV), 709
St. Joseph Hospital (Chicago IL), 234
St. Joseph Hospital (Elgin IL), 234
St. Joseph Hospital (Eureka CA), 122
St. Joseph Hospital (Florence CO), 144
St. Joseph Hospital (Lexington KY), 300
St. Joseph Hospital (Fort Wayne IN), 254
St. Joseph Hospital (Nashua NH), 431
St. Joseph Hospital (Orange CA), 123
St. Joseph Hospital and Health Center (Kokomo IN), 254
St. Joseph Hospital—Augusta (Augusta GA), 199
St. Joseph Hospital of Cheektowaga New York (Cheektowaga NY), 476
St. Joseph Medical Center (Bloomington IL), 234
St. Joseph Medical Center (Houston TX), 659
St. Joseph Medical Center (Kansas City MO), 410
St. Joseph Medical Center (Reading PA), 575
St. Joseph Medical Center (Tacoma WA), 697
St. Joseph Medical Center (Towson MD), 331
St. Joseph Medical Center (Wichita KS), 283

St. Joseph Memorial Hospital (Murphysboro IL), 234
St. Joseph Mercy Hospital (Ypsilanti MI), 363
St. Joseph Mercy Livingston Hospital (Howell MI), 363
St. Joseph Mercy Oakland (Pontiac MI), 363
St. Joseph Mercy Saline Hospital (Saline MI), 363
St. Joseph Regional Health Center (Bryan TX), 659
St. Joseph Regional Medical Center (Lewiston ID), 210
St. Joseph Regional Medical Center (Plymouth IN), 254
St. Joseph Regional Medical Center—South Bend (South Bend IN), 255
St. Joseph's Area Health Services (Park Rapids MN), 379
St. Joseph's Community Health Services (Hillsboro WI), 725
St. Joseph's Community Hospital West Bend (West Bend WI), 725
St. Joseph's Hospital (Alton IL), 235
St. Joseph's Hospital (Asheville NC), 497
St. Joseph's Hospital (Breese IL), 235
St. Joseph's Hospital (Chippewa Falls WI), 725
St. Joseph's Hospital (Elmira NY), 476
St. Joseph's Hospital (Highland IL), 235
St. Joseph's Hospital (Marshfield WI), 725
St. Joseph's Hospital (Parkersburg WV), 709
St. Joseph's Hospital (Philadelphia PA), 575
St. Joseph's Hospital (St. Paul MN), 379
St. Joseph's Hospital (Savannah GA), 199
St. Joseph's Hospital (Tampa FL), 177
St. Joseph's Hospital and Health Center (Dickinson ND), 503
St. Joseph's Hospital and Medical Center (Paterson NJ), 441
St. Joseph's Hospital and Medical Center (Phoenix AZ), 70
Saint Joseph's Hospital of Atlanta (Atlanta GA), 199
St. Joseph's Hospital of Chewelah (Chewelah WA), 697
St. Joseph's Hospital Health Center (Syracuse NY), 476
St. Joseph's Hospital Yonkers (Yonkers NY), 476
St. Joseph's Medical Center (Brainerd MN), 379
St. Joseph's Medical Center of Stockton (Stockton CA), 123
St. Joseph's Mercy Health Center (Hot Springs AR), 82
St. Joseph's Wayne Hospital (Wayne NJ), 441
St. Joseph's Women's Hospital (Tampa FL), 177
St. Jude Medical Center (Fullerton CA), 123
St. Louis, Missouri, 396, 397, 399, 400, 401, 404, 408, 409, 410, 411, 413
St. Louis University Hospital (St. Louis MO), 410
St. Louise Regional Hospital (Gilroy CA), 123
St. Lucie Medical Center (Port St. Lucie FL), 177
St. Luke Hospital East (Fort Thomas KY), 300
St. Luke Hospital West (Florence KY), 300
St. Luke's Baptist Hospital (San Antonio TX), 659
St. Luke's Behavioral Health Center (Phoenix AZ), 71
St. Luke's Boise Medical Center (Boise ID), 210
St. Luke's Cancer Institute (Kansas City MO), 410
St. Luke's Community Medical Center—The Woodlands (The Woodlands TX), 659
St. Luke's Cornwall Hospital (Cornwall NY), 476
St. Luke's Episcopal Hospital (Houston TX), 659
St. Luke's Hospital (Bethlehem PA), 575
St. Luke's Hospital (Cedar Rapids IA), 271
St. Luke's Hospital (Chesterfield MO), 410
St. Luke's Hospital (Columbus NC), 497

St. Luke's Hospital (Crosby ND), 503
St. Luke's Hospital (Duluth MN), 379
St. Luke's Hospital (Jacksonville FL), 177
St. Luke's Hospital (Maumee OH), 525
St. Luke's Hospital (San Francisco CA), 123
St. Luke's Hospital—Allentown Campus (Allentown PA), 575
Saint Luke's Hospital of Kansas City (Kansas City MO), 410
St. Luke's Magic Valley Regional Medical Center
   (Twin Falls ID), 210
St. Luke's Medical Center (Cudahy WI), 726
St. Luke's Medical Center (Phoenix AZ), 71
St. Lukes Memorial Hospital (Spokane WA), 697
St. Luke's Miners Memorial Hospital (Coaldale PA), 575
St. Luke's Northland Hospital (Kansas City MO), 410
St. Luke's Quakertown Hospital (Quakertown PA), 576
St. Luke's Regional Medical Center (Sioux City IA), 271
St. Luke's Roosevelt Hospital (New York NY), 476
St. Luke's South Hospital (Overland Park KS), 283
St. Luke's Wood River Medical Center (Ketchum ID), 210
St. Margaret Mercy Healthcare Center (Dyer IN), 255
St. Margaret Mercy Healthcare Center (Hammond IN), 255
St. Margaret's Hospital (Spring Valley IL), 235
St. Mark's Hospital (Salt Lake City UT), 673
St. Mark's Medical Center (La Grange TX), 660
St. Martin Hospital (Breaux Bridge LA), 316
St. Mary and Elizabeth Medical Center—Claremont
   (Chicago IL), 235
St. Mary and Elizabeth Medical Center—Division
   (Chicago IL), 235
St. Mary Hospital (Quincy IL), 236
St. Mary Medical Center (Apple Valley CA), 123
St. Mary Medical Center (Galesburg IL), 236
St. Mary Medical Center (Langhorne PA), 576
St. Mary Medical Center (Long Beach CA), 124
St. Mary Medical Center (Walla Walla WA), 698
St. Mary Mercy Hospital (Livonia MI), 364
St. Mary Rogers Memorial Hospital (Rogers AR), 82
St. Mary's Duluth Clinic (Duluth MN), 379
St. Mary's Health Care (Grand Rapids MI), 364
St. Mary's Health Center (Jefferson City MO), 411
St. Mary's Hospital (Amsterdam NY), 477
St. Mary's Hospital (Centralia IL), 236
St. Mary's Hospital (Decatur IL), 236
St. Mary's Hospital (Leonardtown MD), 332
St. Mary's Hospital (Passaic NJ), 442
St. Mary's Hospital (Pierre SD), 597
St. Mary's Hospital (Rhinelander WI), 726
St. Marys Hospital (Rochester MN), 379
St. Mary's Hospital (Streator IL), 236
St. Mary's Hospital (Waterbury CT), 150
St. Mary's Hospital and Medical Center
   (Grand Junction CO), 144
St. Mary's Hospital of Athens (Athens GA), 200
St. Mary's Hospital Medical Center (Green Bay WI), 726
St. Mary's Hospital Medical Center (Madison WI), 726
St. Mary's Jefferson Memorial Hospital (Jefferson City TN), 612
St. Mary's Medical Center (Blue Springs MO), 411
St. Mary's Medical Center (Huntington WV), 709

St. Mary's Medical Center (Knoxville TN), 612
St. Mary's Medical Center (San Francisco CA), 124
St. Mary's Medical Center (West Palm Beach FL), 177
St. Mary's Medical Center of Campbell County
   (La Follette TN), 613
St. Mary's Medical Center—Evansville (Evansville IN), 255
St. Mary's Medical Center—Hobart (Hobart IN), 255
St. Mary's of Michigan Medical Center (Saginaw MI), 364
St. Mary's Regional Health Center (Detroit Lakes MN), 380
St. Mary's Regional Medical Center (Enid OK), 543
St. Mary's Regional Medical Center (Lewiston ME), 325
St. Mary's Regional Medical Center (Reno NV), 427
St. Mary's Regional Medical Center (Russellville AR), 82
St. Mary's Warrick (Boonville IN), 255
St. Michael Hospital (Oklahoma City OK), 543
St. Michael's Hospital (Stevens Point WI), 726
St. Michael's Hospital and Nursing Home
   (Sauk Centre MN), 380
St. Michael's Medical Center (Newark NJ), 442
St. Nicholas Hospital (Sheboygan WI), 726
St. Patrick Hospital and Health Sciences Center
   (Missoula MT), 417
St. Peter Community Hospital (St. Peter MN), 380
St. Peter's Hospital (Albany NY), 477
St. Peter's Hospital (Helena MT), 417
St. Peter's University Hospital (New Brunswick NJ), 442
St. Petersburg, Florida, 154, 159, 172, 174, 176, 178
St. Petersburg General Hospital (St. Petersburg FL), 178
St. Rita's Medical Center (Lima OH), 525
St. Rose Dominican Hospital (Henderson NV), 427
St. Rose Dominican Hospital—Siena Campus
   (Henderson NV), 427
St. Rose Hospital (Hayward CA), 124
St. Tammany Parish Hospital (Covington LA), 316
St. Thomas Hospital (Nashville TN), 613
St. Vincent Carmel Hospital (Carmel IN), 256
St. Vincent Charity Hospital (Cleveland OH), 525
St. Vincent Doctors Hospital (Little Rock AR), 82
St. Vincent Frankfort Hospital (Frankfort IN), 256
St. Vincent Health Center (Erie PA), 576
St. Vincent Healthcare (Billings MT), 417
St. Vincent Heart Center of Indiana (Indianapolis IN), 256
St. Vincent Hospital (Green Bay WI), 727
St. Vincent Hospital (Santa Fe NM), 449
St. Vincent Hospital (Worcester MA), 343
St. Vincent Hospital and Health Services (Indianapolis IN),
   256
St. Vincent Infirmary Medical Center (Little Rock AR), 83
St. Vincent Medical Center (Los Angeles CA), 124
St. Vincent Medical Center—North (Sherwood AR), 83
St. Vincent Mercy Hospital (Elwood IN), 256
St. Vincent Mercy Medical Center (Toledo OH), 525
St. Vincent's—Birmingham (Birmingham AL), 59
St. Vincent's—Blount (Oneonta AL), 59
St. Vincent's—East (Birmingham AL), 59
St. Vincent's Hospital—Manhattan (New York NY), 477
St. Vincent's Medical Center (Bridgeport CT), 150
St. Vincent's Medical Center (Jacksonville FL), 178

St. Vincent's—St. Clair (Pell City AL), 60
Ste. Genevieve County Memorial Hospital
   (Ste. Genevieve MO), 411
Sts. Mary and Elizabeth Hospital (Louisville KY), 300
Saints Medical Center (Lowell MA), 344
Salem Community Hospital (Salem OH), 525
Salem Hospital (Salem OR), 552
Salem Township Hospital (Salem IL), 236
Salina Regional Health Center (Salina KS), 284
Salinas Valley Memorial Health Care System
   (Salinas CA), 124
Saline Memorial Hospital (Benton AR), 83
Salt Lake Regional Medical Center (Salt Lake City UT), 673
Sam Houston Memorial Hospital (Houston TX), 660
Samaritan Albany General Hospital (Albany OR), 552
Samaritan Hospital (Lexington KY), 300
Samaritan Hospital (Moses Lake WA), 698
Samaritan Hospital (Troy NY), 477
Samaritan Lebanon Community Hospital (Lebanon OR), 552
Samaritan Medical Center (Watertown NY), 477
Samaritan North Lincoln Hospital (Lincoln City OR), 552
Samaritan Pacific Community Hospital (Newport OR), 553
Samaritan Regional Health System (Ashland OH), 525
Sampson Regional Medical Center (Clinton NC), 497
San Angelo Community Medical Center (San Angelo TX),
   660
San Antonio, Texas, 619, 624, 648, 649, 651, 659, 663,
   664, 666
San Antonio Community Hospital (Upland CA), 124
San Diego, California, 86, 103, 127, 129, 135
San Dimas Community Hospital (San Dimas CA), 125
San Fernando Community Hospital (San Fernando CA), 125
San Francisco, California, 89, 90, 105, 116, 122, 123, 124,
   125, 135
San Francisco General Hospital (San Francisco CA), 125
San Gabriel Valley Medical Center (San Gabriel CA), 125
San Gorgonio Memorial Hospital (Banning CA), 125
San Jacinto Methodist Hospital (Baytown TX), 660
San Joaquin Community Hospital (Bakersfield CA), 125
San Joaquin General Hospital (French Camp CA), 126
San Jose, California, 100, 106, 115, 120, 126
San Juan Regional Medical Center (Farmington NM), 449
San Leandro Hospital (San Leandro CA), 126
San Luis Valley Regional Medical Center (Alamosa CO), 145
San Mateo Medical Center (San Mateo CA), 126
San Ramon Regional Medical Center (San Ramon CA), 126
Sandhills Regional Medical Center (Hamlet NC), 497
Sanford USD Medical Center (Sioux Falls SD), 598
Santa Barbara Cottage Hospital (Santa Barbara CA), 126
Santa Clara Valley Medical Center (San Jose CA), 126
Santa Monica—UCLA Medical Center (Santa Monica CA),
   127
Santa Rosa Medical Center (Milton FL), 178
Santa Rosa Memorial Hospital (Santa Rosa CA), 127
Santiam Memorial Hospital (Stayton OR), 553
Sarah Bush Lincoln Health Center (Mattoon IL), 237
Sarah D. Culbertson Memorial Hospital (Rushville IL), 237
Sarasota Memorial Hospital (Sarasota FL), 178

Saratoga Hospital (Saratoga Springs NY), 477
Sartori Memorial Hospital (Cedar Falls IA), 271
Satilla Regional Medical Center (Waycross GA), 200
Sauk Prairie Memorial Hospital (Prairie De Sac WI), 727
Saunders Medical Center (Wahoo NE), 424
Savoy Medical Center (Mamou LA), 316
SCCI Hospital—San Angelo (San Angelo TX), 660
Scenic Mountain Medical Center (Big Spring TX), 660
Schneck Medical Center (Seymour IN), 256
Schuyler Hospital (Montour Falls NY), 478
Scripps Green Hospital (La Jolla CA), 127
Scotland County Memorial Hospital (Memphis MO), 411
Scotland Memorial Hospital (Laurinburg NC), 497
Scott and White Memorial Hospital (Temple TX), 661
Scott County Hospital (Oneida TN), 613
Scott County Hospital (Scott City KS), 284
Scott Memorial Hospital (Scottsburg IN), 257
Scottsdale Healthcare—Osborn (Scottsdale AZ), 71
Scottsdale Healthcare—Shea (Scottsdale AZ), 71
Screven County Hospital (Sylvania GA), 200
Scripps Memorial Hospital—Encinitas (Encinitas CA), 127
Scripps Memorial Hospital—La Jolla (La Jolla CA), 127
Scripps Mercy Hospital (San Diego CA), 127
Scripps Mercy Hospital—Chula Vista (Chula Vista CA), 128
Seattle, Washington, 693, 695, 699, 700, 701
Sebastian River Medical Center (Sebastian FL), 178
Sebasticook Valley Hospital (Pittsfield ME), 325
Selby General Hospital (Marietta OH), 526
Select Specialty Hospital (Honolulu HI), 207
Select Specialty Hospital Lexington (Lexington KY), 300
Select Specialty Hospital—Saginaw (Saginaw MI), 364
Select Specialty Hospital—Tricities (Bristol TN), 613
Select Specialty Hospital Wichita (Wichita KS), 284
Self Regional Healthcare (Greenwood SC), 592
Selma Community Hospital (Selma CA), 128
Seminole Medical Center (Seminole OK), 543
Sempercare Hospital of Augusta (Augusta GA), 200
Sempercare Hospital of Midland (Midland TX), 661
Sentara Bayside Hospital (Virginia Beach VA), 687
Sentara Careplex Hospital (Hampton VA), 687
Sentara Leigh Hospital (Norfolk VA), 687
Sentara Norfolk General Hospital (Norfolk VA), 687
Sentara Virginia Beach General Hospital
    (Virginia Beach VA), 687
Sentara Williamsburg Regional Medical Center
    (Williamsburg VA), 687
Sequoia Hospital (Redwood City CA), 128
Sequoyah Memorial Hospital (Sallisaw OK), 543
Seton Edgar B. Davis Hospital (Luling TX), 661
Seton Health System—St. Mary's Campus (Troy NY), 478
Seton Highland Lakes (Burnet TX), 661
Seton Medical Center (Austin TX), 661
Seton Medical Center (Daly City CA), 128
Seton Northwest Hospital (Austin TX), 661
Seven Rivers Regional Medical Center (Crystal River FL), 178
Sevier Valley Medical Center (Richfield UT), 674
Sewickley Valley Hospital (Sewickley PA), 576
Shady Grove Adventist Hospital (Rockville MD), 332

Shamokin Area Community Hospital (Coal Township PA), 576
Shands Hospital at the University of Florida
    (Gainesville FL), 179
Shands Jacksonville (Jacksonville FL), 179
Shands Lake Shore (Lake City FL), 179
Shands Starke (Starke FL), 179
Shannon West Texas Medical Center (San Angelo TX), 662
Share Memorial Hospital (Alva OK), 544
Sharon Hospital (Sharon CT), 150
Sharon Regional Health System (Sharon PA), 576
Sharp Chula Vista Medical Center (Chula Vista CA), 128
Sharp Coronado Hospital and Healthcare Center
    (Coronado CA), 128
Sharp Memorial Hospital (San Diego CA), 129
Shasta Regional Medical Center (Redding CA), 129
Shawano Medical Center (Shawano WI), 727
Shawnee Mission Medical Center (Shawnee Mission KS), 284
Shelby County Myrtue Memorial Hospital (Harlan IA), 271
Shelby Memorial Hospital (Shelbyville IL), 237
Shelby Regional Medical Center (Center TX), 662
Shenandoah Memorial Hospital (Shenandoah IA), 271
Shenandoah Memorial Hospital (Woodstock VA), 688
Sheridan Community Hospital (Sheridan MI), 364
Sherman Hospital (Elgin IL), 237
Sherman Oaks Hospital (Sherman Oaks CA), 129
Shoals Hospital (Muscle Shoals AL), 60
Shore Memorial Hospital (Nassawadox VA), 688
Shore Memorial Hospital (Somers Point NJ), 442
Shreveport, Louisiana, 305, 306, 307, 310, 319
Sibley Memorial Hospital (Washington DC), 702
Sid Peterson Memorial Hospital (Kerrville TX), 662
Sidney Health Center (Sidney MT), 417
Sierra Kings District Hospital (Reedley CA), 129
Sierra Medical Center (El Paso TX), 662
Sierra Nevada Memorial Hospital (Grass Valley CA), 129
Sierra View District Hospital (Porterville CA), 129
Sierra Vista Hospital (Truth Or Consequences NM), 450
Sierra Vista Regional Health Center (Sierra Vista AZ), 71
Sierra Vista Regional Medical Center
    (San Luis Obispo CA), 130
Siloam Springs Memorial Hospital (Siloam Springs AR), 83
Silver Cross Hospital (Joliet IL), 237
Silverton Hospital (Silverton OR), 553
Simi Valley Hospital and Health Care Service
    (Simi Valley CA), 130
Simpson General Hospital (Mendanhall MS), 393
Sinai Hospital of Baltimore (Baltimore MD), 332
Sinai-Grace Hospital (Detroit MI), 364
Singing River Hospital System (Pascagoula MS), 393
Sioux Valley Canby Campus (Canby MN), 380
Sisters of Charity Hospital (Buffalo NY), 478
Sisters of Charity Providence Hospitals (Columbia SC), 593
Skaggs Community Health Center (Branson MO), 411
Skagit Valley Hospital (Mount Vernon WA), 698
Skiff Medical Center (Newton IA), 272
Sky Ridge Medical Center (Lone Tree CO), 145
Skyline Madison Campus (Madison TN), 613
Skyline Medical Center (Nashville TN), 613

Slidell Memorial Hospital (Slidell LA), 317
SMC Regional Medical Center (Osceola AR), 83
Smith County Memorial Hospital (Carthage TN), 614
Smith County Memorial Hospital (Smith Center KS), 284
Smith Northview Hospital (Valdosta GA), 200
Smithville Regional Hospital (Smithville TX), 662
Smyth County Community Hospital (Marion VA), 688
Soldiers and Sailors Memorial Hospital (Wellsboro PA), 577
Soldiers and Sailors Memorial Hospital of Yates
    (Penn Yan NY), 478
Somerset Hospital (Somerset PA), 577
Somerset Medical Center (Somerville NJ), 442
Somerville Hospital (Somerville MA), 344
Sonoma Valley Hospital (Sonoma CA), 130
Sonora Regional Medical Center (Sonora CA), 130
Sound Shore Medical Center of Westchester
    (New Rochelle NY), 478
South Austin Hospital (Austin TX), 662
South Baldwin Regional Medical Center (Foley AL), 60
South Bay Hospital (Sun City Center FL), 179
South Beach Community Hospital (Miami Beach FL), 179
South Carolina
    five star rated facilities, 806
    hospitals, 585–94
    procedure, hospital ratings by, 992–95
    top doctors, 1073
South Central Kansas Regional Medical Center
    (Arkansas City KS), 284
South Central Regional Medical Center (Laurel MS), 393
South Coast Medical Center (Laguna Beach CA), 130
South County Hospital (Wakefield RI), 584
South Dakota
    five star rated facilities, 807
    hospitals, 594–98
    procedure, hospital ratings by, 996–97
    top doctors, 1073–74
South Florida Baptist Hospital (Plant City FL), 180
South Fulton Medical Center (East Point GA), 200
South Georgia Medical Center (Valdosta GA), 201
South Haven Community Hospital (South Haven MI), 365
South Jersey Healthcare Regional Medical Center
    (Vineland NJ), 442
South Jersey Hospital—Elmer Division (Elmer NJ), 443
South Lake Hospital (Clermont FL), 180
South Miami Hospital (South Miami FL), 180
South Nassau Communities Hospital (Oceanside NY), 478
South Point Hospital (St. Louis MO), 411
South Pointe Hospital (Warrensville Heights OH), 526
South Shore Hospital (Chicago IL), 237
South Shore Hospital (South Weymouth MA), 344
South Sunflower County Hospital (Indianola MS), 393
South Texas Regional Medical Center (Jourdanton TX), 663
Southampton Hospital (Southampton NY), 479
Southampton Memorial Hospital (Franklin VA), 688
Southcoast Hospitals Group—Charlton Memorial
    (Fall River MA), 344
Southcoast Hospitals Group—St. Luke's Hospital
    (New Bedford MA), 344

Please note that all individual hospital listings provide page numbers for Chapter 6 (Hospital Ratings by Clinical Specialty) only. All other hospital listings can be found under their state listing.

Southcoast Hospitals Group—Tobey Hospital
(Wareham MA), 344
SouthCrest Hospital (Tulsa OK), 544
Southeast Alabama Medical Center (Dothan AL), 60
Southeast Arizona Medical Center (Douglas AZ), 71
Southeast Georgia Regional Medical Center
(Brunswick GA), 201
Southeast Missouri Hospital (Cape Girardeau MO), 412
Southeastern Ohio Regional Medical Center
(Cambridge OH), 526
Southeastern Regional Medical Center (Lumberton NC), 497
Southern Hills Hospital and Medical Center
(Las Vegas NV), 427
Southern Hills Medical Center (Nashville TN), 614
Southern Maine Medical Center (Biddeford ME), 325
Southern Maryland Hospital Center (Clinton MD), 332
Southern New Hampshire Medical Center (Nashua NH), 431
Southern Ocean County Hospital (Manahawkin NJ), 443
Southern Ohio Medical Center (Portsmouth OH), 526
Southern Regional Medical Center (Riverdale GA), 201
Southern Tennessee Medical Center (Winchester TN), 614
Southern Virginia Regional Medical Center (Emporia VA),
688
Southside Community Hospital (Farmville VA), 688
Southside Health Center (Corpus Christi TX), 663
Southside Hospital (Bay Shore NY), 479
Southside Regional Medical Center (Petersburg VA), 689
Southwest Alabama Medical Center (Thomasville AL), 60
Southwest Florida Regional Medical Center
(Fort Myers FL), 180
Southwest General Health Center (Middleburg Heights OH),
526
Southwest General Hospital (San Antonio TX), 663
Southwest Health Center (Platteville WI), 727
Southwest Healthcare System—Inland Valley Med. Ctr.
(Wildomar CA), 130
Southwest Healthcare System—Rancho Springs Med. Ctr.
(Murrieta CA), 131
Southwest Medical Center (Lafayette LA), 317
Southwest Medical Center (Liberal KS), 285
Southwest Memorial Hospital (Cortez CO), 145
Southwest Mississippi Regional Medical Center
(McComb MS), 393
Southwest Regional Medical Center (Little Rock AR), 83
Southwest Regional Medical Center (Waynesburg PA), 577
Southwest Washington Medical Center (Vancouver WA), 698
Southwestern General Hospital (El Paso TX), 663
Southwestern Medical Center (Lawton OK), 544
Southwestern Memorial Hospital (Weatherford OK), 544
Southwestern Vermont Medical Center (Bennington VT), 676
Spalding Regional Medical Center (Griffin GA), 201
Spanish Peaks Regional Health Center (Walsenburg CO),
145
Sparks Regional Medical Center (Fort Smith AR), 84
Sparta Community Hospital (Sparta IL), 238
Spartanburg Regional Medical Center (Spartanburg SC),
593
Speare Memorial Hospital (Plymouth NH), 432

Spearfish Regional Hospital (Spearfish SD), 598
specialty(-ies), xiii, xiv, 7, 11, 15, 17, 28
Spectrum Health Hospitals (Grand Rapids MI), 365
Spectrum Health—Reed City Campus (Reed City MI), 365
Spencer Municipal Hospital (Spencer IA), 272
Spokane, Washington, 691, 693, 696, 697, 700
Spooner Health System (Spooner WI), 727
Spring Branch Medical Center (Houston TX), 663
Spring Valley Hospital (Las Vegas NV), 427
Spring View Hospital (Lebanon KY), 301
Springfield Hospital (Springfield PA), 577
Springfield Hospital (Springfield VT), 676
Springhill Medical Center (Mobile AL), 60
Springhill Medical Center (Springhill LA), 317
Springs Memorial Hospital (Lancaster SC), 593
Spruce Pine Community Hospital (Spruce Pine NC), 498
SSM DePaul Health Center (Bridgeton MO), 412
SSM St. Joseph Health Center (St. Charles MO), 412
SSM St. Joseph Health Center—Wentzville (Wentzville MO),
412
SSM St. Joseph Hospital of Kirkwood (Kirkwood MO), 412
SSM St. Joseph Hospital West (Lake St. Louis MO), 412
SSM St. Mary's Health Center (St. Louis MO), 413
Stamford Hospital (Stamford CT), 150
Standish Community Hospital (Standish MI), 365
Stanford Hospital (Stanford CA), 131
Stanly Memorial Hospital (Albemarle NC), 498
star ratings, xiii
Starke Memorial Hospital (Knox IN), 257
Starr County Memorial Hospital (Rio Grande City TX), 663
Staten Island University Hospital (Staten Island NY), 479
stents, 42
Stephens County Hospital (Toccoa GA), 201
Stephens Memorial Hospital (Breckenridge TX), 664
Stephens Memorial Hospital (Norway ME), 325
Sterling Regional Medical Center (Sterling CO), 145
Stevens Community Medical Center (Morris MN), 380
Stevens Hospital (Edmonds WA), 698
Stewart Memorial Community Hospital (Lake City IA), 272
Stewart Webster Hospital (Richland GA), 201
Stillwater Medical Center (Stillwater OK), 544
Stokes-Reynolds Memorial Hospital (Danbury NC), 498
Stone County Hospital (Wiggins MS), 393
Stone County Medical Center (Mountain View AR), 84
Stonecrest Medical Center (Smyrna TN), 614
Stones River Hospital (Woodbury TN), 614
Stonewall Jackson Hospital (Lexington VA), 689
Stonewall Jackson Memorial Hospital (Weston WV), 709
Stony Brook University Medical Center (Stony Brook NY),
479
Stormont-Vail Healthcare (Topeka KS), 285
Straub Clinic and Hospital (Honolulu HI), 207
Stringfellow Memorial Hospital (Anniston AL), 61
Strong Memorial Hospital (Rochester NY), 479
Stroud Regional Medical Center (Stroud OK), 544
Sturdy Memorial Hospital (Attleboro MA), 345
Sturgis Hospital (Sturgis MI), 365
Sturgis Regional Hospital (Sturgis SD), 598

Stuttgart Regional Medical Center (Stuttgart AR), 84
Suburban Hospital (Bethesda MD), 332
Sullivan County Community Hospital (Sullivan IN), 257
Summa Health Systems Hospitals (Akron OH), 526
Summerlin Hospital Medical Center (Las Vegas NV), 427
Summers County ARH Hospital (Hinton WV), 709
Summersville Memorial Hospital (Summersville WV), 709
Summit Medical Center (Hermitage TN), 614
Summit Medical Center (Van Buren AR), 84
Sumner Regional Medical Center (Gallatin TN), 615
Sumner Regional Medical Center (Wellington KS), 285
Sun Belt Regional Medical Center—East
(Channelview TX), 664
Sun Coast Hospital (Largo FL), 180
Sunbury Community Hospital (Sunbury PA), 577
Sunnyside Community Hospital (Sunnyside WA), 698
Sunrise Hospital and Medical Center (Las Vegas NV), 428
Susan B. Allen Memorial Hospital (El Dorado KS), 285
Sutter Amador Hospital (Jackson CA), 131
Sutter Auburn Faith Hospital (Auburn CA), 131
Sutter Coast Hospital (Crescent City CA), 131
Sutter Davis Hospital (Davis CA), 131
Sutter Delta Medical Center (Antioch CA), 132
Sutter General Hospital (Sacramento CA), 132
Sutter Lakeside Hospital (Lakeport CA), 132
Sutter Maternity and Surgery Center (Santa Cruz CA), 132
Sutter Medical Center of Santa Rosa—Chanate
(Santa Rosa CA), 132
Sutter Memorial Hospital (Sacramento CA), 132
Sutter Roseville Medical Center (Roseville CA), 133
Sutter Solano Medical Center (Vallejo CA), 133
Sutter Tracy Community Hospital (Tracy CA), 133
Sutter Warrack Hospital (Santa Rosa CA), 133
SVCMC—St. Vincent's Hospital Staten Island
(Staten Island NY), 479
Swain County Hospital (Bryson City NC), 498
Swedish American Hospital (Rockford IL), 238
Swedish Covenant Hospital (Chicago IL), 238
Swedish Medical Center (Englewood CO), 145
Swedish Medical Center—Ballard Campus (Seattle WA),
699
Swedish Medical Center—Cherry Hills Campus
(Seattle WA), 699
Swedish Medical Center—First Hill (Seattle WA), 699
Sweetwater Hospital Association (Sweetwater TN), 615
Swift County Benson Hospital (Benson MN), 380
Sycamore Shoals Hospital (Elizabethton TN), 615

T

T. J. Samson Community Hospital (Glasgow KY), 301
Tacoma General Allenmore Hospital (Tacoma WA), 699
Tahlequah City Hospital (Tahlequah OK), 545
Tahoe Forest Hospital District (Truckee CA), 133
Takoma Adventist Hospital (Greeneville TN), 615
Tallahassee Memorial Healthcare (Tallahassee FL), 180
Tampa, Florida, 170, 177, 181
Tampa General Hospital (Tampa FL), 181
Tanner Medical Center—Carrollton (Carrollton GA), 202

Please note that all individual hospital listings provide page numbers for Chapter 6 (Hospital Ratings by Clinical Specialty) only. All other hospital listings can be found under their state listing.

Tanner Medical Center—Villa Rica (Villa Rica GA), 202
Tattnall Community Hospital (Reidsville GA), 202
Taylor Brown Memorial Hospital (Waterloo NY), 480
Taylor Regional Hospital (Campbellsville KY), 301
Taylor Regional Hospital (Hawkinsville GA), 202
Taylorville Memorial Hospital (Taylorville IL), 238
Tazewell Community Hospital (Tazewell VA), 689
TCA of Central Oklahoma (Oklahoma City OK), 545
teaching hospitals, 27–28
Teche Regional Medical Center (Morgan City LA), 317
Tempe St. Luke's Hospital (Tempe AZ), 72
Temple Community Hospital (Los Angeles CA), 133
Temple University Hospital (Philadelphia PA), 577
Tennessee
    five star rated facilities, 808–9
    hospitals, 598–618
    procedure, hospital ratings by, 998–1003
    top doctors, 1074–75
Terre Haute Regional Hospital (Terre Haute IN), 257
Terrebonne General Hospital (Houma LA), 317
tests, diagnostic, 35, 36
Texas
    five star rated facilities, 809–15
    hospitals, 618–69
    procedure, hospital ratings by, 1004–17
    top doctors, 1075–78
Texas County Memorial Hospital (Houston MO), 413
Texas Orthopedic Hospital (Houston TX), 664
Texoma Medical Center (Denison TX), 664
Texsan Heart Hospital (San Antonio TX), 664
Theda Clark Medical Center (Neenah WI), 727
Thibodaux Regional Medical Center (Thibodaux LA), 317
Thomas H. Boyd Memorial Hospital (Carrollton IL), 238
Thomas Hospital (Fairhope AL), 61
Thomas Jefferson University Hospital (Philadelphia PA), 578
Thomas Memorial Hospital (South Charleston WV), 710
Thomasville Medical Center (Thomasville NC), 498
Thorek Memorial Hospital (Chicago IL), 238
Three Rivers Community Hospital (Grants Pass OR), 553
Three Rivers Community Hospital Washington Output Ctr. (Grants Pass OR), 553
Three Rivers Health (Three Rivers MI), 365
Three Rivers Hospital (Waverly TN), 615
Three Rivers Medical Center (Louisa KY), 301
three star rating, xiii, xiv
Tift Regional Medical Center (Tifton GA), 202
Tillamook County General Hospital (Tillamook OR), 553
Timpanogos Regional Hospital (Orem UT), 674
Tioga Medical Center (Tioga ND), 503
Tippah County Hospital (Ripley MS), 394
Tipton Hospital (Tipton IN), 257
Tishomingo Health Services (Iuka MS), 394
Titus County Memorial Hospital (Mt. Pleasant TX), 664
Titusville Hospital (Titusville PA), 578
TLC Health Network (Gowanda NY), 480
Toledo, Ohio, 518, 519, 524, 525, 527
Toledo Hospital (Toledo OH), 527
Tomah Memorial Hospital (Tomah WI), 728

Tomball Regional Hospital (Tomball TX), 665
top performing doctors, xi
Toppenish Community Hospital (Toppenish WA), 699
Torrance Memorial Medical Center (Torrance CA), 134
Touchette Regional Hospital (Centreville IL), 239
Touro Infirmary (New Orleans LA), 318
Town and Country Hospital (Tampa FL), 181
Trace Regional Hospital and Swing Bed (Houston MS), 394
Tracy Area Medical Services (Tracy MN), 381
Transylvania Community Hospital (Brevard NC), 498
traveling nurses, 28
Trego County Lemke Memorial Hospital (WaKeeney KS), 285
Tri-City Medical Center (Oceanside CA), 134
Tri-City Regional Medical Center (Hawaiian Gardens CA), 134
Tri-County Area Hospital District (Lexington NE), 424
Tri-County Hospital (Wadena MN), 381
Trident Medical Center (Charleston SC), 593
Trigg County Hospital (Cadiz KY), 301
Tri-Lakes Medical Center (Batesville MS), 394
Trinitas Hospital—Williamson (Elizabeth NJ), 443
Trinity Community Hospital (Jasper FL), 181
Trinity Health System (Steubenville OH), 527
Trinity Hospital (Erin TN), 615
Trinity Hospitals (Minot ND), 503
Trinity Medical Center (Birmingham AL), 61
Trinity Medical Center (Brenham TX), 665
Trinity Medical Center (Carrollton TX), 665
Trinity Medical Center (Minot ND), 503
Trinity Medical Center—7th Street Campus (Moline IL), 239
Trinity Medical Center—Terrace Park Campus (Bettendorf IA), 272
Trinity Medical Center—West Campus (Moline IL), 239
Trinity Regional Medical Center (Fort Dodge IA), 272
Tri-State Memorial Hospital (Clarkston WA), 699
TRMC of Orangeburg and Calhoun (Orangeburg SC), 593
Trousdale Medical Center (Hartsville TN), 616
Troy Community Hospital (Troy PA), 578
Troy Regional Medical Center (Troy AL), 61
Truman Medical Center—Hospital Hill (Kansas City MO), 413
Truman Medical Center—Lakewood (Kansas City MO), 413
Trumbull Memorial Hospital (Warren OH), 527
trusting your doctor, 2, 10, 12, 15, 35
Tuality Community Hospital (Hillsboro OR), 554
Tuality Forest Grove Hospital (Forest Grove OR), 554
tubes, asking about, 34–35
Tucson, Arizona, 66, 67, 69, 72
Tucson Heart Hospital (Tucson AZ), 72
Tucson Medical Center (Tucson AZ), 72
Tufts-New England Medical Center (Boston MA), 345
Tulane University Hospital (New Orleans LA), 318
Tulare District Hospital (Tulare CA), 134
Tulsa, Oklahoma, 530, 535, 540, 542, 543, 544, 545
Tulsa Regional Medical Center (Tulsa OK), 545
Tuomey Healthcare System (Sumter SC), 593
Twelve Oaks Medical Center (Houston TX), 665
Twin Cities Community Hospital (Templeton CA), 134
Twin Cities Hospital (Niceville FL), 181

Twin City Hospital (Dennison OH), 527
Twin County Regional Hospital (Galax VA), 689
Twin Lakes Regional Medical Center (Leitchfield KY), 301
Twin Rivers Regional Medical Center (Kennett MO), 413
Tyle Memorial Hospital (Tunkhannock PA), 578
Tyler County Hospital (Woodville TX), 665
Tyler Holmes Memorial Hospital (Winona MS), 394
Tyrone Hospital (Tyrone PA), 578

U

UAMS Medical Center (Little Rock AR), 84
UCLA Medical Center (Los Angeles CA), 134
UCSF Medical Center (San Francisco CA), 135
UHHS Bedford Medical Center (Bedford OH), 527
UHHS Brown Memorial Hospital (Conneaut OH), 527
UHHS Geauga Regional Hospital (Chardon OH), 528
UHHS Memorial Hospital of Geneva (Geneva OH), 528
UHHS Richmond Heights Hospital (Richmond Heights OH), 528
Uintah Basin Medical Center (Roosevelt UT), 674
Ukiah Valley Medical Center (Ukiah CA), 135
UMass Memorial Medical Center (Worcester MA), 345
UMass Memorial Medical Center—Memorial Campus (Worcester MA), 345
UMC of Southern Nevada (Las Vegas NV), 428
UMDNJ-University Hospital (Newark NJ), 443
Underwood Memorial Hospital (Woodbury NJ), 443
Unicoi County Memorial Hospital (Erwin TN), 616
Union County General Hospital (Clayton NM), 450
Union County Hospital District (Anna IL), 239
Union General Hospital (Blairsville GA), 202
Union General Hospital (Farmerville LA), 318
Union Hospital (Dover OH), 528
Union Hospital (Terre Haute IN), 257
Union Hospital (Union NJ), 443
Union Hospital of Cecil County (Elkton MD), 332
Union Memorial Hospital (Baltimore MD), 333
Uniontown Hospital (Uniontown PA), 578
United General Hospital (Sedro Woolley WA), 700
United Health Services Hospitals (Binghamton NY), 480
United Hospital Center (Clarksburg WV), 710
United Hospital District (Blue Earth MN), 381
United Hospital System (Kenosha WI), 728
United Hospitals (St. Paul MN), 381
United Memorial Health Center (Greenville MI), 366
United Memorial Medical Center (Batavia NY), 480
United Regional Health Care System (Wichita Falls TX), 665
United Regional Medical Center (Manchester TN), 616
Unity Health Center (Shawnee OK), 545
Unity Hospital (Fridley MN), 381
Unity Hospital (Muscatine IA), 272
Unity Hospital (Rochester NY), 480
Unity St. Mary's Campus (Rochester NY), 480
University Community Hospital (Tampa FL), 181
University Community Hospital at Carrollwood (Tampa FL), 181
University Health System (San Antonio TX), 666
University Hospital (Augusta GA), 203

Please note that all individual hospital listings provide page numbers for Chapter 6 (Hospital Ratings by Clinical Specialty) only. All other hospital listings can be found under their state listing.

University Hospital (Cincinnati OH), 528
University Hospital and Clinics—Holmes County (Lexington MS), 394
University Hospital and Medical Center (Tamarac FL), 182
University Hospital of Brooklyn—Downstate (Brooklyn NY), 481
University Hospital SUNY Upstate Medical University (Syracuse NY), 481
University Hospitals Case Medical Center (Cleveland OH), 528
University Medical Center (Fresno CA), 135
University Medical Center (Lebanon TN), 616
University Medical Center (Lubbock TX), 666
University Medical Center (Tucson AZ), 72
University Medical Center—Mesabi (Hibbing MN), 381
University Medical Center at Princeton (Princeton NJ), 444
University of Alabama Hospital (Birmingham AL), 61
University of Alabama Medical West (Bessemer AL), 61
University of California—Davis Medical Center (Sacramento CA), 135
University of California—Irvine Medical Center (Orange CA), 135
University of California—San Diego Medical Center (San Diego CA), 135
University of Chicago Medical Center (Chicago IL), 239
University of Colorado Hospital Authority (Aurora CO), 146
University of Illinois Medical Center (Chicago IL), 239
University of Iowa Hospital and Clinics (Iowa City IA), 273
University of Kansas Hospital (Kansas City KS), 285
University of Kentucky Hospital (Lexington KY), 302
University of Louisville Hospital (Louisville KY), 302
University of Maryland Medical Center (Baltimore MD), 333
University of Michigan Hospital (Ann Arbor MI), 366
University of Minnesota Hospital and Clinic (Minneapolis MN), 382
University of Minnesota Medical Center—Fairview (Minneapolis MN), 382
University of Mississippi Medical Center (Jackson MS), 395
University of Missouri Hospital and Clinics (Columbia MO), 413
University of New Mexico Hospital (Albuquerque NM), 450
University of North Carolina Hospital (Chapel Hill NC), 499
University of Pittsburgh Medical Center—Bedford (Everett PA), 579
University of Pittsburgh Medical Center—Braddock (Braddock PA), 579
University of Pittsburgh Medical Center—Cranberry (Cranberry Township PA), 579
University of Pittsburgh Medical Center—Horizon (Greenville PA), 579
University of Pittsburgh Medical Center—Lee (Johnstown PA), 579
University of Pittsburgh Medical Center—McKeesport (McKeesport PA), 579
University of Pittsburgh Medical Center—Northwest (Seneca PA), 580
University of Pittsburgh Medical Center—Passavant (Pittsburgh PA), 580

University of Pittsburgh Medical Center—Presbyterian Shadyside (Pittsburgh PA), 580
University of Pittsburgh Medical Center—St. Margaret (Pittsburgh PA), 580
University of Pittsburgh Medical Center—Shadyside (Pittsburgh PA), 580
University of Pittsburgh Medical Center—South Side (Pittsburgh PA), 580
University of South Alabama—Knollwood Hospital (Mobile AL), 62
University of South Alabama Medical Center (Mobile AL), 62
University of Tennessee Memorial Hospital (Knoxville TN), 616
University of Texas Health Center at Tyler (Tyler TX), 666
University of Texas Medical Branch Galveston (GalvestonTX), 666
University of Utah Hospital (Salt Lake City UT), 674
University of Virginia Hospital (Charlottesville VA), 689
University of Washington Medical Center (Seattle WA), 700
University Physicians Healthcare Hospital at Kino (Tucson AZ), 72
Upland Hills Health (Dodgeville WI), 728
Upper Chesapeake Medical Center (Bel Air MD), 333
Upper Valley Medical Center (Piqua OH), 529
Upper Valley Medical Center (Troy OH), 529
Upson Regional Medical Center (Thomaston GA), 203
Upstate Carolina Medical Center (Gaffney SC), 594
U.S. General Accounting Office, 25
USC University Hospital (Los Angeles CA), 136
UT Southwestern Medical Center (Dallas TX), 666
UT Southwestern Zale Lipshy Hospital (Dallas TX), 666
Utah
    five star rated facilities, 816
    hospitals, 670–74
    procedure, hospital ratings by, 1018–19
    top doctors, 1078
Utah Valley Regional Medical Center (Provo UT), 674
Uvalde Memorial Hospital (Uvalde TX), 667
UW Health-UW Hospitals and Clinics (Madison WI), 728

V

Vail Valley Medical Center (Vail CO), 146
Val Verde Regional Medical Center (Del Rio TX), 667
Valdese General Hospital (Valdese NC), 499
Valley Baptist Medical Center (Harlingen TX), 667
Valley Baptist Medical Center—Brownsville (Brownsville TX), 667
Valley Care Medical Center (Pleasanton CA), 136
Valley General Hospital (Monroe WA), 700
Valley Hospital (Ridgewood NJ), 444
Valley Hospital and Medical Center (Spokane WA), 700
Valley Hospital Medical Center (Las Vegas NV), 428
Valley Medical Center (Renton WA), 700
Valley Memorial Hospital (Livermore CA), 136
Valley Memorial Hospital (Sunnyside WA), 700
Valley Presbyterian Hospital (Van Nuys CA), 136
Valley Regional Hospital (Claremont NH), 432
Valley Regional Medical Center (Brownsville TX), 667

Valley View Hospital Association (Glenwood Springs CO), 146
Valley View Medical Center (Cedar City UT), 674
Valley View Regional Hospital (Ada OK), 545
Valley West Community Hospital (Sandwich IL), 240
Van Buren County Hospital (Keosauqua IA), 273
Van Wert County Hospital (Van Wert OH), 529
Vanderbilt University Hospital (Nashville TN), 616
Vassar Brothers Medical Center (Poughkeepsie NY), 481
Vaughan Regional Medical Center—Parkway Campus (Selma AL), 62
Venice Regional Medical Center (Venice FL), 182
Ventura County Medical Center (Ventura CA), 136
Verde Valley Medical Center (Cottonwood AZ), 72
Verdugo Hills Hospital (Glendale CA), 136
Vermont
    five star rated facilities, 817
    hospitals, 675–76
    procedure, hospital ratings by, 1020–21
Vernon Memorial Hospital (Viroqua WI), 728
Veterans Memorial (Waukon IA), 273
Via Christi Regional Medical Center (Wichita KS), 286
Victor Valley Community Hospital (Victorville CA), 137
Victory Memorial Hospital (Brooklyn NY), 481
Villages Regional Hospital (The Villages FL), 182
Ville Platte Medical Center (Ville Platte LA), 318
viral infections, 8
Virginia
    five star rated facilities, 817–19
    hospitals, 677–90
    procedure, hospital ratings by, 1022–25
    top doctors, 1079
Virginia Commonwealth Univeristy Health System (Richmond VA), 689
Virginia Gay Hospital (Vinton IA), 273
Virginia Hospital Center—Arlington (Arlington VA), 690
Virginia Mason Medical Center (Seattle WA), 701
Virginia Regional Medical Center (Virginia MN), 382
Virtua Memorial Hospital—Burlington County (Mount Holly NJ), 444
Virtua West Jersey Hospital—Berlin (Berlin NJ), 444
Virtua West Jersey Hospital—Marlton (Marlton NJ), 444
Vista Medical Center—East (Waukegan IL), 240
volume, xiii, 42, 44
Volunteer Community Hospital (Martin TN), 617

W

W. J. Mangold Memorial Hospital (Lockney TX), 667
W. W. Hastings Indian Hospital (Tahlequah OK), 545
Wa Foote Hospital (Jackson MI), 366
Wabash County Hospital (Wabash IN), 258
Wabash General Hospital (Mount Carmel IL), 240
Waccamaw Community Hospital (Murrells Inlet SC), 594
Wadley Regional Medical Center (Texarkana TX), 668
Wadsworth Rittman Hospital (Wadsworth OH), 529
Wagoner Community Hospital (Wagoner OK), 546
Wahiawa General Hospital (Wahiawa HI), 207
Wakemed Cary Hospital (Cary NC), 499

Please note that all individual hospital listings provide page numbers for Chapter 6 (Hospital Ratings by Clinical Specialty) only. All other hospital listings can be found under their state listing.

Wakemed—Raleigh Campus (Raleigh NC), 499
Waldo County General Hospital (Belfast ME), 325
Walker Baptist Medical Center (Jasper AL), 62
Walla Walla General Hospital (Walla Walla WA), 701
Wallace Thomson Hospital (Union SC), 594
Wallowa Memorial Hospital (Enterprise OR), 554
Walls Regional Hospital (Cleburne TX), 668
Walter O. Boswell Memorial Hospital (Sun City AZ), 73
Walthall County General Hospital (Tylertown MS), 395
Walton Regional Medical Center (Monroe GA), 203
War Memorial Hospital (Berkeley Springs WV), 710
Ward Memorial Hospital (Monahans TX), 668
Warm Springs Medical Center (Warm Springs GA), 203
Warminster Hospital (Warminster PA), 581
Warren General Hospital (Warren PA), 581
Warren Hospital (Phillipsburg NJ), 444
Warren Memorial Hospital (Front Royal VA), 690
Washakie Medical Center (Worland WY), 732
Washington
    five star rated facilities, 819–21
    hospitals, 691–701
    procedure, hospital ratings by, 1026–29
    top doctors, 1079–80
Washington, DC
    five star rated facilities, 821
    hospitals, 702–3
    procedure, hospital ratings by, 1030–31
Washington Adventist Hospital (Takoma Park MD), 333
Washington County Hospital (Hagerstown MD), 333
Washington County Hospital (Plymouth NC), 499
Washington County Hospital (Washington IA), 273
Washington County Memorial Hospital (Potosi MO), 414
Washington County Memorial Hospital (Salem IN), 258
Washington County Regional Medical Center
    (Sandersville GA), 203
Washington Hospital (Washington PA), 581
Washington Hospital Center (Washington DC), 703
Washington Hospital Healthcare System (Fremont CA), 137
Washington Regional Medical Center at North Hills
    (Fayetteville AR), 84
Washington St. Tammany Parish Medical Center
    (Bogalusa LA), 318
Watauga Medical Center (Boone NC), 499
Waterbury Hospital Health Center (Waterbury CT), 151
Watertown Memorial Hospital (Watertown WI), 728
Watonga Municipal Hospital (Watonga OK), 546
Watsonville Community Hospital (Watsonville CA), 137
Waukesha Memorial Hospital (Waukesha WI), 729
Waupun Memorial Hospital (Waupun WI), 729
Waverly Health Center (Waverly IA), 273
Wayne County Hospital (Corydon IA), 274
Wayne County Hospital (Monticello KY), 302
Wayne General Hospital (Waynesboro MS), 395
Wayne Hospital (Greenville OH), 529
Wayne Medical Center (Waynesboro TN), 617
Wayne Memorial Hospital (Goldsboro NC), 500
Wayne Memorial Hospital (Honesdale PA), 581
Wayne Memorial Hospital (Jesup GA), 203

Waynesboro Hospital (Waynesboro PA), 581
Webster General Hospital (Eupora MS), 395
Wedowee Hospital (Wedowee AL), 62
Weeks Medical Center (Lancaster NH), 432
Weirton Medical Center (Weirton WV), 710
Welborn Baptist Hospital (Evansville IN), 258
Welch Community Hospital (Welch WV), 710
Wellington Regional Medical Center (Wellington FL), 182
Wellmont Bristol Regional Medical Center (Bristol TN), 617
Wellmont Hawkins County Memorial Hospital
    (Rogersville TN), 617
Wellmont Holston Valley Medical Center (Kingsport TN), 617
Wellmont Lonesome Pine Hospital (Big Stone Gap VA), 690
Wellstar Cobb Hospital (Austell GA), 204
Wellstar Douglas Hospital (Douglasville GA), 204
Wellstar Kennestone Hospital (Marietta GA), 204
Wellstar Paulding Hospital (Dallas GA), 204
Wentworth-Douglass Hospital (Dover NH), 432
Wesley Long Community Hospital (Greensboro NC), 500
Wesley Medical Center (Hattiesburg MS), 395
Wesley Medical Center (Wichita KS), 286
West Allis Memorial Hospital (West Allis WI), 729
West Anaheim Medical Center (Anaheim CA), 137
West Boca Medical Center (Boca Raton FL), 182
West Branch Regional Medical Center (West Branch MI),
    366
West Calcasieu Cameron Hospital (Sulphur LA), 318
West Carroll Memorial Hospital (Oak Grove LA), 319
West Central Community Hospital (Clinton IN), 258
West Florida Hospital (Pensacola FL), 182
West Georgia Medical Center (Lagrange GA), 204
West Hills Medical Center (West Hills CA), 137
West Houston Medical Center (Houston TX), 668
West Jefferson Medical Center (Marrero LA), 319
West Park Hospital District (Cody WY), 733
West River Regional Medical Center (Hettinger ND), 504
West Shore Hospital (Manistee MI), 366
West Suburban Hospital Medical Center (Oak Park IL), 240
West Valley Hospital (Goodyear AZ), 73
West Valley Medical Center (Caldwell ID), 210
West Virginia
    five star rated facilities, 822
    hospitals, 703–11
    procedure, hospital ratings by, 1032–33
    top doctors, 1080
West Virginia University Hospitals (Morgantown WV), 710
Westbrook Community Hospital (Westbrook ME), 326
Westchester General Hospital (Miami FL), 183
Westchester Medical Center (Valhalla NY), 481
Westerly Hospital (Westerly RI), 585
Western Arizona Regional Medical Center
    (Bullhead City AZ), 73
Western Baptist Hospital (Paducah KY), 302
Western Medical Center Hospital Anaheim (Anaheim CA),
    137
Western Medical Center Santa Ana (Santa Ana CA), 138
Western Missouri Medical Center (Warrensburg MO), 414
Western Pennsylvania Hospital (Pittsburgh PA), 581

Western Pennsylvania Hospital—Forbes Regional Campus
    (Monroeville PA), 582
Western Plains Medical Complex (Dodge City KS), 286
Western Reserve Care System (Youngstown OH), 529
Westfield Memorial Hospital (Westfield NY), 481
Westlake Community Hospital (Melrose Park IL), 240
Westlake Regional Hospital (Columbia KY), 302
Westmoreland Regional Hospital (Greensburg PA), 582
Westpark Medical Center (McKinney TX), 668
Westside Regional Medical Center (Plantation FL), 183
Westview Hospital (Indianapolis IN), 258
Wetzel County Hospital (New Martinsville WV), 711
Wheaton Franciscan Healthcare—Elmbrook Memorial
    (Brookfield WI), 729
Wheaton Franciscan Healthcare—St. Francis
    (Milwaukee WI), 729
Wheaton Franciscan Healthcare—St. Joseph
    (Milwaukee WI), 729
Wheeler County Hospital (Glenwood GA), 204
Wheeling Hospital (Wheeling WV), 711
Whidbey General Hospital (Coupeville WA), 701
Whidden Memorial Hospital (Everett MA), 345
Whispering Oaks Hospital (Jefferson City MO), 414
White County Community Hospital (Sparta TN), 617
White County Medical Center (Carmi IL), 240
White County Medical Center—North Campus
    (Searcy AR), 85
White County Medical Center—South Campus
    (Searcy AR), 85
White County Memorial Hospital (Monticello IN), 258
White Memorial Medical Center (Los Angeles CA), 138
White Plains Hospital Center (White Plains NY), 482
White River Medical Center (Batesville AR), 85
Whitesburg ARH Hospital (Whitesburg KY), 302
Whitman Hospital and Medical Center (Colfax WA), 701
Whittier Hospital (Whittier CA), 138
Wichita, Kansas, 276, 278, 283, 284, 286
Wilbarger General Hospital (Vernon TX), 668
Wilcox Memorial Hospital (Lihue HI), 207
Wilkes Regional Medical Center (North Wilkesboro NC), 500
Wilkes-Barre General Hospital (Wilkes-Barre PA), 582
William N. Wishard Memorial Hospital (Indianapolis IN),
    259
William Newton Hospital (Winfield KS), 286
William W. Backus Hospital (Norwich CT), 151
Willamette Falls Hospital (Oregon City OR), 554
Willamette Valley Medical Center (McMinnville OR), 554
Williamsburg Regional Hospital (Kingstree SC), 594
Williamson ARH Hospital (South Williamson KY), 303
Williamson Medical Center (Franklin TN), 618
Williamson Memorial Hospital (Williamson WV), 711
Williamsport Hospital and Medical Center
    (Williamsport PA), 582
Willis Knighton Bossier Health Center (Bossier City LA), 319
Willis Knighton Medical Center (Shreveport LA), 319
Wills Memorial Hospital (Washington GA), 205
Wilmington Hospital (Wilmington DE), 153
Wilson Medical Center (Wilson NC), 500

Please note that all individual hospital listings provide page numbers for Chapter 6 (Hospital Ratings by Clinical Specialty) only. All other hospital listings can be found under their state listing.

Wilson Memorial Hospital (Sidney OH), 530
Wilson N. Jones Medical Center (Sherman TX), 669
Winchester Hospital (Winchester MA), 345
Winchester Medical Center (Winchester VA), 690
Windber Hospital (Windber PA), 582
Windham Community Memorial Hospital and Hatch
    Hospital (Willimantic CT), 151
Windom Area Hospital (Windom MN), 382
Wing Memorial Hospital and Medical Center
    (Palmer MA), 346
Winkler County Memorial Hospital (Kermit TX), 669
Winn Parish Medical Center (Winnfield LA), 319
Winner Regional Healthcare Center (Winner SD), 598
Winneshiek Medical Center (Decorah IA), 274
Winona Community Memorial Hospital (Winona MN), 382
Winslow Memorial Hospital (Winslow AZ), 73
Winston Medical Center (Louisville MS), 395
Winter Haven Hospital (Winter Haven FL), 183
Winthrop-University Hospital (Mineola NY), 482
Wiregrass Medical Center (Geneva AL), 62
Wisconsin
    five star rated facilities, 823–24
    hospitals, 711–30
    procedure, hospital ratings by, 1034–39
    top doctors, 1080

Wisconsin Heart Hospital (Wauwatosa WI), 730
Wise Regional Health System (Decatur TX), 669
Witham Health Services (Lebanon IN), 259
Woman's Christian Association (Jamestown NY), 482
Woman's Hospital at Dallas Regional Medical Center
    (Mesquite TX), 669
Women's East Pavilion (Chattanooga TN), 618
Wood County Hospital (Bowling Green OH), 530
Woodhull Medical and Mental Health Center
    (Brooklyn NY), 482
Woodland Heights Medical Center (Lufkin TX), 669
Woodland Medical Center (Cullman AL), 63
Woodland Memorial Hospital (Woodland CA), 138
Woodlawn Hospital (Rochester IN), 259
Woods Memorial Hospital (Etowah TN), 618
Woodward Regional Hospital (Woodward OK), 546
Wooster Community Hospital (Wooster OH), 530
World War II Veterans Memorial Hospital (Meriden CT), 151
Worthington Regional Hospital (Worthington MN), 382
Wright Medical Center (Clarion IA), 274
Wuesthoff Medical Center—Melbourne (Melbourne FL), 183
Wuesthoff Medical Center—Rockledge (Rockledge FL), 183
WVHCS Hospital (Wilkes-Barre PA), 582
Wyandot Memorial Hospital (Upper Sandusky OH), 530
Wyckoff Heights Medical Center (Brooklyn NY), 482

Wyoming
    five star rated facilities, 825
    hospitals, 730–33
    procedure, hospital ratings by, 1040–41
Wyoming County Community Hospital (Warsaw NY), 482
Wyoming Medical Center (Casper WY), 733
Wythe County Community Hospital (Wytheville VA), 690

Y

Yakima Regional Medical and Cardiac Center (Yakima
    WA), 701
Yakima Valley Memorial Hospital (Yakima WA), 701
Yale-New Haven Hospital (New Haven CT), 151
Yalobusha General Hospital (Water Valley MS), 396
Yampa Valley Medical Center (Steamboat Springs CO), 146
Yavapai Regional Medical Center (Prescott AZ), 73
Yoakum Community Hospital (Yoakum TX), 669
Yonkers General Hospital (Yonkers NY), 483
York General Hospital (York NE), 425
York Hospital (York ME), 326
York Hospital (York PA), 583
Yukon Kuskokwim Delta Regional Hospital (Bethel AK), 64
Yuma Regional Medical Center (Yuma AZ), 73

Z

Zeeland Community Hospital (Zeeland MI), 366

ACKNOWLEDGMENTS

HealthGrades would like to thank the dedicated and passionate employees who work diligently every day to ensure consumers have access to accurate, independent data on the quality of America's hospitals and physicians. If not for their efforts, this book would not have been possible.

We would also like to thank: Kerry Hicks, HealthGrades' CEO who, one decade ago, developed the idea to rate hospitals based on quality and began the current wave of transparency in healthcare; Scott Shapiro, Vice President of Corporate Communications and Marketing, who had the idea to take HealthGrades' online provider ratings offline and put them into the hands of readers everywhere. We believe, as he would say, that this is literally the most important book your family will ever buy; Dr. Samantha Collier who, with editorial support from Marsha Austin, enhanced the value of this book immensely with her frank, and often humorous, insider's perspective on the world of medicine. Dr. Collier dedicated countless hours and much introspection to this project, all while managing a rigorous travel schedule and performing her duties as HealthGrades' Chief Medical Officer. Special thanks go to Sarah Loughran, Executive Vice President, for providing the strategic direction for this groundbreaking enterprise, and for seeing the book through to fruition; and to Brad Hayes, lead project manager, and his department who made miracles happen to ensure the accuracy and timeliness of the vast amounts of data needed to build this reference guide.

Special thanks also go to the following HealthGrades employees for their contributions:

Mark Bartling, Yvonne Chavez, Allen Dodge, Kelly Engdahl, Steve Duryee, Diamond Folks, Gay Gillespie, Aaron Goddard, Kyle Hansen, Wei He, Jeremy Henderson, Dave Hicks, Cassandra Mondrow, Carol Nicholas, Kristin Reed, Kim Roalson, Jim Strickland, Sheri Suedekum, Harold Taylor, John Tran, Bill Wosilius, and the other HealthGrades experts that contributed their time to this project.

HealthGrades extend particular thanks to Nathaniel Marunas and Devorah Klein at Barnes & Noble, Inc. for seeing the value in getting this information into people's hands. Finally, enormous thanks to Jessica Jones, Laurie Dolphin, and Allison Meierding of D&J Book Packaging, whose care and feeding of this book made it a reality.

ABOUT HEALTHGRADES

HealthGrades, Inc. (Nasdaq: HGRD) is the leading healthcare ratings organization, providing ratings and profiles of hospitals, nursing homes, and physicians. Millions of consumers and many of the nation's largest employers, health plans, and hospitals rely on HealthGrades' independent ratings, advisory services, and decision-support resources to make healthcare decisions based on the quality and cost of care. More information on the company can be found at www.healthgrades.com.

ABOUT THE AUTHOR

Dr. Samantha L. Collier is a board certified internist, former assistant professor of medicine at OUHSC–Tulsa, and currently the chief medical officer at HealthGrades, the leading independent healthcare ratings company.

Her role at HealthGrades has allowed her the opportunity to discuss the importance of healthcare ratings, public profiling, and patient safety to multitudes of national conferences, including the Harvard Quality Colloquium, CMS National Customer Service conference, the American College of Healthcare Executives and the National Association for Healthcare Quality. She also has assisted over one hundred hospital organizations throughout the country with the development of quality improvement initiatives that have improved their public profiling positions and competitive positioning and quality of care.

Dr. Collier has co-authored several studies at HealthGrades, including First Time Preplanned and "Patient Choice" Cesarean Section Rates in the United States, HealthGrades' Annual Hospital Quality in America Study, and Health-Grades' Annual Patient Safety in American Hospitals Study, which have received significant public attention in *The Wall Street Journal*, *The New York Times*, *Newsweek*, *Time*, and on *CNN*, *The Today Show*, and hundreds of other news outlets.

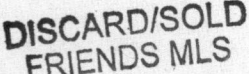